a LANGE medical book

CURRENT
Medical Diagnosis & Treatment 2003

42nd Edition

Edited by

Lawrence M. Tierney, Jr., MD
Professor of Medicine
University of California, San Francisco
Associate Chief of Medical Services
Veterans Affairs Medical Center, San Francisco

Stephen J. McPhee, MD
Professor of Medicine
Division of General Internal Medicine
Department of Medicine
University of California, San Francisco

Maxine A. Papadakis, MD
Professor of Clinical Medicine
Associate Dean for Student Affairs
School of Medicine
University of California, San Francisco

With Associate Authors

Lange Medical Books/McGraw-Hill
Medical Publishing Division

New York   Chicago   San Francisco   Lisbon   London   Madrid   Mexico City
Milan   New Delhi   San Juan   Seoul   Singapore   Sydney   Toronto

The McGraw·Hill Companies

Current Medical Diagnosis & Treatment 2003, Forty-Second Edition

1 2 3 4 5 6 7 8 9 0   DOW/DOW   0 9 8 7 6 5 4 3 2

ISBN 0-07-139593-8

ISSN 0092-8682

Notice

Medicine is an ever-changing science. As new research and clinical experience broaden our knowledge, changes in treatment and drug therapy are required. The authors and the publisher of this work have checked with sources believed to be reliable in their efforts to provide information that is complete and generally in accord with the standards accepted at the time of publication. However, in view of the possibility of human error or changes in medical sciences, neither the authors nor the publisher nor any other party who has been involved in the preparation or publication of this work warrants that the information contained herein is in every respect accurate or complete, and they disclaim all responsibility for any errors or omissions or for the results obtained from use of the information contained in this work. Readers are encouraged to confirm the information contained herein with other sources. For example and in particular, readers are advised to check the product information sheet included in the package of each drug they plan to administer to be certain that the information contained in this work is accurate and that changes have not been made in the recommended dose or in the contraindications for administration. This recommendation is of particular importance in connection with new or infrequently used drugs.

This book was set in Adobe Garamond by Pine Tree Composition
The editors were Isabel Nogueira, Harriet Lebowitz, Jim Ransom, and Barbara Holton.
The production supervisor was Phil Galea.
The illustration manager was Charissa Baker.
The book designer was Eve Siegel.
The illustrator was Linda F. Harris.
The index was prepared by Kathy Pitcoff.

RR Donnelley was printer and binder.

This book is printed on acid-free paper.

Contents

19. Allergic & Immunologic Disorders 759
Jeffrey L. Kishiyama, MD, & Daniel C. Adelman, MD

20. Arthritis & Musculoskeletal Disorders 783
David B. Hellmann, MD, FACP, & John H. Stone, MD, MPH

21. Fluid & Electrolyte Disorders 839
Masafumi Fukagawa, MD, PhD, Kiyoshi Kurokawa, MD, MACP, & Maxine A. Papadakis, MD

22. Kidney 867
Suzanne Watnick, MD, & Gail Morrison, MD

Authors

Daniel C. Adelman, MD
Associate Adjunct Professor of Medicine, Division of Allergy and Immunology, University of California, San Francisco
dadelman@pcyc.com
Allergic & Immunologic Disorders

Joshua S. Adler, MD
Associate Clinical Professor of Medicine, Department of Medicine, University of California, San Francisco; Director of Ambulatory Practices, University of California, San Francisco
jadler@itsa.ucsf.edu
Preoperative Evaluation

Thomas M. Amidon, MD
Clinical Instructor, University of Washington, Bellevue
tamidon@oima.org
Heart

Michael J. Aminoff, MD, DSc, FRCP
Professor of Neurology, University of California, San Francisco; Attending Physician, University of California, San Francisco
aminoff@itsa.ucsf.edu
The Nervous System

David M. Barbour, PharmD, BCPS
Adjoint Clinical Faculty, School of Pharmacy, University of Colorado Health Sciences Center, Denver; Clinical Pharmacy Specialist, Kaiser Permanente, Boulder
dave.barbour@uchsc.edu
Drug References

Robert B. Baron, MD, MS
Professor of Medicine; Associate Dean for Continuing Medical Education; Vice Chief and Director, Educational Programs, Division of General Internal Medicine; Director, Primary Care Internal Medicine Residency Program, University of California, San Francisco
baron@medicine.ucsf.edu
Lipid Abnormalities; Nutrition

Thomas E. Baudendistel, MD
Assistant Clinical Professor of Medicine, University of California, San Francisco
tommyyb@itsa.ucsf.edu
Internet Resources

Timothy G. Berger, MD
Clinical Professor, Department of Dermatology, University of California, San Francisco
tgberger@orca.ucsf.edu
Skin, Hair, & Nails

Brian M. Berman, MD
Professor of Family Medicine and Director, Complementary Medicine Program, University of Maryland School of Medicine, Baltimore
bberman@compmed.umm.edu
Complementary & Alternative Medicine

Mark Bisanzo, MD
Harvard Affiliated Emergency Medicine Residency, Brigham and Women's Hospital, Massachusetts General Hospital, Boston
mbisanzo@partners.org
Internet Resources

Peter R. Carroll, MD, FACS
Professor and Chair, Department of Urology, University of California, San Francisco
pcarroll@urol.ucsf.edu
Urology

Henry F. Chambers, MD
Professor of Medicine, University of California, San Francisco; Chief, Division of Infectious Diseases, San Francisco General Hospital
Infectious Diseases: Bacterial & Chlamydial

Mark S. Chesnutt, MD
Associate Professor of Medicine, Pulmonary & Critical Care Medicine; Director, Medical Critical Care, Oregon Health Science University, Portland
chesnutm@ohsu.edu
Lung

Richard Cohen, MD, MPH
Clinical Professor, Division of Occupational and Environmental Medicine, University of California, San Francisco
rcohenmd@pacbell.net
Disorders Due to Physical Agents

Kenneth E. Covinsky, MD, MPH
Assistant Professor of Medicine, University of California, San Francisco; Staff Physician, San Francisco Veterans Affairs Medical Center
covinsky@medicine.ucsf.edu
Geriatric Medicine

William R. Crombleholme, MD
Professor and Vice Chair, Department of Obstetrics, Gynecology and Reproductive Sciences, University of Pittsburgh, Magee-Women's Hospital
wcrombleholme@mail.magee.edu
Obstetrics

Gurpreet Dhaliwal, MD
Chief Resident, Department of Medicine, University of California, San Francisco
gurpreet@medicine.ucsf.edu
References

Stuart J. Eisendrath, MD
Professor of Clinical Psychiatry, University of California, San Francisco; Director, Ambulatory Services, Langley Porter Psychiatric Hospital and Clinics, San Francisco
eisen@itsa.ucsf.edu
Psychiatric Disorders

Darryl A. Elmouchi, MD
Chief Resident, Department of Medicine, University of California, San Francisco, and San Francisco Veterans Affairs Medical Center
delmouch@medicine.ucsf.edu
References

Paul A. Fitzgerald, MD
Clinical Professor of Medicine, Department of Medicine, Division of Endocrinology, University of California, San Francisco
paulf@itsa.ucsf.edu
Endocrinology

Lawrence S. Friedman, MD
Professor of Medicine, Harvard Medical School; Physician, Gastrointestinal Unit and Chief, Walter Bauer Firm, (Medical Services), Massachusetts General Hospital, Boston
friedman.lawrence@mgh.harvard.edu
Liver, Biliary Tract, & Pancreas

Masafumi Fukagawa, MD, PhD, FJSIM
Associate Professor and Director, Division of Nephrology and Dialysis Center, Kobe University School of Medicine, Japan
fukagawa@med.kobe-u.ac.jp
Fluid & Electrolyte Disorders

Armando E. Giuliano, MD
Director, Joyce Eisenberg Keefer Breast Center; Clinical Professor of Surgery, University of California, Los Angeles; Chief of Surgical Oncology, John Wayne Cancer Institute, Santa Monica, California
giulianoa@jwci.org
Breast

Lee Goldman, MD, MPH
Julius R. Krevans Distinguished Professor and Chair, Department of Medicine; Associate Dean for Clinical Affairs, School of Medicine, University of California, San Francisco
goldman@medicine.ucsf.edu
Preoperative Evaluation

Robert S. Goldsmith, MD, MPH, DTM&H
Professor Emeritus of Tropical Medicine and Epidemiology, Department of Epidemiology and Biostatistics, University of California, San Francisco
rg645@itsa.ucsf.edu
Infectious Diseases: Protozoal & Helminthic

Ralph Gonzales, MD, MSPH
Associate Professor, Division of General Internal Medicine, Department of Medicine, University of California, San Francisco
ralphg@medicine.ucsf.edu
Common Symptoms

Justin V. Graham, MD
Division of Infectious Diseases, Stanford Medical Informatics, Stanford University Medical Center, Stanford, California
jus10@stanford.edu
Information Technology in Patient Care: The Internet, Telemedicine, & Clinical Decision Support; Internet Resources

B. Joseph Guglielmo, PharmD
Professor and Vice Chair, Department of Clinical Pharmacy, School of Pharmacy, University of California, San Francisco
bjg@itsa.ucsf.edu
Anti-infective Chemotherapeutic & Antibiotic Agents

Richard J. Hamill, MD
Professor, Departments of Medicine and Molecular Virology & Microbiology, Baylor College of Medicine; Staff Physician, Veterans Affairs Medical Center, Houston, Texas
richard.hamill@med.va.gov
Infectious Diseases: Mycotic

David B. Hellmann, MD, FACP
Mary Betty Stevens Professor of Medicine; Chairman, Department of Medicine, Johns Hopkins Bayview Medical Center, Johns Hopkins University School of Medicine, Baltimore
hellmann@jhmi.edu
Arthritis & Musculoskeletal Disorders

Harry Hollander, MD
Professor of Clinical Medicine and Director, Categorical Medicine Residency Program, University of California, San Francisco
drwine@itsa.ucsf.edu
HIV Infection

Ellen F. Hughes, MD, PhD
Clinical Professor, Department of Medicine, University of California, San Francisco
ehughes@medicine.ucsf.edu
Complementary & Alternative Medicine

Robert K. Jackler, MD
Professor of Otolaryngology and Neurological Surgery, University of California, San Francisco
rkj@itsa.ucsf.edu
Ear, Nose, & Throat

Bradly P. Jacobs, MD, MPH
Assistant Clinical Professor, Department of Medicine; Medical Director, Clinical Programs, Osher Center for Integrative Medicine, University of California, San Francisco
bradlyj@itsa.ucsf.edu
Complementary & Alternative Medicine

Richard A. Jacobs, MD, PhD
Clinical Professor of Medicine and Clinical Pharmacy, University of California, San Francisco
jacobsd@medicine.ucsf.edu
General Problems in Infectious Diseases; Infectious Diseases: Spirochetal; Anti-infective Chemotherapeutic & Antibiotic Agents

C. Bree Johnston, MD, MPH
Assistant Clinical Professor of Medicine, Division of Geriatrics, Veterans Affairs Medical Center, San Francisco, California, University of California, San Francisco
bree526@itsa.ucsf.edu
Geriatric Medicine

Michael J. Kaplan, MD
Associate Professor of Otolaryngology-Head and Neck Surgery and of Neurological Surgery, University of California, San Francisco
mjkaplan@orca.ucsf.edu
Ear, Nose & Throat

John H. Karam, MD
Professor Emeritus of Medicine, Department of Medicine, University of California, San Francisco
bem69kar@aol.com
Diabetes Mellitus & Hypoglycemia

Mitchell H. Katz, MD
Associate Clinical Professor of Medicine, Epidemiology & Biostatistics, University of California, San Francisco; Director of Health, San Francisco Department of Public Health
mitch.katz@sfdph.org
HIV Infection

Ajay J. Kirtane, MD
Chief Resident, Department of Medicine, Moffitt-Long Hospital, University of California, San Francisco
References

Jeffrey L. Kishiyama, MD
Assistant Clinical Professor of Medicine, University of California, San Francisco
jkish@itsa.ucsf.edu
Allergic & Immunologic Disorders

Rick G. Kulkarni, MD
Clinical Instructor, Department of Emergency Medicine, Beth Israel Deaconess Medical Center, Boston, Massachusetts
Rkulkarn@caregroup.harvard.edu
Information Technology in Patient Care: The Internet, Telemedicine, & Clinical Decision Support; Internet Resources

Kiyoshi Kurokawa, MD, MACP
Professor of Medicine and Director, Institute of Medical Sciences, Tokai University, Isehara, Kanagawa, Japan
kurokawa@is.icc.u-tokai.ac.jp
Fluid & Electrolyte Disorders

Jonathan E. Lichtmacher, MD
Associate Director, Adult Psychiatry Clinic, Langley Porter Hospitals and Clinics, University of California, San Francisco
jonathanl@lppi.ucsf.edu
Psychiatric Disorders

Charles A. Linker, MD
Clinical Professor of Medicine and Director, Adult Leukemia and Hematologic Malignancies Program, University of California, San Francisco
Blood

Jafi Lipson
Medical Student, University of California, San Francisco
Jlipson@itsa.ucsf.edu
Internet Resources

William L. Lyons, MD
Assistant Clinical Professor, University of California, San Francisco
wlyons@itsa.ucsf.edu
Geriatric Medicine

H. Trent MacKay, MD, MPH
Associate Professor of Obstetrics and Gynecology, Uniformed Services, University of the Health Sciences, Bethesda, Maryland; Chief, Obstetrics and Gynecology Service, National Naval Medical Center, Bethesda, Maryland
mackayt@mail.nih.gov
Gynecology

Umesh Masharani, MB, BS; MRCP(UK)
Associate Clinical Professor of Medicine, Department of Endocrinology and Metabolism, University of California, San Francisco
ubm@itsa.ucsf.edu
Diabetes Mellitus & Hypoglycemia

Barry M. Massie, MD
Professor of Medicine, University of California, San Francisco; Chief, Cardiology Division, San Francisco Veterans Affairs Medical Center
barry.massie@med.va.gov
Heart; Systemic Hypertension

Stephen J. McPhee, MD
Professor of Medicine, Division of General Internal Medicine, Department of Medicine, University of California, San Francisco
smcphee@medicine.ucsf.edu
General Approach to the Patient; Health Maintenance & Disease Prevention

Kenneth R. McQuaid, MD
Professor of Clinical Medicine, University of California, San Francisco; Director of Gastrointestinal Endoscopy, San Francisco Veterans Affairs Medical Center
krmcq@itsa.ucsf.edu
Alimentary Tract

Louis M. Messina, MD
Professor and Chief, Division of Vascular Surgery; Vice Chair, Department of Surgery, University of California, San Francisco
messina@surgery.ucsf.edu
Blood Vessels and Lymphatics

Brent R.W. Moelleken, MD, FACS
Plastic and Reconstructive Surgery; Attending Surgeon, University of California, Los Angeles Medical Center; Private Practice, Beverly Hills, California
rijuv@aol.com
Disorders Due to Physical Agents

Gail Morrison, MD, FACP
Vice Dean for Education, Director of Academic Programs, and Professor of Medicine, School of Medicine, University of Pennsylvania, Philadelphia
morrisog@mail.med.upenn.edu
Kidney

C. Diana Nicoll, MD, PhD, MPA
Clinical Professor and Vice Chair, Department of Laboratory Medicine; Associate Dean, University of California, San Francisco; Chief of Staff and Chief, Laboratory Medicine Service, San Francisco Veterans Affairs Medical Center
diana.nicoll@med.va.gov
Diagnostic Testing & Medical Decision Making; Appendix: Therapeutic Drug Monitoring & Laboratory Reference Ranges

Kent R. Olson, MD
Clinical Professor of Medicine and Pharmacy, University of California, San Francisco; Medical Director, San Francisco Division, California Poison Control System, University of California, San Francisco
olson@itsa.ucsf.edu
Poisoning

Laura K. Pak, MD
Assistant Professor of Surgery, Division of Vascular Surgery, University of California, San Francisco
pakl@surgery.ucsf.edu
Blood Vessels & Lymphatics

Steven Z. Pantilat, MD
Assistant Clinical Professor of Medicine, University of California, San Francisco; Project on Death in America Faculty Scholar; Director, Comfort Care Suites and Attending Physician, Moffitt-Long Hospital, San Francisco
stevep@medicine.ucsf.edu
Care at the End of Life

Maxine A. Papadakis, MD
Professor of Clinical Medicine and Associate Dean for Student Affairs, School of Medicine, University of California, San Francisco
papadakm@medsch.ucsf.edu
Fluid & Electrolyte Disorders

Michael Pignone, MD, MPH
Assistant Professor of Medicine, University of North Carolina, Chapel Hill
pignone@med.unc.edu
General Approach to the Patient; Health Maintenance & Disease Prevention; Diagnostic Testing & Medical Decision-Making

Mark J. Pletcher, MD, MPH
Clinical Research Fellow, Division of General Internal Medicine, University of California, San Francisco
markp@itsa.ucsf.edu
References

Thomas J. Prendergast, MD
Associate Professor of Medicine and Anesthesiology, Section of Pulmonary and Critical Care Medicine, Dartmouth-Hitchcock Medical Center, Lebanon, New Hampshire
thomas.j.prendergast@hitchcock.org
Lung

Reed E. Pyeritz, MD, PhD
Professor of Medicine and Genetics; Chief, Division of Medical Genetics, University of Pennsylvania School of Medicine, Philadelphia
reed.pyeritz@uphs.upenn.edu
Medical Genetics

Michael W. Rabow, MD
Assistant Clinical Professor of Medicine, Division of General Internal Medicine, University of California, San Francisco
mrabow@medicine.ucsf.edu
Care at the End of Life

Paul Riordan-Eva, FRCOphth
Consultant Ophthalmologist, King's College Hospital, London; Honorary Consultant Neuro-Ophthalmologist, National Hospital for Neurology and Neurosurgery, London, United Kingdom
paulreva@doctors.org.uk
Eye

Hope S. Rugo, MD
Associate Clinical Professor of Medicine, University of California, San Francisco Comprehensive Cancer Center
hope.rugo@ucsfmedctr.org
Cancer

Wayne X. Shandera, MD
Assistant Professor of Internal Medicine, Baylor College of Medicine, Houston
shandera@bcm.tmc.edu
Infectious Diseases: Viral & Rickettsial

Samuel A. Shelburne III, MD
Chief Resident, Department of Internal Medicine, Baylor College of Medicine, Houston
sshelburne@pdq.net
Infectious Diseases: Viral & Rickettsial

Marshall L. Stoller, MD
Professor, Department of Urology, University of California, San Francisco
Urology

John H. Stone, MD, MPH
Associate Professor of Medicine, Division of Rheumatology, Johns Hopkins Hospital; Director, Johns Hopkins Vasculitis Center, Baltimore
jstone@jhmi.edu
Arthritis & Musculoskeletal Disorders

Lawrence M. Tierney, Jr., MD
Professor of Medicine, University of California, San Francisco; Associate Chief of Medical Service, San Francisco Veterans Affairs Medical Center
vaspa@itsa.ucsf.edu
Blood Vessels & Lymphatics

Sushrut S. Waikar, MD
Chief Resident, Department of Medicine, Moffitt-Long Hospital, University of California, San Francisco
waikarss@medicine.ucsf.edu
References

Suzanne Watnick, MD
Assistant Professor of Medicine, Division of Nephrology and Hypertension, Oregon Health Sciences University, Portland
swatnick@hotmail.com
Kidney

Preface

Current Medical Diagnosis & Treatment 2003 is the 42nd annual volume of this single-source reference for practitioners in both hospital and ambulatory settings. It emphasizes the practical features of clinical diagnosis and patient management in all fields of internal medicine and in specialties of interest to primary care practitioners and subspecialists who provide generalist care.

OUTSTANDING FEATURES

- Medical advances up to the time of publication
- Detailed presentation of all primary care topics, including gynecology, obstetrics, dermatology, ophthalmology, otolaryngology, psychiatry, neurology, toxicology, and urology
- Concise format, facilitating efficient use in any practice setting
- More than 1000 diseases and disorders
- Only text with annual update of HIV infection
- Prevention and cost information
- Easy access to drug dosages, with trade names indexed and prices updated in each edition
- Annotated recent references, with unique identifiers (PubMed, PMID, numbers) for all citations
- Companion Web site featuring direct links to more than 450 selected Web sites
- Inexpensive

INTENDED AUDIENCE

House officers and all students of the healing arts will find the descriptions of diagnostic and therapeutic modalities, with citations to the current literature, of everyday usefulness in patient care.

Internists, family physicians, nurse practitioners, and other primary care providers will appreciate *CMDT* as a ready reference and refresher text. Physicians in other specialties, surgeons, and dentists will find the book a basic internal medicine reference. Nurses and physician's assistants will welcome the format and scope of the book as a means of learning diagnosis and treatment.

Those who are not involved in health care but seek information about the nature of specific diseases and their diagnosis and treatment may also find this book to be a valuable resource.

SPECIAL TO THIS EDITION

- New chapter on common symptoms, including cough, lower extremity edema, fever, involuntary weight loss, fatigue, and upper abdominal pain and dyspepsia
- Updated information on the management of atrial fibrillation; end-of-life care information integrated throughout the text
- Advances in cancer, obesity, hepatitis C, nonalcoholic fatty liver disease
- Developments in thyroid disease, diabetes mellitus, asthma, and HIV infection
- New information on alternative medicine and complementary therapies
- Major revision of chapters on blood vessels and lymphatics, and cancer
- Drug information, bibliographies, and Web sites updated through June 2002
- An update on antibiotics, including new antiviral and antifungal agents
- Expanded information on the clinical presentation and treatment of bioterrorism-related diseases, such as anthrax.
- List of key Internet addresses for peer-reviewed, current medical information, including:
  - Centers for Disease Control and Prevention traveler's and immunization information
  - National Institutes of Health Consensus Statements
  - The Agency for Healthcare Research and Quality of the United States Public Health Service Clinical Guidelines
- Complete list of USA Poison Control Centers with telephone numbers

COMPANION WEB SITE

CMDT's companion Web site, Current-Med.com, contains an annotated list of Web sites selected and revised throughout the year. The entries provide descriptions of sites as well as ratings of them on a six-category scale. All linked Internet addresses are updated monthly. The companion Web site address is provided on the first page of each chapter.

CMDT IS ONLINE IN 2003

In late 2002, the online version of *CMDT* will be available. It will include the content in the book version as well as these valuable features:

• New diagnostic test information
• Up-to-date clinical guidelines for screening, prevention, and disease management
• Hundreds of new color images, graphs, algorithms, and tables
• Patient education materials (printable), including direct links to the *Journal of the American Medical Association's* weekly patient pages
• Relevant Web sites keyed to chapter content
• Web Site of the Week, which features a site of special interest
• Direct PubMed links to abstracts of all references to ensure immediate access to evidence
• Prevention and cost information
• Clinical vignettes linked to chapter content and Internet resources
• An integrated drug database
• Puzzles (What Is This?), updated daily, to improve learners' pattern recognition
• In the News, updated daily and linked to related chapter content
• A forum for readers to communicate items of interest

ORDER OR SUBSCRIBE TO CMDT AND CURRENT-MED.COM (CMDT ONLINE)

It is now possible to receive each year's edition of the only annually updated textbook of medicine automatically upon publication simply by returning the enclosed postcard to McGraw-Hill. You can order *Current Medical Diagnosis and Treatment 2003* and the online version by visiting the McGraw-Hill Web site, www.current-med.com, or calling 1-800-262-4729.

ACKNOWLEDGMENTS

We wish to thank our associate authors for participating once again in the annual updating of this important book. In particular, we wish to thank Dr. Steven A. Schroeder, who served as the book's chief title page editor from 1988 to 1993 and as a chapter author for General Approach to the Patient; Health Maintenance & Disease Prevention; and Common Symptoms from 1987 through 2002. We would also like to recognize the contribution to *CMDT* of several past authors: Dr. Neil M. Resnick, who authored the Geriatric Medicine chapter from 1992 through 2002; Dr. Joseph C. Presti, who coauthored the Urology chapter for the 1994 through 2002 editions; and Dr. Alain R. Bouckenooghe, who coauthored the chapter on Infectious Diseases: Viral and Rickettsial from 2000 through 2002. Their expertise has contributed immeasurably to the excellence of this text.

Many students and physicians have contributed useful suggestions to this and previous editions, and we are grateful. We continue to welcome comments and recommendations for future editions in writing or via electronic mail. The editors' and authors' institutional and Internet e-mail addresses are given in the Authors section.

Lawrence M. Tierney, Jr., MD
Stephen J. McPhee, MD
Maxine A. Papadakis, MD

San Francisco, California
September 2002

Dedication

To

John H. Karam, MD

John H. Karam, MD, a revered figure at the University of California, San Francisco and a contributing author for more than twenty-five editions of this book's chapter on diabetes and hypoglycemia—and a contributor of over one hundred peer-reviewed journal articles—died in San Francisco in an accident on September 23, 2002.

All who knew John Karam drew pleasure and strength from his warm and gentle demeanor, and his stature as one of the world's great diabetologists is known to us all and to our readers around the world. His legacy to countless patients—through his skills in clinical care, his clinical research, and indeed his literary contributions to this and other books—is a remarkable achievement they will understand and acknowledge.

Our profession is made poorer by his sudden absence from our counsels and endeavors. We dedicate this volume of *Current Medical Diagnosis & Treatment* to him in grateful acknowledgment of his extraordinary contributions to medicine and to humankind.

Lawrence M. Tierney, Jr., MD
Stephen J. McPhee, MD
Maxine A. Papadakis, MD
And the Contributing Authors of *CMDT 2003*

General Approach to the Patient; Health Maintenance & Disease Prevention

Stephen J. McPhee, MD, & Michael Pignone, MD, MPH

See www.current-med.com/ch01.html

■ GENERAL APPROACH TO THE PATIENT

The approach to diagnosis begins with the history and pertinent physical examination—both susceptible to errors of omission and commission. The medical interview serves several functions. It is used to collect information of help in diagnosis (the "history" of the present illness), to assess and communicate prognosis, to provide emotional support, and to reach agreement with the patient about further diagnostic procedures and therapeutic options. It also serves as an opportunity to influence patient behavior, such as in motivational discussions about smoking cessation. Interviewing techniques that avoid domination by the physician increase patient satisfaction. Effective physician-patient communication can improve health outcomes.

Patient Compliance

For many illnesses, treatment depends on difficult fundamental behavioral changes, including alterations in diet, taking up exercise, giving up smoking, and cutting down drinking. Compliance is a problem in every practice; up to 50% of patients fail to achieve full compliance, and a third never take their medicines. Compliance rates for short-term, self-administered therapies are higher than for long-term therapies and are inversely correlated with the number of interventions, their complexity and cost, and the patient's perception of overmedication.

Patients seem better able to take prescribed medications than to comply with recommendations to follow a diet, exercise regularly, or perform various self-care activities (such as monitoring blood glucose levels at home). Writing out advice to patients, including changes in medication, may be helpful. Because functional health illiteracy is common, with over 40% of patients unable to read and understand basic written instructions, other forms of communication, such as videotape or oral instructions, may be more effective.

To help improve adherence, clinicians can work with patients to agree on the goals for therapy, prescribe a simple dosage regimen for all medications (preferably one or two doses daily), help the patient devise cues to help in remembering to take doses (time of day, mealtime, alarms), and provide ways to simplify dosing (medication boxes). Single-unit doses supplied in foil-backed wrappers should be avoided for patients who have difficulty opening them. Medication boxes with compartments (eg, Medisets) that are filled weekly are useful. Microelectronic devices can provide feedback to show patients whether they have taken doses as scheduled or to notify patients within a day if doses are skipped.

Compliance is also improved when a trusting doctor-patient relationship has been established. Clinicians can improve patient compliance by inquiring specifically about the behaviors in question. When asked, many patients admit to incomplete compliance with medication regimens, with advice about giving up cigarettes, or with engaging only in "safe sex" practices. Although difficult, sufficient time must be made available for communication of health messages. Other ways of assessing medication compliance include pill counts and refill records; monitoring serum, urine, or saliva levels of drugs or metabolites; or assessing predictable drug effects such as weight changes with diuretics or bradycardia from beta-blockers. Even partial compliance, as with drug treatment of hypertension and diabetes mellitus, improves outcomes compared with noncompliance.

Guiding Principles of Care

Ethical principles that guide the successful approach to diagnosis and treatment are honesty, beneficence, justice, avoidance of conflict of interest, and the pledge to do no harm. Increasingly, Western medicine involves patients in important decisions about medical care, including how far to proceed with treatment of patients who have terminal illnesses (see Chapter 5).

The physician's role does not end with diagnosis and treatment. The importance of the empathic clinician in helping patients and their families bear the burden of serious illness and death cannot be overemphasized. "To cure sometimes, to relieve often, and to comfort always" is a French saying as apt today as it was five centuries ago—as is Francis Peabody's admonition: "The secret of the care of the patient is in caring for the patient."

Braddock CH 3rd et al: Informed decision making in outpatient practice: time to get back to basics. JAMA 1999;282:2313. [PMID: 10612318] (Informed decision-making was incomplete in 91% of 3552 clinical decisions. Discussion of the nature of an intervention occurred most frequently [71%] and assessment of patient understanding least frequently [1.5%].)

Branch WT Jr: The ethics of caring and medical education. Acad Med 2000;75:127. [PMID: 10693842] (Receptivity, taking responsibility, and creating an educational environment that fosters caring help the physician to remain always the patient's advocate and to maintain the therapeutic relationship when dealing with and resolving ethical dilemmas.)

Butler C et al: The practitioner, the patient and resistance to change: Recent ideas on compliance. Can Med Assoc J 1996;154:1357. [PMID: 8616739] (The authors propose a patient-centered, negotiation-based framework that harnesses patients' intrinsic motivation to make their own decisions and promotes clinicians' acceptance of those decisions even if they run counter to current medical wisdom.)

Cegala DJ et al: The effects of patient communication skills training on compliance. Arch Fam Med 2000;9:57. [PMID: 10664643] (A randomized controlled trial demonstrating that training patients in communication skills increased compliance with medications; behavioral treatments including diet, exercise, and smoking cessation; and follow-up appointments.)

Cramer JA: Enhancing patient compliance in the elderly. Role of packaging aids and monitoring. Drugs Aging 1998;12:7. [PMID: 9467683] (Elderly patients are at risk of noncompliance because of deficits in physical dexterity, cognitive skills and memory, and the number of medications typically prescribed.)

■ HEALTH MAINTENANCE & DISEASE PREVENTION

Preventive medicine is categorized as primary, secondary, or tertiary. Primary prevention aims to remove or reduce disease risk factors (eg, immunization, giving up or not starting smoking). Secondary prevention techniques promote early detection of disease or precursor states (eg, routine cervical Papanicolaou screening to detect carcinoma of the cervix). Tertiary prevention measures are aimed at limiting the impact of established disease (eg, partial mastectomy and radiation therapy to remove and control localized breast cancer). Table 1–1 lists deaths from preventable causes in the USA—diseases that in 1990 accounted for 50% of all fatalities. Table 1–2 compares recommendations for periodic health examinations as developed by the United States Preventive Services Task Force, the

Table 1–1. Deaths from preventable causes in the United States in 1990.[1]

Cause	Estimated Number of Deaths	Percentage of Total Deaths
Tobacco	400,000	19
Dietary factors and activity patterns	300,000	14
Alcohol	100,000	5
Microbial agents	90,000	4
Toxic agents	60,000	3
Firearms	35,000	2
High-risk sexual behavior	30,000	1
Motor vehicle injuries	25,000	1
Illicit use of drugs	20,000	< 1
TOTAL	1,060,000	≈50

[1]Reproduced, with permission, from McGinnis JM, Foege WH: Actual causes of death in the United States. JAMA 1993;270:2707.

American College of Physicians, and the Canadian Task Force on the Periodic Health Examination. Despite emerging consensus on many of the services, controversy persists for others. Many effective preventive services are underutilized. A recent analysis found the following services had the most potential for improvement, based on their effectiveness and underuse: counseling about smoking cessation; screening older adults for vision impairment; screening and counseling adults and adolescents about alcohol abuse; screening older adults for colorectal cancer; screening young women for chlamydia infection; and vaccinating older adults against pneumococcal disease.

Coffield AB: Priorities among recommended clinical preventive services. Am J Prev Med 2001;21:1. [PMID:11418251]

PREVENTION OF INFECTIOUS DISEASES

Much of the decline in the incidence and fatality rates of infectious diseases is attributable to public health measures—especially immunization, improved sanitation, and better nutrition.

Immunization remains the best means of preventing many infectious diseases. In the USA, immunization has resulted in near elimination of measles, mumps, rubella, poliomyelitis, diphtheria, pertussis, and tetanus. *Haemophilus influenzae* type b invasive disease has been reduced by more than 95% since introduction of the first conjugate vaccines. Opportunities still exist for reducing morbidity and mortality from vaccine-preventable diseases. For example,

Table 1–2. Expert recommendations for preventive care for asymptomatic, low-risk adults.

Preventive Service	United States Preventive Services Task Force			American College of Physicians			Canadian Task Force on the Periodic Health Examination		
	Sex	Age	Minimum Frequency[1]	Sex	Age	Minimum Frequency[1]	Sex	Age	Minimum Frequency[1]
Physical examination									
Blood pressure	MF	18+	q 2 yrs	MF	18+	q 2 yrs	MF	25–64	q 5 yrs
							MF	65+	q 2 yrs
Clinical breast examination	F	50–69[2]	q 1–2 yrs[3]	F	40+	Annually	F	50–69	Annually
Laboratory tests									
Papanicolaou smear	F	18[4]–65	q 3 yrs	F	20[4]–65[5]	q 3 yrs	F	18[4]–69	q 3 yrs[6]
Stool for occult blood	MF	50+	Annually	MF	50–70/80	Annually[7]	NR	NR	NR
Sigmoidoscopy	MF	50+	q ? yrs	MF	50–70	q 10 yrs	NR	NR	NR
Mammography	F	50–69[2]	q 1–2 yrs	F	50–75	q 2 yrs	F	50–69	Annually
Cholesterol	M	35–65	q ? yrs	M	35–65	Once	M	30–59	q ? yrs
	F	45–65		F	45–65				
Immunizations									
Tetanus-diphtheria booster	MF	18+	q 15–30 yrs	MF	18+	q 10 yrs or once at age 50	MF	18+	q 10 yrs
Influenza vaccination	MF	65+	Annually	MF	65+	Annually	MF	65+	Annually
Pneumococcal vaccination	MF	65+	Once[8]	MF	65+	Once[8]	NR	NR	NR
Counseling[9]	MF	18+	At routine visits	MF	18+	At routine visits	MF	18+	At routine visits

NR = no recommendation; ? = "periodic."

[1]Where question marks appear, the appropriate interval is left to clinical discretion because of lack of evidence.

[2]There is insufficient evidence to recommend for or against routine mammography or clinical breast examination for women age 40–49 or age ≥ 70, though recommendations for high-risk women in these age groups may be made on other grounds.

[3]Combined with mammography. There is insufficient evidence to recommend for or against clinical breast examination alone.

[4]Or following onset of sexual activity.

[5]There is insufficient evidence to recommend for or against an upper age limit for Papanicolaou testing after age 65 in women with regular previous normal smears.

[6]After two normal annual smears.

[7]For persons who decline screening sigmoidoscopy, barium enema, or colonoscopy.

[8]Reimmunize at age 65 those high-risk individuals who are 6 years or more after primary dose.

[9]Regarding tobacco use, nutrition, exercise, sexual behavior, substance abuse, injury prevention, and dental care.

in adults in the USA, there are an estimated 50,000–70,000 deaths annually from influenza, hepatitis B, and invasive pneumococcal disease. Among targeted adult groups, only about 40% have had influenza vaccination, 20% pneumococcal vaccination, and 10% hepatitis B vaccination. The American College of Physicians recommends that clinicians should review each adult's immunization status at age 50; assess risk factors that would indicate a need for pneumococcal vaccination and annual influenza immunizations; reimmunize at age 65 those who received an immunization against pneumococcus more than 6 years before; ensure that all adults have completed a primary diphtheria-tetanus immunization series, and administer a single booster at age 50; and assess the postvaccination serologic response to hepatitis B vaccination in all recipients who have ongoing risks of exposure to blood or body fluids (eg, sharp injuries, blood splashes).

Recently, needle-free jet injectors have been used successfully in administering trivalent inactivated influenza vaccine. In randomized, controlled trials, a novel triple-antigen (S, pre-S1, and pre-S2) recombinant hepatitis B vaccine (Hepacare) appears to be more effective than currently available single-antigen (S only) vaccine (Engerix B, Recombivax-HB). The new triple-antigen vaccine is also effective in more than three-quarters of inadequate responders to current single-antigen vaccines.

Recommended immunization schedules for children and adults are set forth in Table 30–4. Persons traveling to countries where infections are endemic should take precautions described in Chapter 30.

Skin testing for tuberculosis and treating selected patients reduces the risk of reactivation tuberculosis (see Table 9–12). Attention to technique helps separate negative from positive results. Drawing a line on the skin with a medium ballpoint pen, starting

1–2 cm away from the skin reaction and then stopping when resistance is felt, gives a more precise measurement of induration. Patients with HIV infection are at an especially high risk for tuberculosis. This is discussed in Chapter 31, as is multidrug-resistant tuberculosis.

HIV infection is now the major infectious disease problem in the world. Since sexual contact is a common mode of transmission, prevention relies on eliminating unsafe sexual behavior by promoting abstinence, later onset of first sexual activity, decreased number of partners, and use of condoms. Appropriately used, condoms can reduce the rate of HIV transmission by nearly 70%. Couples with one infected partner who used condoms inconsistently had a considerable risk of infection: the rate of seroconversion was 4.8 per 100 persons per year, leading to an estimated cumulative incidence of 12.7% after 24 months. No seroconversions were noted with consistent condom use. Unfortunately, as many as one-third of HIV-positive individuals continue unprotected sexual practices after learning that they are HIV-infected. Tailored group educational intervention focused on practicing "safer sex" can reduce their transmission-risk behaviors with partners who are not HIV-positive. Other approaches to prevent HIV infection include treatment of sexually transmitted diseases, development of vaginal microbicides, and vaccine development. Increasingly, cases of HIV infection are transmitted by intravenous drug use. HIV prevention activities should include provision of sterile injection equipment for these individuals.

In immunocompromised patients, live vaccines are contraindicated but many killed or component vaccines are safe and recommended. *Asymptomatic* HIV-infected patients have not shown adverse consequences when given live MMR and influenza vaccinations as well as tetanus, hepatitis B, *H influenzae* type b, and pneumococcal vaccinations—all should be given. However, if poliomyelitis immunization is required, the inactivated poliomyelitis vaccine is indicated. In *symptomatic* HIV-infected patients, live virus vaccines such as MMR should generally be avoided, but annual influenza vaccination is safe.

Whenever possible, immunizations should be completed before procedures that require or induce immunosuppression (organ transplantation or chemotherapy), or that reduce immunogenic responses (splenectomy). However, if this is not possible, the patient may mount only a partial immune response, yet even this partial response can be of benefit. Patients who undergo allogeneic bone marrow transplantation lose preexisting immunities and should be revaccinated. In many situations, family members should also be vaccinated to protect the immunocompromised patient, though oral live polio vaccine should be avoided because of the risk of infecting the patient.

New cases of poliomyelitis have been reported in Haiti recently, slowing its eradication in the Western Hemisphere.

Avery RK: Immunizations in adult immunocompromised patients: which to use and which to avoid. Cleve Clin J Med 2001;68:337. [PMID: 11326813]

Coyle SL et al: Outreach-based HIV prevention for injecting drug users: a review of published outcome data. Public Health Rep 1998;113(Suppl 1):19. [PMID: 9722807] (Outreach prevention programs can lead to lower HIV incidence rates among program participants.)

Gardner P et al: Recommended schedules for routine immunization of children and adults. Infect Dis Clin North Am 2001;15:1. [PMID: 11301810]

Iseman M: A 52-year-old man with a positive PPD. JAMA 2001;286:2015. [PMID: 11667939]

Kalichman SC et al: Effectiveness of an intervention to reduce HIV transmission risks in HIV-positive people. Am J Prev Med 2001;21:84. [PMID: 11457627]

Wilcox SA et al: Registry-driven, community-based immunization outreach: a randomized controlled trial. Am J Public Health 2001;91:1507. [PMID: 11527789]

Young MD et al: Adult hepatitis B vaccination using a novel triple antigen recombinant vaccine. Hepatology 2001;34:372. [PMID: 11481622] (A two-dose [0, 1 month] regimen of the triple-antigen vaccine provided similar rates of protection as the standard three-dose [0, 1, 6 months] regimen of single-antigen vaccine [91% versus 88% seroprotected by 7 months], and a three-dose [0, 1, 6 months] regimen of the triple-antigen vaccine provided superior protection [98% versus 88%; *P* < .001].)

Zuckerman JN et al: Evaluation of a new hepatitis B triple-antigen vaccine in inadequate responders to current vaccines. Hepatology 2001;34(4 Part 1):798. [PMID: 11584378]

PREVENTION OF CARDIOVASCULAR DISEASE

Cardiovascular diseases, including coronary heart disease and stroke, represent two of the most important causes of morbidity and mortality in developed countries. Several risk factors increase the risk for coronary disease and stroke. They can be divided into those that are modifiable (eg, lipid disorders, hypertension, cigarette smoking) and those that are not (eg, gender, age, family history of early coronary disease). This section considers the role of screening for and treating the former.

Impressive declines in age-specific mortality rates from heart disease and stroke have been achieved in all age groups in North America during the past 2 decades. The chief reasons for this favorable trend appear to be modification of risk factors, especially cigarette smoking and hypercholesterolemia, plus more aggressive detection and treatment of hypertension and better care for patients with heart disease.

Cigarette Smoking

Cigarette smoking remains the most important cause of preventable morbidity and early mortality in developed countries. Nicotine is highly addictive, raises brain levels of dopamine, and produces withdrawal symptoms on discontinuation. Cigarettes are responsible for one in every five deaths in the USA, yet smoking prevalence rates have been increasing among high school and college students. Cigar smoking has also increased; there is also continued use of smokeless tobacco (chewing tobacco and snuff), particularly among young people. Tobacco dependence may have a genetic component.

Smokers have twice the risk of fatal heart disease, ten times the risk of lung cancer, and several times the risk of cancers of the mouth, throat, esophagus, pancreas, kidney, bladder, and cervix; a two- to threefold higher incidence of stroke and peptic ulcers (which heal less well than in nonsmokers); a two- to fourfold greater risk of fractures of the hip, wrist, and vertebrae; four times the risk of invasive pneumococcal disease; and a twofold increase in cataracts. In the United States, over 90% of cases of chronic obstructive pulmonary disease (COPD) occur among current or former smokers. Both active smoking and passive smoking are associated with deterioration of the elastic properties of the aorta and with progression of carotid artery atherosclerosis. Smoking has also been associated with increased risks of leukemia, of colon and prostate cancers, of breast cancer among postmenopausal women who are slow acetylators of N-acetyltransferase-2 enzymes, osteoporosis, and Alzheimer's disease. In cancers of the head and neck, lung, esophagus, and bladder, smoking is linked to mutations of the $P53$ gene, the most common genetic change in human cancer. Patients with head and neck cancer who continue to smoke during radiation therapy have lower rates of response than those who do not smoke. Olfaction and taste are impaired in smokers, facial wrinkles are increased. Heavy smokers have a 2.5 greater risk of age-related macular degeneration. Smokers die 5–8 years earlier than never-smokers.

The children of smokers have lower birth weights, are more likely to be mentally retarded, have more frequent respiratory infections, less efficient pulmonary function, and a higher incidence of chronic ear infections than children of nonsmokers and are more likely to become smokers themselves.

In addition, exposure to environmental tobacco smoke has been shown to increase the risk of cervical cancer, lung cancer, invasive pneumococcal disease, and heart disease; to promote endothelial damage and platelet aggregation; and to increase urinary excretion of tobacco-specific lung carcinogens. The incidence of breast cancer may be increased as well. Of approximately 450,000 smoking-related deaths in the USA, as many as 53,000 are attributable to passive smoking.

Smoking cessation lessens the risks of death and of myocardial infarction in people with coronary artery disease; reduces the rate of death and acute myocardial infarction in patients who have undergone percutaneous coronary revascularization; lessens the risk of stroke; slows the rate of progression of carotid atherosclerosis; and is associated with reversal of chronic bronchitis and improved pulmonary function. Women smokers who quit smoking by age 35 add about 3 years to their life expectancy, and men add more than 2 years to theirs. Smoking cessation can increase

life expectancy even for those who stop after the age of 65.

Fortunately, adult rates are now at an all-time low—23%—but rates are climbing for young people.

Although tobacco use constitutes the most serious common medical problem, it is undertreated. Over 70% of smokers see a physician each year, but only 20% of them receive any medical quitting advice or assistance. (Those whose physicians advise them to quit are 1.6 times as likely to attempt quitting.) About 4% of smokers are able to quit each year.

The five steps for helping smokers quit are summarized in Table 1–3. Common elements of supportive smoking cessation treatments are reviewed in Table 1–4. A system should be implemented to identify smokers and advice to quit should be tailored to the patient's level of readiness to change. All patients trying to quit should be offered pharmacotherapy except those with medical contraindications, those smoking fewer than ten cigarettes per day, women who are pregnant or breast feeding, and adolescents. Nicotine replacement therapy doubles the chance of successful quitting. Guidelines for its use are presented in Table 1–5. Suggestions for the nicotine patch are listed in Table 1–6 and for nicotine gum in Table 1–7. Both patch and gum are now available over-the-counter, and nicotine nasal spray by prescription. When the spray is combined with the patch, cessation rates are substantially higher. The sustained-release antidepressant drug bupropion (150–300 mg/d) is an effective smoking cessation agent and is associated with minimal weight gain. It acts by boosting brain levels of dopamine and norepinephrine, mimicking the effect of nicotine. Bupropion, either alone or in combination with a nicotine patch, has been shown to produce significantly higher abstinence rates (30–35% at 1 year) than either a patch alone or placebo. Weight gain was less in the combined program. (See Table 1–8.)

Weight gain occurs in most patients (80%) following smoking cessation. For many it averages 2 kg, but for others (10–15%) major weight gain—over 13 kg—may occur.

Clinicians should not show disapproval of patients who cannot stop smoking. Thoughtful advice that emphasizes the benefits of cessation and recognizes common barriers to success can increase quit rates. An intercurrent illness such as acute bronchitis or acute myocardial infarction may motivate even the most addicted smoker to quit. Individualized or group counseling are very cost-effective, even more so than treating hypertension. An additional strategy is to recommend that any smoking take place out of doors to limit the effects of passive smoke on housemates and coworkers. This can lead to smoking reduction and quitting. The clinician's role in smoking cessation is summarized in Table 1–4.

Ayanian JZ et al: Perceived risks of heart disease and cancer among cigarette smokers. JAMA 1999;281:1019. [PMID:

Table 1–3. Actions and strategies for the primary care clinician to help patients quit smoking.[1]

Action	Strategies for Implementation
Step 1. Ask—Systematically Identify All Tobacco Users at Every Visit	

Implement an officewide system that ensures that for *every* patient at *every* clinic visit, tobacco-use status is queried and documented[2]	Expand the vital signs to include tobacco use.
	  Data should be collected by the health care team.
	  The action should be implemented using preprinted progress note paper that includes the expanded vital signs, a vital signs stamp, or, for computerized records, an item assessing tobacco-use status.
	Alternatives to the vital signs stamp are to place tobacco-use status stickers on all patients' charts or to indicate smoking status using computerized reminder systems.

Step 2. Advise—Strongly Urge All Smokers to Quit	

In a *clear, strong,* and *personalized* manner, urge every smoker to quit	Advice should be
	  Clear: "I think it is important for you to quit smoking now, and I will help you. Cutting down while you are ill is not enough."
	  Strong: "As your clinician, I need you to know that quitting smoking is the most important thing you can do to protect your current and future health."
	  Personalized: Tie smoking to current health or illness and/or the social and economic costs of tobacco use, motivational level/readiness to quit, and the impact of smoking on children and others in the household.
	Encourage clinic staff to reinforce the cessation message and support the patient's quit attempt.

Step 3. Attempt—Identify Smokers Willing to Make a Quit Attempt	
Ask every smoker if he or she is willing to make a quit attempt at this time	If the patient is willing to make a quit attempt at this time, provide assistance (see step 4). If the patient prefers a more intensive treatment or the clinician believes more intensive treatment is appropriate, refer the patient to interventions administered by a smoking cessation specialist and follow up with him or her regarding quitting (see step 5). If the patient clearly states he or she is not willing to make a quit attempt at this time, provide a motivational intervention.
Step 4. Assist—Aid the Patient in Quitting	

A. Help the patient with a quit plan	*Set a quit date.* Ideally, the quit date should be within 2 weeks, taking patient preference into account.
	Help the patient prepare for quitting. The patient must:
	  Inform family, friends, and coworkers of quitting and request understanding and support.
	  Prepare the environment by removing cigarettes from it. Prior to quitting, the patient should avoid smoking in places where he or she spends a lot of time (eg, home, car).
	  Review previous quit attempts. What helped? What led to relapse?
	  Anticipate challenges to the planned quit attempt, particularly during the critical first few weeks.

B. Encourage nicotine replacement therapy except in special circumstances	Encourage the use of the nicotine patch or nicotine gum therapy for smoking cessation (see Tables 1–5 to 1–7 for specific instructions and precautions).
C. Give key advice on successful quitting	*Abstinence:* Total abstinence is essential. Not even a single puff after the quit date. *Alcohol:* Drinking alcohol is highly associated with relapse. Those who stop smoking should review their alcohol use and consider limiting or abstaining from alcohol use during the quit process. *Other smokers in the household:* The presence of other smokers in the household, particularly a spouse, is associated with lower success rates. Patients should consider quitting with their significant others and/or developing specific plans to maintain abstinence in a household where others still smoke.
D. Provide supplementary materials	*Source:* Federal agencies, including the National Cancer Institute and the Agency for Health Care Policy and Research; nonprofit agencies (American Cancer Society, American Lung Association, American Heart Association); or local or state health departments. *Selection concerns:* The material must be culturally, racially, educationally, and age appropriate for the patient. *Location:* Readily available in every clinic office.

(continued)

Table 1–3. Actions and strategies for the primary care clinician to help patients quit smoking.[1] (continued)

Action	Strategies for Implementation
Step 5. Arrange—Schedule Follow-Up Contact	
Schedule follow-up contact, either in person or via telephone[2]	*Timing:* Follow-up contact should occur soon after the quit date, preferably during the first week. A second follow-up contact is recommended within the first month. Schedule further follow-up contacts as indicated.
	Actions during follow-up: Congratulate success. If smoking occurred, review the circumstances and elicit recommitment to total abstinence. Remind the patient that a lapse can be used as a learning experience and is not a sign of failure. Identify the problems already encountered and anticipate challenges in the immediate future. Assess nicotine replacement therapy use and problems. Consider referral to a more intense or specialized program.

[1]Modified and reproduced, with permission, from: The Agency for Health Care Policy and Research. *Smoking Cessation Clinical Practice Guideline.* JAMA 1996;275:1270.
[2]Repeated assessment is not necessary in the case of the adult who has never smoked or not smoked for many years and for whom the information is clearly documented in the medical record.

Table 1–4. Common elements of supportive smoking treatments.[1]

Component	Examples
Encouragement of the patient in the quit attempt	Note that effective cessation treatments are now available. Note that half the people who have *ever* smoked have now quit. Communicate belief in the patient's ability to quit.
Communication of caring and concern	Ask how the patient feels about quitting. Directly express concern and a willingness to help. Be open to the patient's expression of fears of quitting, difficulties experienced, and ambivalent feelings.
Encouragement of the patient to talk about the quitting process	Ask about Reasons that the patient wants to quit. Difficulties encountered while quitting. Success the patient has achieved. Concerns or worries about quitting.
Provision of basic information about smoking and successful quitting	Inform the patient about The nature and time course of withdrawal. The addictive nature of smoking. The fact that any smoking (even a single puff) increases the likelihood of full relapse.

[1]Modified, with permission, from: The Agency for Health Care Policy and Research. *Smoking Cessation Clinical Practice Guideline.* JAMA 1996;275:1270.

Table 1–5. Clinical guidelines for prescribing nicotine replacement products.[1]

1. **Who should receive nicotine replacement therapy?**
   Available research shows that nicotine replacement therapy generally increases rates of smoking cessation. Therefore, except in special circumstances, the clinician should encourage the use of nicotine replacement with patients who smoke. Little research is available on the use of nicotine replacement with light smokers (ie, those smoking ≤ 10–15 cigarettes/d). If nicotine replacement is to be used with light smokers, a lower starting dose of the nicotine patch or nicotine gum should be considered.

2. **Should nicotine replacement therapy be tailored to the individual smoker?**
   Research does not support the tailoring of nicotine patch therapy (except with light smokers as noted above). Patients should be prescribed the patch dosages outlined in Table 1–6.
   Research supports tailoring nicotine gum treatment. Specifically, research suggests that 4-mg gum rather than 2-mg gum be used with patients who are highly dependent on nicotine (eg, those smoking > 20 cigarettes/d, those who smoke immediately upon awakening, and those who report histories of severe nicotine withdrawal symptoms). Clinicians may also recommend the higher gum dose if patients request it or have failed to quit using the 2-mg gum.

[1]Modified with permission, from: The Agency for Health Care Policy and Research. *Smoking Cessation Clinical Practice Guideline.* JAMA 1996;275:1270.

Table 1–6. Suggestions for the clinical use of the nicotine patch.[1]

Parameter of Clinical Use	Suggestions
Patient selection	Appropriate as a primary pharmacotherapy for smoking cessation.
Precautions	*Pregnancy:* Pregnant smokers should first be encouraged to attempt cessation without pharmacologic treatment. The nicotine patch should be used during pregnancy only if the increased likelihood of smoking cessation, with its potential benefits, outweighs the risk of nicotine replacement and potential concomitant smoking. Similar factors should be considered in lactating women. *Cardiovascular diseases:* While not an independent risk factor for acute myocardial events, the nicotine patch should be used only after consideration of risks and benefits among particular cardiovascular patient groups: those in the immediate (within 2 weeks) post-myocardial infarction period, those with serious arrhythmias, and those with severe or worsening angina pectoris. *Skin reactions:* Up to 50% of patients using the nicotine patch will have a local skin reaction. Skin reactions are usually mild and self-limiting but may worsen over the course of therapy. Local treatment with hydrocortisone cream (2.5%) or triamcinolone cream (0.5%) and rotating patch sites may ameliorate such local reactions. In fewer than 5% of patients do such reactions require the discontinuation of nicotine patch treatment.
Dosage[2]	Treatment of 8 weeks or less has been shown to be as efficacious as longer treatment periods. Based on this finding, we suggest the following treatment schedules as reasonable for most smokers. Clinicians should consult the package insert for other treatment suggestions. Finally, clinicians should consider individualizing treatment based on specific patient characteristics such as previous experience with the patch, number of cigarettes smoked, and degree of addiction.

Brand	Duration (weeks)	Dosage (mg/h)
Nicoderm and Habitrol	4 then 2 then 2	21/24 14/24 7/24
Prostep	4 then 4	22/24 11/24
Nicotrol	4 then 2 then 2	15/16 10/16 5/16

Prescribing instructions	Abstinence from smoking: The patient should refrain from smoking while using the patch. Location: At the start of each day, the patient should place a new patch on a relatively hairless location between the neck and the waist. Activities: There are no restrictions while using the patch. Time: Patches should be applied as soon as patients awaken on their quit day.

[1]Reproduced, with permission, from: The Agency for Health Care Policy and Research. *Smoking Cessation Clinical Practice Guideline.* JAMA 1996;275:1270. Updated and revised, with permission, from *Treating Tobacco Use and Dependence.* U.S. Public Health Service. *www.surgeongeneral.gov/tobacco/default.htm*
[2]These dosage recommendations are based on a review of the published research literature and do not necessarily conform to package insert information.

10086437] (Only 29% and 40% of current smokers—respectively—believed they have a higher than average risk of myocardial infarction or cancer.)

Blonal T et al: Nicotine nasal spray with nicotine patch for smoking cessation: randomized trial with six year follow-up. BMJ 1999;318:285. [PMID: 9924052] (Patch plus spray better than patch alone.)

Howard G et al: Cigarette smoking and progression of atherosclerosis. JAMA 1998;279:119. [PMID: 9440661] (Active smoking, former smoking, and environmental tobacco smoke exposure are associated with accelerated irreversible carotid artery thickening.)

Hughes JR et al: Recent advances in the pharmacotherapy of smoking. JAMA 1999;281:72. [PMID: 9892454] (Reviews nicotine gum and patch, nicotine nasal spray, nicotine inhaler, and bupropion.

JAMA patient page: Secondhand smoke. JAMA 1998;280:1968. [PMID: 9851487]

Jorenby DE et al: A controlled trial of sustained-release bupropion, a nicotine patch, or both for smoking cessation.

Table 1–7. Suggestions for the clinical use of nicotine gum.[1]

Parameter of Clinical Use	Suggestions
Patient selection	Appropriate as a primary pharmacotherapy for smoking cessation.
Precautions	*Pregnancy:* Pregnant smokers should first be encouraged to attempt cessation without pharmacologic treatment. Nicotine gum should be used during pregnancy only if the increased likelihood of smoking cessation, with its potential benefits, outweighs the risk of nicotine replacement and potential concomitant smoking. *Cardiovascular diseases:* Although not an independent risk factor for acute myocardial events, nicotine gum should be used only after consideration of risks and benefits among particular cardiovascular patient groups: those in the immediate (within 2 weeks) post-myocardial infarction period, those with serious arrhythmias, and those with serious or worsening angina pectoris. *Adverse effects:* Common adverse effects of nicotine chewing gum include mouth soreness, hiccups, dyspepsia, and jaw ache. These effects are generally mild and transient and can often be alleviated by correcting the patient's chewing technique (see "Prescribing instructions" below).
Dosage	*Dosage:* Nicotine gum is available in doses of 2 mg and 4 mg per piece. Patients who smoke less than 25 cigarettes per day should be prescribed the 2-mg gum initially. The 4-mg gum should be prescribed to patients who express a preference for it, have failed with the 2-mg gum but remain motivated to quit, and/or smoke greater than 25 cigarettes per day. The gum is most commonly prescribed for the first few months of a quit attempt. Clinicians should tailor the duration of therapy to fit the needs of each patient. Patients using the 2-mg strength should use not more than 30 pieces per day, whereas those using the 4-mg strength should not exceed 20 pieces per day.
Prescribing instructions	*Abstinence from smoking:* The patient should refrain from smoking while using the gum. *Chewing technique:* The gum should be chewed slowly until a "peppery" taste emerges, then "parked" between cheek and gum to facilitate nicotine absorption through the oral mucosa. Gum should be slowly and intermittently chewed and parked for about 30 minutes. *Absorption:* Acidic beverages (eg, coffee, juices, soft drinks) interfere with the buccal absorption of nicotine, so eating and drinking anything except water should be avoided for 15 minutes before and during chewing. *Scheduling of dose:* A common problem is that patients do not use enough gum to get the maximum benefit: they chew too few pieces per day and do not use the gum for a sufficient number of weeks. Instructions to chew the gum on a fixed schedule (at least 1 piece every 1 to 2 hours) for at least 1 to 3 months may be more beneficial than ad lib use.

[1]Reproduced, with permission, from: The Agency for Health Care Policy and Research. *Smoking Cessation Clinical Practice Guideline.* JAMA 1996;275:1270. Updated and revised, with permission, from *Treating Tobacco Use and Dependence.* U.S. Public Health Service. www.surgeongeneral.gov/tobacco/default.htm

N Engl J Med 1999;340:685. [PMID: 10053177] (Abstinence rates were 36% in the combined therapy group, 31% in the bupropion group, 16% in the nicotine patch group, and 16% in the placebo group. Weight gain at 7 weeks was significantly less in the combined-treatment group.)

Seidman DF et al: *Helping the Hardcore Smoker: A Clinician's Guide.* Lawrence Erlbaum Publishers, 1999.

Werner RM et al: What's so passive about passive smoking? Secondhand smoke as a cause of atherosclerotic disease. (Editorial.) JAMA 1998;279:157. [PMID: 9440668] (One-third as much atherosclerotic progression as active smoking.)

Lipid Disorders

Lower LDL cholesterol concentrations and higher HDL levels are associated with a reduced risk of coronary heart disease. Elevated plasma lipoprotein(a) is an independent risk factor for early onset of coronary heart disease in men but has not yet been evaluated clinically. The absolute benefits of screening for—and treating—abnormal lipid levels depend on the presence of other cardiovascular risk factors. If other risk factors are present, cardiovascular risk is higher and the benefits of therapy are greater. Patients with known cardiovascular disease are at still higher risk and benefit from treatment even when lipid levels are only modestly elevated.

Compliance with statin-type drugs is better than for the other classes of lipid-lowering agents. Six major randomized, placebo-controlled trials have convincingly demonstrated significant reductions in total mortality and major coronary events with lowering levels of low-density lipoprotein cholesterol by statin therapy. These results were achieved in a broad range of patients including those with or without a history of coronary artery disease and those with elevated or average LDL-C levels. Statins also appear to reduce the risk of stroke.

Guidelines for therapy are discussed in Chapter 29.

Table 1–8. Suggestions for the clinical use of bupropion SR.

Parameter of Clinical Use	Suggestions
Patient selection	Appropriate as a first-line pharmacotherapy for smoking cessation.
Precautions	*Pregnancy*—Pregnant smokers should be encouraged to quit first without pharmacologic treatment. Bupropion SR should be used during pregnancy only if the increased liklihood of smoking abstinence, with its potential benefits, outweighs the risk of bupropion SR treatment and potential concomitant smoking. Similar factors should be considered in lactating women (FDA Class B). *Cardiovascular diseases*—Generally well tolerated; infrequent reports of hypertension. *Side effects*—The most common side effects reported by bupropion SR users were insomnia (35–40%) and dry mouth (10%). *Contraindications*—Bupropion SR is contraindicated in individuals with a history of seizure disorder, a history of an eating disorder, who are using another form of bupropion (Wellbutrin or Wellbutrin SR), or who have used an MAO inhibitor in the past 14 days.
Dosage	Patients should begin with a dose of 150 mg q AM for 3 days, then increase to 150 mg bid. Dosing at 150 mg bid should continue for 7–12 weeks following the quit date. Unlike nicotine replacement products, patients should begin bupropion SR treatment 1–2 weeks *before* they quit smoking. For maintenance therapy, consider bupropion SR 150 mg bid for up to 6 months.
Prescribing instructions	*Cessation prior to quit date*—Recognize that some patients will lose their desire to smoke prior to their quit date, or will spontaneously reduce the amount they smoke. *Scheduling of dose*—If insomnia is marked, taking the PM dose earlier (in the afternoon, at least 8 hours after the first dose) may provide some relief. *Alcohol*—Use alcohol only in moderation.

Modified, with permission, from *Treating Tobacco Use and Dependence.* U.S. Public Health Service. www.surgeongeneral.gov/tobacco/default.htm

Grundy SM: United States Cholesterol Guidelines 2001: expanded scope of intensive low-density lipoprotein-lowering therapy. Am J Cardiol 2001;88(7B):23J. [PMID: 11595195] (New clinical guidelines of the National Cholesterol Education Program Adult Treatment Panel III report, released in May 2001.)

Hebert PR et al: Cholesterol lowering with statin drugs, risk of stroke, and total mortality: An overview of randomized trials. JAMA 1997;278:313. [PMID: 9228438] (Patients given statin drugs had significant reductions in risk of stroke of 29%, cardiovascular disease deaths of 28%, and total mortality of 22%.)

Hunt D et al: Benefits of pravastatin on cardiovascular events and mortality in older patients with coronary heart disease are equal to or exceed those seen in younger patients: Results from the LIPID trial. Ann Intern Med 2001;134:931. [PMID: 11352694] (Pravastatin therapy reduced the risk for all major cardiovascular events and all-cause mortality in older patients with coronary heart disease and average or moderately elevated cholesterol levels.)

JAMA patient page: Cholesterol. JAMA 1999;281:206. [PMID: 9917126]

Pignone MP et al: Screening and treating adults for lipid disorders: a summary of the evidence for the U.S. Preventive Services Task Force. Am J Prev Med 2001;20(3 Suppl):77. [PMID: 11306236] (Systematic review of the evidence for screening and treating lipid disorders in persons without previously diagnosed heart disease.)

Ramires JA et al: Cholesterol lowering with statins reduces exercise-induced myocardial ischemia in hypercholesterolemic patients with coronary artery disease. Am J Cardiol 2001;88:1134. [PMID: 11703958]

Simon JA et al: Postmenopausal hormone therapy and risk of stroke: The Heart and Estrogen-progestin Replacement Study (HERS). Circulation 2001;103:638. [PMID: 11156873] (No benefit.)

Smilde TJ et al: Effect of aggressive versus conventional lipid lowering on atherosclerosis progression in familial hypercholesterolaemia (ASAP): a prospective, randomised, double-blind trial. Lancet 2001;357:577. [PMID: 11558482] (Aggressive LDL cholesterol reduction with atorvastatin was associated with regression of carotid intimal media thickness in patients with familial hypercholesterolemia, while conventional LDL lowering was not.)

Hyperhomocysteinemia

Elevated plasma homocysteine may be an independent risk factor for coronary artery disease and may impart a risk similar to that associated with cigarette smoking or hyperlipidemia. Elevated levels can be reduced with folate and pyridoxine treatment, but their clinical significance is unknown.

Booth GL et al: Preventive health care, 2000 update: screening and management of hyperhomocysteinemia for the prevention of coronary artery disease events. Canadian Task Force on Preventive Health Care. Can Med Assoc J 2000;163:21. [PMID: 10920726] (There is insufficient evidence to justify screening for elevated serum homocysteine, but patients should be encouraged to maintain an adequate intake of folate and vitamins B_6 and B_{12}.)

Tice JA et al: Cost-effectiveness of vitamin therapy to lower plasma homocysteine levels for the prevention of coronary heart disease: effect of grain fortification and beyond. JAMA 2001;286:936. [PMID: 11509058] (Vitamin fortification of grain appears cost-effective.)

Hypertension

Over 43 million adults in the USA have hypertension. Of these 43 million, 31% are unaware of their elevated blood pressure; 17% are aware but untreated; 29% are being treated but have not controlled their blood pressure (still greater than 140/90 mm Hg); and only 23% are well controlled. In every adult age group, higher values of systolic and diastolic blood pressure carry greater risks of stroke and congestive heart failure. Systolic blood pressure is a better predictor of morbid events than is diastolic blood pressure. Clinicians can apply specific blood pressure criteria, such as those of the Joint National Committee, to decide at what levels treatment should be considered in individual cases. Table 11–1 presents a classification of hypertension based on blood pressures. Primary prevention of hypertension can be accomplished by strategies aimed at both the general population and special high-risk populations. The latter include persons with high-normal blood pressure or a family history of hypertension, blacks, and individuals with various behavioral risk factors such as physical inactivity; excessive consumption of salt, alcohol, or calories; and deficient intake of potassium. Effective interventions for primary prevention of hypertension include reduced sodium and alcohol consumption, weight loss, and regular exercise. Potassium supplementation lowers blood pressure modestly, and a diet high in fresh fruits and vegetables and low in fat, red meats, and sugar-containing beverages also reduces blood pressure. Interventions of unproved efficacy include pill supplementation of potassium, calcium, magnesium, fish oil, or fiber; macronutrient alteration; and stress management. A major cause of the recent impressive decline in stroke deaths has been improved diagnosis and treatment of hypertension. Diets rich in fruits and vegetables may also protect against stroke. Pharmacologic management of hypertension is discussed in Chapter 11.

Conlin PR et al: The effect of dietary patterns on blood pressure control in hypertensive patients: results from the DASH trial. Am J Hypertens 2000;13:949. [PMID: 10981543]

Hyman DJ, Pavlik VN:- Characteristics of patients with uncontrolled hypertension in the United States. N Engl J Med 2001;345:479. [PMID: 11519501] (Examines the factors associated with hypertension control or lack thereof.)

Perry HM Jr et al: Antihypertensive efficacy of treatment regimens used in Veterans Administration hypertension clinics. Department of Veterans Affairs Cooperative Study Group on Antihypertensive Agents. Hypertension 1998;31:771. [PMID: 9495260] (The regimens of diuretic or diuretic plus beta-blocker gave the lowest average pressures and calcium antagonist the highest.)

Chemoprevention

As discussed in Chapters 10 and 24, regular use of low-dose aspirin (81–325 mg) can reduce the incidence of myocardial infarction in patients at increased risk for heart disease.

Hayden M et al: Aspirin for the primary prevention of cardiovascular events: a summary of the evidence for the U.S. Preventive Services Task Force. Ann Intern Med 2002;136:161. [PMID:11790072] (Systematic review of the benefits and adverse effects of aspirin in adults without known cardiovascular disease.)

PREVENTION OF PHYSICAL INACTIVITY & SEDENTARY LIFESTYLE

Dietary factors and the lack of sufficient physical activity are the second most important contributors to preventable deaths, trailing only tobacco use. The prevalence of obesity is increasing in both children and adults in the United States. Reversing these trends will require regular physical activity as well as modification of diet. A sedentary lifestyle has been linked to 28% of deaths from leading chronic diseases. The CDC has recommended that every adult in the United States should engage in 30 minutes or more of moderate-intensity physical activity on most days of the week. This new guideline complements previous advice urging at least 20–30 minutes of more vigorous aerobic exercise three to five times a week.

Patients who engage in regular moderate to vigorous exercise have a lower risk of myocardial infarction, stroke, hypertension, type 2 diabetes mellitus, diverticular disease, and osteoporosis. The benefits of exercise appear to be dose-dependent, with a major difference in benefit between no and mild to moderate exercise and a smaller difference in benefit between moderate and vigorous exercise. The relative risk of stroke was found to be less than one-sixth in men who exercised vigorously compared with those who were inactive; the risk of type 2 diabetes mellitus was about half among men who exercised five or more times weekly compared with those who exercised once a week. Glucose control is improved in diabetics who exercise regularly, even at a modest level. Persons who engage in regular exercise have a lower long-term risk of coronary events, including fatal myocardial infarctions (in both men and women), and in middle-aged and older individuals exercise improves coronary and endothelial and smooth muscle function and confers a decreased risk of hypertension. In older nonsmoking men, walking 2 miles or more per day is associated with an almost 50% lower mortality. Physical activity is associated with a lower risk of colon cancer (though not rectal cancer) in men and women and of breast and reproductive organ cancer in women. Finally, weight-bearing exercise (especially resistance and high-impact activities) increases bone mineral content and retards development of osteoporosis in women and contributes to a reduced risk of falls in older persons.

Exercise may also confer benefits on those with chronic illness. Men and women with chronic symptomatic osteoarthritis of one or both knees benefited from a supervised walking program, with improved self-reported functional status and decreased use of pain medication. Exercise produces sustained lowering of both systolic and diastolic blood pressure in patients with mild hypertension. In addition, physical activity can help patients maintain ideal body weight. individuals who maintain ideal body weight have a 35–55% lower risk for myocardial infarction than with those who are obese. Physical activity reduces depression and anxiety, improves adaptation to stress, improves sleep quality, and enhances mood, self-esteem, and overall performance.

However, physical exertion can rarely trigger the onset of acute myocardial infarction, particularly in persons who are habitually sedentary. Increased activity increases the risk of musculoskeletal injuries, which can be minimized by proper warm-up, stretching, and by gradual rather than sudden increase in activity. Other potential complications of exercise include angina pectoris, arrhythmias, sudden death, and asthma. In insulin-requiring diabetics who undertake vigorous exercise, the need for insulin is reduced; hypoglycemia may be a consequence.

Only about 20% of adults in the USA are active at the moderate level—and only 8% currently exercise at the more vigorous level—recommended for health benefits. Instead, 60% report irregular or no leisure time physical activity.

Clinicians should advise patients about the benefits and risks of exercise, prescribe an exercise program appropriate for each patient, and provide advice that will help to prevent injuries or cardiovascular complications. The value of routine electrocardiography stress testing prior to initiation of an exercise program in middle aged or older adults remains controversial. Patients with ischemic heart disease or other cardiovascular disease require medically supervised, graded exercise programs. Exercise should not be prescribed for patients with decompensated congestive heart failure, complex ventricular arrhythmias, unstable angina pectoris, hemodynamically significant aortic stenosis, aortic aneurysm, or uncontrolled diabetes mellitus. Five- to 10-minute warm-up and cool-down periods, stretching exercises, and gradual increases in exercise intensity help to prevent musculoskeletal and cardiovascular complications.

Physical activity can be incorporated into any person's daily routine. For example, the clinician can advise a patient to take the stairs instead of the elevator, to walk or bike instead of driving, to do housework or yard work, to get off the bus one or two stops earlier and walk the rest of the way, to park at the far end of the parking lot, or to walk during the lunch hour. Table 29–2 shows energy expenditures associated with selected physical activities. The basic message must be: the more the better, and anything is better than nothing.

Dunn AL et al: Comparison of lifestyle and structured interventions to increase physical activity and cardiorespiratory fitness: A randomized trial. JAMA 1999;281:327. [PMID: 9929085] (In previously sedentary healthy adults, a lifestyle of physical activity intervention is as effective as a structured exercise program in improving energy expenditure, cardiorespiratory fitness, and blood pressure.)

Ettinger WH et al: A randomized trial comparing aerobic exercise and resistance training to a health education program on physical disability in older adults with knee osteoarthritis. JAMA 1997;277:25. [PMID: 8980206] (Exercise has beneficial but modest effect on pain, physical performance, and disability.)

Hambrecht R et al: Effect of exercise on coronary and endothelial function in patients with coronary artery disease. N Engl J Med 2000;342:454. [PMID: 10675425]

Hu FB et al: Walking compared with vigorous physical activity and risk of type 2 diabetes in women. JAMA 1999; 282:1433. [PMID: 10535433] (Relative risk of developing type 2 diabetes was inversely proportionate to levels of activity even after adjusting for risk factors, including body mass index.)

JAMA patient page: Exercise. JAMA 1999;281:394. [PMID: 9929097]

Kushi LH et al: Physical activity and mortality in postmenopausal women. JAMA 1997;277:1287. [PMID: 9109466] (Among 40,417 postmenopausal women, those who reported regular physical activity had a significantly reduced risk of death at 7-year follow-up.)

Lyznicki JM et al: Obesity: assessment and management in primary care. Am Fam Physician 2001;63:2185. [PMID: 11417771]

Wannamethee SG et al: Physical activity in the prevention of cardiovascular disease: an epidemiological perspective. Sports Med 2001;31:101. [PMID: 11227978]

CANCER PREVENTION

Primary Prevention

Cigarette smoking is the most important preventable cause of cancer. Primary prevention of skin cancer consists of restricting exposure to ultraviolet light by wearing appropriate clothing and use of sunscreens. In the past 2 decades, there has been a threefold increase in the incidence of squamous cell carcinoma and a fourfold increase in melanoma in the United States. Individuals who engage in regular physical exercise and avoid obesity have lower rates of breast and colon cancer. Prevention of occupationally induced cancers involves minimizing exposure to carcinogenic substances such as asbestos, ionizing radiation, and benzene compounds. Chemoprevention may be an important part of primary cancer prevention (see Chapter 40). Tamoxifen for breast cancer prevention is discussed in Chapters 16 and 40.

Screening & Early Detection

Screening has been shown to prevent death from cancers of the breast, colon, and cervix through cancer screening procedures. Note that Table 1–9, derived from American Cancer Society guidelines, differs in many instances from the recommendations of other authorities as shown previously in Table 1–2, which take a more conservative view of the efficacy of cancer screening maneuvers. For example, the value of screening mammography for women aged 40–49, breast self-examination for women, and serum PSA testing for men are all controversial. A federal consensus panel was unable to agree on the advisability of routine mammography for women aged 40–49, leaving the decision instead to the discretion of individual patients and their clinicians. By contrast, the American Cancer Society mammography screening guidelines were changed to include annual mammograms for women in their 40s.

Single serum PSA measurements appear to offer relatively high sensitivity and specificity to detect prostate cancer. The sensitivity is about 65%, the specificity about 80%, and the positive predictive value for prostate cancer is about 45%. When both the digital rectal examination and serum PSA are abnormal, PSA specificity increases, but sensitivity falls (to 30%) and predictive value rises only slightly. Whether early detection and treatment alters the natural course of the disease remains to be seen. There are still no data on the

Table 1–9. Screening for cancer: American Cancer Society (1999) guidelines for the early detection of cancer in people without symptoms.[1]

Test or Procedure	Sex	Age	Frequency
Sigmoidoscopy, flexible, or— Colonoscopy, or— Air contrast barium enema	MF	50 and over[2]	Every 5 years Every 10 years Every 5–10 years
Stool test for occult blood	MF	50 and over[2]	Every year
Digital rectal examination and serum PSA[3]	M	50 and over[4]	Every year
Papanicolaou test	F	Women who are or have been sexually active or have reached age 18 years	Annually until at least three consecutive satisfactory normal annual examinations, then less often at discretion of physician. Not indicated if cervix has been removed for a nonmalignant condition.
Pelvic examination	F	18–40	Every 1–3 years with Papanicolaou test.
		Over 40	Every year
Endometrial tissue sample	F	At menopause; women at high risk[5]	At menopause and thereafter at the discretion of the physician
Breast self-examination	F	20 and over	Every month
Breast physical examination	F	20–40 40 and over	Every 3 years Every year
Mammography	F	40 and over	Every year
Health counseling and cancer checkup[6]	MF	Over 20 Over 40	Every 3 years Every year
Chest x-ray		Not recommended	
Sputum cytologic examination		Not recommended	

[1]From Update January 1992: The American Cancer Society Guidelines for the Cancer-Related Check-Up. CA Cancer J Clin 1992;42:44; and from the American Cancer Society 1999 update.
[2]People should begin colorectal cancer screening earlier or undergo screening more often (or both) if they have any of the following colorectal cancer risk factors: (1) a personal history of colorectal cancer or adenomatous polyps; (2) a strong family history of colorectal cancer or polyps (cancer or polyps in a first degree relative younger than 60 or in two first-degree relatives of any age); (3) families with hereditary colorectal cancer syndromes (familial adenomatous polyposis and hereditary nonpolyposis colon cancer).
[3]Digital rectal examination and serum prostate-specific antigen: if either is abnormal, further evaluation by transrectal ultrasound and biopsy as indicated.
[4]For men with ≥ 10-year life expectancy. Screening is recommended for younger men if at higher risk (blacks, strong family history of prostate cancer).
[5]History of infertility, obesity, failure of ovulation, abnormal uterine bleeding, or unopposed estrogen or tamoxifen therapy.
[6]To include examination for cancers of the thyroid, testicles, ovaries, lymph nodes, oral region, and skin.

morbidity and mortality benefits of such screening. Unlike the American College of Physicians, the American Cancer Society recommends that providers offer annual PSA testing for men over age 50. Screening is not recommended by any group for men who have estimated life expectancies of less than 10 years. Decision aids have been developed to help men weigh the arguments for and against PSA screening.

Annual or biennial fecal occult blood testing reduces mortality from colorectal cancer by 16–33%. The risk of death from colon cancer among patients undergoing at least one sigmoidoscopic examination is reduced by 60–80% compared with that among those not having sigmoidoscopy. Colonoscopy has been recently advocated as a screening examination. While it is more accurate than flexible sigmoidoscopy for detecting cancer and polyps, its value in reducing colon cancer mortality has not been studied.

Screening for cervical cancer with a Papanicolaou smear is indicated in adolescent and adult women every 1–3 years. Screening for vaginal cancer with a Papanicolaou smear is not indicated in women who have undergone hysterectomies for benign disease with removal of the cervix.

Barry MJ: Health decision aids to facilitate shared decision making in office practice. Ann Intern Med 2002;136:127. [PMID: 11790064] (Examines the effect of decision aids on patients' interest in PSA screening.)

Baxter N: Preventive health care, 2001 update: should women be routinely taught breast self-examination to screen for breast cancer? CMAJ 2001;164:1837. [PMID:11450279] (Breast self-examination appears to be ineffective in reducing breast cancer mortality.)

Coley CM et al: Early detection of prostate cancer: Part II: estimating the risks, benefits, and costs. Ann Intern Med 1997;126:468. [PMID: 9072935] (One-time digital rectal examination and PSA measurement may increase average life expectancy by approximately 2 weeks at a reasonable marginal cost for men aged 50–69.)

Elmore JG et al: Ten-year risk of false positive screening mammograms and clinical breast examinations. N Engl J Med 1998;338:1089. [PMID: 9545356] (Over a 10-year period, one-third of women screened had a false-positive abnormal test result.)

Kerlikowske K et al: Screening mammography in elderly women. JAMA 2000;283:3202. [PMID: 10866866]

Levine M et al: Chemoprevention of breast cancer. A joint guideline from the Canadian Task Force on Preventive Health Care and the Canadian Breast Cancer Initiative's Steering Committee on Clinical Practice Guidelines for the Care and Treatment of Breast Cancer. CMAJ 2001;164:1681. [PMID: 11450210]

Ransohoff DF et al: Clinical practice. Screening for colorectal cancer. N Engl J Med 2002;346:40. [PMID: 11778002] (Clinical review of the effectiveness of colon cancer screening.)

Ringash J: Preventive health care, 2001 update: screening mammography among women aged 40–49 years at average risk of breast cancer. CMAJ 2001;164:469. [PMID: 11233866]

Screening for prostate cancer. American College of Physicians. Ann Intern Med 1997;126:480. [PMID: 9072936] (Instead of routine screening, the ACP recommends that clinicians individualize the decision to screen.)

PREVENTION OF INJURIES & VIOLENCE

Injuries remain the most important cause of loss of potential years of life before age 65. Road traffic injuries, self-inflicted injuries, falls, and interpersonal violence are the major sources of injuries. Injuries affect mostly young people, often causing long-term disability.

Though there has been a steady decline in motor vehicle accident deaths per miles driven, road traffic injuries remain the tenth leading cause of death and the ninth leading cause of the burden of disease. Although seat belt use protects against serious injury and death in motor vehicle accidents, at least one-fourth of adults do not use seat belts routinely. Air bags are protective for adults but not for small children. In 1996, 64% of motorcyclists used helmets, an improvement over previous years. The rate of helmet use by motorcyclists approached 100% in states with helmet laws. Recent data for bicyclists are not available. Young men appear most likely to resist wearing helmets. Clinicians should try to educate their patients about seat belts, safety helmets, the risks of using cellular telephones while driving, drinking and driving—or using other intoxicants or long-acting benzodiazepines and then driving—and the risks of having guns in the home. Chronic alcohol abuse adversely affects outcome from trauma and increases the risk of readmission for new trauma. Males aged 16–35 are at especially high risk for serious injury and death from accidents and violence, with blacks and Latinos at greatest risk. For 16- and 17-year-old drivers, the risk of fatal crashes increases with the number of passengers. Deaths from firearms have reached epidemic levels in the United States and will soon surpass in numbers deaths from motor vehicle accidents. Having a gun in the home increases the likelihood of homicide nearly threefold and of suicide fivefold. Alcohol and illicit drug use are associated with an increased risk of violent death. Physicians should be alert to signs of depression and suicidal ideation and should initiate interventions to prevent suicide.

Finally, clinicians have a critical role in detection, prevention, and management of physical or sexual abuse—in particular, routine assessment of women for risk of domestic violence. Inclusion of a single question about domestic violence in the medical history—"At any time, has a partner ever hit you, kicked you, or otherwise physically hurt you?"—increased identification of this common problem from nil to 11.6%. Another screening device consists of three questions: (1) "Have you ever been hit, kicked, punched, or otherwise hurt by someone within the past year? If so, by whom?" (2) "Do you feel safe in your current relationship?" (3) "Is there a partner from a previous relationship who is making you feel unsafe now?" Use of these questions increased identification of domestic violence to 29.5% of women in an emergency department.

Physical and psychologic abuse, exploitation, and neglect of older adults are serious underrecognized problems. Clues to elder mistreatment include the patient's appearance, recurrent urgent-care visits, missed appointments, suspicious physical findings, and implausible explanations for injuries.

Barrier PA: Domestic violence. Mayo Clin Proc 1998;73:271. [PMID: 9511786]

Chen LH et al: Carrying passengers as a risk factor for crashes fatal to 16- and 17-year-old drivers. JAMA 2000;283:1578. [PMID: 10735394] (Risk steadily increases with increasing number of passengers.)

Conner KR et al: Violence, alcohol, and completed suicide: a case-control study. Am J Psychiatr 2001;158:1701. [PMID: 11579005] (Violent behavior increases the risk of suicide.)

el-Bayoumi G et al: Domestic violence in women. Med Clin North Am 1998;82:391. [PMID: 9531931]

Goodman P: Domestic violence resources on the Internet. JAMA 1998;280:477. [PMID: 9701089]

JAMA patient page: Domestic violence. JAMA 1998;280:488. [PMID: 9701090]

Hirsch CH et al: The management of elder mistreatment: the physician's role. Wien Klin Wochenschr 2001;113:384. [PMID: 11432128]

King EG et al: The global burden of injuries. Am J Public Health 2000;90:523. [PMID: 10754963]

Martin SL et al: Physical abuse of women before, during, and after pregnancy. JAMA 2001;285:1581. [PMID: 11268265] (Among 2648 women, the prevalence of abuse was 6.9% before pregnancy, 6.1% during pregnancy, and 3.2% during the postpartum period.)

Rivara FP et al: Injury prevention. (Two parts.) N Engl J Med 1997;337:543, 613. [PMID: 9262499, 9271485] (Comprehensive review including magnitude of the problem, motor

Table 1–10. Screening for alcohol abuse.

---

1. CAGE screening test[1]

Have you ever felt the need to	Cut down on drinking?
Have you ever felt	Annoyed by criticism of your drinking?
Have you ever felt	Guilty about your drinking?
Have you ever taken a morning	Eye opener?

INTERPRETATION: Two "yes" answers are considered a positive screen. One "yes" answer should arouse a suspicion of alcohol abuse.

---

2. The Alcohol Use Disorder Identification Test (AUDIT).[2] (Scores for response categories are given in parentheses. Scores range from 0 to 40, with a cutoff score of ≥ 5 indicating hazardous drinking, harmful drinking, or alcohol dependence.)

1. How often do you have a drink containing alcohol?

(0) Never	(1) Monthly or less	(2) Two to four times a month	(3) Two or three times a week	(4) Four or more times a week

2. How many drinks containing alcohol do you have on a typical day when you are drinking?

(0) 1 or 2	(1) 3 or 4	(2) 5 or 6	(3) 7 to 9	(4) 10 or more

3. How often do you have six or more drinks on one occasion?

(0) Never	(1) Less than monthly	(2) Monthly	(3) Weekly	(4) Daily or almost daily

4. How often during the past year have you found that you were not able to stop drinking once you had started?

(0) Never	(1) Less than monthly	(2) Monthly	(3) Weekly	(4) Daily or almost daily

5. How often during the past year have you failed to do what was normally expected of you because of drinking?

(0) Never	(1) Less than monthly	(2) Monthly	(3) Weekly	(4) Daily or almost daily

6. How often during the past year have you needed a first drink in the morning to get yourself going after a heavy drinking session?

(0) Never	(1) Less than monthly	(2) Monthly	(3) Weekly	(4) Daily or almost daily

7. How often during the past year have you had a feeling of guilt or remorse after drinking?

(0) Never	(1) Less than monthly	(2) Monthly	(3) Weekly	(4) Daily or almost daily

8. How often during the past year have you been unable to remember what happened the night before because you had been drinking?

(0) Never	(1) Less than monthly	(2) Monthly	(3) Weekly	(4) Daily or almost daily

9. Have you or has someone else been injured as a result of your drinking?

(0) No	(2) Yes, but not in the past year	(4) Yes, during the past year

10. Has a relative or friend or a doctor or other health worker been concerned about your drinking or suggested you cut down?

(0) No	(2) Yes, but not in the past year	(4) Yes, during the past year

---

[1]Modified from Mayfield D et al: The CAGE questionnaire: Validation of a new alcoholism screening instrument. Am J Psychiatry 1974,131:1121.

[2]From Piccinelli M et al: Efficacy of the alcohol use disorders identification test as a screening tool for hazardous alcohol intake and related disorders in primary care: A validity study. BMJ 1997,314:420.

vehicle accidents, bicycling injuries, falls, poisoning, fires and scalding, drowning, injuries from firearms, and injury control strategies.)

Teret SP et al: Support for new policies to regulate firearms. Results of two national surveys. N Engl J Med 1998;339:813. [PMID: 9738090] (Strong public support, even among gun owners, for innovative strategies to regulate firearms.)

Weinbaum Z et al: Female victims of intimate partner physical domestic violence (IPP-DV), California 1998. Am J Prev Med 2001;21:313. [PMID: 11701303] (Overall 6% of 4006 women surveyed reported physical domestic violence during the previous 12 months.)

SUBSTANCE ABUSE: ALCOHOL & ILLICIT DRUGS

Common brain neurotransmitter changes follow regular use of addictive substances such as alcohol, tobacco, and illicit drugs. Substance abuse is a major public health problem in the United States and is estimated to be a factor in 41% of highway fatality accidents. Approximately two-thirds of high school seniors are regular users of alcohol, and the lifetime prevalence of alcoholism is estimated to be between 12% and 16%. Underdiagnosis is substantial, both because of patient denial and lack of detection of clinical clues. A substantial decline in alcohol-related fatalities testifies to the success of educational and law-enforcement efforts to stop drinking and driving. Even so, alcohol-impaired driving remains prevalent, especially among men aged 18–34 years. Binge drinking among college students has recently increased.

As with cigarette use, clinician identification and counseling about alcoholism may improve the chances of recovery. About 10% of all adults seen in medical practices are problem drinkers. An estimated 15–30% of hospitalized patients have problems with alcohol abuse or dependence, but the connection between patients' presenting complaints and their alcohol abuse is often missed. The CAGE test (see Table 1–10) is both sensitive and specific for chronic alcoholism. However, it is less sensitive in detecting heavy or binge drinking in elderly patients and has been criticized for being less applicable to minority groups or to women. Others recommend asking three questions: (1) How many days per week do you drink? (frequency.) (2) On a day when you drink alcohol, how many drinks do you have in one day? (quantity.) (3) On how many occasions in the last month did you drink more than five drinks? (binge drinking.) The Alcohol Use Disorder Identification Test (AUDIT) consists of questions on the quantity and frequency of alcohol consumption, on alcohol dependence symptoms, and on alcohol-related problems (Table 1–10). It has been found to accurately detect hazardous drinking, harmful drinking, and alcohol dependence and does not seem to be affected by ethnic or gender bias. Choice of therapy remains controversial. However, use of screening procedures and brief intervention methods (see Table 1–11 and Chapter 25) can produce a 10–30%

Table 1–11. Basic counseling steps for patients who abuse alcohol.[1]

Establish a therapeutic relationship
Make the medical office or clinic off-limits for substance abuse
Present information about negative health consequences
Emphasize personal responsibility and self-efficacy
Convey a clear message and set goals
Involve family and other supports
Establish a working relationship with community treatment resources
Provide follow-up

[1]From the United States Department of Health and Human Services, U.S. Public Health Service, Office of Disease Prevention and Health Promotion. *Clinician's Handbook of Preventive Services: Put Prevention Into Practice.* U.S. Government Printing Office, 1994.

reduction in long-term alcohol use and alcohol-related problems. Several pharmacologic agents are effective in reducing alcohol consumption.

Use of illegal drugs—including cocaine, methamphetamine, and so-called "designer drugs"—either sporadically or episodically remains an important problem. A disturbing trend is the recent increase in use of marijuana and inhalants among eighth graders and high school students. Many drug users are employed, and many use drugs during pregnancy. Cocaine or tobacco use during early pregnancy substantially increases the risk of miscarriage. Abuse of anabolic-androgenic steroids has been associated with use of other illicit drugs, alcohol, and cigarettes and with violence and criminal behavior. As with alcohol abuse, the recognition of drug abuse presents special problems and requires that the clinician actively consider the diagnosis. Clinical aspects of substance abuse and treatment issues are discussed in Chapter 25.

Bradley KA et al: Screening for problem drinking: Comparison of CAGE and AUDIT. J Gen Intern Med 1998;13:379. [PMID: 9833223] (The self-administered AUDIT was superior to the CAGE.)

Fleming MF et al: Brief physician advice for problem alcohol drinkers: A randomized, controlled trial in community-based primary care practices. JAMA 1997;277:1039. [PMID: 9723864] (Brief biweekly counseling sessions resulted in significant reductions in 7-day alcohol use, episodes of binge drinking, and frequency of excessive drinking at 1 year.)

Friedmann PD et al: Management of adults recovering from alcohol or other drug problems: Relapse prevention in primary care. JAMA 1998;279:1227. [PMID: 9555766]

Fuchs CS et al: Alcohol consumption and mortality among women. N Engl J Med 1995;332:1245. [PMID: 7708067] (Light-to-moderate alcohol consumption is associated with reduced mortality rates in women, largely among those at greatest risk for coronary heart disease.)

Garbutt JC et al: Pharmacologic treatment of alcohol dependency: a review of the evidence. JAMA 1999;281:1318. [PMID: 10208148] (Reviews use of naltrexone, acamprosate, and disulfiram.)

JAMA patient page: Alcohol. JAMA 1999;281:1352. [PMID: 10208153]

Ness RB et al: Cocaine and tobacco use and the risk of spontaneous abortion. N Engl J Med 1999;340:333. [PMID: 9929522] (Both of these vasoconstrictive drugs increased the risk.)

O'Conner PG et al: Patients with alcohol problems. N Engl J Med 1998;338:592. [PMID: 9475768] (Reviews diagnosis, epidemiology, screening, and diagnostic procedures, available treatments, and clinician's role.)

Samet JH et al: Alcohol and other substance abuse. Med Clin North Am 1997;81:831. (Entire issue devoted to the subject. Articles cover general approaches, screening, pharmacologic and nonpharmacologic therapy, gender and geriatric issues, dual diagnosis, and clinician impairment.)

Schuckit MA: New findings in the genetics of alcoholism. JAMA 1999;281.1875. [PMID: 10349877] (Brief review.)

Swift RM: Drug therapy for alcohol dependence. N Engl J Med 1999;340:1482. [PMID: 9924003] (Comprehensive review of the condition and its treatments.)

Common Symptoms

Ralph Gonzales, MD, MSPH

See www.current-med.com/ch02.html

New or unexplained symptoms account for about half of office visits, the remainder for ongoing care of established medical conditions. The evidence-based medicine movement of the last decade has reshaped how illness is diagnosed and treated and promises to improve the cost and quality of health care delivery and patient outcomes.

Evidence-based symptom evaluation combines knowledge of a symptom's clinical epidemiology with disease candidates according to Bayesian principles (see Chapter 42), such that the likelihood of a specific disease is a function of patient demographics, comorbidities, and clinical features. This knowledge can help support decisions about further testing or treatment or whether to perform additional testing before treatment, or to treat without further testing.

In addition to epidemiologic factors, clinicians should recognize that biological, psychological and social factors affect how individual patients process and filter symptoms. Thus, patients vary in deciding when symptoms are sufficiently bothersome or worrisome to cause them to seek medical attention, and interpret these symptoms within a particular social and cultural context. Patients also vary in what they expect from the office visit and how much they will tolerate unexplained symptoms.

Even when all of these factors are properly applied, many symptoms defy diagnosis. If symptom relief is not easily achieved, management of these patients becomes challenging. The shift toward evidence-based principles, which encourage narrow study questions in homogeneous study populations, inadvertently results in syndromes not readily explained by current biomedical models of disease, such as dyspepsia and chronic fatigue syndrome. It has long been known that clinical syndromes due to common respiratory viruses (primarily in college students) illustrate the complexity of how symptoms are manifested, even when the cause is known. Using this example, one must accept five realities about respiratory infections: (1) The same clinical syndrome may be produced by a variety of infectious agents; (2) the same agent may produce a variety of syndromes; (3) the most likely cause of a syndrome may vary by patient age, year, ge-

ography, and setting; (4) diagnosis of the agent is frequently impossible on the basis of clinical findings alone; and (5) the causes of a large proportion of infectious disease syndromes are still unknown.

COUGH

ESSENTIAL INQUIRIES

- *Duration of cough.*
- *Dyspnea (at rest or with exertion).*
- *Constitutional symptoms.*
- *Tobacco use history.*
- *Vital signs (heart rate, respiratory rate, body temperature).*
- *Chest examination.*
- *Chest radiography when cough lasts more than 3–6 weeks.*

General Considerations

Cough adversely affects personal and work-related interactions, disrupts normal sleep, and causes discomfort of the throat and chest wall. Most people seeking medical attention for acute cough desire symptom relief. Few are worried about a serious illness. Cough results from stimulation of mechanical or chemical afferent nerve receptors in the bronchial tree. Effective cough depends on an intact afferent-efferent reflex arc, adequate expiratory and chest wall muscle strength, and normal mucociliary production and clearance.

Clinical Findings

A. SYMPTOMS AND SIGNS

Distinguishing acute (< 3 weeks) and persistent (> 3 weeks) cough illness syndromes is useful as a guide to evaluation. In otherwise healthy adults, most acute cough syndromes are due to viral respiratory tract infections. Additional features of infection such as fever, nasal congestion, and sore throat help confirm the diagnosis. Dyspnea (at rest or with exertion) may reflect a more serious condition, and further evaluation should include assessment of hypoxemia (pulse oximetry or arterial blood gas measurement), airflow obstruction (peak flow or spirometry), and parenchymal disease (chest radiography). The timing and character of the cough have not been found to be useful in establishing the cause of acute or persistent cough syndromes, although cough variant asthma should be considered in adults with prominent nocturnal cough. Uncommon causes of acute cough illness should be suspected in those with a past medical history of heart disease (congestive heart failure), or hay fever (allergic rhinitis).

Cough lasting more than 3 weeks is less likely due to respiratory tract infection. Still, in patients with cough persisting 3–6 weeks following a typical acute respiratory tract infection, it is the most likely cause, and additional evaluation is usually not necessary. Conversely, any of the conditions listed under persistent cough can contribute to or cause an acute cough.

When ACE inhibitor therapy, antecedent upper respiratory tract infection, and chest radiograph abnormalities are absent, up to 90% of cases of persistent cough are due to postnasal drip, asthma, or gastroesophageal reflux disease (GERD). A history of nasal or sinus congestion, wheezing, or heartburn should direct subsequent evaluation and treatment, though these conditions frequently cause persistent cough in the absence of typical symptoms. Bronchogenic carcinoma is suspected when cough is accompanied by unexplained weight loss and fevers with night sweats, particularly in persons with significant tobacco or occupational exposures. Persistent cough accompanied by excessive secretions suggests chronic bronchitis in a smoker, or bronchiectasis in a patient with a history of recurrent or complicated pneumonia; chest x-rays are helpful in diagnosis. Dyspnea at rest or with exertion is not commonly reported among patients with persistent cough. The report of dyspnea requires assessment for other evidence of chronic lung disease or congestive heart failure.

B. PHYSICAL EXAMINATION

Examination can direct subsequent diagnostic testing for acute and persistent cough. Pneumonia is suspected when acute cough is accompanied by vital sign abnormalities (tachycardia, tachypnea, fever) or findings suggestive of airspace consolidation (rales, decreased breath sounds, fremitus, egophony). Purulent sputum predicts neither bacterial bronchitis nor radiographic pneumonia in the otherwise healthy adult. While purulent sputum is a statistically significant risk factor for pneumonia (relative risk about 2.0), this means only that the rate of pneumonia in patients

with purulent sputum is 4% compared with 2% among those without purulent sputum (ie, 95 out of 100 adults with purulent sputum do not have radiographic pneumonia). In addition, antibiotic treatment of adults with purulent sputum production shows no benefit. Wheezing and rhonchi are frequent findings in adults with acute bronchitis, and do not represent adult-onset asthma in most cases.

Physical examination of adults with persistent cough may also reveal evidence of chronic sinusitis, contributing to postnasal drip syndrome or asthma. Chest and cardiac signs may distinguish COPD from congestive heart failure. In patients with cough and dyspnea, a normal match test (ability to blow out a match from 10 inches away) and maximum laryngeal height > 4 cm (measured from the sternal notch to the cricoid cartilage at end-expiration) substantially decreases the likelihood of COPD. Similarly, normal jugular venous pressure and negative hepatojugular reflux decrease the likelihood of new-onset congestive heart failure.

Differential Diagnosis

A. ACUTE COUGH

Acute cough may be a symptom of acute respiratory tract infection, asthma, allergic rhinitis, and congestive heart failure.

B. PERSISTENT COUGH

Possible causes are postnasal drip syndrome, asthma, gastroesophageal reflux disease, chronic bronchitis, bronchiectasis, tuberculosis or other chronic infection, interstitial lung disease, and bronchogenic carcinoma. Persistent cough may also have a psychogenic origin.

Diagnostic Studies
(Table 2–1)

A. ACUTE COUGH

Chest radiography is considered if adults have abnormal vital signs or chest examination. In patients with dyspnea, pulse oximetry and peak flow exclude

Table 2–1. Empiric treatments or tests for persistent cough.

Suspected Condition	Step 1 (Empiric Therapy)	Step 2 (Diagnostic Testing)
Postnasal drip	Therapy for allergy or chronic sinusitis	ENT referral; sinus CT scan
Asthma	Beta$_2$ agonist	Spirometry; consider methacholine challenge if normal
GERD	Proton pump inhibitors	Esophageal pH monitoring

hypoxemia or obstructive airway disease. A normal pulse oximetry (eg, > 93%) does not rule out a significant A–a gradient when patients have effective respiratory compensation.

B. PERSISTENT COUGH

Chest radiography is indicated if ACE inhibitor therapy-related and postinfectious cough are excluded by history. When the chest film is normal, evaluation for postnasal drip, asthma, and GERD should be initiated. The presence of typical symptoms of these conditions directs further evaluation or empiric therapy, though typical symptoms are often absent. Definitive procedures for determining the presence of each are available. However, empiric treatment with a maximum strength regimen for postnasal drip, asthma, or GERD for 2–4 weeks is the recommended approach since documenting the presence of postnasal drip, asthma, and GERD does not mean they are the cause of the cough illness. In about 25% of cases, persistent cough has multiple contributors.

Irwin RS et al: Managing cough as a defense mechanism and symptom. A consensus panel report of the American College of Chest Physicians. Chest 1998;114(2 Suppl):133S. [PMID: 9725800]

Metlay JP et al: National trends in the use of antibiotics by primary care physicians for adult patients with cough. Arch Intern Med 1998;158:1813. [PMID: 9738612] (The characteristics of cough illness visits and the frequency of treatment with antibiotics.)

LOWER EXTREMITY EDEMA

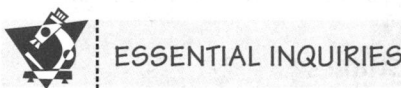 ESSENTIAL INQUIRIES

- *History of venous thromboembolism.*
- *Symmetry.*
- *Pain.*
- *Dependence.*

General Considerations

Acute and chronic lower extremity edema present important diagnostic and treatment challenges. Lower extremities can swell in response to increased venous or lymphatic pressures, decreased intravascular oncotic pressure, increased capillary leak, and local injury or infection. Chronic venous insufficiency is by far the most common cause, affecting up to 2% of the population. The incidence of venous insufficiency has not changed during the past 25 years, suggesting that preventive strategies are needed. Venous insufficiency is a common complication of deep venous thrombosis; however, only a minority of patients with chronic venous insufficiency report a history of this disorder. Venous ulcer formation commonly affects patients with chronic venous insufficiency, and management of venous ulceration is both labor-intensive and expensive as to cost.

Clinical Findings

A. SYMPTOMS AND SIGNS

Normal lower extremity venous pressure (in the erect position: 80 mm Hg in deep veins, 20–30 mm Hg in superficial veins) and cephalad venous blood flow require competent bicuspid venous valves, effective muscle contractions, and normal respirations. When one or more of these components fail, venous hypertension may result. Chronic exposure to elevated venous pressure by the postcapillary venules in the legs leads to leakage of fibrinogen and growth factors into the interstitial space, leukocyte aggregation and activation, and obliteration of the cutaneous lymphatic network. These changes account for the brawny, fibrotic skin changes observed in patients with chronic venous insufficiency, and the predisposition toward skin ulceration, particularly in the medial malleolar area.

Among common causes of lower extremity swelling, deep venous thrombosis (DVT) is the most life-threatening. Historical clues suggesting DVT include a history of cancer, recent limb immobilization, or confinement to bed for at least 3 days following major surgery within the past month (Table 2–2). A search for alternative explanations is equally important in excluding DVT. Bilateral involvement and significant improvement upon awakening favor systemic causes (eg, venous insufficiency, congestive heart failure, and cirrhosis). Pain, particularly if severe, is uncommon in uncomplicated venous insufficiency. Lower extremity swelling and inflammation in a limb previously affected by DVT could represent anticoagulation failure and thrombus recurrence but more often is caused by postphlebitic syndrome with valvular incompetence. Other causes of a painful, swollen calf include ruptured popliteal cyst, calf strain or trauma, and cellulitis. Lower extremity swelling is a familiar complication of therapy with calcium channel blockers (particularly felodipine and amlodipine), thioglitazones, and minoxidil.

Physical examination should include assessment of the heart, lungs, and abdomen for evidence of pulmonary hypertension (primary, or secondary to chronic lung disease), congestive heart failure, or cirrhosis. Some patients with the latter have pulmonary hypertension without lung disease. There is a spectrum of skin findings related to chronic venous insufficiency that depend on the severity and chronicity of the disease, ranging from hyperpigmentation and stasis dermatitis to abnormalities highly specific for

Table 2–2. Risk stratification of adults referred for ultrasound to rule out DVT.

Step 1: Calculate risk factor score
Score 1 point for each Untreated malignancy Paralysis, paresis, or recent plaster immobilization Recently bedridden for > 3 days due to major surgery within 4 weeks Localized tenderness along distribution of deep venous system Entire leg swelling Swelling of one calf > 3 cm more than the other (measured 10 cm below tibial tuberosity) Pitting edema Collateral superficial (nonvaricose) veins **Alternative diagnosis as likely as or more likely than DVT: subtract 2 points**

Step 2: Obtain ultrasound

Score	Ultrasound Positive	Ultrasound Negative
≤ 0	Confirm with venogram	DVT ruled out
1–2	Treat for DVT	Repeat ultrasound in 3–7 days
≥ 3	Treat for DVT	Confirm with venogram

chronic venous insufficiency: lipodermatosclerosis (thick brawny skin; in advanced cases, the lower leg resembles an inverted champagne bottle) and atrophie blanche (small depigmented macules within areas of heavy pigmentation). The size of both calves should be measured 10 cm below the tibial tuberosity and elicitation of pitting and tenderness performed. Swelling of the entire leg or swelling of one leg greater than 3 cm more than the other suggests deep venous obstruction. In normal persons, the left calf is slightly larger than the right as a result of the left common iliac vein coursing under the aorta.

An ulcer located over the medial malleolus is a hallmark of chronic venous insufficiency but can be due to other causes. Shallow, large, modestly painful ulcers are characteristic of venous insufficiency, whereas small, deep, and more painful ulcers are more apt to be due to arterial insufficiency, vasculitis, infections (including cutaneous diphtheria), or cancer. Diabetic vascular ulcers, however, may be painless. When an ulcer is on the foot or above the mid calf, causes other than venous insufficiency should be considered.

B. Imaging Studies

Most causes of lower extremity swelling can be demonstrated with color duplex ultrasonography. Patients without an obvious cause of acute lower extrem-

ity swelling (eg, calf strain) should have an ultrasound performed, since DVT is difficult to exclude on clinical grounds. Assessment of the ankle-brachial pressure index (ABPI) is important in the management of chronic venous insufficiency, since peripheral arterial disease may be exacerbated by compression therapy. This can be performed at the same time as ultrasound. Caution is required in interpreting the results of ABPI in older patients and diabetics due to decreased compressibility of their arteries.

Differential Diagnosis

Possible causes include chronic venous insufficiency, deep venous thrombosis, cellulitis, musculoskeletal disorders (Baker's cyst rupture, gastrocnemius tear or rupture, compartment syndrome), lymphedema, congestive heart failure, cirrhosis, nephrotic syndrome, and calcium channel blocker or thioglitazone side effect.

Treatment

In patients with chronic venous insufficiency without a comorbid volume overload state (eg, congestive heart failure), it is best to avoid diuretic therapy. These patients have relatively decreased intravascular volume, and administration of diuretics may result in acute renal insufficiency and oliguria. The most effective treatment involves (1) leg elevation, above the level of the heart, for 30 minutes three to four times daily, and during sleep; and (2) compression therapy. A wide variety of stockings and devices are effective in decreasing swelling and preventing ulcer formation. They should be put on with awakening, before hydration forces result in edema. Patients with decreased ABPI should be managed in concert with a vascular surgeon.

Heit JA et al: Trends in the incidence of venous stasis syndrome and venous ulcer: a 25-year population-based study. J Vasc Surg 2001;33:1022. [PMID: 11331844]

Valencia IC et al: Chronic venous insufficiency and venous leg ulceration. J Am Acad Dermatol 2001;44:401. [PMID: 11209109]

FEVER & HYPERTHERMIA

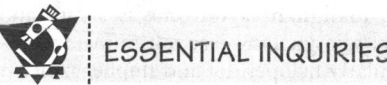 ESSENTIAL INQUIRIES

- *Localizing symptoms.*
- *Weight loss.*
- *Joint pain.*
- *Intravenous substance use.*

- *Immunosuppression or neutropenia.*
- *History of cancer.*
- *Medications.*
- *Travel.*

General Considerations

The average normal oral body temperature taken in mid morning is 36.7 °C (range 36–37.4 °C). This spectrum includes a mean and 2 standard deviations, thus encompassing 95% of a normal population, measured in mid morning. The normal rectal or vaginal temperature is 0.5 °C higher than the oral temperature, and the axillary temperature is correspondingly lower. Rectal temperature is more reliable than oral temperature, particularly in mouth breathers or in tachypneic states.

The normal diurnal temperature variation is 0.5–1 °C, being lowest in the early morning and highest in the evening. There is a slight sustained temperature rise following ovulation, during the menstrual cycle, and in the first trimester of pregnancy.

Fever is a regulated rise to a new "set point" of body temperature. When proper stimuli act on appropriate monocyte-macrophages, these cells elaborate pyrogenic cytokines, causing elevation of the set point through effects in the hypothalamus. These cytokines include interleukin-1 (IL-1), tumor necrosis factor (TNF), interferon-gamma, and interleukin-6 (IL-6). The elevation in temperature results from either increased heat production (eg, shivering) or decreased loss (eg, peripheral vasoconstriction). Body temperature in cytokine-induced fever seldom exceeds 41.1 °C unless there is structural damage to hypothalamic regulatory centers.

Hyperthermia

Hyperthermia—not mediated by cytokines—occurs when body metabolic heat production or environmental heat load exceeds normal heat loss capacity or when there is impaired heat loss; heat stroke is an example. Body temperature may rise to levels (> 41.1 °C) capable of producing irreversible protein denaturation and resultant brain damage; no diurnal variation is observed.

Neuroleptic malignant syndrome is a rare and potentially lethal idiosyncratic reaction to major tranquilizers, particularly haloperidol and fluphenazine. It has clinical and pathophysiologic similarities to malignant hyperthermia of anesthesia. (See Chapters 25 and 39.)

Fever as a symptom provides important information about the presence of illness—particularly infections—and about changes in the clinical status of the patient. The fever pattern, however, is of marginal value for most specific diagnoses except for the relapsing fever of malaria, borreliosis, and occasional cases of lymphoma, especially Hodgkin's disease. Furthermore, the degree of temperature elevation does not necessarily correspond to the severity of the illness. In general, the febrile response tends to be greater in children than in adults; in older persons and neonates and in those receiving certain medications (eg, NSAIDs or corticosteroids), a normal temperature or even hypothermia may be observed.

Markedly elevated body temperature may result in profound metabolic disturbances. High temperature during the first trimester of pregnancy may cause birth defects, such as anencephaly. Fever increases insulin requirements and alters the metabolism and disposition of drugs used for the treatment of the diverse diseases associated with fever.

Prolonged Fever

Most febrile illnesses are due to common infections, are short-lived, and are relatively easy to diagnose. In certain instances, however, the origin of the fever may remain obscure ("fever of undetermined origin"; FUO) even after protracted diagnostic examination. The term FUO has traditionally been reserved for unexplained cases of fever exceeding 38.3 °C on several occasions for at least 3 weeks in patients without neutropenia or immunosuppression (see Chapter 30).

After extensive evaluation, one-fourth of these patients are judged to have chronic or indolent infection, about one-fourth autoimmune diseases, and about one-tenth a malignancy; the remainder have miscellaneous other disorders or no diagnosis is reached. Long-term follow-up of patients with initially undiagnosed FUO demonstrates that half become symptom-free during evaluation. In the remainder, a definitive diagnosis is established in 20%, usually within 2 months after investigation, and 30% have persistent or recurring fever for months or even years.

Approach to the Patient With FUO

Standardized algorithms for FUO are difficult to extrapolate to the individual patient. Nevertheless, the results of a history, physical examination, routine laboratory tests, and blood cultures provide important diagnostic clues that lead to a definitive diagnosis in most cases. In patients without a diagnosis or clues to one, staged diagnostic approaches have been employed for research purposes. Chest radiography and abdominal ultrasound and CT scans, often repeated after previous nondiagnostic studies, are most helpful. Radionuclide agents include labeled leukocytes, gallium-67, and radiolabeled human immunoglobulin; however, these tests appear to be most useful in patients with localizing signs of inflammation. There is little or no value to be derived from undirected immunologic, microbiologic, serologic, or endocrinologic studies. In older patients, a temporal artery biopsy is occasionally of use.

Fever of unknown origin is commonly associated with AIDS and HIV-related infections, though uncomplicated HIV infection is not a cause of prolonged fever. When FUO is observed in HIV-infected individuals, it usually occurs in the late stages. The most common causes are disseminated *Mycobacterium avium* infection, *Pneumocystis carinii* pneumonia, cytomegalovirus infection, disseminated histoplasmosis, and lymphoma.

The differential diagnosis of a febrile illness in the returned traveler is extensive but most commonly includes tropical infections such as malaria, dysentery, hepatitis, and dengue fever. A substantial number of febrile illnesses in travelers are never diagnosed.

Differential Diagnosis

See Table 2–3.

Treatment

Most fever is well tolerated. When the temperature is greater than 40 °C, symptomatic treatment may be required. A reading over 41 °C is likely to be hyperthermia and thus not cytokine-mediated, and emergent management is indicated. (See Heat Stroke, Chapter 38.)

Table 2–3. Differential diagnosis of fever and hyperthermia

Fever—common causes
  Infections: bacterial, viral, rickettsial, fungal, parasitic
  Autoimmune diseases
  Central nervous system disease, including head trauma and mass lesions
  Malignant disease, especially renal cell carcinoma, primary or metastatic liver cancer, leukemia and lymphoma
Fever—less common causes
  Cardiovascular diseases, including myocardial infarction, thrombophlebitis, and pulmonary embolism
  Gastrointestinal diseases, including inflammatory bowel disease, alcoholic hepatitis, granulomatous hepatitis
  Miscellaneous diseases, including drug fever, sarcoidosis, familial Mediterranean fever, tissue injury, hematoma, and factitious fever
Hyperthermia
  Peripheral thermoregulatory disorders, including heat stroke, malignant hyperthermia of anesthesia, and malignant neuroleptic syndrome

---

A. MEASURES FOR REMOVAL OF HEAT

Alcohol sponges, cold sponges, ice bags, ice-water enemas, and ice baths will lower body temperature. They are more useful in hyperthermia, since patients with cytokine-related fever will attempt to override these therapies.

B. ANTIPYRETIC DRUGS

Antipyretic therapy is not needed except for patients with marginal hemodynamic status. Aspirin or acetaminophen, 325–650 mg every 4 hours, is effective in reducing fever. These drugs are best administered continuously rather than as needed, since "prn" dosing results in periodic chills and sweats due to fluctuations in temperature caused by varying levels of drug.

C. ANTIMICROBIAL THERAPY

In most febrile patients, empirical antibiotic therapy should be deferred pending further evaluation. However, persons in whom a clinically significant infection is likely should be started on appropriate antibiotic therapy. Prompt broad-spectrum antimicrobials are also indicated for febrile patients who are clinically unstable, even before infection can be documented. These include patients with hemodynamic instability, those with neutropenia (neutrophils less than 500/µL), others who are asplenic (surgically or secondary to sickle cell disease) or immunosuppressed (including individuals taking systemic corticosteroids, azathioprine, cyclosporine, or other immunosuppressive medications), and those who are HIV-infected (see Chapter 31). For treatment of fever during neutropenia following chemotherapy, outpatient parenteral antimicrobial therapy with an agent such as ceftriaxone can be provided effectively and safely. If a fungal infection is suspected in patients with prolonged fever and neutropenia, fluconazole is an equally effective but less toxic alternative to amphotericin B.

Armstrong WS et al: Human immunodeficiency virus-associated fever of unknown origin: a study of 70 patients in the United States and review. Clin Infect Dis 1999;28:341. [PMID: 10064253]

Cornely OA et al: Ceftriaxone and cefotaxime are equally effective in the treatment of neutropenic fever. Antibiot Chemother 2000;50:37. [PMID: 10874453]

Hopkins PM: Malignant hyperthermia: advances in clinical management and diagnosis. Br J Anaesth 2000;85:118. [PMID: 10928000]

Mackowiak PA: Concepts of fever. Arch Intern Med 1998;158:1871. [PMID: 9759682]

Magill AJ: Fever in the returned traveler. Infect Dis Clin North Am 1998;12:445. [PMID: 9658253] (Causes include malaria, acute schistosomiasis, the enteric fevers, rickettsial diseases, leptospirosis, and dengue fever.)

Marik PE: Fever in the ICU. Chest 2000;117:855. [PMID: 10713016]

Pizzo PA: Fever in immunocompromised patients. N Engl J Med 1999;341:893. [PMID: 10486422]

INVOLUNTARY WEIGHT LOSS

 ESSENTIAL INQUIRIES

- Age.
- Caloric intake.
- Fever.
- Change in bowel habits.
- Secondary confirmation (eg, changes in clothing size).
- Substance use.
- Age-appropriate cancer screening history.

General Considerations

Body weight is determined by a person's caloric intake, absorptive capacity, metabolic rate, and energy losses. The metabolic rate can be affected by a multitude of medical conditions through the release of various cytokines such as cachectin and interleukins. Body weight normally peaks by the fifth or sixth decade and then gradually declines at a rate of 1–2 kg per decade.

Clinical Findings

Involuntary weight loss is regarded as clinically significant when it exceeds 5% or more of usual body weight over a 6- to 12-month period and often indicates serious physical or psychologic illness. Physical causes are usually evident during the initial evaluation. Cancer (about 30%), gastrointestinal disorders (about 15%), and dementia or depression (about 15%) are the most common causes. When an adequately nourished-appearing patient complains of weight loss, inquiry should be made about exact weight changes (with approximate dates) and about changes in clothing size. Family members may provide confirmation of weight loss, as may old documents such as driver's licenses.

Once the weight loss is established, the history, medication profile, physical examination, and conventional laboratory and radiologic investigations such as complete blood count, serologic tests, TSH level, urinalysis, fecal occult blood test, chest x-ray, and upper gastrointestinal series usually reveal the cause. When these tests are normal, the second phase of evaluation should focus on more definitive gastrointestinal investigation (eg, tests for malabsorption; endoscopy) and cancer screening (eg, Pap smear, mammography, PSA).

If the initial evaluation is unrevealing, follow-up is preferable to further diagnostic testing. Death at 2-year follow-up was not nearly as high in patients with unexplained involuntary weight loss (8%) as in those with weight loss due to malignant (79%) and established nonmalignant diseases (19%). Psychiatric consultation should be considered when there is evidence of depression, dementia, anorexia nervosa, or other emotional problems. Ultimately, in approximately 15–25% of cases, no cause for the weight loss can be found.

A mild, gradual weight loss occurs in some older individuals. It is due to changes in body composition, including loss of height and lean body mass and lower basal metabolic rate, leading to decreased energy requirements. However, rapid unintentional weight loss is predictive of morbidity and mortality in any population. In addition to various disease states, causes in older individuals include loss of teeth and consequent difficulty with chewing, alcoholism, and social isolation.

Differential Diagnosis

Consider malignancy, gastrointestinal disorders (eg, malabsorption; pancreatic insufficiency), dementia, depression, anorexia nervosa, hyperthyroidism, alcoholism, and social isolation.

Treatment

Weight stabilization occurs in the majority of surviving patients with both established and unknown causes of weight loss through treatment of the underlying disorder and caloric supplementation. Nutrient intake goals are established in relation to the severity of weight loss, in general ranging from 30 to 40 kcal/kg per day. In order of preference, route of administration options include oral, temporary nasojejunal tube, or percutaneous gastric or jejunal tube. Parenteral nutrition is reserved for patients with serious associated problems. A variety of pharmacologic agents have been proposed for the treatment of weight loss. These can be categorized into appetite stimulants (corticosteroids, progestational agents, dronabinol and serotonin antagonists); anabolic agents (growth hormone and testosterone derivatives); and anticatabolic agents (omega-3 fatty acids, pentoxifylline, hydrazine sulfate, and thalidomide).

Gazewood JD et al: Diagnosis and management of weight loss in the elderly. J Fam Pract 1998;47:19. [PMID: 9673603]

Poehlman ET et al: Energy expenditure, energy intake, and weight loss in Alzheimer disease. Am J Clin Nutr 2000;71:650S. [PMID: 10681274] (Unexplained weight loss and cachexia are common.)

Lankisch P et al: Unintentional weight loss: diagnosis and prognosis. The first prospective follow-up study from a secondary referral centre. J Intern Med 2001;249:41. [PMID: 11168783]

FATIGUE & CHRONIC FATIGUE SYNDROME

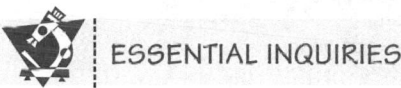

ESSENTIAL INQUIRIES

- *Weight loss.*
- *Fever.*
- *Sleep-disordered breathing.*
- *Medications.*
- *Substance use.*

General Considerations

As an isolated symptom, fatigue accounts for 1–3% of visits to generalists. The symptom of fatigue may be less well defined and explained by patients than symptoms associated with specific functions. Fatigue or lassitude and the closely related complaints of weakness, tiredness, and lethargy are often attributed to overexertion, poor physical conditioning, sleep disturbance, obesity, undernutrition, and emotional problems. A history of the patient's daily living and working habits may obviate the need for extensive and unproductive diagnostic studies.

Clinical Findings

Important diseases that can cause fatigue include hyperthyroidism and hypothyroidism, congestive heart failure, infections (endocarditis, hepatitis), COPD, sleep apnea, anemia, autoimmune disorders, and cancer. Alcoholism, drug side effects such as from sedatives and beta-blockers, and psychologic conditions such as insomnia, depression, and somatization disorder are other causes. The lifetime prevalence of significant fatigue (present for at least 2 weeks) is about 25%. Fatigue of unknown cause or related to psychiatric illness exceeds that due to physical illness, injury, medications, drugs, or alcohol. Psychiatric disorders associated with fatigue include depression, dysthymia, somatoform disorders, panic attack, and alcohol abuse.

Chronic Fatigue Syndrome

A working case definition of chronic fatigue syndrome (Figure 2–1) indicates that it is not a homogeneous abnormality, and there is no single pathogenic mechanism. No physical finding or laboratory test can be used to confirm the diagnosis of this disorder.

Early theories postulated an infectious or immune dysregulation mechanism, and it appears that neurologic, affective, and cognitive symptoms also occur frequently. Neuropsychologic, neuroendocrine, and brain imaging studies have confirmed the occurrence of neurobiologic abnormalities in most patients. Sleep disorders have been reported in 40–80% of patients with chronic fatigue syndrome, but their treatment has provided only modest benefit, suggesting that it is an effect rather than a cause of the fatigue. Magnetic resonance imaging may show brain abnormalities on T2-weighted images—chiefly small, punctate, subcortical white matter hyperintensities, predominantly in the frontal lobes.

After the history and physical examination process is completed, standard investigation of chronic fatigue should include complete blood count, erythrocyte sedimentation rate, serum chemistries—BUN, electrolytes, glucose, creatinine, calcium; liver and thyroid function tests—antinuclear antibody, urinalysis, and tuberculin skin test; and screening questionnaires for psychiatric disorders. Other tests to be performed as clinically indicated are serum cortisol, rheumatoid factor, immunoglobulin levels, Lyme serology in endemic areas, and tests for HIV antibody. More extensive testing is usually unhelpful, including antibody to Epstein-Barr virus. There may be an abnormally high rate of postural hypotension; some of these patients report response to increases in dietary sodium as well as antihypotensive agents such as fludrocortisone, 0.1 mg/d.

A variety of treatments have been tried. Acyclovir, intravenous immunoglobulin, nystatin, and low-dose hydrocortisone do not improve symptoms. There is a greater prevalence of past and current psychiatric diagnoses in patients with this syndrome. Affective disorders are especially common, but fluoxetine alone, 20 mg daily, is not beneficial. Patients with chronic fatigue syndrome have benefited from a comprehensive multidisciplinary intervention, including optimal medical management, treating any ongoing affective or anxiety disorder pharmacologically, and implementing a comprehensive cognitive-behavioral treatment program. Cognitive behavior therapy, a form of nonpharmacologic treatment emphasizing self-help and aiming to change perceptions and behaviors that may perpetuate symptoms and disability, is helpful. Although few patients are cured, the treatment effect is substantial. Graded exercise has been shown to improve functional work capacity and physical function. At present, intensive individual cognitive behavioral therapy administered by a skilled therapist remains the treatment of choice for patients with chronic fatigue syndrome.

Finally, the clinician's sympathetic listening and explanatory responses can help overcome the patient's frustrations and debilitation by this still mysterious illness. All patients should be encouraged to engage in normal activities to the extent possible and should be reassured that full recovery is eventually possible in most cases.

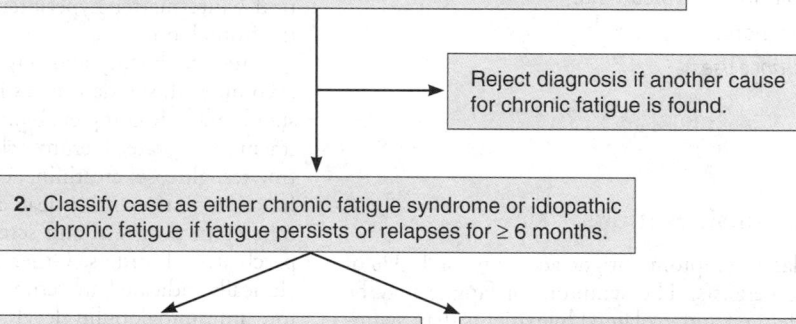

1. Clinically evaluate cases of prolonged or chronic fatigue by:
    A. History and physical examination;
    B. Mental status examination (abnormalities require appropriate psychiatric, psychologic, or neurologic examination);
    C. Tests (abnormal results that strongly suggest an exclusionary condition must be resolved):
        1. Screening lab tests: CBC, ESR, ALT, total protein, albumin, globulin, alkaline phosphatase, Ca²⁺, PO₄³⁻, glucose, BUN, electrolytes, creatinine, TSH and UA.
        2. Additional tests as clinically indicated to exclude other diagnoses.

Reject diagnosis if another cause for chronic fatigue is found.

2. Classify case as either chronic fatigue syndrome or idiopathic chronic fatigue if fatigue persists or relapses for ≥ 6 months.

A. Classify as chronic fatigue syndrome if:
    1. Criteria for severity of fatigue are met, and
    2. Four or more of the following symptoms are concurrently present for ≥ 6 months: (a) impaired memory or concentration, (b) sore throat, (c) tender cervical or axillary lymph nodes, (d) muscle pain, (e) multi-joint pain, (f) new headaches, (g) unrefreshing sleep, and (h) postexertion malaise.

B. Classify as idiopathic chronic fatigue if fatigue severity or symptom criteria for chronic fatigue syndrome are not met.

Figure 2–1. Evaluation and classification of unexplained chronic fatigue. (ALT, alanine aminotransferase; BUN, blood urea nitrogen; CBC, complete blood count; ESR, erythrocyte sedimentation rate; Ca²⁺, calcium; PO₄³⁻, phosphate; TSH, thyroid-stimulating hormone; UA, urinalysis.) (Modified and reproduced, with permission, from Fukuda K et al: The chronic fatigue syndrome: A comprehensive approach to its definition and study. Ann Intern Med 1994;121:953.)

Jason LA et al: A community-based study of chronic fatigue syndrome. Arch Intern Med 1999;159:2129. [PMID: 10527290]

Kulig J: Advances in medical management of asthma, headaches, and fatigue. Med Clin North Am 2000;84:829. [PMID: 10928191]

Lee P: Recent developments in chronic fatigue syndrome. Am J Med 1998;105(Suppl 3A):1S. [PMID: 9790473] (An entire journal issue devoted to chronic fatigue syndrome.)

Liao S et al: Fatigue in an older population. J Am Geriatr Soc 2000;48:426. [PMID: 10798471] (Fatigue is common, underrecognized, and undertreated among older residents in long-term care settings.)

Whiting P et al: Interventions for the treatment and management of chronic fatigue syndrome: a systematic review. JAMA 2001;286:1360. [PMID: 11560542] (Cognitive behavior therapy and graded exercise therapy are the only effective and acceptable treatments for adult outpatients.)

Powell P et al: Randomised controlled trial of patient education to encourage graded exercise in chronic fatigue syndrome. BMJ 2001;322:1. [PMID: 11179154] (Providing patients with physiologic explanations for symptoms was effective in encouraging self-managed graded exercise.)

Reid S et al: Chronic fatigue syndrome. BMJ 2000;320:292. [PMID: 10650029]

UPPER ABDOMINAL PAIN & DYSPEPSIA

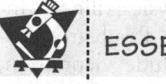 ESSENTIAL INQUIRIES

- *Age.*
- *Weight loss.*
- *Dysphagia.*
- *Heartburn.*
- *Blood in stool.*
- *Pregnancy.*
- *Atherosclerotic disease.*
- *Gastric cancer risk factors.*

General Considerations

Abdominal pain is a frequent reason for seeking medical attention. Acute abdominal pain accounts for 5–10% of emergency department visits in many areas. The most frequent diagnosis assigned to adults with acute abdominal pain is undifferentiated or unexplained abdominal pain (40%), followed distantly by gastroenteritis (7%). A majority of patients discharged with undifferentiated abdominal pain will be pain-free at 2- to 3-week follow-up, and most of the remaining patients will report improvement in symptoms. As the abdominal pain or discomfort becomes recurrent and remains unexplained, most patients fall under the category of dyspepsia.

Clinical Findings

In general, the history and physical examination alone are not sufficient to distinguish pathologic abdominal pain from functional dyspepsia. The duration of pain preceding the emergency department visit does not help distinguish diagnosis or resolution of pain at follow-up. Similarly, the location of pain and the presence or absence of fever should not be used to restrict the differential diagnosis. Peritoneal signs (rebound or cough tenderness) are not sufficiently sensitive to rule out peritonitis or appendicitis (sensitivity 60–80%) and are only modestly specific for these diseases (specificity 50–70%). Administration of opioid analgesics to facilitate diagnostic evaluation is safe, humane, and does not obscure abdominal findings such as tenderness to palpation or localized rigidity.

On the positive side, serial evaluations over several hours improve the diagnostic accuracy in patients with unclear causes of abdominal pain. All patients should have stool occult blood testing performed, female patients of childbearing age a pregnancy test, and female patients of any age a pelvic examination. Atypical presentations of pathologic or life-threatening conditions are more common in older adults (age over 65 years) and those infected with HIV. After routine assessment in older patients, an ECG may help to exclude atypical cardiac ischemia, and abdominal CT scan has consistently been shown to have the highest yield diagnostically.

Differential Diagnosis

Consider dyspepsia, gastroenteritis, peptic ulcer disease, gastroesophageal reflux disease, pancreaticobiliary disease, ischemic bowel, abdominal aortic aneurysm, nephrolithiasis, and pelvic inflammatory disease.

American College of Emergency Physicians: Clinical policy: critical issues for the initial evaluation and management of patients presenting with a chief complaint of nontraumatic acute abdominal pain. Ann Emerg Med 2000;36:406. [PMID: 11020699]

Lukens TW et al: The natural history of clinical findings in undifferentiated abdominal pain. Ann Emerg Med 1993;22:690. [PMID: 8457097]

Talley NJ et al: Functional gastroduodenal disorders. Gut 1999;45(Suppl II):1137. [PMID: 10457043] (International consensus conference on classification of gastrointestinal disorders.)

Preoperative Evaluation

3

Joshua S. Adler, MD, & Lee Goldman, MD, MPH
See www.current-med.com/ch03.html

Each year, tens of millions of patients in the United States undergo a surgical procedure requiring general or spinal-epidural anesthesia. A disproportionate and increasing number of these patients are over age 65. Most patients do not suffer significant morbidity as a result of the surgical procedure or the anesthetic. The rate of major complications varies from 3% to 15% depending on the patient's age and the presence of underlying disease. Cardiac, pulmonary, and neurologic complications account for most of the perioperative morbidity and mortality.

The role of the medical consultant includes clearly defining the patient's medical conditions, evaluating the severity and stability of these conditions, providing a surgical risk assessment, and recommending perioperative measures to reduce surgical risk.

Leung JM et al: Relative importance of preoperative health status versus intraoperative factors in predicting postoperative adverse outcomes in geriatric patients. J Am Geriatr Soc 2001;49:1080. [PMID: 11555070]

Polanczyk CA et al: Impact of age on perioperative complications and length of stay in patients undergoing noncardiac surgery. Ann Intern Med 2001;134:637. [PMID: 11304103]

PHYSIOLOGIC EFFECTS OF ANESTHESIA & SURGERY

The complications of anesthesia and surgery are, for the most part, logical results of their known physiologic effects. Both general and spinal or epidural anesthetic agents usually cause peripheral vasodilation, and most of the commonly used general anesthetic regimens also decrease myocardial contractility. These effects often result in transient mild hypotension or, less frequently, prolonged or more severe hypotension. The decrease in tidal volume caused by general and spinal-epidural anesthesia can close small airways and lead to atelectasis. Epinephrine and norepinephrine levels increase during surgery and remain elevated for a day or two. The serum cortisol level is generally elevated for 1–3 days, and serum antidiuretic hormone levels may be elevated for up to 1 week postoperatively. There is some evidence that general anesthesia may be associated with a relative hypercoagulable state during the perioperative period. This does not occur with spinal or epidural anesthesia. The degree to which this hypercoagulability contributes to perioperative morbidity is not known.

There is no evidence that spinal or epidural anesthesia is preferable to general anesthesia in terms of cardiac outcomes or overall surgical outcomes. Similarly, there is no conclusive evidence that the routine use of invasive hemodynamic monitoring with pulmonary artery catheters improves surgical outcomes. In general, the choice of anesthetic technique or agent and the decision to use invasive hemodynamic monitoring should be left to the anesthesiologist.

EVALUATION OF THE ASYMPTOMATIC PATIENT

Patients without significant medical problems—especially those under age 50—are at very low risk for perioperative complications. The preoperative evaluation of these patients should include a complete history and physical examination. Special emphasis is placed on the assessment of functional status, exercise tolerance, and cardiopulmonary symptoms and signs in an effort to reveal previously unrecognized disease (especially cardiopulmonary disease) that may require further evaluation prior to surgery. Additionally, a directed bleeding history (Table 3–1) should be taken to uncover disorders of hemostasis that could contribute to excessive surgical blood loss.

Routine testing of patients whose history and physical examination does not disclose significant medical problems should include a 12-lead ECG for those over 50 years of age and for any patient with risk factors for coronary artery disease, specifically to look for evidence of silent myocardial ischemia or infarction. Additional testing of asymptomatic healthy patients has not been found to be helpful and is not recommended. However, the preoperative evaluation may provide an opportunity to perform other tests that are recommended as part of routine health maintenance (see Chapter 1).

Schein OD et al: The value of routine preoperative medical testing before cataract surgery. Study of Medical Testing for

Table 3-1. A directed preoperative bleeding history.[1]

1. Have you ever bled for a long time or developed a swollen tongue or mouth after cutting or biting your tongue, cheek, or lip?
2. Do you develop bruises larger than a silver dollar without being able to remember when or how you injured yourself?
3. Has bleeding ever started up again the day after a tooth extraction?
4. Was bleeding after surgery ever hard to stop? Have you ever developed unusual bruising around an area of surgery or injury?
5. Has any blood relative had a problem with unusual bleeding or bleeding after surgery?

[1]Adapted, with permission, from Rapaport SI: Preoperative hemostatic evaluation: which tests, if any? Blood 1983;61:229.

Cataract Surgery. N Engl J Med 2000;342:168. [PMID: 10639542] (Randomized trial of preoperative laboratory testing versus no testing prior to cataract surgery showed no difference in outcomes.)

CARDIAC RISK ASSESSMENT

The cardiac complications of noncardiac surgery are perhaps the major cause of perioperative morbidity and demise. As such, this has been the most extensively studied area of perioperative medicine. The most important perioperative cardiac complications are myocardial infarction, congestive heart failure, and cardiac death. Older age, preexisting coronary artery disease, and congestive heart failure are the principal risk factors for development of these complications.

Major abdominal, thoracic, and vascular surgical procedures (especially abdominal aortic aneurysm repair) tend to carry a higher risk of postoperative cardiac complications than other procedures. Emergency operations are generally associated with more cardiac complications than elective operations. These high-risk procedures are more often associated with major fluid shifts, hemorrhage, and hypoxemia, which may predispose to cardiac complications.

Coronary Artery Disease

Approximately 50,000 patients undergoing surgery each year suffer a perioperative myocardial infarction. Patients without coronary artery disease are at extremely low risk (< 0.5%) for perioperative ischemic cardiac complications. Patients with known or suspected coronary artery disease, as defined in Table 3-2, have a five- to 50-fold increased risk of perioperative cardiac complications.

The estimated risk of cardiac complications in patients with coronary artery disease can be further refined through an assessment of the severity of anginal symptoms, the use of multifactorial indices, and the judicious use of noninvasive tests for ischemia. The

Table 3-2. Characteristics defining patients with known or suspected coronary artery disease.[1]

1. History of myocardial infarction
2. Angiographic evidence of coronary artery disease
3. Evidence of ischemia on prior noninvasive testing
4. Typical angina pectoris
5. Peripheral vascular disease

[1]Adapted, with permission, from Ashton CM et al: The incidence of perioperative myocardial infarction in men undergoing noncardiac surgery. Ann Intern Med 1993;118:504.

severity of anginal symptoms is most accurately assessed using a standardized scale such as that shown in Table 3-3. Multifactorial indices combine several clinical parameters to estimate an overall risk of cardiac complications. A recently updated risk index is presented in Table 3-4. This index more accurately predicts perioperative outcomes using modern surgical techniques.

Preoperative Noninvasive Ischemia Testing

Noninvasive tests for myocardial ischemia such as exercise treadmill testing, dipyridamole-thallium scintigraphy, and dobutamine stress echocardiography have been shown to improve upon the clinical risk assessment and help to optimize preoperative management in selected patients. Most patients, however, can be accurately stratified through an assessment of anginal symptoms. Patients who have mild symptoms, defined as Canadian Cardiovascular Society (CCS) class 1 or 2 angina, and a low or intermediate multifactorial index score are at low risk for cardiac complications. Patients with severe symptoms, CCS class 3 or 4 angina, or a

Table 3-3. Canadian Cardiovascular Society angina class.[1]

I. Ordinary physical activity, such as walking and climbing stairs, does not cause angina. Angina occurs with strenuous or rapid or prolonged exertion at work or recreation.
II. Slight limitation of ordinary activity. Angina occurs with walking or climbing stairs rapidly, walking uphill, walking or stair climbing after meals, or only during the few hours after awakening. Angina occurs when walking more than two blocks on the level or climbing more than one flight of stairs at a normal pace and in normal conditions.
III. Marked limitation of ordinary physical activity. Angina occurs with walking one to two blocks on the level and climbing one flight of stairs in normal conditions and at a normal pace.
IV. Inability to carry on any physical activity without discomfort; angina may be present at rest.

[1]Reproduced, with permission, from Campeau L: Grading of angina pectoris. (Letter.) Circulation 1975;54:522.

Table 3–4. Revised cardiac risk index.[1]

Independent Predictors of Postoperative Cardiac Complications	Scoring (Number of Predictors Present)	Risk of Major Cardiac Complications[2]
1. Intrathoracic, intraperitoneal, or infrainguinal vascular surgery		
2. History of ischemic heart disease	None	0.4%
3. History of congestive heart failure	One	0.9%
4. Insulin treatment for diabetes mellitus	Two	7.0%
5. Serum creatinine level > 2 mg/dL	More than 2	11%
6. History of cerebrovascular disease		

[1]Adapted from Lee TH et al: Derivation and prospective validation of a simple index for prediction of cardiac risk of major noncardiac surgery. Circulation 1999;100:1043.
[2]Myocardial infarction, pulmonary edema, ventricular fibrillation, cardiac arrest, complete heart block.

high multifactorial index score are likely to be at high risk for cardiac complications. Noninvasive ischemia testing in either of these groups of patients is unlikely to improve the accuracy of the clinical risk assessment. However, any patient who is considered a candidate for noninvasive ischemia testing independent of the planned noncardiac surgery should generally have such testing prior to surgery if the test result may lead to coronary revascularization. This is particularly true for patients found to be at high risk on clinical assessment.

Noninvasive cardiac testing may be useful when the patient's medical history is unreliable or when orthopedic or vascular conditions severely limit physical activity. In patients who are able to exercise, exercise electrocardiography may be very helpful. Patients without ischemia at or above 85% of their maximal predicted heart rate are at low risk for perioperative cardiac complications.

For patients who cannot exercise, an assessment of specific clinical criteria can help to identify those most likely to benefit from noninvasive testing. Patients who have no risk factors for coronary artery disease are at low risk for cardiac complications regardless of the results of noninvasive ischemia testing, and patients with clinical evidence of severe coronary artery disease are at high risk regardless of the test result. Dipyridamole-thallium scintigraphy or dobutamine stress echocardiography is most helpful in patients with an intermediate clinical risk. A normal dipyridamole-thallium scan or stress echocardiogram predicts a low risk of complications (comparable to that of patients with a low-risk clinical assessment), whereas evidence of thallium redistribution—or stress-induced echocardiographic wall motion abnormalities—predicts a much higher risk (comparable to that of patients with a high-risk clinical assessment). In the case of peripheral vascular surgery, the absence of a regional wall motion abnormality on stress-echocardiography predicts a low risk of perioperative cardiac death or myocardial infarction even in patients with high-risk clinical criteria. When such patients receive perioperative beta-blocking medications, their risk approximates that of the low clinical risk group.

The predictive powers of dipyridamole-thallium scintigraphy and dobutamine stress echocardiography appear to be comparable. Evidence of ischemia on preoperative continuous electrocardiographic monitoring has been associated with perioperative cardiac complications. However, the practical use of this test is limited by the need for a normal baseline ECG and the minimum 24-hour testing period.

Left ventricular systolic dysfunction, moderate or severe left ventricular hypertrophy, and a peak aortic gradient greater than 40 mm Hg on resting echocardiography are associated with an increased risk of cardiac complications in selected patients. Resting echocardiography, however, is not recommended for routine perioperative risk assessment.

Preoperative Management of Patients With Coronary Artery Disease

A. LOW-RISK PATIENTS WITH CORONARY ARTERY DISEASE

Patients in this group have roughly a 4% risk of myocardial infarction and about a 1% mortality rate. Results from the Coronary Artery Surgery Study trial registry indicate that patients who have undergone prior coronary artery bypass graft surgery are at lower risk for cardiac complications with subsequent noncardiac surgery compared with similar patients treated medically. However, this should not be interpreted as a prescription for the use of prophylactic revascularization. The use of coronary angiography and revascularization in these patients depends on two factors: the urgency of the surgery and whether the patient has indications for such evaluation regardless of the planned surgery. The mortality rate for coronary artery bypass surgery is roughly 1.5%; thus, the routine prophylactic use of this procedure prior to elective noncardiac surgery is unlikely to decrease total morbidity or mortality rates. However, in patients who are candidates for coronary angiography and subsequent revascularization independent of the planned surgery, it seems prudent to proceed with these prior to elective noncardiac surgery when feasible. The data on percutaneous transluminal coronary angioplasty (PTCA) suggest that it is not sufficiently different from coronary artery bypass graft surgery to warrant its routine preoperative use.

Preoperative antianginal medications, including beta-blockers, calcium channel blockers, and nitrates, should be continued preoperatively and during the postoperative period. The institution of prophylactic beta-blockers in the immediate preoperative period has been shown to reduce intraoperative myocardial ischemia and may reduce the incidence of perioperative myocardial infarction. In the first large clinical trial, prophylactic atenolol reduced cardiac morbidity at 6, 12, and 24 months after noncardiac surgery in patients with known or suspected coronary artery disease. The most dramatic results of perioperative beta blockade have been demonstrated in a randomized controlled trial of prophylactic bisoprolol in patients who had known coronary artery disease and abnormal stress echocardiograms and who underwent major noncardiac surgery. The risk of nonfatal myocardial infarction or cardiac death was reduced from 34% to 3.4% in the bisoprolol group compared with the placebo group. Thus, perioperative prophylactic beta blockade is recommended for patients with known or suspected coronary artery disease undergoing major surgery. The dosing schedules for atenolol and bisoprolol are set forth in Table 3–5.

Prophylactic intraoperative intravenous nitroglycerin may decrease the frequency of ischemia but has not been shown to reduce the rate of postoperative complications. This may be considered for high-risk patients. Too little is known about the effects of the prophylactic use of calcium channel blockers to make any recommendations. A recent clinical trial of the prophylactic use of the α_2-adrenergic agonist mivazerol in patients with coronary artery disease found no significant benefit overall but a significant reduction

Table 3–5. Preoperative prophylactic beta-blocker administration.

Atenolol	5–10 mg[1] given intravenously every 12 hours beginning 1 hour before surgery and continued until the patient is eating; followed by 50–100 mg[1] orally daily until postoperative day 7.
Bisoprolol	5–10 mg[1] given orally once daily begun at least 7 days prior to surgery and continued for 30 days postoperatively.[2]

[1]The higher dose is used unless the heart rate is below 60 beats per minute.
[2]Intravenous atenolol or metoprolol may be used during the period when the patient is not eating. The dosage should be adjusted to achieve a target heart rate of 60 beats per minute.

Adapted from Mangano DT et al: Effects of atenolol on mortality and cardiovascular morbidity after noncardiac surgery. N Engl J Med 1996;335:1713; and from Poldermans D et al: The effect of bisoprolol on perioperative mortality and myocardial infarction in high-risk patients undergoing vascular surgery. N Engl J Med 1999;341:1789.

in coronary events and deaths in a preplanned subgroup analysis of patients undergoing vascular surgery; however, recommendations for its routine use cannot yet be made.

B. High-Risk Patients With Coronary Artery Disease

In this group surgery should be postponed, except in emergency situations, to allow for stabilization of ischemic symptoms. For patients with a recent myocardial infarction, delaying surgery for 3–6 months postinfarction to allow for appropriate stabilization and therapy may significantly reduce perioperative mortality and morbidity rates. Patients with unstable angina should be evaluated and treated as indicated by their cardiac status prior to surgery and then reevaluated with respect to severity of symptoms and functional status. Patients with severe stable angina or worsening angina may be managed in a variety of ways. Like patients with less severe angina, those who are potential candidates for coronary revascularization independently of the planned noncardiac surgery should certainly proceed with this evaluation prior to noncardiac surgery. For patients who are not obvious candidates for revascularization, one approach is to optimize their antianginal medications and reevaluate their symptoms. This approach assumes that an improvement in symptoms correlates with a reduction in perioperative cardiac complication rates—an assumption that is without clear validation at present. All high-risk patients should be treated with prophylactic atenolol or bisoprolol if they are not already taking a beta-blocking agent and if it is not otherwise contraindicated. An alternative approach is preoperative PTCA. However, it is not known if such a strategy effectively reduces surgical risk. In a cohort analysis from the BARI (Bypass Angioplasty Revascularization Investigation) trial, patients who underwent multivessel angioplasty (without intracoronary stent placement) for stable coronary artery disease had a 1.6% cardiac complication rate with subsequent noncardiac surgery. It is of note that the complication rate was 0.8% when the interval between the PTCA and noncardiac surgery was less than 4 years compared with a rate of 3.6% when surgery was done more than 4 years following PTCA.

The use of intracoronary stents in the immediate preoperative period, however, may increase the risk of perioperative cardiac complications. In a recent retrospective study, patients who underwent noncardiac surgery within 14 days after intracoronary stenting had extremely high total morbidity and mortality (32%) rates. The complication rates were substantially lower in patients who underwent noncardiac surgery 15–39 days after stenting. The presumed mechanism of this very high mortality is acute stent thrombosis that results from discontinuation of anticoagulant therapy prior to the standard 4 weeks. Therefore, it is prudent to delay elective surgery for at least 4 weeks after intracoronary stenting.

An approach to the assessment and management of patients with known or suspected coronary artery disease is set forth in Table 3–6.

Congestive Heart Failure & Left Ventricular Dysfunction

Decompensated congestive heart failure, manifested by an elevated jugular venous pressure, an audible third heart sound, or evidence of pulmonary edema on physical examination or chest radiography significantly increases the risk of perioperative pulmonary edema (roughly 15%) and cardiac death (2–10%). Preoperative control of congestive heart failure, including the use of diuretics and afterload reducing agents, is likely to reduce the perioperative risk. One must be cautious not to give too much diuretic, since the volume-depleted patient will be much more susceptible to intraoperative hypotension. Although spironolactone, beta-adrenergic blocking agents, and angiotensin receptor-blocking agents have been shown to reduce mortality in patients with heart failure, institution of these agents in the immediate preoperative period has not been studied and is not recommended as routine practice.

Patients with compensated left ventricular dysfunction are at increased risk for developing perioperative pulmonary edema but are not at excess risk for other cardiac complications. One large study found that patients with a left-ventricular ejection fraction of less than 50% had an absolute risk of 12% for postoperative congestive heart failure compared with 3% for patients with an ejection fraction greater than 50%. Such patients should be maintained on all heart failure medications up to and including the day of surgery. Patients receiving digoxin and diuretics should routinely have serum electrolyte and digoxin levels measured prior to surgery because abnormalities in these levels may increase the risk of perioperative arrhythmias. Preoperative echocardiography or radionuclide angiography to assess left ventricular function should

Table 3–6. Assessment and management of patients with known or suspected coronary artery disease undergoing major surgery.

1. Assess functional capacity by history.
2. If the history is reliable and the patient has CCS class I or II angina, surgery is low risk. Administer perioperative beta-blocking medication.
3. If the patient has CCS class III or IV angina or if the history is unreliable, perform noninvasive ischemia testing.
4. If the results of noninvasive testing are negative, administer beta-blocking medications; surgery is low risk.
5. If the results of nonvasive testing are positive, the patient remains at high risk. Administer beta-blocking medications and consider the role of revascularization.

be considered for patients with evidence of left ventricular dysfunction who have not had an objective assessment of left ventricular function, and in patients for whom the cause of left ventricular dysfunction is in question. The surgeon and anesthesiologist should be made aware of the presence and severity of left ventricular dysfunction so that appropriate decisions can be made regarding perioperative fluid management and intraoperative monitoring.

Valvular Heart Disease

There are few data available regarding the perioperative risks of valvular heart disease independent of associated coronary artery disease or congestive heart failure. Patients with severe symptomatic aortic stenosis are clearly at increased risk for cardiac complications. Such patients who are candidates for valve replacement surgery or, if only short-term relief is needed, for balloon valvuloplasty independent of the planned noncardiac surgery should have the corrective procedure performed prior to noncardiac surgery. In the largest recent series of patients with severe aortic stenosis who underwent noncardiac surgery, the mortality rate was less than 5% and the cardiac morbidity rate was approximately 10%. It is noteworthy that all patients had normal or near-normal preoperative left ventricular systolic function and that patients with asymptomatic aortic stenosis appeared to be at lower risk than patients with symptomatic aortic stenosis. The relatively low morbidity and mortality in this series may be due to the recent use of invasive intraoperative monitoring, including pulmonary artery catheterization and transesophageal echocardiography. Nevertheless, noncardiac surgery in patients with severe aortic stenosis must be approached with great caution.

The severity of valvular lesions should be defined prior to surgery to allow for appropriate fluid management and consideration of invasive intraoperative monitoring. Echocardiography should also be considered in patients with a previously unexplained heart murmur for those procedures in which a valvular abnormality would require antibiotic prophylaxis. For specific recommendations regarding antibiotic prophylaxis, see Chapter 33.

Arrhythmias

Several early studies on cardiac risk factors reported that both atrial and ventricular arrhythmias were independent predictors of an increased risk of perioperative complications. Recent data have shown these rhythm disturbances to be frequently associated with underlying structural heart disease, especially coronary artery disease and left ventricular dysfunction. The finding of a rhythm disturbance on preoperative evaluation should prompt consideration of further cardiac evaluation, particularly when the finding of structural heart disease would alter perioperative management. Patients found to have a rhythm disturbance without evidence of underlying heart disease are at very low risk for perioperative cardiac complications.

Management of patients with arrhythmias in the preoperative period should be guided by factors independent of the planned surgery. In patients with atrial fibrillation, adequate rate control should be established. Symptomatic supraventricular and ventricular tachycardia must be controlled prior to surgery. There is no evidence that the use of antiarrhythmic medications to suppress an asymptomatic arrhythmia alters perioperative risk.

It seems prudent for patients who have indications for a permanent pacemaker to have it placed prior to noncardiac surgery. When surgery is urgent, these patients may be managed perioperatively with temporary transvenous pacing. Patients with bundle branch block who do not meet recognized criteria for a permanent pacemaker do not require pacing during surgery.

Hypertension

Severe hypertension, defined as a systolic pressure greater than 180 mm Hg or diastolic pressure greater than 110 mm Hg, appears to be an independent predictor of perioperative cardiac complications, including myocardial infarction and congestive heart failure. Mild to moderate hypertension immediately preoperatively is associated with intraoperative blood pressure lability and asymptomatic myocardial ischemia but does not appear to be an independent risk factor for adverse cardiac outcomes. It seems wise to delay surgery in patients with severe hypertension until blood pressure can be controlled, though it is not known whether the risk of cardiac complications is reduced with this approach. It is unlikely that treatment of mild to moderate hypertension in the immediate preoperative period will significantly reduce the risk of cardiac complications. However, chronic medications for hypertension should be continued up to and including the day of surgery.

Boersma E et al: Predictors of cardiac events after major vascular surgery, role of clinical characteristics, dobutamine echocardiography, and beta-blocker therapy. JAMA 2001;285: 1865. [PMID: 11308400] (Prospective study of vascular surgery patients evaluated the protective effects of beta-blocker therapy in its implications for preoperative noninvasive ischemia testing.)

Fleisher LA et al: Clinical practice. Lowering cardiac risk in non-cardiac surgery. N Engl J Med 2001;345:1677. [PMID: 11759647] (Recommendations for use of perioperative beta-blocker therapy, α_2-agonist therapy, and noninvasive testing.)

Hassan SA et al: Outcomes of noncardiac surgery after coronary artery bypass surgery or coronary angioplasty in the Bypass Angioplasty Revascularization Investigation (BARI). Am J Med 2001;110:260. [PMID: 11239843] (Cardiac complication rates after noncardiac surgery were similarly low in patients who had undergone CABG surgery or multivessel angioplasty.)

Kaluza GL et al: Catastrophic outcomes of noncardiac surgery soon after coronary stenting. J Am Coll Cardiol 2000; 35:1288. [PMID: 10758971] (Patients who underwent noncardiac surgery within 14 days after coronary stenting had a 32% mortality rate.)

Lee TH et al: Derivation and prospective validation of a simple index for prediction of cardiac risk of major noncardiac surgery. Circulation 1999;100:1043. [PMID: 10477528] (Derivation of a new multifactorial cardiac risk index based on surgical outcome data from the 1990s.)

Polanczyk CA et al: Right heart catheterization and cardiac complications in patients undergoing noncardiac surgery. JAMA 2001;286:309. [PMID: 11466096] (A prospective observational study of over 4000 patients who underwent major noncardiac surgery found no reduction in complication rates associated with the use of pulmonary artery catheters.)

Poldermans D et al: The effect of bisoprolol on perioperative mortality and myocardial infarction in high risk patients undergoing vascular surgery. N Engl J Med 1999;341:1789. [PMID: 10588963] (Randomized trial of preoperative oral bisoprolol versus placebo in patients with coronary artery disease showed a substantial reduction in perioperative morbidity and mortality.)

Torsher LC et al: Risk of patients with severe aortic stenosis undergoing noncardiac surgery. Am J Cardiol 1998;81:448. [PMID: 9485135] (Consecutive series of patients with severe aortic stenosis who underwent noncardiac surgery without preoperative correction of the valvular abnormality.)

PULMONARY EVALUATION IN NON-LUNG RESECTION SURGERY

Pneumonia and respiratory failure requiring prolonged mechanical ventilation are the most important postoperative pulmonary complications and occur in 3–19% of surgical procedures.

Risk Factors for the Development of Postoperative Pulmonary Complications

Numerous series have investigated the risk factors for the development of postoperative pulmonary complications. The risk of developing a pulmonary complication is highest in patients undergoing cardiac, thoracic, and upper abdominal surgery, with reported complication rates ranging from 9% to 19%. The risk in patients undergoing lower abdominal or pelvic procedures ranges from 2% to 5%, and for extremity procedures the range is less than 1–3%. The pulmonary complication rate for laparoscopic procedures appears to be much lower than that for open procedures. In one series of over 1500 patients who underwent laparoscopic cholecystectomy, the pulmonary complication rate was less than 1%.

Three patient-specific factors have been repeatedly found to increase the risk of postoperative pulmonary complications: chronic lung disease, morbid obesity, and tobacco use. Patients with chronic obstructive pulmonary disease (COPD) have a two- to fourfold increased risk compared with patients without

COPD. Assessment of the severity of COPD using pulmonary function tests has not been shown to improve upon the clinical risk assessment with the exception that patients with an FEV_1 under 500 mL, an FEV_1 below 50% of the predicted value, or an arterial PCO_2 greater than 45 mm Hg appear to be at particularly high risk. In a single large prospective cohort of United States military veterans, additional risk factors for the development of postoperative pneumonia included: age over 60 years, dependent functional status, impaired sensorium, prior stroke, and neck or intracranial surgery.

Patients with asthma are at increased risk for bronchospasm during tracheal intubation and extubation and during the postoperative period. However, if patients are at their optimal pulmonary function (as determined by symptoms, physical examination, or spirometry) at the time of surgery, they do not appear to be at increased risk for other pulmonary complications.

Morbidly obese patients—those weighing over 113 kg (250 lb)—are approximately twice as likely to develop postoperative pneumonia as patients weighing less. Mild obesity does not appear to increase the risk of clinically important pulmonary complications.

Several studies have shown that current cigarette smoking is associated with an increased risk for developing postoperative atelectasis. In a single study, cigarette smoking was also found to double the risk of developing postoperative pneumonia, even when controlling for underlying lung disease. A summary of the known risk factors for pulmonary complications is presented in Table 3–7.

Pulmonary Function Testing & Arterial Blood Gas Analysis

The vast majority of studies have shown that preoperative pulmonary function testing in unselected patients is not helpful in predicting postoperative pulmonary complications. The data are conflicting regarding the utility of preoperative pulmonary function testing in certain selected groups of patients: the morbidly obese, those with COPD, and those undergoing upper abdominal or cardiothoracic surgery. No single pulmonary function test value places a patient at prohibitive risk for non-lung resection surgery. At

present, definitive recommendations regarding the indications for preoperative pulmonary function testing cannot be made. In general terms, such testing may be helpful to confirm the diagnosis of COPD or asthma, to assess the severity of known pulmonary disease, and perhaps as part of the risk assessment for patients undergoing upper abdominal surgery, cardiac surgery, or thoracic surgery.

Arterial blood gas measurement is not routinely recommended except in patients with known lung disease and suspected hypoxemia or hypercapnia.

Perioperative Management

The goal of perioperative management is to reduce the likelihood of postoperative pulmonary complications. Smoking cessation for at least 4 weeks prior to thoracic surgery reduced the incidence of pulmonary complications by 25%. Incentive spirometry (IS), continuous positive airway pressure (CPAP), intermittent positive-pressure breathing (IPPB), and deep breathing exercises (DBE) have all been shown to reduce the incidence of postoperative atelectasis and, in a small number of studies, to reduce the incidence of postoperative pulmonary complications. In comparative trials, these methods were equally effective. Given the higher cost of CPAP and IPPB, IS and DBE are the preferred methods. IS must be performed for 15 minutes every 2 hours. DBE must be performed hourly and consist of 3-second breath-holding, pursed lip breathing, and coughing. These measures should be started preoperatively and be continued for 1–2 days postoperatively.

There has been recent enthusiasm for the use of postoperative epidural analgesia to improve pain control and perhaps to reduce pulmonary complications. Most studies suggest that postoperative epidural opioid and local anesthetic agents provide excellent pain control but do not appreciably reduce pulmonary complication rates.

There is some evidence that the incidence of postoperative pulmonary complications in patients with COPD or asthma may be reduced by preoperative optimization of pulmonary function. Patients who are wheezing will probably benefit from therapy with bronchodilators and, in certain cases, corticosteroids preoperatively. Antibiotics may be of benefit for patients who cough with purulent sputum if the sputum can be cleared prior to surgery. Patients who take oral theophylline should be maintained on it during the intraoperative and postoperative periods, using intravenous theophylline when necessary.

Table 3–7. Risk factors for postoperative pulmonary complications.

1. Upper abdominal or cardiothoracic surgery
2. Anesthetic time > 4 hours
3. Morbid obesity
4. Chronic obstructive pulmonary disease or asthma
5. Tobacco use > 20 pack-years

Arozullah AM et al: Development and validation of a multifactorial risk index for predicting postoperative pneumonia after major noncardiac surgery. Ann Intern Med 2001;135:847. [PMID: 11712875] (A prospective cohort study of United States veterans confirmed known risk factors for postoperative pneumonia and found additional risk factors, including older age, neurologic disease, and neck or cranial surgery.)

Ferguson MK: Preoperative assessment of pulmonary risk. Chest 1999;115(5 Suppl):58S. [PMID: 10331335] (Systematic review of studies evaluating risk factors for postoperative pulmonary complications.)

Nakagawa M et al: Relationship between the duration of the preoperative smoke-free period and the incidence of postoperative complications after pulmonary surgery. Chest 2001; 120:705. [PMID: 11555496] (A retrospective cohort study of 288 patients demonstrated that smoking cessation of at least 4 weeks' duration was associated with a reduction in pulmonary complications after thoracic surgery. Smoking cessation for less than 4 weeks was not associated with a reduction in adverse outcomes.)

Overend TJ et al: The effect of incentive spirometry on postoperative pulmonary complications. Chest 2001;120:971. [PMID: 11555536] (Systematic review concluded that incentive spirometry may not contribute to a reduction in postoperative pulmonary complications above that obtained with deep breathing exercises alone.)

EVALUATION OF THE PATIENT WITH LIVER DISEASE

Patients with serious liver disease are generally thought to be at increased risk for perioperative morbidity and demise. Appropriate preoperative evaluation requires consideration of the effects of anesthesia and surgery on postoperative liver function and of the complications associated with anesthesia and surgery in patients with preexisting liver disease.

The Effects of Anesthesia & Surgery on Liver Function

Postoperative elevation of serum aminotransferase levels is a relatively common finding after major surgery. Most of these elevations are transient and not associated with hepatic dysfunction. Studies in the 1960s and early 1970s showed that patients with liver disease are at increased relative risk for postoperative deterioration in hepatic function, though the absolute risk is not known. General anesthetic agents may cause deterioration of hepatic function via intraoperative reduction in hepatic blood flow leading to ischemic injury. It is important to remember that agents used for spinal and epidural anesthesia produce similar reductions in hepatic blood flow and thus may be equally likely to lead to ischemic liver injury. Intraoperative hypotension, hemorrhage, and hypoxemia may also contribute to liver injury.

Risk Factors for Surgical Complications

Surgery in the patient with serious liver disease has been associated in several series with a variety of significant complications, including hemorrhage, infection, renal failure, and encephalopathy, and with a substantial mortality rate. A key limitation in interpreting these data is our inability to determine the contribution of the liver disease to the observed complications independent of the surgical procedure.

In three small series of patients with acute viral hepatitis who underwent abdominal surgery, the mortality rate was roughly 10%. Patients undergoing portosystemic shunt surgery who have evidence of alcoholic hepatitis on the preoperative liver biopsy have a significantly increased surgical mortality rate. Although data are quite limited, it seems reasonable to delay elective surgery in patients with acute viral or alcoholic hepatitis, at least until the acute episode has resolved. These data are not sufficient to warrant substantial delays in urgent or emergent surgery.

There are few data regarding the risks of surgery in patients with chronic hepatitis. In a series of 272 patients with chronic hepatitis undergoing a variety of surgical procedures for variceal hemorrhage, the in-hospital mortality rate was less than 2%. It is of note that patients with Child-Pugh class C cirrhosis (see Chapter 15) or with serum aminotransferase levels over 150 units/L were excluded. In a study of patients undergoing hepatectomy for hepatocellular carcinoma, patients with both cirrhosis and active hepatitis on the preoperative liver biopsy had a fourfold increase in mortality (8.7%) compared with patients with cirrhosis alone or active hepatitis alone.

Substantial data exist regarding surgery in patients with cirrhosis. In several series from the 1960s and 1970s, patients with cirrhosis undergoing abdominal surgery had substantial mortality rates. Biliary surgery was especially risky. Patients with Childs-Pugh class A or B cirrhosis who underwent abdominal surgery during the 1990s, however, had relatively low mortality rates (hepatectomy 0–8%, open cholecystectomy 0–1%, laparoscopic cholecystectomy 0–1%). Three recent studies investigated the risk factors for morbidity and mortality in patients with hepatocellular carcinoma and underlying Child-Pugh class A or B cirrhosis who underwent liver resection. An elevation of serum alanine aminotransferase (ALT) above twice-normal, an abnormal indocyanine green test, and an abnormal result on technetium-99m galactosyl-human serum albumin liver scintigraphy all were associated with increased perioperative morbidity or mortality. Patients with Childs-Pugh class C cirrhosis who underwent portosystemic shunt surgery, biliary surgery, or trauma surgery during the 1970s and 1980s had a 50–85% mortality rate. More recent surgical data in these patients are lacking. A conservative approach would be to avoid elective surgery in patients with class C cirrhosis or those with class A or B cirrhosis and concomitant active hepatitis.

Noun R et al: High preoperative serum alanine transferase levels: Effect on the risk of liver resection in Child grade A cirrhotic patients. World J Surg 1997;21:390. [PMID: 9143570] (An ALT level more than twice normal is associated with an increased risk of perioperative complications.)

Poggio JL et al: A comparison of laparoscopic and open cholecystectomy in patients with compensated cirrhosis and symptomatic gallstones. Surgery 2000;127:405. [PMID: 10776431] (A retrospective cohort study of patients with cirrhosis who underwent either open or laparoscopic chole-cystectomy demonstrated a low complication rate for either surgical technique.)

PREOPERATIVE HEMATOLOGIC EVALUATION

Several hematologic disorders may have an impact on the outcomes of surgery. A detailed discussion of the preoperative management of patients with complicated hematologic disorders is beyond the scope of this section. Two of the more common clinical situations faced by the medical consultant are the patient with preexisting anemia and the assessment of bleeding risk.

The key issues in the anemic patient are to determine the need for preoperative diagnostic evaluation and the need for transfusion. When feasible, the diagnostic evaluation of the patient with previously unrecognized anemia should be done prior to surgery because certain types of anemia (particularly sickle cell disease and immune hemolytic anemias) may have implications for perioperative management. Most data suggest that morbidity and mortality increase as the preoperative hemoglobin level decreases, though none of these data were corrected for the presence of preexisting diseases. Hemoglobin levels below 8 or 9 g/dL appear to be associated with significantly more perioperative complications than higher levels. In patients with ischemic heart disease, a preoperative hemoglobin level below 10 g/dL has been associated with an increased perioperative mortality rate. It is not known, however, whether preoperative transfusion reduces the risk for perioperative complications. Determination of the need for preoperative transfusion in an individual patient must consider factors other than the absolute hemoglobin level, including the presence of cardiopulmonary disease, the type of surgery, and the likelihood of surgical blood loss.

The most important component of the bleeding risk assessment is a directed bleeding history (Table 3–1). Patients who are reliable historians and who reveal no suggestion of abnormal bleeding on directed bleeding history and physical examination are at very low risk for having an occult bleeding disorder. Laboratory tests of hemostatic parameters in these patients are generally not needed. When the directed bleeding history is unreliable or incomplete or when abnormal bleeding is suggested, a formal evaluation of hemostasis should be done prior to surgery and should include measurement of the prothrombin time, the activated partial thromboplastin time, the platelet count, and the bleeding time.

Wahr JA: Myocardial ischaemia in anaemic patients. Br J Anaesth 1998;81(Suppl 1):10. [PMID: 10318982] (Review of surgical risks in anemic patients.)

NEUROLOGIC EVALUATION

Delirium occurs after major surgery in approximately 9% of patients over the age of 50 years. Postoperative delirium has been associated with higher rates of major postoperative cardiac and pulmonary complications, poor functional recovery, and increased length of hospital stay. Several preoperative and postoperative factors have been associated with the development of postoperative delirium (Table 3–8). Patients with multiple risk factors are at especially high risk.

Delirium is most common after hip fracture repair, occurring in 35–65% of patients. In a randomized controlled trial of hip fracture surgery patients, those who received daily visits and targeted recommendations from a geriatrician had a lower risk of postoperative delirium (32%) than the control patients (50%). The most frequent interventions to prevent delirium were maintenance of the hematocrit greater than 30%; minimizing the use of benzodiazepines, anticholinergic, and antihistamine medications; maintenance of regular bowel function; and early discontinuation of urinary catheters.

Stroke may occur in 1–6% of patients undergoing cardiac, carotid artery, or peripheral vascular surgery, but it occurs in less than 1% of all other surgical procedures. Most of the available data on postoperative stroke are in cardiac surgery patients. Stroke after cardiac surgery is associated with significantly increased mortality, up to 20% in some studies. The risk factors for stroke after cardiac surgery include age > 60 years, a calcified aorta, prior stroke, carotid stenosis > 50%, peripheral vascular disease, cigarette smoking, diabetes mellitus, and renal failure. Most studies suggest that asymptomatic carotid bruits are associated with little

Table 3–8. Risk factors for the development of postoperative delirium.[1]

Preoperative factors
Age > 70 years
Alcohol abuse
Poor cognitive status
Poor physical function status
Markedly abnormal serum sodium, potassium, or glucose level[2]
Aortic aneurysm surgery
Noncardiac thoracic surgery
Postoperative factors
Use of meperidine or benzodiazepines
Increased pain at rest
Postoperative hematocrit < 30%

[1]Adapted, with permission, from Marcantonio ER et al: A clinical prediction rule for delirium after elective noncardiac surgery. JAMA 1994;271:134; and from Marcantonio ER et al: The relationship of postoperative delirium with psychoactive medications. JAMA 1994;272:1518.
[2]Defined as follows: sodium < 130 or > 150 mmol/L, potassium < 3 or > 6 mmol/L, glucose < 60 or > 300 mg/dL.

or no increased risk of stroke in noncardiac, noncarotid surgery. The importance of asymptomatic carotid artery stenoses > 50% is not known.

Prophylactic carotid endarterectomy in most patients with asymptomatic carotid artery disease is unlikely to be beneficial. On the other hand, patients with carotid disease who are candidates for carotid endarterectomy anyway (Chapter 12) should probably have the carotid surgery prior to the elective surgery. Some patients require both cardiac and carotid surgery. The ideal timing of these two procedures is not certain and must be decided individually for each patient. In general, the more symptomatic and threatening condition should be addressed first. Nonstroke neurologic complications including coma, seizures, memory loss, and diminished intellectual function are also common after cardiac surgery. The risk factors for these complications include a calcified aorta, age > 70 years, pulmonary disease, and neurologic disease.

John R et al: Multicenter review of preoperative risk factors for stroke after coronary artery bypass grafting. Ann Thorac Surg 2000;69:30. [PMID: 10654481] (Multicenter analysis of risk factors for stroke after CABG surgery.)

Marcantonio ER et al: Reducing delirium after hip fracture: a randomized trial. J Am Geriatr Soc 2001;49:516. [PMID: 11380472] (A randomized controlled trial of daily geriatrician consultations and targeted recommendations reduced the occurrence of postoperative delirium in hip fracture patients on the orthopedic surgery service.)

MANAGEMENT OF ENDOCRINE DISEASES

Diabetes Mellitus

Patients with diabetes are at increased risk for postoperative infections. Furthermore, diabetic patients are more likely to have cardiovascular disease and thus are at increased risk for postoperative cardiac complications. The most challenging issue in diabetics, however, is the maintenance of glucose control during the perioperative period.

The increased secretion of cortisol, epinephrine, glucagon, and growth hormone during surgery is associated with insulin resistance and hyperglycemia in diabetic patients. The goal of management is the prevention of severe hyperglycemia or hypoglycemia in the perioperative period.

Although the ideal blood glucose level during surgery is not known, a level between 100 and 250 mg/dL is usually recommended. In vitro studies have shown that cellular immunity may be impaired when the blood glucose level exceeds 250 mg/dL. However, it is not known whether blood glucose levels above 250 mg/dL are associated with more postoperative infections.

All diabetic patients should have serum electrolyte levels measured and abnormalities in any of these levels corrected prior to surgery. Blood urea nitrogen and serum creatinine levels should also be measured to assess renal function. The specific pharmacologic management of diabetes during the perioperative period depends on several factors, including the type of diabetes (insulin-dependent or not), the adequacy of preoperative glucose control, the preoperative diabetes therapy, and the type and length of surgery (Table 3-9).

All diabetic patients require careful management, including blood glucose monitoring to prevent hypoglycemia and to ensure prompt treatment of severe hyperglycemia (Table 3–10). For patients who require intraoperative insulin, no single regimen has been found to be superior in comparative trials. Three commonly used insulin administration methods are shown in Table 3–11. The subcutaneous route is used most often because it is easier to implement and is less expensive. Intravenous insulin, which offers more rapid onset, shorter duration of action, and ease of dose titration, may be preferable in patients with poorly controlled diabetes.

Glucocorticoid Replacement

Perioperative complications (predominantly hypotension) resulting from primary or secondary adrenocortical insufficiency are rare. It is not known whether the administration of high-dose glucocorticoids during the perioperative period in patients at risk for adrenocortical insufficiency decreases the risk of these complications. In a trial comparing high-dose glucocorticoid therapy with simply administering chronic glucocorticoid medications in patients with secondary

Table 3–9. The need for intraoperative insulin.[1]

Insulin Generally Required	Insulin Generally Not Required
Type 1 patients undergoing any surgical procedure Type 2 patients on insulin undergoing any surgical procedure Type 2 patients on oral agents undergoing major surgical procedures[3]	Diet-controlled diabetics undergoing any surgical procedure Type 2 patients well controlled on oral agents undergoing minor surgery[2] requiring general or spinal anesthesia

[1]Adapted, with permission, from Schiff RL, Emanuele MA: The surgical patient with diabetes mellitus: Guidelines for management. J Gen Intern Med 1995;10:154.
[2]Minor surgery = procedures such as laparoscopic surgery and transurethral prostatectomy.
[3]Major surgery = thoracotomy, sternotomy, laparotomy, major vascular surgery.

Table 3–10. Management of patients who do not need insulin during surgery.

Patient	Recommended Management
Diabetes well controlled on diet alone	Avoid glucose-containing solutions during surgery Measure blood glucose level every 4–6 hours during surgery
Diabetes well controlled on an oral sulfonylurea, metformin, or a thiazolidinedione	The last dose of medication should be taken on the evening before surgery. Measure glucose every 6 hours in the perioperative period and give subcutaneous regular insulin as needed to maintain blood sugar below 250 mg/dL While the patient is fasting, infuse 5% glucose-containing solution at approximately 100 mL/h and continue until the patient is eating Measure blood glucose level every 4–6 hours (or more frequently as indicated) during surgery Resume oral hypoglycemic therapy when the patient returns to baseline diet

adrenal suppression, there were no differences in perioperative complications. Therefore, definitive recommendations regarding perioperative glucocorticoid therapy cannot be made. The most conservative approach would be to consider any patient to be at risk for having adrenocortical insufficiency who has received either the equivalent of 20 mg of prednisone daily for 1 week or the equivalent of 7.5 mg of prednisone daily for 1 month within the past year. A com-

monly used regimen is 100 mg of hydrocortisone given intravenously every 8 hours beginning on the morning of surgery and continuing for 48–72 hours. Tapering the dose is not necessary. Patients being maintained on chronic corticosteroids should then resume their usual dose.

Hypothyroidism

Severe symptomatic hypothyroidism has been associated with several perioperative complications, including intraoperative hypotension, congestive heart failure, cardiac arrest, and death. Elective surgery should be delayed in patients with severe hypothyroidism until adequate thyroid hormone replacement can be achieved. Conversely, patients with asymptomatic or mild hypothyroidism generally tolerate surgery well, with only a slight increase in the incidence of intraoperative hypotension; surgery need not be delayed for the month or more required to ensure adequate thyroid hormone replacement.

Glowniak JV et al: A double blind study of perioperative steroid requirements in secondary adrenal insufficiency. Surgery 1997;121:123. [PMID: 9037222]

Hemmerling TM et al: Comparison of a continuous glucose-insulin-potassium infusion versus intermittent bolus application of insulin on perioperative glucose control and hormone status in insulin-treated typed 2 diabetics. J Clin Anesthesia 2001;13:293. [PMID: 11435055] (A randomized controlled trial of continuous versus bolus insulin administration during the perioperative period demonstrated no differences in glycemic control or clinical outcomes.)

Scherpereel PA et al: Perioperative care of diabetic patients. Eur J Anaesthesiol 2001;18:277. [PMID: 11350470] (An extensive review of current issues in perioperative care of patients with diabetes)

Table 3–11. Intraoperative insulin administration methods.

Method	Intravenous Insulin Administration	Glucose Administration	Blood Glucose Monitoring
Subcutaneous insulin	One-half to two-thirds of the usual dose of insulin is administered on the morning of surgery	Infuse 5% glucose-containing solution at a rate of at least 100 mL/h beginning on the morning of surgery and continuing until the patient begins eating	Every 2–4 hours beginning the morning of surgery
Continuous intravenous insulin infusion in glucose-containing solution	On the morning of surgery, infuse 5–10% glucose solution containing 5–15 units regular insulin per liter of solution at a rate of 100 mL/h. This provides 0.5–1.5 units of insulin per hour. Additional insulin may be added as needed to keep blood sugar < 250 mg/dL		Every 2–4 hours during intravenous insulin infusion
Separate intravenous insulin and glucose infusions	Infuse intravenous regular insulin at a rate of 0.5–1.5 units/h, adjusting as needed to keep blood sugar < 250 mg/dL	Infuse 5–10% glucose-containing solution at a rate of 100 mL/h	Every 2–4 hours during intravenous insulin infusion

RENAL DISEASE

The risk for development of a significant reduction in renal function, including dialysis-requiring acute renal failure, after major surgery has been estimated to be between 2% and 20%. The mortality associated with the development of postoperative acute renal failure that requires dialysis after general, vascular, or cardiac surgery exceeds 50%. Risk factors that have been associated with postoperative deterioration in renal function are shown in Table 3–12. Several medications, including "renal dose" dopamine, mannitol, and furosemide, have been evaluated in an attempt to preserve renal function during the perioperative period. None of these, however, have been proved effective in clinical trials. Maintenance of adequate intravascular volume is likely to be the most effective method to reduce the risk of perioperative deterioration in renal function.

Although the mortality rate for elective major surgery is low (1–4%) in patients with dialysis-dependent chronic renal failure, the risk for perioperative complications, including postoperative hyperkalemia, pneumonia, fluid overload, and bleeding, is substantially increased. Postoperative hyperkalemia requiring emergent hemodialysis has been reported to occur in 20–30% of patients, and postoperative pneumonia may occur in up to 20% of patients. Patients should be dialyzed preoperatively within 24 hours before surgery, and their serum electrolyte levels should be measured just prior to surgery and monitored closely during the postoperative period.

Sadovnikoff N: Perioperative acute renal failure. Int Anesthesiol Clin 2001;39:95. [PMID: 11285947] (Review of the current issues in the prevention of perioperative renal deterioration.)

ANTIBIOTIC PROPHYLAXIS OF SURGICAL WOUND INFECTIONS

The development of a postoperative wound infection is a common and extremely important cause of morbidity and prolonged hospital stays. There are an estimated 0.5–1 million postoperative wound infec-

tions annually in the United States. For most major procedures, the use of prophylactic antibiotics has been demonstrated to reduce the incidence of postoperative wound infections significantly. For example, antibiotic prophylaxis in colorectal surgery reduces the incidence of wound infection from 25–50% to below 9%. Prophylactic antibiotics are considered standard care for all but "clean" surgical procedures. Clean procedures are those that are elective, nontraumatic, and not associated with acute inflammation and that do not enter the respiratory, gastrointestinal, biliary, or genitourinary tract. The postoperative wound infection rate for clean procedures is thought to be roughly 2%. However, in certain clean procedures, such as those that involve the insertion of a foreign body, antibiotic prophylaxis is still recommended because the consequences of infection are serious.

Multiple studies have evaluated the effectiveness of different antibiotic regimens for various surgical procedures. In most cases, no single antibiotic regimen has been shown to be superior. Several general conclusions can be drawn from these data. First, there is substantial evidence to suggest that a single dose of an appropriate intravenous antibiotic—or combination of antibiotics—is as effective as multiple-dose regimens that extend into the postoperative period. For longer procedures, the dose should be repeated every 3–4 hours to ensure maintenance of a therapeutic serum level. One important exception is cardiac surgery, in which at least 24 hours of postoperative therapy is recommended. Second, for most procedures, a first-generation cephalosporin is as effective as later-generation agents. Third, with the exception of colorectal surgery, all prophylactic antibiotics should be given intravenously at induction of anesthesia or roughly 30 minutes prior to the skin incision. Although the type of procedure is the main factor determining the risk of developing a postoperative wound infection, certain patient factors have been associated with increased risk, including diabetes, older age, and multiple medical comorbidities. Current antibiotic prophylaxis recommendations for a variety of procedures are shown in Table 3–13.

The most promising intervention to reduce the occurrence of postoperative wound infection may be the administration of supplemental oxygen during and immediately after surgery. In a recent study of patients undergoing colorectal surgery, the administration of 80% oxygen during and for 2 hours after surgery was associated with a 50% reduction in the development of postoperative wound infections compared with the use of 30% oxygen.

Greif R et al: Supplemental perioperative oxygen to reduce the incidence of surgical wound infections. N Engl J Med 2000;342:161. [PMID: 9054745] (A randomized trial demonstrated that the perioperative administration of 80% oxygen reduces the incidence of postoperative wound infections compared with 30% oxygen.)

Table 3–12. Risk factors for the development of postoperative acute renal failure.

Preoperative chronic renal insufficiency
Aortic surgery
Cardiac surgery
Peripheral vascular disease
Severe heart failure
Preoperative jaundice
Age > 70 years

Table 3–13. Recommended antibiotic prophylaxis for selected surgical procedures.

Procedure	Recommended Antibiotic	Adult Dose
Superficial cutaneous	None	
Head and neck	Cefazolin	1–2 g intravenously
Neurologic	Cefazolin	1–2 g intravenously
Thoracic	Cefazolin	1–2 g intravenously
Noncardiac vascular	Cefazolin	1–2 g intravenously
Orthopedic, clean, without implantation of foreign material	None	
Orthopedic, all other	Cefazolin	1–2 g intravenously
Cesarean delivery	Cefazolin	2 g intravenously
Hysterectomy	Cefazolin or cefotetan	1–2 g intravenously
Gastroduodenal	Cefazolin (high risk only)[1]	1–2 g intravenously
Biliary	Cefazolin (high risk only)	1–2 g intravenously
Urologic	Cefazolin (high risk only)[2]	1–2 g intravenously
Appendectomy for uncomplicated appendicitis	Cefotetan or cefoxitin	1–2 g intravenously
Colorectal[3]	Neomycin sulfate plus erythromycin base	1 g of each agent given orally at 19, 18, and 9 hours before surgery
	–or–	
	Cefotetan or cefoxitin	1–2 g intravenously
Breast and hernia	Cefazolin (high-risk only)[1]	1–2 g intravenously

[1]High risk defined as patients with risk factors for wound infection such as older age, diabetes, or multiple medical comorbidities.
[2]High risk defined as prolonged postoperative catheterization or positive urine cultures.
[3]All patients should have mechanical bowel preparation with polyethylene glycol, mannitol, or magnesium citrate.

McDonald M et al: Single versus multiple-dose antimicrobial prophylaxis for major surgery: a systematic review. Aust N Z J Surg 1998;68:388. [PMID: 9623456] (A systematic review of randomized trials comparing single-dose versus multiple-dose regimens. Concludes that single-dose regimens are as effective as multiple-dose regimens.)

Polk HC et al: Prophylactic antibiotics in surgery and surgical wound infections. World J Surg 2000;66:105. [PMID: 10695738] (Expert review of the effectiveness of prophylactic antibiotics in surgery.)

Geriatric Medicine

4

C. Bree Johnston, MD, William L. Lyons, MD, & Kenneth E. Covinsky, MD

See www.current-med.com/ch04.html

GENERAL PRINCIPLES OF GERIATRIC MEDICINE

Human biologic aging is best characterized as the progressive constriction of each organ system's homeostatic reserve. This decline ("homeostenosis") begins around the fifth decade, is progressive, and varies among individuals. Each organ system's decline is largely independent of changes in other organ systems and is influenced by genetic factors, diet, environment, and personal habits.

Several principles follow from these facts: Individuals become more dissimilar as they age, rejecting any stereotype of aging; an abrupt decline in any system or function is almost certainly due to disease and not to "normal (or usual) aging"; "normal aging" can be attenuated to some extent by modification of risk factors (eg, increased blood pressure, smoking, sedentary lifestyle); and "healthy old age" is not an oxymoron. In the absence of disease, the decline in homeostatic reserve should not cause symptoms or impose restrictions on activities of daily living.

These facts may make it easier to understand the striking increases that have occurred in longevity (Table 4–1). The bulk of the years near the end of life is characterized by a lack of significant impairment—only 20% of people over age 85, for example, live in nursing homes, and about half of individuals in this age range are independent in their activities of self care. This has substantial implications for disease screening, patient counseling, and medical decision-making.

Still, as individuals age, they are more likely to suffer from disease, disability, and treatment side effects. Combined with the decrease in physiologic reserve, these added burdens (if present) make the older person more vulnerable to environmental, pathologic, or pharmacologic insults. Understanding these facts is crucial for optimal care of older patients.

The health problems and medical management of elderly patients differ from those of younger ones, as follows.

(1) Disease presentation is often atypical in the elderly. A disorder in one organ system may lead to symptoms in another, especially one compromised by preexisting disease. Because these organ systems are often the brain, the lower urinary tract, or the cardiovascular or musculoskeletal system, a limited number of presenting symptoms predominate—confusion, depression, falling, incontinence, functional decline, and syncope—irrespective of the underlying disease. A 45-year-old may seek care for productive cough, fever, and dyspnea as manifestations of pneumonia, but the same disease may cause an 80-year-old to present with a new problem with falls and difficulty following a conversation. Thus, regardless of the presenting symptom in older people, the differential diagnosis is often the same. The corollary is equally important: The organ system usually associated with a particular symptom is less likely to be the source of that symptom in older individuals than in younger ones. Thus, compared with middle-aged individuals, acute confusion in older patients is less often due to a new brain lesion, incontinence to a bladder disorder, falling to a neuropathy, or syncope to heart disease.

(2) Because of impaired compensatory mechanisms, disease in older patients often presents at an earlier stage (Figure 4–1). Heart failure may be precipitated by slight hyperthyroidism, significant cognitive dysfunction by only mild hyperparathyroidism, urinary retention by only mild prostatic enlargement, and nonketotic hyperosmolar coma by only mild glucose intolerance. Thus, treatment of the underlying disease can be easier in the elderly because it may be less advanced at the time of presentation. Similarly, drug side effects can occur with low doses of drugs that usually produce no side effects in younger people. For instance, a mild anticholinergic agent (eg, diphenhydramine) may cause confusion; diuretics may precipitate urinary incontinence; digoxin may induce anorexia even with normal serum levels; and over-the-counter sympathomimetics may result in urinary retention in older men with mild prostatic obstruction. The predisposition to develop symptoms at an earlier stage of disease is often offset by the change in illness behavior that occurs with age. The current cohort of elderly people may be less likely to seek attention until

41

Table 4–1. Median life expectancy, in years, of older women and men.

Age	Women	Men
70	15	13
75	12	10
80	9	7
85	7	5

symptoms become disabling. Physicians must ask specific questions of their older patients in order to uncover problems in the early stages.

(3) Since many compensatory mechanisms are often compromised concurrently, there are usually multiple abnormalities amenable to treatment. Small improvements in each may yield dramatic benefits overall. Cognitive impairment in patients with Alzheimer's disease may respond much better to interventions that address comorbidity than to prescription of donepezil, as comorbid conditions may interfere with the ability to compensate for cognitive loss. Similar approaches apply to most other common geriatric syndromes, including falls, incontinence, depression, and syncope.

(4) Many abnormal findings in younger patients are relatively common in older people and may not be responsible for a particular symptom. Such findings include bacteriuria, premature ventricular contractions, impaired glucose tolerance, reduced vibratory sense in the toes, and involuntary bladder contractions. These may be only incidental findings resulting in missed diagnoses and misdirected therapy. Bacteriuria should not end the search for a source of fever in

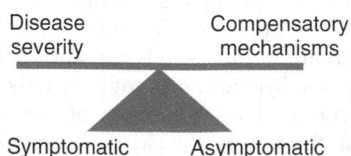

Figure 4–1. Most common symptoms result when the ability to compensate for organ system dysfunction is inadequate. Thus, even mild organ system dysfunction may cause symptoms if compensatory mechanisms are impaired. Because such impairments occur commonly in older patients, evaluation and therapy of most symptoms must extend beyond the organ system usually considered to be the cause. (Reproduced, with permission, from Resnick NM: An 89-year-old woman with urinary incontinence. JAMA 1996;276:1832.)

an acutely ill older patient, nor should an elevated random blood sugar be incriminated as the cause of neuropathy. Some abnormalities must not be dismissed as due to old age. There is no anemia, erectile dysfunction, depression, or confusion of old age.

(5) Symptoms in older people are often due to multiple causes, and the diagnostic "law of parsimony" often does not apply. Fever, anemia, Roth spots, and a heart murmur are almost diagnostic of endocarditis in a younger patient but are more apt to reflect aspirin-induced blood loss, a cholesterol embolus, insignificant aortic sclerosis, and a viral illness in an older patient.

Moreover, even when the diagnosis is correct, treatment of a single disease in an older patient is unlikely to result in cure. In a younger patient, incontinence due to involuntary bladder contractions is treated effectively with a bladder relaxant medication. In an older patient whose incontinence is associated with fecal impaction, who is taking medications that cloud the sensorium, and who has impaired dexterity due to arthritis, treatment of the bladder abnormality is unlikely to restore continence. Disimpaction, discontinuation of the offending medications, and treatment of the arthritis may restore continence without the need for a bladder relaxant.

(6) Because the older patient is more likely than a younger one to suffer the adverse consequences of disease, treatment—and even prevention—may be equally effective. The benefits to survival of exercise, as well as beta-blocker therapy after myocardial infarction, appear to be at least as impressive in older patients as in younger ones; the relative value of immunization against influenza is even greater. Prevention in older patients must be viewed in a broader context. Although interventions to increase bone density may decrease fracture risk, this risk may be reduced further by strategies that improve balance, strengthen legs, ameliorate contributing medical conditions, replete nutritional deficits, and eliminate environmental hazards.

(7) In contrast to the care of younger patients, for whom cure of disease and prolongation of life are usually of paramount concern, the goals of care for older patients may well differ. Although some may seek a focus on life extension, others clearly prefer improved function, comfort, and quality of life.

Resnick NM et al: How should clinical care of the aged differ? Lancet 1997;350:1157. [PMID: 9343515] (Overview of differences required in approaching the elderly patient.)

Rothschild JM et al: Preventable medical injuries in older patients. Arch Intern Med 2000;160:2717. [PMID: 11025781] (Literature review summarizing iatrogenic injuries suffered by older patients as a result of adverse drug events, falls, nosocomial infections, pressure sores, delirium, and surgical or perioperative complications.)

■ GENERAL APPROACH TO THE OLDER PATIENT

Understanding the Patient's Values & Goals

An effective therapeutic encounter calls for a clear understanding of the patient's goals and preferences. Knowing about the patient's goals early will help the physician to focus the patient's visits appropriately. Some patients will not have clear-cut goals and are willing to be guided by the physician's judgment. Goals made explicit at the outset may change after discussion with a physician. The patient's wishes regarding end-of-life care and attempts at resuscitation should emerge from a frank discussion of these goals. When an advance directive has been executed, it should be reviewed and placed in the medical record. The clinician may ask if the patient has granted some individual a durable power of attorney for health, and that individual's name and contact information should be recorded as well. Goals and values for care should be discussed with the surrogate as well as with the patient.

Rosenfeld KE et al: End-of-life decision making: a qualitative study of elderly individuals. J Gen Intern Med 2000;15: 620. [PMID: 11029675] (Discussions with the elderly about advance directives and goals of care should focus on valued life activities and acceptable health status rather than specific medical interventions.)

Tsevat J et al: Health values of hospitalized patients 80 years or older. HELP Investigators. Hospitalized Elderly Longitudinal Project. JAMA 1998;279:371. [PMID: 9459470] (Elderly hospitalized patients, on average, valued 1 year at their current state of health to 9.7 months of excellent health; compared with surrogates, patients were willing to trade having less time for having better health.)

Tulsky JA et al: Opening the black box: how do physicians communicate about advance directives? Ann Intern Med 1998;129:441. [PMID: 9735081] (Physicians' discussions succeed in introducing patients to the concept of advance directives, but, as they rarely dealt with patients' values and attitudes toward uncertainty, discussions were of limited usefulness.)

Weighing Priorities

Optimal care for the older patient is facilitated when the clinician explicitly sets priorities, deciding what specific evaluations and therapies are most likely to provide benefit. Setting these priorities should be based upon the patient's goals for care and life expectancy, the prevalence of specific diseases, the performance characteristics of screening or diagnostic tests, and the effectiveness of therapeutic interventions. The concepts of "number needed to screen" and "number needed to treat" often help put diagnostic tests and interventions into perspective.

Interventions that are likely to help well elders may differ from those that will benefit frail elders or younger people. Tight glucose control in an elderly diabetic who values her independence might be sacrificed if it would require initiation of insulin therapy with placement in a nursing facility. Colon cancer screening might be advised in an 80-year-old man in good health who is highly motivated (number needed to screen to prevent one death over remaining life: about 200), but not for a man of the same age with multiple comorbidities, a life expectancy of less than 5 years, or an aversion to medical care (Table 4–1). Some interventions produce almost immediate benefit, and those may be useful at any age. Even the oldest old people can benefit from beginning an exercise program. Likewise, an 80-year-old person with a limited life expectancy is likely to benefit from a screening for falls and a fall risk reduction program (number needed to screen to prevent one fall over 1 year: about 20).

Caregiver Issues

Providing primary care for a frail elderly person requires attention to the caregiver as well as the patient, since the health and well-being of the two are closely linked. High levels of functional dependency place an enormous burden on a caregiver. Burnout, neglect, and abuse are possible consequences, and stressed caregivers may suffer higher mortality. Likewise, an older patient's need for nursing home placement is often better predicted from assessment of the caregiver characteristics and stress than the severity of the patient's illness. For the stressed caregiver, a social worker may help identify programs such as caregiver support groups, respite programs, adult day care, or hired home health aids.

It is wise to observe and talk with every elderly person alone for at least part of a visit in order to question directly (Table 4–2) about possible abuse and neglect. Clues to the possibility of elder abuse include behavioral changes in the presence of the caregiver, delays between injuries and sought treatment, inconsistencies between an observed injury and associated

Table 4–2. Questions that may elicit a history of elder abuse.

1. Has anyone ever hurt you?
2. Has anyone ever touched you without your consent?
3. Has anyone ever made you do things you didn't want to do?
4. Has anyone taken anything of yours without asking?
5. Has anyone ever scolded or threatened you?
6. Have you signed any papers that you didn't understand?
7. Is there anyone at home you are fearful of?
8. Are you alone much?
9. Has anyone ever refused to help you take care of yourself when you needed help?

explanation, lack of appropriate clothing or hygiene, and not filling prescriptions. The elderly patient who is also a caregiver is at risk for depression and should be screened for it.

Dyer CB et al: The high prevalence of depression and dementia in elder abuse and neglect. J Am Geriatr Soc 2000;48:205. [PMID: 10682951] (Case-control study describing the characteristics of abused or neglected elderly.)

Lachs MS et al: The mortality of elder mistreatment. JAMA 1998;280:428. [PMID: 9701077]

Mahoney JE et al: Problems of older adults living alone after hospitalization. J Gen Intern Med 2000;15:611. [PMID: 11029674] (Older persons who live alone and receive home nursing after hospitalization are less likely to improve in function—and more likely to be institutionalized—than those who live with others.)

Schulz R et al: Caregiving as a risk factor for mortality: The Caregiver Health Effects Study. JAMA 1999;282:2215. [PMID: 10605952] (Prospective cohort study suggests higher mortality in caregivers experiencing strain.)

Using Time Efficiently

Certain strategies can guide a physician in using time wisely with an elderly patient: (1) Identify the patient's goals and values for medical care early in your therapeutic relationship. (2) Use brief assessment instruments when appropriate, and train non-physician personnel in their performance. (3) Employ portable amplifiers, large print information, and magnifying lenses. (4) Involve other professionals (nurses, social workers, dietitians, physical and occupational therapists, psychologists) in complex cases.

ASSESSMENT OF THE ELDERLY

Functional Assessment

Functional assessment gauges a patient's ability to manage tasks of self care, household management, and mobility.

About one-fourth of patients over 65 have impairments in their IADLs (instrumental activities of daily living: transportation, shopping, cooking, using the telephone, managing money, taking medications, housecleaning, laundry) or ADLs (activities of daily living: bathing, dressing, eating, transferring from bed to chair, continence, toileting). Half of those over 85 have these latter impairments. Persons who are unable to perform IADLs independently are far more likely to have dementia than their independent counterparts.

Information about function can be used in a number of ways: (1) as baseline information; (2) as a measure of the patient's need for support services or placement; (3) as an indicator of possible caregiver stress; (4) as a potential marker of specific disease activity; and (5) to determine the need for therapeutic interventions.

In general, persons who need help only with IADLs may be aided by a chore worker, a day program, or placement in a board-and-care home or assisted living situation. While many persons who need help with ADLs may require a nursing home level of care, most live at home with caregivers.

Screening for Vision Impairment

An appreciable minority of elders have severe visual loss. Visual impairment is an independent risk factor for falls; it also has a significant impact on quality of life. Direct visual testing with a Snellen chart or Jaeger card is the most sensitive and specific approach to visual screening, though the performance of these instruments in most primary care settings is uncertain. Referring all older people for a complete eye examination has the advantages of improving the quality of the examination and allowing for cataract and glaucoma screening.

Screening for Hearing Impairment

Over one-third of those over 65 and half of those over 85 have some hearing loss. This deficit is correlated with social isolation and depression. Although the optimal screening method for hearing loss in the elderly is undetermined, the whispered voice test is easy to perform and has sensitivities and specificities ranging from 70% to 100%. To determine the degree to which the impairment interferes with functioning, the physician may ask if the patient becomes frustrated when conversing with family members, is embarrassed when meeting new people, has difficulty listening to the radio or watching TV, or has problems understanding conversations in noisy restaurants.

Compliance with hearing amplification can be a challenge because of the stigma associated with hearing aid use as well as the cost of such devices, which are not paid for under most Medicare plans. High compliance rates can be achieved with a proactive approach such as the use of loaner aids for low-income persons. In addition to standard hearing aids, pocket amplifiers as well as amplifiers to telephone, television, and radio may be useful.

Screening for Falls & Gait Impairment

Falls are the leading cause of nonfatal injuries in older persons, and their complications are the leading cause of death from injury in those over 65. Hip fractures are common precursors to functional impairment and nursing home placement. Furthermore, fear of falling may lead some elders to restrict their activities. About one-third of people over 65 fall each year, and the frequency increases markedly with advancing age.

Every older person should be asked about falls; many will not volunteer such information. One should ask about home hazards that might be remediable. Because gait impairments commonly coexist with falls, its assessment is performed in older people with a fall history and is likely to be more sensitive to abnormalities (commonly multifactorial, due to muscular weakness, arthritis, and neurologic impairments) than other components of the neurologic examination.

Gait and balance can be readily assessed. Is the patient able to rise from a chair without use of his arms in a single, smooth attempt? Is there stability immediately upon standing, or does the patient stagger? Is balance maintained when the patient is pushed lightly on the sternum? Is there steadiness when standing with eyes closed? Can a 360 degree rotation be achieved in a smooth, continuous motion? How is walking initiated, and does each foot swing clear of the floor and pass the opposite foot? Are the steps equal? Is there stopping or discontinuity between steps, or sway of the trunk, flexion of knees or back, spreading out of the arms? Do the heels almost touch during the stride, or is there a wide-based gait? Is a walking aid (cane, walker) necessary or being used properly?

Screening for Cognitive Impairment

The prevalence of dementia doubles every 5 years after age 60, so that by age 85 about 30–50% of individuals have some degree of impairment. Patients with mild or early dementia frequently remain undiagnosed because their social graces are retained.

Although there is no consensus at present on whether older patients should be screened for dementia, the benefits of early detection include the identification of reversible causes, planning for the future (including advance directives), providing support and counseling for the caregiver, and modification of interventions for other diseases as appropriate (eg, simplifying drug regimens, minimizing anticholinergic drug use), and beginning anticholinesterase inhibitor drugs.

The combination of the "clock draw" (in which the patient is asked to sketch a clock face, with all the numerals placed properly, the two clock hands positioned at a specified time) and the "three-item recall" is fairly quick and has reasonable test characteristics. When the patient is able to recall all three items after 3 minutes, the probability of dementia is greatly reduced. Conversely, an abnormally drawn clock markedly increases the probability of dementia. When patients fail either of these screening tests, further testing with the Mini-Mental State questionnaire (Figure 25–1), neuropsychologic testing, or other instruments is warranted.

Manly JJ et al: Cognitive test performance among nondemented elderly African Americans and whites. Neurology 1998;

50:1238. [PMID: 9595969] (Clinicians must use culturally appropriate norms when evaluating ethnically diverse elderly patients for dementia.)

Screening for Incontinence

Incontinence in the elderly is common, and interventions can improve most patients. Many patients fail to tell their providers about it. A simple question about involuntary leakage of urine is a reasonable screen: "Do you have a problem with urine leaks or accidents?"

Screening for Depression

Although major depressive disorder has a slightly lower prevalence in the elderly than in younger populations, depressive symptomatology is actually more common. Its prevalence in ill and hospitalized elders is particularly high. A simple two-question screen (Table 4–3) has shown 96% sensitivity for detecting major depression in a general population and may have even higher sensitivity in those over age 65. Positive responses can be followed up with more comprehensive, structured interviews, eg, Yesavage's Geriatric Depression Scale (Table 4–4).

Steffens DC et al: Prevalence of depression and its treatment in an elderly population: the Cache County study. Arch Gen Psychiatry 2000;57:601. [PMID: 10839339] (Prevalence of major depression in the elderly is higher than in previous reports, and its treatment is suboptimal.)

Screening the High-Functioning Elder

Standard functional screening measures may not be useful in capturing subtle impairments in highly functional independent elders. One technique for these patients is to identify and regularly ask about a target activity, such as playing bridge, bowling, or practicing law. If the patient begins to have trouble with or discontinues such an "advanced activity of daily living," it may indicate early impairment, such as dementia, incontinence, or worsening hearing loss, which additional gentle questioning or assessment may uncover.

Assessment of Decision-Making Capacity

It is common for a cognitively impaired elder to face a serious medical decision and for the clinicians involved in his care to ascertain whether the capacity exists to make the choice. There are four components of a thorough assessment: (1) Ability to express a choice. (2) Understanding relevant information about the risks and benefits of planned therapy and the alternatives, including no treatment. (3) Comprehension of the problem and its consequences. (4) Ability to reason. A patient's choice should follow rationally from an understanding of the consequences.

Table 4–3. Simple geriatric screen.

Assessment Procedure	Abnormal	Action
Do you have difficulty with eyesight? Jaeger Card or Snellen chart Test each eye (with glasses)	Yes Can't read 20/40	Refer
Whisper short sentence from 6–12 inches (out of view) or audiometry	Unable to hear	Cerumen check Refer
"Touch the back of your head with your hands" "Pick up the pencil"	Unable do do either	Further examination Consider occupational therapy?
"Rise from your chair (do not use arms to get up), walk 10 feet, walk back to the chair, and sit down"	Observed problem, or unable to perform in < 15 seconds	Formal balance and gait evaluation; further examination; home evaluation and physical therapy
"Have you had any falls in the last year?" "Do you have trouble with stairs, lighting, bathroom, or other home hazards?"	Yes Yes to any	Formal balance and gait evaluation Home evaluation, physical therapy
Body mass index < 21 or weight loss exceeding 5%	Yes to either	Nutrition evaluation
"Do you have a problem with urine leaks or accidents?"	Yes	Incontinence evaluation
"Over the past month, have you often been bothered by feeling sad, depressed, or hopeless?" "During the last month, have you often been bothered by little interest or pleasure in doing things?"	Yes to either	Geriatric Depression Scale or other depression assessment
Name three objects: ask again in three 3 minutes	Unable to recall	Mini-Mental State Examination

Do you have problems with any of the following areas? Who assists? Do you use devices to help you? (For "yes" answers, consider referral to occupational therapy, physical therapy, social services.)

–Strenuous activities (eg, fast walking, bicycling)	–Transferring out of bed
–Cooking	–Dressing
–Shopping	–Using the toilet
–Heavy housework (eg, washing windows)	–Eating
–Doing laundry	–Walking
–Transportation by driving or bus	–Bathing (sponge bath, tub, shower)
–Managing finances	

In performing such assessments, it is to be remembered that decision-making capacity varies over time: a delirious patient may regain his capacity after an infection is treated, and so reassessments are often appropriate. Furthermore, the capacity to make a decision is a function of the decision in question. A mildly demented woman may lack the capacity to consent to coronary artery bypass grafting yet retain the capacity to allow removal of a suspicious nevus.

Grisso T, Appelbaum PS: *Assessing Competence to Consent to Treatment: A Guide for Physicians and Other Health Professionals.* Oxford Univ Press, 1998. (A practical guide for conducting assessments of decision-making capacity.)

Functional Screening Instrument

Table 4–3 gives a simple functional screening list. In addition to ADL and IADL assessment, it looks for evidence of health problems that affect function: sensory impairment, limited upper extremity range of motion, mobility, falls, weight loss, incontinence, depressed mood, and cognitive impairment.

Kakaiya R et al: Evaluation of fitness to drive: the physician's role in assessing elderly or demented patients. Postgrad Med 2000;107:229. [PMID: 10728147] (An approach to the evaluation, and recommendations on how to advise some patients to stop driving.)

Table 4–4. Yesavage Geriatric Depression Scale (short form).

---

1. Are you basically satisfied with your life? (no)
2. Have you dropped many of your activities and interests? (yes)
3. Do you feel that your life is empty? (yes)
4. Do you often get bored? (yes)
5. Are you in good spirits most of the time? (no)
6. Are you afraid that something bad is going to happen to you? (yes)
7. Do you feel happy most of the time? (no)
8. Do you often feel helpless? (yes)
9. Do you prefer to stay home at night, rather than go out and do new things? (yes)
10. Do you feel that you have more problems with memory than most? (yes)
11. Do you feel it is wonderful to be alive now? (no)
12. Do you feel pretty worthless the way you are now? (yes)
13. Do you feel full of energy? (no)
14. Do you feel that your situation is hopeless? (yes)
15. Do you think that most persons are better off than you are? (yes)

Score one point for each response that matches the yes-or-no answer after the question.
Scores: Normal 3 ± 2; Mildly depressed: 7 ± 3; Very depressed: 12 ± 2

SELECTED PREVENTIVE MEASURES IN GERIATRIC PRACTICE

Exercise

Inactive elders are at greater risk of becoming functionally dependent than their more physically active counterparts. Physical activity is associated with reduced risks of developing diabetes mellitus and future disability. Even sedentary elders should be urged to increase their level of physical activity. By writing out an exercise prescription, a physician demonstrates the importance of the activity and may improve compliance. Components include strength training (isolated muscle group contractions), endurance training (walking, cycling, swimming), flexibility (static stretch of various muscle groups), and balance (tai chi, dance). Ideally, the patient should aim for a total of 30 minutes of activity daily, though any increase in exercise is likely to be beneficial.

Gill TM et al: Exercise stress testing for older persons starting an exercise program. JAMA 2000;284:2591. [PMID: 11086356] (Exercise testing may often be unnecessary prior to initiating a program of graduated exercise.)

Hypertension

Treatment of hypertension is of substantial benefit in the elderly, and the absolute benefit of treatment may be greater in older than in younger patients. Pulse pressure may be a useful marker of risk for heart failure and stroke among elders with systolic hypertension. Antihypertensive treatment of patients over 80—including treatment of isolated systolic hypertension—reduces the incidence of strokes and other cardiovascular events as well as heart failure. Lifestyle modifications (weight loss for overweight patients, alcohol and sodium limitation, increased aerobic physical activity) are reasonable to recommend for all hypertensive patients for whom treatment is appropriate. For those who require pharmacologic treatment, thiazides are the drugs of choice unless a comorbid condition makes another choice preferable.

Stroke Prevention

The incidence of stroke in older adults roughly doubles with each 10 years of age. The greatest risk factor is hypertension. Another is atrial fibrillation, the prevalence of which also increases with age. Many elderly patients with this arrhythmia are not anticoagulated because their physicians fear injuries due to falls. In most instances, the benefits of anticoagulation are likely to outweigh the increased risk of fall-related bleeding unless the patient has multiple falls, high-risk falls, or a very low risk of stroke, such as a person under age 65 with lone atrial fibrillation.

Cancer Screening

Screening elderly men for prostate cancer is not necessary since it does not prolong life and given the risk of incontinence or erectile dysfunction that may accompany surgical therapy or radiation. An older woman should undergo annual mammography and breast examinations until her life expectancy falls below 5–10 years (Table 4–1). Screening for colon cancer (either with colonoscopy every 10 years, or with annual fecal occult blood testing plus flexible sigmoidoscopy every 5 years) can be stopped when a patient's life expectancy is less than 5–10 years.

Osteoporosis

Primary prevention of osteoporosis begins with identification of risk factors (older age, female gender, white or Asian race, low calcium intake, smoking, excessive alcohol use, and chronic glucocorticoid use). Calcium carbonate (500 mg three times daily at meals) and vitamin D (400–800 IU/d, contained in one or two multivitamin tablets) reduce the risk of osteoporotic fractures in both men and women. Measurement of bone mineral density (preferably using dual-energy x-ray absorptiometry of the proximal femur) of women with multiple risk factors may uncover asymptomatic osteoporosis; such women may also be offered hormone replacement therapy or alendronate.

Immunizations

Individuals over age 65—and health-care workers who are in contact with them—should receive annual influenza vaccination. Similarly, persons over 65 should receive at least one pneumococcal immunization; some experts recommend revaccination in those over 75 or with severe chronic disease and who were vaccinated more than 5 years previously. A single booster dose of tetanus and diphtheria vaccine should be given at age 65 or older.

PPD for Congregate Living

The elderly are a significant reservoir of tuberculosis, both primary and reactivation. Over 20% of elderly patients who develop the disease live in nursing homes. Long-term care facilities should routinely perform a tuberculin skin test (PPD) on all entering patients, using the two-step approach in which a second dose is administered to persons whose first was negative. If the second reaction is also negative, the patient is uninfected or anergic; if positive, a boosted response is likely, signifying a tuberculin reactor but not a recent converter. Whether these reactors need treatment is controversial, but their positive-PPD status should be noted. Prophylaxis and treatment regimens are described in Chapter 9. Skin testing is repeated annually in congregate settings or if an active case is identified in the group.

Dawson-Hughes B et al: Effect of calcium and vitamin D supplementation on bone density in men and women 65 years of age or older. N Engl J Med 1997;337:670. [PMID: 9278463] (Randomized study documented efficacy in reducing all fractures in older adults.)

Gill TM et al: Role of exercise stress testing and safety monitoring for older persons starting an exercise program. JAMA 2000;284:342. [PMID: 10891966] (Authors present recommendations to minimize the risk of cardiac events for previously sedentary older persons who wish to start an exercise program.)

Gueyffier F et al: Antihypertensive drugs in very old people: a subgroup meta-analysis of randomised controlled trials. Lancet 1999;353:793. [PMID: 10459960] (Treatment of hypertension reduced rate of strokes, other cardiovascular events, and heart failure in persons over 89, but effect on mortality was inconclusive.)

Ibrahim SA et al: Underutilization of oral anticoagulation therapy for stroke prevention in elderly patients with heart failure. Am Heart J 2000;140:219. [PMID: 10925333] (Only 20% of patients with atrial fibrillation received oral anticoagulation.)

Staessen JA et al: Risks of untreated and treated isolated systolic hypertension in the elderly: meta-analysis of outcome trials. Lancet 2000;355:865. [PMID: 10752701] (Treatment of systolic blood pressure greater than 160 mm Hg, especially in men aged 70 or more, prevented stroke and reduced total and cardiovascular mortality and coronary events.)

Vaccarino V et al: Pulse pressure and risk of cardiovascular events in the systolic hypertension in the elderly program. Am J Cardiol 2001;88:980. [PMID: 11703993] (An increase in pulse pressure was associated with more heart failure and
stroke after controlling for systolic and diastolic blood pressure and other risk factors).

■ COMMON PROBLEMS OF THE FRAIL ELDERLY

DEMENTIA

Older individuals experience occasional difficulty retrieving items from memory (usually manifested as word-finding complaints) and experience a slowing in their rate of information processing. By contrast, dementia is an acquired persistent and progressive impairment in intellectual function, with compromise in multiple cognitive domains at least one of which is memory. The demented patient's deficits must represent a significant decline in function and must be severe enough to interfere with work or social life.

Intellectual impairments in older patients are frequently the result of two other syndromes, each of which frequently coexists with dementia: depression and delirium. Depression is a common concomitant of dementia, but it can also masquerade as dementia. Moreover, a patient with depression and cognitive impairment whose intellectual function improves with treatment of the mood disorder has an almost fivefold greater risk of suffering irreversible dementia later in life. Delirium, characterized by acute confusion, occurs much more commonly in patients with underlying dementia.

General Considerations

Dementia is the fourth leading cause of death in the United States and has a prevalence which doubles every 5 years in the senior population, reaching 30–50% at age 85. Women suffer disproportionately, both as patients (even after age adjustment) and as caregivers. Alzheimer's disease accounts for roughly two-thirds of cases in the USA, with vascular dementia (either alone or combined with Alzheimer's disease) accounting for much of the rest. Risk factors for Alzheimer's disease are older age, family history, and female gender. Some epidemiologic studies suggest that users of NSAIDs, hormone replacement therapy, and HMG-CoA reductase inhibitors, those with moderate alcohol intake, and those with higher education and stronger social supports may have a lower risk of developing dementia. However, these studies should be viewed cautiously since each of these protective factors may be markers for more causative unmeasured protective factors. Risk factors for vascular dementia are those for stroke, ie, older age, male sex, black race, hypertension, cigarette use, previous myocardial infarction, atrial fibrillation, diabetes, and hyperlipidemia.

Causes of potentially reversible cognitive impairment include drug effect, depression, thyroid disease, vitamin B_{12} deficiency, hypercalcemia, subdural hematoma, syphilis, HIV infection, and normal pressure hydrocephalus. The prevalence of fully reversible dementias is well under 5%, and the correction of these suspected causes leads only to partial improvement.

Clinical Features

Demented patients have memory impairment and at least one or more of the following: language impairment (initially just word finding; later, difficulty following a conversation; finally, mutism); apraxia (inability to perform previously learned tasks, such as cutting a loaf of bread, despite intact sensory and motor function); agnosia (inability to recognize objects); and impaired executive function (poor abstraction, mental flexibility, planning, and judgment). Alzheimer's disease typically presents with early problems in memory and visuospatial abilities (eg, becoming lost in familiar surroundings, inability to copy a geometric design on paper), yet social graces may be retained despite advanced cognitive decline. Personality changes and behavioral difficulties (wandering, inappropriate sexual behavior, agitation) may develop as the disease progresses. Hallucinations are not typically observed except in moderate-to-severe dementia. End-stage disease is characterized by near-mutism; inability to sit up, hold up the head, or track objects with the eyes; difficulty with eating and swallowing; weight loss; bowel or bladder incontinence; and recurrent respiratory or urinary infections.

"Subcortical" dementias (eg, the dementia of Parkinson's disease, and most cases of vascular dementia) are characterized by psychomotor slowing, reduced attention, early loss of executive function, personality changes, and benefit from cuing in tests of memory.

Dementia with Lewy bodies may be confused with delirium, as fluctuating cognitive impairment is frequently observed. Rigidity and bradykinesia are primarily noted, and tremor is rare. Response to dopaminergic agonist therapy is poor. Hallucinations—classically visual and bizarre (eg, animals or mythologic creatures)—may occur as well. These patients demonstrate a hypersensitivity to neuroleptic therapy, and attempts to treat the hallucinations may lead to marked worsening of extrapyramidal symptoms.

Frontotemporal dementias are a group of diseases that include Pick's disease, dementia associated with amyotrophic lateral sclerosis, and others. Patients manifest personality change (euphoria, disinhibition, apathy) and compulsive behaviors (often peculiar eating habits or hyperorality). In contrast to Alzheimer's disease, visuospatial function is relatively preserved.

Dementia in association with motor findings, such as extrapyramidal features or ataxia, may represent a less common disorder (eg, progressive supranuclear palsy, corticobasal ganglionic degeneration, olivopontocerebellar atrophy).

Differential Diagnosis

In addition to depression and delirium, apparent cognitive impairment in the elderly may be the result of drug effects or uncorrected sensory deficits; these problems more often exacerbate dementia than mimic it.

Many medications have been associated with diminished mentation in older patients. Anticholinergic agents, hypnotics, neuroleptics, and opioids are well-established causes, but beta-blockers, antiepileptics, antihistamines (including H_2 antagonists), and corticosteroids have been implicated as well.

An elderly patient with intact cognition but with severe impairments in vision or hearing commonly becomes confused in an unfamiliar medical setting and consequently may be falsely labeled as demented. Cognitive testing is best performed after optimal correction of the sensory deficits.

Diagnosis

Historical questions in an evaluation for dementia include those directed at the rate of progression of the deficits, their nature (including any personality or behavioral change), motor problems, risk factors for HIV or syphilis, family history, medication list, functional disabilities, and degree of social support.

The neurologic examination emphasizes assessment of mental status (see Figure 25–1). The remainder of the physical examination should focus on identifying comorbid conditions that may aggravate the individual's disability.

Laboratory studies for most patients are intended to uncover treatable causes of cognitive impairment and include a complete blood count, electrolytes, calcium, creatinine, glucose, TSH, and vitamin B_{12} levels. HIV testing, RPR, and liver function tests may be informative in selected patients.

Although consensus is lacking with respect to which patients benefit from head CT or MRI, those with focal neurologic signs or symptoms, seizures, gait abnormalities, and an acute or subacute onset are most likely to yield positive findings.

Referral for neuropsychologic testing may be helpful in the following circumstances: to distinguish dementia from depression, to diagnose dementia in persons of very poor education or very high premorbid intellect, and to aid diagnosis when impairment is mild.

Treatment

Soon after diagnosis, patients and families should be made aware of the Alzheimer's Association as well as the wealth of helpful publications available for advice in coping with behavioral problems, financial worries, and other matters. Caregiver support, education, and counseling can prevent or delay nursing home placement. Education includes the manifestations and natural history of dementia as well as the availability of local support services such as respite care. Even under the best of circumstances, caregiver stress can be substantial. They are at increased risk of depression, and physicians should be alert for signs of elder abuse when working with stressed caregivers.

Because demented patients have greatly diminished cognitive reserve, they are at high risk of experiencing acute cognitive or functional decline in the setting of new medical illness. Consequently, fragile cognitive status may be best maintained by ensuring that comorbid diseases such as congestive heart failure and infections are detected and treated.

Acetylcholinesterase inhibitors (eg, donepezil, galantamine, rivastigmine) produce statistically significant but clinically modest improvements in cognitive function when used to treat mildly to moderately demented patients. A minority show improvement, while a larger number may experience a less rapid decline in cognition or functional status. Starting doses, respectively, of donepezil, galantamine, and rivastigmine, are 5 mg orally daily (maximum 10 mg daily). 4 mg orally twice daily (maximum 12 mg twice daily), and 1.5 mg orally twice daily (maximum 6 mg twice daily). The doses are increased gradually as tolerated. The most bothersome side effects include diarrhea, nausea, anorexia, and weight loss. It is felt that patients with more advanced dementia may also benefit from this therapy, though donepezil in nursing home residents with dementia has no appreciable benefit in terms of problem behaviors or physical function. When the drugs should be discontinued is unclear, though benefits accrue for up to 1 year. Behavioral problems in demented patients are often best managed with a nonpharmacologic approach. Initially, it should be established that the problem is not unrecognized delirium, pain, urinary obstruction, or fecal impaction. It also helps to inquire whether the caregiver can tolerate the behavior, as it is often easier to find ways to accommodate to the behavior than to modify it. If not, the caregiver is asked to keep a brief, informal journal in which the behavior is described along with antecedent events and consequences. Recurring precipitants of the behavior are often found to be present or it may be that the behavior is rewarded— for example, by increased attention. Caregivers are taught to use simple language when communicating with the patient, to break down activities into simple component tasks, and to employ a "distract, not confront" approach when the patient seems disturbed by a troublesome issue. Additional steps to address behavioral problems include the discontinuation of all medications except those considered absolutely necessary and correction, if possible, of sensory deficits.

There is no clear consensus about a pharmacologic approach to treatment of behavioral problems in pa-tients who have not benefited from nonpharmacologic therapies. The target symptoms—depression, anxiety, psychosis—may suggest which class of medications might be most helpful in a given patient. Patients with depressive symptoms may show improvement with antidepressant therapy, including trazodone (starting with 25–50 mg at night). Anxious behavior may respond to buspirone, starting at 5–7.5 mg twice daily and advancing to 30 mg daily if necessary; this generally requires several weeks to show efficacy.

There is a benefit from use of neuroleptics in a minority of demented patients with hallucinations or delusions. The choice of agent is determined by the side effect profile and the patient's comorbidities. Low-potency typical antipsychotics (eg, thioridazine) tend to be strongly sedating and anticholinergic, whereas high-potency typical drugs (such as haloperidol) are less so but have a higher incidence of associated parkinsonism. The newer, atypical agents (risperidone, olanzapine, quetiapine) have fewer motor side effects, at least at lower doses, but are considerably more expensive. In selected cases, neuroleptics may be needed for treatment of agitated patients without clear psychosis. Federal regulations require that if antipsychotic agents are employed in treatment of a nursing home patient, drug reduction efforts must be made at least every 6 months.

Haloperidol, trazodone, behavioral management techniques, and placebo produce comparable if modest reductions in agitation in patients with dementia.

The efficacy of acetylcholinesterase inhibitors for behavioral disturbances in Alzheimer's dementia is still undetermined. Patients with Lewy body dementia have shown clinically significant improvement in behavioral symptoms when treated with rivastigmine.

Prognosis

Life expectancy after a diagnosis of Alzheimer's disease is typically 3–15 years; it may be shorter than previously reported. Other neurodegenerative dementias, such as dementia with Lewy bodies, show more rapid decline.

Dunkin JJ et al: Dementia caregiver burden: a review of the literature and guidelines for assessment and intervention. Neurology 1998;51(1 Suppl 1):S53. [PMID: 9674763] (Predictors of institutionalization and the effect of the caregiver on the course and symptomatology of dementia.)

Lyketsos CG et al: Mental and behavioral disturbances in dementia: findings from the Cache County Study on Memory in Aging. Am J Psychiatry 2000;157:708. [PMID: 10784462] (Apathy, depression, agitation, and aggression were highly prevalent, occurring in nearly 25% of patients with dementia.)

Mace NL, Rabins PV: *The 36-Hour Day,* 3rd ed. Johns Hopkins Univ Press, 1999. (Practical suggestions and advice for family members caring for persons with dementing illnesses.)

McKeith I et al: Efficacy of rivastigmine in dementia with Lewy bodies: a randomised, double-blind, placebo-controlled international study. Lancet 2000;356:2031. [PMID:

11145488] (Randomized controlled trial showing that 6–12 mg of rivastigmine produced significant behavioral effects in patients with Lewy-body dementia.)

Mohs RC et al. A 1-year placebo-controlled preservation of function survival study of donepezil in AD patients. Neurology 2001;57:1942. [PMID: 11502917] (Decreased functional decline in patients treated with donepezil compared with placebo at 1 year.)

Tariot P et al: 5-month, randomized, placebo controlled trial of galantamine in AD. The Galantamine USA-10 Study Group. Neurology 2000;54:2269. [PMID: 10881251] (Randomized controlled trial showing benefits in cognition, function, and behavior with 16–24 mg daily of galantamine compared with placebo.)

Teri L et al: Treatment of agitation in Alzheimer's disease: A randomized, placebo-controlled clinical trial. Neurology 2000;55:1271. [PMID: 11087767] (No difference noted among placebo, haloperidol, trazodone, and behavioral management in the treatment of agitated, demented patients.)

DEPRESSION

Geriatric patients with depression are more likely than younger ones to have somatic complaints, less likely to report depressed mood or feelings of guilt, and more likely to experience delusions.

Depressive syndromes that arise late in life are a heterogeneous collection, and a significant number may represent individuals with neurodegenerative disorders (eg, dementia). Consequently, close follow-up of a newly diagnosed patient, with frequent assessment of mental status and neurologic examination, may disclose an additional or alternative diagnosis.

Recognizing and treating depression in the elderly is vital, as the syndrome is associated with disability, increased rates of hospitalization and nursing home admission, and higher mortality. Medical illness and disability—more common in the elderly—are risk factors for depression. In particular, stroke and Parkinson's disease appear to predispose to depression. Suicide, the most dreaded complication of depression, has its highest risk in the geriatric age group. Although the presence of comorbid medical illnesses and cognitive disorders may interfere with diagnosis, use of the Geriatric Depression Scale (Table 4–4) with candidate cases may provide the data needed to make a treatment decision.

Elderly patients with depressive symptoms should be questioned about medication use, as many drugs (benzodiazepines, cimetidine, clonidine, and digoxin, to name a few) may contribute to the clinical picture. Similarly, several medical problems can cause fatigue, lethargy, or hypoactive delirium, all of which may be mistaken for depression. Laboratory determination of blood count complete; erythrocyte sedimentation rate; liver, thyroid, and renal function; and calcium may be helpful, as well as urinalysis and electrocardiography.

Many experts recommend longer trials of antidepressants (at least 9 weeks) in elderly patients than in younger ones.

Covinsky KE et al: Depressive symptoms and 3-year mortality in older hospitalized medical patients. Ann Intern Med 1999;130:563. [PMID: 10189325] (Depressive symptoms are associated with long-term mortality in older patients hospitalized with medical illnesses.)

Lebowitz BD et al: Diagnosis and treatment of depression in late life. Consensus statement update. JAMA 1997;278:1186. [PMID: 9326481]

Salzman C: Clinical Geriatric Psychopharmacology, 3rd ed. Williams & Wilkins, 1998. (Perhaps the best text on the topic.)

Schulz R et al: Association between depression and mortality in older adults: the Cardiovascular Health Study. Arch Intern Med 2000;160:1761. [PMID: 10871968] (Depression was an independent risk factor for mortality in community-residing elderly.)

DELIRIUM
(See also Chapter 25)

Delirium is an acute, fluctuating disturbance of consciousness, associated with a change in cognition or the development of perceptual disturbances. It is the pathophysiologic consequence of an underlying general medical condition such as infection, coronary ischemia, hypoxemia, or metabolic derangement. Delirium is associated with worse clinical outcomes (higher in-hospital and postdischarge mortality, longer lengths of stay, greater probability of placement in a nursing facility), though it is unclear if delirium causes worse outcomes or is simply an ominous marker.

Although the acutely agitated, "sundowning" elderly patient often comes to mind when considering delirium, many episodes are more subtle. Such quiet, or hypoactive, delirium may only be suspected if one notices new cognitive slowing or inattention.

Cognitive impairment is an important risk factor for delirium. Approximately 25% of delirious patients are demented, and 40% of demented hospitalized patients are delirious. Other risk factors are male sex, severe illness, hip fracture, fever or hypothermia, hypotension, malnutrition, polypharmacy and use of psychoactive medications, sensory impairment, use of restraints, use of intravenous lines or urinary catheters, metabolic disorders, depression, and alcoholism.

Assessment

A key component of a delirium workup is review of medications, as a large number of drugs, the addition of a new agent, or the discontinuation of an agent known to cause withdrawal symptoms are all associated with the development of delirium. Laboratory evaluation of most patients should include a complete blood count, electrolytes, BUN and serum creatinine, glucose, calcium, albumin, liver function studies, urinalysis, and electrocardiography. In selected cases, serum magnesium, serum drug levels, arterial blood gas measurements, blood cultures, chest radiography, and urinary toxin screens may be helpful.

Management

Prevention is the best approach. Measures include improving cognition (frequent reorientation, activities), sleep (massage, noise reduction), mobility, vision (visual aids and adaptive equipment), hearing (portable amplifiers, cerumen disimpaction), and hydration status (volume repletion). Management of established episodes of delirium entails treatment of the underlying cause, eliminating unnecessary medications, and avoidance of restraints. For refractory cases in which the patient's or others' welfare is at risk, haloperidol may be necessary, starting at 0.5 mg by mouth or intramuscularly and repeating every 30 minutes until the agitation is controlled.

Most episodes of delirium clear in a matter of days after correction of the precipitant, but some patients suffer episodes of longer duration. These individuals merit closer follow-up for the development of dementia if not already diagnosed.

Elie M et al: Delirium risk factors in elderly hospitalized patients. J Gen Intern Med 1998;13:204. [PMID: 9541379] (Strongest predictors were dementia, medical illness, alcohol abuse, depression, and advanced age.)

Inouye SK et al: A multicomponent intervention to prevent delirium in hospitalized older patients. N Engl J Med 1999; 340:669. [PMID: 10053175] (Compares one intervention unit with two usual care units, assessing cognitive impairment, sleep deprivation, immobility, visual impairment, hearing impairment, and dehydration. Delirium developed in 9.9% of the intervention group compared with 15% of usual care group.)

Marcantonio ER et al: Reducing delirium after hip fracture: a randomized trial. J Am Geriatr Soc 2001;49:516. [PMID: 11380742] (Perioperative geriatric management can reduce delirium in elderly hip fracture patients.)

IMMOBILITY

Although common in older people, reduced mobility is never normal and is often treatable if its causes are identified. It is an important cause of hospital-induced functional decline. Among hospitalized medical patients over 70, about 10% experience a decline in their ability to perform activities of daily living, much of which results from preventable reductions in mobility.

The hazards of bed rest in the elderly are multiple, serious, quick to develop, and slow to reverse. Deconditioning of the cardiovascular system occurs within days and involves fluid shifts, fluid loss, decreased cardiac output, decreased peak oxygen uptake, and increased resting heart rate. More striking changes occur in skeletal muscle, with loss of contractile velocity and strength. Pressure sores are a third serious complication; mechanical pressure, moisture, friction, and shearing forces all predispose to their development. Thrombophlebitis and pulmonary embolism are additional serious risks. Within days after being confined to bed, the risk of postural hypotension, falls, skin breakdown, and pulmonary embolism rises rapidly in the older patient. Moreover, recovery from these changes usually takes weeks to months.

The main causes of immobility are weakness, stiffness, pain, imbalance, and psychologic problems. Weakness may result from disuse of muscles, malnutrition, electrolyte disturbances, anemia, neurologic disorders, or myopathies. The commonest cause of stiffness in the elderly is osteoarthritis, but Parkinson's disease, rheumatoid arthritis, and pseudogout also are possible in this age group, and drugs such as haloperidol may also contribute. Polymyalgia rheumatica should be strongly considered in the elderly patient with pain and stiffness, particularly of the pelvic and shoulder girdle, associated with systemic symptoms (see Chapter 20).

Pain, whether from bone (eg, osteoporosis, osteomalacia, Paget's disease, metastatic bone cancer, trauma), joints (eg, osteoarthritis, rheumatoid arthritis, hip fractures, gout), bursae, or muscle (polymyalgia rheumatica, intermittent claudication, or "pseudoclaudication"), may immobilize the patient. Painful foot problems are common as well and include plantar warts, ulcerations, bunions, corns, and ingrown and overgrown toenails. Poorly fitting shoes are a frequent cause of these disorders.

Imbalance and fear of falling are major causes of immobilization. Imbalance often results from several causes concurrently, including neurologic disorders (eg, stroke; cervical myelopathy; peripheral neuropathy due to diabetes or alcohol; and vestibulocerebellar abnormalities), orthostatic or postprandial hypotension, or drugs (eg, diuretics, antihypertensives, sedatives, neuroleptics, and antidepressants). It may also occur following prolonged bed rest.

Psychologic conditions such as severe anxiety or depression may contribute to immobilization.

Prevention & Treatment

When immobilization cannot be avoided, several measures can be employed to minimize its consequences. Adequate nutrition should be ensured, and the skin over pressure points should be inspected frequently. To minimize cardiovascular deconditioning, patients should be positioned as close to the upright position as possible, several times daily. To reduce the risks of contracture and weakness, range of motion exercises should be started immediately and isometric and isotonic exercises performed while the patient is in bed. Whenever possible, patients should assist with their own positioning, transferring, and self-care. As long as the patient remains immobilized, pharmacologic (eg, low-dose heparin) or nonpharmacologic means (eg, graduated compression stockings) should be employed to reduce the risk of thrombosis.

Avoiding restraints and discontinuing invasive devices (intravenous lines, urinary catheters) may increase an elderly patient's prospects for early mobility. Once this becomes feasible, graduated ambulation should begin. Advice from a physical therapist is often helpful. Installing handrails, lowering the bed, and providing chairs of proper height with arms and rubber skid guards may make the patient safely mobile in the home. A properly fitted cane or walker may also be useful.

In treating arthritis, NSAIDs cause more serious gastrointestinal bleeding in the elderly than in younger individuals. Although the newer COX-2 inhibitors result in less serious gastrointestinal toxicity than traditional NSAIDs, it has been suggested that they are associated with higher thrombotic risks. Both classes of drugs may result in confusion, increased blood pressure, and renal toxicity. For many cases of osteoarthritis, acetaminophen or glucosamine may be effective and safer than an NSAID or COX-2 inhibitor. Exercise is effective treatment for both knee and hip osteoarthritis.

If depression is preventing a patient from participating in physical therapy, it may prove necessary to start with a short course of stimulant medication (eg, methylphenidate; see Chapter 25), at least until a more traditional antidepressant has had time to take effect.

van Baar ME et al: Effectiveness of exercise therapy in patients with osteoarthritis of the hip or knee. Arthritis Rheum 1999;42:1361. [PMID: 104032263] (Concludes there is evidence of benefit of exercise therapy in patients with osteoarthritis of the hip or knee, with evidence greater for knee disease.)

FALLS & GAIT DISORDERS

Thirty percent of community-dwelling elderly persons fall each year, including half of people over age 80, and one out of four of those who fall have serious injuries. About 5% of falls result in fracture. Falls are the sixth leading cause of death for older people. Just as important, they are a contributing factor in 40% of admissions to nursing homes. Resultant hip fractures and fear of falls are major causes of loss of independence. Nonetheless, falls are not inevitable or untreatable.

Causes of Falls

Balance and ambulation require a complex interplay of cognitive, neuromuscular, and cardiovascular function. With age, balance becomes impaired and sway increases. This predisposes the older person to a fall when challenged by an additional insult to any of these systems.

A fall may be the clinical manifestation of an occult problem, such as pneumonia or myocardial infarction, but much more commonly falls are due to the interaction between an impaired patient and an environmental risk factor. While a warped floorboard may pose little problem for a vigorous, unmedicated, cognitively intact person, it may be sufficient to precipitate a fall

and hip fracture in the patient with impaired vision, balance, muscle tone, or cognition. Thus, falls in older people are rarely due to a single cause, and effective intervention entails a comprehensive assessment of the patient's intrinsic deficits (usually diseases and medications), the activity engaged in at the time of the fall, and environmental obstacles.

Intrinsic deficits are those that impair sensory input, judgment, blood pressure regulation, reaction time, and balance and gait. Dizziness may be closely related to the deficits associated with falls and gait abnormalities. While it may be impossible to isolate a sole "cause" or a "cure" for falls, gait abnormalities, or dizziness, it is often possible to identify and ameliorate some of the underlying contributory conditions and improve the patient's overall function.

As for most geriatric conditions, medications and alcohol use are among the most common, significant, and reversible causes of falling. Benzodiazepines, opioids, phenothiazines, vasodilators, and diuretics particularly increase fall risk. Other often overlooked but treatable contributors include postprandial hypotension (which peaks 30–60 minutes after a meal), insomnia, urinary urgency, and peripheral edema (which can burden impaired leg strength and gait because of the additional weight).

Since most falls occur in or around the home, a visit by a visiting nurse, physical therapist, or physician reaps substantial benefits in identifying environmental obstacles and is generally reimbursed by third-party payers, including Medicare. Insufficient lighting is an underappreciated factor in many cases. In addition to the number and location of lamps, noting their wattage is also important; because of a loss of contrast sensitivity, older people often need twice the wattage to maximize visual acuity. Replacement of 60-watt bulbs with 100-watt bulbs may be cost-effective.

Complications of Falls

The most common fractures resulting from falls are of the wrist, hip, and vertebrae. There is a high mortality rate (approximately 20% in one year) in elderly women with hip fractures, particularly if they were debilitated prior to the time of the fracture.

Fear of falling again is a common, serious, but treatable factor in the elderly person's loss of confidence and independence. Referral to a physical therapist for gait training with special devices is often all that is required.

Chronic subdural hematoma is an easily overlooked complication of falls that must be considered in any elderly patient presenting with new neurologic symptoms or signs, particularly obtundation. Headache is uncommonly present. In many cases there is no history of trauma.

Dehydration, electrolyte imbalance, pressure sores, rhabdomyolysis, and hypothermia may all complicate a fall.

Prevention & Management

The risk of falling and consequent injury, disability, and potential institutionalization can be reduced by modifying those factors outlined in Table 4–5. Emphasis is placed on treating all contributory medical conditions, minimizing environmental hazards, and reducing the number of medications—particularly those that induce parkinsonism, orthostasis (eg, alpha-blockers, calcium channel blockers, nitrates, antiparkinsonism agents, antipsychotics, tricyclic antidepressants), peripheral edema, and confusion. Also important are strength, balance, and gait training as well as steps to improve bone density (with calcium and vitamin D supplementation).

Patients with repeated falls are often reassured by the availability of phones at floor level, a portable phone, or a lightweight radio call system. Their therapy should also include training in techniques for arising after a fall. Use of an anatomically designed external hip protector may reduce hip fracture risk in frail elders.

Close J et al: Prevention of falls in the elderly trial: a randomised controlled trial. Lancet 1999;353:93. [PMID: 10023893] (Risk of repeat falls was significantly reduced in the intervention group receiving medical and occupational therapy, with odds ratio 0.39.)

Cumming RG et al: Home visits by an occupational therapist for assessment and modification of environmental hazards: A randomized trial of falls prevention. J Am Geriatr Soc 1999;47:1397. [PMID: 10591231] (Intervention consisting of a single home visit by an occupational therapist, with telephone follow-up to encourage adherence to recommendations, led to a significant reduction in falls in patients with a previous fall history.)

Kannus P et al: Fall-induced injuries and death among older adults. JAMA 1999;281:1895. [PMID: 10349892] (Total falls and deaths from falls have dramatically increased over the last two decades, but age-adjusted falls have remained steady.)

Kannus P et al: Prevention of hip fracture in elderly people with use of a hip protector. N Engl J Med 2000;343:1506. [PMID: 11087879] (Randomized, controlled trial of specially designed hip protectors which are placed inside the pockets of stretchy undergarments reduced hip fracture incidence by more than 50%.)

Mahoney JE et al: Temporal association between hospitalization and rate of falls after discharge. Arch Intern Med 2000;160:2788. [PMID: 11025789] (Frequency of elders' falls is substantially increased in the first month after medical hospitalization.)

Ooi WL et al: The association between orthostatic hypotension and recurrent falls in nursing home residents. Am J Med 2000;108:106. [PMID: 11126303] (Prospective study of nursing home residents showed that among subjects with a history of previous falls, those with orthostatic hypotension had an increased risk of recurrent falls.)

URINARY INCONTINENCE

Classification
(Table 4–6)

Because continence requires adequate mobility, mentation, motivation, and manual dexterity, problems outside the bladder often result in geriatric incontinence. These are causes of transient incontinence, though they may cause prolonged incontinence if the problems are not identified and treated. Instances of new-onset incontinence often arise during hospitalization. In contrast to transient incontinence, causes of established, or persistent, incontinence generally can be found in the urinary tract itself.

Table 4–5. Fall risk factors and targeted interventions.

Risk Factor	Targeted Intervention
Postural hypotension (> 20 mm Hg drop in systolic BP, or systolic BP < 90 mm Hg)	Behavioral recommendations, such as hand clenching, elevation of head of bed; discontinuation or substitution of high-risk medications
Use of benzodiazepine or sedative-hypnotic	Education about sleep hygiene, discontinuation or substitution of medications
Use of over three prescription medications	Review of medications
Environmental hazards	Appropriate changes; installation of safety equipment (eg, grab bars)
Gait impairment	Gait training, assistive devices, balance or strengthening exercises
Impairment in transfer or balance	Balance exercises, training in transfers, environmental alterations (eg, grab bars)
Impairment in leg or arm muscle strength or limb range of motion	Excercise with resistance bands or putty, with graduated increases in resistance

Table 4–6. Classification of geriatric incontinence.

Transient
  Delirium or confusional state
  Infection, urinary (symptomatic)
  Atrophic urethritis or vaginitis
  Pharmaceuticals
  Psychologic, especially severe depression
  Excessive urine output (eg, congestive heart failure, hyperglycemia)
  Restricted mobility
  Stool impaction
Established
  Detrusor overactivity (urge incontinence)
  Urethral incompetence (stress incontinence)
  Urethral obstruction
  Detrusor underactivity (eg, neurogenic bladder)

A. Transient Causes

Use of the mnemonic "DIAPPERS" may help one remember the categories of transient incontinence.

1. Delirium—A clouded sensorium impedes recognition of both the need to void and the location of the nearest toilet. Delirium is the most common cause of incontinence in hospitalized patients; once it clears, incontinence resolves.

2. Infection—Symptomatic urinary tract infection commonly causes or contributes to incontinence. Asymptomatic bacteriuria does not.

3. Atrophic urethritis and vaginitis—Because it usually coexists with atrophic vaginitis, atrophic urethritis can be diagnosed presumptively by the presence of vaginal mucosal telangiectasia, petechiae, erosions, erythema, or friability. Urethral inflammation commonly contributes to incontinence in women and responds to treatment for several months with low-dose estrogen (eg, 0.3–0.6 mg conjugated estrogens by mouth; topical administration is more expensive and may be uncomfortable).

4. Pharmaceuticals—Drugs are one of the most common causes of transient incontinence. Typical offending agents include potent diuretics, anticholinergics, psychotropics, opioid analgesics, alpha blockers (in women), alpha agonists (in men), and calcium channel blockers.

5. Psychologic factors—Severe depression with psychomotor retardation may impede the ability or motivation to reach a toilet.

6. Excess urine output—Excess urine output may also overwhelm the ability of an older person to reach a toilet in time. In addition to diuretics, common causes include excess fluid intake; metabolic abnormalities (eg, hyperglycemia, hypercalcemia, diabetes insipidus); and disorders associated with peripheral edema, with its associated heavy nocturia when previously dependent legs assume a horizontal position in bed. Edema may be due to heart failure, venous insufficiency, malnutrition, cirrhosis, and use of calcium channel blockers or NSAIDs.

7. Restricted mobility—(See Immobility section, above.) If mobility cannot be improved, access to a urinal or commode (eg, at the bedside) may improve continence.

8. Stool impaction—This is a common cause of urinary incontinence in hospitalized or immobile patients. Although the mechanism is still unknown, a clinical clue to its presence is the onset of both urinary and fecal incontinence. Disimpaction restores urinary continence.

B. Established Causes

Causes of established incontinence (Figure 4–2) should be addressed after the transient causes have been uncovered and managed appropriately.

1. Detrusor overactivity (urge incontinence)—Detrusor overactivity refers to uninhibitable bladder

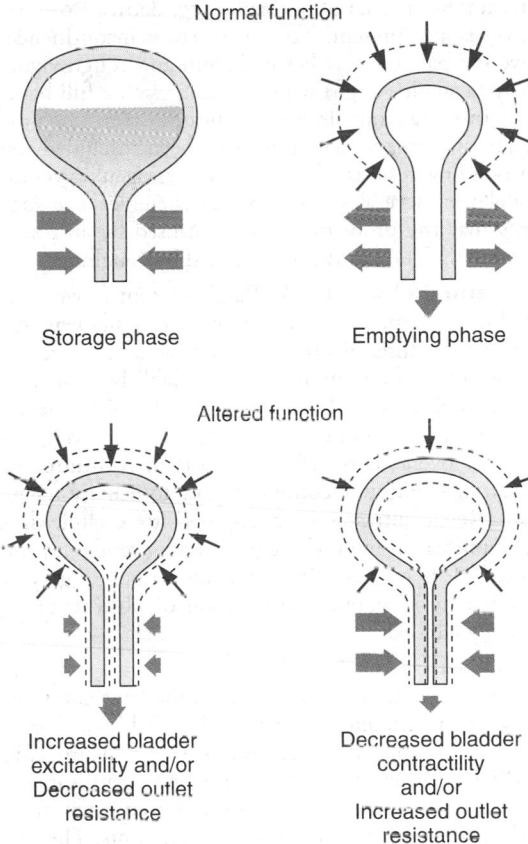

Figure 4–2. **Top:** Normal bladder physiology. **Bottom:** Pathophysiology underlying established causes of urinary incontinence.

contractions that cause leakage. It is the most common cause of established geriatric incontinence, accounting for two-thirds of cases. Women will complain of urinary leakage after the onset of an intense urge to urinate that cannot be forestalled. In men the symptoms are similar, but since detrusor overactivity may be due to coexisting urethral obstruction (typically from prostatic disease), urodynamic testing should be done if prescription of a bladder relaxant is planned, in order to avoid precipitating urinary retention. Because detrusor overactivity also may be due to bladder stones or tumor, the abrupt onset of otherwise unexplained urge incontinence—especially if accompanied by perineal or suprapubic discomfort or sterile hematuria—should be investigated by cystoscopy and cytologic examination of a urine specimen.

2. Urethral incompetence (stress incontinence)—The second most common cause of established incontinence in older women (it is rare in men), stress incontinence is characterized by instantaneous leakage of urine in response to a stress maneuver. It commonly coexists with detrusor overactivity. Typically, urinary loss occurs with laughing, coughing, or lifting heavy objects. Leakage is worse, or occurs only during the day, unless another abnormality (eg, detrusor overactivity) is also present. To test for stress incontinence, have the patient relax her perineum and cough vigorously (a single cough) while standing with a full bladder. Instantaneous leakage indicates stress incontinence if urinary retention has been excluded by postvoiding residual determination using ultrasound. A delay of several seconds or persistent leakage suggests that the problem is instead caused by an uninhibited bladder contraction induced by coughing.

3. Urethral obstruction—Rarely present in women, urethral obstruction (due to prostatic enlargement, urethral stricture, bladder neck contracture, or prostatic cancer) is a common cause of established incontinence in older men. It can present as dribbling incontinence after voiding, urge incontinence due to detrusor overactivity (which coexists in two-thirds of cases), or overflow incontinence due to urinary retention. Renal ultrasound is required to exclude hydronephrosis in men whose postvoiding residual urine exceeds 150 mL. In older men for whom surgery is planned, urodynamic confirmation of obstruction is strongly advised.

4. Detrusor underactivity (overflow incontinence)—Detrusor underactivity is the least common cause of incontinence. It may be idiopathic or due to sacral lower motor nerve dysfunction ("neurogenic bladder"). When it causes incontinence, detrusor underactivity is associated with urinary frequency, nocturia, and frequent leakage of small amounts. The elevated postvoiding residual urine (generally over 450 mL) distinguishes it from detrusor overactivity and stress incontinence, but only urodynamic testing differentiates it from urethral obstruction in men. Such testing usually is not required in women, in whom obstruction is rarely present.

Treatment

A. TRANSIENT CAUSES

Each identified transient cause should be treated regardless of whether an established cause coexists. For patients with urinary retention induced by an anticholinergic agent, discontinuation of the drug should first be considered. If this is not feasible, substituting a less anticholinergic agent (eg, sertraline instead of desipramine for depression) may be useful.

B. ESTABLISHED CAUSES

1. Detrusor overactivity—The cornerstone of treatment is behavioral therapy. Patients are instructed to void every 1–2 hours while awake. Once daytime continence is restored, the interval is increased by 30 minutes until the interval is 4–5 hours. Most patients who become continent during the day on this regimen become continent at night as well. For patients who are unable to manage on their own, caregivers should ask whether they need to void at suitable intervals.

Biofeedback can be extremely helpful in training cognitively intact, motivated patients to exercise their pelvic floor muscles and thus improve continence. Results superior to use of bladder relaxants are possible.

If behavioral approaches prove insufficient, drug therapy to relax the detrusor may be necessary. Regimens should be monitored to avoid inducing urinary retention. Use of oxybutynin (2.5–5 mg three or four times daily), long-acting oxybutynin (5–15 mg daily), or tolterodine (1–2 mg twice daily) may reduce episodes of incontinence. All may cause dry mouth, confusion, or other anticholinergic side effects.

In refractory cases, where intermittent catheterization is feasible, the physician may choose intentionally to induce urinary retention with a bladder relaxant and have the patient empty the bladder three or four times daily. Clean but not sterile technique is required.

2. Urethral incompetence (stress incontinence)—Although a last resort, surgery is the most effective treatment for stress incontinence, resulting in a cure rate of 75–85% even in older women. For women who wish to avoid surgery and who can employ them indefinitely, pelvic muscle exercises are effective for mild to moderate stress incontinence; they can be combined, if necessary, with biofeedback or vaginal cones.

The effectiveness of topical or oral estrogens is likely to be low unless atrophic vaginitis with urethral irritation is present.

Occasionally, a pessary or even a tampon (for women with vaginal stenosis) provides some relief, especially for frail women.

3. Urethral obstruction—Surgical decompression is the most effective treatment for obstruction, especially in the setting of urinary retention. A variety of newer, less invasive techniques make decompression feasible even for frail men. For the nonoperative candidate with urinary retention, intermittent or indwelling catheterization is used. For a man with prostatic obstruction who is not in retention and who wishes to defer surgery or is not a good surgical candidate, treatment with alpha-blocking agents (eg, terazosin, 1–10 mg daily; prazosin, 1–5 mg orally twice daily; tamsulosin, 0.4–0.8 mg daily) may relieve symptoms. Finasteride or the herbal supplement saw palmetto may partially relieve symptoms in a minority of patients, but the onset of effect may take many months.

4. Detrusor underactivity—For the patient with a poorly contractile bladder, augmented voiding techniques (eg, double voiding, suprapubic pressure) often prove effective. If further emptying is needed, intermittent or indwelling catheterization is the only option. Antibiotics should be used only for symptomatic upper urinary tract infection or as prophylaxis against recurrent symptomatic infections in a patient using intermittent catheterization; they should not be used as prophylaxis with an indwelling catheter.

Burgio KL et al: Behavioral vs drug treatment for urge urinary incontinence in older women: a randomized, controlled trial. JAMA 1998;280:1995. [PMID: 9863850] (Episodes of incontinence were reduced over 80% on average with behavioral treatment, compared with 70% reduction from medication and 40% from placebo.)

Fantl JA et al: Urinary incontinence in adults: Acute and chronic management. Clinical Practice Guideline, No. 2, 1996 Update. Rockville, MD: United States Department of Health and Human Services. Public Health Service, AHCPR. Publication No. 96-0682.

Samsioe G: Urogenital aging—a hidden problem. Am J Obstet Gynecol 1998;178:S245. [PMID: 9609599]

WEIGHT LOSS & MALNUTRITION

Undernutrition affects substantial numbers of elderly persons and often precedes hospitalization for "failure to thrive." Unintended weight loss exceeding 5% in 1 month or 10% in 6 months deserves evaluation.

Table 4–7 lists causes of weight loss in older adults and may suggest points of history to explore. Useful laboratory and radiologic studies include complete blood count, serum chemistries (including glucose, TSH, creatinine, calcium), urinalysis, and chest film. These studies are intended to uncover an occult metabolic or neoplastic cause but are not exhaustive.

Treatment with nutritional supplements may lead to weight gain, but they are expensive; use of instant breakfast powder in whole milk (for those who can tolerate dairy products) is a less costly alternative. Megestrol acetate has been employed as an appetite stimulant (primarily in cancer and AIDS patients) but has not been shown to increase body mass or lengthen life in the elderly population.

Table 4–7. Causes of unintended weight loss in the elderly.

Medical
- Chronic heart, lung disease
- Dementia
- Oral problems (eg, poor denture fit)
- Dysphagia
- Mesenteric ischemia
- Cancer
- Diabetes
- Hyperthyroidism

Psychosocial
- Alcoholism
- Depression
- Social isolation
- Limited funds
- Problems with shopping or food preparation
- Inadequate assistance with feeding

Drug-related
- NSAIDs
- Antiepileptics
- Digoxin
- Selective serotonin reuptake inhibitors

For those who have lost the ability to feed themselves, assiduous hand feeding may allow maintenance of weight. Although artificial nutrition and hydration ("tube feeding") may seem a more convenient alternative, it deprives the patient of the taste and texture of food as well as the social milieu typically associated with mealtime; before this option is chosen, the patient or his surrogate will wish to review the benefits and burdens of the treatment in light of overall goals of care. If the patient makes repeated attempts to pull out the tube during a trial of artificial nutrition, the treatment burden becomes substantial, and the utility of tube feeding should be reconsidered. Though commonly employed, there is no evidence that tube feeding prolongs life in patients with end-stage dementia.

"Failure to thrive" is a syndrome lacking a consensus definition but generally represents a constellation of weight loss (due to some combination of causes listed in Table 4–7), weakness, and progressive functional decline. The label is typically applied when some triggering event—loss of social support, a bout of depression or pneumonia, the addition of a new medication—pulls a struggling elderly person below the threshold of successful independent living. Ideally, use of the preventive measures recommended earlier in this chapter will reduce the patient's chances of reaching this stage of frailty.

Covinsky KE et al: The relationship between clinical assessments of nutritional status and adverse outcomes in older hospitalized medical patients. J Am Geriatr Soc 1999;47:532. [PMID: 10323645] (Prospective cohort study shows malnutrition in hospitalized older patients is associated with greater mortality, delayed functional recovery, and higher rates of nursing home use.)

Finucane TE et al: Tube feeding in patients with advanced dementia: a review of the evidence. JAMA 1999;282:1365. [PMID: 10527184] (Authors found no data suggesting that tube feeding of advanced dementia patients reduced risk of pressure sores or infection nor that it improved function or provided palliation.)

Gazewood JD et al: Diagnosis and management of weight loss in the elderly. J Fam Pract 1998;47:19. [PMID: 10527184]

PHARMACOTHERAPY & POLYPHARMACY

There are several reasons for the greater incidence of iatrogenic drug reactions in the elderly population. Drug metabolism is often impaired in this group, due to a decrease in glomerular filtration rate, as well as reduced hepatic clearance. The latter is due to decreased activity of microsomal enzymes and reduced hepatic perfusion with aging. The volume of distribution of drugs is also affected. Since the elderly have a decrease in total body water and a relative increase in body fat, water-soluble drugs become more concentrated, and fat-soluble drugs have longer half lives. In addition, serum albumin levels decrease, especially in sick patients, with reduction in protein binding of some drugs (eg, warfarin, phenytoin), leaving more free (active) drug available.

Older individuals often have varying responses to a given serum drug level. Thus, they are more sensitive to some drugs (eg, opioids) and less sensitive to others (eg, beta-blocking agents).

Finally, the older patient with multiple chronic conditions is likely to be receiving many drugs, including nonprescribed agents. Thus, adverse drug reactions and dosage errors are more likely to occur, especially if the patient has visual, hearing, or memory deficits.

Precautions in Administering Drugs

The following suggestions are designed to reduce the risk of drug toxicity.

A. Drug Selection and Administration

1. The symptom requiring treatment may be due to another drug, leading to a "prescribing cascade," in which adverse drug effects are attributed to new medical conditions, in time resulting in prescription of still more medications.

2. Nonpharmacologic means should be tried before drugs. Pharmacotherapy is not necessarily indicated in some common clinical situations. In asymptomatic bacteriuria, for example, antibiotics need not be given unless the disorder is associated with obstructive uropathy, other anatomic abnormalities, or stones. Ankle edema is often due to venous insufficiency, drugs (NSAIDs, calcium channel blockers), malnutrition, or inactivity in chair-bound patients and need not be treated with diuretics unless associated with heart failure. Leg elevation in the evening or fitted pressure-gradient stockings are often helpful.

3. Therapy is begun with less than the usual adult dosage and the dosage increased slowly, consistent with its pharmacokinetics in older patients. However, age-related changes in drug distribution and clearance are variable among individuals, and some require full doses. After determining acceptable measures of success and toxicity, the dose is increased until one or the other is reached.

Despite the importance of beginning new drugs in a slow, measured fashion, all too often an inadequate trial is permitted (in terms of duration of course, or ultimate dose) before they are discontinued. Angiotensin-converting enzyme inhibitors and antidepressants, in particular, are frequently stopped before therapeutic dosages are reached.

4. Steps are taken to improve adherence to the prescribed medical regimen. The following increase the odds of nonadherence: the patient lives alone; uses more than one pharmacy or provider; is prescribed medications with multiple daily doses; has a drug regimen that is changed frequently; is prescribed a large number of drugs; has difficulty reaching a pharmacy; and has poor cognition, vision, or dexterity. When

possible, the physician should keep the dosing schedule simple, the number of pills low, and the medication changes infrequent.

5. A family member is asked to bring in all medications at each visit for reinforcing instructions regarding reasons for drug use, dosage, frequency of administration, and possible adverse effects.

6. Although serum drug levels may be useful for monitoring certain drugs with narrow therapeutic windows (eg, phenytoin, theophylline, lithium, tricyclic antidepressants), toxicity can still occur even with "normal" therapeutic levels of many drugs.

7. Trials of individual drug discontinuation should be considered (including antihypertensives, digoxin, antiepileptics), particularly in a controlled environment such as a nursing facility.

B. Considerations With Specific Drug Classes

1. Anticoagulants—Many elderly patients with atrial fibrillation are not anticoagulated because physicians fear injuries and secondary bleeding due to falls. Head injuries due to falls are usually of greatest concern, and occur in about 1% of falls. Given that anticoagulation can result in an annual absolute risk reduction in stroke of 3–8%, the benefits of anticoagulation outweigh the risks of falling in most instances.

2. Glaucoma medications—Not only can topical beta-blockers cause systemic side effects (bradycardia, asthma, heart failure), but so too can oral carbonic anhydrase inhibitors. The latter may produce malaise, anorexia, and weight loss.

3. Analgesics—Meperidine is associated with an increased risk of delirium and seizures in the elderly, and should be avoided in this population. Of the NSAIDs, indomethacin carries the highest risk of causing confusion. For treatment of osteoarthritis, use of acetaminophen on a scheduled basis is safer than use of an NSAID, with comparable effectiveness.

4. Antihypertensives—In most instances, the first choice for treating hypertension in older people is a thiazide in low dosage, eg, hydrochlorothiazide 12.5 mg by mouth daily. Thiazides increase the risk of attacks of gout flares, perhaps less so at this dosage. Concomitant use of an NSAID can exacerbate hypertension.

5. Cold remedies—Over-the-counter cold remedies frequently cause adverse effects in elderly people. The anticholinergic properties of many can create confusion (even in nondemented persons), impair bladder emptying, or cause constipation, and decongestants not infrequently cause urinary hesitancy or retention in men.

6. Antiemetics—Prochlorperazine and metoclopramide both can cause drug-induced parkinsonism.

Bedell SE et al: Discrepancies in the use of medications: their extent and predictors in an outpatient practice. Arch Intern Med 2000;160:2129. [PMID: 10904455] (Multivariate analysis shows patient age and number of prescribed medications were the two most significant predictors of medication discrepancy.)

Beers MH: Explicit criteria for determining potentially inappropriate medication use by the elderly. An update. Arch Intern Med 1997;157:1531. [PMID: 9236554]

McLeod PJ et al: Defining inappropriate practices in prescribing for elderly people: A national consensus panel. CMAJ 1997;156:385. [PMID: 9033421]

Care at the End of Life

5

Michael W. Rabow, MD, & Steven Z. Pantilat, MD
See www.current-med.com/ch05.html

◾ THE END OF LIFE

DIAGNOSIS OF THE END OF LIFE

In the United States, approximately 2.3 million people die each year. Despite all the successes of medical progress, death inevitably comes, and clinicians battling to prolong life must recognize when life is ending in order to continue caring properly for their patients. Unfortunately, end-of-life practices do not always meet the standards set by professional organizations. While death itself remains a mystery and while caring for the dying traditionally has not been well researched or adequately taught as part of medical training, caring for patients at the end of life is an important responsibility and a rewarding opportunity for clinicians.

The terms "palliative care," "care of the dying," and "end-of-life care" imply a focus on care of the whole person who is approaching death rather than on an attempt to cure underlying disease. Since it emphasizes that the dying process is part of life, the expression "end-of-life care" is preferable and will be used here. From the medical perspective, the end of life may be defined as that time when death—whether due to terminal illness, acute or chronic illness, or age itself—is expected within weeks to months and can no longer be reasonably forestalled by medical intervention.

Clinicians have an important role in helping patients understand that their lives are ending. This information influences patients' treatment decisions and may change how they spend their remaining time. While certain diseases such as cancer are amenable to prognostic estimates regarding the time course to death, the other common causes of mortality in the United States—including heart disease, stroke, chronic lung disease, and dementia—have variable and difficult to predict prognoses. Even for patients with cancer, clinician estimates of prognosis are often inaccurate and generally overly optimistic. Nonetheless, clinical experience, epidemiologic data, guidelines

from professional organizations,* and formal computer-based modeling and prediction tools† may be employed to help patients identify the end period of their lives. Recognizing that patients may have different levels of comfort with prognostic information, clinicians can introduce the topic by simply saying, "I have information about the likely time course of your illness. Would you like to talk about it now?"

EXPECTATIONS ABOUT THE END OF LIFE

Patients' experiences of the end of life are influenced by their expectations about how they will die and the meaning of death. Many people fear how they will die more than death itself. Patients report fear of dying in pain or of suffocation, of loss of control, indignity, isolation, and being a burden to their families. All of these anxieties can be alleviated with good supportive care provided by an attentive group of caretakers.

For most of human history, death has been regarded as part of the natural process of life. However, with recent technologic advances that serve to forestall the end of life, death has become "medicalized." No longer seen clearly as a profound personal and spiritual event basic to the human condition, death is often regarded as a failure of medical science. The medicalization of death can create or heighten a sense of guilt about the failure to prevent dying. Both the general public and clinicians are complicit in denying death, treating dying persons as patients and death as an enemy to be battled furiously in hospitals rather than as an inevitable outcome to be experienced as a part of life at home. Currently in the United States, approximately 80% of people die in hospitals or long-term care facilities.

For most patients at the end of life, the clinician should continue to pursue cure of potentially re-

---

*For example, the National Hospice Organization.
†For example, the Acute Physiology and Chronic Health Evaluation (APACHE) system or the Study to Understand Prognoses and Preferences for Outcomes and Risks of Treatment (SUPPORT) model.

versible disease, provide comfort, and help the patient prepare for death. Patients at the end of life identify a number of elements as important to quality end-of-life care: adequate pain and symptom management; avoiding inappropriate prolongation of dying; achieving a sense of control; relieving the burden on others; and strengthening relationships with loved ones.

COMMUNICATION & THE ROLE OF THE CLINICIAN AT THE END OF LIFE

Caring for patients at the end of life requires the same skills clinicians employ in other tasks of medical care: eliciting a complete history, examining for signs of physical disease, making careful diagnoses of treatable conditions, providing patient education, sharing in decision-making, and expressing understanding and caring. Communication skills are vitally important. In particular, clinicians must become experts at delivering bad news and then dealing with its consequences (Table 5–1). Higher quality communication is associated with greater satisfaction and increased clinician knowledge of patient wishes.

Three further clinician obligations are central to the clinician's role at this time. First, clinicians must work to identify, understand, and relieve patient suffering. Suffering is experienced by the person as a whole and may include physical, psychologic, social, or spiritual distress. Disease, disability, and disintegration at the end of life can threaten a person's sense of integrity or "intactness" and thereby cause suffering. In assisting with redirection and growth, providing support, assessing meaning, and fostering transcendence, clinicians can help ameliorate their patients' suffering and help the patient and family live fully during this stage of life.

Second, clinicians caring for patients at the end of life have an obligation to serve as a facilitator or catalyst for hope. While a particular outcome may be extremely unlikely (such as cure of advanced cancer following exhaustive conventional and experimental treatments), hope may be defined as the patient's belief in what is still possible. Although hope for a "miraculous cure" may be

Table 5–1. Suggestions for the delivery of bad news.

Prepare an appropriate place and time.
Address basic information needs.
Be direct; avoid jargon and euphemisms.
Allow for silence and emotional ventilation.
Assess and validate patient reactions.
Respond to immediate discomforts and risks.
Listen actively and express empathy.
Achieve a common perception of the problem.
Reassure about pain relief.
Ensure basic follow-up and make specific plans for the future.

---

simplistic and even harmful, hope for relief of pain, for reconciliation with loved ones, for discovery of meaning in the life remaining, and for spiritual transformation is still quite supportable at the end of life. With questions such as "What is still possible for you?"—"What do you wish for before you die?"—"What good might come of this?" clinicians can help patients uncover hope, explore meaningful and realistic goals, and develop strategies to realize them.

Third, patients' feelings of isolation and fear engendered by the prospect of dying demand that clinicians communicate directly to patients that care will continue to be provided throughout the final stage of life. Perhaps the essential principle of care at the end of life is this promise of nonabandonment: a clinician's pledge to an individual patient to serve as a caring partner, a resource for creative problem-solving and relief of suffering, a guide during uncertain times, and a witness to the patient's experiences—no matter what happens. Dying patients need their clinicians to offer their presence—not necessarily the ability to solve all problems but rather a commitment to recognize and receive the patients' difficulties and experiences with respect and empathy. At its best, the patient-clinician relationship can be a covenant of compassion and a recognition of common humanity.

CARING FOR THE FAMILY

In caring for patients at the end of life, clinicians must appreciate the central role played by family, friends, and romantic partners and often must deal with strong emotions of fear, anger, shame, sadness, and guilt experienced by those individuals. While significant others may support and comfort a patient at the end of life, the threatened loss of a loved one may also create or reveal dysfunctional or painful family dynamics. Furthermore, clinicians must be attuned to the potential impact of illness on the patient's family: substantial physical caregiving responsibilities and financial burdens as well as increased rates of anxiety, depression, chronic illness, and even mortality. Family caregivers commonly provide the bulk of care for patients at the end of life, yet their work is often not acknowledged or compensated.

Clinicians can help families confront the imminent loss of a loved one (Table 5–2) and often must negotiate amid complex and changing family needs. Identifying a spokesperson for the family, conducting family meetings, allowing all to be heard, and providing time for consensus may help the clinician work effectively with the family.

THE LIMITS OF CARE AT THE END OF LIFE

Many clinicians find caring for patients at the end of life to be one of the most rewarding aspects of practice. However, working with the dying requires

Table 5–2. Clinician behaviors helpful to families of dying patients.[1]

Timely, frequent, and consistent communication
Adapting communication to need
Focusing on patient's wishes
Attending to the comfort of the patient
Being aware of family conflict
Accommodating family's grief
Refocusing hope
Encouraging planning
Remaining available
Following up with family after death

---

[1]Adapted, with permission, from Bascom PB, Tolle SW: Care of the family when the patient is dying. West J Med 1995;163:292.

tolerance of great uncertainty, ambiguity, and existential challenges. Clinicians must recognize and respect their own limitations and attend to their own needs in order to avoid being overburdened, overly distressed, or emotionally depleted. Open recognition of their own feelings enables clinicians to process their emotions and take steps to care for themselves; conferring and consulting with colleagues, retreating, relaxing and recuperating, obtaining informal or professional support, or even—under extraordinary circumstances—transferring the care of a patient to another clinician when it is no longer possible for the original clinician to meet the patient's needs. Moreover, care of patients at the end of life is not solely the responsibility of physicians. Ideally, physicians, nurses, social workers, psychologists, therapists (physical, occupational, recreational), dietitians, clergy, and volunteers should coordinate their efforts to care for patients and can support one another.

Clinicians may be limited in caring for persons at the end of life not only by their emotional responses but by a sense of moral obligation as well. While the ethical, legal, and professional controversies over clinician-assisted suicide are beyond the scope of this chapter, clinicians should be aware of the "right to die" movement as an expression, at least in part, of patient dissatisfaction with how people are cared for at the end of life. In the United States, clinician-assisted suicide is illegal in every state but Oregon—and legal there only with careful restrictions. While individual clinicians must decide for themselves within the evolving legal context what their personal limits may be in caring for patients who request aid in dying (eg, clinician-assisted suicide), all clinicians can reclaim their long-privileged and universally accepted role of caring for the dying. They can do so by dedicating themselves not to abandon their patients and by providing appropriate attention to symptom management, sensitivity to psychologic and social stresses, and unconditional presence and openness to spiritual challenges at the end of life. Research has demonstrated that palliative care interventions can cause some patients who have requested clinician-assisted suicide to withdraw their request.

Cassell EJ: Diagnosing suffering: a perspective. Ann Intern Med 1999;131:531. [PMID: 10507963]

Christakis NA et al: Extent and determinants of error in doctors' prognoses in terminally ill patients: prospective cohort study. BMJ 2000;320:469. [PMID: 10678857] (In this prospective cohort study, only 20% of prognostic estimates by physicians were accurate, and 63% were overly optimistic.)

Emanuel EJ et al: Assistance from family members, friends, paid care givers, and volunteers in the care of terminally ill patients. N Engl J Med 1999;341:956. [PMID: 10498492]

Fox E et al: Evaluation of prognostic criteria for determining hospice eligibility in patients with advanced lung, heart, or liver disease. JAMA 1999;282:1638. [PMID: 10553790] (Clinical prediction tools underestimate the number of patients eligible for the hospice benefit.)

Ganzini L et al: Physicians experiences with the Oregon Death with Dignity Act. N Engl J Med 2000;342:557. [PMID: 10684915]

Meier DE et al: The inner life of physicians and care of the seriously ill. JAMA 2001;286:3007. [PMID: 11743845] (Many emotions arise in the care of terminally ill patients, and clinicians should actively identify and control these responses.)

Quill TE et al: Nonabandonment: A central obligation for physicians. Ann Intern Med 1995;122:368. [PMID: 7847649]

Singer PA et al Quality end-of-life care. JAMA 1999;281:163. [PMID: 9917120]

■ THE SETTING & STRUCTURE OF CARE

ETHICAL & LEGAL BACKGROUND

Clinicians' care of patients at the end of life is guided by the same ethical and legal principles that inform other types of medical care. Foremost among these are the principles of truth-telling, nonmaleficence, beneficence, autonomy, proportionality, and distributive justice. These are the basic principles that must guide clinicians in helping patients make difficult decisions about care, including decisions about the withdrawal and withholding of support.

Three additional ethical considerations are relevant to care at the end of life. First, important ethical principles may be in conflict. For example, while a patient may desire a particular medical intervention, the clinician may refuse to undertake the intervention if it is of no therapeutic benefit (ie, futile) or violates the clinician's own moral code. In clinical practice, what constitutes a futile intervention is frequently a point of controversy. However, most disagreements can be resolved through repeated discussions between clinicians and families.

Second, although clinicians and family members often feel differently about withholding versus withdrawing support, there is broad consensus among ethicists, supported by legal precedent, of their ethical equivalence. Patients have the same right to stop unwanted medical treatments once begun as they do to refuse those treatments in the first place, including artificial nutrition and hydration.

Third, the ethical principle of "double effect" argues that the potential to hasten imminent death is acceptable if it comes as the unintended consequence of a primary intention to provide comfort and relieve suffering. For example, sufficient doses of morphine should be provided to control pain even if there is the potential unintended secondary effect of depressing respiration. In practice, one can almost always find an effective pain regimen without hastening death.

ADVANCE DIRECTIVES

Well-informed, competent adults have a right to refuse medical intervention even if refusal is likely to result in death. Many people believe that there are fates worse than death and are willing to sacrifice some quantity of life in exchange for protecting a certain quality of life. In order to further patient autonomy, clinicians are obligated to inform patients about the risks, benefits, alternatives, and expected outcomes of end-of-life medical interventions such as cardiopulmonary resuscitation, intubation and mechanical ventilation, vasopressor medication, hospitalization and ICU care, and artificial nutrition and hydration. Advance directives are oral or written statements made by patients when they are competent that are intended to guide care should they become incompetent. Advance directives allow patients to project their autonomy into the future to a time when they are incompetent. While oral statements about these matters are ethically binding, they are not legally binding in all states. Written advance directives are essential in order to give effect to the patient's wishes in these matters. State-specific advance directive forms are available from a number of sources, including the Web site www.partnershipforcaring.org.

In addition to documenting patient preferences for care, the Durable Power of Attorney for Health Care (DPOA-HC) allows the patient to designate a surrogate decision-maker. The DPOA-HC is important since it is often difficult to anticipate what decisions will need to be made. The responsibility of the surrogate is to provide "substituted judgment"—to decide as the *patient* would, not as the *surrogate* wants. In the absence of a designated surrogate, clinicians turn to family members or next of kin under the assumption that they know the patient's wishes. Unfortunately, surveys demonstrate that clinicians and families often are no better than chance at predicting patient wishes, so it is imperative to have these discussions with all patients.

Clinicians should educate all patients—ideally, well before the end of life—about the opportunity to formulate an advance directive. Research shows that most patients have already thought about end-of-life issues, want to discuss these issues with their clinician, want the clinician to bring up the subject, and feel better for having had the discussion. Chart reminders to clinicians can increase the frequency of advance directive completions. It is especially important during discussions about end-of-life care that clinicians reassure patients about the ability to control pain and other symptoms and make an explicit pledge not to abandon the patient. Despite regulations requiring clinicians to inform patients of their rights to formulate an advance directive, only about 10% of people in the United States (including clinicians themselves) actually have executed advance directives, and studies have shown that clinicians are often unaware of or actually ignore their patients' advance directives.

DNAR ORDERS

Clinicians can encourage patients to express their preferences for the use of CPR. Unfortunately, most patients and many clinicians are uninformed or misinformed about the nature and success of CPR. Despite the favorable portrayal of CPR in the popular media, only about 15% of all patients who undergo CPR in the hospital survive to hospital discharge. Moreover, among certain populations of patients—especially those with systemic noncardiac disease—the likelihood of survival to hospital discharge following CPR may be nil or extremely slight (Table 5–3).

Patients may ask their clinician to write an order that CPR not be attempted on them. Although this order initially was referred to as a DNR ("do not resuscitate") order, many clinicians now prefer the term DNAR ("do not attempt resuscitation") to emphasize the low likelihood of successful resuscitation.

Table 5–3. Survival to hospital discharge following cardiopulmonary resuscitation of patients with various underlying diseases.[1]

Conditions with highest survival rates:	
Ventricular fibrillation post-MI	26–46%
Drug reaction or overdose	22–28%
Ventricular arrhythmia	19–50%
Conditions with lowest survival rates:	
Malignancy[2]	0–3.5%
Neurologic disease	0–6.7%
Renal failure	0–10%
Respiratory disease	0–7%
Sepsis	0–7%
Nursing home residence	0–1.7%
Out-of-hospital cardiopulmonary arrest[3]	0.6%

[1]Modified, with permission, from Moss AH: Informing the patient about cardiopulmonary resuscitation: When the risks outweigh the benefits. J Gen Intern Med 1989;4:349.

[2]Survival was 0% in patients with metastatic disease in the first nine studies reported.

[3]If return of spontaneous circulation was not obtained after 25 minutes of standard advanced cardiac life support out-of-hospital.

In addition to mortality statistics, patients deciding about CPR preferences should also be informed about the possible consequences of surviving a CPR attempt. CPR may result in fractured ribs, lacerated internal organs, and neurologic disability, and there is a high likelihood of requiring other aggressive interventions, such as ICU care, if CPR is successful.

For some patients at the end of life, decisions about CPR may be not about whether they will live but about how they will die. Clinicians should correct the misconception that withholding CPR in appropriate circumstances is tantamount to "not doing everything" or "just letting someone die." Frequently, CPR will not improve the quality of a dying patient's life or alter the patient's underlying prognosis. While respecting the patient's right ultimately to make the decision—and keeping in mind their own biases and prejudices—clinicians should offer explicit recommendations about DNAR orders and in that way protect dying patients and their families from feelings of guilt and from the sorrow associated with vain hopes. Finally, clinicians should encourage patients and their families to make proactive decisions about what is wanted in end-of-life care rather than focusing only on what is not to be done.

HOSPICE & OTHER PALLIATIVE CARE INSTITUTIONS

While most patients die in hospitals and long-term care facilities, good care of the dying may not be the central goal of most hospitals and nursing homes. Only a minority of United States hospitals currently have formal palliative care programs. Hospice is an approach to care where the most urgent objective is to provide a caring environment for meeting the physical and emotional needs of the terminally ill. Hospice care focuses on the patient and family rather than the disease and on providing comfort and pain relief rather than on treating illness or prolonging life. Hospices provide intensive caring with the goal of helping people live well until they die.

The hospice philosophy emphasizes individualized attention, human contact, and an interdisciplinary team approach involving clinicians, nurses, health aides, social workers, psychologists, therapists (physical, occupational, recreational), dietitians, chaplains, and volunteers. Hospice care can include arranging for respite for family caregivers and providing legal, financial, and other services. While some hospice care is provided in hospitals and institutional residences, about 80% of patients receiving hospice care remain at home where they can be cared for by the family and visiting hospice staff. Primary care clinicians are strongly encouraged to continue caring for their patients during the time they are receiving hospice care.

Hospice care has been shown to increase patient satisfaction, to ease family anxiety, and even to reduce costs depending on when patients are referred to hospice care. While hospice care may be the appropriate standard of care for the dying, only about 25% of all patients who die receive hospice care, and 63% of these people have end-stage cancer. Hospice care tends to be utilized late in the course of the end of life. The average length of stay in hospices in the United States is just 36 days, with 15% of patients dying within 7 days after beginning hospice care.

Most hospice organizations require clinicians to estimate the patient's probability of survival to be less than 6 months, since this is a criterion for eligibility to receive Medicare coverage (a benefit available since 1982). Unfortunately, as currently structured, the hospice benefit tends to be unavailable to people who are homeless, isolated, or with terminal prognoses that are difficult to quantify.

Many of the goals of hospice care, such as relief of suffering and attention to the patient as a person, are relevant to curative medical care. However, the emphasis on patient well-being rather than on cure, the direct acknowledgment of death and dying issues, and the effort to care for people in their homes make hospice an important alternative to acute hospital care at the end of life. While the initiation of hospice care is often described as a transition from aggressive care to comfort care, hospice care also provides "aggressive" care, though not directed at achieving a cure. It is more appropriate to consider hospice care as one among many health care resources available to patients at the end of life. For the dying, it may be appropriate to "treat" pneumonia with morphine and antipyretics rather than with antibiotics. Helping patients decide when to avail themselves of the resources of hospice care is an important function even for clinicians providing the most aggressive and intensive curative medical interventions.

CULTURAL ISSUES

The individual's experience of dying occurs in the context of a complex interaction of personal, philosophic, and cultural influences. Various religious, ethnic, gender, class, and cultural traditions inform patients' styles of communication, comfort in discussing particular topics, expectations about dying and medical interventions, and attitudes about the appropriate disposition of dead bodies. Studies have shown differences in knowledge and beliefs regarding advance directives, autopsy, organ donation, hospice care, and withdrawal of support among patients of different ethnic groups. While each patient must be considered an individual, understanding cultural assumptions and beliefs and respecting ethnic traditions are important responsibilities of the clinician caring for a patient at the end of life, especially when the cultures of origin of the clinician and patient differ.

Council on Ethical and Judicial Affairs: Medical futility in end-of-life care. JAMA 1999;281:937. [PMID 10078492]

Ebell MH et al: Survival after in-hospital cardiopulmonary resuscitation: a meta-analysis. J Gen Intern Med 1998;13:805. [PMID: 9844078]

Kagawa-Singer M et al: Perspectives on care at the close of life. Negotiating cross-cultural issues at the end of life: "You got to go where he lives." JAMA 2001;286:2993. [PMID: 11743841]

Mebane EW et al: The influence of physician race, age, and gender on physician attitudes toward advance care directives and preferences for end-of-life decision-making. J Am Geriatr Soc 1999;47:579. [PMID: 10323652]

Pan CX et al: How prevalent are hospital-based palliative care programs? Status report and future directions. J Palliat Med 2001;4:315. [PMID: 11596542] (Thirty-six percent of hospitals report having a pain management service, and 15% have an end-of-life care service.)

■ MANAGEMENT OF PAIN & OTHER COMMON SYMPTOMS

For patients at the end of life, maximizing the quality of life—rather than postponing death—is the first priority of care. In this context, symptoms that cause disability and suffering must be considered medical emergencies and managed aggressively by frequent elicitation, continuous reassessment, and individualized treatment. While patients at the end of life may experience a host of bothersome symptoms, pain, dyspnea, and delirium are reported to be among the most feared and burdensome. The palliative care of pain and a selected number of other common symptoms is described below. Throughout, the principles of good end-of-life care dictate that comfort is the main focus of palliative care and that properly informed patients or their surrogates may decide to pursue aggressive symptom relief even if, as a known but unintended consequence, the treatments hasten demise.

PAIN AT THE END OF LIFE

Definition & Prevalence

Pain is a common problem for patients at the end of life—up to 75% of patients dying of cancer experience pain—and it is what many people say they fear most about dying. Pain is a common complaint among patients with noncancer diagnoses as well. Pain is undertreated at the end of life. One study has documented that 50% of severely ill hospitalized patients spent half of their time during the last 3 days of life in moderate to severe pain. The Joint Commission on Accreditation of Healthcare Organizations (JCAHO) has recently promulgated new pain management standards for all patient care organizations accredited by JCAHO.

The experience of pain also includes the patient's emotional reaction to it. The experience of pain is influenced by many factors, including the patient's prior experiences with pain, the meaning of the pain, emotional stresses, and the influence of family and culture. Pain is a subjective phenomenon, and clinicians cannot reliably detect its existence or quantify its severity without asking the patient directly. A useful means of assessing pain and evaluating the effectiveness of analgesia is to ask the patient to rate the degree of pain along a numerical or visual pain scale (Table 5–4).

Barriers to Good Care

Poor management of pain at the end of life has been documented in many settings. Some clinicians refer pain management to others when they believe that a patient's pain is not due to the disease for which they are treating the patient. Studies have shown, however, that oncologists often misperceive the origin of their patients' pain and inappropriately ignore complaints of pain.

Many clinicians have received little formal training in and have limited clinical experience with pain management and thus are understandably reluctant to attempt to manage severe pain. Lack of knowledge about the proper selection and dosing of analgesic medications carries with it attendant and typically exaggerated fears about the side effects of pain medications, including the possibility of respiratory depression with an overdose of opioids. Most clinicians, however, can develop good pain management skills, and nearly all pain, even at the end of life, can be managed without hastening death through respiratory depression.

Fears of the physiologic effects of opioids are often coupled with fears on the part of clinician, patient, or family that patients will become addicted to opioid pain medications. While physiologic **tolerance** (requiring increasing dosage to achieve the same analgesic effect) and **dependence** (requiring continued dosing to prevent symptoms of medication withdrawal) are expected with opioid use, at the end of life the use of opioids for relief of pain and dyspnea is not associated with a risk of psychologic **addiction** (misuse of a substance for purposes other than one for which it was prescribed and despite negative consequences in health, employment, or legal and social spheres). Even patients who demonstrate some of the behaviors sometimes associated with addiction (demand for specific medications and doses, anger and irritability, poor cooperation or disturbed interpersonal reactions) may in fact not be addicted. The term **pseudo-addiction** has been used when patients exhibit behaviors associated with addiction but only because their pain is inadequately treated. Once they achieve pain relief, these behaviors cease. In all cases, clinicians must be willing to use appropriate doses of opioids in order to relieve distressing symptoms for patients at the end of life.

Finally, some clinicians fear legal repercussions from prescribing the high doses of opioids sometimes

Table 5–4. Pain assessment scales.

A. Numeric Rating Scale

No pain   Worst pain

1   2   3   4   5   6   7   8   9   10

B. Numeric Rating Scale Translated into Word and Behavior Scales

Pain intensity	Word scale	Nonverbal behaviors
0	No pain	Relaxed, calm expression
1–2	Least pain	Stressed, tense expression
3–4	Mild pain	Guarded movement, grimacing
5–6	Moderate pain	Moaning, restless
7–8	Severe pain	Crying out
9–10	Excruciating pain	Increased intensity of above

C. Wong Baker FACES Pain Rating Scale[1]

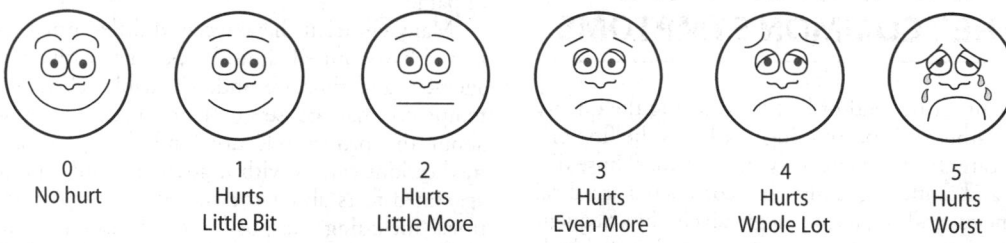

0	1	2	3	4	5
No hurt	Hurts Little Bit	Hurts Little More	Hurts Even More	Hurts Whole Lot	Hurts Worst

[1]Especially useful for patients who cannot read English and for pediatric patients. Wong DL, Hockenberry-Eaton M, Wilson D, Winkelstein ML, Ahmann E, DeVito-Thomas PA: *Whaley and Wong's Nursing Care of Infants and Children,* ed. 6. St. Louis, 1999, Mosby p. 1153. Copyrighted by Mosby-Year Book, Inc. Reprinted by permission.

necessary to control pain at the end of life. Some states have enacted special licensing and documentation requirements for opioid prescribing. However, governmental and professional medical groups and regulators are making it clear that appropriate treatment of pain is a fundamental responsibility of the clinician. While some clinicians nevertheless remain apprehensive about the legal implications of overtreatment, clinicians have recently been successfully sued for undertreatment of pain. Although clinicians may feel trapped between fears about over- or underprescribing opioids, there remains a wide range of practice in which clinicians can appropriately treat pain.

Principles of Pain Management

General guidelines for management of pain are recommended for the treatment of all patients with pain (see Table 5–5). Because pain is so common at the end of life, all patients should be asked about its presence. Clinicians should ask about the nature, severity, timing, location, quality, and aggravating and relieving factors of the pain. The goal of pain management is properly decided by the patient. While some patients may wish to be completely free of pain even at the cost of significant sedation, most will wish to control pain at a level that still allows maximal functioning. Careful attention to pain relief and perseverance in achieving

Table 5–5. Recommended clinical approach to pain management.[1]

Ask about pain regularly. Assess pain systematically (quality, description, location, intensity or severity, aggravating and ameliorating factors, cognitive responses). Ask about goals for pain control, management preferences.

Believe the patient and family in their reports of pain and what relieves it.

Choose pain control options appropriate for the patient, family, and setting. Consider drug type, dosage, route, contraindications, side effects. Consider nonpharmacologic adjunctive measures.

Deliver interventions in a timely, logical, coordinated manner.

Empower patients and their families. Enable patients to control their course to the greatest extent possible.

Follow up to reassess persistence of pain, changes in pain pattern, development of new pain.

[1]Modified, with permission, from Jacox AK et al: *Management of Cancer Pain: Quick Reference Guide No. 9.* AHCPR Publication No. 94–0593. Rockville, MD: Agency for Health Care Policy and Research, Public Health Service, U.S. Department of Health and Human Services. March 1994.

it are indicated for all patients. Hospice clinicians regularly report a success rate higher than 90% in relieving pain in terminally ill patients.

Chronic severe pain should be treated around the clock. For ongoing pain, one can give a long-acting analgesic around the clock plus a short-acting agent as needed for "breakthrough" pain. At the end of life, the oral route of administration is preferred because it is easier to administer at home, is not painful, and imposes no risk from needle exposure. Rectal, transdermal, and subcutaneous administration are also frequently used, as is intravenous administration when necessary. Patient-controlled analgesia (PCA) of intravenous medications is appreciated by patients, may lead to less medication use, and has been adapted for use with oral administration.

Frequent reassessment of pain is essential. Regular communication with patients—and often their families—is necessary to establish goals of care, maintain current records of pain descriptions and levels, and ensure effectiveness of treatment.

When possible, the cause of pain should be diagnosed and treated, assuming that the burden of these efforts does not increase the patient's suffering. Removing the underlying cause of pain can preempt the need for ongoing treatment with analgesic medications along with their side effects. Regardless of decisions about seeking and treating the underlying cause of pain, however, prompt symptomatic relief of pain should be offered to every patient.

Pharmacologic Pain Management Strategies

Typically, pain can be well controlled with analgesic medications—both opioid and nonopioid. The Agency for Healthcare Research and Quality has published useful guidelines for the treatment of both acute and cancer pain. For mild to moderate pain, acetaminophen, aspirin, and nonsteroidal anti-inflammatory drugs (NSAIDs) may be sufficient. For moderate to severe pain, analgesics that include those agents combined with opioids may be helpful. Severe pain typically requires pure opioid agonists.

A. ACETAMINOPHEN AND NSAIDS

Appropriate doses of acetaminophen may be just as effective as an analgesic and antipyretic as NSAIDs but without anti-inflammatory effects and without the risk of gastrointestinal bleeding or ulceration. Acetaminophen can be given at a dosage of 500–1000 mg orally every 6 hours, though it can be taken every 4 hours as long as the risk of hepatotoxicity is kept in mind. Hepatotoxicity is a concern at doses greater than 4 g/d chronically, and doses for elderly patients and those with liver disease generally should not exceed 2 g/d.

Aspirin (325–650 mg orally every 4 hours) is an effective analgesic, antipyretic, and anti-inflammatory medication. Gastrointestinal irritation and bleeding, bleeding from other sources, allergy, and an association with Reye's syndrome in children and teenagers limit its use.

Commonly used NSAIDS and their dosages are listed in Table 5–6. Like aspirin, the other NSAIDs are antipyretic, analgesic, and anti-inflammatory. NSAIDs inhibit prostaglandin synthesis, inhibiting platelet aggregation and consequently increasing the risk of gastrointestinal bleeding by 1.5 times normal. The risks of bleeding and nephrotoxicity from NSAIDs are both increased in the elderly. Gastrointestinal bleeding and ulceration may be decreased with the concurrent use of proton pump inhibitors (eg, omeprazole, 20–40 mg orally daily) or with the new class of NSAIDs that inhibit only cyclooxygenase-2. COX-2 inhibitors include celecoxib (100 mg/d to 200 mg twice daily orally) and rofecoxib (12.5–50 mg/d orally). The NSAIDs, including COX-2 inhibitors, can lead to exacerbations of congestive heart failure and should be used with caution in patients with that disorder.

B. OPIOID MEDICATIONS

For many patients at the end of life, opioids are the mainstay of pain management. Opioids are appropriate for severe pain due to any cause. Opioid medications are listed in Table 5–7. Full opioid agonists such as morphine, hydromorphone, oxycodone, methadone, fentanyl, hydrocodone, and codeine are used most commonly. Hydrocodone and codeine are typically combined with acetaminophen or an NSAID. Short-acting formulations of oral morphine sulfate (starting dosage 4 mg orally every 3–4 hours), hydromorphone (1 mg orally every 3–4 hours), or oxycodone (5 mg orally every 3–4 hours) are useful for acute pain and as rescue treatment for patients experiencing pain that breaks through long-acting medications. For chronic stable pain, one should give sustained-release morphine (two or three times a day) or oxycodone (two or three times a day), methadone (three or four times a day), and transdermal fentanyl (starting dose 25 μg every 3 days, with 24–40 hours required to achieve full analgesia).

Meperidine is not useful for chronic pain because it has a short half-life and a toxic metabolite that can cause irritability and seizures. Partial agonists such as buprenorphine are limited by a dose-related ceiling effect. Mixed agonist-antagonists such as pentazocine and butorphanol tartrate also have a ceiling effect and are contraindicated in patients already receiving full agonist opioids since they may reverse the pain control achieved by the full agonist and cause a withdrawal effect.

A useful technique for opioid management of chronic pain at the end of life is **equianalgesic dosing**. The dosages of any full opioid agonists used to control pain can be translated into an equivalent dose of any other opioid. In this way, 24-hour opioid requirements and dosing regimens established initially using shorter-acting opioid medications can be

Table 5–6. Useful nonsteroidal anti-inflammatory drugs.[1]

Drug	Usual Dose for Adults ≥ 50 kg	Usual Dose for Adults < 50 kg[2]	Cost per Unit	Cost for 30 Days[3]	Comments[4]
Acetaminophen[5] (Tylenol, Datril, etc)	650 mg q4h or 975 mg q6h	10–15 mg/kg q4h (oral); 15–20 mg/kg q4h (rectal)	$0.04/325 mg (oral) OTC $0.50/325 mg (rectal) OTC	$14.40 (oral) $180.00 (rectal)	Not an NSAID because it lacks peripheral anti-inflammatory effects. Equivalent to aspirin as analgesic and antipyretic agent.
Aspirin[6]	650 mg q4h or 975 mg q6h	10–15 mg/kg q4h (oral); 15–20 mg/kg q4h (rectal)	$0.02/325 mg OTC $0.17/300 mg (rectal) OTC	$7.20 (oral) $61.20 (rectal)	Available also in enteric-coated form that is more expensive and more slowly absorbed but better tolerated.
Celecoxib[5] (Celebrex)	200 mg qd (osteoarthritis), 100–200 mg bid (rheumatoid arthritis)	100 mg qd–bid	$1.58/100 mg $2.64/200 mg	$79.20 OA; $158.40 RA	Cyclooxygenase 2 inhibitors. No antiplatelet effects. Lower doses for elderly who weigh < 50 kg. Lower incidence of endoscopic gastrointestinal ulceration. Not known if true lower incidence of gastrointestinal bleeding. Celecoxib contraindicated in sulfonamide allergy.
Valdecoxib (Bextra)	10 mg qd for OA or RA	10 mg qd	$2.92/10 mg or 20 mg	$87.60	
Rofecoxib[5] (Vioxx)	12.5–25 mg qd for OA	12.5 mg qd	$2.64/12.5 mg $2.64/25 mg	$79.20 OA	
Choline magnesium salicylate[7] (Trilasate)	1000–1500 mg tid	25 mg/kg tid	$0.57/500 mg	$153.90	Salicylates cause less gastro-intestinal distress and renal impairment than NSAIDs but are probably less effective in pain management than NSAIDs.
Choline salicylate[7] (Arthropan)	870 mg q3–4h		$48.93/480 mL; 174 mg/mL OTC	$98.00	Minimal antiplatelet effects.
Diclofenac (Voltaren, Cataflam, others)	50–75 mg bid–tid		$0.91/50 mg, $1.06/75 mg	$81.90 $95.40	May impose higher risk of hepatotoxicity. Low incidence of gastrointestinal side effects. Enteric-coated product, slow onset.
Diclofenac Sustained Release (Voltaren-XR)	100–200 mg qd		$3.60/100 mg	$216.00	
Diflunisal[8] (Dolobid)	500 mg q12h		$0.97/500 mg	$58.20	Fluorinated acetylsalicylic acid derivative.
Etodolac (Lodine)	200–400 mg q6–8h		$1.26/300 mg	$151.20	Perhaps less gastrointestinal toxicity.
Fenoprofen calcium (Nalfon)	300–600 mg q6h		$0.47/300 mg or 600 mg	$56.40	Perhaps more side effects than others, including tubulointersti-tial nephritis.
Flurbiprofen (Ansaid)	50–100 mg tid–qid		$0.77/50 mg, $1.08/100 mg	$92.40 $97.20	Adverse gastrointestinal effects may be more common among elderly.

(continued)

Table 5–6. Useful nonsteroidal anti-inflammatory drugs.[1] (continued)

Drug	Usual Dose for Adults ≥ 50 kg	Usual Dose for Adults < 50 kg[2]	Cost per Unit	Cost for 30 Days[3]	Comments[4]
Ibuprofen (Motrin, Advil, Rufen, others)	400–800 mg q6h	10 mg/kg q6–8h	$0.20/400 mg Rx $0.28/600 mg Rx $0.05/200 mg OTC	$48.00 $33.60 $9.00	Relatively well tolerated. Less gastrointestinal toxicity.
Indomethacin (Indocin, Indometh, others)	25–50 mg bid–qid		$0.37/25 mg; $0.63/50 mg	$44.40 $75.60	Higher incidence of dose-related toxic effects, especially gastro-intestinal and bone marrow effects.
Ketoprofen (Orudis, Oruvail, others)	25–50 mg q6–8h (max 300 mg/d)		$0.96/50 mg Rx $1.07/75 mg Rx $0.10/12.5 mg OTC	$172.80 $128.40 $18.00	Lower doses for elderly.
Ketorolac tro-methamine (Toradol)	10 mg q4–6h to a maximum of 40 mg/d PO		$0.93/10 mg	Not recom-mended	Short-term use (< 5 days) only; otherwise, increased risk of gastrointestinal side effects.
Ketorolac tro-methamine[9] (Toradol)	60 mg initially, then 30 mg q6h IM		$7.40/30 mg	Not recom-mended	Intramuscular NSAID as alterna-tive to opioid. Lower doses for elderly. Short-term use (< 5 days) only.
Magnesium salicylate (various)	650 mg q4h		$0.17/325 mg OTC	$40.80	
Meclofenamate sodium[10] (Meclomen)	50–100 mg q6h		$3.40/100 mg	$408.00	Diarrhea more common.
Mefenamic acid (Ponstel)	250 mg q6h		$1.34/250 mg	$160.80	
Nabumetone (Relafen)	500–1000 mg once daily (max dose 2000 mg/d)		$1.30/500 mg $1.53/750 mg	$137.70	May be less ulcerogenic than ibuprofen, but overall side effects may not be less.
Naproxen (Naprosyn, Anaprox, Aleve [OTC], others)	200–500 mg q6–8h	5 mg/kg q8h	$1.16/500 mg Rx $0.10/220 mg OTC	$104.40 $9.00 OTC	Generally well tolerated. Lower doses for elderly.
Oxaprozin (Daypro)	600–1200 mg once daily		$1.51/600 mg	$90.60	Similar to ibuprofen. May cause rash, pruritus, photosensitivity.
Piroxicam (Feldene)	20 mg daily		$2.64/20 mg	$79.20	Single daily dose convenient. Long half-life. May cause higher rate of gastrointestinal bleeding and dermatologic side effects.
Sodium salicylate	325–650 q3–4h		$0.06/650 mg OTC	$14.40	

(continued)

Table 5–6. Useful nonsteroidal anti-inflammatory drugs.[1] (continued)

Drug	Usual Dose for Adults ≥ 50 kg	Usual Dose for Adults < 50 kg[2]	Cost per Unit	Cost for 30 Days[3]	Comments[4]
Sulindac (Clinoril)	150–200 mg bid		$0.98/150 mg; $1.21/200 mg	$58.80 $72.60	May cause higher rate of gastrointestinal bleeding. May have less nephrotoxic potential.
Tolmetin (Tolectin)	200–600 mg qid		$0.65/200 mg; $1.30/600 mg	$78.00 $156.00	Perhaps more side effects than others, including anaphylactic reactions.

OTC = over-the-counter; Rx = prescription; OA = osteoarthritis; RA = rheumatoid arthritis.

[1]Modified from Jacox AK et al: Management of Cancer Pain: Quick Reference Guide for Clinicians No. 9. AHCPR Publication No. 94–0593. Rockville, MD: Agency for Health Care Policy and Research, Public Health Service, U.S. Department of Health and Human Services. March 1994.

[2]Acetaminophen and NSAID dosages for adults weighing less than 50 kg should be adjusted for weight.

[3]Cost to pharmacist (average wholesale price, generic when possible) for quantity listed. Source: *Drug Topics Red Book,* March 2002; Vol. 21, No. 3.

[4]The adverse effects of headache, tinnitus, dizziness, confusion, rashes, anorexia, nausea, vomiting, gastrointestinal bleeding, diarrhea, nephrotoxicity, visual disturbances, etc, can occur with any of these drugs. Tolerance and efficacy are subject to great individual variations among patients. Note: All NSAIDs can increase serum lithium levels.

[5]Acetaminophen, celecoxib, rofecoxib, and valdecoxib lack the antiplatelet activities of other NSAIDs.

[6]May inhibit platelet aggregation for 1 week or more and may cause bleeding.

[7]May have minimal antiplatelet activity.

[8]Administration with antacids may decrease absorption.

[9]Has the same gastrointestinal toxicities as oral NSAIDs.

[10]Coombs-positive autoimmune hemolytic anemia has been associated with prolonged use.

translated into equivalent dosages of longer-acting medications or formulations. Cross-tolerance is often incomplete, however, so less than the full calculated equianalgesic dosage is generally administered initially when switching between opioid formulations.

While some clinicians and patients inexperienced with the management of severe chronic pain may feel more comfortable with combined nonopioid-opioid agents because of the toxicities of acetaminophen and NSAIDS at higher doses, full agonist opioids provide more flexibility in dosing and the dose may be increased as required for more effective analgesia. There is no maximal allowable or effective dose for full opioid agonists. The dose should be increased to whatever is necessary to relieve pain, remembering that certain types of pain may respond better to agents other than opioids.

While physiologic tolerance is possible with opioids, failure of a previously effective opioid dose to adequately relieve pain is almost certainly due to an increase in the underlying pain. In this case, for moderate pain, the dosage of opioid can be increased by 25–50%. For severe pain, a dosage increase of 50–100% may be appropriate. The frequency of dosing should be adjusted so that pain control is continuous. In addition, chronic dosing may be adjusted by adding the amount of short-acting opioid necessary for breakthrough pain over the preceding 24 hours to the long-acting medication dose. In establishing or reestablishing adequate dosing, frequent reassessment

of the patient's pain and medication side effects is necessary.

As dosages of opioids are increased, increasing difficulty with the side effects of opioids is to be expected. Constipation is a common side effect that should be anticipated and prevented in all patients. The prophylaxis and management of opioid-induced constipation are outlined below.

Sedation can be expected with opioids, though tolerance to the sedative effects typically develops within 24–72 hours at a stable dose. Sedation typically appears well before significant respiratory depression. If treatment for sedation is desired, dextroamphetamine (2.5–7.5 mg orally at 8 AM and noon) or methylphenidate (2.5–10 mg orally at 8 AM and noon) may be helpful. Some patients even use caffeinated beverages to help manage minor opioid sedation.

Although sedation is more common, patients may experience euphoria when first taking opioids or when the dosage is increased. However, patients generally develop tolerance to this effect after a few days at a stable dose. At higher doses of opioids, patients may develop multifocal myoclonus. This symptom will typically resolve after lowering the dose or switching opioids. While waiting for the level of the offending medication to fall, low doses of clonazepam or dantrolene may be helpful for treating myoclonus.

Nausea due to opioids may occur with initiation of therapy and resolve after a few days. If it is severe or persistent, it can be treated with prochlorperazine,

Table 5–7. Useful opioid agonist analgesics.[1]

Drug	Approximate Equianalgesic Dose[2]		Usual Starting Dose				Potential Advantages	Potential Disadvantages
			Adults ≥ 50 kg Body Weight		Adults < 50 kg Body Weight			
	Oral	Parenteral	Oral	Parenteral	Oral	Parenteral		
OPIOID AGONISTS[3]								
Morphine[4]	30 mg q3–4h (repeat around-the-clock dosing); 60 mg q3–4h (single or intermittent dosing)	10 mg q3–4h	30 mg q3–4h $0.18/15 mg	10 mg q3–4h $0.65/10 mg	0.3 mg/kg q3–4h	0.1 mg/kg q3–4h	Standard of comparison; multiple dosage forms available.	No unique problems when compared with other opioids.
Morphine controlled-release[4] (MS Contin, Roxanol, Oramorph)	90–120 mg q12h	Not available	90–120 mg q12h $1.69/30 mg	Not available	Not available	Not available		
Hydromorphone[4] (Dilaudid)	7.5 mg q3–4h	1.5 mg q3–4h	2 mg q 3–4h $0.37/2 mg	1.5 mg q3–4h $1.04/2 mg	0.06 mg/kg q3–4h	0.015 mg/kg q3–4h	Similar to morphine. Available in injectable high-potency preparation, rectal suppository.	Short duration.
Levorphanol (Levo Dromoran)	4 mg q6–8h	2 mg q6–8h	4 mg q6–8h $0.87/2 mg	2 mg q6–8h $3.96/2 mg	0.04 mg/kg q6–8h	0.02 mg q6–8h	Longer-acting than morphine sulfate.	
Meperidine[5] (Demerol)	300 mg q2–3h; normal dose 50–150 mg q3–4h	100 mg q3h $0.68/50	Not recommended $0.68/50 mg	100 mg q3h $1.09/100 mg	Not recommended	0.75 mg/kg q2–3h	May be useful for acute pain if the patient is intolerant to morphine.	Short duration. Metabolite in high concentrations may cause seizures.
Methadone (Dolophine, others)	20 mg q6–8h	10 mg q6–8h	20 mg q6–8h $0.15/10 mg	10 mg q6–8h $.80/10 mg	0.2 mg/kg q6–8h	0.1 mg/kg q6–8h	Somewhat longer-acting than morphine. Useful in cases of intolerance to morphine.	Analgesic duration shorter than plasma duration. May accumulate, requiring close monitoring during first weeks of treatment.
Oxymorphone[3] (Numorphan)	Not available	1 mg q3–4h	Not available	1 mg q3–4h $2.95/1 mg				
Codeine [6,7] (with aspirin or acetaminophen)[8]	180–200 mg q3–4h; normal dose, 15–60 mg q4–6h	130 mg q3–4h	60 mg q4–6h $0.46/60 mg	30 mg q4–6h $1.26/30 mg	0.5–1 mg/kg q4–6h	Not recommended	Similar to morphine.	

(continued)

Table 5–7. Useful opioid agonist analgesics.[1] (continued)

Drug	Approximate Equianalgesic Dose[2]		Usual Starting Dose				Potential Advantages	Potential Disadvantages
			Adults ≥ 50 kg Body Weight		Adults < 50 kg Body Weight			
	Oral	Parenteral	Oral	Parenteral	Oral	Parenteral		
COMBINATION OPIOID-NSAID OR ANTIDEPRESSANT PREPARATIONS								
Hydrocodone[6] (in Lorcet, Lortab, Vicodin, others)[8]	30 mg q3–4h	Not available	10 mg q3–4h $0.39/ 5 mg	Not available	0.2 mg/kg q3–4h	Not available		Combination with acetaminophen limits dosage titration.
Oxycodone[6] (Roxicodone, Percocet, Percodan, Tylox, others)[8]	30 mg q3–4h	Not available	10 mg q3–4h $0.26/ 5 mg	Not available	0.2 mg/kg q3–4h	Not available	Similar to morphine.	Combination with acetaminophen and aspirin limits dosage titration.
Oxycodone Controlled Release (Oxycontin)	40 mg q12h	Not available	20–40 mg q12h $2.47/ 20 mg					
Tramadol (Ultram)		Not available	50–100 mg q4–6h $0.81/50 mg $194.00 maximum dose 400 mg/d	Not available	50–100 mg q4–6h maximum dose; 300 mg maximum dose for patients over 75 years of age	Not available	Novel agent. Both opioid and non-opioid (inhibits reuptake of norepinephrine and serotonin)	Withdrawal may occur if abruptly discontinued. Must reduce dose in elderly (age > 75); increase dosing interval in renal insufficiency.

[1]Modified from Jacox AK et al: Management of Cancer Pain: Quick Reference Guide for Clinicians No. 9. AHCPR Publication No. 94–0593. Rockville, MD. Agency for Health Care Policy and Research, Public Health Service, U.S. Department of Health and Human Services. March 1994. Reproduced in part from Hosp Formul 1994;29(8 Part 2):586. (Erstad BL: A rational approach to the management of acute pain states.) Copyright by Advanstar Communications, Inc.

[2]Published tables vary in the suggested doses that are equianalgesic to morphine. Clinical response is the criterion that must be applied for each patient; titration to clinical efficacy is necessary. Because there is not complete cross-tolerance among these drugs, it is usually necessary to use a lower than equianalgesic dose initially when changing drugs and to retitrate to response.

[3]*Caution:* Recommended doses do not apply for adult patients with renal or hepatic insufficiency or other conditions affecting drug metabolism.

[4]*Caution:* For morphine, hydromorphone, and oxymorphone, rectal administration is an alternative route for patients unable to take oral medications. Equianalgesic doses may differ from oral and parenteral doses. A short-acting opioid should normally be used for initial therapy.

[5]Not recommended for chronic pain. Doses listed are for brief therapy of acute pain only. Switch to another opioid for long-term therapy.

[6]*Caution:* Doses of aspirin and acetaminophen in combination products must also be adjusted to the patient's body weight (Table 5–6).

[7]*Caution:* Doses of codeine above 60 mg often are not appropriate because of diminishing incremental analgesia with increasing doses but continually increasing nausea, constipation, and other side effects.

[8]*Caution:* Monitor total acetaminophen dose carefully, including any OTC use. Total acetaminophen dose maximum 4 g/d. If liver impairment or heavy alcohol use, maximum is 2 g/d.

Note: Cost to pharmacist (average wholesale price, generic when possible) for quantity listed. Source: *Drug Topics Red Book,* March 2002; Vol. 21, No. 3.

10 mg orally or intravenously every 8 hours or 25 mg rectally every 6 hours.

Although clinicians may worry about respiratory depression with opioids, that effect is uncommon when a low dose is given initially and titrated upward very slowly. Even patients with pulmonary disease can tolerate low-dose opioids, though they should be monitored carefully. Clinicians should not allow concerns about respiratory depression to prevent them from treating pain adequately.

True allergy (with urticaria) to opioids is rare. More commonly, patients will describe an intolerance due to side effects such as nausea, pruritus, or urinary retention in response to a particular opioid. If such symptoms develop, they can usually be relieved by lowering the dose or switching to another agent.

C. NEUROPATHIC PAIN

Although many types of pain will respond to opioids, neuropathic pain—which patients typically describe as burning, shooting, "pins and needles," or electricity and which is commonly associated with numbness—may respond better to antidepressants (tricyclic antidepressants [TCAs] in particular) and anticonvulsants like gabapentin, clonazepam, and carbamazepine. (Table 5–8) It is therefore critical to ask the patient to describe the pain and to listen for words that suggest neuropathic pain. The TCAs are a good first choice for neuropathic pain and usually have an effect within days and at lower doses than are needed for an antidepressant effect. Desipramine, 25–150 mg/d orally, and nortriptyline, 25–150 mg/d orally, are good first choices as they cause less orthostatic hypotension and have less anticholinergic effects than amitriptyline. One can start with a low dosage (25 mg orally daily) and titrate upward every 4 or 5 days. Other antidepressant medications such as sustained-release bupropion may also be effective for neuropathic pain; however, the selective serotonin reuptake inhibitors (SSRIs) are not.

The anticonvulsants can be used in the same dosages as are used to prevent seizures. Because carbamazepine can cause bone marrow suppression, it is important to periodically order a complete blood count in patients taking this drug. Gabapentin can cause sedation, dizziness, ataxia, and gastrointestinal side effects and therefore should be started at low dosages of 100–300 mg orally three times a day. The dose of gabapentin can be titrated upward by 300 mg/d every 4 or 5 days to a dosage of 3600 mg/d. Gabapentin is relatively safe in accidental overdosage and may be preferred over TCAs for a patient with a history of congestive heart failure or arrhythmia or if there is a risk of suicide.

The lidocaine patch is effective in postherpetic neuralgia and may be effective in other types of neuropathic pain as well. A new patch is applied to the painful region daily. Mexiletine at a starting dosage of 150 mg orally once or twice a day can also be used for treating neuropathic pain but should be avoided in patients with arrhythmias. The dosage can be increased slowly to a maximum of 300 mg orally three times daily if side effects such as nausea, vomiting, tremor, dizziness, unsteadiness, and paresthesias do not limit dosing. Baclofen can be helpful for treating lancinating or paroxysmal neuropathic pain. Side effects including dizziness, somnolence, and gastrointestinal distress can be mitigated by starting at a low dosage (5 mg orally two or three times daily) and titrating slowly upward to a dosage of 30–90 mg/d. Because abrupt withdrawal from baclofen can cause a syndrome that includes delirium and seizures, the drug should be tapered slowly before being discontinued.

D. ADJUVANT PAIN MEDICATIONS AND TREATMENTS

For bone pain, the anti-inflammatory effects of NSAIDs can be helpful. Radiation therapy can also relieve pain from bone metastases. In many situations, a combination of medications such as NSAIDs, opioids, and TCAs may be needed to relieve pain. For some

Table 5–8. Pharmacologic treatment of neuropathic pain.

Drug[1]	Starting Dose	Typical Dose
Tricyclic antidepressants[2]		
Amitriptyline	25 mg orally at bedtime	10–150 mg orally at bedtime
Nortriptyline	25 mg orally at bedtime	10–150 mg orally at bedtime
Desipramine	25 mg orally at bedtime	10–200 orally at bedtime
Nontricyclic antidepressants		
Sustained-release bupropion	150 mg orally qd	150 mg orally bid
Anticonvulsants		
Carbamazepine[1,3]	100 mg orally bid	200 mg orally bid–qid
Clonazepam[1]	0.5 mg orally tid	0.5–1 mg orally tid
Gabapentin	100–300 mg orally tid	300–1200 mg orally tid

[1]Begin at the starting dose and titrate up every 4 or 5 days.
[2]Begin with a low dose. Pain relief can often be achieved at doses far below antidepressant doses, thereby minimizing adverse side effects.
[3]Periodically monitor blood counts, as drug can cause bone marrow suppression.

patients, such as those with pain from pancreatic cancer, a nerve block—in this case of the celiac plexus—can provide dramatic pain relief. Intrathecal pumps may be useful for patients with severe pain responsive to opioids but who require such large doses that systemic side effects such as sedation and constipation become limiting. Neurolysis, rhizotomy, or ablative surgery and neurosurgery may help selected patients. Despite anecdotal reports, cannabinoids have not been proved to work as analgesics.

Corticosteroids such as dexamethasone or prednisone can be helpful for patients with headache due to increased intracranial pressure, pain from spinal cord compression, metastatic bone pain, and neuropathic pain due to invasion or infiltration of nerves by tumor. Because of the side effects of long-term corticosteroid administration, they are most appropriate in patients with end-stage disease.

Nonpharmacologic Treatments

It is important to bear in mind the benefits and patient satisfaction associated with nonpharmacologic therapies in treating pain. Hot or cold packs, massage, and physical therapy can be helpful for musculoskeletal pain. Similarly, biofeedback, acupuncture, chiropractic, meditation, music therapy, cognitive behavioral therapy, guided imagery, cognitive distraction, and framing may be of help in treating pain. Because mood and psychologic issues play an important role in the patient's perception of and response to pain, psychotherapy, support groups, prayer, and pastoral counseling can also help in the management of pain. Major depression, which may be instigated by chronic pain or may alter the response to pain, should be treated aggressively.

DYSPNEA

Dyspnea is the subjective experience of difficulty in breathing and may be characterized by patients as tightness in the chest, shortness of breath, or a feeling of suffocation. Dyspnea is common among dying patients—up to one-half of severely ill patients may experience severe dyspnea.

Treatment of dyspnea is usually first directed at the underlying cause, which may be related to pneumonia, pulmonary embolism, pleural effusion, bronchospasm, tracheal obstruction, neuromuscular disease, restriction of movement of the chest or abdominal walls, cardiac ischemia, congestive heart failure, superior vena cava syndrome, or severe anemia.

At the end of life, dyspnea is often treated nonspecifically with opioids. Immediate-release morphine, preferably via the oral or buccal route, treats dyspnea effectively and typically at doses lower than would be necessary for the relief of moderate pain. Supplemental oxygen may be useful for the dyspneic patient who is hypoxic and may provide subjective benefit to other dyspneic patients as well. However, a nasal cannula and face mask are sometimes not well tolerated, and fresh air from a window or fan may provide relief. Judicious use of nonpharmacologic relaxation techniques such as meditation and guided imagery may be beneficial for some patients. Anxiolytics may be useful for the anxiety associated with dyspnea but do not appear to act directly to relieve dyspnea.

NAUSEA & VOMITING

Nausea and vomiting are common and distressing symptoms. As with pain, the management of nausea may be maximized by around-the-clock dosing. An understanding of the four major inputs to the vomiting center may help direct treatment. (See Chapter 14.)

The chemoreceptor trigger zone may be stimulated by certain drugs (eg, morphine, NSAIDs), metabolic derangements, and chemotherapeutic agents. Vomiting associated with a particular opioid may be avoided by substitution with an equianalgesic dose of another opioid or a sustained-release formulation. In addition to the other dopamine receptor antagonist antiemetics listed in Table 14–2 that block the trigger zone, haloperidol (0.5–5 mg orally every 4–6 hours) is commonly used. Vomiting associated with chemotherapy may respond to agents such as ondansetron, granisetron, and dolasetron.

Vomiting may be due to stimulation of peripheral afferent nerves from the gut. Offering patients small amounts of food only when they are hungry may prevent nausea and vomiting. Nasogastric suction may provide rapid relief for vomiting associated with constipation, gastroparesis, or gastric outlet obstruction, with the addition of laxatives, prokinetic agents (metoclopramide, 10–20 mg orally or intravenously four times a day), scopolamine (1.5 mg patch every 3 days), and high-dose corticosteroids as more definitive treatment. Treatment with high-dose corticosteroids (eg, dexamethasone, 20 mg orally or intravenously) or cyclizine (5 mg orally every 8 hours) may be useful for nausea and vomiting due to disease of intra-abdominal or pelvic organs.

Increased intracranial pressure may cause vomiting and may be relieved with high-dose corticosteroids or palliative cranial radiation. Vomiting due to disturbance of the vestibular apparatus may be treated with anticholinergic and antihistaminic agents (including diphenhydramine, 25 mg orally or intravenously every 8 hours; or scopolamine, 1.5 mg patch every 3 days).

The beneficial effects of benzodiazepines for vomiting may derive less from any primary antiemetic action than from their sedative and amnestic effects in the setting of anticipatory vomiting, and for that reason they should rarely be used alone for the relief of nausea.

Finally, many patients find dronabinol (2.5–20 mg orally every 4–6 hours) helpful in the management of nausea and vomiting.

CONSTIPATION

Given the frequent use of opioids, poor dietary intake, and physical inactivity, constipation is a common problem among the dying. Clinicians must inquire about any difficulty with hard or infrequent stools. Constipation is an easily treatable cause of discomfort and distress. (See Chapter 14.)

Constipation may be prevented or relieved if patients can increase their activity and their intake of dietary fiber and fluids. Simple considerations such as privacy, undisturbed toilet time, and a bedside commode rather than a bedpan may be important for some patients.

For patients taking opioids, anticipating and preventing constipation is important. A prophylactic bowel regimen of stool softeners (docusate) and stimulants (bisacodyl or senna) should be started when opioid treatment is begun. Lactulose, sorbitol, magnesium citrate, and enemas can be added as needed (Table 14–4).

DELIRIUM & AGITATION

Many terminally ill patients die in a state of delirium—a disturbance of consciousness and a change in cognition that develops over a short time and is manifested by misinterpretations, illusions, hallucinations, disturbances in the sleep-wake cycle (eg, sundowning), psychomotor disturbances (eg, lethargy, restlessness), and mood disturbance (eg, fear, anxiety). Delirium complicated by myoclonus or convulsions at the end of life has been called **terminal restlessness.**

Careful attention to patient safety and nonpharmacologic strategies to help the patient remain oriented (clocks, calendars, a familiar environment, reassurance and redirection from caregivers) may be sufficient to prevent or manage minor delirium. Some delirious patients may be "pleasantly confused," and a decision by the patient's family and the clinician not to treat delirium may be justified.

More commonly, however, delirium at the end of life is distressing to patients and family and requires treatment. Delirium may interfere with the family's ability to feel comforting to the patient and may prevent a patient from being able to recognize and report important symptoms.

While there are many reversible causes of delirium (see Chapter 25), identifying and correcting the underlying cause at the end of life is often simply a question of attention to the choice and dosing of psychoactive medications.

When the cause of delirium cannot be identified, treated, or corrected rapidly enough, delirium may be treated symptomatically with neuroleptics. Haloperidol (1–10 mg orally, subcutaneously, intramuscularly, or intravenously twice or three times a day) is used commonly, but significant extrapyramidal adverse effects may occur. Newer agents such as risperidone (1–3 mg orally twice a day) also may be helpful in delirium.

As an adjunct to the above neuroleptics, especially in the setting of anxiety, benzodiazepines such as lorazepam (0.5–2 mg orally, sublingually, subcutaneously, or intravenously every 4–6 hours) may be useful. When delirium is refractory to treatment and remains intolerable, sedation may be required to provide relief and may be achieved rapidly with midazolam (0.5–5 mg/h subcutaneously or intravenously) or barbiturates.

Allan L et al: Randomised crossover trial of transdermal fentanyl and sustained release oral morphine for treating chronic non-cancer pain. BMJ 2001;322:1154. [PMID: 11348910] (Patients with chronic noncancer pain preferred the transdermal patch delivery system over sustained-release oral morphine.)

Dyspnea. Mechanisms, assessment, and management: a consensus statement. American Thoracic Society. Am J Respir Crit Care Med 1999;159:321. [PMID: 9872857]

Laird MA et al: Use of gabapentin in the treatment of neuropathic pain. Ann Pharmacother 2000;34:802. [PMID: 10860142]

Langman MJ et al: Adverse upper gastrointestinal effects of rofecoxib compared with NSAIDs. JAMA 1999;282:1929. [PMID: 10580458]

Luce JM et al: Perspectives on care at the close of life. Management of dyspnea in patients with far-advanced lung disease "once I lose it, it's kind of hard to catch it. . ." JAMA 2001;285:1331. [PMID: 11255389]

Sellick SM et al: Critical review of 5 nonpharmacologic strategies for managing cancer pain. Cancer Prev Control 1998;2:7. [PMID: 9765761] (Assesses the effectiveness of acupuncture, massage therapy, hypnosis, therapeutic touch, and biofeedback; hypnosis can be efficacious, but evidence is less clear for the other therapies.)

Semenchuk MR et al: Double-blind, randomized trial of bupropion SR for the treatment of neuropathic pain. Neurology 2001;57:1583. [PMID: 11706096] (This nontricyclic antidepressant medication was effective for treatment of neuropathic pain of diverse causes.)

Sharia S et al: Nonsteroidal anti-inflammatory drugs in the management of pain and inflammation: a basis for drug selection. Am J Ther 1999;6:3. [PMID: 10423641]

■ OTHER SPECIFIC TASKS OF CARING

NUTRITION & HYDRATION

Tube feedings do not prevent aspiration pneumonia, and there is scientific debate about whether artificial nutrition prolongs life in the terminally ill. In fact, there has been a growing awareness among hospice clinicians of the potential medical benefits of forgoing unwanted or artificial nutrition and hydration (including tube feedings, parenteral nutrition, and intravenous hydration) at the end of life.

At the end of life, eating without hunger and artificial nutrition are associated with a number of potential complications. Force feeding may cause nausea and vomiting in ill patients, and eating will lead to diarrhea in the setting of malabsorption. Nutrition may increase oral and airway secretions and the risk of choking, aspiration, and dyspnea. Nasogastric and gastrostomy tube feeding and total parenteral nutrition impose risks of infection, epistaxis, pneumothorax, electrolyte imbalance, and aspiration—as well as the need to physically restrain the delirious patient to prevent dislodgment of catheters and tubes.

Withholding nutrition at the end of life causes remarkably little hunger or distress. Ill people often have no hunger with total caloric deprivation, and the associated ketonemia produces a sense of well-being, analgesia, and mild euphoria. However, carbohydrate intake even in small amounts (such as that provided by 5% intravenous dextrose solution) blocks ketone production and may blunt the positive effects of total caloric deprivation.

Withholding hydration may lead to death in a few days to a month. The quality of life for those at the end of life may be adversely affected by supplemental hydration because of its contribution to oral and airway secretions (leading to aspiration or the "death rattle"), polyuria, and the development or worsening of ascites, pleural or other effusions, and peripheral and pulmonary edema.

Although it is unclear to what extent withholding hydration at the end of life creates an uncomfortable sensation of thirst, any such sensation is usually relieved by simply moistening the dry mouth. Ice chips, hard candy, swabs, or a solution of equal parts nystatin solution, viscous lidocaine, diphenhydramine, and minted mouthwash are effective.

Individuals at the end of life have a right to refuse nutrition and hydration. However, providing or withholding oral food and water is not simply a medical decision since doing so may have profound social and cultural significance for patients, families, and clinicians themselves. Withholding supplemental enteral or parenteral nutrition and hydration challenges the assumption that offering food is an expression of compassion and love. In fact, individuals at the end of life who choose to forgo nutrition and hydration are unlikely to suffer from hunger or thirst. Family and friends can be encouraged to express their love and caring in ways other than intrusive attempts at forced feeding or artificial nutrition and hydration.

WITHDRAWAL OF CURATIVE EFFORTS

Requests from appropriately informed and competent patients or their surrogates for withdrawal of interventions intended to prolong life must be respected. The clinician receiving such requests should recognize and explore the significance of this change in health care goals. Alternatively, clinicians may determine unilaterally that further intervention is medically inappropriate—eg, continuing renal dialysis in a patient dying of multi-organ failure. In such cases, the clinician's in-

tention to withdraw a specific intervention should be communicated to the patient and family. If differences of opinion exist about the professional propriety of what is being done, the assistance of an institutional ethics committee should be sought.

Limitation of life support prior to death is an increasingly common practice in intensive care units. The withdrawal of life-sustaining interventions such as mechanical ventilation must be approached carefully to avoid needless patient suffering and distress for those in attendance. Clinicians should educate the patient and family about the expected course of events and the difficulty of determining the precise timing of death after withdrawal of support. Sedative and analgesic agents should be administered to ensure patient comfort even at the risk of respiratory depression or hypotension. Scopolamine (10 μg/h subcutaneously or intravenously, or 15 mg patch every 3 days) or atropine (1% ophthalmic solution, 1 or 2 drops sublingually as often as every hour) can be used for controlling airway secretions and the resultant "death rattle." A guideline for withdrawal of mechanical ventilation is provided in Table 5–9.

PSYCHOLOGIC, SOCIAL, & SPIRITUAL ISSUES

Dying is not exclusively or even primarily a biomedical event. It is an intimate personal experience with profound psychologic, interpersonal, and existential

Table 5–9. Guidelines for withdrawal of mechanical ventilation.[1]

---

1. Stop neuromuscular blocking agents.
2. Administer opioids or sedatives to eliminate distress.
    If not already sedated, begin with fentanyl 100 μg (or morphine sulfate 10 mg) by intravenous bolus and infusion of fentanyl 100 μg per hour intravenously (or morphine sulfate 10 mg per hour intravenously).
    Distress is indicated by RR > 24, nasal flaring, use of accessory muscles of respiration, HR increase > 20%, MAP increase > 20%, grimacing, clutching.
3. Discontinue vasoactive agents and other agents unrelated to patient comfort, such as antibiotics, intravenous fluids, and diagnostic procedures.
4. Decrease FIO_2 to room air and PEEP to 0 cm H_2O.
5. Observe patient for distress.
    If patient is distressed, increase opioids by repeating bolus dose and increasing hourly infusion rate by 50 μg fentanyl (or 5 mg morphine sulfate),[2] then return to observation.
    If patient is not distressed, place on T piece and observe.
    If patient continues without distress, extubate patient and continue to observe for distress.

---

[1]Adapted, with permission, from San Francisco General Hospital Guidelines for Withdrawal of Mechanical Ventilation/Life Support.
[2]Ventilatory support may be increased until additional opioids have effect.

meanings. For many people at the end of life, the prospect of impending death stimulates a deep and urgent assessment of their identity, the quality of their relationships, and the meaning and purpose of their existence. As Ira Byock, a national hospice leader, has observed, while the relief of physical symptoms is the "first priority" in caring for patients at the end of life, the "ultimate goal" remains helping patients to die well.

Psychologic Challenges

In 1969, Elisabeth Kübler-Ross identified five psychologic stages or patterns of emotions that patients at the end of life may experience denial and isolation, anger, bargaining, depression, and acceptance. Not every patient will experience these emotions, and not necessarily in an orderly progression. In addition to these five stages are the perpetual challenges of anxiety and fear of the unknown. Simple information, listening, assurance, and support may help patients with these psychologic challenges. In fact, patients and families rank emotional support as one of the most important aspects of good end-of-life care. Psychotherapy and group support may be beneficial as well.

Despite the significant emotional stress of facing death, clinical depression is not normal at the end of life. Signs of depression must be distinguished from normal anticipatory grief, and depression should be treated. Although traditional antidepressant treatments such as selective serotonin reuptake inhibitors are effective, less commonly used but more rapidly acting medications such as dextroamphetamine or methylphenidate may be particularly useful when the end of life is near.

Social Challenges

At the end of life, patients should be encouraged to discharge personal, professional, and business obligations. This might include completing important work or personal projects, distributing possessions, writing a will, and making funeral and burial arrangements.

The prospect of death often prompts patients to examine the quality of their interpersonal relationships, including the relationship with the clinician. Dying may intensify a patient's need to feel cared for by the doctor, highlighting the clinician's obligation of nonabandonment and the need for clinician empathy and compassion.

Concern about estranged relationships or "unfinished business" with significant others and interest in reconciliation may become paramount at this time. At the end of life, even healthy interpersonal relationships must reach completion (Table 5–10).

Spiritual Challenges

Spirituality is the attempt to understand or accept the underlying meaning of life, one's relationships to one-

Table 5–10. Five statements often necessary for the completion of important interpersonal relationships.[1]

(1) "Forgive me."	(An expression of regret)
(2) "I forgive you."	(An expression of acceptance)
(3) "Thank you."	(An expression of gratitude)
(4) "I love you."	(An expression of affection)
(5) "Good-bye."	(Leave-taking)

[1]Courtesy of Ira R. Byock, MD.

self and other people, one's place in the universe, and the possibility of a "higher power" in the universe. Spirituality is distinguished from any particular religious practices or beliefs and is generally considered a universal human concern.

Perhaps because of an inappropriately exclusive attention to the biologic challenge of forestalling death or perhaps from feelings of discomfort or incompetence, clinicians frequently ignore their patients' spiritual concerns or reflexively refer these important issues to psychiatrists or other caretakers (nurses, social workers, clergy). However, the existential challenges of dying are central to the well-being of people at the end of life and are the proper concern of clinicians. Within a biologic, psychosocial, and spiritual model of medical care, clinicians may work to provide more than simple physical comfort and control of bothersome symptoms. Clinicians can help patients to die well by providing care to the whole person—by providing physical comfort and social support and by helping patients discover their own unique meaning in the world and an acceptance of death as a part of life.

Unlike physical ailments such as infections and fractures, which usually require a clinician's intervention to be treated, the patient's spiritual concerns often require only a clinician's attention, listening, and witness. Clinicians should routinely inquire about the patient's spiritual concerns and ask whether the patient wishes to discuss them. For example, asking, "How are you within yourself?" communicates that the clinician is interested in the patient's whole experience and provides an opportunity for the patient to share perceptions about his or her inner life. Questions that might constitute an existential "review of systems" are presented in Table 5–11.

Attending to the spiritual concerns of patients calls for listening carefully to their stories. Story-telling gives patients the opportunity to verbalize what is meaningful to them and to leave something of themselves behind—the promise of being remembered. Story-telling may be facilitated by suggesting that the patient share his or her life story with family members, record it on audio or video tape, assemble a photo album, organize a scrapbook, or write an autobiography.

While dying may be a period of inevitable loss of physical functioning, the end of life also offers an op-

Table 5–11. An existential review of systems.

Intrapersonal

How are you within yourself?[1]

What does your illness/dying mean to you?

What do you think caused your illness?

How have you been healed in the past?

What do you think is needed for you to be healed now?

What is right with you now?

What do you hope for?

Interpersonal

Who is important to you?

To whom does your illness/dying matter?

Do you have any unfinished business with significant others?

Transpersonal

What is your source of strength, help, or hope?

Do you have spiritual concerns or a spiritual practice?

If so, how does your spirituality relate to your illness/dying and how can I help integrate your spirituality into your health care?[1]

What do you think happens after we die?

What purpose might your illness/dying serve?

What do you think is trying to happen here?[1]

[1]Courtesy of IR Byock, MD, DB Larson, MD, and AL Suchman, MD.

portunity for psychologic, interpersonal, and spiritual development. Individuals may grow—even achieve a heightened sense of well-being or transcendence—in the process of dying. Through listening, support, and presence, clinicians may help foster this learning and be a catalyst for this transformation. Rather than thinking of dying simply as the termination of life, clinicians and patients may be guided by a developmental model of dying that recognizes a series of lifelong developmental tasks and landmarks and allows for growth at the end of life.

Block SD: Assessing and managing depression in the terminally ill patient. Ann Intern Med 2000;132:209. [PMID: 10651602]

Block SD: Perspectives on care at the close of life. Psychological considerations, growth, and transcendence at the end of life: the art of the possible. JAMA. 2001;285:2898. [PMID: 11401612]

Ehman JW et al: Do patients want physicians to inquire about their spiritual or religious beliefs if they become gravely ill? Arch Intern Med 1999;159:1803. [PMID: 10448785] (Many patients with lung disease would welcome carefully worded inquiry into their spiritual beliefs by physicians.)

Finucane TE et al: Tube feeding in patients with advanced dementia: a review of the evidence. JAMA 1999;282:1365. [PMID: 10527184] (Tube feeding rarely achieves any of the goals for which it is initiated in patients with dementia.)

Lo B et al: Discussing religious and spiritual issues at the end of life: a practical guide for physicians. JAMA 2002;287:749. [PMID: 11851542]

Prendergast TJ et al: A national survey of end-of-life care for critically ill patients. Am J Respir Crit Care Med 1998; 158:1163. [PMID: 9769276] (Disagreements between clinicians and families can almost always be resolved within a few days.)

■ TASKS AFTER DEATH

After the death of a patient, the clinician is called upon to perform a number of tasks, both required and recommended. The clinician must plainly and directly inform the family of the death. Providing words of sympathy and reassurance, time for questions and initial grief, and a quiet private room for the family at this time are appropriate and much appreciated.

THE PRONOUNCEMENT & DEATH CERTIFICATE

In most states of the USA, clinicians are legally required to confirm the death of a patient in a formal process called "pronouncement." The clinician must verify the absence of spontaneous respirations and cardiac activity and the presence of fixed and dilated pupils. A note describing these findings and the time of death is entered in the patient's chart.

While the pronouncement may often seem like an awkward and unnecessary formality, clinicians may use this time to reassure the patient's loved ones at the bedside that the patient died peacefully and that all appropriate care had been given. Both clinicians and families may use the ritual of the pronouncement as an opportunity to process emotionally the death of the patient.

Accurately reporting the underlying cause of death on the death certificate is also legally required and important both for patients' families (for insurance purposes and the need for an accurate family medical history) and for the epidemiologic study of disease and public health. Unfortunately, recent research has shown that physicians are untrained in and unskilled at correctly completing death certificates. The physician should be specific about the major cause of death (eg, "decompensated cirrhosis") and its contributory cause (eg, "hepatitis B and hepatitis C infections and chronic alcoholic hepatitis") as well as any associated conditions (eg, "acute renal failure")—and not simply put down "cardiac arrest" as the cause of death.

AUTOPSY & ORGAN DONATION

Discussing the options and obtaining consent for autopsy and organ donation with patients themselves prior to death is usually the best practice. This advances the principle of patient autonomy and lessens the responsibilities of distressed family members during the period immediately following the death. Recent research demonstrates that after a patient dies, however, designated organ transplant personnel are more successful than the treating clinicians at obtaining consent for organ donation from surviving family members. Federal regulations now require that a designated representative of an organ procurement organization approach the family about organ donation.

Most people in the United States support the donation of organs for transplants. Currently, however, organ transplantation is severely limited by the availability of donor organs. Many potential donors and the families of actual donors experience a sense of reward in contributing, even through death, to the lives of others.

Clinicians must be sensitive to ethnic and cultural differences in attitudes about autopsy and organ donation. Patients or their families should be reminded of their right to limit autopsy or organ donation in any way they choose. Pathologists can perform autopsies without interfering with funeral plans or the appearance of the deceased.

The results of an autopsy may help surviving family members (and clinicians) understand the exact cause of a patient's death and foster a sense of closure. A clinician-family conference to review the results of the autopsy provides a good opportunity for clinicians to assess how well families are grieving and to answer questions. Unfortunately, despite the advantages of conducting postmortem examinations, autopsy rates have fallen drastically to less than 15% today. Families report refusing autopsies out of fear of disfigurement of the body or delay of the funeral—or say they were simply not asked. They report allowing autopsies in order to advance medical knowledge, to identify the exact cause of their loved one's death, and to be reassured that appropriate care was given. Routinely addressing these issues when discussing autopsy may help increase the autopsy rate.

FOLLOW-UP & GRIEVING

Proper care of patients at the end of life includes following up with surviving family members after the patient has died. Following up enables the clinician to assess how families are grieving, to reassure them about the nature of normal grieving, and to identify complicated grief or depression. Clinicians can recommend support groups and counseling as needed. A card or telephone call from the clinician to the family days to weeks after the patient's death (and perhaps on the anniversary of the death) allows the clinician to express concern for the family and the deceased.

After a patient dies, the clinician too may need to grieve. Although clinicians may be relatively unaffected by the deaths of some patients, other deaths may cause distressing feelings of sadness, loss, and guilt. These emotions should be recognized as the first step toward processing them or preventing them in the future.

For clinicians, grieving the loss of a patient is normal. Each clinician may find personal or communal resources that help with the process of grieving. Shedding tears, the support of colleagues, time for reflection, and traditional or personal mourning rituals all may be effective. Attending the funeral of a patient who has died can be a satisfying personal experience that is almost universally appreciated by families and that may be the final element in caring well for people at the end of life.

Bedell SE et al: The doctor's letter of condolence. N Engl J Med 2001;344:1162 [PMID: 11302139]. (Condolence letters from physicians are important and welcomed by grieving family members.)

Dalen JE: The moribund autopsy: DNR or CPR? Arch Intern Med 1997;157:1633. [PMID: 9250221] (Argues for the continued importance of autopsy.)

Ferris TG et al: When the patient dies: a survey of medical house staff about care after death. J Palliat Med 1998;1:231. (Resident physicians reported little or no training in the tasks that must be undertaken after the death of a patient.)

Prigerson HG et al: Perspectives on care at the close of life. Caring for bereaved patients "all the doctors just suddenly go." JAMA 2001;286:1369. [PMID: 11560543]

Skin, Hair, & Nails

6

Timothy G. Berger, MD

See www.current-med.com/ch06.html

DIAGNOSIS OF SKIN DISORDERS

Morphology

Specific skin diseases cause characteristic lesions. Identifying lesions as pustules, vesicles, or scaly plaques will guide the clinician to the *group* of diseases that will include the correct diagnosis. This chapter will group diseases according to the types of lesions they cause and guide the reader through the history, physical findings, and laboratory tests that discriminate among the differential diagnoses.

History

A detailed history is important, though in the case of skin cancer or moles (nevi) the physical examination takes precedence. Important components of a history include systemic disorders, prescription or OTC systemic and topical medications, and exposure to physical and chemical agents in the home and work environments. If a treatment is not working, ask the patient how they are using it.

Physical Examination

It is best to examine the entire skin surface, including the nails, scalp, palms, soles, and mucous membranes, in bright (preferably natural) light. Total skin examination allows recognition of typical disease patterns (eg, elbow, knee, scalp, and fingernail involvement with psoriasis) while ensuring that no potentially important lesions are overlooked (eg, a small malignant melanoma on the buttock). In examining the face of an elderly individual for nonmelanoma skin cancer, special attention should be given to the lid margins, nose, ears, and lips—areas of sun exposure. Similarly, a rash appearing at the waistline may suggest contact dermatitis due to laundry detergent, fabric, or clothing waistbands.

PRINCIPLES OF DERMATOLOGIC THERAPY

Planning Topical Treatment

In general, it is better to be familiar with a few dermatologic drugs and treatment methods than to attempt to use a great many. When in doubt about the proper method of treatment, one should *undertreat* rather than overtreat: Inappropriate chronic use of a topical corticosteroid may cause irreversible side effects.

Frequently Employed Treatment Measures

A. GENERAL MEASURES

Soap should be used only in the axillae and groin and on the feet by persons with dry or irritated skin. Unless their occupations expose them to oils or soot, most people do not need soaping over all body surfaces.

B. LOCAL MEASURES

In general, topical agents used by prescription are supplied in only one strength, and thus, with the exception of Table 6–1, concentrations will not be listed in this chapter. Exceptions include hydrocortisone (1% and 2.5%); triamcinolone acetonide cream and ointment (0.025% and 0.1%) or solution (0.1%); fluocinolone cream, ointment, or solution (0.01%), or cream and ointment (0.025%). There is little evidence that one concentration has clinical effects that are significantly different from another. Nondermatologists should become familiar with a few agents and use them properly rather than try to master the universe of topical agents. All useful antifungals come in only one strength. Selenium sulfide lotion 2.5% is used to treat tinea versicolor; selenium 1% is used in OTC antidandruff shampoos.

1. Corticosteroids—Representative topical corticosteroid creams, lotions, ointments, gels, and sprays are presented in Table 6–1. Specific indications for topical steroid therapy will be discussed in the context of specific dermatologic entities to follow; however, some basic principles of topical steroid therapy should be mentioned here. Topical steroids are divided into classes based on their potency. There is little (except price) to recommend one agent over another within the same class. For a given agent, an ointment is more potent than a cream; however, ointments are generally more greasy. The potency of a topical steroid may be

Table 6–1. Useful topical dermatologic therapeutic agents.

Agent	Formulations, Strengths, and Prices[1]	Apply	Potency Class	Common Indications	Comments
Corticosteroids					
Hydrocortisone acetate	Cream 1%: $3.22/30 g Ointment 1%: $3.34/30 g Lotion 1%: $18.36/120 mL	bid	Low	Seborrheic dermatitis. Pruritus ani. Intertrigo.	Not the same as hydrocortisone butyrate or valerate! Not for poison oak! OTC lotion (Aquinil HC). OTC solution (Scalpicin, T Scalp).
	Cream 2.5%: $8.84/30 g Ointment 2.5%: $8.84/30 g Lotion 2.5%: $45.64/60 mL	bid	Low	As for 1% hydrocortisone.	Perhaps better for pruritus ani. Not clearly better than 1%. More expensive. Not OTC.
Alclometasone dipropionate (Aclovate)	Cream 0.05%: $15.10/15 g Ointment 0.05%: $31.48/45 g	bid	Low	As for hydrocortisone.	More efficacious than hydrocortisone. Perhaps causes less atrophy.
Desonide	Cream 0.05%: $20.31/15 g Ointment 0.05%: $51.31/60 g Lotion 0.05%: $33.44/60 mL	bid	Low	As for hydrocortisone. For lesions on face or body folds resistant to hydrocortisone.	More efficacious than hydrocortisone. Can cause rosacea or atrophy. Not fluorinated.
Prednicarbate (Dermatop)	Emollient cream 0.1%: $16.81/15 g	bid	Medium	As for triamcinolone.	May cause less atrophy. No generic formulations. Preservative-free.
Triamcinolone acetonide	Cream 0.1%: $2.64/15 g Ointment 0.1%: $2.64/15 g Lotion 0.1%: $10.22/60 mL	bid	Medium	Eczema on extensor areas. Used for psoriasis with tar. Seborrheic dermatitis and psoriasis on scalp.	Caution in body folds, face. Economical in 0.5 lb and 1 lb sizes for treatment of large body surfaces. Economical as solution for scalp.
	Cream 0.025%: $1.82/15 g Ointment 0.025%: $5.52/80 g	bid	Medium	As for 0.1% strength.	Possibly less efficacy and few advantages over 0.1% formulation.
Fluocinolone acetonide	Cream 0.025%: $3.05/15 g Ointment 0.025%: $4.20/15 g	bid	Medium	As for triamcinolone.	
	Solution 0.01%: $11.00/60 mL	bid	Medium	As for triamcinolone solution.	
Mometasone furoate (Elocon)	Cream 0.1%: $22.43/15 g Ointment 0.1%: $22.43/15 g Lotion 0.1%: $46.43/60 mL	qd	Medium	As for triamcinolone.	Often used inappropriately on the face or in children. Not fluorinated.
Diflorasone diacetate	Cream 0.05%: $35.52/15 g Ointment 0.05%: $50.91/30 g	bid	High	Nummular dermatitis. Allergic contact dermatitis. Lichen simplex chronicus.	
Amcinonide (Cyclocort)	Cream 0.1%: $20.58/15 g Ointment 0.1%: $20.58/15 g	bid	High	As for betamethasone.	
Fluocinonide (Lidex)	Cream 0.05%: $8.80/15 g Gel 0.05%: $21.01/15 g Ointment 0.05%: $20.85/15 g Solution 0.05%: $26.08/60 mL	bid	High	As for betamethasone. Gel useful for poison oak.	Economical generics. Lidex cream can cause stinging on eczema. Lidex emollient cream preferred.

(continued)

Table 6–1. Useful topical dermatologic therapeutic agents. (continued)

Agent	Formulations, Strengths, and Prices[1]	Apply	Potency Class	Common Indications	Comments
Betamethasone dipropionate (Diprolene)	Cream 0.05%: $5.57/15 g Ointment 0.05%: $5.57/15 g Lotion 0.05%: $14.23/60 mL	bid	Ultra-high	For lesions resistant to high-potency steroids. Lichen planus. Insect bites.	Economical generics available.
Clobetasol propionate (Temovate)	Cream 0.05%: $23.14/15 g Ointment 0.05%: $23.14/15 g Lotion 0.05%: $69.85/50 mL	bid	Ultra-high	As for betamethasone dipropionate.	Somewhat more potent than diflorasone. Limited to 2 continuous weeks of use. Limited to 50 g or less per week. Cream may cause stinging; use "emollient cream" formulation. Generic available.
Halobetasol propionate (Ultravate)	Cream 0.05%: $30.62/15 g Ointment 0.05%: $30.62/15 g	bid	Ultra-high	As for clobetasol.	Same restrictions as clobetasol. Cream does not cause stinging. Compatible with calcipotriene (Dovonex).
Flurandrenolide (Cordran)	Tape: $18.84/80″ × 30″ roll	q12h	Ultra-high	Lichen simplex chronicus.	Protects the skin and prevents scratching.
Nonsteroidal anti-inflammatory agents					
Tacrolimus (Protopic)	Ointment 0.1%: $64.09/30 g Ointment 0.03%: $59.95/30 g	bid	N/A	Atopic dermatitis.	Steroid substitute not causing atrophy or striae. Burns in 40% (+) of patients with eczema.
Pimecrolimus	Cream 1%	bid	N/A	Atopic dermatitis.	Steroid substitute not causing atrophy or striae. Does not burn.
Antibiotics (for acne)					
Clindamycin phosphate	Solution 1%: $10.51/30 mL Gel 1%: $29.74/30 mL Lotion 1%: $44.68/60 mL Pledget 1%: $42.50/60	bid	N/A	Mild papular acne.	Lotion is less drying for patients with sensitive skin.
Erythromycin	Solution 2%: $7.04/60 mL Gel 2%: $20.69/30 g Pledget 2%: $24.77/60	bid	N/A	As for clindamycin.	Many different manufacturers. Economical.
Erythromycin/ Benzoyl peroxide (Benzamycin)	Gel $58.94/23.3 g Gel $102.53/46.6 g	bid	N/A	As for clindamycin. Can help treat comedonal acne.	No generics. More expensive. More effective than other topical antibiotics. Main jar requires refrigeration.
Clindamycin/ Benzoyl peroxide (Benzeclin)	Gel $52.50/g	bid		As for benzamycin.	No generic. More effective than either agent alone.
Antibiotics (for impetigo)					
Mupirocin (Bactroban)	Ointment 2%: $28.50/15 g	tid	N/A	Impetigo, folliculitis.	Because of cost use limited to tiny areas of impetigo. Used in the nose twice daily for 5 days to reduce staphylococcal carriage.

(continued)

Table 6-1. Useful topical dermatologic therapeutic agents. (continued)

Agent	Formulations, Strengths, and Prices[1]	Apply	Potency Class	Common Indications	Comments
Antifungals					
Clotrimazole	Cream 1%: $4.50/15 g OTC Solution 1%: $15.52/30 mL	bid	N/A	Dermatophyte and candida infections.	Available OTC. Inexpensive generic cream available.
Miconazole	Cream 2%: $3.20/30 g OTC	bid	N/A	As for clotrimazole.	As for clotrimazole.
Other imidazoles					
Econazole (Spectazole)	Cream 1%: $16.25/15 g	qd	N/A	As for clotrimazole.	No generic. Somewhat more effective than clotrimazole and miconazole.
Ketoconazole	Cream 2%: $16.46/15 g	qd	N/A	As for clotrimazole.	No generic. Somewhat more effective than clotrimazole and miconazole.
Oxiconazole (Oxistat)	Cream 1%: $20.94/15 g Lotion 1%: $35.24/30 mL	bid	N/A		
Sulconazole (Exelderm)	Cream 1%: $12.56/15 g Solution 1%: $27.05/30 mL	bid	N/A	As for clotrimazole.	No generic. Somewhat more effective than clotrimazole and miconazole.
Other antifungals					
Butenafine (Mentax)	Cream 1%: $30.74/15 g	qd	N/A	Dermatophytes.	Fast response; high cure rate; expensive.
Ciclopirox (Loprox)	Cream 0.77%: $31.83/30 g Lotion 0.77%: $66.67/60 mL	bid	N/A	As for clotrimazole.	No generic. Somewhat more effective than clotrimazole and miconazole.
Naftifine (Naftin)	Cream 1%: $40.40/30 g Gel 1%: $63.75/60 mL	qd	N/A	Dermatophytes.	No generic. Somewhat more effective than clotrimazole and miconazole.
Terbinafine (Lamisil)	Cream 1%: $6.79/12 g OTC	qd	N/A	For dermatophytes.	Fast clinical response. OTC. Less expensive than butenafine or naftifine.
Antipruritics					
Camphor/ menthol	Compounded lotion (0.5% of each)	bid–tid	N/A	For mild eczema, xerosis, mild contact dermatitis.	
Pramoxine hydrochloride (PRAX)	Lotion 1%: $11.70/120 mL	qid	N/A	Dry skin, varicella, mild eczema, pruritus ani.	OTC formulations (Prax, Aveeno Anti-Itch Cream or Lotion; Itch-X Gel). By prescription mixed with 1% or 2% hydrocortisone.
Doxepin (Zonalon)	Cream 5%: $32.70/30 g	qid	N/A	Topical antipruritic, best used in combination with appropriate topical steroid to enhance efficacy.	Can cause sedation.
Emollients					
Aveeno	Cream, lotion, others	qd–tid	N/A	Xerosis, eczema.	Choice is most often based on personal preference by patient.

(continued)

Table 6–1. Useful topical dermatologic therapeutic agents. (continued)

	Formulations, Strengths, and Prices[1]	Apply	Potency Class	Common Indications	Comments
Aqua glycolic	Cream, lotion, shampoo, others	qd–tid	N/A	Xerosis. Ichthyosis, keratosis pilaris. Mild facial wrinkles. Mild acne or seborrheic dermatitis.	Contains 8% glycolic acid. Available from other makers, eg, Alpha Hydrox, or generic 8% glycolic acid lotion. May cause stinging on eczematous skin.
Aquaphor	Ointment: $3.68/52.5 g	qd–tid	N/A	Xerosis. Eczema. For protection of area in pruritus ani.	Not as greasy as petrolatum.
Carmol	Lotion 10%: $8.25/180 mL Cream 20%: $7.59/90 g	bid	N/A	Contains urea as humectant.	Nongreasy hydrating agent (10%); debrides keratin (20%).
Complex 15	Lotion: $6.48/240 mL Cream: $4.82/75 g	qd–tid	N/A	Xerosis. Lotion or cream recommended for split or dry nails.	Active ingredient is a phospholipid.
DML	Cream, lotion, facial moisturizer	qd–tid	N/A	As for Complex 15.	Face cream has sunscreen.
Dermasil	Lotion, cream	qd–tid	N/A	Xerosis, eczema.	
Eucerin	Cream: $5.10/120 g Lotion: $5.10/240 mL	qd–tid	N/A	Xerosis, eczema.	Many formulations made. Eucerin Plus contains alpha-hydroxy acid and may cause stinging on eczematous skin. Facial moisturizer has SPF 25 sunscreen.
Lac-Hydrin-Five	Lotion: $10.12/240 mL	bid	N/A	Xerosis, ichthyosis, keratosis pilaris.	Expensive, not OTC.
Lubriderm	Lotion: $5.03/300 mL	qd–tid	N/A	Xerosis, eczema.	Unscented usually preferred.
Neutrogena	Cream, lotion, facial moisturizer: $7.39/240 mL	qd–tid	N/A	Xerosis, eczema.	Face cream has titanium-based sunscreen.
SBR Lipocream	Cream: $6.39/30 g	qd–tid	N/A	Xerosis, eczema.	Less greasy but effective moisturizer.
Triceram Cream	Cream: $30.00–$31.50/ 3.4 oz tube	bid	N/A	Xerosis, eczema.	Contains ceramide; anti-inflammatory and non-greasy moisturizer.
U-Lactin	Lotion: $7.13/240 mL	qd	N/A	Hyperkeratotic heels.	Moisturizes and removes keratin.

[1]Cost to pharmacist (average wholesale price, generic when possible) for quantity listed. Source: *Drug Topics Red Book,* March 2002; Vol. 21, No. 3.

dramatically increased by applying an occlusive dressing over the steroid. Such dressings may include gloves, plastic wrap, or plastic occlusive suits for patients with generalized erythroderma or atopy. Caution should be used in applying topical steroids to areas of thin skin (face, scrotum, vulva, skin folds).

For patients using steroids on their eyelids, treatment should be restricted to avoid the risk of glaucoma or cataracts. One may estimate the amount of topical steroid needed by using the "rule of nines" (as in burn evaluation; see Figure 38–4). In general, it takes an average of 20–30 g to cover the body surface of an adult once. Systemic absorption does occur, but adrenal suppression, diabetes, hypertension, osteoporosis, and other complications of systemic steroids are very rare with topical steroid therapy.

2. Emollients for dry skin ("moisturizers")—Dry skin is not related to water intake but to abnormal function of the epidermis. Many types of emollients are available. Petrolatum, mineral oil, Aquaphor, and Eucerin cream are the heaviest and best for very dry skin. Emollients are most effective when applied to wet skin immediately after a bath to trap the moisture. They should be applied with the "grain" of the hairs rather than by rubbing up and down to avoid folliculitis. If the skin is too greasy after application, pat dry again with a damp towel.

In some cases, lotions may be useful and are not as greasy as the creams and ointments listed above. The appearance of dry skin and ichthyosis may be improved by lactic acid products (Lac-Hydrin, U-Lactin) or glycolic acid-containing lotions (Aqua Glycolic) provided no inflammation (erythema) is present. Moisturizers that are similar to the skin's normal lipids and thus feel less greasy than ointments include SBR Lipocream and Triceram cream.

3. Drying agents for weepy dermatoses—If the skin is weepy from infection or inflammation, drying agents may afford relief. The best drying agent is water, and repeated compresses, with or without such agents as aluminum salts (Burow's solution, Domeboro tablets) or colloidal oatmeal (Aveeno) are a good first step. Shake lotions (eg, starch or calamine lotions) and powders (especially if the process is acute) may result in messy crusts and are seldom used by dermatologists.

4. Topical antipruritics—Lotions that contain 0.5% each of camphor and menthol (Sarna) are effective for mild pruritic dermatoses. Pramoxine hydrochloride, 1% cream or lotion, or pramoxine hydrochloride, 1%, with 0.5% menthol, as a surface anesthetic may be an effective antipruritic agent (Prax, PrameGel, Aveeno Anti-Itch lotion). Hydrocortisone, 1% or 2.5%, may be incorporated for its anti-inflammatory effect (Pramosone cream, lotion, or ointment). Doxepin cream 5% may reduce pruritus due to eczematous dermatoses. It appears most effective when applied together with a topical steroid of the appropriate class for the condition or site being treated. Like pramoxine, it is a steroid enhancer, improving response to a given strength of topical steroid. Drowsiness and dry mouth may occur. Monoamine oxidase inhibitors should be discontinued at least 2 weeks before treatment.

5. Systemic antipruritic drugs—

a. Antihistamines—H$_1$ blockers are the agents of choice for pruritus when due to histamine, such as in urticaria. Otherwise, they appear to relieve pruritus only by their sedating and not their antihistamine effects. Thus, less sedating antihistamines may be less effective in non-histamine-related pruritus. Except in the case of urticaria, nonsedating antihistamines are of little or no value in inflammatory skin diseases such as atopic dermatitis and are rarely indicated.

Traditional H$_1$ antihistamines are usually grouped into six classes (Table 19–1). Alkylamines (chlorpheniramine and dexchlorpheniramine) are the least sedating. Ethanolamines (diphenhydramine) are very sedating, as are phenothiazines (promethazine). Piperidines (cyproheptadine), piperazines (hydroxyzine), and ethylenediamines (tripelennamine) cause less sedation. The least sedating antihistamines are loratadine and famotidine. Cetirizine is also relatively nonsedating. Some tricyclic antidepressants, such as doxepin, have potent antihistaminic activity and are useful in urticaria and other forms of pruritus.

b. Systemic corticosteroids—(See Chapter 26.)

Burr S: Emollients for managing dry skin conditions. Prof Nurse 1999;15:43. [PMID: 10595180]

Weisshar E et al: Systemic drugs with antipruritic potency. Skin Therapy Lett 2000;5:1. [PMID: 10854341]

Yosipovitch G et al: The diagnostic and therapeutic approach to idiopathic generalized pruritus. Int J Dermatol 1999;38:881. [PMID: 10632764]

Sunscreens

Protection from ultraviolet light should begin at birth but will reduce the incidence of actinic keratoses and some nonmelanoma skin cancers when initiated at any age. The best protection is shelter, but protective clothing, avoidance of direct sun exposure during the peak hours of the day, and the assiduous use of chemical sunscreens are important. Estimates are that if fair children were to use such sunscreens regularly, their lifetime risk of skin cancer might be reduced by 75%.

A number of highly effective sunscreens are available in cream, lotion, and nongreasy gel and liquid formulations. Fair-complexioned persons should use a sunscreen with an SPF (sun protective factor) of at least 15 and preferably 30–40 every day. For those who are sensitive to PABA (*p* aminobenzoic acid), PABA-free formulations are available. Sunscreens with high SPF values (> 30) afford some protection against UVA as well as UVB light exposure and may be helpful in managing photosensitivity disorders.

Physical blockers (titanium dioxide and zinc oxide [Blue Lizard]) are available in vanishing formulations (Ti-Baby Natural, Ti Screen Natural, Neutrogena Chemical-Free Sun Blocker).

Gasparro FP: Sunscreens, skin photobiology, and skin cancer: the need for UVA protection and evaluation of efficacy. Environ Health Perspect 2000;108(Suppl 1):71. [PMID: 10698724] (UVA protection may be critical to prevent photodamage.)

Green AA et al: Daily sunscreen application and betacarotene supplementation in prevention of basal-cell and squamous-cell carcinomas of the skin: a randomised controlled trial. Lancet 1999;354:723. [PMID: 10475183]

Complications of Topical Dermatologic Therapy

Complications of topical therapy can be largely avoided. They fall into several categories:

A. ALLERGY

Of the topical antibiotics, neomycin has the greatest potential for sensitization. Diphenhydramine, benzocaine, and ethylenediamine are potential sensitizers in topical medications. Preservatives and even the topical steroids themselves can cause allergic contact dermatitis.

B. IRRITATION

Preparations of retinoic acid, benzoyl peroxide, and other acne medications should be applied sparingly to the skin when it is dry. Repeated use of lindane (Kwell, etc) and antiseptic soaps can be irritating. Sunscreens may cause irritation or an acne-like eruption.

C. ABSORPTION

Drugs may be absorbed through the skin, especially near mucous membranes, through broken or inflamed skin, or from under occlusive dressings. The possibility of systemic absorption has special implications for pregnant women or women who may become pregnant while using the topical medication. A few notable examples of topical drugs that may be harmful to a fetus include podophyllum resin, lindane, and tretinoin (Retin-A). In most cases, substitutes are available (eg, permethrin or precipitated sulfur may be substituted for lindane). In general it is always prudent to consult a pharmacology textbook or pharmacist when prescribing medications for pregnant or nursing women.

D. OVERUSE

Fluorinated topical corticosteroids may induce acne-like lesions on the face (steroid rosacea) and atrophic striae in body folds.

Journe F et al: Sunscreen sensitization: a 5-year study. Acta Dermato-Venereologica 1999;79:211. [PMID: 10384919] (A review of allergic reactions to sunscreen.)

■ I. COMMON DERMATOSES

Dermatologic diseases will be classified and discussed here, when possible, according to the types of lesions they cause. Therefore, in order to make a diagnosis, it is best to (1) focus on the type of individual lesion the patient exhibits; (2) choose the morphologic category the lesions seem to fit; and then (3) identify the specific features of the history, physical examination, and laboratory tests that will establish the working diagnosis.

The major morphologic types of skin lesion are listed in Table 6–2 along with the disorders with which they are most prominently associated. Miscellaneous skin, hair, and nail disorders and drug eruptions are discussed at the end of the chapter.

PIGMENTED LESIONS

Deaths from **malignant melanoma** are prevented by early diagnosis followed by excision. The nondermatologist clinician must be able to evaluate pigmented lesions and appropriately refer for evaluation all potential malignant melanomas. In order to avoid missing some malignant melanomas, it is understood that many patients will be referred for what ultimately prove to be benign lesions.

In general, a **benign mole** is a small (< 6 mm), well-circumscribed lesion with a well-defined border and a single shade of pigment from beige or pink to dark brown. The physical examination must take precedence over the history, though a reliable history that a lesion has been present without change for decades is obviously a comfort.

Suspicious moles have an irregular notched border where the pigment appears to be leaking into the normal surrounding skin; the topography may be irregular, ie, partly raised and partly flat. Color variegation is present, and colors such as pink, blue, gray, white, and black are indications for referral. The American Cancer Society has proposed the mnemonic "ABCD = Asymmetry, Border irregularity, Color variegation, and Diameter greater than 6 mm." Bleeding and ulceration are ominous signs. A mole that stands out from the patient's other moles deserves special scrutiny. A patient with a large number of moles is statistically at increased risk for melanoma and deserves careful and periodic examination, particularly if the lesions are atypical.

The history of a changing mole (evolution) is the single most important historical reason for close evaluation and possible referral. Referral of suspicious pigmented lesions is always appropriate.

Moles have their own natural history. In the patient's first decade of life, moles often appear as flat, small, brown lesions. They are called **junctional nevi** because the nevus cells are at the junction of the epidermis and dermis. Over the next 2 decades, these moles grow in size and often become raised, reflecting the appearance of a dermal component, giving rise to **compound nevi.** Moles may darken and grow during pregnancy. As Caucasian patients enter their seventh and eighth decades, most moles have lost their junctional component and dark pigmentation and undergo fibrosis or other degenerative changes. Still, at every stage of life, normal moles should be well-demarcated, symmetric, and uniform in contour and color.

Edman RL et al: Prevention and early detection of malignant melanoma. Am Fam Physician 2000;62:2277. [PMID: 11126854]

Table 6–2. Morphologic categorization of skin lesions and diseases.

Pigmented	Freckle, lentigo, seborrheic keratosis, nevus, blue nevus, halo nevus, dysplastic nevus, melanoma
Scaly	Psoriasis, dermatitis (atopic, stasis, seborrheic, chronic allergic contact or irritant contact), xerosis (dry skin), lichen simplex chronicus, tinea, tinea versicolor, secondary syphilis, pityriasis rosea, discoid lupus erythematosus, exfoliative dermatitis, actinic keratoses, Bowen's disease, Paget's disease, intertrigo
Vesicular	Herpes simplex, varicella, herpes zoster, dyshidrosis (vesicular dermatitis of palms and soles), vesicular tinea, dermatophytid, dermatitis herpetiformis, miliaria, scabies, photosensitivity
Weepy or encrusted	Impetigo, acute contact allergic dermatitis, any vesicular dermatitis
Pustular	Acne vulgaris, acne rosacea, folliculitis, candidiasis, miliaria, any vesicular dermatitis
Figurate ("shaped") erythema	Urticaria, erythema multiforme, erythema migrans, cellulitis, erysipelas, erysipeloid, arthropod bites
Bullous	Impetigo, blistering dactylitis, pemphigus, pemphigoid, porphyria cutanea tarda, drug eruptions, erythema multiforme, toxic epidermal necrolysis
Papular	Hyperkeratotic: warts, corns, seborrheic keratoses Purple-violet: lichen planus, drug eruptions, Kaposi's sarcoma Flesh-colored, umbilicated: molluscum contagiosum Pearly: basal cell carcinoma, intradermal nevi Small, red, inflammatory: acne, miliaria, candidiasis, scabies, folliculitis
Pruritus[1]	Xerosis, scabies, pediculosis, bites, systemic causes, anogenital pruritus
Nodular, cystic	Erythema nodosum, furuncle, cystic acne, follicular (epidermal) inclusion cyst
Photodermatitis (photodistributed rashes)	Drug, polymorphic light eruption, lupus erythematosus
Morbilliform	Drug, viral infection, secondary syphilis
Erosive	Any vesicular dermatitis, impetigo, aphthae, lichen planus, erythema multiforme
Ulcerated	Decubiti, herpes simplex, skin cancers, parasitic infections, syphilis (chancre), chancroid, vasculitis, stasis, arterial disease

[1]Not a morphologic class but included because it is one of the most common dermatologic presentations.

Grob JJ et al: The "ugly duckling" sign. Arch Dermatol 1998;134:103. [PMID: 9449921] (A mole that stands out or looks different than others should be carefully evaluated.)

Kittler H et al: Morphologic changes of pigmented skin lesions: a useful extension of the ABCD rule for dermatoscopy. J Am Acad Dermatol 1999;40:558. [PMID: 10188673]

Egan CL et al: Cutaneous melanoma risk and phenotypic changes in large congenital nevi. J Am Acad Dermatol 1998;39:923. [PMID: 9843003]

Sahin S et al: Risk of melanoma and medium-sized congenital melanocytic nevi. J Am Acad Dermatol 1998;39:428. [PMID: 9738777]

CONGENITAL NEVI

The management of small congenital nevi—less than a few centimeters in diameter—is controversial. The vast majority will never become malignant, but some experts feel that the risk of melanoma in these lesions may be somewhat increased. Since 1% of Caucasians are born with these lesions, management should be conservative and excision advised only for lesions in cosmetically nonsensitive areas where the patient cannot easily see the lesion and note any suspicious changes. Excision should be considered for congenital nevi whose contour (bumpiness, nodularity) or color (different shades) makes it difficult for examiners to note early signs of malignant change. Giant congenital melanocytic nevi (> 5% BSA) are at greater risk for development of melanoma, and surgical removal in stages is often recommended.

ATYPICAL (DYSPLASTIC) NEVI

The term "atypical nevus" or "atypical mole" has supplanted "dysplastic nevus." The diagnosis of atypical moles is made clinically and not histologically, and moles should be removed only if they are suspected to be melanomas. Clinically, these moles are large (> 5 mm in diameter), with an ill-defined, irregular border and irregularly distributed pigmentation. It is estimated that 5–10% of the United States population have one or more atypical nevi. Studies have defined an increased risk of melanoma in the following populations: patients with 50 or more nevi with one or more atypical moles and one mole at least 8 mm or larger, and patients with a few to many definitely atypical moles. These patients deserve education and regular (usually every 6–12 months) follow-up. Kindreds with familial melanoma (numerous atypical nevi and a strong family history) deserve even closer attention, as the risk of developing single or even multiple melanomas in some of these individuals can reach 100%.

Bataille V et al: Genetics of risk factors for melanoma: an adult twin study of nevi and freckles. J Natl Cancer Inst 2000;92:457. [PMID: 10716963]

Marghoob AA: The dangers of atypical mole (dysplastic nevus) syndrome. Teaching at-risk patients to protect themselves from melanoma. Postgrad Med 1999;105:147. [PMID: 10376056] (Guidelines for following patients with atypical nevi.)

Snels DG et al: Risk of cutaneous malignant melanoma in patients with nonfamilial atypical nevi from a pigmented lesions clinic. J Am Acad Dermatol 1999;40(5 Part 1):686. [PMID: 10321594] (Even nonfamilial atypical nevi are associated with a high risk for melanoma [relative risk 35–40].)

BLUE NEVI

Blue nevi are small, slightly elevated, and blue-black lesions. They are common in persons of Asian descent, and an individual patient may have several of them. If present without change for many years, they may be considered benign, since malignant blue nevi are rare. However, blue-black papules and nodules that are new or growing must be evaluated to rule out nodular melanoma.

Knoell KA et al: Familial multiple blue nevi. J Am Acad Dermatol 1998;39(2 Part 2):322. [PMID: 9703144]

FRECKLES & LENTIGINES

Freckles (ephelides) and lentigines are flat brown spots. Freckles first appear in young children, darken with ultraviolet exposure, and fade with cessation of sun exposure. In adults, depending on the fairness of the complexion, flat brown spots (lentigines), often with sharp borders, gradually appear in sun-exposed areas, particularly the dorsa of the hands. They do not fade with cessation of sun exposure. They should be evaluated like all pigmented lesions: If the pigmentation is homogeneous and they are symmetric and flat, they are most likely benign. Solar lentigines, so-called liver spots, improve in over 80% of individuals treated with topical 0.1% tretinoin once nightly for 6–10 months.

SEBORRHEIC KERATOSES

Seborrheic keratoses are benign plaques, beige to brown or even black, 3–20 mm in diameter, with a velvety or warty surface. They appear to be stuck or pasted onto the skin. They are common—especially in the elderly—and may be mistaken for melanomas or other types of cutaneous neoplasms. Although they may be frozen with liquid nitrogen or curetted if they itch or are inflamed, no treatment is needed.

Gill D et al: The prevalence of seborrheic keratoses in persons aged 15 to 30 years. Arch Dermatol 2000;136:759. [PMID: 10871940] (Seborrheic keratoses are common in Caucasians under 30 years of age.)

MALIGNANT MELANOMA

 ESSENTIALS OF DIAGNOSIS

- May be flat or raised.
- Should be suspected in any pigmented skin lesion with recent change in appearance.
- Examination with good light may show varying colors, including red, white, black, and bluish.
- Borders typically irregular.

General Considerations

Malignant melanoma is the leading cause of death due to skin disease. There were 51,400 cases of melanoma in the USA in 2001, with 7800 deaths. One in four cases of melanoma occur before the age of 40. Melanoma is the most common cancer of women between the ages of 25 and 29 and the second most common cause in women ages 30–34. Overall survival for melanomas in Caucasians rose from 60% in 1960–1963 to 85% in 1983–1990, due primarily to earlier detection of lesions.

Tumor thickness is the single most important prognostic factor. Ten-year survival rates—related to thickness in millimeters—are as follows: < 0.76 mm, 96%; 0.76–1.69 mm, 81%; 1.7–3.6 mm, 57%; > 3.6 mm, 31%. With lymph node involvement, the 5-year survival rate is 30%; and with distant metastases, it is less than 10%. More accurate prognoses can be made on the basis of thickness, site, histologic features, and sex of the patient.

Clinical Findings

Primary malignant melanomas may be classified into various clinicohistologic types, including lentigo maligna melanoma (arising on sun-exposed skin of older individuals); superficial spreading malignant melanoma (the most common type, occurring in two-thirds of individuals developing melanoma); nodular malignant melanoma; acral-lentiginous melanomas (arising on palms, soles, and nail beds); malignant melanomas on mucous membranes; and miscellaneous forms such as amelanotic (nonpigmented) melanoma and melanomas arising from blue nevi (rare) and congenital nevi.

While superficial spreading melanoma is largely a disease of Caucasians, persons of other races are at risk for other types of melanoma, particularly acral lentigi-

nous melanoma. These occur as dark, sometimes irregularly shaped lesions on the palms and soles and as
new, often broad and solitary, darkly pigmented longitudinal streaks in the nails. Acral lentiginous
melanoma may be a difficult diagnosis because benign
pigmented lesions of the hands, feet, and nails occur
commonly in more darkly pigmented persons and
clinicians may hesitate to biopsy the palms and especially the soles and nail beds. As a result, the diagnosis
is often delayed until the tumor has become clinically
obvious and histologically thick. Clinicians should
give special attention to new or changing lesions in
these areas.

Melanomas vary from macules to nodules. Variegation of color from flesh tints to pitch black and a frequent admixture of white, blue, purple, and red may
occur. The border tends to be irregular, and growth
may be rapid or indolent. Melanomas are often larger
than 6 mm. Again, one should refer lesions based on a
suspicion of melanoma rather than delay until the diagnosis is certain. Dermoscopy—use of a special magnifying device to evaluate pigmented lesions—helps
select suspicious lesions that require biopsy. In experienced hands, the specificity is 85% and the sensitivity
95%.

Treatment

Treatment of melanoma consists of excision. After histologic diagnosis, the area is usually reexcised with
margins dictated by the thickness of the tumor. Large
margins (radius ≥ 5 cm) are no longer indicated. Thin
low-risk and intermediate-risk tumors require only
conservative margins of 1–3 cm. More specifically,
surgical margins of 0.5 cm for melanoma in situ and 1
cm for lesions less than 1 mm in thickness are most
often recommended.

Sentinel lymph node biopsy (selective lymphadenectomy) using preoperative lymphoscintigraphy
and intraoperative lymphatic mapping is effective for
staging melanoma patients with intermediate risk
without clinical adenopathy and is recommended for
all patients with lesions over 1 mm in thickness or
with high-risk histologic features. Alpha interferon
and vaccine therapy may reduce recurrences in patients with high-risk melanomas. Referral of intermediate-risk and high-risk patients to centers with expertise in melanoma is strongly recommended.

Bafounta M et al: Is dermoscopy (epiluminescence microscopy)
useful for the diagnosis of melanoma? Arch Dermatol
2001;137:1343. [PMID: 11594860]

Balch CM et al: A new American Joint Committee on Cancer
staging system for cutaneous melanoma. Cancer
2000;88:1484. [PMID: 10717634]

Goldstein BG et al: Diagnosis and management of malignant
melanoma. Am Fam Physician 2001;63:1359. [PMID:
11310650]

Rigel DS et al: Malignant melanoma: prevention, early detection,
and treatment in the 21st century. CA Cancer J Clin
2000;50:215. [PMID: 10986965]

White WL et al: Sentinel lymphadenectomy in the management
of primary cutaneous malignant melanoma. An update.
Dermatol Clin 1999;17:645. [PMID: 10410864]

SCALING DISORDERS
ATOPIC DERMATITIS
(Eczema)

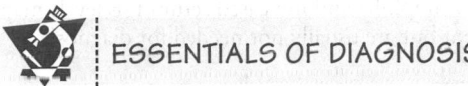 ESSENTIALS OF DIAGNOSIS

- *Pruritic, exudative, or lichenified eruption on
face, neck, upper trunk, wrists, and hands and in
the antecubital and popliteal folds.*
- *Personal or family history of allergic manifestations (eg, asthma, allergic rhinitis, atopic dermatitis).*
- *Tendency to recur.*

General Considerations

Atopic dermatitis looks different at different ages and
in people of different races. Because most patients
have scaly dry skin at some point, this disease is being
discussed under scaly dermatoses. However, acute
flares may present with red patches that are weepy,
shiny, or lichenified (ie, thickened, with more prominent skin markings) and plaques and papules. Diagnostic criteria for atopic dermatitis must include pruritus, typical morphology and distribution (flexural
lichenification in adults), and a tendency toward
chronic or chronically relapsing dermatitis. Also helpful are (1) a personal or family history of atopic disease
(asthma, allergic rhinitis, atopic dermatitis), (2) xero-
sis-ichthyosis, (3) facial pallor with infraorbital darkening, (4) elevated serum IgE, (5) fissures under the
ear lobes, (6) a tendency toward nonspecific hand dermatitis, (7) a tendency toward repeated skin infections, and (8) nipple eczema.

Clinical Findings

A. SYMPTOMS AND SIGNS

Itching may be severe and prolonged. The epidermal
inflammation of acute dermatitis results in rough, red
patches without the thickening and discrete demarca-
tion of a proliferative epidermal disorder such as psoriasis. The distribution of the lesions is characteristic,
with involvement of the face, neck, and upper trunk
("monk's cowl"). The bends of the elbows and knees
are involved. The skin is dry, leathery, and lichenified.
Pigmented persons tend to present with a papular
eruption and poorly demarcated hypopigmented

patches (pityriasis alba) are commonly seen on the cheeks and extremities. In black patients with severe disease, pigmentation may be lost in lichenified areas around the wrists and ankles.

B. Laboratory Findings

Food allergy is an uncommon cause of flares of atopic dermatitis in adults. Blinded food challenges are the most reliable method of diagnosing suspected food allergy. RASTs or skin tests may suggest dust mite allergy. Eosinophilia and increased serum IgE levels may be present but are usually not needed for diagnosis.

Differential Diagnosis

Atopic dermatitis must be distinguished from seborrheic dermatitis (frequent scalp and face involvement, greasy and scaly lesions, and quick response to therapy). Contact dermatitis and impetigo may be in the differential, especially for hyperacute, weepy flares of atopic dermatitis (although typically these diseases do not have a chronic course and characteristic distribution). Patients with active lesions are almost always colonized with *Staphylococcus aureus,* and impetiginization of atopic skin should be considered and treated when the patient presents with an acute flare.

Treatment

Treatment is most effective if the patient is instructed about many aspects of skin care and specific ways to use medications.

A. General Measures

These patients have hyperirritable skin. Anything that dries or irritates the skin will potentially trigger dermatitis. Atopic individuals are sensitive to low humidity and often get worse in the winter, when the air is dry. Adults with atopic disorders should not bathe more than once daily. Soap should be confined to the armpits, groin, and feet and should be used only just before rinsing and ending the bath. Washcloths and brushes should not be used. Soaps should not be drying, and Dove, Eucerin, Aveeno, Basis, Alpha Keri, Purpose, and other soaps or cleansers, such as Cetaphil or Aquanil, may be recommended. After rinsing, the skin should be patted dry (not rubbed) and then immediately—before it dries completely—covered with a thin film of an emollient such as Aquaphor, Eucerin, Vaseline, or a corticosteroid as needed. Triceram cream, a therapeutic moisturizer, will reduce inflammation as well as moisturize without a greasy or occlusive feel. It is much more expensive than traditional moisturizers. Atopic patients may be irritated by scratchy fabrics, including wools and acrylics. Cottons are preferable, but synthetic blends also are tolerated.

Other triggers of eczema in some patients include sweating, ointments, hot bathing, and animal danders.

To determine the potential effect of fluids, the patient may eliminate one food at a time for several months and monitor the severity of the disease. Dairy products and wheat are the most common offenders. Foods that are a problem typically cause itching within minutes to a few hours after eating.

B. Local Treatment

Corticosteroids should be applied sparingly to the dermatitis twice to four times daily and rubbed in well. Their potency should be appropriate to the severity of the dermatitis. In general, one should begin with hydrocortisone or another slightly stronger mild steroid (Aclovate, Desonide) and use triamcinolone 0.1% for short periods of time. It is vital that patients taper corticosteroids and substitute emollients when the dermatitis clears to avoid both tachyphylaxis and the side effects of corticosteroids. Tapering is also important to avoid rebound flares of the dermatitis that may follow their abrupt cessation. Doxepin cream 5% may be used up to four times daily and is best applied simultaneously with the topical steroid. Stinging and drowsiness occur in 25%. Tacrolimus ointment (Protopic) is effective in managing atopic dermatitis as a first-line steroid-sparing agent. It is available in 0.03% and 0.1% concentrations and is applied twice daily. Burning on application occurs in about half of patients but may resolve with continued treatment. The medication does not appear to cause skin atrophy, striae, or other topical steroid-associated side effects and is safe for application on the face and even the eyelids. Pimecrolimus (Elidel) cream 0.1% is another nonsteroidal anti-inflammatory agent with indications similar to those of tacrolimus. It is in a cream base and burns much less frequently than tacrolimus.

Treatment is dictated by the stage of the dermatitis.

1. Acute weeping lesions—Use saline or aluminum subacetate solution (Domeboro tablets, one in a pint of cool water) or colloidal oatmeal (Aveeno; dispense one box, and use as directed on box) as soothing or astringent soaks, baths, or wet dressings for 10–30 minutes two to four times daily. Lesions on extremities particularly may be bandaged for protection at night. Steroid lotions or creams are preferred to ointments for this stage. Use high-potency corticosteroids after bathing but spare the face and body folds. Tacrolimus may not be tolerated at this stage. Systemic corticosteroids may be required (see below).

2. Subacute or scaly lesions—At this stage, the lesions are dry but still red and pruritic. Mid- to high-potency steroids in ointment form if tolerated—creams if not—should be continued until scaling and elevated skin lesions are cleared and itching is decreased substantially. At that point, patients should begin a 2- to 4-week taper from twice-daily to daily to alternate-day dosing with topical steroids to reliance on emollients, with occasional use of steroids on specific itchy areas. Instead of tapering the frequency of usage of a more potent steroid, it may be preferable to switch to a low-potency steroid such as hydrocortisone or alclometasone. Tacrolimus or pimecrolimus may be added if steroids cannot be stopped.

3. Chronic, dry, lichenified lesions—Thickened and usually well-demarcated, they are best treated with high-potency to highest potency steroid ointments. Nightly occlusion for 2–6 weeks may enhance the initial response. Occasionally, tar preparations such as LCD (liquor carbonis detergens) 10% in Aquaphor or 2% crude coal tar (MG-217, an OTC preparation) may be beneficial if corticosteroids are not sufficient.

C. SYSTEMIC AND ADJUVANT THERAPY

Systemic corticosteroids are indicated only in extensive and more severe cases. Oral prednisone dosages should be high enough to suppress the dermatitis quickly, usually starting with 40–60 mg daily for adults. The dosage is then tapered to nil over a period of 2–4 weeks. Owing to the chronic nature of atopic dermatitis and the side effects of chronic systemic corticosteroids, long-term use of these agents is not a good form of maintenance therapy. Classic antihistamines may relieve severe pruritus. Hydroxyzine, brompheniramine, or doxepin may be useful—the dosage increased gradually to avoid drowsiness. Fissures, crusts, erosions, or pustules indicate staphylococcal infection clinically. Therefore, antistaphylococcal antibiotics given systemically—such as dicloxacillin or first-generation cephalosporins—may be helpful in management and are often used during flares. Phototherapy can be an important adjunct for severely affected patients, and the properly selected patient with recalcitrant disease may benefit greatly from therapy with UVB with or without coal tar, UVA, or PUVA.

Complications of Treatment

The clinician should monitor for skin atrophy. **Eczema herpeticum,** a generalized herpes simplex infection manifested by monomorphic vesicles, crusts, or erosions superimposed on atopic dermatitis or other extensive eczematous processes, is treated successfully with oral acyclovir, 200 mg five times daily, or intravenous acyclovir in a dose of 10 mg/kg intravenously every 8 hours (500 mg/m^2 every 8 hours).

Prognosis

The disease runs a chronic or intermittent course. Affected adults may have only hand dermatitis. Poor prognostic factors for persistence into adulthood in atopic dermatitis include onset early in childhood, early generalized disease, and asthma. Only 40–60% of these patients have lasting remissions.

Hanifin JM et al: Update on therapy of atopic dermatitis. J Allergy Clin Immunol 1999;104(3 Part 2):S123. [PMID: 10482863]

Jaffe R: Atopic dermatitis. Prim Care 2000;27:503. [PMID: 10815058]

Reitamo S et al: Safety and efficacy of 1 year of tacrolimus ointment monotherapy in adults with atopic dermatitis. The European Tacrolimus Ointment Study Group. Arch Dermatol 2000;136:999. [PMID: 10926735]

LICHEN SIMPLEX CHRONICUS (Circumscribed Neurodermatitis)

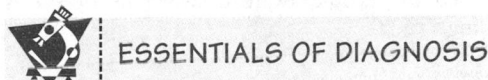 ESSENTIALS OF DIAGNOSIS

- Chronic itching.
- Lichenified lesions with exaggerated skin lines overlying a thickened, well-circumscribed scaly plaque.
- Predilection for nape of neck, wrists, external surfaces of forearms, lower legs, popliteal and antecubital areas.

General Considerations

Lichen simplex chronicus represents a self-perpetuating scratch-itch cycle.

Clinical Findings

Intermittent itching incites the patient to scratch the lesions. Itching may be so intense as to interfere with sleep. Dry, leathery, hypertrophic, lichenified plaques appear on the neck, ankles, perineum, or almost anywhere. The patches are rectangular, thickened, and pigmented. The skin lines are exaggerated.

Differential Diagnosis

This disorder can be differentiated from plaque-like lesions such as psoriasis (redder lesions having whiter scales on the elbows, knees, and scalp and nail findings), lichen planus (violaceous, usually smaller polygonal papules), and nummular (coin-shaped) dermatitis. Similar lesions are seen in chronic atopic dermatitis.

Treatment

Topical corticosteroids give relief. Clobetasol, halobetasol, diflorasone, and betamethasone dipropionate in augmented vehicle are effective without occlusion and are used twice daily for several weeks. In some patients, flurandrenolide (Cordran) tape may be more effective, since it prevents scratching and rubbing of the lesion. These superpotent steroids are probably the treatment of choice but must be used with careful follow-up to avoid local side effects. The injection of triamcinolone acetonide suspension (5–10 mg/mL) into the lesions may occasionally be curative. Use of tars, such as 10% LCD (liquor carbonis detergens) in triamcinolone 0.1% ointment, or continuous occlusion with DuoDerm (occlusive flexible hydrocolloid dressing) for 7 days at a time for 1–2 months, may also be helpful. The area should be protected and the patient encouraged to become aware of when he or she is scratching.

Prognosis

The disease tends to remit during treatment but may recur or develop at another site.

PSORIASIS

 ESSENTIALS OF DIAGNOSIS

- *Silvery scales on bright red, well-demarcated plaques, usually on the knees, elbows, and scalp.*
- *Nail findings including pitting and onycholysis (separation of the nail plate from the bed).*
- *Mild itching (usually).*
- *May be associated with psoriatic arthritis.*
- *Histopathology is not often useful and can be confusing.*

General Considerations

Psoriasis is a common benign, acute or chronic inflammatory skin disease that appears to be based upon a genetic predisposition. Injury or irritation of normal skin tends to induce lesions of psoriasis at the site (Koebner's phenomenon). Psoriasis has several variants—the most common is the plaque type. Eruptive (guttate) psoriasis consisting of myriad lesions 3–10 mm in diameter occurs occasionally after streptococcal pharyngitis. Grave, occasionally life-threatening forms (generalized pustular and erythrodermic psoriasis) may rarely occur. Plaque type or extensive erythrodermic psoriasis with abrupt onset may accompany HIV infection.

Clinical Findings

There are often no symptoms, but itching may occur. Although psoriasis may occur anywhere, one should examine the scalp, elbows, knees, palms and soles, and nails. The lesions are red, sharply defined plaques covered with silvery scales. The glans penis and vulva may be affected. Occasionally, only the flexures (axillae, inguinal areas) are involved. Fine stippling ("pitting") in the nails is highly suggestive of psoriasis. Psoriatics often have a pink or red intergluteal fold. Not all patients have findings in all locations, but the occurrence of a few may help make the diagnosis when other lesions are not typical. Some patients present mainly with hand or foot dermatitis and only minimal findings elsewhere, posing a difficult diagnostic problem. There may be associated arthritis that can resemble the rheumatoid variety but with a negative rheumatoid factor; distal interphalangeal joints are frequently involved, especially if there are nail changes.

Differential Diagnosis

The combination of red plaques with silvery scales on elbows and knees, with scaliness in the scalp or nail findings, is diagnostic. Psoriasis lesions are well demarcated and affect extensor surfaces—in contrast to atopic dermatitis, with poorly demarcated plaques in flexural distribution. In body folds, scraping and culture for candida and examination of scalp and nails will distinguish psoriasis from intertrigo and candidiasis. Dystrophic changes in nails may simulate onychomycosis, but again, the general examination combined with a potassium hydroxide (KOH) or fungal culture will be valuable in diagnosis. The cutaneous features of Reiter's syndrome may mimic psoriasis.

Treatment

There are many therapeutic options in psoriasis, to be chosen according to the extent and severity of disease and with a clear understanding of the risks and benefits of therapy.

A. LIMITED DISEASE

For many patients, the easiest regimen is to use a high-potency to highest-potency topical steroid cream or ointment. It is best to restrict the highest-potency steroids to 2–3 weeks of twice-daily use and then use them in a pulse fashion three or four times on weekends or switch to a midpotency corticosteroid. Topical corticosteroids rarely induce a lasting remission. They may induce tachyphylaxis or cause psoriasis to become unstable. Additional measures are therefore commonly added to topical steroid therapy. Tar preparations such as Fototar cream, LCD (liquor carbonis detergens) 10% in Nutraderm lotion, or mixed directly with triamcinolone 0.1% cream are useful adjuncts when applied twice daily. Occlusion alone has been shown to clear isolated plaques in 30–40% of patients.

Occlusive dressings such as thin Duoderm are placed on the lesions and left undisturbed for as long as possible (a minimum of 5 days, up to 7 days) and then replaced. Responses may be seen within several weeks. Anthralin is another agent for localized disease, but it must be used properly, is irritating, and may stain the skin. Calcipotriene ointment 0.005%, a vitamin D analog, is used twice daily for treatment of moderate-plaque psoriasis. It has become the second most commonly used topical treatment for psoriasis (after topical steroids). Initially, patients are treated with twice-daily steroids to rapidly improve the psoriasis. Calcipotriene is then substituted for one of the steroid applications for several weeks. Eventually the topical steroids are stopped, and once- or twice-daily calcipotriene is continued chronically. Calcipotriene usually cannot be applied to the groin or on the face because of irritation. Treatment of extensive psoriasis with calcipotriene may result in hypercalcemia. Calcipotriene is incompatible with many topical steroids, so if used concurrently it must be applied at a different time.

Tazarotene gel, a topical retinoid, is useful for the treatment of mild to moderate plaque psoriasis. About 50% of patients obtained at least 75% improvement of their skin lesions with twice-daily application, though fewer than 10% of plaques completely clear with 8 weeks of treatment. Tazarotene gel is available in 0.05% and 0.1% formulations. There is no difference between once-daily and twice-daily applications of the 0.1% formulation, but the 0.05% formulation is less effective when used once-daily. This agent appears to be similar to calcipotriene in that it may be used to augment the benefits of other forms of treatment. It is more expensive than calcipotriene and more irritating. Tazarotene gel is compatible with topical steroids and may be applied simultaneously.

For the scalp, start with a tar shampoo, used daily if possible. For thick scales, use 6% salicylic acid gel (eg, Keralyt), P & S solution (phenol, mineral oil, and glycerin), or fluocinolone acetonide 0.01% in oil (Derma-Smoothe/FS) under a shower cap at night, and shampoo in the morning. In order of increasing potency, triamcinolone 0.1%, or fluocinolone, betamethasone dipropionate, fluocinonide or amcinonide, and clobetasol are available in solution form for use on the scalp twice daily. For psoriasis in the body folds, treatment is much more difficult, since potent steroids cannot be used. When mild corticosteroids are not effective and involvement or itch is severe, some of the modalities described immediately below may be required.

B. GENERALIZED DISEASE

If psoriasis involves more than 30% of the body surface, it is difficult to treat with topical agents. The treatment of choice is outpatient UVB light exposure three times weekly. Clearing occurs in an average of 7 weeks, and maintenance may be needed since relapses are frequent. Severe psoriasis unresponsive to outpatient ultraviolet light may be treated in a psoriasis day care center with the Goeckerman regimen, which involves use of crude coal tar for many hours and exposure to UVB light. Such treatment may offer the best chance for prolonged remissions.

PUVA (psoralen plus ultraviolet A, ie, ultraviolet light in the 320- to 400-nm wavelength range) may be effective even in patients who have failed standard UVB treatment. Long-term use of PUVA is associated with an increased risk of skin cancer (especially squamous cell carcinoma and perhaps melanoma), particularly in persons with fair complexions or those who have received ionizing radiation. Thus, periodic examination of the skin is imperative. Atypical lentigines are common. There can be rapid aging of the skin in fair individuals. Cataracts are a threat but have not been reported with proper use of protective glasses. PUVA may be used in combination with other therapy, such as acitretin or methotrexate.

Parenteral corticosteroids should not be used because of the possibility of induction of pustular lesions. Methotrexate is very effective for severe psoriasis in doses up to 25 mg once weekly. It should be used according to published protocols. Liver biopsy is performed initially after methotrexate has been used long enough by the patient to demonstrate that it is effective and well tolerated, and then at intervals depending on the cumulative dose, usually 1.5–2 g. Administration of folic acid, 1–2 mg daily, will eliminate nausea caused by methotrexate without compromising efficacy.

Acitretin, a synthetic retinoid, is most effective for pustular psoriasis in dosages of 0.5–1 mg/kg/d, but it also improves erythrodermic and plaque types and psoriatic arthritis. Liver enzymes and serum lipids must be checked periodically. Because acitretin is a teratogen and persists for long periods in fat, women of childbearing age must wait at least 3 years after completing acitretin treatment before considering pregnancy. When used as single agents, retinoids will flatten psoriatic plaques, but high doses may be required for complete clearing. Retinoids find their greatest use when combined with phototherapy—either UVB or PUVA, with which they are synergistic.

Cyclosporine dramatically improves psoriasis and may be used to control severe cases. Relapses are the rule after cessation of therapy, so another agent must be added if cyclosporine is stopped. Sulfasalazine in dosages of 1 g three times daily markedly improved about one-third of patients in a double-blinded study. Thus, sulfasalazine may be considered for patients who are not candidates for—or who cannot tolerate—more toxic drugs. Thioguanine is another effective alternative for severe disease and is used at doses of 40–80 mg for 2–7 days per week with frequent monitoring of the complete blood count.

Systemic immunomodulators can be effective in treating psoriasis, though the exact indications for the agents discussed below are still unclear. The TNF inhibitors etanercept (Enbrel) and infliximab (Remicade) have both shown substantial antipsoriatic activity comparable to that of the most potent immunosuppressives. Cost and potential toxicity are current limitations in use. Efalizumab, an anti-CD11a monoclonal antibody, is well tolerated and has moderate efficacy and no systemic toxicity has been reported to date. Alefacept (Amevive), a human fusion protein, inhibits activation of T cells by binding to CD2, selectively targeting memory-effector T cells. It does not seem to increase infections, and responses are rapid (within 2 weeks) and durable.

Prognosis

The course tends to be chronic and unpredictable, and the disease may be refractory to treatment.

Chaudhari U et al: Efficacy and safety of infliximab monotherapy for plaque-type psoriasis: a randomised trial. Lancet 2001;357:1842. [PMID: 11410193]

Koo J: Systemic sequential therapy of psoriasis: a new paradigm for improved therapeutic results. J Am Acad Dermatol 1999;41(3 Part 2):S25. [PMID: 10459144]

Lebwohl M et al: Treatment of psoriasis. Part 1. Topical therapy and phototherapy. J Am Acad Dermatol 2001;45:487. [PMID: 11568737] (New radiation sources such as lasers are now available. Newer treatments based on light sources are being examined.)

Lebwohl M et al: Treatment of psoriasis. Part 2. Systemic therapies. J Am Acad Dermatol 200145:649. [PMID: 11606913] (Combinations of different treatments are described. Investigational therapies are reviewed.)

Mease PJ et al: Etanercept in the treatment of psoriatic arthritis and psoriasis: a randomised trial. Lancet 2000;356:385. [PMID: 10972371]

Pardasani AG et al: Treatment of psoriasis: an algorithm-based approach for primary care physicians. Am Fam Phys 2000;61:725. [PMID: 10695585] (Cure is seldom achieved. If control becomes difficult or if psoriasis is generalized, the patient may benefit from phototherapy, systemic therapy, and referral to a physician who specializes in the treatment of psoriasis.)

PITYRIASIS ROSEA

ESSENTIALS OF DIAGNOSIS

- *Oval, fawn-colored, scaly eruption following cleavage lines of trunk.*
- *Herald patch precedes eruption by 1–2 weeks.*
- *Occasional pruritus.*

General Considerations

This is a common mild, acute inflammatory disease which is 50% more common in females. Young adults are principally affected, mostly in the spring or fall. Concurrent household cases have been reported.

Clinical Findings

Itching is common but is usually mild. The diagnosis is made by finding one or more classic lesions. The lesions consist of oval, fawn-colored plaques up to 2 cm in diameter. The centers of the lesions have a crinkled or "cigarette paper" appearance and a collarette scale, ie, a thin bit of scale that is bound at the periphery and free in the center. Only a few lesions in the eruption may have this characteristic appearance, however. Lesions follow cleavage lines on the trunk (so-called Christmas tree pattern), and the proximal portions of the extremities are often involved. Variants that affect the flexures (axillae and groin), so called inverse pityriasis rosea, and papular variants, especially in black patients, also occur. An initial lesion ("herald patch") that is often larger than the later lesions often precedes the general eruption by 1–2 weeks. The eruption usually lasts 4–8 weeks and heals without scarring.

Differential Diagnosis

A serologic test for syphilis should be performed if at least a few perfectly typical lesions are not present and especially if there are palmar and plantar or mucous membrane lesions or adenopathy, features that are suggestive of secondary syphilis. For the nonexpert, an RPR test in all cases is not unreasonable. Tinea corporis may present with red, slightly scaly plaques, but rarely are there more than a few lesions of tinea corporis compared to the many lesions of pityriasis rosea. A scraping of scale for a KOH test will rapidly make the diagnosis. Seborrheic dermatitis on occasion presents on the body with poorly demarcated patches over the sternum, in the pubic area, and in the axillae. The classic lesions of pityriasis rosea are not present. Tinea versicolor lesions, viral exanthems, and drug eruptions may simulate pityriasis rosea.

Treatment

Pityriasis rosea often requires no treatment. In Asians, Hispanics, or blacks, in whom lesions may remain hyperpigmented for some time, more aggressive management may be indicated. The most effective management consists of daily UVB treatments for a week, or prednisone as used for contact dermatitis. Topical steroids of medium strength (triamcinolone 0.1%) may also be used if pruritus is bothersome. Oral erythromycin for 14 days was reported to clear 73% of patients within 2 weeks (compared with none of the patients on placebo).

Prognosis

Pityriasis rosea is usually an acute self-limiting illness that disappears in about 6 weeks.

Sharma PK et al: Erythromycin in pityriasis rosea: A double-blind, placebo-controlled clinical trial. J Am Acad Dermatol 2000;42(2 Part 1):241. [PMID: 10642679]

SEBORRHEIC DERMATITIS & DANDRUFF

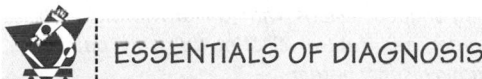

ESSENTIALS OF DIAGNOSIS

- Dry scales and underlying erythema.
- Scalp, central face, presternal, interscapular areas, umbilicus, and body folds.

General Considerations

Seborrheic dermatitis is an acute or chronic papulosquamous dermatitis. Seborrheic dermatitis may represent an inflammatory reaction to *Malassezia furfur* yeasts.

Clinical Findings

Pruritus is an inconstant finding. The scalp, face, chest, back, umbilicus, eyelid margins, and body folds have dry scales or oily yellowish scurf. Fissuring and secondary infection are occasionally present. Patients with Parkinson's disease, patients who become acutely ill and are hospitalized, and patients with HIV infection often have seborrheic dermatitis.

Differential Diagnosis

There is often a clinical spectrum ranging from simple dandruff to seborrheic dermatitis to scalp psoriasis. On the scalp, the presence of well-demarcated red plaques is termed psoriasis, and general erythema without tight, thick, silvery scale is called seborrheic dermatitis. The presence of mild scaling without any erythema is termed simple dandruff. Extensive seborrheic dermatitis may simulate intertrigo in flexural areas, but scalp, face, and sternal involvement suggests seborrheic dermatitis. Scaling of the scalp due to tinea capitis may simulate dandruff or seborrheic dermatitis, but alopecia is usually present in tinea capitis.

Treatment

A. SEBORRHEA OF THE SCALP

The clinician should suggest several shampoos and let the patient decide which is most acceptable. Shampoos that contain tar, zinc pyrithione, or selenium are used daily if possible, while ketoconazole shampoo (1% or 2%) is used twice weekly. Topical corticosteroid solutions or lotions are then added if necessary, and are used twice daily. (See treatment for scalp psoriasis, above.)

B. FACIAL SEBORRHEIC DERMATITIS

Mild soaps are usually used as described under atopic dermatitis. The mainstay of therapy is a mild corticosteroid (hydrocortisone 1%, alclometasone, desonide) used intermittently and not near the eyes. Potent fluorinated corticosteroids used on the face may produce steroid rosacea or atrophy and telangiectasia. These are rarely indicated for seborrheic dermatitis. If the disorder cannot be controlled with intermittent use of a topical steroid alone, ketoconazole (Nizoral) 2% cream is added twice daily.

C. SEBORRHEIC DERMATITIS OF NONHAIRY AREAS

Low-potency steroid creams—ie, 1% or 2.5% hydrocortisone, desonide, or alclometasone dipropionate—are highly effective.

D. SEBORRHEA OF INTERTRIGINOUS AREAS

Avoid greasy ointments. Apply low-potency steroid lotions or creams twice daily for 5–7 days and then once or twice weekly for maintenance as necessary. Ketoconazole shampoo may be a useful adjunct.

E. INVOLVEMENT OF EYELID MARGINS

"Marginal blepharitis" usually responds to gentle cleaning of the lid margins nightly as needed, with undiluted Johnson and Johnson Baby Shampoo using a cotton swab.

Prognosis

The tendency is to lifelong recurrences. Individual outbreaks may last weeks, months, or years.

Johnson BA et al: Treatment of seborrheic dermatitis. Am Fam Phys 2000;61:2703. [PMID: 10821151]

FUNGAL INFECTIONS OF THE SKIN

Mycotic infections are traditionally divided into two principal groups—superficial and deep. In this chapter, we will discuss only the superficial infections: tinea corporis and tinea cruris; dermatophytosis of the feet and dermatophytid of the hands; tinea unguium (onychomycosis); and tinea versicolor. See Chapter 36 for discussion of deep mycoses.

The diagnosis of fungal infections of the skin is usually based on the location and characteristics of the lesions and on the following laboratory examinations: (1) Direct demonstration of fungi in 10% KOH of scrapings from suspected lesions. "If it's scaly, scrape it" is a time-honored maxim. (2) Cultures of organisms from skin scrapings. Histologic sections of nails stained with periodic acid-Schiff (Hotchkiss-McManus) technique may be diagnostic if scrapings and cultures are negative. Serologic and skin tests are of no value in the diagnosis of superficial fungal infections.

Principles of Treatment

In general, treatment follows a diagnosis confirmed by KOH preparation or culture, especially if systemic antifungal therapy is to be used. Many other diseases cause scaling, and use of an antifungal agent without a firm diagnosis makes subsequent diagnosis more difficult. In general, fungal infections are treated topically except for those involving the scalp or nails or those deep in hair follicles on the face or body.

Griseofulvin is safe and effective for treating dermatophyte infections of the skin (except for the scalp and nails). It is more economical than the newer agents and may be used initially when systemic treatment is required for tinea cruris, tinea pedis, or tinea corporis.

Itraconazole, an azole antifungal, rapidly accumulates in the nail plate from the matrix and nail bed and persists for 6 months after oral administration is discontinued.

Terbinafine is an allylamine oral antifungal. It has excellent activity against dermatophytes. In vitro activity against yeast forms is variable, but the drug is active against hyphal forms. It is well delivered to the nail plate and persists in the nail for 6–9 months after treatment has ended.

Fluconazole has excellent activity against yeasts and may be the treatment of choice for many forms of mucocutaneous candidiasis. It is not known whether fluconazole is selectively delivered to the keratin compartment, and there have not been sufficient studies to determine effective doses in treating dermatophytosis. Fluconazole appears to require longer treatment courses and so is more expensive than either itraconazole or terbinafine for the treatment of dermatophytosis.

Itraconazole, fluconazole, and terbinafine can all cause elevation of liver function tests and—though rarely in the dosing regimens used for the treatment of dermatophytosis—clinical hepatitis. Ketoconazole is no longer recommended for the treatment of dermatophytosis (except for tinea versicolor) because of the higher rate of hepatitis when it is used for more than a month.

General Measures & Prevention

Since moist skin favors the growth of fungi, dry the skin carefully after bathing or after perspiring heavily. Talc or other drying powders may be useful. The use of topical corticosteroids for other diseases may be complicated by intercurrent tinea or candidal infection, and topical antifungals are often used in intertriginous areas with steroids to prevent this.

Rupke SJ: Fungal skin disorders. Prim Care 2000;27:407. [PMID: 10815051]

1. Tinea Corporis or Tinea Circinata (Body Ringworm)

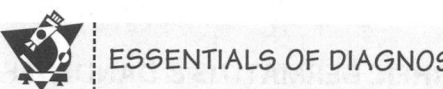 ESSENTIALS OF DIAGNOSIS

- Ring-shaped lesions with an advancing scaly border and central clearing or scaly patches with a distinct border.
- On exposed skin surfaces or the trunk.
- Microscopic examination of scrapings or culture confirms the diagnosis.

General Considerations

The lesions are often on exposed areas of the body such as the face and arms. A history of exposure to an infected cat may occasionally be obtained, usually indicating microsporum infection. All species of dermatophytes may cause this disease, but *Trichophyton rubrum* is the most common pathogen, usually representing extension onto the trunk or extremities of tinea cruris, pedis, or manuum.

Clinical Findings

A. SYMPTOMS AND SIGNS

Itching may be present. In classic lesions, rings of erythema have an advancing scaly border and central clearing, occasionally with hyperpigmentation.

B. LABORATORY FINDINGS

Hyphae can be demonstrated by removing peripheral scale and examining it microscopically using KOH. The diagnosis may be confirmed by culture.

Differential Diagnosis

Positive fungal studies distinguish tinea corporis from other skin lesions with annular configuration, such as the annular lesions of psoriasis, lupus erythematosus, syphilis, erythema multiforme, and pityriasis rosea. Psoriasis has typical lesions on elbows, knees, scalp, and nails. Secondary syphilis is often manifested by characteristic palmar, plantar, and mucous membrane lesions. Tinea corporis rarely has the large number of lesions seen in pityriasis rosea. Granuloma annulare lacks scales.

Complications

Complications include extension of the disease down the hair follicles (in which case it becomes much more difficult to cure), pyoderma, and dermatophytid.

Prevention

Treat infected household pets (microsporum infections).

Treatment

A. LOCAL MEASURES

The following applied topically are effective against dermatophyte infections other than those of the nails: miconazole, 2% cream; clotrimazole, 1% solution, cream, or lotion; ketoconazole, 2% cream; econazole, 1% cream or lotion; sulconazole, 1% cream; oxiconazole, 1% cream; ciclopirox, 1% cream; naftifine, 1% cream or gel; butenafine cream; and terbinafine, 1% cream. Miconazole, clotrimazole, and terbinafine are available OTC. Allylamines (especially terbinafine and butenafine) require shorter courses and lead to the most rapid response and prolonged remissions. Treatment should be continued for 1–2 weeks after clinical clearing. Betamethasone dipropionate with clotrimazole is often overused by nondermatologists. In general, short-term use of betamethasone-clotrimazole (Lotrisone) does not justify the expense, and chronic improper use may result in side effects from the high-potency steroid component, especially in body folds. Cases of tinea that are clinically resistant to this combination have been reported.

B. SYSTEMIC MEASURES

Griseofulvin (ultramicrosize), 250–500 mg twice daily, is used. Typically, only 2–4 weeks of therapy are required. Itraconazole as a single week-long pulse of 200 mg once daily is also effective in tinea corporis. Terbinafine, 250 mg daily for 1 month, is an alternative.

Prognosis

Body ringworm usually responds promptly to conservative topical therapy or to griseofulvin by mouth within 4 weeks.

2. Tinea Cruris
(Jock Itch)

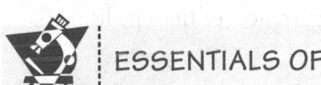

ESSENTIALS OF DIAGNOSIS

- Marked itching in intertriginous areas, usually sparing the scrotum.
- Peripherally spreading, sharply demarcated, centrally clearing erythematous lesions.
- May have associated tinea infection of feet or toenails.
- Laboratory examination with microscope or culture confirms diagnosis.

General Considerations

Tinea cruris lesions are confined to the groin and gluteal cleft. Intractable pruritus ani may occasionally be caused by a tinea infection.

Clinical Findings

A. SYMPTOMS AND SIGNS

Itching may be severe, or the rash may be asymptomatic. The lesions have sharp margins, cleared centers, and active, spreading scaly peripheries. Follicular pustules are sometimes encountered. The area may be hyperpigmented on resolution.

B. LABORATORY FINDINGS

Hyphae can be demonstrated microscopically in potassium hydroxide preparations. The organism may be cultured readily.

Differential Diagnosis

Tinea cruris must be distinguished from other lesions involving the intertriginous areas, such as candidiasis, seborrheic dermatitis, intertrigo, psoriasis of body folds ("inverse psoriasis"), erythrasma, and rarely tinea versicolor. Candidiasis is generally bright red and marked by satellite papules and pustules outside of the main border of the lesion. Candida typically involves the scrotum. Tinea versicolor can be diagnosed by the KOH preparation. Seborrheic dermatitis also often involves the face, sternum, and axillae. Intertrigo tends to be more red, less scaly, and present in obese individuals in moist body folds with less extension onto the thigh. Inverse psoriasis is characterized by distinct plaques. Other areas of typical psoriatic involvement should be checked, and the KOH examination will be negative. Erythrasma is best diagnosed with Wood's light—a brilliant coral-red fluorescence is seen.

Treatment

A. GENERAL MEASURES

Drying powder (eg, miconazole nitrate [Zeasorb-AF]) should be dusted into the involved area in patients with excessive perspiration or occlusion of skin due to obesity. Underwear should be loose-fitting.

B. LOCAL MEASURES

Any of the preparations listed in the section on tinea corporis may be used. There is great variation in expense, with miconazole, clotrimazole, and terbinafine available OTC and usually at a lower price. Terbinafine cream is curative in over 80% of cases after once-daily use for 7 days.

C. Systemic Measures

Griseofulvin ultramicrosize is reserved for severe cases. Give 250–500 mg orally twice daily for 1–2 weeks. One week of either itraconazole, 200 mg daily, or terbinafine, 250 mg daily, is also effective.

Prognosis

Tinea cruris usually responds promptly to topical or systemic treatment. It may leave behind postinflammatory hyperpigmentation.

Crawford F et al: Topical treatments for fungal infections of the skin and nails of the foot. Cochrane Database Syst Rev 2000(2):CD001434. [PMID: 10796792]

3. Tinea Manuum & Tinea Pedis (Dermatophytosis, Tinea of Palms & Soles, "Athlete's Foot")

 ESSENTIALS OF DIAGNOSIS

- *Most often presenting with asymptomatic scaling.*
- *May progress to fissuring or maceration in toe web spaces.*
- *Itching, burning, and stinging of interdigital webs, palms, and soles seen occasionally; deep vesicles in inflammatory cases.*
- *The fungus is shown in skin scrapings examined microscopically or by culture of scrapings.*

General Considerations

Tinea of the feet is an extremely common acute or chronic dermatosis. Certain individuals appear to be more susceptible than others. Most infections are caused by trichophyton species.

Clinical Findings

A. Symptoms and Signs

The presenting symptom may be itching, burning, or stinging. Pain may indicate secondary infection with complicating cellulitis. Interdigital tinea pedis is the most common cause of leg cellulitis in healthy individuals. Tinea pedis has several presentations that vary with the location. On the sole and heel, tinea may appear as chronic noninflammatory scaling, occasionally with thickening and cracking of the epidermis. This

may extend over the sides of the feet in a "moccasin" distribution. The KOH preparation is usually positive. Tinea pedis often appears as a scaling or fissuring of the toe webs, perhaps with sodden maceration. As the web spaces become more macerated, the KOH preparation and fungal culture are less often positive because bacterial species begin to dominate. Finally, there may also be grouped vesicles distributed anywhere on the soles or palms, generalized exfoliation of the skin of the soles, or nail involvement in the form of discoloration and thickening and crumbling of the nail plate.

B. Laboratory Findings

Hyphae can be demonstrated microscopically in skin scales treated with 10% potassium hydroxide. Culture does not always demonstrate pathogenic fungi from macerated areas.

Differential Diagnosis

Differentiate from other skin conditions involving the same areas, such as interdigital erythrasma (use Wood's light). Psoriasis may be a cause of chronic scaling on the palms or soles and may cause nail changes. Repeated fungal cultures should be negative, and the condition will not respond to antifungal therapy. Contact dermatitis (from shoes) will often involve the dorsal surfaces and will respond to topical or systemic corticosteroids. Vesicular lesions should be differentiated from pompholyx (dyshidrosis) and scabies by proper scraping of the roofs of individual vesicles. Rarely, gram-negative organisms may cause toe web infections in the setting of prior tinea or in its absence. Culture is not very specific, because gram-negative organisms can be cultured from normal toe webs. This entity is treated with aluminum salts (see below) and imidazole antifungal agents or ciclopirox.

Prevention

The essential factor in prevention is personal hygiene. Wear open-toed sandals if possible. Use of rubber or wooden sandals in community showers and bathing places is often recommended, though the effectiveness of this practice has not been studied. Careful drying between the toes after showering is essential. A hair dryer used on low setting may be used. Socks should be changed frequently, and absorbent nonsynthetic socks are preferred. Apply dusting and drying powders as necessary. The use of powders containing antifungal agents (eg, Zeasorb-AF) or chronic use of antifungal creams may prevent recurrences of tinea pedis.

Treatment

A. Local Measures

1. Macerated stage—Treat with aluminum subacetate solution soaks for 20 minutes twice daily. Broad-spectrum antifungal creams and solutions (containing imidazoles or ciclopirox instead of tolnaftate and haloprogin) will help combat diphtheroids and other gram-positive organisms present at this stage and alone may be adequate therapy. If topical imidazoles fail, often 1 week of once-daily allylamine treatment (terbinafine or butenafine) will result in clearing.

2. Dry and scaly stage—Use any of the agents listed in the section on tinea corporis. The addition of urea 10% lotion or cream (Carmol) under an occlusive dressing may increase the efficacy of topical treatments in thick ("moccasin") tinea of the soles.

B. SYSTEMIC MEASURES

Griseofulvin should be used only for severe cases or those recalcitrant to topical therapy. If the infection is cleared by systemic therapy, the patient should be encouraged to begin maintenance with topical therapy, since recurrence is common.

Itraconazole, 200 mg daily for 2 weeks or 400 mg daily for 1 week, or terbinafine, 250 mg daily for 2–4 weeks, may be used in refractory cases.

Prognosis

For many individuals, tinea pedis is a chronic affliction, temporarily cleared by therapy only to recur.

Roldan YB et al: Erysipelas and tinea pedis. Mycoses 2000; 43:181. [PMID: 10948816]

Tanuma H et al: Bifonazole (Mycospor cream) in the treatment of moccasin-type tinea pedis. Comparison between combination therapy of bifonazole cream + 10% urea ointment (Urepearl) and occlusive dressing therapy with the same agents. Mycoses 2000;43:129. [PMID: 10907343]

4. Tinea Versicolor (Pityriasis Versicolor)

ESSENTIALS OF DIAGNOSIS

- *Pale macules with fine scales that will not tan, or hyperpigmented macules.*
- *Velvety, tan, pink, whitish, or brown macules that scale with scraping.*
- *Central upper trunk the most frequent site.*
- *Yeast and short hyphae observed on microscopic examination of scales.*

General Considerations

Tinea versicolor is a mild, superficial *Malassezia furfur* infection of the skin (usually of the trunk). This yeast is a colonizer of all humans, which accounts for the high recurrence rate after treatment. It is not understood why some patients manifest the spore and hyphal form of the organism and the clinical disease. The eruption is often called to patients' attention by the fact that the involved areas will not tan, and the resulting hypopigmentation may be mistaken for vitiligo. A hyperpigmented form is not uncommon.

Clinical Findings

A. SYMPTOMS AND SIGNS

Lesions are asymptomatic, but a few patients note itching. The lesions are velvety, tan, pink, white, or brown macules that vary from 4–5 mm in diameter to large confluent areas. The lesions initially do not look scaly, but scales may be readily obtained by scraping the area. Lesions may appear on the trunk, upper arms, neck, face, and groin.

B. LABORATORY FINDINGS

Large, blunt hyphae and thick-walled budding spores ("spaghetti and meatballs") may be seen under the 10× objective when skin scales have been cleared in 10% KOH. Fungal culture is not useful.

Differential Diagnosis

Vitiligo usually presents with periorificial lesions or lesions on the tips of the fingers. Vitiligo (and not tinea versicolor) is characterized by total depigmentation, not just a lessening of pigmentation. Vitiligo does not scale. Pink and red-brown lesions on the chest are differentiated from seborrheic dermatitis of the same areas by the KOH preparation.

Treatment & Prognosis

Topical treatments include selenium sulfide lotion, which may be applied from neck to waist daily and left on for 5–15 minutes for 7 days; this treatment is repeated weekly for a month and then monthly for maintenance. Ketoconazole shampoo lathered on the chest and back and left on for 5 minutes may also be used weekly for maintenance. One must stress to the patient that the raised and scaly aspects of the rash are being treated; the alterations in pigmentation may take months to fade or fill in. Tinver lotion (contains sodium thiosulfate) is effective. Irritation and odor from these agents are common complaints from patients. Relapses are common.

Sulfur-salicylic acid soap or shampoo (Sebulex) or zinc pyrithrone-containing shampoos used on a continuing basis may be effective prophylaxis.

Ketoconazole, 200 mg daily orally for 1 week or 400 mg as a single oral dose, results in short-term cure of 90% of cases. Patients should be instructed not to shower for 12–18 hours after taking ketoconazole, because it is delivered in sweat to the skin. The single dose may not work in more hot and humid areas, and more protracted therapy carries a small but finite risk of drug-induced hepatitis for a completely benign disease. Without maintenance therapy, recurrences will occur in over 80% of "cured" cases over the subsequent 2 years.

Newer imidazole creams, solutions, and lotions are quite effective for localized areas but are too expensive for use over large areas such as the chest and back.

Rogers CJ et al: Diagnosing tinea versicolor: don't scrape, just tape. Pediatr Dermatol 2000;17:68. [PMID: 10720993]

DISCOID LUPUS ERYTHEMATOSUS (Chronic Cutaneous Lupus Erythematosus)

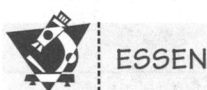 ESSENTIALS OF DIAGNOSIS

- *Localized red plaques, usually on the face.*
- *Scaling, follicular plugging, atrophy, dyspigmentation, and telangiectasia of involved areas.*
- *Histology distinctive.*
- *Photosensitive.*

General Considerations

This type of lupus erythematosus is a localized inflammation of the skin occurring most frequently in areas exposed to solar irradiation. Permanent hair loss and loss of pigmentation are common sequelae. Systemic lupus erythematosus is discussed in Chapter 20.

Clinical Findings

A. SYMPTOMS AND SIGNS

Symptoms are usually mild. The lesions consist of dusky red, well-localized, single or multiple plaques, 5–20 mm in diameter, usually on the face. The scalp, external ears, and oral mucous membranes may be involved. There is atrophy, telangiectasia, depigmentation, and follicular plugging. The lesion may be covered by dry, horny, adherent scales. On the scalp, significant hair loss may occur.

B. LABORATORY FINDINGS

If ANA is positive in high titer or when the clinical picture suggests systemic involvement, the findings of antibody to double-stranded DNA and hypocomplementemia suggest the diagnosis of systemic lupus erythematosus. Rare patients with marked photosensitivity and a picture otherwise suggestive of lupus have negative ANA tests but are positive for antibodies against Ro/SSA. A direct immunofluorescence test reveals basement membrane antibody but may be falsely positive in sun-exposed skin.

Differential Diagnosis

The diagnosis is based on the clinical appearance confirmed by skin biopsy in all cases. The scales are dry and "thumbtack-like" and can thus be distinguished from those of seborrheic dermatitis and psoriasis. Older lesions that have left depigmented scarring (classically in the concha of the ear) or areas of hair loss will also differentiate lupus from these diseases. Ten percent of patients with systemic lupus erythematosus have discoid skin lesions, and 5% of patients with discoid lesions have SLE.

Treatment

A. GENERAL MEASURES

Protect from sunlight. Use high SPF (> 30) sunblock with UVB and UVA coverage daily. *Caution:* Do not use any form of radiation therapy. Avoid using drugs that are potentially photosensitizing (eg, thiazides, piroxicam) where possible.

B. LOCAL TREATMENT

The following should be tried before systemic therapy: high-potency corticosteroid creams applied each night and covered with airtight, thin, pliable plastic film (eg, Saran Wrap); or Cordran tape; or ultra-high-potency corticosteroid cream or ointment applied twice daily without occlusion.

C. LOCAL INFILTRATION

Triamcinolone acetonide suspension, 2.5–10 mg/mL, may be injected into the lesions once a month. This should be tried before systemic therapy.

D. SYSTEMIC TREATMENT

1. Antimalarials—*Caution:* These drugs should be used only when the diagnosis is secure, because they have been associated with flares of psoriasis, which may be in the differential diagnosis. They may also cause ocular changes, and ophthalmologic evaluation is required every 6 months.

   a. Hydroxychloroquine sulfate—0.2–0.4 g orally daily for several months may be effective and is often used prior to chloroquine. A 3-month trial is recommended.

   b. Chloroquine sulfate—250 mg daily may be effective in some cases where hydroxychloroquine is not.

   c. Quinacrine (Atabrine)—100 mg daily may be the safest of the antimalarials, since eye damage has not been reported. It colors the skin yellow and is therefore not acceptable to some patients. It may be added to the above antimalarials for incomplete responses.

2. Isotretinoin—Isotretinoin, 1 mg/kg/d, is effective in chronic or subacute cutaneous lupus erythematosus. Recurrences are prompt and predictable on discontinuation of therapy. Because of teratogenicity, the drug is used with caution in women of childbearing age using effective contraception with negative pregnancy tests before and during therapy.

3. Thalidomide—Thalidomide is a potent teratogen but very effective in refractory cases in doses of 50–100 mg daily. Monitor for neuropathy.

Prognosis

The disease is persistent but not life-endangering unless systemic lupus intervenes, which is uncommon. Treatment with antimalarials is effective in perhaps 60% of cases. Although the only morbidity may be cosmetic, this can be of overwhelming significance in more darkly pigmented patients with widespread disease. Scarring alopecia can be prevented or lessened with close attention and aggressive therapy.

Duong DJ et al: American experience with low-dose thalidomide therapy for severe cutaneous lupus erythematosus. Arch Dermatol 1999;135:1079. [PMID: 10490113]

CUTANEOUS T CELL LYMPHOMA (Mycosis Fungoides)

ESSENTIALS OF DIAGNOSIS

- *Localized or generalized erythematous scaling plaques.*
- *Pruritus.*
- *Lymphadenopathy.*
- *Distinctive histology.*

General Considerations

Mycosis fungoides is a cutaneous T cell lymphoma that begins on the skin and may involve only the skin for years or decades. Certain medications (including SSRIs) may produce eruptions clinically and histologically identical to those of mycosis fungoides, so this possibility must always be considered.

Clinical Findings

A. SYMPTOMS AND SIGNS

Patients present with localized or generalized erythematous patches or plaques, usually on the trunk. Plaques are almost always over 5 cm in diameter. Pruritus is a frequent complaint. The lesions often begin as nondescript or nondiagnostic patches, and it is not unusual for the patient to have skin lesions for more than a decade before the diagnosis can be confirmed. In more advanced cases, tumors appear. Lymphadenopathy may occur locally or widely. Lymph node enlargement may be due to benign expansion of the node (dermatopathic lymphadenopathy) or by specific involvement with mycosis fungoides.

B. LABORATORY FINDINGS

The skin biopsy remains the basis of diagnosis, though at times numerous biopsies are required before the diagnosis can be confirmed. In addition, circulating atypical cells (Sézary cells) can be detected in the blood by sensitive methods. Eosinophilia may be present.

Differential Diagnosis

Mycosis fungoides may be confused with psoriasis, a drug eruption, an eczematous dermatitis, Hansen's disease (leprosy), or tinea corporis. Histologic examination can distinguish these conditions.

Treatment

The treatment of mycosis fungoides is complex. Early and aggressive treatment has not been proved to cure or prevent progression of the disease. Topical mechlorethamine ointment or solution, topical steroids, and PUVA are all used for early patches and plaques. Radiation therapy for local lesions and systemic agents such as retinoids, antitumor chemotherapeutic drugs, and alpha interferon are used alone or in various combinations for more advanced disease or in patients who fail topical therapy.

Prognosis

Mycosis fungoides is usually slowly progressive (over decades). Prognosis is better in patients with patch or plaque stage disease and worse in patients with erythroderma, tumors, and lymphadenopathy. Survival is not reduced in patients with limited patch disease. Elderly patients with patch and plaque stage disease commonly die of other causes. Overly aggressive treatment may lead to complications and premature demise.

Kim YH et al: Mycosis fungoides and the Sézary syndrome. Semin Oncol 1999;26:276. [PMID: 10375085]

Siegel RS et al: Primary cutaneous T-cell lymphoma: review and current concepts. J Clin Oncol 2000;18:2908. [PMID: 10920140]

van Doorn R et al: Mycosis fungoides: disease evolution and prognosis of 309 Dutch patients. Arch Dermatol 2000;136:504. [PMID: 1076864]

EXFOLIATIVE DERMATITIS (Exfoliative Erythroderma)

 ESSENTIALS OF DIAGNOSIS

- Scaling and erythema over most of the body.
- Itching, malaise, fever, chills, weight loss.

General Considerations

A preexisting dermatosis is the cause of exfoliative dermatitis in up to 63% of cases, including psoriasis, atopic dermatitis, contact dermatitis, pityriasis rubra pilaris, and seborrheic dermatitis. Reactions to topical or systemic drugs (eg, sulfonamides) account for perhaps 20–40% of cases and cancer (cutaneous T cell lymphoma, Sézary syndrome) for 10–20%. Causation of the remainder is indeterminable. At the time of acute presentation, without a clear-cut prior history of skin disease or drug exposure, it may be impossible to make a specific diagnosis of the underlying condition, and diagnosis may require follow-up with time.

Clinical Findings

A. Symptoms and Signs

Symptoms may include itching, weakness, malaise, fever, and weight loss. Chills are prominent. Redness and scaling may be generalized and sometimes includes loss of hair and nails. Generalized lymphadenopathy may be due to lymphoma or leukemia or may be part of the clinical picture of the skin disease (dermatopathic lymphadenitis). The mucosa is spared.

B. Laboratory Findings

A skin biopsy is required and may show changes of a specific inflammatory dermatitis or cutaneous T cell lymphoma or leukemia. Peripheral leukocytes may show clonal rearrangements of the T cell receptor in Sézary syndrome.

Differential Diagnosis

It may be impossible to identify the cause of exfoliative dermatitis early in the course of the disease, so careful follow-up is necessary. Psoriasis, severe seborrheic dermatitis, and drug eruptions may have an erythrodermic phase.

Complications

Debility (protein loss) and dehydration may develop in patients with generalized inflammatory exfoliative erythroderma; or sepsis may occur.

Treatment

A. Topical Therapy

Home treatment is with cool to tepid baths and application of mid-potency steroids under wet dressings or with the use of an occlusive plastic suit. If the exfoliative erythroderma becomes chronic and is not manageable in an outpatient setting, hospitalize the patient. Keep the room at a constant warm temperature and provide the same topical treatment as for an outpatient.

B. Specific Measures

Stop all drugs, if possible. Systemic corticosteroids may provide spectacular improvement in severe or fulminant exfoliative dermatitis, but long-term therapy should be avoided (see Chapter 26). In addition, systemic corticosteroids must be used with caution because some patients with erythroderma have psoriasis and could develop pustular psoriasis. For cases of psoriatic erythroderma and pityriasis rubra pilaris, either acitretin or methotrexate may be indicated. Erythroderma secondary to lymphoma or leukemia requires specific topical or systemic chemotherapy. Suitable antibiotic drugs with coverage for staphylococcus should be given when there is evidence of bacterial infection.

Prognosis

Most patients recover completely or improve greatly over time but may require chronic therapy. Deaths are rare in the absence of cutaneous T cell lymphoma. A minority of patients will suffer from undiminished erythroderma for indefinite periods.

Karakayli G et al: Exfoliative dermatitis. Am Fam Physician 1999;59:625. [PMID: 10029788]

Levine N: Exfoliative erythroderma. Skin biopsy is required to determine the cause of this pruritic eruption. Geriatrics 2000;55:25. [PMID: 10953683]

MISCELLANEOUS SCALING DERMATOSES

Isolated scaly patches may represent actinic (solar) keratoses, nonpigmented seborrheic keratoses, or Bowen's or Paget's disease.

Actinic Keratoses

Actinic keratoses are small (0.2–1 cm) patches—flesh-colored, pink, or slightly hyperpigmented—that feel like sandpaper and are tender when the finger is drawn over them. They occur on sun-exposed parts of the body in persons of fair complexion. Actinic keratoses are considered premalignant, but only 1:1000 lesions per year progress to become squamous cell carcinomas.

Application of liquid nitrogen is a rapid and effective method of eradication. The lesions crust and disappear in 10–14 days. An alternative treatment is the use of 1–5% fluorouracil cream. This agent may be rubbed into the lesions morning and night until they become first red and sore and then crusted and eroded (usually 2–3 weeks), and then stopped. Any lesions that persist should be evaluated for possible biopsy.

Chiarello SE: Cryopeeling (extensive cryosurgery) for treatment of actinic keratoses: an update and comparison. Dermatol Surg 2000;26;728 [PMID: 20398588]

Dinehart SM: The treatment of actinic keratoses. J Am Acad Dermatol 2000;42(1 Part 2):25. [PMID: 10607354]

Bowen's Disease & Paget's Disease

Bowen's disease (intraepidermal squamous cell carcinoma) occurs either on sun-exposed or sun-protected cutaneous surfaces. The lesion is a small (1–3 cm), well-demarcated, slightly raised, pink to red, scaly plaque and may resemble psoriasis or a large actinic keratosis. While it may take some time, these lesions may progress to invasive squamous cell carcinoma. Excision or other definitive treatment is indicated.

Extramammary Paget's disease, considered by some to be a manifestation of apocrine sweat gland carcinoma, resembles chronic eczema and may involve apocrine areas such as the genitalia. There seems to be less likelihood of an underlying sweat gland carcinoma if the lesions are on the vulva than if they are on the perianal area. Mammary Paget's disease of the nipple, a unilateral or rarely bilateral red scaling plaque that may ooze, is associated with an underlying intraductal mammary carcinoma.

Mehta NJ et al: Extramammary Paget's disease. South Med J 2000;93:713. [PMID: 10923963]

Zollo JD et al: The Roswell Park Cancer Institute experience with extramammary Paget's disease. Br J Dermatol 2000;142:59. [PMID: 10651695]

INTERTRIGO

Intertrigo is caused by the macerating effect of heat, moisture, and friction. It is especially likely to occur in obese persons and in humid climates. The symptoms are itching, stinging, and burning. The body folds develop fissures, erythema, and sodden epidermis, with superficial denudation. Candidiasis may complicate intertrigo. "Inverse psoriasis," tinea cruris, erythrasma, and candidiasis must be ruled out.

Maintain hygiene in the area, and keep it dry. Compresses may be useful acutely. Hydrocortisone 1% and an imidazole cream or nystatin cream are effective. Recurrences are common.

VESICULAR DERMATOSES

HERPES SIMPLEX
(Cold or Fever Sore; Genital Herpes)

 ESSENTIALS OF DIAGNOSIS

- *Recurrent small grouped vesicles on an erythematous base, especially in the orolabial and genital areas.*
- *May follow minor infections, trauma, stress, or sun exposure; regional lymph nodes may be swollen and tender.*
- *Tzanck smear is positive for multinucleated epithelial giant cells; viral cultures and direct fluorescent antibody tests are positive.*

General Considerations

Over 85% of adults have serologic evidence of herpes simplex type 1 (HSV-1) infections, most often acquired asymptomatically in childhood. Occasionally, primary infections may be manifested as severe gingivostomatitis. Thereafter, the subject may have recurrent self-limited attacks, provoked by sun exposure, orofacial surgery, fever, or a viral infection.

About 25% of the United States population has serologic evidence of infection with herpes simplex type 2 (HSV-2). HSV-2 causes lesions whose morphology and natural history are similar to those caused by HSV-1 on the genitalia of both sexes. The infection is acquired by sexual contact. In monogamous heterosexual couples where one partner has HSV-2 infection, seroconversion of the noninfected partner occurs in 10% over a 1-year period. Up to 70% of such infections appeared to be transmitted during periods of asymptomatic shedding. Uninfected female partners are at greater risk than males. Owing to changes in sexual behavior, up to 40% of newly acquired cases of genital herpes are due to HSV-1.

Clinical Findings

A. SYMPTOMS AND SIGNS

The principal symptoms are burning and stinging. Neuralgia may precede or accompany attacks. The lesions consist of small, grouped vesicles that can occur anywhere but which most often occur on the vermilion border of the lips, the penile shaft, the labia, the perianal skin, and the buttocks. Regional lymph nodes may be swollen and tender. The lesions usually crust and heal in 1 week. Patients can be educated to recognize attacks that they previously did not identify as recurrences of herpes simplex. Herpes simplex is the most common cause of painful genital ulcerations in patients with HIV infection.

B. LABORATORY FINDINGS

Lesions of herpes simplex must be distinguished from chancroid, syphilis, pyoderma, or trauma. Direct immunofluorescent antibody slide tests offer rapid, sensitive diagnosis. Viral culture may also be helpful. The Tzanck smear, which demonstrates multinucleated cells, is the least sensitive test. Herpes simplex and varicella-zoster viruses cannot be distinguished on the Tzanck smear. Herpes serology is not used in the diagnosis of an acute genital ulcer. However, specific HSV 2 serology by Western blot or new ELISA assays can determine who is HSV-infected and potentially infectious. Likewise, a negative serology documents lack of infection, ie, risk for infection. Such testing is very useful in couples in which only one partner reports a history of genital herpes.

Complications

Complications include pyoderma, eczema herpeticum, herpetic whitlow, herpes gladiatorum (epidemic herpes in wrestlers transmitted by contact), esophagitis, neonatal infection, keratitis, and encephalitis.

Prevention

Sunscreens are very useful adjuncts in preventing sun-induced recurrences. Prophylactic use of oral acyclovir may prevent recurrences. Acyclovir should be started at a dosage of 200 mg five times daily beginning 24 hours prior to ultraviolet light exposure, dental surgery, or orolabial cosmetic surgery. Comparable doses are 500 mg twice daily for valacyclovir and 250 mg twice daily for famciclovir.

Treatment

A. SYSTEMIC THERAPY

Three systemic agents are available for the treatment of herpes infections: acyclovir, its valine analog valacyclovir, and famciclovir. All three agents are very effective and, when used properly, virtually nontoxic. Only acyclovir is available for intravenous administration. In the nonimmunocompromised, with the exception of severe orolabial herpes, only genital disease is treated. For first clinical episodes (including primary) herpes simplex, the dosage of acyclovir is 200 mg orally five times daily (or 800 mg three times daily); of valacyclovir, 1000 mg twice daily; and of famciclovir, 250 mg three times daily. The duration of treatment is from 7 to 10 days depending on the severity of the

outbreak. Most cases of recurrent herpes are mild and do not require therapy. In addition, pharmacotherapy is of limited benefit, with studies finding a reduction in the average outbreak by only 12–24 hours. If treatment is desired, recurrent herpes outbreaks may be treated with 5 days of acyclovir, 200 mg five times a day; valacyclovir, 500 mg twice daily; or famciclovir, 125 mg twice daily. The addition of a potent topical steroid three times daily reduces the duration, size, and pain of orolabial herpes treated with an oral antiviral agent.

In patients with frequent or severe recurrences, suppressive therapy is most effective in controlling disease. Suppressive treatment will reduce outbreaks by 85% and reduces viral shedding by more than 90%. The recommended suppressive doses, taken continuously, are acyclovir, 400 mg twice daily; valacyclovir, 500 mg once daily; or famciclovir, 125–250 mg twice daily. Long-term suppression appears very safe, and after 5–7 years a substantial proportion of patients can discontinue treatment. It is unknown if the suppression of outbreaks and asymptomatic shedding will reduce transmission, but given the reduction of viral titers such therapy provides this might be considered as part of patient education. Barrier protection is not completely effective, since shedding occurs from widespread areas of the perineum not covered by condoms.

B. LOCAL MEASURES

In general, topical therapy is not effective. It is strongly urged that 5% acyclovir ointment, if used at all, be limited to the restricted indications for which it has been approved, ie, initial herpes genitalis and mucocutaneous herpes simplex infections in immunocompromised patients. Penciclovir cream, to be applied at the first symptom every 2 hours while awake for 4 days for recurrent orolabial herpes, reduces the average attack duration from 5 days to 4.5 days.

Prognosis

Aside from the complications described above, recurrent attacks last several days, and patients recover without sequelae.

Baker DA et al: Once-daily valacyclovir hydrochloride for suppression of recurrent genital herpes. Obstet Gynecol 1999;94:103. [PMID: 10289727]

Emmert DH: Treatment of common cutaneous herpes simplex virus infections. Am Fam Phys 2000;61:1697. [PMID: 10750877]

Spruance SL et al: Combination treatment with famciclovir and a topical corticosteroid gel versus famciclovir alone for experimental ultraviolet radiation-induced herpes simplex labialis: a pilot study. J Infect Dis 2000;181:1906. [PMID: 10837169]

Wald A: New therapies and prevention strategies for genital herpes. Clin Infect Dis 1999;28(Suppl 1):S4. [PMID: 10028105]

HERPES ZOSTER
(Shingles)

ESSENTIALS OF DIAGNOSIS

- Pain along the course of a nerve followed by painful grouped vesicular lesions.
- Involvement is unilateral; some lesions (< 20) may occur outside the affected dermatome.
- Lesions are usually on face or trunk.
- Tzanck smear positive, especially in vesicular lesions.

General Considerations

Herpes zoster is an acute vesicular eruption due to the varicella-zoster virus. It usually occurs in adults. With rare exceptions, patients suffer only one attack. Dermatomal herpes zoster does not imply the presence of a visceral malignancy. Generalized disease, however, raises the suspicion of an associated immunosuppressive disorder such as Hodgkin's disease or HIV infection. HIV-infected patients are 20 times more likely to develop zoster, often before other clinical findings of HIV disease are present. A history of HIV risk factors and HIV testing when appropriate should be considered, especially in zoster patients under 55 years of age.

Clinical Findings

Pain usually precedes the eruption by 48 hours or more and may persist and actually increase in intensity after the lesions have disappeared. The lesions consist of grouped, tense, deep-seated vesicles distributed unilaterally along a dermatome. The commonest distributions are on the trunk or face. Up to 20 lesions may be found outside the affected dermatomes. Regional lymph glands may be tender and swollen.

Differential Diagnosis

Since poison oak and poison ivy dermatitis can occur unilaterally, they must be differentiated at times from herpes zoster. Allergic contact dermatitis is pruritic; zoster is painful. One must differentiate herpes zoster from lesions of herpes simplex, which occasionally occurs in a dermatomal distribution. One should use doses of antivirals appropriate for zoster in the absence of a clear diagnosis. Facial zoster may simulate erysipelas initially, but zoster is unilateral and shows

vesicles after 24–48 hours. The pain of preeruptive herpes zoster may lead the clinician to diagnose migraine, myocardial infarction, acute abdomen, herniated nucleus pulposus, etc, depending on the dermatome involved.

Complications

Sacral zoster may be associated with bladder and bowel dysfunction. Persistent neuralgia, anesthesia or scarring of the affected area following healing, facial or other nerve paralysis, and encephalitis may occur. Postherpetic neuralgia is most common after involvement of the trigeminal region, and in patients over the age of 55. Early (within 72 hours after onset) and aggressive antiviral treatment of herpes zoster reduces the severity and duration of postherpetic neuralgia. Zoster ophthalmicus (V_1) can result in visual impairment.

Treatment

A. GENERAL MEASURES

1. Immunocompetent host—Since early treatment of zoster reduces postherpetic neuralgia, those with a risk of developing this complication should be treated, ie, those over age 55. In addition, younger patients with acute moderate to severe pain may be benefited by effective antiviral therapy. Treatment can be given with oral acyclovir, 800 mg five times daily; famciclovir, 500 mg three times daily; or valacyclovir, 1 g three times daily—all for 7 days. For reasons of increased bioavailability and ease of dosing schedule, the preferred agents are those given three times daily. Patients should maintain good hydration, and elderly patients with reduced renal function should be followed closely. The dose of antiviral should be adjusted for renal function as recommended. Nerve blocks may be important in the management of initial severe pain. Ophthalmologic consultation is vital for involvement of the first branch of the trigeminal nerve. Systemic corticosteroids are effective in reducing acute pain, improving quality of life, and returning patients to normal activities much more quickly. They do not increase the risk of dissemination in immunocompetent hosts. If not contraindicated, a tapering 3-week course of prednisone, starting at 60 mg/d, should be considered for its adjunctive benefit in immunocompetent patients. Oral corticosteroids do not reduce the prevalence, severity, or duration of postherpetic neuralgia beyond that achieved by effective antiviral therapy.

2. Immunocompromised host—Given the safety and efficacy of currently available antivirals, most immunocompromised patients with herpes zoster are candidates for antiviral therapy. The dosage schedule is as listed above, but treatment should be continued until the lesions have completely crusted and are healed or almost healed (up to 2 weeks).

Corticosteroids should not be given adjunctively in immunosuppressed hosts since they increase the risk of dissemination. Progression of disease may necessitate intravenous therapy with acyclovir, 10 mg/kg intravenously, three times daily. After 3–4 days, oral therapy may be substituted if there has been a good response to intravenous therapy. Adverse effects include decreased renal function from crystallization, nausea and vomiting, and abdominal pain.

Foscarnet, administered in a dosage of 40 mg/kg two or three times daily intravenously, is indicated for treatment of acyclovir-resistant varicella-zoster virus infections.

B. Local Measures

Calamine or starch shake lotions may be of some help.

C. Postherpetic Neuralgia

The most effective treatment is prevention with early and aggressive antiviral therapy. Once established, postherpetic neuralgia may be treated with capsaicin ointment, 0.025–0.075%, or lidocaine (Lidoderm) topical patches. Chronic postherpetic neuralgia may be relieved by regional blocks (stellate ganglion, epidural, local infiltration, or peripheral nerve), with or without corticosteroids added to the injections. Amitriptyline, 25–75 mg as a single nightly dose, is the first-line oral therapy beyond simple analgesics. Gabapentin, up to 3600 mg daily (starting at 300 mg three times daily), may be added for additional pain relief.

Prognosis

The eruption persists 2–3 weeks and usually does not recur. Motor involvement in 2–3% may lead to temporary palsy.

Alper BS et al: Does treatment of acute herpes zoster prevent or shorten postherpetic neuralgia? J Fam Pract 2000;49:255. [PMID: 10735485]

Dworkin RH et al: Prospects for the prevention of postherpetic neuralgia in herpes zoster patients. Clin J Pain 2000;16(2 Suppl):S90. [PMID: 10870747]

Stankus SJ et al: Management of herpes zoster (shingles) and postherpetic neuralgia. Am Fam Phys 2000;61:2437. [PMID: 10794584]

POMPHOLYX (Dyshidrosis, Dyshidrotic Eczema)

 ESSENTIALS OF DIAGNOSIS

- *"Tapioca" vesicles of 1–2 mm on the palms, soles, and sides of fingers, associated with pruritus.*
- *Vesicles may coalesce to form multiloculated blisters.*
- *Scaling and fissuring may follow drying of the blisters.*
- *Appearance in the third decade, with lifelong recurrences.*

General Considerations

"Dyshidrotic eczema" is a misnomer, suggesting that the vesicles of this condition are related to eccrine sweat ducts and sweating, which they are not. This is an extremely common form of hand dermatitis, preferably called pompholyx (Gr "bubble") or vesicular dermatitis of the palms and soles. Patients often have an atopic background and report flares with stress. Clues to a possible cause of pompholyx are suggested by the following observations. In Scandinavia, women with contact allergy to nickel and pompholyx appear to flare when given oral challenges with nickel. Nickel-free diets have given variable results. The chelator disulfiram has been reported to cause a 25% improvement in one controlled study in nickel-sensitive patients, and oral cromolyn sodium has also been shown to be of benefit. Patients with widespread dermatitis due to any cause may develop pompholyx-like eruptions as a part of an autoeczematization response.

Clinical Findings

Small clear vesicles stud the skin at the sides of the fingers and on the palms or soles. They look like the grains in tapioca. They may be associated with intense itching. Later, the vesicles dry and the area becomes scaly and fissured.

Differential Diagnosis

Unroofing the vesicles and scraping the blister roof for a KOH examination will reveal hyphae in cases of vesicular tinea. Blisters extending onto the dorsum of the hands may represent allergic contact dermatitis, and the culprit must be sought by history or by patch testing. Patients with inflammatory tinea pedis may have a vesicular dermatophytid of the palms. NSAIDs may produce an eruption very similar to that of dyshidrosis.

Prevention

There is no known way to prevent attacks.

Treatment

Topical and systemic corticosteroids help some patients dramatically. Since this is a chronic problem, systemic steroids are generally not appropriate therapy. A high-potency topical steroid used early in the attack may help abort the flare and ameliorate pruritus. Topical steroids are also important in treating the scaling and fissuring that are seen after the vesicular phase. It is essential that patients avoid anything that irritates the skin; they should wear cotton gloves inside vinyl gloves when doing dishes or other wet chores, use long-handled brushes instead of sponges, and use a hand cream after washing the hands. If a history of nickel allergy (rashes with costume jewelry or from watchbands) is obtained, nickel-free diets may be considered. Patients respond to PUVA therapy using topical psoralen and special UVA light sources designed to treat hands and feet.

Prognosis

For most patients, the disease is an inconvenience. Even with moderate to severe disease, flares can be controlled with scrupulous care. For some, pompholyx can be incapacitating.

DERMATOPHYTID
(Allergy or Sensitivity to Fungi)

 ESSENTIALS OF DIAGNOSIS

- *Pruritic, grouped vesicular lesions involving the sides and flexor aspects of the fingers and the palms.*
- *Fungal infection elsewhere on the body, usually the feet.*
- *No fungus demonstrable in lesions.*

General Considerations

Dermatophytid must be considered in the differential diagnosis of vesicles on the hands and feet. It is a hypersensitivity reaction to an active focus of inflammatory dermatophytosis elsewhere on the body, usually the feet. Fungi are present in the primary lesions but are not present in the lesions of dermatophytid. The hands are most often affected, but dermatophytid may occur on other areas also.

Clinical Findings

A. SYMPTOMS AND SIGNS

Itching is the only symptom.

B. LABORATORY FINDINGS

This entity is best diagnosed morphologically and by response to treatment.

Differential Diagnosis

Dermatophytid must be distinguished from all diseases causing vesicular eruptions of the hands—especially contact dermatitis, pompholyx, and photosensitive drug eruptions and "id" reactions due to inflammatory rashes.

Treatment

The lesions should be treated according to type of dermatitis. The primary focus of tinea should be treated with an oral antifungal or by local measures as described for dermatophytosis (see above).

Prognosis

Dermatophytid may occur in an explosive series of episodes, and recurrences are not uncommon; however, it clears with adequate treatment of the primary infection elsewhere on the body.

Busch RF: Dermatophytid reaction and chronic otitis externa. Otolaryngol Head Neck Surg 1998;118(3 Part 1):420. [PMID: 9727132]

PORPHYRIA CUTANEA TARDA

 ESSENTIALS OF DIAGNOSIS

- *Noninflammatory blisters on sun-exposed sites, especially the dorsal surfaces of the hands.*
- *Hypertrichosis, skin fragility.*
- *Associated liver disease.*
- *Elevated urine porphyrins.*

General Considerations

Porphyria cutanea tarda is the most common type of porphyria. Cases are sporadic or hereditary. The disease is associated with ingestion of certain medications (eg, estrogens), and liver disease from alcoholism or hepatitis C. In patients with liver disease, hemosiderosis is often present.

Clinical Findings

A. SYMPTOMS AND SIGNS

Patients complain of painless blistering and fragility of the skin of the dorsal surfaces of the hands. Facial hypertrichosis and hyperpigmentation are common.

B. LABORATORY FINDINGS

Urinary uroporphyrins are elevated two- to fivefold above coproporphyrins. Patients may also have abnormal liver function tests, evidence of hepatitis C infection, increased liver iron stores, and hemochromatosis gene mutations. Multiple triggering factors are often discovered.

Differential Diagnosis

Skin lesions identical to those of porphyria cutanea tarda may be seen in patients being maintained on dialysis and with the ingestion of certain medications (tetracyclines and NSAIDs, especially naproxen). In this so-called pseudoporphyria, the biopsy results are identical to those associated with porphyria cutanea tarda, but urine porphyrins are normal.

Prevention

Although the lesions are triggered by sun exposure, the wavelength of light triggering the lesions is beyond that absorbed by sunscreens, which for that reason are ineffective. Barrier sun protection with clothing is required.

Treatment

Stopping all triggering medications and substantially reducing or stopping alcohol consumption may alone lead to improvement. Phlebotomy without oral iron supplementation at a rate of one unit every 2–4 weeks will gradually lead to improvement. Very low dose antimalarials (as low as 200 mg of hydroxychloroquine twice weekly) will increase the excretion of porphyrins, improving the skin disease. Treatment is continued until the patient is asymptomatic. Urine porphyrins may be monitored.

Prognosis

Most patients improve with treatment. Sclerodermoid skin lesions may develop on the trunk, scalp, and face.

Bulaj ZJ et al: Hemochromatosis genes and other factors contributing to the pathogenesis of porphyria cutanea tarda. Blood 2000;95:1565. [PMID: 10688809]

Rich MW: Porphyria cutanea tarda. Don't forget to look at the urine. Postgrad Med 1999;105:208. [PMID: 10223097]

DERMATITIS HERPETIFORMIS

Dermatitis herpetiformis is an uncommon disease manifested by pruritic papules, vesicles, and papulovesicles mainly on the elbows, knees, buttocks, posterior neck, and scalp. It appears to have its highest prevalence in Scandinavia and is associated with HLA antigens -B8, -DR3, and -DQ2. The diagnosis is made by light microscopy, which demonstrates neutrophils at the dermal papillary tips. Direct immunofluorescence studies show granular deposits of IgA along the dermal papillae. Circulating anti-endomysium antibodies and antibod-

ies to tissue transglutaminase are present in 70% of cases. Patients have gluten-sensitive enteropathy, but for the great majority it is subclinical. However, ingestion of gluten plays a role in the exacerbation of skin lesions, and strict long-term avoidance of dietary gluten has been shown to decrease the dose of dapsone (usually 100–200 mg/d) required to control the disease and may even eliminate the need for drug treatment. Although adherence to a gluten-free diet is difficult, the availability of many gluten-free foods makes this easier to accomplish. Patients with dermatitis herpetiformis are at increased risk for development of gastrointestinal lymphoma, and this risk is reduced by a gluten-free diet.

Hervonen K et al: Concordance of dermatitis herpetiformis and celiac disease in monozygous twins. J Invest Dermatol 2000;115:990. [PMID: 11121131]

Stroubou E et al: Ursodeoxycholic acid causing exacerbation of dermatitis herpetiformis. J Am Acad Dermatol 2001; 45:319. [PMID: 11464204]

WEEPING OR ENCRUSTED LESIONS

IMPETIGO

Impetigo is a contagious and autoinoculable infection of the skin caused by staphylococci or streptococci (or both). Classically, two forms have been recognized: (1) a vesiculopustular type, with thick golden-crusted lesions caused by *Staphylococcus aureus* or group A β-hemolytic streptococcus; and (2) a bullous type, associated with phage group II *S aureus*. However, most cases of impetigo of either presentation now appear to be due to staphylococci.

Clinical Findings

A. SYMPTOMS AND SIGNS

Itching is the only symptom. The lesions consist of macules, vesicles, bullae, pustules, and honey-colored gummy crusts that when removed leave denuded red areas. The face and other exposed parts are most often involved. **Ecthyma** is a deeper form of impetigo caused by staphylococci or streptococci, with ulceration and scarring. It occurs frequently on the legs and other covered areas.

B. LABORATORY FINDINGS

Gram stain and culture confirm the diagnosis.

Differential Diagnosis

The main differential diagnosis is between impetigo and acute allergic contact dermatitis. Contact dermatitis may be suggested by the history or by linear distribution of the lesions, and culture should be negative for staphylococci and streptococci. Herpes simplex infection usually presents with grouped vesicles or discrete erosions and may be associated with a history of recurrences. Viral culture and Tzanck smears of the lesions are positive.

Treatment

Topical antibiotics are not as effective as systemic antibiotics. Two percent mupirocin ointment (Bactroban), dispensed as 15 g and used three times daily for 10 days, may be effective for limited disease. If the affected area is large or if there is fever or toxicity—or if there is any concern that a nephritogenic strain of streptococcus may be causative—systemic antibiotics should be given. Dicloxacillin or cephalexin, 250 mg four times daily, is usually effective. Erythromycin, 250 mg four times daily, is a reasonable alternative depending on the prevalence of erythromycin-resistant staphylococci in the community and as determined by culture and sensitivity tests. Recurrent impetigo is associated with nasal carriage of S aureus, treated with rifampin, 600 mg daily, or intranasal mupirocin ointment twice daily for 5 days.

Crusts and weepy areas may be treated with compresses, and washcloths and towels must be segregated and washed separately.

Veien NK: The clinician's choice of antibiotics in the treatment of bacterial skin infection. Br J Dermatol 1998;139(Suppl 53):30. [PMID: 9990410]

ALLERGIC CONTACT DERMATITIS

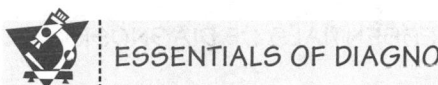

ESSENTIALS OF DIAGNOSIS

- *Erythema and edema, with pruritus, often followed by vesicles and bullae in an area of contact with a suspected agent.*
- *Later, weeping, crusting, or secondary infection.*
- *A history of previous reaction to suspected contactant.*
- *Patch test with agent positive.*

General Considerations

Contact dermatitis is an acute or chronic dermatitis that results from direct skin contact with chemicals or allergens. Eighty percent of cases are due to excessive exposure to or additive effects of primary or universal irritants (eg, soaps, detergents, organic solvents) and are called irritant contact dermatitis. The minority are due to actual contact allergy such as poison ivy or poi-

son oak. The most common topicals causing allergic rashes include antimicrobials (especially neomycin), antihistamines, anesthetics (benzocaine), hair dyes, preservatives (eg, parabens), latex, and adhesive tape. Occupational exposure is an important cause of allergic contact dermatitis. Weeping and crusting are typically due to allergic and not irritant dermatitis, which often appears red and scaly. Contact dermatitis due to latex rubber in gloves is of special concern in health care workers.

Clinical Findings

A. SYMPTOMS AND SIGNS

In allergic contact dermatitis, the acute phase is characterized by tiny vesicles and weepy and crusted lesions, whereas resolving or chronic contact dermatitis presents with scaling, erythema, and possibly thickened skin. Itching, burning, and stinging may be severe. The lesions, distributed on exposed parts or in bizarre asymmetric patterns, consist of erythematous macules, papules, and vesicles. The affected area is often hot and swollen, with exudation and crusting, simulating and at times complicated by infection. The pattern of the eruption may be diagnostic (eg, typical linear streaked vesicles on the extremities in poison oak or ivy dermatitis). The location will often suggest the cause: Scalp involvement suggests hair tints, sprays, or tonics; face involvement, creams, cosmetics, soaps, shaving materials, nail polish; neck involvement, jewelry, hair dyes, etc.

B. LABORATORY FINDINGS

Gram stain and culture will rule out impetigo or secondary infection (impetiginization). If itching is generalized and impetiginized scabies is considered, a scraping for mites should be done. During the acute episode, patch testing cannot be performed. After the episode has cleared, the patch test may be useful, but not all potential allergens are available for testing. In the event of a positive reaction, the clinical relevance of the chemical agent to the dermatitis must be determined. In suspected photocontact dermatitis—involvement of face, "V" of the upper chest, and hands, sparing the skin under the nose, chin, and inner upper eyelid—photopatch tests may be done by exposing the traditional patch test site to ultraviolet light after 24 hours.

Differential Diagnosis

Asymmetric distribution, blotchy erythema around the face, linear lesions, and a history of exposure help distinguish contact dermatitis from other skin lesions. The most commonly confused diagnosis is impetigo. Differentiation may be difficult if the area of involvement is consistent with that seen in other types of skin disorders such as scabies, dermatophytid, atopic dermatitis, pompholyx, and other eczemas.

Prevention

Prompt and thorough removal of allergens by washing with water or solvents or other chemical agents may be effective if done very shortly after exposure to poison oak or ivy. Several barrier creams (eg, Stokogard, Ivy Shield) offer some protection to patients at high risk for poison oak and ivy dermatitis if applied before exposure. Iodoquinol cream (Vioform) may benefit nickel allergic patients in a similar manner. Ingestion of rhus antigen is of limited clinical value for the induction of tolerance.

The mainstay of prevention is identification of agents causing the dermatitis and avoidance of exposure or use of protective clothing and gloves. In industry-related cases, prevention may be accomplished by moving the worker to another part of the workplace with different responsibilities.

Treatment

A. OVERVIEW

While local measures are important, severe or widespread involvement is difficult to manage without systemic corticosteroids because even the highest-potency topical steroids seem not to work well on vesicular and weepy lesions. Localized involvement (except on the face) can often be managed solely with topical agents. Irritant contact dermatitis is treated by protection from the irritant and use of topical steroids as for atopic dermatitis (described above). The treatment of allergic contact dermatitis is detailed below.

B. LOCAL MEASURES

1. Acute weeping dermatitis—Compresses are most often used. It is unwise to scrub lesions with soap and water. Calamine or starch shake lotions may sometimes be used in intervals between wet dressings, especially for involvement of intertriginous areas or when oozing is not marked. Lesions on the extremities may be bandaged with wet dressings for 30–60 minutes several times a day. Potent topical corticosteroids in gel or cream form may help suppress acute contact dermatitis and relieve itching. In cases where weeping is marked or in intertriginous areas, ointments will make the skin even more macerated and should be avoided. Suggested preparations are fluocinonide gel, 0.05%, used two or three times daily with compresses, or clobetasol or halobetasol cream, used twice daily for a maximum of 2 weeks—not in body folds or on the face. This should be followed by tapering of the number of applications per day or use of a mid-potency steroid such as triamcinolone 0.1% cream to prevent rebound of the dermatitis. A soothing formulation is 0.1% triamcinolone acetonide in Sarna lotion (0.5% camphor, 0.5% menthol, 0.5% phenol).

2. Subacute dermatitis (subsiding)—Mid-potency (triamcinolone 0.1%) to high-potency steroids (amcinonide, fluocinonide, desoximetasone) are the mainstays of therapy.

3. Chronic dermatitis (dry and lichenified)—High- to highest-potency steroids are used in ointment form.

C. SYSTEMIC THERAPY

For acute severe cases, one may give prednisone orally for 12–21 days. Prednisone, 60 mg for 4–7 days, 40 mg for 4–7 days, and 20 mg for 4–7 days without a further taper is one useful regimen. Another is to dispense seventy-eight 5 mg pills to be taken 12 the first day, 11 the second day, and so on. The key is to use enough corticosteroid (and as early as possible) to achieve a clinical effect and to taper slowly enough to avoid rebound. A Medrol Dosepak (methylprednisolone) with 5 days of medication is inappropriate on both counts. (See Chapter 26.)

Prognosis

Allergic contact dermatitis is self-limited if reexposure is prevented but often takes 2–3 weeks for full resolution.

Belsito DV: The diagnostic evaluation, treatment, and prevention of allergic contact dermatitis in the new millennium. J Allergy Clin Immunol 2000;105:409. [PMID: 10719287]

Tanner TL: Rhus (Toxicodendron) dermatitis. Prim Care 2000;27:493. [PMID: 10815057]

PUSTULAR DISORDERS
ACNE VULGARIS

 ESSENTIALS OF DIAGNOSIS

- *Occurs often at puberty, though onset may be delayed into the third or fourth decade.*
- *Open and closed comedones are the hallmark of acne vulgaris.*
- *The most common of all skin conditions.*
- *Severity varies from purely comedonal to papular or pustular inflammatory acne to cysts or nodules.*
- *Face and trunk may be affected.*
- *Scarring may be a sequela of the disease or picking and manipulating by the patient.*

General Considerations

Acne vulgaris is polymorphic. Open and closed comedones, papules, pustules, and cysts are found. The disease is activated by androgens in those who are genetically predisposed.

Acne vulgaris is more common and more severe in males. It does not always clear spontaneously when maturity is reached. Twelve percent of women and 3% of men over age 25 have acne vulgaris. This rate does not decrease until after age 44. The skin lesions parallel sebaceous activity. Pathogenic events include plugging of the infundibulum of the follicles, retention of sebum, overgrowth of the acne bacillus (*Propionibacterium acnes*) with resultant release of and irritation by accumulated fatty acids, and foreign body reaction to extrafollicular sebum. The mechanism of antibiotics in controlling acne is not clearly understood, but they may work because of their antibacterial or anti-inflammatory properties. Relapse or resistance may occur after emergence of tetracycline- or erythromycin-resistant strains of *P acnes*. These strains are usually sensitive to minocycline, however.

When a resistant case of acne is encountered in a woman, hyperandrogenism may be suspected. This may or may not be accompanied by hirsutism, irregular menses, or other signs of virilism.

Clinical Findings

There may be mild soreness, pain, or itching. The lesions occur mainly over the face, neck, upper chest, back, and shoulders. Comedones are the hallmark of acne vulgaris. Closed comedones are tiny, flesh-colored, noninflamed bumps that give the skin a rough texture or appearance. Open comedones typically are a bit larger and have black material in them. Inflammatory papules, pustules, ectatic pores, acne cysts, and scarring are also seen.

Acne may have different presentations at different ages. Preteens often present with comedones as their first lesions. Some patients have primarily comedones, with few inflammatory lesions. Inflammatory lesions in young teenagers are often found in the middle of the face, extending outward as the patient becomes older. Women in their third and fourth decades (often with no prior history of acne) commonly present with papular lesions on the chin and around the mouth so-called perioral dermatitis.

Differential Diagnosis

In adults, acne rosacea presents with papules and pustules in the middle third of the face, but telangiectasia, flushing, and the absence of comedones distinguish this disease from acne vulgaris. A pustular eruption on the face in patients receiving antibiotics or with otitis externa should be investigated with culture to rule out an uncommon gram-negative folliculitis. Patients who use systemic steroids or topical fluorinated steroids on the face may develop acne. Acne may be exacerbated or caused by irritating creams or oils. Pustules on the face can also be caused by tinea infections. Lesions on the back are more problematic. When they occur alone, one should suspect staphylococcal folliculitis, miliaria ("heat rash"), or, uncommonly, malassezia

folliculitis. Bacterial culture, trial of an antistaphylococcal antibiotic, and observing the response to therapy, will help in the differential diagnosis. In patients with HIV infection, folliculitis is common and often severe and may be either staphylococcal folliculitis or eosinophilic folliculitis.

Complications

Cyst formation, pigmentary changes in pigmented patients, severe scarring, and psychologic problems may result.

Treatment

A. GENERAL MEASURES

1. Education of the patient—When scarring seems out of proportion to the severity of the lesions, one must suspect that the patient is manipulating the lesions. It is essential that the patient be educated in a supportive way about this complication. Although there are exceptions, it is wise to let the patient know that at least 4–6 weeks will be required to see improvement and that old lesions may take months to fade. Therefore, improvement will be judged according to the number of new lesions forming after 6–8 weeks of therapy. Additional time will be required to see improvement on the back and chest, as these areas are slowest to respond. If hair pomades are used, they should contain glycerin and not oil. Avoid topical exposure to oils, cocoa butter (theobroma oil), and greases.

2. Diet—Foods do not cause or exacerbate acne.

B. COMEDONAL ACNE

Treatment of acne is based on the type and severity of lesions. Comedones require treatment different from that of pustules and cystic lesions. In assessing severity, one must also take the sequelae of the lesions into account. Therefore, one must treat an individual who gets only two new lesions per month that scar or leave postinflammatory hyperpigmentation much more aggressively than a comparable patient whose lesions clear without sequelae. Soaps play little role in acne treatment, and unless the patient's skin is exceptionally oily, a mild soap should be used to avoid irritation that will limit the usefulness of other topicals, all of which are themselves somewhat irritating.

1. Topical retinoids—Tretinoin is very effective for comedonal acne or for treatment of the comedonal component of more severe acne, but its usefulness is limited by irritation. Start with 0.025% cream (not gel) and have the patient use it at first twice weekly at night, then build up to as often as nightly. A few patients cannot use even this low-strength preparation more than three times weekly, but even that may cause improvement. A pea-sized amount is sufficient to cover half the entire face. To avoid irritation, have the patient wait 20 minutes after washing to apply.

Adapalene gel 0.1% and reformulated tretinoin (Renova, Retin A Micro, Avita) are other options for patients irritated by standard tretinoin preparations. Some patients—especially teenagers—do best on 0.01% gel. Although the absorption of tretinoin is minimal, its use during pregnancy is contraindicated. Some patients report photosensitivity with tretinoin. Patients should be warned that they may flare in the first 4 weeks of treatment. Tazarotene gel (0.05% or 0.1%) (Tazorac), a topical retinoid approved for treatment of psoriasis and acne, may also be effective.

2. Benzoyl peroxide—Benzoyl peroxide products are available in concentrations of 2.5%, 4%, 5%, 8%, and 10%, but it appears that 2.5% is as effective as 10% and less irritating. In general, water-based and not alcohol-based gels should be used to decrease irritation.

3. Antibiotics—Use of topical antibiotics (see below) has been demonstrated to decrease comedonal lesions.

4. Comedo extraction—Open and closed comedones may be removed with a comedo extractor but will recur if not prevented by treatment.

C. PAPULAR INFLAMMATORY ACNE

Antibiotics are the mainstay for treatment of inflammatory acne. They may be used topically or orally. The oral antibiotics of choice are tetracycline and erythromycin. Minocycline is often effective in acne unresponsive or resistant to treatment with these antibiotics but it is expensive. Doxycycline is effective, economical, and easy to take. Rarely, other antibiotics such as trimethoprim-sulfamethoxazole (one double-strength tablet twice daily), clindamycin (150 mg twice daily), or a cephalosporin (cefadroxil or cephalexin) may be tried. Topical clindamycin phosphate and erythromycin are also used (see below). Topicals are probably the equivalent of about 500 mg/d of tetracycline given orally, which is half the usual starting dose. Topical antibiotics are used in three situations: for mild papular acne that can be controlled by topicals alone, for patients who refuse or cannot tolerate oral antibiotics, or to wean patients under good control from oral to topical preparations. It has been recommended that switching or rotating antibiotics be avoided to decrease resistance and that courses of benzoyl peroxide be used on occasion.

1. Mild acne—The first choice of topical antibiotics in terms of efficacy and relative lack of induction of resistant *P acnes* is the combination of erythromycin or clindamycin with benzoyl peroxide topical gel. Clindamycin (Cleocin T) lotion (least irritating), gel, or solution, or one of the many brands of topical erythromycin gel or solution may be used twice daily and the benzoyl peroxide in the morning. (A combination of erythromycin or clindamycin with benzoyl peroxide is available as a prescription item.) The addition of tretinoin 0.025% cream or 0.01% gel at night may be effective, since it works via a different mechanism.

2. Moderate acne—Tetracycline, 500 mg twice daily, erythromycin, 500 mg twice daily, doxycycline, 100 mg twice daily, and minocycline, 50–100 mg twice daily, are all effective though minocycline is more expensive. When initiating minocycline therapy, start at 100 mg in the evening for 4–7 days, then 100 mg twice daily, to decrease the incidence of vertigo. Plan a return visit in 6 weeks and at 3–4 months after that. If the patient's skin is quite clear, instructions should be given for tapering the dose by 250 mg for tetracycline and erythromycin, by 100 mg for doxycycline, or by 50 mg for minocycline every 6–8 weeks—while treating with topicals—to arrive at the lowest systemic dose needed to maintain clearing. In general, lowering the dose to zero without other therapy results in prompt recurrence of acne. Tetracycline, minocycline, and doxycycline are contraindicated in pregnancy.

It is important to discuss the issue of contraceptive failure when prescribing antibiotics for women taking oral contraceptives. Women may need to consider using barrier methods as well, and should report breakthrough bleeding. Oral contraceptives or spironolactone (50–100 mg daily) may be added as an antiandrogen in women with antibiotic-resistant acne or in women in whom relapse occurs after isotretinoin therapy.

3. Severe acne—

a. Isotretinoin (Accutane)—A vitamin A analog, isotretinoin is used for the treatment of severe cystic acne that has not responded to conventional therapy. Informed consent must be obtained before its use in women of childbearing age. A dosage of 0.5–1 mg/kg/d for 20 weeks for a cumulative dose of at least 120 mg/kg is usually adequate for severe cystic acne. Patients should be offered isotretinoin therapy before they experience significant scarring if they are not promptly and adequately controlled by antibiotics. The drug is *absolutely contraindicated during pregnancy* because of its teratogenicity; two serum pregnancy tests should be obtained before starting the drug in a female and every month thereafter. Sufficient medication for only 1 month should be dispensed. Two forms of effective contraception must be used. Side effects occur in most patients, usually related to dry skin and mucous membranes (dry lips, nosebleed, and dry eyes). If headache occurs, pseudotumor cerebri must be considered. Depression has been reported. At higher dosage levels, about 25% of patients will develop hypertriglyceridemia, 15% hypercholesterolemia, and 5% a lowering of high-density lipoproteins. Some patients develop minor elevations of liver function tests. Fasting blood sugar may be elevated. Miscellaneous adverse reactions include decreased night vision, musculoskeletal or bowel symptoms, rash, thinning of hair, exuberant granulation tissue in lesions, and bony hyperostoses (seen only with very high doses or with long duration of therapy). Moderate to severe myalgias necessitate decreasing the dosage or stopping the drug. Laboratory tests to be performed in all patients before treatment and after 4 weeks on therapy include cholesterol, triglycerides, and liver function studies.

Elevations of liver enzymes and triglycerides return to normal upon conclusion of therapy. The drug may induce long-term remissions in 30–40%, or acne may recur that is more easily controlled with conventional therapy in 40–50%. Occasionally, acne does not respond or promptly recurs after therapy, but it may clear after a second course.

b. Intralesional injection—In otherwise moderate acne, intralesional injection of dilute suspensions of triamcinolone acetonide (2.5 mg/mL, 0.05 mL per lesion), will often hasten the resolution of deeper papules and occasional cysts.

c. Laser, dermabrasion—Cosmetic improvement may be achieved by excision and punch-grafting of deep scars and by abrasion of inactive acne lesions, particularly flat, superficial scars. The technique is not without untoward effects, since hyperpigmentation, hypopigmentation, grooving, and scarring have been known to occur. Dark-skinned individuals do poorly. Corrective surgery within 12 months after isotretinoin therapy may not be advisable.

Prognosis

Acne vulgaris eventually remits spontaneously, but when this will occur cannot be predicted. The condition may persist throughout adulthood and may lead to severe scarring if left untreated. Patients treated with antibiotics continue to improve for the first 3–6 months of therapy. Relapse during treatment may suggest the emergence of resistant *P acnes*. The disease is chronic and tends to flare intermittently in spite of treatment. Remissions following systemic treatment with isotretinoin may be lasting in up to 60% of cases. Relapses after isotretinoin usually occur within 3 years and require a second course in up to 20% of patients.

Johnson BA et al: Use of systemic agents in the treatment of acne vulgaris. Am Fam Physician 2000;62:1823. [PMID: 11057839]

Shaw JC: Low-dose adjunctive spironolactone in the treatment of acne in women: a retrospective analysis of 85 consecutively treated patients. J Am Acad Dermatol 2000;43:498. [PMID: 10954662]

Thiboutot D: New treatments and therapeutic strategies for acne. Arch Fam Med 2000;9:179. [PMID: 10693736]

ROSACEA

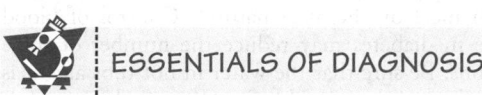

ESSENTIALS OF DIAGNOSIS

- *A chronic facial disorder of middle-aged and older people.*
- *A vascular component (erythema and telangiectasis) and a tendency to flush easily.*
- *An acneiform component (papules and pustules) may also be present.*
- *A glandular component accompanied by hyperplasia of the soft tissue of the nose (rhinophyma).*

General Considerations

No single factor adequately explains the pathogenesis of this disorder. A statistically significant incidence of migraine headaches accompanying rosacea has been reported.

Topical steroids can change trivial dermatoses of the face into **perioral dermatitis** and **steroid rosacea.** These occur predominantly in young women and may be confused with acne rosacea.

Clinical Findings

The cheeks, nose, and chin—at times the entire face—may have a rosy hue. One sees no comedones. Inflammatory papules are prominent, and there may be pustules. Associated seborrhea may be found. The patient often complains of burning or stinging with episodes of flushing. It is not uncommon for patients to have associated ophthalmic disease, including blepharitis and keratitis. This often requires systemic antibiotic therapy.

Differential Diagnosis

Rosacea is distinguished from acne by age, the presence of the vascular component, and the absence of comedones. The rosy hue of rosacea is due to inflammation and telangiectases and generally will pinpoint the diagnosis.

Treatment

Medical management is aimed only at the inflammatory papules and pustules and the erythema that surrounds them. The only satisfactory treatment for the telangiectasias is laser surgery. Rhinophyma (soft tissue and sebaceous hyperplasia of the nose) responds only to surgical debulking. Rosacea is usually a lifelong affliction, so maintenance therapy is required.

A. LOCAL THERAPY

Metronidazole, 0.75% gel applied twice daily or 1% cream once daily, is the topical treatment of choice. If metronidazole is not tolerated, topical clindamycin (solution, gel, or lotion) used twice daily is effective.

Erythromycin as described above may be helpful (see Acne Vulgaris). Five to 8 weeks of treatment are needed for significant response.

B. Systemic Therapy

Tetracycline or erythromycin, 250 or 500 mg orally twice daily on an empty stomach, should be used when topical therapy is inadequate. Minocycline, 50–100 mg daily to twice daily, may work in refractory cases.

Isotretinoin may succeed where other measures fail. A dosage of 0.5–1 mg/kg/d orally for 12–28 weeks is recommended. See precautions above.

Metronidazole, 250 mg twice daily for 3 weeks, may be worth trying but is seldom required. Side effects are few, though metronidazole may produce a disulfiram-like effect when the patient ingests alcohol.

Prognosis

Rosacea tends to be a stubborn and persistent process. With the regimens described above, it can usually be controlled adequately.

Thibodot DM: Acne and rosacea. New and emerging therapies. Dermatol Clin 2000;18:63. [PMID: 10626112]

Zuber TJ: Rosacea. Prim Care 2000;27:309. [PMID: 10815045]

FOLLICULITIS
(Including Sycosis)

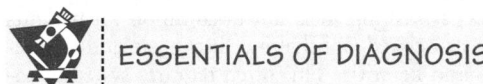

ESSENTIALS OF DIAGNOSIS

- Itching and burning in hairy areas.
- Pustules in the hair follicles.

General Considerations

Folliculitis has multiple causes. It may be caused by staphylococcal infection and may be more common in the diabetic. When the lesion is deep-seated, chronic, and recalcitrant on the head and neck, it is called sycosis. Sycosis is usually propagated by the autoinoculation and trauma of shaving. The upper lip is particularly susceptible to involvement in men.

Gram-negative folliculitis, which may develop during antibiotic treatment of acne, may present as a flare of acne pustules or nodules. Klebsiella, enterobacter, E coli, and proteus have been isolated from these lesions.

"Hot tub folliculitis," caused by Pseudomonas aeruginosa, is characterized by pruritic or tender follicular or pustular lesions occurring within 1–4 days after bathing in a hot tub, whirlpool, or public swimming pool. Rarely, systemic infections may result.

Nonbacterial folliculitis may also be caused by oils that are irritating to the follicle, and these may be encountered in the workplace (machinists) or at home (various cosmetics and cocoa butter or coconut oils).

Folliculitis may also be caused by occlusion, perspiration, and rubbing, such as that resulting from tight jeans and other heavy fabrics on the upper legs.

Folliculitis on the back that looks like acne but does not respond to acne therapy may be caused by the yeast Malassezia furfur. This infection may require biopsy for diagnosis.

Folliculitis—so called "steroid acne"—may be seen during topical or systemic corticosteroid therapy.

A form of sterile folliculitis called eosinophilic folliculitis consisting of urticarial papules with prominent eosinophilic infiltration is common in patients with AIDS.

Pseudofolliculitis is caused by ingrowing hairs in the beard area. In this entity, the papules and pustules are located at the side of and not in follicles. It may be treated by growing a beard, by using chemical depilatories, or by shaving with a foil-guard razor. Laser hair removal is dramatically beneficial in patients with pseudofolliculitis, requires limited maintenance, and can be done on patients of any skin color. Pseudofolliculitis is a true medical indication for such a procedure and should not be considered cosmetic.

Clinical Findings

The symptoms range from slight burning and tenderness to intense itching. The lesions consist of pustules of hair follicles.

Differential Diagnosis

It is important to differentiate bacterial from nonbacterial folliculitis. The history is important for pinpointing the causes of nonbacterial folliculitis, and a Gram stain and culture is indispensable. One must differentiate folliculitis from acne vulgaris or pustular miliaria (heat rash) and from infections of the skin such as impetigo or fungal infections. Pseudomonas folliculitis is often suggested by the history of hot tub use. Eosinophilic folliculitis in AIDS often requires biopsy for diagnosis.

Complications

Abscess formation is the major complication of bacterial folliculitis.

Prevention

Correct any predisposing local causes (eg, irritations of a mechanical or chemical nature). Control of blood glucose in diabetes may reduce the number of these infections. Be sure that the water in hot tubs and spas is treated properly with chlorine. If staphylococcal folliculitis is persistent, treatment of nasal or perineal carriage with rifampin, 600 mg daily for 5 days, or with topical mupirocin ointment 2% twice daily for 5 days, may help. The latter may cause stinging in some patients. Chronic oral clindamycin, 150–300 mg/d, is also effective in preventing recurrent staphylococcal folliculitis and furunculosis.

Treatment

A. LOCAL MEASURES

Cleanse the area gently with chlorhexidine and apply saline or aluminum subacetate soaks or compresses to the involved area for 15 minutes twice daily if very exudative.

Anhydrous ethyl alcohol containing 6.25% aluminum chloride (Xerac AC), applied to lesions and environs and followed by an antibiotic ointment (see above), may be helpful, especially for chronic folliculitis of the buttocks.

B. SPECIFIC MEASURES

Systemic antibiotics may be tried if the skin infection is resistant to local treatment, if it is extensive or severe and accompanied by a febrile reaction, if it is complicated, or if it involves the nose or upper lip. Extended periods of treatment (4–8 weeks or more) with antistaphylococcal antibiotics are required in some cases.

Hot tub pseudomonas folliculitis virtually always resolves without treatment but may be treated in adults with ciprofloxacin, 500 mg twice daily for 5 days.

Gram-negative folliculitis in acne patients may be treated with isotretinoin in compliance with all precautions discussed above (see Acne Vulgaris).

Folliculitis due to *M furfur* is treated with topical 2.5% selenium sulfide, 15 minutes daily for 3 weeks, or with oral ketoconazole, 200 mg daily for 7–14 days.

Irritant folliculitis is best treated by protection from the offending substance and use of drying agents such benzoyl peroxide or Xerac AC.

Eosinophilic folliculitis may be treated initially by the combination of potent topical steroids and oral antihistamines. In more severe cases, treatment is with one of the following: topical permethrin (application for 12 hours every other night for 6 weeks); itraconazole, 200–400 mg daily (tablets); UVB or PUVA phototherapy; or isotretinoin, 0.5 mg/kg/d for up to 5 months. A remission may be induced by some of these therapies, but chronic treatment may be required.

Prognosis

Bacterial folliculitis is occasionally stubborn and persistent, requiring prolonged or intermittent courses of antibiotics. Steroid folliculitis is treatable by acne therapy and resolves as steroids are discontinued.

MILIARIA
(Heat Rash)

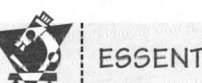 ESSENTIALS OF DIAGNOSIS

- Burning, itching, superficial aggregated small vesicles, papules, or pustules on covered areas of the skin, usually the trunk.
- More common in hot, moist climates.
- Rare forms associated with fever and even heat prostration.

General Considerations

Miliaria is an acute dermatitis that occurs most commonly on the trunk and intertriginous areas. A hot, moist environment is the most frequent cause. Bedridden febrile patients are susceptible. Plugging of the ostia of sweat ducts occurs, with consequent ballooning and ultimate rupture of the sweat duct, producing an irritating, stinging reaction. Increase in numbers of resident aerobes, notably cocci, apparently plays a role.

Clinical Findings

The usual symptoms are burning and itching. In severe cases, fever, heat prostration, and even death may result. The lesions consist of small, superficial, reddened, thin-walled, discrete but closely aggregated vesicles (miliaria crystallina), papules (miliaria rubra), or vesicopustules or pustules (miliaria pustulosa). The reaction occurs most commonly on covered areas of the skin.

Differential Diagnosis

Miliaria is to be distinguished from drug rash and folliculitis.

Prevention

Use of an antibacterial preparation such as chlorhexidine prior to exposure to heat and humidity may help prevent the condition. Susceptible persons should avoid exposure to hot, humid environments.

Treatment

Triamcinolone acetonide, 0.1% in Sarna lotion, or a mid-potency corticosteroid in a lotion or cream—but not ointment—base, should be applied two to four times daily. Alternative measures that have been employed with varying success are drying shake lotions and antipruritic powders or other dusting powders. Secondary infections (superficial pyoderma) are treated with erythromycin or dicloxacillin, 250 mg four times daily by mouth. Anticholinergic drugs given by mouth may be helpful in severe cases, eg, glycopyrrolate, 1 mg twice daily.

Prognosis

Miliaria is usually a mild disorder, but death may occur with the severe forms (tropical anhidrosis and asthenia) as a result of interference with the heat-regulating mechanism.

Wenzel FG et al: Nonneoplastic disorders of the eccrine glands. J Am Acad Dermatol 1998;38:1. [PMID: 9448199]

MUCOCUTANEOUS CANDIDIASIS

 ESSENTIALS OF DIAGNOSIS

- *Severe pruritus of vulva, anus, or body folds.*
- *Superficial denuded, beefy-red areas with or without satellite vesicopustules.*
- *Whitish curd-like concretions on the oral and vaginal mucous membranes.*
- *Yeast on microscopic examination of scales or curd.*

General Considerations

Mucocutaneous candidiasis is a superficial fungal infection that may involve almost any cutaneous or mucous surface of the body. It is particularly likely to occur in diabetics, during pregnancy, and in obese persons who perspire freely. Antibiotics and oral contraceptive agents may be contributory. Oral candidiasis may be the first sign of HIV infection (see Chapter 31).

Clinical Findings

A. SYMPTOMS AND SIGNS

Itching may be intense. Burning is reported, particularly around the vulva and anus. The lesions consist of superficially denuded, beefy-red areas in the depths of the body folds such as in the groin and the intergluteal cleft, beneath the breasts, at the angles of the mouth, and in the umbilicus. The peripheries of these denuded lesions are superficially undermined, and there may be satellite vesicopustules. Whitish, curd-like concretions may be present on the surface of the mucosal lesions. Paronychia and interdigital erosions may occur.

B. LABORATORY FINDINGS

Clusters of budding cells and hyphae can be seen under high power when skin scales or curd-like lesions have been cleared in 10% KOH. The organism may be isolated on Sabouraud's medium.

Differential Diagnosis

Intertrigo, seborrheic dermatitis, tinea cruris, "inverse psoriasis," and erythrasma involving the same areas may mimic mucocutaneous candidiasis.

Complications

Systemic invasive candidiasis with candidemia may be seen with immunosuppression and in patients receiving broad-spectrum antibiotic and hypertonic glucose solutions, as in hyperalimentation. There may or may not be clinically evident mucocutaneous candidiasis.

Treatment

A. GENERAL MEASURES

Affected parts should be kept dry and exposed to air as much as possible. If possible, discontinue systemic antibiotics. For treatment of systemic invasive candidiasis, see Chapter 36.

B. LOCAL MEASURES

1. Nails and skin—Apply ciclopirox cream, nystatin cream, 100,000 units/g, or miconazole, econazole, ketoconazole, or clotrimazole cream three or four times daily. Gentian violet, 1%, or carbolfuchsin paint (Castellani's paint) may be applied once or twice weekly as an alternative, but these preparations are messy.

2. Vulvar and anal mucous membranes—For vaginal candidiasis, single-dose fluconazole (150 mg) is effective. Intravaginal clotrimazole, miconazole, terconazole, or nystatin may also be used. Chronic suppressive therapy may be required for recurrent or "intractable" cases. Non-*albicans* candidal species may be identified by culture in some refractory cases and may respond to oral itraconazole, 200 mg twice daily for 2–4 weeks.

3. Balanitis—This is most frequent in uncircumcised men, and candida usually plays a role. Topical imidazole cream or nystatin ointment is the initial treatment if the lesions are mildly erythematous or superficially erosive. Soaking with dilute aluminum acetate for 15 minutes twice daily may quickly relieve burning or itching. Chronicity and relapses, especially after sexual contact, suggest reinfection from a sexual partner who should be treated. Severe purulent balanitis is usually due to bacteria. If it is so severe that phimosis occurs, oral antibiotics—some with activity against anaerobes—are required; if rapid improvement does not occur, urologic consultation is indicated.

Prognosis

Cases of cutaneous candidiasis range from the easily cured to the intractable and prolonged.

Ringdahl EN: Treatment of recurrent vulvovaginal candidiasis. Am Fam Physician 2000;61:3306. [PMID: 10865926]

FIGURATE ERYTHEMAS

URTICARIA & ANGIOEDEMA

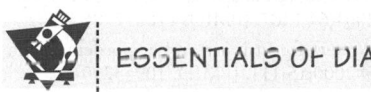 ESSENTIALS OF DIAGNOSIS

- *Eruptions of evanescent wheals or hives.*
- *Itching is usually intense but may on rare occasions be absent.*
- *Special forms of urticaria have special features (dermographism, cholinergic urticaria, solar urticaria, or cold urticaria).*
- *Most incidents are acute and self-limited over a period of 1–2 weeks.*
- *Chronic urticaria (episodes lasting > 6 weeks) may have an autoimmune basis.*

General Considerations

Urticaria can result from many different stimuli on an immunologic or nonimmunologic basis. The most common immunologic mechanism is hypersensitivity mediated by IgE, seen for most patients with acute urticaria; another involves activation of the complement cascade. Some patients with chronic urticaria demonstrate autoantibodies directed against mast cell IgE receptors, with histamine-releasing activity. ACE inhibitor and angiotensin II receptor antagonist therapy may be complicated by urticaria or angioedema. In general, extensive costly workups are not indicated in patients who present with urticaria. A careful history and physical examination are more helpful.

Clinical Findings

A. SYMPTOMS AND SIGNS

Lesions are itchy red swellings of a few millimeters to many centimeters. The morphology of the lesions may vary over a period of minutes to hours, resulting in geographic or bizarre patterns. Individual lesions in true urticaria last less than 24 hours, and often only 2–4 hours. Angioedema is involvement of deeper vessels, with swelling of the lips, eyelids, palms, soles, and genitalia in association with more typical lesions. An-

gioedema is no more likely than urticaria to be associated with systemic complications such as laryngeal edema or hypotension. In cholinergic urticaria, triggered by a rise in core body temperature (hot showers, exercise), wheals are 2–3 mm in diameter with a large surrounding red flare.

B. LABORATORY FINDINGS

Laboratory studies are not likely to be helpful in the evaluation of acute or chronic urticaria unless there are suggestive findings in the history and physical examination. The most common causes of acute urticaria are foods, viral infections, and medications. The cause of chronic urticaria is often not found. In patients with individual slightly purpuric lesions that persist past 24 hours, a skin biopsy may help exclude urticarial vasculitis. Quantitative immunoglobulins, cryoglobulins, cryofibrinogens, and antinuclear antibodies are often sought in cold urticaria but are rarely found. Liver tests may be of interest, since a serum sickness-like prodrome, with urticaria, may be associated with acute hepatitis B infection. An autologous serum is available to detect those patients with an autoimmune basis for their chronic urticaria. They should be considered only in the most difficult cases, since management will not be altered.

Differential Diagnosis

Papular urticaria resulting from insect bites persists for days. A central punctum can usually be seen. Streaked urticarial lesions may be seen in acute allergic plant dermatitis, eg, poison ivy, oak, or sumac. Contact urticaria may be caused by a host of substances, including chemicals, foods, and medications, and may be one type of reaction to latex. Contact urticaria is often limited to areas exposed to the contactant. Urticarial response to heat, sun, water, and pressure are quite rare. Urticaria may be seen as part of serum sickness, associated with fever and arthralgia.

In hereditary angioedema, there is generally a positive family history and gastrointestinal or respiratory symptoms, but urticaria is not part of the syndrome. Lesions are not pruritic.

Treatment

A. GENERAL MEASURES

A detailed search by history for a cause of acute urticaria should be undertaken, and treatment may then be tailored to include the provocative condition. The chief nonallergic causes are drugs, eg, atropine, pilocarpine, morphine, and codeine; arthropod bites, eg, insect bites and bee stings (though the latter may cause anaphylaxis as well as angioedema); physical factors such as heat, cold, sunlight, and pressure; and, presumably, neurogenic factors such as in cholinergic urticaria induced by exercise, excitement, hot showers, etc.

Allergic causes may include penicillins, aspirin, and other medications; inhalants such as feathers and animal danders; ingestion of shellfish, tomatoes, or strawberries; injections of sera and vaccines; external contactants, including various chemicals and cosmetics; and infections such as hepatitis.

B. SYSTEMIC TREATMENT

The mainstay of treatment initially includes H_1 antihistamines (see above). Hydroxyzine, 10 mg twice daily to 25 mg three times daily to even 100 mg three times daily, may be very useful if tolerated. Giving hydroxyzine as one dose of 50–75 mg at night may reduce sedation and other side effects. Cyproheptadine, 4 mg four times daily, may be especially useful for cold urticaria. "Nonsedating" or less sedating antihistamines are added if the generic sedating antihistamines are not effective. Fexofenadine is given in a dosage of 60 mg twice a day. Loratadine in a dosage of 10 mg/d is similar to the other H_1 antihistamines in effectiveness. Cetirizine, a metabolite of hydroxyzine, is less sedating (13% of patients) and is given in a dosage of 10 mg/d.

Doxepin (a tricyclic antidepressant), 25 mg three times daily, or, more commonly, 25–75 mg at bedtime, can be very effective in chronic urticaria. It has anticholinergic side effects.

H_2 antihistamines in combination with H_1 blockers may be helpful in patients with symptomatic dermatographism.

Other agents with some promise as adjuvants include calcium channel blockers (used for at least 4 weeks); terbutaline, 1.25–2.5 mg three times daily; colchicine, 0.6 mg twice daily; danazol; and warfarin. A few patients with chronic urticaria may respond to a salicylate- and tartrazine-free diet. Although salicylates are ubiquitous in nature, drugs and foods are the most obvious sources. One group has reported curing over 60% of chronic urticaria patients with an allergen elimination diet over a 3-month period. This diet proscribes milk products; beer, wine, and cider; mushrooms, soy sauce, canned tomatoes, pickled and smoked meats, shellfish, vinegar, soured breads, melon, dried fruit, diet soda, chocolate, nuts, peanut products, and strawberries. Systemic steroids in a dose of about 40 mg daily will usually suppress acute and chronic urticaria. However, the use of corticosteroids is rarely indicated, since properly selected combinations of agents with less toxicity are usually effective. Once steroids are withdrawn, the urticaria virtually always returns if it had been chronic. Rather than using systemic steroids in difficult cases, consultation should be sought from a dermatologist or allergist with experience in managing severe urticaria. Cyclosporine (3–5 mg/kg/d) may be effective in severe cases of autoimmune chronic urticaria.

C. LOCAL TREATMENT

Local treatment is rarely rewarding.

Prognosis

Acute urticaria usually lasts only a few days to 6 weeks. Half of patients whose urticaria persists for more than 6 weeks will have it for years.

Alper BS: SOAP: Solutions to often-asked problems. Choice of antihistamines for urticaria. Arch Fam Med 2000;9:748. [PMID: 10927716]

Cha YJ et al: Angioedema due to losartan. Ann Pharmacother 1999;33:936. [PMID: 10492494]

Greaves M: Chronic urticaria. J Allergy Clin Immunol 2000; 105:664. [PMID: 10756214]

Hosey RG et al: Exercise-induced anaphylaxis and urticaria. Am Fam Physician 2001;64:1367. [PMID: 11681778]

Kaplan AP: Diagnostic tests for urticaria and angioedema. Clin Allergy Immunol 2000;15:111. [PMID: 10943290]

ERYTHEMA MULTIFORME

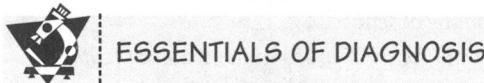

ESSENTIALS OF DIAGNOSIS

- *Sudden onset of symmetric erythematous skin lesions with history of recurrence.*
- *May be macular, papular, urticarial, bullous, or purpuric.*
- *"Target" lesions with clear centers and concentric erythematous rings or "iris" lesions may be noted in erythema multiforme minor. These are rare in drug-associated erythema multiforme major (Stevens-Johnson syndrome).*
- *Erythema multiforme minor on extensor surfaces, palms, soles, or mucous membranes. Erythema multiforme major favors the trunk.*
- *Herpes simplex, systemic infection or disease, and drug reactions are often associated.*

General Considerations

Erythema multiforme is an acute inflammatory skin disease due to multiple causes. Erythema multiforme is divided clinically into minor and major types based on the clinical findings. Approximately 90% of cases of erythema multiforme minor follow outbreaks of herpes simplex. Erythema multiforme major (Stevens-Johnson syndrome) is marked by toxicity and involvement of two or more mucosal surfaces (often oral and conjunctival) and is most often caused by drugs, especially sulfonamides, nonsteroidal anti-inflammatory drugs, and anticonvulsants such as phenytoin. *Mycoplasma pneumoniae* may trigger erythema multiforme major. Erythema multiforme may also present as recurring oral ulceration, with skin lesions present in only half of the cases, and is diagnosed by oral biopsy. Since erythema multiforme may have its own prodrome, many medications taken for such symptoms have been implicated in its pathogenesis without definitive proof. As in all drug eruptions, the exposure to drugs associated with erythema multiforme may be systemic or topical; any agent should be considered a potential offender.

Clinical Findings

A. SYMPTOMS AND SIGNS

A classic target lesion, found most commonly in herpes-associated erythema multiforme, consists of three concentric zones of color change, most often found acrally on the hands and feet. Not all lesions will have this appearance. Drug-associated erythema multiforme is manifested by raised target-like lesions, with only two zones of color change and a central blister, or nondescript reddish or purpuric macules. In erythema multiforme major, mucous membrane ulcerations are present at two or more sites, causing pain on eating, swallowing, and urination.

B. LABORATORY FINDINGS

Blood tests are not useful for diagnosis. Skin biopsy is diagnostic. Direct immunofluorescence studies are negative.

Differential Diagnosis

Urticaria and drug eruptions are the chief entities that must be differentiated from erythema multiforme minor. Individual lesions of true urticaria itch, should come and go within 24 hours, are usually responsive to antihistamines, and do not affect the mucosa. In erythema multiforme major, the main differential diagnosis is toxic epidermal necrolysis, and some investigators regard these entities as variants of the same disease. The presence of blisters is always worrisome and dictates the need for consultation. The differential diagnosis of blisters includes pemphigus, pemphigoid, and bullous drug eruptions. Skin biopsy is the mainstay of diagnosis.

Complications

Visceral lesions are rare complications (eg, pneumonitis, myocarditis, nephritis). The tracheobronchial mucosa and conjunctiva may be involved in severe cases with resultant scarring (Stevens-Johnson syndrome). Ophthalmologic consultation is recommended if ocular involvement is present.

Treatment

A. GENERAL MEASURES

Erythema multiforme major (Stevens-Johnson syndrome) with extensive denudation of skin is best treated in a burn unit. Otherwise, patients need not be admitted unless mucosal involvement interferes with hydration and nutrition. Patients who begin to blister should be seen daily. Immediate discontinuation of the inciting medication (before blistering occurs) improves prognosis and reduces the risk of death in erythema multiforme major.

B. SPECIFIC MEASURES

Although there are no good data to support the use of corticosteroids in erythema multiforme major, they are still often prescribed. If corticosteroids are to be tried in more severe cases, they should be used early, before blistering occurs, and in moderate to high doses (prednisone, 100–250 mg) and stopped within days if there is no dramatic response. In one trial, IGIV (0.75 g/kg/d for 4 days) yielded dramatic benefit in severe cases. Oral and topical corticosteroids are useful in the oral variant of erythema multiforme. Oral acyclovir prophylaxis of herpes simplex infections may be effective in preventing recurrent herpes-associated erythema multiforme minor. Antistaphylococcal antibiotics are used for secondary infection, which is uncommon.

C. LOCAL MEASURES

Topical therapy is not very effective in this disease. For oral lesions, 1% diphenhydramine elixir mixed with Kaopectate or with 1% dyclonine may be used as a mouth rinse several times daily.

Prognosis

Erythema multiforme minor usually lasts 2–6 weeks and may recur. Stevens-Johnson syndrome, in which visceral involvement may occur, may be serious or even fatal in the most severe cases.

Garcia-Doval I et al: Toxic epidermal necrolysis and Stevens-Johnson syndrome: does early withdrawal of causative drugs decrease the risk of death? Arch Dermatol 2000;136:323. [PMID: 10724193]

Katta R: Taking aim at erythema multiforme. How to spot target lesions and less typical presentations. Postgrad Med 2000; 107:87. [PMID: 10649667]

Rzany B et al: Risk of Stevens-Johnson syndrome and toxic epidermal necrolysis during first weeks of antiepileptic therapy: a case-control study. Study Group of the International Case Control Study on Severe Cutaneous Adverse Reactions. Lancet 1999;353:2190. [PMID: 10392983]

Viard I et al: Inhibition of toxic epidermal necrolysis by blockade of CD95 with human intravenous immunoglobulin. Science 1998;282:490. [PMID: 9774279]

ERYTHEMA MIGRANS
(See also Chapter 34.)

Erythema migrans is a unique cutaneous eruption that characterizes the localized or generalized early stage of Lyme disease. Three to 32 days (median: 7 days) after a tick bite, there is gradual expansion of redness around the papule representing the bite site. The advancing border is usually slightly raised, warm, red to bluish-red, and free of any scale. Centrally, the site of the bite may clear, leaving only a rim of peripheral erythema, or it may become indurated, vesicular, or necrotic. The annular erythema usually grows to a median diameter of 15 cm (range: 3–68 cm, but virtually always > 5 cm). It is accompanied by a burning sensation in half of patients; rarely, it is pruritic or painful. Twenty percent of patients will develop multiple secondary annular lesions similar in appearance to the primary lesion but without indurated centers and generally of smaller size. In the southeastern USA, similar lesions are seen in patients without evidence of Lyme borreliosis. The etiology of these cases is unclear, but they are not due to borrelia.

Without treatment, erythema migrans and the secondary lesions fade in a median of 28 days, though some may persist for months. Ten percent of untreated patients experience recurrences over the ensuing months. Treatment with systemic antibiotics (see Table 34–4) is necessary to prevent systemic involvement. However, only 60–70% of those with systemic involvement experience erythema migrans.

Ledbetter LS et al: Large, patchy skin eruptions after a hiking trip. Erythema chronicum migrans hallmarks Lyme disease. Postgrad Med 2000;107:51. [PMID: 10844941]

ERYSIPELAS

 ESSENTIALS OF DIAGNOSIS

- *Edematous, spreading, circumscribed, hot, erythematous area, with or without vesicles or bullae.*
- *Central face frequently involved.*
- *Pain, chills, fever, and systemic toxicity may be striking.*

General Considerations

Erysipelas is a superficial form of cellulitis that occurs classically on the cheek, caused by β-hemolytic streptococci.

Clinical Findings

A. SYMPTOMS AND SIGNS

The symptoms are pain, malaise, chills, and moderate fever. A bright red spot appears first, very often near a fissure at the angle of the nose. This spreads to form a tense, sharply demarcated, glistening, smooth, hot area. The margin characteristically makes noticeable advances in days or even hours. The lesion is some-

what edematous and can be pitted slightly with the finger. Vesicles or bullae occasionally develop on the surface. The lesion does not usually become pustular or gangrenous and heals without scar formation. The disease may complicate any break in the skin that provides a portal of entry for the organism.

B. LABORATORY FINDINGS

Leukocytosis and an increased sedimentation rate are almost invariably present but are not specific; blood cultures may be positive.

Differential Diagnosis

Erysipeloid is a benign bacillary infection producing redness of the skin of the fingers or the backs of the hands in fishermen and meat handlers.

Complications

Unless erysipelas is promptly treated, death may result from extension of the process and systemic toxicity, particularly in the very young and in the aged.

Treatment

Place the patient at bed rest with the head of the bed elevated. Intravenous antibiotics effective against group A beta-hemolytic streptococci and staphylococci are indicated for the first 48 hours in all but the mildest cases. A 7-day course is completed with penicillin VK, 250 mg, dicloxacillin, 250 mg, or a first-generation cephalosporin, 250 mg, orally four times a day. Either erythromycin, 250 mg four times daily for 7–14 days, or clarithromycin, 250 mg twice daily for 7–14 days, is a good alternative in penicillin-allergic patients. Quinolones have poor activity against streptococci and are not recommended.

Prognosis

Erysipelas formerly was a life-threatening infection. It can now usually be quickly controlled with systemic penicillin or erythromycin therapy.

See references next section.

CELLULITIS

Cellulitis, a diffuse spreading infection of the skin, usually on the lower leg, may be due to one of several organisms, usually gram-positive cocci, though gram-negative rods such as *Escherichia coli* may also be responsible. The lesion is hot and red. The major portal of entry for lower leg cellulitis is toe web tinea pedis with fissuring of the skin at this site. The toe webs should be carefully examined in all cases and any associated web space tinea pedis treated aggressively. Attempts to isolate the responsible organism by injecting and then aspirating saline are successful in 20% of cases. In cases of venous stasis, the only clue to cellulitis may be a new localized area of tenderness. Recurrent attacks may sometimes affect lymphatic vessels, producing a permanent swelling called "solid edema."

Two potentially life threatening entities that can mimic cellulitis (ie, present with a painful, red, swollen lower extremity) include deep venous thrombosis and necrotizing fasciitis. The diagnosis of necrotizing fasciitis should be suspected in a patient who has a very toxic appearance, bullae, crepitus or anesthesia of the involved skin, overlying skin necrosis, and laboratory evidence of rhabdomyolysis or DIC. While these findings may be present with severe cellulitis and bacteremia, it is essential to rule out necrotizing fasciitis because rapid surgical debridement is essential. Other skin lesions that may resemble cellulitis include sclerosing panniculitis, an acute, exquisitely tender red plaque on the medial lower legs above the malleolus in patients with venous stasis or varicosities, and acute severe contact dermatitis on a limb, which produces erythema, vesiculation, and edema as seen in cellulitis, but with itching instead of pain. The erythema and edema are also more superficial than in cellulitis.

Intravenous or parenteral antibiotics may be required for the first 24–72 hours. In mild cases or following the initial parenteral therapy, dicloxacillin or cephalexin, 250–500 mg four times daily for 7–10 days, is usually adequate. In patients in whom intravenous treatment is not instituted, the first dose of oral antibiotic can be increased to 750–1000 mg to achieve rapid high blood levels.

Baddour LM: Cellulitis syndromes: an update. Int J Antimicrob Agents 2000;14:113. [PMID: 2018804]

Quartey-Papafio CM: Lesson of the week: importance of distinguishing between cellulitis and varicose eczema of the leg. BMJ 1999;318:1672. [PMID: 10373173]

Roldan YB et al: Erysipelas and tinea pedis. Mycoses 2000; 43:181. [PMID: 10948816]

ERYSIPELOID

Erysipelothrix insidiosa infection must be differentiated from erysipelas and cellulitis. It is usually a benign infection, seen in fishermen and meat handlers. It is characterized by a well-demarcated, purplish, indurated plaque that extends peripherally with central clearing. Lesions are most common on a finger or the dorsal hand surface. Local joint symptoms may be present as the lesions slowly spread over several weeks.

Penicillin V potassium, 250–500 mg orally four times daily for 7–10 days, is usually promptly curative. Some strains are resistant to erythromycin but sensitive to ciprofloxacin. Penicillin G, 2–4 million units

intravenously every 4 hours, may be used instead if the patient appears toxic, with arthritis or endocarditis.

BLISTERING DISEASES
PEMPHIGUS

ESSENTIALS OF DIAGNOSIS

- *Relapsing crops of bullae.*
- *Often preceded by mucous membrane bullae, erosions, and ulcerations.*
- *Superficial detachment of the skin after pressure or trauma variably present (Nikolsky's sign).*
- *Acantholysis on biopsy.*
- *Immunofluorescence studies are confirmatory.*

General Considerations

Pemphigus is an uncommon intraepidermal blistering disease occurring on skin and mucous membranes. It is caused by autoantibodies to adhesion molecules expressed in the skin and mucous membranes (desmoglein 3, sometimes desmoglein I and plakoglobin in pemphigus vulgaris), and to a complex containing desmosomal proteins, including desmoglein I (in pemphigus foliaceus). These autoantibodies cause acantholysis, the separation of epidermal cells from each other. The cause is unknown, and in the preantibiotic, presteroid era the condition, if untreated, was usually fatal within 5 years. The bullae appear spontaneously and are tender and painful when they rupture. If the lesions become extensive, the complications of the disease lead to great toxicity and debility. Drug-induced autoimmune pemphigus from drugs including penicillamine and captopril has been reported. More than 95% of patients with pemphigus vulgaris are positive for HLA-DR4/DQw3 or HLA-DRw6/DQw1, and in one series of 13 patients, all of whom were DQw1-positive, all had a single DQβ allele designated PV6β. Pemphigus may present with atypical features, and repeated reevaluation of clinical findings and changes shown by immunofluorescence and histopathologic studies may be necessary.

There are several forms of pemphigus: **pemphigus vulgaris** and its variant, **pemphigus vegetans;** and the more superficially blistering **pemphigus foliaceus** and its variant, **pemphigus erythematosus.** All forms may occur at any age but most commonly in middle age. The vulgaris form begins in the mouth in over 50% of cases. The foliaceus form is especially apt to be associated with other autoimmune diseases, or it may be drug-induced, eg, by exposure to penicillamine. Paraneoplastic pemphigus, a unique form of the disorder, is associated with numerous types of benign and malignant neoplasms.

Clinical Findings

A. SYMPTOMS AND SIGNS

Pemphigus is characterized by an insidious onset of flaccid bullae in crops or waves. In pemphigus vulgaris, lesions often appear first on the oral mucous membranes, and these rapidly become erosive. In some cases, erosions and crusts predominate over blisters. The scalp is another site of early involvement. Rubbing a cotton swab or finger laterally on the surface of uninvolved skin may cause easy separation of the epidermis (**Nikolsky's sign**).

B. LABORATORY FINDINGS

The diagnosis is made by light microscopy and by direct and indirect immunofluorescence microscopy. Microscopically, acantholysis is the hallmark of pemphigus, but in some patients there may be eosinophilic spongiosis initially. Immunofluorescence microscopy shows deposits of IgG intercellularly in the epidermis. C3 and other immunoglobulins and complement components may be present on occasion. Indirect immunofluorescence microscopy to detect circulating pemphigus antibodies is not necessary for the diagnosis, but antibody titers in some patients may correspond with disease activity and might help in management.

Differential Diagnosis

Blistering diseases include erythema multiforme, drug eruptions, bullous impetigo, contact dermatitis, dermatitis herpetiformis, and bullous pemphigoid, but flaccid blisters are not typical of these diseases, and acantholysis is not seen. In the early stages, pemphigus tends to be treated as impetigo, but bacterial cultures and clinical suspicion leading to early biopsy will clarify the diagnosis. All of these diseases have clinical characteristics and different immunofluorescence test results that distinguish them from pemphigus.

Paraneoplastic pemphigus is clinically, histologically, and immunologically distinct from other forms of the disease. Oral erosions and erythematous plaques resembling erythema multiforme are seen. Survival rates are low because of the underlying malignancy.

Complications

Secondary infection commonly occurs; this is a major cause of morbidity and mortality. Disturbances of fluid and electrolyte balance can occur owing to losses through the involved skin in severe cases.

Treatment

A. GENERAL MEASURES

When the disease is severe, hospitalize the patient at bed rest and provide antibiotics and intravenous feedings as indicated. Anesthetic troches used before eating ease painful oral lesions.

B. SYSTEMIC MEASURES

Pemphigus requires systemic therapy as early in its course as possible. However, the main morbidity in this disease today is generally due to the side effects of such therapy. Initial therapy is with systemic steroids: prednisone, 60–80 mg daily. In all but the most mild cases, a steroid-sparing agent is added from the beginning, since the course of the disease is long and the steroid-sparing agents take several weeks to exert their activity. Azathioprine (100 mg daily or mycophenolate mofetil (1 g twice daily) is used most frequently, the latter seeming to be the most reliable and recommended for most cases. In refractory cases, monthly IGIV at 2 g/kg intravenously over 3 days is useful and has replaced high-dose steroids plus cyclophosphamide and pulse intravenous steroids as rescue therapy. In pemphigus foliaceus and mild cases of pemphigus vulgaris, tetracycline, 500 mg, and nicotinamide, 500 mg, three times daily, may be tried. Dapsone may also be tried as a steroid-sparing agent, especially in pemphigus foliaceus.

C. LOCAL MEASURES

In patients with limited disease, skin and mucous membrane lesions should be treated with topical corticosteroids. Complicating infection requires appropriate systemic and local antibiotic therapy.

Prognosis

The course tends to be chronic in most patients, though some appear to experience remission. Infection is the most frequent cause of death, usually from *Staphylococcus aureus* septicemia.

Cotell S et al: Autoimmune blistering skin diseases. Am J Emerg Med 2000;18:288. [PMID: 10830686]

Engineer L et al: Analysis of current data on the use of intravenous immunoglobulins in management of pemphigus vulgaris. J Am Acad Dermatol 2000;43:1049. [PMID: 11100022]

Nousari HC et al: Pemphigus and bullous pemphigoid. Lancet 1999;354:667. [PMID: 10466686]

Stanley JR: Understanding of the pathophysiology of pemphigus suggests innovative therapeutic approaches. Br J Dermatol 2000;142:208. [PMID: 10730750]

Williams JV et al: Use of mycophenolate mofetil in the treatment of paraneoplastic pemphigus. Br J Dermatol 2000;142:506. [PMID: 10735959]

OTHER BLISTERING DISEASES

Many other skin disorders are characterized by formation of bullae, or blisters. These include bullous pemphigoid, cicatricial pemphigoid, dermatitis herpetiformis, herpes gestationis, and other less common bullous disorders, including the various forms of epidermolysis bullosa, which are due to genetic defects in epidermal keratin and various basement membrane zone components.

Bullous Pemphigoid

Bullous pemphigoid is a relatively benign pruritic disease characterized by tense blisters in flexural areas, usually remitting in 5 or 6 years, with a course characterized by exacerbations and remissions. Most affected persons are over the age of 60 (often in their 70s or 80s), and men are affected twice as frequently as women. The appearance of blisters may be preceded by urticarial or edematous lesions for months. Oral lesions are present in about one-third of affected persons. The disease may occur in various forms, including localized, vesicular, vegetating, erythematous, erythrodermic, and nodular. There is no statistical association with internal malignant disease.

The diagnosis is made by biopsy and direct immunofluorescence examination. Light microscopy shows a subepidermal blister. With direct immunofluorescence, IgG and C3 are found at the dermal-epidermal junction. Circulating anti basement membrane antibodies can be found in the sera of patients in about 70% of cases.

If the patient has only a few blisters, ultrapotent steroids may be adequate. Prednisone at dosages of 60–80 mg/d is often used to achieve rapid control of more widespread disease. Although slower in onset of action, tetracycline or erythromycin, 1–1.5 g/d, alone or combined with nicotinamide—*not nicotinic acid or niacin!*—(up to 1.5 g/d), if tolerated, may control the disease in patients who cannot use corticosteroids or may allow decreasing or eliminating steroids after control is achieved. Dapsone is particularly effective in mucous membrane pemphigoid. If these drugs are not effective, methotrexate, 5–25 mg weekly, or azathioprine, 50 mg one to three times daily, may be used as steroid-sparing agents. Mycophenolate mofetil (1 g twice daily) or IGIV as used for pemphigus vulgaris may be used in refractory cases.

Ahmed AR: Intravenous immunoglobulin therapy for patients with bullous pemphigoid unresponsive to conventional immunosuppressive treatment. J Am Acad Dermatol 2001;45:825. [PMID: 11756944]

Heilborn JD et al: Low-dose oral pulse methotrexate as monotherapy in elderly patients with bullous pemphigoid. J Am Acad Dermatol 1999;40(5 Part 1):741. [PMID: 10321603]

Nousari HC et al: Pemphigus and bullous pemphigoid. Lancet 1999;354:667. [PMID: 10466686]

Herpes (Pemphigoid) Gestationis

Herpes gestationis occurs in about one in 50,000–60,000 pregnancies. The vesicles and bullae often appear first in periumbilical distribution, and there may be erythematous papules and plaques. It usually begins in the fifth or sixth month of pregnancy, or the onset may be delayed to the postpartum period. The disease is self-limited, but it may recur in subsequent pregnancies. Use of estrogens or progesterone or the onset of menses may trigger flare-ups. The risks to mother and fetus appear to be less significant than was formerly thought but include an increase in prematurity and small-for-gestational-age infants. Blisters are subepidermal, with eosinophils present. Direct immunofluorescence shows C3 at the basement membrane zone in most cases. IgG is found less often.

Corticosteroids are the treatment of choice and are sometimes effective when used topically only.

Engineer L et al: Pemphigoid gestationis: a review. Am J Obstet Gynecol 2000;183:483. [PMID: 10942491]

PAPULES

WARTS

 ESSENTIALS OF DIAGNOSIS

- *Verrucous papules anywhere on the skin or mucous membranes, usually no larger than 1 cm in diameter.*
- *Prolonged incubation period (average 2–18 months). Spontaneous "cures" are frequent (50%).*
- *"Recurrences" (new lesions) are frequent.*

General Considerations

Warts are caused by human papillomaviruses. The type of mucocutaneous surface infected and the morphology of the wart are closely related to the HPV type causing the infection. Especially in genital warts, simultaneous infection with numerous wart types is common. Genital HPVs are divided into low-risk and high-risk types depending on the likelihood of their association with cervical and anal cancer.

Clinical Findings

There are usually no symptoms. Tenderness on pressure occurs with plantar warts; itching occurs with anogenital warts. Occasionally a wart will produce mechanical obstruction (eg, nostril, ear canal, urethra).

Warts vary widely in shape, size, and appearance. Flat warts are most evident under oblique illumination. Subungual warts may be dry, fissured, and hyperkeratotic and may resemble hangnails or other nonspecific changes. Plantar warts resemble plantar corns or calluses.

Differential Diagnosis

Some warty-looking lesions are actually hypertrophic actinic keratoses or squamous cell carcinomas. Some genital warty lesions may be due to secondary syphilis (condylomata lata). The lesions of molluscum contagiosum may be mistaken for warts, especially when they are very large in immunocompromised persons. Seborrheic keratosis may also be confused with warts. In AIDS, wart-like lesions may be caused by varicella-zoster virus.

Prevention

The use of condoms may reduce transmission of genital warts. A person with flat warts should be educated about the infectivity of warts and advised not to scratch or traumatize the areas. Using an electric shaver may prevent autoinoculation.

Treatment

Treatment is aimed at inducing "wart-free" intervals for as long as possible without scarring, since no treatment can guarantee a remission or prevent recurrences. In immunocompromised patients, the goal is even more modest, ie, to control the size and number of lesions present.

A. Removal

For common warts of the hands, patients are usually offered liquid nitrogen or keratolytic agents. The former may work in fewer treatments but requires office visits and is painful. Keratolytic agents are irritating but effective and usually painless if used correctly. They can be used at home but must be applied almost daily for 8–12 weeks for maximum effect.

1. Liquid nitrogen is applied to achieve a thaw time of 20–45 seconds. Two freeze-thaw cycles are given every 2–4 weeks for several visits. Scarring will occur if it is used incorrectly or too aggressively. For example, the face, dorsal hands, and legs are more sensitive than the palms. Improper use along the sides of the fingers has been reported to cause nerve damage and paresthesias. Liquid nitrogen may cause permanent depigmentation in darkly pigmented individuals. It is useful on dry penile warts and on filiform warts involving the face and

body. Liquid nitrogen may be used for condylomas, but snipping of lesions followed by light electrodesiccation is more effective.

2. Keratolytic agents—Any of the following salicylic acid products may be used against common warts or plantar warts: Occlusal, Trans-Ver-Sal, and Duofilm. Plantar warts may be treated by applying a 40% salicylic acid plaster (Mediplast) after paring. The plaster may be left on for 5–6 days, then removed, the lesion pared down, and another plaster applied. Although it may take weeks or months to eradicate the wart, the method is safe and effective with almost no side effects.

3. Podophyllum resin—Anogenital warts are often initially treated by painting each wart carefully (protecting normal skin) every 2–3 weeks with 25% podophyllum resin (podophyllin) in compound tincture of benzoin. Pregnant patients should not be so treated. The purified active component of the resin, podofilox, is available for use at home twice daily three consecutive days a week for cycles of 4–6 weeks. It is less irritating and more effective than podophyllum resin. After a single 4-week cycle, 45% of patients were wart-free; but of these, 60% relapsed at 6 weeks. Thus, multiple cycles of treatment are often necessary.

4. Imiquimod—A 5% cream of this local interferon inducer has moderate activity in clearing external genital warts. Seventy-seven percent of women and 40% of men with external genital warts had complete clearing of their lesions, and 90% and 74%, respectively, had greater than 50% reduction in their warts. The superior response in women may relate to enhanced penetration of the moist skin of the vulva as compared with the penile shaft. Treatment is once-daily on 3 alternate days per week. Response may be slow, with patients who eventually cleared having responses at 8 weeks (44%) or 12 weeks (69%). Once cleared, about 13% had recurrences in the short term.

There is less pregnancy risk than with podophyllum resin (category B versus category X with podophyllin). It is more expensive than podophyllotoxin, but given the high rate of response in women and its safety and low relapse rate, it appears to be the "patient-administered" treatment of choice in women. In men, the more rapid response, lower cost, and similar efficacy make podophyllotoxin the initial treatment of choice, with imiquimod used for recurrences or refractory cases. Anecdotally, this agent may also have efficacy in superficial flat warts.

5. Operative removal—Plantar warts may be removed by blunt dissection. Local anesthetic is injected into the base, and the wart is then removed with a curette or scissors or by shaving off at the base of the wart with a scalpel. Trichloroacetic acid or Monsel's solution on a tightly wound cotton-tipped applicator may be painted on the wound, or light electrocautery may be used. Excision of warts, however, may result in a permanent painful scar on the foot and is not recommended. For genital warts, snip biopsy (scissors) removal followed by light electrocautery is more effective than cryotherapy but does scar. It is often preferred by patients with pedunculated or large lesions that require multiple cryotherapy or podophyllin treatments for removal.

6. Laser therapy—The CO_2 laser is effective for treating recurrent warts, periungual warts, plantar warts, and condylomata acuminata. It leaves open wounds which must fill in with granulation tissue over 4–6 weeks and is best reserved for warts resistant to other modalities. Lasers with emissions of 585, 595, or 532 nm may also be used every 3–4 weeks to gradually ablate the wart. This is no more effective than cryotherapy in controlled trials. For genital warts, it has not been shown that laser therapy is more effective than electrosurgical removal.

7. Other agents—Bleomycin diluted to 1 unit/mL may be injected into warts. It has been shown to have a high cure rate for plantar and common warts. It should not be used on digital warts because of the potential complications of Raynaud's phenomenon, nail loss, and terminal digital necrosis.

B. IMMUNOTHERAPY

Cimetidine in doses of 35–50 mg/kg daily may benefit younger patients with common warts. Squaric acid dibutylester may be effective. It is applied in a concentration of 0.2–2% directly to the warts from once weekly to five times weekly to induce a mild contact dermatitis. Between 60% and 80% of warts clear over 10–20 weeks.

C. RETINOIDS

Tretinoin (Retin-A) cream or gel applied topically twice daily may be effective (anecdotally) for facial or beard flat warts. Extensive warts have been reported to disappear when oral retinoids are administered for 4–8 weeks.

D. PHYSICAL MODALITIES

Soaking warts in hot (42.2 °C) water for 10–30 minutes daily for 6 weeks has resulted in dramatic involution in some cases.

Prognosis

There is a striking tendency to the development of new lesions. Warts may disappear spontaneously or may be unresponsive to treatment.

Beutner KR et al: Genital warts and their treatment. Clin Infect Dis 1999;28(Suppl 1):S37. [PMID: 10028109]

McMillan A: The management of difficult anogenital warts. Sex Transm Infect 1999;75:192. [PMID: 10448402]

Plasencia JM: Cutaneous warts: diagnosis and treatment. Prim Care 2000;27:423. [PMID: 10815052]

von Krogh G et al: European course on HPV associated pathology: guidelines for primary care physicians for the diagnosis and management of anogenital warts. Sex Transm Infect 2000;76:162. [PMID: 10961190]

CALLOSITIES & CORNS OF FEET OR TOES

Callosities and corns are caused by pressure and friction due to faulty weight-bearing, orthopedic deformities, improperly fitting shoes, or neuropathies.

Tenderness on pressure and "after-pain" are the only symptoms. The hyperkeratotic well-localized overgrowths always occur at pressure points. Fingerprint lines are preserved over the surface (not so in warts). On paring, a glassy core is found (which differentiates these disorders from plantar warts, which have multiple capillary bleeding points or black dots when pared). A soft corn often occurs laterally on the proximal portion of the fourth toe as a result of pressure against the bony structure of the interphalangeal joint of the fifth toe.

Treatment consists of correcting mechanical abnormalities that cause friction and pressure. Shoes must be properly fitted and orthopedic deformities corrected. Callosities may be removed by careful paring of the callus after a warm water soak or with keratolytic agents as found in various brands of corn pads.

Plantar hyperkeratosis of the heels can be treated successfully by using 20% urea (Ureacin 20) or 12% lactic acid (Lac-Hydrin) nightly and a pumice stone after soaking in water.

Women who tend to form calluses and corns should not wear confining footgear and high-heeled shoes.

Woodburn J et al: Preliminary investigation of debridement of plantar callosities in rheumatoid arthritis. Rheumatology 2000;39:652. [PMID: 10888711]

MOLLUSCUM CONTAGIOSUM

Molluscum contagiosum, caused by a poxvirus, presents as single or multiple rounded, dome-shaped, waxy papules 2–5 mm in diameter that are umbilicated. Lesions at first are firm, solid, and flesh-colored but upon reaching maturity become softened, whitish, or pearly gray and may suppurate. The principal sites of involvement are the face, lower abdomen, and genitals.

The lesions are autoinoculable and spread by wet skin-to-skin contact. In sexually active individuals, they may be confined to the penis, pubis, and inner thighs and are considered a sexually transmitted disease.

Molluscum contagiosum is common in patients with AIDS, usually with a helper T cell count < 100/μL. AIDS patients tend to develop extensive lesions over the face and neck as well as in the genital area.

The diagnosis is easily established in most instances because of the distinctive central umbilication of the dome-shaped lesion. The best treatment is by curettage or applications of liquid nitrogen as for warts—but more briefly, since molluscum contagiosum is more responsive to therapy than warts. When lesions are frozen, the central umbilication often becomes more apparent. Light electrosurgery with a fine needle is also effective. It has been estimated that individual lesions persist for about 2 months. They are difficult to eradicate in patients with AIDS unless immunity improves, in which case spontaneous clearing may occur.

Cattelan AM et al: A complete remission of recalcitrant molluscum contagiosum in an AIDS patient following highly active antiretroviral therapy (HAART). J Infect 1999;38:58. [PMID: 10090515]

BASAL CELL CARCINOMA

Basal cell carcinomas are the most common form of cancer. They occur on sun-exposed skin in otherwise normal fair-skinned individuals. The most common presentation is a papule or nodule that may have a central scab or erosion. Occasionally the nodules have a brown-gray color or have stippled pigment (pigmented basal cell carcinoma). Intradermal nevi without pigment on the face of older white individuals may resemble basal cell carcinomas. Basal cell carcinomas grow slowly, attaining a size of 1–2 cm or more in diameter, often after years of growth. There is a waxy, "pearly" appearance, with telangiectatic vessels easily visible. It is the pearly or translucent quality of these lesions that is most diagnostic, a feature best appreciated if the skin is stretched. Less common types include morpheaform or scar-like lesions. These are hypopigmented, somewhat thickened plaques. On the back and chest, basal cell carcinomas appear as reddish, somewhat shiny, scaly plaques.

Clinicians should examine the skin routinely, looking for bumps, patches, and scabbed lesions. When examining the face, look at the eyelid margins and medial canthi, the nose and alar folds, the lips, and then around and behind the ears. While metastases almost never occur, therapy of basal cell carcinomas may cause significant cosmetic deformity in these areas, particularly for inadequately treated or recurrent lesions. Neglected lesions may ulcerate and produce great destruction. Basal cell carcinomas of the medial canthi are particularly dangerous. Recurrent lesions around the nose and ears may track along cartilage underneath the skin, requiring treatment of much more extensive areas than are apparent from inspection.

Lesions suspected to be basal cell carcinomas should be biopsied, by shave or punch biopsy. Therapy is then aimed at eradication with minimal cosmetic deformity, often by excision and suturing with recurrence rates of 5% or less. The technique of three cycles of curettage and electrodesiccation depends on the skill of the operator and is not recommended for head and neck lesions. After 4–6 weeks of healing, it leaves a broad, hypopigmented, at times hypertrophic scar. Radiotherapy is effective and sometimes appropriate for older individuals (over 65), but recurrent tumors after radiation therapy are more difficult to treat and may be more aggressive. Mohs surgery—removal of the tumor followed by immediate frozen section histopathologic examination of margins with subsequent reexcision of tumor-positive areas and final closure of the defect—gives the highest cure rates (98%) and results in least tissue loss. It is appropriate therapy for tumors of the eyelids or for recurrent lesions, or where tissue sparing is needed for cosmesis. Sun avoidance, particularly in children, is essential to lower the incidence of new basal cell cancers. Patients with basal cell carcinomas must be followed for 5 years to detect new or recurrent lesions.

Garner KL et al: Basal and squamous cell carcinoma. Prim Care 2000;27:447. [PMID: 10815054]

Jerant AF et al: Early detection and treatment of skin cancer. Am Fam Physician 2000;62:357. [PMID: 10929700] (Basic "safe sun" measures: sun avoidance during peak UVB hours, proper use of sunscreen and protective clothing, and avoidance of suntanning.)

SQUAMOUS CELL CARCINOMA

Squamous cell carcinoma usually occurs subsequent to prolonged sun exposure on exposed parts in fair-skinned individuals who sunburn easily and tan poorly. It may arise from an actinic keratosis. The lesions appear as small red, conical, hard nodules that occasionally ulcerate. They are not as distinctive as basal cell carcinomas and are more easily misdiagnosed clinically. The frequency of metastasis is not precisely known, though metastatic spread is said to be less likely with squamous cell carcinoma arising out of actinic keratoses than with those that arise de novo. In actinically induced squamous cell cancers, rates of metastasis are estimated from retrospective studies to be 3–7%. Squamous cell carcinomas of the lip, oral cavity, tongue, and genitalia have much higher rates of metastasis and require special management.

Keratoacanthomas most often act in benign fashion but resemble squamous cell carcinoma histologically and for all practical purposes should be treated as though they were skin cancers.

Examination of the skin and therapy are essentially the same as for basal cell carcinoma. The preferred treatment of squamous cell carcinoma is excision. Electrodesiccation and curettage and x-ray radiation may be used for some lesions, and fresh tissue microscopically controlled excision (Mohs) is recommended for high-risk lesions (lips, temples, ears, nose) and for recurrent tumors. Some keratoacanthomas respond to intralesional injection of fluorouracil or methotrexate, but they must be excised if they do not. Follow-up for squamous cell carcinoma must be more frequent and thorough than for basal cell carcinoma, starting at every 3 months, with careful examination of lymph nodes. In addition, palpation of the lips is essential to detect hard or indurated areas that represent early squamous cell carcinoma. All such cases must be biopsied. Multiple squamous cell carcinomas are very common on the sun-exposed skin of organ transplant patients because of the host's immunosuppressed state. The tumors begin to appear after 5 years of immunosuppression. Biologic behavior may be aggressive, and careful management is required.

Garner KL et al: Basal and squamous cell carcinoma. Prim Care 2000;27:447. [PMID: 10813054]

JAMA patient page: Skin cancer. JAMA 1999;281:676. [PMID: 10029132]

VIOLACEOUS TO PURPLE PAPULES & NODULES

LICHEN PLANUS

ESSENTIALS OF DIAGNOSIS

- *Pruritic, violaceous, flat-topped papules with fine white streaks and symmetric distribution.*
- *Lacy lesions of the buccal mucosa.*
- *Commonly seen along linear scratch marks (Koebner phenomenon) on anterior wrists, penis, legs.*
- *Histopathologic examination is diagnostic.*

General Considerations

Lichen planus is an inflammatory pruritic disease of the skin and mucous membranes characterized by distinctive papules with a predilection for the flexor surfaces and trunk. The three cardinal findings are typical skin lesions, mucosal lesions, and histopathologic features of band-like infiltration of lymphocytes and melanophages in the dermis. Drugs causing lichen planus-like reactions include gold, streptomycin, tetracycline, iodides, chloroquine, quinacrine, quinidine, NSAIDs, phenothiazines, and hydrochlorothiazide. Hepatitis C infection is found with greater frequency in lichen planus patients than in controls in Europe and the USA. Lichen planus has been seen after exposure to color film developing solutions.

Clinical Findings

Itching is mild to severe. The lesions are violaceous, flat-topped, angulated papules, 1–4 mm in diameter, discrete or in clusters, with very fine white streaks on the surface (Wickham's striae) on the flexor surfaces of the wrists and on the penis, lips, tongue, and buccal and vaginal mucous membranes. Mucosal lichen planus has been reported in the genital and anorectal areas, the gastrointestinal tract, the bladder, the larynx, and the conjunctiva. The papules may become bullous or ulcerated. The disease may be generalized. Mucous membrane lesions have a lacy white network overlying them that may be confused with leukoplakia. The Koebner phenomenon (appearance of lesions in areas of trauma) may be seen.

A special form of lichen planus is the erosive or ulcerative variety. On palms and soles, it can be disabling. It is a major problem in the mouth or genitalia, and squamous cell carcinoma may develop.

Differential Diagnosis

Lichen planus must be distinguished from similar lesions produced by medications (see above) and other papular lesions such as psoriasis, lichen simplex chronicus, and syphilis. Lichen planus on the mucous membranes must be differentiated from leukoplakia. Erosive oral lesions require biopsy and often direct immunofluorescence for diagnosis since lichen planus may simulate other erosive diseases. Histologic examination may make the distinction from graft-versus-host disease and in some cases from lichen planus-like drug eruptions.

Treatment

A. TOPICAL THERAPY

Superpotent topical corticosteroids such as betamethasone dipropionate in optimized vehicle, diflorasone diacetate, clobetasol propionate, and halobetasol propionate ointments applied twice daily are most helpful for localized disease in nonflexural areas. Alternatively, high-potency corticosteroid cream or ointment may be used nightly under thin pliable plastic film.

Application of tretinoin cream 0.05% to mucosal lichen planus, followed by a corticosteroid ointment, may be helpful. Topical tacrolimus appears effective in oral and vaginal erosive lichen planus, but chronic therapy is required to prevent relapse. Concern regarding absorption suggests monitoring blood counts when treating mucosal lesions. For disabling hypertrophic lichen planus of the soles, tretinoin cream applied and covered with thin, pliable polyethylene film nightly is said to be effective.

B. SYSTEMIC THERAPY

Corticosteroids (see Chapter 26) may be required in severe cases, or where the most rapid response to treatment is desired. Unfortunately, relapse almost always occurs as the steroids are tapered, making systemic corticosteroid therapy an impractical option for the management of chronic lichen planus.

Isotretinoin and acitretin by mouth appear to be effective in some cases of oral and cutaneous lichen planus.

Psoralens plus long-wave ultraviolet light (PUVA) may be effective treatment for lichen planus.

Prognosis

Lichen planus is a benign disease, but it may persist for months or years and may be recurrent. Hypertrophic lichen planus and oral lesions tend to be especially persistent, and neoplastic degeneration has been described in chronically eroded lesions.

Katta R: Lichen planus. Am Fam Phys 2000;61:3319. [PMID: 10865927]

Mignogna MD et al: Oral lichen planus: different clinical features in HCV-positive and HCV-negative patients. Int J Dermatol 2000;39:134. [PMID: 10692063]

KAPOSI'S SARCOMA

Before 1980 in the USA, this rare malignant skin lesion was seen mostly in elderly white men, had a chronic clinical course, and was rarely fatal. Kaposi's sarcoma occurs endemically in an often aggressive form in young black men of equatorial Africa, but it is rare in American blacks. Epidemic clusters of Kaposi's sarcoma, predominantly in homosexual men with AIDS, have been found in large cities of the USA. A novel herpesvirus, human herpes virus 8 (HHV-8) or Kaposi's sarcoma-associated herpes virus (KSHV), is universally present in all forms of Kaposi's sarcoma (endemic Kaposi's sarcoma in Africa, Kaposi's sarcoma in elderly males, and HIV associated Kaposi's sarcoma). The epidemiology of infection with this virus parallels the incidence of Kaposi's sarcoma in various risk groups and geographic regions. For example, it is a common infection in central Africa, is more common in Italy than in the USA, and is common in HIV-infected homosexual men and rare in HIV-infected hemophiliacs. The virus is present in the skin lesions and circulating B lymphocytes of persons with Kaposi's sarcoma, but uncommonly in their normal skin. A serologic test is available to detect infection with this virus, but its sensitivity is insufficient for commercial use at this time.

Red, purple, or dark plaques or nodules on cutaneous or mucosal surfaces should alert the clinician to the possibility of the disease. Kaposi's sarcoma commonly involves the gastrointestinal tract, but in asymptomatic patients these lesions are not sought or treated. Pulmonary Kaposi's sarcoma may be life-threatening and is managed aggressively. The incidence of AIDS-associated Kaposi's sarcoma is diminishing.

For Kaposi's sarcoma in the elderly, palliative local therapy with intralesional chemotherapy or radiation is usually all that is required. In the setting of iatrogenic immunosuppression, the treatment of Kaposi's sarcoma is primarily reduction of doses of immunosuppressive medications. In AIDS-associated Kaposi's sarcoma, the patient should first be given effective anti-HIV antiretrovirals (including a protease inhibitor), because in most cases this treatment alone is associated with improvement. Other therapeutic options include cryotherapy or intralesional vinblastine (0.1–0.5 mg/mL) for cosmetically objectionable lesions; radiation therapy for accessible and space-occupying lesions; and laser surgery for certain intraoral and pharyngeal lesions. Systemic chemotherapy is indicated in patients with rapidly progressive skin disease (more than ten new lesions per month), with edema or pain, and with symptomatic visceral disease or pulmonary disease. Liposomal doxorubicin is highly effective in controlling these cases and has considerably less toxicity—and greater efficacy—than anthracycline monotherapy or combination chemotherapeutic regimens.

Antman K et al: Kaposi's sarcoma. N Engl J Med 2000;342:1027. [PMID: 10749966]

Dezube BJ: Acquired immunodeficiency syndrome-related Kaposi's sarcoma: clinical features, staging, and treatment. Semin Oncol 2000;27:424. [PMID: 10950369]

Jones JL et al: Incidence and trends in Kaposi's sarcoma in the era of effective antiretroviral therapy. J Acquir Immune Defic Syndr 2000;24:270. [PMID: 10969352]

Schulz TF: Kaposi's sarcoma-associated herpesvirus (human herpesvirus 8): epidemiology and pathogenesis. J Antimicrob Chemother 2000;45(Suppl T3):15. [PMID: 10855768]

PRURITUS (Itching)

Pruritus is a disagreeable sensation that provokes a desire to scratch. It is modulated by central factors, including cortical ones. Not all cases of pruritus are mediated by histamine.

Although many cases of generalized pruritus can be attributed to dry skin—whether naturally occurring and precipitated or aggravated by climatic conditions or arising from disease states—there are many other causes: scabies, dermatitis herpetiformis, atopic dermatitis, pruritus vulvae et ani, miliaria, insect bites, pediculosis, contact dermatitis, drug reactions, urticaria, urticarial eruptions of pregnancy, psoriasis, lichen planus, lichen simplex chronicus, exfoliative dermatitis, folliculitis, bullous pemphigoid, and fiberglass dermatitis.

Persistent pruritus not explained by cutaneous disease should prompt a staged workup for systemic causes. Perhaps the commonest cause of pruritus associated with systemic disease is uremia in conjunction with hemodialysis. Both this condition and the pruritus of obstructive biliary disease may be helped by phototherapy with ultraviolet B or PUVA. Naltrexone and nalmefene have been shown to relieve the pruritus of biliary cholestasis; naltrexone is not effective in pruritus associated with renal failure. Endocrine disorders such as hypo- or hyperthyroidism, psychiatric disturbances, lymphoma, leukemia, and other internal malignant disorders, iron deficiency anemia, and certain neurologic disorders may also cause pruritus. Danazol, 400–800 mg daily, may be tried for pruritus associated with myeloproliferative disorders and other systemic illnesses.

Burning or itching involving the face, scalp, and genitalia may be manifestations of primary depression and treatable with drugs such as tricyclics (amitriptyline, imipramine, doxepin), SSRIs, and other antidepressants.

Prognosis

Elimination of external factors and irritating agents may give complete relief from pruritus. Pruritus accompanying specific skin disease will subside when the disease is controlled. Idiopathic pruritus and that accompanying serious internal disease may not respond to any type of therapy.

Bergasa NV et al: Oral nalmefene therapy reduces scratching activity due to the pruritus of cholestasis: a controlled study. J Am Acad Dermatol 1999;41(3 Part 1):431. [PMID: 10459118]

Metze D et al: Efficacy and safety of naltrexone, an oral opiate receptor antagonist, in the treatment of pruritus in internal and dermatological diseases. J Am Acad Dermatol 1999;41:533. [PMID: 10495371]

Millikan LE: Pruritus: unapproved treatments or indications. Clin Dermatol 2000;18:149. [PMID: 10742622]

ANOGENITAL PRURITUS

ESSENTIALS OF DIAGNOSIS

- *Itching, chiefly nocturnal, of the anogenital area.*
- *Examination is highly variable, ranging from no skin findings to excoriations and inflammation of any degree, including lichenification.*

General Considerations

Most cases have no obvious cause, but multiple specific causes have been identified. Anogenital pruritus may be due to intertrigo, psoriasis, lichen simplex chronicus, or seborrheic or contact dermatitis (from soaps, colognes, douches, contraceptives, and perhaps scented toilet tissue), or it may be due to irritating secretions, as in diarrhea, leukorrhea, or trichomoniasis, or to local disease (candidiasis, dermatophytosis, erythrasma). Oxyuriasis (pinworm) is a rare cause in adults. Psychologic abnormalities are usually not evi-

dent. Lichen sclerosus et atrophicus may at times be the cause. Erythrasma is easily diagnosed by demonstration of coral-red fluorescence with Wood's light; it is easily cured with erythromycin orally and topically.

Uncleanliness may be at fault. In pruritus ani, hemorrhoids are often found, and leakage of mucus and bacteria from the distal rectum onto the perianal skin may be important in cases in which no other skin abnormality is found.

Many women experience pruritus vulvae. In women, pruritus ani by itself is rare, and pruritus vulvae does not usually involve the anal area, though anal itching will usually spread to the vulva. In men, pruritus of the scrotum is most commonly seen in the absence of pruritus ani. When all possible known causes have been ruled out, the condition is diagnosed as idiopathic or essential pruritus—by no means rare.

Clinical Findings

A. SYMPTOMS AND SIGNS

The only symptom is itching, which is chiefly nocturnal. Physical findings are usually not present, but there may be erythema, fissuring, maceration, lichenification, excoriations, or changes suggestive of candidiasis or tinea.

B. LABORATORY FINDINGS

Urinalysis and blood glucose testing may lead to a diagnosis of diabetes mellitus. Microscopic examination or culture of tissue scrapings may reveal yeasts or fungi. Stool examination may show pinworms.

Differential Diagnosis

The etiologic differential diagnosis consists of candida infection, parasitosis, local irritation from contact with drugs and irritants, and other primary skin disorders of the genital area such as psoriasis, seborrhea, intertrigo, or lichen sclerosus et atrophicus.

Prevention

Instruct the patient in proper anogenital hygiene after treating systemic or local conditions.

Treatment

A. GENERAL MEASURES

Treating constipation, preferably with high-fiber management (psyllium), may help. Instruct the patient to use very soft or moistened tissue or cotton after bowel movements and to clean the perianal area thoroughly with cool water if possible. Women should use similar precautions after urinating. Instruct the patient regarding the harmful and pruritus-inducing effects of scratching.

B. LOCAL MEASURES

Pramoxine cream or lotion or hydrocortisone-pramoxine (Pramosone), 1% or 2.5% cream, lotion, or ointment, is helpful in managing pruritus in the anogenital area. The ointment or cream should be applied after a bowel movement. Iodochlorhydroxyquin-hydrocortisone creams are useful also but may stain underwear. Potent fluorinated topical corticosteroids may lead to atrophy and striae if used for more than a few days and should in general be avoided. This includes combinations with antifungals. The use of strong steroids on the scrotum may lead to persistent severe burning upon withdrawal of the drug. Soaks with aluminum subacetate solution, 1:20, are of value if the area is acutely inflamed and oozing. Undercloth-ing should be changed daily. Affected areas may be painted with Castellani's solution. Balneol Perianal Cleansing Lotion or Tucks premoistened pads, ointment, or cream (all Tucks preparations contain witch hazel) may be very useful for pruritus ani.

Prognosis

Although benign, anogenital pruritus may be persistent and recurrent.

Vincent C: Anorectal pain and irritation: anal fissure, levator syndrome, proctalgia fugax, and pruritus ani. Prim Care 1999;26:53. [PMID: 9922294]

SCABIES

 ESSENTIALS OF DIAGNOSIS

- *Generalized itching.*
- *Pruritic vesicles and pustules in "runs" or "galleries," especially on finger webs and the heels of the palms and in wrist creases.*
- *Mites, ova, and brown dots of feces visible microscopically.*
- *Red papules or nodules on the scrotum and on the penile glans and shaft are pathognomonic.*

General Considerations

Scabies is caused by infestation with *Sarcoptes scabiei*. The infestation usually spares the head and neck (though even these areas may be involved in infants, in the elderly, and in patients with AIDS). Scabies is usually acquired by sleeping with or in the bedding of an infested individual or by other close contact. The entire household may be affected.

Clinical Findings

A. SYMPTOMS AND SIGNS

Itching is almost always present and can be quite severe. The lesions consist of more or less generalized excoriations with small pruritic vesicles, pustules, and "runs" or "burrows" in the web spaces and on the heels of the palms, wrists, elbows, and around the axillae. Often, burrows are found only on the feet, as they have been scratched off in other locations. The burrow appears as a short irregular mark, 2–3 mm long and the width of a hair. Characteristic lesions may occur on the nipples in females and as pruritic papules on the scrotum or penis in males. Pruritic papules may be seen over the buttocks.

B. LABORATORY FINDINGS

The diagnosis should be confirmed by microscopic demonstration of the organism, ova, or feces in a mounted specimen. The success of this procedure depends on choosing the best unexcoriated lesions from interdigital webs, wrists, elbows, or feet. A bit of immersion oil is placed on the lesion and a No. 15 blade is used to scrape the lesion until it is flat. Pinpoint bleeding may result from the scraping. The diagnosis can also be confirmed in most cases with the burrow ink test. Apply ink to the burrow and then do a very superficial shave biopsy by sawing off the burrow with a No. 15 blade, painlessly and bloodlessly. The mite, ova, and feces can be seen under the light microscope.

Differential Diagnosis

Scabies must be distinguished from the various forms of pediculosis and from other causes of pruritus.

Treatment & Prognosis

Treatment is aimed at killing scabies mites and controlling the dermatitis, which can persist for months after effective eradication of the mites, with midpotency topical steroids. Bedding and clothing should be laundered or cleaned or set aside for 14 days in plastic bags. Unless the lesions are complicated by severe secondary pyoderma, treatment consists primarily of disinfestation. If secondary pyoderma is present, it should be treated with systemic antibiotics. Unless treatment is aimed at all infected persons in a family or institutionalized group, reinfestations will probably occur. Resistance to 5% permethrin cream is rare.

Disinfestation with lindane (gamma benzene hexachloride), 1% in cream or lotion base, applied from the neck down overnight, may be used in adults. A warning has been issued by the FDA regarding potential neurotoxicity, and any use of lindane in infants and pregnant women or in any patient with widespread excoriations and open skin—as well as overuse in adults—is discouraged. This preparation can be used before secondary infection is controlled.

Permethrin 5% cream is highly effective and safe in the management of scabies. Treatment consists of a single application for 8–12 hours. It may be repeated in 1 week. The drug has been used safely in infants aged 2 months to 5 years and is the treatment of choice in children. An alternative drug is crotamiton cream or lotion, which may be applied in the same way as lindane but is used nightly for 4 nights. It is far less effective if used for only 48 hours.

Pregnant patients should be treated only if they have documented scabies themselves. Permethrin 5% cream once for 12 hours—or 5% or 6% sulfur in petrolatum applied nightly for 3 nights from the collarbones down—may be used.

Benzyl benzoate may be compounded as a lotion or emulsion in strengths from 20% to 35% and used as generalized applications (from collarbones down) overnight for two treatments 1 week apart. The USP formula is 275 mL benzyl benzoate (containing 5 g of triethanolamine and 20 g of oleic acid) in water to make 1000 mL. It is cosmetically acceptable, clean, and not overly irritating. Patients will continue to itch for several weeks after treatment. Use of triamcinolone 0.1% cream will help resolve the dermatitis. Scabies in nursing home patients, institutionalized or mentally impaired (especially Down's syndrome) patients, and AIDS patients may be much more difficult to treat.

Most failures in normal hosts are related to incorrect use or incomplete treatment of the housing unit. In these cases, repeat treatment with permethrin once weekly for two weeks, with reeducation regarding the method and extent of application, is suggested. In immunocompetent individuals, ivermectin in a dose of 200 μg/kg is effective in about 75% of cases with a single dose and 95% of cases with two doses 2 weeks apart. In immunosuppressed hosts and those with crusted (hyperkeratotic) scabies, multiple doses of ivermectin (every 2 weeks for two or three doses) plus topical therapy with permethrin once or twice weekly may be effective when topical treatment and oral therapy alone fail.

Persistent pruritic postscabietic papules may be treated with mid- to high-potency steroids or with intralesional triamcinolone acetonide (2.5–5 mg/mL).

Chosidow O: Scabies and pediculosis. Lancet 2000;355:819. [PMID: 10711939]

Usha V et al: A comparative study of oral ivermectin and topical permethrin cream in the treatment of scabies. J Am Acad Dermatol 2000;42(2 Part 1):236. [PMID: 10642678]

PEDICULOSIS

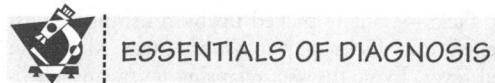

ESSENTIALS OF DIAGNOSIS

- Pruritus with excoriation.
- Nits on hair shafts; lice on skin or clothes.
- Occasionally, sky-blue macules (maculae ceruleae) on the inner thighs or lower abdomen in pubic louse infestation.

General Considerations

Pediculosis is a parasitic infestation of the skin of the scalp, trunk, or pubic areas. Body lice usually occur among people who live in overcrowded dwellings with inadequate hygiene facilities. Pubic lice may be acquired by sexual transmission. Head lice may be transmitted by shared use of hats or combs and are epidemic among children of all socioeconomic classes in elementary schools. Head lice are very uncommon among black children. Adults contacting children with head lice frequently acquire the infestation.

There are three different varieties: (1) pediculosis pubis, caused by *Pthirus pubis* (pubic louse, "crabs"); (2) pediculosis corporis, by *Pediculus humanus* var *corporis* (body louse); and (3) pediculosis capitis, by *Pediculus humanus* var *capitis* (head louse).

Head and body lice are similar in appearance and are 3–4 mm long. The body louse can seldom be found on the body, because the insect comes onto the skin only to feed and must be looked for in the seams of the clothing. Trench fever, relapsing fever, and typhus are transmitted by the body louse in countries where those diseases are endemic.

Clinical Findings

Itching may be very intense in body louse infestations, and scratching may result in deep excoriations, especially over the upper shoulders, posterior flanks, and neck. In some cases, only itching is present, with few excoriations seen. Pyoderma may be the presenting sign in any of these infestations. Head lice can be found on the scalp or may be manifested as small nits resembling pussy willow buds on the scalp hairs close to the skin. They are easiest to see above the ears and at the nape of the neck. Pubic louse infestations are occasionally generalized, particularly in hairy individuals; the lice may even be found on the eyelashes and in the scalp.

Differential Diagnosis

Head louse infestation must be distinguished from seborrheic dermatitis, body louse infestation from scabies, and pubic louse infestation from anogenital pruritus and eczema.

Treatment

Body lice are treated by disposing of the infested clothing. For pubic lice, lindane lotion or cream (Kwell, Scabene) is used. A thin layer is applied to the infested and adjacent hairy areas. It is removed after 8 hours by thorough washing. Permethrin rinse 1% for 10 minutes and permethrin cream 5% applied for 8 hours are effective alternatives. Sexual contacts should be treated. Clothes and bedclothes should be washed and dried at high temperature if possible.

Permethrin 1% cream rinse (Nix) is a topical OTC pediculicide and ovicide and is the treatment of choice for head lice. It is applied to the scalp and hair and left on for 30 minutes to 8 hours before being rinsed off. Treatment should be repeated in 1 week. Five percent permethrin lotion may be used in refractory cases. Permethrin 1% cream (Nix) is more effective than synergized pyrethrins (RID), OTC products that are applied undiluted until the infested areas are entirely wet. After 10 minutes, the areas are washed thoroughly with warm water and soap and then dried. Malathion lotion 1% (Ovide) is very effective, but it is highly volatile and flammable, so application must be done in a well-ventilated room or outdoors. Nits are removed meticulously with a fine-toothed comb under bright illumination. For involvement of eyelashes, petrolatum is applied thickly twice daily for 8 days, and remaining nits are then plucked off. Adults with head lice virtually always acquire their infestation from elementary school-aged children, so a source of infection must always be sought. Head lice are extremely difficult to eradicate in the epidemic setting, probably because the currently available pediculicides are not uniformly ovicidal when applied as directed.

Chosidow O: Scabies and pediculosis. Lancet 2000;355:819. [PMID: 10711939]

Parish LC et al: The saga of ectoparasitoses: scabies and pediculosis. Int J Dermatol 1999;38:432. [PMID: 10397581]

SKIN LESIONS DUE TO OTHER ARTHROPODS

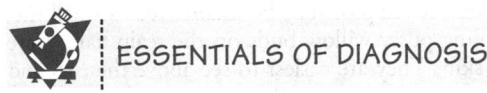

ESSENTIALS OF DIAGNOSIS

- *Localized rash with pruritus.*
- *Furuncle-like lesions containing live arthropods.*
- *Tender erythematous patches that migrate ("larva migrans").*
- *Generalized urticaria or erythema multiforme in some patients.*

General Considerations

Some arthropods (eg, most pest mosquitoes and biting flies) are readily detected as they bite. Many others are not, eg, because they are too small, because there is no immediate reaction, or because they bite during sleep.

Reactions may be delayed for many hours; many are allergic. Patients are most apt to consult a clinician when the lesions are multiple and pruritus is intense.

Many persons will react severely only to their earliest contacts with an arthropod, thus presenting pruritic lesions when traveling, moving into new quarters, etc. Body lice, fleas, bedbugs, and mosquitoes should be considered. Spiders are often incorrectly believed to be the source of bites; they rarely attack humans, though the brown spider (*Loxosceles laeta, Loxosceles reclusa*) may cause severe necrotic reactions and death due to intravascular hemolysis, and the black widow spider (*Latrodectus mactans*) may cause severe systemic symptoms and death. (See also Chapter 39.)

In addition to arthropod bites, the most common lesions are venomous stings (wasps, hornets, bees, ants, scorpions) or bites (centipedes), furuncle-like lesions due to fly maggots or sand fleas in the skin, and a linear creeping eruption due to a migrating larva.

Clinical Findings

The diagnosis may be difficult when the patient has not noticed the initial attack but suffers a delayed reaction. Individual bites are often in clusters and tend to occur either on exposed parts (eg, midges and gnats) or under clothing, especially around the waist or at flexures (eg, small mites or insects in bedding or clothing). The reaction is often delayed for 1–24 hours or more. Pruritus is almost always present and may be all but intolerable once the patient starts to scratch. Secondary infection may follow scratching. Urticarial wheals are common. Papules may become vesicular. The diagnosis is aided by searching for exposure to arthropods and by considering the patient's occupation and recent activities.

The principal arthropods are as follows:

(1) Fleas—Fleas are bloodsucking ectoparasites that feed on dogs, cats, humans, and other species. Flea saliva produces papular urticaria in sensitized individuals. *Ctenocephalides felis* and *Ctenocephalides canis* are the most common species found on cats and dogs, and both species attack humans. The human flea is *Pulex irritans.*

To break the life cycle of the flea, one must treat the home, pets, and outside environment, using quick-kill insecticides, residual insecticides, and a growth regulator. Obviously, this is a repetitive job.

(2) Bedbugs—In crevices of beds or furniture; bites tend to occur in lines or clusters. Papular urticaria is a characteristic lesion of bedbug (*Cimex lectularius*) bites. The closely related kissing bug has a painful bite.

(3) Ticks—Usually picked up by brushing against low vegetation. Ticks may transmit Rocky Mountain spotted fever, Lyme disease, relapsing fever, and ehrlichiosis.

(4) Chiggers or red bugs—These are larvae of trombiculid mites. A few species confined to particular

regions and locally recognized habitats (eg, berry patches, woodland edges, lawns, brush turkey mounds in Australia, poultry farms) attack humans, often around the waist, on the ankles, or in flexures, raising intensely itching erythematous papules after a delay of many hours. The red chiggers may sometimes be seen in the center of papules that have not yet been scratched.

(5) Bird and rodent mites—Larger than chiggers, bird mites infest pigeon lofts or nests of birds in eaves. Bites are multiple anywhere on the body. Room air conditioning units may suck in bird mites and infest the inhabitants of the room. Rodent mites from mice or rats may cause similar effects. Pet gerbils may be infested with bird mites. The diagnosis of bird mites, rodent mites, or carpet mites may easily be overlooked and the patient treated for other dermatoses.

(6) Mites in stored products—These are white and almost invisible and infest products such as copra, vanilla pods, sugar, straw, cottonseeds, and cereals. Persons who handle these products may be attacked, especially on the hands and forearms and sometimes on the feet. Infested bedding may occasionally lead to generalized dermatitis.

(7) Caterpillars of moths with urticating hairs—The hairs are blown from cocoons or carried by emergent moths, causing severe and often seasonally recurrent outbreaks after mass emergence. The gypsy moth is a cause in the eastern USA.

(8) Tungiasis—Tungiasis is due to the burrowing flea known as *Tunga penetrans* and is found in Africa, the West Indies, and South and Central America. The female burrows under the skin, sucks blood, swells to 0.5 cm, and then ejects her eggs onto the ground. Ulceration, lymphangitis, gangrene, and septicemia may result, in some cases with lethal effect. Ethyl chloride spray will kill the insect when applied to the lesion, and disinfestation may be accomplished with insecticide applied to the terrain. Simple surgical excision is usually performed.

Differential Diagnosis

Arthropods should be considered in the differential diagnosis of skin lesions showing any of the above symptoms.

Prevention

Arthropod infestations are best prevented by avoidance of contaminated areas, personal cleanliness, and disinfection of clothing, bedclothes, and furniture as indicated. Chiggers, bedbugs, and mites can be killed by lindane (Kwell, Scabene) applied to the head and clothing. (It is not necessary to remove clothing.) Benzyl benzoate and dimethylphthalate are excellent acaricides; clothing should be impregnated by spray or by dipping in a soapy emulsion.

Treatment

Living arthropods should be removed carefully with tweezers after application of alcohol and preserved in alcohol for identification. In endemic Rocky Mountain spotted fever areas, ticks should not be removed with the bare fingers.

Corticosteroid lotions or creams are helpful. Calamine lotion or a cool wet dressing is always appropriate. Topical antibiotics may be applied if secondary infection is suspected. Localized persistent lesions may be treated with intralesional corticosteroids.

Stings produced by many arthropods may be alleviated by applying papain powder (Adolph's Meat Tenderizer) mixed with water, or aluminum chloride hexahydrate (Xerac AC).

Extracts from venom sacs of bees, wasps, yellow jackets, and hornets are available for immunotherapy of patients at risk for anaphylaxis.

Elston DM et al: What's eating you? Bedbugs. Cutis 2000;65:262. [PMID: 10826083]

INFLAMMATORY NODULES

ERYTHEMA NODOSUM

 ESSENTIALS OF DIAGNOSIS

- *Painful red nodules without ulceration on anterior aspects of legs.*
- *Slow regression over several weeks to resemble contusions.*
- *Women are predominantly affected by a ratio of 4–8:1 over men.*
- *Some cases associated with infection or drug sensitivity.*

General Considerations

Erythema nodosum is a symptom complex characterized by tender, erythematous nodules that appear most commonly on the extensor surfaces of the lower legs. It usually lasts about 6 weeks and may recur. The disease may be associated with various infections—streptococcosis, primary coccidioidomycosis, other deep fungal infections, tuberculosis, *Yersinia pseudotuberculosis* and *Yersinia enterocolitica* infection, or syphilis. It may accompany sarcoidosis and inflammatory bowel disease. Erythema nodosum may be associated with pregnancy or with use of oral contraceptives or other medication.

Clinical Findings

A. SYMPTOMS AND SIGNS

The swellings are exquisitely tender and may be preceded by fever, malaise, and arthralgia. They are most often located on the anterior surfaces of the legs below the knees but may occur (rarely) on the arms, trunk, and face. The lesions, 1–10 cm in diameter, are at first pink to red; with regression, all the various hues seen in a contusion can be observed.

B. LABORATORY FINDINGS

The histologic finding of septal panniculitis is characteristic of erythema nodosum. Evaluation of patients presenting with acute erythema nodosum should include a careful history and physical examination for prior upper respiratory infection or diarrheal illness, symptoms of any deep fungal infection endemic to the area, a chest x-ray, a PPD, and two consecutive ASO titers at 2- to 4-week intervals. If no underlying cause is found, only a small percentage of patients will go on to develop a significant underlying illness (usually sarcoidosis) over the next year.

Differential Diagnosis

Erythema induratum is seen on the posterior surfaces of the legs and may show ulceration. Nodular vasculitis is usually on the calves. Erythema multiforme occurs in generalized distribution. Lupus panniculitis presents as tender nodules on the buttocks and posterior arms that heal with depressed scars. In the late stages, erythema nodosum must be distinguished from simple bruises and contusions.

Treatment

One must first identify and treat the underlying cause. Primary therapy is with nonsteroidal anti-inflammatory agents in usual doses. Saturated solution of potassium iodide, 5–15 drops three times daily, may result in prompt involution in many cases. Side effects of potassium iodide include salivation, swelling of salivary glands, and headache. Complete bed rest may be advisable if the lesions are painful. Systemic therapy directed against the lesions themselves may include corticosteroid therapy (see Chapter 26) unless contraindicated by associated infection; salicylates are helpful for several days during the acute painful stage.

Prognosis

The lesions usually disappear after about 6 weeks, but they may recur.

Garcia-Porrua C et al: Erythema nodosum: etiologic and predictive factors in a defined population. Arthritis Rheum 2000;43:584. [PMID: 10728752]

FURUNCULOSIS (BOILS) & CARBUNCLES

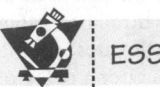 ESSENTIALS OF DIAGNOSIS

- *Extremely painful inflammatory swelling based on a hair follicle that forms an abscess.*
- *Predisposing condition (diabetes mellitus, HIV disease, injection drug use) sometimes present.*
- *Coagulase-positive* Staphylococcus aureus *is the causative organism.*

General Considerations

A furuncle (boil) is a deep-seated infection (abscess) involving the entire hair follicle and adjacent subcutaneous tissue. The most common sites of occurrence are the hairy parts exposed to irritation and friction, pressure, or moisture. Because the lesions are autoinoculable, they are often multiple. Thorough investigation usually fails to uncover a predisposing cause; however, diabetes mellitus (especially if using insulin injections), injection drug use, allergy injections, and HIV disease all increase the risk of staphylococcal infections by increasing the rate of nasal carriage.

A carbuncle consists of several furuncles developing in adjoining hair follicles and coalescing to form a conglomerate, deeply situated mass with multiple drainage points.

Clinical Findings

A. SYMPTOMS AND SIGNS

Pain and tenderness may be prominent. The abscess is either rounded or conical. It gradually enlarges, becomes fluctuant, and then softens and opens spontaneously after a few days to 1–2 weeks to discharge a core of necrotic tissue and pus. The inflammation occasionally subsides before necrosis occurs. Infection of the soft tissue around the nails (paronychia) may be due to staphylococci when it is acute. Other organisms may be involved, including candida and herpes simplex (herpetic whitlow).

B. LABORATORY FINDINGS

There may be slight leukocytosis, but a white blood cell count is rarely required. Although *S aureus* is almost always the cause, pus should be cultured, especially in immunocompromised patients, to rule out methicillin-resistant *S aureus* or other bacteria. Culture of the anterior nares may identify chronic staphylococcal carriage in cases of recurrent cutaneous infection.

Differential Diagnosis

The most common entity in the differential is an inflamed epidermal inclusion cyst that suddenly becomes red, tender, and expands greatly in size over one to a few days. The history of a prior cyst in the same location, the presence of a clearly visible cyst orifice, and the extrusion of malodorous cheesy rather than purulent material helps in the diagnosis. Tinea profunda (deep dermatophyte infection of the hair follicle) may simulate recurrent furunculosis. Furuncle is also to be distinguished from deep mycotic infections such as sporotrichosis (often in gardeners) and blastomycosis, from other bacterial infections such as anthrax and tularemia (rare), and from acne cysts. Hidradenitis suppurativa presents with recurrent tender sterile abscesses in the axillae, groin, on the buttocks, or below the breasts. The presence of old scars or sinus tracts plus negative cultures suggests this diagnosis.

Complications

Serious and sometimes fatal cavernous sinus thrombosis may occur as a complication of a manipulated furuncle on the central portion of the upper lip or near the nasolabial folds. Perinephric abscess, osteomyelitis, and even endocarditis may rarely occur.

Treatment

A. SPECIFIC MEASURES

Incision and drainage is recommended for all loculated suppurations and is the mainstay of therapy. Systemic antibiotics are indicated (chosen on the basis of cultures and sensitivity tests if possible). Sodium dicloxacillin or cephalexin, 1 g daily in divided doses by mouth for 10 days, is usually effective. Erythromycin in similar doses may be used in penicillin-allergic individuals in communities with low populations of erythromycin-resistant staphylococci or if the particular isolate is sensitive. Ciprofloxacin, 500 mg twice daily, is effective against strains of staphylococci resistant to other antibiotics.

Recurrent furunculosis may be effectively treated with a combination of dicloxacillin, 250–500 mg four times daily for 2–4 weeks, and rifampin, 300 mg twice daily for 5 days during this period. Chronic clindamycin, 150–300 mg daily for 1–2 months, may also cure recurrent furunculosis. Family members and intimate contacts may need evaluation for staphylococcal carrier state and perhaps concomitant treatment. Applications of topical 2% mupirocin to the nares, axillae, and anogenital areas twice daily for 5 days eliminates the staphylococcal carrier state.

B. LOCAL MEASURES

Immobilize the part and avoid overmanipulation of inflamed areas. Use moist heat to help larger lesions "localize." Use surgical incision and debridement *after* the lesions are "mature." It is not necessary to incise and drain an acute staphylococcal paronychia. Inserting a flat metal spatula or sharpened hardwood stick into the nail fold where it adjoins the nail will release pus from a mature lesion. Inflamed epidermal cysts may be treated in the initial stages with intralesional injections of triamcinolone acetonide into the borders of the lesions, attempting not to puncture the cyst itself. Drainage of fluctuant lesions results in rapid resolution and reduction of pain.

Prognosis

Recurrent crops may harass the patient for months or years.

Veien NK: The clinician's choice of antibiotics in the treatment of bacterial skin infection. Br J Dermatol 1998;139(Suppl 53):30. [PMID: 9990410]

PHOTODERMATITIS

ESSENTIALS OF DIAGNOSIS

- Painful or pruritic erythema, edema, or vesiculation on sun exposed surfaces: the face, neck, hands, and "V" of the chest.
- Inner upper eyelids spared, as is the area under the chin.

General Considerations

Photodermatitis is an acute or chronic inflammatory skin reaction due to hypersensitivity to sunlight or other sources of actinic rays, photosensitization of the skin by certain drugs, or idiosyncrasy to actinic light as seen in some constitutional disorders including the porphyrias and many hereditary disorders (phenylketonuria, xeroderma pigmentosum, and others). Contact photosensitivity may occur with perfumes, antiseptics, and other chemicals.

Photodermatitis is manifested most commonly as photosensitivity—a tendency for the individual to sunburn more easily than usual—or, more rarely, as photoallergy, a true immunologic reaction that often presents with papular or vesicular lesions.

Clinical Findings

A. SYMPTOMS AND SIGNS

The acute inflammatory skin reaction, if severe enough, is accompanied by pain, fever, gastrointestinal symptoms, malaise, and even prostration, but this is very rare. Signs include erythema, edema, and possibly vesiculation and oozing on exposed surfaces. Peeling of the epidermis and pigmentary changes often result. The key to diagnosis is localization of the rash to photoexposed areas, though these eruptions may become generalized with time to involve even photoprotected areas. The lips are commonly involved in hereditary polymorphous light eruption, a disorder seen in persons of Native American descent.

B. LABORATORY FINDINGS

Blood and urine tests are not helpful in diagnosis unless porphyria cutanea tarda is suggested by the presence of blistering, scarring, milia (white cysts 1–2 mm in diameter) and skin fragility of the dorsal hands, and facial hypertrichosis. Testing for photosensitivity may be necessary to define the wavelengths of light.

Differential Diagnosis

The differential diagnosis is long. If a clear history of the use of a topical or systemic photosensitizer is not available and if the eruption is persistent, then a workup including biopsy and light testing may be required. Photodermatitis must be differentiated from contact dermatitis that may develop from one of the many substances in suntan lotions and oils, as these may often have a similar distribution. Sensitivity to actinic rays may also be part of a more serious condition such as porphyria cutanea tarda, variegate porphyria, or lupus erythematosus. These disorders are diagnosed by appropriate blood or urine tests. Phenothiazines, sulfones, chlorothiazides, griseofulvin, sulfonylureas, nonsteroidal anti-inflammatory agents, and antibiotics (eg, some tetracyclines) may photosensitize the skin. Polymorphous light eruption is a very common idiopathic photodermatitis that affects both sexes equally and often has its onset in the third to fourth decades except in Native Americans, in whom it commonly presents in childhood. Polymorphous light eruption is chronic in nature. Transitory periods of spontaneous remission do occur. The action spectrum usually lies in the short (below 320 nm) ultraviolet wavelengths but may also extend into the long ultraviolet wavelengths (320–400 nm).

Complications

Some individuals continue to be chronic light reactors even when they apparently are no longer exposed to photosensitizing or phototoxic drugs.

Prevention

While sunscreens are useful agents in general and should be used by persons with photosensitivity, patients may react to such low amounts of energy that sunscreens alone may not be sufficient. Sunscreens with an SPF of 30–50, usually containing avobenzone

(Parasol 1789), titanium dioxide, and micronized zinc oxide, are especially useful in patients with photoallergic dermatitis.

Treatment

A. SPECIFIC MEASURES

Drugs should be suspected in cases of photoallergy even if the particular medication (such as hydrochlorothiazide) has been used for months.

B. LOCAL MEASURES

When the eruption is vesicular or weepy, treatment is similar to that of any acute dermatitis, using cooling and soothing wet dressing.

Sunscreens should be used as described above. Mid-potency to high-potency topical steroids are of limited benefit in phototoxic reactions but may help in polymorphous light eruption and photoallergic reactions. Since the face is often involved, close monitoring every 2 weeks is necessary to avoid side effects of potent steroids.

C. SYSTEMIC MEASURES

Aspirin may have some value for fever and pain of acute sunburn, as prostaglandins appear to play a pathogenetic role in the early erythema. Systemic corticosteroids in doses as described for acute contact dermatitis may be required for severe photosensitivity reactions. Otherwise, different photodermatoses may be treated in specific ways.

Patients with severe photosensitivity may require immunosuppressives, such as azathioprine, in the range of 50–150 mg/d; or cyclosporine, 3–5 mg/kg/d.

Prognosis

The most common phototoxic sunburn reactions are usually benign and self-limiting except when the burn is severe or when it occurs as an associated finding in a more serious disorder. Polymorphous light eruption and some cases of photoallergy can persist for years.

Vassileva SG et al: Antimicrobial photosensitive reactions. Arch Intern Med 1998;158:871. [PMID: 9778198]

ULCERS

DECUBITUS ULCERS (BEDSORES, PRESSURE SORES)

Bedsores (pressure sores) are a special type of ulcer caused by impaired blood supply and tissue nutrition resulting from prolonged pressure over bony or cartilaginous prominences. The skin overlying the sacrum and hips is most commonly involved, but bedsores may also be seen over the occiput, ears, elbows, heels, and ankles. They occur most readily in aged, paralyzed, debilitated, and unconscious patients. Low-grade infection may occur as a complication.

Differential Diagnosis

Herpes simplex virus should be suspected in ulcers in immunocompromised patients, particularly if there is a scalloped border, representing the erosions of herpetic vesicles. Rarely, ulcerated lesions in the perianal area represent actual skin cancers. Rapidly expanding ulcers may also represent pyoderma gangrenosum associated with inflammatory bowel disease. Ecthyma gangrenosum is an ulcerating lesion, commonly due to pseudomonas, and observed in neutropenic patients. All ulcerative lesions should be biopsied and cultured if suspicious or if they do not heal properly.

Prevention

Good nursing care, good nutrition, and maintenance of skin hygiene are important preventive measures. The skin and the bed linens should be kept clean and dry. Bedfast, paralyzed, moribund, listless, or incontinent patients who are candidates for the development of decubiti must be turned *frequently* (at least every hour) and must be examined at pressure points for the appearance of small areas of redness and tenderness. Written schedules can be very helpful. Water-filled mattresses, rubber pillows, alternating-pressure mattresses, and thick papillated foam pads are useful in prevention and in the treatment of lesions. "Donut" devices should not be used.

Treatment

A large number of treatments and protocols exist for management of decubiti. Early lesions should be treated with topical antibiotic powders and adhesive absorbent bandage (Gelfoam). Once clean, they may be treated with hydrocolloid dressings such as Duo-Derm. Established lesions require surgery for debridement, cleansing, and dressing. A spongy foam pad placed under the patient may work best in some cases. It must be laundered often. In general, topical antiseptics are not recommended. Systemic antibiotics are required for deep infections.

Theaker C et al: Risk factors for pressure sores in the critically ill. Anaesthesia 2000;55:221. [PMID: 10671839]

LEG ULCERS SECONDARY TO VENOUS INSUFFICIENCY

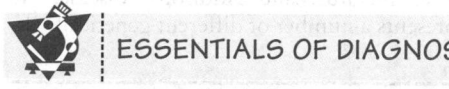

ESSENTIALS OF DIAGNOSIS

- *Past history of varicosities, thrombophlebitis, or postphlebitic syndrome.*
- *Irregular ulceration, often on the medial aspect of the lower legs above the malleolus.*
- *Edema of the legs, varicosities, hyperpigmentation, and red and scaly areas (stasis dermatitis) and scars from old ulcers support the diagnosis.*

General Considerations

Patients at risk may have a history of venous insufficiency, either with obvious varicosities or with a past history of thrombophlebitis, or with immobility of the calf muscle group (paraplegics, etc). Red, pruritic patches of stasis dermatitis often precede ulceration. Because venous insufficiency is the most common cause of lower leg ulceration, testing of venous competence is still a required part of the evaluation even when no changes of venous insufficiency are present.

Clinical Findings

A. SYMPTOMS AND SIGNS

Classically, chronic edema is followed by a dermatitis, which is often pruritic. These changes are followed by hyperpigmentation, skin breakdown, and eventually sclerosis of the skin of the lower leg. The ulcer base may be clean, but it often has a yellow fibrin eschar that often requires surgical treatment. Ulcers that appear on the feet, toes, or above the knees should be approached with other diagnoses in mind.

B. LABORATORY FINDINGS

Thorough evaluation of the patient's vascular system (including measurement of the ankle/brachial index) is essential. Doppler and light rheography examinations as office procedures are usually sufficient (except in the diabetic) to elucidate the cause of most vascular cases of lower leg ulceration.

Differential Diagnosis

The differential includes vasculitis, pyoderma gangrenosum, arterial ulcerations, infection, trauma, arachnid bites, and sickle cell anemia. When the diagnosis is in doubt, a punch biopsy from the border (not base) of the lesion may be helpful.

Prevention

Compression stockings to reduce edema are the most important means of prevention. Compression should achieve a pressure of 30 mm Hg below the knee and 40 mm Hg at the ankle. The stockings should not be used in patients with arterial insufficiency with an ankle-brachial pressure index less than 0.7. Pneumatic sequential compression devices may be of great benefit.

Treatment

A. LOCAL MEASURES

Institution of compression therapy is begun with cleaning of the ulcer. The patient is instructed to clean the base with saline or cleansers such as Saf-clens or Cara-klenz daily. A curette or small scissors can be used to remove the yellow fibrin eschar, under local anesthesia if the areas are very tender.

Once the base is clean, the ulcer is treated with metronidazole gel to reduce bacterial growth and odor. Any red dermatitic skin is treated with a medium- to high-potency steroid ointment. The ulcer is then covered with an occlusive hydroactive dressing (Duoderm or Cutinova) or a polyurethane foam (Allevyn) followed by an Unna zinc paste boot. This is changed weekly. The ulcer should begin to heal within weeks, and healing should be complete within 2–3 months. If the patient is diabetic, becaplermin (Regranex) may be applied to the ulcer along with good local treatment in those ulcers which are not becoming smaller or developing a granulating base. Some ulcerations require grafting. Full- or split-thickness grafts often do not take, and pinch grafts (small shaves of skin laid onto the bed) may be more effective. Cultured epidermal cell grafts—or Apligraf, a bilayered skin construct—may accelerate wound healing, but they are very expensive. They should be considered in refractory ulcers, especially those which have not healed after a year or more of conservative therapy.

B. SYSTEMIC THERAPY

Pentoxifylline, 400 mg three times daily administered with compression, is beneficial in accelerating healing of leg ulcers. Zinc supplementation is occasionally beneficial in patients with low serum zinc levels. If cellulitis accompanies the ulcer, systemic antibiotics are recommended: dicloxacillin, 250 mg orally four times a day; ciprofloxacin, 500 mg orally twice a day; or levofloxacin, 500 mg once daily.

Prognosis

The combination of compression stockings and newer dressings enables venous stasis ulcers to heal within weeks or months. Topical growth factors, antibiotics, debriding agents, and xenografts and autografts have been shown to be effective in recalcitrant cases. Ongoing control of edema is essential to prevent recurrent ulceration.

Jull AB et al: Oral pentoxifylline for treatment of venous leg ulcers. Cochrane Database Syst Rev 2000(2):CD001733. [PMID: 10796661]

McMullin GM: Improving the treatment of leg ulcers. Med J Aust 2001;175:375. [PMID: 11700817]

■ II. MISCELLANEOUS DERMATOLOGIC DISORDERS*

PIGMENTARY DISORDERS

Although the color of skin may be altered by many diseases and agents, the vast majority of patients have either an increase or decrease in pigment secondary to some inflammatory disease such as acne or atopic dermatitis.

Other pigmentary disorders include those resulting from exposure to exogenous pigments such as carotenemia, argyria, deposition of other metals (such as gold when given chronically for rheumatoid arthritis), and tattooing. Other endogenous pigmentary disorders are attributable to metabolic substances—including hemosiderin (iron)—in purpuric processes; or to homogentisic acid in ochronosis; bile pigments; and carotenes.

Classification

One should first determine whether the disorder is hyper- or hypopigmentation, ie, an increase or decrease in normal skin colors. Each may be considered to be primary or to be secondary to other disorders.

A. PRIMARY PIGMENTARY DISORDERS

1. Hyperpigmentation—The disorders in this category are nevoid, congenital or acquired, and include pigmented nevi, ephelides (juvenile freckles), and lentigines (senile freckles). Hyperpigmentation occurs also in arsenical melanosis or in association with Addison's disease (due to lack of the inhibitory influence of cortisol on the production of MSH by the pituitary gland). Axillary freckling and café au lait spots may be seen in neurofibromatosis. **Melasma (chloasma)** occurs as patterned hyperpigmentation of the face, usually as a direct effect of estrogens. It occurs not only during pregnancy but also in 30–50% of women taking oral contraceptives, and rarely in men. One report suggests that such men have low testosterone and elevated LH levels.

2. Hypopigmentation and depigmentation—The disorders in this category are vitiligo, albinism, and piebaldism. In vitiligo, pigment cells (melanocytes) are destroyed. The greater the pigment loss, the fewer the number of melanocytes. Vitiligo, present in approximately 1% of the population, may be associated with hyperthyroidism and hypothyroidism, pernicious anemia, diabetes mellitus, and Addison's disease. Albinism represents a number of different genetically de-

---

*Hirsutism is discussed in Chapter 26.

termined traits, with different phenotypes. These often affect the eye and vision. Piebaldism, a localized hypomelanosis manifested by a white forelock, is an autosomal dominant trait that in some cases may be associated with neurologic abnormalities. Hypopigmented ash leaf spots may be seen in tuberous sclerosis. Hypopigmented halos are common around nevi and may occur around melanomas.

B. SECONDARY PIGMENTARY DISORDERS

Any damage to the skin (irritation, allergy, infection, excoriation, burns, or dermatologic therapy such as chemical peels and freezing with liquid nitrogen) may result in hyper- or hypopigmentation. Several disorders of clinical importance are as described below:

1. Hyperpigmentation—The most common type of secondary hyperpigmentation occurs after another dermatologic condition, such as acne, and is most commonly seen in dark-skinned persons. It is called postinflammatory hyperpigmentation.

Berloque hyperpigmentation is the pigmentation due to phototoxicity from chemicals in the rinds of limes and other citrus fruits and to celery. Pigmentation may be produced by certain drugs, eg, chloroquine, chlorpromazine, minocycline, and amiodarone. Irritation from benzoyl peroxide and tretinoin can result in hyperpigmentation, as may topical fluorouracil. Fixed drug eruptions to phenolphthalein in laxatives, to trimethoprim-sulfamethoxazole, to NSAIDs, and to tetracyclines, for example, are further causes.

2. Hypopigmentation—Leukoderma is a disorder that may complicate atopic dermatitis, lichen planus, psoriasis, discoid lupus erythematosus, and lichen simplex chronicus. Practitioners must exercise special care in using liquid nitrogen on any patient with olive or darker complexions, since doing so may result in hypopigmentation or depigmentation, at times permanent. Intralesional or intra-articular injections of high concentrations of corticosteroids may also cause localized temporary hypopigmentation.

Differential Diagnosis

One must distinguish true lack of pigment from pseudoachromia, such as occurs in tinea versicolor, pityriasis simplex, and seborrheic dermatitis. The evaluation of pigmentary disorders in Caucasians is helped by Wood's light, which accentuates epidermal pigmentation and highlights hypopigmentation.

Complications

Actinic keratoses and skin cancers are more likely to develop in persons with vitiligo and albinism. There may be severe emotional trauma in extensive vitiligo and other types of hypo- and hyperpigmentation, par-

ticularly when they occur in naturally dark-skinned persons.

Treatment & Prognosis

A. HYPERPIGMENTATION

Therapeutic bleaching preparations generally contain hydroquinone. Hydroquinone has occasionally caused unexpected hypopigmentation, hyperpigmentation, or even secondary ochronosis and pigmented milia, particularly with prolonged use.

The role of exposure to ultraviolet light cannot be overstressed as a factor promoting or contributing to most disorders of hyperpigmentation, and such exposure should be minimized. Melasma, ephelides, and postinflammatory hyperpigmentation may be treated with varying success with 3–4% hydroquinone cream, gel, or solution and a sunscreen containing UVA photoprotectants (Avobenzone, zinc oxide, titanium dioxide). Tretinoin cream, 0.025–0.05%, may be added. Superficial melasma responds well, but if there is predominantly dermal deposition of pigment (does *not* enhance with Wood's light), the prognosis is poor. Response to therapy takes months and requires avoidance of sunlight. Hyperpigmentation often recurs after treatment if the skin is exposed to ultraviolet light. Solar lentigines respond to liquid nitrogen application. Tretinoin, 0.1% cream used over 10 months, will fade solar lentigines (liver spots), hyperpigmented facial macules in Asians, and postinflammatory hyperpigmentation in blacks. New laser systems for the removal of epidermal and dermal pigments are available, and referral should be considered for patients whose responses to medical treatment are inadequate.

B. HYPOPIGMENTATION

The pigment dilution is stable in various forms of albinism; spontaneous return of pigment is rare in vitiligo; in secondary hypopigmentation, repigmentation may occur spontaneously. Cosmetics such as Covermark and Dermablend are highly effective for concealing disfiguring patches. Therapy of vitiligo is long and tedious, and the patient must be strongly motivated. If less than 20% of the skin is involved (most cases), topical methoxsalen, 0.1% in ethanol and propylene glycol or in Acid Mantle cream or Unibase, is used, with cautious exposure to long-wavelength ultraviolet light (UVA), followed by thorough washing and sun avoidance. With 20–25% involvement, oral PUVA is best. Severe phototoxic response (sunburn) may occur with topical or oral psoralens plus UVA. The face and upper chest respond best, and the fingertips and the genital areas do not respond to this treatment. Years of treatment are often required. Newer techniques of using epidermal autografts and cultured epidermis combined with PUVA therapy give hope for surgical correction of vitiligo. Potent topical corticosteroids have been advocated for treatment of vitiligo, with daily use for 10 days followed by 10 days of rest, then repetition.

Kim NY et al: Pigmentary diseases. Med Clin North Am 1998;82:1185. [PMID: 9769800]

Sialy R et al: Melasma in men: a hormonal profile. J Dermatol 2000;27:64. [PMID: 10692830]

Westerhof W: Vitiligo management update. Skin Therapy Lett 2000;5:1. [PMID: 10889569]

BALDNESS
(Alopecia)

Baldness Due to Scarring

Cicatricial baldness may occur following chemical or physical trauma, lichen planopilaris, severe bacterial or fungal infections, severe herpes zoster, chronic discoid lupus erythematosus, scleroderma, and excessive ionizing radiation. The specific cause is often suggested by the history, the distribution of hair loss, and the appearance of the skin, as in lupus erythematosus. Biopsy is useful in the diagnosis of scarring alopecia, but specimens must be taken from the active border and not from the scarred central zone.

Scarring alopecias are irreversible and permanent. It is important to diagnose and treat the scarring process as early in its course as possible.

Baldness Not Due to Scarring

Nonscarring alopecia may occur in association with various systemic diseases such as systemic lupus erythematosus, secondary syphilis, hyper- or hypothyroidism, iron deficiency anemia, and pituitary insufficiency. The only treatment necessary is prompt and adequate control of the underlying disorder, in which case hair loss may be reversible.

Androgenetic (pattern) baldness, the most common form of alopecia, is of genetic predetermination. The earliest changes occur at the anterior portions of the calvarium on either side of the "widow's peak" and on the crown (vertex) of the scull. The extent of hair loss is variable and unpredictable. Rogaine Extra Strength, a solution containing 50 mg/mL of minoxidil, is available over the counter. The best results are achieved in persons with recent onset (< 5 years) and smaller areas of alopecia. Approximately 40% of patients treated twice daily for a year will have moderate to dense growth. Finasteride (Propecia), 1 mg orally daily, has similar efficacy and may be additive to minoxidil. As opposed to minoxidil, finasteride is used only in males.

Hair loss or thinning of the hair in women results from the same cause as common baldness in men (androgenetic alopecia) and may be treated with minoxidil (Rogaine). A workup consisting of determination of serum testosterone, DHEAS, iron, total iron binding capacity, and thyroid function tests and a complete blood count will identify most other causes of hair thinning in premenopausal women. Women who complain

of thin hair but show little evidence of alopecia need follow-up, because more than 50% of the scalp hair can be lost before the clinician can perceive it.

Telogen effluvium is transitory increase in the number of hairs in the telogen (resting) phase of the hair growth cycle. This may occur spontaneously, may appear at the termination of pregnancy, may be precipitated by "crash dieting," high fever, stress from surgery or shock, or malnutrition, or may be provoked by hormonal contraceptives. Whatever the cause, telogen effluvium usually has a latent period of 2–4 months. The prognosis is generally good. The condition is diagnosed by the presence of large numbers of hairs with white bulbs coming out upon gentle tugging of the hair. Counts of hairs lost by the patient on combing or shampooing often exceed 150 per day, compared to an average of 70–100. In one study, a major cause of telogen effluvium was found to be iron deficiency, and the hair counts bore a clear relationship to serum iron levels.

Alopecia areata is of unknown cause but is believed to be an immunologic process. Typically, there are patches that are perfectly smooth and without scarring. Tiny hairs 2–3 mm in length, called "exclamation hairs," may be seen. Telogen hairs are easily dislodged from the periphery of active lesions. The beard, brows, and lashes may be involved. Involvement may extend to all of the scalp hair (alopecia totalis) or to all scalp and body hair (alopecia universalis). Severe forms may be treated by systemic corticosteroid therapy, although recurrences follow discontinuation of therapy. Alopecia areata is occasionally associated with Hashimoto's thyroiditis, pernicious anemia, Addison's disease, and vitiligo.

Intralesional corticosteroids are frequently effective for alopecia areata. Triamcinolone acetonide in a concentration of 2.5–10 mg/mL is injected in aliquots of 0.1 mL at approximately 1- to 2-cm intervals, not exceeding a total dose of 30 mg per month for adults. Alternatively, anthralin 0.5% ointment used daily, may help some patients. Alopecia areata is usually self-limiting, with complete regrowth of hair in 80% of patients, but some mild cases are resistant, as are the extensive totalis and universalis types. Both topical diphencyprone and squaric acid dibutylester, have been used to treat persistent alopecia areata. The principle is to sensitize the skin, then intermittently apply weaker concentrations to produce and maintain a slight dermatitis. Hair regrowth in 3–6 months in some patients has been reported to be remarkable. Long-term safety and efficacy have not been established. Support groups for patients with extensive alopecia areata are very beneficial. In **trichotillomania** (the pulling out of one's own hair), the patches of hair loss are irregular and growing hairs are always present, since they cannot be pulled out until they are long enough. The patches are often unilateral, occurring on the same side as the patient's dominant hand. The patient may be unaware of the habit.

Drug-induced alopecia is becoming increasingly important. Incriminated drugs include thallium, excessive and prolonged use of vitamin A, retinoids, antimitotic agents, anticoagulants, antithyroid drugs, oral contraceptives, trimethadione, allopurinol, propranolol, indomethacin, amphetamines, salicylates, gentamicin, and levodopa. While chemotherapy-induced alopecia is very distressing, it must be emphasized to the patient before treatment that it is invariably reversible.

Bertolino AP: Alopecia areata. A clinical overview. Postgrad Med 2000;107:81. [PMID: 10887448]

Madani S et al: Alopecia areata update. J Am Acad Dermatol 2000;42:549. [PMID: 10727299]

Price VH: Treatment of hair loss. N Engl J Med 1999;341:964. [PMID: 10498493]

NAIL DISORDERS

1. Morphologic Abnormalities of the Nails

Classification

Nail disorders may be classified as (1) local, (2) congenital or genetic, and (3) those associated with systemic or generalized skin diseases.

A. LOCAL NAIL DISORDERS

1. Onycholysis (distal separation of the nail plate from the nail bed, usually of the fingers) is caused by excessive exposure to water, soaps, detergents, alkalies, and industrial keratolytic agents. Candidal infection of the nail folds and subungual area, nail hardeners, and drug-induced photosensitivity may cause onycholysis, as may hyper- and hypothyroidism and psoriasis.

2. Distortion of the nail occurs as a result of chronic inflammation of the nail matrix underlying the eponychial fold. Such changes may also be caused by warts, tumors, nevi, synovial and mucous cysts, etc, impinging on the nail matrix.

3. Discoloration and crumbly thickened nails are noted in dermatophyte infection and psoriasis.

4. Allergic reactions (to formaldehyde and resins in undercoats and polishes or to nail glues) are characterized by onycholysis or by grossly distorted, hypertrophic, and misshapen nails.

B. CONGENITAL AND GENETIC NAIL DISORDERS

1. A longitudinal single nail groove may occur as a result of a genetic or traumatic defect in the nail matrix.

2. Nail atrophy may be congenital.

3. Clubbed fingers may be congenital.

C. NAIL CHANGES ASSOCIATED WITH SYSTEMIC OR GENERALIZED SKIN DISEASES

1. Beau's lines (transverse furrows) may follow any serious systemic illness.

2. Atrophy of the nails may be related to trauma or to vascular or neurologic disease.

3. Clubbed fingers may be due to the prolonged hypoxemia associated with cardiopulmonary disorders. (See Chapter 9.)

4. Spoon nails may be seen in anemic patients.

5. Stippling or pitting of the nails is seen in psoriasis, alopecia areata, and hand eczema.

6. Nail hyperpigmentation may be caused by zidovudine, doxorubicin, cyclophosphamide, bleomycin, daunorubicin, fluorouracil, hydroxyurea, melphalan, mechlorethamine, and nitrosoureas.

Differential Diagnosis

It is important to distinguish congenital and genetic disorders from those caused by trauma and environmental disorders. Onychomycosis may cause nail changes identical to those seen in psoriasis. Careful examination for more characteristic lesions elsewhere on the body is essential to the diagnosis of the nail disorders. Cancer should be suspected (eg, Bowen's disease or squamous cell carcinoma) as the cause of any persistent solitary subungual or periungual lesion.

Complications

Secondary bacterial infection occasionally occurs in onychodystrophies and leads to considerable pain and disability and more serious consequences if circulation or innervation is impaired. Toenail changes may lead to an ingrown nail—in turn often complicated by bacterial infection and occasionally by exuberant granulation tissue. Poor manicuring and poorly fitting shoes may contribute to this complication. Cellulitis may result.

Treatment & Prognosis

Treatment consists usually of careful debridement and manicuring and, above all, reduction of exposure to irritants (soaps, detergents, alkali, bleaches, solvents, etc). Congenital or genetic nail disorders are usually uncorrectable. Longitudinal grooving due to temporary lesions of the matrix, such as warts, synovial cysts, and other impingements, may be cured by removal of the offending lesion. Intradermal triamcinolone acetonide suspension, 2.5 mg/mL, may be injected in the area of the nail matrix at intervals of 2–4 weeks for the successful management of various types of inflammatory nail dystrophies (psoriasis, lichen planus) but is painful.

If it is necessary to remove dystrophic nails for any reason (eg, fungal nails or severe psoriasis), a nonsurgical method is to apply urea 40%, anhydrous lanolin 20%, white wax 5%, white petrolatum 25%, and silica gel type H. The nail folds are painted with compound tincture of benzoin and covered with cloth adhesive tape. The urea ointment is applied generously to the nail surface and covered with plastic film, and then adhesive tape. The ointment is left on for 5–10 days; then the nail plate may be curetted off. Medication can then be applied that is appropriate for the condition being treated.

2. Tinea Unguium (Onychomycosis)

Tinea unguium is a trichophyton infection of one or more (but rarely all) fingernails or toenails. The species most commonly found is *Trichophyton rubrum*. "Saprophytic" fungi may rarely (< 5%) cause onychomycosis.

The nails are lusterless, brittle, and hypertrophic, and the substance of the nail is friable. Laboratory diagnosis is mandatory since only 50% of dystrophic nails are due to dermatophytosis. Portions of the nail should be cleared with 10% potassium hydroxide and examined under the microscope for hyphae. Fungi may also be cultured. Periodic acid-Schiff stain of a histologic section of the nail plate will also demonstrate the fungus readily.

Onychomycosis is difficult to treat because of the long duration of therapy required and the frequency of recurrences. Fingernails respond more readily than toenails. For toenails, it is in some situations best to discourage therapy and to control discomfort by paring the thickened nail plate.

Topical treatment has relatively low efficacy (10% or less), but in well-motivated patients with minimally thickened nails it can be useful. Naftifine gel 1% or ciclopirox nail lacquer (Penlac) 8% applied twice daily may clear fingernails in 4–6 months and toenails in 12–18 months.

In general, systemic therapy is required for the treatment of nail onychomycosis. Fingernails can virtually always be cleared, whereas toenails respond in about 60% of cases. For fingernails, ultramicrosize griseofulvin, 750 mg or more daily for 6 months, is often effective. Treatment alternatives are itraconazole, 200 mg daily for 3 months; itraconazole, 400 mg the first 7 days of each month for 2 months; and terbinafine, 250 mg daily for 6 weeks. Once clear, fingernails often remain free of disease for years. The efficacy of griseofulvin for toenails is too low to be considered a therapeutic option in most cases. Ketoconazole, with its risk of hepatotoxicity with long-term use, is also not recommended. Itraconazole may be given as 200 mg daily for 3 months or 400 mg for the first 7 days of each month for 3 months for toenail onychomycosis. It is not FDA-approved for treatment of toenail onychomycosis. About 60% of patients will have substantial improvement, and 25–35% will be mycologically and clinically cured at 1 year. It interacts with numerous other medications and requires gastric acid to be absorbed.

In comparative trials, terbinafine, 250 mg daily for 3 months, has efficacy equal to or superior to that of itraconazole. About 75% of patients have significant clinical improvement, and 35–50% are cured at 1 year. The combination of a topical antifungal nail lacquer for 1 year and oral terbinafine for 3 months was superior to the oral agent alone, doubling the cure rate. Terbinafine is associated with fewer drug interactions than itraconazole (but may result in prolonged prothrombin times in patients taking warfarin). Also unlike itraconazole, terbinafine is absorbed in patients with low gastric acid (those receiving H$_2$ blockers). The rate of long-term recurrences following these forms of treatment is unknown. No matter which therapy is used, constant topical treatment for any coexistent tinea pedis is mandatory and should probably be continued for life to attempt to prevent recurrence.

Ciclopirox (Penlac) nail lacquer for onychomycosis. Med Lett Drugs Ther 2000;42:51. [PMID: 10859733]

Evans EG et al: Double blind, randomised study of continuous terbinafine compared with intermittent itraconazole in treatment of toenail onychomycosis. The LION Study Group. BMJ 1999;318:1031. [PMID: 10205099]

Mayeaux EJ Jr: Nail disorders. Prim Care 2000;27:333. [PMID: 10815047]

Piraccini BM et al: Drug-induced nail disorders: incidence, management and prognosis. Drug Saf 1999;21:187. [PMID: 10487397]

DERMATITIS MEDICAMENTOSA (Drug Eruption)

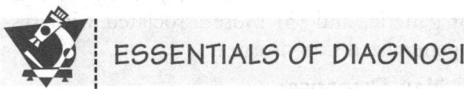

ESSENTIALS OF DIAGNOSIS

- *Usually, abrupt onset of widespread, symmetric erythematous eruption.*
- *May mimic any inflammatory skin condition.*
- *Constitutional symptoms (malaise, arthralgia, headache, and fever) may be present.*

General Considerations

As is well recognized, only a minority of cutaneous drug reactions result from allergy. True allergic drug reactions involve prior exposure, an "incubation" period, reactions to doses far below the therapeutic range, manifestations different from the usual pharmacologic effects of the drug, involvement of only a small portion of the population at risk, restriction to a limited number of syndromes (anaphylactic and anaphylactoid, urticarial, vasculitic, etc), and reproducibility.

Rashes are among the most common adverse reactions to drugs and occur in 2–3% of hospitalized patients. Amoxicillin, trimethoprim-sulfamethoxazole, and ampicillin or penicillin are the commonest causes of urticarial and maculopapular reactions. Toxic epidermal necrolysis and Stevens-Johnson syndrome are most commonly produced by sulfonamides and anticonvulsants. Phenolphthalein, pyrazolone derivatives, tetracyclines, NSAIDs, trimethoprim-sulfamethoxazole, and barbiturates are the major causes of fixed drug eruptions.

Clinical Findings

A. SYMPTOMS AND SIGNS

The onset is usually abrupt, with bright erythema and often severe itching, but may be delayed. Fever and

Table 6–3. Skin reactions due to systemic drugs.

Reaction	Appearance	Distribution and Comments	Common Offenders
Toxic erythema	Morbilliform, maculo-papular, exanthematous reactions.	The commonest skin reaction to drugs. Often more pronounced on the trunk than on the extremities. In previously exposed patients, the rash may start in 2–3 days. In the first course of treatment, the eruption often appears about the seventh to ninth days. Fever may be present.	Antibiotics (especially ampicillin and trimethoprim sulfamethoxazole), sulfonamides and related compounds (including thiazide diuretics, furosemide, and sulfonylurea hypoglycemic agents), and barbiturates.
Erythema multiforme major	Target-like lesions. Bullae may occur. Mucosal involvement.	Mainly on the extensor aspects of the limbs.	Sulfonamides, penicillamine, barbiturates, and NSAIDs.
Erythema nodosum	Inflammatory cutaneous nodules.	Usually limited to the extensor aspects of the legs. May be accompanied by fever, arthralgias, and pain.	Oral contraceptives.
Allergic vasculitis	Inflammatory changes may present as urticaria that lasts over 24 hours, hemorrhagic papules ("palpable purpura"), vesicles, bullae, or necrotic ulcers.	Most severe on the legs.	Sulfonamides, indomethacin, phenytoin, allopurinol, and ibuprofen.
Purpura	Itchy, petechial macular rash.	Dependent areas. Results most typically from thrombocytopenia.	Thiazides, sulfonamides, sulfonylureas, barbiturates, quinine, and sulindac.
Eczema	Similar to contact dermatitis.	A rare epidermal reaction in patients previously sensitized by external exposure who are given the same or a related substance systemically.	Penicillin, neomycin, phenothiazines, and local anesthetics.
Exfoliative dermatitis and erythroderma	Red and scaly.	Entire skin surface.	Allopurinol, sulfonamides, isoniazid, gold, or carbamazepine.
Photosensitivity: Increased sensitivity to light, often of ultraviolet A wavelengths, but may be due to UVB or visible light as well	Sunburn, vesicles, papules in photodistributed pattern.	Exposed skin of the face, the neck, and the backs of the hands and, in women, the lower legs. Exaggerated response to ultraviolet light. On occasion, ultraviolet emission from fluorescent lighting may be sufficient.	Sulfonamides and sulfonamide-related compounds (thiazide diuretics, furosemide, sulfonylureas), tetracyclines (especially demeclocycline), phenothiazines, sulindac, amiodarone, and NSAIDs.
Drug-related lupus erythematosus	May present with a photosensitive rash accompanied by fever, polyarthritis, myalgia, and serositis.	Less severe than systemic lupus erythematosus, sparing the kidneys and central nervous system. Recovery often follows drug withdrawal.	Most commonly hydralazine and procainamide; less often, isoniazid and phenytoin.

(continued)

Table 6–3. Skin reactions due to systemic drugs. (continued)

Reaction	Appearance	Distribution and Comments	Common Offenders
Lichenoid and lichen planus-like eruptions	Pruritic, erythematous to violaceous polygonal papules that coalesce or expand to form plaques.	May be in photo- or nonphoto-distributed pattern.	Bismuth, carbamazepine, chlordiazepoxide, chloroquine, chlorpropamide, dapsone, ethambutol, furosemide, gold salts, hydroxychloroquine, levamisole, meprobamate, methyldopa, paraphenylenediamine salts, penicillamine, phenothiazines, pindolol, propranolol, quinidine, quinine, quinacrine, streptomycin, sulfonylureas, tetracyclines, thiazides, and triprolidine.
Fixed drug eruptions	Single or multiple demarcated, round, erythematous plaques that often become hyperpigmented.	Recur at the same site when the drug is repeated. Hyperpigmentation, if present, remains after healing.	Numerous drugs, including antimicrobials, analgesics, barbiturates, cardiovascular drugs, heavy metals, antiparasitic agents, antihistamines, phenolphthalein, ibuprofen, and naproxen.
Toxic epidermal necrolysis	Large sheets of erythema, followed by separation, which looks like scalded skin.	Rare.	In adults, the eruption has occurred after administration of many classes of drugs, particularly barbiturates, phenytoin, sulfonamides, and NSAIDs.
Urticaria	Red, itchy wheals that vary in size from < 1 cm to many centimeters. May be accompanied by angioedema.	Chronic urticaria is rarely caused by drugs.	Acute urticaria: penicillins, NSAIDs, sulfonamides, opiates, and salicylates. Angioedema is common in patients receiving ACE inhibitors.
Pruritus	Itchy skin without rash.		Pruritus ani may be due to overgrowth of candida after systemic antibiotic treatment. NSAIDs may cause pruritus without a rash.
Hair loss		Hair loss most often involves the scalp, but other sites may be affected.	A predictable side effect of cytotoxic agents and oral contraceptives. Diffuse hair loss also occurs unpredictably with a wide variety of other drugs, including anticoagulants, antithyroid drugs, newer antimicrobials, cholesterol-lowering agents, heavy metals, corticosteroids, androgens, NSAIDs, retinoids (isotretinoin, etretinate), and beta-blockers.
Pigmentary changes	Flat hyperpigmented areas.	Forehead and cheeks (chloasma, melasma). The most common pigmentary disorder associated with drug ingestion. Improvement is slow despite stopping the drug.	Oral contraceptives are the usual cause.
	Blue-gray discoloration.	Light-exposed areas.	Chlorpromazine and related phenothiazines.
	Brown or blue-gray pigmentation.	Generalized.	Heavy metals (silver, gold, bismuth, and arsenic). Arsenic, silver, and bismuth are not used therapeutically, but patients who receive gold for rheumatoid arthritis may show this reaction.

(continued)

Table 6-3. Skin reactions due to systemic drugs. (continued)

Reaction	Appearance	Distribution and Comments	Common Offenders
Pigmentary changes (continued)	Yellow color.	Generalized.	Usually quinacrine.
	Blue-black patches on the shins.		Minocycline, chloroquine.
	Blue-black pigmentation of the nails and palate and depigmentation of the hair		Chloroquine.
	Slate-gray color.	Primarily in photoexposed areas.	Amiodarone.
	Brown discoloration of the nails.	Especially in more darkly pigmented patients.	Zidovudine (azidothymidine; AZT), hydroxyurea.
Psoriasiform eruptions	Scaly red plaques.	May be located on trunk and extremities. Palms and soles may be hyperkeratotic. May cause psoriasiform eruption or worsen psoriasis.	Chloroquine, lithium, beta-blockers, and quinacrine.
Pityriasis rosea-like eruptions	Oval, red, slightly raised patches with central scale.	Mainly on the trunk.	Barbiturates, bismuth, captopril, clonidine, gold salts, methopromazine, metoprolol, metronidazole, and tripelennamine.
Seborrheic dermatitis-like eruptions	Diffuse redness and loose scale.	On scalp, face, mid chest, axillae, groin.	Cimetidine, gold salts, and methyldopa.
Bullous eruptions	Tense blisters > 1 cm.	Hands, feet, genital areas common; other sites possible.	Aspirin, barbiturates, bromides, chlorpromazine, warfarin, phenytoin, sulfonamides and related compounds, and promethazine.

other constitutional symptoms may be present. The skin reaction usually occurs in symmetric distribution.

Table 6–3 summarizes the types of skin reactions, their appearance and distribution, and the common offenders in each case.

B. Laboratory Findings

Routinely ordered blood work is of no value in the diagnosis of drug eruptions. However, skin biopsies may be helpful in making the diagnosis.

Differential Diagnosis

Observation after discontinuation, which may be a slow process, helps establish the diagnosis. Rechallenge, though of theoretical value, may pose a danger to the patient and is best avoided.

Complications

Some cutaneous drug reactions may be associated with a clinical complex involving other organs (complex drug reactions). The organ systems involved depend on the individual medication or drug class. Most common is an infectious mononucleosis-like illness and hepatitis associated with administration of anticonvulsants.

Treatment

A. General Measures

Systemic manifestations are treated as they arise (eg, anemia, icterus, purpura). Antihistamines may be of value in urticarial and angioneurotic reactions. Epinephrine 1:1000, 0.5–1 mL intravenously or subcutaneously, should be used as an emergency measure. In severe cases, corticosteroids may be used at doses similar to those used for acute contact dermatitis.

B. Local Measures

The varieties and stages of dermatitis are treated according to the major dermatitis present. Extensive blistering eruptions resulting in erosions and superficial ulcerations demand hospitalization and nursing care as for burn patients.

Prognosis

Drug rash usually disappears upon withdrawal of the drug and proper treatment.

Mishriki YY: Two different lesions, same reason. Fixed drug eruption. Postgrad Med 2000;107:191. [PMID: 10887455]

Eye

7

Paul Riordan-Eva, FRCOphth

See www.current-med.com/ch07.html

SYMPTOMS OF OCULAR DISEASE

Redness

Redness is the most frequently encountered symptom of ocular disorders. It is due to hyperemia of the conjunctival, episcleral, or ciliary vessels; erythema of the eyelids; or subconjunctival hemorrhage. The major differential diagnoses are conjunctivitis, corneal disorders, acute glaucoma, and acute uveitis (Table 7–1).

Leibowitz HM: The red eye. N Engl J Med 2000;343:345. [PMID: 10922425] (Clinical review of the approach to the patient complaining of unilateral or bilateral red eye.)

Ocular Discomfort

Ocular pain may be caused by trauma (chemical, mechanical, or physical), infection, inflammation, or sudden increase in intraocular pressure.

Foreign body sensation is most commonly due to corneal or conjunctival foreign bodies. Other causes are disturbances of the corneal epithelium and rubbing of eyelashes against the cornea (trichiasis).

Photophobia is commonly due to corneal inflammation, aphakia, iritis, or albinism. A less common cause is fever associated with viral infections.

Itching is characteristically associated with allergic eye disease.

Scratching and burning due to dryness of the eyes are common complaints of older people but may occur at any age. Deficiency of tear film components may be due to dry environment, local ocular disease, systemic disorders (eg, Sjögren's disease), or drugs (eg, atropine-like agents).

Watering (epiphora) is usually due to inadequate tear drainage through obstruction of the lacrimal drainage system or malposition of the lower lid. Reflex tearing occurs with any disturbance of the corneal epithelium.

"Eyestrain" & Headache

Eyestrain is discomfort associated with prolonged reading or close work. Refractive error, presbyopia, inadequate illumination, and latent ocular deviation are causes, as are corneal inflammation, iritis, and acute glaucoma. Headache is only occasionally due to ocular disorders. Headache is a major symptom of giant cell arteritis, a cause of visual loss.

Conjunctival Discharge

Purulent discharge usually indicates bacterial infection of the conjunctiva, cornea, or lacrimal sac. Viral conjunctivitis or keratitis produces watery discharge. Allergic conjunctivitis usually results in tearing and ropy discharge associated with itching.

Visual Loss

The most important causes of blurred vision are refractive error, cataract, macular degeneration, diabetic retinopathy, vitreous hemorrhage, retinal detachment involving the macula, central retinal vein occlusion, central retinal artery occlusion, corneal opacities, and optic nerve disorders.

Monocular field loss indicates disease of the retina or optic nerve. Important causes are retinal detachment, chronic glaucoma, branch retinal artery or vein occlusion, optic neuritis, and anterior ischemic optic neuropathy, which also produce bilateral visual loss. Lesions of the optic chiasm due to pituitary tumors result in bitemporal field loss. Retrochiasmal lesions cause contralateral homonymous field defects. The more posterior the lesion in the visual pathway, the more congruous are the defects in the two eyes. Cerebrovascular disease and tumors are responsible for most lesions of the retrochiasmal visual pathways.

Visual Impairment & Blindness

An individual is visually impaired if the best corrected distant visual acuity in the better eye is 20/80 or less or if visual fields are significantly restricted. Legal blindness is defined as visual acuity for distant vision of 20/200 or less in the better eye with best correction or widest diameter of the visual field subtending an angle of less than 20 degrees. There are 500,000 legally blind people in the USA; half are over 65. The leading causes of blindness are glaucoma, diabetic

Table 7-1. The inflamed eye: Differential diagnosis of common causes.

	Acute Conjunctivitis	Acute Uveitis	Corneal Trauma or Acute Glaucoma[1]	Infection
Incidence	Extremely common	Common	Uncommon	Common
Discharge	Moderate to copious	None	None	Watery or purulent
Vision	No effect on vision	Often blurred	Markedly blurred	Usually blurred
Pain	Mild	Moderate	Severe	Moderate to severe
Conjunctival injection	Diffuse; more toward fornices	Mainly circumcorneal	Mainly circumcorneal	Mainly circumcorneal
Cornea	Clear	Usually clear	Steamy	Clarity change related to cause
Pupil size	Normal	Small	Moderately dilated and fixed	Normal
Pupillary light response	Normal	Poor	None	Normal
Intraocular pressure	Normal	Commonly low but may be elevated	Elevated	Normal
Smear	Causative organisms	No organisms	No organisms	Organisms found only in corneal ulcers due to infection

[1]Angle-closure glaucoma.

retinopathy, and macular degeneration. Most states require best corrected visual acuity with both eyes of 20/40 for an unrestricted driving license.

WHO estimates that 30 million of the world's population have vision of 10/200 or less. The most frequent causes of blindness worldwide are cataract, trachoma, leprosy, onchocerciasis, and xerophthalmia.

Diplopia

Double vision typically results from extraocular muscle imbalance. This may be caused by head injury, vascular disturbance, intracranial tumors, or intraorbital lesions; myasthenia gravis; Wernicke's syndrome; Graves' ophthalmopathy; or muscle entrapment as a result of orbital blowout fracture. Monocular diplopia, which persists when the fellow eye is covered, is usually due to refractive error or lens opacities.

"Spots Before the Eyes" & "Flashing Lights"

Spots before the eyes (floaters) are often caused by benign vitreous opacities. However, they may also be caused by posterior vitreous detachment, vitreous hemorrhage, or posterior uveitis. Sudden onset of floaters, particularly when associated with flashing lights (photopsia), necessitates dilated fundal examination to exclude a retinal tear or detachment.

Tanner V et al: Acute posterior vitreous detachment: the predictive value of vitreous pigment and symptomatology. Br J Ophthalmol 2000;84:1264. [PMID: 11049952]

OCULAR EXAMINATION

Abbreviations and symbols commonly used in ophthalmology are listed in the accompanying box.

Visual Acuity (VA)

Corrected distant visual acuity should be tested for each eye in turn, using a Snellen chart, annotated according to the distance at which each line can be read by a normal individual. Visual acuity is expressed as a fraction—the test distance over the figure assigned to the lowest line the patient can read. If the patient is unable to read the top line of the chart, acuity is recorded as counting fingers (CF), hand movements (HM), perception of light (LP), or no light perception (NLP). Distant acuity is usually measured at 20 feet. A corrected acuity of less than 20/30 is abnormal.

If assessment of distant visual acuity is not possible, near acuity can be tested with a reduced Snellen chart or standardized reading test types. The patient must be wearing an appropriate reading correction.

Visual Fields

Confrontation testing, preferably using a 5 mm red target, is valuable for rapid assessment of field defects. Amsler charts are the easiest method of detecting central field abnormalities due to macular disease.

Pandit RJ et al: Effectiveness of testing visual fields by confrontation. Lancet 2001;358:1339. [PMID: 11684217] (Examination of the central visual field with a 5 mm red target, the

ABBREVIATIONS & SYMBOLS USED IN OPHTHALMOLOGY

A or Acc	Accommodation
Ax or x	Axis of cylindric lens
BI or BO	Base-in or base-out (prism)
CF	Counting fingers
Cyl	Cylindric lens or cylinder
D	Diopter (lens strength)
E	Esophoria
EOG	Electro-oculography
EOM	Extraocular muscles or movements
ERG	Electroretinography
H	Hyperphoria
HM	Hand movements
HT	Hypertropia
IOP	Intraocular pressure
J1–J20	Test types (Jaeger) for testing reading vision
KP	Keratic precipitates
LP	Light perception
L proj	Light projection
NLP	No light perception
NPC	Near point of convergence
OD (R, or RE)	Oculus dexter (right eye)
OS (L, or LE)	Oculus sinister (left eye)
OU	Oculi unitas (both eyes)
PD	Interpupillary distance
PH	Pinhole
PRRE	Pupils round, regular, and equal
S or Sph	Spherical lens
ET	Esotropia (with L or R)
VA	Visual acuity
VER	Visual evoked response
X	Exophoria
XT	Exotropia
+	Plus or convex lens
−	Minus or concave lens
( )	Combined with
∞	Infinity (6 meters [20 feet] or more distance)
°	Degree (measurement of strabismus angle)
Δ	Prism diopter

most sensitive method of confrontation field testing in 138 patients.)

Pupils

The pupils are examined for absolute and relative size and reactions to both light and accommodation. A large, poorly reacting pupil may be due to third nerve palsy, iris damage caused by acute glaucoma, or pharmacologic mydriasis. A small, poorly reacting pupil is observed in Horner's syndrome, inflammatory adhesions between iris and lens (posterior synechiae), or neurosyphilis (Argyll Robertson pupils). Physiologic anisocoria is a common cause of unequal pupils that react normally.

A relative afferent pupillary defect, in which the pupillary light reaction is of reduced intensity when light is shined into the affected eye compared with the normal eye, indicates optic nerve disease. (It is detected with the "swinging light test," in which the pupillary light reactions are compared as a bright light is moved from one eye to the other.)

Extraocular Movements

Examination of extraocular movements begins with an assessment of whether the two eyes are correctly aligned. A misalignment of the visual axes under binocular viewing conditions is known as a manifest deviation, or **tropia.** A deviation when binocular function is disrupted is known as a latent deviation, or **phoria.** A manifest deviation may be apparent by comparing the relative positions of the corneal light reflexes. A more reliable test is the **cover test,** in which the deviated eye moves to take up fixation when the other eye is occluded. The correctional movement is in the opposite direction to that of the original manifest deviation. If no manifest deviation is present, occlusion of one eye will elicit any latent deviation because binocular function will have been disrupted. As the occluder is removed **(uncover test),** latent deviation is then detected by any correctional movement that occurs to reestablish the normal alignment of the eyes. Latent deviation is common among normal individuals.

Horizontal diplopia indicates dysfunction of the medial and lateral rectus muscles; vertical diplopia results from dysfunction of the superior and inferior recti and the obliques. The false outer image arises from the affected eye. If a muscle is underacting, the image separation will be greatest in its normal direction of action. If a muscle is prevented from relaxing, image separation will be greatest in the direction opposite to its normal action. For example, a paretic lateral rectus or a tethered medial rectus of the right eye will cause maximal image separation on looking to the right.

Nystagmus in the primary position is always abnormal. Minor degrees of nystagmus at the extremes of gaze are normal. Other forms of physiologic nystagmus include optokinetic nystagmus and that induced by rotation or caloric stimulation. Exaggerated gaze-evoked nystagmus may be due to drugs or posterior fossa disease.

Proptosis (Exophthalmos)

Proptosis is suspected when there is widening of the palpebral aperture, with exposure of sclera both superiorly and inferiorly. (Eyelid retraction generally causes more exposure superiorly than inferiorly.) By viewing from above while the patient is asked to look down and the upper lids are lifted by the examiner, a further estimate of the degree of proptosis can be made. Exophthalmometry provides objective assessment. In nonaxial proptosis, there is also horizontal or vertical displacement of the globe, indicating the presence of a mass lesion outside the extraocular muscle cone.

The most frequent cause of proptosis in adults is dysthyroid eye disease. Other causes include cellulitis, tumors, and pseudotumor of the orbit.

Ptosis

Neurologic causes of ptosis include Horner's syndrome, in which the pupil is constricted, and third nerve palsy, in which there are abnormalities of eye movements and the pupil may be dilated. Myasthenia gravis is always considered; pupils are normal.

Anterior Segment Examination

Although slitlamp examination is recommended for accurate documentation of anterior segment abnormalities, examination with a flashlight and loupe usually provides sufficient information for initial diagnosis. Patterns of redness indicate the site of the problem. In conjunctivitis, it extends diffusely across the globe and the inner surface of the lids. Keratitis, intraocular inflammation, and acute glaucoma lead to predominantly circumcorneal injection. Episcleritis and scleritis cause localized or diffuse deep injection, which in the case of scleritis is associated with blue discoloration.

Focal lesions of the cornea due to infection or trauma can be differentiated from the diffuse corneal haze of acute glaucoma and from the cloudiness of the anterior chamber and perhaps hypopyon (white cells within the anterior chamber) of iritis. Instillation of fluorescein and examination with a blue light aids in detection of corneal epithelial defects.

Direct Ophthalmoscopy

Direct ophthalmoscopy with dilation provided by tropicamide 0.5–1% is principally used for examining the retina, but other useful information can be gained. It only rarely induces angle-closure glaucoma (see below). Assessment of the red reflex and clarity of fundal details indicate the degree of media opacity. Abnormalities may then be localized to the cornea, lens, or vitreous by variations of focus of the ophthalmoscope and use of parallax.

The optic disk is examined for swelling, pallor, and glaucomatous cupping. Macular lesions causing poor central vision are usually apparent. The retinal vessels are scrutinized for caliber and wall changes. Retinal hemorrhages, exudates, and cotton-wool spots are noted. In hospital patients, dilation should be noted in the record to avoid confusion on neurologic examination.

OPHTHALMOLOGIC REFERRALS

Sudden loss of vision requires emergency ophthalmologic consultation. Important causes in an uninflamed eye are vitreous hemorrhage, retinal detachment, exudative age-related macular degeneration, retinal artery or vein occlusions, anterior ischemic optic neuropathy, giant cell arteritis, and optic neuritis. Sudden visual loss in an inflamed eye may be due to acute anterior uveitis, acute glaucoma, or corneal ulcer. Other emergencies include orbital cellulitis, gonococcal keratoconjunctivitis, and major ocular trauma.

Patients developing gradual loss of vision should also be referred. The principal causes are cataract, atrophic age-related macular degeneration, chronic glaucoma, chronic uveitis, and intraorbital and intracranial tumors.

Patients with diabetes must undergo annual examination through dilated pupils. Any myopic patient should be warned of the increased risk of retinal detachment and made aware of the importance of reporting relevant symptoms. First-degree adult relatives of patients with glaucoma are screened annually.

Shields SR: Managing eye disease in primary care. Part 1. How to screen for occult disease. Postgraduate Medicine 2000; 108:69. [PMID: 20497570] (First of three articles reviewing screening, management, and referral of ophthalmologic disease in primary care.)

Shields SR: Managing eye disease in primary care. Part 2. How to recognize and treat common eye problems. Postgrad Med 2000;108:83. [PMID: 11043082] (Overview of common eye complaints.)

Shields SR: Managing eye disease in primary care. Part 3. When to refer for ophthalmologic care. Postgrad Med 2000; 108:99. [PMID: 11043083] (Outlines need for specialty referral with emphasis on five acute eye problems in which emergency management by primary care physicians can be critical to visual outcome.)

REFRACTIVE ERRORS

Refractive errors are the most common cause of blurred vision. In emmetropia (the normal state), objects at infinity are seen clearly with the unaccommodated eye. Objects nearer than infinity are seen with the aid of accommodation, which increases the refractive power of the lens. In hyperopia, objects at infinity are not seen clearly unless accommodation is used, and near objects may not be seen because accommodative capacity is finite. Hyperopia is corrected with plus (convex) lenses. In myopia, the unaccommodated eye brings to a focus images of objects closer than infinity, the distance of such objects from the patient becoming progressively shorter with increasing myopia. Thus, the high myope is able to focus on very near objects without glasses. Objects beyond this distance cannot be seen without the aid of corrective (minus, concave) lenses. In **astigmatism,** the refractive errors in the horizontal and vertical axes differ.

Various surgical techniques are available for the correction of refractive errors, particularly myopia, including photorefractive keratectomy (PRK), in which the excimer laser is used to reshape the anterior cornea; laser in situ keratomileusis (LASIK), in which a portion of the corneal stroma undergoes laser remodeling and is then replaced under an anterior corneal flap; and extraction of the clear crystalline lens.

Presbyopia is the natural loss of accommodative capacity with age. Emmetropes usually notice inability to focus on objects at a normal reading distance at about age 45. Hyperopes experience symptoms at an earlier age. Presbyopia is corrected with plus lenses for near work.

Use of a pinhole will overcome most refractive errors and thus allows their exclusion as a cause of visual loss. Transient refractive errors occur in diabetes—typically when diabetic control is erratic—and may be the presenting feature. Autoinoculation of scopolamine from seasickness patches or atropine from vials for parenteral use leads to inadvertent pupillary dilation and loss of accommodation.

Mannis MJ et al: Making sense of refractive surgery in 2001: why, when, for whom, and by whom? Mayo Clinic Proc 2001;76: 823. [PMID: 11499822] (Overview of refractive surgery—indications, contraindications, and complications—with a commentary on the economics and the ethical questions attending this rapidly proliferating technology.)

McDonnell PJ: Emergence of refractive surgery. Arch Ophthalmol 2000;118:1119. [PMID: 10922209] (Discussion of the rapid growth and benefits.)

Contact Lenses

Contact lenses are used mostly for correction of refractive errors but also in the management of diseases of the cornea, conjunctiva, or lids. The various types are hard lenses made of polymethylmethacrylate (PMMA), rigid gas-permeable lenses made of cellulose acetate butyrate (CAB) or silicone acrylates, and soft or hydrogel lenses based on hydroxyethylmethacrylate (HEMA). Hard lenses are much more durable and easier to care for than soft lenses but are more difficult to tolerate. Rigid gas-permeable lenses are an effective compromise.

Contact lens care includes cleaning and sterilization whenever the lenses are removed and removal of protein deposits as required. Sterilization is accomplished by thermal or chemical methods. For individuals developing reactions to preservatives in contact lens solutions, preservative-free systems are available. All contact lenses can be inserted in the morning and removed at night. Soft lenses are also available for extended wear. Disposable soft lenses to avoid the neces-

sity for lens cleaning and sterilization are available for daily wear or extended wear.

The major risk from contact lens wear is corneal ulceration, potentially a blinding condition. Soft lenses present the major hazard, particularly with extended wear, for which there is an approximately eightfold increase in risk of corneal ulceration compared with daily wear. The increased risk from extended wear begins with the first night of overnight wear and increases progressively thereafter. Disposable lenses are also associated with corneal ulceration.

Contact lens wearers should be made aware of the risks they face and ways to minimize them, such as avoiding extended-wear soft lenses and maintaining meticulous lens hygiene. Whenever there is ocular discomfort or redness, contact lenses should be removed. Ophthalmologic care is sought if symptoms persist.

Suchecki JK et al: A comparison of contact lens-related complications in various daily wear modalities. CLAO J 2000; 26:204. [PMID: 11071345] (Daily disposable lenses—rather than less frequently disposable or conventional daily wear lenses—were associated with the lowest complication rate among 138 contact lens patients.)

Tabbara KF et al: Extended wear contact lens related bacterial keratitis. Br J Ophthalmol 2000;84:327. [PMID: 10684847] (Small series of bacterial keratitis associated with extended-wear contact lenses, predominantly due to *Pseudomonas aeruginosa*.)

DISORDERS OF THE LIDS & LACRIMAL APPARATUS

Hordeolum

Hordeolum is a common staphylococcal abscess that is characterized by a localized red, swollen, acutely tender area on the upper or lower lid. Internal hordeolum is a meibomian gland abscess that points onto the conjunctival surface of the lid; external hordeolum or sty is smaller and on the margin. The chief symptom is pain of an intensity directly related to the amount of swelling.

Warm compresses are helpful. Incision may be indicated if resolution does not begin within 48 hours. An antibiotic ointment (bacitracin or erythromycin) applied to the eyelid every 3 hours may be beneficial during the acute stage. Internal hordeolum may lead to generalized cellulitis of the lid.

Chalazion

Chalazion is a common granulomatous inflammation of a meibomian gland that may follow an internal hordeolum. It is characterized by a hard, nontender swelling on the upper or lower lid. The conjunctiva in the region of the chalazion is red and elevated. If the chalazion is large enough to impress the cornea, vision will be distorted.

Tumors

Verrucae and papillomas of the skin of the lids can often be excised by the general physician if they do not involve the lid margin; otherwise, surgery should be performed by an ophthalmologist so as to avoid permanent notching of the lid. Cancer—including basal cell epithelioma, squamous cell carcinoma, meibomian gland carcinoma, and malignant melanoma should be ruled out by microscopic examination of the excised material, since 2% of lesions thought to be benign clinically are found to be malignant. Basal cell epithelioma is the most common of these lesions. Mohs' technique of intraoperative examination of excised tissue is particularly valuable in ensuring complete excision of eyelid tumors.

Kersten RC et al: Accuracy of clinical diagnosis of cutaneous eyelid lesions. Ophthalmology 1997;104:479. [PMID: 9082276] (Two percent of eyelid lesions thought clinically to be benign were found to be malignant, mostly basal cell carcinoma, on histopathologic examination.)

Shuttleworth G et al: Management of acute eye conditions. Practitioner 2000;244:138. [PMID: 10892047]

Blepharitis

Blepharitis is a common chronic bilateral inflammation of the lid margins. Anterior blepharitis involves the eyelid skin, eyelashes, and associated glands. It may be ulcerative, because of infection by staphylococci; or seborrheic, and associated with seborrhea of the scalp, brows, and ears. Both types are commonly present. Posterior blepharitis is inflammation of the eyelids secondary to dysfunction of the meibomian glands. There may be bacterial infection, particularly with staphylococci, or a primary glandular dysfunction, in which there is a strong association with acne rosacea.

Symptoms are irritation, burning, and itching. In anterior blepharitis, the eyes are "red-rimmed," and scales or granulations can be seen clinging to the lashes. In posterior blepharitis, the lid margins are hyperemic with telangiectasias; the meibomian glands and their orifices are inflamed, with dilation of the glands, plugging of the orifices, and abnormal secretions. The lid margin is frequently rolled inward to produce a mild entropion, and the tears may be frothy or abnormally greasy.

Both anterior and, more particularly, posterior blepharitis may be complicated by hordeola or chalazions; abnormal lid or lash positions, producing trichiasis; recurrent conjunctivitis, epithelial keratitis of the lower third of the cornea, marginal corneal infiltrates, and inferior corneal vascularization and thinning.

In anterior blepharitis, cleanliness of the scalp, eyebrows, and lid margins is effective local therapy. Scales must be removed from the lids daily with a damp cotton applicator and baby shampoo. An antistaphylococcal antibiotic eye ointment such as bacitracin or erythromycin is applied daily to the lid margins with a cotton-tipped applicator. Antibiotic sensitivity studies may be required in severe staphylococcal blepharitis.

In mild posterior blepharitis, regular meibomian gland expression may be sufficient to control symptoms. Inflammation of the conjunctiva and cornea indicates a need for more active treatment, including long-term low-dose systemic antibiotic therapy, usually with tetracycline (250 mg twice daily), doxycycline (100 mg daily), or erythromycin (250 mg three times daily), and short-term topical steroids, eg, prednisolone, 0.125% twice daily. Topical therapy with antibiotics such as ciprofloxacin 0.3% ophthalmic solution twice daily may be helpful but should be restricted to short courses.

Entropion & Ectropion

Entropion (inward turning of usually the lower lid) occurs occasionally in older people as a result of degeneration of the lid fascia, or may follow extensive scarring of the conjunctiva and tarsus. Surgery is indicated if the lashes rub on the cornea. Botulinum toxin injections may also be used for temporary correction of the involutional lower eyelid entropion of older people.

Ectropion (outward turning of the lower lid) is fairly common in elderly people. Surgery is indicated if ectropion causes excessive tearing, exposure keratitis, or a cosmetic problem.

Steel DH et al: Botulinum toxin for the temporary treatment of involutional lower lid entropion: a clinical and morphological study. Eye 1997;11:472. [PMID: 9425409]

Dacryocystitis

Dacryocystitis is infection of the lacrimal sac due to obstruction of the nasolacrimal system. It may be acute or chronic and occurs most often in infants and in persons over 40. It is usually unilateral.

In acute dacryocystitis, the usual infectious organisms are S aureus and β-hemolytic streptococci; in chronic dacryocystitis, S epidermidis, anaerobic streptococci, or Candida albicans.

Acute dacryocystitis is characterized by pain, swelling, tenderness, and redness in the tear sac area; purulent material may be expressed. In chronic dacryocystitis, tearing and discharge are the principal signs, and mucus or pus may also be expressed.

Acute dacryocystitis responds well to systemic antibiotic therapy, but recurrences are common if the obstruction is not removed. The chronic form may be kept latent with antibiotics, but relief of the obstruction is the only cure. In adults, the standard procedure for obstruction of the lacrimal drainage system is dacryocystorhinostomy, which involves surgical exploration of the lacrimal sac and formation of a fistula into the nasal cavity. Laser-assisted endoscopic dacryocystorhinostomy and balloon dilation or probing of the nasolacrimal system are alternatives. Congenital nasolacrimal duct obstruction often resolves spontaneously but if necessary can be treated by probing of the nasolacrimal system.

Fenton S et al: Balloon dacryocystoplasty study in the management of adult epiphora. Eye 2001;15:67. [PMID: 11318299] (Ninety-four percent initial success but 29% reobstruction at 1 year in 52 eyes treated by balloon dilation of the nasolacrimal system.)

Onerci M et al: Long-term results and reasons for failure of intranasal endoscopic dacryocystorhinostomy. Acta Otolaryngol 2000;120:319. [PMID: 11603798] (Long-term relief of symptoms in 94% of cases treated by experienced surgeons and in 58% of cases treated by inexperienced surgeons.)

CONJUNCTIVITIS

Conjunctivitis is the most common eye disease. It may be acute or chronic. Most cases are due to bacterial (including gonococcal and chlamydial) or viral infection. Other causes include keratoconjunctivitis sicca, allergy, and chemical irritants. The mode of transmission of infectious conjunctivitis is usually direct contact via fingers, towels, handkerchiefs, etc, to the fellow eye or to other persons.

Conjunctivitis must be differentiated from acute uveitis, acute glaucoma, and corneal disorders (Table 7–1).

Morrow GL et al: Conjunctivitis. Am Fam Physician 1998; 57:735. [PMID: 9490996] (General review of management.)

Bacterial Conjunctivitis

The organisms isolated most commonly in bacterial conjunctivitis are staphylococci, streptococci (particularly *S pneumoniae*), *Haemophilus* spp, *Pseudomonas* spp, and *Moraxella* spp. All may produce a copious purulent discharge. There is no blurring of vision and only mild discomfort. In severe cases, examination of stained conjunctival scrapings and cultures are recommended.

The disease is usually self-limited, lasting about 10–14 days if untreated. A sulfonamide (eg, sulfacetamide, 10% ophthalmic solution or ointment) instilled locally three times daily will usually clear the infection in 2–3 days.

A. Gonococcal Conjunctivitis

Gonococcal conjunctivitis, usually acquired through contact with infected genital secretions, is manifested by a copious purulent discharge. It is an ophthalmologic emergency because corneal involvement may rapidly lead to perforation. The diagnosis should be confirmed by stained smear and culture of the discharge. If the cornea is not involved, a single intra-

muscular dose of ceftriaxone, 1 g, is effective. When the cornea is involved, a 5-day course of parenteral ceftriaxone, 1–2 g daily, is required. Topical antibiotics, such as erythromycin and bacitracin, may also be used. In such patients, other sexually transmitted diseases, including chlamydiosis, syphilis, and HIV infection, should be considered.

B. Chlamydial Keratoconjunctivitis

1. Trachoma—(*Chlamydia trachomatis* serotypes A–C.) Trachoma is a major cause of blindness worldwide. Recurrent episodes of infection in childhood are manifest as bilateral follicular conjunctivitis, epithelial keratitis, and corneal vascularization (pannus). Cicatrization of the tarsal conjunctiva leads to entropion and trichiasis in adulthood, with secondary central corneal scarring.

The specific diagnosis can be made in Giemsa-stained conjunctival scrapings. Treatment should be started on the basis of clinical findings without waiting for laboratory confirmation. Oral tetracycline or erythromycin, 250 mg six times a day, or doxycycline, 100 mg twice a day, is given for 3–5 weeks. Single-dose therapy with azithromycin, 20 mg/kg, may also be effective. Local treatment is not necessary. Surgical treatment includes correction of eyelid deformities and corneal transplantation.

2. Inclusion conjunctivitis—(*C trachomatis* serotypes D–K.) The agent of inclusion conjunctivitis is a common cause of genital tract disease in adults. The eye is usually involved following accidental contact with genital secretions. Adult inclusion conjunctivitis thus occurs most frequently in sexually active young adults. The disease starts with acute redness, discharge, and irritation. The eye findings consist of follicular conjunctivitis with mild keratitis. A nontender preauricular lymph node can often be palpated. Healing usually leaves no sequelae. Cytologic examination of conjunctival scrapings shows a picture similar to that of trachoma. Treatment is with oral tetracycline or erythromycin, 250–500 mg four times a day, or doxycycline, 300 mg initially followed by 100 mg once a day, for 2 weeks. Before treatment, all cases should be assessed for genital tract infection so that management can be adjusted accordingly.

Bowman RJ et al: Natural history of trachomatous scarring in The Gambia: results of a 12-year longitudinal follow-up. Ophthalmology 2001;108:2219. [PMID: 11733262] (Demonstration of the link between trichiasis and subsequent corneal opacity.)

Ezz al Arab G et al: The burden of trachoma in the rural Nile Delta of Egypt: a survey of Menofiya governorate. Br J Ophthalmol 2001;85:1406. [PMID: 11734509] (Reiteration of the serious problem of trachoma in the Nile delta of Egypt.)

Robert PY et al: Comparative review of topical ophthalmic antibacterial preparations. Drugs 2001;61:175. [PMID: 11270936] (Overview of the efficacy, costs, and toxicities of commonly available topical antibacterial preparations.)

Viral Conjunctivitis

One of the most common causes of viral conjunctivitis is adenovirus type 3. Conjunctivitis due to this agent is usually associated with pharyngitis, fever, malaise, and preauricular adenopathy (pharyngoconjunctival fever). Locally, the palpebral conjunctiva is red, and there is a copious watery discharge and scanty exudate. Children are more often affected than adults, and contaminated swimming pools are sometimes the source of infection. Epidemic keratoconjunctivitis is caused by adenovirus types 8 and 19. It is more likely to be complicated by visual loss due to corneal subepithelial infiltrates. Local sulfonamide therapy may prevent secondary bacterial infection, hot compresses reduce the discomfort of the associated lid edema, and weak topical steroids (eg, prednisolone, 0.125% four times daily) may be necessary to treat the corneal infiltrates. The disease usually lasts at least 2 weeks.

Keratoconjunctivitis Sicca (Dry Eyes)

This is a common disorder, particularly in elderly women. A wide range of conditions predispose to or are characterized by dry eyes. Hypofunction of the lacrimal glands, causing loss of the aqueous component of tears, may be due to aging, hereditary disorders, systemic disease (eg, Sjögren's syndrome), or systemic and topical drugs. Excessive evaporation of tears may be due to environmental factors (eg, a hot, dry, or windy climate) or abnormalities of the lipid component of the tear film, as in blepharitis. Mucin deficiency may be due to malnutrition, infection, burns, or drugs.

The patient complains of dryness, redness, or a scratchy feeling of the eyes. In severe cases there is persistent marked discomfort, with photophobia, difficulty in moving the eyelids, and often excessive mucus secretion. In many cases, gross examination reveals no abnormality, but on slitlamp examination there are subtle abnormalities of tear film stability and reduced volume of the tear film meniscus along the lower lid. In more severe cases, damaged corneal and conjunctival cells stain with 1% rose bengal. (Rose bengal staining should be avoided in severe cases because of the intense pain it may cause.) In the most severe cases there is marked conjunctival injection, loss of the normal conjunctival and corneal luster, epithelial keratitis that may progress to frank ulceration, and mucous strands. Schirmer's test, which measures the rate of production of the aqueous component of tears by the amount of wetting of filter paper strips during a 5-minute period, may be helpful when the diagnosis is in doubt, but false-positive and false-negative results are frequent.

Treatment depends upon the cause. In most early cases, the corneal and conjunctival epithelial changes are reversible. Aqueous deficiency can be treated by replacement of the aqueous component of tears with various types of artificial tears. The simplest preparations are physiologic (0.9%) or hypo-osmotic (0.45%) solutions of sodium chloride. Balanced salt solution is a more physiologic but also more expensive preparation. All these drop preparations can be used as frequently as every half-hour but in most cases are needed only three or four times a day. More prolonged duration of action can be achieved with drop preparations containing methylcellulose (eg, Isopto Plain) or polyvinyl alcohol (eg, Liquifilm Tears or Hypo Tears) or by using petrolatum ointment (Lacri-Lube). Such mucomimetics are particularly indicated when there is mucin deficiency. Artificial tear preparations are generally very safe and without side effects. However, the preservatives necessary to maintain their sterility are potentially toxic and allergenic and may cause keratitis and cicatrizing conjunctivitis in frequent users. Furthermore, the development of such reactions may be misinterpreted by both the patient and the doctor as a worsening of the dry eye state requiring more frequent use of the artificial tears and leading in turn to further deterioration, rather than being recognized as a need to change to a preservative-free preparation. If the mucus is tenacious, mucolytic agents (eg, acetylcysteine, 20% six times a day) may provide some relief. Blepharitis should be treated appropriately (see above).

Pflugfelder SC et al: The diagnosis and management of dry eye: a twenty-five-year review. Cornea 2000;19:644. [PMID: 11009316] (Review of the advances in the diagnosis, pathogenesis, and management of dry eye disease in the past 25 years.)

Yazdani C et al: Prevalence of treated dry eye disease in a managed care population. Clin Ther 2001;23:1672. [PMID: 11726003] (Prevalence in the USA is 0.5%.)

Allergic Eye Disease

Allergic eye disease takes a number of different forms, but all are expressions of an atopic diathesis, which may also be manifested as atopic asthma, atopic dermatitis, or allergic rhinitis. Symptoms include itching, tearing, redness, stringy discharge, and, in the more severe forms, photophobia and visual loss.

Allergic conjunctivitis is a benign disease, occurring usually in late childhood and early adulthood. It may be seasonal (hay fever conjunctivitis), developing usually during the spring or summer, or perennial. Clinical signs are limited to conjunctival hyperemia and edema (chemosis), the latter occasionally being so marked and sudden in onset as to cause alarm. Vernal keratoconjunctivitis also tends to occur in late childhood and early adulthood. It is usually seasonal, with a predilection for the spring. The conjunctivitis is characterized by large "cobblestone" papillae on the upper tarsal conjunctiva. There may be lymphoid follicles at the limbus. Atopic keratoconjunctivitis is a more chronic disorder of adulthood. Both the upper and the lower tarsal conjunctiva exhibit a fine papillary conjunctivitis with fibrosis, resulting in forniceal shortening and entropion with trichiasis. Staphylococcal blepharitis is a frequent complicating factor. Corneal involvement, including refractory ulceration, is frequent during acute exacerbations of both vernal and atopic keratoconjunctivitis. They are also commonly complicated by herpes simplex keratitis.

For mild and moderately severe allergic eye disease, topical levocabastine, a histamine H_1-receptor antagonist, or ketorolac, a nonsteroidal anti-inflammatory agent, applied topically four times daily, reduces symptoms. Topical lodoxamide, a mast cell stabilizer, applied four times daily, produces longer-term prophylaxis, but the therapeutic response takes a few days to develop. Topical vasoconstrictors and antihistamines are advocated in hay fever conjunctivitis but are of limited efficacy and may produce rebound hyperemia and follicular conjunctivitis. Systemic antihistamines may be useful in prolonged, severe atopic keratoconjunctivitis. Topical corticosteroids are essential to the control of acute exacerbations of both vernal and atopic keratoconjunctivitis. Steroid-induced side effects, including cataracts, glaucoma, and exacerbation of herpes simplex keratitis, are major problems. Systemic steroid therapy and even plasmapheresis may be required in severe atopic keratoconjunctivitis. In allergic conjunctivitis specific allergens may be identifiable and thus avoidable. In vernal keratoconjunctivitis, a cooler climate often provides significant benefit.

Bielory L et al: Allergic ocular disease. A review of pathophysiology and clinical presentations. Clin Rev Allergy Immunol 2001;20:183. [PMID: 11349609]

New drugs for allergic conjunctivitis: Med Lett Drugs Ther 2000;42:39. [PMID: 10825920] (Review of treatments for allergic eye disease.)

PINGUECULA & PTERYGIUM

Pinguecula is a yellow elevated nodule on either side of the cornea (more commonly on the nasal side) in the area of the palpebral fissure. It is common in persons over age 35.

Pterygium is a fleshy, triangular encroachment of the conjunctiva onto the nasal side of the cornea and is usually associated with constant exposure to wind, sun, sand, and dust. Pterygium may be either unilateral or bilateral. There may be a genetic predisposition, but no hereditary pattern has been described. Of the two, pinguecula is more common. Both show elastoid degeneration of the conjunctival substantia propria.

Pingueculae rarely grow, but inflammation (pingueculitis) may occur. No treatment is usually required for pingueculitis or episodes of inflammation of pterygium, but artificial tears are often beneficial, and short courses of topical nonsteroidal anti-inflammatory agents or weak steroids (prednisolone, 0.125% three times a day) may sometimes be necessary.

Excision of a pterygium is indicated if the growth threatens to interfere with vision by approaching the visual axis. Recurrences are frequent and often more aggressive than the primary lesion.

CORNEAL ULCER

Corneal ulcers are most commonly due to infection, which may involve bacteria, viruses, fungi, or amebas. Noninfectious causes—all of which may be complicated by infection—include neurotrophic keratitis (resulting from loss of corneal sensation), exposure keratitis (due to inadequate eyelid closure), severe dry eyes, severe allergic eye disease, and various inflammatory disorders that may be purely ocular or part of a systemic vasculitis.

Delayed or ineffective treatment of corneal infection may lead to devastating consequences through intraocular infection or corneal scarring. Prompt referral is essential.

Patients present with pain, photophobia, tearing, and reduced vision. The eye is red, with predominantly circumcorneal injection, and there may be purulent or watery discharge. The corneal appearance varies according to the organisms involved.

Ladas JG et al: Systemic disorders associated with peripheral corneal ulceration. Curr Opin Ophthalmol 2000;11:468. [PMID: 11141643] (Review of corneal involvement in systemic autoimmune diseases.)

Lekskul M et al: Nontraumatic corneal perforation. Cornea 2000;19:313. [PMID: 10832690] (Retrospective study highlighting the importance of dry eyes and exposure keratitis, as well as bacterial keratitis, in the development of corneal perforation.)

Bacterial Keratitis

Bacterial keratitis tends to pursue an aggressive course. Precipitating factors include contact lens wear, especially soft contact lenses worn overnight, and corneal trauma. The pathogens most commonly isolated are *Pseudomonas aeruginosa,* pneumococcus, moraxella species, and staphylococci. The cornea is hazy, with usually a central ulcer and adjacent stromal abscess. Hypopyon is often present. The ulcer should be scraped to recover material for Gram's stain and culture prior to starting treatment with high-concentration (fortified) topical antibiotics, given at least every hour night and day for the first 24 hours. The initial choice of antibiotics is based on the Gram stain result. Gram-positive cocci are treated with a cephalosporin, such as cefazolin, 100 mg/mL; and gram-negative bacilli are treated with an aminoglycoside, such as tobramycin, 15 mg/mL. If no organisms are seen, these two agents are used together. A fluoroquinolone such as ciprofloxacin, 3 mg/mL, or ofloxacin, 3 mg/mL, may be used instead of an aminoglycoside.

Gangopadhyay N et al: Fluoroquinolone and fortified antibiotics for treating bacterial corneal ulcers. Br J Ophthalmol 2000;84:378. [PMID: 10729294] (Commercially available fluoroquinolone drops as effective as fortified tobramycin and cefazolin.)

Schaefer F et al: Bacterial keratitis: a prospective clinical and microbiological study. Br J Ophthalmol 2001;85:842. [PMID: 11423460] (Contact lens wear, blepharitis, and trauma are the most common risk factors for bacterial keratitis.)

Herpes Simplex Keratitis

Herpes simplex keratitis is an important cause of ocular morbidity in adults. The ability of the virus to colonize the trigeminal ganglion leads to recurrences that may be precipitated by fever, excessive exposure to sunlight, or immunodeficiency (eg, HIV infection).

The dendritic (branching) ulcer is the most characteristic manifestation of epithelial keratitis due to the herpes simplex virus. More extensive ("geographic") ulcers may also occur, particularly if topical corticosteroids have been used. These ulcers are most easily seen after instillation of sterile fluorescein and examination with a blue light. Epithelial disease in itself does not lead to corneal scarring. It responds well to simple debridement and patching. More rapid healing can be achieved by the addition of topical antivirals such as trifluridine drops, vidarabine ointment, acyclovir ointment, or ganciclovir gel. Long-term oral acyclovir reduces the rate of recurrent epithelial disease. Topical corticosteroids must not be used.

Stromal herpes simplex keratitis produces increasingly severe corneal opacity and irregularity with each recurrence. Topical antivirals alone are usually insufficient to control stromal disease. Thus, topical corticosteroids are frequently used in combination, but steroid dependence is a common consequence. Corticosteroids may also enhance viral replication, leading to severe epithelial disease. Oral acyclovir, 200–400 mg five times a day, may be helpful in the treatment of severe herpetic keratitis and for prophylaxis against recurrences, particularly in atopic or HIV-infected individuals. Corneal grafting is sometimes necessitated by severe stromal scarring, but the overall outcome is relatively poor. *Caution:* For patients with known or possible herpetic disease, topical corticosteroids should be prescribed only under strict ophthalmologic supervision.

Oral acyclovir for herpes simplex virus eye disease: effect on prevention of epithelial keratitis and stromal keratitis. Herpetic Eye Disease Study Group. Arch Ophthalmol 2000;118: 1030. [PMID: 10922194] (Long-term oral acyclovir 800 mg/d reduced the rate of recurrent HSV epithelial keratitis and stromal keratitis.)

Wilhelmus KR: Interventions for herpes simplex virus epithelial keratitis. Cochrane Database Syst Rev 2001;1:CD002898. [PMID: 11279774] (Topical vidarabine, trifluridine, or acyclovir increased the rate of healing of epithelial keratitis.)

Fungal Keratitis

Fungal keratitis tends to occur after corneal injury involving plant material or in an agricultural setting, in eyes with chronic ocular surface disease, and in contact lens wearers. There is often an indolent course.

The cornea characteristically has multiple stromal abscesses with relatively little epithelial loss. Intraocular infection is common. Corneal scrapings must be cultured on media suitable for fungi whenever the history or corneal appearance is suggestive of fungal disease.

Acanthamoeba Keratitis

Acanthamoeba has become a more commonly recognized cause of suppurative keratitis in contact lens wearers. Although severe pain and perineural and ring infiltrates in the corneal stroma are characteristic features, earlier forms of the disease with changes confined to the corneal epithelium are identifiable. Culture requires specialized media. Treatment is severely hampered by the organism's ability to encyst within the corneal stroma. Various agents have been used, including neomycin-polymyxin-gramicidin, chlorhexidine, the investigational agents propamidine isethionate and polyhexamethyl biguanide, and various oral and topical imidazoles such as ketoconazole, miconazole, and itraconazole. Epithelial debridement may be useful in early infections. Corneal grafting may be required in the acute stage to arrest the progression of infection or after resolution of the infection to restore vision.

McCulley JP et al: The diagnosis and management of Acanthamoeba keratitis. CLAO J 2000;26:47. [PMID: 10656311]

O'Day DM et al: Advances in the management of keratomycosis and Acanthamoeba keratitis. Cornea 2000;19:681. [PMID: 11009320] (Discusses the well-defined therapeutic approach of keratoplasty and the controversial role of corticosteroids for these initially devastating infections.)

Herpes Zoster Ophthalmicus

Herpes zoster frequently involves the ophthalmic division of the trigeminal nerve. It presents with malaise, fever, headache, and burning and itching in the periorbital region. These symptoms may precede the eruption by a day or more. The rash is initially vesicular, quickly becoming pustular and then crusting. Involvement of the tip of the nose or the lid margins indicates a high likelihood of involvement of the eye. Ocular signs include conjunctivitis, keratitis, episcleritis, and anterior uveitis, often with elevated intraocular pressure. Recurrent anterior segment inflammation, neurotrophic keratitis, and posterior subcapsular cataract are possible long-term effects. Optic neuropathy, cranial nerve palsies, acute retinal necrosis, and cerebral angiitis are infrequent complications of the acute stage. HIV infection and AIDS are important risk factors for herpes zoster ophthalmicus and increase the chance of development of complications.

Treatment with high-dose oral acyclovir (800 mg five times a day) or valaciclovir (500 mg three times a day), started within 72 hours after appearance of the rash, reduces the incidence of ocular complications but not of postherpetic neuralgia. Anterior uveitis requires topical steroids and cycloplegics.

Colin J et al: Comparison of the efficacy and safety of valaciclovir and acyclovir for the treatment of herpes zoster ophthalmicus. Ophthalmology 2000;107:1507. [PMID: 10919899] (Oral valaciclovir as effective as oral acyclovir in preventing ocular complications of herpes zoster ophthalmicus.)

ACUTE (ANGLE-CLOSURE) GLAUCOMA

 ESSENTIALS OF DIAGNOSIS

- *Rapid onset in older age groups, particularly hyperopes and Asians.*
- *Severe pain and profound visual loss.*
- *Red eye, steamy cornea, dilated pupil.*
- *Hard eye.*

General Considerations

Primary acute angle-closure glaucoma can occur only with closure of a preexisting narrow anterior chamber angle, as is found in elderly persons (owing to physiologic enlargement of the lens), hyperopes, and Asians. In the USA, about 1% of people over age 35 have narrow anterior chamber angles, but many of these never develop acute glaucoma; thus, the condition is uncommon. Rarely angle closure is associated with pupillary dilation and thus might occur from sitting in a darkened movie theater, at times of stress (owing to increased circulating epinephrine), from pharmacologic mydriasis for ophthalmoscopic examination, or from systemic anticholinergic medications such as atropine (eg, preoperative medication), antidepressants, or nebulized bronchodilators. The selective serotonin reuptake agent paroxetine has been associated with several cases.

Acute angle-closure glaucoma may also occur secondary to long-standing anterior uveitis or dislocation of the lens. Symptoms are the same as in primary acute angle-closure glaucoma, but differentiation is important because of differences in management. Chronic angle-closure glaucoma is particularly common in eastern Asia. It presents in the same way as open-angle glaucoma (see below).

Clinical Findings

Patients with acute glaucoma usually seek treatment immediately because of extreme pain and blurred vision, though there are subacute cases in which presentation is delayed. The blurred vision is characteristically associated with halos around lights. Nausea and even abdominal pain may occur, and acute glaucoma must be remembered in the differential diagnosis of

abdominal discomfort and vomiting. The eye is red, the cornea steamy, and the pupil moderately dilated and nonreactive to light. Tonometry reveals elevated intraocular pressure.

Differential Diagnosis

Acute glaucoma must be differentiated from conjunctivitis, acute uveitis, and corneal disorders (Table 7–1).

Treatment

A. PRIMARY

In primary acute angle-closure glaucoma, laser peripheral iridotomy will usually result in permanent cure. Intraocular pressure must be lowered beforehand. A single 500 mg intravenous dose of acetazolamide, followed by 250 mg orally four times a day, is usually sufficient. Osmotic diuretics, such as oral glycerol and intravenous urea or mannitol—the dosage of all three being 1–2 g/kg—can be used if necessary. Once the intraocular pressure has started to fall, topical 4% pilocarpine, 1 drop every 15 minutes for 1 hour and then four times a day, is used to treat the underlying angle closure. The fellow eye should undergo prophylactic iridectomy.

B. SECONDARY

In secondary acute angle-closure glaucoma, systemic acetazolamide is also used, with or without osmotic agents, to control intraocular pressure. Further treatment is determined by the cause.

Prognosis

Untreated acute glaucoma results in severe and permanent visual loss within 2–5 days after onset of symptoms.

Banta JT et al: Presumed topiramate-induced bilateral acute angle-closure glaucoma. Am J Ophthalmol 2001;132:112. [PMID: 11438067] (Secondary angle-closure glaucoma due to topiramate.)

Pandit RJ et al: Mydriasis and glaucoma: exploding the myth. A systematic review. Diabet Med 2000;17:693. [PMID: 11110501] (Mydriasis with tropicamide is safe—almost never precipitates acute angle-glaucoma even in people with chronic glaucoma.)

OPEN-ANGLE GLAUCOMA

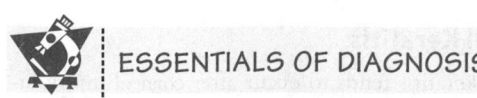 **ESSENTIALS OF DIAGNOSIS**

- *Insidious onset in older age groups.*
- *No symptoms in early stages.*

- *Gradual loss of peripheral vision over a period of years, resulting in tunnel vision.*
- *Persistent elevation of intraocular pressure associated with pathologic cupping of the optic disks.*
- *"Halos around lights" are present only in severe cases.*

General Considerations

In open-angle glaucoma, the intraocular pressure is elevated due to abnormal drainage of aqueous through the trabecular meshwork. Over a period of months or years, this results in excavation ("cupping") and pallor of the optic disk with loss of vision varying from slight constriction of the peripheral fields to complete blindness.

The cause of the decreased rate of aqueous outflow in primary open-angle glaucoma has not been clearly established. However a number of mutations, such as in the myocilin gene on chromosome 1, have been identified in a small proportion of cases. The disease is bilateral, and there is an increased prevalence in first-degree relatives of affected individuals and in diabetics. Primary open-angle glaucoma occurs at an earlier age, is more frequent in blacks, and may result in more severe optic nerve damage. There is increasing evidence that factors other than the level of intraocular pressure—particularly vascular abnormalities—may play a role in the pathogenesis of glaucomatous optic nerve damage. Open-angle glaucoma may also develop secondary to other eye disease, such as uveitis or the effects of trauma. Elevation of intraocular pressure is also a complication of steroid therapy, whether it be topical, systemic, inhaled, or administered by nasal spray.

In the USA, it is estimated that 1–2% of people over 40 have glaucoma; about 25% of these cases are undetected. Over 90% of all cases of glaucoma are of the open-angle type. Worldwide, about 50% of all glaucoma is due to angle closure. This is due to the high prevalence of angle closure in eastern Asia, resulting either in acute angle-closure glaucoma (see above) or in chronic angle-closure glaucoma, which presents in the same was as open-angle glaucoma.

Clinical Findings

Patients with open-angle glaucoma have no symptoms initially. On examination, there may be slight cupping of the optic disk observed as an absolute increase—or an asymmetry between the two eyes—of the ratio of the diameter of the optic cup to the diameter of the whole optic disk (cup-disk ratio). (Cup-disk ratio of greater than 0.3 or asymmetry of cup-disk ratio of 0.2

or more is suggestive of glaucoma.) Changes in the retinal nerve fiber layer may be observed as an earlier finding in some patients. The visual fields gradually constrict, but central vision remains good until late in the disease.

Tonometry, ophthalmoscopic visualization of the optic nerve, and central visual field testing are the best studies for the diagnosis and follow up. The diagnosis of glaucoma generally depends upon identification of consistent abnormalities in at least two of these parameters. The normal range of intraocular pressure is 10–24 mm Hg. Except in acute cases, the diagnosis of glaucoma is not made on the basis of one tonometric measurement. Intraocular pressure is influenced by various factors, including posture and diurnal variation. In many individuals, elevated intraocular pressure is not associated with optic disk or visual field abnormalities. These ocular hypertensives are at increased risk of developing glaucomatous damage. Treatment to reduce intraocular pressure may be justified if there is a moderate to high risk of the development of glaucoma. The level of risk is determined by several factors including age, optic disk appearance, level of intraocular pressure, and corneal thickness. Conversely, a significant proportion of patients with glaucoma have normal intraocular pressure when it is first measured, and it is only repeated measurement which identifies the abnormally high pressure. Furthermore, there are patients with normal tension glaucoma, in which the intraocular pressure is always within the normal range despite repeated measurement even though they have glaucomatous optic disk and visual field abnormalities. There are many other causes of optic disk abnormalities or visual field changes that mimic glaucomatous damage, and visual field testing may prove unreliable in some patients, particularly the elderly. Taken together, these factors mean that the diagnosis of glaucoma is not always straightforward, which greatly hampers the effectiveness of screening programs.

Prevention

All persons over age 40, particularly blacks, should have tonometric and ophthalmoscopic examinations every 3–5 years. In diabetics and in individuals with a family history of glaucoma, annual examination is indicated.

Treatment

Topical β-adrenergic blocking agents, such as timolol 0.25% or 0.5%, carteolol 1%, levobunol 0.5%, and metipranolol 0.3% solutions twice daily, or timolol 0.5% gel once daily, are still the most commonly used antiglaucoma agents. They are contraindicated in patients with reactive airway disease or heart failure. Betaxolol, 0.25% or 0.5%, a β1-receptor selective blocking agent, is theoretically safer in patients with reactive airway disease but is less effective at reducing intraocular pressure. Brimonidine 0.2%, a selective α_2 agonist, dorzolamide 2%, a topical carbonic anhydrase inhibitor, and a prostaglandin analog (latanoprost 0.005%, bimatoprost 0.03%, or travoprost 0.004%) can all be used in addition to a β-blocker (brimonidine and dorzolamide twice daily and a prostaglandin analog once daily) or as initial therapy when β-blockers are contraindicated (brimonidine twice daily, dorzolamide three times daily and a prostaglandin analog once daily). Brimonidine and dorzolamide are associated with allergic reactions. Latanoprost may produce permanent darkening of iris and eyebrow color, uveitis, macular edema, and exacerbation of angina. Whether these adverse effects occur with other prostaglandin analogs has yet to be determined.

Apraclonidine, 0.5–1%, another α_2 agonist, can be used three times a day to postpone the need for surgery in patients receiving maximal medical therapy, but long-term use is limited by a high incidence of allergic reactions. It is more commonly used to control acute rises in intraocular pressure, such as after laser therapy. Epinephrine, 0.5–1%, and the prodrug dipiverin, 0.1%, are being used much less frequently, particularly because of allergic reactions and their adverse effects on the outcome of subsequent glaucoma surgery. Pilocarpine 1–4% (and sometimes higher concentrations in patients with dark irides) four times a day is little used because of the induced myopia in younger patients and the pupillary constriction that compromises vision in patients with cataract. Oral carbonic anhydrase inhibitors (eg, acetazolamide) may still be used on a long-term basis if topical therapy is inadequate and surgical or laser therapy is inappropriate.

Laser trabeculoplasty is used as an adjunct to topical therapy to defer surgery and is also advocated as primary treatment. Surgery is generally undertaken when intraocular pressure is inadequately controlled by medical and laser therapy, but it may also be used as primary treatment. Trabeculectomy is the standard procedure. Adjunctive treatment with subconjunctival fluorouracil or mitomycin is used peri- or postoperatively in difficult cases. Viscocanalostomy and deep sclerectomy, two alternative procedures under investigation, have the advantage of avoiding a full-thickness incision into the eye.

Prognosis

Untreated chronic glaucoma that begins at age 40–45 will probably cause complete blindness by age 60–65. Early diagnosis and treatment will preserve useful vision throughout life in most cases.

Edmunds B et al: The National Survey of Trabeculectomy. II. Variations in operative technique and outcome. Eye 2001;15:441. [PMID: 11767016] (United Kingdom survey establishing success rates of trabeculectomy for open-angle glaucoma.)

Gandolfi S et al: Three-month comparison of bimatoprost and latanoprost in patients with glaucoma and ocular hypertension. Adv Ther 2001;18:110. [PMID: 11571823] (Bimatoprost 0.03% more effective than latanoprost 0.005% at controlling intraocular pressure.)

Gordon MO et al: The Ocular Hypertension Treatment Study: baseline factors that predict the onset of primary open-angle glaucoma. Arch Ophthalmol 2002;120:714. [PMID: 12049575] (Age, optic disk appearance, level of intraocular pressure and corneal thickness determine risk of progression from ocular hypertension to glaucoma.)

Grierson I: The patient with primary open-angle glaucoma. Practitioner 2000;244:654. [PMID: 10954981]

Hattenhauer MG et al: The probability of blindness from open-angle glaucoma. Ophthalmology 1998;105:2099. [PMID: 9818612] (Among 295 patients with glaucoma or ocular hypertension, 25% overall and 55% of the glaucoma patients were blind in at least one eye at 20 years follow-up and 10% overall were blind in both eyes.)

Kass MA et al: The Ocular Hypertension Treatment Study: a randomized trial determines that topical ocular hypotensive medication delays or prevents the onset of primary open-angle glaucoma. Arch Ophthalmol 2002;120:701. [PMID: 12049574] (Treatment of ocular hypertension recommended if there is moderate to high risk of the development of glaucoma.)

Netland PA et al: Travoprost compared with latanoprost and timolol in patients with open-angle glaucoma or ocular hypertension. Am J Ophthalmol 2001;132:472. [PMID: 11589866] (Travoprost 0.004% as good as or better than either latanoprost or timolol in lowering intraocular pressure and significantly better in black patients.)

UVEITIS

Uveitis means inflammation of the uveal tract, which is formed by the iris (iritis), ciliary body (cyclitis), and choroid (choroiditis). Inflammatory eye disease may also originate primarily in the retina (retinitis) or retinal blood vessels (retinal vasculitis).

Intraocular inflammation is classified as anterior uveitis, posterior uveitis, or panuveitis. Uveitis may also be categorized as acute or chronic and granulomatous or nongranulomatous. In most cases the pathogenesis of uveitis is primarily immunologic, but in AIDS or other immunodeficiency states, infection may be the primary cause.

Clinical Findings

Anterior uveitis is characterized by inflammatory cells and flare within the aqueous. Cells may also be seen on the corneal endothelium as keratic precipitates (KPs). In granulomatous uveitis, these are large "mutton-fat" KPs, and iris nodules may be seen. In nongranulomatous uveitis, the KPs are smaller and iris nodules are not seen. Occasionally, granulomatous uveitis may initially masquerade as nongranulomatous disease. In severe anterior uveitis, there may be hypopyon (layered collection of white cells) and fibrin within the anterior chamber. In virtually all forms of anterior uveitis, the pupil is small, and with the development of posterior synechiae (adhesions between the iris and anterior lens capsule), it also becomes irregular.

Nongranulomatous anterior uveitis tends to present acutely with unilateral pain, redness, photophobia, and visual loss. Granulomatous anterior uveitis is more likely to present less acutely with blurred vision in a mildly inflamed eye.

In posterior uveitis, there are cells in the vitreous. Inflammatory lesions may be present in the retina or choroid. Fresh lesions are yellow, with indistinct margins, whereas older lesions have more definite margins and are commonly pigmented. Retinal vessel sheathing may occur adjacent to such lesions or more diffusely. In severe cases, vitreous opacity precludes visualization of retinal details.

Posterior uveitis tends to present with gradual visual loss in a relatively quiet eye. Bilateral involvement is common. Visual loss may be due to vitreous haze and opacities, inflammatory lesions involving the macula, macular edema, retinal vein occlusion, or, rarely, associated optic neuropathy.

Etiology

The systemic disorders associated with acute nongranulomatous anterior uveitis are the HLA-B27-related conditions sacroiliitis, ankylosing spondylitis, Reiter's syndrome, psoriasis, ulcerative colitis, and Crohn's disease. Behçet's syndrome produces both anterior uveitis with recurrent hypopyon and posterior uveitis with retinal vein occlusions. Both herpes simplex and herpes zoster infections may cause nongranulomatous anterior uveitis.

Diseases producing granulomatous anterior uveitis also tend to be causes of posterior uveitis. These include sarcoidosis, which is commonly bilateral; tuberculosis; syphilis; toxoplasmosis; Vogt-Koyanagi-Harada syndrome (bilateral uveitis associated with alopecia, poliosis [depigmented eyelashes, eyebrows, or hair], vitiligo, and hearing loss); and sympathetic ophthalmia. Syphilis produces a characteristic "salt and pepper" fundus, often with surprisingly little visual loss unless there is also primary syphilitic optic atrophy. In congenital toxoplasmosis, there is usually evidence of previous episodes of retinochoroiditis. The principal agents responsible for ocular inflammation in AIDS and other immunodeficiency states are cytomegalovirus, herpes simplex and herpes zoster viruses, mycobacteria, cryptococcus, toxoplasma, and candida.

Autoimmune retinal vasculitis and pars planitis (intermediate uveitis) are idiopathic conditions that produce posterior uveitis.

Retinal detachment, intraocular tumors, and central nervous system lymphoma may all masquerade as uveitis.

Treatment

Anterior uveitis will usually respond to topical corticosteroids. Occasionally, periocular steroid injections or even systemic steroids may be required. Dilation of the pupil is important to relieve discomfort and prevent posterior synechiae.

Posterior uveitis more commonly requires systemic corticosteroid therapy and occasionally systemic immunosuppression with azathioprine or cyclosporine. Pupillary dilation is not usually necessary.

In all cases if an infectious cause is identified, specific antimicrobial therapy is indicated. In general, the prognosis for anterior uveitis, particularly the nongranulomatous type, is better than that for posterior uveitis.

Boyd SR et al: Immunopathology of the noninfectious posterior and intermediate uveitides. Surv Ophthalmol 2001;46:209. [PMID: 11738429] (Review of the pathogenesis of various types of uveitis.)

Cunningham ET Jr: Uveitis in HIV-positive patients. Br J Ophthalmol 2000;84:233. [PMID: 10684829]

Jabs DA et al: Guidelines for the use of immunosuppressive drugs in patients with ocular inflammatory disorderss: Recommendations of an expert panel. Am J Ophthalmol 2000; 130:492. [PMID: 11024423] (Recommendations of a multidisciplinary panel on the optimal use of immunosuppressive agents in uveitis.)

Lightman S et al: Developments in the treatment of uveitis. Expert Opin Investig Drugs 2002;11:59. [PMID: 11772321] (Review of new treatments for uveitis.)

McCluskey PJ et al: Management of chronic uveitis. BMJ 2000; 320:555. [PMID: 10688564]

Power WJ et al: Outcomes in anterior uveitis associated with the HLA-B27 haplotype. Ophthalmology 1998;105:1646. [PMID: 9754172] (The HLA-B27 haplotype increased the incidence of complications, the need for greater levels of immunosuppression, and the prevalence of blindness.)

CATARACT

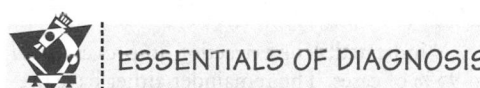

ESSENTIALS OF DIAGNOSIS

- *Blurred vision, progressive over months or years.*
- *No pain or redness.*
- *Lens opacities (may be grossly visible).*

General Considerations

A cataract is a lens opacity. Cataracts are usually bilateral. They may be congenital (owing to intrauterine infections such as rubella and cytomegalovirus, or inborn errors of metabolism such as galactosemia); traumatic; or secondary to systemic disease (diabetes, myotonic dystrophy, atopic dermatitis), systemic or inhaled corticosteroid treatment, or uveitis. Senile cataract is by far the most common type; most persons over age 60 have some degree of lens opacity. Cigarette smoking increases the risk of cataract formation.

Clinical Findings

Even in its early stages, a cataract can be seen through a dilated pupil with an ophthalmoscope, a slitlamp, or an ordinary hand illuminator. As the cataract matures, the retina will become increasingly more difficult to visualize, until finally the fundus reflection is absent and the pupil is white.

Treatment

Functional visual impairment is the prime criterion for surgery. The cataract is usually removed by one of the techniques in which the delicate posterior lens capsule remains (extracapsular). This may, however, call for subsequent laser treatment if the posterior capsule opacifies. With the development of ultrasonic fragmentation (phacoemulsification) of the lens nucleus, it is now possible to perform cataract surgery through a small incision and without suturing the wound, thus reducing the postoperative complication rate and accelerating the patient's visual rehabilitation.

It is routine practice to implant an intraocular lens at the time of surgery. This dispenses with the need for heavy cataract glasses or contact lenses. With improved intraocular lenses, the success rate is high. Multifocal intraocular lenses have been used with some success to reduce the need for both distance and reading glasses.

Prognosis

If surgery is indicated, lens extraction improves visual acuity in 95% of cases. The remainder either have preexisting retinal damage or develop perioperative or postoperative complications.

Foster A: Cataract—a global perspective: output, outcome and outlay. Eye 1999;13:449. [PMID: 10627823] (Review of cataract as a world-wide blinding disease and methods to provide cost-effective surgery in developing countries.)

Mamalis N et al. Endophthalmitis following cataract surgery. Ophthalmol Clin North Am 2001;14:661. [PMID: 11787745] (Review of intraocular infection following cataract surgery.)

Superstein R: Indications for cataract surgery. Curr Opin Ophthalmol 2001;12:58. [PMID: 11150082] (Highlights factors that help determine the indications for cataract surgery.)

RETINAL DETACHMENT

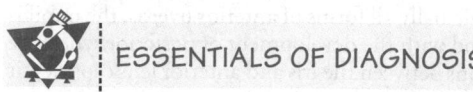

ESSENTIALS OF DIAGNOSIS

- *Blurred vision in one eye becoming progressively worse. ("A curtain came down over my eye.")*
- *No pain or redness.*
- *Detachment seen by ophthalmoscopy.*

General Considerations

Detachment of the retina is usually spontaneous but may be secondary to trauma. Spontaneous detachment occurs most frequently in persons over 50 years of age. Cataract extraction and myopia are the two most common predisposing causes.

Clinical Findings

As soon as the retina is torn, fluid vitreous is able to pass through the tear and lodge behind the sensory retina. This, combined with vitreous traction and the pull of gravity, results in progressive detachment. The superior temporal area is the most common site of detachment. The area involved rapidly increases, causing corresponding progressive visual loss. Central vision remains intact until the macula becomes detached.

On ophthalmoscopic examination, the retina is seen hanging in the vitreous like a gray cloud. One or more retinal tears, usually crescent-shaped and red or orange, are usually present and can be seen by an experienced examiner.

Treatment

All cases of retinal detachment should be referred immediately to an ophthalmologist. During transportation, the patient's head should be positioned so that the detached portion of the retina will fall back with the aid of gravity.

Treatment is directed primarily at closing the retinal tears. A permanent adhesion between the neurosensory retina, the retinal pigment epithelium, and the choroid is produced in the region of the tears by applying cryotherapy to the sclera or laser photocoagulation to the retina. In order to achieve apposition of the neurosensory retina to the retinal pigment epithelium while this adhesion is developing, an indentation may be made in the sclera with a silicone sponge or buckle, the fluid between the neurosensory retina and the retinal pigment epithelium (subretinal fluid) may be drained via an incision in the sclera, and an expansile gas may be injected into the vitreous cavity. Certain types of uncomplicated retinal detachment may be treated by the technique of pneumatic retinopexy, in which an expansile gas is initially injected into the vitreous cavity followed by careful positioning of the patient's head to facilitate reattachment of the retina. Once the retina is repositioned, the retinal tear is sealed by laser photocoagulation or cryotherapy. All the stages of pneumatic retinopexy can be performed under local anesthesia as an office procedure. The last stage is the same as is used to seal retinal tears without associated detachment as prophylaxis against detachment.

In complicated retinal detachments—particularly those in which fibroproliferative tissue has developed on the surface of the retina or within the vitreous cavity—retinal reattachment can be accomplished only by removal of the vitreous, direct manipulation of the retina, and internal tamponade of the retina with air, expansile gases, or even silicone oil. (The presence of an expansile gas within the eye is a contraindication to air travel. Such gases may persist in the globe for weeks after surgery.) (See Chapter 38.)

Prognosis

About 80% of uncomplicated cases can be cured with one operation; an additional 15% will need repeated operations; and the remainder never reattach. The prognosis is worse if the macula is detached or if the detachment is of long duration. Without treatment, retinal detachment often becomes total within 6 months. Spontaneous detachments are ultimately bilateral in 2–25% of cases.

Eter N et al: Long-term results of pneumatic retinopexy. Graefes Arch Clin Exp Ophthalmol 2000;238:677. [PMID: 11011688] (Nearly all eyes treated initially by pneumatic retinopexy were found to have successful retinal reattachment at average follow-up of more than 6 years; 30% required more than one procedure.)

Lincoff H et al: Changing patterns in the surgery for retinal detachment: 1929 to 2000. Klin Monatsbl Augenheilkd 2000;216:352. [PMID: 10919114] (Historical and literature review of retinal detachment surgery by one of the principal contributors to its development.)

VITREOUS HEMORRHAGE

Patients with vitreous hemorrhage complain of sudden visual loss, sudden onset of floaters that may progressively increase in severity, or, occasionally, "bleeding within the eye." Visual acuity ranges from 20/20 to light perception only. The eye is not inflamed, and the clue to diagnosis is the inability to see fundal details clearly despite the presence of a clear lens. Causes of vitreous hemorrhage include diabetic retinopathy, retinal tears (with or without retinal detachment), retinal vein occlusions, exudative age-related macular degeneration, blood dyscrasias, trauma, and subarachnoid hemorrhage (Terson's syndrome). In all cases,

examination by an ophthalmologist is essential. Retinal tears and detachments necessitate urgent treatment (see above).

AGE-RELATED MACULAR DEGENERATION

Age-related macular degeneration is the leading cause of permanent visual loss in the elderly. The exact cause is unknown, but the incidence increases with each decade over age 50 (to almost 30% by age 75). Other associations besides age include race (usually white), sex (slight female predominance), family history, and a history of cigarette smoking.

Age-related macular degeneration includes a broad spectrum of clinical and pathologic findings that can be classified into two groups: atrophic ("dry") and exudative ("wet"). Although both types are progressive and usually bilateral, they differ in manifestations, prognosis, and management. The precursor to age-related macular degeneration is age-related maculopathy, of which the hallmark is the development of retinal drusen. Hard drusen appear ophthalmoscopically as discrete yellow deposits, usually in the macular region. Soft drusen are larger, paler, and less distinct. Large, confluent soft drusen are particularly associated with the development of exudative age-related macular degeneration.

Atrophic degeneration is characterized by gradually progressive bilateral visual loss of moderate severity due to atrophy and degeneration of the outer retina, retinal pigment epithelium, Bruch's membrane, and choriocapillaris. In exudative degeneration, visual loss is of more rapid onset and greater severity, and the two eyes are frequently affected sequentially over a period of a few years. The exudative form accounts for about 90% of all cases of legal blindness due to this disorder. Impairment of the barrier function of Bruch's membrane (between the retinal pigment epithelium and the choriocapillaris) allows serous fluid or blood to leak into the retina to produce elevation of the retinal pigment epithelium from Bruch's membrane (retinal pigment epithelial detachment) or separation of the neurosensory retina from the retinal pigment epithelium (serous retinal detachment). These changes may resolve spontaneously, with variable visual outcome, but are often associated with neovascularization arising from the choroidal vessels and extending between the retinal pigment epithelium and Bruch's membrane (subretinal neovascular membrane). This membrane produces permanent visual loss.

Sudden visual loss in patients with exudative age-related macular degeneration occurs at the time of pigment epithelial or sensory retinal detachment or hemorrhage from a subretinal neovascular membrane. All these changes may occur in previously undiagnosed patients, in patients known to have atrophic changes, and in the other eye of patients with exudative disease. Laser photocoagulation of subretinal neovascular membranes may delay the onset of permanent visual loss but only when the membrane is far enough away from the fovea to permit such treatment. Conventional laser photocoagulation of subfoveal neovascular membranes is associated with an inevitable immediate reduction in vision because of associated retinal damage. Photodynamic laser therapy (PDT) produces selective vascular damage, which may thus limit the degree of visual loss, but repeated treatments are usually necessary and the high cost may not be justifiable. Various surgical techniques to excise subfoveal neovascular membranes—or to reposition the macula away from them—continue to be investigated. The value of radiotherapy for subretinal neovascular membranes remains uncertain. Older patients developing sudden visual loss due to macular disease—particularly paracentral distortion or scotoma with preservation of central acuity—should be referred urgently to an ophthalmologist for assessment.

There is no specific treatment for atrophic age-related macular degeneration, but—as with the exudative form—patients often benefit from low vision aids. The disorder results in loss of central vision only. Peripheral fields and hence navigational vision are always maintained, though these may become impaired by cataract formation for which surgery may be helpful. The value of oral antioxidants and zinc in preventing visual loss in age-related macular degeneration continues to be assessed.

Berglin L et al: The Swedish national survey of surgical excision for submacular choroidal neovascularization (CNV). Acta Ophthalmol Scand 2001;79:580. [PMID: 11782223] (Surgical removal of submacular CNV did not appear to improve visual acuity in patients over 50 years of age.)

Fine SL et al: Age-related macular degeneration. N Engl J Med 2000;342:483. [PMID: 10675430]

Fong DS: Age-related macular degeneration: update for primary care. Am Fam Physician 2000;61:3035. [PMID: 10839553]

Ohji M et al: Comparison of three techniques of foveal translocation in patients with subfoveal choroidal neovascularization resulting from age-related macular degeneration. Am J Ophthalmol 2001;132:888. [PMID: 11730654] (Foveal translocation improved or maintained visual acuity in a significant proportion of treated eyes and was best associated with 360-degree retinotomy in the case of larger choroidal neovascular membranes.)

A randomized, placebo-controlled, clinical trial of high-dose supplementation with vitamins C and E, beta carotene, and zinc for age-related macular degeneration and vision loss: AREDS report no. 8. Arch Ophthalmol 2001;119:1417. [PMID: 11594942] (Oral antioxidants—vitamin C 500 mg, vitamin E 400 IU, and beta-carotene 15 mg)—plus oral zinc 80 mg and copper 2 mg may reduce the risk of visual loss in nonsmokers with age-related macular degeneration.)

Sharma S et al: The cost-effectiveness of photodynamic therapy for fellow eyes with subfoveal choroidal neovascularization secondary to age-related macular degeneration. Ophthalmology 2001;108:2051. [PMID: 11713079] (Photodynamic therapy provides only minimal cost-effectiveness for patients with good visual acuity in their better-seeing eye

and is not cost-effective in those with poor visual acuity in their better-seeing eye.)

Wormald R et al: Photodynamic therapy for neovascular age-related macular degeneration (Cochrane Review). Cochrane Database Syst Rev 2001;3:CD002030. [PMID: 11687007] (Photodynamic therapy effective for well-demarcated but not for poorly-demarcated choroidal neovascular membranes.)

CENTRAL & BRANCH RETINAL VEIN OCCLUSIONS

The severity of visual loss in central retinal vein occlusion is variable. The visual impairment is commonly first noticed upon waking in the morning. Ophthalmoscopic signs include disk swelling, venous dilation and tortuosity, retinal hemorrhages, and cotton-wool spots.

In those with initially good acuity (20/60 or better), the visual prognosis is good. In those with poor initial acuity (20/200 or worse), extensive hemorrhages and multiple cotton-wool spots indicate widespread retinal ischemia, which can be confirmed by demonstrating extensive areas of capillary closure on fluorescein angiography. These eyes are at high risk of developing neovascular (rubeotic) glaucoma, typically within 3 months after venous occlusion, and should be monitored by an ophthalmologist so that laser panretinal photocoagulation can be undertaken if neovascularization occurs. The visual prognosis in these cases is poor.

Branch retinal vein occlusions may present in a variety of ways. Sudden loss of vision may occur at the time of occlusion if the fovea is involved or some time afterward from vitreous hemorrhage due to retinal new vessels. More gradual visual loss may occur with development of macular edema or exudate. In a significant proportion, the occlusion is noted incidentally in patients with glaucoma, systemic hypertension, diabetes mellitus, or uveitis.

In acute branch retinal vein occlusion there are signs similar to those of central retinal vein occlusion but affecting only the retina drained by the obstructed vein. There is no specific treatment, but if retinal neovascularization develops, the area of retina affected by the initial occlusion should be laser-photocoagulated. Macular edema may also respond to laser treatment.

All patients with retinal vein occlusion should be referred urgently to an ophthalmologist and investigated for glaucoma, hypertension, diabetes, and hyperlipidemia. In younger patients, an assessment for thrombophlebitis is indicated. Hyperhomocystinemia and antiphospholipid antibodies may also be risk factors. Hyperviscosity syndromes are rarely associated with retinal vein occlusions but may worsen their prognosis. Branch retinal vein occlusion is an important feature of Behçet's syndrome.

Hayreh SS et al: Systemic diseases associated with various types of retinal vein occlusion. Am J Ophthalmol 2001;131:61.

[PMID: 11162981] (Systemic hypertension and diabetes mellitus are associated with branch and central retinal vein occlusion, though to different extents.)

Lahey JM et al: Laboratory evaluation of hypercoagulable states in patients with central retinal vein occlusion who are less than 56 years of age. Ophthalmology 2002;109:126. [PMID: 11772591] (See annotation Marcucci reference, below.)

Marcucci R et al: Thrombophilic risk factors in patients with central retinal vein occlusion. Thromb Haemost 2001;86:772. [PMID: 11583306] (Two papers implicating hyperhomocysteinemia and circulating antiphospholipid antibodies as risk factors for central retinal vein occlusion.)

CENTRAL & BRANCH RETINAL ARTERY OCCLUSIONS

Central retinal artery occlusion presents as sudden profound visual loss. Visual acuity is reduced to counting fingers or worse, and visual field is commonly restricted to an island of vision in the temporal field. Ophthalmoscopy reveals pallid swelling of the retina, most obvious in the posterior segment, with a cherry-red spot at the fovea. The retinal arteries are attenuated, and "box-car" segmentation of blood in the veins may be seen. Occasionally, emboli are seen in the central retinal artery or its branches. The retinal swelling subsides over a period of 4–6 weeks, leaving a relatively normal retinal appearance but a pale optic disk and attenuated arterioles.

The patient should be referred as an emergency to an ophthalmologist. If seen within a few hours after onset, emergency treatment—including laying the patient flat, ocular massage, high concentrations of inhaled oxygen, intravenous acetazolamide, and anterior chamber paracentesis—may influence the visual outcome. Thrombolysis, particularly by local intra-arterial but also intravenously, is being used but may not improve overall outcome.

The main management problem is identifying any treatable underlying disorder. Giant cell arteritis must be excluded in all older patients, especially because of the risk—highest in the first few days—of involvement of the other eye. If giant cell arteritis is suspected, one should institute high-dose corticosteroids immediately and proceed promptly to temporal artery biopsy. Carotid and cardiac sources of emboli must also be considered in retinal artery occlusion and appropriate treatment given to reduce the risk of stroke (see Chapter 12). Internal carotid artery dissection should be considered when central retinal artery occlusion is associated with head or neck pain.

Branch retinal artery occlusion may also present with sudden loss of vision if the fovea is involved, but more commonly sudden loss of visual field is the presenting complaint. Fundal signs of retinal swelling and adjacent cotton-wool spots are limited to the area of retina supplied by the occluded vessel. Embolic causes are proportionately more common than in central retinal artery occlusion. Migraine, oral contraceptives, and vasculitis must also be considered. Congenital or acquired thrombophilia has been identified in patients with central and branch retinal artery occlusions. Patients with branch retinal artery occlusions should be referred urgently to an ophthalmologist.

Beatty S et al: Local intra-arterial fibrinolysis for acute occlusion of the central retinal artery: a meta-analysis of the published data. Br J Ophthalmol 2000;84:914. [PMID: 10906103] (Marginal visual benefit compared with conventional management; a randomized comparative trial is necessary.)

Riordan-Eva P et al: Temporal artery biopsy in the management of giant cell arteritis with neuro-ophthalmic complications. Br J Ophthalmol 2001;85:1248. [PMID: 11567973] (Discussion of the importance of temporal artery biopsy in the diagnosis of giant cell arteritis.)

Salomon O et al: Thrombophilia as a cause for central and branch retinal artery occlusion in patients without an apparent embolic source. Eye 2001;15:511. [PMID: 11767028] (Congenital or acquired thrombophilia in 43% of patients with retinal artery occlusion and no carotid or cardiac source of emboli.)

AMAUROSIS FUGAX

Amaurosis fugax ("fleeting blindness") is characteristically caused by retinal emboli from ipsilateral carotid disease. The visual loss is usually described as a curtain passing vertically across the visual field with complete monocular visual loss lasting a few minutes and a similar curtain effect as the episode passes. In order to reduce the risk of stroke, patients with high-grade stenosis (70–99%) of the ipsilateral internal carotid artery should be considered for carotid endarterectomy. Patients with medium-grade (30–69%) or low-grade (up to 29%) stenosis are better treated medically with aspirin or other antiplatelet drugs. The most reliable method of evaluating carotid stenosis is intra-arterial angiography, but this is associated with a number of complications including stroke. The noninvasive techniques of duplex ultrasonography and magnetic resonance angiography are suitable screening methods. Emboli from cardiac sources may also be responsible for amaurosis fugax. Echocardiography should be undertaken in young patients and in any patient with clinical evidence of a potential cardiac source of emboli. In younger patients without carotid or cardiac disease, amaurosis fugax may be due to choroidal or retinal vascular spasm, in which case calcium channel blockers such as slow-release nifedipine, 60 mg/d, appear to be effective.

Similar obscurations of vision may occur with poor ocular perfusion due to severe occlusive carotid disease or to aortic dissection. More transient obscurations (lasting only a few seconds to 1 minute) affecting both eyes occur in patients with raised intracranial pressure. In all cases of episodic visual loss, early ophthalmologic consultation is advisable.

Benavente O et al: Prognosis after transient monocular blindness associated with carotid-artery stenosis. N Engl J Med 2001;345:1084. [PMID: 11596587] (Better prognosis in internal carotid artery stenosis presenting with transient monocular blindness than those presenting with hemispheric transient ischemic attack.)

RETINAL DISORDERS ASSOCIATED WITH SYSTEMIC DISEASES

Many systemic diseases are associated with retinal manifestations. These include diabetes mellitus, essential hypertension, preeclampsia-eclampsia of pregnancy, blood dyscrasias, and AIDS. The retinal changes caused by these disorders can be easily observed with an ophthalmoscope.

Diabetic Retinopathy

Diabetic retinopathy is the leading cause of new blindness among US adults aged 20–65. It is broadly classified as nonproliferative and proliferative.

Nonproliferative retinopathy is characterized by dilation of veins, microaneurysms, retinal hemorrhages, retinal edema, and hard exudates. A major subgroup are those patients in which visual loss develops owing to edema, exudates, or ischemia at the macula (diabetic maculopathy). This is the most common cause of legal blindness in maturity-onset diabetes.

Proliferative retinopathy is characterized by neovascularization, arising either from the optic disk or the major vascular arcades. Vitreous hemorrhage is a common sequela. Proliferation into the vitreous of blood vessels, with their associated fibrous component, leads to tractional retinal detachment. Without treatment, the visual prognosis with proliferative retinopathy is generally much worse than that with nonproliferative retinopathy. Severe proliferative retinopathy is often complicated by maculopathy.

Nonproliferative retinopathy is occasionally present at the time of diagnosis in maturity-onset diabetes and may be the presenting feature. Treatment includes optimizing control of blood glucose and any associated hypertension or hyperlipidemia. Institution of intensive insulin therapy can be associated with temporary exacerbation of retinopathy, particularly characterized by multiple cotton-wool spots. Laser photocoagulation is particularly helpful in the treatment of focal macular edema but may also be used when there is diffuse macular edema. The presence of macular edema can be detected only by stereoscopic examination of the retina or by fluorescein angiography. The level of visual acuity is a poor guide to the presence of treatable maculopathy—hence the need for regular ophthalmologic follow-up.

Proliferative retinopathy must be recognized early and treated by panretinal laser photocoagulation to prevent blindness. Neovascularization is all too often diagnosed only at the time of vitreous hemorrhage. In some patients, a "preproliferative" retinopathy may be identified. Whether panretinal laser photocoagulation should be undertaken at this time can be determined by the degree of retinal ischemia as assessed by fluorescein angiography.

Surgical treatment (vitrectomy) is being used increasingly either to remove vitreous hemorrhage and thus allow perioperative panretinal laser photocoagulation for the underlying retinal neovascularization, to deal with retinal detachments involving the macula, to manage rapidly progressive proliferative disease, or to treat persistent macular edema.

Patients with diabetes mellitus should have at least yearly ophthalmoscopic examination through dilated pupils. Examination by an ophthalmologist is usually advisable in juvenile-onset diabetes of more than 5 years' duration; at the time of diagnosis in maturity-onset diabetes; in early pregnancy, or prior to conception in women contemplating pregnancy, and every 4–8 weeks throughout pregnancy; if ocular symptoms develop; or if there are suspicious findings of retinopathy, especially neovascularization or macular exudates. Failure to diagnose diabetic retinopathy by ophthalmoscopic examination is common, particularly if the pupils are not dilated. The severity of diabetic retinopathy can be lessened by careful control of blood glucose levels, but good diabetic control is more important in preventing the development of retinopathy than in influencing its subsequent course. Proliferative diabetic retinopathy, especially after successful laser treatment, is not a contraindication to treatment with thrombolytic agents, aspirin, or warfarin unless there has been recent vitreous or preretinal hemorrhage.

Aiello LP et al: Systemic considerations in the management of diabetic retinopathy. Am J Ophthalmol 2001;132:760. [PMID: 11704039] (Literature review highlighting the importance of optimal diabetic control and management of concomitant systemic disorders in preventing development and progression of diabetic retinopathy.)

Bresnick GH et al: A screening approach to the surveillance of patients with diabetes for the presence of vision-threatening retinopathy. Ophthalmology 2000;107:19. [PMID: 10647713] (Guidelines for identification in primary care of diabetics requiring ophthalmologic referral.)

Early worsening of diabetic retinopathy in the Diabetes Control and Complications Trial. Arch Ophthalmol 1998;116:874. [PMID: 9682700] (Intensive insulin therapy was associated with worsening of retinopathy in 15% of patients, but the long-term outcome was better.)

Kohner EM et al: United Kingdom Prospective Diabetes Study, 30. Diabetic retinopathy at diagnosis of non-insulin dependent diabetes mellitus and associated risk factors. Arch Ophthalmol 1998;116:297. [PMID: 9514482] (Thirty-five percent of men and 40% of women with newly diagnosed type 2 diabetes mellitus had diabetic retinopathy.)

Neely KA et al: Diabetic retinopathy. Med Clin North Am 1998;82:847. [PMID: 9706124] (Review of screening and management of diabetic retinopathy.)

Sharma S et al. The cost-effectiveness of early vitrectomy for the treatment of vitreous hemorrhage in diabetic retinopathy. Curr Opin Ophthalmol 2001;12:230. [PMID: 11389353] (Early vitrectomy for the treatment of vitreous hemorrhage secondary to diabetic retinopathy shown to be highly cost-effective.)

Hypertensive Retinochoroidopathy

Systemic hypertension affects both the retinal and choroidal circulations. The clinical manifestations vary according to the degree and rapidity of rise in blood pressure and the underlying state of the ocular circulation. The most florid disease occurs in young patients with abrupt elevations of blood pressure, such as may occur in pheochromocytoma, malignant essential hypertension, acute renal failure, or preeclampsia-eclampsia.

Chronic hypertension accelerates the development of atherosclerosis. The retinal arterioles become more tortuous and narrow and develop abnormal light reflexes ("silver-wiring" and "copper-wiring"). There is increased venous compression at the retinal arteriovenous crossings ("arteriovenous nicking"), which is an important factor predisposing to branch retinal vein occlusions. Flame-shaped hemorrhages occur in the nerve fiber layer of the retina.

Acute elevations of blood pressure result in loss of autoregulation in the retinal circulation, leading to the breakdown of endothelial integrity and occlusion of precapillary arterioles and capillaries. These pathologic changes are manifested as cotton-wool spots, retinal hemorrhages, retinal edema, and retinal exudates, often in a stellate appearance at the macula. In the choroid, vasoconstriction and ischemia result in serous retinal detachments and retinal pigment epithelial infarcts. These infarcts later develop into pigmented lesions that may be focal, linear, or wedge-shaped. The abnormalities in the choroidal circulation may also affect the optic nerve head, producing ischemic optic neuropathy with optic disk swelling. Malignant hypertensive retinopathy was the term previously used to describe the constellation of clinical signs resulting from the combination of abnormalities in the retinal, choroidal, and optic disk circulation. When there is such severe disease, there is likely to be permanent retinal, choroidal, or optic nerve damage. Precipitous reduction of blood pressure may exacerbate such damage.

Schubert HD: Ocular manifestations of systemic hypertension. Curr Opin Ophthalmol 1998;9:69. [PMID: 10387339] (A general review of hypertensive retinochoroidopathy.)

Blood Dyscrasias

In conditions characterized by thrombocytopenia or severe anemia, various types of hemorrhages are present in both the retina and choroid and may lead to visual loss. If macular hemorrhages have not occurred, it is possible to regain normal vision with treatment.

Proliferative retinopathy (sickle cell retinopathy) is particularly common in hemoglobin SC disease but may also occur with other hemoglobin S variants. Severe visual loss is rare. Retinal photocoagulation reduces the frequency of vitreous hemorrhage. Surgery is occasionally needed for unresolving vitreous hemorrhage or tractional retinal detachment.

AIDS

Cotton-wool spots, retinal hemorrhages, and microaneurysms are the most common ophthalmic abnormalities in AIDS patients.

Cytomegalovirus retinitis occurs in many AIDS patients, generally when CD4 counts are below $50/\mu L$. It is characterized by progressively enlarging yellowish-white patches of retinal opacification, which are accompanied by retinal hemorrhages; they usually begin adjacent to the major retinal vascular arcades. Patients are often asymptomatic until there is involvement of the fovea or optic nerve or until retinal detachment develops.

The agents effective in cytomegalovirus retinitis are ganciclovir, foscarnet, and the nucleotide analog cidofovir, formerly known as HPMPC, which has the significant advantage of a prolonged intracellular half-life such that no more than weekly administration is required. Major side effects are neutropenia with systemic ganciclovir due to bone marrow suppression, and limiting therapy with zidovudine (AZT), and nephrotoxicity with foscarnet and cidofovir. Dosage of both ganciclovir and foscarnet needs to be adjusted in renal failure. Oral probenecid and intravenous hydration are used to minimize nephrotoxicity from cidofovir. All three agents are only virostatic. Reactivation of disease and hence eventually complete loss of vision can only be delayed rather than prevented.

Initial therapy is either intravenous—ganciclovir, 5 mg/kg twice a day, foscarnet 60 mg/kg three times a day, or cidofovir 5 mg/kg once weekly, usually for 2 weeks—or by local administration, using either intravitreal injection of ganciclovir or foscarnet or the sustained-release ganciclovir intravitreal implant. Intravitreal cidofovir is effective, but there is a high incidence of uveitis, low intraocular pressure, and ciliary body necrosis. Maintenance therapy can be undertaken with lower-dose intravenous therapy (ganciclovir, 3.75 mg/kg/d, or foscarnet, 60 mg/kg/d, for 5 days each week; or cidofovir, 5 mg/kg once every 2 weeks), oral ganciclovir (3 g/d), or intravitreal therapy. Local therapy tends to be more effective than systemic therapy and avoids systemic side effects, but there is a risk of intraocular complications, and the incidences of retinitis in the fellow eye and of extraocular cytomegalovirus infection are higher. Unresponsive disease or reactivation during maintenance therapy can be managed by changing to a different agent or by use of combination therapy. Retinal detachment, either directly due to retinitis or as a complication of intravitreal therapy, generally requires vitrectomy and intravitreal silicone oil. The use of oral ganciclovir as prophylaxis against cytomegalovirus retinitis in patients with low CD4 counts or high CMV burdens has not been found to be worthwhile.

Antiretroviral therapy may result in reduction of HIV virus load and increase in CD4 counts, and even regression of CMV retinitis without the use of anticytomegalovirus therapy. If the CD4 count is maintained above 100/μL, it may be possible to discontinue maintenance anticytomegalovirus therapy. Highly active antiretroviral therapy (HAART) occasionally leads to "immune recovery" uveitis, which may lead to severe visual loss.

Other opportunistic ophthalmic infections occurring in AIDS patients include herpes simplex retinitis, toxoplasmic and candidal chorioretinitis, and herpes zoster ophthalmicus. Kaposi's sarcoma of the conjunctiva and orbital lymphoma may also be seen on rare occasions.

MacDonald JC et al: Highly active antiretroviral therapy-related immune recovery in AIDS patients with cytomegalovirus retinitis. Ophthalmology 2000;107:877. [PMID: 10811078] (Lack of reactivation of cytomegalovirus retinitis in 19 out of 22 patients with persistent elevation of CD4 cell count over 50/μL after highly active antiretroviral therapy.)

Robinson MR et al: Ocular manifestations of HIV infection. Curr Opin Ophthalmol 1999;10:431. [PMID: 10662248] (Review of recent advances in the diagnosis and management of HIV-associated ocular disease.)

ANTERIOR ISCHEMIC OPTIC NEUROPATHY

Anterior ischemic optic neuropathy—due to inadequate perfusion of the posterior ciliary arteries that supply the anterior portion of the optic nerve—produces sudden visual loss, usually with an altitudinal field defect, and optic disk swelling. In older patients, it is often caused by giant cell arteritis, which necessitates emergency high-dose systemic steroid treatment to prevent visual loss in the fellow eye. (See Central and Branch Retinal Artery Occlusion, above.) The predominant factor predisposing to nonarteritic anterior ischemic optic neuropathy is congenitally small optic disks. Other causative factors include systemic hypertension, diabetes mellitus, systemic vasculitis, and possibly hyperhomocystinemia.

Chan CC et al: Steroid management in giant cell arteritis. Br J Ophthalmol 2001;85:1061. [PMID: 11520757] (Retrospective review of patients with arteritic anterior ischemic optic neuropathy indicating better outcome with initial intravenous rather than oral steroid therapy.)

Pianka P et al: Hyperhomocystinemia in patients with nonarteritic anterior ischemic optic neuropathy, central retinal artery occlusion, and central retinal vein occlusion. Ophthalmology 2000;107:1588. [PMID: 10919914] (Found in 45% of patients with nonarteritic anterior ischemic optic neuropathy.)

OPTIC NEURITIS

Optic neuritis is characterized by unilateral loss of vision which usually develops suddenly and may increase during the following few days. At its worst, the level of vision may vary from 20/30 to no perception of light. Visual acuity usually then improves within 2–3 weeks and frequently returns to normal. Commonly there is pain in the region of the eye, particularly on eye movements. Field loss is usually a central scotoma, but a wide range of monocular field defects are possible. There is marked loss of color vision and a relative afferent pupillary defect. In about two-thirds of cases, the optic nerve is normal during the acute stage (retrobulbar optic neuritis). In the remainder, the optic disk is swollen (papillitis) with occasional flame-shaped peripapillary hemorrhages. In all cases, optic atrophy subsequently develops if there has been destruction of sufficient optic nerve fibers.

Optic neuritis is particularly associated with demyelinative disease, occurring in patients known to have multiple sclerosis and as a first manifestation of the disease in others. In patients with clinically isolated optic neuritis, as many as 75% will have developed clinically definite multiple sclerosis within 15 years. The presence of white matter lesions on brain MRI at presentation correlates with subsequent development of this disorder. Long-term therapy with interferon beta may reduce the risk of developing it.

Optic neuritis may also occur in association with viral infections (including measles, mumps, influenza, and those caused by the varicella-zoster virus), with various autoimmune disorders, particularly systemic lupus erythematosus, and by spread of inflammation from meninges, orbital tissues, or paranasal sinuses.

Prednisolone alone has no beneficial effect on the visual outcome in acute demyelinative optic neuritis and may increase the risk of recurrent disease. Intravenous methylprednisolone (250 mg every 6 hours for 3 days) followed by oral prednisolone (1 mg/kg for 11 days, then tapered off over 4 days) accelerates visual recovery, but with a small risk of systemic side effects. This regimen reduces the risk of development of multiple sclerosis during the first 2 years after the episode of optic neuritis, particularly in patients with multiple white matter lesions on brain MRI. Whether such therapy is to be used in an individual patient should be determined by the degree of visual loss, the state of the fellow eye, the patient's visual requirements, the results of brain MRI, and the patient's susceptibility to systemic side effects from steroid therapy. Optic neuritis due to herpes zoster or systemic lupus erythematosus generally has a poorer prognosis than other forms of optic neuritis and also requires high-dose intravenous corticosteroid therapy. All patients with optic neuritis should be referred urgently for neuro-ophthalmologic assessment. Any patient with a clinical diagnosis of isolated optic neuritis in which visual recovery does not occur requires further investigation, particularly to exclude a compressive lesion or an intrinsic optic nerve tumor.

Comi G et al: Effect of early interferon treatment on conversion to definite multiple sclerosis: a randomised study. Lancet 2001;357:1576. [PMID: 11377645] (Two randomized controlled studies showing reduced risk of clinically definite multiple sclerosis and progression of brain MRI abnormalities with interferon beta-1a therapy initiated after first episode of demyelinative optic neuritis.)

Interferon beta-1a for optic neuritis patients at high risk for multiple sclerosis. Am J Ophthalmol 2001;132:463. [PMID: 11589865] (See annotation Comi reference, above.)

OPTIC DISK SWELLING

Optic disk swelling may result from intraocular disease, orbital and optic nerve lesions, severe hypertensive retinochoroidopathy, or raised intracranial pressure. Intraocular causes include central retinal vein occlusion, posterior uveitis, and posterior scleritis. Optic nerve lesions causing disk swelling include optic neuritis, anterior ischemic optic neuropathy; optic disk drusen (pseudopapilledema); optic nerve sheath meningioma; and optic nerve infiltration by sarcoidosis, leukemia, or lymphoma. Any orbital lesion causing optic nerve compression may produce disk swelling.

Papilledema (optic disk swelling due to raised intracranial pressure) is usually bilateral and most commonly produces enlargement of the blind spot without loss of acuity. Chronic papilledema, as occurs in idiopathic intracranial hypertension (previously known as benign intracranial hypertension) and dural venous sinus occlusion, may be associated with progressive visual field loss and occasionally profound loss of acuity. All patients with chronic papilledema must be monitored carefully, especially their visual fields, and optic nerve sheath fenestration (also known as optic nerve sheath decompression) or lumboperitoneal shunt should be considered in those with progressive visual failure not controlled by medical therapy (weight loss where appropriate and acetazolamide).

Optic disk drusen should be considered when disk swelling is not associated with any visual disturbance or symptoms of raised intracranial pressure. Exposed optic disk drusen may be obvious clinically or can be demonstrated by their autofluorescence. Buried drusen are best detected by orbital ultrasound or CT scanning. Other family members may be similarly affected.

Banta JT et al: Pseudotumor cerebri and optic nerve sheath decompression. Ophthalmology 2000;107:1907. [PMID: 11013197] (Stabilization or improvement of visual field in 90% of eyes undergoing optic nerve sheath fenestration.)

Johnson LN et al: The role of weight loss and acetazolamide in the treatment of idiopathic intracranial hypertension (pseudotumor cerebri). Ophthalmology 1998;105:2313. [PMID: 9855165] (Weight loss of approximately 6% resulted in complete resolution of papilledema, whereas acetazolamide therapy without weight loss did not result in any improvement in papilledema.)

OCULAR MOTOR PALSIES

In complete **third nerve paralysis,** there is complete ptosis and the eye is divergent and slightly depressed. Extraocular movements are restricted in all directions except laterally (preserved lateral rectus function). Intact fourth nerve (superior oblique) function is detected by the presence of inward rotation on attempted depression of the eye.

Pupillary involvement (dilated pupil that does not react to accommodation or to light shined in either eye) is an important sign differentiating "surgical" from "medical" causes of isolated third nerve palsy. (Compressive lesions of the third nerve, such as aneurysm of the posterior communicating artery and uncal herniation due to a supratentorial mass lesion, characteristically have pupillary involvement.) It is crucial that patients presenting with painful isolated third nerve palsy with pupillary involvement be assumed to have a posterior communicating artery aneurysm until this has been excluded, at which time they should be referred immediately for neurosurgical assessment. Medical causes of isolated third nerve palsy include diabetes, systemic hypertension, syphilis, and giant cell arteritis.

Fourth nerve paralysis causes upward deviation of the eye with failure of depression on adduction. There is vertical diplopia that becomes most apparent on attempted reading and descending stairs. Many cases of isolated fourth nerve palsy are due to decompensation of a congenital lesion. Trauma is a major cause of acquired—particularly bilateral—fourth nerve palsy, but cerebral neoplasms and medical causes such as in third nerve palsies should also be considered.

Sixth nerve paralysis causes convergent squint in the primary position with failure of abduction of the affected eye, producing horizontal diplopia that increases on gaze to the affected side and on looking into the distance. It is an important sign of raised intracranial pressure, particularly in children. Sixth nerve palsy may also be due to trauma, neoplasms, brain stem lesions, or medical causes (see above).

An intracranial or intraorbital mass lesion should be considered in any patient presenting with an isolated ocular motor palsy. In patients with isolated ocular motor nerve palsies presumed to be due to medical causes, brain MRI must be performed if recovery has not begun within 3 months.

Ocular motor nerve palsies occurring in association with other neurologic signs may be due to lesions in the brain stem, around the cavernous sinus, or in the orbit. Lesions around the cavernous sinus involve the upper divisions of the trigeminal nerve, the ocular motor nerves, and occasionally the optic chiasm. Orbital apex lesions involve the optic nerve and the ocular motor nerves.

Myasthenia and dysthyroid eye disease must always be considered in the differential diagnosis of disordered extraocular movements.

DYSTHYROID EYE DISEASE

Dysthyroid eye disease is a clinical syndrome caused by deposition of mucopolysaccharides and infiltration with chronic inflammatory cells of the orbital tissues, particularly the extraocular muscles. Patients may have clinical or laboratory evidence of thyroid dysfunction, elevated thyroid autoantibodies, or no detectable abnormality outside the orbit. Radioiodine therapy and cigarette smoking increase the severity of dysthyroid eye disease.

The primary clinical features are proptosis, lid retraction and lid lag, conjunctival chemosis and episcleral inflammation, and extraocular muscle abnormalities due to restriction of their actions. Resulting symptoms are cosmetic abnormalities, surface irritation, which usually responds to artificial tears, and diplopia, which should be treated conservatively (eg, with prisms) in the active stages of the disease and only by surgery when the disease has been static for at least 6 months.

The important complications are corneal exposure and optic nerve compression, both of which may lead to profound visual loss. Treatment is by urgent orbital decompression, either medically, with high-dose systemic steroids (prednisolone 80–100 mg/d)—although this is often of only short-term benefit—by radiotherapy, or by surgery, usually consisting of extensive removal of bone from the medial, inferior, and lateral walls of the orbit.

The optimal management of moderately severe dysthyroid eye disease without visual loss is controversial. Oral steroids, radiotherapy, and surgical decompression have all been advocated, but there is a risk of serious local or systemic side-effects from all three. Lateral tarsorrhaphy may be used for moderately severe corneal exposure. Other lid procedures are particularly useful for correcting lid retraction but should not be undertaken until the orbital disease is quiescent and orbital decompression or extraocular muscle surgery has been undertaken if necessary.

Bartalena L et al: Cigarette smoking and treatment outcomes in Graves ophthalmopathy. Ann Intern Med 1998;129:632. [PMID: 9786811] (Cigarette smoking increased the risk of progression of dysthyroid eye disease after radioiodine therapy and reduced the rate of response to orbital radiotherapy and systemic steroid therapy.)

Gorman CA et al: A prospective, randomized, double-blind, placebo-controlled study of orbital radiotherapy for Graves' ophthalmopathy. Ophthalmology 2001;108:1523. [PMID: 11535445] (No beneficial effect from radiotherapy for dysthyroid eye disease without visual loss.)

Mourits MP et al: Radiotherapy for Graves' orbitopathy: randomised placebo-controlled study. Lancet 2000;355:1505. [PMID: 10801172] (Radiotherapy produced a beneficial effect on ocular motility but not on proptosis or eyelid swelling.)

Van Stavern GP et al: Optic neuropathies. An overview. Ophthalmol Clin North Am 2001;14:61. [PMID: 11370572] (Reviews the diverse group of pathologic processes that may affect the optic nerve.)

ORBITAL CELLULITIS

Orbital cellulitis is manifested by an abrupt onset of fever, proptosis, restriction of extraocular movements, and swelling and redness of the lids, usually in a child.

Infection of the paranasal sinuses is the usual underlying cause. Immediate treatment with intravenous antibiotics is necessary to prevent optic nerve damage and spread of infection to the cavernous sinuses—manifested as increased restriction of extraocular movements, impaired visual acuity, diminished pupillary reflexes, and papilledema, all of which may be bilateral—meninges, and brain. The response to antibiotics is usually excellent, but abscess formation may necessitate surgical drainage.

Ambati BK et al: Periorbital and orbital cellulitis before and after the advent of *Haemophilus influenzae* type B vaccination. Ophthalmology 2000;107:1450. [PMID: 10919886] (Sharp decline in cases of periorbital and orbital cellulitis coinciding with the introduction of the vaccine.)

Ferguson MP et al: Current treatment and outcome in orbital cellulitis. Aust N Z J Ophthalmol 1999;27:375. [PMID: 10641894] (Highlights the importance of paranasal sinus disease as a predisposing factor and the good outcome with adequate treatment.)

OCULAR TRAUMA

Conjunctival & Corneal Foreign Bodies

If a patient complains of "something in my eye" and gives a consistent history, a foreign body is usually present on the cornea or under the upper lid even though it may not be readily visible. Visual acuity should be tested before treatment is instituted, as a basis for comparison in the event of complications.

After a local anesthetic (eg, proparacaine, 0.5%) is instilled, the eye is examined with the aid of a hand flashlight, using oblique illumination, and loupe. Corneal foreign bodies may be made more apparent by the instillation of sterile fluorescein. They are then removed with a sterile wet cotton-tipped applicator. Polymyxin-bacitracin ophthalmic ointment should be instilled. It is not necessary to patch the eye, but the patient must be examined 24 hours later for secondary infection of the crater. If a corneal foreign body cannot be removed in this manner, the patient should be referred to an ophthalmologist.

Steel foreign bodies usually leave a diffuse rust ring. This requires excision of the affected tissue and is best done under local anesthesia using a slitlamp. **Caution:** Anesthetic drops should not be given to the patient for self-administration.

If there is no infection, a layer of corneal epithelial cells will line the crater within 24 hours. It should be emphasized that the intact corneal epithelium forms an effective barrier to infection, but once it is disturbed the cornea becomes extremely susceptible to infection. Early infection is manifested by a white necrotic area around the crater and a small amount of gray exudate. These patients should be referred immediately to an ophthalmologist, since untreated corneal infection may lead to loss of the eye.

In the case of a foreign body under the upper lid, a local anesthetic is instilled and the lid is everted by grasping the lashes gently and exerting pressure on the mid portion of the outer surface of the upper lid with an applicator. If a foreign body is present, it can easily be removed by passing a wet sterile cotton-tipped applicator across the conjunctival surface.

Intraocular Foreign Body

Intraocular foreign body requires emergency treatment by an ophthalmologist. Patients giving a history of "something hitting the eye"—particularly if it happens while hammering on metal or using grinding equipment—must be carefully assessed for the possibility of an intraocular foreign body, especially when no corneal foreign body is seen, a corneal or scleral wound is apparent, or there is marked visual loss or media opacity. Such patients must be treated as for corneal laceration (see below) and referred without delay to an ophthalmologist. Intraocular foreign bodies significantly increase the risk of intraocular infection.

Corneal Abrasions

A patient with a corneal abrasion complains of severe pain and photophobia. There is often a history of trauma to the eye, commonly involving a fingernail, piece of paper, or contact lens. Visual acuity is recorded, and the cornea and conjunctiva are examined with a light and loupe to rule out a foreign body. If an abrasion is suspected but cannot be seen, sterile fluorescein is instilled into the conjunctival sac: the area of corneal abrasion will stain a deeper green than the surrounding cornea.

Treatment includes polymyxin-bacitracin ophthalmic ointment and application of a bandage with firm pressure to prevent movement of the lid. The patient should rest at home, keeping the fellow eye closed, and should be observed the following day to be certain the cornea has healed. Recurrent corneal erosion may follow corneal abrasions.

Contusions

Contusion injuries of the eye and surrounding structures may cause ecchymosis ("black eye"), subconjunctival hemorrhage, edema or rupture of the cornea, hemorrhage into the anterior chamber (hyphema), rupture of the root of the iris (iridodialysis), paralysis of the pupillary sphincter, paralysis of the muscles of accommodation, cataract, dislocation of the lens, vitreous hemorrhage, retinal hemorrhage and edema (most common in the macular area), detachment of the retina, rupture of the choroid, fracture of the orbital floor ("blowout fracture"), or optic nerve injury. Many of these injuries are immediately obvious; others may not become apparent for days or weeks. Patients with moderate to severe contusions should be seen by an ophthalmologist.

Any injury severe enough to cause hyphema involves the danger of secondary hemorrhage, which may cause intractable glaucoma with permanent visual loss. Any patient with traumatic hyphema should be advised to rest quietly until complete resolution has occurred. Daily ophthalmologic assessment is essential. Aspirin and related drugs increase the risk of secondary hemorrhage and must be avoided.

Ashar A et al: Blindness associated with midfacial fractures. J Oral Maxillofac Surg 1998;56:1146. [PMID: 9766539] (Ten out of 49 patients with midfacial fractures lost vision in one eye.)

Lacerations

A. Lids

If the lid margin is lacerated, the patient should be referred for specialized care, since permanent notching may result. Lacerations of the lower eyelid near the inner canthus often sever the lower canaliculus. Lid lacerations not involving the margin may be sutured just like any other skin laceration.

B. Conjunctiva

In lacerations of the conjunctiva, sutures are not necessary. In order to prevent infection, sulfonamides or other antibiotics are instilled into the eye until the laceration is healed.

C. Cornea or Sclera

Patients with suspected corneal or scleral lacerations must be seen by an ophthalmologist as soon as possible. Manipulation is kept to a minimum, since pressure may result in extrusion of the intraocular contents. The eye is bandaged lightly and covered with a metal shield that rests on the orbital bones above and below. The patient should be instructed not to squeeze the eye shut and to remain as quiet as possible. The eye is routinely studied by x-ray, and CT scanning if necessary, to identify and localize any metallic intraocular foreign body. MRI is contraindicated owing to the risk of movement of the foreign body in the magnetic field.

Ultraviolet Keratitis (Actinic Keratitis)

Ultraviolet burns of the cornea are usually caused by use of a sunlamp without eye protection, exposure to a welding arc, or exposure to the sun when skiing ("snow blindness"). There are no immediate symptoms, but about 6–12 hours later the patient complains of agonizing pain and severe photophobia. Slitlamp examination after instillation of sterile fluorescein shows diffuse punctate staining of both corneas.

Treatment consists of binocular patching and instillation of 1–2 drops of 1% cyclopentolate (to relieve the discomfort of ciliary spasm). All patients recover within 24–48 hours without complications. Local anesthetics should not be prescribed.

Chemical Conjunctivitis & Keratitis

Chemical burns are treated by irrigation of the eyes with saline solution or plain water as soon as possible after exposure. Neutralization of an acid with an alkali or vice versa generates heat and may cause further damage. Alkali injuries are more serious and require prolonged irrigation, since alkalies are not precipitated by the proteins of the eye as are acids. It is important to remove any retained particulate matter such as is typically present in injuries involving cement and building plaster. This may require double eversion of the upper lid. The pupil should be dilated with 1% cyclopentolate, 1 drop twice a day, to relieve discomfort and prophylactic topical antibiotics should be started. In moderate to severe injuries, intensive topical corticosteroids and topical and systemic vitamin C are also necessary. Complications include mucus deficiency, scarring of the cornea and conjunctiva, symblepharon (adhesions between the tarsal and bulbar conjunctiva), tear duct obstruction, and secondary infection.

Brodovsky SC et al: Management of alkali burns—an 11-year retrospective review. Ophthalmology 2000;107:1829. [PMID: 11013181] (Treatment with intensive topical steroids, ascorbate, citrate, and antibiotics—compared with a short course of topical steroids and antibiotics—was beneficial only in moderately severe alkali burns. Mild burns did not require such intensive treatment, and severe burns had a poor outcome whatever treatment was given.)

May DR et al: The epidemiology of serious eye injuries from the United States Eye Injury Registry. Graefes Arch Clin Exp Ophthalmol 2000;238:153. [PMID: 10766285] (Predominance of males under the age of 30.)

PRINCIPLES OF TREATMENT OF OCULAR INFECTIONS

Before one can determine the drug of choice, the causative organisms must be identified, but in most instances empirical treatment, based on clinical experience, is used in the first instance. In the treatment of conjunctivitis and for prophylaxis against ocular infection, it is preferable to use a drug that is not given systemically. Of the available local antibacterial agents, the sulfonamides are effective and inexpensive. Two reliable sulfonamides for ophthalmic use are sulfisoxazole and sodium sulfacetamide. The sulfonamides have the added advantages of low allergenicity and effectiveness against the chlamydial group of organisms. They are available in ointment or solution form. Combined bacitracin-polymyxin ointment is often used prophylactically after corneal foreign body removal for the protection it affords against both gram-positive and gram-negative organisms.

Among the most effective broad-spectrum antibiotics for ophthalmic use are gentamicin, tobramycin, neomycin, and ciprofloxacin. These drugs have some effect against gram-negative as well as gram-positive organisms but are generally not effective against the pneumococcus, for which penicillin G or nafcillin (if beta-lactamase resistance is present) is required. Allergic reactions to neomycin are common. Other antibiotics frequently used are erythromycin, the tetracyclines, and the cephalosporins.

Method of Administration

Most ocular anti-infective drugs are administered locally. Ointments have greater therapeutic effectiveness than solutions, since contact can be maintained longer. However, they do cause blurring of vision; if this must be avoided, solutions should be used.

Systemic administration is required for all intraocular infections, orbital cellulitis, dacryocystitis, gonococcal keratoconjunctivitis, inclusion conjunctivitis, and severe external infection that does not respond to local treatment.

TECHNIQUES USED IN THE TREATMENT OF OCULAR DISORDERS

Table 7–2 lists commonly used ophthalmic drugs and their indications and costs.

Instilling Medications

The patient is placed in a chair with head tilted back, both eyes open, and looking up. The lower lid is retracted slightly, and 2 drops of liquid are instilled into the lower cul-de-sac. The patient looks down while finger contact is maintained, so that the eyes are not squeezed shut. Ointments are instilled in the same general manner.

For self-medication, the same techniques are used except that medications are usually better instilled with the patient lying down.

Eye Bandage

Most eye bandages should be applied firmly enough to hold the lid securely against the cornea. An ordinary patch consisting of gauze-covered cotton is usually sufficient. Tape is applied from the cheek to the forehead.

PRECAUTIONS IN MANAGEMENT OF OCULAR DISORDERS

Use of Local Anesthetics

Unsupervised self-administration of local anesthetics is dangerous because the patient may further injure an anesthetized eye without knowing it. The drug may also interfere with the normal healing process.

Pupillary Dilation

Dilating the pupil can very occasionally precipitate acute glaucoma if the patient has a narrow anterior chamber angle and should be undertaken with caution if the anterior chamber is obviously shallow (readily determined by oblique illumination of the anterior

Table 7–2. Topical ophthalmic agents.

Agent	Representative Cost/Size[1]	Sig	Indications
AGENTS FOR GLAUCOMA AND INTRAOCULAR HYPERTENSION			
Sympathomimetics			
Apraclonidine HCl 0.5% solution (Iopidine)	$57.60/5 mL	1 drop three times daily	Reduction of intraocular pressure. Expensive. Reserve for treatment of resistant cases.
Apraclonidine HCl 1% solution (Iopidine)	$8.58/unit dose 0.1 mL	1 drop 1 hour before and immediately after anterior segment laser surgery	To control or prevent elevations of intraocular pressure after laser trabeculoplasty or iridotomy.
Brimonidine tartrate 0.2% solution (Alphagan)	$36.28/5 mL	1 drop two or three times daily	Reduction of Intraocular pressure.
Dipivefrin HCl 0.1% solution (various)[2]	$14.07/5 mL	1 drop every 12 hours	Open-angle glaucoma.
Epinephrine HCl 0.25%, 0.5% (Epifrin), 1% and 2% solution (various)[3]	1%: $47.33/15 mL 2%: $51.78/15 mL	1 drop twice daily	
Beta-adrenergic blocking agents			
Betaxolol HCl 0.5% solution (Betoptic) and 0.25% suspension (Betoptic S)[4]	0.5%: $50.64/10 mL	1 drop twice daily	Reduction of intraocular pressure.
Carteolol HCl 1% solution (Ocupress)[5]	$37.07/10 mL	1 drop twice daily	
Levobunolol HCl 0.25% and 0.5% solution (Betagan)[5]	0.5%: $32.29/10 mL	1 drop once or twice daily	
Metipranolol HCl 0.3% solution (OptiPranolol)[5]	$16.61/5 mL	1 drop twice daily	
Timolol 0.25% and 0.5% solution (Betimol)[5]	0.5%: $33.38/10 mL	1 drop once or twice daily	
Timolol maleate 0.25% and 0.5% solution (Timoptic) and 0.25% and 0.5% gel (Timoptic-XE)[5]	0.5% solution: $17.00/5 mL 0.5% gel: $30.90/5 ml	1 drop once or twice daily	
Miotics			
Pilocarpine HCl (various)[6] (1–4%, 6%, 8%, 10%)	2%: $11.79/15 mL	1 drop three or four times daily	Reduction of intraocular pressure, treatment of acute or chronic angle-closure glaucoma, and pupillary constriction.
Pilocarpine HCl 4% gel (Pilopine HS)	$37.86/4 g	Apply 0.5-inch ribbon in lower conjunctival sac at bedtime.	
Pilocarpine 20 μg/h for 7 days, and 40 μg/h for 7 days ocular therapeutic system (Ocusert Pilo-20 and Ocusert Pilo-40)[7]	40 μg/h: $45.13/8 each	Replace each unit every 7 days.	
Carbonic anhydrase inhibitor			
Dorzolamide HCl 2% solution (Trusopt)	$26.94/5 mL $53.91/10 mL	1 drop three times daily	Reduction of intraocular pressure.
Brinzolamide 1% suspension (Azopt)	$26.40/5 mL $52.80/10 mL	1 drop three times daily	

(continued)

Table 7–2. Topical ophthalmic agents. (continued)

Agent	Representative Cost/Size[1]	Sig	Indications
Prostaglandin analogs			
Bimatoprost 0.003% solution (Lumigan)	$50.13/2.5 mL	1 drop once daily in the evening	Reduction of intraocular pressure.
Latanoprost 0.005% solution (Xalatan)	$50.05/2.5 mL	1 drop once or twice daily in the evening	
Travoprost 0.004% solution (Travatan)	$45.54/2.5 mL	1 drop once daily in the evening	
ANTI-INFLAMMATORY AGENTS			
Nonsteroidal anti-inflammatory agents[8]			
Diclofenac sodium 0.1% solution (Voltaren)	$49.81/5 mL	1 drop to affected eye four times daily beginning 24 hours after cataract surgery and continuing through first 2 postoperative weeks.	Treatment of postoperative inflammation following cataract extraction, and laser corneal surgery.
Flurbiprofen sodium 0.03% solution (various)	$8.73/2.5 mL	1 drop every half hour beginning 2 hours before surgery.	Inhibition of intraoperative miosis. Treatment of cystoid macular edema and inflammation after cataract surgery.
Ketorolac tromethamine 0.5% solution (Acular)	$53.59/5 mL	1 drop four times daily	Relief of ocular itching due to seasonal allergic conjunctivitis.
Corticosteroids[9]			
Dexamethasone sodium phosphate 0.1% solution (various)	$16.51/5 mL	1 or 2 drops as often as indicated by severity. Use every hour during the day and and every 2 hours during the night in severe inflammation. Taper off as inflammation decreases.	Treatment of steroid-responsive inflammatory conditions of anterior segment.
Dexamethasone sodium phosphate 0.05% ointment (various)	$6.34/3.5 g	Apply thin coating on lower conjunctival sac three or four times daily.	
Fluorometholone 0.1% suspension (various)[10]	$26.16/10 mL	1 or 2 drops as often as indicated by severity. Use every hour during the day and every 2 hours during the night in severe inflammation. Taper off as inflammation decreases.	
Fluorometholone 0.25% suspension (FML Forte)[10]	$37.60/10 mL		
Fluorometholone 0.1% ointment (FML S.O.P.)	$32.38/3.5 g	Apply thin coating on lower conjunctival sac three or four times daily.	
Medrysone 1% suspension (HMS)	$31.65/10 mL	1 or 2 drops as often as indicated by severity of inflammation. Use every hour during the day and every 2 hours during the night in severe inflammation. Taper off as inflammation decreases.	
Prednisolone acetate 0.12% suspension (Pred Mild)	$34.41/10 mL		
Prednisolone acetate 0.125% suspension (various)	$23.94/5 mL $35.88/10 mL		
Prednisolone sodium phosphate 0.125% solution (various)	$18.38/5 mL		

(continued)

Table 7–2. Topical ophthalmic agents. (continued)

Agent	Representative Cost/Size[1]	Sig	Indications
Corticosteroids[9] (continued)			
Prednisolone acetate 1% suspension (various)	$37.26/10 mL		
Prednisolone sodium phosphate 1% solution (various)	$27.03/10 mL		
Rimexolone 1% suspension (Vexol)	$25.74/5 mL		
Mast cell stabilizers			
Cromolyn sodium 4% solution (Crolom)	$44.56/10 mL	1 drop four to six times daily	Allergic conjunctivitis.
Lodoxamide tromethamine 0.1% solution (Alomide)	$58.02/10 mL	1 or 2 drops four times daily (up to 3 months)	Vernal keratoconjunctivitis.
ANTIBIOTIC OINTMENTS AND SOLUTIONS			
Bacitracin 500 units/g ointment (various)[11]	$3.79/3.5 g	Refer to package insert (instructions vary)	Infections involving lid, conjunctiva, or cornea.
Chloramphenicol 0.5% (5 mg/mL) solution (various)[12]	$22.15/7.5 mL		As above, with both gram-positive and gram-negative coverage.
Chloramphenicol 1% (10 mg/g) ointment (various)[12]	$20.53/3.5 g		
Ciprofloxacin HCl (various)	0.3% solution $36.24/5 mL 0.3% ointment $40.56/3.5 g		
Erythromycin 0.5% ointment (various)[13]	$5.00/3.5 g		
Gentamicin sulfate 0.3% solution (various)	$8.17/5 mL		
Gentamicin sulfate 0.3% ointment (various)	$14.56/3.5 g		
Norfloxacin 0.3% solution (Chibroxin)	$21.49/5 mL		
Ofloxacin 0.3% solution (Ocuflox)	$37.66/5 mL		
Polymyxin B sulfate 500,000 units, powder for solution (Polymyxin B Sulfate Sterile)[14]	$8.64/500,000 units		
Tobramycin 0.3% solution (various)	$15.00/5 mL		
Tobramycin 0.3% ointment (Tobrex)	$40.20/3.5 g		
SULFONAMIDES			
Sulfacetamide sodium 10% solution (various)	$5.08/15 mL	1 or 2 drops every 1–3 hours	Conjunctivitis, corneal ulcer, and other superficial ocular infections due to susceptible microorganisms. Used as adjunct to systemic sulfonamide therapy in treatment of trachoma.

(continued)

Table 7–2. Topical ophthalmic agents. (continued)

Agent	Representative Cost/Size[1]	Sig	Indications
SULFONAMIDES (continued)			
Sulfacetamide sodium 10% ointment (various)	$6.95/3.5 g	Apply small amount (0.5 inch) into lower conjunctival sac once to four times daily and at bedtime.	

Note: Many combination products containing antibiotics, antibiotics and steroids, or sulfonamides and steroids are available as solutions, suspensions, or ointment.

TOPICAL ANTIFUNGAL AGENTS			
Natamycin 5% suspension (Natacyn)	$120.00/15 mL	1 drop every 1–2 hours.	Fungal blepharitis, conjunctivitis, and keratitis caused by susceptible organisms. Drug of choice for *Fusarium solani* keratitis.
TOPICAL ANTIVIRAL AGENTS			
Ganciclovir 4.5 mg surgical insert (Vitrasert)	$5000.00 each	1 implant every 5–8 months	Treatment of CMV retinitis in patients with AIDS.
Trifluridine 1% solution (Viroptic)	$91.68/7.5 mL	1 drop onto cornea every 2 hours while awake for a maximum daily dose of 9 drops until resolution occurs. Then an additional 7 days of 1 drop every 4 hours while awake (minimum five times daily)	Primary keratoconjunctivitis and recurrent epithelial keratitis due to HSV types 1 or 2.[15]
Vidarabine monohydrate 3% ointment (Vira-A)	$27.05/3.5 g	0.5 inch of ointment into the lower conjunctival sac five times daily at 3-hour intervals.	Acute keratoconjunctivitis and recurrent epithelial keratitis due to HSV types 1 or 2.[15]
TOPICAL ANTIHISTAMINICS[16]			
Levocabastine HCl 0.05% ophthalmic solution (Livostin)	$73.90/10 mL	1 drop four times daily (up to 2 weeks)	Allergic conjunctivitis; temporary relief of seasonal allergic conjunctivitis.

[1]Cost to pharmacist (average wholesale price, generic when possible) for quantity listed. Source: *Drug Topics Red Book,* March 2002; Vol. 21, No. 3.
[2]Macular edema occurs in 30% of patients.
[3]May (rarely) increase blood pressure. **Caution:** Avoid in patients with sulfite hypersensitivity (some brands contain sulfite).
[4]Cardioselective (β_1) beta-blocker.
[5]Nonselective (β_1 and β_2) beta-blocker. Monitor all patients for systemic side effects, particularly exacerbation of asthma.
[6]Decreased night vision, headaches possible.
[7]Sustained-release preparation. Refrigerate.
[8]Cross-sensitivity to aspirin and other NSAIDs.
[9]Long-term use may increase intraocular pressure or cause cataracts.

[10]May be less likely to elevate intraocular pressure.
[11]Little efficacy against gram-negative organisms (except neisseria).
[12]Aplastic anemia has been reported with prolonged ophthalmic use. Use only in serious infections for which less toxic drugs are ineffective or contraindicated.
[13]Also indicated for prophylaxis of ophthalmia neonatorum due to *N gonorrhoeae* or *C trachomatis*. Increasing resistance of *S pneumoniae* and *P aeruginosa* has been noted.
[14]No gram-positive coverage.
[15]Recurrences are common and call for additional 7-day treatment.
[16]Antihistamines (topical) are potential sensitizers and may produce local reactions.

Table 7–3. Adverse ocular effects of systemic drugs.

Drug	Possible Side Effects
Respiratory drugs	
Oxygen	Retinopathy of prematurity.
Anticholinergic bronchodilators	Angle-closure glaucoma.
Cardiovascular system drugs	
Digitalis	Disturbances of color vision, scotomas, photopsia.
Quinidine	Optic neuritis (rare).
Thiazides (Diuril, etc)	Xanthopsia (yellow vision), myopia.
Carbonic anhydrase inhibitors (acetazolamide)	Ocular hypotony, transient myopia.
Amiodarone	Corneal deposits, optic neuropathy, thyroid ophthalmopathy.
Oxyprenolol	Photophobia, ocular irritation.
Gastrointestinal drugs	
Anticholinergic agents	Risk of angle-closure glaucoma due to mydriasis. Blurring of vision due to cycloplegia (occasional).
Central nervous system drugs	
Barbiturates	Extraocular muscle palsies with diplopia, nystagmus, ptosis, cortical blindness.
Chloral hydrate	Diplopia, ptosis, miosis.
Phenothiazines	Deposits of pigment in conjunctiva, cornea, lens and retina. Oculogyric crises.
Amphetamines	Widening of palpebral fissure. Dilation of pupil, paralysis of ciliary muscle with loss of accommodation.
Monoamine oxidase inhibitors	Nystagmus, extraocular muscle palsies, optic atrophy.
Tricyclic agents	Dilation of pupil (risk of angle-closure glaucoma), cycloplegia.
Phenytoin	Nystagmus, diplopia, ptosis, slight blurring of vision (rare).
Neostigmine	Nystagmus, miosis.
Morphine	Miosis.
Haloperidol	Capsular cataract.
Lithium carbonate	Exophthalmos, oculogyric crisis, nystagmus.
Diazepam	Nystagmus.
Topiramate	Angle-closure glaucoma.
Paroxetine	Angle-closure glaucoma.
Hormonal agents	
Corticosteroids	Cataract (posterior subcapsular), local immunologic suppression, causing susceptibility to viral (herpes simplex), bacterial, and fungal infections; steroid-induced glaucoma.
Female sex hormones	Retinal artery occlusion, retinal vein occlusion, papilledema, ocular palsies with diplopia, nystagmus, optic neuropathy.
Tamoxifen	Crystalline retinal deposits.
Antibiotics	
Chloramphenicol	Optic neuritis and atrophy.
Streptomycin	Optic neuritis.
Tetracycline	Pseudotumor cerebri, transient myopia.
Antimalarial agents	
Chloroquine, etc	Macular changes, central scotomas, pigmentary degeneration of the retina, chloroquine keratopathy, ocular palsies, ptosis, ERG depression.
Amebicides	
Iodochlorhydroxyquin	Optic atrophy.
Chemotherapeutic agents	
Sulfonamides	Stevens-Johnson syndrome.
Ethambutol	Optic neuritis and atrophy.
Isoniazid	Optic neuritis and atrophy.

(continued)

Table 7–3. Adverse ocular effects of systemic drugs. (continued)

Drug	Possible Side Effects
Heavy metals	
Gold salts	Deposits in the cornea and conjunctiva.
Lead compounds	Optic atrophy, papilledema, ocular palsies.
Chelating agents	
Penicillamine	Ocular pemphigoid, optic neuritis, ocular myasthenia.
Oral hypoglycemic agents	
Chlorpropamide	Transient change in refractive error, diplopia, Stevens-Johnson syndrome.
Vitamins	
Vitamin A	Papilledema, retinal hemorrhages, loss of eyebrows and eyelashes, nystagmus, diplopia, blurring of vision.
Vitamin D	Band-shaped keratopathy.
Antirheumatic agents	
Salicylates	Nystagmus, retinal hemorrhages, cortical blindness (rare).
Indomethacin	Corneal deposits.
Phenylbutazone	Retinal hemorrhages.

segment of the eye). A short-acting mydriatic such as tropicamide should be used and the patient warned to report immediately if ocular discomfort or redness develops. Angle closure is more likely to occur if pilocarpine is used to overcome pupillary dilation than if the pupil is allowed to constrict naturally.

Local Corticosteroid Therapy

Repeated use of local corticosteroids presents several hazards: herpes simplex (dendritic) keratitis, fungal infection, open-angle glaucoma, and cataract formation. Furthermore, perforation of the cornea may occur when the corticosteroids are used for herpes simplex keratitis.

Contaminated Eye Medications

Ophthalmic solutions are prepared with the same degree of care as fluids intended for intravenous administration, but once bottles are opened there is always a risk of contamination, particularly with solutions of tetracaine, proparacaine, fluorescein, and any preservative-free preparations. The most dangerous is fluorescein, as this solution is frequently contaminated with *P aeruginosa,* an organism that can rapidly destroy the eye. Sterile fluorescein filter paper strips are now available and are recommended for use in place of fluorescein solutions.

Whether in plastic or glass containers, eye solutions should not remain in use for long periods after the bottle is opened. Four weeks after opening is an absolute maximal time to use a solution containing preservatives before discarding. Preservative-free preparations should be kept refrigerated and discarded within 1 week after opening. Any solution should of course be checked for signs of bacterial contamination prior to use.

If the eye has been injured accidentally or by surgical trauma, it is of the greatest importance to use freshly opened bottles of sterile medications or single-use eyedropper units.

Toxic & Hypersensitivity Reactions to Topical Therapy

Patients receiving long-term topical therapy may develop local toxic or hypersensitivity reactions to the active agent or preservatives, especially if there is inadequate tear secretion. Preservatives in contact lens cleaning solutions may produce similar problems. Burning and soreness are exacerbated by drop instillation or contact lens insertion; occasionally, fibrosis and scarring of the conjunctiva and cornea may occur.

An antibiotic instilled into the eye can sensitize the patient to that drug and cause a hypersensitivity reaction upon subsequent systemic administration.

Systemic Effects of Ocular Drugs

The systemic absorption of certain topical drugs (through the conjunctival vessels and lacrimal drainage system) must be considered when there is a systemic medical contraindication to the use of the drug. Ophthalmic solutions of the nonselective beta-blockers, eg, timolol, may worsen patients with congestive heart failure or asthma. Atropine ointment should be prescribed for children rather than the drops, since absorption of the 1% topical solution may be toxic. Phenylephrine eye drops can precipitate hypertensive crises and angina. Also to be considered are adverse interactions between systemically administered and ocular drugs. Using only 1 or 2 drops at a time and a few minutes of nasolacrimal occlusion or eyelid closure ensure maximum efficacy and decrease systemic side effects of topical agents.

ADVERSE OCULAR EFFECTS OF SYSTEMIC DRUGS

Systemically administered drugs produce a wide variety of adverse effects on the visual system. Table 7–3 lists the major examples.

Fraunfelder FT, Mayer SM: Ocular and systemic side effects of drugs. In: *General Ophthalmology,* 15th ed. Vaughan D, Asbury T, Riordan-Eva P (editors). Appleton & Lange, 1999.

Ear, Nose, & Throat

Robert K. Jackler, MD, & Michael J. Kaplan, MD

See www.current-med.com/ch08.html

8

■ DISEASES OF THE EAR

HEARING LOSS

Classification & Epidemiology

A. CONDUCTIVE HEARING LOSS

Conductive hearing loss results from dysfunction of the external or middle ear. There are four mechanisms, each resulting in impairment of the passage of sound vibrations to the inner ear: (1) obstruction (eg, cerumen impaction), (2) mass loading (eg, middle ear effusion), (3) stiffness effect (eg, otosclerosis), and (4) discontinuity (eg, ossicular disruption). Conductive losses in adults are most commonly due to cerumen impaction or transient auditory tube dysfunction associated with upper respiratory tract infection. Persistent conductive losses usually result from chronic ear infection, trauma, or otosclerosis. Conductive hearing loss is generally correctable with medical or surgical therapy—or in some cases both.

B. SENSORY HEARING LOSS

Sensory hearing loss results from deterioration of the cochlea, usually due to loss of hair cells from the organ of Corti. Sensorineural losses in adults are common. A gradually progressive, predominantly high-frequency loss with advancing age (presbyacusis) is typical. Other than aging effects, common causes of sensorineural loss include excessive noise exposure, head trauma, and systemic diseases such as diabetes mellitus. Sensory hearing loss is not correctable with medical or surgical therapy but often may be prevented or stabilized.

C. NEURAL HEARING LOSS

Neural hearing loss occurs with lesions involving the eighth nerve, auditory nuclei, ascending tracts, or auditory cortex. It is the least common clinically recognized cause of hearing loss. Causes include acoustic neuroma, multiple sclerosis, and cerebrovascular disease.

Blanchfield BB et al: The severely to profoundly hearing-impaired population in the United States: prevalence estimates and demographics. J Am Acad Audiol 2001;12:183. [PMID: 11763876]

Karlsmose B et al: A randomised controlled trial of screening for adult hearing loss during preventive health checks. Br J Gen Pract 2001;51:351. [PMID: 11360697]

Morris DP et al: The common causes of hearing loss in adults. Practitioner 2000;244:70. [PMID: 10892040]

Evaluation of Hearing (Audiology)

In a quiet room, the hearing level may be estimated by having the patient repeat aloud words presented in a soft whisper, a normal spoken voice, or a shout. Tuning forks are useful in differentiating conductive from sensorineural losses. A 512-Hz tuning fork is employed, since frequencies below this level elicit a tactile response. In the **Weber test,** the tuning fork is placed on the forehead or front teeth. In conductive losses, the sound appears louder in the poorer-hearing ear, whereas in sensorineural losses it radiates to the better side. In the **Rinne test,** the tuning fork is placed alternately on the mastoid bone and in front of the ear canal. In conductive losses, bone conduction exceeds air conduction; in sensorineural losses, the opposite is true.

Formal audiometric studies are performed in a soundproofed room. Pure-tone thresholds in decibels (dB) are obtained over the range of 250–8000 Hz (the main speech frequencies are between 500 and 3000 Hz) for both air and bone conduction. Conductive losses create a gap between the air and bone thresholds, whereas in sensorineural losses both air and bone thresholds are equally diminished. The threshold of normal hearing is from 0 to 20 dB, which corresponds to the loudness of a soft whisper. Mild hearing loss is indicated by a threshold of 20–40 dB (soft spoken voice), moderate loss by a threshold of 40–60 dB (normal spoken voice), severe loss by a threshold of 60–80 dB (loud spoken voice), and profound loss by a threshold of 80 dB (shout). The clarity of hearing is often impaired in sensorineural hearing loss. This is evaluated by speech discrimination testing, which is reported as percentage correct (90–100% is normal). The site of the lesion responsible for sensorineural loss—whether it lies in the cochlea or in the central auditory system—may be determined with auditory brain stem-evoked responses.

Every patient who complains of a hearing loss should be referred for audiologic evaluation unless the cause is easily remediable (eg, cerumen impaction, otitis media). Audiologic screening is not recommended for adults with apparently normal hearing unless they are exposed to potentially injurious levels of noise or have reached the age of 65, after which screening evaluations should be done every few years.

Smith PA et al: Hearing assessment in general practice, schools and health clinics: guidelines for professionals who are not qualified audiologists. Education Committee of the British Society of Audiology. Br J Audiol 2000;34:57. [PMID: 10759078]

Zadeh MH et al: Evaluation of hearing impairment. Compr Ther 2001;27:302. [PMID: 1765688]

Hearing Rehabilitation

Patients with hearing loss not correctable by medical therapy may benefit from hearing amplification. Contemporary hearing aids are comparatively free of distortion and have been miniaturized to the point where they often may be contained entirely within the ear canal. To optimize the benefit, a hearing aid must be carefully selected to conform to the nature of the hearing loss. Digitally programmable hearing aids are now becoming available that allow optimization of speech intelligibility and may be tuned to deal with difficult listening circumstances.

Much current interest is focused upon the development of semi-implantable and even fully implantable hearing aids. A variety of devices are under development that deliver vibrations—usually via either a rare earth magnet or a piezoceramic crystal—directly to the ossicular chain. Some of these devices are in clinical trials.

Aside from hearing aids, many assistive devices are available to improve comprehension in individual and group settings, to help with hearing television and radio programs, and for telephone communication. In individuals with profound sensory hearing loss, the cochlear implant—an electronic device that is surgically implanted to stimulate the auditory nerve—offers socially beneficial auditory rehabilitation to most adults with acquired deafness.

Clark GM: Cochlear implants in the third millennium. Am J Otol 1999;20:4. [PMID: 9918163] (Futuristic view of high-technology innovations with potential use in the rehabilitation of deafness.)

Klein AJ, Weber PC: Hearing aids. Med Clin North Am 1999; 83:139. [PMID: 9927966] (Reviews new digital technology.)

Maniglia AJ et al: Implantable electronic otologic devices—state of the art. Otolaryngol Clin North Am 2001;34:No. 2. (Entire issue.)

DISEASES OF THE AURICLE

Disorders of the external ear are for the most part dermatologic. Skin cancers due to sun exposure are common and may be treated with standard techniques. Traumatic auricular hematoma must be recognized and drained to prevent significant cosmetic deformity (cauliflower ear) resulting from dissolution of supporting cartilage. Similarly, cellulitis of the auricle must be treated promptly to prevent development of perichondritis and its resultant deformity. Relapsing polychondritis is a systemic disorder often associated with recurrent, frequently bilateral, painful episodes of auricular erythema and edema. Treatment with corticosteroids may help forestall cartilage dissolution. Respiratory compromise may occur as a result of progressive involvement of the tracheobronchial tree. Chondritis and perichondritis may be differentiated from auricular cellulitis by sparing of involvement of the lobule, which does not contain cartilage.

Ahmad I et al: Epidemiology of basal cell carcinoma and squamous cell carcinoma of the pinna. J Laryngol Otol 2001; 115:85. [PMID: 11320842]

Chen S et al: Painful erythematous ear. Arch Dermatol 2000; 136:418. [PMID: 10724211]

DISEASES OF THE EAR CANAL

1. Cerumen Impaction

Cerumen is a protective secretion produced by the outer portion of the ear canal. In most individuals, the ear canal is self-cleansing. Recommended hygiene consists of cleaning the external opening with a washcloth over the index finger without entering the canal itself. In most cases, cerumen impaction is self-induced through ill-advised attempts at cleaning the ear. It may be relieved with detergent ear drops (eg, 3% hydrogen peroxide; 6.5% carbamide peroxide), mechanical removal, suction, or irrigation. Irrigation is performed with water at body temperature to avoid a vestibular caloric response. The stream should be directed at the ear canal wall adjacent to the cerumen plug. Irrigation should be performed only when the tympanic membrane is known to be intact.

Use of jet irrigators designed for cleaning teeth (eg, WaterPik) for wax removal should be avoided since they may result in tympanic membrane perforations. Following irrigation, the ear canal should be thoroughly dried (eg, by instilling isopropyl alcohol or using a hair blow-dryer on low-power setting) to reduce the likelihood of inducing external otitis. Specialty referral for cleaning under microscopic guidance is indicated when the impaction has not responded to routine measures or if the patient has a history of chronic otitis media or tympanic membrane perforation.

Grossan M: Safe, effective techniques for cerumen removal. Geriatrics 2000;55:80. [PMID: 10659076]

2. Foreign Bodies

Foreign bodies in the ear canal are more frequent in children than in adults. Firm materials may be removed with a loop or a hook, taking care not to displace the object medially toward the tympanic membrane; microscopic guidance is helpful. Aqueous irrigation should not be performed for organic foreign bodies (eg, beans, insects), because water may cause them to swell. Living insects are best immobilized before removal by filling the ear canal with lidocaine.

3. External Otitis

External otitis presents with otalgia, frequently accompanied by pruritus and purulent discharge. There is often a history of recent water exposure or mechanical trauma (eg, scratching, cotton applicators). External otitis is usually caused by gram-negative rods (eg, pseudomonas, proteus) or fungi (eg, aspergillus), which grow in the presence of excessive moisture.

Examination reveals erythema and edema of the ear canal skin, often with a purulent exudate. Manipulation of the auricle often elicits pain. Because the lateral surface of the tympanic membrane is ear canal skin, it is often erythematous. However, in contrast to acute otitis media, it moves normally with pneumatic otoscopy. When the canal skin is very edematous, it may be impossible to visualize the tympanic membrane.

Fundamental to the treatment of external otitis is protection of the ear from additional moisture and avoidance of further mechanical injury by scratching. Otic drops containing a mixture of aminoglycoside antibiotic and anti-inflammatory corticosteroid in an acid vehicle are generally very effective (eg, neomycin sulfate, polymyxin B sulfate, and hydrocortisone). Purulent debris filling the ear canal should be gently removed to permit entry of the topical medication. Drops should be used abundantly (5 or more drops three or four times a day) to penetrate the depths of the canal. When substantial edema of the canal wall prevents entry of drops into the ear canal, a wick is placed to facilitate entry of the medication. In recalcitrant cases—particularly when cellulitis of the periauricular tissue has developed—oral fluoroquinolones (eg, ciprofloxacin, 500 mg twice daily for 1 week) are the drugs of choice because of their effectiveness against pseudomonas species.

Holten KB et al: Management of the patient with otitis externa. J Fam Pract 2001;50:353. [PMID: 11300988]

Roland PS: Chronic external otitis. Ear Nose Throat J 2001;80(6 Suppl):12. [PMID: 11488077]

4. Pruritus

Pruritus of the external auditory canal, particularly at the meatus, is a common problem. While it may be associated with external otitis or with dermatologic conditions such as seborrheic dermatitis and psoriasis, most cases are self-induced either from excoriation or by overly zealous ear cleaning. To permit regeneration of the protective cerumen blanket, patients should be instructed to avoid use of soap and water or cotton swabs in the ear canal. Patients with excessively dry canal skin may benefit from application of mineral oil, which helps to counteract dryness and repel moisture. When an inflammatory component is present, topical application of a corticosteroid (eg, 0.1% triamcinolone) may be beneficial. It is axiomatic in persistent pruritus that the patient must cease scratching the ear. In stubborn cases, the fingernails must be kept short and the patient may need to wear cotton gloves at night to avoid manipulation during sleep. Symptomatic reduction of pruritus may be obtained by use of oral antihistamines (eg, diphenhydramine, 25 mg orally at bedtime). Topical application of isopropyl alcohol promptly relieves ear canal pruritus in many patients.

5. Malignant External Otitis

Persistent external otitis in the diabetic or immunocompromised patient may evolve into osteomyelitis of the skull base, often called malignant external otitis. Usually caused by *Pseudomonas aeruginosa*, osteomyelitis begins in the floor of the ear canal and may extend into the middle fossa floor, the clivus, and even the contralateral skull base. The patient usually presents with persistent foul aural discharge, granulations in the ear canal, deep otalgia, and progressive cranial nerve palsies involving nerves VI, VII, IX, X, XI, or XII. Diagnosis is confirmed by the demonstration of osseous erosion on CT and radionuclide scanning.

Treatment is chiefly medical, requiring prolonged antipseudomonal antibiotic administration, often for several months. Although intravenous therapy is often required, selected patients may be managed with the oral agent ciprofloxacin (500–1000 mg orally twice daily), which has proved effective against many of the causative pseudomonas strains. To avoid relapse, antibiotic therapy should be continued, even in the asymptomatic patient, until gallium scanning indicates a marked reduction in the inflammatory process. Surgical debridement of infected bone is reserved for cases of deterioration despite medical therapy.

6. Exostoses & Osteomas

Bony overgrowths of the ear canal are a frequent incidental finding and occasionally have clinical significance. Clinically, they present as skin-covered mounds in the medial ear canal obscuring the tympanic membrane to a variable degree. Solitary osteomas are of no significance as long as they do not cause obstruction or infection. Multiple exostoses, which are generally acquired from repeated exposure to cold water, often progress and require surgical removal.

Wong BJ et al: Prevalence of external auditory canal exostoses in surfers. Arch Otolaryngol Head Neck Surg 1999;125:969. [PMID: 10488981] (Prolonged and frequent water exposure contributes to exostosis formation.)

7. Neoplasia

The most common neoplasm of the ear canal is squamous cell carcinoma. When an apparent otitis externa does not resolve on therapy, this should be suspected and biopsy performed. This disease carries a very high 5-year mortality rate because the tumor tends to invade the lymphatics of the cranial base and must be treated with wide surgical resection and radiation therapy. Adenomatous tumors, originating from the ceruminous glands, generally follow a more indolent course.

Barrs DM: Temporal bone carcinoma. Otolaryngol Clin North Am 2001;34:1197. [PMID: 11728941]

Roland PS: Chronic external otitis. Ear Nose Throat J 2001;80(6 Suppl):12. [PMID: 11488077]

DISEASES OF THE AUDITORY TUBE

1. Auditory Tube Dysfunction

The tube that connects the middle ear to the nasopharynx— the auditory tube, or eustachian tube - provides ventilation and drainage for the middle ear cleft. It is normally closed, opening only during the act of swallowing or yawning. When auditory tube function is compromised, air trapped within the middle ear becomes absorbed and negative pressure results. The most common causes of auditory tube dysfunction are diseases associated with edema of the tubal lining, such as viral upper respiratory tract infections and allergy. The patient usually reports a sense of fullness in the ear and mild to moderate impairment of hearing. When the tube is only partially blocked, swallowing or yawning may elicit a popping or crackling sound. Examination reveals retraction of the tympanic membrane and decreased mobility on pneumatic otoscopy. Following a viral illness, this disorder is usually transient, lasting days to weeks. Treatment with systemic and intranasal decongestants (eg, pseudoephedrine, 60 mg orally every 4 hours; oxymetazoline, 0.05% spray every 8–12 hours) combined with autoinflation by forced exhalation against closed nostrils may hasten relief. Autoinflation should not be recommended to patients with active intranasal infection, since this maneuver may precipitate middle ear infection. Allergic patients may also benefit from desensitization or intranasal corticosteroids (eg, beclomethasone dipropionate, two sprays in each nostril twice daily for 2–6 weeks). Air travel, rapid altitudinal change, and underwater diving should be avoided.

An overly patent auditory tube is a relatively uncommon problem that may be quite distressing. Typical complaints include fullness in the ear and autophony, an exaggerated ability to hear oneself breathe and speak. A patulous auditory tube may develop during rapid weight loss, or may be idiopathic. In contrast to a hypofunctioning auditory tube, the aural pressure is often made worse by exertion and may diminish during an upper respiratory tract infection. Although physical examination is usually normal, respiratory excursions of the tympanic membrane may occasionally be detected during vigorous breathing. Treatment includes avoidance of decongestant products, insertion of a ventilating tube to reduce the outward stretch of the ear drum during phonation, and, rarely, surgical narrowing of the auditory tube.

Derebery MJ et al: Allergic eustachian tube dysfunction: Diagnosis and treatment. Am J Otol 1997;18:160. [PMID: 9093670] (Patients who do not respond well to conventional pharmacotherapy may benefit from specific allergic therapy.)

Monsell EM et al: Eustachian tube dysfunction. Otolaryngol Clin North Am 1996;29:437. [PMID: 8743342] (Management of both hypo- and hyperfunction.)

2. Serous Otitis Media

When the auditory tube remains blocked for a prolonged period, the resultant negative pressure will result in transudation of fluid. This condition, known as serous otitis media, is especially common in children because their auditory tubes are narrower and more horizontal in orientation than adults. It is less common in adults, in whom it usually follows an upper respiratory tract infection or barotrauma. In an adult with persistent unilateral serous otitis media, nasopharyngeal carcinoma must be excluded. The tympanic membrane in serous otitis media is dull and hypomobile, occasionally accompanied by air bubbles in the middle ear and conductive hearing loss. The treatment of serous otitis media is similar to that for auditory tube dysfunction. A short course of oral corticosteroids (eg, prednisone, 40 mg/d for 7 days) has been advocated by some in the management of serous otitis media, as have oral antibiotics (eg, amoxicillin, 250 mg orally three times daily for 7 days)—or even a combination of the two. The role of these regimens remains controversial, but they are probably of little lasting benefit.

When medication fails to bring relief after several months, a ventilating tube placed through the tympanic membrane may restore hearing and alleviate the sense of aural fullness.

Morris MS: Tympanostomy tubes: types, indications, techniques, and complications. Otolaryngol Clin North Am 1999;32:385. [PMID: 10393774]

Slack R et al: Current management of glue ear. Practitioner 1998;242:455. [PMID: 10492959]

3. Barotrauma

Individuals with auditory tube dysfunction due either to congenital narrowness or to acquired mucosal edema may be unable to equalize the barometric stress exerted on the middle ear by air travel, rapid altitudinal change, or underwater diving. The problem is generally most acute during airplane descent, since the negative middle ear pressure tends to collapse and lock the auditory tube. Several measures are useful to enhance auditory tube function and avoid otic barotrauma. The patient should be advised to swallow, yawn, and autoinflate frequently during descent, which may be painful if the auditory tube collapses. Systemic decongestants (eg, pseudoephedrine, 60–120 mg) should be taken several hours before anticipated arrival time so that they will be maximally effective during descent. Topical decongestants such as 1% phenylephrine nasal spray should be administered 1 hour before arrival.

The treatment of acute negative middle ear pressure that persists on the ground is with decongestants and attempts at autoinflation. Myringotomy (creation of a small eardrum perforation) provides immediate relief and is appropriate in the setting of severe otalgia and hearing loss. Repeated episodes of barotrauma in persons who must fly frequently may be alleviated by insertion of ventilating tubes.

Underwater diving represents even a greater barometric stress to the ear than flying. The problem occurs most commonly during the descent phase, when pain develops within the first 15 feet if inflation of the middle ear via the auditory tube has not occurred. Divers must descend slowly and equilibrate in stages to avoid the development of severely negative pressures in the tympanum that may result in hemorrhage (hemotympanum) or perilymphatic fistulization. In the latter, the oval or round window ruptures, resulting in sensory hearing loss and acute vertigo. Emesis due to acute labyrinthine dysfunction can be very dangerous during an underwater dive. Sensory hearing loss or vertigo, which develops during the ascent phase of a saturation dive, may be the first (or only) symptom of decompression sickness. Immediate recompression will return intravascular gas bubbles to solution and restore the inner ear microcirculation. Patients should be warned to avoid diving when they have upper respiratory infections or episodes of nasal allergy. Tympanic membrane perforation is an absolute contraindication to diving, as the patient will experience an unbalanced thermal stimulus to the semicircular canals and may experience vertigo, disorientation, and even emesis. Finally, individuals with only one hearing ear should be discouraged from diving because of the significant risk of otologic injury.

Becker GD et al: Barotrauma of the ears and sinuses after scuba diving. Eur Arch Otorhinolaryngol 2001;258:159. [PMID: 11407445]

Newbegin C et al: Ear barotrauma after flying and diving. Practitioner 2000;244:96. [PMID: 10892042]

DISEASES OF THE MIDDLE EAR

1. Acute Otitis Media

Acute otitis media is a bacterial infection of the mucosally lined air-containing spaces of the temporal bone. Purulent material forms not only within the middle ear cleft but also within the mastoid air cells and petrous apex when they are pneumatized. Acute otitis media is usually precipitated by a viral upper respiratory tract infection that causes auditory tube edema. This results in accumulation of fluid and mucus, which becomes secondarily infected by bacteria. The most common pathogens both in adults and in children are *Streptococcus pneumoniae, Haemophilus influenzae,* and *Streptococcus pyogenes.*

Acute otitis media is most common in infants and children, though it may occur at any age. The patient presents with otalgia, aural pressure, decreased hearing, and often fever. The typical physical findings are erythema and decreased mobility of the tympanic membrane. Occasionally, bullae will be seen on the tympanic membrane. Although it is taught that this represents infection with *Mycoplasma pneumoniae,* most cases involve more common pathogens.

Rarely, when middle ear empyema is severe, the tympanic membrane can be seen to bulge outward. In such cases, tympanic membrane rupture is imminent. Rupture is accompanied by a sudden decrease in pain, followed by the onset of otorrhea. With appropriate therapy, spontaneous healing of the tympanic membrane occurs in most cases. When perforation persists, chronic otitis media frequently evolves. Mastoid tenderness often accompanies acute otitis media and is due to the presence of pus within the mastoid air cells. This alone does not indicate suppurative (surgical) mastoiditis.

The treatment of acute otitis media is specific antibiotic therapy, often combined with nasal decongestants. The first-choice antibiotic treatment is either amoxicillin (20–40 mg/kg/d) or erythromycin (50 mg/kg/d) plus sulfonamide (150 mg/kg/d) for 10 days. Alternatives useful in resistant cases are cefaclor (20–40 mg/kg/d) or amoxicillin-clavulanate (20–40 mg/kg/d) combinations.

Tympanocentesis for bacterial (aerobic and anaerobic) and fungal culture may be performed by any experienced physician. A 20-gauge spinal needle bent 90 degrees to the hub attached to a 3 mL syringe is inserted through the inferior portion of the tympanic membrane. Interposition of a pliable connecting tube between the needle and syringe permits an assistant to aspirate without inducing movement of the needle. Tympanocentesis is useful for otitis media in immunocompromised patients and when infection persists or recurs despite multiple courses of antibiotics.

Surgical drainage of the middle ear (myringotomy) is reserved for patients with severe otalgia or when complications of otitis (eg, mastoiditis, meningitis) have occurred.

Recurrent acute otitis media may be managed with long-term antibiotic prophylaxis. Single daily doses of sulfamethoxazole (500 mg) or amoxicillin (250 or 500 mg) are given over a period of 1–3 months. Failure of this regimen to control infection is an indication for insertion of ventilating tubes.

Aronovitz GH: Antimicrobial therapy of acute otitis media: review of treatment recommendations. Clin Ther 2000;22: 29. [PMID: 10688388]

Pelton SI et al: The promise of immunoprophylaxis for prevention of acute otitis media. Pediatr Infect Dis J 1999;18:926. [PMID: 10530543]

Pichichero ME: Acute otitis media: Part I. Improving diagnostic accuracy. Am Fam Phys 2000;61:2051. [PMID: 10779248]

2. Chronic Otitis Media & Cholesteatoma

Chronic infection of the middle ear and mastoid generally develops as a consequence of recurrent acute otitis media, although it may follow other diseases and trauma. Perforation of the tympanic membrane is usually present. This may be accompanied by mucosal changes such as polypoid degeneration and granulation tissue and osseous changes such as osteitis and sclerosis. The bacteriology of chronic otitis media differs from that of acute otitis media. Common organisms include *P aeruginosa*, proteus species, *Staphylococcus aureus*, and mixed anaerobic infections. The clinical hallmark of chronic otitis media is purulent aural discharge. Drainage may be continuous or intermittent, with increased severity during upper respiratory tract infection or following water exposure. Pain is uncommon except during acute exacerbations. Conductive hearing loss results from destruction of the tympanic membrane and ossicular chain. The medical treatment of chronic otitis media includes regular removal of infected debris, use of earplugs to protect against water exposure, and topical antibiotic drops for exacerbations. The activity of ciprofloxacin against pseudomonas may help to dry a chronically discharging ear when given in a dosage of 500 mg orally twice a day for 1–6 weeks.

Definitive management is surgical in most cases. Tympanic membrane repair may be accomplished with temporalis muscle fascia or with homograft middle ear structures. Successful reconstruction of the tympanic membrane may be achieved in about 90% of cases, often with elimination of infection and significant improvement in hearing. When the mastoid air cells are involved by irreversible infection, they should be exenterated through mastoidectomy.

Cholesteatoma is a special variety of chronic otitis media. The most common cause is prolonged auditory tube dysfunction, with resultant chronic negative middle ear pressure that draws inward the upper flaccid portion of the tympanic membrane. This creates a squamous epithelium-lined sac, which—when its neck becomes obstructed—may fill with desquamated keratin and become chronically infected. Cholesteatomas typically erode bone, with early penetration of the

mastoid and destruction of the ossicular chain. Over time they may erode the inner ear, involve the facial nerve, and on rare occasions spread intracranially. Physical examination reveals an epitympanic retraction pocket or marginal tympanic membrane perforation that exudes keratin debris. The treatment of cholesteatoma is surgical marsupialization of the sac or its complete removal. This often requires creation of a "mastoid bowl" in which the ear canal and mastoid are joined into a large common cavity that must be periodically cleaned.

Hamilton J: Current trends in managing chronic middle ear disease. Hosp Med 2001;62:673. [PMID: 11762097]

Holten KB et al: Management of the patient with otitis externa. J Fam Pract 2001;50:353. [PMID:11300988]

Indudharan R et al: Antibiotics in chronic suppurative otitis media: a bacteriologic study. Ann Otol Rhinol Laryngol 1999;108:440. [PMID: 10335703] (Among the available topical antibiotic preparations, ciprofloxacin and gentamicin appear to be the best choices.)

Sakagami M et al: Long-term observation on hearing change in patients with chronic otitis media. Auris Nasus Larynx 2000;27:117. [PMID: 10733188] (Early operation improves long-term hearing prognosis.)

3. Complications of Otitis Media

Mastoiditis

Acute suppurative mastoiditis usually evolves following several weeks of inadequately treated acute otitis media. It is characterized by postauricular pain and erythema accompanied by a spiking fever. Radiography reveals coalescence of the mastoid air cells due to destruction of their bony septa. Initial treatment consists of intravenous antibiotics and myringotomy for culture and drainage. Failure of medical therapy indicates the need for surgical drainage (mastoidectomy).

Lee ES et al: Clinical experiences with acute mastoiditis—1988 through 1998. Ear Nose Throat J 2000;79:884. [PMID: 11107691]

Petrous Apicitis

The medial portion of the petrous bone between the inner ear and clivus may become a site of persistent infection when the drainage of its pneumatic cell tracts becomes blocked. This may cause foul discharge, deep ear and retro-orbital pain, and sixth nerve palsy (Gradenigo's syndrome); meningitis may be a complication. Treatment is with prolonged antibiotic therapy (based on culture results) and surgical drainage via petrous apicectomy.

Otogenic Skull Base Osteomyelitis

Infections originating in the external or middle ear may result in osteomyelitis of the skull base, usually due to *P aeruginosa*. The diagnosis and management of this disease are discussed in the section on malignant external otitis.

Facial Paralysis

Facial palsy may be associated with either acute or chronic otitis media. In the acute setting, it results from inflammation of the seventh nerve in its middle ear segment, perhaps mediated through bacterially secreted neurotoxins. Treatment consists of myringotomy for drainage and culture, followed by intravenous antibiotics (based on culture results). The use of corticosteroids is controversial. The prognosis is excellent, with complete recovery in the vast majority of cases.

Facial palsy associated with chronic otitis media usually evolves slowly due to chronic pressure on the seventh nerve in the middle ear or mastoid by cholesteatoma. Treatment requires surgical correction of the underlying disease. The prognosis is less favorable than for facial palsy associated with acute otitis media.

White N et al: Facial paralysis secondary to acute otitis media. Pediatr Emerg Care 2000;16:343. [PMID: 11063365]

Sigmoid Sinus Thrombosis

Trapped infection within the mastoid air cells adjacent to the sigmoid sinus may cause septic thrombophlebitis. This is heralded by signs of systemic sepsis (spiking fevers, chills), at times accompanied by signs of increased intracranial pressure (headache, lethargy, nausea and vomiting, papilledema). Diagnosis can be made noninvasively by magnetic resonance venography. Treatment is with intravenous antibiotics (based on culture results), surgical drainage, and—when embolization is suspected—ligation of the internal jugular vein in the neck.

Syms MJ et al: Management of lateral sinus thrombosis. Laryngoscope 1999;109:1616. [PMID: 10522931] (Conservative operation and intravenous antibiotics are usually successful.)

Central Nervous System Infection

Otogenic meningitis is by far the most common intracranial complication of ear infection. In the setting of acute suppurative otitis media, it arises from hematogenous spread of bacteria, most commonly *H influenzae* and *S pneumoniae*. In chronic otitis media, it results either from passage of infections along preformed pathways such as the petrosquamous suture line or from direct extension of disease through the dural plates of the petrous pyramid.

Epidural abscesses arise from direct extension of disease in the setting of chronic infection. They are usually asymptomatic but may present with deep local pain, headache, and low-grade fever. They are often discovered as an incidental finding at surgery. Brain abscess may arise in the temporal lobe or cerebellum as a result of septic thrombophlebitis adjacent to an epidural abscess. The predominant causative organisms are *S aureus, S pyogenes,* and *S pneumoniae.* Rupture into the subarachnoid space results in meningitis and often death.

Osma U et al: The complications of chronic otitis media: report of 93 cases. J Laryngol Otol 2000;114:97. [PMID: 10748823] (In developing nations, intracranial complications still result in a 26% mortality rate.)

Sennaroglu L et al: Otogenic brain abscess: review of 41 cases. Otolaryngol Head Neck Surg 2000;123:751. [PMID: 112974]

4. Otosclerosis

Otosclerosis is a progressive disease with a marked familial tendency that affects bone surrounding the inner ear. Lesions involving the footplate of the stapes result in increased impedance to the passage of sound through the ossicular chain, producing conductive hearing loss. This may be corrected through surgical replacement of the stapes with a prosthesis (stapedectomy). When otosclerotic lesions impinge on the cochlea, permanent sensory hearing loss occurs. Some evidence suggests that this level of hearing loss may be stabilized by treatment with oral sodium fluoride over prolonged periods of time (Florical—8.3 mg sodium fluoride and 364 mg calcium carbonate—two tablets orally each morning). Fluorides have minimal adverse effects other than occasional mild gastric irritation, which may be eliminated by ingesting the drug with meals.

Chole RA et al: Pathophysiology of otosclerosis. Otol Neurotol 2001;22:249. [PMID: 11300278]

de Bruijn AJ et al: Efficacy of evaluation of audiometric results after stapes surgery in otosclerosis. The effects of using different audiologic parameters and criteria on success rates. Otolaryngol Head Neck Surg 2001;124:76. [PMID: 11228458]

5. Trauma to the Middle Ear

Tympanic membrane perforation may result from impact injury or explosive acoustic trauma. Spontaneous healing occurs in the great majority of cases. Persistent perforation may result from secondary infection brought on by exposure to water. Patients should be advised to wear earplugs while swimming or bathing during the healing period. Hemorrhage behind an intact tympanic membrane (hemotympanum) may follow blunt trauma or extreme barotrauma. Spontaneous resolution over several weeks is the usual course. When a conductive hearing loss greater than 30 dB persists for more than 3 months following trauma, disruption of the ossicular chain should be suspected. Middle ear exploration with reconstruction of the ossicular chain, combined with repair of the tympanic membrane when required, will usually restore hearing.

Brodie HA et al: Management of complications from 820 temporal bone fractures. Am J Otol 1997;18:188. [PMID: 9093676]

6. Middle Ear Neoplasia

Primary middle ear tumors are rare. Glomus tumors arise either in the middle ear (glomus tympanicum) or in the jugular bulb with upward erosion into the hypotympanum (glomus jugulare). They present clinically with pulsatile tinnitus and hearing loss. A vascular mass may be visible behind an intact tympanic membrane. Large glomus jugulare tumors are often associated with multiple cranial neuropathies, especially involving nerves VII, IX, X, XI, and XII. Treatment may require surgery, radiotherapy, or both.

Jackler RK, Driscoll C: *Tumors of the Ear and Temporal Bone.* Lippincott Williams & Wilkins, 2000.

EARACHE

External otitis and acute otitis media are the two most common causes of earache. In external otitis, there is often a recent history of swimming, Q-tip use, or physical trauma, while in acute otitis media there is usually an antecedent or concurrent upper respiratory infection. The physical findings also differ. In external otitis, the ear canal skin is erythematous, while in acute otitis media this generally occurs only if the tympanic membrane has ruptured, spilling purulent material into the ear canal. Also, in external otitis the tympanic membrane may be erythematous, but it retains its mobility owing to the normal aeration of the middle ear cavity. Pain out of proportion to the physical findings may be due to herpes zoster oticus, especially when vesicles appear in the ear canal or concha. Chronic otitis media is usually not painful except during acute exacerbations. Persistent pain and discharge from the ear suggest osteomyelitis of the skull base or cancer.

The sensory innervation of the ear is derived from the trigeminal, facial, glossopharyngeal, vagal, and upper cervical nerves. Because of this rich innervation, referred otalgia is quite frequent. Temporomandibular joint dysfunction is a common cause of ear pain. It is often made worse by chewing or psychogenic grinding of the teeth (bruxism) and may be associated with dental malocclusion. Management includes soft diet, local heat to the masticatory muscles, massage, analgesics, and dental referral. Repeated episodes of severe lancinating otalgia may occur in glossopharyngeal neuralgia. Treatment with carbamazepine (100–300 mg orally every 8 hours) often confers substantial symptomatic relief. Severe glossopharyngeal neuralgia, which is refractory to medical management, may respond to microvascular decompression of the ninth nerve. Infections and neoplasia that involve the oropharynx, hypopharynx, and larynx frequently cause otalgia. Persistent earache demands specialty referral to exclude cancer of the upper aerodigestive tract.

Kuttila S et al: Aural symptoms and signs of temporomandibular disorder in association with treatment need and visits to a physician. Laryngoscope 1999;109:1669. [PMID: 10522940] (Temporomandibular joint dysfunction is the most common nonotologic cause of otalgia.)

Leonetti JP et al: An isolated symptom of malignant infratemporal tumors. Am J Otol 1998;19:486. [PMID: 9661761] (Emphasizes that unexplained chronic ear pain may be a symptom of occult malignancy.)

DISEASES OF THE INNER EAR

1. Sensory Hearing Loss

Diseases of the cochlea result in sensory hearing loss, a condition that is usually irreversible. Most cochlear diseases result in bilateral symmetric hearing loss. The presence of unilateral or asymmetric sensorineural hearing loss suggests a lesion proximal to the cochlea. Lesions affecting the eighth nerve and central auditory system are discussed in the section on neural hearing loss. The primary goals in the management of sensory hearing loss are prevention of further losses and functional improvement with amplification and auditory rehabilitation.

Presbyacusis

Presbyacusis, the most frequent cause of sensory hearing loss, is the progressive, predominantly high-frequency symmetric hearing loss of advancing age. It is difficult to separate the various etiologic factors (eg, noise trauma) that may contribute to presbyacusis, but genetic predisposition appears to play a role. Most patients notice a loss of speech discrimination that is especially pronounced in noisy environments. About 25% of people between the ages of 65 and 75 years and almost 50% of those over 75 experience hearing difficulties.

Fook L et al: Hearing impairment in older people: a review. Postgrad Med J 2000;76:537. [PMID: 10964114]

Willot JF et al: Modulation of presbycusis: current status and future directions. Audiol Neurootol 2001;6:231. [PMID: 11729326]

Noise Trauma

Noise trauma is the second most common cause of sensory hearing loss. Sounds exceeding 85 dB are potentially injurious to the cochlea, especially with prolonged exposures. The loss typically begins in the high frequencies (especially 4000 Hz) and progresses to involve the speech frequencies with continuing exposure. Among the more common sources of injurious noise are industrial machinery, weapons, and excessively loud music. In recent years, monitoring of noise levels in the workplace by regulatory agencies has led to preventive programs that have reduced the frequency of occupational losses. Individuals of all ages, especially those with existing hearing losses, should wear earplugs when exposed to moderately loud noises and specially designed earmuffs when exposed to explosive noises.

May JJ: Occupational hearing loss. Am J Industrial Med 2000; 37:112. [PMID: 10573600]

Physical Trauma

Head trauma has effects on the inner ear similar to those of severe acoustic trauma. Some degree of sensory hearing loss may occur following simple concussion and is frequent after skull fracture. Deployment of air bags during an automobile accident has been associated with hearing loss.

Yaremchuk K et al: Otologic injuries from airbag deployment. Otolaryngol Head Neck Surg 2001;125:130. [PMID: 11555742]

Ototoxicity

Ototoxic substances may affect both the auditory and vestibular systems. The most common ototoxic medications are salicylates, aminoglycosides, loop diuretics, and several antineoplastic agents, notably cisplatin. The latter three categories may cause irreversible hearing loss even when administered in therapeutic doses. When using these medications, it is important to identify high-risk patients such as those with preexisting hearing losses or renal insufficiency. Patients simultaneously receiving multiple ototoxic agents are at particular risk owing to ototoxic synergy. Useful measures to reduce the risk of ototoxic injury include serial audiometry and monitoring of serum peak and trough levels and substitution of equivalent nonototoxic drugs whenever possible.

It is possible for topical agents that enter the middle ear to be absorbed into the inner ear via the round window. When the tympanic membrane is perforated, use of potentially ototoxic ear drops (eg, neomycin, gentamicin) is best avoided.

Palomar Garcia V et al: Drug-induced otoxicity: current status. Acta Otolaryngol 2001;121:569. [PMID: 11583387]

Tange RA: Eardrops and aminoglycoside ototoxicity revisited. Adverse Drug React Toxicol Rev 2001;20:164. [PMID: 11668866]

Sudden Sensory Hearing Loss

Sudden loss of hearing in one ear may occur at any age but is more common in the elderly. It most probably is the result of sudden vascular occlusion of the internal auditory artery or of a viral inner ear infection. Prognosis is mixed, with many patients suffering permanent deafness in the involved ear while others have complete recovery. Although the subject is controversial, oral corticosteroids are felt by many to improve the odds of recovery. A common regimen is prednisone, 80 mg/d, followed by a tapering dose over a 10-day period.

Haberkamp TJ et al: Management of idiopathic sudden sensorineural hearing loss. Am J Otol 1999;20:587. [PMID: 10503580]

Hereditary Hearing Loss

Sensory hearing loss with onset during adult life often runs in families. The mode of inheritance may be either autosomal dominant or recessive. The age at onset, the rate of progression of hearing loss, and the audiometric pattern (high-frequency, low-frequency, or flat) can often be predicted by studying family members. In recent years, great strides have been made in identifying the molecular genetic errors associated with hereditary hearing loss, and several dozen specific mutations have now been characterized.

Petit C et al: Molecular genetics of hearing loss. Annu Rev Genet 2001;35:589.

Tekin M et al: Advances in hereditary deafness. Lancet 2001; 358:1082. [PMID: 11589958]

Autoimmune Hearing Loss

Sensory hearing loss may be associated with a wide array of systemic autoimmune disorders such as systemic lupus erythematosus, Wegener's granulomatosis, and Cogan's syndrome (hearing loss, keratitis, aortitis). The loss is most often bilateral and progressive. The hearing level often fluctuates, with periods of deterioration alternating with partial or even complete remission. The tendency is for the gradual evolution of permanent hearing loss, which usually stabilizes with some remaining auditory function but occasionally proceeds to complete deafness. Vestibular dysfunction, particularly dysequilibrium and postural instability, may accompany the auditory symptoms. A syndrome resembling Meniere's disease may also occur with intermittent attacks of severe vertigo.

In the majority of cases, the autoimmune pattern of audiovestibular dysfunction presents in the absence of recognized systemic autoimmune disease. Use of laboratory tests to screen for autoimmune disease (eg, antinuclear antibody, rheumatoid factor, erythrocyte sedimentation rate) may be informative. Specific tests of immune reactivity against inner ear antigens (anticochlear antibodies, lymphocyte transformation tests) are available but are currently of interest for research purposes only. Responsiveness to oral corticosteroid treatment is helpful in making the diagnosis and constitutes first-line therapy. If stabilization of hearing becomes dependent on long term corticosteroid use, steroid-sparing immunosuppressive regimens (eg, methotrexate, 7.5 mg three times a week) may become necessary.

Rahman MU et al: Autoimmune vestibulo-cochlear disorders. Curr Opin Rheumatol 2001;13:184. [PMID: 11333346]

Raut VV et al: Hearing loss in rheumatoid arthritis. J Otolaryngol 2001;30:289.

Other Causes of Sensory Hearing Loss

There are numerous less common causes of sensory hearing loss. Metabolic derangements (eg, diabetes, hypothyroidism, hyperlipidemia, and renal failure), infections (eg, measles, mumps, syphilis), and physical factors (eg, radiation therapy) are some of the chief examples. Identification of metabolic or infectious sensory hearing losses is especially important, as these may occasionally be reversible with medical therapy. Meniere's syndrome and labyrinthitis are discussed in the section on vestibular disorders.

Duck SW et al: Interaction between hypertension and diabetes mellitus in the pathogenesis of sensorineural hearing loss. Laryngoscope 1997;107(12 Part 1):1596. [PMID: 9396671] (Both animal and human studies implicate these as potential causes of inner ear decline.)

2. Tinnitus

Tinnitus is the perception of abnormal ear or head noises. Persistent tinnitus usually indicates the presence of sensory hearing loss. Intermittent periods of mild, high-pitched tinnitus lasting for several minutes are common in normal-hearing persons. When severe and persistent, tinnitus may interfere with sleep and the ability to concentrate, resulting in considerable psychologic distress.

The most important treatment of tinnitus is avoidance of exposure to excessive noise, ototoxic agents, and other factors that may cause cochlear damage. Masking the tinnitus with music or through amplification of normal sounds with a hearing aid may also bring some relief. Although intravenous treatment with antiarrhythmic drugs (eg, lidocaine) suppresses tinnitus in some individuals, evidence suggests no benefit with oral agents that are potentially suitable for long-term symptom relief. Among the numerous drugs that have been tried, oral antidepressants (eg, nortriptyline at an initial dosage of 50 mg orally at bedtime) have proved to be the most efficacious.

Pulsatile tinnitus—often described by the patient as listening to one's own heartbeat—should be distinguished from tonal tinnitus. Though often ascribed to conductive hearing loss, this symptom may be far more serious and indicates a vascular abnormality such as glomus tumor, carotid vaso-occlusive disease, arteriovenous malformation, or aneurysm. MR angiography should be considered to establish the diagnosis.

A staccato "clicking" tinnitus may result from middle ear muscle spasm, sometimes associated with palatal myoclonus. The patient typically perceives a rapid series of popping noises, lasting seconds to a few minutes, accompanied by a fluttering feeling in the ear.

Jastreboff PJ et al: Tinnitus Retraining Therapy (TRT) as a method for treatment of tinnitus and hyperacusis patients. J Am Acad Audiol 2000;11:162. [PMID: 10755812] (A neurophysiologically based therapy to improve coping with troublesome tinnitus.)

Laurikainen E et al: Treatment of severe tinnitus. Acta Otolaryngol Suppl 2000;543:77. [PMID: 10908984]

3. Hyperacusis

Excessive sensitivity to sound may occur in normal-hearing individuals either for psychologic reasons or in association with ear disease. Patients with cochlear dysfunction commonly experience recruitment, an abnormal sensitivity to loud sounds despite a reduced sensitivity to softer ones. Fitting hearing aids and other amplification devices to patients with recruitment requires use of compression circuitry to avoid uncomfortable overamplification. For normal-hearing individuals with hyperacusis, use of an earplug in noisy environments is often beneficial.

Katzenell U et al: Hyperacusis: review and clinical guidelines. Otol Neurotol 2001;22:321. [PMID: 11347634]

4. Vertigo
(Table 8–1)

Vertigo is the cardinal symptom of vestibular disease. It is either a sensation of motion when there is no motion or an exaggerated sense of motion in response to a

Table 8–1. Common vestibular disorders: Differential diagnosis based on classic presentations.

Duration of Typical Vertiginous Episodes	Auditory Symptoms Present	Auditory Symptoms Absent
Seconds	Perilymphatic fistula	Positioning vertigo (cupulolithiasis), vertebrobasilar insufficiency, cervical vertigo
Hours	Endolymphatic hydrops (Meniere's syndrome, syphilis)	Recurrent vestibulopathy, vestibular migraine
Days	Labyrinthitis, labyrinthine concussion	Vestibular neuronitis
Months	Acoustic neuroma, ototoxicity	Multiple sclerosis, cerebellar degeneration

given bodily movement. Thus, vertigo is not just "spinning" but may present, for example, as a sense of tumbling, of falling forward or backward, or of the ground rolling beneath one's feet ("earthquake-like"). It should be distinguished from imbalance, light-headedness, and syncope, all of which are usually nonvestibular in origin. The vertigo that results from peripheral vestibulopathy is usually of sudden onset, may be so severe that the patient is unable to walk or stand, and is frequently accompanied by nausea and vomiting. Tinnitus and hearing loss may be associated and provide strong support for a peripheral origin.

A minimal physical examination of the patient with vertigo includes the Romberg test, an evaluation of gait, and observation for the presence of nystagmus. In peripheral lesions, nystagmus is usually horizontal with a rotatory component; the fast phase usually beats away from the diseased side. Visual fixation tends to inhibit nystagmus except in very acute peripheral lesions or with central nervous system disease. The Nylen-Bárány maneuvers are performed as follows: Put the patient in a sitting position on the examination table with the head turned to the right. Quickly lower the patient to the supine position with the head extending over the edge and placed 30 degrees lower than the body. Watch for nystagmus for 30 seconds. Repeat with the head turned to the left. Lastly, perform the maneuver without turning the head.

These maneuvers are intended to induce positioning nystagmus but are of limited use when the patient is able to visually fixate. This objection may be overcome either by placing +2-diopter lenses (Fresnel glasses) over the eyes or by making observations in the dark by means of electronystagmographic recording. The Fukuda test, in which the patient walks in place with eyes closed, is useful for detecting subtle defects. A positive response is observed when the patient rotates, usually toward the side of the diseased labyrinth. Vertigo arising from central lesions tends to develop gradually and then become progressively more severe and debilitating. Nystagmus is not always present but can occur in any direction and may be dissociated in the two eyes. The associated nystagmus is often nonfatigable, vertical rather than horizontal in orientation, without latency, and unsuppressed by visual fixation. Electronystagmography is useful in documenting these characteristics. The evaluation of central audiovestibular dysfunction usually requires imaging of the brain with MRI.

Episodic vertigo can occur in patients with diplopia from external ophthalmoplegia and is maximal when the patient looks in the direction where the separation of images is greatest. Cerebral lesions involving the temporal cortex may also produce vertigo, which is sometimes the initial symptom of a seizure. Finally, vertigo may be a feature of a number of systemic disorders and can occur as a side effect of certain anticonvulsant, antibiotic, hypnotic, analgesic, and tranquilizing drugs or of alcohol.

Laboratory investigations such as audiologic evaluation, caloric stimulation, electronystagmography, CT scan or MRI, and brain stem auditory evoked potential studies are indicated in patients with persistent vertigo or when central nervous system disease is suspected. These studies will help to distinguish between central and peripheral lesions and to identify causes requiring specific therapy. Electronystagmography consists of objective recording of the nystagmus induced by head and body movements, gaze, and caloric stimulation. It is helpful in quantifying the degree of vestibular hypofunction and may help with the differentiation between peripheral and central lesions. Computer-driven rotatory chairs and posturography platforms offer improved diagnostic abilities but are not widely available.

Bakr MS et al: Electronystagmography: how useful is it? J Laryngol 2000;114:178. [PMID: 10829104] (Useful only when the cause of dizziness is central or uncertain. Electronystagmography does not significantly aid in the diagnosis of peripheral lesions except as confirmation.)

Bath AP et al: Experience from a multidisciplinary "dizzy" clinic. Am J Otol 2000;21:92. [PMID: 10651441] (Peripheral causes predominate with fewer than 10% of cases having a CNS cause.)

Hanley K et al: A systematic review of vertigo in primary care. Br J Gen Pract 2001;51:666. [PMID: 11510399]

Magnusson M et al: Peripheral vestibular disorders with acute onset of vertigo. Curr Opin Neurol 2002;15:5. [PMID: 11796944]

Oas JG: Benign paroxysmal positional vertigo: a clinician's perspective. Ann N Y Acad Sci 2001;942:201. [PMID: 11710462]

Vertigo Syndromes Due to Peripheral Lesions

A. ENDOLYMPHATIC HYDROPS (MENIERE'S SYNDROME)

Meniere's syndrome results from distention of the endolymphatic compartment of the inner ear. The primary lesion appears to be in the endolymphatic sac, which is thought to be responsible for endolymph filtration and excretion. Although a precise cause of hydrops cannot be established in most cases, two known causes are syphilis and head trauma. The classic syndrome consists of episodic vertigo, usually lasting 1–8 hours; low-frequency sensorineural hearing loss, often fluctuating; tinnitus, usually low-tone and "blowing" in quality; and a sensation of aural pressure. Symptoms wax and wane as the endolymphatic pressure rises and falls. Caloric testing commonly reveals loss or impairment of thermally induced nystagmus on the involved side.

Episodic vertigo resembling that of Meniere's syndrome but without accompanying auditory symptoms is known as recurrent vestibulopathy. The pathogenic mechanism of this symptom complex is unknown in most cases, though a few patients suffer from a variant of migraine. Others will go on to develop the classic syndrome of endolymphatic hydrops.

B. LABYRINTHITIS

Patients with labyrinthitis suffer from acute onset of continuous, usually severe vertigo lasting several days to a week, accompanied by hearing loss and tinnitus. During a recovery period that lasts for several weeks, rapid head movements may bring on transient vertigo. Hearing may return to normal or remain permanently impaired in the involved ear. The cause of labyrinthitis is unknown, although it frequently follows an upper respiratory tract infection.

C. POSITIONING VERTIGO

This form of vertigo is usually peripheral in origin. Transient vertigo following changes in head position is a frequent complaint. The term "positioning vertigo" is more accurate than "positional vertigo" because it is provoked by changes in head position rather than by the maintenance of a particular posture. Use of the term "*benign* positional vertigo" is discouraged except for cases known to be unassociated with central nervous system disorders. True positional vertigo suggests either vertebrobasilar insufficiency or dysfunction of the cervical spine.

The typical symptoms of positioning vertigo occur in clusters that persist for several days. Typically with peripheral lesions, there is a latency period of several seconds following a head movement before symptoms develop, and they subside within 10–60 seconds. Constant repetition of the positional change leads to habituation. In central lesions, there is no latent period, fatigability, or habituation of the sign and symptoms. Single-session physical therapy protocols, based on the theory that peripheral positioning vertigo results from free-floating otoconia within a semicircular canal, have recently been developed. These strive to reposition the offending crystals through a series of head manipulations. New surgical procedures are also being explored which, by interrupting the posterior semicircular canal, attempt to prevent the exaggerated response to angular head motion.

D. VESTIBULAR NEURONITIS

In vestibular neuronitis, a paroxysmal, usually single attack of vertigo occurs without accompanying impairment of auditory function and may persist for several days to weeks before clearing. Examination reveals nystagmus and absent responses to caloric stimulation on one or both sides. The cause of the disorder is unclear. Treatment is symptomatic.

E. TRAUMATIC VERTIGO

The most common cause of vertigo following head injury is labyrinthine concussion. Symptoms generally diminish within several days but may linger for a month or more. Basilar skull fractures that traverse the inner ear usually result in severe vertigo lasting several days to a week and deafness in the involved ear.

Chronic posttraumatic vertigo may result from cupulolithiasis. This occurs when traumatically detached statoconia (otoconia) settle on the ampulla of the posterior semicircular canal and cause an excessive degree of cupular deflection in response to head motion. Clinically, this presents as episodic positioning vertigo.

F. PERILYMPHATIC FISTULA

Leakage of perilymphatic fluid from the inner ear into the tympanic cavity via the round or oval window is often discussed as a cause of vertigo and sensory hearing loss but is actually very rare. Most cases result from either physical injury (eg, blunt head trauma, hand slap to ear), extreme barotrauma during airflight, scuba diving, etc, or vigorous Valsalva maneuver (eg, during weight lifting). Treatment may require middle ear exploration and window sealing with a tissue graft; however, this is seldom indicated without a clear-cut history of a precipitating traumatic event.

G. CERVICAL VERTIGO

Position receptors located in the facets of the cervical spine are important physiologically in the coordination of head and eye movements. Cervical proprioceptive dysfunction is a common cause of vertigo triggered by neck movements. This disturbance often commences after neck injury, particularly hyperextension. An association also exists with degenerative cervical spine disease. Although symptoms vary, vertigo may be triggered by assuming a particular head position as opposed to moving to a new head position (the latter typical of labyrinthine dysfunction). Management consists of neck movement exercises to the extent permitted by orthopedic considerations.

Friedland DR et al: A critical appraisal of spontaneous perilymphatic fistulas of the inner ear. Am J Otol 1999;20:261. [PMID: 10100535] (Most experts consider perilymphatic fistula to be an overdiagnosed entity.)

Furman JM et al: Benign paroxysmal positional vertigo. N Engl J Med 1999;341:1590. [PMID: 10564690]

Kotimaki J et al: Prognosis of hearing impairment in Meniere's disease. Acta Otolaryngol Suppl 2001;545:14. [PMID: 11677728]

Thai-Van H et al: Meniere's disease: pathophysiology and treatment. Drugs 2001;61:1089. [PMID: 11465871]

Vertigo Syndromes Due to Central Lesions

Central nervous system causes of vertigo include brain stem vascular disease, arteriovenous malformations, tumor of the brain stem and cerebellum, multiple sclerosis, and vertebrobasilar migraine. Vertigo of central origin often becomes unremitting and disabling. The associated nystagmus is often nonfatigable, vertical rather than horizontal in orientation, without latency, and unsuppressed by visual fixation. Electronystagmography is useful in documenting these characteristics. There are commonly other signs of brain stem dysfunction (eg, cranial nerve palsies; motor, sensory, or cerebellar deficits in the limbs) or of increased intracranial pressure. Auditory function is generally spared. The underlying cause should be treated.

Baloh RW: Episodic vertigo: central nervous system causes. Curr Opin Neurol 2002;15:17. [PMID: 11796946]

Management of the Patient With Vertigo

Few specific treatments for labyrinthine disorders have been designed to reverse a known pathogenic mechanism. In Meniere's disease, treatment is intended to lower endolymphatic pressure. A low-salt diet (< 2 g sodium daily), at times supplemented by diuretics, adequately controls symptoms in the great majority of patients. A typical diuretic regimen is hydrochlorothiazide, 50–100 mg daily. Other specific treatments are antibiotics as required and surgical repair of perilymphatic fistulas.

Symptomatic treatment is useful in the vertiginous patient to lessen the abnormal sensation and to alleviate vegetative symptoms such as nausea and vomiting. The most common drug classes employed are the antihistamines, anticholinergics, and sedative-hypnotics. Ample evidence exists that vestibular suppressant medications adversely affect the process of central compensation following acute vestibular disease. For this reason, these drugs should be used only for brief periods. Generally, they are best administered to patients with prominent vegetative symptoms and are best tapered and halted when symptoms are resolved, usually within 1–2 weeks.

In acute severe vertigo, vestibular suppressants such as diazepam, 2.5–5 mg sublingually, orally, or intravenously, may abate an attack. Relief from nausea and vomiting usually requires an antiemetic delivered intramuscularly or by rectal suppository (eg, prochlorperazine, 10 mg intramuscularly, or 25 mg rectally every 6 hours). Less severe vertigo may often be successfully alleviated with antihistamines such as meclizine, 25 mg, or cyclizine or dimenhydrinate, 25–50 mg, orally every 6 hours. Scopolamine, administered in low dosage transdermally (0.5 mg/d), has proved beneficial to many patients with recurrent vertigo, although side effects (dry mouth, blurred vision, urinary obstruction) often limit its utility. Sometimes employing one-half or even one-fourth of a patch may allow therapeutic effect without the usual adverse consequences. A combination of drugs sometimes helps when the response to one drug is disappointing.

Bed rest may reduce the severity of acute vertigo. Conversely, in chronic or recurrent vertigo, one of the most important therapies is exercise. Physical activity substantially enhances the central nervous system's ability to compensate for labyrinthine dysfunction and should be encouraged once nausea and vomiting have resolved. In general, the patient should be instructed to repeatedly perform maneuvers that provoke vertigo—up to the point of nausea or fatigue—in an ef-

fort to habituate them. Patients with vertigo and imbalance refractory to conventional therapy may benefit from a formal rehabilitation program under the guidance of a physical therapist. Substantial success has been reported in such patients through use of customized habituation protocols and specialized equipment, including tilt tables. Recently, use of a series of head maneuvers (theoretically intended to reposition free-floating otolithic particles) has gained popularity in the management of positioning vertigo. Such protocols have been shown to be at least as effective as vestibular habituation exercises, and they are less time-consuming.

For patients with recalcitrant vertigo or clusters of attacks, specialty referral may be useful. Prednisone has been used for clusters refractory to diuretics, low-salt diet, and vestibular suppressants.

Permanent therapy in medically refractory unilateral peripheral vestibular dysfunction is selective chemical destruction of the vestibular hair cell population by infusion of ototoxins transtympanically into the middle ear. Absorption into perilymph occurs via the round window. The most frequently used drug is gentamicin (80 mg/mL diluted 50:50 with bicarbonate), which is injected into the middle ear via a spinal needle. Results in patients with Meniere's syndrome have been impressive, with about 80–90% of patients relieved of severe episodic vertigo.

Surgical remedies are reserved for those who remain substantially disabled despite a prolonged and varied trial of medical therapy and exercises. Selective section of the vestibular portion of the eighth nerve brings relief of vertigo in over 90% of such patients. Surgical removal of the semicircular canals (labyrinthectomy) is also highly effective but is appropriate only for patients with little or no hearing in the involved ear.

Bamiou DE et al: Symptoms, disability and handicap in unilateral peripheral vestibular disorders. Effects of early presentation and initiation of balance exercises. Scand Audiol 2000; 29:238. [PMID: 11195943]

Bracher ES et al: A combined approach for the treatment of cervical vertigo. J Manipulative Physiol Ther 2000;23:96. [PMID: 10728930] (A program of exercises usually improves symptoms.)

Brantberg K et al: Symptoms, findings and treatment in patients with dehiscence of the superior semicircular canal. Acta Otolaryngol 2001;121:68. [PMID: 11270498]

Devaiah AK et al: Clinical indicators useful in predicting response to the medical management of Meniere's disease. Laryngoscope 2000;110:1861. [PMID: 11081600]

Epley JM: Human experience with canalith repositioning maneuvers. Ann N Y Acad Sci 2001;942:179. [PMID: 11710460]

Harner SG et al: Long term followup of transtympanic gentamicin for Meniere's disease. Otol Neurotol 2001;22:210. [PMID: 11300271]

Smith PF: Pharmacology of the vestibular system. Curr Opin Neurol 2000;13:31. [PMID: 10719647]

Strupp M et al: Exercise and drug therapy alter recovery from labyrinth lesion in humans. Ann N Y Acad Sci 2001; 942:79. [PMID: 11710505]

Welling DB et al: Endolymphatic mastoid shunt: a reevaluation of efficacy. Otolaryngol Head Neck Surg 2000;122:340. [PMID: 10699806] (Favorable results in selected medically refractory patients.)

DISEASES OF THE CENTRAL AUDITORY & VESTIBULAR SYSTEMS (Table 8–1)

Lesions of the eighth cranial nerve and central audiovestibular pathways produce neural hearing loss and vertigo. One characteristic of neural hearing loss is deterioration of speech discrimination out of proportion to the decrease in pure tone thresholds. Another is auditory adaptation, wherein a steady tone appears to the listener to decay and eventually disappear. Auditory evoked responses are useful in distinguishing cochlear from neural losses and may give insight into the site of lesion within the central pathways.

The evaluation of central audiovestibular dysfunction usually requires imaging of the brain with CT scans or MRI. The paramagnetic contrast agent gadolinium-DTPA, when used with MRI scanning, substantially improves diagnostic sensitivity in the detection of central audiovestibular lesions.

Davidson HC: Imaging evaluation of sensorineural hearing loss. Semin Ultrasound CT MR 2001;22:229. [PMID: 11451098]

Griffiths TD: Central auditory processing disorders. Curr Opin Neurol 2002;15:31. [PMID: 11796948]

Solomon D: Distinguishing and treating causes of central vertigo. Otolaryngol Clin North Am 2000;33:579. [PMID: 10815038]

1. Vestibular Schwannoma (Acoustic Neuroma)

Eighth nerve schwannomas are among the most common of intracranial tumors. These benign lesions arise within the internal auditory canal and gradually grow to involve the cerebellopontine angle, eventually compressing the pons and resulting in hydrocephalus. Their typical auditory symptoms are unilateral hearing loss with a deterioration of speech discrimination exceeding that predicted by the degree of pure tone loss. Nonclassic presentations, such as sudden unilateral hearing loss, are fairly common. Any individual with a unilateral or asymmetric sensorineural hearing loss should be evaluated for an intracranial mass lesion. Vestibular dysfunction more often takes the form of continuous dysequilibrium than episodic vertigo. Other lesions of the cerebellopontine angle such as meningioma and epidermoids may have similar audiovestibular manifestations. Diagnosis is made by enhanced MRI, though auditory evoked responses may have a role in screening. Microsurgical excision is most often indicated, though small tumors in older individuals may be managed with stereotactic radiotherapy or simply followed with serial imaging studies.

Daniels RL et al: Causes of unilateral sensorineural hearing loss screened by high resolution fast spin echo magnetic resonance imaging: review of 1070 consecutive cases. Am J Otol 2000;21:173. [PMID: 10733160] (Vestibular schwannoma identified in approximately 5% of those screened.)

Hoistad DL et al: Update on conservative management of acoustic neuroma. Otol Neurotol 2001;22:682. [PMID: 11568679]

Slattery WH 3rd et al: Perioperative morbidity of acoustic neuroma surgery. Otol Neurotol 2001;22:895. [PMID: 11698815]

2. Vascular Compromise

Vertebrobasilar insufficiency is a common cause of vertigo in the elderly. It is often triggered by changes in posture or extension of the neck. Reduced flow in the vertebrobasilar system may be demonstrated noninvasively through magnetic resonance angiography. Empirical treatment is with vasodilators and aspirin.

Migraine may cause vertiginous attacks. The diagnosis is obvious when vertigo accompanies a typical headache pattern, but this is not always the case. In patients with a history of both migraine headaches and recurrent vertigo, a therapeutic trial of β-adrenergic blocking drugs (propranolol, 80–240 mg orally every 12–24 hours) and ergots (ergotamine, 1 mg orally every 4–6 hours) is reasonable.

Vascular loops that impinge upon the brain stem root entry zone of cranial nerves have been shown to cause dysfunction. Widely recognized examples are hemifacial spasm and tic douloureux. It has been suggested that hearing loss, tinnitus, and disabling positioning vertigo may result from a vascular loop abutting the eighth nerve.

Neuhauser H et al: The interrelations of migraine, vertigo, and migrainous vertigo. Neurology 2001;56:436. [PMID: 11222783]

Welsh LW et al: Vertigo: analysis by magnetic resonance angiography. Ann Otol Rhinol Laryngol 2000;109:248. [PMID: 10747304] (Abnormalities of the vertebrobasilar system were detected in 52% of older adults.)

3. Multiple Sclerosis

Patients with multiple sclerosis may suffer from episodic vertigo and chronic imbalance. Hearing loss in this disease is most commonly unilateral and of rapid onset. Spontaneous recovery may occur.

Alpini D et al: Vertigo and multiple sclerosis: aspects of differential diagnosis. Neurol Sci 2001;22(Suppl 2):S84. [PMID: 11794485]

OTOLOGIC MANIFESTATIONS OF AIDS

The otologic manifestations of AIDS are protean. The pinna and external auditory canal may be affected by Kaposi's sarcoma as well as persistent and potentially invasive fungal infections, particularly due to *Aspergillus fumigatus*. The most common middle ear manifestation of AIDS is serous otitis media due to auditory tube dysfunction arising from adenoidal hypertrophy (HIV lymphadenopathy), recurrent mucosal viral infections, or an obstructing nasopharyngeal tumor (eg, lymphoma). For middle ear effusions, ventilating tubes are seldom helpful and may trigger profuse watery otorrhea. Acute otitis media is usually caused by the typical bacterial organisms that occur in nonimmunocompromised patients, though *Pneumocystis carinii* otitis has been reported. Sensorineural hearing loss is common and in some cases appears to result from viral central nervous system infection. In cases of progressive hearing loss, it is important to evaluate for cryptococcal meningitis and syphilis. Acute facial paralysis due to herpes zoster infection (Ramsay Hunt's syndrome) is quite common and follows a clinical course similar to that in nonimmunocompromised patients. Treatment is primarily with high-dose acyclovir. Corticosteroids may also be effective.

Chandrasekhar SS et al: Otologic and audiologic evaluation of human immunodeficiency virus-infected patients. Am J Otolaryngol 2000;21:1. [PMID: 10668670] (Ear disease affects up to 33% of HIV-infected patients. Otitis media is a frequent finding. Sensorineural hearing loss is more severe in patients with advanced HIV infection.)

McNaghten AD et al: Prevalence of hearing loss in a cohort of HIV-infected patients. Arch Otolaryngol Head Neck Surg 2001;127:1516. [PMID: 11735832]

Truitt TO et al: Otolaryngologic manifestations of human immunodeficiency virus infection. Med Clin North Am 1999;83:303. [PMID: 9927976]

■ DISEASES OF THE NOSE & PARANASAL SINUSES

INFECTIONS OF THE NOSE & PARANASAL SINUSES

1. Viral Rhinitis (Common Cold)

The nonspecific symptoms of the ubiquitous common cold are present in the early phases of many diseases that affect the upper aerodigestive tract. Because there are numerous serologic types of rhinoviruses, adenoviruses, and other viruses, patients remain susceptible throughout life. Headache, nasal congestion, watery rhinorrhea, sneezing, and a scratchy throat accompanied by general malaise are typical in viral infections. Nasal examination usually shows reddened, edematous mucosa and a watery discharge. The presence of purulent nasal discharge suggests bacterial infection.

There is no curative treatment for a cold. There is a common misperception among patients that antibiotics are helpful. Supportive measures such as decon-

gestants (pseudoephedrine, 30–60 mg every 4–6 hours or 120 mg twice daily) may provide some relief of rhinorrhea and nasal obstruction.

Nasal sprays such as oxymetazoline or phenylphrine are rapidly effective. They should not be used for more than a few days at a time, since chronic use leads to a rebound congestion that is often worse than the original symptoms. This chronic nasal stuffiness is known as rhinitis medicamentosa. Treatment requires complete cessation of the sprays. This triggers a period of severe nasal congestion that usually lasts 1–2 weeks. Topical intranasal corticosteroids (flunisolide, two sprays in each nostril twice daily) or a short tapering course of oral prednisone may help during the process of withdrawal.

Other than transient middle ear effusion, complications of viral rhinitis are unusual. Secondary bacterial infection may occur and is suggested by persistence of symptoms beyond a week accompanied both by purulent green or yellow nasal secretions and unilateral facial or tooth pain. The most common pathogens are the same as those responsible for acute otitis media, ie, *Streptococcus pneumoniae*, other streptococci, *Haemophilus influenzae*, *Staphylococcus aureus*, and *Moraxella catarrhalis*. (See Acute Sinusitis, below.)

Hickner JM et al: Principles of appropriate antibiotic use for acute rhinosinusitis in adults: background. Ann Emerg Med 2001;37:703. [PMID: 11385344] (Also discusses distinguishing sinusitis from a cold.)

Hueston WJ et al: Criteria used by clinicians to differentiate sinusitis from viral upper respiratory tract infection. J Fam Pract 1998;46:487. [PMID: 9638113] (The use of unreliable criteria may lead to misdiagnoses and inappropriate prescriptions for antibiotics.)

JAMA patient page: The common cold. JAMA 1998;279:2066. [PMID: 9643869]

McKee MD et al: Antibiotic use for the treatment of upper respiratory infections in a diverse community. J Fam Pract 1999;48:993. [PMID: 10628580] (Members of some ethnic communities believed that antibiotics are effective for colds, indicated that they are likely to seek care for them, and had obtained antibiotics from sources other than a physician's prescription, such as directly from pharmacists or a supplier outside the United States.)

2. Acute Sinusitis

Acute sinus infections are uncommon compared with viral rhinitis, but they still affect over 14% of the population, accounting for over 2 billion dollars in health care expenditures for sinusitis annually. Because sinusitis usually has followed an acute respiratory infection and because media advertisements often use the term "sinusitis" when "rhinitis" would be more accurate, it is understandable that patients and clinicians alike sometimes confuse these entities. Sinusitis is suggested when symptoms have persevered for more than a week and pain is reported unilaterally, either as toothache or as pain over the maxillary sinus. Objective signs include a change of secretions from watery or mucoid to purulent green or yellow, or (occasionally) visible swelling or erythema over a sinus.

Sinusitis usually is a result of impaired mucociliary clearance and obstruction of the osteomeatal complex. Diseases that swell the nasal mucous membrane, such as viral or allergic rhinitis, are usually the underlying cause. Edematous mucosa causes obstruction of the sinus drainage tract, resulting in the accumulation of mucous secretion in the sinus cavity that becomes secondarily infected by bacteria. The typical pathogens of bacterial sinusitis are the same as those that cause acute otitis media: *S pneumoniae,* other streptococci, *H influenzae,* and, less commonly, *S aureus* and *M catarrhalis.* It should be kept in mind that about 25% of healthy asymptomatic individuals may, if sinus aspirates are cultured, harbor such bacteria as well.

Clinical Findings

A. SYMPTOMS AND SIGNS

Because the maxillary sinus is the largest of the paranasal sinuses and its ostia into the nose is superiorly placed, thereby failing to take advantage of gravity, it is the most commonly affected sinus. Pain and pressure over the cheek are the usual symptoms. Pain may refer to the upper incisor and canine teeth via branches of the trigeminal nerve, which traverse the floor of the sinus. It is not uncommon for maxillary sinusitis to result from dental infection, and teeth that are tender should be carefully examined for signs of abscess. Discolored nasal discharge and poor response to decongestants may also suggest sinusitis. Other possible causes for facial pain, such as trigeminal neuralgia and optic neuritis, should be kept in mind as well.

Acute ethmoiditis in adults is usually accompanied by maxillary sinusitis. In such cases, the symptoms of maxillary sinusitis generally predominate. Ethmoidal infection presents with pain and pressure over the high lateral wall of the nose that may radiate to the orbit. Periorbital cellulitis may be present.

Sphenoid sinusitis is usually seen in the setting of pansinusitis. The patient may complain of a headache "in the middle of the head" and often points to the vertex. Sixth nerve palsy may occur as the abducens nerve courses just lateral to the sinus.

Acute frontal sinusitis usually causes pain and tenderness of the forehead. This is most easily elicited by palpation of the orbital roof just below the medial end of the eyebrow. Palpation here is more accurate than percussion of the supraorbital area or forehead.

B. IMAGING

It is usually possible to make the diagnosis of sinusitis on clinical grounds alone. Although more sensitive than clinical examination, routine radiographs are not cost-effective and are not recommended by the Agency for Health Care Policy and Research. However, they may be helpful when clinically based criteria are difficult to evaluate. The hallmarks of acute sinusitis radiologically are soft tissue density without bone destruction. An air-fluid level may also be seen.

Limited coronal CT scans have largely replaced conventional sinus films. CT is no more expensive, is more sensitive to both inflammatory changes and bone destruction (which would raise the possibility of an underlying tumor), and by identifying anatomic blockage of the osteomeatal complex may also help guide endoscopic sinus surgery in recurrent or chronic sinusitis. In critically ill intubated patients, where the prevalence of nosocomial sinusitis is as high as 40%, CT identification and subsequent antibiotic treatment appear to reduce the incidence of bronchopneumonia. Occasionally, a CT scan may be indicated to demonstrate that a patient with midface pain does *not* have sinusitis.

While reasonably sensitive, CT scans are not specific. Sinus abnormalities can be seen in the majority of patients with an upper respiratory infection, while only 2% develop bacterial sinusitis. Thus, sinusitis is a clinical diagnosis for which CT may be helpful in confirming, denying, or monitoring.

If malignancy is suspected, MRI with gadolinium should be ordered instead of CT. MRI will distinguish tumor from inflammation and inspissated mucus far better than CT, as well as better delineating tumor extent with respect to adjacent structures such as the orbit, skull base, and palate. Bone destruction can be demonstrated as well by MRI as by CT.

Treatment

Two-thirds of untreated patients will improve symptomatically within 2 weeks. Administration of antibiotics does, however, reduce by 50% the incidence of clinical failure and, coupled with clinical criteria-based diagnosis, represents the most cost-effective treatment strategy. Symptoms may be improved with oral or nasal decongestants (or both)—eg, oral pseudoephedrine, 30–120 mg per dose, up to 240 mg/d; nasal oxymetazoline, 0.05%, or xylometazoline, 0.05–0.1%, one or two sprays in each nostril every 6–8 hours for up to 3 days.

Double-blinded studies exist to support any of the following antibiotic choices:

Amoxicillin (500 mg orally three times a day), possibly with clavulanate (125 mg three times a day)

Trimethoprim-sulfamethoxazole (4 mg/kg TMP and 20 mg/kg SMZ twice daily; available as tablets with 80 or 160 mg TMP and 160 or 800 mg SM)

Cephalexin (250–500 mg orally four times a day)

Cefuroxime (250 mg orally twice daily)

Cefaclor (250 mg orally three times a day)

Cefixime (400 mg orally daily)

Quinolones, such as ciprofloxacin (500 mg twice daily), levofloxacin (500 mg once daily), moxifloxacin (400 mg once daily), and sparfloxacin (200 mg once daily after an initial dose of 400 mg).

Macrolides, such as azithromycin (500 mg once daily, possibly for only three days) or clarithromycin (500 mg orally twice daily, for 14 days)

Usually, amoxicillin or trimethoprim-sulfamethoxazole is adequate and most cost-effective and covers the common pathogens discussed earlier. Treatment is usually for 10 days (or as stated above), though longer courses are sometimes required to prevent relapses. Recurrent sinusitis or sinusitis that does not appear to respond clinically warrants evaluation by a specialist. Selection of antibiotics is usually empiric, but if symptoms persist, obtaining a culture endoscopically or via maxillary sinus puncture may help narrow the choice based on culture and sensitivity tests. Resistance by *Haemophilus influenzae* and *Streptococcus pneumoniae* is a public health concern. Culture may also be helpful in nosocomial sinusitis, where the bacterial spectrum may be less typical and the potential complications greater.

Failure of sinusitis to resolve after an adequate course of oral antibiotics may necessitate hospital admission for intravenous antibiotics and possible surgical drainage. Frontal sinusitis that does not promptly respond to outpatient care should be managed aggressively, because the posterior sinus wall is adjacent to the dura and because undertreated infection may lead to intracranial extension. If intravenous antibiotics fail to ameliorate symptoms, it may be necessary to surgically drill a small opening into the floor of the frontal sinus to drain and irrigate the sinus. Persistent maxillary empyema may be cultured and relieved with a needle inserted through the lateral wall of the nose or anterior wall of the antrum through the gingivobuccal sulcus.

Complications

Local complications of sinusitis include osteomyelitis and mucocele. Mucoceles, a consequence of longstanding ductal obstruction, are more common in the supraorbital ethmoids and frontal sinuses and may become secondarily infected. They appear radiologically as a smoothly expanded sinus filled with homogeneous soft tissue density. Treatment is surgical, requiring either drainage of the mucocele intranasally or its complete excision with fat ablation of the sinus cavity.

Osteomyelitis requires prolonged antibiotics as well as removal of necrotic bone. The frontal sinus is most commonly affected, with bone involvement suggested by a tender puffy swelling of the forehead. Following treatment, secondary cosmetic reconstructive procedures may be necessary.

Intracranial complications of sinusitis occur either through hematogenous spread, as in cavernous sinus thrombosis and meningitis, or by direct extension, as in epidural and intraparenchymal brain abscesses. Fortunately, they are rare today. Cavernous sinus thrombosis is heralded by ophthalmoplegia, chemosis, and visual loss. Frontal epidural abscess is usually quiescent. It may be detected on CT scan, a study recommended in all cases of atypical or complicated sinusitis.

It should always be kept in mind that paranasal sinus cancer is in the differential diagnosis of sinusitis. The presence of bone destruction radiologically, cranial neuropathies (especially V_2), persistent pain, epistaxis, or a prolonged clinical course should raise the suspicion of possible cancer.

Antimicrobial treatment guidelines for acute bacterial rhinosinusitis. Sinus and Allergy Health Partnership. Otolaryngol Head Neck Surg 2000;123(1 Part 2):5. [PMID: 10887346] (One of several committee publications in 2000 to review in detail this topic and suggest treatment algorithms.)

Benninger MS et al: Diagnosis and treatment of uncomplicated acute bacterial rhinosinusitis: summary of the Agency for Health Care Policy and Research evidence-based report. Otolaryngol Head Neck Surg 2000;122:1. [PMID: 10629474]

Brooks I et al: Medical management of acute bacterial sinusitis. Recommendations of a clinical advisory committee on pediatric and adult sinusitis. Ann Otol Rhinol Laryngol 2000;182(Suppl):2. [PMID: 10823486] (One of several committee publications in 2000 to review in detail this topic and suggest treatment algorithms.)

Gwaltney JM Jr: Acute community acquired bacterial sinusitis: To treat or not to treat. Can Respir J 1999;6(Suppl A):46A. [PMID: 10202234] (Abnormalities of the sinuses can be seen in 90% of healthy adults with URIs, but only 2% develop bacterial sinusitis. Evidence supports antibiotic treatment of sinusitis to eradicate infection and reduce symptoms, but there is insufficient evidence that antibiotic treatment reduces serious complications or reduces progression to chronic sinus disease.)

Holzapfel L et al: A randomized study assessing the systematic search for maxillary sinusitis in nasotracheally mechanically ventilated patients. Influence of nosocomial maxillary sinusitis on the occurrence of ventilator-associated pneumonia. Am J Respir Crit Care Med 1999;159:695. [PMID: 10051239] (Treatment of sinusitis of nasotracheally intubated patients with fever and purulent aspirate within an aspirated sinus and confirmatory CT resulted in a decreased incidence of bronchopneumonia in this study of 399 patients.)

Nadel DM et al: Endoscopically guided sinus cultures in normal subjects. Am J Rhinol 1999;13:87. [PMID: 10219435] (Seven of 25 normal volunteers had positive cultures.)

Piccirillo JF et al: Impact of first-line vs second-line antibiotics for the treatment of acute uncomplicated sinusitis. JAMA 2001;286:1849. [PMID: 11597286] (Cost is the sole difference.)

Williams JW Jr et al: Antibiotics for acute maxillary sinusitis. Cochrane Database Syst Rev 2000:CD000243. [PMID: 10796515] (A comprehensive review of potentially relevant studies concluding that penicillin or amoxicillin for 7–14 days is usually sufficient, but noting that clinicians should weigh whether the moderate benefits of antibiotic use are worth the potential for side effects.)

3. Nasal Vestibulitis

Inflammation of the nasal vestibule commonly results from folliculitis of the hairs that line this orifice. Systemic antibiotics effective against *S aureus* (such as dicloxacillin, 250 mg orally four times daily for 7–10 days) are indicated. Topical mupirocin (applied two or three times daily) may be a helpful addition. If recurrent, the addition of rifampin (10 mg/kg orally twice daily for the last 4 days of treatment) may eliminate the *S aureus* carrier state. If a furuncle exists, it should be incised and drained, preferably intranasally. Adequate treatment of these infections is important to prevent retrograde spread of infection through valveless veins into the cavernous sinus and intracranial structures.

4. Rhinocerebral Mucormycosis

Although mucormycosis is rare, any clinician seeing patients in a primary care setting must be aware of its presenting signs and symptoms. The fungus (mucor, absidia, rhizopus) spreads rapidly through vascular channels and may be lethal if not detected early. Patients with mucormycosis almost invariably have an underlying disease, often diabetes mellitus or end-stage renal disease. It also occurs following bone marrow transplantation, in patients with lymphoma, in patients who are immunosuppressed for other reasons, and in patients receiving deferoxamine (a metal chelator). Occasional cases have been reported in patients with AIDS, though aspergillus is more common in this setting. The initial symptoms may be similar to those of bacterial sinusitis, although facial pain is often more severe. Examination of the nasal mucosa is likely to show black, necrotic eschar adherent to the inferior turbinate, though this may not be present in early stages. Cranial neuropathies and black necrotic skin overlying the ethmoid sinuses are advanced signs. Early diagnosis requires suspicion of the disease and nasal or sinus biopsy, which reveals broad nonseptate hyphae within tissues. Because CT or MRI may initially show only soft tissue changes, intervention should be based on the clinical setting and not on radiologic demonstration of bony destruction or intracranial changes.

Mucormycosis represents a medical and surgical emergency. Once recognized, prompt wide surgical debridement and amphotericin B by intravenous infusion are indicated. Liposomal amphotericin B may be used in patients with renal insufficiency. When there appears to be sufficiently little orbital involvement that orbital preservation is a realistic therapeutic objective, conservative debridement of the orbit may be supplemented with adjunctive amphotericin B irrigation. Close management of the underlying disease is also of great importance. Even with early diagnosis and immediate appropriate intervention, the prognosis is guarded. In diabetics, the mortality rate is about 20%; in patients with renal failure, it is over 50%; in AIDS, it is close to 100%.

Case records of the Massachusetts General Hospital. Weekly clinicopathological exercises. Case 22-1999. A 68-year-old woman with multiple myeloma, diabetes mellitus, and an inflamed eye. N Engl J Med 1999;41:265. [PMID: 10413740]

Seiff SR et al: Role of local amphotericin B therapy for sino-orbital fungal infections. Ophthal Plast Reconstr Surg 1999; 15:28. [PMID: 9949426]

ALLERGIC RHINITIS

The symptoms of "hay fever" are similar to those of viral rhinitis but are usually persistent and show seasonal variation. Nasal symptoms are often accompanied by eye irritation, which causes pruritus, erythema, and excessive tearing. Numerous allergens may cause these symptoms: pollens are most common in the spring, grasses in the summer, and ragweed in the fall. Dust and household mites may produce year-round symptoms.

On physical examination, the mucosa of the turbinates is usually pale or violaceous because of venous engorgement. This is in contrast to the erythema of viral rhinitis. Nasal polyps, which are yellowish boggy masses of hypertrophic mucosa, may be seen.

Treatment of allergic and perennial rhinitis has improved in recent years. Numerous over-the-counter antihistamines, such as brompheniramine or chlorpheniramine (4 mg orally every 6–8 hours, or 8–12 mg orally every 8–12 hours as a sustained-release tablet) and clemastine (1.34–2.68 mg orally twice daily) offer the benefit of reduced cost though usually associated with higher rates of drowsiness compared with the newer prescription antihistamines. These oral H_1 receptor antagonists include cetirizine (10 mg orally once daily), fexofenadine (60 mg orally twice daily or 120 mg once daily), and loratadine (10 mg orally once daily). Fexofenadine appears to be nonsedating; the other two minimally sedating. Also shown to be effective in randomized trials are ebastine (10–20 mg orally once daily) and misolastine (10 mg once daily). Two H_1 receptor antagonist antihistamine nasal sprays have also been shown to be effective in randomized trials: levocabastine (0.2 mg twice daily) and azelastine (two sprays per nostril, 1.1 mg/d).

Intranasal corticosteroid sprays are a mainstay of treatment of allergic rhinitis. Evidence-based literature reviews show that these are more effective—and frequently less expensive—than nonsedating antihistamines. Patients should be reminded that there may be a delay in onset of relief of 1–2 weeks. Steroid sprays may also shrink nasal polyps, thereby providing an improved nasal airway and delaying or eliminating the indications for endoscopic sinus surgery. Available preparations include beclomethasone (42 μg/spray twice daily each nostril), flunisolide (25 μg/spray twice daily each nostril), mometasone furoate (200 μg once daily per nostril), and fluticasone propionate (200 μg once daily per nostril). The latter two synthetic glucocorticoids appear to have higher topical potencies and lipid solubility and reduced systemic bioavailability, suggesting possible practical advantages.

Maintaining an allergen-free environment by covering pillows and mattresses with plastic covers, substituting synthetic materials (foam mattress, acrylics) for animal products (wool, horsehair), and removing dust-collecting household fixtures (carpets, drapes, bedspreads, wicker) is worth the attempt to help more troubled patients. Air purifiers and dust filters (such as Bionaire models) may also aid in maintaining an allergen-free environment. When symptoms are extremely bothersome, a search for offending allergens may prove helpful. This can either be done by skin testing or by serum RAST testing. Desensitization by gradually increasing subdermal exposure to identified allergens may be tried in selected patients, with variable results.

Adjunctive options include intranasal anticholinergic agents such as ipratropium bromide 0.03% sprays (42 μg per nostril three times daily) when rhinorrhea is a major symptom and intranasal cromolyn spray prior to the onset of seasonal symptoms.

For more information on allergic rhinitis, see Chapter 19.

Corren J: Intranasal corticosteroids for allergic rhinitis: how do different agents compare? J Allergy Clin Immunol 1999;104(4 Part 1):S144. [PMID: 10518811] (Newer intranasal steroids such as mometasone and fluticasone appear to have practical advantages over older agents in terms of higher topical potencies and lipid solubilities and lower systemic bioavailabilities. All the available intranasal corticosteroids appear to be equally effective in controlling symptoms.)

Dockhorn R et al: Ipratropium bromide nasal spray 0.03% and beclomethasone nasal spray alone and in combination for the treatment of rhinorrhea in perennial rhinitis. Ann Allergy Asthma Immunol 1999;82:349. [PMID: 10227333] (Ipratropium bromide nasal spray 0.03% is useful in troublesome rhinorrhea.)

Hadley JA: Evaluation and management of allergic rhinitis. Med Clin North Am 1999;83:13. [PMID: 9927957] (An overview.)

OLFACTORY DYSFUNCTION

The physiology of olfaction is less well understood than that of the other special senses. The taste of foods is strongly affected by our sense of smell, and studies have shown a moderate correlation between taste discrimination ability and odor discrimination ability. In the past few years, discovery of the family of odor-receptor genes as well as inositol phosphate and cyclic nucleotide signaling pathways have led to a molecular basis of olfactory reception. Clinically, odorant molecules traverse the nasal vault to reach the cribriform area and become soluble in the mucus overlying the exposed dendrites of receptor cells. Anatomic blockage of the nares is the most common cause of olfactory dysfunction (hyposmia or anosmia). Polyps, septal deformities, and nasal tumors may prevent air from reaching the area of the cribriform plate high in the nose where these receptors are located. Transient olfactory dysfunction often accompanies the common cold, nasal allergies, and perennial rhinitis. About 20% of olfactory dysfunction is idiopathic, although it often follows a viral illness. Some have suggested administering large doses of vitamin A and zinc to such patients, although little evidence supports their use. Central nervous system neoplasms, especially those that involve the olfactory groove or temporal lobe, may affect olfaction. Head trauma accounts for less than 5% of cases of hyposmia. Absent, diminished, or distorted smell or taste has been reported in a wide variety of endocrine, nutritional, and nervous disorders. In particular, olfactory dysfunction in Parkinson's disease and Alzheimer's disease has been the subject of recent research. A great many medications have also been implicated.

Evaluation of olfactory dysfunction should include a thorough history of systemic illnesses and medication use as well as a physical examination focusing on the nose and nervous system. Most clinical offices are not set up to test olfaction, but such feats may at times be worthwhile if only to assess whether a patient possesses any sense of smell at all. Odor identification and discrimination can be tested using standardized choices (see references). Odor threshold can be tested using increasing concentrations of various materials. In permanent hyposmia, counseling should be offered about seasoning foods with spices (eg, pepper) that stimulate the trigeminal as well as olfactory chemoreceptors and about safety issues such as the use of smoke alarms and electric rather than gas home appliances.

Axel R: The molecular logic of smell. Sci Am 1995 Oct;273:154. [PMID: 7481719]

Bromley SM: Smell and taste disorders: a primary care approach. Am Fam Phys 2000;61:427. [PMID: 10670508]

Kaneda H et al: Decline in taste and odor discrimination abilities with age, and relationship between gustation and olfaction. Chem Senses 2000;25:331. [PMID: 10866991] (There is a moderate but significant correlation between taste discrimination ability and odor discrimination ability.)

Kobal G et al: Multicenter investigation of 1,036 subjects using a standardized method for the assessment of olfactory function combining tests of odor identification, odor discrimination, and olfactory thresholds. Eur Arch Otorhinolaryngol 2000;257:205. [PMID: 10867835] ("Sniffin' Sticks" is a standardized test of chemosensory performance based on odor-dispensing devices. It tests threshold, discrimination, and identification.)

McCaffrey RJ et al: Olfactory dysfunction discriminates probable Alzheimer's dementia from major depression: a cross-validation and extension. J Neuropsychiatry Clin Neurosci

2000;12:29. [PMID: 10678509] (Olfactory assessment may help distinguish Alzheimer's disease from depression in elderly patients.)

EPISTAXIS

Bleeding from Kiesselbach's plexus, a vascular plexus on the anterior nasal septum, is by far the most common type of epistaxis encountered. Predisposing factors include nasal trauma (nose picking, foreign bodies, forceful nose blowing), rhinitis, drying of the nasal mucosa from low humidity, deviation of the nasal septum, alcohol use, and antiplatelet medications. Most cases of anterior epistaxis may be successfully treated by direct pressure on the bleeding site. The nasal alae should be firmly compressed for at least 10 minutes. Venous pressure is reduced in the sitting position, and leaning forward lessens the swallowing of blood. Short-acting topical nasal decongestants (eg, phenylephrine, 0.125–1% solution, one or two sprays), which act as vasoconstrictors, may also be helpful. When the bleeding does not readily subside, the nose should be examined, using good illumination and suction, in an attempt to locate the bleeding site. Topical 4% cocaine applied either as a spray or on a cotton strip serves both as an anesthetic and as a vasoconstricting agent. If cocaine is unavailable, a topical decongestant (eg, oxymetazoline) and a topical anesthetic (eg, tetracaine) provide equivalent results. When visible, the bleeding site may be cauterized with silver nitrate, diathermy, or electrocautery. A supplemental patch of Surgicel or Gelfoam may be helpful.

Occasionally, a site of bleeding may be inaccessible to direct control, or attempts at direct control may be unsuccessful. In such cases, nasal packing is necessary. A properly placed anterior pack requires several feet of half-inch iodoform packing lubricated with bacitracin or petroleum ointment. The packing is carefully and systematically placed along the floor and then the vault of the nose. If the equipment necessary to place a pack is not available, various manufactured nasal balloons may serve as either a temporizing or definitive solution.

About 5% of nasal bleeding originates in the posterior nasal cavity. This requires placement of a pack to occlude the choana before placement of a pack anteriorly. Because this is uncomfortable for the patient and because it requires oxygen supplementation to prevent hypoxia, hospitalization for several days is indicated. Narcotic analgesics are needed to reduce the considerable discomfort and elevated blood pressure caused by a posterior pack. Ligation of the nasal arterial supply (internal maxillary artery and ethmoid arteries) is a possible alternative to posterior nasal packing, as is endovascular embolization of the internal maxillary artery. This is certainly necessary when packing fails to control life-threatening hemorrhage. On rare occasions, ligation of the external carotid artery may be necessary.

After control of epistaxis, the patient is advised to avoid vigorous exercise for several days. Avoidance of hot or spicy foods and tobacco is also advisable, as they may cause vasodilation. Avoiding nasal trauma, including nose picking, is an obvious necessity. Lubrication with petroleum jelly or bacitracin ointment and increased home humidity may also be useful ancillary measures.

It is important in all patients with epistaxis to consider underlying causes of the bleeding. Laboratory assessment of bleeding parameters may be indicated, especially in recurrent cases. Other causes of recurrent epistaxis, such as hereditary hemorrhagic telangiectasia (Osler-Weber-Rendu syndrome), should also be considered. Similarly, once the acute episode has passed, careful examination of the nose and paranasal sinuses to rule out neoplasia is wise.

Patients presenting with epistaxis often have higher blood pressures than control patients. Continued management of patients with epistaxis should therefore include follow-up investigation of possible hypertension.

Cullen MM et al: Comparison of internal maxillary artery ligation versus embolization for refractory posterior epistaxis. Otolaryngol Head Neck Surg 1998;118:636. [PMID: 9591862] (Internal maxillary artery ligation is more expensive, but embolization is usually unavailable in nonurban areas. Complication rates for ligation are the same or higher, but major complications of embolization are more serious.)

Herkner H et al: Hypertension in patients presenting with epistaxis. Ann Emerg Med 2000;35:126. [PMID: 10650229] (Patients with epistaxis who have elevated blood pressure need follow-up to see if the hypertension is sustained and hence requires treatment.)

Leppanen M et al: Microcatheter embolization of intractable idiopathic epistaxis. Cardiovasc Intervent Radiol 1999;22:499. [PMID: 10556410] (Embolization is safe and effective. It should be considered the primary treatment for intractable idiopathic epistaxis.)

Pond F et al: Epistaxis. Strategies for management. Aust Fam Physician 2000;29:933. [PMID: 11059081]

Tan LK et al: Epistaxis. Med Clin North Am 1999;83:43. [PMID: 9927959] (In shifting management philosophy of epistaxis toward targeting the bleeding point, endoscopic evaluation may have a significant impact on decreasing length of stay and blood transfusion rates. Advances in interventional radiology have also reduced the risk of embolization. Patient education, especially teaching first-aid measures to patients at high risk for nosebleeds, also encourages more effective use of health care resources.)

Thaha MA et al: Routine coagulation screening in the management of emergency admission for epistaxis—is it necessary? J Laryngol Otol 2000;114:38. [PMID: 10789409] (The only patients who had abnormal studies were those on warfarin, or warfarin and aspirin. The authors suggest therefore that a good history should be sufficient.)

NASAL TRAUMA

The nasal pyramid is the most frequently fractured bone in the body. Fracture is suggested by crepitance or palpably mobile bony segments. Epistaxis and pain are common, as are soft tissue hematomas ("black eye"). It is important to make certain that there is no palpable step-off of the infraorbital rim, which would indicate the presence of a zygomatic complex fracture. Radiologic confirmation may at times be helpful but is not necessary in uncomplicated nasal fractures.

Treatment is aimed at maintaining long-term nasal airway patency and nasal aesthetics. Closed reduction, using topical 4% cocaine and locally injected 1% lidocaine, should be attempted within 1 week of injury. In the presence of marked nasal swelling, it is best to wait several days for the edema to subside before undertaking reduction. Persistent functional or cosmetic defects may be repaired by delayed reconstructive nasal surgery.

Intranasal examination should be performed in all cases to rule out septal hematoma, which appears as a widening of the anterior septum, visible just posterior to the columella. The septal cartilage receives its only nutrition from its closely adherent mucoperichondrium. An untreated subperichondrial hematoma will result in loss of the nasal cartilage with resultant saddlenose deformity. Septal hematomas may become infected, with *S aureus* the predominant organism. Treatment consists of incision and drainage via an intranasal septal mucosal incision. It is important to be sure that both sides of the septal cartilage are adequately drained. A small Penrose drain sutured in place is helpful. Antibiotics should be given and the drained fluid sent for culture.

Ashoor AJ et al: Nasal bone fracture. Saudi Med J 2000;21:471. [PMID: 11500684]

Green KM: Reduction of nasal fractures under local anaesthetic. Rhinology 2001;39:43. [PMID: 11340695] (About a third require revision.)

Gur E et al: Walk-through injuries: glass door facial injuries. Ann Plast Surg 2001;46:613. [PMID: 11405360]

Rohrich RJ et al: Nasal fracture management: minimizing secondary nasal deformities. Plast Reconstr Surg 2000;106:266. [PMID: 10946923]

TUMORS & GRANULOMATOUS DISEASE

1. Benign Nasal Tumors

Nasal Polyps

Nasal polyps are pale, edematous, mucosally covered masses commonly seen in patients with allergic rhinitis, but compelling evidence argues against a purely allergic pathogenesis. They may result in chronic nasal obstruction and a diminished sense of smell. In patients with nasal polyps and a history of asthma, aspirin should be avoided as it may precipitate a severe episode of bronchospasm. The presence of polyps in children should suggest the possibility of cystic fibrosis.

Initial treatment with topical nasal steroids (see Allergic Rhinitis section for specific drugs) for 1–3 months is usually successful for small polyps and may reduce the need for operation. A short course of oral corticosteroids (eg, prednisone, 6-day course using twenty-one 5 mg tablets: 30 mg on day 1 and tapering by 5 mg each day) may also be of benefit. When medical management is unsuccessful, polyps should be removed surgically. In healthy persons, this is a minor outpatient procedure. In recurrent cases or when surgery itself is associated with increased risk (such as in asthmatics), a more complete procedure, such as ethmoidectomy, may be advisable. In recurrent polyposis, it may be necessary to remove polyps from the ethmoid, sphenoid, and maxillary sinuses to provide longer-lasting relief.

Badia L et al: Topical corticosteroids in nasal polyposis. Drugs 2001;61:573. [PMID: 11368283]

Mygind N: Advances in the medical treatment of nasal polyps. Allergy 1999;54(Suppl 53):12. [PMID: 10442545] (An overview of medical management.)

Norlander T et al: The relationship of nasal polyps, infection, and inflammation. Am J Rhinol 1999;13:349. [PMID: 10582112] (An overview of current understanding of pathogenesis, with implications for treatment.)

Stammberger H: Surgical treatment of nasal polyps: past, present, and future. Allergy 1999;54(Suppl 53):7. [PMID: 10442544] (An overview of treatment when medical intervention is inadequate.)

Voegels RL et al: Nasal polyposis and allergy: is there a correlation? Am J Rhinol 2001;15:9. [PMID: 11258659]

Inverted Papilloma

Inverted papillomas are benign tumors that usually arise in the common wall between the nose and maxillary sinus. They present with unilateral nasal obstruction and occasionally hemorrhage. Because squamous cell carcinomas are seen in 5–10% of inverted papillomas, complete excision is necessary. All excised tissue (not just a portion) should be carefully reviewed by the pathologist to be sure no carcinoma is present.

Dammann F et al: Inverted papilloma of the nasal cavity and the paranasal sinuses: using CT for primary diagnosis and follow-up. AJR Am J Roentgenol 1999;172:543. [PMID: 9930821]

Dictor M et al: Association of inverted sinonasal papilloma with non-sinonasal head-and-neck carcinoma. Int J Cancer 2000;85:11. [PMID: 10709101] (Five percent of inverted papillomas developed sinus carcinoma. Interestingly, there was also an increased incidence of other head and neck carcinomas.)

Nachtigal D et al: Unique characteristics of malignant schneiderian papilloma. Otolaryngol Head Neck Surg 1999;121:766. [PMID: 10580235] (Some of the features that might arouse clinical concern that an inverted papilloma might harbor a malignancy.)

Lawson W et al: Inverted papilloma: A report of 112 cases. Laryngoscope 1995;105(3 Part 1):282. [PMID: 7877417] (Clinical course and management.)

Sham CL et al: Endoscopic resection of inverted papilloma of the nose and paranasal sinuses. J Laryngol Otol 1998;112:758. [PMID: 9850318] (A retrospective study of 22 patients with inverted papillomas resected endoscopically is presented with a follow-up of 33–96 months. The authors conclude that the role of an endoscopic approach is restricted to carefully selected patients with limited nasoethmoid and maxillary disease.)

Juvenile Angiofibroma

These highly vascular tumors arise in the nasopharynx, typically in adolescent males. Initially, they cause nasal obstruction and hemorrhage. Any adolescent male with recurrent epistaxis should be evaluated for an angiofibroma. Though benign, these tumors expand locally from the pterygopalatine fossa at the pterygoid canal and extend to the pterygoid base, the greater wing of the sphenoid, the nasal cavity and the paranasal sinuses. They may involve the skull base, usually extradurally, and extend into the superior clivus. Treatment consists of preoperative embolization followed by surgical excision via an approach appropriate for the tumor extent. Small angiofibromas may occasionally be resected endoscopically. Extensive ones may require skull base approaches. Recurrences are not uncommon and should be resected if possible. Unresectable recurrences that do not appear to grow significantly may be followed radiologically with serial MR scans in expectation of possible eventual involution stabilization or involution of tumor. Low-dose (30 Gy) irradiation may be helpful in nonresectable, continually growing tumors.

Danesi G et al: Anterior approaches in juvenile nasopharyngeal angiofibromas with intracranial extension. Otolaryngol Head Neck Surg 2000;122:277. [PMID: 10652407] (Anterior extradural approaches usually suffice even for larger lesions with intracranial extension.)

Herman P et al: Long-term follow up of juvenile nasopharyngeal angiofibromas: analysis of recurrences. Laryngoscope 1999;109:140. [PMID: 9917056] (Recurrences may be followed radiologically as they may involute. Radiation to 30 Gy may at times be needed.)

Tewfik TL et al: Juvenile nasopharyngeal angiofibroma. J Otolaryngol 1999;28:145. [PMID: 10410346]

2. Malignant Nasopharyngeal & Paranasal Sinus Tumors

Unfortunately, malignant tumors of the nose, nasopharynx, and paranasal sinuses tend to remain asymptomatic until late in their course. Although the prognosis is poor for advanced tumors, results of treatment of resectable tumors of paranasal sinus origin have improved with the wider use of skull base resections and intensity-modulated radiation therapy. Cure rates are often 45–60%. Early symptoms are nonspecific, mimicking those of rhinitis or sinusitis. Unilateral nasal obstruction and discharge are common, with pain and recurrent hemorrhage often clues to the diagnosis of cancer. Any patient with unilateral or persistent nasal symptoms should be thoroughly evaluated.

A high index of suspicion remains a key to the earlier diagnosis of these tumors. Patients often present with advanced symptoms such as proptosis, expansion of a cheek, or ill-fitting maxillary dentures. Malar hypesthesia, due to involvement of the infraorbital nerve, is common in maxillary sinus tumors. Biopsy is necessary for definitive diagnosis, and MRI is the best imaging study to delineate the extent of disease and plan appropriate surgery and radiation.

Squamous cell carcinoma is the most common cancer found. It is especially common in the nasopharynx, where it obstructs the auditory tube and results in serous otitis media. Nasopharyngeal carcinoma (poorly differentiated squamous cell carcinoma, nonkeratinizing squamous cell carcinoma, or lymphoepithelioma) is usually associated with elevated IgA antibody to the viral capsid antigen of the Epstein-Barr virus. It is particularly common in patients of southern Chinese descent. Any adult with persistent serous otitis media, especially when unilateral, requires careful evaluation of the nasopharynx. Adenocarcinomas, mucosal melanomas, sarcomas, and non-Hodgkin's lymphomas are less commonly encountered neoplasms of this area.

Treatment depends on the tumor type and the extent of disease. Nasopharyngeal carcinoma at this time is best treated by concomitant radiation and cisplatin followed by adjuvant chemotherapy with cisplatin and fluorouracil—this protocol significantly decreased local, nodal, and distant failures and increased progression-free and overall survival. Other squamous cell carcinomas are best treated—when resectable—with a combination of surgery and irradiation. Numerous protocols investigating the role of chemotherapy are under evaluation. Cranial base surgery appears to be an effective modality in improving the overall prognosis in paranasal sinus malignancies eroding the ethmoid roof.

Benninger MS: The impact of cigarette smoking and environmental tobacco smoke on nasal and sinus disease: a review of the literature. Am J Rhinol 1999;13:435. [PMID: 10631398]

Cantau G et al: Anterior craniofacial resection for malignant ethmoid tumors—a series of 91 patients. Head Neck 1999;21:185. [PMID: 10208659]

Cheng SH et al:. Examining prognostic factors and patterns of failure in nasopharyngeal carcinoma following concomitant radiotherapy and chemotherapy: impact on future clinical trials. Int J Radiat Oncol Biol Phys 2001;50:717. [PMID: 11395240] (Concomitant radiation plus chemotherapy has increased control rates. Patients with intracranial extension or extensive nodal involvement fail more often than those with less extensive disease.)

Chien YC et al: Serologic markers of Epstein-Barr virus infection and nasopharyngeal carcinoma in Taiwanese men. N Engl J Med 2001;345:1877. [PMID: 11756578]

Claus F et al: Postoperative radiotherapy of paranasal sinus tumours: a challenge for intensity modulated radiotherapy. Acta Otorhinolaryngol Belg 1999;53:263. [PMID: 10635406] (Intensity-modulated radiotherapy is helpful in administering a high tumor dose while sparing surrounding organs in anatomically complex areas such as the paranasal sinuses and skull base.)

Fu KK: Combined radiotherapy and chemotherapy for nasopharyngeal carcinoma. Semin Radiat Oncol 1998;8:247. [PMID: 9873102] (Reviews the results of randomized trials of combined chemotherapy and radiotherapy for nasopharyngeal carcinoma to date.)

Sanguineti G et al: Treatment of nasopharyngeal carcinoma: state of the art and new perspectives (review). Oncol Rep 1999;6:377. [PMID: 10023009] (An overview of treatment advances.)

Wei WI: Nasopharyngeal cancer: current status of management: a New York Head and Neck Society lecture. Arch Otolaryngol Head Neck Surg 2001;127:766. [PMID: 11448346]

3. Wegener's Granulomatosis, NK Cell & T Cell EBV-Positive Lymphoma, & Sarcoidosis

The nose and paranasal sinuses are involved in over 90% of cases of Wegener's granulomatosis. It is often not realized that involvement at these sites is more common than involvement of lungs or kidneys. Examination shows bloodstained crusts and friable mucosa. Biopsy classically shows necrotizing granulomas and vasculitis, but the diagnosis may be difficult. Sarcoidosis also commonly involves the paranasal sinuses and is clinically similar to other chronic sinonasal inflammatory processes. Biopsy shows noncaseating granulomas.

Polymorphic reticulosis (midline malignant reticulosis, idiopathic midline destructive disease, lethal midline granuloma), as the multitude of apt descriptive terms suggest, is not well understood but appears to be a nasal lymphoma. In contrast to Wegener's granulomatosis, involvement is limited to the mid face, and there may be extensive bone destruction. Its progression in time to a lymphoma is being described with increasing frequency.

Many destructive lesions of the mucosa and nasal structures labeled as polymorphic reticulosis are in fact non-Hodgkin's lymphoma of either NK cell or T cell origin. Immunophenotyping, especially for CD56 expression, is essential in the histologic evaluation. Even when apparently localized, these lymphomas have a poor prognosis, with progression and death within a year the rule.

For treatment of Wegener's granulomatosis, see Chapter 20.

Cheung MM et al: Primary non-Hodgkin's lymphoma of the nose and nasopharynx: Clinical features, tumor immunophenotype, and treatment outcome in 113 patients. J Clin Oncol 1998;16:70. [PMID: 9440725] (As immunophenotype and stage correlate with prognosis, CD56 expression should be analyzed. NK and T cell lymphomas have a very poor prognosis.)

DeShazo RD et al: Diagnostic criteria for sarcoidosis of the sinuses. J Allergy Clin Immunol 1999;103(5 Part 1):789. [PMID: 10329811]

Duffy M: Advances in diagnosis, treatment, and management of orbital and periocular Wegener's granulomatosis. Curr Opin Ophthalmol 1999;10:352. [PMID: 10621551] (Trimethoprim-sulfamethoxazole or methotrexate may be useful in selected patients with limited forms of Wegener's granulomatosis.)

Hasni SA et al: Sarcoidosis presenting as necrotizing sinus destruction mimicking Wegener's granulomatosis. J Rheumatol 2000;27:512. [PMID: 10685824]

Hausdorff J et al: Non-Hodgkin's lymphoma of the paranasal sinuses: Clinical and pathological features, and response to combined-modality therapy. Cancer J Sci Am 1997;3:303. [PMID: 9327155] (Combined modality therapy with central nervous system prophylaxis improves outcome compared with radiotherapy, and autologous bone marrow transplantation as initial therapy is a consideration.)

Knecht K et al: More than a mouth ulcer. Oral ulcer due to Wegener's granulomatosis. Postgrad Med 1999;105:200. [PMID: 10335330]

Magliulo G et al: Wegener's granulomatosis presenting as facial palsy. Am J Otolaryngol 1999;20:43. [PMID: 9950112]

O'Devaney K et al: Wegener's granulomatosis of the head and neck. Ann Otol Rhinol Laryngol 1998;107(5 Part 1):439. [PMID: 9596226] (Manifestations and differential diagnosis.)

Perry SR et al: The clinical and pathologic constellation of Wegener granulomatosis of the orbit. Ophthalmology 1997;104:683. [PMID: 9111264] (Reviews ophthalmologic symptoms such as decreased vision, redness, and ocular-facial pain; signs such as proptosis, scleritis, and lid inflammation; serologic tests; and treatment.)

Rinaldo A et al: Wegener's granulomatosis presenting with otologic manifestations. J Otolaryngol 1999;28:347. [PMID: 10604165]

■ DISEASES OF THE ORAL CAVITY & PHARYNX

LEUKOPLAKIA, ERYTHROPLAKIA, ORAL LICHEN PLANUS, & ORAL CANCER

Leukoplakia is any white lesion that, unlike oral candidiasis, cannot be removed by rubbing the mucosal surface. These areas are usually small but may be several centimeters in diameter. Histologically, they are often hyperkeratoses occurring in response to chronic irritation (eg, from dentures, tobacco, lichen planus); about 2–6%, however, represent either dysplasia or early invasive squamous cell carcinoma.

Erythroplakia is similar to leukoplakia except that it has a definite erythematous component. The distinction is important, since about 90% of cases of erythroplakia are either dysplasia or carcinoma. Squamous cell carcinoma accounts for 90% of oral cancer. Alcohol and tobacco are the major epidemiologic risk factors. The differential diagnosis may include oral candidiasis, necrotizing sialometaplasia, pseudoepitheliomatous hyperplasia, median rhomboid glossitis, and vesiculoerosive inflammatory disease such as erosive lichen planus. This should not be confused with the brown-black gingival melanin pigmentation—diffuse or speckled common in nonwhites, blue-black embedded fragments of dental amalgam, or other systemic disorders associated with general pigmentation (neurofibromatosis, familial polyposis, Addison's disease). Intraoral melanoma is extremely rare.

Oral lichen planus is a relatively common (0.5–2% of the population) chronic inflammatory autoimmune disease that may be difficult to diagnose clinically because of its numerous distinct phenotypic subtypes. For example, the reticular pattern may mimic candidiasis or hyperkeratosis, while the erosive pattern may mimic squamous cell carcinoma. Management begins with distinguishing it from other oral lesions; this usually requires biopsy. Therapy is aimed at managing pain and discomfort. Steroids have been used widely both locally and systemically. Cyclosporines and retinoids have also been used. Many think there is a low rate (1%) of squamous cell carcinoma arising within lichen planus (in addition to the possibility of clinical misdiagnosis).

Any erythroplakic or enlarging leukoplakic area should have an incisional biopsy or an exfoliative cytologic examination. Specialty referral should be sought early both for diagnosis and treatment. Intraoral staining with 1% toluidine blue may aid in selection of the most suspicious biopsy site. A systematic intraoral examination—including the lateral tongue, floor of the mouth, gingiva, buccal area, palate, and tonsillar fossae—and palpation of the neck for enlarged lymph nodes should be part of any general physical examination, especially in patients over 45 who smoke tobacco or drink immoderately. Indirect or fiberoptic examination of the nasopharynx, oropharynx, hypopharynx, and larynx by an otolaryngologist–head and neck surgeon or radiation oncologist should also be considered for such patients when there is unexplained or persistent throat or ear pain, oral or nasal bleeding, or oral erythroplakia. Fine-needle aspiration biopsy may be indicated if an enlarged lymph node is found.

Early detection of squamous cell carcinoma is the key to successful management. Lesions less than 4 mm in depth have a low propensity to metastasize. Most patients in whom the tumor is detected before it is 2 cm in diameter are cured. Small lesions are best treated with surgical excision, often with a laser. Radiation is an alternative but is associated with xerostomia, osteonecrosis of the mandible, and inability to use a curative dose again in the treatment field. Large tumors nevertheless are usually treated with a combination of resection and irradiation. Reconstruction, if required, is done at the time of resection and can involve the use of myocutaneous flaps or vascularized free flaps with or without bone.

Molecular analyses of premalignant and malignant tissues have produced strong evidence that clonal genetic alterations, such as loss of retinoic acid beta-receptor expression, occur during the early stage of aerodigestive tract carcinogenesis. These molecular and epidemiologic studies provide the foundation on which clinical trials have been designed to evaluate the role of retinoids and other compounds in the reversal of premalignancy and the possible reduction in the 4–7% annual rate of second primary tumors.

A number of clinical trials have suggested a role for beta-carotene, vitamin E, and retinoids in producing regression of leukoplakia and reducing the incidence of recurrent squamous cell carcinomas. Retinoids suppress head and neck and lung carcinogenesis in animal models and inhibit carcinogenesis in individuals with premalignant lesions. They also seem to reduce the incidence of second primary cancers in head and neck and lung cancer patients previously treated for a primary.

Chan ES et al: Interventions for treating oral lichen planus. Cochrane Database Syst Rev 2000;CD001168. [PMID: 10796611] (Concludes there is only weak evidence to support any intervention; there is a need for larger placebo-controlled trials.)

Garewal HS et al: Beta-carotene produces sustained remissions in patients with oral leukoplakia: results of a multicenter prospective trial. Arch Otolaryngol Head Neck Surg 1999; 125:1305. [PMID: 10604407]

Geyer C et al: Chemoprevention in head and neck cancer: basic science and clinical application. Semin Radiat Oncol 1998;8:292. [PMID: 9873107] (The rationale of retinoid chemoprevention of second head and neck cancers, based on the concepts of field cancerization and multistep carcinogenesis.)

Martin GC et al: Oral leukoplakia status six weeks after cessation of smokeless tobacco use. J Am Dent Assoc 1999;130:945. [PMID: 1042398] (Most leukoplakic lesions resolved clinically. If a young patient will stop using smokeless tobacco, delaying a biopsy of a minimally suspicious lesion may be reasonable.)

Mellott A et al: Chemoprevention in head and neck cancer. Cancer Treat Res 2001;106:221. [PMID: 11225004]

Sciubba JJ: Oral cancer. The importance of early diagnosis and treatment. Am J Clin Dermatol 2001;2:239. [PMID: 11705251]

Scully C et al: ABC of oral health. Swellings and red, white, and pigmented lesions. BMJ 2000;321225. [PMID: 10903660]

Sudbo J et al: DNA content as a prognostic marker in patients with oral leukoplakia. N Engl J Med 2001;344:1270. [PMID: 11320386] (Higher risk in aneuploid cells.)

CANDIDIASIS

Oral candidiasis (thrush) is usually painful and looks like creamy-white curd-like patches overlying erythematous mucosa. Because these white areas are easily rubbed off (eg, by a tongue depressor)—unlike leukoplakia or lichen planus—only the underlying irregular erythema may be seen. Oral candidiasis is commonly encountered among denture wearers; in debilitated patients, diabetes patients, anemia patients, patients undergoing chemotherapy or local irradiation; and in patients receiving corticosteroids or broad-spectrum antibiotics. Candidiasis is often seen as the first manifestation of HIV infection. Angular cheilitis is another manifestation of candidiasis, though it is also seen in nutritional deficiencies.

The diagnosis is made clinically. A wet preparation using potassium hydroxide will reveal spores and may show nonseptate mycelia. Biopsy will show intraepithelial pseudomycelia of *Candida albicans.*

Effective antifungal therapy may be achieved with any of the following: fluconazole (100 mg daily for 7–14 days), ketoconazole (200–400 mg with breakfast [requires acidic gastric environment for absorption] for 7–14 days), clotrimazole troches (10 mg dissolved orally five times daily), or nystatin vaginal troches (100,000 units dissolved orally five times daily) or mouth rinses (500,000 units [5 mL of 100,000 units/mL] held in the mouth before swallowing three times daily). Shorter-duration therapy has proved effective, using fluconazole. In patients with HIV infection, however, longer courses may be needed, and itraconazole (200 mg orally daily) may be indicated in fluconazole-refractory cases. In addition, 0.12% chlorhexidine or half-strength hydrogen peroxide mouth rinses may provide local relief. Nystatin powder (100,000 units/g) applied to dentures three or four times daily for several weeks may help denture wearers.

Epstein JB et al: Oropharyngeal candidiasis: A review of its clinical spectrum and current therapies. Clin Ther 1998;20:40. [PMID: 9522103] (In immunocompetent patients, topical agents often suffice in uncomplicated cases. Amphotericin B is now available as an oral suspension, adding another option, though systemic agents are often necessary in severe and recurrent cases.)

Graybill JR et al: Randomized trial of itraconazole oral solution for oropharyngeal candidiasis in HIV/AIDS patients. Am J Med 1998;104:33. [PMID: 9528717] (There were few adverse reactions to either itraconazole or fluconazole. About half of patients in all groups relapsed by 1 month.)

Laskaris G: Oral manifestations of infectious diseases. Dent Clin North Am 1996;40:395. [PMID: 8621529] (Presents the clinical features of the most common and important oral infectious diseases.)

Patton LL et al: A systematic review of the effectiveness of antifungal drugs for the prevention and treatment of oropharyngeal candidiasis in HIV-positive patients. Oral Surg Oral Med Oral Pathol Oral Radiol Endod 2001;92:170. [PMID: 11505264]

Smith D et al: A randomised, double-blind study of itraconazole versus placebo in the treatment and prevention of oral or oesophageal candidosis in patients with HIV infection. Int J Clin Pract 1999;53:349. [PMID: 10695098] (Itraconazole, 200 mg daily, is effective and well-tolerated for treatment and subsequent prophylaxis.)

GLOSSITIS & GLOSSODYNIA

Inflammation of the tongue with loss of filiform papillae leads to a red, smooth-surfaced tongue (glossitis). Rarely painful, it may be secondary to nutritional deficiencies (eg, niacin, riboflavin, iron or vitamin E),

drug reactions, dehydration, irritants, and possibly autoimmune reactions or psoriasis. If the primary cause cannot be identified and corrected, empirical nutritional replacement therapy may be of value.

Glossodynia is burning and pain of the tongue; it may occur with or without glossitis. It has been associated with diabetes, drugs (eg, diuretics), tobacco, xerostomia, and candidiasis as well as the listed causes of glossitis. Periodontal disease is not apt to be a factor. Treating possible underlying causes, changing chronic medications to alternative ones, and smoking cessation may resolve symptoms. Glossodynia is benign, and reassurance that there is no infection or tumor is likely to be appreciated. Anxiolytic medications and evaluation of possible psychologic status may be considered as well.

Bohmer T et al: The association between atrophic glossitis and protein-calorie malnutrition in old age. Age Aging 2000;29:47. [PMID: 10690695] (Atrophic glossitis is common in elderly people and is a marker for malnutrition and reduced muscle function.)

Grinspan D et al: Burning mouth syndrome. Int J Dermatol 1995;34:483. [PMID: 7591412] (After eliminating patients with local or systemic illnesses, this study reviews the definition of psychosomatic processes causing oral dysesthesia.)

Miyaoka H et al: A psychiatric appraisal of "glossodynia." Psychosomatics 1996;37:346. [PMID: 8701012] (The psychopathology of patients felt to have these pain symptoms without a clear etiology may be more associated with personality trait characteristics than with neurotic or depressive symptoms.)

Osaki T et al: Candidiasis may induce glossodynia without objective manifestation. Am J Med Sci 2000;319:100. [PMID: 10698094]

INTRAORAL ULCERATIVE LESIONS

1. Necrotizing Ulcerative Gingivitis (Trench Mouth, Vincent's Infection)

Necrotizing ulcerative gingivitis, often caused by an infection of both spirochetes and fusiform bacilli, is common in young adults under stress (classically at examination time). Underlying systemic diseases may also predispose to this disorder. Clinically, there is painful acute gingival inflammation and necrosis, often with bleeding, halitosis, fever, and cervical lymphadenopathy. Warm half-strength peroxide rinses and oral penicillin (250 mg three times daily for 10 days) may help. Dental gingival curettage may prove necessary.

Necrotizing ulcerative periodontitis is discussed later in this chapter in the section on AIDS.

Worle B et al: Chronic ulcerative stomatitis. Br J Dermatol 1997;137:262. [PMID: 9292078] (Chronic ulcerative stomatitis has recently been described as an entity characterized by chronic ulceration of oral mucosa that responds to treatment with hydroxychloroquine.)

2. Aphthous Ulcer (Canker Sore, Ulcerative Stomatitis)

Aphthous ulcers are very common and easy to recognize. Their cause remains uncertain, though an association with human herpesvirus 6 has been suggested. Found on nonkeratinized mucosa (eg, buccal and labial mucosa and not gingiva or palate), they may be single or multiple, are usually recurrent, and appear as painful small (usually 1–2 mm, but sometimes 1–2 cm) round ulcerations with yellow-gray fibrinoid centers surrounded by red halos. The painful stage lasts 7–10 days; healing is completed in 1–3 weeks.

Treatment is nonspecific. Topical steroids (triamcinolone acetonide, 0.1%, or fluocinonide ointment, 0.05%) in an adhesive base (Orabase Plain) do appear to provide symptomatic relief. Other topical therapies shown to be effective in controlled studies include diclofenac 3% in hyaluronan 2.5%, doxymycine-cyanoacrylate, mouthwashes containing the enzymes amyloglucosidase and glucose oxidase, and amlexanox 5% oral paste. A 1-week tapering course of prednisone (40–60 mg/d) has also been used successfully.

Large or persistent areas of ulcerative stomatitis may be secondary to erythema multiforme or drug allergies, acute herpes simplex, pemphigus, pemphigoid, bullous lichen planus, Behçet's disease, or inflammatory bowel disease. Squamous cell carcinoma may occasionally present in this fashion. When the diagnosis is not clear, incisional biopsy is indicated.

Chandrasekhar J et al: Oxypentifylline in the management of recurrent aphthous oral ulcers: an open clinical trial. Oral Surg Oral Med Oral Pathol Oral Radiol Endod 1999; 87:564. [PMID: 10348513] (Available in UK.)

Krause I et al: Recurrent aphthous stomatitis in Behçet's disease: clinical features and correlation with systemic disease expression and severity. J Oral Pathol Med 1999;28:193. [PMID: 10226940]

Landow K: Help for canker sores? Postgrad Med 2000;107:255. [PMID: 10649679]

MacPhail L: Topical and systemic therapy for recurrent aphthous stomatitis. Semin Cutan Med Surg 1997;16: 301. [PMID: 9421222] (The most effective treatments involve systemic or topical steroids or thalidomide.)

McBride DR: Management of aphthous ulcers. Am Fam Phys 2000;62:149. [PMID: 10905785]

Muzio LL et al: The treatment of oral aphthous ulceration or erosive lichen planus with topical clobetasol propionate in three preparations: a clinical and pilot study on 54 patients. J Oral Pathol Med 2001;30:611. [PMID: 11722711]

3. Herpetic Stomatitis

Herpetic gingivostomatitis is common, mild, and short-lived and requires no intervention in most adults. In immunocompromised individuals, however, reactivation of herpes simplex virus infection is frequent and may be severe. Clinically, there is initial burning, followed by typical small vesicles that rupture and form scabs. Acyclovir (200–800 mg five times daily for 7–14 days) may shorten the course and reduce postherpetic pain. Differential diagnosis includes ulcerative stomatitis (see above), erythema multiforme, syphilitic chancre, and carcinoma. Coxsackievirus-caused lesions (grayish white tonsillar and palatal ulcers of herpangina or buccal and lip ulcers in hand-foot-and-mouth disease) are seen more commonly in children under age 6.

Holbrook WP et al: Herpetic gingivostomatitis in otherwise healthy adolescents and young adults. Acta Otol Scand 2001;59.113. [PMID: 11501077]

Woo SB, Lee SF: Oral recrudescent herpes simplex virus infection. Oral Surg Oral Med Oral Pathol Oral Radiol Endod 1997;83:239. [PMID: 9117756] (Since acyclovir is available for treatment, the authors recommend all oral ulcers in immunocompromised patients be cultured for herpes simplex virus.)

PHARYNGITIS & TONSILLITIS

Pharyngitis and tonsillitis account for over 10% of all office visits to primary care clinicians and 50% of outpatient antibiotic use. The most appropriate management continues to be debated because some of the issues are deceptively complex, but consensus has increased in recent years. The main concern is determining who is likely to have a group A β-hemolytic streptococcal infection (GABHS), as this can lead to subsequent complications such as rheumatic fever and glomerular nephritis. A second public health policy concern is reducing the extraordinary cost (both in dollars and in the development of antibiotic-resistant *Streptococcus pneumoniae*) in the United States associated with unnecessary and unrecommended antibiotic use. Questions now being asked: Is there still a role for culturing a sore throat, or have the rapid antigen tests supplanted this procedure under most circumstances? Are clinical criteria alone a sufficient basis for decisions about which patients should be given antibiotics? Should any patient receive any antibiotic other than penicillin (or erythromycin if penicillin-allergic)? For how long should treatment be continued? Numerous well-done studies in the past few years as well as increasing experience with rapid laboratory tests for detection of streptococci (eliminating the delay caused by culturing) appear to make a consensus approach more possible.

The clinical features most suggestive of group A β-hemolytic streptococcal pharyngitis include fever over 38 °C, tender anterior cervical adenopathy, lack of a cough, and a pharyngotonsillar exudate. These four features (the Centor criteria), when present, strongly suggest GABHS, and some would treat regardless of laboratory results. When three of the four are present, laboratory sensitivity of rapid antigen testing exceeds 90%. When only one criterion is present, GABHS is unlikely. Sore throat may be severe, with odynophagia, tender adenopathy, and a scarlatiniform rash. An elevated white count and left shift are also possible. Hoarseness, cough, and coryza are not suggestive of this disease.

Marked lymphadenopathy and a shaggy white-purple tonsillar exudate, often extending into the nasopharynx, suggest mononucleosis, especially if present in a young adult. Hepatosplenomegaly and a positive heterophil agglutination test or elevated anti-EBV titer are corroborative. However, about one-third of patients with infectious mononucleosis have secondary streptococcal tonsillitis, requiring treatment. Ampicillin should routinely be avoided if mononucleosis is suspected because it induces a rash. Diphtheria (extremely rare but described in the alcoholic population) presents with low-grade fever and an ill patient with a gray tonsillar pseudomembrane.

The most common pathogens other than group A β-hemolytic streptococci in the differential diagnosis of "sore throat" are viruses, *Neisseria gonorrhoeae*, mycoplasma, and *Chlamydia trachomatis*. Rhinorrhea and lack of exudate would suggest a virus, but in practice it is not possible to confidently distinguish viral upper respiratory infection from group A β-hemolytic streptococcal infection on clinical grounds alone. Infections with *Corynebacterium diphtheriae*, anaerobic streptococci, and *Corynebacterium haemolyticum* (which responds better to erythromycin than penicillin) may also mimic pharyngitis due to group A β-hemolytic streptococci.

Treatment strategies for pharyngitis and tonsillitis range from "treat all comers" to "test all comers, reserving treatment for those with positive results." Issues that affect this decision include the reliability of cultures and rapid tests for streptococci (latex agglutination antigen tests and solid-phase enzyme immunoassays [ELISA]), the incidence of pharyngitis not due to group A β-hemolytic streptococci in the community, patient follow-up and medical compliance, and cost. The advantage of the "treat all" approach is the initial short-term cost, savings from elimination of diagnostic tests, and prevention of rheumatic fever, but such an approach necessarily causes the highest rate of antibiotic use and side effects and therefore overall the highest cost. At the other extreme is the "culture all" approach, which is associated with the fewest side effects but is dependent on excellent and rapid follow-up to prevent postinfectious complications. The sensitivity of current GABHS rapid antigen tests is now excellent, exceeding 90% in appropriately selected patients. It thus appears appropriate to screen for the four Centor criteria and use them in one of the following ways: (1) test patients who satisfy two or more criteria, and treat only those with positive results; (2) test those who satisfy two or three criteria, and treat both those with positive results and all patients who satisfy all four criteria without testing them; or (3) test nobody and treat all who satisfy three or four criteria. Routine cultures are not needed. Webb and colleagues, using this approach, found no increase in rates of complications among 7500 patients annually, about 75% of whom had high-specificity antigen tests without culture confirmation of negative results.

Thirty years ago, a single injection of benzathine penicillin or procaine penicillin was standard antibiotic treatment. This remains effective, but the injections are painful. If compliance is an issue, it may be the best choice. Oral treatment is also effective. Antibiotic choice aims to reduce the already low (10–20%) incidence of treatment failures (positive culture after treatment despite symptomatic resolution) and recurrences. A review of recent controlled studies suggests that penicillin V potassium (250 mg orally three times daily or 500 mg twice daily for 10 days) or cefuroxime axetil (250 mg orally twice daily for 5–10 days) are both effective. The efficacy of a 5-day regimen of penicillin V appears to be similar to a that of a 10-day course, with a 94% clinical response rate and an 84% streptococcal eradication rate. Erythromycin (active against mycoplasma and chlamydia) is a reasonable alternative to penicillin in allergic patients. Cephalosporins are somewhat more effective than penicillin in producing bacteriologic cures; 5-day administration has been successful for cefpodoxime and cefuroxime. The macrolide antibiotics have also been reported to be successful in shorter-duration regimens. Azithromycin (500 mg once daily) because of its long half-life, need be taken for only 3 days.

Adequate antibiotic treatment usually avoids the streptococcal complications of scarlet fever, glomerulonephritis, rheumatic myocarditis, and local abscess formation.

Antibiotics for treatment failures are also somewhat controversial. Surprisingly, penicillin-tolerant strains are not isolated more frequently in those who fail treatment than in those treated successfully with penicillin. The reasons for failure appear to be complex, and a second course of treatment with the same drug is not unreasonable. Alternatives to penicillin include cefuroxime and other cephalosporins, dicloxacillin (which is β-lactamase-resistant), and amoxicillin with clavulanate. When there is a history of penicillin allergy, alternatives should be used, such as erythromycin. Erythromycin resistance—with failure rates of about 25%—is an increasing problem in many areas. In cases of severe penicillin allergy, cephalosporins should be avoided as the cross-reaction is common (8% or more).

Ancillary treatment of pharyngitis includes analgesics and anti-inflammatory agents, such as aspirin or acetaminophen. Some patients find that salt water gargling is soothing. In severe cases, anesthetic gargles and lozenges (eg, benzocaine) may provide additional symptomatic relief. Occasionally, odynophagia is so intense that hospitalization for intravenous hydration and antibiotics is necessary.

Cooper RJ et al: Principles of appropriate antibiotic use for acute pharyngitis in adults: background. Ann Intern Med 2001;134:509. [PMID: 11255530] (Overview of issues and recommendations.)

Dimatteo LA et al: The relationship between the clinical features of pharyngitis and the sensitivity of a rapid antigen test: evidence of spectrum bias. Ann Emerg Med 2001;38:648.

[PMID: 11719744] (The sensitivity of rapid antigen tests is over 90% when three or four of the following clinical criteria are present: fever, absence of cough, pharyngeal exudate, and enlarged lymph nodes.)

Gonzales R et al: Excessive antibiotic use for acute respiratory infections in the. United States. Clin Infect Dis 2001;33:757. [PMID. 11512079] (Over $700 million annually appears to be spent in the United States unnecessarily.)

Gonzales R et al: Principles of appropriate antibiotic use for treatment of acute respiratory tract infections in adults: background, specific aims, and methods. Ann Intern Med 2001;134:479. [PMID: 11233324]

Linder JA et al: Antibiotic treatment of adults with sore throat by community primary care physicians: a national survey, 1989–1999. JAMA 2001;286:1181. [PMID: 11559262] (Although less than 20% of adult sore throats culture group A beta-hemolytic streptococci, over two-thirds of the 6.7 million United States visits in this decade for sore throat resulted in antibiotic prescriptions. Over half of the antibiotics prescribed were other than those recommended for first-line use.)

Ressel G: Principles of appropriate antibiotic use: Part IV. Acute pharyngitis. Am Fam Physician 2001;64:870. [PMID: 11563576]

Snow V et al: Principles of appropriate antibiotic use for acute pharyngitis in adults. Ann Intern Med 2001;134:506. [PMID: 11255529]

Sonnad SS et al: Issues in the development, dissemination, and effect of an evidence-based guideline for managing sore throat in adults. Jt Comm J Qual Improv 1999;25:630. [PMID: 10605653] (Had the guidelines been followed, the amount of testing would have been reduced by 17% and the appropriateness of testing improved for 32%.)

Webb KH et al: Use of a high-sensitivity rapid strep test without culture confirmation of negative results: 2 years' experience. J Fam Pract 2000;49:34. (Erratum in J Fam Practice 2000;49:378.) [PMID: 10678338] (In two years' experience, use of a high-sensitivity antigen test without culture confirmation of all negative results was not associated with an increase in complications of group A beta-hemolytic streptococci.)

PERITONSILLAR ABSCESS & CELLULITIS

When infection penetrates the tonsillar capsule and involves the surrounding tissues, peritonsillar cellulitis results. Peritonsillar abscess and cellulitis present with severe sore throat, odynophagia, trismus, medial deviation of the soft palate and peritonsillar fold, and an abnormal muffled ("hot potato") voice. Following therapy, peritonsillar cellulitis usually either resolves over several days or evolves into peritonsillar abscess. The existence of an abscess may be confirmed by aspirating pus from the peritonsillar fold just superior and medial to the upper pole of the tonsil. A No. 19 or No. 21 needle should be passed no deeper than 1 cm, because the internal carotid artery passes posterior and deep to the tonsillar fossa. There is controversy about the best way to treat peritonsillar abscesses. Some incise and drain the area and continue with parenteral antibiotics, whereas others aspirate only and follow as an outpatient. To drain the abscess and avoid recurrence, it may be appropriate to consider immediate tonsillectomy (quinsy tonsillectomy). About 10% of patients with peritonsillar abscess exhibit relative indications for tonsillectomy. All three approaches are rational and have support in the literature. Regardless, one must be sure the abscess is adequately drained, since complications such as extension to the retropharyngeal, deep neck, and posterior mediastinal spaces are possible. Bacteria may also be aspirated into the lungs, resulting in pneumonia. While there is controversy about whether a single abscess is sufficient indication for tonsillectomy, most would agree that patients with recurrent abscesses should have their tonsils removed.

Kieff DA et al: Selection of antibiotics after incision and drainage of peritonsillar abscesses. Otolaryngol Head Neck Surg 1999;120:57. [PMID: 9913550] (Retrospective review. Penicillin was an excellent choice in cases requiring parenteral antibiotics.)

TONSILLECTOMY

Despite the frequency with which tonsillectomy is performed, the indications for the procedure remain controversial. Most would agree that airway obstruction causing sleep apnea or cor pulmonale is an absolute indication for tonsillectomy. Similarly, persistent marked tonsillar asymmetry should prompt an excisional biopsy to rule out lymphoma. Relative indications include recurrent streptococcal tonsillitis, causing considerable loss of time from school or work, recurrent peritonsillar abscess, and chronic tonsillitis.

Tonsillectomy is not an entirely benign procedure. The pros and cons of tonsillectomy need to be discussed with each prospective patient. Postoperative bleeding occurs in 2–4% of cases and on rare occasions can lead to laryngospasm and airway obstruction. Pain may be considerable, especially in the adult. Protracted emesis or fever may also occasionally occur. Secondary bleeding 5–8 days postoperatively is far more common than bleeding in the first 24 hours. There is increasing economic pressure for these procedures to be done as outpatient surgery. At present it seems clear that outpatient tonsillectomy is usually safe when followed by a 6-hour period of uneventful observation, but individual circumstances may mandate hospitalization.

Although reports in the 1970s suggested an association of tonsillectomy with Hodgkin's disease, careful review of this literature reveals no conclusively causative association.

Bhattacharyya N et al: Efficacy and quality-of-life impact of adult tonsillectomy. Arch Otolaryngol Head Neck Surg 2001; 127:1347. [PMID: 11701072]

Boot H et al: Long-term results of uvulopalatopharyngoplasty for obstructive sleep apnea syndrome. Laryngoscope 2000; 110(3 Part 1):469. [PMID: 10718440] (The response to UPPP for obstructive sleep apnea syndrome decreases progressively over the years after surgery. UPPP in combination with tonsillectomy was more effective than UPPP alone.)

Peeters A et al: Tonsillectomy and adenotomy as a one day procedure? Acta Otorhinolaryngol Belg 1999;53:91. [PMID: 10427360] (Because of a postoperative major bleeding frequency between 2.6% and 3%, the authors prefer an overnight postoperative stay.)

Randall DA et al: Complications of tonsillectomy and adenoidectomy. Otolaryngol Head Neck Surg 1998;118:61. [PMID: 9450830] (Review of common and rare potential complications.)

Raut VV et al: Peritonsillar abscess: the rationale for interval tonsillectomy. Ear Nose Throat J 2000;79:206. [PMID 10743768] (Reviews practices among 571 practicing otolaryngologists in the United Kingdom. Most recommend interval tonsillectomy following a peritonsillar abscess only for patients with a history of tonsillitis.)

Wei JL et al: Evaluation of posttonsillectomy hemorrhage and risk factors. Otolaryngol Head Neck Surg 2000;123:229. [PMID: 10964296] (Two percent bled, usually between postoperative days 5 and 7. Adults age 21–30 bled about twice as often—3.6%—as children. Half of patients who bled returned to the operating room for control.)

DEEP NECK INFECTIONS

Deep neck abscesses usually present with marked neck pain and swelling in a toxic febrile patient. They are emergencies because they may rapidly compromise the airway. They may also spread to the mediastinum or cause septicemia. Most commonly, they originate from odontogenic infections. Other causes include suppurative lymphadenitis, direct spread of pharyngeal infection, penetrating trauma, pharyngoesophageal foreign bodies, cervical osteomyelitis, and intravenous injection of the internal jugular vein, especially in drug abusers. Recurrent deep neck infection may suggest an underlying congenital lesion such as a branchial cleft cyst.

Fundamentals of treatment include securing the airway, intravenous antibiotics, and incision and drainage. In highly selected patients without airway compromise, needle aspiration and catheter drainage or even conservative management without antibiotics alone has been reported to be successful in uniloculated abscesses. The airway may be secured either by intubation or tracheotomy. Tracheotomy is preferable in the patients with substantial pharyngeal edema, since attempts at intubation may precipitate acute airway obstruction. Bleeding in association with a deep neck abscess suggests the possibility of carotid artery or internal jugular vein involvement and requires prompt neck exploration both for drainage of pus and for vascular control.

Contrast-enhanced CT usually augments the clinical examination in defining the extent of the infection. It often will distinguish inflammation (requiring antibiotics) from abscess (requiring drainage) and define for the surgeon the extent of an abscess. CT with MRI may also identify thrombophlebitis of the internal jugular vein secondary to oropharyngeal inflammation. This condition, known as Lemierre's syndrome, may be associated with septic emboli and requires prompt institution of antibiotics appropriate for *Fusobacterium necrophorum* as well as the more usual upper airway pathogens.

Ludwig's angina is the most commonly encountered neck space infection. It is a cellulitis of the sublingual and submaxillary spaces, often arising from infection of the tooth roots that extend below the mylohyoid line of the mandible. Clinically, there is edema and erythema of the upper neck under the chin and often of the floor of the mouth. The tongue may be displaced upward and backward by the posterior spread of cellulitis. This may lead to occlusion of the airway and necessitate tracheotomy. Microbiologic isolates include streptococci, staphylococci, bacteroides, and fusobacterium. Usual doses of penicillin plus metronidazole, ampicillin-sulbactam, clindamycin, or selective cephalosporins are good initial choices. Culture and sensitivity data will then refine the choice. Dental consultation is advisable. External drainage via bilateral submental incisions is required if the airway is threatened or when medical therapy has not reversed the process.

Agarwal R et al: Lemierre's syndrome: a complication of acute oropharyngitis. J Laryngol Otol 2000;114:545. [PMID: 10992941]

Gidley PW et al: Contemporary management of deep neck space infections. Otolaryngol Head Neck Surg 1997;116:16. [PMID: 9018251] (Operative drainage, bacteriology, and complications.)

Miller WD et al: A prospective, blinded comparison of clinical examination and computed tomography in deep neck infections. Laryngoscope 1999;109:1873. [PMID: 10569425] (They complement each other in assessing suspected deep neck infection.)

Nusbaum AO et al: Recurrence of a deep neck infection: a clinical indication of an underlying congenital lesion. Arch Otolaryngol Head Neck Surg 1999;125:1379. [PMID: 10604419]

Wong TY: A nationwide survey of deaths from oral and maxillofacial infections: the Taiwanese experience. J Oral Maxillofacial Surg 1999;57:1297. [PMID: 10555793] (Two-thirds of deaths occurred in patients with diabetes. The death rate was about 1:150, usually associated with sepsis.)

Yeow KM et al: US-guided needle aspiration and catheter drainage as an alternative to open surgical drainage for uniloculated neck abscesses. J Vasc Interv Radiol 2001; 12:589. [PMID: 11340137]

■ DISEASES OF THE SALIVARY GLANDS

The salivary glands are divided into the two large parotid glands, two submandibular glands, several sublingual glands, and 600–1000 minor salivary glands located throughout the upper aerodigestive tract.

ACUTE INFLAMMATORY SALIVARY GLAND DISORDERS

1. Sialadenitis

Acute bacterial sialadenitis in the adult most commonly affects either the parotid or submandibular gland. It typically presents with acute swelling of the gland, increased pain and swelling with meals, and tenderness and erythema of the duct opening. Pus often can be massaged from the duct. Sialadenitis often occurs in the setting of dehydration or in association with chronic illness. Underlying Sjögren's syndrome may contribute. Ductal obstruction, often by an inspissated mucous plug, is followed by salivary stasis and secondary infection. The most common organism recovered from purulent draining saliva is *S aureus*. Treatment consists of intravenous antibiotics such as nafcillin (1 g intravenously every 4–6 hours) and measures to increase salivary flow, including hydration, warm compresses, sialagogues (eg, lemon drops), and massage of the gland. Usually one can switch to an oral agent based on clinical and microbiologic improvement to complete a 10-day course. Failure of the process to resolve on this regimen suggests abscess formation, ductal stricture, stone, or tumor causing obstruction. Ultrasound or CT scan may be helpful in establishing the diagnosis. Sialography is best avoided in acute cases.

Bates D et al: Parotid and submandibular sialadenitis treated by salivary gland excision. Aust N Z J Surg 1998;68:120. [PMID: 9494003] (In recurrent cases with prolonged symptoms, surgical excision of the affected gland is effective.)

Nahlieli O et al: Long-term experience with endoscopic diagnosis and treatment of salivary gland inflammatory diseases. Laryngoscope 2000;110:988. [PMID: 10852519] (Among 236 procedures since 1994, 83% were successful, 75% showed obstruction, and 25% showed sialadenitis without obstruction.)

Yousem DM et al: Major salivary gland imaging. Radiology 2000;216:19. [PMID: 10887223] (A tutorial review.)

2. Sialolithiasis

Calculus formation is more common in Wharton's duct (draining the submandibular glands) than in Stensen's duct (draining the parotid glands). Clinically, a patient may note postprandial pain and local swelling, often with a history of recurrent acute sialadenitis. Stones in Wharton's duct are usually large and radiopaque, whereas those in Stensen's duct are usually radiolucent and smaller. Those very close to the orifice of Wharton's duct may be palpated manually in the anterior floor of the mouth and removed intraorally by dilating or incising the distal duct. The duct proximal to the stone must be temporarily clamped (using, for instance, a single throw of a suture) to keep manipulation of the stone from pushing it back toward the submandibular gland. Those more than 1.5–2 cm from the duct are too close to the lingual nerve to be removed safely in this manner. Similarly, dilation of Stensen's duct, located on the buccal surface opposite the second maxillary molar, may relieve distal stricture or allow a small stone to pass. The location of the facial nerve makes intraoral retrieval of more proximal parotid stones unsafe.

Repeated episodes of sialadenitis invariably lead to stricture and chronic infection. If the obstruction cannot be safely removed or dilated, excision of the gland may be necessary. In recent years there has been increased success with endoscopic techniques both to diagnose and remove salivary stones, with success rates for calculus removal in excess of 80%.

Bull PD: Salivary gland stones: diagnosis and treatment. Hosp Med 2001;62:396. [PMID: 11480125]

Nahlieli O et al: Endoscopic technique for the diagnosis and treatment of obstructive salivary gland diseases. J Oral Maxillofac Surg 1999;57:1394. [PMID: 10596658] (Endoscopy was possible in 145 of 154, of which 112 were obstructed. The success rate was 82% for calculus removal. Thirty-two percent of the submandibular and 63% of the parotid sialoliths were undetected prior to the procedure.)

Williams MF: Sialolithiasis. Otolaryngol Clin North Am 1999; 32:819. [PMID: 10477749]

CHRONIC INFLAMMATORY & INFILTRATIVE DISORDERS OF THE SALIVARY GLANDS

Numerous infiltrative disorders may cause unilateral or bilateral parotid gland enlargement. Sjögren's disease and sarcoidosis are examples of lymphoepithelial and granulomatous diseases that may affect the salivary glands. Metabolic disorders, including alcoholism, diabetes mellitus, and vitamin deficiencies, may also cause diffuse enlargement. Several drugs have been associated with parotid enlargement, including thioureas, iodine, and drugs with cholinergic effects (eg, phenothiazines), which stimulate salivary flow and cause more viscous saliva.

SALIVARY GLAND TUMORS

Approximately 80% of salivary gland tumors occur in the parotid gland. In adults, about 80% of these are benign. In the submandibular triangle, it is sometimes difficult to distinguish a primary submandibular gland tumor from a metastatic submandibular space node. Only 50–60% of primary submandibular tumors are benign. Tumors of the minor salivary glands are most likely to be malignant, with adenoid cystic carcinoma predominating.

Most parotid tumors present as an asymptomatic mass in the superficial part of the gland. Their presence may have been noted by the patient for months or years. Facial nerve involvement correlates strongly with malignancy. Tumors may extend deep to the plane of the facial nerve or may originate in the parapharyngeal space. In such cases, medial deviation of the soft palate is visible on intraoral examination. MRI and CT scans have largely replaced sialography in defining the extent of tumor.

When the clinician encounters a patient with an otherwise asymptomatic salivary gland mass where tumor is the most likely diagnosis, the choice is whether to simply excise the mass via a parotidectomy with facial nerve dissection or submandibular gland excision or to obtain a fine-needle aspiration (FNA) biopsy first. Although the accuracy of FNA biopsy for malignancy has been reported to be quite high, results vary among institutions. If a negative FNA biopsy would lead to a decision not to proceed to surgery, then it should be considered. Poor overall health of the patient and the possibility of inflammatory disease as the cause of the mass are situations where FNA biopsy might be helpful. In otherwise straightforward nonrecurrent cases, excision is indicated. In benign and small low-grade malignant tumors, no additional treatment is needed. Postoperative irradiation is required for larger and high-grade cancers.

Hocwald E et al: Prognostic factors in major salivary gland cancer. Laryngoscope 2001;111:1434. [PMID: 11568581]

Vaughan ED: Management of malignant salivary gland tumours. Hosp Med 2001;62:400. [PMID: 11480126]

■ DISEASES OF THE LARYNX

DYSPHONIA, HOARSENESS, & STRIDOR

The primary symptoms of laryngeal disease are hoarseness and stridor. Hoarseness is caused by an abnormal flow of air past the vocal cords. The voice is "breathy" when too much air passes incompletely apposed vocal cords, as in unilateral vocal cord paralysis. The voice is harsh when turbulence is created by irregularity of the vocal cords, as in laryngitis or a mass lesion. Stridor, a high-pitched sound, is produced by lesions that narrow the airway. Airway narrowing above the vocal cords produces predominantly inspiratory stridor. Airway narrowing below the vocal cord level produces either expiratory or mixed stridor.

Evaluation of an abnormal voice begins with obtaining a history of the circumstances preceding its onset and an examination of the airway. This may include indirect or flexible laryngoscopy and at times videostrobolaryngoscopy. Especially when the patient has a history of tobacco use, laryngeal cancer or lung cancer (leading to paralysis of a recurrent laryngeal nerve) must be strongly considered. Laryngitis, voice abuse, and vocal cord nodules are among the most common causes of hoarseness.

Garrett CG et al: Hoarseness. Med Clin North Am 1999;83:115. [PMID: 9927964] (Describes normal vocal anatomy and physiology and outlines a practical approach in evaluating patients with voice disorders.)

Hagen P et al: Dysphonia in the elderly: Diagnosis and management of age-related voice changes. South Med J 1996;89:204. [PMID: 8578351]

MacKenzie K et al: Is voice therapy an effective treatment for dysphonia? A randomised controlled trial. BMJ 2001;323:658. [PMID: 11566828]

Rosen CA et al: Evaluating hoarseness: keeping your patient's voice healthy. Am Fam Physician 1998;57:2775. [PMID: 9636340] (In the absence of an upper respiratory tract infection, any patient with hoarseness persisting for more than 2 weeks requires evaluation. Voice therapy is helpful in many non-cancer-related cases of hoarseness.)

COMMON LARYNGEAL DISORDERS

1. Epiglottitis

Epiglottitis (or, more correctly, supraglottitis) in adults should be suspected when a patient presents with a rapidly developing sore throat or when odynophagia (pain on swallowing) is out of proportion to apparently minimal oropharyngeal findings on examination. It may be viral or bacterial in origin. Unlike in children, indirect laryngoscopy is generally safe and may demonstrate a swollen, erythematous epiglottis. Initial treatment is hospitalization for intravenous antibiotics—eg, ceftizoxime, 1–2 g intravenously every 8–12 hours; or cefuroxime, 750–1500 mg intravenously every 8 hours; and dexamethasone, usually 4–10 mg as initial bolus, then 4 mg intravenously every 6 hours—and observation of the airway. Steroids may be tapered as signs and symptoms resolve. Similarly, substitution of oral antibiotics may be appropriate to complete a 10-day course. When epiglottitis is recognized early in the adult, it is usually possible to avoid intubation. Indications for intubation are dyspnea or rapid pace of sore throat (where progression to airway compromise may occur before the effects of steroids and antibiotics take hold). If the patient is not intubated, prudence would suggest monitoring oxygen saturation with continuous pulse oximetry and initial admission to an intensive care unit.

Ducic Y et al: Description and evaluation of the vallecula sign: a new radiologic sign in the diagnosis of adult epiglottitis. Ann Emerg Med 1997;30:1. [PMID: 9209217] (Radiologic exclusion of epiglottitis may have merit compared with direct inspection in adults, but in children strong clinical suspicion should trigger a protocol that includes intraoperative inspection and airway control.)

Garpenholt O et al: Epiglottitis in Sweden before and after introduction of vaccination against Haemophilus influenzae type b. Pediatr Infect Dis J 1999;18:490. [PMID: 10391176] (Interestingly, there was a tendency toward fewer cases of epiglottitis in adults even though only children were vaccinated. The incidence in children was reduced 20-fold.)

Hebert PC et al: Adult epiglottitis in a Canadian setting. Laryngoscope 1998;108(1 Part 1):64. [PMID: 9432069] (Only the presence of dyspnea [noted in 29% of patients] at the time of admission predicted the need for intubation.)

Park KW et al: Airway management for adult patients with acute epiglottitis: a 12-year experience at an academic medical center (1984–1995). Anesthesiology 1998;88:254. [PMID: 9447879]

2. Laryngeal Papillomas

Papillomas are common lesions of the larynx and other sites where ciliated and squamous epithelia meet. Unlike oral papillomas, laryngeal papillomas are likely to be symptomatic, with hoarseness that progresses to stridor over weeks to months. The disease is more common in children. Repeated laser excisions via microdirect laryngoscopy are often needed to control the disease. Tracheotomy should be avoided, if possible, since it introduces an additional squamociliary junction where papillomas appear to preferentially grow. Interferon treatment has been under investigation.

Dedo HH et al: CO2 laser treatment in 244 patients with respiratory papillomas. Laryngoscope 2001;111:1639. [PMID: 11568620]

Derkay CS: Recurrent respiratory papillomatosis. Laryngoscope 2001;111:57. [PMID: 11192901]

3. Acute Laryngitis

Acute laryngitis is probably the most common cause of hoarseness, which may persist for a week or so after other symptoms of an upper respiratory infection have cleared. The patient should be warned to avoid vigorous use of the voice (singing, shouting) while laryngitis is present, since this may foster the formation of vocal nodules. Although thought to be usually viral in origin, both *Moraxella catarrhalis* and *Haemophilus influenzae* may be isolated from the nasopharynx at higher than expected frequencies. Erythromycin may reduce the severity of hoarseness and cough.

Spiegel JR et al: Acute laryngitis. Ear Nose Throat J 2000;79:488. [PMID: 10935296]

4. Gastroesophageal Reflux & Hoarseness

Gastroesophageal reflux into the larynx (laryngopharyngeal reflux) should be considered a possible cause of chronic hoarseness if other causes of abnormal laryngeal airflow (such as tumor) have been excluded by indirect or direct laryngoscopy. Gastroesophageal reflux disease (GERD) has also been implicated as a contributing factor to other symptoms such as throat clearing, throat discomfort, chronic cough, a sensation of postnasal drip, and esophageal spasm; as well as in many cases of posterior laryngitis and some cases of asthma. As less than half of patients with documented laryngopharyngeal reflux have typical symptoms of heartburn and regurgitation, the lack of such symptoms should not be construed as eliminating this cause.

Management should initially exclude other causes of hoarseness, laryngitis, or chronic cough; consultation with an otolaryngologist is advisable. Many next advocate an empiric trial of a proton pump inhibitor at twice-daily dosing (eg, omeprazole 20 mg twice daily) for 2–3 months as a practical alternative to an initial pH study. If symptoms improve and cessation of therapy leads to symptoms again, then a proton pump inhibitor is resumed at the lowest dose effective for remission, usually daily but at times on a demand basis. Although H_2 receptor antagonists are an alternative to proton pump inhibitors, they are generally both less clinically effective and less cost-effective. Nonresponders should undergo pH testing and manometry. Twenty-four-hour pH monitoring of the pharynx should best document laryngopharyngeal reflux and is advocated by some as the initial management step but it is costly, more difficult, and less available than lower esophageal monitoring alone. Lower esophageal pH monitoring does not correlate well with laryngopharyngeal reflux symptoms.

Berardi RR: A critical evaluation of proton pump inhibitors in the treatment of gastroesophageal reflux disease. Am J Manag Care 2000;6(9 Suppl):S491. [PMID: 10977489] (Proton pump inhibitors are more cost-effective than H2 receptor antagonists.)

Fraser AG et al: Presumed laryngo-pharyngeal reflux: investigate or treat? J Laryngol Otol 2000;114:441. [PMID: 10962677] (Fifty-five percent responded to omeprazole. Reflux symptoms were not a predictor of response.)

Gerson LB et al: A cost-effectiveness analysis of prescribing strategies in the management of gastroesophageal reflux disease. Am J Gastroenterol 2000;95:395. [PMID: 10685741] (Initial treatment with proton pump inhibitors followed by on-demand dosing is more cost-effective treatment for GERD.)

Giacchi RJ et al: Compliance with anti-reflux therapy in patients with otolaryngologic manifestations of gastroesophageal reflux disease. Laryngoscope 2000;110:19. [PMID: 10646709] (A review of otolaryngologic symptoms of GERD, sore throat, throat clearing, sensation of postnasal drip, hoarseness, and esophageal spasm; with suggestions on management.)

Klinkenberg-Knol EC: Otolaryngologic manifestations of gastro-oesophageal reflux disease. Scand J Gastroenterol Suppl 1998;225:24. [PMID: 9515748] (Documents that only 25% of patients with laryngopharyngeal symptoms felt to be secondary to GERD have esophagitis endoscopically—hence pH monitoring with a dual pH probe is necessary for diagnosis.)

Knight RE, Wells JR, Parrish RS: Esophageal dysmotility as an important co-factor in extraesophageal manifestations of gastroesophageal reflux. Laryngoscope 2000;110:1462-6. [PMID: 10983943] (About 75% of patients with extraesophageal manifestations [such as hoarseness, chronic cough, paroxysmal laryngospasm or dysphagia/globus pharyngeus] had dysmotility. Of note is that there is no statistically significant association between dysmotility and abnormal acid reflux in these patients.)

Ulualp SO et al: Laryngopharyngeal reflux: state of the art diagnosis and treatment. Otolaryngol Clin North Am 2000;33:785. [PMID: 10918661]

Wong RK et al: ENT manifestations of gastroesophageal reflux. Am J Gastroenterol 2000;95(8 Suppl):S15. [PMID: 10950101] (Presents a thoughtful algorithm for treatment: After excluding other causes of hoarseness and laryngitis, advocates treating empirically for 2–3 months with a proton pump inhibitor twice daily, reserving testing for nonresponders. This supplement also contains a number of other closely related articles on this subject.)

TUMORS OF THE LARYNX

1. Benign Tumors of the Larynx

Vocal cord nodules are smooth, paired lesions that form at the junction of the anterior one-third and posterior two-thirds of the vocal cords. They are a common cause of hoarseness resulting from vocal abuse. In adults, they are referred to as "singer's nodules"; in children, "screamer's nodules." Treatment requires modification of voice habits, and referral to a speech therapist is indicated. Recalcitrant nodules may require surgical excision.

Polypoid changes in the vocal cords may result from vocal abuse, smoking, chemical industrial irritants, or hypothyroidism. Attention to the underlying problem may resolve the polypoid changes. Inhaled steroid spray (eg, beclomethasone, 42 µg/spray, or dexamethasone, 84 µg/spray, two or three times a day) may hasten resolution. At times, removal of the hyperplastic vocal cord mucosa may be indicated.

A common but often unrecognized cause of hoarseness is contact ulcers on the vocal processes of the arytenoid cartilages secondary to esophageal reflux. Treatment may be with H_2-receptor blockers or proton pump inhibitors (see Gastroesophageal Reflux and Hoarseness, above). Intubation granulomas may also be seen posteriorly between the vocal processes.

2. Laryngeal Leukoplakia

Leukoplakia is a frequent cause of hoarseness, most commonly arising in smokers. Direct laryngoscopy with biopsy is advised. Histologic examination usually demonstrates mild, moderate, or severe dysplasia. Cessation of smoking may reverse dysplastic changes. A certain percentage of patients—estimated to be less than 5% of those with mild dysplasia and about 35–60% of those with severe dysplasia—will subsequently develop squamous cell carcinoma. In some cases, invasive squamous cell carcinoma is present in the initial biopsy.

3. Squamous Cell Carcinoma of the Larynx

Squamous cell carcinoma is the most common cancer seen in the larynx. It occurs predominantly in heavy smokers, with alcohol an apparent cocarcinogen. It is most common between ages 50 and 70. Hoarseness is the usual presenting symptom. Any patient with hoarseness that has persisted beyond 2–3 weeks should be evaluated by indirect laryngoscopy. Odynophagia, hemoptysis, weight loss, referred otalgia, vocal cord immobility, and cervical adenopathy suggest more advanced disease.

Early squamous cell carcinoma is best treated with radiation, with cure rates in excess of 85–95%. For larger tumors, organ preservation approaches, usually consisting of irradiation and concomitant chemotherapy, are often recommended. Total laryngectomy is necessary for many large tumors and for most irradiation failures. A number of partial laryngectomy procedures are sometimes considered for selected smaller and intermediate-sized tumors. Treatment of glottic (vocal cord) tumors in which a cord is paralyzed and for supraglottic tumors includes treatment of the neck because of the high risk of neck node involvement. The use of tracheoesophageal valves following total laryngectomy restores useful speech for most patients.

Garden AS: Organ preservation for carcinoma of the larynx and hypopharynx. Hematol Oncol Clin North Am 2001;15:243. [PMID: 11370491]

Sasaki CT et al: Cancer of the pharynx and larynx. Am J Med 2001;111(Suppl 8A):118S. [PMID: 11749936]

VOCAL CORD PARALYSIS

Most cases of vocal cord paralysis result from involvement of a recurrent laryngeal nerve; others arise more proximally along the vagus nerve itself. Common causes of recurrent laryngeal nerve involvement include thyroid surgery (and occasionally thyroid cancer), other neck surgery (anterior discectomy and carotid endarterectomy), and mediastinal or apical involvement by lung cancer. Skull base tumors often involve cranial nerves IX, X, and XI. Occasionally, no cause can be identified. When either no cause is found or the paresis follows surgical trauma in which the nerve was not divided, spontaneous recovery commonly occurs, usually within a year.

Unlike unilateral cord paralysis, which produces a breathy hoarseness, bilateral cord paralysis usually causes inspiratory and expiratory stridor if acute, in which case intervention to create an emergency airway may be needed. If insidious in onset, it may be asymptomatic at rest, including a normal voice, though there is usually dyspnea on exertion. Causes of bilateral cord paralysis include thyroid surgery, esophageal cancer, and ventricular shunt malfunction. Unilateral or bilateral cord immobility may also be seen in cricoarytenoid arthritis secondary to advanced rheumatoid arthritis, intubation injuries, glottic and subglottic stenosis, and, of course, laryngeal cancer. The goal of intervention is the creation of a safe airway with minimal reduction in voice quality and airway protection from aspiration. A number of cord lateralization procedures have been advocated as a means of removing the tracheotomy tube.

Surgical management of persistent or irrecoverable symptomatic unilateral vocal cord paralysis has evolved over the last several decades. The primary goal is medialization of the paralyzed cord in order to rehabilitate the voice. Additional goals include eliminating aspiration, improving diet, and aiding in the subsequent decannulation of individuals with glottic insufficiency. Success has been reported for years with injection medialization using predominantly Teflon, but other materials as well have been used, such as fat or Gelfoam. An alternative to injection medialization of the vocal fold is to medialize the soft tissue and arytenoid via a small incision overlying the thyroid cartilage under local anesthesia. A section of the cartilage is removed, providing access to the soft tissue of the larynx and the arytenoid cartilage. An implant is inserted that displaces this soft tissue and arytenoid medially.

Carrau RL et al: Laryngeal framework surgery for the management of aspiration. Head Neck 1999;21:139. [PMID: 1091982] (In addition to rehabilitation of the voice, medialization laryngoplasty with silicone with or without arytenoid adduction is usually helpful for aspiration as well.)

Crumley RL: Laryngeal synkinesis revisited. Ann Otol Rhinol Laryngol 2000;109:365. [PMID: 10778890] (A good discussion of the finer points of the problem.)

Espinoza FI et al: Vocal fold paralysis following carotid endarterectomy. J Laryngol Otol 1999;113:439. [PMID: 10505157] (Ten percent noted hoarseness postoperatively; in 4%, examination confirmed vocal cord paralysis.)

Hughes CA et al: Unilateral true vocal fold paralysis: cause of right-sided lesions. Otolaryngol Head Neck Surg 2000;122:678. [PMID: 10793345]

Lo CY et al. A prospective evaluation of recurrent laryngeal nerve paralysis during thyroidectomy. Arch Surg 2000;135:204. [PMID: 10668882] (Of 33 cases of unilateral cord paralysis, only five had recognizable nerve damage intraoperatively. Complete recovery occurred in 26 of the remaining 28.)

McLean-Muse A et al: Montgomery Thyroplasty Implant for vocal fold immobility: phonatory outcomes. Ann Otol Rhinol Laryngol 2000;109:393. [PMID: 10778895] (Unilateral vocal cord immobility can be treated with a commercially available implant system.)

Morpeth JF et al: Vocal fold paralysis after anterior cervical diskectomy and fusion. Laryngoscope 2000;110:43. [PMID: 10646714] (Twenty-one [5%] of 441 developed vocal cord paralysis; 15 of 18 reviewed at 1 year had recovered.)

■ TRACHEOTOMY & CRICOTHYROTOMY

There are two primary indications for tracheotomy: airway obstruction at or above the level of the larynx and respiratory failure requiring prolonged mechanical ventilation. In an acute emergency, cricothyrotomy secures an airway more rapidly than tracheotomy, with fewer potential immediate complications such as pneumothorax and hemorrhage. Although classically it has been recommended that one should change a cricothyrotomy to a tracheotomy as soon as it is convenient and safe, recent studies have questioned this if decannulation can be expected soon. Percutaneous dilation tracheotomy as an elective bedside (or ICU) procedure has undergone scrutiny in recent years as an alternative to tracheotomy. In experienced hands the various methods of percutaneous dilation tracheotomy have been documented to be safe, though complications do occur. When a patient is not intubated, simultaneous bronchoscopy may reduce complications. The major cost reduction comes from not using the main operating room. Bedside tracheotomy (in the ICU) achieves similar cost reduction and is advocated by some as slightly less costly than the percutaneous dilation procedure.

The most common indication for elective tracheotomy is the need for prolonged mechanical ventilation. There is no firm rule about how many days a patient must be intubated before conversion to tracheotomy should be advised. The incidence of serious complications such as subglottic stenosis increases with extended endotracheal intubation. As soon as it is apparent that the patient will require protracted ventilatory support, tracheotomy should replace the endotracheal tube. Less frequent indications for tracheotomy are life-threatening aspiration pneumonia, the need to improve pulmonary toilet to correct problems related to insufficient clearing of tracheobronchial secretions, and sleep apnea.

Posttracheotomy care requires humidified air to prevent secretions from crusting and occluding the inner cannula of the tracheotomy tube. The tracheotomy tube should be cleaned several times daily. The most frequent early complication of tracheotomy is dislodgment of the tracheotomy tube. Surgical creation of an inferiorly based tracheal flap sutured to the inferior neck skin may make reinsertion of a dislodged tube easier. It should be recalled that the act of swallowing requires elevation of the larynx, which is prevented by tracheotomy. Therefore, frequent tracheal and bronchial suctioning is often required to clear the aspirated saliva as well as the increased tracheobronchial secretions. Care of the skin around the stoma is important to prevent maceration and secondary infection.

Freeman BD et al: A prospective, randomized study comparing percutaneous with surgical tracheostomy in critically ill patients. Crit Care Med 2001;29:926. [PMID: 11378598]

Maziak DE et al: The timing of tracheotomy: a systematic review. Chest 1998;114:605. [PMID: 9726751] (Insufficient evidence that the timing of tracheotomy for critically ill patients in the ICU influences the duration of mechanical ventilation or the extent of airway injury.)

Rosenbower TJ et al: The long-term complications of percutaneous dilatational tracheostomy. Am Surg 1998;64:82. [PMID: 9457043]

■ FOREIGN BODIES IN THE UPPER AERODIGESTIVE TRACT

FOREIGN BODIES OF THE TRACHEA & BRONCHI

Aspiration of foreign bodies occurs less frequently in adults than in children. The elderly and denture wearers appear to be at greatest risk. Wider familiarity with the Heimlich maneuver has reduced deaths. If the maneuver is unsuccessful, cricothyrotomy may be necessary. Plain chest radiographs may reveal a radiopaque foreign body. Detection of radiolucent foreign bodies may be aided by inspiration-expiration films that demonstrate air trapping distal to the obstructed segment. Atelectasis and pneumonia may occur later.

Tracheal and bronchial foreign bodies should be removed under general anesthesia by a skilled endoscopist working with an experienced anesthesiologist.

Debeljak A et al: Bronchoscopic removal of foreign bodies in adults: experience with 62 patients from 1974–1998. Eur Respir J 1999;14:792. [PMID: 10573222] (Flexible or rigid bronchoscopy is effective.)

Friedman EM: Tracheobronchial foreign bodies. Otolaryngol Clin North Am 2000;33:179. [PMID: 10637351]

Zaytoun GM et al: Endoscopic management of foreign bodies in the tracheobronchial tree: predictive factors for complications. Otolaryngol Head Neck Surg 2000;123:311. [PMID: 10964313] (A review of 504 cases and 42 complications in Beirut over 10 years.)

ESOPHAGEAL FOREIGN BODIES

Foreign bodies in the esophagus create urgent but not life-threatening situations as long as the airway is not compromised. There is probably time to consult an experienced clinician for management. Patients are likely to have difficulty handling secretions and may be spitting out their saliva. It is a useful diagnostic sign of complete obstruction if the patient is drooling or cannot handle secretions. They may often point to the exact level of the obstruction. Indirect laryngoscopy often shows pooling of saliva at the esophageal inlet. Plain films may detect radiopaque foreign bodies such as chicken bones. Coins tend to align in the coronal plane in the esophagus and sagittally in the trachea. If a foreign body is suspected, a barium swallow may help make the diagnosis.

The treatment of an esophageal foreign body depends very much on identification of its nature. In children, swallowed nonfood objects are common, and treatment options include esophageal bougienage dislodgment or Foley catheter displacement for coins, endoscopic removal under general anesthesia, and observation insofar as about 20% of objects will pass spontaneously. The cost and the complications associated with each of these approaches has been studied, suggesting that bougienage is most appropriate for coins, but considerable debate exists. In adults, however, food foreign bodies are more common, and there is the greater possibility of underlying esophageal pathology. Endoscopic removal and examination is usually best, via flexible esophagoscopy or rigid laryngoscopy-esophagoscopy. Obstruction may sometimes occur from a metal stent placed in the treatment of esophageal cancer.

Lam HC et al: Management of ingested foreign bodies: a retrospective review of 5240 patients. J Laryngol Otol 2001;115:954. [PMID: 11779322]

Mayoral W et al: Nonmalignant obstruction is a common problem with metal stents in the treatment of esophageal cancer. Gastrointest Endosc 2000;51:556. [PMID: 10805841] (Obstruction can be secondary to tumor ingrowth or to nonmalignant causes such as granulation tissue or fibrosis.)

Mosca S et al. Endoscopic management of foreign bodies in the upper gastrointestinal tract: report on a series of 414 adult patients. Endoscopy 2001;33(8):692. [PMID: 11490386] (Thirty-one percent had an underlying cause, such as stricture.)

Soprano JV et al: Four strategies for the management of esophageal coins in children. Pediatrics 2000;105:e5. [PMID: 10617742] (Although this article is about children, the cost analysis and consideration of alternatives is worth reading as background for a discussion of foreign bodies in adults.)

■ DISEASES PRESENTING AS NECK MASSES

The differential diagnosis of neck masses is heavily dependent on the location in the neck, the age of the patient, and the presence of associated disease processes. Rapid growth and tenderness suggest an inflammatory process, while firm, painless, and slowly enlarging masses are often neoplastic. In young adults, most neck masses are benign (branchial cleft cyst, thyroglossal duct cyst, reactive lymphadenitis), though malignancy should always be considered (lymphoma, metastatic thyroid carcinoma). Lymphadenopathy is common in HIV-positive individuals, but a growing or dominant mass may well be malignant. In adults over 40, cancer is the most common cause of persistent neck mass. A metastasis from squamous cell carcinoma arising within the mouth, pharynx, larynx, or upper esophagus should be suspected, especially if there is a history of tobacco or significant alcohol use. Especially among patients younger than 30 or older than 70, lymphoma should be considered. In any case, a comprehensive otolaryngologic examination is needed. Cytologic evaluation of the neck mass via fine-needle aspiration biopsy is likely to be the next step if an obvious primary tumor is not visible or palpable on physical examination.

CONGENITAL LESIONS PRESENTING AS NECK MASSES IN ADULTS

1. Branchial Cleft Cysts

Branchial cleft cysts usually present as a soft cystic mass along the anterior border of the sternocleidomastoid muscle. These lesions are usually recognized in the second or third decades of life, often when they suddenly swell or become infected. To prevent recurrent infection and possible carcinoma, they should be completely excised, along with their fistulous tracts.

First branchial cleft cysts present high in the neck, sometimes just below the ear. A fistulous connection with the floor of the external auditory canal may be present. Second branchial cleft cysts, which are far more common, may communicate with the tonsillar fossa. Third branchial cleft cysts, which may communicate with the piriform sinus, are rare.

Enepekides DJ: Management of congenital anomalies of the neck. Facial Plast Surg Clin North Am 2001;9:131. [PMID: 11465000] (An overview.)

Palacios E et al: Branchial cleft cyst. Ear Nose Throat J 2001;80:302.[PMID: 11393908]

Triglia JM et al: First branchial cleft anomalies: A study of 39 cases and a review of the literature. Arch Otolaryngol Head Neck Surg 1998;124:291. [PMID: 9525513] (Three types of presentation are seen: chronic purulent drainage from the ear [n = 12], periauricular periparotid swelling [n = 18], and abscess or persistent fistula in the neck superior to the axial plane of the hyoid [n = 21]. There were four cases of membranous attachment between the floor of the external auditory canal and the tympanic membrane. Complications were 11 fistulas, 20 sinuses, and 8 cysts.)

2. Thyroglossal Duct Cysts

Thyroglossal duct cysts occur along the embryologic course of the thyroid's descent from the tuberculum impar of the tongue base to its usual position in the low neck. Although they may occur at any age, they are commonest before age 20. They present as a midline neck mass, often just below the hyoid bone, that moves with swallowing. Surgical excision is recommended to prevent recurrent infection. This requires removal of the entire fistulous tract along with the middle portion of the hyoid bone.

Maddalozzo J et al: Complications associated with the Sistrunk procedure. Laryngoscope 2001;111:119. [PMID: 11192879] (This is the procedure of choice; complications are few.)

Ahuja AT et al: Thyroglossal duct cysts: sonographic appearances in adults. AJNR Am J Neuroradiol 1999;20:579. [PMID: 10319964] (Variable appearance on ultrasound.)

Ewing CA et al: Presentations of thyroglossal duct cysts in adults. Eur Arch Otorhinolaryngol 1999;256:136. [PMID: 10234482]

INFECTIOUS & INFLAMMATORY NECK MASSES

1. Reactive Cervical Lymphadenopathy

Normal lymph nodes in the neck are usually less than 1 cm in length. Infections involving the pharynx, salivary glands, and scalp often cause tender enlargement of neck nodes. Enlarged nodes are common in HIV-infected persons. Except for the occasional node that suppurates and requires incision and drainage, treatment is directed against the underlying infection. An enlarged node unassociated with an obvious infection should be further evaluated, especially if the patient has a history of smoking or alcohol use (common etiologic factors in head and neck squamous cell carcinoma) or a history of cancer. Other common indications for fine-needle aspiration biopsy of a node include its persistence or continued enlargement. Common causes of cervical adenopathy include tumor (squamous cell carcinoma, lymphoma, occasional metastases from non-head and neck sites) and infection (eg, reactive nodes, mycobacteria [discussed below], and cat scratch disease). Rare causes of adenopathy include Kikuchi's disease (histiocytic necrotizing lymphadenitis) and autoimmune adenopathy.

Amedee RG et al: Fine-needle aspiration biopsy. Laryngoscope 2001;111:1551. [PMID: 11568593]

2. Tuberculous & Nontuberculous Mycobacterial Lymphadenitis

Granulomatous neck masses are not uncommon. The differential diagnosis includes mycobacterial adenitis, sarcoidosis, and cat-scratch disease due to *Bartonella henselae*. Although mycobacterial adenitis can extend to the skin and drain externally (as described for atypical mycobacteria and referred to as scrofula), this late presentation is no longer common. The usual presentation of granulomatous disease in the neck is simply single or matted nodes. Fine-needle aspiration is usually the best initial diagnostic approach: cytology, smear for acid-fast bacilli, culture, and sensitivity test; and polymerase chain reaction (PCR) can all be done.

Mycobacterial lymphadenitis is on the rise both in immunocompromised and immunocompetent individuals. Identification of *Mycobacterium tuberculosis* can usually be confirmed by a combination of FNA smear and culture in a suspected patient, but excisional biopsy of a node may be needed. PCR from FNA (or from excised tissue) is the single most sensitive test and is particularly useful when conventional methods have not been diagnostic but clinical impression remains consistent for tuberculous infection. Short-course therapy (6 months) consisting of an initial 4 months of streptomycin, isoniazid, rifampin, and pyrazinamide followed by 2 months of rifampin is the current recommended treatment for tuberculous lymphadenopathy. For atypical (nontuberculous) lymphadenopathy, treatment depends on sensitivity results of culture, but antibiotics likely to be useful include 6 months of isoniazid and rifampin and, for at least the first 2 months, ethambutol—all in standard dosages (see Table 9-14). Some would totally excise the involved nodes prior to chemotherapy, depending on location and other factors.

Ellison E et al: Fine needle aspiration diagnosis of mycobacterial lymphadenitis. Sensitivity and predictive value in the United States. Acta Cytol 1999;43:153. [PMID: 10097702] (Interpreting nondiagnostic granulomatous inflammation should be done with caution.)

Goel MM et al: Polymerase chain reaction vs. conventional diagnosis in fine needle aspirates of tuberculous lymph nodes. Acta Cytol 2001;45:333. [PMID: 11393063] (Fine-needle aspirate, smears, culture, biopsy, and PCR were evaluated in 142 patients. The authors feel that in developing countries PCR can be reserved for problem cases as the diagnosis can usually be made without it. The sensitivity and negative predictive value of PCR was > 90%.)

Jha BC et al: Cervical tuberculous lymphadenopathy: changing clinical pattern and concepts in management. Postgrad Med J 2001;77:185. [PMID: 11222827] (FNA yielded the diagnosis in 52 of 56 patients. Short-course chemotherapy was adequate. Abscesses were treated with aspiration.)

Kanlikama M et al: Management strategy of mycobacterial cervical lymphadenitis. J Laryngol Otol 2000;114:274. [PMID: 10845042]

King AD et al: MRI of tuberculous cervical lymphadenopathy. J Comput Assist Tomogr 1999;23:244. [PMID: 1096332] (Reviews the spectrum of findings.)

Singh KK et al: Comparison of in house polymerase chain reaction with conventional techniques for the detection of *Mycobacterium tuberculosis* DNA in granulomatous lymphadenopathy. J Clin Pathol 2000;53:355. [PMID: 10889817] (PCR is the most sensitive single test available. It is particularly valuable as an adjunctive test when conventional methods of diagnosis fail but the clinical impression remains strong. Although most patients have a positive skin test, fewer than 20% today have an abnormal chest radiograph.)

Thongsuksai P et al: Histiocytic necrotizing lymphadenitis (Kikuchi's disease): clinicopathologic characteristics of 23 cases and literature review. J Med Assoc Thai 1999;82:812. [PMID: 10511791] (More common in young women than men, this rare cause of fever and lymphadenopathy follows a self-limited course. Even more rarely, it may be associated with hemophagocytic syndrome, which may be more severe and for which bone marrow aspiration is indicated for diagnosis.)

van Loenhout-Rooyackers JH et al: Shortening the duration of treatment for cervical tuberculous lymphadenitis. Eur Respir J 2000;15:192. [PMID: 10678645] (Six months is probably sufficient.)

3. Lyme Disease

Lyme disease, caused by the spirochete *Borrelia burgdorferi* and transmitted by ticks of the *Ixodes* genus, may have protean manifestation, but over 75% of patients have symptoms involving the head and neck. Facial paralysis, dysesthesias, dysgeusia, or other cranial neuropathies are most common. Headache, pain, and cervical lymphadenopathy may occur. See Chapter 34 for a more thorough discussion.

Hu LT et al: Update on the prevention, diagnosis, and treatment of Lyme disease. Adv Intern Med 2001;46:247.[PMID: 11270961]

Poland GA: Prevention of Lyme disease: a review of the evidence. Mayo Clin Proc 2001;76:713. [PMID: 11444404]

Rahn DW: Lyme vaccine: issues and controversies. Infect Dis Clin North Am 2001;15:171. [PMID: 11301814]

Sigal LH: Lyme disease: a clinical update. Hosp Pract (Off Ed) 2001;36:31. [PMID: 11446598]

Steere AC: Lyme disease. N Engl J Med 2001;345:115. [PMID: 11450660]

TUMOR METASTASES

In older adults, 80% of firm, persistent, and enlarging neck masses are metastatic in origin. The great majority of these arise from squamous cell carcinoma of the upper aerodigestive tract. A complete head and neck examination may reveal the tumor of origin, but examination under anesthesia with direct laryngoscopy, esophagoscopy, and bronchoscopy is usually required to fully evaluate the tumor and exclude second primaries.

It is often helpful to obtain a cytologic diagnosis if initial head and neck examination fails to reveal the primary tumor. An open biopsy should be done only when neither physical examination by an experienced clinician specializing in head and neck cancer nor fine-needle aspiration biopsy performed by an experienced cytopathologist yields a diagnosis. In such a setting, one should strongly consider obtaining an MRI or PET scan prior to open biopsy, as these methods may yield valuable information about a possible presumed primary site or another site for FNA.

Other than thyroid carcinoma, non-squamous cell metastases to the neck are infrequent. While tumors not involving the head and neck seldom metastasize to the middle or upper neck, the supraclavicular region is quite often involved by lung and breast tumors. Infradiaphragmatic tumors, with the exception of renal cell carcinoma, rarely metastasize to the neck.

LYMPHOMA

About 10% of lymphomas present in the head and neck. Lymphoma arising in AIDS patients is an increasing concern. Multiple rubbery nodes, especially in the young adult, are suggestive of this disease. A thorough physical examination may demonstrate other sites of nodal or organ involvement. Fine needle aspiration may be diagnostic, but open biopsy is often required.

Jayaram G et al: Fine needle aspiration cytology of lymph nodes in HIV-infected individuals. Acta Cytol 2000;44:960. [PMID: 11127753]

■ OTOLARYNGOLOGIC MANIFESTATIONS OF HIV INFECTION (See also Chapter 31.)

ORAL CAVITY & PHARYNX

The evaluation of oral lesions is critically important in HIV-infected individuals and in patients at risk for HIV infection. Oral candidiasis and hairy leukoplakia, each occurring in 10–20% of HIV-infected patients, are frequently the presenting signs of HIV disease. Kaposi's sarcoma (prevalence about 1%) may similarly be the first indication of HIV infection—as may necrotizing ulcerative periodontitis (occurring in 2–5%), but less predictively. The course of candidiasis and hairy leukoplakia in known HIV-infected patients may correlate with the degree of immune suppression and overall disease progression, heralding the subsequent development of AIDS. For these reasons, oral lesions are useful in staging HIV disease and in designing entry criteria and end points for antiretroviral clinical trials. The United States Department of Health Services Clinical Practice Guideline for Evaluation and Management of Early HIV Infection recommends examination of the oral mucosa with each physician visit as well as dental examination at least every 6 months.

When CD4 cell counts drop below 200/μL, the incidence of intraoral lesions rises dramatically. In the past few years, the severity of these lesions has lessened, but their incidence has increased. Candidiasis is common and may require treatment for longer than the usual 1-week course with fluconazole (100 mg daily) or ketoconazole (200–400 mg daily). Clotrimazole and topical nystatin are less effective. Itraconazole (200 mg daily) is often helpful in fluconazole-resistant cases, or some cases due to non-albicans species, which are frequently azole-unresponsive. Giant intraoral ulcers have been seen in some patients.

Hairy leukoplakia occurring on the lateral border of the tongue is another common early finding. It may develop quickly and appears as slightly raised leukoplakic areas with a corrugated or "hairy" surface. Histologically, parakeratosis and koilocytes are seen with little or no underlying inflammation. Among HIV-positive patients with oral lesions, hairy leukoplakia was seen in 19% in one study. Clinical response following administration of zidovudine or acyclovir has been reported, and treatment is under active investigation. The appearance of hairy leukoplakia may herald subsequent more ominous manifestations of AIDS.

Kaposi's sarcoma is most common on the hard palate but may be seen anywhere in the oral cavity and pharynx. It usually appears as a raised violaceous lesion beneath an intact mucosa, although it may be ulcerated, erythematous, and bleeding. Radiation therapy may control the tumor. A brisk mucositis can be expected following radiation therapy.

In addition to Kaposi's sarcoma, an increased incidence of non-Hodgkin's lymphoma is seen in AIDS. An increase in squamous cell carcinoma is also seen in the homosexual population, perhaps related to HIV infection.

Cartledge JD et al: Non-albicans oral candidosis in HIV-positive patients. J Antimicrob Chemother 1999;43:419. [PMID: 10223601] (Ten percent of candidal cultures also included non-albicans species, predominantly from patients with low CD4 lymphocyte counts. About 90% of non-albicans isolates were resistant to fluconazole in vitro, and 60% of such patients treated with azole therapy failed to clear these isolates clinically.)

Laskaris G: Oral manifestations of HIV disease. Clin Dermatol 2000;18:447.[PMID: 11024312]

Margiotta V et al: HIV infection: oral lesions, CD4+ cell count and viral load in an Italian study population. J Oral Pathol Med 1999;28:173. [PMID: 10235371] (Confirms correlation with CD4 depletion and high level of viral load. Monitoring oral lesions is a useful tool for identifying progression of HIV infection and is of possible value in monitoring antiretroviral therapy.)

Patton LL. Sensitivity, specificity, and positive predictive value of oral opportunistic infections in adults with HIV/AIDS as markers of immune suppression and viral burden. Oral Surg Oral Med Oral Pathol Oral Radiol Endod 2000;90:182. [PMID: 10936837] (Several presentations of candidiasis, Kaposi's sarcoma, linear gingival erythema, and hairy leukoplakia all are > 65% predictive.)

Ryder MI: Periodontal management of HIV-infected patients. Periodontol 2000;23:85. [PMID: 11276769]

Vazquez JA: Therapeutic options for the management of oropharyngeal and esophageal candidiasis in HIV/AIDS patients. HIV Clin Trials 2000;1:47 [PMID: 11590489]

THE NECK

Persistent generalized lymphadenopathy is extremely common in HIV infection. A tender or growing node may represent secondary infection, lymphoma, or other tumor. Fine-needle aspiration for culture and cytology is the best initial diagnostic step. Open biopsy will often be needed if granulomatous disease or lymphoma is suspected, though fine-needle aspiration biopsy may be diagnostic of *M tuberculosis* infection in seropositive patients.

Parotid cysts and benign lymphoepithelial lesions in HIV-positive patients may be seen, often in association with cervical adenopathy.

Craven DE et al: Response of lymphoepithelial parotid cysts to antiretroviral treatment in HIV-infected adults. Ann Intern Med 1998;128:455. [PMID: 9488329] (In six of nine patients, cysts resolved completely with combination antiretroviral therapy. Surgical resection should be reserved for patients in whom medical therapy has failed or those who refuse or are poorly compliant with medical therapy.)

Engels EA: Human immunodeficiency virus infection, aging, and cancer. J Clin Epidemiol 2001;54(Suppl 1):S29. [PMID: 11750207]

Kersten MJ: Management of AIDS-related non-Hodgkin's lymphomas. Drugs 2001;61:1301.[PMID: 11511024] (Antiretroviral therapy appears to have decreased the incidence of lymphoma; reviews current management)

Mandel L: Ultrasound findings in HIV-positive patients with parotid gland swellings. J Oral Maxillofac Surg 2001; 59:283. [PMID: 11243610]

Moazzez AH et al: Head and neck manifestations of AIDS in adults. Am Fam Physician 1998;57:1813. [PMID: 9575321] (Common manifestations and current treatment recommendations.)

Singh B et al: Head and neck manifestations of non-Hodgkin's lymphoma in human immunodeficiency virus-infected patients. Am J Otolaryngol 2000;21:10. [PMID: 10668671]

Singh B et al: Alterations in head and neck cancer occurring in HIV-infected patients—results of a pilot, longitudinal, prospective study. Acta Oncologica 1999;38:1047. [PMID: 10665761] (Squamous cell carcinoma in HIV-infected individuals has a particularly poor prognosis.)

PARANASAL SINUSES

Sinusitis is common in HIV infection and the causative organisms are diverse. The same pathogens encountered in nonimmunocompromised patients remain the most common. Early sinus irrigation, with aspirates sent for cytologic examination as well as fungal, viral, legionella, and aerobic and anaerobic culture may be helpful in severe cases. Guaifenesin (600 mg orally four times daily), a mucolytic agent, may offer some adjunctive symptomatic relief. Functional endoscopic surgery to provide sinus drainage is often helpful.

Invasive aspergillus sinusitis is an increasingly reported complication in AIDS. Though this infection is more indolent than mucormycosis, most patients with AIDS and aspergillus sinusitis die as a result of intracranial extension.

Friedman M et al: Endoscopic sinus surgery in patients infected with HIV. Laryngoscope 2000;110(10 Part 1):1613. [PMID: 11037812]

Murphy C et al: Sinonasal disease and olfactory impairment in HIV disease: endoscopic sinus surgery and outcome measures. Laryngoscope 2000;110(10 Part 1):1707. [PMID: 11037830]

General References for Otolaryngologic Manifestations of HIV Infection

Fischbein NJ et al: Imaging of otolaryngologic manifestations of HIV infection. Neuroimaging Clin North Am 1997;7:375. [PMID: 9113696] (Most patients have abnormalities on head and neck examination at some point in their disease. The authors review the spectrum of imaging findings in this population.)

Moazzez AH et al: Head and neck manifestations of AIDS in adults. Am Fam Physician 1998;57:1813. [PMID: 9575321] (An overview.)

Reisacher WR et al: Manifestations of AIDS in the head and neck. South Med J 1999;92:684. [PMID: 10414477]

Lung

9

Mark S. Chesnutt, MD, & Thomas J. Prendergast, MD
See www.current-med.com/ch09.html

■ COMMON MANIFESTATIONS OF LUNG DISEASE

DYSPNEA

Dyspnea is a common symptom. It is analogous to pain in that sensory input from multiple sites in the respiratory system is integrated in the cerebral cortex. In general, dyspnea increases with the level of functional impairment as measured by spirometry. However, there is only a weak correlation between airflow limitation or exercise tolerance and the severity of dyspnea.

Several pathophysiologic processes contribute to dyspnea. The most important is the increased respiratory effort that accompanies many different diseases: airflow obstruction (asthma; chronic obstructive pulmonary disease [COPD]), changes in pulmonary compliance (interstitial fibrosis, congestive heart failure) or chest wall compliance (obesity, pleural disease), intrinsic respiratory muscle weakness (inanition, neuromuscular disease, chronic respiratory failure), or the weakness conveyed by the mechanical disadvantage of hyperinflation (asthma or emphysema). Dyspnea is magnified by increased respiratory drive. Acute hypercapnia is therefore a potent stimulus to dyspnea, hypoxemia a weak one. In mechanically ventilated patients, failure to provide adequate inspiratory flow rates to patients with heightened respiratory drive commonly results in dyspnea that may present as agitation. Stimulation of irritant receptors in the airways intensifies dyspnea, while stimulation of pulmonary stretch receptors decreases it.

Clinical Findings

The history should focus on onset and timing of symptoms, the patient's position at onset of symptoms, the relationship of symptoms to activity, and any factors that may improve or exacerbate symptoms. The clinician can assess dyspnea and response to treatment with a ten-point numeric rating scale by asking the patient, "On a scale of zero to ten, with zero being no shortness of breath and ten being the worst shortness of breath you can imagine, how short of breath are you?" Exertional dyspnea should be quantified, but the absolute level of exertion that precipitates dyspnea is less important than acute changes in the threshold level of activity. A complete allergic, occupational, and smoking history is essential.

Acute dyspnea has a short list of causes, most of which are readily identified: asthma, pulmonary infection, pulmonary edema, pneumothorax, pulmonary embolus, metabolic acidosis, or acute respiratory distress syndrome (ARDS). Panic attacks may present as a respiratory complaint. Orthopnea (dyspnea on recumbency) and nocturnal dyspnea suggest asthma, gastroesophageal reflux disease (GERD), left ventricular dysfunction, or obstructive sleep apnea. Rapid onset of severe dyspnea when supine suggests phrenic nerve impairment and diaphragmatic paralysis. Platypnea (dyspnea that worsens in the upright position) is a rare complaint associated with arteriovenous malformations at the lung bases, resulting in increased shunting and hypoxemia in the upright position (orthodeoxia).

Chronic dyspnea is invariably progressive. Symptoms often first appear during exertion; patients learn to limit their activity to accommodate their diminished pulmonary reserve until dyspnea occurs with minimal activity or at rest. Episodic dyspnea suggests congestive heart failure, asthma, acute or chronic bronchitis, or recurrent pulmonary emboli. Constant dyspnea is most commonly due to COPD but may indicate interstitial lung disease (eg, pulmonary fibrosis), pulmonary vascular disease, or fixed airflow obstruction from severe asthma.

Dyspnea is increasingly being recognized as a major issue in the care of dying patients, and clinicians typically undertreat this symptom.

Evaluation should include a complete blood count, renal function tests, chest radiograph, spirometry, and noninvasive oximetry. Patients over 40 years of age or with a family history of early coronary disease should have an electrocardiogram. Arterial blood gases, measurement of lung volumes, ventilation/perfusion scanning, echocardiography, and cardiopulmonary exercise testing are reserved for cases that elude diagnosis on initial evaluation.

Treatment

In patients with advanced lung disease, the responsible condition may be easily identified but treatment only partially effective. Oxygen improves survival in those who are hypoxemic and can improve the exercise tolerance of all patients. Its effect on dyspnea is variable. Anxiety can play an important role in the distress caused by dyspnea and may be relieved by judicious use of benzodiazepines such as lorazepam, 0.5–1 mg orally every 4–6 hours. Pulmonary rehabilitation can improve respiratory function and train patients in energy conservation and breathing techniques that help moderate their sense of respiratory effort. Opioids reduce respiratory drive and blunt dyspnea. They can be titrated safely even in patients with advanced lung disease. Finally, fresh air or a fan may offer additional relief. Smokers with progressive exertional dyspnea should know that they can limit future loss of function through smoking cessation.

Alhamad EH et al: Evaluating chronic dyspnea: A step-wise approach. J Respir Dis 2001;22:79. (Basic review with a logical approach to the difficult diagnostic referral.)

Dyspnea. Mechanisms, assessment, and management: a consensus statement. American Thoracic Society. Am J Respir Crit Care Med. 1999;159:321. [PMID: 9872857] (Exhaustive review of mechanisms and management with extensive bibliography.)

Luce JM et al: Management of dyspnea in patients with far-advanced lung disease: "once I lose it, it's kind of hard to catch it . . .". JAMA 2001;285:1331. [PMID: 11255389] (Case-based review of pathophysiology and treatment of dyspnea in advanced lung disease, with particular attention to palliative care.)

COUGH

Cough is an important physiologic mechanism that defends against respiratory pathogens and helps to clear the tracheobronchial tree of mucus, foreign particles, and noxious aerosols. Excessive cough is one of the most common symptoms for which patients seek medical care and may represent up to one-third of a pulmonologist's outpatient practice referrals. Persistent severe cough, seen in interstitial lung disease or bronchiectasis, may impair respiration as well as disrupt sleep and social functioning. Bronchospasm (brought on by repetitive forced exhalation), syncope, rib fractures, and urinary incontinence are all potential complications. A reduced or absent cough, seen in some postoperative patients or those with neuromuscular disease, will reduce clearance of secretions and may impair oxygenation.

Cough may be voluntary or involuntary. Involuntary cough is stimulated by vagal afferent receptors in the trachea, especially at the carina, and the larynx but also from others throughout the head and neck. Stimulation of cough receptors may be mechanical, as in cases of aspiration, or irritative.

Clinical Findings

It is important to distinguish acute (< 3 weeks) from chronic cough. Acute cough most commonly follows viral or bacterial upper respiratory tract infection. Within 2 days after onset of the common cold, 85% of untreated patients cough; 26% are still coughing 14 days later; in a few, cough will persist for 6–8 weeks. Many patients with persistent cough following upper respiratory tract infection have underlying asthma. Other causes of acute cough include aspiration, pneumonia, pulmonary embolism, and pulmonary edema.

The most common cause of chronic cough is a low-grade chronic bronchitis secondary to exposure to tobacco smoke, though smokers do not commonly seek medical attention for this problem. Over 90% of nonsmokers presenting for evaluation of chronic cough suffer from postnasal drip, gastroesophageal reflux disease, or asthma (even without other symptoms). Angiotensin-converting enzyme (ACE) inhibitors have become another common cause. In primary care settings, single causes predominate.

The character and timing of chronic cough and the presence or absence of sputum production do not permit an etiologic diagnosis and should not be used as the sole basis for empirical therapy. The history and physical examination should attempt to identify anatomic locations of the afferent limb of the cough reflex in light of the common causes listed above. A nasal discharge, frequent need to clear the throat, and mucoid or mucopurulent secretions in the posterior pharynx suggest postnasal drip. Sinus radiographs may be diagnostic of acute or chronic sinusitis. Wheezing on chest auscultation or airflow obstruction on pulmonary function tests suggest asthma. In cough-variant asthma, methacholine bronchoprovocation testing may be positive in the absence of clinical findings of asthma. Gastroesophageal reflux disease is an important cause of chronic cough but is associated with the fewest clinical clues. Patients may complain of heartburn or regurgitation, but cough may be the only symptom. Barium swallow is specific but insensitive, and esophageal pH monitoring may be necessary. Chest radiographs are best reserved for cough in smokers and patients with hemoptysis or constitutional symptoms such as fever and weight loss.

Treatment

The first step is to eliminate irritant exposures such as tobacco smoke (primary or secondary) and occupational agents and to discontinue medications such as ACE inhibitors or beta-blockers, including eyedrops. Cough due to ACE inhibitors should subside within

1–4 days after discontinuing the medication, though it may take weeks to months. Postnasal drip syndrome due to allergic rhinitis that does not respond to antihistamines should be treated with intranasal steroids. Chronic sinusitis may require prolonged antibiotics directed against *Haemophilus influenzae*. Cough caused by asthma that does not respond after 2 weeks of bronchodilators and corticosteroids suggests another contributing condition. Cough due to gastroesophageal reflux disease is difficult to treat, since H_2 blockers may not be adequate. Most practitioners now initiate antitussive therapy for gastroesophageal reflux disease with proton pump inhibitors. Patients whose cough began after an upper respiratory tract infection usually respond to treatment with an antihistamine-decongestant combination or treatment for asthma.

Irwin RS et al: The diagnosis and treatment of cough. N Engl J Med 2000;343:1715. [PMID: 11106722] (Current review directed at primary care physicians.)

HEMOPTYSIS

Hemoptysis is the expectoration of blood that originates below the vocal cords. It is commonly classified as trivial, mild, or massive, the last defined as more than 200–600 mL in 24 hours. The dividing lines are arbitrary, since the amount of blood is rarely quantified with precision. Massive hemoptysis can be usefully defined as any amount that is hemodynamically significant or threatens ventilation, in which case the initial management goal is not diagnostic but therapeutic.

The lungs are supplied with a dual circulation. The pulmonary arteries arise from the right ventricle to supply the pulmonary parenchyma in a low-pressure circuit. The bronchial arteries arise from the aorta or intercostal arteries and carry blood under systemic pressure to the airways, blood vessels, hila, and visceral pleura. The bronchial arterial circulation represents only 1–2% of total pulmonary blood flow but is frequently the source of hemoptysis: It is a high-pressure circuit; it provides the blood supply to the airways and lesions within those airways; and flow can increase dramatically under conditions of chronic inflammation—eg, chronic bronchiectasis.

The causes of hemoptysis can be classified anatomically. Blood may arise from the airways in chronic bronchitis, bronchiectasis, and bronchogenic carcinoma; from the pulmonary vasculature in left ventricular failure, mitral stenosis, pulmonary emboli, and arteriovenous malformations; or from the pulmonary parenchyma in pneumonia, inhalation of crack cocaine, or autoimmune diseases such as Goodpasture's disease or Wegener's granulomatosis. Iatrogenic hemorrhage may follow transbronchial lung biopsies, anticoagulation, or pulmonary artery rupture due to distal placement of a balloon-tipped catheter.

Clinical Findings

Blood-tinged sputum in the setting of acute bronchitis in an otherwise healthy nonsmoker does not warrant an extensive diagnostic evaluation if the hemoptysis subsides with resolution of the infection. However, hemoptysis is frequently a sign of serious disease, especially in patients with a high prior probability of underlying pulmonary pathology. The goal of the history is to identify patients at risk for one of the disorders listed above. Pertinent features are tobacco use, duration of symptoms, and the presence of respiratory infection. Nonpulmonary sources of hemorrhage—from the nose or the gastrointestinal tract—should be ruled out.

Laboratory evaluation should include a chest radiograph and complete blood count, including platelet count. Renal function tests, urinalysis, and coagulation studies are appropriate in specific circumstances. Flexible bronchoscopy reveals endobronchial cancer in 3–6% of patients with hemoptysis who have a normal (nonlateralizing) chest radiograph. Nearly all of these patients are smokers over the age of 40, and most will have had symptoms for more than a week. Bronchoscopy is indicated in such patients. High-resolution CT of the chest is complementary to bronchoscopy. It can diagnose unsuspected bronchiectasis and arteriovenous malformations and will show central endobronchial lesions in many cases. It is the test of choice for suspected small peripheral malignancies.

Treatment

The management of mild hemoptysis consists of identifying and treating the specific cause. Massive hemoptysis is life-threatening. The airway must be protected, ventilation ensured, and effective circulation maintained. If the location of the bleeding site is known, the patient should be placed in the decubitus position with the involved lung dependent. Uncontrollable hemorrhage warrants rigid bronchoscopy and surgical consultation. In stable patients, flexible bronchoscopy may localize the site of bleeding, and angiography can embolize the involved bronchial arteries. Embolization is effective initially in 85% of cases, though rebleeding may occur in up to 20% of patients over the following year. The anterior spinal artery arises from the bronchial artery in up to 5% of people, and paraplegia may result if it is inadvertently cannulated.

Colice GL: Detecting lung cancer as a cause of hemoptysis in patients with a normal chest radiograph: bronchoscopy vs CT. Chest 1997;111:877. [PMID: 9106564] (Hypothetical protocol comparing different diagnostic strategies to identify the most efficient evaluation.)

Hirshberg B et al: Hemoptysis: etiology, evaluation and outcome in a tertiary referral hospital. Chest 1997;112:440. [PMID: 9266882] (Bronchiectasis, bronchitis, lung cancer, and infections caused 73% of cases; bronchoscopy and CT were complementary.)

Jean-Baptiste E: Clinical assessment and management of massive hemoptysis. Crit Care Med 2000;28:1642. [PMID: 10834728] (Description of an approach to massive hemoptysis.)

■ APPROACH TO THE PATIENT

PHYSICAL EXAMINATION

Examination of the patient with suspected pulmonary disease includes inspection, palpation, percussion, and auscultation of the chest. An efficient approach begins with observing the pattern of breathing, auscultation of the chest, and inspection for extrapulmonary signs of pulmonary disease. More detailed examination follows from initial findings.

The pattern of breathing refers to the respiratory rate and rhythm, the depth of breathing or tidal volume, and the relative amount of time spent in inspiration and expiration. Normal values are a rate of 12–14 breaths per minute, tidal volumes of 5 mL/kg, and a ratio of inspiratory to expiratory time of 2:3. **Tachypnea** is an increased rate of breathing and is commonly associated with a decrease in tidal volume. The rhythm is normally regular, with a sigh (1.5–2 times normal tidal volume) every 90 breaths or so to prevent collapse of alveoli and atelectasis. Alterations in the rhythm of breathing include rapid, shallow breathing, seen in restrictive lung disease and as a precursor to respiratory failure; Kussmaul breathing, rapid large-volume breathing indicating intense stimulation of the respiratory center, seen in metabolic acidosis; and Cheyne-Stokes respirations, a rhythmic waxing and waning of both rate and tidal volumes that includes regular periods of apnea. This pattern is seen in patients with end-stage left ventricular failure or neurologic disease and in many normal subjects at high altitude, especially during sleep.

During normal quiet breathing, the primary muscle of respiration is the diaphragm. Movement of the chest wall is minimal. The use of accessory muscles of respiration, the intercostal and sternocleidomastoid muscles, indicates high work of breathing. At rest, the use of accessory muscles is a sign of significant pulmonary impairment. As the diaphragm contracts, it pushes the abdominal contents down. Hence, the chest and abdominal wall normally expand simultaneously. Expansion of the chest but collapse of the abdomen on inspiration indicates weakness of the diaphragm. The chest normally expands symmetrically. Asymmetric expansion suggests unilateral volume loss, as in atelectasis or pleural effusion, unilateral airway obstruction, asymmetric pulmonary or pleural fibrosis, or splinting from chest pain.

The examiner may palpate as follows: the trachea at the suprasternal notch, to detect shifts in the mediastinum; on the posterior chest wall, to gauge fremitus and the transmission through the lungs of vibrations of spoken words; and on the anterior chest wall to assess the cardiac impulse. All these maneuvers are characterized by low interobserver agreement.

Chest percussion identifies dull areas that correspond to lung consolidation or pleural effusion or hyperresonant areas suggesting emphysema or pneumothorax. Percussion has a low sensitivity (10–20% in several studies) compared with chest radiographs to detect abnormalities. Specificity is high (85–99%). Since an insensitive test is a poor screening examination, percussion and palpation are not necessary in every patient. These techniques do serve as important confirmatory tests in specific patients when the prior probability of a finding is increased. For example, in a patient with a suspected tension pneumothorax, the finding of tracheal shift and hyperresonance can be lifesaving, permitting immediate decompression of the affected side.

Auscultation of the chest depends on a reliable and consistent classification of auditory findings. Normal lung sounds heard over the periphery of the lung are called **vesicular.** They have a gentle, rustling quality heard throughout inspiration that fades during expiration. Normal sounds heard over the suprasternal notch are called tracheal or **bronchial** lung sounds. They are louder, higher-pitched, and have a hollow quality that tends to be louder on expiration. Bronchial lung sounds heard over the periphery of the lung are abnormal and imply consolidation. Globally diminished lung sounds are an important finding predictive of significant airflow obstruction.

Abnormal lung sounds ("adventitious" breath sounds) may be continuous (> 80 ms in duration) or discontinuous (< 20 ms). Continuous lung sounds are divided into **wheezes,** which are high-pitched, musical, and have a distinct whistling quality; and **rhonchi,** which are lower-pitched, sonorous, and may have a gurgling quality. Wheezes occur in the setting of bronchospasm, mucosal edema, or excessive secretions. In each, the airway is narrowed to the point where adjacent airway walls flutter as airflow is limited. Rhonchi originate in the larger airways when excessive secretions and abnormal airway collapsibility cause repetitive rupture of fluid films. Rhonchi frequently clear after cough.

Discontinuous lung sounds are called **crackles**— brief, discrete, nonmusical sounds with a popping quality. Fine crackles are soft, high-pitched, and crisp (< 10 ms in duration). They are formed by the explosive opening of small airways previously held closed by surface forces and are heard in interstitial diseases or early pulmonary edema. Coarse crackles are louder, lower-pitched, and slightly longer in duration (< 20 ms) and probably result from gas bubbling through fluid. Coarse crackles are heard in pneumonia, obstructive lung disease, and late pulmonary edema.

Interobserver agreement regarding auscultatory findings is good. The clinical usefulness of these findings is also well established. The presence of wheezes on physical examination is a powerful predictor of obstructive lung disease. The absence of wheezes is not helpful since patients may have significant airflow limitation without wheezing. Such patients will have globally diminished lung sounds as the clinical clue to their obstructive lung disease. Normal lung sounds exclude significant airway obstruction. The timing and character of crackles can reliably distinguish different pulmonary disorders. Fine, late inspiratory crackles suggest pulmonary fibrosis, while early coarse crackles suggest pneumonia or heart failure.

Extrapulmonary signs of intrinsic pulmonary disease include digital clubbing, cyanosis, elevation of central venous pressures, and lower extremity edema.

Digital clubbing refers to structural changes at the base of the nails that include softening of the nail bed and loss of the normal 150-degree angle between the nail and the cuticle. The distal phalanx is convex and enlarged: its thickness is equal to or greater than the thickness of the distal interphalangeal joint. Symmetric clubbing may be a normal variant but more commonly is a sign of underlying disease. Clubbing is seen in patients with chronic infections of the lungs and pleura (lung abscess, empyema, bronchiectasis, cystic fibrosis), malignancies of the lungs and pleura, chronic interstitial lung disease (idiopathic pulmonary fibrosis), and arteriovenous malformations. It does not normally accompany asthma or COPD; when seen in the latter, one should suspect concomitant lung cancer. It is observed less often in small-cell cancer than in other histologic types. Clubbing is not specific to pulmonary disorders; it is also seen in cyanotic congenital heart disease, infective endocarditis, cirrhosis, and inflammatory bowel disease. Hypertrophic pulmonary osteoarthropathy is a syndrome of digital clubbing, chronic proliferative periostitis of the long bones, and synovitis. It is seen in the same conditions as digital clubbing but is particularly common in bronchogenic carcinoma. The cause of clubbing and hypertrophic osteoarthropathy is not known with certainty, but the disorder may reflect platelet clumping and local release of platelet-derived growth factor at the nail bed. Both clubbing and osteoarthropathy may resolve with appropriate treatment of the underlying disease.

Cyanosis is a blue or bluish-gray discoloration of the skin and mucous membranes caused by increased amounts (> 5 g/dL) of unsaturated hemoglobin in capillary blood. Since the oxygen saturation at which cyanosis becomes clinically apparent is a function of hemoglobin concentration, anemia may prevent cyanosis from appearing while polycythemia may lead to cyanosis in the setting of mild hypoxemia. Cyanosis is therefore not a reliable indicator of hypoxemia but should prompt direct measurement of arterial PO_2 or oxyhemoglobin saturation.

Estimation of **central venous pressure** (CVP) and assessment of lower extremity edema are indirect measures of pulmonary hypertension, the major cardiovascular complication of chronic lung disease. Estimation of CVP can be done with precision. Elevated CVP is a pathologic finding associated with impaired ventricular function, pericardial effusion or restriction, valvular heart disease, and chronic obstructive or restrictive lung disease. Peripheral edema is a nonspecific finding that, in the setting of chronic lung disease, suggests right ventricular failure.

Bettencourt PE et al: Clinical utility of chest auscultation in common pulmonary diseases. Am J Respir Crit Care Med 1994;150:1291. [PMID: 7952555] (Acoustic analysis of crackles in COPD, congestive heart failure, idiopathic pulmonary fibrosis, and pneumonia demonstrates that the examination can identify specific diagnoses.)

Metlay JP et al: Does this patient have community-acquired pneumonia? Diagnosing pneumonia by history and physical examination. JAMA 1997;278:1440. [PMID: 9356004] (A review of the usefulness of physical examination compared with chest radiography in the diagnosis of pneumonia.)

Myers KA et al:Does this patient have clubbing? JAMA 2001;286:341. [PMID: 11466101] (Systematic literature review on the precision and accuracy of the physical examination for digital clubbing.)

Straus SE et al: The accuracy of patient history, wheezing, and laryngeal measurements in diagnosing obstructive airway disease. CARE-COAD1 Group. JAMA 2000;283:1853. [PMID: 10770147] (Advocates less emphasis on the presence of individual symptoms or signs in the diagnosis of chronic airflow obstruction.)

Welsby PD et al: Some high pitched thoughts on chest examination. Postgrad Med J 2001;77:617. [PMID: 11571368] (Reviews evidence supporting the use of the stethoscope diaphragm to detect and characterize abnormal lung sounds.)

PULMONARY FUNCTION TESTS

Standard pulmonary function tests measure airflow rates, lung volumes, and the ability of the lung to transfer gas across the alveolar-capillary membrane. Indications for pulmonary function testing include the following: assessment of the type and extent of lung dysfunction; diagnosis of causes of dyspnea and cough; detection of early evidence of lung dysfunction; longitudinal surveillance in occupational settings; follow-up of response to therapy; preoperative assessment; and disability evaluation.

Contraindications to pulmonary function testing include acute severe asthma, respiratory distress, angina aggravated by testing, pneumothorax, ongoing hemoptysis, and active tuberculosis. Many test results are effort-dependent, and some patients may be too impaired to make a maximal effort. Suboptimal effort limits validity and is a common cause of misinterpretation of results. All pulmonary function tests are measured against predicted values derived from large studies of healthy subjects. In general, these predictions vary with age, gender, height and, to a lesser extent, weight and ethnicity.

Spirometry (see box) and measurement of lung volumes allow measurement of the presence and severity of obstructive and restrictive pulmonary dysfunction.

LUNG VOLUMES, CAPACITIES, AND THE NORMAL SPIROGRAM[1]

The volume of gas in the lungs is divided into volumes and capacities as shown in the bars to the left of the figure below. Lung volumes are primary: they do not overlap each other. Tidal volume (V_T) is the amount of gas inhaled and exhaled with each resting breath. Residual volume (RV) is the amount of gas remaining in the lungs at the end of a maximal exhalation. The vital capacity (VC) is the total amount of gas that can be exhaled following a maximal inhalation. The vital capacity and the residual volume together constitute the total lung capacity (TLC), or the total amount of gas in the lungs at the end of a maximal inhalation. The functional residual capacity (FRC) is the amount of gas

in the lungs at the end of a resting tidal breath. (IC, inspiratory capacity; IRV, inspiratory reserve volume; ERV, expiratory reserve volume.)

The forced vital capacity (FVC) maneuver begins with an inhalation from FRC to TLC (lasting about 1 second) followed by a forceful exhalation from TLC to RV (lasting about 5 seconds). The amount of gas exhaled during the first second of this maneuver is the forced expiratory volume in 1 second (FEV_1). Normal subjects expel approximately 80% of the FVC in the first second. The ratio of the FEV_1 to the FVC (often referred to as the FEV_1%) is diminished in patients with obstructive lung disease. It may be increased in patients with restrictive physiology.

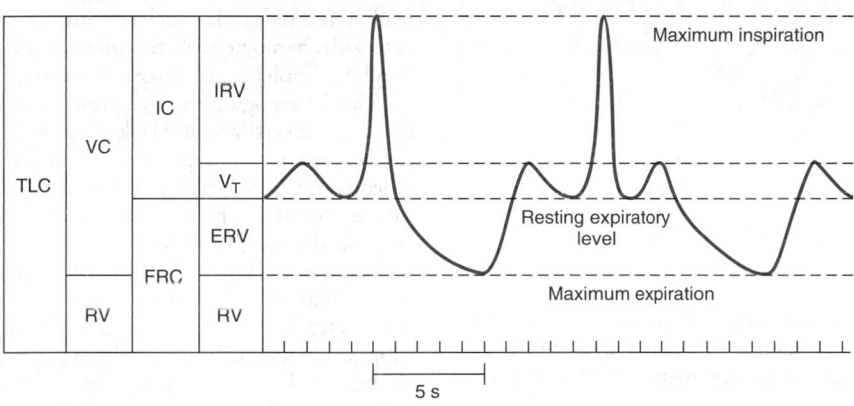

Modified, with permission, from Staub NC: *Basic Respiratory Physiology.* Churchill Livingstone, 1991.

Obstructive dysfunction is marked by a reduction in airflow rates judged by a fall in the ratio of FEV_1 (forced expiratory volume in the first second) to FVC (forced vital capacity). Causes include asthma, COPD (chronic bronchitis and emphysema), bronchiectasis, bronchiolitis, and upper airway obstruction. Restrictive dysfunction is marked by a reduction in lung volumes with a normal to increased FEV_1/FVC ratio. Severity is graded by the reduction in total lung capacity. A reduced FVC suggests pulmonary restriction but is not diagnostic. Causes include decreased lung compliance from infiltrative disorders such as pulmonary fibrosis; reduced muscle strength from phrenic nerve injury, diaphragm dysfunction, or neuromuscular disease; pleural disease, including large pleural effusion or marked pleural thickening; and prior lung resection. The flow-volume loop combines the maximal expiratory and inspiratory flow-volume curves and is especially helpful in determining the site of airway obstruction. (See Figure 9–1.)

Spirometry is adequate for evaluation of most patients with suspected respiratory disease. If airflow obstruction is evident, spirometry is repeated 10–20 minutes after an inhaled bronchodilator is administered. This doubles the cost of the study. The absence of improvement in spirometry after inhaled bronchodilator in the pulmonary function laboratory does *not* preclude a successful clinical response to bronchodilator therapy. Measurements of lung volumes and diffusing capacity are useful in selected patients, but these tests are expensive and should not be ordered routinely with spirometry.

Measurement of the single-breath **diffusing capacity** for carbon monoxide (D_LCO), which reflects the ability of the lung to transfer gas across the alveolar/capillary interface, is particularly helpful in evaluation of patients with diffuse infiltrative lung disease or emphysema. The total pulmonary diffusing capacity (D_L) depends upon the diffusion properties of the alveolar-capillary membrane and the amount of

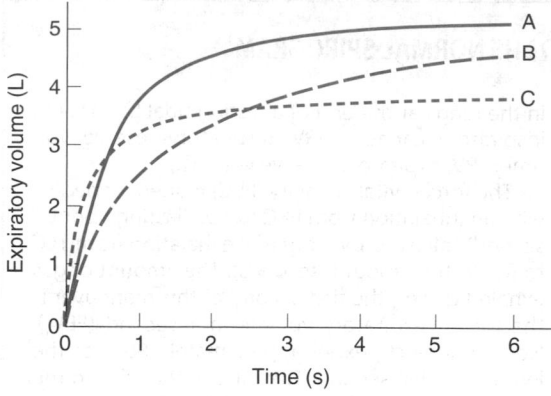

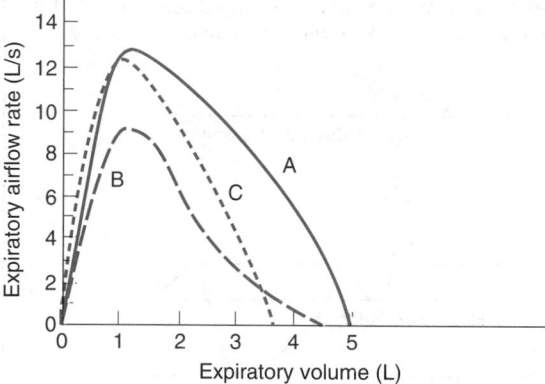

Figure 9–1. Representative spirograms (upper panel) and expiratory flow-volume curves (lower panel) for normal *(A)*, obstructive *(B)*, and restrictive *(C)* patterns.

hemoglobin occupying the pulmonary capillaries. The diffusing capacity should therefore be corrected for the blood hemoglobin concentration.*

Elevated $D_L CO$ is observed in pulmonary hemorrhage and may be seen in acute congestive heart failure and asthma due to an increase in pulmonary capillary blood volume. A diffusing capacity of 6 mL CO/mm Hg or more below the predicted value in women or 8.1 mL CO/mm Hg in men is considered abnormally low (Intermountain Thoracic Society guidelines). Reporting the ratio of measured diffusing capacity to alveolar volume ($D_L CO/V_A$) is helpful, because a diminished diffusing capacity may only reflect a reduction in lung volume. In patients with emphysema, the diffusing capacity is characteristically low, the alveolar volume normal or increased, and the $D_L CO/V_A$ ratio is low. In patients with diffuse infiltrative lung disease, both the diffusing capacity and the alveolar volume are characteristically reduced, and the $D_L CO/V_A$ ratio is normal or low.

*Corrected $D_L CO$ = Measured $D_L CO \times \dfrac{[Hb] + 10.22}{1.7\,[Hb]}$

where [Hb] is the measured hemoglobin concentration (g/dL).

In patients with AIDS, $D_L CO$ is a highly sensitive screening test for the presence of pulmonary disease, especially *Pneumocystis carinii* pneumonia, but it lacks specificity. A normal $D_L CO$ in an AIDS patient is strong evidence against pneumocystis pneumonia. An abnormal result indicates the need for further diagnostic evaluation. Routine measurement of $D_L CO$ and other pulmonary function tests in AIDS patients with pulmonary disease is not advised, because of expense and lack of specificity.

Arterial blood gas analysis is indicated whenever a clinically important acid-base disturbance, hypoxemia, or hypercapnia is suspected. **Oximetry** provides an inexpensive, noninvasive alternative means of monitoring hemoglobin saturation with oxygen. Oximeters monitor oxygen saturation and not oxygen tension. Figure 9–2 displays the normal relationship between oxygen saturation and partial pressure of oxygen in blood. This relationship is not linear. The clinical accuracy of pulse oximeters is reduced in such conditions as severe anemia (< 5 g/dL hemoglobin), the presence of abnormal hemoglobin moieties (carboxyhemoglobin, methemoglobin, fetal hemoglobin), the presence of intravascular dyes, motion artifact, and lack of pulsatile arterial blood flow (hypotension, hypothermia, cardiac arrest, simultaneous use of a blood pressure cuff, and cardiopulmonary bypass). The normal arterial P_{O_2} falls with increasing altitude (Table 9–1).

Nonspecific bronchial provocation testing may aid the evaluation of suspected asthma, when baseline spirometry is normal, and in unexplained cough. The subject inhales a nebulized solution containing methacholine or histamine. These agents cause bronchial smooth muscle constriction in asthmatics at much lower doses than in nonasthmatics. If the FEV_1 falls by more than 20% at a dose of 16 mg/mL or less, the

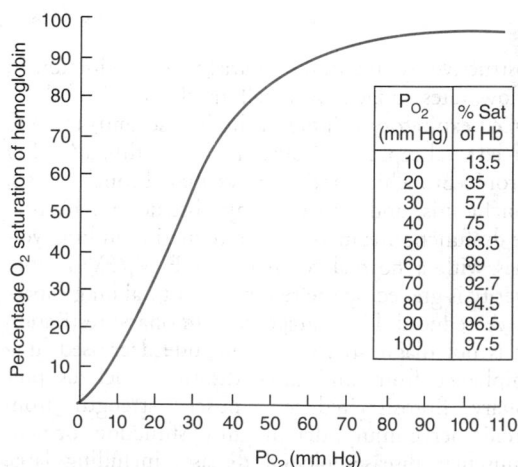

Figure 9–2. Oxygen-hemoglobin dissociation curve, pH 7.40, temperature 38 °C. (Reproduced, with permission, from Comroe JH Jr et al: *The Lung: Clinical Physiology and Pulmonary Function,* 2nd ed. Year Book, 1962.)

Table 9–1. The effect of altitude on Po₂ in normal adults.

Altitude (feet)	Barometric Pressure (mm Hg)	Atmospheric[1] Po₂ (mm Hg)	Tracheal[2] Po₂ (mm Hg)	Arterial[3] Po₂ (mm Hg)
Sea level	760	159	149	99
2000	707	148	138	88
4000	656	137	127	77
6000	609	127	118	68
8000	564	118	108	58
10,000	523	109	100	50
15,000	426	90	80	30

[1]Dry gas.
[2]Saturated with water vapor.
[3]Actual values at altitude will be higher, depending on the degree of adaptation (ventilatory response to hypoxia).

test is positive. Bronchial provocation testing is 95% sensitive for the diagnosis of asthma. A negative result therefore makes asthma unlikely. Specificity is lower—about 70%—since false positives may occur in several common conditions, including COPD, congestive heart failure, recent viral respiratory infection, cystic fibrosis, and sarcoidosis.

Crapo RO: Pulmonary-function testing. N Engl J Med 1994; 331:25. [PMID: 8202099]

Ferguson GT: Office spirometry for lung health assessment in adults: A consensus statement from the National Lung Health Education Program. Chest 2000;117:1146. [PMID: 10767253] (Consensus statement recommends the widespread use of office spirometry by primary care providers for smokers over 45 years of age.)

Cardiopulmonary Exercise Stress Testing

Cardiopulmonary exercise testing is usually performed to evaluate patients with unexplained exertional dyspnea. A bicycle ergometer or treadmill is used. Minute ventilation, expired oxygen and carbon dioxide tension, heart rate, blood pressure, and respiratory rate are monitored. The exercise protocol is determined by the indications for the test and the ability of the patient to exercise. Complications are rare.

Mottram CD: Exercise testing. Respir Care Clin N Am 1997; 3:247. [PMID: 9390911]

Bronchoscopy

Flexible fiberoptic bronchoscopy is an essential tool in the diagnosis and management of many pulmonary diseases. Bronchoscopy is indicated for evaluation of the airway, diagnosis and staging of bronchogenic carcinoma, evaluation of hemoptysis, and diagnosis of pulmonary infections. It allows transbronchial lung biopsy, bronchoalveolar lavage, and removal of re-

tained secretions and foreign bodies from the airway. The procedure is contraindicated in severe bronchospasm and a bleeding diathesis. Complications include hemorrhage, fever, and a transient hypoxemia. The rate of major complications is less than 1%, and deaths are rare. The rate of major complications jumps to about 7% when transbronchial lung biopsy is performed. Hospitalization for fiberoptic bronchoscopy is not necessary.

Rigid bronchoscopy is performed for massive bleeding, extraction of large obstructing objects (foreign bodies, blood clots, tumor masses, broncholiths), biopsy of tracheal or main stem bronchus tumors and bronchial carcinoids, and facilitation of laser therapy. Unlike fiberoptic bronchoscopy, which can usually be performed with only topical anesthesia and low-dose conscious sedation (a narcotic or a benzodiazepine, or both), rigid bronchoscopy usually requires general anesthesia.

Liebler JM et al: Fiberoptic bronchoscopy for diagnosis and treatment. Crit Care Clin 2000;16:83. [PMID: 10650501]

Seijo LM et al: Interventional pulmonology. N Engl J Med 2001;344:740. [PMID: 11236779] (Thorough overview.)

■ DISORDERS OF THE AIRWAYS

Airway disorders have diverse causes but share certain common pathophysiologic and clinical features. Airflow limitation is characteristic and frequently causes dyspnea and cough. Other symptoms are common and typically disease-specific. Disorders of the airways can be classified as those which involve the upper airways—loosely defined as those above and including the vocal cords—and those which involve the lower airways.

DISORDERS OF THE UPPER AIRWAYS

Upper airway obstruction may occur acutely or present as a chronic condition. Acute upper airway obstruction can be immediately life-threatening and must be relieved promptly to avoid asphyxia. Causes of acute upper airway obstruction include foreign body aspiration, laryngospasm, laryngeal edema from airway burns, angioedema, trauma to the larynx or pharynx, infections (Ludwig's angina, pharyngeal or retropharyngeal abscess, acute epiglottis), and acute allergic laryngitis.

Chronic obstruction of the upper airway may be caused by carcinoma of the pharynx or larynx, laryngeal or subglottic stenosis, laryngeal granulomas or webs, or bilateral vocal cord paralysis. Laryngeal or subglottic stenosis may become evident weeks or months following a period of translaryngeal endotracheal intubation. Inspiratory stridor, intercostal retractions on inspiration, a palpable inspiratory thrill over the larynx, and wheezing localized to the neck or trachea on auscultation are characteristic findings. Flow-volume loops may show flow limitations characteristic of obstruction. Soft tissue radiographs of the neck may show supra- or infraglottic narrowing. CT and MRI scans can reveal exact sites of obstruction. Flexible endoscopy may be diagnostic, but caution is necessary to avoid exacerbating upper airway edema and precipitating critical airway narrowing.

Vocal cord dysfunction syndrome is a condition characterized by paradoxical vocal cord adduction, resulting in both acute and chronic upper airway obstruction. It can cause dyspnea and wheezing that may present as asthma; it may be distinguished from asthma by the lack of response to bronchodilator therapy, normal spirometry immediately after an attack, spirometric evidence of upper airway obstruction, a negative bronchial provocation test, or direct visualization of adduction of the vocal cords on both inspiration and expiration. Bronchodilators are of no therapeutic benefit. Treatment consists of speech therapy.

Bacharier LB et al: Vocal cord dysfunction: A practical approach to diagnosis. J Respir Dis 2001;22:93. (Good clinical review of this often enigmatic syndrome.)

Morris MJ et al: Vocal cord dysfunction in patients with exertional dyspnea. Chest 1999;116:1676. [PMID: 10593794] (Vocal cord abnormalities are a frequent occurrence in patients with symptoms of exertional dyspnea and should be strongly considered in their evaluation.)

Noble VE et al: Stridor. J Emerg Med 2000;19:183.[PMID: 10903470] (Upper airway complaint commonly seen in emergency care settings.)

DISORDERS OF THE LOWER AIRWAYS

Tracheal obstruction may be intrathoracic (below the suprasternal notch) or extrathoracic. Fixed tracheal obstruction may be caused by acquired or congenital tracheal stenosis, primary or secondary tracheal neoplasms, extrinsic compression (tumors of the lung, thymus, or thyroid; lymphadenopathy; congenital vascular rings; aneurysms, etc), foreign body aspiration, tracheal granulomas and papillomas, and tracheal trauma.

Acquired **tracheal stenosis** is usually secondary to previous tracheotomy or endotracheal intubation. Dyspnea, cough, and inability to clear pulmonary secretions occur weeks to months after tracheal decannulation or extubation. Physical findings may be absent until tracheal diameter is reduced 50% or more, when wheezing, a palpable tracheal thrill, and harsh breath sounds may be detected. The diagnosis is usually confirmed by plain films or CT of the trachea. Complications include recurring pulmonary infection and life-threatening respiratory failure. Management is directed toward ensuring adequate ventilation and oxygenation and avoiding manipulative procedures that may increase edema of the tracheal mucosa. Surgical reconstruction, endotracheal stent placement, or laser photoresection may be required.

Bronchial obstruction may be caused by retained pulmonary secretions, aspiration, foreign bodies, bronchogenic carcinoma, compression by extrinsic masses, and tumors metastatic to the airway. Clinical and radiographic findings vary depending on the location of the obstruction and the degree of airway narrowing. Symptoms include dyspnea, cough, wheezing, and, if infection is present, fever and chills. A history of recurrent pneumonia in the same lobe or segment or slow resolution (> 3 months) of pneumonia on successive radiographs suggests the possibility of bronchial obstruction and the need for bronchoscopy. Complete obstruction of a main stem bronchus may be obvious on physical examination (asymmetric chest expansion, mediastinal shift, absence of breath sounds on the affected side, and dullness to percussion), but partial obstruction is often difficult or impossible to detect. Prolonged expiration and localized wheezing may be the only clues. Segmental or subsegmental bronchial obstruction may produce no abnormalities on physical examination.

Roentgenographic findings include **atelectasis** (local parenchymal collapse), postobstructive infiltrates, and air trapping caused by unidirectional expiratory obstruction. CT scanning may demonstrate the nature and the exact location of obstruction of the central bronchi. MRI may be superior to CT for delineating the extent of the underlying disease in the hilum, but it is usually reserved for cases in which CT findings are equivocal. Bronchoscopy is the definitive diagnostic study, particularly if tumor or foreign body aspiration is suspected. The finding of tubular breath sounds on physical examination or an air bronchogram on chest radiograph in an area of atelectasis rules out complete airway obstruction. Bronchoscopy is unlikely to be of therapeutic benefit in this situation.

Right middle lobe syndrome is recurrent or persistent atelectasis of the right middle lobe. This collapse is related to the relatively long length and narrow diameter of the right middle lobe bronchus and the oval ("fish mouth") opening to the lobe, in the setting of impaired collateral ventilation. Fiberoptic bronchoscopy or CT scan is often necessary to rule out obstructing tumor. Foreign body or other benign causes are common.

Kwon KY et al: Middle lobe syndrome: A clinicopathological study of 21 patients. Hum Pathol 1995;26:302. [PMID: 7890282] (Detailed description of clinical characteristics and pathologic findings in patients who had surgical resections.)

ASTHMA

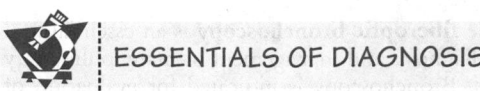 ESSENTIALS OF DIAGNOSIS

- *Episodic or chronic symptoms of airflow obstruction: breathlessness, cough, wheezing, and chest tightness.*

- Symptoms frequently worse at night or in the early morning.
- Prolonged expiration and diffuse wheezes on physical examination.
- Limitation of airflow on pulmonary function testing or positive bronchoprovocation challenge.
- Complete or partial reversibility of airflow obstruction, either spontaneously or following bronchodilator therapy.

General Considerations

Asthma is a common disease, affecting approximately 5% of the population. Men and women appear to be equally affected. Each year, approximately 470,000 hospital admissions and 5000 deaths in the USA are attributed to asthma. Hospitalization rates have been highest among blacks and children, and death rates for asthma are consistently highest among blacks aged 15–24 years. Prevalence, hospitalizations, and fatal asthma have all increased in the United States over the past 20 years.

Definition & Pathogenesis

Asthma is a chronic inflammatory disorder of the airways. The histopathologic features include denudation of airway epithelium, collagen deposition beneath the basement membrane, airway edema, mast cell activation, and inflammatory cell infiltration with neutrophils, eosinophils, and lymphocytes (especially T lymphocytes). Hypertrophy of bronchial smooth muscle and hypertrophy of mucous glands with plugging of small airways with thick mucus can occur. This airway inflammation underlies disease chronicity and contributes to airway hyperresponsiveness, airflow limitation, and respiratory symptoms (including recurrent episodes of wheezing, breathlessness, chest tightness, and cough, particularly during the nighttime and early morning hours).

A genetic predisposition to asthma is recognized. The strongest identifiable predisposing factor for the development of asthma is atopy. Exposure of sensitive patients to inhaled allergens increases airway inflammation, airway hyperresponsiveness, and symptoms. Patients may develop symptoms immediately (immediate asthmatic response) or 4–6 hours after their exposures (late asthmatic response). Common aeroallergens include house dust mites (often found in pillows, mattresses, upholstered furniture, carpets, and drapes), cockroaches, cats, and seasonal pollens. Substantially reducing exposure reduces pathologic findings and clinical symptoms.

Nonspecific precipitants of asthma include exercise, upper respiratory tract infections, rhinitis, sinusitis, postnasal drip, aspiration, gastroesophageal reflux, changes in the weather, and stress. Exposure to environmental tobacco smoke increases asthma symptoms and the need for medications and reduces lung function. Increased air levels of respirable particles, ozone, SO_2, and NO_2 precipitate asthma symptoms and increase emergency department visits and hospitalizations. Selected individuals may experience asthma symptoms after exposure to aspirin, nonsteroidal anti-inflammatory drugs, or tartrazine dyes. Certain other medications may also precipitate asthma symptoms (Table 9–28). Occupational asthma is triggered by various agents in the workplace and may occur weeks to years after initial exposure and sensitization. Women may experience catamenial asthma at predictable times during the menstrual cycle. Exercise-induced bronchoconstriction usually begins within 3 minutes after the end of exercise, peaks within 10–15 minutes and then resolves by 60 minutes. This phenomenon is thought to be a consequence of the airways' attempt to warm and humidify an increased volume of expired air during exercise. "Cardiac asthma" is wheezing precipitated by uncompensated congestive heart failure.

Clinical Findings

Symptoms and signs vary widely from patient to patient as well as individually over time. General clinical findings in stable asthma patients are listed below; findings seen during asthma exacerbations are listed in Table 9–3.

A. SYMPTOMS AND SIGNS

Asthma is characterized by episodic wheezing, difficulty in breathing, chest tightness, and cough. The frequency of asthma symptoms is highly variable. Some patients may have only a chronic dry cough and others a productive cough. Some patients have infrequent, brief attacks of asthma and others may suffer nearly continuous symptoms. Asthma symptoms may occur spontaneously or may be precipitated or exacerbated by many different triggers as discussed above. Asthma symptoms are frequently worse at night; circadian variations in bronchomotor tone and bronchial reactivity reach their nadir between 3 and 4 AM, increasing symptoms of bronchoconstriction.

Some physical findings increase the probability of asthma. Nasal mucosal swelling, increased nasal secretions, and nasal polyps are often seen in patients with allergic asthma. Eczema, atopic dermatitis, or other manifestations of allergic skin disorders may also be present. Hunched shoulders and use of accessory muscles of respiration suggest an increased work of breathing. Chest examination may be normal between exacerbations in patients with mild asthma. Wheezing during normal breathing or a prolonged forced expiratory phase correlates well with the presence of airflow obstruction. Wheezing during forced expiration does not. During severe asthma exacerbations, airflow may be too limited to produce wheezing, and the only diagnostic clue on auscultation may be globally reduced breath sounds with prolonged expiration.

B. PULMONARY FUNCTION TESTING

Clinicians are able to identify airflow obstruction on examination, but they have limited ability to assess it or to predict whether it is reversible. The evaluation for asthma should therefore include spirometry (FEV_1, FVC, FEV_1/FVC) before and after the administration of a short-acting bronchodilator. These measurements help determine the presence and extent of airflow obstruction and whether it is immediately reversible. Airflow obstruction is indicated by a reduced FEV_1/FVC ratio ($< 75\%$). In severe airflow obstruction with significant air trapping, the FVC may also be reduced, resulting in a pattern that suggests a restrictive ventilatory defect. Significant reversibility of airflow obstruction is defined by an increase of $\geq 12\%$ and 200 mL in FEV_1 or $\geq 15\%$ and 200 mL in FVC after inhaling a short-acting bronchodilator. However, the absence of improvement in airflow after administration of a bronchodilator is not proof of irreversible airflow obstruction.

Peak expiratory flow (PEF) meters are handheld devices designed as home monitoring tools. PEF monitoring can establish peak flow variability, quantify asthma severity, and provide both the patient and the clinician with objective measurements on which to base treatment decisions. There are conflicting data about whether measuring PEF improves asthma outcomes, but doing so is recommended as part of a comprehensive approach to asthma management in Expert Panel Report 2 of the National Asthma Education and Prevention Program (NAEPP) of the National Heart, Lung and Blood Institute.

Predicted values for PEF vary with age, height, and gender but are poorly standardized. Comparison with reference values is less helpful than comparison with the patient's best baseline. PEF shows diurnal variation. It is generally lowest on first awakening and highest several hours before the midpoint of the waking day. PEF should be measured in the morning before the administration of a bronchodilator and in the afternoon after taking a bronchodilator. A 20% change in PEF values from morning to afternoon or from day to day suggests inadequately controlled asthma. PEF values less than 200 L/min indicate severe airflow obstruction.

Bronchial provocation testing with histamine or methacholine—or exercise challenge testing—may be useful when asthma is suspected and spirometry is nondiagnostic. Bronchial provocation is not generally recommended if the FEV_1 is less than 65% of predicted. A positive test is defined as a decrease in FEV_1 of at least 20% at exposure to a concentration of 16 mg/mL or less. A negative test has a negative predictive value for asthma of 95%.

Arterial blood gas measurements may be normal during a mild asthma exacerbation, but respiratory alkalosis and an increase in the alveolar-arterial oxygen difference (A–a DO_2) are common. During severe exacerbations, hypoxemia develops and the $PaCO_2$ returns to normal. The combination of an increased $PaCO_2$ and respiratory acidosis is a harbinger of respiratory failure and may indicate the need for mechanical ventilation.

C. ADDITIONAL TESTING

Routine chest radiographs in patients with asthma usually show only hyperinflation. Other findings may include bronchial wall thickening and diminished peripheral lung vascular shadows. Chest radiographs are indicated when pneumonia, another disorder mimicking asthma, or a complication of asthma such as pneumothorax is suspected. The diagnostic usefulness of measurements of biologic markers of inflammation such as cell counts and mediator titers in blood and sputum is being investigated. Skin testing or in vitro testing to assess sensitivity to relevant environmental allergens may be useful in patients with persistent asthma. Evaluations for paranasal sinus disease or gastroesophageal reflux should be considered in patients with pertinent symptoms and in those who have severe or refractory asthma.

Complications

Complications of asthma include exhaustion, dehydration, airway infection, cor pulmonale, and tussive syncope. Pneumothorax occurs but is rare. Acute hypercapnic and hypoxic respiratory failure occurs in severe disease.

Differential Diagnosis

Disorders that mimic asthma typically fall into one of three categories: upper and lower airway disorders, systemic vasculitides, and psychiatric disorders. It is prudent to consider these conditions in patients who have atypical asthma symptoms or response to therapy. Upper airway disorders that mimic asthma include vocal cord paralysis, vocal cord dysfunction syndrome, foreign body aspiration, laryngotracheal masses, tracheal narrowing, tracheomalacia, and airway edema as in the setting of angioedema or inhalation injury. Lower airway disorders include nonasthmatic chronic obstructive pulmonary disease (chronic bronchitis or emphysema), bronchiectasis, allergic bronchopulmonary mycosis, cystic fibrosis, eosinophilic pneumonia, and bronchiolitis obliterans. Systemic vasculitides that often have an asthmatic component include Churg-Strauss syndrome and other systemic vasculitides with pulmonary involvement. Psychiatric causes include conversion disorders, which have been variably referred to as functional asthma, emotional laryngeal wheezing, vocal cord dysfunction, or episodic laryngeal dyskinesis. Munchausen syndrome or malingering may rarely explain the patient's complaints.

Classification of Asthma Severity

The Expert Panel of the NAEPP has developed asthma classification schemes which are useful in directing asthma therapy and identifying patients at high risk of developing life-threatening asthma attacks. Table 9–2 is used to classify the severity of chronic, stable asthma; Table 9–3 to classify severity of asthma exacerbations. A patient's clinical features before treatment are used to classify the patient. The presence of only one of the severity features is sufficient to place a patient in that category; patients should be assigned to the most severe grade in which any feature occurs.

Approach to Long-Term Treatment

The goals of asthma therapy are to minimize chronic symptoms that impair normal activity (including exercise), to prevent recurrent exacerbations, to minimize the need for emergency department visits or hospitalizations, and to maintain near-normal pulmonary function. These goals should be met while providing optimal pharmacotherapy with the fewest adverse effects and while meeting patients' and families' expectations of satisfaction with asthma care.

Current approaches to persistent asthma focus on daily anti-inflammatory therapy with inhaled corticosteroids. Treatment algorithms are based on both the severity of a patient's baseline asthma and the severity of asthma exacerbations. Expert Panel Report 2 from the NAEPP recommends a stepwise approach to therapy (Table 9–4). The amount of medication and frequency of dosing are dictated by asthma severity and directed toward suppression of increasing airway inflammation. To establish prompt control, therapy should be initiated early at higher intensity than anticipated for chronic therapy. Pharmacotherapy can then be cautiously stepped down once asthma control is achieved and sustained; this allows for identification of the minimum medication necessary to maintain long-term control.

Pharmacologic Agents for Asthma

Asthma medications can be divided into long-term control and quick-relief medications. Long-term control medications are taken daily to achieve and maintain control of persistent asthma. These agents—also known as maintenance, controller, or preventive medications—act primarily to attenuate airway inflammation. Quick-relief medications are taken to promote prompt reversal of acute airflow obstruction and relief of accompanying symptoms by direct relaxation of bronchial smooth muscle.

Many asthma medications can be administered orally or by inhalation. Inhalation of an appropriate agent offers the advantage of delivery of high concentrations of medication directly to the target organ. This results in a more rapid onset of pulmonary effects as well as fewer systemic effects compared with oral administration of the same dose. Metered-dose inhalers (MDIs) propelled by chlorofluorocarbons (CFCs) have been the most widely used delivery system, but non-CFC propellent systems and dry powder inhalers are available. These alternatives are effective and well tolerated. Proper MDI technique and the use of an inhalation chamber improve drug delivery to the lung and decrease oropha-

Table 9–2. Classification of severity of chronic stable asthma.[1]

	Symptoms	Nighttime Symptoms	Lung Function
Mild intermittent	Symptoms ≤ 2 times a week Asymptomatic and normal PEF between exacerbations Exacerbations brief (few hours to few days); intensity may vary	≤ 2 times a month	FEV_1 or PEF ≥ 80% predicted PEF variability ≤ 20%
Mild persistent	Symptoms > 2 times a week but < 1 time a day Exacerbations may affect activity	> 2 times a month	FEV_1 or PEF > 80% predicted PEF variability 20–30%
Moderate persistent	Daily symptoms Daily use of inhaled short-acting β_2-agonist Exacerbations affect activity Exacerbations ≥ 2 times a week; may last days	> 1 time a week	FEV_1 or PEF > 60% to < 80% predicted PEF variability > 30%
Severe persistent	Continual symptoms Limited physical activity Frequent exacerbations	Frequent	FEV_1 or PEF ≤ 60% predicted PEF variability > 30%

[1]Adapted from National Asthma Education and Prevention Program. Expert Panel Report 2: Guidelines for the Diagnosis and Management of Asthma. National Institutes of Health Pub No. 97-4051. Bethesda, MD, 1997.

Table 9–3. Classification of severity of asthma exacerbations[1]

	Mild	Moderate	Severe	Impending Respiratory Failure
Symptoms				
Breathlessness	With activity	With talking	At rest	At rest
Speech	Sentences	Phrases	Words	Mute
Signs				
Body position	Able to recline	Prefers sitting	Unable to recline	Unable to recline
Respiratory rate	Increased	Increased	Often > 30/min	> 30/min
Use of accessory respiratory muscles	Usually not	Commonly	Usually	Paradoxical thoracoabdominal movement
Breath sounds	Moderate wheezing at mid- to end-expiration	Loud wheezes throughout expiration	Loud inspiratory and expiratory wheezes	Little air movement without wheezes
Heart rate (beats/min)	< 100	100–120	> 120	Relative bradycardia
Pulsus paradoxus (mm Hg)	< 10	10–25	Often > 25	Often absent
Mental status	May be agitated	Usually agitated	Usually agitated	Confused or drowsy
Functional assessment				
PEF (% predicted or personal best)	> 80	50–80	< 50 or response to therapy lasts < 2 hours	< 50
Sao_2 (%, room air)	> 95	91–95	< 91	< 91
Pao_2 (mm Hg, room air)	Normal	> 60	< 60	< 60
$Paco_2$ (mm Hg)	< 42	< 42	≥ 42	≥ 42

[1] Adapted from National Asthma Education and Prevention Program. Expert Panel Report 2: Guidelines for the Diagnosis and Management of Asthma. National Institutes of Health Pub No. 97-4051. Bethesda, MD, 1997.

ryngeal deposition. Nebulizer therapy is reserved for acutely ill patients and those who cannot use MDIs because of difficulties with coordination or cooperation.

A. LONG-TERM CONTROL MEDICATIONS

Anti-inflammatory agents, long-acting bronchodilators, and leukotriene modifiers comprise the important medications in this group of agents (see Table 9–5). Other classes of agents are mentioned briefly below.

1. Corticosteroids—Corticosteroids are the most potent and consistently effective anti-inflammatory agents currently available. They reduce both acute and chronic inflammation, resulting in fewer asthma symptoms, improvement in airflow, decreased airway hyperresponsiveness, fewer asthma exacerbations, and less airway remodeling. These agents may also potentiate the action of beta-adrenergic agonists.

Inhaled corticosteroids are preferred for the long-term control of asthma and are first-line agents for patients with persistent asthma. Patients with persistent symptoms or asthma exacerbations who are not taking inhaled corticosteroids should be started on an inhaled

corticosteroid; symptomatic patients already taking an inhaled corticosteroid should have the dose increased. Dosages for inhaled corticosteroids vary depending on the specific agent and delivery device. Because of limited data directly comparing the currently available inhaled corticosteroids and individual patient variability, the most important determinants of agent selection and appropriate dosing are the patient's status and response to treatment. For most patients, twice-daily dosing provides adequate control of asthma. Once-daily dosing may be sufficient in selected patients with mild persistent asthma. Maximum responses from inhaled corticosteroids may not be observed for months. The use of an inhalation chamber coupled with mouth washing after inhalation decreases local side effects (cough, dysphonia, oropharyngeal candidiasis) and systemic absorption. Systemic effects (adrenal suppression, osteoporosis, skin thinning, easy bruising, and cataracts) may occur with high-dose inhalation therapy.

Systemic corticosteroids (oral or parenteral) are most effective in achieving prompt control of asthma during exacerbations or when initiating long-term asthma therapy. In patients with severe persistent asthma, systemic corticosteroids are often required for

Table 9–4. Stepwise approach for managing asthma.[1,2]

	Long-Term Control	Quick Relief	Education
Step 1: Mild intermittent	No daily medication needed.	Short-acting bronchodilator: **inhaled β_2-agonists** as needed for symptoms. Intensity of treatment will depend on severity of exacerbation. Use of short-acting inhaled β_2-agonists > 2 times a week may indicate the need for long-term control therapy.	Teach basic facts about asthma Teach inhaler/inhalation chamber technique Discuss roles of medications Develop self-management & action plans Discuss appropriate environmental control measures
Step 2: Mild persistent	One daily medication: **Anti-Inflammatory**: either **inhaled corticosteroid (low doses)** or **cromolyn** or **nedocromil** Less desirable alternatives: sustained-release theophylline or leukotriene modifier	Short-acting bronchodilator: **inhaled β_2-agonists** as needed for symptoms. Intensity of treatment will depend on severity of exacerbation. Use of short-acting inhaled β_2-agonists on a daily basis, or increasing use, indicates the need for additional long-term control therapy.	Step 1 actions plus: Teach self-monitoring Refer to group education if available Review and update self-management plan
Step 3: Moderate persistent	Daily medication: Either **Anti-inflammatory**: **inhaled corticosteroid (medium dose)** or **Inhaled corticosteroid (low-medium dose)** and a long-acting bronchodilator (**long-acting inhaled β_2-agonist**, sustained-release theophylline or long-acting β_2-agonist tablets) If needed: **Anti-inflammatory**: inhaled **corticosteroid (medium-high dose)** and **Long-acting bronchodilator (long-acting inhaled β_2-agonist**, sustained-release theophylline or long-acting β_2-agonist tablets)	Short-acting bronchodilator: **inhaled β_2-agonists** as needed for symptoms. Intensity of treatment will depend on severity of exacerbation. Use of short-acting inhaled β_2-agonists on a daily basis, or increasing use, indicates the need for additional long-term control therapy.	Step 1 actions plus: Teach self-monitoring Refer to group education if available Review and update self-management plan

(continued)

Table 9–4. Stepwise approach for managing asthma.[1,2] (continued)

	Long-Term Control	Quick Relief	Education
Step 4: Severe persistent	Daily medication: **Anti-inflammatory: inhaled corticosteroid (high dose)** and **Long-acting bronchodilator (long-acting inhaled β₂-agonist,** sustained-release theophylline or long-acting β₂-agonist tablets) and Corticosteroid tablets or syrup (2 mg/kg/d, generally not to exceed 60 mg/d)	Short-acting bronchodilator: **inhaled β₂-agonists** as needed for symptoms. Intensity of treatment will depend on severity of exacerbation. Use of short-acting inhaled β₂-agonists on a daily basis, or increasing use, indicates the need for additional long-term control therapy.	Step 2 and 3 actions plus: Refer to individual education, counseling

Step down: Review treatment every 1–6 months; a gradual stepwise reduction in treatment may be possible.

Step up: If asthma control is not maintained, consider step up to next treatment level after reviewing medication technique, adherence, and environmental control.

[1]Modified from National Asthma Education and Prevention Program. Expert Panel Report 2: Guidelines for the Diagnosis and Management of Asthma. National Institutes of Health Pub. No. 97-4051. Bethesda, MD, 1997.

[2]Preferred treatments are in colored text; however, specific medication plans should be tailored to individual patients.

the long-term suppression of symptoms. Repeated efforts should be made to reduce the dose to the minimum needed to control symptoms. Alternate-day treatment is preferred to daily treatment. Rapid discontinuation of systemic corticosteroids after chronic use may precipitate adrenal insufficiency. Concurrent treatment with calcium supplements and vitamin D should be initiated to prevent steroid-induced bone mineral loss in long-term administration. Bisphosphonates may offer additional protection to these patients (see Table 26–18).

2. Long-acting bronchodilators—

a. Mediator inhibitors—Cromolyn sodium and nedocromil are long-term control medications that prevent asthma symptoms and improve airway function in patients with mild persistent asthma or exercise-induced asthma. Both of these agents modulate mast cell mediator release and eosinophil recruitment and inhibit both early and late asthmatic responses to allergen challenge and exercise-induced bronchospasm. The clinical response to these agents is less predictable than the response to inhaled corticosteroids. Nedocromil may help reduce the dose requirements for inhaled corticosteroids. Both agents have excellent safety profiles.

b. Beta-adrenergic agents—Long-acting β₂ agonists provide bronchodilation for up to 12 hours after a single dose. However, because their onset of action is delayed, they are not effective—and should not be used—in the treatment of acute bronchoconstriction. The only agent of this class available in the United States is salmeterol, indicated for long-term prevention of asthma symptoms, nocturnal symptoms, and prevention of exercise-induced bronchospasm. Salmeterol should not be used in place of anti-inflammatory therapy. When added to standard doses of inhaled corticosteroids, salmeterol provides equivalent control when compared with doubling the inhaled corticosteroid dose. Side effects are minimal at the standard dose of two puffs twice a day.

c. Phosphodiesterase inhibitors—Theophylline provides mild bronchodilation in asthmatics. This drug may also have anti-inflammatory properties, enhance mucociliary clearance, and strengthen diaphragmatic contractility. Sustained-release theophylline preparations are effective in controlling nocturnal asthma and are usually reserved for use as adjuvant therapy in patients with moderate or severe persistent asthma. They can also be used as alternative long-term preventive therapy in patients with mild persistent asthma. Theophylline serum concentrations need to be monitored closely owing to the drug's narrow toxic-therapeutic range, individual differences in metabolism, and the effects of many factors on drug absorption and metabolism. Decreases in theophylline clearance accompany the use of cimetidine, macrolide and quinolone antibiotics, and oral contraceptives. Increases in theophylline clearance are caused by rifampin, phenytoin, barbiturates, and tobacco.

Adverse effects at therapeutic doses include insomnia, upset stomach, aggravation of dyspepsia and gastroesophageal reflux symptoms, and urination difficulties in elderly men with prostatism. Dose-related toxicities are common and include nausea, vomiting, tachyarrhythmias, headache, seizures, hyperglycemia and hypokalemia.

Table 9-5. Long-term control medications for asthma.[1]

Drug	Important Formulations	Usual Adult Dosage	Cost[2]	Comments
Inhaled corticosteroids:[3]				
Beclomethasone dipropionate (QVAR)	40 μg/puff	Two or three puffs BID	$41.32/7.30 g	Chlorofluorocarbon-free; hydrofluoralkane propellant
	80 μg/puff	One to two puffs BID	$52.04/7.30 g	
Beclomethasone dipropionate (Vanceril)	MDI: 42 μg/puff; 200 puffs/inhaler	Two or three puffs four times a day, or four to six puffs twice daily	$46.52/16.80 g	Chlorofluorocarbon propellant
	84 μg/puff; 120 puffs/inhaler	Two puffs twice a day	$53.33/12.20 g	
Budesonide (Pulmicort Turbuhaler)	Dry powder delivery system: 200 μg/puff; 200 puffs/inhaler	One inhalation twice a day	$129.43/inhaler	Dry powder
Flunisolide (AeroBid)	MDI: 250 μg/puff; 100 puffs/inhaler	Two to four puffs twice a day	$67.01/7 g	Chlorofluorocarbon propellant
Fluticasone (Flovent)	MDI: 44, 110 or 220 μg/puff; 120 puffs/inhaler	Two or three puffs (of 110 μg) twice a day	$70.58/13 g	Chlorofluorocarbon propellant
(Flovent Rotadisk)	Dry powder delivery system: 44, 88, 220 μg/blister; 4 blisters/Rotadisk, 15 Rotadisks per tube	One or two puffs (of 88 μg) twice a day	$53.30/60 88 μg disks	Dry powder
Triamcinolone acetonide (Azmacort)	MDI: 100 μg/puff; 240 puffs/inhaler	Two or three puffs four times a day, or four to six puffs twice daily	$68.58/20 g	Chlorofluorocarbon propellant
Systemic corticosteroids				
Methylprednisolone (many)	Tablets: 4 mg	5–60 mg daily to every other day as needed	$0.54/4 mg	
Prednisolone (many)	Tablets: 5 mg	5–60 mg daily to every other day as needed	$0.04/5 mg	
Prednisone (many)	Tablets: 1, 2.5, 5, 10, 20, 50 mg	5–60 mg daily to every other day as needed	$0.04/5 mg	
Combination Inhaled corticosteroid and long-acting β_2 agonist				
Fluticasone and salmeterol (Advair Diskus)	Dry powder delivery system 100, 250, or 500 μg fluticasone per dose and 50 μg salmeterol per dose	One puff twice a day of 250/50; cannot use more than one puff twice a day due to salmeterol component.	$135.52/60 250/50 disks	Dry powder

Table 9–5. Long-term control medications for asthma.[1] (continued)

Drug	Important Formulations	Usual Adult Dosage	Cost[2]	Comments
Cromolyn (Intal)	MDI: 800 μg per puff: 200 puffs/inhaler	2–4 puffs 4 times a day	$77.95/14.2 g	Chlorofluorocarbon propellant
	Nebulizer solution, 20 mg/2 mL ampule	20 mg (2 mL) four times a day	$0.77/2 mL	Administer with powered nebulizer
Nedocromil (Tilade)	MDI: 1.75 mg/puff; 112 puffs/inhaler	Two puffs four times a day	$42.72/16.2 g	Chlorofluorocarbon propellant
Long-acting β_2-agonists[4] Salmeterol (Serevent)	MDI: 21 μg/puff; 120 puffs/inhaler	Two puffs every 12 hours	$76.64/13 g	Chlorofluorocarbon propellant
(Serevent Diskus)	Dry powder: 50 μg/blister; 60 blisters per pack	One blister every 12 hours	$80.02/60	Dry powder
Sustained-release albuterol (Proventil Repetab)	Sustained-release tablet, 4 mg	One tablet every 12 hours	$0.88/4 mg	Usually reserved for nocturnal symptoms not improved with other therapies
Theophylline (many)	Sustained-release tablets and capsules	Initially 10 mg/kg/d up to 300 mg maximum; then 200–600 mg every 8–24 hours	$0.21/200 mg	Maintenance dose guided by serum drug level. Absorption and dosing vary with brand
Leukotriene modifiers Montelukast (Singulair)	Tablet, 10 mg	One tablet each evening	$2.64/10 mg $79.26/mo	
Zafirlukast (Accolate)	Tablet, 20 mg	One tablet twice a day	$1.18/20 mg $70.86/mo	Administration with meals decreases bioavailability; take at least 1 hour before or 2 hours after meals
Zileuton (Zyflo)	Tablet, 600 mg	One tablet four times a day	$0.86/600 mg $103.19/mo	Monitor hepatic enzymes

[1] Only drugs available in the United States are listed.
[2] Cost to pharmacist (average wholesale price, generic when possible) for quantity listed. Source: *Drug Topics Red Book*, March 2002; Vol. 21, No. 3.
[3] Dosing should be individualized. See text.
[4] Not for acute relief of symptoms.

3. Leukotriene modifiers—This is the newest class of medications for long-term control of asthma. Leukotrienes are potent biochemical mediators that contribute to airway obstruction and asthma symptoms by contracting airway smooth muscle, increasing vascular permeability and mucus secretion, and attracting and activating airway inflammatory cells. Zileuton is a 5-lipoxygenase inhibitor that decreases leukotriene production, and zafirlukast and montelukast are cysteinyl leukotriene receptor antagonists. They cause modest improvements in lung function and reductions in asthma symptoms and lessen the need for beta-agonist rescue therapy. These agents may be considered as alternatives to low-dose inhaled corticosteroids in patients with mild persistent asthma. Zileuton can cause reversible elevations in plasma aminotransferase levels, and a small number of patients who have taken montelukast or zafirlukast subsequently have been diagnosed with Churg-Strauss syndrome.

4. Desensitization—Immunotherapy for specific allergens may be considered in selected asthma patients who have exacerbations of asthma symptoms when exposed to allergens to which they are sensitive and who do not respond to environmental control measures or other forms of conventional therapy. Studies show a reduction in asthma symptoms in patients treated with single-allergen immunotherapy. Because of the risk of immunotherapy-induced bronchoconstriction, it should be administered only in a setting where such complications can be treated.

5. Miscellaneous agents—Oral sustained-release β_2 agonists are reserved for patients with bothersome nocturnal asthma symptoms or moderate to severe persistent asthma who do not respond to other therapies. Corticosteroid-sparing anti-inflammatory agents such as troleandomycin, methotrexate, cyclosporine, intravenous immunoglobulin, and gold should be used only in selected severe asthmatics. These and other agents have variable benefit and worrisome toxicities.

B. QUICK-RELIEF MEDICATIONS

Short-acting bronchodilators and systemic corticosteroids comprise the important medications in this group of agents (Table 9–6).

1. Beta-adrenergic agents—Short-acting inhaled beta-adrenergic agonists are clearly the most effective bronchodilators during exacerbations. Beta-adrenergic agonists should be used in all patients to treat acute symptoms. These agents relax airway smooth muscle and cause a prompt increase in airflow and reduction of symptoms. Administration before exercise effectively prevents exercise-induced bronchoconstriction. There is no convincing evidence to support the use of one agent over another. However, β_2-selective agents produce less cardiac stimulation than those with mixed β_1 and β_2 activities. Currently available short-acting β_2-selective adrenergic agonists include albuterol, bitolterol, pirbuterol, and terbutaline.

Inhaled β agonist therapy is as effective as oral or parenteral therapy in relaxing airway smooth muscle and improving acute asthma and offers the advantages of rapid onset of action (< 5 minutes) with fewer systemic side effects. Repetitive administration produces incremental bronchodilation. Intravenous and subcutaneous routes of administration should be reserved for patients who because of age or mechanical factors are unable to inhale medications.

One or two inhalations of a short-acting inhaled β_2 agonist from a metered-dose inhaler is usually sufficient for mild to moderate symptoms; severe exacerbations may require up to four inhalations every few hours. Administration by wet nebulization does not offer more effective delivery than metered-dose inhalers; it is perceived to be more effective because it is given in higher doses. With most β_2 agonists, the recommended dose by nebulizer for acute asthma (albuterol, 2.5 mg) is 25–30 times that delivered by a single activation of the metered-dose inhaler (albuterol, 0.09 mg). This difference suggests that the standard use of inhalations from a metered-dose inhaler will often be insufficient in the setting of an acute exacerbation. Equivalent bronchodilation can be achieved by either high doses (6–12 puffs) of a β_2 agonist by metered-dose inhaler with an inhalation chamber or by nebulizer therapy. Nebulizer therapy may be more effective in patients who are unable to coordinate inhalation of medication from a metered-dose inhaler because of age, agitation, or severity of the exacerbation.

Scheduled daily use of β_2 agonists is not generally recommended. Increased use (more than one canister a month) or lack of expected effect indicates diminished asthma control and dictates the need for additional long-term control therapy.

2. Anticholinergics—Anticholinergic agents reverse vagally mediated bronchospasm but not allergen- or exercise-induced bronchospasm. They may decrease mucus gland hypersecretion seen in asthma. Ipratropium bromide, a quaternary derivative of atropine free of atropine's side-effects, is the only available agent. This drug reverses acute bronchospasm and is the inhaled alternative for patients with intolerance to β_2 agonists. Ipratropium bromide may be a useful adjunct to inhaled short-acting β_2 agonists and considered in patients with moderate to severe asthma exacerbations. High doses of inhaled ipratropium bromide (0.5 mg) cause additional bronchodilation in some patients with severe airway obstruction, but the long-term role in management of asthma has not been clarified. It is the drug of choice for bronchospasm due to beta-blocker medications.

3. Phosphodiesterase inhibitors—Methylxanthines are not recommended for therapy of asthma exacerbations. Aminophylline has clearly been shown to be less effective than β_2 agonists when used as single-drug therapy for acute asthma and adds little except toxicity to the acute bronchodilator effects achieved by nebulized metaproterenol alone. In patients currently taking a theophylline-containing preparation, the serum

Table 9–6. Quick-relief medications for asthma.[1]

Drug	Important Formulations	Usual Adult Dosage	Cost[2]	Comments
Short-acting Inhaled β_2-agonists				
Albuterol (Proventil, Ventolin)	MDI: 90 μg/puff, 200 puffs/canister	Two puffs 5 minutes before exercise Two puffs every 4–6 hours as needed	$21.70/17 g	Preferred formulation in most cases. Chlorofluorocarbon propellant.
	Nebulizer solutions: 5 mg/mL (0.5%)	1.25–5 mg (0.25–1 mL) in 2–3 mL of normal saline every 4–8 hours as needed	$14.95/20 mL	Administer with powered nebulizer. More frequent dosing is acceptable for acute or severe exacerbations.
	Unit dose: 0.083%, 3 mL	One dose every 4–8 hours as needed	$1.25/unit	May mix with cromolyn or ipratropium nebulizer solutions.
	Dry powder (Ventolin Rotocaps): 200 μg/capsule	One or two capsules every 4–6 hours as needed	$32.15/100 200-μg capsules	Rotohaler required for inhalation.
	Tablets: 2 mg, 4 mg	2–4 mg orally every 6–8 hours	$31.14/100 2-mg tablets	Extended-release 4 mg tablet (Proventil Repetab) available for use every 12 hours.
Albuterol HFA (Proventil HFA)	MDI: 90 μg/puff, 200 puffs/canister	Two puffs 5 minutes before exercise Two puffs every 4–6 hours as needed	$35.06/6.7 g	Nonchlorofluorocarbon propellant.
Bitolterol (Tornalate)	Nebulizer solution, 2 mg/mL (0.2%)	0.5–2 mg (0.25–1 mL) in 2–3 mL of normal saline every 4–8 hours as needed	$16.54/30 mL	Administer with powered nebulizer. May not mix with other nebulizer solutions.
Pirbuterol (Maxair)	MDI: 200 μg/puff, 300 puffs/canister	Two puffs every 4–6 hours as needed	$50.52/25 g	Chlorofluorocarbon propellant.
(Maxair Autoinhaler)	MDI 200 μg/puff, 400 puffs/canister	Two puffs every 4–6 hours as needed	$56.76/14 g	Breath-activated MDI system. Chlorofluorocarbon propellant.
Terbutaline (Brethine)	Tablets: 2.5 mg, 5 mg	2.5–5 mg orally three times a day	$49.79/100 5-mg tablets	Tremor, nervousness, palpitations common; therefore not recommended.
	Injection solution, 1 mg/mL	0.25 mg (0.25 mL) subcutaneously; may be repeated once in 30 minutes	$2.82/1 mg	Onset of action 30 minutes. Not limited to β_2-agonist effects.
Anticholinergics Ipratropium bromide (Atrovent)	MDI: 18 μg/puff, 200 puffs/canister	Two to four puffs every 6 hours	$44.56/14 g	Chlorofluorocarbon propellant.
	Unit dose nebulizer solution, 0.2 mg/mL (0.02%), 2.5 mL (0.5 mg)	0.25–0.5 mg (1–2 mL) every 6 hours	$1.76/unit	

(continued)

Table 9–6. Quick-relief medications for asthma.[1] (continued)

Drug	Important Formulations	Usual Adult Dosage	Cost[2]	Comments
Systemic corticosteroids				
Methylprednisolone (many)	Tablets: 4 mg	40–60 mg/d as single dose or in two divided doses for 3–10 days	$11.00/4 mg dose-pack	
Methylprednisolone sodium succinate (many)	Intravenous injection solution vials: 40, 125, 500 mg	0.5–1 mg/kg every 6 hours	$3.41/125 mg vial	
Prednisolone (many)	Tablets: 5 mg	40–60 mg/d as single dose or in two divided doses for 3–10 days	$0.04/5 mg tablet	
	Syrup: 15 mg/5 mL		$74.50/240 mL syrup	
Prednisone (many)	Tablets: 1, 2.5, 5, 10, 20, 50 mg	40–60 mg/d as single dose or in two divided doses for 3–10 days	$0.04/5 mg	

[1]Only drugs available in the United States are listed.
[2]Cost to pharmacist (average wholesale price, generic when possible) for quantity listed. Source: *Drug Topics Red Book*, March 2002; Vol. 21, No. 3.

theophylline concentration should be determined to exclude theophylline toxicity.

4. Glucocorticoids—Systemic corticosteroids are effective primary treatment for patients with moderate to severe exacerbations or for patients who fail to respond promptly and completely to inhaled β_2-agonist therapy. They are one of the mainstays of the treatment of patients with severe asthma. These medications speed the resolution of airflow obstruction and reduce the rate of relapse. Delays in administering corticosteroids may result in delayed benefits from these important agents. Therefore, oral corticosteroids should be available for early administration at home in many patients with moderate to severe asthma.

It may be prudent to administer corticosteroids to critically ill patients via the intravenous route in order to avoid concerns about altered gastrointestinal absorption in these patients. The minimal effective dose of systemic corticosteroids for asthma patients has not been identified. Outpatient prednisone "burst" therapy is 0.5–1 mg/kg/d (typically 40–60 mg) as a single or in two divided doses for 3–10 days. Severe exacerbations requiring hospitalization typically require 1 mg/kg of prednisone equivalent every 6–12 hours for 48 hours or until the FEV_1 (or PEFR) returns to 50% of predicted (or 50% of baseline). The dose is then decreased to 60–80 mg/d until the PEF reaches 70% of predicted or personal best. No clear advantage has been found for higher doses of corticosteroids in severe exacerbations.

5. Antimicrobials—Antibiotics have no role in routine asthma exacerbations. They may be useful if bacterial respiratory tract infections are thought to contribute. Thus, patients with fever and purulent sputum and evidence of pneumonia or bacterial sinusitis are reasonable candidates.

Approach to Treatment of Asthma Exacerbations

The principal goals in the treatment of asthma exacerbations are correction of hypoxemia, reversal of airflow obstruction, and reduction of the likelihood of recurrence of obstruction. Early intervention may lessen the severity and duration of an exacerbation. Of paramount importance is correction of hypoxemia through the use of supplemental oxygen. At the same time, rapid reversal of airflow obstruction should be attempted by repetitive or continuous administration of an inhaled short-acting β_2 agonist and the early administration of systemic corticosteroids to patients with moderate to severe asthma exacerbations or to patients who fail to respond promptly and completely to an inhaled short-acting β_2 agonist.

Serial measurements of lung function to quantify the severity of airflow obstruction and its response to treatment are especially useful. The improvement in FEV_1 after 30 minutes of treatment correlates significantly with a broad range of indices of the severity of asthma exacerbations. Serial measurement of airflow in the emergency department is an important factor in disposition and may reduce the rate of hospital admissions for asthma exacerbations.

The postexacerbation care plan is an important aspect of management. Regardless of the severity, all patients should be provided with necessary medications and education in how to use them, instruction in self-assessment, a follow-up appointment, and instruction in an action plan for managing recurrence.

Approach to Treatment of Mild Asthma Exacerbations

Mild asthma exacerbations are characterized by only minor changes in airway function (PEF > 80%) and minimal symptoms and signs of airway dysfunction (Table 9–3). The majority of exacerbations can be managed with home-based therapies. Most patients respond quickly and fully to an inhaled short-acting β_2 agonist alone. However, an inhaled short-acting β_2 agonist may need to be continued every 3–4 hours for 24–48 hours. For mild exacerbations in patients already taking an inhaled corticosteroid, authorities recommend doubling the dose until peak flow returns to predicted or personal best. In patients not already taking an inhaled corticosteroid, initiation of this agent should be considered. A course of oral corticosteroids may be necessary for mild exacerbations that persist despite an increase in the dose of inhaled corticosteroids.

Approach to Treatment of Moderate & Severe Asthma Exacerbations

Some patients with moderate asthma exacerbations can be managed at home with the telephone assistance of a clinician. However, most such patients require a more comprehensive evaluation and treatment program such as that outlined below for severe asthma exacerbations. A course of oral corticosteroids is usually necessary.

Owing to the life-threatening nature of severe exacerbations of asthma, treatment should be started immediately once the exacerbation is recognized. All patients with a severe exacerbation should immediately receive oxygen, high doses of an inhaled short-acting β_2 agonist, and systemic corticosteroids. A brief history pertinent to the exacerbation can be completed while treatment is given. More detailed assessments, including laboratory studies, usually add little in the early phase of evaluation and management and should be delayed until after initial therapy has been completed.

Asphyxia is a common cause of death, and oxygen therapy is therefore very important. Supplemental oxygen should be given to maintain an SaO_2 > 90% or a PaO_2 > 60 mm Hg. Oxygen-induced hypoventilation is very rare, and concern for hypercapnia should never delay correction of hypoxemia.

Frequent high-dose delivery of an inhaled short-acting β_2 agonist is indicated and is usually well tolerated in the setting of severe airway obstruction. Some studies suggest that continuous therapy is more efficacious than intermittent administration of these agents, but there is no clear consensus as long as similar doses are administered. At least three metered-dose inhaler or nebulizer treatments should be given in the first hour of therapy. Thereafter, the frequency of administration varies according to the improvement in airflow and associated symptoms and the occurrence of side effects.

Systemic corticosteroids are administered as detailed above. Mucolytic agents (eg, acetylcysteine, potassium iodide) may worsen cough or airflow ob-

struction. Anxiolytic and hypnotic drugs are contraindicated in critically ill asthma patients because of their respiratory depressant effects.

Repeat assessment of patients with severe exacerbations should be made after the initial dose of inhaled bronchodilator and after three doses of inhaled bronchodilators (60–90 minutes after initiating treatment). The response to initial treatment is a better predictor of the need for hospitalization than is the severity of an exacerbation on presentation. The decision to hospitalize a patient should be based on the duration and severity of symptoms, severity of airflow obstruction, course and severity of prior exacerbations, medication use at the time of the exacerbation, access to medical care and medications, adequacy of social support and home conditions, and presence of psychiatric illness. In general, discharge to home is appropriate if the PEF or FEV_1 has returned to $\geq$ 70% of predicted or personal best and symptoms are minimal or absent. Patients with a rapid response to treatment should be observed for 30 minutes after the most recent dose of bronchodilator to ensure stability of response before discharge to home.

A small minority of patients will not respond well to treatment and will show signs of impending respiratory failure due to a combination of worsening airflow obstruction and respiratory muscle fatigue (Table 9–3). Such patients can deteriorate rapidly and thus should be monitored in a critical care setting. Intubation of an acutely ill asthma patient is technically difficult and is best done semielectively, before the crisis of a respiratory arrest. At the time of intubation, close attention should be given to maintaining intravascular volume because hypotension commonly accompanies the administration of sedation and the initiation of positive-pressure ventilation in patients dehydrated due to poor recent oral intake and high insensible losses.

The main goals of mechanical ventilation are to ensure adequate oxygen and avoid barotrauma. Controlled hypoventilation with permissive hypercapnia is often required to limit airway pressures. Frequent high-dose delivery of inhaled short-acting β_2 agonists should be continued along with anti-inflammatory agents as discussed above. Many questions remain regarding the optimal delivery of inhaled β_2 agonists to intubated, mechanically ventilated patients. Further studies are needed to determine the comparative efficacy of metered-dose inhalers and nebulizers, optimal ventilator settings to use during drug delivery, ideal site along the ventilator circuit for introduction of the delivery system, and maximal acceptable drug doses. Unconventional therapies such as magnesium sulfate, helium-oxygen mixtures, and inhalational anesthetic agents are of unclear benefit but may be appropriate in selected patients.

Assessment, Monitoring, & Prevention

Periodic assessments and ongoing monitoring of asthma are essential to determine if the goals of therapy are being met. Clinical assessment and patient self-assessment are the primary methods for monitoring asthma. Patients should be given a written action plan based on signs and symptoms or expiratory flow rates. An action plan is especially important for patients with moderate to severe asthma or those with a history of severe exacerbations. Patients should be taught to recognize symptoms—especially patterns indicating inadequate asthma control or predicting the need for additional therapy. The written asthma action plan should direct the asthma patient to adjust medications in response to particular signs, symptoms, and peak flow measurements and should state when to seek medical help.

Spirometry is recommended at the time of initial assessment, once treatment is initiated and symptoms and peak flows have stabilized, and at least every 1–2 years thereafter. Regular follow-up visits (at least every 6 months, or more frequently based on patient status) are essential to help maintain asthma control and to reevaluate medication requirements. Patients with persistent asthma should receive the pneumococcal vaccine (Pneumovax) and annual influenza vaccinations.

Busse WW et al: Asthma. N Engl J Med 2001;344:350. [PMID: 11172168] (Review of latest findings in asthma pathophysiology.)

Drazen JM et al: Treatment of asthma with drugs modifying the leukotriene pathway. N Engl J Med 1999;340:197. [PMID: 9895400] (Evidence-based review of this new class of agents from leading researchers in the field.)

National Asthma Education and Prevention Program: Expert Panel Report 2: Guidelines for the diagnosis and management of asthma. National Institutes of Health, Pub No. 97-4051, Bethesda, MD, 1997. (Basic recommendations for the diagnosis and management of asthma based on exhaustive review of scientific literature and expert opinion.)

Naureckas ET et al. Clinical practice. Mild asthma. N Engl J Med 2001; 345:1257. [PMID: 11680447] (Clinical review of a common outpatient problem.)

Suissa S et al: Low-dose inhaled corticosteroids and the prevention of death from asthma. N Engl J Med 2000;343:332. [PMID: 10922423] (Canadian population-based cohort study from 1975 through 1991 suggests that regular use of low-dose inhaled corticosteroids is associated with a decreased risk of death from asthma.)

Woodruff PG et al: Asthma: prevalence, pathogenesis, and prospects for novel therapies. JAMA 2001;286:395. [PMID: 11466111] (Discussion of implications for therapy of recent insights into asthma pathophysiology.)

CHRONIC OBSTRUCTIVE PULMONARY DISEASE (COPD)

ESSENTIALS OF DIAGNOSIS

- *History of cigarette smoking.*
- *Chronic cough and sputum production (in chronic bronchitis) and dyspnea (in emphysema).*
- *Rhonchi, decreased intensity of breath sounds, and prolonged expiration on physical examination.*
- *Airflow limitation on pulmonary function testing.*

General Considerations

Chronic obstructive pulmonary disease (COPD) is a disease state characterized by the presence of airflow obstruction due to chronic bronchitis or emphysema; the airflow obstruction is generally progressive, may be accompanied by airway hyperreactivity, and may be partially reversible (American Thoracic Society). Although emphysema and chronic bronchitis must be diagnosed and treated as specific diseases, most patients with COPD have features of both conditions. The National Heart, Lung, and Blood Institute (NHLBI) estimates that 14 million Americans have been diagnosed with COPD; an equal number is thought to be afflicted but remains undiagnosed. Grouped together, COPD and asthma now represent the fourth leading cause of death in the United States, with over 100,000 deaths reported annually. The death rate from COPD is increasing rapidly, especially among elderly men.

Chronic bronchitis is characterized by excessive secretion of bronchial mucus and is manifested by productive cough for 3 months or more in at least 2 consecutive years in the absence of any other disease that might account for this symptom. **Emphysema** denotes abnormal, permanent enlargement of air spaces distal to the terminal bronchiole, with destruction of their walls and without obvious fibrosis. It is worthwhile to note that chronic bronchitis is defined in clinical terms, whereas emphysema is defined in pathologic terms. Cigarette smoking is clearly the most important cause of COPD. Nearly all smokers suffer an accelerated decline in lung function that is dose- and duration-dependent. Fifteen percent develop progressively disabling symptoms in their 40s and 50s. It is estimated that 80% of patients seen for COPD have significant exposure to tobacco smoke. Air pollution, airway infection, familial factors, and allergy have also been implicated in chronic bronchitis, and hereditary factors (deficiency of α_1-antiprotease) have been implicated in emphysema. The pathogenesis of emphysema may involve excessive lysis of elastin and other structural proteins in the lung matrix by elastase and other proteases derived from lung neutrophils, macrophages, and mononuclear cells. Atopy and the tendency for bronchoconstriction to develop in response to nonspecific airway stimuli may be important risks for COPD.

Clinical Findings

A. SYMPTOMS AND SIGNS

Patients with COPD characteristically present in the fifth or sixth decade of life complaining of excessive cough, sputum production, and shortness of breath. Symptoms have often been present for 10 years or more. Dyspnea is noted initially only on heavy exertion, but as the condition progresses it occurs with mild activity. In severe disease, dyspnea occurs at rest. Frequent exacerbations of illness are common and result in absence from work and eventual disability. Pneumonia, pulmonary hypertension, cor pulmonale, and chronic respiratory failure characterize the late stage of COPD. Death usually occurs during an exacerbation of illness in association with acute respiratory failure.

Clinical findings may be completely absent early in the course of COPD. As the disease progresses, two symptom patterns tend to emerge, historically referred to as "pink puffers" and "blue bloaters" (Table 9–7). These patterns have been thought to represent pure forms of emphysema and bronchitis, respectively, but this is a simplification of the anatomy and pathophysiology. Most COPD patients have pathologic evidence of both disorders, and their clinical course may reflect other factors such as central control of ventilation and concomitant sleep-disordered breathing.

B. LABORATORY FINDINGS

Examination of the sputum may reveal *Streptococcus pneumoniae, Haemophilus influenzae,* or *Moraxella catarrhalis.* Positive sputum cultures are poorly correlated with acute exacerbations, and research techniques demonstrate evidence of preceding viral infection in a majority of patients with exacerbations. The ECG may show sinus tachycardia, and in advanced disease, chronic pulmonary hypertension may produce electrocardiographic abnormalities typical of cor pulmonale. Supraventricular arrhythmias (multifocal atrial tachycardia, atrial flutter, and atrial fibrillation) and ventricular irritability also occur.

Arterial blood gas measurements characteristically show no abnormalities early in COPD other than an

Table 9–7. Patterns of disease in advanced COPD.

	Type A: Pink Puffer (Emphysema Predominant)	Type B: Blue Bloater (Bronchitis Predominant)
History and physical examination	Major complaint is dyspnea, often severe, usually presenting after age 50. Cough is rare, with scant clear, mucoid sputum. Patients are thin, with recent weight loss common. They appear uncomfortable, with evident use of accessory muscles of respiration. Chest is very quiet without adventitious sounds. No peripheral edema.	Major complaint is chronic cough, productive of mucopurulent sputum, with frequent exacerbations due to chest infections. Often presents in late 30s and 40s. Dyspnea usually mild, though patients may note limitations to exercise. Patients frequently overweight and cyanotic but seem comfortable at rest. Peripheral edema is common. Chest is noisy, with rhonchi invariably present; wheezes are common.
Laboratory studies	Hemoglobin usually normal (12–15 g/dL). Pa_{O_2} normal to slightly reduced (65–75 mm Hg) but Sa_{O_2} normal at rest. Pa_{CO_2} normal to slightly reduced (35–40 mm Hg). Chest radiograph shows hyperinflation with flattened diaphragms. Vascular markings are diminished, particularly at the apices.	Hemoglobin usually elevated (15–18 g/dL). Pa_{O_2} reduced (45–60 mm Hg) and Pa_{CO_2} slightly to markedly elevated (50–60 mm Hg). Chest radiograph shows increased interstitial markings ("dirty lungs"), especially at bases. Diaphragms are not flattened.
Pulmonary function tests	Airflow obstruction ubiquitous. Total lung capacity increased, sometimes markedly so. $D_{L}CO$ reduced. Static lung compliance increased.	Airflow obstruction ubiquitous. Total lung capacity generally normal but may be slightly increased. $D_{L}CO$ normal. Static lung compliance normal.
Special evaluations V/Q matching	Increased ventilation to high V/Q areas, ie, high dead space ventilation.	Increased perfusion to low V/Q areas.
Hemodynamics	Cardiac output normal to slightly low. Pulmonary artery pressures mildly elevated and increase with exercise.	Cardiac output normal. Pulmonary artery pressures elevated, sometimes markedly so, and worsen with exercise.
Nocturnal ventilation	Mild to moderate degree of oxygen desaturation not usually associated with obstructive sleep apnea.	Severe oxygen desaturation, frequently associated with obstructive sleep apnea.
Exercise ventilation	Increased minute ventilation for level of oxygen consumption. Pa_{O_2} tends to fall, Pa_{CO_2} rises slightly.	Decreased minute ventilation for level of oxygen consumption. Pa_{O_2} may rise; Pa_{CO_2} may rise signficantly.

increased A a DO_2. Indeed, they are unnecessary unless hypoxemia or hypercapnia is suspected. Hypoxemia occurs in advanced disease, particularly when chronic bronchitis predominates. Compensated respiratory acidosis occurs in patients with chronic respiratory failure, particularly in chronic bronchitis, with worsening of acidemia during acute exacerbations.

Spirometry provides objective information about pulmonary function and assesses the results of therapy. Pulmonary function tests early in the course of COPD reveal only evidence of abnormal closing volume and reduced midexpiratory flow rate. Reductions in FEV_1 and in the ratio of forced expiratory volume to (FEV_1/FVC) occur later. In severe disease, the forced vital capacity is markedly reduced. Lung volume measurements reveal an increase in the total lung capacity (TLC), a marked increase in the residual volume (RV), and an elevation of the RV/TLC ratio, indicative of air trapping, particularly in emphysema.

C. Imaging

When emphysema is the main clinical feature, hyperinflation is apparent. Parenchymal bullae or subpleural blebs are pathognomonic of emphysema. Radiographs of patients with chronic bronchitis may show only nonspecific peribronchial and perivascular markings. Pulmonary hypertension becomes evident as enlargement of central pulmonary arteries in advanced disease. Doppler echocardiography is an effective way to estimate pulmonary artery pressure if pulmonary hypertension is suspected.

Differential Diagnosis

Clinical, roentgenographic, and laboratory findings should enable the clinician to distinguish COPD from other obstructive pulmonary disorders such as bronchial asthma, bronchiectasis, cystic fibrosis, bronchopulmonary mycosis, and central airflow obstruction. Bronchiectasis is distinguished from COPD by features such as recurrent pneumonia and hemoptysis, digital clubbing, and radiographic abnormalities. Patients with severe α_1-antiprotease deficiency are recognized by the appearance of panacinar bibasilar emphysema early in life, usually in the third or fourth decade, and hepatic cirrhosis and hepatocellular carcinoma may occur. Cystic fibrosis occurs in children and younger adults. Rarely, mechanical obstruction of the central airways simulates COPD. Flow-volume loops may help separate patients with central airway obstruction from those with diffuse intrathoracic airway obstruction characteristic of COPD.

Complications

Acute bronchitis, pneumonia, pulmonary thromboembolism, and concomitant left ventricular failure may worsen otherwise stable COPD. Pulmonary hypertension, cor pulmonale, and chronic respiratory failure are common in advanced COPD. Spontaneous pneumothorax occurs in a small fraction of patients with emphysema. Hemoptysis may result from chronic bronchitis or may signal bronchogenic carcinoma.

Prevention

COPD is largely preventable through elimination of chronic exposure to tobacco smoke. Smokers with early evidence of airflow limitation can alter their disease by smoking cessation. Smoking cessation slows the decline in FEV_1 in middle-aged smokers with mild airways obstruction. Vaccination against influenza and pneumococcal infection may also be of benefit.

Treatment

Standards for the management of patients with COPD have been published by the American Thoracic Society. See Chapter 38 for a discussion of air travel in patients with lung disease.

A. Ambulatory Patients

1. Smoking cessation—The single most important intervention in smokers with COPD is to encourage smoking cessation. Simply telling a patient to quit succeeds 5% of the time. The Lung Health Study reported 22% sustained abstinence at 5 years in their intervention group (behavior modification plus nicotine gum). Nicotine transdermal patch, nicotine gum, and bupropion increase cessation rates in motivated smokers (see Chapter 1).

2. Oxygen therapy—The only drug therapy that is documented to alter the natural history of COPD is supplemental oxygen in those patients with resting hypoxemia. Requirements for Medicare coverage for a patient's home use of oxygen and oxygen equipment are listed in Table 9–8. Arterial blood gas analysis is preferable to ear or pulse oximetry to guide initial oxygen therapy. Hypoxemic patients with pulmonary hypertension, chronic cor pulmonale, erythrocytosis, impaired cognitive function, exercise intolerance, nocturnal restlessness, or morning headache are particularly likely to benefit from home oxygen therapy. Proved benefits of home oxygen therapy in advanced COPD include longer survival, reduced hospitalization needs, and better quality of life. Oxygen by nasal prongs must be given at least 15 hours a day unless therapy is intended only for exercise or sleep. In patients treated with continuous oxygen, the survival after 36 months is about 65%—significantly better than the survival rate of about 45% in those who are treated with only nocturnal oxygen. Survival in hypoxemic patients with COPD treated with supplemental oxygen therapy is directly proportionate to the number of hours per day oxygen is administered.

Home oxygen may be supplied by liquid oxygen systems (LOX), compressed gas cylinders, or oxygen concentrators. Most patients benefit from having both stationary and portable systems. For most patients, a flow rate of 1–3 L/min achieves a PaO_2 greater than 55

Table 9–8. Home oxygen therapy: requirements for Medicare coverage.[1]

Group I (any of the following):

1. $Pao_2 \leq 55$ mm Hg or $Sao_2 \leq 88\%$ taken at rest breathing room air, while awake.
2. During sleep (prescription for nocturnal oxygen use only):
   a. $Pao_2 \leq 55$ mm Hg or $Sao_2 \leq 88\%$ for a patient whose awake, resting, room air Pao_2 is ≥ 56 mm Hg or $Sao_2 \geq 89\%$,

   or

   b. Decrease in $Pao_2 > 10$ mm Hg or decrease in $Sao_2 > 5\%$ associated with symptoms or signs reasonably attributed to hypoxemia (eg, impaired cognitive processes, nocturnal restlessness, insomnia).
3. During exercise (prescription for oxygen use only during exercise):
   a. $Pao_2 \leq 55$ mg Hg or $Sao_2 \leq 88\%$ taken during exercise for a patient whose awake, resting, room air Pao_2 is ≥ 56 mm Hg or $Sao_2 \geq 89\%$.

   and

   b. There is evidence that the use of supplemental oxygen during exercise improves the hypoxemia that was demonstrated during exercise while breathing room air.

Group II:[2]

$Pa\,O_2 = 56–59$ mm Hg or $Sao_2 = 89\%$ if there is evidence of any of the following:

1. Dependent edema suggesting congestive heart failure.
2. P pulmonale on ECG (P wave > 3 mm in standard leads II, III, or aVF).
3. Hematocrit > 56%.

---

[1]Health Care Financing Administration, 1989.
[2]Patients in this group must have a second oxygen test 3 months after the initial oxygen set-up.

---

mm Hg. The monthly cost of home oxygen therapy ranges from $300.00 to $500.00 or more, being higher for liquid oxygen systems. Medicare covers approximately 80% of home oxygen expenses. **Transtracheal oxygen** is an alternative method of delivery and may be useful for patients who require higher flows of oxygen than can be delivered via the nose or who are experiencing troublesome side effects such as nasal drying or epistaxis from nasal delivery of oxygen. Reservoir nasal cannulas or "pendants" and demand (pulse) oxygen delivery systems are also available to conserve oxygen.

3. Bronchodilators—Bronchodilators are the most important agents in the pharmacologic management of patients with COPD. Bronchodilators do not alter the inexorable decline in lung function that is the hallmark of the disease, but they offer improvement in symptoms, exercise tolerance, and overall health status. Aggressiveness of bronchodilator therapy should be matched to the severity of the patient's disease. In patients who experience no symptomatic improvement, bronchodilators should be discontinued.

The two most commonly prescribed bronchodilators are the anticholinergic ipratropium bromide and

the short-acting β_2 agonists (eg, albuterol, metaproterenol), delivered by metered-dose inhaler or as an inhalation solution by nebulizer. Ipratropium bromide is generally preferred to the short-acting β_2 agonists as a first line agent because of its longer duration of action and absence of sympathomimetic side effects. Some studies have suggested that ipratropium achieves superior bronchodilation in COPD patients. Typical doses are two to four puffs (36–72 μg) every 6 hours. There is a dose response above this level without additional side effects. Short-acting β_2 agonists are less expensive and have a more rapid onset of action, commonly leading to greater patient satisfaction. At maximal doses, β_2 agonists have bronchodilator action equivalent to that of ipratropium but may cause tachycardia, tremor, or hypokalemia. There does not appear to be any advantage of scheduled use of short-acting β_2 agonists compared with as-needed administration. Use of both short-acting β_2 agonists and anticholinergics at submaximal doses leads to improved bronchodilation compared with either agent alone but does not improve dyspnea.

Long-acting β_2 agonists (eg, formoterol, salmeterol) and anticholinergics (tiotropium) appear to achieve bronchodilation that is equivalent or superior to what is experienced with ipratropium in addition to similar improvements on health status. Their role in management of stable COPD is an area of active research.

Oral **theophylline** is a third-line agent in COPD patients who fail to achieve adequate symptom control with anticholinergics and β_2 agonists. Sustained-release theophylline improves hemoglobin saturation during sleep in COPD patients and is a first-line agent for those with sleep-related breathing disorders. Theophylline has fallen out of favor because of its narrow therapeutic window and the availability of potent inhaled bronchodilators. Nonetheless, theophylline does improve dyspnea, exercise performance, and pulmonary function in many stable COPD patients. Its benefits may result from anti-inflammatory properties and extrapulmonary effects on myocardial contractility and renal function.

4. Corticosteroids—Apart from acute exacerbations, COPD is not generally a steroid-responsive disease. Only 10% of stable outpatients with COPD given oral corticosteroids have a greater than 20% increase in FEV_1 compared with patients receiving placebo. Since there are no clear predictors of which patients will respond, empirical trials of oral and inhaled corticosteroids are common. Such trials should be guided by the following principles. The baseline FEV_1 should be (1) stable—not measured during an exacerbation—and (2) documented on maximal bronchodilator therapy, and (3) the postbronchodilator FEV_1 value is considered the appropriate baseline. Corticosteroid therapy equivalent to 0.5 mg/kg/d of prednisone is given for 14–21 days. The drug should be discontinued unless there is a 20% or greater increase in FEV_1. Patients who feel better without spirometric evidence of improvement or a clear change in functional status are nonresponders. Responders are usually switched to inhaled corticosteroids, but there are few data to guide this practice. COPD patients should not be treated with inhaled corticosteroids for the sole reason that these agents lack the toxicity of oral preparations.

Several large clinical trials have reported no evidence of a change in decline in lung function in patients treated with inhaled corticosteroids. Some clinical trials have reported a small reduction in the frequency of COPD exacerbations and an increase in self reported functional status in treated patients. Typically, these effects are small and occur with long-term, high-dose inhaled therapy.

5. Antibiotics—Antibiotics are commonly prescribed to outpatients with COPD for the following indications: (1) to treat an acute exacerbation, (2) to treat acute bronchitis, and (3) to prevent acute exacerbations of chronic bronchitis (prophylactic antibiotics). There is evidence from clinical studies that antibiotics improve outcomes slightly in the first two situations. There is no convincing evidence to support the use of prophylactic antibiotics in patients with COPD. Patients with a flare of COPD associated with dyspnea and a change in the quantity or character of sputum benefit the most from antibiotic therapy. Common agents include trimethoprim-sulfamethoxazole (160/800 mg every 12 hours), amoxicillin or amoxicillin-clavulanate (500 mg every 8 hours), or doxycycline (100 mg every 12 hours) given for 7–10 days. There are few controlled trials of antibiotics in severe COPD exacerbations; prompt administration of parenteral antibiotics seems reasonable as long as the decision is reevaluated frequently.

6. Other measures—In patients with chronic bronchitis, increased mobilization of secretions may be accomplished through the use of adequate systemic hydration, effective cough training methods, or use of a hand-held flutter device and postural drainage, sometimes with chest percussion or vibration. Postural drainage and chest percussion should be used only in selected patients with excessive amounts of retained secretions that cannot be cleared by coughing and other methods; these measures are of no benefit in pure emphysema. Expectorant-mucolytic therapy has generally been regarded as unhelpful in patients with chronic bronchitis. Cough suppressants and sedatives should be avoided as routine measures.

Human α_1-antitrypsin is available for replacement therapy in emphysema due to congenital deficiency of α_1-antitrypsin. Patients over 18 years of age with airflow obstruction by spirometry and levels less than 11 μmol/L are potential candidates for replacement therapy. α_1-Antitrypsin is administered intravenously in a dose of 60 mg/kg body weight once weekly.

Graded aerobic physical exercise programs (eg, walking 20 minutes three times weekly, or bicycling) are helpful to prevent deterioration of physical condition and to improve the patient's ability to carry out daily activities. Training of inspiratory muscles by inspiring against progressively larger resistive loads improves exercise tolerance in some but not all patients. Pursed-lip breathing to slow the rate of breathing and abdominal breathing exercises to relieve fatigue of accessory muscles of respiration may reduce dyspnea in some patients.

Severe dyspnea in spite of optimal medical management may warrant a clinical trial of an opioid. Sedative-hypnotic drugs (eg, diazepam, 5 mg three times daily) are controversial in intractable dyspnea but may benefit very anxious patients. Intermittent negative-pressure (cuirass) ventilation and transnasal positive-pressure ventilation at home to rest the respiratory muscles are promising approaches to improve respiratory muscle function and reduce dyspnea in patients with severe COPD. A bilevel transnasal ventilation system has been reported to reduce dyspnea in ambulatory patients with severe COPD, but the long-term benefits of this approach and compliance with it have not been defined.

B. Hospitalized Patients

Hospitalization is indicated for acute worsening of COPD that fails to respond to measures for ambulatory patients. Patients with acute respiratory failure or complications such as cor pulmonale and pneumothorax should also be hospitalized.

Management of the hospitalized patient with an acute exacerbation of COPD includes supplemental oxygen, inhaled ipratropium bromide and inhaled β_2 agonists, and broad-spectrum antibiotics, corticosteroids, and, in selected cases, chest physiotherapy. Theophylline should not be initiated in the acute setting, but patients taking theophylline prior to acute hospitalization should have their theophylline serum levels measured and maintained in the therapeutic range. Oxygen therapy should not be withheld for fear of worsening respiratory acidemia; hypoxemia is more detrimental than hypercapnia. Cor pulmonale usually responds to measures that reduce pulmonary artery pressure, such as supplemental oxygen and correction of acidemia; bed rest, salt restriction, and diuretics may add some benefit. Cardiac arrhythmias, particularly multifocal atrial tachycardia, usually respond to aggressive treatment of COPD itself. Atrial flutter may require DC cardioversion after initiation of the above therapy. If progressive respiratory failure ensues, tracheal intubation and mechanical ventilation are necessary. In clinical trials of COPD patients with hypercapnic acute respiratory failure, noninvasive positive-pressure ventilation (NPPV) delivered via face mask reduced the need for intubation and shortened ICU lengths of stay. Other studies have suggested a lower risk of nosocomial infections and less use of antibiotics in COPD patients treated with NPPV. These benefits do not appear to extend to hypoxemic respiratory failure or to patients with acute lung injury or ARDS.

C. Surgery for COPD

1. Lung transplantation—Experience with both single and bilateral sequential lung transplantation for severe COPD is accumulating rapidly. Requirements for lung transplantation are severe lung disease, limited activities of daily living, exhaustion of medical therapy, ambulatory status, potential for pulmonary rehabilitation, limited life expectancy without transplantation, adequate function of other organ systems, and a good social support system. Average total charges for lung transplantation through the end of the first postoperative year exceed $250,000. The two-year survival rate after lung transplantation for COPD is 75%. Complications include rejection, opportunistic infection, and obliterative bronchiolitis. Substantial improvements in pulmonary function and exercise performance have been noted after transplantation.

2. Lung volume reduction surgery (reduction pneumoplasty)—This is an experimental surgical approach to relief of dyspnea and improvement in exercise tolerance in patients with advanced diffuse emphysema and lung hyperinflation. Bilateral resection of 20–30% of lung volume in selected patients results in modest improvements in pulmonary function, exercise performance, and dyspnea. The duration of any improvement as well as any mortality benefit remains uncertain. Prolonged air leaks occur in up to one-half of patients postoperatively. Mortality rates in centers with the largest experience with lung volume reduction surgery range from 4% to 10%.

The National Emphysema Treatment Trial (NETT) is an ongoing randomized, multicenter clinical trial comparing lung volume reduction surgery with medical treatment. In October 2001, the safety monitoring board closed enrollment in the trial to patients with an $FEV_1 < 20\%$ predicted *and* either a homogeneous distribution of emphysema or a $D_{L}CO < 20\%$ of predicted due to excess mortality in the patients randomized to surgery. Additional results await completion of the trial.

3. Bullectomy—Bullectomy is an older surgical procedure for palliation of severe dyspnea in patients with severe bullous emphysema. In this procedure, the surgeon removes a very large emphysematous bulla that demonstrates no ventilation or perfusion on lung scanning and compresses adjacent lung that has preserved function. Bullectomy can now be performed with a CO_2 laser via thoracoscopy.

Prognosis

The outlook for patients with clinically significant COPD is poor. The median survival time of patients with severe COPD ($FEV_1 \leq 1$ L) is about 4 years. The degree of pulmonary dysfunction (as measured by FEV_1) at the time the patient is first seen is probably the most important predictor of survival. Comprehensive care programs, cessation of smoking, and supplemental oxygen may reduce the rate of decline of pulmonary function, but therapy with bronchodilators and other approaches probably has little, if any, impact on the natural course of COPD.

Dyspnea at the end of life can be extremely uncomfortable and distressing to the patient and family.

Dyspnea can be effectively managed with a combination of medications and mechanical interventions (see Dyspnea, Treatment, above). As patients near the end of life, meticulous attention to palliative care is essential. (See Chapter 5.)

Bach PB et al: Management of acute exacerbations of chronic obstructive pulmonary disease: a summary and appraisal of published evidence. Ann Intern Med 2001;134:600. [PMID: 11296189] (A critical review of the available data on diagnostic evaluation, risk stratification, and therapeutic management of patients with acute exacerbations of COPD.)

Barnes PJ: Chronic obstructive pulmonary disease. N Engl J Med 2000;343:269. [PMID: 10911010] (Current review by a leading researcher in the field.)

Crockett AJ et al: Domiciliary oxygen for chronic obstructive pulmonary disease. Cochrane Database of Systematic Reviews 2000;(2):CD001744. [PMID: 10796666] (Meta-analysis of clinical trials of oxygen therapy in COPD. One of several such analyses of issues in COPD within the Cochrane Database.)

Effect of inhaled triamcinolone on the decline in pulmonary function in chronic obstructive pulmonary disease. The Lung Health Study Research Group. N Engl J Med 2000; 343:1902. [PMID: 11136260] (Inhaled corticosteroids offered a small symptomatic benefit but did not alter long-term decline in lung function among smokers with COPD. Bone density in the steroid treatment group was reduced at the lumbar spine and the femur.)

Niewoehner DE: Effect of systemic glucocorticoids on exacerbations of chronic obstructive pulmonary disease. N Engl J Med 2000;340:1941. [PMID: 10379017] (Steroid naïve patients hospitalized with acute exacerbations of COPD were discharged an average 1.2 days sooner when given systemic corticosteroids.)

Patients at high risk of death after lung-volume-reduction surgery. N Engl J Med 2001;345:1075. [PMID: 11596586] (Unacceptably high mortality seen in enrollees with low $D_{L}CO$ or homogeneous distribution of emphysema randomized to surgery.)

Seemungal T et al: Respiratory viruses, symptoms, and inflammatory markers in acute exacerbations and stable chronic obstructive pulmonary disease. Am J Respir Crit Care Med 2001;164:1618. [PMID: 11719299] (Careful observational study documenting viral infections prior to 64% of COPD exacerbations in stable outpatients.)

BRONCHIECTASIS

Bronchiectasis is a congenital or acquired disorder of the large bronchi characterized by permanent, abnormal dilation and destruction of bronchial walls. It may be caused by recurrent inflammation or infection of the airways and may be localized or diffuse. Cystic fibrosis causes about half of all cases of bronchiectasis. Other causes include lung infection (tuberculosis, fungal infections, lung abscess, pneumonia), abnormal lung defense mechanisms (humoral immunodeficiency, α_1-antiprotease deficiency with cigarette smoking, mucociliary clearance disorders, rheumatic diseases), and localized airway obstruction (foreign body, tumor, mucoid impaction). Immunodeficiency states that may lead to bronchiectasis include congenital or acquired panhypogammaglobulinemia; common variable immunodeficiency; selective IgA, IgM, and IgG subclass deficiencies; and acquired immunodeficiency from cytotoxic therapy, AIDS, lymphoma, multiple myeloma, leukemia, and chronic renal and hepatic diseases. However, most patients with bronchiectasis have panhypergammaglobulinemia, presumably reflecting an immune system response to chronic airway infection. Acquired primary bronchiectasis is now uncommon in the USA because of improved control of bronchopulmonary infections.

Symptoms of bronchiectasis include chronic cough, production of copious amounts of purulent sputum, hemoptysis, and recurrent pneumonia. Weight loss, anemia, and other systemic manifestations are common. Physical findings are nonspecific, but persistent crackles at the lung bases are common. Clubbing is infrequent in mild cases but is common in severe disease. Copious, foul-smelling, purulent sputum is characteristic. Obstructive pulmonary dysfunction with hypoxemia is seen in moderate or severe disease. Radiographic abnormalities include crowded bronchial markings related to peribronchial fibrosis and small cystic spaces at the base of the lungs. High-resolution CT is the diagnostic study of choice.

Treatment of acute exacerbations consists of antibiotics (selected on the basis of sputum smears and cultures), daily chest physiotherapy with postural drainage and chest percussion, and inhaled bronchodilators. Hand-held flutter valve devices may be as effective as chest physiotherapy in clearing secretions. Empirical oral antibiotic therapy for 10–14 days with amoxicillin or amoxicillin-clavulanate (500 mg every 8 hours), ampicillin or tetracycline (250–500 mg four times daily), or trimethoprim-sulfamethoxazole (160/800 mg every 12 hours) is reasonable therapy in an acute exacerbation if a specific bacterial pathogen cannot be isolated. Preventive or suppressive treatment is sometimes given to stable outpatients with bronchiectasis who have copious purulent sputum. Clinical trial data to guide this practice are scant. Common regimens include high-dose (3 g/d) amoxicillin or alternating cycles of the antibiotics listed above given orally for 2–4 weeks. Inhaled aerosolized aminoglycosides clearly reduce colonization by pseudomonas species. In patients with underlying cystic fibrosis, inhaled antibiotics improve FEV_1 and reduce hospitalizations, but these benefits are not consistently seen in the non-cystic fibrosis population. Complications of bronchiectasis include hemoptysis, cor pulmonale, amyloidosis, and secondary visceral abscesses at distant sites (eg, brain). Bronchoscopy is sometimes necessary to evaluate hemoptysis, remove retained secretions, and rule out obstructing airway lesions. Surgical resection is reserved for the few patients with localized bronchiectasis and adequate pulmonary function who fail to respond to conservative management. Surgery is also indicated for massive hemoptysis.

Barker AF et al: Tobramycin solution for inhalation reduces sputum *Pseudomonas aeruginosa* density in bronchiectasis. Am J Respir Crit Care Med 2000;162:481. [PMID: 10934074] (Placebo-controlled, double-blind, randomized trial of inhaled tobramycin in patients with bronchiectasis and *P aeruginosa* infection showed impressive reduction of colonization but no improvement in FEV_1.)

Hansell DM: Bronchiectasis. Radiol Clin North Am 1998;36:107. [PMID: 9465870] (Thorough review of clinical and radiographic features of bronchiectasis with special emphasis on CT scanning.)

Mysliwiec V et al: Bronchiectasis: the "other" obstructive lung disease. Postgrad Med 1999;106:123. [PMID: 10418580] (Clinical review by a general practitioner.)

ALLERGIC BRONCHOPULMONARY MYCOSIS

Allergic bronchopulmonary mycosis is a pulmonary hypersensitivity disorder caused by allergy to fungal antigens that colonize the tracheobronchial tree. It usually occurs in atopic asthmatic individuals who are 20–40 years of age, in response to antigens of aspergillus species. For this reason, the disorder is commonly referred to as allergic bronchopulmonary aspergillosis. Primary criteria for the diagnosis include (1) a clinical history of asthma, (2) peripheral eosinophilia, (3) immediate skin reactivity to aspergillus antigen, (4) precipitating antibodies to aspergillus antigen, (5) elevated serum IgE levels, (6) pulmonary infiltrates (transient or fixed), and (7) central bronchiectasis. If the first six of these seven primary criteria are present, the diagnosis is almost certain. Secondary diagnostic criteria include identification of aspergillus in sputum, a history of brown-flecked sputum, and late skin reactivity to aspergillus antigen. High-dose prednisone (0.5–1 mg/kg orally per day) for at least 2 months is the treatment of choice, and the response in early disease is usually excellent. Depending on the overall clinical situation, prednisone can then be cautiously tapered. Relapses are frequent, and protracted or repeated treatment with corticosteroids is not uncommon. Patients with corticosteroid-dependent disease may benefit from itraconazole (200 mg orally once or twice daily) without added toxicity. Bronchodilators (Table 9–6) are also helpful. Complications include hemoptysis, severe bronchiectasis, and pulmonary fibrosis.

Stevens DA et al: A randomized trial of itraconazole in allergic bronchopulmonary aspergillosis. N Engl J Med 2000; 342:756. [PMID: 10717010] (Itraconazole may benefit patients with corticosteroid-dependent allergic bronchopulmonary aspergillosis.)

Vlahakis NE et al: Diagnosis and treatment of allergic bronchopulmonary aspergillosis. Mayo Clinic Proc 2001; 76:930. [PMID: 11560305]. (Comprehensive review.)

CYSTIC FIBROSIS

ESSENTIALS OF DIAGNOSIS

- *Chronic or recurrent cough, sputum production, dyspnea, and wheezing.*
- *Recurrent infections or chronic colonization of the airways with nontypeable* Haemophilus influenzae, *mucoid and nonmucoid* Pseudomonas aeruginosa, Staphylococcus aureus, *or* Burkholderia cepacia.
- *Pancreatic insufficiency, recurrent pancreatitis, distal intestinal obstruction syndrome, chronic hepatic disease, nutritional deficiencies, or male urogenital abnormalities.*
- *Bronchiectasis and scarring on chest radiographs.*
- *Airflow obstruction on spirometry.*
- *Sweat chloride concentration above 60 meq/L on two occasions or mutations in genes known to cause cystic fibrosis.*

General Considerations

Cystic fibrosis is the most common cause of severe chronic lung disease in young adults and the most common fatal hereditary disorder of Caucasians in the USA. It is an autosomal recessive disorder affecting about one in 3200 Caucasians; one in 25 is a carrier. Cystic fibrosis is caused by abnormalities in a membrane chloride channel (the cystic fibrosis transmembrane conductance regulator [CFTR] protein) that results in altered chloride transport and water flux across the apical surface of epithelial cells. Almost all exocrine glands produce an abnormal mucus that obstructs glands and ducts. Obstruction results in glandular dilation and damage to tissue. In the respiratory tract, inadequate hydration of the tracheobronchial epithelium impairs mucociliary function. High concentrations of DNA in airway secretions (due to chronic airways inflammation and autolysis of neutrophils) increase sputum viscosity. Over 800 mutations in the gene that encodes CFTR have been described, and at least 230 mutations are known to be associated with clinical abnormalities. The mutation referred to as ΔF508 accounts for about 60% of cases of cystic fibrosis.

About one-third of the nearly 30,000 cystic fibrosis patients in the USA are adults. Because of the wide range of alterations seen in the CFTR protein structure and function, adults with cystic fibrosis may present with a variety of pulmonary and nonpulmonary manifestations. Pulmonary manifestations in adults include acute and chronic bronchitis, bronchiectasis, pneumonia, atelectasis, and peribronchial and parenchymal scarring. Pneumothorax and hemoptysis are common. Hypoxemia, hypercapnia, and cor pulmonale occur in advanced cases. Biliary cirrhosis and gallstones may occur. Nearly all men with cystic fibrosis have congenital bilateral absence of the vas deferens with azoospermia. Patients with cystic fibrosis have an increased risk of malignancies of the gastrointestinal tract, osteopenia, and arthropathies.

Clinical Findings

A. SYMPTOMS AND SIGNS

Cystic fibrosis should be suspected in a young adult presenting with a history of chronic lung disease (especially bronchiectasis), pancreatitis, or infertility. Cough, sputum production, decreased exercise tolerance, and recurrent hemoptysis are typical complaints. Patients also often complain of facial (sinus) pain or pressure and purulent nasal discharge. Steatorrhea, diarrhea, and abdominal pain are also common. Digital clubbing, increased anteroposterior chest diameter, hyperresonance to percussion, and apical crackles are noted on physical examination. Sinus tenderness, purulent nasal secretions, and nasal polyps may also be seen.

B. LABORATORY FINDINGS

Arterial blood gas studies often reveal hypoxemia and, in advanced disease, a chronic, compensated respiratory acidosis. Pulmonary function studies show a mixed obstructive and restrictive pattern. There is a reduction in forced vital capacity, airflow rates, and total lung capacity. Air trapping (high ratio of residual volume to total lung capacity) and reduction in pulmonary diffusing capacity are common.

C. IMAGING

Hyperinflation is seen early in the disease process. Peribronchial cuffing, mucus plugging, bronchiectasis (ring shadows and cysts), increased interstitial markings, small rounded peripheral opacities, and focal atelectasis may be seen separately or in various combinations. Pneumothorax can also be seen. Thin-section CT scanning may confirm the presence of bronchiectasis.

D. DIAGNOSIS

The quantitative pilocarpine iontophoresis sweat test reveals elevated sodium and chloride levels (> 60 meq/L) in the sweat of patients with cystic fibrosis. Two tests on different days are required for accurate diagnosis. Facilities must perform enough tests to maintain laboratory proficiency and quality. A normal sweat chloride test does not exclude the diagnosis. Genotyping or other alternative diagnostic studies (such as measurement of nasal membrane potential difference, semen analysis, or assessment of pancreatic function) should be pursued if the test is repeatedly negative but there is a high clinical suspicion of cystic fibrosis. Standard genotyping is a limited diagnostic tool because it screens for only a fraction of the known cystic fibrosis mutations.

Treatment

Early recognition and comprehensive multidisciplinary therapy improve symptom control and the chances of survival and amelioration of symptoms. Referral to a regional cystic fibrosis center is strongly recommended. Conventional treatment programs focus on the following areas: clearance and reduction of lower airway secretions, reversal of bronchoconstriction, treatment of respiratory tract infections and airway bacterial burden, pancreatic enzyme replacement, and nutritional and psychosocial support (including genetic and occupational counseling).

Clearance of lower airway secretions can be promoted by postural drainage, chest percussion or vibration techniques, positive expiratory pressure (PEP) or flutter valve breathing devices, directed cough, and other breathing techniques; these approaches require detailed patient instruction by experienced personnel. Sputum viscosity in cystic fibrosis is increased by the large quantities of extracellular DNA that result from chronic airways inflammation and autolysis of neutrophils. Inhaled recombinant human deoxyribonuclease (rhDNase) cleaves extracellular DNA in sputum. When administered chronically at a daily nebulized dose of 2.5 mg, this therapy leads to improved FEV_1 and reduces the risk of cystic fibrosis-related respiratory exacerbations and the need for intravenous antibiotics. Pharyngitis, laryngitis, and voice alterations are common adverse effects. Annual cost exceeds $12,000. Antibiotics are used to treat active airway infections based on results of culture and susceptibility testing of sputum. *S aureus* (including methicillin-resistant strains) and a mucoid variant of *P aeruginosa* are commonly present. *Haemophilus influenzae, Stenotrophomonas maltophilia,* and *Burkholderia cepacia*—the latter a highly drug-resistant organism—are occasionally isolated. The use of aerosolized antibiotics (inhalational tobramycin solution and others) for prophylaxis or treatment of lower respiratory tract infections is sometimes helpful. Although some studies of inhaled antibiotics demonstrate reduced exacerbations and increased FEV_1 in patients chronically infected with *P aeruginosa,* there is concern about the emergence of drug-resistant organisms, equipment contamination with *B cepacia,* and side effects such as bronchospasm.

Inhaled bronchodilators (eg, albuterol, two puffs every 4 hours as needed) should be considered in patients who demonstrate an increase of at least 12% in FEV_1 after an inhaled bronchodilator. Vaccination against pneumococcal infection and annual influenza vaccination are advised. Screening of family members and genetic counseling are suggested.

Lung transplantation is currently the only definitive treatment for advanced cystic fibrosis. Double-lung or heart-lung transplantation is required. A few transplant centers offer living lobar lung transplantation to selected patients. The 3-year survival rate following transplantation for cystic fibrosis is about 55%.

Investigational therapies for cystic fibrosis include anti-inflammatory agents (eg, ibuprofen, pentoxifylline, antiproteases), protein modification agents (eg, milrinone, phenylbutyrate), ion transport agents (eg, amiloride), and gene therapy.

Prognosis

The longevity of patients with cystic fibrosis is increasing, and the median survival age is now 31 years. Death occurs from pulmonary complications (eg, pneumonia, pneumothorax, or hemoptysis) or as a result of terminal chronic respiratory failure and cor pulmonale.

Liou TG et al: Survival effect of lung transplantation among patients with cystic fibrosis. JAMA 2001;286:2683. [PMID: 11730443] (In the majority of patients with cystic fibrosis, lung transplantation has an equivocal or negative impact on survival.)

Rosenstein BJ et al: The diagnosis of cystic fibrosis: a consensus statement. J Pediatr 1998;132:589. [PMID: 9580754] (Cystic Fibrosis Foundation Consensus Panel guidelines for use of CF diagnostic tests.)

Rubin BK: Emerging therapies for cystic fibrosis lung disease. Chest 1999;115: 1120. [PMID: 10208218] (Comprehensive review article.)

Ryan G et al: Nebulised anti-pseudomonal antibiotics for cystic fibrosis. Cochrane Database of Systematic Reviews. 2000(2):CD001021. [PMID: 10796732] (Meta-analysis of clinical trials of inhaled antibiotics. One of several analyses within the Cochrane Database of key issues in management of cystic fibrosis.)

BRONCHIOLITIS

Bronchiolitis is nonspecific inflammation of terminal and respiratory bronchioles. In children, bronchiolitis is a common and often severe acute respiratory illness, usually caused by respiratory syncytial virus. Acute infectious bronchiolitis is rare in adults. In adults, bronchiolitis is a chronic, frequently progressive nonspecific response to injury of the distal small airways.

Bronchiolitis has two pathologic variants, either of which may be associated with obliteration of bronchioles (bronchiolitis obliterans). **Constrictive bronchiolitis** is characterized by chronic inflammation, concentric scarring, and smooth muscle hypertrophy causing luminal obstruction. These patients have airflow obstruction on spirometry, minimal radiographic abnormalities, and a progressive clinical course unresponsive to corticosteroids. **Proliferative bronchiolitis** occurs when intraluminal polyps consisting of fibroblasts, foamy macrophages, and lymphocytes partially or completely obstruct the bronchioles. When this exudate extends to the alveolar space, the pattern is referred to as bronchiolitis obliterans with organizing pneumonia; (BOOP). Patients with proliferative bronchiolitis may have obstruction or restriction on pulmonary function testing. Radiographic infiltrates are common. The disease is frequently responsive to corticosteroids.

The most common clinical patterns are described below.

Toxic fume bronchiolitis obliterans follows 1–3 weeks after exposure to oxides of nitrogen, phosgene, and other noxious gases. The chest radiograph shows diffuse nonspecific alveolar or "ground-glass" densities.

Postinfectious bronchiolitis obliterans is a late response to mycoplasmal or viral lung infection in adults and has a highly variable radiographic appearance.

Bronchiolitis obliterans may also occur in association with rheuatoid arthritis, polymyositis, and dermatomyositis. Penicillamine therapy has been implicated as a possible cause of bronchiolitis obliterans in patients with rheumatoid arthritis. Bronchiolitis obliterans occurs in up to 70% of patients following lung transplantation and 10% of patients undergoing allogeneic bone marrow transplantation, the latter occurring in the setting of chronic graft-versus-host disease.

Idiopathic bronchiolitis obliterans with organizing pneumonia (BOOP), also referred to as **cryptogenic organizing pneumonia,** affects men and women equally. Most patients are between the ages of 50 and 70. Dry cough, dyspnea, and a flu-like illness, ranging in duration from a few days to several months, are typical. Fever and weight loss are common. Physical examination demonstrates crackles in most patients, and wheezing is present in about a third. Clubbing is uncommon. Pulmonary function studies demonstrate restrictive dysfunction and hypoxemia. The chest radiograph typically shows patchy, bilateral, ground glass or alveolar infiltrates. Solitary pneumonia-like infiltrates and a diffuse interstitial pattern have also been described (see Table 9–19).

BOOP is usually a difficult diagnosis to make on clinical grounds alone. The presence of fever and weight loss, abrupt onset of symptoms (often following an upper respiratory tract infection), a relatively short duration of symptoms, the absence of clubbing, and the presence of alveolar infiltrates help the clinician distinguish this entity from idiopathic interstitial pneumonia. However, open lung biopsy may be necessary. Buds of loose connective tissue and inflammatory cells fill alveoli and distal bronchioles. Corticosteroid therapy is effective in two-thirds of cases, often abruptly. Relapses are common if corticosteroids are stopped prematurely, and most patients require at least 6 months of therapy. Prednisone is usually given initially in doses of 1 mg/kg/d for 2–3 months. The dose is then tapered slowly to 20–40 mg/d, depending on response, and eventually to an alternate-day regimen.

Two well-described disorders are not usually associated with obliteration of bronchioles. Respiratory bronchiolitis is a disorder of small airways in cigarette smokers. Clinically and radiographically, this disorder resembles desquamative interstitial pneumonia (DIP). (See Table 9–19.) Cough, dyspnea, and crackles on chest auscultation are typical. However, the reduction in lung compliance seen in pulmonary fibrosis is not found in this disorder. The condition may be recognized only on open lung biopsy, which demonstrates characteristic metaplasia of terminal and respiratory bronchioles and filling of respiratory and terminal bronchioles, alveolar ducts, and alveoli by pigmented alveolar macrophages. The prognosis is good if the patient stops smoking.

Diffuse panbronchiolitis is an idiopathic disorder of respiratory bronchioles frequently diagnosed in Japan. The condition appears to be rare in the United States or Europe. Men are affected about twice as often as women and are most often between ages 20 and 80. About two-thirds of patients are nonsmokers. The large majority have a history of chronic pansinusitis. Marked dyspnea, cough, and sputum production are cardinal features. Crackles and rhonchi are noted on physical examination. Pulmonary function tests reveal obstructive abnormalities. The chest radiograph shows a distinct pattern of diffuse small nodular shadows and hyperinflation. Open lung biopsy is necessary for diagnosis.

Colby TV: Bronchiolitis. Pathologic considerations. Am J Clin Pathol 1998;109:101. [PMID: 9426525] (Classification of multiple clinical and radiographic patterns of bronchiolitis from an anatomic pathologist.)

Epler GR: Bronchiolitis obliterans organizing pneumonia. Arch Intern Med 2001;161:158. [PMID: 11176728] (Review of clinical findings and management of BOOP.)

Paradis I: Bronchiolitis obliterans: pathogenesis, prevention, and management. Am J Med Sci 1998;315:161.[PMID: 9519929] (Detailed review with emphasis on lung transplantation.)

■ PULMONARY INFECTIONS

PNEUMONIA

Lower respiratory tract infections continue to be a major health problem despite advances in the identification of etiologic organisms and the availability of potent new antimicrobial drugs. In addition, there is still much controversy regarding diagnostic approaches and treatment choices for pneumonia.

Microorganisms gain access to the lower respiratory tract by aspiration of oropharyngeal secretions and associated bacterial flora, inhalation of infected aerosols, and hematogenous dissemination. The consequences of seeding the lower respiratory tract with microorganisms depend on the size of the inoculum, the virulence of the microorganism, and host susceptibility. Characteristics of pneumonia caused by specific agents and appropriate antimicrobial therapy are presented in Table 9–9. Pneumonias are typically classi-

Table 9-9. Characteristics and treatment of selected pneumonias.

Organism; Appearance on Smear of Sputum	Clinical Setting	Complications	Laboratory Studies	Antimicrobial Therapy [1,2]
Streptococcus pneumoniae (pneumococcus). Gram-positive diplococci.	Chronic cardiopulmonary disease; follows upper respiratory tract infection.	Bacteremia, meningitis, endocarditis, pericarditis, empyema.	Gram stain and culture of sputum, blood, pleural fluid	Preferred:[3] Penicillin G, amoxicillin. Alternative: Macrolides, cephalosporins, doxycycline, fluoroquinolones, clindamycin vancomycin.
Haemophilus influenzae. Pleomorphic gram-negative coccobacilli.	Chronic cardiopulmonary disease; follows upper respiratory tract infection.	Empyema, endocarditis.	Gram stain and culture of sputum, blood, pleural fluid.	Preferred:[3] Cefotaxime, ceftriaxone cefuroxime, doxycycline, azithromycin, TMP-SMZ.[4] Alternative: Fluoroquinolones, clarithromycin.
Staphylococcus aureus. Plump gram-positive cocci in clumps.	Residence in chronic care facility, nosocomial, influenza epidemics; cystic fibrosis, bronchiectasis, injection drug use.	Empyema, cavitation.	Gram stain and culture of sputum, blood, pleural fluid.	For methicillin-susceptible strains: Preferred: A penicillinase-resistant penicillin with or without rifampin, or gentamicin. Alternative: A cephalosporin; clindamycin, TMP-SMZ,[4] vancomycin. For methicillin-resistant strains: Vancomycin with or without gentamicin or rifampin.
Klebsiella pneumoniae. Plump gram-negative encapsulated rods.	Alcohol abuse, diabetes mellitus; nosocomial.	Cavitation, empyema.	Gram stain and culture of sputum, blood, pleural fluid.	Preferred: Third-generation cephalosporin. For severe infections, add an aminoglycoside. Alternative: Aztreonam, imipenem, beta-lactam/beta-lactamase inhibitor, or a fluoroquinolone.
Escherichia coli. Gram-negative rods.	Nosocomial; rarely, community-acquired.	Empyema.	Gram stain and culture of sputum, blood, pleural fluid.	Same as for *Klebsiella pneumoniae.*
Pseudomonas aeruginosa. Gram-negative rods.	Nosocomial; cystic fibrosis, bronchiectasis.	Cavitation.	Gram stain and culture of sputum, blood.	Preferred: An antipseudomonal beta-lactam plus an aminoglycoside. Alternative: Ciprofloxacin plus an aminoglycoside or an antipseudomonal beta-lactam.
Anaerobes. Mixed flora.	Aspiration, poor dental hygiene.	Necrotizing pneumonia, abscess empyema.	Culture of pleural fluid or of material obtained by transtracheal or transthoracic aspiration.	Preferred: Clindamycin, beta-lactam/beta-lactamase inhibitor, imipenem.

(continued)

247

Table 9–9. Characteristics and treatment of selected pneumonias. (continued)

Organism; Appearance on Smear of Sputum	Clinical Setting	Complications	Laboratory Studies	Antimicrobial Therapy [1,2]
Mycoplasma pneumoniae. PMNs and monocytes; no bacteria.	Young adults; summer and fall.	Skin rashes, bullous myringitis; hemolytic anemia.	PCR. Culture.[6] Complement fixation titer.[5] Cold agglutinin serum titers are not helpful as they lack sensitivity and specificity.	Preferred: Doxycycline or erythromycin. Alternative: Clarithromycin; azithromycin, or a fluoroquinolone.
Legionella species. Few PMNs; no bacteria.	Summer and fall; exposure to contaminated construction site, water source, air conditioner; community-acquired or nosocomial.	Empyema, cavitation, endocarditis, pericarditis.	Direct immunofluorescent examination or PCR of sputum or tissue; culture of sputum or tissue.[6] Urinary antigen assay for *L pneumophila* serogroup 1.	Preferred: A macrolide with or without rifampin; a fluoroquinolone. Alternative: Doxycycline with or without rifampin.
Chlamydia pneumoniae. Nonspecific.	Clinically similar to *M pneumoniae*, but prodromal symptoms last longer (up to 2 weeks). Sore throat with hoarseness common. Mild pneumonia in teenagers and young adults.	Reinfection in older adults with underlying COPD or heart failure may be severe or even fatal.	Isolation of the organism is very difficult. Serologic studies include microimmunofluorescence with TWAR antigen. PCR at selected laboratories.	Preferred: Doxycycline. Alternative: Erythromycin, clarithromycin, azithromycin, or a fluoroquinolone.
Moraxella catarrhalis. Gram-negative diplococci.	Preexisting lung disease; elderly; corticosteroid or immunosuppressive therapy.	Rarely, pleural effusions and bacteremia.	Gram stain and culture of sputum, blood, pleural fluid.	Preferred: TMP-SMZ,[4] a second- or third-generation cephalosporin, amoxicillin–clavulanic acid, or a macrolide. Alternative: A fluoroquinolone.
Pneumocystis carinii. Nonspecific.	AIDS, immunosuppressive or cytotoxic drug therapy, cancer.	Pneumothorax, respiratory failure, ARDS, death.	Methenamine silver, Giemsa, or DFA stains of sputum or bronchoalveolar lavage fluid.	Preferred: TMP-SMZ[4] or pentamidine isethionate plus prednisone. Alternative: Dapsone plus trimethoprim; clindamycin plus primaquine; trimetrexate plus folinic acid.

[1]Antimicrobial sensitivities should guide therapy when available. (Modified from: The choice of antibacterial drugs. Med Lett Drugs Ther 1999;41:95, and from Bartlett JG et al: Practice guidelines for the management of community-acquired pneumonia in adults. Clin Infect Dis 2000;31:347).

[2]For additional antimicrobial therapy information, see Chapter 37: Tables 37–1 (drugs of choice), 37–5 and 37–7 (doses per day), and 37–4, 37–7, and 37–9 (pharmacology and dosage adjustment for renal dysfunction).

[3]Consider penicillin resistance when choosing therapy. See text.

[4]Trimethoprim-sulfamethoxazole.

[5]Fourfold rise in titer is diagnostic.

[6]Selective media are required.

fied as being either community-acquired or hospital-acquired (nosocomial). Anaerobic pneumonias and lung abscess can occur in both settings and warrant separate consideration.

This section sets forth the evaluation and management of immunocompetent hosts separately from the approach to the evaluation and management of pulmonary infiltrates in immunocompromised hosts—defined as patients with HIV disease, absolute neutrophil counts < 1000/μL, current or recent exposure to myelosuppressive or immunosuppressive drugs, or those currently taking prednisone in a dosage of over 5 mg/d.

1. Community-Acquired Pneumonia

ESSENTIALS OF DIAGNOSIS

- Symptoms and signs of an acute lung infection: fever or hypothermia, cough with or without sputum, dyspnea, chest discomfort, sweats or rigors.
- Bronchial breath sounds or rales are frequent auscultatory findings.
- Parenchymal infiltrate on chest radiograph.
- Occurs outside of the hospital or less than 48 hours after admission in a patient who is not hospitalized or residing in a long-term care facility for more than 14 days before the onset of symptoms.

General Considerations

Community-acquired pneumonia is a common disorder, with approximately 2–3 million cases diagnosed each year in the United States. It is the most deadly infectious disease in the United States and the sixth leading cause of death. Mortality is estimated to be approximately 14% among hospitalized patients and less than 1% for patients who do not require hospitalization. Important risk factors for increased morbidity and mortality from community-acquired pneumonia include advanced age, alcoholism, comorbid medical conditions, altered mental status, respiratory rate ≥ 30 breaths/min, hypotension (defined by systolic blood pressure < 90 mm Hg or diastolic blood pressure < 60 mm Hg), and BUN > 30 mg/dL.

A predictor of patient risk and mortality from community-acquired pneumonia has been developed and validated by the Pneumonia Patient Outcomes Research Team (PORT). The PORT prediction scheme utilizes 19 clinical variables to stratify patients into five mortality risk classes. (See Table 9–10.) Patients under 50 years of age without those comorbid conditions and specific physical examination abnor-

malities listed in Table 9–10 are assigned to risk class I. All other patients are assigned to risk categories based on the scoring system in Table 9–11. Thirty-day mortality by category is listed in Table 9–11. The PORT model can be used along with clinical judgment in the initial decision about whether to hospitalize a patient with community-acquired pneumonia.

In immunocompetent patients, the history, physical examination, radiographs, and sputum examination are neither sensitive nor specific for identifying the microbiologic cause of community-acquired pneumonia. While helpful in selected patients, these modalities do not consistently differentiate bacterial from viral causes or distinguish "typical" from "atypical" causes. As a result, the American Thoracic Society recommends empirical treatment based on epidemiologic data. In contrast, practice guidelines proposed by the Infectious Disease Society of America advocate systematic use of the microbiology laboratory in an attempt to administer pathogen-directed antimicrobial therapy whenever possible, especially in hospitalized patients.

Definition & Pathogenesis

Community-acquired pneumonia begins outside of the hospital or is diagnosed within 48 hours after admission to the hospital in a patient who has not resided in a long-term care facility for 14 days or more before the onset of symptoms.

Pulmonary defense mechanisms (cough reflex, mucociliary clearance system, immune responses) normally prevent the development of lower respiratory tract infections following aspiration of oropharyngeal secretions containing bacteria or inhalation of infected aerosols. Community-acquired pneumonia occurs when there is a defect in one or more of the normal host defense mechanisms or when a very large infectious inoculum or a highly virulent pathogen overwhelms the host.

Prospective studies have failed to identify the cause of community-acquired pneumonia in 40–60% of cases; two or more causes are identified in up to 5% of cases. Bacteria are more commonly identified than viruses. The most common bacterial pathogen identified in most studies of community-acquired pneumonia is *Streptococcus pneumoniae*, accounting for approximately two-thirds of bacterial isolates. Other common bacterial pathogens include *Haemophilus influenzae, Mycoplasma pneumoniae, Chlamydia pneumoniae, Staphylococcus aureus, Neisseria meningitidis, Moraxella catarrhalis, Klebsiella pneumoniae,* other gram-negative rods, and legionella species. Common viral causes of community-acquired pneumonia include influenza virus, respiratory syncytial virus, adenovirus, and parainfluenza virus. A detailed assessment of epidemiologic risk factors may aid in diagnosing pneumonias due to the following causes: *Chlamydia psittaci* (psittacosis), *Coxiella burnetii* (Q fever), *Francisella tularensis* (tularemia), endemic fungi (blasto-

Table 9–10. Scoring system for risk class assignment for PORT prediction rule.[1]

Patient Characteristic	Points Assigned[2]
Demographic factor	
Age: men	Number of years
Age: women	Number of years minus 10
Nursing home resident	10
Comorbid illnesses	
Neoplastic disease[3]	30
Liver disease[4]	20
Congestive heart failure[5]	10
Cerebrovascular disease[6]	10
Renal disease[7]	10
Physical examination finding	
Altered mental status[8]	20
Respiratory rate > 30 breaths/min	20
Systolic blood pressure < 90 mm Hg	20
Temperature < 35 +°C or > 40+°C	15
Pulse > 125 beats/min	10
Laboratory or radiographic finding	
Arterial pH < 7.35	30
Blood urea nitrogen > 30 mg/dL	20
Sodium < 130 meq/L	20
Glucose > 250 mg/dL	10
Hematocrit < 30%	10
Arterial P_{O_2} < 60 mm Hg	10
Pleural effusion	10

[1]Modified and reproduced, with permission, from Fine MJ et al: A prediction rule to identify low-risk patients with community-acquired pneumonia. N Engl J Med 1997;336:243. Copyright © 1997 Massachusetts Medical Society. All rights reserved.
[2]A total point score for a given patient is obtained by summing the patient's age in years (age minus 10 for women) and the points for each applicable characteristic.
[3]Any cancer except basal or squamous cell of the skin that was active at the time of presentation or diagnosed within 1 year before presentation.
[4]Clinical or histologic diagnosis of cirrhosis or another form of chronic liver disease.
[5]Systolic or diastolic dysfunction documented by history, physical examination and chest radiograph, echocardiogram, MUGA scan, or left ventriculogram.
[6]Clinical diagnosis of stroke or transient ischemic attack or stroke documented by MRI or CT scan.
[7]History of chronic renal disease or abnormal blood urea nitrogen and creatinine concentration documented in the medical record.
[8]Disorientation (to person, place, or time, not known to be chronic), stupor, or coma.

Table 9–11. PORT risk class 30-day mortality rates and recommendations for site of care.[1]

Number of Points	Risk Class	Mortality at 30 days (%)	Recommended Site of Care
Absence of predictors	I	0.1–0.4	Outpatient
≤ 70	II	0.6–0.7	Outpatient
71–90	III	0.9–2.8	Outpatient or brief inpatient
91–130	IV	8.2–9.3	Inpatient
≥ 130	V	27.0–31.1	Inpatient

[1]Data from Fine MJ et al: A prediction rule to identify low-risk patients with community-acquired pneumonia. N Engl J Med 1997;336:243. Copyright © 1997 Massachusetts Medical Society. All rights reserved.

myces, coccidioides, histoplasma), and sin nombre virus (hantavirus pulmonary syndrome).

Clinical Findings

A. SYMPTOMS AND SIGNS

Most patients with community-acquired pneumonia experience an acute or subacute onset of fever, cough with or without sputum production, and dyspnea. Other common symptoms include rigors, sweats, chills, chest discomfort, pleurisy, fatigue, myalgias, anorexia, headache, and abdominal pain.

Common physical findings include fever or hypothermia, tachypnea, tachycardia, and mild arterial oxygen desaturation. Many patients will appear acutely ill. Chest examination is often remarkable for altered breath sounds and rales. Dullness to percussion may be present if a parapneumonic pleural effusion is present.

The differential diagnosis of lower respiratory tract symptoms and signs is extensive and includes upper respiratory tract infections, reactive airway diseases, congestive heart failure, bronchiolitis obliterans organizing pneumonia, lung cancer, pulmonary vasculitis, pulmonary thromboembolic disease, and atelectasis.

B. LABORATORY FINDINGS

Controversy surrounds the role of Gram stain and culture analysis of expectorated sputum in patients with community-acquired pneumonia. Most reports suggest that these tests have poor positive and negative predictive value in most patients. Some argue, however, that the tests should still be performed to try to identify etiologic organisms in the hope of reducing microbial resistance to drugs, unnecessary drug costs, and avoidable side effects of empirical antibiotic therapy. Expert panel guidelines suggest that sputum Gram stain should be attempted in all patients with community-acquired pneumonia and that sputum culture should be obtained for all patients who require hospitalization. Sputum should be obtained before antibiotics are initiated except in a case of suspected antibiotic failure. The specimen is obtained by deep cough and should be grossly purulent. Culture should be performed only if the specimen meets strict cytologic criteria (except for detection of legionella or mycobacteria).

Additional testing is generally recommended for patients who require hospitalization: preantibiotic blood cultures (at least two sets with needle sticks at separate sites), arterial blood gases, complete blood count with differential, and a chemistry panel (including serum glucose, electrolytes, urea nitrogen, creatinine, bilirubin, and liver enzymes). The results of these tests help assess the severity of the disease and guide evaluation and therapy. HIV serology should be obtained from all hospitalized patients.

C. Imaging

Chest radiography may confirm the diagnosis and detect associated lung diseases. It can also be used to help assess severity and response to therapy over time. Radiographic findings can range from patchy airspace infiltrates to lobar consolidation with air bronchograms to diffuse alveolar or interstitial infiltrates. Additional findings can include pleural effusions and cavitation. No pattern of radiographic abnormalities is pathognomonic of a specific cause of pneumonia.

Progression of pulmonary infiltrates during antibiotic therapy or lack of radiographic improvement over time are poor prognostic signs and also raise concerns about secondary or alternative pulmonary processes. Clearing of pulmonary infiltrates in patients with community-acquired pneumonia can take 6 weeks or longer and is usually fastest in young patients, nonsmokers, and those with only single lobe involvement.

D. Special Examinations

Sputum induction is reserved for patients who cannot provide expectorated sputum samples or who may have *Pneumocystis carinii* or *Mycobacterium tuberculosis* pneumonia. Transtracheal aspiration, fiberoptic bronchoscopy, and transthoracic needle aspiration techniques to obtain samples of lower respiratory secretions or tissues are reserved for selected patients.

Thoracentesis with pleural fluid analysis (stains, cultures; glucose, lactate dehydrogenase, and total protein levels; leukocyte count with differential; pH determination) should be performed on most patients with pleural effusions to assist in diagnosis of the etiologic agent and assess for empyema or complicated parapneumonic process. Serologic assays, polymerase chain reaction tests, specialized culture tests, and other new diagnostic tests for organisms such as legionella, *Mycoplasma pneumoniae,* and *Chlamydia pneumoniae* are performed when these diagnoses are suspected. Limitations of many of these tests include delay in obtaining test results and poor sensitivity and specificity.

Treatment

Antimicrobial therapy should be initiated promptly after the diagnosis of pneumonia is established and appropriate specimens are obtained, especially in patients who require hospitalization. Delays in obtaining diagnostic specimens or the results of testing should not preclude the early administration of antibiotics to acutely ill patients. Decisions regarding hospitalization should be based on prognostic criteria as outlined above in the section on general considerations. Treatment recommendations can be divided into those for patients who can be treated as outpatients and those for patients who require hospitalization.

Special consideration must be given to emerging resistance of *Streptococcus pneumoniae* strains to penicillin. Intermediate resistance to penicillin is defined as an MIC of 0.1–1 μg/mL. Strains with high-level resistance usually require an MIC ≥ 2 μg/mL for penicillin. Resistance to other antibiotics (beta-lactams, trimethoprim-sulfamethoxazole, macrolides, others) often accompanies resistance to penicillin. The prevalence of resistance varies by patient group, geographic region, and over time. Local resistance pattern data should therefore guide empirical therapy of suspected or documented *S pneumoniae* infections until specific susceptibility test results are available.

A. Treatment of Outpatients

Empirical antibiotic options for patients with community-acquired pneumonia who do not require hospitalization include the following: (1) Macrolides (clarithromycin, 500 mg orally twice a day, or azithromycin, 500 mg orally as a first dose and then 250 mg once a day for 4 days). (2) Doxycycline (100 mg orally twice a day). (3) Fluoroquinolones (with enhanced activity against *S pneumoniae,* such as gatifloxacin, 400 mg orally once a day, levofloxacin 500 mg orally once a day, or moxifloxacin 400 mg orally once a day). Some experts prefer doxycycline or macrolides for patients under 50 years of age without comorbidities and a fluoroquinolone for patients with comorbidities or who are older than 50 years of age. Alternatives include erythromycin (250–500 mg orally four times daily), amoxicillin-potassium clavulanate—especially for suspected aspiration pneumonia—500 mg orally three times a day or 875 mg orally twice a day, and some second- and third-generation cephalosporins such as cefuroxime axetil (250–500 mg orally twice a day), cefpodoxime proxetil (100–200 mg orally twice a day), or cefprozil (250–500 mg orally twice a day).

There are limited data to guide recommendations for duration of treatment. The decision is influenced by the severity of illness, the etiologic agent, response to therapy, other medical problems, and complications. Therapy until the patient is afebrile for at least 72 hours is usually sufficient for pneumonia due to *S pneumoniae.* A minimum of 2 weeks of therapy is appropriate for pneumonia due to *S aureus, P aeruginosa,* klebsiella, anaerobes, *M pneumoniae*, *C pneumoniae*, or legionella species.

B. Treatment of Hospitalized Patients

Empirical antibiotic options for patients with community-acquired pneumonia who require hospitalization can be divided into those for patients who can be cared for on a general medical ward and those for patients who require care in an intensive care unit. Patients who only require general medical ward care usually respond to an extended-spectrum beta-lactam (such as ceftriaxone or cefotaxime) with a macrolide (clarithromycin or azithromycin is preferred if *H influenzae* infection is suspected) or a fluoroquinolone (with enhanced activity against *S pneumoniae*) such as gatifloxacin, levofloxacin, or moxifloxacin. Alternatives include a beta-lactam/beta-lactamase inhibitor (ampicillin-sulbactam or piperacillin-tazobactam) with a macrolide.

Patients requiring admission to the intensive care unit require a macrolide or a fluoroquinolone (with enhanced activity against *S pneumoniae*) plus an extended-spectrum cephalosporin (ceftriaxone, cefotaxime) or a beta-lactam/beta-lactamase inhibitor (ampicillin-sulbactam or piperacillin-tazobactam). Patients with penicillin allergies can be treated with a fluoroquinolone (with enhanced activity against *S pneumoniae*) with or without clindamycin. Patients with suspected aspiration pneumonia should receive a fluoroquinolone (with enhanced activity against *S pneumoniae*) with or without clindamycin, metronidazole, or a beta-lactam/beta-lactamase inhibitor. Patients with structural lung diseases such as bronchiectasis or cystic fibrosis benefit from empirical therapy with an antipseudomonal penicillin, carbapenem, or cefepime plus a fluoroquinolone (including high-dose ciprofloxacin) until sputum culture and sensitivity results are available. Expanded discussions of specific antibiotics are provided in Chapter 37.

Although almost all patients who are admitted to a hospital for therapy of community-acquired pneumonia receive intravenous antibiotics, no studies demonstrate superior outcomes when these patients are treated intravenously instead of orally if patients can tolerate oral therapy and the drug is well absorbed. Duration of antibiotic treatment is the same as for outpatients with community-acquired pneumonia.

Prevention

Polyvalent pneumococcal vaccine (containing capsular polysaccharide antigens of 23 common strains of *S pneumoniae*) has the potential to prevent or lessen the severity of the majority of pneumococcal infections in immunocompetent patients. Indications for pneumococcal vaccination include the following: age ≥ 65 years or any chronic illness that increases the risk of community-acquired pneumonia (see Chapter 30). Immunocompromised patients and those at highest risk of fatal pneumococcal infections should receive a single revaccination 6 years after the first vaccination. Immunocompetent persons 65 years of age or older should receive a second dose of vaccine if the patient first received the vaccine 6 or more years previously and was under 65 years old at the time of vaccination.

The influenza vaccine is effective in preventing severe disease due to influenza virus with a resulting positive impact on both primary influenza pneumonia and secondary bacterial pneumonias. The influenza vaccine is administered annually to persons at risk for complications of influenza infection (age ≥ 65 years, residents of chronic care facilities, patients with pulmonary or cardiovascular disorders, patients recently hospitalized with chronic metabolic disorders) as well as health care workers and others who are able to transmit influenza to high-risk patients.

Hospitalized patients who would benefit from pneumococcal and influenza vaccines should be vaccinated during hospitalization. The vaccines can be given simultaneously, and there are no contraindications to use immediately after an episode of pneumonia.

Bartlett JG et al: Practice guidelines for the management of community-acquired pneumonia in adults. Clin Infect Dis 2000;31:347. [PMID: 10987697] (Expert panel, peer-reviewed, evidence-based practice guidelines commissioned by the Infectious Diseases Society of America and designed to assist primary care practitioners in the diagnosis and treatment of community-acquired pneumonia in immunocompetent adults.)

Fine MJ et al: A prediction rule to identify low-risk patients with community-acquired pneumonia. N Engl J Med 1997;336:243. [PMID: 8995086] (Stratification based on age, coexisting disease, abnormal physical findings, and abnormal laboratory values may help decision-making regarding need for hospitalization for patients with pneumonia.)

Niederman MS et al: Guidelines for the management of adults with community-acquired pneumonia. Diagnosis, assessment of severity, antimicrobial therapy, and prevention. Am J Respir Crit Care Med 2001;163:1730. [PMID: 11401897] (Evidence-based revision of the American Thoracic Society's 1993 paper on community-acquired pneumonia.)

Singh N et al: Rational empiric antibiotic prescription in the ICU. Chest 2000;117:1496. [PMID: 10807841] (An attempt to show how existing data can guide antibiotic choices.)

2. Hospital-Acquired Pneumonia

 ESSENTIALS OF DIAGNOSIS

- *Occurs more than 48 hours after admission to the hospital and excludes any infection present at the time of admission.*
- *At least two of the following: fever, cough, leukocytosis, purulent sputum.*

- New or progressive parenchymal infiltrate on chest radiograph.
- Especially common in patients requiring intensive care or mechanical ventilation.

General Considerations

Hospital-acquired (nosocomial) pneumonia is an important cause of morbidity and mortality despite the widespread use of preventive measures, advances in diagnostic testing, and potent new antimicrobial agents. Nosocomial pneumonia is the second most common cause of hospital-acquired infection and is the leading cause of deaths due to nosocomial infections with mortality rates ranging from 20% to 50%. While the majority of cases occur in patients who are not in the intensive care unit, the highest risk patients are those in such units or who are being mechanically ventilated; these patients also experience higher morbidity and mortality from nosocomial pneumonias.

Definition & Pathogenesis

Hospital-acquired pneumonia is defined as pneumonia developing more than 48 hours after admission to the hospital. Ventilator-associated pneumonia develops in a mechanically ventilated patient more than 48 hours after intubation.

Colonization of the pharynx and possibly the stomach with bacteria is the most important step in the pathogenesis of nosocomial pneumonia. Pharyngeal colonization is promoted by exogenous factors (instrumentation of the upper airway with nasogastric and endotracheal tubes, contamination by dirty hands and equipment, and treatment with broad-spectrum antibiotics that promote the emergence of drug-resistant organisms) and patient factors (malnutrition, advanced age, altered consciousness, swallowing disorders, and underlying pulmonary and systemic diseases). Aspiration of infected pharyngeal or gastric secretions delivers bacteria directly to the lower airway. Impaired cellular and mechanical defense mechanisms in the lungs of hospitalized patients raise the risk of infection after aspiration has occurred. Tracheal intubation increases the risk of lower respiratory infection by mechanical obstruction of the trachea, impairment of mucociliary clearance, trauma to the mucociliary escalator system, and interference with coughing. Tight adherence of bacteria such as pseudomonas to the tracheal epithelium and the biofilm that lines the endotracheal tube makes clearance of these organisms from the lower airway difficult. Less important pathogenetic mechanisms of nosocomial pneumonia include inhalation of contaminated aerosols and hematogenous dissemination of microorganisms.

The role of the stomach in the pathogenesis of nosocomial pneumonia remains controversial. Observational studies have suggested that elevations of gastric pH due to antacids, H_2-receptor antagonists or enteral feeding is associated with gastric microbial overgrowth, tracheobronchial colonization, and nosocomial pneumonia. Sucralfate, a cytoprotective agent that does not alter gastric pH, is associated with a trend toward a lower incidence of ventilator-associated pneumonia.

The most common organisms responsible for nosocomial pneumonia are *Pseudomonas aeruginosa, Staphylococcus aureus,* enterobacter, *Klebsiella pneumoniae,* and *Escherichia coli.* Proteus, *Serratia marcescens, H influenzae,* and streptococci account for most of the remaining cases. Infection by *P aeruginosa* and acinetobacter tend to cause pneumonia in the most debilitated patients, those with previous antibiotic therapy, and those requiring mechanical ventilation. Anaerobic organisms (bacteroides, anaerobic streptococci, fusobacterium) may also cause pneumonia in the hospitalized patient; when isolated, they are commonly part of a polymicrobial flora. Mycobacteria, fungi, chlamydiae, viruses, rickettsiae, and protozoal organisms are uncommon causes of nosocomial pneumonia.

Clinical Findings

A. SYMPTOMS AND SIGNS

The signs and symptoms associated with nosocomial pneumonia are non-specific; however, one or more clinical findings (fever, leukocytosis, purulent sputum, and a new or progressive pulmonary infiltrate on chest radiograph) are present in most patients. Other findings associated with nosocomial pneumonia include those listed above for community-acquired pneumonia.

The differential diagnosis of new lower respiratory tract symptoms and signs in hospitalized patients includes congestive heart failure, atelectasis, aspiration, acute respiratory distress syndrome, pulmonary thromboembolism, pulmonary hemorrhage, and drug reactions.

B. LABORATORY FINDINGS

The minimum evaluation for suspected nosocomial pneumonia includes blood cultures from two different sites and an arterial blood gas or pulse oximetry determination. Blood cultures can identify the pathogen in up to 20% of all patients with nosocomial pneumonia; positivity is associated with increased risk for complications and other sites of infection. The assessment of oxygenation helps define the severity of illness and determines the need for supplemental oxygen. Blood counts and clinical chemistry tests are not helpful in establishing a specific diagnosis of nosocomial pneumonia; however, they can help define the severity of illness and identify complications. Thoracentesis for pleural fluid analysis (stains, cultures; glucose, lactate dehydrogenase, and total protein levels; leukocyte count with differential; pH determination) should be performed in patients with pleural effusions.

Examination of sputum is attended by the same disadvantages as in community-acquired pneumonia. Gram stains and cultures of sputum are neither sensitive nor specific in the diagnosis of nosocomial pneumonia. The identification of a bacterial organism by culture of sputum does not prove that the organism is a lower respiratory tract pathogen. However, it can be used to help identify antibiotic sensitivity patterns of bacteria and as a guide to therapy. If nosocomial pneumonia from *Legionella pneumophila* is suspected, direct fluorescent antibody staining can be performed. Sputum stains and cultures for mycobacteria and certain fungi may be diagnostic.

C. IMAGING

Radiographic findings are nonspecific and can range from patchy airspace infiltrates to lobar consolidation with air bronchograms to diffuse alveolar or interstitial infiltrates. Additional findings can include pleural effusions and cavitation. Progression of pulmonary infiltrates during antibiotic therapy and lack of radiographic improvement over time are poor prognostic signs and also raise concerns about secondary or alternative pulmonary processes. Clearing of pulmonary infiltrates can take 6 weeks or longer.

D. SPECIAL EXAMINATIONS

Endotracheal aspiration using a sterile suction catheter and fiberoptic bronchoscopy with bronchoalveolar lavage or a protected specimen brush can be used to obtain lower respiratory tract secretions for analysis, most commonly in patients with ventilator-associated pneumonias. Endotracheal aspiration cultures have significant negative predictive value but limited positive predictive value in the diagnosis of specific etiologic agents in patients with nosocomial pneumonia. A recent clinical trial of an invasive diagnostic approach using quantitative culture of bronchoalveolar lavage samples or protected specimen brush samples in patients suspected of having ventilator-associated pneumonia reported significantly less antibiotic use, earlier attenuation of organ dysfunction, and fewer deaths at 14 days in the invasive management group.

Treatment

Treatment of nosocomial pneumonia, like treatment of community-acquired pneumonia, is usually empirical. Because of the high mortality rate, therapy should be started as soon as pneumonia is suspected. Initial regimens must be broad in spectrum and tailored to the specific clinical setting. There is no uniform consensus on the best regimens.

Recommendations for the treatment of hospital-acquired pneumonia have been proposed by many organizations, including the American Thoracic Society. Initial empirical therapy with antibiotics is determined by the severity of illness, risk factors, and the length of hospitalization. Empirical therapy for mild to moderate nosocomial pneumonia in a patient without unusual risk factors or a patient with severe early-onset (within 5 days after hospitalization) hospital-acquired pneumonia may consist of a second-generation cephalosporin, a nonantipseudomonal third-generation cephalosporin, or a combination of a beta-lactam and beta-lactamase inhibitor.

Empirical therapy for patients with severe, late-onset ($\geq$ 5 days after hospitalization) hospital-acquired pneumonia or with ICU- or ventilator-associated pneumonia should include a combination of antibiotics directed against the most virulent organisms, particularly *P aeruginosa,* acinetobacter species, and enterobacter species. The antibiotic regimen should include an aminoglycoside or fluoroquinolone plus one of the following: an antipseudomonal penicillin, an antipseudomonal cephalosporin, imipenem-cilastatin, or aztreonam—aztreonam alone with an aminoglycoside will be inadequate if coverage for gram-positive organisms or *H influenzae* is required. Vancomycin is added if infection with methicillin-resistant *S aureus* infection is of concern (especially in patients with coma, head trauma, diabetes mellitus, or renal failure, or who are in the ICU). Anaerobic coverage with clindamycin or a beta-lactam/beta-lactamase inhibitor combination may be added for patients who have risk factors for anaerobic pneumonia, including aspiration, recent thoracoabdominal surgery, or an obstructing airway lesion. A macrolide is added when patients are at risk for legionella infection, such those receiving high-dose corticosteroids. After results of sputum, blood, and pleural fluid cultures have been obtained, it may be possible to switch to a regimen with a narrower spectrum. Duration of antibiotic therapy should be individualized based on the pathogen, severity of illness, response to therapy, and comorbid conditions. Therapy for gram-negative bacterial pneumonia should continue for at least 14–21 days.

Expanded discussions of specific antibiotics are provided in Chapter 37. Antibiotic dosage suggestions are provided in Chapter 37.

Arozullah AM et al: Development and validation of a multifactorial risk index for predicting postoperative pneumonia after major noncardiac surgery. Ann Intern Med 2001;135:847. [PMID: 11712875] (Prospective multicenter Veterans Administration cooperative study attempts to establish a prediction index for the development of postoperative pneumonia.)

Fagon JY et al: Invasive and noninvasive strategies for management of suspected ventilator-associated pneumonia. A randomized trial. Ann Intern Med 2000;132:621. [PMID: 10766680] (An invasive management strategy using bronchoscopic techniques was associated with fewer deaths at 14 days, earlier attenuation of organ dysfunction, and less antibiotic use.)

Morehead RS et al: Ventilator-associated pneumonia. Arch Intern Med 2000;160:1926 [PMID: 10888967] (Comprehensive review.)

3. Anaerobic Pneumonia & Lung Abscess

ESSENTIALS OF DIAGNOSIS

- History of or predisposition to aspiration.
- Indolent symptoms, including fever, weight loss, malaise.
- Poor dentition.
- Foul-smelling purulent sputum (in many patients).
- Infiltrate in dependent lung zone, with single or multiple areas of cavitation or pleural effusion.

General Considerations

Aspiration of small amounts of oropharyngeal secretions occurs during sleep in normal individuals but rarely causes disease. Sequelae of aspiration of larger amounts of material include nocturnal asthma, chemical pneumonitis, mechanical obstruction of airways by particulate matter, bronchiectasis, and pleuropulmonary infection. Individuals predisposed to disease induced by aspiration include those with depressed levels of consciousness due to drug or alcohol use, seizures, general anesthesia, or central nervous system disease; those with impaired deglutition due to esophageal disease or neurologic disorders; and those with tracheal or nasogastric tubes, which disrupt the mechanical defenses of the airways.

Periodontal disease and poor dental hygiene, which increase the number of anaerobic bacteria in aspirated material, is associated with a greater likelihood of anaerobic pleuropulmonary infection. Aspiration of infected oropharyngeal contents initially leads to pneumonia in dependent lung zones, such as the posterior segments of the upper lobes and superior and basilar segments of the lower lobes. Body position at the time of aspiration determines which lung zones are dependent. The onset of symptoms is insidious. By the time the patient seeks medical attention, necrotizing pneumonia, lung abscess, or empyema may be apparent.

Most aspiration patients with necrotizing pneumonia, lung abscess, and empyema are found to be infected with multiple species of anaerobic bacteria. Most of the remainder are infected with both anaerobic and aerobic bacteria. *Prevotella melaninogenica*, peptostreptococcus, *Fusobacterium nucleatum*, and bacteroides species are commonly isolated anaerobic bacteria.

Clinical Findings

A. SYMPTOMS AND SIGNS

Patients with anaerobic pleuropulmonary infection usually present with constitutional symptoms such as fever, weight loss, and malaise. Cough with expectoration of foul-smelling purulent sputum suggests anaerobic infection, though the absence of productive cough does not rule out such an infection. Dentition is often poor. Patients are rarely edentulous; if so, an obstructing bronchial lesion is usually present.

B. LABORATORY FINDINGS

Expectorated sputum is inappropriate for culture of anaerobic organisms because of contaminating mouth flora. Representative material for culture can be obtained only by transthoracic aspiration, thoracentesis, or bronchoscopy with a protected brush. Transthoracic aspiration is rarely indicated, because drainage occurs via the bronchus and anaerobic pleuropulmonary infections usually respond well to empirical therapy.

C. IMAGING

The different types of anaerobic pleuropulmonary infection are distinguished on the basis of their radiographic appearance. **Lung abscess** appears as a thick-walled solitary cavity surrounded by consolidation. An air-fluid level is usually present. Other causes of cavitary lung disease (tuberculosis, mycosis, cancer, infarction, Wegener's granulomatosis) should be excluded. **Necrotizing pneumonia** is distinguished by multiple areas of cavitation within an area of consolidation. **Empyema** is characterized by the presence of purulent pleural fluid and may accompany either of the other two radiographic findings. Ultrasonography is of value in locating fluid and may also reveal pleural loculations.

Treatment

Penicillins have been the standard treatment for anaerobic pleuropulmonary infections. However, an increasing number of anaerobic organisms produce beta-lactamases, and up to 20% of patients do not respond to penicillins. Improved responses have been documented with clindamycin (600 mg intravenously every 8 hours until improvement, then 300 mg orally every 6 hours) or amoxicillin-clavulanate (875 mg orally every 12 hours). Penicillin (amoxicillin, 500 mg every 8 hours, or penicillin G, 1–2 million units intravenously every 4–6 hours) plus metronidazole (500 mg orally or intravenously every 8–12 hours) is another option. Antibiotic therapy should be continued until the chest radiograph improves, a process that may take a month or more; patients with lung abscesses should be treated until radiographic resolution of the abscess cavity is demonstrated. Anaerobic pleuropulmonary disease requires adequate drainage with tube thoracostomy for the treatment of empyema. Open pleural drainage is sometimes necessary because of the propensity of these infections to produce loculations in the pleural space.

PULMONARY INFILTRATES IN THE IMMUNOCOMPROMISED HOST

Pulmonary infiltrates in immunocompromised patients may arise from infectious or noninfectious causes. Infection may be due to bacterial, mycobacterial, fungal, protozoal, helminthic, or viral pathogens. Noninfectious processes such as pulmonary edema, alveolar hemorrhage, drug reactions, pulmonary thromboembolic disease, malignancy, and radiation pneumonitis may mimic infection.

Although almost any pathogen can cause pneumonia in a compromised host, two clinical tools help the clinician narrow the differential diagnosis. The first is knowledge of the underlying immunologic defect. Specific immunologic defects are associated with particular infections. Defects in humoral immunity predispose to bacterial infections; defects in cellular immunity lead to infections with viruses, fungi, mycobacteria, and protozoa. Neutropenia and impaired granulocyte function predispose to infections from S aureus, aspergillus, gram-negative bacilli, and candida. The time course of infection also provides clues to the etiology of pneumonia in immunocompromised patients. A fulminant pneumonia is often caused by bacterial infection, whereas an insidious pneumonia is more apt to be caused by viral, fungal, protozoal, or mycobacterial infection. Pneumonia occurring within 2–4 weeks after organ transplantation is usually bacterial, whereas several months or more after transplantation P carinii, viruses (eg, CMV), and fungi (eg, aspergillus) are encountered more often.

Chest radiography is rarely helpful in narrowing the differential diagnosis. Examination of expectorated sputum for bacteria, fungi, mycobacteria, legionella, and P carinii is important and may preclude the need for expensive, invasive diagnostic procedures. Sputum induction is often necessary for diagnosis. The sensitivity of induced sputum for detection of P carinii depends upon institutional expertise, number of specimens analyzed, and detection methods.

Routine evaluation frequently fails to identify a causative organism. The clinician may begin empirical antimicrobial therapy and proceed to invasive procedures such as bronchoscopy, transthoracic needle aspiration, or open lung biopsy. The approach to management must be based on the severity of the pulmonary infection, the underlying disease, the risks of empirical therapy, and local expertise and experience with diagnostic procedures. Bronchoalveolar lavage using the flexible bronchoscope is a safe and effective method for obtaining representative pulmonary secretions for microbiologic studies. It involves less risk of bleeding and other complications than bronchial brushing and transbronchial biopsy. Bronchoalveolar lavage is especially suitable for the diagnosis of P carinii pneumonia in patients with AIDS when induced sputum analysis is negative. Open lung biopsy, now often performed by video-assisted thoracoscopy, provides the best opportunity for diagnosis of pulmonary infiltrates in the immunocompromised host. However, a specific diagnosis is obtained in only about two-thirds of cases, and the information obtained rarely affects the outcome. Therefore, empirical treatment is often preferred.

Baughman RP: The lung in the immunocompromised patient. Infectious complications. Part 1. Respiration 1999;66:95. [PMID: 10202312] (Heavily referenced article reviews infections, their frequency of occurrence, and their clinical presentation in various immunosuppressed groups.)

Hilbert G et al: Noninvasive ventilation in immunosuppressed patients with pulmonary infiltrates, fever, and acute respiratory failure. N Engl J Med 2001;344:481. [PMID: 11172189] (In a prospective, randomized trial of intermittent noninvasive ventilation in 52 immunosuppressed patients, early initiation of noninvasive ventilation was associated with significant reductions of endotracheal intubations and an improved likelihood of survival to hospital discharge.)

PULMONARY TUBERCULOSIS

 ESSENTIALS OF DIAGNOSIS

- Fatigue, weight loss, fever, night sweats, and cough.
- Pulmonary infiltrates on chest radiograph, most often apical.
- Positive tuberculin skin test reaction (most cases).
- Acid-fast bacilli on smear of sputum or sputum culture positive for Mycobacterium tuberculosis.

General Considerations

Tuberculosis is one of the world's most widespread and deadly illnesses. Mycobacterium tuberculosis, the organism that causes tuberculosis infection and disease, infects an estimated 20–43% of the world's population. Each year, 3 million people worldwide die from the disease. In the United States, it is estimated that 15 million people are infected with M tuberculosis. Tuberculosis occurs disproportionately among disadvantaged populations such as the malnourished, homeless, and those living in overcrowded and substandard housing. There is an increased occurrence of tuberculosis among HIV-positive individuals.

Infection with *M tuberculosis* begins when a susceptible person inhales airborne droplet nuclei containing viable organisms. Tubercle bacilli that reach the alveoli are ingested by alveolar macrophages. Infection follows if the inoculum escapes alveolar macrophage microbicidal activity. Once infection is established, lymphatic and hematogenous dissemination of tuberculosis typically occurs before the development of an effective immune response. This stage of infection, **primary tuberculosis,** is usually clinically and radiographically silent. In most persons with intact cell-mediated immunity, T cells and macrophages surround the organisms in granulomas that limit their multiplication and spread. The infection is contained but not eradicated, since viable organisms may lie dormant within granulomas for years to decades.

Individuals with this **latent tuberculosis infection** do not have active disease and cannot transmit the organism to others. However, reactivation of disease may occur if the host's immune defenses are impaired. Approximately 10% of individuals with latent tuberculosis infection who are not given preventive therapy will develop active tuberculosis in their lifetime; half of these cases occur in the 2 years following primary infection. Up to 50% of HIV-infected patients will develop active tuberculosis within 2 years after infection with tuberculosis. Diverse conditions such as gastrectomy, silicosis, and diabetes mellitus and disorders associated with immunosuppression (eg, HIV infection or therapy with corticosteroids or other immunosuppressive drugs) are associated with an increased risk of reactivation.

In approximately 5% of cases, the immune response is inadequate and the host develops **progressive primary tuberculosis,** accompanied by both pulmonary and constitutional symptoms that are described below. Standard teaching has held that 90% of tuberculosis in adults represents activation of latent disease. New diagnostic technologies such as DNA fingerprinting suggest that as many as one-third of new cases of tuberculosis in urban populations are primary infections resulting from person-to-person transmission.

The percentage of patients with atypical presentations—particularly elderly patients, patients with HIV infection, and those in nursing homes—has increased. Extrapulmonary tuberculosis is especially common in patients with HIV infection, who often display lymphadenitis or miliary disease.

Strains of *M tuberculosis* resistant to one or more first-line antituberculous drugs are being encountered with increasing frequency. Risk factors for drug resistance include immigration from parts of the world with a high prevalence of drug-resistant tuberculosis, close and prolonged contact with individuals with drug-resistant tuberculosis, unsuccessful previous therapy, and patient noncompliance. Resistance to one or more antituberculosis drugs has been found in 15% of

tuberculosis patients in the United States. Outbreaks of multidrug-resistant tuberculosis in hospitals and correctional facilities in Florida and New York have been associated with mortality rates of 70–90% and median survival rates of 4–16 weeks.

Clinical Findings

A. Symptoms and Signs

The patient with pulmonary tuberculosis typically presents with slowly progressive constitutional symptoms of malaise, anorexia, weight loss, fever, and night sweats. Chronic cough is the most common pulmonary symptom. It may be dry at first but typically becomes productive of purulent sputum as the disease progresses. Blood-streaked sputum is common, but significant hemoptysis is rarely a presenting symptom; life-threatening hemoptysis may occur in advanced disease. Dyspnea is unusual unless there is extensive disease. Rarely, the patient is asymptomatic. On physical examination, the patient appears chronically ill and malnourished. On chest examination, there are no physical findings specific for tuberculosis infection. The examination may be normal or may reveal classic findings such as posttussive apical rales.

B. Laboratory Findings

Definitive diagnosis depends on recovery of *M tuberculosis* from cultures or identification of the organism by DNA or RNA amplification techniques. Three consecutive morning sputum specimens are advised. Sputum induction may be helpful in patients who cannot voluntarily produce satisfactory specimens. Fluorochrome staining with rhodamine-auramine of concentrated, digested sputum specimens is performed initially as a screening method, with confirmation by the Kinyoun or Ziehl-Neelsen stains. Demonstration of acid-fast bacilli on sputum smear does not confirm a diagnosis of tuberculosis, since saprophytic nontuberculous mycobacteria may colonize the airways and rarely may cause pulmonary disease.

In patients thought to have tuberculosis despite negative sputum smears, fiberoptic bronchoscopy can be considered. Bronchial washings are helpful; however, transbronchial lung biopsies increase the diagnostic yield. Postbronchoscopy expectorated sputum specimens may also be useful. Early morning aspiration of gastric contents after an overnight fast is an alternative to bronchoscopy but is suitable only for culture and not for stained smear, because nontuberculous mycobacteria may be present in the stomach in the absence of tuberculous infection. *M tuberculosis* may be cultured from blood in up to 15% of patients with tuberculosis.

Cultures on solid media to identify *M tuberculosis* may require 12 weeks. Liquid medium culture systems allow detection of mycobacterial growth in several days. Once mycobacteria have been grown in culture, nucleic acid probes or high-performance liquid chromatography can be used to identify the species within hours. The results of nucleic acid (DNA and RNA) amplification tests for tuberculosis should be interpreted in the clinical context and on the basis of local laboratory performance. Drug susceptibility testing of culture isolates is considered routine for the first isolate of *M tuberculosis,* when a treatment regimen is failing, and when sputum cultures remain positive after 2 months of therapy.

DNA fingerprinting using the restriction fragment length polymorphism analysis is available to identify individual strains of *M tuberculosis,* thereby revealing if infection has been transmitted from person to person. In addition, this method can be used to detect laboratory cross-contamination.

Needle biopsy of the pleura reveals granulomatous inflammation in approximately 60% of patients with pleural effusions caused by *M tuberculosis.* Pleural fluid cultures for *M tuberculosis* are positive in less than 25% of cases of pleural tuberculosis. Culture of three pleural biopsy specimens combined with microscopic examination of a pleural biopsy yields a diagnosis in up to 90% of patients with pleural tuberculosis.

C. IMAGING

Radiographic abnormalities in primary tuberculosis include small homogeneous infiltrates, hilar and paratracheal lymph node enlargement, and segmental atelectasis. Pleural effusion may be present, especially in adults, sometimes as the sole radiographic abnormality. Cavitation may be seen with progressive primary tuberculosis. Ghon (calcified primary focus) and Ranke (calcified primary focus and calcified hilar lymph node) complexes are seen in a minority of patients and represent residual evidence of healed primary tuberculosis.

Reactivation tuberculosis is associated with various radiographic manifestations, including fibrocavitary apical disease, nodules, and pneumonic infiltrates. The usual location is in the apical or posterior segments of the upper lobes or in the superior segments of the lower lobes; up to 30% of patients may present with radiographic evidence of disease in other locations. This is especially true in elderly patients, in whom lower lobe infiltrates with or without pleural effusion are encountered with increasing frequency. Lower lung tuberculosis may masquerade as pneumonia or lung cancer. A "miliary" pattern (diffuse small nodular densities) can be seen with hematologic or lymphatic dissemination of the organism. Resolution of reactivation tuberculosis leaves characteristic radiographic findings. Dense nodules in the pulmonary hila, with or without obvious calcification, upper lobe fibronodular scarring, and bronchiectasis with volume loss are common findings.

In patients with early HIV infection, the radiographic features of tuberculosis resemble those in patients without HIV infection. In contrast, atypical radiographic features predominate in patients with late stage HIV infection. These patients often display lower lung zone, diffuse, or miliary infiltrates, pleural effusions, and involvement of hilar and, in particular, mediastinal lymph nodes.

D. SPECIAL EXAMINATIONS

The **tuberculin skin test** identifies individuals who have been infected with *M tuberculosis* but does not distinguish between active and latent infection. The test is used to evaluate a person who has symptoms of tuberculosis, an asymptomatic person who may be infected with *M tuberculosis* (eg, after contact exposure), or to establish the prevalence of tuberculous infection in a population. Routine testing of individuals at low risk for tuberculosis is not recommended. The Mantoux test is the preferred method: 0.1 mL of purified protein derivative (PPD) containing 5 tuberculin units is injected intradermally on the volar surface of the forearm using a 27-gauge needle on a tuberculin syringe. The transverse width in millimeters of induration at the skin test site should be measured after 48–72 hours. Table 9–12 summarizes the CDC criteria for interpretation of the Mantoux tuberculin skin test. A **tuberculin skin test conversion** is defined as an increase of ≥ 10 mm of induration within a 2-year period regardless of patient age.

In general, it takes 2–10 weeks after tuberculosis infection for a person to develop an immune response to PPD. Both false-positive and false-negative results occur. False-positive tuberculin skin test reactions occur in persons previously vaccinated against MTB with BCG (extract of *Mycobacterium bovis*) and in those infected with nontuberculous mycobacteria. False-negative tuberculin skin test reactions may result from improper testing technique, concurrent infections, malnutrition, advanced age, immunologic disorders, lymphoreticular malignancies, corticosteroid therapy, chronic renal failure, HIV infection, and fulminant tuberculosis. Some individuals with latent tuberculosis infection may have a negative skin test reaction when tested many years after exposure.

Serial testing may create a false impression of skin test conversion. Dormant mycobacterial sensitivity is sometimes restored by the antigenic challenge of the initial skin test. This phenomenon is called "boosting." A two-step testing procedure is used to reduce the likelihood that a boosted tuberculin reaction will be misinterpreted as a recent infection. Following a negative tuberculin skin test, the person is retested in 1–3 weeks. If the second test is negative, the person is uninfected or anergic; if positive, a boosted reaction is likely. Two-step testing should be used for the initial tuberculin skin testing of individuals who will be tested repeatedly, such as health care workers. Anergy testing is not recommended for routine use to distinguish a true-negative result from anergy. Poor anergy test standardization and lack of outcome data limit the evaluation of its effectiveness. Interpretation of the tuberculin skin test in persons who have previously received BCG vaccination is the same as in those who have not had BCG.

Table 9–12. Classification of positive tuberculin skin test reactions.[1,2]

Reaction Size	Group
> 5 mm	1. HIV-positive persons. 2. Recent contacts of individuals with active tuberculosis. 3. Persons with fibrotic changes on chest x-rays suggestive of prior tuberculosis. 4. Patients with organ transplants and other immunosuppressed patients (receiving the equivalent of > 15 mg/d of prednisone for 1 month or more).
≥ 10 mm	1. Recent immigrants (< 5 years) from countries with a high prevalence of tuberculosis (eg, Asia, Africa, Latin America). 2. HIV-negative injection drug users. 3. Mycobacteriology laboratory personnel. 4. Residents of and employees[3] in the following high-risk congregate settings: correctional institutions; nursing homes and other long-term facilities for the elderly; hospitals and other health care facilities; residential facilities for AIDS patients; and homeless shelters. 5. Persons with the following medical conditions that increase the risk of tuberculosis: gastrectomy, ≥ 10% below ideal body weight, jejunoileal bypass, diabetes mellitus, silicosis, chronic renal failure, some hematologic disorders, (eg leukemias, lymphomas), and other specific malignancies (eg, carcinoma of the head or neck and lung). 6. Children < 4 years of age or infants, children, and adolescents exposed to adults at high risk.
≥ 15 mm	1. Persons with no risk factors for tuberculosis.

[1]Adapted from: Screening for tuberculosis and tuberculosis infection in high-risk populations: recommendations of the Advisory Council for the Elimination of Tuberculosis. MMWR Morb Mortal Wkly Rep 1995;44(RR-11):19.

[2]A tuberculin skin test reaction is considered positive if the transverse diameter of the indurated area reaches the size required for the specific group. All other reactions are considered negative.

[3]For persons who are otherwise at low risk and are tested at entry into employment, a reaction of > 15 mm induration is considered positive.

Novel in vitro methods promise significant changes in the identification of persons with latent *M tuberculosis* infection. Potential advantages of in vitro testing include reduced variability and subjectivity associated with placing and reading the PPD, fewer false-positive results from prior BCG vaccination, and better discrimination of positive responses due to nontuberculous mycobacteria.

Persons with concomitant HIV and tuberculosis infection usually respond best when the HIV infection is treated concurrently. In some cases, prolonged antituberculous therapy may be warranted. Therefore, all patients with tuberculosis infection should be tested for HIV within 2 months after diagnosis.

Treatment

A. GENERAL MEASURES

The goals of therapy are to eliminate all tubercle bacilli from an infected individual while avoiding the emergence of clinically significant drug resistance. The basic principles of antituberculosis treatment are (1) to administer multiple drugs to which the organisms are susceptible; (2) to add at least two new antituberculous agents to a regimen when treatment failure is suspected; (3) to provide the safest, most effective therapy in the shortest period of time; and (4) to ensure adherence to therapy.

All suspected and confirmed cases of tuberculosis should be reported promptly to local and state public health authorities. Public health departments will perform case investigations on sources and patient contacts to determine if other individuals with untreated, infectious tuberculosis are present in the community. They can identify infected contacts eligible for treatment of latent tuberculous infection, and ensure that a plan for monitoring adherence to therapy is established for each patient with tuberculosis. Patients with tuberculosis should be treated by physicians who are skilled in the management of this infection. Clinical expertise is especially important in cases of drug-resistant tuberculosis.

Nonadherence to antituberculous treatment is a major cause of treatment failure, continued transmission of tuberculosis, and the development of drug resistance. Adherence to treatment can be improved by providing detailed patient education about tuberculosis and its treatment in addition to a case manager who oversees all aspects of an individual patient's care. **Directly observed therapy (DOT),** which requires that a health care worker physically observe the patient ingest antituberculous medications in the home, clinic, hospital, or elsewhere, also improves adherence to treatment. The importance of direct observation of therapy cannot be overemphasized. The Centers for Disease Control and Prevention recommends DOT for all patients with drug-resistant tuberculosis and for those receiving intermittent (twice- or thrice-weekly) therapy.

Hospitalization for initial therapy of tuberculosis is not necessary for most patients. It should be considered if a patient is incapable of self-care or is likely to expose new, susceptible individuals to tuberculosis. Hospitalized patients with active disease require a private room with appropriate ventilation until tubercle bacilli are no longer found in their sputum ("smear-negative") on three consecutive smears taken on separate days.

Table 9–13. Characteristics of antituberculous drugs.[1]

Drug	Most Common Side Effects	Tests for Side Effects	Drug Interactions	Remarks
Isoniazid	Peripheral neuropathy, hepatitis, rash, mild CNS effects.	AST and ALT; neurologic examination.	Phenytoin (synergistic); disulfiram.	Bactericidal to both extracellular and intracellular organisms. Pyridoxine, 10 mg orally daily as prophylaxis for neuritis; 50–100 mg orally daily as treatment.
Rifampin	Hepatitis, fever, rash, flu-like illness, gastrointestinal upset, bleeding problems, renal failure.	CBC, platelets, AST and ALT.	Rifampin inhibits the effect of oral contraceptives, quinidine, corticosteroids, warfarin, methadone, digoxin, oral hypoglycemics; aminosalicyclic acid may interfere with absorption of rifampin. Significant interactions with protease inhibitors and nonnucleoside reverse transcriptase inhibitors.	Bactericidal to all populations of organisms. Colors urine and other body secretions orange. Discoloring of contact lenses.
Pyrazinamide	Hyperuricemia, hepatotoxicity, rash, gastrointestinal upset, joint aches.	Uric acid, AST, ALT.	. . .	Bactericidal to intracellular organisms.
Ethambutol	Optic neuritis (reversible with discontinuance of drug; rare at 15 mg/kg); rash.	Red-green color discrimination and visual acuity (difficult to test in children under 3 years of age).	. . .	Bacteriostatic to both intracellular and extracellular organisms. Mainly used to inhibit development of resistant mutants. Use with caution in renal disease or when ophthalmologic testing is not feasible.
Streptomycin	Eighth nerve damage, nephrotoxicity.	Vestibular function (audiograms); BUN and creatinine.	Neuromuscular blocking agents may be potentiated and cause prolonged paralysis.	Bactericidal to extracellular organisms. Use with caution in older patients or those with renal disease.

[1]See also Chapter 37.

Additional treatment considerations can be found in Chapter 33. Characteristics of antituberculous drugs are provided in Table 9–13 and in Chapter 37. More complete information can be obtained from the Centers for Disease Control and Prevention's Division of Tuberculosis Elimination Web site at http://www.cdc.gov/nchstp/tb/.

B. TREATMENT OF TUBERCULOSIS FOR HIV-NEGATIVE PERSONS

Most patients with previously untreated pulmonary tuberculosis can be effectively treated with either a 6-month or a 9-month regimen, though the 6-month regimen is preferred. The initial phase of a 6-month regimen consists of 2 months of daily isoniazid, rifampin, and pyrazinamide. In areas where the prevalence of isoniazid resistance is 4% or higher, ethambutol or streptomycin should also be administered daily

to prevent the development of drug resistance. If the MTB isolate is susceptible to isoniazid and rifampin, the second phase of therapy consists of isoniazid and rifampin for a minimum of 4 additional months, with treatment to extend at least 3 months beyond documentation of conversion of sputum cultures to negative for MTB. If directly observed therapy is used, medications may be given intermittently using one of the following regimens:

(1) Daily isoniazid, rifampin, pyrazinamide, and ethambutol or streptomycin for 2 months, followed by isoniazid and rifampin two or three times each week for 4 months if susceptibility to isoniazid and rifampin is demonstrated.

(2) Daily isoniazid, rifampin, pyrazinamide, and ethambutol or streptomycin for 2 weeks, then administration of the same agents twice weekly for

6 weeks followed by administration of isoniazid and rifampin twice each week for 4 months if susceptibility to isoniazid and rifampin is demonstrated.

(3) Thrice-weekly administration of isoniazid, rifampin, pyrazinamide, and ethambutol or streptomycin for 6 months.

Patients who cannot or should not (eg, pregnant women) take pyrazinamide should receive daily isoniazid and rifampin along with streptomycin (except in pregnant women) or ethambutol for 4–8 weeks. If susceptibility to isoniazid and rifampin is demonstrated or drug resistance is unlikely, then streptomycin or ethambutol can be discontinued and isoniazid and rifampin may be given two times a week for a total of 9 months therapy. If drug resistance is a concern, patients should receive isoniazid, rifampin, and either streptomycin (except in pregnant women) or ethambutol for 9 months. Patients with smear- and culture-negative disease (ie, pulmonary tuberculosis diagnosed on clinical grounds) and patients for whom drug susceptibility testing is not available can be treated with 6 months of isoniazid and rifampin combined with pyrazinamide for the first 2 months. This regimen assumes low prevalence of drug resistance.

When a twice-weekly or thrice-weekly regimen is used instead of a daily regimen, the dosages of isoniazid, pyrazinamide, and ethambutol or streptomycin must be increased. Recommended dosages for the initial treatment of tuberculosis are listed in Table 9–14. Fixed-dose combinations of isoniazid and rifampin (Rifamate) and of isoniazid, rifampin, and pyrazinamide (Rifater) are available to simplify treatment. Single tablets improve compliance but are more expensive than the individual drugs purchased separately.

C. Treatment of Tuberculosis in HIV-Positive Persons

Management of tuberculosis is rendered even more complex in patients with concomitant HIV disease. Experts in the management of both tuberculosis and HIV disease should be involved in the care of such patients. The Centers for Disease Control and Prevention (CDC) has published detailed recommendations for the treatment of tuberculosis in HIV-positive patients. This document can be obtained by calling 800-843-6356 or by accessing the CDC Web site at http://www.cdc.gov/epo/mmwr/preview/mmwrhtml/00055357.htm.

The basic approach to HIV-positive patients with tuberculosis is similar to that detailed above for patients without HIV disease. Additional considerations in HIV-positive patients include (1) longer duration of therapy and (2) drug interactions between rifamycin derivatives such as rifampin and rifabutin, used to treat tuberculosis, and some of the protease inhibitors and nonnucleoside reverse transcriptase inhibitors (NNRTIs), used to treat HIV. Directly observed therapy should be used for all HIV-positive tuberculosis patients. Pyridoxine (vitamin B_6), 25–50 mg orally each day, should be administered to all HIV-positive patients being treated with isoniazid to reduce central and peripheral nervous system side effects.

D. Treatment of Drug-Resistant Tuberculosis

Patients with drug-resistant MTB infection require careful supervision and management. Clinicians who are unfamiliar with the treatment of drug-resistant tuberculosis should seek expert advice. Tuberculosis resistant only to isoniazid can be successfully treated with a 6-month regimen of rifampin, pyrazinamide, and ethambutol or streptomycin or a 12-month regi-

Table 9–14. Recommended dosages for the initial treatment of tuberculosis.

Drugs	Daily	Cost[1]	Twice a Week[2]	Cost[1]/wk	Three Times a Week[2]	Cost[1]/wk
Isoniazid	5 mg/kg Max: 300 mg/dose	$0.08/300 mg	15 mg/kg Max: 900 mg/dose	$0.48	15 mg/kg Max: 900 mg/dose	$0.72
Rifampin	10 mg/kg Max: 600 mg/dose	$3.80/600 mg	10 mg/kg Max: 600 mg/dose	$7.60	10 mg/kg Max: 600 mg/dose	$11.40
Pyrazinamide	15–30 mg/kg Max: 2 g/dose	$3.68/2 g	50–70 mg/kg Max: 4 g/dose	$14.72	50–70 mg/kg Max: 3 g/dose	$16.56
Ethambutol	5–25 mg/kg Max: 2.5 g/dose	$8.95/2.5 g	50 mg/kg Max: 2.5 g/dose	$17.90	25–30 mg/kg Max: 2.5 g/dose	$26.85
Streptomycin	15 mg/kg Max: 1 g/dose	$6.90/1 g	25–30 mg/kg Max: 1.5 g/dose	$27.60	25–30 mg/kg Max: 1.5 g/dose	$41.40

[1]Cost to pharmacist (average wholesale price, generic when possible) for quantity listed. Source: *Drug Topics Red Book,* March 2002; Vol. 21, No. 3.
[2]All intermittent dosing regimens should be used with directly observed therapy.

men of rifampin and ethambutol. When isoniazid resistance is documented during a 9-month regimen without pyrazinamide, isoniazid should be discontinued. If ethambutol was part of the initial regimen, rifampin and ethambutol should be continued for a minimum of 12 months. If ethambutol was not part of the initial regimen, susceptibility tests should be repeated and two other drugs to which the organism is susceptible should be added. Treatment of MTB isolates resistant to agents other than isoniazid and treatment of drug resistance in HIV patients require expert consultation.

Multidrug-resistant tuberculosis (MDRTB) calls for an individualized daily directly observed treatment plan under the supervision of a clinician experienced in the management of this entity. Treatment regimens are based on the patient's overall status and the results of susceptibility studies. Most MDRTB isolates are resistant to at least isoniazid and rifampin and require a minimum of three drugs to which the organism is susceptible. These regimens are continued until culture conversion is documented, and then a two-drug regimen is then continued for at least another 12 months. Some experts recommend at least 18–24 months of a three-drug regimen.

E. Treatment of Extrapulmonary Tuberculosis

In most cases, regimens that are effective for treating pulmonary tuberculosis are also effective for treating extrapulmonary disease. However, many experts recommend 9 months of therapy when miliary, meningeal, or bone and joint disease is present. Treatment of skeletal tuberculosis is enhanced by early surgical drainage and debridement of necrotic bone. Corticosteroid therapy has been shown to help prevent cardiac constriction from tuberculous pericarditis and to reduce neurologic complications from tuberculous meningitis.

F. Treatment of Pregnant or Lactating Women

Tuberculosis in pregnancy is usually treated with isoniazid, rifampin, and ethambutol. Ethambutol can be excluded if isoniazid resistance is unlikely. Therapy is continued for 9 months. Since the risk of teratogenicity with pyrazinamide has not been clearly defined, pyrazinamide should be used only if resistance to other drugs is documented and susceptibility to pyrazinamide is likely. Streptomycin is contraindicated in pregnancy because it may cause congenital deafness. Pregnant women taking isoniazid should receive pyridoxine (vitamin B_6), 10–25 mg orally once a day, to prevent peripheral neuropathy.

Small concentrations of antituberculous drugs are present in breast milk and are not known to be harmful to nursing newborns. Therefore, breast feeding is not contraindicated while receiving antituberculosis therapy.

G. Treatment Monitoring

Adults should have measurements of serum bilirubin, hepatic enzymes, urea nitrogen, creatinine, and a complete blood count (including platelets) before starting chemotherapy for tuberculosis. Visual acuity and red-green color vision tests are recommended before initiation of ethambutol and serum uric acid before starting pyrazinamide. Audiometry should be performed if streptomycin therapy is initiated.

Routine monitoring of laboratory tests for evidence of drug toxicity during therapy is not recommended. Monthly questioning for symptoms of drug toxicity is advised. Patients should be educated about common side effects of antituberculous medications and instructed to seek medical attention should these symptoms occur. Monthly follow-up of outpatients is recommended, including sputum smear and culture for *M tuberculosis* until cultures convert to negative. Patients with negative sputum cultures after 2 months of treatment should have at least one additional sputum smear and culture performed at the end of therapy. Patients with MDRTB should have sputum cultures performed monthly during the entire course of treatment. A chest radiograph at the end of therapy provides a useful baseline for any future films.

Patients whose cultures do not become negative or whose symptoms do not resolve despite 3 months of therapy should be evaluated for drug-resistant organisms and for nonadherence to the treatment regimen. Directly observed therapy is required for the remainder of the treatment regimen, and the addition of at least two drugs not previously given should be considered pending repeat drug susceptibility testing. The clinician should seek expert assistance if drug resistance is newly found, if the patient remains symptomatic, or if smears or cultures remain positive.

Patients with only a clinical diagnosis of pulmonary tuberculosis (smears and cultures negative for *M tuberculosis*) whose symptoms and radiographic abnormalities are unchanged after 3 months of treatment usually either have another process or have had tuberculosis in the past.

H. Treatment of Latent Tuberculosis

Treatment of latent tuberculous infection is essential to controlling and eliminating tuberculosis in the United States. Treatment of latent tuberculous infection substantially reduces the risk that infection will progress to active disease. Targeted testing is used to identify persons who are at high risk for tuberculosis and who stand to benefit from treatment of latent infection. Table 9–12 defines high-risk groups and gives the tuberculin skin test criteria for treatment of latent tuberculous infection. It is essential that each person who meets the criteria for treatment of latent tuberculous infection undergo a careful assessment to exclude active disease. A history of past treatment for tuberculosis and contraindications to treatment should be sought. All patients at risk for HIV infection should be tested for HIV. Patients suspected of having tuberculosis should receive one of the recommended multidrug regimens for active disease until the diagnosis is confirmed or excluded.

Some close contacts of persons with active tuberculosis should be evaluated for treatment of latent tuberculous infection despite a negative tuberculin skin test reaction (< 5 mm induration). These include immunosuppressed persons and those who may develop disease quickly after tuberculous infection. Close contacts who have a negative tuberculin skin test reaction on initial testing should be retested 10–12 weeks later.

Several treatment regimens for both HIV-negative and HIV-positive persons are available for the treatment of latent tuberculous infection:

(1) Isoniazid: A 9-month regimen (minimum of 270 doses administered within 12 months) is considered optimal. Dosing options include a daily dose of 300 mg or twice-weekly doses of 15 mg/kg. Persons at risk of developing isoniazid-associated peripheral neuropathy (diabetes mellitus, uremia, malnutrition, alcoholism, HIV infection, pregnancy, seizure disorder) may be given supplemental pyridoxine (vitamin B_6), 10–50 mg/d.

(2) Rifampin and pyrazinamide: A 2-month regimen (60 doses administered within 3 months) of daily rifampin (10 mg/kg up to a maximum dose of 600 mg) and pyrazinamide (15–20 mg/kg up to a maximum dose of 2 g) is recommended.

(3) Rifampin: Patients who cannot tolerate isoniazid or pyrazinamide can be considered for a 4-month regimen (minimum of 120 doses administered within 6 months) of rifampin. HIV-positive patients given rifampin who are receiving protease inhibitors or nonnucleoside reverse transcriptase inhibitors require management by experts in both tuberculosis and HIV disease (see Treatment of Tuberculosis for HIV-Positive Persons, above).

Contacts of persons with isoniazid-resistant, rifampin-sensitive tuberculosis should receive a 2-month regimen of rifampin and pyrazinamide or a 4 month regimen of daily rifampin alone. Contacts of persons with MDRTB should receive two drugs to which the infecting organism has demonstrated susceptibility. Tuberculin skin test-negative and HIV-negative contacts may be observed without treatment or treated for 6 months. HIV-positive contacts should be treated for 12 months. All contacts of persons with MDRTB should have 2 years of follow up regardless of treatment.

Persons with a positive tuberculin skin test (≥ 5 mm of induration) and fibrotic lesions suggestive of old tuberculosis on chest radiographs who have no evidence of active disease and no history of treatment for tuberculosis should receive 9 months of isoniazid—or 2 months of rifampin and pyrazinamide—or 4 months of rifampin (with or without isoniazid). Pregnant or breast feeding women with latent tuberculosis should receive either daily or twice-weekly isoniazid with pyridoxine (vitamin B_6).

Baseline laboratory testing is indicated for patients at risk for liver disease, patients with HIV infection, women who are pregnant or within 3 months of delivery, and persons who use alcohol regularly. Patients receiving treatment for latent tuberculous infection should be evaluated once a month to assess for signs and symptoms of active tuberculosis and hepatitis and for adherence to their treatment regimen. Routine laboratory testing during treatment is indicated for those with abnormal baseline laboratory tests and for those at risk for developing liver disease.

Vaccine bacillus Calmette-Guérin (BCG) is an antimycobacterial vaccine developed from an attenuated strain of *Mycobacterium bovis*. Millions of individuals worldwide have been vaccinated with BCG. However, it is not generally recommended in the United States because of the low prevalence of tuberculous infection, the vaccine's interference with the ability to determine latent tuberculous infection using tuberculin skin test reactivity, and its variable effectiveness against pulmonary tuberculosis. BCG vaccination in the United States should only be undertaken after consultation with local health officials and experts in the management of tuberculosis. Vaccination of health care workers should be considered on an individual basis in settings in which a high percentage of tuberculosis patients are infected with strains resistant to both isoniazid and rifampin; in which transmission of such drug-resistant *M tuberculosis* and subsequent infection are likely; and in which comprehensive tuberculous infection-control precautions have been implemented but have not been successful. The BCG vaccine is contraindicated in persons with impaired immune responses due to disease or medications.

Prognosis

Almost all properly treated patients with tuberculosis can be cured. Relapse rates are less than 5% with current regimens. The main cause of treatment failure is nonadherence to therapy.

Diagnostic standards and classification of tuberculosis in adults and children. American Thoracic Society and The Centers for Disease Control and Prevention. Am J Respir Crit Care Med 2000;161(4 Part 1):1376. [PMID: 10764337]

Horsburgh CR et al: Practice guidelines for the treatment of tuberculosis. Clin Infect Dis 2000;31:633. [PMID: 11017808] (Guidelines for treatment of active and latent tuberculosis from the Infectious Disease Society of America.)

Mazurek GH et al: Comparison of a whole-blood interferon gamma assay with tuberculin skin testing for detecting latent *Mycobacterium tuberculosis* infection. JAMA 2001; 286:1740. [PMID: 11594899]

Small PM et al: Management of tuberculosis in the United States. N Engl J Med 2001;345:189. [PMID: 11463015] (Current review.)

Targeted tuberculin testing and treatment of latent tuberculosis infection. Am J Respir Crit Care Med 2000;161(4 Part 2):S221. [PMID: 10764341] (Joint Statement of the American Thoracic Society and the Centers for Disease Control and Prevention, endorsed by the Council of the Infectious Diseases Society of America.)

Volmink J et al: Directly observed therapy and treatment adherence. Lancet 2000;355:1345. [PMID: 10776760] (Meta-analysis confirms efficacy of directly observed therapy but raises a question about how it works.)

PULMONARY DISEASE CAUSED BY NONTUBERCULOUS MYCOBACTERIA

ESSENTIALS OF DIAGNOSIS

- Chronic cough, sputum production, and fatigue; less commonly: malaise, dyspnea, fever, hemoptysis, and weight loss.
- Parenchymal infiltrates on chest radiograph, often with thin-walled cavities, that spread contiguously and often involve overlying pleura.
- Isolation of nontuberculous mycobacteria in a sputum culture.

General Considerations

Mycobacteria other than *M tuberculosis*—"atypical" mycobacteria, or nontuberculous mycobacteria (NTM)—are ubiquitous in water and soil and have been isolated from tap water. There appears to be a continuing increase in the number and prevalence of NTM species. Marked geographic variability exists, both in the NTM species responsible for disease and in the prevalence of disease. These organisms are not considered communicable from person to person, have distinct laboratory characteristics, and are often resistant to most antituberculous drugs. See Chapter 33 for further information.

Definition & Pathogenesis

The diagnosis of lung disease caused by NTM is based on a combination of clinical, radiographic, and bacteriologic criteria and the exclusion of other diseases that can resemble the condition. Specific diagnostic criteria are discussed below. Complementary data are important for diagnosis because NTM organisms can reside in or colonize the airways without causing clinical disease, especially in patients with AIDS, and many patients have preexisting lung disease that may make their chest radiographs abnormal.

Mycobacterium avium complex (MAC) is the most frequent cause of NTM pulmonary disease in humans in the United States. *M kansasii* is the next most frequent pulmonary pathogen. Other NTM causes of pulmonary disease include *M abscessus, M xenopi,* and *M malmoense;* the list of more unusual etiologic NTM species is long. Most NTM cause a chronic, slowly progressive pulmonary infection that resembles tuberculosis but tends to progress more slowly. Disseminated disease is rare in immunocompetent hosts; however, disseminated MAC disease is common in patients with AIDS.

Clinical Findings

A. SYMPTOMS AND SIGNS

Most patients with NTM infection experience a chronic cough, sputum production, and fatigue. Less common symptoms include malaise, dyspnea, fever, hemoptysis, and weight loss. Symptoms from coexisting lung disease (commonly COPD, bronchiectasis, previous mycobacterial disease, cystic fibrosis, and pneumoconiosis) may confound the evaluation.

Common physical findings include fever and altered breath sounds, including rales or rhonchi.

B. LABORATORY FINDINGS

The diagnosis of NTM infection rests on recovery of the pathogen from cultures. Sputum cultures positive for atypical mycobacteria do not in themselves prove infection because NTM may exist as saprophytes colonizing the airways or may be environmental contaminants. Bronchial washings are considered to be more sensitive than expectorated sputum samples; however, their specificity for clinical disease is not known.

Bacteriologic criteria have been proposed based on studies of patients with cavitary disease with MAC or *M kansasii.* Diagnostic criteria in HIV-seronegative or immunocompetent hosts include the following: (1) at least three sputum or bronchial wash samples within a 1-year period with the following findings: three positive cultures with negative AFB smears or two positive cultures and one positive AFB smear; (2) if expectorated sputum samples are not available, a single bronchial wash culture with 2+ to 4+ growth or any positive culture plus a 2+ to 4+ AFB smear. The diagnosis can also be established by demonstrating NTM in a lung biopsy or bronchial wash plus histopathologic changes such as granulomatous inflammation in a lung biopsy. Rapid species identification of some NTM is possible using DNA probes or high-pressure liquid chromatography. Criteria are less stringent for patients with severe immune suppression. HIV-infected patients may show significant MAC growth on culture of bronchial washings without clinical infection, and, therefore, HIV patients being evaluated for MAC infection must be considered individually.

In general, drug susceptibility testing on cultures of NTM is not recommended except for the following NTM: (1) *M kansasii* and rifampin; (2) rapid growers (such as *M fortuitum, M chelonei, M abscessus*) and amikacin, doxycycline, imipenem, fluoroquinolones, clarithromycin, cefoxitin, and a sulfonamide.

C. IMAGING

Chest radiographic findings include infiltrates that are progressive or persist for at least 2 months, cavitary lesions, and multiple nodular densities. The cavities are often thin-walled and have less surrounding parenchymal infiltrate than is commonly seen with MTB infections. Evidence of contiguous spread and pleural involvement is often present. High-resolution computed tomography of the chest may show multiple small nodules with or without multifocal bronchiectasis. Progression of pulmonary infiltrates during therapy or lack of radiographic improvement over time are poor prognostic signs and also raise concerns about secondary or alternative pulmonary processes. Clearing of pulmonary infiltrates due to NTM is slow.

Treatment

Treatment regimens and responses vary with the species of NTM. Disease caused by *M kansasii* responds well to drug therapy. A daily regimen of rifampin, isoniazid, and ethambutol for at least 18 months with a minimum of 12 months of negative cultures is usually successful.

The treatment of the immunocompetent patient with MAC infection is controversial and largely empirical. Traditional chemotherapeutic regimens have taken an aggressive approach using a combination of agents, but these have been associated with a high incidence of drug-induced side effects. Adherence to such regimens is also difficult. Non-HIV-infected patients with MAC pulmonary disease usually receive a combination of daily clarithromycin or azithromycin, rifampin or rifabutin, and ethambutol. Streptomycin is considered for the first 2 months as tolerated. The optimal duration of treatment is unknown, but therapy should be continued for 12 months after sputum conversion. Medical treatment is initially successful in about two-thirds of cases, but relapses after treatment are common; long-term benefit is demonstrated in about half of all patients. Those who do not respond favorably generally have active but stable disease. Surgical resection is an alternative for the patient with progressive disease that responds poorly to chemotherapy; the success rate with surgical therapy is good.

Diagnosis and treatment of disease caused by nontuberculous mycobacteria. Am J Respir Crit Care Med 1997;156(2 Part 2):S1. [PMID: 9279284] (Reviews diagnostic criteria and treatment approaches for nontuberculous mycobacterial disease.)

Holland SM. Nontuberculous mycobacteria. Am J Med Sci 2001;321:49. [PMID: 11202480] (Current review.)

■ PULMONARY NEOPLASMS

SCREENING FOR LUNG CANCER

Periodic evaluation of asymptomatic people at high risk for lung cancer is an attractive strategy without demonstrated benefit. Available evidence from the Mayo Lung Project suggests that serial chest radiographs can identify a significant number of early stage malignancies and that screened patients have an improved 5-year survival from their lung cancers. However, neither disease-specific mortality from lung cancer nor all-cause mortality is affected by screening. Three large randomized clinical trials published between 1984 and 1986 came to similar conclusions. Since then, screening for lung cancer has not been recommended by any major advisory group. The illusory benefits of screening have been attributed to lead time, length, and overdiagnosis biases.

The availability of rapid acquisition, low-dose spiral computed tomography (CT) has rekindled enthusiasm for lung cancer screening. CT is a very sensitive test. Compared with chest radiography, chest CT identifies between four and ten times the number of asymptomatic lung malignancies. CT may also increase the number of false-positive tests, unnecessary diagnostic procedures, and overdiagnosis. A mortality benefit remains to be proved.

Black WC: Should this patient be screened for cancer? Eff Clin Pract 1999;2:86. [PMID: 10538481] (A review of the principles of screening using helical CT and lung cancer as the clinical setting in which to apply a decision analysis model. Addresses the importance of mortality as an end point and the difficulty in designing such studies.)

Marcus PM. Lung cancer screening: an update. J Clin Oncol 2001;19(18 Suppl):83. [PMID: 11560979] (Review of issues with description of the current Lung Screening Study.)

Patz EF et al: Screening for lung cancer. N Engl J Med 2000;343:1627. [PMID: 11096172] (Detailed, scholarly analysis of a controversial topic.)

SOLITARY PULMONARY NODULE

A solitary pulmonary nodule, sometimes referred to as a "coin lesion," is a < 3 cm isolated, rounded opacity on the chest radiograph outlined by normal lung and not associated with infiltrate, atelectasis, or adenopathy. Most are asymptomatic and represent an unexpected finding on chest radiography. The finding is important because it carries a significant risk of malignancy. The frequency of malignancy in surgical series ranges from 10% to 68% depending on patient population. Most benign nodules are infectious granulomas. **Benign neoplasms** such as hamartomas account for less than 5% of solitary nodules.

The goal of evaluation is to identify and resect malignant tumors in patients who stand to benefit from resection while avoiding invasive procedures in benign disease. The task is to identify nodules with a sufficiently high probability of malignancy to warrant biopsy or resection or a sufficiently low probability of malignancy to justify observation.

Symptoms alone rarely establish etiology, but clinical and radiographic data can be used to assess the probability of malignancy. The patient's age is important. Malignant nodules are rare in persons under age 30. Above age 30, the likelihood of malignancy increases with age. Smokers are at increased risk, and the likelihood of malignancy increases with the number of cigarettes smoked daily. Patients with a prior malignancy have a higher likelihood of having a malignant solitary nodule.

The first and most important step in the radiographic evaluation is to review old radiographs. Comparison with prior studies allows estimation of doubling time, which is an important marker for malignancy. Rapid progression (doubling time less than 30 days) suggests infection; long-term stability (doubling time over 465 days) suggests benignity. Certain radiographic features help in estimating the probability of malignancy. Increasing size is correlated with malignancy. A recent study of solitary nodules identified by CT scan showed a 1% malignancy rate in those 2–5 mm, 24% in 6–10 mm, 33% in 11–20 mm and 80% in 21–45 mm. The appearance of a smooth, well-defined edge is characteristic of a benign process. Ill defined margins or a lobular appearance suggest malignancy. A high-resolution computed tomographic (HRCT) finding of spiculated margins or a peripheral halo are both highly associated with malignancy. Calcification and its pattern are also helpful clues. Benign lesions tend to have dense calcification in a central or laminated pattern. Malignant lesions are associated with sparser calcification that is typically stippled or eccentric. Cavitary lesions with thick (> 16 mm) walls are much more likely to be malignant. HRCT offers better resolution of these characteristics than chest radiography and is more likely to detect lymphadenopathy or the presence of multiple lesions. HRCT is indicated in any suspicious solitary pulmonary nodule.

Treatment

Based on clinical and radiologic data, the clinician should assign a specific probability of malignancy to the lesion. The decision whether and how to obtain a diagnostic biopsy depends on the interpretation of this probability in light of the patient's unique clinical situation. The probabilities in parentheses below represent guidelines only and should not be interpreted as prescriptive.

In the case of solitary pulmonary nodules, a continuous probability function may be grouped into three categories. In patients with a low probability (< 8%) of malignancy (eg, age under 30, lesions stable for more than 2 years, characteristic pattern of benign calcification), watchful waiting is appropriate. Management consists of serial radiographs every 3 months for 1 year and then every 6 months for a second year. Three-dimensional reconstruction of HRCT images may provide a more sensitive test for growth. These techniques are in research trials.

Patients with a high probability (> 70%) of malignancy should proceed directly to resection provided there are no contraindications to surgery. Biopsies rarely yield a specific benign diagnosis and are not indicated.

Optimal management of patients with an intermediate probability of malignancy (8–70%) remains controversial. The traditional approach is to obtain a diagnostic biopsy either through transthoracic needle aspiration (TTNA) or bronchoscopy. Bronchoscopy yields a diagnosis in 10–80% of procedures depending on the size of the nodule and its location. Complications are generally rare. TTNA has a higher diagnostic yield, reported to be between 50% and 97%. The yield is strongly operator-dependent, however, and is affected by the location and size of the lesion. Complications are higher than bronchoscopy, with pneumothorax occurring in up to 30% of patients.

Disappointing diagnostic yields and a high false-negative rate (up to 25–30% in TTNA) have prompted alternative approaches. Several new imaging techniques may help to improve the specificity of HRCT in excluding malignancy. Malignant nodules tend to be more highly vascularized and therefore show increased enhancement on HRCT following the intravenous infusion of iodine-containing contrast media. Sensitivity and specificity appear promising but await validation. Positron emission tomography (PET) detects increased glucose metabolism within malignant lesions with high sensitivity (85–95%) and specificity (70–85%). Many diagnostic algorithms have incorporated PET into the assessment of patients with inconclusive HRCT findings. PET has several drawbacks, however: resolution below 1 cm is poor, the test is expensive, and availability remains limited. Sputum cytology is highly specific but lacks sensitivity. It is used in central lesions and in patients who are poor candidates for invasive diagnostic procedures. Researchers have attempted to improve the sensitivity of sputum cytology through the use of monoclonal antibodies to proteins that are up-regulated in pulmonary malignancies. Such tests offer promise but remain research tools at this time.

Video-assisted thoracoscopic surgery (VATS) offers a more aggressive approach to diagnosis. VATS is more invasive than bronchoscopy or TTNA but is associated with less postoperative pain, shorter hospital stays, and more rapid return to function than traditional thoracotomy. These advantages have led some centers to recommend VATS resection of all solitary pulmonary nodules with intermediate probability of malignancy. In some cases, surgeons will remove the nodule and evaluate it in the operating room with frozen section. If the nodule is malignant, they will proceed to lobectomy and lymph node sampling, either thoracoscopically or through conversion to standard thoracotomy.

Gould MK et al: Accuracy of positron emission tomography for diagnosis of pulmonary nodules and mass lesions. A meta-analysis. JAMA 2001;285:914. [PMID: 11180735] (Detailed review concludes that PET scanning has high sensitivity and intermediate specificity for malignancy but that few data exist for nodules smaller than 1 cm.)

Gurney JW: Determining the likelihood of malignancy in solitary pulmonary nodules with Bayesian analysis. Part I. Theory.

Radiology 1993;186:405. [PMID: 8421743] (A classic article that provides a detailed quantitative review of clinical and radiographic factors affecting the likelihood of malignancy in solitary pulmonary nodules.)

Lacasse Y et al: Transthoracic needle aspiration biopsy for the diagnosis of localised pulmonary lesions: a meta-analysis. Thorax 1999;54:884. [PMID: 10491450] (A review from noted Canadian researchers concludes that transthoracic needle biopsy of intermediate-probability lung nodules is usually accurate enough to determine further therapy.)

Ost D et al: Evaluation and management of the solitary pulmonary nodule. Am J Respir Crit Care Med 2000;162:782. [PMID: 10988081] (Succinct, up-to-date review of epidemiology and management of solitary pulmonary nodules.)

BRONCHOGENIC CARCINOMA

ESSENTIALS OF DIAGNOSIS

- New cough, or change in chronic cough.
- Dyspnea, hemoptysis, anorexia, weight loss.
- Enlarging nodule or mass; persistent infiltrate, atelectasis, or pleural effusion on chest radiograph or CT scan.
- Cytologic or histologic findings of lung cancer in sputum, pleural fluid, or biopsy specimen.

General Considerations

Lung cancer is the leading cause of cancer deaths in both men and women. The American Cancer Society estimates 169,400 new diagnoses and 154,900 deaths from lung cancer in the USA in 2002, accounting for 13% of new cancer diagnoses and 28% of all cancer deaths. More Americans now die of lung cancer than of colon, breast, and prostate cancers combined. This dramatic increase in a previously reportable disease is causally related to exposure to carcinogens through inhalation of tobacco smoke. The causal connection between cigarettes and lung cancer is now established not only epidemiologically but also through identification of carcinogens in tobacco smoke and analysis of the effect of these carcinogens on specific oncogenes expressed in lung cancer. Even cigarette manufacturers no longer dispute the role of tobacco in this epidemic. Ninety percent of cases of lung cancer in men and 79% in women are directly attributable to cigarette smoking. Through the 1990s, mortality from lung cancer fell among men while it increased among women, reflecting changing patterns of tobacco use over the past 30 years (see Chapter 1). Other environmental risk factors for the development of lung cancer include exposure to environmental tobacco smoke, radon gas (among uranium miners and in areas where radium in the soil causes significant indoor air contamination), asbestos (60- to 100-fold increased risk in smokers with asbestos exposure), metals (arsenic, chromium, nickel, iron oxide), and industrial carcinogens (bischloromethyl ether). A familial predisposition to lung cancer is recognized. Certain diseases are associated with an increased risk of lung cancer, including pulmonary fibrosis, COPD, and sarcoidosis. Second primary lung cancers are more frequent in patients who survive their initial lung cancer.

The mean age at diagnosis of lung cancer is 60; it is unusual under the age of 40. Forty-one percent of patients diagnosed with lung cancer in 1997 survived for 1 year, compared with 34% in 1975. The combined 5-year survival rate for all stages of lung cancer was 15% in 1997, compared with 12% in 1974–76.

Four histologic types of bronchogenic carcinoma account for more than 90% of cases of primary lung cancer. **Squamous cell carcinoma** (25–35% of cases) arises from the bronchial epithelium, typically as a centrally located, intraluminal sessile or polypoid mass. Squamous cell tumors are more likely to present with hemoptysis and more frequently are diagnosed by sputum cytology. They spread locally and may be associated with hilar adenopathy and mediastinal widening on chest radiography. **Adenocarcinoma** (35–40% of cases) arises from mucus glands or, in the case of the **bronchioloalveolar cell carcinoma** (2% of cases), from any epithelial cell within or distal to the terminal bronchioles. Adenocarcinomas usually present as peripheral nodules or masses. Bronchioloalveolar cell carcinoma spreads intra-alveolarly and may present as an infiltrate or as single or multiple pulmonary nodules. **Large cell carcinoma** (5–10% of cases) is a heterogeneous group of relatively undifferentiated tumors that share large cells and do not fit into other categories. Large cell carcinomas typically have rapid doubling times and an aggressive clinical course. They present as central or peripheral masses. **Small cell carcinoma** (15–20% of cases) is a tumor of bronchial origin that typically begins centrally, infiltrating submucosally to cause narrowing or obstruction of the bronchus without a discrete luminal mass. Hilar and mediastinal abnormalities are common on chest radiography.

For purposes of staging and treatment, bronchogenic carcinoma is divided into small cell lung cancer (SCLC) and the other three types, conveniently labeled non-small cell lung cancer (NSCLC). This practical classification reflects different natural histories and different treatment. SCLC is prone to early hematogenous spread. It is rarely amenable to surgical resection and has a very aggressive course with a median survival (untreated) of 6–18 weeks. The three histologic categories comprising NSCLC spread more slowly. They may be cured in the early stages following resection, and they respond similarly to chemotherapy.

Clinical Findings

Lung cancer is symptomatic at diagnosis in 75–90% of patients. The clinical presentation depends on the type and location of the primary tumor, the extent of local spread, and the presence of distant metastases and any paraneoplastic syndromes.

A. Symptoms and Signs

Anorexia, weight loss, or asthenia occurs in 55–88% of patients presenting with a new diagnosis of lung cancer. Up to 60% of patients have a new cough or a change in a chronic cough; 6–31% have hemoptysis; and 25–40% complain of pain, sometimes nonspecific chest pain but often referable to bony metastases to the vertebrae, ribs, or pelvis. Local spread may cause endobronchial obstruction with atelectasis and postobstructive pneumonia, pleural effusion (12–33%), change in voice (compromise of the recurrent laryngeal nerve), superior vena cava syndrome (obstruction of the SVC with supraclavicular venous engorgement), and Horner's syndrome (ipsilateral ptosis, miosis, and anhidrosis from involvement of the inferior cervical ganglion and the paravertebral sympathetic chain). Distant metastases to the liver are associated with asthenia and weight loss. Brain metastases (10%; more common in adenocarcinoma) may present with headache, nausea, vomiting, seizures, or altered mental status.

Paraneoplastic syndromes are incompletely understood patterns of organ dysfunction related to immune-mediated or secretory effects of neoplasms (see Chapter 40). These syndromes occur in 10–20% of lung cancer patients. They may precede, accompany, or follow the diagnosis of lung cancer. They do not necessarily indicate metastatic disease. Digital clubbing is seen in up to 20% of patients at diagnosis. Fifteen percent of patients with small cell carcinoma will develop SIADH; 10% of patients with squamous cell carcinoma will develop hypercalcemia. Other common paraneoplastic syndromes include increased ACTH production, anemia, hypercoagulability, peripheral neuropathy, and the Eaton-Lambert myasthenia syndrome. Their recognition is important because treatment of the primary tumor may improve or resolve symptoms even when the cancer is not curable.

B. Laboratory Findings

The diagnosis of lung cancer rests on examination of a tissue or cytology specimen. Sputum cytology is highly specific but insensitive; the yield is highest when there are lesions in the central airways. Thoracentesis (sensitivity 50–65%) can be used to establish a diagnosis of lung cancer in patients with malignant pleural effusions. If cytologic examination of an adequate sample (50–100 mL) of pleural fluid is nondiagnostic, the procedure should be repeated once. If results remain negative, thoracoscopy is preferred to blind pleural biopsy. Fine needle aspiration of palpable supraclavicular or cervical lymph nodes is frequently diagnostic. Serum tumor markers are neither sensitive enough nor specific enough to aid in diagnosis.

Fiberoptic bronchoscopy allows visualization of the major airways, cytology brushing of visible lesions or lavage of lung segments with cytologic evaluation of specimens, direct biopsy of endobronchial abnormalities, blind transbronchial biopsy of the pulmonary parenchyma or peripheral nodules, and fine needle aspiration biopsy of mediastinal lymph nodes. Diagnostic yield varies widely (10–90%) depending on the size of the lesion and its location. Recent advances include fluorescence bronchoscopy, which improves the ability to identify early endobronchial lesions; and endoscopic ultrasound, which permits more accurate direction of fine needle aspiration. Transthoracic needle aspiration (TTNB) has a sensitivity between 50% and 97%. Mediastinoscopy, video-assisted thoracoscopic surgery (VATS), and thoracotomy are necessary in cases where less invasive techniques fail to yield a diagnosis.

C. Imaging

Nearly all patients with lung cancer have abnormal findings on chest radiography or CT scan. These findings are rarely specific for a particular diagnosis. Interpretation of characteristic findings in isolated nodules is described above (see Solitary Pulmonary Nodule).

D. Special Examinations

1. Staging—Accurate staging (Table 9–15) is crucial (1) to provide the clinician with information to guide treatment, (2) to provide the patient with accurate information regarding prognosis, and (3) to standardize entry criteria for clinical trials to allow interpretation of results.

There are two essential principles of staging NSCLC. First, the more extensive the disease, the worse the prognosis; and second, surgical resection offers the best and perhaps the only realistic hope for cure. Staging of NSCLC uses two integrated systems. The **TNM international staging system** attempts a physical description of the neoplasm: T describes the size and location of the primary tumor; N describes the presence and location of nodal metastases; and M refers to the presence or absence of distant metastases. These TNM stages are grouped into prognostic categories (stages I–IV) using the results of clinical trials. This classification is used to guide therapy. Many patients with stage I and stage II disease are cured through surgery. Patients with stage IIIB and stage IV disease do not benefit from surgery. Patients with stage IIIA disease have locally invasive disease that may benefit from surgery in certain circumstances.

Small cell lung cancer is not staged using the TNM system because micrometastases are assumed to be present on diagnosis. SCLC is divided into two categories: **limited disease** (30%), when the tumor is limited to the unilateral hemithorax (including contralateral mediastinal nodes); or **extensive disease**

Table 9–15. TNM staging for lung cancer.[1]

Stage	T	N	M	Description
0	Tis			Carcinoma in situ
IA	T1	N0	M0	Limited local disease without nodal or distant metastases
IB	T2	N0	M0	
IIA	T1	N1	M0	Limited local disease with ipsilateral hilar or peribronchial nodal involvement but not distant
IIB	T2	N1	M0	metastases *or*
	T3	N0	M0	Locally invasive disease without nodal or distant metastases
IIIA	T3	N1	M0	Orally invasive disease with ipsilateral or peribronchial nodal involvement but not distant metastases *or*
	T1–3	N2	M0	Limited or locally invasive disease with ipsilateral mediastinal or subcarinal nodal involvement but not distant metastases
IIIB	Any T	N3	M0	Any primary with contralateral mediastinal or hilar nodes, or ipsilateral scalene or supraclavicular nodes *or*
	T4	Any N	M0	Unresectable local invasion with any degree of adenopathy but no distant metastases; malignant pleural effusion
IV	Any T	Any N	M1	Distant metastases
Primary Tumor (T)				
TX				Primary tumor cannot be assessed; or tumor proved by the presence of malignant cells in sputum or bronchial washings but not visualized by imaging or bronchoscopy.
T0				No evidence of primary tumor.
Tis				Carcinoma in situ.
T1				A tumor ≤ 3 cm in greatest dimension, surrounded by lung or visceral pleura, and without evidence of invasion proximal to a lobar bronchus at bronchoscopy.
T2				A tumor > 3.0 cm in greatest dimension, or a tumor of any size that either involves a main bronchus (but is ≥ 2 cm distal to the carina), invades the visceral pleura, or has associated atelectasis or obstructive pneumonitis extending to the hilar region. Any associated atelectasis or obstructive pneumonitis must involve less than an entire lung.
T3				A tumor of any size with direct extension into the chest wall (including superior sulcus tumors), the diaphragm, the mediastinal pleura, or the parietal pericardium; or a tumor in the main bronchus < 2 cm distal to the carina without involving the carina; or associated atelectasis or obstructive pneumonitis of the entire lung.
T4				A tumor of any size with invasion of the mediastinum, heart, great vessels, trachea, esophagus, vertebral body, or carina; or with a malignant pleural or pericardial effusion; or with satellite tumor nodules within the ipsilateral lobe of the lung containing the primary tumor.
Regional Lymph Nodes (N)				
NX				Regional lymph nodes cannot be assessed.
N0				No demonstrable metastasis to regional lymph nodes.
N1				Metastasis to lymph nodes in the peribronchial or the ipsilateral hilar region, or both, including direct extension.
N2				Metastasis to ipsilateral mediastinal lymph nodes and/or subcarinal lymph nodes.
N3				Metastasis to contralateral mediastinal lymph nodes, contralateral hilar lymph nodes, ipsilateral or contralateral scalene or supraclavicular lymph nodes.
Distant Metastases (M)				
MX				Presence of distant metastasis cannot be assessed.
M0				No (known) distant metastasis.
M1				Distant metastasis present.

[1]Adapted from Mountain CF: Revisions in the international system for staging lung cancer. Chest 1997;111:1710.

(70%), when the tumor extends beyond the hemithorax (including pleural effusion). This scheme also guides therapy. Patients with limited SCLC benefit from thoracic radiation therapy in addition to chemotherapy and may benefit from prophylactic cranial radiation therapy.

For both SCLC and NSCLC, staging begins with a thorough history and physical examination. A complete examination is essential to exclude obvious metastatic disease to lymph nodes, skin, and bone. A detailed history is essential because the patient's performance status is a powerful predictor of disease course. All patients should have measurement of a complete blood count, electrolytes including calcium, creatinine, liver tests including LDH and alkaline phosphatase, and a chest radiograph. Further evaluation will follow the results of these tests. In general, screening asymptomatic lung cancer patients with CT and MRI imaging of the brain, radionuclide bone imaging, and abdominal CT imaging does not change patient outcomes. These tests should be targeted to specific symptoms and signs (see Table 9–16).

NSCLC patients being considered for surgery require meticulous evaluation to identify those with resectable disease. CT imaging is the most important modality for staging candidates for resection. A chest CT scan precisely defines the size of parenchymal lesions and identifies atelectatic lung or pleural effusions. However, CT imaging is less accurate at determining invasion of the chest wall (sensitivity 62%) or mediastinum (sensitivity 60–75%). The sensitivity and specificity of CT imaging for identifying metastatic lung cancer to the mediastinal lymph nodes have been reported to be between 64–79% and 62–78%, respectively. Therefore, chest CT scan does not provide definitive information on staging. CT imaging does inform the decision about whether to proceed to resection of the primary tumor and sample the mediastinum at thoracotomy (common if there are no lymph nodes > 1 cm), or to employ TTNB, mediastinoscopy, or limited thoracotomy to biopsy suspected metastatic disease (common where there are lymph nodes > 1–2 cm).

Positron emission tomography (PET) using fluoro-2-deoxyglucose (FDG) is a noninvasive alternative for identifying metastatic foci in the mediastinum or distant sites. Sensitivity and specificity for the detection of mediastinal metastases are 91% and 86%, respectively, which is superior to CT imaging. PET is a very promising modality whose advocates hope will reduce the need for mediastinal surgery. Disadvantages include limited resolution below 1 cm, the expense of FDG, and limited availability. It is probable that PET will be introduced into algorithms for staging NSCLC, but its precise role remains to be defined.

2. Preoperative assessment—See Chapter 2.

3. Pulmonary function testing—Many patients with NSCLC have moderate to severe chronic lung disease that increases the risk of perioperative complications as well as long-term pulmonary insufficiency following lung resection. All patients considered for surgery re-

Table 9–16. Approach to staging of patients with lung cancer.[1]

Part A: Recommended tests for all patients
    Complete blood count
    Electrolytes, calcium, alkaline phosphatase, albumin, AST, ALT, total bilirubin, creatinine
    Chest radiograph
    CT of chest through the adrenal glands[2,3]
    Pathologic confirmation of malignancy[4]
Part B: Recommended tests for selected but not all patients

Test	Indication
CT of liver with contrast or liver ultrasound	Elevated liver function tests; abnormal non-contrast-enhanced CT of liver or abnormal clinical evaluation
CT of brain with contrast or MRI brain	CNS symptoms or abnormal clinical evaluation
Radionuclide bone scan	Elevated alkaline phosphatase (bony fraction), elevated calcium, bone pain, or abnormal clinical evaluation
Pulmonary function tests	If lung resection or thoracic radiotherapy planned
Quantitative radionuclide perfusion lung scan or exercise testing to evaluate maximum oxygen consumption	Patients with borderline resectability due to limited cardiovascuar status

[1]Modified and reproduced, with permission, from: Pretreatment evaluation of non-small cell lung cancer. Consensus Statement of the American Thoracic Society and the European Respiratory Society. Am J Respir Crit Care Med 1997;156:320.
[2]May not be necessary if patient has obvious M1 disease on chest x-ray or physical examination.
[3]Intravenous iodine contrast enhancement is not essential but is recommended in probable mediastinal invasion.
[4]While optimal in most cases, tissue diagnosis may not be necessary prior to surgery in some cases where the lesion is enlarging or the patient will undergo surgical resection regardless of the outcome of a biopsy.

quire spirometry. In the absence of other comorbidities, patients with good lung function (preoperative FEV_1 > 2 L) are at low risk for complications from lobectomy or pneumonectomy. If the FEV_1 is less than 2 L, then an estimated postoperative FEV_1 should be calculated. The postresection FEV_1 may be estimated from considering preoperative spirometry and the amount of lung to be resected; in severe obstructive disease, a quantitative lung perfusion scan may improve the estimate. A predicted post-lung resection FEV_1 > 800 mL (or > 40% of predicted FEV_1) is associated with a low incidence of perioperative complications. High-risk patients include those with a predicted postoperative FEV_1 < 700 mL (or < 40% of predicted FEV_1). In these patients—and in those with borderline spirometry—cardiopulmonary exercise testing may be helpful. A maximal oxygen uptake (MVO_2) of > 15 mL/kg/min identifies patients with an acceptable incidence of complications and mortality. Patients with an MVO_2 of < 10 mL/kg/min have a very high mortality rate at thoracotomy. Hypoxemia and hypercapnia are not independent predictors of outcome.

Treatment.

A. NON-SMALL CELL CARCINOMA

In NSCLC, cure is unlikely without resection. Therefore, the initial approach to the patient is determined by the answers to two questions: (1) Is complete surgical resection technically feasible? (2) If yes, is the patient able to tolerate the surgery with acceptable morbidity and mortality? Clinical features that preclude complete resection include extrathoracic metastases or a malignant pleural effusion; or tumor involving the heart, pericardium, great vessels, esophagus, recurrent laryngeal or phrenic nerves, trachea, main carina, or contralateral mediastinal lymph nodes. Accordingly, stage I and stage II patients are treated with surgical resection where possible. Stage IIIA patients have poor outcomes when treated with resection alone. They should be referred to multimodality protocols, including chemotherapy and radiotherapy. Stage IIIB patients treated with combined chemotherapy and radiation therapy have improved survival. Selected stage IIIB patients taken to resection following multimodality therapy have shown long-term survival and may be cured. Stage IV patients are treated with symptom-based palliative therapy, which may include outpatient chemotherapy (see below).

The surgical approach affects the outcome. In a prospective trial of stage I patients randomized to lobectomy versus limited resection, there was a three-fold increased rate of local recurrence in the limited resection group and a trend toward mortality benefit at 5 years in the lobectomy patients (56% versus 73% mortality, P = .09). There are inadequate outcome data on which to base a comparison of VATS with standard thoracotomy. Radiation therapy following surgery improves local control but does not improve survival.

Neoadjuvant chemotherapy consists of giving antineoplastic drugs in advance of surgery or radiation therapy. There is no consensus on the impact of neoadjuvant therapy on survival in stage I and stage II NSCLC. Such therapy is not recommended outside of ongoing clinical trials. Neoadjuvant therapy is more widely used in selected patients with stage IIIA or stage IIIB disease. Some studies suggest a survival advantage. This remains an area of active research.

Adjuvant chemotherapy consists of administering antineoplastic drugs following surgery or radiation therapy. Adjuvant chemotherapy with alkylating agents such as cyclophosphamide increases mortality. In stage I and N0 stage II disease, patients treated with multidrug platinum-based chemotherapy show a trend toward improved survival—on the order of 3 months (5%) at 5 years. Toxicity may be significant, however, and such therapy is not widely recommended. Newer antineoplastic agents with less toxicity are in clinical trials in these patients. In patients with stage IIIA disease and node positive stage II disease, the data are conflicting whether chemotherapy following surgery improves survival. Patients with locally advanced disease (stages IIIA and IIIB) who are not surgical candidates have improved survival when treated with combination chemotherapy and radiation therapy compared with no therapy or radiation alone.

In patients with advanced disease (stage IIIB and stage IV) but good performance status (WHO performance status 0–1, < 5% weight loss in the past 6 months; see Chapter 4), multidrug platinum-based chemotherapy is associated with an increase in survival equivalent to a mean gain of 6 weeks at 1 year. There is no evidence of a survival benefit in patients with poor performance status.

Multiple clinical trials evaluating quality of life suggest that there is better overall performance status and symptom control in patients with stage IIIB and stage IV NSCLC receiving chemotherapy plus good supportive care versus supportive care alone. Several trials suggest an increase in median survival of from 5 months to 7 months. These trials compare small numbers of patients; they are unblinded; and they are supported by the pharmaceutical companies that make the drugs used—all of which suggests caution in interpreting the results. Nonetheless, the reported findings are consistent. Furthermore, newer antineoplastic agents such as paclitaxel, gemcitabine, and navelbine show increased effectiveness in advanced NSCLC along with favorable side effect profiles. It remains to be seen which patients stand to benefit most from what combination of agents. At this time, outpatient chemotherapy for advanced NSCLC should be offered on protocol to patients with good performance status.

B. SMALL CELL CARCINOMA

In SCLC, response rates to cisplatin and etoposide are excellent: 80–100% response in limited-stage disease (50–70% complete response), and 60–80% response in extensive stage disease (15–40% complete response). However, remissions tend to be short-lived with a median duration of 6–8 months. Once the disease has recurred, median survival is 3–4 months. Overall 2-year survival is 20% in limited-stage disease and 5% in extensive-stage disease. Thoracic radiation therapy improves survival in patients with limited SCLC but not those with extensive disease. Whole brain radiation therapy decreases the incidence of central nervous system disease but does not affect survival. Its effect on symptoms is controversial.

Occasionally, a patient may have a peripheral nodule resected that turns out to be SCLC. Five-year survival following resection of the equivalent of stage I and stage II SCLC is higher than in patients treated with chemotherapy.

C. Palliative therapy: Photoresection with the Nd:YAG laser is sometimes performed on central tumors to relieve endobronchial obstruction, improve dyspnea, and control hemoptysis. External beam radiation therapy is also used to control dyspnea and hemoptysis in addition to pain from bony metastases, obstruction from superior vena cava syndrome, and symptomatic brain metastases. Resection of *solitary* brain metastases does not affect survival but may improve quality of life when combined with radiation therapy. Intraluminal radiation (brachytherapy) is an alternative approach to endobronchial disease. Pain syndromes are very common in advanced disease. As patients approach the end of life, meticulous efforts at pain control are essential (see Chapter 5). Consultation with or referral to a palliative care specialist is recommended in advanced disease to aid in symptom management and to facilitate referrals to hospice programs.

Prognosis

The overall 5-year survival rate for lung cancer is 15%. Predictors of survival are the type of tumor (SCLC versus NSCLC), the stage of the tumor, and the patient's performance status, including weight loss in the past 6 months. These are independent predictors in both early and late stage disease. Most data suggest that there is no difference among non-small cell carcinomas when adjusted for stage and performance status. However, squamous cell carcinoma may have a better prognosis than adenocarcinoma or large cell carcinoma at the same TNM stage. (See Table 9–17.)

Hoffman PC et al: Lung cancer. Lancet 2000;355:479. [PMID: 10841143] (Up to date review from medical oncologists with emphasis on recent chemotherapy trials.)

Pieterman RM et al: Preoperative staging of non-small-cell lung cancer with positron-emission tomography. N Engl J Med 2000;343:254. [PMID: 10911007] (PET improves the rate of detection of local and distant metastases in patients with non-small-cell lung cancer compared to CT imaging.)

Pretreatment evaluation of non-small-cell lung cancer. Consensus Statement of the American Thoracic Society and the European Respiratory Society. Am J Respir Crit Care Med 1997;156:320. [PMID: 9230769] (Detailed review of diagnosis and staging from two major American and European professional societies.)

Reif MS et al: Evidence-based medicine in the treatment of non-small cell lung cancer. Clin Chest Med 2000;21:107. [PMID: 10763093] (Excellent review of a large and conflicting data base of clinical studies.)

Rom WN et al: Molecular and genetic aspects of lung cancer. Am J Respir Crit Care Med 2000;161:1355.[PMID: 10764334] (State of the art review of molecular biology of lung cancer.)

Smith RA et al: Epidemiology of lung cancer. Radiol Clin North Am 2000;38:453. [PMID: 10855253] (Review of risk factors, incidence trends and mortality.)

Table 9–17. Approximate survival rates following treatment for lung cancer.[1]

Non-Small Cell Lung Cancer: Mean 5-Year Survival Following Resection		
Stage	**Clinical Staging**	**Surgical Staging**
IA (T1N0M0)	60%	74%
IB (T2N0M0)	38%	61%
IIA (T1N1M0)	34%	55%
IIB (T2N1M0, T3N0M0)	23%	39%
IIIA	9–13%	22%
IIIB[2]	3–7%	
IV[2]	1%	

Small Cell Lung Cancer: 2-Year Survival Following Chemotherapy		
Stage	**Mean**	**Median**
Limited	15–20%	14–20 months
Extensive	< 3%	8–13 months

[1]Data from multiple sources. Modified and reproduced, with permission, from Reif MS et al: Evidence-based medicine in the treatment of non-small cell cancer. Clin Chest Med 2000;21:107.
[2]Independent of therapy, generally not surgical patients.

BRONCHIAL CARCINOID TUMORS

Carcinoid and bronchial gland tumors are sometimes termed bronchial adenomas. This term should be avoided because it implies that the lesions are benign, when in fact carcinoid tumors and bronchial gland carcinomas are low-grade malignant neoplasms.

Carcinoid tumors are about six times more common than bronchial gland carcinomas, and most of them occur as pedunculated or sessile growths in central bronchi. Men and women are equally affected. Most patients are under 60 years of age. Common symptoms of bronchial carcinoid tumors are hemoptysis, cough, focal wheezing, and recurrent pneumonia. Peripherally located bronchial carcinoid tumors are rare and present as asymptomatic solitary pulmonary nodules. Carcinoid syndrome (flushing, diarrhea, wheezing, hypotension) is rare. Fiberoptic bronchoscopy may reveal a pink or purple tumor in a central airway. These lesions have a well-vascularized stroma, and biopsy may be complicated by significant bleeding. CT scanning is helpful to localize the lesion and to follow its growth over time. Octreotide scintigraphy is also available for localization of these tumors.

Bronchial carcinoid tumors grow slowly and rarely metastasize. Complications involve bleeding and airway obstruction rather than invasion by tumor and metastases. Surgical excision is necessary in some cases, and the prognosis is generally favorable. Most bronchial carcinoid tumors are resistant to radiation and chemotherapy.

Kulke MH et al: Carcinoid tumors. N Engl J Med. 1999; 340:858. [PMID: 10080850] (Exhaustive review.)

SECONDARY LUNG CANCER

Secondary lung cancers represent metastases from extrapulmonary malignant neoplasms that spread to the lungs through vascular or lymphatic channels or by direct extension. Almost any cancer can metastasize to the lung. Metastases usually occur via the pulmonary artery and typically present as multiple nodules or masses on chest radiography. The radiographic differential diagnosis of multiple pulmonary nodules also includes pulmonary arteriovenous malformation, pulmonary abscesses, granulomatous infection, sarcoidosis, rheumatoid nodules, and Wegener's granulomatosis. Metastases to the lungs are found in 20–55% of patients dying of various malignancies. Most are intraparenchymal. Endobronchial metastases occur in fewer than 5% of patients dying of nonpulmonary cancer; carcinoma of the kidney, breast, colon, and cervix and malignant melanoma are the most likely primary tumors.

Lymphangitic carcinoma denotes diffuse involvement of the pulmonary lymphatic network by primary or secondary lung cancer, probably a result of extension of tumor from lung capillaries to the lymphatics. **Tumor embolization** from extrapulmonary cancer (renal cell carcinoma, hepatocellular carcinoma, choriocarcinoma) is an uncommon route for tumor spread to the lungs. Secondary lung cancer may also present as malignant pleural effusion (see below).

Clinical Findings

A. SYMPTOMS AND SIGNS

Symptoms are uncommon but include cough, hemoptysis, and, in advanced cases, dyspnea. Symptoms are more often referable to the site of the primary tumor.

B. LABORATORY FINDINGS

The diagnosis of secondary lung cancer is usually established by identifying a primary tumor. Appropriate studies should be ordered if there is a suspicion of any primary cancer, such as breast, thyroid, testis, or prostate, for which specific treatment is available.

Mammography should be considered unless one has been performed recently. If the history and physical examination fail to reveal the site of the primary tumor, attention is better focused on the lung, where tissue samples obtained by bronchoscopy, percutaneous needle biopsy, or thoracotomy may establish the histologic diagnosis and suggest the most likely primary. Occasionally, cytologic studies of pleural fluid or pleural biopsy reveal the diagnosis. Sputum cytology is rarely helpful.

C. IMAGING

Chest radiographs usually show multiple spherical densities with sharp margins. The size of metastatic lesions varies from a few millimeters (miliary densities) to large masses. Nearly all are less than 5 cm in diameter. The lesions are usually bilateral, pleural or subpleural in location, and more common in lower lung zones. Cavitation suggests primary squamous cell tumor; calcification suggests osteosarcoma. Lymphangitic spread and solitary pulmonary nodule are less common radiographic presentations of secondary lung cancer. Conventional chest radiography is less sensitive than CT scan in detecting pulmonary metastases.

Treatment

Once the diagnosis has been established, management consists of treatment of the primary neoplasm and any pulmonary complications. Surgical resection of a *solitary* pulmonary nodule is often prudent in the patient with known current or previous extrapulmonary cancer. Local resection of one or more pulmonary metastases is feasible in a few carefully selected patients with various sarcomas and carcinomas (breast, testis, colon, kidney, and head and neck). Surgical resection should be considered only if the primary tumor is under control, if the patient is a good surgical risk, if all of the metastatic tumor can be resected, if nonsurgical approaches are not available, and if there are no metastases elsewhere in the body. Relative contraindications to resection of pulmonary metastases include (1) malignant melanoma primary, (2) requirement for pneumonectomy, (3) pleural involvement, and (4) simultaneous appearance of two or more metastases. The overall 5-year survival rate in secondary lung cancer treated surgically is 20–35%. For patients with progressive disease, diligent attention to palliative care is essential (see Chapter 5).

Greelish JP et al: Secondary pulmonary malignancy. Surg Clin North Am 2000;80:633. [PMID: 10836010] (Detailed review advocates for more aggressive surgical approach to secondary pulmonary malignancies.)

MESOTHELIOMA

Mesotheliomas are primary tumors arising from the surface lining of the pleura (80% of cases) or peritoneum (20% of cases). About three-fourths of pleural mesotheliomas are diffuse (usually malignant) tumors, and the remaining one-fourth are localized (usually benign). Men outnumber women by a 3:1 ratio. Numerous studies have confirmed the association of **malignant pleural mesothelioma** with exposure to asbestos (particularly the crocidolite form). The lifetime risk to asbestos workers of developing malignant pleural mesothelioma is about 8%. The clinician should inquire about asbestos exposure through mining, milling, manufacturing, shipyard work, insulation, brake linings, building construction and demolition, roofing materials, and a variety of asbestos products (pipe, textiles, paint, tile, gaskets, panels). Sixty to 80 percent of patients with malignant mesothelioma report a history of asbestos exposure. Although cigarette smoking significantly increases the risk of bronchogenic carcinoma in asbestos workers and aggravates asbestosis, there is no association between smoking and mesothelioma.

The mean age at onset of symptoms of malignant pleural mesothelioma is about 60 years. The latent period between exposure and onset of symptoms ranges from 20 to 40 years. Symptoms include the insidious onset of shortness of breath, nonpleuritic chest pain, and weight loss. Physical findings include dullness to percussion, diminished breath sounds, and, in some cases, finger clubbing. Radiographic abnormalities consist of nodular, irregular, unilateral pleural thickening and varying degrees of unilateral pleural effusion. CT scan helps demonstrate the extent of pleural involvement.

Pleural fluid is exudative and often hemorrhagic. Open pleural biopsy is usually necessary to obtain an adequate specimen for histologic diagnosis; even then, distinction from benign inflammatory conditions and from metastatic adenocarcinoma may be difficult. The histologic variants of malignant pleural mesothelioma are epithelial and fibrous (sarcomatous). Special stains and electron microscopy may be needed to confirm the diagnosis.

Malignant pleural mesothelioma progresses rapidly as the tumor spreads quickly along the pleural surface to involve the pericardium, mediastinum, and contralateral pleura. The tumor may eventually extend beyond the thorax to involve abdominal lymph nodes and organs. Progressive pain and dyspnea are characteristic. Median survival time from onset of symptoms ranges from 5 months in extensive disease to 16 months in localized disease, and about 75% of patients are dead within 1 year after diagnosis. Treatment with surgery, radiotherapy, chemotherapy, and a combination of methods has been attempted but is generally unsuccessful. Some surgeons believe that extrapleural pneumonectomy is the preferred surgical approach for patients with early stage disease. Drainage of pleural effusions, pleurodesis, radiation therapy, and even resectional surgery may offer palliative benefit in some patients.

Sterman DH et al: Advances in the treatment of malignant pleural mesothelioma. Chest 2000;116:504. [PMID: 10453882] (Review of current therapies.)

Sugarbaker DJ et al: Multimodality management of malignant pleural mesothelioma. Chest 1998;113(Suppl):61S. [PMID: 9438692] (Extrapleural pneumonectomy plus combination chemotherapy.)

MEDIASTINAL MASSES

Various developmental, neoplastic, infectious, traumatic, and cardiovascular disorders may cause masses that appear in the mediastinum on chest radiograph. A useful convention arbitrarily divides the mediastinum into three compartments—anterior, middle, and posterior—in order to classify mediastinal masses and assist in differential diagnosis. Specific mediastinal masses have a predilection for one or more of these compartments; most are located in the anterior or middle compartment. The differential diagnosis of an anterior mediastinal mass includes thymoma, teratoma, thyroid lesions, lymphoma, and mesenchymal tumors (lipoma, fibroma). The differential diagnosis of a middle mediastinal mass includes lymphadenopathy, pulmonary artery enlargement, aneurysm of the aorta or innominate artery, developmental cyst (bronchogenic, enteric, pleuropericardial), dilated azygous or hemiazygous vein, and foramen of Morgagni hernia. The differential diagnosis of a posterior mediastinal mass includes hiatus hernia, neurogenic tumor, meningocele, esophageal tumor, foramen of Bochdalek hernia, thoracic spine disease, and extramedullary hematopoiesis. The neurogenic tumor group includes neurilemmoma, neurofibroma, neurosarcoma, ganglioneuroma, and pheochromocytoma.

Symptoms and signs of mediastinal masses are nonspecific and are usually caused by the effects of the mass on surrounding structures. Insidious onset of retrosternal chest pain, dysphagia, or dyspnea is often an important clue to the presence of a mediastinal mass. In about half of cases, symptoms are absent, and the mass is detected on routine chest radiograph. Physical findings vary depending upon the nature and location of the mass.

CT scanning is helpful in management; additional radiographic studies of benefit include barium swallow if esophageal disease is suspected, Doppler sonography or venography of brachiocephalic veins and the superior vena cava, and arteriography. MRI is useful; its advantages include distinction between vessels and masses, no need for contrast media, and better delineation of hilar structures. MRI also allows imaging in multiple planes, whereas CT permits only axial imaging. Tissue diagnosis is necessary if a neoplastic disorder is suspected. Treatment and prognosis depend on the underlying cause of the mediastinal mass.

Aquino SL et al: Reconciliation of the anatomic, surgical, and radiographic classifications of the mediastinum. J Comp Assist Tomogr 2001;25:489. [PMID: 11351204] (Review and analysis of subdivisions of the mediastinum by radiologists, surgeons, and anatomists.)

Ronson RS et al: Embryology and surgical anatomy of the mediastinum with clinical implications. Surg Clin North Am 2000;80:157. [PMID: 10685147] (Reviews general mediastinal embryology and anatomy and provides algorithms for the investigation of mediastinal masses.)

■ INTERSTITIAL LUNG DISEASE (Diffuse Parenchymal Lung Disease)

Interstitial lung disease, or diffuse parenchymal lung disease, comprises a heterogeneous group of disorders that share a common response of the lung to injury: alveolitis, or inflammation, and fibrosis of the interalveolar septum. The term "interstitial" is misleading since the pathologic process usually begins with injury to the alveolar epithelial or capillary endothelial cells. Persistent alveolitis may lead to obliteration of alveolar capillaries and reorganization of the lung parenchyma, accompanied by irreversible fibrosis. The process does not affect the airways proximal to the respiratory bronchioles. At least 180 disease entities may present as interstitial lung disease (Table 9–18). In the majority of patients, no specific cause can be identified. In the remainder, drugs and a variety of organic and inorganic dusts are the principal causes.

The clinical consequence of widespread lung fibrosis is diminished lung compliance, which presents as restrictive lung disease. Patients usually describe an insidious onset of exertional dyspnea and cough. Sputum production is minimal. Chest examination reveals fine, late inspiratory crackles at the lung bases. Digital clubbing is seen in 25–50% of patients at diagnosis. Pulmonary function testing shows a loss of lung volume with normal to increased airflow rates. The diffusing capacity for carbon monoxide is decreased, and hypoxemia with exercise is common. In advanced cases, resting hypoxemia may be present. The chest radiograph is normal on presentation in up to 10% of patients. More typically, it shows patchy distribution of ground-glass, reticular, or reticulonodular infiltrates. In advanced disease there are multiple small, thick-walled cystic spaces in the lung periphery ("honeycomb lung"). Honeycombing indicates the presence of locally advanced fibrosis with destruction of normal lung architecture. Conventional and high-resolution CT scanning (HRCT) reveal in greater detail the findings described on chest radiograph. In some cases, HRCT may be strongly suggestive of a specific pathologic process.

The history—particularly the occupational and medication history—may provide evidence of a specific cause. Serologic tests for antinuclear antibodies and rheumatoid factor are positive in 20–40% of pa-

Table 9-18. Differential diagnosis of interstitial lung disease.

Drug-related
  Antiarrhythmic agents (amiodarone)
  Antibacterial agents (nitrofurantoin, sulfonamides)
  Antineoplastic agents (bleomycin, cyclophosphamide, methotrexate, nitrosoureas)
  Antirheumatic agents (gold salts, penicillamine)
  Phenytoin
Environmental and occupational (inhalation exposures)
  Dust, inorganic (asbestos, silica, hard metals, beryllium)
  Dust, organic (thermophilic actinomycetes, avian antigens, aspergillus species)
  Gases, fumes, and vapors (chlorine, isocyanates, paraquat, sulfur dioxide)
  Ionizing radiation
  Talc (injection drug users)
Infections
  Fungus, disseminated (*Coccidioides immitis, Blastomyces dermatitidis, Histoplasma capsulatum*)
  Mycobacteria, disseminated
  Pneumocystis carinii
  Viruses
Primary pulmonary disorders
  Bronchiolitis obliterans-organizing pneumonia (BOOP)
  Idiopathic fibrosing interstitial pneumonia: Acute interstitial pneumonitis, desquamative interstitial pneumonitis, nonspecific interstitial pneumonitis, usual interstitial pneumonitis, respiratory bronchiolitis-associated interstitial lung disease
  Pulmonary alveolar proteinosis
Systemic disorders
  Acute respiratory distress syndrome (ARDS)
  Amyloidosis
  Ankylosing spondylitis
  Autoimmune disease: Dermatomyositis, polymyositis, rheumatoid arthritis, systemic sclerosis (scleroderma), systemic lupus erythematosus
  Chronic eosinophilic pneumonia
  Goodpasture's syndrome
  Idiopathic pulmonary hemosiderosis
  Inflammatory bowel disease
  Langerhans cell histiocytosis (eosinophilic granuloma)
  Lymphangitic spread of cancer (lymphangitic carcinomatosis)
  Lymphangioleiomyomatosis
  Pulmonary edema
  Pulmonary venous hypertension, chronic
  Sarcoidosis
  Wegener's granulomatosis

tients but are rarely diagnostic. Antineutrophil cytoplasmic antibodies (ANCAs) may be diagnostic in some clinical settings. Invasive diagnostic testing is frequently necessary to make a specific diagnosis. Three diagnostic techniques are in common use: bronchoalveolar lavage, transbronchial biopsy, and surgical lung biopsy, either through an open procedure or using video-assisted thoracoscopic surgery.

Bronchoalveolar lavage may provide a specific diagnosis in cases of infection, particularly with *Pneumocystis carinii* or mycobacteria, or when cytologic examination reveals the presence of malignant cells. The findings may be suggestive if not diagnostic of eosinophilic pneumonia, Langerhans cell histiocytosis (eosinophilic granuloma), and alveolar proteinosis. Analysis of the cellular constituents of lavage fluid may suggest a specific disease, but these findings are not diagnostic.

Transbronchial biopsy through the flexible bronchoscope is easily performed in most patients. The risks of pneumothorax (5%) and hemorrhage (1–10%) are low. However, the tissue specimens recovered are small, sampling error is common, and crush artifact may complicate diagnosis. Transbronchial biopsy can make a definitive diagnosis of sarcoidosis, lymphangitic spread of carcinoma, pulmonary alveolar proteinosis, miliary tuberculosis, and Langerhans cell histiocytosis. Transbronchial biopsy cannot establish a specific diagnosis of idiopathic interstitial pneumonia. These patients generally require surgical lung biopsy.

Surgical lung biopsy is the standard for diagnosis of interstitial lung disease. Two or three biopsies taken from multiple sites in the same lung, including apparently normal tissue, may yield a specific diagnosis as well as prognostic information regarding the extent of fibrosis versus active inflammation. Patients under age 60 without a specific diagnosis generally should undergo surgical lung biopsy. In older and sicker patients, the risks and benefits must be weighed carefully for three reasons: (1) the morbidity of the procedure can be significant; (2) a definitive diagnosis may not be possible even with surgical lung biopsy; and (3) when a specific diagnosis is made, there may be no effective treatment. Empirical therapy or no treatment may be preferable to surgical lung biopsy in some patients.

Known causes of interstitial lung disease are dealt with in their specific sections. The important idiopathic forms are discussed below.

IDIOPATHIC FIBROSING INTERSTITIAL PNEUMONIA (Formerly: Idiopathic Pulmonary Fibrosis)

The most common diagnosis among patients presenting with interstitial lung disease is idiopathic pulmonary fibrosis, known in Britain as cryptogenic fibrosing alveolitis. Historically, this diagnosis was based on clinical and radiographic criteria with only a minority of patients undergoing surgical lung biopsy. When biopsies were obtained, several histologic patterns were grouped together under the category idiopathic pulmonary fibrosis because of the common element of fibrosis. We now recognize that these distinct histopathologic features are associated with different

natural histories and responses to therapy (see Table 9–19). Therefore, in the evaluation of patients with idiopathic interstitial lung disease, one should attempt to identify specific disorders and use the terms idiopathic pulmonary fibrosis or cryptogenic fibrosing alveolitis to denote only the histologic pattern of usual interstitial pneumonitis (UIP).

Patients with idiopathic fibrosing interstitial pneumonia may present with any of the histologic patterns described in Table 9–19. The first step in evaluation is to identify patients whose disease is truly idiopathic. As indicated in Table 9–18, most identifiable causes of interstitial lung disease are either infectious, drug-related, or environmental or occupational agents. Interstitial lung diseases associated with other medical conditions (pulmonary-renal syndromes, collagen-vascular disease) may be identified through a careful medical history. Apart from acute interstitial pneumonia, the clinical presentations of the idiopathic interstitial pneumonias are sufficiently similar to preclude a specific diagnosis. Chest radiographs and HRCT scans are occasionally diagnostic. Ultimately, many patients with apparently idiopathic disease require surgical lung biopsy to make a definitive diagnosis. The importance of accurate diagnosis is twofold. First, it allows the clinician to provide accurate information about the cause and natural history of the illness. Second, accurate diagnosis helps to distinguish patients most likely to benefit from therapy. Surgical lung biopsy may spare patients with usual interstitial pneumonia treatment with potentially morbid therapies.

The diagnosis of usual interstitial pneumonia can be made on clinical grounds alone in selected patients. A diagnosis of UIP can be made with 90% confidence in patients over 65 who present with idiopathic disease by history, demonstrate inspiratory crackles on physical examination and restrictive physiology on pulmonary function testing, characteristic radiographic evidence of progressive fibrosis over several years, and diffuse, patchy fibrosis with pleural-based honeycombing on high-resolution CT scan. Such patients do not need surgical lung biopsy. Note that the diagnosis of UIP cannot be confirmed on transbronchial lung biopsy since the histologic diagnosis requires a pattern of changes rather than a single pathognomonic finding. Transbronchial biopsy may exclude UIP by confirming a specific alternative diagnosis.

Treatment of idiopathic fibrosing interstitial pneumonia is controversial. No randomized study has demonstrated that any treatment improves survival or quality of life compared with no treatment. Clinical experience suggests that patients with desquamative interstitial pneumonia (DIP; or respiratory bronchiolitis-associated interstitial lung disease, RB-ILD), nonspecific interstitial pneumonia (NSIP), or bronchiolitis obliterans-organizing pneumonia (BOOP) (see Table 9–19) frequently respond to corticosteroids and should be given a trial of therapy—typically pred-

Table 9–19. Idiopathic fibrosing interstitial pneumonias.

Name and Clinical Presentation	Histopathology	Radiographic Pattern	Response to Therapy and Prognosis
Usual interstitial pneumonia (UIP) Age 55–60, slight male predominance. Insidious dry cough and exertional dyspnea lasting months to years. Clubbing present at diagnosis in 25–50%. Diffuse fine late inspiratory crackles on lung auscultation. Restrictive ventilatory defect and reduced diffusing capacity on pulmonary function tests. ANA and RF positive in 25% in the absence of documented collagen-vascular disease.	Patchy, temporally and geographically nonuniform distribution of fibrosis, honeycomb change, and normal lung. Type I pneumocytes are lost, and there is proliferation of alveolar type II cells. "Fibroblast foci" of actively proliferating fibroblasts and myofibroblasts. Inflammation is generally mild and consists of small lymphocytes. Intra-alveolar macrophage accumulation is present but is not a prominent feature.	Diminished lung volume. Increased linear or reticular bibasilar and subpleural opacities. Unilateral disease is rare. HRCT shows minimal ground-glass and variable honeycomb change. Areas of normal lung may be adjacent to areas of advanced fibrosis. Between 2% and 10% have normal chest radiographs and HRCT scans on diagnosis.	No randomized study has demonstrated improved survival compared with untreated patients. Inexorably progressive. Response to corticosteroids and cytotoxic agents at best 15%, and these probably represent misclassification of histopathology. Median survival approximately 3 years, depending on stage at presentation. Current interest in antifibrotic agents.
Respiratory bronchiolitis-associated interstitial lung disease (RB-ILD)[1] Age 40–45. Presentation similar to that of UIP though in younger patients. Similar results on pulmonary function tests, but less severe abnormalities. Patients with respiratory bronchiolitis are invariably heavy smokers.	Increased numbers of macrophages evenly dispersed within the alveolar spaces. Rare fibroblast foci, little fibrosis, minimal honeycomb change. In RB-ILD the accumulation of macrophages is localized within the peribronchiolar air spaces; in DIP, it is diffuse. Alveolar architecture is preserved.	May be indistinguishable from UIP. More often presents with a nodular or reticulonodular pattern. Honeycombing rare. HRCT more likely to reveal diffuse ground glass opacities and upper lobe emphysema.	Spontaneous remission occurs in up to 20% of patients, so natural history unclear. Smoking cessation is essential. Prognosis clearly better than that of UIP: median survival greater than 10 years. Corticosteroids thought to be effective, but there are no randomized clinical trials to support this view.
Acute interstitial pneumonitis (AIP) Clinically known as Hamman-Rich syndrome. Wide age range, many young patients. Acute onset of dyspnea followed by rapid development of respiratory failure. Half of patients report a viral syndrome preceding lung disease. Clinical course indistinguishable from that of idiopathic ARDS.	Pathologic changes reflect acute response to injury within days to weeks. Resembles organizing phase of diffuse alveolar damage. Fibrosis and minimal collagen deposition. May appear similar to UIP but more homogeneous and there is no honeycomb change—though this may appear if the process persists for more than a month in a patient on mechanical ventilation.	Diffuse bilateral airspace consolidation with areas of ground-glass attenuation on HRCT scan.	Supportive care (mechanical ventilation) critical but effect of specific therapies unclear. High initial mortality: Fifty to 90 percent die within 2 months after diagnosis. Not progressive if patient survives. Lung function may return to normal or may be permanently impaired.

(continued)

nisone, 1–2 mg/kg/d for a minimum of 2 months. The same therapy is almost uniformly ineffective in patients with UIP. Since this therapy carries significant morbidity, the pulmonary community is shifting away from the routine use of corticosteroids in patients with usual interstitial pneumonia. A small but well-designed clinical study has reported promising preliminary results with recombinant interferon gamma-1b. A large follow-up study is in progress.

Gross TJ et al: Idiopathic pulmonary fibrosis. N Engl J Med 2001;345:517. [PMID: 11519507] (Review article.)

Idiopathic pulmonary fibrosis: diagnosis and treatment. American Thoracic Society International consensus statement. Am J Respir Crit Care Med 2000;161:646. [PMID: 10673212]

Table 9–19. Idiopathic fibrosing interstitial pneumonias. (continued)

Name and Clinical Presentation	Histopathology	Radiographic Pattern	Response to Therapy and Prognosis
Nonspecific interstitial pneumonitis (NSIP) Age 45–55. Slight female predominance. Similar to UIP but onset of cough and dyspnea over months, not years.	Nonspecific in that histopathology does not fit into better-established categories. Varying degrees of inflammation and fibrosis, patchy in distribution but uniform in time, suggesting response to single injury. Most have lymphocytic and plasma cell inflammation without fibrosis. Honeycombing present but scant. Some have advocated division into cellular and fibrotic subtypes.	May be indistinguishable from UIP. Most typical picture is bilateral areas of ground-glass attenuation and fibrosis on HRCT. Honeycombing is rare.	Treatment thought to be effective, but no prospective clinical studies have been published. Prognosis overall good but depends on the extent of fibrosis at diagnosis. Median survival greater than 10 years.
Bronchiolitis obliterans organizing pneumonia (BOOP) Typically age 50–60 but wide variation. Abrupt onset, frequently weeks to a few months following a flu-like illness. Dyspnea and dry cough prominent, but constitiutional symptoms are common: fatigue, fever, and weight loss. Pulmonary function tests usually show restriction, but up to 25% show concomitant obstruction.	Included in the idiopathic interstitial pneumonias on clinical grounds. Buds of loose connective tissue (Masson bodies) and inflammatory cells fill alveoli and distal bronchioles.	Lung volumes normal. Chest radiograph typically shows interstitial and parenchymal disease with discrete, peripheral alveolar and ground-glass infiltrates. Nodular opacities common. HRCT shows subpleural consolidation and bronchial wall thickening and dilation.	Rapid response to corticosteroids in two-thirds of patients. Long-term prognosis generally good for those who respond. Relapses are common.

[1]Includes desquamative interstitial pneumonia (DIP).

(Comprehensive joint consensus statement from the ATS and its European counterpart, the European Respiratory Society.)

Katzenstein AL et al: Idiopathic pulmonary fibrosis: Clinical relevance of pathologic classification. Am J Respir Crit Care Med 1998;157:1301. [PMID: 9563754] (Focuses on clinical and pathologic characteristics of four distinct forms of idiopathic interstitial pneumonia formerly grouped together as pulmonary fibrosis.)

Lynch JP et al: Idiopathic pulmonary fibrosis: Is lung biopsy essential? J Respir Dis 2000;21:197. (A careful attempt to distinguish the specific clinical, radiographic, and pathologic features of the idiopathic interstitial pneumonias.)

Raghu G et al: The accuracy of the clinical diagnosis of new-onset idiopathic pulmonary fibrosis and other interstitial lung disease. Chest 1999;116:1168. [PMID: 10559072] (A prospective assessment of selected referral patients comparing expert clinical and radiographic assessment with biopsy findings.)

Selman M et al: Idiopathic pulmonary fibrosis: prevailing and evolving hypotheses about its pathogenesis and implications for therapy. Ann Intern Med 2001;134:136. [PMID: 11177318]

SARCOIDOSIS

Sarcoidosis is a systemic disease of unknown etiology characterized in about 90% of patients by granulomatous inflammation of the lung. The incidence is highest in North American blacks and northern European whites; among blacks, women are more frequently affected than men. Onset of disease is usually in the third or fourth decade.

Patients may present with malaise, fever, and dyspnea of insidious onset. Symptoms referable to the skin, eyes, peripheral nerves, liver, kidney, or heart may also cause the patient to seek care. Some individuals are asymptomatic and come to medical attention after abnormal findings (typically bilateral hilar and right paratracheal lymphadenopathy) on chest radiographs. Physical findings are atypical of interstitial lung disease: crackles are uncommon on chest examination. Other findings may include erythema nodosum, parotid gland enlargement, hepatosplenomegaly, and lymphadenopathy. Laboratory tests may show leukopenia, an elevated erythrocyte sedimentation rate, and hypercalcemia (about 5% of patients) or hypercalciuria (20%). Angiotensin-converting enzyme (ACE) levels are elevated in 40–80% of patients with active disease. This finding is neither sensitive nor specific enough to have diagnostic significance. Physiologic testing may reveal evidence of airflow obstruction, but restrictive changes with decreased lung volumes and diffusing capacity are more common. Skin test anergy is present in 70%.

Radiographic findings are variable and include bilateral hilar adenopathy alone (stage I), hilar adenopathy and parenchymal involvement (stage II), or parenchymal involvement alone (stage III). Parenchymal involvement is usually manifested radiographically by diffuse reticular infiltrates, but focal infiltrates, acinar shadows, nodules, and, rarely, cavitation may be seen. Pleural effusion is noted in fewer than 10% of patients.

The diagnosis of sarcoidosis generally requires histologic demonstration of noncaseating granulomas in biopsies from a patient with other typical associated manifestations. Other granulomatous diseases (eg, berylliosis, tuberculosis) must be excluded. Biopsy of easily accessible sites (eg, palpable lymph nodes, skin lesions, or salivary glands) is likely to be positive. Transbronchial lung biopsy has a high yield (75–90%) as well, especially in patients with radiographic evidence of parenchymal involvement. Some clinicians believe that tissue biopsy is not necessary when stage I radiographic findings are detected in a clinical situation that strongly favors the diagnosis of sarcoidosis (eg, a young black woman with erythema nodosum). Biopsy is essential whenever clinical and radiographic findings suggest the possibility of an alternative diagnosis such as lymphoma. Bronchoalveolar lavage fluid in sarcoidosis is usually characterized by an increase in lymphocytes and a high CD4/CD8 cell ratio. Bronchoalveolar lavage is useful in following the activity of sarcoidosis in selected patients but does not establish a diagnosis.

Indications for treatment with oral corticosteroids include constitutional symptoms, hypercalcemia, iritis, arthritis, central nervous system involvement, cardiac involvement, granulomatous hepatitis, cutaneous lesions other than erythema nodosum, and symptomatic pulmonary lesions. Long-term therapy is usually required over months to years. ACE serum levels usually fall with clinical improvement. Immunosuppressive drugs and cyclosporine have been tried, primarily when corticosteroid therapy has been exhausted, but experience with these drugs is limited.

About 20% of patients with lung involvement suffer irreversible lung impairment, characterized by progressive fibrosis, bronchiectasis, and cavitation. Pneumothorax, hemoptysis, mycetoma formation in lung cavities, and respiratory failure often complicate this advanced stage. Myocardial sarcoidosis occurs in about 5% of patients, sometimes leading to restrictive cardiomyopathy, cardiac arrhythmias and conduction disturbances. The outlook is best for patients with hilar adenopathy alone; radiographic involvement of the lung parenchyma is associated with a worse prognosis. Erythema nodosum portends a good outcome. Death due to pulmonary insufficiency occurs in about 5% of patients.

Statement on sarcoidosis. American Thoracic Society International consensus statement. Am J Respir Crit Care Med 1999;160:736. [PMID: 10430755] (Comprehensive consensus statement on epidemiology, pathogenesis, pathology, clinical features, and treatment.)

PULMONARY ALVEOLAR PROTEINOSIS

Pulmonary alveolar proteinosis is a disease in which phospholipids accumulate within alveolar spaces. The condition may be primary (idiopathic) or secondary (occurring in immune deficiency, hematologic malignancies, inhalation of mineral dusts, or following lung infections, including tuberculosis and viral infections). Progressive dyspnea is the usual presenting symptom, and chest radiograph shows bilateral alveolar infiltrates suggestive of pulmonary edema. The diagnosis is based on demonstration of characteristic findings on bronchoalveolar lavage (milky appearance and PAS-positive lipoproteinaceous material) in association with typical clinical and radiographic features. In some cases, transbronchial or open lung biopsy (revealing amorphous intra-alveolar phospholipid) is necessary.

The course of the disease varies. Some patients experience spontaneous remission; others develop progressive respiratory insufficiency. Pulmonary infection with nocardia or fungi may occur. Therapy for alveolar proteinosis consists of periodic whole lung lavage.

Shah PL et al: Pulmonary alveolar proteinosis: clinical aspects and current concepts on pathogenesis. Thorax 2000;55:67. [PMID: 10607805] (Comprehensive review.)

EOSINOPHILIC PULMONARY SYNDROMES

Eosinophilic pulmonary syndromes are a diverse group of disorders typically characterized by eosinophilic pulmonary infiltrates, peripheral blood eosinophilia, and pulmonary symptoms such as dyspnea and cough. Many patients have constitutional symptoms, including fever. **Chronic eosinophilic pneumonia** is predominantly a disorder of women characterized by fever, night sweats, weight loss, and dyspnea. Pulmonary infiltrates on chest radiography are invariably peripheral. Therapy with oral prednisone (1 mg/kg daily for 1–2 weeks followed by a gradual taper over many months) usually results in dramatic improvement; however, most patients require at least 10–15 mg of prednisone every other day for a year or more (sometimes indefinitely) to prevent relapses.

Other eosinophilic pulmonary syndromes demonstrate a variety of patterns of pulmonary infiltrates associated with exposure to various drugs (common drugs include nitrofurantoin, phenytoin, ampicillin, acetaminophen, and ranitidine) or infection with helminths (eg, ascaris, hookworms, strongyloides) or filariae (eg, *Wuchereria bancrofti, Brugia malayi,* tropical pulmonary eosinophilia). Löffler's syndrome is acute eosinophilic pneumonia with transient pulmonary infiltrates. Pulmonary eosinophilia can also be a feature of many other processes, including allergic bronchopulmonary aspergillosis, Churg-Strauss syndrome, systemic hypereosinophilic syndromes, eosinophilic granuloma of the lung (also referred to as pulmonary Langerhans cell granulomatosis or primary pulmonary histocytosis X), neoplasms, and numerous interstitial lung diseases. No precipitating cause may be apparent in as many as one-third of cases. If an extrinsic cause is identified, therapy consists of removal of the offending drug or treatment of the underlying parasitic infection. Corticosteroid treatment (prednisone, 1 mg/kg body weight orally per day) should be instituted if no treatable extrinsic cause is discovered. The response to corticosteroids is usually dramatic. Recurrences are common.

Johkoh T et al: Eosinophilic lung diseases: diagnostic accuracy of thin-section CT in 111 patients. Radiology 2000;216:773. [PMID: 10966710]

Milbrandt EB et al: Progressive infiltrates and eosinophilia with multiple possible causes. Chest 2000;118:230. [PMID: 10893384]

■ DISORDERS OF THE PULMONARY CIRCULATION

PULMONARY THROMBOEMBOLISM

 ESSENTIALS OF DIAGNOSIS

- *Predisposition to venous thrombosis, usually of the lower extremities.*
- *Usually one of the following: dyspnea, chest pain, hemoptysis, syncope.*
- *Tachypnea and a widened alveolar-arterial P_{O_2} difference.*
- *Characteristic defects on ventilation-perfusion lung scan, spiral CT scan of the chest, or pulmonary angiogram.*

General Considerations

Pulmonary thromboembolism, often referred to as pulmonary embolism, is a common, serious and potentially fatal complication of thrombus formation within the deep venous circulation. Pulmonary thromboembolism is estimated to cause 50,000 deaths each year in the United States and is the third leading cause of death among hospitalized patients. Despite this prevalence, the majority of cases are not recognized antemortem, and fewer than 10% of patients with fatal emboli have received specific treatment for the condition. Management demands a vigilant systematic approach to diagnosis and an understanding of risk factors so that appropriate preventive therapy can be given.

Many substances can embolize to the pulmonary circulation, including air (during neurosurgery, as a complication of central venous catheters), amniotic fluid (during active labor), fat (as a complication of long bone fractures), foreign bodies (talc in intravenous drug users), parasite eggs (schistosomiasis), septic emboli (as a complication of acute infectious endocarditis), and tumor cells (renal cell carcinoma). The most common embolus is thrombus, which may arise anywhere in the venous circulation or heart but most often originates in the deep veins of the major calf muscles. Thrombi confined to the calf rarely embolize to the pulmonary circulation. However, about 20% of calf vein thrombi propagate proximally to the popliteal and ileofemoral veins, at which point they may break off and embolize to the pulmonary circulation. Fifty to 60 percent of patients with proximal deep venous thrombosis (DVT) will develop pulmonary emboli; half of these embolic events will be asymptomatic. Nearly 70% of patients who present with symptomatic pulmonary emboli will have lower extremity DVT when evaluated.

Pulmonary embolism and deep venous thrombosis are two manifestations of the same disease. The risk factors for pulmonary emboli are the risk factors for thrombus formation within the venous circulation: venous stasis, injury to the vessel wall, and hypercoagulability. Venous stasis increases with immobility (bed rest—especially postoperative—obesity, stroke), hyperviscosity (polycythemia), and increased central venous pressures (low cardiac output states, pregnancy). Vessels may be damaged by prior episodes of thrombosis, orthopedic surgery, or trauma. Hypercoagulability can be caused by medications (oral contraceptives, hormonal replacement therapy) or disease (malignancy, extensive surgery) or may be the result of inherited gene defects. The most common inherited cause in Caucasian populations is resistance to activated protein C, also known as factor V Leiden. The trait is present in approximately 3% of healthy American men and in 20–40% of patients with idiopathic venous thrombosis. Other major risks for hypercoagulability include the following: deficiencies or dysfunction of protein C, protein S, and antithrombin III;

prothrombin gene mutation; and the presence of antiphospholipid antibodies (lupus anticoagulant and anticardiolipin antibody).

Pulmonary thromboembolism has multiple physiologic effects. Physical obstruction of the vascular bed and vasoconstriction from neurohumoral reflexes both increase pulmonary vascular resistance. Massive thrombus may cause right ventricular failure. Vascular obstruction increases physiologic dead space (wasted ventilation) and leads to hypoxemia through right-to-left shunting, decreased cardiac output, and surfactant depletion causing atelectasis. Reflex bronchoconstriction promotes wheezing and increased work of breathing.

Clinical Findings

A. SYMPTOMS AND SIGNS

The clinical diagnosis of pulmonary thromboembolism is notoriously difficult for two reasons. First, the clinical findings depend on both the size of the embolus and the patient's preexisting cardiopulmonary status. Second, common symptoms and signs of pulmonary emboli are not specific to this disorder (Table 9–20).

Indeed, no single symptom or sign or combination of clinical findings is specific to pulmonary thromboembolism. Some findings are fairly sensitive: dyspnea and pain on inspiration occur in 75–85% and 65–75% of patients, respectively. Tachypnea is the only sign reliably found in more than half of patients. A common clinical strategy is to use combinations of clinical findings to identify patients at low risk for pulmonary thromboembolism. For example, 97% of patients in the Prospective Investigation of Pulmonary Embolism Diagnosis (PIOPED) study with angiographically proved pulmonary emboli had one or more of three findings: dyspnea, chest pain with breathing, or tachypnea. Such a sensitive screen allows exclusion of the diagnosis on clinical grounds in a small number of patients. To establish the diagnosis or to exclude it definitively, further testing is required in the majority of patients.

B. LABORATORY FINDINGS

The ECG is abnormal in 70% of patients with pulmonary thromboembolism. However, the most common abnormalities are sinus tachycardia and nonspecific ST and T wave changes, each seen in approximately 40% of patients. Five percent or less of patients in the PIOPED study had P pulmonale, right ventricular hypertrophy, right axis deviation, and right bundle branch block.

Arterial blood gases usually reveal acute respiratory alkalosis due to hyperventilation. The arterial P_{O_2} and the alveolar-arterial oxygen difference (A–a D_{O_2}) are most often abnormal in patients with pulmonary thromboembolism compared with healthy, age-matched controls. However, arterial blood gases are not diagnostic: among patients who presented for evaluation in the PIOPED study, neither the P_{O_2} nor the A–a D_{O_2} differentiated between those with and those without pulmonary emboli. Profound hypoxia with a normal chest radiograph in the absence of preexisting lung disease is highly suspicious for pulmonary thromboembolism.

Plasma levels of D-dimer, a degradation product of cross-linked fibrin, are elevated in the presence of thrombus. Using a D-dimer threshold between 300 and 500 ng/mL, the quantitative enzyme-linked immunosorbent assay (ELISA) has shown a sensitivity for venous thromboembolism of 97% and a specificity of 45%. Therefore, the absence of D-dimer using the ELISA assay provides strong evidence against venous thromboembolism. Two considerations have delayed widespread inclusion of plasma D-dimer assays into diagnostic algorithms. First, the accurate quantitative ELISA assay used in multiple studies takes several hours to perform and is not widely available. Commonly used latex agglutination assays are much less sensitive and are difficult to standardize. Second, the D-dimer is elevated in most hospitalized patients, particularly those with malignancies or following surgery. Appropriate diagnostic thresholds are not yet established for inpatients.

C. IMAGING AND SPECIAL EXAMINATIONS

1. **Chest radiography**—The chest radiograph is necessary to exclude other common lung diseases and to permit interpretation of the ventilation-perfusion scan, but it does not establish the diagnosis by itself. The chest radiograph was normal in only 12% of patients with confirmed pulmonary thromboembolism in the PIOPED study. The most frequent findings were atelectasis, parenchymal infiltrates, and pleural effusions. However, the prevalence of these findings was the same in hospitalized patients without pulmonary thromboembolism. A prominent central pulmonary artery with local oligemia (Westermark's sign) or pleural-based areas of increased opacity that represent intraparenchymal hemorrhage (Hampton's hump) are uncommon. Paradoxically, the chest radiograph may be most helpful when normal in the setting of hypoxemia.

2. **Lung scanning**—A perfusion scan is performed by injecting radiolabeled microaggregated albumin into the venous system, allowing the particles to embolize to the pulmonary capillary bed. To perform a ventilation scan, the patient breathes a radioactive gas or aerosol while the distribution of radioactivity in the lungs is recorded.

A defect on perfusion scanning represents diminished blood flow to that region of the lung. This finding is not specific for pulmonary embolism. Defects in the perfusion scan are interpreted in conjunction with the ventilation scan to give a high, low, or intermediate (indeterminate) probability that pulmonary thromboembolism is the cause of the abnormalities. Criteria for the combined interpretation of ventilation and perfusion scans (commonly referred to as a single

Table 9–20. Frequency of specific symptoms and signs in patients at risk for pulmonary thromboembolism.

	UPET[1] PE+ (n = 327)	PIOPED[2] PE+ (n = 117)	PIOPED[2] PE''' (n = 248)
Symptoms			
Dyspnea	84%	73%	72%
Respirophasic chest pain	74%	66%	59%
Cough	53%	37%	36%
Leg pain	nr	26%	24%
Hemoptysis	30%	13%	8%
Palpitations	nr	10%	18%
Wheezing	nr	9%	11%
Anginal pain	14%	4%	6%
Signs			
Respiratory rate ≥ 16 UPET, ≥ 20 PIOPED	92%	70%	68%
Crackles (rales)	58%	51%	40%[3]
Heart rate ≥ 100/min	44%	30%	24%
Fourth heart sound (S_4)	nr	24%	13%[3]
Accentuated pulmonary component of second heart sound (S_2P)	53%	23%	13%[3]
T ≥ 37.5 °C UPET, ≥ 38.5 °C PIOPED	43%	7%	12%
Homans' sign	nr	4%	2%
Pleural friction rub	nr	3%	2%
Third heart sound (S_3)	nr	3%	4%
Cyanosis	19%	1%	2%

[1]Data from the Urokinase-Streptokinase Pulmonary Embolism Trial, as reported in Bell WR, Simon TL, DeMets DL: The clinical features of submassive and massive pulmonary emboli. Am J Med 1977;62:355.
[2]Data from patients enrolled in the PIOPED Study, as reported in Stein PD et al: Clinical, laboratory, roentgenographic, and electrocardiographic findings in patients with acute pulmonary embolism and no preexisting cardiac or pulmonary disease. Chest 1991;100:598.
PE+ = confirmed diagnosis of pulmonary embolism; PE– = diagnosis of pulmonary embolism ruled out; nr = not reported.
[3]$P < .05$ comparing patients in the PIOPED Study.

test, the V/Q scan) are complex, confusing, and not completely standardized. A normal perfusion scan excludes the diagnosis of clinically significant pulmonary thromboembolism (negative predictive value of 91% in the PIOPED study). A high-probability V/Q scan is most often defined as having two or more segmental perfusion defects in the presence of normal ventilation and is sufficient to make the diagnosis of pulmonary thromboembolism in most instances (positive predictive value of 88% among PIOPED patients). In the presence of abnormal pulmonary vasculature, as commonly happens in prior pulmonary thromboembolism, or if the clinical pretest probability for embolism is low, angiography may be indicated even in the presence of a high-probability V/Q scan.

Ventilation-perfusion scans are most helpful when they are either normal or indicate a high probability of pulmonary thromboembolism. Such readings are reliable—interobserver agreement is best for normal and high-probability scans, and they carry predictive power. The likelihood ratios associated with normal and high-probability scans are 0.10 and 18, respectively, indicating significant and frequently conclusive changes from pretest to posttest probability.

However, 75% of PIOPED V/Q scans were nondiagnostic, ie, of low or intermediate probability. At angiography, these patients had an overall incidence of pulmonary thromboembolism of 14% and 30%, respectively. The likelihood ratios associated with low-probability and intermediate scans are 0.36 and 1.2, respectively, confirming the clinical impression that these studies add little diagnostic information. One of the most important findings of PIOPED was that the clinical assessment of pretest probability could be used to aid the interpretation of the V/Q scan. For those patients with low-probability V/Q scans and a low (20% or less) clinical pretest probability of pulmonary thromboembolism, the diagnosis was confirmed in only 4%. Such patients may reasonably be observed without angiography. All other patients with nondiagnostic V/Q scans require further testing to determine the presence of venous thromboembolism.

3. CT—Spiral CT angiography requires administration of intravenous radiocontrast dye but is otherwise noninvasive. It is very sensitive for the detection of thrombus in the proximal pulmonary arteries but less so in the segmental and subsegmental arteries. Test results vary widely by study and facility. Factors influencing results include patient size and cooperation, the quality of the scanner, the imaging protocol, and the experience of the radiologist. One report comparing spiral CT with angiography reported sensitivity of 53–60% and specificity of 81–97%. Reviewing spiral CT scanning as an alternative to the V/Q scan as the initial test for pulmonary thromboembolism, detection of thrombi was comparable, but more nonthromboembolism pulmonary diagnoses were made with CT scanning. Independent of cost and availability, spiral CT may offer advantages as a screening examination in hospitalized patients and in patients with significant comorbidities. Some centers now use spiral CT as the initial screening test for pulmonary thromboembolism in patients likely to have indeterminate V/Q scans, ie, those with abnormal chest radiographs. A contentious issue is whether a negative result requires any further evaluation. False-negative results may occur in up to 20% of spiral CTs. Advocates of spiral CT contend that these false-negatives represent small peripheral thromboemboli and that such patients can be followed off anticoagulation without undue risk. Further study is required to clarify the role of this diagnostic modality, this is especially true in view of ongoing advances in CT technology and the increasing availability of multi-detector-row spiral CT scanners.

4. Venous thrombosis studies—Seventy percent of patients with pulmonary thromboembolism will have deep venous thrombosis on evaluation, and approximately half of patients with DVT will have pulmonary thromboembolism on angiography. Since the history and physical examination are neither sensitive nor specific for pulmonary thromboembolism and since the results of V/Q scanning are frequently equivocal, documentation of DVT in a patient with suspected pulmonary thromboembolism establishes the need for treatment and may preclude pulmonary angiography.

Commonly available diagnostic techniques include venous ultrasonography, impedance plethysmography, and contrast venography. In most centers, venous ultrasonography is the test of choice to detect proximal DVT. Inability to compress the common femoral or popliteal veins in symptomatic patients is diagnostic of first-episode DVT (positive predictive value of 97%); full compressibility of both sites excludes proximal DVT (negative predictive value of 98%). The test is less accurate in distal thrombi, recurrent thrombi, or in asymptomatic patients. Impedance plethysmography relies on changes in electrical impedance between patent and obstructed veins to determine the presence of thrombus. Accuracy is comparable though not quite as high as ultrasonography. Both ultrasonography and impedance plethysmography are useful in the serial examination of patients with high clinical suspicion of venous thromboembolism but negative leg studies. In patients with suspected first-episode DVT and a negative ultrasound or impedance plethysmography examination, multiple studies have confirmed the safety of withholding anticoagulation while conducting two sequential studies on days 1–3 and 7–10. Similarly, patients with nondiagnostic V/Q scans and an initial negative venous ultrasound or impedance plethysmography examination may be followed off therapy with serial leg studies over 2 weeks. When serial examinations are negative for proximal DVT, the risk of subsequent venous thromboembolism over the following 6 months is less than 2%.

Contrast venography remains the reference standard for the diagnosis of DVT. An intraluminal filling defect is diagnostic of venous thrombosis. However, venography has significant shortcomings and has been replaced by venous ultrasound as the diagnostic procedure of choice. Difficulties include patient discomfort, expense, allergic reactions to radiocontrast media, contrast-induced phlebitis, and technical difficulties in cannulation of dorsal foot veins and in the interpretation of studies. There is a significant (2–4%) risk of developing venous thrombosis from the procedure—a risk that may be higher than the false-negative rate of noninvasive studies. Venography is used principally in complex situations where there is discrepancy between clinical suspicion and noninvasive testing.

5. Pulmonary angiography—Pulmonary angiography remains the reference standard for the diagnosis of pulmonary thromboembolism. An intraluminal filling defect in more than one projection establishes a definitive diagnosis. Secondary findings highly suggestive of pulmonary thromboembolism include abrupt arterial cutoff, asymmetry of blood flow—especially segmental oligemia—or a prolonged arterial phase with slow filling. Pulmonary angiography was performed in 755 patients in the PIOPED study. A definitive diagnosis was established in 97%; in 3% the studies were nondiagnostic; and four patients (0.8%) with negative angiograms subsequently had pulmonary thromboemboli at autopsy. Serial angiography has demonstrated minimal resolution of thrombus prior to day 7. Thus, negative angiography prior to day 7 for practical purposes excludes the diagnosis.

Pulmonary angiography is a safe but invasive procedure with well-defined morbidity and mortality. Minor complications occur in approximately 5% of patients. Most are allergic contrast reactions, transient renal dysfunction, or related to percutaneous catheter insertion; cardiac perforation and arrhythmias are reported but rare. Among the PIOPED patients who underwent angiography, there were five deaths (0.7%) directly related to the procedure. Pulmonary hypertension is thought to increase the risk of serious complications, though a study of patients with average pulmonary arterial pressures of 74/34 mm Hg developed no major complications or deaths associated with pulmonary angiography.

The appropriate role of pulmonary angiography in the diagnosis of pulmonary thromboembolism remains a subject of active debate. There is wide agreement that angiography is indicated in several specific situations: In patients with nondiagnostic V/Q scans, intermediate or high clinical pretest probability of pulmonary thromboembolism and negative noninvasive leg studies; in any patient in whom the diagnosis is in doubt when there is a high clinical pretest probability of pulmonary thromboembolism; and when the diagnosis of pulmonary thromboembolism must be established with certainty, as when anticoagulation is contraindicated or placement of an inferior vena cava filter is contemplated.

6. MRI—MRI has sensitivity and specificity equivalent to contrast venography in the diagnosis of deep venous thrombosis. It has improved sensitivity when compared with venous ultrasound in the diagnosis of DVT, without loss of specificity. The test is noninva-sive and avoids the use of potentially nephrotoxic radiocontrast dye. However, it remains expensive and not widely available. Artifacts introduced by respiratory and cardiac motion have limited the use of MRI in the diagnosis of pulmonary thromboembolism. New techniques have improved sensitivity and specificity to levels comparable with spiral CT, but MRI remains primarily a research tool for pulmonary thromboembolism.

7. Integrated approach—The integrated approach uses the clinical likelihood of venous thromboembolism along with the overlapping results of noninvasive testing to come to one of three decision points: to establish venous thromboembolism (pulmonary thromboembolism or DVT) as the diagnosis; to exclude venous thromboembolism with sufficient confidence to follow the patient without therapy; or to refer the patient for pulmonary angiography. An ideal diagnostic algorithm would proceed in a stepwise fashion to come to these decision points in a cost-effective way at minimal risk to the patient. One such algorithm is offered in Figure 9–3.

The most innovative developments in systematic diagnosis have suggested three changes to this standard model. First are attempts to refine the clinical pretest probability to identify a subset of patients at low likelihood for venous thromboembolism. Second, some investigators have used negative D-dimer determinations (to exclude venous thromboembolism) in combination with venous ultrasonography (to estab-

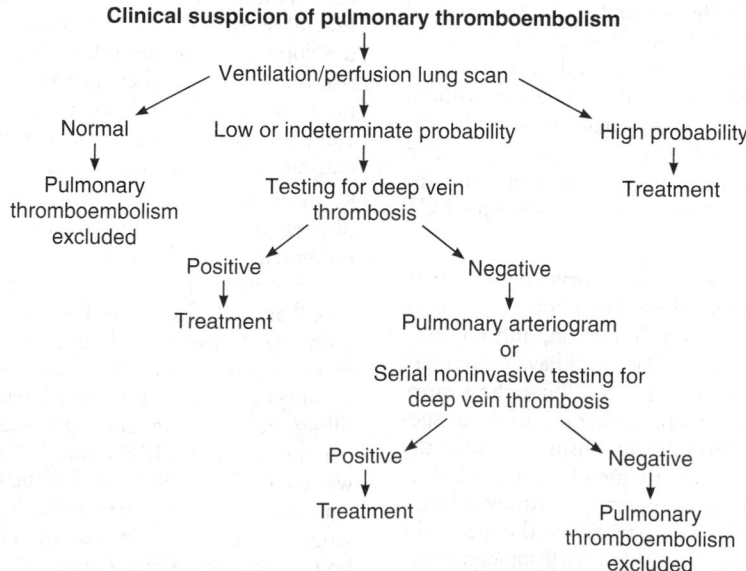

Figure 9–3. A simple algorithm for the management of venous thromboembolism based on the results of ventilation/perfusion lung scanning. The algorithm starts with a clinical suspicion of pulmonary thromboembolism. Management of patients with ventilation/perfusion lung scans of low or indeterminate probability must always be guided by clinical judgment based upon cumulative clinical information and the degree of suspicion of pulmonary thromboembolism.

lish the diagnosis of DVT) to evaluate a majority of outpatients *before* proceeding to ventilation-perfusion scanning. The increasing availability of improved and rapid D-dimer assays may result in significant changes to these algorithms in the future. Third, there is active debate about the role of spiral CT in the initial evaluation of suspected pulmonary thromboembolism; clarification should come from studies using multi-detector-row spiral CT scanners.

Prevention

Venous thromboembolism is often clinically silent until it presents with significant morbidity or mortality. It is a prevalent disease, clearly associated with identifiable risk factors. For example, the incidence of proximal DVT, pulmonary thromboembolism, and fatal pulmonary thromboembolism in untreated patients undergoing hip fracture surgery is reported to be 10–20%, 4–10%, and 0.2–5%, respectively. There is unambiguous evidence of the efficacy of prophylactic therapy in this and other clinical situations, yet it remains underused. Only about 50% of surgical deaths from pulmonary thromboembolism had received any form of preventive therapy. Tables 9–21 and 9–22 provide overviews of strategies for the prevention of venous thromboembolism.

Options for therapy begin with mechanical devices such as graduated-compression stockings and intermittent pneumatic compression. The latter improves venous return and may increase endogenous fibrinolysis by stimulating the vascular endothelium. Standard pharmacologic therapy in medical patients is low-dose unfractionated heparin, 5000 units subcutaneously every 8–12 hours. Low-molecular-weight heparins are more expensive but have several advantages compared with unfractionated heparin: better bioavailability, once- or twice-daily dosing, and a lower incidence of heparin-associated thrombocytopenia. In high-risk surgical patients, low-molecular-weight heparins can be administered without the need for coagulation monitoring and dose adjustments, as would be the case with unfractionated heparin.

Treatment

A. ANTICOAGULATION

Anticoagulation is not definitive therapy but a form of secondary prevention. Heparin binds to and accelerates the ability of antithrombin III to inactivate thrombin, factor Xa, and factor IXa. It thus retards additional thrombus formation, allowing endogenous fibrinolytic mechanisms to lyse existing clot. The standard regimen of heparin followed by 6 months of oral warfarin results in an 80–90% reduction in the risk of both recurrent venous thrombosis and death from pulmonary thromboembolism.

Heparin has troublesome pharmacokinetics. Its clearance is dose-dependent; it is highly protein-bound; and a minimum or threshold level is necessary to achieve an antithrombotic effect. It is necessary to monitor the activated partial thromboplastin time (aPTT) and adjust dosing to maintain the aPTT 1.5–2.5 times control. In patients with a moderate to high clinical likelihood of pulmonary thromboembolism and no contraindications, full anticoagulation with heparin should begin with the diagnostic evaluation. Once the diagnosis of proximal DVT or pulmonary thromboembolism is established, it is critical to ensure adequate therapy. Failure to achieve therapeutic heparin levels within 24 hours is associated with a fivefold-increased risk of clot propagation. The weight-based regimen in Table 9–23 is superior to standard dosing. Heparin causes immune-mediated thrombocytopenia in 3% of patients; therefore, the platelet count should be determined frequently for the first 14 days of therapy.

Low-molecular-weight heparins are depolymerized preparations of heparin with multiple advantages over unfractionated heparin. They exhibit less binding to cells and proteins and have superior bioavailability, a longer plasma half-life, and more predictable dose-response characteristics. They appear to carry an equivalent or lower risk of hemorrhage, and immune-mediated thrombocytopenia is less common. LMW heparins appear to be at least as effective as unfractionated heparin in the treatment of venous thromboembolism. They are administered in dosages determined by body weight once or twice daily without the need for coagulation monitoring, and subcutaneous administration appears to be as effective as the intravenous route. This profile makes LMW heparins ideal for home-based therapy of venous thromboembolism. Home-based therapy appears safe and efficacious in a small number of selected patients. Table 9–24 sets forth selected LMW heparin anticoagulation regimens.

Anticoagulation therapy for venous thromboembolism is continued for a minimum of 3 months, so oral anticoagulant therapy with warfarin is usually initiated concurrently with heparin. Warfarin affects hepatic synthesis of vitamin K-dependent coagulant proteins. It usually requires 5–7 days to become therapeutic; therefore, heparin is generally continued for 5 days. Warfarin is safe if begun concurrently with heparin, initially at a dose of 5–10 mg/d. The lower dose is preferred in older patients. Maintenance therapy usually requires 2–15 mg/d. Adequacy of therapy must be monitored by following the prothrombin time, most often adjusted for differences in reagents and reported as the international normalized ratio, or INR. The target INR is 2.5, with the acceptable range from 2.0 to 3.0; below 2.0, there is an increased risk of thrombosis; above 4.0, there is an increased risk of hemorrhage. Warfarin has interactions with many drugs. Meticulous attention to medications is part of the routine management of every patient receiving warfarin. Warfarin is a pregnancy category X medication, indi-

Table 9–21. Selected methods for the prevention of venous thromboembolism.[1]

Risk Group	Recommendations for Prophylaxis
Surgical patients	
General surgery	Early ambulation
Low-risk: Minor procedures, age under 40, and no clinical risk factors	
Moderate risk: Minor procedures with additional thrombosis risk factors; age 40–60, and no other clinical risk factors; or major operations with age under 40 without additional clinical risk factors	ES, or LDUH, or LMWH, or IPC; plus early ambulation if possible
Higher risk: Major operation, over age 40 or with additional risk factors	LDUH, or LMWH, or IPC
Higher risk plus increased risk of bleeding	ES or IPC
Very high risk: Multiple risk factors	LDUH, or higher-dose LMWH, plus ES or IPC
Selected very high risk	Consider ADPW, INR 2.0–3.0, or postdischarge LMWH
Orthopedic surgery	
Elective total hip replacement surgery	Subcutaneous LMWH, or ADPW, or adjusted-dose heparin started preoperatively; plus IPC or ES
Elective total knee replacement surgery	LMWH, or ADPW, or IPC
Hip fracture surgery	LMWH or ADPW
Neurosurgery	
Intracranial neurosurgery	IPC with or without ES; LDUH and postoperative LMWH are acceptable alternatives; IPC or ES plus LDUH or LMWH may be more effective than either modality alone in high-risk patients.
Acute spinal cord injury	LMWH; IPC and ES may have additional benefit when used with LMWH. In the rehabilitation phase, conversion to full-dose warfarin may provide ongoing protection.
Trauma	
With an identifiable risk factor for thromboembolism	LMWH; IPC or ES if there is a contraindication to LMWH; consider duplex ultrasound screening in very high risk patients; IVC filter insertion if proximal DVT is identified and anticoagulation is contraindicated.
Medical patients	
Acute myocardial infarction	Subcutaneous LDUH, or full-dose heparin; if heparin is contraindicated, IPC and ES may provide some protection.
Ischemic stroke with impaired mobility	LMWH or LDUH or danaparoid; IPC or ES if anticoagulants are contraindicated
General medical patients with clinical risk factors; especially patients with cancer, congestive heart failure, or severe pulmonary disease	Low-dose LMWH, or LDUH
Cancer patients with indwelling central venous catheters	Warfarin, 1 mg/d, or LMWH

[1]Recommendations assembled from Geerts WH et al: Prevention of venous thromboembolism. Chest 2001;119(Suppl):132.

Key:
ADPW = adjusted-dose perioperative warfarin: begin 5–10 mg the day of or the day following surgery; adjust dose to INR 2.0–3.0
DVT = deep venous thrombosis
ES = elastic stockings
IPC = intermittent pneumatic compression
IVC = inferior vena cava
LDUH = low-dose unfractionated heparin: 5000 units subcutaneously every 8–12 hours starting 1–2 hours before surgery.
LMWH = low-molecular weight heparin. See Table 9–24 for dosing regimens.

Table 9–22. Selected low-molecular-weight heparin and heparinoid regimens to prevent venous thromboembolism.[1]

Risk Group	Drug	Dose[2]	Administration Regimen	Cost[3]
General surgery, moderate risk	Dalteparin (Fragmin)	2500 units	1–2 h preop and qd postop	$15.35/dose
	Enoxaparin (Lovenox)	20 mg	1–2 h preop and qd postop	$17.47/dose
	Nadroparin (Fraxiparin)	2850 units	2–4 h preop and qd postop	
	Tinzaparin (Innohep)	3500 units	2 h preop and qd postop	$29.40/dose
General surgery, high risk	Dalteparin (Fragmin)	5000 units	8–12 preop and qd postop	$24.90/dose
	Danaparoid (Organon)	750 units	1–4 h preop and Q 12 h postop	$141.31/dose
	Enoxaparin (Lovenox)	40 mg	1–2 h preop and qd postop	$24.46/dose
	Enoxaparin (Lovenox)	30 mg	q 12 h starting 8–12 h postop	$18.35/dose
Orthopedic surgery	Dalteparin (Fragmin)	5000 units	8–12 h preop and qd starting 12–24 h postop	$24.90/dose
	Dalteparin (Fragmin)	2,500 units	6–8 h postop then 5,000 units qd	$15.35/dose
	Danaparoid (Organon)	750 units	1–4 preop and q 12 h postop	$141.31/dose
	Enoxaparin (Lovenox)	30 mg	q 12 h starting 12–24 h postop	$18.35/dose
	Enoxaparin (Lovenox)	40 mg	qd starting 10–12 h preop	$24.46/dose
	Nadroparin (Fraxiparin)	38 units/kg	12 h preop, 12 h postop, and qd on postop days 1, 2, 3; then increase to 57 units/kg qd	No price available: Not available in USA.
	Tinzaparin (Innohep)	75 units/kg	qd starting 12–24 h postop	$74.67/dose (60 kg pt).
	Tinzaparin (Innohep)	4500 units	12 h preop and qd postop	$74.67/dose
Major trauma	Enoxaparin (Lovenox)	30 mg	q12h starting 12–36 h postinjury if hemostatically stable	$18.35/dose
Acute spinal cord injury	Enoxaparin (Lovenox)	30 mg	q12h	$18.35/dose
Medical conditions	Dalteparin (Fragmin)	2500 units	qd	$15.35/dose
	Danaparoid (Organon)	750 units	q12h	$141.31/dose
	Enoxparin (Lovenox)	40 mg	qd	$24.46/dose
	Nadroparin (Fraxiparin)	2850 units	qd	No price available: not available in USA.

[1]Modified and reproduced with permission, from Geerts WH et al: Prevention of venous thromboembolism. Chest 2001;119:132S.
[2]Dose expressed in anti-Xa units; for enoxaparin, 1 mg = 100 anti-Xa units. All doses are to be administered subcutaneously.
[3]Cost to pharmacist (average wholesale price, generic when possible) for quantity listed. Source: *Drug Topics Red Book,* March 2002; Vol. 21, No. 3.
Preop = preoperatively; Postop = postoperatively; qd = once daily.

cating known fetopathic and teratogenic effects. When oral anticoagulation with warfarin is contraindicated, LMW heparin is a convenient alternative.

The optimal duration of anticoagulation therapy for venous thromboembolism is unknown. There appears to be a protective benefit to continued anticoagulation in first-episode venous thromboembolism (twice the rate of recurrence in 6 weeks compared with 6 months of therapy) and recurrent disease (eightfold risk of recurrence in 6 months compared with 4 years of therapy). These studies do not distinguish patients with reversible risk factors, such as surgery or transient immobility, from patients who have a nonreversible hypercoagulable state such as factor V Leiden, inhibitor deficiency, antiphospholipid syndrome, or ma-

Table 9–23. Intravenous heparin dosing based on body weight.[1]

Initial dosing

1. Load with 80 units/kg IV, then
2. Initiate a maintenance infusion at 18 units/kg/h
3. Check activated partial thromboplastin time (aPTT) in 6 hours

Dose adjustment schedule based on aPTT results

< 35 s (< 1.25 × control)	Rebolus with 80 units/kg; increase infusion by 4 units/kg/h
35–45 s (1.2– 1.5 × control)	Rebolus with 40 units/kg; increase infusion by 2 units/kg/h
46–70 s (1.5– 2.3 × control)	No change
71–90 s (2.3–3 × control)	Decrease infusion rate by 2 units/kg/h
> 90 s (> 3 × control)	Stop infusion for 1 hour, then decrease infusion by 3 units/kg/h

Repeat aPTT every 6 hours for the first 24 hours. If the aPTT is 46–70 s after 24 hours, then recheck once daily every morning. If the aPTT is outside this therapeutic range at 24 hours, continue checking every 6 hours until it is 46–70 s. Once it has been in the therapeutic range on two consecutive measurements after 24 hours, check once daily every morning.

[1]Adapted from Raschke RA et al: The weight-based heparin dosing nomogram compared with a "standard care" nomogram. Ann Intern Med 1993;119:874.

lignancy. Patients with idiopathic venous thromboembolism may benefit most from prolonged therapy. For many patients, venous thrombosis is a recurrent disease, and continued therapy will result in a lower rate of recurrence at the cost of an increased risk of hemorrhage. Therefore, the appropriate duration of therapy will need to take into consideration potentially reversible risk factors, the individual's age, the likelihood and potential consequences of hemorrhage, and patient preferences for continued therapy. It is reason-

Table 9–24. Selected low-molecular-weight heparin anticoagulation regimens.[1,2]

Drug	Suggested Treatment Dose
Dalteparin	200 units/kg once daily (not to exceed 18,000 units/dose)
Enoxaparin	1.5 mg/kg once daily (single dose not to exceed 180 mg)
Nadroparin	86 units/kg twice daily for 10 days, or 171 units/kg once daily (single dose not to exceed 17,000 units)
Tinzaparin	175 units/kg once daily

[1]Modified and reproduced with permission, from Hyers TM et al: Antithrombotic therapy for venous thromboembolic disease. Chest 2001;119(Suppl):176S.
[2]Dose expressed in anti-Xa units; for enoxaparin, 1 mg = 100 anti-Xa units. All doses are to be administered subcutaneously.

able to continue therapy for 6 months after a first episode when there is a reversible risk factor, 12 months after a first-episode idiopathic thrombus, and 6–12 months to indefinitely in patients with nonreversible risk factors or recurrent disease.

The major complication of anticoagulation is hemorrhage. Risk factors for hemorrhage include the intensity of the anticoagulant effect; the duration of therapy; concomitant administration of drugs such as aspirin that interfere with platelet function; and patient characteristics, particularly increased age, previous gastrointestinal hemorrhage, and coexistent renal insufficiency.

The reported incidence of major hemorrhage following intravenous administration of unfractionated heparin is nil to 7%; that of fatal hemorrhage is nil to 2%. The incidence with LMW heparins is not statistically different. There is no information comparing hemorrhage rates at different doses of heparin. The risk of subtherapeutic heparin administration in the first 24–48 hours after diagnosis is significant; it appears to outweigh the risk of short-term supratherapeutic heparin levels. The incidence of hemorrhage during therapy with warfarin is reported to be between 3% and 4% per patient year. The frequency varies with the target INR and is consistently higher when the INR exceeds 4.0. There is no apparent additional antithrombotic benefit in venous thromboembolism with a target INR above 2.0–3.0.

B. THROMBOLYTIC THERAPY

Streptokinase, urokinase, and recombinant tissue plasminogen activator (rt-PA; alteplase) increase plasmin levels and thereby directly lyse intravascular thrombi. In patients with established pulmonary thromboembolism, thrombolytic therapy accelerates resolution of emboli within the first 24 hours compared with standard heparin therapy. This is a consistent finding using angiography, V/Q scanning, echocardiography, and direct measurement of pulmonary artery pressures. However, at 1 week and 1 month after diagnosis, these agents show no difference in outcome compared with heparin and warfarin. There is no evidence that thrombolytic therapy improves mortality. Subtle improvements in pulmonary function, including improved single-breath diffusing capacity and a lower incidence of exercise-induced pulmonary hypertension, have been observed. The reliability and clinical importance of these findings is unclear. The major disadvantages of thrombolytic therapy compared with heparin are its greater cost and a significant increase in major hemorrhagic complications. The incidence of intracranial hemorrhage in patients with pulmonary thromboemboli treated with alteplase is 2.1% compared with 0.2% in patients treated with heparin.

Current evidence supports thrombolytic therapy for pulmonary thromboembolism in patients at high risk for death in whom the more rapid resolution of thrombus may be lifesaving. Such patients are usually hemodynamically unstable despite heparin therapy.

Absolute contraindications to thrombolytic therapy include active internal bleeding and stroke within the past 2 months. Major contraindications include uncontrolled hypertension and surgery or trauma within the past 6 weeks.

C. ADDITIONAL MEASURES

Interruption of the inferior vena cava may be indicated in patients with a major contraindication to anticoagulation who have or are at high risk for development of proximal deep vein thrombosis or pulmonary embolus. Placement of an inferior vena cava filter is also recommended for recurrent thromboembolism despite adequate anticoagulation, for chronic recurrent embolism with pulmonary hypertension, and with the concurrent performance of surgical pulmonary embolectomy or pulmonary thromboendarterectomy. Percutaneous transjugular placement of a mechanical filter is the preferred mode of inferior vena cava interruption. These devices reduce the short-term incidence of pulmonary thromboemboli in patients presenting with proximal lower extremity deep venous thrombosis. However, they are associated with a two-fold increased risk of recurrent deep venous thrombosis in the first 2 years following placement.

In rare critically ill patients for whom thrombolytic therapy is contraindicated or unsuccessful, mechanical or surgical extraction of thrombus may be indicated. Pulmonary embolectomy is an emergency procedure of last resort with a very high mortality rate. It is now performed only in a few specialized centers. Several catheter devices to fragment and extract thrombus through a transvenous approach have been reported in small numbers of patients. Comparative outcomes with surgery, thrombolytic therapy, or heparin have not been studied.

Prognosis

Pulmonary thromboembolism is estimated to cause more than 50,000 deaths annually. In the majority of deaths, pulmonary thromboembolism is not recognized antemortem or death occurs before specific treatment can be initiated. These statistics highlight the importance of preventive therapy in high-risk patients. The outlook for patients with diagnosed and appropriately treated pulmonary thromboembolism is generally good. Overall prognosis depends on the underlying disease rather than the pulmonary thromboembolism itself. Death from recurrent thromboemboli is uncommon, occurring in less than 3% of cases. Perfusion defects resolve in most survivors. Approximately 1% of patients develop chronic thromboembolic pulmonary hypertension. Selected patients may benefit from pulmonary endarterectomy.

Decousus H et al: A clinical trial of vena caval filters in the prevention of pulmonary embolism in patients with proximal deep-vein thrombosis. N Engl J Med 1998;338:409. [PMID: 9459643] (Initial beneficial effects of filter placement were counterbalanced by excess recurrence of deep vein thrombosis without mortality difference.)

Geerts WH et al: Prevention of venous thromboembolism. Chest 2001;119(1 Suppl):132. [PMID: 1115/647] (Exhaustive review of all aspects of prophylactic therapy.)

Goodman LR et al: Subsequent pulmonary embolism: risk after a negative helical CT pulmonary angiogram—prospective comparison with scintigraphy. Radiology 2000;215:535. [PMID: 10796937] (With 90% follow-up in 3 months, authors report 1% subsequent diagnosis of pulmonary embolism in patients with negative helical CT. Mortality higher in CT group and no autopsy confirmation of cause of death. Highlights need for further study.)

Hyers TM et al: Antithrombotic therapy for venous thromboembolic disease. Chest 2001;119:176S. [PMID: 11157648] (Detailed evidence-based recommendations.)

Kearon C et al: A comparison of three months of anticoagulation with extended anticoagulation for a first episode of idiopathic venous thromboembolism. N Engl J Med 1999; 340:901. [PMID: 10089183] (Randomized to 3 versus 24 months of therapy. Trial halted early due to increased recurrence in control group.)

Perrier A et al: Performance of helical computed tomography in unselected outpatients with suspected pulmonary embolism. Ann Intern Med 2001;135:88. [PMID: 11453707] (Sensitivity and specificity of helical CT for the diagnosis of venous thromboembolism were 70% and 91%, respectively, suggesting that helical CT is not adequate as the sole screening test for outpatients.)

Tapson VF et al: The diagnostic approach to acute venous thromboembolism. Clinical practice guideline. American Thoracic Society. Am J Respir Crit Care Med 1999;160:1043. [PMID: 10471639]

Value of the ventilation/perfusion scan in acute pulmonary embolism. Results of the prospective investigation of pulmonary embolism diagnosis (PIOPED). The PIOPED Investigators. JAMA 1990;263:2753. [PMID: 2332219] (Classic article defining the additive utility of clinical judgment with ventilation-perfusion scanning in the diagnostic evaluation of pulmonary embolism.)

Wells PS et al: Excluding pulmonary embolism at the bedside without diagnostic imaging: management of patients with suspected pulmonary embolism presenting to the emergency department by using a simple clinical model and d-dimer. Ann Intern Med 2001;135:98. [PMID: 11453709] (Use of clinical assessment of prior probability of venous thromboembolism and quantitative measurement of D-dimer levels allowed safe and efficient triage and decreased the need for diagnostic imaging.)

White RH et al: A population-based study of the effectiveness of inferior vena caval filter use among patients with venous thromboembolism. Arch Intern Med 2000;160:2033. [PMID: 10888977]

PULMONARY HYPERTENSION

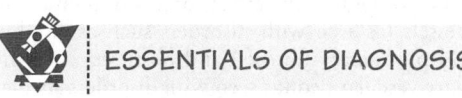

ESSENTIALS OF DIAGNOSIS

- *Dyspnea, fatigue, chest pain, and syncope on exertion.*
- *Narrow splitting of second heart sound with loud pulmonary component; findings of right*

ventricular hypertrophy and cardiac failure in advanced disease.

- Hypoxemia and increased wasted ventilation on pulmonary function tests.
- Electrocardiographic evidence of right ventricular strain or hypertrophy and right atrial enlargement.
- Enlarged central pulmonary arteries on chest radiograph.

General Considerations

The pulmonary circulation is unique because of its high blood flow, low pressure (normally 25/8 mm Hg, mean 12), and low resistance (normally 200–250 dynes/sec/cm^{-5}). It can accommodate large increases in blood flow during exercise with only modest increases in pressure because of its ability to recruit and distend lung blood vessels. The normal pulmonary circulation is largely passive, since its pressures are determined mainly by the function of the right and left ventricles. Contraction of smooth muscle in the walls of pulmonary arteriolar resistance vessels becomes an important factor in numerous pathologic states. Pulmonary hypertension is present when pulmonary artery pressure rises to a level inappropriate for a given cardiac output. Once present, pulmonary hypertension is self-perpetuating. It introduces secondary structural abnormalities in pulmonary vessels, including smooth muscle hypertrophy and intimal proliferation, and these may eventually stimulate atheromatous changes and in situ thrombosis, leading to further narrowing of the arterial bed.

Primary (idiopathic) pulmonary hypertension (see Chapter 10) is a rare disorder of the pulmonary circulation occurring mostly in young and middle-aged women. It is characterized by progressive dyspnea, a rapid downhill course, and an invariably fatal outcome. This condition is also called plexogenic pulmonary arteriopathy, in reference to the characteristic histopathologic plexiform lesion found in muscular pulmonary arteries. It has been observed in occasional patients with HIV infection.

Selected mechanisms responsible for **secondary pulmonary hypertension** and examples of corresponding clinical conditions are set forth in Table 9–25. Pulmonary arteriolar vasoconstriction due to chronic hypoxemia may complicate any chronic lung disease and compound the effects of loss of pulmonary blood vessels (as seen with disorders such as emphysema and pulmonary fibrosis) and obstruction of the pulmonary vascular bed (as seen with disorders such as chronic pulmonary thromboembolic disease). Sustained increases in pulmonary venous pressure from disorders such as left ventricular failure (systolic, diastolic, or both), mitral stenosis, and pulmonary veno-occlusive disease may cause "postcapillary" pulmonary

Table 9–25. Mechanisms of pulmonary hypertension and examples of corresponding clinical conditions.

Reduction in cross-sectional area of pulmonary arterial bed
  Vasoconstriction
    Hypoxia from any cause (chronic lung disease, sleep-disordered breathing, etc)
    Acidosis
  Loss of vessels
    Lung resection
    Emphysema
    Vasculitis
    Intestitial lung disease
    Collagen-vascular disease
  Obstruction of vessels
    Pulmonary embolism (thromboemboli, tumor emboli, etc)
    In situ thrombosis
    Schistosomiasis
    Sickle cell disease
  Narrowing of vessels
    Secondary structural changes due to pulmonary hypertension
Increased pulmonary venous pressure
  Constrictive pericarditis
  Left ventricular failure or reduced compliance
  Mitral stenosis
  Left atrial myxoma
  Pulmonary veno-occlusive disease
  Mediastinal diseases compressing pulmonary veins
Increased pulmonary blood flow
  Congenital left-to-right intracardiac shunts
Increased blood viscosity
  Polycythemia
Miscellaneous
  Pulmonary hypertension occurring in association with hepatic cirrhosis and portal hypertension
  HIV infection

---

hypertension. Increased pulmonary blood flow due to intracardiac shunts and increased blood viscosity due to polycythemia can also cause pulmonary hypertension. Pulmonary hypertension has also been associated with hepatic cirrhosis and portal hypertension.

Pulmonary veno-occlusive disease is a rare cause of postcapillary pulmonary hypertension occurring in children and young adults. The cause is unknown, but associations with various conditions such as viral infection, bone marrow transplantation, chemotherapy, and malignancy have been described. The disease is characterized by progressive fibrotic occlusion of pulmonary veins and venules, along with secondary hypertensive changes in the pulmonary arterioles and muscular pulmonary arteries. Nodular areas of pulmonary congestion, edema, hemorrhage, and hemosiderosis are found. Chest radiography reveals prominent, symmetric interstitial markings, Kerley B lines, pulmonary artery dilation, and normally sized left atrium and left ventricle. Premortem diagnosis is often difficult but is occasionally established by open lung biopsy. There is no effective therapy, and most patients die within 2 years as a result of progressive pulmonary hypertension.

Clinical Findings

A. Symptoms and Signs

Secondary pulmonary hypertension is difficult to recognize clinically in the early stages, when symptoms and signs are primarily those of the underlying disease. Pulmonary hypertension may cause or contribute to dyspnea, present initially on exertion and later at rest. Dull, retrosternal chest pain resembling angina pectoris may be present. Fatigue and syncope on exertion also occur, presumably a result of reduced cardiac output related to elevated pulmonary artery pressures or bradycardia.

The signs of pulmonary hypertension include narrow splitting of the second heart sound, accentuation of the pulmonary component of the second heart sound, and a systolic ejection click. In advanced cases, tricuspid and pulmonary valve insufficiency and signs of right ventricular failure and cor pulmonale are found.

B. Laboratory Findings

Polycythemia is found in many cases of pulmonary hypertension that are associated with chronic hypoxemia. Electrocardiographic changes are those of right axis deviation, right ventricular hypertrophy, right ventricular strain, or right atrial enlargement.

C. Imaging and Special Examinations

Chest radiographs (plain films as well as high-resolution CT scans) can assist in the diagnosis of pulmonary hypertension as well as determination of the cause. Radiographic findings depend on the cause of pulmonary hypertension. In chronic disease, dilation of the right and left main and lobar pulmonary arteries and enlargement of the pulmonary outflow tract are seen; in advanced disease, right ventricular and right atrial enlargement are seen. Peripheral "pruning" of large pulmonary arteries is characteristic of pulmonary hypertension in severe emphysema.

Echocardiography is helpful in evaluating patients thought to have mitral stenosis, left atrial myxoma, and pulmonary valvular disease and may also reveal right ventricular enlargement and paradoxical motion of the interventricular septum. Doppler ultrasonography is a reliable noninvasive means of estimating pulmonary artery systolic pressure. However, precise hemodynamic measurements can only be obtained with right heart catheterization, which is helpful when postcapillary pulmonary hypertension, intracardiac shunting, or thromboembolic disease is considered as part of the differential diagnosis.

Routine pulmonary function tests reveal no findings diagnostic of pulmonary hypertension. However, they may help identify the cause. Diminution of the pulmonary capillary bed may cause reduction in the single breath diffusing capacity.

The following studies may be useful to exclude causes of secondary pulmonary hypertension: liver function tests, HIV test, collagen-vascular serologic studies, polysomnography ventilation-perfusion lung scanning, pulmonary angiography, and surgical lung biopsy. Ventilation-perfusion lung scanning is very helpful in identifying patients with pulmonary hypertension caused by recurrent pulmonary thromboemboli, a condition that is often very difficult to recognize clinically.

Treatment

Treatment of primary pulmonary hypertension is discussed in Chapter 10. Treatment of secondary pulmonary hypertension consists mainly of treating the underlying disorder. Early recognition of pulmonary hypertension is crucial to interrupt the self-perpetuating cycle responsible for rapid clinical progression. By the time most patients present with signs and symptoms of pulmonary hypertension, however, the condition is far advanced. If hypoxemia or acidosis is detected, corrective measures should be started immediately. Inhaled nitric oxide has been found to be effective in lowering the pulmonary artery pressure in critically ill patients with pulmonary hypertension, asthma, and acute respiratory distress syndrome. This benefit is only temporary, however. Supplemental oxygen administered for at least 15 hours per day has been demonstrated to slow the progression of pulmonary hypertension in patients with hypoxemic COPD.

Some clinicians employ permanent anticoagulation therapy in pulmonary hypertension of unknown cause, since multiple small pulmonary emboli or in situ thrombosis may produce this picture and be difficult to recognize clinically. Vasodilator therapy using various pharmacologic agents (eg, calcium antagonists, hydralazine, isoproterenol, diazoxide, nitroglycerin) has been tried in primary pulmonary hypertension and a few patients with secondary pulmonary hypertension with disappointing results. Patients most likely to benefit from long-term pulmonary vasodilator therapy are those who respond favorably to a vasodilator challenge at right heart catheterization. It is clear that long-term oral vasodilator therapy should be employed only if hemodynamic benefit is documented. Complications of pulmonary vasodilator therapy have occurred, including systemic hypotension, hypoxemia, and even death.

Continuous long-term intravenous infusion (using a portable pump) of prostacyclin (PGI_2; epoprostenol), a potent pulmonary vasodilator, has been shown to confer hemodynamic and symptomatic benefits in selected patients with primary or secondary pulmonary hypertension. Continuous infusion prostacyclin is the first therapy to demonstrate improved survival of patients with primary pulmonary hypertension. Drawbacks of therapy are difficulties in titration, technical problems with portable delivery systems, and the high cost of the drug.

Patients with marked polycythemia (hematocrit > 60%) should undergo repeated phlebotomy in an attempt to reduce blood viscosity. Cor pulmonale complicating pulmonary hypertension is treated by managing the underlying pulmonary disease and by using diuretics, salt restriction, and, in appropriate patients, supplemental oxygen. The use of digitalis in cor pulmonale remains controversial. Pulmonary thromboendarterectomy may benefit selected patients with pulmonary hypertension secondary to chronic thrombotic obstructions of major pulmonary arteries.

Single or double lung transplantation may be performed on patients with end-stage primary pulmonary hypertension. The two-year survival rate is 50%. Bronchiolitis obliterans is common in those who survive the operation.

Prognosis

The prognosis in secondary pulmonary hypertension depends on the course of the underlying disease. Patients with pulmonary hypertension due to fixed obliteration of the pulmonary vascular bed generally respond poorly to therapy; development of cor pulmonale in these cases implies a poor prognosis. The prognosis is favorable when pulmonary hypertension is detected early and the conditions leading to it are readily reversed.

Fedullo PF et al: Chronic thromboembolic pulmonary hypertension. N Engl J Med 2001;345:1465. [PMID: 11794196] (Review article.)

Krowka MJ: Pulmonary hypertension: diagnostics and therapeutics. Mayo Clin Proc 2000;75:625. [PMID: 10852424] (Concise review for clinicians.)

Peacock AJ: Primary pulmonary hypertension. Thorax 1999; 54:1107. [PMID: 10567632] (Comprehensive review.)

PULMONARY VASCULITIS

Wegener's granulomatosis is an idiopathic disease manifested by a combination of glomerulonephritis, necrotizing granulomatous vasculitis of the upper and lower respiratory tracts, and varying degrees of small vessel vasculitis (see Chapter 20). Chronic sinusitis, arthralgias, fever, skin rash, and weight loss are frequent presenting symptoms. Pulmonary complaints occur less often. The most common sign of lung disease is nodular pulmonary infiltrates, often with cavitation, seen on chest radiography. Tracheal stenosis and endobronchial disease are sometimes seen.

Normochromic, normocytic anemia, mild leukocytosis, and thrombocytosis are common, and virtually all patients have an elevated erythrocyte sedimentation rate. Serum anti-neutrophil cytoplasmic antibodies (ANCAs) that display a cytoplasmic immunofluorescent staining pattern (c-ANCAs) are elevated in 90% of patients with active Wegener's granulomatosis and

in 40% of patients in remission. The specificity of c-ANCA is about 90% for the diagnosis of Wegener's granulomatosis. ANCAs that display a perinuclear immunofluorescent staining pattern (p-ANCAs) are not specific for Wegener's granulomatosis but may be seen in Wegener's variants such as microscopic polyangiitis and other types of vasculitis, rheumatoid arthritis, liver disease, and inflammatory bowel disease. The diagnosis is most often based on biopsy of lung, sinus tissue, or kidney with demonstration of necrotizing granulomatous vasculitis.

Allergic angiitis and granulomatosis (Churg-Strauss syndrome) is an idiopathic multisystem vasculitis of small and medium-sized arteries that occurs in patients with asthma. Histologic features include fibrinoid necrotizing epithelioid and eosinophilic granulomas. The skin and lungs are most often involved, but other organs, including the heart, gastrointestinal tract, liver, and peripheral nerves, may also be affected. Marked peripheral eosinophilia is the rule. Abnormalities on chest radiographs range from transient infiltrates to multiple nodules. This illness may be part of a spectrum that includes polyarteritis nodosa.

Treatment of pulmonary vasculitis consists of combination therapy with corticosteroids and cyclophosphamide. Oral prednisone (1 mg/kg ideal body weight per day initially, tapering slowly to alternate-day therapy over 3–6 months) is the corticosteroid of choice; in Wegener's granulomatosis, some clinicians may omit the use of steroids. For fulminant vasculitis, therapy may be initiated with intravenous methylprednisolone (up to 1 g intravenously per day) for several days. Cyclophosphamide (1–2 mg/kg ideal body weight per day initially, with dosage adjustments to avoid neutropenia) is given daily by mouth for at least 1 year after complete remission is obtained and then is slowly tapered.

Five-year survival rates in patients with these vasculitis syndromes have been improved by the combination therapy. Complete remissions can be achieved in over 90% of patients with Wegener's granulomatosis. The addition of trimethoprim-sulfamethoxazole (one double-strength tablet by mouth twice daily) to standard therapy may help prevent relapses, but its role as sole therapy or as part of combination therapy in patients with active disease remains uncertain.

Harper L et al: Pathogenesis of ANCA-associated systemic vasculitis. J Pathol 2000;190:349. [PMID: 10685069] (Review of pathophysiology of autoimmune vasculitides including Wegener's disease.)

Schwarz MI et al: Small vessel vasculitis of the lung. Thorax 2000;55:502. [PMID: 10817800] (Comprehensive expert review.)

ALVEOLAR HEMORRHAGE SYNDROMES

Diffuse alveolar hemorrhage may occur in a variety of immune and nonimmune disorders. Hemoptysis, alveolar infiltrates on chest radiograph, anemia, dyspnea, and occasionally fever are characteristic. Rapid clearing of diffuse lung infiltrates within 2 days is a clue to the diagnosis of diffuse alveolar hemorrhage. Pulmonary hemorrhage is associated with an increased $D_{L}CO$.

Causes of **immune alveolar hemorrhage** have been classified as anti-basement membrane antibody disease (Goodpasture's syndrome), vasculitis and collagen vascular disease (systemic lupus erythematosus, Wegener's granulomatosis, systemic necrotizing vasculitis, and others), and pulmonary capillaritis associated with idiopathic rapidly progressive glomerulonephritis. **Nonimmune causes** of diffuse hemorrhage include coagulopathy, mitral stenosis, necrotizing pulmonary infection, drugs (penicillamine), toxins (trimellitic anhydride), and idiopathic pulmonary hemosiderosis.

Goodpasture's syndrome is idiopathic recurrent alveolar hemorrhage and rapidly progressive glomerulonephritis. The disease is mediated by anti-glomerular basement membrane antibodies. Goodpasture's syndrome occurs mainly in men who are in their 30s and 40s. Hemoptysis is the usual presenting symptom, but pulmonary hemorrhage may be occult. Dyspnea, cough, hypoxemia, and diffuse bilateral alveolar infiltrates are typical features. Iron deficiency anemia and microscopic hematuria are usually present. The diagnosis is based on characteristic linear IgG deposits in glomeruli or alveoli by immunofluorescence and on the presence of anti-glomerular basement membrane antibody in serum. Combinations of immunosuppressive drugs (initially methylprednisolone, 30 mg/kg intravenously over 20 minutes every other day for three doses, followed by daily oral prednisone, 1 mg/kg/d; with cyclophosphamide, 2 mg/kg by mouth per day) and plasmapheresis have yielded excellent results.

Idiopathic pulmonary hemosiderosis is a disease of children or young adults characterized by recurrent pulmonary hemorrhage; in contrast to Goodpasture's syndrome, renal involvement and anti-glomerular basement membrane antibodies are absent, but iron deficiency is typical. Treatment of acute episodes of hemorrhage with corticosteroids may be useful. Recurrent episodes of pulmonary hemorrhage may result in interstitial fibrosis and pulmonary failure.

■ ENVIRONMENTAL & OCCUPATIONAL LUNG DISORDERS

SMOKE INHALATION

The inhalation of products of combustion may cause serious respiratory complications. As many as one-third of patients admitted to burn treatment units have pulmonary injury from smoke inhalation. Morbidity and mortality due to smoke inhalation exceed those attributed to the burns themselves. The death rate of patients with both severe burns and smoke inhalation exceeds 50%.

All patients suspected of having significant smoke inhalation must be assessed for three consequences of smoke inhalation: impaired tissue oxygenation, thermal injury to the upper airway, and chemical injury to the lung. Impaired tissue oxygenation results from inhalation of carbon monoxide or cyanide and is an immediate threat to life. The management of patients with carbon monoxide and cyanide poisoning is discussed in Chapter 39. The clinician must recognize that patients with carbon monoxide poisoning display a normal partial pressure of oxygen in arterial blood (PaO_2) but have a low measured (ie, not oximetric) oxyhemoglobin saturation (SaO_2). Immediate treatment with 100% oxygen is essential and should be continued until the measured carboxyhemoglobin level falls to less than 10% and concomitant metabolic acidosis has resolved.

Thermal injury to the mucosal surfaces of the upper airway occurs from inhalation of hot gases. Complications become evident by 18–24 hours. These include edema, impaired ability to clear oral secretions, and upper airway obstruction, producing inspiratory stridor. Respiratory failure occurs in severe cases. Early management (see also Chapter 38) includes the use of a high-humidity face mask with supplemental oxygen, gentle suctioning to evacuate oral secretions, elevation of the head 30 degrees to promote clearing of secretions, and topical epinephrine to reduce edema of the oropharyngeal mucous membrane. Helium-oxygen gas mixtures (Heliox) may reduce labored breathing due to upper airway narrowing. Close monitoring with arterial blood gases and later with oximetry is important. Examination of the upper airway with a fiberoptic laryngoscope or bronchoscope is superior to routine physical examination. Endotracheal intubation is often necessary to establish airway patency and is likely to be necessary in patients with deep facial burns or oropharyngeal or laryngeal edema. Tracheotomy should be avoided if possible because of an increased risk of pneumonia and death from sepsis.

Chemical injury to the lung results from inhalation of toxic gases and products of combustion, including aldehydes and organic acids. The site of lung injury depends upon the solubility of the gases inhaled, the duration of exposure, and the size of inhaled particles that transport noxious gases to distal lung units. Bronchorrhea and bronchospasm are seen early after exposure along with dyspnea, tachypnea, and tachycardia. Labored breathing and cyanosis may follow. Physical examination at this stage reveals diffuse wheezing and rhonchi. Bronchiolar edema and high-permeability pulmonary edema (ARDS) may develop within 1–2 days after exposure. Sloughing of the bronchiolar mucosa may occur within 2–3 days, leading to airway obstruction, atelectasis and worsening hypoxemia.

Bacterial colonization and pneumonia are common by 5–7 days after the exposure.

Treatment of smoke inhalation consists of supplemental oxygen, bronchodilators, suctioning of mucosal debris and mucopurulent secretions via an indwelling endotracheal tube, chest physical therapy to aid clearance of secretions, and adequate humidification of inspired gases. Positive end-expiratory pressure (PEEP) has been advocated to treat bronchiolar edema. Judicious fluid management and close monitoring for secondary bacterial infection with daily sputum Gram stains round out the management protocol.

The routine use of corticosteroids for chemical lung injury from smoke inhalation has been shown to be ineffective and may even be harmful. Routine or prophylactic use of antibiotics is not recommended.

Those patients who survive should be watched for the development of late bronchiolitis obliterans.

Lee-Chiong TL Jr: Smoke inhalation injury. Postgrad Med 1999;105:55. [PMID: 10026703] (Review of basic mechanisms of injury with discussion of how to assess and manage complications caused by smoke inhalation.)

PULMONARY ASPIRATION SYNDROMES

Aspiration of foreign material into the tracheobronchial tree results from various disorders that impair normal deglutition, especially disturbances of consciousness and esophageal dysfunction.

Aspiration of Inert Material

Aspiration of inert material may cause asphyxia if the amount aspirated is massive and if cough is impaired, in which case immediate tracheobronchial suctioning is necessary. Most patients suffer no serious sequelae from aspiration of inert material.

Aspiration of Toxic Material

Aspiration of toxic material into the lung usually results in clinically evident pneumonia. **Hydrocarbon pneumonitis** is caused by aspiration of ingested petroleum distillates, eg, gasoline, kerosene, furniture polish, and other household petroleum products. Lung injury results mainly from vomiting and secondary aspiration. Therapy is supportive. The lung should be protected from repeated aspiration with a cuffed endotracheal tube if necessary. **Lipoid pneumonia** is a chronic syndrome related to the repeated aspiration of oily materials, eg, mineral oil, cod liver oil, and oily nose drops; it often occurs in elderly patients with impaired swallowing. Patchy infiltrates in dependent lung zones and lipid-laden macrophages in expectorated sputum are characteristic findings.

"Café Coronary"

Acute obstruction of the upper airway by food is associated with difficulty in swallowing, old age, dental problems that impair chewing, and use of alcohol and sedative drugs. The Heimlich procedure is lifesaving in many cases.

Retention of an Aspirated Foreign Body

Retention of an aspirated foreign body in the tracheobronchial tree may produce both acute and chronic conditions, including recurrent pneumonia, bronchiectasis, lung abscess, atelectasis, and postobstructive hyperinflation. Occasionally, a misdiagnosis of asthma, COPD, or lung cancer is made in adult patients who have aspirated a foreign body. The plain chest radiograph usually suggests the site of the foreign body. In some cases, an expiratory film, demonstrating regional hyperinflation due to a check-valve effect, is helpful. Bronchoscopy is usually necessary to establish the diagnosis and attempt removal of the foreign body.

Baharloo F et al: Tracheobronchial foreign bodies: presentation and management in children and adults. Chest 1999; 115:1357. [PMID: 10334153]

Chronic Aspiration of Gastric Contents

Chronic aspiration of gastric contents may result from primary disorders of the larynx or the esophagus, such as achalasia, esophageal stricture, scleroderma, esophageal carcinoma, esophagitis, and gastroesophageal reflux. In the last condition, relaxation of the tone of the lower esophageal sphincter allows reflux of gastric contents into the esophagus and predisposes to chronic pulmonary aspiration, especially at night. Cigarette smoking, consumption of alcohol, and use of theophylline are known to relax the lower esophageal sphincter. Pulmonary disorders linked to gastroesophageal reflux and chronic aspiration include bronchial asthma, pulmonary fibrosis, and bronchiectasis. Even in the absence of aspiration, acid in the esophagus may trigger bronchospasm through reflex mechanisms.

The diagnosis of chronic aspiration is difficult. Ambulatory monitoring of esophageal pH for 24 hours detects esophageal reflux. Esophagogastroscopy and barium swallow are sometimes necessary to rule out esophageal disease. Management consists of elevation of the head of the bed, cessation of smoking, weight reduction, and antacids, H_2 receptor antagonists (eg, cimetidine, 300–400 mg), or proton pump inhibitors (eg, omeprazole, 20 mg) at night. Metoclopramide (10–15 mg orally four times daily or 20 mg at bedtime),or bethanechol (10–25 mg at bedtime) may also be helpful in some patients with gastroesophageal reflux.

Acute Aspiration of Gastric Contents (Mendelson's Syndrome)

Acute aspiration of gastric contents is often catastrophic. The pulmonary response depends on the characteristics and amount of the gastric contents aspirated. The more acidic the material, the greater the degree of chemical pneumonitis. Aspiration of pure gastric acid (pH < 2.5) causes extensive desquamation of the bronchial epithelium, bronchiolitis, hemorrhage, and pulmonary edema. Acute gastric aspiration is one of the commonest causes of adult respiratory distress syndrome. The clinical picture is one of abrupt onset of respiratory distress, with cough, wheezing, fever, and tachypnea. Crackles are audible at the bases of the lungs. Hypoxemia may be noted immediately after aspiration occurs. Radiographic abnormalities, consisting of patchy alveolar infiltrates in dependent lung zones, appear within a few hours. If particulate food matter has been aspirated along with gastric acid, radiographic features of bronchial obstruction may be observed. Fever and leukocytosis are common even in the absence of superinfection.

Treatment of acute aspiration of gastric contents consists of supplemental oxygen, measures to maintain the airway, and the usual measures for treatment of acute respiratory failure. There is no evidence to support the routine use of corticosteroids or prophylactic antibiotics after gastric aspiration has occurred. Secondary pulmonary infection, which occurs in about one-fourth of patients, typically appears 2–3 days after aspiration. Management of this complication depends upon the observed flora of the tracheobronchial tree. Hypotension secondary to alveolocapillary membrane injury and intravascular volume depletion is common and is managed with the judicious administration of intravenous fluids.

OCCUPATIONAL PULMONARY DISEASES

Many acute and chronic pulmonary diseases are directly related to inhalation of noxious substances encountered in the workplace. Disorders that are due to chemical agents may be classified as follows: (1) pneumoconioses, (2) hypersensitivity pneumonitis, (3) obstructive airway disorders, (4) toxic lung injury, (5) lung cancer, (6) pleural diseases, and (7) miscellaneous disorders.

Pneumoconioses

Pneumoconioses are chronic fibrotic lung diseases caused by the inhalation of coal dust and various other inert, inorganic, or silicate dusts (Table 9–26). Pneumoconioses due to inhalation of inert dusts may be asymptomatic disorders with diffuse nodular infiltrates on chest radiograph. Clinically important pneu-

Table 9–26. Selected pneumoconioses.

Disease	Agent	Occupations
Metal dusts		
Siderosis	Metallic iron or iron oxide	Mining, welding, foundry work
Stannosis	Tin, tin oxide	Mining, tin-working, smelting
Baritosis	Barium salts	Glass and insecticide manufacturing
Coal dust		
Coal worker's pneumoconiosis	Coal dust	Coal mining
Inorganic dusts		
Silicosis	Free silica (silicon dioxide)	Rock mining, quarrying, stone cutting, tunneling, sandblasting, pottery, diatomaceous earth
Silicate dusts		
Asbestosis	Asbestos	Mining, insulation, construction, shipbuilding
Talcosis	Magnesium silicate	Mining, insulation, construction, shipbuilding
Kaolin pneumoconiosis	Sand, mica, aluminum silicate	Mining of china clay; pottery and cement work
Shaver's disease	Aluminum powder	Manufacture of corundum

moconioses include coal workers' pneumoconiosis, silicosis, and asbestosis. Treatment for each is supportive.

A. COAL WORKER'S PNEUMOCONIOSIS

In coal worker's pneumoconiosis, ingestion of inhaled coal dust by alveolar macrophages leads to the formation of coal macules, usually 2–5 mm in diameter, which appear on chest radiograph as diffuse small opacities that are especially prominent in the upper lung. Simple coal worker's pneumoconiosis is usually asymptomatic; pulmonary function abnormalities are unimpressive. Cigarette smoking does not increase the prevalence of coal worker's pneumoconiosis but may have an additive detrimental effect on ventilatory function. In complicated coal worker's pneumoconiosis ("progressive massive fibrosis"), conglomeration and contraction in the upper lung zones occur, with radiographic features resembling complicated silicosis. **Caplan's syndrome** is a rare condition characterized by the presence of necrobiotic rheumatoid nodules

(1–5 cm in diameter) in the periphery of the lung in coal workers with rheumatoid arthritis.

B. SILICOSIS

In silicosis, extensive or prolonged inhalation of free silica (silicon dioxide) particles in the respirable range (0.3–5 μm) causes the formation of small rounded opacities (silicotic nodules) throughout the lung. Calcification of the periphery of hilar lymph nodes ("eggshell" calcification) is an unusual finding that strongly suggests silicosis. Simple silicosis is usually asymptomatic and has no effect on routine pulmonary function tests; in complicated silicosis, large conglomerate densities appear in the upper lung and are accompanied by dyspnea and obstructive and restrictive pulmonary dysfunction. The incidence of pulmonary tuberculosis is increased in patients with chronic silicosis. All patients with silicosis should have a tuberculin skin test and a current chest radiograph. If old, healed pulmonary tuberculosis is suspected, multidrug treatment for tuberculosis (not single-agent preventive therapy) should be instituted.

C. ASBESTOSIS

Asbestosis is a nodular interstitial fibrosis occurring in asbestos workers and miners is characterized by inexorably progressive dyspnea, inspiratory crackles, and in some cases, clubbing and cyanosis. The radiographic features include interstitial fibrosis, thickened pleura, and calcified plaques (pleural) on the diaphragms or lateral chest wall. The lower lungs are more often involved than the upper. High-resolution CT scanning is the best imaging method in asbestosis because of its ability to detect parenchymal fibrosis and define the presence of coexisting pleural plaques. Cigarette smoking in asbestos workers increases the prevalence of radiographic pleural and parenchymal changes and markedly increases the incidence of lung carcinoma. It may also interfere with the clearance of short asbestos fibers from the lung. Pulmonary function studies show restrictive dysfunction and reduced diffusing capacity.

Hypersensitivity Pneumonitis

Hypersensitivity pneumonitis (extrinsic allergic alveolitis) is a nonatopic, nonasthmatic allergic pulmonary disease. It is manifested mainly as occupational disease (Table 9–27), in which exposure to inhaled organic agents leads to acute and eventually chronic pulmonary disease. Acute illness is characterized by sudden onset of malaise, chills, fever, cough, dyspnea, and nausea 4–8 hours after exposure to the offending agent. This may occur after the patient has left work or even at night and thus may mimic paroxysmal nocturnal dyspnea. Bibasilar crackles, tachypnea, tachycardia, and (occasionally) cyanosis are noted. Small nodular densities sparing the apices and bases of the lungs are noted on chest radiograph. Pulmonary function studies reveal restrictive dysfunction and reduced

Table 9–27. Selected causes of hypersensitivity pneumonitis.

Disease	Antigen	Source
Farmer's lung	*Micropolyspora faeni, Thermoactinomyces vulgaris*	Moldy hay
"Humidifier" lung	Thermophilic actinomycetes	Contaminated humidifiers, heating systems, or air conditioners
Bird fancier's lung ("pigeon-breeder's disease")	Avian proteins	Bird serum and excreta
Bagassosis	*Thermoactinomyces sacchari* and *T vulgaris*	Moldy sugar cane fiber (bagasse)
Sequoiosis	Graphium, aureobasidium, and other fungi	Moldy redwood sawdust
Maple bark stripper's disease	*Cryptostroma (Coniosporium) corticale*	Rotting maple tree logs or bark
Mushroom picker's disease	Same as farmer's lung	Moldy compost
Suberosis	*Penicillium frequentans*	Moldy cork dust
Detergent worker's lung	*Bacillus subtilis* enzyme	Enzyme additives

diffusing capacity. Laboratory studies reveal an increase in the white blood cell count with a shift to the left, hypoxemia, and the presence of precipitating antibodies to the offending agent in serum. Hypersensitivity pneumonitis antibody panels against common offending antigens are available.

Acute hypersensitivity pneumonitis is characterized by interstitial infiltrates of lymphocytes and plasma cells, with noncaseating granulomas in the interstitium and air spaces. A subacute hypersensitivity pneumonitis syndrome (15% of cases) has been described that is characterized by the insidious onset of chronic cough and slowly progressive dyspnea, anorexia, and weight loss. Chronic respiratory insufficiency and the appearance of pulmonary fibrosis on radiographs may occur after repeated exposure to the offending agent. Surgical lung biopsy is occasionally necessary for diagnosis. Diffuse fibrosis is the hallmark of the subacute and chronic phases.

Treatment of hypersensitivity pneumonitis consists of identification of the offending agent, avoidance of further exposure, and, in severe acute or protracted cases, oral corticosteroids (prednisone, 0.5 mg/kg daily as a single morning dose, tapered to nil over 4–6 weeks). Change in occupation is often unavoidable.

Obstructive Airway Disorders

Occupational pulmonary diseases manifested as obstructive airway disorders include occupational asthma, industrial bronchitis, and byssinosis.

A. OCCUPATIONAL ASTHMA

It has been estimated that from 2% to 5% of all cases of asthma are related to occupation. Offending agents in the workplace are numerous; they include grain dust, wood dust, tobacco, pollens, enzymes, gum arabic, synthetic dyes, isocyanates (particularly toluene diisocyanate), rosin (soldering flux), inorganic chemicals (salts of nickel, platinum, and chromium), trimellitic anhydride, phthalic anhydride, formaldehyde, and various pharmaceutical agents. Diagnosis of occupational asthma depends on a high index of suspicion, an appropriate history, spirometric studies before and after exposure to the offending substance, and peak flow rate measurements in the workplace. Bronchial provocation testing may be helpful in some cases. Treatment consists of avoidance of further exposure to the offending agent and bronchodilators, but symptoms may persist for years after workplace exposure has been terminated.

B. INDUSTRIAL BRONCHITIS

Industrial bronchitis is chronic bronchitis found in coal miners and others exposed to cotton, flax, or hemp dust. Chronic disability from industrial bronchitis is infrequent.

C. BYSSINOSIS

Byssinosis is an asthma-like disorder in textile workers caused by inhalation of cotton dust. The pathogenesis is obscure. Chest tightness, cough, and dyspnea are characteristically worse on Mondays or the first day back at work, with symptoms subsiding later in the week. Repeated exposure leads to chronic bronchitis.

Toxic Lung Injury

Toxic lung injury from inhalation of irritant gases is discussed in the section on smoke inhalation. **Silo-filler's disease** is acute toxic high-permeability pulmonary edema caused by inhalation of nitrogen dioxide encountered in recently filled silos. Bronchiolitis obliterans is a common late complication, which may be prevented by early treatment of the acute reaction with corticosteroids. Extensive exposure to silage gas may be fatal.

Lung Cancer

Many industrial pulmonary carcinogens have been identified, including asbestos, radon gas, arsenic, iron, chromium, nickel, coal tar fumes, petroleum oil mists, isopropyl oil, mustard gas, and printing ink. Cigarette smoking acts as a cocarcinogen with asbestos and radon gas to cause bronchogenic carcinoma. Asbestos alone causes malignant mesothelioma. Almost all histologic types of lung cancer have been associated with these carcinogens. Chloromethyl methyl ether specifically causes small cell carcinoma of the lung.

Pleural Diseases

Occupational diseases of the pleura may result from exposure to asbestos (see above) or talc. Inhalation of talc causes pleural plaques that are similar to those caused by asbestos. Benign asbestos pleural effusion occurs in some asbestos workers and may cause chronic blunting of the costophrenic angle on chest radiograph.

Other Occupational Pulmonary Diseases

Occupational agents are also responsible for other pulmonary disorders. These include **berylliosis,** an acute or chronic pulmonary disorder related to exposure to beryllium, which is absorbed through the lungs or skin and widely disseminated throughout the body. Acute berylliosis is a toxic, ulcerative tracheobronchitis and chemical pneumonitis following intense and severe exposure to beryllium. Chronic berylliosis, a systemic disease closely resembling sarcoidosis, is more common. Chronic pulmonary beryllium disease is thought to be an alveolitis mediated by the proliferation of beryllium-specific helper-inducer T cells in the lung. Exposure to beryllium now occurs in machining and handling of beryllium products and alloys. Beryllium miners are not at risk for berylliosis. Beryllium is no longer used in fluorescent lamp production, which was a source of exposure before 1950.

Newman LS: Occupational illness. N Engl J Med 1995; 333:1128. [PMID: 7565952] (Clinical assessment and management of occupational disease.)

Schwartz DA et al: Occupational lung disease. Adv Intern Med 1997;42:269. [PMID: 9048122] (Review with 161 references.)

Wagner GR: Asbestosis and silicosis. Lancet 1997;349: 1311. [PMID: 9142077] (Review with emphasis on accurate diagnosis and disease reporting.)

DRUG-INDUCED LUNG DISEASE

Typical patterns of pulmonary response to drugs implicated in drug-induced respiratory disease are summarized in Table 9–28. Pulmonary injury due to drugs occurs as a result of allergic reactions, idiosyncratic reactions, overdose, or undesirable side effects. In most patients, the mechanism of pulmonary injury is unknown.

Precise diagnosis of drug-induced pulmonary disease is often difficult, because results of routine laboratory studies are not helpful and radiographic findings

Table 9–28. Pulmonary manifestations of selected drug toxicities.

Asthma	**Pulmonary edema**
Beta-blockers	Noncardiogenic
Aspirin	Aspirin
Nonsteroidal anti-	Chlordiazepoxide
inflammatory drugs	Cocaine
Histamine	Ethchlorvynol
Methacholine	Heroin
Acetylcysteine	Cardiogenic
Aerosolized pentamidine	Beta-blockers
Any nebulized medication	**Pleural effusion**
Chronic cough	Bromocriptine
Angiotensin-converting en-	Nitrofurantoin
zyme inhibitors	Any drug inducing sys-
Pulmonary infiltration	temic lupus erythe-
Without eosinophilia	matosus
Amitriptyline	Methysergide
Azathioprine	Chemotherapeutic
Amiodarone	agents
With eosinophilia	**Mediastinal widening**
Sulfonamides	Phenytoin
L-Tryptophan	Corticosteroids
Nitrofurantoin	Methotrexate
Penicillin	**Respiratory failure**
Methotrexate	Neuromuscular blockade
Crack cocaine	Aminoglycosides
Drug-induced systemic	Succinylcholine
lupus erythematosus	Gallamine
Hydralazine	Dimethyltubocurarine
Procainamide	(metocurine)
Isoniazid	Central nervous system
Chlorpromazine	depression
Phenytoin	Sedatives
Interstitial pneumonitis/	Hypnotics
fibrosis	Opioids
Nitrofurantoin	Alcohol
Bleomycin	Tricyclic antidepres-
Busulfan	sants
Cyclophosphamide	Oxygen
Methysergide	
Phenytoin	

are not specific. A high index of suspicion and a thorough medical history of drug usage are critical to establishing the diagnosis of drug-induced lung disease. The clinical response to cessation of the suspected offending agent is also helpful. Acute episodes of drug-induced pulmonary disease usually disappear 24–48 hours after the drug has been discontinued, but chronic syndromes may take longer to resolve. Challenge tests to confirm the diagnosis are risky and rarely performed.

Treatment of drug-induced lung disease consists of discontinuing the offending agent immediately and managing the pulmonary symptoms appropriately.

Inhalation of crack cocaine may cause a spectrum of acute pulmonary syndromes, including pulmonary infiltration with eosinophilia, pneumothorax and pneumomediastinum, bronchiolitis obliterans, and acute respiratory failure associated with diffuse alveolar damage and alveolar hemorrhage. Corticosteroids have been used with variable success to treat alveolar hemorrhage.

Ozkan M et al: Drug-induced lung disease. Cleve Clin J Med 2001;68:782. [PMID: 11563482] (Review of various drugs known to induce injury along with common patterns of injury.)

RADIATION LUNG INJURY

The lung is an exquisitely radiosensitive organ that can be affected by external beam radiation therapy. The degree of pulmonary injury is determined by the volume of lung irradiated, the dose and rate of exposure, and potentiating factors (eg, concurrent chemotherapy, previous radiation therapy in the same area, and simultaneous withdrawal of corticosteroid therapy). Symptomatic radiation lung injury occurs in about 10% of patients treated for carcinoma of the breast, 5–15% of patients treated for carcinoma of the lung, and 5–35% of patients treated for lymphoma. Two phases of the pulmonary response to radiation are apparent: an acute phase (radiation pneumonitis) and a chronic phase (radiation fibrosis).

Radiation Pneumonitis

Radiation pneumonitis usually occurs 2–3 months (range 1–6 months) after completion of radiotherapy and is characterized by insidious onset of dyspnea, intractable dry cough, chest fullness or pain, weakness, and fever. The pathogenesis of acute radiation pneumonitis is unknown, but there is speculation that hypersensitivity mechanisms are involved. The dominant histopathologic finding is that of a lymphocytic interstitial pneumonitis. Inspiratory crackles may be heard in the involved area. In severe disease, respiratory distress and cyanosis occur that are characteristic of acute respiratory distress syndrome (ARDS). An increased white blood cell count and elevated sedimentation rate are common. Pulmonary function studies reveal reduced lung volumes, reduced lung compliance, hypoxemia, reduced diffusing capacity, and reduced maximum voluntary ventilation. Chest radiograph, which correlates poorly with the presence of symptoms, usually demonstrates an alveolar or nodular infiltrate limited to the irradiated area. Air bronchograms are often observed. Sharp borders of the infiltrate may help distinguish radiation pneumonitis from other conditions such as infectious pneumonia, lymphangitic spread of carcinoma, and recurrent tumor. Treatment consists of aspirin, cough suppressants, and bed rest. Acute respiratory failure, if present, is treated appropriately. Although there is no proof that corticosteroids are effective in radiation pneumonitis, prednisone (1 mg/kg/d orally) is usually given immediately for about 1 week. The dose is then reduced and maintained at 20–40 mg/d for several weeks, then slowly tapered. Radiation pneumonitis usually resolves in 2–3 weeks. Death from ARDS is unusual.

Pulmonary Radiation Fibrosis

Pulmonary radiation fibrosis occurs in nearly all patients who receive a full course of radiation therapy for cancer of the lung and breast. Patients who experience radiation pneumonitis develop pulmonary fibrosis after an intervening period (6–12 months) of well-being. Most patients are asymptomatic, though slowly progressive dyspnea may occur. Radiation fibrosis may occur with or without antecedent radiation pneumonitis. Cor pulmonale and chronic respiratory failure are rare. Radiographic findings include obliteration of normal lung markings, dense interstitial and pleural fibrosis, reduced lung volumes, tenting of the diaphragm, and sharp delineation of the irradiated area. No specific therapy is proved effective, and corticosteroids have no value.

Other Complications of Radiation Therapy

Other complications of radiation therapy directed to the thorax include pericardial effusion, constrictive pericarditis, tracheoesophageal fistula, esophageal candidiasis, radiation dermatitis, and rib fractures. Small pleural effusions, radiation pneumonitis outside the irradiated area, spontaneous pneumothorax, and complete obstruction of central airways are unusual occurrences.

Abid SH et al: Radiation-induced and chemotherapy-induced pulmonary injury. Curr Opinion Oncol 2001;13:242. [PMID: 11429481] (Review of clinically important chemotherapy and radiation-induced pulmonary injuries, the pathologic mechanisms, and recent treatment.)

Abratt RP et al: Lung toxicity following chest irradiation in patients with lung cancer. Lung Cancer 2002;35:103. [PMID: 11804681] (Careful review of clinical issues in pulmonary toxicity from therapeutic radiation therapy.)

■ PLEURAL DISEASES

PLEURITIS

Pain due to acute pleural inflammation is caused by irritation of the parietal pleura. Such pain is localized, sharp, and fleeting and is made worse by cough, sneezing, deep breathing, or movement. When the central portion of the diaphragmatic parietal pleura is irritated, pain may be referred to the ipsilateral shoulder. There are numerous causes of pleuritis. The setting in

which pleuritic pain develops helps to narrow the differential diagnosis. In young, otherwise healthy individuals, pleuritis is usually caused by viral respiratory infections or pneumonia. The presence of pleural effusion, pleural thickening, or air in the pleural space requires further diagnostic and therapeutic measures. Simple rib fracture may cause severe pleurisy.

Treatment of pleuritis consists of treating the underlying disease. Analgesics and anti-inflammatory drugs (eg, indomethacin, 25 mg orally two or three times daily) are often helpful for pain relief. Codeine (30–60 mg orally every 8 hours) may be used to control cough associated with pleuritic chest pain if retention of airway secretions is not a likely complication. Intercostal nerve blocks are sometimes helpful.

PLEURAL EFFUSION

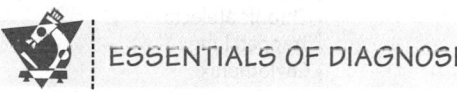 ESSENTIALS OF DIAGNOSIS

- *May be asymptomatic; chest pain seen in the setting of pleuritis, trauma, or infection; dyspnea common with large effusions.*
- *Dullness to percussion and decreased breath sounds over the effusion.*
- *Radiographic evidence of pleural effusion.*
- *Diagnostic findings on thoracentesis.*

General Considerations

There is constant movement of fluid from parietal pleural capillaries into the pleural space at a rate of 0.01 mL/kg body weight/h. Absorption of pleural fluid occurs through parietal pleural lymphatics. The resultant homeostasis leaves 5–15 mL of fluid in the normal pleural space. A pleural effusion is an abnormal accumulation of fluid in the pleural space. Pleural effusions may be classified by differential diagnosis (Table 9–29) or by underlying pathophysiology. Five pathophysiologic processes account for most pleural effusions: increased production of fluid in the setting of normal capillaries due to increased hydrostatic or decreased oncotic pressures (transudates); increased production of fluid due to abnormal capillary permeability (exudates); decreased lymphatic clearance of fluid from the pleural space (exudates); infection in the pleural space (empyema); and bleeding into the pleural space (hemothorax).

Diagnostic thoracentesis should be performed whenever there is a new pleural effusion and no clinically apparent cause. Observation is appropriate in some situations (eg, symmetric bilateral pleural effusions in the setting of congestive heart failure), but an

Table 9–29. Causes of pleural fluid transudates and exudates.

Transudates	Exudates
Congestive heart failure (≈90% of cases)	Pneumonia (parapneumonic effusion)
Cirrhosis with ascites	Cancer
Nephrotic syndrome	Pulmonary embolism
Peritoneal dialysis	Empyema
Myxedema	Tuberculosis
Acute atelectasis	Connective tissue disease
Constrictive pericarditis	Viral infection
Superior vena cava obstruction	Fungal infection
Pulmonary embolism	Rickettsial infection
	Parasitic infection
	Asbestos
	Meigs' syndrome
	Pancreatic disease
	Uremia
	Chronic atelectasis
	Trapped lung
	Chylothorax
	Sarcoidosis
	Drug reaction
	Post-myocardial infarction syndrome

atypical presentation or failure of an effusion to resolve as expected warrants thoracentesis. Sampling allows visualization of the fluid in addition to chemical and microbiologic analyses to identify the pathophysiologic processes listed above. A definitive diagnosis is made through positive cytology or identification of a specific causative organism in approximately 25% of cases. In another 50–60% of patients, identification of relevant pathophysiology in the appropriate clinical setting greatly narrows the differential diagnosis and leads to a presumptive diagnosis.

Clinical Findings

A. SYMPTOMS AND SIGNS

Patients with pleural effusions most often report dyspnea, cough, or respirophasic chest pain. Symptoms are more common in patients with existing cardiopulmonary disease. Small pleural effusions are less likely to be symptomatic than larger effusions. Physical findings are usually absent in small effusions. Larger effusions may present with dullness to percussion and diminished or absent breath sounds over the effusion. Compressive atelectasis may cause bronchial breath sounds and egophony just above the effusion. A massive effusion with increased intrapleural pressure may cause contralateral shift of the trachea and bulging of the intercostal spaces. A pleural friction rub indicates infarction or pleuritis.

B. LABORATORY FINDINGS

The gross appearance of pleural fluid helps to identify several types of pleural effusion. Grossly purulent fluid signifies empyema, an infection of the pleural space. Milky white pleural fluid should be centrifuged. A clear supernatant above a pellet of white cells indicates empyema, whereas a persistently turbid supernatant suggests a chylous effusion. Analysis of this supernatant reveals chylomicrons and a high triglyceride level (> 100 mg/dL), often from traumatic disruption of the thoracic duct. Hemorrhagic pleural effusion is a mixture of blood and pleural fluid. Ten thousand red cells per milliliter create blood-tinged pleural fluid; 100,000/mL create grossly bloody pleural fluid. Hemothorax is the presence of gross blood in the pleural space, usually following chest trauma or instrumentation. It is defined as a ratio of pleural fluid hematocrit to peripheral blood hematocrit > 0.5.

Pleural fluid samples should be sent for measurement of protein, glucose, and LDH in addition to total and differential white blood cell counts. Chemistry determinations are used to classify effusions as transudates or exudates. This classification is important because the differential diagnosis for each entity is vastly different (Table 9–29). A pleural exudate is an effusion that has *one or more* of the following laboratory features: (1) ratio of pleural fluid protein to serum protein > 0.5; (2) ratio of pleural fluid LDH to serum LDH > 0.6; (3) pleural fluid LDH greater than two-thirds the upper limit of normal serum LDH.

Transudates have none of these features. Transudates occur in the setting of normal capillary integrity and suggest the *absence* of local pleural disease. Distinguishing laboratory findings include a glucose equal to serum glucose, pH between 7.40 and 7.55, and fewer than 1000 wbc/μL with a predominance of mononuclear cells. Causes include increased hydrostatic pressure (congestive heart failure accounts for 90% of transudates), decreased oncotic pressure (hypoalbuminemia, cirrhosis), and greater negative pleural pressure (acute atelectasis). Exudates form as a result of pleural disease associated with increased capillary permeability or reduced lymphatic drainage. Bacterial pneumonia and cancer are the most common causes of exudative effusion, but there are many other causes with characteristic laboratory findings. These findings are summarized in Table 9–30.

Pleural fluid pH is useful in the assessment of parapneumonic effusions. A pH below 7.30 suggests the need for drainage of the pleural space. An elevated amylase level in pleural fluid suggests pancreatitis, pancreatic pseudocyst, adenocarcinoma of the lung or pancreas, or esophageal rupture.

Thoracentesis with culture and pleural biopsy is indicated in suspected tuberculous pleural effusion. Pleural fluid culture is 44% sensitive, and the combination of closed pleural biopsy with culture and histologic examination for granulomas is 70–90% sensitive for the diagnosis of pleural tuberculosis.

Pleural fluid specimens should be sent for cytologic examination in all cases of exudative effusions in patients suspected of harboring an underlying malig-

Table 9–30. Characteristics of important exudative pleural effusions.

Etiology or Type of Effusion	Gross Appearance	White Blood Cell Count (cells/μL)	Red Blood Cell Count (cells/μL)	Glucose	Comments
Malignant effusion	Turbid to bloody; occasionally serous	1000 to < 100,000 M	100 to several hundred thousand	Equal to serum levels; < 60 mg/dL in 15% of cases	Eosinophilia uncommon; positive results on cytologic examination
Uncomplicated parapneumonic effusion	Clear to turbid	5000–25,000 P	< 5000	Equal to serum levels	Tube thoracostomy unnecessary
Empyema	Turbid to purulent	25,000–100,000 P	< 5000	Less than serum levels; often very low	Drainage necessary; putrid odor suggests anaerobic infection
Tuberculosis	Serous to serosanguineous	5000–10,000 M	< 10,000	Equal to serum levels; occasionally < 60 mg/dL	Protein 4.0 g/dL and may exceed 5 g/dL; eosinophils (> 10%) or mesothelial cells (> 5%) make diagnosis unlikely
Rheumatoid effusion	Turbid; greenish-yellow	1000–20,000 M or P	< 1000	< 40 mg/dL	Secondary empyema common; high LDH, low complement, high rheumatoid factor, cholesterol crystals are characteristic
Pulmonary infarction	Serous to grossly bloody	1000–50,000 M or P	100 to > 100,000	Equal to serum levels	Variable findings; no pathognomonic features
Esophageal rupture	Turbid to purulent; red-brown	< 5000 to > 50,000 P	1000–10,000	Usually low	High amylase level (salivary origin); pneumothorax in 25% of cases; effusion usually on left side; pH < 6.0 strongly suggests diagnosis
Pancreatitis	Turbid to serosanguineous	1000–50,000 P	1000–10,000	Equal to serum levels	Usually left-sided; high amylase level

M = mononuclear cell predominance; P = polymorphonuclear leukocyte predominance.

nancy. The diagnostic yield depends on the nature and extent of the underlying malignancy. Sensitivity is between 50% and 65%. A negative cytologic examination in a patient with a high prior probability of malignancy should be followed by one repeat thoracentesis. If that examination is negative, thoracoscopy (by a pulmonologist or by video-assisted thoracoscopic surgery) is preferred to closed pleural biopsy. The sensitivity of thoracoscopy is 92–96%.

C. IMAGING

The lung is less dense than water and floats on pleural fluid that accumulates in dependent regions. Subpulmonary fluid may appear as lateral displacement of the apex of the diaphragm with an abrupt slope to the costophrenic sulcus or a greater than 2 cm separation between the gastric air bubble and the lung. On a standard upright chest radiograph, approximately 75–100 mL of pleural fluid must accumulate in the posterior costophrenic sulcus to be visible on the lateral view, and 175–200 mL must be present in the lateral costophrenic sulcus to be visible on the frontal view. Chest CT scans may identify as little as 10 mL

of fluid. At least 1 cm of fluid on the decubitus view is necessary to permit blind thoracentesis. Ultrasonography is useful to guide thoracentesis in the setting of smaller effusions.

Pleural fluid may become trapped (loculated) by pleural adhesions, thereby forming unusual collections along the lateral chest wall or within lung fissures. Round or oval fluid collections in fissures that resemble intraparenchymal masses are called pseudotumors. Massive pleural effusion causing opacification of an entire hemithorax is most commonly caused by cancer but may be seen in tuberculosis and other diseases.

Treatment

A. TRANSUDATIVE PLEURAL EFFUSION

Transudative pleural effusions characteristically occur in the absence of pleural disease. Treatment is directed at the underlying condition. Therapeutic thoracentesis for severe dyspnea may offer only transient benefit. Pleurodesis and tube thoracostomy are rarely indicated.

B. MALIGNANT PLEURAL EFFUSION

Approximately 15% of patients dying of cancer are reported to have malignant pleural effusions. Almost any form of cancer may cause effusions, but the most common causes are lung cancer (one-third of cases) and breast cancer. In 5–10% of malignant pleural effusions, no primary tumor is identified.

Between 40% and 80% of exudative pleural effusions are malignant, while over 90% of malignant pleural effusions are exudative. The most common mechanisms contributing to the formation of malignant effusions include direct tumor involvement of the pleura, local inflammation in response to tumor spread, and impairment or disruption of lymphatics. The term "paramalignant pleural effusion" attaches to an effusion in a patient with cancer when repeated attempts to identify tumor cells in the pleura or pleural fluid are nondiagnostic but when there is a presumptive relation to the underlying malignancy. For example, superior vena caval syndrome with elevated systemic venous pressures causing a transudative effusion would be "paramalignant."

Most patients with malignant effusions have advanced disease and multiple symptoms. Dyspnea occurs in over half of patients with malignant pleural effusions. The cause of dyspnea is probably related to mechanical distortion of the lung and chest wall. Hypoxemia from intrapulmonary shunting and ventilation-perfusion mismatching is common and may be severe. Treatment may be systemic, with therapy for the underlying malignancy; or local, to address specific symptoms related to the effusion itself. Local treatment usually involves drainage through repeated thoracentesis or placement of a chest tube. Pleurodesis is a procedure by which an irritant is placed into the pleural space following chest tube drainage and lung reexpansion. The goal is to form fibrous adhesions between the visceral and parietal pleura, resulting in obliteration of the pleural space to prevent or significantly reduce reaccumulation of pleural fluid. Multiple agents have been used for pleurodesis, but the two in most common use are doxycycline (500 mg in 50–100 mL saline) and sterile, asbestos-free talc (by poudrage at thoracoscopy using 5 g or instillation of talc slurry through a chest tube using 4–5 g in 50 mL). Doxycycline and talc are associated with a 70–75% and a 90% success rate, respectively. Major side effects are pain and fever, which appear to be less common with talc. Pain associated with pleurodesis can be extreme. Patients should be premedicated with an anxiolytic-anamnestic agent in addition to opioid analgesics.

C. PARAPNEUMONIC PLEURAL EFFUSION

Parapneumonic pleural effusions are exudates that accompany approximately 40% of bacterial pneumonias. They are divided into three categories: simple or uncomplicated, complicated, and empyema. Uncomplicated parapneumonic effusions are free-flowing sterile exudates of modest size that resolve quickly with antibiotic treatment of pneumonia. They do not need drainage. Empyema is gross infection of the pleural space indicated by positive Gram stain or culture. Empyema should always be drained by tube thoracostomy to facilitate clearance of infection and to reduce the probability of fibrous encasement of the lung, causing permanent pulmonary impairment.

Complicated parapneumonic effusions present the most difficult management decisions. They tend to be larger than simple parapneumonic effusions and to show more evidence of inflammatory stimuli such as low glucose level, low pH, or evidence of loculation. Inflammation probably reflects ongoing bacterial invasion of the pleural space despite rare positive bacterial cultures. The morbidity associated with complicated effusions is due to their tendency to form a fibropurulent pleural "peel," trapping otherwise functional lung and leading to permanent impairment. Tube thoracostomy is indicated when pleural fluid glucose is < 60 mg/dL or the pH is < 7.2. These thresholds have not been prospectively validated and should not be interpreted strictly. The clinician should consider drainage of a complicated effusion if the pleural fluid pH is between 7.2 and 7.3 or the LDH is > 1000 units/mL. Pleural fluid cell count and protein have little diagnostic value in this setting.

Tube thoracostomy drainage of empyema or parapneumonic effusions is frequently complicated by loculation that prevents adequate drainage. Intrapleural injection of fibrinolytic agents (streptokinase, 250,000 units, or urokinase, 100,000 units, in 100 mL of normal saline once or twice daily) has been reported to improve drainage, shorten hospitalization, and reduce the need for surgery. Reported success rates in small studies are between 70% and 90%.

D. HEMOTHORAX

A small-volume hemothorax that is stable or improving on chest radiographs may be managed by close observation. In all other cases, hemothorax is treated by immediate insertion of a large-bore thoracostomy tube to (1) drain existing blood and clot, (2) quantify the amount of bleeding, (3) reduce the risk of fibrothorax, and (4) permit apposition of the pleural surfaces in an attempt to reduce hemorrhage. Thoracotomy may be indicated to control hemorrhage, remove clot, and treat complications such as bronchopleural fistula formation.

Antony VB et al: American Thoracic Society Guidelines: Management of malignant pleural effusions. Am J Respir Crit Care Med 2000;162:1987. [PMID: 11069845] (Exhaustive review of etiology, pathogenesis, and management of malignant pleural effusions.)

Colice GL et al: Medical and surgical treatment of parapneumonic effusions: an evidence-based guideline. Chest 2000;118:1158. [PMID: 11035692] (Expert panel convened by the ACCP to develop an evidence-based clinical practice guideline on the medical and surgical treatment of parapneumonic effusions.)

Muthuswamy P et al: Clinical problem-solving. The effusion that would not go away. N Engl J Med 2001;345:756. [PMID:

11547746] (Detailed review of a common management problem.)

SPONTANEOUS PNEUMOTHORAX

 ESSENTIALS OF DIAGNOSIS

- *Acute onset of unilateral chest pain and dyspnea.*
- *Minimal physical findings in mild cases; unilateral chest expansion, decreased tactile fremitus, hyper-resonance, diminished breath sounds, mediastinal shift, cyanosis and hypotension in tension pneumothorax.*
- *Presence of pleural air on chest radiograph.*

General Considerations

Pneumothorax, or accumulation of air in the pleural space, is classified as spontaneous (primary or secondary) or traumatic. Primary spontaneous pneumothorax occurs in the absence of an underlying lung disease, whereas secondary spontaneous pneumothorax is a complication of preexisting pulmonary disease. Traumatic pneumothorax results from penetrating or blunt trauma. Iatrogenic pneumothorax may follow procedures such as thoracentesis, pleural biopsy, subclavian or internal jugular vein catheter placement, percutaneous lung biopsy, bronchoscopy with transbronchial biopsy, and positive-pressure mechanical ventilation. Tension pneumothorax usually occurs in the setting of penetrating trauma, lung infection, cardiopulmonary resuscitation, or positive-pressure mechanical ventilation. In tension pneumothorax, the pressure of air in the pleural space exceeds ambient pressure throughout the respiratory cycle. A check-valve mechanism allows air to enter the pleural space on inspiration and prevents egress of air on expiration.

Primary pneumothorax affects mainly tall, thin boys and men between the ages of 10 and 30 years. It is thought to occur from rupture of subpleural apical blebs in response to high negative intrapleural pressures. Family history and cigarette smoking may also be important factors.

Secondary pneumothorax occurs as a complication of COPD, asthma, cystic fibrosis, tuberculosis, pneumocystis pneumonia, menstruation (catamenial pneumothorax), and a wide variety of interstitial lung diseases including sarcoidosis, lymph-angioleiomyomatosis, Langerhans cell histiocytosis, and tuberous sclerosis. Aerosolized pentamidine and a prior history of pneumocystis pneumonia are considered risk factors for the development of pneumothorax. One-half of patients with pneumothorax in the setting of recurrent pneumocystis pneumonia will develop pneumothorax on the contralateral side. The mortality rate of pneumothorax in pneumocystis pneumonia is high.

Clinical Findings

A. SYMPTOMS AND SIGNS

Chest pain ranging from minimal to severe on the affected side and dyspnea occur in nearly all patients. Symptoms usually begin during rest and usually resolve within 24 hours even if the pneumothorax persists. Alternatively, pneumothorax may present with life-threatening respiratory failure if underlying COPD or asthma is present.

If pneumothorax is small (less than 15% of a hemithorax), physical findings, other than mild tachycardia, are unimpressive. If pneumothorax is large, diminished breath sounds, decreased tactile fremitus, and decreased movement of the chest are often noted. Tension pneumothorax should be suspected in the presence of marked tachycardia, hypotension, and mediastinal or tracheal shift.

B. LABORATORY FINDINGS

Arterial blood gas analysis is often unnecessary but reveals hypoxemia and acute respiratory alkalosis in most patients. Left-sided primary pneumothorax may produce QRS axis and precordial T wave changes on the ECG that may be misinterpreted as acute myocardial infarction.

C. IMAGING

Demonstration of a visceral pleural line on chest radiograph is diagnostic and may only be seen on an expiratory film. A few patients have secondary pleural effusion that demonstrates a characteristic air-fluid level on chest radiography. In supine patients, pneumothorax on a conventional chest radiograph may appear as an abnormally radiolucent costophrenic sulcus (the "deep sulcus" sign). In patients with tension pneumothorax, chest radiographs show a large amount of air in the affected hemithorax and contralateral shift of the mediastinum.

Differential Diagnosis

If the patient is a young, tall, thin, cigarette-smoking man, the diagnosis of primary spontaneous pneumothorax is usually obvious and can be confirmed by chest radiograph. In secondary pneumothorax, it is sometimes difficult to distinguish loculated pneumothorax from an emphysematous bleb. Occasionally, pneumothorax may mimic myocardial infarction, pulmonary embolization, or pneumonia.

Complications

Tension pneumothorax may be life-threatening. Pneumomediastinum and subcutaneous emphysema may occur as complications of spontaneous pneumothorax. If pneumomediastinum is detected, rupture of the esophagus or a bronchus should be considered.

Treatment

Treatment depends upon the severity of pneumothorax and the nature of the underlying disease. In a reliable patient with a small (< 15% of a hemithorax), stable spontaneous primary pneumothorax, observation alone may be appropriate. Many small pneumothoraces resolve spontaneously as air is absorbed from the pleural space; supplemental oxygen therapy may increase the rate of reabsorption. Simple aspiration drainage of pleural air with a small-bore catheter (eg, 16 gauge angiocatheter or larger drainage catheter) can be performed for spontaneous primary pneumothoraces that are large or progressive. Placement of a small-bore chest tube (7F to 14F) attached to a one-way Heimlich valve provides protection against development of tension pneumothorax and may permit observation from home. The patient should be treated symptomatically for cough and chest pain, and followed with serial chest radiographs every 24 hours.

Patients with secondary pneumothorax, large pneumothorax, tension pneumothorax, or severe symptoms or those who have a pneumothorax on mechanical ventilation should undergo chest tube placement (tube thoracostomy). The chest tube is placed under water-seal drainage, and suction is applied until the lung expands. The chest tube can be removed after the air leak subsides.

All patients who smoke should be advised to discontinue smoking and warned that the risk of recurrence is 50%. Future exposure to high altitudes, flying in unpressurized aircraft, and scuba diving should be avoided.

Indications for thoracoscopy or open thoracotomy include recurrences of spontaneous pneumothorax, any occurrence of bilateral pneumothorax, and failure of tube thoracostomy for the first episode (failure of lung to reexpand or persistent air leak). Surgery permits resection of blebs responsible for the pneumothorax and pleurodesis by mechanical abrasion and insufflation of talc.

Management of pneumothorax in patients with pneumocystis pneumonia is challenging because of a tendency toward recurrence, and there is no consensus on the best approach. Use of a small chest tube attached to a Heimlich valve has been proposed to allow the patient to leave the hospital. Some clinicians favor its insertion early in the course.

Prognosis

An average of 30% of patients with spontaneous pneumothorax experience recurrence of the disorder after either observation or tube thoracostomy for the first episode. Recurrence after surgical therapy is less frequent. Following successful therapy, there are no long-term complications.

Sahn SA et al: Spontaneous pneumothorax. N Engl J Med 2000;342:868. [PMID: 10727592] (Comprehensive review.)

Weissberg D et al: Pneumothorax. Chest 2000;117:1279. [PMID: 10807811] (Retrospective review of 1199 patients with pneumothorax summarizes one institution's approach to treatment.)

■ DISORDERS OF CONTROL OF VENTILATION

The principal influences on ventilatory control are arterial PCO_2, pH, PO_2, and brainstem tissue pH. These variables are monitored by peripheral and central chemoreceptors. Under normal conditions, the ventilatory control system maintains arterial pH and PCO_2 within narrow limits; arterial PO_2 is more loosely controlled.

Abnormal control of ventilation can be seen with a variety of conditions ranging from rare disorders such as Ondine's curse, neuromuscular disorders, myxedema, starvation, and carotid body resection to more common disorders such as asthma, COPD, obesity, congestive heart failure, and sleep-related breathing disorders. A few of these disorders will be discussed in this section.

Caruana-Montaldo B et al: The control of breathing in clinical practice. Chest 2000;117:205. [PMID: 10631221] (Outline of clinically relevant aspects of control of ventilation plus instructive case presentations.)

PRIMARY ALVEOLAR HYPOVENTILATION

Primary alveolar hypoventilation ("Ondine's curse") is a rare syndrome of unknown cause characterized by inadequate alveolar ventilation despite normal neurologic function and normal airways, lungs, chest wall, and ventilatory muscles. Hypoventilation is even more marked during sleep. Individuals with this disorder are usually nonobese males in their third or fourth decades who present with lethargy, headache, and somnolence. Dyspnea is absent. Physical examination may reveal cyanosis and evidence of pulmonary hypertension and cor pulmonale. Hypoxemia and hypercapnia are present and improve with voluntary hyperventilation. Erythrocytosis is common. Treatment with ventilatory stimulants is usually unrewarding. Augmentation of ventilation by mechanical methods (phrenic nerve stimulation, rocking bed, mechanical ventilators) has been helpful to some patients. Adequate oxygenation should be maintained with supplemental oxygen, but nocturnal oxygen therapy should be prescribed only if diagnostic nocturnal polysomnography has demonstrated its efficacy and safety. Primary alveolar hypoventilation resembles—but should be distinguished from—**central alveolar hypoventilation,** in which impaired ventilatory drive with chronic respiratory acidemia and hypoxemia follows an insult to the brain stem (eg, bulbar poliomyelitis, infarction, meningitis, encephalitis, trauma).

Krachman S et al: Hypoventilation syndromes. Clin Chest Med 1998;19:139. [PMID: 9554224] (Reviews the diverse group of hypoventilation disorders.)

OBESITY-HYPOVENTILATION SYNDROME (Pickwickian Syndrome)

Some obese individuals display symptoms and findings of alveolar hypoventilation. In obesity-hypoventilation syndrome, hypoventilation appears to result from a combination of blunted ventilatory drive and increased mechanical load imposed upon the chest by obesity. Voluntary hyperventilation returns the PCO_2 and the PO_2 toward normal values, a correction not seen in lung diseases causing chronic respiratory failure such as COPD. Most patients with obesity-hypoventilation syndrome also suffer from obstructive sleep apnea (see below), which must be treated aggressively if identified as a comorbid disorder. Therapy of obesity-hypoventilation syndrome consists mainly of weight loss, which improves hypercapnia and hypoxemia as well as the ventilatory responses to hypoxia and hypercapnia. Noninvasive positive-pressure ventilation is helpful in some patients. Respiratory stimulants may be helpful and include theophylline, acetazolamide, and medroxyprogesterone acetate, 10–20 mg every 8 hours orally. Improvement in hypoxemia, hypercapnia, erythrocytosis, and cor pulmonale are goals of therapy.

SLEEP-RELATED BREATHING DISORDERS

Abnormal ventilation during sleep is manifested by apnea (breath cessation for at least 10 seconds) or hypopnea (decrement in airflow with drop in oxyhemoglobin saturation of at least 4%). Episodes of apnea are **central** if ventilatory effort is absent for the duration of the apneic episode, **obstructive** if ventilatory effort persists throughout the apneic episode but no airflow occurs because of transient obstruction of the upper airway, and **mixed** if absent ventilatory effort precedes upper airway obstruction during the apneic episode. Pure central sleep apnea is uncommon; it may be an isolated finding or may occur in patients with primary alveolar hypoventilation or with lesions of the brain stem. Obstructive and mixed sleep apneas are more common and may be associated with life-threatening cardiac arrhythmias, severe hypoxemia during sleep, daytime somnolence, pulmonary hypertension, cor pulmonale, systemic hypertension, and secondary erythrocytosis.

Definitive diagnostic evaluation for suspected sleep apnea should include otolaryngologic examination and overnight polysomnography (the monitoring of multiple physiologic factors during sleep). Electroencephalography, electro-oculography, electromyography, electrocardiography, pulse oximetry, and measurement of respiratory effort and airflow are performed in a complete evaluation. Screening may be performed using home nocturnal pulse oximetry, which when normal has a high negative predictive value in ruling out significant sleep apnea.

Obstructive Sleep Apnea

Upper airway obstruction during sleep occurs when loss of normal pharyngeal muscle tone allows the pharynx to collapse passively during inspiration. Patients with anatomically narrowed upper airways (eg, micrognathia, macroglossia, obesity, tonsillar hypertrophy) are predisposed to the development of obstructive sleep apnea. Ingestion of alcohol or sedatives before sleeping or nasal obstruction of any type, including the common cold, may precipitate or worsen the condition. Hypothyroidism and cigarette smoking are additional risk factors for obstructive sleep apnea. Before making the diagnosis of obstructive sleep apnea, a drug history should be obtained and a seizure disorder, narcolepsy, or psychiatric depression excluded.

Most patients with obstructive or mixed sleep apnea are obese middle-aged men. Systemic hypertension is common. Patients may complain of excessive daytime somnolence, morning sluggishness and headaches, daytime fatigue, cognitive impairment, recent weight gain, and impotence. Bed partners usually report loud cyclical snoring, breath cessation, witnessed apneas, restlessness, and thrashing movements of the extremities during sleep. Personality changes, poor judgment, work-related problems, depression, and intellectual deterioration (memory impairment, inability to concentrate) may also be observed.

Physical examination may be normal or may reveal systemic and pulmonary hypertension with cor pulmonale. The patient may appear sleepy or even fall asleep during the evaluation. The oropharynx is frequently found to be narrowed by excessive soft tissue folds, large tonsils, pendulous uvula, or prominent tongue. Nasal obstruction by a deviated nasal septum, poor nasal air flow, and a nasal twang to the speech may be observed. A "bull neck" appearance is common.

Erythrocytosis is common. A hemoglobin level and thyroid function tests should be obtained. Observation of the sleeping patient reveals loud snoring interrupted by episodes of increasingly strong ventilatory effort that fail to produce airflow. A loud snort often accompanies the first breath following an apneic episode. Polysomnography reveals apneic episodes lasting as long as 60 seconds. Oxygen saturation falls, often to very low levels. Bradyarrhythmias such as sinus bradycardia, sinus arrest, or atrioventricular block may occur. Tachyarrhythmias, including paroxysmal supraventricular tachycardia, atrial fibrillation, and ventricular tachycardia, may be seen once airflow is reestablished.

Weight loss and strict avoidance of alcohol and hypnotic medications are the first steps in management. Weight loss may be curative, but most patients are unable to lose the 10–20% of body weight required. Nasal continuous positive airway pressure (nasal CPAP) at night is curative in many patients. Polysomnography is frequently necessary to determine the level of CPAP (usually 5–15 cm H_2O) necessary to abolish obstructive apneas. Unfortunately, only about 75% of patients continue to use nasal CPAP after 1 year. Pharmacologic therapy for obstructive sleep apnea is disappointing. Supplemental oxygen may lessen the severity of nocturnal desaturation but may also lengthen apneas. Polysomnography is necessary to assess the effects of oxygen therapy; it should not be routinely prescribed. Mechanical devices inserted into the mouth at bedtime to hold the jaw forward and prevent pharyngeal occlusion have modest effectiveness in relieving apnea; however, patient compliance is not optimal.

Uvulopalatopharyngoplasty, a procedure consisting of resection of pharyngeal soft tissue and amputation of approximately 15 mm of the free edge of the soft palate and uvula, is helpful in approximately 50% of selected patients. It is more effective in eliminating snoring than apneic episodes. Uvulopalatopharyngoplasty may now be performed on an outpatient basis with a laser. **Nasal septoplasty** is performed if gross anatomic nasal septal deformity is present. **Tracheostomy** relieves upper airway obstruction and its physiologic consequences and represents the definitive treatment for obstructive sleep apnea. However, it has numerous adverse effects, including granuloma formation, difficulty with speech, and stoma and airway infection. Furthermore, the long-term care of the tracheostomy, especially in obese patients, can be difficult. Tracheostomy and other maxillofacial surgery approaches are reserved for patients with life-threatening arrhythmias or severe disability who have failed to respond to conservative therapy.

Some patients with sleep apnea have nocturnal bradycardia. A pilot study in 15 patients with either central or obstructive sleep apnea showed some improvement in oxygen saturation with atrial pacing. This single study must be considered preliminary.

Exar EN et al: The upper airway resistance syndrome. Chest 1999;115:1127. [PMID: 10208219] (Review of pathophysiology and diagnostic and therapeutic approaches.)

Fogel RB et al: Obstructive sleep apnea. Adv Intern Med 2000;45:351. [PMID: 10635055] (Review article.)

Garrigue S et al: Benefit of atrial pacing in sleep apnea syndrome. N Engl J Med 2002;346:404. [PMID: 11832528]

Loube DI et al: Indications for positive airway pressure treatment of adult obstructive sleep apnea patients: consensus statement. Chest 1999;115: 863. [PMID: 100-84504]

Wright J et al: Continuous positive airways pressure for obstructive sleep apnea. Cochrane Database Syst Rev 2000;2:CD001106. [PMID: 10796595] (Systematic analysis of therapeutic trials.)

HYPERVENTILATION SYNDROMES

Hyperventilation is an increase in alveolar ventilation that leads to hypocapnia. It may be caused by a variety of conditions, such as pregnancy, hypoxemia, obstructive and infiltrative lung diseases, sepsis, hepatic dysfunction, fever, and pain. The term "central neurogenic hyperventilation" denotes a monotonous, sustained pattern of rapid and deep breathing seen in comatose patients with brain stem injury of multiple causes. Functional hyperventilation may be acute or chronic. Acute hyperventilation presents with hyperpnea, paresthesias, carpopedal spasm, tetany, and anxiety. Chronic hyperventilation may present with various nonspecific symptoms, including fatigue, dyspnea, anxiety, palpitations, and dizziness. The diagnosis of chronic hyperventilation syndrome is established if symptoms are reproduced during voluntary hyperventilation. Once organic causes of hyperventilation have been excluded, treatment of acute hyperventilation consists of rebreathing expired gas from a paper bag held over the face in order to decrease respiratory alkalemia and its associated symptoms. Anxiolytic drugs are also useful.

Foster GT et al: Respiratory alkalosis. Respir Care 2001;46:384. [PMID: 11262557] (Review of a common clinical problem.)

Gardner WN: The pathophysiology of hyperventilation disorders. Chest 1996;109:516. [PMID: 8620731] (Concise review.)

■ ACUTE RESPIRATORY FAILURE

Respiratory failure is defined as respiratory dysfunction resulting in abnormalities of oxygenation or ventilation (CO_2 elimination) severe enough to threaten the function of vital organs. Arterial blood gas criteria for respiratory failure are not absolute but may be arbitrarily established as a P_{O_2} under 60 mm Hg or a P_{CO_2} over 50 mm Hg. Acute respiratory failure may occur in a variety of pulmonary and nonpulmonary disorders (Table 9–31). A complete discussion of treatment of acute respiratory failure is beyond the scope of this chapter. Only a few selected general principles of management will be reviewed here.

Table 9–31. Selected causes of acute respiratory failure in adults.

Airway disorders	Neuromuscular and related disorders
Asthma	Primary neuromuscular diseases
Acute exacerbation of chronic bronchitis or emphysema	Guillain-Barré syndrome
Obstruction of pharynx, larynx, trachea, main stem	Myasthenia gravis
bronchus, or lobar bronchus by edema, mucus, mass,	Poliomyelitis
or foreign body	Polymyositis
Pulmonary edema	Drug- or toxin-induced
Increased hydrostatic pressure	Botulism
Left ventricular dysfunction (eg, myocardial ischemia,	Organophosphates
heart failure)	Neuromuscular blocking agents
Mitral regurgitation	Aminoglycosides
Left atrial outflow obstruction (eg, mitral stenosis)	Spinal cord injury
Volume overload states	Phrenic nerve injury or dysfunction
Increased pulmonary capillary permeability	Electrolyte disturbances: hypokalemia, hypophosphatemia
Acute respiratory distress syndrome	Myxedema
Acute lung injury	**Central nervous system disorders**
Unclear etiology	Drugs: sedative, hypnotic, opioid, anesthetics
Neurogenic	Brain stem respiratory center disorders: trauma, tumor,
Negative pressure (inspiratory airway obstruction)	vascular disorders, hypothyroidism
Reexpansion	Intracranial hypertension
Tocolytic-associated	Central nervous system infections
Parenchymal lung disorders	**Increased CO_2 production**
Pneumonia	Fever
Interstitial lung diseases	Infection
Diffuse alveolar hemorrhage syndromes	Hyperalimentation with excess caloric and carbohydrate
Aspiration	intake
Lung contusion	Hyperthyroidism
Pulmonary vascular disorders	Seizures
Thromboembolism	Rigors
Air embolism	Drugs
Amniotic fluid embolism	
Chest wall, diaphragm and pleural disorders	
Rib fracture	
Flail chest	
Pneumothorax	
Pleural effusion	
Massive ascites	
Abdominal distention and abdominal compartment syndrome	

Clinical Findings

Symptoms and signs of acute respiratory failure are those of the underlying disease combined with those of hypoxemia or hypercapnia. The chief symptom of hypoxemia is dyspnea, though profound hypoxemia may exist in the absence of complaints. Signs of hypoxemia include cyanosis, restlessness, confusion, anxiety, delirium, tachypnea, tachycardia, hypertension, cardiac dysrhythmias, and tremor. Dyspnea and headache are the cardinal symptoms of hypercapnia. Signs of hypercapnia include peripheral and conjunctival hyperemia, hypertension, tachycardia, tachypnea, impaired consciousness, papilledema, and asterixis. The symptoms and signs of acute respiratory failure are both insensitive and nonspecific; therefore, the physician must maintain a high index of suspicion and obtain arterial blood gas analysis if respiratory failure is suspected.

Treatment

Treatment of the patient with acute respiratory failure consists of (1) specific therapy directed toward the underlying disease; (2) respiratory supportive care directed toward the maintenance of adequate gas exchange; and (3) general supportive care. Only the last two aspects are discussed below.

A. RESPIRATORY SUPPORT

Respiratory support has both nonventilatory and ventilatory aspects.

1. Nonventilatory aspects—The main therapeutic goal in acute hypoxemic respiratory failure is to ensure adequate oxygenation of vital organs. Inspired oxygen concentration should be the lowest value that results in an arterial oxygen saturation of $\geq 90\%$ ($PO_2 \geq 60$ mm Hg). Higher arterial oxygen tensions are of no proven benefit. Restoration of normoxia may cause hypoventilation in patients with chronic hypercapnia; however, *oxygen therapy should not be withheld for fear of causing progressive respiratory acidemia.* Hypoxemia in patients with obstructive airway disease is usually easily corrected by administering low-flow oxygen by nasal cannula (1–3 L/min) or Venturi mask (24–28%). Higher concentrations of oxygen are necessary to correct hypoxemia in patients with acute respiratory distress syndrome (ARDS), pneumonia, and other parenchymal lung diseases.

2. Ventilatory aspects—Ventilatory support consists of maintaining patency of the airway and ensuring adequate alveolar ventilation. Mechanical ventilation may be provided via face mask (noninvasive) or through tracheal intubation.

a. Noninvasive positive-pressure ventilation (NPPV)—NPPV delivered via a full face mask or nasal mask has become first-line therapy in COPD patients with hypercapnic respiratory failure who can protect and maintain the patency of their airway, handle their own secretions, and tolerate the mask apparatus. Several studies have demonstrated the effectiveness of this therapy in reducing intubation rates and ICU stays in patients with ventilatory failure. Patients with acute lung injury or ARDS or those who suffer from severely impaired oxygenation do not benefit and should be intubated if they require mechanical ventilation. A bilevel positive pressure ventilation mode is preferred for most patients.

b. Tracheal intubation—Indications for tracheal intubation include (1) hypoxemia despite supplemental oxygen, (2) upper airway obstruction, (3) impaired airway protection, (4) inability to clear secretions, (5) respiratory acidosis, (6) progressive general fatigue, tachypnea, use of accessory respiratory muscles, or mental status deterioration, and (7) apnea. In general, orotracheal intubation is preferred to nasotracheal intubation in urgent or emergency situations because it is easier, faster, and less traumatic. The position of the tip of the endotracheal tube at the level of the aortic arch should be verified by chest radiograph immediately following intubation, and auscultation should be performed to verify that both lungs are being inflated. Only tracheal tubes with high-volume, low-pressure air-filled cuffs should be used. Cuff inflation pressure should be kept below 20 mm Hg if possible to minimize tracheal mucosal injury.

c. Mechanical ventilation—Indications for mechanical ventilation include (1) apnea, (2) acute hypercapnia that is not quickly reversed by appropriate specific therapy, (3) severe hypoxemia, and (4) progressive patient fatigue despite appropriate treatment.

Several modes of positive-pressure ventilation are available. Controlled mechanical ventilation (CMV), or assist/control (A/C), is a ventilatory mode in which the ventilator is set to deliver a minimum number of breaths each minute; the patient may trigger the ventilator to deliver additional breaths at the prescribed

tidal volume. Synchronized intermittent mandatory ventilation (SIMV) is a ventilatory mode in which the ventilator may deliver a set number of breaths each minute. The patient may take additional breaths; however, these breaths are not supported by the ventilator unless the pressure support mode is added. Numerous alternative modes of mechanical ventilation now exist, the most popular being pressure support ventilation (PSV), pressure control ventilation (PCV), and continuous positive airway pressure (CPAP).

Positive end-expiratory pressure (PEEP) is useful in improving oxygenation in patients with diffuse parenchymal lung disease such as ARDS. It should be used cautiously in patients with localized parenchymal disease, hyperinflation, or very high airway pressure requirements during mechanical ventilation.

d. Complications of mechanical ventilation—Potential complications of mechanical ventilation are numerous. Migration of the tip of the endotracheal tube into a main bronchus can cause atelectasis of the contralateral lung and overdistention of the intubated lung. **Barotrauma** (alternatively referred to as "volutrauma"), manifested by subcutaneous emphysema, pneumomediastinum, subpleural air cysts, pneumothorax, or systemic gas embolism, may occur in patients whose lungs are overdistended by excessive tidal volumes, especially those with hyperinflation caused by airflow obstruction. Subtle parenchymal lung injury due to overdistention of alveoli is another potential hazard. Strategies to avoid barotrauma include deliberate hypoventilation through the use of low mechanical tidal volumes and respiratory rates, resulting in "permissive hypercapnia."

Acute respiratory alkalosis caused by overventilation is common. Hypotension induced by elevated intrathoracic pressure that results in decreased return of systemic venous blood to the heart may occur in patients treated with PEEP, those with severe airflow obstruction, and those with intravascular volume depletion. Ventilator-associated pneumonia is another serious complication of mechanical ventilation.

B. GENERAL SUPPORTIVE CARE

Maintenance of adequate nutrition is vital; parenteral nutrition should be used only when conventional enteral feeding methods are not possible. Overfeeding, especially with carbohydrate-rich formulas, should be avoided, because it can increase CO_2 production and may potentially worsen or induce hypercapnia in patients with limited ventilatory reserve. However, failure to provide adequate nutrition is more common. Hypokalemia and hypophosphatemia may worsen hypoventilation due to respiratory muscle weakness. Sedative-hypnotics and opioid analgesics are frequently used. They should be titrated carefully to avoid oversedation, leading to prolongation of intubation. Temporary paralysis with a nondepolarizing neuromuscular blocking agent is occasionally used to facilitate mechanical ventilation and to lower oxygen consumption. Prolonged muscle weakness due to an acute myopathy is a potential complication of these agents. It is more common in patients with renal dysfunction and in those given concomitant corticosteroids.

Psychologic and emotional support of the patient and family, skin care to avoid decubitus ulcers, and meticulous avoidance of nosocomial infection and complications of tracheal tubes are vital aspects of comprehensive care for patients with acute respiratory failure.

Attention must also be paid to preventing complications associated with serious illness. Stress gastritis and ulcers may be avoided by administering sucralfate, antacids, or histamine H_2 receptor antagonists. There is some concern that the latter two agents, which raise the gastric pH, may permit increased growth of gram-negative bacteria in the stomach, predisposing to pharyngeal colonization and ultimately nosocomial pneumonia; many clinicians prefer sucralfate. The risk of deep venous thrombosis and pulmonary embolism may be reduced by subcutaneous administration of heparin (5000 units every 12 hours) or placement of a sequential compression device on an extremity.

Course & Prognosis

The course and prognosis of acute respiratory failure vary and depend on the underlying disease. The prognosis of acute respiratory failure caused by uncomplicated sedative or narcotic drug overdose is excellent. Acute respiratory failure in patients with COPD who do not require intubation and mechanical ventilation has a good immediate prognosis. On the other hand, ARDS associated with sepsis has an extremely poor prognosis, with mortality rates of about 90%. Overall, adults requiring mechanical ventilation for all causes of acute respiratory failure have survival rates of 62% to weaning, 43% to hospital discharge, and 30% to 1 year after hospital discharge.

Mehta S et al: Noninvasive ventilation: State of the Art. Am J Respir Crit Care Med 2001;163:540. [PMID: 11179136] (Comprehensive review of all aspects of noninvasive ventilation, with 341 references.)

Raju P et al: The pathogenesis of respiratory failure: an overview. Respir Clin N Am 2000;6:195. [PMID: 10757961]

Tobin MJ. Advances in mechanical ventilation. N Engl J Med 2001;344:1986. [PMID: 11430329]

■ ACUTE RESPIRATORY DISTRESS SYNDROME (ARDS)

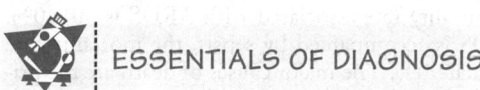

ESSENTIALS OF DIAGNOSIS

- *Acute onset of respiratory failure.*
- *Bilateral radiographic pulmonary infiltrates.*
- *Absence of elevated left atrial pressure (if measured, pulmonary capillary wedge pressure ≤ 18 mm Hg).*
- *Ratio of partial pressure of oxygen in arterial blood (Pa_{O_2}) to fractional concentration of inspired oxygen (F_{IO_2}) < 200, regardless of the level of positive end-expiratory pressure (PEEP).*

General Considerations

Acute respiratory distress syndrome (ARDS; formerly called adult respiratory distress syndrome) denotes acute hypoxemic respiratory failure following a systemic or pulmonary insult without evidence of heart failure. ARDS is the most severe form of acute lung injury and is characterized by bilateral, widespread radiographic pulmonary infiltrates, normal pulmonary capillary wedge pressure (≤ 18 mm Hg) and a PaO_2/FIO_2 ratio < 200. ARDS may follow a wide variety of clinical events (Table 9–32). Common risk factors for ARDS include sepsis, aspiration of gastric contents, shock, infection, lung contusion, nonthoracic trauma, toxic inhalation, near-drowning, and multiple blood transfusions. About one-third of ARDS patients initially have sepsis syndrome. Pro-inflammatory cytokines released from stimulated inflammatory cells appear to be pivotal in lung injury. Although the

Table 9–32. Selected disorders associated with ARDS.

Systemic Insults	Pulmonary Insults
Trauma	Aspiration of gastric contents
Sepsis	Embolism of thrombus, fat,
Pancreatitis	air, or amniotic fluid
Shock	Miliary tuberculosis
Multiple transfusions	Diffuse pneumonia
Disseminated intravascular	Acute eosinophilic pneumo-
coagulation	nia
Burns	Bronchiolitis obliterans
Drugs and drug overdose	organizing pneumonia
Opioids	Upper airway obstruction
Aspirin	Free-base cocaine smoking
Phenothiazines	Near-drowning
Tricyclic antidepressants	Toxic gas inhalation
Amiodarone	Nitrogen dioxide
Chemotherapeutic agents	Chlorine
Nitrofurantoin	Sulfur dioxide
Protamine	Ammonia
Thrombotic thrombocyto-	Smoke
penic purpura	Oxygen toxicity
Cardiopulmonary bypass	Lung contusion
Head injury	Radiation exposure
Paraquat	High-altitude exposure
	Lung reexpansion or reper-
	fusion

mechanism of lung injury varies with the cause, damage to capillary endothelial cells and alveolar epithelial cells is common to ARDS regardless of cause. Damage to these cells causes increased vascular permeability and decreased production and activity of surfactant; these abnormalities lead to interstitial and alveolar pulmonary edema, alveolar collapse, and hypoxemia.

Clinical Findings

ARDS is marked by the rapid onset of profound dyspnea that usually occurs 12–48 hours after the initiating event. Labored breathing, tachypnea, intercostal retractions, and crackles are noted on physical examination. Chest radiography shows diffuse or patchy bilateral infiltrates that rapidly become confluent; these characteristically spare the costophrenic angles. Air bronchograms occur in about 80% of cases. Upper lung zone venous engorgement is distinctly uncommon. Heart size is normal, and pleural effusions are small or nonexistent. Marked hypoxemia occurs that is refractory to treatment with supplemental oxygen. Many patients with ARDS demonstrate multiple organ failure, particularly involving the kidneys, liver, gut, central nervous system, and cardiovascular system.

Differential Diagnosis

Since ARDS is a physiologic and radiographic syndrome rather than a specific disease, the concept of differential diagnosis does not strictly apply. Normal-permeability ("cardiogenic" or hydrostatic) pulmonary edema must be excluded, however, because specific therapy is available for that disorder. Measurement of pulmonary capillary wedge pressure by means of a flow-directed pulmonary artery catheter may be required in selected patients with suspected cardiac dysfunction. Routine use of the Swan-Ganz catheter in ARDS is discouraged.

Prevention

No measures that effectively prevent ARDS have been identified; specifically, prophylactic use of PEEP in patients at risk for ARDS has not been shown to be effective. Intravenous methylprednisolone does not prevent ARDS when given early to patients with sepsis syndrome or septic shock.

Treatment

Treatment of ARDS must include identification and specific treatment of the underlying precipitating and secondary conditions (eg, sepsis). Meticulous supportive care must then be provided to compensate for the severe dysfunction of the respiratory system associated with ARDS and to prevent complications (see above). Treatment of the hypoxemia seen in ARDS usually requires tracheal intubation and positive-pressure mechanical ventilation. The lowest levels of PEEP (used to recruit atelectatic alveoli) and supplemental oxygen required to maintain the PaO$_2$ above 60 mm Hg or the SaO$_2$ above 90% should be used. Efforts should be made to decrease FiO$_2$ to less than 60% as soon as possible in order to avoid oxygen toxicity. PEEP can be increased as needed as long as cardiac output and oxygen delivery do not decrease and airway pressures do not increase excessively. Prone positioning may improve oxygenation in selected patients by helping recruit atelectatic alveoli; however, great care must be taken during the maneuver to avoid dislodging catheters and tubes.

A variety of mechanical ventilation strategies are available. A multicenter study of 800 patients demonstrated that the use of a detailed volume ventilation protocol that employs small tidal volumes (6 mL/kg of ideal body weight) resulted in a 10% absolute mortality reduction over standard therapy; this trial reported the lowest mortality (31%) of any intervention to date for ARDS.

Cardiac output that falls when PEEP is used may be improved by reducing the level of PEEP or by the judicious use of inotropic drugs (eg, dopamine); administering fluids to increase intravascular volume should be done only with great caution, because increases in pulmonary capillary pressure worsen pulmonary edema in the presence of increased capillary permeability. Therefore, the goal of fluid management is to maintain pulmonary capillary wedge pressure at the lowest level compatible with adequate cardiac output. Crystalloid solutions should be used when intravascular volume expansion is necessary. Diuretics should be used to reduce intravascular volume if pulmonary capillary wedge pressure is elevated.

Oxygen delivery can be increased in anemic patients by ensuring that hemoglobin concentrations are at least 8 g/dL; patients are not likely to benefit from higher levels. Increasing oxygen delivery to supranormal levels through the use of inotropes and high hemoglobin concentrations is not clinically useful and may be harmful in some circumstances. Strategies to decrease oxygen consumption include the appropriate use of sedatives, analgesics, and antipyretics.

A large number of innovative therapeutic interventions to improve outcomes in ARDS patients have been or are being investigated. Unfortunately, to date, none have consistently shown benefit in clinical trials. Systemic corticosteroids have been studied extensively with variable and inconsistent results. While recent studies suggest a benefit in late-phase ARDS, confirmatory studies are required before they can be recommended for use on a routine basis.

Course & Prognosis

The mortality rate associated with ARDS is 30–40%. If ARDS is accompanied by sepsis, the mortality rate may reach 90%. The major causes of death are the primary illness and secondary complications such as multiple organ system failure or sepsis. Median survival is about 2 weeks. Many patients who succumb to ARDS and its complications die after withdrawal of support (see Withdrawal of Support in Chapter 5). Most survivors of ARDS are left with some pulmonary symptoms (cough, dyspnea, sputum production) which tend to improve over time. Mild abnormalities of oxygenation, diffusing capacity, and lung mechanics persist in some individuals.

Artigas A et al. The American-European Consensus Conference on ARDS, Part 2: Ventilatory, pharmacologic, supportive therapy, study design strategies, and issues related to recovery and remodeling. Acute respiratory distress syndrome. Am J Respir Crit Care Med 1998;157:1332. [PMID: 9563759] (Expert panel discussion of standards for the ICU care of patients with acute lung injury.)

Valta P et al: Acute respiratory distress syndrome: frequency, clinical course, and costs of care. Crit Care Med 1999;27:2367. [PMID: 10579250]

Ventilation with lower tidal volumes as compared with traditional tidal volumes for acute lung injury and the acute respiratory distress syndrome. The Acute Respiratory Distress Syndrome Network: N Engl J Med 2000;342:1301. [PMID: 10793162] (In patients with acute lung injury and ARDS, mechanical ventilation with a lower tidal volume than is traditionally used results in decreased mortality and increases the number of days without ventilator use.)

Ware LB et al: The acute respiratory distress syndrome. N Engl J Med 2000;342:1334. [PMID: 10793167] (State of the art review.)

Heart

Barry M. Massie, MD, & Thomas M. Amidon, MD
See www.current-med.com/ch10.html

10

■ SYMPTOMS & SIGNS

COMMON SYMPTOMS

The most common symptoms of heart disease are dyspnea, chest pain, palpitations, presyncope or syncope, and fatigue. None are specific, and interpretation depends on the entire clinical picture and, in many cases, diagnostic testing.

Dyspnea

Dyspnea due to heart disease is precipitated or exacerbated by exertion and results from elevated left atrial and pulmonary venous pressures or from hypoxia. The former are most commonly caused by left ventricular systolic dysfunction, left ventricular diastolic dysfunction (due to hypertrophy, fibrosis, or pericardial disease), or valvular obstruction. The acute onset or worsening of left atrial hypertension may result in **pulmonary edema. Hypoxia** may be due to pulmonary edema or intracardiac shunting. Dyspnea should be quantified by the amount of activity that precipitates it. Dyspnea is also a common symptom of pulmonary disease, and the etiologic distinction may be difficult. Shortness of breath is also found in sedentary or obese individuals, anxiety states, anemia, and many other illnesses.

Orthopnea is dyspnea that occurs in recumbency and results from an increase in central blood volume. Orthopnea may also result from pulmonary disease and obesity. **Paroxysmal nocturnal dyspnea** is shortness of breath that occurs abruptly 30 minutes to 2 hours after going to bed and is relieved by sitting up or standing up; this symptom is more specific for cardiac disease. Both are more specific for cardiac diseases than exertional dyspnea, but neither is diagnostic of heart failure.

Chest Pain or Discomfort

Chest pain and other forms of discomfort are common symptoms that can occur as a result of pulmonary, pleural, or musculoskeletal disease, esophageal or other gastrointestinal disorders, cervicothoracic nerve root irritation, or anxiety states, as well as many cardiovascular diseases. Myocardial ischemia is the most frequent cause of cardiac chest pain, but it is often experienced more as a sensation of discomfort than actual pain, thereby increasing the potential for neglect on the part of the patient and misdiagnosis by the physician. This is usually described as dull, aching, or as a sensation of "pressure," "tightness," "squeezing," or "gas," rather than as sharp or spasmodic. **Ischemic symptoms** usually subside within 5–20 minutes but may last longer. Protracted episodes often represent **myocardial infarction.** The pain is commonly accompanied by a sense of anxiety or uneasiness. The location is usually retrosternal or left precordial. Though the pain may radiate to or be localized in the throat, lower jaw, shoulders, inner arms, upper abdomen, or back, it nearly always also involves the sternal region. Ischemic pain is often precipitated by exertion, cold temperature, meals, stress, or combinations of these factors and is usually relieved by rest, but many episodes do not conform to these patterns. It is not related to position or respiration and is usually not elicited by chest palpation. In myocardial infarction, a precipitating factor is frequently not apparent.

Hypertrophy of either ventricle and aortic valvular disease may also give rise to ischemic pain or pain with less typical features. Myocarditis, cardiomyopathy, primary pulmonary hypertension, and mitral valve prolapse are associated with chest pain atypical for angina pectoris. Pericarditis may produce pain that changes with position or respiration. Aortic dissection produces an instantaneous onset of tearing pain of great intensity that often radiates to the back.

Lee TH et al: Evaluation of the patient with acute chest pain. N Engl J Med 2000;342:1187. [PMID: 10770985] (Clinical decision-making includes clinical evaluation, laboratory testing, noninvasive imaging, and observation in short-stay chest pain units. Algorithm included.)

Palpitations, Dizziness, Syncope

Awareness of the heartbeat may be a normal phenomenon or may reflect increased cardiac or stroke output in patients with many noncardiac conditions (eg, exercise, thyrotoxicosis, anemia, anxiety). It may also be due to cardiac abnormalities that increase stroke volume (regurgitant valvular disease, bradycardia) or may be a manifestation of cardiac arrhythmias. Ventricular premature beats may be sensed as extra or "skipped" beats. Supraventricular or ventricular tachycardia may be felt as rapid, regular or irregular palpitations or "fluttering"; many patients are asymptomatic, however.

If the abnormal rhythm is associated with a sufficient decline in arterial pressure or cardiac output, it may—especially in the upright position—impair cerebral blood flow, causing dizziness, blurring of vision, loss of consciousness (syncope), or other symptoms.

Cardiogenic syncope most commonly results from sinus node arrest or exit block, atrioventricular conduction block, or ventricular tachycardia or fibrillation. It is associated with few prodromal symptoms and may thus be an occasion for injuries. The absence of premonitory symptoms helps distinguish cardiogenic syncope from vasovagal faints, postural hypotension, or seizure but is not a reliable screening tool. Although recovery is often immediate, some patients may exhibit seizure-like movements. Aortic valve disease and hypertrophic obstructive cardiomyopathy may also cause syncope, which is usually exertional or postexertional. Another form of syncope is termed **neurocardiogenic syncope,** commonly known as vasovagal syncope. In this syndrome, there is an inappropriate increase in vagal efferent activity, often resulting from a precedent increase in sympathetic cardiac stimulation. Syncope may follow a brief period of diaphoresis and presyncopal symptoms, or it may be abrupt in onset, mimicking arrhythmia-induced syncope.

Barsky AJ: Palpitations, arrhythmias, and awareness of cardiac activity. Ann Intern Med 2001;134:832. [PMID: 11346318] (Discusses symptom perception in patients with palpitations.)

Kapoor WN: Syncope. N Engl J Med 2000;343:1856. [PMID: 11117979] (Reviews differential diagnosis, management.)

Schnipper JL et al: Diagnostic evaluation and management of patients with syncope. Med Clin North Am 2001;85:423, xi. [PMID: 11233954]

Sloane PD et al: Dizziness: state of the science. Ann Intern Med 2001;134:823. [PMID: 11346317] (An overview of etiologies with discussion of chronic causes of dizziness as well.)

See also references in section on syncope.

FUNCTIONAL CLASSIFICATION OF HEART DISEASE

As a means of quantifying the limitation on activity of cardiac patients imposed by their symptoms, the classification system of the New York Heart Association is commonly employed. In following individual patients, it is important to document specific activities that produce symptoms.

Class I: No limitation of physical activity. Ordinary physical activity does not cause undue fatigue, dyspnea, or anginal pain.

Class II: Slight limitation of physical activity. Ordinary physical activity results in symptoms.

Class III: Marked limitation of physical activity. Comfortable at rest, but less than ordinary activity causes symptoms.

Class IV: Unable to engage in any physical activity without discomfort. Symptoms may be present even at rest.

SIGNS OF HEART DISEASE

Although the cardiovascular examination centers on the heart, peripheral signs are often invaluable.

Appearance

While cardiac patients may appear healthy and comfortable at rest, many with acute myocardial infarction appear anxious and restless. **Diaphoresis** suggests hypotension or a hyperadrenergic state, such as during pericardial tamponade, tachyarrhythmias, or myocardial infarction. Patients with severe congestive heart failure or other chronic low cardiac output states may appear **cachectic.**

Cyanosis may be central, due to arterial desaturation, or peripheral, reflecting impaired tissue delivery of adequately saturated blood in low-output states, polycythemia, or peripheral vasoconstriction. Central cyanosis may be caused by pulmonary disease, left heart failure, or right-to-left shunting; the latter will not be improved by increasing the inspired oxygen concentration. **Pallor** usually indicates anemia but may be a sign of low cardiac output.

Vital Signs

Although the normal **heart rate** usually ranges from 50 to 90 beats/min, both slower and more rapid rates may occur in normal individuals or may reflect noncardiac conditions such as anxiety or pain, medication effect, fever, thyroid disease, pulmonary disease, anemia, or hypovolemia. If symptoms or clinical suspicion warrants, an electrocardiogram (ECG) should be performed to diagnose arrhythmia, conduction disturbance, or other abnormality. The range of normal

blood pressure is wide, but even in asymptomatic individuals systolic pressures below 90 mm Hg or above 140 mm Hg and diastolic pressures above 90 mm Hg warrant further clinical evaluation and follow-up. Initially elevated pressures may decline if the patient is allowed to relax and rest comfortably. **Tachypnea** is also nonspecific, but pulmonary disease and heart failure should be considered when respiratory rates exceed 16/min under resting conditions. **Periodic breathing** (Cheyne-Stokes respiration) is not uncommon in severe heart failure.

Peripheral Pulses & Venous Pulsations

Diminished peripheral pulses most commonly result from arteriosclerotic peripheral vascular disease and may be accompanied by localized **bruits.** Asymmetry of pulses should also arouse suspicion of coarctation of the aorta or aortic dissection. **Exaggerated pulses** may indicate aortic regurgitation, coarctation, patent ductus arteriosus, or other conditions that increase stroke volume. The carotid pulse is a valuable aid to assessment of left ventricular ejection. It has a **delayed upstroke** in aortic stenosis and a **bisferiens** quality (two palpable peaks) in mixed aortic stenosis and regurgitation or hypertrophic obstructive cardiomyopathy. **Pulsus paradoxus** (a decrease in systolic blood pressure during inspiration greater than the normal 10 mm Hg) is a valuable sign of pericardial tamponade, though it also occurs in asthma and chronic obstructive pulmonary disease. **Pulsus alternans,** in which the amplitude of the pulse alternates every other beat during sinus rhythm, occurs when cardiac contractility is very depressed or with large pericardial effusions.

Jugular venous pulsations provide insight into right atrial pressure. They indicate (1) **elevated central venous pressure** if they are more than 3 vertical centimeters above the angle of Louis, (2) increased central blood volume if they rise more than 1 cm with sustained (30 seconds) right upper quadrant abdominal pressure (**hepatojugular reflux**), (3) tricuspid obstruction or pulmonary hypertension if the *a* wave is exaggerated, and (4) tricuspid regurgitation if **large *cv*** waves are seen. The latter may be associated with hepatic pulsations. Atrioventricular dissociation due to conduction block or ventricular arrhythmia can be recognized by intermittent **cannon *a* waves.**

Constant J: Using internal jugular pulsations as a manometer for right atrial pressure measurements. Cardiology 2000;93:26. [PMID: 10894903] (Overview of the use of jugular venous pulsations.)

Drazner MH et al: Prognostic importance of elevated jugular venous pressure and a third heart sound in patients with heart failure. N Engl J Med 2001;345:574. [PMID: 11529211] (SOLVD investigators demonstrated that elevated jugular venous pressure and S_3 were independently associated with pump failure, hospitalization, and death in patients with congestive heart failure.)

Pulmonary Examination

Rales heard at the lung bases are a sign of congestive heart failure but may be caused by similarly localized pulmonary disease. **Wheezing** and **rhonchi** suggest obstructive pulmonary disease but may occur in left heart failure. **Pleural effusions** with bibasilar percussion dullness and reduced breath sounds are common in congestive heart failure.

Precordial Pulsations

A **parasternal lift** usually indicates right ventricular hypertrophy, pulmonary hypertension (pulmonary artery systolic pressure > 50 mm Hg), or left atrial enlargement; pulmonary artery pulsations may also be visible. The left ventricular **apical impulse,** if sustained and enlarged, suggests myocardial hypertrophy or dysfunction. If it is very prominent but not sustained, the apical impulse may indicate volume overload or high-output states. Additional precordial pulsations may reflect regional abnormalities of left ventricular contraction.

Heart Sounds & Murmurs

Auscultation is diagnostic of—or helpful in diagnosis of—many heart diseases, including cardiac failure. Specific findings are discussed under diagnostic headings.

The **first heart sound (S_1),** the closing of the mitral valve and tricuspid valve, may be diminished with severe left ventricular dysfunction or accentuated with mitral stenosis or short PR intervals. S_2, the closing of the atrioventricular valve and pulmonary valve, is usually split, with the two components (aortic preceding pulmonary) being separated more during inspiration; **splitting** is *fixed* in atrial septal defect, *wide* with right bundle branch block, and *absent* or *reversed* (**paradoxic splitting**) with aortic stenosis, left ventricular failure, or left bundle branch block. With normal splitting, an accentuated P_2 is an important sign of pulmonary hypertension. **Third and fourth heart sounds** (ventricular and atrial gallops, respectively) indicate ventricular volume overload or impaired compliance and may be heard over either ventricle. An apical S_3 is a normal finding in younger individuals and in pregnancy. Additional auscultatory findings include sharp, high-pitched sounds classified as **"clicks."** These may be early systolic and represent **ejection sounds** (as with a bicuspid aortic valve or pulmonary stenosis) or may occur in mid or late systole, indicating myxomatous changes in the mitral valve.

While many **murmurs** indicate valvular disease, a soft, short systolic murmur, usually localized along the left sternal border or toward the apex, may be innocent, reflecting pulmonary flow. **Innocent murmurs** often vary with inspiration, diminish in the upright position, and are most frequently heard in thin individuals. **Systolic murmurs** are **pansystolic (holosystolic)** when they merge with the first sound and persist through all of systole or **"ejection" murmurs** when they begin after the first sound and end before the second sound, with a peak in early or mid systole. The former represent mitral regurgitation if maximal at the apex or in the axilla and tricuspid regurgitation or ventricular septal defect if best heard at the sternal border. Short aortic ejection murmurs with a preserved A_2 are common in older individuals, especially when hypertension has been present, and even if they are moderately loud they usually reflect thickening (sclerosis) of the valve rather than stenosis. Association of murmurs with palpable vibrations (**"thrills"**) is always clinically significant, as are **diastolic murmurs.** Further evaluation is warranted when the patient has symptoms of possible cardiac origin. Some studies suggest that one should have a low threshold for evaluating murmurs with echocardiograms.

Attenhofer Jost CG et al: Echocardiography in the evaluation of systolic murmurs of unknown cause. Am J Med 2000;108: 614. [PMID: 10856408] (Although in adults a functional murmur can usually be differentiated from an organic murmur, echocardiography is helpful in identifying the lesion and determining its severity.)

Drazner MH et al: Prognostic importance of elevated jugular venous pressure and a third heart sound in patients with heart failure. N Engl J Med 2001;345:574. [PMID: 11529211] (SOLVD investigators demonstrated that elevated jugular venous pressure and S_3 were independently associated with pump failure, hospitalization, and death in patients with congestive heart failure.)

Richardson TR et al: Bedside cardiac examination: constancy in a sea of change. Curr Probl Cardiol 2000;25:783. [PMID: 11082789] (Discussion of cardiac auscultation including a historical perspective.)

Edema

Subcutaneous fluid collections appear first in the lower extremities in ambulatory patients or in the sacral region of bedridden individuals. In heart disease, edema results from elevated right atrial pressures. Right heart failure most commonly results from left heart failure, although the right-sided signs may predominate. Other cardiogenic causes of edema include pericardial disease, right-sided valve lesions, and cor pulmonale. Edema may also be due to peripheral venous insufficiency, venous obstruction, nephrotic syndrome, cirrhosis, premenstrual fluid retention, drugs (especially vasodilators such as calcium channel blockers or salt-retaining medications such as nonsteroidal anti-inflammatory agents), or it may be idiopathic.

Brater DR: Diuretic therapy. N Engl J Med 1998;339:387. [PMID: 9691107] (Clinical pharmacology and use in hepatic, renal, and cardiac disorders.)

Rasool A et al: Treatment of edematous disorders with diuretics. Am J Med Sci 2000;319:25. [PMID: 10653442]

■ DIAGNOSTIC TESTING

The **chest x-ray** provides information about heart size, the pulmonary circulation (with characteristic signs suggesting both pulmonary artery or pulmonary venous hypertension), primary pulmonary disease, and aortic abnormalities. The **echocardiogram** provides much more reliable information about chamber size, hypertrophy, pericardial effusions, valvular abnormalities, and congenital abnormalities and has replaced the x-ray for evaluation of cardiac disease. The **electrocardiogram (ECG)** indicates cardiac rhythm, reveals conduction abnormalities, and provides evidence of ventricular hypertrophy, myocardial infarction, or ischemia. Nonspecific ST segment and T wave changes may reflect these processes but are also noted with electrolyte imbalance, drug effects, and many other conditions. Routine x-rays and ECGs are not recommended to screen for heart disease and have a limited role in the follow-up of patients with known heart disease. However, a baseline ECG is helpful in older patients.

NONINVASIVE DIAGNOSTIC TESTING

Noninvasive diagnostic procedures are growing in number and application. However, they are frequently overutilized. The clinician should carefully consider what question is being asked and how the results will alter patient management before ordering these tests. They have limited applicability in screening for asymptomatic disease and should not be substituted for a careful clinical evaluation.

The most versatile and generally informative noninvasive technique is **echocardiography,** which plays a crucial role in the evaluation of patients with most cardiac symptoms and conditions, including congenital, valvular, coronary, and cardiomyopathic heart disease. An overview of echocardiography and its applications is presented below, as is a brief discussion of the evolving role of cardiac MRI. Other specialized noninvasive cardiac testing procedures, such as stress testing, ambulatory electrocardiography, cardiac nuclear medicine tests, and cardiac computed tomography are discussed in conjunction with their major applications.

Echocardiography

M-mode and **two-dimensional echocardiograms** provide measurements of left ventricular size, function, and thickness. Left ventricular segmental wall motion can be assessed, and the size of all four cardiac chambers can be determined. The morphology of the heart valves can be examined. Hypertrophic cardiomyopathy, pericardial effusion, mitral valve prolapse, valvular vegetations, and cardiac tumors may all be diagnosed. **Doppler ultrasound** provides a quantitative estimation of transvalvular gradients and pulmonary artery pressure and qualitative evaluation of valvular regurgitation and intraventricular shunts. **Color Doppler** visually demonstrates patterns and directionality of flow; it has been particularly useful in evaluating congenital heart disease. However, Doppler studies frequently detect *clinically insignificant* valvular regurgitation; care should be taken not to overinterpret those findings.

Transesophageal echocardiography is used to improve the quality of echocardiograms, to derive information about posterior structures (especially the atria and atrioventricular valves) and prosthetic valves, and to monitor patients during surgery. It is superior to surface echocardiography in diagnosing left atrial thrombi, valvular vegetations, and eccentric mitral regurgitant jets (especially with prosthetic valves). The absence of mural thrombi identifies patients in atrial fibrillation at low risk for embolization, thus facilitating early cardioversion. It is also quite sensitive in detecting aortic dissection and severe atherosclerosis of the ascending aorta, which may be the source for transient ischemic attacks or embolic strokes.

Stress echocardiography is used to enhance the information available from ECGs and as an alternative to nuclear medicine procedures. Echocardiograms may be performed during or immediately following exercise. Transient depression of segmental wall motion during or following stress suggests ischemia. Improvement in wall motion during low-dose dobutamine infusions is an indicator of myocardial viability. Dobutamine infusions can also be utilized as a form of stress testing in patients unable to exercise.

ACC/AHA Guidelines for Clinical Applications of Echocardiography. J Am Coll Cardiol 1997;29:862. [PMID: 9091535] (Extensive discussion and recommendations.)

Gottdiener JS: Overview of stress echocardiography: uses, advantages, and limitations. Prog Cardiovasc Dis 2001;43:315. [PMID: 11235847]

Kadish AH et al: ACC/AHA clinical competence statement on electrocardiography and ambulatory electrocardiography: a report of the American College of Cardiology/American Heart Association/American College of Physicians American Society of Internal Medicine Task Force on Clinical Competence (ACC/AHA Committee to Develop a Clinical Competence Statement on Electrocardiography and Ambulatory Electrocardiography). Circulation 2001;104:3169. [PMID: 11738321]

Stewart WJ et al: Echocardiography in emergency medicine: a policy statement by the American Society of Echocardiography and the American College of Cardiology. Task Force on Echocardiography in Emergency Medicine of the American Society of Echocardiography and the Echocardiography and Technology and Practice Executive Committees of the American College of Cardiology. J Am Coll Cardiol 1999;33:586. [PMID: 9973044]

Magnetic Resonance Imaging (MRI)

Cardiac MRI continues to evolve rapidly. Currently available systems provide high-quality and high-resolution images of cardiac and adjacent vascular structures, making this a preferred technique to evaluate many cardiac conditions, including pericardial and congenital abnormalities. MRI also provides excellent images that can be used to quantify cardiac function and structure. With the use of gadolinium contrast agents, MRI has been used to assess myocardial perfusion and viability.

Botnar RM et al: Coronary magnetic resonance angiography. Cardiol Rev 2001;9:77. [PMID: 11209146]

CARDIAC CATHETERIZATION & ANGIOGRAPHY

Although cardiac catheterization and angiography remain the standard tests for assessment of many hemodynamic and anatomic abnormalities of the heart, they have often been supplanted by echocardiography and other imaging modalities for the initial and serial evaluation of many conditions. Nonetheless, "invasive" procedures (ie, those involving the use of intravascular and intracardiac catheters), when appropriately employed, remain invaluable in the management of most patients with congenital, valvular, and coronary heart disease.

Right heart catheterization is convenient to perform in the laboratory, at the bedside, or in the operating room. It allows measurement of right atrial, right ventricular, pulmonary artery and pulmonary capillary wedge pressures (the latter an indicator of left atrial pressure), oxygen saturation, and cardiac output. These data may diagnose intracardiac shunts, physiologically significant pericardial disease, and right-sided valve lesions and can distinguish between cardiac and pulmonary disease. Hemodynamic monitoring may be very helpful in the assessment and treatment of shock, heart failure, complicated myocardial infarction, respiratory failure, and postoperative hemodynamic instability. However, this procedure is not without risk—complications include pneumothorax, bleeding, arrhythmias, pulmonary artery rupture, pulmonary emboli, and infection. Therefore, the role of this procedure remains unsettled, though the available evidence indicates that appropriate use of pulmonary artery catheters to guide therapy may reduce morbidity. Bedside echocardiography can be used to assess left ventricular function, pericardial effusion, valvular abnormalities, intracardiac shunts, and pulmonary artery and central venous pressures when the need for continuous monitoring is not anticipated.

Left heart catheterization is performed to assess the cardiac valves and left ventricular function. Mitral stenosis and aortic stenosis are quantified by measuring the pressure gradients across the valves and, taking flow into account, the estimated valve areas. Mitral and aortic regurgitation are assessed semiquantitatively from contrast injections in the left ventricle and aorta, respectively. The ejection fraction and regional wall motion are assessed by contrast left ventriculograms. The severity of stenotic valve lesions can usually also be measured by echocardiography, though regurgitant lesions may be more difficult to quantify. Left ventricular function can also be assessed by echocardiography and nuclear scintigraphy. Therefore, the main indications for left heart catheterization are for confirmation of the need for valve surgery and for obtaining coronary angiograms. Increasingly, the catheterization laboratory is used for performing coronary interventions.

Bernard GR et al: Pulmonary artery catheterization and clinical outcomes: National Heart, Lung, and Blood Institute and Food and Drug Administration Workshop Report. Consensus Statement. JAMA 2000;283:2568. [PMID: 10815121] (Describes indications and areas that further study is needed.)

Ivanov R et al: The incidence of major morbidity in critically ill patients managed with pulmonary artery catheters: a meta-analysis. Crit Care Med 2000;28:615. [PMID: 10752803] (Meta-analysis of 12 randomized controlled trials shows that there is a significant reduction in morbidity using pulmonary artery catheter-guided strategies.)

Scanlon PJ et al: ACC/AHA guidelines for coronary angiography. A report of the American College of Cardiology/American Heart Association Task Force on practice guidelines (Committee on Coronary Angiography). Developed in collaboration with the Society for Cardiac Angiography and Interventions. J Am Coll Cardiol 1999;33:1756. [PMID: 10334456]

■ CONGENITAL HEART DISEASE

Congenital lesions account for only about 2% of heart disease that present in adulthood. Only the most common acyanotic lesions are discussed here. The review articles cited below provide further discussion of the major congenital conditions that affect adults.

Brickner ME et al: Congenital heart disease in adults. N Engl J Med 2000;342:256 and 334. [PMID: 10648769 and 10655533] (Two-part series covering acyanotic and cyanotic conditions, surgical interventions, and late complications. Excellent diagrams accompany text.)

Corno AF: Surgery for congenital heart disease. Curr Opin Cardiol 2000;15:238. [PMID: 11139086]

Moodie DS: Diagnosis and management of congenital heart disease in the adult. Cardiol Rev 2001;9:276. [PMID: 11520451]

Perloff JK et al: Challenges posed by adults with repaired congenital heart disease. Circulation 2001;103:2637. [PMID: 11382736]

PULMONARY STENOSIS

ESSENTIALS OF DIAGNOSIS

- No symptoms in patients with mild or moderately severe lesions.
- Severe cases may present with right-sided heart failure and cause sudden death.
- High-pitched systolic ejection murmur maximal in the second left interspace. P_2 delayed and soft or absent. Ejection click often present. Increased right ventricular impulse.
- Palpable thrill at second left intercostal space.
- Right ventricular hypertrophy on ECG; pulmonary artery dilation on x-ray. Echo-Doppler diagnostic.

General Considerations

Stenosis of the pulmonary valve or infundibulum increases the resistance to outflow, raises the right ventricular pressure, and limits pulmonary blood flow. In the absence of associated shunts, arterial saturation is normal, but severe stenosis causes peripheral cyanosis by reducing cardiac output. Clubbing and polycythemia do not develop unless a patent foramen ovale or atrial septal defect is present, permitting right-to-left shunting.

Clinical Findings

A. SYMPTOMS AND SIGNS

Mild cases (right ventricular-pulmonary artery gradient < 30 mm Hg) are asymptomatic. Moderate to severe stenosis (gradients 50 to > 80 mm Hg) may cause dyspnea on exertion, syncope, chest pain, and eventually right ventricular failure.

There is a palpable parasternal lift. A loud, harsh systolic murmur and a prominent thrill are present in the left second and third interspaces parasternally; the murmur is in the third and fourth interspaces in infundibular stenosis. The second sound is obscured by the murmur in severe cases; the pulmonary component is diminished, delayed, or absent. Both components are audible in mild cases. A right-sided S_4 and a prominent a wave in the venous pulse are present in severe cases.

B. ELECTROCARDIOGRAPHY AND CHEST X-RAY

Right axis deviation or right ventricular hypertrophy is noted; peaked P waves provide evidence of right atrial overload. Heart size may be normal on radiographs, or there may be a prominent right ventricle and atrium or gross cardiac enlargement, depending upon the severity. There is often poststenotic dilation of the main and left pulmonary arteries. Pulmonary vascularity is normal or diminished.

C. DIAGNOSTIC STUDIES

Echocardiography usually demonstrates the anatomic abnormality and assesses right ventricular size and function. Doppler ultrasound can estimate the gradient accurately; its findings are usually confirmed by cardiac catheterization.

Prognosis & Treatment

Patients with mild pulmonary stenosis may have a normal life span. Moderate stenosis may be asymptomatic in childhood and adolescence, but symptoms may appear as patients grow older. Severe stenosis is associated with sudden death and can cause heart failure in the 20s and 30s.

Symptomatic patients or those with evidence of right ventricular hypertrophy and resting gradients over 75–80 mm Hg require correction in most cases. Percutaneous balloon valvuloplasty has proved successful and is usually the treatment of choice. Surgery can be performed with an operative mortality rate of 2–4% and an excellent long-term result in most cases.

Gibbs JL: Interventional catheterisation. Opening up I: the ventricular outflow tracts and great arteries. Heart 2000;83:111. [PMID: 10618351] (Review of interventional strategies for pulmonary stenosis as well as left-sided lesions.)

COARCTATION OF THE AORTA

ESSENTIALS OF DIAGNOSIS

- Infants may have severe heart failure; children and adults are usually asymptomatic, presenting with hypertension.
- Absent or weak femoral pulses.
- Systolic pressure higher in upper extremities than in lower extremities; diastolic pressures are similar.
- Harsh systolic murmur heard in the back.
- ECG shows left ventricular hypertrophy; chest x-ray shows rib notching; echo-Doppler is diagnostic.

General Considerations

Coarctation of the aorta consists of localized narrowing of the aortic arch just distal to the origin of the left subclavian artery. Collateral circulation develops through the intercostal arteries and the branches of the subclavian arteries. Coarctation is one of the causes of secondary hypertension and should be considered in young patients with elevated blood pressure. A bicuspid aortic valve is also present in 25% of cases.

Clinical Findings

A. SYMPTOMS AND SIGNS

If cardiac failure does not occur in infancy, there are usually no symptoms until the hypertension produces left ventricular failure or cerebral hemorrhage; the latter may also occur from associated cerebral aneurysms. Strong arterial pulsations are seen in the neck and suprasternal notch. Hypertension is present in the arms, but the pressure is normal or low in the legs. This difference is exaggerated by exercise. Femoral pulsations are weak and are delayed in comparison with the brachial pulse. Patients with large collaterals may have relatively small gradients but still have severe coarctation. Late systolic ejection murmurs at the base are often heard better posteriorly, especially over the spinous processes. There may be an associated aortic insufficiency murmur due to a bicuspid aortic valve.

B. ELECTROCARDIOGRAPHY AND CHEST X-RAY

The ECG usually shows left ventricular hypertrophy. Radiography shows scalloping of the ribs due to enlarged collateral intercostal arteries, dilation of the left subclavian artery and poststenotic aortic dilation, and left ventricular enlargement.

C. DIAGNOSTIC STUDIES

Measurement of the gradient across the lesion by catheterization and aortography remain the primary methods of diagnosis. MRI is a useful imaging adjunct, and Doppler ultrasound can also estimate the severity of obstruction.

Prognosis & Treatment

Cardiac failure is common in infancy and in older untreated patients; it is uncommon in late childhood and young adulthood. Most untreated patients with the adult form of coarctation die before age 50 from the complications of hypertension, rupture of the aorta, infective endarteritis, or cerebral hemorrhage (associated in some cases with congenital cerebral aneurysms). Aortic dissection also occurs with increased frequency in coarctation.

Resection of the coarcted site has a surgical mortality rate of 1–4%. The risks of the disease are such, however, that all coarctations in patients up to age 20 years should be resected. In patients under 40 years of age, surgery is advisable if the patient has refractory hypertension or significant left ventricular hypertrophy. The surgical mortality rate rises considerably in patients over age 50, making surgery of doubtful value. Balloon angioplasty of the stenosis has been accomplished successfully and may become the procedure of choice, but aortic tears have been described. About one-fourth of corrected patients continue to be hypertensive years after surgery and they have all the complications associated with hypertension.

Harrison DA et al: Endovascular stents in the management of coarctation of the aorta in the adolescent and adult: one year follow up. Heart 2001;85:561. [PMID: 11303011] (Good results in series of 27 patients.)

Koertschman J et al: Balloon angioplasty of coarctation of the aorta a safe alternative for surgery in adults: immediate and mid-term results. Catheter Cardiovasc Interv 2000;50:28. [PMID: 10816276] (Percutaneous balloon dilation provides excellent results, including substantial reductions in blood pressure.)

ATRIAL SEPTAL DEFECT

ESSENTIALS OF DIAGNOSIS

- *Usually asymptomatic until middle age.*
- *Right ventricular lift; S_2 widely split and fixed*
- *Grade I–III/VI systolic ejection murmur at pulmonary area.*
- *ECG shows right ventricular conduction delay; x-ray shows dilated pulmonary arteries and increased vascularity; echo-Doppler usually diagnostic.*

General Considerations

The most common form of atrial septal defect (80% of cases) is persistence of the ostium secundum in the mid septum; less commonly, the ostium primum (which is low in the septum) persists, in which case mitral or tricuspid abnormalities may also be present. A third form is the sinus venosus defect of the upper part of the septum. This is often associated with partial anomalous drainage of the pulmonary veins into the superior vena cava. In all cases, normally oxygenated blood from the higher pressure left atrium passes into the right atrium, increasing right ventricular output and pulmonary blood flow.

As a result of the prolonged high flow through the pulmonary circulation, some patients develop severe pulmonary hypertension due to irreversible pulmonary vascular disease. This may then lead to Eisenmenger's syndrome, which is characterized by right-to-left shunting and cyanosis.

Clinical Findings

A. SYMPTOMS AND SIGNS

Most patients with small or moderate defects are asymptomatic. With large shunts, exertional dyspnea or cardiac failure may develop, most commonly in the fourth decade or later. Prominent right ventricular and pulmonary artery pulsations are readily visible and palpable. A moderately loud systolic ejection murmur can be heard in the second and third interspaces parasternally as a result of increased pulmonary artery flow. S_2 is widely split and does not vary with breathing.

B. ELECTROCARDIOGRAPHY AND CHEST X-RAY

Right axis deviation or right ventricular hypertrophy may be present in ostium secundum defects. Incomplete or complete right bundle branch block is present in nearly all cases of atrial septal defect, and superior axis deviation is noted in ostium primum defect. With sinus venosus defects, the P axis is leftward of +15 degrees. The chest radiograph shows large pulmonary arteries, increased pulmonary vascularity, an enlarged right atrium and ventricle, and a small aortic knob.

C. DIAGNOSTIC STUDIES

Echocardiography can demonstrate right ventricular volume overload with a large right ventricle and atrium, and sometimes the defect itself. Echocardiography with saline bubble contrast and Doppler flow studies can demonstrate shunting. A transesophageal echo is helpful when transthoracic echo quality is not optimal, and it improves the sensitivity for small shunts and patent foramen ovale. Radionuclide flow studies quantify left-to-right shunting, and MRI can also elucidate the anatomy. Cardiac catheterization remains the definitive diagnostic procedure, since it can demonstrate an increase in oxygen saturation between the venae cavae and right ventricle due to the admixture of oxygenated blood from the left atrium, quantify the shunt, and measure pulmonary vascular resistance. Right and left ventricular contrast angiography may demonstrate associated valvular abnormalities or anomalous pulmonary venous drainage.

Prognosis & Treatment

Patients with small shunts may live a normal life span. Large shunts cause disability by age 40. Raised pulmonary vascular resistance secondary to pulmonary hypertension rarely occurs in childhood or young adult life in secundum defects but is more common in primum defects. After age 40, pulmonary hypertension, cardiac arrhythmias (especially atrial fibrillation), and heart failure may occur in secundum defects. Paradoxic systemic arterial embolization is a concern, especially in patients with pulmonary hypertension or venous thrombosis. A patent foramen ovale is present in 20–30% of adults and is the lesion responsible for most paradoxic emboli. However, the risk for such events is relatively low except in patients with associated atrial septal aneurysms, who require aggressive anticoagulation or closure of the defect. Infective endocarditis does not occur with increased frequency.

Small atrial septal defects do not require surgery. The risks are now sufficiently low so that patients with left-to-right shunts and pulmonary-to-systemic flow ratios between 1.5 and 2.0 may be operated on if the total clinical picture warrants. Ratios exceeding 2.0 are an indication for surgical closure of the defect.

Transcatheter techniques for closing atrial septal defects have been developed. These involve the deployment of an umbrella-like occlusion device from a femoral venous approach. The devices work best in patients with centrally located secundum defects.

Surgery should be withheld from patients with pulmonary hypertension with reversed (right-to-left) shunting (Eisenmenger's syndrome) because of the risk of acute right heart failure. Relocation of pulmonary veins is required in patients with partial anomalous venous drainage. In ostium primum defects, in addition to closure of the defect, suture of the valve clefts—especially those of the mitral valve—is advisable if mitral regurgitation of any significant degree is present. The surgical mortality rate is low (< 1%) in patients under age 45 who are not in cardiac failure and those who have systolic pulmonary artery pressures less than 60 mm Hg. It increases to 5–10% in patients over age 40 with cardiac failure or with systolic pulmonary artery pressures greater than 60 mm Hg.

Attie F et al: Surgical treatment for secundum atrial septal defects in patients > 40 years old. A randomized clinical trial. J Am Coll Cardiol 2001;38:2035. [PMID: 11738312] (Randomized trial showing that surgical closure was superior to medical therapy in preventing major complications. Closure is recommended for patients with a pulmonary:systemic flow ratio ± 1.7 if pulmonary artery systolic pressure is < 70 mm Hg.)

Ebeid MR: Percutaneous catheter closure of secundum atrial septal defects: a review. J Invas Cardiol 2002;14:25. [PMID: 1173692] (Design, delivery, results, and complications of six different devices are reviewed.)

Mas JL et al: Recurrent cerebrovascular events associated with patent foramen ovale, atrial septal aneurysm, or both. N Engl J Med 2001;345:1740. [PMID: 11742048] (Patients with patent foramen ovale or atrial septal aneurysm and prior stroke are at high risk for recurrence and should be treated with aggressive anticoagulation.)

VENTRICULAR SEPTAL DEFECT

ESSENTIALS OF DIAGNOSIS

- *Adults asymptomatic if defect is small to moderate.*
- *Grade II–VI/VI pansystolic murmur maximal at the left sternal border; associated thrill common.*
- *ECG may show left ventricular hypertrophy—or right ventricular hypertrophy if shunt is reversed; x-ray shows increased pulmonary vascularity. Echo-Doppler is diagnostic.*

General Considerations

In this lesion, a persistent opening in the upper interventricular septum resulting from failure of fusion with the aortic septum permits blood to pass from the high-pressure left ventricle into the low-pressure right ventricle. The subsequent natural history and pathophysiology depend on the size of the defect and the magnitude of left-to-right shunting. Large defects are associated with early left ventricular failure. Chronic but more moderate left-to-right shunts may lead to pulmonary vascular disease and right-sided failure. Many ventricular defects close spontaneously in early childhood.

Clinical Findings

A. SYMPTOMS AND SIGNS

The clinical features are dependent upon the size of the defect and the presence or absence of a raised pulmonary vascular resistance. Large shunts are associated with loud, harsh holosystolic murmurs in the left third and fourth interspaces along the sternum and, in some cases, middiastolic flow murmurs and an S_3 at the apex. Smaller shunts may produce only an early systolic murmur or a diamond-shaped murmur. A systolic thrill is common. Clinical evidence of pulmonary hypertension is often more informative than the murmur itself. High defects may be associated with aortic regurgitation owing to prolapse of a valve leaflet.

B. ELECTROCARDIOGRAPHY AND CHEST X-RAY

The ECG may be normal or may show right, left, or biventricular hypertrophy, depending on the size of the defect and the pulmonary vascular resistance. With large shunts, the right or left ventricle (or both), the left atrium, and the pulmonary arteries are enlarged, and pulmonary vascularity is increased on chest radiographs. If pulmonary vascular disease evolves, an enlarged pulmonary artery with diminished distal vascularity is seen.

C. DIAGNOSTIC STUDIES

Echocardiography can demonstrate chamber size and may demonstrate the defect. Doppler ultrasound can qualitatively assess the magnitude of shunting and the pulmonary artery pressure. Magnetic resonance imaging can often visualize the defect, while radionuclide flow studies quantify pulmonary-to-systemic flow ratios. Cardiac catheterization permits definitive diagnosis in all but the most trivial defects; it is the only technique that can measure pulmonary vascular resistance.

Prognosis & Treatment

Patients with the typical murmur as the only abnormality have a normal life expectancy except for the threat of infective endocarditis. Endocarditis is more typical of smaller shunts. Antibiotic prophylaxis is mandatory. With large shunts, congestive heart failure may develop early in life, and survival beyond age 40 is unusual. Shunt reversal occurs in an estimated 25% of patients, producing Eisenmenger's syndrome.

Small shunts (pulmonary to systemic flow ratio < 1.5) in asymptomatic patients do not require surgery. Defects causing large shunts should be repaired to prevent pulmonary hypertension or late heart failure. Once pulmonary hypertension is present (systolic pulmonary arterial pressures > 85 mm Hg), the surgical mortality risk is at least 50%. If right-to-left shunting is present (Eisenmenger's syndrome), surgery is contraindicated. Many defects (up to 40%) close spontaneously. Therefore, surgery should be deferred until late childhood unless there are signs of heart failure or pulmonary hypertension. Surgical mortality rates are low (2–3%). Some defects can be closed percutaneously.

Turner SW et al: The natural history of ventricular septal defects. Arch Dis Child 1999;81:413. [PMID: 10519715]

Vongpatanasin W et al: The Eisenmenger syndrome in adults. Ann Intern Med 1998;128:745. [PMID: 9556469] (Physiology and management.)

PATENT DUCTUS ARTERIOSUS

 ESSENTIALS OF DIAGNOSIS

- Adults with small or moderately large patent ductus are usually asymptomatic at least until middle age.
- Widened pulse pressure; loud S_2.
- Continuous murmur over pulmonary area; thrill common.
- Echo-Doppler is helpful, but the lesion is best visualized by aortography.

General Considerations

The embryonic ductus arteriosus fails to close normally and persists as a shunt connecting the left pulmonary artery and aorta, usually near the origin of the left subclavian artery. Prior to birth, the ductus is kept patent by the effect of circulating prostaglandins; in early infancy, a patent ductus can often be closed by administration of intravenous indomethacin (0.2 mg/kg intravenously). If the defect is not closed, blood flows continuously from the aorta through the ductus into the pulmonary artery in both systole and diastole; the defect is a form of arteriovenous fistula, increasing the work of the left ventricle. If it remains open, obliterative changes in the pulmonary arterioles can cause pulmonary hypertension, with reversal of the direction of shunting. Then the shunt is bidirectional or right-to-left (Eisenmenger's syndrome). This complication does not correlate with shunt size.

Clinical Findings

A. SYMPTOMS AND SIGNS

There are no symptoms unless left ventricular failure or pulmonary hypertension develops. The heart is of normal size or slightly enlarged, with a hyperdynamic apical impulse. The pulse pressure is wide, and diastolic pressure is low. A continuous rough "machinery" murmur, accentuated in late systole at the time of S_2, is heard best in the left first and second interspaces at the left sternal border. Thrills are common.

B. ELECTROCARDIOGRAPHY AND CHEST X-RAY

A normal tracing or left ventricular hypertrophy is found, depending upon the magnitude of shunting. On chest radiographs, the heart is normal in size and contour, or there may be left ventricular and left atrial enlargement. The pulmonary artery, aorta, and left atrium are prominent.

C. DIAGNOSTIC STUDIES

Echocardiography quantifies left ventricular and atrial size. MRI can demonstrate the abnormality, and the magnitude of the shunt can also be determined by radionuclide flow studies. Cardiac catheterization establishes the presence and severity of a left-to-right shunt and whether pulmonary hypertension is present; angiography can define its anatomy.

Prognosis & Treatment

Large shunts cause a high mortality rate from cardiac failure early in life. Smaller shunts are compatible with long survival, congestive heart failure being the most common complication. Infective endocarditis or endarteritis may also occur, and antibiotic prophylaxis is required. A small percentage of patients develop pulmonary hypertension and reversal of shunt (right-to-left shunting), such that the lower legs, especially the toes, appear cyanotic and clubbed in contrast to normally pink fingers. At this stage, the patient is inoperable.

Surgical ligation of the patent ductus can be accomplished with excellent results in uncomplicated patients. Recent experience with transcatheter closure has also been favorable, indicating that where available, this newer option is the procedure of choice for most patients. Closure is recommended for children or adults with symptoms or large shunts. Asymptomatic adults with no left ventricular hypertrophy and small left-to-right shunts are at low risk of developing pulmonary hypertension or congestive heart failure. The indications for closure of a patent ductus arteriosus in the presence of pulmonary hypertension are controversial. Opinion favors closure whenever the pulmonary vascular resistance is low and the flow through the ductus is from left to right.

Bilkis AA et al: The Amplatzer duct occluder: experience in 209 patients. J Am Coll Cardiol 2001;37:258. [PMID: 11153748] (Transcatheter closure is safe and effective.)

■ VALVULAR HEART DISEASE

While most cases of valvular disease in the United States were at one time due to rheumatic heart disease (still true in developing countries), other causes are now more common. The typical findings of each lesion are described in Table 10–1. Table 10–2 shows how to use bedside maneuvers to distinguish murmurs.

Echocardiography yields information about valve morphology, left ventricular mass and function, and atrial and ventricular chamber size. Doppler ultrasound provides quantitative measurements of transvalvular gradients and pulmonary artery pressure and gives more qualitative estimates of valvular regurgitation. The prevalence of mild or even moderate valvular regurgitation is not small, and care must be taken not to overestimate the importance of these findings. Transesophageal echo (TEE) often provides improved image quality. Valve morphology (particularly with prosthetic valves), vegetations, thrombi, and eccentric regurgitant jets are more easily identified with TEE.

The now withdrawn diet medications fenfluramine and dexfenfluramine may be associated with valvular heart disease, but whether these agents cause clinically significant valvular abnormalities remains controversial. Recent data suggest that this is, if anything, a rare occurrence.

Bonow RO et al: Guidelines for the management of patients with valvular heart disease. Circulation 1998;98:1949. [PMID: 9799219] (Task force summary offers extensive recommendations for diagnosis and for medical and surgical management of valve disease.)

Hayek E et al: Current medical management of valvular heart disease. Cleve Clin J Med 2001; 68:881. [PMID: 11596627] (Drug therapy may stabilize but often does not alter or delay the natural history of valve disease or the need for surgery. Drug therapy lowers the risk of endocarditis and rheumatic fever.)

Jollis JG et al: Fenfluramine and phentermine and cardiovascular findings: effect of treatment duration on prevalence of valve abnormalities. Circulation 2000;101:2071. [PMID: 10790349] (This is the largest study to demonstrate a relation between the length of treatment with fenfluramine-phentermine and the prevalence of valvular abnormalities. Regurgitation was associated with treatment periods of more than 6 months and was not severe or accompanied by significant differences in cardiovascular symptoms.)

Prêtre R et al: Cardiac valve surgery in the octogenarian. Heart 2000;83:116. [PMID: 10618352] (As the population ages, surgery for degenerative aortic and mitral valve disease is becoming increasingly common. Results in appropriately selected patients are quite good.)

Shipton B et al: Valvular heart disease: review and update. Am Fam Physician 2001;63:2201. [PMID: 11417772]

MITRAL STENOSIS

ESSENTIALS OF DIAGNOSIS

- *Dyspnea, orthopnea, and paroxysmal nocturnal dyspnea.*
- *Symptoms often precipitated by onset of atrial fibrillation or pregnancy.*
- *Prominent mitral first sound, opening snap (usually), and apical diastolic crescendo rumble.*
- *ECG shows left atrial abnormality and, commonly, atrial fibrillation. Echo-Doppler confirms diagnosis and quantitates severity.*

General Considerations

Nearly all patients with mitral stenosis have underlying rheumatic heart disease, though a history of rheumatic fever is often absent.

Clinical Findings

A. SYMPTOMS AND SIGNS

A characteristic finding of mitral stenosis is a localized middiastolic murmur low in pitch whose duration varies with the severity of the stenosis and the heart rate (Table 10–1). Because it is thickened, the valve opens in early diastole with an opening snap. The sound is sharp, is widely distributed over the chest, and occurs early after A_2 in severe and later in milder varieties of mitral stenosis. In severe mitral stenosis with low flow across the mitral valve, the murmur may be soft and difficult to find, but the opening snap can usually be heard. If the patient has both mitral stenosis and mitral regurgitation, the dominant features may be the systolic murmur of mitral regurgitation with or without a short diastolic murmur and a delayed opening snap.

When the valve has narrowed to less than 1.5 cm^2 (normal, 4–6 cm^2), the left atrial pressure must rise to maintain normal flow across the valve and a normal cardiac output. This results in a pressure difference between the left atrium and left ventricle during diastole. The pressure gradient and the length of the diastolic murmur reflect the severity of mitral stenosis; they persist throughout diastole when the lesion is severe or when the ventricular rate is rapid.

In mild cases, left atrial pressure and cardiac output may be essentially normal and the patient asymptomatic, but in moderate stenosis (valve area < 1.5 cm^2)—

Table 10–1. Differential diagnosis of valvular heart disease.

	Mitral Stenosis	Mitral Regurgitation	Aortic Stenosis	Aortic Regurgitation	Tricuspid Stenosis	Tricuspid Regurgitation
Inspection	Malar flush, precordial bulge, and diffuse pulsation in young patients.	Usually prominent and hyperdynamic apical impulse to left of MCL.	Sustained PMI, prominent atrial filling wave.	Hyperdynamic PMI to left of MCL and down. Visible carotid pulsations.	Giant a wave in jugular pulse with sinus rhythm. Often olive-colored skin (mixed jaundice and local cyanosis).	Large v wave in jugular pulse.
Palpation	"Tapping" sensation over area of expected PMI. Middiastolic or presystolic thrill at apex. Small pulse. Right ventricular pulsation left third to fifth ICS parasternally when pulmonary hypertension is present.	Forceful, brisk PMI; systolic thrill over PMI. Pulse normal, small, or slightly collapsing.	Powerful, heaving PMI to left and slightly below MCL. Systolic thrill over aortic area, sternal notch, or carotids. Small and slowly rising carotid pulse.	Apical impulse forceful and displaced significantly to left and down. Prominent carotid pulses. Rapidly rising and collapsing pulses.	Middiastolic thrill between lower left sternal border and PMI. Presystolic pulsation of liver (sinus rhythm only).	Right ventricular pulsation. Occasionally systolic thrill at lower left sternal edge. Systolic pulsation of liver.
Heart sounds, rhythm, and blood pressure	Loud snapping M_1. Opening snap following S_2 along left sternal border or at apex. Atrial fibrillation common. Blood pressure normal.	M_1 normal or buried in murmur. Prominent third heart sound. Atrial fibrillation common. Blood pressure normal. Midsystolic clicks may be present.	A_2 normal, soft, or absent. Paradoxic splitting of S_2 if A_2 is audible. Prominent S_4. Blood pressure normal, or systolic pressure normal with high diastolic.	S_1 normal or reduced, A_2 loud. Wide pulse pressure with diastolic pressure < 60 mm Hg.	S_1 often loud.	Atrial fibrillation is usually present.
Murmurs						
Location and transmission	Localized at or near apex. Rarely, short diastolic (Graham Steell) murmur along lower left sternal border in severe pulmonary hypertension.	Loudest over PMI; transmitted to left axilla left infrascapular area. With posterior papillary muscle dysfunction, may transmit to base.	Right second ICS parasternally or at apex, heard in carotids and occasionally in upper interscapular area.	Diastolic: louder along left sternal border in third to fourth interspace. Heard over aortic area and apex. May be associated with low-pitched middiastolic murmur at apex (Austin Flint) in nonrheumatic disease.	Third to fifth ICS along left sternal border out to apex.	As for tricuspid stenosis.
Timing	Onset at opening snap ("middiastolic") with presystolic accentuation if in sinus rhythm. Graham Steell begins with P_2 (early diastole).	Pansystolic: begins with M_1 and ends at or after A_2. May be late systolic in papillary muscle dysfunction.	Midsystolic: begins after M_1, ends before A_2, reaches maximum intensity in mid systole.	Begins immediately after aortic second sound and ends before first sound.	As for mitral stenosis.	As for mitral regurgitation.

(continued)

Table 10–1. Differential diagnosis of valvular heart disease. (cont.)

	Mitral Stenosis	Mitral Regurgitation	Aortic Stenosis	Aortic Regurgitation	Tricuspid Stenosis	Tricuspid Regurgitation
Murmurs (cont'd)						
Character	Low-pitched, rumbling; presystolic murmur merges with loud M_1 and ends at or after A_2. May be late systolic in papillary muscle dysfunction.	Blowing, high-pitched; occasionally harsh or musical.	Harsh, rough.	Blowing, often faint.	As for mitral regurgitation.	Blowing, coarse, or musical.
Optimum auscultatory conditions	After exercise, left lateral recumbency. Bell chest piece lightly applied.	After exercise; diaphragm chest piece. In prolapse, findings most prominent while standing.	Patient resting, leaning forward, breath held in full expiration.	Patient leaning forward, breath held in expiration.	Murmur usually louder and at peak during inspiration. Patient recumbent.	Murmur usually becomes louder during inspiration.
X-ray	Straight left heart border. Large left atrium sharply indenting esophagus. Elevation of left main stem bronchus. Large right ventricle and pulmonary artery if pulmonary hypertension is present. Calcification occasionally seen in mitral valve.	Enlarged left ventricle and left atrium.	Concentric left ventricular hypertrophy. Prominent ascending aorta, small knob. Calcified valve common.	Moderate to severe left ventricular enlargement. Prominent aortic knob.	Enlarged right atrium only.	Enlarged right atrium and ventricle.
Electrocardiography	Broad P waves in standard leads; broad negative phase of diphasic P in V_1. If pulmonary hypertension is present, tall peaked P waves, right axis deviation, or right ventricular hypertrophy appears.	Left axis deviation or frank left ventricular hypertrophy. P waves broad, tall, or notched in standard leads. Broad negative phase of diphasic P in V_1.	Left ventricular hypertrophy.	Left ventricular hypertrophy.	Tall, peaked P waves. Normal axis.	Right axis usual.
Echocardiography M mode	Thickened, immobile mitral valve with anterior and posterior leaflets moving together. Slow early diastolic filling slope, left atrial enlargement, normal to small left ventricle.	Thickened mitral valve in rheumatic disease; mitral valve prolapse; flail leaflet or vegetations may be seen. Enlarged left ventricle with above-normal, normal, or decreased function.	Dense persistent echoes from the aortic valve with poor leaflet excursion, left ventricular hypertrophy with preserved contractile function.	Diastolic vibrations of the anterior leaflet of the mitral valve and septum, early closure of the mitral valve when severe, dilated left ventricle with normal or decreased contractility.	Tricuspid valve thickening, decreased early diastolic filling slope of the tricuspid valve. Mitral valve also usually abnormal.	Enlarged right ventricle prolapsing valve, mitral valve often abnormal.

(continued)

324

Echocardiography (cont.)

Two-dimensional	Maximum diastolic orifice size reduced, subvalvular apparatus foreshortened, variable thickening of other valves.	Same as M mode but more reliable.	Above plus poststenotic dilation of the aorta, restricted opening of the aortic leaflets, bicuspid aortic valve in about 30%.	Above plus may show vegetations in endocarditis, bicuspid valve, root dilation.	Above plus enlargement of the right atrium.	Same as above.
Doppler	Prolonged pressure half-time across mitral valve; indirect evidence of pulmonary hypertension.	Regurgitant flow mapped into left atrium; indirect evidence of pulmonary hypertension.	Increased transvalvular flow velocity, yielding calculated gradient. Valve area estimate using continuity equation.	Demonstrates regurgitation and qualitatively estimates severity.	Prolonged pressure half-time across tricuspid valve.	Regurgitant flow mapped into right atrium and venae cavae; right ventricular systolic pressure estimated.

A_2 = Aortic second sound
ICS = Intercostal space
M_1 = Mitral first sound

MCL = Midclavicular line
P_2 = Pulmonary second sound
PMI = Point of maximal impulse

S_2 = Second heart sound
S_4 = Fourth heart sound
V_1 = Chest ECG lead 1

Table 10–2. Effect of various interventions on systolic murmurs.[1]

Intervention	Hypertrophic Obstructive Cardiomyopathy	Aortic Stenosis	Mitral Regurgitation	Mitral Prolapse
Valsalva	↑	↓	↓ or ↔	↑ or ↓
Standing	↑	↑ or ↔	↓ or ↔	↑
Handgrip or squatting	↓	↓ or ↔	↑	↓
Supine position with legs elevated	↓	↑ or ↔	↔	↓
Exercise	↑	↑ or ↔	↓	↑
Amyl nitrite	↑↑	↑	↓	↑
Isoproterenol	↑↑	↑	↓	↑

Key: ↑ = increased; ↑↑ = markedly increased; ↓ = decreased; ↔ = unchanged
[1]Modified from Paraskos JA: Combined valvular disease. In: *Valvular Heart Disease*. Dalen JE, Alpert JS (editors). Little, Brown, 1987.

especially with tachycardia, which shortens diastole and increases mitral flow rate—dyspnea and fatigue appear as the left atrial pressure rises. With severe stenosis, the left atrial pressure is high enough to produce pulmonary venous congestion at rest and reduce cardiac output, with resulting dyspnea, fatigue, and right heart failure. Recumbency at night further increases the pulmonary blood volume, causing orthopnea and paroxysmal nocturnal dyspnea. Severe pulmonary congestion may also be initiated by any acute respiratory infection, excessive salt and fluid intake, endocarditis, or recurrence of rheumatic carditis. As a result of long-standing pulmonary venous hypertension, anastomoses develop between the pulmonary and bronchial veins in the form of bronchial submucosal varices. These often rupture, producing mild or severe hemoptysis. In a few patients, the pulmonary arterioles become narrowed; this greatly increases the pulmonary artery pressure and accelerates the development of right ventricular hypertrophy and failure. These patients have relatively little dyspnea but experience fatigue on exertion.

Fifty to 80 percent of patients develop paroxysmal or chronic atrial fibrillation that, until the ventricular rate is controlled, may precipitate dyspnea or pulmonary edema.

B. DIAGNOSTIC STUDIES

Echocardiography is the most valuable technique for assessing mitral stenosis. The valve is thickened, opens poorly, and closes slowly. The anterior and posterior leaflets are fixed and move together, rather than in opposite directions. Left atrial size can be determined by echocardiography: increased size denotes an increased likelihood of atrial fibrillation or systemic emboli. The mitral valve area can be measured, and the gradient and pulmonary artery pressure can be estimated by Doppler techniques. Echocardiography also detects

atrial myxoma, which sometimes presents clinically in a fashion resembling mitral stenosis.

Because echocardiography and careful symptom evaluation provide most of the needed information, cardiac catheterization is employed primarily to detect associated valve, coronary, or myocardial disease—usually after the decision to intervene has been made.

Treatment & Prognosis

Mitral stenosis may be present for a lifetime with few or no symptoms, or it may become severe in a few years. In most cases, there is a long asymptomatic phase, followed by subtle limitation of activity. Pregnancy and its associated increase in cardiac output and the transmitral pressure gradient often precipitates symptoms. The onset of atrial fibrillation often precipitates more severe symptoms, which usually improve with control of the ventricular rate or restoration of sinus rhythm. Conversion to and subsequent maintenance of sinus rhythm is most commonly successful when the duration of atrial fibrillation is brief (< 6–12 months) and the left atrium is not severely dilated (diameter < 4.5 cm). Once atrial fibrillation occurs, the patient should receive warfarin anticoagulation therapy even if sinus rhythm is restored, since atrial fibrillation often recurs even with antiarrhythmic therapy and 20–30% of these patients will have systemic embolization if untreated. Systemic embolization in the presence of only mild to moderate disease is not an indication for surgery but should be treated with warfarin anticoagulation.

Indications for relieving the stenosis include the following: (1) uncontrollable pulmonary edema; (2) limiting dyspnea and intermittent pulmonary edema; (3) evidence of pulmonary hypertension with right ventricular hypertrophy or hemoptysis; (4) limitation of activity despite ventricular rate control and medical therapy; and (5) recurrent systemic emboli despite anticoagulation with moderate or severe stenosis.

Open mitral commissurotomy may be effective in patients without substantial mitral regurgitation. Replacement of the valve is indicated when combined stenosis and insufficiency are present or when the mitral valve is so distorted and calcified that a satisfactory valvulotomy is not possible. Operative mortality rates are low: 1–3% in most institutions. Balloon valvuloplasty is effective in patients without accompanying regurgitation. Initial success rates are high, especially if valve calcification is not excessive. The rate of restenosis is lower than that with aortic stenosis. As a result, this option appears to be a suitable alternative to surgery for many patients in experienced centers.

Problems associated with prosthetic valves are thrombosis (especially at the mitral position), paravalvular leak, endocarditis, and degenerative changes in tissue valves. Warfarin anticoagulant therapy is mandatory with mechanical prostheses and is usually employed for at least the initial 3 months with bioprostheses, especially if the patient has significant left atrial enlargement. If atrial fibrillation persists postoperatively, ongoing anticoagulation is required.

Bruce CJ et al: Newer advances in the diagnosis and treatment of mitral stenosis. Curr Probl Cardiol 1998;23:130. [PMID: 9568404] (Etiology, pathophysiology, and clinical examination are discussed. Diagnostic challenges using echo or invasive techniques are covered. Treatment algorithms include balloon valvotomy and surgical intervention.)

Vahanian A: Balloon valvuloplasty. Heart 2001;85:223. [PMID: 11156680]

MITRAL REGURGITATION
(Mitral Insufficiency)

ESSENTIALS OF DIAGNOSIS

- *Variable causes determine clinical presentation.*
- *May be asymptomatic for many years (or for life) or may cause left-sided heart failure.*
- *Pansystolic murmur at the apex, radiating into the axilla; associated with S_3.*
- *ECG shows left atrial abnormality or atrial fibrillation and left ventricular hypertrophy; x-ray shows left atrial and ventricular enlargement. Echo-Doppler confirms diagnosis and estimates severity.*

General Considerations

Mitral regurgitation may result from many processes. Rheumatic disease is associated with a thickened valve with reduced mobility and often a mixed picture of stenosis and regurgitation. In developed countries, more common causes of mitral regurgitation include myxomatous degeneration (eg, **mitral valve prolapse** with or without connective tissue diseases such as Marfan's syndrome), infective endocarditis, and subvalvular dysfunction (due to papillary muscle dysfunction or ruptured chordae tendineae). Cardiac tumors, chiefly left atrial myxoma, are a rare cause of mitral regurgitation.

Clinical Findings

A. SYMPTOMS AND SIGNS

During left ventricular systole, the mitral leaflets do not close normally, and blood is ejected into the left atrium as well as through the aortic valve. The net effect is an increased volume load on the left ventricle, and the presentation depends on the rapidity with which the lesion develops. In acute regurgitation, left atrial pressure rises abruptly, leading to pulmonary edema if severe. When it is chronic, the left atrium enlarges progressively, but the pressure in pulmonary veins and capillaries rises only transiently during exertion. Exertional dyspnea and fatigue progress gradually over many years.

Mitral regurgitation leads to left atrial enlargement and may cause subsequent atrial fibrillation. Systemic embolization is relatively unusual compared with other conditions causing atrial fibrillation. Mitral regurgitation may predispose to infective endocarditis.

Clinically, mitral regurgitation is characterized by a pansystolic murmur maximal at the apex, radiating to the axilla and occasionally to the base; a hyperdynamic left ventricular impulse and a brisk carotid upstroke; and a prominent third heart sound. Left atrial enlargement is usually considerable in chronic mitral regurgitation; the degree of left ventricular enlargement usually reflects the severity of regurgitation. Calcification of the mitral valve is less common than in pure mitral stenosis. Hemodynamically, left ventricular volume overload may ultimately lead to left ventricular failure and reduced cardiac output, but for many years the left ventricular end-diastolic pressure and the cardiac output may be normal at rest, even with considerable increase in left ventricular volume.

Nonrheumatic mitral regurgitation may develop abruptly, such as with papillary muscle dysfunction following myocardial infarction, valve perforation in infective endocarditis, or ruptured chordae tendineae in mitral valve prolapse. In acute mitral regurgitation, patients are in sinus rhythm rather than atrial fibrillation, have little or no enlargement of the left atrium, no calcification of the mitral valve, no associated mitral stenosis, and in many cases little left ventricular dilation.

Myxomatous mitral valve ("floppy" or "billowing" mitral valve, or mitral valve prolapse) is usually asymptomatic but may be associated with nonspecific chest pain, dyspnea, fatigue, or palpitations. Most patients are female, many are thin, and some have minor chest wall deformities. There are characteristic midsystolic clicks, which may be multiple, often but not always followed by a late systolic murmur. These findings are accentuated in the standing position. The diagnosis is primarily clinical but can be confirmed echocardiographically. Its significance is in dispute because of the frequency with which it is diagnosed in healthy young women (up to 10%), but in occasional patients this lesion is not benign. Patients who have only a midsystolic click usually have no sequelae, but patients with a late or pansystolic murmur may develop significant mitral regurgitation, often due to rupture of chordae tendineae. The need for valve replacement is commonest in men and increases with aging, so that approximately 2% of patients with clinically significant regurgitation over age 60 will require surgery. Infective endocarditis may occur, chiefly in patients with murmurs; such patients should have antibiotic prophylaxis prior to dental work and surgical procedures. β-Adrenergic blocking agents are often effective for supraventricular arrhythmias. Sudden death is rare in mitral prolapse, but when symptomatic ventricular tachycardia is present, aggressive management with an implantable cardioverter-defibrillator is usually indicated. An association between mitral prolapse and embolic cerebrovascular events has also been reported but not confirmed in subsequent studies. Echocardiographic evidence of marked thickening or redundancy of the valve is associated with a higher incidence of most complications.

Papillary muscle dysfunction or infarction following acute myocardial infarction is less common. When mitral regurgitation is due to papillary dysfunction, it may subside as the infarction heals or left ventricular dilation diminishes. If severe regurgitation persists, these patients have a poor prognosis with or without surgery. Transient—but sometimes severe—mitral regurgitation may occur during episodes of myocardial ischemia. Patients with dilated cardiomyopathies of any origin may have **secondary mitral regurgitation** due to papillary muscle dysfunction or dilation of the mitral annulus. In these, mitral valve replacement has been considered contraindicated because of the poor risk:benefit ratio and deterioration of left ventricular function postoperatively. However, several groups have reported good results with mitral valve repair in patients with left ventricular ejection fractions greater than 30% and secondary mitral insufficiency.

B. DIAGNOSTIC STUDIES

Echocardiography is useful in demonstrating the underlying pathologic process (rheumatic, prolapse, flail leaflet), and Doppler techniques provide qualitative and semiquantitative estimates of the severity of mitral regurgitation. It should be noted that Doppler also detects clinically insignificant regurgitation in many normal individuals, and this finding must be interpreted in the context of the clinical presentation. The accompanying information concerning left ventricular size and function, left atrial size, pulmonary artery pressure, and right ventricular function can be invaluable in planning treatment as well as in recognizing associated lesions. Transesophageal echocardiography may reveal the cause of regurgitation and identify candidates for valvular repair. Nuclear medicine techniques as well as MRI permit measurement of left ventricular function and estimation of the severity of regurgitation.

Cardiac catheterization provides accurate assessment of regurgitation and, additionally, of left ventricular function and pulmonary artery pressure. Coronary angiography is often indicated to determine the presence of coronary artery disease prior to valve surgery.

Treatment & Prognosis

Acute mitral regurgitation due to endocarditis, myocardial infarction, and ruptured chordae tendineae often requires emergency surgery. Some patients can be stabilized with vasodilators or intra-aortic balloon counterpulsation, which reduce the amount of regurgitant flow by lowering systemic vascular resistance. Patients with chronic lesions may remain asymptomatic for many years. Operation is usually necessary when patients develop symptoms. However, because progressive and irreversible deterioration of left ventricular function may occur prior to the onset of symptoms, early operation is indicated even in asymptomatic patients with a declining ejection fraction (< 55–60%) or marked left ventricular dilation (end-systolic dimension > 4.5–5 cm on echocardiography).

There has been growing success with valve repair in nonrheumatic lesions, which avoids the complications of prosthetic valves described earlier. In addition, left ventricular function is better preserved when the subvalvular structures can be maintained intact by valve repair. Selected patients with poor left ventricular function and severe mitral regurgitation may benefit from this intervention. Mitral valve surgery is increasingly being performed using the appreciably less invasive thoracoscopic approach.

Jacobs W et al: Mitral valve prolapse: a review of the literature. Am J Med Sci 2001;321:401. [PMID: 11419477]

Otto CM: Clinical practice. Evaluation and management of chronic mitral regurgitation. N Engl J Med 2001;345:740. [PMID: 11547744] (Review discussing workup as well as timing of interventions, with an algorithmic approach.)

AORTIC STENOSIS

ESSENTIALS OF DIAGNOSIS

- *In adults, usually asymptomatic until middle or old age.*
- *Delayed and diminished carotid pulses.*

- *Soft, absent, or paradoxically split S₂.*
- *Harsh systolic murmur, sometimes with thrill along left sternal border, often radiating to the neck; may be louder at apex in older patients.*
- *ECG usually shows left ventricular hypertrophy; calcified valve on x-ray or fluoroscopy; echo-Doppler is diagnostic in most cases.*

General Considerations

Aortic valvular stenosis may follow rheumatic fever but is more commonly caused by progressive valvular calcification. This may occur in younger patients with a congenitally bicuspid valve or in elderly individuals with normal three-cusp valves. In the latter group, the aortic valve becomes sclerotic and, with further calcification, stenotic. Approximately 25% of patients over age 65 and 35% of those over age 70 have echocardiographic evidence of sclerosis, which appears to be related to atherosclerotic vascular disease and is associated with a higher rate of vascular events. About 10–20% of these will progress to hemodynamically significant aortic stenosis over a period of 10–15 years. Thus, aortic stenosis has become the most common surgical valve lesion in developed countries. Degenerative valve disease is three to four times more frequent in men than in women and is more common in smokers and hypertensives. Valvular stenosis must be distinguished from supravalvular obstruction and from outflow obstruction of the left ventricular infundibulum, both relatively rare.

Clinical Findings

A. Symptoms and Signs

Slightly narrowed, thickened, or roughened valves (aortic sclerosis) or aortic dilation may produce the typical murmur and thrill without causing significant hemodynamic effects. In mild or moderate cases, the characteristic signs are a systolic ejection murmur at the aortic area transmitted to the neck and apex; in severe cases, a palpable left ventricular heave or thrill, a weak to absent aortic second sound, or reversed splitting of the second sound are present (see Table 10–1). When the valve area is less than 0.8–1 cm² (normal, 3–4 cm²), ventricular systole becomes prolonged and the typical carotid pulse pattern of delayed upstroke and low amplitude is present, but this may be an unreliable finding in older patients with extensive arteriosclerotic vascular disease. Left ventricular hypertrophy increases progressively, with resulting elevations in ventricular end-diastolic pressure. (Cardiac output is maintained until the stenosis is severe (with a valve area < 0.8 cm²). Patients may present with left ventricular failure, angina pectoris, or syncope.

Symptoms of failure may be sudden in onset or may progress gradually. Angina pectoris frequently oc-

curs in aortic stenosis. One-half of patients with calcific aortic stenosis and angina have significant associated coronary artery disease, whereas coronary disease is noted at only half this rate in the absence of angina. Syncope is typically exertional and may be due to arrhythmias (usually ventricular tachycardia but sometimes sinus bradycardia), hypotension, or decreased cerebral perfusion resulting from increased blood flow to exercising muscle without compensatory increase in cardiac output. Sudden death may occur but is rarely the initial manifestation of aortic stenosis in previously asymptomatic patients.

B. Diagnostic Studies

The clinical assessment of aortic stenosis may be difficult, especially in older patients. The ECG reveals left ventricular hypertrophy or suggestive repolarization changes in most patients but may be normal in up to 10%. The chest radiograph may show a normal or enlarged cardiac silhouette, calcification of the aortic valve, and dilation and calcification of the ascending aorta. The echocardiogram provides useful data about aortic valve calcification and opening and left ventricular thickness and function, while Doppler can estimate the aortic valve gradient. These data can reliably exclude or diagnose severe stenosis. In patients with moderate obstruction, especially with low cardiac output or concomitant regurgitation, these evaluations may be inaccurate.

Cardiac catheterization is the definitive diagnostic procedure. The valve gradient is measured and the valve area calculated; a valve area below 0.8 cm² indicates severe stenosis. Aortic regurgitation can be quantified by aortic root angiography. Coronary arteriography should be performed in most adults with aortic stenosis to assess for concomitant coronary disease.

Prognosis & Treatment

Following the onset of heart failure, angina, or syncope, the prognosis without surgery is poor (50% 3-year mortality rate). Medical treatment may stabilize patients in heart failure, but surgery is indicated for all symptomatic patients, including those with left ventricular dysfunction, which often improves postoperatively. Valve replacement is usually not indicated in asymptomatic individuals. Exceptions are those with declining left ventricular function, very severe left ventricular hypertrophy, and very high gradients (> 80 mm Hg) or severely reduced valve areas (≤ 0.7 cm²).

The surgical mortality rate for valve replacement is 2–5%, but it rises to 10% above the age of 75. Mortality rates are substantially higher when left ventricular function is depressed or when severe coronary disease and prior myocardial infarctions are present. Severe coronary lesions are usually bypassed at the same time. Anticoagulation with warfarin is required for mechanical prostheses but is not essential with bioprostheses. Although bioprosthetic valves have hitherto undergone degenerative changes and required replacement within 7–10 years (sometimes within 3 years), newer ones may be more durable. Some centers have begun performing the Ross procedure, which entails switching the patient's pulmonary valve to the aortic position and placing a bioprosthesis in the pulmonary position. Because bioprostheses do not deteriorate as fast on the right side of the heart, this procedure has produced excellent long-term results without anticoagulation.

Although percutaneous balloon valvuloplasty can produce short-term reductions in the severity of aortic stenosis, restenosis occurs rapidly in most adults who have calcified valves. Except in adolescents, balloon valvuloplasty should be reserved for individuals who are poor candidates for surgery or as an intermediate procedure to stabilize high-risk patients prior to surgery.

Aikawa K et al: Timing of surgery in aortic stenosis. Prog Cardiovasc Dis 2001;43:477. [PMID: 11431802]

Palta S et al: New insights into the progression of aortic stenosis: implications for secondary prevention. Circulation 2000;101:2497. [PMID: 10831524] (Identifies risk factors for faster progression of aortic stenosis such as initial valve area, hypercholesterolemia, smoking, and serum calcium.)

Rosenhek R et al: Predictors of outcome in severe, asymptomatic aortic stenosis. N Engl J Med 2000;343:611. [PMID: 10965007] (In asymptomatic patients with aortic stenosis, it appears to be relatively safe to delay surgery until symptoms develop. However, outcomes vary widely. The presence of moderate to severe valvular calcification—together with a rapid increase in aortic jet velocity—identifies patients with a very poor prognosis who may benefit from early surgery.)

AORTIC REGURGITATION
(Aortic Insufficiency)

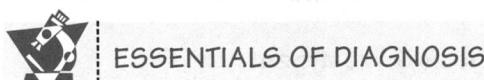

ESSENTIALS OF DIAGNOSIS

(Chronic Regurgitation)

- *Usually asymptomatic until middle age; presents with left-sided failure or chest pain.*
- *Wide pulse pressure with associated peripheral signs.*
- *Hyperactive, enlarged left ventricle.*
- *Diastolic murmur along left sternal border.*
- *ECG shows left ventricular hypertrophy; x-ray shows left ventricular dilation. Echo-Doppler confirms diagnosis and estimates severity.*

General Considerations

Rheumatic aortic regurgitation has become less common than in the preantibiotic era, but nonrheumatic causes are frequent and are the major cause of isolated aortic regurgitation. These include congenitally bicuspid valves, infective endocarditis, and hypertension. Many patients have aortic regurgitation secondary to aortic root diseases such as cystic medial necrosis, Marfan's syndrome, aortic dissection, ankylosing spondylitis, Reiter's syndrome, and syphilis.

Clinical Findings

A. SYMPTOMS AND SIGNS

The clinical presentation is determined by the rapidity with which regurgitation develops. In chronic regurgitation, the only sign for many years may be a soft aortic diastolic murmur. As the valve deformity increases, larger amounts regurgitate, diastolic blood pressure falls, and the left ventricle progressively enlarges. Most patients remain asymptomatic even at this point, and an often prolonged plateau phase, characterized by stable left ventricular dilation, occurs. Left ventricular failure is a late event and may be sudden in onset. Exertional dyspnea and fatigue are the most frequent symptoms, but paroxysmal nocturnal dyspnea and pulmonary edema may also occur. Angina pectoris or atypical chest pain may be present. Associated coronary artery disease and syncope are less common than in aortic stenosis.

Hemodynamically, because of compensatory left ventricular dilation, patients eject a large stroke volume which is adequate to maintain forward cardiac output until late in the course of the disease. Left ventricular diastolic pressure remains normal also but may abruptly rise when heart failure occurs. Abnormal left ventricular systolic function, as manifested by reduced ejection fraction and increasing end-systolic left ventricular volume, is a late sign.

The major physical findings relate to the wide arterial pulse pressure. The pulse has a rapid rise and fall (water-hammer pulse or Corrigan's pulse), with an elevated systolic and low diastolic pressure, owing to the large stroke volume and rapid diastolic runoff back into the left ventricle, respectively. The large stroke volume is also responsible for characteristic findings such as Quincke's pulses (subungual capillary pulsations), Duroziez's sign (diastolic murmur over a partially compressed peripheral artery, commonly the femoral), and Musset's sign (head bob with each pulse). The apical impulse is prominent, laterally displaced, and usually hyperdynamic and may be sustained. The murmur itself may be quite soft and localized; the aortic diastolic murmur is high-pitched and decrescendo. A mid or late diastolic low-pitched mitral murmur (Austin Flint murmur) may be heard in advanced aortic regurgitation, owing to obstruction of mitral flow produced by partial closure of the mitral valve by the regurgitant jet.

When aortic regurgitation develops acutely (as in aortic dissection or infective endocarditis), left ventricular failure, manifested primarily as pulmonary edema, may develop rapidly, and surgery is urgently required. Patients with acute aortic regurgitation do not have the dilated left ventricle of chronic aortic regurgitation. In the same way, the diastolic murmur is shorter and may be minimal in intensity, and the pulse pressure may not be widened, making clinical diagnosis difficult.

B. DIAGNOSTIC STUDIES

The ECG usually shows moderate to severe left ventricular hypertrophy. Radiographs show cardiomegaly with left ventricular prominence.

Echocardiography can demonstrate whether the lesion involves the aortic root or if valvular disease is present. Serial assessments of left ventricular size and function are critical in determining the timing for valve replacement. Doppler techniques can qualitatively estimate the severity of regurgitation, though it should be noted that "mild" regurgitation is not uncommon and should not be overinterpreted. Scintigraphic studies can quantify left ventricular function and functional reserve during exercise a useful predictor of prognosis.

Cardiac catheterization can help quantify severity and is used to evaluate the coronary and aortic root anatomy preoperatively.

Treatment & Prognosis

Aortic regurgitation that appears or worsens during or after an episode of infective endocarditis or aortic dissection may lead to acute severe left ventricular failure or subacute progression over weeks or months. The former usually presents as pulmonary edema; surgical replacement of the valve is indicated even during active infection. These patients may be transiently improved or stabilized by vasodilators.

Chronic regurgitation has a long natural history, but the prognosis without surgery becomes poor when symptoms occur. Vasodilators, such as hydralazine, nifedipine, and angiotensin-converting enzyme inhibitors, can reduce the severity of regurgitation, and prophylactic treatment may postpone or avoid surgery in asymptomatic patients with severe regurgitation and dilated left ventricles. Beta-blocker therapy may slow the rate of aortic dilation in Marfan's syndrome. Surgery is usually indicated once aortic regurgitation causes symptoms. Surgery is also indicated for those with few or no symptoms who present with significant left ventricular dysfunction (ejection fraction < 45–50%) or who exhibit progressive deterioration of left ventricular function, irrespective of symptoms. Although the operative mortality rate is higher when left ventricular function is severely impaired, valve replacement or repair is still indicated, since left ventricular function often improves somewhat and the long-term prognosis is thereby enhanced.

The operative mortality rate is usually in the 3–5% range. Aortic regurgitation due to aortic root disease requires repair or replacement of the root, a more difficult operation. Following surgery, left ventricular size usually decreases and left ventricular function improves, except where dysfunction has been present chronically.

Carabello BA: Progress in mitral and aortic regurgitation. Prog Cardiovasc Dis 2001;43:457. [PMID: 11431801] (Discussion of pathophysiology as well as treatment options.)

Dujardin KS et al: Mortality and morbidity of aortic regurgitation in clinical practice: a long term follow-up study. Circulation 1999;99:1851. [PMID: 10199882] (Patients with low ejection fractions, dilated ventricles, or heart failure symptoms should undergo valve replacement surgery.)

Underwood MJ et al: The aortic root: structure, function, and surgical reconstruction. Heart 2000;83:376. [PMID: 10722531] (Reviews anatomy and surgical issues of aortic root abnormalities that are responsible for a growing proportion of aortic regurgitation cases.)

TRICUSPID STENOSIS

Tricuspid stenosis is usually rheumatic in origin. It should be suspected when "right heart failure" appears in the course of mitral valve disease, marked by hepatomegaly, ascites, and dependent edema. It may also occur in carcinoid syndrome. The typical diastolic rumble along the lower left sternal border mimics mitral stenosis. In sinus rhythm, a presystolic liver pulsation may be found.

Hemodynamically, a diastolic pressure gradient of 5–15 mm Hg is found across the tricuspid valve in conjunction with raised pressure in the right atrium and jugular veins, with prominent a waves and with a slow y descent because of slow right ventricular filling.

Echocardiography usually demonstrates the lesion, and Doppler flow studies can measure the gradient; accompanying valve lesions can also be detected. Right heart catheterization is diagnostic.

Acquired tricuspid stenosis may be amenable to valvotomy under direct vision, but it usually requires a prosthetic valve replacement. Although experience is limited, balloon valvuloplasty may be the initial procedure of choice in many patients.

TRICUSPID REGURGITATION

Tricuspid regurgitation may occur in a variety of situations other than disease of the tricuspid valve itself. The most common is right ventricular overload resulting from left ventricular failure due to any cause. Tricuspid regurgitation occurs in association with right ventricular and inferior myocardial infarction. Tricuspid valve endocarditis and resulting regurgitation are common in intravenous drug users. Other causes include the carcinoid syndrome, lupus erythematosus, and myxomatous degeneration of the valve (associated with mitral valve prolapse). Ebstein's anomaly, a congenital defect of the tricuspid valve, often presents in adults as massive right-sided cardiomegaly due to tricuspid regurgitation.

The symptoms and signs of tricuspid regurgitation are identical to those resulting from right ventricular failure due to any cause. In the presence of mitral valve disease, the tricuspid valvular lesion can be suspected on the basis of early onset of right heart failure and a harsh systolic murmur along the lower left sternal border which is separate from the mitral murmur and which often increases in intensity during and just after inspiration.

Hemodynamically, tricuspid regurgitation is characterized by a prominent regurgitant systolic (v) wave in the right atrium and jugular venous pulse, with a rapid y descent and a small or absent x descent. The regurgitant wave, like the systolic murmur, is increased with inspiration, and its size depends upon the size of the right atrium. In tricuspid regurgitation, especially with right ventricular failure, an inspiratory S_3 may be present.

Tricuspid regurgitation secondary to severe mitral valve disease or other left-sided lesions may regress when the underlying disease is corrected. When surgery is required, valve repair or valvuloplasty of the tricuspid ring is often preferable to valve replacement. Replacement of the tricuspid valve is infrequently done now.

Singh JP et al: Prevalence and clinical determinants of mitral, tricuspid, and aortic regurgitation. Am J Cardiol 1999;83:897. [PMID: 10190406] (Up to 20% of patients undergoing routine echo examination had some valve regurgitation, with age being the most common clinical predictor.)

CHOICE & MANAGEMENT OF PROSTHETIC VALVES

Valve repair may be useful for tricuspid, mitral, and occasionally aortic regurgitation. Likewise, percutaneous or open valvulotomy may be indicated in mitral, pulmonary, and tricuspid stenosis. Nonetheless, the number of valve replacement procedures continues to increase as a result of the aging of the population. The choice of a mechanical device versus a bioprosthesis is often a difficult one, balancing the risk of chronic anticoagulation and thromboembolism (mechanical) versus the need for eventual reoperation (bioprosthesis). In general, otherwise healthy patients below age 65 should receive mechanical valves unless anticoagulation is contraindicated, because their life expectancy is greater than the durability of tissue prostheses. Furthermore, deterioration of bioprostheses is accelerated in younger patients. In patients with a small left ventricular cavity or aortic annulus, mechanical disk valves have significant hemodynamic advantages. Finally, patients who will require anticoagulation in any case, such as those in atrial fibrillation, should receive mechanical valves. Bioprostheses are preferable in older patients with life expectancies less than 10 years and when anticoagulation is contraindicated. However, hemodialysis patients should not receive tissue valves because they have a high failure rate. As noted previously, the Ross procedure offers another option in younger patients with aortic stenosis.

The identification of valve dysfunction may be difficult, but Doppler echocardiography, especially via the transesophageal approach, can identify regurgita-

tion and stenosis in most cases. In patients with mechanical valves, careful anticoagulation is required with a target INR of 3.0–4.0. Anticoagulation should rarely be discontinued. For elective surgery, oral warfarin can be stopped 2–3 days preoperatively with heparin coverage until effective anticoagulation is resumed. Management of anticoagulation during pregnancy is difficult, since warfarin may be teratogenic in the first trimester and should be discontinued in advance of delivery. Some experts recommend substitution with low-molecular-weight heparin in the first trimester. In one controlled study, aspirin, 100 mg daily, in addition to warfarin, reduced emboli and the mortality rate.

Salem DN et al: Antithrombotic therapy in valvular heart disease. Chest 2001;119:207S. [PMID: 11157650]

Sapirstein JS et al: The "ideal" replacement heart valve. Am Heart J 2001;141:856. [PMID: 11320378] (Discussion of current replacement valves as well as ideal characteristics for a designer valve.)

■ CORONARY HEART DISEASE (Arteriosclerotic Coronary Artery Disease; Ischemic Heart Disease)

Coronary atherosclerotic heart disease is the commonest cause of cardiovascular disability and death in the USA. Men are more often affected than women by an overall ratio of 4:1, but before age 40 the ratio is 8:1, and beyond age 70 it is 1:1. In men, the peak incidence of clinical manifestations is at age 50–60; in women, at age 60–70.

Risk Factors for Coronary Heart Disease

Epidemiologic studies have identified a number of important risk factors for premature coronary heart disease. These include a positive family history (particularly when onset is before age 50), age, male gender, blood lipid abnormalities, diabetes mellitus, hypertension, physical inactivity, cigarette smoking, elevated blood homocysteine levels, markers of inflammation such as C-reactive protein and hyperfibrinogenemia, and hypoestrogenemia in women. Interventions to lessen some of these risk factors, such as lipid abnormalities, hypertension, and smoking, reduce the risk for subsequent coronary events. However, the benefits of intervening for other risk factors, including estrogen replacement and reducing homocysteine levels, are less clear.

Overwhelming evidence indicates that abnormalities of lipid metabolism play a direct role in the pathophysiology of this condition. Risk increases progressively with higher levels of LDL cholesterol and declines with higher levels of HDL cholesterol. Therefore, the ratio of LDL to HDL cholesterol provides a composite marker of risk, with ratios below 3 indicating a lower risk and ratios above 5 indicating a higher risk. Patients with clinical manifestations of coronary disease before age 50 often have predisposing risk factors, though many do not. These risk factors are less closely linked to the onset of coronary disease in later years.

It is now apparent that other abnormalities of lipid metabolism may also play a role in the pathogenesis of coronary artery disease, and these should be sought in individuals with otherwise unexplained premature coronary atherosclerosis. Among the patterns associated with increased atherosclerosis are elevated levels of apolipoprotein(a) and of small, dense LDL lipoprotein particles. These lipoproteins and their accompanying lipids appear more likely to pass into the vessel wall and may be more difficult to clear. Accumulating evidence suggests that hypertriglyceridemia is an independent risk factor for coronary artery disease as well. Elevated triglyceride levels often occur in association with other lipid abnormalities, including low levels of HDL cholesterol and elevated concentrations of lipoprotein(a) and small, dense LDL particles. Some experts advocate the use of non-HDL cholesterol, which accounts for several atherogenic lipids, as the preferred risk indicator.

Elevated levels of serum homocysteine and nonspecific markers of inflammation such as C-reactive protein, fibrinogen, and ferritin correlate with the occurrence of coronary disease. Although hyperhomocysteinemia may increase the risk of thrombosis, it may also simply be a marker of inflammatory activity in coronary disease (see below).

Pathophysiology

Knowledge concerning the pathophysiology of atherosclerosis and the clinical presentations of coronary artery disease is accumulating rapidly. Abnormal lipid metabolism or excessive intake of cholesterol and saturated fats—especially when superimposed on a genetic predisposition—initiates the atherosclerotic process. The initial step is the "fatty streak," or subendothelial accumulation of lipids and lipid-laden monocytes (macrophages). Low-density lipoproteins (LDLs) are the major atherogenic lipid. High-density lipoproteins (HDLs), in contrast, are protective and probably assist in the mobilization of LDLs. The pathogenetic role of other lipids, including triglycerides, is less clear. LDLs undergo in situ oxidation, which makes them more difficult to mobilize as well as locally cytotoxic.

Macrophages migrate into the subendothelial space and take up lipids, giving them the appearance of "foam" cells. As the plaque progresses, smooth muscle cells also migrate into the lesion. At this stage, the lesion may be hemodynamically insignificant, but endothelial function is abnormal and its ability to limit the entry of lipoproteins into the vessel wall is impaired. If the plaque remains stable, a fibrous cap forms, the lesion becomes calcified, and the vessel lumen slowly becomes narrowed.

Although many atherosclerotic plaques remain stable or progress only gradually, others may rupture, with a resulting extrusion of lipids and tissue factors that result in a cascade of events culminating in intravascular thrombosis. The outcome of these events is determined by whether the vessel becomes occluded or whether thrombolysis occurs, either spontaneously or as the result of treatment, and whether the plaque subsequently becomes stabilized. The result may be partial or complete vessel occlusion (causing the symptoms of unstable angina or myocardial infarction), or the plaque may become restabilized, often with more severe stenosis.

Several features are associated with enhanced plaque vulnerability, including a higher lipid content, a higher concentration of macrophages, and a very thin fibrous cap. Lesions with these characteristics are often the culprit lesions in young individuals, in whom acute myocardial infarction or sudden death is the first manifestation of coronary disease; and this abrupt progression explains why most infarctions do not occur at the site of preexisting critical stenosis. Conversely, the relatively greater reduction in clinical events than in lesion severity in lipid-lowering treatment trials is probably explained by the regression or prevention of these early nonfibrotic lesions.

Recent observations have resurrected an old theory that atherosclerosis progresses as the result of an inflammatory response in the vessel wall, perhaps initiated or worsened by an infectious agent. A high circulating level of C-reactive protein, a nonspecific inflammatory marker, is associated with a higher rate of ischemic events. Agents as diverse as *Chlamydia pneumoniae*, cytomegalovirus, and *Helicobacter pylori* have been indirectly implicated. However, two recently presented randomized trials indicate no benefit from azithromycin, an agent effective for chlamydia.

Christen WG et al: Blood levels of homocysteine and increased risks of cardiovascular disease. Causal or casual. Arch Intern Med 2000;160:422. [PMID: 10695683] (Presents a strong case that homocysteine is elevated nonspecifically as an acute phase reactant.)

Kullo IJ et al: Novel risk factors for atherosclerosis. Mayo Clin Proc 2000;75:369. [PMID: 10761492] (Focus on homocysteine, infection, inflammation, and lipoprotein subparticles with discussion of clinical relevance.)

Libby P: Current concepts of the pathogenesis of the acute coronary syndromes. Circulation 2001;104:365. [PMID: 11457759] (Reviews the role of inflammation, plaque stabilization, and thrombosis in acute coronary syndromes.)

Muhlestein JB: Chronic infection and coronary artery disease. Med Clin North Am 2000;84:123. [PMID: 10685131] (Discusses the role of chronic infection in the pathogenesis of atherosclerosis.)

Ridker PM et al: Novel risk factors for systemic atherosclerosis. JAMA 2001;285:2481. [PMID: 11368701] (Of 11 biomarkers evaluated, the ratio of total cholesterol to HDL and the C-reactive protein were the best predictors of peripheral arterial disease.)

Tsang TSM et al: Risks of coronary heart disease in women: current understanding and evolving concepts. Mayo Clin Proc 2000;75:1289. [PMID: 11126839] (Focus on modifiable risk factors includes estrogen status, homocysteine, and chronic infection or inflammation.)

Wood D: Established and emerging cardiovascular risk factors. Am Heart J 2001;141:S49. [PMID: 11174359] (Reviews risk factors and potential management strategies.)

Primary & Secondary Prevention of Ischemic Heart Disease

Although many risk factors for coronary artery disease are not modifiable, it is now clear that interventions such as smoking cessation, treatment of dyslipidemia, and lowering of blood pressure can both prevent coronary disease and delay its progression and complications after it is manifest. Treatment of lipid abnormalities delays the progression of atherosclerosis and in some cases produces regression. Even in the absence of regression, fewer new lesions develop, endothelial function may be restored, and coronary event rates are markedly reduced in patients with clinical evidence of atherosclerosis.

A series of clinical trials has demonstrated the efficacy of lowering LDL cholesterol with HMG-CoA reductase inhibitors (statins) in preventing death, coronary events, and strokes. Beneficial results have been found in patients who have already experienced coronary events (secondary prevention), in those at particularly high risk for events (diabetics and patients with peripheral artery disease), and those with elevated LDL cholesterol without multiple risk factors. Benefits occurred regardless of age, race, or the presence of hypertension. Therefore, aggressive lipid-lowering therapy should be implemented in all patients with dyslipidemia and coronary artery, cerebrovascular, or peripheral vascular disease. Furthermore, there is now clear evidence that reduction of LDL cholesterol can prevent coronary events and stroke in patients without clinically manifest atherosclerosis (primary prevention) and LDL levels as low as 130 mg/dL. The recently reported Heart Protection Study demonstrated more than 20% reductions in vascular events in patients with prior myocardial infarction, stroke, peripheral vascular disease, or diabetes with total cholesterol levels as low as 135 mg/dL, a substantial number of whom had LDL cholesterol levels under 100 mg/dL. This result suggests that all patients at significant risk for vascular events should receive a statin regardless of their cholesterol level—and, by implication, that these agents may work by additional mechanisms that are unrelated to lipid lowering.

Treatment of abnormally low HDL levels or elevations of lipoprotein(a) and small, dense LDL particles is more difficult, but oral niacin in high dosages (2–3 g/d or more) may be effective. A trial in postinfarction patients has demonstrated that an increase in HDL levels with gemfibrozil (600 mg twice daily) in patients with relatively low LDL levels prolongs reinfarction-free survival. The value of reducing elevated triglyceride levels is less clear, but since elevated triglycerides are often associated with other lipid abnormalities, treatment of high-risk patients with niacin, gemfibrozil, or fenofibrate for levels above 400 mg/dL is appropriate.

Since LDL oxidation appears to play a role in the atherogenicity of lipid molecules that have passed into the vessel wall, antioxidant therapy has been advocated as a preventive measure. Thus far, however, there are few data to support this popular concept, and many large, well-controlled studies have failed to demonstrate a benefit with vitamin E therapy. Indeed, there have been no positive prospective trials with any antioxidant agent. Antioxidant therapy may hinder the effectiveness of niacin and statin therapy.

Elevated plasma homocysteine levels are associated with an increased risk of vascular events. Although homocysteine levels can be reduced with dietary supplements of folic acid (1 mg/d) in combination with vitamin B_6 and vitamin B_{12}, it is not clear that this reduces clinical events in individuals with coronary artery disease.

Antiplatelet therapy is another very effective preventive measure. Aspirin (325 mg every other day) in males over the age of 50 reduces the incidence of myocardial infarction. Whether this approach should be employed in the general population or only in those at higher risk is unclear, and the optimal dosage is not known. A prudent approach would be to administer 81–325 mg daily to men with multiple coronary risk factors or concomitant diabetes starting at age 45–50 if no contraindication is present. The same approach is probably warranted for women, commencing 5–10 years later. The previously mentioned GISSI Prevention Trial found a significant mortality reduction with omega-3 fatty acid administration (1 g daily)—which has an antiplatelet effect—in postinfarction patients.

The effect of hormone replacement therapy in postmenopausal women is uncertain. Although observational data suggest that estrogen replacement protects against the development of coronary artery disease, prospective controlled trials have not confirmed a benefit. The HERS trial, a prospective evaluation of estrogen use in women with coronary artery disease, showed no benefit in reducing mortality or preventing subsequent cardiac events. An analysis from the Women's Health Initiative also suggested a possible early increase in coronary events with estrogen replacement, but this and other trials are ongoing, and this issue should be considered unresolved.

Control of blood pressure has now been shown to prevent infarctions in older patients. Although unproved, it seems likely that control of blood pressure in younger individuals also prevents subsequent coronary events. The role of exercise remains controversial. Although individuals who exercise for at least 30 minutes a week are at lower risk for subsequent coronary events, it is difficult to be certain that this outcome relates specifically to exercise rather than a generally healthy lifestyle.

The Heart Outcomes Prevention Evaluation (HOPE) trial demonstrated that the ACE inhibitor ramipril reduces fatal and nonfatal vascular events (cardiovascular deaths, nonfatal myocardial infarctions, and nonfatal strokes) by 20–25% in patients at high risk, including diabetics with additional risk factors or patients with clinical coronary, cerebral, or peripheral arterial atherosclerotic disease. Thus, the role of ACE inhibitors in secondary prevention appears to be expanding beyond patients with heart failure or left ventricular systolic dysfunction.

The decrease in number of coronary deaths over the last 2 decades may be due to a decrease in the prevalence of risk factors but probably also reflects improvements in medical therapy, the role of coronary care units, better treatment of angina, arrhythmias, and heart failure, and improved survival after coronary revascularization in some patient subsets.

Ades PA: Cardiac rehabilitation and secondary prevention of coronary heart disease. N Engl J Med 2001;345:892. [PMID: 11565523] (Addresses issues related to cardiac rehabilitation, including indications and level of activity for different disease states.)

Awtry EH et al: Aspirin. Circulation 2000;101:1206. [PMID: 10715270] (Pharmacology, toxicity, and utility in both primary and secondary prevention are discussed, and other antiplatelet agents are compared.)

Brown BG et al: Simvastatin and niacin, antioxidant vitamins, or the combination for the prevention of coronary disease. N Engl J Med 2001;345:1583. [PMID: 11757504] (Combination of statin and niacin reduced cardiac events in patients with coronary artery disease and low HDL levels. Antioxidants attenuated the beneficial rise in HDL.)

Collaborative meta-analysis of randomised trials of antiplatelet therapy for prevention of death, myocardial infarction, and stroke in high-risk patients. BMJ 2002;324:71. [PMID: 11786451]

Dagenais GR et al: Effects of ramipril on coronary events in high-risk persons: results of the Heart Outcomes Prevention Evaluation Study. Circulation 2001;104:522. [PMID: 11479247] (Secondary outcomes from the HOPE trial, which demonstrated better outcomes in high-risk patients treated with ramipril.)

Executive Summary of The Third Report of The National Cholesterol Education Program (NCEP) Expert Panel on Detection, Evaluation, And Treatment of High Blood Cholesterol In Adults (Adult Treatment Panel III). JAMA 2001 285:2486. [PMID: 11368702]

Grodstein F et al: Postmenopausal hormone use and secondary prevention of coronary events in the Nurses' Health Study. Ann Intern Med 2001;135:1. [PMID: 11434726] (Recurrent coronary events were more frequent with short term hormone replacement but less frequent with long-term use.)

JAMA patient page: Cholesterol. JAMA 1999;281:206. [PMID: 9917126]

Mosca L et al: Hormone replacement therapy and cardiovascular disease. Circulation 2001;104:499. [PMID: 11468217] (Discourages use for secondary prevention whereas primary prevention trials are still ongoing.)

Pruthi S et al: Vitamin E supplementation in the prevention of coronary heart disease. Mayo Clin Proc 2001;76:1131. [PMID: 11702901] (Three trials with over 25,000 patients failed to demonstrate benefit of vitamin E in preventing coronary heart disease.)

Ridker PM et al: Measurement of C-reactive protein for the targeting of statin therapy in the primary prevention of acute coronary events. N Engl J Med 2001;344:1959. [PMID: 11430324] (Treatment with a statin benefited patients with elevated C-reactive protein levels who had a normal ratio of total cholesterol to HDL cholesterol.)

Rubins HB et al: Gemfibrozil for the secondary prevention of coronary heart disease in men with low levels of high-density lipoprotein cholesterol. Veterans Affairs High-Density Lipoprotein Cholesterol Intervention Trial Study Group. N Engl J Med 1999;341:410. [PMID: 10438259] (Therapy with gemfibrozil reduced the risk of cardiovascular events in patients with low HDL and normal LDL.)

Skegg DC: Hormone therapy and heart disease after the menopause. Lancet 2001;358:1196. [PMID: 11675050]

van den Hoogen PC et al: The relation between blood pressure and mortality due to coronary heart disease among men in different parts of the world. Seven Countries Study Research Group. N Engl J Med 2000;342:1. [PMID: 10620642] (Relative increases in blood pressure resulted in increased risk of cardiovascular events in different parts of the world, but the same absolute blood pressures resulted in different risks in the various countries.)

Yusuf S et al: Effects of an angiotensin-converting enzyme inhibitor, ramipril, on cardiovascular events in high-risk patients. The Heart Outcomes Prevention Evaluation Study Investigators. N Engl J Med 2000;342:145. [PMID: 10639539] (In a placebo-controlled randomized trial, ramipril reduced the risk of death, myocardial infarction, and stroke in patients aged 55 or older with known vascular disease or diabetes plus one other vascular risk factor. Of note is the accompanying article by the same HOPE investigators showing that vitamin E supplementation had no effect on cardiovascular events in the same population.)

Pathophysiology of Myocardial Ischemia & Acute Coronary Syndromes

Advanced coronary atherosclerosis and even complete occlusion may remain clinically silent. There is only a modest correlation between the clinical symptoms and the anatomic extent of disease. At present, the only means of determining the location and extent of narrowing is coronary arteriography, although ischemia can be recognized by other less invasive studies. Myocardial ischemia may be provoked by either increased myocardial oxygen requirements (exercise, mental stress, or spontaneous fluctuations in heart rate and blood pressure) or by decreased oxygen supply (caused by coronary vasospasm, platelet plugging, or partial thrombosis). Abnormal endothelial function appears to play a role in the fluctuating threshold for ischemia; impaired release of nitric oxide (endothelium-derived relaxing factor) may permit unopposed vasoconstriction and facilitate platelet adhesion.

In angina pectoris, increased oxygen demand is the most frequent mechanism. In contrast, the acute coronary syndromes of unstable angina and myocardial infarction are caused by plaque disruption, platelet plugging, and coronary thrombosis. Of interest is the predilection for these episodes to occur in the early morning or shortly after arising. The outcome of this series of events is determined by whether the vessel becomes occluded or whether thrombolysis occurs, either spontaneously or as a result of treatment, and whether the plaque subsequently becomes stabilized. Thus, therapy is primarily directed toward inhibition of platelet activity (aspirin, clopidogrel, IIb/IIIa receptor antagonists), antithrombotic agents (the heparins), and thrombolysis in acute syndromes and toward minimizing myocardial oxygen requirements—as well as preventive measures—in chronic angina.

Some episodes of myocardial ischemia are painful, causing angina pectoris; others are completely silent. Many silent episodes are brought on by emotional and mental stress. In patients with diagnosed coronary disease, as evidenced by prior myocardial infarction or angina, silent ischemic episodes have the same prognostic import as painful ones. The prognosis for patients with only silent ischemia is not well established, nor is the potential benefit of preventing silent ischemia.

Rauch U et al: Thrombus formation on atherosclerotic plaques: Pathogenesis and clinical consequences. Ann Intern Med 2001;134:224. [PMID: 11177336] (Comprehensive review of pathophysiology of thrombus formation in atherosclerosis and focus on antithrombotic and antiplatelet treatments.)

Myocardial Hibernation & Stunning

Areas of myocardium that are persistently underperfused but still viable may develop sustained contractile dysfunction. This phenomenon, which is termed myocardial hibernation, appears to represent an adaptive response but may lead to left ventricular failure. It is important to recognize this phenomenon, since this form of dysfunction is reversible following coronary revascularization. Hibernating myocardium can be identified by radionuclide testing, positron emission tomography, contrast-enhanced MRI, or its retained response to inotropic stimulation with dobutamine. A related phenomenon, termed myocardial stunning, is the occurrence of persistent contractile dysfunction following prolonged or repetitive episodes of myocardial ischemia.

Wijns W et al: Hibernating myocardium. N Engl J Med 1998; 339:173. [PMID: 0664095] (Mechanisms, diagnosis, and management.)

ANGINA PECTORIS

ESSENTIALS OF DIAGNOSIS

- *Precordial chest pain, usually precipitated by stress or exertion, relieved rapidly by rest or nitrates.*

- *Electrocardiographic or scintigraphic evidence of ischemia during pain or stress testing.*

- *Angiographic demonstration of significant obstruction of major coronary vessels.*

General Considerations

Angina pectoris is usually due to atherosclerotic heart disease. Coronary vasospasm may occur at the site of a lesion or, less frequently, in apparently normal vessels. Other unusual causes of coronary artery obstruction such as congenital anomalies, emboli, arteritis, or dissection may cause ischemia or infarction. Angina may also occur in the absence of coronary artery obstruction as a result of severe myocardial hypertrophy, severe aortic stenosis or regurgitation, or in response to increased metabolic demands, as in hyperthyroidism, marked anemia, or paroxysmal tachycardias with rapid ventricular rates. Rarely, angina occurs with angiographically normal coronary arteries and without other identifiable causes. This presentation has been labeled syndrome X and is most likely due to inadequate flow reserve in the resistance vessels (microvasculature). Although treatment is often not very successful in relieving symptoms, the prognosis of syndrome X is good.

Clinical Findings

A. HISTORY

The diagnosis of angina pectoris depends principally upon the history, which should specifically include the following information.

1. Circumstances that precipitate and relieve angina—Angina occurs most commonly during activity and is relieved by resting. Exertion that involves straining the thoracic or upper extremity muscles (eg, lifting) or walking rapidly uphill precipitates attacks most consistently. Patients prefer to remain upright rather than lie down. The amount of activity required to produce angina may be relatively consistent under comparable physical and emotional circumstances or may vary from day to day. It is usually less after meals, during excitement, or on exposure to cold. The threshold for angina is often lower in the morning or after strong emotion; the latter can provoke attacks in the absence of exertion. In addition, discomfort may occur during sexual activity, at rest, or at night as a result of coronary spasm.

2. Characteristics of the discomfort—Patients often do not refer to angina as "pain" but as a sensation of tightness, squeezing, burning, pressing, choking, aching, bursting, "gas," indigestion, or an ill-characterized discomfort. It is often characterized by clenching a fist over the mid chest. The distress of angina is rarely sharply localized and is not spasmodic.

3. Location and radiation—The distribution of the distress may vary widely in different patients but is usually the same for each patient unless unstable angina or myocardial infarction supervenes. In 80–90% of cases, the discomfort is felt behind or slightly to the left of the mid sternum. When it begins farther to the left or, uncommonly, on the right, it characteristically moves centrally substernally. Although angina may radiate to any dermatome from C8 to T4, it radiates most often to the left shoulder and upper arm, frequently moving down the inner volar aspect of the arm to the elbow, forearm, wrist, or fourth and fifth fingers. Radiation to the right shoulder and distally is less common, but the characteristics are the same. Occasionally, angina may be felt initially in the lower jaw, the back of the neck, the interscapular area, high in the left back, or in the volar aspect of the wrist. If the patient identifies the site of pain by pointing to the area of the apical impulse with one finger, angina is unlikely.

4. Duration of attacks—Angina is of short duration and subsides completely without residual discomfort. If the attack is precipitated by exertion and the patient promptly stops to rest, it usually lasts less than 3 minutes. Attacks following a heavy meal or brought on by anger often last 15–20 minutes. Attacks lasting more than 30 minutes are unusual and suggest the development of unstable angina, myocardial infarction, or an alternative diagnosis.

5. Effect of nitroglycerin—The diagnosis of angina pectoris is strongly supported if sublingual nitroglycerin invariably shortens an attack and if prophylactic nitrates permit greater exertion or prevent angina entirely.

6. Risk factors—The presence of risk factors described previously makes the diagnosis of angina more likely, but their absence does not exclude angina since most patients do not have a risk profile markedly different from that of the general population.

B. SIGNS

Examination during a spontaneous or induced attack frequently reveals a significant elevation in systolic and diastolic blood pressure, although hypotension may also occur. Occasionally, a gallop rhythm and an apical systolic murmur due to transient mitral regurgitation from papillary muscle dysfunction are present during pain only. Supraventricular or ventricular arrhythmias may be present, either as the precipitating factor or as a result of ischemia.

It is important to detect signs of diseases that may contribute to or accompany atherosclerotic heart disease, eg, diabetes mellitus (retinopathy or neuropathy), xanthelasma, tendinous xanthomas, hypertension, thyrotoxicosis, myxedema, or peripheral vascular disease. Aortic stenosis or regurgitation, hypertrophic

cardiomyopathy, and mitral valve prolapse should be sought, since they may produce angina or other forms of chest pain.

Differential Diagnosis

Angina can usually be diagnosed from a proper history. When atypical features are present—such as prolonged duration (hours or days); or darting, knifelike pains at the apex or over the precordium—ischemia is less likely.

Anterior chest wall syndrome is characterized by sharply localized tenderness of intercostal muscles. Inflammation of the chondrocostal junctions, which may be warm, swollen, and red, may result in diffuse chest pain that is also reproduced by local pressure (Tietze's syndrome). Intercostal neuritis (due to herpes zoster, diabetes mellitus, etc) also mimics angina.

Cervical or thoracic spine disease involving the dorsal roots produces sudden sharp, severe chest pain suggesting angina in location and "radiation" but related to specific movements of the neck or spine, recumbency, and straining or lifting. Pain due to cervical or thoracic disk disease involves the outer or dorsal aspect of the arm and the thumb and index fingers rather than the ring and little fingers.

Peptic ulcer, chronic cholecystitis, esophageal spasm, and functional gastrointestinal disease may produce pain suggestive of angina pectoris. Reflux esophagitis is characterized by lower chest and upper abdominal pain after heavy meals, occurring in recumbency or upon bending over. The pain is relieved by antacids, sucralfate, H_2 receptor antagonists or proton pump inhibitors. The picture may be especially confusing because ischemic pain may also be associated with upper gastrointestinal symptoms, and esophageal motility disorders may be improved by nitrates and calcium channel blockers. Assessment of esophageal motility may be necessary.

Degenerative and inflammatory lesions of the left shoulder and thoracic outlet syndromes may cause chest pain due to nerve irritation or muscular compression; the symptoms are usually precipitated by movement of the arm and shoulder and are associated with paresthesias.

Spontaneous pneumothorax may cause chest pain as well as dyspnea and may create confusion with angina as well as myocardial infarction. Even the ECG may resemble infarction because of changes in voltage from the pneumothorax. The same is true of pneumonia and pulmonary embolization. Dissection of the thoracic aorta can cause severe chest pain that is commonly felt in the back; it is sudden in onset, reaches maximum intensity immediately, and may be associated with changes in pulses. Other cardiac disorders such as mitral valve prolapse, hypertrophic cardiomyopathy, myocarditis, pericarditis, aortic valve disease, or right ventricular hypertrophy may cause atypical chest pain or even myocardial ischemia. Noninvasive testing and, in many cases, cardiac catheterization may be required to establish the diagnosis.

Evaluation of Patients With Angina Pectoris

A. LABORATORY FINDINGS

Serum lipid levels should be determined in all patients with suspected angina. Anemia and diabetes may also be investigated if clinically appropriate.

B. ELECTROCARDIOGRAPHY

The resting ECG is normal in about a quarter of patients with angina. In the remainder, abnormalities include old myocardial infarction, nonspecific ST–T changes, atrioventricular or intraventricular conduction defects, and changes of left ventricular hypertrophy. During anginal episodes, the characteristic electrocardiographic change is horizontal or downsloping ST segment depression that reverses after the ischemia disappears. T wave flattening or inversion may also occur. Less frequently, ST segment elevation is observed; this finding suggests severe (transmural) ischemia and often occurs with coronary spasm.

C. EXERCISE ELECTROCARDIOGRAPHY

Exercise testing is the most useful noninvasive procedure for evaluating the patient with angina. Ischemia that is not present at rest is detected by precipitation of typical chest pain or ST segment depression (or, rarely, elevation). Exercise testing is often combined with scintigraphic studies or echocardiography (see below), but in patients without baseline ST segment abnormalities or in whom anatomic localization is not necessary, the exercise ECG should be the initial procedure because of considerations of cost and convenience.

Exercise testing can be done on a motorized treadmill or with a bicycle ergometer. A variety of exercise protocols are utilized, the most common being the Bruce protocol, which increases the treadmill speed and elevation every 3 minutes until limited by symptoms. At least two electrocardiographic leads should be monitored continuously.

1. Precautions and risks—The usually quoted risk of exercise testing is one infarction or death per 1000 tests, but individuals who continue to have pain at rest or minimal activity are at higher risk and should not be tested. Many of the traditional exclusions, such as recent myocardial infarction or congestive heart failure, are no longer employed *if the patient is stable and ambulatory,* but aortic stenosis remains a contraindication. While most tests are carried to a symptom-limited end point (except submaximal testing early postinfarction), the test should be terminated when hypotension, significant ventricular or supraventricular arrhythmias, more than mild to moderate angina, or more than 3- to 4-mm ST segment depression occurs.

2. Indications—Exercise testing is employed (1) to confirm the diagnosis of angina; (2) to determine the severity of limitation of activity due to angina; (3) to assess prognosis in patients with known coronary disease, including those recovering from myocardial infarction, by detecting groups at high or low risk; (4) to evaluate responses to therapy; and (5) less successfully, to screen asymptomatic populations for silent coronary disease. The latter application is controversial. Because false-positive tests often exceed true positives, leading to much patient anxiety and self-imposed or mandated disability, exercise testing of asymptomatic individuals should be done only for those at high risk (usually a strong family history of premature coronary disease or hyperlipidemia), those whose occupations place them or others at special risk (eg, airline pilots), and older individuals commencing strenuous activity.

3. Interpretation—The usual electrocardiographic criterion for a positive test is 1 mm (0.1 mV) horizontal or downsloping ST segment depression (beyond baseline) measured 80 ms after the J point. By this criterion, 60–80% of patients with anatomically significant coronary disease will have a positive test, but 10–30% of those without significant disease will also be positive. False-positives are uncommon when a 2-mm depression is present. Additional information is inferred from the time of onset and duration of the electrocardiographic changes, their magnitude and configuration, blood pressure and heart rate changes, the duration of exercise, and the presence of associated symptoms. In general, patients exhibiting more severe ST segment depression (> 2 mm) at low workloads (< 6 minutes on the Bruce protocol) or heart rates (< 70% of age-predicted maximum)—especially when the duration of exercise and rise in blood pressure are limited or when hypotension occurs during the test— have more severe disease and a poorer prognosis. Depending on symptom status, age, and other factors, such patients should be referred for coronary arteriography and possible revascularization. On the other hand, less impressive positive tests in asymptomatic patients are often "false-positives." Therefore, exercise testing results that do not conform to the clinical picture should be confirmed by stress scintigraphy or echocardiography.

D. SCINTIGRAPHIC ASSESSMENT OF ISCHEMIA

Two nuclear medicine studies provide additional information about the presence, location, and extent of coronary artery disease.

1. Myocardial perfusion scintigraphy—This test provides images in which radionuclide uptake is proportionate to blood flow at the time of injection. Thallium-201, technetium-99m sestamibi, and tetrafosmin are most frequently used. Areas of diminished uptake reflect relative hypoperfusion (compared to other myocardial regions). If the radiotracer is injected during exercise or dipyridamole- or adenosine-induced coronary vasodilation, scintigraphic defects indicate a zone of hypoperfusion that may represent either ischemia or scar. If the myocardium is viable, as relative blood flow equalizes over time or during a scintigram performed under resting conditions, these defects tend to "fill in" or reverse, indicating reversible ischemia. Defects observed when the radiotracer is injected at rest or still present 3–4 hours after an injection during exercise or pharmacologic vasodilation (intravenous adenosine or dipyridamole) usually indicate myocardial infarction (old or recent) but may be present with severe ischemia. Occasionally, other conditions, including infiltrative diseases (sarcoidosis, amyloidosis), left bundle branch block, and dilated cardiomyopathy, may produce resting or persistent perfusion defects.

In experienced laboratories, stress perfusion scintigraphy is positive in 75–90% of patients with anatomically significant coronary disease and in 20–30% of those without it. False-positive tests may occur as a result of diaphragmatic attenuation or, in women, attenuation through breast tissue. Tomographic imaging (SPECT) can reduce the severity of artifacts. Gated imaging allows for analysis of ventricular size, ejection fraction, and regional wall motion.

Myocardial scintigraphy is indicated (1) when the resting ECG makes an exercise ECG difficult to interpret (LBBB, baseline ST–T changes, low voltage, etc); (2) for confirmation of the results of the exercise ECG when they are contrary to the clinical impression (eg, a positive test in an asymptomatic patient); (3) to localize the region of ischemia; (4) to distinguish ischemic from infarcted myocardium; (5) to assess the completeness of vascularization following bypass surgery or coronary angioplasty; or (6) as a prognostic indicator in patients with known coronary disease.

2. Radionuclide angiography—This procedure images the left ventricle and measures its ejection fraction and wall motion. In coronary disease, resting abnormalities usually represent infarction, and those that occur only with exercise usually indicate stress-induced ischemia. Normal subjects usually exhibit an increase in ejection fraction with exercise or no change; patients with coronary disease may exhibit a decrease. Exercise radionuclide angiography has approximately the same sensitivity as thallium-201 scintigraphy, but it is less specific in older individuals and those with other forms of heart disease. The indications are similar to those for thallium-201 scintigraphy.

3. Positron emission tomography (PET)—PET utilizes positron emitting agents to demonstrate either perfusion or metabolism of myocardium. PET can accurately distinguish transiently dysfunctional ("stunned") myocardium from scar by showing persistent glycolytic metabolism with the tracer fluorodeoxyglucose (FDG) in regions with reduced blood flow. A nearby cyclotron is required to produce this tracer, but the newer SPECT camera can provide acceptable images without the more expensive PET technology.

E. ECHOCARDIOGRAPHY

Echocardiography can image the left ventricle and reveal segmental wall motion abnormalities, which may indicate ischemia or prior infarction. It is a convenient technique for assessing left ventricular function, which is an important indicator of prognosis and determinant of therapy. Echocardiograms performed during supine exercise or immediately following upright exercise may demonstrate exercise-induced segmental wall motion abnormalities as an indicator of ischemia. This technique requires considerable expertise; however, in experienced laboratories, the test accuracy is comparable to that obtained with scintigraphy—though a higher proportion of tests are technically inadequate. Pharmacologic stress with high-dose (20–40 μg/kg/ min) dobutamine can be used as an alternative to exercise. Echo contrast agents allow for perfusion imaging and may improve the diagnostic accuracy of this form of testing.

F. NEWER IMAGING MODALITIES

Many new imaging techniques have been developed, but their application in cardiovascular disease remains to be determined. **Computed tomography (CT scan)** can image the heart and, with contrast medium, the vascular system, but the relatively slow speed of most instruments limits its utility. The main application of CT is the evaluation of pericardial disease. **Ultrafast or electron beam CT (EBCT)** involves a specially designed instrument with high temporal resolution. Its availability is limited, but it provides excellent assessments of cardiac structure and function. EBCT is increasingly being used to detect and quantify coronary artery calcification, but proper application of this highly sensitive test is uncertain. False-negative studies may occur in patients under 50 years of age, and positive studies in older patients do not necessarily provide a quantitative assessment of the severity of coronary arteriosclerosis. Thus, although this test can stratify patients into lower and higher risk groups, the appropriate management of individual patients with asymptomatic coronary artery calcification—beyond aggressive risk factors modification—is unclear.

Cardiac magnetic resonance imaging (MRI) is an evolving modality that provides high-resolution images of the heart and great vessels without radiation exposure or use of iodinated contrast media. It provides excellent anatomic definition, permitting assessment of pericardial disease, neoplastic disease of the heart, myocardial thickness, chamber size, and many congenital heart defects. It is the best noninvasive test for nonemergently evaluating dissection of the aorta. Rapid acquisition sequences can produce excellent cine-mode images demonstrating left ventricular function and wall motion, and it is thus a useful alternative when the echocardiogram is suboptimal. Recent advances have been made in imaging the proximal coronary arteries and assessing myocardial perfusion with paramagnetic contrast agents, but these applications remain investigational.

G. Ambulatory Electrocardiographic Monitoring

With current ambulatory electrocardiographic recorders and with trained technicians, episodes of ischemic ST segment depression can be monitored. In patients with coronary artery disease, these episodes usually signify ischemia, even when asymptomatic ("silent"). In many, silent episodes are more frequent than symptomatic ones. In most cases, they occur in patients with other evidence of ischemia, and they respond to the same treatments, so that the role of ambulatory monitoring is unclear, as is the benefit of abolishing all such episodes in patients who are otherwise being managed properly.

H. Coronary Angiography

Selective coronary arteriography is the definitive diagnostic procedure for coronary artery disease. It can be performed with low mortality (about 0.1%) and morbidity (1–5%), but the cost is high, and with currently available noninvasive techniques it is usually not indicated solely for diagnosis.

Coronary arteriography should be performed in the following groups:

(1) Patients being considered for coronary artery revascularization because of limiting stable angina who have failed to improve on an adequate medical regimen.

(2) Patients in whom coronary revascularization is being considered because the clinical presentation (unstable angina, postinfarction angina, etc) or noninvasive testing suggests high-risk disease (see Indications for Revascularization).

(3) Patients with aortic valve disease who also have angina pectoris, in order to determine whether the angina is due to accompanying coronary disease. Coronary angiography is also performed in asymptomatic older patients undergoing valve surgery so that concomitant bypass may be done if the anatomy is propitious.

(4) Patients who have had coronary revascularization with subsequent recurrence of symptoms, to determine whether bypass grafts or native vessels are occluded.

(5) Patients with cardiac failure in whom a surgically correctable lesion, such as left ventricular aneurysm, mitral regurgitation, or reversible ischemic dysfunction, is suspected.

(6) Patients surviving sudden death or with symptomatic or life-threatening arrhythmias in whom coronary artery disease may be a correctable cause.

(7) Patients with chest pain of uncertain cause or cardiomyopathy of unknown cause.

Coronary arteriography visualizes the location and severity of stenoses. Narrowing greater than 50% of the luminal diameter is considered clinically significant, although most lesions producing ischemia are associated with narrowing in excess of 70%. This information has important prognostic value, since mortality rates are progressively higher in patients with one-, two-, and three-vessel disease and those with left main coronary artery obstruction (ranging from 1% per year to 25% per year). In those with strongly positive exercise ECGs or scintigraphic studies, three-vessel or left main disease may be present in 75–95% depending upon the criteria employed. Coronary arteriography also shows whether the obstructions are amenable to bypass surgery or percutaneous transluminal coronary angioplasty (PTCA).

Coronary angiography may underestimate the degree of atherosclerosis because it images only the lumen of the vessel. If there is concentric plaque with arterial enlargement (remodeling), then the lumen may appear relatively normal. Intravascular ultrasound (IVUS) utilizes a small ultrasound transducer that can be positioned within the artery and image beneath the endothelial surface. This technique is useful when the angiogram is equivocal as well as for assessing the results of angioplasty or stenting.

I. Left Ventricular Angiography

Left ventricular angiography is usually performed at the same time as coronary arteriography. Global and regional left ventricular function are visualized, as well as mitral regurgitation if present. Left ventricular function is the major determinant of prognosis in stable coronary disease and of the risk of bypass surgery.

Beller GA et al: Contributions of nuclear cardiology to diagnosis and prognosis of patients with coronary artery disease. Circulation 2000;101:1465. [PMID: 10736294] (Review with emphasis on role of newer techniques.)

Camici PG: Positron emission tomography and myocardial imaging. Heart 2000;83:475. [PMID: 10722554] (This technique has been valuable in elucidating the pathophysiology of ischemic heart disease, but cost is high and availability is limited.)

Gottdiener JS: Overview of stress echocardiography: uses, advantages, and limitations. Prog Cardiovasc Dis 2001;43:315. [PMID: 11235847]

Kim WY et al: Coronary magnetic resonance angiography for the detection of coronary stenoses. N Engl J Med 2001;345: 1863. [PMID: 11756576] (Left main, three-vessel, and proximal coronary disease can be reliably detected by this noninvasive technique.)

Lee TH et al: Clinical practice. Noninvasive tests in patients with stable coronary artery disease. N Engl J Med 2001;344: 1840. [PMID: 11407346] (Review article covering different clinical scenarios and modalities of testing.)

Nissen SE et al: Intravascular ultrasound. Circulation 2001;103: 604. [PMID: 11157729] (Intravascular ultrasound has contributed to our understanding of atherosclerosis and is useful in assessing ambiguous angiography and guiding intervention and in brachytherapy.)

O'Rourke RA et al: American College of Cardiology/American Heart Association Expert Consensus Document on electron-beam computed tomography for the diagnosis and prognosis of coronary artery disease. J Am Coll Cardiol 2000;36:326. [PMID: 10898458] (Sensitivity for detecting coronary artery disease is 94%, but predictability of clinical outcome and clinical role are still in question.)

Scanlon PJ et al: ACC/AHA guidelines for coronary angiography: executive summary and recommendations. A report of the American College of Cardiology/American Heart Association Task Force on Practice Guidelines (Committee on Coronary Angiography) developed in collaboration with the Society for Cardiac Angiography and Interventions. Circulation 1999;99:2345. [PMID: 10226103]

Tavel ME: Stress testing in cardiac evaluation: current concepts with emphasis on the ECG. Chest 2001;119:907. [PMID: 11243976] (Overview of ECG-based stress testing.)

Williams SV et al: Guidelines for the management of patients with chronic stable angina: diagnosis and risk stratification. Ann Intern Med 2001;135:530. [PMID: 11578158] (Discusses a staged approach to risk stratification of patients.)

Coronary Vasospasm & Angina With Normal Coronary Arteriograms

Although most symptoms of myocardial ischemia result from fixed stenosis of the coronary arteries or intraplaque hemorrhage or thrombosis at the site of lesions, some ischemic events may be precipitated or exacerbated by coronary vasoconstriction.

Spasm of the large coronary arteries with resulting decreased coronary blood flow may occur spontaneously or may be induced by exposure to cold, emotional stress, or vasoconstricting medications, such as ergot derivative drugs. Spasm may occur both in normal and in stenosed coronary arteries and may be silent or result in angina pectoris. Even myocardial infarction may occur as a result of spasm in the absence of visible obstructive coronary heart disease, although most instances of such coronary spasm occur in the presence of coronary stenosis.

Cocaine can induce myocardial ischemia and infarction by causing coronary artery vasoconstriction or by increasing myocardial energy requirements.

Prinzmetal's (variant) angina is a clinical syndrome in which chest pain occurs without the usual precipitating factors and is associated with ST segment elevation rather than depression. It often affects women under 50 years of age. It characteristically occurs in the early morning, awakening patients from sleep, tends to involve the right coronary artery, and is apt to be associated with arrhythmias or conduction defects. There may be no fixed stenoses. Ischemia usually results from coronary vasoconstriction and may be diagnosed by challenge with ergonovine (a vasoconstrictor).

Patients with this pattern of pain or any chest pain syndrome associated with ST segment elevation should undergo coronary arteriography to determine whether fixed stenotic lesions are present. If they are, aggressive medical therapy or revascularization is indicated, since this may represent an unstable phase of the disease. If significant lesions are not seen and spasm is suspected, ergonovine may be administered intravenously to precipitate vasospasm. This must be done cautiously and with nitroglycerin prepared for intracoronary administration, since irreversible spasm may lead to infarction. Episodes respond well to nitrates or calcium channel blockers, and both drugs are effective prophylactically. By allowing unopposed α_1-mediated vasoconstriction, beta-blockers have exacerbated coronary vasospasm, but they may have a role in management of patients in whom spasm is associated with fixed stenoses.

There is a growing consensus that myocardial ischemia may also occur in patients with normal coronary arteries as a result of disease of the coronary microcirculation or abnormal vascular reactivity. This has been termed syndrome X.

Al Suwaidi J et al: Pathophysiology, diagnosis, and current management strategies for chest pain in patients with normal findings on angiography. Mayo Clin Proc 2001;76:813. [PMID: 11499821] (Accurate history and good physical examination are vital in assessment of chest pain.)

Ammann P et al: Characteristics and prognosis of myocardial infarction in patients with normal coronary arteries. Chest 2000;117:333. [PMID: 10669671] (Myocardial infarction with normal coronary arteries may result from inflammation and spasm.)

Lange RA et al: Cardiovascular complications of cocaine use. N Engl J Med 2001;345:351. [PMID: 11484693] (Cocaine-related angina, myocardial infarction cardiomyopathy, and sudden death rate is on the rise.)

Treatment

A. TREATMENT OF ACUTE ATTACK

Sublingual nitroglycerin is the drug of choice; it acts in about 1–2 minutes. Nitrates decrease arteriolar and venous tone, reduce preload and afterload, and lower the oxygen demand of the heart. Nitrates may also improve myocardial blood flow by dilating collateral channels and, in the presence of increased vasomotor tone, coronary stenoses. As soon as the attack begins, one fresh tablet is placed under the tongue. This may be repeated at 3- to 5-minute intervals. The dosage (0.3, 0.4, or 0.6 mg) and the number of tablets to be used before seeking further medical attention must be individualized. Nitroglycerin buccal spray is also available as a metered (0.4 mg) delivery system. It has the advantage of being more convenient for patients who have difficulty handling the pills and of being more stable. Nitroglycerin should also be used prophylactically before activities likely to precipitate angina. Pain not responding to three tablets or lasting more than 20 minutes may represent evolving infarction, and the patient should be instructed to seek immediate medical attention.

B. PREVENTION OF FURTHER ATTACKS

1. Aggravating factors—Angina may be aggravated by hypertension, left ventricular failure, arrhythmia (usually tachycardias), strenuous activity, cold temperatures, and emotional states. These factors should be identified and treated or avoided where possible.

2. Nitroglycerin—Nitroglycerin, 0.3–0.6 mg sublingually or 0.4–0.8 mg translingually by spray, should be taken 5 minutes before any activity likely to precipitate angina. Sublingual isosorbide dinitrate (2.5–10 mg) is only slightly longer-acting than sublingual nitroglycerin.

3. Long-acting nitrates—A number of longer-acting nitrate preparations are available. These include isosorbide dinitrate, 10–40 mg orally three times daily; isosorbide mononitrate, 10–40 mg orally twice daily or 60–120 mg once daily in a sustained-release preparation; oral sustained-release nitroglycerin preparations, 6.25–12.5 mg two to four times daily; nitroglycerin ointment, 6.25–25 mg applied two to four times daily; and transdermal nitroglycerin patches that deliver nitroglycerin at a predetermined rate (usually 5–20 mg/24 h). The main limitation to chronic nitrate therapy is tolerance, which occurs to some degree in most patients. The degree of tolerance can be limited by utilizing a regimen which includes a minimum 8- to 10-hour period per day without nitrates. Isosorbide dinitrate given three times daily, with the last dose after dinner, is the most commonly used approach, but longer-acting isosorbide mononitrate is becoming more popular. Because it is the active metabolite of the dinitrate, isosorbide mononitrate has more consistent bioavailability. Transdermal nitrate preparations should be removed overnight in most patients.

Nitrate therapy is often limited by headache. Other side effects include nausea, light-headedness, and hypotension.

4. Beta-blockers—Beta-blockers prevent angina by reducing myocardial oxygen requirements during exertion and stress. This is accomplished by reducing the heart rate, myocardial contractility, and, to a lesser extent, blood pressure. The beta-blockers are the only antianginal agents that have been demonstrated to prolong life in patients with coronary disease (postmyocardial infarction). They are at least as effective at relieving angina as alternative agents in studies employing exercise testing, ambulatory monitoring, and symptom assessment. As a result, they should be considered for first-line therapy in most patients with chronic angina.

In the United States, only propranolol, metoprolol, nadolol, and atenolol are approved for angina. Nonetheless, all available beta-blockers appear to be effective for angina, though those with intrinsic sympathomimetic activity, such as pindolol, are less desirable because they may exacerbate angina in some individuals and have not been effective in secondary prevention trials. The pharmacology and side effects of the beta-blockers are discussed in Chapter 11 (Table 11–6). The dosages of all these drugs when given for angina are similar. The major contraindications are bronchospastic disease, bradyarrhythmias, and overt heart failure.

5. Calcium channel blocking agents—Verapamil, diltiazem, and the dihydropyridine group of calcium blockers are chemically and pharmacologically heterogeneous agents that prevent angina by reducing myocardial oxygen requirements and by inducing coronary artery vasodilation. Myocardial oxygen demand is lessened by reducing blood pressure, left ventricular wall stress, and, in the case of verapamil and diltiazem, resting or exercise heart rate. Though these agents are all potent coronary vasodilators, it is unclear whether they improve myocardial blood flow in most patients with stable exertional angina. In those with coronary vasospasm, the calcium channel blockers may be the agents of choice.

Most calcium channel blockers have negative inotropic, chronotropic, and dromotropic properties in vitro, but the reflex sympathetic response may obscure these effects in vivo (except in the presence of beta blockade or severely depressed left ventricular function). Unlike the beta-blockers, calcium channel blockers have not reduced mortality postinfarction and in some cases have increased ischemia and mortality rates. This appears to be the case with some dihydropyridines and with diltiazem and verapamil in patients with clinical heart failure or moderate to severe left ventricular dysfunction. A recent meta-analysis suggested that short-acting nifedipine in moderate to high doses causes an increase in mortality in patients early after myocardial infarction or with unstable angina. It is uncertain whether these findings are relevant to longer-acting dihydropyridines, and data with verapamil and diltiazem suggest that these latter agents are safe in postinfarction patients with preserved left ventricular function. Nevertheless, considering the uncertainties and the lack of demonstrated favorable effect on outcomes, calcium channel blockers should be considered third-line anti-ischemic drugs in the postinfarction patient. Similarly, with the exception of amlodipine, which in the PRAISE trial proved safe in patients with heart failure, these agents should be avoided in patients with congestive heart failure or low ejection fractions.

The pharmacologic effects and side effects of the calcium channel blockers are discussed in Chapter 11 and summarized in Table 11–8. Although all have been shown to be efficacious for angina, not all preparations and agents are approved for this indication. By and large, diltiazem and verapamil are preferable as first-line agents because they produce less reflex tachycardia and because the former, at least, may cause fewer side effects. Nifedipine, nicardipine, and amlodipine are also approved agents for angina. Isradipine, felodipine, and nisoldipine are not approved for angina but probably are as effective as the other dihydropyridines.

6. Alternative and combination therapies—Patients who do not respond to one class of antianginal medication often respond to another. It may, therefore, be worthwhile to use an alternative agent before progressing to combinations. If the patient remains symptomatic, a beta-blocker and a long-acting nitrate or a beta-blocker and a calcium channel blocker (other than verapamil, where the risk of atrioventricular block or heart failure is higher) are the most appropriate combinations. A few patients will have a further response to a regimen including all three agents.

7. Platelet-inhibiting agents—Coronary thrombosis is responsible for most episodes of myocardial infarction and many unstable ischemic syndromes. Several studies have demonstrated the benefit of anti-platelet drugs following unstable angina and infarction. Therefore, unless contraindicated, small doses of aspirin (81–325 mg daily or 325 mg every other day) should be prescribed for patients with angina. Clopidogrel is an antiplatelet agent that acts by inhibiting ADP-induced platelet aggregation. Unlike its older congener ticlopidine, clopidogrel does not cause agranulocytosis but may rarely induce thrombotic thrombocytopenic purpura. It can reduce cardiac events in patients with acute coronary syndromes and is an appropriate alternative in aspirin-intolerant patients.

8. Risk reduction—As discussed above, patients with coronary disease should undergo aggressive risk factor modification. This approach, with a particular focus on lowering LDL cholesterol to ≤ 100 mg/dL, not only prevents future events but may markedly improve symptomatic angina. Indeed, the Atorvastatin Versus Revascularization Treatment (AVERT) trial showed that patients randomized to aggressive lipid-lowering and medical therapy tended to have fewer subsequent ischemic events.

9. Revascularization—The indications for coronary artery revascularization and the choice of procedure are discussed below.

Prognosis

The prognosis of angina pectoris has improved with advances in the understanding of its pathophysiology and in pharmacologic therapy. Mortality rates vary depending on the number of vessels diseased, the severity of obstruction, the status of left ventricular function, and the presence of complex arrhythmias. In patients with stable symptoms and normal ejection fractions (> 55%, depending on the laboratory), the mortality rate is 1–2% per year. However, the outlook in individual patients is unpredictable, and nearly half of the deaths are sudden. Therefore, risk stratification is often attempted. Patients with accelerating symptoms have a poorer outlook. Among stable patients, those whose exercise tolerance is severely limited by ischemia (less than 6 minutes on the Bruce treadmill protocol) and those with extensive ischemia by exercise electrocardiography or scintigraphy have more severe anatomic disease and a poorer prognosis.

Fihn SD et al: Guidelines for the management of patients with chronic stable angina: treatment. Ann Intern Med 2001; 135:616. [PMID: 11601935] (Covers medical as well as percutaneous interventional and surgical management.)

Gibbons RJ et al: ACC/AHA/ACP-ASIM guidelines for the management of patients with chronic stable angina: a report of the American College of Cardiology/American Heart Association Task Force on Practice Guidelines (Committee on Management of Patients With Chronic Stable Angina). J Am Coll Cardiol 1999;33:2092. [PMID: 10362225]

Heidenreich PA et al: Meta-analysis of trial comparing β-blockers, calcium antagonists, and nitrates for stable angina. JAMA 1999;281:1927. [PMID: 10349897] (Meta-analysis of 97 studies over 30 years suggests that beta-blockers are associated with fewer adverse events than calcium antagonists.)

Williams SV et al: Guidelines for the management of patients with chronic stable angina: diagnosis and risk stratification. Ann Intern Med 2001;135:530. [PMID: 11578158] (Two-part review that covers diagnostic testing and treatment of coronary artery disease. Strategy for selection of medical therapy, percutaneous intervention, or CABG is outlined.)

REVASCULARIZATION PROCEDURES FOR PATIENTS WITH ANGINA PECTORIS

Indications

The indications for coronary artery revascularization in patients with angina pectoris are often debated. There is general agreement that otherwise healthy patients in the following groups should undergo revascularization. (1) Patients with unacceptable symptoms despite medical therapy to its tolerable limits. (2) Patients with left main coronary artery stenosis greater than 50% with or without symptoms. (3) Patients with three-vessel disease with left ventricular dysfunction (ejection fraction < 50% or previous transmural infarction). (4) Patients with unstable angina who after symptom control by medical therapy continue to exhibit ischemia on exercise testing or monitoring. (5) Post-myocardial infarction patients with continuing angina or severe ischemia on noninvasive testing. (See sections on Unstable Angina and Myocardial Infarction.)

In addition, many cardiologists feel that patients with less severe symptoms should be revascularized if they have two-vessel disease associated with underlying left ventricular dysfunction, anatomically critical lesions (> 90% proximal stenoses, especially of the proximal left anterior descending artery) or physiologic evidence of severe ischemia (early positive exercise tests, large exercise-induced thallium scintigraphic defects, or frequent episodes of ischemia on ambulatory monitoring). This trend toward aggressive intervention has accelerated as a result of the growing use of coronary angioplasty and stenting. While such patients are at increased risk, it has not been proved that their prognosis is better after coronary revascularization by either surgery or angioplasty.

Type of Procedure

A. CORONARY ARTERY BYPASS GRAFTING (CABG)

CABG can be accomplished with a very low mortality rate (1–3%) in otherwise healthy patients with preserved cardiac function. However, the mortality rate of this procedure rises to 4–8% in older individuals and in patients who have had a prior CABG. Increasingly, younger individuals with focal lesions of one or several vessels are undergoing coronary angioplasty as the initial revascularization procedure.

Grafts employing one or both internal mammary arteries (usually to the left anterior descending artery or its branches) provide the best long-term results in terms of patency and flow. Segments of the saphenous vein (or, less optimally, other veins) or the radial artery interposed between the aorta and the coronary arteries distal to the obstructions are also utilized. One to five distal anastomoses are commonly performed. After successful surgery, symptoms generally abate. The need for antianginal medications diminishes, and left ventricular function may improve.

Minimally invasive surgical techniques utilize different approaches to the heart than standard sternotomy and cardiopulmonary bypass. The surgical approach may involve a limited sternotomy, lateral thoracotomy (MIDCAB), or thoracoscopy (port-access). These approaches may be used in conjunction with standard cardiopulmonary bypass, with peripheral cardiopulmonary bypass, or with operating on the beating heart utilizing a mechanical coronary stabilizer. Avoiding bypass may lessen the risk of cerebral complications. These techniques allow earlier postoperative mobilization and discharge. They are more technically demanding, usually not suitable for more than two grafts, and do not have established durability.

The operative mortality rate is increased in patients with poor left ventricular function (left ventricular ejection fraction < 35%) or those requiring additional procedures (valve replacement or ventricular aneurysmectomy). Patients over 70 years of age, patients undergoing repeat procedures, or those with important noncardiac disease (especially renal insufficiency, and diabetes) or poor general health also have higher operative mortality and morbidity rates, and full recovery is slow. Thus, CABG should be reserved for more severely symptomatic patients in this group. Early (1–6 months) graft patency rates average 85–90% (higher for internal mammary grafts), and subsequent graft closure rates are about 4% annually. Early graft failure is common in vessels with poor distal flow, while late closure is more frequent in patients who continue smoking and those with untreated hyperlipidemia. Antiplatelet therapy with aspirin improves graft patency rates. Smoking cessation and vigorous treatment of blood lipid abnormalities is necessary, with a goal for LDL cholesterol of ≤ 100 mg/dL and of HDL cholesterol ≥ 45 mg/dL. Repeat revascularization (see below) is often necessitated by progressive native vessel disease and graft occlusions.

Reoperation is technically demanding and less often fully successful than the initial operation.

B. PERCUTANEOUS TRANSLUMINAL CORONARY ANGIOPLASTY (PTCA) AND STENTING

Coronary artery stenoses can be effectively dilated by inflation of a balloon under high pressure. This procedure is performed in the cardiac catheterization laboratory under local anesthesia either at the same time as diagnostic coronary arteriography or at a later time. The mechanism of dilation involves both rupture of the atheromatous plaque and remodeling of the vessel.

This procedure was at one time reserved for proximal single-vessel disease, but now it is widely employed in multivessel disease with multiple lesions, though only rarely in left main disease. PTCA is possible but often less successful in bypass graft stenoses. Bypass graft patients with multivessel disease have lower mortality rates and fewer nonfatal myocardial infarctions with surgery than with percutaneous interventions. Optimal lesions for PTCA are relatively proximal, noneccentric, free of significant calcification or plaque dissection, and removed from the origin of large branches. With improved catheter systems, experienced operators are able to successfully dilate 90% of lesions attempted. The major early complication is intimal dissection with vessel occlusion. This can usually be treated by repeat PTCA or by deployment of an intracoronary stent. The use of platelet glycoprotein IIb/IIIa inhibitors (abciximab, tirofiban) has markedly reduced the rate of acute vessel closure. Placement of intracoronary stents improves initial results, especially with complex and long lesions. Although the early experience with stents was complicated by an unacceptable rate of acute thrombosis, this problem has largely been prevented by aggressive antithrombotic therapy (chronic aspirin plus clopidogrel for 30 days, with acute use of platelet glycoprotein IIb/IIIa inhibitors in high-risk patients). Restenosis rates have fallen with the use of stents. Stents are now used in the majority of patients undergoing percutaneous revascularization.

The major limitation with PTCA has been restenosis, which occurs in the first 6 months in 30–40% of vessels dilated, though it can often be treated successfully by repeat PTCA. The use of stents has reduced the restenosis rate by half, and preliminary data indicate that coated stents which elute antiproliferative agents may prevent most cases of restenosis. Currently, recurrent in-stent restenosis is treated with brachytherapy.

The number of PTCA and stent procedures now exceeds that of CABG operations, but the justification for many of the procedures performed in patients with stable angina is unclear. Several studies have shown PTCA to be superior to medical therapy for symptom relief but not in preventing infarction or death. In patients with no or only mild symptoms, aggressive lipid-lowering and antianginal therapy may be preferable to PTCA.

Several studies of PTCA versus CABG in patients with multivessel disease have been reported. The consistent finding has been comparable mortality and infarction rates over follow-up periods of 1–3 years but a high rate (approximately 40%) of repeat procedures following PTCA. As a result, the choice of revascularization procedure is often a matter of patient preference. However, it should be noted that less than 20% of patients with multivessel disease met the entry criteria, so these results cannot be generalized to all multivessel disease patients. Outcomes with percutaneous revascularization in diabetics have been inferior to those with CABG. However, these trials preceded the widespread use of stenting.

C. Experimental Approaches

Several experimental approaches have been studied in patients with refractory angina who are not candidates for percutaneous or surgical revascularization procedures. Lasers have been used either from the epicardial surface of the left ventricle during surgery or from the ventricular cavity by catheter-based techniques. Several studies have reported an improvement in symptoms, but this has not been associated with objective evidence of improved perfusion, raising the possibility of a placebo effect. Other studies have evaluated intracoronary injections of growth factors such as vascular endothelial growth factor (VEGF) or fibroblast growth factors, but thus far there is little evidence of benefit. Lastly, mechanical extracorporeal counterpulsation, which entails repetitive inflation of a high-pressure chamber surrounding the lower half of the body during the diastolic phase of the cardiac cycle for daily 1-hour sessions over a period of 7 weeks, has been advocated. Although modest increases in exercise tolerance have been reported, the response has been variable, often time-limited, and not shown to be associated with improved myocardial perfusion—so again, a placebo effect may be responsible.

Summary of Results of Treatment

Several randomized trials have shown that over follow-up periods of several years, the mortality and infarction rates with percutaneous revascularization and CABG are generally comparable. An exception may be diabetic patients, who have had better outcomes with CABG. Recovery after PTCA is obviously faster, but the intermediate-term success rate of CABG is higher both because of the high restenosis rate with PTCA and, less importantly, with stenting. The increasing popularity of PTCA and stenting primarily reflects the lower cost and, shorter hospitalization, the perception that CABG is best done only once and can be reserved for later and the preference of patients for less invasive treatment. These arguments make PTCA the procedure of choice for revascularization of single-vessel disease, though this is not usually indicated except when symptoms are refractory. The situation is less clear with multivessel disease. It should also be noted that the excellent outcome of patients treated medically has made it difficult to show an advantage with either revascularization approach except in patients who remain symptom-limited or have left main lesions or three-vessel disease and left ventricular dysfunction. The expected availability of drug-eluting stents may shift the balance toward percutaneous revascularization in the future.

Bucher HC et al: Percutaneous transluminal coronary angioplasty versus medical treatment for non-acute coronary heart disease: meta-analysis of randomised controlled trials. BMJ 2000;321:73. [PMID: 10884254] (PTCA may lead to a greater reduction in angina than medical treatment but at the cost of more coronary artery bypass grafting. Trials have not included enough patients to permit informative estimates of the effect of PTCA on myocardial infarction, death, or subsequent revascularization, though trends so far do not favor PTCA.)

Eagle KA et al: ACC/AHA Guidelines for Coronary Artery Bypass Graft Surgery: A Report of the American College of Cardiology/American Heart Association Task Force on Practice Guidelines (Committee to Revise the 1991 Guidelines for Coronary Artery Bypass Graft Surgery). American College of Cardiology/American Heart Association. J Am Coll Cardiol 1999;34:1262. [PMID: 10520819]

Freedman SB et al: Therapeutic angiogenesis for coronary artery disease. Ann Intern Med 2002;136:54. [PMID: 11777364] (Growth factors such as VEGF and FGF may reduce angina and increase exercise time in patients with coronary artery disease. Optimal drug dose and route of administration are not yet known.)

Lincoff AM et al: Platelet glycoprotein IIb/IIIa receptor blockade in coronary disease. J Am Coll Cardiol 2000;35:1103. [PMID: 10758948] (Use of these agents with stenting and in acute coronary syndromes is becoming standard. Data from 11 trials and 323,000 patients are reviewed.)

O'Shea JC et al: Platelet glycoprotein IIb/IIIa integrin blockade with eptifibatide in coronary stent intervention. JAMA 2001; 285:2468. [PMID: 11368699] (Eptifibatide is superior to placebo in patients undergoing nonurgent stent implantation.)

Serruys PW et al: Comparison of coronary-artery bypass surgery and stenting for the treatment of multivessel disease. N Engl J Med 2001;344:1117. [PMID: 11297702] (Stenting offers same protection against death, stroke and myocardial infarction as CABG and is less expensive, but it more often requires repeat revascularization.)

Trial of invasive versus medical therapy in elderly patients with chronic symptomatic coronary-artery disease (TIME): a randomised trial. Lancet 2001;358:951. [PMID: 11583747] (Trial showing that elderly patients may benefit more from an invasive management strategy.)

Urano H et al: Enhanced external counterpulsation improves exercise tolerance, reduces exercise-induced myocardial ischemia and improves left ventricular diastolic filling in patients with coronary artery disease. J Am Coll Cardiol 2001;37:93. [PMID: 11153780] (Trial demonstrating benefit in refractory patients.)

UNSTABLE ANGINA

Most clinicians use the term "unstable angina" to denote an accelerating or "crescendo" pattern of pain in cases where previously stable angina occurs with less exertion or at rest, lasts longer, and is less responsive to medication. Coronary angioscopy has shown that a high proportion of patients with this pattern of symptoms have "complex" coronary stenoses characterized by plaque rupture, ulceration, or hemorrhage with subsequent thrombus formation. This inherently unstable situation may progress to complete occlusion and infarction or may heal, with reendothelialization and a return to a stable though possibly more severe pattern of ischemia. New-onset angina is sometimes considered unstable, but if it is exertional and responsive to rest and medication, it does not carry the same poor prognosis.

Diagnosis

Most patients with unstable angina will exhibit electrocardiographic changes during pain—commonly ST segment depression or T wave flattening or inversion but sometimes, and more ominously, ST segment elevation. They may exhibit signs of left ventricular dysfunction during pain and for a time thereafter.

Chest pain is one of the most frequent reasons for emergency department visits, and the consequences of misdiagnosis are significant (clinically for false-negative diagnoses and economically for false-positives). Up to half of patients have noncardiac diagnoses, and even many of those with coronary disease are at low risk for early events (< 1% 30-day event rate). However, those with recent, prolonged, or recurrent episodes and accompanying electrocardiographic changes indicative of ischemia (ST segment depression > 1 mm, ischemic ST segment elevation, T wave inversions, or new LBBB) may have much higher event rates. Many hospitals have developed **chest pain observation units** to provide a longer period of observation and immediate testing in patients determined to be at low risk in order to improve the triage process. In many cases those who have not experienced new chest pain and have no electrocardiographic changes or cardiac enzyme elevations undergo treadmill exercise tests or imaging procedures to exclude ischemia at the end of a 6–24 hour period and are discharged directly from the emergency department if these tests are negative.

Treatment

A. General Measures

Treatment of unstable angina should be multifaceted and vigorous. Patients should be hospitalized, maintained at bed rest or at very limited activity, monitored, and given supplemental oxygen. Sedation with a benzodiazepine agent may help if anxiety is present. The systolic blood pressure is usually maintained at 100–120 mm Hg, except in previously severe hypertensives, and the heart rate should be lowered to 60/min.

B. Anticoagulation, Antiplatelet, and Thrombolytic Therapy

Because intravascular thrombosis plays a prominent role in the pathophysiology of unstable angina and its progression to myocardial infarction, antithrombotic therapy is an important part of treatment for unstable angina. Most patients should receive a combination of two or more agents. Aspirin, 325 mg daily , should be commenced on admission, and intravenous heparin should be started if symptoms have been recent (past 24 hours) or if they recur. Heparin therapy, when necessary, should be continued for at least 2 days. Several trials have shown that low-molecular-weight heparin is marginally superior to unfractionated heparin in preventing recurrent ischemic events in the setting of acute coronary syndromes. Enoxaparin (1 mg/kg subcutaneously every 12 hours) is the best-studied member of this class of agents. The Clopidogrel in Unstable Angina to Prevent Recurrent Events (CURE) trial demonstrated a 20% reduction in the composite end point of cardiovascular death, myocardial infarction, and stroke with the addition of clopidogrel (300 mg loading dose, 75 mg daily for 12 months) in patients with non-ST segment elevation acute coronary syndromes.

The administration of drugs that block monoclonal antibodies to the platelet glycoprotein IIb/IIIa receptor is a useful adjunct in high-risk patients (usually defined by fluctuating ST segment depression or positive biomarkers) with unstable angina, particularly when they are undergoing PTCA or stenting. The short-acting small molecule inhibitors have been the best-studied agents in the nonintervention setting. Tirofiban, 0.4 μg/kg/min for 30 minutes, followed by 0.1 μg/kg/min, and eptifibatide, 180 μg/kg bolus followed by a continuous infusion of 0.1 μg/kg/min, have both have been shown to be effective in unstable angina and non-Q wave myocardial infarction when added to heparin. Downward dose adjustments are required in patients with reduced renal function.

Since in unstable angina the vessel usually remains patent and the thrombi are undergoing continuous spontaneous formation and thrombolysis, thrombolytic therapy has not been effective in improving the outcome.

C. Nitroglycerin

The nitrates are first-line anti-ischemic therapy for unstable angina. Nonparenteral therapy with sublingual or oral agents or nitroglycerin ointment is usually sufficient. If pain persists or recurs, intravenous nitroglycerin should be started. The usual initial dosage is 10 μg/min. The dosage should be titrated to 1 μg/kg/min over 30–60 minutes and further increased as tolerated if pain recurs. Dosages up to 10 μg/kg/min or higher may be used. Tolerance to continuous nitrate infusion is common. Careful—usually continuous—blood pressure monitoring is required when intravenous nitroglycerin is used.

D. BETA-BLOCKERS

These agents are also a part of the initial treatment of unstable angina unless otherwise contraindicated. If the patient has no physical findings of heart failure, these agents can usually be started without measurements of left ventricular function. Patients with evidence of large or multiple old infarctions are an exception. The pharmacology of these agents is discussed in Chapter 11 and summarized in Table 11–6. Use of agents with intrinsic sympathomimetic activity should be avoided in this setting. The goal of acute treatment is to reduce the heart rate below 60–70/min. Oral medication is adequate in most patients, but intravenous treatment with metoprolol, given as three 5 mg doses 5 minutes apart, achieves a more rapid effect. Oral therapy should be aggressively titrated upward as blood pressure permits.

E. CALCIUM CHANNEL BLOCKERS

Calcium channel blockers have not been shown to favorably affect outcome in unstable angina, and they should be used primarily as third-line therapy in patients with continuing symptoms on nitrates and beta-blockers or those who are not candidates for these drugs. In the presence of nitrates and without accompanying beta-blockers, diltiazem or verapamil is preferred, since nifedipine and the other dihydropyridines are more likely to cause reflex tachycardia or hypotension. The initial dosage should be low, but upward titration should proceed rapidly.

F. INTRA-AORTIC BALLOON COUNTERPULSATION (IABC)

IABC can both reduce myocardial energy requirements (systolic unloading) and improve diastolic coronary blood flow. This approach is sometimes employed to stabilize patients prior to angiography or revascularization, but with modern techniques it is rarely necessary.

Prognosis & Indications for Revascularization

Over 90% of patients can be rendered pain-free with these measures. Patients who do not become ischemia-free on medical therapy should have early coronary arteriography and revascularization. Controlled trials have reported mixed results as to whether a strategy of routine coronary angiography and revascularization is superior to aggressive medical therapy and selective revascularization in patients with recurrent ischemia or very positive stress tests. Recent trials that have employed both platelet glycoprotein IIb/IIIa antagonists and stents in the majority of patients have favored an early but not necessarily immediate invasive strategy (eg, within several days and prior to discharge). Depending on the stringency of the definition of unstable angina, 10–30% of patients will have an early infarction, and the 1-year mortality rate is 10–20%. Elevated troponin I or T concentrations and "silent" ST segment shifts have both identified patients at higher risk for subsequent myocardial infarction or recurrence of severe ischemia. These markers identify a subset of patients who benefit from the early use of glycoprotein IIb/IIIa receptor antagonists and, most likely, early revascularization.

Because recurrent episodes, infarction, and sudden death may occur following relief of unstable angina, additional evaluations should be performed in patients who have been stabilized, consisting of either (1) early exercise or pharmacologic stress testing to identify high-risk subsets for further invasive evaluation, or (2) coronary arteriography. The choice of approach should be individualized based on the patient's age and general health as well as the severity of symptoms and signs of ischemia. The artery responsible for the ischemia can usually be determined from electrocardiographic or scintigraphic changes during pain, and the lesion is often amenable to PTCA. If revascularization is not performed, long-term management is the same as that outlined for stable angina pectoris.

Ambrose JA et al: Unstable angina: current concepts of pathogenesis and treatment. Arch Intern Med 2000;160:25. [PMID: 10632302] (Review article covering pathogenesis and treatment with an emphasis on trials supporting the use of newer antithrombotic and antiplatelet therapy.)

Antman EM et al: The TIMI risk score for unstable angina/non-ST elevation MI: A method for prognostication and therapeutic decision. JAMA 2000;284:835. [PMID: 10938172] (A scoring system using age, risk factors, symptoms, electrocardiographic changes, and serum markers can accurately predict outcome and allow tailoring of interventions.)

Bhatt DL et al: Current role of platelet glycoprotein IIb/IIIa inhibitors on acute coronary syndromes. JAMA 2000;284:1549. [PMID: 11000650] (Use of these drugs merits a prominent role in the management of patients with acute coronary syndromes.)

Braunwald E et al: ACC/AHA guidelines for the management of patients with unstable angina and non-ST-segment elevation myocardial infarction. J Am Coll Cardiol 2000;36:970. [PMID: 10987629]

Cannon CP et al: Comparison of early invasive and conservative strategies in patients with unstable coronary syndromes treated with the glycoprotein IIb/IIIa inhibitor tirofiban. N Engl J Med 2001;344:1879. [PMID: 11419424] (Early invasive strategy in patients with unstable coronary syndrome was associated with 22% reduction in death, myocardial infarction, or rehospitalization.)

Eikelboom JW et al: Unfractionated heparin and low-molecular-weight heparin in acute coronary syndrome without ST elevation: a meta-analysis. Lancet 2000;355:1936. [PMID: 10859038] (Meta-analysis of over 17,000 patients shows that unfractionated or low-molecular-weight heparin halves the rate of myocardial infarction in patients with unstable angina.)

Hamm CW et al: Acute coronary syndrome without ST elevation: Implementation of new guidelines. Lancet 2001;358:1533. [PMID: 11705583] (Updated guidelines emphasize use of troponin assays, low-molecular-weight heparins, glycoprotein IIb/IIIa antagonists, and invasive management strategies in patients with unstable angina and non-ST elevation myocardial infarction.)

Levine GN et al: Antithrombotic therapy in patients with acute coronary syndromes. Arch Intern Med 2001;161:937. [PMID: 11295956]

O'Rourke RA et al: New approaches to diagnosis and management of unstable angina and non-ST-segment elevation myocardial infarction. Arch Intern Med 2001;161:674. [PMID: 11231699] (Discussion of glycoprotein IIb/IIIa antagonists, LMWH, and invasive strategies. A practical treatment algorithm is included.)

Schwartz GG et al: Effects of atorvastatin on early recurrent ischemic events in acute coronary syndromes: the MIRACL study: a randomized controlled trial. JAMA 2001;285:1711. [PMID: 11277825] (Trial showing early benefit in treating patients with an acute coronary syndrome with high-dose atorvastatin.)

Wallentin L et al: Outcome at 1 year after an invasive compared with a non-invasive strategy in unstable coronary-artery disease: the FRISC II invasive randomized trial. Lancet 2000;356:9. [PMID: 10892758] (The Invasive strategy saves 1:7 lives and prevents two myocardial infarctions and 20 readmissions for every 100 patients treated.)

Yeghiazarians Y et al: Unstable angina pectoris. N Engl J Med 2000;342:101. [PMID: 10631280] (Comprehensive review covering pharmacologic therapy, revascularization, and risk stratification.)

Yusuf S et al: Effects of clopidogrel in addition to aspirin in patients with acute coronary syndromes without ST-segment elevation. N Engl J Med 2001;345:494. [PMID: 11519503] (Large-scale trial demonstrated that patients with acute coronary syndrome who received the antiplatelet drug clopidogrel had a lower incidence of cardiovascular death, myocardial infarction, or stroke but more bleeding.)

ACUTE MYOCARDIAL INFARCTION

 ESSENTIALS OF DIAGNOSIS

- *Sudden but not instantaneous development of prolonged (> 30 minutes) anterior chest discomfort (sometimes felt as "gas" or pressure) that may produce arrhythmias, hypotension, shock, or cardiac failure.*

- *Rarely painless, masquerading as acute congestive heart failure, syncope, stroke, or shock.*

- *Electrocardiography: ST segment elevation or depression, evolving Q waves, symmetric inversion of T waves.*

- *Elevation of cardiac enzymes (CK-MB, troponin T, or troponin I).*

- *Appearance of segmental wall motion abnormality by imaging techniques.*

General Considerations

Myocardial infarction results from prolonged myocardial ischemia, precipitated in most cases by an occlusive coronary thrombus at the site of a preexisting (though not necessarily severe) atherosclerotic plaque.

More rarely, infarction may result from prolonged vasospasm, inadequate myocardial blood flow (eg, hypotension), or excessive metabolic demand. Very rarely, myocardial infarction may be caused by embolic occlusion, vasculitis, aortic root or coronary artery dissection, or aortitis. Cocaine is a cause of infarction, which should be considered in young individuals without risk factors.

The location and extent of infarction depend upon the anatomic distribution of the occluded vessel, the presence of additional stenotic lesions, and the adequacy of collateral circulation. Thrombosis in the anterior descending branch of the left coronary artery results in infarction of the anterior left ventricle and interventricular septum. Occlusion of the left circumflex artery produces anterolateral or posterolateral infarction. Right coronary thrombosis leads to infarction of the posteroinferior portion of the left ventricle and may involve the right ventricular myocardium and interventricular septum. The arteries supplying the atrioventricular node and the sinus node more commonly arise from the right coronary; thus, atrioventricular block at the nodal level and sinus node dysfunction occur more frequently during inferior or right-sided infarctions. Individual variation in coronary anatomy and the presence of collateral vessels can make the prediction of coronary anatomy from infarct location imperfect.

Infarctions are often classified as transmural, if the classic electrocardiographic evolution of ST segment elevation to Q waves was observed; or nontransmural or subendocardial, if pain, enzyme elevations, and ST–T wave changes occurred in the absence of new Q waves. However, on pathologic examination, most infarctions involve the subendocardium predominantly, and some transmural extension is common even in the absence of Q waves. Thus, a better classification is Q wave versus non-Q wave infarction. The latter generally results from incomplete occlusion or spontaneous lysis of the thrombus and often signifies the presence of additional jeopardized myocardium; it is associated with a higher incidence of reinfarction and recurrent ischemia.

The size and anatomic location of an infarction determine the acute course, the early complications, and the long-term prognosis. Hemodynamic stability is related to extent of necrosis. In small infarctions, cardiac function is normal, whereas with more extensive damage, early heart failure and hypotension (cardiogenic shock) may appear. Preventing extension of an infarct and subsequent myocardial injury is a major goal of early management. The complications of acute infarction are discussed below.

Myocardial infarction redefined—a consensus document of The Joint European Society of Cardiology/American College of Cardiology Committee for the redefinition of myocardial infarction. J Am Coll Cardiol 2000;36:959. [PMID: 10987628] (Consensus statement redefining myocardial infarction in the light of new serum tests and with emphasis on implications for prognosis and management.)

Tavazzi L: Clinical epidemiology of acute myocardial infarction. Am Heart J 1999;138(2 Part 2):S48. [PMID: 10426859] (The decline in mortality from acute myocardial infarction is due as much to primary and secondary prevention as to improved therapeutic intervention. Half of myocardial infarction survivors are rehospitalized within 1 year.)

Clinical Findings

A. SYMPTOMS

1. Premonitory pain—One-third of patients give a history of alteration in the pattern of angina, recent onset of typical or atypical angina, or unusual "indigestion" or pressure or squeezing felt in the chest.

2. Pain of infarction—Most infarctions occur at rest unlike anginal episodes, and more commonly in the early morning. The pain is similar to angina in location and radiation but is more severe, and it builds up rapidly or in waves to maximum intensity over a few minutes or longer. Nitroglycerin has little effect; even opioids may not relieve the pain.

3. Associated symptoms—Patients may break out in a cold sweat, feel weak and apprehensive, and move about, seeking a position of comfort. They prefer not to lie quietly. Light-headedness, syncope, dyspnea, orthopnea, cough, wheezing, nausea and vomiting, or abdominal bloating may be present singly or in any combination.

4. Painless infarction—In a minority of cases, pain is absent or minor and is overshadowed by the immediate complications. As many as 25% of infarctions are detected on routine ECG without there having been any recallable acute episode.

5. Sudden death and early arrhythmias—Approximately 20% of patients with acute infarction will die before reaching the hospital; these deaths are usually in the first hour and are chiefly due to ventricular fibrillation.

B. SIGNS

1. General—Patients usually appear anxious and are often sweating profusely. The heart rate may range from marked bradycardia (most commonly in inferior infarction) to tachycardia resulting from increased sympathetic nervous system activity, low cardiac output, or arrhythmia. The blood pressure may be high, especially in former hypertensives, or low in patients with shock. Respiratory distress usually indicates heart failure. Fever, usually low-grade, may appear after 12 hours and persist for several days.

2. Chest—Clear lung fields are a good prognostic sign, but basilar rales are common and do not necessarily indicate heart failure. More extensive rales or diffuse wheezing suggests pulmonary edema.

3. Heart—The cardiac examination may be unimpressive or very abnormal. An abnormally located ventricular impulse often represents the dyskinetic infarcted region. Jugular venous distention reflects right atrial hypertension, which may indicate right ventricular infarction or elevated left ventricular filling pressures. The absence of elevated central venous pressure, however, does not indicate normal left atrial or left ventricular diastolic pressures. Soft heart sounds may indicate left ventricular dysfunction. Atrial gallops (S_4) are the rule, whereas ventricular gallops (S_3) are less common and indicate significant left ventricular dysfunction. Mitral regurgitation murmurs are not uncommon and usually indicate papillary muscle dysfunction or, rarely, rupture. Pericardial friction rubs are uncommon in the first 24 hours but may appear later.

4. Extremities—Edema is usually not present. Cyanosis and cold temperature indicate low output. The peripheral pulses should be noted, since later shock or emboli may alter the examination.

C. LABORATORY FINDINGS

The most valuable laboratory tests are cardiac-specific markers of myocardial damage, including quantitative determinations of CK-MB, troponin I, and troponin T. All are relatively specific for necrosis (the troponins somewhat more so), though they may be elevated following severe ischemic episodes. Each of these tests may become positive as early as 4–6 hours after the onset of a myocardial infarction and should be abnormal by 8–12 hours. Circulating levels of troponins may remain elevated for 5–7 days or longer and should obviate the use of less specific LDH isoenzyme assays.

D. ELECTROCARDIOGRAPHY

Most patients with acute infarction have ECG changes, and a normal tracing is rare. The extent of the electrocardiographic abnormalities provides only a crude estimate of the magnitude of infarction. The classic evolution of changes is from peaked ("hyperacute") T waves, to ST segment elevation, to Q wave development, to T wave inversion. This may occur over a few hours to several days. The evolution of new Q waves (> 30 ms in duration and 25% of the R wave amplitude) is diagnostic, but Q waves do not occur in 30–50% of acute infarctions (subendocardial or non-Q wave infarctions). If these patients have an appropriate clinical presentation, characteristic cardiac enzymes, and ST segment changes (usually depression) or T wave inversion lasting at least 48 hours, they are classified as having non-Q wave infarctions.

E. CHEST X-RAY

The chest x-ray may demonstrate signs of congestive heart failure, but these changes often lag behind the clinical findings. Signs of aortic dissection should be sought as a possible alternative diagnosis.

F. ECHOCARDIOGRAPHY

Echocardiography provides convenient bedside assessment of left ventricular global and regional function. This can help with the diagnosis and management of infarction; echocardiography has been used successfully to make judgments about admission and management of patients with suspected infarction, since normal wall motion makes an infarction unlikely. Doppler echocardiography is probably the most convenient procedure for diagnosing postinfarction mitral regurgitation or ventricular septal defect.

G. Scintigraphic Studies

Technetium-99m pyrophosphate scintigraphy can be used to diagnose acute myocardial infarction. When injected at least 18 hours postinfarction, the radiotracer complexes with calcium in necrotic myocardium to provide a "hot spot" image of the infarction. This test is insensitive to small infarctions, and false-positive studies occur, so its use is limited to patients in whom the diagnosis by electrocardiography and enzymes is not possible—principally those who present several days after the event or have intraoperative infarctions. Radiolabeled antimyosin antibody fragments are more sensitive and specific imaging agents, but scintigraphy must be performed 24 and 48 hours postinjection, so this test has limited clinical utility in the diagnosis of acute myocardial infarction.

Scintigraphy with thallium-201 or the newer technetium-based perfusion tracers will demonstrate "cold spots" in regions of diminished perfusion, which usually represent infarction when the radio-tracer is administered at rest, but abnormalities do not distinguish recent from old damage.

Radionuclide angiography demonstrates akinesis or dyskinesis in areas of infarction and also measures ejection fraction, which can be valuable. Right ventricular dysfunction may indicate infarction of this chamber.

H. Hemodynamic Measurements

These can be invaluable in managing the complicated patient. Their use is described below and in Table 10–3.

Myocardial infarction redefined—a consensus document of The Joint European Society of Cardiology/American College of Cardiology Committee for the redefinition of myocardial infarction. J Am Coll Cardiol 2000;36:959. [PMID: 10987628] (Consensus statement redefining myocardial infarction in the light of new serum tests and with emphasis on implications for prognosis and management.)

Serum marker analysis in acute myocardial infarction. American College of Emergency Physicians. Ann Emerg Med 2000;35:534. [PMID: 10783422] (Use and interpretation of serum markers.)

Sgarbossa EB et al: Electrocardiographic diagnosis of acute myocardial infarction: Current concepts for the clinician. Am Heart J 2001;141:507. [PMID: 11275913]

See also see references following Unstable Angina section.

Treatment

A. Aspirin

All patients with definite or suspected myocardial infarction should receive aspirin at a dose of 162 mg or 325 mg at once regardless of whether thrombolytic therapy is being considered or the patient has been taking aspirin. Chewable aspirin provides more rapid blood levels. Patients with a definite aspirin allergy may be treated with clopidogrel 300 mg, though the onset of its effectiveness will be slower.

B. Thrombolytic Therapy

Thrombolytic therapy reduces mortality and limits infarct size in patients with acute myocardial infarction associated with ST segment elevation (defined as ≥ 0.1 mV in two inferior or lateral leads or two contiguous precordial leads), or with new-onset LBBB. The greatest benefit occurs if treatment is initiated within the first 3 hours, when a 50% or greater reduction in mortality rate can be achieved. The magnitude of benefit declines rapidly thereafter, but a 10% relative mortality reduction can be achieved up to 12 hours after the

Table 10–3. Hemodynamic subsets in acute myocardial infarction.

Category	CI or SWI	PCWP	Treatment	Comment
Normal	> 2.2, < 30	< 15	None	Mortality rate < 5%.
Hyperdynamic	> 3.0, > 40	< 15	Beta-blockers	Characterized by tachycardia; mortality rate < 5%.
Hypovolemic	< 2.5, < 30	< 10	Volume expansion	Hypotension, tachycardia, but preserved left ventricular function by echocardiography; mortality rate 4–8%.
Left ventricular failure	< 2.2, < 30	> 15	Diuretics	Mild dyspnea, rales, normal blood pressure; mortality rate 10–20%.
Severe failure	< 2.0, < 20	> 18	Diuretics, vasodilators	Pulmonary edema, mild hypotension; inotropic agents, IABC may be required; mortality rate 20–40%.
Shock	< 1.8, < 30	> 20	Inotropic agents, IABC	IABC early unless rapid reversal occurs; mortality rate > 60%.

CI = cardiac index (L/min/m^2); SWI = stroke work index (g-m/m^2, calculated as [mean arterial pressure – PCWP] × stroke volume index × 0.0136); PCWP = pulmonary capillary wedge pressure (in mm Hg; pulmonary artery diastolic pressure may be used instead); IABC = intra-aortic balloon counterpulsation.

onset of chest pain. The survival benefit is greatest in patients with large—usually anterior—infarctions. Patients without ST-segment elevation (previously labeled "non-Q wave" infarctions) generally have incomplete or partially recanalized occlusions and have not benefited from thrombolysis. Thrombolytic therapy has also not been shown to improve the prognosis of patients with prior coronary artery bypass grafting, presumably because it is ineffective in opening bypass grafts.

Major bleeding complications occur in 0.5–5% of patients, the most serious of which is intracranial hemorrhage. The major risk factors for intracranial bleeding are age over 65 years, hypertension at presentation, low body weight (< 70 kg), and the use of clot-specific thrombolytic agents (t-PA, reteplase, tenecteplase). Although patients over age 75 have a much higher mortality rate with acute myocardial infarction and, therefore, potentially greater benefit, the risk of severe bleeding is also much higher and the net benefit is less clear. Patients presenting more than 12 hours after the onset of chest pain may also derive a small benefit, particularly if pain and ST segment elevation persist, but rarely does this benefit outweigh the attendant risk.

Therefore, the current recommendation is to administer thrombolytic therapy to patients with ST segment elevation infarctions who are under 75 years of age and present within 6–12 hours of the onset of symptoms. Contraindications include previous hemorrhagic stroke, other strokes, or cerebrovascular events within 1 year, known intracranial neoplasm, current blood pressure > 180 mm Hg systolic or 110 mm Hg diastolic, active internal bleeding (excluding menstruation), or suspected aortic dissection. Relative contraindications are blood pressure > 180/110 mm Hg at presentation, other intracerebral pathology not listed above as a contraindication, known bleeding diathesis, trauma within 2–4 weeks, major surgery within 3 weeks, prolonged (> 10 minutes) or traumatic cardiopulmonary resuscitation, recent (within 2–4 weeks) internal bleeding, noncompressible vascular punctures, active diabetic retinopathy, pregnancy, active peptic ulcer disease, a history of severe hypertension, current use of anticoagulants (INR > 2.0–3.0), and prior allergic reaction or exposure within 2 years to streptokinase or anistreplase.

Five thrombolytic agents are available for acute myocardial infarction and are characterized in Table 10–4.

Streptokinase was the first thrombolytic agent to be extensively evaluated. It is less clot-specific and has subsequently proved to produce rapid but less effective coronary artery reopening than the newer agents, although the mortality differences are small. Streptokinase has a tendency to induce sometimes severe hypotension, particularly if infused rapidly. This can be managed by slowing or interrupting the infusion and administering fluids. There is little evidence that adjunctive heparin is beneficial in patients given streptokinase, unlike when it is administered with the more clot-specific agents. Allergic reactions, including anaphylaxis, occur in 1–2% of patients, and this agent should generally not be administered to patients with prior exposure.

Anistreplase (anisolyated plasminogen streptokinase activator complex; APSAC) is a conjugate of streptokinase that is inactive until the anisoyl group is hydrolyzed, which occurs gradually after injection (half-time 90 minutes). Thus, it can be injected as a bolus but will provide continuing thrombolytic activity. Otherwise, it has most of the same features of streptokinase, including the potential to produce allergic reactions and hypotension. Newer agents that can also be administered as boluses have largely supplanted it.

Alteplase (recombinant tissue plasminogen activator; t-PA) is a naturally occurring thrombolytic factor that is theoretically thrombus-specific. In the first GUSTO trial, which compared t-PA with streptokinase, the 30-day mortality rate with t-PA was one absolute percentage point lower (one additional life saved per 100 patients treated), though there was also a small *increase* in the rate of intracranial hemorrhage. An angiographic substudy confirmed a higher 90-minute patency rate and a higher rate of normal (TIMI grade 3) flow in patients. Alteplase has a shorter half-life than streptokinase and is associated with a higher rate of early reocclusion, thus necessitating the concomitant use of intravenous heparin. Alteplase has since become the most widely used thrombolytic therapy in the United States despite its considerably higher price than that of streptokinase.

Two additional clot-specific agents are now available. **Reteplase** is a recombinant plasminogen activator closely related to t-PA. In comparative trials it appears to have efficacy similar to that of alteplase, but it has a longer duration of action and can be administered as two boluses 30 minutes apart. **Tenecteplase** (TNK-t-PA) is a genetically engineered mutant of native t-PA that has reduced plasma clearance, increased fibrin sensitivity, and increased resistance to plasminogen activator inhibitor-1. It can be given as a single weight-adjusted bolus. In a large comparative trial, this agent was quite comparable to t-PA with regard to both efficacy and safety.

Selection of a thrombolytic agent: Although there continues to be heated discussion about which agent to use, the relatively small differences in efficacy between them are minor compared with the potential benefit of treating a greater proportion of appropriate candidates in a more prompt manner. The principal objective should be to administer a thrombolytic agent within 30 minutes of presentation—or even during transport. The evidence does suggest that the clot-specific agents (alteplase, reteplase, and tenecteplase) are marginally more effective than streptokinase, and thus they are generally favored by most cardiologists. These agents do produce slightly higher rates of intracranial bleeding and require intravenous coadministration of

Table 10–4. Thrombolytic therapy for acute myocardial infarction.

	Streptokinase	Alteplase; Tissue Plasminogen Activator (t-PA)	Reteplase	Tenecteplase (TNK-t-PA)
Source	Group C streptococcus	Recombinant DNA	Recombinant DNA	Recombinant DNA
Half-life	20 minutes	5 minutes	15 minutes	20 minutes
Usual dose	1.5 million units	100 mg	20 units	40 mg
Administration	750,000 units over 20 minutes followed by 750,000 units over 40 minutes	Initial bolus of 15 mg, followed by 50 mg infused over next 30 minutes and 35 mg over the following 60 minutes	10 units as a bolus over 2 minutes, repeated after 30 minutes	Single bolus weight-adjusted 0.5 mg/kg
Anticoagulation after infusion	Aspirin, 325 mg daily. There is no evidence that adjunctive heparin improves outcome following streptokinase.	Aspirin, 325 mg daily. Heparin, 5000 units as bolus, followed by 1000 units per hour infusion, subsequently adjusted to maintain PTT 1½–2 times control.	Aspirin, 325 mg; heparin as with t-PA	Aspirin 325 mg daily
Clot selectivity	Low	High	High	High
Fibrinogenolysis	+++	+	+	+
Bleeding	+	+	+	+
Hypotension	+++	+	+	+
Allergic reactions	++	0	0	+
Reocclusion	5–20%	10–30%	—	5–20%
Approximate cost[1]	$567.65	$2750.00	$2750.00	$2750.00

[1]Cost to pharmacist (average wholesale price, generic when possible) for quantity listed. Source: *Drug Topics Red Book*, March 2002; Vol. 21, No.3.

heparin, which also increases bleeding risk. As a result, streptokinase may be preferable in patients at higher risk of this complication, particularly older patients with elevated blood pressures. Streptokinase and anistreplase should be avoided in patients with previous allergic reactions or recent exposure to either. Because of their potential for substantially lowering blood pressure, they should also be avoided in patients who present with hypotension. The ability to administer tenecteplase as a single bolus is an attractive feature that may facilitate earlier treatment. The combination of reduced-dose thrombolytic given with a platelet glycoprotein IIb/IIa antagonist is under investigation.

Postthrombolytic management: After completion of the thrombolytic infusion, aspirin should be continued. Anticoagulation with intravenous heparin (60 units/kg bolus to a maximum of 4000 units, followed by an infusion of 12 units/kg/min adjusted to maintain an aPTT of 50–75 seconds) is continued for at least 24 hours after alteplase, reteplase, or tenecteplase but is optional in patients receiving streptokinase. Pro-

phylactic treatment with antacids and an H_2 blocker is indicated.

Reperfusion rates of 40–80% can be expected, determined primarily by the interval between onset of the infarction and treatment. Reperfusion is recognized clinically by the abrupt cessation of pain, the occurrence of ventricular arrhythmias (most characteristically accelerated idioventricular rhythm), the rapid evolution of the ECG to Q waves, and an early peak of CK (by 12 hours); however, all of these signs may be misleading. Even with anticoagulation, 10–20% of reperfused vessels will reocclude during hospitalization. This is usually recognized by the recurrence of pain and ST segment elevation and is treated by readministration of a thrombolytic agent or immediate angiography and PTCA.

The optimal management of myocardial infarction after thrombolysis is controversial but has been clarified considerably by the TIMI 2 trial. Patients with recurrent ischemic pain prior to discharge should undergo catheterization and, if indicated, revascularization. Asymptomatic, clinically stable patients should undergo predischarge evaluation to determine whether residual jeopardized myocardium is present. This can be accomplished by submaximal exercise or pharmacologic stress scintigraphy. Those with significantly positive tests or a low threshold for symptomatic ischemia should undergo angiography and revascularization where feasible. Patients with negative tests have an excellent prognosis without intervention, though they may require revascularization for symptoms at a later time.

C. Acute PTCA and Stenting for ST Segment Elevation Myocardial Infarction

Immediate coronary angiography and PTCA or stenting of the infarct-related artery is an increasingly utilized alternative to thrombolysis. It is the approach of choice in patients with absolute and many relative contraindications to thrombolytic therapy. The results of this approach in specialized centers are excellent, exceeding those obtainable by thrombolytic therapy even in good candidates, but this experience may not be generalizable to centers and operators with less experience or expertise. Stenting—in conjunction with platelet glycoprotein IIb/IIIa antagonists—is now widely used in acute myocardial infarction patients. In the subgroup of patients with cardiogenic shock, early catheterization and percutaneous or surgical revascularization is the preferred management, because thrombolysis has not improved their dismal prognosis. Because an acute interventional approach carries a lower risk of hemorrhagic complications, it may also be the preferred strategy in older patients.

D. Initial Management of Non-ST-Segment Elevation Myocardial Infarction

Patients presenting with an acute myocardial infarction without ST segment elevation or evolving Q waves generally do not have persistent thrombotic coronary occlusions (with the exception of LBBB or anterior ST segment depressions that may represent reciprocal changes from a true posterior infarction). Thrombolytic therapy is not appropriate in these patients, and in general their management should be similar to that of patients with unstable angina, who usually have the same underlying pathophysiology. This is described in the previous section, and includes aspirin, heparin, platelet glycoprotein IIb/IIIa antagonists, beta-blockers, and nitrates. As is the case with unstable angina, controversy continues over whether there is an advantage to a routine strategy of early coronary angiography, but patients with continuing or recurrent ischemia or very positive stress tests should undergo angiography and revascularization when appropriate.

E. General Measures

CCU monitoring should be instituted as soon as possible. Uncomplicated patients can be transferred to a telemetry unit after 24–48 hours. Activity should initially be limited to bed rest but can be advanced within 24 hours. Progressive ambulation should be started after 24–72 hours if tolerated. Low-flow oxygen therapy (2–4 L/min) should be given if oxygen saturation is reduced.

F. Analgesia

An initial attempt should be made to relieve pain with sublingual nitroglycerin. However, if no response occurs after two or three tablets, intravenous opioids provide the most rapid and effective analgesia and may also reduce pulmonary congestion. Morphine sulfate, 4–8 mg, or meperidine, 50–75 mg, should be given. Subsequent small doses can be given every 15 minutes until pain abates.

G. Beta-Adrenergic Blocking Agents

Several studies have shown modestly improved short-term survival when intravenous beta-blockers (metoprolol, 5 mg intravenously every 5 minutes for three doses) are given immediately after acute myocardial infarction. These agents reduce the duration of ischemic pain and the incidence of ventricular fibrillation. A favorable effect appears to persist even after thrombolytic therapy. Beta-blockade should be avoided in patients with decompensated heart failure, asthma, or high degrees of atrioventricular block.

H. Nitrates

Nitroglycerin is the agent of choice for recurrent ischemic pain and is useful in lowering blood pressure or relieving pulmonary congestion. However, routine nitrate administration is not recommended, since no improvement in outcome has been observed in the ISIS-4 or GISSI-3 trials, in which a total of over 70,000 patients were randomized to nitrate treatment or placebo.

I. Angiotensin-Converting Enzyme (ACE) Inhibitors

A series of trials (SAVE, AIRE, SMILE, TRACE, GISSI-III, and ISIS-IV) have shown both short- and long-term improvement in survival with ACE inhibitor therapy. The benefits are greatest in patients with low ejection fractions, large infarctions, or clinical evidence of heart failure, and only these patients should receive chronic ACE inhibitor therapy for postinfarction indications. Acute short-term treatment may improve survival in a broader group of patients, but this is uncertain. Treatment should be commenced carefully in the first postinfarction day if the patient is not hypotensive. When there is no evidence of heart failure or when a very large infarction is not present, ACE inhibitors should be considered only after the administration of thrombolytic therapy, aspirin, beta-blockers, and, if the patient has evidence of continuing ischemia, nitrates.

J. Antiarrhythmic Prophylaxis

The incidence of ventricular fibrillation in hospitalized patients is approximately 5%, with 80% of episodes occurring in the first 12–24 hours. Prophylactic lidocaine infusions (1–2 mg/min) prevent most episodes, but this therapy has not reduced the mortality rate and it increases the risk of asystole, so this approach is no longer recommended except in patients with nonsustained ventricular tachycardia. Intravenous magnesium sulfate has been effective in one study, but ISIS-4 did not report a benefit with routine magnesium administration.

K. CALCIUM CHANNEL BLOCKERS

There are no studies to support the use of calcium channel blockers in most acute myocardial infarction patients—and indeed, they have the potential to exacerbate ischemia and cause death from reflex tachycardia or myocardial depression. One exception is that diltiazem and verapamil appear to prevent reinfarction and ischemia in the subset of patients with non-Q wave infarction. Diltiazam is preferable because it causes less myocardial depression. The dosage is 240–360 mg daily. Otherwise, long-acting calcium channel blockers should be reserved for management of hypertension or ischemia as second- or third-line drugs after beta-blockers and nitrates.

L. ANTICOAGULATION

With the exception of patients undergoing thrombolysis and subsequent heparin therapy, the use of full anticoagulation in the acute setting remains controversial. Patients who will be at bed rest or on limited activity status for some time should be given prophylaxis for deep vein thrombosis (5000 units of heparin subcutaneously every 12 hours) unless contraindicated. Aspirin, 325 mg daily, should be continued also unless contraindicated.

Armstrong PW et al: Fibrinolysis for acute myocardial infarction: current status and new horizons for pharmacological reperfusion, part 1. Circulation 2001;103:2862. [PMID: 11401946] (Reviews history as well as various agents for fibrinolysis.)

Armstrong PW et al: Fibrinolysis for acute myocardial infarction: current status and new horizons for pharmacological reperfusion, part 2. Circulation 2001;103:2987. [PMID: 11413091] (Reviews ancillary therapies, indications, and risks as well as future directions.)

Califf RM: Combination therapy for acute myocardial infarction: fibrinolytic therapy and glycoprotein IIb/IIIa inhibition. Am Heart J 2000;139:S33. [PMID: 10650314] (Discusses current status of combination fibrinolysis with IIb/IIIa inhibitors.)

Efficacy and safety of tenecteplase in combination with enoxaparin, abciximab, or unfractionated heparin: the ASSENT-3 randomised trial in acute myocardial infarction. Lancet 2001;358:605. [PMID: 11530146] (A study of 6095 patients with acute MI demonstrated fewer ischemic endpoints with tenecteplase and either enoxaparin or abciximab than with tenecteplase and unfractionated heparin.)

Llevadot J et al: Bolus fibrinolytic therapy in acute myocardial infarction. JAMA 2001;286:442. [PMID: 11466123] (Bolus thrombolytics are as safe and effective as accelerated TPA but more convenient to administer.)

Miller WL et al: Adjunctive therapies in the treatment of acute coronary syndromes. Mayo Clin Proc 2001;76:391. [PMID: 11322355] (Current knowledge supporting adjunctive and emerging strategies in acute coronary syndromes focuses on aspirin, beta blockers, ACE inhibitors, and statins.)

Montalescot G et al: Platelet glycoprotein IIb/IIIa inhibition with coronary stenting for acute myocardial infarction. N Engl J Med 2001;344:1895. [PMID: 11419426] (Addition of abciximab to stenting in patients with acute myocardial infarction improves procedural and clinical outcome.)

Ryan TJ: Percutaneous coronary intervention in ST-elevation myocardial infarction. Curr Cardiol Rep 2001;3:273. [PMID: 11406084]

Thiemann DR et al: Lack of benefit for intravenous thrombolysis in patients with myocardial infarction who are older than 75 years. Circulation 2000;101:2239. [PMID: 10811589] (In a retrospective cohort study, thrombolytic therapy in patients aged 76–86 years was associated with a survival disadvantage.)

Topol EJ: Acute myocardial infarction: thrombolysis. Heart 2000;83:122. [PMID: 10618353]

Zahn R et al: Primary angioplasty versus intravenous thrombolysis in acute myocardial infarction: Can we define subgroups of patients benefiting most from primary angioplasty? J Am Coll Cardiol 2001;37:1827. [PMID: 11401118] (Pooled registry of almost 10,000 patients demonstrates benefit of primary angioplasty over thrombolysis in patients with acute myocardial infarction.)

Complications

A variety of complications can occur after myocardial infarction even when treatment is initiated promptly.

A. POSTINFARCTION ISCHEMIA

Approximately 30% of patients will have angina postinfarction. This is more common in patients with angina prior to infarction and in non-ST segment elevation infarction. Postinfarction angina is associated with increased short- and long-term mortality. The underlying mechanism is usually inadequate blood flow through a recanalized vessel or reocclusion. Vigorous medical therapy should be instituted, including nitrates and beta-blockers as well as aspirin, heparin, and platelet glycoprotein IIb/IIIa antagonists. Most patients with postinfarction angina—and all who are refractory to medical therapy—should undergo early catheterization and revascularization by PTCA or CABG.

B. ARRHYTHMIAS

Abnormalities of rhythm and conduction are common.

1. Sinus bradycardia—This is most common in inferior infarctions or may be precipitated by medications. Observation or withdrawal of the offending agent is usually sufficient. If accompanied by signs of low cardiac output, atropine, 0.5–1 mg intravenously, is usually effective. Temporary pacing is rarely required.

2. Supraventricular tachyarrhythmias—Sinus tachycardia is common and may reflect either increased adrenergic stimulation or hemodynamic compromise due to hypovolemia or pump failure. In the latter, beta blockade is contraindicated. Supraventricular premature beats are common and may be premonitory for atrial fibrillation. Electrolyte abnormalities and hypoxia should be corrected and causative agents (especially aminophylline) stopped. Atrial fibrillation should be rapidly controlled or converted to sinus rhythm. Intravenous beta-blockers such as metoprolol (2.5–5 mg/h) or short-acting esmolol (50–200 μg/kg/min) are the agents of choice if cardiac function is adequate. Intravenous diltiazem (5–15 mg/h) may be used if beta-blockers are contraindicated or ineffective. Digoxin (0.5 mg as initial dose, then 0.25 mg every 90–120 minutes [up to 1–1.25 mg] for a loading dose, followed by 0.25 mg daily if renal function is normal) is preferable if heart failure is present with atrial fibrillation, but the onset of action is delayed. Electrical cardioversion (commencing with 100 J) may be necessary if atrial fibrillation is complicated by hypotension, heart failure, or ischemia, but the arrhythmia often recurs. A short course of a class Ia agent such as procainamide or quinidine may be required in addition to digoxin, a beta-blocker, or a calcium channel blocker to maintain sinus rhythm. Amiodarone (150 mg intravenous bolus and then 15–30 mg/h intravenously, or rapid oral loading with 400 mg three times daily) may be helpful to restore or maintain sinus rhythm.

3. Ventricular arrhythmias—Ventricular arrhythmias are most common in the first few hours after infarction. Ventricular premature beats may be premonitory for ventricular tachycardia or fibrillation but generally should not be treated in the absence of nonsustained ventricular tachycardia (usually more than six consecutive beats). In the latter case, prophylactic lidocaine has been shown to prevent subsequent sustained ventricular tachycardia or fibrillation but does not improve survival in patients who are being monitored. Prophylactic lidocaine may be started as a 1 mg/kg bolus followed by an infusion of 2 mg/min. Toxicity (tremor, anxiety, confusion, seizures) is common, especially in older patients and those with hypotension, heart failure, or liver disease.

Ventricular tachycardia should be treated with a 1 mg/kg bolus of lidocaine if the patient is stable or by electrical cardioversion (100–200 J) if not. If the arrhythmia cannot be suppressed with lidocaine, procainamide (100 mg boluses over 1–2 minutes every 5 minutes to a cumulative dose of 750–1000 mg), or intravenous amiodarone (150 mg over 10 minutes, which may be repeated as needed, followed by 360 mg over 6 hours and then 540 mg over 18 hours) should be initiated, followed by an infusion of 20–80 mg/kg/min. Ventricular fibrillation is treated electrically (300–400 J). Unresponsive ventricular fibrillation should be treated with additional amiodarone and repeat cardioversion while CPR is administered.

Accelerated idioventricular rhythm is a regular, wide complex rhythm at a rate of 70–100/min. It often follows reperfusion and usually does not require specific therapy.

4. Conduction disturbances—All degrees of atrioventricular block may occur in the course of acute myocardial infarction. Block at the level of the atrioventricular node is more common than infranodal block and occurs in approximately 20% of inferior myocardial infarctions. First-degree block is the most common and requires no treatment. Second-degree block is usually of the Mobitz type I form (Wenckebach), is often transient, and requires treatment only if associated with a heart rate slow enough to cause symptoms. Complete atrioventricular block occurs in up to 5% of acute inferior infarctions, usually is preceded by Mobitz I second-degree block, and generally resolves spontaneously, though it may persist for hours to several weeks. The escape rhythm originates in the distal atrioventricular node or atrioventricular junction and hence has a narrow QRS complex and is reliable, albeit often slow (30–50 beats/min). Treatment is often necessary because of resulting hypotension and low cardiac output. Intravenous atropine (1 mg) usually restores atrioventricular conduction temporarily, but if the escape complex is wide or if repeated atropine treatments are needed, temporary ventricular pacing is indicated. The prognosis for these patients is only slightly worse than that of patients who do not develop atrioventricular block.

In anterior infarctions, the site of block is distal, below the atrioventricular node, and usually a result of extensive damage of the His-Purkinje system and bundle branches. New first-degree block (prolongation of the PR interval) is unusual in anterior infarction; Mobitz type II atrioventricular block or complete heart block may be preceded by intraventricular conduction defects or may occur abruptly. The escape rhythm, if present at all, is an unreliable wide-complex idioventricular rhythm. Urgent ventricular pacing is mandatory, but even with successful pacing, morbidity and mortality are high because of the extensive myocardial damage. New conduction abnormalities such as right or left bundle branch block or fascicular blocks may presage progression, often sudden, to second- or third-degree atrioventricular block. Temporary ventricular pacing is recommended for new-onset alternating bilateral bundle branch block, bifascicular block, or bundle branch block with worsening first-degree atrioventricular block. Patients with anterior infarction who progress to second- or third-degree block even transiently should be considered for insertion of a prophylactic permanent ventricular pacemaker before discharge.

C. MYOCARDIAL DYSFUNCTION

The severity of cardiac dysfunction is proportionate to the extent of myocardial necrosis but is exacerbated by preexisting dysfunction and ongoing ischemia. Patients who have normal blood pressure, no signs of heart failure, and normal urine output have a good prognosis. Those with hypotension or evidence of more than mild heart failure should have bedside right heart catheterization and continuous measurements of arterial pressure. These measurements permit the accurate assessment of cardiac function, facilitate the correct choice of therapy, and provide important prognostic information. Table 10–3 categorizes patients based upon these hemodynamic findings.

1. Acute left ventricular failure—Basilar rales are common in acute myocardial infarction, but dyspnea, more diffuse rales, and arterial hypoxemia usually indicate left ventricular failure. Since both the physical examination and chest x-ray correlate poorly with hemodynamic measurements and since the central venous pressure does not correlate with the pulmonary capillary wedge pressure (PCWP), right heart catheterization may be essential in monitoring therapy. General measures include supplemental oxygen to increase arterial saturation to above 95% and elevation of the trunk. Diuretics are usually the initial therapy unless right ventricular infarction is present. Intravenous furosemide (10–40 mg) or bumetanide (0.5–1 mg) is preferred because of the reliably rapid onset and short duration of action of these drugs. Higher dosages can be given if an inadequate response occurs. Morphine sulfate (4 mg intravenously followed by increments of 2 mg) is valuable in acute pulmonary edema.

Diuretics are usually effective; however, since most patients with acute infarction are not volume overloaded, the hemodynamic response may be limited and may be associated with hypotension. Vasodilators will reduce PCWP and improve cardiac output by a combination of venodilation (increasing venous capacitance) and arteriolar dilation (reducing afterload and left ventricular wall stress). In mild heart failure, sublingual isosorbide dinitrate (2.5–10 mg every 2 hours) or nitroglycerin ointment (6.25–25 mg every 4 hours) may be adequate to lower PCWP. In more severe failure, especially if cardiac output is reduced, sodium nitroprusside is the preferred agent. It should be initiated only with hemodynamic monitoring; the initial dosage should be low (0.25 µg/kg/min) to avoid excessive hypotension, but the dosage can be increased by increments of 0.5 µg/kg/min every 5–10 minutes up to 5–10 µg/kg/min until the desired hemodynamic response (PCWP < 18 mm Hg, CI > 2.5) is obtained. Excessive hypotension (mean blood pressure < 65–75 mm Hg) or tachycardia (> 10/min increase) should be avoided. Combination of nitroprusside with inotropic agents may be necessary to preserve blood pressure or maximize benefit.

Intravenous nitroglycerin (starting at 10 µg/min) is usually less effective but may lower PCWP with less hypotension. Oral or transdermal vasodilator therapy with nitrates or angiotensin-converting enzyme inhibitors is often necessary after the initial 24–48 hours (see below).

Inotropic agents should be avoided if possible, because they often increase heart rate and myocardial oxygen requirements. Dobutamine has the best hemodynamic profile, increasing cardiac output and modestly lowering PCWP, usually without excessive tachycardia, hypotension, or arrhythmias. The initial dosage is 2.5 µg/kg/min, and it may be increased by similar increments up to 15–20 µg/kg/min at intervals of 5–10 minutes. Dopamine is more useful in the presence of hypotension (see below), since it produces peripheral vasoconstriction, but it has a less beneficial effect on PCWP. Amrinone is a positive inotrope and vasodilator that produces hemodynamic effects similar to those of dobutamine but with a greater decrease in PCWP. However, its longer duration of action makes it less useful in unstable situations. Milrinone is a more potent and newer congener of amrinone with fewer side effects. It should be commenced in a loading dose of 50 µg/kg over 10 minutes, followed by an infusion of 0.375–0.75 µg/kg/min. Digoxin has not been helpful in acute infarction except to control the ventricular response in atrial fibrillation, but it may be beneficial if chronic heart failure persists.

2. Hypotension and shock—Patients with hypotension (systolic blood pressure < 100 mm Hg, individualized depending on prior blood pressure) and signs of diminished perfusion (low urine output, confusion, cold extremities) should be hemodynamically monitored. Up to 20% will have findings indicative of intravascular hypovolemia (due to diaphoresis, vomiting, decreased venous tone, medications—such as diuretics, nitrates, morphine, beta-blockers, calcium channel blockers, and thrombolytic agents—and lack of oral intake). These should be treated with successive boluses of 100 mL of normal saline until PCWP reaches 15–18 mm Hg to determine whether cardiac output and blood pressure respond. Pericardial tamponade due to hemorrhagic pericarditis (especially after thrombolytic therapy or cardiopulmonary resuscitation) or ventricular rupture should be considered and excluded by echocardiography if clinically indicated. Right ventricular infarction, characterized by a normal PCWP but elevated right atrial pressure, can produce hypotension. This is discussed below.

Most hypotensive patients will have moderate to severe left ventricular dysfunction; pathologic studies indicate that more than 20% of the left ventricle is infarcted (> 40% in cardiogenic shock). If hypotension is only modest (systolic pressure > 90 mm Hg) and the PCWP is elevated, diuretics and an initial trial of nitroprusside (see above for dosing) are indicated. If the blood pressure falls, inotropic support will need to be added or substituted. Such patients may also be treated with intra-aortic balloon counterpulsation (IABC). This device unloads the left ventricle during systole and increases diastolic coronary artery filling pressure. It often facilitates the use of vasodilators in patients who previously did not tolerate them.

Dopamine is the most appropriate pressor for cardiogenic hypotension. It should be initiated at a rate of 2–4 µg/kg/min and increased at 5-minute intervals to the appropriate hemodynamic end point. At low dosages (< 5 µg/kg/min), it improves renal blood flow; at intermediate dosages (2.5–10 µg/kg/min), it stimulates myocardial contractility; at higher dosages (> 8 μg/kg/min), it is a potent α_1-adrenergic agonist. In general, blood pressure and cardiac index rise, but PCWP does not fall. Dopamine may be combined with nitroprusside or dobutamine (see above for dosing), or the latter may be used in its place if hypotension is not severe. Amrinone and milrinone have hemodynamic effects similar to those of dobutamine, but their longer duration of action precludes rapid dosage adjustment. Norepinephrine (0.1–0.5 μg/kg/min) is the usual pressor of last resort, since isoproterenol and epinephrine produce less vasoconstriction, do not increase coronary perfusion pressure (aortic diastolic pressure), and both tend to worsen the balance between myocardial oxygen delivery and utilization.

Patients with cardiogenic shock not due to hypovolemia have a poor prognosis, with 30-day mortality rates of 50–80%. If they do not respond rapidly, IABC should be instituted. Surgically implanted ventricular assist devices may be used in extreme cases. Early cardiac catheterization and coronary angiography followed by percutaneous or surgical revascularization offer the best chance of survival, particularly in patients under 75 years of age.

D. RIGHT VENTRICULAR INFARCTION

Right ventricular infarction is present in one-third of patients with inferior wall infarction but is clinically significant in less than 50% of these. It presents as hypotension with relatively preserved left ventricular function and should be considered whenever patients with inferior infarction exhibit signs of low cardiac output and raised venous pressure. Hypotension is often exacerbated by medications that decrease intravascular volume or produce venodilation, such as diuretics, nitrates, and narcotics. Right atrial pressure and jugular venous pulsations are high, while PCWP is normal or low and the lungs are clear. The diagnosis is suggested by ST segment elevation in right-sided anterior chest leads. The diagnosis can be confirmed by echocardiography or hemodynamic measurements. When hypotension is present, hemodynamic measurements are necessary to monitor therapy. Treatment consists of fluid loading to improve left ventricular filling; inotropic agents may also be useful.

E. MECHANICAL DEFECTS

Partial or complete rupture of a papillary muscle or of the interventricular septum occurs in less than 1% of acute myocardial infarctions and carries a poor prognosis. These complications occur in both anterior and inferior infarctions, usually 3–7 days after the acute event. They are detected by the appearance of a new systolic murmur and clinical deterioration, often with pulmonary edema. The two lesions are distinguished by the location of the murmur (apical versus parasternal) and by Doppler echocardiography. Hemodynamic monitoring is essential for appropriate management and demonstrates an increase in oxygen saturation between the right atrium and pulmonary artery in ventricular septal defect and, often, a large v

wave with mitral regurgitation. Treatment by nitroprusside and, preferably, IABC reduces the regurgitation or shunt, but surgical correction is mandatory. In patients remaining hemodynamically unstable or requiring continuous parenteral pharmacologic treatment or counterpulsation, early surgery is recommended, though mortality rates are high (15% to nearly 100%, depending on residual ventricular function and clinical status). Patients who are stabilized medically can have delayed surgery with lower risks (10–25%).

F. MYOCARDIAL RUPTURE

Complete rupture of the left ventricular free wall occurs in less than 1% of patients and usually results in immediate death. It occurs 2–7 days postinfarction, usually involves the anterior wall, and is more frequent in older women. Incomplete or gradual rupture may be sealed off by the pericardium, creating a **pseudoaneurysm.** This may be recognized by echocardiography, radionuclide angiography, or left ventricular angiography, often as an incidental finding. It demonstrates a narrow-neck connection to the left ventricle. Early surgical repair is indicated, since delayed rupture is common.

G. LEFT VENTRICULAR ANEURYSM

Ten to 20 percent of patients surviving an acute infarction develop a left ventricular aneurysm, a sharply delineated area of scar that bulges paradoxically during systole. This usually follows anterior Q wave infarctions. Aneurysms are recognized by persistent ST segment elevation (beyond 4–8 weeks), and a wide neck from the left ventricle can be demonstrated by echocardiography, scintigraphy, or contrast angiography. They rarely rupture but may be associated with arterial emboli, ventricular arrhythmias, and congestive heart failure. Surgical resection may be performed for these indications if other measures fail. The best results (mortality rates of 10–20%) are obtained when the residual myocardium contracts well and when significant coronary lesions supplying adjacent regions are bypassed.

H. PERICARDITIS

The pericardium is involved in approximately 50% of infarctions, but pericarditis is often not clinically significant. Twenty percent of patients with Q wave infarctions will have an audible friction rub if examined repetitively. Pericardial pain occurs in approximately the same proportion after 2–7 days and is recognized by its variation with respiration and position (improved by sitting). Often, no treatment is required, but aspirin (650 mg every 4–6 hours) or indomethacin (25 mg three or four times daily) will usually relieve the pain. Anticoagulation should be avoided, since hemorrhagic pericarditis may result.

From 1 to 12 weeks after infarction, Dressler's syndrome (post-myocardial infarction syndrome) occurs in less than 5% of patients. This is an autoimmune phenomenon and presents as pericarditis with associated fever, leukocytosis, and, occasionally, pericardial or pleural effusion. It may recur over months. Treatment is the same as for other forms of pericarditis. A short course of corticosteroids may help if nonsteroidal agents do not relieve symptoms.

I. MURAL THROMBUS

Mural thrombi are common in large anterior infarctions but not in infarctions at other locations. Arterial emboli occur in approximately 2% of patients with known infarction, usually within 6 weeks. Anticoagulation with heparin followed by short-term (3-month) warfarin therapy prevents most emboli and should be considered in all patients with large anterior infarctions. Mural thrombi can be detected by echocardiography or CT scan (MRI has yielded frequent false-positive results) but with only moderate reliability, and only a small percentage (up to 25%) embolize, so these procedures should not be relied upon for determining the need for anticoagulation.

Crenshaw BS et al: Risk factors, angiographic patterns, and outcomes in patients with ventricular septal defect complicating acute myocardial infarction. Circulation 2000;101:27. [PMID: 10618300] (Although this complication appears less common in patients treated with thrombolysis, it continues to have a high mortality rate.)

Haji SA et al: Right ventricular infarction—diagnosis and treatment. Clin Cardiol 2000;23:473. [PMID: 1089443]

Hasdai D et al: Cardiogenic shock complicating acute coronary syndromes. Lancet 2000;356:749. [PMID: 11085707] (Review that includes unstable angina and non-Q wave myocardial infarction.)

Hochman JS et al: Early revascularization in acute myocardial infarction complicated by cardiogenic shock. SHOCK Investigators. Should We Emergently Revascularize Occluded Coronaries for Cardiogenic Shock. N Engl J Med 1999;341:625. [PMID: 10460813] (In this trial, 152 patients with myocardial infarction and cardiogenic shock were randomized to early revascularization or initial medical stabilization prior to revascularization. There was a trend toward improved survival in the early revascularization group at 30 days, which was significant at 6 months in patients under 75 years of age. In patients 75 or older, there was a strong trend toward poorer outcomes with revascularization.)

Mangrum JM: Tachyarrhythmias associated with acute myocardial infarction. Emerg Med Clin North Am 2001;19:385. [PMID: 11373985]

Mehta SR et al: Impact of right ventricular involvement of mortality and morbidity in patients with inferior myocardial infarction. J Am Coll Cardiol 2001;37:37. [PMID: 11153770] (More than threefold increase in death, shock, and arrhythmia when patients with inferior myocardial infarction have right ventricular involvement.)

Prieto A et al: Nonarrhythmic complications of acute myocardial infarction. Emerg Med Clin North Am 2001;19:397. [PMID: 11373986] (Review. Includes right ventricular infarction.)

Rathore SS et al: Acute myocardial infarction complicated by heart block in the elderly: prevalence and outcomes. Am Heart J 2001;141:47. [PMID: 11136486] (Trial demonstrating that heart block is a common complication of MI in elderly patients.)

Sayer JW et al: Prognostic implications of ventricular fibrillation in acute myocardial infarction: new strategies required for mortality reduction. Heart 2000;84:258. [PMID: 10956285] (Most episodes occurred early after admission and were associated with increased early mortality, but survivors did not have a worse long-term prognosis.)

Postinfarction Management

Twenty percent of patients with acute myocardial infarction die before they reach the hospital. Mortality rates in hospitalized patients range from 5% to 15% and are determined chiefly by the size of the infarction and the age and general condition of the patient. Patients developing heart failure or hypotension have high early mortality rates. Several classification criteria have been developed to estimate early prognosis for survival. The most accurate is hemodynamic subsetting (Table 10–3). The prognosis after discharge is determined by three major factors: the degree of left ventricular dysfunction, the extent of residual ischemic myocardium, and the presence of ventricular arrhythmias. The mortality rate in the first year after discharge is approximately 6–8%, with over half of deaths occurring in the first 3 months, chiefly in patients with postinfarction heart failure. Subsequently, the mortality rate averages 4% per year.

A. RISK STRATIFICATION

A number of findings indicate increased risk after infarction. These include: (1) postinfarction angina; (2) non-Q wave infarction; (3) heart failure; (4) left ventricular ejection fraction less than 40%; (5) stress-induced ischemia, diagnosed by electrocardiography, scintigraphy, or echocardiography; and (6) ventricular ectopy (> 10 VPB/h). Patients with postinfarction angina should undergo coronary arteriography. Authorities differ about which tests should be performed routinely in other patients, but in most a noninvasive assessment of left ventricular function and residual ischemia is appropriate. Significant left ventricular dysfunction is most likely with anterior infarction or multiple infarctions. In such patients, noninvasive assessment of left ventricular function by echocardiography or scintigraphy will help assess prognosis and facilitate medical management. If the ejection fraction is less than 40%, coronary angiography may be indicated, as this is a high-risk subset in which revascularization may improve prognosis. ACE inhibitor therapy is also indicated in patients with reduced ejection fractions. Submaximal exercise or pharmacologic stress testing before discharge or a maximal test after 3–6 weeks (the latter being more sensitive for ischemia) helps patients and physicians plan the return to normal activity. Imaging in conjunction with stress testing adds additional sensitivity for ischemia and provides localizing information. Both exercise and pharmacologic stress imaging have successfully predicted subsequent outcome. One of these tests should usually be employed prior to discharge in patients who have received thrombolytic therapy as a means of selecting appropriate candidates for coronary angiography.

Ambulatory electrocardiographic monitoring for arrhythmias is of less clear value; though it has some prognostic value beyond measurements of left ventricular function, no benefit from antiarrhythmic therapy for asymptomatic patients has been demonstrated. Ischemia detected during ambulatory monitoring is an indicator of poor prognosis, but it is unclear how much additional information is obtained in patients who have also undergone exercise testing or scintigraphic studies. The role of other procedures such as assessment of heart rate variability or baroreceptor testing is uncertain.

A conservative approach to postinfarction evaluation would include measurement of left ventricular function in patients with signs of heart failure or large infarctions and a test for ischemia in patients without recurrent chest pain. The latter should occur before discharge if the patient has undergone thrombolytic therapy but may be delayed for 3–6 weeks in most other patients.

B. Secondary Prevention

Postinfarction management should begin with identification and modification of risk factors. Treatment of hyperlipidemia and smoking cessation both prevent recurrent infarction and death. LDL cholesterol levels should be lowered below 100 mg/dL with drug therapy (usually a statin) commencing prior to discharge. Blood pressure control and exercise are also recommended.

Beta-blockers improve survival rates, primarily by reducing the incidence of sudden death in high-risk subsets of patients, though their value may be less in uncomplicated patients with small infarctions and normal exercise tests. No advantage of one preparation over another has been demonstrated except that those with intrinsic sympathomimetic activity have not proved beneficial in postinfarction patients.

Antiplatelet agents are beneficial; aspirin (325 mg daily) is recommended, but clopidogrel (75 mg daily) is also effective. Warfarin anticoagulation for 3 months reduces the incidence of arterial emboli after large anterior infarctions, and according to the results of at least one study it improves long-term prognosis. An advantage to combining aspirin and warfarin has not been demonstrated except perhaps in patients with atrial fibrillation.

Calcium channel blockers have not been shown to improve prognoses overall and should not be prescribed purely for secondary prevention. Antiarrhythmic therapy other than with beta-blockers has not been shown to be effective except in patients with symptomatic arrhythmias. Amiodarone has been studied in several trials of postinfarct patients with either left ventricular dysfunction or frequent ventricular ectopy. Although survival was not improved, amiodarone was not harmful—unlike other agents in this setting. Therefore it is the agent of choice for individuals with symptomatic postinfarction supraventricular arrhythmias, although emerging data suggest that implantable defibrillators are the preferred option for ventricular arrhythmias.

Cardiac rehabilitation programs and exercise training can be of considerable psychologic benefit, but it is not known whether they alter prognosis.

C. ACE Inhibitors in Patients With Left Ventricular Dysfunction

Patients who sustain substantial myocardial damage often experience subsequent progressive left ventricular dilation and dysfunction, leading to clinical heart failure and reduced long-term survival. In patients with ejection fractions less than 40%, long-term ACE inhibitor therapy prevents left ventricular dilation and the onset of heart failure and prolongs survival. The Heart Outcomes Prevention Evaluation (HOPE) also demonstrated a reduction of approximately 20% in mortality rates and the occurrence of nonfatal myocardial infarction and stroke with ramipril treatment of postinfarction patients without confirmed left ventricular systolic dysfunction. Therefore, ACE inhibitor therapy should be strongly considered in this broader group of patients—and especially in diabetics and patients with even mild systolic hypertension, in whom the greatest benefit was observed.

D. Revascularization

Because of the increasing use of thrombolytic therapy and accumulating experience with PTCA, the indications for revascularization are rapidly evolving. Postinfarction patients who appear likely to benefit from early revascularization if the anatomy is appropriate are (1) those who have undergone thrombolytic therapy and have residual symptoms or laboratory evidence of ischemia; (2) patients with left ventricular dysfunction (ejection fraction < 30–40%) and evidence of ischemia; (3) patients with non-Q wave infarction and evidence of more than mild ischemia; and (4) patients with markedly positive exercise tests and multivessel disease. The value of revascularization in the following groups is less clear: (1) patients treated with thrombolytic agents, with little evidence of reperfusion or residual ischemia; (2) patients with left ventricular dysfunction but no detectable ischemia; and (3) patients with preserved left ventricular function who have mild ischemia and are not symptom-limited. Patients who survive infarctions without complications, have preserved left ventricular function (ejection fraction > 50%), and have no exercise-induced ischemia have an excellent prognosis and do not require invasive evaluation.

Ades PA: Cardiac rehabilitation and secondary prevention of coronary heart disease. N Engl J Med 2001;345:892. [PMID: 11565523] (Review of clinical trials suggests that rehabilitation is indicated after myocardial infarction, percutaneous intervention, or CABG or transplant, and potentially in chronic coronary artery disease and congestive heart failure.)

Dargie HJ et al: Effect of carvedilol on outcome after myocardial infarction in patients with left ventricular dysfunction: the CAPRICORN randomized trial. Lancet 2001;357:1385. [PMID: 11356434] (Patients with acute myocardial infarction and LVEF less than 40% demonstrated decreased mortality and reinfarction when carvedilol is added to ACE inhibitor therapy.)

JAMA patient page: Heart attack. JAMA 1998;280:1462. [PMID: 9801010]

Michaels AD et al: Risk stratification after acute myocardial infarction in the reperfusion era. Prog Cardiovasc Dis 2000;42:273. [PMID: 10661780]

Sutton MGS et al: Left ventricular remodeling after myocardial infarction: pathophysiology and therapy. Circulation 2000;101:2981. [PMID: 10869273] (Mechanisms of myocardial fibrosis and ventricular dilation are reviewed. Opening the artery and ACE inhibition are most beneficial.)

■ DISTURBANCES OF RATE & RHYTHM

Abnormalities of cardiac rhythm and conduction can be lethal (sudden cardiac death), symptomatic (syncope, near syncope, dizziness, or palpitations), or asymptomatic. They are dangerous to the extent that they reduce cardiac output, so that perfusion of the brain or myocardium is impaired, or tend to deteriorate into more serious arrhythmias with the same consequences. Stable supraventricular tachycardia is generally well tolerated in patients without underlying heart disease but may lead to myocardial ischemia or congestive heart failure in patients with coronary disease, valvular abnormalities, and systolic or diastolic myocardial dysfunction. Ventricular tachycardia, if prolonged (lasting more than 10–30 seconds), often results in hemodynamic compromise and is more likely to deteriorate into ventricular fibrillation.

Whether slow heart rates produce symptoms at rest or on exertion depends upon whether cerebral perfusion can be maintained, which is generally a function of whether the patient is upright or supine and whether left ventricular function is adequate to maintain stroke volume. If the heart rate abruptly slows, as with the onset of complete heart block or sinus arrest, syncope or convulsions may result.

Arrhythmias are detected either because they present with symptoms or because they are detected during the course of monitoring. Arrhythmias causing sudden death, syncope, or near syncope require further evaluation and treatment unless they are related to conditions that are unlikely to recur (eg, electrolyte abnormalities or acute myocardial infarction). In contrast, there is controversy over when and how to evaluate and treat rhythm disturbances that are not symptomatic but are possible markers for more serious abnormalities (eg, nonsustained ventricular tachycardia). This uncertainty reflects two issues: (1) the difficulty of reliably stratifying patients into high-risk and low-risk groups; and (2) the lack of treatments which are both effective and safe. Thus, screening patients for these so-called "premonitory" abnormalities is often not productive.

A number of procedures are employed to evaluate patients with symptoms who are felt to be at risk for life-threatening arrhythmias, including in-hospital and ambulatory electrocardiographic monitoring, event recorders (instruments that can be worn for prolonged periods in order to record or transmit rhythm tracings when infrequent episodes occur), exercise testing, intracardiac electrophysiologic studies (to assess sinus node function, atrioventricular conduction, and inducibility of arrhythmias), signal-averaged ECGs, and tests of autonomic nervous system function (especially tilt-table testing). These are discussed below and in the subsequent sections on individual rhythm disturbance and symptomatic presentation. In general, these techniques are more successful in diagnosing symptomatic arrhythmias than in predicting the outcome of asymptomatic ones.

MECHANISMS OF ARRHYTHMIAS

Susceptibility to arrhythmias results from genetic abnormalities (most often affecting ion channels) and acquired structural heart disease. Susceptibility may be increased by electrolyte abnormalities, hormonal imbalances (thyrotoxicosis, hypercatecholamine states), hypoxia, drug effects (such as QT interval prolongation or changes in automaticity, conduction, and refractoriness), and myocardial ischemia. Most arrhythmias can be classified as (1) disorders of impulse formation or automaticity, (2) abnormalities of impulse conduction, (3) reentry, and (4) triggered activity.

Altered automaticity is the mechanism for sinus node arrest, many premature beats, and automatic rhythms as well as an initiating factor in reentry arrhythmias.

Abnormalities of impulse conduction can occur at the sinus or atrioventricular node, in the intraventricular conduction system, and within the atria or ventricles. These are responsible for sinoatrial exit block, for atrioventricular block at the node or below, and for establishing reentry circuits.

Reentry is the underlying mechanism for many arrhythmias, including premature beats, most paroxysmal supraventricular tachycardias, and atrial flutter. For reentry to occur, there must be an area of unidirectional block with an appropriate delay to allow repeat depolarization at the site of origin. Reentry is confirmed if the arrhythmia can be terminated by interruption of the circuit by a spontaneous or induced premature beat.

Triggered activity occurs when afterdepolarizations (abnormal electrical activity persisting after repolarization) reach the threshold level required to trigger a new depolarization. This may be the mechanism of ventricular tachycardia in the prolonged QT syndrome and in some cases of digitalis toxicity.

Priori SG et al: Genetic and molecular basis of cardiac arrhythmias: impact on clinical management. Parts I and II. Circulation 1999;99:518. [PMID: 9927398] (Consensus statement on the genetics of inherited arrhythmias and practical advice on the role of genetic testing in these syndromes.)

TECHNIQUES FOR EVALUATING RHYTHM DISTURBANCES

Electrocardiographic Monitoring

The ideal way of establishing a causal relationship between a symptom and a rhythm disturbance is to demonstrate the presence of the rhythm during the symptom. Unfortunately, this is not always easy because symptoms are usually sporadic.

Patients with aborted sudden death and recent or recurrent syncope are often monitored in the hospital. Those with less ominous symptoms may be monitored as outpatients. When episodes are infrequent, use of an event recorder is preferable to 24-hour continuous monitoring. Exercise testing may be helpful when the symptoms are associated with exertion or stress. If symptomatic bradyarrhythmias or supraventricular tachyarrhythmias are detected, therapy can usually be initiated without additional diagnostic studies. Further electrophysiologic studies may be useful in evaluating ventricular tachyarrhythmias.

Caution is required before attributing a patient's symptom to rhythm or conduction abnormalities observed during monitoring without concomitant symptoms. In many cases, the symptoms are due to a different arrhythmia or to noncardiac causes. For instance, dizziness or syncope in older patients may be unrelated to concomitantly observed bradycardia, sinus node abnormalities, and ventricular ectopy. Ambulatory monitoring is frequently used to quantify ventricular ectopy and detect asymptomatic ventricular tachycardia in post-myocardial infarction or heart failure patients. Unfortunately, while asymptomatic ventricular arrhythmias have concerning prognostic implications, there are few data to support specific therapeutic intervention. Thus, monitoring in asymptomatic individuals is usually not indicated.

Crawford MH at al: ACC/AHA Guidelines for Ambulatory Electrocardiography. A report of the American College of Cardiology/American Heart Association Task Force on Practice Guidelines (Committee to Revise the Guidelines for Ambulatory Electrocardiography). Developed in collaboration with the North American Society for Pacing and Electrophysiology. J Am Coll Cardiol 1999;34:912. [PMID: 10483977] (Consensus statement on methodology and applications.)

Heart Rate Variability

Although it has long been appreciated that there are periodical fluctuations in heart rate even under basal conditions, considerable recent interest has been focused on measurements of **heart rate variability.** These measurements can be made under controlled conditions in the electrocardiography laboratory or from recordings obtained during ambulatory monitoring. Greater fluctuations in heart rate correspond to greater parasympathetic activity, and several studies have indicated that greater heart rate variability is associated with a better prognosis and fewer life-threatening arrhythmias in a variety of cardiac conditions. More recently, analyses have employed frequency transformation of RR cycle length variability to provide indices of the relative balance between parasympathetic and sympathetic activity, with the greater contribution of the parasympathetic system being considered to confer a better prognosis. In studies of postinfarction patients and patients with symptomatic arrhythmias, these indices have had some prognostic value. However, adequate data are not yet available to support routine use of this technique in clinical practice.

Huikuri HV et al: Measurement of heart rate variability: a clinical tool or a research toy? J Am Coll Cardiol 1999;34: 1878. [PMID: 10588197] (Although there are significant associations between reduced heart rate variability and mortality, there is lack of consensus on what are the most useful measurements and how to utilize them in clinical practice.)

Signal-Averaged ECG

Another technique is the **signal-averaged ECG.** Most commonly, an orthogonal three-lead system is employed to record 300 consecutive beats during basal conditions. Using appropriate electrical filtering and computer averaging of the signal, very low frequency signals called "late potentials" can be identified in the period following the QRS complex. Abnormal late potentials are considered markers for potential ventricular arrhythmias. Adequate data are not yet available to define the role of this technique with confidence, but it may be useful in detecting groups of patients at increased risk for arrhythmic events after myocardial infarction. Approximately one-third of post-myocardial infarction patients will have abnormal late potentials, and these individuals are at higher risk for arrhythmic events, though the positive predictive value of this finding is relatively low (10–15%). More importantly, the absence of late potentials identifies a group of patients at low risk for arrhythmic events, so post-myocardial infarction patients found to have frequent ventricular ectopy or nonsustained ventricular tachycardia in the absence of late potentials may not require further investigation or treatment. The prognostic value of late potentials in patients with chronic ischemic heart disease who are more than 6–12 months removed from myocardial infarction and in patients with other forms of heart disease is not yet known.

Gomes JA et al. Prediction of long-term outcomes by signal-averaged electrocardiography in patients with unsustained ventricular tachycardia, coronary artery disease and left ventricular dysfunction. Circulation 2001;104:436. [PMID: 11468206] (In a prospective study of 1925 patients with unsustained ventricular tachycardia, coronary artery disease, and left ventricular dysfunction, the signal-averaged ECG was a significant multivariate predictor of sudden death, cardiac death, and total mortality.)

Electrophysiologic Testing

Electrophysiologic testing employing intracardiac electrocardiographic recordings and programmed atrial or ventricular (or both) stimulation is useful in the diagnosis and management of complex arrhythmias. The primary indications for electrophysiologic testing are (1) evaluation of recurrent syncope of possible cardiac origin, when the ambulatory ECG has not provided the diagnosis; (2) differentiation of supraventricular from ventricular arrhythmias; (3) evaluation of therapy in patients with accessory atrioventricular pathways; (4) evaluation of the efficacy of pharmacotherapy in survivors of aborted sudden death or other patients with symptomatic or life-threatening ventricular tachycardia; and (5) evaluation of patients for catheter ablation procedures or antitachycardia devices.

Sheahan RG: Syncope and arrhythmias: role of the electrophysiological study. Am J Med Sci 2001;322:37. [PMID: 11465245]

Autonomic Testing (Tilt Table Testing)

In many patients with recurrent syncope or near syncope, arrhythmias are not the cause. This is particularly true when the patient has no evidence of associated heart disease by history, examination, standard ECG, or noninvasive testing. Syncope may be neurocardiogenic in origin, mediated by excessive vagal stimulation or an imbalance between sympathetic and parasympathetic autonomic activity. With assumption of upright posture, there is venous pooling in the lower limbs. However, instead of the normal response, which consists of an increase in heart rate and vasoconstriction, a sympathetically mediated increase in myocardial contractility activates mechanoreceptors that trigger reflex bradycardia and vasodilation. Autonomic testing is an important component of the evaluation in these individuals and should usually precede invasive electrophysiologic procedures. Carotid sinus massage in patients who do not have carotid bruits or a history of cerebral vascular disease can precipitate sinus node arrest or atrioventricular block in patients with carotid sinus hypersensitivity. Head-up tilt-table testing can identify patients whose syncope may be on a vasovagal basis. Although different testing protocols are employed, passive tilting to at least 70 degrees for 10–40 minutes—in conjunction with isoproterenol infusion, if necessary—is typical. Syncope due to bradycardia, hypotension, or both will occur in approximately one-third of patients with recurrent syncope. Some recent studies have suggested that, at least with some of the more extreme protocols, false-positive responses may occur.

Fitzpatrick AP et al: Tilt methodology in reflex syncope: emerging evidence. J Am Coll Cardiol 2000;36:179. [PMID: 10898431] (How to perform and interpret tilt tests.)

Antiarrhythmic Drugs (Table 10–5)

Antiarrhythmic drugs have limited efficacy and produce frequent side effects. They are often divided into four classes based upon their electropharmacologic actions. Some have multiple actions.

Class I agents block membrane sodium channels. Three subclasses are further defined by the effect of agents on the Purkinje fiber action potential. Class Ia drugs slow the rate of rise of the action potential (V_{max}) and prolong its duration, thus slowing conduction and increasing refractoriness. Class Ib agents shorten action potential duration; they do not affect conduction or refractoriness. Class Ic agents prolong V_{max} and slow repolarization, thus slowing conduction and prolonging refractoriness, but more so than class Ia drugs.

Class II agents are the beta-blockers, which decrease automaticity, prolong atrioventricular conduction, and prolong refractoriness.

Class III agents block potassium channels and prolong repolarization, widening the QRS and prolonging the QT interval. They decrease automaticity and conduction and prolong refractoriness.

Class IV agents are the calcium channel blockers, which decrease automaticity and atrioventricular conduction.

Although the in vitro electrophysiologic effects of most of these agents have been defined, their use remains largely empirical. All can exacerbate arrhythmias (proarrhythmic effect), and most depress left ventricular function.

The risk of antiarrhythmic agents has been highlighted by the Coronary Arrhythmia Suppression Trial (CAST), in which two class Ic agents (flecainide, encainide) and a class Ia agent (moricizine) increased mortality rates in patients with asymptomatic ventricular ectopy after myocardial infarction. A similar result has been reported with D-sotalol, a class III agent without the beta-blocking activity of D,L-sotalol, the currently marketed formulation. Therefore, these agents (and perhaps any antiarrhythmic drug) should not be used except for life-threatening ventricular arrhythmias and symptomatic supraventricular tachyarrhythmias.

Table 10–5. Antiarrhythmic drugs.

Agent	Intravenous Dosage	Oral Dosage	Therapeutic Plasma Level	Route of Elimination	Side Effects
Class Ia: Action: Sodium channel blockers: Depress phase 0 depolarization; slow conduction; prolong repolarization. **Indications:** Supraventricular tachycardia, ventricular tachycardia, prevention of ventricular fibrillation, symptomatic ventricular premature beats.					
Quinidine	6–10 mg/kg (IM or IV) over 20 min (rarely used parenterally)	200–400 mg every 4–6 h or every 8 h (long acting)	2–5 mg/mL	Hepatic	GI, ↓LVF, ↑Dig
Procainamide	100 mg/1–3 min to 500–1000 mg; maintain at 2–6 mg/min	50 mg/kg/d in divided doses every 3–4 h or every 6 h (long-acting)	4–10 mg/mL; NAPA (active metabolite), 10–20 μg/mL	Renal	SLE, hypersensitivity, ↓LVF
Disopyramide		100–200 mg every 6–8 h	2–8 mg/mL	Renal	Urinary retention, dry mouth, markedly ↓LVF
Moricizine		200–300 mg every 8 h	**Note:** Active metabolites	Hepatic	Dizziness, nausea, headache, ↓theophylline level, ↓LVF
Class Ib: Action: Shorten repolarization. **Indications:** Ventricular tachycardia, prevention of ventricular fibrillation, symptomatic ventricular beats.					
Lidocaine	1–2 mg/kg at 50 mg/min; maintain at 1–4 mg/min		1–5 mg/mL	Hepatic	CNS, GI
Mexiletine		100–300 mg every 6–12 h. Maximum: 1200 mg/d	0.5–2 mg/mL	Hepatic	CNS, GI, leukopenia
Phenytoin	50 mg/5 min to 1000 mg (12 mg/kg); maintain at 200–400 mg/d	200–400 mg every 12–24 h	5–20 mg/mL	Hepatic	CNS, GI
Class Ic: Action: Depress phase 0 repolarization; slow conduction. *Propafenone* is a weak calcium channel- and beta-blocker and prolongs action potential and refractoriness. **Indications:** Life-threatening ventricular tachycardia or fibrillation; refractory supraventricular tachycardia.					
Flecainide		100–200 mg twice daily	0.2–1 mg/mL	Hepatic	CNS, GI, ↓↓LVF, incessant VT, sudden death
Propafenone		150–300 mg every 8–12 h	**Note:** Active metabolites	Hepatic	CNS, GI, ↓↓LVF, ↑Dig
Class II: Action: Beta-blocker, slows AV conduction. **Note:** Other beta-blockers may also have antiarrhythmic effects but are not yet approved for this indication in the USA. **Indications:** Supraventricular tachycardia; may prevent ventricular fibrillation.					
Esmolol	500 mg/kg over 1–2 min; maintain at 25–200 mg/kg/min	Other beta-blockers may be used concomitantly	0.15–2 mg/mL	Hepatic	↓LVF, bronchospasm
Propranolol	1–5 mg at 1 mg/min	40–320 mg in 1–4 doses daily (depending on preparation)	Not established	Hepatic	↓LVF, bradycardia, AV block, bronchospasm
Metoprolol	2.5–5 mg	50–200 mg daily	Not established	Hepatic	↓LVF, bradycardia, AV block

(continued)

Table 10–5. Antiarrhythmic drugs (continued).

Agent	Intravenous Dosage	Oral Dosage	Therapeutic Plasma Level	Route of Elimination	Side Effects
Class III: Action: Prolong action potential. **Indications:** *Amiodarone:* refractory ventricular tachycardia, supraventricular tachycardia, prevention of ventricular tachycardia, atrial fibrillation, ventricular fibrillation; *dofetilide:* atrial fibrillation and flutter; *sotalol:* ventricular tachycardia; atrial fibrillation; *bretylium:* ventricular fibrillation, ventricular tachycardia; *ibutilide:* conversion of atrial fibrillation and flutter.					
Amiodarone	150 mg infused rapidly, followed by 1 mg/min infusion for 6 hours (360 mg) and then 0.5 mg/min. Additional 150 mg as needed	800–1600 mg/d for 7–21 days; maintain at 100–400 mg/d (higher doses may be needed)	1–5 mg/mL	Hepatic	Pulmonary fibrosis, hypothyroidism, hyperthyroidism, corneal and skin deposits, hepatitis, ↑Dig, neurotoxicity, GI
Sotalol		80–160 mg every 12 h (higher doses may be used for life-threatening arrhythmias)		Renal (dosing interval should be extended if creatinine clearance is < 60 mL/min)	Early incidence of torsade de pointes, ↓LVF, bradycardia, fatigue (and other side effects associated with beta-blockers)
Dofetilide		500 mg twice daily		Renal (dose must be reduced with renal dysfunction)	Torsade de pointes in 3%; interaction with cytochrome P450 inhibitors
Ibutilide	1 mg over 10 minutes, followed by a second infusion of 0.5–1 mg over 10 minutes			Hepatic and renal	Torsade de pointes in up to 5% of patients within 3 hours after administration. Patients must be monitored with defibrillator nearby.
Bretylium	5–10 mg/kg over 5–10 min; maintain at 0.5–2 mg/min. Maximum: 30 mg/kg		0.5–1.5 mg/mL	Renal	Hypotension, nausea
Class IV: Action: Slow calcium channel blockers. **Indications:** Supraventricular tachycardia.					
Verapamil	10–20 mg over 2–20 min; maintain at 5 mg/kg/min	80–120 mg every 6–8 h; 240–360 mg once daily with sustained-release preparation	0.1–0.15 mg/mL	Hepatic	↓LVF, constipation, ↑Dig, hypotension
Diltiazem	0.25 mg/kg over 2 min; second 0.35 mg/kg bolus after 15 min if response is inadequate; infusion rate, 5–15 mg/h	180–360 mg daily in 1–3 doses depending on preparation (oral forms not approved for arrhythmias)		Hepatic metabolism, renal excretion	Hypotension, ↓LVF

(continued)

Table 10–5. Antiarrhythmic drugs (continued).

Agent	Intravenous Dosage	Oral Dosage	Therapeutic Plasma Level	Route of Elimination	Side Effects
Class V: Indications: Supraventricular tachycardia.					
Adenosine	6 mg rapidly followed by 12 mg after 1–2 min if needed. Use half these doses if administered via central line.			Adenosine receptor stimulation, metabolized in blood	Transient flushing, dyspnea, chest pain, AV block, sinus bradycardia; effect ↓ by theophylline, ↑ by dipyridamole
Digoxin	0.5 mg over 20 min followed by increment of 0.25 or 0.125 mg to 1–1.5 mg over 24 hours	1–1.5 mg over 24–36 hours in 3 or 4 doses; maintenance, 0.125–0.5 mg/d	0.7–2 mg/mL	Renal	AV block, arrhythmias, GI, visual changes

Key: AV = atrioventricular; CNS = central nervous system; ↑Dig = elevation of serum digoxin level; GI = gastrointestinal (nausea, vomiting, diarrhea); ↓LVF = reduced left ventricular function; NAPA = N-acetylprocainamide; SLE = systemic lupus erythematosus; VT = ventricular tachycardia

The use of antiarrhythmic agents for specific arrhythmias is discussed below.

Guidelines 2000 for Cardiopulmonary Resuscitation and Emergency Cardiovascular Care Part 6: advanced cardiovascular life support: section 5: pharmacology I: agents for arrhythmias. The American Heart Association in collaboration with the International Liaison Committee on Resuscitation. Circulation 2000;102(8 Suppl):I112. [PMID: 10966669]

Goldschlager N et al: Practical guidelines for clinicians who treat patients with amiodarone. Arch Intern Med 2000;160: 1741. [PMID: 10871966] (Amiodarone has become the most important antiarrhythmic agent in cardiac practice.)

Kowey PR et al: Classification and pharmacology of antiarrhythmic drugs. Am Heart J 2000;140:12. [PMID: 10874257] (Understanding the pharmacology of these agents is critical to their proper use.)

Roden DM: Antiarrhythmic drugs: from mechanisms to clinical practice. Heart 2000;84:339. [PMID: 10956304]

Radiofrequency Ablation for Cardiac Arrhythmias

Catheter ablation techniques have become the primary modality for treatment of many arrhythmias. This growing trend reflects the increasing ability to localize the origin or conduction pathways of many arrhythmias, the improved technology for delivering radiofrequency energy, and growing dissatisfaction with the efficacy and safety of pharmacologic therapy. Ablation has become the primary modality of therapy for many symptomatic supraventricular arrhythmias, including atrioventricular nodal reentry tachycardia, reentry tachycardias involving accessory pathways, paroxysmal atrial tachycardia, inappropriate sinus tachycardia, and automatic junctional tachycardia. Many laboratories have achieved reasonable success rates in preventing atrial flutter with radiofrequency techniques, and experience with atrial fibrillation is accumulating as well.

Catheter ablation of ventricular arrhythmias has proved more difficult. Three specific forms of ventricular tachycardia, however, have proved to be amenable to radiofrequency ablation. These include bundle-branch reentry, tachycardia originating in the right ventricular outflow tract, and some tachycardias originating in the left side of the interventricular septum. Other forms of ventricular tachycardia, particularly in patients with coronary artery disease, may be amenable to ablation, but experience thus far is limited.

These procedures are generally safe, though there is a low incidence of perforation of the atria or right ventricle that results in pericardial tamponade and sufficient damage to the atrioventricular node to require permanent cardiac pacing in less than 5% of patients. In addition, some procedures involve transseptal or retrograde left ventricular catheterization, with the attendant potential complications of aortic perforation, damage to the heart valves, or left-sided emboli.

Calkins H: Catheter ablation for cardiac arrhythmias. Med Clin North Am 2001;85:473. [PMID: 11233956]

SUPRAVENTRICULAR ARRHYTHMIAS

1. Sinus Arrhythmia, Bradycardia, & Tachycardia

Sinus arrhythmia is a cyclic increase in normal heart rate with inspiration and decrease with expiration. It results from reflex changes in vagal influence on the normal pacemaker and disappears with breath holding or increase of heart rate due to any cause. It has no clinical significance. It is common in both the young and the elderly.

Sinus bradycardia is a heart rate slower than 50/min due to increased vagal influence on the normal pacemaker or organic disease of the sinus node. The rate usually increases during exercise or administration of atropine. In healthy individuals, and especially in patients who are in excellent physical condition, sinus bradycardia to a rate of 50 or even lower is a normal finding. However, severe sinus bradycardia may be an indication of sinus node pathology (see below), especially in elderly patients and individuals with heart disease. It may cause weakness, confusion, or syncope if cerebral perfusion is impaired. Atrial and ventricular ectopic rhythms are more apt to occur with slow sinus rates. Pacing may be required if symptoms correlate with the bradycardia.

Sinus tachycardia is defined as a heart rate faster than 100 beats/min that is caused by rapid impulse formation from the normal pacemaker; it occurs with fever, exercise, emotion, pain, anemia, heart failure, shock, thyrotoxicosis, or in response to many drugs. Alcohol and alcohol withdrawal are common causes of sinus tachycardia and other supraventricular arrhythmias. The onset and termination are usually gradual, in contrast to paroxysmal supraventricular tachycardia due to reentry. The rate infrequently exceeds 160/min but may reach 180/min in young persons. The rhythm is basically regular, but serial 1-minute counts of the heart rate indicate that it varies five or more beats per minute with changes in position, with breath holding or with sedation. Rare individuals have persistent or episodic "inappropriate" sinus tachycardia that may be very symptomatic or may lead to left ventricular contractile dysfunction. Radiofrequency modification of the sinus node has mitigated this problem.

Mangrum JM et al: The evaluation and management of bradycardia. N Engl J Med 2000;342:703. [PMID: 10706901] (Evaluation and management of sinus node dysfunction and AV node conduction block with a comprehensive differential diagnosis and electrocardiographic examples.)

2. Atrial Premature Beats (Atrial Extrasystoles)

Atrial premature beats occur when an ectopic focus in the atria fires before the next sinus node impulse or a reentry circuit is established. The contour of the P wave usually differs from the patient's normal complex. The subsequent R–R cycle length is usually unchanged or only slightly prolonged. Such premature beats occur frequently in normal hearts and are never a sufficient basis for a diagnosis of heart disease. Speeding of the heart rate by any means usually abolishes most premature beats. Early atrial premature beats may cause aberrant QRS complexes (wide and bizarre) or may be nonconducted to the ventricles because the latter are still refractory.

3. Differentiation of Aberrantly Conducted Supraventricular Beats From Ventricular Beats

This distinction can be very difficult in patients with a wide QRS complex; it is important because of the differing prognostic and therapeutic implications of each type. Findings favoring a ventricular origin include (1) atrioventricular dissociation; (2) a QRS duration exceeding 0.14 s; (3) capture or fusion beats (infrequent); (4) left axis deviation with right bundle branch block morphology; (5) monophasic (R) or biphasic (qR, QR, or RS) complexes in V_1; and (6) a qR or QS complex in V_6. Supraventricular origin is favored by (1) a triphasic QRS complex, especially if there was initial negativity in leads I and V_6; (2) ventricular rates exceeding 170/min; (3) QRS duration longer than 0.12 s but not longer than 0.14 s; and (4) the presence of preexcitation syndrome.

The relationship of the P waves to the tachycardia complex is helpful. A 1:1 relationship usually means a supraventricular origin, except in the case of ventricular tachycardia with retrograde P waves. If the P waves are not clearly seen, Lewis leads (in which the right arm electrode is placed in the V_1 position two interspaces higher than usual and the left arm electrode is placed in the usual V_1 position) may be employed. This accentuates the size of the P waves. Esophageal leads, in which the electrode is placed directly posterior to the left atrium, achieve the same effect even more clearly. Right atrial electrograms may also help to clarify the diagnosis by accentuating the P waves.

4. Paroxysmal Supraventricular Tachycardia

This is the commonest paroxysmal tachycardia and often occurs in patients without structural heart disease. Attacks begin and end abruptly and may last a few seconds to several hours or longer. The heart rate may be 140–240/min (usually 160–220/min) and is perfectly regular (despite exercise or change in position). The P wave usually differs in contour from sinus beats. Patients may be asymptomatic except for awareness of rapid heart action, but some experience mild chest pain or shortness of breath, especially when episodes are prolonged, even in the absence of associated cardiac abnormalities. Paroxysmal supraventricular tachycardia may result from digitalis toxicity and then is commonly associated with atrioventricular block.

The most common mechanism for paroxysmal supraventricular tachycardia is reentry, which may be initiated or terminated by a fortuitously timed atrial or ventricular premature beat. The reentry circuit most commonly involves dual pathways (a slow and a fast pathway) within the atrioventricular node. This is referred to as AV nodal reentry tachycardia (AVNRT). Less commonly, reentry is due to an accessory pathway between the atria and ventricles (AVRT). Approximately one-third of patients with supraventricular tachycardia have aberrant pathways to the ventricles. The pathophysiology and management of arrhythmias due to accessory pathways differs in important ways and is discussed separately below.

Treatment of the Acute Attack

In the absence of heart disease, serious effects are rare, and most attacks break spontaneously. Particular effort should be made to terminate the attack quickly if cardiac failure, syncope, or anginal pain develops or if there is underlying cardiac or (particularly) coronary disease. Because reentry is the most common mechanism for paroxysmal atrial tachycardia, effective therapy requires that conduction be interrupted at some point in the reentry circuit.

A. MECHANICAL MEASURES

A variety of methods have been used to interrupt attacks, and patients may learn to perform these themselves. These include Valsalva's maneuver, stretching the arms and body, lowering the head between the knees, coughing, and breath holding. Carotid sinus massage is often performed by physicians but should be avoided if the patient has carotid bruits or a history of transient cerebral ischemic attacks. Firm but gentle pressure and massage are applied first over the right carotid sinus for 10–20 seconds and, if unsuccessful, then over the left carotid sinus. *Pressure should not be exerted on both sides at the same time!* Continuous electrocardiographic or auscultatory monitoring of the heart rate is essential so that pressure can be relieved as soon as the rhythm is broken or if excessive bradycardia occurs. Carotid sinus pressure will interrupt up to half of the attacks, especially if the patient has received a digitalis glycoside or other agent (such as adenosine or a calcium channel blocker) that delays atrioventricular conduction. These maneuvers stimulate the vagus nerve, delay atrioventricular conduction, and block the reentry mechanism, terminating the arrhythmia.

B. DRUG THERAPY

If mechanical measures fail, two rapidly acting intravenous agents will terminate more than 90% of episodes. Intravenous adenosine has a very brief duration of action and minimal negative inotropic activity. A 6 mg bolus is administered. If no response is observed after 1–2 minutes, a second 12 mg bolus should be given, followed by a third if necessary. Since the half-life of adenosine is less than 10 seconds, the drug must be given rapidly (in 1–2 seconds from a peripheral intravenous line); use half the dose if given through a central line. Adenosine is very well tolerated, but nearly 20% of patients will experience transient flushing, and some patients experience severe chest discomfort.

Calcium channel blockers also rapidly induce atrioventricular block and break most episodes of reentry supraventricular tachycardia. Intravenous verapamil may be given as a 2.5 mg-bolus, followed by additional doses of 2.5 mg to 5 mg every 1–3 minutes up to a total of 20 mg if blood pressure and rhythm are stable. If the rhythm recurs, further doses can be given. Oral verapamil, 80–120 mg every 4–6 hours, can be used as well in stable patients who are tolerating the rhythm without difficulty, but avoid it if there is any concern that the arrhythmia may be ventricular in origin. Intravenous diltiazem (0.25 mg/kg over 2 minutes, followed by a second bolus of 0.35 mg/kg if necessary and then an infusion of 5–15 mg/h) may cause less hypotension and myocardial depression.

Esmolol, a short-acting beta-blocker, may also be effective; the initial dose is 500 μg/kg intravenously over 1 minute followed by an infusion of 25–200 μg/min. Parasympathetic stimulating drugs such as edrophonium, 5–10 mg intravenously, which delay atrioventricular conduction, may break the reentry mechanism. Because it frequently causes nausea and vomiting, it should be used only if the previously discussed agents fail. Metaraminol or phenylephrine, alpha-adrenergic stimulants that activate the baroreceptors by raising the blood pressure and causing vagal stimulation, can break attacks but should be used cautiously because they may provoke excessive hypertension. Digoxin is effective, but it often requires several hours to safely administer an adequate dose. An initial dose of 0.5–0.75 mg intravenously over 20 minutes, followed by 0.25-mg or 0.125-mg increments every 2–4 hours up to a total of 1–1.25 mg, is used. Intravenous procainamide may terminate supraventricular tachycardia; however, since it facilitates atrioventricular conduction and an initial increase in rate may occur, it is usually not given until after digoxin, verapamil, or a beta-blocker has been administered.

C. CARDIOVERSION

If the patient is hemodynamically stable or if adenosine and verapamil are contraindicated or ineffective, synchronized electrical cardioversion (beginning at 100 J) is almost universally successful. If digitalis toxicity is present or strongly suspected, as in the case of paroxysmal tachycardia with block, electrical cardioversion should be avoided.

Prevention of Attacks

A. RADIOFREQUENCY ABLATION

Because of concerns about the safety and the intolerability of antiarrhythmic medications, radiofrequency ablation is the preferred approach to patients with recurrent symptomatic reentry supraventricular tachycardia, whether it is due to dual pathways within the atrial ventricular node or to accessory pathways.

B. DRUGS

Digoxin orally is the usual drug of first choice because of its convenience and efficacy. Verapamil, alone or in combination with digitalis, is a second choice. (*Note:* Verapamil increases digoxin serum levels.) Beta-blockers are also effective. Patients who do not respond to agents that increase refractoriness of the atrioventricular node may be treated with class Ia (disopyramide, quinidine, procainamide), class Ic (propafenone), or class III (sotalol, amiodarone) drugs. In patients with evidence of structural heart disease, either sotalol or amiodarone is probably a better choice because of the lower incidence of ventricular proarrhythmia during chronic therapy.

Chauhan VS et al: Supraventricular tachycardia. Med Clin North Am 2001;85:193. [PMID: 11233946]

Trohman RG: Supraventricular tachycardia: implications for the intensivist. Crit Care Med 2000;28:N129. [PMID: 11055681] (Discusses acute management of supraventricular arrhythmias.)

5. Supraventricular Tachycardias Due to Accessory Atrioventricular Pathways (Preexcitation Syndromes)

Pathophysiology & Clinical Findings

Accessory pathways between the atria and the ventricle which avoid the conduction delay of the atrioventricular node predispose to reentry tachycardias, such as AVRT and atrial flutter, and to atrial fibrillation. These may be wholly or partly within the node (Mahaim fibers), yielding a short PR interval and normal QRS morphology (**Lown-Ganong-Levine syndrome**). More commonly, they make direct connections between the atria and ventricle through Kent bundles (**Wolff-Parkinson-White syndrome**). This produces a short PR interval but an early delta wave at the onset of the wide, slurred QRS complex owing to early ventricular depolarization of the region adjacent to the pathway. While the morphology and polarity of the delta wave can suggest the location of the bypass tract, mapping by intracardiac recordings is required for precise anatomic localization.

Accessory pathways occur in 0.1–0.3% of the population and facilitate reentry arrhythmias owing to the disparity in refractory periods of the atrioventricular node and accessory pathway. Whether the tachycardia is associated with a narrow or wide QRS complex is determined by whether antegrade conduction is through the node (narrow) or the bypass tract (wide). Many patients with Wolff-Parkinson-White syndrome never conduct in an antegrade direction through the bypass tract which is therefore "concealed." Orthodromic tachycardia is a reentrant rhythm that conducts antegrade down the AV node and retrograde up the accessory pathway, resulting in a narrow QRS complex. Antidromic tachycardia conducts down the accessory pathway and retrograde through the AV node, resulting in a wide QRS complex. Since accessory pathways are less refractory than specialized conduction tissue, tachycardias proceeding in this direction have the potential to be more rapid. Up to 30% of patients with Wolff-Parkinson-White syndrome will develop atrial fibrillation or flutter with antegrade conduction down the accessory pathway and a rapid ventricular response.

Treatment

Some patients have a delta wave found incidentally on electrocardiography. In the absence of palpitations, lightheadedness, or syncope, these patients do not require specific therapy. They should be advised to report the onset of any of these symptoms.

A. RADIOFREQUENCY ABLATION

As with AVNRT, radiofrequency ablation has become the procedure of choice in patients with accessory pathways and recurrent symptoms. Patients with preexcitation syndromes who have episodes of atrial fibrillation or flutter should be tested by induction of atrial fibrillation in the electrophysiologic laboratory, noting duration of the RR cycle; if it is less than 220 ms, a short refractory period is present. These individuals are at highest risk for sudden death, and prophylactic ablation is indicated. Success rates for ablation of accessory pathways with radiofrequency catheters exceed 90% in appropriate patients.

B. PHARMACOLOGIC THERAPY

Narrow complex reentry rhythms involving a bypass tract can be managed as discussed for AVNRT. Atrial fibrillation and flutter must be managed differently, since agents such as digoxin, calcium channel blockers, and even beta-blockers may decrease the refractoriness of the accessory pathway or increase that of the AV node, leading to sometimes faster ventricular rates. Therefore, these agents should be avoided. The class Ia antiarrhythmics, as well as the newer class Ic and class III agents, will increase the refractoriness of the bypass tract and are the drugs of choice for wide-complex tachycardias. If hemodynamic compromise is present, electrical cardioversion is warranted.

Long-term therapy often involves a combination of agents that increase refractoriness in the bypass tract (class Ia or Ic agents) and in the atrioventricular node (verapamil, digoxin, and beta-blockers), provided that atrial fibrillation or flutter with short RR cycle lengths is not present (see above). Sotalol and amiodarone are effective in refractory cases. Patients who are difficult to manage should undergo electrophysiologic evaluation.

Al-Khatib SM et al: Clinical features of Wolff-Parkinson-White syndrome. Am Heart J 1999;138:403. [PMID: 10467188] (History, pathology, epidemiology, genetics, and various dysrhythmias are reviewed. Asymptomatic patients may be treated conservatively unless there is family history of sudden death or they are in a high-risk profession.)

Fitzsimmons PJ et al: The natural history of Wolff-Parkinson-White syndrome in 228 military aviators: a long-term follow-up of 22 years. Am Heart J 2001;142:530. [PMID: 11526369] (Prospective study demonstrating low risk of sudden death and 1% patient-year risk of supraventricular tachycardia.)

Goudevenos JA et al: Ventricular pre-excitation in the general population: a study on the mode of presentation and clinical course. Heart 2000;83:29. [PMID: 10618331] (Population-based study from Greece showing that Wolff-Parkinson-White syndrome is more common and diagnosed at a younger age in men than in women. About half of patients with the WPW pattern on electrocardiography are asymptomatic at diagnosis and remain so. Sudden death is rare.)

6. Atrial Fibrillation

Atrial fibrillation is the commonest chronic arrhythmia, with an incidence and prevalence that rise with age, so that it affects nearly 10% of individuals over age 80. It occurs in rheumatic and other forms of valvular heart disease, dilated cardiomyopathy, atrial septal defect, hypertension, and coronary heart disease as well as in patients with no apparent cardiac disease; it may be the initial presenting sign in thyrotoxicosis, and this condition should be excluded with the initial episode. Atrial fibrillation often appears paroxysmally before becoming the established rhythm. Pericarditis, chest trauma, thoracic or cardiac surgery, or pulmonary disease (as well as medications such as theophylline and beta-adrenergic agonists) may cause attacks in patients with normal hearts. Acute alcohol excess and alcohol withdrawal—and, in predisposed individuals, even consumption of small amounts of alcohol—may precipitate atrial fibrillation. This latter presentation, which is often termed "holiday heart," is usually transient and self-limited. Short-term rate control usually suffices as treatment.

Atrial fibrillation is the only common arrhythmia in which the ventricular rate is rapid and the rhythm very irregular. The atrial rate is 400–600/min, but most impulses are blocked at the atrioventricular node. The ventricular response is completely irregular, ranging from 80 to 180/min in the untreated state. Because of the varying stroke volumes resulting from varying periods of diastolic filling, not all ventricular beats produce a palpable peripheral pulse. The difference between the apical rate and the pulse rate is the "pulse deficit"; this deficit is greater when the ventricular rate is high.

Atrial fibrillation itself is rarely life-threatening; however, it can have serious consequences if the ventricular rate is sufficiently rapid to precipitate hypotension, myocardial ischemia, or tachycardia-induced myocardial dysfunction. Although many patients—particularly older or inactive individuals—have relatively few symptoms if the rate is controlled, some patients are aware of the irregular rhythm and may experience it as very uncomfortable. Perhaps the most serious consequence of atrial fibrillation is the propensity for thrombus formation due to stasis in the atria (particularly the atrial appendages) and consequent embolization, most devastatingly to the cerebral circulation. Overall, the rate of stroke is approximately five events per 100 patient-years of follow-up. However, patients with significant obstructive valvular disease, chronic heart failure or left ventricular dysfunction, diabetes, hypertension, or age over 75 years and those with a history of prior embolic events are at substantially higher risk (up to nearly 20 events per 100 patient-years in patients with multiple risk factors). Patients with one or more of these risk factors for stroke should be treated with warfarin. Patients with none of these factors may be treated with aspirin if conditions are present that increase the risk of warfarin. Patients below the age of 60–65 years without any of these stroke risk factors ("lone atrial fibrillation") may be treated with aspirin or no antithrombotic therapy.

Newly Diagnosed Atrial Fibrillation

A. INITIAL MANAGEMENT

The approach to the initial management of atrial fibrillation depends on the clinical presentation. If, as is often the case—particularly in older individuals—the patient presents without symptoms, hemodynamic instability, or evidence of important precipitating conditions (such as silent myocardial infarction or ischemia, decompensated heart failure, pulmonary embolus, or hemodynamically significant valvular disease), hospitalization is usually not necessary. In most such cases, atrial fibrillation is an unrecognized chronic or paroxysmal condition and should be managed accordingly (see below).

In contrast, if the patient is hemodynamically unstable—usually as a result of a rapid ventricular rate or associated cardiac or noncardiac conditions—hospitalization and immediate treatment of atrial fibrillation are required. Urgent cardioversion is usually indicated in patients with shock or severe hypotension, pulmonary edema, or ongoing myocardial infarction or ischemia. Although if atrial fibrillation has been present for more than 48 hours there is a potential risk of thromboembolism, the need for immediate rate control in these very unstable patients outweighs that risk. Electrical cardioversion is usually preferred in unstable patients. An initial shock with 100–200 J is administered in synchrony with the R wave. If sinus rhythm is not restored, an additional attempt with 360 J is indicated. If this fails, cardioversion may be successful after loading with intravenous ibutilide (1 mg over 10 minutes, repeated in 10 minutes if necessary) or intravenous procainamide (500–1000 mg administered at a rate of 20 mg/min with careful monitoring of blood pressure).

In less unstable patients or those at particularly high risk for embolism (underlying mitral stenosis, a history of prior emboli, or severe heart failure), a strategy of rate control is appropriate. A rate control strategy is appropriate both when the conditions that precipitated atrial fibrillation are likely to persist (such as following cardiac or noncardiac surgery, respiratory failure, or pericarditis) and when these conditions might resolve spontaneously over a period of hours to days (such as alcohol-induced atrial fibrillation, electrolyte or fluid imbalances, excessive exposure to theophylline or sympathomimetic agents, or some of the same previously cited conditions). The choice of agent is guided by the hemodynamic status of the patient, associated conditions, and the urgency of achieving rate control. Although both hypotension and heart failure may improve when the ventricular rate is slowed, calcium channel blockers and beta-blockers may themselves precipitate hemodynamic deterioration. Digoxin is less risky, but even when used aggressively (0.5 mg intravenously over 30 minutes, followed by increments of 0.25 mg every 1–2 hours to a total dose of 1–1.5 mg over 24 hours in patients not previously receiving this agent), rate control is rather slow and may be inadequate, particularly in patients with sympathetic activation. In the setting of myocardial infarction or ischemia, beta-blockers are the preferred agent. The most frequently used agents are either metoprolol (administered as a 5 mg intravenous bolus, repeated twice at intervals of 5 minutes and then given as needed by repeat boluses or orally at total daily doses of 50–400 mg) or, in very unstable patients, esmolol (0.5 mg/kg intravenously, repeated if necessary, followed by a titrated infusion of 0.05–0.2 mg/kg/min). If hypertension is present or beta-blockers are contraindicated, calcium channel blockers are immediately effective. Diltiazem (20 mg bolus, repeated after 15 minutes if necessary, followed by a maintenance infusion of 5–15 mg/h) is the preferred calcium blocker if hypotension or left ventricular dysfunction is present. Otherwise, verapamil (5–10 mg intravenously over 2–3 minutes, repeated after 30 minutes if necessary) may be used. Amiodarone, even when administered intravenously, has a relatively slow onset but is often a useful adjunct when rate control with the previously cited agents is incomplete or contraindicated or when cardioversion is planned in the near future.

If rate control proves unsuccessful or early cardioversion is considered necessary and the duration of atrial fibrillation exceeds 2–3 days or is unknown, a strategy of transesophageal echo-guided cardioversion should be considered. By this approach, the presence of atrial thrombus is excluded and electrical cardioversion is attempted while the patient remains under sedation. If thrombus is present, the cardioversion is delayed until after a 3- to 4-week period of therapeutic anticoagulation. In any case, because atrial contractile activity may not recover for several weeks after restoration of sinus rhythm in patients who have been in atrial fibrillation for more than several days, cardioversion is usually followed by anticoagulation for at least 1 month unless it is contraindicated.

B. Subsequent Management

Up to two-thirds of patients experiencing a first episode of atrial fibrillation will spontaneously revert to sinus rhythm within 24 hours. If atrial fibrillation persists or has been present for more than a week, spontaneous conversion is unlikely. In most such cases early cardioversion is not required, so management consists of rate control and anticoagulation whether or not the patient has been admitted to hospital. Rate control is usually relatively easy to achieve with beta-blockers, rate-slowing calcium blockers, and digoxin, used as single agents or more often in combination. Good rate control should consist of a ventricular rate between 50 and 100 beats/min with usual daily activities and a ventricular rate not exceeding 120 beats/min except with moderate to strenuous activity. In older patients, who often have diminished atrioventricular nodal function and relatively limited activity, this can often be achieved with a single agent. Most younger or more active individuals require a combination of two agents. Choice of the initial medication is best based on the presence of accompanying conditions: Hypertensive patients should be given beta-blockers or calcium blockers; coronary patients should usually receive a beta-blocker; and patients with heart failure should be given digoxin or a beta-blocker. Adequacy of rate control should be evaluated by recording the apical pulse rate both at rest and with an appropriate level of activity (such as after brisk walking around the corridor or climbing stairs).

Anticoagulation with warfarin to an INR target of 2.0–3.0 should be established and maintained as long as the patient is in atrial fibrillation. The only exception is the patient with "lone atrial fibrillation" (eg, no evidence of associated heart disease, hypertension, atherosclerotic vascular disease, or diabetes) who is under age 60. Cardioversion, if planned, should be performed after at least 3 weeks of anticoagulation at a therapeutic level. Except in patients with mitral stenosis or a history of prior embolic events or those with demonstrated thrombus on transesophageal echocardiography, it is not necessary to achieve therapeutic anticoagulation levels in hospital, so the use of intravenous heparin or low-molecular-weight heparin while transitioning to oral warfarin is not necessary.

C. Rate Control or Elective Cardioversion

Two recent large randomized controlled trials (the 4060 patient Atrial Fibrillation Follow-up Investigation of Rhythm Management, or AFFIRM trial; and the Rate Control Versus Electrical Cardioversion for Persistent Atrial Fibrillation, or RACE trial) compared strategies of rate control and rhythm control. In both, a strategy of rate control and chronic anticoagulation was associated with no higher rates of death or stroke—both, if anything, favored rate control—and only a modestly increased risk of hemorrhagic events than a strategy of restoring sinus rhythm and maintaining it with antiarrhythmic drug therapy. Of note is that exercise tolerance and quality of life were not significantly better in the rhythm control group. Nonetheless, the decision as to whether to attempt to restore sinus rhythm following the initial episode remains controversial. Elective cardioversion following an appropriate period of anticoagulation is generally recommended for the initial episode in patients in whom atrial fibrillation is thought to be of recent onset and when there is an identifiable precipitating factor. Similarly, cardioversion is appropriate in patients who remain symptomatic from the rhythm despite aggressive efforts to achieve rate control. However, it should be noted that even in patients for whom this is the initial episode of atrial fibrillation, the recurrence rate is sufficiently high that longer-term anticoagulation is generally appropriate until persistence of sinus rhythm can be confirmed for at least 6 months.

In cases where elective cardioversion is required, it may be accomplished electrically (as described above) or pharmacologically. Intravenous ibutilide may also be used as described above in a setting where the patient can undergo continuous electrocardiographic monitoring for at least 3 hours following administration. In patients in whom a decision has been made to continue antiarrhythmic therapy to maintain sinus rhythm (see next paragraph), cardioversion can be attempted with an agent that is being considered for long-term use. For instance, after therapeutic anticoagulation has been established, amiodarone can be initiated on an outpatient basis (300–400 mg twice daily for 2 weeks, followed by 200 mg twice daily for at least a 2–4 weeks and then a chronic dose of 200 mg daily). Since amiodarone increases the prothrombin time in patients taking warfarin and digoxin levels, careful monitoring of anticoagulation and drug levels is required. Other agents that may be used for both cardioversion and maintenance therapy include propafenone (150–300 mg twice daily; should be avoided in patients with structural heart disease); flecainide (50–150 mg twice daily; should be avoided in patients with structural heart disease); and dofetilide (0.5 mg twice daily; downward dose adjustment is required with renal dysfunction and dosing must be initiated in hospital because of risk of torsade de pointes). Sotalol (80–160 mg twice daily; should be initiated in hospital in patients with structural heart disease because of risk of torsade de pointes) is not very effective for converting atrial fibrillation but can be used to maintain sinus rhythm following cardioversion.

Unfortunately, sinus rhythm will persist in only 25% of patients who have had a sustained (lasting more than several days) or recurrent episode of atrial fibrillation. However, if the patient is treated chronically with an antiarrhythmic agent, sinus rhythm will persist in approximately 50%. The most commonly employed medications are amiodarone, sotalol, propafenone, flecainide, and dofetilide, but the latter four agents are associated with a clear risk of proarrhythmia, and amiodarone frequently causes other adverse effects. Therefore, it may be prudent to determine whether atrial fibrillation recurs during a period of 6 months without antiarrhythmic drugs during which anticoagulation is maintained. If it does recur, the decision as to whether to restore sinus rhythm and initiate chronic antiarrhythmic therapy can be based on how well the patient tolerates atrial fibrillation. In such a patient, chronic anticoagulation is probably indicated in any case, because of the high rate of recurrence and the likely occurrence of asymptomatic paroxysmal episodes.

Paroxysmal & Refractory Atrial Fibrillation

A. RECURRENT PAROXYSMAL ATRIAL FIBRILLATION

It is now well established that patients with recurrent paroxysmal atrial fibrillation are at similar stroke risk as those who are in atrial fibrillation chronically. While these episodes may be apparent to the patient, many are not recognized and may be totally asymptomatic. Thus, ambulatory electrocardiographic monitoring or event recorders are indicated in those in whom paroxysmal atrial fibrillation is suspected. Antiarrhythmic agents are usually not successful in preventing paroxysmal atrial fibrillation episodes. However, immediate self-administered treatment with an antiarrhythmic agent (experience is perhaps greatest with propafenone, 300 mg orally, repeated once after 2–3 hours if necessary) may interrupt symptomatic episodes, and chronic use of a beta-blocker or rate-slowing calcium channel blocker may reduce the severity of symptoms. In any case, chronic anticoagulation is indicated except in those who are under 60–65 years of age and have no additional stroke risk factors (see above).

B. REFRACTORY ATRIAL FIBRILLATION

Because of trial results indicating that important adverse clinical outcomes (death, stroke, hemorrhage, heart failure) are no more common with rate control than rhythm control, atrial fibrillation should generally be considered refractory if it causes persistent symptoms or limits activity. This is much more likely in younger individuals and those who are very active or engage in strenuous exercise. Even in such individuals, 2- or 3-drug combinations of a beta-blocker, rate-slowing calcium blocker, and digoxin usually can prevent excessive ventricular rates, though in some cases they are associated with excessive bradycardia during sedentary periods. If rapid ventricular rates persist, amiodarone may be substituted for or added to these agents.

If no drug works, radiofrequency AV node ablation and permanent pacing ensures rate control and may facilitate a more physiologic rate response to activity. There is growing experience with focal ablation of foci in the pulmonary veins that initiate atrial fibrillation, following which sinus rhythm may be restored or maintained. A surgical approach called the Maze procedure can also be used to eliminate the multiple re-entry circuits that cause atrial fibrillation, and implantable atrial defibrillators can be used to convert paroxysmal episodes. The role of these latter procedures is limited, however.

Albers GW et al: Antithrombotic therapy in atrial fibrillation. Chest 2001;119:194S. [PMID: 11157649]

Chugh SS et al: Epidemiology and natural history of atrial fibrillation: clinical implications. J Am Coll Cardiol 2001;37:371. [PMID: 11216949]

Falk RH: Atrial fibrillation. N Engl J Med 2001;344:1067. [PMID: 11287978]

Fuster V et al: ACC/AHA/ESC guidelines for the management of patients with atrial fibrillation: executive summary. A Report of the American College of Cardiology/American Heart Association Task Force on Practice Guidelines and the European Society of Cardiology Committee for Practice Guidelines and Policy Conferences (Committee to Develop Guidelines for the Management of Patients With Atrial Fibrillation): developed in Collaboration With the North American Society of Pacing and Electrophysiology. J Am Coll Cardiol 2001;38:1231. [PMID: 11583910]

Klein AL et al: Use of transesophageal echocardiography to guide cardioversion in patients with atrial fibrillation. N Engl J Med 2001;344:1411. [PMID: 11346805] (Multicenter randomized trial involving 1222 patients compared a TEE-guided strategy for cardioversion with a conventional approach and found no difference in rates of death, maintenance of sinus rhythm, or functional status after 8 weeks—but did find a somewhat lower rate of hemorrhagic events.)

Maisel WH et al: Atrial fibrillation after cardiac surgery. Ann Intern Med 2001;135:1061. [PMID: 11747385] (Atrial fibrillation occurs in 10–65% of patients after heart surgery. Beta-blockers and amiodarone can lower the incidence. Most patients revert to sinus rhythm with rate control.)

Mounsey JP et al: Cardiovascular drugs. Dofetilide. Circulation 2000;102:2665. [PMID: 11085972] (Reviews pharmacology of this pure class III potassium channel blocker recently approved for the treatment of atrial fibrillation. Although the drug is effective, proarrhythmia, metabolism, and drug interactions require special caution.)

Pappone C et al: Atrial electroanatomic remodeling after circumferential radiofrequency pulmonary vein ablation. Circulation 2001;104:2539. [PMID: 11714647] (Radiofrequency ablation around the pulmonary veins eliminated recurrence in 85% of patients with paroxysmal and 68% of patient with permanent atrial fibrillation at 10-month follow-up.)

Roy D et al: Amiodarone to prevent recurrence of atrial fibrillation. Canadian Trial of Atrial Fibrillation Investigators. N Engl J Med 2000;30;342:913. [PMID: 10738049] (Amiodarone was more effective than sotalol or propafenone in a prospective trial.)

Scheinman MM: Mechanisms of atrial fibrillation: is a cure at hand? J Am Coll Cardiol 2000;35:1687. [PMID: 10807477] (Discusses mechanisms of this arrhythmia with implications for therapy.)

7. Atrial Flutter

Atrial flutter is less common than fibrillation. It occurs most often in patients with COPD but may be seen also in those with rheumatic or coronary heart disease, congestive heart failure, atrial septal defect, or surgically repaired congenital heart disease. Ectopic impulse formation occurs at atrial rates of 250–350/min, with transmission of every second, third, or fourth impulse through the atrioventricular node to the ventricles. Ventricular rate control is accomplished using the same agents utilized in atrial fibrillation, but it is much more difficult with atrial flutter than with atrial fibrillation. Conversion of atrial flutter to sinus rhythm with class I antiarrhythmic agents is also difficult to achieve, and administration of these drugs has been associated with slowing of the atrial flutter rate to the point where 1:1 atrioventricular conduction can occur at rates in excess of 200/min, with subsequent hemodynamic collapse. The intravenous class III antiarrhythmic agent ibutilide has been significantly more successful in converting atrial flutter. About 50–70% of patients return to sinus rhythm within 60–90 minutes following the infusion of 1–2 mg of this agent. Electrical cardioversion is also very effective for atrial flutter, with approximately 90% of patients converting following shocks of as little as 25–50 J.

The persistence of atrial contractile function in this arrhythmia provides some protection against thrombus formation, though the risk of systemic embolization remains slightly increased. Precardioversion anticoagulation is not necessary for atrial flutter of less than 48 hours' duration except in the setting of mitral valve disease. However, anticoagulation is prudent in chronic atrial flutter, particularly since transient periods of atrial fibrillation are common in these patients.

Chronic atrial flutter is often a difficult management problem, since rate control is difficult. Amiodarone is probably the pharmacologic agent of choice, since it has the potential of both maintaining sinus rhythm and helping with rate control when flutter recurs.

Atrial flutter can follow a typical or atypical reentry circuit around the atrium. The anatomy of the typical circuit has been well defined and allows for radiofrequency ablation within the atrium to interrupt the circuit and eliminate atrial flutter. This technique should be considered in patients refractory to drug therapy.

Natale A et al: Prospective randomized comparison of antiarrhythmic therapy versus first-line radiofrequency ablation in patients with atrial flutter. J Am Coll Cardiol 2000;35:1898. [PMID: 10841241] (Randomized trial of 61 patients showing that radiofrequency ablation could potentially be used as first-line therapy in carefully selected patients.)

Niebauer MJ et al: Management of atrial flutter. Cardiol Rev 2001;9:253. [PMID: 11520448]

8. Multifocal (Chaotic) Atrial Tachycardia

This is a rhythm characterized by varying P-wave morphology (by definition, three or more foci) and markedly irregular PP intervals. The rate is usually between 100 and 140/min, and atrioventricular block is unusual. Most patients have severe associated COPD. Treatment of the underlying condition is the most effective approach; verapamil, 240–480 mg daily in divided doses, is also of value in some patients.

McCord J et al: Multifocal atrial tachycardia. Chest 1998;113:203. [PMID: 9440591] (Focus on patients with pulmonary disease; role for antiarrhythmic treatment unclear.)

9. Atrioventricular Junctional Rhythm

The atrial-nodal junction or the nodal-His bundle junctions may assume pacemaker activity for the heart, usually at a rate of 40–60/min. This may occur in patients with myocarditis, coronary artery disease, and digitalis toxicity as well as in individuals with normal hearts. The rate responds normally to exercise, and the diagnosis is often an incidental finding on electrocardiographic monitoring, but it can be suspected if the jugular venous pulse shows cannon *a* waves. Junctional rhythm is often an escape rhythm because of depressed sinus node function with sinoatrial block or delayed conduction in the atrioventricular node. **Nonparoxysmal junctional tachycardia** results from increased automaticity of the junctional tissues in digitalis toxicity or ischemia and is associated with a narrow QRS complex and a rate usually less than 120–130/min. It is usually considered benign when it occurs in acute myocardial infarction, but the ischemia that induces it may also cause ventricular tachycardia and ventricular fibrillation.

VENTRICULAR ARRHYTHMIAS

1. Ventricular Premature Beats (Ventricular Extrasystoles)

Ventricular premature beats are characterized by wide QRS complexes that differ in morphology from the patient's normal beats. They are usually not preceded by a P wave, although retrograde ventriculoatrial conduction may occur. Unless the latter is present, there is a fully compensatory pause (ie, without change in the PP interval). Bigeminy and trigeminy are arrhythmias in which every second or third beat is premature; these patterns confirm a reentry mechanism for the ectopic beat. Exercise generally abolishes premature beats in normal hearts, and the rhythm becomes regular. The patient may or may not sense the irregular beat, usually as a skipped beat. Ambulatory electrocardiographic monitoring or monitoring during graded exercise may reveal more frequent and complex ventricular premature beats than occur in a single routine ECG. An increased frequency of ventricular premature beats during exercise is associated with a higher risk of cardiovascular mortality, though there is no evidence that specific therapy has a role.

Sudden death occurs more frequently (presumably as a result of ventricular fibrillation) when ventricular premature beats occur in the presence of organic heart disease but not in individuals with no known cardiac disease. If no associated cardiac disease is present and if the ectopic beats are asymptomatic, no therapy is indicated. If they are frequent, electrolyte abnormalities (especially hypo- or hyperkalemia and hypomagnesemia), hyperthyroidism, and occult heart disease should be excluded. Pharmacologic treatment is indicated only for patients who are symptomatic. Because of concerns about worsening arrhythmia and sudden death with most antiarrhythmic agents, beta-blockers are the agents of first choice. If the underlying condition is mitral prolapse, hypertrophic cardiomyopathy, left ventricular hypertrophy, or coronary disease—or if the QT interval is prolonged—beta-blocker therapy is appropriate. The class I and III agents (see Table 10–5) are all effective in reducing ventricular premature beats but often cause side effects and may exacerbate serious arrhythmias in 5–20% of patients. Therefore, every attempt should be made to avoid using class I or III antiarrhythmic agents in patients without symptoms.

Jouven X et al: Long-term outcome in asymptomatic men with exercise-induced premature ventricular depolarizations. N Engl J Med 2000;343:826. [PMID:10995861] (In asymptomatic middle-aged men, exercise-induced ventricular premature depolarization is associated with a 2.5-fold increase in risk of cardiovascular death as a positive test for ischemia.)

Simpson RJ Jr et al: Association of ventricular premature complexes with electrocardiographic-estimated left ventricular mass in a population of African-American and white men and women. (The Atherosclerosis Risk in Communities.) Am J Cardiol 2001;07:19. [PMID: 11137833] (Study demonstrating a correlation between Cornell Voltage-based estimation of left ventricular mass and ventricular premature complexes.)

2. Ventricular Tachycardia

Ventricular tachycardia is defined as three or more consecutive ventricular premature beats. The usual rate is 160–240/min and is moderately regular but less so than atrial tachycardia. The distinction from aberrant conduction of supraventricular tachycardia may be difficult. The usual mechanism is reentry, but abnormally triggered rhythms occur. Ventricular tachycardia is either nonsustained (lasting less than 30 seconds) or sustained. It may be asymptomatic or associated with syncope or milder symptoms of impaired cerebral perfusion.

Ventricular tachycardia is a frequent complication of acute myocardial infarction and dilated cardiomyopathy but may occur in chronic coronary disease, hypertrophic cardiomyopathy, mitral valve prolapse, myocarditis, and in most other forms of myocardial disease. **Torsade de pointes,** a form of ventricular tachycardia in which QRS morphology twists around the baseline, may occur spontaneously in the setting of hypokalemia or hypomagnesemia or after any drug that prolongs the QT interval; it has a particularly poor prognosis. In nonacute settings, most patients with ventricular tachycardia have known or easily detectable cardiac disease, and the finding of ventricular tachycardia is an unfavorable prognostic sign.

Treatment

A. ACUTE VENTRICULAR TACHYCARDIA

The treatment of acute ventricular tachycardia is determined by the degree of hemodynamic compromise and the duration of the arrhythmia. The management of ventricular tachycardia in acute infarction has been discussed. In other patients, if ventricular tachycardia causes hypotension, heart failure, or myocardial ischemia, synchronized DC cardioversion with 100–360 J should be performed immediately. If the patient is tolerating the rhythm, lidocaine, 1 mg/kg as an intravenous bolus injection, may terminate it. If the patient is stable and lidocaine is not effective, a trial of intravenous procainamide, 20 mg/min intravenously (up to 1000 mg), followed by an infusion of 20–80 μg/kg/min. Intravenous amiodarone is often effective when these approaches are not. This formulation is much more bioavailable than the oral form, so more rapid loading can be achieved. It is usually initiated with a rapid loading infusion of 150 mg over 10 minutes, followed by a slow infusion of 1 mg/min for 6 hours and then a maintenance infusion of 0.5 mg/min for an additional 18–42 hours. Supplemental infusions of 150 mg over 10 minutes can be given for recurrent ventricular tachycardia. Bretylium, 5 mg/kg intravenously over 3–5 minutes, repeated after 20 minutes if necessary, followed by an infusion of 1–2 mg/min, is also an alternative. Empiric magnesium replacement (1 g intravenously) may help. Ventricular tachycardia can also be terminated by ventricular overdrive pacing, and this approach is useful when the rhythm is recurrent.

B. CHRONIC RECURRENT VENTRICULAR TACHYCARDIA

1. Sustained ventricular tachycardia—Patients with symptomatic or sustained ventricular tachycardia in the absence of a reversible precipitating cause (acute myocardial infarction or ischemia, electrolyte imbalance, drug toxicity, etc) are at high risk for recurrence. In those with significant left ventricular dysfunction, subsequent sudden death is common. Several trials, including the Antiarrhythmic Drug Versus Implantable Defibrillator (AVID) and the Canadian Implantable Defibrillator trials, strongly suggest that these patients should be managed with implantable cardioverter-defibrillator devices (ICDs). In those with preserved left ventricular function, the mortality rate is lower and treatment with amiodarone, optimally in combination with a beta-blocker, may be adequate. Sotalol may be an alternative, though there is less supporting evidence. The role of electrophysiologic studies in this group is less clear than was previously thought, but they may help identify patients who are candidates for radiofrequency ablation of a ventricular tachycardia focus. This is particularly the case for arrhythmias that originate in the right ventricular outflow tract (appearing as LBBB with inferior axis on the surface ECG), the posterior fascicle (RBBB, superior axis morphology), or sustained bundle branch reentry. As experience accumulates, it is likely that other forms of ventricular tachycardia will be amenable to radiofrequency ablation.

2. Nonsustained ventricular tachycardia (NSVT)— NSVT is defined as runs of three or more ventricular beats lasting less than 30 seconds. These may be symptomatic (usually experienced as light-headedness) or asymptomatic. In individuals without heart disease, NSVT is not clearly associated with a poor prognosis. However, in patients with structural heart disease, particularly when they have reduced ejection fractions, there is an increased risk of subsequent symptomatic ventricular tachycardia or sudden death. Beta-blockers reduce these risks in patients who have coronary disease with significant left ventricular systolic dysfunction (ejection fractions < 35–40%), but if sustained ventricular tachycardia has been induced during electrophysiologic testing, an implantable defibrillator may be indicated. In patients with chronic heart failure and reduced ejection fractions—whether due to coronary disease or primary cardiomyopathy and regardless of the presence of asymptomatic ventricular arrhythmias—beta-blockers reduce the incidence of sudden death by 40–50% and should be routine therapy (see section on Heart Failure).

Although there are no definitive data with amiodarone in this group, trends from a number of studies suggest that it may be beneficial. Other antiarrhythmic agents should generally be avoided because their proarrhythmic risk appears to outweigh any benefit, even in patients with inducible arrhythmias that are successfully suppressed in the electrophysiology laboratory.

Gemayel C et al: Arrhythmogenic right ventricular cardiomyopathy. J Am Coll Cardiol 2001;38:1773. [PMID: 11738273] (Etiology, diagnosis, and management of this in-patient cause of sudden death in young individuals.)

Gupta AK et al: Wide QRS complex tachycardias. Med Clin North Am 2001;85:245. [PMID: 11233948] (Discusses a clinical approach to the diagnosis of wide-complex tachycardia.)

Saliba WI et al: Ventricular tachycardia syndromes. Med Clin North Am 2001;85:267. [PMID: 11233949]

Weigner MJ et al: Nonsustained ventricular tachycardia. A guide to the clinical significance and management. Med Clin North Am 2001;85:305. [PMID: 11233950] (Discusses symptomatic and asymptomatic NSVT.)

3. Ventricular Fibrillation & Sudden Death

Sudden cardiac death is defined as unexpected nontraumatic death in clinically well or stable patients who die within 1 hour after onset of symptoms. The causative rhythm in most cases is ventricular fibrillation, which is usually preceded by ventricular tachycardia except in the setting of acute ischemia or infarction. Complete heart block and sinus node arrest may also cause sudden death. A disproportionate number of sudden deaths occur in the early morning hours. Over 75% of victims of sudden cardiac death have severe coronary artery disease. Many have old infarctions. Sudden death may be the initial manifestation of coronary disease in up to 20% of patients and accounts for approximately 50% of deaths from coronary disease. When ventricular fibrillation occurs in the initial 24 hours after infarction, long-term management is no different from that of other patients with acute infarction. Other conditions that predispose to sudden death include severe left ventricular hypertrophy, hypertrophic cardiomyopathy, congestive cardiomyopathy, aortic stenosis, pulmonary stenosis, primary pulmonary hypertension, cyanotic congenital heart disease, atrial myxoma, mitral valve prolapse, hypoxia, electrolyte abnormalities, prolonged QT interval syndrome, and conduction system disease. Late potentials (after the QRS complex) on a signal-averaged surface ECG in patients with prior myocardial infarction may identify a group of patients at risk of ventricular arrhythmias and sudden death.

Unless ventricular fibrillation occurred shortly after myocardial infarction, is associated with ischemia, or is seen with an unusual correctable process (such as an electrolyte abnormality, drug toxicity, or aortic stenosis), surviving patients require evaluation and intervention since recurrences are frequent. Exercise testing or coronary arteriography should be performed to exclude coronary disease as the underlying cause, since revascularization may prevent recurrence. Conduction disturbances should be managed as described in the next section. If prodromal supraventricular arrhythmias or ventricular arrhythmias, such as sustained or nonsustained ventricular tachycardia, are found by ambulatory electrocardiographic monitoring, their elimination by pharmacologic therapy or ablation may prevent further episodes. There is growing consensus that if myocardial infarction or ischemia, other precipitating causes of ventricular fibrillation, or bradyarrhythmias and conduction disturbances are not found to be the cause of the sudden death episode, an implantable defibrillator is the treatment of choice for appropriate patients.

Eisenberg MS et al: Cardiac resuscitation. N Engl J Med 2001;344:1304. [PMID: 11320390]

Fogel RI et al: Management of malignant arrhythmias and cardiac arrest. Crit Care Med 2000;28:N165. [PMID: 11055686] (Discusses trials and implications for therapy.)

Glikson M et al: The implantable cardioverter defibrillator. Lancet 2001;357:1107. [PMID: 11297981] (Review of mechanics, indications.)

Huikuri HV et al: Sudden death due to cardiac arrhythmias. N Engl J Med 2001;345:1473. [PMID: 11794197] (Epidemiology and causes of sudden death reviewed with a focus on methods of predicting risk. Implantable defibrillators are more effective treatment than drug therapy.)

JAMA patient page: CPR. JAMA 1998;281:1244. [PMID: 10199440]

Jones JL et al: Electrophysiology of ventricular fibrillation and defibrillation. Crit Care Med 2000;28:N219. [PMID: 11098951] (Discusses pathophysiology as well as implications for defibrillation.)

Josephson ME et al: The role of the implantable cardioverter-defibrillator for prevention of sudden cardiac death. Ann Intern Med 2000;133:901. [PMID: 11103061] (Randomized trials suggest ICD is the treatment of choice for survivors of sudden cardiac death and may have a preventive role in patients with coronary artery disease, left ventricular dysfunction, and inducible ventricular tachycardia.)

Marenco JP et al: Improving survival from sudden cardiac arrest: the role of the automated external defibrillator. JAMA 2001;285:1193. [PMID: 11231750] (MEDLINE Review and data synthesis of the literature on the defibrillators.)

4. Accelerated Idioventricular Rhythm

Accelerated idioventricular rhythm is a regular wide complex rhythm with a rate of 60–120/min, usually with a gradual onset. Because the rate is often similar to the sinus rate, fusion beats and alternating rhythms are common. Two mechanisms have been invoked: (1) an escape rhythm due to suppression of higher pacemakers resulting from sinoatrial and atrioventricular block or from depressed sinus node function; and (2) slow ventricular tachycardia due to increased automaticity or, less frequently, reentry. It occurs commonly in acute infarction and following reperfusion after thrombolytic drugs. The incidence of associated ventricular fibrillation is much less than that of ventricular tachycardia with a rapid rate, and treatment is not indicated unless there is hemodynamic compromise or more serious arrhythmias. This rhythm also is common in digitalis toxicity.

Accelerated idioventricular rhythm must be distinguished from the idioventricular or junctional rhythm with rates less than 40–45/min that occurs in the presence of complete atrioventricular block. Atrioventricular dissociation—where ventricular rate exceeds sinus—but not atrioventricular block occurs in most cases of accelerated idioventricular rhythm.

5. Long QT Syndrome

Congenital long QT syndrome is an uncommon disease that is characterized by recurrent syncope, a long QT interval (usually 0.5–0.7 s), documented ventricular arrhythmias, and sudden death. It may occur in the presence (Jervell syndrome, Lange-Nielsen syndrome) or absence (Romano-Ward syndrome) of congenital deafness. Inheritance may be autosomal recessive or autosomal dominant (Romano-Ward). Specific genetic mutations affecting membrane potassium and sodium channels have been identified and help delineate the mechanisms of susceptibility to arrhythmia.

Beta-blockers are the most effective therapy for congenital long QT syndrome and are often used in conjunction with permanent pacemakers, since low heart rates predispose to ventricular arrhythmias. Agents that prolong the QT (classes Ia, Ic, and III) are contraindicated. ICDs are effective in patients who continue to have life-threatening ventricular arrhythmias while taking beta-blockers. Refractory acute arrhythmic episodes may be treated by local anesthetic block of the left stellate ganglion, and recurrent episodes can be treated by resection of this ganglion as well as of the first three to five thoracic ganglia.

Acquired long QT interval secondary to use of antiarrhythmic agents or antidepressant drugs, electrolyte abnormalities, myocardial ischemia, or significant bradycardia may result in ventricular tachycardia (particularly torsade de pointes, ie, twisting about the baseline into varying QRS morphology). Notably, many drugs that are in some settings effective for the treatment of ventricular arrhythmias prolong the QT interval. Prudence dictates that drug therapy which prolongs the QT interval beyond 500 ms be discontinued.

The management of **torsade de pointes** differs from that of other forms of ventricular tachycardia. Class I, Ic, or III antiarrhythmics, which prolong the QT interval, should be avoided—or withdrawn immediately if being used. Intravenous beta-blockers may be effective, especially in the congenital form; intravenous magnesium should be given acutely. An effective approach is temporary ventricular or atrial pacing, which can both break and prevent the rhythm.

Moss AJ et al: Effectiveness and limitations of beta-blocker therapy in congenital long-QT syndrome. Circulation 2000; 101:616. [PMID: 10673253] (Study demonstrating reduction in event rate in treated patients with congenital long QT syndrome.)

Passman R et al: Polymorphic ventricular tachycardia, long Q-T syndrome, and torsades de pointes. Med Clin North Am 2001;85:321. [PMID: 11233951] (Reviews specifics of polymorphic ventricular tachycardia.)

Towbin JA et al: Molecular biology and the prolonged QT syndromes. Am J Med 2001;110:385. [PMID: 11286954] (Discusses molecular basis of the long QT syndromes with implications for genetic testing.)

■ BRADYCARDIAS & CONDUCTION DISTURBANCES

Abnormalities of conduction can occur between the sinus node and atrium, within the atrioventricular node, and in the intraventricular conduction pathways.

SICK SINUS SYNDROME

This imprecise diagnosis is applied to patients with sinus arrest, sinoatrial exit block (recognized by a pause equal to a multiple of the underlying PP interval or progressive shortening of the PP interval prior to a pause), or persistent sinus bradycardia. These rhythms are often caused or exacerbated by drug therapy (digitalis, calcium channel blockers, beta-blockers, sympatholytic agents, antiarrhythmics), and agents that may be responsible should be withdrawn prior to making the diagnosis. Another presentation is of recurrent supraventricular tachycardias (paroxysmal reentry tachycardias, atrial flutter, and atrial fibrillation), associated with bradyarrhythmias ("tachy-brady syndrome"). The long pauses that often follow the termination of tachycardia cause the associated symptoms.

Sick sinus syndrome occurs most commonly in elderly patients. The pathologic changes are usually nonspecific, characterized by patchy fibrosis of the sinus node and cardiac conduction system. Sick sinus syndrome may be caused by other conditions, including sarcoidosis, amyloidosis, Chagas' disease, and various cardiomyopathies. Coronary disease is an uncommon cause.

Most patients with electrocardiographic evidence of sick sinus syndrome are asymptomatic, but rare individuals may experience syncope, dizziness, confusion, palpitations, heart failure, or angina. Because these symptoms are either nonspecific or are due to other causes, it is essential that they be demonstrated to coincide temporally with arrhythmias. This may require prolonged ambulatory monitoring or the use of an event recorder. Pharmacologic therapy for sick sinus syndrome has been difficult, but recent studies have indicated that oral theophylline may be effective, especially when sinus bradycardia is the major manifestation. Most symptomatic patients will require permanent pacing. Dual-chamber pacing is preferred because ventricular pacing is associated with a higher incidence of subsequent atrial fibrillation, and subsequent atrioventricular block occurs at a rate of 2% per year. Treatment of associated tachyarrhythmias is often difficult without first instituting pacing, since digoxin and other antiarrhythmic agents may exacerbate the bradycardia. Unfortunately, symptomatic relief following pacing has not been consistent, largely because of inadequate documentation of the etiologic role of bradyarrhythmias in producing the symptom. Furthermore, many of these patients may have associated ventricular arrhythmias that may require treatment; however, carefully selected patients may become asymptomatic with permanent pacing alone.

Mangrum JM et al: The evaluation and management of bradycardia. N Engl J Med 2000;342:703. [PMID: 10706901] (Reviews bradycardia and management strategies.)

ATRIOVENTRICULAR BLOCK

Atrioventricular block is categorized as first-degree (PR interval > 0.21 s with all atrial impulses conducted), second-degree (intermittent blocked beats), or third-degree (complete heart block, in which no supraventricular impulses are conducted to the ventricles).

Second-degree block is subclassified. In **Mobitz type I (Wenckebach)** atrioventricular block, the atrioventricular conduction time (PR interval) progressively lengthens, with the RR interval shortening, before the blocked beat; this phenomenon is almost always due to abnormal conduction within the atrioventricular node. In **Mobitz type II** atrioventricular block there are intermittently nonconducted atrial beats not preceded by lengthening AV conduction. It is usually due to block within the His bundle system.

The classification as Mobitz type I or Mobitz type II is only partially reliable, because patients may appear to have both types on the surface ECG, and one cannot predict the site of origin of the 2:1 atrioventricular block from the ECG. The width of the QRS complexes assists in determining whether the block is nodal or infranodal. When they are narrow, the block is usually nodal; when they are wide, the block is usually infranodal. Electrophysiologic studies may be necessary for accurate localization. Management of atrioventricular block in acute myocardial infarction has already been discussed. This section deals with patients in the nonischemic setting.

First-degree and **Mobitz type I block** may occur in normal individuals with heightened vagal tone. They may also occur as a drug effect (especially digitalis, calcium channel blockers, beta-blockers, or other sympatholytic agents), often superimposed on organic disease. These disturbances also occur transiently or chronically due to ischemia, infarction, inflammatory processes, fibrosis, calcification, or infiltration. The prognosis is usually good, since reliable alternative pacemakers arise from the atrioventricular junction below the level of block if higher degrees of block occur.

Mobitz type II block is almost always due to organic disease involving the infranodal conduction system. In the event of progression to complete heart block, alternative pacemakers are not reliable. Thus, prophylactic ventricular pacing is required.

Complete (third-degree) heart block is a more advanced form of block often due to a lesion distal to the His bundle and associated with bilateral bundle branch block. The QRS is wide and the ventricular rate is slower, usually less than 50/min. Transmission of atrial impulses through the atrioventricular node is completely blocked, and a ventricular pacemaker maintains a slow, regular ventricular rate, usually less than 45/min. Exercise does not increase the rate. The first heart sound varies in intensity; wide pulse pressure, a changing systolic blood pressure level, and cannon venous pulsations in the neck are also present. Patients may be asymptomatic or may complain of weakness or dyspnea if the rate is less than 35/min; symptoms may occur at higher rates if the left ventricle cannot increase its stroke output. During periods of transition from partial to complete heart block, some patients have ventricular asystole that lasts several seconds to minutes. Syncope occurs abruptly.

Patients with episodic or chronic infranodal complete heart block require permanent pacing, and temporary pacing is indicated if implantation of a permanent pacemaker is delayed.

Barold SS et al: Second-degree atrioventricular block: a reappraisal. Mayo Clin Proc 2001;76:44. [PMID: 11155413] (Careful definition of various types of atrioventricular block with evaluation and management recommendations.)

ATRIOVENTRICULAR DISSOCIATION

When a ventricular pacemaker is firing at a rate faster than or close to the sinus rate (accelerated idioventricular rhythm, ventricular premature beats, or ventricular tachycardia), atrial impulses arriving at the atrioventricular node when it is refractory may not be conducted. This phenomenon is atrioventricular dissociation but does not necessarily indicate atrioventricular block. No treatment is required aside from management of the causative arrhythmia.

INTRAVENTRICULAR CONDUCTION DEFECTS

Intraventricular conduction defects, including bundle branch block, are common in individuals with otherwise normal hearts and in many disease processes, including ischemic heart disease, inflammatory disease, infiltrative disease, cardiomyopathy, and postcardiotomy. Below the atrioventricular node and bundle of His, the conduction system trifurcates into a right bundle and anterior and posterior fascicles of the left bundle. Conduction block in each of these fascicles can be recognized on the surface ECG. Although such conduction abnormalities are often seen in normal hearts, they are more commonly due to organic heart disease—either an isolated process of fibrosis and calcification or more generalized myocardial disease. Bifascicular block is present when two of these—right bundle, left anterior and posterior hemibundle—are involved. Trifascicular block is defined as right bundle branch block with alternating left hemiblock, alternating right and left bundle branch block, or bifascicular block with documented prolonged infranodal conduction (long His-ventricular interval).

The prognosis of intraventricular block is generally that of the underlying myocardial process. Patients with no apparent heart disease have an overall survival rate similar to that of matched controls. However, left bundle branch block—but not right—is associated with a higher risk of development of overt cardiac disease and cardiac mortality. Even in bifascicular block, the incidence of occult complete heart block or progression to it is low, and pacing is not usually warranted. In patients with symptoms (eg, syncope) consistent with heart block and intraventricular block, pacing should be reserved for those with documented concomitant complete heart block on monitoring or those with a very prolonged HV interval (> 90 ms) with no other cause for symptoms. Even in the latter group, prophylactic pacing has not improved the prognosis significantly, probably because of the high incidence of ventricular arrhythmias in the same population.

PERMANENT PACING

The indications for permanent pacing have been discussed: symptomatic bradyarrhythmias, asymptomatic

Mobitz II atrioventricular block, or complete heart block. The versatility of pacemaker generator units has increased markedly, and dual-chamber multiple programmable units are being implanted with increasing frequency. A standardized nomenclature for pacemaker generators is employed, usually consisting of four letters. The first letter refers to the chamber which is stimulated (A = atrium, V = ventricle, D = dual, for both). The second letter refers to the chamber where sensing occurs (also A, V, or D). The third position refers to the sensory mode (I = inhibition by a sensed impulse, T = triggering by a sensed impulse, D = dual modes of response). The fourth letter refers to the programmability or rate modulation capacity (usually P for programming for two functions, M for programming more than two, and R for rate modulation).

A pacemaker that senses and paces in both chambers is the most physiologic approach to pacing patients who remain in sinus rhythm. Atrioventricular synchrony is particularly important in patients in whom atrial contraction produces a substantial increment in stroke volume and in those in whom sensing the atrial rate to provide rate-responsive ventricular pacing is useful. Dual-chamber pacing is most useful for individuals with left ventricular systolic or—perhaps more importantly—diastolic dysfunction and for physically active individuals. In patients with single-chamber pacemakers, the lack of an atrial kick may lead to the so-called pacemaker syndrome, in which the patient experiences signs of low cardiac output while upright. Uncontrolled data suggest that chronic dual-chamber pacing is associated with a lower incidence of chronic atrial fibrillation than single-chamber ventricular pacing. However, patients with intermittent or potential bradyarrhythmias or conduction disturbances in whom pacing is primarily prophylactic should undergo ventricular pacing.

Pulse generators are also available that can increase their rate in response to motion or respiratory rate when the atrial rate is not an indication of the optimal heart rate. These are most useful in active individuals. Follow-up after pacemaker implantation, usually by telephonic monitoring, is essential. All pulse generators and lead systems have an early failure rate that is now below 5% and an expected battery life varying from 4 years to 10 years.

Bryce M et al: Evolving indications for permanent pacemakers. Ann Intern Med 2001;134:1130. [PMID: 11412054] (Controversial indications such as hypertrophic and dilated cardiomyopathy, neurocardiogenic syncope, and atrial fibrillation are discussed.)

Connolly SJ et al: Effects of physiologic pacing versus ventricular pacing on the risk of stroke and death due to cardiovascular causes. Canadian Trial of Physiologic Pacing Investigators. N Engl J Med 2000;342:1385. [PMID: 10805823] (Randomized trial of over 2500 patients comparing ventricular pacing with dual-chamber "physiologic" pacing. Only a small difference in the incidence of atrial fibrillation and no difference in stroke rates were observed over a 3-year follow-up period. This trial argues for more selective use of physiologic pacing.)

Gregoratos G et al: ACC/AHA Guidelines for Implantation of Cardiac Pacemakers and Arrhythmia Devices: Executive Summary—a report of the American College of Cardiology/American Heart Association Task Force on Practice Guidelines (Committee on Pacemaker Implantation). Circulation 1998; 97:1325. [PMID: 9570207]

Glikson M et al: Cardiac pacing. A review. Med Clin North Am 2001;85:369. [PMID: 11233953] (Reviews indications as well as types of pacemakers.)

Gold MR et al: Permanent pacing: New indications. Heart 2001;86:355. [PMID: 11514497]

JAMA patient page. Heart pacemakers. JAMA 2001;286:878. [PMID: 11519499]

EVALUATION OF SYNCOPE

Syncope, defined as a transient loss of consciousness and postural tone due to inadequate cerebral blood flow with prompt recovery without resuscitative measures, is a common clinical problem, especially in the elderly. Thirty percent of the adult population will experience at least one episode, and syncope accounts for approximately 3% of emergency room visits. Causes include cardiac abnormalities (either disturbances of rhythm or hemodynamics), vascular disorders, or neurologic processes. A specific cause is identified in about 50% of cases during the initial evaluation. The prognosis is relatively benign except when accompanying cardiac disease is present. Syncope is more likely to occur in patients with known heart disease, older men, and young women (who are prone to vasovagal episodes). Syncope is characteristically abrupt in onset, often resulting in injury, transient (lasting for seconds to a few minutes), and followed by prompt recovery or full consciousness.

Vasomotor syncope may be due to excessive vagal tone or impaired reflex control of the peripheral circulation. The most frequent type of vasodepressor syncope is vasovagal hypotension or the "common faint," which is often initiated by stressful, painful, or claustrophobic experience, especially in young women. Premonitory symptoms, such as nausea, diaphoresis, tachycardia, and pallor, are usual. Episodes can be aborted by lying down or removing the inciting stimulus. Enhanced vagal tone with resulting hypotension is the cause of syncope in carotid sinus hypersensitivity and postmicturition syncope; vagal-induced sinus bradycardia, sinus arrest, and atrioventricular block are common accompaniments and may themselves be the cause of syncope. Carotid sinus massage under carefully monitored conditions or tilt-table testing may be diagnostic (see above under Autonomic Testing). Treatment consists largely of counseling patients to avoid predisposing situations. Paradoxically, beta-blockers may be helpful in patients with altered autonomic function uncovered by head-up tilt testing. Permanent pacing may benefit patients with documented bradycardiac responses.

Orthostatic (postural) hypotension is another common cause of vasomotor syncope, especially in the elderly, in diabetics or other patients with autonomic neuropathy, in patients with blood loss or hypovolemia, and in patients taking vasodilators, diuretics, and adrenergic blocking drugs. In addition, a syndrome of chronic idiopathic orthostatic hypotension exists primarily in older men. In most of these conditions, the normal vasoconstrictive response to assuming upright posture, which compensates for the abrupt decrease in venous return, is impaired. A greater than normal decline (20 mm Hg) in blood pressure immediately upon arising from the supine to the standing position is observed, with or without tachycardia depending on the status of autonomic (baroreceptor) function. Studying patients with a tilt table can establish the diagnosis with more certainty. Autonomic function can be assessed by observing blood pressure and heart rate responses to Valsalva's maneuver and by tilt testing. In older patients, vasoconstrictor abnormalities and autonomic insufficiency are perhaps the most common causes of syncope. Thus, tilt testing should be employed before proceeding to invasive studies unless clinical and ambulatory electrocardiographic evaluation suggests a cardiac abnormality.

Cardiogenic syncope can occur on a mechanical or arrhythmic basis. Mechanical problems that can cause syncope include aortic stenosis (where syncope may occur from autonomic reflex abnormalities or ventricular tachycardia), pulmonary stenosis, hypertrophic obstructive cardiomyopathy, congenital lesions associated with pulmonary hypertension or right-to-left shunting, and left atrial myxoma obstructing the mitral valve. Episodes are commonly exertional or postexertional. More commonly, cardiac syncope is due to disorders of automaticity (sick sinus syndrome), conduction disorders (atrioventricular block), or tachyarrhythmias (especially ventricular tachycardia and supraventricular tachycardia with rapid ventricular rate).

The evaluation for syncope depends on findings from the history and physical examination (especially orthostatic blood pressure evaluation, examination of carotid and other arteries, cardiac examination, and, if appropriate, carotid sinus massage). The resting ECG may reveal arrhythmias, evidence of accessory pathways, prolonged QT interval, and other signs of heart disease (such as infarction or hypertrophy). If the history is consistent with syncope, ambulatory electrocardiographic monitoring is essential. This may need to be repeated several times, since yields increase with longer periods of monitoring, at least up to 3 days. Event recorder and transtelephone electrocardiographic monitoring may be helpful in patients with intermittent presyncopal episodes. Electrophysiologic studies to assess sinus node function and atrioventricular conduction and to induce supraventricular or ventricular tachycardia are indicated in patients with recurrent episodes and nondiagnostic ambulatory ECGs. They reveal an arrhythmic cause in 20–50% of patients, depending on the study criteria, and are most often diagnostic when the patient has had multiple episodes and has identifiable cardiac abnormalities.

Kapoor WN: Syncope. N Engl J Med 2000;343:1856. [PMID: 11117979] (Differential diagnosis, evaluation, and management of this common but often elusive condition.)

Schnipper JL et al: Diagnostic evaluation and management of patients with syncope. Med Clin North Am 2001;85:423. [PMID: 11233954]

RECOMMENDATIONS FOR RESUMPTION OF DRIVING

An important management problem in patients who have experienced syncope, symptomatic ventricular tachycardia, or aborted sudden death is to provide recommendations concerning automobile driving. According to a survey published in 1991, only eight states had specific laws dealing with this issue, whereas 42 had laws restricting driving in patients with seizure disorders. There are not adequate data to support driving restrictions in patients with asymptomatic arrhythmias, though patients with frequent nonsustained ventricular tachycardia, associated heart disease, and significant left ventricular dysfunction are at high enough risk to warrant cautioning. Patients with syncope or aborted sudden death thought to have been due to temporary factors (acute myocardial infarction, bradyarrhythmias subsequently treated with permanent pacing, drug effect, electrolyte imbalance) should be strongly advised after recovery not to drive for at least 1 month. Other patients with symptomatic ventricular tachycardia or aborted sudden death, whether treated pharmacologically, with antitachycardia devices, or with ablation therapy, should not drive for at least 6 months. Longer restrictions are warranted in many such patients if spontaneous arrhythmias persist. The physician should comply with local regulations and consult local authorities concerning individual cases.

Akiyama T et al: Resumption of driving after life-threatening ventricular tachyarrhythmia. N Engl J Med 2001;345:391. [PMID: 11496849] (Study assessing risk of ventricular arrhythmias in patients in the AVID trial.)

Carr DB: The older adult driver. Am Fam Phys 2000;61:141. [PMID: 10643955] (Review with suggestions for how to deal with a major social and very personal issue.)

■ CARDIAC FAILURE

 ESSENTIALS OF DIAGNOSIS

- *Left ventricular failure: Exertional dyspnea, cough, fatigue, orthopnea, paroxysmal nocturnal dyspnea, cardiac enlargement, rales, gallop rhythm, and pulmonary venous congestion.*

- *Right ventricular failure: Elevated venous pressure, hepatomegaly, dependent edema; usually due to left ventricular failure.*

- *Assessment of left ventricular function is a crucial part of diagnosis and management.*

General Considerations

Systolic function of the heart is governed by four major determinants: the contractile state of the myocardium, the preload of the ventricle (the end-diastolic volume and the resultant fiber length of the ventricles prior to onset of the contraction), the afterload applied to the ventricles (the impedance to left ventricular ejection), and the heart rate.

Cardiac function may be inadequate as a result of alterations in any of these determinants. In most instances, the primary derangement is depression of myocardial contractility caused either by loss of functional muscle (due to myocardial infarction, etc) or by processes diffusely affecting the myocardium. However, the heart may fail as a pump because preload is excessively elevated, such as in valvular regurgitation, or when afterload is excessive, such as in aortic stenosis or in severe hypertension. Pump function may also be inadequate when the heart rate is too slow or too rapid. While the normal heart can tolerate wide variations in preload, afterload, and heart rate, the diseased heart often has limited reserve for such alterations. Finally, cardiac pump function may be supranormal but nonetheless inadequate when metabolic demands or requirements for blood flow are excessive. This situation is termed **high-output heart failure** and, though uncommon, tends to be specifically treatable. Causes of high output include thyrotoxicosis, beriberi, severe anemia, arteriovenous shunting, and Paget's disease of bone.

Manifestations of cardiac failure can also occur as a result of isolated or predominant **diastolic dysfunction** of the heart. In these cases, filling of the left or right ventricle is abnormal, either because myocardial relaxation is impaired or because the chamber is noncompliant ("stiff") due to excessive hypertrophy or changes in composition of the myocardium. Even though contractility may be preserved, diastolic pressures are elevated and cardiac output may be reduced, potentially causing fluid retention, dyspnea, and exercise intolerance.

Pathophysiology

When the heart fails, a number of adaptations occur both in the heart and systemically. If the stroke volume of either ventricle is reduced by depressed contractility or excessive afterload, end-diastolic volume and pressure in that chamber will rise. This increases end-diastolic myocardial fiber length, resulting in a greater systolic shortening (Starling's law of the heart). If the condition is chronic, ventricular dilation will occur. While this may restore resting cardiac output, the resulting chronic elevation of diastolic pressures will be transmitted to the atria and to the pulmonary and systemic venous circulation. Ultimately, increased capillary pressure may lead to transudation of fluid with resulting pulmonary or systemic edema. Reduced cardiac output, particularly if associated with reduced arterial pressure or perfusion of the kidneys, will also activate several neural and humoral systems. Increased activity of the sympathetic nervous system will stimulate myocardial contractility, heart rate, and venous tone; the latter change results in a rise in the effective central blood volume, which serves to further elevate preload. Though these adaptations are designed to increase cardiac output, they may themselves be deleterious. Thus, tachycardia and increased contractility may precipitate ischemia in patients with underlying coronary artery disease, and the rise in preload may worsen pulmonary congestion. Sympathetic nervous system activation also increases peripheral vascular resistance; this adaptation is designed to maintain perfusion to vital organs, but when it is excessive it may itself reduce renal and other tissue blood flow. Peripheral vascular resistance is also a major determinant of left ventricular afterload, so that excessive sympathetic activity may further depress cardiac function.

One of the more important effects of lower cardiac output is reduction of renal blood flow and glomerular filtration rate, which leads to sodium and fluid retention. The renin-angiotensin-aldosterone system is also activated, leading to further increases in peripheral vascular resistance and left ventricular afterload as well as sodium and fluid retention. Heart failure is associated with increased circulating levels of arginine vasopressin, which also serves as a vasoconstrictor and inhibitor of water excretion. While release of atrial natriuretic peptide is increased in heart failure owing to the elevated atrial pressures, there is evidence of resistance to its natriuretic and vasodilating effects.

Hemodynamic Alterations

Myocardial failure is characterized by two hemodynamic derangements, and the clinical presentation is determined by their severity. The first is reduction in cardiac reserve, ie, the ability to increase cardiac output in response to increased demands imposed by exercise or even ordinary activity. The second abnormality, elevation of ventricular diastolic pressures, is primarily a result of the compensatory processes.

Heart failure may be right-sided or left-sided. Patients with the picture of **left heart failure** have symptoms of low cardiac output and elevated pulmonary venous pressure; dyspnea is the predominant feature. Signs of fluid retention predominate in **right heart failure,** with the patient exhibiting edema, hepatic congestion, and, on occasion, ascites. Most patients exhibit symptoms or signs of both right- and left-sided failure, and left ventricular dysfunction is the primary cause of right ventricular failure. Surprisingly, some individuals with severe left ventricular dysfunction will display few signs of left heart failure and appear to have isolated right heart failure. Indeed, they may be clinically indistinguishable from patients with cor pulmonale, who have right heart failure secondary to pulmonary disease.

Although this section primarily concerns cardiac failure due to systolic left ventricular dysfunction, patients with **diastolic dysfunction** experience many of the same symptoms and may be difficult to distinguish clinically. Diastolic pressures are elevated even though diastolic volumes are normal or small. These pressures are transmitted to the pulmonary and systemic venous systems, resulting in dyspnea and edema. The most frequent cause of diastolic cardiac dysfunction is left ventricular hypertrophy, commonly resulting from hypertension, but conditions such as hypertrophic or restrictive cardiomyopathy, diabetes, and pericardial disease can produce the same clinical picture. While diuretics are often useful in these patients, the other therapies discussed in this section (digitalis, vasodilators, inotropic agents) may be inappropriate.

Causes & Prevention of Cardiac Failure

The syndrome of cardiac failure can be produced by many diseases. In developed countries, coronary artery disease with resulting myocardial infarction and loss of functioning myocardium (ischemic cardiomyopathy) is the commonest cause. In the 4S study, aggressive lipid-lowering therapy in patients with known coronary disease reduced the incidence of heart failure by 30%. A number of processes may present with dilated or congestive cardiomyopathy, which is characterized by left ventricular or biventricular dilation and generalized systolic dysfunction. These are discussed elsewhere in this chapter, but the most common are alcoholic cardiomyopathy, viral myocarditis (including infections by HIV), and dilated cardiomyopathies with no obvious underlying cause (idiopathic cardiomyopathy). Rare causes of dilated cardiomyopathy include infiltrative diseases (hemochromatosis, sarcoidosis, amyloidosis, etc), other infectious agents, metabolic disorders, cardiotoxins, and drug toxicity.

Systemic hypertension remains an important cause of congestive heart failure and, even more commonly in the USA, an exacerbating factor in patients with cardiac dysfunction due to other causes. In several trials, antihypertensive therapy—particularly when directed to the systolic blood pressure—has been effective in reducing the incidence of new-onset heart failure by 40–60%. Valvular heart disease has become a less frequent cause of heart failure with the declining incidence and severity of rheumatic fever. However, aortic stenosis remains a common and reversible cause. Patients with chronic volume overload of the left ventricle, such as mitral or aortic regurgitation, may develop progressive myocardial dysfunction and have a picture of cardiomyopathy even after the underlying condition is corrected. This form of congestive heart failure is preventable by early diagnosis and treatment of the valvular lesion.

Cohn JN et al: Cardiac remodeling concepts and clinical implications: a consensus paper from an international forum on cardiac remodeling. Behalf of an International Forum on Cardiac Remodeling. J Am Coll Cardiol 2000;35:569. [PMID: 10716457]

Davis RC et al: ABC of heart failure. History and epidemiology. BMJ 2000;320;39. [PMID: 10617530] (Historical perspectives and epidemiology.)

Eichhorn EJ: Prognosis determination in heart failure. Am J Med 2001;110 (Suppl 7A):14S. [PMID: 11334772] (Reviews data regarding prognosticating in patients with heart failure.)

Francis GS: Pathophysiology of chronic heart failure. Am J Med 2001;110 (Suppl 7A):37S. [PMID: 11334774]

Lip GY et al: ABC of heart failure: aetiology. BMJ 2000;320:104. [PMID: 10625270] (Discusses causes.)

Massie BM: Pathophysiology of heart failure. In: *Cecil Textbook of Medicine*, 21st ed. Saunders, 2001.

McMurray JJ et al: Epidemiology, aetiology, and prognosis of heart failure. Heart 2000;83:596. [PMID: 10768918]

Schrier RW et al: Hormones and hemodynamics in heart failure. N Engl J Med 1999;341:577. [PMID: 10451464] (Physiologic review covers the role of the sympathetic nervous system, renin-angiotensin-aldosterone system, vasopressin, and natriuretic peptides.)

Senni M et al: Heart failure with preserved systolic function. A different natural history? J Am Coll Cardiol 2001;38:1277. [PMID: 11691495]

Clinical Findings

A. SYMPTOMS

The symptoms of cardiac failure have been discussed in part in earlier sections. The most common complaint is shortness of breath, chiefly exertional dyspnea at first and then progressing to orthopnea, paroxysmal nocturnal dyspnea, and rest dyspnea. A more subtle and often overlooked symptom of heart failure is a chronic nonproductive cough, which is often worse in the recumbent position. Nocturia due to excretion of fluid retained during the day and increased renal perfusion in the recumbent position is a common nonspecific symptom of heart failure. Patients with heart failure also complain of fatigue and exercise intolerance. These symptoms correlate poorly with the degree of cardiac dysfunction and result in part from changes in peripheral blood flow and blood flow to skeletal muscle which are part of the syndrome of heart failure. Patients with right heart failure may experience right upper quadrant pain due to passive congestion of the liver, loss of appetite and nausea due to edema of the gut or impaired gastrointestinal perfusion, and peripheral edema.

Cardiac failure may present acutely in a previously asymptomatic patient. Causes include myocardial infarction, myocarditis, and acute valvular regurgitation due to endocarditis or other conditions. These patients usually present with pulmonary edema. The management of acute heart failure has been discussed under myocardial infarction and centers around initial stabilization with diuretics and parenteral vasodilators or inotropic agents.

Patients with episodic symptoms may be having left ventricular dysfunction due to intermittent ischemia. This potentially reversible form of heart failure should be considered, especially in patients with angina pectoris and those with diabetes mellitus. Patients may also present with acute exacerbations of chronic, stable heart failure. Exacerbations are usually caused by alterations in therapy (or patient noncompliance), excessive salt and fluid intake, arrhythmias, excessive activity, pulmonary emboli, intercurrent infection, or progression of the underlying disease.

Patients with heart failure are often categorized by the New York Heart Association classification as class I (asymptomatic), class II (symptomatic with moderate activity), class III (symptomatic with mild activity), or class IV (symptomatic at rest). However, this classification has major limitations in that patient reports are highly subjective and in that symptoms vary from day to day. In any case, the classification is insufficiently sensitive to be useful in predicting outcomes or assessing the results of treatment.

B. SIGNS

Many patients with heart failure, including some with severe symptoms, appear comfortable at rest. Others will be dyspneic during conversation or minor activity, and those with long-standing severe heart failure may appear cachectic or cyanotic. The vital signs may be normal, but tachycardia, hypotension, and reduced pulse pressure may be present. Patients often show signs of increased sympathetic nervous system activity, including cold extremities and diaphoresis. Important peripheral signs of heart failure can be detected by examination of the neck, the lungs, the abdomen, and the extremities. Right atrial pressure may be estimated through the height of the pulsations in the jugular venous system. In addition to the height of the venous pressure, abnormal pulsations such as regurgitant v waves should be sought. Examination of the carotid pulse may allow estimation of pulse pressure as well as detection of aortic stenosis. The thyroid examination is important, since occult hyperthyroidism and hypothyroidism are readily treatable causes of heart failure. In the lungs, crackles at the lung bases reflect transudation of fluid into the alveoli. Pleural effusions may cause bibasilar dullness to percussion. Expiratory wheezing and rhonchi may be signs of heart failure. Patients with severe right heart failure may have hepatic enlargement—tender or nontender—due to passive congestion. Systolic pulsations may be felt in tricuspid regurgitation. Sustained moderate pressure on the liver may increase jugular venous pressure (a positive hepatojugular reflux is an increase of > 1 cm). Ascites may also be present. Peripheral pitting edema is a common sign in patients with right heart failure and may extend into the thighs and abdominal wall.

The cardiac examination has been discussed. Cardinal signs in heart failure are a parasternal lift, indicating pulmonary hypertension; an enlarged and sustained left ventricular impulse, indicating left ventricular dilation and hypertrophy; a diminished first heart sound, suggesting impaired contractility; and S_3 gallops originating in the left and sometimes the right ventricle. An S_4 is usually present in diastolic heart failure. Murmurs should be sought to exclude primary valvular disease; secondary mitral regurgitation and tricuspid regurgitation murmurs are common in patients with dilated ventricles. In chronic heart failure, many of the expected signs of heart failure may be absent despite markedly abnormal cardiac function and hemodynamic measurements.

C. LABORATORY FINDINGS

A blood count may reveal anemia, a cause of high-output failure and an exacerbating factor in other forms of cardiac dysfunction. Biochemical studies may show renal insufficiency as a possible compounding factor. Renal function tests also determine whether cardiac failure is associated with prerenal azotemia. Serum electrolytes may disclose hypokalemia, which increases the risk of arrhythmias; hyperkalemia, which may limit the use of inhibitors of the renin-angiotensin system; or hyponatremia, an indicator of marked activation of the renin-angiotensin system and a poor prognostic sign. Thyroid function should be assessed in older patients to detect occult thyrotoxicosis or myxedema. In unexplained cases, appropriate biopsies may lead to a diagnosis of amyloidosis, and additional assessment should include iron studies to exclude hemochromatosis. Myocardial biopsy may exclude specific causes of dilated cardiomyopathy but rarely reveals specific reversible diagnoses.

Assays of serum "B-type" natriuretic peptide (BNP) may be a useful adjunct to the clinical history and physical examination in the diagnosis of heart failure. BNP is expressed primarily in the ventricles and is elevated when ventricular filling pressures are high. It is quite sensitive in patients with symptomatic heart failure—whether due to systolic or to diastolic dysfunction—but less specific in older patients, women, and patients with COPD.

D. ELECTROCARDIOGRAPHY AND CHEST X-RAY

Electrocardiography may indicate an underlying or secondary arrhythmia, myocardial infarction, or nonspecific changes that often include low voltage, intraventricular conduction defects, left ventricular hypertrophy, and nonspecific repolarization changes. Chest radiographs provide information about the size and shape of the cardiac silhouette. Cardiomegaly is an important finding. Evidence of pulmonary venous hypertension includes relative dilation of the upper lobe veins, perivascular edema (haziness of vessel outlines), interstitial edema, and alveolar fluid. In acute heart failure, these findings correlate moderately well with pulmonary venous pressure. However, patients with chronic heart failure may show relatively normal pulmonary vasculature despite markedly elevated pressures. Pleural effusions are common and tend to be bilateral or right-sided.

E. ADDITIONAL STUDIES

Many studies have indicated that the clinical diagnosis of systolic myocardial dysfunction is often inaccurate. The primary confounding conditions are diastolic dysfunction of the heart with decreased relaxation and filling of the left ventricle (particularly in hypertension and in hypertrophic states) and pulmonary disease. Since heart failure patients usually have significant resting electrocardiographic abnormalities, stress imaging procedures such as perfusion scintigraphy or dobutamine echocardiography are often indicated.

The most useful test is the echocardiogram. This will reveal the size and function of both ventricles and of the atria. It will also allow detection of pericardial effusion, valvular abnormalities, intracardiac shunts, and segmental wall motion abnormalities suggestive of old myocardial infarction as opposed to more generalized forms of dilated cardiomyopathy.

Radionuclide angiography measures left ventricular ejection fraction and permits analysis of regional wall motion. This test is especially useful when echocardiography is technically suboptimal, such as in patients with severe pulmonary disease. When myocardial ischemia is suspected as a cause of left ventricular dysfunction, stress testing should be performed.

F. CARDIAC CATHETERIZATION

In most patients with heart failure, clinical examination and noninvasive tests can determine left ventricular size and function well enough to confirm the diagnosis. Left heart catheterization is necessary when significant valvular disease must be excluded and when the presence and extent of coronary artery disease must be determined. The latter is particularly important when left ventricular dysfunction may be partially reversible by revascularization. The combination of angina or noninvasive evidence of significant myocardial ischemia with symptomatic heart failure is often an indication for coronary angiography if the patient is a potential candidate for revascularization. Right heart catheterization may be useful to select and monitor therapy in patients refractory to standard therapy.

Dao Q et al: Utility of B-type natriuretic peptide in the diagnosis of congestive heart failure in an urgent-care setting. J Am Coll Cardiol 2001;37:379. [PMID: 11216950] (BNP results in 250 patients presenting to an urgent care clinic or emergency room with dyspnea, showing a very high negative predictive value. Retrospective analysis indicates that this test could have corrected most of the diagnoses missed by urgent care physicians.)

Davies MK et al: ABC of heart failure. BMJ 2000;320:297. [PMID: 10650030] (Brief overview of diagnostic tools for heart failure.)

Struthers AD: The diagnosis of heart failure. Heart 2000;84:334. [PMID: 10956303]

Drazner MH et al: Prognostic importance of elevated jugular venous pressure and a third heart sound in patients with heart failure. N Engl J Med 2001;345:574. [PMID: 11529211] (Retrospective study demonstrating the poor prognosis of these findings.)

Zile MR et al: Heart failure with a normal ejection fraction: is measurement of diastolic function necessary to make the diagnosis of diastolic heart failure? Circulation 2001;104:779. [PMID: 11502702] (Catheterization is not necessary to make the diagnosis of diastolic dysfunction.)

Pharmacologic Treatment

The treatment of chronic heart failure is discussed here. Acute pulmonary edema is discussed in the next section.

A. CORRECTION OF REVERSIBLE CAUSES

The major reversible causes of chronic heart failure include valvular lesions, myocardial ischemia, arrhythmias (especially persistent tachycardias), alcohol- or drug-induced myocardial depression, intracardiac shunts, and high-output states. Calcium channel blockers, antiarrhythmic drugs, and nonsteroidal anti-inflammatory agents are important causes of worsening heart failure. Some metabolic and infiltrative cardiomyopathies may be partially reversible, or their progression may be slowed; these include hemochromatosis, sarcoidosis, and amyloidosis. Acute myocarditis may respond to immunosuppressive therapy and corticosteroids. Reversible causes of diastolic dysfunction include pericardial disease and left ventricular hypertrophy due to hypertension. Once it is established that there is no reversible component, the measures outlined below are appropriate.

B. DIET AND ACTIVITY

Patients should routinely practice moderate salt restriction (2–2.5 g sodium or 5–6 g salt per day). More severe sodium restriction is usually difficult to achieve and unnecessary because of the availability of potent diuretic agents. In severe heart failure, restriction of activity may facilitate temporary recompensation. However, in stable patients, a prudent increase in activity or a regular exercise regimen can be encouraged. Indeed, a gradual exercise program is associated with diminished symptoms and substantial increases in exercise capacity.

C. DIURETIC THERAPY

Diuretics are the most effective means of providing symptomatic relief to patients with moderate to severe congestive heart failure. Few patients with symptoms or signs of fluid retention can be optimally managed without a diuretic. However, excessive diuresis can lead to electrolyte imbalance and neurohormonal activation. A combination of a diuretic and an ACE inhibitor should be the initial treatment in most symptomatic patients. When fluid retention is mild, thiazide diuretics or a similar type of agent (hydrochlorothiazide, 25–50 mg; metolazone, 2.5–5 mg; chlorthalidone, 25–50 mg; etc) may be sufficient. These agents block sodium reabsorption in the cortical diluting segment at the terminal portion of the loop of Henle and in the proximal portion of the distal convoluted tubule. The result is natriuresis and kaliuresis.

These agents also have weak carbonic anhydrase inhibitor activity, which results in proximal tubule inhibition of sodium reabsorption. Thiazide or related diuretics often provide better control of hypertension than short-acting loop agents.

The thiazides are generally ineffective when the glomerular filtration rate falls below 30 mL/min, a not infrequent occurrence in patients with severe heart failure. Metolazone maintains its efficacy down to a glomerular filtration rate of approximately 10–20 mL/min. Adverse reactions include hypokalemia and intravascular volume depletion with resulting prerenal azotemia, skin rashes, neutropenia and thrombocytopenia, hyperglycemia, hyperuricemia, and hepatic dysfunction.

Patients with more severe heart failure should be treated with one of the loop diuretics. These include furosemide (20–320 mg daily), bumetanide (1–8 mg daily), and torsemide (20–200 mg daily). These agents have a rapid onset and a relatively short duration of action. In patients with preserved renal function, two or more doses are preferable to a single larger dose. In acute situations or when gastrointestinal absorption is in doubt, they should be given intravenously. The loop diuretics inhibit chloride reabsorption in the ascending limb of the loop of Henle, which results in natriuresis, kaliuresis, and metabolic alkalosis. They are active even in severe renal insufficiency, but larger doses (up to 500 mg of furosemide or equivalent) may be required. The major adverse reactions include intravascular volume depletion, prerenal azotemia, and hypotension. Hypokalemia, particularly with accompanying digitalis therapy, is a major problem. Less common side effects include skin rashes, gastrointestinal distress, and ototoxicity (the latter more common with ethacrynic acid and possibly less common with bumetanide).

The potassium-sparing agents spironolactone, triamterene, and amiloride are often useful in combination with the loop diuretics and thiazides. Triamterene and amiloride act on the distal tubule to reduce potassium secretion. Their diuretic potency is only mild and not adequate for most patients with heart failure, but they may minimize the hypokalemia induced by more potent agents. Side effects include hyperkalemia, gastrointestinal symptoms, and renal dysfunction. Spironolactone is a specific inhibitor of aldosterone, which is often increased in congestive heart failure and has important effects beyond potassium retention (see below). Its onset of action is slower than the other potassium-sparing agents, and its side effects include gynecomastia. Combinations of potassium supplements or angiotensin converting enzyme inhibitors and potassium-sparing drugs can produce hyperkalemia but have been used with success in patients with persistent hypokalemia.

Patients with refractory edema may respond to combinations of a loop diuretic and thiazide-like agents. Metolazone, because of its maintained activity with renal insufficiency, is the most useful agent for such a combination. Extreme caution must be observed with this approach, since massive diuresis and electrolyte imbalances often occur; 2.5 mg of metolazone should be added to the previous dosage of loop diuretic. In many cases this is necessary only once or twice a week, but dosages up to 10 mg daily have been used in some patients.

D. INHIBITORS OF THE RENIN-ANGIOTENSIN-ALDOSTERONE SYSTEM

The renin-angiotensin-aldosterone system is activated early in the course of heart failure and plays an important role in the progression of this syndrome. Inhibition of this system with ACE inhibitors should be considered part of the initial therapy of this syndrome based on their favorable effects on prognosis.

1. Angiotensin-converting enzyme inhibitors— ACE inhibitors block the renin-angiotensin-aldosterone system by inhibiting the conversion of angiotensin I to angiotensin II, producing vasodilation by limiting angiotensin II-induced vasoconstriction, and decreasing sodium retention by reducing aldosterone secretion. Since angiotensin-converting enzyme is also involved in the degradation of bradykinin, ACE inhibitors result in higher bradykinin levels, which in turn stimulate the synthesis of prostaglandins and nitric oxide. Experimental data and hemodynamic studies in patients indicate that these latter actions may be important. Although the other vasodilators tend to stimulate the renin-angiotensin system and often lose part of their effect due to the resulting fluid retention, tolerance to the ACE inhibitors is uncommon.

Many ACE inhibitors are available (see Table 11–7), and at least seven have been shown to be effective for the treatment of heart failure or the related indication of postinfarction left ventricular dysfunction. ACE inhibitors reduce mortality by approximately 20% in patients with symptomatic heart failure and have been shown also to prevent hospitalizations, increase exercise tolerance, and reduce symptoms in these patients. As a result, ACE inhibitors should be part of first-line treatment of patients with symptomatic left ventricular systolic dysfunction (ejection fraction < 40%), usually in combination with a diuretic. They are also indicated for the management of patients with reduced ejection fractions without symptoms because they prevent the progression to clinical heart failure.

Because ACE inhibitors may induce significant hypotension, particularly following the initial doses, they must be started with caution. Hypotension is most prominent in patients with already low blood pressures (systolic pressure < 100 mm Hg), hypovolemia, prerenal azotemia (especially if it is diuretic-induced), and hyponatremia (an indicator of activation of the renin-angiotensin system). These patients should generally be started at low dosages (captopril 6.25 mg three times daily, enalapril 2.5 mg daily, or the equivalent), but other patients may be started at twice these dosages. Within several days (for those with the markers of higher risk) or at most 2 weeks, patients should be questioned about symptoms of hypotension, and both renal function and K^+ levels should be monitored.

ACE inhibitors should be titrated to the dosages proved effective in clinical trials (captopril 50 mg three times daily, enalapril 10 mg twice daily, lisinopril 10 mg daily, or the equivalent) over a period of 1–3 months. The large majority of patients will tolerate these doses. Asymptomatic hypotension is not a contraindication to up-titrating or continuing ACE inhibitors. Some patients exhibit rises in serum creatinine or K^+, but they do not require discontinuation if the levels stabilize—even at values as high as 3 mg/dL and 5.5 meq/L, respectively. Renal dysfunction is more frequent in diabetics, older patients, and those with low systolic pressures, and these groups should be monitored more closely. The most common side effects of ACE inhibitors in heart failure patients are dizziness (often not related to the level of blood pressure) and cough, though the latter is as often due to heart failure or intercurrent pulmonary conditions as to the ACE inhibitor.

2. Angiotensin II receptor blockers—Another approach to inhibiting the renin-angiotensin-aldosterone system is the use of specific angiotensin II receptor blockers (see Table 11–7), which will block or decrease most of the effects of the system. In addition, since there are alternative pathways of angiotensin II production in many tissues, the receptor blockers may provide more complete system blockade.

However, these agents do not share the effects of ACE inhibitors on other potentially important pathways that produce increases in bradykinin, prostaglandins, and nitric oxide in the heart, blood vessels, and other tissues. The recently completed Valsartan in Heart Failure Trial (Val-HeFT) examined the efficacy of adding valsartan to ACE inhibitor therapy. No benefit in survival was observed and only a modest reduction in hospitalizations; however, in the small subset of patients without background ACE inhibitor therapy, valsartan significantly reduced both mortality and hospitalizations for heart failure. Therefore, angiotensin receptor blockers may be considered as alternatives to ACE inhibitors in ACE-intolerant patients.

3. Spironolactone—There is growing evidence that aldosterone may mediate some of the major effects of renin-angiotensin-aldosterone system activation, such as myocardial remodeling and fibrosis, as well as sodium retention and potassium loss at the distal tubules. Thus, spironolactone should be considered as a neurohormonal antagonist rather than narrowly as a potassium-sparing diuretic. The RALES trial compared spironolactone 25 mg daily with placebo in patients with advanced heart failure already receiving ACE inhibitors and diuretics and showed a 29% reduction in mortality as well as similar decreases in other clinical end points. Hyperkalemia was uncommon in this severe heart failure population, which was

maintained on high doses of diuretic, but potassium levels should be monitored closely (after 1 and 4 weeks of therapy) in patients receiving ACE inhibitors. Neither the efficacy nor the safety of spironolactone has been established in the large majority of patients with mild or moderate heart failure who are taking low doses of diuretics, though this agent may be considered in patients who require potassium supplementation.

E. Beta-Blockers

Although beta-blockers have traditionally been considered contraindicated in patients with heart failure because they may block the compensatory actions of the sympathetic nervous system, there is now strong evidence that these agents have important beneficial effects in this patient population. The mechanism of this benefit remains unclear, but it is likely that chronic elevations of catecholamines and sympathetic nervous system activity cause progressive myocardial damage, leading to worsening left ventricular function and dilation. The primary evidence for this hypothesis is that over a period of 3–6 months, beta-blockers produce consistent substantial rises in ejection fraction (averaging 10% absolute increase) and reductions in left ventricular size and mass.

Clinical trial results have been reported in over 10,000 patients, primarily those with mild to moderate heart failure (NYHA class II and class III, ejection fraction < 35–40%) receiving ACE inhibitors and diuretics randomized to beta-blockers or placebo. Carvedilol, a nonselective β_1 and β_2 receptor blocker with additional weak alpha-blocking activity, was the first beta-blocker approved for heart failure in the United States after showing a reduction in death and hospitalizations in four smaller studies with a total of nearly 1100 patients. Subsequently, trials with two β_1-selective agents, bisoprolol (CIBIS II, with 2647 patients) and sustained-release metoprolol (MERIT, with nearly 4000 patients), both showed 35% reductions in mortality as well as fewer hospitalizations. Recently, a trial using carvedilol in 2200 patients with severe (NYHA class III/IV) heart failure was terminated ahead of schedule because of a 35% reduction in mortality. In these trials, there were reductions in sudden deaths and deaths from worsening heart failure, and benefits were seen in patients with underlying coronary disease and those with primary cardiomyopathies. In all these studies, the beta-blockers were generally well tolerated, with similar numbers of withdrawals in the active and placebo groups. This has led to a strong recommendation that *stable* patients (defined as having no recent deterioration or evidence of volume overload) with mild, moderate, and even severe heart failure should be treated with a beta-blocker unless there is a noncardiac contraindication. In the COPERNICUS trial, carvedilol was both well tolerated and highly effective in reducing both mortality and heart failure hospitalizations in a group of patients with severe (NYHA class III or IV) symptoms, but care was taken to ensure that they were free of fluid retention at the time of initiation. In this study, one death was prevented for every 13 patients treated for 1 year—as dramatic an effect as has been seen with a pharmacologic therapy in the history of cardiovascular medicine. It is not known whether there are differences between beta-blockers, but a trial comparing carvedilol and metoprolol (COMET) is ongoing and should be reported in 2003.

Since even apparently stable patients may deteriorate when beta-blockers are initiated, this must be done gradually and with great care. Carvedilol is initiated at a dosage of 3.125 mg twice daily and may be increased to 6.25, 12.5, and 25 mg twice daily at intervals of approximately 2 weeks. The protocols for sustained-release metoprolol use were started at 12.5 or 25 mg daily and doubled at intervals of 2 weeks to a target dose of 200 mg daily (using the Toprol XL sustained-release preparation). Bisoprolol was administered at a dosage of 1.25, 2.5, 3.75, 5, 7.5, and 10 mg daily, with increments at 1- to 4-week intervals. More gradual up-titration is often more convenient and may be better tolerated.

Patients should be instructed to monitor their weights at home as an indicator of fluid retention and to report any increase or change in symptoms immediately. Before each dose increase, the patient should be seen and examined to ensure that there has not been fluid retention or worsening of symptoms. If heart failure worsens, this can usually be managed by increasing diuretic doses and delaying further increases in beta-blocker doses, though downward adjustments or discontinuation is sometimes required. Carvedilol, because of its alpha-blocking activity, may cause dizziness or hypotension. This can usually be managed by reducing the doses of other vasodilators and by slowing the pace of dose increases.

F. DIGITALIS GLYCOSIDES

The digitalis glycosides (primarily digoxin) are the only orally active positive inotropic agents currently available. They bind to the sodium-potassium ATPase on the sarcolemmal membrane, inhibiting the sodium pump and thereby increasing intracellular sodium. This facilitates sodium-calcium exchange, with a resultant increase in cytosolic calcium, which enhances contractile protein cross-bridge formation and force generation. The digitalis glycosides also have electrophysiologic effects that may be beneficial or deleterious in individual patients. The primary therapeutic effect is an enhancement of cardiac parasympathetic tone, which delays atrioventricular conduction and reduces sinus node automaticity, thereby decreasing the ventricular response in patients with atrial fibrillation and slightly slowing the rate of patients in sinus rhythm. However, the increase in intracellular calcium and sodium may enhance automaticity of latent pacemakers, increasing the excitability of ventricular myocytes and inducing ventricular arrhythmias, especially when hypokalemia or myocardial ischemia is present.

Although the digitalis glycosides were once the mainstay of congestive heart failure treatment, their use in patients who are in sinus rhythm has declined because they lack the benefits of the neurohormonal antagonists on prognosis and because safety concerns persist. However, their efficacy in reducing the symptoms of heart failure has been established in at least four multicenter trials which have demonstrated that digoxin withdrawal is associated with worsening symptoms and signs of heart failure, more frequent hospitalizations for decompensation, and reduced exercise tolerance. This was also seen in the 6800-patient Digitalis Investigators Group (DIG) trial, though that study found no benefit (or harm) with regard to survival. A reduction in deaths due to progressive heart failure was balanced by an increase in deaths due to ischemic and arrhythmic events. Based on these results, digoxin should be used for patients who remain symptomatic when taking diuretics and ACE inhibitors as well as for heart failure patients who are in atrial fibrillation and require rate control.

Digoxin, the only widely employed digitalis preparation, has a half-life of 24–36 hours and is eliminated almost entirely by the kidneys. The oral maintenance dose may range from 0.125 mg three times weekly to 0.5 mg daily. It is lower in patients with renal dysfunction, in older patients, and in those with smaller lean body mass. Although a loading dose of 0.75–1.25 mg (depending primarily on lean body size) over 24–48 hours may be given if an early effect is desired, in most patients with chronic heart failure it is sufficient to begin with the expected maintenance dose (usually 0.125–0.25 mg daily). Amiodarone, quinidine, propafenone, and verapamil are among the drugs that may increase digoxin levels up to 100%. It is prudent to measure a blood level after 7–14 days (and at least 6 hours after the last dose was administered). Most of the positive inotropic effect is apparent with serum digoxin levels between 0.7 ng and 1.2 ng/mL, and levels above this range may be associated with a higher risk of arrhythmias, though toxicity is rare with levels below 1.8 ng/mL. Once an appropriate maintenance dose is established, subsequent levels are usually not indicated unless there is a change in renal function or medications that affect digoxin levels or a significant deterioration in cardiac status that may be associated with reduced clearance.

Digoxin toxicity has become less frequent as there has been a better appreciation of its pharmacology, but the therapeutic-to-toxic ratio is quite narrow. Symptoms of digitalis toxicity include anorexia, nausea, headache, blurring or yellowing of vision, and disorientation. Cardiac toxicity may take the form of atrioventricular conduction or sinus node depression; junctional, atrial, or ventricular premature beats or tachycardias; or ventricular fibrillation. Potassium administration (following serum potassium measurement, since severe toxicity may be associated with hyperkalemia) is usually indicated for the tachyarrhythmias even when levels are in the normal range, but may worsen conduction disturbances. Lidocaine or phenytoin may be useful for ventricular arrhythmias, as is overdrive pacing, but quinidine, amiodarone, and propafenone should be avoided because they will increase digoxin levels. Electrical cardioversion should be avoided if possible, since it may cause intractable ventricular fibrillation or cardiac standstill. Pacing is indicated for third-degree AV block (complete heart block) and symptomatic or severe block (heart rate < 40/min) if they persist after treatment with atropine. Digoxin immune fab (ovine) are available for life-threatening toxicity or large overdoses, but it should be remembered that their half-life is shorter than that of digoxin and so repeat administration may be required.

G. Vasodilators

Agents that dilate arteriolar smooth muscle and lower peripheral vascular resistance reduce left ventricular afterload. Medications that diminish venous tone and increase venous capacitance reduce the preload of both ventricles as their principal effect. Since most patients with moderate to severe heart failure have both elevated preload and reduced cardiac output, the maximum benefit of vasodilator therapy can be achieved by an agent or combination of agents with both actions. Many patients with heart failure have mitral or tricuspid regurgitation; agents that reduce resistance to ventricular outflow tend to redirect regurgitant flow in a forward direction.

Although vasodilators that are also neurohumoral antagonists—specifically, the ACE inhibitors—improve prognosis, such a benefit is less clear with the direct-acting vasodilators. The combination of hydralazine and isosorbide dinitrate has also improved survival, but to a lesser extent than ACE inhibitors.

The intravenous vasodilating drugs and their dosages have been discussed elsewhere in this chapter (in the section on complications in acute myocardial infarction).

1. Nitrates—Intravenous vasodilators (sodium nitroprusside or nitroglycerin) are used primarily for acute or severely decompensated chronic heart failure, especially when accompanied by hypertension or myocardial ischemia. If neither of the latter is present, therapy is best initiated and adjusted based on hemodynamic measurements. Starting dosages of both agents are 10–20 μg/kg/min with upward titration by increments of 10 μg/kg/min as frequently as every 5–10 minutes. Dosages above 200 μg/kg/min are usually not required.

Isosorbide dinitrate, 20–80 mg orally three times daily, has proved effective in several small studies. Nitroglycerin ointment, 12.5–50 mg (1–4 in) every 6–8 hours, appears to be equally effective although somewhat inconvenient for long-term therapy. The nitrates are moderately effective in relieving shortness of breath, especially in patients with mild to moderate symptoms, but less successful—probably because they have little effect on cardiac output—in advanced heart failure. Nitrate therapy is generally well tolerated, but

headaches and hypotension may limit the dose of all agents. The development of tolerance to chronic nitrate therapy is now generally acknowledged. This is minimized by intermittent therapy, especially if a daily 8- to 12-hour nitrate-free interval is employed, but probably develops to some extent in most patients receiving these agents. Transdermal nitroglycerin patches have no sustained effect in patients with heart failure and should not be employed for this indication.

2. Nesiritide—This new agent, a recombinant form of human brain natriuretic peptide, is a potent vasodilator that reduces ventricular filling pressures and improves cardiac output. Its hemodynamic effects resemble those of intravenous nitroglycerin with a more predictable dose response curve and a longer duration of action. In clinical studies, nesiritide (administered as 2 μg/kg by intravenous bolus injection followed by an infusion of 0.01 μg/kg/min, which may be uptitrated if needed) produced a rapid improvement in both dyspnea and hemodynamics. The primary adverse effect is hypotension, which may be symptomatic and sustained. Since most patients with acute heart failure respond well to conventional therapy, the role of nesiritide may be primarily in patients who continue to be symptomatic after initial treatment with diuretics and nonparenteral nitrates.

3. Hydralazine—Oral hydralazine is a potent arteriolar dilator and markedly increases cardiac output in patients with congestive heart failure. However, as a single agent, it has not been shown to improve symptoms or exercise tolerance during chronic treatment. The combination of nitrates and oral hydralazine produces greater hemodynamic effects.

Hydralazine therapy is frequently limited by side effects. Approximately 30% of patients are unable to tolerate the relatively high doses required to produce hemodynamic improvement in heart failure (200–400 mg daily in divided doses). The major side effect is gastrointestinal distress, but headaches, tachycardia, and hypotension are relatively common. Angiotensin receptor blockers have largely supplanted the use of the hydralazine-isosorbide dinitrate combination in ACE-intolerant patients.

H. Positive Inotropic Agents

The digitalis derivatives are the only available oral inotropic agents in the USA. A number of other oral positive inotropic agents have been investigated for the chronic treatment of heart failure, but all have increased mortality without convincing evidence of improvement in symptoms. Intravenous agents, such as the β_1 agonist dobutamine and the phosphodiesterase inhibitor milrinone, are sometimes employed on a long-term or intermittent basis. The limited available data suggest that continuous therapy is also likely to increase mortality; intermittent inotropic therapy has never been evaluated in controlled trials, and its use is largely based on anecdotal experience. A recent randomized placebo-controlled trial of 950 patients evaluating intravenous milrinone in patients admitted for decompensated heart failure who had no definite indications for inotropic therapy showed no benefit in terms of survival, decreasing length of admission, or preventing readmission—and significantly increased rates of sustained hypotension and atrial fibrillation. Thus, the role of positive inotropic agents appears to be limited to patients with symptoms and signs of low cardiac output (primarily hypoperfusion and deteriorating renal function) and those who fail to respond to intravenous diuretics. In some cases, dobutamine or milrinone may help maintain patients who are awaiting cardiac transplantation.

I. Calcium Channel Blockers

First-generation calcium channel blockers may accelerate the progression of congestive heart failure. However, two trials with amlodipine in patients with severe heart failure showed that this agent was safe, though not superior to placebo. These agents should be avoided unless they are being utilized to treat associated angina or hypertension, and for these indications amlodipine is the drug of choice.

J. Anticoagulation

Patients with left ventricular failure and reduced ejection fractions are at somewhat increased risk of developing intracardiac thrombi and systemic arterial emboli. However, this risk appears to be primarily in patients who are in atrial fibrillation or who have large recent (within 3–6 months) myocardial infarctions. These groups should be anticoagulated. Other heart failure patients have embolic rates of approximately two per 100 patient-years of follow-up, which approximates the rate of major bleeding, and routine anticoagulation does not appear warranted except in patients with prior embolic events or mobile left ventricular thrombi.

K. Antiarrhythmic Therapy and Implantable Cardioverter Defibrillators (ICDs)

Patients with moderate to severe heart failure have a high incidence of both symptomatic and asymptomatic arrhythmias. Although fewer than 10% of patients have syncope or presyncope resulting from ventricular tachycardia, ambulatory monitoring reveals that up to 70% of patients have asymptomatic episodes of nonsustained ventricular tachycardia. These arrhythmias indicate a poor prognosis independent of the severity of left ventricular dysfunction, but many of the deaths are probably not arrhythmia-related. Beta-blockers, because of their marked favorable effect on prognosis in general and on the incidence of sudden death specifically, should be initiated in these as well as other heart failure patients. Empiric antiarrhythmic therapy has not proved beneficial in patients with asymptomatic ventricular arrhythmias, and most other agents are contraindicated because of their proarrhythmic effects in this population and their adverse effect on cardiac function.

Patients with aborted sudden death, hemodynamically unstable ventricular arrhythmias, and unexplained cardiogenic syncope are at high risk for fatal ventricular arrhythmias. If these patients have a reasonable life expectancy and stable, nonrefractory heart failure, an implantable defibrillator is the approach of choice (again in conjunction with beta blockade). There are not sufficient data on which to base firm recommendations for the management of patients with asymptomatic nonsustained ventricular arrhythmias. Beta-blockers are the first line of therapy, but there is no evidence that antiarrhythmic drugs are beneficial, and they carry substantial risk (with the exception of amiodarone). In the second Multicenter Automatic Defibrillator Implantation Trial (MADIT II), 1232 patients with prior myocardial infarction and an ejection fraction ≤ 30% without a history of symptomatic ventricular arrhythmias were randomized to an ICD or a control group. Mortality was 31% lower in the ICD group, which translated into nine lives saved for each 100 patients who received a device and were followed for 3 years. The potential implications of this result are enormous, since this translates into an estimated cost of $300,000 per life saved. Before acting on this result, corroborative data should be awaited from the ongoing Sudden Cardiac Death in Heart Failure Trial (SCD-HeFT). Patients in this larger trial appear to be more symptomatic and more aggressively treated. Importantly, it includes a third arm in which patients have been randomized to amiodarone.

Nonpharmacologic Treatment

A. Case Management and Exercise Training

Thirty to 50 percent of congestive heart failure patients who are hospitalized will be readmitted within 3–6 months. Strategies to prevent clinical deterioration, such as case management, home monitoring of weight and clinical status, and patient adjustment of diuretics, can prevent rehospitalizations and should be part of the treatment regimen of advanced heart failure.

Exercise training improves activity tolerance in significant part by reversing the peripheral abnormalities associated with heart failure and deconditioning. Whether formal exercise programs are more beneficial than individual activity prescriptions is unknown, but stable patients should be encouraged to remain active and engage in appropriate aerobic exercise.

B. Coronary Revascularization

Since underlying coronary artery disease is the cause of heart failure in the majority of patients, coronary revascularization may both improve symptoms and prevent progression. However, trials have not been performed in patients with symptomatic heart failure. Nonetheless, patients with angina who are candidates for surgery should be evaluated for revascularization, usually by coronary angiography. Noninvasive testing for ischemic but viable myocardium may be a more appropriate first step in patients with known coronary disease but no current clinical evidence of ischemia. The benefit of evaluating patients with heart failure of new onset without angina or prior myocardial infarction is limited. In general, bypass surgery is preferable to PTCA in the setting of heart failure because it provides more complete revascularization.

C. BIVENTRICULAR PACING

Many patients with heart failure due to systolic dysfunction have abnormal intraventricular conduction that results in dyssynchronous and hence inefficient contractions. Several studies have evaluated the efficacy of "multisite" pacing, using leads that stimulate the right ventricle from the apex and the left ventricle from the lateral wall via the coronary sinus. Patients with wide QRS complexes (generally ≥ 140 ms), reduced ejection fractions, and severe symptoms have been evaluated. Results from studies with up to 6 months of follow-up have reported an increase in ejection fraction and improvement in symptoms and exercise tolerance. Definitive data on mortality or morbidity are not yet available. Nonetheless, this appears to be a promising therapeutic approach in patients who remain symptomatic despite aggressive medical therapy. Devices that combine biventricular pacing and ICD capabilities are also available.

D. CARDIAC TRANSPLANTATION

Because of the poor prognosis of patients with advanced heart failure, cardiac transplantation has become widely used. Since the advent of cyclosporine immunosuppressive therapy and more careful screening of donor hearts, the survival of patients after cardiac transplantation has increased considerably. Many centers now have 1-year survival rates exceeding 80–90%, and 5-year survival rates above 70%. Infections, hypertension and renal dysfunction caused by cyclosporine, rapidly progressive coronary atherosclerosis, and immunosuppressant-related cancers have been the major complications. The high cost and limited number of donor organs require careful patient selection early in the course.

E. OTHER SURGICAL TREATMENT OPTIONS

Several surgical procedures for severe heart failure have received considerable publicity. Cardiomyoplasty is a procedure in which the latissimus dorsi muscle is wrapped around the heart and stimulated to contract synchronously with it. In ventricular reduction surgery, a large part of the anterolateral wall is resected to make the heart function more efficiently. Both approaches are too risky in end-stage patients and have not been shown to improve prognosis or symptoms in controlled studies, and for these reasons they have largely been dropped. Externally powered and implantable ventricular assist devices can be used in patients who require ventricular support either to allow the heart to recover or as a bridge to transplantation. The latest generation devices are small enough to allow patients unrestricted mobility and even discharge from the hospital. However, complications are frequent, including bleeding, thromboembolism, and infection, and the cost is very high, exceeding $150,000 in the initial 1–3 months.

Long-Term Prognosis

Despite advances in treatment of patients with congestive heart failure, their prognosis remains poor, with annual mortality rates ranging from 5% in stable patients with mild symptoms to 30–50% in patients with advanced, progressive symptoms. Poorer prognosis is associated with severe left ventricular dysfunction (ejection fractions < 20%), prominent symptoms and limitation of exercise capacity (maximal oxygen consumption < 10 mL/kg/min), secondary renal insufficiency, hyponatremia, and elevated plasma catecholamine levels. About 40–50% of deaths in heart failure patients are sudden. Although many of these are due to ventricular arrhythmias, many others are the result of undiagnosed acute myocardial infarction or bradyarrhythmias. The remainder of deaths are due to progressive heart failure or comorbid conditions. Patients who develop end-stage heart failure may suffer severe dyspnea and require meticulous efforts at palliative care (see Chapter 5).

Brater DC: Diuretic therapy. N Engl J Med 1998;339:387. [PMID: 9691107] (A clear presentation of pharmacology, with a focus on diuretic resistance.)

Brophy JM et al: Beta-blockers in congestive heart failure. Ann Intern Med 2001;134:550. [PMID: 11281737] (Analysis of 22 trials and 10,000 patients shows four lives saved and four hospitalizations avoided for every 100 congestive heart failure patients treated with beta-blockers.)

Burnier M et al: Angiotensin II type 1 receptor blockers. Circulation 2001;103:904. [PMID: 11171802] (In-depth review establishes role of these agents in hypertension with an emerging role for myocardial infarction, congestive heart failure, and renal protection.)

Cohn JN et al: A randomized trial of the angiotensin-receptor blocker valsartan in chronic heart failure. N Engl J Med 2001;345:1667. [PMID: 11759645] (Most interesting finding is the dramatic improvement in survival and reduction in heart failure hospitalizations in the 366 patients who were not receiving ACE inhibitors, suggesting that these agents should be utilized in ACE inhibitor-intolerant patients.)

Cuffe MS, et al. Short-term intravenous milrinone for acute exacerbation of chronic heart failure: a randomized controlled trial. JAMA 2002;27;287:1541. [PMID: 11911756] (Randomized trial of milrinone versus placebo in 950 patients with acute decompensated heart failure showing no benefit and a relatively high incidence of adverse events.)

Felker GM et al: Inotropic therapy for heart failure: An evidence-based approach. Am Heart J 2001;142:393. [PMID: 11526351] (Routine use of inotropes is not supported, and they should be reserved for diuretic-refractory patients or as a bridge to more definitive therapy.)

Gerber TC et al. Left ventricular and biventricular pacing in congestive heart failure. Mayo Clin Proc 2001;76:803. [PMID: 1149982] (Review article covering this new approach.)

Hauptman PJ et al: Digitalis. Circulation 1999;99:1265. [PMID: 10069797] (Review of the molecular and clinical pharmacology and focus on Digoxin Investigation Group data set still warrants the use of this drug in patients with heart failure.)

Hunt SA et al: ACC/AHA guidelines for the evaluation and management of chronic heart failure in the adult: executive summary. Circulation 2001;104:2996. [PMID: 11834347]

Hunt SA: Current status of cardiac transplantation. JAMA 1998;280:1692. [PMID: 9832002] (Indications, patient selection, surgical technique, and immunosuppression are reviewed. Early and late limitations are outlined. Improved immunosuppression and better mechanical assist devices will improve future therapy.)

Moss AJ et al: Prophylactic implantation of a defibrillator in patients with myocardial infarction and reduced ejection fraction. N Engl J Med 2002;346:877. [PMID: 11907286] (Randomized trial showing improved survival with an ICD in patients with prior myocardial infarctions and ejection fractions ≤ 30%.)

Packer M et al: Effect of carvedilol on survival in severe chronic heart failure. N Engl J Med 2001;344:1651. [PMID: 11386263] (Carvedilol was associated with a 35% decrease in deaths among patients with severe chronic heart failure.)

Pitt B et al: The effect of spironolactone on morbidity and mortality in patients with severe heart failure. Randomized Aldactone Evaluation Study Investigators. N Engl J Med 1999;341:709. [PMID: 10471456] (Spironolactone therapy was associated with a 30% decrease in mortality attributed to reductions in both sudden death and progression of heart failure.)

Rose EA et al: Long-term use of a left ventricular assist device for end-stage heart failure. N Engl J Med 2001;345:1435. [PMID: 11794191] (Long-term use of LVAD in selected patients with advanced congestive heart failure led to survival benefit and improved quality of life, but few patients survived beyond 2 years.)

Westaby S: Non-transplant surgery for heart failure. Heart 2000;83:603. [PMID: 10768919] (Role of revascularization and antiremodeling therapy.)

Young JB et al: Intravenous nesiritide vs nitroglycerin for treatment of decompensated congestive heart failure: a randomized controlled trial. JAMA. 2002;287:1531. [PMID: 11911755] (Trial showing early improvement in symptoms and hemodynamics with nesiritide in patients with acute heart failure.)

ACUTE PULMONARY EDEMA

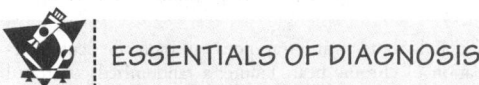

ESSENTIALS OF DIAGNOSIS

- *Acute onset or worsening of dyspnea at rest.*
- *Tachycardia, diaphoresis, cyanosis.*
- *Pulmonary rales, rhonchi; expiratory wheezing.*
- *X-ray shows interstitial and alveolar edema with or without cardiomegaly.*
- *Arterial hypoxemia.*

General Considerations

Typical causes of acute cardiogenic pulmonary edema include acute myocardial infarction or severe ischemia, exacerbation of chronic heart failure, acute volume overload of the left ventricle (valvular regurgitation or ventricular septal defect), and mitral stenosis.

Clinical Findings

Acute pulmonary edema presents with a characteristic clinical picture of severe dyspnea, the production of pink, frothy sputum, and diaphoresis and cyanosis. Rales are present in all lung fields, as are generalized wheezing and rhonchi. Pulmonary edema may appear suddenly in the setting of chronic heart failure or may be the first manifestation of cardiac disease, usually acute myocardial infarction, which may be painful or silent.

A number of noncardiac conditions can also produce pulmonary edema. This occurs either because of imbalance in the Starling forces (either a decrease in plasma proteins or an increase in pulmonary venous pressure) or a functional or anatomic abnormality of the alveolar-capillary membrane. Causes include intravenous narcotics, increased intracerebral pressure, high altitude, sepsis, several medications, inhaled toxins, transfusion reactions, shock, and disseminated intravascular coagulation. These are distinguished from cardiogenic pulmonary edema by the clinical setting, the history, and the physical examination. Conversely, in most patients with cardiogenic pulmonary edema, an underlying cardiac abnormality can usually be detected clinically or by the ECG, chest x-ray, or echocardiogram.

The chest radiograph reveals signs of pulmonary vascular redistribution, blurriness of vascular outlines, increased interstitial markings, and, characteristically, the butterfly pattern of distribution of alveolar edema. The heart may be enlarged or normal in size depending on whether heart failure was previously present. Assessment of cardiac function by echocardiography is important, since a substantial proportion of patients have normal ejection fractions with elevated atrial pressures due to diastolic dysfunction. In cardiogenic pulmonary edema, the pulmonary capillary wedge pressure is invariably elevated, usually over 25 mm Hg. In noncardiogenic pulmonary edema, the wedge pressure may be normal or even low.

Treatment

The patient should be placed in a sitting position with legs dangling over the side of the bed; this facilitates respiration and reduces venous return. Oxygen is delivered by mask to obtain an arterial PO_2 greater than 60 mm Hg. Noninvasive pressure support ventilation may improve oxygenation and prevent severe CO_2 retention while pharmacologic interventions take effect. However, if respiratory distress remains severe, endotracheal intubation and mechanical ventilation may be necessary.

Morphine is highly effective in pulmonary edema. The initial dosage is 4–8 mg intravenously (subcutaneous administration is effective in milder cases) and may be repeated after 2–4 hours. Morphine increases venous capacitance, lowering left atrial pressure, and relieves anxiety, which can reduce the efficiency of ventilation. However, morphine may lead to CO_2 retention by reducing the ventilatory drive. It should be avoided in patients with narcotic-induced pulmonary edema, who may improve with narcotic antagonists, and in those with neurogenic pulmonary edema.

Intravenous diuretic therapy (furosemide, 40 mg, or bumetanide, 1 mg—or higher doses if the patient has been receiving chronic diuretic therapy) is usually indicated even if the patient has not exhibited prior fluid retention. These agents produce venodilation prior to the onset of diuresis. Nitrate therapy accelerates clinical improvement by reducing both blood pressure and left ventricular filling pressures. Bronchospasm may occur in response to pulmonary edema and may itself exacerbate hypoxemia and dyspnea. Treatment with inhaled beta-adrenergic agonists or intravenous aminophylline may be helpful, but both may also provoke tachycardia and supraventricular arrhythmias. Particularly in patients with elevated arterial pressures, parenteral vasodilators such as intravenous nitroprusside or nesiritide may be worthwhile. In patients with low-output states, particularly when hypotension is present, positive inotropic agents are indicated. These approaches to treatment have been discussed previously.

Gandhi SK et al: The pathogenesis of acute pulmonary edema associated with hypertension. N Engl J Med 2001;344:17. [PMID: 11136955] (Trial showing that diastolic dysfunction alone may be the cause of pulmonary edema in these patients.)

Sacchetti AD et al: Acute cardiogenic pulmonary edema. What's the latest in emergency treatment? Postgrad Med 1998;103:145. [PMID: 9479313] (Clinical examples illustrate the use of drugs and noninvasive ventilatory support to treat acute pulmonary edema.)

■ MYOCARDITIS & THE CARDIOMYOPATHIES

ACUTE MYOCARDITIS

Acute myocarditis causes focal or diffuse inflammation of the myocardium. Most cases are infectious, caused by viral, bacterial, rickettsial, spirochetal, fungal, or parasitic agents; but toxins, drugs, and immunologic disorders can also cause myocarditis.

1. Infectious Myocarditis

 ESSENTIALS OF DIAGNOSIS

- *Often follows an upper respiratory infection.*
- *May present with chest pain (pleuritic or non-specific) or signs of heart failure.*
- *ECG may show sinus tachycardia, other arrhythmias, nonspecific repolarization changes, intraventricular conduction abnormalities.*
- *Echocardiogram documents cardiomegaly and contractile dysfunction.*
- *Myocardial biopsy, though not sensitive, may reveal a characteristic inflammatory pattern.*

General Considerations

Viral myocarditis is the most common form and is usually caused by coxsackieviruses, but a host of other agents have also been responsible. Rickettsial myocarditis occurs with scrub typhus, Rocky Mountain spotted fever, and Q fever. Diphtheritic myocarditis is caused by the exotoxin and often is manifested by conduction abnormalities as well as heart failure.

Chagas' disease, caused by the insect-borne protozoan *Trypanosoma cruzi,* is a common form of myocarditis in Central and South America; the major clinical manifestations appear after a latent period of more than a decade. At this stage, patients present with cardiomyopathy, conduction disturbances, and sudden death. Associated gastrointestinal involvement (megaesophagus and megacolon) is the rule. Toxoplasmosis causes myocarditis that is usually asymptomatic but can lead to heart failure. Among parasitic infections, trichinosis is the most common cause of cardiac involvement. The potential for the HIV virus to cause myocarditis is now well recognized, though the prevalence of this complication is not known. In addition, other infectious myocarditides are more common in patients with AIDS.

Giant cell myocarditis is a rare idiopathic disorder characterized by giant cell and lymphocyte infiltration of the heart muscle. Patients usually die from ventricular arrhythmias or heart failure but occasionally respond to immunosuppressive therapy or early transplantation.

Clinical Findings

A. SYMPTOMS AND SIGNS

Patients may present several days to a few weeks after the onset of an acute febrile illness or a respiratory infection or with heart failure without antecedent symptoms. The onset of heart failure may be gradual or may be abrupt and fulminant. Pleural-pericardial chest pain is common. Examination reveals tachycardia, gallop rhythm, and other evidence of heart failure or conduction defect. It is likely that most myocardities are subclinical, though they may present later as idiopathic cardiomyopathy or with ventricular arrhythmias.

B. ELECTROCARDIOGRAPHY AND CHEST X-RAY

Nonspecific ST–T changes and conduction disturbances are common. Ventricular ectopy may be the initial and only clinical finding. Chest x-ray is nonspecific, but cardiomegaly is frequent.

C. DIAGNOSTIC STUDIES

Echocardiography provides the most convenient way of evaluating cardiac function and can exclude many other processes. Gallium-67 scintigraphy has been reported to yield cardiac uptake in acute or subacute myocarditis. Paired serum viral titers and serologic tests for other agents may indicate the cause.

D. ENDOMYOCARDIAL BIOPSY

Pathologic examinations may reveal a lymphocytic inflammatory response with necrosis, but the patchy distribution of abnormalities makes the test relatively insensitive. This picture defines an "active" inflammatory stage and may persist for many months.

Treatment & Prognosis

Specific antimicrobial therapy is indicated when an infecting agent is identified. Immunosuppressive therapy with corticosteroids and other agents have been felt by some to improve the outcome when the process is acute (< 6 months) and if the biopsy suggests ongoing inflammation. However, controlled trials have not been positive, so the value of routine myocardial biopsies in patients presenting with an acute myocarditic picture is uncertain; immunosuppressive therapy without histologic confirmation is unwise. Otherwise, treatment is directed toward the manifestations of heart failure and arrhythmias.

Many cases resolve spontaneously, but in others cardiac function deteriorates progressively and may lead to dilated cardiomyopathy. Many cases of dilated cardiomyopathy may represent the end stage of viral myocarditis.

Feldman AM et al: Myocarditis. N Engl J Med 2000;343:1388. [PMID: 11070105] (Etiology and pathophysiology are reviewed. Treatment is primarily supportive care.)

Garg A et al: The ineffectiveness of immunosuppressive therapy in lymphocytic myocarditis: An overview. Ann Intern Med 1998;129:317. [PMID: 9729186] (Prednisone, either alone or in combination with azathioprine or cyclosporine, did not improve survival or left ventricular function in patients with biopsy-proved lymphocytic myocarditis.)

Liu PP et al: Advances in the understanding of myocarditis. Circulation 2001;104:1076. [PMID: 11524405] (Myocarditis is defined in terms of viral, autoimmune, and dilated cardiomyopathy stages.)

Rassi A et al: Chagas' heart disease. Clin Cardiol 2000;23:883. [PMID: 11129673] (Infection with the parasite *T cruzi* can cause myocardial inflammation and lead to sudden death or heart failure. Eighteen million South Americans are infected.)

Rerkpattanapipat P et al: Cardiac manifestations of acquired immunodeficiency syndrome. Arch Intern Med 2000; 160; 602. [PMID: 10724045] (Review of diverse presentations, including myocarditis, cardiomyopathy, and pericarditis.)

2. Drug-Induced & Toxic Myocarditis

A variety of medications, illicit drugs, and toxic substances can produce acute or chronic myocardial injury; the clinical presentation varies widely. Doxorubicin and other cytotoxic agents, emetine, and catecholamines (especially with pheochromocytoma) can produce a pathologic picture of inflammation and necrosis together with clinical heart failure and arrhythmias; toxicity of the first two is dose-related. The phenothiazines, lithium, chloroquine, disopyramide, antimony-containing compounds, and arsenicals can also cause electrocardiographic changes, arrhythmias, or heart failure. Hypersensitivity reactions to sulfonamides, penicillins, and aminosalicylic acid as well as other drugs can result in cardiac dysfunction. Radiation can cause an acute inflammatory reaction as well as a chronic fibrosis of heart muscle, usually in conjunction with pericarditis.

The incidence of cocaine cardiotoxicity has increased markedly. Cocaine can cause coronary artery spasm, myocardial infarction, arrhythmias, and myocarditis. Because many of these processes are believed to be mediated by cocaine's inhibitory effect on norepinephrine reuptake by sympathetic nerves, beta-blockers have been used therapeutically. In coronary spasm, calcium channel blockers are more appropriate.

Pai VB et al: Cardiotoxicity of chemotherapeutic agents: incidence, treatment and prevention. Drug Saf 2000;22:263. [PMID: 10789823]

THE CARDIOMYOPATHIES

The cardiomyopathies are a heterogeneous group of entities affecting the myocardium primarily and not associated with the major causes of cardiac disease, ie, ischemic heart disease, hypertension, valvular disease, or congenital defects. While some have specific causes, many cases are idiopathic. There is now general agreement on a classification based upon general features of presentation and pathophysiology (Table 10–6).

Davies MJ: The cardiomyopathies: an overview. Heart 2000;83: 469. [PMID: 10722553]

Table 10–6. Classification of the cardiomyopathies.

	Dilated	Hypertrophic	Restrictive
Frequent causes	Idiopathic, alcoholic, myocarditis, postpartum, doxorubicin, endocrinopathies, genetic diseases	Hereditary syndrome, possibly chronic hypertension	Amyloidosis, post radiation, post open heart surgery, diabetes, endomyocardial fibrosis
Symptoms	Left or biventricular congestive heart failure	Dyspnea, chest pain, syncope	Dyspnea, fatigue, right-sided congestive heart failure
Physical examination	Cardiomegaly, S_3, elevated jugular venous pressure, rales	Sustained point of maximal impulse, S_4, variable systolic murmur, bisferiens carotid pulse	Elevated jugular venous pressure, Kussmaul's sign
ECG	ST–T changes, conduction abnormalities, ventricular ectopy	Left ventricular hypertrophy, exaggerated septal Q waves	ST–T changes, conduction abnormalities, low voltage
Chest x-ray	Enlarged heart, pulmonary congestion	Mild cardiomegaly	Mild to moderate cardiomegaly
Echocardiogram, nuclear studies	Left ventricular dilation and dysfunction	Left ventricular hypertrophy, asymmetric septal hypertrophy, small left ventricular size, normal or supranormal function, systolic anterior mitral motion, diastolic dysfunction	Small or normal left ventricular size, normal or mildly reduced left ventricular function
Cardiac catheterization	Left ventricular dilation and dysfunction, high diastolic pressures, low cardiac output	Small, hypercontractile left ventricle, dynamic outflow gradient, diastolic dysfunction	High diastolic pressure, "square root" sign, normal or mildly reduced left ventricular function

Franz WM et al: Cardiomyopathies: from genetics to the prospect of treatment. Lancet 2001;358:1627. [PMID: 11716909]

1. Primary Dilated Cardiomyopathy

ESSENTIALS OF DIAGNOSIS

- *Symptoms and signs of heart failure.*
- *ECG may show low QRS voltage, nonspecific repolarization abnormalities, intraventricular conduction abnormalities.*
- *X-ray shows cardiomegaly.*
- *Echocardiogram confirms left ventricular dilation, thinning, and global dysfunction.*

General Considerations

Dilated cardiomyopathies usually present with symptoms and signs of congestive heart failure (most commonly dyspnea). Occasionally, symptomatic ventricular arrhythmias are the presenting event. Left ventricular dilation and systolic dysfunction are essential for diagnosis. A growing number of cardiomyopathies due to genetic abnormalities are being recognized, but these still represent a small minority of cases. Often no cause can be identified, but chronic alcohol abuse and unrecognized myocarditis are probably frequent causes. Amyloidosis, sarcoidosis, hemochromatosis, and diabetes all may present as dilated cardiomyopathies as well as with a restrictive picture. Histologically, the picture is one of extensive fibrosis unless a specific diagnosis is established.

Clinical Findings

A. SYMPTOMS AND SIGNS

In most patients, symptoms of heart failure develop gradually. They may be recognized because of asymptomatic cardiomegaly or electrocardiographic abnormalities, including arrhythmias. The initial presentation may be severe biventricular failure. The physical examination reveals cardiomegaly, S_3 gallop rhythm, and often a murmur of functional mitral regurgitation. Signs of left- and right-sided failure may be present on initial examination, a clue to a process involving the heart diffusely.

B. ELECTROCARDIOGRAPHY AND CHEST X-RAY

The major findings are listed in Table 10–6.

C. DIAGNOSTIC STUDIES

An echocardiogram is indicated to exclude unsuspected valvular or other lesions and confirm the presence of dilated cardiomyopathy. Exercise thallium-201 scintigraphy may suggest the possibility of underlying coronary disease if a large reversible defect is found, but false-positives occur in cardiomyopathy. Cardiac catheterization is seldom of specific value unless myocardial ischemia or left ventricular aneurysm is suspected. The serum ferritin is an adequate screening study for hemochromatosis.

Treatment

Few cases of cardiomyopathy are amenable to specific therapy. Alcohol use should be discontinued. There is often marked recovery of cardiac function following a period of abstinence in alcoholic cardiomyopathy. Endocrine causes (thyroid dysfunction, acromegaly, pheochromocytoma) should be treated. Immunosuppressive therapy is not indicated in chronic dilated cardiomyopathy. The management of congestive heart failure is outlined in the section on heart failure.

Prognosis

The prognosis of dilated cardiomyopathy without clinical heart failure is variable, with some patients remaining stable, some deteriorating gradually, and others declining rapidly. Once heart failure is manifest, the natural history is similar to that of other causes of heart failure. Arterial and pulmonary emboli are more common in dilated cardiomyopathy than in ischemic cardiomyopathy; suitable candidates may benefit from chronic anticoagulation. Those patients whose disease progresses may require treatment for severe dyspnea (see above) and ultimately need high-quality palliative care (see Chapter 5).

Corrado D et al: Arrhythmogenic right ventricular cardiomyopathy: diagnosis, prognosis, and treatment. Heart 2000;83: 588. [PMID: 10768917] (An inherited condition that frequently presents with ventricular arrhythmias. The characteristic electrocardiographic and echocardiographic features are described, and management approaches, including use of the implantable cardioverter-defibrillator, are discussed.)

Elliott P: Cardiomyopathy. Diagnosis and management of dilated cardiomyopathy. Heart 2000;84:106. [PMID: 10862601]

Felker GM et al: Underlying causes and long-term survival in patients with initially unexplained cardiomyopathy. N Engl J Med 2000;342:1077. [PMID: 10760308] (Series of 1230 patients with cardiomyopathy who underwent extensive work-up, including coronary angiography and endomyocardial biopsy, showing that the prognosis varies with the underlying cause.)

Gavazzi A et al: Alcohol abuse and dilated cardiomyopathy in men. Am J Cardiol 2000; 85:1114. [PMID: 10781762] (A frequent and sometimes unrecognized cause of dilated cardiomyopathy.)

Wu LA et al: Current role of endomyocardial biopsy in the management of dilated cardiomyopathy and myocarditis. Mayo Clin Proc 2001;76:1030. [PMID: 11605687] (Biopsy may guide therapy in acute myocarditis but should not be routinely employed in dilated cardiomyopathy.)

2. Hypertrophic Cardiomyopathy

ESSENTIALS OF DIAGNOSIS

- *May present with dyspnea, chest pain, syncope.*
- *Examination shows sustained apical impulse, S_4, systolic ejection murmur.*
- *ECG shows left ventricular hypertrophy, occasionally septal Q waves in the absence of infarction.*
- *Echocardiogram shows hypertrophy, which may be asymmetric; usually shows normal or enhanced contractility and signs of dynamic obstruction.*

General Considerations

Myocardial hypertrophy unrelated to any pressure or volume overload tends to impinge upon the left ventricular cavity. The interventricular septum may be disproportionately involved (asymmetric septal hypertrophy), but in some cases the hypertrophy is localized to the apex. The left ventricular outflow tract is often narrowed during systole between the bulging septum and an anteriorly displaced anterior mitral valve leaflet, causing a dynamic obstruction (hence the name idiopathic hypertrophic subaortic stenosis; IHSS). The obstruction is worsened by factors that increase myocardial contractility (sympathetic stimulation, digoxin, postextrasystolic beat) or that decrease left ventricular filling (Valsalva's maneuver, peripheral vasodilators).

Hypertrophic cardiomyopathy is in some cases inherited as an autosomal dominant trait with variable penetrance caused by mutations of a number of genes, most of which code for myosin heavy chains or proteins regulating calcium handling. It is becoming clear that the prognosis is related to the specific gene mutation. These patients usually present in early adulthood. Others are elderly, and many of those patients have a long history of hypertension. Some cases occur sporadically.

Except in late stages, hypertrophic cardiomyopathy is characterized by a small, hypercontractile left ventricle. Although dyspnea is a common symptom, it results mainly from markedly impaired diastolic compliance rather than systolic dysfunction or outflow obstruction.

Clinical Findings

A. SYMPTOMS AND SIGNS

The most frequent symptoms are dyspnea and chest pain. Syncope is also common and is typically postexertional, when diastolic filling diminishes and outflow obstruction increases. Arrhythmias are an important problem. Atrial fibrillation is a long-term consequence of chronically elevated left atrial pressures and is a poor prognostic sign. Ventricular arrhythmias are also common, and sudden death may occur, often in athletes after extraordinary exertion.

Features on physical examination are a bisferiens carotid pulse, triple apical impulse (due to the prominent atrial filling wave and early and late systolic impulses), and a loud S_4. In cases with outflow obstruction, a loud systolic murmur is present that increases with upright posture or Valsalva's maneuver and decreases with squatting.

B. Electrocardiography and Chest X-Ray

Left ventricular hypertrophy is nearly universal. Exaggerated septal Q waves inferolaterally may suggest myocardial infarction. The chest x-ray is often unimpressive.

C. Diagnostic Studies

The echocardiogram is diagnostic, revealing asymmetric left ventricular hypertrophy, systolic anterior motion of the mitral valve, early closing followed by reopening of the aortic valve, a small and hypercontractile left ventricle, and delayed relaxation and filling of the left ventricle during diastole. Doppler ultrasound reveals turbulent flow and a dynamic gradient across the aortic valve and, commonly, mitral regurgitation. Cardiac catheterization may confirm the gradient but adds little to echocardiographic studies.

Treatment

Beta-blockers should be the initial drug in symptomatic individuals, especially when dynamic outflow obstruction is noted on the echocardiogram. Dyspnea, angina, and arrhythmias respond in about 50% of patients. Calcium channel blockers, especially verapamil, have also been effective in symptomatic patients. Their effect may be due primarily to improved diastolic function, but their vasodilating actions may also increase outflow obstruction. Excision of part of the myocardial septum has been successful in patients with severe symptoms when performed by surgeons experienced with the procedure. Dual-chamber pacing may prevent the progression of hypertrophy and obstruction. Nonsurgical septal ablation has been performed by injection of alcohol into septal branches of the left coronary artery. Patients with malignant ventricular arrhythmias and unexplained syncope in the presence of a positive family history for sudden death are probably best managed with an implantable defibrillator.

Prognosis

The natural history of hypertrophic cardiomyopathy is highly variable. Several specific mutations are associated with a higher incidence of early malignant arrhythmias and sudden death, and definition of the genetic abnormality provides the best estimate of prognosis. Some patients remain asymptomatic for many years or for life. Sudden death, especially during exercise, may be the initial event. Indeed, hypertrophic cardiomyopathy is the pathologic feature most frequently associated with sudden death in athletes. Other patients have a history of gradually progressive symptoms. A final stage may be a transition into dilated cardiomyopathy.

Elliott PM et al: Sudden death in hypertrophic cardiomyopathy: identification of high-risk patients. J Am Coll Cardiol 2000;36:2212. [PMID: 11127463] (A family history of sudden death and marked increases in left ventricular thickness identify high-risk patients.)

Erwin JP et al: Dual chamber pacing for patients with hypertrophic obstructive cardiomyopathy. Mayo Clin Proc 2000;75:173. [PMID: 10683657] (Little objective evidence of benefit, although some patients report improvement.)

Maron BJ et al: Efficacy of implantable cardioverter-defibrillators for the prevention of sudden death in patients with hypertrophic cardiomyopathy. N Engl J Med 2000;342:365. [PMID: 10666426] (Ventricular tachycardia and ventricular fibrillation are the primary mechanisms of sudden death in patients with hypertrophic cardiomyopathy, and implantable cardioverter-defibrillators are effective for their treatment.)

Maron BJ et al: Epidemiology of hypertrophic cardiomyopathy-related death: revisited in a large non-referral-based patient population. Circulation 2000;102:858. [PMID: 10952953] (Cause of death in 86 patients who were not from the usual tertiary care institutions specializing in this condition were reviewed. Fifty-one percent, mostly younger patients, died suddenly; 36% died of progressive heart failure and 13% from stroke, with these groups being older.)

Maron BJ: Role of alcohol septal ablation in treatment of obstructive hypertrophic cardiomyopathy. Lancet 2000;355:425. [PMID: 10841119] (Concise review.)

Merrill WH et al: Long-lasting improvement after septal myectomy for hypertrophic obstructive cardiomyopathy. Ann Thorac Surg 2000;69:1732. [PMID: 10892916] (Describes follow-up of a series of surgically treated patients.)

Qin JX et al: Outcome of patients with hypertrophic obstructive cardiomyopathy after percutaneous transluminal septal myocardial ablation and septal myectomy surgery. J Am Coll Cardiol 2001;38:1994. [PMID: 11738306] (Ethanol ablation and surgical myectomy can both be effective in reducing gradient and symptoms in patients with hypertrophic obstructive cardiomyopathy.)

Roberts R et al: New concepts in hypertrophic cardiomyopathies. Circulation 2001;104:2113, 2249. [PMID: 11673355, 11684639] (Two-part review covers clinical features, molecular and genetic basis, and pharmacologic, surgical, and pacing treatments.)

3. Restrictive Cardiomyopathy

Restrictive cardiomyopathy is characterized by impaired diastolic filling with preserved contractile function. This condition is relatively uncommon, with the most frequent causes being amyloidosis, radiation, and myocardial fibrosis after open heart surgery. In Africa, endomyocardial fibrosis, a specific entity in which there is severe fibrosis of the endocardium, often with eosinophilia (Löffler's syndrome) is common. Other causes of a restrictive picture are infiltrative cardiomyopathies (eg, sarcoidosis, hemochromatosis, carcinoid syndrome) and connective tissue diseases (eg, scleroderma).

Amyloidosis can affect the heart in several ways. Although it is a frequent cause of restrictive cardiomyopathy, it more often produces dilated cardiomyopathy with congestive heart failure. Almost invariably, conduction disturbances are present. Low voltages on the ECG combined with ventricular hypertrophy by echo are suggestive. Rectal, abdominal fat, or gingival biopsies—as well as myocardial biopsy—can be diagnostic.

The primary diagnostic problem with restrictive cardiomyopathy is differentiation from constrictive pericarditis. The clinical picture often strongly suggests the diagnosis, but the status of left ventricular function (usually normal with pericarditis, slightly depressed with restrictive cardiomyopathy) can be helpful, as can be evidence of a thickened pericardium. Myocardial biopsies are usually negative with pericarditis but not in restrictive cardiomyopathy. In some cases, only surgical exploration can make the diagnosis.

Unfortunately, little useful therapy is available for either the causative conditions or restrictive cardiomyopathy itself. Diuretics can help, but excessive diuresis can produce worsening symptoms. Steroids may be helpful in sarcoidosis but relieve conduction abnormalities more often than heart failure.

Ammash NM et al: Clinical profile and outcome of idiopathic restrictive cardiomyopathy. Circulation 2000;101:2490. [PMID: 10831523] (Clinical, echo, and hemodynamic features are described. Treatment is supportive and prognosis is poor.)

Hancock EW: Differential diagnosis of restrictive cardiomyopathy and constrictive pericarditis. Heart 2001;86:343. [PMID: 11514495] (Reviews differential diagnosis.)

McCarthy RE et al: A review of the amyloidoses that infiltrate the heart. Clin Cardiol 1998;21:547. [PMID: 9702380] (Review of the pathogenesis and presentation of the most frequent cause of restrictive cardiomyopathy.)

■ ACUTE RHEUMATIC FEVER & RHEUMATIC HEART DISEASE

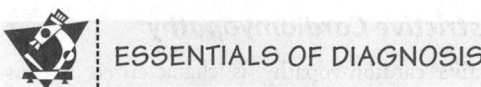

ESSENTIALS OF DIAGNOSIS

- *Uncommon in USA but may be overlooked.*
- *Peak incidence ages 5–15 years.*
- *Diagnosis based on Jones criteria and confirmation of streptococcal infection.*
- *May involve mitral and other valves acutely, rarely leading to heart failure.*

General Considerations

Rheumatic fever is a systemic immune process which is a sequela to beta-hemolytic streptococcal infection of the pharynx. Pyodermic infections are not associated with rheumatic fever. Signs of rheumatic fever usually commence 2–3 weeks after infection but may appear as early as 1 week or as late as 5 weeks. It had become quite uncommon in the USA, except in recent immigrants. However, there have been recent reports of new outbreaks in several regions of the USA. The peak incidence is between ages 5 and 15; rheumatic fever is rare before age 4 and after age 40. Rheumatic carditis and valvulitis may be self-limited or may lead to slowly progressive valvular deformity. The characteristic lesion is a perivascular granulomatous reaction with vasculitis. The mitral valve is attacked in 75–80% of cases, the aortic valve in 30% (but rarely as the sole valve), and the tricuspid and pulmonary valves in under 5%.

Clinical Findings

Diagnostic criteria first described by Jones are still employed. The presence of two major criteria—or one major and two minor criteria—establishes the diagnosis.

A. MAJOR CRITERIA

1. Carditis—Carditis is most likely to be evident in children and adolescents. Any of the following suggests the presence of carditis. (1) Pericarditis. (2) Cardiomegaly, detected by physical signs, radiography, or echocardiography. (3) Congestive failure, right- or left-sided—the former perhaps more prominent in children, with painful liver engorgement due to tricuspid regurgitation. (4) Mitral or aortic regurgitation murmurs, indicative of dilation of a valve ring with or without associated valvulitis. The Carey-Coombs short middiastolic mitral murmur may be present.

In the absence of any of the above definitive signs, the diagnosis of carditis depends upon the following less specific abnormalities: (1) electrocardiographic changes, including changing contour of P waves or inversion of T waves; (2) changing quality of heart sounds; (3) sinus tachycardia, arrhythmia, or ectopic beats.

2. Erythema marginatum and subcutaneous nodules—The former begin as rapidly enlarging macules that assume the shape of rings or crescents with clear centers. They may be raised, confluent, and either transient or persistent.

Subcutaneous nodules are uncommon except in children. They are small (≤ 2 cm in diameter), firm, and nontender and are attached to fascia or tendon sheaths over bony prominences. They persist for days or weeks, are recurrent, and are indistinguishable from rheumatoid nodules.

3. Sydenham's chorea—Sydenham's chorea—involuntary choreoathetoid movements primarily of the face, tongue, and upper extremities—may be the sole manifestation; only half of cases have other overt signs of rheumatic fever. Girls are more frequently affected, and occurrence in adults is rare. This is the least common (3% of cases) but most diagnostic of the manifestations of rheumatic fever.

4. Arthritis—This is a migratory polyarthritis that involves the large joints sequentially. In adults, only a single joint may be affected. The arthritis lasts 1–5 weeks and subsides without residual deformity. Prompt response of arthritis to therapeutic doses of salicylates or nonsteroidal agents is characteristic.

B. MINOR CRITERIA

These include fever, polyarthralgias, reversible prolongation of the PR interval, rapid erythrocyte sedimentation rate, and evidence of an antecedent β-hemolytic streptococcal infection or a history of rheumatic fever.

C. LABORATORY FINDINGS

There is nonspecific evidence of inflammatory disease, as shown by a rapid sedimentation rate. High or increasing titers of antistreptococcal antibodies (antistreptolysin O and anti-DNAse B) are used to confirm recent infection; 10% of cases lack this serologic evidence.

Differential Diagnosis

Rheumatic fever may be confused with the following: rheumatoid arthritis, osteomyelitis, endocarditis, chronic meningococcemia, systemic lupus erythematosus, Lyme disease, sickle cell anemia, "surgical abdomen," and many other diseases.

Complications

Congestive heart failure occurs in severe cases. In the longer term, the development of rheumatic heart disease is the major problem. Other complications include arrhythmias, pericarditis with effusion, and rheumatic pneumonitis.

Treatment

A. GENERAL MEASURES

The patient should be kept at strict bed rest until the temperature returns to normal without medications, the sedimentation rate is normal, the resting pulse rate is normal (< 100/min in adults), and the ECG has returned to baseline.

B. MEDICAL MEASURES

1. Salicylates—The salicylates markedly reduce fever and relieve joint pain and swelling. They have no effect on the natural course of the disease. Adults may require aspirin, 0.6–0.9 g every 4 hours; children are treated with lower doses. Toxicity includes tinnitus, vomiting, and gastrointestinal bleeding.

2. Penicillin—Penicillin (benzathine penicillin, 1.2 million units intramuscularly once, or procaine penicillin, 600,000 units intramuscularly daily for 10 days) is employed to eradicate streptococcal infection if present. Erythromycin may be substituted.

3. Corticosteroids—There is no proof that cardiac damage is prevented or minimized by corticosteroids. A short course of corticosteroids (prednisone, 40–60 mg orally daily, with tapering over 2 weeks) usually causes rapid improvement of the joint symptoms and is indicated when response to salicylates has been inadequate.

Prevention of Recurrent Rheumatic Fever

The initial episode of rheumatic fever can usually be prevented by early treatment of streptococcal pharyngitis. (See Chapter 33.) Prevention of recurrent episodes is critical. Recurrences of rheumatic fever are most common in patients who have had carditis during their initial episode and in children, 20% of whom will have a second episode within 5 years. Recurrences are uncommon after 5 years and in patients over 25 years of age. Prophylaxis is usually discontinued after these times except in groups with a high risk of streptococcal infection—parents or teachers of young children, nurses, military recruits, etc.

A. PENICILLIN

The preferred method of prophylaxis is with benzathine penicillin G, 1.2 million units intramuscularly every 4 weeks. Oral penicillin (200,000–250,000 units twice daily) is less reliable.

B. SULFONAMIDES OR ERYTHROMYCIN

If the patient is allergic to penicillin, sulfadiazine (or sulfisoxazole), 1 g daily, or erythromycin, 250 mg orally twice daily, may be substituted.

Prognosis

Initial episodes of rheumatic fever may last months in children and weeks in adults. The immediate mortality rate is 1–2%. Persistent rheumatic carditis with cardiomegaly, heart failure, and pericarditis imply a poor prognosis; 30% of children thus affected die within 10 years after the initial attack. After 10 years, two-thirds of patients will have detectable valvular abnormalities (usually thickened valves with limited mobility), but significant symptomatic valvular heart disease or persistent cardiomyopathy occurs in less than 10% of patients with a single episode. In developing countries, acute rheumatic fever occurs earlier in life, recurs more frequently, and the evolution to chronic valvular disease is both accelerated and more severe.

Rheumatic Heart Disease

Chronic rheumatic heart disease results from single or repeated attacks of rheumatic fever that produce rigidity and deformity of valve cusps, fusion of the commissures, or shortening and fusion of the chordae tendineae. Stenosis or insufficiency results, and the two often coexist. The mitral valve alone is affected in 50–60% of cases; combined lesions of the aortic and mitral valves occur in 20%; pure aortic lesions are less common. Tricuspid involvement occurs only in association with mitral or aortic disease in about 10% of cases. The pulmonary valve is rarely affected. A history of rheumatic fever is obtainable in only 60% of patients with rheumatic heart disease.

The first clue to organic valvular disease is a murmur. Physical examination permits accurate diagnosis in many cases, but echocardiography will reveal valve cusp thickening with decreased opening in stenosis, estimate the magnitude of regurgitation, and demonstrate the earliest stages of specific chamber enlargement.

Recurrences of acute rheumatic fever can be prevented (see above). The patient should also receive prophylactic antibiotics preceding dental extraction, urologic and surgical procedures, etc, to prevent endocarditis (Table 33–4). With mitral valve disease, it is important to identify the onset of atrial fibrillation in order to institute anticoagulation. The important findings in each of the major valve lesions are summarized in Table 10–1. The hemodynamic changes, symptoms, associated findings, and course have been discussed previously.

Narula J et al: Diagnosis of active rheumatic carditis. Circulation 1999;100:1576. [PMID: 10510063] (Argues for the incorporation of echocardiographic data into the classic Jones criteria for diagnosis of rheumatic carditis.)

Stollerman GH: Rheumatic fever. Lancet 1997;349:935. [PMID: 9093263] (Clinical manifestations, pathogenesis, changing epidemiology, and prevention.)

■ DISEASES OF THE PERICARDIUM

ACUTE PERICARDITIS

The pericardium consists of two layers: the inner visceral layer, which is attached to the epicardium; and an outer parietal layer. The pericardium stabilizes the heart in anatomic position and reduces contact between the heart and surrounding structures. It is composed of fibrous tissue, and while it will permit moderate changes in cardiac size, it cannot stretch rapidly enough to accommodate rapid dilation of the heart or accumulation of fluid without increasing intrapericardial (and, therefore, intracardiac) pressure.

The pericardium is often involved by processes that affect the heart, but it may also be affected by diseases of adjacent tissues and may itself be a primary site of disease.

INFLAMMATORY PERICARDITIS

Acute inflammation of the pericardium may be infectious in origin or may be due to systemic diseases (autoimmune syndromes, uremia), neoplasm, radiation, drug toxicity, hemopericardium, or contiguous inflammatory processes in the myocardium or lung. In many of these conditions, the pathologic process involves both the pericardium and the myocardium.

The presentation and course of inflammatory pericarditis depend on its cause, but all syndromes are often (not always) associated with chest pain, which is usually pleuritic and postural (relieved by sitting). The pain is substernal but may radiate to the neck, shoulders, back, or epigastrium. Dyspnea may also be present. A pericardial friction rub is characteristic, with or without evidence of fluid accumulation or constriction (see below). Fever and leukocytosis are often present. The ECG usually shows generalized ST and T wave changes and may manifest a characteristic progression beginning with diffuse ST elevation, followed by a return to baseline and then to T wave inversion. The chest x-ray may show cardiac enlargement if fluid has collected, as well as signs of related pulmonary disease. The echocardiogram may disclose pericardial effusions and indicate their hemodynamic significance, but it is often normal in inflammatory pericarditis.

Several of the specific pericarditis syndromes are discussed below.

Viral Pericarditis

Viral infections (especially infections with coxsackieviruses and echoviruses but also influenza, Epstein-Barr, varicella, hepatitis, mumps, and HIV viruses) are the commonest cause of acute pericarditis and probably are responsible for many cases classified as idiopathic. Males—usually under age 50—are most commonly affected. Pericardial involvement often follows upper respiratory infection. The diagnosis is usually clinical, but rising viral titers in paired sera may be obtained for confirmation. Cardiac enzymes may be slightly elevated, reflecting a myocarditic component. The differential diagnosis is primarily with myocardial infarction.

Treatment is generally symptomatic. Aspirin (650 mg every 3–4 hours) or other nonsteroidal agents (eg, indomethacin, 100–150 mg daily in divided doses) are usually effective. Corticosteroids may be beneficial in unresponsive cases. In general, symptoms subside in several days to weeks. The major early complication is tamponade, which occurs in fewer than 5% of patients. There may be recurrences in the first few weeks or months. Rare patients will continue to experience recurrences chronically, sometimes leading to constrictive pericarditis, when pericardial resection may be required.

Tuberculous Pericarditis

Tuberculous pericarditis has become rare in developed countries but remains common in other areas. It results from direct lymphatic or hematogenous spread; clinical pulmonary involvement may be absent or minor, although associated pleural effusions are common. The presentation tends to be subacute, but nonspecific symptoms (fever, night sweats, fatigue) may be present for days to months. Pericardial effusions are usually small or moderate but may be large. The diagnosis can be inferred if acid-fast bacilli are found elsewhere. The yield of organisms by pericardiocentesis is low; pericardial biopsy has a higher yield but may also be negative, and pericardiectomy may be required. Standard antituberculous drug therapy is usually successful (see Chapter 9), but constrictive pericarditis can occur.

Other Infectious Pericarditides

Bacterial pericarditis has become rare and usually results from direct extension from pulmonary infections. Symptoms and signs are similar to those of other types of inflammatory pericarditides, but patients appear toxic and are often critically ill. *Borrelia burgdorferi,* the organism responsible for Lyme disease, can also cause myopericarditis.

Uremic Pericarditis

This syndrome is a common complication of renal failure. The pathogenesis is uncertain; it occurs both with untreated uremia and in otherwise stable dialysis patients. The pericardium is characteristically "shaggy," and the effusion is hemorrhagic and exudative. Uremic pericarditis can present with or without symptoms; fever is absent. The pericarditis usually resolves with the institution of—or with more aggressive—dialysis. Tamponade is fairly common, and partial pericardiectomy (pericardial window) may be necessary. While anti-inflammatory agents may relieve the pain and fever associated with uremic pericarditis, indomethacin and systemic glucocorticoids do not affect the natural history of uremic pericarditis.

Neoplastic Pericarditis

Spread of adjacent lung cancer as well as invasion by breast cancer, renal cell carcinoma, Hodgkin's disease, and lymphomas are the commonest neoplastic processes involving the pericardium and have become the most frequent cause of pericardial tamponade in many countries. Often the process is painless, and the presenting symptoms relate to hemodynamic compromise or the primary disease. The diagnosis can usually be made by cytologic examination of the effusion or by biopsy, but it may be difficult to establish clinically if the patient has received mediastinal radiation within the previous year. MRI and CT scan can visualize neighboring tumor when present. The prognosis with neoplastic effusion is dismal, with only a small minority surviving 1 year. If it is compromising the patient, the effusion is initially drained. Instillation of chemotherapeutic agents or tetracycline may also prevent recurrence. Pericardial windows are rarely effective, but partial pericardiectomy from a subxiphoid incision may be successful; patients may be too ill to tolerate this.

Postmyocardial Infarction or Postcardiotomy Pericarditis (Dressler's Syndrome)

Pericarditis may occur 2–5 days after infarction due to an inflammatory reaction to transmural myocardial necrosis. It usually presents as a recurrence of pain with pleural-pericardial features. A rub is often audible, and repolarization changes may be confused with ischemia. Large effusions are uncommon, and spontaneous resolution usually occurs in a few days. Aspirin or nonsteroidal agents in the dosages given in the section on viral pericarditis provide symptomatic relief.

Dressler's syndrome occurs weeks to several months after myocardial infarction or open heart surgery, may be recurrent, and probably represents an autoimmune syndrome. Patients present with typical pain, fever, malaise, and leukocytosis. The sedimentation rate is usually high. Large pericardial effusions and accompanying pleural effusions are frequent. Tamponade is rare with Dressler's syndrome after infarction but not when it occurs postoperatively. Nonsteroidal agents may be given, but recurrences are common; corticosteroids are effective but may be difficult to withdraw without relapse.

Radiation Pericarditis

Radiation can initiate a fibrinous and fibrotic process in the pericardium, presenting as subacute pericarditis or constriction. The clinical onset is usually within the first year but may be delayed for many years. Radiation pericarditis usually follows treatments of more than 4000 cGy delivered to ports including more than 30% of the heart. Symptomatic therapy is the initial approach, but recurrent effusions and constriction often require surgery.

Other Causes of Pericarditis

These include connective tissue diseases, such as lupus erythematosus and rheumatoid arthritis, drug-induced pericarditis (minoxidil, penicillins), and myxedema.

Aikat S et al: A review of pericardial diseases: Clinical, ECG and hemodynamic features and management. Cleve Clin J Med 2000;67:903. [PMID: 11127986] (Practical review of acute and constrictive pericardial disease.)

Oakley CM: Myocarditis, pericarditis and other pericardial diseases. Heart 2000;84:449. [PMID: 10995424]

Wood JE et al: Pericarditis associated with renal failure: evolution and management. Semin Dial 2001;14:61. [PMID: 11208042]

PERICARDIAL EFFUSION

Pericardial effusion can develop during any of the processes discussed in the preceding paragraphs. The speed of accumulation determines the physiologic importance of the effusion. Because the pericardium stretches, large effusions (> 1000 mL) that develop slowly may produce no hemodynamic effects. Smaller effusions that appear rapidly can cause tamponade. Tamponade is characterized by elevated intrapericardial pressure (> 15 mm Hg), which restricts venous return and ventricular filling. As a result, the stroke volume and pulse pressure fall, and the heart rate and venous pressure rise. Shock and death may result.

Clinical Findings

A. SYMPTOMS AND SIGNS

Pericardial effusions may be associated with pain if they occur as part of an acute inflammatory process or may be painless, as is often the case with neoplastic or uremic effusion. Dyspnea and cough are common, especially with tamponade. Other symptoms may result from the primary disease.

A pericardial friction rub may be present even with large effusions. In cardiac tamponade, tachycardia, tachypnea, a narrow pulse pressure, and a relatively preserved systolic pressure are characteristic. Pulsus paradoxus—a greater than 10 mm Hg decline in systolic pressure during inspiration due to further impairment of left ventricular filling—is the classic finding, but it may also occur with obstructive lung disease. Central venous pressure is elevated, and edema or ascites may be present; these signs favor a more chronic process.

B. LABORATORY FINDINGS

Laboratory tests tend to reflect the underlying processes.

C. DIAGNOSTIC STUDIES

Chest x-ray can suggest effusion by an enlarged cardiac silhouette with a globular configuration but may appear normal. The ECG often reveals nonspecific T wave changes and low QRS voltage. Electrical alternans is present uncommonly but is pathognomonic. Echocardiography is the primary method for demonstrating pericardial effusion. Tamponade presents a characteristic picture of inadequate ventricular filling (diastolic collapse of the right ventricle or right atrium). The echocardiogram readily discriminates pericardial effusion from congestive heart failure. MRI also demonstrates pericardial fluid and lesions. Diagnostic pericardiocentesis or biopsy is often indicated for microbiologic and cytologic studies; a pericardial biopsy may be performed relatively simply through a small subxiphoid incision.

Treatment

Small effusions can be followed clinically and with the aid of echocardiograms. When tamponade is present, urgent pericardiocentesis is required. Removal of a small amount of fluid often produces immediate hemodynamic benefit, but complete drainage with a catheter is preferable. Continued drainage may be indicated.

Additional therapy is determined by the nature of the primary process. Recurrent effusion in neoplastic disease and uremia, in particular, may require partial pericardiectomy.

Karam N et al: Diagnosis and management of chronic pericardial effusions. Am J Med Sci 2001;322:79. [PMID: 11525201]

Sagrista-Sauleda J et al: Long-term follow-up of idiopathic chronic pericardial effusion. N Engl J Med 1999;341:2042. [PMID: 10615077] (Large pericardial effusions are often well tolerated but may cause tamponade unexpectedly. Pericardiectomy should be considered in patients in whom effusion recurs after pericardiocentesis.)

Soler-Soler J et al: Management of pericardial effusion. Heart 2001;86:235. [PMID: 11454853]

Tsang TS: Outcomes of primary and secondary treatment of pericardial effusion in patients with malignancy. Mayo Clin Proc 2000;75:248. [PMID: 10725950] (Review of 275 patients who underwent pericardioceteses for malignant disease. Effusion recurrence was strongly predicted by absence of extended drainage and large effusion size. Median survival was 135 days, but 26% survived beyond a year.)

CONSTRICTIVE PERICARDITIS

Inflammation can lead to a thickened, fibrotic, adherent pericardium that restricts diastolic filling and produces chronically elevated venous pressures. In the past, tuberculosis was the most common cause of constrictive pericarditis, but the process now more often occurs after radiation therapy, cardiac surgery, or viral pericarditis; histoplasmosis is another uncommon cause.

The principal symptoms are slowly progressive dyspnea, fatigue, and weakness. Chronic edema, hepatic congestion, and ascites are usually present. The examination reveals these signs and a characteristically elevated jugular venous pressure with a rapid y descent. Kussmaul's sign—an increase in jugular venous pressure during inspiration—occurs in constrictive pericarditis and restrictive cardiomyopathy. Pulsus paradoxus is unusual. Atrial fibrillation is common.

The chest x-ray may show normal heart size or cardiomegaly. Pericardial calcification is best seen on the lateral view and is common. Echocardiography can demonstrate a thick pericardium and small chambers. CT scans and MRI are helpful in revealing pericardial thickening and may be more sensitive than echocardiography.

The primary differential diagnoses are restrictive cardiomyopathy and tamponade. The former distinction can be difficult and is best made by evaluating left ventricular function (more consistently depressed in cardiomyopathy), measuring hemodynamics (which show more complete equalization of diastolic pressures in all four chambers in constrictive pericarditis), and demonstrating pericardial thickening and calcification.

Initial treatment consists of gentle diuresis. Surgical removal of the pericardium, which should be complete, is usually required in symptomatic patients but is associated with a relatively high mortality rate.

Myers RB et al: Constrictive pericarditis: clinical and pathophysiologic characteristics. Am Heart J 1999;138:219. [PMID: 10426832] (This article reviews constrictive pericarditis, including epidemiology, mechanism, clinical findings, diagnosis, and treatment, and offers a discussion of differentiation from restrictive cardiomyopathy.)

Osterberg L et al: Case presentation and review: Constrictive pericarditis. West J Med 1998;169:232. [PMID: 9795593] (Pathophysiology, diagnosis, and treatment are reviewed. Etiology, physical findings, and hemodynamic waveforms are included. Surgical pericardiectomy is the treatment of choice.)

■ PULMONARY HYPERTENSION & HEART DISEASE

PRIMARY PULMONARY HYPERTENSION

Primary pulmonary hypertension is defined as pulmonary hypertension and elevated pulmonary vascular resistance in the absence of other disease of the lungs or heart. Pathologically, it is characterized by diffuse narrowing of the pulmonary arterioles. Circumstantial evidence suggests that unrecognized recurrent pulmonary emboli or in situ thrombosis may play a role in some cases. However, the latter may well be an exacerbating factor (precipitated by local endothelial injury) rather than a cause of the syndrome. Primary pulmonary hypertension must be distinguished from chronic pulmonary heart disease (cor pulmonale), recurrent pulmonary emboli, mitral stenosis, and congenital heart disease; cirrhosis of the liver is another cause. The diet pills fenfluramine, dexfenfluramine, and phentermine may cause a picture indistinguishable from that of primary pulmonary hypertension, which is frequently irreversible. Exclusion of secondary causes by echocardiography and lung scanning—and, if necessary, pulmonary angiography—is essential.

The clinical picture is similar to that of pulmonary hypertension from other causes. Patients—characteristically young women—present with evidence of right heart failure that is usually progressive, leading to death in 2–8 years. Patients have manifestations of low cardiac output, with weakness and fatigue, as well as edema and ascites as right heart failure advances. Peripheral cyanosis is present, and syncope on effort may occur.

The chest x-ray shows enlarged main pulmonary arteries with reduced peripheral branches. The right ventricle is enlarged. The ECG shows right ventricular and atrial hypertrophy.

Some authorities advocate chronic oral anticoagulation. The efficacy of vasodilator drugs is controversial. They may lower systemic arterial pressure more than pulmonary arterial pressure, resulting in hypotension that may be life-threatening. The calcium channel blockers nifedipine and diltiazem may be effective early in the course of the disease but offer little in advanced stages. More advanced disease has been managed successfully with chronic infusions of prostacyclin, a potent pulmonary vasodilator. This agent often improves symptoms, sometimes dramatically, in patients who have not responded to other vasodilators. An oral endothelin antagonist, bosentan, has proved very effective in treating moderate to severe primary pulmonary hypertension and may become the treatment of choice for all stages of the disease. Inhaled nitric oxide has been used in patients who do not respond to prostacyclin.

Even with prostacyclin therapy, the symptoms usually progress, and most patients will ultimately require heart-lung transplantation.

Archer S et al: Primary pulmonary hypertension: a vascular biology and translational research "work in progress." Circulation 2000;102:2781. [PMID: 11094047] (The growing understanding of the pathophysiology of this condition is paying off in new therapies.)

Gaine S: Pulmonary hypertension. JAMA 2000;284:3160. [PMID: 11135781] (Treatment-based classification is outlined. Continuous epoprostenol infusion and lung transplantation are the most effective current treatment options.)

Rubin LJ et al: Bosentan therapy for pulmonary arterial hypertension. N Engl J Med 2002;346:806. [PMID: 11907289] (Randomized trial showing improvement in exercise tolerance and preventing deterioration.)

PULMONARY HEART DISEASE (Cor Pulmonale)

ESSENTIALS OF DIAGNOSIS

- *Symptoms and signs of chronic bronchitis and pulmonary emphysema.*
- *Elevated jugular venous pressure, parasternal lift, edema, hepatomegaly, ascites.*
- *ECG shows tall, peaked P waves (P pulmonale), right axis deviation, and right ventricular hypertrophy.*
- *Chest x-ray: Enlarged right ventricle and pulmonary artery.*
- *Echocardiogram or radionuclide angiography excludes primary left ventricular dysfunction.*

General Considerations

The term "cor pulmonale" denotes right ventricular hypertrophy and eventual failure resulting from pulmonary disease and attendant hypoxia or from pulmonary vascular disease. Its clinical features depend upon both the primary underlying disease and its effects on the heart.

Cor pulmonale is most commonly caused by chronic obstructive pulmonary disease. Less frequent causes include pneumoconiosis, pulmonary fibrosis, kyphoscoliosis, primary pulmonary hypertension, repeated episodes of subclinical or clinical pulmonary embolization, Pickwickian syndrome, schistosomiasis, and obliterative pulmonary capillary or lymphangitic infiltration from metastatic carcinoma.

Clinical Findings

A. SYMPTOMS AND SIGNS

The predominant symptoms of compensated cor pulmonale are related to the pulmonary disorder and include chronic productive cough, exertional dyspnea, wheezing respirations, easy fatigability, and weakness. When the pulmonary disease causes right ventricular failure, these symptoms may be intensified. Dependent edema and right upper quadrant pain may also appear. The signs of cor pulmonale include cyanosis, clubbing, distended neck veins, right ventricular heave or gallop (or both), prominent lower sternal or epigastric pulsations, an enlarged and tender liver, and dependent edema.

B. LABORATORY FINDINGS

Polycythemia is often present in cor pulmonale secondary to COPD. The arterial oxygen saturation is often below 85%; PCO_2 may or may not be elevated.

C. ELECTROCARDIOGRAPHY AND CHEST X-RAY

The ECG may show right axis deviation and peaked P waves. Deep S waves are present in lead V_6. Right axis deviation and low voltage may be noted in patients with pulmonary emphysema. Frank right ventricular hypertrophy is uncommon except in primary pulmonary hypertension. The ECG often mimics myocardial infarction; Q waves may be present in leads II, III, and aVF because of the vertically placed heart, but they are rarely deep or wide, as in inferior myocardial infarction. Supraventricular arrhythmias are frequent and nonspecific.

The chest radiograph discloses the presence or absence of parenchymal disease and a prominent or enlarged right ventricle and pulmonary artery.

D. DIAGNOSTIC STUDIES

Pulmonary function tests usually confirm the underlying lung disease. The echocardiogram should show normal left ventricular size and function but right ventricular dilation. Perfusion lung scans are rarely of value, but, if negative, they help to exclude pulmonary emboli, an occasional cause of cor pulmonale. Pulmonary angiography is the most specific method of diagnosis for the pulmonary emboli, but it carries increased risk when performed in patients with pulmonary hypertension.

Differential Diagnosis

In its early stages, cor pulmonale can be diagnosed on the basis of radiologic, echocardiographic, or electrocardiographic evidence. Catheterization of the right heart will establish a definitive diagnosis but is usually performed to exclude left-sided heart failure, which may in some patients be an inapparent cause of right-sided failure. Differential diagnostic considerations relate chiefly to the specific pulmonary disease that has produced right ventricular failure (see above).

Treatment

The details of the treatment of chronic pulmonary disease (chronic respiratory failure) are discussed in Chapter 9. Otherwise, therapy is directed at the pulmonary process responsible for right heart failure. Oxygen, salt and fluid restriction, and diuretics are mainstays; digitalis has no place in right heart failure unless atrial fibrillation is present.

Prognosis

Compensated cor pulmonale has the same prognosis as the underlying pulmonary disease. Once congestive signs appear, the average life expectancy is 2–5 years, but survival is significantly longer when uncomplicated emphysema is the cause.

Krowka MJ: Pulmonary hypertension: diagnostics and therapeutics. Mayo Clin Proc 2000;75:625. [PMID: 10852424] (Covers secondary as well as primary causes. Etiology, screening tests, and treatment options are reviewed.)

Vizza CD et al: Right and left ventricular dysfunction in patients with severe pulmonary disease. Chest 1998;113:576. [PMID: 9515827] (In patients with advanced pulmonary disease, left ventricular dysfunction is less common than right ventricular dysfunction, but problems with the left ventricle may be due in part to ventricular interdependence.)

■ NEOPLASTIC DISEASES OF THE HEART

Primary cardiac tumors are rare and constitute only a small fraction of all tumors that involve the heart or pericardium. Metastases from malignant tumors elsewhere are more frequent. Tumors involving the heart are bronchogenic carcinoma, carcinoma of the breast, malignant melanoma, the lymphomas, renal cell carcinoma, and, in patients with AIDS, Kaposi's sarcoma. These are often clinically silent but may lead to pericardial tamponade, arrhythmias and conduction disturbances, heart failure, and peripheral emboli. The diagnosis is often made by echocardiography, but MRI and CT scanning are also helpful. Electrocardiography may reveal regional Q waves. The prognosis is dismal; effective treatment is not available.

The commonest primary tumors of the heart are atrial myxomas. These tend to occur in middle age, more often in women than in men. They usually originate in the intraventricular septum, with over 80% growing into the left atrium. Myxomas are benign tumors but can embolize systemically.

Patients with myxoma can present with a picture of a systemic illness, obstruction of blood flow through the heart, or signs of peripheral embolization. The characteristic picture includes fever, malaise, weight loss, leukocytosis, elevated sedimentation rate, and emboli (peripheral or pulmonary, depending on the location of the tumor). This picture is often confused with infective endocarditis, lymphoma, other cancers, or autoimmune diseases. In other cases, the tumor may grow to considerable size and produce symptoms by obstructing mitral flow. Episodic pulmonary edema (classically occurring when an upright posture is assumed) and signs of low output may result. Physical examination may reveal a diastolic sound related to motion of the tumor ("tumor plop") or a diastolic murmur similar to that of mitral stenosis. Right-sided myxomas may cause symptoms of right-sided failure. The diagnosis is established by echocardiography or by pathologic study of embolic material. MRI is also useful. Contrast angiography is usually not necessary. Surgical excision is usually curative.

Other primary cardiac tumors include rhabdomyomas, fibrous histiocytomas, hemangiomas, and a variety of unusual sarcomas. The diagnosis may be supported by an abnormal cardiac contour on x-ray. Echocardiography is usually helpful but may miss tumors infiltrating the ventricular wall. It is likely that MRI will be useful as well.

Roberts WC: Primary and secondary neoplasms of the heart. Am J Cardiol 1997;80:671. [PMID: 9295010] (Review of primary and metastatic cardiac tumors, including pathologic specimens.)

■ CARDIAC INVOLVEMENT IN MISCELLANEOUS SYSTEMIC DISEASES

The heart may be involved in a number of systemic syndromes. Many of these have been mentioned briefly in prior subsections of this chapter. The pericardium, myocardium, heart valves, and coronary arteries may be involved either singly or in various combinations. In most cases the cardiac manifestations are not the dominant feature, but in some it is the primary cause of symptoms and may be fatal.

The most common type of myocardial involvement is an infiltrative cardiomyopathy, such as systemic amyloidosis, sarcoidosis, hemochromatosis, or glycogen storage disease. Cardiac calcinosis can occur in hyperparathyroidism (usually the secondary form) and in primary oxalosis. A number of muscular dystrophies can cause a cardiomyopathic picture (particularly Duchenne's, less frequently myotonic dystrophy, and several rarer forms). In addition to left ventricular dysfunction and heart failure, all of these conditions frequently cause conduction abnormalities, which may be the presenting or only feature. The myocardium may also be involved in inflammatory and autoimmune diseases. It is commonly affected in polymyositis and dermatomyositis, but usually this is subclinical. Systemic lupus erythematosus, scleroderma, and mixed connective tissue disease may cause myocarditis, but these commonly also involve the pericardium, coronary arteries, or valves. Several endocrinopathies, including acromegaly, thyrotoxicosis, myxedema, and pheochromocytoma, can produce cardiomyopathies, though again they are usually not isolated features.

Pericardial involvement is quite common in many of the connective tissue diseases. Systemic lupus erythematosus may present with pericarditis, and pericardial involvement is not uncommon (but is less frequently symptomatic) in active rheumatoid arthritis, systemic sclerosis, and mixed connective tissue disease. Endocardial involvement takes the form of patchy fibrous—predominantly on the right side—or inflammatory or sclerotic changes of the heart valves. Carcinoid heart disease typically is manifested as tricuspid regurgitation, and the same may be the case in systemic lupus erythematosus. The hypereosinophilic syndromes involve the endocardium, leading to restrictive cardiomyopathy. A variety of arthritic syndromes are associated with aortic valvulitis or aortitis, including ankylosing spondylitis, rheumatoid arthritis, and Reiter's syndrome, as is tertiary syphilis also. Disorders of elastic tissue (Marfan's syndrome is the most frequent) often affect the ascending aorta, with resulting aneurysmal dilation and aortic regurgitation.

Virtually any vasculitic syndrome can involve the coronary arteries, leading to myocardial infarction. This is most common with polyarteritis nodosa and systemic lupus erythematosus. Two vasculitic syndromes have a particular predilection for the coronary arteries—Kawasaki's disease and Takayasu's disease. In these, myocardial infarction may be the presenting symptom.

Kulke MH et al: Carcinoid tumors. N Engl J Med 1999;340:858. [PMID: 10080850] (Discusses carcinoid tumors with specific discussion of carcinoid heart disease.)

Moder KG et al: Cardiac involvement in systemic lupus erythematosus. Mayo Clin Proc 1999;74:275. [PMID: 10089998] (SLE is the connective tissue disease that most frequently involves the heart [more than 50% of cases]. Pericarditis is most common, but myocarditis, endocarditis, and coronary arteritis all occur with moderate frequency.)

■ TRAUMATIC HEART DISEASE

Penetrating wounds to the heart are, of course, usually lethal unless surgically repaired. Stab wounds to the right ventricle occasionally lead to hemopericardium without progressing to tamponade. The clinical result may be constrictive pericarditis, so surgery is recommended even if the patient presents in a stable condition.

Blunt trauma is a more frequent cause of cardiac injuries, particularly outside of the emergency room setting. This type of injury is quite frequent in motor vehicle accidents and may occur with any form of chest trauma. The most common injuries are myocardial contusions or hematomas. These may be asymptomatic (particularly in the setting of more severe injuries) or may present with chest pains of a nonspecific nature or, not uncommonly, with a pericardial component. A minority of patients will develop left or, less commonly, right ventricular aneurysm. Elevations of cardiac enzymes are frequent, and echocardiography may reveal an akinetic segment. Heart failure is uncommon if there are no associated cardiac or pericardial injuries, and conservative management is usually sufficient.

Severe trauma may also cause cardiac or valvular rupture. Cardiac rupture may involve any chamber, but survival is most likely if injury is to one of the atria or the right ventricle. Hemopericardium or pericardial tamponade is the usual clinical presentation, and surgery is almost always necessary. Mitral and aortic valve rupture may occur during severe blunt trauma—the former presumably if the impact occurs during systole and the latter if during diastole. Patients reach the hospital in shock or severe heart failure. Immediate surgical repair is essential. The same types of injuries may result in transection of the aorta, either at the level of the arch or distal to the takeoff of the left subclavian artery. Transthoracic and transesophageal echocardiography are the most helpful and immediately available diagnostic techniques.

Blunt trauma may also result in damage to the coronary arteries. Acute or subacute coronary thrombosis is the most common presentation. The clinical syndrome is one of acute myocardial infarction with attendant electrocardiographic, enzymatic, and contractile abnormalities. Emergent revascularization is sometimes feasible, either by the percutaneous route or by coronary artery bypass surgery. Left ventricular aneurysms are common outcomes of traumatic coronary occlusions. Coronary artery dissection or rupture may also occur in the setting of blunt cardiac trauma.

Orliaguet G et al: The heart in blunt trauma. Anesthesiology 2001;95:544. [PMID: 11506131]

Prêtre R et al: Blunt trauma to the heart and great vessels. N Engl J Med 1997;336:626. [PMID: 9032049]

■ THE CARDIAC PATIENT & SURGERY

Patients with known or suspected cardiac disease undergoing general surgery present a common management problem. Anesthesia and surgery are often associated with marked fluctuations of heart rate and blood pressure, changes in intravascular volume, myocardial ischemia or depression, arrhythmias, decreased oxygenation, increased sympathetic nervous system activity, and alterations in medical regimens and pharmacokinetics. Even with careful monitoring and management, the perioperative period can be very stressful to cardiac patients.

The risk of surgery in patients with heart disease depends primarily on three factors: the type of operation, the nature of the heart disease, and the degree of preoperative stability. The type of anesthesia is less important, though halothane, enflurane, and barbiturates are more severe myocardial depressants, while narcotics have little depressive effect. Spinal and epidural anesthesia were previously thought to be preferable in patients with heart disease, but this has not proved to be the case.

The highest-risk procedures are surgery of the aorta and vascular procedures, in part because these patients often have associated severe coronary disease but also because marked blood pressure and volume changes are common. Major abdominal and thoracic surgery are also associated with substantial cardiovascular risk, especially in older patients with associated cardiovascular disease.

Numerous studies have evaluated the excess risk of surgery in patients with various cardiac diseases. Recent (within 3 months) myocardial infarction, unstable angina, congestive heart failure, and significant aortic stenosis are associated with substantial increases in operative morbidity and mortality rates. Any degree of instability in these conditions magnifies the potential risk. Stable angina, especially in an inactive individual, is also associated with a higher operative risk. Although less common, cyanotic congenital heart disease and severe primary or secondary pulmonary hypertension pose great risks during major surgery. In patients with any of these problems, the risk-to-benefit ratio of the planned surgery should be carefully examined. If the procedure is necessary but elective, consideration should be given to delaying it until full recovery postinfarction and correction or optimal stabilization of the other conditions are achieved. Hypertension should be at least moderately controlled. Patients with severe angina should have increased medical therapy or be considered for revascularization before noncardiac surgery. Symptomatic arrhythmias, nonsustained ventricular tachycardia, or high-grade atrioventricular block and cardiac failure should be treated optimally.

Clinical assessment provides the most useful guidance in determining the risk of noncardiac surgery. Important indicators of high risk have been discussed above. A multifactorial cardiac risk index is included in Chapter 3 (Table 3–4). Patients with known but clinically stable heart disease, such as angina pectoris or prior myocardial infarction, are at intermediate risk, particularly for major operations such as vascular surgery. If a history or symptoms of heart failure are present, assessment of left ventricular function can be very helpful in perioperative management. Although frequently advocated, further noninvasive testing for myocardial ischemia for the purpose of risk stratification is probably overutilized. Tests such as stress myocardial perfusion scintigraphy or dobutamine echocardiography should be reserved for situations in which the results may alter patient management. There is no evidence that prophylactic revascularization by either PTCA or coronary artery bypass surgery alters long-term outcome in patients undergoing noncardiac surgical procedures without the usual indications for PTCA or CABG. Only in the case of major vascular operations is perioperative mortality and morbidity high enough that prophylactic PTCA or CABG should be considered.

However, it should be noted that many patients undergoing surgery have not had recent medical follow-up, and this may be an appropriate opportunity to perform a more complete evaluation. Thus, stress testing may be indicated for selected patients with symptomatic angina or prior myocardial infarction with a view to instituting more comprehensive medical management or performing coronary revascularization to reduce long-term (rather than perioperative) mortality and morbidity. At the least, such patients should not be discharged without a plan for an appropriate follow-up and institution of antihyperlipidemic, aspirin, and beta-blocker therapy as indicated.

Once the decision to operate is made, careful management is essential. Most cardiac medications should be continued preoperatively and postoperatively. In patients judged to be at high risk or medium risk, beta-blockers should be initiated preoperatively unless contraindicated. If practical, oral therapy with atenolol or metoprolol should be started several days prior to surgery and gradually increased to 100 mg in single or divided doses. Otherwise, 15 mg of metoprolol or 10 mg of atenolol may be administered intravenously in 5 mg increments separated by 5–10 minutes prior to induction. These doses should be repeated every 12 hours—or more frequently if excessive tachycardia occurs—until oral therapy can be commenced. Monitoring is an important prophylactic measure in high-risk individuals; hemodynamic monitoring can facilitate early intervention in patients with heart failure, severe valve disease, or easily induced myocardial ischemia. Excessive hypertension, hypotension, and myocardial ischemia should be identified and appropriately treated using rapidly acting agents. Transesophageal echocardiography can also be used for intraoperative monitoring of ischemia, but its value has never been established in well-designed studies. Ischemic events, whether symptomatic or silent, should be vigorously treated.

Auerbach AD et al: Beta-blockers and reduction of cardiac events in noncardiac surgery: scientific review. JAMA 2002;287: 1435. [PMID: 11903031]

Boersma E et al: Predictors of cardiac events after major vascular surgery: Role of clinical characteristics, dobutamine echocardiography, and beta-blocker therapy. JAMA 2001;285: 1865. [PMID: 11308400] (Study investigating the role of stress echocardiography and clinical predictors especially in relation to beta-blocker therapy.)

Eagle KA et al: Guidelines for perioperative cardiovascular evaluation for noncardiac surgery. Report of the American College of Cardiology/American Heart Association Task Force on Practice Guidelines (Committee on Perioperative Cardiovascular Evaluation for Noncardiac Surgery). J Am Coll Cardiol 1996;27:910. [PMID: 8613622] (Most extensive, evidence-based review and guideline.)

Fleisher LA et al: Clinical Practice. Lowering cardiac risk in noncardiac surgery. N Engl J Med 2001;345:1677. [PMID: 11759647] (Concise algorithmic approach.)

■ THE CARDIAC PATIENT & PREGNANCY

The management of cardiac disease in pregnancy is discussed in detail in the references listed below. Only a few major points can be covered in this brief section.

CARDIOVASCULAR CHANGES DURING PREGNANCY

Normal physiologic changes during pregnancy can exacerbate symptoms of underlying cardiac disease even in previously asymptomatic individuals. Maternal blood volume rises progressively until the end of the sixth or seventh month. Stroke volume increases over the same time course as a result of the volume change and an increase in ejection fraction. The latter reflects predominantly a decline in peripheral resistance due to vasodilation and the low-resistance shunting through the placenta. The heart rate tends to rise in the third trimester. Overall, cardiac output increases by 30–50%; systolic blood pressure tends to rise slightly or remain unchanged, but diastolic pressure falls significantly.

High cardiac output causes alterations in the cardiac examination. A third heart sound is prominent and normal, and a pulmonary flow murmur is common. Electrocardiographic changes include rate-related decreases in PR and QT intervals, a leftward axis shift, inferior Q waves due to the more horizontal position of the heart, and nonspecific ST–T wave changes.

MANAGEMENT OF PREEXISTING CONDITIONS

The physiologic changes imposed by pregnancy can cause cardiac decompensation in patients with any significant cardiac abnormality, but the most severe problems are encountered in patients with valvular stenosis (especially mitral and aortic stenosis), congenital or acquired abnormalities associated with pulmonary hypertension or right-to-left shunting, congestive heart failure due to any cause, coronary heart disease, and hypertension. Valvular insufficiency or left-to-right shunting often diminishes because of the fall in peripheral resistance and is better tolerated.

Mitral stenosis becomes more hemodynamically severe owing to the increase in diastolic flow and the rate-related shortening of diastole. Left atrial pressures rise, and dyspnea or pulmonary edema can occur in previously asymptomatic individuals. The onset of atrial fibrillation often leads to acute decompensation. Patients with moderate to severe stenosis should have the condition corrected prior to becoming pregnant if possible. Patients who become symptomatic can undergo successful surgery, preferably in the third trimester. Balloon valvuloplasty is an attractive alternative, though radiation exposure to the fetus is unavoidable. Coarctation is usually well tolerated, but patients with symptoms should have corrective surgery before pregnancy. Patients with severe pulmonary hypertension and cyanotic congenital heart disease and those with severe aortic stenosis are at extremely high risk and should attempt to avoid pregnancy.

Asymptomatic arrhythmias should be closely observed unless underlying heart disease is present, in which case they should be treated with drugs. Paroxysmal supraventricular arrhythmias are quite common. Patients with Wolff-Parkinson-White syndrome may have more problems during pregnancy. Therapy is similar to that required for nonpregnant women.

Preexisting systemic hypertension is usually well tolerated and controllable, though the fetal morbidity rate is slightly increased. The incidence of preeclampsia and eclampsia (see Chapter 18) is increased.

Hydralazine and methyldopa are the antihypertensive agents for which there has been the greatest experience during pregnancy. Diuretics have also been used frequently, but concern has been raised that intravascular hypovolemia might impair uterine blood flow. Nonetheless, these agents are relatively safe. More recently, there has been considerable use of the combined alpha-beta-blocker labetalol and of calcium channel blockers, which have been proved effective and safe to both the mother and fetus. On the other hand, atenolol has been associated with lower fetal weights. ACE inhibitors and angiotensin II blockers are contraindicated in pregnancy because of the risk of fetal injury. Beta-blockers may retard fetal growth, but experience with them has been generally favorable. Little is known about the safety of most other antihypertensive agents.

CARDIOVASCULAR COMPLICATIONS OF PREGNANCY

Pregnancy-related hypertension (eclampsia and preeclampsia) is discussed in Chapter 18.

Cardiomyopathy of Pregnancy (Peripartum Cardiomyopathy)

In approximately one out of 4000–15,000 patients, dilated cardiomyopathy develops in the final month of pregnancy or within 6 months after delivery. The cause is unclear, but immune and viral causes have been postulated. The course of the disease is variable; many cases improve or resolve completely over several months, but others progress to refractory heart failure. Immunosuppressive therapy has been advocated, but few supportive data are available. Recently, beta-blockers have been administered judiciously to these patients, with at least anecdotal success. Recurrence in subsequent pregnancies is common, particularly if cardiac function has not recovered.

Coronary Artery & Other Vascular Abnormalities

There have been a number of reports of myocardial infarction during pregnancy. It is known that pregnancy predisposes to dissection of the aorta and other arteries, perhaps because of the accompanying connective tissue changes. However, coronary artery dissection is responsible for only a minority of the infarctions, with the majority being caused by atherosclerotic coronary artery disease or coronary emboli. Most of the events occur near term or shortly following delivery. Clinical management is essentially similar to that of other patients with acute infarction.

SPECIAL PROBLEMS

Prophylaxis for Infective Endocarditis

Although there is not universal agreement, many authorities recommend antibiotic prophylaxis during labor for patients at risk for endocarditis, especially if forceps or an episiotomy is employed. Ampicillin (2 g intravenously or intramuscularly) plus gentamicin (1.5 mg/kg intravenously or intramuscularly [up to 80 mg]) followed by amoxicillin, 1.5 g orally every 6 hours, is the recommended regimen.

Management of Labor

While vaginal delivery is usually well tolerated, unstable patients (including patients with severe hypertension and worsening heart failure) should have cesarean section. An increased risk of aortic rupture has been noted during delivery in patients with coarctation of the aorta and severe aortic root dilation with Marfan's syndrome, and vaginal delivery should be avoided in these conditions.

Cardiovascular Drugs During Pregnancy

Experience during pregnancy with many drugs is limited, and the effect on the fetus is often not well defined. Drugs with known potential for teratogenicity or fetal injury include phenytoin and the ACE inhibitors. Warfarin also presents a risk, but—at least in patients with prosthetic heart valves—many recommend that it be continued until the final 2 weeks. Self-injected low-molecular-weight heparin may be a good alternative, but data regarding efficacy and safety are lacking. Other than antihypertensive agents, which have been discussed above, cardiac drugs that appear safe during pregnancy include the digitalis glycosides, quinidine, procainamide, lidocaine, and short-term verapamil.

Elkayam U et al: Maternal and fetal outcomes of subsequent pregnancies in women with peripartum cardiomyopathy. N Engl J Med 2001;344:1567. [PMID: 11372007] (Study demonstrating that subsequent pregnancies can result in worsening of cardiac function and significant morbidity.)

Ginsberg JS et al: Use of antithrombotic agents during pregnancy. Chest 2001;119:122S. [PMID: 11157646]

Mosca L et al: Guide to preventive cardiology for women. AHA/ACC Scientific Statement Consensus panel statement. Circulation 1999;99:2480. [PMID: 10318674]

Pearson GD et al: Peripartum cardiomyopathy: NHLBI workshop recommendations and review. JAMA 2000;283:1183. [PMID: 10703781] (Reviews available literature on epidemiology, diagnosis, and management, including subsequent pregnancies.)

Report of the National High Blood Pressure Education Program Working Group on High Blood Pressure in Pregnancy. Am J Obstet Gynecol 2000;183:S1. [PMID: 10920346] (When and how to treat as well as counseling for future pregnancies in affected patients.)

Sadler L et al: Pregnancy outcomes and cardiac complications in women with mechanical, bioprosthetic and homograft valves. Br J Obstet Gynaecol 2000;107:245. [PMID: 10688509] (Retrospective study of 147 pregnancies in 79 women. Pregnancy loss was high in patients with mechanical mitral valves treated with warfarin throughout pregnancy, whereas thromboembolic cardiac complications were associated with heparin. Pregnancy outcome was good with bioprosthetic valves.)

Siu SC et al: Heart disease and pregnancy. Heart 2001;85:710. [PMID: 11359761]

Siu SC et al: Prospective multicenter study of pregnancy outcomes in women with heart disease. Circulation 2001;104:515. [PMID: 11479246] (Describes outcomes in 562 patients and suggests use of a risk index.)

CARDIOVASCULAR SCREENING OF ATHLETES

The sudden death of a competitive athlete inevitably becomes an occasion for local if not national publicity. On each such occasion, the public and the medical community ask whether such events could be prevented by more careful or complete screening. Although each such event is tragic, it must be appreciated that there are approximately 5 million competitive athletes at the high school level or above in any given year. The number of cardiac deaths occurring during athletic participation is unknown, but estimates at the high school level range from one in 300,000 to one in 100,000 participants. Death rates among more mature athletes increase as the prevalence of coronary artery disease rises. These numbers highlight the problem of how to screen individual participants. Even an inexpensive test such as an ECG would generate an enormous cost if required of all athletes, and it is likely that few at-risk individuals would be detected. Echocardiography, either as a routine test or as a follow-up examination for abnormal ECGs, would be prohibitively expensive.

Thus, the most feasible approach is that of a careful medical history and cardiac examination performed by personnel aware of the conditions responsible for most sudden deaths in competitive athletes. In a series of 158 athletic deaths in the United States between 1985 and 1995, hypertrophic cardiomyopathy (36%) and coronary anomalies (19%) were by far the most frequent underlying conditions. Left ventricular hypertrophy was present in another 10%, ruptured aorta (presumably due to Marfan's syndrome or cystic medial necrosis) in 6%, myocarditis or dilated cardiomyopathy in 6%, aortic stenosis in 4%, and arrhythmogenic right ventricular dysplasia in 3%.

It is likely that a careful family and medical history and cardiovascular examination will identify some individuals at risk. A family history of premature sudden death or cardiovascular disease or of any of these predisposing conditions should mandate further workup, including an echocardiogram and ECG. Symptoms of chest pain, syncope, or near-syncope also warrant further evaluation. A Marfan-like appearance, significant elevation of blood pressure or abnormalities of heart rate or rhythm, and pathologic heart murmurs or heart sounds should also be investigated before clearance for athletic participation is given. Such an evaluation is recommended before participation at the high school and college levels and every 2 years during athletic competition. Selective use of routine electrocardiography and stress testing is recommended in men above age 40 and women above age 50 who continue to participate in vigorous exercise and at earlier ages when there is a positive family history for premature coronary artery disease or multiple risk factors.

Corrado D et al: Screening for hypertrophic cardiomyopathy in young athletes. N Engl J Med 1998;339:364. [PMID: 9691102] (Screening resulted in detection of hypertrophic cardiomyopathy in 0.07% of screened athletes, and its detection may have explained the relatively low incidence of sudden death due to that disorder in these young Italian athletes.)

Maron BJ: Cardiovascular risks to young persons on the athletic field. Ann Intern Med 1998;129:379. [PMID: 9735066] (Comprehensive review by a leading authority.)

Pelliccia A et al: Clinical significance of abnormal electrocardiographic patterns in trained athletes. Circulation 2000;102:278. [PMID: 10899089] (Study demonstrating abnormal ECGs in 40% of athletes, usually associated with physiologic cardiac remodeling.)

Pfister GC et al: Preparticipation cardiovascular screening for US collegiate student-athletes. JAMA 2000;283:1597. [PMID: 10735397] (Survey of current practices, concluding that the potential to detect or suspect cardiovascular abnormalities

capable of causing sudden death in competitive student athletes is limited.)

Pluim BM et al: The athlete's heart. A meta-analysis of cardiac structure and function. Circulation 2000;101:336. [PMID: 10645932] (Discusses types of cardiac adaptation differing by specific athletic activity.)

Systemic Hypertension

11

Barry M. Massie, MD

See www.current-med.com/ch11.html

Fifty million Americans have elevated blood pressure (systolic blood pressure ≥ 140 mm Hg or diastolic blood pressure ≥ 90 mm Hg); of these, 70% are aware of their diagnosis, but only 50% are receiving treatment and only 25% are under control by the 140/90 mm Hg threshold. Hypertension increases with age and is more common in blacks than in whites. The mortality rates for stroke and coronary heart disease, the major complications of hypertension, have declined by up to 60% over the past 3 decades but have recently leveled off. The incidence of end-stage renal disease and of heart failure, two other conditions in which hypertension plays a major causative role, continues to rise.

Cardiovascular morbidity and mortality increase as both systolic and diastolic blood pressures rise, but in individuals over age 50 the systolic pressure and pulse pressure are better predictors of complications than diastolic pressure. As shown in Table 11–1, hypertension is diagnosed based upon elevations of *either* the systolic or diastolic blood pressure, and the objective of management is to achieve normalization of both.

Blood pressure should be measured with a well-calibrated sphygmomanometer with a cuff of proper size (the bladder width within the cuff should encircle at least 80% of the arm circumference) after the patient has been resting comfortably, back supported in the sitting or supine position, for a least 5 minutes and at least 30 minutes after smoking or coffee ingestion. Because blood pressure readings in many individuals are highly variable—especially in the office setting—the diagnosis of hypertension should be made only after elevation is noted on three readings on different occasions, over a period of several months unless the elevations are severe or associated with symptoms (see Table 11–1). Transient elevation of blood pressure caused by excitement or apprehension does not constitute hypertensive disease but may indicate a propensity toward its evolution. Ambulatory 24-hour blood pressure monitoring may be helpful in evaluating patients with borderline or variable office blood pressure, approximately 20% of whom will have no evidence of hypertension elsewhere, as well as in assessing resistant hypertension and possible treatment-related hypotensive symptoms. This technique is employed only to address specific management problems because of cost ($200–$300).

Continued hypertension does not necessarily indicate the need for pharmacologic treatment. Nonpharmacologic approaches and individualized assessment of the benefit-to-risk ratio of drug therapy should precede pharmacologic management in patients with stage I hypertension (diastolic pressure < 100 mm Hg; systolic < 160 mm Hg). Some patients with pressure in these ranges do not require therapy if they have no evidence of target organ damage or concomitant cardiovascular disease or diabetes.

Conversely, as a group, patients with high-normal blood pressures are at increased risk for future cardiovascular events. Treatment of high-risk individuals (those with diabetes, chronic renal insufficiency, atherosclerotic vascular disease) who have high-normal pressures is often indicated, particularly when agents that favorably modify risk factors are employed.

Guidelines Subcommittee. 1999 World Health Organization—International Society of Hypertension guidelines for the management of hypertension. J Hypertens 1999;17:151. [PMID: 10067796] (Recent comprehensive guidelines.)

JAMA patient page: Blood pressure. JAMA 1999;281:484. [PMID: 9952215]

Kaplan NM: *Clinical Hypertension*, 7th ed. Williams & Wilkins, 1998. (Concise, practical monograph covering epidemiology, mechanisms, diagnosis, and treatment.)

Vasan RS et al: Impact of high normal blood pressure on the risk of cardiovascular events. N Engl J Med 2001;345:1291. [PMID: 11794147] (Compared with those whose blood pressures are < 130/85 mm Hg, women and men with high-normal pressures have a hazard ratio for cardiovascular events of 2.5 and 1.6, respectively. Whether treatment is warranted except in those with other major risk factors is uncertain.)

MANAGEMENT OF HYPERTENSION

Etiology & Classification

A. PRIMARY (ESSENTIAL) HYPERTENSION

Essential hypertension is the term applied to the 95% of cases in which no cause can be identified. This occurs in 10–15% of white adults and 20–30% of black

Table 11–1. Classification and follow-up of blood pressure measurements.[1]

Category[2]	Systolic Blood Pressure (mm Hg)	Diastolic Blood Pressure (mm Hg)	Follow-Up Recommended
Optimal	< 120	< 80	Recheck in 2 years
Normal	< 130	< 85	Recheck in 2 years
High normal	130–139	85–90	Recheck in 1 year[3]
Hypertension[4] Stage 1 (mild)	140–159	90–99	Confirm within 2 months
Stage 2 (moderate)	160–179	100–109	Evaluate or refer within 1 month
Stage 3 (severe)	> 180	> 110	Evaluate or refer within 1 week

[1]From: The sixth report of the Joint National Committee on detection, education, and treatment of high blood pressure (JNC VI). Arch Intern Med 1997;157:2413.
[2]When systolic and diastolic pressures fall into different categories, the higher category should be selected to classify the individual's blood pressure. Isolated systolic hypertension is defined as a systolic blood pressure of 140 mm Hg or more and a diastolic blood pressure of less than 90 mm Hg.
[3]Consider offering counseling about lifestyle modifications (Table 11–2).
[4]In individuals aged 18 years or older not taking antihypertensive drugs and not acutely ill. Based on the average of two or more readings on two or more occasions after initial screening.

adults in the USA. The onset is usually between ages 25 and 55; it is uncommon before age 20. In young people, secondary hypertension resulting from renal insufficiency, renal artery stenosis, or coarctation of the aorta makes up a greater—but still relatively small—proportion of cases.

Elevations in pressure are often intermittent early in the course. Even in established cases, the blood pressure fluctuates widely in response to emotional stress and physical activity. Blood pressures taken by the patient at home or during daily activities using a portable apparatus are often lower than those recorded in the office, clinic, or hospital and may be more reliable in estimating prognosis. Patients with daytime average pressures less than 135/85 mm Hg have a low rate of cardiovascular complications and a low prevalence of left ventricular hypertrophy, suggesting that this is an appropriate ambulatory blood pressure criterion for diagnosing hypertension.

The pathogenesis of essential hypertension is multifactorial. Genetic factors play an important role. Children with one—and more so with two—hypertensive parents have higher blood pressures. Environmental factors also are significant. Increased salt intake has long been incriminated. It alone is probably not sufficient to elevate blood pressure to abnormal levels; a combination of too much salt plus a genetic predisposition is required. Other factors that may be involved in the pathogenesis of essential hypertension are the following:

1. Sympathetic nervous system hyperactivity— This is most apparent in younger hypertensives, who may exhibit tachycardia and an elevated cardiac output. However, correlations between plasma catecholamines and blood pressure are poor. Insensitivity of the baroreflexes may play a role in the genesis of adrenergic hyperactivity.

2. Renin-angiotensin system—Renin, a proteolytic enzyme, is secreted by the juxtaglomerular cells surrounding afferent arterioles in response to a number of stimuli, including reduced renal perfusion pressure, diminished intravascular volume, circulating catecholamines, increased sympathetic nervous system activity, increased arteriolar stretch, and hypokalemia. Renin acts on angiotensinogen to cleave off the ten-amino-acid peptide angiotensin I. This peptide is then acted upon by angiotensin-converting enzyme to create the eight-amino-acid peptide angiotensin II, a potent vasoconstrictor and a major stimulant of aldosterone release from the adrenal glands. The incidence of hypertension and its complications may be increased in individuals with the DD genotype of the allele coding for angiotensin-converting enzyme. Despite the role of this system in the regulation of blood pressure, it probably does not play a primary role in the pathogenesis of most essential hypertension. Patients with low plasma renin activity may have higher intravascular volumes. Black hypertensives and older patients tend to have lower plasma renin activity; plasma levels are classified in relation to dietary sodium intake or urinary sodium excretion. Approximately 10% of essential hypertension patients have high levels, 60% normal, and 30% low.

3. Defect in natriuresis—Normal individuals increase their renal sodium excretion in response to elevations in arterial pressure and to a sodium or volume load. Hypertensive patients, particularly when their blood pressure is normal, exhibit a diminished ability to excrete a sodium load. This defect may result in increased plasma volume and hypertension. During chronic hypertension, a sodium load is usually handled normally.

4. Intracellular sodium and calcium—Intracellular Na^+ is elevated in blood cells and other tissues in essential hypertension. This may result from abnormalities in Na^+-K^+ exchange and other Na^+ transport mechanisms. An increase in intracellular Na^+ may lead to increased intracellular Ca^{2+} concentrations as a result of facilitated exchange and might explain the increase in vascular smooth muscle tone that is characteristic of established hypertension.

5. Exacerbating factors—A number of conditions elevate blood pressure, especially in predisposed individuals. **Obesity** is associated with an increase in intravascular volume and an elevated cardiac output. Weight reduction lowers blood pressure modestly. The relationship between **sodium intake** and hypertension remains controversial, and some—not all—hypertensives respond to high salt intake with substantial blood pressure increases. Hypertensive patients should consume no more than 100 mmol/d of salt (2.4 g of sodium, 6 g of sodium chloride daily).

Excessive use of **alcohol** also raises blood pressure, perhaps by increasing plasma catecholamines. Hypertension can be difficult to control in patients who consume more than 40 g of ethanol (two drinks) daily or drink in "binges." **Cigarette smoking** raises blood pressure, again by increasing plasma norepinephrine. Although the long-term effect of smoking on blood pressure is less clear, the synergistic effects of smoking and high blood pressure on cardiovascular risk are well documented. The relationship of **exercise** to hypertension is variable. Aerobic exercise lowers blood pressure in previously sedentary individuals, but increasingly strenuous exercise in already active subjects has less effect. The relationship between stress and hypertension is not established. **Polycythemia,** whether primary or due to diminished plasma volume, increases blood viscosity and may raise blood pressure. **Nonsteroidal anti-inflammatory agents** produce increases in blood pressure averaging 5 mm Hg, and are best avoided in patients with borderline or elevated blood pressures. Low **potassium intake** is associated with higher blood pressure in some patients; an intake of 90 mmol/d is recommended.

B. SECONDARY HYPERTENSION

Approximately 5% of patients with hypertension have specific causes. The history, examination, and routine laboratory tests may identify such patients. In particular, patients who develop hypertension at an early age without a positive family history, those who first exhibit hypertension when over age 50, or those previously well-controlled who become refractory to treatment are more likely to have secondary hypertension. Causes include the following.

1. Estrogen use—A small increase in blood pressure occurs in most women taking oral contraceptives, but considerable rises are noted occasionally. This is caused by volume expansion due to increased activity of the renin-angiotensin-aldosterone system. The primary abnormality is an increase in the hepatic synthesis of renin substrate. Five percent of women taking oral contraceptives chronically will exhibit a rise in blood pressure above 140/90 mm Hg, twice the expected prevalence. Contraceptive-related hypertension is more common in women over 35 years of age, in those who have taken contraceptives for more than 5 years, and in obese individuals. It is less common in those taking low-dose estrogen tablets. In most, hypertension is reversible by discontinuing the contraceptive, but it may take several weeks. Postmenopausal estrogen does not cause hypertension. These agents maintain endothelium-mediated vasodilation.

2. Renal disease—Renal parenchymal disease is the most common cause of secondary hypertension. Hypertension may result from glomerular diseases, tubular interstitial disease, and polycystic kidneys. Most cases are related to increased intravascular volume or increased activity of the renin-angiotensin-aldosterone system. Hypertension accelerates progression of renal insufficiency, and rigorous control to target blood pressure of 130/85 or lower will retard this progression. Diabetic nephropathy is another cause of chronic hypertension. This process is exacerbated by intraglomerular hypertension, itself worsened by systemic hypertension. Dilation of the efferent arterioles by angiotensin-converting enzyme inhibition reduces the rate of progression.

3. Renal vascular hypertension—Renal artery stenosis is present in 1–2% of hypertensive patients. Its cause in most younger individuals is fibromuscular hyperplasia, which is most common in women under 50. The remainder of renal vascular disease is due to atherosclerotic stenoses of the proximal renal arteries. The mechanism of hypertension is excessive renin release due to reduction in renal blood flow and perfusion pressure. Renal vascular hypertension may occur when a single branch of the renal artery is stenotic, but in as many as 25% of patients both arteries are obstructed.

Renal vascular hypertension should be suspected in the following circumstances: (1) if the documented onset is below age 20 or after age 50; (2) if there are epigastric or renal artery bruits; (3) if there is atherosclerotic disease of the aorta or peripheral arteries (15–25% of patients with symptomatic lower limb atherosclerotic vascular disease have renal artery stenosis); or (4) if there is abrupt deterioration in renal function after administration of angiotensin-converting enzyme inhibitors. Additional evaluation is indicated in such patients, especially if hypertension is difficult to control.

There is no ideal screening test for renal vascular hypertension. If the suspicion of renal vascular hypertension is sufficiently high, renal arteriography, the definitive diagnostic test, is the best approach. Where suspicion is moderate to low, radioisotope renography, duplex ultrasound, and MR or CT angiography have all been used successfully, but the results vary greatly between institutions. Except when stenosis is critical (> 80–90%) and unifocal, its significance may be assessed by measuring differences in renin activity between the renal veins. If the lesion is not associated with an increase in renin activity, hypertension often persists despite correction.

Young individuals and low-risk patients of any age who have not responded to medical therapy should have the lesion corrected. Percutaneous intervention with stent placement is the preferred approach for fibromuscular hyperplasia and for discrete stenotic arteriosclerotic lesions that do not involve the renal artery ostium. In older individuals with arteriosclerosis, only a minority experience complete normalization without continued drug therapy. Thus, it is reasonable to manage these patients medically if renal function does not deteriorate. Although ACE inhibitors have improved the success rate of medical therapy of hypertension due to renal artery stenosis, they have been associated with marked hypotension and renal dysfunction in individuals with bilateral renal artery stenosis. Thus, renal function and blood pressure should be closely monitored during the first weeks of therapy in patients in whom this is a consideration.

4. Primary hyperaldosteronism and Cushing's syndrome—Patients with excess aldosterone secretion make up less than 0.5% of all cases of hypertension. The usual lesion is an adrenal adenoma, though some patients have bilateral adrenal hyperplasia. The diagnosis should be suspected when patients present with hypokalemia prior to diuretic therapy associated with excessive urinary potassium excretion (usually > 40 meq/L on a spot specimen) and suppressed levels of plasma renin activity; serum sodium usually exceeds 140 meq/L. Aldosterone concentrations in urine and blood are elevated. The lesion can be demonstrated by CT scanning or MRI. Less commonly, patients with Cushing's syndrome (glucocorticoid excess) may present with hypertension (see Chapter 26).

5. Pheochromocytoma—Although hypertension due to pheochromocytoma may be episodic, most patients have sustained elevations. The majority of patients have orthostatic falls in blood pressure, the converse of essential hypertension; some develop glucose intolerance. The diagnosis and treatment are discussed in Chapter 26.

6. Coarctation of the aorta—This uncommon cause of hypertension is discussed in Chapter 10.

7. Hypertension associated with pregnancy—Hypertension occurring de novo or worsening during pregnancy is one of the commonest causes of maternal and fetal morbidity and mortality (see Chapter 18).

8. Other causes of secondary hypertension—Hypertension has also been associated with hypercalcemia due to any cause, acromegaly, hyperthyroidism, hypothyroidism, and a variety of neurologic disorders causing increased intracranial pressure. A number of medications may cause or exacerbate hypertension—most importantly cyclosporine and NSAIDs.

Dosh SA: The diagnosis of essential and secondary hypertension in adults. J Fam Pract 2001;50:707. [PMID: 11509166] (Concise review with probability tables and recommendations for diagnostic testing.)

Krijnen P et al: A clinical prediction rule for renal artery stenosis. Ann Intern Med 1998;129:705. [PMID: 9841602] (Study provides a clinical prediction model to help select patients for further diagnostic procedures.)

Zarnke KB et al: The 2000 Canadian recommendations for the management of hypertension: part two—diagnosis and assessment of people with high blood pressure. Can J Cardiol 2001;17:249. [PMID: 11773936] (Well-referenced consensus statement.)

Complications of Untreated Hypertension

Complications of hypertension are related either to sustained elevations of blood pressure, with consequent changes in the vasculature and heart, or to atherosclerosis that accompanies and is accelerated by long-standing hypertension. The excess morbidity and mortality related to hypertension are progressive over the whole range of systolic and diastolic blood pressures; the risk approximately doubles for each 6 mm Hg increase in diastolic blood pressure. However, target-organ damage varies markedly between individuals with similar levels of office hypertension. Ambulatory pressures are more closely related to end-organ damage.

A. HYPERTENSIVE CARDIOVASCULAR DISEASE

Cardiac complications are the major causes of morbidity and mortality in essential hypertension, and preventing them is a major goal of therapy. Electrocardiographic evidence of left ventricular hypertrophy is found in up to 15% of chronic hypertensives. It is an indication of increased risk for morbidity and mortality; for any level of blood pressure, its presence is associated with incremental risk. Echocardiographic left ventricular hypertrophy is a powerful predictor of prognosis. Left ventricular hypertrophy may cause or facilitate many cardiac complications of hypertension, including congestive heart failure, ventricular arrhythmias, myocardial ischemia, and sudden death.

Left ventricular diastolic dysfunction, which may present with all of the signs and symptoms of congestive heart failure, is common in patients with long-standing hypertension. The occurrence of heart failure is reduced by 50% with antihypertensive therapy. Hypertensive left ventricular hypertrophy regresses with therapy and is most closely related to the degree of systolic blood pressure reduction. Diuretics have produced equal or greater reductions of left ventricular mass when compared with other drug classes.

B. HYPERTENSIVE CEREBROVASCULAR DISEASE AND DEMENTIA

Hypertension is the major predisposing cause of stroke, especially intracerebral hemorrhage but also ischemic cerebral infarction. Cerebrovascular complications are more closely correlated with systolic than diastolic blood pressure. The incidence of these complications is markedly reduced by antihypertensive therapy. Preceding hypertension is associated with a higher incidence of subsequent dementia, both the vascular and the Alzheimer types. Effective blood pressure control may modify the risk or rate of progression of cognitive dysfunction.

C. HYPERTENSIVE RENAL DISEASE

Chronic hypertension leads to nephrosclerosis, a common cause of renal insufficiency; aggressive blood pressure control attenuates the process. In patients with hypertensive nephropathy, the blood pressure should be 130/85 mm Hg or lower when proteinuria is present. Secondary renal disease is more common in blacks, particularly when accompanying diabetes is present. Hypertension also plays an important role in accelerating the progression of other forms of renal disease, most commonly diabetic nephropathy. Angiotensin-converting enzyme inhibitors are particularly effective in preventing the latter complication, but these agents appear to prevent the progression of other forms of nephropathy.

D. AORTIC DISSECTION

Hypertension is a contributing factor in many patients with dissection of the aorta. Its diagnosis and treatment are discussed in Chapter 12.

E. ATHEROSCLEROTIC COMPLICATIONS

Most Americans with hypertension die of complications of atherosclerosis, but the linkage between hypertension and atherosclerotic cardiovascular disease is much less close than that with the previously discussed complications. Effective antihypertensive therapy is thus less successful in preventing complications of coronary heart disease.

Berkin KE et al: Essential hypertension: The heart and hypertension. Heart 2001;86:407. [PMID: 11559694] (Review of effects of hypertension and antihypertensive therapy on the heart.)

Birkenhager WH et al: Blood pressure, cognitive functions, and prevention of dementia in older persons with hypertension. Arch Intern Med 2001;161:152. [PMID: 11176727] (Suggests that antihypertensive therapy prevents dementia, providing another reason to treat systolic hypertension in older persons.)

Clinical Findings

The clinical and laboratory findings are mainly referable to involvement of the target organs: heart, brain, kidneys, eyes, and peripheral arteries.

A. SYMPTOMS

Mild to moderate essential hypertension is asymptomatic for many years. Suboccipital pulsating headaches, characteristically occurring early in the morning and subsiding during the day, are said to be characteristic, but any type of headache may occur. Accelerated hypertension is associated with somno-lence, confusion, visual disturbances, and nausea and vomiting (hypertensive encephalopathy).

Patients with pheochromocytomas that secrete predominantly norepinephrine usually have sustained hypertension but may have episodic hypertension. Attacks (lasting minutes to hours) of anxiety, palpitation, profuse perspiration, pallor, tremor, and nausea and vomiting occur; blood pressure is markedly elevated, and angina or acute pulmonary edema may occur. In primary aldosteronism, patients may have muscular weakness, polyuria, and nocturia due to hypokalemia; malignant hypertension is rare.

Chronic hypertension often leads to left ventricular hypertrophy, which may be associated with diastolic or, in late stages, systolic dysfunction. Exertional and paroxysmal nocturnal dyspnea may result, and ischemic heart disease is more common (especially when concomitant coronary artery disease is present).

Cerebral involvement causes (1) stroke due to thrombosis or (2) small or large hemorrhage from microaneurysms of small penetrating intracranial arteries, and focal symptoms depend upon which vessels are involved. Hypertensive encephalopathy is probably caused by acute capillary congestion and exudation with cerebral edema. The findings are usually reversible if adequate treatment is given promptly. There is no strict correlation of diastolic blood pressure with hypertensive encephalopathy; it usually exceeds 130 mm Hg.

B. SIGNS

Like symptoms, physical findings depend upon the cause of hypertension, its duration and severity, and the degree of effect on target organs.

1. Blood pressure—On initial examination, pressure is taken in both arms and, if lower extremity pulses are diminished or delayed, in the legs to exclude coarctation of the aorta. An orthostatic drop is present in pheochromocytoma. Older patients may have falsely elevated readings by sphygmomanometry because of noncompressible vessels. This may be suspected in the presence of Osler's sign—a palpable brachial or radial artery when the cuff is inflated above systolic pressure. Occasionally, it may be necessary to make direct measurements of intra-arterial pressure, especially in patients with apparent severe hypertension who do not tolerate therapy.

2. Retinas—Narrowing of arterial diameter to less than 50% of venous diameter, copper or silver wire appearance, exudates, hemorrhages, or papilledema are associated with a worse prognosis.

3. Heart and arteries—Left ventricular enlargement with a left ventricular heave indicates severe or long-standing hypertrophy. Older patients frequently have systolic ejection murmurs resulting from calcific aortic sclerosis, and these may evolve to significant aortic stenosis in some individuals. Aortic insufficiency may be auscultated in up to 5% of patients, and hemodynamically insignificant aortic insufficiency can be detected by Doppler echocardiography in 10–20%. A presystolic (S_4) gallop due to decreased compliance of the left ventricle is quite common in patients with sinus rhythm.

4. Pulses—The timing of upper and lower extremity pulses should be compared to exclude coarctation of the aorta. All major peripheral pulses should be evaluated to exclude aortic dissection and peripheral atherosclerosis, which may be associated with renal artery involvement.

C. LABORATORY FINDINGS

Recommended testing includes the following: hemoglobin; urinalysis and renal function studies, to detect hematuria, proteinuria, and casts, signifying primary renal disease or nephrosclerosis; serum K^+, to seek mineralocorticoid excess; fasting blood sugar level, since hyperglycemia is noted in diabetes and pheochromocytoma; plasma lipids, as an indicator of atherosclerosis risk and an additional target for therapy; and serum uric acid, since if elevated it is a relative contraindication to diuretic therapy.

D. ELECTROCARDIOGRAPHY AND CHEST X-RAY

Electrocardiographic criteria are highly specific but not very sensitive for left ventricular hypertrophy. The "strain" pattern of ST–T wave changes is a sign of more advanced disease and is associated with a poor prognosis. A chest x-ray is not necessary in the workup for uncomplicated hypertension since it usually does not yield additional information.

E. ECHOCARDIOGRAPHY

Although echocardiography has been advocated to determine the need for drug therapy in patients with borderline or mildly elevated pressures, it is unusual to find left ventricular mass readings above the upper 75% confidence limits in the absence of systolic hypertension. The primary role of echocardiography should be to evaluate patients with clinical symptoms or signs of cardiac disease.

F. DIAGNOSTIC STUDIES

Only if the clinical presentation or routine tests suggest secondary or complicated hypertension are additional diagnostic studies indicated. These may include tests for endocrine causes of hypertension, renal ultrasound to diagnose primary renal disease (polycystic kidneys, obstructive uropathy) and testing for renal artery stenosis. Further evaluation may include abdominal imaging studies (ultrasound, CT scan, or MRI) or renal arteriography.

G. SUMMARY

Since most hypertension is "primary," few studies are necessary beyond those listed above. If conventional therapy is unsuccessful or if symptoms suggest a secondary cause, further studies are indicated.

Reeves RA: Does this patient have hypertension? How to measure blood pressure. JAMA 1995;273:1211. [PMID: 7707630]

(Still the most accessible information on the technique of measuring blood pressure.)

Nonpharmacologic Therapy

Lifestyle modification may have an impact on morbidity and mortality. A diet rich in fruits, vegetables, and low-fat dairy foods and low in saturated and total fats (DASH diet) has been shown to lower blood pressure. Additional measures can prevent or mitigate hypertension or its cardiovascular consequences as shown in Table 11–2.

All patients with high-normal or elevated blood pressures, those who have a family history of cardiovascular complications of hypertension, and those who have multiple coronary risk factors should be counseled about nonpharmacologic approaches to lowering blood pressure. Approaches of proved but modest value include weight reduction, reduced alcohol consumption, and in some patients reduced salt intake. Gradually increasing activity levels should be encouraged in previously sedentary patients, but strenuous exercise training programs in already active individuals may have less benefit. Calcium and potassium supplements have been advocated, but their ability to lower blood pressure is limited.

Smoking cessation will reduce overall cardiovascular risk.

Burgess E et al: Lifestyle modifications to prevent and control hypertension. 6. Recommendations on potassium, magnesium and calcium. Canadian Hypertension Society, Canadian Coalition for High Blood Pressure Prevention and Control, Laboratory Centre for Disease Control at Health Canada, Heart and Stroke Foundation of Canada. CMAJ 1999;160:S35. [PMID: 10333852] (Guidelines recommending a daily dietary intake of 60 mmol of potassium both for the prevention and for the treatment of hyperten-

Table 11–2. Lifestyle modifications for hypertension prevention and management.[1]

Lose weight if overweight
Limit alcohol intake to no more than 1 oz (30 mL) of ethanol (eg, 24 oz [720 mL] of beer, 10 oz [300 mL] of wine, or 2 oz [60 mL] of 100-proof whiskey) per day for men or 0.5 oz (15 mL) of ethanol per day for women and lighter-weight men
Increase aerobic physical activity (30–45 minutes most days of the week)
Reduce sodium intake to no more than 100 mmol/d (2.4 g of sodium or 6 g of sodium chloride)
Maintain adequate intake of dietary potassium (approximately 90 mmol/d)
Maintain adequate intake of dietary calcium and magnesium for general health
Stop smoking and reduce intake of dietary saturated fat and cholesterol for overall cardiovascular health

[1]From: The sixth report of the Joint National Committee on detection, education, and treatment of high blood pressure (JNC VI). Arch Intern Med 1997;157:2413.

sion; magnesium and calcium supplementation is not recommended.)

Campbell NR et al: Lifestyle modifications to prevent and control hypertension. 3. Recommendations on alcohol consumption. Canadian Hypertension Society, Canadian Coalition for High Blood Pressure Prevention and Control, Laboratory Centre for Disease Control at Health Canada, Heart and Stroke Foundation of Canada. CMAJ 1999;160:S13. [PMID: 10333049] (Guidelines recommending that alcohol consumption should not exceed 14 drinks per week for men and 9 drinks per week for women.)

Cleroux J et al: Lifestyle modifications to prevent and control hypertension. 4. Recommendations on physical exercise training. Canadian Hypertension Society, Canadian Coalition for High Blood Pressure Prevention and Control, Laboratory Centre for Disease Control at Health Canada, Heart and Stroke Foundation of Canada. CMAJ 1999;160:S21. [PMID: 10333850] (Recommendation that patients with mild hypertension should engage in 50–60 minutes of moderate exercise, such as brisk walking or cycling, three or four times per week.)

Fodor JD et al: Lifestyle modifications to prevent and control hypertension. 5. Recommendations on dietary salt. Canadian Hypertension Society, Canadian Coalition for High Blood Pressure Prevention and Control, Laboratory Centre for Disease Control at Health Canada, Heart and Stroke Foundation of Canada. CMAJ 1999;160:S29. [PMID: 10333851]

Reisin E: Nonpharmacologic approaches to hypertension: Weight, sodium, alcohol, exercise, and tobacco cessation. Med Clin North Am 1997;81:1289. [PMID: 9356599]

Who Should Be Treated With Medications? (Tables 11–3 and 11–4)

Many excellent trials have shown that drug therapy of patients with stage II and III hypertension reduces the incidence of stroke by 30–50%, congestive heart failure by 40–50%, and progression to accelerated hypertension syndromes. The decreases in fatal and nonfatal coronary heart disease and cardiovascular and total mortality have been less dramatic, ranging from 10% to 15%. This lesser decrease in coronary heart disease has generated controversy. Some have attributed the lesser benefit to characteristics of the drugs (primarily diuretics and beta-blockers), such as their adverse effect on lipid profiles and electrolyte balance. Others believe it is due to the more chronic and multifactorial nature of coronary artery disease, the generally low-risk populations included in trials, and the large number of crossovers from placebo to active therapy. Several studies in older persons with predominantly systolic hypertension have confirmed that antihypertensive therapy prevents fatal and nonfatal myocardial infarction and overall cardiovascular mortality. These trials have also placed the focus on control of systolic blood pressure—in contrast to the historical emphasis on diastolic blood pressures.

Goals of Treatment

The decision to initiate drug therapy should be based upon the assessment of overall cardiovascular risk rather

Table 11–3. Components of cardiovascular risk stratification in patients with hypertension.[1]

Major risk factors
Smoking
Dyslipidemia
Diabetes mellitus
Age > 60 years
Sex (men and postmenopausal women)
Family history of cardiovascular disease: women < 65 years or men < 55 years
Target organ damage/clinical cardiovascular disease
Heart disease
Left ventricular hypertrophy
Angina or prior myocardial infarction
Prior coronary revascularization
Heart failure
Stroke or transient ischemic attack
Nephropathy
Peripheral arterial disease
Retinopathy

[1]From: The sixth report of the Joint National Committee on detection, education, and treatment of high blood pressure (JNC VI). Arch Intern Med 1997;157:2413.

than the level of blood pressure alone. Table 11–3 lists the major risk factors for cardiovascular morbidity and mortality and the cardiovascular manifestations that predispose to further complications. Table 11–4 sets forth the criteria used to institute therapy. Thus, patients with systolic blood pressure over 160 mm Hg with diastolic blood pressure over 90 mm Hg after repeated measurements should be treated to a goal blood pressure below 140 mm Hg systolic and below 90 mm Hg diastolic. Those with stage I hypertension and at least one additional indicator of increased risk should be treated also. Very high risk groups, such as diabetics, patients with nephropathy, and (most likely) patients with heart failure and coronary disease benefit from antihypertensives even when their blood pressure is in the high-normal range. There has been concern that excessive lowering of diastolic blood pressures may induce myocardial ischemia. On balance, a lower target blood pressure (130/85 mm Hg) is indicated in high-risk individuals, such as patients with diabetes or renal dysfunction, and in selected individuals with clinical cardiovascular disease.

Hansson L et al: Effects of intensive blood-pressure lowering and low-dose aspirin in patients with hypertension: principal results of the Hypertension Optimal Treatment (HOT) randomized trial. Lancet 1998;351:1755. [PMID: 9635947] (Large study showing more intensive therapy reduced cardiovascular events, especially in diabetics.)

Kaplan NM: What is goal blood pressure for the treatment of hypertension? Arch Intern Med 2001;161:1480. [PMID: 11427094] (An expert's perspective.)

Tight blood pressure control and risk of macrovascular and microvascular complications in type 2 diabetes. Prospective

Table 11–4. Risk stratification and treatment.[1,2]

Blood Pressure Stages (mm Hg)	Risk Group A (No Risk Factors; No TOD/CCD[3])	Risk Group B (At Least 1 Risk Factor, Not Including Diabetes; No TOD/CCD)	Risk Group C (TOD/CCD and/or Diabetes, With or Without Other Risk Factors)
High-normal (130–139/85–89)	Lifestyle modification	Lifestyle modification	Drug therapy[4]
Stage 1 (140–159/80–99)	Lifestyle modification (up to 12 mo)	Lifestyle modification[5] (up to 6 mo)	Drug therapy
Stages 2 and 3 (≥ 160/≥ 100)	Drug therapy	Drug therapy	Drug therapy

[1]From: The sixth report of the Joint National Committee on detection, education, and treatment of high blood pressure (JNC VI). Arch Intern Med 1997;157:2413.
[2]***Note:*** For example, a patient with diabetes and blood pressure of 142/94 mm Hg plus left ventricular hypertrophy should be classified as having stage 1 hypertension with target organ disease (left ventricular hypertrophy) and with another major risk factor (diabetes). This patient would be categorized as "Stage 1, Risk Group C," and recommended for immediate initiation of pharmacologic treatment. Lifestyle modification should be adjunctive therapy for all patients recommended for pharmacologic therapy.
[3]TOD/CCD indicates target organ disease/clinical cardiovascular disease (see Table 11–3).
[4]For those with heart failure, renal insufficiency, or diabetes.
[5]For patients with multiple risk factors, clinicians should consider drugs as initial therapy plus lifestyle modifications.

Diabetes Study Group. BMJ 1998;317:703. [PMID: 9732337] (Aggressive control reduces complications; choice of drug may not be as important.)

DRUG THERAPY

General Principles

There are now many classes of potentially antihypertensive drugs of which five (diuretics, beta-blockers, ACE inhibitors, calcium channel blockers, and angiotensin II receptor antagonists) are suitable for initial or single-drug therapy. A number of considerations enter into the selection of the initial drug for a given patient. These include the weight of evidence for beneficial effects on clinical outcomes, the safety and the tolerability of the drug, its cost, demographic differences in response, concomitant medical conditions, and lifestyle issues. The specific classes of antihypertensive medications are discussed below, and guidelines for the choice of the initial medications are offered thereafter.

Current Antihypertensive Agents (See Tables 11–5 to 11–9 for dosages.)

A. DIURETICS

(Table 11–5.) Diuretics are the antihypertensives that have been most extensively studied and most consistently effective in clinical trials. They lower blood pressure initially by decreasing plasma volume (by suppressing tubular reabsorption of sodium, thus increasing the excretion of sodium and water) and cardiac output, but during chronic therapy their major hemodynamic effect is reduction of peripheral vascular resistance. Most of the antihypertensive effect of these agents is achieved at lower dosages than used previously (typically, 12.5 or 25 mg of hydrochlorothiazide or equivalent), but their biochemical and metabolic ef-

fects are dose-related. The thiazide diuretics are the most widely used. During chronic therapy, hydrochlorothiazide may be administered every other day with undiminished efficacy. The loop diuretics (such as furosemide) may lead to electrolyte and volume depletion more readily than the thiazides and have short durations of action; therefore, they should not be used in hypertension except in the presence of renal dysfunction (serum creatinine above 2.5 mg/dL). Relative to the beta-blockers and the ACE inhibitors, diuretics are more potent in blacks, older individuals, the obese, and other subgroups with increased plasma volume or low plasma renin activity. Interestingly, they are relatively more effective in smokers than in nonsmokers. Chronic diuretic administration also mitigates the loss of bone mineral content in older women at risk for osteoporosis.

Overall, diuretics administered alone control blood pressure in 50% of patients and can be used effectively in combination with all other agents. They are also useful for lowering isolated or predominantly systolic hypertension. Some observations suggest that the use of thiazide diuretics as initial therapy has been associated with greater reductions in stroke than beta-blockers.

The adverse effects of diuretics relate chiefly to the metabolic changes listed in Table 11–5. Impotence, skin rashes, and photosensitivity are less frequent. Hypokalemia has been a concern but is uncommon at the recommended dosages (12.5–25 mg hydrochlorothiazide). The risk can be minimized by limiting salt intake or a high-potassium diet; potassium replacement is not required to maintain serum K^+ at > 3.5 mmol/L. Higher serum levels are prudent in patients at special risk from intracellular potassium depletion, such as those taking digoxin or who have a history of ventricular arrhythmias. Insulin release and insulin sensitivity are reduced by hypokalemia in diabetic hypertensives. Diuretic therapy is most beneficial when combina-

Table 11–5. Antihypertensive drugs: Diuretics.

Drug	Proprietary Name	Initial Dosage	Dosage Range	Cost per Unit	Cost for 30 Days' Treatment[1] (Average Dosage)	Adverse Effects	Comments
THIAZIDES AND RELATED DIURETICS							
Hydrochlorothiazide	Esidrix, Hydro-Diuril	12.5 or 25 mg once daily	12.5–50 mg once daily	$0.08/25 mg	$2.40	$\downarrow K^+, \downarrow Mg^{2+} ? Ca^{2+}, \downarrow Na^+, ?$ uric acid, ? glucose, ? LDL cholesterol, ? triglycerides; rash, erectile dysfunction.	Low dosages effective in many patients without associated metabolic abnormalities; metolazone more effective with concurrent renal insufficiency; indapamide does not alter serum lipid levels.
Chlorthalidone	Hygroton, Thaliton	12.5 or 25 mg once daily	12.5–50 mg once daily	$0.16/25 mg	$4.80		
Metolazone	Zaroxolyn	1.25 or 2.5 mg once daily	1.25–5 mg once daily	$1.07/5 mg	$32.10		
	Mykrox	0.5 mg once daily	0.5–1 mg once daily	$0.94/0.5 mg	$28.20		
Indapamide	Lozol	2.5 mg once daily	2.5–5 mg once daily	$0.83/2.5 mg	$24.90		
LOOP DIURETICS							
Furosemide	Lasix	20 mg bid	40–320 mg in 2 or 3 doses	$0.16/40 mg	$9.60	Same as thiazides, but higher risk of excessive diuresis and electrolyte imbalance. Increases calcium excretion.	**Furosemide:** Short duration of action a disadvantage; should be reserved for patients with renal insufficiency or fluid retention. Poor antihypertensive. **Torsemide:** Effective blood pressure medication at low dosage.
Bumetanide	Bumex	0.25 mg bid	0.5–10 mg in 2 or 3 doses	$0.40/1 mg	$24.00		
Torsemide	Demadex	2.5 mg once daily	5–10 mg once daily	$0.72/10 mg	$21.60		

417

Table 11–5. Antihypertensive drugs: Diuretics. (continued)

Drug	Proprietary Name	Initial Dosage	Dosage Range	Cost per Unit	Cost for 30 Days' Treatment[1] (Average Dosage)	Adverse Effects	Comments
COMBINATION PRODUCTS							
Hydrochlorothiazide and triamterene	Dyazide (25/50 mg) Maxzide (37.5/25 mg)	1 tab once daily	1 or 2 tabs once daily	$0.34	$10.20	Same as thiazides plus GI disturbances, hyperkalemia rather than hypokalemia; headache; triamterene can cause kidney stones and renal dysfunction; spironolactone causes gynecomastia. Hyperkalemia can occur if this combination is used in patients with renal failure or those taking ACE inhibitors.	Use should be limited to patients with demonstrable need for a potassium-sparing agent.
Hydrochlorothiazide and amiloride	Moduretic (50/5 mg)	½ tab once daily	1 or 2 tabs once daily	$0.33	$9.90		
Hydrochlorothiazide and spironolactone	Aldactazide (25/25 mg)	1 tab once daily	1 or 2 tabs once daily	$0.50	$15.00		

[1]Cost to pharmacist (average wholesale price, generic when possible) for quantity listed. Source: *Drug Topics Red Book*, March 2002; Vol. 21, No. 3.

Table 11–6. Antihypertensive drugs: Beta-adrenergic blocking agents.

Drug	Proprietary Name	Initial Dosage	Dosage Range	Cost per Unit	Cost for 30 Days' Treatment (Based on Average Dosage)[1]	β_1 Selectivity[2]	ISA[3]	MSA[4]	Lipid Solubility	Renal vs Hepatic Elimination	Comments[5]
Acebutolol	Sectral	200 mg once daily	200–1200 mg in 1 or 2 doses	$1.34/400 mg	$40.20	+	+	+	+	H > R	Positive ANA; rare LE syndrome; also indicated for arrhythmias. Doses > 800 mg have β_1 and β_2 effects.
Atenolol	Tenormin	25 mg once daily	25–200 mg once daily	$0.74/50 mg	$22.20	+	0	0	0	R	Also indicated for angina pectoris and post-MI. Doses > 100 mg have β_1 and β_2 effects.
Betaxolol	Kerlone	10 mg once daily	10–40 mg once daily	$0.95/10 mg	$28.50	+	0	0	+	H > R	
Bisoprolol and hydrochlorothiazide	Ziac	5 mg/6.25 mg	2.5–10 mg plus 6.25 mg	$1.14/2.5/6.25 mg	$34.20	+	0	0	0	R = H	Low-dose combination approved for initial therapy. Bisoprolol also effective for heart failure.
Carteolol	Cartrol	2.5 mg once daily	2.5–10 mg once daily	$1.27/5 mg	$38.10	0	+	0	+	R > H	
Carvedilol	Coreg	6.25 mg	12.5–100 mg in 2 doses	$1.65/25 mg	$99.00 (25 mg bid)	0	0	0	+++	H > R	α;β blocking activity 1:3; may cause orthostatic symptoms; effective for congestive heart failure.
Labetalol	Normodyne, Trandate	100 mg bid	200–1200 mg in 2 doses	$0.68/200 mg	$40.80	0	0/+	0	++	H	α;β blocking activity 1:3; more orthostatic hypotension, fever, hepatotoxicity.

(continued)

Table 11–6. Antihypertensive drugs: Beta-adrenergic blocking agents. (continued)

Drug	Proprietary Name	Initial Dosage	Dosage Range	Cost per Unit	Cost for 30 Days' Treatment (Based on Average Dosage)[1]	Special Properties					Comments[5]
						β1 Selectivity[2]	ISA[3]	MSA[4]	Lipid Solubility	Renal vs Hepatic Elimination	
Metoprolol	Lopressor	50 mg in 1 or 2 doses	50–200 mg in 1 or 2 doses	$0.44/50 mg	$26.40	+	0	+	+++	H	Also indicated for angina pectoris and post-MI. Approved for heart failure. Doses > 100 mg have β1 and β2 effects.
	Toprol XL (SR preparation)	50 mg once daily	50–200 mg once daily	$0.98/100 mg	$29.40						
Nadolol	Corgard	20 mg once daily	20–160 mg once daily	$1.00/40 mg	$30.00	0	0	0	0	R	
Penbutolol	Levatol	20 mg once daily	20–80 mg once daily	$1.47/20 mg	$44.10	0	+	0	++	R > H	
Pindolol	Visken	5 mg bid	10–60 mg in 2 doses	$0.69/5 mg	$41.40	0	++	+	+	H > R	In adults, 35% renal clearance.
Propranolol	Inderal	20 mg bid	40–320 mg in 2 doses	$0.18/40 mg	$10.80	0	0	++	+++	H	Once-daily SR preparation also available. Also indicated for angina pectoris and post-MI.
Timolol	Blocadren	5 mg bid	10–40 mg in 2 doses	$0.29/10 mg	$17.40	0	0	0	++	H > R	Also indicated post-MI. 80% hepatic clearance.

ISA = intrinsic sympathomimetic activity; MSA = membrane-stabilizing activity; 0 = no effect; +, ++, +++ = some, moderate, most effect.

[1]Cost to pharmacist (average wholesale price, generic when possible) for quantity listed. Source: *Drug Topics Red Book*, March 2002; Vol. 21, No. 3.

[2]Agents with β1 selectivity are less likely to precipitate bronchospasm and decreased peripheral blood flow *in low doses*, but selectivity is only relative.

[3]Agents with ISA cause less resting bradycardia and lipid changes.

[4]MSA generally occurs at concentrations greater than those necessary for beta-adrenergic blockade. The clinical importance of MSA by beta-blockers has not been defined.

[5]Adverse effects of all beta-blockers: bronchospasm, fatigue, sleep disturbance and nightmares, bradycardia and atrioventricular block, worsening of congestive heart failure, cold extremities, gastrointestinal disturbances, impotence, ↑triglycerides, ↓HDL cholesterol, rare blood dyscrasias.

Table 11–7. Antihypertensive drugs: ACE inhibitors and angiotensin II blockers.

Drug	Proprietary Name	Initial Dosage	Dosage Range	Cost per Unit	Cost of 30 Days' Treatment (Average Dosage)[1]	Adverse Effects	Comments
ACE inhibitors							
Benazepril	Lotensin	10 mg once daily	5–40 mg in 1 or 2 doses	$0.94/20 mg	$28.20	Cough, hypotension, dizziness, renal dysfunction, hyperkalemia, angioedema; taste alteration and rash (may be more frequent with captopril); rarely, proteinuria, blood dyscrasia. Contraindicated in pregnancy.	More fosinopril is excreted by the liver in patients with renal dysfunction (dose reduction may or may not be necessary). Captopril and lisinopril are active without metabolism. Captopril, enalapril, lisinopril, and quinapril are approved for congestive heart failure.
Captopril	Capoten	25 mg bid	50–300 mg in 2 or 3 doses	$0.65/25 mg	$39.00		
Enalapril	Vasotec	5 mg once daily	5–40 mg in 1 or 2 doses	$1.47/20 mg	$44.10		
Fosinopril	Monopril	10 mg once daily	10–80 mg in 1 or 2 doses	$1.10/20 mg	$33.00		
Lisinopril	Prinivil, Zestril	5–10 mg once daily	5–40 mg once daily	$1.07/20 mg	$32.10		
Moexipril	Univasc	7.5 mg once daily	7.5–30 mg in 1 or 2 doses	$0.74/7.5 mg	$22.20		
Perindopril	Aceon	4 mg once daily	4–16 mg in 1 or 2 doses	$1.56/8 mg	$46.80		
Quinapril	Accupril	10 mg once daily	10–80 mg in 1 or 2 doses	$1.13/20 mg	$33.90		
Ramipril	Altace	2.5 mg once daily	2.5–20 mg in 1 or 2 doses	$1.27/5 mg	$38.10		
Trandolapril	Mavik	1 mg once daily	1–8 mg once daily	$0.88/4 mg	$26.40		
Angiotensin II blockers							
Candesartan cilexitil	Atacand	16 mg once daily	8–32 mg once daily	$1.34/16 mg	$40.20	Hyperkalemia, renal dysfunction, rare angioedema. Combinations have additional side effects. Contraindicated in pregnancy.	Losartan has a very flat dose-response curve. Valsartan and Irbesartan have wider dose-response ranges and longer durations of action. Addition of low-dose diuretic (separately or as combination pills) increases the response.
Candesartan cilexitil/HCTZ	Atacand HCT	16 mg/12.5 mg once daily	8–32 mg of candesartan once daily	$1.81/16 mg/12.5 mg	$54.30		
Eprosartan	Teveten	600 mg once daily	400–800 mg in 1–2 doses	$1.37/600 mg	$41.10		
Irbesartan	Avapro	150 mg once daily	150–300 mg once daily	$1.44/150 mg	$43.20		
Irbesartan and hydrochlorothiazide	Avalide	150 mg/12.5 mg once daily	150–300 mg irbesartan daily	$1.73/tablet	$51.90		
Losartan	Cozaar	50 mg once daily	25–100 mg in 1 or 2 doses	$1.43/50 mg	$42.90		

(continued)

Table 11–7. Antihypertensive drugs: ACE inhibitors and angiotensin II blockers. (continued)

Drug	Proprietary Name	Initial Dosage	Dosage Range	Cost per Unit	Cost of 30 Days' Treatment (Average Dosage)[1]	Adverse Effects	Comments
Angiotensin II blockers (continued)							
Losartan and hydrochlorothiazide	Hyzaar	50 mg/ 12.5 mg once daily	One or 2 tablets once daily	$1.43/50 mg/12.5 mg/ tablet	$42.90		
Telmisartan	Micardis	40 mg once daily	20–80 mg once daily	$1.40/40 mg	$42.00		
Telmisartan and HCTZ	Micardis HCT	40 mg/ 12.5 mg once daily	20–80 mg telmisartan daily	$1.50/40 mg/12.5 mg	$45.00		
Valsartan	Diovan	80 mg once daily	80–320 mg once daily	$1.52/160 mg	$45.60		
Valsartan and HCTZ	Diovan HCT	80 mg/ 12.5 mg once daily	80–320 mg valsartan daily	$1.65/160 mg/12.5 mg	$49.50		

[1]Cost to pharmacist (average wholesale price, generic when possible) for quantity listed. Source: *Drug Topics Red Book,* March 2002; Vol. 21, No. 3.

tions of thiazide and potassium-sparing agents, such as triamterene or amiloride, are used. Although these medications have additional side effects (primarily gastrointestinal), and may be dangerous in the presence of oliguria it is reasonable to use them in appropriate patients receiving higher doses of diuretics and in place of potassium supplements. Diuretics also increase serum uric acid and may precipitate gout. Increases in blood glucose, triglycerides, low-density lipoprotein cholesterol, and plasma insulin may occur but are relatively minor during long-term low-dose therapy.

B. BETA-ADRENERGIC BLOCKING AGENTS

(Table 11–6.) These drugs are effective in hypertension because they decrease the heart rate and cardiac output. Even after continued use of beta-blockers, cardiac output remains lower and systemic vascular resistance higher with agents that do not have intrinsic sympathomimetic or alpha-blocking activity. The beta-blockers also decrease renin release and are more efficacious in populations with elevated plasma renin activity, such as younger white patients. They neutralize the reflex tachycardia caused by vasodilators and are especially useful in patients with associated conditions that benefit from this therapy. These include individuals with angina pectoris, chronic previous myocardial infarction, stable congestive heart failure, and those with migraine headaches and somatic manifestations of anxiety.

Although all beta-blockers appear to be similar in antihypertensive potency, controlling approximately 50% of patients, they differ in a number of pharmacologic properties (these differences are summarized in Table 11–6), including those relatively specific to the cardiac β_1 receptors (cardioselectivity) and whether they also block the β_2 receptors in the bronchi and vasculature; at higher dosages, however, all agents are nonselective. The beta-blockers also differ in their pharmacokinetics and lipid solubility—which determines whether they cross the blood-brain barrier and affect the incidence of central nervous system side effects—and route of metabolism. Labetalol and carvedilol are combined alpha- and beta-blockers and, unlike most beta-blockers, decrease peripheral vascular resistance.

The side effects of all beta-blockers include inducing or exacerbating bronchospasm in predisposed patients (asthmatics, some COPD patients); sinus node and atrioventricular conduction depression (resulting in bradycardia or AV block); precipitating or worsening clinically important left ventricular failure; nasal congestion; Raynaud's phenomenon; and central nervous system symptoms with nightmares, excitement, depression, and confusion. Fatigue, lethargy, and impotence may occur. All beta-blockers tend to increase plasma triglycerides. The nonselective and, to a lesser extent, the cardioselective (β_1-selective) beta-blockers tend to depress the protective HDL fraction of plasma cholesterol. This is not seen in agents with intrinsic

Table 11–8. Antihypertensive drugs: Calcium channel-blocking agents.

Drug	Proprietary Name	Initial Dosage	Dosage Range	Cost for 30 Days' Treatment (Average Dosage)[1]	Special Properties Peripheral Vasodilation	Special Properties Cardiac Automaticity and Conduction	Special Properties Contractility	Adverse Effects	Comments
Nondihydropyridine agents									
Diltiazem	Cardizem SR	90 mg bid	180–360 mg in 2 doses	$90.60 (120 mg bid)	++	↓↓	↓↓	Edema, headache, bradycardia, GI disturbances, dizziness, AV block congestive heart failure, urinary frequency.	Also approved for angina.
	Cardizem CD	180 mg qd	180–360 mg qd	$68.45 (240 mg qd)					
	Cartia XT	180 mg qd	120–300 mg qd	$61.53 (240 mg qd)					
	Dilacor XR	180 or 240 mg qd	180–480 mg daily	$39.30 (240 mg qd)					
	Tiazac SA	240 mg qd	180–540 mg qd	$48.90 (240 mg qd)					
Verapamil	Calan SR	180 mg qd	180–480 mg in 1 or 2 doses	$56.40	++	↓↓↓	↓↓↓	Same as diltiazem but more likely to cause constipation and congestive heart failure.	Also approved for angina and arrhythmias.
	Isoptin SR			$59.10					
	Verelan			$59.40					
	Covera-HS			$57.30					
	Generic Verapamil extended release			$38.10 (240 mg qd)					

(continued)

123

Table 11–8. Antihypertensive drugs: Calcium channel-blocking agents. (continued)

Drug	Proprietary Name	Initial Dosage	Dosage Range	Cost for 30 Days' Treatment (Average Dosage)[1]	Special Properties			Adverse Effects	Comments
					Peripheral Vasodilation	Cardiac Automaticity and Conduction	Contractility		
				DIHYDROPYRIDINES					
Amlodipine	Norvasc	5 mg qd	5–20 mg qd	$65.23 (10 mg qd)	+++	↓/0	↓/0	Edema, dizziness, palpitations, flushing, headache, hypotension, tachycardia, GI disturbances, urinary frequency, worsening of congestive heart failure (may be less common with felodipine, amlodipine).	Amlodipine, nicardipine, and nifedipine also approved for angina.
Felodipine	Plendil	5 mg qd	5–20 mg qd	$60.60 (10 mg qd)	+++	↓/0	↓/0		
Isradipine	DynaCirc	2.5 mg bid	2.5–5 mg bid	$93.60 (5 mg bid)	+++	↓/0	→		
	DynaCirc CR	5 mg qd	5–10 mg qd	$66.90 (10 mg qd)					
Nicardipine	Cardene	20 mg tid	20–40 mg tid	$35.10 (20 mg tid)	+++	↓/0	→		
	Cardene SR	30 mg bid	30–60 mg bid	$52.31 (30 mg bid)					
Nifedipine	Adalat CC	30 mg qd	30–120 mg qd	$69.30 (60 mg qd)	+++	→	↓↓		
	Procardia XL	30 mg qd	30–120 mg qd	$78.60 (60 mg qd)	+++	→	↓↓		
Nisoldipine	Sular	20 mg/d	20–60 mg/d	$31.50 (40 mg qd)	+++	↓/0	→		

[1]Cost to pharmacist (average wholesale price, generic when possible) for quantity listed. Source: *Drug Topics Red Book*, March 2002; Vol. 21, No. 3.

Table 11–9. Alpha-adrenoceptor blocking agents, sympatholytics, and vasodilators.

Drug	Proprietary Name	Initial Dosage	Dosage Range	Cost per Unit	Cost for 30 Days' Treatment (Average Dosage)[1]	Adverse Effects	Comments
ALPHA-ADRENOCEPTOR BLOCKERS							
Prazosin	Minipress	1 mg hs	2–20 mg in 2 or 3 doses	$0.64/5 mg	$38.40 (5 mg bid)	Syncope with first dose; postural hypotension, dizziness, palpitations, headache, weakness, drowsiness, sexual dysfunction, anticholinergic effects, urinary incontinence; first-dose effects may be less with doxazosin.	May ↑HDL and ↓LDL cholesterol. May provide short-term relief of obstructive prostatic symptoms. Less effective in preventing cardiovascular events than diuretics.
Terazosin	Hytrin	1 mg hs	1–20 mg in 1 or 2 doses	$1.60/1, 2, 5, 10 mg	$48.00 (5 mg qd)		
Doxazosin	Cardura	1 mg hs	1–16 mg qd	$0.97/4 mg	$29.10 (4 mg qd)		
CENTRAL SYMPATHOLYTICS							
Clonidine	Catapres	0.1 mg bid	0.2–0.6 mg in 2 doses	$0.22/0.1 mg	$13.20 (0.1 mg bid)	Sedation, dry mouth, sexual dysfunction, headache, bradyarrhythmias; side effects may be less with guanfacine. Contact dermatitis with clonidine patch. Methyldopa also causes hepatitis, hemolytic anemia, fever.	"Rebound" hypertension may occur even after gradual withdrawal. Methyldopa should be avoided in favor of safer agents.
	Catapres TTS	0.1 mg/d patch weekly	0.1–0.3 mg/d patch weekly	$17.37/0.2 mg	$69.47 (0.2 mg weekly)		
Guanabenz	Wytensin	4 mg bid	8–64 mg in 2 doses	$0.66/4 mg	$39.60 (4 mg bid)		
Guanfacine	Tenex	1 mg once daily	1–3 mg qd	$0.87/1 mg	$26.10 (1 mg qd)		
Methyldopa	Aldomet	250 mg bid	500–2000 mg in 2 doses	$0.65/500 mg	$39.00 (500 mg bid)		
PERIPHERAL NEURONAL ANTAGONISTS							
Guanadrel	Hylorel	5 mg bid	10–70 mg in 2 doses	$1.82/10 mg	$109.20 (10 mg bid)	Orthostatic hypotension, diarrhea, exercise hypotension, sexual dysfunction, salt and water retention.	
Reserpine	Serpasil	0.05 mg once daily	0.05–0.25 mg qd	$0.18/0.1 mg	$5.40 (0.1 mg qd)	Depression (less likely at low dosages, ie, < 0.25 mg), night terrors, nasal stuffiness, drowsiness, peptic disease, gastrointestinal disturbances, bradycardia.	

(continued)

425

Table 11–9. Alpha-adrenoceptor blocking agents, sympatholytics, and vasodilators. (continued)

Drug	Proprietary Name	Initial Dosage	Dosage Range	Cost per Unit	Cost for 30 Days' Treatment (Average Dosage)[1]	Adverse Effects	Comments
				DIRECT VASODILATORS			
Hydralazine	Apresoline	25 mg bid	50–300 mg in 2–4 doses	$0.05/25 mg	$3.00 (25 mg bid)	GI disturbances, tachycardia, headache, nasal congestion, rash, LE-like syndrome.	May worsen or precipitate angina.
Minoxidil	Loniten	5 mg once daily	5–40 mg qd	$0.54/10 mg	$16.20 (10 mg qd)	Tachycardia, fluid retention, headache, hirsutism, pericardial effusion, thrombocytopenia.	Should be used in combination with beta-blocker and diuretic.

[1]Cost to pharmacist (average wholesale price, generic when possible) for quantity listed. Source: *Drug Topics Red Book,* March 2002; Vol. 21, No. 3.

sympathomimetic activity, and as with diuretics, the changes are blunted with time and dietary changes.

Beta-blockers have traditionally been considered contraindicated in patients with congestive heart failure. Evolving experience suggests that they have a propitious effect on the natural history of patients with chronic stable heart failure and reduced ejection fractions (see Chapter 10). Beta blockers are used cautiously in patients with type 1 diabetes, since they can mask the symptoms of hypoglycemia and prolong these episodes by inhibiting gluconeogenesis. Although they may increase blood glucose levels in type 2 diabetics, the prognosis of these patients on balance is improved. These drugs should also be used with caution in patients with advanced peripheral vascular disease associated with rest pain or nonhealing ulcers, but they are generally well tolerated in patients with mild claudication.

C. ANGIOTENSIN-CONVERTING ENZYME (ACE) INHIBITORS

(Table 11–7.) These drugs are being increasingly used as the initial medication in mild to moderate hypertension. Their primary mode of action is inhibition of the renin-angiotensin-aldosterone system, but they also inhibit bradykinin degradation, stimulate the synthesis of vasodilating prostaglandins, and, sometimes, reduce sympathetic nervous system activity. These latter actions may explain why they exhibit some effect even in patients with low plasma renin activity. The ACE inhibitors appear to be more effective in younger whites. They are relatively less effective in blacks and older persons and in predominantly systolic hypertension. While as single therapy they achieve adequate antihypertensive control in only about 40–50% of patients, the combination of an ACE inhibitor and a diuretic or calcium channel blocker is potent.

The ACE inhibitors are the agents of choice in type I diabetics with frank proteinuria or evidence of renal dysfunction, because they delay the progression to end-stage renal disease. Many authorities have expanded this indication to include type II diabetics and type I diabetics with microalbuminuria, even when they do not meet the usual criteria for antihypertensive therapy. The Heart Outcomes Prevention Evaluation (HOPE) trial demonstrated that the ACE inhibitor ramipril reduces the number of cardiovascular deaths, nonfatal myocardial infarctions and nonfatal strokes, and instances of new-onset heart failure in a population of patients at high risk for vascular events. This study included diabetics with at least one additional risk factor and patients with coronary artery disease, peripheral artery disease, and prior stroke. Although this was not specifically a hypertensive population, the results inferentially support the use of ACE inhibitors in similar hypertensive patients. ACE inhibitors may also delay the progression of other forms of renal disease. They are a drug of choice (usually in conjunction with a diuretic) in patients with congestive heart failure and are indicated also in asymptomatic patients with reduced ejection fractions, whether due to myocardial infarction or to other causes.

ACE inhibitors have effects on mortality and most cardiovascular outcomes similar to those achieved with diuretics and beta-blockers. However, compared with calcium channel blockers, ACE inhibitors are associated with lower incidences of coronary events and heart failure.

An advantage of the ACE inhibitors is their relative freedom from troublesome side effects. Severe hypotension can occur in patients with bilateral renal artery stenosis; acute renal failure may ensue. Hyperkalemia may develop in patients with intrinsic renal disease and type IV renal tubular acidosis (commonly seen in diabetics) and in the elderly. A chronic dry cough is common, seen in 10% of patients or more, and may require stopping the drug. Dizziness occurs but may not be related to the degree of blood pressure lowering. Skin rashes are observed with any ACE inhibitor. Taste alterations are seen more often with captopril than with the non-sulfhydryl-containing agents (enalapril and lisinopril) but often disappear with continued therapy. Angioedema is an uncommon but potentially dangerous side effect of all agents of this class because of their inhibition of kininase.

D. ANGIOTENSIN II RECEPTOR BLOCKERS

(Table 11–7.) Although losartan, the first member of this group, was less potent in reducing blood pressure than the ACE inhibitors, the newer angiotensin II antagonists (valsartan, irbesartan, candesartan, telmisartan, and eprosartan) appear to be equipotent. Much less is known about their ability to prevent cardiovascular events in hypertensive patients and in other clinical settings. Although angiotensin II receptor blockers and ACE inhibitors both inhibit the renin-angiotensin system, ACE inhibitors also interfere with the degradation of kinins and thus may stimulate prostaglandin and nitric oxide production. Whether these actions improve vascular protection is uncertain. However, it appears that angiotensin II receptor blockers prevent the progression of diabetic nephropathy in type 2 diabetics, and the Valsartan in Heart Failure trial suggests that these agents can reduce mortality and morbidity in heart failure patients.

Unlike ACE inhibitors, the angiotensin II receptor blockers do not cause cough and are only infrequently associated with skin rashes, the most common side effects of the ACE inhibitors. However, they still present a risk of hypotension and renal failure in patients with bilateral renal artery stenosis and hyperkalemia, and, rarely, angioedema. Because of their higher costs, limited long-term experience, and unproved benefits in heart failure and diabetes, the angiotensin II blockers should be reserved primarily for patients who develop cough when taking ACE inhibitors.

E. CALCIUM CHANNEL BLOCKING AGENTS

(Table 11–8.) These agents act by causing peripheral vasodilation, which is associated with less reflex tachycardia and fluid retention than other vasodilators. They are effective as single-drug therapy in approximately 60% of patients in all demographic groups and all grades of hypertension. As a result, they may be preferable to beta-blockers and ACE inhibitors in blacks and older subjects. Calcium channel blockers and diuretics are less additive when given together than when either is combined with beta-blockers or ACE inhibitors. However, verapamil and diltiazem should be combined cautiously with beta-blockers because of their potential for depressing atrioventricular conduction and sinus node automaticity as well as contractility.

Concerns have been raised about increased risk of myocardial infarction in hypertensive patients and of higher mortality in acute coronary syndromes. Comparative studies using calcium channel blockers as initial therapy have been associated with trends toward a higher risk of myocardial infarction and heart failure than is the case with diuretics or beta-blockers; the numbers of cardiovascular events and all-cause mortality did not differ. Diabetic patients receiving calcium channel blockers appear to have higher rates of heart failure and myocardial infarction than those receiving ACE inhibitors. Whether these outcomes reflect beneficial effects of ACE inhibitors or specific risks of calcium channel blockers is uncertain. Nonetheless, ACE inhibitors are the drugs of choice for diabetic patients, and current calcium channel blockers, despite their neutral metabolic effects, should not be used as initial therapy. On the other hand, it has been suggested that calcium channel blockers may be more effective in preventing stroke.

The most common side effects of calcium channel blockers are headache, peripheral edema, bradycardia, and constipation (especially with verapamil in the elderly). The dihydropyridine agents—nifedipine, nicardipine, isradipine, felodipine, and amlodipine—are more likely to produce symptoms of vasodilation, such as headache, flushing, palpitations, and peripheral edema. Calcium channel blockers have negative inotropic effects and may cause or exacerbate heart failure in patients with cardiac dysfunction. Amlodipine is the only calcium channel blocker with established safety in patients with severe heart failure. Most calcium blockers are now available in preparations that can be administered once daily.

F. ALPHA-ADRENOCEPTOR ANTAGONISTS

(Table 11–9.) Prazosin, terazosin, and doxazosin block postsynaptic alpha receptors, relax smooth muscle, and reduce blood pressure by lowering peripheral vascular resistance. These agents are effective as single-drug therapy in some individuals, but tachyphylaxis may appear during long-term therapy and side effects are relatively common. These include marked hypotension and syncope after the first dose, which,

therefore, should be small and be given at bedtime. Postdosing palpitations, headache, and nervousness may continue to occur during chronic therapy; they may be less frequent or severe with doxazosin because of its more gradual onset of action.

Unlike the beta-blockers and diuretics, the alpha-blockers have no adverse effect on serum lipid levels—in fact, they increase high-density lipoprotein cholesterol while reducing total cholesterol. Whether this is beneficial in the long term has not been established. In the ongoing Antihypertensive Lipid Lowering Heart Attack Trial (ALLHAT), subjects receiving doxazosin as initial therapy had a significant increase in heart failure hospitalizations and a higher incidence of stroke relative to the subjects receiving diuretics and were removed from the study. In sum, alpha-blockers should generally not be used as initial agents to treat hypertension—except perhaps in men with symptomatic prostatism.

G. DRUGS WITH CENTRAL SYMPATHOLYTIC ACTION

(Table 11–9.) Methyldopa, clonidine, guanabenz, and guanfacine lower blood pressure by stimulating alpha-adrenergic receptors in the central nervous system, thus reducing efferent peripheral sympathetic outflow. These agents are effective as single therapy in some patients, but they are usually employed as second- or third-line agents because of the high frequency of drug intolerance, including sedation, fatigue, dry mouth, postural hypotension, and impotence. An important concern is rebound hypertension following withdrawal. Methyldopa also causes hepatitis and hemolytic anemia and is avoided except in individuals who have already tolerated chronic therapy. There is considerable experience with methyldopa in pregnant women, and it is still used for this population. Clonidine is available in patches and may have particular value in patients in whom compliance is a troublesome issue.

H. ARTERIOLAR DILATORS

(Table 11–9.) Hydralazine and minoxidil relax vascular smooth muscle and produce peripheral vasodilation. When given alone, they stimulate reflex tachycardia, increase myocardial contractility, and cause headache, palpitations, and fluid retention. They are usually given in combination with diuretics and beta-blockers in resistant patients. Hydralazine produces frequent gastrointestinal disturbances and may induce a lupus-like syndrome. Minoxidil causes hirsutism and marked fluid retention; this agent is reserved for the most refractory of patients.

I. PERIPHERAL SYMPATHETIC INHIBITORS

(Table 11–9.) These agents are now used infrequently and usually in refractory hypertension. Reserpine remains a cost-effective antihypertensive agent. Its reputation for inducing mental depression and its other side effects—sedation, nasal stuffiness, sleep disturbances, and peptic ulcers—has made it unpopular, though these problems are uncommon at low dosages. Guanethidine and guanadrel inhibit catecholamine release from peripheral neurons but frequently cause orthostatic hypotension (especially in the morning or after exercise), diarrhea, and fluid retention.

Developing an Antihypertensive Regimen

Because the most extensive and most favorable experience in randomized control trials has been with diuretic-based and, to a lesser extent, beta-blocker-based regimens, these should be the initial agents for the majority of uncomplicated hypertensives. Figure 11–1 summarizes results achieved with these agents in clinical trials. However, many patients—perhaps the majority in middle-aged and older populations—will have associated medical conditions that become important determinants of drug selection. In some con-

ditions, specific medications have shown major benefits in randomized controlled trials and should therefore be the initial agents of choice for these populations. The favored agents include ACE inhibitors in patients with type 1 diabetes and proteinuria and probably in type 2 diabetics with microalbuminuria or atherosclerotic vascular disease; ACE inhibitors, beta-blockers, and diuretics in patients with congestive heart failure; beta-blockers in patients who have experienced a myocardial infarction; and ACE inhibitors in postinfarction patients with documented left ventricular systolic dysfunction (ejection fraction < 40%). ACE inhibitors may also prevent fatal and nonfatal vascular events, including myocardial infarction, stroke, and heart failure in normotensive or treated hypertensive patients at high risk for these problems. However, in the hypertensive population, it is not certain whether they are more effective in reducing these end points than diuretics or beta-block-

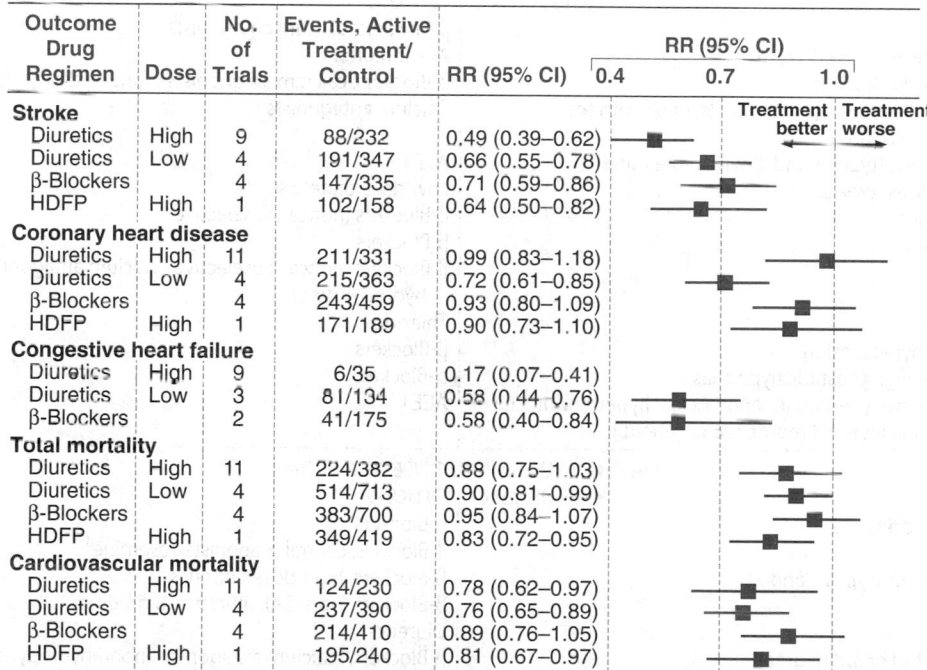

Figure 11–1. Meta-analysis of randomized, placebo-controlled clinical trials in hypertension according to first-line treatment strategy. For these comparisons, the numbers of participants randomized to active treatment and placebo, respectively, were 7768 and 12,075 for high-dose diuretic therapy, 4305 and 5116 for low-dose diuretic therapy, and 6736 and 12,147 for beta-blocker therapy. Because the Medical Research Council trials included two active arms, the placebo group is included twice in these totals (for diuretic comparison and for beta-blocker comparison). The total number of participants randomized to active and control therapy were 24,294 and 23,926, respectively. RR indicates relative risk; CI, confidence interval; and HDFP, Hypertension Detection and Follow-Up Program. (Data from Psaty et al. Reproduced, with permission, from: The sixth report of the Joint National Committee on prevention, detection, evaluation, and treatment of high blood pressure. Arch Intern Med 1997;157.2413. Copyright © 1997 by American Medical Association.)

ers except perhaps in diabetics. When ACE inhibitors have been compared with calcium antagonists in diabetic patients, there has been a lower incidence of myocardial infarction and heart failure with the ACE inhibitors.

Diuretics have consistently proved effective (even more so than beta-blockers) in trials of older patients with isolated or predominantly systolic hypertension,

but the Syst-Eur Trial showed that calcium channel blockers appear to achieve similar benefits, and this class should therefore be considered a second-line alternative to diuretics in these patients. Table 11–10 also lists a number of conditions for which there is evidence of an advantage of one class—as well as conditions in which certain antihypertensive drugs should be avoided.

Table 11–10. Considerations for individualizing antihypertensive drug therapy.[1]

Indication	Drug Therapy
COMPELLING INDICATIONS UNLESS CONTRAINDICATED	
Diabetes mellitus (type 1) with proteinuria	ACE I
Heart failure	ACE I, diuretics, β-blockers
Post-myocardial infarction	β-Blockers (non-ISA), ACE I (with systolic dysfunction)
Isolated systolic hypertension (older patients)	Diuretics (preferred), calcium antagonists
MAY HAVE FAVORABLE EFFECTS ON COMORBID CONDITIONS[2]	
Angina	β-Blockers, calcium antagonists
Atherosclerotic vascular disease	ACE inhibitors
Atrial tachycardia, fibrillation	β-Blockers, calcium antagonists (nondihydropyridine)
Cyclosporine-induced hypertension (caution with the dose of cyclosporine)	Calcium antagonists
Diabetes mellitus (types 1 and 2) with proteinuria	ACE I
Diabetes mellitus (type 2)	Low-dose diuretics
Essential tremor	β-Blockers (noncardioselective)
Hyperthyroidism	β-Blockers
Migraine	β-Blockers (noncardioselective), calcium antagonists (nondihydropyridine)
Osteoporosis	Thiazides
Preoperative hypertension	β-Blockers
Prostatism (benign prostatic hyperplasia)	α-Blockers
Renal insufficiency (caution in renovascular hypertension and creatinine level ≥ 3 mg/dL [265.2 μmol/L])	ACE I
MAY HAVE UNFAVORABLE EFFECTS ON COMORBID CONDITIONS[2,3]	
Bronchospastic disease	β-Blockers[4]
Depression	β-Blockers, central α-agonists, reserpine[4]
Diabetes mellitus (types 1 and 2)	β-Blockers, high-dose diuretics
Dyslipidemia	β-Blockers (non-ISA), diuretics (high-dose)
Gout	Diuretics
Heart block (2nd or 3rd degree)	β-Blockers,[4] calcium antagonists (nondihydropyridine)[4]
Heart failure	Calcium antagonists (except amlodipine), α–blockers, β-blockers[5]
Liver disease	Labetalol hydrochloride, methyldopa[4]
Peripheral vascular disease	β-Blockers
Pregnancy	ACE I,[4] angiotensin II receptor blockers[4]
Renal insufficiency	Potassium-sparing agents
Renovascular disease	ACE I, angiotensin II receptor blockers

ACE I, angiotensin-converting enzyme inhibitors; ISA, intrinsic sympathomimetic activity.
[1]Modified from: The sixth report of the Joint National Committee on detection, education, and treatment of high blood pressure (JNC VI). Arch Intern Med 1997;157:2413.
[2]Conditions and drugs are listed in alphabetical order.
[3]These drugs may be used with special monitoring unless contraindicated.
[4]Contraindicated.
[5]β-Blockers may worsen heart failure initially but are indicated in stable patients.

When an initial agent is selected, the patient should be informed of common side effects and the need for diligent compliance. Treatment should start at a low dose, and unless the initial blood pressure is very high (> 180/110 mm Hg), follow-up visits should usually be at 4- to 6-week intervals to allow for full medication effects to be established (especially with diuretics) before further titration or adjustment. If, after titration to usual doses, the patient has shown a discernible but incomplete response and a good tolerance of the initial drug, the second agent should be added. If the initial medication was a diuretic or a calcium channel blocker, the second agent should be a beta-blocker, ACE inhibitor, or angiotensin II blocker, since these combinations are generally complementary. If the initial drug was a beta-blocker, ACE inhibitor, or angiotensin II blocker, the second drug should be a diuretic. On the other hand, if the first agent showed no effect, another should be substituted. Again, if the first drug was a diuretic or a calcium channel blocker, the substituted drug should be a beta-blocker, ACE inhibitor, or angiotensin II blocker; if a beta-blocker, ACE inhibitor, or angiotensin II blocker, the substituted agent should be a diuretic or a calcium channel blocker. Low-dose combinations of complementary antihypertensive drugs are another approach to initial therapy.

Most patients with hypertension can be controlled with one-drug or two-drug regimens that combine complementary agents. A minority of patients require three, four, or even more medications in combination. The need for multidrug regimens is more frequent in patients with high systolic pressures and in diabetics. Unless absolutely contraindicated, one of these components should be a diuretic. Particularly useful multidrug regimens are (1) a diuretic plus a beta-blocker plus a vasodilator or a calcium channel blocker; (2) a diuretic plus an ACE inhibitor plus either a calcium channel blocker or a sympatholytic (or both); and (3) a calcium channel blocker plus an ACE inhibitor plus either a sympatholytic or a beta-blocker (or both). Patients who are compliant with their medications and who do not respond to these combinations should usually be evaluated for secondary hypertension before proceeding to more complex regimens.

Special Considerations in the Treatment of Diabetic Hypertensive Patients

Hypertensive patients with diabetes are at particularly high risk for cardiovascular events. More aggressive treatment of hypertension in these patients prevents progressive nephropathy, myocardial infarction, and stroke. Treatment recommendations suggest a target of < 130/85 mm Hg. Because of their beneficial effects in diabetic nephropathy, ACE inhibitors (and angiotensin II receptor blockers in intolerant patients) should be part of the initial treatment regimen. However, most diabetics require combinations of three to five agents to achieve these goals, usually including a diuretic and a calcium channel blocker or beta-blocker. In addition to rigorous blood pressure control, management of diabetics should include aggressive treatment of other risk factors and early intervention for coronary disease and left ventricular dysfunction.

Treatment of Additional Cardiovascular Risk Factors

Since the goal is to reduce cardiovascular morbidity and mortality, attention must be paid to the management of other risk factors. Aggressive reduction of elevated LDL-cholesterol levels reduces the risk of myocardial infarction and death in patients with multiple risk factors. Thus, if LDL-cholesterol levels remain over 130 mg/dL following an attempt at dietary intervention, drug therapy is indicated in most hypertensives. Levels under 100 mg/dL should be achieved in patients with coronary artery disease, cerebrovascular disease, peripheral arterial disease, or diabetes. Smoking cessation, regular exercise, and weight loss when indicated are other important features of hypertension management.

Follow-Up of the Treated Hypertensive

Once blood pressure is controlled on a well-tolerated regimen, follow-up visits can be infrequent and laboratory testing limited to tests appropriate for the patient and the medications utilized. Yearly monitoring of blood lipids is recommended, and an ECG should be repeated at 2- to 4-year intervals depending on whether initial abnormalities are present, the presence of coronary risk factors, and age.

Patients who have had excellent blood pressure control for several years, especially if they have lost weight and initiated favorable lifestyle modifications, should be considered for "step-down" of therapy to determine if lower doses or discontinuing of medications is feasible.

Bakris GL et al: Angiotensin-converting enzyme inhibitor-associated elevations in serum creatinine: is this a cause for concern? Arch Intern Med 2000;160:685. [PMID: 10724055] (Patients with rises in creatinine up to 30% during the first 2 months of therapy experience the greatest long-term preservation of renal function.)

Blood Pressure Lowering Treatment Trialists' Collaboration. Effects of ACE inhibitors, calcium antagonists, and other blood-pressure-lowering drugs: Results of prospectively designed overviews of randomized trials. Lancet 2000; 356:1955. [PMID: 11130523] (Diuretics, beta-blockers, ACE inhibitors, and calcium antagonists all prevent major cardiovascular events, but some differences were observed in the effects of calcium antagonists compared with other agents.)

Drugs for hypertension. Med Lett Drugs Ther 2001 (1099):17. [PMID: 11242494]

Garovic VD: Hypertension in pregnancy: Diagnosis and treatment. Mayo Clin Proc 2000;75:1071. [PMID: 11040855]

Graves JW: Management of difficult to control hypertension. Mayo Clin Proc 2000;75:278. [PMID: 10725955] (Practical step-by-step approach.)

Kaplan NM: Management of hypertension in patients with type 2 diabetes mellitus: guidelines based on current evidence. Ann Intern Med 2001;135:1079. [PMID: 11747387] (Concise review and recommendations.)

Staessen JA et al: Cardiovascular protection and blood pressure reduction: a meta-analysis. Lancet 2001;358:1305. [PMID: 11684211] (As opposed to the Blood Pressure Lowering Trialists meta-analysis referenced above, this study suggests that the magnitude of blood pressure lowering rather than the specific agent utilized may be the most important factor in reducing the incidence of vascular events.)

Weir MR et al: Diuretics and beta-blockers: is there a risk for dyslipidemia? Am Heart J 2000;139:174. [PMID: 10618579] (A review of the minimal effects of low-dose thiazides or cardioselective beta-blockers on the lipid profile.)

Yusuf S et al: Effects of an angiotensin-converting-enzyme inhibitor, ramipril, on cardiovascular events in high-risk patients. The Heart Outcomes Prevention Evaluation Investigators. N Engl J Med 2000;342:145. [PMID: 10639539] (Ramipril prevented fatal and nonfatal events in diabetes patients with cardiovascular disease; not all patients had elevated blood pressure, but extrapolation of these findings to the hypertensive population is reasonable.)

HYPERTENSIVE URGENCIES & EMERGENCIES

Hypertensive emergencies have become less frequent in recent years but still require prompt recognition and aggressive but careful management. A spectrum of acute presentations exists, and the appropriate therapeutic approach varies accordingly.

Hypertensive urgencies are situations in which blood pressure must be reduced within a few hours. These include patients with asymptomatic severe hypertension (systolic blood pressure > 220 mm Hg, or diastolic pressure > 125 mm Hg that persist after a period of observation) and with optic disk edema, progressive target organ complications, and severe perioperative hypertension. Elevated blood pressure levels alone—in the absence of symptoms or new or progressive target organ damage—rarely require emergency therapy. Parenteral drug therapy is not usually required, and partial reduction of blood pressure with relief of symptoms is the goal.

Hypertensive emergencies require substantial reduction of blood pressure within 1 hour to avoid the risk of serious morbidity or death. Although blood pressure is usually strikingly elevated (diastolic pressure > 130 mm Hg), the correlation between pressure and end-organ damage is often poor. It is the latter that determines the seriousness of the emergency and the approach to treatment. Emergencies include hypertensive encephalopathy (headache, irritability, confusion, and altered mental status due to cerebrovascular spasm), hypertensive nephropathy (hematuria, proteinuria, and progressive renal dysfunction due to arteriolar necrosis and intimal hyperplasia of the interlobular arteries), intracranial hemorrhage, aortic dissection, preeclampsia-eclampsia, pulmonary edema,

unstable angina, or myocardial infarction. **Malignant hypertension** is by historical definition characterized by encephalopathy or nephropathy with accompanying papilledema. Progressive renal failure usually ensues if treatment is not provided. The therapeutic approach is identical to that employed with other antihypertensive emergencies.

Parenteral therapy is indicated in most hypertensive emergencies, especially if encephalopathy is present. The initial goal in hypertensive emergencies is to reduce the pressure by no more than 25% (within minutes to 1 or 2 hours) and then toward a level of 160/100 mm Hg within 2–6 hours. Excessive reductions in pressure may precipitate coronary, cerebral, or renal ischemia. To avoid such declines, the use of agents that have a predictable, dose-dependent, transient, and not precipitous antihypertensive effect is preferable. In that regard, the use of sublingual or oral fast-acting nifedipine preparations is best avoided.

Pharmacologic Management

A. PARENTERAL AGENTS

A growing number of agents are available for management of acute hypertensive problems. (Table 11–11 lists drugs, dosages, and adverse effects.) Sodium nitroprusside is the agent of choice for the most serious emergencies because of its rapid and easily controllable action, but continuous monitoring is essential when this agent is used. In the presence of myocardial ischemia, intravenous nitroglycerin or an intravenous beta-blocker, such as labetalol or esmolol, is preferable.

1. Nitroprusside sodium—This agent is given by controlled intravenous infusion gradually titrated to the desired effect. It lowers the blood pressure within seconds by direct arteriolar and venous dilatation. Monitoring with an intra-arterial line avoids hypotension. Nitroprusside—in combination with a beta-blocker—is especially useful in patients with aortic dissection.

2. Nitroglycerin, intravenous—This agent is a less potent antihypertensive than nitroprusside and should be reserved for patients with accompanying acute ischemic syndromes.

3. Labetalol—This combined beta- and alpha-blocking agent is the most potent adrenergic blocker for rapid blood pressure reduction. Other beta-blockers are far less potent. Excessive blood pressure drops are unusual. Experience with this agent in hypertensive syndromes associated with pregnancy has been favorable.

4. Esmolol—This rapidly acting beta-blocker is approved only for treatment of supraventricular tachycardia but is often used for lowering blood pressure. It is less potent than labetalol and should be reserved for patients in whom there is particular concern about serious adverse events related to beta-blockers.

Table 11–11. Drugs for hypertensive emergencies and urgencies.

Agent	Action	Dosage	Onset	Duration	Adverse Effects	Comments
PARENTERAL AGENTS (INTRAVENOUSLY UNLESS NOTED)						
Nitroprusside (Nipride)	Vasodilator	0.25–10 µg/kg/min	Seconds	3–5 minutes	GI, CNS; thiocyanate and cyanide toxicity, especially with renal and hepatic insufficiency; hypotension.	Most effective and easily titratable treatment. Use with beta-blocker in aortic dissection.
Nitroglycerin	Vasodilator	0.25–5 µg/kg/min	2–5 minutes	3–5 minutes	Headache, nausea, hypotension, bradycardia.	Tolerance may develop. Useful primarily with myocardial ischemia
Labetalol (Normodyne, Trandate)	Beta- and alpha-blocker	20–40 mg every 10 minutes to 300 mg; 2 mg/min infusion	5–10 minutes	3–6 hours	GI, hypotension, bronchospasm, bradycardia, heart block.	Avoid in congestive heart failure, asthma. May be continued orally.
Esmolol (Brevibloc)	Beta-blocker	Loading dose 500 µg/kg over 1 minute; maintenance, 25–200 µg/kc/min	1–2 minutes	10–30 minutes	Bradycardia, nausea.	Avoid in congestive heart failure, asthma. Weak antihypertensive.
Fenoldopam (Corlopam)	Dopamine receptor agonist	0.1–1.6 µg/kg/min	4–5 minutes	< 10 minutes	Reflex tachycardia, hypotension, ↑ intraocular pressure.	May protect renal function.
Nicardipine (Cardene)	Calcium channel blocker	5 mg/h; may increase by 1–2.5 mg/h every 15 minutes to 15 mg/h	1–5 minutes	3–6 hours	Hypotension, tachycardia, headache	May precipitate myocardial ischemia.
Enalaprilat (Vasotec)	ACE inhibitor	1.25 mg every 6 hours	15 minutes	6 hours or more	Excessive hypotension.	Additive with diuretics; may be continued orally.
Furosemide (Lasix)	Diuretic	10–80 mg	15 minutes	4 hours	Hypokalemia, hypotension.	Adjunct to vasodilator.
Hydralazine (Apresoline)	Vasodilator	5–20 mg IV or IM (less desirable); may repeat after 20 minutes	10–30 minutes	2–6 hours	Tachycardia, headache, GI.	Avoid in coronary artery disease, dissection. Rarely used except in pregnancy.
Diazoxide (Hyperstat)	Vasodilator	50–150 mg repeated at intervals of 5–15 minutes, or 15–30 mg/min by IV infusion to a maximum of 600 mg	1–2 minutes	4–24 hours	Excessive hypotension, tachycardia, myocardial ischemia, headache, nausea, vomiting, hyperglycemia. Necrosis with extravasation.	Avoid in coronary artery disease and dissection. Use with beta-blocker and diuretic. Mostly obsolete.
Trimethaphan (Arfonad)	Ganglionic blocker	0.5–5 mg/min	1–3 minutes	10 minutes	Hypotension, ileus, urinary retention, respiratory arrest. Liberates histamine; use caution in allergic individuals.	Useful in aortic dissection. Otherwise rarely used.
ORAL AGENTS						
Nifedipine (Adalat, Procardia)	Calcium channel blocker	10 mg initially; may be repeated after 30 minutes	15 minutes	2–6 hours	Excessive hypotension, tachycardia, headache, angina, myocardial infarction, stroke.	Response unpredictable.
Clonidine (Catapres)	Central sympatholytic	0.1–0.2 mg initially; then 0.1 mg every hour to 0.8 mg	30–60 minutes	6–8 hours	Sedation.	Rebound may occur.
Captopril (Capoten)	ACE inhibitor	12.5–25 mg	15–30 minutes	4–6 hours	Excessive hypotension.	

5. Nicardipine—Intravenous nicardipine is the most potent antihypertensive agent and the longest-acting of the parenteral calcium channel blockers. As a primarily arterial vasodilator, it has the potential to precipitate reflex tachycardia, and for that reason it should not be used without a beta-blocker in patients with coronary artery disease.

6. Fenoldopam—Fenoldopam is a new peripheral dopamine-1 (DA_1) receptor agonist that causes a dose-dependent reduction in arterial pressure without evidence of tolerance, rebound, or withdrawal or deterioration of renal function. In higher dosage ranges, tachycardia may occur.

7. Enalaprilat—This is the active form of the oral ACE inhibitor enalapril. The onset of action is usually within 15 minutes, but the peak effect may be delayed for up to 6 hours. Thus, enalaprilat is used primarily as an adjunctive agent.

8. Diazoxide—Diazoxide acts promptly as a vasodilator without decreasing renal blood flow. To avoid hypotension, it should be given in small boluses or as an infusion rather than as the previously recommended large bolus. One use of diazoxide has been in preeclampsia-eclampsia. Hyperglycemia and sodium and water retention may occur. The drug should be used only for short periods and is best combined with a loop diuretic.

9. Hydralazine—Hydralazine can be given intravenously or intramuscularly, but its effect is less predictable than that of other drugs in this group. It produces reflex tachycardia and should not be given without beta-blockers in patients with possible coronary disease or aortic dissection. Hydralazine is now used primarily in pregnancy and in children, but even in these situations, newer agents are supplanting it.

10. Trimethaphan—The ganglionic blocking agent trimethaphan is titrated with the patient sitting; its activity depends upon this. The patient can be placed supine if the hypotensive effect is excessive. The effect occurs within a few minutes and persists for the duration of the infusion. This agent has largely been replaced by nitroprusside and newer medications.

11. Diuretics—Intravenous loop diuretics can be very helpful when the patient has signs of heart failure or fluid retention, but the onset of their hypotensive response is slow, making them an adjunct rather than a primary agent for hypertensive emergencies. Low dosages should be used initially (furosemide, 20 mg; or bumetanide, 0.5 mg). They facilitate the response to vasodilators, which often stimulate fluid retention.

B. ORAL AGENTS

Patients with less severe acute hypertensive syndromes can often be treated with oral therapy. Abrupt blood pressure lowering is not usually necessary in asymptomatic individuals, and the use of agents such as rapid-acting nifedipine probably causes more adverse effects than benefits.

1. Clonidine—Clonidine, 0.2 mg orally initially, followed by 0.1 mg every hour to a total of 0.8 mg, will usually lower blood pressure over a period of several hours. Sedation is frequent, and rebound hypertension may occur if the drug is stopped.

2. Captopril—Captopril, 12.5–25 mg orally, will also lower blood pressure in 15–30 minutes. The response is variable and may be excessive.

3. Nifedipine—Fast-acting nifedipine capsules are commonly employed in the emergency room or urgent care setting because they usually provide a rapid reduction in blood pressure. However, the nifedipine effect is unpredictable and may be excessive, resulting in hypotension and reflex tachycardia. Because myocardial infarction and stroke have been reported in this setting, the use of nifedipine without concomitant beta-blocker therapy is not advised.

C. SUBSEQUENT THERAPY

When the blood pressure has been brought under control, combinations of oral antihypertensive agents can be added as parenteral drugs are tapered off over a period of 2–3 days. Most subsequent regimens should include a diuretic.

Elliott WJ: Hypertensive emergencies. Crit Care Clin 2001; 17:435. [PMID: 11450325] (Current review article.)

Murphy MB et al: Fenoldopam: a selective peripheral dopamine receptor agonist for the treatment of severe hypertension. N Engl J Med 2001;345:1548. [PMID: 11794223] (Preserves renal blood flow while effectively lowering blood pressure; questionable if it is superior to the more rapidly acting nitroprusside.)

12

Blood Vessels & Lymphatics

Louis M. Messina, MD, Laura K. Pak, MD, & Lawrence M. Tierney, Jr., MD
See www.current-med.com/ch12.html

Most arterial occlusive disease is produced by atherosclerosis. Atherosclerosis is a generalized response of the artery wall to injury. Atherosclerotic plaques are characterized by smooth muscle migration into the intima and subsequent proliferation and extracellular lipid deposition. Complex lesions are composed of a fibrous cap containing smooth muscle and inflammatory cells overlying a central core of lipid-rich necrotic debris. Clinical symptoms are produced by progressive stenosis, calcification, intraplaque hemorrhage, distal embolization, and luminal thrombosis after cap rupture. Atherosclerosis is a systemic disease, associated with some degree of involvement of all major arteries, but its most common clinical manifestations involve a limited number of arteries at areas of turbulent flow and low sheer stress: the carotid bifurcation, the infrarenal aorta and the iliac, superficial femoral, and tibial arteries, and the ostia of the renal and visceral arteries.

Most arterial aneurysms are classified as atherosclerotic or degenerative, because atheromas are found in the aneurysm wall and many patients have typical atherosclerotic risk factors. Both occlusive disease and aneurysms may be present in the same individual. However, the exact role of atherosclerosis in the causation of aneurysms is poorly defined. An imbalance of tissue metalloproteinases and metalloproteinase inhibitors is responsible for elastin and collagen degradation. Genetic predisposition, inflammation, and hemodynamic factors may also play a permissive role in aneurysm formation.

Atherosclerosis has been associated with increasing age, hypercholesterolemia, diabetes mellitus, smoking, a positive family history, hypertension, elevated levels of lipoprotein(a) and C-reactive protein, sedentary lifestyle, obesity, and homocystinuria. Control of risk factors by use of antihypertensive and lipid-lowering medications, regulation of blood sugar, tobacco cessation, and regular exercise remain the mainstays of treatment. Aspirin and clopidogrel (and potentially glycoprotein IIb/IIIa inhibitors) may prevent microemboli by impairing platelet aggregation; clopidogrel reduces the relative risk of stroke, myocardial infarction, and vascular death by 24% over aspirin alone in at-risk patients. Preliminary studies suggest that antioxidants, particularly dietary vitamin E, may also be beneficial in slowing the progression of disease. More recently, research has focused on the use of macrolide antibiotics in atherosclerotic disease, based on the finding of *Chlamydia pneumoniae* in symptomatic atheromas. Gene transfer of vascular endothelial growth factor (VEGF) and endothelial nitric oxide synthetase (eNOS), as well as specifically targeted gene therapy for risk factor management represent active area of investigation.

Frangos SG et al: Vascular drugs in the new millennium. J Am Coll Surg 2000,191:76. [PMID: 10898187]

Hodis HN et al: Estrogen in the prevention of atherosclerosis: A randomized, double-blind, placebo-controlled trial. Ann Intern Med 2001;135:939. [PMID: 11730394]

Khurana R et al: Gene therapy for cardiovascular disease: A case for cautious optimism. Hypertension 2001;38:1210. [PMID: 11711525]

Kilaru S et al: Nicotine: A review of its role in atherosclerosis. J Am Coll Surg 2001;193:538. [PMID: 11708512]

Lusis AJ et al: Atherosclerosis. Nature 2000;407:233. [PMID: 11001066]

McQuillan BM et al: Antioxidant vitamins and the risk of carotid atherosclerosis. J Am Coll Cardiol 2001;38:1788. [PMID: 11738275]

Ridker PM et al: Novel risk factors for systemic atherosclerosis. JAMA 2001;285:2481. [PMID: 11368701]

ARTERIAL ANEURYSMS

ANEURYSMS OF THE ABDOMINAL AORTA

 ESSENTIALS OF DIAGNOSIS

- *Most aortic aneurysms are asymptomatic, detected during a routine physical examination or sonography.*

- *Severe back or abdominal pain and hypotension indicate rupture.*
- *Concomitant atherosclerotic occlusive disease of lower extremities is present in 25%.*

General Considerations

Over 90% of abdominal aneurysms originate below the renal arteries, and many extend into the common iliac arteries. The infrarenal aorta is normally 2 cm in diameter; an aneurysm is defined as an aortic diameter exceeding 3 cm. An aortic aneurysm is present in 5–8% of the population over the age of 65. The reported incidence has tripled over the last 30 years. Half of all newly detected aneurysms are under 5 cm in diameter and require routine ultrasound surveillance. Two-thirds will increase sufficiently in size to require repair. Beta-blockers and, more recently, oral roxithromycin (300 mg daily for 30 days) have been shown to decrease the expansion rate of small aneurysms. Patients with chronic obstructive pulmonary disease appear more likely to rupture smaller aneurysms.

Clinical Findings

A. Symptoms and Signs

1. Asymptomatic aneurysms—An aneurysm may be suspected on routine physical examination by detection of a prominent aortic pulsation. More often, asymptomatic aneurysms are discovered as incidental findings on abdominal ultrasound or CT scan performed for other reasons. Peripheral pulses are often normal, but coexisting renal or lower extremity arterial occlusive disease is present in 25%. Popliteal artery aneurysms are present in 15% of patients with aneurysms of the abdominal aorta, and, conversely, more than one-third of patients with popliteal aneurysms have abdominal aortic aneurysms.

2. Symptomatic aneurysms—Midabdominal or lower back pain (or both) in the presence of a prominent aortic pulsation may indicate rapid aneurysmal growth, rupture, or inflammatory aortic aneurysm. Inflammatory aneurysms account for fewer than 5% of aortic aneurysms and are characterized by extensive periaortic and retroperitoneal inflammation of unknown cause. These patients may have low-grade fever, elevated sedimentation rate, and a history of recent upper respiratory tract infection; they are often active smokers. Infected aortic aneurysms (either caused by septic emboli to a normal aorta or bacterial colonization of an existing aneurysm) are rare but should be suspected in patients with saccular aneurysms or aneurysms in conjunction with fever of unknown origin, particularly if blood cultures are positive for salmonella. Peripheral emboli can also be a symptom of aneurysmal disease.

3. Ruptured aneurysms—Patients with ruptured aortic aneurysms present with severe back, abdominal, or flank pain and hypotension. Posterior rupture confined to the retroperitoneum carries a better prognosis than anterior rupture into the peritoneal cavity. As many as 90% of patients die either before they reach the hospital or in the immediate perioperative period. The only chance for survival is emergent surgical repair.

B. Laboratory Findings

Electrocardiogram, serum creatinine, hematocrit and hemoglobin, and type and crossmatch should be obtained routinely in all patients.

C. Imaging

Abdominal ultrasonography is the screening study of choice and is valuable also for following aneurysm growth in patients with small (< 5 cm) aneurysms. Aneurysms typically grow by about 10% of their diameter per year; annual ultrasound examinations are recommended for aneurysms greater than 3.5 cm. In about three-fourths of patients, size can be estimated by measurement of curvilinear calcifications in the aneurysm wall on an abdominal radiograph, but this is much less accurate than ultrasonography.

Contrast-enhanced CT scanning not only precisely sizes the aneurysm but also defines its relationship to the renal arteries. MRI is as sensitive and specific as CT and is useful if renal insufficiency precludes contrast-enhanced CT. Aortography is indicated prior to elective aneurysm repair when arterial occlusive disease of the visceral or lower extremity arteries is suspected or when endograft repair is being considered.

Treatment

A. Standard Therapy

Surgical excision and synthetic graft replacement is the treatment of choice for most aneurysms of the infrarenal abdominal aorta greater than 5 cm. The maximum diameter of the aneurysm correlates best with the risk of rupture. Yearly rupture risk is 2% for 4–5.9 cm aneurysms, 7% for 6–6.9 cm aneurysms, and 25% for 7 cm aneurysms. Recommendation of an elective repair must be balanced with the risk of rupture. In asymptomatic good-risk patients, surgery is advised when the aneurysm exceeds 5 cm, while poor-risk patients may not be considered for repair until the aneurysm exceeds 6 cm. Urgent repair is indicated for symptomatic patients irrespective of aneurysm size.

Preoperative evaluation must include a detailed assessment of cardiac risk and examination of the carotid arteries since acute myocardial infarction, arrhythmia, and stroke remain among the most frequent perioperative complications. In patients with asymptomatic aneurysms and a history of angina or of carotid stenosis greater than 80%, coronary angioplasty, coronary bypass grafting, or carotid endarterectomy may be indicated before repair of the aneurysm.

B. ENDOVASCULAR REPAIR

Endovascular stent grafts, or "covered stents," have evolved over the last decade for treatment of aortic aneurysms. Aortic stent grafts are configured to be uni-iliac or bifurcated depending on the particular anatomy of the aneurysm. Uni-iliac grafts are combined with endovascular occlusion of the contralateral common iliac artery and femoral-femoral bypass grafting. Both types of grafts are deployed via the common femoral arteries; in most cases, this involves bilateral inguinal incisions. The operation can be performed under epidural anesthesia, often in less than 2 hours and with minimal blood loss, which has made repair of aortic aneurysms feasible in high-risk patients previously deemed inoperable. Additional advantages include reduced incisional pain, fewer cardiopulmonary complications, and avoidance of postoperative ileus; most patients are discharged from the hospital on the second postoperative day. Endografts have been used successfully for repair of ruptured aneurysms, using balloon catheter control of the supraceliac aorta to facilitate intraoperative angiography and stent deployment.

Not all patients are candidates for standard endovascular repair. The proximal neck of the aneurysm must be adequate (at least 1.5 cm in length and less than 3 cm in width) to allow fixation and sufficient tissue apposition below the renal arteries. Iliac artery aneurysms, iliac stenoses, and iliac tortuosity or calcification all increase the complexity of stent deployment. The newest technology includes use of smaller introducer sheaths intended for eventual percutaneous deployment. Long-term durability of endovascular grafts needs to be established before comparison can be made with open repair for use in the good-risk patient with asymptomatic aortic aneurysm. Objective comparison with open surgical repair has been complicated by the multiplicity of continually evolving stent graft designs.

Complications

Complications after aneurysm resection include myocardial infarction, bleeding, respiratory insufficiency, ischemic colitis, limb ischemia, renal insufficiency, and stroke. Bowel infarction, liver dysfunction, acalculous cholecystitis, and renal failure are more common with emergent aneurysm repair or when repair of the aneurysm requires supraceliac or suprarenal cross-clamping. However, renal insufficiency can occur even when the clamp is infrarenal and there is no reported intraoperative hypotension, presumably because of renal artery vasoconstriction, atheroemboli, preoperative contrast administration for CT scan, and dehydration from fasting or bowel preparation. For this reason, mannitol (25 g intravenous bolus) is given as a diuretic and free-radical scavenger prior to cross-clamping, and dopamine (3 μg/kg/min) or fenoldopam (0.05–0.1 μg/kg/min) continued in the immediate postoperative period to increase renal perfusion and glomerular filtration rate. Rarely (0.1% of cases), lower extremity paralysis complicates repair of abdominal aortic aneurysm because of occlusion of the spinal artery from atheroemboli, shock, or aortic cross clamping. Graft infection and graft-enteric fistulas are well described as fatal late complications, occurring more often after emergent aneurysm repair. One complication specific to endovascular repair is persistent filling of the aneurysm (endoleak). Endoleaks are classified as type 1 (leak around the top or bottom of the stent graft), type 2 (leak from a back-bleeding patent lumbar artery or inferior mesenteric artery), and type 3 (leak through the graft material). They are detected by contrast CT obtained routinely on postoperative days 2 and 30, and at 6-month or yearly intervals thereafter. Type 1 endoleaks are restented to allow adequate proximal or distal fixation. Type 2 endoleaks are not uncommon (20–30% of patients) in the immediate postoperative period but usually disappear by the 1-month CT scan. Persistent type 2 endoleaks occur in 5% of patients and are correlated with the use of warfarin and the presence of a patent inferior mesenteric artery preoperatively. They can be eliminated by endovascular coil embolization of the feeding arteries.

Renal failure from contrast nephropathy, intraoperative atheroemboli, or graft impingement on the main or accessory renal arteries is another possible complication of endovascular repair. Conversion to open repair because of aortic or iliac rupture, inability to gain access, error in positioning, inadequate fixation, or stent malfunction is rare (1–3%) if patients are properly screened preoperatively.

Prognosis

Mortality following elective open or endovascular repair is 1–5%. In general, a patient with an aortic aneurysm greater than 5 cm has a threefold greater chance of dying as a consequence of rupture of the aneurysm than of dying from surgical resection. Five-year survival after surgical repair is 60–80%. Five to 10 percent of patients will develop another aortic aneurysm adjacent to the graft or in the thoracic aorta.

Chuter TAM et al: Endoleak after endovascular repair of abdominal aortic aneurysm. J Vasc Surg 2001;34:98. [PMID: 11436081]

Newman AB et al: Cardiovascular disease and mortality in older adults with small abdominal aortic aneurysms detected by ultrasonography: The cardiovascular health study. Ann Intern Med 2001;134:182. [PMID: 11177330]

Ohki T et al: Endovascular grafts and other image-guided catheter-based adjuncts to improve the treatment of ruptured aortoiliac aneurysms. Ann Surg 2000;232:466. [PMID: 10998645]

Ohki T et al: Increasing incidence of midterm and long-term complications after endovascular graft repair of abdominal aortic aneurysms: A note of caution based on a 9-year experience. Ann Surg 2001;234:323. [PMID: 11524585]

Vammen S et al: Randomized double-blind controlled trial of roxithromycin for prevention of abdominal aortic aneurysm expansion. Br J Surg 2001;88:1066. [PMID: 11488791]

ANEURYSMS OF THE THORACIC AORTA

Aneurysms of the thoracic aorta account for fewer than 10% of aortic aneurysms. Medial degeneration, chronic dissection, vasculitis, and collagen-vascular disease (Marfan's syndrome or Ehlers-Danlos syndrome) are common causes; syphilis is now a rare cause of thoracic aneurysm. Traumatic aneurysms occur at the ligamentum arteriosus just beyond the left subclavian artery and result from shearing injury during rapid-deceleration automobile accidents.

Thoracoabdominal aneurysms are categorized by the Crawford classification: Type 1 extends from left subclavian artery to the renal arteries, type 2 from the left subclavian artery to the iliac bifurcation, type 3 from the midthoracic to the infrarenal region, and type 4 from the diaphragmatic hiatus to the infrarenal region. The prevalence of each type of thoracoabdominal aneurysm is roughly equal, but type 4 aneurysms have the lowest operative mortality (2–5%) and the lowest risk of postoperative neurologic deficits (2–10%).

Clinical Findings

A. SYMPTOMS AND SIGNS

Clinical manifestations depend largely on the size and position of the aneurysm and its rate of growth. Most are asymptomatic and are discovered during a diagnostic procedure undertaken for other reasons. Some patients present with substernal, back, or neck pain. Others develop dyspnea, stridor, or a brassy cough from pressure on the trachea, dysphagia from pressure on the esophagus, hoarseness from pressure on the left recurrent laryngeal nerve, or neck and arm edema from external compression of the superior vena cava. Aortic regurgitation due to distortion of the aortic valve annulus may occur with aneurysms of the ascending aorta.

B. IMAGING

An aneurysm suspected on chest radiography must be differentiated from other anterior mediastinal masses, including lung neoplasm, thymoma, cyst, and substernal goiter. CT scan and MRI are the most sensitive and accurate means of imaging thoracic aneurysms. Aortography may be necessary to assess involvement of the arch vessels. The coronary vessels and the aortic valve should also be studied if aortic root replacement is anticipated.

Treatment

Control of hypertension and use of beta-blockers may slow aneurysmal growth. Indications for surgical treatment include the presence of symptoms, rapid expansion, or size greater than 5 cm. Operative risk from comorbid medical conditions must be considered when recommending repair of asymptomatic aneurysms. Morbidity and mortality are higher than with abdominal aortic aneurysms; the 30-day operative mortality is 8–20% with repair of type 1 and type 2 thoracoabdominal aneurysms. The thoracotomy incision is associated with a higher risk of pulmonary complications and more challenging postoperative pain management. Proximity to the recurrent laryngeal nerve, the phrenic nerve, and the carotid and subclavian arteries makes injury to these structures possible. The great radicular artery (artery of Adamkiewicz) arises from an intercostal artery between T8 and L1 and is the dominant artery to the spinal cord in 80% of patients, imposing a 5–30% risk of paraplegia during thoracic aneurysm repair. Use of left heart bypass or femoral bypass to preserve retrograde perfusion below the level of the cross-clamp or antegrade perfusion by direct cannulation of selected arteries reduces end-organ ischemia. Lumbar drains, spinal cord cooling, naloxone infusion, and administration of corticosteroids are also described as techniques for spinal cord protection.

Endovascular repair of thoracic aortic aneurysms reduces cardiopulmonary risk, but the location of the aneurysm may preclude endovascular repair by current methods. Recent investigations involve development of branched stent grafts for repair of arch aneurysms.

Prognosis

Five-year survival for patients with unrepaired thoracic aneurysms greater than 6 cm is 20–25%. Most deaths are due to rupture or to the complications of generalized atherosclerosis.

Chuter TAM et al: Multi-branched stent-graft for type III thoracoabdominal aortic aneurysm. J Vasc Interv Radiol 2001; 12:391. [PMID: 11287522]

Griepp RB et al: Natural history of descending thoracic and thoracoabdominal aneurysms. Ann Thorac Surg 1999;67:1927. [PMID: 10391340]

Wada T et al: Prevention and detection of spinal cord injury during thoracic and thoracoabdominal aortic repairs. Ann Thorac Surg 2001;72:80. [PMID: 11465235]

PERIPHERAL ARTERY ANEURYSMS (Popliteal & Femoral)

Atherosclerosis is the main cause of nonmycotic femoral and popliteal aneurysms. Most lower extremity aneurysms occur in men over age 50. Half are bilateral. One-third of patients with popliteal aneurysms and one-half of those with femoral aneurysms have an associated aortoiliac aneurysm.

Popliteal Aneurysms

Popliteal aneurysms account for approximately 85% of all peripheral artery aneurysms. Symptoms are rarely due to rupture but result rather from arterial thrombosis, peripheral embolization, or compression of adjacent structures with resultant venous thrombosis or neuropathy. Arterial thrombosis can be limb-threatening if all outflow vessels are occluded, leading to amputation in up to 30% of patients.

Ultrasound is the diagnostic study of choice to measure the diameter of the aneurysm as well as to search for other arterial aneurysms. MRA or conventional arteriography is required to define the anatomy of the outflow arteries in preparation for operative repair.

Surgery is recommended for all asymptomatic aneurysms larger than 2 cm and for all symptomatic aneurysms regardless of size. If preoperative angiography reveals no patent distal vessels for bypass, catheter-directed thrombolysis can be attempted. If a patent outflow vessel is identified or is recanalized with thrombolytic therapy, a saphenous vein bypass graft with proximal and distal ligation of the aneurysm is performed. In large aneurysms producing popliteal vein or nerve compression, resection of the aneurysm in addition to grafting is required.

Femoral Aneurysms

Femoral aneurysms present as pulsatile groin masses. They have the potential for the same complications as popliteal aneurysms. Because the incidence of complications is lower than with popliteal aneurysms, patients with combined disease undergo repair of aortoiliac and popliteal aneurysms before repair of the femoral aneurysm.

Femoral pseudoaneurysms may result from injury produced by intravenous drug abuse, femoral artery puncture for angiography, or femoral line insertion. Mycotic aneurysms must be widely debrided with proximal and distal ligation or interposition grafting using autologous vein. Uninfected, small (< 5 cm) traumatic pseudoaneurysms can often be treated by ultrasound-guided compression of the neck of the aneurysm or by thrombin injection, which has a reported success rate of 90%. If these techniques are not successful, open repair is required. Pseudoaneurysms may also develop at the distal anastomosis of an aortofemoral bypass graft. They should be repaired if graft infection is suspected or if their diameter exceeds 2 cm.

Calton WC et al: Ultrasound-guided thrombin injection is a safe and durable treatment for femoral pseudoaneurysms. Vasc Surg 2001;35:379. [PMID: 11565042]

Dangas G et al: Vascular complications after percutaneous coronary interventions following hemostasis with manual compression versus arteriotomy closure devices. J Am Coll Cardiol 2001;38:638. [PMID: 11527609]

Diwan A et al: Incidence of femoral and popliteal artery aneurysms in patients with abdominal aortic aneurysms. J Vasc Surg 2000;31:863. [PMID: 10805875]

Steinmetz E et al: Preoperative intraarterial thrombolysis before surgical revascularization for popliteal artery aneurysm with acute ischemia. Ann Vasc Surg 2000;14:360. [PMID: 10943788]

VISCERAL ANEURYSMS

Mesenteric, Hepatic, and Splenic Artery Aneurysms

Historically, mesenteric aneurysms had a high mortality rate because of failures of diagnosis. High-resolution CT scanning has increased the capability to detect incidental mesenteric aneurysms and has broadened our understanding of the disease. In the last decade, hepatic artery aneurysms have become the most common of the visceral artery aneurysms, superseding splenic artery aneurysms, which now comprise less than 40% of the total. Superior mesenteric, celiac, gastric, and gastroepiploic artery aneurysms each represent about 5% of visceral aneurysms. Aneurysms of mesenteric branch vessels are rare and often associated with connective tissue disease or vasculitis.

Medial degeneration is the most commonly cited cause of hepatic aneurysms. Increasingly, however, injury during cholangiography, hepatic biopsy, or blunt abdominal trauma is implicated—particularly in intrahepatic aneurysms, which account for about half of all hepatic aneurysms. Splenic artery aneurysms are most commonly related to medial fibroplasia, though portal hypertension, splenomegaly, pregnancy, amphetamine use, and local inflammation (eg, pancreatitis) have all been implicated as possible risk factors. These aneurysms occur four times more frequently in women than in men, underscoring possible hormonal influences. Most superior mesenteric artery aneurysms are associated with infective endocarditis and suspected septic emboli. Atherosclerosis may play a role in the pathogenesis of celiac artery aneurysms—and a secondary role in development of other mesenteric aneurysms.

Surgical (aneurysmectomy or aneurysmorrhaphy with ligation of branches) or endovascular (embolization) management is warranted for symptomatic aneurysms and aneurysms over 2 cm in circumference. Asymptomatic splenic aneurysms less than 2 cm in diameter rarely rupture, and treatment is not generally advised unless the patient is pregnant since the highest risk of rupture is in young women during pregnancy.

Kasirajan K et al: Endovascular management of visceral artery aneurysm. J Endovasc Ther 2001;8:150. [PMID: 11357975]

O'Driscoll D et al: Hepatic artery aneurysm. Br J Radiol 1999;72:1018. [PMID: 10673957]

Renal Artery Aneurysms

Renal artery aneurysms have a reported incidence of about 1% in the adult population. Many are asymptomatic and diagnosed as an incidental finding on CT scan or angiography performed for another purpose. Others are found during evaluation for hematuria, renal infarct, flank pain, or suspected renovascular hypertension. Five percent present with rupture. Fibromuscular dysplasia is present in about 40% of patients; another 25% have atherosclerosis. Medial degeneration, trauma, and injury after renal biopsy or percutaneous nephrolithostomy are other potential causes. Indications for treatment include size greater than 2 cm, local symptoms, renovascular hypertension, distal embolization, growth on serial imaging, or aneurysms in women of childbearing age.

The standard surgical approach for renal artery aneurysms is excision with interposition grafting; infrequently, the aneurysm extends into the branch vessels, and ex vivo reconstruction may be required. Autologous and prosthetic materials have been equally effective for interposition grafting of main renal arteries greater than 5 mm in diameter, with a 5-year primary patency rate approaching 70%. Recently, polytetrafluoroethylene-covered stent grafts have been used for treatment of saccular aneurysms of the main renal artery. Interlobar aneurysms can be treated by endovascular embolization with microcoils.

Reiher L et al: Reconstruction for renal artery aneurysms and its effect on hypertension. Eur J Vasc Endovasc Surg 2000;20:454. [PMID: 11112464]

Rundback JH et al: Percutaneous stent-graft management of renal artery aneurysms. J Vasc Interv Radiol 2000;11:1189. [PMID: 11041477]

AORTIC DISSECTION

ESSENTIALS OF DIAGNOSIS

- *A history of hypertension or Marfan's syndrome is often present.*
- *Sudden severe chest pain with radiation to the back, occasionally migrating to the abdomen and hips.*
- *Patient appears to be in shock, but blood pressure is normal or elevated; pulse discrepancy in many patients.*
- *Acute aortic regurgitation may develop.*

General Considerations

Aortic dissection is the most common aortic catastrophe requiring admission to a hospital. It is caused by an intimal tear, which allows creation of a false lumen between the media and adventitia. Over 95% of intimal tears occur either in the ascending aorta just distal to the aortic valve (Stanford type A) or just distal to the left subclavian artery (Stanford type B). These are points where the aorta is fixed and allow for intimal injury during shear stress. The false lumen can rupture into the left pleural space, retroperitoneum, or abdominal cavity. More commonly, the dissection propagates distally to involve aortic branch vessels, producing acute spinal cord (3%), visceral (9%), renal (12%), or lower extremity (9%) ischemia. Antegrade extension of a type B dissection can stretch the aortic annulus or occlude a coronary artery orifice, producing acute aortic regurgitation, myocardial infarction, and intrapericardial rupture with tamponade. Both blood pressure and the rate of acceleration of pulsatile flow (dP/dt) are important in propagation of dissection; 80% of patients with acute dissection are hypertensive. Other risk factors for dissection are Marfan's syndrome, pregnancy, bicuspid aortic valve, and coarctation of the aorta.

When not appropriately diagnosed and treated, aortic dissection is a lethal disease. Untreated type A dissections are associated with 50% mortality at 48 hours and 90% mortality at 1 month—due to free rupture, tamponade, or acute left ventricular failure. Mortality with untreated type B dissection is 10–20%, usually secondary to free rupture into the pleural space, acute mesenteric ischemia, or renal failure.

Clinical Findings

A. SYMPTOMS AND SIGNS

Eighty-five percent of patients report sudden excruciating ("ripping") pain in the chest or upper back. The pain may radiate into the abdomen, neck, or groin. Most patients are hypertensive at presentation. Some present with syncope, hemiplegia, or lower extremity paralysis. On physical examination, peripheral pulses and blood pressures may be diminished or unequal. A diastolic murmur of aortic insufficiency may be heard.

B. LABORATORY FINDINGS

The ECG may be normal but often reveals left ventricular hypertrophy from long-standing hypertension. Acute ischemic changes suggest coronary artery involvement. Because dissections preferentially extend into the right coronary ostium, inferior wall abnormalities predominate.

C. IMAGING

Chest radiographs often reveal—in comparison with previous films—an abnormal aortic contour or a widened superior mediastinum. Pleural or pericardial effusion may be present. Dynamic CT scanning, angiography, MRI, and transesophageal echocardiography (TEE) have all been used to diagnose acute dissection. TEE is favored because of its high sensitivity (98%) and specificity (99%) and because it can be performed rapidly and at the bedside. The best initial study is the one most readily available that can be interpreted accurately in a given hospital setting. MRI has not played a major role in the initial diagnosis but is useful for serial follow-up.

Differential Diagnosis

Acute myocardial infarction, pulmonary embolus, esophageal disruption, strangulated paraesophageal hernia, mesenteric ischemia, and symptomatic aortic aneurysm may all be considered in the differential diagnosis of the patient presenting with acute aortic dissection.

Treatment

A. MEDICAL TREATMENT

Aggressive blood pressure control should be initiated immediately. The patient is placed at bed rest and given opioids for pain relief. An arterial line is placed for continuous blood pressure monitoring. Treatment is targeted to reductions in aortic pressure and pulsatile flow (dP/dt). This is accomplished by lowering systemic vascular resistance and cardiac output (primarily heart rate).

Systemic vascular resistance is reduced by means of a rapid-acting antihypertensive agent titrated by intravenous infusion to maintain a systolic blood pressure 100–120 mm Hg. Possible medications include nitroprusside (0.3–10 μg/kg/min), which causes direct vasodilation by its action on smooth muscle nitric oxide receptors; or fenoldopam (0.1–1.6 μg/kg/min), which acts as an agonist of D_1-dopamine receptors. When nitroprusside is continued for 48 hours or more, thiocyanate levels should be checked and the infusion stopped if the level is over 10 mg/dL (to avoid toxicity).

The heart rate is decreased by administering the selective β_1-adrenergic antagonist esmolol (50–300 μ/kg/min intravenously); by intermittent administration of metoprolol (5–10 mg intravenously every 15 minutes); or the α_1 and nonselective beta-antagonist labetalol (20–80 mg intravenously every 10 minutes or 1–2 mg/min).

Chronic medical management of aortic dissections involves use of a beta-antagonist (eg, metoprolol, 25–100 mg orally twice daily; atenolol, 50–100 mg orally daily), often in combination with another antihypertensive agent such as the centrally-acting α_2 agonist clonidine (0.1–0.3 mg orally twice daily or 0.1–0.3 mg transdermal patch topically every 24 hours) or the direct vasodilator hydralazine (10–50 mg orally four times daily), the calcium channel blocker amlodipine (2.5–10 mg orally daily), or the angiotensin-converting enzyme inhibitor enalapril, 2.5–20 mg orally daily).

B. SURGICAL TREATMENT

All patients with type A dissection should undergo emergent surgical repair. Most patients with type B dissection can be managed initially with aggressive drug therapy. Indications for surgical treatment of type B dissections are aortic rupture; severe intractable pain; mesenteric, renal, or limb ischemia; and progression of the dissection. For type A dissection, the ascending aorta and, if necessary, the aortic valve and arch are replaced with reimplantation of the coronary and brachiocephalic vessels. The mortality rate for such operations approaches 20%. Type B dissection with ischemic complications is treated by obliteration

of the false lumen and secondary arterial bypass if this fails to restore blood flow to the ischemic organs. Several different techniques have been described for obliteration of the false lumen: resection of the entry point of the dissection and prosthetic tube graft interposition, open or endovascular fenestration of the dissection flap, or stent graft deployment to cover the entry point. Use of felt strips or instillation of tissue glue into the false lumen during open repair are described as methods for strengthening the dissected aortic wall.

Surgical indications and risks for chronic type B dissections are the same as for degenerative thoracoabdominal aneurysms. Repair is considered in symptomatic patients or patients with aneurysms larger than 5 cm. Reported surgical mortality is 5–30%. For this reason, long-term medical management may be the preferred treatment for patients with significant comorbidities.

Prognosis

Because of comorbid illnesses, operative mortality of patients with type B dissection is twice that of patients with type A dissection. After hospital discharge, 5-year survival is 70–80% for repaired type A and 50–70% for repaired type B dissections. In some medically-treated type B dissections, the false lumen thromboses and eventually heals with minimal dilation. In others, a chronic dissection results in a progressively enlarging aneurysm requiring eventual repair in up to 30% of patients. For this reason, all unoperated patients should be followed with annual CT scan or MRI.

Beregi J-P et al: Endovascular treatment for dissection of the descending aorta. Lancet 2000;356:482. [PMID: 10981895]

Coady MA et al: Natural history, pathogenesis, and etiology of thoracic aortic aneurysms and dissections. Cardiol Clin 1999;17:615. [PMID: 10589336]

Dake MD et al: Endovascular stent-graft placement for the treatment of acute aortic dissection. N Engl J Med 1999; 340:1546. [PMID: 10332016]

Genoni M et al: Chronic beta-blocker therapy improves outcome and reduces treatment costs in chronic type B aortic dissection. Eur J Cardiothorac Surg 2001;19:606. [PMID: 11343940]

Hagan P et al: The international registry of acute aortic dissection (IRAD): New insights into an old disease. JAMA 2000; 283:897. [PMID: 10685714]

■ LOWER EXTREMITY OCCLUSIVE DISEASE

Occlusive disease of the lower extremities is a common cause of disability. It is also a predictor of cardiovascular morbidity and mortality; patients with intermittent claudication have a 2.5 times higher risk of cardiac events than that of an age-matched population. Severe triple-vessel coronary artery disease is found in almost

30% of patients undergoing routine coronary catheterization prior to peripheral bypass. Vascular endothelial dysfunction may be a systemic phenomenon and a marker for atherosclerosis; impairment of flow-mediated dilation in the peripheral arteries has been shown to correlate with the presence of coronary artery disease. It is essential for the primary care clinician to emphasize prevention of disease, particularly in light of what is known about etiologic factors.

DeBakey first characterized the distribution of atherosclerotic disease in the lower extremity. Plaque formation predominates at the aortic bifurcation, at the tibial trifurcation, and in the superficial femoral artery at the adductor hiatus. Interestingly, occlusive disease often spares the internal iliac, profunda, and peroneal arteries. Three distinct patterns of disease have since been described. Type 1 disease affects about 10–15% of patients and is limited to the aorta and common iliac arteries. It is most commonly found in younger men and women (ages 40–55) who are heavy smokers or who have hyperlipidemia. Type 2 disease (25% of patients) involves the aorta, the common iliac artery, and the external iliac artery. Type 3 disease is the most common (60–70% of patients) and is multilevel disease, affecting the aorta and the iliac, femoral, popliteal, and tibial arteries. Patients with type 2 and type 3 patterns of disease have typical risk factors for atherosclerosis: older age, male gender, diabetes, and hypertension. They also have a high incidence of coexisting cerebrovascular and coronary artery disease.

Clinical Findings

A. SYMPTOMS AND SIGNS

Lower extremity occlusive disease is manifested by several different clinical presentations: impotence, claudication, rest pain, and gangrene. The symptoms and physical examination predict the location and severity of disease. Occlusive disease of the iliac arteries can produce male erectile dysfunction. The triad of bilateral hip and buttock claudication, erectile dysfunction, and absent femoral pulses is known as Leriche's syndrome.

Claudication is characterized by pain, numbness, or weakness in the calves, thighs, or buttocks brought on by walking and completely relieved after a few minutes of rest. These reproducible symptoms help to differentiate claudication from other causes of leg pain such as radiculopathy and musculoskeletal disorders. Ischemic rest pain, defined as pain in the absence of exertion, is usually described as a nocturnal pain located across the dorsum of the foot at the metatarsal heads. It is ameliorated by placing the legs in the dependent position, usually by hanging them over the side of the bed. Rest pain implies impending or gangrene.

Examination of the pulses indicates the level of disease. Absent or weak femoral pulses or the presence of an iliac or femoral bruit suggests inflow disease. Similarly, normal femoral pulses but a diminished or ab-

sent popliteal pulse is indicative of superficial femoral artery stenosis; and normal femoral and popliteal pulses and nonpalpable dorsalis pedis or posterior tibial pulse indicate tibial disease. An ankle-brachial index (ABI) is useful in gauging the degree of arterial insufficiency. A normal ratio of ankle to brachial systolic blood pressures is 1.0; less than 0.8 is consistent with claudication. Exercise, which lowers the ABI by exaggerating the difference in brachial and ankle blood pressures, can sometimes aid in detection of occlusive disease. Rest pain and nonhealing ulcers are common with an ABI less than 0.4. A toe-brachial index (TBI) can be used in diabetic or renal failure patients when an ABI cannot be obtained because the tibial arteries are calcified and noncompressible. A penile-brachial index (PBI) is obtained when vasogenic impotence is suspected. A PBI less than 0.6 suggests significant arterial disease. These measurements can also be used to monitor progression of disease and to assess the effect of therapeutic intervention.

Other findings on physical examination include atrophy of the skin, subcutaneous tissues, and muscles of the calf. Dependent rubor, hair loss, and coolness of the skin are signs of advanced ischemia. Ulcers from arterial occlusive disease are painful, well-circumscribed lesions generally located over pressure points, such as the first metatarsal head or heel. Ulcers that have failed to heal with 3 months of appropriate local wound care and ulcers associated with an ABI less than 0.3 are unlikely to heal without treatment to improve arterial blood flow and tissue perfusion.

B. IMAGING

Angiography demonstrates the extent of the disease and the condition of the distal target vessels for potential bypass operation. The standard study images the infrarenal aorta and iliacs (including oblique views of the pelvis and groin to visualize the origins of the hypogastric and profunda arteries), the runoff vessels, and the foot in a lateral position. Angiography is undertaken only for percutaneous treatment or in preparation for surgical intervention. Gadolinium-enhanced MRA and duplex ultrasound are noninvasive imaging modalities occasionally used in evaluation of lower extremity occlusive disease, particularly in workup of popliteal occlusion and in identification of tibial target vessels poorly visualized by conventional angiography. Ultrasound is also used in routine follow-up of infrainguinal bypass grafts to screen for graft stenoses amenable to prophylactic angioplasty. Radiographs of the lower leg and foot are often obtained to rule out osteomyelitis underlying an infected ulcer or to identify calcification of potential runoff vessels.

Treatment

A. CONSERVATIVE MEASURES

Treatment of claudication begins with identification and control of risk factors and initiation of an exercise program. Tobacco cessation slows the rate of progression of arterial occlusive disease and reduces cardiovascular mortality. Lipid-lowering medications have been shown to produce a 40% risk reduction for new-onset claudication or worsening of claudication. A supervised, dedicated walking program sustained over 3–6 months has been shown to increase pain-free walking distance by as much as 150%. Exercise improves symptoms by increasing muscle anaerobic metabolism rather than by increasing collateral flow as previously thought; the ABI does not change appreciably. A standard program is structured as a 30-minute daily session: walking along flat ground until discomfort occurs, resting until it subsides, and then resuming walking.

Some medications are available for use in the treatment of claudication. Pentoxifylline (400 mg orally three times daily), which theoretically works by causing deformation of red blood cells, has been used with variable therapeutic success. More recently, the phosphodiesterase inhibitor cilostazol (100 mg orally twice daily), which impairs platelet aggregation and increases calcium-mediated vasodilation, has been shown to increase walking distance by 34% more than placebo. It is contraindicated in patients with heart failure and is not well tolerated in about 20% of patients due to side effects of headache, dizziness, and diarrhea. Propionyl-L-carnitine (1000 mg orally twice daily) has also been correlated with increased walking distance in patients with claudication. Its mechanism of action is unknown; it may improve skeletal muscle metabolism. Ginkgo biloba extract (120 mg/d) is a herbal medication with some reported benefit in claudication (see Chapter 44). It has been correlated with an increased risk of bleeding and so should be used with caution in patients on anticoagulation. Aspirin (325 mg orally daily) is routinely prescribed for all patients who do not have drug allergy or intolerance. It is continued indefinitely after angioplasty or surgery in order to decrease thrombotic complications and impede progression of intimal hyperplasia. Clopidogrel (75 mg orally daily) or warfarin (dosed to maintain an INR of 2.0–3.0) may be selected for postoperative patients perceived to have a higher risk of graft thrombosis due to a hypercoagulable state, suboptimal conduit, or poor distal runoff.

Treatment of male erectile dysfunction requires evaluation of its possible causes (medications, diabetes mellitus, psychogenic factors, and arterial occlusive disease). Iliac artery revascularization can be beneficial in some cases of vasculogenic impotence. Other patients may respond to sildenafil, 25–50 mg 30 minutes to 4 hours prior to sexual activity. It is contraindicated in patients taking nitroglycerin because of the risk of myocardial ischemia due to hypotension (see Chapter 23).

B. SURGERY

Percutaneous or open operation is considered for good-risk patients with short-distance (less than two blocks) claudication that impairs their ability to work or perform activities of daily living. Development of rest pain or tissue loss indicates progression of disease and also warrants evaluation for possible surgery.

Because many of these patients have coexisting ischemic heart disease, medical management should be optimized preoperatively. The roles of exercise testing and coronary angiography are discussed in Chapter 3 and Chapter 10. The carotid arteries should be imaged by ultrasound; endarterectomy may be indicated to minimize perioperative stroke risk.

1. Endovascular techniques—Common iliac artery stenoses are often amenable to percutaneous treatment. Stent angioplasty has been shown to decrease recurrence rates seen with angioplasty alone; most recent studies report a 70–80% 3-year patency rate with self-expanding (Wall) stents or balloon-expandable (Palmaz) stents. Stenting of distal lesions (external iliac or infrainguinal arteries) is not as successful, with reported 3-year primary patency rates of 55–60%. Stents do not appear to confer added benefits over angioplasty alone for femoral-popliteal lesions except in cases of postangioplasty arterial dissection or successfully recanalized short-segment arterial occlusion. Ideal lesions for angioplasty are discrete, short-segment (< 5 cm in length), concentric lesions in noncalcified large-diameter vessels. Often, endovascular techniques are used in conjunction with surgery for treatment of multifocal lower extremity occlusive disease such as an iliac stent being placed at the time of an ipsilateral femoral popliteal bypass. Some surgeons are evaluating long-segment closed superficial femoral artery endarterectomy combined with distal stenting as an alternative to femoral popliteal bypass in high-risk surgical patients with suboptimal vein available for bypass conduit. Few groups have achieved favorable results with percutaneous atherectomy devices or laser probes.

2. Open surgery—Aortobifemoral bypass grafting using a synthetic prosthesis is the standard treatment for complex aortoiliac occlusive disease. In general, a bifurcated polytetrafluoroethylene or Dacron graft is anastomosed end-to-end with the infrarenal abdominal aorta and end-to-side to each common femoral artery. If both external iliac arteries are occluded, an end-to-side aortic anastomosis preserves inflow into the internal iliac arteries. For high-risk patients, an axillary-femoral or femoral-femoral bypass graft can be considered, though such extra-anatomic grafts have lower long-term patency than bypass grafting (50% versus 80% at 10 years).

For infrainguinal occlusive disease, the bypass conduit of choice is autogenous greater saphenous vein. Five-year patency rates of 75–80% can be achieved with vein bypasses to the dorsalis pedis artery or the posterior tibial artery at the ankle. By contrast, the 5-year patency of femoral-tibial bypasses performed with synthetic conduit is less than 40%. Some surgeons prefer prosthetic graft for femoral-to-above-knee-popliteal artery bypasses, as the reported long-term patency in this position is almost equivalent to that of vein graft. Others maintain an "all autogenous" policy for all infrainguinal bypass grafts. In as many as 30% of patients, the greater saphenous vein is inadequate because it is sclerotic, thrombosed, or less than 3 mm in diameter or because the patient has undergone varicose vein stripping or saphenous vein harvesting for coronary artery bypass or previous leg bypass. Alternative conduits in these patients include lesser saphenous vein, arm vein, cryopreserved homologous vein, or prosthetic graft with a distal vein cuff.

Other determinants of long-term graft patency include quality of arterial inflow, patency of runoff arteries, and length of the bypass conduit. It is imperative to address any flow-limiting aortoiliac disease before performing any infrainguinal bypass.

Thomboendarterectomy involves resecting the thickened intima and media from the diseased vessel and is an alternative to bypass for short-segment lesions in larger arteries. It can be used in type 1 disease to obviate the need for prosthetic graft. Common femoral or profunda femoral thromboendarterectomy is combined with distal bypass to improve inflow.

Lumbar sympathectomy, once a common procedure, is now reserved for symptomatic patients with unreconstructable disease. Hyperbaric oxygen has also achieved successful healing of ischemic ulcers in selected patients who are not candidates for revascularization.

Operative mortality is 2–5% for open aortic surgery and 1–3% for infrainguinal bypass, largely attributable to cardiac complications. Risks specific to aortic surgery include renal insufficiency, bowel ischemia, impotence or retrograde ejaculation, and blue toe syndrome secondary to distal emboli. Late complications include graft thrombosis, graft infection, and aortoduodenal fistula. Particular concerns of percutaneous techniques include puncture site complications (hematoma, pseudoaneurysm, arteriovenous fistula, retroperitoneal hemorrhage, occlusion), dissection or rupture of the vessel during angioplasty, distal emboli from catheter manipulation, and contrast nephropathy. Patients with chronic renal insufficiency (serum creatinine > 1.5 mg/dL) undergoing angiography may be pretreated with intravenous hydration and acetylcysteine, 400 mg orally twice daily for 48 hours before and after contrast administration.

Prognosis

Twenty-five percent of patients with claudication will eventually develop ischemic rest pain or ulceration, though fewer than 10% will require amputation. In part, the high rate of limb salvage reflects a high mortality rate from comorbid disease. Because of coronary artery disease, patients with claudication have a 5-year survival of 50%. For this reason, operation is generally deferred until failure of medical management, impair-ment of activities of daily living, or clear progression of disease is documented. Almost 80% of patients with mild to moderate claudication will have relatively stable symptoms and will go for years without much progression. Some may improve as collateral circulation develops.

The overall 5-year patency rate for infrainguinal saphenous vein grafts is 60–80%. Higher graft patency and limb salvage rates are achieved with suprageniculate bypasses and with patients presenting with claudication rather than rest pain or gangrene. Graft occlusion may convert a patient with claudication to one with limb-threatening ischemia because of loss of collateral flow. Conversely, a diabetic with sensory deficit from peripheral neuropathy who undergoes bypass for distal gangrene may have a clinically silent graft occlusion after the ulcer heals. Surveillance duplex ultrasound is advised at 6-month intervals to detect stenotic, or "threatened," grafts before they progress to occlusion.

Conte MS et al: Impact of increasing comorbidity on infrainguinal reconstruction: A 20-year perspective. Ann Surg 2000;233:445. [PMID: 11224635]

Hiatt WR: Medical treatment of peripheral arterial disease and claudication. N Engl J Med 2001;344:1608. [PMID: 11372014]

Hirsch AT et al: Peripheral arterial disease detection, awareness, and treatment in primary care. JAMA 2001;286:1317. [PMID: 11560536]

Jensen J et al: Prevalence and etiology of impotence in 101 male hypertensive outpatients. Am J Hypertens 1999;12:271. [PMID: 10192229]

Kuvin JT et al: Peripheral vascular endothelial function testing as a noninvasive indicator of coronary artery disease. J Am Coll Cardiol 2001;38:1843. [PMID: 11743920]

Muradin GSR et al: Balloon dilation and stent implantation for treatment of femoropopliteal arterial disease: Meta-analysis. Radiology 2001;221:137. [PMID: 11568332]

Ouriel K: Peripheral arterial disease. Lancet 2001;358:1257. [PMID: 11675083]

UNUSUAL CAUSES OF POPLITEAL ARTERY OCCLUSION

The most common cause of popliteal artery occlusion is athero-occlusive disease. Thrombosis of a popliteal aneurysm can also cause popliteal occlusion and acute leg ischemia. Claudication in a young, athletic individual with no risk factors for atherosclerosis and normal pulses on the unaffected leg suggests popliteal entrapment syndrome, popliteal adventitial cystic disease, trauma, or extrinsic compression by a Baker cyst.

Popliteal entrapment syndrome is a group of anatomic anomalies that lead to arterial compression in the popliteal space. Type 1 (20% of patients) is produced by an abnormal course of the popliteal artery, passing medial to the medial head of the gastrocnemius muscle. Type 2 (25%) is caused by medial insertion of the medial head of the gastrocnemius muscle,

The popliteal artery is compressed by an abnormal accessory slip of gastrocnemius muscle in type 3 (30%) or popliteus muscle in type 4 (8%). Almost 30% of patients have bilateral disease. Claudication symptoms may be atypical, such as pain with walking but not with running. Diagnosis is made by MRA or by positional angiography; the patent artery becomes impinged with passive dorsiflexion or active plantar flexion of the ankle. Treatment is surgical and involves transection of the abnormal muscle; if the artery is occluded, short-segment bypass with greater or lesser saphenous vein is also required.

Popliteal adventitial disease is a rare disorder of unknown cause characterized by formation of cysts within the wall of the popliteal artery. The cysts compress the arterial lumen, causing stenosis or occlusion. Their contents resemble synovial fluid, and some may be in continuity with the joint space. The disease most often affects healthy men 40–50 years of age. Larger cysts are amenable to ultrasound-guided aspiration, but most are small and appear only as a thickening of the popliteal artery wall on MRA. In these cases, bypass or interposition grafting is curative.

Lambert AW et al: Popliteal artery entrapment syndrome. Br J Surg 1999;86:1365. [PMID: 10583279]

Levien LJ et al: Adventitial cystic disease: a unifying hypothesis. J Vasc Surg 1998;28:193. [PMID: 9719314]

OCCLUSIVE CEREBROVASCULAR DISEASE

Every year, half a million people in the United States suffer a stroke. Fifteen to 30 percent of these episodes are fatal, making stroke the third leading cause of death in this country. Initially, hypoperfusion of the brain secondary to high-grade carotid stenosis or occlusion was thought to be the cause of stroke. However, carotid thromboendarterectomy (TEA) performed in awake patients revealed that only 10–15% of patients become symptomatic during carotid occlusion by cross-clamping. Most neurologic events are in fact caused by emboli occluding small cerebral arteries. Emboli from the carotid bifurcation may consist of platelet aggregates that form on irregular or ulcerated surfaces or plaque debris liberated by turbulent flow and intraplaque hemorrhage. Less commonly (fewer than 10% of cases), emboli arise from the heart (eg, mural thrombus or atrial myxoma) or from the aortic arch. Stroke can also be caused by intracerebral hemorrhage (from trauma or a ruptured cerebral aneurysm) or by small vessel occlusive disease in the pons, basal ganglia, and internal capsule of the brain (lacunar infarcts).

A transient ischemic attack (TIA) is defined as the sudden onset of a neurologic deficit that resolves completely within 24 hours. A stroke is a neurologic deficit that persists beyond 24 hours. A single TIA is associated with a 30% risk of subsequent stroke.

Risk of neurologic events increases with the degree of carotid artery stenosis. For stenoses less than 60%, risk of stroke is 1.6% per year; this doubles for stenoses over 60%. At 80% stenosis, the annual ipsilateral stroke risk is 5–10%. Increased stroke risk is also associated with rapid progression of carotid disease and with plaque heterogeneity or ulceration. Risk factors for carotid disease include hypertension, diabetes mellitus, hypercholesterolemia, advanced age, smoking, and coronary artery disease.

Clinical Findings

A. SYMPTOMS

Typical manifestations of carotid artery occlusive disease include contralateral weakness or sensory loss, expressive aphasia, and amaurosis fugax (transient partial or complete loss of vision in the ipsilateral eye). Vertebrobasilar TIAs are characterized by brain stem and cerebellar symptoms, including dysarthria, diplopia, vertigo, ataxia, and hemiparesis or quadriparesis.

Dizziness and unsteadiness, particularly when associated with a quick change in position, are nonspecific symptoms and more often the result of postural hypotension than of vertebrobasilar insufficiency. Atypical neurologic symptoms, personality changes, and dementia are not typical symptoms of carotid disease.

B. SIGNS

Occlusive disease of the brachiocephalic arteries may be accompanied by cervical bruits, diminished or absent pulses in the neck or arms, Hollenhorst plaques (bright, refractile cholesterol emboli) in the retinal arteries, or a blood pressure difference between the two arms of more than 10 mm Hg. The common carotid pulsation can be examined qualitatively by palpation at the base of the neck. The presence of superficial temporal artery pulsation confirms patency of the ipsilateral external carotid artery. A carotid bruit is a high-pitched, blowing noise sharply localized high in the lateral neck close to the angle of the mandible. Heart sounds must be auscultated to make certain that the bruit is not caused by a referred murmur of aortic stenosis. Only 30% of patients with cervical bruits have carotid stenosis greater than 60%. The absence of a bruit also does not preclude the possibility of a hemodynamically significant lesion—thus, bruits are neither sensitive nor specific for carotid occlusive disease. In fact, asymptomatic carotid bruits are stronger predictors of death from coronary artery disease than of death from stroke.

IMAGING STUDIES

Duplex ultrasonography has become the study of choice for evaluation of carotid occlusive disease. It provides both physiologic and anatomic information. Percent stenosis is derived from measurement of blood flow velocities, with sensitivity and specificity greater than 90%. Ultrasound also provides some characterization of the plaque itself, including its location and the presence of calcification, ulceration, and intraplaque hemorrhage. Patients with adequate ultrasound studies may be offered surgery without further imaging. Patients with suboptimal ultrasound studies or in whom intracranial tandem lesions are suspected are referred for gadolinium-enhanced magnetic resonance angiography, which provides more detailed information about plaque composition and characterizes the intracranial circulation and the brain parenchyma. When compared with en bloc resected specimens, correlation of percent stenosis is better with ultrasound and MRA than with conventional angiography. This can be explained by the fact that MRA and ultrasound both produce cross-sectional imaging of vessels whose stenotic regions may be eccentric. Symptomatic patients with ipsilateral carotid occlusion by ultrasound should be referred for conventional or CT angiography before electing nonoperative management because a small percentage of these patients will have an internal carotid artery "string sign" and should be revascularized. Catheter angiography carries a 1% risk of procedure-related stroke and is reserved for patients with greatly disparate ultrasound and MRA findings, those suspected of vertebrobasilar insufficiency or intracranial lesions unable to undergo MRA, and those potentially requiring endovascular intervention. As ultrasound is highly operator-dependent, MRA is highly equipment-dependent; selection of the most accurate imaging modality may vary by institution.

Treatment

A. Medical Measures

Acute or evolving strokes and strokes associated with major neurologic deficits are initially managed medically, delaying surgery for 5–8 weeks until the deficit is stable, as discussed in the section on cerebrovascular accidents in Chapter 24. Patients with transient ischemic attacks may be treated with an oral antiplatelet medication (aspirin, 325 mg daily; ticlopidine, 250 mg twice daily; or clopidogrel, 75 mg twice daily) to reduce the likelihood of thrombosis and microemboli. However, if the attacks are of increasing frequency, the patient is admitted and placed on a heparin drip while being evaluated for surgery. Postoperatively, most patients are maintained on aspirin indefinitely to reduce the incidence of thrombosis or recurrent disease in the newly endarterectomized vessel.

For patients in whom neurologic symptoms are thought to be secondary to intracerebral disease not amenable to surgical reconstruction, warfarin or clopidogrel may be indicated.

B. Surgery

1. Transient ischemic attacks and stroke—Carotid endarterectomy plus optimal drug therapy and risk factor modification are highly effective in preventing stroke and death in symptomatic patients with carotid stenosis greater than 70%—as demonstrated by the North American Symptomatic Carotid Endarterectomy Trial (NASCET). A more modest risk:benefit ratio has been demonstrated for carotid endarterectomy in symptomatic 50–69% stenoses. Surgical success is maximized when preoperative symptoms are related to ischemia of the ipsilateral hemisphere and when the surgery is done by a vascular surgeon who performs carotid endarterectomies regularly with a mortality-complication rate less than 5%. Placement of a temporary carotid shunt during surgery allows cerebral perfusion during cross-clamping; however, the shunt may increase the technical complexity of the operation. Indications for intraoperative shunting vary by surgeon. Most surgeons shunt patients with previous stroke; some selectively shunt for a measured stump pressure (internal carotid back pressure) under 50 mm Hg or for patients with EEG changes; and others shunt all patients.

2. Asymptomatic carotid stenosis—Approximately 5% of patients per year with asymptomatic carotid stenosis greater than 80% suffer a stroke. This statistic helps form the basis for the American Heart Association's recommendation of upper limits of acceptable combined morbidity and mortality for carotid endarterectomy: 3% for asymptomatic patients, 5–7% for those with TIAs or stroke, and 10% for those with recurrent carotid stenosis. The Asymptomatic Carotid Artery Stenosis (ACAS) trial demonstrated that in good-risk asymptomatic patients with greater than 60% stenosis, surgery afforded an overall risk reduction of 53% over aspirin alone. These findings are supported by a smaller Veterans Administration Hospital study of patients with asymptomatic carotid artery stenosis. Most vascular surgeons offer surgery to asymptomatic patients with greater than 80% stenosis in the ipsilateral carotid artery.

3. Percutaneous techniques—Patients who are not good candidates for surgery because of medical comorbidities can be considered for carotid angioplasty and stenting. This option is also explored in patients with a history of previous neck surgery or irradiation, in whom there is a higher risk of cranial nerve injury because of fibrosis and scarring. Stenting has also recently been shown to be safe and effective treatment for immediate postoperative stroke, particularly when the neurologic event is due to dissection of the vessel. Carotid stenting is associated with a 5–18% risk of periprocedural stroke or transient ischemic attack, which is not significantly improved with various cerebral protection devices, and an 8–14% per year incidence of recurrent stenosis (compared with less than 4% per year with surgery). This makes it a seldom-favored approach for most carotid disease.

Prognosis

Prognosis is related to the difficulty of surgery and the collateral flow in the circle of Willis. Surgery carries a reported average 1–2% mortality rate and a 1–4% risk of neurologic complication, though wide institutional variation exists. In symptomatic patients, endarterectomy reduces stroke risk fivefold to tenfold at 5 years. The 5–15% incidence of late stroke after uncomplicated endarterectomy is often related to contralateral carotid or intracranial disease.

Restenosis occurring less than 2 years after carotid endarterectomy is usually not symptomatic because it is due to intimal hyperplasia, which produces a smooth, nonfriable luminal surface. These lesions respond well to angioplasty and stenting, and the risk of procedural neurologic events is lower than for atherosclerotic lesions. After 2 years, restenosis is more often related to progression of atherosclerotic disease. These lesions can be friable and prone to intraplaque hemorrhage, just like the original plaque. In general, repeat surgery or stenting is advised for symptomatic restenoses or stenoses greater than 80%.

Barnett HJM et al: Causes and severity of ischemic stroke in patients with internal carotid artery stenosis. JAMA 2000; 283:1429. [PMID: 10732932]

Endovascular versus surgical treatment in patients with carotid stenosis in the Carotid and Vertebral Artery Transluminal Angioplasty Study (CAVATAS): A randomised trial. Lancet 2001;357:1729. [PMID: 11403808]

La Biche R et al: Presence of *Chlamydia pneumonia* in human symptomatic and asymptomatic carotid atherosclerotic plaque. Stroke 2001;32:855. [PMID: 11283382]

Rapp J et al: Atheroemboli to the brain: Size threshold for causing acute neuronal cell death. J Vasc Surg 2000;32:68. [PMID: 10876208]

Sacco RL: Extracranial carotid stenosis. N Engl J Med 2001; 345:1113. [PMID: 11596592]

OTHER DISEASES OF THE CAROTID ARTERY

Carotid Dissection

Carotid dissection is a false channel in the wall of the carotid artery produced by a tear in the intima. The classic triad of symptoms is unilateral neck pain or headache, stroke or transient ischemic attack, and an incomplete Horner syndrome (miosis and ptosis without anhidrosis). Dissections can be spontaneous or traumatic, caused by shearing of the internal carotid artery between the C2 and C3 transverse processes during deceleration injuries such as car accidents, wrestling, chiropractic maneuvers, and "head-banging" dancing. The primary treatment of dissection is medical. With warfarin anticoagulation (to an INR of 2.0–3.0), 60–85% of carotid dissections will heal in 3–6 months with complete or near-complete neurologic recovery. Recurrent dissection is estimated at 3% at 3 years and 12% at 10 years and most often involves a different cervical vessel, which justifies the use of long-term aspirin. Surgery (usually carotid interposition) or carotid stenting is indicated for ongoing symptoms with residual stenosis or aneurysm.

Carotid Body Tumors

The carotid body is a chemoreceptor derived from embryonic neural crest cells located at the carotid bifurcation. Carotid body tumors (also called paraganglionomas or chemodectomas) are rare and usually present as painless neck masses. Most of these tumors are slow-growing and benign, but lymph node metastases have been reported. If untreated, they are locally invasive; a large tumor may cause vagus or hypoglossal nerve deficit from mass effect or may encircle the internal carotid artery to the skull base. The tumor is hypervascular and splays the internal and external carotid arteries, giving it a classic angiographic appearance of a tumor blush in the center of a widened carotid bifurcation. Biopsy is contraindicated; diagnosis is made by angiography or MRA. Preoperative angiography for tumor embolization and test occlusion of the internal carotid artery are advised for tumors over 4 cm in diameter. Using the same approach as for carotid endarterectomy, the tumor is resected off the carotid artery, with care to preserve the artery wall adventitia. Many small arteries arising from the external and internal carotid arteries supply the tumor and must be individually ligated. The incidence of cranial nerve injury with resection of large tumors approaches 40%. Prognosis after complete resection is excellent, with survival equal to that of age-matched controls and long-term recurrence of 6%.

Carotid Artery Aneurysms

Carotid aneurysms are much more common in the intracerebral than in the cervical portion of the carotid arteries. Most often, cervical aneurysms arise in the common carotid artery and are fusiform; these are associated with atherosclerosis. Traumatic aneurysms can be related to healing of an internal carotid dissection or to penetrating trauma. Mycotic aneurysms can be caused by staphylococcal, *Escherichia coli,* or tuberculous infections. Many other vasculitides are associated with carotid aneurysms, such as Behçet's disease, Takayasu's disease, fibromuscular dysplasia, and segmental arterial mediolysis. Anytime a mass in the neck is pulsatile, an aneurysm should be considered and diagnosis confirmed by angiography. Other symptoms include neck pain, cranial nerve dysfunction, and transient ischemic attack or stroke. Surgery should be considered for aneurysms resulting from penetrating trauma, aneurysms associated with neurologic deficit, mycotic aneurysms, and aneurysms over 2 cm in diameter. Primary repair of the artery may be accomplished for most penetrating injuries. Carotid resection and interposition grafting or simple carotid ligation is performed for most other aneurysms.

Hertzer NR: Extracranial carotid aneurysms: A new look at an old problem. J Vasc Surg 2000;31:823. [PMID: 10753296]

van der May AG et al: Management of carotid body tumors. Otolaryngol Clin North Am 2001;34:907. [PMID: 11557446]

VISCERAL ARTERY INSUFFICIENCY

Chronic intestinal ischemia results from atherosclerotic occlusive lesions at the origins of the superior mesenteric, celiac, and inferior mesenteric arteries. Because of collateral flow via the marginal artery of

Drummond, the pancreaticoduodenal arteries, and the hemorrhoidal arteries, bowel ischemia does not occur until two of the three main visceral arteries are severely diseased. In fact, almost 30% of patients with peripheral vascular disease have asymptomatic occlusive disease of the mesenteric arteries. Symptoms consist of epigastric or periumbilical postprandial pain, often accompanied by bloating or diarrhea and, at later stages, food avoidance (sitophobia), resulting in weight loss. Chronic intestinal ischemia is usually a diagnosis of exclusion, derived after a negative work-up for peptic ulcer disease, gastroesophageal reflux, pancreatitis, irritable bowel syndrome, and malignancy. A suggestive history in a person over 45 years of age who appears chronically ill, has risk factors for arterial occlusive disease, and has no other identifiable cause for abdominal symptoms is an indication for arteriography. Intravenous hydration must be provided to avoid acute bowel ischemia from catheter-induced or contrast-associated arterial spasm. Surgical or endovascular management is directed toward restoration of antegrade visceral arterial flow. Transaortic endarterectomy and mesenteric artery bypass are associated with a 5–9% mortality rate and a 10–25% recurrence rate at long-term follow-up. A higher recurrence rate is observed with stenting of short-segment lesions; these patients require routine angiographic follow-up. Perioperative nutritional supplementation is essential to the successful management of these patients.

Celiac axis compression syndrome (stenosis of the celiac artery caused by external compression of the arcuate ligament) has been described as a variant of chronic mesenteric ischemia. As an isolated entity, it is occasionally associated with cramping abdominal pain, nausea, vomiting, and diarrhea. Division of the arcuate ligament may be combined with mesenteric reconstruction for multivessel occlusive disease, but it is seldom performed as an isolated procedure, because of poorly defined symptoms and variable postoperative result.

Acute intestinal ischemia may result from (1) embolic occlusion of a visceral branch of the abdominal aorta, generally in patients with mitral valvular disease, atrial fibrillation, or left ventricular mural thrombus; (2) thrombosis of an atherosclerotic mesenteric vessel; or (3) low flow or shock state due to cardiac failure or arterial spasm induced by ergot or cocaine intoxication; or (4) postcoarctectomy syndrome, producing nonocclusive mesenteric vascular insufficiency. Emboli are responsible for almost half of all cases. Symptoms include sudden onset of severe epigastric and periumbilical abdominal pain with minimal appreciable findings on abdominal examination ("pain out of proportion to physical findings") and a high leukocyte count. Lactic acidosis, hypotension, and abdominal distention indicate bowel infarction. Mortality approaches 80% despite aggressive surgical management.

Visceral angiography can be performed in the stable patient; duplex ultrasound is of less diagnostic value in this setting. Mesenteric thrombosis causes occlusion at the origin of the vessel, while emboli most often lodge within the superior mesenteric artery at the first jejunal branch. In hypoperfusion-related mesenteric ischemia, the vessels are pruned but patent. Angiography also allows delivery of catheter-directed therapy: thrombolytics (alteplase, 0.5–1 mg/h) for thrombotic disease or vasodilators (papaverine, 30–60 mg/h) for nonocclusive disease. Broad-spectrum antibiotics are administered to all patients. Embolic disease, acidosis, hemodynamic instability, or severe or progressive abdominal pain mandate emergent laparotomy. Mesenteric flow is first reestablished with thromboembolectomy or bypass, and the bowel resection margins are then determined by gross inspection or examination with fluorescein. A second-look operation is planned if any bowel is of questionable viability at the close of the case.

Mesenteric vein occlusion is responsible for 5–15% of cases of acute mesenteric ischemia. Risk factors include hypercoagulable state (malignancy; protein C, protein S, or antithrombin III deficiency; presence of anticardiolipin or antiphospholipid antibody, polycythemia vera), intra-abdominal sepsis, previous splenectomy or portal angiography or sclerotherapy, portal hypertension, and cirrhosis. Diagnosis is made by contrast-enhanced abdominal CT scan or arterial portography. Patients should be treated with long-term anticoagulation. Surgery is reserved for those suspected of having bowel infarction and consists of bowel resection and occasionally venous thrombectomy. In some cases, percutaneous transhepatic administration of thrombolytics has been successful.

Ischemic colitis can develop as a result of acute or chronic colonic ischemia and is characterized by bouts of crampy lower abdominal pain and mild—often bloody—diarrhea. This picture may be indistinguishable from inflammatory bowel disease. Colonoscopy reveals segmental inflammatory changes, most prominent in the watershed areas of the rectosigmoid junction and splenic flexure. Conservative management is usually adequate. Surgery may be indicated for progressive symptoms or stricture formation.

Kasirajan K et al: Chronic mesenteric ischemia: Open surgery versus percutaneous angioplasty and stenting. J Vasc Surg 2001;33:63. [PMID: 11137925]

Klotz S et al: Diagnosis and treatment of nonocclusive mesenteric ischemia after open heart surgery. Ann Thorac Surg 2001; 72:1583. [PMID: 11722048]

RENAL ARTERY STENOSIS

Renal artery stenosis is produced predominantly by atherosclerotic occlusive disease (80–90% of patients) or fibromuscular dysplasia (10–15% of patients). Characteristically, patients with occlusive disease have common risk factors for atherosclerosis, and their lesions are focal proximal or ostial calcific plaques, often described as "spillover" aortic disease. Patients with fibromuscular dysplasia tend to be women 30–50 years of age with distal renal artery disease that often extends into the branch vessels in a classic "string of beads" pattern of alternating stenoses and dilations.

Renal artery stenosis has two important clinical manifestations: renovascular hypertension and ischemic nephropathy. Renovascular hypertension accounts for only about 5% of all cases of hypertension. In certain subsets of patients, the incidence is much higher. Seventy percent of patients over 60 years of age with diastolic blood pressure greater than 105 mm Hg and serum creatinine greater than 2 mg/dL have renovascular hypertension. In hypertensive children under 5 years of age, the incidence of this disease approaches 80%. Evaluation should be considered in patients with poorly controlled or acutely worsening hypertension on a seemingly adequate medical regimen (three or more antihypertensive medications), particularly when presenting in conjunction with renal insufficiency, lateral abdominal bruit, or noncardiogenic "flash" pulmonary edema. A history of acute renal failure when starting an angiotensin-converting enzyme inhibitor is highly suggestive.

An incidental finding of renal artery stenosis greater than 50% is noted in as many as 45% of patients undergoing angiography for aortoiliac occlusive disease. Infrequently, it is associated with progressive renal insufficiency. High-grade (over 70%) bilateral stenoses or stenosis in a solitary kidney warrant close follow-up. Renal artery occlusive disease is suspected in patients with rapidly progressive renal insufficiency and no evidence of obstructive uropathy or intrinsic renal disease (no proteinuria on urinalysis, no polycystic disease on ultrasound).

Initial screening tests include duplex ultrasound, captopril renal scintigraphy, and MRA. Sensitivity and specificity of detecting renal artery stenosis greater than 60% are over 90% for each of these modalities, but the tests are highly operator-dependent and equipment-dependent—the most reliable examination varies by institution. An assessment should also be made of the kidney parenchyma: renal size, cortical thickness, and presence of infarcts. One pitfall of these modalities is failure to identify small accessory renal arteries, which when diseased can contribute to renovascular hypertension.

Indications for treatment include renovascular hypertension refractory to aggressive medical management or renal artery stenosis with progressive renal failure or sudden-onset noncardiogenic pulmonary edema. Percutaneous endovascular or open surgical procedures do not confer added benefit over medical therapy alone in patients with well-controlled hypertension and no ischemic nephropathy.

Angiography is generally required for planning an operative strategy and in many cases discloses a lesion amenable to angioplasty and stenting. Ideal lesions for endovascular treatment are focal, proximal, nonostial plaques that do not extend into the branch vessels.

Primary stenting is advised for stenoses in renal arteries greater than 6 mm in diameter because of improved patency over angioplasty alone. One exception to this rule is fibromuscular dysplasia, in which a durable clinical effect is often produced by angioplasty alone. In patients with renal insufficiency, use of nonionized contrast, preprocedure intravenous hydration, and administration of the antioxidant acetylcysteine, 600 mg orally twice daily for 2 days before and 2 days after examination, is advised. The long-term patency of renal artery stents is yet undefined, but a 20–44% restenosis rate from intimal hyperplasia is noted at 6–36 months. Overall, 3–13% of initially stented patients ultimately require surgery.

Surgery is indicated for treatment of progressive renal failure or uncontrolled renovascular hypertension in patients with lesions refractory to angioplasty, complex lesions extending into the branch vessels, or concomitant aortic disease requiring surgical reconstruction. Because of superior long-term patency, surgery may be preferred over angioplasty for primary treatment of renal artery occlusive disease in good-risk surgical candidates. Surgical options include transaortic renal endarterectomy, renal artery bypass, or extra-anatomic (hepatorenal, splenorenal, or iliorenal) bypass. Mannitol (25 g intravenously) and fenoldopam (0.5–1 µg/kg/min) have been beneficial in the perioperative management of these patients. Nephrectomy is considered for patients with renovascular hypertension and irreversible renal atrophy (kidney length less than 5 cm, severe cortical thinning, less than 10% of total renal function by split function testing). Endarterectomy and aortorenal bypass have 5-year patency greater than 80%, with beneficial blood pressure response in 70–90% of patients and improvement or stabilization in renal function in 70–80%.

Iglesias JI et al: The natural history of incidental renal artery stenosis in patients with aortoiliac vascular disease. Am J Med 2000;109:642. [PMID: 11099684]

Paty PS et al: Is prosthetic renal artery reconstruction a durable procedure? An analysis of 489 bypass grafts. J Vasc Surg 2001;34:127. [PMID: 11436085]

Safian R: Renal-artery stenosis. N Engl J Med 2001;344:431. [PMID: 11172181]

Tepel M et al: Prevention of radiographic-contrast-agent-induced reductions in renal function by acetylcysteine. N Engl J Med 2000;343:180. [PMID: 10900277]

van de Ven PJ et al: Arterial stenting and balloon angioplasty in ostial atherosclerotic renovascular disease: A randomised trial. Lancet 1999;353:282. [PMID: 9929021]

ACUTE LIMB ISCHEMIA

Acute limb ischemia can be embolic, thrombotic, or traumatic. Symptoms and signs are related to the location of the occlusion, the duration of ischemia, and the degree of development of collateral circulation. Baseline pulse examination and assessment of motor and sensory function are imperative. Characteristically, acute ischemia is described by the six Ps: pain, pallor, pulselessness, paresthesias, poikilothermia, and paralysis. Pain and paresthesias are the most common early symptoms.

The following differential points should be considered: (1) Are there manifestations of advanced occlusive arterial disease in other areas, especially the opposite extremity (bruit, absent pulses, secondary skin changes), and is there a history of intermittent claudication? These findings suggest primary arterial thrombosis. (2) Is there a history of rheumatic heart disease, atrial fibrillation or myocardial infarction? These findings suggest embolism.

1. Arterial Embolism

Eighty to 90 percent of arterial emboli arise from the heart. Atrial fibrillation is present in 60–70% of patients with arterial emboli and is associated with formation of thrombus in the left atrial appendage. Thrombus within a postinfarct ventricular aneurysm may also be a potential embolic source. Emboli arising from rheumatic heart disease are decreasing in incidence and now comprise less than 20% of arterial emboli. Cardiac valvular prostheses and cardiac tumors (myxomas) can also produce emboli. Noncardiac emboli arise from atherosclerotic lesions in proximal vessels, tumors, and foreign bodies. Paradoxical emboli deriving from deep venous thrombosis in the leg can also occur.

Emboli tend to lodge at the bifurcation of major arteries, with 40% going to the aortic bifurcation or the infrainguinal vessels. Thirty percent lodge in the cerebrovascular vessels, 10% in the visceral vessels, and 15% in the upper extremity vessels. Noncardiac emboli from arterial ulcerations are usually small, giving rise to peripheral ulceration and digital ischemia or occasionally to a systemic illness resembling vasculitis.

Treatment

Heparin sodium should be given as soon as the diagnosis of acute arterial occlusion is made and continued intraoperatively in order to prevent distal thrombosis. Emergent embolectomy is performed by introducing a balloon catheter through a small arteriotomy. An embolus at the aortic bifurcation or in the iliac artery can often be removed under local anesthesia through unilateral or bilateral common femoral arteriotomies. Smaller balloon catheters passed distally from the femoral artery can be used to extract popliteal or tibial emboli, though these often require popliteal arteriotomy. Percutaneous catheter techniques (aspiration, mechanical thrombolysis, or thrombolytic therapy) have some reported success in treatment of peripheral embolic disease. Lifelong anticoagulation is recommended because of the high frequency of recurrent emboli. Surface or transesophageal echocardiography should be performed to exclude the possibility of atrial thrombus, valvular disease, or cardiac tumor.

Embolectomy performed more than 6 hours following onset of symptoms is often accompanied by development of a compartment syndrome. In mild cases, fasciotomy performed at the time of embolectomy can result in full functional recovery of the limb. The most common persistent major neurologic deficit is foot drop secondary to peroneal nerve ischemia. Myoglobinuria and renal failure can result from rhabdomyolysis and can be minimized with aggressive hydration, forced diuresis, and alkalinization of the urine. These measures decrease the risk of myoglobin precipitation in the renal tubules. One regimen involves initial infusion of 250 mL/h of crystalloid, half as 0.45 normal saline and the rest as D_5W with two ampules of sodium bicarbonate and 12.5 g of mannitol per liter of fluid. Severe cases of compartment syndrome may result in anuric renal failure and systemic inflammatory response syndrome. In these patients, primary amputation may be life-saving.

Prognosis

Arterial embolism is associated with a 5–25% risk of limb loss and a 25–30% in-hospital mortality. Heart disease is responsible for over half of these deaths.

In patients with atrial fibrillation, mechanical or pharmacologic cardioversion or long-term anticoagulant therapy may decrease the risk of further emboli.

If no heart disease exists, prognosis is dependent on identification and exclusion of the embolic source. Cholesterol emboli from proximal arterial aneurysm or ulceration may occlude small distal vessels, producing digital ischemia or "trash foot." One common scenario is "blue toes" after aortography or aortic cross-clamping for coronary artery bypass or aneurysm repair. However, atheroemboli can also produce transient ischemic attacks, acute renal insufficiency, or bowel ischemia depending on their location. Microhematuria, eosinophilia, and an elevated sedimentation rate are detectable transiently on laboratory testing. Biopsy of the infarcted tissue reveals cholesterol clefts in the small vessels under polarized light. These lesions are not treatable by embolectomy because the vessels involved are so small, and heparinization may worsen the problem by liberating more fragments from an ulcerated atherosclerotic plaque. Aortic or iliac lesions can be treated by endarterectomy, by resection and interposition graft, or by placement of a covered stent.

2. Acute Arterial Thrombosis

Acute arterial thrombosis is most commonly a complication of chronic atherosclerotic occlusive disease but can also occur as a consequence of trauma, low-flow states such as hypovolemic or cardiogenic shock, or an inflammatory arteritis. Polycythemia, dehydration, and hypercoagulable states also increase the risk of thrombosis. Generally, thrombus starts at the point of greatest stenosis and propagates distally to the next open branch point, such as a patent collateral vessel.

Treatment

Nonoperative treatment is the initial approach for many patients with acute arterial thrombosis. Because thrombosis develops in the setting of chronic occlusive disease, there are usually well-developed collaterals and little arterial spasm. The extremity is able to tolerate the longer periods of ischemia required for catheter-directed thrombolysis. Instillation of alteplase (0.5–1 mg/h) directly into the thrombus through a multi-side-holed catheter may allow recanalization of distal vessels that are less amenable to surgical thrombectomy. It also helps to disclose the underlying stenotic lesion, which can then be treated with angioplasty, endarterectomy, or bypass grafting. Thrombolysis is successful in 50–80% of cases, with a limb salvage rate approaching 90%.

Less commonly, arterial thrombosis follows penetrating trauma, such as arterial transection and foreign body embolization; or blunt trauma, such as posterior knee dislocation and crush injury. These patients require surgical treatment. The vessel involved may be previously undiseased, with only a few small collaterals. Thrombolysis is generally not indicated because of the more advanced state of limb ischemia on presentation and the high incidence of bleeding complications.

Prognosis

Limb salvage is usually possible with acute thrombosis of the iliac or superficial femoral arteries but is less likely with popliteal thrombosis because of the paucity of available collaterals. Acute thrombosis of a popliteal aneurysm is associated with a 10–25% risk of amputation.

Canova CR et al: Long-term results of percutaneous thrombo-embolectomy in patients with infrainguinal embolic occlusions. Int Angiol 2001;20:66. [PMID: 11342998]

Frost L et al: Incident thromboembolism in the aorta and the renal, mesenteric, pelvic, and extremity arteries after discharge from the hospital with a diagnosis of atrial fibrillation. Arch Intern Med 2001;161:272. [PMID: 11176743]

■ OTHER ARTERIOPATHIES

THROMBOANGIITIS OBLITERANS (Buerger's Disease)

Buerger's disease is an episodic and segmental inflammatory and thrombotic process of the peripheral arteries and veins. The cause is not known. It is seen most commonly in men under 40 who smoke, and particularly in those of Eastern European or Asian background. It is characterized by occlusion of distal arteries, producing claudication, rest pain, and tissue necrosis. The inflammatory process is intermittent, with quiescent periods lasting weeks, months, or years.

Different arterial segments may become occluded in successive episodes; recanalization can occur during periods of disease remission.

There are no pathognomonic signs, but several findings are characteristic of Buerger's disease. (1) The typical patient is a man under 40 who smokes. Fewer than 20% of patients are women. (2) There is a history of migratory superficial segmental thrombophlebitis, eg, red, tender nodules in the branches of the saphenous vein. Biopsy of the affected vein may show inflammatory infiltrate in the vessel wall, microabscesses, and thrombus or recanalization with perivascular fibrosis, depending on the stage of disease. (3) Intermittent claudication typically begins in the arch of the foot and progresses to the calf; instep claudication is not typical of atherosclerotic occlusive disease. Rest pain and diminished sensation from ischemic neuropathy are present in over 70% of patients at presentation. (4) Proximal pulses are normal, while distal pulses are diminished or absent. Digital disease is often asymmetric: not all of the toes are affected to the same degree. The affected digits may be pale or cyanotic or erythematous. (5) Ulcers are present in 75% of patients and are typically located at the nail margins. (6) The disease is never confined to one limb. Although not all limbs may be symptomatic, an abnormal Allen test or distal pulse examination can usually be demonstrated. (7) There is often a history of cold sensitivity or Raynaud's phenomenon. (8) The clinical course is usually episodic, with acute exacerbations followed by rather definite remissions. By contrast, steadily progressive symptoms are typical in atherosclerotic occlusive disease.

Atherosclerotic occlusive disease, emboli, and autoimmune disorders are included in the differential diagnosis. Several angiographic findings can be helpful in making these distinctions. Buerger's disease involves the distal arteries and spares the proximal arteries; it is segmental in appearance, with skip areas of disease; there is no vascular calcification; and extensive collateralization via tortuous "corkscrew" vessels is typical. Peripheral ultrasound or angiography and echocardiography are helpful in excluding an embolic source. Blood tests (complete blood count, coagulation studies, sedimentation rate, antinuclear antibody, lupus anticoagulant, rheumatoid factor, anticentromere antibody, and antiphospholipid antibody) are obtained to rule out vasculitis, lupus erythematosus, scleroderma, rheumatoid vascular disease, or a hypercoagulable state due to antiphospholipid antibody syndrome. A careful history is generally sufficient to exclude other rare disorders that may mimic Buerger's disease, such as ergotamine intoxication, cannabis arteritis, or small vessel occlusive disease secondary to the use of vibratory tools (hypothenar hammer syndrome).

Smoking cessation is imperative. The disease can remain active with as little as a single cigarette a day; chewing tobacco, marijuana, nicotine patches, nicotine gum, and exposure to second-hand smoke must all be eliminated to arrest the disease process. Local wound care of ulcers consists of limited debridement, appropriate dressings, and intravenous antibiotics for cellulitis. Nonulcerated skin should be kept moisturized. Lamb's wool between the toes and heel protectors or sheepskin-lined boots (Rooke boots) help to reduce further trauma to the skin. Warming pads must be used judiciously, as burns are possible in patients with diminished sensation from peripheral neuropathy. Supplementary oxygen by nasal cannula is often used to increase oxygen supply to the wound. Some ulcers may respond to hyperbaric oxygen.

Nonsteroidal anti-inflammatory medications and opioids are used for pain control. Aspirin (325 mg daily) or another antiplatelet agent is generally prescribed to reduce thrombotic complications. Calcium channel blockers are often used to promote vasodilation. Preliminary trials have shown intravenous infusion of the prostaglandin analog iloprost to be efficacious in healing of ischemic ulcers, but the drug is not yet available in the United States. Vascular endothelial growth factor (VEGF) is also being investigated for use in Buerger's disease.

Rarely do distal target vessels exist for arterial bypass. Sympathectomy may at least transiently reduce the vasospastic manifestations of the disease and aid in the establishment of collateral circulation to the skin. It is indicated for relief of intractable rest pain and healing of ulcers refractory to other treatment. Sympathectomy is often performed in conjunction with digital amputation. Amputation is reserved for patients with wet gangrene or severe rest pain.

Prognosis is dependent on the success of smoking cessation. Over 90% of patients who quit smoking avoid further amputation.

Olin JW: Current concepts: Thromboangiitis obliterans (Buerger's disease). N Engl J Med 2000;343:864. [PMID: 10995867]

IDIOPATHIC ARTERITIS OF TAKAYASU ("Pulseless Disease")

Takayasu's disease is a rare polyarteritis of unknown cause with a special predilection for the branches of the aortic arch. It results in segmental stenoses, occlusions, and aneurysms. It predominantly affects Asian women under the age of 40. There are a myriad of clinical presentations depending on the stage of disease (early "inflammatory" or late "occlusive") and the vessels involved. Early stages of disease are often accompanied by fever, myalgias, arthralgias, and pain over the involved artery as well as leukocytosis and elevated sedimentation rate. Other symptoms are related to arterial insufficiency: syncope, dizziness, amaurosis fugax, stroke, angina, pulmonary hypertension, and claudication. Hypertension related to proximal renal artery stenosis or aortic coarctation is present in over one-quarter of patients. Vascular bruits, diminished peripheral pulses, or asymmetric blood pressure measurements are common findings on physical examination.

Angiography is essential for diagnosis and most often will reveal combined occlusive and aneurysmal disease. The most commonly involved vessels are the subclavian artery, descending thoracic aorta, renal artery, carotid artery, and mesenteric arteries, although the ascending and abdominal aorta and the vertebral, coronary, pulmonary, iliac, and brachial arteries can also be affected. In cases of upper extremity stenoses, aortic root pressure should be measured by manometry at the time of angiography to assess for essential hypertension. MRA can also be used for routine surveillance of patients with suspected Takayasu's disease.

Pulseless disease must be differentiated from vascular lesions of the aortic arch due to atherosclerosis, though in the latter instance concomitant lower extremity disease is invariably present. Histologically, the arterial lesions are indistinguishable from those of giant cell arteritis. In the early, active stage, corticosteroids (prednisone, 1 mg/kg/d) are used to control symptoms and limit the progression of disease; cytotoxic agents may be added if steroids are ineffectual. Surgical or percutaneous intervention is not advised until the disease becomes indolent. Bypass of the occluded or aneurysmal segments is the usual surgical approach. Histologic examination of the resected artery may show nonspecific transmural inflammation or chronic fibrosis. Percutaneous angioplasty or stenting is possible for short-segment stenoses, but there is a high recurrence rate in these usually noncompliant vessels.

Kerr GS et al: Takayasu arteritis. Ann Intern Med 1994;120:919. [PMID: 7909656] (A balanced clinical review.)

FIBROMUSCULAR DYSPLASIA

Fibromuscular dysplasia is a nonatherosclerotic, noninflammatory disease of unknown cause characterized by segmental irregularity of small and medium-sized muscular arteries. Typically, it affects white women 30–50 years of age; a family history of disease is not unusual. The most frequently involved vessels (in descending order) are the renal, carotid, and common iliac arteries. Patients present with renovascular hypertension and, less often, with renal insufficiency, transient ischemic attacks or claudication. Angiography reveals a "string of beads" pattern of disease. There are four recognized histologic types of fibromuscular dysplasia: medial fibrodysplasia, intimal fibroplasia, medial hyperplasia, and perimedial dysplasia, though the first type is responsible for over 80% of all cases. Aspirin is advised for most patients. Percutaneous or surgical intervention is reserved for symptomatic patients. Most lesions respond well to percutaneous angioplasty; stents do not appear to offer any advantage over angioplasty alone. More complex lesions extending into branch vessels may require interposition grafting. It is important to recognize that intracranial aneurysms are present in as many as half of patients with internal carotid fibromuscular dysplasia.

VASCULITIS

The term vasculitis describes a diverse group of inflammatory disorders characterized by multi-organ system vascular involvement, systemic markers of disease (fever, malaise, weight loss, elevated white blood cell count and sedimentation rate), and suspected immunologic origin. Often there are accompanying rheumatologic or cutaneous manifestations such as arthralgias, conjunctivitis, or erythema nodosum. Drugs (amphetamines, cocaine, hydralazine, procainamide), infections (hepatitis B, gonococcus, streptococcus), chronic inflammatory diseases, and cancer are cited as inciting causes for vasculitis. These diseases can be grouped into disorders that affect medium and large blood vessels (polyarteritis nodosa, scleroderma, systemic lupus erythematosus, temporal arteritis, Behçet's disease, Kawasaki syndrome, rheumatoid arteritis, relapsing polychondritis) and those that affect smaller vessels (Churg-Strauss syndrome, Wegener's granulomatosis, Henoch-Schönlein purpura, essential mixed cryoglobulinemia). These are discussed in detail in Chapter 20. In general, the vascular lesions are treated with anti-inflammatory medications. Surgery is indicated for acute complications (bowel infarction, gangrene, or aneurysm rupture) and for chronic ischemic symptoms or large aneurysms in patients with quiescent disease.

■ VASOMOTOR DISORDERS

RAYNAUD'S DISEASE & RAYNAUD'S PHENOMENON

ESSENTIALS OF DIAGNOSIS

- *Episodic bilateral digital pallor, cyanosis, and rubor.*
- *Precipitated by cold or emotional stress; relieved by warmth.*
- *Seventy to 80 percent of patients are women.*

General Considerations

Raynaud's syndrome is an episodic vasospastic disorder characterized by digital color change (white-blue-red) with exposure to cold environment or emotional stress. If idiopathic, it is called Raynaud's disease. If associated with a possible precipitating systemic or regional disorder (autoimmune diseases, myeloproliferative disorders, multiple myeloma, cryoglobulinemia, myxedema, macroglobulinemia, or arterial occlusive disease), it is

called Raynaud's phenomenon. The incidence of disease is estimated to be as high as 10% in the general population. Other vasospastic disorders, such as variant angina and migraine headache, are common in patients with Raynaud's syndrome. An abnormality of the sympathetic nervous system has long been implicated in the etiology of Raynaud's disease; recently, research has focused on the theory of up-regulation of vascular smooth muscle α_2-adrenergic receptors.

Clinical Findings

Classically, Raynaud's disease and Raynaud's phenomenon are characterized by intermittent attacks of pallor of the hands or fingers brought on by cold or emotional stress, progressing to cyanosis and then rubor on rewarming. Mild discomfort, paresthesias, numbness, and trace edema often accompany the color changes. In Raynaud's disease, the disease is symmetric, by rule; in Raynaud's phenomenon, the changes may be most noticeable in one hand or even in one or two fingers only. Infrequently, the feet and toes are involved. Between attacks, the affected extremities may be entirely normal.

The distinction between Raynaud's disease and Raynaud's phenomenon is meant to reflect a difference in prognosis. While Raynaud's disease is benign and entirely reversible, Raynaud's phenomenon may progress to atrophy of the terminal fat pads and development of fingertip gangrene. However, because many inciting diseases may not be clinically suspected at the time the diagnosis of Raynaud's disease is made, there is a large degree of crossover between groups. The diagnosis is based on clinical criteria. Raynaud's disease appears first between ages 15 and 45, almost always in women. A patient with suggestive symptoms that persist for over 3 years without evidence of an associated disease is given the diagnosis of Raynaud's disease.

Differential Diagnosis

A patient with Raynaud's syndrome must be evaluated for possible inciting systemic disorders. Directed history and physical examination and serologic testing may be helpful in excluding the collagen-vascular disorders, which include scleroderma, systemic lupus erythematosus, dermatomyositis, and rheumatoid arthritis. It is estimated that 80% of patients with scleroderma ultimately develop Raynaud's phenomenon. Likewise, cryoglobulinemia can be excluded by appropriate testing. Raynaud's phenomenon is also occasionally seen in patients with neurogenic thoracic outlet syndrome or carpal tunnel syndrome; nerve conduction studies can be obtained if warranted by examination. Frostbite, ergotamine toxicity, and use of chemotherapeutic agents, which can also be associated with Raynaud's phenomenon, can usually be excluded by a careful history; up to one-third of patients receiving combined bleomycin and vincristine (such as for testicular cancer) develop symptomatic vasospastic disease. An abnormal or asymmetric pulse examination, differential blood pressure cuff measurements, gangrene, or a positive Allen test—any of these are suggestive of arterial occlusive disease and should prompt upper extremity angiography to exclude stenosis or occlusion from atherosclerosis, Buerger's disease, arterial thoracic outlet syndrome, embolic disease, or repetitive motion injury of the small vessels of the hand. Even undiseased upper extremity vessels often show intense vasospasm with contrast injection, so the arm is wrapped for warmth and prophylactic use of a vasodilator (papaverine or nitroglycerin, 30 mg, injected through the angiography catheter) is advised; both arms are imaged for side-by-side comparison.

Other vasospastic disorders that should be included in the differential but are usually easily distinguishable by physical examination are acrocyanosis and livedo reticularis.

Treatment

A. GENERAL MEASURES

Warmth and protection of the hands are the basic tenets of therapy. In Raynaud's phenomenon, wounds heal slowly, and infections are consequently hard to control. Gloves should be worn in cold environments and during activities that may cause trauma to the skin, such as dishwashing, gardening, woodworking, or office filing. Moisturizing lotion should be applied frequently to avoid fissured dry skin. Smoking cessation is imperative, as nicotine is a known vasoconstrictor. Stress management should be addressed. Oral contraceptives, beta-blockers, and ergotamines are associated with exacerbation of symptoms and ideally should be discontinued. Aspirin is prescribed to decrease the risk of thrombotic complications.

B. VASODILATORS

Vasodilator drugs may be of some benefit in patients whose symptoms are not adequately controlled with simpler measures. Low-dose nifedipine (sustained-release, 30 mg/d) or diltiazem (sustained-release, 30 mg/d) has superseded topical or oral nitroglycerin for treatment of vasospasm. Use of prostaglandins has been disappointing, but the serotonin reuptake inhibitor and antidepressant fluoxetine (20 mg daily) shows some promise in reduction of the frequency and severity of attacks.

C. SURGERY

Bypass should be considered for severe Raynaud's phenomenon associated with reconstructible arterial occlusive disease. Sympathectomy is indicated for unreconstructible occlusive disease or pure vasospastic disease refractory to medical management. In the lower extremity, sympathectomy may produce complete and permanent relief of symptoms; but for unclear reasons, the beneficial effects are often transient in the upper extremity. Limited improvement is seen in advanced ischemia, particularly if significant digital artery obstructive disease is present.

Prognosis

Raynaud's disease is usually benign, causing mild discomfort on exposure to cold and progressing very slightly over the years. The prognosis of Raynaud's phenomenon is that of the associated disease.

Coleiro B et al: Treatment of Raynaud's phenomenon with the selective serotonin reuptake inhibitor fluoxetine. Rheumatology (Oxford) 2001;40:1038. [PMID: 11561116]

Pache M et al: Cold feet and prolonged sleep-onset latency in vasospastic syndrome. Lancet 2001;358:125. [PMID: 11463418]

Spencer-Green G: Outcomes in primary Raynaud's phenomenon: A meta-analysis of the frequency, rates, and predictors of transition to secondary disease. Arch Intern Med 1998; 158:595. [PMID: 9521223]

LIVEDO RETICULARIS

Livedo reticularis is an uncommon vasospastic disorder of unknown cause that results in a painless, mottled discoloration on large areas of the extremities, generally in a fishnet pattern with reticulated cyanotic areas surrounding a paler central core. It occurs in men and women of all ages. In most instances, livedo reticularis is entirely benign; infrequently, it is associated with an occult malignancy, polyarteritis nodosa, atherosclerotic microemboli, or antiphospholipid antibody syndrome. The disorder is characterized by arteriolar vasoconstriction with capillary and venous dilation; the particular pattern is believed to represent arborization of capillaries surrounding the feeding arteriole.

Livedo reticularis is most apparent on the thighs but can occur on the forearms or lower abdomen and is most pronounced in cold weather. In warm environments, the reticular pattern may fade but does not entirely disappear. A few patients report paresthesias, coldness, or numbness in the involved areas. Peripheral pulses are normal. The affected regions may be cool. Skin ulceration is rare. Treatment consists of protection from exposure to cold; use of vasodilators is seldom indicated. In the rare patient who develops ulcerations or gangrene, an underlying systemic disease should be excluded.

ACROCYANOSIS

Acrocyanosis is an uncommon vasospastic disorder characterized by persistent cyanosis of the hands and feet and, to a lesser degree, the forearms and legs. It is associated with arteriolar vasoconstriction combined with dilation of the subcapillary venous plexus of the skin, through which deoxygenated blood slowly circulates. It is worse in cold weather but does not completely disappear during the warm season. It occurs primarily in women, is most common in the teens and twenties, and may improve with advancing age or during pregnancy.

It is characterized by symmetric coldness, sweating, slight edema, and cyanotic discoloration of the hands or feet. Peripheral pulses are normal, and pain, trophic lesions, and disability do not occur.

Naldi L et al: Cutaneous manifestations associated with antiphospholipid antibodies in patients with suspected primary antiphospholipid syndrome: a case-control study. Ann Rheum Dis 1993;52:219. [PMID: 8484676] (Livedo reticularis and acrocyanosis were significantly associated with antiphospholipid antibodies.)

ERYTHROMELALGIA

Erythromelalgia is a paroxysmal bilateral vasodilatory disorder of unknown cause. Idiopathic (primary) erythromelalgia occurs in otherwise healthy persons and affects men and women equally. A secondary type is occasionally seen in patients with polycythemia vera, hypertension, gout, and neurologic diseases.

The chief symptoms are erythema, warmth, and bilateral burning pain that lasts minutes to hours, at first involving circumscribed areas on the balls of the feet or palms and often progressing to involve the entire extremity. Symptoms occur in response to vasodilation produced by exercise or heat and can be prominent at night when the extremities are warmed under bedclothes. Relief may be obtained by cooling and elevating the affected extremity.

No findings are generally present between attacks. With onset of an attack, skin temperature and arterial pulsations are increased and the involved areas are warm, erythematous, and sweaty.

In primary erythromelalgia, aspirin (650 mg every 4–6 hours) often provides excellent relief and may in fact be diagnostic. Warm environments are avoided. Beta-blockers, epidural corticosteroid injections, and lidocaine patches have reported anecdotal success. Secondary erythromelalgia may improve with treatment of the primary disease process.

Davis MD et al: Lidocaine patch for pain of erythromelalgia. Arch Dermatol 2002;138:17. [PMID: 11790162]

Stricker LJ et al: Resolution of refractory symptoms of secondary erythermalgia with intermittent epidural bupivacaine. Reg Anesth Pain Med 2001;26:488. [PMID: 11561273]

COMPLEX REGIONAL PAIN SYNDROME TYPE 1 (REFLEX SYMPATHETIC DYSTROPHY)

ESSENTIALS OF DIAGNOSIS

- Burning or aching pain of greater severity and longer duration than expected following trauma to an extremity.

- Manifestations of localized vasomotor instability are generally present.

General Considerations

The syndrome is characterized by burning or aching pain in an injured extremity which is more severe than would be expected given the inciting trauma. It occurs in all age groups and equally in both sexes and can involve either the arms or the legs. The degree of trauma is in some cases surprisingly minor (phlebotomy), but most cases follow crushing injuries with lacerations and soft tissue destruction. Closed fractures, simple lacerations, burns (especially electric burns), elective operative procedures, and myocardial infarction with referred left arm pain are other reported causes.

Clinical Findings

In the early stages, the pain, tenderness, and hyperesthesia are localized to the injured area and the extremity is warm, dry, swollen, and red or slightly cyanotic. With time, muscle spasm and joint stiffness limit mobility, and the nails may become ridged. In advanced stages, the pain is more diffuse, and nocturnal pain may become extreme; the extremity becomes cool and clammy and intolerant of temperature changes (particularly cold); and the skin becomes glossy and atrophic. The patient's dominant concern is to avoid external stimuli, particularly in trigger point areas. Pain and disuse lead to loss of function. Radiographs reveal asymmetric osteopenia more severe than anticipated from immobility alone.

Prevention

Trauma to peripheral nerves during surgery is avoided by knowledge of their anatomy and careful mobilization by handling of the perineural tissue only. Splinting and adequate analgesia followed by early mobilization of an injured extremity minimizes the occurrence of reflex sympathetic dystrophy.

Treatment & Prognosis

A. CONSERVATIVE MEASURES

Early recognition and treatment are essential to preserve function of the limb. In the early stages, when major secondary changes have not yet developed, physical therapy involving active and passive exercises combined with a mild anxiolytic (diazepam, 2 mg twice daily; or alprazolam, 0.125–0.25 mg twice daily) may relieve symptoms. Opioids have been a mainstay of treatment; recently, however, gabapentin (beginning at 200 mg twice daily) has been used with success. Sympathetic blocks (stellate ganglion or lumbar) can be combined with intensive physical therapy for cases refractory to more conservative treatment. Protection from further injury and avoidance of irritating stimuli are imperative.

B. SURGERY

Patients who achieve significant temporary relief of symptoms after sympathetic blocks may be cured by sympathectomy. With advanced disease and in cases with significant psychologic overlay, however, the prognosis for improvement with sympathectomy is poor. Implantable spinal cord biostimulator devices have had limited success.

Kemmler MA et al: Impact of spinal cord stimulation on sensory characteristics in complex regional pain syndrome type 1: A randomized trial. Anesthesiology 2001;95:72. [PMID: 11465587]

Wasner G et al: Vascular abnormalities in reflex sympathetic dystrophy (CPRS 1): Mechanisms and diagnostic value. Brain 2001;124:587. [PMID: 11222458]

THORACIC OUTLET SYNDROME

Thoracic outlet syndrome can be subdivided into neurogenic, venous, and arterial types depending on which structures are compressed in the interscalene triangle or costoclavicular space.

Neurogenic thoracic outlet syndrome is the most common (over 90% of patients) and often the most difficult to diagnose and treat effectively. Patients most often present with supraclavicular and anterior chest wall burning pain and with segmental pain and paresthesias of the arm in an ulnar nerve distribution. Weakness of the intrinsic muscles of the hand is not uncommon. Thenar or hypothenar muscle wasting is rare. There is usually a history of whiplash trauma (motor vehicle accident, fall, assault) or repetitive activity of the upper extremity (word processing, filing), particularly overhead activities (lifting). Physical examination will often disclose supraclavicular tenderness and positive brachial plexus tension testing. A positive Adson test (obliteration of the radial pulse on inspiration while turning the head away from the affected side) or a positive Roos test (reproduction of symptoms with rapid opening and closing of the hand with the arm 90 degrees abducted at the shoulder and 90 degrees flexed at the elbow); or a positive Tinel sign (tingling in the distribution of the nerve produced by tapping in the supraclavicular interscalene region) may also be elicited. Presence of a cervical rib or other bony anomalies should be excluded by chest film. Electrophysiologic testing is usually negative. The cornerstone of treatment is specific physical therapy treatment such as the Edgelow Neurovascular Entrapment Self-Treatment (ENVEST) program, beginning with breathing exercises and attention to posture. Transcutaneous electrical nerve stimulation (TENS) is often helpful. Surgery may be indicated in severe refractory cases and involves resection of the hypertrophied anterior and middle scalene muscles, brachial plexus neurolysis, and resection of bony abnormalities.

Although in carefully selected patients the initial surgical outcome is excellent, symptoms return within a year in as many as 25%, presumably due to late postoperative scarring around the nerve roots.

Venous thoracic outlet syndrome involves external compression of the subclavian vein by the first rib, anterior scalene muscle, clavicle, and costocoracoid ligament. A history of repetitive upper arm exercises or clavicular fracture is common. Positional venography is essential in the diagnosis of venous thoracic outlet syndrome; external compression of the vein and filling of venous collaterals is demonstrated by abduction of the arm. Thrombosis of the involved vein segment is known as Paget-Schroetter syndrome, or effort thrombosis, and often presents as acute unilateral arm edema, axillary fullness, hand cyanosis, and enlarged shoulder and chest wall collateral veins in an otherwise healthy patient. Evaluation for hypercoagulable state, including plasma levels of antithrombin III, factor V Leiden, cardiolipin antibody, and proteins C and S, is recommended, as an abnormality is detected in 56% of patients presenting with acute axillary-subclavian vein thrombosis. Treatment for symptomatic venous thoracic outlet syndrome involves anterior scalene and first rib resection with venolysis, which can be performed through a supraclavicular, a combined supra- and infraclavicular, or a transaxillary approach. If the vein is thrombosed, multimodality therapy is employed: preoperative thrombolysis followed immediately by surgery with intraoperative angioplasty of any residual venous stenosis. If the vein cannot be recannulated preoperatively, surgical thrombectomy may be required. The prognosis is excellent with appropriate treatment.

Arterial thoracic outlet syndrome is the least common of these disorders and involves compression of the subclavian artery between the anterior and middle scalene muscles. It most often produces subclavian artery aneurysms, which result in digital ischemia due to atheroemboli. Arm claudication is a less common presentation. The Wylie-Allen test (performed by exsanguinating the arm with elevation, occluding the radial and ulnar arteries at the wrist, and observing capillary refill of the hand when these arteries are released) may reveal occult digital artery occlusions that can be confirmed by angiography. Treatment involves removal of anterior and middle scalene muscles and resection of the aneurysm with polytetrafluoroethylene interposition graft.

Alexrod DA et al: Outcomes after surgery for thoracic outlet syndrome. J Vasc Surg 2001;33:1220. [PMID: 11389421]

Schneider D et al: Management of vascular thoracic outlet syndrome. Chest Surg Clin North Am 1999;9:781.

Hingorani A et al: Upper extremity deep venous thrombosis: An underrecognized manifestation of a hypercoagulable state. Ann Vasc Surg 2000;14:421. [PMID: 10990549]

Pascarelli EF et al: Understanding work-related upper-extremity disorders: Clinical findings in 485 computer users, musicians, and others. J Occup Rehabil 2001;11:1. [PMID: 11706773]

■ VENOUS DISEASES

VARICOSE VEINS

ESSENTIALS OF DIAGNOSIS

- Dilated, tortuous superficial veins in the lower extremities.
- May be asymptomatic or associated with fatigue, aching discomfort, bleeding, or localized pain.
- Edema, pigmentation, and ulceration suggest concomitant venous stasis disease.
- Increased frequency after pregnancy.

General Considerations

Abnormally dilated veins develop in several locations, giving rise to varicoceles, esophageal varices, and hemorrhoids. However, varicose veins are most commonly found in the legs as abnormally dilated, elongated, and tortuous alterations in the saphenous veins and their tributaries. Fifteen percent of adults develop saphenous vein varicosities. Risk factors include female gender, pregnancy, family history, prolonged standing, and history of phlebitis.

The long saphenous vein and its tributaries are most commonly involved, but the short saphenous vein may also be affected. These vessels lie immediately beneath the skin and superficial to the deep fascia.

An inherited vein wall or valvular defect appears to play a role in the development of most primary varicosities. Secondary varicosities may result from valve damage following thrombophlebitis, trauma, deep venous thrombosis, arteriovenous fistula, or nontraumatic proximal venous obstruction (pregnancy, pelvic tumor). Venous reflux caused by valvular incompetence is characteristic of both primary and secondary varicose veins. At the saphenofemoral junction and the perforating veins of the medial calf and thigh, the superficial and deep veins of the leg communicate; valve incompetence in these segments permits blood flow to be bidirectional. Thus, high venous pressures (> 300 mm Hg) from within the deep system that occur during calf compression associated with walking are transmitted to these superficial veins, which dilate. With long-standing disease, the surrounding tissue and skin may develop secondary changes such as fibrosis, chronic edema, and skin pigmentation and atrophy.

Clinical Findings

A. SYMPTOMS

The severity of the symptoms is not necessarily correlated with the number and size of the varicosities. Dull, aching heaviness or a feeling of fatigue brought on by periods of standing is the most common complaint. Itching from an associated eczematoid dermatitis may occur above the ankle.

B. SIGNS

Dilated, tortuous, elongated veins on the medial aspect of the thigh and leg are usually readily visible with the patient standing, though in very obese patients palpation may be necessary to detect their presence and location. Smaller, flat, blue-green reticular veins, telangiectasias, and spider veins may accompany varicose veins and are further evidence of venous dysfunction. Secondary tissue changes may be absent even in the presence of extensive large varicosities; but with deep venous insufficiency and long-standing varicose veins signs of chronic venous insufficiency appear. These may include brownish pigmentation and thinning of the skin above the ankle, edema, fibrosis, scaling dermatitis, and venous ulceration. Duplex ultrasonography is used to detect the precise location of incompetent valves. The Brodie-Trendelenburg test is less accurate but can help differentiate saphenofemoral valve incompetence from perforator vein incompetence. With the patient lying supine, the leg is elevated until all varicosities collapse. A tourniquet is placed at the mid thigh to exclude reflux secondary to incompetence at the saphenofemoral junction. With the tourniquet in place, the patient is asked to stand. If the varicosities stay collapsed, this implies valvular insufficiency at the saphenofemoral junction. However, if the varicosities rapidly refill, perforator vein incompetence is implicated. The tourniquet can then be moved more distally to identify the location of the incompetent perforator.

Differential Diagnosis

Primary varicose veins should be differentiated from secondary varicose veins in order to exclude the possibility of chronic venous insufficiency of the deep system of veins, obstruction of the pelvic veins, arteriovenous fistula (congenital or acquired), or congenital venous malformation. If extensive varicose veins are encountered in a young patient—especially if unilateral and in an atypical distribution (lateral leg)—Klippel-Trenaunay syndrome must be considered. The classic triad of Klippel-Trenaunay syndrome is varicose veins, limb hypertrophy, and a cutaneous birth-mark (port wine stain or venous malformation). Because the deep veins are often anomalous or absent, saphenous vein stripping can be hazardous. Standard treatment for patients with Klippel-Trenaunay syndrome is graduated support stockings, surgery for correction of leg length discrepancy, and limited stab avulsion (excision through 1 cm long incisions) of symptomatic varices after thorough duplex ultrasound vein mapping.

Pain or discomfort secondary to arthritis, radiculopathy, or arterial insufficiency should be distinguished from symptoms associated with coexistent varicose veins.

Complications

Complications of varicose veins include secondary ulceration, bleeding, chronic stasis dermatitis, superficial venous thrombosis, and thrombophlebitis.

Treatment

A. NONSURGICAL MEASURES

Knee-high or thigh-high elastic graduated compression stockings give external support to the superficial veins. For most patients, a gradient of compression of 20–30 mm Hg is appropriate. The stockings are worn all day to reduce venous hypertension due to pooling of blood and are removed at night. Periodic leg elevation and regular exercise are encouraged. In many patients, this program may provide relief of symptoms and discourage progression of disease sufficient to avoid surgery.

Small venous ulcers generally heal with leg elevation and compression bandages (Ace wrap or Unna boot). Varicose vein excision should be postponed until infection and edema are controlled.

B. SURGICAL MEASURES

Indications for surgical treatment include persistent or disabling pain, recurrent superficial thrombophlebitis, erosion of the overlying skin with bleeding, and manifestations of chronic venous insufficiency (particularly ulceration).

The operative plan is dependent on determination of the competency of the deep and perforating veins and the location of sites of venous reflux. Preoperative duplex ultrasound is essential in identification of incompetent perforating veins and in assessment of the saphenofemoral junction. Surgery can then be tailored to the pattern of disease. Stab avulsion surgery is combined with prevention of reflux by high ligation of the saphenofemoral junction or ligation of perforator branches. Stripping of the entire saphenous system is rarely required and may be complicated by hematoma formation, infection, and saphenous nerve irritation.

C. COMPRESSION SCLEROTHERAPY

Compression sclerotherapy can be used for telangiectasias, spider veins, and small (< 4 mm) varicosities that persist after vein stripping. With patients in supine position, small volumes of a sclerosing solution (23.4% hypertonic saline or 2.5% sodium morrhuate) are injected and direct pressure is then maintained with compression stockings. The goal is to obliterate the abnormal vein by inducing localized endothelial destruction and fibrosis. More than one treatment is often required. Complications—including allergic reactions, thrombophlebitis, neoangiogenesis, skin necrosis, or hyperpigmentation—are rare.

Prognosis

With careful patient selection and properly selected operative techniques, most patients experience relief of symptoms and the recurrence rate is about 10%. Patients should be informed that this is a chronic disease and that prevention of new varicosities is dependent on continued use of the compression stockings, leg elevation, and exercise. If extensive varicosities reappear after surgery, the completeness of the high ligation should be questioned, and reexploration of the saphenofemoral area may be necessary. Even after adequate treatment, secondary tissue changes may not regress.

Belcaro G et al: Endovascular sclerotherapy, surgery, and surgery plus sclerotherapy in superficial venous incompetence: A randomized, 10 year follow-up trial—Final results. Angiology 2000;51:529. [PMID: 10917577]

Bradbury A et al: The relationship between lower limb symptoms and superficial and deep venous reflux on duplex ultrasonography: The Edinburgh Vein Study. J Vasc Surg 2000;32:921. [PMID: 11054224]

1. Thrombophlebitis of the Deep Veins

 ESSENTIALS OF DIAGNOSIS

- *Pain in the calf or thigh, often associated with edema. Fifty percent of patients are asymptomatic.*
- *History of congestive heart failure, recent surgery, trauma, neoplasia, oral contraceptive use, or prolonged inactivity.*
- *Physical signs unreliable.*
- *Duplex ultrasound is diagnostic.*

General Considerations

Acute deep venous thrombosis (DVT) affects as many as 800,000 new patients per year. Treatment of this disease is estimated to cost $1–2.5 billion per year, not including costs associated with long-term sequelae.

Although the cause is often multifactorial, Virchow's triad (stasis, vascular injury, and hypercoagulability) defines the events that predispose a vein to the development of thrombophlebitis. Trauma to the endothelium of the vein wall results in exposure of subendothelial tissues to platelets. With venous stasis, platelet aggregates form on the vein wall and deposition of fibrin, leukocytes, and erythrocytes results in a free-floating thrombus. Within 7–10 days, this thrombus becomes adherent to the vein wall and secondary inflammatory changes develop, though a free-floating tail may persist. The thrombus is ultimately invaded by fibroblasts, resulting in neovascularization and scarring of the vein wall and destruction of the valves. Central recanalization usually follows, with restoration of flow through the vein; however, because the valves are damaged irreparably, chronic venous insufficiency with postphlebitis syndrome occurs in approximately 35% of patients. In 80% of cases, the thrombosis begins in the deep veins of the calf. Propagation into the popliteal and femoral veins takes place in approximately 25% of these cases.

About 3% of patients undergoing major general surgical procedures will develop clinical manifestations of thrombophlebitis, and up to 30% develop asymptomatic deep vein thrombosis. Certain operations, such as total hip replacement, are associated with appreciably higher incidences of thromboembolic complications. Prolonged bed rest or immobility caused by cardiac failure, stroke, ventilatory support, pelvic bone or limb fracture, paralysis, extended air travel, or a lengthy operative procedure is one contributing factor. A hypercoagulable state resulting from malignancy, nephrotic syndrome, inherited deficiency in protein C or S or antithrombin III, homocystinuria, factor V Leiden mutation, or paroxysmal nocturnal hemoglobinuria may also play a role. An estimated 20% of patients with new deep venous thrombosis have an underlying occult or known malignancy. One-fourth of these are lung cancer, though cancers of the pancreas, prostate, breast, and ovary are not uncommon. Most are associated with increased fibrinogen or thrombocytosis. Other risk factors for deep venous thrombosis include advanced age, type A blood group, obesity, previous thrombosis, multiparity, use of oral contraceptives, inflammatory bowel disease, and lupus erythematosus. Oral contraceptives should be avoided in women who smoke or who have a history of phlebitis because of the high associated risk of thrombotic disease.

Clinical Findings

A. SYMPTOMS AND SIGNS

Fifty percent of patients with thrombophlebitis and 60–70% with acute pulmonary embolism have no symptoms or signs in the involved extremity. Symptomatic patients with deep venous thrombosis may complain of a dull ache, tightness, or pain in the calf or leg, especially when walking. Physical examination may disclose slight edema of the involved calf, a palpable cord, distention of the superficial venous collaterals, or low-grade fever and tachycardia. Homans' sign (pain on passive dorsiflexion of the ankle) is positive in only 50% of cases. Iliofemoral venous thrombosis can result in cyanosis of the skin (phlegmasia cerulea dolens) or a pale, cool extremity if reflex arterial spasm is superimposed (phlegmasia alba dolens).

B. DIAGNOSTIC TECHNIQUES

Because of the difficulty in making a precise diagnosis by history and physical examination and because of the morbidity associated with treatment, diagnostic studies are essential.

1. Duplex ultrasonography—Duplex ultrasonography, because of its high sensitivity, specificity, and reproducibility, has supplanted venography as the most widely used diagnostic test in the initial evaluation of patients suspected of having this disorder. The examination includes both a B mode image and Doppler flow analysis. Each venous segment is assessed for the presence of thrombosis, indicated by venous dilation and incompressibility during light probe pressure. Doppler findings suggestive of acute thrombosis are absence of spontaneous flow, loss of flow variation with respiration, and failure to increase flow velocity with distal augmentation. The criteria for the presence of chronic venous thrombosis are less well established. The chronically occluded vein is often narrowed, and there are prominent nearby collaterals. Chronic thrombi are highly echogenic, while acute thrombi are anechoic (and therefore not visible) on the B mode image. Duplex ultrasound is less accurate in detection of calf DVTs and is highly operator-dependent.

2. Ascending contrast venography—This study is rarely used because it is invasive and exposes the patient to ionizing radiation and the risks of contrast allergy, contrast-induced nephropathy, and phlebitis. Patients in whom deep venous thrombosis is strongly suspected but ultrasound is equivocal are now being referred for gadolinium-enhanced magnetic resonance venography. In experienced hands, this examination has a sensitivity of 100% and a specificity of 96% and may provide some information about the age of the thrombus.

Differential Diagnosis

Localized muscle strain or contusion or Achilles tendon rupture can often mimic thrombophlebitis. Cellulitis can have a similar clinical presentation: edema, localized pain, and erythema. Other causes of unilateral leg edema (lymphedema, rupture of a Baker cyst, obstruction of the popliteal vein by a Baker cyst, obstruction of the iliac vein by tumor or fibrosis, or external compression of the left iliac vein by the right common iliac artery, known as May-Thurner syndrome) and bilateral leg edema (heart, liver, or kidney failure, or vena caval obstruction by tumor, retroperitoneal fibrosis, or pregnancy) must be excluded.

Complications

Complications of deep venous thrombosis include pulmonary embolism (see Chapter 9), varicose veins, and chronic venous insufficiency.

Prevention

Prophylactic measures may diminish the incidence of venous thrombosis in hospitalized patients. Choice of therapy is dependent on stratification of individual patient risk factors.

A. Nonpharmacologic Measures

Venous stasis can be minimized by several simple maneuvers. Elevation of the foot of the bed 15–20 degrees encourages venous outflow. Slight flexion of the knees is desirable. A footboard enables the patient to perform leg exercises (ankle flexion and extension) while in bed. Sitting in a chair for long periods in the early postoperative period should be avoided. Early ambulation is ideal. Graduated compression stockings and sequential compression devices have proven efficacy in reducing risk of calf vein thrombosis and are particularly useful in moderate-risk and high-risk patients in whom anticoagulation is contraindicated. They function by increasing venous flow, decreasing venous stasis, and increasing the release of endothelial fibrinolytic factors and are safe for use on almost all patients. They have not been shown to decrease the incidence of pulmonary emboli.

B. Anticoagulation

Low-dose unfractionated heparin, 5000 units subcutaneously twice daily, and low-molecular-weight heparin (LMWH), eg, with enoxaparin, 30 mg subcutaneously twice daily, have both been shown to reduce significantly the incidence of postoperative deep venous thrombosis and pulmonary embolus. LMWH appears to be more effective in the orthopedic surgery patient and is associated also with a lower risk of bleeding complications (1–5% with enoxaparin versus 2–12% with unfractionated heparin). Use of heparin products is contraindicated in patients with recent craniotomy, intracranial bleeding, or severe gastrointestinal bleeding. Either medication must be withheld 12 hours prior to placement or removal of an epidural catheter to avoid epidural hematoma. Coagulation studies are unaffected with prophylactic dosing, but the platelet count must be monitored for early detection of heparin-induced thrombocytopenia, which occurs with peak incidence at 5–10 days of treatment. Warfarin is seldom used for perioperative deep venous thrombosis prophylaxis but may be indicated for long-term management of minimally ambulatory patients. Lifetime anticoagulation with low-dose warfarin or prophylactic vena caval filter placement is considered in patients with hypercoagulable state or paralysis.

Treatment

The standard treatment of deep venous thrombosis is systemic anticoagulation with heparin (initial bolus 100 units/kg followed by 10 units/kg/h, dosed to goal partial thromboplastin time of 1.5–2 times normal). This reduces the risk of pulmonary embolism and decreases the rate of thrombophlebitis recurrence by 80%. Systemic anticoagulation does not directly lyse thrombi but stops propagation and allows natural fibrinolysis to occur.

Warfarin is started after therapeutic heparinization. The two therapies should overlap to diminish the possibility of a hypercoagulable state, which can occur during the first few days of warfarin administration because warfarin also inhibits synthesis of the natural anticoagulant proteins C and S. The recommended treatment for the first episode of uncomplicated deep venous thrombosis is 3–6 months of warfarin to maintain a goal INR of 2.0–3.0. After a second episode, warfarin is continued indefinitely. The risk for recurrent venous thrombosis is increased markedly in the presence of factor V Leiden mutations, homozygous activated protein C resistance, antiphospholipid antibody, and deficiencies of antithrombin III and of protein C or protein S, so lifelong anticoagulation is also recommended for these conditions.

Recently, enoxaparin at therapeutic dosing (1 mg/kg subcutaneously twice daily) has been shown to be equally safe and effective for treatment of deep venous thrombosis. Enoxaparin does not require monitoring of its anticoagulant effect because of its predictable dose-response relationship, so it has been promoted for use in outpatient treatment. Unfractionated heparin inhibits thrombin by complexing thrombin and antithrombin III. The enoxaparin molecule is too small to inhibit thrombin in this manner; its main therapeutic effect comes from inhibition of factor Xa activity, which accounts for its lower risk of bleeding complications and thrombocytopenia. It has also demonstrated less protein C and S inhibition, less complement activation, and a lower risk of osteoporosis.

Current research efforts are directed toward creation of an oral thrombin inhibitor. This is expected to have a more favorable dose-response curve and side-effect profile than warfarin.

Many studies have evaluated the efficacy of fibrinolytic agents in the treatment of acute deep venous thrombosis. Although faster clot lysis and increased venous patency are observed with alteplase versus heparin, this has not translated to a decreased incidence of postphlebitis syndrome. Risk of bleeding complications is higher with alteplase and does not appear to be reduced by selective catheterization for local administration. To be effective, it is felt that alteplase should be instituted within 1 week after clot formation, before extensive fibrin cross-linking can occur. One possible application for alteplase is acute iliofemoral venous thrombosis complicated by massive extremity edema and cyanosis. In this setting, iliofemoral thrombectomy is unsuccessful in as many as 50% of patients, often because of inability to effectively treat distal thrombosis.

Treatment of isolated calf vein thrombosis is controversial, as they are associated with a low risk of pulmonary emboli. However, if untreated, 25% progress to the proximal deep veins, where the incidence of chronic venous insufficiency is 25% and that of fatal pulmonary embolism is 10%. Patients with symptomatic calf vein thrombosis should be anticoagulated; asymptomatic patients may be followed expectantly with serial ultrasound examination.

Prognosis

With early and effective treatment, prognosis in most cases is good. Mortality is related to pulmonary embolus, which occurs in 60% of patients with inadequately treated proximal lower extremity thrombosis.

Breddin HK et al: Effects of a low-molecular weight heparin on thrombus regression and recurrent thromboembolism in patients with deep-vein thrombosis. N Engl J Med 2001; 344:626. [PMID: 11228276]

Forster A et al: Tissue plasminogen activator for the treatment of deep venous thrombosis of the lower extremity: A systematic review. Chest 2001;119:572. [PMID: 11171740]

Heit JA et al: Comparison of the oral direct thrombin inhibitor ximelagatran with enoxaparin as prophylaxis against venous thromboembolism after total knee replacement: A phase 2 dose-finding study. Arch Intern Med 2001;161:2215. [PMID: 11575978]

Hirsh J et al: Clinical trials that have influenced the treatment of venous thromboembolism: A historical perspective. Ann Intern Med 2001;134:409. [PMID: 11242501]

Lopez-Beret P et al: Systematic study of occult pulmonary thromboembolism in patients with deep venous thrombosis. J Vasc Surg 2001;33:515. [PMID: 11241121]

Scurr JH et al: Frequency and prevention of symptomless deep-vein thrombosis in long-haul flights: A randomised trial. Lancet 2001;12:1461. [PMID: 11377600]

2. Thrombophlebitis of the Superficial Veins

ESSENTIALS OF DIAGNOSIS

- *Induration, redness, and tenderness along a superficial vein.*
- *Often a history of recent intravenous line or trauma. No significant swelling of the extremity.*

General Considerations

Superficial thrombophlebitis may occur spontaneously in patients with varicose veins, in pregnant or postpartum women, or in patients with thromboangiitis obliterans or Behçet's disease. It can also occur after trauma, such as a blow to the leg, or after intravenous infusion. A migratory thrombophlebitis may be a manifestation of abdominal cancer such as carcinoma of the pancreas (Trousseau's syndrome). The long saphenous vein and its tributaries are most often involved. Superficial thrombophlebitis is associated with occult deep vein thrombosis in about 20% of cases. Pulmonary emboli are rare unless extension into the deep venous system occurs.

Clinical Findings

The patient usually experiences a dull pain in the region of the involved vein. Induration, redness, and tenderness correspond to dilated, thrombosed superficial veins. Edema of the extremity and deep calf tenderness are absent unless the deep veins are involved. Chills and high fever suggest septic or suppurative phlebitis, which is most often encountered as a complication of an indwelling intravenous catheter. Plastic intravenous catheters should be observed daily for signs of local inflammation and removed if a local reaction develops to avoid serious thrombotic or septic complications.

Differential Diagnosis

The linear rather than circular nature of the lesion and the distribution along the course of a superficial vein help to differentiate superficial phlebitis from cellulitis, erythema nodosum, erythema induratum, panniculitis, and fibrositis. Lymphangitis and deep thrombophlebitis must also be considered.

Treatment

The primary treatment of superficial venous thrombophlebitis is the administration of nonsteroidal anti-inflammatory drugs, local heat, and elevation. Ambulation is encouraged. In the majority of circumstances, symptoms will resolve within 7 to 10 days. Excision of the involved vein is recommended for symptoms that persist over 2 weeks on treatment, or for recurrent phlebitis in the same vein segment. If there is progressive proximal extension to the saphenofemoral junction or cephalic-subclavian junction, ligation and resection of the vein at the junction should be performed. Anticoagulation is reserved for rapidly progressing disease or extension into the deep system.

Septic thrombophlebitis requires treatment with intravenous antibiotics. As the causative organism is often staphylococcus or a gram-negative rod, broad-spectrum antibiotic coverage should be instituted until blood culture results become available. If rapid resolution of the phlebitis occurs, no treatment beyond a 7- to 10-day course of antibiotics is required. However, if the patient becomes septic, immediate excision of the infected vein is required.

Prognosis

The course is generally benign and brief, and the prognosis depends on the underlying pathologic process. Phlebitis of a saphenous vein occasionally extends to the deep veins, in which case pulmonary emboli may occur.

Belcaro G et al: Superficial thrombophlebitis of the legs: A randomized, controlled, follow-up study. Angiology 1999;50: 523. [PMID: 10431991]

CHRONIC VENOUS INSUFFICIENCY

 ESSENTIALS OF DIAGNOSIS

- *History of phlebitis or leg injury.*
- *Ankle edema is the earliest sign.*
- *Late signs are stasis pigmentation, dermatitis, subcutaneous induration, varicosities, and ulceration.*

General Considerations

Chronic venous insufficiency is most often secondary to deep venous thrombosis, although a history of phlebitis is not obtainable in about 25% of patients. Other possible causes are leg trauma, varicose veins, neoplastic obstruction of the pelvic veins, or congenital or acquired arteriovenous fistula.

The basic physiologic abnormality in patients with chronic venous insufficiency is chronic elevation in venous pressure. The normal venous capacitance can accommodate large-volume changes that occur during exercise with only minimal changes in venous pressure. However, when valves in the deep and perforating veins are destroyed by thrombophlebitis, valvular reflux and bidirectional blood flow result in abnormally high ambulatory venous pressures. Proximal venous obstruction also results in venous hypertension. High ambulatory venous pressure transmitted through perforating veins of the calf and ankle results in superficial varicosities, edema and fibrosis of the subcutaneous tissue and skin, hyperpigmentation, and, later, dermatitis and ulceration.

Clinical Findings

Chronic venous insufficiency is characterized by progressive edema of the leg that begins at the ankle and calf and is accompanied by a dull aching discomfort. Typically, the edema is worst at the end of the day and improves with leg elevation. Varicosities are often present. Stasis dermatitis, brownish pigmentation, brawny induration, and ulceration develop with long-standing disease. The skin is usually thin, shiny, atrophic, and cyanotic. Cellulitis may appear in scaly, dry, itchy regions with skin breakdown; in other areas, a weeping dermatitis may develop. Venous stasis ulcers are large, painless, and irregular in outline. They have a shallow, moist granulation bed and occur in the gaiter area on the medial or lateral aspects of the ankle. Healing of these ulcers results in a thin scar on a fibrotic base that often breaks down with minor trauma.

Differential Diagnosis

Congestive heart failure and chronic renal disease may result in bilateral edema of the lower extremities. Lymphedema is associated with a brawny thickening in the subcutaneous tissue that does not respond readily to elevation; edema is particularly prominent on the dorsum of the feet and in the toes; varicosities are absent, and there is often a history of recurrent cellulitis.

Primary varicose veins or acute deep venous thrombosis may be difficult to differentiate from chronic venous insufficiency without diagnostic tests.

Other conditions associated with chronic ulcers of the leg include autoimmune diseases (eg, Felty's syndrome), arterial insufficiency (often painful, well circumscribed, and located over pressure points), sickle cell anemia, erythema induratum (bilateral and usually on the posterior aspect of the lower part of the leg), and fungal infections (cultures specific; no chronic swelling or varicosities).

Prevention

The irreversible tissue changes that accompany chronic venous stasis disease can be minimized by early and aggressive management of conditions associated with deep venous reflux such as acute deep venous thrombosis and varicose veins.

Treatment

A. GENERAL MEASURES

The key to successful management of chronic venous stasis disease is the realization that it is an incurable but manageable problem. Most patients respond to a conservative treatment program. The causes of complications of chronic venous insufficiency are largely mechanical, and so the solutions are mechanical. Bed rest with leg elevation is fundamental in the treatment of the acute complications. Similarly, chronic care of the leg includes (1) intermittent elevation of the legs during the day and elevation of the legs at night (kept above the level of the heart with pillows under the mattress); (2) avoidance of long periods of sitting or standing; (3) the daily use of fitted knee-high or thigh-high graduated compression stockings (20–30 mm Hg); and (4) regular exercise.

B. MANAGEMENT OF STASIS DERMATITIS

Eczematous eruption may be acute or chronic; treatment varies accordingly. The simplest treatment for acute weeping dermatitis is strict bed rest, leg elevation, and wet saline compresses. Antiseptic solutions containing peroxide, boric acid, or buffered aluminum acetate (Burow's solution) are not recommended because they impede wound healing. Cadexomer iodine is an iodine-containing starch powder dressing that has been shown to speed healing of weepy ulcers. Alginate dressings are also effective in this setting. In general, however, no definitive advantage has emerged of occlusive over semiocclusive dressings or of topical antibiotics, growth factors, or free radical scavengers over simple inert dressings.

Systemic antibiotics and topical antifungal agents (1% clotrimazole or 2% miconazole cream) are indicated only if active infection is suspected. With reduction of the acute edema, 0.5% hydrocortisone cream is applied to the area for 1–2 weeks or until no further improvement is noted. Cordran tape, a plastic tape impregnated with flurandrenolide, is a convenient way to apply both medication and dressing. Zinc oxide ointment with ichthammol, 3%, applied once or twice daily, is an alternative treatment for chronic dermatitis.

C. ULCERATION

Venous ulcerations can be treated by wet-to-dry normal saline dressings and Ace wrap compression, or with an Unna boot. The Unna boot is a layered dressing composed of a medicated bandage (such as the original Dome paste composed of calamine, zinc oxide, glycerin, sorbitol, gelatin, and magnesium aluminum silicate), followed by a gauze dressing, followed by an elastic wrap. It must be kept dry and is usually changed weekly. Occasionally, the ulcer is so large and chronic that wide debridement and skin grafting is the best approach. This can be combined with open or endoscopic ligation of incompetent perforating veins contributing to elevated venous pressure in the ulcer bed. Venous reconstructive surgery is performed in some centers for intractable chronic venous stasis disease. The goal of the surgery is to increase venous outflow and decrease venous hypertension in the limb by repairing or replacing incompetent valves in the deep system. Valvuloplasty, venous segment transposition, and valvular transplantation have been performed with variable reported success rates.

Prognosis

Recurrent venous stasis ulcers and progressive venous stasis changes of the skin are not uncommon, particularly if patients do not adhere to a lifelong routine of intermittent leg elevation, regular exercise, and use of graduated compression stockings.

Mohr DN et al: The venous stasis syndrome after deep venous thrombosis or pulmonary embolism: A population-based study. Mayo Clin Proc 2000;75:1249. [PMID: 11126832]

SUPERIOR VENA CAVA OBSTRUCTION

Superior vena cava syndrome is a rare disorder caused by partial or complete obstruction of the superior vena cava. The most frequent causes are (1) superior mediastinal tumors (responsible for over 80% of cases), such as adenocarcinoma of the lung, lymphoma, thyroid carcinoma, thymoma, teratoma, synovial cell carcinoma, or angiosarcoma; (2) chronic fibrotic mediastinitis, either idiopathic or secondary to tuberculosis, histoplasmosis, pyogenic infections, or drugs (such as methysergide); (3) thrombophlebitis secondary to indwelling central venous catheters or pacemaker wires; (4) aneurysm of the aortic arch; and (5) constrictive pericarditis.

Clinical Findings

A. SYMPTOMS AND SIGNS

Symptoms include swelling of the neck and face, headache, dizziness, visual disturbances, stupor, and syncope related to progressive obstruction of the venous drainage of the head, neck, and upper extremities. Bending over or lying down accentuates the symptoms; sitting quietly is generally preferred. The severity of symptoms is dependent on the degree and duration of stenosis and the development of venous collateral circulation. Dilated anterior chest wall veins and facial flushing ultimately can progress to brawny edema and cyanosis of the face and arms. Cerebral and laryngeal edema result in impaired mental status and respiratory insufficiency.

B. DIAGNOSIS

Diagnosis is usually suggested by the history and physical examination. Duplex ultrasound can be suggestive, but more specific anatomic information is obtained with CT scan or MRA, which can also disclose etiologic causes. Contrast venography is reserved for cases in which surgical or endoscopic treatment is anticipated.

Treatment

Therapy is dictated by the cause of the disease and the severity of symptoms. Benign thrombosis is treated with central venous catheter removal, head elevation, and short-course warfarin anticoagulation or thrombolysis and venous angioplasty. Venous bypass (left atrial appendage to internal jugular or innominate vein) has good patency rates in selected patients refractory to more conservative measures. Surgical excision of the fibrous tissue encasing the great vessels may reestablish flow in patients with mediastinal fibrosis or pericardial constriction. Unless concomitant tumor resection is planned, superior vena cava syndrome secondary to malignant disease is preferentially treated by endovascular stenting. Chemotherapy or external beam radiation may also achieve symptomatic improvement in patients with malignancy.

Lanciego C et al: Stenting as first option for endovascular treatment of malignant superior vena cava syndrome. AJR Am J Roentgenol 2001;177:585. [PMID: 11517051]

■ DISEASES OF THE LYMPHATIC CHANNELS

LYMPHANGITIS & LYMPHADENITIS

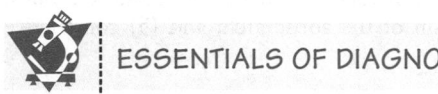
ESSENTIALS OF DIAGNOSIS

- *Red streak extending from an infected area toward enlarged, tender regional lymph nodes.*
- *Chills, fever, and malaise may be present.*

General Considerations

Lymphangitis and lymphadenitis frequently accompany a streptococcal or staphylococcal infection in the distal arm or leg. The inciting wound may be a superficial scratch with cellulitis, an insect bite, or an established abscess. A prominent red streak extending toward tender, enlarged regional lymph nodes is diagnostic. Systemic manifestations include fever, chills, tachycardia, and malaise. If untreated, the infection can progress rapidly, often in a matter of hours.

Clinical Findings

A. SYMPTOMS AND SIGNS

Throbbing pain at the site of the inciting wound is usually present. Malaise, anorexia, sweating, chills, and fever of 37.8–40 °C develop rapidly. The red streak may be faint initially and easily missed, especially in dark-skinned patients. The involved regional lymph nodes may be significantly enlarged and tender.

B. LABORATORY FINDINGS

Leukocytosis with a left shift is usually present. Blood cultures are often positive for staphylococcal or streptococcal species. Wound cultures may be helpful in treatment of the more severe or refractory infections but are often difficult to interpret because of skin contaminants.

Differential Diagnosis

Superficial thrombophlebitis is distinguished from lymphangitis by the pattern of erythema (localized to an indurated thrombosed vein) and the lack of lymphadenitis. Cat-scratch disease caused by *Bartonella*

henselae typically presents with enlarged but non-tender lymph nodes. Lymphangitis must also be differentiated from cellulitis and from severe soft tissue infections such as acute streptococcal hemolytic gangrene and necrotizing fasciitis requiring emergent debridement. These infections are nonlinear and are characterized by induration and subcutaneous crepitus.

Treatment

The extremity is elevated, and warm compresses are applied to the involved area. Analgesics and intravenous antibiotics (penicillin G, 4 million units every 6 hours; or cephazolin, 1 g every 8 hours) should be instituted immediately. Examination of the wound will determine the need for debridement or incision and drainage of an abscess.

Prognosis

Early institution of appropriate antibiotic therapy and wound care will usually control the infection in 48–72 hours. Delayed or inadequate therapy can result in rapidly progressive infection, septicemia, and death.

LYMPHEDEMA

ESSENTIALS OF DIAGNOSIS

- *Painless edema of upper or lower extremities.*
- *Involves the dorsal surfaces of the hands and fingers or the feet and toes.*
- *Developmental or acquired, unilateral or bilateral.*
- *Edema is pitting initially and becomes brawny and nonpitting with time.*
- *Ulceration, varicosities, and stasis pigmentation do not occur. There may be episodes of lymphangitis and cellulitis.*

General Considerations

The underlying mechanism in lymphedema is impairment of the flow of lymph from an extremity. When due to congenital developmental abnormalities consisting of hypo- or hyperplastic changes of the proximal or distal lymphatics, it is referred to as primary lymphedema. Familial lymphedema developing before 1 year of age is called Milroy's disease; it is usually bilateral and affects boys more often than girls. More often, lymphedema develops during adolescence (lymphedema praecox) and is unilateral; there is a 3.5:1 female predominance. Lymphedema occurring after age 35 is referred to as lymphedema tarda. The secondary form of lymphedema results from an inflammatory or mechanical obstruction of the lymphatics following trauma, regional lymph node resection, irradiation, bacterial or fungal infections, lymphoproliferative diseases, or filariasis.

Lymphatic obstruction results in stasis of a protein-rich fluid, with slowly progressive, painless edema and secondary fibrosis that may be exacerbated by superimposed episodes of acute infection. The edema is usually centered around the ankle and involves the toes and the dorsum of the foot. Hypertrophy of the limb results, with markedly thickened skin and subcutaneous tissue. Rarely, lymphangiosarcoma or angiosarcoma may develop as a complication of chronic lymphedema. This neoplastic transformation of blood vessels and lymphatics is called the Stewart-Treves syndrome.

Diagnosis is usually made on the basis of clinical findings. Venous duplex ultrasonography is performed to exclude venous insufficiency or vascular malformations. Lymphangiography and radioactive isotope studies are indicated only if surgical reconstruction is anticipated.

Treatment

Lymphedema is a chronic disease for which there is no complete cure. However, a variety of conservative measures can substantially reduce the risk of further complications and disability. No drug therapy is effective. Use of benzopyrones (eg, dicumarol) and corticosteroid injections to increase lymphatic transport has not shown consistent benefit. Diuretics can be useful for acute exacerbation of edema secondary to infection or for coexisting venous stasis disease but are not recommended for long-term use.

The mainstay of treatment is external compression and meticulous skin care. Mechanical reduction of lymphedema can best be achieved with a program of frequent leg elevation, manual lymphatic drainage massage, and external compression. Sequential pneumatic compression devices are traditionally the first line of treatment for limb reduction. Many different devices are available for use on the leg, and Reid sleeves can be custom fit for patients with postmastectomy arm lymphedema. Graduated compression stockings (20–30 mm Hg) maintain the limb after reduction by pneumatic compression.

Good skin care is imperative in order to prevent infection. Moisturizing lotions should be applied regularly, especially after showering or bathing. Drying and cracking of the skin can create portals of entry for bacteria. Infection is difficult to eradicate because of disordered lymphatic drainage and can be a threat to limb survival.

In carefully selected cases, surgery may improve limb function. The goal is to reduce limb bulk, either by ablative techniques (excision of excess tissue) or by physiologic techniques (lymphatic reconstruction). Microsurgical lymphaticovenous anastomosis has yielded some satisfactory cosmetic and functional results, though long-term efficacy is as yet unknown.

Campisi C et al: Long-term results after lymphatic-venous anastomoses for the treatment of obstructive lymphedema. Microsurgery 2001;21:135. [PMID: 11494379]

Ko DS et al: Effective treatment of lymphedema of the extremities. Arch Surg 1998;133:452. [PMID: 9565129]

■ HYPOTENSION & SHOCK

ESSENTIALS OF DIAGNOSIS

- *Hypotension, tachycardia, oliguria, altered mental status.*
- *Peripheral hypoperfusion and hypoxia.*

General Considerations

Shock occurs when the rate of arterial blood flow is inadequate to meet tissue metabolic needs. Tissue oxygen delivery is dependent on cardiac output, hemoglobin saturation, and peripheral microcirculation—some or all of these factors are altered in the shock state. The physiologic response to shock is mediated by the neuroendocrine system through release of catecholamines, renin, antidiuretic hormone, glucagon, cortisol, and growth hormone. These hormones are responsible for many of the clinical manifestations of shock: tachycardia, oliguria, delayed capillary refill, increasing agitation, and insulin resistance. Treatment must be directed both at the manifestations of shock and at its cause.

Classification
(Table 12–1)

A. HYPOVOLEMIC SHOCK

Decreased intravascular volume resulting from loss of blood, plasma, or fluids and electrolytes may be obvious (eg, external hemorrhage) or subtle (eg, sequestration in a "third space"). Compensatory vasoconstriction temporarily reduces the size of the vascular bed and may transiently maintain the blood pressure, but unreplaced ongoing losses of over 15% of the blood volume result in hypotension, increased peripheral resistance, collapse of capillary and venous beds, and progressive tissue hypoxia. Even a moderate sudden loss of circulating fluids can result in severe damage to vital organs.

Table 12–1. Classification of shock by mechanism and common causes.[1]

Hypovolemic shock
    Loss of blood (hemorrhagic shock)
        External hemorrhage
            Trauma
            Gastrointestinal tract bleeding
        Internal hemorrhage
            Hematoma
            Hemothorax or hemoperitoneum
    Loss of plasma
        Burns
        Exfoliative dermatitis
    Loss of fluid and electrolytes
        External
            Vomiting
            Diarrhea
            Excessive sweating
            Hyperosmolar states (diabetic ketoacidosis,
                hyperosmolar nonketotic coma)
        Internal ("third spacing")
            Pancreatitis
            Ascites
             Bowel obstruction
Cardiogenic shock
    Dysrhythmia
        Tachyarrhythmia
        Bradyarrhythmia
    "Pump failure" (secondary to myocardial infarction or
        other cardiomyopathy)
    Acute valvular dysfunction (especially regurgitant lesions)
    Rupture of ventricular septum or free ventricular wall
Obstructive shock
    Tension pneumothorax
    Pericardial disease (tamponade, constriction)
    Disease of pulmonary vasculature (massive pulmonary
        emboli, pulmonary hypertension)
    Cardiac tumor (atrial myxoma)
    Left atrial mural thrombus
    Obstructive valvular disease (aortic or mitral stenosis)
Distributive shock
    Septic shock
    Anaphylactic shock
    Neurogenic shock
    Vasodilator drugs
    Acute adrenal insufficiency

[1]Reproduced, with permission, from Saunders CE, Ho MT (editors): *Current Emergency Diagnosis & Treatment*, 4th ed. McGraw-Hill, 1992

B. CARDIOGENIC SHOCK

Pump failure can be related to myocardial infarction, cardiomyopathy, myocardial contusion, valvular incompetence or stenosis, or arrhythmias. See discussion in Chapter 10.

C. OBSTRUCTIVE SHOCK

Cardiac tamponade, tension pneumothorax, and massive pulmonary embolism can cause acute decrease in cardiac output resulting in shock. These are medical emergencies requiring prompt diagnosis and treatment. Pericardiocentesis or pericardial window, chest tube placement, or catheter-directed thrombolytic therapy can be lifesaving.

D. DISTRIBUTIVE SHOCK

Reduction in systemic vascular resistance from sepsis, anaphylaxis, systemic inflammatory response syndrome (SIRS) produced by severe pancreatitis or burns, or acute adrenal insufficiency may result in inadequate cardiac output despite normal circulatory volume. Elevated nitric oxide levels may explain many of the physiologic aspects of the disease.

1. Septic shock—Sepsis is the most common cause of distributive shock and carries a mortality of 40–80%. Typically, patients present with fever, chills, hypotension, hyperglycemia, and altered mental status due to gram-negative bacteremia (*Escherichia coli,* klebsiella, proteus, and pseudomonas). Gram-positive cocci and gram-negative anaerobes (bacteroides) are less often implicated. Risk factors include extremes of age, diabetes, immunosuppression, and recent urinary, biliary, or gynecologic manipulation, such as placement of a percutaneous nephrostomy or biliary drain in an obstructed system.

2. Neurogenic shock—Neurogenic shock is caused by traumatic spinal cord injury or effects of an epidural or spinal anesthetic. Reflex vagal parasympathetic stimulation evoked by pain, gastric dilation, or fright may simulate neurogenic shock, producing hypotension, bradycardia, and syncope.

Diagnosis of Shock & Impending Shock

The different types of shock are characterized by the same clinical signs.

A. HYPOTENSION

Hypotension in adults is traditionally defined as a systolic blood pressure of 90 mm Hg or less but must be evaluated relative to the patient's normal blood pressure. While a systolic blood pressure of 90 mm Hg may be normal in a healthy, athletic adult, a pressure of 100 mm Hg may indicate shock in a patient who is normally hypertensive. A drop in systolic pressure of more than 10–20 mm Hg and an increase in pulse of more than 15 with positional change suggests depleted intravascular volume. Orthostatic hypotension resulting from peripheral neuropathy or use of beta-blockers is usually not associated with an increase in pulse rate.

B. End Organ Hypoperfusion

Patients in shock often have cool or mottled extremities and weak or absent peripheral pulses. Splanchnic vasoconstriction leads to oliguria, bowel ischemia, and hepatic dysfunction, which can ultimately result in multiorgan failure.

C. Altered Mental Status

Patients may demonstrate normal mental status or may be restless, agitated, confused, lethargic, or comatose as a result of inadequate perfusion of the brain.

Treatment

A. General Measures

Treatment depends upon prompt diagnosis and an accurate appraisal of inciting conditions. Initial therapy consists of basic life support: airway maintenance, oxygen, cardiopulmonary resuscitation, intravenous access and fluid resuscitation. Cardiac monitoring can detect myocardial ischemia requiring cardiac catheterization and thrombolytic therapy or malignant arrhythmias treated by standard advanced cardiac life support (ACLS) protocols. A thorough history and physical examination, including stool guaiac testing, is helpful in locating potential sources of sepsis or hemorrhage and excluding immediately reversible causes such as tamponade or tension pneumothorax. Unresponsive or minimally responsive patients are immediately given 50% dextrose (one ampule intravenously) and naloxone (2 mg intravenously or intramuscularly) followed by neurologic assessment (Glasgow Coma Scale) and are then intubated for airway protection. Specimens should be sent for complete blood count, electrolytes, glucose, arterial blood gas determinations, coagulation parameters, and typing and cross matching. An arterial line is placed for continuous blood pressure measurement and a Foley catheter for assessment of urine volume. Urine output should be maintained at > 0.5 mL/kg/h.

Early consideration is given to placement of a pulmonary artery catheter for hemodynamic pressure measurements. This is helpful in distinguishing cardiogenic and septic shock and in monitoring the effects of volume resuscitation or pressor medications. Because of the attendant risks associated with pulmonary artery catheters (infection, arrhythmias, vein thrombosis, pulmonary artery rupture), the value of the information they might provide must be carefully weighed in each patient. They are useful in management of patients with cardiogenic shock; in other types of shock, a central venous line may be adequate. Central lines may also be useful in the administration of medications and in measurement of central venous oxygen saturation. In general, a central venous pressure (CVP) or pulmonary capillary wedge pressure (PCWP) under 5 mm Hg suggests hypovolemia and over 18 mm Hg suggests volume overload, cardiac failure, tamponade, or pulmonary hypertension. A cardiac index < 2 L/min/m^2 indicates a need for phar-

macologic or mechanical pressor support. A high cardiac index (> 4 L/min/m^2) in a hypotensive patient is consistent with early septic shock. The systemic vascular resistance (SVR) is a derived value and is low (< 800 dyn·s/cm^{-5}) in early sepsis and neurogenic shock and high (> 1500 dyne·s/cm^{-5}) in hypovolemic and cardiogenic shock. Treatment is directed at maintaining a central venous pressure of 8–12 mm Hg, a mean arterial pressure of 65–90 mm Hg, a cardiac index of 2–4 L/min/m^2, and central venous oxygen saturation of greater than 70%.

B. Volume Replacement

Hypovolemic shock is treated with fluid resuscitation. Initial response is gauged after bolus administration of 2 L of crystalloid, and additional fluid requirements are then estimated from measurement of ongoing losses, CVP or PCWP, and urine output.

Selection of the proper fluid for restoration and maintenance of hemodynamic stability is controversial. Blood products are indicated in hemorrhagic shock; type-specific or type O negative packed red blood cells (PRBC) are given to maintain the hematocrit above 30%. Whole blood provides extra volume and clotting factors. Each unit of PRBC or whole blood is expected to raise the hematocrit by 3%. With abnormal coagulation studies, platelet count less than 10,000/μL, or transfusion of over six units of PRBC, fresh frozen plasma and platelets should be administered. When hematocrit is greater than 30% and CVP is less than 8 mm Hg, crystalloid solutions are generally the preferred resuscitation fluid. Isotonic (0.9%) sodium chloride or lactated Ringer's solution (which contains potassium, calcium, and bicarbonate as well as sodium chloride) is given in boluses of 500 or 1000 mL. Dextrose-containing solutions are generally not needed initially except in the treatment of hypoglycemic shock. Hypertonic (7.5%) saline is being investigated for use in the prehospital setting and in the hypotensive patient with closed head injury.

Plasma expanders—or colloids such as albumin, dextran, and hetastarch—are high-molecular-weight substances that increase plasma oncotic pressure. Increased capillary permeability in the lung accompanying septic shock or SIRS may result in increased pulmonary edema in patients administered colloids, so use of these agents warrants careful consideration. Side effects include coagulopathy and anaphylaxis. Oxygen-carrying synthetic plasma expanders ("artificial blood") has been used with success in some trauma centers for treatment of hypovolemic shock.

Large volume resuscitation with unwarmed fluids produces hypothermia, which must be treated to avoid hypothermia-induced coagulopathy.

C. Medications

Calcium should be administered to maintain an ionized calcium level greater than 1. Sodium bicarbonate may be considered in patients with arterial pH less than 7.20.

Pressors are administered only after adequate fluid resuscitation. Dopamine hydrochloride has variable effects according to dosage. At low doses (2–3 μg/kg/min), stimulation of dopaminergic and beta-agonist receptors produces increased glomerular filtration rate, heart rate, and contractility. At higher doses (> 5 μg/kg/min), alpha-adrenergic effects predominate, resulting in peripheral vasoconstriction.

Dobutamine (2–20 μg/kg/min), a synthetic catecholamine with greater inotropic effect and afterload reduction than dopamine, is the first-line drug for cardiogenic shock. Because tachyphylaxis can occur after 48 hours, the phosphodiesterase inhibitor amrinone (5–15 μg/kg/min) is often substituted. Diuretics, thrombolytics, morphine, nitroglycerin, antiarrhythmics, and antiplatelet agents may be part of a multimodality approach to treatment of cardiogenic shock secondary to acute myocardial infarction.

Distributive shock or neurogenic shock may require peripheral vasoconstrictors such as epinephrine (2–10 μg/min) or norepinephrine (0.5–30 μg/min). Phenylephrine is avoided in neurogenic shock because of the potential for reflex bradycardia.

Vasopressin (antidiuretic hormone [ADH]) is gaining widespread acceptance in treatment of distributive shock and has been added to the ACLS algorithm for ventricular fibrillation cardiac arrest. Shock due to sepsis or SIRS is associated with low levels of endogenous vasopressin; in hemorrhagic shock, vasopressin is initially elevated and then drops to subnormal levels. Vasopressin has multiple therapeutic effects: peripheral vasoconstriction, decreased heart rate, hemostasis, increased serum cortisol, and coronary, cerebral, and pulmonary vasodilation. It is shown also to potentiate the effects of other peripheral vasoconstrictors. Paradoxically, at low doses (0.01–0.04 units/min), it acts as a diuretic. The dose is regulated to maintain normal physiologic serum levels of 20–30 pg/mL. The effect on mortality rate in septic shock is yet unknown. Vasopressin-induced vasoconstriction may be mediated by effects on nitric oxide synthesis.

Methylene blue is another inhibitor of the nitric oxide pathway being investigated for use in distributive shock.

Broad-spectrum antibiotics are administered in septic shock until blood cultures and sensitivities become available. Sedation, anxiolytics, and pain medications are tailored for each individual case. Corticosteroids are lifesaving in the treatment of shock associated with acute adrenal insufficiency (see Chapter 26) and decrease inflammation associated with acute spinal shock, but they are of no benefit in other types of shock. Research has focused on regulation of specific inhibitors of the inflammatory response. Protein C levels are diminished in septic shock, and recombinant protein C (drotrecogin alfa) is now in phase 3 trials. It has been shown to significantly decrease 28-day mortality in septic shock when given as a continuous infusion of 24 μg/kg/h for 96 hours. Its mechanism of action is reduction of systemic inflammation by inhibition of thrombosis. Administration of recombinant protein C has been correlated with lower D-dimer and interleukin-6 levels in this setting.

Other Treatment Modalities

Cardiac failure may require use of transcutaneous or transvenous pacing or placement of an intra-arterial balloon pump. Emergent revascularization by stent angioplasty or coronary artery bypass appears to improve long-term outcome. Urgent hemodialysis or continuous venovenous hemofiltration may be indicated for maintenance of fluid and electrolyte balance during acute renal insufficiency resulting from shock.

Bernard GR et al: Efficacy and safety of recombinant human activated protein C for severe sepsis. N Engl J Med 2001; 344:699. [PMID: 11236773]

Hochman JS et al: One-year survival following early revascularization for cardiogenic shock. JAMA 2001;285:190. [PMID: 11176812]

Holmes CL et al: Physiology of vasopressin relevant to management of septic shock. Chest 2001;120:989. [PMID: 11555538]

Landry DW et al: The pathogenesis of vasodilatory shock. N Engl J Med 2001;345:588. [PMID: 11529214]

Orlinsky M et al: Current controversies in shock and resuscitation. Surg Clin North Am 2001;81:1217. [PMID: 11766174]

Rivers E et al: Early goal-directed therapy in the treatment of severe sepsis and septic shock. N Engl J Med 2001;345:1368. [PMID: 11794169]

Blood

13

Charles A. Linker, MD
See www.current-med.com/ch13.html

■ ANEMIAS

General Approach to Anemias

Anemia is present in adults if the hematocrit is less than 41% (hemoglobin < 13.5 g/dL) in males or 37% (hemoglobin < 12 g/dL) in females. Congenital anemia is suggested by the patient's personal and family history. Poor diet results in folic acid deficiency and contributes to iron deficiency. Bleeding is present universally in iron deficiency in adults. Physical examination includes attention to signs of primary hematologic diseases (lymphadenopathy, hepatosplenomegaly, or bone tenderness). Mucosal changes such as a smooth tongue suggest megaloblastic anemia.

Anemias are classified according to their pathophysiologic basis, ie, whether related to diminished production or accelerated loss of red blood cells (Table 13–1); or according to cell size (Table 13–2). The diagnostic possibilities in microcytic anemia are iron deficiency, thalassemia, and anemia of chronic disease. A severely microcytic anemia (MCV < 70 fL) is due either to iron deficiency or thalassemia. Macrocytic anemia may be due to megaloblastic (folate or vitamin B_{12} deficiency) or nonmegaloblastic causes, especially antiretrovirals. A severely macrocytic anemia (MCV > 125 fL) is almost always megaloblastic; exceptions are the myelodysplastic syndromes.

IRON DEFICIENCY ANEMIA

ESSENTIALS OF DIAGNOSIS

- *Both pathognomonic: absent bone marrow iron stores or serum ferritin < 12 μg/L.*
- *Caused by bleeding in adults unless proved otherwise.*
- *Response to iron therapy.*

General Considerations

Iron deficiency is the most common cause of anemia worldwide. The causes are listed in Table 13–3. Iron is necessary for the formation of heme and other enzymes. Total body iron ranges between 2 g and 4 g: approximately 50 mg/kg in men and 35 mg/kg in women. Most (70–95%) of iron is present in hemoglobin in circulating red blood cells. One milliliter of packed red blood cells (not whole blood) contains approximately 1 mg of iron. In men, red blood cell volume is approximately 30 mL/kg. A 70-kg man will therefore have approximately 2100 mL of packed red blood cells and consequently 2100 mg of iron in his circulating blood. In women, the red cell volume is about 27 mL/kg; a 50-kg woman will thus have 1350 mg of iron circulating in her red blood cells. Only 200–400 mg of iron is present in myoglobin and nonheme enzymes. Aside from circulating red blood cells, the major location of iron in the body is the storage pool, as ferritin or as hemosiderin and in macrophages. The range for storage iron is wide (0.5–2 g); approximately 25% of women in the USA have none.

The average American diet contains 10–15 mg of iron per day. About 10% of this amount is absorbed. Absorption occurs in the stomach, duodenum, and upper jejunum. Dietary iron present as heme is efficiently absorbed (10–20%) but nonheme iron less so (1–5%), largely because of interference by phosphates, tannins, and other food constituents. Small amounts of iron—approximately 1 mg/d—are normally lost though exfoliation of skin and mucosal cells. There is no physiologic mechanism for increasing normal body iron losses.

Menstrual blood loss in women plays a major role in iron metabolism. The average monthly menstrual blood loss is approximately 50 mL, or about 0.7 mg/d. However, menstrual blood loss may be five times the average. In order to maintain adequate iron stores, women with heavy menstrual losses must absorb 3–4 mg of iron from the diet each day. This strains the upper limit of what may reasonably be absorbed, and women with menorrhagia of this degree will almost always become iron-deficient.

Table 13–1. Classification of anemias by pathophysiology.

Decreased production
Hemoglobin synthesis: iron deficiency, thalassemia, anemia of chronic disease
DNA synthesis: megaloblastic anemia
Stem cell: aplastic anemia, myeloproliferative leukemia
Bone marrow infiltration: carcinoma, lymphoma
Pure red cell aplasia
Increased destruction
Blood loss
Hemolysis (intrinsic)
Membrane: hereditary spherocytosis, elliptocytosis
Hemoglobin: sickle cell, unstable hemoglobin
Glycolysis: pyruvate kinase deficiency, etc.
Oxidation: G6PD deficiency
Hemolysis (extrinsic)
Immune: warm antibody, cold antibody
Microangiopathic: thrombotic thrombocytopenic purpura, hemolytic-uremic syndrome, mechanical cardiac valve, paravalvular leak
Infection: clostridial
Hypersplenism

In general, iron metabolism is balanced between absorption of 1 mg/d and loss of 1 mg/d. Pregnancy may also upset the iron balance, since requirements increase to 2–5 mg of iron per day during pregnancy and lactation. Normal dietary iron cannot supply these requirements, and medicinal iron is needed during pregnancy and lactation. Repeated pregnancy (especially with breast feeding) may cause iron deficiency if increased requirements are not met with supplemental medicinal iron. Decreased iron absorption can on very rare occasions cause iron deficiency and usually occurs after gastric surgery, though concomitant bleeding is frequent.

By far the most important cause of iron deficiency anemia is blood loss, especially gastrointestinal blood

Table 13–2. Classification of anemias by MCV.

Microcytic
Iron deficiency
Thalassemia
Anemia of chronic disease
Macrocytic
Megaloblastic
Vitamin B_{12} deficiency
Folate deficiency
Nonmegaloblastic
Myelodysplasia, chemotherapy
Liver disease
Increased reticulocytosis
Myxedema
Normocytic
Many causes

Table 13–3. Causes of iron deficiency.

Deficient diet
Decreased absorption
Increased requirements
Pregnancy
Lactation
Blood loss
Gastrointestinal
Menstrual
Blood donation
Hemoglobinuria
Iron sequestration
Pulmonary hemosiderosis

loss. Chronic aspirin use may cause it even without a documented structural lesion. Iron deficiency demands a search for a source of gastrointestinal bleeding if other sites of blood loss (menorrhagia, other uterine bleeding, and repeated blood donations) are excluded.

Chronic hemoglobinuria may lead to iron deficiency, since more than 1 mg/d of iron can be lost by this route; traumatic hemolysis due to a prosthetic cardiac valve and other causes of intravascular hemolysis (eg, paroxysmal nocturnal hemoglobinuria) should also be considered.

Clinical Findings

A. SYMPTOMS AND SIGNS

As a rule, the only symptoms of iron deficiency anemia are those of the anemia itself (easy fatigability, tachycardia, palpitations and tachypnea on exertion). Severe deficiency causes skin and mucosal changes, including a smooth tongue, brittle nails, and cheilosis. Dysphagia because of the formation of esophageal webs (Plummer-Vinson syndrome) also occurs. Many iron-deficient patients develop pica, craving for specific foods (ice chips, lettuce, etc), often not rich in iron.

B. LABORATORY FINDINGS

Iron deficiency develops in stages. The first is depletion of iron stores. At this point, there is anemia and no changes in red blood cell size. The serum ferritin will become abnormally low. A ferritin value less than 30 μg/L is a highly reliable indicator of iron deficiency. The serum total iron-binding capacity (TIBC) rises.

After iron stores have been depleted, red blood cell formation will continue with deficient supplies of iron. Serum iron values decline to less than 30 μg/dL and transferrin saturation to less than 15%.

In the early stages, the MCV remains normal. Subsequently, the MCV falls and the blood smear shows hypochromic microcytic cells. With further progression, anisocytosis (variations in red blood cell size) and poikilocytosis (variation in shape of red cells) develop. Severe iron deficiency will produce a bizarre peripheral blood smear, with severely hypochromic cells, target cells, hypochromic pencil-shaped cells, and occasionally small numbers of nucleated red blood cells. The platelet count is commonly increased.

Differential Diagnosis

Other causes of microcytic anemia include anemia of chronic disease, thalassemia, and (less commonly) sideroblastic anemia. Anemia of chronic disease is characterized by normal or increased iron stores in the bone marrow and a normal or elevated ferritin level; the serum iron is low, often drastically so; the TIBC is either normal or low. Thalassemia produces a greater degree of microcytosis for any given level of anemia than does iron deficiency. Red blood cell morphology on the peripheral smear becomes abnormal earlier in the course of thalassemia.

Treatment

To make the diagnosis of iron deficiency anemia, one can either demonstrate an iron-deficient state or evaluate the response to a therapeutic trial of iron replacement.

Since the anemia itself is rarely life-threatening, the most important part of treatment is identification of the cause—especially a source of occult blood loss.

A. Oral Iron

There is no better treatment than ferrous sulfate, 325 mg three times daily, which provides 180 mg of iron daily of which up to 10 mg is absorbed (though absorption may exceed this amount in cases of severe deficiency). Compliance is improved by introducing the medicine more slowly in a gradually escalating dose with food. An appropriate response is a return of the hematocrit level halfway toward normal within 3 weeks with full return to baseline after 2 months. Iron therapy should continue for 3–6 months after restoration of normal hematologic values in order to replenish iron stores. Failure of response to iron therapy is usually due to noncompliance, although occasional patients may absorb iron poorly. Other reasons for failure to respond include incorrect diagnosis (anemia of chronic disease, thalassemia) and ongoing gastrointestinal blood loss that exceeds the rate of new erythropoiesis.

B. Parenteral Iron

The indications are intolerance to oral iron, refractoriness to oral iron, gastrointestinal disease (usually inflammatory bowel disease) precluding the use of oral iron, and continued blood loss that cannot be corrected. Because of the possibility of anaphylactic reactions, parenteral iron therapy should be used only in cases of persistent anemia after a reasonable course of oral therapy.

The dose (total 1.5–2 g) may be calculated by estimating the decrease in volume of red blood cell mass and then supplying 1 mg of iron for each milliliter of volume of red blood cells below normal. One should then add approximately 1 g for storage iron. The entire dose may be given as an intravenous infusion over 4–6 hours. A test dose of a dilute solution is given first, and the patient should be observed during the entire infusion for anaphylaxis.

Goddard AF et al: Guidelines for the management of iron deficiency anaemia. British Society of Gastroenterology. Gut 2000;46(Suppl 3–4):IV1. [PMID: 10862605]

Goodnough LT et al: Erythropoietin, iron, and erythropoiesis. Blood 2000;96:823. [PMID: 10910892]

ANEMIA OF CHRONIC DISEASE

Many chronic systemic diseases are associated with mild or moderate anemia. Common causes include chronic infection or inflammation, cancer, and liver disease. The anemia of chronic renal failure is somewhat different in pathophysiology and is usually more severe.

Red blood cell survival is modestly reduced, and the bone marrow fails to compensate adequately by increasing red blood cell production. Failure to increase red cell production is largely due to sequestration of iron within the reticuloendothelial system. Decrease in erythropoietin is rarely an important cause of underproduction of red cells except in renal failure.

Clinical Findings

A. Symptoms and Signs

The clinical features are those of the anemia, which is usually modest. The diagnosis should be suspected in patients with known chronic diseases; it is confirmed by the findings of low serum iron, low TIBC, and normal or increased serum ferritin (or normal or increased bone marrow iron stores). In cases of significant anemia, coexistent iron deficiency or folic acid deficiency should be suspected. Decreased dietary intake of folate or iron is common in these ill patients, and many will also have ongoing gastrointestinal blood losses. Patients undergoing hemodialysis regularly lose both iron and folate during dialysis.

B. Laboratory Findings

The hematocrit rarely falls below 25% (except in renal failure). The MCV is usually normal or slightly reduced. Red blood cell morphology is nondiagnostic, and the reticulocyte count is neither strikingly reduced nor increased. Serum iron values may be unmeasurable, and transferrin saturation may be extremely low, leading to an erroneous diagnosis of iron deficiency. In contrast to iron deficiency, serum ferritin values should be normal or increased. A serum ferritin value of less than 30 μg/L should suggest coexistent iron deficiency.

Treatment

In most cases no treatment is necessary. Purified recombinant erythropoietin has been shown to be effective for treatment of the anemia of renal failure and other secondary anemias such as anemia related to cancer or inflammatory disorders (eg, rheumatoid arthritis). In renal failure, optimal response to erythropoietin requires adequate intensity of dialysis. Erythropoietin must be injected subcutaneously and is very expensive. One effective schedule is 30,000 units once weekly. This agent is used only when the patient is transfusion-dependent or when the quality of life is clearly improved by the hematologic response.

Cazzola M et al: Use of recombinant human erythropoietin outside the setting of uremia. Blood 1997;89:4248. [PMID: 9192747]

Goodnough LT: Erythropoietin therapy. N Engl J Med 1997;336:933. [PMID: 9070475]

THE THALASSEMIAS

ESSENTIALS OF DIAGNOSIS

- *Microcytosis out of proportion to the degree of anemia.*
- *Positive family history or lifelong personal history of microcytic anemia.*
- *Abnormal red blood cell morphology with microcytes, acanthocytes, and target cells.*
- *In beta thalassemia, elevated levels of hemoglobin A_2 or F.*

General Considerations

The thalassemias are hereditary disorders characterized by reduction in the synthesis of globin chains (alpha or beta). Reduced globin chain synthesis causes reduced hemoglobin synthesis and eventually produces a hypochromic microcytic anemia because of defective hemoglobinization of red blood cells. Thalassemias can be considered among the hypoproliferative anemias, the hemolytic anemias, and the anemias related to abnormal hemoglobin, since all of these factors may play a role in pathogenesis.

Normal adult hemoglobin is primarily hemoglobin A, which represents approximately 98% of circulating hemoglobin. Hemoglobin A is formed from a tetramer—two alpha chains and two beta chains—and can be designated $\alpha_2\beta_2$. Two copies of the α-globin gene are located on chromosome 16, and there is no substitute for α-globin in the formation of hemoglobin. The β-globin gene resides on chromosome 11 adjacent to genes encoding the beta-like globin chains,

delta and gamma. The tetramer of $\alpha_2\delta_2$ forms hemoglobin A_2, which normally comprises 1–2% of adult hemoglobin. The tetramer $\alpha_2\gamma_2$ forms hemoglobin F, which is the major hemoglobin of fetal life but which comprises less than 1% of normal adult hemoglobin.

Alpha thalassemia is due primarily to gene deletion causing reduced α-globin chain synthesis (Table 13–4). Since all adult hemoglobins are alpha-containing, alpha thalassemia produces no change in the percentage distribution of hemoglobins A, A_2, and F. In severe forms of alpha thalassemia, excess beta chains may form a β_4 tetramer called hemoglobin H.

Beta thalassemias are usually caused by point mutations rather than deletions (Table 13–5). These mutations result in premature chain termination or in problems with transcription of RNA and ultimately result in reduced or absent β-globin chain synthesis. The molecular defects leading to beta thalassemia are numerous and heterogeneous. Defects that result in absent globin chain expression are termed β^0, whereas those causing reduced synthesis are termed β^+. The reduced β-globin chain synthesis in beta thalassemia results in a relative increase in the percentages of hemoglobins A_2 and F compared to hemoglobin A, as the beta-like globins (gamma and delta) substitute for the missing beta chains. In the presence of reduced beta chains, the excess alpha chains are unstable and precipitate, leading to damage of red blood cell membranes. This leads to intramedullary and peripheral hemolysis. The bone marrow becomes hyperplastic under the drive of anemia and ineffective erythropoiesis resulting from destruction of the developing erythroid cells. This marked expansion of the erythroid element in the bone marrow causes severe bony deformities, osteopenia, and pathologic fractures.

Clinical Findings

A. Symptoms and Signs

The alpha thalassemia syndromes are seen primarily in persons from southeast Asia and China, and, less commonly, in blacks. Normally, adults have four copies of the α-globin chain. When three α-globin genes are present, the patient is hematologically normal and is called a silent carrier. When two α-globin genes are present, the patient is said to have alpha thalassemia trait, one form of thalassemia minor. These patients

Table 13–4. Alpha thalassemia syndromes.

Alpha Globin Genes	Syndrome	Hematocrit	MCV
4	Normal	Normal	
3	Silent carrier	Normal	
2	Thalassemia minor	32–40%	60–75 fL
1	Hemoglobin H disease	22–32%	60–70 fL
0	Hydrops fetalis		

Table 13–5. Beta thalassemia syndromes.

	Beta Globin Genes	Hb A	Hb A$_2$	Hb F
Normal	Homozygous β	97–99%	1–3%	< 1%
	Homozygous β^0	0%	4–10%	90–96%
	Homozygous β$^+$	0–10%	4–10%	90–96%
Thalassemia intermedia	Homozygous β$^+$ (mild)	0–30%	0–10%	6–100%
Thalassemia minor	Heterozygous β^0	80–95%	4–8%	1–5%
	Heterozygous β$^+$	80–95%	4–8%	1–5%

are clinically normal and have normal life expectancy and performance status, with a mild microcytic anemia. When only one α-globin chain is present, the patient has hemoglobin H disease. This is a chronic hemolytic anemia of variable severity (thalassemia minor or intermedia). Physical examination will reveal pallor and splenomegaly. Although affected individuals do not usually require transfusions, they may do so during periods of hemolytic exacerbation caused by infection or other stresses. When all four α-globin genes are deleted, the affected fetus is stillborn as a result of hydrops fetalis.

Beta thalassemia affects persons of Mediterranean origin (Italian, Greek) and to a lesser extent Chinese, other Asians, and blacks. Patients homozygous for beta thalassemia have thalassemia major. Affected children are normal at birth but after 6 months, when hemoglobin synthesis switches from hemoglobin F to hemoglobin A, develop severe anemia requiring transfusion. Numerous clinical problems ensue, including growth failure, bony deformities (abnormal facial structure, pathologic fractures), hepatosplenomegaly, and jaundice. The clinical course is modified significantly by transfusion therapy, but the transfusional iron overload (hemosiderosis) results in a clinical picture similar to hemochromatosis, with heart failure, cirrhosis, and endocrinopathies, usually after more than 100 units. These problems develop because of the body's inability to excrete the iron (see above) from transfused red cells. Death from cardiac failure usually occurs between ages 20 and 30.

Patients homozygous for a milder form of beta thalassemia (allowing a higher rate of globin gene synthesis) have thalassemia intermedia. These patients have chronic hemolytic anemia but do not require transfusions except under periods of stress. They also may develop iron overload because of periodic transfusion. They survive into adult life but with hepatosplenomegaly and bony deformities. Patients heterozygous for beta thalassemia have thalassemia minor and a clinically insignificant microcytic anemia.

Prenatal diagnosis is available, and genetic counseling should be offered and the opportunity for prenatal diagnosis discussed.

B. LABORATORY FINDINGS

1. Alpha thalassemia trait—Patients with two α-globin genes have mild anemia, with hematocrits between 28% and 40%. The MCV is strikingly low (60–75 fL) despite the modest anemia, and the red blood count is normal or increased. The peripheral blood smear shows mild abnormalities, including microcytes, hypochromia, occasional target cells, and acanthocytes (cells with irregularly spaced bulbous projections). The reticulocyte count and iron parameters are normal. Hemoglobin electrophoresis will show no increase in the percentage of hemoglobins A$_2$ or F and no hemoglobin H. Alpha thalassemia trait is thus usually diagnosed by exclusion.

2. Hemoglobin H disease—These patients have a variably severe hemolytic anemia, with hematocrits between 22% and 32%. The MCV is remarkably low (60–70 fL) and the peripheral blood smear markedly abnormal, with hypochromia, microcytosis, target cells, and poikilocytosis. The reticulocyte count is elevated. Hemoglobin electrophoresis will show the presence of a fast migrating hemoglobin (hemoglobin H), which comprises 10–40% of the hemoglobin. A peripheral blood smear can be stained with supravital dyes to demonstrate the presence of hemoglobin H.

3. Beta thalassemia minor—As in alpha thalassemia trait, these patients have a modest anemia with hematocrit between 28% and 40%. The MCV ranges from 55 to 75 fL, and the red blood cell count is normal or increased. The peripheral blood smear is mildly abnormal, with hypochromia, microcytosis, and target cells. In contrast to alpha thalassemia, basophilic stippling may be present. The reticulocyte count is normal or slightly elevated. Hemoglobin electrophoresis (using quantitative techniques) may show an elevation of hemoglobin A$_2$ to 4–8% and occasional elevations of hemoglobin F to 1–5%.

4. Beta thalassemia major—Beta thalassemia major produces severe anemia, and without transfusion the hematocrit may fall to less than 10%. The peripheral blood smear is bizarre, showing severe poikilocytosis, hypochromia, microcytosis, target cells, basophilic stippling, and nucleated red blood cells. Little or no hemoglobin A is present. Variable amounts of hemoglobin A$_2$ are seen, and the major hemoglobin present is hemoglobin F.

Differential Diagnosis

Mild forms of thalassemia must be differentiated from iron deficiency. Compared to iron deficiency anemia, patients with thalassemia have a lower MCV, a more normal red blood count, and a more abnormal peripheral blood smear at modest levels of anemia. Iron studies are normal. Severe forms of thalassemia may be confused with other hemoglobinopathies. The diagnosis is made by hemoglobin electrophoresis.

Treatment

Patients with mild thalassemia (alpha thalassemia trait or beta thalassemia minor) require no treatment and should be identified so that they will not be subjected to repeated evaluations for iron deficiency and inappropriately given supplemental iron. Patients with hemoglobin H disease should take folate supplementation and avoid medicinal iron and oxidative drugs such as sulfonamides. Patients with severe thalassemia are maintained on a regular transfusion schedule and receive folate supplementation. Splenectomy is performed if hypersplenism causes a marked increase in the transfusion requirement. Deferoxamine is routinely given as an iron-chelating agent to avoid or postpone hemosiderosis. A diet low in iron may help in all of these patients.

Allogeneic bone marrow transplantation has been introduced as treatment for beta thalassemia major. Children who have not yet experienced iron overload and chronic organ toxicity do well, with long-term survival in more than 80% of cases.

Aessopos A et al: Cardiac involvement in thalassemia intermedia: a multicenter study. Blood 2001;97:3411. [PMID: 11369631]

Lucarelli G: Bone marrow transplantation in adult thalassemia patients. Blood 1999;93:1164. [PMID: 9949158]

Olivieri NF: The beta-thalassemias. N Engl J Med 1999;341:99. [PMID: 10395636]

SIDEROBLASTIC ANEMIA

The sideroblastic anemias are a heterogeneous group of disorders in which hemoglobin synthesis is reduced because of failure to incorporate heme into protoporphyrin to form hemoglobin. Iron accumulates, particularly in the mitochondria. A Prussian blue stain of the bone marrow will reveal ringed sideroblasts, cells with iron deposits (in the mitochondria) encircling the red cell nucleus. The disorder is usually acquired. Sometimes it represents a stage in evolution of a generalized bone marrow disorder (myelodysplasia) that may ultimately terminate in acute leukemia. Other causes include chronic alcoholism and lead poisoning.

Patients have no specific clinical features other than those related to anemia. The anemia is usually moderate, with hematocrits of 20–30%, but transfusions may occasionally be required. Although the MCV is usually normal or slightly increased, it may occasionally be low, leading to confusion with iron deficiency. The peripheral blood smear characteristically shows a dimorphic population of red blood cells, one normal and one hypochromic. In cases of lead poisoning, coarse basophilic stippling of the red cells is seen.

The diagnosis is made by examination of the bone marrow. Characteristically, there is marked erythroid hyperplasia, a sign of ineffective erythropoiesis (expansion of the erythroid compartment of the bone marrow that does not result in the production of reticulocytes in the peripheral blood). The iron stain of the bone marrow shows a generalized increase in iron stores and the presence of ringed sideroblasts. Other characteristic laboratory features include a high serum iron and a high transferrin saturation. In lead poisoning, serum lead levels will be elevated.

Occasionally, the anemia is so severe that support with transfusion is required. These patients usually do not respond to erythropoietin therapy.

VITAMIN B₁₂ DEFICIENCY

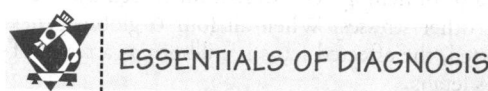

■ ESSENTIALS OF DIAGNOSIS

- *Macrocytic anemia.*
- *Macro-ovalocytes and hypersegmented neutrophils on peripheral blood smear.*
- *Serum vitamin B$_{12}$ level less than 100 pg/mL.*

General Considerations

Vitamin B$_{12}$ belongs to the family of cobalamins and serves as a cofactor for two important reactions in humans. As methylcobalamin, it is a cofactor for methionine synthetase in the conversion of homocysteine to methionine and as adenosylcobalamin for the conversion of methylmalonyl-CoA to succinyl-CoA. All vitamin B$_{12}$ comes from the diet and is present in all foods of animal origin. The daily absorption of vitamin B$_{12}$ is 5 μg.

After being ingested, vitamin B$_{12}$ is bound to intrinsic factor, a protein secreted by gastric parietal cells. Other cobalamin-binding proteins (called R factors) compete with intrinsic factor for vitamin B$_{12}$. Vitamin B$_{12}$ bound to R factors cannot be absorbed. The vitamin B$_{12}$–intrinsic factor complex travels through the intestine and is absorbed in the terminal ileum by cells with specific receptors for the complex. It is then transported through plasma and stored in the liver. Three plasma transport proteins have been identified. Transcobalamins I and III (differing only in carbohydrate structure) are secreted by white blood cells. Although approximately 90% of plasma vitamin B$_{12}$ circulates bound to these proteins, only transcobalamin II is capable of transporting vitamin B$_{12}$ into cells. The liver contains 2000–5000 μg of stored vitamin B$_{12}$.

Since daily losses are 3–5 μg/d, the body usually has sufficient stores of vitamin B_{12} so that vitamin B_{12} deficiency develops more than 3 years after vitamin B_{12} absorption ceases.

Since vitamin B_{12} is present in all foods of animal origin, dietary vitamin B_{12} deficiency is extremely rare and seen only in vegans—strict vegetarians who avoid all dairy products as well as meat and fish (Table 13–6). Abdominal surgery may lead to vitamin B_{12} deficiency in several ways. Gastrectomy will eliminate that site of intrinsic factor production; blind loop syndrome will cause competition for vitamin B_{12} by bacterial overgrowth in the lumen of the intestine; and surgical resection of the ileum will eliminate the site of vitamin B_{12} absorption. Rare causes of vitamin B_{12} deficiency include fish tapeworm (*Diphyllobothrium latum*) infection, in which the parasite uses luminal vitamin B_{12}, pancreatic insufficiency (with failure to inactivate competing cobalamin-binding proteins), and severe Crohn's disease, causing sufficient destruction of the ileum to impair vitamin B_{12} absorption.

The most common cause of vitamin B_{12} deficiency is that associated with **pernicious anemia.** Although the disease is hereditary, it is rare clinically before age 35. Pernicious anemia produces a number of clinical findings in addition to vitamin B_{12} deficiency. Atrophic gastritis is invariably present and results in histamine-fast achlorhydria. These patients may also have a number of other autoimmune diseases, including IgA deficiency, as well as polyglandular endocrine insufficiency. The atrophic gastritis is associated with an increased risk of gastric carcinoma.

Clinical Findings

A. SYMPTOMS AND SIGNS

The hallmark of vitamin B_{12} deficiency is megaloblastic anemia. The anemia may be severe, with hematocrits as low as 10–15%. The megaloblastic state also produces changes in mucosal cells, leading to glossitis, as well as other vague gastrointestinal disturbances such as anorexia and diarrhea. Vitamin B_{12} deficiency also leads to a complex neurologic syndrome. Peripheral nerves are usually affected first, and patients complain initially of paresthesias. The posterior columns next become impaired, and patients complain of difficulty with balance. In more advanced cases, cerebral function may be altered as well, and on occasion dementia and other neuropsychiatric changes may precede hematologic changes.

Patients are usually pale and may be mildly icteric. Neurologic examination may reveal decreased vibration and position sense but is more commonly normal in early stages of the disease.

B. LABORATORY FINDINGS

The megaloblastic state produces an anemia of variable severity that on occasion may be very severe. The MCV is usually strikingly elevated, between 110 and 140 fL. However, it is possible to have vitamin B_{12} deficiency with a normal MCV. Occasionally, the normal MCV may be explained by coexistent thalassemia or iron deficiency, but in other cases the reason is obscure. Patients with neurologic symptoms and signs that suggest possible vitamin B_{12} deficiency should be evaluated for that deficiency despite a normal MCV and the absence of anemia. The peripheral blood smear is usually strikingly abnormal, with anisocytosis and poikilocytosis. A characteristic finding is the macro-ovalocyte, but numerous other abnormal shapes are usually seen. The neutrophils are hypersegmented. Typical features include a mean lobe count greater than four or the finding of six-lobed neutrophils. The reticulocyte count is reduced. Because vitamin B_{12} deficiency affects all hematopoietic cell lines, in severe cases the white blood cell count and the platelet count are reduced, and pancytopenia is present.

Bone marrow morphology is characteristically abnormal. Marked erythroid hyperplasia is present as a response to defective red blood cell production (ineffective erythropoiesis). Megaloblastic changes in the erythroid series include abnormally large cell size and asynchronous maturation of the nucleus and cytoplasm—ie, cytoplasmic maturation continues while impaired DNA synthesis causes retarded nuclear development. In the myeloid series, giant metamyelocytes are characteristically seen.

Other laboratory abnormalities include elevated serum LDH and a modest increase in indirect bilirubin. These two findings are a reflection of intramedullary destruction of developing abnormal erythroid cells and are similar to those observed in peripheral hemolytic anemias.

The diagnosis of vitamin B_{12} deficiency is made by finding an abnormally low vitamin B_{12} serum level. Whereas the normal vitamin B_{12} level is 150–350 pg/mL, most patients with overt vitamin B_{12} deficiency will have serum levels less than 100 pg/mL. When the serum level of vitamin B_{12} is borderline, the diagnosis can be confirmed by an elevated serum level

Table 13–6. Causes of vitamin B_{12} deficiency.

Dietary deficiency (rare)
Decreased production of intrinsic factor
Pernicious anemia
Gastrectomy
Helicobacter pylori infection
Competition for vitamin B_{12} in gut
Blind loop syndrome
Fish tapeworm (rare)
Pancreatic insufficiency
Decreased ileal absorption of vitamin B_{12}
Surgical resection
Crohn's disease
Transcobalamin II deficiency (rare)

of methylmalonic acid or homocysteine. The Schilling test has been the traditional test used to document the decreased absorption of oral vitamin B_{12} that is characteristic of pernicious anemia. A large intramuscular dose of vitamin B_{12} is given to saturate plasma transport proteins. Thereafter, radiolabeled vitamin B_{12} is administered orally, and a 24-hour urine collection is performed to determine how much vitamin B_{12} is absorbed and subsequently excreted. Normally, more than 7% of a dose is present in the urine; most patients with impaired absorption will have less than 3% present in the urine. The second stage of the Schilling test is to give radiolabeled vitamin B_{12} together with intrinsic factor. If pernicious anemia (a lack of intrinsic factor) is the cause of vitamin B_{12} deficiency, the combined use of vitamin B_{12} and intrinsic factor should correct the abnormally low absorption. However, the full-blown megaloblastic state causes abnormalities in intestinal epithelium that may lead to generalized malabsorption. In these cases, the second stage of the Schilling test will remain abnormal until the intestinal mucosal defect is first corrected by vitamin B_{12} replacement (in approximately 2 months). The repeat evaluation should thus be deferred until there has been time for correction. If the deficiency is caused by bacterial overgrowth in a blind loop (eg, jejunal diverticula), a course of antibiotics will reverse the abnormal second stage of the Schilling test. If the deficiency has been produced by pancreatic insufficiency, a course of pancreatic enzymes will reverse the abnormality. If a fish tapeworm is responsible, an anthelmintic agent is indicated (see Chapter 35).

Differential Diagnosis

Vitamin B_{12} deficiency should be differentiated from folic acid deficiency, the other common cause of megaloblastic anemia, in which red blood cell folate is low while vitamin B_{12} levels are normal. The distinction between vitamin B_{12} deficiency and myelodysplasia (the other common cause of macrocytic anemia with abnormal morphology) is based on the characteristic morphology and the low vitamin B_{12} level. Peripheral neuropathy and dementia of other cause may be similar clinically to nonhematologic pernicious anemia.

Treatment

Patients with pernicious anemia are often treated with parenteral therapy. Intramuscular injections of 100 μg of vitamin B_{12} are adequate for each dose. Replacement is usually given daily for the first week, weekly for the first month, and then monthly for life. It is a lifelong disorder, and if patients discontinue their monthly therapy the vitamin deficiency will recur. Oral cobalamin may be used instead of parenteral therapy in a dose of 1000 μg/d and must be continued indefinitely.

Patients respond to therapy with an immediate improvement in their sense of well-being. Hypokalemia may complicate the first several days of therapy, par-

ticularly if the anemia is severe. A brisk reticulocytosis occurs in 5–7 days, and the hematologic picture normalizes in 2 months. Central nervous system symptoms and signs are reversible if they are of relatively short duration (less than 6 months) but become permanent if treatment is not initiated promptly.

Kaptan K et al: *Helicobacter pylori*—is it a novel causative agent in vitamin B_{12} deficiency? Arch Intern Med 2000;160:1349. [PMID: 10809040] (Eradication of *H pylori* infection improved anemia and vitamin B_{12} levels in many patients.)

FOLIC ACID DEFICIENCY

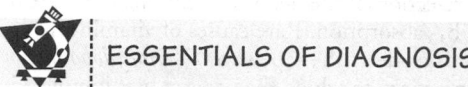

ESSENTIALS OF DIAGNOSIS

- *Macrocytic anemia.*
- *Macro-ovalocytes and hypersegmented neutrophils on peripheral blood smear.*
- *Normal serum vitamin B_{12} levels.*
- *Reduced folate levels in red blood cells or serum.*

General Considerations

Folic acid is the term commonly used for pteroylmonoglutamic acid. In its reduced form of tetrahydrofolate, it serves as an important mediator of many reactions involving one-carbon transfers. Important reactions include the conversion of homocysteine to methionine and of deoxyuridylate to thymidylate, an important step in DNA synthesis.

Folic acid is present in most fruits and vegetables (especially citrus fruits and green leafy vegetables) and daily requirements of 50–100 μg/d are usually met in the diet. Total body stores of folate are approximately 5000 μg, enough to supply requirements for 2–3 months.

By far the most common cause of folate deficiency is inadequate dietary intake (Table 13–7). Alcoholics,

Table 13–7. Causes of folate deficiency.

Dietary deficiency
Decreased absorption
Tropical sprue
Drugs: phenytoin, sulfasalazine, trimethoprim-sulfamethoxazole
Increased requirement
Chronic hemolytic anemia
Pregnancy
Exfoliative skin disease
Loss: dialysis
Inhibition of reduction to active form
Methotrexate

anorectic patients, persons who do not eat fresh fruits and vegetables, and those who overcook their food are candidates for folate deficiency. Reduced folate absorption is rarely seen, since absorption occurs from the entire gastrointestinal tract. However, drugs such as phenytoin, trimethoprim-sulfamethoxazole, or sulfasalazine may interfere with folate absorption. Folic acid requirements are increased in pregnancy, hemolytic anemia, and exfoliative skin disease, and in these cases the increased requirements (five to ten times normal) may not be met by a normal diet. Patients with increased folate requirements should receive supplementation with 1 mg/d of folic acid.

Clinical Findings

A. SYMPTOMS AND SIGNS

The features are similar to those of vitamin B_{12} deficiency, with megaloblastic anemia and megaloblastic changes in mucosa. However, there are none of the neurologic abnormalities associated with vitamin B_{12} deficiency.

B. LABORATORY FINDINGS

The megaloblastic anemia is identical to that resulting from vitamin B_{12} deficiency (see above). However, the serum vitamin B_{12} level is normal. A red blood cell folate level of less than 150 ng/mL is diagnostic of folate deficiency.

Differential Diagnosis

The megaloblastic anemia of folate deficiency should be differentiated from vitamin B_{12} deficiency by the finding of a normal vitamin B_{12} level and a reduced red blood cell folate or serum folate level. Alcoholics, who often have folate deficiency, may also have anemia of liver disease. This latter macrocytic anemia does not cause megaloblastic morphologic changes but rather produces target cells in the peripheral blood. Hypothyroidism is associated with mild macrocytosis but also with pernicious anemia.

Treatment

Folic acid deficiency is treated with folic acid, 1 mg/d orally. The response is similar to that seen in the treatment of vitamin B_{12} deficiency, with rapid improvement and a sense of well-being, reticulocytosis in 5–7 days, and total correction of hematologic abnormalities within 2 months. Large doses of folic acid may produce hematologic responses in cases of vitamin B_{12} deficiency but will allow neurologic damage to progress.

PURE RED CELL APLASIA

Adult acquired pure red cell aplasia is rare. It appears to be an autoimmune disease mediated either by T lymphocytes or (rarely) by an IgG antibody against erythroid precursors. In adults, the disease is usually idiopathic. However, cases have been seen in association with systemic lupus erythematosus, chronic lymphocytic leukemia, lymphomas, or thymoma. Some drugs (phenytoin, chloramphenicol) may cause red cell aplasia. Transient episodes of red cell aplasia are probably common in response to viral infections, especially parvovirus infections. However, these acute episodes will go unrecognized unless the patient has a chronic hemolytic disorder, in which case the hematocrit may fall precipitously.

The only signs are those of anemia unless the patient has an associated autoimmune or lymphoproliferative disorder. The anemia is often severe, normochromic, with low or absent reticulocytes. Red blood cell morphology is normal, and the myeloid and platelet lines are unaffected. The bone marrow is normocellular. All elements present are normal, but erythroid precursors are markedly reduced or absent. In some cases, chest imaging studies will reveal a thymoma.

The disorder is distinguished from aplastic anemia (in which the marrow is hypocellular and cell lines affected) and from myelodysplasia. This latter disorder is recognized by the presence of morphologic abnormalities that should not be present in pure red cell aplasia.

Possible offending drugs should be stopped. With thymoma, resection results in amelioration of anemia in some instances. High-dose intravenous immune globulin has produced excellent responses in a small number of cases, especially in parvovirus-related cases. For most cases, the treatment of choice is immunosuppressive therapy with a combination of antithymocyte globulin and cyclosporine—similar to therapy of aplastic anemia.

Casadevall N et al: Pure red-cell aplasia and antierythropoietin antibodies in patients treated with recombinant erythropoietin. N Engl J Med 2002;346:469. [PMID: 11844847]

Fisch P et al: Pure red cell aplasia. Br J Haematol 2000;111:1010. [PMID: 11167735]

HEMOLYTIC ANEMIAS

The hemolytic anemias are a group of disorders in which red blood cell survival is reduced, either episodically or continuously. The bone marrow has the ability to increase erythroid production up to eightfold in response to reduced red cell survival, so anemia will be present only when the ability of the bone marrow to compensate is outstripped. This will occur when red cell survival is extremely short or when the ability of the bone marrow to compensate is impaired for some second reason.

Since red blood cell survival is normally 120 days, in the absence of red cell production the hematocrit will fall at the rate of approximately 1/100 of the hematocrit per day, which translates to a decrease in the hematocrit reading of approximately 3% per week. For example, a fall of hematocrit from 45% to 36%

over 3 weeks' time need not indicate hemolysis, since this rate of fall would result simply from cessation of red blood cell production. If the hematocrit is falling at a faster rate than that due to decreased production, blood loss or hemolysis is the cause.

Reticulocytosis is an important clue to the presence of hemolysis, since in most hemolytic disorders the bone marrow will respond with increased red blood cell production. However, hemolysis can be present without reticulocytosis when a second disorder (infection, folate deficiency) is superimposed on hemolysis; in these circumstances, the hematocrit will fall rapidly. However, reticulocytosis also occurs during recovery from hypoproliferative anemia or bleeding. Hemolysis is correctly diagnosed (when bleeding is excluded) if the hematocrit is either falling or stable despite reticulocytosis.

Hemolytic disorders are generally classified according to whether the defect is intrinsic to the red cell or due to some external factor (Table 13–8). Intrinsic defects have been described in all components of the red blood cell, including the membrane, enzyme systems, and hemoglobin; most of these disorders are hereditary. Hemolytic anemias due to external factors are the immune hemolytic anemias.

Certain laboratory features are common to all the hemolytic anemias. Haptoglobin, a normal plasma protein that binds and clears hemoglobin released into plasma, may be depressed in hemolytic disorders. However, haptoglobin levels are influenced by many factors and, by themselves, are not a reliable indicator of hemolysis. When intravascular hemolysis occurs, transient hemoglobinemia occurs. Hemoglobin is filtered through the glomerulus and usually reabsorbed by tubular cells. Hemoglobinuria will be present only when the capacity for reabsorption of hemoglobin by these cells is exceeded. In the absence of hemoglobin-

uria, evidence for prior intravascular hemolysis is the presence of hemosiderin in shed renal tubular cells (positive urine hemosiderin). With severe intravascular hemolysis, hemoglobinemia and methemalbuminemia may be present. Hemolysis increases the indirect bilirubin, and the total bilirubin may rise to 4 mg/dL. Bilirubin levels higher than this may indicate some degree of hepatic dysfunction. Serum LDH levels are strikingly elevated in cases of microangiopathic hemolysis (thrombotic thrombocytopenic purpura, hemolytic-uremic syndrome) and may be elevated in other hemolytic anemias.

HEREDITARY SPHEROCYTOSIS

ESSENTIALS OF DIAGNOSIS

- *Positive family history.*
- *Splenomegaly.*
- *Spherocytes and increased reticulocytes on peripheral blood smear.*
- *Microcytic, hyperchromic indices.*

General Considerations

Hereditary spherocytosis is a disorder of the red blood cell membrane, leading to chronic hemolytic anemia. Normally, the red blood cell is a biconcave disk with a diameter of 7–8 μm. The red blood cells must be both strong and deformable—strong to withstand the stress of circulating for 120 days and deformable so as to pass through capillaries 3 μm in diameter and splenic fenestrations in the cords of the red pulp of approximately 2 μm. The red blood cell skeleton, made up primarily of the proteins spectrin and actin, gives the red cells these characteristics of strength and deformability.

The membrane defect in hereditary spherocytosis is an abnormality in spectrin, the protein providing most of the scaffolding for the red blood cell membranes. The result is a decrease in surface-to-volume ratio that results in a spherical shape of the cell. These spherical cells are less deformable and unable to pass through 2-μm fenestrations in the splenic red pulp. Hemolysis takes place because of trapping of red blood cells within the spleen.

Clinical Findings

A. SYMPTOMS AND SIGNS

Hereditary spherocytosis is an autosomal dominant disease of variable severity. It is often diagnosed dur-

Table 13–8. Classification of hemolytic anemias.

Intrinsic
 Membrane defects: hereditary spherocytosis, hereditary elliptocytosis, paroxysmal nocturnal hemoglobinuria
 Glycolytic defects: pyruvate kinase deficiency, severe hypophosphatemia
 Oxidation vulnerability: G6PD deficiency, methemoglobinemia
 Hemoglobinopathies: sickle cell syndromes, unstable hemoglobins, methemoglobinemia
Extrinsic
 Immune: autoimmune, lymphoproliferative disease, drug toxicity
 Microangiopathic: thrombotic thrombocytopenic purpura, hemolytic-uremic syndrome, disseminated intravascular coagulation, valve hemolysis, metastatic adenocarcinoma, vasculitis
 Infection: plasmodium, clostridium, borrelia
 Hypersplenism
 Burns

ing childhood, but milder cases may be discovered incidentally late in adult life. Anemia may or may not be present, since the bone marrow may be able to compensate for shortened red cell survival. Severe anemia (aplastic crisis) may occur in folic acid deficiency or when bone marrow compensation is temporarily impaired by infection. Chronic hemolysis causes jaundice and pigment (calcium bilirubinate) gallstones, leading to attacks of cholecystitis. Examination may reveal icterus and a palpable spleen.

B. LABORATORY FINDINGS

The anemia is of variable severity, and the hematocrit may be normal. Reticulocytosis is always present. The peripheral blood smear shows the presence of spherocytes, small cells that have lost their central pallor. Spherocytes usually make up only a small percentage of red blood cells on the peripheral smear. Hereditary spherocytosis is the only important disorder associated with microcytosis and an increased MCHC, often greater than 36 g/dL. As with other hemolytic disorders, there may be an increase in indirect bilirubin. The Coombs test is negative.

Because spherocytes are red cells that have lost some membrane surface, they are abnormally vulnerable to swelling induced by hypotonic media. Increased osmotic fragility merely reflects the presence of spherocytes and does not distinguish hereditary spherocytosis from other spherocytic hemolytic disorders such as autoimmune hemolytic anemia.

Treatment

These patients should receive uninterrupted supplementation with folic acid, 1 mg/d. The treatment of choice is splenectomy, which will not correct the membrane defect or correct the spherocytosis but will eliminate the site of hemolysis. In very mild cases discovered late in adult life, splenectomy may not be necessary.

Bader-Meunier B et al: Long-term evaluation of the beneficial effect of subtotal splenectomy for management of hereditary spherocytosis. Blood 2001;97:399. [PMID: 11154215] (May be preferable to splenectomy to avoid infectious complications associated with asplenia.)

Bolton-Maggs PH: The diagnosis and management of hereditary spherocytosis. Baillieres Best Pract Res Clin Haematol 2000;13:327. [PMID: 11030038]

PAROXYSMAL NOCTURNAL HEMOGLOBINURIA

Paroxysmal nocturnal hemoglobinuria is an acquired clonal stem cell disorder that results in abnormal sensitivity of the red blood cell membrane to lysis by complement. The defect involves both increased binding of C3b and increased vulnerability to lysis by complement, and is expressed as a deficiency in proteins normally linked to the cell by phosphoinositol. Paroxysmal nocturnal hemoglobinuria should be suspected in confusing cases of hemolytic anemia or pancytopenia. The best screening test is the sucrose hemolysis test.

Clinical Findings

A. SYMPTOMS AND SIGNS

Classically, patients report episodic hemoglobinuria resulting in reddish brown urine. Hemoglobinuria may be present in the first morning urine, since the mild respiratory acidosis of sleep leads to enhanced complement activity. In addition to anemia, these patients are prone to thrombosis, especially mesenteric and hepatic vein thromboses. This hypercoagulopathy may be related to platelet activation by complement. As this is a stem cell disorder, paroxysmal nocturnal hemoglobinuria may progress either to aplastic anemia, to myelodysplasia, or to acute myelogenous leukemia.

B. LABORATORY FINDINGS

Anemia is of variable severity, and reticulocytosis may or may not be present. Abnormalities on the blood smear are nondiagnostic and may include macro-ovalocytes. Since the episodic hemolysis in paroxysmal nocturnal hemoglobinuria is intravascular, the finding of urine hemosiderin is a useful test. Serum LDH is characteristically elevated. Iron deficiency is commonly present and is related to chronic iron loss from hemoglobinuria, since hemolysis is primarily intravascular.

The white blood cell count and platelet count may be decreased. A decreased leukocyte alkaline phosphatase—evidence for qualitative abnormality in the myeloid series—may be seen. Bone marrow morphology is variable and may show either generalized hypoplasia or erythroid hyperplasia. Flow cytometric assays may confirm the diagnosis by demonstrating the absence of CD59.

Treatment

Iron replacement is often indicated for treatment of iron deficiency. This may improve the anemia but may also cause a transient increase in hemolysis. For unclear reasons, prednisone is effective in decreasing hemolysis, and some patients can be managed effectively with alternate-day steroids. In severe cases and cases of transformation to myelodysplasia, allogeneic bone marrow transplantation has been used to treat the disorder.

Karadimitris A et al: The cellular pathogenesis of paroxysmal nocturnal haemoglobinuria. Leukemia 2001;15:1148. [PMID: 11480554]

Raiola AM et al: Bone marrow transplantation for paroxysmal nocturnal hemoglobinuria. Haematologica 2000;85:59. [PMID: 10629593]

GLUCOSE-6-PHOSPHATE DEHYDROGENASE DEFICIENCY

 ESSENTIALS OF DIAGNOSIS

- X-linked recessive disorder seen commonly in American black men.
- Episodic hemolysis in response to oxidant drugs or infection.
- Minimally abnormal peripheral blood smear.
- Reduced levels of G6PD between hemolytic episodes.

General Considerations

Glucose-6-phosphate dehydrogenase (G6PD) deficiency is a hereditary enzyme defect that causes episodic hemolytic anemia because of decreased ability of red blood cells to deal with oxidative stresses. The hexose monophosphate shunt is not an important source of energy in red cells but is important in generating reduced glutathione, which protects hemoglobin from oxidative denaturation. The first step in this pathway is the production of NADPH by the action of G6PD on glucose 6-phosphate. NADPH serves as a cofactor for glutathione reductase in generating reduced glutathione, which detoxifies hydrogen peroxide. In the absence of reduced glutathione, hemoglobin may become oxidized. Oxidized hemoglobin denatures and forms precipitants called Heinz bodies. These Heinz bodies cause membrane damage, which leads to removal of these cells by the spleen.

Numerous types of G6PD enzymes have been described. The normal type found in Caucasians is designated G6PD-B. Most American blacks have G6PD-A, which is normal in function. Ten to 15 percent of American blacks have the variant G6PD designated A⁻, in which there is only 15% of normal enzyme activity, and enzyme activity declines rapidly as the red blood cell ages past 40 days, a fact that explains many of the clinical findings in this disorder. Many other G6PD variants have been described, including some Mediterranean variants with extremely low enzyme activity.

Clinical Findings

G6PD deficiency is an X-linked recessive disorder affecting 10–15% of American black males. Female carriers are rarely affected—only when an unusually high percentage of cells producing the normal enzyme are inactivated.

A. SYMPTOMS AND SIGNS

Patients are usually healthy, without chronic hemolytic anemia or splenomegaly. Hemolysis occurs as a result of oxidative stress on the red blood cells, generated either by infection or exposure to certain drugs. Common drugs initiating hemolysis include dapsone, primaquine, quinidine, quinine, sulfonamides, and nitrofurantoin. Even with continuous use of the offending drug, the hemolytic episode is self-limited because older red blood cells (with low enzyme activity) are removed and replaced with a population of young red blood cells with adequate functional levels of G6PD. Severe G6PD deficiency (as in Mediterranean variants) may produce a chronic hemolytic anemia.

B. LABORATORY FINDINGS

Between hemolytic episodes, the blood is normal. During episodes of hemolysis, there is reticulocytosis and increased serum indirect bilirubin. The red blood cell smear is not diagnostic but may reveal a small number of "bite" cells—cells that appear to have had a bite taken out of their periphery. This indicates pitting of hemoglobin aggregates by the spleen. Heinz bodies may be demonstrated by staining a peripheral blood smear with crystal violet. (They are not visible on the usual Wright-stained blood smear.) Specific enzyme assays for G6PD may reveal a low level but may be misleading if they are performed shortly after a hemolytic episode when the enzyme-deficient cohort of cells has been removed. In these cases, the enzyme assays should be repeated weeks after hemolysis has resolved. In severe cases of G6PD deficiency, enzyme levels are always low.

Treatment

No treatment is necessary except to avoid known oxidant drugs.

Mehta A et al: Glucose-6-phosphate dehydrogenase deficiency. Baillieres Best Pract Res Clin Haematol 2000;13:21. [PMID: 10916676]

SICKLE CELL ANEMIA & RELATED SYNDROMES

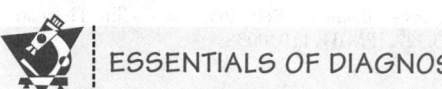 ESSENTIALS OF DIAGNOSIS

- Irreversibly sickled cells on peripheral blood smear.
- Positive family history and lifelong history of hemolytic anemia.
- Recurrent painful episodes.
- Hemoglobin S is the major hemoglobin seen on electrophoresis.

General Considerations

Sickle cell anemia is an autosomal recessive disorder in which an abnormal hemoglobin leads to chronic hemolytic anemia with numerous clinical consequences. A single DNA base change leads to an amino acid substitution of valine for glutamine in the sixth position on the β-globin chain. The abnormal beta chain is designated β[s] and the tetramer of $\alpha_2\beta^S_2$ is designated hemoglobin S.

When in the deoxy form, hemoglobin S forms polymers that damage the red blood cell membrane. Both polymer formation and early membrane damage are reversible. However, red blood cells that have undergone repeated sickling are damaged beyond repair and become irreversibly sickled.

The rate of sickling is influenced by a number of factors, most importantly by the concentration of hemoglobin S in the individual red blood cell. Red cell dehydration makes the cell quite vulnerable to sickling. Sickling is also strongly influenced by the presence of other hemoglobins within the cell. Hemoglobin F cannot participate in polymer formation, and its presence markedly retards sickling. Other factors that increase sickling are those which lead to formation of deoxyhemoglobin S, eg, acidosis and hypoxemia, either systemic or locally in tissues.

Prenatal diagnosis is now available for couples at risk of producing a child with sickle cell anemia. DNA from fetal cells can be directly examined, and the presence of the sickle cell mutation can be accurately and definitively diagnosed. Genetic counseling should be made available to such couples.

Clinical Findings

A. SYMPTOMS AND SIGNS

The hemoglobin S gene is carried in 8% of American blacks, and one birth out of 400 in American blacks will produce a child with sickle cell anemia. The disorder has its onset during the first year of life, when hemoglobin F levels fall as a signal is sent to switch from γ-globin to β-globin production.

Chronic hemolytic anemia produces jaundice, pigment (calcium bilirubinate) gallstones, splenomegaly, and poorly healing ulcers over the lower tibia. The chronic anemia may become life-threatening when severe anemia is produced by hemolytic or aplastic crises. The latter occur when the ability of the bone marrow to compensate is reduced by viral or other infection or by folate deficiency. Hemolytic crises may be related to splenic sequestration of sickled cells (primarily in childhood, before the spleen has been infarcted as a result of repeated sickling) or with coexistent disorders such as G6PD deficiency.

Acute painful episodes due to acute vaso-occlusion may occur spontaneously or be provoked by infection, dehydration, or hypoxia. Clusters of sickled red cells occlude the microvasculature of the organs involved.

These episodes last hours to days and produce acute pain and low-grade fever. Common sites of acute painful episodes include the bones (especially the back and long bones) and the chest. Acute vaso-occlusion may also cause strokes due to sinus thrombosis and priapism. Vaso-occlusive episodes are not associated with increased hemolysis.

Repeated episodes of vascular occlusion affect a large number of organs, especially the heart and liver. Ischemic necrosis of bone occurs, rendering the bone susceptible to osteomyelitis due to staphylococci or (less commonly) salmonellae. Infarction of the papillae of the renal medulla causes renal tubular concentrating defects and gross hematuria, more often encountered in sickle cell trait than in sickle cell anemia. Retinopathy similar to that noted in diabetes is often present and may lead to blindness.

These patients are prone to delayed puberty. An increased incidence of infection is related to hyposplenism as well as to defects in the alternative pathway of complement.

On examination, patients are often chronically ill and jaundiced. There is hepatomegaly, but the spleen is not palpable in adult life. The heart is enlarged, with a hyperdynamic precordium and systolic murmurs. Nonhealing ulcers of the lower leg and retinopathy may be present.

Sickle cell anemia becomes a chronic multisystem disease, with death from organ failure. With improved supportive care, average life expectancy is now between ages 40 and 50.

B. LABORATORY FINDINGS

Chronic hemolytic anemia is present. The hematocrit is usually 20–30%. The peripheral blood smear is characteristically abnormal, with irreversibly sickled cells comprising 5–50% of red cells. Other findings include reticulocytosis (10–25%), nucleated red blood cells, and hallmarks of hyposplenism such as Howell-Jolly bodies and target cells. The white blood cell count is characteristically elevated to 12,000–15,000/μL, and thrombocytosis may occur. Indirect bilirubin levels are high.

Most clinical laboratories offer a screening test for sickle cell hemoglobin, and the diagnosis of sickle cell anemia is then confirmed by hemoglobin electrophoresis (Table 13–9). Hemoglobin S has an abnormal migration pattern on electrophoresis and will usually comprise 85–98% of hemoglobin. In homozygous S disease, no hemoglobin A will be present. Hemoglobin F levels are variably increased, and high hemoglobin F levels are associated with a more benign clinical course.

Treatment

No specific treatment is available for the primary disease. Patients are maintained on folic acid supplemen-

Table 13–9. Hemoglobin distribution in sickle cell syndromes.

Genotype	Clinical Diagnosis	Hb A	Hb S	Hb A$_2$	Hb F
AA	Normal	97–99%	0	1–2%	< 1%
AS	Sickle trait	60%	40%	1–2%	< 1%
SS	Sickle cell anemia	0	86–98%	1–3%	5–15%
S β^0 thalassemia	Sickle β thalassemia	0	70–80%	3–5%	10–20%
S β$^+$ thalassemia	Sickle β thalassemia	10–20%	60–75%	3–5%	10–20%
AS, α thalassemia	Sickle trait	70–75%	25–30%	1–2%	< 1%

tation and given transfusions for aplastic or hemolytic crises. Pneumococcal vaccination reduces the incidence of infections with this pathogen.

When acute painful episodes occur, precipitating factors should be identified and infections treated if present. The patient should be kept well hydrated, and oxygen should be given if the patient is hypoxic.

Acute vaso-occlusive crises can be treated with exchange transfusion. These are primarily indicated for the treatment of intractable pain crises, priapism, and stroke.

Cytotoxic agents increase hemoglobin F levels by stimulating erythropoiesis in more primitive erythroid precursors. Hydroxyurea (500–750 mg/d) reduces the frequency of painful crises in patients whose quality of life is disrupted by frequent pain crises. Long-term safety is uncertain, and concern remains about the potential of secondary malignancies. Allogeneic bone marrow transplantation is being studied as a possible curative option for severely affected young patients.

Steinberg MH: Management of sickle cell disease. N Engl J Med 1999;340:1021. [PMID: 10099145]

Vichinsky EP et al: Causes and outcomes of the acute chest syndrome in sickle cell disease. National Acute Chest Syndrome Study Group. N Engl J Med 2000;342:1855. [PMID: 10861320] (Fat embolism and infection were the most frequently identified causes. The most common causes of death were pulmonary embolism and pneumonia.)

Walters MC et al: Impact of bone marrow transplantation for symptomatic sickle cell disease: an interim report. Blood 2000;95:1918. [PMID: 10706855]

SICKLE CELL TRAIT

Patients with the heterozygous genotype (AS) have sickle cell trait. These persons are clinically normal and have acute painful episodes only under extreme conditions such as vigorous exertion at high altitudes (or in unpressurized aircraft). The patients are hematologically normal, with no anemia and normal red blood cells on peripheral blood smear. They may, however, have a defect in renal tubular function, causing an inability to concentrate the urine, and experience episodes of gross hematuria. A screening test for sickle hemoglobin will be positive, and hemoglobin electrophoresis will reveal that approximately 40% of hemoglobin is hemoglobin S (Table 13–9).

No treatment is necessary. Genetic counseling is a reasonable strategy.

SICKLE THALASSEMIA

Patients with homozygous sickle cell anemia and alpha thalassemia have a somewhat milder form of hemolysis because of a slower rate of sickling related to reduced hemoglobin concentration (MCHC) within the red blood cell.

Patients who are double heterozygotes for sickle cell anemia and beta thalassemia are clinically affected with sickle cell syndromes. Sickle β^0 thalassemia is clinically very similar to homozygous SS disease. Vaso-occlusive crises may be somewhat less severe, and the spleen is usually not infarcted. Hematologically, the MCV is usually low, in contrast to the normal MCV of sickle cell anemia. Hemoglobin electrophoresis (Table 13–9) reveals no hemoglobin A but will show an increase in hemoglobin A$_2$ which is not present in sickle cell anemia.

Sickle β$^+$ thalassemia is a milder disorder than homozygous SS disease, with fewer crises. The spleen is usually palpable. The hemolytic anemia is less severe, and the hematocrit is usually 30–38%, with reticulocytes of 5–10%. Hemoglobin electrophoresis shows the presence of some hemoglobin A.

HEMOGLOBIN C DISORDERS

Hemoglobin C is formed by a single amino acid substitution at the same site of substitution as in sickle hemoglobin but with lysine instead of valine substituted for glutamine at the β$_6$ position. Hemoglobin C is nonsickling but may participate in polymer formation in association with hemoglobin S. Homozygous hemoglobin C disease produces a mild hemolytic anemia with splenomegaly, mild jaundice, and pigment (calcium bilirubinate) gallstones. The peripheral blood smear shows generalized red cell targeting and occasional cells with rectangular crystals of hemoglobin C. Persons heterozygous for hemoglobin C are clinically normal.

Patients with hemoglobin SC disease are double heterozygotes for beta S and beta C. These patients, like those with sickle β$^+$ thalassemia, have a milder hemolytic anemia and milder clinical course than those with homozygous SS disease. There are fewer vaso-occlusive events, and the spleen remains palpable in adult life. However, persons with hemoglobin SC disease have more retinopathy and more ischemic necrosis of bone than those with SS disease. The hematocrit is usually 30–38%, with 5–10% reticulocytes and few irreversibly sickled cells on the blood smear. Target cells are more numerous than in SS disease. Hemoglobin electrophoresis will show approximately 50% hemoglobin C, 50% hemoglobin S, and no increase in hemoglobin F levels.

UNSTABLE HEMOGLOBINS

Unstable hemoglobins are prone to oxidative denaturation even in the presence of a normal G6PD system. The disorder is autosomal dominant and of variable severity. Most patients have a mild chronic hemolytic anemia with splenomegaly, mild jaundice, and pigment (calcium bilirubinate) gallstones. Less severely affected patients are not anemic except under conditions of oxidative stress.

The diagnosis is made by the finding of Heinz bodies and a normal G6PD level. Hemoglobin electrophoresis is usually normal, since these hemoglobins characteristically do not have a change in their migration pattern. These hemoglobins precipitate in isopropanol. Usually no treatment is necessary. Patients with chronic hemolytic anemia should receive folate supplementation and avoid known oxidative drugs. In rare cases, splenectomy may be required.

AUTOIMMUNE HEMOLYTIC ANEMIA

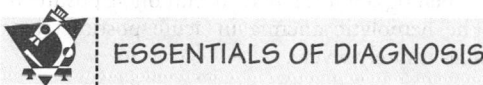

ESSENTIALS OF DIAGNOSIS

- *Acquired anemia caused by IgG autoantibody.*
- *Spherocytes and reticulocytosis on peripheral blood smear.*
- *Positive Coombs test.*

General Considerations

Autoimmune hemolytic anemia is an acquired disorder in which an IgG autoantibody is formed that binds to the red blood cell membrane. The antibody is most commonly directed against a basic component of the Rh system present on virtually all human red blood cells. When IgG antibodies coat the red blood cell, the Fc portion of the antibody is recognized by macrophages present in the spleen and other portions of the reticuloendothelial system. The interaction between splenic macrophage and the antibody-coated red blood cell results in removal of red blood cell membrane and the formation of a spherocyte because of the decrease in surface-to-volume ratio of the red blood cell. These spherocytic cells have decreased deformability and become trapped in the red pulp of the spleen because of their inability to squeeze through the 2-μm fenestrations. When large amounts of IgG are present on red blood cells, complement may be fixed. Direct lysis of cells is rare, but the presence of C3b on the surface of red blood cells allows Kupffer cells in the liver to participate in the hemolytic process because of the presence of C3b receptors on Kupffer cells.

Approximately half of all cases of autoimmune hemolytic anemia are idiopathic. The disorder may also be seen in association with systemic lupus erythematosus, chronic lymphocytic leukemia, or lymphomas. It must be distinguished from drug-induced hemolytic anemia. Penicillin (and other drugs) coat the red blood cell membrane, and the antibody is directed against the membrane-drug complex.

The Coombs antiglobulin test forms the basis for diagnosis of these immune hemolytic disorders. The Coombs reagent is a rabbit IgM antibody raised against human IgG or human complement. The direct Coombs test is performed by mixing the patient's red blood cells with the Coombs reagent and looking for agglutination, which indicates the presence of antibody on the red blood cell surface. The indirect Coombs test is performed by mixing the patient's serum with a panel of type O red blood cells. After incubation of the test serum and panel red blood cells, the Coombs reagent is added. Agglutination in this system indicates the presence of free antibody in the patient's serum. Because the traditional Coombs test relies on visible agglutination as an end point, the test is not very sensitive and will not detect immune hemolytic anemias in which only a small amount of IgG is present on red blood cells. More sensitive tests (micro-Coombs) are now available.

Clinical Findings

A. Symptoms and Signs

Autoimmune hemolytic anemia typically produces an anemia of rapid onset that may be life-threatening in severity. Patients complain of fatigue and may present with angina or congestive heart failure. On examination, jaundice and splenomegaly are usually present.

B. Laboratory Findings

The anemia is of variable severity but may be severe, with hematocrit of less than 10%. Reticulocytosis is usually present, and spherocytes are seen on the peripheral blood smear. In cases of severe hemolysis, the stressed bone marrow may also release nucleated red blood cells. As with other hemolytic disorders, indirect bilirubin is increased. Approximately 10% of patients with autoimmune hemolytic anemia have coincident immune thrombocytopenia (Evans's syndrome).

The direct Coombs test is positive, and the indirect Coombs test may or may not be positive. A positive indirect Coombs test indicates the presence of a large amount of autoantibody that has saturated binding sites in the red blood cell and consequently appears in the serum. A patient with acquired spherocytic hemolytic anemia that may be of the autoimmune variety who has a negative Coombs test should be tested with a micro-Coombs test (which is necessary to make the diagnosis in approximately 10% of cases). Because the patient's serum usually contains the autoantibody, it may be difficult to obtain a compatible cross-match with donor's cells.

Treatment

Initial treatment consists of prednisone, 1–2 mg/kg/d in divided doses. Most transfused blood will survive similarly to the patient's own red blood cells. Because of difficulty in performing the cross-match, incompatible blood may be given. Decisions regarding transfusions should be made in consultation with a hematologist. If prednisone is ineffective or if the disease recurs on tapering the dose, splenectomy should be performed. Patients with autoimmune hemolytic anemia refractory to prednisone and splenectomy may be treated with a variety of immunosuppressive agents, including cyclophosphamide, azathioprine, or cyclosporine. Danazol, 600–800 mg/d, is less often effective than in immune thrombocytopenia.

High-dose intravenous immune globulin (1 g daily for 1 or 2 days) may be highly effective in controlling hemolysis. The benefit is short-lived (1–3 weeks), and the drug is very expensive. Treatment with rituximab, a monoclonal antibody against the B cell antigen CD20, works in some cases. The suggested dose is 375 mg/m^2 intravenously weekly for 4 weeks.

The long-term prognosis for patients with this disorder is good, especially if there is no underlying autoimmune disorder or lymphoma. Splenectomy is often successful in controlling the disorder.

Kokori SI et al: Autoimmune hemolytic anemia in patients with systemic lupus erythematosus. Am J Med 2000;108:198. [PMID: 10723973]

Mauro FR et al: Autoimmune hemolytic anemia in chronic lymphocytic leukemia: clinical, therapeutic, and prognostic features. Blood 2000;95:2786. [PMID: 10779422]

Zecca M et al. Anti-CD20 monoclonal antibody for the treatment of severe, immune-mediated, pure red cell aplasia and hemolytic anemia. Blood 2001;97:3995. [PMID: 11389047]

COLD AGGLUTININ DISEASE

ESSENTIALS OF DIAGNOSIS

- *Increased reticulocytes and spherocytes on peripheral blood smear.*
- *Coombs test positive only for complement.*
- *Positive cold agglutinin test.*

General Considerations

Cold agglutinin disease is an acquired hemolytic anemia due to an IgM autoantibody usually directed against the I antigen on red blood cells. These IgM autoantibodies characteristically will not react with cells at 37 °C but only at lower temperatures. Since the blood temperature (even in the most peripheral parts of the body) rarely goes lower than 20 °C, only antibodies active at higher temperatures than this will produce clinical effects. Hemolysis results indirectly from attachment of IgM, which in the cooler parts of the circulation (fingers, nose, ears) binds and fixes complement. When the red blood cell returns to a warmer temperature, the IgM antibody dissociates, leaving complement on the cell. Lysis of cells rarely occurs. Rather, C3b present on the red cells is recognized by Kupffer cells (which have receptors for C3b), and red blood cell sequestration ensues.

Most cases of chronic cold agglutinin disease are idiopathic. Others occur in association with Waldenström's macroglobulinemia, in which a monoclonal IgM paraprotein is produced. Acute postinfectious cold agglutinin disease occurs following mycoplasmal pneumonia or infectious mononucleosis (with antibody directed against antigen i rather than I).

Clinical Findings

A. SYMPTOMS AND SIGNS

In chronic cold agglutinin disease, symptoms related to red blood cell agglutination occur on exposure to cold, and patients may complain of mottled or numb fingers or toes. Hemolytic anemia is rarely severe, but episodic hemoglobinuria may occur on exposure to cold. The hemolytic anemia in acute postinfectious syndromes is rarely severe.

B. LABORATORY FINDINGS

Mild anemia is present with reticulocytosis and spherocytes. The direct Coombs test will be positive for complement only. Occasionally, a micro-Coombs test is necessary to reveal bound complement (low-titer cold agglutinin disease). A bedside cold agglutinin test may be performed by placing a glass slide in ice and then putting a few drops of heparinized blood on it. Inspection may reveal small clumps of agglutinated blood.

Treatment

Treatment is largely symptomatic, based on avoiding exposure to cold. Patients with severe involvement may be treated with alkylating agents such as cyclophosphamide or with immunosuppressive agents such as cyclosporine. Splenectomy and prednisone are usually ineffective since hemolysis takes place in the liver. High-dose intravenous immunoglobulin (2 g/kg) may be effective temporarily.

There is some evidence that treatment with rituximab, a monoclonal antibody directed against B lymphocytes, may be effective. The dose is 375 mg/m^2 intravenously weekly for 4 weeks.

MICROANGIOPATHIC HEMOLYTIC ANEMIAS

The microangiopathic hemolytic anemias are a group of disorders in which red blood cell fragmentation takes place. The anemia is intravascular, producing hemoglobinemia, hemoglobinuria, and, in severe cases, methemalbuminemia. The hallmark of the disorder is the finding of fragmented red blood cells (schistocytes, helmet cells) on the peripheral blood smear.

These fragmentation syndromes can be caused by a variety of disorders (Table 13–8). Thrombotic thrombocytopenic purpura is the most important of these and is discussed below. Clinical features are variable and depend on the underlying disorder. Coagulopathy and thrombocytopenia are variably present.

Chronic microangiopathic hemolytic anemia (such as is present with a malfunctioning cardiac valve prosthesis) may cause iron deficiency anemia because of continuous low-grade hemoglobinuria.

APLASTIC ANEMIA

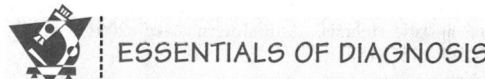

ESSENTIALS OF DIAGNOSIS

- *Pancytopenia.*
- *No abnormal cells seen.*
- *Hypocellular bone marrow.*

General Considerations

All hematopoietic cells are derived from a pluripotent stem cell that gives rise to precursors of erythroid, myeloid, and platelet forms. Injury to or suppression of this hematopoietic stem cell will result in pancytopenia. Aplastic anemia is a condition of bone marrow failure that arises from injury to or abnormal expression of the stem cell. The bone marrow becomes hypoplastic, and pancytopenia develops.

There are a number of causes of aplastic anemia (Table 13–10). Direct stem cell injury may be caused by radiation, chemotherapy, toxins, or pharmacologic agents. Systemic lupus erythematosus may rarely cause suppression of the hematopoietic stem cell by an IgG autoantibody directed against the stem cell. However, the most common pathogenesis of aplastic anemia appears to be autoimmune suppression of hematopoiesis by a T cell-mediated cellular mechanism.

Clinical Findings

A. SYMPTOMS AND SIGNS

Patients come to medical attention because of the consequences of bone marrow failure. Anemia leads to symptoms of weakness and fatigue; neutropenia causes

Table 13–10. Causes of aplastic anemia.

Congenital (rare)
"Idiopathic" (probably autoimmune)
Systemic lupus erythematosus
Chemotherapy, radiotherapy
Toxins: benzene, toluene, insecticides
Drugs: chloramphenicol, phenylbutazone, gold salts, sulfonamides, phenytoin, carbamazepine, quinacrine, tolbutamide
Posthepatitis
Pregnancy
Paroxysmal nocturnal hemoglobinuria

vulnerability to bacterial infections; and thrombocytopenia results in mucosal and skin bleeding. Physical examination may reveal signs of pallor, purpura, and petechiae. Other abnormalities such as hepatosplenomegaly, lymphadenopathy, or bone tenderness should *not* be present, and their presence should lead one to question the diagnosis.

B. LABORATORY FINDINGS

The hallmark of aplastic anemia is pancytopenia. However, early in the evolution of aplastic anemia, only one or two cell lines may be reduced.

Anemia may be severe and is always associated with decreased reticulocytes. Red blood cell morphology is unremarkable. The MCV is usually normal but occasionally may be increased. Neutrophils and platelets are reduced in number, and no immature or abnormal forms are seen. The bone marrow aspirate and the bone marrow biopsy appear hypocellular, with only scant amounts of normal hematopoietic progenitors. No abnormal cells are seen.

Differential Diagnosis

The diagnosis of aplastic anemia is made in cases of pancytopenia with a hypocellular marrow biopsy containing no abnormal cells. Aplastic anemia must be differentiated from other causes of pancytopenia (Table 13–11). Myelodysplastic disorders or acute leukemia may occasionally be confused with aplastic anemia. These are differentiated by the presence of morphologic abnormalities or increased blasts. Hairy cell leukemia has been misdiagnosed as aplastic anemia and should be recognized by the presence of splenomegaly and by abnormal lymphoid cells on the bone marrow biopsy. Pancytopenia with a normocellular bone marrow is usually due to systemic lupus erythematosus, disseminated infection, or hypersplenism. Isolated thrombocytopenia may occur early as aplastic anemia develops and be confused with immune thrombocytopenia.

Treatment

Mild cases of aplastic anemia may be treated with supportive care. Red blood cell transfusions and platelet

Table 13–11. Causes of pancytopenia.

Bone marrow disorders
  Aplastic anemia
  Myelodysplasia
  Acute leukemia
  Myelofibrosis
  Infiltrative disease: lymphoma, myeloma, carcinoma,
    hairy cell leukemia
  Megaloblastic anemia
Nonmarrow disorders
  Hypersplenism
  Systemic lupus erythematosus
  Infection: tuberculosis, AIDS, leishmaniasis, brucellosis

---

transfusions are given as necessary, and antibiotics are used to treat infections.

Severe aplastic anemia is defined by the presence of neutrophils less than 500/μL, platelets less than 20,000/μL, reticulocytes less than 1%, and bone marrow cellularity less than 20%. When this constellation of features is present (or three of the four), the median survival without treatment is approximately 3 months, and only 20% of patients survive for 1 year. The treatment of choice for young adults (under age 50) who have HLA-matched siblings is allogeneic bone marrow transplantation. Children or very young adults (under age 30) may benefit from allogeneic transplantation using an unrelated donor.

For adults over age 50 or those without HLA-matched siblings, the treatment of choice for severe aplastic anemia is immunosuppression with antithymocyte globulin (ATG) plus cyclosporine. ATG is given in the hospital in conjunction with transfusion and antibiotic support. A useful regimen is 40 mg/kg/d for 4 days in combination with cyclosporine, 6 mg/kg orally twice daily. ATG must be used in combination with corticosteroids (prednisone 1–2 mg/kg/d initially, followed by a rapid taper) to avoid complications of serum sickness. Responses usually occur in 4–12 weeks and are usually only partial, but the blood counts rise high enough to give patients a safe and transfusion-free life.

High-dose immunosuppression with cyclophosphamide, 200 mg/kg, has produced remissions in refractory cases and should be considered for patients without suitable bone marrow donors. Results employing this as primary therapy are promising, but prolonged pancytopenia (median 7 weeks of neutropenia) requiring antibiotic and transfusion support is a major concern.

Androgens have been widely used in the past, with a low response rate. However, a few patients can be maintained successfully with this form of treatment. One regimen is oxymetholone, 2–3 mg/kg orally daily.

Course & Prognosis

Patients with severe aplastic anemia have a rapidly fatal illness if left untreated. Allogeneic bone marrow transplantation is highly successful in children and young adults with HLA-matched siblings. For this group of patients, the durable complete response rate exceeds 80%. ATG treatment leads to partial response in approximately 60% of adults, and the long-term prognosis of responders appears to be good. There is increasing evidence that some fraction (as many as 25%) of these nontransplanted patients may develop clonal hematologic disorders such as paroxysmal nocturnal hemoglobinuria or myelodysplasia after many years of follow-up.

Bacigalupo A et al: Antilymphocyte globulin, cyclosporine, prednisolone, and granulocyte colony-stimulating factor for severe aplastic anemia: an update of the GITMO/EBMT study on 100 patients. European Group for Blood and Marrow Transplantation (EBMT) Working Party on Severe Aplastic Anemia and the Gruppo Italiano Trapianti di Midollo Osseo (GITMO). Blood 2000;95:1931. [PMID: 10706857]

Brodsky RA et al: Durable treatment-free remission after high-dose cyclophosphamide therapy for previously untreated severe aplastic anemia. Ann Intern Med 2001;135:477. [PMID: 11578150]

Deeg HJ: Long-term outcome after marrow transplantation for severe aplastic anemia. Blood 1998;91:3637. [PMID: 9572999]

■ NEUTROPENIA

Neutropenia is defined as a count below 1500/μL. However, blacks and other specific population groups may normally have neutrophil counts as low as 1200/μL. The neutropenic patient is increasingly vulnerable to infection by gram-positive and gram-negative bacteria and by fungi. The risk of infection is related to the severity of neutropenia. Patients with "chronic benign neutropenia" are free of infection for years despite very low neutrophil levels.

A variety of bone marrow disorders and nonmarrow conditions may cause neutropenia (Table 13–12). All the causes of aplastic anemia (Table 13–10) and pancytopenia (Table 13–11) may cause neutropenia. Isolated neutropenia is often due to an idiosyncratic reaction to a drug, and agranulocytosis (complete absence of neutrophils in the peripheral blood) is almost always due to a drug reaction. In these cases, examination of the bone marrow shows virtual absence of myeloid precursors, with other cell lines undisturbed. **Felty's syndrome**—immune neutropenia associated with seropositive nodular rheumatoid arthritis and splenomegaly—is another cause. Neutropenia in the presence of a normal bone marrow may be due to immunologic peripheral destruction, sepsis, or hyper-

Table 13–12. Causes of neutropenia.

Bone marrow disorders
    Aplastic anemia
    Pure white cell aplasia
    Congenital (rare)
    Cyclic neutropenia
    Drugs: sulfonamides, chlorpromazine, procainamide,
        penicillin, cephalosporins, cimetidine, methimazole,
        phenytoin, chlorpropamide, antiretroviral medications
    Benign chronic
Peripheral disorders
    Hypersplenism
    Sepsis
    Immune
    Felty's syndrome
    HIV infection
    Large granular lymphocytosis

splenism. Severe neutropenia may be associated with clonal disorders of T lymphocytes, often with the morphology of large granular lymphocytes.

Clinical Findings

Neutropenia results in stomatitis and in infections due to gram-positive or gram-negative aerobic bacteria or to fungi such as candida or aspergillus. The most common infections are septicemia, cellulitis, and pneumonia. In the presence of severe neutropenia, the usual signs of inflammatory response to infection may be absent. Nevertheless, fever in the neutropenic patient should always be assumed to be of infectious origin.

Treatment

Potential causative drugs are discontinued. Infections are treated with broad-spectrum antibiotics, but particular attention should be paid to enteric gram-negative bacteria. Effective antibiotics include the quinolones such as levofloxacin, 500 mg orally or intravenously daily, or new cephalosporins such as cefipime, 2 g intravenously every 8 hours.

Many cases of idiopathic or autoimmune neutropenia respond to myeloid growth factors such as G-CSF. Once- or twice-weekly dosage will often be sufficient to produce a protective neutrophil count.

When Felty's syndrome leads to repeated bacterial infections, splenectomy is the treatment of choice. It usually leads to healing of leg ulcers and to reduction in the rate of infection whether or not the neutrophil count rises.

The prognosis of patients with neutropenia depends on the underlying cause. Most patients with drug-induced agranulocytosis can be supported with broad-spectrum antibiotics and will recover completely. The myeloid growth factors G-CSF (filgrastim) and GM-CSF (sargramostim) may be useful in shortening the duration of neutropenia associated with chemotherapy. The neutropenia associated with large granular lymphocytes responds to cyclosporine therapy.

Klastersky J et al: The multi-national association for supportive care in cancer risk index. A multinational scoring system for identifying low-risk, febrile neutropenic cancer patients. J Clin Oncol 2000;18:3038. [PMID: 10944139]

Pizzo PA: Fever in immunocompromised patients. N Engl J Med 1999;341:893. [PMID: 10486422]

■ LEUKEMIAS & OTHER MYELOPROLIFERATIVE DISORDERS

Myeloproliferative disorders are due to acquired clonal abnormalities of the hematopoietic stem cell. Since the stem cell gives rise to myeloid, erythroid, and platelet cells, one sees qualitative and quantitative changes in all these cell lines. In some disorders (chronic myelogenous leukemia), specific characteristic chromosomal changes are seen. In others, no characteristic cytogenetic abnormalities are seen.

Classically, the myeloproliferative disorders produce characteristic syndromes with well-defined clinical and laboratory features (Tables 13–13 and 13–14). However, these disorders are grouped together because the disease may evolve from one form into another and because hybrid disorders are commonly seen. All of the myeloproliferative disorders may progress to acute myelogenous leukemia.

POLYCYTHEMIA VERA

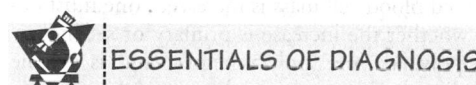 ESSENTIALS OF DIAGNOSIS

- *Increased red blood cell mass.*
- *Splenomegaly.*

Table 13–13. Classification of myeloproliferative disorders.

Myeloproliferative syndromes
    Polycythemia vera
    Myelofibrosis
    Essential thrombocytosis
    Chronic myeloid leukemia
Myelodysplastic syndromes
Acute myeloid leukemia

Table 13–14. Laboratory features of myeloproliferative disorders.

	White Count	Hematocrit	Platelet Count	Red Cell Morphology
Chronic myeloid leukemia	↑↑	N	N or ↑	N
Myelofibrosis	N or ↓ or ↑	N or ↓	↓ or N or ↑	Abn
Polycythemia vera	N or ↑	↑	N or ↑	N
Essential thrombocytosis	N or ↑	N	↑↑	N

- *Normal arterial oxygen saturation.*
- *Usually elevated white blood count and platelet count.*

General Considerations

Polycythemia vera is an acquired myeloproliferative disorder that causes overproduction of all three hematopoietic cell lines, most prominently the red blood cells. The hematocrit is elevated (at sea level) when values exceed 54% in males or 51% in females (Table 13–15).

When the hematocrit is elevated, the red blood cell mass should be measured to determine whether true polycythemia or relative polycythemia exists. Normal values for red blood cell mass are 26–34 mL/kg in men and 21–29 mL/kg in women. Relative ("spurious") polycythemia presents in middle-aged men who are overweight and hypertensive (often on diuretic therapy); the hematocrit is almost always less than 60%; they have a high normal red cell mass and a low-normal plasma volume.

If the red blood cell mass is increased, one must determine whether the increase is primary or secondary. Primary polycythemia (polycythemia vera) is a bone marrow disorder characterized by autonomous overproduction of erythroid cells. Erythroid production is independent of erythropoietin, and the serum erythropoietin level is low. In vitro, erythroid progenitor cells grow without added erythropoietin, a finding not seen in normal individuals.

Clinical Findings

A. SYMPTOMS AND SIGNS

Most patients present with symptoms related to expanded blood volume and increased blood viscosity. Common complaints include headache, dizziness, tinnitus, blurred vision, and fatigue. Generalized pruritus, especially that occurring following a warm shower or bath, may be a striking symptom and is related to histamine release from the increased number of basophils present. Patients may also initially complain of epistaxis. This is probably related to engorgement of mucosal blood vessels in combination with abnormal hemostasis due to qualitative abnormalities in platelet function. Sixty percent of patients are men, and the median age at presentation is 60 years. Polycythemia rarely occurs in persons under age 40.

Physical examination reveals plethora and engorged retinal veins. The spleen is palpable in 75% of cases but nearly always enlarged when imaged.

Thrombosis is the most common complication of polycythemia vera and the major cause of morbidity and death in this disorder. Thrombosis appears to be related to increased blood viscosity and abnormal platelet function. Uncontrolled polycythemia leads to a very high incidence of thrombotic complications of surgery, and elective surgery should be deferred until the condition has been treated. Paradoxically, in addition to thrombosis, increased bleeding also occurs. There is a high incidence of peptic ulcer disease.

B. LABORATORY FINDINGS

The hallmark of polycythemia vera is a hematocrit above normal, at times greater than 60%. Red blood cell morphology is normal. By definition, the red blood cell mass is elevated. The white blood count is elevated to 10,000–20,000/μL and the platelet count is variably increased, sometimes to counts exceeding 1,000,000/μL. Platelet morphology is usually normal. White blood cells are usually normal, but basophilia and eosinophilia are frequently present.

Table 13–15. Causes of polycythemia.

Spurious polycythemia
Secondary polycythemia
  Hypoxia: cardiac disease, pulmonary disease, high altitude
  Carboxyhemoglobin: smoking
  Renal lesions
  Erythropoietin-secreting tumors (rare)
  Abnormal hemoglobins (rare)
Polycythemia vera

The bone marrow is hypercellular, with panhyperplasia of all hematopoietic elements. Iron stores are usually absent from the bone marrow, having been transferred to the increased circulating red blood cell mass. Iron deficiency may also result from chronic gastrointestinal blood loss. Bleeding may lower the hematocrit to the normal range (or lower), creating diagnostic confusion.

Vitamin B_{12} levels are strikingly elevated because of increased levels of transcobalamin III (secreted by white blood cells). Overproduction of uric acid may lead to hyperuricemia.

Although red blood cell morphology is usually normal at presentation, microcytosis, hypochromia, and poikilocytosis may result from iron deficiency following treatment by phlebotomy (see below). Progressive hypersplenism may also lead to elliptocytosis.

Differential Diagnosis

Spurious polycythemia, in which an elevated hematocrit is due to contracted plasma volume rather than increased red cell mass, may be related to diuretic use or may occur without obvious cause.

A secondary cause of polycythemia should be suspected if splenomegaly is absent and the high hematocrit is not accompanied by increases in other cell lines. Arterial oxygen saturation should be measured to determine if hypoxia is the cause. A smoking history should be taken; carboxyhemoglobin levels may be elevated in smokers. A renal sonogram may be considered to look for an erythropoietin-secreting cyst or tumor. A positive family history should lead to investigation for congenital high-oxygen-affinity hemoglobin.

Polycythemia vera should be differentiated from other myeloproliferative disorders (Table 13–14). Marked elevation of the white blood count (above 30,000/µL) suggests chronic myelogenous leukemia. This disorder is confirmed by the presence of the Philadelphia chromosome. Abnormal red blood cell morphology and nucleated red blood cells in the peripheral blood are seen in myelofibrosis. This condition is diagnosed by bone marrow biopsy showing fibrosis of the marrow. Essential thrombocytosis is diagnosed when the platelet count is strikingly elevated and the red blood cell mass is normal.

Treatment

The treatment of choice is phlebotomy. One unit of blood (approximately 500 mL) is removed weekly until the hematocrit is less than 45%; the hematocrit is maintained at less than 45% by repeated phlebotomy as necessary. Because repeated phlebotomy worsens iron deficiency, the requirement for phlebotomy should gradually decrease. It is important to avoid medicinal iron supplementation, as this can thwart the goals of a phlebotomy program. Maintaining the hematocrit at normal levels has been shown to decrease the incidence

of thrombotic complications. A diet low in iron may also increase the intervals between phlebotomies.

Occasionally, myelosuppressive therapy is indicated. Indications include a high phlebotomy requirement, thrombocytosis, and intractable pruritus. There is evidence that reduction of the platelet count to less than 600,000/µL will reduce the risk of thrombotic complications. Alkylating agents have been shown to increase the risk of conversion of this disease to acute leukemia and should be avoided. Hydroxyurea is now being widely used when myelosuppressive therapy is indicated because of the established leukemogenic potential of alkylating agents. The usual dose is 500–1500 mg/d orally, adjusted to keep platelets < 500,000/µL without reducing the neutrophil count to < 2000/µL. Anagrelide is used in treatment of thrombocytosis and may prove valuable.

The role of antiplatelet agents such as aspirin in preventing thrombotic complications is controversial. High doses of aspirin (325 mg three times daily) plus dipyridamole (25 mg three times daily) cause a marked increase in gastrointestinal bleeding and should be avoided. Low-dose aspirin (81–325 mg daily) may reduce the risk of thrombosis without excessive bleeding risk.

Allopurinol may be indicated for hyperuricemia. Antihistamine therapy with diphenhydramine or other H_1 blockers may be helpful for control of pruritus.

Prognosis

Polycythemia is an indolent disease with median survival of 11–15 years. The major cause of morbidity and mortality is arterial thrombosis. Over time, polycythemia vera may convert to myelofibrosis or to chronic myelogenous leukemia. In approximately 5% of cases, the disorder progresses to acute myelogenous leukemia, which is usually refractory to therapy.

Streiff MB et al. The diagnosis and management of polycythemia vera in the era since the Polycythemia Vera Study Group: a survey of an American Society of Hematology members' practice patterns. Blood 2002;99:1144. [PMID: 11830459]

Tefferi A et al: A clinical update in polycythemia vera and essential thrombocythemia. Am J Med 2000;109:141. [PMID: 10967156]

ESSENTIAL THROMBOCYTOSIS

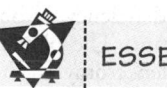

ESSENTIALS OF DIAGNOSIS

- *Elevated platelet count in absence of other causes.*
- *Normal red blood cell mass.*
- *Absence of Philadelphia chromosome.*

General Considerations

Essential thrombocytosis is an uncommon myeloproliferative disorder of unknown cause in which marked proliferation of the megakaryocytes in the bone marrow leads to elevation of the platelet count.

Clinical Findings

A. SYMPTOMS AND SIGNS

The median age at presentation is 50–60 years, and there is a slightly increased incidence in women. The disorder is commonly suspected because of the finding of an elevated platelet count. Less commonly, the first sign is thrombosis.

The most common clinical problem is thrombosis. The risk of thrombosis rises with age. Venous thromboses may occur in unusual sites such as the mesenteric, hepatic, or portal vein. Some patients experience erythromelalgia, painful burning of the hands accompanied by erythema; this symptom is reliably relieved by aspirin. Bleeding, typically mucosal, is less common and is related to a concomitant qualitative platelet defect. Splenomegaly is present in at least 25% of patients.

B. LABORATORY FINDINGS

An elevated platelet count is the hallmark of this disorder, and the count may be markedly elevated to over 2,000,000/μL. The white blood cell count is often mildly elevated, usually not above 30,000/μL, but with some immature myeloid forms. The hematocrit is normal. The peripheral blood smear reveals large platelets, but giant degranulated forms seen in myelofibrosis are not observed. Red blood cell morphology is normal. The bleeding time is prolonged in 20% of patients.

The bone marrow shows increased numbers of megakaryocytes but no other morphologic abnormalities. The Philadelphia chromosome is absent but should be assayed in all suspected cases to differentiate the disorder from chronic myeloid leukemia.

Differential Diagnosis

Essential thrombocytosis must be distinguished from secondary causes of an elevated platelet count. In reactive thrombocytosis, the platelet count seldom exceeds 1,000,000/μL. Inflammatory disorders such as rheumatoid arthritis and ulcerative colitis cause significant elevations of the platelet count, as may chronic infection. The thrombocytosis of iron deficiency is observed only when anemia is significant. The platelet count is temporarily elevated after splenectomy.

Regarding other myeloproliferative disorders, the lack of elevated hematocrit and red blood cell mass distinguishes it from polycythemia vera. Unlike myelofibrosis, red blood cell morphology is normal, nucleated red blood cells are absent, and giant degranulated platelets are not seen. In chronic myeloid leukemia, the Philadelphia chromosome establishes the diagnosis.

Treatment

The risk of thrombosis can be reduced by control of the platelet count, and one should aim to keep it less than 500,000/μL. Standard therapy has consisted of hydroxyurea in a dose of 0.5–2 g/d. In some cases this is not effective because of dose-limiting neutropenia. Anagrelide is highly effective in a dose of 2–4 mg/d but may cause headache, mild anemia, and peripheral edema, and in high doses congestive heart failure.

Vasomotor symptoms such as erythromelalgia and paresthesias respond rapidly to aspirin and eventually to control of the platelet count. The role of chronic low-dose aspirin therapy to reduce the risk of thrombosis remains unsettled. In the unusual event of severe bleeding, the platelet count can be *lowered* rapidly with plateletpheresis.

Course & Prognosis

Essential thrombocytosis is an indolent disorder and allows long-term survival. Average survival is longer than 15 years from diagnosis. The major source of morbidity—thrombosis—can be reduced by appropriate platelet control. Late in the course of the disease, the bone marrow may become fibrotic, and massive splenomegaly may occur, sometimes with splenic infarction. There is a 5% risk of transformation to acute leukemia over 20 years.

Storen EC et al: Long-term use of anagrelide in young patients with essential thrombocytopenia. Blood 2001;97:893. [PMID: 11159509]

Tefferi A et al: A long-term retrospective study of young women with essential thrombocythemia. Mayo Clin Proc 2001;76:22. [PMID: 11155408] (Survival similar to that of an age- and sex-matched cohort.)

MYELOFIBROSIS

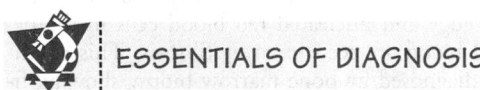 ESSENTIALS OF DIAGNOSIS

- *Striking splenomegaly.*
- *Teardrop poikilocytosis on peripheral smear.*
- *Leukoerythroblastic blood picture; giant abnormal platelets.*
- *Hypercellular bone marrow with reticulin or collagen fibrosis.*

General Considerations

Myelofibrosis (myelofibrosis with myeloid metaplasia, agnogenic myeloid metaplasia) is a myeloproliferative disorder characterized by fibrosis of the bone marrow, splenomegaly, and a leukoerythroblastic peripheral blood picture with teardrop poikilocytosis. It is widely believed that fibrosis occurs in response to increased secretion of platelet-derived growth factor (PDGF) and possibly other cytokines. In response to bone marrow fibrosis, extramedullary hematopoiesis takes place in the liver, spleen, and lymph nodes. In these sites, mesenchymal cells responsible for fetal hematopoiesis can be reactivated.

Clinical Findings

A. SYMPTOMS AND SIGNS

Myelofibrosis develops in adults over age 50 and is usually insidious in onset. Patients most commonly present with fatigue due to anemia or abdominal fullness related to splenomegaly. Uncommon presentations include bleeding and bone pain. On examination, splenomegaly is almost invariably present and is commonly massive. The liver is enlarged in more than half of cases.

Later in the course of the disease, progressive bone marrow failure takes place as it becomes progressively more fibrotic. Anemia becomes severe, requiring transfusion. Progressive thrombocytopenia leads to bleeding. The spleen continues to enlarge, which leads to early satiety. Painful episodes of splenic infarction may occur. Late in the course, the patient becomes cachectic and may experience severe bone pain, especially in the upper legs. Hematopoiesis in the liver leads to portal hypertension with ascites, esophageal varices, and occasionally transverse myelitis caused by myelopoiesis in the epidural space.

B. LABORATORY FINDINGS

Patients are almost invariably anemic at presentation. The white blood count is variable—either low, normal, or elevated—and may be increased to 50,000/μL. The platelet count is variable. The peripheral blood smear is dramatic, with significant poikilocytosis and numerous teardrop forms in the red cell line. Nucleated red blood cells are present and the myeloid series is shifted, with immature forms including a small percentage of promyelocytes or myeloblasts. Platelet morphology may be bizarre, and giant degranulated platelet forms (megakaryocyte fragments) may be seen. The triad of teardrop poikilocytosis, leukoerythroblastic blood, and giant abnormal platelets is highly suggestive of myelofibrosis.

The bone marrow usually cannot be aspirated (dry tap), though early in the course of the disease it is hypercellular, with a marked increase in megakaryocytes. Fibrosis at this stage is detected by a silver stain demonstrating increased reticulin fibers. Later, biopsy reveals more severe fibrosis, with eventual replacement of hematopoietic precursors by collagen. There is no characteristic chromosomal abnormality.

Differential Diagnosis

A leukoerythroblastic blood picture from other causes may be seen in response to severe infection, inflamma-

tion, or infiltrative bone marrow processes. However, teardrop poikilocytosis and giant abnormal platelet forms will not be present. Bone marrow fibrosis may be seen in metastatic carcinoma, Hodgkin's disease, and hairy cell leukemia. These disorders are diagnosed by characteristic morphology of involved tissues.

Concerning other myeloproliferative disorders, chronic myelogenous leukemia is diagnosed when there is marked leukocytosis, normal red blood cell morphology, and the presence of the Philadelphia chromosome. Polycythemia vera is characterized by an elevated red blood cell mass. Essential thrombocytosis shows predominant and consistent platelet count elevations.

Treatment

There is no specific treatment for this disorder. Anemic patients are supported with transfusion. Androgens such as oxymetholone, 200 mg orally daily, or testosterone reduce the transfusion requirement in one-third of cases but are poorly tolerated by women. Splenectomy is not routinely performed but is indicated for splenic enlargement causing recurrent painful episodes, severe thrombocytopenia, or an unacceptable transfusion requirement. Allogeneic bone marrow transplantation has been performed successfully with 50% long-term survival and should be considered in younger patients. The use of less toxic, nonmyeloablative regimens for allogeneic transplantation is likely to increase.

Course & Prognosis

It is difficult to date the onset of myelofibrosis, but the median survival from time of diagnosis is approximately 5 years. End-stage myelofibrosis is characterized by generalized debility, liver failure, and bleeding from thrombocytopenia, with some cases terminating in acute myelogenous leukemia.

Anderson JE et al: Myeloablation and autologous peripheral blood stem cell rescue results in hematologic and clinical responses in patients with myeloid metaplasia with myelofibrosis. Blood 2001;98:586. [PMID: 11468154]

Tefferi A: Myelofibrosis with myeloid metaplasia. N Engl J Med 2000;342:1255. [PMID: 10781623]

CHRONIC MYELOGENOUS LEUKEMIA

ESSENTIALS OF DIAGNOSIS

- *Strikingly elevated white blood count.*
- *Markedly left-shifted myeloid series but with a low percentage of promyelocytes and blasts.*
- *Presence of Philadelphia chromosome or bcr-abl gene.*

General Considerations

Chronic myelogenous leukemia is a myeloproliferative disorder characterized by overproduction of myeloid cells. These myeloid cells retain the capacity for differentiation, and normal bone marrow function is retained during the early phases. The disease usually remains stable for years and then transforms to a more overtly malignant disease.

Chronic myelogenous leukemia is associated with a characteristic chromosomal abnormality, the Philadelphia chromosome, a reciprocal translocation between the long arms of chromosomes 9 and 22. A large portion of 22q is translocated to 9q, and a smaller piece of 9q is moved to 22q. The portion of 9q that is translocated contains *abl*, a proto-oncogene that is the cellular homolog of the Ableson murine leukemia virus. The *abl* gene is received at a specific site on 22q, the break point cluster (bcr). The fusion gene *bcr/abl* produces a novel protein that differs from the normal transcript of the *abl* gene in that it possesses tyrosine kinase activity (a characteristic activity of transforming genes). Evidence that the *bcr/abl* fusion gene is pathogenic is provided by transgenic mouse models in which introduction of the gene almost invariably leads to leukemia.

Usually at the time of diagnosis, the Philadelphia chromosome-positive clone dominates and may be the only one detected. However, a normal clone is present and may express itself either in vivo, after certain forms of therapy, or in vitro, in long-term bone marrow cultures. Approximately 5% of cases of chronic myelogenous leukemia are Philadelphia chromosome-negative at the level of light microscope cytogenetics, though molecular studies demonstrate the *bcr/abl* fusion gene. The entity formerly known as Philadelphia chromosome-negative CML is now recognized as chronic myelomonocytic leukemia (CMML), a subtype of myelodysplasia.

Early chronic myelogenous leukemia ("chronic phase") does not behave like a malignant disease. Normal bone marrow function is retained, white blood cells differentiate, and, despite some qualitative abnormalities (low leukocyte alkaline phosphatase), the neutrophils combat infection normally. However, chronic myelogenous leukemia is inherently unstable, and the disease progresses to accelerated phase and finally after several years, to blast crisis. This progression of the disease is often associated with added chromosomal defects superimposed on the Philadelphia chromosome. Blast crisis chronic myelogenous leukemia is morphologically indistinguishable from acute leukemia.

Clinical Findings

A. Symptoms and Signs

Chronic myelogenous leukemia is a disorder of middle age (median age at presentation is 42 years). Patients usually present with fatigue, night sweats, and low-grade fever related to the hypermetabolic state caused by overproduction of white blood cells. At other times, the patient complains of abdominal fullness related to splenomegaly, or an elevated white blood count is discovered incidentally. Rarely, the patient will present with a clinical syndrome related to leukostasis with blurred vision, respiratory distress, or priapism. The white blood count in these cases is usually greater than 500,000/μL.

On examination, the spleen is enlarged (often markedly so), and sternal tenderness may be present as a sign of marrow overexpansion.

Acceleration of the disease is often associated with fever in the absence of infection, bone pain, and splenomegaly. In blast crisis, patients may experience bleeding and infection related to bone marrow failure.

B. Laboratory Findings

The hallmark of chronic myelogenous leukemia is an elevated white blood count; the median white blood count at diagnosis is 150,000/μL. The peripheral blood is characteristic. The myeloid series is left-shifted, with mature forms dominating and with cells usually present in proportion to their degree of maturation. Blasts are usually less than 5%. Basophilia and eosinophilia of granulocytes may be present. At presentation, the patient is usually not anemic. Red blood cell morphology is normal, and nucleated red blood cells are rarely seen. The platelet count may be normal or elevated (sometimes to strikingly high levels). Platelet morphology is usually normal, but abnormally large forms may be seen.

The bone marrow is hypercellular, with left-shifted myelopoiesis. Myeloblasts comprise less than 5% of marrow cells.

The leukocyte alkaline phosphatase score is invariably low and is a sign of qualitative abnormalities in neutrophils. The vitamin B_{12} level is usually elevated because of increased secretion of transcobalamin III, and uric acid levels may be high. The Philadelphia chromosome may be detected in either the peripheral blood or the bone marrow. The *bcr/abl* gene may be reliably found in peripheral blood by molecular techniques.

With progression to the accelerated and blast phases, progressive anemia and thrombocytopenia occur, and the percentage of blasts in the blood and bone marrow increases. Blast phase chronic myelogenous leukemia is diagnosed when blasts comprise more than 30% of bone marrow cells.

Differential Diagnosis

Early chronic myelogenous leukemia must be differentiated from the reactive leukocytosis associated with infection. In such cases, the white blood count is usually less than 50,000/μL, splenomegaly is absent, the leukocyte alkaline phosphatase is increased, and the Philadelphia chromosome is not present.

Chronic myelogenous leukemia must be distinguished from other myeloproliferative disease (Table 13–14). The hematocrit should not be elevated, the red blood cell morphology is normal, and nucleated red blood cells are rare or absent. Definitive diagnosis is made by finding the Philadelphia chromosome or *bcr/abl*.

Treatment

Treatment is usually not emergent even with white blood counts over 200,000/μL, since the majority of circulating cells are mature myeloid cells that are smaller and more deformable than primitive leukemic blasts. In the rare instances in which symptoms result from extreme hyperleukocytosis (priapism, respiratory distress, visual blurring, altered mental status), emergent leukapheresis is performed in conjunction with myelosuppressive therapy.

The treatment of CML has changed with the introduction of imatinib mesylate. This drug is a specifically designed inhibitor of the tyrosine kinase activity of the *bcr/abl* oncogene. It is well tolerated and results in nearly universal (98%) hematologic control of chronic phase disease. It has now replaced both interferon and hydroxyurea as standard therapy. For patients with the chronic phase of CML, the dose is 400 mg orally daily. The most common toxicities are nausea, periorbital swelling, rash, and myalgia, but most of these are modest. The best outcomes are seen in patients in whom the drug produces both hematologic and cytogenetic remission. The latter is assessed by testing bone marrow cytogenetics after 6 months of treatment. Patients with major (< 35% abnormal metaphases) or complete cytogenetic response appear to have an excellent prognosis, with over 95% remaining in control for longer than 2 years. Since almost all clinical experience with imatinib began in early 2000, long-term outcome is uncertain. The addition of either alpha interferon or low-dose chemotherapy with cytarabine holds promise for even better results.

Hydroxyurea was formerly the standard treatment for this disease and can be used for patients who do not tolerate imatinib. Hydroxyurea is oral and very well tolerated. The usual dose is 0.5–2.5 g/d, adjusted to keep the white blood cell count ideally near 5000/μL but in any case above 2000/μL. It is given without interruption because of rapid white blood count rebound.

Recombinant alpha interferon had largely replaced hydroxyurea as the treatment of choice for chronic phase CML before the development of imatinib. In comparison with hydroxyurea, it prolongs the chronic phase of the disease and survival. However, interferon has the disadvantages of being given by subcutaneous injection and has pronounced side effects. These include fatigue, myalgias, and anorexia. The best results are seen with the full dose of 5×10^6 units/m²/d, continued for 5 years and then reduced to a lower dose. Many patients will be unable to tolerate this dose. The role of this agent is likely to be that of adjunct to imatinib.

The only available curative therapy for CML is allogeneic bone marrow transplantation. This treatment is indicated for adults under 60 who have HLA-matched siblings. Sixty percent of patients have long-term disease-free survival following transplantation. The best results (70–80% success rate) are obtained in patients who are under 40 and transplanted within 1 year after diagnosis. The introduction of imatinib has changed the approach to allogeneic transplant for CML. Patients with the best transplant outcomes (under 40 with matched sibling donors) may be offered allogeneic transplant. An alternative approach is to initiate imatinib and to recommend transplant if there is no cytogenetic response after 6 months. These recommendations are in flux and may change as long-term experience with imatinib accumulates. For young patients without sibling donors whose disease is not controlled by imatinib, HLA-matched unrelated donors may be located through registries such as the National Marrow Donors Program. Results are inferior to those achieved with matched sibling transplants but offer a cure rate of 40–60% in an otherwise invariably fatal disease.

Allogeneic transplantation cures chronic myeloid leukemia by initial cytoreduction followed by long-term immunologic control mediated by the donor's immune system. This alloimmune phenomenon has been called the "graft-versus-leukemia" effect. The most compelling evidence for its importance is that chronic phase disease which has recurred after allogeneic transplantation can usually be reversed without additional chemotherapy by the infusion of T lymphocytes from the initial bone marrow donor. This donor lymphocyte infusion can lead to long-term remission in 50–70% of cases. In response to appreciation of the importance of the graft-versus-leukemia effect, less toxic forms of allogeneic transplantation (nonmyeloablative) have been developed that require much less initial cytoreductive therapy and rely exclusively on the immune effect for long-term disease control. This approach has been encouraging and is likely to further expand the role of allogeneic transplant for CML.

Course & Prognosis

In the past, median survival was 3–4 years. With interferon-based therapies, this was increased to 5–6 years. It is anticipated that imatinib will lead to marked improvements in survival rates, but this remains to be proved.

Bonifazi F et al: Chronic myeloid leukemia and interferon-a: a study of complete cytogenetic responders. Blood 2001; 98:3074. [PMID: 11698293]

Druker BJ et al: Efficacy and safety of a specific inhibitor of the BCR-ABL tyrosine kinase in chronic myeloid leukemia. N Engl J Med 2001;344:1031. [PMID: 11287972] (The landmark paper in the field.)

Kalidas M et al: Chronic myelogenous leukemia. JAMA 2001; 286:895. [PMID: 11509034]

Radich JP et al: The significance of *brc-abl* molecular detection in chronic myeloid leukemia patients "late," 18 months or more after transplantation. Blood 2001;98:1701. [PMID: 11535500]

MYELODYSPLASTIC SYNDROMES

 ESSENTIALS OF DIAGNOSIS

- Cytopenias with a hypercellular bone marrow.
- Morphologic abnormalities in two or more hematopoietic cell lines.

General Considerations

The myelodysplastic syndromes are a group of acquired clonal disorders of the hematopoietic stem cell. They are characterized by the constellation of cytopenias, a hypercellular marrow, and a number of morphologic and cytogenetic abnormalities. The disorders are usually idiopathic but may be seen after cytotoxic chemotherapy—especially mechlorethamine procarbazine for Hodgkin's disease and melphalan for multiple myeloma or ovarian carcinoma.

Despite the presence of adequate numbers of hematopoietic progenitor cells, "ineffective hematopoiesis" occurs, resulting in various cytopenias. Ultimately, the disorder may evolve into acute myelogenous leukemia, and the term "preleukemia" has been used to describe these disorders. Although no specific chromosomal abnormality is seen in myelodysplasia, there are frequently abnormalities involving the long arm of chromosome 5 (which contains a number of genes encoding both growth factors and receptors involved in myelopoiesis) as well as deletions of chromosomes 5 and 7.

Myelodysplasia encompasses several heterogeneous syndromes. Those without excess bone marrow blasts are termed "refractory anemia," with or without ringed sideroblasts. Those with excess blasts are diagnosed as "refractory anemia with excess blasts" (RAEB 5–19% blasts). Those with a proliferative syndrome including peripheral blood monocytosis greater than 1000/μL are termed chronic myelomonocytic leukemia (CMML).

Clinical Findings

A. SYMPTOMS AND SIGNS

Patients are usually over age 60. Many are diagnosed while asymptomatic because of the finding of abnormal blood counts. Patients usually present with fatigue, infection, or bleeding related to bone marrow failure. The course may be indolent, and the disease may present as a wasting illness with fever, weight loss, and general debility. On examination, splenomegaly may be present in combination with pallor, bleeding, and various signs of infection.

B. LABORATORY FINDINGS

Anemia may be marked and may require transfusion support. The MCV is normal or increased, and macro-ovalocytes may be seen on the peripheral blood smear. The reticulocyte count is usually reduced. The white blood cell count is usually normal or reduced, and neutropenia is common. The neutrophils may exhibit morphologic abnormalities, including deficient numbers of granules or a bilobed nucleus (Pelger-Huet). The myeloid series may be left-shifted, and small numbers of promyelocytes or blasts may be seen. The platelet count is normal or reduced, and hypogranular platelets may be present.

The bone marrow is characteristically hypercellular. Erythroid hyperplasia is common, and signs of abnormal erythropoiesis include megaloblastic features, nuclear budding, or multinucleated erythroid precursors. The Prussian blue stain may demonstrate ringed sideroblasts. The myeloid series is often left-shifted, with variable increases in blasts. Deficient or abnormal granules may be seen. A characteristic abnormality is the presence of dwarf megakaryocytes with a unilobed nucleus.

Differential Diagnosis

In subtle cases, cytogenetic evaluation of the bone marrow may help distinguish this clonal disorder from other causes of cytopenias. As the number of blasts increases in the bone marrow, myelodysplasia is arbitrarily separated from acute myelogenous leukemia by the presence of less than 20% blasts.

Treatment

Patients affected primarily by anemia are supported with red blood cell transfusions. Those with severe neutropenia may benefit from the use of myeloid growth factors such as G-CSF or GM-CSF. Erythropoietin (epoetin alfa), 30,000 units subcutaneously weekly, reduces the red cell transfusion requirement in some patients. The response rate is 20% or less, but a 4-week trial of erythropoietin is reasonable since it will be of benefit and cost-effective for the subgroup of responders. The combination of myeloid growth factors and high doses of erythropoietin produces a higher response rate, but the cost is prohibitive. Azacitidine (5-azacytidine) improves both symptoms and blood counts and appears to prolong the time to conversion to acute leukemia.

Patients under age 60 with matched sibling donors can be treated with allogeneic bone marrow transplantation. Cure rates are 30–50%. The use of less toxic allogeneic transplant regimens is being explored and may increase the role of this therapy in patients with less aggressive forms of the disease (without excess blasts).

Course & Prognosis

Myelodysplasia is an ultimately fatal disease. Patients most commonly succumb to infections or bleeding. The risk of transformation to acute myelogenous leukemia depends on the percentage of blasts in the bone marrow. Patients with refractory anemia may survive many years, and the risk of leukemia is low (< 10%). Those with excess blasts or CMML have short survivals (usually < 2 years) and have a higher (20–50%) risk of developing acute leukemia. The finding of deletions of chromosomes 5 and 7 is associated with a poor prognosis.

Deeg HJ et al: Allogeneic and syngeneic marrow transplantation for myelodysplastic syndrome in patients 55–66 years of age. Blood 2000;95:1188. [PMID: 10666189]

Heaney ML et al: Myelodysplasias. N Engl J Med 1999;340:1649. [PMID: 10341278]

Nösslinger T et al: Myelodysplastic syndromes, from French-American-British to World Health Organization: comparison of classifications on 431 unselected patients from a single institution. Blood 2001;98:2935. [PMID: 11698274]

ACUTE LEUKEMIA

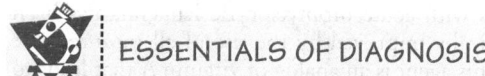

ESSENTIALS OF DIAGNOSIS

- *Short duration of symptoms, including fatigue, fever, and bleeding.*
- *Cytopenias or pancytopenia.*
- *More than 20% blasts in the bone marrow.*
- *Blasts in peripheral blood in 90%.*

General Considerations

Acute leukemia is a malignancy of the hematopoietic progenitor cell. The malignant cell loses its ability to mature and differentiate. These cells proliferate in an uncontrolled fashion and replace normal bone marrow elements. Most cases arise with no clear cause. However, radiation and some toxins (benzene) are leukemogenic. In addition, a number of chemotherapeutic agents (especially procarbazine, melphalan, other alkylating agents, and etoposide) may cause leukemia. The leukemias seen after toxin or chemotherapy exposure often develop from a myelodysplastic prodrome and are associated with abnormalities in chromosomes 5 and 7.

Much as been learned about the molecular biology of the leukemias. One subtype, acute promyelocytic leukemia, is characterized by chromosomal translocation t(15;17), which produces fusion gene *PML-RARα*. This change in the retinoic acid receptor produces a block in differentiation that can be overcome with pharmacologic doses of retinoic acid (see below).

Most of the clinical findings in acute leukemia are due to replacement of normal bone marrow elements by the malignant cell. Less common manifestations result from organ infiltration (skin, gastrointestinal tract, meninges). Acute leukemia is potentially curable with combination chemotherapy.

Acute lymphoblastic leukemia (ALL) comprises 80% of the acute leukemias of childhood. The peak incidence is between 3 and 7 years of age. It is also seen in adults, causing approximately 20% of adult acute leukemias. Acute myelogenous leukemia (AML) is chiefly an adult disease with a median age at presentation of 60 years and an increasing incidence with advanced age.

Clinical Findings

A. SYMPTOMS AND SIGNS

Most patients have been ill for days or weeks. Bleeding (usually due to thrombocytopenia) occurs in the skin and mucosal surfaces, with gingival bleeding, epistaxis, or menorrhagia. Less commonly, widespread bleeding is seen in patients with disseminated intravascular coagulation (in acute promyelocytic leukemia and monocytic leukemia). Infection is due to neutropenia, with the risk of infection rising as the neutrophil count falls below 500/μL; with neutrophil counts less than 100/μL, infection within days is the rule. The most common pathogens are gram-negative bacteria (*E coli*, klebsiella, pseudomonas) or fungi (candida, aspergillus). Common presentations include cellulitis, pneumonia, and perirectal infections; death within a few hours may occur if treatment with appropriate antibiotics is delayed.

Patients may also seek medical attention because of gum hypertrophy and bone and joint pain. The most dramatic presentation is hyperleukocytosis, in which a markedly elevated circulating blast count (usually > 200,000/μL) leads to impaired circulation, presenting as headache, confusion, and dyspnea. Such patients require emergent leukapheresis and chemotherapy.

On examination, patients appear pale and have purpura and petechiae; signs of infection may not be present. Stomatitis and gum hypertrophy may be seen in patients with monocytic leukemia, as may rectal fissures. There is variable enlargement of the liver, spleen, and lymph nodes. Bone tenderness may be present, particularly in the sternum, tibia, and femur.

B. LABORATORY FINDINGS

The hallmark of acute leukemia is the combination of pancytopenia with circulating blasts. However, blasts may be absent from the peripheral smear in as many as 10% of cases ("aleukemic leukemia").

The bone marrow is hypercellular and dominated by blasts. More than 20% blasts are required to make a diagnosis of acute leukemia.

A number of other laboratory abnormalities are noted. Hyperuricemia may be seen. If disseminated intravascular coagulation is present, the fibrinogen level will be reduced, the prothrombin time prolonged, and fibrin degradation products or fibrin D-dimers present. Patients with acute lymphoblastic leukemia (especially T cell) may have a mediastinal mass visible on chest radiograph. Meningeal leukemia will have blasts present in the spinal fluid, seen in approximately 5% of cases at diagnosis; it is more common in monocytic types of acute myelogenous leukemia.

Acute leukemia should be classified as either acute lymphoblastic or acute myelogenous leukemia. The Auer rod, an eosinophilic needle-like inclusion in the cytoplasm, is pathognomonic of acute myelogenous leukemia. To confirm the myeloid nature of the cells, histochemical stains demonstrating myeloid enzymes such as peroxidase may be useful. Monocytic lineage can be established by the finding of butyrate esterase. Acute lymphoblastic leukemia is considered when there is no morphologic or histochemical evidence of myeloid or monocytic lineage. The diagnosis is confirmed by demonstrating surface markers characteristic of primitive lymphoid cells; terminal deoxynucleotidal transferase (TdT) is present in 95% of cases of acute lymphoblastic leukemia. A variety of monoclonal antibodies have been used to define other phenotypes of acute lymphoblastic leukemia. Primitive B lymphocyte antigens include CD19 and sometimes CD10. T cell acute lymphoblastic leukemia is diagnosed by the finding of CD2, CD5, and CD7.

Acute myelogenous leukemia is usually categorized on the basis of morphology and histochemistry as follows: acute undifferentiated leukemia (M0), acute myeloblastic leukemia (M1), acute myeloblastic leukemia with differentiation (M2), acute promyelocytic leukemia (M3), acute myelomonocytic leukemia (M4), acute monoblastic leukemia (M5), erythroleukemia (M6), and megakaryoblastic leukemia (M7). The World Health Organization (WHO) has sponsored a new classification of the leukemias and other hematologic malignancies that incorporates cytogenetic, molecular, and immunophenotype information.

Acute lymphoblastic leukemia is most usefully classified by immunologic phenotype as follows: common, early B lineage, and T cell.

Cytogenetic studies are the most powerful prognostic factors in the acute leukemias. Favorable cytogenetics in acute myeloid leukemia include t(8;21), t(15;17), and inv(16)(p13;q22). These patients have a higher chance of achieving both short- and long-term disease control. Favorable cytogenetics in acute lymphoblastic leukemia are the hyperdiploid states. Unfavorable cytogenetics in AML are monosomy 5 and 7 and complex abnormalities; unfavorable cytogenetics in ALL are the Philadelphia chromosome t(9;22) and t(4;11).

Differential Diagnosis

Acute myelogenous leukemia must be distinguished from other myeloproliferative disorders, chronic myelogenous leukemia, and myelodysplastic syndromes. Acute leukemia also resembles a left-shifted bone marrow recovering from a previous toxic insult. If the question is in doubt, a bone marrow study should be repeated in several days to see if maturation has taken place. Acute lymphoblastic leukemia must be separated from other lymphoproliferative disease such as chronic lymphocytic leukemia, lymphomas, and hairy cell leukemia. It may also be confused with the atypical lymphocytosis of mononucleosis and pertussis.

Treatment

Most young patients with acute leukemia are treated with the objective of effecting a cure. The first step in treatment is to obtain complete remission, defined as normal peripheral blood with resolution of cytopenias, normal bone marrow with no excess blasts, and normal clinical status. The type of initial chemotherapy depends on the subtype of leukemia. Most patients with acute myeloid leukemia are treated with a combination of an anthracycline (daunorubicin or idarubicin) plus cytarabine. This therapy will produce complete remissions in 70–80% of patients under age 60 and in 40–60% of older patients. The treatment of patients with acute promyelocytic leukemia has been dramatically improved by the use of all-*trans*-retinoic acid. This agent is an analog of vitamin A that leads to terminal differentiation of acute promyelocytic leukemia cells through an interaction with the abnormal retinoic acid receptor created by a specific chromosomal translocation which is the hallmark of the subtype of leukemia. Patients with acute promyelocytic leukemia should be treated with anthracyclines plus all-*trans*-retinoic acid, and more than 90% will achieve complete remission. Adults with acute lymphoblastic leukemia are treated with combination chemotherapy, including daunorubicin, vincristine, prednisone, and asparaginase. This treatment produces complete remissions in 80–90% of patients.

Once a patient has entered remission, postremission therapy is given with curative intent. Options include standard chemotherapy and autologous and allogeneic transplantation. The optimal treatment strategy depends on the patient's age and clinical status and the risk factor profile of the leukemia. Acute promyelocytic leukemia is generally treated with chemotherapy plus retinoic acid, and 60–70% of patients remain in long-term remission. For average-risk patients with acute myeloid leukemia, cure rates for postremission therapy are 25–30% for chemotherapy, 50% for autologous transplantation, and 50–60% for allogeneic transplantation. Some types of acute myeloid leukemia have a more favorable prognosis, with cure rates of 40–60% with chemotherapy and

70% with autologous transplantation. Patients who do not enter remission or who have high-risk cytogenetics (such as monosomy 7) do far more poorly. Allogeneic transplantation is the treatment of choice, but cure rates are only 20%.

Once leukemia has recurred after initial chemotherapy, the prognosis is much more guarded. For patients in second remission, transplantation (autologous or allogeneic) offers a 30–50% chance of cure. For those patients with acute promyelocytic leukemia who relapse, arsenic trioxide is a novel therapy which can produce second remissions. The role of arsenic trioxide in primary treatment may hold promise.

Acute lymphoblastic leukemia is treated initially with combination chemotherapy, including daunorubicin, vincristine, prednisone, and asparaginase. Remission induction therapy for acute lymphoblastic leukemia is less myelosuppressive than treatment for acute myelogenous leukemia and does not necessarily produce marrow aplasia. After achieving complete remission, patients receive central nervous system prophylaxis so that meningeal sequestration of leukemic cells does not develop. As with acute myelogenous leukemia, patients may be treated with either chemotherapy or high-dose chemotherapy plus bone marrow transplantation. Treatment decisions are made based on patient age and risk factors of the disease. High-risk patients with adverse cytogenetics or poor responses to chemotherapy are best treated with allogeneic transplantation. Autologous transplantation is a possibility in high-risk patients who lack a suitable donor.

Prognosis

Approximately 70–80% of adults with acute myelogenous leukemia under age 60 achieve complete remission. High-dose postremission chemotherapy leads to cure in 30–40% of these patients, and high-dose cytarabine has been shown to be superior to therapy with lower doses. Allogeneic bone marrow transplantation (for younger adults with HLA-matched siblings) is curative in approximately 60% of cases. Autologous bone marrow transplantation is a promising new form of therapy that may cure 50–70% of patients in first remission; it may be superior to nonablative chemotherapy. Older adults with acute myelogenous leukemia achieve complete remission in up to 50% of instances.

Champlin RE et al: Blood stem cells compared with bone marrow as a source of hematopoietic cells for allogeneic transplantation. IBMTR Histocompatibility and Stem Cell Sources Working Committee and the European Group for Blood and Marrow Transplantation (EBMT). Blood 2000; 95:3702. [PMID: 10845900] (Treatment-related mortality rates were lower and leukemia-free survival rates were higher with blood stem cell transplants in advanced disease.)

Linker CA et al: Autologous stem cell transplantation for acute myeloid leukemia in first remission. Biol Blood Marrow Transplant 2000;6:50. [PMID: 10707999]

Ohnishi K et al: Prolongation of the QT interval and ventricular tachycardia in patients treated with arsenic trioxide for acute promyelocytic leukemia. Ann Intern Med 2000;133:881. [PMID: 1103958]

Slovak ML et al: Karyotypic analysis predicts outcome of pre-remission and post-remission therapy in adult acute myeloid leukemia. The Southwest Oncology Group/Eastern Cooperative Oncology Group study. Blood 2000;96:4075. [PMID: 11110676]

Soignet SL et al: United States multicenter study of arsenic trioxide in relapsed acute promyelocytic leukemia. J Clin Oncol 2001;19:3852. [PMID: 11559723]

CHRONIC LYMPHOCYTIC LEUKEMIA

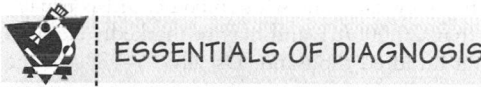

ESSENTIALS OF DIAGNOSIS

- *Most patients asymptomatic at presentation.*
- *Splenomegaly typical.*
- *Lymphocytosis > 5000/μL.*
- *Mature appearance of lymphocytes.*
- *Co-expression of CD19, CD5.*

General Considerations

Chronic lymphocytic leukemia (CLL) is a clonal malignancy of B lymphocytes. The disease is usually indolent, with slowly progressive accumulation of long-lived small lymphocytes. These cells are immunoincompetent and respond poorly to antigenic stimulation.

Chronic lymphocytic leukemia is manifested clinically by immunosuppression, bone marrow failure, and organ infiltration with lymphocytes. Immunodeficiency is also related to inadequate antibody production by the abnormal B cells. With advanced disease, chronic lymphocytic leukemia may cause damage by direct tissue infiltration.

Clinical Findings

A. SYMPTOMS AND SIGNS

Chronic lymphocytic leukemia is a disease of older patients, with 90% of cases occurring after age 50 and a median age at presentation of 65. Many patients will be incidentally discovered to have lymphocytosis. Others present with fatigue or lymphadenopathy. On examination, 80% of patients will have lymphadenopathy and half will have enlargement of the liver or spleen.

A prognostically useful staging system (Rai system) has been developed as follows: stage 0, lymphocytosis only; stage I, lymphocytosis plus lymphadenopathy; stage II, organomegaly; stage III, anemia; stage IV, thrombocytopenia.

Chronic lymphocytic leukemia usually pursues an indolent course. A variant of CLL, prolymphocytic leukemia, often pursues a more aggressive course. The morphology of the latter cases is different, characterized by larger and more immature cells. In 5–10% of cases, chronic lymphocytic leukemia may be complicated by autoimmune hemolytic anemia or autoimmune thrombocytopenia. In approximately 5% of cases, while the systemic disease remains stable, an isolated lymph node transforms into an aggressive large cell lymphoma **(Richter's syndrome).**

B. LABORATORY FINDINGS

The hallmark of chronic lymphocytic leukemia is isolated lymphocytosis. The white blood count is usually greater than 20,000/μL and may be markedly elevated to several hundred thousand. Usually 75–98% of the circulating cells are lymphocytes. Lymphocytes appear small and mature, with condensed nuclear chromatin, and are morphologically indistinguishable from normal small lymphocytes. The hematocrit and platelet count are usually normal at presentation. The bone marrow is variably infiltrated with small lymphocytes. The malignant cells weakly express surface immunoglobulin, and the monoclonal nature of the cells can be demonstrated by the finding of a single light chain type on the surface. The immunophenotype of CLL is unique in that it co-expresses the B lymphocyte lineage marker CD19 with the T lymphocyte marker CD5.

Hypogammaglobulinemia is present in half and becomes more common with advanced disease. In some, a small amount of IgM paraprotein is present in the serum. Pathologic changes in lymph nodes are the same as in diffuse small cell lymphocytic lymphoma.

Differential Diagnosis

Few syndromes can be confused with chronic lymphocytic leukemia. Viral infections producing lymphocytosis should be obvious from the presence of fever and other clinical findings; however, fever may occur in CLL from concomitant bacterial infection. Pertussis may cause a particularly high total lymphocyte count. Other lymphoproliferative diseases such as Waldenström's macroglobulinemia, hairy cell leukemia, or lymphoma in the leukemic phase are distinguished on the basis of the morphology and immunophenotype of circulating lymphocytes and bone marrow.

Treatment

Most cases of early indolent chronic lymphocytic leukemia require no specific therapy. Indications for treatment include progressive fatigue, symptomatic lymphadenopathy, or anemia or thrombocytopenia. These patients have either symptomatic and progressive stage II disease or stage III/IV disease. The best initial treatment of CLL has changed. Standard treatment had been chlorambucil, 0.6–1 mg/kg orally every 3 weeks for approximately 6 months. This treatment is convenient, well-tolerated, and usually effective and remains a reasonable first choice for older patients. Fludarabine has now replaced chlorambucil as front-line therapy. It has been shown to produce a higher response rate and responses that are more complete and long-lasting. Fludarabine requires intravenous infusion 5 days a week once a month for 4–6 months and causes immunosuppression that is often long-lasting. Combination therapy with fludarabine plus either rituximab or cyclophosphamide (or both) produces better rates of response and complete response. Whether combination therapy will improve remission duration or survival is as yet uncertain. The monoclonal antibody alemtuzumab has been approved for treatment of refractory CLL.

Associated autoimmune hemolytic anemia or immune thrombocytopenia may require treatment with prednisone or splenectomy. Fludarabine should be avoided in patients with autoimmune hemolytic anemia since it may exacerbate this condition.

Allogeneic transplantation offers potentially curative treatment for patients with CLL, but it should be used only in patients whose disease cannot be controlled by standard therapies. Nonmyeloablative allogeneic transplant has produced encouraging results and may expand the role of transplant in CLL.

Prognosis

Median survival is approximately 6 years, and 25% of patients live more than 10 years. Patients with stage 0 or stage I disease have a median survival of 10 years, and these patients may be reassured that they can live a normal life for many years. Patients with stage III or stage IV disease have a median survival of less than 2 years, and allogeneic transplant offers a possibility of improving the outcome.

Del Poeta G et al: Clinical significance of CD38 expression in chronic lymphocytic leukemia. Blood 2001;98: 2633. [PMID: 11675331]

Dighiero G et al: When and how to treat chronic lymphocytic leukemia. N Engl J Med 2000;343:1799. [PMID: 11114321]

Rai KR et al: Fludarabine compared with chlorambucil as primary therapy for chronic lymphocytic leukemia. N Engl J Med 2000;343:1750. [PMID: 11114313]

HAIRY CELL LEUKEMIA

ESSENTIALS OF DIAGNOSIS

- *Pancytopenia.*
- *Splenomegaly, often massive.*
- *Hairy cells present on blood smear and especially in bone marrow biopsy.*

General Considerations

Hairy cell leukemia, an uncommon form of leukemia, is an indolent cancer of B lymphocytes.

Clinical Findings

A. SYMPTOMS AND SIGNS

The disease characteristically presents in middle-aged men. The median age at presentation is 55 years, and there is a striking 5:1 male predominance. Most patients present with gradual onset of fatigue, others complain of symptoms related to markedly enlarged spleen, and some come to attention because of infection.

Splenomegaly is almost invariably present and may be massive. The liver is enlarged in half of cases; lymphadenopathy is uncommon.

Hairy cell leukemia is usually an indolent disorder whose course is dominated by pancytopenia and recurrent infections, including mycobacterial infections.

B. LABORATORY FINDINGS

The hallmark of hairy cell leukemia is pancytopenia. Anemia is nearly universal, and 75% have thrombocytopenia and neutropenia. Nearly all patients have striking monocytopenia, which is encountered in almost no other condition. The "hairy cells" are usually present in small numbers on the peripheral blood smear and have a characteristic appearance with numerous cytoplasmic projections. The bone marrow is usually inaspirable (dry tap), and the diagnosis is made by characteristic morphology on bone marrow biopsy. The hairy cells have a characteristic histochemical staining pattern, with tartrate-resistant acid phosphatase (TRAP). On immunophenotyping, the cells co-express the antigens CD11c and CD22. Pathologic examination of the spleen shows marked infiltration of the red pulp with hairy cells. This is in contrast to the usual predilection of lymphomas to involve the white pulp of the spleen.

Differential Diagnosis

Hairy cell leukemia should be distinguished from other lymphoproliferative diseases such as Waldenström's macroglobulinemia and non-Hodgkin's lymphomas. It also may be confused with other causes of pancytopenia, including hypersplenism due to any cause and paroxysmal nocturnal hemoglobinuria.

Treatment

The treatment of choice is cladribine (2-chlorodeoxyadenosine; CdA), 0.14 mg/kg daily for 7 days. This is a relatively nontoxic drug that produces benefit in 95% of cases and complete remission in more than 80%. Responses are long-lasting, with few patients relapsing in the first few years. Treatment with pentostatin produces similar results, but that drug is more cumbersome to administer.

Course & Prognosis

The development of new therapies has changed the prognosis of this disease. Formerly, median survival was 6 years, and only one-third of patients survived longer than 10 years. It now appears that most patients with hairy cell leukemia will live longer than 10 years. With current trends in treatment, the prognosis appears open-ended at this time.

Flinn IW et al: Long-term follow-up for remission duration, mortality, and second malignancies in hairy cell leukemia patients treated with pentostatin. Blood 2000;96:2981. [PMID: 11049974]

Kreitman RJ et al: Efficacy of the anti-CD22 recombinant immunotoxin BL22 in chemotherapy-resistant hairy-cell leukemia. N Engl J Med 2001;345:241. [PMID: 11474661] (This agent induced complete remission in a small number of patients with resistant hairy cell leukemia.)

■ LYMPHOMAS

NON-HODGKIN'S LYMPHOMAS

The non-Hodgkin's lymphomas are a heterogeneous group of cancers of lymphocytes. The disorders vary in clinical presentation and course from indolent to rapidly progressive.

Molecular biology has provided clues to the pathogenesis of these disorders. The best-studied example is Burkitt's lymphoma, in which a characteristic cytogenetic abnormality of translocation between the long arms of chromosomes 8 and 14 has been identified. The proto-oncogene c-myc is translocated from its normal position on chromosome 8 to the heavy chain locus on chromosome 14. Cells committed to B cell differentiation are likely to have enhanced expression of this heavy chain locus, and it is likely that overexpression of c-myc (in its new anomalous position) is related to malignant transformation. In the follicular lymphomas, translocations of a possible oncogene bcl-2 from chromosome 8 to the heavy chain locus on chromosome 14 causes over-expression of bcl-2, which appears to protect the lymphoma cell against apoptosis, the normal pathway to cell death.

Classification of the lymphomas is a controversial area still undergoing evolution. The most recent grouping (see Table 13–16) separates diseases based on both clinical and pathologic features.

Clinical Findings

A. SYMPTOMS AND SIGNS

Patients with indolent lymphomas usually present with painless lymphadenopathy, which may be isolated or widespread. Involved lymph nodes may be present in the retroperitoneum, mesentery, and pelvis. The indolent lymphomas are often disseminated at

Table 13–16. REAL/WHO proposed classification of non-Hodgkin's lymphoma.

B cell lymphomas
    Precursor B cell lymphoblastic lymphoma
    Small lymphocytic lymphoma/chronic lymphocytic
       leukemia
    Marginal zone lymphomas
       Nodal marginal zone lymphoma
       Extranodal MALT
       Splenic
    Hairy cell leukemia
    Follicular lymphoma
    Mantle cell lymphoma
    Diffuse large B cell lymphoma
    Burkitt's lymphoma
T cell lymphomas
    Anaplastic large cell lymphoma
    Peripheral T cell lymphoma
    Mycosis fungoides

the time of diagnosis, and bone marrow involvement is frequent. Patients with intermediate and high-grade lymphomas also have constitutional symptoms such as fever, drenching night sweats, or weight loss.

On examination, lymphadenopathy may be isolated, or extranodal sites of disease (skin, gastrointestinal tract) may be found. Patients with Burkitt's lymphoma are noted to have abdominal pain or abdominal fullness because of the predilection of the disease for the abdomen.

Once a pathologic diagnosis is established, the patient is staged. Chest x-ray and CT scan of the abdomen and pelvis, bone marrow biopsy, and—in selected cases with high-risk morphology—a lumbar puncture are performed.

B. LABORATORY FINDINGS

The peripheral blood is usually normal, but a number of lymphomas may present in a leukemic phase.

Bone marrow involvement is manifested as paratrabecular lymphoid aggregates. In some high-grade lymphomas, the meninges are involved and malignant cells are found with cerebrospinal fluid cytology. The chest radiograph may show a mediastinal mass in lymphoblastic lymphoma. The serum LDH has been shown to be a useful prognostic marker and is now incorporated in risk stratification of treatment.

The diagnosis of lymphoma is made by tissue biopsy. Needle aspiration may yield suspicious results, but a lymph node biopsy (or biopsy of involved extranodal tissue) is required for diagnosis and staging.

Treatment

The treatment of indolent lymphoma depends on the stage of disease and the clinical status of the patient. A small number of patients have limited disease with only one abnormal lymph node and are treated with localized irradiation. Most patients with indolent lym-

phoma have disseminated disease at the time of diagnosis. If the disease is not bulky and the patient not symptomatic, no initial therapy may be required. Some patients will have spontaneous remissions and may defer treatment for 1–3 years. In the past, standard chemotherapy for patients requiring treatment has been alkylators such as chlorambucil, 0.6–1 mg/kg every 3 weeks, or combination therapy with cyclophosphamide, vincristine, and prednisone (CVP). However, fludarabine may produce equivalent results. A monoclonal antibody (rituximab) directed against the B cell surface antigen CD20 is effective as salvage therapy for relapsed low-grade B cell lymphomas and may improve outcomes when added to initial chemotherapy. Radioimmunoconjugates which fuse anti-B cell antibodies with radiation may produce improved results with modest increases in toxicity compared with antibody alone, and one such agent (yttrium-90 ibritumomab) is in use. The preferred approach is as yet not established. Some patients with clinically aggressive low-grade lymphomas may be appropriate candidates for allogeneic transplantation. As in other hematologic malignancies, the use of less toxic nonmyeloablative regimens for allogeneic transplant may expand the role of transplant in this disease. The role of autologous transplantation remains uncertain, but some patients with recurrent disease appear to have prolonged remissions.

Patients with intermediate-grade lymphomas such as diffuse large cell lymphoma are treated with curative intent. Those with localized disease receive short-course chemotherapy (such as three courses of cyclophosphamide, doxorubicin [hydroxydaunomycin; Adriamycin], vincristine [Oncovin], and prednisone [CHOP]) plus localized radiation. Most patients who have more advanced disease are treated with six to eight cycles of chemotherapy such as CHOP. Older patients with diffuse large cell lymphomas may benefit from the addition of rituximab to CHOP. Individuals with high-risk lymphoma are best treated with autologous stem cell transplantation early in the course. Patients with intermediate-grade lymphoma who relapse after initial chemotherapy may still be cured by autologous stem cell transplantation if their disease remains responsive to chemotherapy.

Persons with special forms of lymphoma require individualized therapy. Burkitt's lymphoma is treated with intensive regimens specifically tailored for this histologic type. Those with lymphoblastic lymphoma receive regimens similar to those used for T cell acute lymphoblastic leukemia. Mantle cell lymphoma is not effectively treated with standard chemotherapy regimens. The role of high-dose therapy with allogeneic or autologous transplantation is under study.

Prognosis

The median survival of patients with indolent lymphomas is 6–8 years. These diseases ultimately become refractory to chemotherapy. This often occurs at the time of histologic progression of the disease to a more aggressive form of lymphoma.

The International Prognostic Index is now widely used to categorize patients with intermediate grade lymphoma into risk groups. Factors that confer adverse prognosis are age over 60 years, elevated serum LDH, stage III or stage IV disease, and poor performance status. Patients with no risk factors or one risk factor have high complete response rates (80%) to standard chemotherapy, and most responses (80%) are durable. Patients with two risk factors have a 70% complete response rate, 70% being long-lasting. Patients with higher-risk disease have lower response rates and poor survival with standard regimens, and alternative treatments are needed. Early treatment with high-dose therapy and autologous stem cell transplantation improves the outcome.

For patients who relapse after initial chemotherapy, the prognosis depends on whether the lymphoma is still partially sensitive to chemotherapy. If it is, autologous transplantation offers a 50% chance of long-term salvage.

The treatment of older patients with lymphoma has been difficult because of poorer tolerance of aggressive chemotherapy. The use of myeloid growth factors and prophylactic antibiotics to reduce neutropenic complications may improve outcomes.

Armitage JO: New approach to classifying non-Hodgkin's lymphomas: clinical features of the major histologic subtypes. J Clin Oncol 1998;16:2780. [PMID: 9704731]

Khouri IF et al: Nonablative allogeneic hematopoietic transplantation as adoptive immunotherapy for indolent lymphoma: low incidence of toxicity, acute graft-versus-host disease, and treatment-related mortality. Blood 2001;98:3595. [PMID: 11739162]

Kouroukis CT et al: Chemotherapy for older patients with newly diagnosed advanced-stage, aggressive-histology non-Hodgkin lymphoma: a systematic review. Ann Intern Med 2002;136: 144. [PMID: 11790067]

McCune SL et al: Monoclonal antibody therapy in the treatment of non-Hodgkin lymphoma. JAMA 2001;286:1149. [PMID: 11559240]

HODGKIN'S DISEASE

ESSENTIALS OF DIAGNOSIS

- *Painless lymphadenopathy.*
- *Constitutional symptoms may or may not be present.*
- *Pathologic diagnosis by lymph node biopsy.*

General Considerations

Hodgkin's disease is a group of cancers characterized by Reed-Sternberg cells in an appropriate reactive cellular background. The nature of the malignant cell is a subject of controversy.

Clinical Findings

There is a bimodal age distribution, with one peak in the 20s and a second over age 50. Most patients present because of a painless mass, commonly in the neck. Others may seek medical attention because of constitutional symptoms such as fever, weight loss, or drenching night sweats, or because of generalized pruritus. An unusual symptom of Hodgkin's disease is pain in an involved lymph node following alcohol ingestion.

An important feature of Hodgkin's disease is its tendency to arise within single lymph node areas and spread in an orderly fashion to contiguous areas of lymph nodes. Only late in the course of the disease will vascular invasion lead to widespread hematogenous dissemination.

Hodgkin's disease is divided into several subtypes: lymphocyte predominance, nodular sclerosis, mixed cellularity, and lymphocyte depletion. Hodgkin's disease should be distinguished pathologically from other malignant lymphomas and may occasionally be confused with reactive lymph nodes seen in infectious mononucleosis, cat-scratch disease, or drug reactions (eg, phenytoin).

Patients undergo a staging evaluation to determine the extent of disease. The staging nomenclature (Ann Arbor) is as follows: stage I, one lymph node region involved; stage II, involvement of two lymph node areas on one side of the diaphragm; stage III, lymph node regions involved on both sides of the diaphragm; stage IV, disseminated disease with bone marrow or liver involvement. In addition, patients are designated stage A if they lack constitutional symptoms and stage B if 10% weight loss over 6 months, fever, or night sweats are present. If symptoms indicate careful evaluation for higher numerical stage, clinical stage IB (for example) is highly likely to emerge as stage II or stage IIIB.

Treatment

The treatment of Hodgkin's disease has evolved, with radiation therapy used as initial treatment only for patients with low-risk stage IA and IIA disease. Staging is usually clinical, and laparotomy is no longer routinely performed. The addition of limited chemotherapy for some patients treated with radiation appears promising.

Most patients with Hodgkin's disease (including all with stage IIIB and IV disease) are best treated with combination chemotherapy using doxorubicin (Adriamycin), bleomycin, vincristine, and dacarbazine (ABVD). New shorter and more intensive regimens have produced promising results and may supplant ABVD in the treatment of advanced disease.

Prognosis

All patients with both localized and disseminated disease should be treated with curative intent. The prognosis of patients with stage IA or IIA disease treated by radiotherapy is excellent, with 10-year survival rates in excess of 80%. Patients with disseminated disease (IIIB, IV) have 5-year survival rates of 50–60%. Poorer results are seen in patients who are older, those who have bulky disease, and those with lymphocyte depletion or mixed cellularity on histologic examination. Others whose disease recurs after initial radiotherapy treatment may still be curable with chemotherapy. The treatment of choice for patients who relapse after initial chemotherapy is high-dose chemotherapy with autologous stem cell transplantation. This offers a 35–50% chance of cure when disease is still chemotherapy-sensitive.

Aisenberg AC: Problems in Hodgkin's disease management. Blood 1999;93:761. [PMID: 9920825]

Josting A et al: Prognostic factors and treatment outcome in primary progressive Hodgkin lymphoma: a report from the German Hodgkin Lymphoma Study Group. Blood 2000;96:1280. [PMID: 10942369]

Moskowitz CH et al: A 2-step comprehensive high-dose chemoradiotherapy second line program for relapsed and refractory Hodgkin disease: analysis by intent to treat and development of a prognostic model. Blood 2001;97:616. [PMID: 11157476]

MULTIPLE MYELOMA

ESSENTIALS OF DIAGNOSIS

- Bone pain, often in the lower back.
- Monoclonal paraprotein by serum and urine protein electrophoresis or immunoelectrophoresis.
- Replacement of bone marrow by malignant plasma cells.

General Considerations

Multiple myeloma is a malignancy of plasma cells characterized by replacement of the bone marrow, bone destruction, and paraprotein formation. There is evidence that a new herpesvirus may be implicated in pathogenesis. Myeloma causes clinical symptoms and signs through a variety of mechanisms.

Replacement of the bone marrow (and perhaps humoral suppression of myelopoiesis) leads initially to anemia and later to general bone marrow failure. Malignant plasma cells can form tumors (plasmacytomas) that may cause spinal cord compression. Bone involvement causes bone pain, osteoporosis, lytic lesions, pathologic fractures, and hypercalcemia. The pathogenesis of osteoclast activation in myeloma appears to involve osteoprotegerin ligand, and the decoy receptor osteoprotegerin may be able to interfere with this pathway.

The paraproteins secreted by the malignant plasma cells may cause problems in their own right. Very high paraprotein levels (either IgG or IgA) may cause hyperviscosity, though this is more often caused by IgM in Waldenström's macroglobulinemia. The light chain component of the immunoglobulin often leads to renal failure (often aggravated by hypercalcemia). Light chain components may be deposited in tissues as amyloid, worsening renal failure with albuminuria and causing a vast array of systemic symptoms.

Myeloma patients are prone to recurrent infections for a number of reasons, including neutropenia and the immunosuppressive effects of chemotherapy. More often, there is a failure of antibody production in response to antigen challenge, and myeloma patients are especially prone to infections with encapsulated organisms such as *Streptococcus pneumoniae* and *Haemophilus influenzae*.

Clinical Findings

A. SYMPTOMS AND SIGNS

Myeloma is a disease of older adults (median age at presentation, 65 years). The most common presenting complaints are those related to anemia, bone pain, and infection. Bone pain is most common in the back or ribs or may present as a pathologic fracture, especially of the femoral neck. Patients may also come to medical attention because of renal failure; spinal cord compression, or the hyperviscosity syndrome (mucosal bleeding, vertigo, nausea, visual disturbances, alterations in mental status). Equally as often, patients are diagnosed because of laboratory findings of hypercalcemia, proteinuria, elevated sedimentation rate, or abnormalities on serum protein electrophoresis obtained for symptoms or in routine screening studies. A few patients come to medical attention because of amyloidosis.

Examination may reveal pallor, bone tenderness, and soft tissue masses. Patients may have neurologic signs related to neuropathy and spinal cord compression. Patients with amyloidosis may have an enlarged tongue, neuropathy, congestive heart failure, or hepatomegaly. Splenomegaly is absent unless amyloidosis is present. Fever occurs only with infection.

B. LABORATORY FINDINGS

Anemia is nearly universal. Red blood cell morphology is normal, but rouleau formation is common and may be marked. The neutrophil and platelet counts are usually normal at presentation. Only rarely will plasma cells be visible on peripheral smear (plasma cell leukemia).

The hallmark of myeloma is the finding of a paraprotein on serum protein electrophoresis (SPEP). The majority of patients will have a monoclonal spike visible in the beta or gamma globulin region. Immunoelectrophoresis (IEP) will reveal this to be a monoclonal protein. Approximately 15% of patients will have no demonstrable paraprotein in the serum. In these, IEP of the urine will reveal either complete immunoglobulin or light chains. Overall, approximately 60% of myeloma patients will have an IgG paraprotein, 25% an IgA, and 15% light chains only. In sporadic cases, no paraprotein is present ("nonsecretory myeloma"); these patients have particularly aggressive disease.

The bone marrow will be infiltrated by variable numbers of plasma cells ranging from 5% to 100%. Occasionally the plasma cells will appear normal but more commonly are not. Many benign processes can result in highly atypical plasma cells; the most useful feature is the appearance of sheets of these cells. Bone radiographs are important in establishing the diagnosis of myeloma. Lytic lesions are most commonly seen in the axial skeleton: skull, spine, proximal long bones, and ribs. At other times, only generalized osteoporosis is seen. The radionuclide bone scan is not useful in detecting bone lesions in myeloma, as there is usually no osteoblastic component.

The level of β_2-microglobulin has strong prognostic significance in myeloma, with levels > 3 mg/L associated with poor survival. Bone marrow cytogenetic characteristics have greater prognostic significance, with deletions of chromosome 13q associated with a dismal outcome. Other laboratory features include hypercalcemia, renal failure, and an elevated erythrocyte sedimentation rate; alkaline phosphatase is not elevated despite extensive bony involvement. Some patients have proximal renal tubular acidosis, with phosphaturia, glycosuria, uricosuria, and aminoaciduria. The urinalysis may reveal proteinuria, but the dipstick test (which detects primarily albumin) is unreliable for light chains. Often there is a narrow anion gap when the paraprotein is cationic (70% of cases).

Differential Diagnosis

When a patient is discovered to have a monoclonal paraprotein, the distinction between myeloma and monoclonal gammopathy of unknown significance (MGUS) must be made. MGUS is present in 1% of all adults and 3% of adults over age 70. Thus, if one considers all patients with paraproteins, MGUS is far more common than myeloma. Most commonly, patients with MGUS will have a monoclonal IgG spike less than 2.5 g/dL, and the height of the spike remains stable. In approximately 25% of cases, MGUS progresses to overt malignant disease, but this may take many years.

Myeloma is distinguished from MGUS by findings of replacement of the bone marrow, bone destruction, and progression. Although the height of the paraprotein spike should not be used by itself to distinguish benign from malignant disease, nearly all patients with IgG spikes greater than 3.5 g/dL prove to have myeloma; an IgA spike of > 2 g/dL is similarly suggestive. If there is doubt about whether paraproteinemia is benign or malignant, the patient should be observed without therapy, since there is no advantage to early treatment of asymptomatic multiple myeloma.

Myeloma must be distinguished from reactive polyclonal hypergammaglobulinemia. Myeloma may also be similar to other malignant lymphoproliferative diseases such as Waldenström's macroglobulinemia, lymphomas, and primary amyloidosis (with which it is commonly associated).

Treatment

Patients with minimal disease or in whom the diagnosis of malignancy is in doubt should be observed without treatment. Most commonly, patients require treatment at diagnosis because of bone pain or other symptoms related to the disease. The best chemotherapy regimen has not been determined. The combination of vincristine, doxorubicin (Adriamycin), and dexamethasone (VAD) has replaced oral melphalan as primary treatment in younger patients because of the lack of bone marrow and stem cell damage.

The optimal initial therapy for patients under age 70 with myeloma is autologous stem cell transplantation. Early aggressive treatment prolongs both remission duration and overall survival. Autologous transplantation is also useful in management of patients with relapsed disease if the disease is still chemotherapy-sensitive. The height of the paraprotein spike on SPEP is a useful marker for monitoring response to therapy. Thalidomide has emerged in the treatment of myeloma, and responses have been seen even in patients whose disease no longer responds to chemotherapy. Derivatives of thalidomide with improved in vitro potency may prove to be effective, and the experimental agents CC-5013 and PS-341, the latter a protease inhibitor, have also produced promising results in patients with refractory disease.

Allogeneic transplantation is potentially curative in myeloma, but its role has been limited because of the unusually high mortality rate (40–50%) in myeloma patients. Newer and less toxic forms of allogeneic transplantation using nonmyeloablative regimens have produced encouraging results and may broaden the applications of the allogeneic approach.

A number of other ancillary measures are important in the treatment of myeloma. Localized radiotherapy may be useful for palliation of bone pain or for eradicating tumor at the site of pathologic fracture. Hypercalcemia should be treated aggressively and immobilization and dehydration avoided. The bisphosphonates (pamidronate 90 mg or zolidronate 4 mg intravenously monthly) reduce pathologic fractures in patients with significant bony disease and are an important adjunct in this subset of patients.

Prognosis

The median survival of patients with myeloma is 3 years. The prognosis is markedly affected by a number of prognostic features, with shorter survivals in those with high paraprotein spikes, renal failure, hypercalcemia, or extensive bony disease. Patients are said to have a low tumor burden if the IgG spike is less than 5 g/dL, there is no more than one lytic bone lesion, and no evidence of hypercalcemia or renal failure. Such patients have a median survival of 5–6 years. Conversely, patients with a high tumor burden have an IgG spike greater than 7 g/dL, hematocrit less than 25%, calcium greater than 12 mg/dL, or more than three lytic bone lesions. Median survival for this group was formerly 1 year, but early intervention with autologous stem cell transplantation prolongs median survival to 3 years in this group. Broader use of immunotherapy with allogeneic transplantation may improve the outlook further, as may new agents under investigation.

Badros A et al: High response rate in refractory and poor-risk multiple myeloma after allotransplantation using a nonmyeloablative conditioning regimen and donor lymphocyte infusions. Blood 2001;97:2574. [PMID: 11313244]

Croucher PI et al: Osteoprotegerin inhibits the development of osteolytic bone disease in multiple myeloma. Blood 2001;98:3534. [PMID: 11739154]

Desikan R et al: Results of high-dose therapy for 1000 patients with multiple myeloma, durable complete remissions and superior survival in the absence of chromosome 13 abnormalities. Blood 2000;95:4008. [PMID: 10845942]

Kanis JA et al: Bisphosphonates in multiple myeloma. Cancer 2000;88:3022. [PMID: 10898347]

Kyle RA et al: A long-term study of prognosis in monoclonal gammopathy of undetermined significance. N Engl J Med 2002;346:564. [PMID: 11856795]

WALDENSTRÖM'S MACROGLOBULINEMIA

ESSENTIALS OF DIAGNOSIS

- *Symptoms nonspecific: splenomegaly common on examination.*
- *Monoclonal IgM paraprotein.*
- *Infiltration of bone marrow by plasmacytic lymphocytes.*
- *Absence of lytic bone disease.*

General Considerations

Waldenström's macroglobulinemia is a malignant disease of B cells that appear to be a hybrid of lymphocytes and plasma cells. These cells characteristically secrete an IgM paraprotein, and many clinical manifestations of the disease are related to this macroglobulin.

Clinical Findings

A. SYMPTOMS AND SIGNS

This disease characteristically develops insidiously in patients in their 60s or 70s. Patients usually present with fatigue related to anemia. Hyperviscosity of serum may be manifested in a number of ways. Mucosal and gastrointestinal bleeding is related to engorged blood vessels and platelet dysfunction. Other complaints include nausea, vertigo, and visual disturbances. Alterations in consciousness vary from mild lethargy to stupor and coma. The IgM paraprotein may also cause symptoms of cold agglutinin disease or peripheral neuropathy.

On examination, there may be hepatosplenomegaly or lymphadenopathy. The retinal veins are engorged. Purpura may be present. There should be no bone tenderness.

B. LABORATORY FINDINGS

Anemia is nearly universal, and rouleau formation is common. The anemia is related in part to expansion of the plasma volume by 50–100% due to the presence of the paraprotein. Other blood counts are usually normal. The abnormal plasmacytic lymphocytes usually appear in small numbers on the peripheral blood smear. The bone marrow is characteristically infiltrated by the plasmacytic lymphocytes.

The hallmark of macroglobulinemia is the presence of a monoclonal IgM spike seen on serum protein electrophoresis (SPEP) in the beta or gamma globulin region. The serum viscosity is usually increased above the normal of 1.4–1.8 times that of water. Symptoms of hyperviscosity usually develop when the serum viscosity is over four times that of water, and marked symptoms usually arise when the viscosity is over six times that of water. Because paraproteins vary in their physicochemical properties, there is no strict correlation between the concentration of paraprotein and serum viscosity.

The IgM paraprotein may cause a positive Coombs test or have cold agglutinin or cryoglobulin properties. If one suspects macroglobulinemia but the SPEP shows only hypogammaglobulinemia, one should repeat the test while taking special measures to maintain the blood at 37 °C, since the paraprotein may precipitate out at room temperature if it is cryoprecipitatable.

Bone radiographs are normal, and there is no evidence of renal failure.

Differential Diagnosis

Waldenström's macroglobulinemia is differentiated from monoclonal gammopathy of unknown significance by the finding of bone marrow infiltration. It is distinguished from chronic lymphocytic leukemia and multiple myeloma by bone marrow morphology and the finding of the characteristic IgM spike, and also on clinical grounds.

Treatment

Patients who present with marked hyperviscosity syndrome (stupor or coma) should be treated on an emergency basis with plasmapheresis. On a chronic basis, some patients can be managed with periodic plasmapheresis alone. Others are treated with intermittent chemotherapy with chlorambucil or cyclophosphamide. New agents such as cladribine and rituximab have produced encouraging results.

As with multiple myeloma, autologous stem cell transplantation is playing a more important role in management and is considered in younger patients with more aggressive disease.

Prognosis

Waldenström's macroglobulinemia is an indolent disease with a median survival rate of 3–5 years. However, patients may survive 10 years or longer.

Dhodapkar MV et al: Prognostic factors and response to fludarabine therapy in patients with Waldenström macroglobulinemia: results of United States intergroup trial (Southwest Oncology Group S9003). Blood 2001;98:41. [PMID: 11418461] (Serum β_2-microglobulin the best predictor of survival and need for therapy.)

Dimopoulos MA et al: Waldenström's macroglobulinemia: clinical features, complications, and management. J Clin Oncol 2000;18:214. [PMID: 10623712]

Morel P et al: Prognostic factors in Waldenstrom's macroglobulinemia. A report on 232 patients with the description of a new scoring system and its validation on 253 other patients. Blood 2000;96:852. [PMID: 10910896]

■ DISORDERS OF HEMOSTASIS

Disorders of hemostasis may be due to defects in either platelet number or function or to problems in formation of a fibrin clot (coagulation). Bleeding due to platelet disorders is typically mucosal or dermatologic. Common problems include epistaxis, gum bleeding, menorrhagia, gastrointestinal bleeding, purpura, and petechiae. Petechiae are seen almost exclusively in conditions of thrombocytopenia and not platelet dysfunction. Bleeding due to coagulopathy may occur as deep muscle hematomas as well as skin bleeding. Spontaneous hemarthroses are seen only in severe hemophilia.

IDIOPATHIC (AUTOIMMUNE) THROMBOCYTOPENIC PURPURA

ESSENTIALS OF DIAGNOSIS

- *Isolated thrombocytopenia.*
- *Other hematopoietic cell lines normal.*
- *No systemic illness.*
- *Spleen not palpable.*
- *Normal bone marrow with normal or increased megakaryocytes.*

General Considerations

Idiopathic thrombocytopenic purpura is an autoimmune disorder in which an IgG autoantibody is formed that binds to platelets. It is not clear which antigen on the platelet surface is involved. Although the antiplatelet antibody may bind complement, platelets are not destroyed by direct lysis. Rather, destruction takes place in the spleen, where splenic macrophages with Fc receptors bind to antibody-coated platelets. Since the spleen is the major site both of antibody production and platelet sequestration, splenectomy is highly effective therapy.

Clinical Findings

A. SYMPTOMS AND SIGNS

Idiopathic thrombocytopenic purpura occurs commonly in childhood, frequently precipitated by viral infection and usually self-limited. In contrast, the adult form is usually a chronic disease and only infrequently follows a viral infection. It is a disease of young persons, with peak incidence between ages 20 and 50, and there is a 2:1 female predominance.

Patients are systemically well and usually not febrile. The presenting complaint is mucosal or skin bleeding. Common types of bleeding are epistaxis, oral bleeding, menorrhagia, purpura, and petechiae. On examination, the patient appears well, and there are no abnormal findings other than those related to bleeding. An enlarged spleen should lead one to doubt the diagnosis. Common signs of bleeding are purpura, petechiae, and hemorrhagic bullae in the mouth.

B. LABORATORY FINDINGS

The hallmark of the disease is thrombocytopenia, which may be less than 10,000/μL. Other counts are usually normal except for occasional mild anemia, which can be explained by bleeding or associated hemolysis. Peripheral blood cell morphology is normal except that platelets are slightly enlarged (megathrombocytes). These larger platelets are young platelets produced in response to enhanced platelet destruction. Approximately 10% of patients will have coexistent autoimmune hemolytic anemia **(Evans's syndrome),** and in these cases one will see anemia, reticulocytosis, and spherocytes on peripheral smear. Red blood cell fragmentation should not be seen.

The bone marrow will appear normal, with a normal or increased number of megakaryocytes. Coagulation studies will be entirely normal.

Differential Diagnosis

Thrombocytopenia may be produced either by abnormal bone marrow function or by peripheral destruction (Table 13–17). Although most bone marrow disorders produce abnormalities in addition to isolated thrombocytopenia, diagnoses such as myelodysplasia can only be excluded by examining the bone marrow. Most causes of thrombocytopenia resulting from peripheral destruction can be ruled out by initial evaluation. Disorders such as disseminated intravascular coagulation, thrombotic thrombocytopenic purpura, hemolytic-uremic syndrome, hypersplenism, and sepsis are easily excluded by the absence of systemic illness. Thus, patients with isolated thrombocytopenia with no other abnormal findings almost certainly have immune thrombocytopenia. Patients should be questioned regarding drug use, especially sulfonamides, quinine, thiazides, cimetidine, gold, and heparin. Heparin is now the most common cause of drug-induced thrombocytopenia in hospitalized patients. Systemic lupus erythematosus and chronic lymphocytic leukemia are common causes of secondary thrombocytopenic purpura, hematologically identical to idiopathic thrombocytopenic purpura.

Treatment

Few adults with idiopathic thrombocytopenic purpura will have spontaneous remissions, and most will require treatment. Initial treatment is with prednisone, 1–2 mg/kg/d. Prednisone works primarily by decreasing the affinity of splenic macrophages for antibody-coated platelets. High-dose prednisone therapy also reduces the binding of antibody to the platelet surface, and long-term therapy may decrease antibody production. Bleeding will often diminish within 1 day after beginning prednisone—even before the platelet count begins to rise. This effect has been attributed to enhanced vascular stability. The platelet count will usually begin to rise within a week, and responses are almost always seen within 3 weeks. About 80% of patients will respond, and the platelet count will usually return to normal. High-dose therapy should be continued until the platelet count is normal, and the dose should then be gradually tapered. In most, thrombocytopenia will recur if prednisone is completely withdrawn, and one aims to find a dose that will maintain an adequate platelet count. It is not necessary for the platelet count to be entirely normal; the risk of bleeding is small with platelet counts above 50,000/μL.

Splenectomy is the most definitive treatment for idiopathic thrombocytopenic purpura, and most adult patients will ultimately undergo splenectomy. High-dose prednisone therapy should not be continued indefinitely in an attempt to avoid surgery. Splenectomy is indicated if patients do not respond to prednisone initially or require unacceptably high doses to maintain an adequate platelet count. Other patients may be intolerant of prednisone or may simply prefer the surgical alternative. Splenectomy can be performed safely even with platelet counts less than 10,000/μL. Eighty percent of patients benefit from splenectomy with either complete or partial remission.

High-dose intravenous immunoglobulin, 1 g/kg for 1 or 2 days, is highly effective in rapidly raising the platelet count. The response rate is 90%, and the platelet count rises within 1–5 days. However, this treatment is expensive, and the beneficial effect lasts only 1–2 weeks. Immunoglobulin treatment should be reserved for bleeding emergencies or situations such as preparing a severely thrombocytopenic patient for surgery.

For patients who fail to respond to prednisone and splenectomy, danazol, 600 mg/d, has been used, with responses obtained in about half of cases. Immunosuppressive agents employed in refractory cases include vincristine, azathioprine, cyclosporine, and cyclophosphamide. Rituximab has been reported to produce good responses in some patients with refractory disease. Rare patients with severe and refractory disease are now being treated with high-dose immunosuppression and autologous stem cell transplantation.

Table 13–17. Causes of thrombocytopenia.

Bone marrow disorders
Aplastic anemia
Hematologic malignancies
Myelodysplasia
Megaloblastic anemia
Chronic alcoholism
Nonmarrow disorders
Immune disorders
Idiopathic thrombocytopenic purpura
Drug-induced
Secondary (CLL, SLE)
Posttransfusion purpura
Hypersplenism
Disseminated intravascular coagulation
Thrombotic thrombocytopenic purpura
Hemolytic-uremic syndrome
Sepsis
Hemangiomas
Viral infections, AIDS
Liver failure

Platelet transfusions are rarely used in the treatment of idiopathic thrombocytopenic purpura, since exogenous platelets will survive no better than the patient's own and will survive less than a few hours. Platelet transfusion should be reserved for cases of life-threatening bleeding in which even fleeting hemostasis may be of benefit.

Prognosis

The prognosis for remission is good. In most cases, the disease is initially controlled with prednisone, and splenectomy offers definitive therapy. The major concern during the initial phases is cerebral hemorrhage, which becomes a risk when the platelet count is less than 5000/μL. These patients usually exhibit warning signs of mucosal bleeding. However, even at these very low platelet counts, fatal bleeding is rare.

Portielje JE et al: Morbidity and mortality in adults with idiopathic thrombocytopenic purpura. Blood 2001;97:2549. [PMID: 11313240] (Most adults with ITP have a good outcome with infrequent hospitalization and no excess mortality compared with the general population.)

Warkentin TE et al: Temporal aspects of heparin-induced thrombocytopenia. N Engl J Med 2001;344:1286. [PMID: 11320387]

THROMBOTIC THROMBOCYTOPENIC PURPURA

 ESSENTIALS OF DIAGNOSIS

- *Thrombocytopenia*
- *Microangiopathic hemolytic anemia.*
- *Neurologic and renal abnormalities, fever.*
- *Normal coagulation tests.*
- *Elevated serum LDH.*

General Considerations

Thrombotic thrombocytopenic purpura (TTP) is an uncommon syndrome with microangiopathic hemolytic anemia, thrombocytopenia, and a markedly elevated serum LDH. Noninfectious fever, neurologic disorders, and renal abnormalities are less commonly seen. The pathogenesis of TTP appears to be a deficiency of a von Willebrand factor-cleaving protease, in some cases due to an antibody directed against the protease.

Thrombotic thrombocytopenic purpura is seen primarily in young adults between ages 20 and 50, and there is a slight female predominance. The syndrome is occasionally precipitated by estrogen use, pregnancy, drugs, or infections and may occur in association with HIV disease.

Clinical Findings

A. SYMPTOMS AND SIGNS

Patients come to medical attention because of anemia, bleeding, or neurologic abnormalities. The neurologic symptoms and signs are unusual in that they may wax and wane over minutes. Neurologic symptoms include headache, confusion, aphasia, and alterations in consciousness from lethargy to coma. With more advanced disease, one may see hemiparesis and seizures.

On examination, the patient appears acutely ill and is usually febrile. One may detect pallor, purpura, petechiae, and signs of neurologic dysfunction. Patients may have abdominal pain and tenderness due to pancreatitis.

B. LABORATORY FINDINGS

Anemia is universal and may be marked. There is usually marked reticulocytosis and occasional circulating nucleated red blood cells. The hallmark is a microangiopathic blood picture with fragmented red blood cells (schistocytes, helmet cells, triangle forms) on the smear. One cannot make the diagnosis without significant red blood cell fragmentation. Thrombocytopenia is invariably present and may be severe.

Hemolysis may be manifested by increasing indirect bilirubin and occasionally hemoglobinemia and hemoglobinuria; methemalbuminemia may impart a brown color to the plasma. The LDH is markedly elevated in proportion to the severity of hemolysis; the Coombs test is negative.

Coagulation tests (prothrombin time, partial thromboplastin time, fibrinogen) are normal unless ischemic tissue damage causes secondary DIC. Elevated fibrin degradation products may be seen, as in other acutely ill patients. Renal insufficiency may be present, with an abnormal urinalysis.

Pathologically, one may see thrombi in capillaries and small arteries, with no evidence of inflammation.

Differential Diagnosis

The normal values of coagulation tests differentiate thrombotic thrombocytopenic purpura from disseminated intravascular coagulation (DIC). Other conditions causing microangiopathic hemolysis (Table 13–18) should be excluded. Evans's syndrome is the

Table 13–18. Causes of microangiopathic hemolytic anemia.

Thrombotic thrombocytopenic purpura
Hemolytic-uremic syndrome
Disseminated intravascular coagulation
Prosthetic valve hemolysis
Metastatic adenocarcinoma
Malignant hypertension
Vasculitis

combination of autoimmune thrombocytopenia and autoimmune hemolytic anemia, but the peripheral smear will show spherocytes and not red blood cell fragments. Skin biopsy is usually not necessary for diagnosis but may be helpful when vasculitis is a consideration. Thrombotic thrombocytopenic purpura and hemolytic-uremic syndrome are not distinct disease entities—rather, there is a spectrum of disease, with thrombotic thrombocytopenic purpura characterized by more neurologic findings and more severe thrombocytopenia and hemolytic-uremic syndrome with more renal failure.

Treatment

Thrombotic thrombocytopenic purpura should be treated emergently with large-volume plasmapheresis. Sixty to 80 mL/kg of plasma should be removed and replaced with fresh-frozen plasma. Treatment should be continued daily until the patient is in complete remission. The optimal duration of plasmapheresis after remission in unknown. Prednisone and antiplatelet agents (aspirin [325 mg three times daily] and dipyridamole [75 mg three times daily]) have been used in addition to plasmapheresis, but their role is unclear.

The management of patients who do not respond to plasmapheresis or who have rapid recurrences is controversial. The combination of splenectomy, corticosteroids, and dextran has been used with success. Splenectomy performed in remission may prevent subsequent relapses. Immunosuppression with drugs such as cyclophosphamide has also been effective.

Prognosis

With the advent of plasmapheresis, the formerly dismal prognosis of thrombotic thrombocytopenic purpura has been dramatically changed. Eighty to 90 percent of patients now recover completely. Neurologic abnormalities are almost always completely reversed. Most complete responses are durable, but in 20% of cases the disease will be chronic and relapsing.

Allford SL et al: Current understanding of the pathophysiology of thrombotic thrombocytopenic purpura. J Clin Pathol 2000;53:497. [PMID: 10961171]

Elliott MA et al: Thrombotic thrombocytopenic purpura and hemolytic uremic syndrome. Mayo Clin Proc 2001;76:1154. [PMID: 11702904]

Veyradier A et al: Specific von Willebrand factor-cleaving protease in thrombotic microangiopathies: a study of 111 cases. Blood 2001;98:1765.[PMID: 11535510]

HEMOLYTIC-UREMIC SYNDROME

 ESSENTIALS OF DIAGNOSIS

- *Microangiopathic hemolytic anemia.*
- *Thrombocytopenia and renal failure.*
- *Elevated serum LDH.*
- *Normal coagulation tests.*
- *Absence of neurologic abnormalities.*

General Considerations

Hemolytic-uremic syndrome is an uncommon disorder consisting of microangiopathic hemolytic anemia, thrombocytopenia, and renal failure due to microangiopathy (with decreased glomerular filtration, proteinuria, and hematuria). The cause is unclear. The disease is similar to thrombotic thrombocytopenic purpura except that different vascular beds are involved. The pathogenesis of the two disorders is probably similar, and a platelet-agglutinating factor found in plasma may be involved. In children, hemolytic-uremic syndrome frequently occurs after a diarrheal illness secondary to infections with shigella, salmonella, *E coli* strain O157:H7, or viral agents. The mortality rate of this form is low (< 5%). In adults, this syndrome is often precipitated by estrogen use or by the postpartum state. Hemolytic-uremic syndrome may be seen as a delayed complication of high-dose corticosteroid therapy and autologous bone marrow or stem cell transplantation, or of the use of cyclosporine or tacrolimus as immunosuppression in allogeneic transplantation. A familial (hereditary) type has been identified in which members of a family have recurrent episodes over several years.

Clinical Findings

A. SYMPTOMS AND SIGNS

Patients present with anemia, bleeding, or renal failure. The renal failure may or may not be oliguric. In contrast to thrombotic thrombocytopenic purpura, there are no neurologic manifestations other than those due to the uremic state.

B. LABORATORY FINDINGS

As in thrombotic thrombocytopenic purpura, there is microangiopathic hemolytic anemia and thrombocytopenia, but the thrombocytopenia is often less severe. The peripheral blood smear should show striking red blood cell fragmentation, and the diagnosis is untenable without this finding. The LDH is usually elevated out of proportion to the degree of hemolysis, and the Coombs test is negative. Coagulation tests are normal with the exception of elevated fibrin degradation products.

Kidney biopsy will show endothelial hyaline thrombi in the afferent arterioles and glomeruli. Ischemic necrosis in the renal cortex may occur with obstruction from intravascular coagulation.

Differential Diagnosis

Disseminated intravascular coagulation is excluded by normal coagulation results. Other causes of microangiopathic hemolytic anemia (Table 13–18) should be entertained. Occasionally, vasculitis or acute glomerulonephritis is considered, and in these cases renal biopsy may be necessary to establish the diagnosis if the platelet count will allow it.

Hemolytic-uremic syndrome is arbitrarily distinguished from thrombotic thrombocytopenic purpura by the consistent presence of renal failure and the lack of neurologic findings.

Treatment

In children, hemolytic-uremic syndrome is almost always self-limited and requires only conservative management of acute renal failure. In adults, however, without treatment, there is a high rate of permanent renal insufficiency and death. The treatment of choice (as in thrombotic thrombocytopenic purpura) is large-volume plasmapheresis with fresh-frozen replacement (exchange of up to 80 mL/kg), repeated daily until remission is achieved.

Prognosis

The prognosis of hemolytic-uremic syndrome in adults remains unclear. Without effective therapy, up to 40% of patients have died, and 80% have had chronic renal insufficiency. Early institution of aggressive therapy with plasmapheresis promises to be beneficial. Survival and correction of hematologic abnormalities are the rule, but restoration of renal function requires that treatment be initiated early.

Banatvala N et al: The United States National Prospective Hemolytic Uremic Syndrome Study: microbiologic, serologic, clinical, and epidemiologic findings. J Infect Dis 2001;183:1063. [PMID: 11237831]

Chandler WL et al: Prothrombotic coagulation abnormalities preceding the hemolytic-uremic syndrome. N Engl J Med 2002;346:23.[PMID: 11777799]

CONGENITAL QUALITATIVE PLATELET DISORDERS

Bleeding disorders characterized by prolonged bleeding times despite a normal platelet count are called qualitative platelet disorders. Patients have a family history or lifelong personal history of the defect. The disorders may be classified as (1) von Willebrand's disease, a congenital disorder of a plasma protein necessary for platelet adhesion; and (2) congenital disorders intrinsic to the platelet (Table 13–19). When an intrinsic qualitative platelet disorder is suspected, platelet aggregation studies should be evaluated to make a specific diagnosis.

1. Von Willebrand's Disease

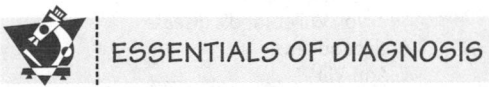

ESSENTIALS OF DIAGNOSIS

- *Family history with autosomal dominant pattern of inheritance.*

Table 13–19. Qualitative platelet disorders.

Congenital
Glanzmann's thrombasthenia
Bernard-Soulier syndrome
Storage pool disease
Acquired
Myeloproliferative disorders
Uremia
Drugs: aspirin, anti-inflammatory agents
Autoantibody
Paraproteins
Acquired storage pool disease
Fibrin degradation products
Von Willebrand's disease

- *Prolonged bleeding time, either at baseline or after challenge with aspirin.*
- *Reduced levels of factor VIII antigen or ristocetin cofactor.*
- *Reduced levels of factor VIII coagulant activity in some patients.*

General Considerations

Von Willebrand's disease is the most common congenital disorder of hemostasis. It is transmitted in an autosomal dominant pattern. It is a group of disorders characterized by deficient or defective von Willebrand factor (vWF), a protein that mediates platelet adhesion. Adhesion is a process separate from platelet aggregation. Platelets adhere to the subendothelium via vWF, which is bound to a specific receptor on the platelet composed of glycoprotein Ib (and missing in Bernard-Soulier syndrome). Platelets aggregate via fibrinogen, which binds to a different receptor composed of glycoproteins IIb and IIIa (deficient in Glanzmann's thrombasthenia). The platelet aggregation system is entirely normal in von Willebrand's disease.

Von Willebrand factor is synthesized in megakaryocytes and endothelial cells and circulates in plasma as multimers of varying size. Only the large multimeric forms are functional in mediating platelet adhesion. Von Willebrand factor has a separate function of binding the factor VIII coagulant protein and protecting it from degradation. The factor VIII coagulant protein (factor VIII:C), a protein encoded by a gene on the X chromosome, is the protein deficient in classic hemophilia. Any of the multimeric forms of vWF can bind and protect factor VIII:C. Von Willebrand's disease, although primarily a disorder of platelet function, may secondarily cause a coagulation disturbance because of deficient levels of factor VIII:C. However, this coagulopathy is rarely severe.

There are several subtypes of von Willebrand's disease. The most common type (type I, 80% of all cases) is caused by a quantitative decrease in vWF. Type IIa is caused by a qualitative abnormality in protein that prevents multimer formation. Only small multimers are present, and both intermediate and large forms that mediate platelet adhesion are missing. Type IIb von Willebrand's disease is caused by a qualitative abnormality in the protein that causes rapid clearance of the large multimeric forms. Type III von Willebrand's disease is a rare autosomal recessive disorder in which vWF is nearly absent. Pseudo-von Willebrand disease is a rare disorder manifested as an abnormal platelet membrane with excessive avidity for the large multimeric forms of vWF, causing their clearance from plasma.

Clinical Findings

A. SYMPTOMS AND SIGNS

Von Willebrand's disease is a common disorder affecting both men and women. Most cases are mild. Most bleeding is mucosal (epistaxis, gingival bleeding, menorrhagia), but gastrointestinal bleeding may occur. In most cases, incisional bleeding occurs after surgery or dental extractions. Von Willebrand's disease is rarely as severe as hemophilia, and spontaneous hemarthroses do not occur. The bleeding tendency is exacerbated by aspirin. Characteristically, bleeding decreases during pregnancy or estrogen use.

B. LABORATORY FINDINGS

Platelet number and morphology are normal, and the bleeding time is usually (not always) prolonged. The bleeding time should be ascertained whenever this diagnosis is considered; it correlates most closely with clinical bleeding. When the bleeding time is normal, it is prolonged markedly by aspirin. Normal persons will prolong their bleeding time to a minor extent with aspirin but rarely out of the normal range. In the most common form of von Willebrand's disease (type I), vWF levels in plasma are reduced. This may be measured by factor VIII antigen, which measures the immunologic presence of vWF, or by ristocetin cofactor activity, which measures functional properties of vWF in mediating platelet adhesion.

When factor VIII antigen is reduced, one may also see a decrease in factor VIII coagulant (factor VIII:C) levels. When factor VIII:C levels are less than 25%, the partial thromboplastin time (PTT) will be prolonged. Platelet aggregation studies with standard agonists (ADP, collagen, thrombin) are normal, but platelet aggregation in response to ristocetin may be subnormal.

In difficult cases, it may be helpful to assay directly the multimeric composition of vWF.

Differential Diagnosis

When patients present with a prolonged bleeding time, one must distinguish von Willebrand's disease from other qualitative platelet disorders (Table 13–19). Acquired qualitative disorders are suggested by recent onset of the bleeding tendency. Congenital intrinsic platelet disorders may present with a positive family history and lifelong history of bleeding episodes. Von Willebrand's disease is diagnosed by the finding of abnormal measurements of vWF and by normal results of platelet aggregation.

When patients present with a prolonged PTT, measurements of factor VIII:C will distinguish von Willebrand's disease from all disorders except hemophilia (Table 13–20). Hemophilia is diagnosed when factor VIII:C is reduced but all measurements of vWF (factor VIII antigen, ristocetin cofactor activity) are normal.

Patients with a suspicious bleeding history but with normal bleeding time and PTT pose a diagnostic problem. On occasion, the postaspirin bleeding time can be used to unmask a bleeding disorder. At other times, one must perform further plasma assays of vWF to make the diagnosis. Von Willebrand's disease waxes and wanes in severity and may be difficult to diagnose, especially in a woman taking estrogens, which raise vWF levels.

It is often useful to distinguish between subtypes of von Willebrand's disease (Table 13–21), because type I usually responds to desmopressin and type IIb may be aggravated by its use.

Treatment

The bleeding disorder is characteristically mild, and no treatment is routinely given other than avoidance of aspirin. However, patients often need to be prepared for surgical or dental procedures. The bleeding time is probably the best indicator of the likelihood of bleeding, and prophylactic therapy may be reasonably withheld if the procedure is minor and the bleeding time is normal.

Desmopressin acetate is useful for mild type I von Willebrand's disease and should be considered first. The dose is 0.3 μg/kg, after which vWF levels usually

Table 13–20. Causes of prolonged partial thromboplastin time.

Congenital factor deficiencies
Contact factors
Factor XII
Factor XI
Factor IX (hemophilia B)
Factor VIII
Hemophilia A
von Willebrand's disease
Anticoagulants
Anti-VIII
Lupus
Heparin

Table 13–21. Types of von Willebrand's disease.

	Bleeding Time	Factor VIII Antigen	Ristocetin Cofactor Activity	Factor VIII Coagulant Activity	Multimer
Type I	↑ or N[1]	↓ or N	↓ or N	↓ or N	N
Type IIa	↑	↓ or N	0	↓ or N	Abn
Type IIb	↑	↓ or N	↓ or N	↓ or N	Abn
Type III	↑	0	0	0	...
Pseudo-vW disease	↑	↓ or N	↓ or N	↓	Abn
Hemophilia A	N	N	N		N

[1]Increases with aspirin.

rise two- to threefold in 30–90 minutes. Desmopressin acetate appears to cause release of stored vWF from endothelial cells. The treatment can be given only every 24 hours as stores of vWF become depleted. The drug is not effective in type IIa von Willebrand's disease, in which no endothelial stores are present, and may be harmful in type IIb, leading to thrombocytopenia and increased bleeding.

Factor VIII concentrates are available that replace cryoprecipitate as the treatment of choice for von Willebrand's disease if factor replacement is required. Some (not all) of these products now contain functional vWF and do not transmit HIV or hepatitis. One appropriate product is Humate-P (Armour). The dose is 20–50 units/kg depending on disease severity.

The antifibrinolytic agent tranexamic acid is useful as adjunctive therapy during dental procedures. After either cryoprecipitate or desmopressin acetate, the patient is given 25 mg/kg three times daily for 5–7 days to reduce the likelihood of bleeding.

Prognosis

The prognosis is excellent. In most cases, the bleeding disorder is mild, and in the more serious cases replacement therapy is effective.

Hambleton J: Diagnosis and incidence of inherited von Willebrand disease. Curr Opin Hematol 2001;8:306. [PMID: 11604566]

Sadler JE et al: Impact, diagnosis and treatment of von Willebrand disease. Thromb Haemost 2000;84:160. [PMID: 10959685]

2. Disorders Intrinsic to the Platelets

Glanzmann's Thrombasthenia

This is a rare autosomal recessive intrinsic platelet disorder causing bleeding. Platelets are unable to aggregate because of lack of receptors (containing glycoproteins IIb and IIIa) for fibrinogen, which form the bridges between platelets during aggregation. Clini-

cally, it is manifested chiefly as mucosal (epistaxis, gingival bleeding, menorrhagia) and postoperative bleeding. The defect is of variable severity but may be severe.

Platelet numbers and morphology are normal, but the bleeding time is markedly prolonged. Platelets fail to aggregate in response to typical agonists (ADP, collagen, thrombin) but aggregate normally in response to ristocetin, which causes platelet clumping by a separate mechanism.

Patients are treated with platelet transfusions when necessary. Platelet transfusion therapy is limited by the tendency of these patients to develop multiple alloantibodies.

Bernard-Soulier Syndrome

This is a rare autosomal recessive intrinsic platelet disorder causing bleeding. Platelets cannot adhere to subendothelium because they lack receptors (composed of glycoprotein Ib) for von Willebrand factor, which mediates platelet adhesion. This is often a severe bleeding disorder with mucosal and postoperative bleeding.

Thrombocytopenia may be present, and platelets on smear are abnormally large. The bleeding time is markedly prolonged. Platelet aggregation is normal in response to standard agonists (collagen, ADP, thrombin), but platelets fail to aggregate in response to ristocetin. Measurements of von Willebrand factor in the plasma are normal. Patients are treated with platelet transfusion when necessary.

Storage Pool Disease

This is a group of mild bleeding disorders characterized by defective secretion of platelet granule contents (especially ADP) that stimulate platelet aggregation. Most patients are mildly affected and have increased bruising and postoperative bleeding.

Platelets are normal in number and morphology, but the bleeding time is slightly prolonged. In some cases, the baseline bleeding time is normal, but it becomes markedly prolonged after aspirin. There are variable abnormalities in platelet aggregation studies.

Most patients do not require treatment but should avoid aspirin. Platelet transfusions transiently correct the bleeding tendency. Some patients respond to desmopressin acetate, 0.3 μg/kg every 24 hours.

Peretz H et al: Glanzmann's thrombasthenia associated with deletion-insertion and alternative splicing in the glycoprotein IIb gene. Blood 1995;85:414. [PMID: 7529063]

ACQUIRED QUALITATIVE PLATELET DISORDERS

A number of acquired disorders lead to abnormal platelet function (Table 13–19).

Uremia

Uremia causes abnormal platelet function by unknown mechanisms. The severity of the bleeding tendency is roughly proportionate to the degree of renal insufficiency. Bleeding is most commonly mucosal and gastrointestinal and may occasionally be severe. Dialysis is effective in reducing the bleeding tendency but may not completely eliminate it. Patients respond to desmopressin acetate, 0.3 μg/kg every 24 hours.

Myeloproliferative Disorders

All the myeloproliferative disorders can produce abnormalities in platelet function. A number of biochemical abnormalities are present in these platelets, but the cause of the bleeding tendency is unclear. The severity of the bleeding tendency correlates roughly with the height of the platelet count, although conditions causing reactive thrombocytosis of normal platelets are not associated with abnormal function. Bleeding decreases when the platelet count is controlled with myelosuppressive therapy. In cases of life-threatening bleeding with high platelet counts, plateletpheresis may be necessary.

Other Disorders

Aspirin causes a mild bleeding tendency by irreversibly acetylating cyclooxygenase, an enzyme that participates in platelet aggregation. The effect lasts for the life of the platelet and may be manifest for 7–10 days, although the major effect lasts 3–5 days. The effect is not dose-dependent, and 65 mg of aspirin is sufficient.

Aspirin by itself does not cause significant bleeding, but it may unmask bleeding disorders such as mild von Willebrand's disease or mild thrombocytopenia. Certain antibiotics (ticarcillin, some cephalosporins) cause a mild bleeding tendency, presumably by coating the surface of platelets. Nonsteroidal anti-inflammatory drugs cause an aspirin-like effect that disappears when the drug leaves the system.

Patients with autoantibodies against platelets may have prolonged bleeding times even in the absence of thrombocytopenia. Platelet-associated IgG levels should be high, and the bleeding tendency responds quickly to modest doses of prednisone, eg, 20 mg/d. Acquired storage pool disease refers to the circulation of "exhausted platelets" that have been stimulated to release their granule contents and hence are no longer functional. Such granule release occurs in response to cardiopulmonary bypass and severe vasculitis.

Noris M et al: Uremic bleeding: closing the circle after 30 years of controversies? Blood 1999;94:2569. [PMID: 10515859]

HEMOPHILIA A

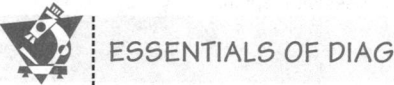 ESSENTIALS OF DIAGNOSIS

- *X-linked recessive pattern of inheritance with only males affected.*
- *Low factor VIII coagulant (VIII:C) activity.*
- *Normal factor VIII antigen.*
- *Spontaneous hemarthroses.*

General Considerations

Hemophilia A (classic hemophilia, factor VIII deficiency hemophilia) is a hereditary disorder in which bleeding is due to deficiency of the coagulation factor VIII (VIII:C). In most cases, the factor VIII coagulant protein is quantitatively reduced, but in a small number of cases the coagulant protein is present by immunoassay but defective.

Hemophilia is an X-linked recessive disease, and as a rule only males are affected. In rare instances, female carriers are clinically affected if their normal X chromosomes are disproportionately inactivated. Females may also become affected if they are the offspring of a hemophiliac father and carrier mother.

Hemophilia is classified as severe if factor VIII:C levels are less than 1%, moderate if levels are 1–5%, and mild if levels are greater than 5%. Families tend to breed true in the severity of hemophilia produced.

Clinical Findings

A. SYMPTOMS AND SIGNS

Hemophilia A is the most common severe bleeding disorder and after von Willebrand's disease is the most common congenital bleeding disorder overall. Approximately one in 10,000 males is affected. The bleeding tendency is related to factor VIII:C levels. Bleeding may occur anywhere. The most common sites of bleeding are into joints (knees, ankles, elbows), into muscles, and from the gastrointestinal tract. Spontaneous hemarthroses are so characteristic of hemophilia that they are virtually diagnostic of the disorder. Patients with mild hemophilia bleed only after major trauma or surgery; those with moderately severe hemophilia bleed with mild trauma or surgery; and those with severe disease bleed spontaneously.

Many hemophiliacs are now seropositive for HIV infection transmitted via factor VIII concentrate, and many have already developed AIDS. HIV-associated immune thrombocytopenia may aggravate the bleeding tendency.

B. LABORATORY FINDINGS

The partial thromboplastin time (PTT) is prolonged, and other measures of coagulation, including prothrombin time, bleeding time, and fibrinogen level, are normal. Levels of factor VIII:C are reduced, but measurements of von Willebrand factor are normal (Table 13–21).

If one mixes plasma from a hemophiliac patient with normal plasma, the PTT will become normal. Failure of the PTT to normalize in such a mixing test is diagnostic of the presence of a factor VIII inhibitor.

A low platelet count should raise a suspicion of HIV-associated immune thrombocytopenia.

Differential Diagnosis

The finding of a reduced factor VIII:C level will distinguish this disorder from other causes of prolonged PTT (Table 13–20). Clinically, factor VIII hemophilia is indistinguishable from factor IX hemophilia, and only specific factor assays can distinguish these disorders. In cases of mild hemophilia, the disorder needs to be distinguished from von Willebrand's disease by VIII:A assay, which shows normal levels of factor VIII antigen in the former.

An important issue for the families of hemophiliac patients is identifying which females are carriers. They can usually be identified by the presence of low or normal levels of factor VIII:C with normal levels of factor VIII antigen.

Treatment

Standard treatment is based on infusion of factor VIII concentrates, now heat-treated to reduce the likelihood of transmission of HIV. Recombinant factor VIII appears safe and effective, though expensive, and should impose no risk of transmitting HIV or other viruses. The level of factor VIII one aims to achieve in plasma depends on the severity of the bleeding problem. In response to minor bleeding, it may be necessary only to raise factor VIII:C levels to 25% with one infusion. For moderate bleeding (such as deep muscle hematomas), it is adequate to raise the level initially to 50% and maintain the level at greater than 25% with repeated infusion for 2–3 days. When major surgery is to be performed, one raises the factor VIII:C level to 100% and then maintains the factor level at greater than 50% continuously for 10–14 days. Head injuries (with or without neurologic signs)

should be emergently treated as though major bleeding were present.

The dose of factor VIII concentrate is calculated assuming that one unit of factor VIII is the amount present in 1 mL of plasma. Plasma volume is 40 mL/kg, and the volume of distribution of factor VIII:C is 1.5 times the plasma volume. Thus, to raise the level 100%, the dose should be $40 \times 1.5 = 60$ units/kg, or approximately 4000 units for a 70-kg individual. To raise the levels to 25% would require 1000 units. The half-life of factor VIII:C is approximately 12 hours. Thus, during major surgery, to achieve an initial level of 100% and maintain it continuously at greater than 50%, a dose of 60 units/kg (approximately 4000 units) initially followed by 30 units/kg (approximately 2000 units) every 12 hours should be adequate. During surgery, one should initially verify that these doses give the anticipated factor VIII levels. If factor VIII levels fail to rise as expected, one should suspect an inhibitor.

For mild hemophiliacs, desmopressin acetate, 0.3 μg/kg every 24 hours, may be useful in preparing for minor surgical procedures. Desmopressin acetate causes release of factor VIII:C and will raise the factor VIII:C levels two- to threefold for several hours. In the management of persistent bleeding following use of either desmopressin acetate or factor VIII concentrate, patients may be treated with aminocaproic acid (EACA; Amicar), 4 g orally every 4 hours for several days.

Aspirin should be avoided in these patients.

Prognosis

The prognosis of patients with hemophilia has been transformed by the availability of factor VIII replacement. The major limiting factor is disability from recurrent joint bleeding. Hepatitis B and C and HIV infection from recurrent transfusion are diminishing in incidence. Approximately 15% of patients develop inhibitors to factor VIII, and these patents cannot be adequately supported with factor VIII.

Mannucci PM et al: The hemophilias—from royal genes to gene therapy. N Engl J Med 2001;344:1773. [PMID: 11396445]

ACQUIRED FACTOR VIII ANTIBODIES

Antibodies to factor VIII may develop either postpartum or with no underlying illness. Factor VIII antibodies also occur in 15% of patients with factor VIII hemophilia who have received infusions of plasma concentrates.

Factor VIII antibodies usually produce a severe bleeding disorder. The PTT is prolonged, and the fibrinogen level, prothrombin time, and platelet count are not affected. A plasma mixing test will usually reveal the presence of an inhibitor by the failure of normal plasma to correct the prolonged PTT. However, the mixing test may require incubation for 2–4 hours to reveal the inhibitor. Factor VIII coagulant levels are low.

Factor VIII antibodies should be suspected in any acquired severe bleeding disorder associated with a prolonged PTT. Factor VIII antibodies are distinguished from lupus anticoagulants both by the presence of clinical bleeding and more importantly by the reduced factor VIII:C level. The diagnosis is confirmed by mixing tests and in vivo by the failure of factor VIII concentrates to raise the factor VIII:C levels by the expected amount.

The treatment of choice is cyclophosphamide, usually combined with prednisone. In the interim, aggressive factor VIII replacement may be necessary. Products that bypass factor VIII such as activated factor VII may be effective but are expensive.

Colowick AB et al: Immunotolerance induction in hemophilia patients with inhibitors: costly can be cheaper. Blood 2000; 96:1698. [PMID: 10961866]

HEMOPHILIA B

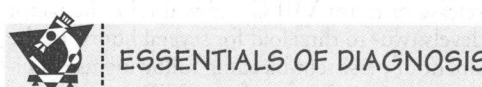

ESSENTIALS OF DIAGNOSIS

- *X-linked recessive inheritance, with only males affected.*
- *Low levels of factor IX coagulant activity.*
- *Spontaneous hemarthroses.*

General Considerations

Hemophilia B (Christmas disease, factor IX hemophilia) is a hereditary bleeding disorder due to deficiency of coagulation factor IX. Most commonly, factor IX is quantitatively reduced, but in one-third of cases an abnormally functioning molecule is immunologically present. Factor IX deficiency is one-seventh as common as factor VIII deficiency hemophilia but is otherwise clinically and genetically identical.

The PTT is prolonged, and factor IX levels are reduced when measured by specific factor assays. Other laboratory features are the same as for factor VIII hemophilia.

Treatment

Factor IX hemophilia is managed with factor IX concentrates. Factor VIII concentrates are ineffective in this type of hemophilia. The same dosing considerations apply as in factor VIII hemophilia, with the exception that the volume of distribution of factor IX is twice the plasma volume, so that 80 units/kg are necessary to achieve a 100% level. In addition, the half-life of factor IX is 18 hours. Thus, to maintain a pa-

tient through major surgery, the dosage should be 80 units/kg (approximately 6000 units) initially followed by 40 units/kg (3000 units) every 18 hours. Factor IX levels should be measured to ensure that expected levels are achieved and that an inhibitor is not present.

Unlike factor VIII concentrates, factor IX concentrates contain a number of other proteins, including activated coagulating factors that appear to contribute to a risk of thrombosis with recurrent usage of factor IX concentrates. Because of the risk of thrombosis, more care is needed in deciding to use these concentrates. Desmopressin acetate is not useful in this disorder, and patients should be cautioned to avoid aspirin.

Prognosis

The prognosis for these patients is the same as for those with factor VIII hemophilia.

Roth DA et al: Human recombinant factor IX: safety and efficacy studies in hemophilia B patients previously treated with plasma-derived factor IX concentrates. Blood 2001;98: 3600. [PMID: 11739163] (Recombinant human factor IX is safe, effective, and free of the potential for transmission of blood-borne pathogens.)

OTHER CONGENITAL COAGULATION DISORDERS

Factor XI Deficiency

This disorder is seen primarily among Ashkenazi Jews and is autosomal recessive. The PTT may be markedly prolonged, and specific assays of factor XI will show reduced levels. This is usually a mild bleeding disorder manifested primarily by postoperative bleeding. Factor replacement is given with fresh-frozen plasma when necessary.

Afibrinogenemia

In this rare disorder, fibrinogen is absent and both prothrombin time and partial thromboplastin time are markedly prolonged. These patients may have a severe bleeding disorder similar to hemophilia. Fibrinogen is replaced with cryoprecipitate.

Other Coagulation Disorders

Bleeding disorders due to isolated deficiency of factors II, V, X, or VII are extremely rare. Deficiencies of factor XII and the contact pathway factors cause a markedly prolonged PTT but are not associated with any increased bleeding.

Factor XIII deficiency results in delayed bleeding after trauma or surgery. All coagulation tests are normal. The disorder is diagnosed by showing instability of the fibrin clot in 8-molar urea. Factor XIII is replaced with cryoprecipitate or plasma. A rare cause of bleeding is deficiency of the normal inhibitors of fibrinolytic activity: α_2-antiplasmin and plasminogen activator inhibitor.

COAGULOPATHY OF LIVER DISEASE

 ESSENTIALS OF DIAGNOSIS

- Clinical picture usually typical of advanced liver disease.
- Prothrombin time more prolonged than PTT.
- No response to vitamin K.

General Considerations

The liver is the site of synthesis of all the coagulation factors except factor VIII. As hepatic insufficiency develops, the vitamin K-dependent factors (factors II, VII, IX, X) and factor V are the first to be affected. Because of its rapid turnover (half-life 6 hours), factor VII levels are the first to decline. Conversely, fibrinogen levels are remarkably well conserved, and decreased fibrinogen synthesis does not occur unless liver disease is very severe.

Liver disease has a number of other effects on the hemostatic system. Increased fibrinolysis occurs because the liver synthesizes α_2-antiplasmin (the main inhibitor of fibrinolysis), which is responsible for the clearance of plasminogen activator. Biliary tract disease may lead to malabsorption of vitamin K, and congestive splenomegaly may produce mild thrombocytopenia. A variety of chronic liver diseases cause abnormal posttranslation modification of fibrinogen with resultant dysfibrinogenemia. The majority of patients with cirrhosis have very low levels of thrombopoietin, and this may contribute to the thrombocytopenia.

Clinical Findings

A. SYMPTOMS AND SIGNS

The coagulopathy of liver disease may lead to bleeding at any site. Excessive fibrinolysis may lead to oozing at venipuncture sites. Most patients have clinically obvious serious liver disease.

B. LABORATORY FINDINGS

Hepatic coagulopathy produces a more marked abnormality in the prothrombin time (PT) than in the partial thromboplastin time (PTT). Early in the course of liver disease, only the PT will be affected. Fibrinogen levels and thrombin time should be normal unless dysfibrinogenemia is present. The platelet count is usually normal but may be reduced by low levels of thrombopoietin, by hypersplenism, by bone marrow suppression by alcohol, and by folic acid deficiency. The peripheral blood smear may show target cells.

Differential Diagnosis

Hepatic coagulopathy can be distinguished from vitamin K deficiency by demonstrating the failure of vitamin K to correct the abnormal values. Liver disease is distinguished from disseminated intravascular coagulation by the normal fibrinogen level and lack of thrombocytopenia. End-stage liver disease almost invariably leads to some element of disseminated intravascular coagulation, and the disorders overlap (Tables 13–22 and 13–23).

Treatment

Long-term treatment of hepatic coagulopathy with factor replacement is usually ineffective. Fresh-frozen plasma is the treatment of choice, and volume overload will limit one's ability to maintain hemostatic factor levels. For example, to maintain factor levels greater than 25%, one must initially raise the level to 50% with 50% of the plasma volume (20 mL/kg) and then replace 10 mL/kg every 6 hours to maintain adequate factor VII levels. In average-sized persons, this will require transfusion of 1400 mL of plasma initially followed by 700 mL every 6 hours. Factor IX concentrates are contraindicated in liver disease because of their tendency to cause disseminated intravascular coagulation. If thrombocytopenia is present, platelet transfusion may be of some help, but platelet recovery is usually disappointing because of hypersplenism.

Prognosis

The prognosis is that of the underlying liver disease.

VITAMIN K DEFICIENCY

 ESSENTIALS OF DIAGNOSIS

- Underlying dietary deficiency or antibiotic use.
- Prothrombin time more prolonged than PTT.
- Rapid correction with vitamin K replacement.

General Considerations

Vitamin K plays a role in coagulation by acting as a cofactor for the posttranslational γ-carboxylation of zymogens II, VII, IX, and X. The modified zymogens (with γ-carboxyglutamic acid residues) are able to bind to platelets in a calcium-dependent reaction and con-

Table 13–22. Causes of isolated prolonged prothrombin time.

Liver disease
Vitamin K deficiency
Warfarin therapy
Factor VII deficiency

Table 13–23. Causes of prolonged prothrombin time and partial thromboplastin time.

Liver disease
Vitamin K deficiency
Disseminated intravascular coagulation
Heparin
Warfarin
Isolated factor deficiencies (rare): II, V, X, I

sequently better participate in the complex reactions that activate factors X and II. Without γ-carboxylation, these reactions on the platelet surface occur slowly and hemostasis is impaired.

Vitamin K is supplied in the diet primarily in leafy vegetables and endogenously from synthesis by intestinal bacteria. Factors that contribute to vitamin K deficiency include poor diet, malabsorption, and broad-spectrum antibiotics suppressing colonic flora. A characteristic setting for vitamin K deficiency is a postoperative patient who is not eating and who is receiving antibiotics. Body stores of vitamin K are small, and deficiency may develop in as little as 1 week.

Clinical Findings

A. Symptoms and Signs

There are no specific clinical features, and bleeding may occur at any site.

B. Laboratory Findings

The prothrombin time is prolonged to a greater extent than the PTT, and with mild vitamin K deficiency only the PT is defective (Tables 13–22 and 13–23). Fibrinogen level, thrombin time, and platelet count are not affected.

Differential Diagnosis

Vitamin K deficiency can be distinguished from hepatic coagulopathy only by assessing the response to vitamin K therapy. Surreptitious warfarin use will produce laboratory features indistinguishable from those of vitamin K deficiency.

Vitamin K deficiency differs from disseminated intravascular coagulation by normal platelet count and fibrinogen levels in the former.

Treatment

Vitamin K deficiency responds rapidly to subcutaneous vitamin K, and a single dose of 15 mg will completely correct laboratory abnormalities in 12–24 hours.

Prognosis

The prognosis is excellent, as vitamin K deficiency can be completely corrected with replacement.

DISSEMINATED INTRAVASCULAR COAGULATION (DIC)

 ESSENTIALS OF DIAGNOSIS

- *Underlying serious illness.*
- *Microangiopathic hemolytic anemia may be present.*
- *Hypofibrinogenemia, thrombocytopenia, fibrin degradation products, and prolonged prothrombin time.*

General Considerations

Coagulation is usually confined to a localized area by the combination of blood flow and circulating inhibitors of coagulation, especially antithrombin III. If the stimulus to coagulation is too great, these control mechanisms can be overwhelmed, leading to the syndrome of disseminated intravascular coagulation. In pathophysiologic terms, disseminated intravascular coagulation can be thought of as the consequence of the presence of circulating thrombin (normally confined to a localized area). The effects of thrombin are to cleave fibrinogen to fibrin monomer, stimulate platelet aggregation, activate factors V and VIII, and release plasminogen activator, which generates plasmin. Plasmin in turn cleaves fibrin, generating fibrin degradation products, and further inactivates factors V and VIII. Thus, the excess thrombin activity produces hypofibrinogenemia, thrombocytopenia, depletion of coagulation factors, and fibrinolysis.

Disseminated intravascular coagulation can be caused by a number of serious illnesses, including sepsis (especially with gram-negative bacteria but possible with any widespread bacterial or fungal infection), severe tissue injury (especially burns and head injury), obstetric complications (amniotic fluid embolus, septic abortion, retained fetus), cancer (acute promyelocytic leukemia, mucinous adenocarcinomas), and major hemolytic transfusion reactions.

Clinical Findings

A. Symptoms and Signs

Disseminated intravascular coagulation leads to both bleeding and thrombosis. Bleeding is far more common than thrombosis, but the latter may dominate if coagulation is activated to a far greater extent than fibrinolysis. Bleeding may occur at any site, but spontaneous bleeding and oozing at venipuncture sites or wounds are important clues to the diagnosis. Thrombosis is most commonly manifested by digital ischemia and gangrene, but catastrophic events such as renal cortical necrosis and hemorrhagic adrenal infarction may occur. Disseminated intravascular coagulation may also secondarily produce microangiopathic hemolytic anemia.

Subacute disseminated intravascular coagulation is seen primarily in cancer patients and is manifested primarily as recurrent superficial and deep venous thromboses (**Trousseau's syndrome**).

B. LABORATORY FINDINGS

Disseminated intravascular coagulation produces a complex coagulopathy with the characteristic constellation of hypofibrinogenemia, elevated fibrin degradation products, thrombocytopenia, and a prolonged prothrombin time. Of the fibrin degradation products, the D-dimer is the most sensitive, since its cross-linking implies origin from fibrin in a clot. All fibrin degradation products are cleared by the liver and thus may be elevated in hepatic dysfunction. Hypofibrinogenemia is another important diagnostic laboratory feature, because only a few other disorders (congenital hypofibrinogenemia, severe liver disease) will lower the fibrinogen level. In some cases of disseminated intravascular coagulation, when the patient's baseline fibrinogen level is markedly elevated, the initial fibrinogen level may be normal. However, since the half-life of fibrinogen is approximately 4 days, a declining fibrinogen level will confirm the diagnosis of disseminated intravascular coagulation.

Other laboratory abnormalities are variably present. The partial thromboplastin time may or may not be prolonged. In approximately one-fourth of cases, a microangiopathic hemolytic anemia is present, and fragmented red blood cells are seen on the peripheral smear. Antithrombin III levels may be markedly depleted. When fibrinolysis is activated, levels of plasminogen and α_2-antiplasmin may be low.

Subacute disseminated intravascular coagulation produces a very different laboratory picture. Thrombocytopenia and elevated D-dimer are usually the only abnormalities. Fibrinogen levels are normal, and the PTT may be normal.

Differential Diagnosis

Liver disease may prolong both the PT and PTT, but fibrinogen levels are usually normal, and the platelet count is usually normal or only slightly reduced. However, severe liver disease may be difficult to distinguish from disseminated intravascular coagulation. Vitamin K deficiency will not affect the fibrinogen level or platelet count and will be completely corrected by vitamin K replacement.

Sepsis may produce thrombocytopenia and digital ischemia, and coagulopathy may be present because of vitamin K deficiency. However, in these cases, the fibrinogen level should be normal.

Thrombotic thrombocytopenic purpura may produce fever and microangiopathic hemolytic anemia. However, fibrinogen levels and other coagulation studies should be normal.

Treatment

The primary focus should be the diagnosis and treatment of the underlying disorder that has given rise to disseminated intravascular coagulation. In many cases, disseminated intravascular coagulation will produce laboratory abnormalities with only mild clinical manifestations, and in these cases no specific therapy is required.

When the underlying cause of disseminated intravascular coagulation is rapidly reversible (such as in obstetric cases), replacement therapy alone may be indicated. The role of heparin in the treatment of disseminated intravascular coagulation is controversial. In some cases, when any increase in bleeding is unacceptable (neurosurgical procedures), heparin therapy is contraindicated. However, when disseminated intravascular coagulation is producing serious clinical consequences and the underlying cause is not rapidly reversible, heparin may be necessary. Such therapy is routinely used in the treatment of acute promyelocytic leukemia.

In replacement therapy, platelet transfusion should be used to maintain a platelet count greater than 30,000/μL, and 50,000/μL if possible. Fibrinogen is replaced with cryoprecipitate, and one should aim for a plasma fibrinogen level of 150 mg/dL. One unit of cryoprecipitate usually raises the fibrinogen level by 6–8 mg/dL, so that 15 units of cryoprecipitate will raise the level from 50 to 150 mg/dL. Coagulation factor deficiency may require replacement with fresh-frozen plasma.

Heparin must be used in combination with replacement therapy, since heparin alone will lead to an unacceptable increase in bleeding. A dose of 500–750 units per hour is necessary. Heparin cannot be effective if antithrombin III levels are markedly depleted. Antithrombin III levels should be measured, and fresh-frozen plasma used to raise levels to greater than 50%. In using heparin, it is not necessary to prolong the PTT. Successful therapy is indicated by a rising fibrinogen level. Fibrin degradation products will decline over 1–2 days. Improvement in the platelet count may lag as much as 1 week behind control of the coagulopathy.

In some cases, when disseminated intravascular coagulation is complicated by excessive fibrinolysis, even the combination of heparin and replacement therapy may not be adequate to control bleeding. In these cases, aminocaproic acid, 1 g intravenously per hour, or tranexamic acid, 10 mg/kg intravenously every 8 hours, should be added to decrease the rate of fibrinolysis, raise the fibrinogen level, and control bleeding. Aminocaproic acid can *never* be used without heparin in disseminated intravascular coagulation because of the risk of thrombosis.

Prognosis

The prognosis is that of the underlying disease.

Levi M et al: Novel approaches to the management of disseminated intravascular coagulation. Crit Care Med 2000; 28:S20. [PMID: 11007192]

Schmaier AH: Disseminated intravascular coagulation. N Engl J Med 1999;341:1937. [PMID: 10610481]

■ HYPERCOAGULABLE STATES

In many cases, thrombosis is related to local factors causing stasis of blood flow or damage to a blood vessel. Common examples are deep venous thrombosis in the legs following prolonged sitting in one position and thrombosis in the femoral and iliac veins following hip surgery. However, in other cases a systemic disorder causes a general increase in the risk of thrombosis (Table 13–24).

Cancer is associated with an increased risk of both venous and arterial thrombosis. In some cases, low-grade disseminated intravascular coagulation appears to be responsible. In unusual cases, a unique cancer procoagulant stimulates the clotting system. Myeloproliferative disorders such as polycythemia vera, essential thrombocytosis, and paroxysmal nocturnal hemoglobinuria are associated with a high incidence of thrombosis, caused by qualitative platelet abnormalities. Venous thrombosis may occur in unusual locations such as the mesenteric, hepatic, or splenic venous beds. Arterial thrombosis occurs as well and may be manifested as large vessel occlusion (stroke, myocardial infarction) or as microvascular events with burning in the hands and feet.

Heparin is an uncommon but important cause of hypercoagulability. Heparin has been associated with thrombocytopenia in about 10% of treatment courses. Often the thrombocytopenia is modest and resolves spontaneously. However, in some cases severe thrombocytopenia occurs. It is most often in this setting that arterial thrombosis occurs as a complication. The arteries involved are often large ones, such as the iliac artery or even the aorta. Heparin is discontinued in this setting, as death may occur otherwise.

A number of congenital biochemical defects have also been associated with hypercoagulability (Table 13–24). A family history is usually present. The thromboses are almost always venous and may occur in the large veins of the abdomen. Thromboses often occur during early adulthood rather than in childhood and are often precipitated by factors such as trauma or pregnancy. The most common of these disorders is an abnormal factor V (factor V Leiden), which is resistant to degradation by activated protein C. Dysfibrinogenemia is diagnosed by a prolonged reptilase time.

The syndrome of **warfarin-induced skin necrosis** may occur in patients with undiagnosed protein C deficiency. Protein C is vitamin K-dependent and has a shorter half-life than the coagulation proteins. Warfarin, by creating a vitamin K-dependent state, will transiently deplete protein C before it leads to anticoagulation. During the period of hypercoagulability due to unopposed protein C depletion, thrombosis of skin vessels may lead to infarction and necrosis. The syndrome can be prevented by the use of heparin for 5–7 days until warfarin induces anticoagulation.

Treatment

If a patient is recognized to be at increased risk of thrombosis, effective prophylactic therapy is usually available. Preoperatively, minidose heparin (5000 units every 8–12 hours) may be useful in reducing the risk of thrombosis in the perioperative period. The hypercoagulable state associated with cancer may benefit from treatment with heparin, 10,000 units subcutaneously every 12 hours. Low-molecular-weight heparin is a more convenient agent which is equally effective and requires less laboratory monitoring. Warfarin is usually ineffective in preventing thrombosis in this situation, most likely because low-grade disseminated intravascular coagulation is the cause. In patients with myeloproliferative disease who have had symptoms of thrombosis, antiplatelet therapy may be helpful. However, such therapy should not be used indiscriminately, because these patients are also at increased risk of bleeding. For patients with **erythromelalgia** (painful redness and burning of the hands), aspirin, 325 mg daily, is effective.

In congenital biochemical defects such as deficiency of antithrombin III or the vitamin K-dependent proteins C and S, warfarin is effective and is given indefinitely. Family members are screened for the presence of the defect.

Table 13–24. Causes of hypercoagulability.

Acquired
Cancer
Inflammatory disorders: ulcerative colitis
Myeloproliferative disorders
Postoperative
Estrogens, pregnancy
Lupus anticoagulant
Heparin-induced thrombocytopenia
Anticardiolipin antibodies
Poroxysmal nocturnal hemoglobinuree
Congenital
Antithrombin III deficiency
Factor V Leiden
Protein C deficiency
Protein S deficiency
Dysfibrinogenemia
Abnormal plasminogen
Activated protein C resistance

Federman DG et al: An update on hypercoagulable disorders. Arch Intern Med 2001;161:1051. [PMID: 11322838]

Meijers JC et al: High levels of coagulation factor XI as a risk factor for venous thrombosis. N Engl J Med 2000;342:696. [PMID: 10706899]

LUPUS ANTICOAGULANT

The lupus anticoagulant is an IgM or IgG immunoglobulin that produces a prolonged PTT by binding to the phospholipid used in the in vitro PTT assay. As such, it is a laboratory artifact and does not cause a clinical bleeding disorder. The "lupus anticoagulant" is seen in 5–10% of patients with systemic lupus erythematosus. More commonly, it is seen without an underlying disorder or in patients taking phenothiazines.

There is no bleeding defect unless a second disorder such as thrombocytopenia, hypoprothrombinemia, or a prolonged bleeding time is present. In fact, the lupus anticoagulant has been associated with an increased risk of thrombosis and of recurrent spontaneous abortions.

The PTT is prolonged and fails to correct when the patient's plasma is mixed in a 1:1 dilution with normal plasma. The PT is either normal or slightly prolonged. The fibrinogen level and thrombin time are normal. The Russell viper venom (RVV) time is a more sensitive assay and is specifically designed to demonstrate the presence of a lupus anticoagulant. An antiphospholipid, the lupus anticoagulant will cause a false-positive VDRL test for syphilis. A related autoantibody, anticardiolipin, can be detected by separate assays.

Lupus anticoagulant should be suspected in cases of a markedly prolonged PTT without clinical bleeding (other causes are factor XII or contact factor deficiency). The plasma mixing test will demonstrate the presence of an inhibitor by the failure of normal plasma to correct the PTT. When acquired factor VIII inhibitors are being considered, a factor VIII:C level may be measured; this will be normal in patients with lupus anticoagulant.

No specific treatment is necessary. Prednisone will usually rapidly eliminate the lupus anticoagulant, and it has been suggested that prednisone therapy reduces spontaneous abortions in this syndrome. It is not clear whether prednisone has any effect on the thrombotic tendency associated with lupus anticoagulant. Patients with thromboses should be treated with anticoagulation in standard doses. Because of the artificially prolonged PTT, heparin therapy is difficult to monitor properly, and low-molecular-weight heparin may be preferred. The dose of warfarin administered may also be inadequate if the baseline PT is prolonged.

Shapiro SS: The lupus anticoagulant/antiphospholipid syndrome. Annu Rev Med 1996;47:533. [PMID: 8712801]

■ BLOOD TRANSFUSIONS

RED BLOOD CELL TRANSFUSIONS

Red blood cell transfusions are given to raise the hematocrit levels in patients with anemia or to replace losses after acute bleeding episodes. Several types of components containing red blood cells are available.

(1) Fresh whole blood—The advantage of this component is the simultaneous presence of red blood cells, plasma, and fresh platelets. Fresh whole blood is never absolutely necessary, since all the above components are available separately. The major indications for use of whole blood are cardiac surgery or massive hemorrhage when more than ten units of blood are required in a 24-hour period.

(2) Packed red blood cells—Packed red cells are the component most commonly used to raise the hematocrit. Each unit has a volume of about 300 mL, of which approximately 200 mL consists of red blood cells. One unit of packed red cells will usually raise the hematocrit by approximately 4%. The expected rise in hematocrit can be calculated using an estimated red blood cell volume of 200 mL/unit and a total blood volume of about 70 mL/kg. For example, a 70-kg man will have a total blood volume of 4900 mL, and each unit of packed red blood cells will raise the hematocrit by $200 \div 4900$ equals 4%.

(3) Leukopoor blood—Patients with severe leukoagglutinin reactions to packed red blood cells may require depletion of white blood cells and platelets from transfused units. White blood cells can be removed either by centrifugation or by washing. Preparation of leukopoor blood is expensive and leads to some loss of red cells.

(4) Frozen blood—Red blood cells can be frozen and stored for up to 3 years, but the technique is cumbersome and expensive, and frozen blood should be used sparingly. The major application is for the purpose of maintaining a supply of rare blood types. Patients with such types may donate units for autologous transfusion should the need arise. Frozen red cells are also occasionally needed for patients with severe leukoagglutinin reactions or anaphylactic reactions to plasma proteins, since frozen blood has essentially all white blood cells and plasma components removed.

(5) Autologous packed red blood cells—Patients scheduled for elective surgery may donate blood for autologous transfusion. These units may be stored for up to 35 days.

Compatibility Testing

Before transfusion, the recipient's and the donor's blood are cross-matched to avoid hemolytic transfusion reactions. Although many antigen systems are present on red blood cells, only the ABO and Rh systems are specifically tested prior to all transfusions. The A and B antigens are the most important, because everyone who lacks one or both red cell antigens has isoantibodies against the missing antigen or antigens in his or her plasma. These antibodies activate complement and can cause rapid intravascular lysis of the incompatible red cells. In emergencies, type O blood can be given to any recipient, but only packed cells should be given to avoid transfusion of donor plasma containing anti-A or anti-B antibodies.

The other important antigen routinely tested for is the D antigen of the Rh system. Approximately 15% of the population lack this antigen. In patients lacking the antigen, anti-D antibodies are not naturally present, but the antigen is highly immunogenic. A recipient whose red cells lack D and who receives D-positive blood may develop anti-D antibodies that can cause severe lysis of subsequent transfusions of D-positive red cells.

Blood typing includes assay of recipient serum for unusual antibodies by mixing the serum with panels of red cells representing commonly occurring weak antigens. The screening is particularly important if the recipient has had previous transfusions.

Hemolytic Transfusion Reactions

The most severe reactions are those involving mismatches in the ABO system. Most of these cases are due to clerical errors and mislabeled specimens. Hemolysis is rapid and intravascular, releasing free hemoglobin into the plasma. The severity of these reactions depends on the dose of red blood cells given. The most severe reactions are those seen in surgical patients under anesthesia.

Hemolytic transfusion reactions caused by minor antigen systems are typically less severe. The hemolysis usually takes place at a slower rate and is extravascular. Sometimes these transfusion reactions may be delayed for 5–10 days after transfusion. In such cases, the recipient has received blood containing an immunogenic action, and in the time since transfusion, a new alloantibody has been formed. The most common antigens involved in such reactions are Duffy, Kidd, Kell, and C and E loci of the Rh system.

A. SYMPTOMS AND SIGNS

Major hemolytic transfusion reactions cause fever and chills, with backache and headache. In severe cases, there may be apprehension, dyspnea, hypotension, and vascular collapse. *The transfusion must be stopped immediately.* In severe cases, disseminated intravascular coagulation, acute renal failure from tubular necrosis, or both can occur.

Patients under general anesthesia will not give such signs, and the first indication may be generalized bleeding and oliguria.

B. LABORATORY FINDINGS AND MANAGEMENT

Identification of the recipient and of the blood should be checked. The donor transfusion bag with its pilot tube must be returned to the blood bank, and a fresh sample of the recipient's blood must accompany the donor bag for retyping of donor and recipient blood samples and for repeat of the cross-match.

The hematocrit will fail to rise by the expected amount. Coagulation studies may reveal evidence of renal failure and disseminated intravascular coagulation. Hemoglobinemia will turn the plasma pink and eventually result in hemoglobinuria. In cases of delayed hemolytic reactions, the hematocrit will fall and the indirect bilirubin will rise. In these cases, the new offending alloantibody is easily detected in the patient's serum.

C. TREATMENT

If a hemolytic transfusion reaction is suspected, the transfusion should be stopped at once. A sample of anticoagulated blood from the recipient should be centrifuged to detect free hemoglobin in the plasma. If hemoglobinemia is present, the patient should be vigorously hydrated to prevent acute tubular necrosis. Forced diuresis with mannitol may help prevent renal damage.

Leukoagglutinin Reactions

Most transfusion reactions are not hemolytic but represent reactions to antigens present on white blood cells in patients who have been sensitized to the antigens through previous transfusions or pregnancy. Most commonly, patients will develop fever and chills within 12 hours after transfusion. In severe cases, cough and dyspnea may occur and the chest x-ray may show transient pulmonary infiltrates. Because no hemolysis is involved, the hematocrit rises by the expected amount despite the reaction.

Leukoagglutinin reactions may respond to acetaminophen and diphenhydramine; corticosteroids are also of value. Removal of leukocytes by filtration before blood storage will reduce the incidence of these reactions.

Anaphylactic Reactions

Rarely, patients will develop urticaria or bronchospasm during a transfusion. These reactions are almost always due to plasma proteins rather than white blood cells. Patients who are IgA-deficient may develop these reactions because of antibodies to IgA. Patients with such reactions may require transfusion of washed or even frozen red blood cells to avoid future severe reactions.

Contaminated Blood

Rarely, blood is contaminated with gram-negative bacteria. Transfusion can lead to septicemia and shock from endotoxin. If this is suspected, the offending unit should be cultured and the patient treated with antibiotics as indicated.

Diseases Transmitted Through Transfusion

Despite the use of only volunteer blood donors and the routine screening of blood, transfusion-associated viral diseases remain a problem. All blood products (red blood cells, platelets, plasma, cryoprecipitate) can transmit viral diseases. All blood donors are screened with questionnaires designed to detect donors at high risk of transmitting diseases. All blood is now screened for hepatitis B surface antigen, antibody to hepatitis B core antigen, syphilis, p24 antigen and antibody to HIV, antibody to HCV, and antibody to HTLV.

With improved screening, the risk of posttransfusion hepatitis has steadily decreased. The risk of hepatitis B is 1:200,000 per unit and of HIV 1:250,000 per unit. The risk of seroconversion to HTLV is 1:70,000, but clinical sequelae when this occurs are rare. The major infectious risk of blood products is hepatitis C, with a seroconversion rate of 1:3300 per unit transfused. Most of these cases are clinically silent, but there is a high incidence of chronic hepatitis.

Platelet Transfusion

Platelet transfusions are indicated in cases of thrombocytopenia due to decreased platelet production. They are not useful in immune thrombocytopenia, since transfused platelets will last no longer than the patient's endogenous platelets. The risk of spontaneous bleeding rises when the platelet count falls to less than 10,000/μL, and the risk of life-threatening bleeding increases when the platelet count is less than 5000/μL. Because of this, prophylactic platelet transfusions are often given at these very low levels. Platelet transfusions are also given prior to invasive procedures or surgery, and the goal should be to raise the platelet count to over 50,000/μL.

Platelets are most commonly derived from donated blood units. One unit of platelets (derived from 1 unit of blood) usually contains $5-7 \times 10^{10}$ platelets suspended in 35 mL of plasma. Ideally, 1 platelet unit will raise the recipient's platelet count by 10,000/μL, and transfused platelets will last for 2 or 3 days. However, responses are often suboptimal, with poor platelet increments and short survival times. This may be due to sepsis, splenomegaly, or alloimmunization. Most alloantibodies causing platelet destruction are directed at HLA antigens. Patients requiring long periods of platelet transfusion support should be monitored to document adequate responses to transfusions so that the most appropriate product can be used. Patients may benefit from HLA-matched platelets derived from either volunteer donors or family members, with platelets obtained by plateletpheresis. Techniques of cross-matching platelets have been developed and appear to identify suitable platelet donors (nonreactive with the patient's serum) without the need for HLA typing. Such single-donor platelets usually contain the equivalent of six units of random platelets, or $30-50 \times 10^{10}$ platelets suspended in 200 mL of plasma. Ideally, these platelet concentrates will raise the recipient's platelet count by 60,000/μL. Leukocyte depletion of platelets has been shown to delay the onset of alloimmunization.

Granulocyte Transfusions

Granulocyte transfusions are seldom indicated and have largely been replaced by the use of myeloid growth factors (G-CSF and GM-CSF) that speed neutrophil recovery. However, they may be beneficial in patients with profound neutropenia (< 100/μL) who have gram-negative sepsis or progressive soft tissue infection despite optimal antibiotic therapy. In these cases, it is clear that progressive infection is due to failure of host defenses. In such situations, daily granulocyte transfusions should be given and continued until the neutrophil count rises to above 500/μL. Such granulocytes must be derived from ABO-matched donors. Although HLA matching is not necessary, it is preferred, since patients with alloantibodies to donor white blood cells will have severe reactions and no benefit.

The donor cells usually contain some immunocompetent lymphocytes capable of producing graft-versus-host disease in HLA-incompatible hosts whose immunocompetence may be impaired. Irradiation of the units of cells with 1500 cGy will destroy the lymphocytes without harm to the granulocytes or platelets.

Goodnough LT: Transfusion medicine. (Two parts.) N Engl J Med 1999;340:438, 525. [PMID: 9971869 and 10021474]

Kuter DJ et al: Thrombopoietin therapy increases platelet yields in healthy platelet donors. Blood 2001;98:1339. [PMID: 11520780]

Schiffer CA et al: Platelet transfusion for patients with cancer: clinical practice guidelines of the American Society of Clinical Oncology. J Clin Oncol 2001;19:1519.

TRANSFUSION OF PLASMA COMPONENTS

Fresh-frozen plasma is available in units of approximately 200 mL. Fresh plasma contains normal levels of all coagulation factors (about 1 unit/mL). Fresh frozen plasma is used to correct coagulation factor deficiencies and to treat thrombotic thrombocytopenic purpura. The risk of transmitting viral disease is comparable to that associated with transfusion of red blood cells.

Cryoprecipitate is made from fresh plasma. One unit has a volume of approximately 20 mL and contains approximately 250 mg of fibrinogen and between 80 and 100 units of factor VIII and von Willebrand factor. Cryoprecipitate is used to supplement fibrinogen in cases of congenital deficiency of fibrinogen or disseminated intravascular coagulation. One unit of cryoprecipitate will raise the fibrinogen level by about 8 mg/dL.

Alimentary Tract

14

Kenneth R. McQuaid, MD

See www.current-med.com/ch14.html

■ SYMPTOMS & SIGNS OF GASTROINTESTINAL DISEASE

DYSPEPSIA

A recent working team defines dyspepsia as pain or discomfort centered in the upper abdomen. The discomfort may be characterized by or associated with upper abdominal fullness, early satiety, burning, bloating, belching, nausea, retching, or vomiting. Heartburn (retrosternal burning) should be distinguished from dyspepsia. Patients with dyspepsia often have heartburn as an additional symptom. When heartburn is the dominant complaint, gastroesophageal reflux is nearly always present and should be distinguished from dyspepsia. Dyspepsia occurs in one-fourth of the adult population and accounts for 3% of general medical office visits.

Etiology

A. FOOD OR DRUG INTOLERANCE

Acute, self-limited "indigestion" may be caused by overeating, eating too quickly, eating high-fat foods, eating during stressful situations, or drinking too much alcohol or coffee. Many medications cause dyspepsia, including aspirin, NSAIDs, antibiotics (metronidazole, macrolides), corticosteroids, digoxin, theophylline, iron, and narcotics.

B. LUMINAL GASTROINTESTINAL TRACT DYSFUNCTION

Peptic ulcer disease is present in 15–25% of patients with dyspepsia. Gastroesophageal reflux disease is present in up to 20% of patients with dyspepsia, even without significant heartburn. Gastric cancer is identified in 1% but is rare in persons under age 45. Other causes include gastroparesis (especially in diabetes mellitus), lactose intolerance or malabsorptive conditions, and parasitic infection (giardia, strongyloides).

C. *HELICOBACTER PYLORI* INFECTION

Chronic gastric infection with *H pylori* as a cause of dyspepsia remains controversial. Without peptic ulcer disease, the prevalence of *H pylori*-associated chronic gastritis is 30–60%, the same as the general population. *H pylori* eradication treatment seldom helps.

D. PANCREATIC DISEASE

Pancreatic carcinoma, chronic pancreatitis.

E. BILIARY TRACT DISEASE

The abrupt onset of epigastric or right upper quadrant pain due to cholelithiasis or choledocholithiasis should be readily distinguished from dyspepsia.

F. OTHER CONDITIONS

Diabetes, thyroid disease, renal insufficiency, myocardial ischemia, intraabdominal malignancy, gastric volvulus or paraesophageal hernia, and pregnancy are sometimes accompanied by dyspepsia.

G. FUNCTIONAL OR "NONULCER" DYSPEPSIA

This is the most common cause of chronic dyspepsia. Up to two-thirds of patients have no obvious organic cause for their symptoms after evaluation. Symptoms may arise from a complex interaction of increased visceral afferent sensitivity, gastric delayed emptying or impaired accommodation to food, or psychosocial stressors. While benign, these symptoms may be chronic and difficult to treat.

Clinical Findings

A. SYMPTOMS AND SIGNS

Given the nonspecific nature of dyspeptic symptoms, the history has limited diagnostic utility. It should clarify the chronicity, location, and quality of the discomfort. Concomitant weight loss, persistent vomiting, dysphagia, hematemesis, or melena warrant endoscopy or abdominal imaging. Potentially offending medications and excessive alcohol use should be identified and discontinued if possible. The patient's reason for seeking care should be determined. Many patients report a fear of a serious underlying condition. Recent changes in employment, marital discord, physical and sexual abuse, anxiety, and depression may all contribute to the development and reporting of symptoms.

The symptom profile alone does not differentiate between nonulcer dyspepsia and peptic ulcer disease. Nevertheless, patients with peptic ulcer disease are more likely to be older (> 45 years), to smoke, and to have pain relieved by food or antacids. Patients with nonulcer dyspepsia are younger, report a variety of abdominal and extragastrointestinal complaints, show signs of anxiety or depression, or have a history of use of psychotropic medications.

The physical examination is rarely helpful. Signs of serious organic disease such as weight loss, organomegaly, abdominal mass, or fecal occult blood are further evaluated. In patients over age 45, initial laboratory work should include a blood count, electrolytes, liver enzymes, calcium, and thyroid function tests.

B. SPECIAL EXAMINATIONS

Upper endoscopy is the study of choice to diagnose gastroduodenal ulcers, erosive esophagitis, and upper gastrointestinal malignancy. Upper gastrointestinal barium radiography is inferior to endoscopy for the evaluation of dyspepsia.

The optimal cost-effective approach to dyspepsia is controversial. Upper endoscopy is indicated in all patients over age 45 years with new-onset dyspepsia and in all patients with weight loss, dysphagia, recurrent vomiting, evidence of bleeding, or anemia. It is also helpful for patients who are concerned about serious underlying disease.

Recognition of the role of *H pylori* in peptic ulcer disease has altered the approach to younger patients with uncomplicated dyspepsia, in whom gastric cancer is rare. Consensus guidelines recommend an initial noninvasive test for *H pylori* (IgG serology, fecal antigen test, or urea breath test) in most young, uncomplicated patients with dyspepsia. If negative in a patient not taking NSAIDs, peptic ulcer disease is virtually excluded. The majority of these *H pylori*-negative patients have functional dyspepsia or atypical gastroesophageal reflux disease and can be treated with an antisecretory agent (H_2 antagonist or proton pump inhibitor) for 2–4 weeks. If symptoms fail to respond or rapidly recur after stopping treatment, endoscopy is recommended. In patients testing positive for *H pylori*, antibiotic therapy proves definitive for over 90% of peptic ulcers and may improve symptoms in a small subset (4–9%) of infected patients with functional dyspepsia. Endoscopic evaluation is warranted when symptoms fail to respond.

Abdominal ultrasonography is performed only when pancreatic or biliary tract disease is suspected. Gastric emptying studies are valuable only in patients with recurrent vomiting. Ambulatory esophageal pH testing may be of value when atypical gastroesophageal reflux is suspected.

Treatment of Functional Dyspepsia

In patients with functional dyspepsia, the following should be considered.

A. GENERAL MEASURES

A stable physician-patient interaction is the most important aspect of therapy. Patients require reassurance that the condition is not serious but may be chronic. Alcohol and caffeine intake should be reduced or discontinued. A food diary, in which patients record their food intake, symptoms, and daily events, may reveal dietary or psychosocial precipitants of pain.

B. PHARMACOLOGIC AGENTS

One-third of patients derive relief from placebo. Antisecretory therapy for 2–4 weeks with either H_2-receptor antagonists (ranitidine or nizatidine, 150 mg twice daily; famotidine, 20 mg twice daily; or cimetidine, 400–800 mg twice daily) or proton pump inhibitors (omeprazole or rabeprazole 20 mg, lansoprazole 30 mg, or pantoprazole 40 mg) may benefit 10–20% of patients, particularly those with dyspepsia and heartburn ("reflux-like dyspepsia") or epigastric pain. Superiority of proton pump inhibitors to H_2-antagonists has not been established. Low doses of antidepressants (eg, desipramine or nortriptyline, 10–50 mg at bedtime) are believed to benefit some patients, possibly by moderating visceral afferent sensitivity. However, side effects are common and response is patient-specific. Doses should be increased slowly. Prokinetic agents (cisapride or metoclopramide, 10 mg three times daily) improve symptoms in up to 60%. Symptomatic improvement does not correlate with the presence or absence of gastric emptying delay. However, owing to their side effects, neither agent is recommended for treatment of functional dyspepsia. Cisapride has been withdrawn from the market by the manufacturer in the United States as a result of its association with life-threatening ventricular arrhythmias. Long-term metoclopramide use is associated with a high incidence of neuropsychiatric side effects.

C. ANTI-*H PYLORI* TREATMENT

A meta-analysis has suggested that a small number of patients (5–15%) may derive benefit from *H pylori* eradication therapy.

Alpers D: Why should psychotherapy be a useful approach to management of patients with nonulcer dyspepsia? Gastroenterology 2000;119:869. [PMID: 10982781] (Patients with refractory nonulcer dyspepsia, have a high prevalence of depression, anxiety disorders, hypochondriasis, physical and sexual abuse, and health care-seeking behavior.)

American Gastroenterological Association medical position statement: evaluation of dyspepsia. Gastroenterology 1998; 114:579. [PMID: 9496949] (An evidenced-based review of evaluation and management of dyspepsia.)

Moayyedi P et al: Effect of population screening and treatment for *Helicobacter pylori* on dyspepsia and quality of life in the community: a randomized controlled trial. Lancet 2000; 355:1655. [PMID: 10905240] (Screening and empirical treatment for *H pylori* is marginally cost-effective for patients under age 45–50 without impact upon quality of life.)

Moayyedi P et al: Systematic review and economic evaluation of *Helicobacter pylori* eradication treatment for non-ulcer dyspepsia. BMJ 2000;321:659. [PMID: 10987767]

Soo S et al: Pharmacological interventions for non-ulcer dyspepsia. Cochrane Database Syst Rev 2000;2:CD001960. [PMID: 10796840]

Talley NJ et al: Functional gastroduodenal disorders. Gut 1999;45(Suppl 2):II37. [PMID: 10457043] (Concise summary of criteria for functional disorders, including functional dyspepsia.)

NAUSEA & VOMITING

Nausea is a vague, intensely disagreeable sensation of sickness or "queasiness" that may or may not be followed by vomiting and is distinguished from anorexia. Vomiting often follows, as does retching (spasmodic respiratory and abdominal movements). Vomiting should be distinguished from regurgitation, the effortless reflux of liquid or food stomach contents; and from rumination, the chewing and swallowing of food that is regurgitated volitionally after meals.

The medullary vomiting center may be stimulated by four different sources of afferent input: (1) Afferent vagal fibers (rich in serotonin 5-HT$_3$ receptors) and splanchnic fibers from the gastrointestinal viscera; these may be stimulated by biliary or gastrointestinal distention, mucosal or peritoneal irritation, or infections. (2) Fibers of the vestibular system, which have high concentrations of histamine H$_1$ and muscarinic cholinergic receptors. (3) Higher central nervous system centers; here, certain sights, smells, or emotional experiences may induce vomiting. For example, patients receiving chemotherapy may develop vomiting in anticipation of its administration. (4) The chemoreceptor trigger zone, located outside the blood-brain barrier in the area postrema of the medulla, which may be stimulated by drugs and chemotherapeutic agents, toxins, hypoxia, uremia, acidosis, and radiation therapy. Although the causes of vomiting are many, a simplified list is provided in Table 14–1.

Complications of vomiting include dehydration, hypokalemia, metabolic alkalosis, aspiration, rupture of the esophagus (Boerhaave's syndrome), and bleeding secondary to a mucosal tear at the gastroesophageal junction (Mallory-Weiss syndrome).

Clinical Findings

A. SYMPTOMS AND SIGNS

Acute symptoms without abdominal pain are typically caused by food poisoning, infectious gastroenteritis, or drugs. Inquiry should be made into recent changes in medications, diet, other intestinal symptoms, or similar illnesses in family members. The acute onset of severe pain and vomiting suggests peritoneal irritation, acute gastric or intestinal obstruction, or pancreaticobiliary disease. Examination may reveal fever, focal tenderness or rigidity, guarding, or rebound tenderness. Persistent vomiting suggests pregnancy, gastric outlet obstruction, gastroparesis, intestinal dysmotility, psychogenic disorders, and central nervous system or systemic disorders. Vomiting immediately after meals strongly suggests bulimia or psychogenic causes. Vomiting of undigested food one to several hours after meals is characteristic of gastroparesis or a gastric outlet obstruction; physical examination may reveal a succussion splash. Patients with acute or chronic symptoms should be asked about neurologic symptoms such as headaches, stiff neck, vertigo, and focal paresthesias or weakness.

B. SPECIAL EXAMINATIONS

In vomiting of acute onset, flat and upright abdominal radiographs are obtained in patients with severe pain or suspicion of mechanical obstruction to look for free intraperitoneal air or dilated loops of small bowel. If mechanical small intestinal or gastric obstruction is thought likely, a nasogastric tube is placed for relief of symptoms. Aspiration of more than 200 mL of residual material in a fasting patient suggests obstruction or gastroparesis. This may be confirmed by a saline load test showing more than 400 mL residual on gastric aspiration performed 30 minutes after nasogastric instillation of 750 mL of 0.9% saline. The cause of gastric outlet obstruction is best demonstrated by upper endoscopy. Gastroparesis is confirmed by nuclear scintigraphic studies, which show delayed gastric emptying and either upper endoscopy or barium upper GI series showing no evidence of mechanical gastric outlet obstruction. Abnormal liver function tests or elevated amylase suggests pancreaticobiliary disease, which may be investigated with an abdominal sonogram or CT scan.

Treatment

A. GENERAL MEASURES

Most causes of acute vomiting are mild, self-limited, and require no specific treatment. Patients should ingest clear liquids (broths, tea, soups, carbonated beverages) and small quantities of dry foods (soda crackers). For more severe acute vomiting, hospitalization may be required. Owing to inability to eat and loss of gastric fluids, patients may become dehydrated and develop hypokalemia with metabolic alkalosis. Intravenous 0.45% saline solution with 20 meq/L of potassium chloride is given in most cases to maintain hydration. A nasogastric suction tube for gastric decompression improves patient comfort and permits monitoring of fluid loss.

B. ANTIEMETIC MEDICATIONS

Medications may be given either to prevent or to control vomiting (see above). Combinations of drugs from different classes may provide better control of symptoms with less toxicity in some patients. All of these medications should be avoided in pregnancy. (For dosages, see Table 14–2.)

1. Serotonin 5-HT$_3$ receptor antagonists—Ondansetron, granisetron, and dolasetron, when initiated

Table 14-1. Causes of nausea and vomiting.

Visceral afferent stimulation	**Mechanical obstruction** Gastric outlet obstruction: peptic ulcer disease, malignancy; gastric volvulus Small intestinal obstruction: adhesions, hernias, volvulus, Crohn's disease, carcinomatosis **Dysmotility** Gastroparesis: diabetic, medications, postviral, postvagotomy Small intestine: scleroderma, amyloidosis, chronic intestinal pseudo-obstruction, familial myoneuropathies **Peritoneal irritation** Peritonitis: perforated viscus, appendicitis, spontaneous bacterial peritonitis **Infections** Viral gastroenteritis: Norwalk agent, rotavirus "Food poisoning": toxins from *B cereus, S aureus, C perfringens* Hepatitis A or B Acute systemic infections **Hepatobiliary or pancreatic disorders** Acute pancreatitis Cholecystitis or choledocholithiasis **Topical gastrointestinal irritants** Alcohol, NSAIDs, oral antibiotics **Other** Cardiac disease: acute myocardial infarction, congestive heart failure Urologic disease: stones, pyelonephritis
Central nervous system disorders	**Vestibular disorders** Labyrinthitis, Meniere's syndrome, motion sickness, migraine **Increased intracranial pressure** CNS tumors, subdural or subarachnoid hemorrhage **Infections** Meningitis, encephalitis **Psychogenic** Anticipatory vomiting, bulimia, psychiatric disorders
Irritation of chemoreceptor trigger zone	**Antitumor chemotherapy** **Drugs and Medications** Alcohol Calcium channel blockers Opioids **Radiation therapy** **Systemic disorders** Diabetic ketoacidosis Uremia Adrenocortical crisis Parathyroid disease Hypothyroidism Pregnancy Paraneoplastic syndrome

prior to treatment, are effective in the prevention of chemotherapy-induced emesis. Single-dose administration schedules are as effective as multiple-dose regimens. The serotonin antagonists are also effective for the treatment of postoperative nausea and vomiting.

2. Dopamine antagonists—The phenothiazines, butyrophenones, and substituted benzamides have antiemetic properties which are due to dopaminergic blockade as well as to their sedative effects. High doses of these agents are associated with antidopaminergic side effects, including extrapyramidal reactions and

Table 14–2. Common antiemetic dosing regimens.

	Dosage	Route
Serotonin 5-HT₃ antagonists		
Ondansetron	8 mg or 0.15 mg/kg once daily	IV
	8 mg twice daily	PO
Granisetron	1 mg or 0.01 mg/kg once daily	IV
	2 mg once daily	PO
Dolasetron	100 mg or 1.8 mg/kg once daily	IV
	100–200 mg once daily	PO
Corticosteroids		
Dexamethasone	8–20 mg once	IV
	4–20 mg once or twice daily	PO
Methylprednisolone	40–100 mg once	IV
Dopamine receptor antagonists		
Metoclopramide	10–30 mg or 0.5 mg/kg every 6–8 hours	IV
	10–20 mg every 6–8 hours	PO
Prochlorperazine	5–20 mg every 4–6 hours	PO, IM, IV
	25 mg suppository every 6 hours	PR
Promethazine	25 mg every 4–6 hours	PO, PR, IM
Droperidol	1–2.5 mg every 4–6 hours	IV
Sedatives		
Diazepam	2–5 mg every 4–6 hours	PO, IV
Lorazepam	1–2 mg every 4–6 hours	PO, IV

depression. These agents are used in a variety of situations. Cases of QT prolongation leading to ventricular tachycardia (torsade de pointes) have been reported in several patients receiving droperidol. Electrocardiographic monitoring should be performed before and for 2–3 hours after injection. Droperidol should not be administered to patients with known QT prolongation.

3. Antihistamines and anticholinergics—These drugs (eg, meclizine, dimenhydrinate, transdermal scopolamine) may be valuable in the prevention of vomiting arising from stimulation of the labyrinth, ie, motion sickness, vertigo, and migraines. They may induce drowsiness.

4. Sedatives—Benzodiazepines are used in psychogenic and anticipatory vomiting.

5. Corticosteroids—The combination of corticosteroids and serotonin receptor antagonists provides the best antiemetic protection with a low incidence of adverse effects for the prevention and treatment of chemotherapy-associated nausea and vomiting.

6. Cannabinoids—Marijuana has been used widely as an appetite stimulant and antiemetic. Pure Δ^9-tetrahydrocannabinol (THC) is the major active ingredient in marijuana and is available by prescription as dronabinol. In doses of 5–15 mg/m², oral dronabinol is effective in treating nausea associated with chemotherapy, but it is associated with central nervous system side effects in most patients.

American Gastroenterological Association Medical Position Statement: Nausea and Vomiting. Gastroenterology 2001; 120:261. [PMID: 11208735]

Graumlich J et al: Pharmaceutical care of postoperative nausea and vomiting: balanced scorecard and outcomes. Pharmacotherapy 2000;20:1365. [PMID: 11079285]

Hornbuckle K et al: The diagnosis and work-up of the patient with gastroparesis. J Clin Gastroenterol 2000;30:117. [PMID: 10730917]

Rabine J et al: Management of the patient with gastroparesis. J Clin Gastroenterol 2001;32:11. [PMID: 11154162]

HICCUPS (Singultus)

Though usually a benign and self-limited annoyance, hiccups may be persistent and a sign of serious underlying illness. In patients being maintained on mechanical ventilation, hiccups can trigger a full respiratory cycle and result in respiratory alkalosis.

Causes of benign, self-limited hiccups include gastric distention (carbonated beverages, air swallowing, overeating), sudden temperature changes (hot then cold liquids, hot then cold shower), alcohol ingestion, and states of heightened emotion (excitement, stress, laughing). There are over 100 causes of recurrent or persistent hiccups, grouped into the following categories:

(1) Central nervous system: Neoplasms, infections, cerebrovascular accident, trauma.

(2) Metabolic: Uremia, hypocapnia (hyperventilation).

(3) Irritation of the vagus or phrenic nerve: (a) Head, neck: Foreign body in ear, goiter, neoplasms. (b) Thorax: Pneumonia, empyema, neoplasms, myocardial infarction, pericarditis, aneurysm, esophageal obstruction, reflux esophagitis. (c) Abdomen: Subphrenic abscess, hepatomegaly, hepatitis, cholecystitis, gastric distention, gastric neoplasm, pancreatitis, or pancreatic malignancy.

(4) Surgical: General anesthesia, postoperative.

(5) Psychogenic and idiopathic.

Clinical Findings

Evaluation of the patient with persistent hiccups should include a detailed neurologic examination, serum creatinine, liver chemistry tests, and a chest radiograph. When the cause remains unclear, CT of the head, chest, and abdomen, echocardiography, bronchoscopy, and upper endoscopy may help. On occasion, hiccups may be unilateral; chest fluoroscopy will make the diagnosis.

Treatment

A number of simple remedies may be helpful in patients with acute benign hiccups. (1) Irritation of the nasopharynx by tongue traction, lifting the uvula with a spoon, catheter stimulation of the nasopharynx, and eating 1 tsp of dry granulated sugar. (2) Interruption of the respiratory cycle by breath holding, Valsalva's maneuver, sneezing, gasping (fright stimulus), or rebreathing into a bag. (3) Stimulation of the vagus, carotid massage. (4) Irritation of the diaphragm by holding knees to chest or by continuous positive airway pressure during mechanical ventilation. (5) Relief of gastric distention by belching or insertion of a nasogastric tube.

A number of drugs have been promoted as being useful in the treatment of hiccups. Chlorpromazine, 25–50 mg orally or intramuscularly, is most commonly used. Other agents reported to be effective include anticonvulsants (phenytoin, carbamazepine), benzodiazepines (lorazepam, diazepam), metoclopramide, baclofen, and occasionally general anesthesia.

Friedman L: Hiccups: a treatment review. Pharmacotherapy 1996;16:986. [PMID: 8946969]

Petroianu G et al: Idiopathic chronic hiccup: Combination therapy with cisapride, omeprazole, and baclofen. Clin Ther 1997;19:1031. [PMID: 9385490]

CONSTIPATION

The first step in evaluating the patient is to determine what is meant by "constipation." In the general population, the "normal" frequency of bowel movements is broad, ranging from three to twelve per week. The complaint may reflect a mistaken perception of what constitutes a normal bowel pattern. Constipation is present when a patient has two or fewer bowel movements per week or excessive difficulty and straining at defecation. The many causes of constipation may be classified as discussed below and summarized in Table 14–3.

Common Identifiable Causes of Constipation

A. POOR DIETARY AND BEHAVIORAL HABITS

The majority of constipated patients have mild symptoms that cannot be attributed to any structural abnormalities, intestinal motility disorders, or systemic disease. Dietary review will reveal that most of these patients do not consume adequate fiber and fluids. Ingestion of 10–12 g of fiber per day either by dietary changes or the addition or commercial fiber supplementation is often all that is needed. At least one or two glasses of fluid should be taken with meals. The elderly are predisposed because of poor eating habits, a variety of medications, decreased colonic motility, and, in some cases, inability to sit on a toilet (bedbound patients).

Table 14–3. Causes of constipation in adults.

Most common
  Inadequate fiber or fluid intake
  Poor bowel habits
Systemic disease
  Endocrine: hypothyroidism, hyperparathyroidism, diabetes mellitus
  Metabolic: hypokalemia, hypercalcemia, uremia, porphyria
  Neurologic: Parkinson's, multiple sclerosis, sacral nerve damage (prior pelvic surgery, tumor), paraplegia, autonomic neuropathy
Medications
  Narcotics
  Diuretics
  Calcium channel blockers
  Anticholinergics
  Psychotropic
  Calcium and iron supplements
  NSAIDs
  Clonidine
  Sucralfate
  Cholestyramine
Structural abnormalities
  Anorectal: rectal prolapse, rectocoele, rectal intussusception, anorectal stricture, anal fissure, solitary rectal ulcer syndrome
  Perineal descent
  Colonic mass with obstruction: adenocarcinoma
  Colonic stricture: radiation, ischemia, diverticulosis
  Hirschsprung's disease
  Idiopathic megarectum
Slow colonic transit
  Idiopathic: isolated to colon
  Psychogenic
  Eating disorders
  Chronic intestinal pseudo-obstruction
Pelvic floor dysfunction
Irritable bowel syndrome

B. STRUCTURAL ABNORMALITIES

Colonic lesions that obstruct fecal passage must be excluded in patients with constipation. Particular concern is raised in patients with lifelong constipation (Hirschsprung's disease) and patients over age 50 with new-onset constipation, progressive thinning of stool, or associated weight loss or hematochezia (suggesting colon carcinoma).

C. SYSTEMIC DISEASES

Medical diseases can cause constipation due to neurologic gut dysfunction, myopathies, endocrine disorders, and electrolyte abnormalities such as hypercalcemia or hypokalemia.

D. MEDICATIONS

Anticholinergic and opioid agents are common causes of constipation.

Causes of Severe or Refractory Constipation

Patients whose constipation cannot be attributed to the above causes and who do not respond to conservative dietary management present difficult management problems. Conceptually, these patients can be divided into three classes.

A. SLOW COLONIC TRANSIT

Normal colonic transit time is approximately 35 hours; more than 72 hours is significantly abnormal. Colonic inertia is more common in women, some of whom have a history of psychosocial problems or sexual abuse. It may be part of a more generalized gastrointestinal dysmotility syndrome or may be attributable to years of cathartic use.

B. PELVIC FLOOR DYSFUNCTION (OUTLET DISORDERS)

Patients with disorders of the rectum or pelvic floor—women more often than men—may have difficulty in moving stool out of the rectum. They may complain of excessive straining with a sense of incomplete evacuation, the need for digital pressure on the vagina or perineum, or even the need for digital disimpaction. Defecatory difficulties can be due to a variety of anatomic problems that impede or obstruct flow, some of which may benefit from surgery.

C. IRRITABLE BOWEL SYNDROME

Patients with primary complaints of abdominal pain, bloating, or a sense of incomplete evacuation may have irritable bowel syndrome. (See below.)

Evaluation

A. INITIAL MANAGEMENT

All patients should undergo a history and physical examination, including stool testing for occult blood. Laboratory studies should include a complete blood count, serum electrolytes including calcium, and serum TSH. In otherwise healthy patients with mild symptoms who are under age 50, a trial of fiber is reasonable. In patients over age 50, those who have failed conservative treatment, or those with anemia or occult blood in the stools, colonoscopy or flexible sigmoidoscopy and barium enema are obtained. Patients without structural, medical, or neurologic disease can be treated initially with fiber supplementation (and osmotic laxatives, if needed).

B. SECOND LEVEL OF INVESTIGATION

Patients with refractory constipation not responding to conservative measures may require further investigation by means of colonic transit and pelvic floor function studies.

Standard Treatment of Chronic Constipation

A. DIETARY MEASURES

Proper dietary fluid and fiber intake should be emphasized. Fiber may be given by means of dietary alterations or fiber supplements (Table 14–4). Increased dietary fiber may cause temporary distention or flatulence, which often diminishes over several days. Response to fiber therapy is not immediate, and increases in dosage should be made gradually over 7–10 day. Whereas fiber may benefit the majority of patients, it normally does not benefit patients with severe colonic inertia or outlet disorders.

B. STOOL SURFACTANT AGENTS

Docusate sodium, 50–200 mg/d, or mineral oil, 14–45 mL/d, may be given orally or rectally to promote softening of stools. Aspiration of mineral oil can cause lipoid pneumonia.

C. OSMOTIC LAXATIVES

These agents, used to soften stools, may be given alone or in combination with fiber supplements (Table 14–4). They are commonly employed in older nonambulatory patients to prevent constipation and fecal impaction. They are safe and are titrated to a dose that results in soft to semiliquid stools. The less expensive saline laxatives should be tried first before using more expensive osmotic agents, such as nonabsorbable carbohydrates or polyethylene glycol solution.

D. SALINE LAXATIVES

Magnesium-containing saline laxatives (milk of magnesia, magnesium sulfate) are the most commonly used agents for the prevention and treatment of chronic constipation. These agents should not be used in patients with renal insufficiency. Sodium phosphate or magnesium citrate may be used for aggressive treatment of acute constipation or as a purgative prior to surgical, endoscopic, or radiographic procedures.

E. NONABSORBABLE CARBOHYDRATES

Either sorbitol (70%) or lactulose, 15–30 mL once or twice daily, is efficacious for the prevention or treatment of chronic constipation. These malabsorbed sugars are often limited by their propensity to induce bloating, cramps, and flatulence.

F. POLYETHYLENE GLYCOL SOLUTION

Polyethylene glycol is a component of solutions traditionally used for colonic lavage prior to colonoscopy (CoLyte, GoLYTELY, NuLytely). Polyethylene glycol 3350 powder (Miralax) is now available for the treatment of acute or chronic constipation. Seventeen grams of powder may be mixed in water or juice and taken once or twice daily.

Table 14–4. Pharmacologic management of constipation

Agent	Dosage	Onset of Action	Comments
Fiber laxatives			
Bran powder	1–4 tbsp orally twice daily	Days	Inexpensive. May cause gas, flatulence
Psyllium	1 tsp once or twice daily	Days	(Metamucil; Perdiem)
Methylcellulose	1 tsp once or twice daily	Days	(Citrucel) Less gas, flatulence
Calcium polycarbophil	1 or 2 tablets once or twice	12–24 hours	(FiberCon) Does not cause gas; pill form
Stool surfactants			
Docusate sodium	100 mg once or twice daily	12–72 hours	(Colace) Marginal benefit
Mineral oil	15–45 mL once or twice daily	6–8 hours	May cause lipoid pneumonia, if aspirated
Osmotic laxatives			
Magnesium hydroxide; magnesium sulfate	15–30 mL orally once or twice	3–12 hours	(Milk of magnesia; Epsom salts)
Lactulose or 70% sorbitol	15–60 mL orally once daily to three times daily	24–48 hours	Cramps, bloating flatulence
Polyethylene glycol (PEG 3350)	17 g in 8 oz liquid once or twice daily	3–24 hours	(Miralax) Less bloating than lactulose, sorbitol
Stimulant laxatives			
Bisacodyl	5–15 mg orally as needed	6–8 hours	May cause cramps; avoid daily use, if possible
Bisacodyl	10 mg per rectum as needed	1 hour	
Cascara	4–8 mL or 2 tablets as needed	8–12 hours	(Nature's Remedy); may cause cramps; avoid daily use, if possible
Senna	5–15 mg orally up to three times daily	8–12 hours	(ExLax; Senekot) May cause cramps, avoid daily use, if possible
Enemas			
Tap water	500 mL per rectum	5–15 minutes	
Phosphate enema	120 mL per rectum	5–15 minutes	Commonly used for acute constipation or to induce movement prior to medical procedures
Soapsuds enema	Up to 1500 mL per rectum	5–15 minutes	Impaction
Mineral oil enema	100–250 mL per rectum	Up to hours	To soften and lubricate fecal impaction
Agents used to clean bowel prior to medical procedures			
Polyethylene glycol (PEG)	4 L orally administered over 2–4 hours	<4 hours	(GoLYTELY; CoLYTE; NuLYTE) Used to cleanse bowel before colonoscopy
Sodium phosphate	45 mL in 12 oz water May repeat in 10–12 hours	1–6 hours	Used before colonoscopy.
Magnesium citrate	10 oz	3–6 hours	Lemon-flavored
Combination kits: sodium phosphate and bisacodyl			(Fleet) Commonly used prior to barium enema

G. Stimulant Agents

These agents stimulate fluid secretion and colonic contraction, resulting in a bowel movement within 6–12 hours after oral ingestion or 15–60 minutes after rectal administration. Common preparations include bisacodyl, senna, cascara, and castor oil (Table 14–4). Phenolphthalein has been removed from the market in the United States because of concerns related to carcinogenicity.

Treatment of Fecal Impaction

Severe impaction of stool in the rectal vault may result in obstruction to further fecal flow, leading to partial or complete large bowel obstruction. Predisposing factors include severe psychiatric disease, prolonged bed rest and debility, neurogenic disorders of the colon, and spinal cord disorders. Clinical presentation includes decreased appetite, nausea, and vomiting, and abdominal pain and distention. There may be paradoxical "diarrhea" as liquid stool leaks around the impacted feces. Firm feces are palpable on digital examination of the rectal vault. Initial treatment is directed at relieving the impaction with enemas (saline, mineral oil, or diatrizoate) or digital disruption of the impacted fecal material. Long-term care is directed at maintaining soft stools and regular bowel movements (as above).

American Gastroenterological Association Medical Position Statement: guidelines on constipation. Gastroenterology 2000; 119:1761. [PMID: 11113098]

De Lillo AR et al: Functional bowel disorders in the geriatric patient: constipation, fecal impaction, and fecal incontinence. Am J Gastroenterol 2000;95:901. [PMID: 10763934]

Mertz H et al: Physiology of refractory chronic constipation. Am J Gastroenterol 1999;94:609. [PMID: 10086639] Slow colonic transit and visceral hypersensitivity were most commonly associated with refractory constipation; pelvic floor dysfunction may be overemphasized as a cause of chronic constipation.)

GASTROINTESTINAL GAS

Belching

Belching (eructation) is the involuntary or voluntary release of gas from the stomach or esophagus. It occurs most frequently after meals, when gastric distention results in transient lower esophageal sphincter relaxation. Belching is a normal reflex and does not itself denote gastrointestinal dysfunction. Virtually all stomach gas comes from swallowed air. With each swallow, 2–5 mL of air are ingested, and excessive amounts may result in distention, flatulence, and abdominal pain. This may occur with rapid eating, gum chewing, smoking, and the ingestion of carbonated beverages. Chronic excessive belching is almost always caused by aerophagia, common in anxious individuals and institutionalized patients. Evaluation should be restricted to patients with other complaints such as dysphagia, heartburn, early satiety, or vomiting.

Once patients understand the relationship between aerophagia and belching, most can deal with the problem by behavioral modification. Physical defects that hamper normal swallowing (ill-fitting dentures, nasal obstruction) should be corrected. Antacids and simethicone are of no value.

Flatus

The rate and volume of expulsion of flatus is highly variable. Flatus is derived from two sources: swallowed air and bacterial fermentation of undigested carbohydrate. The majority of swallowed air not belched passes through the gut and leaves as flatus. Swallowed air may contribute up to 500 mL of flatus per day (primarily nitrogen). Bacterial fermentation of undigested carbohydrates leads to the additional production of gas, particularly H_2, CO_2, and methane. The majority of this fermentation takes place in the colon. Under normal circumstances, a small substrate of fermentable substrates reaches the colon. These substances include fructose, lactose, sorbitol, trehalose (mushrooms), raffinose, and stachyose (legumes, cruciferous vegetables). Complex starches and fiber may also cause gas. Gas production may be increased with ingestion of these carbohydrates or with malabsorption.

Determining abnormal from normal amounts of flatus is difficult. An initial trial of a lactose-free diet is recommended. Common gas-producing foods should be reviewed and the patient given an elimination trial. These include beans of all kinds, peas, lentils, broccoli, brussels sprouts, cauliflower, cabbage, parsnips, leeks, onions, beer, and coffee. Foul odor may be caused by garlic, onion, eggplant, mushrooms, and certain herbs and spices. For patients with persistent complaints, fructose, complex starches, and fiber may be eliminated, but such restrictive diets are unacceptable to most patients. Of refined flours, only rice flour is gas-free.

The nonprescription agent Beano (α-D-galactosidase enzyme) reduces gas caused by foods containing raffinose and stachyose, ie, cruciferous vegetables, legumes, nuts, and some cereals. Activated charcoal may afford relief. Simethicone is of no proved benefit.

Complaints of chronic abdominal distention or bloating are common but do not correlate with increased intra-abdominal gas volumes. Many such patients have an underlying functional gastrointestinal disorder such as irritable bowel syndrome or nonulcer dyspepsia.

Levitt M et al: Evaluation of an extremely flatulent patient. Case report and proposed diagnostic and therapeutic approach. Am J Gastroenterol 1998;93:2276. [PMID: 9820415] (Outstanding review by experts in the field.)

Suarez F: Intestinal gas. Clin Perspect Gastroenterol July/August 2000:209.

DIARRHEA

Diarrhea can range in severity from an acute self-limited episode to a severe, life threatening illness. To properly evaluate the complaint, the physician must determine the patient's normal bowel pattern and the nature of the current symptoms.

Approximately 10 L of fluid enter the duodenum daily, of which all but 1.5 L are absorbed by the small intestine. The colon absorbs most of the remaining fluid, with only 100 mL lost in the stool. Diarrhea is defined as a stool weight of more than 250 g/24 h, but quantification of stool weight is necessary only in some patients with chronic diarrhea. In most cases, the physician's working definition of diarrhea is increased stool frequency (more than two or three bowel movements per day) or liquidity of feces.

The causes of diarrhea are myriad. In clinical practice, it is helpful to distinguish acute from chronic diarrhea, as the evaluation and treatment are entirely different (Tables 14–5 and 14–7).

Table 14–5. Causes of acute infectious diarrhea.

Noninflammatory Diarrhea	Inflammatory Diarrhea
Viral	**Viral**
Norwalk virus	Cytomegalovirus
Norwalk-like virus	
Rotavirus	
Protozoal	**Protozoal**
Giardia lamblia	Entamoeba histolytica
Cryptosporidium	
Bacterial	**Bacterial**
1. Preformed enterotoxin production	1. Cytotoxin production
Staphylococcus aureus	Enterohemorrhagic E coli O157:H5 (EHEC)
Bacillus cereus	Vibrio parahaemolyticus
Clostridium perfringens	Clostridium difficile
2. Enterotoxin production	2. Mucosal invasion
Enterotoxigenic E coli (ETEC)	Shigella
Vibrio cholerae	Campylobacter jejuni
	Salmonella
	Enteroinvasive E coli (EIEC)
	Aeromonas
	Plesiomonas
	Yersinia enterocolitica
	Chlamydia
	Neisseria gonorrhoeae
	Listeria monocytogenes

1. Acute Diarrhea

Etiology & Clinical Findings

Diarrhea acute in onset and persisting for less than 3 weeks is most commonly caused by infectious agents, bacterial toxins (either preformed or produced in the gut), or drugs. Similar recent illnesses in family members suggests an infectious origin. Ingestion of improperly stored or prepared food implicates food poisoning. Exposure to unpurified water (camping, swimming) or contaminated produce may result in infection with giardia, cryptosporidium, or cyclospora. Recent travel abroad suggests "traveler's diarrhea" (see Chapter 30). Antibiotic administration within the preceding several weeks increases the likelihood of *Clostridium difficile* colitis. Finally, risk factors for HIV infection or sexually transmitted diseases should be determined. (AIDS-associated diarrhea is discussed in Chapter 31.) Persons practicing unprotected anal intercourse are at risk for a variety of infections that cause proctitis and rectal discharge, including gonorrhea, syphilis, lymphogranuloma venereum, and herpes simplex.

The nature of the diarrhea helps distinguish among different infectious causes (Table 14–5).

A. NONINFLAMMATORY DIARRHEA

Watery, nonbloody diarrhea associated with periumbilical cramps, bloating, nausea, or vomiting suggests a small bowel source caused by either a toxin-producing bacterium (enterotoxigenic *E coli* [ETEC], *Staphylococcus aureus, Bacillus cereus, Clostridium perfringens*) or other agents (viruses, giardia) that disrupt normal absorption and secretory process in the small intestine. Prominent vomiting suggests viral enteritis or *S aureus* food poisoning. Though typically mild, the diarrhea (which originates in the small intestine) can be voluminous and result in dehydration with hypokalemia and metabolic acidosis (eg, cholera). Because tissue invasion does not occur, fecal leukocytes are not present.

B. INFLAMMATORY DIARRHEA

The presence of fever and bloody diarrhea (dysentery) indicates colonic tissue damage caused by invasion (shigellosis, salmonellosis, campylobacter or yersinia infection, amebiasis) or a toxin (*C difficile, E coli* O157:H7). Because these organisms involve predominantly the colon, the diarrhea is small in volume (< 1 L/d) and associated with left lower quadrant cramps, urgency, and tenesmus. Fecal leukocytes usually are present in infections with invasive organisms. *E coli* O157:H7 is a toxigenic noninvasive organism that may be acquired from contaminated meat or unpasteurized apple juice and has resulted in several outbreaks of an acute, often severe hemorrhagic colitis. In immunocompromised and HIV-infected patients, cytomegalovirus can cause intestinal ulceration with watery or bloody diarrhea.

Infectious dysentery must be distinguished from acute ulcerative colitis, which may also present acutely with fever, abdominal pain, and bloody diarrhea. Diarrhea that persists for more than 14 days is not attributable to bacterial pathogens (except for *C difficile*) and should be evaluated as chronic diarrhea.

Evaluation (Figure 14–1)

In over 90% of patients with acute diarrhea, the illness is mild and self-limited, responding within 5 days to simple rehydration therapy or antidiarrheal agents; diagnostic investigation is unnecessary. The isolation rate of bacterial pathogens from stool cultures in patients with acute diarrhea is under 3%. Thus, the goal of initial evaluation is to distinguish patients with mild disease from those with more serious illness. If diarrhea worsens or persists for more than 7–10 days, stool should be sent for fecal leukocyte determination, ovum and parasite evaluation, and bacterial culture.

Prompt medical evaluation is indicated in the following situations: (1) Signs of inflammatory diarrhea manifested by any of the following: fever (> 38.5 °C), bloody diarrhea, or abdominal pain. (2) The passage of six or more unformed stools in 24 hours. (3) Profuse watery diarrhea and dehydration. (4) Frail older patients. (5) Immunocompromised patients (AIDS, posttransplantation).

Physical examination pays note to mental status and the presence of abdominal tenderness or peritonitis. Peritoneal findings may be present in infection with *C difficile* or enterohemorrhagic *E coli*. Hospitalization is required in patients with severe dehydration, toxicity, or marked abdominal pain, and stool specimens should be sent for examination for fecal leukocytes and bacterial cultures (Table 14–6). The rate of positive bacterial cultures in such patients is 60–75%. A stool wet mount examination for amebiasis is performed in sexually active homosexuals, those with a history of recent travel to amebiasis-endemic areas, and those whose bacterial cultures are negative. With a history of antibiotic exposure, a stool sample should be tested for *C difficile* toxin. If *E coli* O157:H7 is suspected, serotyping is indicated. Special culture media are required for yersinia, aeromonas, and plesiomonas. In patients with diarrhea that persists for more than 10 days, three stool examinations for ova and parasites should also be performed. The stool giardia antigen assay is more sensitive than stool microscopy for detection of this organism. Rectal swabs may be sent for culture of chlamydia, *Neisseria gonorrhoeae,* and herpes simplex virus in sexually active patients with suspected proctitis.

Prompt sigmoidoscopy is warranted for symptoms of severe proctitis (tenesmus, discharge, rectal pain) or for suspected *C difficile* colitis patients who appear ill. It may also be helpful in distinguishing infectious diarrhea from ulcerative colitis or ischemic colitis.

Treatment

A. DIET

Most mild diarrhea will not lead to dehydration provided the patient takes adequate oral fluids containing carbohydrates and electrolytes. Patients find it more comfortable to rest the bowel by avoiding high-fiber foods, fats, milk products, caffeine, and alcohol. Frequent feedings of fruit drinks, tea, "flat" carbonated beverages, and soft, easily digested foods (eg, soups, crackers) are encouraged.

B. REHYDRATION

In more severe diarrhea, dehydration can occur quickly, especially in children. Oral rehydration with fluids containing glucose, Na^+, K^+, Cl^-, and bicarbonate or citrate is preferred when feasible. A convenient mixture is ½ tsp salt (3.5 g), 1 tsp baking soda (2.5 g $NaHCO_3$), 8 tsp sugar (40 g), and 8 oz orange juice (1.5 g KCl), diluted to 1 L with water. Alternatively, oral electrolyte solutions (eg, Pedialyte, Gatorade) are readily available. Fluids should be given at rates of 50–200 mL/kg/24 h depending on the hydration status. Intravenous fluids (lactated Ringer's injection) are preferred in patients with severe dehydration.

C. ANTIDIARRHEAL AGENTS

Antidiarrheal agents may be used safely in patients with mild to moderate diarrheal illnesses to improve patient comfort. Opioid agents help decrease the stool number and liquidity and control fecal urgency. However, they should not be used in patients with bloody diarrhea, high fever, or systemic toxicity or discontinued in patients whose diarrhea is worsening despite therapy. With these provisos, such drugs provide excellent symptomatic relief. Loperamide is preferred, in a dosage of 4 mg initially, followed by 2 mg after each loose stool (maximum: 16 mg/24 h).

Bismuth subsalicylate (Pepto-Bismol), two tablets or 30 mL four times daily, reduces symptoms in patients with traveler's diarrhea by virtue of its anti-inflammatory and antibacterial properties. It also reduces vomiting associated with viral enteritis. Anticholinergic agents (eg, diphenoxylate with atropine) are contraindicated in acute diarrhea because of the rare precipitation of toxic megacolon.

D. ANTIBIOTIC THERAPY

1. Empirical treatment—Empirical antibiotic treatment of all patients with acute diarrhea is not indicated. Even patients with inflammatory diarrhea caused by invasive pathogens usually have symptoms that will resolve within several days without antimicrobials. Empirical treatment is recommended with moderate to severe fever, tenesmus, or bloody stools or the presence of fecal leukocytes while the stool bacterial culture is incubating. The drugs of choice are the fluoroquinolones (eg, ciprofloxacin 500 mg, ofloxacin

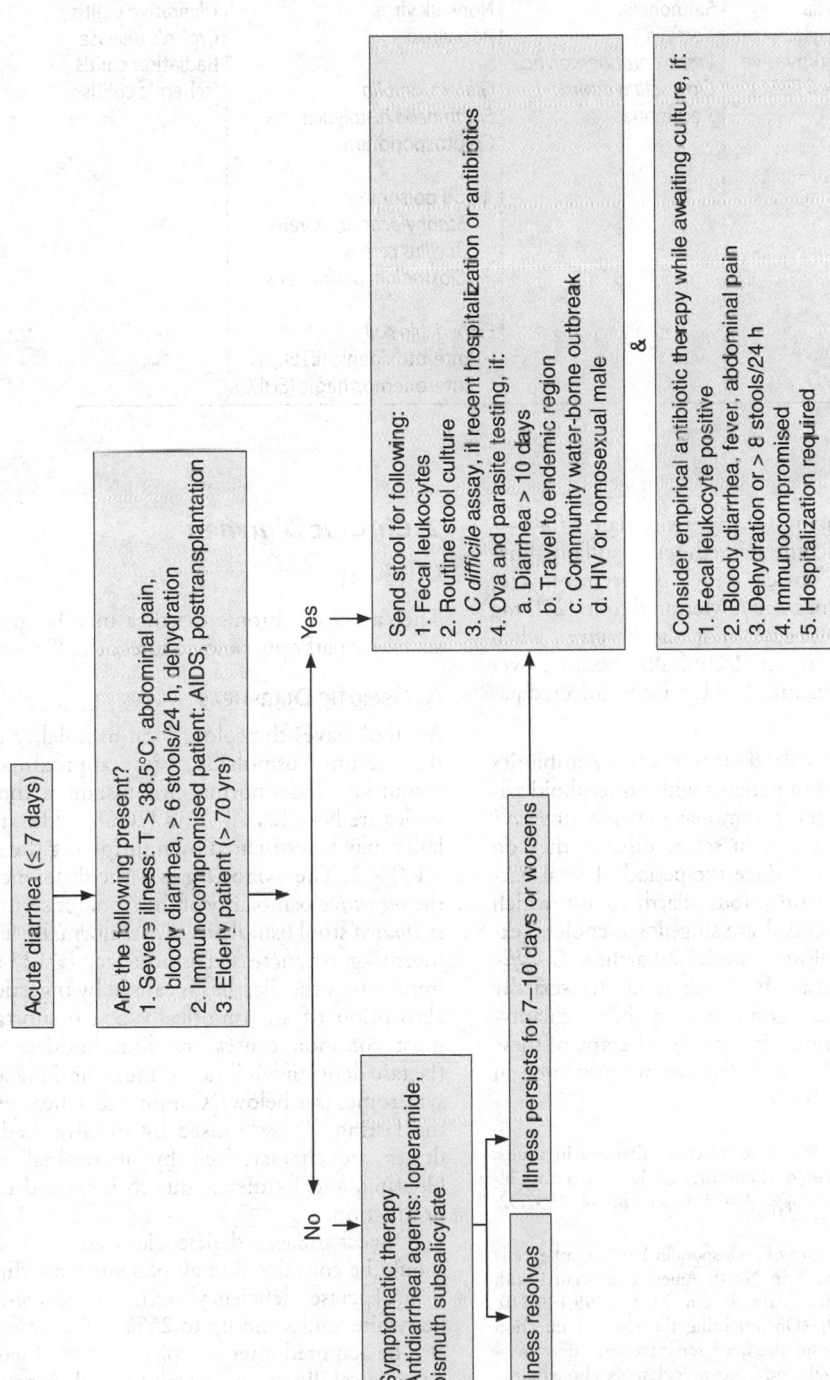

Figure 14–1. Evaluation of acute diarrhea.

Acute diarrhea (≤ 7 days)

Are the following present?
1. Severe illness: T > 38.5°C, abdominal pain, bloody diarrhea, > 6 stools/24 h, dehydration
2. Immunocompromised patient: AIDS, posttransplantation
3. Elderly patient (> 70 yrs)

No

Symptomatic therapy
Antidiarrheal agents: loperamide, bismuth subsalicylate

Illness resolves

Illness persists for 7–10 days or worsens

Yes

Send stool for following:
1. Fecal leukocytes
2. Routine stool culture
3. *C difficile* assay, if recent hospitalization or antibiotics
4. Ova and parasite testing, if:
   a. Diarrhea > 10 days
   b. Travel to endemic region
   c. Community water-borne outbreak
   d. HIV or homosexual male

&

Consider empirical antibiotic therapy while awaiting culture, if:
1. Fecal leukocyte positive
2. Bloody diarrhea, fever, abdominal pain
3. Dehydration or > 8 stools/24 h
4. Immunocompromised
5. Hospitalization required

Table 14–6. Fecal leukocytes in intestinal disorders.

Infectious			Noninfectious
Present	**Variable**	**Absent**	**Present**

Shigella
Campylobacter
Enteroinvasive
  E coli (EIEC)
	Salmonella
	Yersinia
	Vibrio parahaemolytica
	Clostridium difficile
	Aeromonas
		Norwalk virus
		Rotavirus
		
		Giardia lamblia
		Entamoeba histolytica
		Cryptosporidium
		
		"Food poisoning"
		  Staphylococcus aureus
		  Bacillus cereus
		  Clostridium perfringens
		
		Escherichia coli
		  Enterotoxigenic (ETEC)
		  Enterohemorrhagic (EHEC)
			Ulcerative colitis
			Crohn's disease
			Radiation colitis
			Ischemic colitis

400 mg, or norfloxacin 400 mg, twice daily) for 5–7 days. Alternatives include trimethoprim-sulfamethoxazole, 160/800 mg twice daily, or erythromycin, 250–500 mg four times daily. Metronidazole (250 mg three times daily for 7 days) may also be given when giardia infection is suspected clinically, because over half of stool specimens may be negative in infected patients.

2. Specific antimicrobial treatment—Antibiotics are not recommended in patients with nontyphoid salmonella, campylobacter, aeromonas, yersinia, or *E coli* O157:H7 infection except in severe disease; they do not hasten recovery or reduce the period of fecal bacterial excretion. The infectious diarrheas for which treatment is recommended are shigellosis, cholera, extraintestinal salmonellosis, traveler's diarrhea, *C difficile* infection, giardiasis, amebiasis, and the sexually transmitted infections (gonorrhea, syphilis, chlamydiosis, and herpes simplex infection). Therapy of these infections and AIDS-related diarrhea are presented in other chapters of this book.

Du Pont HL: Guidelines on acute infectious diarrhea in adults. The Practice Parameters Committee of the American College of Gastroenterology. Am J Gastroenterol 1997;92: 1962. [PMID: 9362174]

Herwaldt BL et al: The return of cyclospora in 1997; another outbreak of cyclosporiasis in North America associated with imported raspberries. Ann Intern Med 1999;130:210. [PMID: 10049199] (Documenting the risks of infection from food sources and the need for increased safety measures from our federal food safety agencies. See also editorial by Osterholm M: Ann Intern Med 1999;130:233.)

Wong CS et al: The risk of the hemolytic-uremic syndrome after antibiotic treatment of *Escherichia coli* O157 infections. N Engl J Med 2000;342:1930. [PMID: 10874060] (Antibiotic treatment increases the risk for hemolytic-uremic syndrome.)

2. Chronic Diarrhea

Etiology

The causes of chronic diarrhea may be grouped into six major pathophysiologic categories (Table 14–7):

A. OSMOTIC DIARRHEAS

As stool leaves the colon, fecal osmolality is equal to the serum osmolality, ie, approximately 290 mosm/kg. Under normal circumstances, the major osmoles are Na^+, K^+, Cl^-, and HCO_3^-. The stool osmolality may be estimated by multiplying the stool (Na^+ + K^+) × 2. The **osmotic gap** is the difference between the *measured* osmolality of the stool (or serum) and the *estimated* stool osmolality and is normally less than 50 mosm/kg. An increased osmotic gap (> 125 mosm/kg) implies that the diarrhea is caused by ingestion or malabsorption of an osmotically active substance. The most common causes are disaccharidase deficiency (lactase deficiency), laxative abuse, and malabsorption syndromes (see below). Osmotic diarrheas resolve during fasting. Those caused by malabsorbed carbohydrates are characterized by abdominal distention, bloating, and flatulence due to increased colonic gas production.

Disaccharidase deficiencies are common and should be considered in all patients with chronic diarrhea. Lactase deficiency occurs in three-fourths of nonwhite adults and up to 25% of Caucasians. It may also be acquired after an episode of viral gastroenteritis, medical illness, or gastrointestinal surgery. Sorbitol is commonly used as a sweetener in gums, candies, and some medications that may cause diarrhea in some patients. The diagnosis of sorbitol or lactose malabsorption may be established by an elimination trial for 2–3 weeks.

Table 14–7. Causes of chronic diarrhea.

Osmotic diarrhea
CLUES: Stool volume decreases with fasting; increased stool osmotic gap
 1. Medications: antacids, lactulose, sorbitol
 2. Disaccharidase deficiency: lactose intolerance
 3. Factitious diarrhea: magnesium (antacids, laxatives)
Secretory diarrhea
CLUES: Large volume (> 1 L/d); little change with fasting; normal stool osmotic gap
 1. Hormonally mediated: VIPoma, carcinoid, medullary carcinoma of thyroid (calcitonin), Zollinger-Ellison syndrome (gastrin)
 2. Factitious diarrhea (laxative abuse); phenolphthalein, cascara, senna
 3. Villous adenoma
 4. Bile salt malabsorption (ileal resection; Crohn's ileitis; postcholecystectomy)
 5. Medications
Inflammatory conditions
CLUES: Fever, hematochezia, abdominal pain
 1. Ulcerative colitis
 2. Crohn's disease
 3. Microscopic colitis
 4. Malignancy: lymphoma, adenocarcinoma (with obstruction and pseudodiarrhea)
 5. Radiation enteritis

Malabsorption syndromes
CLUES: Weight loss, abnormal laboratory values; fecal fat > 10 g/24 h
 1. Small bowel mucosal disorders: celiac sprue, tropical sprue, Whipple's disease, eosinophilic gastroenteritis, small bowel resection (short bowel syndrome), Crohn's disease
 2. Lymphatic obstruction: lymphoma, carcinoid, infectious (tuberculosis, MAI),[1] Kaposi's sarcoma, sarcoidosis, retroperitoneal fibrosis
 3. Pancreatic disease: chronic pancreatitis, pancreatic carcinoma
 4. Bacterial overgrowth: motility disorders (diabetes, vagotomy), scleroderma, fistulas, small intestinal diverticula
Motility disorders
CLUES: Systemic disease or prior abdominal surgery
 1. Postsurgical: vagotomy, partial gastrectomy, blind loop with bacterial overgrowth
 2. Systemic disorders: scleroderma, diabetes mellitus, hyperthyroidism
 3. Irritable bowel syndrome
Chronic infections
 1. Parasites: *Giardia lamblia, Entamoeba histolytica*
 2. AIDS-related:
 Viral: Cytomegalovirus, HIV infection (?)
 Bacterial: *Clostridium difficile, Mycobacterium avium* complex
 Protozoal: Microsporida (*Enterocytozoon bieneusi*), cryptosporidium, *Isospora belli*

[1]MAI = *Mycobacterium avium-intracellulare.*

Ingestion of magnesium- or phosphate-containing compounds (laxatives, antacids) should be considered in enigmatic chronic diarrhea. Surreptitious use should be considered, especially in patients with a long history of undiagnosed medical ailments or employment in the medical field. The fat substitute olestra is also believed to cause diarrhea and cramps in occasional patients.

B. MALABSORPTIVE CONDITIONS

The major causes of malabsorption are small mucosal intestinal diseases, intestinal resections, lymphatic obstruction, small intestinal bacterial overgrowth, and pancreatic insufficiency. Its characteristics are weight loss, osmotic diarrhea, and nutritional deficiencies. Significant diarrhea in the absence of weight loss is not likely to be due to malabsorption. The physical and laboratory abnormalities related to deficiencies of vitamins or minerals are discussed in Chapter 29.

C. SECRETORY CONDITIONS

Increased intestinal secretion or decreased absorption results in a high-volume watery diarrhea with a normal osmotic gap. There is little change in stool output during the fasting state, and dehydration and electrolyte imbalance may develop. Causes include en-docrine tumors (stimulating intestinal or pancreatic secretion), bile salt malabsorption (stimulating colonic secretion), and laxative abuse.

D. INFLAMMATORY CONDITIONS

Diarrhea is present in most patients with inflammatory bowel disease (ulcerative colitis, Crohn's disease, microscopic colitis). A variety of other symptoms may be present, including abdominal pain, fever, weight loss, and hematochezia. (See Inflammatory Bowel Disease, below.)

E. MOTILITY DISORDERS

Abnormal intestinal motility secondary to systemic disorders or surgery may result in diarrhea due to rapid transit or to stasis of intestinal contents with bacterial overgrowth, resulting in malabsorption.

F. IRRITABLE BOWEL

Probably the most common cause of chronic diarrhea is irritable bowel syndrome (see Irritable Bowel Syndrome, below).

G. CHRONIC INFECTIONS

Chronic parasitic infections may cause diarrhea through a number of mechanisms. Agents most commonly associated with diarrhea include the protozoans giardia, *Entamoeba histolytica,* and cyclospora as well as the intestinal nematodes.

Immunocompromised patients are susceptible to infectious agents that can cause acute or chronic diarrhea (see Chapter 31), including Microsporida, cryptosporidium, cytomegalovirus, *Isospora belli,* cyclospora, and *Mycobacterium avium* complex.

H. FACTITIOUS DIARRHEA

Fifteen percent of patients have factitious diarrhea caused by surreptitious laxative abuse or dilution of stool.

Evaluation

The history and physical examination commonly suggest the underlying pathophysiology that guides the subsequent diagnostic workup (Figure 14–2). Important tests are described here. AIDS-associated diarrhea is discussed in Chapter 31.

A. STOOL ANALYSIS

1. Twenty-four-hour stool collection for weight and quantitative fecal fat—A stool weight of more than 300 g/24 h confirms diarrhea. A weight greater than 1000–1500 g suggests a secretory process. A fecal fat determination in excess of 10 g/24 h indicates a malabsorptive disorder. (See Celiac Sprue and specific tests for malabsorption, below.)

2. Stool osmolality—Stool osmolality less than serum osmolality implies that water or urine has been added to the specimen (factitious diarrhea). A stool pH less than 5.6 is consistent with carbohydrate malabsorption.

3. Stool laxative screen—In cases of suspected laxative abuse, stool magnesium, phosphate, and sulfate levels may be measured. Phenolphthalein and bisacodyl can be analyzed in stool water, using chromatographic techniques. Anthraquinones and bisacodyl are sought for in the urine.

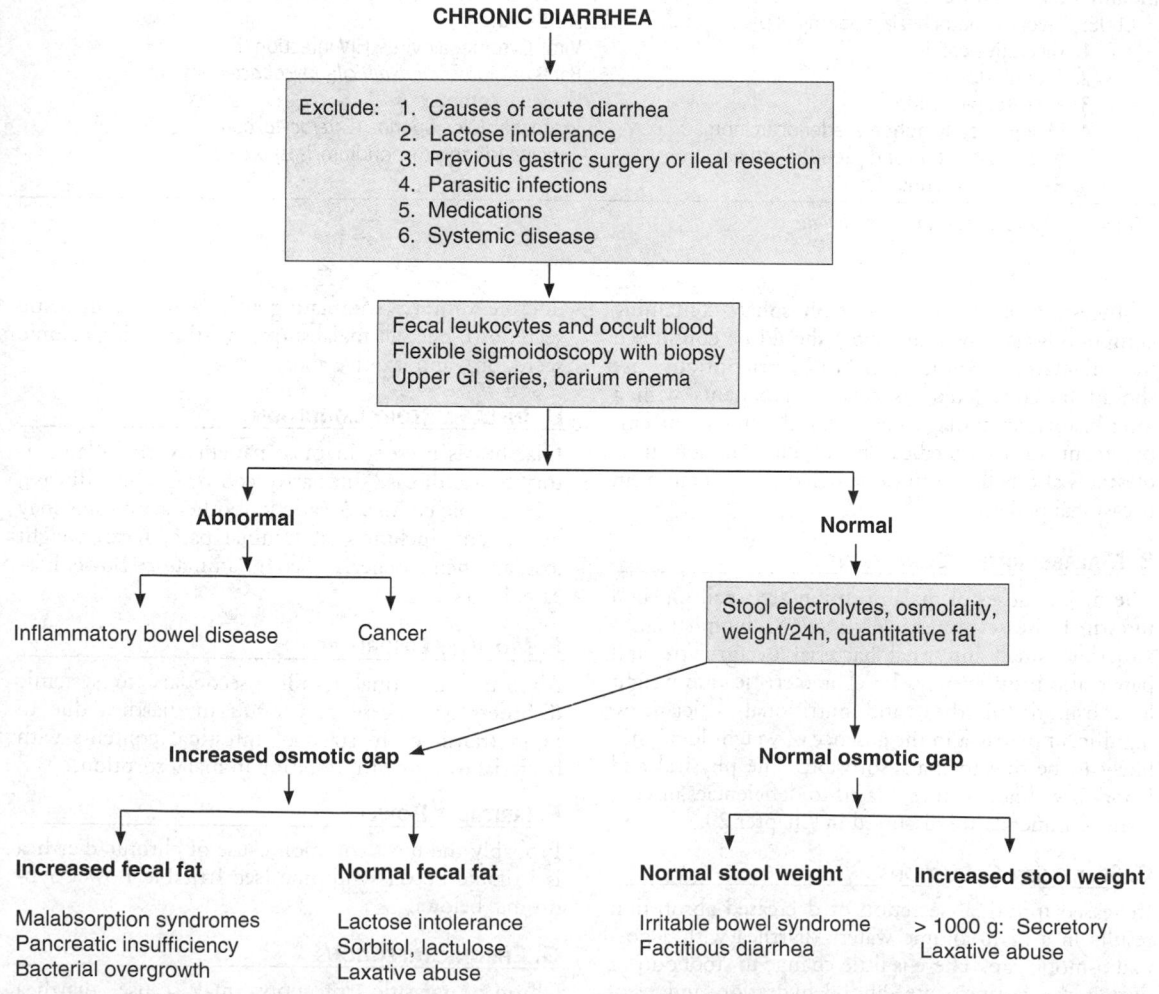

Figure 14–2. Decision diagram for diagnosis of causes of chronic diarrhea.

4. Fecal leukocytes—The presence of fecal leukocytes implies inflammatory diarrhea.

5. Stool for ova and parasites—The presence of giardia and *E histolytica* may be detected in wet mounts. A fecal ELISA for giardia-specific antigen is a more sensitive and specific method of detection. Cryptosporidium and cyclospora are found with modified acid-fast staining.

B. BLOOD TESTS

1. Routine laboratory tests—CBC, serum electrolytes, liver function tests, calcium, phosphorus, albumin, TSH, beta-carotene, and prothrombin time may be of value. Anemia occurs in malabsorption syndromes (folate, iron deficiency [rare], or vitamin B_{12}) as well as inflammatory conditions. Hypoalbuminemia is present in malabsorption, protein-losing enteropathies, and inflammatory diseases. Hyponatremia and non-anion gap metabolic acidosis occur in secretory diarrheas.

2. Other laboratory tests—In patients with suspected malabsorption, serologic testing for celiac sprue includes IgG and IgA antigliadin or antiendomysial antibodies. Secretory diarrheas due to neuroendocrine tumors are rare. When this is suspected, serum VIP (VIPoma), calcitonin (medullary thyroid carcinoma), gastrin (Zollinger-Ellison syndrome), and glucagon determinations may be diagnostic. Urine should be sent for 5-HIAA (carcinoid), VMA, metanephrines, and histamine determinations.

3. Endoscopic examination and mucosal biopsy—Either sigmoidoscopy or colonoscopy with mucosal biopsy is helpful in the detection of inflammatory bowel disease (including microscopic colitis), and melanosis coli (indicative of chronic anthraquinone laxative use). Upper endoscopy with small bowel biopsy is performed when a small intestinal malabsorptive disorder is suspected (celiac sprue, Whipple's disease) and in patients with AIDS to document cryptosporidium, Microsporida, and *M avium-intracellulare* infection. An aspirate of small intestinal contents may be sent for quantitative aerobic and anaerobic bacterial culture if bacterial overgrowth is suspected.

4. Other imaging studies—Calcification on a plain abdominal radiograph confirms a diagnosis of chronic pancreatitis, though abdominal CT is more sensitive for the diagnosis of chronic pancreatitis as well as pancreatic cancer. Small intestinal barium radiography is helpful in the diagnosis of Crohn's disease, small bowel lymphoma, carcinoid, and jejunal diverticula. Neuroendocrine tumors may be localized using somatostatin receptor scintigraphy.

Treatment

A number of antidiarrheal agents may be used in certain patients with chronic diarrheal conditions and are listed below. Opioids are safe in most patients with chronic, stable symptoms.

Loperamide: 4 mg initially, then 2 mg after each loose stool (maximum: 16 mg/d).

Diphenoxylate with atropine: one tablet three or four times daily as needed.

Codeine and deodorized tincture of opium: Because of potential habituation, these drugs are avoided except in cases of chronic, intractable diarrhea. Codeine may be given in a dosage of 15–60 mg every 4 hours; tincture of opium, 10–25 drops every 6 hours as needed.

Clonidine: α_2-Adrenergic agonists inhibit intestinal electrolyte secretion. Clonidine, 0.1–0.6 mg twice daily, or a clonidine patch, 0.1–0.2 mg/d, may help in some patients with secretory diarrheas, diabetic diarrhea, and cryptosporidiosis.

Octreotide: This somatostatin analog stimulates intestinal fluid and electrolyte absorption and inhibits intestinal fluid secretion and the release of gastrointestinal peptides. It is given for secretory diarrheas due to neuroendocrine tumors (VIPomas, carcinoid) and in some cases of AIDS-related diarrhea. Effective doses range from 50 μg to 250 μg subcutaneously three times daily.

Cholestyramine: This bile salt-binding resin may be useful in patients with bile salt-induced diarrhea secondary to intestinal resection or ileal disease. A dosage of 4 g once to three times daily is recommended.

American Gastroenterological Association medical position statement: Guidelines for the evaluation and management of chronic diarrhea. Gastroenterology 1999;116:1461. [PMID: 10348831]

Chassany O et al: Drug-induced diarrhoea. Drug Saf 2000;22:53. [PMID: 10647976] (Excellent review of drugs associated with diarrhea.)

Balasekaran R: Positive results on tests for steatorrhea in persons consuming olestra potato chips. Ann Intern Med 2000; 132:279. [PMID: 10681282]

GASTROINTESTINAL BLEEDING

1. Acute Upper Gastrointestinal Bleeding

 ESSENTIALS OF DIAGNOSIS

- *Hematemesis (bright red blood or "coffee grounds").*
- *Melena in most cases; hematochezia in massive upper gastrointestinal bleeds.*
- *Volume status to determine severity of blood loss; hematocrit is a poor early indicator of blood loss.*
- *Endoscopy diagnostic and may be therapeutic.*

General Considerations

There are over 350,000 hospitalizations a year in the USA for acute upper gastrointestinal bleeding, with a mortality rate of 10%. Approximately half of patients are over 60 years of age, and in this age group the mortality rate is even higher. Patients seldom die of exsanguination but rather from complications of an underlying disease.

The most common presentation of upper gastrointestinal bleeding is hematemesis or melena. Hematemesis may be either bright red blood or brown "coffee grounds" material. Melena develops after as little as 50–100 mL of blood loss in the upper gastrointestinal tract, whereas hematochezia requires a loss of more than 1000 mL. Although hematochezia generally suggests a lower bleeding source (eg, colonic), upper gastrointestinal bleeding may present with hematochezia in 10% of cases.

Upper gastrointestinal bleeding is self-limited in 80% of patients; urgent medical therapy and endoscopic evaluation are obligatory in the rest. Patients with bleeding more than 48 hours prior to presentation have a low risk of recurrent bleeding.

Etiology

Acute upper gastrointestinal bleeding may originate from a number of sources. These are listed in order of the frequency and discussed in detail below.

A. Peptic Ulcer Disease

Peptic ulcers account for half of major upper gastrointestinal bleeding with an overall acute mortality rate of 6–10%.

B. Portal Hypertension

Portal hypertension causes bleeding from varices (most commonly esophageal; rarely, gastric or duodenal) or portal hypertensive gastropathy. Less than one-third of patients with portal hypertension and varices will develop acute bleeding. However, these lesions account for 10–20% of significant gastrointestinal hemorrhages, with a hospital mortality rate of 15–40%. If untreated, half will rebleed during hospitalization. A mortality rate of 60–80% is expected at 1–4 years. Bleeding from the gastric mucosa in portal hypertensive gastropathy is responsible for 20% of cases of upper gastrointestinal bleeding in patients with cirrhosis.

C. Mallory-Weiss Tears

Lacerations of the gastroesophageal junction cause 5–10% of cases of upper gastrointestinal bleeding. Many patients report a history of heavy alcohol use or retching. Less than 10% have continued or recurrent bleeding.

D. Vascular Anomalies

Vascular anomalies are found throughout the gastrointestinal tract and may be the source of chronic or acute gastrointestinal bleeding. They account for 7% of cases of acute upper tract bleeding. **Vascular ectasias** (angiodysplasias) have a bright red stellate appearance. They may be part of systemic conditions (hereditary hemorrhagic telangiectasia, CREST syndrome) or may occur sporadically. There is an increased incidence in patients with chronic renal failure.

E. Gastric Neoplasms

Gastric neoplasms result in 1% of upper gastrointestinal hemorrhages.

F. Erosive Gastritis

Because this process is superficial, it is a relatively unusual cause of severe gastrointestinal bleeding (< 5% of cases) and more commonly results in chronic blood loss. Gastric mucosal erosions are due to NSAIDs, alcohol, or severe medical or surgical illness (stress gastritis).

G. Erosive Esophagitis

Severe erosive esophagitis due to chronic gastroesophageal reflux may rarely cause significant upper gastrointestinal bleeding.

H. Others

An aortoenteric fistula complicates 2% of abdominal aortic grafts or can occur as the initial presentation of a previously untreated aneurysm. Usually located between the graft or aneurysm and the third portion of the duodenum, these fistulas characteristically present with a herald nonexsanguinating initial hemorrhage, with melena and hematemesis, or with chronic intermittent bleeding. The diagnosis may be suspected by upper endoscopy or abdominal CT. Surgery is mandatory to prevent exsanguinating hemorrhage; patients are at very high risk, especially those with graft-enteric fistulas in whom graft infection is always present. Other rare causes of upper gastrointestinal bleeding include hemobilia (from hepatic tumor, angioma, penetrating trauma), pancreatic malignancy, pseudoaneurysm (hemosuccus pancreaticus), and Dieulafoy's lesion (aberrant gastric submucosal artery).

Initial Evaluation & Management

A. Stabilization

The initial step is assessment of the hemodynamic status. A systolic blood pressure less than 100 mm Hg (irrespective of heart rate) identifies a high-risk patient with severe acute bleeding. A heart rate over 100/min with a systolic blood pressure over 100 mm Hg signifies moderate acute blood loss. A normal systolic blood pressure and heart rate suggests relatively minor hemorrhage. Postural hypotension and tachycardia are useful when present but may be due to causes other than blood loss. Because the hematocrit may take 24–72 hours to equilibrate with the extravascular fluid, it is not a reliable indicator of the severity of acute bleeding.

In patients with significant bleeding, two 18-gauge or larger intravenous lines should be started prior to further diagnostic tests. Blood is sent for complete blood count, prothrombin time with INR, serum creatinine, liver enzymes and serologies, and cross-matching for 2–4 units or more of packed red blood cells. In patients without hemodynamic compromise or overt active bleeding, aggressive fluid repletion can be delayed until the extent of the bleeding is further clarified. Patients with evidence of hemodynamic compromise are given 0.9% saline or lactated Ringer's injection and crossmatched blood. It is rarely necessary to administer type-specific or O-negative blood. Central venous pressure monitoring is desirable in some cases, but line placement should not interfere with rapid volume resuscitation.

A nasogastric tube should be placed in all patients with suspected upper tract bleeding. The aspiration of red blood or "coffee grounds" confirms an upper gastrointestinal source of bleeding, though 10% of patients with confirmed upper tract sources of bleeding have nonbloody aspirates—especially when bleeding originates in the duodenum. An aspirate of bright red blood indicates active bleeding and is associated with the highest risk of further bleeding, and complications, while a clear aspirate identifies patients at lower initial risk. Efforts to stop or slow bleeding by gastric lavage with large volumes of fluid are of no benefit and expose the patient to an increased risk of aspiration. Periodic reaspiration of the nasogastric tube serves as an indicator of ongoing bleeding or rebleeding.

B. Blood Replacement

The amount of fluid and blood products required is based upon assessment of vital signs, evidence of active bleeding from nasogastric aspirate, and laboratory tests. Sufficient packed red blood cells should be given to maintain a hematocrit of 25–30%. In the absence of continued bleeding, the hematocrit should rise 3% for each unit of transfused packed red cells. Transfusion of blood should not be withheld from patients with brisk active bleeding regardless of the hematocrit. It is desirable to transfuse blood in anticipation of the nadir hematocrit. In actively bleeding patients, platelets are transfused if the platelet count is under 50,000/μL and considered if there is impaired platelet function due to aspirin use (regardless of the platelet count). Uremic patients (who also have dysfunctional platelets) with active bleeding are given one or two doses of desmopressin (DDAVP), 0.3 μg/kg intravenously, at 12- to 24-hour intervals. Fresh frozen plasma is administered for actively bleeding patients with a coagulopathy and an INR > 1.5. The INR is intended to guide warfarin therapy and is not a reliable marker of bleeding risk in the setting of liver disease. In the face of massive bleeding, 1 unit of fresh frozen plasma should be given for each 5 units of packed red blood cells transfused.

C. Initial Triage

A preliminary assessment of risk based upon several clinical factors aids in the resuscitation as well as the rational triage of the patient.

1. Very low risk—Reliable patients without serious comorbid medical illnesses or advanced liver disease who have normal hemodynamics, no evidence of overt bleeding (hematemesis or melena) within 48 hours, a negative nasogastric lavage, and normal laboratory tests do not require hospital admission and can undergo further evaluation as outpatients as indicated.

2. Low to moderate risk—Patients in this category are admitted after appropriate stabilization for further evaluation and treatment. In some centers, these patients undergo upper endoscopy. Based upon the findings at endoscopy, patients deemed to be at low risk of rebleeding may be discharged and followed as outpatients.

3. High risk—Patients with active bleeding manifested by hematemesis or bright red blood on nasogastric aspirate, an estimated loss of more than 5 units of blood, persistent hemodynamic derangement despite fluid resuscitation, serious comorbid medical illness, or evidence of advanced liver disease require ICU admission.

Subsequent Evaluation & Treatment

Specific treatment of the various causes of upper gastrointestinal bleeding is discussed elsewhere in this chapter. The following general comments apply to most patients with bleeding:

A. History and Physical Examination

The physician's impression of the bleeding source is correct in only 40% of cases. Signs of chronic liver disease implicate bleeding due to portal hypertension, but a different lesion is identified in 25–50% of patients with cirrhosis. A history of dyspepsia, NSAID use, or peptic ulcer disease suggests peptic ulcer. Acute bleeding preceded by heavy alcohol ingestion or retching suggests a Mallory-Weiss tear, though most of these patients have neither.

B. Upper Endoscopy

Virtually all patients with upper tract bleeding should undergo upper endoscopy, performed after the patient is hemodynamically stable, usually within 12 hours after admission. Patients with continued active bleeding require more urgent endoscopic evaluation. The benefits of endoscopy in this setting are threefold.

1. To identify the source of bleeding—The appropriate acute and long-term medical therapy is determined by the cause of bleeding. Patients with portal hypertension will be treated differently from those with ulcer disease. If surgery is required for uncontrolled bleeding, the source of bleeding as determined at endoscopy will determine the approach.

2. To determine the risk of rebleeding—Patients with a nonbleeding Mallory-Weiss tear, esophagitis, gastritis, and ulcers that have a clean, white base have a very low risk of rebleeding. It may be safe and cost-effective to discharge such patients from the emergency room without admission. Patients with ulcers that are actively bleeding or have a visible vessel or who have variceal bleeding require initial management in an ICU setting.

3. To render endoscopic therapy—Hemostasis can be achieved in actively bleeding lesions with endoscopic modalities such as cautery or injection. About 90% of actively bleeding varices can be effectively treated acutely with injection of a sclerosant or application of a rubber band to the bleeding varix. Similarly, 90% of actively bleeding ulcers, angiomas, or Mallory-Weiss tears can be controlled with either injection of epinephrine or direct cauterization of the vessel by a heater probe or multipolar electrocautery probe. Certain nonbleeding lesions such as esophageal varices, ulcers with visible blood vessels, and angiomas are also treated with these therapies. Specific endoscopic therapy of varices, peptic ulcers, and Mallory-Weiss tears is dealt with elsewhere in this chapter.

C. ACUTE PHARMACOLOGIC THERAPIES

1. Acid inhibitory therapy—H_2 receptor antagonists do not stop acute bleeding or reduce the incidence of rebleeding. Intravenous proton pump inhibitors (omeprazole, 80 mg bolus, followed by 8 mg/h continuous infusion for 72 hours) to reduce the risk of rebleeding in patients with peptic ulcers with high-risk features (active bleeding, visible vessel, or adherent clot) after endoscopic treatment. High doses of oral proton pump inhibitors (omeprazole 40 mg or lansoprazole 60 mg, twice daily for 5 days) may also be effective. Pending the results of endoscopic examination, it may be reasonable to initiate therapy with a high-dose proton pump inhibitor (intravenously or orally) in patients with suspected peptic ulcer bleeding.

2. Octreotide—Continuous intravenous infusion of octreotide (100 μg bolus, followed by 50–100 μg/h) reduces splanchnic blood flow and portal blood pressures and is effective in the initial control of bleeding related to portal hypertension. It is administered promptly to all patients with active upper gastrointestinal bleeding and evidence of liver disease or portal hypertension until the source of bleeding can be determined by endoscopy.

3. Vasopressin—Intravenous vasopressin is not used in the treatment of upper gastrointestinal bleeding. Octreotide has superior efficacy and is virtually devoid of short-term side effects.

D. OTHER TREATMENT

1. Intra-arterial embolization or vasopressin—Angiographic treatment is used rarely in patients with persistent bleeding from ulcers, angiomas, or Mallory-

Weiss tears who have failed endoscopic therapy and are poor operative risks.

2. Transvenous intrahepatic portosystemic shunts (TIPS)—Placement of a wire stent from the hepatic vein through the liver to the portal vein provides effective decompression of the portal venous system and control of acute variceal bleeding. It is indicated in patients in whom endoscopic modalities have failed to control acute variceal bleeding.

Lau JYW et al: Effect of intravenous omeprazole on recurrent bleeding after endoscopic treatment of bleeding peptic ulcers. N Engl J Med 2000;343:310. [PMID: 10922420]

Longstreth GM et al: Successful outpatient management of acute upper gastrointestinal hemorrhage: use of practice guidelines in a large patient series. Gastrointest Endosc 1998;47:219. [PMID: 9540873] (Clinical guidelines and endoscopic findings can be used to stratify patients with acute upper gastrointestinal bleeding, and low-risk patients can be managed as outpatients.)

Van Dam J et al: Endoscopy of the upper gastrointestinal tract. N Engl J Med 1999;341:1738. [PMID: 10580074]

2. Acute Lower Gastrointestinal Bleeding

 ESSENTIALS OF DIAGNOSIS

- Hematochezia usually present.
- 10% of cases of hematochezia due to upper gastrointestinal source.
- Evaluation with colonoscopy in stable patients.
- Massive active bleeding calls for evaluation with sigmoidoscopy, upper endoscopy, angiography, or nuclear bleeding scan.

General Considerations

Lower gastrointestinal bleeding is defined as that arising below the ligament of Treitz, ie, the small intestine or colon; however, over 95% of cases arise from the colon. The severity of lower gastrointestinal bleeding ranges from mild anorectal bleeding to massive, large-volume hematochezia. Bright red blood that drips into the bowl after a bowel movement or is mixed with solid brown stool signifies mild bleeding, usually from an anorectosigmoid source, and can be evaluated in the outpatient setting. Serious lower gastrointestinal bleeding is more common in older men. In patients hospitalized with gastrointestinal bleeding, lower tract bleeding is one-fourth as common as upper gastrointestinal hemorrhage and tends to have a more benign course. Patients hospitalized with lower gastrointestinal tract bleeding are less likely to present with shock or orthostasis (< 20%) or to require transfusions (< 40%). Spontaneous cessation of bleeding occurs in over 85% of cases, and hospital mortality is less than 3%.

Etiology

The cause of these lesions is dependent both upon the age of the patient and the severity of the bleeding. In patients under 50 years of age, the most common causes are infectious colitis, anorectal disease, and inflammatory bowel disease. In older patients, significant hematochezia is most often seen with diverticulosis, vascular ectasias, malignancy, or ischemia. In 20% of acute bleeding episodes, no source of bleeding can be identified.

A. DIVERTICULOSIS

Hemorrhage occurs in 3-5% of all patients with diverticulosis and is the most common cause of major lower tract bleeding, accounting for 50% of cases. A significant percentage of cases are associated with the use of nonsteroidal anti-inflammatory agents. Although diverticula are more prevalent on the left side of the colon, bleeding more commonly originates on the right side. Diverticular bleeding usually presents as acute, painless, large-volume maroon or bright red hematochezia in patients over age 50. More than 95% of cases require less than 4 units of blood transfusion. Bleeding subsides spontaneously in 80% but may recur in up to 25% of patients.

B. VASCULAR ECTASIAS

Vascular ectasias (or angiodysplasias) occur throughout the upper and lower intestinal tracts and cause painless bleeding ranging from melena or hematochezia to occult blood loss. They are responsible for 5–10% of cases of lower gastrointestinal bleeding, where they are most often seen in the cecum and ascending colon. They are flat, red lesions (2–10 mm) with ectatic peripheral vessels radiating from a central vessel, and are most common in patients over 70 and in those with chronic renal failure. Bleeding in younger patients more commonly arises from the small intestine.

Most colonic ectasias are degenerative lesions that are felt to arise from chronic colonic mucosal contraction obstructing venous mucosal drainage. Over time, the mucosal capillaries dilate and become incompetent. The cause of gastric and small intestinal ectasias is unknown. Some are congenital, part of an inherited syndrome such as hereditary hemorrhagic telangiectasia, or related to autoimmune disorders, typically scleroderma. Ectasias can be identified in up to 25% of subjects over age 60, so their mere presence does not prove that the lesion is the source of bleeding, as active bleeding is seldom seen.

C. NEOPLASMS

Benign polyps and carcinoma are associated with chronic occult blood loss or intermittent anorectal hematochezia. However, colonic neoplasms may cause up to 10% of acute lower gastrointestinal hemorrhage. After endoscopic removal of colonic polyps, important bleeding may occur up to 2 weeks later in 0.3% of patients. Delayed bleeding can be managed conservatively (ie, without repeat colonoscopy) in 70% of cases.

D. INFLAMMATORY BOWEL DISEASE

Patients with inflammatory bowel disease (especially ulcerative colitis) often have diarrhea with variable amounts of hematochezia. Bleeding varies from occult blood loss to recurrent hematochezia usually mixed with stool. Symptoms of abdominal pain, tenesmus, and urgency are often present.

E. ANORECTAL DISEASE

Anorectal disease commonly results in small amounts of bright red blood noted on the toilet paper, streaking of the stool, or dripping into the toilet bowl. The bleeding is slight and seldom results in significant blood loss. Painless bleeding is commonly caused by internal hemorrhoids. Bleeding associated with pain during bowel movements suggests an anal fissure.

F. ISCHEMIC COLITIS

This entity is seen commonly in older patients, most of whom have atherosclerotic disease. Most cases occur spontaneously due to transient episodes of nonocclusive ischemia. Ischemic colitis may also occur in 5% of patients after surgery for ileoaortic or abdominal aortic aneurysm. Young patients may develop colonic ischemia due to vasculitis, coagulation disorders, estrogen therapy, and long distance running. Ischemic colitis results in hematochezia or bloody diarrhea associated with mild cramps. In most, the bleeding is mild and self-limited.

G. OTHERS

Radiation-induced proctitis causes anorectal bleeding that may develop months to years after pelvic radiation. Endoscopy reveals multiple rectal telangiectasias. Acute infectious colitis (see Acute Diarrhea, above) commonly causes bloody diarrhea. Rare causes of lower tract bleeding include vasculitic ischemia, solitary rectal ulcer, NSAID-induced ulcers in the small bowel or right colon, small bowel diverticula, and colonic varices.

Evaluation & Management

The color of the stool helps distinguish upper from lower gastrointestinal bleeding, especially when observed by the physician. Brown stools mixed or streaked with blood predict a source in the rectosigmoid or anus. Large volumes of bright red blood suggest a colonic source; maroon stools imply a lesion in the right colon or small intestine; and black stools (melena) predict a source proximal to the ligament of Treitz. Although 10% of patients admitted with self-reported hematochezia have an upper gastrointestinal source of bleeding (eg, peptic ulcer), bright red blood per rectum occurs uncommonly with upper tract bleeding and almost always in the setting of massive hemorrhage with shock. Painless large-volume bleeding usually suggests diverticular bleeding or vascular ectasias. Bloody diarrhea associated with cramping abdominal pain, urgency, or tenesmus is characteristic of inflammatory bowel disease, infectious colitis, or ischemic colitis.

Important considerations in management include the following:

A. EXCLUSION OF AN UPPER TRACT SOURCE

A nasogastric tube aspirating red blood or dark brown ("coffee grounds") guaiac-positive material strongly implicates an upper gastrointestinal source of bleeding. If blood is not seen and bile is aspirated, an upper source is found in only 1% of patients.

B. ANOSCOPY AND SIGMOIDOSCOPY

In otherwise healthy patients under age 45 with small-volume bleeding, anoscopy and sigmoidoscopy are performed to look for evidence of anorectal disease, inflammatory bowel disease, or infectious colitis. If a lesion is found, no further evaluation is needed immediately unless the bleeding persists or is recurrent. In patients over age 45 with small-volume hematochezia, the entire colon must be evaluated with either colonoscopy or sigmoidoscopy and barium enema, to exclude tumor.

C. COLONOSCOPY

In order to determine the probable site of bleeding, colonoscopy should be performed within 6–24 hours of admission after adequate resuscitation and colonic lavage in all patients with lower gastrointestinal bleeding that appears to have ceased. For patients with severe or active lower gastrointestinal bleeding, many physicians choose first to obtain a nuclear bleeding scan or angiogram in an attempt to localize the site of active bleeding. Increasingly it is recommended that urgent colonoscopy be performed in patients with severe or ongoing hemorrhage within 1 hour after administration of a rapid, high-volume colonic lavage solution, given until the effluent is clear of blood and clots (GoLYTELY; CoLYTE, NuLYTE; 4–8 L given orally or by nasogastric tube over 3–5 hours). In most cases in which bleeding has stopped, a diagnosis of diverticular hemorrhage is made presumptively after identification of diverticula at colonoscopy with no other source of blood loss. At urgent colonoscopy, the probable site of bleeding can be identified in 70–85% of patients, and a high-risk lesion can be identified and treated in up to 20%.

D. SMALL INTESTINE PUSH ENTEROSCOPY OR CAPSULE IMAGING

Less than 5% of acute episodes of lower gastrointestinal bleeding arise from the small intestine, eluding diagnostic evaluation with upper endoscopy and colon-oscopy. Because of the difficulty of examining the small intestine and its relative rarity as a source of acute bleeding, evaluation of the small bowel is not usually pursued in patients during the initial episode of acute lower gastrointestinal bleeding. However, the small intestine is investigated in patients with unexplained recurrent hemorrhage of obscure origin. "Push enteroscopy" consists of passage of a long, small-diameter endoscope that may reach from the proximal to the distal jejunum. Vascular ectasias identified within reach of the enteroscope can be cauterized. Likewise, a wireless video capsule device allows video imaging of the entire small bowel. The small capsule (about 2 cm in diameter) is ingested and reaches the small intestine in a matter of hours. Video images are transmitted to a portable recorder. This technique allows identification of vascular ectasias and other bleeding lesions but does not permit precise localization or therapy.

E. NUCLEAR BLEEDING SCANS AND ANGIOGRAPHY

Significant continued bleeding occurs in only 15% of patients but may limit the diagnostic effectiveness of endoscopy. In such patients, either angiographic embolization or surgery may become necessary to control the bleeding. Localization of the site guides the surgical approach. Technetium-labeled red blood cell scanning can detect significant active bleeding and localize it to the small intestine, right colon, or left colon. Because bleeding may be slow or intermittent, less than half of studies are diagnostic, and the accuracy of a positive study is only 78%. Nuclear bleeding studies are more apt to be positive in patients passing bright red or maroon stools at the time of the scan. Selective mesenteric angiography requires more brisk bleeding (0.5–1 mL/min) for a positive result than technetium scans and leads to major complications in up to 3% of patients. Accordingly, angiograms are performed only in patients with massive bleeding or positive technetium scans. Localization of an actively bleeding vessel is possible in up to 50%.

Treatment

A. DISCONTINUE ASPIRIN AND NSAIDs

Up to 80% of patients with lower gastrointestinal tract bleeding have recently ingested aspirin or NSAIDs, which may potentiate bleeding through inhibition of platelet function. These agents should be discontinued.

B. THERAPEUTIC COLONOSCOPY

Until recently, colonoscopy served a largely diagnostic role in the patient with lower gastrointestinal bleeding. High-risk lesions (eg, diverticulum with active bleeding or a visible vessel, or a vascular ectasia) may now be treated endoscopically with saline or epinephrine injection, cautery (bipolar or heater probe), or application of metallic clips. In severe diverticular hemorrhage with high-risk lesions identified at colonoscopy, rebleeding occurs in half of untreated patients compared with virtually no rebleeding in patients treated endoscopically. Radiation proctitis is effectively treated with one to five applications of cautery therapy to the rectal telangiectasias, preferably with an argon plasma coagulator.

C. INTRA-ARTERIAL VASOPRESSIN OR EMBOLIZATION

Selective mesenteric arterial infusion of vasoconstrictors (eg, vasopressin) may arrest bleeding in up to 80% of patients with active bleeding from a diverticulum or vascular ectasia, but bleeding recurs in up to 50%. Intra-arterial embolization, which provides definitive control of bleeding in up to 90%, now is preferred by many angiographers. Embolization may be associated with abdominal pain, fever, and ischemic infarction in up to 15%, though use of microcoils appears to be safer than other embolic agents. Embolization may be preferred to surgery in patients with continued bleeding who are poor operative candidates.

D. SURGICAL TREATMENT

Surgery is indicated in patients with ongoing bleeding that requires more than 4–6 units of blood within 24 hours or more than 10 total units. Most such hemorrhages are caused by a bleeding diverticulum or vascular ectasia. With increasing experience with urgent colonoscopy and angiographic embolization, the need for surgical treatment appears to be decreasing. Preoperative localization of the bleeding site by nuclear scan or angiography allows limited resection of the bleeding segment of small intestine or colon. When accurate localization is not possible or when emergency surgery is required for massive hemorrhage, total abdominal colectomy with ileorectal anastomosis is required—with significantly higher morbidity and mortality than limited resections.

Surgery may also be indicated in patients with two or more hospitalizations for diverticular hemorrhage depending upon the severity of bleeding and the patient's other comorbid conditions.

AGA Technical Review on Intestinal Ischemia. Gastroenterology 2000;118:954. [PMID: 10784596]

Bloomfeld RS et al. Endoscopic therapy of acute diverticular hemorrhage. Am J Gastroenterol 2001;96:2367. [PMID: 11515176]

Bloomfeld RS et al: Provocative angiography in patients with gastrointestinal hemorrhage of obscure origin. Am J Gastroenterol 2000;95:2807. [PMID: 11051352] (A small number of patients have recurrent gastrointestinal bleeding for which no source can be found after detailed study; anticoagulants [heparin], thrombolytics [urokinase] or vasodilators during angiography can provoke an acute episode of bleeding that can be identified and treated with embolization or surgery.)

Enns R: Acute lower gastrointestinal bleeding: Part 1. Can J Gastroenterol 2001;15:509. [PMID: 11544535]

Enns R: Acute lower gastrointestinal bleeding: Part 2. Can J Gastroenterol 2001;15:517. [PMID: 11544534]

Gostout C: The role of endoscopy in managing lower gastrointestinal bleeding. N Engl J Med 2000;342:125. [PMID: 10631283]

Jensen D et al: Urgent colonoscopy for the diagnosis and treatment of severe diverticular hemorrhage. N Engl J Med 2000;342:78. [PMID: 10631275]

Kramer S et al: Embolization for gastrointestinal hemorrhages. Eur Radiol 2000;10:802. [PMID: 10823636]

Taieb S et al: Effective use of argon plasma coagulation in the treatment of severe radiation proctitis. Dis Colon Rectum 2001;44:1766. [PMID: 11742159]

3. Occult Gastrointestinal Bleeding

Occult gastrointestinal bleeding is the presence of a positive fecal occult blood test (FOBT) or of iron deficiency anemia in an adult in the absence of visible fecal blood loss. FOBT may be performed in patients with gastrointestinal symptoms or as a screening test for colorectal neoplasia (see Colorectal Cancer Screening, below). From 1–2.5% of patients in screening programs have a positive FOBT.

In the United States, 2% of men and 5% of women have iron deficiency anemia (serum ferritin < 30–45 μg/L). In premenopausal women, iron deficiency anemia is most commonly attributable to menstrual and pregnancy-associated iron loss; however a gastrointestinal source of chronic blood loss is present in 10%. Among men and postmenopausal women, a potential gastrointestinal cause of blood loss can be identified in the colon in 15–30% and in the upper gastrointestinal tract in 35–55%; and a malignancy is present in 10%. Iron deficiency on rare occasions is caused by malabsorption (especially celiac disease) or malnutrition.

Causes of Occult Gastrointestinal Blood Loss

The most common lesions include: (1) neoplasms; (2) vascular abnormalities (vascular ectasias, portal hypertensive gastropathy); (3) acid-peptic lesions; (4) infections (nematodes, especially hookworm; tuberculosis); (5) medications (especially NSAIDs or aspirin); and (6) other causes such as inflammatory bowel disorder or malabsorption disorders. After complete gastrointestinal evaluation with colonoscopy and upper endoscopy, the origin of positive FOBT or iron deficiency anemia remains unexplained in 30–50% of patients.

Evaluation

All adults over age 40–45 with positive FOBTs or iron deficiency anemia should undergo colonoscopy or upper endoscopy. Endoscopic evaluation is also recommended in premenopausal women and younger men with gastrointestinal symptoms (abdominal pain, dyspepsia or heartburn, change in bowel habits, weight loss), a positive family history of gastrointestinal cancer, or anemia that is disproportionate to the estimated menstrual blood loss. The presence and nature of gastrointestinal symptoms help guide the choice of initial study.

A. COLONOSCOPY

Unless patients have symptoms referable to the upper gastrointestinal tract, the colon should be evaluated first. Colonoscopy detects over 95% of colorectal polyps and cancer and permits polypectomy, tumor biopsy, or endoscopic cautery of vascular ectasias. The finding on colonoscopy of a significant lesion clearly consistent with chronic bleeding (mass lesion, large ulceration, bleeding ectasias) obviates the need for upper endoscopy. Barium enema examinations are less accurate than colonoscopy, missing up to half of significant adenomas. Furthermore, up to 30–40% of patients with a positive FOBT will have a polyp or mass lesion detected on barium enema, which then necessitates colonoscopic evaluation. For these reasons, barium enema can no longer be recommended except in patients in whom colonoscopy is contraindicated or where expertise in colonoscopy is not available.

B. UPPER ENDOSCOPY

Upper endoscopy should be performed first in patients with symptoms referable to the upper gastrointestinal tract (heartburn, dyspepsia, dysphagia, vomiting, weight loss). Upper endoscopy should also be performed in patients with iron deficiency anemia after colonoscopy. In asymptomatic patients with a positive FOBT without iron deficiency anemia whose colonoscopic examination is negative, significant abnormalities are found in almost half of patients on upper endoscopy. Although the cost-effectiveness of evaluation of the upper gastrointestinal tract in this setting is uncertain, upper endoscopy is recommended by many experts. Owing to its lower diagnostic accuracy, upper gastrointestinal radiography should be performed only in patients in whom upper endoscopy is contraindicated or where a gastroenterologist is unavailable.

C. SMALL INTESTINAL EVALUATION

Patients with occult bleeding who have a negative endoscopic evaluation of the colon and upper gastrointestinal tract may be given a trial of iron supplementation and closely observed. Most require no further evaluation. If there is persistent chronic gastrointestinal blood loss or anemia that responds poorly to iron supplementation, further evaluation for a small intestinal source is indicated. Small bowel enteroscopy permits visualization of the upper one-third to one-half of the small intestine for vascular ectasias. If enteroscopy is unrevealing, a small bowel series or enteroclysis is performed to look for mass lesions; however, barium studies cannot identify small intestinal vascular ectasias. The video capsule device described above captures up to 8 hours of video images of the small intestine which are transmitted to a portable recorder for subsequent viewing. Capsule endoscopy appears to be most useful in the detection of small bowel vascular ectasias; its role relative to push enteroscopy is under investigation.

Rarely, angiography or intraoperative endoscopy of the entire small intestine is indicated in patients with transfusion-dependent chronic or recurrent bleeding that cannot be localized by other means.

American Gastroenterological Association Medical Position Statement: Evaluation and management of occult and obscure gastrointestinal bleeding. Gastroenterology 2000;118:197. [PMID: 10611169]

Rossini FP et al: Small-bowel endoscopy. Endoscopy 2002;34:13. [PMID: 11778126]

■ DISEASES OF THE PERITONEUM

APPROACH TO THE PATIENT WITH ASCITES

Etiology of Ascites

The term "ascites" denotes the pathologic accumulation of fluid in the peritoneal cavity. Healthy men have little or no intraperitoneal fluid, but women normally may have up to 20 mL depending on the phase of the menstrual cycle. The causes of ascites may be classified into two broad pathophysiologic categories: that which is associated with a normal peritoneum and that which occurs due to a diseased peritoneum (Table 14–8). The most common cause of ascites is portal hypertension secondary to chronic liver disease, which accounts for over 80% of patients with ascites. The management of portal hypertensive ascites is discussed in Chapter 15. The most common causes of non-portal hypertensive ascites include infections (tuberculous peritonitis), intra-abdominal malignancy, inflammatory disorders of the peritoneum, and ductal disruptions (chylous, pancreatic, biliary).

Clinical Features

A. SYMPTOMS AND SIGNS

The history usually is one of increasing abdominal girth, with the presence of abdominal pain depending on the cause. Because most ascites is secondary to chronic liver disease with portal hypertension, patients should be asked about risk factors for liver disease, especially ethanol consumption, transfusions, tattoos, intravenous drug use, a history of viral hepatitis or jaundice, and birth in an area endemic for hepatitis. A history of cancer or marked weight loss arouses suspicion of malignant ascites. Fevers may suggest infected peritoneal fluid, including bacterial peritonitis (spontaneous or secondary). Patients with chronic liver disease and ascites are at greatest risk of developing spontaneous bacterial peritonitis. In immigrants, immunocompromised hosts, or severely malnourished alcoholics, tuberculous peritonitis should be considered.

Physical examination should emphasize signs of portal hypertension and chronic liver disease. Elevated jugular venous pressure may suggest right-sided con-

Table 14–8. Causes of ascites.

NORMAL PERITONEUM

Portal hypertension (SAAG ≥ 1.1 g/dL)
1. **Hepatic congestion[1]**
   Congestive heart failure
   Constrictive pericarditis
   Tricuspid insufficiency
   Budd-Chiari syndrome
   Veno-occlusive disease
2. **Liver disease[2]**
   Cirrhosis
   Alcoholic hepatitis
   Fulminant hepatic failure
   Massive hepatic metastases
   Hepatic fibrosis
   Acute fatty liver of pregnancy
3. **Portal vein occlusion**

Hypoalbuminemia (SAAG < 1.1 g/dL)
   Nephrotic syndrome
   Protein-losing enteropathy
   Severe malnutrition with anasarca

Miscellaneous conditions (SAAG < 1.1 g/dL)
   Chylous ascites
   Pancreatic ascites
   Bile ascites
   Nephrogenic ascites
   Urine ascites
   Myxedema (SAAG ≥ 1.1 g/dL)
   Ovarian disease

DISEASED PERITONEUM (SAAG < 1.1 g/dL[2])

Infections
   Bacterial peritonitis
   Tuberculous peritonitis
   Fungal peritonitis
   HIV-associated peritonitis

Malignant conditions
   Peritoneal carcinomatosis
   Primary mesothelioma
   Pseudomyxoma peritonei
   Massive hepatic metastases
   Hepatocellular carcinoma

Other conditions
   Familial Mediterranean fever
   Vasculitis
   Granulomatous peritonitis
   Eosinophilic peritonitis

SAAG = serum-ascites albumin gradient.
[1]Hepatic congestion usually associated with SAAG ≥ 1.1 g/dL and ascitic fluid total protein > 2.5 g/dL.
[2]There may be cases of "mixed ascites" in which portal hypertensive ascites is complicated by a secondary process such as infection. In these cases, the SAAG is ≥ 1.1 g/dL.

gestive heart failure or constrictive pericarditis. A large tender liver is characteristic of acute alcoholic hepatitis or Budd-Chiari syndrome. The presence of large abdominal wall veins with cephalad flow also suggests portal hypertension; inferiorly directed flow implies hepatic vein obstruction. Signs of chronic liver disease include palmar erythema, cutaneous spider angiomas,

gynecomastia, and Dupuytren's contracture. Asterixis secondary to hepatic encephalopathy may be present. Anasarca results from cardiac failure or nephrotic syndrome with hypoalbuminemia. Finally, firm lymph nodes in the left supraclavicular region or umbilicus may suggest intra-abdominal malignancy.

The physical examination is relatively insensitive for detecting ascitic fluid. In general, patients must have at least 1500 mL of fluid to be detected reliably by this method. Even the experienced clinician may find it difficult to distinguish between obesity and small-volume ascites. Abdominal ultrasound establishes the presence of fluid.

B. LABORATORY TESTING

1. Abdominal paracentesis—Abdominal paracentesis is performed as part of the diagnostic evaluation in all patients with new onset of ascites to help determine the cause. It should also be performed to diagnose bacterial peritonitis in all patients admitted to the hospital with cirrhosis and ascites (in whom the prevalence of bacterial peritonitis is 10–30%) and when patients with known ascites develop clinical deterioration (fever, abdominal pain, rapid worsening of renal function, or worsened hepatic encephalopathy).

a. Inspection—Cloudy fluid suggests infection. Milky fluid is seen with chylous ascites due to high triglyceride levels. Bloody fluid is most commonly attributable to a traumatic paracentesis, but up to 20% of cases of malignant ascites are bloody.

b. Routine studies—

(1) Cell count—A white blood cell count is the most important test. Normal ascitic fluid contains < 500 leukocytes/μL and < 250 PMNs/μL. Any inflammatory condition can cause an elevated ascitic white count. A polymorphonuclear neutrophil count of > 250/μL (neutrocytic ascites), with a percentage of > 75% of all white cells is highly suggestive of bacterial peritonitis, either spontaneous primary peritonitis or secondary peritonitis (ie, caused by an intra-abdominal source of infection, such as a perforated viscus or appendicitis). An elevated white count with a predominance of lymphocytes arouses suspicion of tuberculosis or peritoneal carcinomatosis.

(2) Albumin and total protein—The serum-ascites albumin gradient (SAAG) is the best single test for the classification of ascites into portal hypertensive and non-portal hypertensive causes (Table 14–8). Calculated by subtracting the ascitic fluid albumin from the serum albumin, the gradient correlates directly with the portal pressure. An SAAG ≥ 1.1 g/dL suggests underlying portal hypertension, while gradients < 1.1 g/dL implicate non-portal hypertensive causes.

The accuracy of the SAAG exceeds 95% in classifying ascites. It should be recognized, however, that approximately 4% of patients have "mixed ascites," ie, underlying cirrhosis with portal hypertension complicated by a second cause for ascites formation (such as malignancy or tuberculosis). Thus, a high SAAG is indicative of portal hypertension but does not exclude concomitant malignancy.

The ascitic fluid total protein provides some additional clues to the cause. An elevated SAAG and a high protein level (> 2.5 g/dL) are seen in most cases of hepatic congestion secondary to cardiac disease or Budd-Chiari syndrome. However, an increased ascitic fluid protein is also found in up to 20% of cases of uncomplicated cirrhosis. Two-thirds of patients with malignant ascites have a total protein level > 2.5 g/dL.

(3) Culture and Gram stain—The best technique consists of the inoculation of aerobic and anaerobic blood culture bottles with 5–10 mL of ascitic fluid at the patient's bedside, which increases the sensitivity for detecting bacterial peritonitis to over 85% in patients with neutrocytic ascites (> 250 PMNs/μL), compared with approximately 50% sensitivity by conventional agar plate or broth cultures.

c. Optional studies—Other laboratory tests are of utility in some specific clinical situations. Glucose and LDH may be helpful in distinguishing spontaneous from secondary bacterial peritonitis (see below). Glucose levels are reduced in patients with tuberculous peritonitis. An elevated amylase may suggest pancreatic ascites or a perforation of the gastrointestinal tract with leakage of pancreatic secretions into the ascitic fluid. Perforation of the biliary tree is suspected with an ascitic bilirubin concentration that is greater than the serum bilirubin. An elevated ascitic creatinine suggests leakage of urine from the bladder or ureters. Ascitic fluid cytologic examination is ordered if peritoneal carcinomatosis is suspected.

C. IMAGING

Abdominal ultrasound is useful in confirming the presence of ascites and in the guidance of paracentesis. Both ultrasound and CT imaging are useful in distinguishing between causes of portal and non-portal hypertensive ascites. Doppler ultrasound and CT can detect thrombosis of the hepatic veins (Budd-Chiari syndrome) or portal veins. In patients with non-portal hypertensive ascites, these studies are useful in detecting lymphadenopathy and masses of the mesentery and of solid organs such as the liver, ovaries, and pancreas. Furthermore, they permit directed percutaneous needle biopsies of these lesions. Ultrasound and CT are poor procedures for the detection of peritoneal carcinomatosis.

D. LAPAROSCOPY

Laparoscopy is an important test in the evaluation of some patients with non-portal hypertensive ascites (low SAAG) or mixed ascites. It permits direct visualization and biopsy of the peritoneum, liver, and some intra-abdominal lymph nodes. Cases of suspected peritoneal tuberculosis or suspected malignancy with nondiagnostic CT imaging and ascitic fluid cytology are best evaluated by this method.

Jeffrey J et al: Ascitic fluid analysis: the role of biochemistry and haematology. Hosp Med (May) 2001;62:282. [PMID: 11885888]

Runyon BA: Ascites. Clin Liver Dis 2000;4:151. [PMID: 11232182]

Runyon BA: Management of adult patients with ascites caused by cirrhosis. Hepatology 1998;27:264. [PMID: 9425946]

SPONTANEOUS BACTERIAL PERITONITIS

 ESSENTIALS OF DIAGNOSIS

- *A history of chronic liver disease and ascites.*
- *Fever and abdominal pain.*
- *Peritoneal finding on examination uncommonly encountered.*
- *Neutrocytic ascites (> 250 WBCs/μL) with neutrophilic predominance.*

General Considerations

"Spontaneous" bacterial infection of ascitic fluid occurs in the absence of an apparent intra-abdominal source of infection. It is seen with few exceptions in patients with ascites caused by chronic liver disease. Translocation of enteric bacteria across the gut wall or mesenteric lymphatics leads to seeding of the ascitic fluid, as may bacteremia from other sites. Approximately 20–30% of cirrhotic patients with ascites develop spontaneous peritonitis; however, the incidence is greater than 40% in patients with ascitic fluid total protein < 1 g/dL, probably due to decreased ascitic fluid opsonic activity.

Virtually all cases of spontaneous bacterial peritonitis are caused by a monomicrobial infection. The most common pathogens are enteric gram-negative bacteria (*Escherichia coli, Klebsiella pneumoniae,* enterococcus species) or gram-positive bacteria (*Streptococcus pneumoniae,* viridans streptococci). Anaerobic bacteria are not associated with spontaneous bacterial peritonitis.

Clinical Findings

A. SYMPTOMS AND SIGNS

Eighty to 90 percent of patients with spontaneous bacterial peritonitis are symptomatic; in many cases the presentation is subtle. Spontaneous bacterial peritonitis may be present in 20% of patients hospitalized with chronic liver disease in the absence of any suggestive symptoms or signs.

The most common symptoms are fever and abdominal pain, present in two-thirds of patients. Spontaneous bacterial peritonitis may also present with a change in mental status due to exacerbation or precipitation of hepatic encephalopathy, or sudden worsening of renal function. Physical examination typically demonstrates signs of chronic liver disease with ascites. Abdominal tenderness is present in less than half of patients, and its presence suggests other processes.

B. LABORATORY FINDINGS

The most important diagnostic test is abdominal paracentesis. Ascitic fluid should be sent for cell count, and blood culture bottles should be inoculated at the bedside; Gram stain is insensitive. An ascitic fluid total protein of more than 1 g/dL is evidence against spontaneous bacterial peritonitis.

In the proper clinical setting, an ascitic fluid PMN count of > 250 cells/μL (neutrocytic ascites) is presumptive evidence of bacterial peritonitis. The percentage of PMNs is greater than 50–70% of the ascitic fluid white blood cells and commonly approximates 100%. Patients with neutrocytic ascites are presumed to be infected and should be started—regardless of symptoms—on antibiotics. Although 10–30% of patients with neutrocytic ascites have negative ascitic bacterial cultures ("culture-negative neutrocytic ascites"), it is presumed nonetheless that these patients have bacterial peritonitis and should be treated empirically. Occasionally, a positive blood culture identifies the organism when ascitic fluid is sterile.

Differential Diagnosis

Spontaneous bacterial peritonitis must be distinguished from secondary bacterial peritonitis, in which ascitic fluid has become secondarily infected by an intra-abdominal infection. Even in the presence of perforation, clinical symptoms and signs of peritonitis may be lacking in up to 30% of patients owing to the separation of the visceral and parietal peritoneum by the ascitic fluid. Causes of secondary bacterial peritonitis include appendicitis, diverticulitis, perforated peptic ulcer, and perforated gallbladder. Secondary bacterial infection accounts for 3% of cases of infected ascitic fluid.

Ascitic fluid total protein, LDH, and glucose are useful in distinguishing spontaneous bacterial peritonitis from secondary infection. Up to two-thirds of patients with secondary bacterial peritonitis have at least two of the following: decreased glucose level (< 50 mg/dL), an elevated LDH level (greater than serum), and total protein > 1 g/dL. Ascitic neutrophil counts > 10,000/μL also are suspicious; however, most patients with secondary peritonitis have neutrophil counts within the range of spontaneous peritonitis. The presence of multiple organisms on ascitic fluid Gram stain or culture is diagnostic of secondary peritonitis.

If secondary bacterial peritonitis is suspected, plain films, abdominal CT imaging, and water-soluble contrast studies of the upper and lower gastrointestinal tracts should be obtained to look for evidence of an intra-abdominal source of infection. If these studies are negative and secondary peritonitis still is suspected, repeat paracentesis should be performed after 48 hours of antibiotic therapy to confirm that the polymorphonuclear neutrophil count is decreasing. Secondary bacterial peritonitis should be suspected in patients in whom the polymorphonuclear neutrophil count is not below the pretreatment value at 48 hours.

Neutrocytic ascites may also be seen in some patients with peritoneal carcinomatosis, pancreatic ascites, or tuberculous ascites. In these circumstances, however, polymorphonuclear neutrophils account for less than 50% of the ascitic white blood cells.

Prevention

Up to 70% of patients who survive an episode of spontaneous bacterial peritonitis will have another episode within 1 year. Prophylactic therapy—with norfloxacin, 400 mg/d; ciprofloxacin, 750 mg weekly; or trimethoprim-sulfamethoxazole, one double-strength tablet daily—has been shown to reduce the rate of recurrent infections to less than 20% and is recommended. Prophylaxis should be considered also in patients who have not had prior bacterial peritonitis but are at increased risk of infection due to low-protein ascites (total ascitic protein < 1 g/dL). Although improvement in survival in cirrhotic patients with ascites treated with prophylactic antibiotics has not been shown, decision analytic modeling suggests that in patients with prior bacterial peritonitis or low ascitic fluid protein, the use of prophylactic antibiotics is a cost-effective strategy.

Treatment

Empirical therapy for spontaneous bacterial peritonitis should be initiated with a third-generation cephalosporin such as cefotaxime (dosage: 2 g intravenously every 8–12 hours depending on renal function), which covers 98% of causative agents of this disorder. If enterococcus infection is suspected, ampicillin may be added. Because of a high risk of nephrotoxicity in patients with chronic liver disease, aminoglycosides should not be used. Although the optimal duration of therapy is unknown, a course of 5 days is sufficient in most patients, or until the ascites fluid polymorphonuclear neutrophil count decreases to < 250 cells/μL. Renal failure develops in up to 40% of patients and is a major cause of death. In patients given intravenous albumin, 1.5 g/kg on day 1 and 1 g/kg on day 3, the incidence of renal failure and mortality are reduced both during hospitalization and at follow-up. Patients with suspected secondary bacterial peritonitis should be given broad-spectrum coverage for enteric aerobic and anaerobic flora with a third-generation cephalosporin and metronidazole pending identification and definitive (usually surgical) treatment of the cause. In fact, the most effective treatment for spontaneous bacterial peritonitis is liver transplant.

Prognosis

The mortality rate of spontaneous bacterial peritonitis exceeds 30%. However, if the disease is recognized and treated early, the rate is less than 10%. As the majority of patients have underlying severe liver disease, many may die of liver failure, hepatorenal syndrome, or bleeding complications from portal hypertension.

Garcia-Tsao G: Current management of the complications of cirrhosis and portal hypertension: variceal hemorrhage, ascites, and spontaneous bacterial peritonitis. Gastroenterology 2001;1220:726. [PMID: 11179247]

Rimola A et al: Diagnosis, treatment and prophylaxis of spontaneous bacterial peritonitis: a consensus document. J Hepatol 2000;32:142. [PMID: 10673079]

TUBERCULOUS PERITONITIS

Tuberculosis occurs in extrapulmonary sites in 10% of non-HIV-infected people and up to 70% of those infected with HIV. Although tuberculous involvement of the peritoneum accounts for less than 2% of all causes of ascites in the United States, it remains a significant problem in the developing world. In Western countries, its incidence is higher among those with HIV disease, immigrants from underdeveloped countries, the urban poor, and nursing home residents.

The presenting symptoms include low-grade fever, abdominal pain, anorexia, and weight loss. Most patients have abdominal swelling with clinically apparent ascites; over 95% have ascites evident on ultrasound examination. In patients without ascites, there may be a doughy consistency to the abdomen. In Western societies, half of patients have underlying cirrhosis and ascites from portal hypertension. In such patients, a diagnosis of tuberculous peritonitis may go unsuspected because symptoms are attributed to the underlying liver disease. A high index of suspicion is required for prompt diagnosis and treatment.

The diagnosis thus can be difficult to establish, particularly in patients with underlying cirrhosis with ascites. Chest radiographs are abnormal in over 70%, but active tuberculous pulmonary disease is evident in less than one-fourth of patients. Skin tests are positive in half. Smears of ascitic fluid for acid-fast bacilli are usually negative, and cultures are positive in only 20%. Other findings are an ascitic fluid total protein > 3.5 g/dL, LDH > 90 units/L, or mononuclear cell-predominant leukocytosis > 500/μL—each has a sensitivity of 70–80% but limited specificity. Although these values have excellent predictive value in patients with isolated tuberculous peritonitis, their accuracy declines in patients with underlying cirrhotic ascites, nephrogenous ascites, malignant ascites (in whom concomitant infection is rare), and pancreatic ascites. Ascitic fluid adenosine deaminase activity, initially believed to be a valuable study, has been shown to have limited predictive value in the presence of cirrhotic ascites.

In patients with suspected tuberculous peritonitis, laparoscopy establishes the diagnosis. In over 90% of patients, characteristic peritoneal nodules are visible, and granulomas are seen on peritoneal biopsy. Ascitic fluid cultures increase in sensitivity to about 85% with high-volume paracenteses. Peritoneal cultures require at least 4–6 weeks and are positive in less than two-thirds of patients.

Treatment of tuberculosis is discussed in Chapter 9, though improvement is noted if laparotomy is performed for diagnostic reasons.

Inadomi J et al: The laparoscopic evaluation of ascites. Gastrointest Endosc Clin N Am 2001;11:79. [PMID: 11175976]

MALIGNANT ASCITES

Two thirds of cases of malignant ascites are caused by peritoneal carcinomatosis. The most common tumors causing carcinomatosis are primary adenocarcinomas of the ovary, uterus, pancreas, stomach, colon, lung, or breast. The remaining one-third are due to lymphatic obstruction or portal hypertension due to hepatocellular carcinoma or diffuse hepatic metastases. Patients present with nonspecific abdominal discomfort and weight loss associated with increased abdominal girth. Nausea or vomiting may be caused by partial or complete intestinal obstruction. Abdominal CT may be useful to demonstrate the primary malignancy or hepatic metastases but seldom confirms the diagnosis of peritoneal carcinomatosis. In patients with carcinomatosis, paracentesis demonstrates a low serum ascites-albumin gradient (< 1.1 mg/dL), an increased total protein (> 2.5 g/dL), and an elevated white cell count (often both neutrophils and mononuclear cells) but with a lymphocyte predominance. Cytology is positive in over 95%, but laparoscopy may be required in patients with negative cytology to confirm the diagnosis and to exclude tuberculous peritonitis, with which it may be confused. Malignant ascites attributable to portal hypertension usually is associated with an increased serum ascites-albumin gradient (> 1.1 g/dL), a variable total protein, and negative ascitic cytology. Ascites caused by peritoneal carcinomatosis does not respond to diuretics.

Patients may be treated with periodic large-volume paracentesis for symptomatic relief. Intraperitoneal chemotherapy is sometimes used to shrink the tumor, but the overall prognosis is extremely poor, with only 10% survival at 6 months. Ovarian cancers represent an exception to this rule. With newer treatments consisting of surgical debulking and intraperitoneal chemotherapy, long-term survival from ovarian cancer is possible.

Aslam N et al: Malignant ascites: new concepts in pathophysiology, diagnosis, and management. Arch Intern Med 2001; 161:2733. [PMID: 11732940]

FAMILIAL MEDITERRANEAN FEVER

This is a rare autosomal recessive disorder of unknown pathogenesis that almost exclusively affects people of Mediterranean ancestry, especially Sephardic Jews, Armenians, Turks, and Arabs. Patients lack a protease in serosal fluids that normally inactivates interleukin-8 and the chemotactic complement factor 5A. Most patients present with symptoms before the age of 20. It is characterized by episodic bouts of acute peritonitis that may be associated with serositis involving the joints and pleura. Peritoneal attacks are marked by the sudden onset of fever, severe abdominal pain, and abdominal tenderness with guarding or rebound tenderness. If left untreated, attacks resolve within 24–48 hours. Because symptoms resemble those of surgical peritonitis, patients may undergo unnecessary exploratory laparotomy. Colchicine, 0.6 mg two or three times daily, has been shown to decrease the frequency and severity of attacks. Secondary amyloidosis (AA protein) with renal or hepatic involvement may occur in 25% of cases and is the main cause of death. Colchicine prevents or arrests further progression of amyloidosis development. In the absence of amyloidosis, the prognosis is excellent. The gene responsible for familial Mediterranean fever (MEFV) has been identified and cloned, and the diagnosis can be established by genetic testing.

Drenth J et al: Hereditary periodic fever. N Engl J Med 2001; 345:1748. [PMID: 11742050]

MESOTHELIOMA

Primary malignant mesothelioma is a rare tumor. Over 70% of cases have a history of asbestos exposure. Patients present with abdominal pain or bowel obstruction, increased abdominal girth, and small to moderate ascites. The chest x-ray reveals pulmonary asbestosis in over 50%. The ascitic fluid is hemorrhagic, with a low serum-ascites albumin gradient. Cytology is often negative. Abdominal CT may reveal sheet-like masses involving the mesentery and omentum. Diagnosis is made at laparotomy or laparoscopy. The prognosis is extremely poor, but long-term survivors have been described with a combination of radiation therapy and systemic or intraperitoneal chemotherapy.

Sebbag G et al: Results of treatment of 33 patients with peritoneal mesothelioma. Br J Surg 2000;87:1587. [PMID: 11091251]

MISCELLANEOUS PERITONEAL DISEASES

Chylous ascites is the accumulation of lipid-rich lymph in the peritoneal cavity. The ascitic fluid is characterized by a milky appearance with a triglyceride level > 1000 mg/dL. The usual cause in adults is lymphatic obstruction or leakage caused by malignancy, especially lymphoma. Nonmalignant causes include postoperative trauma, cirrhosis, tuberculosis, pancreatitis, and filariasis.

Pancreatic ascites is the intraperitoneal accumulation of massive amounts of pancreatic secretions due either to disruption of the pancreatic duct or to a pancreatic pseudocyst. It is most commonly seen in patients with chronic pancreatitis and complicates up to 3% of cases of acute pancreatitis. Because the pancreatic enzymes are not activated, pain often is absent. The ascitic fluid is characterized by a high protein level (> 2.5 g/dL) but a low SAAG. Ascitic fluid amylase levels are in excess of 1000 units/L. In nonsurgical cases, initial treatment consists of bowel rest, total parenteral nutrition, and octreotide to decrease pancreatic secretion. Persistent leakage requires treatment with either endoscopic placement of stents into the pancreatic duct or surgical drainage.

Bile ascites is caused most commonly by complications of biliary tract surgery, percutaneous liver biopsy, or abdominal trauma. Unless the bile is infected, bile ascites usually does not cause abdominal pain, fever, or leukocytosis. Paracentesis reveals yellow fluid with a ratio of ascites bilirubin to serum bilirubin greater than 1.0. Treatment is dependent upon the location and rate of bile leakage. Postcholecystectomy cystic duct leaks may be treated with endoscopic sphincterotomy or biliary stent placement to facilitate bile flow across the sphincter of Oddi. Other leaks may be treated with percutaneous drainage by interventional radiologists or with surgical closure.

Godil A et al: Endoscopic management of benign pancreatic disease. Pancreas 2000;20:1. [PMID: 10630377]

■ DISEASES OF THE ESOPHAGUS

EVALUATION OF ESOPHAGEAL DISORDERS

Symptoms

Heartburn, dysphagia, and odynophagia virtually always indicate a primary esophageal disorder.

A. HEARTBURN

Heartburn (pyrosis) is the feeling of substernal burning, often radiating to the neck. Caused by the reflux of acidic (or, rarely, alkaline) material into the esophagus, it is highly specific for gastroesophageal reflux disease.

B. DYSPHAGIA

Difficulties in swallowing may arise from problems in transferring the food bolus from the oropharynx to the upper esophagus (oropharyngeal dysphagia) or from impaired transport of the bolus through the body of the esophagus (esophageal dysphagia). The history usually leads to the correct diagnosis.

1. Oropharyngeal dysphagia—The oropharyngeal phase of swallowing is a complex process requiring elevation of the tongue, closure of the nasopharynx, relaxation of the upper esophageal sphincter, closure of the airway, and pharyngeal peristalsis. A variety of mechanical and neuromuscular conditions can disrupt this process (Table 14–9). Problems with the oral phase of swallowing cause drooling or spillage of food from the mouth, inability to chew or initiate swallowing, or dry mouth. Pharyngeal dysphagia is characterized by an immediate sense of the bolus catching in the neck, the need to swallow repeatedly to clear food from the pharynx, or coughing or choking during meals. There may be associated dysphonia, dysarthria, or other neurologic symptoms.

2. Esophageal dysphagia—Esophageal dysphagia may be caused by **mechanical lesions** obstructing the esophagus or by **motility disorders** (Table 14–10). Patients with mechanical obstruction experience dysphagia, primarily for solids. This is recurrent, predictable, and, if the lesion progresses, will worsen as the lumen narrows. Patients with **motility disorders** have dysphagia for both solids and liquids. It is episodic, unpredictable, and nonprogressive.

C. ODYNOPHAGIA

Odynophagia is sharp substernal pain on swallowing that may limit oral intake. It usually reflects severe erosive disease. It is most commonly associated with

Table 14–9. Causes of oropharyngeal dysphagia.

Neurologic disorders
 Brainstem cerebrovascular accident, mass lesion
 Amyotrophic lateral sclerosis, multiple sclerosis, pseudobulbar palsy, post-polio syndrome, Guillain-Barré syndrome
 Parkinson's disease, Huntington's disease, dementia
 Tardive dyskinesia
Muscular and rheumatologic disorders
 Myopathies, polymyositis
 Oculopharyngeal dystrophy
 Sjögren's syndrome
Metabolic disorders
 Thyrotoxicosis, amyloidosis, Cushing's disease, Wilson's disease
 Medication side effects: anticholinergics, phenothiazines
Infectious disease
 Polio, diphtheria, botulism, Lyme disease, syphilis, mucositis (candida, herpes)
Structural disorders
 Zenker's diverticulum
 Cervical osteophytes, cricopharyngeal bar, proximal esophageal webs
 Oropharyngeal tumors
 Postsurgical or radiation changes
 Pill-induced injury
Motility disorders
 Upper esophageal sphincter dysfunction

Table 14–10. Causes of esophageal dysphagia.

Cause	Clues
Mechanical obstruction	**Solid foods worse than liquids**
Schatzki's ring	Intermittent dysphagia; not progressive
Peptic stricture	Chronic heartburn; progressive dysphagia
Esophageal cancer	Progressive dysphagia; age over 50
Motility disorder	**Solid and liquid foods**
Achalasia	Progressive dysphagia
Diffuse esophageal spasm	Intermittent; not progressive; may have chest pain
Scleroderma	Chronic heartburn; Raynaud's phenomenon

infectious esophagitis due to candida, herpesviruses, or cytomegalovirus, especially in immunocompromised patients. It may also be caused by corrosive injury due to caustic ingestions and by pill-induced ulcers.

Diagnostic Studies

A. UPPER ENDOSCOPY

Endoscopy is the study of choice for evaluating persistent heartburn, odynophagia, and structural abnormalities detected on barium esophagography. In addition to direct visualization, it allows biopsy of mucosal abnormalities and dilation of strictures.

B. VIDEOESOPHAGOGRAPHY

Oropharyngeal dysphagia is best evaluated with rapid-sequence videoesophagography.

C. BARIUM ESOPHAGOGRAPHY

Patients with esophageal dysphagia often are evaluated first with a radiographic barium study to differentiate between mechanical lesions and motility disorders, providing important information about the latter in particular. In patients in whom there is a high suspicion of a mechanical lesion, many clinicians will proceed first to endoscopic evaluation without a barium study. In patients with esophageal dysphagia and a suspected motility disorder, barium esophagoscopy should be obtained first.

D. ESOPHAGEAL MANOMETRY

Esophageal motility may be assessed using manometric techniques. It is indicated (1) to determine the location of the lower esophageal sphincter to allow precise placement of a pH probe; (2) to assess peristaltic function in the esophageal body in patients being considered for antireflux surgery; and (3) to establish the diagnosis of achalasia or diffuse esophageal spasm in patients with dysphagia in whom these diagnoses have been first suggested by endoscopy or barium study.

E. ESOPHAGEAL pH RECORDING

Esophageal pH may be monitored continuously by means of a small pH probe placed 5 cm above the lower esophageal sphincter. The probe is attached to a portable pH device capable of recording pH for up to 24 hours. The recording provides information about the amount of acid esophageal reflux and on the temporal correlations between symptoms and reflux.

American Gastroenterological Association Medical Position Statement. Guidelines on the use of esophageal pH recording. Gastroenterology 1996;110:1981. [PMID: 8964427]

American Gastroenterological Association Medical Position Statement on Management of Oropharyngeal Dysphagia. Gastroenterology 1999;116:452. [PMID: 9922327]

Hila A et al: Pharyngeal and upper esophageal sphincter manometry in the evaluation of dysphagia. J Clin Gastroenterol 2001;33:355. [PMID: 11606849]

INFLAMMATORY ESOPHAGEAL CONDITIONS

1. Gastroesophageal Reflux Disease

 ESSENTIALS OF DIAGNOSIS

- *Heartburn; may be exacerbated by meals, bending, or recumbency.*
- *Typical uncomplicated cases do not require diagnostic studies.*
- *Endoscopy demonstrates abnormalities in < 50% of patients.*
- *Barium esophagography seldom helpful.*

General Considerations

Gastroesophageal reflux disease affects 20% of adults, who report at least weekly episodes of heartburn, and up to 10% complain of daily symptoms. Though most patients have mild disease, up to 50% develop esophageal mucosal damage (reflux esophagitis) and a few develop more serious complications. Several factors may contribute to gastroesophageal reflux disease.

A. INCOMPETENT LOWER ESOPHAGEAL SPHINCTER

The antireflux barrier at the gastroesophageal junction is dependent upon intrinsic lower esophageal sphincter pressure, the intra-abdominal location of the sphincter, and the extrinsic compression of the sphincter by the crural diaphragm. In most patients, baseline lower esophageal sphincter pressures are normal (10–30 mm Hg). In patients without hiatal hernias, about 70% of reflux episodes occur during relaxations of the lower esophageal sphincter that occur spontaneously ("transient relaxations") or as prolonged relax-

ation after swallowing. The remaining events occur during periods of low sphincter pressure ("hypotensive" sphincter). A small number of patients with more severe involvement (especially those with strictures) have chronically incompetent sphincters (< 10 mm Hg), resulting in free reflux or stress reflux during lifting, bending, or abdominal straining.

B. HIATAL HERNIA

Hiatal hernias are common and usually cause no symptoms. In patients with gastroesophageal reflux, however, they are associated with higher amounts of acid reflux and delayed esophageal acid clearance leading to more severe esophagitis, especially Barrett's esophagus. Increased reflux episodes occur during normal swallowing-induced relaxation, periods of sphincter hypotension, and straining due to reflux of acid from the hiatal hernia sac into the esophagus.

C. IRRITANT EFFECTS OF REFLUXATE

Esophageal mucosal damage is related to the potency of the refluxate and the amount of time it is in contact with the mucosa. Acidic gastric fluid (pH < 4.0) is extremely caustic to the esophageal mucosa and is the major injurious agent in the majority of cases. In some patients, reflux of bile or alkaline pancreatic secretions may be contributory.

D. ABNORMAL ESOPHAGEAL CLEARANCE

Acid refluxate normally is cleared and neutralized by esophageal peristalsis and salivary bicarbonate. During sleep, swallowing-induced peristalsis is infrequent, prolonging acid exposure to the esophagus. One-third of patients with severe gastroesophageal reflux disease also have diminished peristaltic clearance. Certain medical conditions such as scleroderma are associated with diminished peristalsis. Sjögren's syndrome, anticholinergic medications, and oral radiation therapy may exacerbate gastroesophageal reflux disease due to impaired salivation.

E. DELAYED GASTRIC EMPTYING

Impaired gastric emptying due to gastroparesis or partial gastric outlet obstruction potentiates gastroesophageal reflux disease.

Clinical Findings

A. SYMPTOMS AND SIGNS

The typical symptom is heartburn. This most often occurs 30–60 minutes after meals and upon reclining. Patients often report relief from taking antacids or baking soda. When this symptom is dominant, the diagnosis is established with a high degree of reliability. Many patients, however, have less specific dyspeptic symptoms with or without heartburn. Overall, a clinical diagnosis of gastroesophageal reflux has a sensitivity of 80% but a specificity of only 70%. Severity is not correlated with the degree of tissue damage. In fact, some patients with severe esophagitis are only mildly symptomatic. Patients may complain of regurgitation—the spontaneous reflux of sour or bitter gastric contents into the mouth. Less common symptoms include dysphagia, which may be due to abnormal peristalsis or the development of complications such as stricture or Barrett's metaplasia.

"Atypical" manifestations of gastroesophageal disease are being recognized with increasing frequency. These include asthma, chronic cough, chronic laryngitis, sore throat, and noncardiac chest pain. Gastroesophageal reflux may be either a causative or an exacerbating factor in up to 50% of these patients, especially those with refractory symptoms. Because many of these patients do not have heartburn or regurgitation, the diagnosis often is overlooked.

Physical examination and laboratory data are normal in uncomplicated disease.

B. SPECIAL EXAMINATIONS

Uncomplicated patients with typical symptoms of heartburn and regurgitation may be treated empirically for 4 weeks for gastroesophageal reflux disease without the need for diagnostic studies. Further investigation is required in patients with complicated disease and those unresponsive to empirical therapy.

1. Upper endoscopy—Upper endoscopy with biopsy is the standard procedure for documenting the type and extent of tissue damage in gastroesophageal reflux. Fifty percent of patients with proved acid reflux will have visible mucosal abnormalities such as erythema and friability of the squamocolumnar junction and erosions, known as reflux esophagitis. However, endoscopy is normal in up to half of symptomatic patients and does not exclude mild disease. Esophageal abnormalities are graded on a scale of I (mild) to IV (severe erosions, stricture, or Barrett's esophagus). Initial medical therapy for gastroesophageal reflux disease is guided by the presence of symptoms, not the endoscopic findings. Hence, endoscopy is not warranted for most patients with typical symptoms suggesting uncomplicated reflux disease. Endoscopy should be performed in patients whose symptoms have not responded after initial empirical therapy and patients with symptoms suggesting complicated disease (dysphagia, odynophagia, occult or overt bleeding, or iron deficiency anemia). Endoscopy also may be warranted in patients with long-standing symptoms (over 5 years) or patients requiring continuous maintenance therapy, to look for Barrett's esophagus.

2. Barium esophagography—This study plays a limited role. In patients with severe dysphagia, it is sometimes obtained prior to endoscopy to identify a stricture.

3. Ambulatory esophageal pH monitoring—Ambulatory pH monitoring is the best study for documenting acid reflux, but it is unnecessary in most patients. It is useful and indicated in the following situations: (1) to document abnormal esophageal acid exposure in a patient being considered for antireflux surgery who has a normal endoscopy (ie, no evidence of reflux esophagitis); (2) to evaluate patients with a normal endoscopy who have reflux symptoms unresponsive to therapy with a proton pump inhibitor; (3) to detect either abnormal amounts of reflux or an association between reflux episodes and atypical symptoms such as noncardiac chest pain, asthma, chronic cough, laryngitis, and sore throat. It is recommended that most patients with atypical symptoms first be given an empirical trial of antireflux therapy with a high-dose proton pump inhibitor for 2–3 months. If symptoms fail to improve, a pH study is then performed.

Differential Diagnosis

Symptoms of gastroesophageal reflux disease may be similar to those of other diseases such as esophageal motility disorders, peptic ulcer, cholelithiasis, nonulcer dyspepsia, and angina pectoris. Reflux erosive esophagitis may be confused with pill-induced damage, radiation esophagitis, or infections (CMV, herpes, candida).

Complications

A. BARRETT'S ESOPHAGUS

This is a condition in which the squamous epithelium of the esophagus is replaced by metaplastic columnar epithelium containing goblet and columnar cells (specialized intestinal metaplasia). Present in up to 10% of patients with chronic reflux, it arises from chronic reflux-induced injury to the esophageal squamous epithelium. Barrett's esophagus is suspected at endoscopy from the presence of orange, gastric type epithelium that extends upward from the stomach into the distal tubular esophagus in a tongue-like or circumferential fashion. Biopsies obtained at endoscopy confirm the diagnosis. Three types of columnar epithelium may be identified: gastric cardiac, gastric fundic, and specialized intestinal metaplasia. Only the latter is believed to carry an increased risk of neoplasia.

Barrett's esophagus does not provoke specific symptoms but gastroesophageal reflux does. Most patients have a long history of reflux symptoms, such as heartburn and regurgitation. Dysphagia due to impaired motility is common. Paradoxically, one-third of patients report minimal or no symptoms of gastroesophageal reflux disease, suggesting decreased acid sensitivity of Barrett's epithelium. Indeed, over 90% of individuals with Barrett's esophagus in the general population do not seek medical attention. Barrett's esophagus may be complicated by stricture formation or acid-peptic ulceration, which can bleed.

Barrett's esophagus should be treated with long-term proton pump inhibitors. Surgical fundoplication may be desirable in some situations. Medical or surgical therapy may prevent progression, but there is no convincing evidence that regression occurs in most patients. Endoscopic ablation of Barrett's epithelium with cautery probes or photodynamic therapy (using photosensitizers and laser energy) has anecdotally resulted in partial or complete regression of columnar epithelium.

The most serious complication of Barrett's esophagus is esophageal adenocarcinoma, which has an estimated annual incidence of 0.8%, representing a 40-fold risk compared with patients without Barrett's esophagus. Virtually all adenocarcinomas of the esophagus and many such tumors of the gastric cardia arise from Barrett's metaplasia. Thus, patients with Barrett's esophagus who are operative candidates undergo endoscopic surveillance with mucosal biopsies every 2–3 years. Patients with low-grade dysplasia are treated with aggressive medical management and endoscopic surveillance every 6–12 months. The management of high-grade dysplasia is controversial. Since 30–40% may progress to (or already contain) invasive adenocarcinoma, surgery is usually recommended. Otherwise, photodynamic ablation or endoscopic mucosal resection may be considered.

Barrett's epithelium of any length carries an increased risk of neoplasia. Although a clinical distinction is sometimes made between "short-segment" (< 3 cm length) and long-segment Barrett's esophagus, both warrant periodic endoscopic surveillance. Specialized intestinal metaplasia is present at the gastroesophageal junction in up to 20% of patients undergoing endoscopy in the absence of visible Barrett's esophagus, but the significance of this entity is unclear.

B. PEPTIC STRICTURE

Stricture formation occurs in about 10% of patients with esophagitis. It is manifested by the gradual development of solid food dysphagia progressive over months to years. Often there is a reduction in heartburn because the stricture acts as a barrier to reflux. Most strictures are located at the gastroesophageal junction. Strictures located above this level usually occur with Barrett's metaplasia. Endoscopy with biopsy is mandatory in all cases to differentiate peptic stricture from other benign or malignant causes of esophageal stricture (Schatzki's ring, esophageal carcinoma). Active erosive esophagitis is often present. Up to 90% of symptomatic patients are effectively treated with dilation. Dilation is continued over one to several sessions. A luminal diameter of 16–17 mm is usually sufficient to relieve dysphagia. Chronic therapy with a proton pump inhibitor (omeprazole or lansoprazole) is required to decrease the likelihood of stricture recurrence. Some patients require intermittent stricture dilation to maintain luminal patency, but operative management for strictures that do not respond to dilation is seldom required.

Treatment

A. MEDICAL TREATMENT

The goal of treatment is to provide symptomatic relief, to heal esophagitis (if present), and to prevent complications. In the majority of patients with uncomplicated disease, empirical treatment is initiated based upon a compatible history without the need for further confirmatory studies. Patients not responding and those with suspected complications undergo further evaluation with upper endoscopy or esophageal pH recording.

Patients with known erosive esophagitis, complications (such as a peptic stricture or Barrett's esophagus), or suspected atypical manifestations (such as asthma or laryngitis) are treated initially with a proton pump inhibitor (see below). In most other patients, treatment may proceed in the following stepwise fashion.

1. Mild, intermittent symptoms—Gastroesophageal reflux is a lifelong disease that requires lifestyle modifications as well as medical intervention. The best advice is to avoid lying down within 3 hours after meals, the period of greatest reflux. Elevating the head of the bed on 6-inch blocks or a foam wedge to reduce reflux and enhance esophageal clearance is recommended, especially for patients with nocturnal and atypical symptoms. Patients should be advised to avoid acidic foods (tomato products, citrus fruits, spicy foods, coffee) and agents that relax the lower esophageal sphincter or delay gastric emptying (fatty foods, peppermint, chocolate, alcohol, and smoking). Weight loss, avoidance of bending after meals, and reduction of meal size may also be helpful.

Antacids are the mainstay for rapid relief of occasional heartburn; however, their duration of action is less than 2 hours. Many are available over the counter. Those containing magnesium should not be used in renal failure, and patients with this condition should be cautioned appropriately. Gaviscon is an alginate-antacid combination that decreases reflux in the upright position.

All H_2 receptor antagonists are available in over-the-counter formulations: cimetidine 200 mg, ranitidine and nizatidine 75 mg, famotidine 10 mg—all of which are half of the typical prescription strength. When taken for active heartburn, these agents have a delay in onset of at least 30 minutes; antacids provide more immediate relief. However, once these agents take effect, they provide heartburn relief for up to 8 hours. When taken before meals known to provoke heartburn, these agents reduce the symptom.

2. Moderate symptoms—Uncomplicated patients with typical reflux symptoms that occur several times per week or daily should be treated empirically with an H_2 receptor antagonist. Standard prescription doses of these agents are ranitidine or nizatidine 150 mg, famotidine 20 mg, or cimetidine 400–800 mg, twice daily. These agents reduce 24-hour acidity by over 60%. Ranitidine and cimetidine are available in less expensive generic formulations. Treatment twice daily affords improvement in up to two-thirds of patients. Given their superior efficacy and once-daily dosing, proton pump inhibitors increasingly are prescribed as first-line therapy for mild to moderate symptoms in preference to beginning with an H_2 receptor antagonist. However, generic H_2 receptor antagonists are significantly less expensive than proton pump inhibitors and provide effective symptomatic relief in most patients with mild to moderate reflux symptoms.

For patients whose symptoms persist despite 6 weeks of standard doses of H_2 receptor antagonist therapy, continued therapy or an increase in dosage of H_2 receptor antagonists is seldom effective in providing symptom relief. These patients should be treated with a proton pump inhibitor (omeprazole or rabeprazole 20 mg, lansoprazole 30 mg, or esomeprazole or pantoprazole 40 mg) once daily (see below). The decision to prescribe proton pump inhibitors is based upon the presence of persistent symptoms, not endoscopic findings.

In those who achieve good symptom relief with either an H_2 receptor antagonist or a proton pump inhibitor, therapy should be discontinued after 8–12 weeks. Patients whose symptoms relapse may be treated with either continuous or intermittent courses of therapy depending upon symptom frequency and patient preference. Many patients are controlled adequately with intermittent courses of therapy rather than continuous maintenance treatment.

Promotility drugs (metoclopramide, cisapride, bethanechol) reduce reflux by increasing lower esophageal sphincter pressure and enhancing esophageal peristalsis and gastric emptying. Side effects preclude the use of these agents for reflux disease. Cisapride causes QT prolongation, leading to serious cardiac arrhythmias, and has been withdrawn from the market in the United States. Metoclopramide is a dopamine antagonist that may cause neuropsychiatric side effects in up to one-third of patients, limiting it to short-term use only.

3. Severe symptoms and erosive disease—For patients with severe symptoms and for patients who undergo endoscopy and have documented erosive esophagitis, the optimal initial therapy is a proton pump inhibitor (omeprazole or rabeprazole 20 mg, lansoprazole 30 mg, pantoprazole or esomeprazole 40 mg) once daily. Proton pump inhibitors given once daily provide symptom relief and healing of esophagitis in over 80% and given twice daily provide relief in over 95% of patients—compared with under 50% with standard doses of H_2 receptor antagonists—and are therefore the drugs of choice for severe or erosive disease. Because there appears to be little difference between these agents in efficacy or side effect profiles, the choice of agent is determined by cost. Esomeprazole, the S-isomer of omeprazole, provides slightly greater inhibition of 24-hour gastric acidity than the other agents, resulting in a small (5%) therapeutic advantage over omeprazole. Approximately 10–20% of patients fail to achieve symptom relief with a once-daily dose within 2–4 weeks and require a higher dosage (twice-daily) proton pump inhibitor. There-

fore, some recommend initiating therapy with a twice-daily dose of proton pump inhibitor, reducing therapy after 2–4 weeks to a once-daily dose. The initial course of therapy is usually 8–12 weeks. As tissue healing correlates well with symptom resolution, repeat endoscopy is warranted in patients only if they fail to respond to once-daily or twice-daily proton pump inhibitor therapy.

After discontinuation of proton pump inhibitor therapy, relapse of symptoms occurs in 80% of patients within 1 year—the majority of relapses occurring within the first 3 months. Therefore, chronic therapy to maintain symptom remission is required in most but not all patients. Patients with severe erosive esophagitis, Barrett's esophagus, or peptic stricture should be maintained on chronic therapy with a proton pump inhibitor at a dose sufficient to provide complete symptom relief. In other patients, a trial off proton pump inhibitors should be considered. Patients with prolonged symptomatic remissions (over 3 months) may be treated effectively with intermittent 4- to 8-week courses of acute proton pump inhibitor therapy. Patients with prompt recurrence of symptoms (within 3 months) require chronic maintenance therapy with either a proton pump inhibitor or an H_2 receptor antagonist. The therapy should be stepped down to the lowest dose that is effective in controlling reflux symptoms.

The maintenance doses of proton pump inhibitors may escalate over time, with over 20% of patients eventually requiring double or triple doses of proton pump inhibitors to control symptoms.

4. Extraesophageal reflux manifestations—Establishing a causal relationship between gastroesophageal reflux and extraesophageal symptoms (eg, asthma, hoarseness, cough) can be difficult. Although ambulatory esophageal pH testing can document the presence of increased acid esophageal reflux, it does not prove a causative connection. A trial of a twice-daily proton pump inhibitor for 2–3 months helps determine whether these symptoms improve after acid suppression.

5. Unresponsive disease—Approximately 10–20% of patients with gastroesophageal reflux symptoms do not respond to once-daily doses of proton pump inhibitors, and 5% do not respond to twice-daily doses. These patients undergo endoscopy prior to escalation of therapy. Patients without endoscopically visible esophagitis should undergo esophageal pH monitoring to determine the amount of esophageal acid reflux and to assess whether the refractory symptoms are truly acid-related. The presence of active erosive esophagitis usually is indicative of inadequate acid suppression and can almost always be treated successfully with higher proton pump inhibitor doses (eg, omeprazole 40 mg twice daily). Breakthrough acid production appears to occur at night in patients with severe disease. A twice-daily proton pump inhibitor (before breakfast and dinner) and a bedtime dose of an

H_2 receptor antagonist may be more effective (and less expensive) in controlling nocturnal acid than a proton pump inhibitor given three times daily. Truly refractory esophagitis may be caused by gastrinoma with gastric acid hypersecretion (Zollinger-Ellison syndrome), pill-induced esophagitis, resistance to proton pump inhibitors, and medical noncompliance.

B. SURGICAL TREATMENT

Surgical fundoplication affords good to excellent relief of symptoms and healing of esophagitis in over 85% of properly selected patients and may now be performed laparoscopically with low complication rates in most instances. Cost-effectiveness studies suggest that aggregate medical costs exceed surgical costs after 10 years. The longevity of the beneficial effects of fundoplication are debated. Different surgical centers report 10-year success rates ranging from 60% to 90%. However, over half of patients require continued acid-suppression medication after fundoplication. Furthermore, over 30% of patients develop new symptoms of dysphagia, bloating, increased flatulence, or dyspepsia. Surgical treatment is not recommended for patients who are well controlled with medical therapies but should be considered (1) for otherwise healthy patients with extraesophageal manifestations of reflux, as these symptoms often require high doses of proton pump inhibitors and may be more effectively controlled with antireflux surgery; (2) for those with severe reflux disease who are unwilling to accept lifelong medical therapy due to its expense, inconvenience, or theoretical risks; and (3) for patients with erosive disease who are intolerant of or resistant to proton pump inhibitors.

C. ENDOSCOPIC THERAPY

There are two endoscopic devices for the treatment of mild to moderate gastroesophageal reflux disease. The first uses an endoscopic "sewing machine" to place sutures below the gastroesophageal junction in the region of the gastric cardia, creating a mucosal plication that may mimic a surgical fundoplication. The second employs an intraesophageal balloon catheter from which needle electrodes are inserted through the mucosa and into the muscularis at multiple levels of the distal esophagus and cardia, permitting application of radiofrequency wave current. It is believed that this current may disrupt neural reflex pathways from the stomach to the esophagus, resulting in a decrease in relaxations of the lower esophageal sphincter. Reports of success come from uncontrolled studies; routine use is not yet advised.

Ell C et al: Endoscopic mucosal resection of early cancer and high-grade dysplasia in Barrett's esophagus. Gastroenterology 2000;118:670. [PMID: 10734018] (Should be considered as alternative to esophageal resection in selected patients.)

Extraesophageal presentations of gastroesophageal reflux disease. Am J Gastroenterol 2000;No. 8, Supplement. [PMID: 10950098]

Fass R et al: Nonerosive reflux disease—current concepts and dilemmas. Am J Gastroenterol 2001;96:303. [PMID: 11232668]

Filipi C et al: Transoral, flexible endoscopic suturing for the treatment of GERD: a multicenter trial. Gastrointest Endosc 2001;53:416. [PMID: 11275879]

Gerson L et al: A cost-effectiveness analysis of prescribing strategies in the management of gastroesophageal reflux disease. Am J Gastroenterol 2000;95:395. [PMID: 10685741]

Inadomi J et al: Step-down management of gastroesophageal reflux disease. Gastroenterology 2001;121:1095. [PMID: 11677201]

Klinkenberg-Knol EC et al: Long-term omeprazole treatment in resistant gastroesophageal reflux disease: efficacy, safety, and influence on gastric mucosa. Gastroenterology 2000;118:661. [PMID: 10734017]

Sampliner R et al: Effective and safe endoscopic reversal of nondysplastic Barrett's esophagus with thermal electrocoagulation combined with high-dose acid inhibition: a multicenter study. Gastrointest Endosc 2001;53:554. [PMID: 11323578]

Schnell T et al: Long-term nonsurgical management of Barrett's esophagus with high-grade dysplasia. Gastroenterology 2001;120:1607. [PMID: 11375943]

Sharma P: Short segment Barrett esophagus and specialized columnar mucosa at the gastroesophageal junction. Mayo Clin Proc 2001;76:331. [PMID: 11243283]

Spechler S et al: Long-term outcomes of medical and surgical therapies for gastroesophageal reflux disease. JAMA 2001; 285:2331. [PMID: 11343480]

Triadifilopoulos G et al: Radiofrequency energy delivery to the gastroesophageal junction for the treatment of GERD. Gastrointest Endosc 2001;53:407. [PMID: 11275878]

Weston A et al: Long-term follow up of Barrett's high grade dysplasia. Am J Gastroenterol 2000;95:1888. [PMID: 10950031]

INFECTIOUS ESOPHAGITIS

ESSENTIALS OF DIAGNOSIS

- *Immunosuppressed patient.*
- *Odynophagia, dysphagia, and chest pain.*
- *Endoscopy with biopsy establishes diagnosis.*

General Considerations

Infectious esophagitis occurs most commonly in immunosuppressed patients. Patients with AIDS, solid organ transplants, leukemia, lymphoma, and those receiving immunosuppressive drugs are at particular risk for opportunistic infections. *Candida albicans,* herpes simplex, and cytomegalovirus are the most common pathogens. Candida infection may occur also in patients who have uncontrolled diabetes and those being treated with systemic corticosteroids, radiation therapy, or systemic antibiotic therapy. Herpes simplex can affect normal hosts, in which case the infection is generally self-limited.

Clinical Findings

A. Symptoms and Signs

The most common symptoms are odynophagia and dysphagia. Substernal chest pain occurs in some patients. Patients with candidal esophagitis are sometimes asymptomatic. Oral thrush is present in only 75% of patients with candidal esophagitis and 25–50% of patients with viral esophagitis and is therefore an unreliable indicator of the cause of esophageal infection. Patients with esophageal CMV infection may have infection at other sites such as the colon and retina. Oral ulcers (herpes labialis) are often associated with herpes simplex esophagitis.

B. Special Examinations

Treatment may be empirical. For diagnostic certainty, endoscopy with biopsy and brushings (for microbiologic and histopathologic analysis) is preferred because of its high diagnostic accuracy. The endoscopic signs of candidal esophagitis are diffuse, linear, yellow-white plaques adherent to the mucosa. Cytomegalovirus esophagitis is characterized by one to several large, shallow, superficial ulcerations. Herpes esophagitis results in multiple small, deep ulcerations.

Treatment

A. Candidal Esophagitis

Treatment depends on the immune status of the patient and the severity of the illness. Topical therapy is used initially in patients with a normal immune system. Options include topical agents (nystatin, 500,000 units "swish and swallow" five times daily; clotrimazole troches, 10 mg dissolved in mouth five times daily) for 7–14 days. Initial therapy for immunocompromised patients (including AIDS) generally is with fluconazole, 100–200 mg/d orally. Ketoconazole should no longer be used because of its lower efficacy, unpredictable absorption, and greater risk of adverse effects. Patients not responding to oral therapy are treated with low-dose amphotericin B, 0.3–0.5 mg/kg/d. The duration of therapy is not standardized.

B. Cytomegalovirus Esophagitis

Initial therapy is with ganciclovir, 5 mg/kg intravenously every 12 hours for 3–6 weeks. Neutropenia is a frequent dose-limiting side effect. If resolution of symptoms occurs, the drug may be discontinued. If the condition has improved but not resolved, full-dose therapy may be continued for an additional 2–3 weeks. In some cases (especially in patients with AIDS), continuous ganciclovir, 5 mg/kg intravenously daily, is required for suppressive therapy. The role of oral ganciclovir in the maintenance treatment of CMV gastrointestinal disease is not established. Patients who either do not respond to or cannot tolerate

ganciclovir are treated acutely with foscarnet, 90 mg/kg intravenously every 12 hours for 3–6 weeks. The principal toxicity is renal failure. In patients with HIV infection, immune restoration with highly active antiretroviral therapy (HAART) is the most effective means of controlling CMV disease.

C. Herpetic Esophagitis

Immune-competent patients may be treated symptomatically and generally do not require specific antiviral therapy. Immunosuppressed patients may be treated with oral acyclovir, 200 mg orally five times daily, or 250 mg/m² intravenously every 8–12 hours, usually for 7–10 days. Famciclovir, 250 mg three times daily, and valacyclovir, 1 g twice daily, are effective but significantly more expensive than generic acyclovir. Nonresponders require therapy with foscarnet, 40 mg/kg intravenously every 8 hours for 21 days.

Prognosis

Most patients with infectious esophagitis can be effectively treated with complete symptom resolution. Depending on the patient's underlying immunodeficiency, relapse of symptoms off therapy can raise difficulties. Chronic suppressive therapy is sometimes required.

Darouiche RO: Oropharyngeal and esophageal candidiasis in immunocompromised patients: treatment issues. Clin Infect Dis 1998;26:259. [PMID: 9502438]

Ramanathan J et al: Herpes simplex esophagitis in the immunocompetent host: an overview. Am J Gastroenterol 2000; 95:2171. [PMID: 11007213]

Whitley RJ et al: Guidelines for the treatment of cytomegalovirus diseases in patients with AIDS in the era of potent retroviral therapy; recommendations of an international panel. Arch Intern Med 1998;158:957. [PMID: 9588429]

PILL-INDUCED ESOPHAGITIS

A number of different medications may injure the esophagus, presumably through direct, prolonged mucosal contact. The most commonly implicated are the NSAIDs, potassium chloride pills, quinidine, zalcitabine, zidovudine, alendronate and risedronate, iron, vitamin C, and antibiotics (doxycycline, tetracycline, clindamycin, trimethoprim-sulfamethoxazole). Because injury is most likely to occur if pills are swallowed without water or while supine, hospitalized or bed-bound patients are at greater risk. Symptoms include severe retrosternal chest pain, odynophagia, and dysphagia, often beginning several hours after taking a pill. These may occur suddenly and persist for days. Some patients (especially the elderly) have relatively little pain, presenting with dysphagia. Endoscopy may reveal one to several discrete ulcers that may be shallow or deep. Chronic injury may result in severe esophagitis with stricture, hemorrhage, or perforation. Healing occurs rapidly when the offending agent is eliminated. To prevent pill-induced damage, patients should take pills with 4 oz of water and remain upright for 30 minutes after ingestion. Known offending agents should not be given to patients with esophageal dysmotility, dysphagia, or strictures.

Kikendall J: Pill esophagitis. J Clin Gastroenterol 1999;28:298. [PMID: 10372925]

Lanza F et al: Endoscopic comparison of esophageal and gastroduodenal effects of risedronate and alendronate in postmenopausal women. Gastroenterology 2000;119:631. [PMID: 10982755] (Endoscopic studies suggest that risedronate is less harmful to the gastrointestinal mucosa.)

CAUSTIC ESOPHAGEAL INJURY

Caustic esophageal injury occurs from accidental (usually children) or deliberate (suicidal) ingestion of liquid or crystalline alkali (drain cleaners, etc) or acid. Ingestion is followed almost immediately by severe burning and varying degrees of chest pain, gagging, dysphagia, and drooling. Aspiration results in stridor and wheezing. Initial examination should be directed to circulatory status and to prompt assessment of airway patency, including laryngoscopy. Subsequently, chest and abdominal radiographs are obtained looking for pneumonitis or free perforation. Initial treatment is supportive, with intravenous fluids and analgesics. Nasogastric lavage and oral antidotes may be dangerous and should generally not be administered. Most patients may be managed medically. Endoscopy is usually performed within the first 24 hours to assess the extent of injury. Many patients are discovered to have no mucosal injury to the esophagus or stomach, allowing prompt discharge and psychiatric referral. Patients with evidence of mild damage (edema, erythema, exudates or superficial ulcers) recover quickly, have low risk of developing stricture, and may be advanced from liquids to a regular diet over 24–48 hours. Nasoenteric feedings should be initiated after 24–48 hours and subsequent oral feedings when the patient is tolerating oral secretions. Patients with signs of severe injury—deep or circumferential ulcers or necrosis (black discoloration) have a high risk (up to 65%) of acute complications, including perforation with mediastinitis or peritonitis, bleeding, stricture, or esophageal-tracheal fistulas. These patients must be kept fasting and monitored closely for signs of deterioration that warrant emergency surgery with possible esophagectomy and colonic or jejunal interposition. A nasoenteric feeding tube is placed after 24 hours. Oral feedings of liquids may be initiated after 2–3 days if the patient is able to tolerate secretions. Neither steroids nor antibiotics are recommended. Esophageal strictures develop in up to 70% of patients with serious esophageal injury weeks to months after the initial injury, requiring recurrent dilations. The risk of esophageal squamous carcinoma is 2–3%, warranting endoscopic surveillance 15–20 years after the caustic ingestion.

Battle WM, Codella M: Caustic injury to the upper gastrointestinal tract. In: *Consultations in Gastroenterology*. Snape WM (editor). Saunders, 1996.

BENIGN ESOPHAGEAL LESIONS

1. Mallory-Weiss Syndrome (Mucosal Laceration of Gastroesophageal Junction)

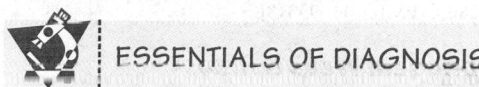

■ ESSENTIALS OF DIAGNOSIS

- *Hematemesis; usually self-limited.*
- *Prior history of vomiting, retching in 50%.*
- *Endoscopy establishes diagnosis.*

General Considerations

Mallory-Weiss syndrome is characterized by a nonpenetrating mucosal tear at the gastroesophageal junction which is hypothesized to arise from events that suddenly raise transabdominal pressure, such as lifting, retching, or vomiting. Alcoholism is a strong predisposing factor. Mallory-Weiss tears are responsible for approximately 5% of cases of upper gastrointestinal bleeding.

Clinical Findings

A. SYMPTOMS AND SIGNS

Patients usually present with hematemesis with or without melena. A history of retching, vomiting, or straining is obtained in about 50% of cases.

B. SPECIAL EXAMINATIONS

As with other causes of upper gastrointestinal hemorrhage, upper endoscopy should be performed after the patient has been appropriately resuscitated. The diagnosis is established by identification of a 0.5–4 cm linear mucosal tear usually located either at the gastroesophageal junction or, more commonly, just below the junction in the gastric mucosa.

Differential Diagnosis

At endoscopy, other potential causes of upper gastrointestinal hemorrhage are found in over 35% of patients with Mallory-Weiss tears, including peptic ulcer disease, erosive gastritis, arteriovenous malformations, and esophageal varices. Patients with underlying portal hypertension are at higher risk of continued or recurrent bleeding.

Treatment

Patients are initially treated as needed with fluid resuscitation and blood transfusions. Most patients stop bleeding spontaneously and require no therapy. Endoscopic hemostatic therapy is employed in patients who have continuing active bleeding. Injection with epinephrine (1:10,000) or cautery with a bipolar or heater probe coagulation device is effective in 90–95% of cases. Angiographic arterial embolization or operative intervention is required in patients who fail endoscopic therapy.

Kortas D et al: Mallory-Weiss tear: predisposing factors and predictors of a complicated course. Am J Gastroenterol 2001; 96:2863. [PMID: 11693318]

2. Esophageal Webs & Rings

Esophageal webs are thin, diaphragm-like membranes of squamous mucosa that typically occur in the mid or upper esophagus and may be multiple. They may be congenital but also occur with graft-versus-host disease, pemphigoid, epidermolysis bullosa, pemphigus vulgaris—and, rarely, in association with iron deficiency anemia (Plummer-Vinson syndrome). Esophageal rings are smooth, circumferential, thin (< 4 mm in thickness) mucosal structures located in the distal esophagus at the squamocolumnar junction. Their pathogenesis is controversial. They are associated in nearly all cases with a hiatal hernia, and reflux symptoms are common, suggesting that acid gastroesophageal reflux may be contributory in some cases. "Ringed esophagus" is characterized by multiple rings, giving the esophagus a corrugated appearance. Some cases may be related to chronic gastroesophageal reflux disease. Most webs and rings are over 20 mm in diameter and are asymptomatic. Solid food dysphagia most often occurs with rings less than 13 mm in diameter. Characteristically, dysphagia is intermittent and not progressive. Large poorly chewed food boluses such as beefsteak are most likely to cause symptoms. Obstructing boluses may pass by drinking extra liquids or after regurgitation. In some cases, an impacted bolus must be extracted endoscopically. Esophageal webs and rings are best visualized using a barium esophagogram with full esophageal distention. Endoscopy is less sensitive than barium esophagography.

The majority of symptomatic patients with a single ring or web can be effectively treated with the passage of a large (> 16 mm diameter) bougie dilator to disrupt the lesion. A single dilation may suffice, but repeat dilations are required in many patients. Graduated dilation is recommended for ringed esophagus due to increased risk of perforation and postprocedural pain. Patients who have heartburn or who require repeated dilation should receive acid suppressive therapy with a chronic proton pump inhibitor.

AGA technical review on treatment of patients with dysphagia caused by benign disorders of the distal esophagus. Gastroenterology 1999;117:233. [PMID: 10381933]

Morrow JG et al: The ringed esophagus: histological features of GERD. Am J Gastroenterol 2001;96:984. [PMID: 11316216]

3. Esophageal Diverticula
Zenker's Diverticulum

Zenker's diverticulum is a protrusion of pharyngeal mucosa that develops at the pharyngoesophageal junction between the inferior pharyngeal constrictor and the cricopharyngeus. The cause is believed to be loss of elasticity of the upper esophageal sphincter, resulting in restricted opening during swallowing. Symptoms of dysphagia and regurgitation tend to develop insidiously over years in older patients. Initial symptoms include vague oropharyngeal dysphagia with coughing or throat discomfort. As the diverticulum enlarges and retains food, patients may note halitosis, spontaneous regurgitation of undigested food, nocturnal choking, gurgling in the throat, or a protrusion in the neck. Complications include aspiration pneumonia, bronchiectasis, and lung abscess. The diagnosis is best established by a barium esophagogram.

Symptomatic patients require upper esophageal myotomy and, in most cases, surgical diverticulectomy. Significant improvement occurs in over 90% of patients treated surgically. Small asymptomatic diverticula may be observed.

American Gastroenterology Association medical position statement on management of oropharyngeal dysphagia. Gastroenterology 1999;116:452. [PMID: 9922327]

Esophageal Diverticula

Diverticula may occur in the mid or distal esophagus. These may arise secondary to motility disorders (diffuse esophageal spasm, achalasia) or may develop above esophageal strictures. Diverticula are seldom symptomatic, and treatment is directed at the underlying disorder. On rare occasions they may be entered at endoscopy, with the associated risk of perforation.

Ferraro P et al: Esophageal diverticula. Chest Surg Clin North Am 1994;4:741. [PMID: 7859008]

4. Benign Esophageal Neoplasms

Benign tumors of the esophagus are quite rare. They are submucosal, the most common being leiomyoma. Most are asymptomatic and picked up incidentally on endoscopy or barium esophagography. Larger lesions can cause dysphagia. The major clinical importance of these lesions is to distinguish them from malignant neoplasms. At endoscopy, a smooth, sessile nodule is observed with normal overlying mucosa. Because the lesion is submucosal, endoscopic biopsies are generally nonrevealing. Endoscopic ultrasonography is extremely helpful to confirm the submucosal origin of the tumor.

5. Esophageal Varices

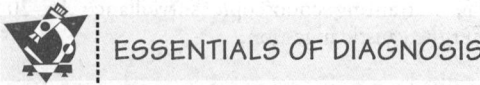

ESSENTIALS OF DIAGNOSIS

- *Develop secondary to portal hypertension.*
- *Found in 50% of patients with cirrhosis.*

- *One-third of patients with varices develop upper gastrointestinal bleeding.*
- *Diagnosis established by upper endoscopy.*

General Considerations

Esophageal varices are dilated submucosal veins that develop in patients with underlying portal hypertension and may result in serious upper gastrointestinal bleeding. The causes of portal hypertension are discussed elsewhere (Chapter 15). Under normal circumstances, there is a 2–6 mm Hg pressure gradient between the portal vein and the inferior vena cava. When the gradient exceeds 12 mm Hg, significant portal hypertension exists. Esophageal varices are the most common cause of important gastrointestinal bleeding due to portal hypertension, though gastric varices and, rarely, intestinal varices may also bleed. Bleeding from esophageal varices most commonly occurs in the distal 5 cm of the esophagus.

The most common cause of portal hypertension is cirrhosis. While approximately 50% of patients with cirrhosis have esophageal varices, only one-third of patients with varices develop serious bleeding from the varices. Bleeding esophageal varices have a higher morbidity and mortality rate than any other source of upper gastrointestinal bleeding. The mortality rate within 2 weeks after an acute bleeding episode is 30%. Of people who survive beyond 2 weeks, recurrent hemorrhage occurs in 70% within 1 year (half within 6 weeks) and the mortality rate is 60% at 2 years.

A number of factors have been identified that may portend an increased risk of bleeding from esophageal varices. The most important are (1) the size of the varices; (2) the presence at endoscopy of red wale markings on the varix (longitudinal markings that resemble whip marks or red spots); (3) the severity of liver disease (as assessed by Child scoring); and (4) active alcohol abuse—alcoholic cirrhotics who continue to drink have an extremely high risk of bleeding. The risk of bleeding correlates poorly with the absolute portosystemic pressure gradient, though bleeding almost never occurs with a gradient under 12 mm Hg.

Clinical Findings

A. SYMPTOMS AND SIGNS

Patients with bleeding esophageal varices present with symptoms and signs of acute gastrointestinal hemorrhage. (See Acute Upper Gastrointestinal Bleeding, above.) In some cases, there may be preceding retching or dyspepsia attributable to alcoholic gastritis or withdrawal. Varices per se do not cause symptoms of dyspepsia, dysphagia, or retching. Variceal bleeding usually is severe, resulting in hypovolemia manifested by postural vital signs or shock. Twenty percent of patients with chronic liver disease who develop bleed-ing—despite findings such as spider angiomas, asterixis, and ascites—do so from some other source.

B. LABORATORY FINDINGS

These are identical to those listed above in the section on acute upper gastrointestinal tract bleeding.

Initial Management

A. ACUTE RESUSCITATION

The initial management of patients with acute upper gastrointestinal bleeding is also discussed in the section on acute upper gastrointestinal bleeding (see above). Variceal hemorrhage is life-threatening; rapid assessment and resuscitation with fluids or blood products are essential. Overtransfusion should be avoided as it leads to increased central and portal venous pressures, increasing the risk of rebleeding. Many patients with bleeding esophageal varices have coagulopathy due to underlying cirrhosis; fresh frozen plasma or platelets should be administered to patients with INRs > 1.8–2.0 (20 mL/kg loading dose, then 10 mg/kg every 6 hours) or with platelet counts < 50,000/µL in the presence of active bleeding. Patients with advanced liver disease are at high risk for poor outcome regardless of the bleeding source and should be transferred to an ICU. In half of cases, variceal hemorrhage stops spontaneously; without therapy, over half of these will rebleed within 1 week.

B. EMERGENT ENDOSCOPY

Emergent endoscopy is performed after the patient's hemodynamic status has been appropriately stabilized (usually within 2–12 hours). In patients with active bleeding, endotracheal intubation is commonly performed to protect against aspiration during endoscopy. A vigorous gastric lavage through a large-bore tube is performed prior to endoscopy to facilitate visualization. An endoscopic examination is then performed to exclude other or associated causes of upper gastrointestinal bleeding such as Mallory-Weiss tears, peptic ulcer disease, and portal hypertensive gastropathy. In many patients, variceal bleeding has stopped spontaneously by the time of endoscopy, and the diagnosis of variceal bleeding is made presumptively. Acute endoscopic treatment of the varices is performed with either banding or sclerotherapy. These techniques arrest active bleeding in 90% of patients and reduce by half (from 70%) the chance of early recurrent bleeding, but their impact upon in-hospital mortality is less clear.

If banding is chosen, repeat sessions are scheduled at intervals of 1–2 weeks until the varices are obliterated or reduced to a small size. Banding achieves lower rates of rebleeding, complications, and death than sclerotherapy and should be considered the endoscopic treatment of choice.

Sclerotherapy is performed by injecting the variceal trunks with a sclerosing agent (eg, ethanolamine, tetradecyl sulfate). A repeat session is conducted at

3–7 days, followed by sessions at 1- to 3-week intervals until the varices are obliterated. Complications occur in 20–30% and include chest pain, fever, bacteremia, esophageal ulceration, stricture, and perforation. However, sclerotherapy is still preferred by some endoscopists in the actively bleeding patient (in whom visualization for banding may be difficult).

C. PHARMACOLOGIC THERAPY

1. Antibiotic prophylaxis—Cirrhotic patients admitted with upper gastrointestinal bleeding have a greater than 50% chance of developing a severe bacterial infection during hospitalization—such as bacterial peritonitis, pneumonia, urinary tract infection—with or without sepsis. Most organisms causing infections are of gut origin. Prophylactic therapy by either oral or intravenous administration of antibiotics may reduce the risk of serious infection to 10–20% as well as hospital mortality. Prophylactic treatment with norfloxacin, 400 mg (or another quinolone) orally or per nasogastric tube twice daily for at least 7 days, is recommended routinely.

2. Somatostatin or octreotide—Somatostatin and octreotide infusions reduce portal pressures in ways that are poorly understood. Somatostatin (250 µg/h)—not available in the United States—or octreotide (50 µg intravenous bolus followed by 50 µg/h) reduces splanchnic and hepatic blood flow and portal pressures in cirrhotic patients. Both agents appear to provide acute control of variceal bleeding in up to 80% of patients; however, data about the absolute efficacy of both are conflicting, but they may be comparable in efficacy to endoscopic therapy. Combined treatment with octreotide or somatostatin infusion and endoscopic therapy (band ligation or sclerotherapy) is superior to either modality alone in controlling acute bleeding and early rebleeding, and it may improve survival. In patients with advanced liver disease and upper gastrointestinal hemorrhage, it is reasonable to initiate therapy with octreotide or somatostatin on admission and continue for 5 days. If bleeding is determined by endoscopy not to be secondary to portal hypertension, the infusion can be discontinued.

3. Vitamin K—In cirrhotic patients with an abnormal prothrombin time, vitamin K (10 mg) should be administered subcutaneously.

4. Lactulose—Encephalopathy may complicate an episode of gastrointestinal bleeding in patients with severe liver disease. In patients with encephalopathy, lactulose should be administered in a dosage of 30–45 mL/h orally until evacuation occurs, then reduced to 15–45 mL/h every 8–12 hours as needed to promote two or three bowel movements daily. (See Chapter 15.)

D. BALLOON TUBE TAMPONADE

Mechanical tamponade with specially designed nasogastric tubes containing large gastric and esophageal balloons (Minnesota or Sengstaken-Blakemore tubes) provides initial control of active variceal hemorrhage in 60–90% of patients; rebleeding occurs in 50%. The gastric balloon is inflated first, followed by the esophageal balloon if bleeding continues. After balloon inflation, tension is applied to the tube to directly tamponade the varices. Complications of prolonged balloon inflation include esophageal and oral ulcerations, perforation, aspiration, and airway obstruction (due to a misplaced balloon). Endotracheal intubation is recommended before placement. Given its high rate of complications, mechanical tamponade is used as a temporizing measure only in patients with bleeding that cannot be controlled with pharmacologic or endoscopic techniques until more definitive decompressive therapy (eg, TIPS; see below) can be provided.

E. PORTAL DECOMPRESSIVE PROCEDURES

In patients with variceal bleeding that cannot be controlled with pharmacologic or endoscopic therapy, emergency portal decompression is necessary.

1. Transvenous intrahepatic portosystemic shunts (TIPS)—Over a wire that is passed through the catheter inserted in the jugular vein, an expandable wire mesh stent (8–12 mm in diameter) is passed through the liver parenchyma, creating a portosystemic shunt from the portal vein to the hepatic vein. TIPS can control acute hemorrhage in over 90% of patients actively bleeding from gastric or esophageal varices. However, posttreatment encephalopathy occurs in 35%, and in patients with decompensated liver disease it may precipitate hepatic failure. Therefore, TIPS is indicated in the 5–10% of patients with acute variceal bleeding who cannot be controlled with pharmacologic and endoscopic therapy—but it is not indicated as initial therapy.

2. Emergency portosystemic shunt surgery—Emergency portosystemic shunt surgery is associated with a 40–60% mortality rate. At centers where TIPS is available, that procedure has become the preferred means of providing emergency portal decompression.

Prevention of Rebleeding

Once the initial bleeding episode has been controlled, the risk of rebleeding is 60–80% without further therapy. The highest incidence of rebleeding is in the first 6 weeks. Several options are available to decrease the likelihood of rebleeding, though their relative merits are controversial. Use of these approaches varies in different medical centers.

A. ENDOSCOPIC TECHNIQUES

Long-term treatment with sclerotherapy or band ligation reduces the incidence of rebleeding to 20–40%; the mortality rate may also be reduced. Band ligation of the varix appears to be equal or superior to sclerotherapy in preventing rebleeding and is associated with a significantly lower complication rate. In most patients, four to six treatment sessions are needed to eradicate the varices. Where expertise is available, endoscopic therapy is generally the preferred approach to long-term therapy of esophageal varices.

B. BETA-BLOCKERS AND NITRATES

Nonselective beta-adrenergic blockers (propranolol, nadolol) are effective in reducing the incidence of rebleeding from esophageal varices and portal hypertensive gastropathy compared with placebo and comparable to that of sclerotherapy. Combination therapy with beta-blockers and sclerotherapy does not appear to be superior to sclerotherapy alone, though it is not known if banding plus beta-blockers confers an advantage. Thus, the choice between beta-blockers and endoscopic therapy to prevent recurrent variceal bleeding is not established and depends upon local experience. Compliant patients with well-compensated liver disease may be optimal candidates for therapy with beta-blockers alone. Most others may be offered endoscopic variceal banding where available. Patients without contraindications to beta-blockers may be started on propranolol, 20 mg twice daily, or nadolol, 40 mg once daily, gradually increasing the dosage until the heart rate falls by 25% or reaches 55 beats/min. The average dosage of propranolol or nadolol is 80 mg daily.

Up to 25% of patients with cirrhosis are intolerant of beta-blockers. Long-acting nitrates such as isosorbide mononitrate also reduce portal pressures but have not demonstrated efficacy in reducing the risk of variceal bleeding when used alone. Combination therapy with isosorbide mononitrate and beta-blockers is more effective and better tolerated than beta-blockers alone in reducing portal pressures and rebleeding. Isosorbide mononitrate is initiated at a dosage of 10 mg daily and gradually increased to 20–40 mg twice daily as tolerated. Side effects include hypotension or headache. Combination therapy with nadolol and isosorbide has been found to be more effective than band ligation alone for the prevention of recurrent variceal bleeding. Whether combined endoscopic and pharmacologic therapies (beta-blockers with or without nitrates) are superior to endoscopic or pharmacologic therapy alone has not yet been determined.

C. TRANSVENOUS INTRAHEPATIC PORTOSYSTEMIC SHUNT (TIPS)

TIPS has resulted in a significant reduction in recurrent bleeding compared with endoscopic sclerotherapy or band ligation—either alone or in combination with beta-blocker therapy. At 1 year, rebleeding rates in patients treated with TIPS versus various endoscopic therapies average 20% and 40%, respectively. However, TIPS was also associated with a higher incidence of encephalopathy (35% versus 15%) and did not result in a decrease in mortality. Another limitation of TIPS is that stenosis and thrombosis of the stents occurs in the majority of patients over time with a consequent risk of rebleeding. Therefore, periodic monitoring with Doppler ultrasonography or hepatic venography is required. Stent patency usually can be maintained by balloon angioplasty or additional stent placement. Given these problems, TIPS should be reserved for patients who have recurrent (two or more) episodes of variceal bleeding that have failed endoscopic or pharmacologic therapies. TIPS is also useful in patients with recurrent bleeding from gastric varices or portal hypertensive gastropathy (for which endoscopic therapies cannot be used). TIPS is likewise considered in patients who are noncompliant with other therapies or who live in remote locations (without access to emergency care).

D. SURGICAL PORTOSYSTEMIC SHUNTS

Shunt surgery has a significantly lower rate of rebleeding compared with endoscopic therapy but also a higher incidence of encephalopathy. Selective (distal splenorenal) shunts have a lower incidence of encephalopathy than portacaval shunts but are more difficult to perform. In most centers, shunt surgery has been reserved for patients who have failed sclerotherapy or for noncompliant patients. With the advent of TIPS, the role of surgical shunts is unclear.

E. LIVER TRANSPLANTATION

Candidacy for orthotopic liver transplantation should be assessed in all patients with chronic liver disease and bleeding due to portal hypertension. Transplant candidates should be treated with band ligation or TIPS to control bleeding pretransplant.

Prevention of First Episodes of Variceal Bleeding

Because of the high mortality rate associated with variceal hemorrhage, prevention of the initial bleeding episode is desirable. All patients with cirrhosis should undergo diagnostic endoscopy to determine whether varices are present. Nonselective beta-adrenergic blockers (nadolol, propranolol) in multiple trials decrease the long-term risk of bleeding to less than 15% (compared with about 25% in placebo-treated patients). Because variceal bleeding occurs in only one-third of cirrhotics, it may be reasonable to use beta-blockers in compliant higher-risk patients, ie, patients with large varices or red color markings. Up to one-third of patients do not tolerate beta-blocker therapy. Combination therapy with propranolol and isosorbide mononitrate may be superior to propranolol alone in primary prevention of variceal bleeding. Prophylactic sclerotherapy in those who have never had a variceal hemorrhage results in a higher mortality rate than placebo or treatment with beta-blockers and should not be done. In contrast, a reduction in the incidence of first episodes of variceal bleeding has been noted in patients treated with variceal ligation (banding). At this time, however, prophylactic variceal ligation is not widely employed in patients with varices without prior bleeding.

Corley D et al: Octreotide for acute esophageal variceal bleeding: a meta-analysis. Gastroenterology 2001;120:946. [PMID: 11231948]

Garcia-Pagan JC et al: Isosorbide mononitrate in the prevention of first variceal bleed in patients who cannot receive β-blockers. Gastroenterology 2001;121:908. [PMID: 11606504]

Garcia-Tsa G: Current management of the complications of cirrhosis and portal hypertension: variceal hemorrhage, ascites, and spontaneous bacterial peritonitis. Gastroenterology 2001;120:726. [PMID: 11179247]

Sharara A et al: Gastroesophageal variceal hemorrhage. N Engl J Med 2001;345:669. [PMID: 11547722]

Vlachogiannakos J et al: Review article: primary prophylaxis for portal hypertensive bleeding in cirrhosis. Aliment Pharmacol Ther 2000;14:851. [PMID: 10886040]

MALIGNANT ESOPHAGEAL LESIONS (Cancer of the Esophagus)

 ESSENTIALS OF DIAGNOSIS

- *Progressive solid food dysphagia.*
- *Weight loss common.*
- *Endoscopy with biopsy establishes diagnosis.*

General Considerations

Esophageal cancer usually develops in persons between 50 and 70 years of age. The overall ratio of men to women is 3:1. There are two histologic types: squamous cell carcinoma and adenocarcinoma. In the United States, squamous cell cancer is much more common in blacks than in whites. Chronic alcohol and tobacco use are strongly associated with an increased risk of squamous cell carcinoma. The risk of squamous cell cancer is also increased in patients with tylosis (a rare disease transmitted by autosomal dominant inheritance and manifested by hyperkeratosis of the palms and soles), achalasia, caustic-induced esophageal stricture, and other head and neck cancers. Squamous cell cancer has a high incidence in certain regions of China and Southeast Asia. Half of cases occur in the distal third of the esophagus. Adenocarcinoma is more common in whites. It is increasing dramatically in incidence and now is as common as squamous carcinoma. The majority of adenocarcinomas develop as a complication of Barrett's metaplasia due to chronic gastroesophageal reflux. Thus, most adenocarcinomas arise in the distal third of the esophagus.

Clinical Findings

A. SYMPTOMS AND SIGNS

Most patients with esophageal cancer present with advanced, incurable disease. Over 90% have solid food dysphagia, which progresses over weeks to months. Odynophagia is sometimes present. Significant weight loss is common. Local tumor extension into the tracheobronchial tree may result in a tracheoesophageal fistula, characterized by coughing on swallowing or pneumonia. Chest or back pain suggests mediastinal extension. Recurrent laryngeal involvement may produce hoarseness. Physical examination is often unrevealing. The presence of supraclavicular or cervical lymphadenopathy or of hepatomegaly implies metastatic disease.

B. LABORATORY FINDINGS

Laboratory findings are nonspecific. Anemia related to chronic disease or occult blood loss is common. Elevated aminotransferase or alkaline phosphatase concentrations suggest hepatic or bony metastases. Hypoalbuminemia may result from malnutrition.

C. IMAGING

Chest x-rays may show adenopathy, a widened mediastinum, pulmonary or bony metastases, or signs of tracheoesophageal fistula such as pneumonia. A barium esophagogram is obtained as the first study to evaluate dysphagia. The appearance of a polypoid, infiltrative, or ulcerative lesion is suggestive of carcinoma and requires endoscopic evaluation. However, even lesions felt to be benign by radiography warrant endoscopic evaluation.

D. UPPER ENDOSCOPY

Endoscopy with biopsy establishes the diagnosis of esophageal carcinoma with a high degree of reliability. In some cases, significant submucosal spread of the tumor may yield nondiagnostic mucosal biopsies. Repeated biopsy may be necessary.

Differential Diagnosis

Esophageal carcinoma must be distinguished from other causes of progressive dysphagia, including peptic stricture, achalasia, and adenocarcinoma of the gastric cardia with esophageal involvement. Benign-appearing peptic strictures should be biopsied at presentation to exclude occult malignancy.

Staging of Disease

After confirmation of the diagnosis of esophageal carcinoma, the stage of the disease should be determined since doing so influences the choice of therapy. Patients should undergo evaluation with CT of the chest and liver to look for evidence of pulmonary or hepatic metastases, lymphadenopathy, and local tumor extension. If there is no evidence of distant metastases or extensive local spread on CT, endoscopic ultrasonography should be performed, which is superior to CT in demonstrating the level of local mediastinal extension and local lymph node involvement. Bronchoscopy is sometimes required in proximal esophageal cancer to exclude tracheobronchial extension.

Apart from distant metastasis, the two most important predictors of poor survival are lymph node involvement and adjacent mediastinal spread.

Stages are determined by the TNM classification as set forth in the accompanying box.

STAGING CRITERIA FOR ESOPHAGEAL CANCER

Primary Tumor (T)

T1: Invasion of lamina propria or submucosa
T2: Invasion of muscularis propria
T3: Invasion of adventitia
T4: Invasion of adjacent structures

Regional Lymph Nodes (N)

N0: No regional lymph node involvement
N1: Regional lymph node involvement

Distant Metastasis (M)

M0: No metastasis
M1: Distant metastasis

Based upon these parameters, the tumor is classified as:

Stage I: T1, N0, M0
Stage IIA: T2 or T3, and N0, M0
Stage IIB: T1 or T2, and N1, M0
Stage III: T3, N1, M0 or T4, any N, M0
Stage IV: Any T or N, M1

Treatment

The approach to esophageal cancer depends upon the tumor stage, patient preference, and the expertise of the attending surgeons, oncologists, and radiotherapists. There is no consensus about the optimal treatment approach. It is helpful, however, to classify patients into two general categories.

A. PALLIATIVE THERAPY

Patients with extensive local tumor spread (T4) or distant metastases (M1) are incurable, ie, most patients with stage III and all with stage IV tumors. The goal in these patients is to provide relief from dysphagia and pain. The optimal palliative approach depends upon the patient's expected survival, patient prefer-

ence, and local institutional experience. None of these modalities prolong survival, and many patients may prefer concerted efforts at pain relief (see Chapter 1) and care directed at symptom management (see Chapter 5).

1. Resection—Palliative resection of the esophagus provides the most rapid and durable relief of dysphagia. For well-nourished patients without comorbid medical problems (ie, suitable surgical candidates) who have an expected survival of more than 6–12 months, this may be recommended provided there is no significant involvement of mediastinal structures.

2. Radiation therapy—For patients with unresectable disease and for poor operative candidates, radiation therapy may afford significant short-term palliation of pain and dysphagia. During therapy, esophagitis may lead to worsening of dysphagia and odynophagia. Combined radiation therapy and chemotherapy may achieve palliation in two-thirds of patients.

3. Local tumor therapy—Patients with advanced esophageal cancer may be quite ill, with an average survival of less than 12 weeks from diagnosis. Palliation of dysphagia may be achieved by peroral placement of expandable, permanent wire stents, application of endoscopic laser therapy, or photodynamic therapy. Although dysphagia and quality of life are improved significantly, patients can seldom eat normally. Complications of stents occur in 20–40% and include perforation, migration, and tumor ingrowth. These are most suitable for patients with a short life expectancy; patients with tracheoesophageal fistula; patients who have failed radiation therapy; or patients in locations where optimal surgical or radiation modalities are not available. Laser therapy (Nd:YAG laser) maintains luminal patency in up to 90% of patients but involves multiple treatment sessions and can be difficult to administer. Photodynamic therapy has been shown to be superior to laser therapy. A photosensitizing agent (porfimer sodium) in combination with low-power 630 nm laser results in significant tumor necrosis. Side effects include sun sensitivity of the skin for 4–6 weeks and the development of esophageal stricture. Both laser therapy and photodynamic therapy require expensive equipment that is not available at many institutions.

B. "CURABLE" DISEASE

There are three broad categories of therapy that may be considered depending upon institutional experience.

1. Surgery alone—Patients with stage I and stage IIA cancer have high cure rates with surgery alone. There is controversy over the optimal surgical approach. The procedure with the lowest morbidity is transhiatal esophagectomy with anastomosis of the stomach to the cervical esophagus. Critics of this approach note that because it does not involve sampling or removal of mediastinal lymph nodes, it is not suitable as a "curative" approach for node-positive disease. Alternatively, many surgeons recommend transthoracic excision of the esophagus with nodal resection. They believe that it has a higher morbidity and no better survival than the transhiatal approach. Regardless of the approach elected, overall 3-year survival after surgery is less than 15% in most series. Patients with small early-stage tumors who are too ill to undergo esophagectomy may be treated with endoscopic mucosal resection of the tumor at qualified centers.

2. Chemotherapy plus radiation therapy—Combined therapy with chemotherapy and radiation therapy is superior to radiation therapy alone and has achieved overall survival rates that equal or exceed those of historical surgical cohorts, though there have been no trials specifically comparing these approaches. However, severe side effects occur commonly with combined therapy. The most promising chemotherapeutic agents have been cisplatin and fluorouracil.

3. Surgery with neoadjuvant chemotherapy and radiation therapy—If lymph node metastases have occurred (stage IIB and stage III), the rate of cure with surgery alone is reduced to less than 10%. Trials of adjuvant (postoperative) or neoadjuvant (preoperative) radiation therapy or chemotherapy have not shown convincing benefits over surgery alone. Patients have been treated with combination radiation therapy and chemotherapy (cisplatin and fluorouracil) prior to resection. A complete pathologic remission (no evidence of tumor at the time of surgery) is seen in up to 25% of patients treated with combination neoadjuvant therapy. However, neoadjuvant chemoradiotherapy in patients with squamous cell cancer shows no mortality benefit, though there is prolonged disease-free survival. Multimodal treatment versus surgery should not be used outside of clinical trials.

Prognosis

The overall 5-year survival rate of esophageal carcinoma is less than 15%. Despite improvements in surgical mortality and increased surgical resectability rates, the prognosis of this disease has not changed for years, in part because most patients present with advanced disease. This suggests that surgical approaches alone are inadequate for most patients. For those patients whose disease progresses despite chemotherapy, meticulous effects at palliative care are essential (see Chapter 5).

Bossett JF et al: Chemoradiotherapy followed by surgery compared with surgery alone in squamous-cell cancer of the esophagus. N Engl J Med 1997;337:161. [PMID: 9219702]

Ell C et al: Endoscopic mucosal resection of early cancer and high-grade dysplasia in Barrett's esophagus. Gastroenterology 2000;118:670. [PMID: 10734018]

Kelsen D: Multimodality therapy for adenocarcinoma of the esophagus. Gastroenterol Clin North Am 1997;26:635. [PMID: 9309410]

Lightdale CJ: Esophageal cancer. Am J Gastroenterol 1999;94:20. [PMID: 9934727]

Siersema P et al: A comparison of 3 types of covered metal stents for the palliation of patients with dysphagia caused by esophagogastric carcinoma: a prospective, randomized study. Gastrointest Endosc 2001;54:145. [PMID: 11474382]

ESOPHAGEAL MOTILITY DISORDERS

1. Achalasia

ESSENTIALS OF DIAGNOSIS

- *Gradual, progressive dysphagia for solids and liquids.*
- *Regurgitation of undigested food.*
- *Barium esophagogram with "bird's beak" distal esophagus.*
- *Esophageal manometry confirms diagnosis.*

General Considerations

Achalasia is an idiopathic motility disorder characterized by loss of peristalsis in the distal two-thirds (smooth muscle) of the esophagus and impaired relaxation of the lower esophageal sphincter. There appears to be denervation of the esophagus resulting primarily from loss of nitric oxide-producing inhibitory neurons in the myenteric plexus. The cause of the neuronal degeneration is unknown.

Clinical Findings

A. SYMPTOMS AND SIGNS

There is a steady increase in the incidence of achalasia with age; however, it can be seen in individuals as young as 25 years. Patients complain of the gradual onset of dysphagia for solid foods and, in the majority, of liquids also. Symptoms at presentation may have persisted for months to years. Substernal discomfort or fullness may be noted after eating. Many patients eat more slowly and adopt specific maneuvers such as lifting the neck or throwing the shoulders back in order to enhance esophageal emptying. Regurgitation of undigested food is common and may occur during meals or up to several hours later. Nocturnal regurgitation can provoke coughing or aspiration. Up to half of patients report substernal chest pain that is unrelated to meals or exercise and may last up to hours. Weight loss is common. Physical examination is unhelpful.

B. IMAGING

Chest x-rays may show an air-fluid level in the enlarged, fluid-filled esophagus. Barium esophagography discloses characteristic findings, including esophageal dilation, loss of esophageal peristalsis, poor esophageal emptying, and a smooth, symmetric "bird's beak" tapering of the distal esophagus. Without treatment, the esophagus may become markedly dilated ("sigmoid esophagus").

C. SPECIAL EXAMINATIONS

After esophagography, endoscopy is always performed to evaluate the distal esophagus and gastroesophageal junction in order to exclude a distal stricture or a submucosal infiltrating carcinoma. The diagnosis is confirmed by esophageal manometry. The typical manometric features are as follows: (1) Complete absence of peristalsis; swallowing results in simultaneous waves which are usually of low amplitude. (2) Incomplete lower esophageal sphincteric relaxation with swallowing. Whereas the normal sphincter relaxes by over 90%, relaxation with most swallows in patients with achalasia is less than 50%. In many patients, the baseline lower esophageal sphincteric pressure is quite elevated. (3) Intraesophageal pressures are greater than gastric pressures due to a fluid- and food-filled esophagus.

Differential Diagnosis

Chagas' disease is associated with esophageal dysfunction that is indistinguishable from idiopathic achalasia and should be considered in patients from endemic regions (Central and South America); it is becoming more common in the southern United States. Primary or metastatic tumors can invade the gastroesophageal junction, resulting in a picture resembling that of achalasia, called "pseudoachalasia." Endoscopic ultrasonography and chest CT may be required to examine the distal esophagus in suspicious cases. Achalasia must be distinguished from other motility disorders such as diffuse esophageal spasm and scleroderma esophagus with a peptic stricture.

Treatment

A. BOTULINUM TOXIN INJECTION

Endoscopically guided injection of botulinum toxin directly into the lower esophageal sphincter results in a marked reduction in lower esophageal sphincter pressure with initial improvement in symptoms in 85% of patients. However, symptom relapse occurs in over 50% of patients within 6–9 months. Twenty-five percent of patients have a sustained response (lasting more than a year). Three-fourths of initial responders who relapse have improvement with repeated injections. The role of botulinum toxin injection relative to other therapies is debated. Because it is inferior to pneumatic dilation therapy and surgery in producing sustained symptomatic relief, this therapy may be most appropriate for elderly patients or those who are poor candidates for more invasive procedures.

B. PNEUMATIC DILATION

Over three-fourths of patients derive good to excellent relief of dysphagia after one or two sessions of pneumatic dilation of the lower esophageal sphincter. Perforations occur in less than 3% of dilations and may require operative repair.

C. SURGICAL MYOTOMY

A modified Heller cardiomyotomy of the lower esophageal sphincter and cardia results in good to excellent symptomatic improvement in over 85% of patients. Because gastroesophageal reflux may develop in up to 20% of patients after myotomy, most surgeons also perform an antireflux procedure (fundoplication). Myotomy is now performed with a laparoscopic approach and is preferred to the open surgical approach. Indeed, the low morbidity of laparoscopic surgery has led some experts to recommend it for initial treatment. In experienced hands, the efficacy of pneumatic dilation and laparoscopic myotomy are nearly equivalent. Pneumatic dilation appears to be a more cost-effective strategy than either botulinum toxin injection or laparoscopic myotomy. The success of laparoscopic surgery is not compromised by prior therapy with either botulinum injection or pneumatic dilation.

Imperiale TR et al: A cost-minimization analysis of alternative treatment strategies in achalasia. Am J Gastroenterol 2000; 95:2737. [PMID: 11051342]

Vaezi M et al: Diagnosis and management of achalasia. Am J Gastroenterol 1999;94:3406. [PMID: 10606295]

2. Other Primary Esophageal Motility Disorders

Abnormalities in esophageal motility may cause dysphagia or chest pain. Dysphagia for liquids as well as solids tends to be intermittent and nonprogressive. Periods of normal swallowing may alternate with periods of dysphagia, which usually is mild though bothersome—rarely severe enough to result in significant alterations in lifestyle or weight loss. Dysphagia may be provoked by stress, large boluses of food, or hot or cold liquids. Some patients may experience anterior chest pain that may be confused with angina pectoris but usually is nonexertional. The pain generally is unrelated to eating. (See Chest Pain of Undetermined Origin, below.)

The evaluation of suspected esophageal motility disorders includes barium esophagography, upper endoscopy, and, in some cases, esophageal manometry. Barium esophagography is useful to exclude mechanical obstruction and to evaluate esophageal motility. The presence of simultaneous contractions (spasm), disordered peristalsis, or failed peristalsis supports a diagnosis of esophageal dysmotility. Upper endoscopy also is performed to exclude a mechanical obstruction (as a cause of dysphagia) and to look for evidence of erosive reflux esophagitis (a common cause of chest pain).

The further evaluation of noncardiac chest pain is discussed in a subsequent section. For patients with disabling symptoms of dysphagia, stationary esophageal manometry should be performed. Manometry should not be routinely used for mild to moderate symptoms because the findings seldom influence further medical management. Based upon the findings of esophageal manometry, patients may be diagnosed with the following conditions: (1) Diffuse esophageal spasm: normal primary peristalsis with more than 20% simultaneous contractions. (2) Nutcracker esophagus: normal peristalsis but increased duration and high amplitude of distal contractions (> 180 mm Hg). (3) Hypertensive lower esophageal sphincter: elevated lower esophageal sphincter pressure (> 45 mm Hg) with normal peristalsis. (4) Nonspecific esophageal motility disorder: intermittent normal peristalsis with any of a number of abnormalities that do not allow classification into one of the above (> 20% nontransmitted peristaltic waves, prolonged duration of contractions, abnormal-appearing wave forms, low amplitude of peristaltic waves).

For patients with mild symptoms, therapy is directed at symptom reduction and reassurance. Patients with dysphagia should be instructed to eat more slowly and take smaller boluses of food. In some cases, a warm liquid at the start of a meal may facilitate swallowing. Treatment of more severe cases with nitrates (isosorbide, 10–30 mg four times daily) or nitroglycerin (0.4 mg sublingually as needed) and calcium channel blockers (nifedipine, 30–60 mg, or diltiazem, 60–90 mg, four times daily) may be tried; their efficacy is unproved. Injection of botulinum toxin may also be helpful. For unclear reasons, dilation with esophageal Maloney bougies provides symptomatic relief in some cases. In debilitated patients, a long surgical myotomy (which may be performed via a thoracoscopic approach) may lead to improvement in 70–80% of cases.

Adler D et al: Primary esophageal motility disorders. Mayo Clin Proc 2001;76:195. [PMID: 11213308]

Spechler S et al: Classification of oesophageal motility abnormalities. Gut 2001;49:145. [PMID: 11413123]

CHEST PAIN OF UNDETERMINED ORIGIN

One-third of patients with chest pain undergo negative cardiac evaluation. Patients with recurrent noncardiac chest pain thus pose a difficult clinical problem. Because coronary artery disease is common and can present atypically, it must be excluded prior to evaluation for other causes.

Causes of noncardiac chest pain may include the following.

A. CHEST WALL AND THORACIC SPINE DISEASE

These are easily diagnosed by history and physical examination.

B. GASTROESOPHAGEAL REFLUX

Up to 25% of patients have increased amounts of gastroesophageal acid reflux. An empirical 7-day trial of acid suppressive therapy with a high-dose proton pump inhibitor is recommended (eg, omeprazole or rabeprazole, 20 mg twice daily; lansoprazole, 30 mg twice daily; or pantoprazole, 40 mg twice-daily), especially in patients with reflux symptoms. Symptomatic improvement strongly suggests that the pain is due to acid esophageal reflux. The sensitivity and specificity of this treatment are 78% and 86%, respectively, compared with therapy based on results of esophageal pH testing. In some cases, an ambulatory esophageal pH study may document a relationship between acid reflux episodes and chest pain events.

C. HEIGHTENED VISCERAL SENSITIVITY

Studies suggest that many patients with noncardiac chest pain report pain in response to a variety of minor noxious stimuli such as intraesophageal acid infusion, inflation of balloons within the esophageal lumen, injection of intravenous edrophonium (a cholinergic stimulus), or intracardiac catheter manipulation. Low doses of antidepressants such as trazodone 50 mg or imipramine 50 mg reduce chest pain symptoms and are thought to reduce visceral afferent awareness.

D. PSYCHOLOGIC DISORDERS

A significant number of patients have underlying depression, anxiety, and panic disorder. Patients reporting dyspnea, sweating, tachycardia, suffocation, or fear of dying should be evaluated for panic disorder.

E. ESOPHAGEAL DYSMOTILITY

Esophageal motility abnormalities such as diffuse esophageal spasm or nutcracker esophagus are rare causes of noncardiac chest pain. Stationary or ambulatory manometry is not recommended because of low specificity and the unlikelihood of finding a clinically significant disorder. In patients with chest pain and dysphagia, barium swallow x-ray should be obtained to look for evidence of achalasia or diffuse esophageal spasm.

Achem SR et al: Unexplained chest pain at the turn of the century. Am J Gastroenterol 1999;94:5. [PMID: 9934722]

Mujica V et al: Pathophysiology of chest pain in patients with nutcracker esophagus. Am J Gastroenterol 2001;96:1371. [PMID: 11374670]

Rao S et al: Functional chest pain of esophageal origin: hyperalgesia or motor dysfunction. Am J Gastroenterol 2001;96: 2584. [PMID: 11569679]

■ DISEASES OF THE STOMACH & DUODENUM

GASTRITIS & GASTROPATHY

The term "gastropathy" is used increasingly to denote conditions in which there is epithelial or endothelial damage without inflammation. Gastritis may be divided into three categories: (1) erosive and hemorrhagic gastritis; (2) nonerosive, nonspecific (histologic) gastritis; and (3) specific types of gastritis, characterized by distinctive histologic and endoscopic features diagnostic of specific disorders.

1. Erosive & Hemorrhagic Gastritis

 ESSENTIALS OF DIAGNOSIS

- Most commonly seen in alcoholics, critically ill patients, or patients taking NSAIDs.
- Often asymptomatic; may cause epigastric pain, nausea, and vomiting.
- May cause hematemesis; usually not significant bleeding.

General Considerations

The most common causes of erosive gastritis are drugs (especially NSAIDs), alcohol, stress due to severe medical or surgical illness, and portal hypertension ("portal gastropathy"). Uncommon causes include caustic ingestion and radiation. Erosive gastritis and hemorrhagic gastritis typically are diagnosed at endoscopy, often being performed because of dyspepsia or upper gastrointestinal bleeding. Endoscopic findings include subepithelial hemorrhages, petechiae, and erosions. These lesions are superficial, vary in size and number, and may be focal or diffuse. There usually is no significant inflammation on histologic examination, though gastropathy may be present.

Clinical Findings

A. SYMPTOMS AND SIGNS

Erosive gastritis is usually asymptomatic. Symptoms, when they occur, include anorexia, epigastric pain, nausea, and vomiting. There is poor correlation between symptoms and the number or severity of endoscopic abnormalities. The most common clinical manifestation of erosive gastritis is upper gastrointestinal bleeding, which presents as hematemesis, "coffee grounds" emesis, or bloody aspirate in a patient receiving nasogastric suction, or as melena. Because erosive gastritis is superficial, hemodynamically significant bleeding is rare.

B. LABORATORY FINDINGS

The laboratory findings are nonspecific. The hematocrit is low if significant bleeding has occurred; iron deficiency may be found.

C. SPECIAL EXAMINATIONS

Upper endoscopy is the most sensitive method of diagnosis. Although bleeding from gastritis is usually insignificant, it cannot be distinguished on clinical grounds from more serious lesions such as peptic ulcers or esophageal varices. Hence, endoscopy is generally performed within 24 hours in patients with upper gastrointestinal bleeding to identify the source. An upper gastrointestinal series is sometimes obtained in lieu of endoscopy in patients with hemodynamically insignificant upper gastrointestinal bleeds to exclude serious lesions but is insensitive for the detection of gastritis.

Differential Diagnosis

Epigastric pain may be due to peptic ulcer, gastroesophageal reflux, gastric cancer, biliary tract disease, food poisoning, viral gastroenteritis, and functional dyspepsia. With severe pain, one should consider a perforated or penetrating ulcer, pancreatic disease, esophageal rupture, ruptured aortic aneurysm, gastric volvulus, and myocardial colic. Causes of upper gastrointestinal bleeding include peptic ulcer disease, esophageal varices, Mallory-Weiss tear, and arteriovenous malformations.

Specific Causes & Treatment

A. STRESS GASTRITIS

1. Prophylaxis—Stress-related mucosal erosions and subepithelial hemorrhages develop within 18 hours in the majority of critically ill patients. Clinically overt bleeding occurs in 6% but clinically important bleeding in less than 2–3%. Bleeding is associated with a higher mortality rate but is seldom the cause of death. Major risk factors include trauma, burns, hypotension, sepsis, central nervous system injury, coagulopathy, mechanical respiration, hepatic or renal failure, and multiorgan failure. The use of enteral nutrition reduces the risk of stress-related bleeding.

Pharmacologic prophylaxis with sucralfate or H_2 receptor antagonists in critically ill patients has been shown to reduce the incidence of clinically overt and significant bleeding by 50%. Prophylaxis should be routinely administered upon admission to critically ill patients with risk factors for significant bleeding. Two of the most important risk factors are coagulopathy and respiratory failure with the need for mechanical ventilation for over 48 hours. When these two risk factors are absent, the risk of significant bleeding is only 0.1%.

It is suggested that sucralfate suspension (1 g orally every 4–6 hours) is comparable in efficacy to H_2 receptor antagonists in the prevention of stress-related bleeding and is associated with a 20% reduction of nosocomial pneumonia. However, some investigators believe ranitidine reduces clinically significant bleeding compared with sucralfate. Infusions of H_2 receptor antagonists at a dose sufficient to maintain intragastric pH above 4.0 are thus recommended for prophylaxis. Sucralfate should be used in patients intolerant of the H_2 receptor antagonists. Cimetidine (900–1200 mg), ranitidine (150 mg), or famotidine (20 mg) by continuous intravenous infusion over 24 hours is adequate to control pH in most patients. After 4 hours of infusion, the pH should be checked by nasogastric aspirate and the dose doubled if the pH is under 4.0. Oral proton pump inhibitors are not be used in the ICU for prophylaxis owing to their unpredictable absorption and the need for high doses in such patients.

2. Treatment—Once bleeding occurs, patients should receive continuous infusions of an H_2 receptor antagonist or proton pump inhibitor as well as sucralfate suspension. Because bleeding is diffuse, endoscopic hemostasis techniques are not helpful. Nevertheless, endoscopy is often performed in such patients to look for other treatable causes of upper gastrointestinal bleeding.

B. NSAID Gastritis

Although half of patients receiving NSAIDs on a chronic basis have gastritis at endoscopy, symptoms of dyspepsia develop in less than one-fourth. Furthermore, of patients with dyspepsia, up to half do not have significant mucosal abnormalities. Given the frequency of dyspeptic symptoms in patients taking NSAIDs, it is neither feasible nor desirable to investigate all such patients. Symptoms may improve with discontinuation of the agent, reduction to the lowest effective dose, or administration with meals. Patients with persistent symptoms despite conservative measures or patients at high risk for NSAID-induced ulcers (see section on peptic ulcer disease) should undergo diagnostic endoscopy. Those without significant NSAID ulceration may be treated symptomatically with sucralfate (1 g four times daily), with H_2 receptor antagonists given twice daily (cimetidine 400 mg, ranitidine 150 mg, or famotidine 20 mg), or with proton pump inhibitors once daily (omeprazole 20 mg, rabeprazole 20 mg, pantoprazole 40 mg, or lansoprazole 30 mg). Upper gastrointestinal bleeding due to NSAID gastritis is usually not severe.

C. Alcoholic Gastritis

Erosive gastritis and hemorrhagic gastritis account for 20% of episodes of upper gastrointestinal bleeding in chronic alcoholics. Therapy with H_2 receptor antago-

nists or sucralfate for 2–4 weeks often is prescribed. On occasion, bleeding may be brisk.

D. Portal Hypertensive Gastropathy

Portal hypertension results in gastric mucosal and submucosal congestion of capillaries and venules. Bleeding from congestive gastropathy accounts for 25% of episodes of upper gastrointestinal bleeding in patients with portal hypertension. It may present suddenly with hematemesis or insidiously with iron deficiency anemia. Recurrent acute bleeding is common. Treatment with propranolol or nadolol reduces the incidence of recurrent acute bleeding by lowering portal pressures. Patients who fail propranolol therapy may be successfully treated with portal decompressive procedures (see section on treatment of esophageal varices).

Wolfe MM et al: Acid suppression: optimizing therapy for gastroduodenal ulcer healing, gastroesophageal reflux disease, and stress-related erosive syndrome. Gastroenterology 2000;118 (2 Suppl 1):S9. [PMID: 10868896]

2. Nonerosive, Nonspecific Gastritis

The diagnosis of nonerosive gastritis is based upon histologic assessment of mucosal biopsies. Endoscopic findings are normal in many cases and do not reliably predict the presence of histologic inflammation. The main types of nonerosive gastritis are those due to *H pylori* infection, those associated with pernicious anemia, and lymphocytic gastritis. (See Specific Types of Gastritis.)

Helicobacter pylori Gastritis

H pylori is a spiral gram-negative rod that resides beneath the gastric mucus layer adjacent to gastric epithelial cells. Although not invasive, it causes gastric mucosal inflammation with polymorphonuclear neutrophils and lymphocytes. The mechanisms of injury and inflammation may in part be related to the products of two genes, *vacA* and *cagA*.

In the United States, the prevalence of infection rises from less than 10% in Caucasians under age 30 to over 50% in those over age 60. The prevalence is higher in non-Caucasians and immigrants from developing countries and is correlated inversely with socioeconomic status. Transmission is from person to person, and an important mode of spread may be gastro-oral (ie, through exposure to vomitus). The majority of infections are probably acquired in childhood.

Acute infection with *H pylori* may cause a transient clinical illness characterized by nausea and abdominal pain that may last for several days and is associated with acute histologic gastritis with polymorphonuclear neutrophils. After these symptoms resolve, the majority progress to chronic infection with chronic, diffuse mucosal inflammation characterized by polymorphonuclear neutrophils and lymphocytes. Inflammation may be confined to the superficial gastric epithelium or may extend deeper into the gastric glands, resulting in varying degrees of gland atrophy (atrophic gastritis) and metaplasia of the gastric epithelium to intestinal type epithelium. Eradication of *H pylori* may be achieved with antibiotics in over 85% of patients and leads to resolution of the chronic gastritis (see section on peptic ulcer disease).

Although chronic *H pylori* infection with gastritis is present in 30–50% of the population, the majority are asymptomatic and suffer no sequelae. *H pylori* infection is strongly associated with peptic ulcer disease; however, only 15% of people with chronic infection develop a peptic ulcer (see section on peptic ulcer disease). Chronic *H pylori* gastritis is associated with a two- to sixfold increased risk of gastric adenocarcinoma and low-grade B cell gastric lymphoma (mucosa-associated lymphoid tissue lymphoma; MALToma). There is little evidence that chronic *H pylori*-associated gastritis is a cause of dyspeptic symptoms. (See Dyspepsia at the beginning of this chapter.)

Testing is indicated for patients with either active or a past history of documented peptic ulcer disease or gastric MALToma and probably for patients with a family history of gastric carcinoma, especially if they are of Asian descent. Testing and empirical treatment may also be cost-effective in young patients (< 45 years) with uncomplicated dyspepsia prior to further medical evaluation. The role of testing and treating *H pylori* in patients with nonulcer dyspepsia remains controversial (See Dyspepsia, above). Because *H pylori* is a common organism but infrequently causes disease, screening of the general population is not indicated.

A. NONINVASIVE TESTING FOR *H PYLORI*

Either serologic tests or fecal antigen tests are recommended as the most cost-effective initial tests for *H pylori*. Laboratory-based quantitative serologic ELISA tests have sensitivity and specificity of over 90% and cost $40–$75. Qualitative office-based kits using whole blood from a finger-stick have a lower (80%) sensitivity and specificity but can be performed within 10 minutes at a cost of $10. Positive serologic tests do not necessarily imply ongoing active infection. After *H pylori* eradication with antibiotics, antibody levels decline to undetectable levels in 50% of patients by 12–18 months. A fecal antigen immunoassay has excellent sensitivity and specificity (90%) at a cost of $60. Because a positive test is indicative of active infection, the fecal antigen assay may be the preferred noninvasive screening test for *H pylori*. However, the cost-effectiveness of each diagnostic test is dependent upon the prevalence of infection and the cost of the tests, which vary greatly.

The ^{13}C-urea and ^{14}C-urea breath tests also have excellent sensitivity and specificity (90%), and a positive test is indicative of active infection. However, their greater cost ($60–$300) make them less attractive than other noninvasive tests in most clinical settings. In cir-

cumstances where testing is clinically indicated (complicated peptic ulcer disease, MALT lymphoma), either a urea breath test (or, where urea testing is not available, a fecal antigen test) should be used to confirm *H pylori* eradication. Proton pump inhibitors significantly reduce the sensitivity of urea breath tests and fecal antigen assays (but not serologic tests) and should be discontinued 7–14 days prior to testing.

B. ENDOSCOPIC TESTING FOR *H PYLORI*

Endoscopy is not indicated to diagnose *H pylori* infection in most circumstances. However, when it is performed for another reason, gastric biopsy specimens can be obtained for detection of *H pylori* and tested for active infection by urease production. This simple, inexpensive ($10) test has excellent sensitivity and specificity (90%). In patients with active upper gastrointestinal bleeding or patients taking proton pump inhibitors, histologic assessment for *H pylori* is preferred. Histologic assessment of biopsies from the gastric antrum and body is more definitive but more expensive ($150–$250) than a rapid urease test. Histologic assessment is also indicated in patients with suspected MALTomas and, possibly, in patients with suspected infection whose rapid urease test is negative. However, serologic testing is the most cost-effective means of confirming *H pylori* infection in patients with a negative rapid urease test.

Hahn M et al: Noninvasive tests as a substitute for histology in the diagnosis of *Helicobacter pylori* infection. Gastrointest Endosc 2000;52:20. [PMID: 10882957]

Peterson WL et al: *Helicobacter pylori*-related disease: guidelines for testing and treating. Arch Intern Med 2000;160:1285. [PMID: 10809031]

Pernicious Anemia Gastritis

Pernicious anemia gastritis is an autoimmune disorder involving the fundic glands with resultant achlorhydria and vitamin B_{12} malabsorption. Fundic histology is characterized by severe gland atrophy and intestinal metaplasia. Parietal cell antibodies directed against the H^+-K^+ ATPase pump are present in 90% of patients. Inflammation and autoimmune destruction of the acid-secreting parietal cells leads to secondary loss of fundic zymogen cells, which secrete intrinsic factor. Achlorhydria leads to pronounced hypergastrinemia (> 1000 pg/mL) due to loss of acid inhibition of gastrin G cells. Hypergastrinemia may induce hyperplasia of gastric enterochromaffin-like cells that may lead to the development of small, multicentric carcinoid tumors in 5% of patients. Metastatic spread is uncommon in lesions smaller than 2 cm. The risk of adenocarcinoma is increased threefold, with a prevalence of 1–3%. Endoscopy with biopsy is indicated in patients with pernicious anemia at the time of diagnosis. Patients with dysplasia or small carcinoids require periodic endoscopic surveillance. Pernicious anemia is discussed in detail in Chapter 13.

Case records of the Massachusetts General Hospital. Weekly clinicopathological exercises. Case 40–2000. A 38-year-old woman with gastric adenocarcinoma. N Engl J Med 2000; 343:1951. [PMID: 11136267]

3. Specific Types of Gastritis

A number of disorders are associated with specific mucosal histologic features.

Infections

Acute bacterial infection of the gastric submucosa and muscularis with a variety of aerobic or anaerobic organisms produces a rare, rapidly progressive, life-threatening condition known as phlegmonous or necrotizing gastritis which requires emergency gastric resection and antibiotic therapy. Viral infection with CMV is commonly seen in patients with AIDS and after bone marrow or solid organ transplantation. Endoscopic findings include thickened gastric folds and ulcerations. Fungal infection with candida may occur in immunocompromised patients. Larvae of *Anisakis marina* ingested in raw fish or sushi may become embedded in the gastric mucosa, producing severe abdominal pain. Pain persists for several days until the larvae die. Endoscopic removal of the larvae provides rapid symptomatic relief.

Granulomatous Gastritis

Chronic granulomatous inflammation may be caused by a variety of systemic diseases, including tuberculosis, syphilis, fungal infections, sarcoidosis, or Crohn's disease. These may be asymptomatic or associated with a variety of gastrointestinal complaints.

Eosinophilic Gastritis

This is a rare disorder in which eosinophils infiltrate the antrum and sometimes the proximal intestine. Infiltration may involve the mucosa, muscularis, or serosa. Peripheral eosinophilia is prominent. Symptoms include anemia from mucosal blood loss, abdominal pain, early satiety, and postprandial vomiting. Treatment with corticosteroids is beneficial in the majority of patients.

Lymphocytic Gastritis

This is an idiopathic condition characterized by fluctuating abdominal pain, nausea, and vomiting. Endoscopic features include mucosal erosions and a varioliform ("pox-like") appearance. Biopsies reveal a diffuse lymphocytic gastritis. There is no established effective therapy.

Ménétrier's Disease (Hypertrophic Gastropathy)

This is an idiopathic entity characterized by giant thickened gastric folds involving predominantly the body of the stomach. Patients complain of nausea, epigastric pain, weight loss, and diarrhea. Because of chronic protein loss, patients may develop severe hypoproteinemia and anasarca. The cause is unknown. Treatment is directed at symptoms. Gastric resection is required in severe cases. There are case reports of resolution of symptoms and improvement in histologic appearance after *H pylori* eradication.

Kawasaki M et al: Ménétrier's disease associated with *Helicobacter pylori* infection: Resolution of enlarged gastric folds and hypoproteinemia after antibacterial treatment. Am J Gastroenterol 1997;92:1909. [PMID: 9382064]

PEPTIC ULCER DISEASE

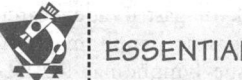 ESSENTIALS OF DIAGNOSIS

- *History of nonspecific epigastric pain present in 80–90% of patients with variable relationship to meals.*
- *Ulcer symptoms characterized by rhythmicity and periodicity.*
- *Ten to 20 percent of patients present with ulcer complications without antecedent symptoms.*
- *Of NSAID-induced ulcers, 30–50% are asymptomatic.*
- *Upper endoscopy with antral biopsy for H pylori is diagnostic procedure of choice in most patients.*
- *Gastric ulcer biopsy or documentation of complete healing necessary to exclude gastric malignancy.*

General Considerations

Peptic ulcer is a break in the gastric or duodenal mucosa that arises when the normal mucosal defensive factors are impaired or are overwhelmed by aggressive luminal factors such as acid and pepsin. By definition, ulcers extend through the muscularis mucosae and are usually over 5 mm in diameter. In the United States, there are about 500,000 new cases per year of peptic ulcer and 4 million ulcer recurrences; the lifetime prevalence of ulcers in the adult population is approximately 10%. Ulcers occur five times more commonly in the duodenum, where over 95% are in the bulb or pyloric channel. In the stomach, benign ulcers are located most commonly in the antrum (60%) and at the junction of the antrum and body on the lesser curvature (25%).

Ulcers occur slightly more commonly in men than in women (1.3:1). Although ulcers can occur in any age group, duodenal ulcers most commonly occur between the ages of 30 and 55, whereas gastric ulcers are more common between the ages of 55 and 70. Ulcers are more common in smokers and in patients taking NSAIDs on a chronic basis (see below). Alcohol and dietary factors do not appear to cause ulcer disease. The role of stress is uncertain. The incidence of duodenal ulcer disease has been declining dramatically for the past 30 years, but the incidence of gastric ulcers appears to be increasing, perhaps as a result of the widespread use of NSAIDs.

Etiology

Three major causes of peptic ulcer disease are now recognized: NSAIDs, chronic *H pylori* infection, and acid hypersecretory states such as Zollinger-Ellison syndrome. Evidence of *H pylori* infection or NSAID ingestion should be sought in all patients with peptic ulcer. NSAID- and *H pylori*-associated ulcers will be considered in the present section; Zollinger-Ellison syndrome will be discussed subsequently. Up to onefourth of ulcers are idiopathic.

A. *H PYLORI*-ASSOCIATED ULCERS

H pylori appears to be a necessary cofactor for the majority of duodenal and gastric ulcers not associated with NSAIDs. The prevalence of *H pylori* infection in duodenal ulcer patients is about 70–75%. Many *H pylori*-infected patients have increased gastric acid secretion. It is hypothesized that increased acid exposure can engender small islands of gastric metaplasia in the duodenal bulb. Colonization of these islands by *H pylori* may lead to duodenitis or duodenal ulcer. The association with gastric ulcers is lower, but *H pylori* is found in the majority in whom NSAIDs cannot be implicated. Overall, it is estimated that one in six infected patients will develop ulcer disease.

The natural history of *H pylori*-associated peptic ulcer disease is well defined. In the absence of specific antibiotic treatment to eradicate the organism, 85% of patients will have an endoscopically visible recurrence within 1 year. Half of these will be symptomatic. After successful eradication of *H pylori* with antibiotics, ulcer recurrence rates are reduced dramatically to 5–20% at 1 year. Some of these ulcer recurrences may be due to NSAID use or reinfection with *H pylori*.

B. NSAID-INDUCED ULCERS

There is a 10–20% prevalence of gastric ulcers and a 2–5% prevalence of duodenal ulcers in chronic NSAID users. The relative risk of gastric ulcers is increased 40-fold, but the risk of duodenal ulcers is only slightly increased. Users of NSAIDs are at least three times more likely than nonusers to suffer serious gastrointestinal complications from these ulcers such as bleeding, perforation, or death. It is noteworthy that gastric ulcers and duodenal ulcers cause about the same number of complications. Approximately 1–2% of chronic NSAID users will have a major complication within 1 year. Aspirin is the most ulcerogenic

NSAID. The risk appears to be dose-related, with some risk even at doses as low as 81 mg every other day. The risk of NSAID complications is greater with higher NSAID dosage, during the first 3 months of administration, with advanced age, and with a prior history of ulcer disease, concomitant corticosteroid administration, or serious medical illness. Celecoxib and rofecoxib are the first members of a new class of NSAIDs that selectively inhibit cyclooxygenase-2 (COX-2)—the principal enzyme involved in prostaglandin production at sites of inflammation—while sparing cyclooxygenase-1 (COX-1), the principal enzyme involved with prostaglandin production in the gastroduodenal mucosa and gastric cytoprotection. The incidence of endoscopically visible ulcers after 6–12 weeks of COX-2 therapy (4%) is not increased compared with patients treated with placebo and significantly lower than the incidence among those receiving nonselective NSAIDs (15–25%). Likewise, the risk of significant clinical events (obstruction, perforation, or severe bleeding) was 0.6–0.76% in patients taking COX-2 selective agents and 1.4% in patients taking nonselective NSAIDs—a relative risk reduction of 0.4–0.5. Among patients taking low-dose aspirin, the risk of a serious event was not significantly different. Other NSAIDs—etodolac, nabumetone, and meloxicam—appear to be partially selective for COX-2 at lower doses and may be safer than nonselective NSAIDs. These less expensive NSAIDs have not been compared with celecoxib or rofecoxib.

Clinical Findings

A. SYMPTOMS AND SIGNS

Epigastric pain (dyspepsia), the hallmark of peptic ulcer disease, is present in 80–90% of patients. However, this complaint is not sensitive or specific enough to serve as a reliable diagnostic criterion for peptic ulcer disease. The clinical history cannot accurately distinguish duodenal from gastric ulcers. Less than one-fourth of patients with dyspepsia have ulcer disease at endoscopy. Twenty percent of patients with ulcer complications such as bleeding have no antecedent symptoms ("silent ulcers"). In patients with NSAID-induced ulcers, half are asymptomatic. Nearly 60% of patients with NSAID complications do not have prior symptoms.

Pain is typically well localized to the epigastrium and not severe. It is described as gnawing, dull, aching, or "hunger-like." Approximately half of patients report relief of pain with food or antacids (especially duodenal ulcers) and a recurrence of pain 2–4 hours later. However, many patients deny any relationship to meals or report worsening of pain. Two-thirds of duodenal ulcers and one-third of gastric ulcers cause nocturnal pain that awakens the patient. A change from a patient's typical rhythmic discomfort to constant or radiating pain may reflect ulcer penetration or perforation. Most patients have symptomatic periods lasting up to several weeks with intervals of months to years in which they are pain-free (periodicity).

Nausea and anorexia may occur with gastric ulcers. Significant vomiting and weight loss are unusual with uncomplicated ulcer disease and suggest gastric outlet obstruction or gastric malignancy.

The physical examination is often normal in uncomplicated peptic ulcer disease. Mild, localized epigastric tenderness to deep palpation may be present. Fecal occult blood testing is positive in one-third of patients.

B. LABORATORY FINDINGS

Laboratory tests are normal in uncomplicated peptic ulcer disease but are ordered to exclude ulcer complications or confounding disease entities. Anemia may occur with acute blood loss from a bleeding ulcer or less commonly from chronic blood loss. Leukocytosis suggests ulcer penetration or perforation. An elevated serum amylase in a patient with severe epigastric pain suggests ulcer penetration into the pancreas. A fasting serum gastrin level to screen for Zollinger-Ellison syndrome is obtained in some patients (see below). Because acid inhibition may raise serum gastrin levels, H_2 receptor antagonists should be withheld for 24 hours and proton pump inhibitors for 1 week before a gastrin level is measured.

C. ENDOSCOPY

Upper endoscopy is the procedure of choice for the diagnosis of duodenal and gastric ulcers. Endoscopy provides better diagnostic accuracy than barium radiography and the ability to biopsy for the presence of malignancy and *H pylori* infection. Duodenal ulcers are virtually never malignant and do not require biopsy. Three to 5 percent of benign-appearing gastric ulcers prove to be malignant. Hence, cytologic brushings and biopsies of the ulcer margin are almost always performed. Provided that the gastric ulcer appears benign to the endoscopist and adequate biopsy specimens reveal no evidence of cancer, dysplasia or atypia, the patient may be followed without further endoscopy. If these conditions are not fulfilled, follow-up endoscopy should be performed 12 weeks after the start of therapy to document complete healing; non-healing ulcers are suspicious for malignancy.

D. IMAGING

Barium upper gastrointestinal series is an acceptable alternative to screening of uncomplicated patients with dyspepsia. However, because it has limited accuracy in distinguishing benign from malignant gastric ulcers, all gastric ulcers diagnosed by x-ray should be reevaluated with endoscopy after 8–12 weeks of therapy.

E. TESTING FOR *H PYLORI*

In patients in whom an ulcer is diagnosed by endoscopy, gastric mucosal biopsies should be obtained both for a rapid urease test and for histologic examination. The specimens for histology are discarded if the urease test is positive. Alternatively, serologic testing may be the most cost-effective means of confirming *H pylori* infection in patients with a negative rapid urease test. (See section on *H pylori* gastritis, above.)

In patients with a history of peptic ulcer or when an ulcer is diagnosed by upper gastrointestinal series, noninvasive assessment for *H pylori* with fecal antigen assay, serologic testing, or urea breath testing should be done. Proton pump inhibitors may cause false-negative urea breath tests and fecal antigen tests and should be withheld for at least 7 days before testing.

Differential Diagnosis

Peptic ulcer disease must be distinguished from other causes of epigastric distress (dyspepsia). Over half of patients with dyspepsia have no obvious organic explanation for their symptoms and are classified as having functional dyspepsia (see sections above on dyspepsia and functional dyspepsia). Atypical gastroesophageal reflux may be manifested by epigastric symptoms. Biliary tract disease is characterized by discrete, intermittent episodes of pain that should not be confused with other causes of dyspepsia. Severe epigastric pain is atypical for peptic ulcer disease unless complicated by a perforation or penetration. Other causes include acute pancreatitis, acute cholecystitis or choledocholithiasis, esophageal rupture, gastric volvulus, and ruptured aortic aneurysm.

Pharmacologic Agents

The pharmacology of several agents that enhance the healing of peptic ulcers is briefly discussed here. They may be divided into three categories: (1) acid-antisecretory agents, (2) mucosal protective agents, and (3) agents that promote healing through eradication of *H pylori*. Recommendations for their use are provided in subsequent sections.

A. ACID-ANTISECRETORY AGENTS

1. Proton pump inhibitors—Proton pump inhibitors covalently bind the acid-secreting enzyme H^+-K^+ ATPase, or "proton pump," permanently inactivating it. Restoration of acid secretion requires synthesis of new pumps, which have a half-life of 18 hours. Thus, although these agents have a serum half-life of less than 60 minutes, their duration of action exceeds 24 hours. The four available agents, omeprazole or rabeprazole 20 mg, lansoprazole 15–30 mg, and pantoprazole 40 mg, inhibit over 90% of 24-hour acid secretion, compared with under 65% for H_2 receptor antagonists in standard dosages. Proton pump inhibitors should be administered 30 minutes before meals (usually breakfast).

Each of the four proton pump inhibitors results in over 90% healing of duodenal ulcers after 4 weeks and 90% of gastric ulcers after 8 weeks when given once daily. Compared with H_2 receptor antagonists, proton pump inhibitors provide faster pain relief and more rapid ulcer healing. However, nearly equivalent overall healing rates may be achieved with longer courses of H_2 receptor antagonists.

The proton pump inhibitors are remarkably safe in short-term therapy. Serum gastrin levels rise significantly (> 500 pg/mL) in 10% of patients receiving chronic therapy, which is associated with the development of gastric enterochromaffin-like cell hyperplasia in humans and gastric carcinoid tumors in rats. Clinical experience with these agents for over 10 years has not detected any significant toxicity in humans. Long-term use may lead to a mild decrease in vitamin B_{12} and iron absorption of unclear significance. Long-term use is unnecessary in peptic ulcer disease but is frequently required in gastroesophageal reflux disease.

2. H_2 receptor antagonists—Although H_2 receptor antagonists are effective in the treatment of peptic ulcer disease, proton pump inhibitors are now the preferred agents because of their ease of use and superior efficacy. Four H_2 receptor antagonists are available: cimetidine, ranitidine, famotidine, and nizatidine. All four agents effectively inhibit nocturnal acid output, but they are less effective at inhibiting meal-stimulated acid secretion. For uncomplicated peptic ulcers, H_2 receptor antagonists may be administered once daily at bedtime as follows: ranitidine and nizatidine 300 mg, famotidine 40 mg, and cimetidine 800 mg. Ulcer symptom relief usually occurs within 2 weeks. Duodenal and gastric ulcer healing rates of 85–90% are obtained within 6 weeks and 8 weeks, respectively. All four agents are well tolerated, and serious adverse effects are rare. Cimetidine is uncommonly used because it inhibits hepatic cytochrome P450 metabolism (raising the serum concentration of theophylline, warfarin, lidocaine, and phenytoin) and may cause gynecomastia or impotence. Ranitidine binds P450 with one-tenth the avidity of cimetidine; famotidine and nizatidine have negligible effects.

B. AGENTS ENHANCING MUCOSAL DEFENSES

Sucralfate, bismuth, misoprostol, and low doses of aluminum-containing antacids all have been shown to promote ulcer healing through the enhancement of mucosal defensive mechanisms. Given the greater efficacy and safety of antisecretory agents and better compliance of patients, sucralfate and these other agents are no longer used as first-line therapy for active ulcers in most clinical settings. Because of the rapid relief of ulcer symptoms they provide, antacids are commonly used as needed to supplement antisecretory agents during the first few days of treatment. Sucralfate, 1 g four times daily, is sometimes added to antisecretory therapy in patients with refractory ulcers. Bismuth has direct antibacterial action against *H pylori* and may be used in combination with antibiotics for eradication (see below). Misoprostol is a prostaglandin analog that stimulates gastroduodenal mucus and bicarbonate secretion. It is effective as a prophylactic agent in reducing the incidence of gastroduodenal ulcers in patients taking nonselective NSAIDs but must be given three or four times daily and causes diarrhea in 10–20% of patients. With the advent of proton pump inhibitors and COX-2 selective NSAIDs, it is now less commonly used for this indication.

C. *H PYLORI* ERADICATION THERAPY

Eradication of *H pylori* has proved difficult. Combination regimens that employ two antibiotics with a proton pump inhibitor or bismuth are required to achieve adequate rates of eradication and to reduce the number of failures due to antibiotic resistance. Therapies employing only one or two antibiotics cannot be recommended. Resistance develops rapidly to metronidazole and clarithromycin but not to amoxicillin or tetracycline. In the United States, up to 50% of strains are resistant to metronidazole and 7% are resistant to clarithromycin. It is advisable to include amoxicillin in first-line therapy in most patients, reserving metronidazole for penicillin-allergic patients. Recommended regimens are listed in Table 14–11. All currently recommended regimens achieve rates of eradication greater than 85% after 10–14 days of treatment. Proton pump inhibitors have direct antimicrobial action against *H pylori;* furthermore, by raising intragastric pH, they suppress bacterial growth and optimize antibiotic efficacy. In most centers in the United States, the preferred regimen is with a 10-day to 14-day course of treatment with a proton pump inhibitor (omeprazole or rabeprazole, 20 mg twice daily; lansoprazole, 30 mg twice daily; or pantoprazole, 40 mg twice daily); amoxicillin, 1 g twice daily; and clarithromycin, 500 mg twice daily. In patients whose infection persists after an initial course of antibiotic therapy, the optimal regimen may be quadruple therapy with a proton pump inhibitor, bismuth subsalicylate, tetracycline, and metronidazole for 14 days (Table 14–11).

Medical Treatment

Patients should be encouraged to eat balanced meals at regular intervals. There is no justification for bland or restrictive diets. Moderate alcohol intake is not harmful. Smoking retards the rate of ulcer healing and increases the frequency of recurrences and should be discouraged.

A. TREATMENT OF *H PYLORI*-ASSOCIATED ULCERS

1. Treatment of active ulcer—The goals of treatment of active *H pylori*-associated ulcers are to relieve dyspeptic symptoms, to promote ulcer healing, and to eradicate *H pylori* infection. Uncomplicated *H pylori*-associated ulcers should be treated for the first 10–14 days with one of the proton pump inhibitor-based *H pylori* eradication regimens listed in Table 14–11. An antisecretory agent must be administered for an additional 2–4 weeks (duodenal ulcer) or 4–6 weeks (gas-

Table 14–11. Treatment options for peptic ulcer disease.

Active *Helicobacter pylori*-associated ulcer:
1. Treat with anti-*H pylori* regimen for 10–14 days. Treatment options:

   Proton pump inhibitor twice daily[1]
   Clarithromycin 500 mg twice daily
   Amoxicillin 1 g twice daily (OR metronidazole 500 mg twice daily, if penicillin allergic)

   Proton pump inhibitor twice daily[1]
   Bismuth subsalicylate two tablets four times daily
   Tetracycline 500 mg four times daily
   Metronidazole 250 mg four times daily

   Ranitidine bismuth citrate 400 mg twice daily
   Clarithromycin 500 mg twice daily
   Amoxicillin 1 g OR tetracycline 500 mg OR metronidazole 500 mg twice daily

   (Proton pump inhibitors administered before meals. Avoid metronidazole regimens in areas of known high resistance or in patients who have failed a course of treatment that included metronidazole).

2. After completion of 10–14 day course of *H pylori* eradication therapy, continue treatment with proton pump inhibitor[1] once daily or H_2 receptor antagonist (as below) for 4–8 weeks to promote healing.

Active ulcer not attributable to *H pylori*:

1. Consider other causes: NSAIDs, Zollinger-Ellison syndrome, gastric malignancy. Treatment options:

   Proton pump inhibitors[1]:
      Uncomplicated duodenal ulcer: treat for 4 weeks
      Uncomplicated gastric ulcer: treat for 8 weeks
   H_2 receptor antagonists:
      Uncomplicated duodenal ulcer: cimetidine 800 mg, ranitidine or nizatidine 300 mg, famotidine 40 mg, once daily at bedtime for 6 weeks
      Uncomplicated gastric ulcer: cimetidine 400 mg, ranitidine or nizatidine 150 mg, famotidine 20 mg, twice daily for 8 weeks
      Complicated ulcers: proton pump inhibitors are preferred drugs

Prevention of ulcer relapse:

1. NSAID-induced ulcer: prophylactic therapy for high-risk patients (prior ulcer disease or ulcer complications, use of corticosteroids or anticoagulants, age > 70 with serious comorbid illnesses).
   Treatment options:

   Proton pump inhibitor once daily
   COX-2 selective NSAID (rofecoxib, celecoxib, valdecoxib)
   (In special circumstances: misoprostol 200 μg 3–4 times daily)

2. Chronic "maintenance" therapy indicated in patients with recurrent ulcers who either are *H pylori*-negative or who have failed attempts at eradication therapy: once daily proton pump inhibitor[1] or H_2 receptor antagonist at bedtime (cimetidine 400–800 mg, nizatidine or ranitidine 150–300 mg, famotidine 20–40 mg)

---

[1]Proton pump inhibitors: omeprazole 20 mg, rabeprazole 20 mg, lansoprazole 30 mg, pantoprazole 40 mg.

tric ulcer) after completion of the antibiotic regimen to ensure complete ulcer healing. A once-daily proton pump inhibitor (omeprazole or rabeprazole 20 mg; lansoprazole 30 mg; pantoprazole 40 mg) is most convenient, but H_2-receptor antagonists may be chosen as less expensive therapy. Confirmation of *H pylori* eradication in patients with uncomplicated ulcers is not necessary. Confirmation is required in all patients with ulcers complicated by bleeding, perforation, or obstruction.

2. Therapy to prevent recurrence—Successful eradication reduces ulcer recurrences to less than 20% after 1–2 years. Therefore, antisecretory therapy can be discontinued after 4–8 weeks in patients with uncomplicated ulcers and the patient observed for recurrence of symptoms. The most common cause of recurrence after antibiotic therapy is failure to achieve successful eradication, which must be evaluated. Once cure has been achieved, reinfection rates are less than 0.5% per year. Although H pylori has reduced the need for chronic maintenance antisecretory therapy to prevent ulcer recurrences, there remains a subset of patients who require chronic therapy with either a proton pump inhibitor once daily or an H_2 receptor antagonist at bedtime. This subset includes patients with H pylori-positive ulcers who have failed recurrent attempts at eradication therapy, patients with a history of H pylori-positive ulcers who have recurrent ulcers despite successful eradication, and patients with idiopathic ulcers (ie, H pylori-negative and not taking NSAIDs). In all patients with recurrent ulcers, NSAID usage (unintentional or surreptitious) and hypersecretory states (including gastrinoma) should be excluded.

B. Treatment of NSAID-Associated Ulcers

1. Treatment of active ulcers—In patients with NSAID-induced ulcers, the offending agent should be discontinued whenever possible. Both gastric and duodenal ulcers respond rapidly to therapy with H_2 receptor antagonists or proton pump inhibitors (Table 14–11) once NSAIDs are eliminated. In some patients with severe inflammatory diseases, it may not be feasible to discontinue NSAIDs. These patients should be treated with proton pump inhibitors once daily, which result in ulcer healing rates of approximately 80% at 8 weeks in patients continuing to take NSAIDs.

H pylori infection does not appear to increase the risk of NSAID-induced ulcers. Nevertheless, about half of patients who develop ulcers while using NSAIDs are infected with H pylori, and in such cases it is impossible to be certain which is the primary pathogenetic factor. Therefore, antibiotic eradication therapy should be given for NSAID-induced ulcers when H pylori tests are positive.

2. Prevention of NSAID-induced ulcers—The goal of prophylactic therapy is to prevent ulcer complications, which occur in only 1–2% of NSAID-treated patients per year. Therefore, prophylactic therapy should be reserved for patients at high risk for developing complications. High-risk factors include a history of ulcer disease or complications, concurrent therapy with corticosteroids or anticoagulants, serious underlying medical illness, and age over 60. Such patients have a greater than 5% chance per year of developing a complicated ulcer from taking a nonselective NSAID. Whenever possible, NSAIDs should be avoided in this high-risk population. If NSAIDs must be given, the following options can be considered. (At this time, the optimal cost-effective approach has not been determined.)

a. COX-2 selective agent—For most patients at high risk of NSAID-induced complications, therapy with a COX-2 selective agent is recommended. The relative risk of significant clinical events (obstruction, perforation, or severe bleeding) in patients taking COX-2 selective agents (celecoxib, rofecoxib) is 0.5 compared with patients taking nonselective NSAIDs. Patients with multiple risk factors have a relative risk reduction but still have a significant risk of complications. In patients who require concurrent therapy with low dose aspirin for cardiovascular prophylaxis, the safety of a COX-2 selective agent may be partially negated.

b. Proton pump inhibitor—Treatment with a proton pump inhibitor given once-daily (omeprazole or rabeprazole 20 mg, lansoprazole 30 mg, or pantoprazole 40 mg) appears to be effective in the prevention of NSAID-induced gastric and duodenal ulcers and is approved by the FDA for this indication. For patients taking a daily proton pump inhibitor for another indication (such as gastroesophageal reflux disease), a nonselective NSAID may be given.

c. Misoprostol—The prostaglandin analog misoprostol is effective in the prevention of NSAID-induced gastric and duodenal ulcers when given at a dosage of 100–200 µg three or four times daily. It is less commonly used as a prophylactic agent against NSAID-induced complications than either COX-2 selective agents or concurrent therapy with a proton pump inhibitor.

d. Multiple NSAID risk factors—Patients with multiple risk factors are at particularly high risk of NSAID-induced complications. The optimal cost-effective approach to management of these patients is unknown. Options include a COX-2 selective agent alone, a COX-2 selective agent and a proton pump inhibitor, and a COX-2 selective agent and misoprostol.

D. Refractory Ulcers

Ulcers that are truly refractory to medical therapy are now uncommon. Less than 5% of ulcers are unhealed after 8 weeks of therapy with proton pump inhibitors. Noncompliance is the most common cause of ulcer nonhealing. Cigarettes retard ulcer healing and should be proscribed. NSAID and aspirin use, sometimes surreptitious, are commonly implicated in refractory ulcers and must be stopped. H pylori eradication enhances healing and decreases the high recurrence rates of refractory ulcers. Therefore, evidence of H pylori infection should be sought and the infection treated, if present, in all refractory ulcer patients. Fasting serum gastrin levels should be obtained to exclude gastrinoma with acid hypersecretion (Zollinger-Ellison syndrome). Nonhealing gastric ulcers raise concerns that an undiagnosed gastric malignancy may be masquerading as a benign gastric ulcer. Repeat ulcer biopsies are mandatory after 2–3 months of therapy in all nonhealed gastric ulcers, and they should be followed with serial endoscopies to verify complete healing. Almost all benign refractory ulcers heal within 8 weeks with a proton pump inhibitor twice daily (omeprazole or rabeprazole 20 mg twice daily, lansoprazole 30 mg twice daily). Patients with persistent nonhealing ulcers are referred for surgical therapy after exclusion of NSAID use and persistent *H pylori* infection.

Bombardier C et al: Comparison of upper gastrointestinal toxicity of rofecoxib and naproxen in patients with rheumatoid arthritis. N Engl J Med 2000;343:1520. [PMID: 11087881]

Chan F et al: Preventing recurrent upper gastrointestinal bleeding in patients with *Helicobacter pylori* infection who are taking low-dose aspirin or naproxen. N Engl J Med 2001;344:967. [PMID: 11274623] (*H pylori* eradication therapy is recommended for all patients with peptic ulcer disease, but patients requiring larger doses of aspirin or chronic NSAIDs should be placed on chronic proton pump inhibitor therapy.)

Feldman M et al: Do cyclooxygenase-2 inhibitors provide benefits similar to those of traditional nonsteroidal anti-inflammatory drugs, with less gastrointestinal toxicity? Ann Intern Med 2000;132:134. [PMID: 10644275]

Fitzgerald G et al: The coxibs, selective inhibitors of cyclooxygenase-2. N Engl J Med 2001;345:433. [PMID: 11496855]

Graham D: Therapy of *Helicobacter pylori:* current status and issues. Gastroenterology 2000;118:S2. [PMID: 10868895]

Huang JQ et al: Role of *Helicobacter pylori* infection and nonsteroidal anti-inflammatory drugs in peptic-ulcer disease: a meta-analysis. Lancet 2002;359:14. [PMID: 11809181] (This meta-analysis reports synergism between these two factors.)

Kearney D: Retreatment of *Helicobacter pylori* infection after initial treatment failure. Am J Gastroenterol 2001;96:1335. [PMID: 11374665]

Laine L: Approaches to nonsteroidal anti-inflammatory drug use in the high-risk patient. Gastroenterology 2001;120:594. [PMID: 11179238]

Silverstein FE et al: Gastrointestinal toxicity with celecoxib vs nonsteroidal anti-inflammatory drugs for osteoarthritis and rheumatoid arthritis. The CLASS study: a randomized controlled trial. JAMA 2000;284:1247. [PMID: 10979111]

Wolfe MM et al: Acid suppression: optimizing therapy for gastroduodenal ulcer healing, gastroesophageal reflux disease, and stress-related mucosal disease. Gastroenterology 2000;118: S9. [PMID: 1086889]

COMPLICATIONS OF PEPTIC ULCER DISEASE

1. *Gastrointestinal Hemorrhage*

ESSENTIALS OF DIAGNOSIS

- *"Coffee grounds" emesis, hematemesis, melena, or hematochezia.*
- *Emergent upper endoscopy is diagnostic and therapeutic.*

General Considerations

Approximately 50% of all episodes of upper gastrointestinal bleeding are due to peptic ulcer. Clinically significant bleeding occurs in 10–20% of ulcer patients. About 80% of patients stop bleeding spontaneously and generally have an uneventful recovery; the remainder have more severe bleeding. The overall mortality rate for ulcer bleeding is 6–10%, but it is higher in the elderly, in patients with comorbid medical problems, and in patients with nosocomial bleeding. Mortality is also higher in patients who present with persistent hypertension or shock, bright red blood in the vomitus or nasogastric lavage fluid, or severe coagulopathy.

Clinical Findings

A. SYMPTOMS AND SIGNS

Up to 20% of patients have no antecedent symptoms of pain; this is particularly true of patients receiving NSAIDs. Common presenting signs include melena and hematemesis. Massive upper gastrointestinal bleeding or rapid gastrointestinal transit may result in hematochezia rather than melena; this may be misinterpreted as signifying a lower tract bleeding source. Nasogastric lavage that demonstrates "coffee grounds" or bright red blood confirms an upper tract source. Recovered nasogastric lavage fluid that is negative for blood does not exclude active bleeding from a duodenal ulcer.

B. LABORATORY FINDINGS

The hematocrit may fall as a result of bleeding or expansion of the intravascular volume with intravenous fluids. The BUN may rise as a result of absorption of blood nitrogen from the small intestine and prerenal azotemia.

Treatment

The assessment and initial management of upper gastrointestinal tract bleeding is discussed elsewhere in this chapter. Specific issues pertaining to peptic ulcer bleeding are described below.

A. MEDICAL THERAPY

A number of pharmacologic agents have been used in patients with peptic ulcer bleeding in an attempt to arrest active bleeding and prevent rebleeding. Since ulcer bleeding abates spontaneously in at least 80% of patients, it has been difficult to demonstrate the benefit of any agent, in part due to inadequate study sample sizes and in part because these agents were given to all patients admitted with ulcer bleeding rather than just those at highest risk of rebleeding.

1. Antisecretory agents—Intravenous H_2-receptor antagonists have not been demonstrated to be of any benefit in the treatment of acute ulcer bleeding. However, intravenous proton pump inhibitors or oral proton pump inhibitors, with or without endoscopic therapy, have been associated with a reduction in rebleeding, transfusions, and the need for further endoscopic therapy. The potential benefit and minimal cost support the use of intravenous proton pump inhibitors (where available) or high-dose oral proton pump inhibitors (eg, omeprazole, 40 mg twice daily) for 5 days in patients with ulcers whose endoscopic appearance suggests a high risk of rebleeding. Many physicians choose to administer a high-dose proton pump inhibitor prior to endoscopy in all patients admitted to the hospital with a gastrointestinal hemorrhage which is suspected to be due to peptic ulcer, discontinuing therapy after endoscopy in patients with ulcers deemed to be at low risk of rebleeding.

2. Somatostatin and octreotide—Intravenous somatostatin (250 μg/h; not available in the United States) and its long-acting analog, octreotide (100 μg bolus; 25–50 μg/h) reduce splanchnic blood flow and inhibit gastric acid secretion. The efficacy of these agents has not been demonstrated convincingly except by meta-analysis showing reduction in rebleeding. Their role at this time is unclear. They may be useful adjunctive agents in patients in whom endoscopic therapy is unsuccessful in controlling bleeding or when endoscopy is not available.

3. Long-term prevention of rebleeding—One-third of patients develop recurrent ulcer bleeding within 3 years if no specific therapy is given. Unblinded studies have demonstrated that in patients with bleeding ulcers who are *H pylori*-positive, successful eradication effectively prevents recurrent ulcer bleeding in virtually all cases. It is therefore recommended that all patients with bleeding ulcers be tested for *H pylori* infection and treated if positive. Four to 8 weeks after completion of antibiotic therapy, a urea breath test should be administered or endoscopy performed with biopsy for histologic confirmation of successful eradication. In patients in whom *H pylori* persists or those whose ulcers are not associated with NSAIDs or *H pylori*, chronic acid suppression with a bedtime dose of an H2 antagonist (ranitidine 150 mg) or a once daily proton pump inhibitor should be prescribed to reduce the likelihood of recurrence of bleeding.

B. ENDOSCOPY

Endoscopy is the preferred diagnostic procedure in virtually all cases of upper gastrointestinal bleeding because of its high diagnostic accuracy, its ability to predict the likelihood of recurrent bleeding, and its availability for therapeutic intervention in high-risk lesions. Endoscopy should be performed within 12–24 hours in virtually all cases. In cases of severe active bleeding, endoscopy is performed as soon as patients have been appropriately resuscitated and are hemodynamically stable.

On the basis of clinical and endoscopic criteria, it is possible to predict which patients are at a higher risk of rebleeding and therefore to make more rational use of hospital resources. Nonbleeding ulcers under 2 cm in size with a base that is clean have a less than 5% chance of rebleeding. Most young (under age 60), otherwise healthy patients with clean-based ulcers may be monitored in the emergency room or on the hospital ward for 24 hours before discharge. Low-risk patients can be safely discharged from the hospital or emergency room immediately after endoscopy. Ulcers that have only a flat red or black spot have a less than 10% chance of significant rebleeding, and those with a firmly adherent clot have a 12–33% rebleeding risk. Patients who are hemodynamically stable with these findings should be admitted to a hospital ward for 48–72 hours and may begin immediate oral feedings and antiulcer (or anti-*H pylori*) medication.

By contrast, the risk of rebleeding or continued bleeding in ulcers with a nonbleeding visible vessel is 50%, and with active bleeding it is 80–90%. Endoscopic therapy with injection or thermocoagulation techniques now is the standard of care for such lesions because it reduces the risk of rebleeding, the number of transfusions, and the need for subsequent surgery. Injection is performed into and around the ulcer vessel with epinephrine (1:10,000). Thermocoagulation is achieved with contact cautery probes applied directly to the ulcer vessel. Using any of these techniques, successful hemostasis of actively bleeding lesions is achieved in 90%. For actively bleeding ulcers, a combination of epinephrine injection followed by thermocoagulation yields better control of bleeding than either modality alone. Significant rebleeding occurs in 10–20% of cases, of which over 70% can be managed successfully with repeat endoscopic treatment. After endoscopic therapy, the risk of rebleeding declines significantly over 3 days to less than 3%. Patients with these high-risk lesions should be monitored in an ICU setting for a minimum period of 24 hours and should remain hospitalized for at least 72 hours.

C. SURGICAL TREATMENT

Patients with high-risk endoscopic lesions and those whose condition warrants ICU admission should be evaluated by a surgeon. However, less than 10% of patients treated with hemostatic therapy require surgery for continued or recurrent bleeding. Overall surgical mortality for emergency ulcer bleeding is less than 6%. The prognosis is poorer for patients over age 60, those with serious underlying medical illnesses or chronic renal failure, and those who require more than 10 units of blood transfusion.

2. Ulcer Perforation

Perforations develop in 5% of ulcer patients, usually from ulcers on the anterior wall of the stomach or duodenum. The incidence of perforations may be increasing, perhaps as a consequence of using NSAIDs or crack cocaine. Zollinger-Ellison disease should be considered in patients who present with ulcer perforation.

Perforation results in a chemical peritonitis that causes sudden, severe generalized abdominal pain that prompts most patients to seek immediate attention. Elderly or debilitated patients and those receiving chronic steroid therapy may experience minimal initial symptoms, presenting late with bacterial peritonitis, sepsis, and shock. On physical examination, patients appear ill, with a rigid, quiet abdomen and rebound tenderness. Hypotension develops later after bacterial peritonitis has developed. If hypotension is present early with the onset of pain, one should consider other abdominal emergencies such as a ruptured aortic aneurysm, mesenteric infarction, or acute pancreatitis. Leukocytosis is almost always present. A mildly elevated serum amylase (less than twice normal) is sometimes seen. Upright or decubitus films of the abdomen reveal free intraperitoneal air in 75% of cases, and in most cases this establishes the diagnosis without need for further studies. The absence of free air may lead to a misdiagnosis of pancreatitis, cholecystitis, or appendicitis. Upper gastrointestinal radiography with water-soluble contrast may be useful in this setting. Barium studies are contraindicated in patients with possible perforation.

Traditional surgical dogma held that the majority of patients with perforated ulcers should undergo emergency laparotomy. Closure of the perforation was performed with an omental ("Graham") patch and, in stable patients, a proximal gastric vagotomy was performed to decrease the chance of ulcer recurrence. This approach is changing as a result of two factors. The first is minimally invasive surgical technique. Laparoscopic perforation closure can be performed in many centers, significantly reducing operative morbidity. Second is the recognition that *H pylori* infection is associated with most ulcers and ulcer perforations. Postoperative treatment of *H pylori* reduces the risk of ulcer recurrence, obviating the need for intraoperative vagotomy. The overall mortality rate in patients treated surgically is 5%.

Up to 40% of ulcer perforations seal spontaneously by the adherence of omentum or adjacent organs to the lesion and do not have significant intraperitoneal spillage. Thus, some centers advocate initial nonoperative management for patients whose onset of symptoms is less than 12 hours and whose upper gastrointestinal series with water-soluble contrast medium does not demonstrate leakage. At present, such conservative therapy is most appropriate for patients who are poor operative candidates. Patients should be monitored closely while receiving fluids, nasogastric suction, antisecretory agents, and broad-spectrum antibiotics. If their condition deteriorates over the first 12 hours (as evidenced by increasing pain, rising pulse or temperature, or worsening peritonitis), they should be taken to the operating room.

3. Ulcer Penetration

An ulcer located along the posterior wall of the duodenum or stomach may perforate into contiguous structures such as the pancreas, liver, or biliary tree. Patients complain of a change in the intensity and rhythmicity of their ulcer symptoms. The pain becomes more severe and constant, may radiate to the back, and is unresponsive to antacids or food. Physical examination and laboratory tests are nonspecific. Mild amylase elevations may sometimes occur. Endoscopy and barium x-ray studies confirm the ulceration but are not diagnostic of an actual penetration. Patients should be given intravenous H_2 receptor antagonists (as above) or omeprazole, 40 mg/d, and followed closely. Those who fail to improve should be considered for surgical therapy.

4. Gastric Outlet Obstruction

Gastric outlet obstruction occurs in 2% of patients with ulcer disease and is due to edema or cicatricial narrowing of the pylorus or duodenal bulb. Most patients have a prior known history of ulcer disease. Obstruction is less commonly caused by gastric neoplasms or extrinsic duodenal obstruction by intra-abdominal neoplasms. The most common symptoms are early satiety, vomiting, and weight loss. Early symptoms are epigastric fullness or heaviness after meals. Later, vomiting may develop that typically occurs one to several hours after eating and consists of partially digested food contents. Chronic obstruction may result in a grossly dilated, atonic stomach, severe weight loss, and malnutrition. Patients may develop dehydration, metabolic alkalosis, and hypokalemia. On physical examination, a succussion splash may be heard in the epigastrium. In most cases, nasogastric aspiration will result in evacuation of a large amount (> 200 mL) of foul-smelling fluid, which establishes the diagnosis. More subtle obstruction is diagnosed by a saline load test or by a nuclear gastric emptying study. Patients are treated initially with intravenous isotonic saline and KCl to correct fluid and electrolyte disorders, intravenous H_2 receptor antagonists (see treatment of stress gastritis, above), and nasogastric decompression of the stomach. Severely malnourished patients should receive total parenteral nutrition. Upper endoscopy is performed after 24–72 hours to define the nature of the obstruction and to exclude gastric neoplasm. At 72 hours, all patients should be evaluated with a saline load test. A positive test consists of more than 400 mL of residual volume 30 minutes after instillation of 750 mL of 0.9% saline into the stomach by nasogastric tube. Patients with a negative load test may be started on clear liquids and their diet advanced as tolerated. The remainder should remain on nasogastric suction for 5–7 days. Traditionally, patients unimproved after that time have been recommended for surgical treatment with vagotomy and either pyloroplasty or antrectomy. However, upper endoscopy with dilation of the gastric obstruction by hydrostatic balloons passed through the instrument has achieved success in two-thirds of patients. It may be reasonable to pursue dilation first in patients with milder symptoms, reserving surgery for those who fail to respond.

Donovan A et al: Perforated duodenal ulcer. Arch Surg 1998; 133:1166. [PMID: 9820345]

Lau JY et al: Effect of intravenous omeprazole on recurrent bleeding after endoscopic treatment of bleeding peptic ulcers. N Engl J Med 2000;343:310. [PMID: 10922429]

Lau JY et al: Endoscopic retreatment compared with surgery in patients with recurrent bleeding after initial endoscopic control of bleeding ulcers. N Engl J Med 1999;340:751. [PMID: 10072409]

Longstreth G et al: Successful outpatient management of acute gastrointestinal hemorrhage: use of practice guidelines in a large patient series. Gastrointest Endosc 1998;47:219. [PMID: 9540873]

ZOLLINGER-ELLISON SYNDROME (Gastrinoma)

 ESSENTIALS OF DIAGNOSIS

- Peptic ulcer disease; may be severe and atypical.
- Gastric acid hypersecretion.
- Diarrhea common, relieved by nasogastric suction.
- Most cases are sporadic; 25% with MEN 1.

General Considerations

Zollinger-Ellison syndrome is caused by gastrin-secreting gut neuroendocrine tumors (gastrinomas), which result in hypergastrinemia and acid hypersecretion. Less than 1% of peptic ulcer disease is caused by gastrinomas. Primary gastrinomas may arise in the pancreas (25%), duodenal wall (45%), or lymph nodes (5–15%), and in other locations or of unknown primary in 20%. Approximately 80% arise within the "gastrinoma triangle" bounded by the porta hepatis, the neck of the pancreas, and the third portion of the duodenum. Most gastrinomas are solitary or multifocal nodules that are potentially resectable. Over two-thirds of gastrinomas are malignant, and one-third have already metastasized to the liver at initial presentation. Approximately 25% of patients have small multicentric gastrinomas associated with MEN 1 that are more difficult to resect.

Clinical Findings

A. SYMPTOMS AND SIGNS

Over 90% of patients with Zollinger-Ellison syndrome develop peptic ulcers. In most cases, the symptoms are indistinguishable from other causes of peptic ulcer disease and therefore may go undetected for years. Ulcers usually are solitary and located in the duodenal bulb, but they may be multiple or occur more distally in the duodenum. Isolated gastric ulcers do not occur. Gastroesophageal reflux symptoms occur often. Diarrhea occurs in one-third of patients, in some cases in the absence of peptic symptoms. Gastric acid hypersecretion can cause direct intestinal mucosal injury and pancreatic enzyme inactivation, resulting in diarrhea, steatorrhea, and weight loss; nasogastric aspiration of stomach acid stops the diarrhea. Screening for Zollinger-Ellison syndrome with fasting gastrin levels should be obtained in patients with ulcers that are refractory to standard therapies, giant ulcers (> 2 cm), ulcers located distal to the duodenal bulb, multiple duodenal ulcers, frequent ulcer recurrences, ulcers associated with diarrhea, ulcers occurring after ulcer surgery, and patients with ulcer complications. Ulcer patients with hypercalcemia or family histories of ulcers (suggesting MEN 1) should also be screened. Finally, patients with peptic ulcers who are *H pylori*-negative and who are not taking NSAIDs should be screened.

B. LABORATORY FINDINGS

The most sensitive and specific method for identifying Zollinger-Ellison syndrome is demonstration of an increased fasting serum gastrin concentration (> 150 pg/mL). Levels should be obtained with patients not taking H_2 receptor antagonists for 24 hours or omeprazole for 6 days. The median gastrin level is 500–700 pg/mL, and 60% have levels less than 1000 pg/mL. Hypochlorhydria with increased gastric pH is a much more common cause of hypergastrinemia than is gastrinoma. Therefore, a measurement of gastric pH (and, where available, gastric secretory studies) is performed in patients with fasting hypergastrinemia. Most patients have a basal acid output of over 15 meq/h. A gastric pH of > 3.0 implies hypochlorhydria and excludes gastrinoma. In a patient with a serum gastrin level of > 1000 pg/mL and acid hypersecretion, the diagnosis of Zollinger-Ellison syndrome is established. With lower gastrin levels (150–1000 pg/mL) and acid secretion, a secretin stimulation test is performed to distinguish Zollinger-Ellison syndrome from other causes of hypergastrinemia. Intravenous secretin (2 units/kg) produces a rise in serum gastrin of over 200 pg/mL within 2–30 minutes in 85% of patients with gastrinoma. An elevated serum calcium suggests hyperparathyroidism and MEN 1 syndrome. In all patients with Zollinger-Ellison syndrome, a serum PTH, prolactin, LH-FSH, and GH level should be obtained to exclude MEN 1.

C. IMAGING

Imaging studies are obtained in an attempt to determine whether there is metastatic disease and, if not, to identify the site of the primary tumor. Although conventional radiologic studies such as CT, MRI, and transabdominal ultrasound are commonly obtained, their sensitivity is less than 50–70% for hepatic metastases and 35% for primary tumors. These studies are being supplanted by somatostatin receptor scintigraphy (SRS) and endoscopic ultrasonography (EUS).

The former should be the first study obtained because of its high sensitivity (> 90%) for detecting hepatic metastases, though its sensitivity for detecting the primary gastrinoma is much lower. If SRS is positive for tumor localization, further imaging studies are not necessary. In patients with negative SRS, EUS is indicated. This study has a sensitivity of > 90% for tumors of the pancreatic head and can visualize half of tumors in the duodenal wall or adjacent lymph nodes. With a combination of SRS and EUS, more than 90% of primary gastrinomas now can be localized preoperatively.

Differential Diagnosis

Gastrinomas are one of several gut neuroendocrine tumors that have similar histopathologic features and arise either from the gut or pancreas. These include carcinoid, insulinoma, VIPoma, glucagonoma, and somatostatinoma. These tumors usually are differentiated by the gut peptides that they secrete; however, poorly differentiated neuroendocrine tumors may not secrete any hormones. Patients may present with symptoms caused by tumor metastases (jaundice, hepatomegaly) rather than functional symptoms. Once a diagnosis of a neuroendocrine tumor is established from the liver biopsy, the specific type of tumor can subsequently be determined. Both carcinoids and gastrinomas may be detected incidentally during endoscopy after biopsy of a submucosal nodule and must be distinguished by subsequent studies.

Hypergastrinemia due to gastrinoma must be distinguished from other causes of hypergastrinemia. Atrophic gastritis with decreased acid secretion is detected by gastric secretory analysis. Other conditions associated with hypergastrinemia (eg, gastric outlet obstruction, vagotomy, chronic renal failure) are associated with a negative secretin stimulation test.

Treatment

A. METASTATIC DISEASE

The most important predictor of survival is the presence of hepatic metastases. In patients with multiple hepatic metastases, initial therapy should be directed at controlling hypersecretion. Proton pump inhibitors (omeprazole, rabeprazole, pantoprazole, or lansoprazole) are given at a dose of 40–120 mg/d, titrated to achieve a basal acid output of < 10 meq/h. At this level, there is complete symptomatic relief and ulcer healing. In patients with isolated hepatic metastases, surgical resection may decrease the need for antisecretory medications and may prolong survival. Owing to the slow growth of these tumors, 30% of patients with hepatic metastases have a survival of 10 years.

B. LOCALIZED DISEASE

Cure can be achieved only if the gastrinoma can be resected before hepatic metastatic spread has occurred. Lymph node metastases do not adversely affect prognosis. Laparotomy should be considered in all patients in whom preoperative studies fail to demonstrate hepatic or other distant metastases. A combination of preoperative studies and intraoperative palpation and sonography allows successful localization and resection in the majority of cases. The 15-year survival of patients who do not have liver metastases at initial presentation is over 80%.

Proye C et al: Noninvasive imaging of insulinomas and gastrinomas with endoscopic ultrasonography and somatostatin receptor scintigraphy. Surgery 1998;124:1143. [PMID: 9854595]

BENIGN TUMORS OF THE STOMACH

Gastric epithelial polyps are usually detected incidentally at endoscopy. The majority are hyperplastic polyps, which are small, single or multiple, have no malignant potential, and do not require removal or endoscopic surveillance. Adenomatous polyps account for 10–20% of gastric polyps. They are usually solitary lesions. In rare instances they ulcerate, causing chronic blood loss. Because of their premalignant potential, endoscopic removal is indicated. Annual endoscopic surveillance is recommended to screen for further polyp development. Submucosal gastric polypoid lesions include benign gastric stromal tumors (commonly known as leiomyomas) and pancreatic rests.

MALIGNANT TUMORS OF THE STOMACH

1. Gastric Adenocarcinoma

 ESSENTIALS OF DIAGNOSIS

- *Dyspeptic symptoms with weight loss in patients over age 40.*
- *Iron deficiency anemia; occult blood in stools.*
- *Abnormality detected on upper gastrointestinal series or endoscopy.*

General Considerations

Although gastric adenocarcinoma is the most common cancer (other than skin cancer) worldwide, its incidence in the United States has declined by two-thirds over the last 30 years to 20,000 cases annually. Gastric cancer is uncommon under age 40; the mean age at diagnosis is 63 years. Men are affected twice as often as women. The incidence is higher in Latinos, African-Americans, and Asian-Americans. Certain regions such as Chile, Colombia, Central America, and Japan have rates as high as 80 per 100,000 population. Although most gastric cancers arise in the antrum, the incidence of proximal tumors of the cardia and fundus is increasing dramatically.

Chronic *H pylori* gastritis is a strong risk factor for gastric carcinoma of the distal (but not proximal) stomach, increasing the relative risk four- to sixfold. It is estimated that 35–90% of cases of distal gastric carcinoma may be attributable to *H pylori*. Less than 1% of chronically infected individuals will develop carcinoma. Other risk factors for gastric cancer include chronic atrophic gastritis with intestinal metaplasia (often secondary to chronic *H pylori* infection), pernicious anemia, and a history of partial gastric resection more than 15 years previously.

Gastric cancer may occur in a variety of morphologic types: (1) polypoid or fungating intraluminal masses; (2) ulcerating masses; (3) diffusely spreading (linitis plastica), in which the tumor spreads through the submucosa, resulting in a rigid, atonic stomach with thickened folds (prognosis dismal); and (4) superficially spreading or "early" gastric cancer—confined to the mucosa or submucosa (with or without lymph node metastases) and associated with an excellent prognosis.

Clinical Findings

A. SYMPTOMS AND SIGNS

Gastric carcinoma is generally asymptomatic until the disease is quite advanced. Symptoms are nonspecific and are determined in part by the location of the tumor. Dyspepsia, vague epigastric pain, anorexia, early satiety, and weight loss are the presenting symptoms in most patients. Patients may derive initial symptomatic relief from over-the-counter remedies, further delaying diagnosis. Ulcerating lesions can lead to acute gastrointestinal bleeding with hematemesis or melena. Pyloric obstruction results in postprandial vomiting. Lower esophageal obstruction causes progressive dysphagia. Physical examination is rarely helpful. A gastric mass is palpated in less than one-fifth of patients. Signs of metastatic spread include a left supraclavicular lymph node (Virchow's node), an umbilical nodule (Sister Mary Joseph nodule), a rigid rectal shelf (Blumer's shelf), and ovarian metastases (Krukenberg tumor). Guaiac-positive stools may be detectable.

B. LABORATORY FINDINGS

Iron deficiency anemia due to chronic blood loss or anemia of chronic disease is common. Liver function test abnormalities may be present if there is metastatic liver spread. Other tumor markers are of no value.

C. ENDOSCOPY

Upper endoscopy should be obtained in all patients over age 45 with new onset of epigastric symptoms (dyspepsia) and in anyone with dyspepsia that is persistent or fails to respond to a short trial of antisecretory therapy. Endoscopy with cytologic brushings and biopsies of suspicious lesions is highly sensitive for detecting gastric carcinoma. It can be difficult to obtain adequate biopsy specimens in linitis plastica lesions. Because of the high incidence of gastric carcinoma in Japan, screening upper endoscopy is performed to detect early gastric carcinoma. Approximately 40% of tumors detected by screening are early, with a 5-year survival rate of almost 90%. Screening programs are not recommended in the USA.

D. IMAGING

A barium upper gastrointestinal series is an acceptable alternative when endoscopy is not readily available but may not detect small or superficial lesions and cannot reliably distinguish benign from malignant ulcerations. Any abnormalities detected with this procedure require endoscopic confirmation.

Once a gastric cancer is diagnosed, preoperative evaluation with abdominal CT and endoscopic ultrasonography is indicated to delineate the local extent of the primary tumor as well as nodal or distant metastases. Abdominal CT is valuable in identifying distant metastases and direct invasion of adjacent structures. Endoscopic ultrasound imaging is superior to CT in determining the depth of tumor penetration and nodal metastases.

E. STAGING

Staging is defined according to the TNM system, in which T1 tumors invade to the submucosa, T2 invade the muscularis propria, T3 penetrate the serosa, and T4 invade adjacent structures. Nodes are graded as N0 if there is no involvement, N1 if there are metastases to perigastric nodes, and N2 if regional lymph nodes are involved. M1 signifies the presence of metastatic disease. The stages are defined as shown in the accompanying box.

Differential Diagnosis

Ulcerating gastric adenocarcinomas are distinguished from benign gastric ulcers by biopsies. Approximately 3% of gastric ulcers initially believed to be benign later prove to be malignant. To exclude malignancy, all gastric ulcers identified at endoscopy should be biopsied. Ulcers that are suspicious for malignancy to the endoscopist or that have atypia or dysplasia on histologic examination warrant repeat endoscopy in 2–3 months to verify healing and exclude malignancy. Nonhealing

---

STAGING CRITERIA FOR GASTRIC ADENOCARCINOMA

Stage I: T1N0, T1N1, T2N0, all M0
Stage II: T1N2, T2N1, T3N0, all M0
Stage III: T2N2, T3N1, T4N0, all M0
Stage IV: T4N2M0, any M1

ulcers should be considered for resection. Infiltrative carcinoma with thickened gastric folds must be distinguished from lymphoma and other hypertrophic gastropathies such as Ménétrier's disease.

Treatment

A. CURATIVE SURGICAL RESECTION

Surgical resection is the only therapy with curative potential. After preoperative staging, about two-thirds of patients will be found to have localized disease (ie, stages I–III) and should undergo surgical exploration. At surgery, approximately one-fourth of these patients will be found to have locally unresectable tumors or peritoneal, hepatic, or distant lymph node metastases for which "curative" surgical resection is not warranted (see below). The remaining patients with confirmed localized disease should undergo radical surgical resection with curative intent. For adenocarcinoma localized to the distal two-thirds of the stomach, a subtotal distal gastrectomy should be performed. For proximal gastric cancer or diffusely infiltrating disease, total gastrectomy is necessary. Although lymph node dissection should be performed for curative resections, there has been ongoing debate about whether an extended (perigastric and regional) lymph node dissection or a limited (perigastric) dissection is needed. A recent study has demonstrated greater short-term morbidity and no long-term survival advantage for extended lymph node dissection. Adjuvant therapy following curative resection has not conferred a survival benefit for postoperative chemotherapy.

B. PALLIATIVE MODALITIES

Many patients will be found either preoperatively or at the time of surgical exploration to have advanced disease that is not amenable to "curative" surgery due to peritoneal or distant metastases or local invasion of other organs. In many of these cases, palliative resection of the tumor nonetheless may be indicated. Such resection removes the risk of bleeding and obstruction, leads to improved quality of life, and improves survival. For patients with unresectable disease, gastrojejunostomy may be indicated to prevent obstruction. Bleeding or obstruction from unresected tumors may be treated with endoscopic laser or stent therapy, radiation therapy, or angiographic embolization. Although chemotherapy has not been shown to prolong life, single-agent or combination therapies with fluorouracil, doxorubicin, and cisplatin or mitomycin may provide palliation in up to 30%.

Prognosis

The long-term survival of gastric carcinoma is less than 15%. However, 5-year survival in patients who undergo successful curative resection is over 45%. Survival is related to tumor stage, location, and histologic features. Stage I and stage II tumors resected for cure have a greater than 50% long-term survival. Patients

with stage III tumors have a poor prognosis (< 20% long-term survival) and should be considered for enrollment in clinical trials. Tumors of the diffuse and signet ring type have a worse prognosis than the intestinal type. Tumors of the proximal stomach (fundus and cardia) carry a far worse prognosis than distal lesions. Even with apparently localized disease, proximal tumors have a 5-year survival of less than 15%. For those whose disease progresses despite therapy, meticulous efforts at palliative care are essential (see Chapter 5).

Bonenkamp JJ et al: Extended lymph-node dissection for gastric cancer. N Engl J Med 1999;340:908. [PMID: 10089184]

De Vivo R et al: The role of chemotherapy in the management of gastric cancer. J Clin Gastroenterol 2000;30:364. [PMID: 10875463]

2. Lymphoma

Lymphoma is the second most common gastric malignancy, accounting for 3–6% of gastric cancers. More than 95% of these are non-Hodgkin's B cell lymphomas. Gastric lymphomas may be primary (arising from the gastric mucosa) or may represent a site of secondary involvement in patients with nodal lymphomas. About 60% of primary gastric lymphomas are believed to arise from mucosa-associated lymphoid tissue (MALT). Distinguishing advanced primary gastric lymphoma with adjacent nodal spread from advanced nodal lymphoma with secondary gastric spread can be problematic. Because the prognosis and treatment of primary and secondary gastric lymphomas are entirely different, the distinction is important. B cells of nodal origin may be distinguished from those derived from MALT (CD19- and CD20-positive).

Infection with *H pylori* may be an important risk factor for the development of primary gastric lymphoma. Chronic infection with *H pylori* causes an intense lymphocytic inflammatory response that may lead to the development of lymphoid follicles. Over 85% of low-grade primary gastric lymphomas and 40% of high-grade lymphomas are associated with *H pylori* infection. The risk of developing lymphoma is increased sevenfold in patients with chronic *H pylori* infection. It is hypothesized that chronic antigenic stimulation may result in a monoclonal lymphoproliferation that may culminate in a low-grade MALT lymphoma. At present, the relationship between high-grade primary lymphomas, MALT, and *H pylori* infection is unclear.

The clinical presentation and endoscopic appearance of gastric lymphoma are similar to those of adenocarcinoma. The majority of patients present with abdominal pain, weight loss, or bleeding. Night sweats are absent in primary lymphoma. At endoscopy, lymphoma may appear as an ulcer, mass, or diffusely infiltrating lesion. The diagnosis is established with endoscopic biopsy. All patients should undergo staging with abdominal and chest CT. Endoscopic ultrasonography is the most sensitive test for determining the presence of perigastric lymphadenopathy.

Nodal lymphomas with secondary gastrointestinal involvement usually present at an advanced stage with widely disseminated disease and are seldom curable. Their treatment is addressed in Chapter 13. By contrast, primary low-grade gastric lymphomas usually are localized to the stomach wall (stage IE) or adjacent lymph nodes (stage IIE) and have an excellent prognosis. Patients with primary low-grade gastric MALT-lymphoma should be tested for *H pylori* infection and treated if positive. Complete lymphoma regression after successful *H pylori* eradication occurs in 75% of cases of stage IE low-grade lymphoma. Remission may take as long as a year. Patients with stage IE or IIE low-grade lymphomas who either are not infected with *H pylori* or fail to respond to eradication therapy can be treated successfully with surgical resection, local radiation therapy, or combination therapy. Stage IEE or 2EE high-grade lymphomas may be treated with resection and CHOP chemotherapy. Stage III and stage IV primary lymphomas are treated with combination chemotherapy. Because of a low risk of perforation with either radiation therapy or chemotherapy, surgical resection is no longer recommended. The long-term survival of primary gastric lymphoma for stage I is over 85% and for stage II is 35–65%.

Fischbach W et al: Primary gastric B-cell lymphoma: results of a prospective multicenter study. The German-Austrian Gastrointestinal Lymphoma Study Group. Gastroenterology 2000;119:1191. [PMID: 11054376]

Steinbach G et al: Antibiotic treatment of gastric lymphoma of mucosa-associated lymphoid tissue. Ann Intern Med 1999;131:88. [PMID: 10419446] (Fifty percent achieved complete remission after antibiotic therapy when *H pylori*-positive; the incidence of remission was 70% in patients with T1N0 disease.)

3. Carcinoid Tumors

Gastric carcinoids are rare tumors that make up less than 1% of gastric neoplasms. They may occur sporadically or secondary to chronic hypergastrinemia that results in hyperplasia and transformation of enterochromaffin cells in the gastric fundus. Sporadic carcinoids account for 20% of gastric carcinoids. Most are solitary, over 2 cm in size, and have a strong propensity for metastatic spread. Most sporadic carcinoids already have carcinoid syndrome and hepatic or pulmonary metastatic involvement at initial presentation. Localized sporadic carcinoids should be treated with radical gastrectomy.

The majority of carcinoids caused by hypergastrinemia occur in association with either pernicious anemia (75%) or Zollinger-Ellison syndrome (5%). Carcinoids associated with Zollinger-Ellison syndrome occur almost exclusively in patients with MEN 1, in which loss of 11q13 has been reported. Carcinoids caused by hypergastrinemia tend to be multi-

centric, less than 1 cm in size, and have a low potential for metastatic spread or development of carcinoid syndrome. Small lesions may be successfully treated with endoscopic resection followed by periodic endoscopic surveillance. Antrectomy reduces serum gastrin levels and may lead to regression of small tumors. Patients with large or multiple carcinoids should undergo surgical tumor resection.

Kulke M et al: Carcinoid tumors. N Engl J Med 1999;340:858. [PMID: 10080850]

4. Stromal Tumors

Gastrointestinal stromal tumors (leiomyomas and leiomyosarcomas) occur throughout the gastrointestinal tract, but approximately two-thirds occur in the stomach. They derive from mesenchymal stem cells and have an epithelioid or spindle cell histologic pattern, resembling smooth muscle. Most have a mutation in the proto-oncogene *c-kit* tyrosine kinase and stain positively for CD117 and CD34. Tumors may grow quite large before causing symptoms, mainly acute or chronic bleeding due to central ulceration within the tumor. At endoscopy, they appear as a submucosal mass that may have central umbilication or ulceration. Endoscopic ultrasound with fine-needle aspiration is the optimal study for assessing these tumors. It is difficult to distinguish benign ("leiomyoma") from malignant ("leiomyosarcoma") stromal tumors on clinical or histologic grounds. Surgery is therefore recommended for tumors over 3–5 cm in size, those that have an irregular border or cystic spaces, and those that have increased mitotic activity (more than two mitoses per high-power field). Mitotic activity may be more accurately assessed by nuclear immunohistochemical staining with Ki-67. Surgical resection is the only effective therapy for localized malignant stromal tumors. Overall 5-year survival is 30%. Metastatic tumors are aggressive and carry a poor prognosis. The tyrosine kinase inhibitor imatinib has recently been found to induce partial remission and clinical improvement in patients with metastatic disease.

Joensuu H et al: Effect of the tyrosine kinase inhibitor STI571 in a patient with metastatic gastrointestinal stromal tumor. N Engl J Med 2001;344:1052. [PMID: 11287975]

■ DISEASES OF THE SMALL INTESTINE

MALABSORPTION

The term "malabsorption" denotes disorders in which there is a disruption of digestion and nutrient absorption. The clinical and laboratory manifestations of malabsorption are summarized in Table 14–12.

Table 14–12. Clinical and laboratory manifestations of malabsorption.[1]

Manifestation	Laboratory Findings	Malabsorbed Nutrients
Steatorrhea (bulky, light-colored stools)	Increased fecal fat; decreased serum cholesterol	Fat
Diarrhea (increased fecal water)	Increased fecal fat or positive bile salt breath test	Fatty acids or bile salts
Weight loss; malnutrition (muscle wasting); weakness, fatigue, abdominal distention	Increased fecal fat and nitrogen; decreased glucose and xylose absorption	Calories (fat, protein, carbohydrates)
Iron deficiency anemia	Hypochromic anemia; low serum iron	Iron
Megaloblastic anemia	Macrocytosis; decreased vitamin B_{12} absorption (^{67}Co-labeled B_{12}); decreased serum vitamin B_{12} and red cell folate	Vitamin B_{12} or folic acid
Paresthesia; tetany; positive Trousseau and Chvostek signs	Decreased serum calcium, magnesium, and potassium	Calcium, vitamin D, magnesium, potassium
Bone pain; pathologic fractures; skeletal deformities	Osteoporosis on x-ray; osteomalacia on biopsy	Calcium, protein
Bleeding tendency (ecchymoses, melena, hematuria)	Prolonged prothrombin time	Vitamin K
Edema	Decreased serum albumin; increased fecal loss of α_1-antitrypsin (antiprotease)	Protein (or protein-losing enteropathy)
Nocturia; abdominal distention	Increased small bowel fluid on x-ray	Water
Milk intolerance (cramps, bloating, diarrhea)	Flat lactose tolerance test; decreased mucosal lactase levels	Lactose

[1]Modified from Bayless TM: Malabsorption in the elderly. Hosp Pract (Aug) 1979;14:67.

Normal Digestion

Normal digestion and absorption may be divided into three phases:

A. INTRALUMINAL PHASE

Dietary fats, proteins, and carbohydrates are hydrolyzed and solubilized by pancreatic and biliary secretions. Fats are broken down by pancreatic lipase to monoglycerides and fatty acids that form micelles with bile salts. Micelles are important for the solubilization and absorption of fat-soluble vitamins (A, D, E, K). Proteins are hydrolyzed by pancreatic proteases to di- and tripeptides and amino acids. Impaired intraluminal digestion may be caused by insufficient intraluminal concentrations of pancreatic enzymes or bile salts. These conditions will not be covered in detail here (see Chapter 15).

Pancreatic insufficiency may be caused by chronic pancreatitis, cystic fibrosis, or pancreatic cancer. Pancreatic enzymes may also be inactivated within the intestinal lumen by acid hypersecretion (Zollinger-Ellison syndrome). Significant pancreatic enzyme insufficiency generally results in significant steatorrhea (due to malabsorption of triglycerides)—often more than 20–40 g/24 h—resulting in weight loss, gaseous distention and flatulence, and large, greasy, foul-smelling stools. The digestion of proteins and carbohydrates is affected to a far lesser degree and is generally not clinically significant. Because micellar function and intestinal absorption are normal, signs of other nutrient or vitamin deficiencies are rare.

Decreased bile salt concentrations may be due to biliary obstruction or cholestatic liver diseases. Because bile salts are resorbed in the terminal ileum, resection or disease of this area (eg, Crohn's disease) can lead to insufficient intraluminal bile salts. Finally, destruction or loss of bile salts may be caused by bacterial overgrowth, massive acid hypersecretion, or medications that bind bile salts (eg, cholestyramine). (Bacterial overgrowth is discussed below.) Insufficient concentrations of intraluminal bile salts lead to mild steatorrhea (due to malabsorption of fatty acids and monoglycerides), though generally less than 20 g/d. Weight loss is minimal. Impaired absorption of fat-soluble vitamins (A, D, E, K) is common, resulting in bleeding tendencies, osteoporosis, and hypocalcemia (Table 14–12). Other nutrient absorption is intact. Intestinal loss of bile salts into the colon may cause a watery secretory diarrhea.

B. MUCOSAL PHASE

The mucosal phase requires a sufficient surface area of intact small intestinal epithelium. Brush border enzymes are important in the hydrolysis of disaccharides and di- and tripeptides. Malabsorption of specific nutrients may occur as a result of deficiency in an isolated brush border enzyme. With the exception of lactase deficiency, these are rare congenital disorders that are evident in childhood. Malabsorption due to primary mucosal diseases, extensive intestinal resections (short bowel syndrome), or lymphoma is discussed below. These disorders result in malabsorption of all nutrients: fats, proteins, and amino acids. Depending upon the severity of malabsorption, patients may manifest a number of symptoms and signs, as outlined in Table 14–12.

C. ABSORPTIVE PHASE

Obstruction of the lymphatic system results in impaired absorption of chylomicrons and lipoproteins. This may lead to steatorrhea and significant enteric protein losses or "protein-losing enteropathy," discussed below.

1. Celiac Disease

ESSENTIALS OF DIAGNOSIS

- Typical symptoms: weight loss, chronic diarrhea, abdominal distention, growth retardation.
- Atypical symptoms: dermatitis herpetiformis, iron deficiency anemia, osteoporosis.
- Abnormal serologic test results.
- Abnormal small bowel biopsy.
- Clinical improvement on gluten-free diet.

General Considerations

Also known as gluten enteropathy or celiac sprue, celiac disease is characterized by diffuse damage to the proximal small intestinal mucosa that results in malabsorption of most nutrients. Although typical symptoms commonly manifest between 6 months and 24 months of age after the introduction of weaning foods, up to half of cases present with atypical symptoms in childhood or adulthood. Population screening with serologic tests suggests that the disease is present in 1:250 whites of Northern European ancestry but is rare in Africans and Asians. A clinical diagnosis of celiac disease is made in only 1:5000 people in the United States, suggesting that most cases are undiagnosed. Celiac disease is strongly associated with selected HLA class II molecules, particularly the DQA1*0501 and DQB1*0201 alleles. While the precise mechanism of damage is unknown, it is clear that removal of gluten from the diet results in resolution of symptoms and intestinal healing in most patients.

Gluten is a storage protein that is present in certain grains such as wheat, rye, and barley but not oats, rice, or corn. It is hypothesized that in a genetically susceptible host, gluten stimulates an inappropriate T cell-mediated immune response in the intestinal submucosa that results in destruction of mucosal enterocytes. One target of this autoimmune response is tissue transglutaminase.

Clinical Findings

A. SYMPTOMS AND SIGNS

The symptoms and signs of malabsorption depend upon the length of small intestine involved and the age at which the patient presents. Infants (< 2 years) are more likely to present with typical symptoms of malabsorption, including diarrhea, weight loss, abdominal distention, weakness, muscle wasting, or growth retardation. The stools are characteristically loose to soft, large, floating, oily or greasy, and foul-smelling. However, they may also be watery and frequent in number (up to 10–12 daily). Children and adults are less likely to manifest these signs of serious malabsorption. Most patients report chronic diarrhea or flatulence due to colonic bacterial digestion of malabsorbed nutrients, but the severity of weight loss is variable. Some patients have no gastrointestinal symptoms but present with fatigue, short stature, osteoporosis, dental enamel hypoplasia, and iron deficiency anemia. Physical examination may be normal in mild cases or may reveal signs of malabsorption, such as loss of muscle mass or subcutaneous fat, pallor due to anemia, easy bruising due to vitamin K deficiency, hyperkeratosis due to vitamin A deficiency, or bone pain due to osteomalacia. Abdominal examination may reveal distention with hyperactive bowel sounds.

Dermatitis herpetiformis is regarded as a cutaneous variant of celiac disease. It is a characteristic skin rash consisting of pruritic papulovesicles over the extensor surfaces of the extremities and over the trunk, scalp, and neck. Dermatitis herpetiformis occurs in less than 10% of patients with celiac disease; however, almost all patients who present with dermatitis herpetiformis have evidence of celiac disease on intestinal mucosal biopsy, though it may not be clinically evident.

B. LABORATORY FINDINGS

1. Routine laboratory tests—Laboratory abnormalities depend upon the extent of intestinal involvement. A complete blood count, serum iron or ferritin, red cell folate, vitamin B_{12} level, serum calcium, alkaline phosphatase, albumin, beta-carotene, and prothrombin time should be obtained in all patients with suspected malabsorption. Limited proximal involvement may result only in microcytic anemia due to iron deficiency. More than 10% of adults with iron deficiency not due to gastrointestinal blood loss may have undiagnosed celiac disease. More extensive involvement results in a megaloblastic anemia due to folate or vitamin B_{12} deficiency. Low serum calcium or elevated alkaline phosphatase may reflect impaired calcium or vitamin D absorption with osteomalacia or osteoporosis. Dual-energy x-ray densitometry scanning is recommended for all patients with sprue to screen for osteoporosis. Elevations of prothrombin time or a decreased serum beta-carotene reflect impaired fat-soluble vitamin absorption. Severe diarrhea may result in a non-anion gap acidosis and hypokalemia.

2. Specific tests for malabsorption—Steatorrhea is usually present but may be absent in mild disease. It may be detected by a qualitative (Sudan stain) or quantitative stool assessment for fecal fat. A positive Sudan stain is strong evidence of steatorrhea and usually obviates the need for quantitative analysis, but it is falsely negative in 25%. A quantitative 72-hour stool collection taken while patients are consuming a 100 g fat diet is a more sensitive means of detecting fat malabsorption. Excretion of more than 10 g/d of fat is abnormal and warrants further evaluation for malabsorption. Other tests of malabsorption such as the D-xylose test to provide evidence of mucosal malabsorption are no longer required with the availability of serologic screening for celiac disease.

3. Serologic tests—A number of serologic tests can be used to screen for celiac disease and to monitor for patient adherence to the gluten-free diet. IgG and IgA antigliadin antibodies are present in over 90% of patients with celiac sprue but are elevated also in other mucosal diseases. The IgG antibody is more sensitive, and the IgA antibody is more specific. Because up to 10% of celiac patients have IgA deficiency, both tests should be obtained. A combination of the two tests provides sensitivity and specificity of over 95%. The IgA endomysial antibody test has over 90% sensitivity and specificity for the diagnosis of celiac disease; however, its use is limited by cost and by variability of results from different laboratories. An assay for tissue transglutaminase antibody with a reported sensitivity and specificity of over 95%, if confirmed, may become the preferred serologic test for screening for celiac disease. Serologic tests become negative after 6–12 months of dietary gluten withdrawal and may be used to monitor dietary compliance, especially in patients whose symptoms fail to resolve after institution of a gluten-free diet.

C. MUCOSAL BIOPSY

Endoscopic mucosal biopsy of the distal duodenum or proximal jejunum is the standard method for confirmation of the diagnosis in patients with a positive serologic test for celiac disease. Rarely, mucosal biopsy may be pursued in patients with negative serologies when symptoms are suggestive of celiac disease. Duodenal mucosal biopsy is also commonly performed in patients with iron deficiency anemia who are undergoing upper and lower endoscopy to exclude a source of gastrointestinal blood loss. At endoscopy, atrophy or scalloping of the duodenal folds may be observed. Histology reveals loss or blunting of intestinal villi, hyper-

trophy of the intestinal crypts, and extensive infiltration of the lamina propria with lymphocytes and plasma cells. An adequate normal biopsy excludes the diagnosis. Reversion of these abnormalities on repeat biopsy after a patient is placed on a gluten-free diet establishes the diagnosis. However, if a patient with a compatible biopsy demonstrates prompt clinical improvement on a gluten-free diet and a decrease in antigliadin antibodies, a repeat biopsy is unnecessary.

Differential Diagnosis

Because of its protean manifestations, celiac disease is underdiagnosed in the adult population. Many patients with chronic diarrhea or flatulence are erroneously diagnosed as having irritable bowel syndrome. Symptoms are present for more than 10 years in most patients before the correct diagnosis is established. Celiac sprue must be distinguished from other causes of malabsorption, as outlined above. Severe panmalabsorption of multiple nutrients is almost always caused by mucosal disease. In a patient with steatorrhea, a normal D-xylose test points to pancreatic insufficiency, reduced bile salts, or lymphatic obstruction. If the D-xylose test, however, is also abnormal, it strongly implicates mucosal disorders or bacterial overgrowth. The histologic appearance of celiac sprue may resemble other mucosal diseases such as tropical sprue, bacterial overgrowth, cow's milk intolerance, viral gastroenteritis, eosinophilic gastroenteritis, and mucosal damage caused by acid hypersecretion associated with gastrinoma. Documentation of clinical response to gluten withdrawal therefore is essential to the diagnosis.

Treatment

Removal of all gluten from the diet is essential to therapy—all wheat, rye, and barley must be eliminated. Although oats previously were felt to be toxic to these patients, moderate amounts are without adverse effects. Rice, soybean, potato, and corn flours are safe. Because of the pervasive use of gluten products in manufactured foods and additives, in medications, and by restaurants, it is imperative that patients and their families confer with a knowledgeable dietitian in order to comply satisfactorily with this lifelong diet. Several excellent dietary guides are available. Most patients with celiac disease also have lactose intolerance either temporarily or permanently and should avoid dairy products until the intestinal symptoms have improved on the gluten-free diet. Nutrient supplements (folate, iron, vitamin B_{12}, calcium, vitamin D) should be provided in the initial stages of therapy but usually are not required long-term with a gluten-free diet. Patients with confirmed osteoporosis may require chronic calcium, vitamin D, and bisphosphonate therapy.

Improvement in symptoms should be evident within a few weeks on the gluten-free diet. The most common reason for treatment failure is incomplete removal of gluten.

Prognosis & Complications

If appropriately diagnosed and treated, patients with celiac disease have an excellent prognosis. Celiac disease may be associated with other autoimmune disorders, including Addison's disease, Graves' disease, type 1 diabetes mellitus, myasthenia gravis, scleroderma, Sjögren's syndrome, atrophic gastritis, and pancreatic insufficiency. In some patients, celiac disease may evolve and become refractory to the gluten-free diet. The most common cause is intentional or unintentional dietary noncompliance, which may be suggested by positive serologic tests. Celiac disease that is truly refractory to gluten withdrawal generally carries a poor prognosis. It may be caused by the development of ulcerative jejunitis or enteropathy or by associated T cell lymphoma, which occurs in up to 10% of patients. These conditions should be considered in patients previously responsive to the gluten-free diet who develop new weight loss, abdominal pain, and malabsorption. Many other patients with refractory symptoms have a "cryptic" intestinal lymphoma, ie, a monoclonal expansion of the intraepithelial T lymphocyte that may or may not progress. Patients with refractory sprue who do not have intestinal T cell lymphoma or ulcerative jejunitis may respond to corticosteroids or immunosuppression with azathioprine or cyclosporine.

American Gastroenterological Association Medical Position Statement: Celiac Sprue. Gastroenterology 2001;120:1522. [PMID: 11313323]

Cellier C et al: Refractory sprue, celiac disease, and enteropathy-associated T-cell lymphoma. Lancet 2000;356:203. [PMID: 10963198]

Fasano A et al: Current approaches to diagnosis and treatment of celiac disease. Gastroenterology 2001;120:636. [PMID: 11179241]

Green P et al: Characteristics of adult celiac disease in the USA: results of a national survey. Am J Gastroenterol 2001; 96:126. [PMID: 11197241]

Ryan B et al: Refractory celiac disease. Gastroenterology 2000; 119:243. [PMID: 10889175]

Celiac Disease Foundation, 13251 Ventura Blvd, Suite #1, Studio City, CA 91604-1838. http://www.celiac.org. (Excellent source for patient information, newsletters, dietary guidelines.)

2. Whipple's Disease

ESSENTIALS OF DIAGNOSIS

- *Multisystemic disease.*
- *Fever, lymphadenopathy, arthralgias.*
- *Malabsorption.*
- *Duodenal biopsy with PAS-positive macrophages with characteristic bacillus.*

General Considerations

Whipple's disease is a rare multisystemic illness caused by infection with the bacillus *Tropheryma whippelii*. It may occur at any age but most commonly affects white men in the fourth to sixth decades. The source of infection is unknown, but no cases of human-to-human spread have been documented.

Clinical Findings

A. Symptoms and Signs

The clinical manifestations are protean. Arthralgias or a migratory, nondeforming arthritis occur in 80% and are typically the first symptom experienced. Gastrointestinal symptoms occur in approximately 75% of cases. They include abdominal pain, diarrhea, and some degree of malabsorption with distention, flatulence, and steatorrhea. Weight loss, present in almost all patients, is the most common presenting symptom. Loss of protein due to intestinal or lymphatic involvement may result in protein-losing enteropathy with hypoalbuminemia and edema. In the absence of gastrointestinal symptoms, the diagnosis often is delayed for several years. Intermittent low-grade fever occurs in over 50% of cases. Chronic cough is common. There may be generalized lymphadenopathy that resembles sarcoidosis. Myocardial or valvular involvement may lead to congestive failure or valvular regurgitation. Ocular findings include uveitis, vitreitis, keratitis, retinitis, and retinal hemorrhages. Central nervous system involvement in approximately 10% of cases is manifested by a variety of findings such as dementia, lethargy, coma, seizures, myoclonus, or hypothalamic signs. Cranial nerve findings include ophthalmoplegia or nystagmus.

Physical examination may reveal hypotension (a late finding), low-grade fever, and evidence of malabsorption (see Table 14-12). Lymphadenopathy is present in 50%. Heart murmurs due to valvular involvement may be evident. Peripheral joints may be enlarged or warm, and peripheral edema may be present. Neurologic findings are cited above. Hyperpigmentation on sun-exposed areas is evident in up to 40%.

B. Laboratory Findings

If significant malabsorption is present, patients may have laboratory abnormalities as outlined in Table 14-12. There may be steatorrhea.

C. Histologic Evaluation

The diagnosis of Whipple's disease is established by histologic evaluation of the involved tissues. In most cases, the diagnosis is established by endoscopic biopsy of the duodenum, which demonstrates infiltration of the lamina propria with PAS-positive macrophages that contain gram-positive bacilli (which are not acid-fast) and dilation of the lacteals. The Whipple bacillus has a characteristic electron microscopic appearance.

In some patients who present with nongastrointestinal symptoms, the duodenal biopsy may be normal, and biopsy of other involved organs or lymph nodes may be necessary. Because the PAS stain is less sensitive and specific for extraintestinal Whipple's disease, PCR is used to confirm the diagnosis by demonstrating the presence of 16S ribosomal RNA of *T whippelii* in blood, cerebrospinal fluid, vitreous fluid, synovial fluid, or cardiac valves. The sensitivity of PCR is 97% and the specificity 100%.

Differential Diagnosis

Whipple's disease should be considered in patients who present with signs of malabsorption, fever of unknown origin, lymphadenopathy, seronegative arthritis, culture-negative endocarditis, or multisystemic disease. Small bowel biopsy readily distinguishes Whipple's disease from other mucosal malabsorptive disorders, such as celiac sprue. Patients with AIDS and infection of the small intestine with *Mycobacterium avium* complex may have a similar clinical and histologic picture; although both conditions are characterized by PAS-positive macrophages, they may be distinguished by the acid-fast stain, which is positive for MAC and negative for the Whipple bacillus. Other conditions that may be confused with Whipple's disease include sarcoidosis, Reiter's syndrome, familial Mediterranean fever, systemic vasculitides, Behçet's disease, intestinal lymphoma, and subacute infective endocarditis.

Treatment

Antibiotic therapy results in a dramatic clinical improvement within several weeks, even in some patients with neurologic involvement. The optimal regimen is unknown. Complete clinical response usually is evident within 1–3 months; however, relapse may occur in up to one-third of patients after discontinuation of treatment. Therefore, prolonged treatment for at least 1 year is required. Drugs that cross the blood-brain barrier are preferred. Trimethoprim-sulfamethoxazole (one double-strength tablet twice daily for 1 year) is recommended as first-line therapy. In patients allergic to sulfonamides, ceftriaxone or chloramphenicol may be reasonable; there is an anecdotal report of a patient with central nervous system disease refractory to antibiotics treated successfully with interferon gamma. After treatment, repeat biopsies may be obtained for PCR. Negative results predict a low likelihood of clinical relapse.

Prognosis

If untreated, the disease is fatal. Because some neurologic signs may be permanent, the goal of treatment is to prevent this progression. Patients must be followed closely after treatment for signs of symptom recurrence.

Raoult D et al: Cultivation of the bacillus of Whipple's disease. N Engl J Med 2000;342:620. [PMID: 10699161]

Ratnaike RN: Whipple's disease. Postgrad Med J 2000;76:760. [PMID: 11085766]

3. Bacterial Overgrowth

The small intestine normally contains a small number of bacteria. Bacterial overgrowth in the small intestine of whatever cause may result in malabsorption via a number of mechanisms. Bacterial deconjugation of bile salts may lead to inadequate micelle formation, resulting in decreased fat absorption with steatorrhea. Microbial uptake of specific nutrients reduces absorption of vitamin B_{12} and carbohydrates. Bacterial proliferation also causes direct damage to intestinal epithelial cells and the brush border, further impairing absorption of proteins and carbohydrates. Passage of the malabsorbed bile acids and carbohydrates into the colon leads to an osmotic and secretory diarrhea.

Causes of bacterial overgrowth include the following: (1) gastric achlorhydria (especially if other predisposing conditions present); (2) anatomic abnormalities of the small intestine with stagnation (afferent limb of Billroth II gastrojejunostomy, small intestine diverticula, obstruction, blind loop, radiation enteritis); (3) small intestine motility disorders (scleroderma, diabetic enteropathy, chronic intestinal pseudo-obstruction); (4) gastrocolic or coloenteric fistula (Crohn's disease, malignancy, surgical resection); and (5) miscellaneous disorders (AIDS, chronic pancreatitis). Bacterial overgrowth is an important cause of malabsorption in the elderly, perhaps because of decreased gastric acidity or impaired intestinal motility.

Clinical Findings

Many patients with bacterial overgrowth are asymptomatic. Patients with severe overgrowth have symptoms and signs of malabsorption, including distention, weight loss, and steatorrhea (Table 14–12). Watery diarrhea is common. Megaloblastic anemia or neurologic signs due to vitamin B_{12} deficiency are common findings and may be manifest at presentation. In patients with vitamin B_{12} deficiency, the Schilling test is diagnostic of bacterial overgrowth if it is abnormal in phase I and II (without and with intrinsic factor) but normalizes after a course of antibiotics. Qualitative or quantitative fecal fat assessment typically is abnormal. D-Xylose absorption is also abnormal due to bacterial uptake of the carbohydrate.

Bacterial overgrowth should be considered in any patient with diarrhea, steatorrhea, weight loss, or macrocytic anemia, especially if the patient has a predisposing cause (such as prior gastrointestinal surgery). A stool collection should be obtained to corroborate the presence of steatorrhea. Small bowel barium radiography may be helpful to document conditions predisposing to intestinal stasis. Where indicated, a small intestinal biopsy may be necessary to exclude other mucosal malabsorptive conditions. A specific diagnosis can be established firmly only by an aspirate and culture of proximal jejunal secretion that demonstrates over 10^5 organisms/mL. However, this is an invasive and laborious test, not done in some clinical settings. A number of noninvasive breath tests have been developed but lack sufficient sensitivity and specificity to be of great utility. The ^{13}C- or ^{14}C-xylose breath test is the most reliable. In this test, bacterial uptake and degradation of the isotope lead to the release of $^{13}CO_2$ or $^{14}CO_2$, which can be measured in exhaled breath.

Owing to the lack of an optimal test for bacterial overgrowth, many clinicians employ an empirical antibiotic trial as a diagnostic and therapeutic maneuver in patients with predisposing conditions for bacterial overgrowth who develop unexplained diarrhea or steatorrhea.

Treatment

Where possible, the anatomic defect that has potentiated bacterial overgrowth should be corrected. Otherwise, treatment as follows for 1–2 weeks with broad-spectrum antibiotics effective against enteric aerobes and anaerobes usually leads to dramatic improvement: twice daily ciprofloxacin 500 mg, norfloxacin 400 mg, or amoxicillin clavulanate 875 mg, or a combination of metronidazole 250 mg three times daily plus either trimethoprim-sulfamethoxazole (one double-strength tablet) twice daily or cephalexin 250 mg four times daily.

In patients in whom symptoms recur off antibiotics, cyclic therapy (eg, 1 week out of 4) may be sufficient. Continuous antibiotics should be avoided, if possible, to avoid development of bacterial antibiotic resistance.

In patients with severe intestinal dysmotility, treatment with small doses of octreotide may prove to be of benefit.

Bailey L et al: Bacterial overgrowth syndrome. Clin Perspect Gastroenterol 2000; Jul/Aug: 225.

Meyers JS et al: Small intestinal bacterial overgrowth syndrome. Current Treat Options Gastroenterol 2001;4:7. [PMID: 11177677]

4. Short Bowel Syndrome

Short bowel syndrome is the malabsorptive condition that arises secondary to removal of significant segments of the small intestine. The most common causes in adults are Crohn's disease, mesenteric infarction, radiation enteritis, and trauma. The type and degree of malabsorption depend upon the length and site of the resection and the degree of adaptation of the remaining bowel.

Terminal Ileal Resection

Resection of the terminal ileum results in malabsorption of bile salts and vitamin B_{12}, which are normally absorbed in this region. Patients with low serum vitamin B_{12} levels, an abnormal Schilling test, or resection of over 50 cm of ileum require monthly intramuscular vitamin B_{12} injections. In patients with less than 100 cm of ileal resection, bile salt malabsorption stimulates fluid secretion from the colon, resulting in watery diarrhea. This may be treated with bile salt binding resins (cholestyramine, 2–4 g three times daily with meals). Resection of over 100 cm of ileum leads to a reduction in the bile salt pool that results in steatorrhea and malabsorption of fat-soluble vitamins. Treatment is with a low fat diet and vitamins supplemented with medium-chain triglycerides, which do not require micellar solubilization. Unabsorbed fatty acids bind with calcium, reducing its absorption and enhancing the absorption of oxalate. Oxalate kidney stones may develop. Calcium supplements should be administered to bind oxalate and increase serum calcium. Cholesterol gallstones due to decreased bile salts are common also. In patients with resection of the ileocolonic valve, bacterial overgrowth may occur in the small intestine, further complicating malabsorption (as outlined above).

Extensive Small Bowel Resection

Resection of 40–50% of the total length of small intestine usually is well tolerated. A more massive resection may result in "short-bowel syndrome," characterized by weight loss and diarrhea due to nutrient, water, and electrolyte malabsorption. After resection, the remaining small intestine has a remarkable ability to adapt, gradually increasing its absorptive capacity up to fourfold over 1 year. The colon also plays an important role in absorption of fluids, electrolytes, and digestion of complex carbohydrates (through bacterial fermentation to short-chain fatty acids) after small bowel resection. If the colon is preserved, 100 cm of proximal jejunum may be sufficient to maintain adequate oral nutrition with a low-fat, high complex-carbohydrate diet, though fluid and electrolyte losses may still be significant. In patients in whom the colon has been removed, at least 200 cm of proximal jejunum is typically required to maintain oral nutrition. Duodenal resection may result in folate, iron, or calcium malabsorption. Levels of other minerals such as zinc and magnesium should be monitored. Parenteral vitamin supplementation may be necessary. Antidiarrheal agents (loperamide, 2–4 mg three times daily) slow transit and reduce diarrheal volume. Octreotide reduces intestinal transit time and fluid and electrolyte secretion. Gastric hypersecretion usually complicates intestinal resection and should be treated with H_2 receptor antagonists.

Patients with less than 100–200 cm of proximal jejunum remaining almost always require parenteral nutrition. Of patients who do, the estimated annual mortality rate is 2–5% per year. Death is most commonly due to TPN-induced liver disease, sepsis, or loss of venous access. Small intestine transplantation is now being performed with reported 5-year graft survival rates of 40%. Currently, it is performed chiefly in patients who develop serious problems due to parenteral nutrition.

Scolapio JS: Treatment of short-bowel syndrome. Curr Opin Clin Nutr Metab Care 2001;4:557. [PMID: 11706294]

5. Lactase Deficiency

Lactase is a brush border enzyme that hydrolyzes the disaccharide lactose into glucose and galactose. The concentration of lactase enzyme levels is high at birth but declines steadily in most people of non-European ancestry during childhood and adolescence and into adulthood. Thus, approximately 50 million people in the USA have partial to complete lactose intolerance. As many as 90% of Asian-Americans, 70% of African-Americans, 95% of Native Americans, 50% of Mexican-Americans, and 60% of Jewish Americans are lactose-intolerant compared with less than 25% of Caucasian adults. Lactase deficiency may also arise secondary to other gastrointestinal disorders that affect the proximal small intestinal mucosa. These include Crohn's disease, sprue, viral gastroenteritis, giardiasis, short bowel syndrome, and malnutrition. Malabsorbed lactose is fermented by intestinal bacteria, producing gas and organic acids. The nonmetabolized lactose and organic acids result in an increased stool osmotic load with an obligatory fluid loss.

Clinical Findings

A. SYMPTOMS AND SIGNS

Patients have great variability in clinical symptoms, depending both on the severity of lactase deficiency and the amount of lactose ingested. Because of the nonspecific nature of these symptoms, there is a tendency for both lactose-intolerant and lactose-tolerant individuals to mistakenly attribute a variety of abdominal symptoms to lactose intolerance. Most patients with lactose intolerance can drink one or two 8 oz glasses of milk daily without symptoms if taken with food at wide intervals, though rare patients have almost complete intolerance. With mild to moderate amounts of lactose malabsorption, patients may experience bloating, abdominal cramps, and flatulence. With higher lactose ingestions, an osmotic diarrhea will result. Isolated lactase deficiency does not result in other signs of malabsorption or weight loss. If these findings are present, other gastrointestinal disorders should be pursued. Diarrheal specimens reveal an increased osmotic gap and a pH of less than 6.0.

B. LABORATORY FINDINGS

The most widely available test for the diagnosis of lactase deficiency is the hydrogen breath test. After ingestion of 50 g of lactose, a rise in breath hydrogen of greater than 20 ppm within 90 minutes is a positive test, indicative of bacterial carbohydrate metabolism. In clinical practice, many physicians prescribe an empirical trial of a lactose-free diet for 2 weeks. Resolution of symptoms (bloating, flatulence, diarrhea) is highly suggestive of lactase deficiency (though a placebo response cannot be excluded) and may be confirmed, if necessary, with a breath hydrogen study.

Differential Diagnosis

The symptoms of late-onset lactose intolerance are nonspecific and may mimic a number of gastrointestinal disorders, such as inflammatory bowel disease, mucosal malabsorptive disorders, irritable bowel syndrome, and pancreatic insufficiency. Furthermore, lactase deficiency frequently develops secondary to other gastrointestinal disorders (as listed above). Concomitant lactase deficiency should always be considered in these gastrointestinal disorders.

Treatment

The goal of treatment in patients with isolated lactase deficiency is achieving patient comfort. Patients usually find their "threshold" of intake at which symptoms will occur. Foods that are high in lactose include milk (12 g/cup), ice cream (9 g/cup), and cottage cheese (8 g/cup). Aged cheeses have a lower lactose content (0.5 g/oz). Unpasteurized yogurt contains bacteria that produce lactase and is generally well tolerated.

Many patients will choose simply to restrict or eliminate milk products. By spreading dairy product intake throughout the day in quantities of less than 12 g of lactose (one cup of milk), most patients can take dairy products without symptoms and do not require lactase supplements. Calcium supplementation should be considered in susceptible patients to prevent osteoporosis. Most food markets provide milk that has been pretreated with lactase, rendering it 70–100% lactose-free. Lactase enzyme replacement is commercially available as a nonprescription formulation (Lactaid). Caplets of lactase may be taken with milk products, improving lactose absorption and eliminating symptoms. The number of caplets ingested depends upon the degree of lactose intolerance.

Jackson KA et al: Lactose maldigestion, calcium intake and osteoporosis in African-, Asian-, and Hispanic-Americans. J Am Coll Nutr 2001;20(Suppl 2):198S. [PMID: 11349943]

INTESTINAL MOTILITY DISORDERS

1. Acute Paralytic Ileus

 ESSENTIALS OF DIAGNOSIS

- *Precipitating factors: surgery, peritonitis, electrolyte abnormalities, severe medical illness.*

- *Nausea, vomiting, obstipation, distention.*
- *Minimal abdominal tenderness; decreased bowel sounds.*
- *Plain abdominal radiography with gas and fluid distention in small and large bowel.*

General Considerations

Ileus is a condition in which there is neurogenic failure or loss of peristalsis in the intestine in the absence of any mechanical obstruction. It is commonly seen in hospitalized patients as a result of (1) intra-abdominal processes such as recent gastrointestinal or abdominal surgery or peritoneal irritation (peritonitis, pancreatitis, ruptured viscus, hemorrhage); (2) severe medical illness such as pneumonia, respiratory failure requiring intubation, sepsis or severe infections, uremia, diabetic ketoacidosis, and electrolyte abnormalities (hypokalemia, hypercalcemia, hypomagnesemia, hypophosphatemia); and (3) medications that affect intestinal motility (opioids, anticholinergics, phenothiazines).

Clinical Findings

A. Symptoms and Signs

Patients who are conscious report mild diffuse, continuous abdominal discomfort with nausea and vomiting. Generalized abdominal distention is present with minimal abdominal tenderness but no signs of peritoneal irritation (unless due to the primary disease). Bowel sounds are diminished to absent.

B. Laboratory Findings

The laboratory abnormalities are attributable to the underlying condition. Serum electrolytes, including potassium, magnesium, phosphorus, and calcium, should be obtained to exclude abnormalities as contributing factors.

C. Imaging

Plain film radiography of the abdomen demonstrates distended gas-filled loops of small and large intestine. Air-fluid levels may be seen. Under some circumstances, it may be difficult to distinguish ileus from partial small bowel obstruction. A limited barium small bowel series or a CT scan may be useful in such instances to exclude mechanical obstruction, especially in postoperative patients.

Differential Diagnosis

Ileus must be distinguished from mechanical obstruction of the small bowel or proximal colon. Pain from small bowel mechanical obstruction is usually intermittent, cramping, and associated initially with profuse vomiting. Acute gastroenteritis, acute appendicitis, and acute pancreatitis may all present with ileus.

Treatment

The primary medical or surgical illness that has precipitated adynamic ileus should be treated. Most cases of ileus respond to restriction of oral intake with gradual liberalization of diet as bowel function returns. Severe or prolonged ileus requires nasogastric suction and parenteral administration of fluids and electrolytes.

Bungard TJ et al: Prokinetic agents for the treatment of postoperative ileus in adults: a review of the literature. Pharmacotherapy 1999;19:416. [PMID: 10212012]

Taguchi A et al: Selective postoperative inhibition of gastrointestinal opioid receptors. N Engl J Med 2001;345:935. [PMID: 11575284] (An investigational oral μ-opioid receptor antagonist has been found to reduce the time to first passage of flatus and bowel movement.)

2. Acute Colonic Pseudo-obstruction (Ogilvie's Syndrome)

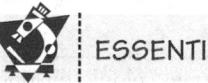 ESSENTIALS OF DIAGNOSIS

- *Severe abdominal distention.*
- *Arises in postoperative state or with severe medical illness.*
- *May be precipitated by electrolyte imbalances, medications.*
- *Absent to mild abdominal pain; minimal tenderness.*
- *Massive dilation of cecum or right colon.*

General Considerations

Spontaneous massive dilation of the cecum and proximal colon may occur in a number of different settings in hospitalized patients. Progressive cecal dilation may lead to spontaneous perforation with dire consequences. The risk of perforation correlates poorly with absolute cecal size. Colonic pseudo-obstruction is most commonly detected in surgical patients after trauma or burns or in the postoperative period and in medical patients with respiratory failure, metabolic imbalance, malignancy, myocardial infarction, congestive heart failure, pancreatitis, or a recent neurologic event (stroke, subarachnoid hemorrhage, trauma). Liberal use of narcotics or anticholinergic agents may precipitate colonic pseudo-obstruction in susceptible patients. It may also occur as a manifestation of colonic ischemia. The etiology of colonic pseudo-obstruction is unknown, but an imbalance between gut sympathetic activity and sacral parasympathetic innervation of the distal colon is hypothesized.

Clinical Findings

A. SYMPTOMS AND SIGNS

Many patients are on ventilatory support or are unable to report symptoms due to altered mental status. Abdominal distention is frequently noted by the clinician as the first sign, often leading to a plain film radiograph that demonstrates colonic dilation. Some patients are asymptomatic, though most report constant but mild abdominal pain. Nausea and vomiting may be present. Bowel movements usually are absent. Abdominal tenderness with some degree of guarding or rebound tenderness may be detected; however, signs of peritonitis are absent unless perforation has occurred. Bowel sounds may be normal or decreased.

B. LABORATORY FINDINGS

Laboratory findings reflect the underlying medical or surgical problems. Serum sodium, potassium, magnesium, phosphorus, and calcium should be obtained. Significant fever or leukocytosis raises concern for colonic perforation.

C. IMAGING

Plain film radiographs demonstrate colonic dilation, usually confined to the cecum and proximal colon. The upper limits of normal for cecal size is 9 cm. A cecal diameter greater than 10–12 cm is associated with an increased risk of colonic perforation. Varying amounts of small intestinal dilation and air-fluid levels due to adynamic ileus may be seen.

Differential Diagnosis

The dilated appearance of the colon may raise concern that there is a distal colonic mechanical obstruction due to malignancy, volvulus, or fecal impaction. In many centers a Hypaque (diatrizoate meglumine) enema is performed both to exclude colonic obstruction and in an attempt to decompress the colon and evacuate distal fecal material. Colonic pseudo-obstruction should be distinguished from toxic megacolon, which is acute dilation of the colon due to inflammation (inflammatory bowel disease) or infection (*Clostridium difficile*-associated colitis, cytomegalovirus). Patients with toxic megacolon manifest fever, dehydration, significant abdominal pain, leukocytosis, and diarrhea, which is often bloody.

Treatment

Conservative treatment is the appropriate first step for patients with no or minimal abdominal tenderness, no fever, no leukocytosis, and a cecal diameter less than 12 cm. The underlying illness is treated appropriately. A nasogastric tube and a rectal tube should be placed. Patients should not remain in one position but should be periodically rolled from side to side and to the prone position in an effort to promote expulsion of colonic gas. All drugs that reduce intestinal motility, such as narcotics, anticholinergics, and calcium channel blockers, are discontinued if possible. Enemas may be administered judiciously if large amounts of stool are evident on radiography. Oral laxatives are not helpful and may cause perforation, pain, or electrolyte abnormalities.

Conservative treatment is successful in over 80% of cases. Patients must be watched for signs of worsening distention or abdominal tenderness. Cecal size should be assessed by abdominal radiographs every 12 hours. Intervention should be considered in patients with sustained or progressive cecal dilation to 10–12 cm or more despite 24 hours of conservative treatment and in those showing signs of clinical deterioration. Neostigmine injection should be given unless contraindicated. A single dose (2 mg intravenously) results in rapid (within 30 minutes) colonic decompression in 75–90% of patients. Cardiac monitoring during neostigmine infusion is indicated for possible bradycardia that may require atropine administration. Colonoscopic decompression is indicated in patients who fail to respond to neostigmine. Colonic decompression with aspiration of air or placement of a decompression tube is successful in up to 90% of patients. However, the procedure is technically difficult in an unprepared bowel and has been associated with perforations in the distended colon. Dilation recurs in up to half of patients. In patients in whom colonoscopy is unsuccessful, a tube cecostomy can be created through a small laparotomy or with percutaneous radiologically guided placement.

Prognosis

In most cases, the prognosis is related to the underlying illness. With aggressive therapy, the development of perforation is unusual.

De Giorgio R et al: Review article: the pharmacologic treatment of acute colonic pseudo-obstruction. Aliment Pharmacol Ther 2001;15:1717. [PMID: 11683685]

CHRONIC INTESTINAL PSEUDO-OBSTRUCTION & GASTROPARESIS

Gastroparesis and chronic intestinal pseudo-obstruction are chronic conditions characterized by intermittent, waxing and waning symptoms and signs of gastric or intestinal obstruction in the absence of any mechanical lesions to account for the findings. They are caused by a heterogeneous group of endocrine disorders (diabetes mellitus, hypothyroidism, cortisol deficiency), postsurgical conditions (vagotomy, partial gastric resection, fundoplication, gastric bypass, Whipple procedure), neurologic conditions (Parkinson's disease, muscular and myotonic dystrophy, autonomic dysfunction, multiple sclerosis, postpolio syndrome, porphyria), rheumatologic syndromes (progressive systemic sclerosis), infections (postviral, Chagas' disease), amyloidosis, paraneoplastic syndromes, medications, and eating disorders (anorexia); a cause may not always be identified. Gastric involvement leads to chronic or intermittent symptoms of gastroparesis with early satiety, nausea, and postprandial vomiting (1–3 hours after meals).

Patients with predominantly small bowel involvement may have abdominal distention, vomiting, diarrhea, and varying degrees of malnutrition. Abdominal pain is not common and should prompt investigation for structural causes of obstruction. Bacterial overgrowth in the stagnant intestine may result in malabsorption. Colonic involvement may result in constipation or alternating diarrhea and constipation.

Plain film radiography may demonstrate dilation of the esophagus, stomach, small intestine, or colon resembling ileus or mechanical obstruction. Mechanical obstruction of the stomach, small intestine, or colon is much more common than gastroparesis or intestinal pseudo-obstruction and must be excluded with endoscopy or barium radiography (upper gastrointestinal series with small bowel follow-through), especially in patients with prior surgery, recent onset of symptoms, or abdominal pain. In cases of unclear origin, studies based on the clinical picture are obtained to exclude underlying systemic disease. Gastric scintigraphy with a low-fat solid meal is the optimal means for assessing gastric emptying. Gastric retention of 60% after 2 hours or more than 10% after 4 hours is abnormal. Small bowel manometry is useful for distinguishing visceral from myopathic disorders and for excluding cases of mechanical obstruction that are otherwise difficult to diagnose by endoscopy or radiographic studies.

There is no specific therapy for gastroparesis or pseudo-obstruction. Acute exacerbations are treated with nasogastric suction and intravenous fluids. Chronic treatment is directed at maintaining nutrition. Patients should eat small, frequent meals that are low in fiber, milk, gas-forming foods, and fat. Some patients may require liquid enteral supplements. Agents that reduce gastrointestinal motility (opioids, anticholinergics) should be avoided. In diabetics, glucose levels should be maintained below 200 mg/dL, as hyperglycemia may slow gastric emptying even in the absence of diabetic neuropathy. Metoclopramide (5–20 mg orally or 5–10 mg intravenously or subcutaneously four times daily before meals) and erythromycin (125–250 mg orally twice daily or 1–2 mg/kg intravenously every 6 hours) are of benefit in treatment of gastroparesis but not small bowel dysmotility. Bacterial overgrowth should be treated with intermittent antibiotics (see above). Patients with predominant small bowel distention may require a venting gastrostomy to relieve distress. Some patients may require surgical placement of a jejunostomy for long-term enteral nutrition. Gastric pacing with internally implanted neurostimulators is being clinically tested for patients with gastroparesis. Patients unable to maintain adequate enteral nutrition require total par-

enteral nutrition or small bowel transplantation. Difficult cases should be referred to centers with expertise in this area.

Hornbuckle K et al: The diagnosis and work-up of the patient with gastroparesis. J Clin Gastroenterol 2000;30:117. [PMID: 10730917]

Pandolfino JE et al: Motility-modifying agents and management of disorders of gastrointestinal motility. Gastroenterology 2000;118(Suppl):S32. [PMID: 10868897]

Rabine J et al: Management of the patient with gastroparesis. J Clin Gastroenterol 2001;32:11. [PMID: 11154162]

TUMORS OF THE SMALL INTESTINE

Benign and malignant tumors of the small intestine are rare. They often cause no symptoms or signs. However, they may cause acute gastrointestinal bleeding with hematochezia or melena or chronic gastrointestinal blood loss resulting in fatigue and iron deficiency anemia. Small bowel tumors may cause obstruction due to luminal narrowing or intussusception of a polypoid mass. Small bowel tumors usually are identified by barium radiographic studies, either enteroclysis or a small bowel series. Visualization and biopsy of duodenal and proximal jejunal mass lesions are performed with a long upper endoscope known as an enteroscope.

1. Benign Tumors of Small Intestine

Benign polyps may be symptomatic or may be incidental findings detected on endoscopy or radiographic study. Most occur singly, and the presence of multiple polyps is suggestive of hereditary polyposis syndrome (discussed under Diseases of the Colon and Rectum). With the exception of lipomas, surgical or endoscopic excision usually is recommended. Adenomatous polyps are the most common benign mucosal tumor. The majority are asymptomatic, though acute or chronic bleeding may occur. Because malignant transformation does occur, endoscopic or surgical resection is warranted. Villous adenomas occur most commonly in the periampullary region of the duodenum (especially in patients with familial adenomatous polyposis) and carry a high risk for development of invasive cancer. Periodic endoscopic or surveillance to detect early ampullary neoplasms is recommended in patients with familial adenomatous polyposis. Evaluation with ERCP and endoscopic ultrasound is required to exclude invasive carcinoma. Ampullary adenomas may be removed by endoscopic or surgical techniques. Lipomas occur commonly in the ileum. Most are asymptomatic and identified incidentally at endoscopy or radiography; however, they rarely may cause obstruction with intussusception. Benign stromal tumors (formerly called leiomyomas) are found at all levels of the intestine. These submucosal mesenchymal lesions may be intraluminal, intramural, or extraluminal. Although most are asymptomatic, they may ulcerate and cause acute or chronic bleeding or obstruction. It is difficult to distinguish benign from malignant stromal tumors (leiomyosarcomas) except by excision.

2. Malignant Tumors of Small Intestine

Malignant tumors of the small intestine are extremely rare, accounting for less than 2% of all gastrointestinal malignancies. They may present with anemia, bleeding, obstruction, or evidence of metastatic disease.

Adenocarcinoma

These are aggressive tumors that occur most commonly in the duodenum or proximal jejunum. The ampulla of Vater is the most common site of small bowel carcinoma, and the incidence of ampullary carcinoma is increased more than 200-fold in patients with familial adenomatous polyposis. Ampullary carcinoma may present with jaundice due to bile duct obstruction or bleeding. Surgical resection of early lesions is curative in up to 40% of patients. Periodic endoscopic surveillance to detect early ampullary neoplasms therefore is recommended in patients with this disorder. Nonampullary adenocarcinoma of the small intestine accounts for 30–40% of small bowel cancers. Most present with symptoms of obstruction, acute or chronic bleeding, or weight loss. Eighty percent have already metastasized at the time of diagnosis. Resection is recommended for control of symptoms. Patients with Crohn's disease have an increased risk of small intestine adenocarcinoma, most commonly in the ileum, which may be difficult to distinguish from disease-related fibrous strictures.

Lymphoma

Gastrointestinal lymphomas may arise in the gastrointestinal tract or involve it secondarily with disseminated disease. In Western countries, primary gastrointestinal lymphomas account for 5% of lymphomas and 20% of small bowel malignancies. They occur most commonly in the distal small intestine. The majority are non-Hodgkin's intermediate or high-grade B cell lymphomas. However, T cell lymphomas may arise in patients with celiac sprue. In the Middle East, lymphomas may arise also in the setting of immunoproliferative small intestinal disease. In this condition, there is diffuse lymphoplasmacytic infiltration with IgA-secreting B lymphocytes of the mucosa and submucosa that results in weight loss, diarrhea, and malabsorption which may lead to lymphomatous transformation. A characteristic feature of the disease is the presence of alpha heavy chains in the serum in 70% produced by clones of IgA plasma cells. The early, premalignant phase may respond to antibiotic therapy alone.

Presenting symptoms or signs of primary lymphoma include abdominal pain, weight loss, nausea and vomiting, distention, anemia, and occult blood in the stool. Fevers are unusual. Protein-losing enteropathy may result in hypoalbuminemia, but other signs of malabsorption are unusual. Barium radiography helps to localize the site of the lesion. The diagnosis requires endoscopic, percutaneous, or laparoscopic biopsy. In order to determine tumor stage, patients must undergo chest and abdominal CT, bone marrow biopsy, and, in some cases, lymphangiography.

Treatment depends on the stage of disease. Resection of primary intestinal lymphoma, if feasible, is usually recommended. Even in cases of stage III or stage IV disease, surgical debulking may improve survival. In patients with limited disease (stage IE) that is resected, the role of adjuvant chemotherapy is unclear. Most patients with more extensive disease are treated with systemic chemotherapy with or without radiation therapy (see Chapter 4).

Carcinoid Tumors

Carcinoids are the most common neuroendocrine tumors arising from the gastrointestinal tract. They derive from a variety of neuroendocrine cells, but the term "carcinoid" usually refers to tumors that secrete serotonin or its precursors. Although many behave in an indolent fashion, the overall 5-year survival rate for patients with carcinoids is 50%, suggesting that most are malignant. The risk of metastatic spread is closely related to tumor size and tumor location. Many small carcinoids are detected incidentally at endoscopy or autopsy. It is not possible by histologic examination to distinguish benign from malignant disease. The best indicator of prognosis is evidence of invasive growth and the presence of regional or distant metastasis.

Over 95% of gastrointestinal carcinoids occur in one of three sites: the rectum, the appendix, or the small intestine. Carcinoids account for up to one-third of small intestinal tumors. Rectal carcinoids are usually detected incidentally as submucosal nodules during proctoscopic examination. Similarly, appendiceal carcinoids are identified in 0.3% of appendectomies. Almost 80% of these tumors are less than 1 cm in size, and 90% are less than 2 cm. Rectal carcinoids less than 1 cm and appendiceal carcinoids less than 2 cm virtually never metastasize and are treated effectively with local excision or simple appendectomy. Tumors larger than 2 cm are associated with the development of metastasis in over 20% of appendiceal carcinoids and 10% of rectal carcinoids. Hence, in younger patients who are good operative risks, a more extensive cancer resection operation is warranted.

Small intestinal carcinoids most commonly arise in the ileum. Up to one-third are multicentric. Although 60% are less than 2 cm in size, even these small carcinoids may metastasize. Almost all tumors over 2 cm are associated with metastasis. Most smaller lesions are asymptomatic, though intussusception with obstruction occurs rarely. Carcinoids may extend locally into the muscularis, serosa, and mesentery, where they engender a fibroblastic reaction with contraction and kinking of the bowel. This may lead to symptoms of partial small bowel obstruction with intermittent abdominal pain or obstruction. Small bowel barium studies may reveal kinking, but because the lesion is extraluminal the diagnosis may be overlooked for several years. Encasement of the mesenteric vessels can lead to bowel infarction. Further extension occurs to the local lymph nodes and to the liver. Abdominal CT may demonstrate a mesenteric mass with tethering of the bowel, lymphadenopathy, and hepatic metastasis. Carcinoid involvement of the heart (resulting in right-sided valvular lesions) is a late manifestation of metastatic disease. Carcinoid syndrome occurs in less than 10% of patients (see Chapter 4) and only in patients with hepatic metastasis. It is caused by tumor secretion of hormonal mediators that cause cramps, flushing, diarrhea, cyanosis, or bronchospasm. Virtually all patients with carcinoid syndrome have obvious signs of cancer with liver metastasis on abdominal imaging. The optimal initial hepatic imaging study is somatostatin receptor scintigraphy, which is positive in over 90% of patients with metastatic carcinoid. A urinary 5-HIAA > 10 mg/24 h or an elevated serum serotonin confirms the diagnosis of carcinoid syndrome.

Small intestinal carcinoids are extremely indolent tumors with slow spread. Patients with disease confined to the small intestine should have local excision, for which the cure rate exceeds 85%. In patients with resectable disease who have lymph node involvement, the 5-year disease-free survival is 80%; however, by 25 years, less than 25% remain disease-free. Even patients with hepatic metastases may have an indolent course with a median survival of 3 years. In patients with advanced disease, therapy should be deferred until the patient is symptomatic. Surgery should be directed toward palliation of obstructive symptoms. In patients with carcinoid syndrome or diarrhea, resection of hepatic metastases may provide dramatic improvement. The somatostatin analog octreotide (150–500 μg subcutaneously three times daily) inhibits hormone secretion from the carcinoid tumor, resulting in dramatic relief of diarrhea and symptoms of carcinoid syndrome in 90% of patients for a median period of 1 year. Thereafter, many patients escape from octreotide control. Hepatic artery occlusion and chemotherapy may provide symptomatic improvement in some patients with hepatic metastases.

Sarcoma

Malignant stromal tumors (commonly called leiomyosarcomas) occur most commonly in the jejunum. Histologically, they resemble smooth muscle cells, but most are believed to arise from precursors to the interstitial cell of Cajal. (See Malignant Tumors of the Stomach: Stromal Tumors.) Tumors may grow quite large before causing symptoms due to obstruction, intussusception, or bleeding due to central ulceration within the tumor. Surgery should be performed for symptomatic tumors and asymptomatic tumors more

than 3–5 cm in size (in which the risk of malignancy is increased). Overall 5-year survival after surgical resection is 30%. The tyrosine kinase inhibitor imatinib induces partial remission and clinical improvement in patients with metastatic disease.

Kaposi's sarcoma was at one time a common complication in AIDS, but the incidence is declining with highly active antiretroviral therapy (HAART). It is strongly associated with infection with human herpesvirus 8. Lesions may be present anywhere in the intestinal tract. Visceral involvement usually is associated with cutaneous disease. Most lesions are clinically silent; however, large lesions may be symptomatic. Lesions of the gingiva, palate, and hypopharynx can lead to painful mastication and dysphagia. Lesions of the stomach or small intestine may lead to bleeding, obstruction, or even perforation. The diagnosis may be confirmed at endoscopy by the characteristic visual appearance and by biopsy. Oral complications can be treated with the CO_2 laser or radiation. Limited bleeding or obstructing lesions in the stomach or anus can be treated with the YAG laser or radiation therapy. Interferon alfa induces regression in up to one-third of patients who have a CD4 cell count of > 200/μL. Widespread involvement may be best treated by systemic chemotherapy using combinations of vincristine, bleomycin, or doxorubicin, to which the tumor is very responsive.

Gill S et al: Small intestinal neoplasms. J Clin Gastroenterol 2001;33:267. [PMID: 11588539]

Hermans P: Kaposi's sarcoma in HIV-infected patients: treatment options. HIV Medicine 2000;1:137. [PMID: 11737340]

Kulke M et al: Carcinoid tumors. N Engl J Med 1999;340:858. [PMID: 10080850].

APPENDICITIS

 ESSENTIALS OF DIAGNOSIS

- Early: periumbilical pain; later: right lower quadrant pain and tenderness.
- Anorexia, nausea and vomiting, obstipation.
- Tenderness or localized rigidity at McBurney's point.
- Low-grade fever and leukocytosis.

General Considerations

Appendicitis is the most common abdominal surgical emergency, affecting approximately 10% of the population. It occurs most commonly between the ages of 10 and 30 years. It is initiated by obstruction of the appendix by a fecalith, inflammation, foreign body, or neoplasm. Obstruction leads to increased intraluminal pressure, venous congestion, infection, and thrombosis of intramural vessels. If untreated, gangrene and perforation develop within 36 hours.

Clinical Findings

A. SYMPTOMS AND SIGNS

Appendicitis usually begins with vague, often colicky periumbilical or epigastric pain. Within 12 hours the pain shifts to the right lower quadrant, manifested as a steady ache that is worsened by walking or coughing. Almost all patients have nausea with one or two episodes of vomiting. Protracted vomiting or vomiting that begins before the onset of pain suggests another diagnosis. A sense of constipation is typical, and some patients administer cathartics in an effort to relieve their symptoms—though some report diarrhea. Low-grade fever (< 38 °C) is typical; high fever or rigors suggest another diagnosis or appendiceal perforation.

On physical examination, localized tenderness with guarding in the right lower quadrant can be elicited with gentle palpation with one finger. When asked to cough, patients may be able to precisely localize the painful area, a sign of peritoneal irritation. Light percussion may also elicit pain. Although rebound tenderness is also present, it is unnecessary to elicit this finding if the above signs are present. The psoas sign (pain on passive extension of the right hip) and the obturator sign (pain with passive flexion and internal rotation of the right hip) are indicative of adjacent inflammation and strongly suggestive of appendicitis.

B. LABORATORY FINDINGS

Moderate leukocytosis (10,000–20,000/μL) with neutrophilia is common. Microscopic hematuria and pyuria are present in one-fourth of patients.

C. IMAGING

No imaging studies are necessary in patients with typical appendicitis. Studies may be useful in patients in whom the diagnosis is uncertain. Abdominal or transvaginal ultrasound has a diagnostic accuracy of over 85% and is especially useful in the exclusion of adnexal disease in younger women. Abdominal CT is useful in cases of suspected appendiceal perforation to diagnose a periappendiceal abscess.

Atypical Presentations of Appendicitis

Owing to the variable location of the appendix, there are a number of "atypical" presentations. Because the retrocecal appendix does not touch the anterior abdominal wall, the pain remains less intense and poorly localized; abdominal tenderness is minimal and may be elicited in the right flank. The psoas sign may be positive. With pelvic appendicitis there is pain in the lower abdomen, often on the left, with an urge to urinate or defecate. Abdominal tenderness is absent, but tenderness is evident on pelvic or rectal examination; the obturator sign may be present. In the elderly, the

diagnosis of appendicitis is often delayed because patients present with minimal, vague symptoms and mild abdominal tenderness. Appendicitis in pregnancy may present with pain in the right lower quadrant, periumbilical area, or right subcostal area owing to displacement of the appendix by the uterus.

Differential Diagnosis

Given its frequency and myriad presentations, appendicitis should be considered in the differential diagnosis of all patients with abdominal pain. It is difficult to reliably diagnose the disease in some cases. A several-hour period of close observation with reassessment usually clarifies the diagnosis. Absence of the classic migration of pain (from the epigastrium to the right lower abdomen), right lower quadrant pain, fever, or guarding makes appendicitis less likely. Ten to 20 percent of patients with suspected appendicitis have either a negative examination at laparotomy or an alternative surgical diagnosis. The widespread use of ultrasonography and CT has reduced the number of incorrect diagnoses. Still, in some cases diagnostic laparotomy or laparoscopy is required. The most common causes of diagnostic confusion are gastroenteritis and gynecologic disorders. Viral gastroenteritis presents with nausea, vomiting, low-grade fever, and diarrhea and can be difficult to distinguish from appendicitis. The onset of vomiting before pain makes appendicitis less likely. As a rule, the pain of gastroenteritis is more generalized and the tenderness less well localized. Acute salpingitis or tubo-ovarian abscess should be considered in young, sexually active women with fever and bilateral abdominal or pelvic tenderness. A twisted ovarian cyst may also cause sudden severe pain. The sudden onset of lower abdominal pain in the middle of the menstrual cycle suggests mittelschmerz. Sudden severe abdominal pain with diffuse pelvic tenderness and shock suggests a ruptured ectopic pregnancy. A positive pregnancy test and pelvic ultrasonography are diagnostic. Retrocecal or retroileal appendicitis (often associated with pyuria or hematuria) may be confused with ureteral colic or pyelonephritis. Other conditions that may resemble appendicitis are diverticulitis, Meckel's diverticulitis, carcinoid of the appendix, perforated colonic cancer, Crohn's ileitis, perforated peptic ulcer, cholecystitis, and mesenteric adenitis. It is virtually impossible to distinguish appendicitis from Meckel's diverticulitis, but both require surgical treatment.

Complications

Perforation occurs in 20% of patients and should be suspected in patients with pain persisting for over 36 hours, high fever, diffuse abdominal tenderness or peritoneal findings, a palpable abdominal mass, or marked leukocytosis. Localized perforation results in a contained abscess, usually in the pelvis. A free perforation leads to suppurative peritonitis with toxicity. Septic thrombophlebitis (pylephlebitis) of the portal venous system is rare and suggested by high fever, chills, bacteremia, and jaundice.

Treatment

The treatment of uncomplicated appendicitis is surgical appendectomy. This may be performed through a laparotomy or by laparoscopy. Prior to surgery, patients should be given systemic antibiotics, which reduce the incidence of postoperative wound infections. Emergency appendectomy is also required in patients with perforated appendicitis with generalized peritonitis.

The optimal treatment of stable patients with perforated appendicitis and a contained abscess is controversial. Surgery in this setting can be difficult. Many recommend percutaneous CT-guided drainage of the abscess with intravenous fluids and antibiotics to allow the inflammation to subside. An interval appendectomy may be performed after 6 weeks to prevent recurrent appendicitis.

Prognosis

The mortality rate from uncomplicated appendicitis is extremely low. Even with perforated appendicitis, the mortality rate in most groups is only 0.2%, though it approaches 15% in the elderly.

Jones PF: Suspected acute appendicitis: trends in management over 30 years. Br J Surg 2001;88:1570. [PMID: 11736966]

Kraemer M et al: Acute appendicitis in late adulthood: incidence, presentation, and outcome. Results of a prospective multicenter acute abdominal pain study and review of the literature. Langenbecks Arch Surg 2000;385:470. [PMID: 11131250]

INTESTINAL TUBERCULOSIS

Intestinal tuberculosis is common in underdeveloped countries. Previously rare in the United States, its incidence has been rising in immigrant groups and patients with AIDS. It is caused by both *Mycobacterium tuberculosis* and *M bovis*. Active pulmonary disease is present in less than 50% of patients. The most frequent site of involvement is the ileocecal region; however, any region of the gastrointestinal tract may be involved. Intestinal tuberculosis may cause mucosal ulcerations or scarring and fibrosis with narrowing of the lumen. Patients may complain of chronic abdominal pain, obstructive symptoms, weight loss, and diarrhea. An abdominal mass may be palpable. Complications include intestinal obstruction, hemorrhage, and fistula formation. The PPD skin test may be negative, especially in patients with weight loss or AIDS. Barium radiography may demonstrate mucosal ulcerations, thickening, or stricture formation. Colonoscopy may demonstrate an ulcerated mass, multiple ulcers with steep edges and adjacent small sessile polyps, or small diverticula, most commonly in the ileocecal region. The differential diagnosis includes Crohn's disease, carcinoma, and intestinal amebiasis. The diagnosis is established by either endoscopic or surgical biopsy revealing acid-fast bacilli, caseating granuloma, or positive cultures from the organism. Detection of tubercle bacilli in biopsy specimens by PCR is now the most sensitive means of diagnosis.

Treatment with standard antituberculous regimens is effective.

Naga M et al: Endoscopic diagnosis of colonic tuberculosis. Gastrointest Endosc 2001;53:789. [PMID: 11375593]

PROTEIN-LOSING ENTEROPATHY

Protein-losing enteropathy comprises a number of conditions that result in excessive loss of serum proteins into the gastrointestinal tract. The essential diagnostic features are hypoalbuminemia and an elevated fecal α_1-antitrypsin level.

The normal intact gut epithelium prevents the loss of serum proteins. Proteins may be lost through one of three mechanisms: (1) mucosal disease with ulceration, resulting in the loss of proteins across the disrupted mucosal surface; (2) lymphatic obstruction, resulting in the loss of protein-rich chylous fluid from mucosal lacteals; and (3) idiopathic change in permeability of mucosal capillaries and conductance of interstitium, resulting in "weeping" of protein-rich fluid from the mucosal surface (Table 14–13).

Table 14–13. Causes of protein-losing enteropathy.

Mucosal disease with ulceration
Chronic gastric ulcer
Gastric carcinoma
Lymphoma
Inflammatory bowel disease
Idiopathic ulcerative jejunoileitis
Lymphatic obstruction
Primary intestinal lymphangiectasia
Secondary obstruction
Cardiac disease: constrictive pericarditis, congestive heart failure
Infections: tuberculosis, Whipple's disease
Neoplasms: lymphoma, Kaposi's sarcoma
Retroperitoneal fibrosis
Sarcoidosis
Idiopathic mucosal transudation
Ménétrier's disease
Zollinger-Ellison syndrome
Acute viral gastroenteritis
Celiac sprue
Eosinophilic gastroenteritis
Allergic protein-losing enteropathy
Parasite infection: giardiasis, hookworm
Amyloidosis
Common variable immunodeficiency
Systemic lupus erythematosus

Hypoalbuminemia is the sine qua non of protein-losing enteropathy. However, a number of other serum proteins such as α_1-antitrypsin also are lost from the gut epithelium. In protein-losing enteropathy caused by lymphatic obstruction, loss of lymphatic fluid commonly results in lymphocytopenia (< 1000/μL), hypoglobulinemia, and hypocholesterolemia.

In most cases, protein-losing enteropathy is recognized as a sequela of a known gastrointestinal disorder. In patients in whom the cause is unclear, evaluation is indicated and is guided by the clinical suspicion. Protein-losing enteropathy must be distinguished from other causes of hypoalbuminemia, which include liver disease and nephrotic syndrome; and from congestive heart failure. Protein-losing enteropathy is confirmed by determining the gut α_1-antitrypsin clearance (24-hour volume of feces × stool concentration of α_1-antitrypsin ÷ serum α_1-antitrypsin concentration). A clearance of more than 13 mL/24 h is abnormal.

Laboratory evaluation of protein-losing enteropathy includes serum protein electrophoresis, lymphocyte count, and serum cholesterol to look for evidence of lymphatic obstruction. Serum ANA and C3 levels are useful to screen for autoimmune disorders. Stool samples should be examined for ova and parasites. Evidence of malabsorption is evaluated by means of a stool qualitative fecal fat determination. Intestinal imaging is performed with an upper endoscopy with small bowel biopsy and a small bowel barium series. Colonic diseases are excluded with barium enema or colonoscopy. A CT scan of the abdomen is performed to look for evidence of neoplasms or lymphatic obstruction. Rarely, lymphangiography is helpful. In some situations, laparotomy with full-thickness intestinal biopsy is required to establish a diagnosis.

Treatment is directed at the underlying cause. Patients with lymphatic obstruction benefit from low-fat diets supplemented with medium-chain triglycerides. Case reports suggest that octreotide may lead to symptomatic and nutritional improvement in some patients.

Landzberg BR et al: Protein-losing enteropathy and gastropathy. Curr Treat Options Gastroenterol 2001;4:39. [PMID: 11177680]

■ DISEASES OF THE COLON & RECTUM

IRRITABLE BOWEL SYNDROME

ESSENTIALS OF DIAGNOSIS

- *Chronic functional disorder characterized by abdominal pain or discomfort with alterations in bowel habits.*
- *Symptoms usually begin in late teens to early 20s.*
- *Limited evaluation to exclude organic causes of symptoms.*

General Considerations

The functional gastrointestinal disorders are characterized by a variable combination of chronic or recurrent gastrointestinal symptoms *not explicable by the presence of structural or biochemical abnormalities*. Several clinical entities are included under this broad rubric, including chest pain of unclear origin (noncardiac chest pain), functional dyspepsia, and biliary dyskinesia (sphincter of Oddi dysfunction). There is a large overlap among these entities. For example, over half of patients with noncardiac chest pain and over one-third with functional dyspepsia also have symptoms compatible with irritable bowel syndrome. In none of these disorders is there a definitive diagnostic study. Rather, the diagnosis is a subjective one based upon the presence of a compatible profile and the exclusion of similar disorders.

Irritable bowel syndrome can be defined, therefore, as an idiopathic clinical entity characterized by some combination of chronic (more than 3 months) lower abdominal symptoms and bowel complaints that may be continuous or intermittent. Consensus definition of irritable bowel syndrome is abdominal discomfort or pain that has two of the following three features: (1) relieved with defecation, (2) onset associated with a change in frequency of stool, (3) onset associated with a change in form (appearance) of stool. Other symptoms supporting the diagnosis include abnormal stool frequency (more than three bowel movements per day or fewer than three per week); abnormal stool form (lumpy or hard; loose or watery); abnormal stool passage (straining, urgency, or feeling of incomplete evacuation); passage of mucus; and bloating or a feeling of abdominal distention.

Patients may have other somatic or psychologic complaints such as dyspepsia, heartburn, chest pain, fatigue, urologic dysfunction, gynecologic symptoms, anxiety, or depression.

The disorder is a common problem presenting to both gastroenterologists and primary care physicians. Up to 20% of the adult population have symptoms compatible with the diagnosis, but most never seek medical attention.

Pathogenesis

A number of pathophysiologic mechanisms have been identified and may have varying importance in different individuals.

A. ABNORMAL MOTILITY

A variety of abnormal myoelectrical and motor abnormalities have been identified in the colon and small intestine. In some cases, these are temporally correlated with episodes of abdominal pain or emotional stress. Whether they represent a primary motility disorder or are secondary to psychosocial stress is debated. Differences between patients with constipation-predominant and diarrhea-predominant syndromes are reported.

B. Heightened Visceral Nociception

Patients often have a lower visceral pain threshold, reporting abdominal pain at lower volumes of colonic gas insufflation or colonic balloon inflation than controls. Although many patients complain of bloating and distention, their absolute intestinal gas volume is normal. Many patients report rectal urgency despite small rectal volumes of stool.

C. Psychosocial Abnormalities

More than half of patients with irritable bowel who seek medical attention have underlying depression, anxiety, or somatization. By contrast, those who do not seek medical attention are similar psychologically to normal individuals. Psychologic abnormalities may influence how the patient perceives or reacts to illness and minor visceral sensations.

Clinical Findings

A. Symptoms and Signs

Irritable bowel is a chronic condition. Symptoms usually begin in the late teens to twenties. Symptoms should be present for at least 3 months before the diagnosis can be considered. The diagnosis is established in the presence of compatible symptoms and after the exclusion of organic disease. Although patients report a variety of symptoms, four in particular are more common in this disorder than in organic disease: (1) abdominal distention, (2) abdominal pain relieved by defecation, (3) more frequent stools with the onset of abdominal pain, and (4) looser stools with the onset of pain. Over 90% of patients have two or more of these symptoms, compared with 30% with organic disorders. In patients over age 60, however, in whom organic disease is more common, the predictive value of these criteria is much lower.

Abdominal pain usually is intermittent, crampy, and in the lower abdominal region. It may be relieved by defecation, worsened by stress, and worse for 1–2 hours after meals. It does not usually occur at night or interfere with sleep. Patients may report predominant problems with constipation, diarrhea, or alternating constipation and diarrhea. It is important to clarify what the patient means by these complaints. The patient may use the term constipation to refer to hard or small stools, straining, or reduced stool frequency. Diarrhea may refer to loose stools, frequent stools, urgency, or fecal incontinence. Many patients report that they have a firm stool in the morning followed by progressively looser movements. Mucus is commonly

seen. Complaints of visible distention and bloating are common, though these are not clinically evident.

The acute onset of symptoms raises the likelihood of organic disease. Nocturnal diarrhea, hematochezia, weight loss, and fever are incompatible with a diagnosis of irritable bowel syndrome and warrant investigation for underlying disease.

A physical examination should be performed to look for evidence of organic disease and to allay the patient's anxieties. The physical examination usually is normal. Abdominal tenderness, especially in the lower abdomen, is common but not pronounced. A new onset of symptoms in a patient over age 40 warrants further examination.

B. Laboratory Findings and Special Examinations

In a patient 20–50 years of age with a presumptive clinical diagnosis of irritable bowel syndrome, a limited series of examinations is warranted to screen for organic disease. The complete blood count, serum albumin, erythrocyte sedimentation rate, and stool occult blood test all should be normal. In patients with diarrhea, thyroid function tests and stool examination for ova and parasites are performed. If diarrhea is predominant, a 24-hour stool collection is useful. Stool weight in excess of 300 g/d is atypical of irritable bowel and warrants further evaluation. In patients under age 40, flexible sigmoidoscopy should be performed. In patients over age 40 who have not had a previous evaluation, barium enema or colonoscopy should be considered.

Differential Diagnosis

These common symptoms have multiple causes. Examples include colonic neoplasia, inflammatory bowel disease, causes of chronic constipation, causes of chronic diarrhea (especially celiac disease, bacterial overgrowth, and lactase deficiency), and endometriosis. Psychiatric disorders such as depression and anxiety must be considered as well. Women with refractory symptoms have an increased incidence of prior sexual and physical abuse.

Treatment

A. General Measures

As with other functional disorders, the most important interventions the physician can offer are reassurance and a forthright explanation of the functional nature of the symptoms. Indeed, an ongoing therapeutic relationship may be the most important factor in successful management of this disorder. Patients should be told that their symptoms arise from either increased sensitivity to minor stimuli or increased reactivity resulting in spasm or abnormal motility. Although the "mind-gut" interaction should be mentioned, it should be emphasized that the symptoms are real. Physicians will earn the confidence of their patients by being nonjudgmental and attentive. Fears that the symptoms will progress, require surgery, or degenerate into serious illness should be allayed. The patient should understand that irritable bowel syndrome is a chronic disorder characterized by periods of exacerbation and quiescence. The physician can help but cannot "cure" such a disorder. The emphasis should be shifted from finding the cause of the symptoms to finding a way to cope with them. Physicians must resist the temptation to chase chronic complaints with new or repeated diagnostic studies.

B. DIETARY THERAPY

Patients commonly report dietary intolerances, though the role of dietary triggers in irritable bowel syndrome has never been convincingly proved. Nevertheless, the physician should be open to the idea that dietary changes may provide symptomatic benefit. In some patients, a food diary, in which symptoms, food intake, and life events are recorded, may reveal dietary or psychosocial factors that precipitate symptoms. Malabsorption of lactose, fructose, and sorbitol may cause bloating, distention, flatulence, and diarrhea. Lactose intolerance should be excluded in patients with predominant diarrhea with a breath hydrogen test or a trial of a lactose-free diet. Sorbitol and fructose are present in a number of fruits, artificially sweetened foods, and some medications. A variety of foods are flatulogenic, producing pain and distention in some patients. These include brown beans, Brussels sprouts, cabbage, cauliflower, raw onions, grapes, plums, raisins, coffee, red wine, and beer. Caffeine is poorly tolerated by most patients with irritable bowel syndrome.

A trial of a high-fiber diet (20–30 g/d) should be recommended for patients with predominant constipation. This may be accomplished by giving 1 tbsp of bran powder two or three times daily with food or in 8 oz of liquid. Some patients report increased gas and distention from fiber supplementation with bran. Fiber supplements with psyllium, methylcellulose, or polycarbophil may be better tolerated (see section on constipation).

C. PHARMACOLOGIC MEASURES

More than two-thirds of patients with irritable bowel syndrome have mild symptoms that respond readily to education, reassurance, and dietary interventions. Drug therapy should be reserved for patients with more severe symptoms that do not respond to these conservative measures. These agents should be viewed as being adjunctive rather than curative. Given the wide spectrum of symptoms, no single agent is expected to provide relief in all or even most patients. Indeed, there is no convincing evidence that any of these agents are superior to placebo, which results in symptomatic improvement in up to 70% of patients. Nevertheless, therapy targeted at the specific dominant symptom (pain, constipation, or diarrhea) may be beneficial.

1. Antispasmodic agents—Anticholinergic agents may be used as needed for acute episodes of pain or bloating or may be given 30–60 minutes before meals to reduce postprandial pain. Side effects include urinary retention, tachycardia, and dry mouth. Available agents include dicyclomine, 10–20 mg orally three or four times daily; hyoscyamine, 0.125 mg orally (or sublingually as needed), or sustained-release, 0.037 mg or 0.75 mg orally twice daily. Although calcium channel blockers relax gastrointestinal smooth muscle, they have not been well tested in patients with irritable bowel syndrome.

2. Antidiarrheal agents—Opioid and other antidiarrheal agents may be useful in patients with frequent loose stools (see section on chronic diarrhea). They may best be used "prophylactically" in situations where diarrhea is anticipated (such as stressful situations) or would be inconvenient (social engagements). Agents include loperamide, 2 mg orally three or four times daily, and diphenoxylate with atropine, 2.5 mg orally four times daily.

Serotonin 5-HT$_3$ receptors are involved in sensory, secretory, and motor processes in the gastrointestinal tract. A 5-HT$_3$ antagonist (alosetron) caused ischemic colitis and was removed from the market.

3. Anticonstipation agents—A trial of fiber supplementation with bran, psyllium, methylcellulose, or polycarbophil is beneficial in most cases. Patients who are unresponsive to fiber may benefit from treatment with osmotic laxatives (milk of magnesia or polyethylene glycol). Patients with intractable constipation should undergo further assessment for slow colonic and pelvic floor dysfunction (see Constipation).

4. Psychotropic agents—Patients with predominant pain, bloating, or diarrhea may benefit from low doses of tricyclic-type antidepressants, which are believed to have central and peripheral neuromodulatory actions independent of their psychotropic effects. Nortriptyline, desipramine, imipramine, or trazodone may be started at a low dosage of 25 mg at bedtime and increased gradually to 50–100 mg as tolerated. Side effects are common, and lack of efficacy with one agent does not preclude benefit from another. Serotonin reuptake inhibitors (sertraline, 50–150 mg daily, or fluoxetine, 20–40 mg daily) are commonly used in patients with constipation-predominant symptoms. Improvement should be evident within 4 weeks.

5. Other agents—Anxiolytics and narcotics should not be used chronically in irritable bowel syndrome because of their habituation potential.

D. OTHER THERAPIES

Behavioral modification with relaxation techniques and hypnotherapy may be beneficial in some patients. Patients with underlying psychologic abnormalities may benefit from evaluation by a psychiatrist or psychologist. Patients with severe disability should be referred to a pain treatment center.

Prognosis

The majority of patients with irritable bowel syndrome learn to cope with their symptoms and lead productive lives.

Camilleri M: Management of the irritable bowel syndrome. Gastroenterology 2001;120:652. [PMID: 11179242]

Drossman D: Irritable bowel syndrome: how far do you go in the workup? Gastroenterology 2001;121:1512. [PMID: 11729133] (The importance of celiac disease and bacterial overgrowth in unselected patients with irritable bowel syndrome requires further study.)

ANTIBIOTIC-ASSOCIATED COLITIS

ESSENTIALS OF DIAGNOSIS

- *Most cases of antibiotic-associated diarrhea are not attributable to* Clostridium difficile *and are usually mild and self-limited.*
- *Symptoms of antibiotic-associated colitis vary from mild to fulminant; almost all colitis is attributable to* C difficile.
- *Diagnosis in mild to moderate cases established by stool toxin assay.*
- *Flexible sigmoidoscopy provides most rapid diagnosis in severe cases.*

General Considerations

Antibiotic-associated diarrhea is a common clinical occurrence. Characteristically, the diarrhea occurs during the period of antibiotic exposure, is dose-related, and resolves spontaneously after discontinuation of the antibiotic. In most cases, this diarrhea is mild, self-limited, and does not require any specific laboratory evaluation or treatment. Stool examination usually reveals no fecal leukocytes, and stool cultures reveal no pathogens. Although *C difficile* is identified in the stool of 15–25% of cases of antibiotic-associated diarrhea, it is also identified in 5–10% of patients treated with antibiotics who do not have diarrhea. Most cases of antibiotic-associated diarrhea are due to changes in colonic bacterial fermentation of carbohydrates and are not due to *C difficile*.

Antibiotic-associated colitis is a significant clinical problem almost always caused by *C difficile*. Hospitalized patients are most susceptible, especially those who are severely ill or malnourished or who are receiving chemotherapy. This anaerobic bacterium colonizes the colon of 5% of healthy adults. In hospitalized patients, however, it is present in over 20% of patients, most of whom have received antibiotics that disrupt the normal bowel flora and thus allow the bacterium

to flourish. Most of these patients are asymptomatic. Recently, patients receiving enteral tube feedings have been found to have a higher risk for acquisition of *C difficile* and the development of *C difficile*-associated diarrhea. The organism is spread in a fecal-oral fashion. It is found throughout hospitals in patient rooms and bathrooms and is readily transmitted from patient to patient by hospital personnel. Fastidious hand washing and use of disposable gloves are helpful in minimizing transmission.

In one-third of colonized patients, *C difficile*-induced colitis may develop. *C difficile* colitis is the major cause of diarrhea in patients hospitalized for more than 3 days, affecting 7:1000 patients. Although virtually all antibiotics have been implicated, colitis most commonly develops after use of ampicillin, clindamycin, and third-generation cephalosporins. Symptoms usually begin during or shortly after antibiotic therapy but may be delayed for up to 8 weeks. All patients with acute diarrhea should be questioned about recent antibiotic exposure.

Clinical Findings

A. Symptoms and Signs

Most patients report mild to moderate greenish, foul-smelling watery diarrhea with lower abdominal cramps. Physical examination is normal or reveals mild left lower quadrant tenderness. With more serious illness, there is abdominal pain and profuse watery diarrhea with up to 30 stools per day. The stools may have mucus but seldom gross blood. There may be fever up to 40 °C, abdominal tenderness, and leukocytosis as high as 50,000/μL. *C difficile* colitis should be considered in all hospitalized patients with unexplained leukocytosis. In most patients, colitis is most severe in the distal colon and rectum. When colitis is more severe in the right side of the colon, there may be little or no diarrhea. In such cases, fever, abdominal distention, pain and tenderness, and leukocytosis suggest the presence of infection.

B. Special Examinations

1. Stool studies—Pathogenic strains of *C difficile* produce two toxins: toxin A is an enterotoxin and toxin B a cytotoxin. In most patients, the diagnosis of antibiotic-associated colitis is established by the demonstration of *C difficile* toxins in the stool. A cytotoxicity assay (toxin B) performed in cell cultures has a specificity of 90% and a sensitivity of 95%. This is the definitive test, but it is expensive and takes at least 24 hours. Rapid enzyme immunoassays (EIA) (2–4 hours) for toxins A and B have been developed that have a 70–85% sensitivity with a single stool specimen but 90% with two specimens. Some toxic strains of *C difficile* do not produce a functional toxin A (and therefore have a negative EIA). When *C difficile* is suspected but the EIA is negative, a cytotoxicity assay should be performed. Culture for *C difficile* is the most sensitive test, but 25% of isolates are not pathogenic. Because it is slower (2–3 days), more costly, and less specific than toxin assays, it is not used in most clinical settings. Fecal leukocytes are present in only 50% of patients with colitis.

2. Flexible sigmoidoscopy—Flexible sigmoidoscopy is performed in patients with more severe symptomatology when a rapid diagnosis is desired so that therapy can be initiated. In patients with mild to moderate symptoms, there may be no abnormalities or only patchy or diffuse, nonspecific colitis indistinguishable from other causes. In patients with severe illness, true **pseudomembranous colitis** is seen. This has a characteristic appearance, with yellow adherent plaques 2–10 mm in diameter scattered over the colonic mucosa interspersed with hyperemic mucosa. Biopsies reveal epithelial ulceration with a classic "volcano" exudate of fibrin and neutrophils. In 10% of cases, pseudomembranous colitis is confined to the proximal colon and may be missed at sigmoidoscopy.

3. Imaging studies—Abdominal radiographs are obtained in patients with fulminant symptoms to look for evidence of toxic dilation or megacolon but are of no value in mild disease. Mucosal edema or "thumbprinting" may be evident. Abdominal CT scan may be very useful in detecting colonic edema, especially in patients with predominantly right-sided colitis or abdominal pain without significant diarrhea (in whom the diagnosis may be unsuspected). CT is also useful in the evaluation of possible complications.

Differential Diagnosis

In the hospitalized patient who develops acute diarrhea after admission, the differential diagnosis includes simple antibiotic-associated diarrhea (not related to *C difficile*), enteral feedings, medications, and ischemic colitis. Other infectious causes are unusual in hospitalized patients who develop diarrhea more than 72 hours after admission, and it is not cost-effective to obtain stool cultures unless tests for *C difficile* are negative. Rarely, other organisms (staphylococci, *Clostridium perfringens*) have been associated with pseudomembranous colitis.

Complications

Fulminant disease may result in dehydration, electrolyte imbalance, toxic megacolon, perforation, and death. Chronic untreated colitis may result in weight loss and protein-losing enteropathy.

Treatment

A. ACUTE THERAPY

If possible, antibiotic therapy should be discontinued. In patients with mild symptoms, doing so may result in prompt resolution of symptoms without specific treatment. If diarrhea is severe or persistent, specific therapy is warranted. The drug of choice is metronida-

zole, 500 mg orally three times daily. The duration of therapy is usually 10–14 days. However, in patients requiring long-term systemic antibiotics, it may be appropriate to continue metronidazole therapy until the antibiotics can be discontinued. Vancomycin, 125 mg orally four times daily, is equally effective as metronidazole but significantly more expensive, and it promotes the emergence of vancomycin-resistant nosocomial infections. Therefore, metronidazole is the preferred first-line therapy in most patients. Vancomycin should be reserved for patients who are intolerant of metronidazole, pregnant women, and children. Symptomatic improvement occurs in most patients within 72 hours. For patients with severe disease who do not respond rapidly to initial metronidazole therapy, therapy should be switched to vancomycin, 125 mg orally four times daily, escalating the dose to 500 mg four times daily if diarrhea and leukocytosis fail to improve. In patients who are unable to take oral medications and those with toxic megacolon, intravenous metronidazole, 500–750 mg every 6 hours, should be given—sometimes supplemented by oral vancomycin administered per nasoenteric tube or enema. Intravenous vancomycin does not penetrate the bowel and should not be used. Total abdominal colectomy may be required in patients with toxic megacolon, perforation, sepsis, or hemorrhage.

B. TREATMENT OF RELAPSE

Up to 20% of patients have a relapse of diarrhea from *C difficile* within 1 or 2 weeks after stopping initial therapy. This may be due to reinfection or failure to eradicate the organism. Most relapses respond promptly to a second course of metronidazole therapy. Some patients have recurrent relapses that can be difficult to treat. The optimal treatment regimen for recurrent relapses is unknown. Many authorities recommend a 6-week tapering regimen of vancomycin (125 mg orally four times daily for 7 days; twice daily for 7 days; once daily for 7 days; every other day for 7 days; and every third day for 2 weeks). Oral administration of a live yeast, *Saccharomyces boulardii*, has been shown to reduce the incidence of relapse by 50% in one United States trial. However, this agent is not yet available in the United States.

Buchner A et al: Medical diagnoses and procedures associated with Clostridium difficile colitis. Am J Gastroenterol 2001; 96:766. [PMID: 11280548]

Yassin S et al: *Clostridium difficile*-associated diarrhea and colitis. Mayo Clin Proc 2001;76:725. [PMID: 11444405]

INFLAMMATORY BOWEL DISEASE

The term "inflammatory bowel disease" includes ulcerative colitis and Crohn's disease. Ulcerative colitis is a chronic, recurrent disease characterized by diffuse mucosal inflammation involving only the colon. Ulcerative colitis invariably involves the rectum and may extend proximally in a continuous fashion to involve part or all of the colon. Crohn's disease is a chronic, recurrent disease characterized by patchy transmural inflammation involving any segment of the gastrointestinal tract from the mouth to the anus.

Drug Therapies for Inflammatory Bowel Disease

Although ulcerative colitis and Crohn's disease appear to be distinct entities, the same pharmacologic agents are used to treat both. Despite extensive research, there are still no specific therapies for these diseases. The mainstays of therapy remain 5-aminosalicylic acid derivatives, corticosteroids, and mercaptopurine or azathioprine.

A. 5-Aminosalicylic Acid (5-ASA)

5-Aminosalicylic acid is a topically active agent that has a variety of anti-inflammatory effects. It is used in the active treatment of ulcerative colitis and Crohn's disease and during disease inactivity in order to maintain remission. It is readily absorbed from the small intestine but demonstrates minimal colonic absorption. A number of oral and topical compounds have been designed to target delivery of 5-ASA to the colon or small intestine while minimizing absorption. Commonly used formulations of 5-ASA are sulfasalazine, mesalamine, and balsalazide.

1. Sulfasalazine—Sulfasalazine consists of 5-aminosalicylic acid linked by an azo bond to a sulfapyridine moiety. It is largely unabsorbed in the small intestine. In the colon, bacterial azoreductases cleave 5-ASA from the sulfapyridine group. It is unclear whether the sulfapyridine group has any anti-inflammatory effects. One gram of sulfasalazine contains 400 mg of 5-ASA. The 5-ASA works topically and is largely unabsorbed. The sulfapyridine group, however, is absorbed and may cause side effects in 15–30% of patients. Dose-related side effects include nausea, headaches, leukopenia, oligospermia, and impaired folate metabolism. Allergic and idiosyncratic side effects are fever, rash, hemolytic anemia, neutropenia, worsened colitis, hepatitis, pancreatitis, and pneumonitis. Despite its side effects, sulfasalazine continues to be used because it is significantly less expensive than other 5-aminosalicylic acid agents. It should always be administered in conjunction with folate.

2. Oral mesalamine agents—These 5-ASA agents are coated in various pH-sensitive resins (Asacol) or packaged in timed-release capsules (Pentasa). Mesalamine tablets dissolve at pH 7.0, releasing 5-ASA in the terminal small bowel and proximal colon. Pentasa releases 5-ASA slowly throughout the small intestine and colon. Side effects of these compounds are uncommon but include nausea, headache, pancreatitis, and nephropathy. Eighty percent of patients intolerant of sulfasalazine can tolerate mesalamine.

3. Azo compounds—Balsalazide and olsalazine are 5-ASA prodrugs released almost entirely in the colon.

They contain 5-ASA linked to an azo bond that requires cleavage by colonic bacterial azoreductases in order to release 5-ASA. Absorption of the prodrugs or 5-ASA from the small intestine is negligible. Compared with mesalamine, there is less systemic absorption of 5-ASA and lower systemic side effects. Balsalazide contains 5-ASA linked to an inert carrier (4-aminobenzoyl-β-alanine). It is as effective as or more effective than other 5-ASA compounds for the treatment of ulcerative colitis.

4. Topical mesalamine—5-Aminosalicylic acid is provided in the form of suppositories (500 mg) and enemas (Rowasa; 4 g/60 mL). These formulations can deliver much higher concentrations of 5-aminosalicylic acid to the distal colon than oral compounds. Side effects are uncommon.

B. Corticosteroids

A variety of intravenous, oral, and topical steroid formulations have been used in inflammatory bowel disease. They have utility in the short-term treatment of moderate to severe disease. However, long-term use is associated with serious, potentially irreversible side effects and is to be avoided. The agents, route of administration, duration of use, and tapering regimens employed are based more upon personal bias and experience than upon data from rigorous clinical trials. The most commonly used intravenous formulations have been hydrocortisone or methylprednisolone, which are given by continuous infusion or every 6 hours. Oral formulations are prednisone or methylprednisolone. Topical preparations are provided as hydrocortisone suppositories (100 mg), foam (90 mg), and enemas (100 mg). Budesonide is an oral glucocorticoid with high topical anti-inflammatory activity but low systemic activity due to high first-pass hepatic metabolism.

C. Mercaptopurine and Azathioprine

Mercaptopurine and azathioprine are used in 10–15% of patients with refractory Crohn's disease and, increasingly, in ulcerative colitis. Side effects occur in 10%, including pancreatitis, bone marrow suppression, infections, hepatitis or cholestatic jaundice, allergies, and, potentially, a higher risk of neoplasm. After therapy is started, complete blood counts should be obtained weekly for 1 month and then once a month to monitor for myelosuppression. About one person in ten has a genetically acquired deficiency in the enzyme thiopurine methyltransferase (TPMT) that metabolizes these thiopurine medications, placing them at risk of profound immunosuppression. Levels of TPMT and mercaptopurine metabolites now are available clinically; their proper use is debated.

Social Support for Patients With Inflammatory Bowel Disease

Inflammatory bowel disease is a lifelong illness that can have profound emotional and social impacts on the individual. Patients should be encouraged to become involved in the Crohn's and Colitis Foundation of America (CCFA). National headquarters may be contacted at 444 Park Avenue South, 11th Floor, New York, NY 10016-7374; phone 212-685-3440. Internet address: http://www.ccfa.org.

1. Crohn's Disease

 ESSENTIALS OF DIAGNOSIS

- Insidious onset.
- Intermittent bouts of low-grade fever, diarrhea, and right lower quadrant pain.
- Right lower quadrant mass and tenderness.
- Perianal disease with abscess, fistulas.
- Radiographic evidence of ulceration, stricturing, or fistulas of the small intestine or colon.

General Considerations

One-third of cases of Crohn's disease involve only the small bowel, most commonly the terminal ileum (ileitis). Half of cases involve the small bowel and colon, most often the terminal ileum and adjacent proximal ascending colon (ileocolitis). In 20% of cases, the colon alone is affected. Unlike ulcerative colitis, Crohn's disease is a transmural process that can result in mucosal inflammation and ulceration, stricturing, fistula development, and abscess formation.

Clinical Findings

A. SYMPTOMS AND SIGNS

Because of the variable location of involvement and severity of inflammation, Crohn's disease may present with a variety of symptoms and signs. In eliciting the history, the clinician should take particular note of fevers, the patient's general sense of well-being, the presence of abdominal pain, the number of liquid bowel movements per day, and prior surgical resections. Physical examination should focus upon the patient's temperature, weight, and nutritional status, the presence of abdominal tenderness or an abdominal mass, rectal examination, and extraintestinal manifestations. Most commonly, there is one or a combination of the following clinical constellations.

1. Chronic inflammatory disease—This is the most common presentation and is often seen in patients with ileitis or ileocolitis. Patients report low-grade fever, malaise, weight loss, and loss of energy. There may be diarrhea, which is nonbloody and often intermittent. Cramping or steady right lower quadrant or periumbilical pain is present. Physical examination re-

veals focal tenderness, usually in the right lower quadrant. A palpable, tender mass that represents thickened or matted loops of inflamed intestine may be present in the lower abdomen.

2. Intestinal obstruction—Narrowing of the small bowel may occur as a result of inflammation, spasm, or fibrotic stenosis. Patients report postprandial bloating, cramping pains, and loud borborygmi. This sometimes occurs in patients with active inflammatory symptoms (as above). More commonly, however, it occurs later in the disease from chronic fibrosis without other systemic symptoms or signs of inflammation.

3. Fistulization with or without infection—A subset of patients develop sinus tracts that penetrate through the bowel and form fistulas to a number of locations. Fistulas to the mesentery are usually asymptomatic but can result in intra-abdominal or retroperitoneal abscesses manifested by fevers, chills, a tender abdominal mass, and leukocytosis. Fistulas from the colon to the small intestine or stomach can result in bacterial overgrowth with diarrhea, weight loss, and malnutrition. Fistulas to the bladder or vagina produce recurrent infections. Enterocutaneous fistulas usually occur at the site of surgical scars.

4. Perianal disease—One-third of patients with either large or small bowel involvement develop perianal disease manifested by anal fissures, perianal abscesses, and fistulas.

5. Extraintestinal manifestations—The extracolonic manifestations (described in the section on ulcerative colitis) may also be seen with Crohn's disease, particularly Crohn's colitis. Other problems may also arise. Oral aphthous lesions are common. There is an increased prevalence of gallstones due to malabsorption of bile salts from the terminal ileum. Nephrolithiasis with urate or calcium oxalate stones may occur.

B. LABORATORY FINDINGS

There is a poor correlation between laboratory studies and the patient's clinical picture. Laboratory values may reflect inflammatory activity or nutritional complications of disease. A complete blood count and serum albumin should be obtained in all patients. Anemia may reflect chronic inflammation, mucosal blood loss, iron deficiency, or vitamin B_{12} malabsorption secondary to terminal ileal inflammation or resection. Leukocytosis may reflect inflammation or abscess formation or may be secondary to corticosteroid therapy. Hypoalbuminemia may be due to intestinal protein loss (protein-losing enteropathy), malabsorption, or chronic inflammation. The sedimentation rate or C-reactive protein level is elevated in many patients during active inflammation. Stool specimens are sent for examination for routine pathogens, ova and parasites, and *C difficile* toxin.

C. SPECIAL DIAGNOSTIC STUDIES

In most patients, the initial diagnosis of Crohn's disease is based upon a compatible clinical picture with supporting radiographic findings. An upper gastrointestinal series with small bowel follow-through is obtained in all patients. Suggestive findings include ulcerations, strictures, and fistulas. To evaluate the colon, a barium enema or colonoscopy is obtained. Colonoscopy offers the advantage of obtaining mucosal biopsies of the colon or terminal ileum. Typical endoscopic findings include aphthoid ulcers, linear or stellate ulcers, strictures, and segmental involvement with areas of normal-appearing mucosa adjacent to inflamed mucosa. In 10% of cases, it may be difficult to distinguish ulcerative colitis from Crohn's disease. When the diagnosis remains uncertain, two serologic tests may be useful in further distinguishing these two diseases. Antineutrophil cytoplasmic antibodies with perinuclear staining (p-ANCA) are found in 50–70% of patients with ulcerative colitis and 5–10% of patients with Crohn's disease. Antibodies to the yeast *S cerevisiae* (ASCA) are found in 60–70% of patients with Crohn's disease and 10–15% of patients with ulcerative colitis. A combination of p-ANCA negativity and ASCA positivity has a 95% positive predictive value and 92% specificity for a diagnosis of Crohn's disease. Conversely, p-ANCA positivity and ASCA negativity has an 88% positive predictive value and 98% specificity for the diagnosis of ulcerative colitis. The presence of granulomas on biopsy are seen in less than 25% of patients but are highly suggestive of Crohn's disease.

Complications

A. Abscess

The presence of a tender abdominal mass with fever and leukocytosis suggests an abscess. Emergent CT of the abdomen is necessary to confirm the diagnosis. Patients should be given broad-spectrum antibiotics and, if malnourished, maintained on TPN. Percutaneous drainage or surgery is usually required.

B. Obstruction

Small bowel obstruction may develop secondary to active inflammation or chronic fibrotic stricturing and is often acutely precipitated by dietary indiscretion. Patients should be given intravenous fluids with nasogastric suction for several days. Systemic steroids are indicated in patients with symptoms or signs of active inflammation but are unhelpful in patients with inactive, fixed disease. Patients unimproved on medical management require surgical resection of the stenotic area or stricturoplasty.

C. Fistulas

The majority of enteromesenteric and enteroenteric fistulas are asymptomatic and require no specific therapy. Most symptomatic fistulas require surgical therapy, particularly when there is evidence of intestinal stricturing below the fistula. Medical therapy is effective in a subset of patients and is usually tried before surgery. Although fistulas may close temporarily in response to TPN or oral elemental diets, they recur when oral feedings are resumed. Azathioprine or mercaptopurine heals fistulas in 30–40% of patients but requires 3–6 months. The anti-TNF antibody infliximab is the most effective medical therapy for chronic fistulizing Crohn's disease. Infliximab injections (5 mg/kg) given at 0, 2, and 6 weeks result in complete closure of fistulas (both perianal and abdominal) in up to half of patients and improvement in up to 75%. In patients treated with infliximab, it is recommended that mercaptopurine or azathioprine also be given to reduce the otherwise high likelihood of fistula recurrence. Rapid closure of perianal fistulas may lead to abscess in patients with active perianal infection. Although cyclosporine has demonstrated some value for fistulous disease, high relapse rates and the risk of toxicity have limited its use.

D. Perianal Disease

Patients with fissures, fistulas, and skin tags commonly have perianal discomfort. Severe pain should suggest a perianal abscess. The treatment of perianal problems can be very difficult. Initial conservative treatment with sitz baths, attempts to control diarrhea, and application of perianal cotton balls to absorb irritating drainage are warranted. Metronidazole, 250 mg three times daily, or ciprofloxacin, 500 mg twice daily, are commonly given but have not been proved to be efficacious. Aminosalicylates are of no benefit. Steroids are of no value and may retard healing. The role of mercaptopurine or azathioprine and infliximab is discussed in the section on fistulas. Patients with abscesses require conservative incision and drainage. Surgical fistulotomy should be avoided in the presence of active Crohn's disease because there is a risk of poor wound healing or incontinence. Patients may benefit from placement of noncutting drains, which allows drainage and improves comfort while medical treatment with antibiotics, azathioprine, or infliximab is instituted.

E. Carcinoma

Patients with extensive colonic Crohn's disease are at increased risk of developing colon carcinoma. Screening colonoscopy to detect dysplasia or cancer is recommended by most authorities for patients with a history of 8 or more years of Crohn's colitis.

F. Hemorrhage

Unlike ulcerative colitis, severe hemorrhage is unusual in Crohn's disease.

G. Malabsorption

Malabsorption may arise from bacterial overgrowth in patients with enterocolonic fistulas, strictures and stasis, extensive jejunal inflammation, and prior surgical resections.

Differential Diagnosis

Chronic cramping abdominal pain and diarrhea are typical of both irritable bowel syndrome and Crohn's disease, but x-ray examinations are normal in the former. Acute fever and right lower quadrant pain may resemble appendicitis or *Yersinia enterocolitica* enteritis. Intestinal lymphoma causes fever, pain, weight loss, and abnormal small bowel radiographs that may mimic Crohn's disease. Patients with undiagnosed AIDS may present with fever and diarrhea. Segmental colitis may be caused by tuberculosis, *Entamoeba histolytica,* chlamydia, or ischemic colitis. Diverticulitis with abscess formation may be difficult to distinguish acutely from Crohn's disease. NSAID-induced colitis may cause diarrhea with or without bleeding, abdominal pain, and anemia. They cause strictures or colitis characterized by erosions or ulcers that tend to be most severe in the right colon.

Treatment of Active Disease

Crohn's disease is a chronic lifelong illness characterized by exacerbations and periods of remission. As no specific therapy exists, current treatment is directed toward symptomatic improvement and controlling the disease process. The treatment must address the specific problems of the individual patient.

A. Nutrition

1. Diet—Patients should eat a well-balanced diet with as few restrictions as possible. There is no convincing evidence of specific food allergy in disease pathogenesis. Because lactose intolerance is common, a trial off dairy products is warranted if flatulence or diarrhea is a prominent complaint. Patients with mainly colonic involvement benefit from fiber supplementation. Conversely, patients with obstructive symptoms should be placed on a low-roughage diet, ie, no raw fruits or vegetables, popcorn, nuts, etc. Resection of more than 100 cm of terminal ileum results in fat malabsorption. A low-fat diet with medium-chain triglyceride supplementation is used. Iron supplements may be necessary in patients with chronic intestinal blood loss. Parenteral vitamin B_{12} (100 μg intramuscularly per month) commonly is needed for patients with previous ileal resection or extensive terminal ileal disease.

2. Enteral therapy—Enteral therapy for 4 weeks is less effective than corticosteroids in inducing remission, and the relapse rate after return to a normal diet is high. Nevertheless, it may be considered in patients (especially children) who are refractory in an attempt to avoid chronic corticosteroids.

3. Total parenteral nutrition—TPN is used short-term in patients with active disease and progressive weight loss or those awaiting surgery who have malnutrition but cannot tolerate enteral feedings because of high-grade obstruction, high-output fistulas, severe diarrhea, or abdominal pain. It is required long-term in a small subset of patients with extensive intestinal resections resulting in short bowel syndrome with malnutrition.

B. Symptomatic Medications

1. Symptomatic treatment of diarrhea—There are several potential mechanisms by which diarrhea may occur in Crohn's disease in addition to active Crohn's disease. A rational empirical treatment approach often yields therapeutic improvement that may obviate the need for corticosteroids or immunosuppressive agents. Involvement of the terminal ileum with Crohn's disease or prior ileal resection may lead to reduced absorption of bile acids that may induce secretory diarrhea from the colon. This diarrhea commonly responds to cholestyramine 2–4 g or colestipol 5 g two or three times daily before meals to bind the malabsorbed bile salts. Patients with extensive ileal disease or more than 100 cm of ileal resection have such severe bile salt malabsorption that steatorrhea may arise. Such patients may benefit from a low-fat diet; bile salt binding agents will exacerbate the diarrhea and should not be given. Patients with Crohn's disease are at risk for the development of small intestinal bacterial overgrowth due to enteral fistulas, ileal resection, and impaired motility and may benefit from a course of broad-spectrum antibiotics (see Bacterial Overgrowth, above). Other causes of diarrhea include lactase deficiency and short bowel syndrome (described in other sections). Use of antidiarrheals may provide benefit in some patients. Loperamide (2–4 mg), diphenoxylate with atropine (one tablet), or tincture of opium (5–15 drops) may be given as needed up to four times daily. Because of the risk of toxic megacolon, these drugs should not be used in patients with active severe colitis.

C. Specific Drug Therapy

1. 5-Aminosalicylic acid agents—Sulfasalazine, 1.5–2 g twice daily, is effective in reducing clinical signs of disease activity in patients with colonic involvement but confers little benefit in small intestine disease. Although mesalamine (Asacol) and its slow-release form (Pentasa) are approved only for the treatment of ulcerative colitis, their release in the small intestine offers usefulness in the treatment of small bowel Crohn's disease. Remission rates of over 40% are reported in patients with mild to moderate small bowel and ileocecal disease, particularly when these agents are used at high dosages (Pentasa 1 g four times daily; Asacol 0.8–1.2 g four times daily).

2. Antibiotics—For patients with mild disease who do not respond to aminosalicylates, antibiotic therapy with metronidazole (10 mg/kg/d) or ciprofloxacin (500 mg twice daily) appears to be as effective as aminosalicylates in controlled trials. Ciprofloxacin may be better for ileitis and metronidazole for ileocolitis or colitis.

3. Corticosteroids—Corticosteroids dramatically suppress the acute clinical symptoms or signs in most patients with both small and large bowel disease. However, steroids do not appear to alter the underlying disease. Prednisone, 40–60 mg/d, is generally administered to patients with an active flare-up of Crohn's disease. After improvement at 2–3 weeks, tapering proceeds at 5 mg/wk until a dosage of 20 mg/d is being given. Thereafter, very slow tapering of 2.5 mg/wk or every other week is recommended. Some patients cannot be completely withdrawn from steroids without experiencing a symptomatic flare-up. Use of chronic low corticosteroid doses (2.5–10 mg/d) should be avoided, if possible, because of associated complications including aseptic necrosis of the hips, osteoporosis, cataracts, diabetes, and hypertension. Patients requiring chronic corticosteroid treatment should be given 5-ASA derivatives or immunomodulatory drugs (as described below) in an effort to wean them from corticosteroids. Alendronate should be considered to prevent osteoporosis in patients requiring chronic corticosteroids. An ileal-release preparation of the oral topically active compound budesonide, 9 mg once daily for 8 weeks, induces remission in 50–70% of patients with mild to moderate Crohn's disease involving the terminal ileum or ascending colon. It is superior to that of mesalamine and comparable to prednisone, with fewer steroid-related adverse effects and less suppression of the pituitary-adrenal axis. Its role relative to other steroids for treatment of acute disease is unclear at present.

Patients with persisting symptoms despite oral steroids or those with high fever, persistent vomiting, evidence of intestinal obstruction, severe weight loss, severe abdominal tenderness, or suspicion of an abscess should be hospitalized. In patients with a tender, palpable inflammatory abdominal mass, CT scan of the abdomen should be obtained prior to administering steroids in order to rule out an abscess. If no abscess is identified, parenteral steroids should be administered (as described for ulcerative colitis). Nutritional support with enteral elemental feedings or parenteral nutrition is indicated for patients unable to tolerate an oral diet after 5 days.

4. Immunomodulatory drugs—Azathioprine (2–2.5 mg/kg) and mercaptopurine (1–1.5 mg/kg) are effective in the long-term treatment of Crohn's disease. They are most useful in the management of patients with unresponsive disease, those requiring chronic corticosteroids, and those with symptomatic fistulas. These agents permit elimination or reduction of steroids in over 75% and fistula closure in 30%. Blood counts should be monitored weekly for the first month, then monthly. Drug dosages should be monitored to maintain a white blood cell count > 3000/μL. Side effects requiring withdrawal of the drug occur in about 10%. The mean time to symptomatic response is 4 months, so these agents are not useful for acute exacerbations. Once patients achieve remission, these drugs reduce the 3-year relapse rate from over 60% to less than 25%. Methotrexate (25 mg intramuscularly weekly for 12 weeks, followed by 12.5–15 mg intramuscularly once weekly) probably is less efficacious but is used in patients who are unresponsive to or intolerant of mercaptopurine or azathioprine. Other immunosuppressive agents have been investigated in the treatment of Crohn's disease, including cyclosporine and thalidomide; however, efficacy has been modest and toxicity greater than with the thiopurines.

A chimeric IgG anti-TNF antibody, infliximab, is increasingly being used for the treatment of active moderate to severe Crohn's disease. After a single dose of 5 mg/kg, improvement occurs in two-thirds and remission in one-third of patients. Maximal response is seen within 2 weeks in most patients and gradually diminishes over 3 months. Antinuclear antibodies and human antichimeric antibodies may develop, leading to a risk of infusion-related reactions, hypersensitivity reactions, and a lupus-like syndrome. Infliximab appears to be most useful in patients with moderate to severe Crohn's disease to promote rapid initial improvement while other immunosuppressives that take weeks to months to achieve therapeutic results, such as azathioprine or mercaptopurine, are being initiated. Re-treatment with infliximab every 8 weeks is required in some patients. Limited experience suggests that efficacy is maintained during long-term treatment. Serious infections may occur in patients taking infliximab, including sepsis, disseminated tuberculosis, invasive fungal infections, listeriosis, pneumocystosis, and other opportunistic infections. All patients should be evaluated with a tuberculin skin test prior to initiation of infliximab therapy.

Maintenance of Remission

Crohn's disease is characterized by exacerbations and remissions. Meta-analysis confirms a modest (6.3%) but significant reduction in disease recurrence in patients treated with mesalamine (Asacol, 800 mg three times daily; or Pentasa, 500–750 mg four times daily). The benefit appears to be greatest in patients with ileal disease or recent surgical resection of active disease. Corticosteroids should not be used in patients with inactive disease to maintain remission. The topically active steroid budesonide has not demonstrated convincing efficacy or safety as maintenance therapy at 1 year. The purine analogs (azathioprine, mercaptopurine) and methotrexate have had a definite impact on maintaining remission and should be used in patients with frequent recurrences and in those who require chronic corticosteroid therapy.

Indications for Surgery

Over half of patients will require at least one surgical procedure. The main indications for surgery are intractability to medical therapy, intra-abdominal abscess, massive bleeding, and obstruction with fibrous stricture. Patients with active inflammation who are unresponsive to medical therapy or who require chronic prednisone in doses exceeding 15 mg/d may achieve dramatic relief from limited excision for 5–15 years before disease recurs.

Prognosis

With proper medical and surgical treatment, the majority of patients are able to cope with this chronic disease and its complications and lead productive lives. Few patients die as a direct consequence of the disease.

Blam M et al: Integrating anti-tumor necrosis factor therapy in inflammatory bowel disease: current and future perspectives. Am J Gastroenterol 2001;96:1977. [PMID: 11467623]

Cosnes J et al: Smoking cessation and the course of Crohn's disease: an intervention study. Gastroenterology 2001;120:1093. [PMID: 11266373] (Patients with Crohn's disease who stopped smoking had a 65% reduction in disease relapse compared with continuing smokers.)

Feagan B et al: A comparison of methotrexate with placebo for the maintenance of remission in Crohn's disease. N Engl J Med 2000;343:1627. [PMID: 10833208] (Methotrexate has modest efficacy in the treatment of active Crohn's disease and maintenance of Crohn's remission.)

Lemann M et al: Methotrexate in Crohn's disease: long-term efficacy and toxicity. Am J Gastroenterol 2000;95:1730. [PMID: 10925976]

Regueiro M. Update in medical treatment of Crohn's disease. J Clin Gastroenterol 2000;31:282. [PMID: 11129268]

Ricart E et al: Infliximab in Crohn's disease in clinical practice at the Mayo Clinic: the first 100 patients. Am J Gastroenterol 2001;96:722. [PMID: 11280541]

Schwartz D et al: Diagnosis and treatment of perianal fistulas in Crohn disease. Ann Intern Med 2001;135:906. [PMID: 11712881]

Valentine JF et al: Prevention and treatment of osteoporosis in patients with inflammatory bowel disease. Am J Gastroenterol 1999;94:878. [PMID: 10201450]

2. Ulcerative Colitis

 ESSENTIALS OF DIAGNOSIS

- Bloody diarrhea.
- Lower abdominal cramps and fecal urgency.
- Anemia, low serum albumin.
- Negative stool cultures.
- Sigmoidoscopy is the key to diagnosis.

General Considerations

Ulcerative colitis is an idiopathic inflammatory condition that involves the mucosal surface of the colon, resulting in diffuse friability and erosions with bleeding. Approximately 50% of patients have disease confined to the rectosigmoid region (proctosigmoiditis); 30% extend to the splenic flexure (left-sided colitis); and less than 20% extend more proximally (extensive colitis). There is some correlation between disease extent and symptom severity. In the majority of patients, the extent of colonic involvement does not progress over time. In most patients, the disease is characterized by periods of symptomatic flare-ups and remissions. Ulcerative colitis is more common in nonsmokers and former smokers. Disease severity may be lower in active smokers and may worsen in patients who stop smoking. Appendectomy before the age of 20 for acute appendicitis is associated with a reduced risk of developing ulcerative colitis.

Clinical Findings

A. SYMPTOMS AND SIGNS

The clinical profile in ulcerative colitis is highly variable. Bloody diarrhea is the hallmark. On the basis of several clinical and laboratory parameters, it is clinically useful to classify patients as having mild, moderate, or severe disease (Table 14–14). Patients should be asked about stool frequency, the presence and amount of rectal bleeding, cramps, abdominal pain, fecal urgency, and tenesmus. Physical examination should focus upon the patient's volume status as determined by orthostatic blood pressure and pulse measurements and by nutritional status. On abdominal examination, the clinician should look for tenderness and evidence of peritoneal inflammation. Red blood may be present on digital rectal examination.

1. Mild to moderate disease—Patients with mild disease have a gradual onset of infrequent diarrhea (less than five movements per day) with intermittent rectal bleeding and mucus. Stools may be formed too loose in consistency. Because of rectal inflammation, there is fecal urgency and tenesmus. Left lower quadrant cramps relieved by defecation are common, but there is no significant abdominal tenderness. Patients with moderate disease have more severe diarrhea with frequent bleeding. Abdominal pain and tenderness may be present but are not severe. There may be mild fever, anemia, and hypoalbuminemia.

2. Severe disease—Patients with severe disease have more than six to ten bloody bowel movements per day, resulting in severe anemia, hypovolemia, and impaired nutrition with hypoalbuminemia. Abdominal pain and tenderness are present. "Fulminant colitis" is a subset of severe disease characterized by rapidly worsening symptoms with signs of toxicity.

Table 14–14. Ulcerative colitis: Assessment of disease activity.

	Mild	Moderate	Severe
Stool frequency (per day)	< 4	4–6	> 6 (mostly bloody)
Pulse (beats/min)	< 90	90–100	> 100
Hematocrit (%)	Normal	30–40	< 30
Weight loss (%)	None	1–10	> 10
Temperature (°F)	Normal	99–100	> 100
ESR (mm/h)	< 20	20–30	> 30
Albumin (g/dL)	Normal	3–3.5	< 3

3. Extracolonic manifestations—Ulcerative colitis is associated with extraintestinal manifestations in 25% of cases. Some extracolonic signs are associated with disease activity. These include erythema nodosum, pyoderma gangrenosum, episcleritis, thromboembolic events, and an oligoarticular, nondeforming arthritis. In patients who are HLA B27-seropositive, there may be anterior uveitis or ankylosing spondylitis which is independent of colitis activity. Sclerosing cholangitis can occur in colitis patients even after total colectomy. Patients with this entity are at higher risk of developing cholangiocarcinoma.

B. Laboratory Findings

The degree of abnormality of the hematocrit, sedimentation rate, and serum albumin reflect disease severity.

C. Endoscopy

In acute colitis, the diagnosis is readily established by sigmoidoscopy. The mucosal appearance is characterized by edema, friability, mucopus, and erosions. Colonoscopy should not be performed in patients with severe disease because of the risk of perforation. After patients have demonstrated improvement on therapy, colonoscopy is sometimes performed to determine the extent of disease, which will dictate the need for subsequent cancer surveillance.

D. Imaging

Plain abdominal radiographs are obtained in patients with severe colitis to look for significant colonic dilation. Barium enemas are of little utility in the evaluation of acute ulcerative colitis and may precipitate toxic megacolon in patients with severe disease.

Differential Diagnosis

The initial presentation of ulcerative colitis is indistinguishable from other causes of colitis, clinically as well as endoscopically. Thus, the diagnosis of idiopathic ulcerative colitis is reached after excluding other known causes of colitis. Infectious colitis should be excluded by sending stool specimens for routine bacterial cultures (to exclude salmonella, shigella, and campylobacter), ova and parasites (to exclude amebiasis), and stool toxin assay for *C difficile*. Mucosal biopsy can distinguish amebic colitis from ulcerative colitis. Enteroinvasive *E coli* and *E coli* O157:H7 will not be detected on routine bacterial cultures. CMV colitis occurs in immunocompromised patients (especially those with AIDS) and is diagnosed on mucosal biopsy. Gonorrhea, chlamydial infection, herpes, and syphilis are considerations in sexually active patients with proctitis. In elderly patients with cardiovascular disease, ischemic colitis may involve the rectosigmoid. A history of radiation to the pelvic region can result in proctitis months to years later. Crohn's disease involving the colon but not the small intestine may be confused with ulcerative colitis. In 10% of patients, a distinction between Crohn's disease and ulcerative colitis may not be possible. The utility of ANCA and ASCA antibodies in these difficult patients is discussed in the section on Crohn's disease.

Treatment
(Table 14–15)

There are two main treatment objectives: (1) to terminate the acute, symptomatic attack and (2) to prevent recurrence of attacks. The treatment of acute ulcerative colitis is dependent upon the extent of colonic involvement and the severity of illness.

Patients with mild to moderate disease should eat a regular diet but limit their intake of caffeine and gas producing vegetables. Fiber supplements decrease diarrhea and rectal symptoms (psyllium, 3.4 g twice daily; methylcellulose, 2 g twice daily; bran powder, 1 tbsp twice daily). Antidiarrheal agents should not be given in the acute phase of illness but are safe and helpful in patients with mild chronic symptoms. Loperamide (2 mg), diphenoxylate with atropine (one tablet), or tincture of opium (8–15 drops) may be given up to four times daily. Such remedies are particularly useful at nighttime and when taken prophylactically for occasions when patients may not have reliable access to toilet facilities.

A. Distal Colitis

Patients with disease confined to the rectum or rectosigmoid region generally have mild but distressing symptoms. Acute therapy is best approached with topical agents. Topical mesalamine is the drug of choice and is superior to topical corticosteroids. Mesalamine is administered as a suppository, 500 mg twice daily for proctitis, and as an enema, 4 g at bedtime for proctosigmoiditis, for 3–12 weeks, with 75% of patients

Table 14–15. Treatment of ulcerative colitis.

Distal colitis
  Proctitis
    Mesalamine suppositories, 500 mg per rectum twice daily, or—
    Hydrocortisone foam, 90 mg per rectum daily, or—
    Hydrocortisone suppositories, 100 mg per rectum daily
  Proctosigmoiditis
    Mesalamine enema, 4 g per rectum daily, or—
    Hydrocortisone enema, 100 mg per rectum daily
Extensive colitis
  Mild to moderate
    Sulfasalazine, 1.5–3 g orally twice daily, or—
    Mesalamine tablets (delayed release), 2.4–4 g/d, or—
    Olsalazine, 0.75–1.5 g orally twice daily
    If no response after 2–4 weeks, add prednisone, 40–60 mg/d (taper by 5 mg/wk)
  Severe
    Methylprednisolone, 48–60 mg IV daily

improving. Topical steroids are a less expensive alternative to mesalamine but are also less effective. Hydrocortisone suppository or foam is prescribed for proctitis and hydrocortisone enema (80–100 mg) for proctosigmoiditis. Systemic effects from short-term use are very slight. It is not known whether combination therapy with mesalamine and hydrocortisone is advantageous. Patients with distal disease who fail to improve with topical therapy should be considered for systemic steroids or immunosuppressives as described below.

Patients whose acute symptoms resolve with acute therapy have an 80–90% chance of a symptomatic relapse within 1 year. Maintenance therapy with mesalamine suppositories (500 mg daily) or with oral agents (see below) reduce the relapse rate to less than 20% per year.

B. Mild to Moderate Colitis

Disease extending above the sigmoid colon is best treated with oral agents. The currently available agents, derivatives of 5-aminosalicylic acid (5-ASA: sulfasalazine, mesalamine, balsalazide), result in symptomatic improvement in 50–75% of patients. Balsalazide, 2.25 g three times daily, appears to be as effective as or more effective than other 5-ASA agents and soon may become the drug of first choice for treatment of mild to moderate ulcerative colitis. Mesalamine, 800 mg three times daily (Asacol) or 1 g four times daily (Pentasa), is also approved for active disease. Higher doses (4–6 g daily) may be required in some patients. Because it is significantly less expensive than balsalazide or mesalamine, sulfasalazine is still commonly used as a first-line agent by many providers. To minimize side effects, sulfasalazine is begun at a dosage of 500 mg twice daily and increased gradually over 1–2 weeks to 2 g twice daily. Most patients improve within 3 weeks, though some require 2–3 months. Total doses of 5–6 g/d may have greater efficacy but are poorly tolerated. Folic acid, 1 mg/d, should be administered to all patients taking sulfasalazine. Balsalazide or mesalamine should be used in patients intolerant of sulfasalazine. It has been suggested that a nicotine patch (22 mg) is effective in symptom improvement in patients with mild to moderate ulcerative colitis, but this is not yet be recommended for routine clinical use.

Patients with mild to moderate disease who fail to improve after 2–3 weeks of 5-ASA therapy should have the addition of corticosteroid therapy. Topical therapy with hydrocortisone foam or enemas (80–100 mg twice daily) may be tried first. Patients who fail to improve after 2 more weeks require systemic steroid therapy. Prednisone and methylprednisolone are most commonly used. Depending on the severity of illness, the initial oral dose of prednisone is 20–30 mg twice daily. Rapid improvement is observed in most cases. One can usually begin to taper prednisone after 2 weeks. Tapering of prednisone should proceed by no more than 5 mg/wk. After tapering to 15 mg/d, slower tapering is sometimes required. Complete tapering without symptomatic flare-ups is possible in the majority of patients.

C. Severe Colitis

About 10–15% of ulcerative colitis patients have a more severe course. Because they may deteriorate rapidly, hospitalization is generally required.

1. General measures—
a. Discontinue all oral intake. Total parenteral nutrition is indicated in patients with poor nutritional status.
b. Avoid all opiate or anticholinergic agents.
c. Restore circulating volume with fluids and blood as needed. Correct electrolyte abnormalities.
d. Perform frequent abdominal examinations to look for evidence of worsening distention or pain.
e. Obtain a plain abdominal radiograph on admission to look for evidence of colonic dilation.
f. Obtain surgical consultation in all patients with severe disease.
g. Send stools for bacterial (including *C difficile*) culture and examination for ova and parasites.

2. Corticosteroid therapy—Methylprednisolone, 48–64 mg, or hydrocortisone, 300 mg, is administered in four divided doses or by continuous infusion over 24 hours. Higher or "pulse" doses are of no benefit. Hydrocortisone enemas may also be administered twice daily as a drip, 100 mg over 30 minutes. In patients who have not previously received corticosteroids, administration of ACTH, 120 units/24 h, may be superior to corticosteroids. Approximately 50–75% of patients achieve remission with systemic steroids within 7–10 days. Once symptomatic improvement has occurred, oral fluids are reinstituted. If fluids are well tolerated, intravenous steroids are discontinued and the patient is started on oral prednisone (as described for moderate disease).

3. Cyclosporine—Intravenous cyclosporine (4 mg/kg/d) benefits 60–75% of patients with severe colitis who have not improved after 7–10 days of corticosteroids. This therapy may be considered in patients with severe steroid-resistant colitis who are reluctant to undergo colectomy. Up to two thirds of responders may be maintained in remission with a combination of oral cyclosporine for 3 months and long-term therapy with mercaptopurine or azathioprine.

4. Surgical therapy—Patients with severe disease who fail to improve after 7–10 days of corticosteroid or cyclosporine therapy are unlikely to respond to further medical therapy, and surgery is recommended.

D. Fulminant Colitis and Toxic Megacolon

A subset of patients with severe disease have a more fulminant course with rapid progression of symptoms over 1–2 weeks and signs of severe toxicity. These patients appear quite ill, with prominent hypovolemia, hemorrhage requiring transfusion, and abdominal distention with tenderness. They are at a higher risk of perforation or development of toxic megacolon and must be followed closely. Broad-spectrum antibiotics should be administered to cover anaerobes and gram-negative bacteria.

Toxic megacolon develops in less than 2% of cases of ulcerative colitis. It is characterized by colonic dilation of more than 6 cm on plain films with signs of toxicity. In addition to the therapies outlined above, nasogastric suction should be initiated. Patients should be instructed to roll from side to side and onto the abdomen in an effort to decompress the distended colon. Serial abdominal plain films should be obtained to look for worsening dilation or ischemia. Patients with fulminant disease or toxic megacolon who worsen or fail to improve within 48–72 hours should undergo surgery to prevent perforation. If operation is performed before perforation, the mortality rate should be low.

Maintenance of Remission

Without chronic therapy, 75% of patients who initially go into remission on medical therapy will experience a symptomatic relapse within 1 year. Chronic maintenance therapy with sulfasalazine, 1–1.5 g twice daily; olsalazine, 500 mg twice daily; and mesalamine, 800 mg three times daily or 500 mg four times daily has been shown to reduce relapse rates to less than 33%.

Refractory Disease

A subset of patients either do not respond to aminosalicylates or corticosteroids or have symptomatic flares during attempts at steroid tapering. Surgical resection is traditionally recommended for patients with refractory disease. However, some patients may wish to avoid surgery and others have moderately severe disease for which surgery might not otherwise be warranted. Limited trials suggest that immunosuppressive therapy with mercaptopurine or azathioprine are of benefit in 60% of patients, allowing tapering of steroids and maintenance of remission. The risks of these agents and chronic immunosuppression must be weighed against the certainty of cure with surgical resection. A single intravenous infusion of infliximab (5 mg/kg) has resulted anecdotally in rapid and sustained clinical and endoscopic improvement in 50–100% of patients with refractory ulcerative colitis.

Risk of Colon Cancer

In ulcerative colitis patients with disease proximal to the sigmoid colon, there is a markedly increased risk of developing colon carcinoma. In patients who have had colitis for more than 10 years, the risk of developing colon cancer increases approximately 0.5–1% per year. Ingestion of folic acid, 1 mg/d, is associated with a decreased risk of cancer development. Colonoscopies are recommended every 1–2 years in patients with extensive colitis, beginning 8–10 years after diagnosis. At colonoscopy, multiple (at least 32) random mucosal biopsies are taken throughout the colon at 10-cm intervals as well as biopsies of mass lesions to look for dysplasia or carcinoma. Because of the relatively high incidence of concomitant carcinoma in patients with dysplasia (either low- or high-grade) in flat mucosa or mass lesions, colectomy is recommended. When low-grade dysplasia is detected only in flat mucosa, some authorities recommend a repeat colonoscopy in 3–6 months to confirm the presence of dysplasia before proceeding with colectomy.

Surgery in Ulcerative Colitis

Surgery is required in 25% of patients. Severe hemorrhage, perforation, and documented carcinoma are absolute indications for surgery. Surgery is indicated also in patients with fulminant colitis or toxic megacolon that does not improve within 48–72 hours, in patients with dysplasia on surveillance colonoscopy, and in patients with refractory disease requiring chronic steroids to control symptoms.

Although total proctocolectomy (with placement of an ileostomy) provides complete cure of the disease, most patients seek to avoid it out of concern for the impact it may have upon their bowel function, their self-image, and their social interactions. After complete colectomy, patients may have a standard ileostomy with an external appliance, a continent ileostomy, or an internal ileal pouch which is anastomosed to the anal canal (ileoanal anastomosis). The latter maintains intestinal continuity, thereby obviating an ostomy. Under optimal circumstances, patients have five to seven loose bowel movements per day without incontinence. Endoscopic or histologic inflammation in the ileal pouch ("pouchitis") develops in over one-fourth of patients, resulting in increased stool frequency, fecal urgency, cramping, and bleeding, but usually resolves with a 2-week course of metronidazole (20 mg/kg/d) or ciprofloxacin (1000 mg/d). Oral therapy with nonpathogenic bacteria ("probiotics") is effective in maintaining remission in patients with recurrent pouchitis. Refractory cases of proctitis can be disabling and may require conversion to a standard ileostomy.

Prognosis

Ulcerative colitis is a lifelong disease characterized by exacerbations and remissions. For most patients, the disease is readily controlled by medical therapy without need for surgery. The majority never require hospitalization. A subset of patients with more severe disease will require surgery, which results in complete cure of the disease. Properly managed, most ulcerative colitis patients lead close to normal productive lives.

Andersson R et al: Appendectomy and protection against ulcerative colitis. N Engl J Med 2001;344:808. [PMID: 11248156]

Beaugerie L et al: Impact of cessation of smoking on the course of ulcerative colitis. Am J Gastroenterol 2001;96:2113. [PMID: 11467641]

Chey W et al: Infliximab therapy for refractory ulcerative colitis. Am J Gastroenterol 2001;96:2373. [PMID: 11513177]

Cottone M et al: Prevalence of cytomegalovirus infection in severe refractory ulcerative and Crohn's colitis. Am J Gastroenterol 2001;96:773. [PMID: 11280549]

D'Haens G et al: Intravenous cyclosporine versus intravenous corticosteroids as single therapy for severe attacks of ulcerative colitis. Gastroenterology 2001;120:1323. [PMID: 11313301]

Marshall JK et al: Putting rectal 5-amino salicylate acid in its place: the role in distal ulcerative colitis. Am J Gastroenterol 2000;95:1628. [PMID: 10925961]

Provenzale D et al: Surveillance issues in inflammatory bowel disease. J Clin Gastroenterol 2001;32:99. [PMID: 11205664]

Shen B et al: Endoscopic and histologic evaluation together with symptom assessment are required to diagnose pouchitis. Gastroenterology 2001;121:261. [PMID: 11487535]

3. Microscopic Colitis

Microscopic colitis is an idiopathic condition in which patients have chronic watery diarrhea with normal-appearing mucosa at endoscopy. Histologic evaluation of mucosal biopsies, however, reveals lymphocytic inflammation in the lamina propria. It occurs much more commonly in women, especially in the fifth to sixth decades. Symptoms tend to be chronic or recurrent but may remit spontaneously after many years. Chronic NSAID therapy has been implicated as a causative factor in up to half of cases. There appear to be two subtypes—lymphocytic colitis and collagenous colitis—the latter distinguished by the presence of a thickened band of collagen below the epithelium. Mild disease may be treated with bulking agents or antidiarrheal agents (loperamide, cholestyramine). Treatment with 5-aminosalicylates (sulfasalazine, mesalamine) is of unproved benefit. Bismuth subsalicylate (two tablets four times daily) for 2 months may proved to be effective.

Fiedler LM et al: Treatment responses in collagenous colitis. Am J Gastroenterol 2001;96:818. [PMID: 11280557]

Pardi D et al: Treatment of refractory microscopic colitis with azathioprine and 6-mercaptopurine. Gastroenterology 2001;120:148. [PMID: 11313319]

DIVERTICULAR DISEASE OF THE COLON

Colonic diverticulosis increases with age, ranging from 5% in those under age 40, to 30% at age 60, to more than 50% over age 80 in Western societies. In contrast, it is very uncommon in developing countries with much lower life expectancies. Most are asymptomatic, discovered incidentally at endoscopy or on barium enema. Complications in one-third include lower gastrointestinal bleeding and diverticulitis.

Colonic diverticula may vary in size from a few millimeters to several centimeters and in number from one to several dozen. Almost all patients with diverticulosis have involvement in the sigmoid colon; however, only 15% have proximal colonic disease.

In most patients, diverticulosis is believed to arise after many years of a diet deficient in fiber. The undistended, contracted segments of colon have higher intraluminal pressures. Over time, the contracted colonic musculature, working against greater pressures to move small, hard stools, develops hypertrophy, thickening, rigidity, and fibrosis. Diverticula may develop more commonly in the sigmoid because intraluminal pressures are highest in this region. The extent to which abnormal motility and hereditary factors contribute to diverticular disease is unknown. Patients with diffuse diverticulosis may have an inherent weakness in the colonic wall. Patients with abnormal connective tissue are also disposed to development of diverticulosis, including Ehlers-Danlos syndrome, Marfan's syndrome, and scleroderma.

1. Uncomplicated Diverticulosis

More than two-thirds of patients with diverticulosis have uncomplicated disease and no specific symptoms. In some, diverticulosis may be an incidental finding detected during colonoscopic examination or barium enema examination. Some patients have nonspecific complaints of chronic constipation, abdominal pain, or fluctuating bowel habits. It is unclear whether these symptoms are due to alterations in the colonic musculature or underlying irritable bowel syndrome. Physical examination is usually normal but may reveal mild left lower quadrant tenderness with a thickened, palpable sigmoid and descending colon. Screening laboratory studies should be normal in uncomplicated diverticulosis.

There is no reason to perform imaging studies for the purpose of diagnosing uncomplicated disease. Diverticula are best seen on barium enema. Involved segments of colon may also be narrowed and deformed. Colonoscopy is a less sensitive means of detecting diverticula.

Asymptomatic patients in whom diverticulosis is discovered and patients with a history of complicated disease (see below) should be treated with a high-fiber diet or fiber supplements (bran powder, 1–2 tbsp twice daily; psyllium or methylcellulose) (see section on constipation). Retrospective studies suggest that such treatment may decrease the likelihood of subsequent complications.

2. Diverticulitis

 ESSENTIALS OF DIAGNOSIS

- *Acute abdominal pain and fever.*
- *Left lower abdominal tenderness and mass.*
- *Leukocytosis.*

Clinical Findings

A. SYMPTOMS AND SIGNS

Perforation of a colonic diverticulum results in an intra-abdominal infection that may vary from microperforation (most common) with localized paracolic inflammation to macroperforation with either abscess or generalized peritonitis. Thus, there is a range from mild to severe disease. Most patients with localized inflammation or infection report mild to moderate aching abdominal pain, usually in the left lower quadrant. Constipation or loose stools may be present. Nausea and vomiting are frequent. In many cases, symptoms are so mild that the patient may not seek medical attention until several days after onset. Physical findings include a low-grade fever, left lower quadrant tenderness, and a palpable mass. Stool occult blood is common, but hematochezia is rare. Leukocytosis is mild to moderate. Patients with free perforation present with a more dramatic picture of generalized abdominal pain and peritoneal signs.

B. IMAGING

Plain abdominal films are obtained in all patients to look for evidence of free abdominal air (signifying free perforation), ileus, and small or large bowel obstruction. In patients with mild symptoms and a presumptive diagnosis of diverticulitis, empirical medical therapy is started without further imaging in the acute phase. Patients who respond to acute medical management should undergo complete colonic evaluation with colonoscopy or barium enema after resolution of clinical symptoms to corroborate the diagnosis or exclude other disorders such as colonic neoplasms. In patients who do not improve rapidly after 2–4 days of empirical therapy and in those with severe disease, CT scan of the abdomen is obtained to look for evidence of diverticulitis, including colonic diverticula and wall thickening, pericolic fat infiltration, abscess formation, or extraluminal air or contrast. Endoscopy and barium enema are contraindicated during the initial stages of an acute attack because of the risk of free perforation, though sigmoidoscopy with minimal air insufflation is sometimes required to exclude other diagnoses.

Differential Diagnosis

Localized diverticulitis must be distinguished from perforated colonic carcinoma, Crohn's disease, appendicitis, ischemic colitis, *C difficile*-associated colitis, and gynecologic disorders (ectopic pregnancy, ovarian cyst or torsion).

Complications

Fistula formation may involve the bladder, ureter, vagina, uterus, bowel, and abdominal wall. Diverticulitis may result in stricturing of the colon with partial or complete obstruction.

Treatment

A. MEDICAL MANAGEMENT

Most patients can be managed with conservative measures. Patients with mild symptoms and no peritoneal signs may be managed initially as outpatients on a clear liquid diet and broad-spectrum oral antibiotics with anaerobic activity. Reasonable regimens include amoxicillin and clavulanate potassium (875 mg/ 125 mg) twice daily; or metronidazole, 500 mg three times daily; plus either ciprofloxacin, 500 mg twice daily, or trimethoprim-sulfamethoxazole, 160/800 mg twice daily orally, for 7–10 days or until the patient is afebrile for 3–5 days. Symptomatic improvement usually occurs within 3 days, at which time the diet may be advanced. Patients with increasing pain, fever, or inability to tolerate oral fluids require hospitalization. Patients with severe diverticulitis (high fevers, leukocytosis, or peritoneal signs) and patients who are elderly or immunosuppressed or who have serious comorbid disease require hospitalization acutely. Patients should be given nothing by mouth and should receive intravenous fluids. If ileus is present, a nasogastric tube should be placed. Intravenous antibiotics should be given to cover anaerobic and gram-negative bacteria. Single-agent therapy with either a second-generation cephalosporin (eg, cefoxitin), piperacillin-tazobactam, or ticarcillin clavulanate appears to be as effective as combination therapy (eg, metronidazole or clindamycin plus an aminoglycoside or third-generation cephalosporin (eg, ceftazidime, cefotaxime). Symptomatic improvement should be evident within 2–3 days. The antibiotics should be continued for 7–10 days, after which time elective evaluation with colonoscopy or barium enema should be performed.

B. SURGICAL MANAGEMENT

Approximately 20–30% of patients with diverticulitis will require surgical management. Surgical consultation should be obtained on all patients with severe disease or those who fail to improve after 72 hours of medical management. Indications for emergent surgical management include free peritonitis and large abscesses. Patients with fistulas or colonic obstruction due to chronic disease will require elective surgery.

Patients with a localized abdominal abscess can be treated acutely with a percutaneous catheter drain placed by an interventional radiologist. This permits control of the infection and resolution of the immediate infectious inflammatory process. In this manner, a subsequent single-stage elective surgical operation can be performed in which the diseased segment of colon is removed and primary colonic anastomosis performed. In patients in whom catheter drainage is not possible or helpful or in cases requiring emergency surgery, it is necessary to perform surgery in two stages. In the first stage, the diseased colon is resected and the proximal colon brought out to form a temporary colostomy. The distal colonic stump is either closed (forming a Hartmann pouch) or exteriorized as a mucous fistula. Weeks later, after inflammation and infection have completely subsided, the colon can be reconnected electively.

Prognosis

Diverticulitis recurs in one-third of patients treated with medical management. Recurrent attacks warrant elective surgical resection, which carries a lower morbidity and mortality risk than emergency surgery.

Stollman NH et al: Diagnosis and management of diverticular disease of the colon in adults. Am J Gastroenterol 1999; 94:1310. [PMID: 10566700]

3. Diverticular Bleeding

Half of cases of acute lower gastrointestinal bleeding are attributable to diverticulosis. For a full discussion, see the section on Acute Lower Gastrointestinal Bleeding.

POLYPS OF THE COLON & SMALL INTESTINE

Polyps are discrete mass lesions that protrude into the intestinal lumen. Although most commonly sporadic, they may be inherited as part of familial polyposis syndrome. Polyps may be divided into three major pathologic groups: mucosal neoplastic (adenomatous) polyps, mucosal nonneoplastic polyps (hyperplastic, juvenile polyps, hamartomas, inflammatory polyps), and submucosal lesions (lipomas, lymphoid aggregates, carcinoids, pneumatosis cystoides intestinalis). The nonneoplastic mucosal polyps have no malignant potential and usually are discovered incidentally at colonoscopy or barium enema. Only the adenomatous polyps have significant clinical implications and will be considered further here. Of polyps removed at colonoscopy, over 70% are adenomatous; most of the remainder are hyperplastic. Hyperplastic polyps are generally small (< 5 mm) and of no consequence. Their only importance is that they cannot be reliably distinguished from adenomatous lesions except by biopsy.

NONFAMILIAL ADENOMATOUS POLYPS

Histologically, adenomas are classified as tubular, villous, or tubulovillous. They may be sessile or pedunculated (containing a stalk). They are present in 35% of adults over 50 years of age. Their significance is that over 95% of cases of adenocarcinoma of the colon are believed to arise from adenomas. It is proposed that there is an adenoma → carcinoma sequence whereby colorectal cancer develops through a continuous process from normal mucosa to adenoma to carcinoma. Most adenomas are small (< 1 cm) and have a low risk of becoming malignant; fewer than 4% of these enlarge with time. Fifteen percent of adenomas are (≥ 1 cm) or contain villous features and have a much higher risk (> 10%) of harboring malignancy or high-grade dysplasia. It has been estimated from longitudinal studies that it takes an average of 5 years for a medium-sized polyp to develop from normal-appearing mucosa and 10 years for a gross cancer to arise. In an asymptomatic population of male veterans over age 50 undergoing screening with colonoscopy, invasive cancer was detected in 1%, adenomas containing high-grade dysplasia in 1.7%, and other adenomas ≥ 1 cm in size in 7.2%.

Clinical Findings

A. Symptoms and Signs

Most patients with adenomatous polyps are completely asymptomatic. Chronic occult blood loss may lead to iron deficiency anemia. Large polyps may ulcerate, resulting in intermittent hematochezia.

B. Fecal Occult Blood Testing

Fecal occult blood tests are commonly performed as part of colorectal cancer screening programs. Unfortunately, these tests detect less than 40% of adenomas larger than 1 cm. Of patients with positive tests, approximately one-third have adenomas—only slightly higher than the expected prevalence in the adult population. (See section on colorectal cancer screening, below.) Thus, these tests are insensitive and nonspecific for adenomas.

C. Special Tests

Polyps are identified by means of barium enema examinations, flexible sigmoidoscopy, or colonoscopy. Barium enema examinations (either single- or double-contrast) as currently performed have unacceptable sensitivity and specificity for the detection of colorectal polyps. A recent comparative study with colonoscopy demonstrated that barium enemas failed to detect approximately half of polyps over 1 cm in size. Spiral CT colonography with computer-enabled luminal image reconstruction ("virtual colonoscopy") detects over 80–90% of clinically significant neoplasms. The clinical role of CT colography is being defined in ongoing studies. At this time, barium enema and CT colography may be best suited for patients with significant cardiac or pulmonary comorbidities—for whom colonoscopy is deemed unsafe—or in clinical settings in which endoscopic expertise is not readily available.

Flexible sigmoidoscopy is commonly performed as part of colorectal screening programs. Approximately one-half to two-thirds of colonic adenomas are within the reach of a flexible sigmoidoscope. Polyps are seen in 10–20% of patients undergoing screening sigmoidoscopy, and polyps less than 8 mm in size should removed by excisional biopsy. Patients with hyperplastic polyps require no further evaluation. Patients with advanced neoplasms (as defined above) have an increased risk of harboring other advanced neoplasms in the proximal colon and should undergo colonoscopy. At present, the management of patients with small adenomas without villous features or high-grade dysplasia is controversial. Opinions are conflicting about whether such lesions found on sigmoidoscopy are predictive of finding an increased prevalence of advanced neoplasms (> 1 cm or containing villous features or high grade dysplasia) in the colon proximal to the splenic flexure during colonoscopy. Some physicians have not routinely performed colonoscopy in patients found to have a single small (< 5–8 mm) polyp in the distal colon on screening sigmoidoscopy. However, most gastroenterologists routinely recommend colonoscopy for all patients with adenomas found in the distal colon at sigmoidoscopy irrespective of size. In patients with no adenomas detected in the distal colon, the prevalence of advanced proximal adenomas is 2.7%; among patients with a distal adenoma less than 10 mm in size, the prevalence of advanced proximal neoplasia was 6.8%.

Colonoscopy allows evaluation of the entire colon and is the best means of detecting and removing adenomatous polyps. It should be performed in all patients who have positive fecal occult blood tests or iron deficiency anemia (see Occult Gastrointestinal Bleeding, above), as the prevalence of colonic neoplasms is increased in these patients. Colonoscopy should also be performed in patients with polyps detected on radiologic imaging studies or adenomas detected on flexible sigmoidoscopy in order to remove these polyps and to fully evaluate the entire colon.

Treatment

A. Colonoscopic Polypectomy

Most adenomatous polyps are amenable to colonoscopic removal with biopsy forceps or snare cautery. Large sessile polyps (> 2–3 cm) may be removed in piecemeal fashion or may require primary surgical resection. Complications after colonoscopic polypectomy include perforation in 0.2% and clinically significant bleeding in 1%.

A malignant polyp is an adenoma that appears grossly benign at endoscopy but on histologic assessment is found to contain cancer that has penetrated through the muscularis mucosae into the submucosa. Malignant polyps may be considered to be adequately treated by polypectomy alone if (1) the polyp is completely excised and submitted for pathologic examination, (2) it is well differentiated, (3) the margin is not involved, and (4) there is no vascular or lymphatic invasion. The risk of residual cancer or nodal metastasis with these favorable histologic features is 0.3% for pedunculated polyps and 1.5% for sessile polyps. The excision site of these "favorable" malignant polyps should be checked in 3 months for residual tissue. In patients with malignant polyps that have unfavorable histologic features, cancer resection is advisable if the patient is a good operative candidate.

B. Postpolypectomy Surveillance

Adenomas can be found in 30–40% of patients when another colonoscopy is performed within 3 years after the initial examination. Periodic colonoscopic surveillance is therefore recommended to detect these "metachronous" adenomas, which either may be new or may have been overlooked during the initial examination. Most of these adenomas are small, without high-risk features and of little immediate clinical significance. The probability of detecting advanced neoplasms at surveillance colonoscopy is increased significantly if the polyps found on initial (index) colonoscopy were advanced (≥ 1 cm, villous features, or high-grade dysplasia) or multiple (more than two polyps) or if the patient's family includes a first-degree member with colorectal cancer. In these higher-risk patients, repeat or "surveillance" colonoscopy should be performed 3 years after the initial colonoscopy and polypectomy. For patients with adenomatous polyps who had low-risk features on initial colonoscopy and polypectomy (ie, one or two polyps less than 10 mm in size without villous features or high-grade dysplasia) or for higher-risk patients whose follow-up surveillance colonoscopy is negative for further polyps after 3 years, repeat colonoscopy to check for metachronous adenomas should be performed in 5 years.

Bond JH: Polyp guideline: diagnosis, treatment, and surveillance for patients with colorectal polyps. Practice Parameters Committee of the American College of Gastroenterology: Am J Gastroenterol 2000;95:3053. [PMID: 11095318]

Lieberman D et al: Use of colonoscopy to screen asymptomatic adults for colorectal cancer. N Engl J Med 2000;343:162. [PMID: 10900274]

Winawer S et al: A comparison of colonoscopy and double-contrast barium enema for surveillance after polypectomy. N Engl J Med 2000;342:1766. [PMID: 10852998]

HEREDITARY COLORECTAL CANCER & POLYPOSIS SYNDROMES

Approximately 1–3% of all colorectal cancers are caused by germline genetic mutations that impose on carriers a high lifetime risk of developing colorectal cancer. Because the diagnosis of these disorders has important implications for treatment of affected members and for screening of family members, it is important to consider these disorders in patients with a family history of colorectal cancer that has affected more than one family member, those with a personal or family history of colorectal cancer developing at an early age (≤ 50 years), those with a personal or family history of multiple polyps (> 20), and those with a personal or family history of multiple extracolonic malignancies.

1. Familial Adenomatous Polyposis

Familial adenomatous polyposis is an autosomal dominant syndrome affecting 1:10,000 people and characterized by the development of multiple (> 100) colonic adenomatous polyps and by other extracolonic features. It is due to an inherited mutation in the adenomatous polyposis coli *(APC)* gene on chromosome 5q21 that leads to frameshifts or premature stop codons, most of which result in truncation of the APC gene product, a protein important in the regulation of cell adhesion and apoptosis. More than 300 different mutations have been reported. The location of the mutation affects the number of polyps formed and the type of extracolonic features seen. Approximately 25% of cases appear to involve spontaneous germline mutations, ie, to occur in the absence of a family history of inherited colon cancer.

Polyps develop by a mean age of 15 years, and almost all affected individuals develop adenomatous polyps by age 35. Unless prophylactic colectomy is performed, colorectal cancer is inevitable by age 50. An attenuated variant of familial adenomatous polyposis has been recognized in which affected family members develop an average of only 30 polyps and therefore have a lower risk of cancer that occurs an average of 12 years later than the classic disease. These families have mutations on either the 5′ or 3′ end of the *APC* gene.

Adenomatous polyps of the duodenum and periampullary area develop in over 90% of patients, resulting in a 5–8% lifetime risk of adenocarcinoma. Adenomas occur less frequently in the gastric antrum and small bowel and in those locations have a lower risk of malignant transformation. Gastric fundus gland polyps occur in over 50% but have no malignant potential.

In addition to gastrointestinal polyps, some patients with familial adenomatous polyposis develop a variety of other benign extraintestinal manifestations, including soft tissue tumors of the skin, desmoid tumors, osteomas, and congenital hypertrophy of the retinal pigment. They may also develop malignancies of the central nervous system (Turcot's syndrome) and tumors of the thyroid and liver (hepatoblastomas). These extraintestinal manifestations vary among families, depending in part upon the type or site of mutation in the *APC* gene.

Genetic counseling and testing should be offered to patients with a diagnosis of familial adenomatous polyposis established by endoscopy and to first-degree family members of patients with the disease; testing should be done also to confirm a diagnosis of attenuated disease in patients with 20 or more adenomas. First-degree relatives of patients with familial adenomatous polyposis should undergo genetic screening after age 10. Genetic testing is also commercially available for Ashkenazic Jews with a personal or family history of colorectal cancer (see Colorectal Cancer: Family History). A protein truncation assay is commercially available that has a sensitivity of 80% for the diagnosis of familial adenomatous polyposis. Therefore, a negative result can be considered to be a true negative only if an affected family member has a positive test result. If the assay cannot be done or is not informative, family members at risk should undergo yearly sigmoidoscopy beginning at 12 years of age. Once the diagnosis has been established, complete proctocolectomy with ileoanal anastomosis or colectomy with ileorectal anastomosis is recommended, usually before age 20. Ileorectal anastomosis affords superior bowel function but has a 10% risk of development of rectal cancer, and for that reason frequent sigmoidoscopy with fulguration of polyps is required. Sulindac and COX-2 selective agents (celecoxib, rofecoxib) have been shown to decrease the number and size of polyps in the rectal stump but not the duodenum. Upper endoscopic evaluation of the stomach, duodenum, and periampullary area should be performed every 1–3 years to look for adenomas or carcinoma. Large (> 2 cm) periampullary adenomas require surgical resection.

2. Hamartomatous Polyposis Syndromes

Hamartomatous polyposis syndromes are rare and account for less than 0.1% of colorectal cancers.

Peutz-Jeghers syndrome is an autosomal dominant condition characterized by hamartomatous polyps throughout the gastrointestinal tract (most notably in the small intestine) as well as mucocutaneous pigmented macules on the lips, buccal mucosa, and skin. The hamartomas may become large, leading to bleeding, intussusception, or obstruction. Although hamartomas are not malignant, up to 13% of patients develop malignancies (especially of the stomach and duodenum) of nonintestinal organs (breast, gonads, pancreas). The defect has been localized to the serine threonine kinase 11 gene, and genetic testing is available.

Familial juvenile polyposis is also autosomal dominant and characterized by several (more than ten) juvenile hamartomatous polyps located most commonly in the colon. There is an increased risk (up to 50%) of adenocarcinoma due to synchronous adenomatous polyps or mixed hamartomatous-adenomatous polyps. Genetic defects have been identified in several genes. Genetic testing is available.

Cowden's syndrome is characterized by juvenile and hamartomatous polyps throughout the gastrointestinal tract. An increased rate of malignancy has not been demonstrated, but the condition must be distinguished from other hamartomatous syndromes.

3. Hereditary Nonpolyposis Colorectal Cancer (HNPCC)

HNPCC is an autosomal dominant condition in which there is a markedly increased risk of developing colorectal cancer as well as a host of other cancers, including endometrial, ovarian, renal or vesical, hepatobiliary, gastric, and small intestinal cancers. It is estimated to account for 1–3% of all colorectal cancers. Affected individuals have a 70–80% lifetime risk of developing colorectal carcinoma and an over 30% life-time risk of endometrial cancer. Unlike individuals with familial adenomatous polyposis, HNPCC patients develop only a few adenomas, which may be flat and more often contain villous features or high-grade dysplasia. In contrast to the traditional polyp → cancer progression (which may take over 10 years), these polyps are believed to undergo rapid transformation from normal tissue → adenoma → cancer. HNPCC tends to develop at an earlier age than sporadic colorectal cancers (mean age: 44 years), and over two-thirds arise proximal to the splenic flexure. Compared with patients with sporadic tumors of similar pathologic stage, those with HNPCC tumors have markedly improved survival. Synchronous or metachronous cancers occur within 10 years in up to 45% of patients.

HNPCC is caused by a defect in one of several genes that are important in the detection and repair of DNA base-pair mismatches: *hMLH1, hMSH2, hMSH6, pPMS1,* and *hPMS2*. Germline mutations in *hMLH1* and *hMSH2* account for more than 90–95% of the known mutations in families with HNPCC. Mutations in any of these mismatch repair genes results in a characteristic phenotypic abnormality known as microsatellite instability. In over 90% of cancers in HNPCC patients, microsatellite instability is readily demonstrated by expansion or contraction of DNA microsatellites (short, repeated DNA sequences). Microsatellite instability also occurs in 15% of sporadic colorectal cancers, over 85% of which do not have demonstrated mutations in mismatch repair genes.

A thorough family cancer history is essential to identify families that may be affected with HNPCC so that appropriate genetic and colonoscopic screening can be offered. The ability to find mutations in one of the known HNPCC genes is not nearly as great as with the inherited polyposis syndromes. Owing to the limitations of genetic testing for HNPCC and the medical, psychologic, and social implications that such testing may have, families with suspected HNPCC should be evaluated first by a genetic counselor and should give informed consent in writing before genetic testing is performed. Patients whose families fulfill the "Amsterdam criteria" have a high likelihood (45–64%) of harboring a germline mutation in one of the mismatch repair genes and should be considered for genetic testing: (1) three or more first-degree family members with colorectal cancer (or one of the other associated cancers); (2) colon cancer involving at least two generations; and (3) at least one colon cancer diagnosed before age 50. These stringent criteria may, however, fail to identify many families with HNPCC. Therefore, genetic testing should be considered also (4) for individuals with colorectal cancer or endometrial cancer diagnosed before age 50 years (especially if right-sided, undifferentiated, or signet ring) or adenoma before age 40 years; (5) for those with colorectal cancer who have a first-degree relative with colorectal cancer or extracolonic cancer diagnosed before age 50 years; and (6) for those with a personal history of two HNPCC-associated cancers. Before proceeding with germline testing of family members, tumor tissues of affected individuals or family members should be tested first for microsatellite instability. Individuals whose tumors do not have microsatellite instability are unlikely to have germline mutations in mismatch repair genes, and further genetic testing is not warranted. Germline testing for gene mutations is warranted in individuals whose tumors demonstrate a high level of microsatellite instability. Germline testing is also warranted in families with a strong history consistent with HNPCC when tumors are unavailable for assessment. If a mutation is detected in a patient with cancer in one of the known mismatch genes, genetic testing of other first-degree family members is indicated. If a mutation in one of the known HNPCC genes is not identified, further genetic testing is of no value and all family members must still be considered to be at increased risk of developing neoplasia and screened accordingly.

If genetic testing documents an HNPCC gene mutation, affected relatives should be screened with colonoscopy every 1–2 years beginning at age 25 (or 5 years younger than the earliest diagnosed family cancer). In families that fulfill the Amsterdam criteria or that have tumors with proved microsatellite instability but who do not have a documented gene mutation in one of the known HNPCC genes, colonoscopic screening (as above) is recommended for all family members. If cancer is found, subtotal colectomy with ileorectal anastomosis (followed by annual surveillance of the rectal stump) should be performed. Women should undergo screening for endometrial cancer beginning at age 25–35 with endometrial aspiration or transvaginal ultrasound. Prophylactic hysterectomy and oophorectomy may be considered, especially in women of post-childbearing age.

American Gastroenterological Association Medical Position Statement: Hereditary colorectal cancer and genetic testing. Gastroenterology 2001;121:195. [PMID: 11438508]

Steinbach G et al: The effect of celecoxib, a cyclooxygenase-2 inhibitor in familial adenomatous polyposis. N Engl J Med 2000;342:1946. [PMID: 10874062]

Terdiman J et al. Efficient detection of hereditary nonpolyposis colorectal cancer gene carriers by screening for tumor microsatellite instability before germline genetic testing. Gastroenterology 2001;120:21. [PMID: 11208710]

Terdiman J: HNPCC: an uncommon but important diagnosis. Gastroenterology 2001;121:1005. [PMID: 11606514]

COLORECTAL CANCER

ESSENTIALS OF DIAGNOSIS

- *Symptoms or signs dependent upon tumor location.*
- *Proximal colon: fecal occult blood, anemia.*

- *Distal colon: change in bowel habits, hematochezia.*
- *Characteristic findings on barium enema.*
- *Diagnosis established with colonoscopy.*

General Considerations

Colorectal cancer is the second leading cause of death due to malignancy in the United States. Approximately 6% of Americans will develop colorectal cancer and 40% of those will die of the disease. An estimated 134,000 new cases and 55,000 deaths occur annually. Colorectal cancers are almost all adenocarcinomas, which tend to form bulky exophytic masses or annular constricting lesions. Approximately half of cancers are located within the rectosigmoid region; one-fourth are located proximally in the cecum and ascending colon. It is currently believed that the majority of colorectal cancers arise from malignant transformation of an adenomatous polyp.

Risk Factors

A number of factors increase the risk of developing colorectal cancer. Recognition of these has impact upon screening strategies. However, 75% of all cases occur in people with no known predisposing factors.

A. Age

The incidence of colorectal cancer rises sharply after age 45, and 90% of cases occur in persons over the age of 50.

B. Personal History of Neoplasia

A personal history of colorectal cancer or adenomatous polyps increases the risk of developing metachronous adenomas or carcinoma and therefore requires periodic colonoscopic surveillance (see Adenomatous Polyps, above). Patients with a family or personal history of breast, uterine, or ovarian cancer have a slightly increased risk.

C. Family History

A family history of colorectal cancer is present in 25% of patients with colon cancer. Patients with a family history of colorectal cancer have a significantly increased risk of developing colorectal cancer and deserve more intensive screening. Approximately 3% of colorectal cancers are caused by inherited autosomal dominant germline mutations resulting in polyposis syndromes or hereditary nonpolyposis colorectal cancer, which are reviewed elsewhere in this chapter. Genetic testing is now available for the diagnosis of most of these syndromes. (See Hereditary Colorectal Cancer and Polyposis Syndromes, above.)

The reason for the familial risk in the remainder of patients is still not well understood. The risk of colon cancer is proportionate to the number and age of affected first-degree family members with colon cancer. A person with one family member with colon cancer has a twofold increased risk; if the affected member was under age 60 years at diagnosis, the risk is greater. People with two first-degree relatives have a fivefold— or 25–30% lifetime—risk of developing colon cancer. First-degree relatives of patients with adenomas diagnosed before age 60 are also at increased risk. Cancers arise at an earlier age in patients with a positive family history, meriting screening at an earlier age. The risk of a 40-year old person with a positive family history is comparable to that of an average-risk 50-year-old.

Approximately 6% of the Ashkenazic Jewish population has a missense mutation in the *APC* gene *(APC I1307K)* which confers a modestly increased lifetime risk of developing colorectal cancer (OR 1.4–1.9) but phenotypically resembles sporadic colorectal cancer rather than familial adenomatous polyposis. Genetic screening is available, and patients harboring the mutation merit intensive screening.

D. Inflammatory Bowel Disease

The risk of adenocarcinoma of the colon begins to rise 7–10 years after disease onset in patients with ulcerative colitis and Crohn's colitis. The cumulative risk approaches 5–10% after 20 years and 20% after 30 years.

E. Dietary Factors and Chemoprevention

In case-control studies, diets rich in fats and red meat are associated with an increased risk of colorectal adenomas and cancer, whereas diets high in fruits, vegetables, and fiber are associated with a decreased risk. However, two prospective, randomized controlled trials failed to demonstrate a risk reduction in the recurrence of adenomas after treatment with a diet low in fat and high in fiber, fruits, and vegetables or with fiber supplementation over a 3- to 4-year period. Both calcium carbonate (3 g/d) and folate therapy have been shown in prospective trials to yield a modest but significant reduction in the relative risk of developing colorectal neoplasia. In women, hormone replacement therapy may also be beneficial. The antioxidant vitamins A, C, and E have not been shown to be of benefit in prospective controlled studies.

Prolonged regular use of aspirin (at least 325 mg twice weekly) and NSAIDs is associated with a 30–50% decrease in the incidence of colorectal cancer and adenomas. Pending the results of prospective, placebo controlled studies of aspirin and other NSAIDs, the relative risks and benefits of these agents as chemopreventive agents for colorectal neoplasia are unclear. Chronic administration of these agents may be considered in patients with a personal or family history of colorectal cancer or advanced adenomas.

F. Race

The incidence of colon adenocarcinoma is higher in blacks than in whites. It is unclear whether this is due to genetic or socioeconomic factors (eg, diet or reduced access to screening).

Clinical Findings

A. SYMPTOMS AND SIGNS

Adenocarcinomas grow slowly and may be present for several years before symptoms appear. However, asymptomatic tumors may still be detected by the presence of fecal occult blood (see Colorectal Cancer Screening, below). Symptoms depend upon the location of the carcinoma. Chronic blood loss from right-sided colonic cancers may cause iron deficiency anemia, manifested by fatigue and weakness. Obstruction, however, is uncommon because of the large diameter of the right colon and the liquid consistency of the fecal material. Lesions of the left colon often involve the bowel circumferentially. Because the left colon has a smaller diameter and the fecal matter is solid, obstructive symptoms may develop with colicky abdominal pain and a change in bowel habits. Constipation may alternate with periods of increased frequency and loose stools. The stool may be streaked with blood, though marked bleeding is unusual. With rectal cancers, patients note tenesmus, urgency, and recurrent hematochezia. Physical examination is usually normal except in advanced disease. A mass may be palpable in the abdomen. The liver should be examined for hepatomegaly, suggesting metastatic spread.

B. LABORATORY FINDINGS

A complete blood count is obtained to look for evidence of anemia. Elevated liver function tests are suspicious for metastatic disease. Carcinoembryonic antigen (CEA) should be measured in all patients with proved colorectal cancer. Levels are elevated in 70% of patients but are poorly correlated with cancer stage. After complete surgical resection, CEA levels should normalize; persistently elevated levels portend a poor prognosis. A rise in CEA levels that had normalized initially after surgery is suggestive of cancer recurrence.

C. INSPECTION OF THE COLON

Cancers may be detected with a high degree of reliability with either barium enema, CT colonography ("virtual colonoscopy"), or colonoscopy. Colonoscopy is the diagnostic procedure of choice in patients with a clinical history suggestive of colon cancer or in patients with an abnormality suspicious for cancer detected on barium enema. Colonoscopy permits biopsy for pathologic confirmation of malignancy. In patients in whom colonoscopy is unable to reach the cecum (5% of cases) or when a nearly obstructing tumor precludes passage of the colonoscope, barium enema or CT colonography examination should be performed.

D. IMAGING

Chest x-ray is obtained to look for evidence of metastatic disease. Some clinicians prefer to obtain an abdominal CT scan to assist in preoperative staging. However, this seldom changes surgical management and is deemed unnecessary by most surgeons for the evaluation of colon cancer. Conversely, for rectal cancer, pelvic MRI and endorectal ultrasonography provide important accurate information about the depth of penetration of the cancer through the rectal wall and pararectal lymph nodes that may guide operative management.

Differential Diagnosis

The nonspecific symptoms of colon cancer may be confused with those of irritable bowel syndrome, diverticular disease, ischemic colitis, inflammatory bowel disease, infectious colitis, and hemorrhoids. Neoplasm must be excluded in any patient over age 45 who reports a change in bowel habits or hematochezia or who has an unexplained iron deficiency anemia or occult blood in the stools.

Staging

Determination of the stage of colorectal cancer is important not only because it correlates with the patient's long-term survival but also because it is used to determine which patients should receive adjuvant therapy (Table 14–16). Although the Dukes classification has been widely employed in the past, the TNM system is now more commonly used.

Treatment

Resection of the primary colonic or rectal cancer is the treatment of choice for virtually all patients who have resectable lesions and can tolerate general anesthesia. Regional lymph node dissection should be performed to determine staging, which guides decisions about adjuvant therapy. Even patients with extensive metastatic disease may benefit from resection of the colonic tumor to reduce the likelihood of intestinal obstruction or serious bleeding.

For rectal carcinoma, the operative approach depends upon the level of the tumor above the anal verge, the size and depth of penetration, and the patient's overall condition. In carefully selected patients with small (< 3 cm), well-differentiated rectal tumors that are less than 7.5 cm from the anal verge and that appear on endosonography to be localized to the rectal wall, transanal excision may be performed. This approach avoids laparotomy and spares the rectum and anal sphincter, preserving normal bowel continence. All other patients will require either a low anterior resection with a colorectal anastomosis or an abdominoperineal resection with a colostomy, depending upon how far above the anal verge the tumor is located and the extent of local tumor spread. With unresectable rectal cancer, the patient may be palliated with a diverting colostomy, laser fulguration, or placement of an expandable wire stent.

A. ADJUVANT THERAPY FOR COLON CANCER

Adjuvant chemotherapy and radiotherapy have been demonstrated to improve overall and tumor-free survival in selected patients with colorectal cancer.

Table 14–16. Staging of colorectal cancer.

American Joint Committee Classification	TNM			Dukes Class[1]
Stage 0				
Carcinoma in situ	Tis	N0	M0	
Stage I				
Tumor invades submucosa	T1	N0	M0	Dukes A
Tumor invades muscularis propria	T2	N0	M0	Dukes B_1
Stage II				
Tumor invades into subserosa or into nonperitonealized pericolic or perirectal tissues	T3	N0	M0	Dukes B_1 or B_2
Tumor perforates the visceral peritoneum or directly invades other organs or structures	T4	N0	M0	Dukes B_2
Stage III				
Any degree of bowel wall perforation with lymph node metastasis				
One to three pericolic or perirectal lymph nodes involved	Any T	N1	M0	Dukes C_1
Four or more pericolic or perirectal lymph nodes involved	Any T	N2	M0	Dukes C_2
Metastasis to lymph nodes along a vascular trunk	Any T	N3	M0	
Stage IV				
Presence of distant metastasis	Any T	Any N	M1	Dukes D

[1]Gastrointestinal Tumor Study Group modification of Dukes classification.

1. Stage I—Because of the excellent 5-year survival rate (80–100%), no adjuvant therapy is recommended.

2. Stage II (node-negative disease)—The expected 5-year survival rate is 50–75%. A benefit from adjuvant chemotherapy has not been demonstrated in controlled trials for stage II colon cancer. Patients with advanced local stage II disease (T3–T4) should be considered for study protocols looking at the role of adjuvant chemotherapy or radiotherapy for control of local recurrence.

3. Stage III (node-positive) disease—The expected 5-year survival rate is 30–50%. Patients with one to three involved nodes have better survival than those with more than three involved nodes. Postoperative adjuvant chemotherapy reduces mortality by 33% and is recommended for all patients. Currently, a combination of fluorouracil and leucovorin for 6 months may be recommended and improves 5-year disease-free survival to 64%. Alternatively, a combination of fluorouracil and levamisole for 1 year may be used, though one trial has shown this to be an inferior strategy. Selected patients with locally advanced (T_3 or T_4) cancer may benefit from radiotherapy to reduce the risk of local recurrence.

4. Stage IV (metastatic disease)—Approximately 20% of patients have metastatic disease at the time of initial diagnosis, and another 30% eventually develop metastasis. The long-term survival of these patients is only 5%. Resection of isolated (one to three) liver or lung metastases may result in long-term (over 5 years) survival in 20–40% of cases. For those with unresectable hepatic metastases, local ablative techniques (cryosurgery, embolization) may provide long-term tumor control. Chemotherapy with fluorouracil with or without leucovorin has been widely used for palliation but does not improve survival. Combination therapy with fluorouracil, leucovorin, and irinotecan (a topoisomerase inhibitor) provides significant improvement in tumor response rate (40%) and overall survival (mean: 15 months) compared with fluorouracil and leucovorin alone but is associated with significantly higher toxicity (diarrhea and neutropenia).

B. Adjuvant Therapy for Rectal Cancer

In the United States, combined postoperative adjuvant therapy with pelvic radiation and chemotherapy with fluorouracil is recommended for both stage II and stage III rectal cancers. Such therapy has been shown to improve both the overall and the disease-free survival rate and to decrease pelvic recurrences. In Europe, radiation is used preoperatively and chemotherapy typically is not used. The merits of these approaches are debated. Preoperative radiation may shrink tumor, permitting low anterior resection or transanal excision of some cases previously thought to need abdominoperineal resection with colostomy. However, it may lead to higher surgical complication rates and unnecessary treatment of some patients who are "over-staged" by clinical criteria. Postoperative therapy allows accurate staging but may lead to inadvertent radiation of small intestines as well as the surgical anastomosis. To date, therapy is individualized. Preoperative radiotherapy may be warranted in patients with known extensive disease or lymph node involvement. When staging suggests stage I or stage II disease, surgery may be performed first, followed by postoperative radiotherapy in patients found to have transmural extension or lymph node involvement. Where possible, patients should be enrolled in clinical trials that seek to identify the optimal combined-modality regimen.

Follow-Up After Surgery

Patients who have undergone resections for cure are followed closely to look for evidence of tumor recurrence. The optimal cost-effective strategy is not clear and varies in different medical centers. Two randomized trials reported that intense follow-up with yearly colonoscopy, abdominal CT, and chest radiography did not improve overall outcome compared with most standard follow-up protocols. In the absence of consensus guidelines, the following may be recommended. Patients should be evaluated every 3–6 months for 3–5 years with history, physical examination, fecal occult blood testing, liver function tests, and CEA determinations. Colonoscopy is performed within 6–12 months after operation to look for evidence of recurrence and then every 3–5 years to look for metachronous polyps or cancer. Because of the high incidence of local tumor recurrence in patients with rectal cancer, sigmoidoscopy should be performed every 6–12 months for 3 years. A change in the patient's clinical picture, abnormal liver function tests, or a rising CEA warrant investigation with chest radiography and abdominal CT to look for recurrent or metastatic disease that may be amenable to therapy.

Prognosis

The stage of disease at presentation is the most important determinant of long-term survival: stage I, > 90%; stage II, > 70%; stage III with fewer than four positive lymph nodes, 67%; stage III with more than four positive lymph nodes, 33%; and stage IV, < 5%. For each stage, rectal cancers have a worse prognosis. Although molecular markers (eg, *P53* mutation, 18q deletion, Ki-*ras* mutation) may be independent risk factors for the development of metastatic disease, these are not yet used clinically to guide therapy or follow-up. Tumors that have microsatellite instability, suggesting inactivation of mismatch repair genes (HNPCC and 15% of sporadic cancers), appear to have a more favorable prognosis.

For those patients whose disease progresses despite therapy, meticulous efforts at palliative care are essential (see Chapter 5).

Screening for Colorectal Neoplasms

Colorectal cancer is ideal for screening because it is a common disease affecting 6% of men and women which is fatal in almost half of cases yet is curable if detected at an earlier stage. Furthermore, the vast majority of cases arise from benign adenomas that progress over many years to cancer; and removal of adenomas has been shown to prevent the vast majority of cancers. Colorectal cancer screening has now been endorsed by the United States Preventive Services Task Force, the Agency for Health Care Policy and Research, the American Cancer Society, and every professional gastroenterology and colorectal surgery society. Although there is continued debate about the optimal cost-effective means of providing population screening, there is unanimous consent that screening *of some kind* should be offered to every patient over the age of 50. Several analyses suggest that the cost of screening is approximately $25,000 per year of life saved for all recommended screening strategies, which is well below the range of $40,000–$50,000 per year generally considered to be cost-effective.

A number of options for screening are available and reimbursed by third-party payers and by Medicare. The recommendations of a multidisciplinary consensus panel are listed in Table 14–17 for patients at average-risk of developing colorectal cancer. Patients with first-degree relatives with colorectal cancer are at increased risk, and for these individuals more intensive screening recommendations are recommended. Recommendations for screening in families with inherited cancer syndromes or inflammatory bowel disease are provided in separate sections. (See Hereditary Colorectal Cancer and Polyposis Syndromes; Inflammatory Bowel Disease.) The advantages and disadvantages of the various options are discussed below. It is important for primary care providers to understand the relative merits of various options and to discuss them with their patients. Despite growing awareness of the importance of screening on the part of medical professionals and the public, less than half of patients have undergone screening of any kind. Discussion and encouragement by the primary care provider is the most important factor in achieving patient compliance with screening programs.

A. Fecal Occult Blood Test (FOBT)

Most colorectal cancers and some large adenomas result in increased chronic blood loss that may be detectable. A variety of tests have been developed that have varying sensitivities for fecal occult blood, some of which are in clinical testing. A guaiac-based test (Hemoccult II) has undergone the most extensive testing and has had the greatest clinical use. Two slides must be prepared from three consecutive bowel movements. To reduce the likelihood of false-positive tests, patients should abstain from aspirin (in doses greater than 325 mg/d), NSAIDs, red meat, poultry, fish, and vegetables with peroxide activity (turnips, horseradish) for 72 hours. Vitamin C may cause a false-negative test. Slides should be developed within 7 days after preparation.

When fecal occult blood testing is administered to the general population as part of a screening program, 1–5% of tests are positive. Patients with positive tests should undergo colonoscopy accompanied by removal of any polyps identified. If colonoscopy reveals no colorectal neoplasm, further screening for colorectal cancer can be deferred for 10 years. Of those with positive

Table 14–17. Recommendations for colorectal cancer screening.[1]

Average-risk individuals ≥ 50 years old[2]
    Annual fecal occult blood testing
    Flexible sigmoidoscopy every 5 years
    Annual fecal occult blood testing *and* flexible sigmoidoscopy every 5 years
    Colonoscopy every 10 years
    Barium enema every 5–10 years
Individuals with a family history of a first-degree member with colorectal neoplasia[3]
    Single first-degree relative with colorectal cancer diagnosed at age ≥ **60 years:**
        Begin screening at age 40. Screening guidelines same as average risk individual; however preferred method is colonoscopy every 10 years.
    Single first-degree relative with colorectal cancer diagnosed at age < **60 years,** or multiple first-degree relatives: Begin screening at age 40 or at age 10 years younger than age at diagnosis of the youngest affected relative, whichever is first in time. Recommended screening: colonoscopy every 3–5 years

[1]For recommendations for families with inherited polyposis syndromes or hereditary nonpolyposis colon cancer, see separate section.
[2]Colorectal Cancer Screening and Rationale. Gastroenterology 1997; 112:5.
[3]Screening Recommendations of American College of Gastroenterology. Am J Gastroenterol 2000;95:868.

tests, 5–18% have colorectal cancer, more likely to be at an earlier stage (Dukes A or B). Adenomatous polyps are identified in 25–50% of patients with positive tests. Finding these polyps is somewhat fortuitous since most are less than 1 cm in size and unlikely to cause occult bleeding. The estimated sensitivity of a fecal occult blood test for colorectal cancer is only 30–50%—ie, a negative test does not exclude the possibility of a significant neoplasm. Sensitivity may be increased in patients who are compliant with annual testing. In several large prospective studies, fecal occult blood testing has been demonstrated to reduce mortality from colorectal cancer by 15–33%. Higher risk reductions are obtained with annual versus biennial testing.

B. Flexible Sigmoidoscopy

Use of a 60 cm flexible sigmoidoscope permits visualization of the rectosigmoid and descending colon. It requires no sedation and in many centers is performed by a nurse specialist or physician's assistant. Adenomatous polyps are identified in 10–20% and colorectal cancers in 1% of patients. Polyps less than 5–8 mm in diameter should be removed by biopsy to determine the histology. Patients found to have adenomatous polyps should undergo pancolonoscopy to look for synchronous neoplasms in the proximal colon. (See Adenomatous Polyps, above.) Up to 80% of cases of advanced neoplasia will be detected in flexible sigmoidoscopy screening programs provided that all patients in whom an adenoma is identified at sigmoidoscopy undergo subsequent colonoscopy. The risk of serious complications (perforation) associated with flexible sigmoidoscopy is less than 1:10,000 patients.

C. Screening Colonoscopy

Colonoscopy permits examination of the entire colon. Approximately 40% of advanced neoplasms (cancer, adenomas ≥ 1 cm, polyps with villous histology, or high-grade dysplasia) are proximal to the splenic flexure, ie, above the reach of a flexible sigmoidoscopic examination. Up to 50–60% of such patients do not have an adenomatous polyp distal to the splenic flexure at sigmoidoscopy. Therefore, screening programs that employ flexible sigmoidoscopy will miss approximately 20–30% of patients with advanced colonic neoplasia. To alleviate discomfort, intravenous sedation is used for most patients. For this reason, screening colonoscopy is the preferred screening test in patients deemed to be at higher risk due to a positive family history of colorectal cancer. Colonoscopy has been advocated by the American College of Gastroenterology as the preferred screening modality in average-risk patients as well. In a population of asymptomatic veterans between the ages of 50 and 75 years of age undergoing screening colonoscopy, the prevalence of advanced adenomas or cancer was 10.7%. The incidence of serious complications after colonoscopy (perforation, bleeding, cardiopulmonary events) is 0.3%.

D. Double Contrast Barium Enema

Like colonoscopy, barium enema permits examination of the entire colon. However, the sensitivity of barium enema is 70–90% for polyps ≥ 1 cm and only 55–85% for early-stage colorectal cancers. Therefore, most authorities do not recommend this examination for screening of asymptomatic patients. It may be used when screening of the entire colon is desired and the patient is unable or unwilling to undergo colonoscopy, or when colonoscopic expertise is unavailable.

E. CT Colonography (Virtual Colonoscopy)

Using computer-assisted image reconstruction and rapid helical CT, three-dimensional views can be generated of the colon lumen that simulate the view of colonoscopy. This technique is performed rapidly, requires no radiation or intravenous contrast, and is without risk. Compared with conventional colonoscopy, the sensitivity of virtual colonoscopy for the detection of polyps ≥ 1 cm is 90%. Virtual colonoscopy is costly, not available at most centers, and not as yet recommended for routine screening.

American Gastroenterological Association Medical Position Statement: Impact of dietary fiber on colon cancer occurrence. Gastroenterology 2000;118:1233. [PMID: 10833498]

Burt R: Colon cancer screening. Gastroenterology 2000;119: 837.[PMID: 10982778]

Chung D: The genetic basis of colorectal cancer: insights into critical pathways of tumorigenesis. Gastroenterology 2000; 119:854. [PMID: 10982779

Colon Cancer—National Cancer Institute—Cancer Net. http:// cancernet.nci.nih.gov

Janne P et al: Chemoprevention of colorectal cancer. N Engl J Med 2000:342:1960. [PMID: 10874065]

Johns L et al: A systematic review and meta-analysis of familial colorectal cancer risk. Ann Intern Med 2001;96:2992. [PMID: 11693338]

Lieberman D et al: One-time screening for colorectal cancer with combined fecal occult-blood testing and examination of the distal colon. N Engl J Med 2001;345:555. [PMID: 11529208]

Mandel J et al: The effect of fecal occult-blood screening on the incidence of colorectal cancer. N Engl J Med 2000;343: 1603.[PMID: 10096167]

Rectal Cancer—National Cancer Institute—Cancer Net http:// cancernet.nci.nih.gov

Rex D et al: Colorectal cancer prevention 2000: Screening recommendations of the American College of Gastroenterology. Am J Gastroenterol 2000;95:868. [PMID: 10763931]

Traverso G et al: Detection of *APC* mutations in fecal DNA from patients with colorectal tumors. N Engl J Med 2002; 346:311.

Yee J et al: Colorectal neoplasia: performance characteristics of CT colonography for detection in 300 patients. Radiology 2001;219:685. [PMID: 11376255]

■ ANORECTAL DISEASES

HEMORRHOIDS

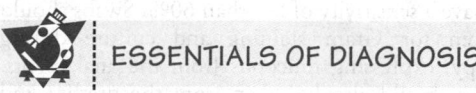

ESSENTIALS OF DIAGNOSIS

- *Bright red blood per rectum*
- *Protrusion, discomfort*

- *Characteristic findings on external anal inspection and anoscopic examination*

General Considerations

Internal hemorrhoids are a plexus of superior hemorrhoidal veins located above the dentate line which are covered by mucosa. They are a normal anatomic entity, occurring in all adults. Internal hemorrhoids form a vascular cushion in the lower rectum that may contribute to normal continence. They occur in three primary locations—right anterior, right posterior, and left lateral—though smaller hemorrhoids may occur between these primary locations. External hemorrhoids arise from the inferior hemorrhoidal veins located below the dentate line and are covered with squamous epithelium of the anal canal or perianal region.

Hemorrhoids may become symptomatic as a result of activities that increase venous pressure, resulting in distention and engorgement. Straining at stool, constipation, prolonged sitting, pregnancy, obesity, and low-fiber diets all may contribute. With time, redundancy and enlargement of the venous cushions may develop and result in bleeding or protrusion.

Clinical Findings

A. Symptoms and Signs

Patients often attribute a variety of perianal complaints to "hemorrhoids." However, the principal problems attributable to internal hemorrhoids are bleeding and mucoid discharge. Bleeding is manifested by bright red blood that may range from streaks of blood visible on toilet paper or stool to bright red blood that drips into the toilet bowl after a bowel movement. Rarely is bleeding severe enough to result in anemia. Initially, internal hemorrhoids are confined to the anal canal (stage I). Over time, the internal hemorrhoids may gradually enlarge and protrude from the anal opening. At first, this prolapse occurs during straining and reduces spontaneously (stage II). With progression over time, the prolapsed hemorrhoids may require manual reduction after bowel movements (stage III) or may remain chronically protruding (stage IV). Chronically prolapsed hemorrhoids may result in mucoid perianal discharge, resulting in irritation and soiling of underclothes. Discomfort and pain are unusual with internal hemorrhoids, occurring only when there is extensive inflammation and thrombosis of irreducible tissue or with thrombosis of an external hemorrhoid (see below).

B. Examination

External hemorrhoids are readily visible on perianal inspection. Nonprolapsed internal hemorrhoids are not visible but may protrude through the anus with gentle straining while the physician spreads the buttocks. Prolapsed hemorrhoids are visible as protuberant purple nodules covered by mucosa. The perianal region should also be examined for other signs of disease such as fistulas, fissures, skin tags, or dermatitis. On digital examination, uncomplicated internal hemorrhoids are neither palpable nor painful. Anoscopic evaluation, best performed in the prone jackknife position, provides optimal visualization of internal hemorrhoids.

Differential Diagnosis

Rectal bleeding may be caused by colorectal neoplasms, ulcerative colitis or Crohn's colitis, infectious proctitis, and diverticular disease. Rectal prolapse, in which a full thickness of rectum protrudes concentrically from the anus, is readily distinguished from mucosal hemorrhoidal prolapse. Proctosigmoidoscopy should be performed in all patients with hematochezia to exclude disease in the rectum or sigmoid colon that could be misinterpreted in the presence of hemorrhoidal bleeding. Patients with iron deficiency anemia should undergo colonoscopy or barium enema to exclude disease proximal to the sigmoid colon.

Treatment

A. CONSERVATIVE MEASURES

Most patients with early (stage I and stage II) disease can be managed with conservative treatment. To decrease straining with defecation, patients should be given instructions for a high-fiber diet and told to increase fluid intake with meals. Dietary fiber may be supplemented with bran powder (1–2 tbsp twice daily added to food or in 8 oz of liquid) or with commercial psyllium bulk laxatives (eg, Metamucil, Citrucel). Suppositories and rectal ointments have no demonstrated utility in the management of mild disease. Mucoid discharge may be treated effectively by the local application of a cotton ball tucked next to the anal opening after bowel movements. For edematous, prolapsed hemorrhoids, gentle manual reduction may be supplemented by suppositories (eg, Anusol with or without hydrocortisone) that have anesthetic and astringent properties and by warm sitz baths.

B. SURGICAL TREATMENT

Patients with stage I or stage II hemorrhoids and recurrent bleeding despite conservative measures may be treated with injection sclerotherapy or rubber band ligation. However, recurrence is common unless patients alter their dietary habits. Surgical excision (hemorrhoidectomy) is reserved for patients with chronic severe bleeding due to stage III or stage IV hemorrhoids or patients with acute thrombosed stage IV hemorrhoids.

Thrombosed External Hemorrhoid

Thrombosis of the external hemorrhoidal plexus results in a perianal hematoma. It most commonly occurs in otherwise healthy young adults and may be precipitated by coughing, heavy lifting, or straining at stool. The condition is characterized by the relatively acute onset of an exquisitely painful, tense and bluish perianal nodule covered with skin that may be up to several centimeters in size. Pain is most severe within the first few hours but gradually eases over 2–3 days as edema subsides. Symptoms may be relieved with warm sitz baths, analgesics, and ointments. If the patient is evaluated in the first 24–48 hours, removal of the clot may hasten symptomatic relief. With the patient in the lateral position, the skin around and over the lump is injected subcutaneously with 1% lidocaine using a tuberculin syringe with a 30-gauge needle. An ellipse of skin is then excised and the clot evacuated. A dry gauze dressing is applied for 12–24 hours, and daily sitz baths are then begun.

Komborozos VA et al: Rubber band ligation of symptomatic internal hemorrhoids: results of 500 cases. Dig Surg 2000; 17:71. [PMID: 10720835]

Pfenninger JL et al: Common anorectal conditions: Part I. Symptoms and complaints. Am Fam Physician 2001;63:2391. [PMID: 11430454]

Pfenninger JL et al: Common anorectal conditions: Part II. Lesions. Am Fam Physician 2001;64:77. [PMID: 11456437]

Thomson WH. Banding and injection of piles. Ann R Coll Surg Engl 2001;83:361. [PMID: 11806568]

ANORECTAL INFECTIONS

A number of organisms can cause inflammation of the anal and rectal mucosa. Proctitis is defined as inflammation of the distal 15 cm of rectum and is characterized by anorectal discomfort, tenesmus, constipation, and discharge. Most cases of proctitis are sexually transmitted, especially by anal-receptive intercourse. Proctocolitis implies inflammation that extends above the rectum to the sigmoid colon or more proximally and is caused by entirely different organisms such as campylobacter, *Entamoeba histolytica,* shigella, and enteroinvasive *E coli.* These organisms are discussed earlier in the section on diarrhea. Symptoms include frequent, small-volume, bloody or watery diarrhea, urgency, cramps, and tenesmus.

Etiology & Management

Several organisms may cause infectious proctitis.

A. NEISSERIA GONORRHOEAE

Gonorrhea may cause itching, burning, tenesmus, and a mucopurulent discharge. Blind swabs of the anal canal have a sensitivity of less than 60%. Swabs should be taken for Gram staining and culture during anoscopy, expressing mucopus from the anal crypts. Cultures should also be taken from the urethra and pharynx in men and from the cervix in women. Complications of untreated infections include strictures, fissures, fistulas, and perirectal abscesses.

B. TREPONEMA PALLIDUM

Anal syphilis may be asymptomatic or may lead to perianal pain and discharge. With primary syphilis, the chancre may be at the anal margin or within the anal canal and may mimic a fissure, fistula, or ulcer. Proctitis or inguinal lymphadenopathy may be present. With secondary syphilis, condylomata lata (pale-brown, flat verrucous lesions) may be seen, with secretion of foul-smelling mucus. The diagnosis is established with dark-field microscopy of scrapings from the chancre or condylomas. The VDRL test is positive in 75% of primary cases and in 99% of secondary cases.

C. CHLAMYDIA TRACHOMATIS

Chlamydial infection may cause proctitis similar to gonorrheal proctitis or may cause lymphogranuloma venereum, characterized by proctocolitis with fever and bloody diarrhea, painful perianal ulcerations, anorectal strictures and fistulas, and inguinal adenopathy (buboes). The diagnosis is established by culture of rectal discharge or rectal biopsy, which is over 80% sensitive.

D. HERPES SIMPLEX TYPE 2

HSV is a common cause of anorectal infection. Symptoms occur 4–21 days after exposure and include severe pain, itching, constipation, tenesmus, urinary retention, and radicular pain from involvement of lumbar or sacral nerve roots. Small vesicles or ulcers may be seen in the perianal area or anal canal. Sigmoidoscopy is not usually necessary but may reveal vesicular or ulcerative lesions in the distal rectum. Diagnosis is established by viral culture or antigen detection assays of vesicular fluid. Symptoms resolve within 2 weeks, but viral shedding may continue for several weeks. Patients may remain asymptomatic with or without viral shedding or may have recurrent mild relapses. Treatment of acute infection with acyclovir, 400 mg orally five times daily for 5–10 days, has been shown to reduce the duration of symptoms and viral shedding. Patients with AIDS and recurrent relapses may benefit from chronic suppressive therapy (see Chapter 32).

E. VENEREAL WARTS

Venereal warts (condylomata acuminata) are a significant cause of anorectal symptoms. Caused by the human papillomavirus, they are seen in up to 50% of homosexual men. HIV-positive individuals with condylomas have a higher relapse rate after therapy and a higher rate of progression to high-grade dysplasia or anal cancer. The warts are located on the perianal skin and extend within the anal canal up to 2 cm above the dentate line. Patients may have no symptoms or may report itching, bleeding, and pain. The warts may form a confluent mass that may obscure the anal opening. Treatment can be difficult. Sexual partners should also be examined and treated. Topical application of podophyllum resin is effective for small perianal lesions. Anal lesions and large lesions may require CO_2 laser surgery or cryosurgery. HIV-positive individuals with condylomas who have detectable serum HIV RNA warrant anoscopic surveillance every 3–6 months.

Sobhani I et al: Prevalence of high-grade dysplasia and cancer in the anal canal in human papillomatosis-infected individuals. Gastroenterology 2001;120:857. [PMID: 11231940]

RECTAL PROLAPSE & SOLITARY RECTAL ULCER SYNDROME

Rectal prolapse is protrusion through the anus of some or all of the layers of the rectum. It is most commonly seen in the elderly. Although surgical and traumatic injuries are causative in some patients, in most cases rectal prolapse arises from chronic, excessive straining at stool in conjunction with weakening of pelvic support structures. Although prolapse initially reduces spontaneously after defecation, with time the rectal mucosa becomes chronically prolapsed, resulting in mucous discharge, bleeding, incontinence, and sphincteric damage. Patients with complete prolapse require surgical correction.

The term solitary rectal ulcer syndrome is a misnomer. The syndrome is characterized by anal pain, excessive straining at stool, and passage of mucus and blood. It is most commonly seen in young adults, especially women. Proctoscopic examination reveals either shallow ulcerations (single or multiple) or a nodular mass located anteriorly 6–10 cm above the anal verge. Biopsy is diagnostic. The disorder may be caused by rectal intussusception with straining. Treatment is directed at decreasing straining through education of the patient and use of bulking agents.

Felt-Bersma RJ et al: Rectal prolapse, rectal intussusception, rectocele, and solitary rectal ulcer syndrome. Gastroenterol Clin North Am 2001;30:199. [PMID: 11394031]

Malouf A et al: Results of behavioral treatment (biofeedback) for solitary rectal ulcer syndrome. Dis Colon Rectum 2001; 44:72. [PMID: 11805566]

FECAL INCONTINENCE

Fecal incontinence is present in up to 10% of the elderly. There are five general requirements for bowel continence: (1) solid or semisolid stool (even healthy young adults have difficulty maintaining continence with liquid rectal contents); (2) a distensible rectal reservoir (as sigmoid contents empty into the rectum, the vault must expand to accommodate); (3) a sensation of rectal fullness (if the patient cannot sense this, overflow may occur before the patient can take appropriate action); (4) intact pelvic nerves and muscles; and (5) the ability to reach a toilet in a timely fashion.

Minor Incontinence

Many patients complain of slight soilage of undergarments that tends to occur after bowel movements or with straining or coughing. This may be due to local anal problems such as hemorrhoids and skin tags that make it difficult to form a tight anal seal, especially if stools are somewhat loose. Patients should be treated with fiber supplements to provide greater stool bulk. Loose application of a cotton ball near the anal opening may absorb small amounts of fecal leakage. Seepage may be improved by Kegel perineal strengthening exercises. Conditions such as ulcerative proctitis that cause tenesmus and urgency, chronic diarrheal conditions, and irritable bowel syndrome may result in difficulty in maintaining complete continence, especially if a toilet is not readily available. Similarly, the elderly may require more time or assistance to reach a toilet, which may lead to incontinence. Elderly patients with chronic constipation may develop stool impaction leading to "overflow" incontinence.

Major Incontinence

Complete uncontrolled loss of stool reflects a significant problem with sphincteric or neurologic damage. Causes of sphincteric damage include traumatic childbirth (especially forceps delivery), episiotomy, prolapse, prior anal surgery, and physical trauma. Neurologic disruption may be caused by obstetric trauma (with pudendal nerve damage), aging, diabetes mellitus, dementia, multiple sclerosis, spinal cord injury, and cauda equina syndrome.

Physical examination should include careful inspection of the perianal area for hemorrhoids, rectal prolapse, fissures, and fistulas. The perianal skin should be stimulated to confirm an intact anocutaneous reflex. Digital examination during relaxation and squeezing gives valuable information about resting tone (due to the internal sphincter) and external sphincter function and excludes fecal impaction. Anoscopy is required to evaluate for hemorrhoids, fissures, and fistulas. Proctosigmoidoscopy is useful to exclude rectal carcinoma or proctitis. Anal ultrasonography is the most reliable test for definition of anatomic defects in the external and internal anal sphincters. Anal manometry and surface electromyography may also be useful to define the severity of weakness, to diagnose nerve injury, and to predict response to biofeedback training.

Patients who are incontinent only of loose or liquid stools are treated with bulking agents and antidiarrheal drugs (eg, loperamide, 2 mg before meals and prophylactically before social engagements, shopping trips, etc). Patients with incontinence of solid stool benefit from scheduled toilet use after glycerin suppositories or tap water enemas. Biofeedback training with anal sphincter exercises is helpful in motivated patients to lower the threshold for awareness of rectal filling, or to improve anal sphincter squeeze function, or both. Operative management is seldom needed but should be considered in patients with major incontinence who have failed medical therapy.

Barnett JL et al: American Gastroenterological Association medical position statement on anorectal testing techniques. Gastroenterology 1999;116:732. [PMID: 10029631]

Soffer E et al: Fecal incontinence: a practical approach to evaluation and treatment. Am J Gastroenterol 2000;95:1873. [PMID: 10950029]

OTHER ANAL CONDITIONS

Anal Fissures

Anal fissures are linear or rocket-shaped ulcers that are usually less than 5 mm in length. They occur most commonly in the posterior midline, but 10% occur anteriorly. Fissures are believed to arise from trauma to the anal canal during defecation, perhaps caused by straining, constipation, or high internal sphincter tone. Patients complain of severe, tearing pain during defecation followed by throbbing discomfort that may lead to constipation due to fear of recurrent pain. There may be mild associated hematochezia, with blood on the stool or toilet paper. Anal fissures are confirmed by visual inspection of the anal verge while gently separating the buttocks. Acute fissures look like cracks in the epithelium. Chronic fissures result in fibrosis and the development of a skin tag at the outermost edge (sentinel pile). Digital and anoscopic examinations may cause severe pain and may not be possible. Medical management is directed at promoting effortless, painless bowel movements. Fiber supplements and sitz baths should be prescribed. Suppositories are of no benefit. Topical agents such as 1% hydrocortisone ointment may be helpful. Topical 0.2–0.5% nitroglycerin ointment applied by cotton swab to the anus and anal canal twice daily for 6–8 weeks results in healing in up to 80% of patients; however, headaches may occur. Injection of botulinum toxin (20 units) into the internal anal sphincter has been shown to cause healing in 90% of patients with chronic anal fissure. Chronic or recurrent fissures may benefit from partial lateral internal sphincterotomy; however, minor incontinence may complicate this procedure.

Altomare DF et al: Glyceryl trinitrate for chronic anal fissure—healing or headache? Results of a multicenter, randomized, placebo-controlled, double-blind trial. Dis Colon Rectum 2000;43:174. [PMID: 10696890]

Argov S et al: Open lateral sphincterotomy is still the best treatment for chronic anal fissure. Am J Surg 2000;179:201. [PMID: 10827320]

McCallion K et al: Progress in the understanding and treatment of chronic anal fissure. Postgrad Med J 2001;77:753. [PMID: 11723312]

Qureshi W: Gastrointestinal uses of botulinum toxin. J Clin Gastroenterol 2002;34:126. [PMID: 11782604]

Perianal Abscess & Fistula

The anal glands located at the base of the anal crypts at the dentate line may become infected, leading to abscess formation. Other causes of abscess include anal fissure and Crohn's disease. Abscesses may extend upward or downward through the intersphincteric plane. Symptoms of perianal abscess are throbbing, continuous perianal pain. Erythema, fluctuance, and swelling may be found in the perianal region on external examination or in the ischiorectal fossa on digital rectal examination. Perianal abscesses are treated with local incision and drainage, while ischiorectal abscesses require drainage in the operating room. After drainage of an abscess, most patients are found to have a fistula in ano.

Fistula in ano most often arises in an anal crypt and is usually preceded by an anal abscess. In patients with fistulas that connect to the rectum, other disorders such as Crohn's disease, lymphogranuloma venereum, rectal tuberculosis, and cancer should be considered. Fistulas are associated with purulent discharge that may lead to itching, tenderness, and pain. Treatment is by surgical incision or excision under anesthesia. Care must be taken to preserve the anal sphincters.

Pruritus Ani

Pruritus ani is characterized by perianal itching and discomfort. It may be caused by poor anal hygiene associated with fistulas, fissures, prolapsed hemorrhoids, skin tags, and minor incontinence. Conversely, overzealous cleansing with soaps may contribute to local irritation or contact dermatitis. Pinworms, candidal infection (especially in diabetics), scabies, and condylomata acuminata must be excluded. In patients with idiopathic pruritus ani, examination may reveal erythema, excoriations, or lichenified, eczematous skin. Education is vital to successful therapy. After bowel movements, the perianal area should be cleansed with nonscented wipes premoistened with lanolin followed by gentle drying. A piece of cotton ball should be tucked next to the anal opening to absorb perspiration or fecal seepage. Anal ointments and lotions may exacerbate the condition and should be avoided.

CARCINOMA OF THE ANUS

These tumors are relatively rare, comprising only 1–2% of all cancers of the anus and large intestine. Squamous (epidermoid) cancers make up the majority of anal cancers; the remainder are cloacogenic tumors arising from the transitional cells in the upper anus. Anal cancer is increased among people practicing receptive anal intercourse and those with a history of other sexually transmitted diseases. In over 80% of cases, human papillomavirus (HPV) may be detected, suggesting that this virus may be a causal factor. Anal cancer is increased in HIV-infected individuals. Combined HIV and HPV infection markedly increases the risk of anal carcinoma. Bleeding, pain, and local tumor are the commonest symptoms. The lesion is often confused with hemorrhoids or other common anal disorders. These tumors tend to become annular, invade the sphincter, and spread upward via the lymphatics into the perirectal mesenteric lymphatic nodes.

Treatment depends upon the tumor stage. MR scan and endoluminal ultrasound assist in determining the depth of penetration and local spread. Small superficial lesions of the perianal skin may be treated by local excision. Larger tumors invading the sphincter or rectum are treated with combined-modality therapy that includes external radiation with simultaneous chemotherapy (fluorouracil and either mitomycin or cisplatin). Local control is achieved in 80% of patients. Radical surgery (abdominoperineal resection) is now performed in patients who fail chemotherapy and radiation therapy. The 5-year survival rate is 60–70% for localized tumors and over 25% for metastatic (stage IV) disease.

Anal Cancer (PDQ) Treatment—National Cancer Institute—Cancer Net. http://cancernet.nci.nih.gov

Goldstone SE et al: High prevalence of anal squamous intraepithelial lesions and squamous-cell carcinoma in men who have sex with men as seen in a surgical practice. Dis Colon Rectum 2001;44:690. [PMID: 11357031]

Whiteford MH et al: The evolving treatment of anal cancer: How are we doing? Arch Surg 2001;136:886. PMID: 11485523]

Liver, Biliary Tract, & Pancreas 15

Lawrence S. Friedman, MD
See www.current-med.com/ch15.html

JAUNDICE
(Icterus)

Jaundice results from the accumulation of bilirubin—a reddish pigment product of heme metabolism—in the body tissues; the cause may be hepatic or nonhepatic. Hyperbilirubinemia may be due to abnormalities in the formation, transport, metabolism, and excretion of bilirubin. Total serum bilirubin is normally 0.2–1.2 mg/dL, and jaundice may not be recognizable until levels are about 3 mg/dL.

Jaundice is caused by predominantly unconjugated or conjugated bilirubin in the serum (Table 15–1). Unconjugated hyperbilirubinemia may result from overproduction of bilirubin because of hemolysis; impaired hepatic uptake of bilirubin due to certain drugs; or impaired conjugation of bilirubin by glucuronide, as in Gilbert's syndrome, due to mild decreases in glucuronyl transferase, or Crigler-Najjar syndrome, caused by moderate decreases or absence of glucuronyl transferase. In the absence of liver disease, hemolysis rarely elevates the serum bilirubin level to more than 7 mg/dL. Predominantly conjugated hyperbilirubinemia may result from impaired excretion of bilirubin from the liver due to hepatocellular disease, drugs, sepsis, hereditary disorders such as Dubin-Johnson syndrome, or extrahepatic biliary obstruction. Features of some hyperbilirubinemic syndromes are summarized in Table 15–2. The term "cholestasis" denotes retention of bile in the liver, and the term "cholestatic jaundice" is often used when conjugated hyperbilirubinemia results from impaired bile flow.

Manifestations of Diseases Associated With Jaundice

A. UNCONJUGATED HYPERBILIRUBINEMIA

Stool and urine color are normal, and there is mild jaundice and indirect (unconjugated) hyperbilirubinemia with no bilirubin in the urine. Splenomegaly occurs in hemolytic disorders except in sickle cell anemia. Abdominal or back pain may occur with acute hemolytic crises.

B. CONJUGATED HYPERBILIRUBINEMIA

1. Hereditary cholestatic syndromes or intrahepatic cholestasis—The patient may be asymptomatic; intermittent cholestasis is often accompanied by pruritus, light-colored stools, and, occasionally, malaise.

2. Hepatocellular disease—Malaise, anorexia, low-grade fever, and right upper quadrant discomfort are frequent. Dark urine, jaundice, and, in women, amenorrhea occur. An enlarged, tender liver; vascular spiders; palmar erythema; ascites; gynecomastia; sparse body hair; fetor hepaticus; and asterixis may be present, depending on the cause, severity, and chronicity of liver dysfunction.

C. BILIARY OBSTRUCTION

There may be right upper quadrant pain, weight loss (suggesting carcinoma), jaundice, dark urine, and light-colored stools. Symptoms and signs may be intermittent if caused by stone, carcinoma of the ampulla, or cholangiocarcinoma. Pain may be absent early in pancreatic cancer. Occult blood in the stools suggests cancer of the ampulla. Hepatomegaly and a palpable gallbladder (Courvoisier's sign) are characteristic, but neither specific nor sensitive of pancreatic head tumor. Fever and chills are far more common in benign obstruction and associated cholangitis.

Diagnostic Methods for Evaluation of Liver Disease & Jaundice (Table 15–3)

A. LABORATORY STUDIES

Elevated serum aspartate and alanine aminotransferase levels (AST, ALT) result from hepatocellular necrosis or inflammation, as in hepatitis; ALT is more specific for the liver than AST, but an AST level at least twice that of the ALT is typical of alcoholic liver injury. In contrast, the ALT level is greater than the AST level in nonalcoholic fatty liver disease prior to the development of cirrhosis. In addition to signaling underlying liver disease, an isolated elevation of the serum ALT level may be the only clue to the diagnosis of celiac disease. Elevated alkaline phosphatase levels are seen

Table 15–1. Classification of jaundice.

Type of Hyperbilirubinemia	Location and Cause
Unconjugated hyperbilirubinemia (predominant indirect-acting bilirubin)	Increased bilirubin production (eg, hemolytic anemias, hemolytic reactions, hematoma, pulmonary infarction)
	Impaired bilirubin uptake and storage (eg, posthepatitis hyperbilirubinemia, Gilbert's syndrome, Crigler-Najjar syndrome, drug reactions)
Conjugated hyperbilirubinemia (predominant direct-acting bilirubin)	**HEREDITARY CHOLESTATIC SYNDROMES** Faulty excretion of bilirubin conjugates (eg, Dubin-Johnson syndrome, Rotor's syndrome) **HEPATOCELLULAR DYSFUNCTION** Biliary epithelial damage (eg, hepatitis, hepatic cirrhosis) Intrahepatic cholestasis (eg, certain drugs, biliary cirrhosis, sepsis, postoperative jaundice) Hepatocellular damage or intrahepatic cholestasis resulting from miscellaneous causes (eg, spirochetal infections, infectious mononucleosis, cholangitis, sarcoidosis, lymphomas, industrial toxins) **BILIARY OBSTRUCTION** Choledocholithiasis, biliary atresia, carcinoma of biliary duct, sclerosing cholangitis, choledochal cyst, external pressure on common duct, pancreatitis, pancreatic neoplasms

in cholestasis or infiltrative liver disease (such as tumor or granuloma). Alkaline phosphatase elevations of hepatic rather than bone, intestinal, or placental origin are confirmed by concomitant elevation of γ-glutamyl transpeptidase or 5′-nucleotidase levels.

B. LIVER BIOPSY

Percutaneous liver biopsy is the definitive study for determining the cause and histologic severity of hepatocellular dysfunction or infiltrative liver disease. In patients with suspected metastatic disease or a hepatic mass, it is performed under ultrasound or CT guidance. A transjugular route can be used in patients with coagulopathy or ascites.

C. IMAGING

Demonstration of dilated bile ducts by ultrasonography or CT scan indicates biliary obstruction (90–95% sensitivity). Ultrasonography, CT scan, and MRI may also demonstrate hepatomegaly, intrahepatic tumors, and portal hypertension. Spiral arterial-phase CT scanning, in which the liver is imaged during peak hepatic enhancement while the patient holds one or two breaths, improves diagnostic accuracy. Dual-phase spiral CT, CT arterial portography, in which imaging follows intravenous contrast infusion via a catheter placed in the superior mesenteric artery, MRI with use of ferumoxides as contrast agents, and intraoperative ultrasonography are the most sensitive techniques for detection of individual small hepatic lesions in patients eligible for resection of metastases. Use of color Doppler ultrasound or contrast agents that produce microbubbles increases the sensitivity of transcutaneous ultrasound for detecting small neoplasms. MRI is the most accurate technique for identifying isolated liver lesions such as hemangiomas, focal nodular hyperplasia, or focal fatty infiltration and for detecting hepatic iron overload. Because of its much lower cost, ultrasonography ($350) is preferable to CT ($1200–$1400) or MRI ($2000) as a screening test. Ultrasonography can detect gallstones with a sensitivity of 95%.

Endoscopic retrograde cholangiopancreatography (ERCP) or percutaneous transhepatic cholangiography (PTC) identifies the cause, location, and extent of biliary obstruction. Magnetic resonance cholangiopancreatography (MRCP) appears to be a sensitive, noninvasive method of detecting bile duct stones, strictures, and dilation. ERCP requires a skilled endoscopist and may be utilized to demonstrate pancreatic or ampullary causes of jaundice, to carry out papillotomy and stone extraction, or to insert a stent through an

Table 15–2. Hyperbilirubinemic disorders.

	Nature of Defect	Type of Hyper-bilirubinemia	Clinical and Pathologic Characteristics
Gilbert's syndrome	Glucuronyl transferase deficiency	Unconjugated (indirect bilirubin)	Benign, asymptomatic hereditary jaundice. Hyperbilirubinemia increased by 24- to 36-hour fast. No treatment required. Prognosis excellent.
Dubin-Johnson syndrome (familial chronic idiopathic jaundice)[1]	Faulty excretory function of hepatocytes	Conjugated (direct) bilirubin	Benign, asymptomatic hereditary jaundice. Gallbladder does not visualize on oral cholecystography. Liver darkly pigmented on gross examination. Biopsy shows centrilobular brown pigment. Prognosis excellent.
Rotor's syndrome			Similar to Dubin-Johnson syndrome, but liver is not pigmented and the gallbladder is visualized on oral cholecystography. Prognosis excellent.
Benign recurrent intrahepatic cholestasis[2]	Cholestasis, often on a familial basis	Unconjugated plus conjugated (total) bilirubin	Episodic attacks of jaundice, itching and malaise. Onset in early life and may persist for a lifetime. Alkaline phosphatase increased. Cholestasis found on liver biopsy. (Biopsy is normal during remission.) Prognosis excellent.
Recurrent jaundice of pregnancy			Benign cholestatic jaundice of unknown cause, usually occurring in the third trimester of pregnancy. Itching, gastrointestinal symptoms, and abnormal liver excretory function tests. Cholestasis noted on liver biopsy. Prognosis excellent, but recurrence with subsequent pregnancies or use of birth control pills is characteristic.

[1]The Dubin-Johnson syndrome is caused by a point mutation in the gene coding for an organic anion transporter in bile canaliculi on chromosome 10q23–24.
[2]Mutations in genes which control hepatocellular transport systems that are involved in the formation of bile and inherited as autosomal recessive traits are on chromosomes 18q21–22, 2q24, and 7q21 in families with progressive familial intrahepatic cholestasis. A gene mutation on chromosome 18q21–22 alters a P-type ATPase expressed in the small intestine and liver and causes benign recurrent intrahepatic cholestasis.

Table 15–3. Liver function tests: Normal values and changes in two types of jaundice.

Tests	Normal Values	Hepatocellular Jaundice	Uncomplicated Obstructive Jaundice
Bilirubin Direct Indirect	0.1–0.3 mg/dL 0.2–0.7 mg/dL	Increased Increased	Increased Increased
Urine bilirubin	None	Increased	Increased
Serum albumin/total protein	Albumin, 3.5–5.5 g/dL	Albumin decreased Total protein, 6.5–8.4 g/dL	Unchanged
Alkaline phosphatase	30–115 units/L	Increased (+)	Increased (++++)
Prothrombin time	INR[1] of 1.0–1.4. After vitamin K, 10% increase in 24 hours	Prolonged if damage severe and does not respond to parenteral vitamin K	Prolonged if obstruction marked, but responds to parenteral vitamin K
ALT, AST	ALT, 5–35 units/L; AST, 5–40 units/L	Increased in hepatocellular damage, viral hepatitis	Minimally increased

[1]INR = International Normalized Ratio.

obstructing lesion. Complications of ERCP include pancreatitis in 5% of cases and, less commonly, cholangitis, bleeding, or duodenal perforation after papillotomy. Severe complications of PTC occur in 3% of cases and include fever, bacteremia, bile peritonitis, and intraperitoneal hemorrhage. Endoscopic ultrasonography is the most sensitive test for detecting small lesions of the ampulla or pancreatic head and for detecting portal vein invasion by pancreatic cancer. It is also accurate in detecting or excluding bile duct stones.

Federle MP (guest editor): Imaging of the liver. Semin Liver Dis 2001;21:133. (Entire issue devoted to all aspects of liver imaging.)

Janssen PL et al: Genes and cholestasis. Hepatology 2001; 34:1067. [PMID: 11731993] (Review of recently identified molecular defects in hepatocellular membrane transporters that account for various genetic hyperbilirubinemic disorders.)

Pratt DS et al: Evaluation of abnormal liver-enzyme results in asymptomatic patients. N Engl J. Med 2000;342:1266. [PMID: 10781624] (Useful review of causes and evaluation of elevated aminotransferase, alkaline phosphatase, and γ-glutamyl transpeptidase levels.)

Rothschild JM et al: Abdominal cross-sectional imaging for inpatients with abnormal liver function test results: yield and usefulness. Arch Intern Med 2001;161:583. [PMID: 11252119] (Clinically significant findings were identified in 35% of cases and included biliary obstruction [25%], cholecystitis [20%], malignancy [20%], and cirrhosis [15%].)

Skelly MM et al: Findings on liver biopsy to investigate abnormal liver function tests in the absence of diagnostic serology. J Hepatol 2001;35:195. [PMID: 11580141] (With unexplained liver test abnormalities after a biochemical serologic evaluation, 35% had nonalcoholic steatohepatitis and 30% had fatty liver on liver biopsy; 5% had cirrhosis.)

■ DISEASES OF THE LIVER

VIRAL HEPATITIS

ESSENTIALS OF DIAGNOSIS

- *Prodrome of anorexia, nausea, vomiting, malaise, aversion to smoking.*
- *Fever, enlarged and tender liver, jaundice.*
- *Normal to low white cell count; abnormal liver tests, especially markedly elevated aminotransferases early in the course.*
- *Liver biopsy shows hepatocellular necrosis and mononuclear infiltrate but is rarely indicated.*

General Considerations

Hepatitis can be caused by many drugs and toxic agents as well as by numerous viruses, the clinical manifestations of which may be quite similar. Viruses causing hepatitis are (1) hepatitis A virus (HAV); (2) hepatitis B virus (HBV); (3) hepatitis C virus (HCV); (4) hepatitis D virus (delta agent); and (5) hepatitis E virus (an enterically transmitted hepatitis seen in epidemic form in Asia, North Africa, and Mexico). The designation hepatitis G virus (HGV) applies to an agent that rarely, if ever, causes frank hepatitis. A DNA virus designated the TT virus (TTV) has been identified in up to 7.5% of blood donors and found to be transmitted readily by blood transfusions, but an association between this virus and liver disease has not been established. A related virus known as SEN-V has been found in 2% of United States blood donors, is transmitted by transfusion, and may account for some cases of transfusion-associated non-ABCDE hepatitis. In immunocompromised and rare immunocompetent hosts, cytomegalovirus, Epstein-Barr virus, and herpes simplex virus should be considered in the differential diagnosis of hepatitis. As yet unidentified agents account for a small percentage of cases of apparent acute viral hepatitis.

A. HEPATITIS A

(Figure 15–1) HAV is a 27-nm RNA hepatovirus (in the picornavirus family) causing epidemics or sporadic cases of hepatitis. Transmission is by the fecal-oral route, and spread is favored by crowding and poor sanitation. Common source outbreaks result from contaminated water or food. The incubation period averages 30 days. Hepatitis A virus is excreted in feces

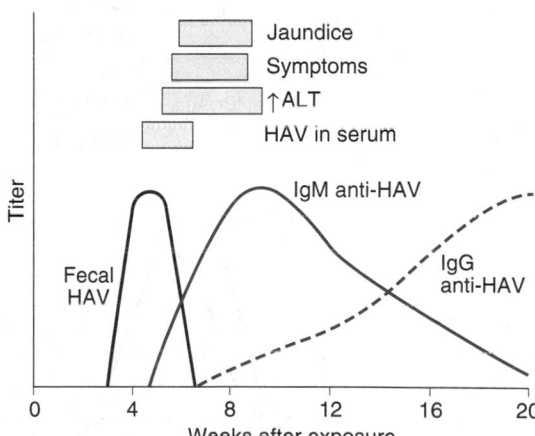

Figure 15–1. The typical course of acute type A hepatitis. (HAV, hepatitis A virus; anti-HAV, antibody to hepatitis A virus; ALT, alanine aminotransferase.) (Reproduced, with permission, from Koff RS: Acute viral hepatitis. In: *Handbook of Liver Disease.* Friedman LS, Keeffe EB [editors]. Churchill Livingstone, 1998.)

for up to 2 weeks before clinical illness. Virus is rarely demonstrated in feces after the first week of illness. The mortality rate for hepatitis A is low, and fulminant hepatitis A is uncommon save for rare instances in which hepatitis A occurs in a patient with chronic hepatitis C. Chronic hepatitis A does not occur, and there is no carrier state. Clinical illness is more severe in adults than in children, in whom it is typically asymptomatic. It is the only viral hepatitis causing spiking fevers.

Antibody to hepatitis A (anti-HAV) appears early in the course of the illness. Both IgM and IgG anti-HAV are detectable in serum soon after the onset. Peak titers of IgM anti-HAV occur during the first week of clinical disease and disappear within 3–6 months. Detection of IgM anti-HAV is an excellent test for diagnosing acute hepatitis A. Titers of IgG anti-HAV peak after 1 month of the disease and may persist for years. IgG anti-HAV indicates previous exposure to HAV, noninfectivity, and immunity. In the USA, about 33% of the population have serologic evidence of previous infection.

B. HEPATITIS B

(Figure 15–2) Hepatitis B virus (HBV) is a 42-nm hepadnavirus with a partially double-stranded DNA genome, inner core protein (hepatitis B core antigen, HBcAg) and outer surface coat (hepatitis B surface antigen, HBsAg). It is usually transmitted by inoculation of infected blood or blood products or by sexual contact and is present in saliva, semen, and vaginal secretions. HBsAg-positive mothers may transmit HBV to neonates at delivery; the risk of chronic infection in the infant is as high as 90%.

Hepatitis B virus (HBV) is prevalent in homosexuals and intravenous drug users, but most cases result from heterosexual transmission; the incidence has decreased by 70% since the late 1980s. Groups at high risk include patients and staff at hemodialysis centers, physicians, dentists, nurses, and personnel working in clinical and pathology laboratories and blood banks. The risk of HBV infection from a blood transfusion is less than one in 60,000 units transfused in the USA. The incubation period of hepatitis B is 6 weeks to 6 months (average 12–14 weeks).

The onset of hepatitis B is more insidious and the aminotransferase levels higher than in HAV infection. The risk of fulminant hepatitis is less than 1%, with a mortality rate of up to 60%. Following acute hepatitis B, HBV infection persists in 1–2% of immunocompetent adults but in a higher percentage of immunocompromised adults or children. Persons with chronic hepatitis B, particularly when HBV infection is acquired early in life and viral replication persists, are at substantial risk of cirrhosis and hepatocellular carcinoma (up to 25–40%). Men are more at risk. Infection caused by HBV may be associated with serum sickness, glomerulonephritis, and polyarteritis nodosa.

There are three distinct antigen-antibody systems that relate to HBV infection and a variety of circulating markers that are useful in diagnosis. Interpretation of common serologic patterns is shown in Table 15–4.

1. HBsAg—The appearance of HBsAg is the first evidence of infection, appearing before biochemical evi-

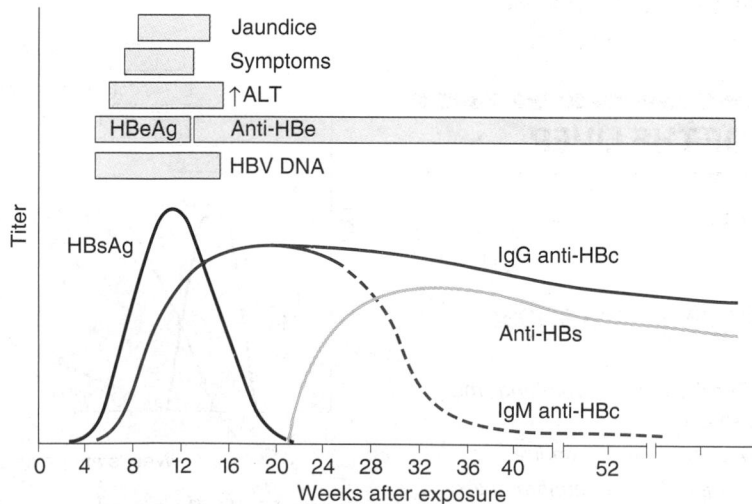

Figure 15–2. The typical course of acute type B hepatitis. (HBsAg, hepatitis B surface antigen; anti-HBs, antibody to HBsAg; HBeAg, hepatitis Be antigen; anti-HBe, antibody to HBeAg; anti-HBc, antibody to hepatitis B core antigen; ALT, alanine aminotransferase.) (Reproduced, with permission, from Koff RS: Acute viral hepatitis. In: *Handbook of Liver Disease.* Friedman LS, Keeffe EB [editors]. Churchill Livingstone, 1998.)

Table 15–4. Common serologic patterns in hepatitis B virus infection and their interpretation.

HBsAg	Anti-HBs	Anti-HBc	HBeAg	Anti-HBe	Interpretation
+	–	IgM	+	–	Acute hepatitis B
+	–	IgG[1]	+	–	Chronic hepatitis B with active viral replication
+	–	IgG	–	+	Chronic hepatitis B with low viral replication
+	+	IgG	+ or –	+ or –	Chronic hepatitis B with heterotypic anti-HBs (about 10% of cases)
–	–	IgM	+ or –	–	Acute hepatitis B
–	+	IgG		+ or –	Recovery from hepatitis B (immunity)
–	+	–	–	–	Vaccination (immunity)
–	–	IgG	–	–	False-positive; less commonly, infection in remote past

[1]Low levels of IgM anti-HBc may also be detected.

dence of liver disease, and persists throughout the clinical illness. Persistence of HBsAg after the acute illness may be associated with clinical and laboratory evidence of chronic hepatitis for variable periods of time. The detection of HBsAg establishes infection with HBV and implies infectivity.

2. Anti-HBs—Specific antibody to HBsAg (anti-HBs) appears in most individuals after clearance of HBsAg and after successful vaccination against hepatitis B. Disappearance of HBsAg and the appearance of anti-HBs signals recovery from HBV infection, noninfectivity, and immunity.

3. Anti-HBc—IgM anti-HBc appears shortly after HBsAg is detected. (HBcAg alone does not appear in serum.) Its presence in the setting of acute hepatitis indicates a diagnosis of acute hepatitis B, and it fills the serologic gap in patients who have cleared HBsAg but do not yet have detectable anti-HBs. IgM anti-HBc can persist for 3–6 months or more. IgM anti-HBc may also reappear during flares of previously inactive chronic hepatitis B. IgG anti-HBc also appears during acute hepatitis B but persists indefinitely, whether the patient recovers (with the appearance of anti-HBs in serum) or develops chronic hepatitis B (with persistence of HBsAg). In asymptomatic blood donors, an isolated anti-HBc with no other positive HBV serologic results may represent a falsely positive result or latent infection in which HBV DNA is detectable only by polymerase chain reaction testing.

4. HBeAg—HBeAg is a soluble protein found only in HBsAg-positive serum. It is a secretory form of HBcAg appearing during the incubation period shortly after the detection of HBsAg. HBeAg indicates viral replication and infectivity. Persistence of HBeAg in serum beyond 3 months indicates an increased likelihood of chronic hepatitis B. Its disappearance is often followed by the appearance of anti-HBe, signifying diminished viral replication and decreased infectivity.

5. HBV DNA—The presence of HBV DNA in serum generally parallels the presence of HBeAg, though HBV DNA is a more sensitive and precise marker of viral replication and infectivity. Very low levels of HBV DNA, detectable only by PCR, may persist in serum after a patient has recovered from acute hepatitis B, but the HBV DNA is bound to IgG and rarely infectious. In some patients with chronic hepatitis B, HBV DNA is present in high levels without HBeAg in serum because of a mutation that prevents synthesis of HBeAg in infected hepatocytes. This "pre-core mutant" appears during the course of chronic wild-type HBV infection, presumably as a result of immune pressure. When additional mutations in the core gene are present, the pre-core mutant enhances the severity of HBV and increases the risk of cirrhosis.

C. HEPATITIS D (DELTA AGENT)

Hepatitis D virus (HDV) is a defective RNA virus that causes hepatitis only in association with hepatitis B infection and specifically only in the presence of HBsAg; it is cleared when the latter is cleared.

HDV may co-infect with HBV or may superinfect a person with chronic hepatitis B, usually by percutaneous exposure. When acute hepatitis D is coincident with acute HBV infection, the infection is generally similar in severity to acute hepatitis B alone. In chronic hepatitis B, superinfection by HDV appears to carry a worse short-term prognosis, often resulting in fulminant hepatitis or severe chronic hepatitis that progresses rapidly to cirrhosis. In the 1970s and early 1980s, HDV was endemic in some areas, such as the

Mediterranean countries, where up to 80% of HBV carriers were superinfected with it. In the United States, HDV occurred primarily among intravenous drug users. However, new cases of hepatitis D are now infrequent, and cases seen today are usually from cohorts infected years ago who survived the initial impact of hepatitis D and now have inactive cirrhosis. These patients have a threefold increased risk of hepatocellular carcinoma. Diagnosis is made by detection of antibody to hepatitis D antigen (anti-HDV) or, where available, HDV RNA in serum.

Hepatitis D is best prevented by prevention of hepatitis B (eg, with HBV vaccine).

D. HEPATITIS C (HCV)

(Figure 15–3) The hepatitis C virus is a single-stranded RNA virus with properties similar to those of flavivirus. At least six major genotypes of HCV have been identified. In the past, HCV was responsible for over 90% of cases of posttransfusion hepatitis, yet only 4% of cases of hepatitis C were attributable to blood transfusions. Over 50% of cases are transmitted by intravenous drug use. Intranasal cocaine use and body piercing also are risk factors. The risk of sexual and maternal-neonatal transmission is low and may be greatest in a subset of patients with high circulating levels of HCV RNA. Having multiple sexual partners may increase the risk of HCV infection. Transmission via breast feeding has not been documented. An outbreak of hepatitis C in patients with immune deficiencies occurred in some recipients of intravenous immune globulin, and nosocomial transmission via multidose vials of saline used to flush Portacaths has occurred. Coinfection with HCV is found in 30–50%

of persons infected with HIV. Covert transmission during bloody fisticuffs has even been reported. In many patients, the source of infection is unknown. There are about 2.7 million HCV carriers in the USA and another 1.3 million previously exposed persons who have cleared the virus.

The incubation period averages 6–7 weeks, and clinical illness is often mild, usually asymptomatic, and characterized by waxing and waning aminotransferase elevations and a high rate (> 80%) of chronic hepatitis. In pregnant patients, serum aminotransferase levels frequently normalize despite persistence of viremia, only to increase again after delivery. HCV is a pathogenetic factor in cryoglobulinemia and glomerulonephritis and may be related to autoimmune thyroiditis, lymphocytic sialadenitis, idiopathic pulmonary fibrosis, sporadic porphyria cutanea tarda, monoclonal gammopathies, and probably lymphoma. The risk of type 2 diabetes mellitus appears to be increased in persons with chronic hepatitis C.

Diagnosis of hepatitis C is based on an enzyme immunoassay that detects antibodies to HCV. Anti-HCV is not protective, and in patients with acute or chronic hepatitis its presence in serum generally signifies that HCV is the cause. Limitations of the enzyme immunoassay include moderate sensitivity (false-negatives) for the diagnosis of acute hepatitis C early in the course and in healthy blood donors and low specificity (false-positives) in some persons with elevated gamma globulin levels. In these situations, a diagnosis of hepatitis C may be confirmed by use of an assay for HCV RNA and, in some cases, a supplemental recombinant immunoblot assay (RIBA) for anti-HCV. Most RIBA-positive persons are potentially infectious, as confirmed by use of polymerase chain reaction-based tests to detect HCV RNA. Occasional persons are found to have anti-HCV in serum, confirmed by RIBA, without HCV RNA in serum, suggesting recovery from HCV infection in the past. Testing of donated blood for HCV has helped reduce the risk of transfusion-associated hepatitis C from 10% a decade ago to less than one per 100,000 units today.

E. HEPATITIS E (HEV)

HEV is a 29- to 32-nm RNA virus similar to calicivirus and responsible for waterborne hepatitis outbreaks in India, Burma, Afghanistan, Algeria, and Mexico. It is rare in the USA but should be considered in patients with acute hepatitis after a trip to an endemic area. Illness is self-limited (no carrier state) with a high mortality rate (10–20%) in pregnant women.

F. HEPATITIS G

The designation hepatitis G virus (HGV) has been applied to a flavivirus that is percutaneously transmitted and associated with chronic viremia lasting at least 10 years. HGV has been detected in 1.5% of blood donors, 50% of intravenous drug users, 30% of hemodialysis patients, 20% of hemophiliacs, and 15% of

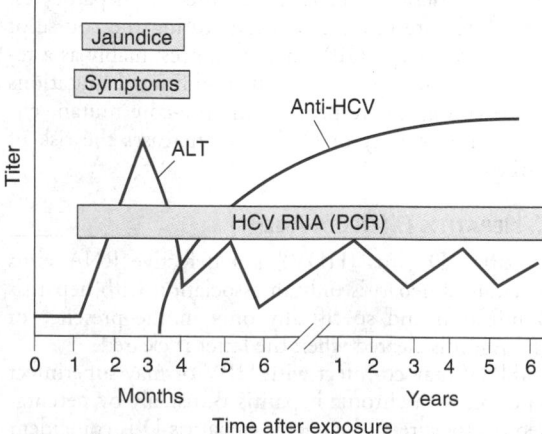

Figure 15–3. The typical course of acute and chronic hepatitis C. (ALT, alanine aminotransferase; Anti-HCV, antibody to hepatitis C virus by enzyme immunoassay; HCV RNA [PCR], hepatitis C viral RNA by polymerase chain reaction.)

patients with chronic hepatitis B or C, but it does not appear to cause important liver disease or affect the response of patients with chronic hepatitis B or C to antiviral therapy. HGV coinfection may improve survival in patients with HIV infection.

Clinical Findings

The clinical picture of viral hepatitis is extremely variable, ranging from asymptomatic infection without jaundice to a fulminating disease and death in a few days.

A. SYMPTOMS

1. Prodromal phase—The onset may be abrupt or insidious, with general malaise, myalgia, arthralgia, easy fatigability, upper respiratory symptoms, and anorexia. A distaste for smoking, paralleling anorexia, may occur early. Nausea and vomiting are frequent, and diarrhea or constipation may occur. Serum sickness may be seen early in acute hepatitis B. Fever is generally present but is low-grade save in occasional cases of hepatitis A. Defervescence and a fall in pulse rate often coincide with the onset of jaundice.

Abdominal pain is usually mild and constant in the right upper quadrant or epigastrium, often aggravated by jarring or exertion, and rarely may be severe enough to simulate cholecystitis.

2. Icteric phase—Jaundice occurs after 5–10 days but may appear at the same time as the initial symptomatology. Most never develop it. With the onset of jaundice, there is often worsening of the prodromal symptoms, followed by progressive clinical improvement.

3. Convalescent phase—There is an increasing sense of well-being, return of appetite, and disappearance of jaundice, abdominal pain and tenderness, and fatigability.

4. Course and complications—The acute illness usually subsides over 2–3 weeks with complete clinical and laboratory recovery by 9 weeks in hepatitis A and by 16 weeks in hepatitis B. In 5–10% of cases, the course may be more protracted, but less than 1% will have a fulminant course. In some cases of acute hepatitis A, clinical, biochemical, and serologic recovery may be followed by one or two relapses, but recovery is the rule. A protracted course of hepatitis A has been reported to be associated with HLA *DRB1*1301*. Hepatitis B, D, and C (and G) may become chronic (see below).

B. SIGNS

Hepatomegaly—rarely marked—is present in over half of cases. Liver tenderness is usually present. Splenomegaly is reported in 15% of patients, and soft, enlarged lymph nodes—especially in the cervical or epitrochlear areas—may occur. Systemic toxicity is most often encountered in hepatitis A.

C. LABORATORY FINDINGS

The white blood cell count is normal to low, especially in the preicteric phase. Large atypical lymphocytes may occasionally be seen. Rarely, aplastic anemia follows an episode of acute hepatitis not caused by any of the known hepatitis viruses. Mild proteinuria is common, and bilirubinuria often precedes the appearance of jaundice. Acholic stools are often present during the icteric phase. Strikingly elevated AST or ALT occurs early, followed by elevations of bilirubin and alkaline phosphatase; in a minority of patients, the latter persist after aminotransferase levels have normalized. Cholestasis is occasionally marked in acute hepatitis A. Marked prolongation of the prothrombin time in severe hepatitis correlates with increased mortality.

Differential Diagnosis

The differential diagnosis includes other viral diseases such as infectious mononucleosis, cytomegalovirus infection, and herpes simplex virus infection; spirochetal diseases such as leptospirosis and secondary syphilis; brucellosis; rickettsial diseases such as Q fever; drug-induced liver disease; and shock liver (ischemic hepatitis). Occasionally, autoimmune hepatitis (see below) may have an acute onset mimicking acute viral hepatitis. Rarely, metastatic cancer of the liver may present with a hepatitis-like picture.

The prodromal phase of viral hepatitis must be distinguished from other infectious disease such as influenza, upper respiratory infections, and the prodromal stages of the exanthematous diseases. Cholestasis may mimic obstructive jaundice.

Prevention

Strict isolation of patients is not necessary, but hand washing after bowel movements is required. Thorough hand washing by medical staff who may contact contaminated utensils, bedding, or clothing is essential. Careful handling of disposable needles—including not recapping used needles—is routine for medical personnel. Screening of donated blood for HBsAg, anti-HBc, and anti-HCV has reduced the risk of transfusion-associated hepatitis markedly. All pregnant women should undergo testing for HBsAg. HBV- and HCV-infected persons should practice safe sex, but there is little evidence that HCV is spread easily by sexual contact. Vaccination against HAV and HBV is recommended for patients with chronic hepatitis C, and vaccination against HAV for patients with chronic hepatitis B.

A. HEPATITIS A

Immune globulin should be given to all *close* (eg, household) personal contacts of patients with hepatitis A. The recommended dose of 0.02 mL/kg intramuscularly is protective if administered during incubation.

Two effective inactivated hepatitis A vaccines are available and recommended for persons living in or traveling to endemic areas, patients with chronic liver disease upon diagnosis, persons with clotting-factor disorders who are treated with concentrates, homosexual and bisexual men, animal handlers, illicit drug users, sewage workers, food handlers, and children and caregivers in day care centers and institutions. Routine vaccination of all children has been recommended in states with a high incidence of hepatitis A. HAV vaccine is also effective in the prevention of secondary spread to household contacts of primary cases. The recommended dose for adults is 1 mL (1440 ELISA units) of Havrix (GlaxoSmithKline) or 0.5 mL (50 units) of Vaqta (Merck) intramuscularly, followed by a booster dose at 6–12 months. A combined hepatitis A and B vaccine (Twinrix, GlaxoSmithKline) is available.

B. HEPATITIS B

Hepatitis B immune globulin (HBIG) may be protective—or may attenuate the severity of illness—if given in large doses within 7 days after exposure (adult dose is 0.06 mL/kg body weight) followed by initiation of the HBV vaccine series (see below). This approach is currently recommended for individuals exposed to hepatitis B surface antigen-contaminated material via mucous membranes or through breaks in the skin and for individuals who have had sexual contact with persons with HBV infection. HBIG is also indicated for newborn infants of HBsAg-positive mothers followed by initiation of the vaccine series (see below).

The currently used vaccines are recombinant-derived. Initially, the vaccine was targeted to persons at high risk, including renal dialysis patients and attending personnel, patients requiring repeated transfusions, spouses of HBsAg-positive individuals, gay men, intravenous drug users, newborns of HBsAg-positive mothers, beginning medical and nursing students, and all medical technologists. Because this strategy failed to lower the incidence of hepatitis B, the CDC recommended universal vaccination of infants and children in the USA. Over 90% of recipients of the vaccine mount protective antibody to hepatitis B. The standard regimen for adults is 10–20 μg initially (depending on the formulation) repeated again at 1 and 6 months, but alternative schedules have been approved. For greatest reliability of absorption, the deltoid muscle is the preferred site. Vaccine formulations free of the mercury-containing preservative thimerosal are given in infants less than 6 months of age. When documentation of seroconversion is considered desirable, postimmunization anti-HBs titers may be checked. Protection appears to be excellent even if the titer wanes—at least for 10 years—and booster reimmunization is not routinely recommended but is advised for immunocompromised persons in whom anti-HBs titers fall below 10 mIU/mL. Universal vaccination of neonates in countries endemic for HBV reduces the incidence of hepatocellular carcinoma.

Treatment

Bed rest is recommended only if symptoms are marked. If nausea and vomiting are pronounced or if oral intake is substantially decreased, intravenous 10% glucose is indicated. Encephalopathy or severe coagulopathy indicates impending acute hepatic failure, and hospitalization is mandatory (see below).

Dietary management consists of palatable meals as tolerated, without overfeeding; breakfast is usually best tolerated. Strenuous physical exertion, alcohol, and hepatotoxic agents are avoided. Small doses of oxazepam are safe, as metabolism is not hepatic; morphine sulfate is avoided.

Corticosteroids have no benefit in patients with viral hepatitis, including those with fulminant disease. Treatment of acute hepatitis C patients with interferon alfa for 6–24 weeks appreciably decreases the risk of chronic hepatitis. Because 20% of patients with acute hepatitis C clear the virus without such treatment, reserving it for patients with persistent infection after 6 months may be advisable.

Prognosis

In the majority, clinical recovery is complete in 3–16 weeks. Laboratory evidence of liver dysfunction may persist for a longer period, but most patients recover completely. The overall mortality rate is less than 1%, but the rate is reportedly higher in older people.

Hepatitis A does not cause chronic liver disease, though it may persist for up to 1 year, and clinical and biochemical relapses may occur before full recovery. The mortality rate is less than 0.2%. The mortality rate for acute hepatitis B is 0.1–1%, but higher with superimposed hepatitis D. Fulminant hepatitis C is rare in the USA. For unknown reasons, the mortality rate for hepatitis E is especially high in pregnant women (10–20%).

Chronic hepatitis, characterized by elevated aminotransferase levels for more than 6 months, develops in 1–2% of immunocompetent adults with acute hepatitis B but in as many as 90% of infected neonates and infants and a substantial proportion of immunocompromised adults. Over 80% of all persons with acute hepatitis C develop chronic hepatitis, which in many cases progresses very slowly. Ultimately, cirrhosis develops in up to 30% of those with chronic hepatitis C and 40% of those with chronic hepatitis B; the risk of cirrhosis is even higher in patients coinfected with both viruses or with HIV. Patients with cirrhosis are at risk with a rate of 3–5% per year of hepatocellular carcinoma. Even in the absence of cirrhosis, patients with chronic hepatitis B—particularly those with active viral replication—are at increased risk.

Branch AD et al: Hepatitis C: state of the art at the millennium. (Parts 1 and 2.) Semin Liver Dis 2000;20:1, 127. (Detailed reviews covering epidemiology, virology, immunology, diagnosis, treatment, and prevention.)

Di Bisceglie A: Natural history of hepatitis C: its impact on clinical management. Hepatology 2000;31:1014. [PMID: 10733560] (Over a 20-year period, 6% of patients with chronic hepatitis C develop decompensated cirrhosis.)

Dodig M et al: Hepatitis C and human immunodeficiency virus coinfections. J Clin Gastroenterol 2001;33:367. [PMID: 11606851] (Estimates are that 30–50% of patients with HIV infection are coinfected with HCV; HCV infection is more severe and progresses more rapidly to cirrhosis in these persons.)

Gaeta GB et al: Chronic hepatitis D: a vanishing disease? An Italian multicenter study. Hepatology 2000;32:824. [PMID: 11003629] (Since 1987 the frequency of anti-HDV antibodies in HBV carriers in Italy has declined from 25% to 10%, with most of the decline in persons under age 50.)

Germer JJ et al: Advances in the molecular diagnosis of hepatitis C and their clinical implications. Mayo Clin Proc 2001;76:911. [PMID: 11560302] (Thorough review of second- and third-generation antibody tests, quantitative and qualitative HCV RNA assays, and techniques for HCV genotyping.)

Jaeckel E et al: Treatment of acute hepatitis C with interferon alfa-2b. N Engl J Med 2001;345:1452. [PMID: 11794193] (Of 44 patients treated within a mean of 89 days from infection, chronic hepatitis developed in only 1.)

Lauer GM et al: Hepatitis C virus infection. N Engl J Med 2001;345:41. [PMID: 11439948] (Reviews epidemiology, pathogenesis, clinical features, course, diagnostic tests, and treatment.)

Liang TJ et al: Pathogenesis, natural history, treatment, and prevention of hepatitis C. Ann Intern Med 2000;132:296. [PMID: 10681285]

Umemura T et al: SEN virus infection and its relationship to transfusion-associated hepatitis. Hepatology 2001;33:1303. [PMID: 11343260] (SEN virus is associated with transfusion-associated non-ABCDE hepatitis.)

Updated U.S. Public Health Service guidelines for the management of occupational exposures to HBV, HCV, and HIV and recommendations for post-exposure prophylaxis. MMWR Morb Mortal Wkly Rep 2001;50(RR-11). [PMID: 11442299]

ACUTE HEPATIC FAILURE

Acute hepatic failure may be fulminant or subfulminant. Fulminant hepatic failure is characterized by the development of hepatic encephalopathy within 8 weeks after the onset of acute liver disease. Coagulopathy is invariably present. Subfulminant hepatic failure occurs when these findings appear between 8 weeks and 6 months after the onset of acute liver disease and carries an equally poor prognosis.

Until recently about 70% of all cases of acute hepatic failure in the USA were caused by acute viral hepatitis, with up to 50% of cases due to hepatitis B—in some cases detectable only by polymerase chain reaction (PCR) methodology—and most of the remainder due to hepatitis A or unknown (non-ABCDE) viruses. In endemic areas, hepatitis D and hepatitis E cause acute hepatic failure. Hepatitis C appears to be a rare cause of acute hepatic failure in the USA, but acute hepatitis A or B superimposed on chronic hepatitis C is associated with a high risk of fulminant hepatitis.

Acetaminophen toxicity is the most common cause of acute hepatic failure in the USA, as it has been in England for some time, accounting for up to 40% of cases. Other causes include idiosyncratic drug reactions, poisonous mushrooms, shock, hyper- or hypothermia, Budd-Chiari syndrome, malignancy (most commonly lymphomas), Wilson's disease, Reye's syndrome, fatty liver of pregnancy and other disorders of fatty acid oxidation, and parvovirus B19 infection.

In acute hepatic failure due to hepatitis or drug toxicity, extensive necrosis of large areas of the liver gives a typical pathologic picture of acute liver atrophy. A systemic inflammatory response, gastrointestinal symptoms, and hemorrhagic phenomena are common. Jaundice may be absent or minimal early, but laboratory tests show severe hepatocellular damage. In acute hepatic failure due to microvesicular steatosis (eg, Reye's syndrome), serum aminotransferase elevations may be modest (< 300 units/L).

The treatment of acute hepatic failure is directed toward correcting metabolic abnormalities. These include coagulation defects; electrolyte and acid-base disturbances; renal failure; hypoglycemia; and encephalopathy. Prophylactic antibiotic therapy decreases the risk of infection, observed in up to 90%, but has no effect on survival and is not routinely recommended. For suspected sepsis, broad coverage is indicated. The most frequent isolates are *Staphylococcus aureus*, streptococcus species, coliforms, and, later in the course, candida species. Early administration of acetylcysteine (140 mg/kg orally followed by 70 mg/kg orally every 4 hours for an additional 17 doses) is indicated for acetaminophen toxicity and improves cerebral blood flow and oxygenation in patients with fulminant hepatic failure due to any cause. Early transfer to a liver transplantation center is essential. Extradural sensors are placed to monitor intracranial pressure for impending cerebral edema, thought to be mediated in part by high arterial ammonia concentrations and decreased cerebral perfusion.

Mannitol 100–200 mL of a 20% solution by intravenous infusion over 10 minutes, may decrease cerebral edema but should be used with caution in patients with renal failure. The value of hyperventilation, intravenous prostaglandin E_1, and hypothermia is uncertain. Indeed, patients may already be hypothermic. Hepatic-assist devices using living hepatocytes, extracorporeal whole liver perfusion, hepatocyte transplantation, and liver xenografts have shown promise experimentally. The mortality rate of fulminant hepatitis with severe encephalopathy is as high as 80%. The outlook is especially poor in patients younger than 10 and older than 40 years of age and in those with an idiosyncratic drug reaction. Other adverse prognostic factors are a serum bilirubin level > 18 mg/dL, INR > 6.5, onset of encephalopathy more than 7 days after the onset of jaundice, and a low factor V level (< 20% of normal). For acetaminophen-induced fulminant hepatic failure, indicators of a poor outcome (which is uncommon) are acidosis (pH < 7.3), INR > 6.5, and azotemia (serum creatinine ≥ 3.4 mg/dL). Emergency liver transplantation is considered for patients with stage II to stage III encephalopathy and is associated with an 80% survival rate at 1 year. Compared with chronic hepatitis B, liver transplantation for fulminant hepatitis B is less likely to result in reinfection of the graft with HBV.

Allen JW et al: Advances in bioartificial liver devices. Hepatology 2001;34:447. [PMID: 11526528] (Primary hepatocytes, which express the broad array of liver functions, are preferred in the design of bioartificial livers but are less plentiful than either cell lines or xenogenic cells.)

Blei AT: Medical therapy of brain edema in fulminant hepatic failure. Hepatology 2000;32:666. [PMID: 10960467]

Gill RQ et al: Acute liver failure. J Clin Gastroenterol 2001; 33:191. [PMID: 11500606] (Concise review.)

Shakil AO et al: Acute liver failure. Liver Transplant 2000;6:163. (Of 177 patients with acute liver failure admitted to a single center, 14% recovered without medical management, 49% underwent liver transplantation, and 37% died without transplantation.)

CHRONIC HEPATITIS

Chronic hepatitis is defined as a chronic inflammatory reaction of the liver of more than 3–6 months' duration, demonstrated by persistently abnormal serum aminotransferase levels and characteristic histologic findings. In many cases, the diagnosis of chronic hepatitis may be based on initial presentation. The causes of chronic hepatitis include HBV, HCV, and HDV, autoimmune hepatitis, chronic hepatitis associated with certain medications (particularly isoniazid), Wilson's disease, and α_1-antiprotease deficiency. Traditionally, chronic hepatitis has been categorized histologically as chronic persistent hepatitis and chronic active hepatitis. However, with improved serologic and autoimmune markers, more specific categorization is possible, based on etiology; the grade of portal, periportal, and lobular inflammation (minimal, mild, moderate, or severe); and the stage of fibrosis (none, mild, moderate, severe, cirrhosis).

Clinical Findings & Diagnosis

A. AUTOIMMUNE HEPATITIS

Though usually a disease of young women, it can occur in either sex at any age. Affected younger persons are often positive for HLA-B8 and -DR3; in older patients, HLA-DR4. The principal susceptibility allele among white Americans and northern Europeans is HLA *DRB1*0301;* HLA *DRB1*0401* is a secondary but independent risk factor. The onset is usually insidious, but up to 40% present with an acute attack of hepatitis and some cases follow a viral illness such as hepatitis A, Epstein-Barr infection, measles, or exposure to a drug or toxin such as nitrofurantoin. The serum bilirubin is usually increased, but 20% are anicteric. Typically, examination reveals a healthy-appearing young woman with multiple spider nevi, cuta-

neous striae, acne, hirsutism, and hepatomegaly. Amenorrhea may be a presenting feature. Extrahepatic features include arthritis, Sjögren's syndrome, thyroiditis, nephritis, ulcerative colitis, and Coombs-positive hemolytic anemia. In classic (type I) autoimmune hepatitis, antinuclear antibody (ANA) or smooth muscle antibody (either or both) is detected in serum. Serum gamma globulin levels are typically elevated (up to 5–6 g/dL). In patients with the latter, the enzyme immunoassay for antibody to HCV may be falsely positive. Other antibodies, including antineutrophil cytoplasmic antibodies (ANCA), may be found. A second type, seen more often in Europe, is characterized by circulating antibody to liver-kidney microsomes (anti-LKM1)—directed against cytochrome P450 2D6—without anti-smooth muscle antibody or ANA. This type can be seen in patients with autoimmune polyglandular syndrome type 1. A third variant is characterized by antibodies to soluble liver antigen/liver pancreas (anti-SLA/LP) and may represent a variant of type I autoimmune hepatitis characterized by severe disease, high relapse rate after treatment, and absence of the usual antibodies (ANA and smooth muscle antibody). Anti-SLA/LP appear to be directed against a transfer RNA complex responsible for incorporating selenocysteine into peptide chains. Concurrent primary biliary cirrhosis or primary sclerosing cholangitis has been recognized in up to 15% of patients with autoimmune hepatitis.

B. CHRONIC HEPATITIS B

Chronic hepatitis B chiefly affects males and afflicts nearly 400 million people worldwide and 1.25 million in the USA. It may be noted as a continuum of acute hepatitis or diagnosed because of persistently elevated aminotransferase levels.

Early in the course, HBeAg and HBV DNA are present in serum, indicative of active viral replications. Low-level IgM anti-HBc is also present in about 70%. In some patients, clinical and biochemical improvement coincides with disappearance of HBeAg and HBV DNA from serum, appearance of anti-HBe, and integration of the HBV genome into the host genome in infected hepatocytes. Such patients may remain at increased risk for cirrhosis and hepatocellular carcinoma. As noted, infection by a pre-core mutant of HBV or spontaneous mutation of the pre-core or pre-core promoter region of the HBV genome during the course of chronic hepatitis caused by wild-type HBV may result in particularly severe chronic hepatitis with rapid progression to cirrhosis, particularly when additional mutations in the core gene of HBV are present.

C. HEPATITIS D

Acute hepatitis D infection superimposed on chronic HBV infection may result in severe chronic hepatitis, which may progress rapidly to cirrhosis and may be fatal. The diagnosis is confirmed by detection of anti-HDV in serum.

D. CHRONIC HEPATITIS C

At least 80% of patients with acute hepatitis C develop chronic hepatitis C. It is clinically indistinguishable from chronic hepatitis due to other causes and may be the most common. In up to 40% of cases, serum aminotransferase levels are persistently normal. The diagnosis is confirmed by detection of anti-HCV by enzyme immunoassay (EIA). In rare cases of suspected chronic hepatitis C but a negative EIA, HCV RNA is detected by PCR. Progression to cirrhosis occurs in 20% of affected patients after 20 years, with an increased risk in men, those who drink more than 50 g of alcohol daily, and possibly those who acquire HCV infection after age 40. Immunosuppressed persons—including patients with hypogammaglobulinemia, HIV infection with a low CD4 count, or with organ transplants receiving immunosuppressants—appear to progress more rapidly to cirrhosis than immunocompetent persons with chronic hepatitis C. Affected persons with persistently normal serum aminotransferase levels usually have mild chronic hepatitis with slow or absent progression to cirrhosis; however, cirrhosis is present in 10–20% of these patients.

Treatment

Activity is modified according to symptoms; bed rest is not necessary. The diet should be well balanced, without limitations other than sodium or protein restriction if dictated by fluid overload or encephalopathy.

A. AUTOIMMUNE HEPATITIS

Prednisone with or without azathioprine improves symptoms, decreases the serum bilirubin, aminotransferase, and gamma globulin levels, and reduces hepatic inflammation. Symptomatic patients with aminotransferase levels elevated tenfold (or fivefold if the serum globulins are elevated at least twofold) are optimal for therapy, and asymptomatic patients with modest enzyme elevations may be considered for therapy depending on the clinical circumstances.

Prednisone or an equivalent drug is given initially in doses of 30 mg orally daily with azathioprine or mercaptopurine, 50 mg/d orally, which are generally well tolerated and permit the use of lower corticosteroid doses. Blood counts are monitored weekly for the first 2 months of therapy and monthly thereafter because of the small risk of bone marrow suppression. The dose of prednisone is lowered from 30 mg/d after 1 week to 20 mg/d and again after 2 or 3 weeks to 15 mg/d. Ultimately, a maintenance dose of 10 mg/d is achieved. While symptomatic improvement is often prompt, biochemical improvement is more gradual, with normalization of serum aminotransferase levels after several months in many cases. Histologic resolution of inflammation may require 18–24 months, the time at which repeat liver biopsy is recommended.

Failure of aminotransferase levels to normalize invariably predicts lack of histologic resolution.

The response rate to therapy with prednisone and azathioprine is 80–90%. Cirrhosis, however, does not reverse with therapy and may even develop after apparent biochemical and histologic remission. Once remission is achieved, therapy may be withdrawn, but the subsequent relapse rate is 50–90%. Relapses may again be treated in the same manner as the initial episode, with the same remission rate. After successful treatment of a relapse, the patient may be kept indefinitely on azathioprine up to 2 mg/kg and the lowest dose of prednisone needed to maintain aminotransferase levels as close to normal as possible. Budesonide, a corticosteroid with less toxicity than prednisone, does not appear to be effective in maintaining remission. Nonresponders to prednisone and azathioprine may be considered for a trial of cyclosporine, tacrolimus, or methotrexate. Mycophenolate mofetil appears to be an effective alternative to azathioprine in patients who cannot tolerate or do not respond to it. Bone density should be monitored, particularly in patients being maintained on corticosteroids, and measures undertaken to prevent or treat osteoporosis. Liver transplantation may be required for treatment failures, and the disease has been recognized to recur in up to one-third of transplanted livers (and rarely to develop de novo) as immunosuppression is reduced.

B. CHRONIC HEPATITIS B

Patients with active viral replication (HBeAg and HBV DNA in serum; elevated aminotransferase levels) may be treated with recombinant human interferon alfa-2b in a dose of 5 million units a day or 10 million units three times a week intramuscularly for 4 months. About 40% of treated patients will respond with sustained normalization of aminotransferase levels, disappearance of HBeAg and HBV DNA from serum, appearance of anti-HBe, and improved survival. A response is most likely in patients with an HBV DNA level under 200 pg/mL and high aminotransferase levels. Moreover, over 60% of these responders may eventually clear HBsAg from serum and liver, develop anti-HBs in serum, and thus be cured. Relapses are uncommon in such complete responders. Patients with HBeAg-negative chronic hepatitis B (pre-core mutant) have a durable sustained response rate of only 15–25% after 12 months of interferon therapy.

The nucleoside analog lamivudine, 100 mg orally daily as a single dose, may be used instead of interferon for the treatment of chronic hepatitis B and is much better tolerated. This agent reliably suppresses HBV DNA in serum, improves liver histology in 40% of patients, and leads to normal ALT levels in over 40% and HBeAg seroconversion in 20% of patients after 1 year of therapy. However, 15–30% of responders experience a mild relapse during treatment as a result of mutation in HBV DNA that confers resistance to lamivudine. Moreover, hepatitis activity may recur when the drug is stopped, and long-term, perhaps indefinite treatment despite a high rate of resistance over time may be required to suppress the disease when HBeAg seroconversion does not ensue. Rates of complete response—as well as resistance to lamivudine—increase with increasing duration of therapy. The drug is well tolerated even in patients with decompensated cirrhosis and may be effective in patients with rapidly progressive hepatitis B ("fibrosing cholestatic hepatitis") following organ transplantation. Although lamivudine therapy leads to biochemical, virologic, and histologic improvement in patients with HBeAg-negative chronic hepatitis B (pre-core mutant), relapse is frequent when therapy is stopped, and long-term treatment is associated with a high rate of viral resistance. Combined use of interferon and lamivudine offers no advantage over the use of either drug alone. Other antiviral agents such as adefovir dipivoxil, emtricitabine, and entecavir are under study, and strategies employing multiple drugs are likely to be studied.

Recombinant interferon alfa-2a (9 million units three times a week for 48 weeks) may lead to normalization of serum aminotransferase levels, histologic improvement, and elimination of HDV RNA from serum in about 50% of patients with chronic hepatitis D, but relapse is common after therapy is stopped. Lamivudine is not effective in chronic hepatitis D.

C. Chronic Hepatitis C

Treatment of chronic hepatitis C is generally considered in patients under age 70 with elevated serum aminotransferase levels and more than minimal inflammation or fibrosis on liver biopsy. Until recently, standard therapy was with a combination of interferon alfa and ribavirin. Recombinant human interferon alfa-2b or alfa-2a in a dose of 3 million units three times a week for 24 weeks and "consensus" interferon (a synthetic recombinant interferon derived by assigning the most commonly observed amino acid at each position of several alpha interferon subtypes) in a dose of 9 mg three times a week have been shown to induce biochemical, virologic, and histologic improvement in up to 50% of patients—return of ALT to normal, loss of HCV RNA from serum for at least 6 months after therapy is stopped, decrease in hepatic inflammation, and occasionally regression of fibrosis. Most experience has been with interferon alfa-2b. Factors predicting an increased chance of response include the absence of cirrhosis on liver biopsy (though treatment is not contraindicated by compensated cirrhosis), low serum HCV RNA levels as assessed by quantitative assays, and infection by genotypes of HCV other than 1a, 1b, or 4. After stopping the medication at 24 weeks, only 30–50% of the treated responders will maintain the improvement. More prolonged treatment (eg, for 12–18 months) has been shown to increase the durability of remission. The use of higher doses of interferon alfa-2b (eg, 6 million units three times a week) increases toxicity and does not appear to increase the rate of sustained responses substantially.

Response rates among blacks appear to be lower than those among whites, in part because of a higher rate of genotype 1 among infected black patients.

A slow-release, long-acting "pegylated" formulation of interferon (peginterferon) taken only once a week is more effective than standard interferon—presumably because of sustained high blood levels—and is now the preferred form of interferon for treatment of chronic hepatitis C. With one formulation of peginterferon administered in a dose of 180 mg once per week for 48 weeks, a sustained biochemical and virologic response was achieved in 38% of patients with chronic hepatitis C compared with 17% of those treated with standard interferon. The dose of peginterferon alfa-2b is 1.5 mg/kg weekly.

Addition of the nucleoside analog ribavirin, 1000–1200 mg daily in two divided doses, results in higher sustained response rates than interferon alone in previously untreated patients with chronic hepatitis C or patients who have had a relapse after an initial response to interferon alfa alone. Long-term response rates are 40% and 50%, respectively, following combination therapy consisting of standard interferon and ribavirin. Rates with a combination of peginterferon and ribavirin are as high as 55% (and up to 90% for HCV genotypes 2 or 3). When used with peginterferon, the dose of ribavirin is also based on the patient's weight and may range from 800 mg to 1400 mg daily in two divided doses.

Interferon alfa with ribavirin may be beneficial in the treatment of cryoglobulinemia associated with chronic hepatitis C. On the other hand, treatment of asymptomatic "chronic carriers" is of uncertain benefit. Patients with both HCV and HIV infections may benefit from treatment of HCV if the CD4 count is not low. Treatment with interferon alfa plus ribavirin is costly ($8000 for a 24-week supply), and side effects, which include flu-like symptoms, are almost universal; more serious toxicity includes psychiatric symptoms (irritability, depression), thyroid dysfunction, and bone marrow suppression. A blood count is obtained at weeks 1, 2, and 4 after therapy is started and monthly thereafter. Interferon is contraindicated in patients with decompensated cirrhosis, profound cytopenias, psychiatric disorders, and autoimmune diseases. Patients taking ribavirin must be monitored for hemolysis, and, because of teratogenic effects in animals, men and women taking the drug must practice strict contraception until 6 months after conclusion of therapy. Ribavirin should be avoided in persons over age 65 and in others in whom hemolysis could pose a risk of angina or stroke. Rash, itching, headache, cough, and shortness of breath also occur with the drug. Rarely, erythropoietin and granulocyte colony-stimulating factor are used to treat therapy-induced anemia and leukopenia, respectively.

In nonresponders to interferon-based therapy treatment with interleukin-10 may normalize aminotransferase levels, improve liver histology, and even reduce fibrosis.

Prognosis

The course of chronic hepatitis is variable and unpredictable. Untreated severe autoimmune hepatitis has a 5-year mortality rate of 50%, which decreases markedly with treatment. The sequelae of chronic hepatitis secondary to hepatitis B include cirrhosis, liver failure, and hepatocellular carcinoma. Up to 40–50% of patients with chronic hepatitis B and cirrhosis die within 5 years after the onset of symptoms, though interferon may improve the prognosis in responders. Chronic hepatitis C is an indolent, often subclinical disease that may lead to cirrhosis and hepatocellular carcinoma after decades. Indeed, the mortality rate from transfusion-associated hepatitis C may be no different from that of an age-matched control population. Nevertheless, mortality rates clearly rise once cirrhosis develops, and mortality from cirrhosis and hepatocellular carcinoma due to hepatitis C is expected to triple in the next 10–20 years. Interferon plus ribavarin appear to have a beneficial effect on survival and quality of life, is cost-effective, and in responders may reduce the risk of hepatocellular carcinoma.

Al Khalidi JA et al: Current concepts in the diagnosis, pathogenesis, and treatment of autoimmune hepatitis. Mayo Clin Proc 2001;76:1237. [PMID: 11761505] (Lucid and comprehensive review.)

Ben-Ari Z et al: Autoimmune hepatitis and its variant syndromes. Gut 2001;49:589. [PMID: 11559660] (Reviews autoimmune hepatitis, overlap with primary biliary cirrhosis, primary sclerosing cholangitis, and viral hepatitis; and autoimmune cholangitis.)

Cummings KJ et al: Interferon and ribavirin vs. interferon alone in the re-treatment of chronic hepatitis C previously non-responsive to interferon: A meta-analysis of randomized trials. JAMA 2001;285:193. [PMID: 11176813] (Sustained virologic response with re-treatment was achieved in 15% of cases. The best results were achieved with use of interferon alfa-2a or -2b and standard rather than reduced doses of ribavirin.)

Gow PJ et al: Treatment of chronic hepatitis. BMJ 2001;323: 1164. [PMID: 11711410] (Terse review.)

Heneghan MA et al: Management and outcome of pregnancy in autoimmune hepatitis. Gut 2001;48:97. [PMID: 11115829] (Because autoimmune hepatitis affects young women, conception is not uncommon when the disease is in remission. Corticosteroids can be used to treat rare flares during pregnancy, and maintenance azathioprine does not need to be discontinued.)

Kjaergard LL et al: Interferon alfa with or without ribavirin for chronic hepatitis C: systematic review of randomized trials. BMJ 2001;323:1151. [PMID: 11711405] (Treatment with interferon and ribavirin has significant beneficial virologic and histologic effects regardless of prior treatment.)

Koff RS (guest editor): Advances in hepatitis C. Clin Liver Dis 2001;5:873. (Entire issue devoted to virology, epidemiology, pathogenesis, clinical features, natural history, treatment, and prevention of hepatitis C.)

Lok AS et al: Chronic hepatitis B. Hepatology 2001;34:1225. [PMID: 11732013] (Practice guidelines emphasizing treatment with interferon and lamivudine.)

Lok AS et al: Management of hepatitis B: 2000—summary of a workshop. Gastroenterology 2001;120:1828. [PMID: 11375963] (Overviews of all aspects of hepatitis B.)

Manns MP et al: Autoimmune hepatitis: clinical challenges. Gastroenterology 2001;120:1502. [PMID: 11313321] (Reviews definition, diagnostic scoring systems, histology, clinical presentation, natural history, prognosis, autoantibodies, differential diagnosis, and treatment.)

Walsh K et al: Update on chronic viral hepatitis. Postgrad Med 2001;77:498. [PMID: 11470928] (Lucid overview.)

ALCOHOLIC HEPATITIS

Alcoholic hepatitis is characterized by acute or chronic inflammation and parenchymal necrosis of the liver induced by alcohol. While alcoholic hepatitis is often a reversible disease, it is the most common precursor of cirrhosis in the USA and is associated with four to five times the number of hospitalizations and deaths as hepatitis C, which is the second most common cause of cirrhosis.

The frequency of alcoholic cirrhosis is estimated to be 10–15% among persons who consume over 50 g of alcohol (4 oz of 100-proof whiskey, 15 oz of wine, or four 12-oz cans of beer) daily for over 10 years. The risk of cirrhosis is lower (5%) in the absence of other cofactors such as chronic viral hepatitis. Genetic factors may also account in part for differences in susceptibility, and there are associations with polymorphisms of the genes encoding for tumor necrosis factor-α and cytochrome P450 2E1. Women appear to be more susceptible than men, in part because of lower gastric mucosal alcohol dehydrogenase levels. Although alcoholic hepatitis may not develop in many patients even after several decades of alcohol abuse, it appears in a few individuals within a year after onset of excessive drinking. In general, over 80% of patients with alcoholic hepatitis have been drinking 5 years or more before developing any symptoms that can be attributed to liver disease; the longer the duration of drinking (10–15 or more years) and the larger the alcoholic consumption, the greater the probability of developing alcoholic hepatitis and cirrhosis. In individuals who drink alcohol excessively, the rate of ethanol metabolism can be sufficiently high to permit the consumption of large quantities of spirits without raising the blood alcohol level over 80 mg/dL, the concentration at which the conventional breath analyzer begins to detect ethanol.

The role of deficiencies in vitamins and calories in the development of alcoholic hepatitis or in the progression of this lesion to cirrhosis remains controversial but is at least contributory. Ethanol-induced elevation of circulating endotoxin levels is thought to play a critical role in the pathogenesis of alcoholic liver disease by inducing release of tumor necrosis factor-α and other cytokines by Kupffer cells. Many of the adverse effects of alcohol on the liver are thought to be mediated by the oxidative metabolite acetaldehyde, which contributes to lipid peroxidation and induction of an immune response following covalent binding to proteins in the liver. Concurrent HBV or HCV infection and heterozygosity for the *HFE* gene mutation for hemochromatosis increase the severity of alcoholic liver disease.

Clinical Findings

A. SYMPTOMS AND SIGNS

The clinical presentation of alcoholic hepatitis can vary from an asymptomatic patient with an enlarged liver to a critically ill individual who dies quickly. A recent period of heavy drinking, complaints of anorexia and nausea, and the demonstration of hepatomegaly and jaundice strongly suggest the diagnosis. Abdominal pain and tenderness, splenomegaly, ascites, fever, and encephalopathy may be present.

B. LABORATORY FINDINGS

Anemia (usually macrocytic) may be present; several mechanisms are possible. Leukocytosis with shift to the left is common in patients with severe disease. Leukopenia is occasionally seen and disappears after cessation of drinking. About 10% of patients have thrombocytopenia related to a direct toxic effect of alcohol on megakaryocyte production or to hypersplenism.

AST is usually elevated but rarely above 300 units/L. AST is greater than ALT, usually by a factor of 2 or more. Serum alkaline phosphatase is generally elevated, but seldom more than three times the normal value. Serum bilirubin is increased in 60–90% of patients. Serum γ-glutamyl transpeptidase, carbohydrate-deficient transferrin, and mitochondrial AST also may be elevated in alcoholics, but these tests lack both sensitivity and specificity. Serum bilirubin levels greater than 10 mg/dL and marked prolongation of the prothrombin time (≥ 6 seconds above control) indicate severe alcoholic hepatitis with a mortality rate as high as 50%. The serum albumin is depressed, and the gamma globulin level is elevated in 50–75% of individuals, even in the absence of cirrhosis. Increased transferrin saturation and hepatic iron stores are found in many alcoholic patients due to sideroblastic anemia. Folic acid deficiency may coexist.

C. LIVER BIOPSY

Liver biopsy is usually diagnostic and demonstrates macrovesicular fat, PMN infiltration with hepatic necrosis, and Mallory bodies (alcoholic hyaline). Micronodular cirrhosis may be present as well.

D. OTHER STUDIES

Ultrasound helps exclude biliary obstruction and identifies subclinical ascites. CT scanning with intravenous contrast or MRI may be indicated in selected cases to evaluate patients for collateral vessels, space-occupying lesions of the liver, or concomitant disease of the pancreas.

Differential Diagnosis

Alcoholic hepatitis may be closely mimicked by cholecystitis and cholelithiasis and by drug toxicity. Other causes of hepatitis or chronic liver disease may be excluded by serologic or biochemical testing, by imaging studies, or by liver biopsy. However, liver biopsy findings are identical to those of nonalcoholic steatohepatitis.

Treatment

A. GENERAL MEASURES

Abstinence from alcohol is essential and must be emphasized repeatedly. Every effort should be made to provide sufficient amounts of carbohydrates and calories in anorectic patients to reduce endogenous protein catabolism, promote gluconeogenesis, and prevent hypoglycemia. Nutritional support (40 kcal/kg with 1.5–2 g/kg as protein) improves survival in patients with malnutrition. Use of liquid formulas rich in branched-chain amino acids does not improve survival beyond that achieved with less expensive caloric supplementation. The administration of vitamins, particularly folic acid and thiamine, is indicated, especially when deficiencies are noted; glucose administration increases the vitamin B_1 requirement and can precipitate Wernicke-Korsakoff syndrome if thiamine is not coadministered.

B. CORTICOSTEROIDS

Methylprednisolone, 32 mg/d for 1 month or the equivalent, may reduce short-term mortality in patients with alcoholic hepatitis and either encephalopathy or a greatly elevated bilirubin concentration and prolonged prothrombin time (specifically, when a discriminant function defined by the patient's prothrombin time minus the control prothrombin time times 4.6 plus the total bilirubin in mg/dL is > 32).

C. EXPERIMENTAL THERAPIES

A recent study has suggested that pentoxifylline—an inhibitor of tumor necrosis factor—400 mg orally three times daily for 4 weeks, reduces 1-month mortality rates in patients with severe alcoholic hepatitis, primarily by decreasing the risk of hepatorenal syndrome. Other experimental therapies include propylthiouracil, oxandrolone, and S-adenosyl-l-methionine.

Prognosis

A. SHORT-TERM

When the prothrombin time is short enough to permit liver biopsy (< 3 seconds above control), the 1-year mortality rate is 7%, rising to 20% if there is progressive prolongation of the prothrombin time during hospitalization. Individuals in whom the prothrombin time prohibits liver biopsy have a 42% mortality rate at 1 year. Other unfavorable prognostic factors are a serum bilirubin greater than 10 mg/dL, hepatic encephalopathy, and azotemia.

B. LONG-TERM

In the USA, the 3-year mortality rate of persons who recover from acute alcoholic hepatitis is ten times greater than that of control individuals of comparable age. Histologically severe disease is associated with continued excessive mortality rates after 3 years, whereas the death rate is not increased after the same period in those whose liver biopsies show only mild alcoholic hepatitis. Complications of portal hypertension (ascites, variceal bleeding, hepatorenal syndrome), coagulopathy, and severe jaundice following recovery from acute alcoholic hepatitis also suggest a poor long-term prognosis.

The most important prognostic consideration is continued excessive drinking. A 6-month period of abstinence is required before liver transplantation can be considered.

Menon KV et al: Pathogenesis, diagnosis, and treatment of alcoholic liver disease. Mayo Clin Proc 2001;76:1021. [PMID: 11605686] (Excellent review.)

Tilg H et al: Cytokines in alcoholic and nonalcoholic steatohepatitis. N Engl J Med 2000;343:1467. [PMID: 11078773] (Reviews central role of tumor necrosis factor-α in both disorders.)

Walsh K et al: Alcoholic liver disease. Postgrad Med J 2000;76:280. [PMID: 10775280] (Epidemiology, spectrum, pathogenesis, clinical features, diagnosis, and treatment.)

DRUG- & TOXIN-INDUCED LIVER DISEASE

The continuing synthesis, testing, and introduction of new drugs into clinical practice has resulted in an increase in toxic reactions of many types. Many widely used therapeutic agents, including over-the-counter "natural" and "herbal" products, may cause hepatic injury. Drug-induced liver disease can mimic viral hepatitis, biliary tract obstruction, or other types of liver disease. In any patient with liver disease, the clinician must inquire carefully about the use of potentially hepatotoxic drugs or exposure to hepatotoxins. In some cases, coadministration of a second agent may increase the toxicity of the first (eg, isoniazid and rifampin, acetaminophen and alcohol). Drug toxicity may be categorized on the basis of pathogenesis or histologic appearance.

Direct Hepatotoxic Group

The liver lesion caused by this group of drugs is characterized by (1) dose-related severity, (2) a latent period following exposure, and (3) susceptibility in all individuals. Examples include acetaminophen, alcohol, carbon tetrachloride, chloroform, heavy metals, mercaptopurine, niacin, plant alkaloids, phosphorus, tetracyclines, valproic acid, and vitamin A.

Idiosyncratic Reactions

Reactions of this type are sporadic, not related to dose, and occasionally associated with features suggesting an allergic reaction, such as fever and eosinophilia. In some, toxicity results directly from a metabolite that is produced only in certain individuals on a genetic basis. Examples include amiodarone, aspirin, carbamazepine, chloramphenicol, diclofenac, flutamide, halothane, isoniazid, ketoconazole, lamotrigine, methyldopa, oxacillin, phenytoin, pyrazinamide, quinidine, streptomycin, troglitazone (withdrawn from the market in the United States), and perhaps tacrine.

Cholestatic Reactions

A. NONINFLAMMATORY

Direct effect of agent on bile secretory mechanisms: azathioprine, estrogens, or anabolic steroids containing an alkyl or ethinyl group at carbon 17, indinavir, mercaptopurine, methyltestosterone, cyclosporine.

B. INFLAMMATORY

Inflammation of portal areas with bile duct injury (cholangitis), often with allergic features such as eosinophilia: amoxicillin-clavulanic acid, chlorothiazide, chlorpromazine, chlorpropamide, erythromycin, penicillamine, prochlorperazine, semisynthetic penicillins (eg, cloxacillin), and sulfadiazine.

Acute or Chronic Hepatitis

Histologically and in some cases clinically indistinguishable from autoimmune hepatitis: aspirin, isoniazid (increased risk in HBV carriers), methyldopa, minocycline, nitrofurantoin, nonsteroidal anti-inflammatory drugs, and propylthiouracil. Hepatitis can occur with also cocaine, ecstasy, efavirenz, nevirapine, ritonavir, sulfonamides, troglitazone (withdrawn from the market in the United States), and zafirlukast.

Other Reactions

A. FATTY LIVER

1. **Macrovesicular**—Alcohol, amiodarone, corticosteroids, methotrexate.

2. **Microvesicular (often resulting from mitochondrial injury)**—Didanosine, stavudine, tetracyclines, valproic acid, zidovudine.

B. GRANULOMAS

Allopurinol, quinidine, quinine, phenylbutazone, phenytoin.

C. FIBROSIS AND CIRRHOSIS

Methotrexate, vitamin A.

D. PELIOSIS HEPATIS (BLOOD-FILLED CAVITIES)

Anabolic steroids, azathioprine, oral contraceptive steroids.

E. NEOPLASMS

Oral contraceptive steroids, estrogens (hepatic adenoma but not focal nodular hyperplasia); vinyl chloride (angiosarcoma).

Bissell DM et al: Drug-induced liver injury: mechanisms and test syndromes. Hepatology 2001;33:1009. [PMID: 11283870] (Overview of pathogenetic mechanisms of hepatotoxicity.)

Hernandez LV et al: Antiretroviral hepatotoxicity in human immunodeficiency virus-infected patients. Aliment Pharmacol Ther 2001;15:1627. [PMID: 11564003] (Hepatotoxicity occurred in 24 of 65 patients taking antiretroviral therapy; risk factors were age over 40, CD4 count less than 310/µL, and coexisting hepatitis C infection.)

Seeff LB et al: Complementary and alternative medicine in chronic liver disease. Hepatology 2001;34:595. [PMID: 11526548] (Reviews extent of use, reported efficacy rates, and reported toxicity.)

Sulkowski MS et al: Hepatotoxicity associated with nevirapine- or efavirenz-containing antiretroviral therapy: Role of hepatitis C and B infections. Hepatology 2002;35:182. [PMID: 11786975] (Severe hepatotoxicity occurred in 15% and 8%, respectively, often after at least 12 weeks of therapy, and was especially common in patients coinfected with HCV or HBV and those also taking protease inhibitors.)

ALCOHOLIC & NONALCOHOLIC FATTY LIVER DISEASE

Ethanol can cause hepatic steatosis (fatty liver) in the absence of malnutrition, although inadequate diets—specifically, those deficient in choline, methionine, and protein—can contribute to liver damage caused by ethanol. Other nonalcoholic causes of steatosis, or nonalcoholic fatty liver disease (NAFLD), are obesity (present in ≥ 40%), diabetes mellitus (in ≥ 20%), hypertriglyceridemia (in ≥ 20%), corticosteroids, poisons (carbon tetrachloride and yellow phosphorus), endocrinopathies such as Cushing's syndrome, hypobetalipoproteinemia, starvation, and total parenteral nutrition. Steatosis is nearly universal in obese alcoholics. In addition to macrovesicular steatosis, histologic features may include focal infiltration by polymorphonuclear neutrophils and Mallory's hyalin, a picture indistinguishable from that of alcoholic hepatitis and referred to as nonalcoholic steatohepatitis (NASH). In patients with nonalcoholic fatty liver disease, older age, obesity, and diabetes are risk factors for advanced hepatic fibrosis and cirrhosis.

Microvesicular steatosis is seen with Reye's syndrome, valproic acid toxicity, high-dose tetracycline, or acute fatty liver of pregnancy and may result in fulminant hepatic failure.

There are several factors, presumably resulting from impaired responsiveness of fat cells to insulin, that are responsible for the accumulation of fat in the liver in patients with nonalcoholic fatty liver disease: (1) increased mobilization of fatty acids from peripheral adipose depots; (2) decreased utilization or oxidation of fatty acids by the liver; (3) increased hepatic fatty acid synthesis; (4) increased esterification of fatty acids into triglycerides; and (5) decreased secretion or liberation of fat from the liver. High serum leptin levels in obese persons may contribute to hepatic steatosis by promoting insulin resistance and altering insulin signaling in hepatocytes. Leptin may also stimulate proinflammatory cytokines and thereby influence progression from hepatic steatosis to steatohepatitis.

The exact stimulus that causes progression of steatosis to steatohepatitis and fibrosis is unclear. The leading possibility is lipid peroxidation and oxidative stress. Some patients with nonalcoholic fatty liver disease have hepatic iron overload, and some of these patients are heterozygous for the *C282Y* gene for hemochromatosis *(HFE);* increased hepatic iron as well as severe steatosis (both attributed to insulin resistance) have been associated with hepatic fibrosis. Hepatic concentrations of cytochrome P450 2E1 are increased in patients with nonalcoholic steatohepatitis, as they are in alcoholic liver disease, and patients with nonalcoholic steatohepatitis appear to replenish depleted hepatic adenosine triphosphate (ATP) stores more slowly than healthy subjects after an ATP-depleting challenge. Increased circulating levels of tumor necrosis factor-α due to obesity and to impaired macrophage function may contribute to the development of nonalcoholic steatohepatitis. Mitochondrial structural abnormalities are associated with nonalcoholic steatohepatitis but not nonalcoholic fatty liver disease alone. Women in whom fatty liver of pregnancy develops often have a defect in fatty acid oxidation due to reduced long-chain 3-hydroxyacyl-CoA dehydrogenase activity.

Hepatomegaly is present in up to 75% of patients with nonalcoholic fatty liver disease, but the stigmas of chronic liver disease are rare.

Laboratory studies may show mildly elevated aminotransferase and alkaline phosphatase levels. In contrast to alcoholic liver disease, the ratio of ALT to AST is almost always greater than 1 in nonalcoholic fatty liver disease, but it decreases to less than 1 as advanced fibrosis and cirrhosis develop. Macrovascular steatosis may be demonstrated on MRI and often on ultrasound and CT. Percutaneous liver biopsy is diagnostic and is the only way to assess the degree of fibrosis.

Treatment consists of removing or modifying the offending factor. Weight loss, dietary fat restriction, and exercise often lead to improvement in liver tests and steatosis in obese patients with fatty liver, but the benefit of such measures is less clear in patients with steatohepatitis. Ursodeoxycholic acid, 13–15 mg/kg/ d, may also improve liver function test results, but the benefit of this agent on liver histology requires further study. Hepatic steatosis due to total parenteral nutrition may be ameliorated—and perhaps prevented—with supplemental choline. Vitamin E and phlebotomy (to reduce oxidative stress), thiazolidinediones (to reverse insulin resistance), gemfibrozil (to lower serum triglyceride levels), and betaine (a methyl donor) may have some benefit. Metformin has been shown to reduce insulin resistance and reverse fatty liver in obese leptin-deficient mice and—in preliminary clinical trials—in humans.

Fatty liver is readily reversible with discontinuation of alcohol or treatment of other underlying conditions. Nonalcoholic fatty liver disease may be associated with hepatic fibrosis in 40% of cases; cirrhosis develops in only 10% (those with steatonecrosis and fibrosis on initial liver biopsy); and decompensated cirrhosis occurs in 2–5% of patients. Nonalcoholic steatohepatitis can recur following liver transplantation.

Angulo P: Nonalcoholic fatty liver disease. N Engl J Med 2002;346:1221. [PMID: 11961152]

Clark JM et al: Nonalcoholic fatty liver disease. Gastroenterology 2002;122:1649. [PMID: 12016429]

Dixon JB et al: Nonalcoholic fatty liver disease: predictors of nonalcoholic steatohepatitis and liver fibrosis in the severely obese. Gastroenterology 2001;121:91. [PMID: 11438497] (Predictors of nonalcoholic steatohepatitis were a raised index of insulin resistance, elevated serum ALT level, and systemic hypertension.)

Fong DG et al: Metabolic and nutritional considerations in nonalcoholic fatty liver. Hepatology 2000;32:3. [PMID: 10869282] (Reviews the pathophysiology of nonalcoholic fatty liver disease, including the central role of insulin resistance.)

Gores GJ, Lindor KD (guest editors): Nonalcoholic steatosis syndromes. Semin Liver Dis 2001;21:1. (Entire issue devoted to the topic of nonalcoholic fatty liver disease.)

CIRRHOSIS

Cirrhosis is the end result of hepatocellular injury that leads to both fibrosis and nodular regeneration throughout the liver. Cirrhosis is a serious and generally irreversible disease and is the tenth leading cause of death in the USA. The clinical features result from hepatic cell dysfunction, portosystemic shunting, and portal hypertension.

The most common histologic classification divides cirrhosis into micronodular, macronodular, and mixed forms. These are descriptive terms rather than separate diseases, and each form may be seen in the same patient at different stages of the disease.

(1) In micronodular cirrhosis, typical of alcoholic liver disease (Laennec's cirrhosis), the regenerating nodules are no larger than the original lobules, ie, approximately 1 mm in diameter or less.

(2) Macronodular cirrhosis is characterized by larger nodules, which can measure several centimeters in diameter and may contain central veins. This form corresponds more or less to postnecrotic (posthepatitic) cirrhosis but does not necessarily follow episodes of massive necrosis and stromal collapse.

Clinical Findings

A. SYMPTOMS AND SIGNS

Cirrhosis may cause no symptoms for long periods. The onset of symptoms may be insidious or, less often, abrupt. Weakness, fatigability, disturbed sleep muscle cramps, and weight loss are common. In advanced cirrhosis, anorexia is usually present and may be extreme, with associated nausea and occasional vomiting. Abdominal pain may be present and is related either to hepatic enlargement and stretching of Glisson's capsule or to the presence of ascites. Menstrual abnormalities (usually amenorrhea), impotence, loss of libido, sterility, and gynecomastia in men may occur. Hematemesis is the presenting symptom in 15–25%.

In 70% of cases, the liver is enlarged, palpable, and firm if not hard and has a sharp or nodular edge; the left lobe may predominate. Skin manifestations consist of spider nevi (invariably on the upper half of the body), palmar erythema (mottled redness of the thenar and hypothenar eminences), and Dupuytren's contractures. Evidence of vitamin deficiencies (glossitis and cheilosis) is common. Weight loss, wasting, and the appearance of chronic illness are present. Jaundice—usually not an initial sign—is mild at first, increasing in severity during the later stages of the disease. Ascites, pleural effusions, peripheral edema, and ecchymotic lesions are late findings. Encephalopathy characterized by day-night reversal, asterixis, tremor, dysarthria, delirium, drowsiness, and ultimately coma also occur late except when precipitated by an acute hepatocellular insult or an episode of gastrointestinal bleeding. Fever may be a presenting symptom in up to 35% of patients and usually reflects associated alcoholic hepatitis, spontaneous bacterial peritonitis, or intercurrent infection. Splenomegaly is present in 35–50% of cases. The superficial veins of the abdomen and thorax are dilated, reflecting the intrahepatic obstruction to portal blood flow, as do rectal varices. The veins fill from below when compressed.

B. LABORATORY FINDINGS

Laboratory abnormalities are either absent or minimal in latent or quiescent cirrhosis. Anemia, a frequent finding, is often macrocytic; causes include suppression of erythropoiesis by alcohol as well as folate deficiency, hemolysis, hypersplenism, and insidious or overt blood loss from the gastrointestinal tract. The white blood cell count may be low, reflecting hypersplenism, or high, suggesting infection; thrombocytopenia is secondary to alcoholic marrow suppression, sepsis, folate deficiency, or splenic sequestration. Prolongation of the prothrombin time may result from failure of hepatic synthesis of clotting factors.

Blood chemistries reflect hepatocellular injury and dysfunction, manifested by modest elevations of AST and alkaline phosphatase and progressive elevation of the bilirubin. Serum albumin is low; gamma globulin is increased and may be as high as in autoimmune hepatitis. The risk of diabetes mellitus is increased in patients with cirrhosis, particularly when associated with HCV infection, alcoholism, hemochromatosis, and nonalcoholic fatty liver disease. Patients with alcoholic cirrhosis may have elevated serum cardiac troponin I levels of uncertain significance.

Liver biopsy may show inactive cirrhosis (fibrosis with regenerative nodules) with no specific features to suggest the underlying cause. Alternatively, there may be additional features of alcoholic liver disease, chronic hepatitis, or other specific causes of cirrhosis.

C. IMAGING

Plain films of the abdomen are seldom helpful. Barium studies of the upper gastrointestinal tract may reveal the presence of esophageal or gastric varices, though endoscopy is more sensitive. Ultrasound is helpful for assessing liver size and detecting ascites or hepatic nodules, including small hepatocellular carcinomas. Together with Doppler studies, it may establish patency of the splenic, portal, and hepatic veins. Hepatic nodules are characterized further by contrast-enhanced CT scan or MRI. Nodules suspicious for malignancy may be biopsied under ultrasound or CT guidance.

D. SPECIAL EXAMINATIONS

Esophagogastroduodenoscopy confirms the presence of varices and detects specific causes of bleeding in the esophagus, stomach, and proximal duodenum. Liver biopsy may be performed by laparoscopy. In selected cases, wedged hepatic vein pressure measurement may establish the presence and cause of portal hypertension.

Differential Diagnosis

Determining the cause of cirrhosis is important prognostically and therapeutically. The most common causes of cirrhosis are chronic hepatitis C and B and alcohol. Many cases of cirrhosis are "cryptogenic," in which unrecognized nonalcoholic fatty liver disease may play a role. Mutations in the keratin 8 gene have been associated with some cases of cryptogenic cirrhosis. In advanced cases, hemochromatosis may be associated with bronzing of the skin, arthritis, heart failure, and diabetes; greater than 60% saturation of serum transferrin or serum ferritin level above the upper limit of normal, detection of the mutated *HFE* gene (see below), and special staining for iron and quantitation of the iron on liver biopsy to confirm the diagnosis. Other metabolic diseases that may lead to cirrhosis include Wilson's disease and α_1-antiprotease (α_1-antitrypsin) deficiency. Primary biliary cirrhosis occurs more frequently in women and is associated with pruritus, significant elevation of alkaline phosphatase, elevated immunoglobulin (IgM) and hypercholesterolemia, and antimitochondrial antibody. Secondary biliary cirrhosis may result from chronic biliary obstruction due to a stone, stricture, or neoplasm and is not associated with antimitochondrial antibody. Congestive heart failure and constrictive pericarditis may lead to hepatic fibrosis ("cardiac cirrhosis") complicated by ascites and may be mistaken for other causes of cirrhosis. Hereditary hemorrhagic telangiectasia can lead to portal hypertension because of portosystemic shunting and nodular transformation of the liver.

Complications

Upper gastrointestinal tract bleeding may occur from varices, portal hypertensive gastropathy, or gastroduodenal ulcer (see Chapter 14). Hemorrhage may be massive, resulting in fatal exsanguination or en-

cephalopathy. Varices may also result from portal vein thrombosis. Liver failure may be precipitated by alcoholism, surgery, and infection. The risk of carcinoma of the liver is increased in patients with cirrhosis. Hepatic Kupffer cell (reticuloendothelial) dysfunction and decreased opsonic activity lead to an increased risk of systemic infection.

Treatment

A. GENERAL MEASURES

The most important principle of treatment is abstinence from alcohol. The diet should be palatable, with adequate calories and protein (75–100 g/d) and, if there is fluid retention, sodium restriction. In the presence of hepatic encephalopathy, protein intake should be reduced to 60–80 g/d. Vitamin supplementation is desirable.

B. TREATMENT OF COMPLICATIONS

1. Ascites and edema—Diagnostic paracentesis is indicated for new ascites. It is rarely associated with serious complications such as bleeding, infection, or bowel perforation even in patients with severe coagulopathy. In addition to a cell count and culture, the ascitic albumin level should be determined; a serum-ascites albumin gradient (serum albumin minus ascitic albumin) > 1.1 suggests portal hypertension. An elevated ascitic adenosine deaminase level is suggestive of tuberculous peritonitis, but the sensitivity of the test is reduced in patients with portal hypertension.

Ascites in patients with results from portal hypertension (increased hydrostatic pressure); hypoalbuminemia (decreased oncotic pressure); peripheral vasodilation, perhaps mediated by endotoxin-induced release of nitric oxide, with resulting increases in renin and angiotensin levels and sodium retention by the kidneys; impaired liver inactivation of aldosterone; and increased aldosterone secretion secondary to increased renin production. Free water excretion is also impaired in cirrhosis, and hyponatremia may develop.

In all patients with cirrhotic ascites, dietary sodium intake may initially be restricted to 400–800 mg/d; the intake of sodium may be liberalized slightly after diuresis ensues. Restriction of fluid intake (800–1000 mL/d) is required for patients with hyponatremia (serum sodium < 125 meq/L). In some patients, there is a rapid diminution of ascites on bed rest and dietary sodium restriction alone. In individuals with ascites, the urinary excretion of sodium is usually less than 10 meq/L.

a. Diuretics—Spironolactone, generally in combination with furosemide, should be used in patients who do not respond to salt restriction. The initial dose of spironolactone is 100 mg daily and may be increased by 100 mg every 3–5 days (up to a maximal conventional daily dose of 400 mg/d, though higher doses have been used) until diuresis is achieved, typically preceded by a rise in the urinary sodium concentration. Monitoring for hyperkalemia is important. In patients who cannot tolerate spironolactone because of side effects such as painful gynecomastia, amiloride, another potassium-sparing diuretic, may be used in a dose of 5–10 mg daily. Diuresis is augmented by the addition of a loop diuretic such as furosemide. This potent diuretic, however, will maintain its effect even with a falling glomerular filtration rate, with resultant prerenal azotemia. The dose of furosemide ranges from 40 to 160 mg/d, and the drug should be administered while monitoring blood pressure, urine output, mental status, and serum electrolytes, especially potassium.

The goal of weight loss in the ascitic patient without associated peripheral edema should be no more than 1–1.5 lb/d (0.5–0.7 kg/d).

b. Large-volume paracentesis—In patients with massive ascites and respiratory compromise, ascites refractory to diuretics, or intolerable diuretic side effects, large-volume paracentesis (4–6 L) is effective. Intravenous albumin concomitantly at a dosage of 10 g/L of ascites fluid removed protects the intravascular volume, though the utility of this practice is debated. Moreover, use of albumin at approximately 15 dollars per gram adds considerable expense to the procedure. Large-volume paracentesis can be repeated daily until ascites is largely resolved and may decrease the need for hospitalization. If possible, diuretics should be continued in the hope of preventing recurrent ascites.

c. Transjugular intrahepatic portosystemic shunt (TIPS)—TIPS has emerged as an alternative to surgical portosystemic shunting in selected cases of variceal bleeding refractory to standard therapy (eg, endoscopic band ligation or sclerotherapy) and has shown benefit in the treatment of severe refractory ascites. The technique involves insertion of an expandable metal stent between a branch of the hepatic vein and portal vein over a catheter inserted via the internal jugular vein. Increased renal sodium excretion and control of ascites refractory to diuretics can be achieved in about 75% of selected cases. The success rate is lower in patients with underlying renal insufficiency. TIPS appears to be the treatment of choice for refractory hepatic hydrothorax (translocation of ascites across the diaphragm to the pleural space). Complications include hepatic encephalopathy in 20–30% of cases, infection, shunt stenosis in up to 60%, and shunt occlusion in up to 30% of cases. Long-term patency usually requires periodic shunt revisions. In most cases, patency can be maintained by balloon dilation, local thrombolysis, or placement of an additional stent. Because of the complications associated with TIPS and uncertainty about its long-term efficacy (reduced hepatic perfusion as a result of TIPS may conceivably shorten a patient's survival), it is currently preferred in patients who require short-term control of variceal bleeding or ascites until liver transplantation can be performed—as opposed to patients in need of definitive control of bleeding or ascites but in whom liver transplantation is not a consideration. Nevertheless, in patients with refractory ascites, long-term survival may be greater with TIPS than with repeated large-volume paracentesis.

d. Peritoneovenous shunts—In the past, peritoneovenous shunts were advocated for use in patients with refractory ascites. These shunts may be effective but carry a considerable complication rate: disseminated intravascular coagulation in 65% of patients (25% symptomatic; 5% severe), bacterial infections in 4–8%, congestive heart failure in 2–4%, and variceal bleeding from sudden expansion of intravascular volume. TIPS is now preferred for refractory ascites.

2. Spontaneous bacterial peritonitis—Spontaneous bacterial peritonitis is heralded by abdominal pain, increasing ascites, fever, and progressive encephalopathy in a patient with cirrhotic ascites; symptoms are typically mild. Paracentesis reveals an ascitic fluid with, most commonly, a total white cell count of up to 500 cells/μL with a high percentage of PMNs and a protein concentration of 1 g/dL or less, corresponding to decreased ascitic opsonic activity. Cultures of ascites give the highest yield—80–90% positive—using blood culture bottles inoculated at the bedside. Common isolates are *E coli* and pneumococci. (Gram-positive cocci are the most common isolates in patients who have undergone invasive procedures such as central venous line placement.) Anaerobes are rare. Pending culture results, if there are 250 or more PMN/μL, intravenous antibiotic therapy should be initiated with cefotaxime, 2 g intravenously every 8–12 hours for at least 5 days. Ceftriaxone or amoxicillin-clavulanic acid are alternatives. A 2-day course of intravenous ciprofloxacin, 200 mg twice daily, followed by oral ciprofloxacin, 500 mg twice daily for 5 days, may be effective in selected patients. Supplemental administration of intravenous albumin may reduce mortality. Response to therapy can be documented by a decrease in the PMN count of at least 50% on repeat paracentesis 48 hours after initiation of therapy. The overall mortality rate is high—up to 70% by 1 year. In survivors, the risk of recurrent peritonitis may be decreased by long-term norfloxacin, 400 mg orally daily (although in recurrence the causative organism is often resistant to quinolones). In high-risk cirrhotics (eg, ascitic protein < 1 g/dL, acute variceal bleeding), first episodes of peritonitis may be prevented by prophylactic norfloxacin or trimethoprim-sulfamethoxazole (one double-strength tablet five times a week).

3. Hepatorenal syndrome—Hepatorenal syndrome is characterized by azotemia in the absence of shock or significant proteinuria in a patient with end-stage liver disease in whom renal function fails to improve following intravenous infusion of 1.5 L of isotonic saline. Oliguria, hyponatremia, and low urinary sodium are typical features. Hepatorenal syndrome is diagnosed only when other causes of renal failure have been excluded. Type I hepatorenal syndrome is characterized by doubling of the serum creatinine to a level greater than 2.5 mg/dL or by halving of the creatinine clearance to less than 20 mL/min in less than 2 weeks. Type II hepatorenal syndrome is more slowly progressive and chronic. The cause is unknown, but the pathogenesis involves intense renal vasoconstriction, possibly because of impaired synthesis of renal vasodilators such as prostaglandin E_2 and decreased total renal blood flow; histologically, the kidneys are normal. Treatment is generally ineffective. Improvement may follow intravenous infusion of the long-acting vasoconstrictor ornipressin and albumin (but with a high rate of ischemic side effects), ornipressin and dopamine, or the somatostatin analog octreotide and midodrine, an alpha-adrenergic drug. Prolongation of survival has been associated with use of the molecular adsorbent recirculating system (MARS), a modified dialysis method that selectively removes albumin-bound substances. Improvement may also follow placement of a TIPS. Mortality is high without liver transplantation, death being due to complicating infection or hemorrhage.

4. Hepatic encephalopathy—Hepatic encephalopathy is a state of disordered central nervous system function resulting from failure of the liver to detoxify noxious agents of gut origin because of hepatocellular dysfunction and portosystemic shunting. Ammonia is the most readily identified toxin but is not solely responsible for the disturbed mental status. Pathogenic factors may include production of false neurotransmitters, increased sensitivity of central nervous system neurons to the inhibitory neurotransmitter γ-aminobutyric acid (GABA), an increase in circulating levels of endogenous benzodiazepines, decreased activity of urea-cycle enzymes due to zinc deficiency, deposition of manganese in the basal ganglia, and swelling of astrocytes in the brain. Bleeding into the intestinal tract may significantly increase the amount of protein in the bowel and precipitate rapid development of encephalopathy. Other precipitants include constipation, alkalosis, potassium deficiency induced by diuretics, opioids, hypnotics, and sedatives; medications containing ammonium or amino compounds; paracentesis with attendant hypovolemia; hepatic or systemic infection; and portosystemic shunts (including TIPS).

Dietary protein should be withheld during acute episodes. When the patient resumes oral intake, protein intake is started at 20 g/d and increased by 10 g every 3–5 days to 60–80 g/d as tolerated, and vegetable protein is better tolerated than meat protein. Gastrointestinal bleeding should be controlled and blood purged from the gastrointestinal tract. This can be accomplished with 120 mL of magnesium citrate by mouth or nasogastric tube every 3–4 hours until the stool is free of gross blood, or by administration of lactulose.

Lactulose, a nonabsorbable synthetic disaccharide, is digested by bacteria in the colon to short-chain fatty acids, resulting in acidification of colon contents. This acidification favors the formation of ammonium ion in the $NH_4^+ \leftrightarrow NH_3 + H^+$ equation; NH_4^+ is not absorbable, whereas NH_3 is absorbable and thought to be neurotoxic. Lactulose also leads to a change in bowel flora so that less ammonia-forming organisms are present. When given orally, the initial dose of lactulose for acute hepatic encephalopathy is 30 mL three or four times daily. The dose should then be titrated so that two or three soft stools per day are produced. When rectal use is indicated because of the patient's inability to take medicines orally, the dose is 300 mL of lactulose in 700 mL of saline or sorbitol as a retention enema for 30–60 minutes; it may be repeated every 4–6 hours.

The ammonia-producing intestinal flora may also be controlled with neomycin sulfate, 0.5–1 g orally every 6 or 12 hours for 7 days. Side effects of neomycin include diarrhea, malabsorption, superinfection, ototoxicity, and nephrotoxicity, usually only after prolonged use. Alternative antibiotics are vancomycin, 1 g orally twice daily, or metronidazole, 250 mg orally three times daily. Patients who do not respond to lactulose alone may improve with a 1-week course of an antibiotic in addition to lactulose.

Avoid opioids, tranquilizers, and sedatives metabolized or excreted by the liver. If agitation is marked, oxazepam, 10–30 mg, which is not metabolized by the liver, may be given cautiously by mouth or by nasogastric tube. Zinc deficiency should be corrected, if present, with oral zinc sulfate, 600 mg/d in divided doses. Eradication of *Helicobacter pylori*, which generates ammonia in the stomach, may improve encephalopathy. Sodium benzoate, 10 g daily, and ornithine aspartate, 9 g three times daily, may lower blood ammonia levels, but there is less experience with these drugs than with lactulose. The benzodiazepine competitive antagonist flumazenil is effective in a minority of patients with severe hepatic encephalopathy, but the drug is short-acting and intravenous administration is required. Use of special dietary supplements enriched with branched-chain amino acids is usually unnecessary except in occasional patients who are intolerant of standard protein supplements.

5. Anemia—For iron deficiency anemia, ferrous sulfate, 0.3 g enteric-coated tablets, one tablet three times daily after meals is effective. Folic acid, 1 mg/d orally, is indicated in the treatment of macrocytic anemia associated with alcoholism. Transfusions with packed red blood cells may be necessary to replace blood loss.

6. Hemorrhagic tendency—Severe hypoprothrombinemia may be treated with vitamin K (eg, phytonadione, 5 mg orally or subcutaneously daily). This treatment is ineffective when synthesis of coagulation factors is impaired because of severe hepatic disease. In such cases, correcting the prolonged prothrombin time requires large volumes of fresh frozen plasma. Because the effect is transient, plasma infusions are not indicated except for active bleeding or before an invasive procedure.

7. Hemorrhage from esophageal varices—See Chapter 14.

8. Hepatopulmonary syndrome—The hepatopulmonary syndrome is the triad of chronic liver disease, an increased alveolar-arterial gradient while the patient is breathing room air, and intrapulmonary vascular dilations or arteriovenous communications that result in a right-to-left intrapulmonary shunt. The syndrome is presumed to result from failure of the diseased liver to clear circulating pulmonary vasodilators. Patients often have dyspnea and arterial deoxygenation in the upright position (orthodeoxia) and relieved by recumbency. The diagnosis should be suspected in a cirrhotic patient with a pulse oximetry level ≤ 92%. Contrast-enhanced echocardiography is a sensitive screening test for detecting pulmonary vascular dilations, whereas macroaggregated albumin lung perfusion scanning is more specific and is used to confirm the diagnosis. High-resolution CT may be useful for detecting dilated pulmonary vessels in affected patients and is under study. Medical therapy has been disappointing; however, intravenous methylene blue may improve oxygenation in patients by inhibiting nitric oxide-induced vasodilation. The syndrome may reverse with liver transplantation, which is contraindicated in patients with moderate to severe pulmonary hypertension (mean pulmonary pressure > 35 mm Hg), though in some cases treatment with epoprostenol may reduce pulmonary hypertension and thereby facilitate liver transplantation. TIPS may provide palliation in patients with hepatopulmonary syndrome awaiting transplantation.

C. Liver Transplantation

Liver transplantation is indicated in selected cases of irreversible, progressive chronic liver disease, acute hepatic failure, and certain metabolic diseases in which the metabolic defect is in the liver. Absolute contraindications include malignancy (except small hepatocellular carcinomas in a cirrhotic liver), advanced cardiopulmonary disease (except pulmonary arteriovenous shunting due to portal hypertension and cirrhosis), and sepsis. Relative contraindications include age over 70, portal and mesenteric vein thrombosis, active alcohol or drug abuse, HIV infection, severe malnutrition, and lack of patient understanding. Alcoholics should be abstinent for 6 months. Liver transplantation should be considered in patients with worsening functional status, rising bilirubin, decreasing albumin, worsening coagulopathy, refractory ascites, recurrent variceal bleeding, or worsening encephalopathy. The major impediment to more widespread use of liver transplantation is a shortage of donor organs. Increasingly, adult living donor liver transplantation is an option for some patients. Five-year survival rates as high as 80% are now reported. Hepatocellular carcinoma, hepatitis B and C, and some cases of Budd-Chiari syndrome may recur in the transplanted liver. The incidence of recurrence of hepatitis B can be reduced by pre- and postoperative treatment with lamivudine and perioperative administration of hepatitis B immune globulin. Immunosuppression is achieved with a combination of cyclosporine or tacrolimus, corticosteroids, azathioprine, and mycophenolate mofetil and may be complicated by infections, renal failure, neurologic disorders, and drug toxicity as well as graft rejection, vascular occlusion, or bile leaks. Patients are at risk of obesity, diabetes, and hyperlipidemia.

Prognosis

The prognosis of cirrhosis has shown little change over the years. Factors determining survival include the patient's ability to stop the intake of alcohol as well as the Child-Turcotte-Pugh class (Table 15–5). Other prognostic scoring systems have been devised, and there is current interest in the Model for End-Stage Liver Disease (MELD), which incorporates the serum bilirubin and creatinine levels, international normalized ratio (INR), and etiology of liver disease as a mea-

Table 15–5. Modified Child-Pugh classification for cirrhosis.

Parameter	Numerical Score		
	1	2	3
Ascites	None	Slight	Moderate to severe
Encephalopathy	None	Slight to moderate	Moderate to severe
Bilirubin (mg/dL)	< 2.0	2–3	> 3.0
Albumin (g/dL)	> 3.5	2.8–3.5	< 2.8
Prothrombin time (seconds increased)	1–3	4–6	> 6.0

Total numerical score	Child-Pugh class
5–6	A
7–9	B
10–15	C

sure of mortality risk in patients with end-stage liver disease and as a tool for determining allocation priorities for donor livers. Hematemesis, jaundice, and ascites are unfavorable signs. In established cases with severe hepatic dysfunction (serum albumin < 3 g/dL, bilirubin > 3 mg/dL, ascites, encephalopathy, cachexia, and upper gastrointestinal bleeding), only 50% survive 6 months. The risk of death in this subgroup of patients with advanced cirrhosis is associated with renal insufficiency, cognitive dysfunction, ventilatory insufficiency, age ≥ 65 years, and prothrombin time ≥ 16 seconds. Liver transplantation has markedly improved the outlook for patients who are acceptable candidates and are referred for evaluation early.

Blei AT et al: Hepatic encephalopathy. Am J Gastroenterol 2001;96:1968. [PMID: 11467622] (Practice guidelines.)

Dagher L et al: The hepatorenal syndrome. Gut 2001;49:729. [PMID: 11600480] (Diagnostic criteria, pathogenesis, and established and emerging treatment options.)

Keeffe EB: Liver transplantation: current status and novel approaches to liver replacement. Gastroenterology 2001;120:749. [PMID: 11179248] (Concise overview of the field.)

Seaman DS: Adult living donor liver transplantation: Current status. J Clin Gastroenterol 2001;33:97. [PMID: 11468434] (Technical aspects, patient and donor evaluation, results, and ethical issues.)

Sorrell MF et al (guest editors): Long-term management of the liver transplant patient. Liver Tranpl 2001;7(Suppl 1):51. (Spectrum of long-term complications.)

PRIMARY BILIARY CIRRHOSIS

Primary biliary cirrhosis is a chronic disease of the liver characterized by autoimmune destruction of intrahepatic bile ducts and cholestasis. It is insidious in onset, occurs usually in women aged 40–60, and is often detected by the chance finding of elevated alkaline phosphatase levels. Estimated incidence and prevalence rates in the USA are 4.5 and 65.4 per 100,000, respectively, in women, and 0.7 and 12.1 per 100,000, respectively, in men. The disease is progressive and is complicated by steatorrhea, xanthomas, xanthelasma, osteoporosis, osteomalacia, and portal hypertension. It may be associated with Sjögren's syndrome, autoimmune thyroid disease, Raynaud's syndrome, scleroderma, hypothyroidism, and celiac disease.

Clinical Findings

A. SYMPTOMS AND SIGNS

Many patients are asymptomatic for years. The onset of clinical illness is insidious and is heralded by pruritus. With progression, physical examination reveals hepatosplenomegaly. Xanthomatous lesions may occur in the skin and tendons and around the eyelids. Jaundice and signs of portal hypertension are late findings. The risk of osteoporosis is increased in patients with primary biliary cirrhosis, as in patients with other forms of chronic liver disease.

B. LABORATORY FINDINGS

Blood counts are normal early in the disease. Liver function tests reflect cholestasis with elevation of alkaline phosphatase, cholesterol (especially high-density lipoproteins), and, in later stages, bilirubin. Antimitochondrial antibodies (directed against pyruvate dehydrogenase or other 2-oxo-acid enzymes in mitochondria) are present in 95% of patients, and serum IgM levels are elevated.

Diagnosis

The diagnosis of primary biliary cirrhosis is based on the detection of cholestatic liver chemistries (often an isolated elevation of the alkaline phosphatase) and antimitochondrial antibodies in serum in combination with characteristic histology on liver biopsy. Liver biopsy also permits histologic staging: I, portal inflammation with granulomas; II, bile duct proliferation, periportal inflammation; III, interlobular fibrous septa; and IV, cirrhosis.

Differential Diagnosis

The disease must be differentiated from chronic biliary tract obstruction (stone or stricture), carcinoma of the bile ducts, primary sclerosing cholangitis, sarcoidosis, cholestatic drug toxicity (eg, chlorpromazine), and in some cases chronic hepatitis. Patients with a clinical and histologic picture of primary biliary cirrhosis but no antimitochondrial antibodies are said to have "autoimmune cholangitis," which has been associated with lower serum IgM levels and a greater frequency of smooth muscle and antinuclear antibodies. Some patients have overlapping features of primary biliary cirrhosis and autoimmune hepatitis.

Treatment

Treatment is primarily symptomatic. Cholestyramine (4 g) or colestipol (5 g) in water or juice three times daily may be beneficial for the pruritus. Rifampin, 150–300 mg orally twice daily, is inconsistently beneficial. Opioid antagonists (eg, naloxone, 0.2 µg/kg/min by intravenous infusion, or naltrexone, 50 mg/d by mouth) show promise in the treatment of pruritus. The 5-HT$_3$ serotonin receptor antagonist ondansetron may also provide some benefit. Deficiencies of vitamins A, K, and D may occur if steatorrhea is present and is aggravated when cholestyramine or colestipol is administered. Calcium supplementation (500 mg three times daily) may help prevent osteomalacia but is of uncertain benefit in osteoporosis.

Because of its lack of toxicity, ursodeoxycholic acid (10–15 mg/kg/d in one or two doses) is the preferred medical treatment and has been shown to slow the progression of disease, improve long-term survival, reduce the risk of developing esophageal varices, and delay the need for liver transplantation. Colchicine (0.6 mg twice daily) and methotrexate (15 mg/wk) have had some reported benefit in improving symptoms and serum levels of alkaline phosphatase and bilirubin. Methotrexate may also improve liver histology. Penicillamine, corticosteroids, and azathioprine have proved to be of no benefit. For patients with advanced disease, liver transplantation is the treatment of choice.

Prognosis

Without liver transplantation, survival averages 7–10 years once symptoms develop. In advanced disease, adverse prognostic markers are older age, high serum bilirubin, edema, low albumin, prolonged prothrombin time, and variceal hemorrhage. Among asymptomatic patients, about one-third will become symptomatic within 15 years. The risk of hepatobiliary malignancies appears to be increased in patients with primary biliary cirrhosis. Liver transplantation for advanced primary biliary cirrhosis is associated with a 1-year survival rate of 85–90%. The disease recurs in the graft in 20% of patients by 3 years, but this does not seem to affect survival.

Collier JD et al: Guidelines on the management of osteoporosis associated with chronic liver disease. Gut 2002;50(Suppl 1):i1. [PMID: 11788576] (Prevalence, pathogenesis, biochemical markers, diagnosis, and management.)

Heathcote EJ: Management of primary biliary cirrhosis. The American Association for the Study of Liver Diseases practice guidelines. Hepatology 2000;31:1005. [PMID: 10733559]

Lazaridis K et al: Ursodeoxycholic acid "mechanisms of action and clinical use in hepatobiliary disorders." J Hepatol 2001;35:134. [PMID: 11495032] (Review of the mechanisms of action and data suggesting that this agent slows the progression of primary biliary cirrhosis and reduces the need for liver transplantation.)

Rouillard S et al: Hepatic osteodystrophy. Hepatology 2001;33:301. [PMID: 11124849] (Dual-energy x-ray absorptiometry can be used for periodic screening.)

Van de Water J et al: Molecular mimicry and primary biliary cirrhosis: Premises not promises. Hepatology 2001;33:771. [PMID: 11283838] (Reviews evidence for a possible infectious cause of primary biliary cirrhosis.)

HEMOCHROMATOSIS

Hemochromatosis is an autosomal recessive disease with linkage in many cases to HLA-A3. The principal genetic defect has been identified as a mutation in the HFE gene on chromosome 6. The alteration leads to substitution of tyrosine for cysteine at position 282 (C282Y) in a region of the gene product involved in interaction with β_2-microglobulin. The HFE protein is thought to play an important role in the process by which duodenal crypt cells sense body iron stores. The presence of the mutation apparently reduces surface expression of an HFE-β_2 microglobulin complex on duodenal crypt cells, decreasing the affinity of the transferrin receptor for transferrin. This impairs transferrin-mediated uptake of iron from the circulation into crypt cells and results in up-regulation of duodenal metal-transporter-1 and ferroportin-1 expression on the luminal side of villous cells, leading in turn to increased iron absorption from the intestine. About 85% of persons with well-established hemochromatosis are homozygous for the C282Y mutation. The frequency of the gene mutation averages 7% in Northern European and North American white populations, resulting in a 0.5% frequency of homozygotes (of whom 40–70% will develop iron overload). By contrast, the gene mutation and hemochromatosis are uncommon in African-American and Asian-American populations. A second genetic mutation leading to substitution of aspartic acid for histidine at position 63 (H63D) of the same protein may contribute to the development of hemochromatosis in a small percentage (1.5%) of persons who are compound heterozygotes for C282Y and H63D.

The disorder is characterized by increased accumulation of iron as hemosiderin in the liver, pancreas, heart, adrenals, testes, pituitary, and kidneys. Eventually the patient may develop hepatic and pancreatic insufficiency, congestive heart failure, and hypogonadism. The disease is rarely recognized clinically before the fifth decade. Heterozygotes do not develop cirrhosis in the absence of associated disorders such as viral hepatitis or nonalcoholic fatty liver disease.

Clinical Findings

The onset is usually after age 50—earlier in men than in women; however, because of widespread liver biochemical testing and iron screening, the diagnosis can be made long before symptoms develop. Clinical manifestations include arthropathy, hepatomegaly and evidence of hepatic insufficiency (late finding), skin pigmentation (combination of slate gray due to iron and brown due to melanin, sometimes resulting in bronze color), cardiac enlargement with or without heart failure or conduction defects, diabetes mellitus with its complications, and impotence in men. Bleeding from esophageal varices may occur, and in patients who develop cirrhosis, there is a 15–20% incidence of hepatocellular carcinoma. Affected patients are at increased risk of infection with *Vibrio vulnificus, Listeria monocytogenes, Yersinia enterocolitica,* and other siderophilic organisms. A variant presentation in young patients is characterized by cardiac dysfunction, hypogonadotropic hypogonadism, and a high mortality rate and is not associated with the C282Y mutation.

Laboratory findings include mildly abnormal liver tests (AST, alkaline phosphatase), an elevated plasma iron with greater than 50% saturation of the transferrin (after an overnight fast), and an elevated serum ferritin (although a normal iron saturation and normal ferritin does not exclude the diagnosis). CT and MRI may show changes consistent with iron overload of the liver, but these techniques are not sensitive enough for screening. Testing for *HFE* mutations is indicated in any patient with evidence of iron overload and in siblings of patients with confirmed hemochromatosis. In patients who are homozygous for *C282Y*, liver biopsy is often indicated to determine whether cirrhosis is present. Biopsy can be deferred, however, in patients under age 40 in whom the serum ferritin level is < 1000 μg/L, serum AST level is normal, and no hepatomegaly is present. The likelihood of cirrhosis is low in these individuals. Liver biopsy is also indicated when iron overload is suspected even though the patient is not homozygous for *C282Y*. In patients with hemochromatosis, the liver biopsy characteristically shows extensive iron deposition in hepatocytes and in bile ducts and the hepatic iron index—hepatic iron content per gram of liver converted to micromoles and divided by the patient's age—is generally greater than 1.9.

Treatment

Early diagnosis and treatment in the precirrhotic phase of hemochromatosis is of great importance. Affected patients should avoid foods rich in iron (such as red meat), alcohol, vitamin C, raw shellfish, and supplemental iron. Treatment consists initially of weekly phlebotomies of 500 mL of blood (about 250 mg of iron), continued for up to 2–3 years to achieve depletion of iron stores. This process is monitored by hematocrit and serum iron determinations. When iron store depletion is achieved (iron saturation < 50% and serum ferritin level < 50 μg/L), maintenance phlebotomies (every 2–4 months) are continued. The chelating agent deferoxamine is indicated for patients with hemochromatosis and anemia or in those with secondary iron overload due to thalassemia who cannot tolerate phlebotomies. The drug is administered intravenously or subcutaneously in a dose of 20–40 mg/kg/d infused over 24 hours and can mobilize 30 mg of iron per day. However, treatment is painful and time-consuming. Complications of hemochromatosis—arthropathy, diabetes, heart disease, portal hypertension, and hypopituitarism—also require treatment.

The course of the disease is favorably altered by phlebotomy therapy. In precirrhotic patients, cirrhosis may be prevented. Cardiac conduction defects and insulin requirements improve with treatment. In patients with cirrhosis, varices may reverse, and the risk of variceal bleeding declines. However, cirrhotic patients must be monitored for the development of hepatocellular carcinoma. Liver transplantation for advanced cirrhosis associated with severe iron overload, including hemochromatosis, has been reported to lead to survival rates that are lower than those for other types of liver disease because of cardiac complications

and an increased risk of infections. Genetic testing is recommended for all first-degree family members of the proband. Screening all white men over age 30 or all adults over age 20 by measurement of the transferrin saturation or possibly the unbound iron-binding capacity has been recommended by some.

Bacon BR: Hemochromatosis: Diagnosis and management. Gastroenterology 2001;120:718. [PMID: 11179246]

El-Serag HB et al: Screening for hereditary hemochromatosis in siblings and children of affected patients: A cost-effectiveness analysis. Ann Intern Med 2000;132:261. [PMID: 10681280] (Screening relatives of patients with *C282Y* homozygous hemochromatosis is cost-effective; siblings of an affected patient should undergo genetic testing, while children should undergo genetic testing if the patient's spouse is heterozygous for *C282Y*.)

Hanson EH et al: *HFE* gene and hereditary hemochromatosis: A HuGE review. Human Genome Epidemiology. Am J Epidemiol 2001;154:193. [PMID: 11479183] (The genetic abnormality and variants, gene frequencies, clinical manifestations, treatment, and screening.)

Tavill AS: Diagnosis and management of hemochromatosis. Hepatology 2001;33:1321. [PMID: 11343262] (Current practice guidelines.)

WILSON'S DISEASE

Wilson's disease (hepatolenticular degeneration) is a rare autosomal recessive disorder that usually occurs between the first and third decades. The condition is characterized by excessive deposition of copper in the liver and brain. The genetic defect, localized to chromosome 13, has been shown to affect a copper-transporting adenosine triphosphatase (ATP7B) in the liver and leads to oxidative damage of hepatic mitochondria. Over 200 different mutations in the Wilson disease gene have been identified, making genetic diagnosis impractical.

The major physiologic aberration in Wilson's disease is excessive absorption of copper from the small intestine and decreased excretion of copper by the liver, resulting in increased tissue deposition, especially in the liver, brain, cornea, and kidney. Serum ceruloplasmin, the plasma copper-carrying protein, is low. Urinary excretion of copper is high.

Clinical Findings

Wilson's disease tends to present as liver disease in adolescents and neuropsychiatric disease in young adults, but there is great variability. The diagnosis should always be considered in any child or young adult with hepatitis, splenomegaly with hypersplenism, hemolytic anemia, portal hypertension, and neurologic or psychiatric abnormalities. Wilson's disease should also be considered in persons under 40 years of age with chronic or fulminant hepatitis.

Hepatic involvement may range from elevated liver tests (although the alkaline phosphatase may be low) to cirrhosis and portal hypertension. The neurologic manifestations are related to basal ganglia dysfunction and include a resting, postural, or kinetic tremor and dystonia of the bulbar musculature with resulting dysarthria and dysphagia. Psychiatric features include behavioral and personality changes and emotional lability. The pathognomonic sign of the condition is the brownish or gray-green Kayser-Fleischer ring, which represents fine pigmented granular deposits in Descemet's membrane in the cornea close to the endothelial surface. The ring is usually most marked at the superior and inferior poles of the cornea. It can frequently be seen with the naked eye and almost invariably by slit lamp examination. It may be absent in patients with hepatic manifestations only but is usually present in those with neuropsychiatric disease. Renal calculi, the Fanconi defect, renal tubular acidosis, hypoparathyroidism, and hemolytic anemia may occur in patients with Wilson's disease.

The diagnosis can be challenging and is based on demonstration of increased urinary copper excretion (> 100 μg/24 h) or low serum ceruloplasmin levels (< 20 μg/dL), and elevated hepatic copper concentration (> 250 μg/g of dry liver). However, increased urinary copper and low serum ceruloplasmin levels are not specific for Wilson's disease. In equivocal cases (when the serum ceruloplasmin level is normal), the diagnosis may require demonstration of low radiolabeled copper incorporation into ceruloplasmin or urinary copper determination after a penicillamine challenge. Liver biopsy may show acute or chronic hepatitis or cirrhosis.

Treatment

Early treatment to remove excess copper is essential before it can produce neurologic or hepatic damage. Early in the treatment phase, restriction of dietary copper (shellfish, organ foods, and legumes) may be of value. Oral penicillamine (0.75–2 g/d in divided doses) is the drug of choice, making possible urinary excretion of chelated copper. Pyridoxine, 50 mg per week, is added, since penicillamine is an antimetabolite of this vitamin. If penicillamine treatment cannot be tolerated because of gastrointestinal, hypersensitivity, or autoimmune reactions, consider the use of trientine, 250–500 mg three times a day. Oral zinc acetate, 50 mg three times a day, promotes fecal copper excretion and may be used as maintenance therapy after decoppering with a chelating agent or as first-line therapy in presymptomatic or pregnant patients. Ammonium tetrathiomolybdate has shown promise as initial therapy for neurologic Wilson's disease.

Treatment should continue indefinitely. Once the serum nonceruloplasmin copper level is within the normal range, the dose of chelating agent can be reduced to the minimum necessary for maintaining that level. The prognosis is good in patients who are effectively treated before liver or brain damage has occurred. Liver transplantation is indicated for fulminant hepatitis (often after plasma exchange as a stabilizing measure), end-stage cirrhosis, and, in se-

lected cases, intractable neurologic disease. Family members, especially siblings, require screening with serum ceruloplasmin, liver function tests, and slit-lamp examination.

Emre S et al: Orthotopic liver transplantation for Wilson's disease: A single-center experience. Transplantation 2001;72: 1232. [PMID: 11602847] (One-year survival rate was 87.5% following transplantation; renal failure was present in 45% of patients with fulminant Wilson's disease but resolved posttransplant.)

Gow PJ et al: Diagnosis of Wilson's disease: An experience over three decades. Gut 2000;46:415. [PMID: 10673307] (In patients with nonfulminant presentations, the combination of a low serum ceruloplasmin and Kayser-Fleischer rings establishes the diagnosis but is present in only 55%; the rest require liver biopsy to demonstrate an elevated hepatic copper.)

Riordan SM et al: The Wilson's disease gene and phenotypic diversity. J Hepatol 2001;34:165. [PMID: 11211896] (Reviews genetic defect, epidemiology, clinical manifestations, and diagnosis; there is no clear association between genotype and presentation or course.)

HEPATIC VEIN OBSTRUCTION (Budd-Chiari Syndrome)

Occlusion of the hepatic veins may occur from a variety of causes. Many cases are associated with polycythemia vera or other myeloproliferative diseases, which may be subclinical. Hepatovenous obstructions may be associated with caval webs, right-sided heart failure or constrictive pericarditis, neoplasms causing hepatic vein occlusions, paroxysmal nocturnal hemoglobinuria, Behçet's syndrome, blunt abdominal trauma, use of birth control pills, and pregnancy. In some cases, an underlying predisposition to thrombosis (eg, hyperprothrombinemia, [factor II G20210A mutation], activated protein C resistance [factor V Leiden mutation], protein C or S or antithrombin deficiency, antiphospholipid antibodies) can be identified. Some cytotoxic agents and pyrrolizidine alkaloids ("bush teas") may cause hepatic veno-occlusive disease (occlusion of terminal venules), which mimics Budd-Chiari syndrome clinically. Veno-occlusive disease is common in patients who have undergone bone marrow transplantation, particularly those with pretransplant aminotransferase elevations or fever during cytoreductive therapy with cyclophosphamide, azathioprine, carmustine, busulfan, or etoposide or those receiving high-dose cytoreductive therapy or high-dose total body irradiation. In India, China, and South Africa, Budd-Chiari syndrome is often the result of occlusion of the hepatic portion of the inferior vena cava, presumably due to prior thrombosis, and the clinical presentation is mild but the course is frequently complicated by hepatocellular carcinoma.

Clinical manifestations may include tender, painful hepatic enlargement; jaundice; splenomegaly; and ascites. With advanced disease, bleeding varices and hepatic coma may be evident. Hepatic imaging studies may show a prominent caudate lobe, since its venous drainage may not be occluded. The screening test of choice is duplex Doppler ultrasonography, which has a sensitivity of 85% for detecting evidence of hepatic venous or inferior vena caval thrombosis. Caval venography can delineate caval webs and occluded hepatic veins. Percutaneous liver biopsy frequently shows a characteristic centrilobular congestion.

Ascites should be treated with fluid and salt restriction and diuretics. Treatable causes of Budd-Chiari syndrome should be sought. Prompt recognition and treatment of an underlying hematologic disorder may avoid the need for surgery. Surgical decompression (side-to-side portacaval, mesocaval, or mesoatrial shunt) of the congested liver may be required to relieve persistent hepatic congestion. In some cases, placement of a transjugular intrahepatic portosystemic shunt (TIPS) may be feasible, although late TIPS dysfunction is common. Balloon angioplasty, in some cases with placement of an intravascular metallic stent, is preferred in patients with an inferior vena caval web and may be feasible in patients with a short segment of thrombosis in the hepatic vein. Rarely, thrombolytic therapy may be attempted within 2 weeks of acute hepatic vein thrombosis. Liver transplantation is considered in patients with cirrhosis and hepatocellular dysfunction. Patients often require lifelong anticoagulation and treatment of the underlying myeloproliferative disease.

Espinosa G et al: Budd-Chiari syndrome secondary to antiphospholipid syndrome: Clinical and immunologic characteristics of 43 patients. Medicine (Baltimore) 2001;80:345. [PMID: 11704712] (Includes four new cases of Budd-Chiari syndrome of twenty-two seen by the authors plus others from the literature.)

Mohanty D et al: Hereditary thrombophilia as a cause of Budd-Chiari syndrome: A study from Western India. Hepatology 2001;34:666. [PMID: 11584361] (In this series of 33 patients, 59% had at least one coagulation disorder, including factor V Leiden [26.4%], protein C deficiency [13.2%], and antiphospholipid antibody [21%].)

Perelló A et al: TIPS is a useful long-term derivative therapy for patients with Budd-Chiari syndrome uncontrolled by medical therapy. Hepatology 2002;35:132. [PMID: 11786969] (Although late TIPS dysfunction is common in this setting, portal hypertension may not recur after TIPS occlusion.)

Slakey DB et al: Budd-Chiari syndrome: Current management options. Ann Surg 2001;233:522. [PMID: 11303134] (Review of 54 patients seen at Johns Hopkins Hospital over 20 years; 80% were treated with a mesocaval or mesoatrial shunt, with 78% of these patients surviving 5 years.)

THE LIVER IN HEART FAILURE

Shock liver, or ischemic hepatopathy, results from an acute fall in cardiac output due, for example, to acute myocardial infarction or arrhythmia, usually in a patient with passive congestion of the liver. Clinical hypotension may be absent (or unwitnessed). In some cases, the precipitating event is arterial hypoxemia due to respiratory failure. The hallmark is a rapid and striking elevation of serum aminotransferase levels (often > 5000 units/L); an early rapid rise in the serum lactate dehydrogenase level is also typical, but elevations of serum alkaline phosphatase and bilirubin are usually mild. The prothrombin time may be prolonged, and encephalopathy may develop. The mortality rate due to the underlying disease is high, but in patients who recover, the aminotransferase levels return to normal quickly, usually within 1 week—in contrast to viral hepatitis.

In patients with passive congestion of the liver due to right-sided heart failure, the serum bilirubin level may be elevated, occasionally as high as 40 mg/dL, due in part to hypoxia of perivenular hepatocytes. Serum alkaline phosphatase levels are normal or slightly elevated. Hepatojugular reflux is present, and with tricuspid regurgitation the liver may be pulsatile. Ascites may be out of proportion to peripheral edema, with a high serum ascites-albumin gradient (> 1.1) and a protein content of more than 2.5 g/dL. In severe cases, signs of encephalopathy may develop.

Henrion J et al: Hypoxic hepatitis caused by acute exacerbation of chronic respiratory failure: A case-controlled, hemodynamic study of 17 consecutive cases. Hepatology 1999;29:427. [PMID: 9918919] (Of 142 consecutive episodes of ischemic hepatitis, 17 were attributed to a combination of severe arterial hypoxemia and elevated central venous pressure, without left cardiac failure, in patients with chronic respiratory failure.)

Seeto RK et al: Ischemic hepatitis: clinical presentation and pathogenesis. Am J Med 2000;109:109. [PMID: 10967151] (Of 31 patients with ischemic hepatitis, all had underlying heart disease and 29 had right-sided heart failure.)

NONCIRRHOTIC PORTAL HYPERTENSION

Noncirrhotic portal hypertension must be considered in the differential diagnosis of splenomegaly or upper gastrointestinal bleeding due to esophageal or gastric varices in patients with normal liver function. This syndrome may be due to portal vein thrombosis, splenic vein obstruction (presenting as gastric varices without esophageal varices), schistosomiasis, noncirrhotic intrahepatic portal sclerosis, or arterial-portal vein fistula. Aside from splenomegaly, the physical findings are not remarkable. Endoscopy shows esophageal or gastric varices. The liver tests are usually normal, but there may be findings of hypersplenism. Magnetic resonance angiography (MRA) of the portal system is generally confirmatory. Needle biopsy of the liver may be indicated to diagnose schistosomiasis and noncirrhotic intrahepatic portal sclerosis. An underlying hypercoagulable state is found in many patients; these include mutation G20210A of prothrombin, factor V Leiden mutation, protein C and S deficiency, antiphospholipid syndrome, and mutation TT677 of methylenetetrahydrofolate reductase. It is possible, however, that deficiency of protein C and S—as well as of antithrombin—is a secondary phenomenon due to portosystemic shunting and reduced hepatic blood flow.

If splenic vein thrombosis is the cause, splenectomy is curative. In other cases, band ligation or sclerotherapy is initiated for variceal bleeding and portosystemic shunting is reserved for failures of endoscopic therapy. Anticoagulation may be indicated for isolated acute portal vein thrombosis if a hypercoagulable disorder is identified.

Amitrano L et al: Inherited coagulation disorders in cirrhotic patients with portal vein thrombosis. Hepatology 2000;31: 345. [PMID: 10655256] (Among the 8% of cirrhotic patients with portal vein thrombosis, 70% had an inherited disorder of coagulation: factor V Leiden mutation [13%], mutation G20210A of prothrombin [35%], or mutation TT677 of methylenetetrahydrofolate reductase [44%].)

Condat B et al: Current outcome of portal view thrombosis in adults: Risk and benefit of anticoagulant therapy. Gastroenterology 2001;120:490. [PMID: 11159889] (Retrospective experience in 136 adult patients with nonmalignant, noncirrhotic portal vein thrombosis suggesting that anticoagulant therapy reduced the risk of recurrence or extension of thrombosis without increasing the risk if variceal bleeding.)

Janssen HL et al: Extrahepatic portal vein thrombosis: aetiology and determinants of survival. Gut 2001;49:720. [PMID: 11600478] (In the absence of cirrhosis, cancer, or mesenteric vein thrombosis, long-term survival is excellent.)

Valla D-C et al: Portal vein thrombosis in adults: Pathophysiology, pathogenesis and management. J Hepatol 2000;32: 865. [PMID: 10845677] (Thorough review.)

PYOGENIC HEPATIC ABSCESS

The liver can be invaded by bacteria via (1) the portal vein (pyelephlebitis); (2) the common duct (ascending cholangitis); (3) the hepatic artery, secondary to bacteremia; (4) direct extension from an infectious process; and (5) traumatic implantation of bacteria through the abdominal wall.

Ascending cholangitis resulting from biliary obstruction due to a stone, stricture, or neoplasm is the most common identifiable cause of hepatic abscess in the USA. In 10% of cases, liver abscess is secondary to appendicitis or diverticulitis. Up to 40% of abscesses have no demonstrable cause and are classified as cryptogenic. The most frequently encountered organisms are *Escherichia coli, Proteus vulgaris, Enterobacter aerogenes,* and multiple anaerobic species. Hepatic candidiasis is seen in immunocompromised patients and those with hematologic malignancies. Rarely, hepatocellular carcinoma can present as a pyogenic abscess because of tumor necrosis, biliary obstruction, and superimposed bacterial infection.

Clinical Findings

The presentation is often insidious. Fever is almost always present and may antedate other symptoms or signs. Pain may be a prominent complaint and is localized to the right hypochondrium or epigastric area.

Jaundice, tenderness in the right upper abdomen, and either steady or swinging fever are the chief physical findings.

Laboratory examination reveals leukocytosis with a shift to the left. Liver function studies are nonspecifically abnormal. Chest roentgenograms usually reveal elevation of the diaphragm if the abscess is on the right side. Ultrasound, CT, or MRI may reveal the presence of intrahepatic defects. On MRI, characteristic findings include high signal intensity on T2-weighted images and rim enhancement. Hepatic candidiasis is seen usually in the setting of systemic candidiasis, and on CT scan the characteristic appearance is that of multiple "bulls-eyes," but imaging studies may be negative in neutropenic patients.

Treatment

Treatment should consist of antimicrobial agents (a third-generation cephalosporin and metronidazole) that are effective against coliform organisms and anaerobes. If the abscess is at least 5 cm in diameter or the response to antibiotic therapy is not rapid, catheter or surgical (eg, laparoscopic) drainage should be undertaken. The mortality rate is still substantial (≥ 8%) and is highest in patients with underlying biliary malignancy or severe multiorgan dysfunction. Hepatic candidiasis often responds to intravenous amphotericin B (total dose of 2–9 g). Fungal abscesses are associated with mortality rates of up to 50% and are treated with intravenous amphotericin B and drainage.

Rockey DC: Hepatobiliary infections. Curr Opin Gastroenterol 2001;17:257. (State-of-the-art review.)

NEOPLASMS OF THE LIVER

1. Hepatocellular Carcinoma

Malignant neoplasms of the liver that arise from parenchymal cells are called hepatocellular carcinomas; those that originate in the ductular cells are called cholangiocarcinomas.

Hepatocellular carcinomas are associated with cirrhosis in general and hepatitis B or C in particular. Incidence rates are rising in the USA and other western countries, presumably because of the high prevalence of chronic hepatitis C infection over the past 2–3 decades. In Africa and most of Asia, hepatitis B is of major etiologic significance, whereas in western countries and Japan hepatitis C and alcoholic cirrhosis are the most common causes. Other associations include hemochromatosis, aflatoxin exposure (associated with mutation of the *P53* gene), α_1-antiprotease (α_1-antitrypsin) deficiency, and tyrosinemia. The fibrolamellar variant of hepatocellular carcinoma occurs in young women and is characterized by a distinctive histologic picture, absence of risk factors, and indolent course.

Histologically, hepatocellular carcinoma is made up of cords or sheets of cells that roughly resemble the hepatic parenchyma. Blood vessels such as portal or hepatic veins are commonly involved by tumor.

The presence of a hepatocellular carcinoma may be unsuspected until there is deterioration in the condition of a cirrhotic patient who was formerly stable. Cachexia, weakness, and weight loss are associated symptoms. The sudden appearance of ascites, which may be bloody, suggests portal or hepatic vein thrombosis by tumor or bleeding from the necrotic tumor.

Physical examination may show tender enlargement of the liver, with an occasionally palpable mass. In Africa, young patients typically present with a rapidly expanding abdominal mass. Auscultation may reveal a bruit over the tumor or a friction rub when the process has extended to the surface of the liver.

Laboratory tests may reveal leukocytosis, as opposed to the leukopenia that is frequently encountered in cirrhotic patients. Anemia is common, but a normal or elevated hematocrit may be found in up to one-third of patients owing to elaboration of erythropoietin by the tumor. Sudden and sustained elevation of the serum alkaline phosphatase in a patient who was formerly stable is a common finding. Hepatitis B surface antigen is present in a majority of cases in endemic areas, whereas in the United States anti-HCV is found in up to 40% of cases. Alpha-fetoprotein levels are elevated in up to 70% of patients with hepatocellular carcinoma in Western countries; however, mild elevations are also often seen in patients with chronic hepatitis. Serum levels of des-gamma-carboxy prothrombin are elevated in up to 90% of patients with hepatocellular carcinoma, but they may also be elevated in patients with vitamin K deficiency, chronic hepatitis, and metastatic cancer. Cytologic study of ascitic fluid rarely reveals malignant cells.

Arterial phase helical CT scanning with and without intravenous contrast or MRI are the preferred imaging studies to characterize the location and vascularity of the tumor. Ultrasound is less sensitive but is used to screen for hepatic nodules in high-risk patients. Contrast-enhanced ultrasound has a sensitivity and specificity approaching those of arterial phase helical CT. Liver biopsy is diagnostic, though seeding of the needle tract by tumor is a potential risk (≤ 5%), and biopsy can be deferred if surgical resection is planned. Staging in the TNM classification includes the following definitions: T0: no evidence of primary tumor; T1: solitary tumor ≤ 2.0 cm; T2: solitary tumor ≤ 2.0 cm with vascular invasion or > 2.0 cm without vascular invasion or ≤ 2.0 cm and multiple in one lobe; T3: solitary tumor > 2.0 cm with vascular invasion or ≤ 2.0 cm and multiple in one lobe with vascular invasion or multiple in one lobe with any > 2.0 cm with or without vascular invasion; and T4: multiple tumors in more than one lobe or involving a major branch of the portal or hepatic veins. Staging systems are under study that also incorporate liver function, tumor aggressiveness and growth rate, general health of the patient, and treatment.

In the USA, overall 1- and 5-year survival rates for patients with hepatocellular carcinoma are 23% and 5%, respectively. Attempts at surgical resection are usually fruitless if concomitant cirrhosis is present and if the tumor is multifocal. Surgical resection of solitary hepatocellular carcinomas may result in cure if liver function is preserved (Child class A or possibly B). Five-year survival rates rise to 56% for patients with localized resectable disease (T1, T2, T3, selected T4; N0; M0) but are virtually nil for those with localized unresectable or advanced disease. Preliminary studies suggest that adaptive immunotherapy and treatment of underlying chronic viral hepatitis may lower postsurgical recurrence rates. Liver transplantation may be appropriate for small unresectable tumors in a patient with advanced cirrhosis, with reported 5-year survival rates of up to 75%. Liver transplantation may achieve a better recurrence-free survival than resection in patients with well-compensated cirrhosis and small tumors (one tumor < 5 cm or three or fewer tumors each < 3 cm in diameter) but is often impractical because of the donor organ shortage. Chemotherapy has not been shown to prolong life, but chemoembolization via the hepatic artery may be palliative. Injection of absolute ethanol into, radiofrequency ablation of, or cryotherapy of small tumors (< 3 cm) may prolong survival, and these are reasonable alternatives to surgical resection in some patients. For patients whose disease progresses despite treatment, meticulous efforts at palliative care are essential (see Chapter 5). Such patients may develop severe pain due to expansion of the liver capsule by the tumor and require concerted efforts at pain management, including the use of opioids (see Chapter 1).

In the patient with chronic hepatitis B or cirrhosis caused by HCV or alcohol, surveillance for the development of hepatocellular carcinoma should be considered with regular (eg, every 6 months) alpha-fetoprotein testing and ultrasonography. The risk of hepatocellular carcinoma in a patient with cirrhosis is 3–5% a year.

2. Benign Liver Neoplasms

Two distinct benign entities with characteristic clinical, radiologic, and histopathologic features have been described in women taking oral contraceptives. **Focal nodular hyperplasia** occurs at all ages but is probably not caused by oral contraceptives. It is often asymptomatic and appears as a hypervascular mass, occasionally with a central hypodense "stellate" scar on CT scan or MRI. Microscopically, focal nodular hyperplasia consists of hyperplastic units of hepatocytes with a central stellate scar containing proliferating bile ducts.

It is not a true neoplasm but a nonspecific reaction to vascular abnormalities. **Liver cell adenoma** occurs most commonly in the third and fourth decades of life and is usually caused by oral contraceptives; the clinical presentation is often one of acute abdominal pain due to necrosis of the tumor with hemorrhage. The tumor is hypovascular and reveals a cold defect on liver scan. Grossly, the cut surface appears structureless. As seen microscopically, the liver cell adenoma consists of sheets of hepatocytes without portal tracts or central veins. The only physical finding in focal nodular hyperplasia or liver cell adenoma is a palpable abdominal mass in a minority of cases. Liver function is usually normal. Arterial phase helical CT and MRI can distinguish an adenoma from focal nodular hyperplasia in 80–90% of cases.

Treatment of focal nodular hyperplasia is resection only in the symptomatic patient. The prognosis is excellent. Liver cell adenoma often undergoes necrosis and rupture, and resection is advised even in asymptomatic persons. In selected cases, laparoscopic resection may be feasible. Regression of benign hepatic tumors may follow cessation of oral contraceptives.

The most common benign neoplasm of the liver is the **cavernous hemangioma,** often an incidental finding on ultrasound or CT scan. This lesion must be differentiated from other space-occupying intrahepatic lesions, usually by MRI. Rarely, fine-needle biopsy is necessary to differentiate these lesions and does not appear to carry an increased risk of bleeding. Cavernous hemangiomas rarely require treatment.

Bioulac-Sage P et al: Diagnosis of focal nodular hyperplasia: not so easy. Am J. Surg Pathol 2001;25:1322. [PMID: 11688469] (Pitfalls in diagnosis.)

Bruix J et al: Clinical management of hepatocellular carcinoma. Conclusions of the Barcelona-2000 EASL Conference. European Association for the Study of the Liver. J Hepatol 2001;35:421. [PMID: 11592607] (Incidence and risk factors, surveillance, diagnosis and staging, prognosis, and treatment.)

DiBisceglie AM (guest editor): Liver tumors. Clin Liver Dis 2001;5:1. (Entire issue devoted to all aspects of benign and malignant liver tumors.)

Hussain SA et al: Hepatocellular carcinoma. Ann Oncol 2001; 12:161. [PMID: 11300318] (Epidemiology, causes, pathology, clinical features, tumor markers, prevention, and treatment.)

Llovet J et al: Increased risk of tumor seeding after percutaneous radiofrequency ablation for single hepatocellular carcinoma. Hepatology 2001;33:1124. [PMID: 11343240] (A cautionary study showing that radiofrequency ablation with a cooled- tip needle was associated with a 12.5% risk of neoplastic seeding of the needle track; risk factors included subcapsular tumor location and poorly differentiated tumor.)

McMahon BJ et al: Screening for hepatocellular carcinoma in Alaska natives infected with chronic hepatitis B: A 16-year population-based study. Hepatology 2000;32:842. [PMID: 11003632] (Screening of HBV carriers with serum alpha-fetoprotein every 6 months led to detection of most tumors at a resectable stage and prolonged survival rates when compared with historical controls.)

■ DISEASES OF THE BILIARY TRACT

CHOLELITHIASIS (Gallstones)

Gallstones are more common in women than in men and increase in incidence in both sexes and all races with aging. In the USA, over 10% of men and 20% of women have gallstones by age 65; the total exceeds 20 million people. Although cholesterol gallstones are less common in black people, cholelithiasis attributable to hemolysis occurs in over a third of individuals with sickle cell anemia. Native Americans of both the Northern and Southern Hemispheres have a high rate of cholesterol cholelithiasis, probably because of a genetic predisposition. As many as 75% of Pima women over the age of 25 years have cholelithiasis. Obesity is a risk factor for gallstones, especially in women. Rapid weight loss also increases the risk of symptomatic gallstone formation. There is evidence that glucose intolerance and elevated serum insulin levels (insulin resistance syndrome) are risk factors for gallstones. A low-carbohydrate diet and physical activity may help prevent gallstones. The incidence of gallstones is high in individuals with Crohn's disease; approximately one-third of individuals with inflammatory involvement of the terminal ileum have gallstones due to disruption of bile salt resorption that results in decreased solubility of the bile. The incidence of cholelithiasis is also increased in patients with diabetes mellitus and in those with cirrhosis. Drugs such as clofibrate, octreotide, and ceftriaxone can cause gallstones. In contrast, aspirin and other nonsteroidal anti-inflammatory drugs may protect against gallstones. Prolonged fasting (over 5–10 days) can lead to formation of biliary "sludge" (microlithiasis), which usually resolves with refeeding but can lead to gallstones or biliary symptoms. Pregnancy is associated with an increased risk of gallstones and of symptomatic gallbladder disease. Hormone replacement therapy appears to have only a slight risk for biliary tract surgery.

Pathogenesis of Gallstones

Gallstones are classified according to their predominant chemical composition as cholesterol or calcium bilirubinate stones. The latter comprise less than 20% of the stones found in Europe or the USA but 30–40% of stones found in Japan.

Three compounds comprise 80–95% of the total solids dissolved in bile: conjugated bile salts, lecithin, and cholesterol. Cholesterol is a neutral sterol, and lecithin is a phospholipid; both are almost completely insoluble in water. However, bile salts in combination with lecithin are able to form multimolecular aggregates (and micelles) or vesicles that solubilize cholesterol in an aqueous solution. Precipitation of cholesterol micro-crystals may come about because of increased biliary secretion of cholesterol, defective formation of vesicles, an excess of factors promoting the nucleation of cholesterol crystals (or deficiency of antinucleating factors), or delayed emptying of the gallbladder.

Presentation (Table 15–6)

Cholelithiasis is frequently asymptomatic and is discovered in the course of routine radiographic study, operation, or autopsy. There is generally no need for prophylactic cholecystectomy in an asymptomatic person unless the gallbladder is calcified or gallstones are over 3 cm in diameter. Ultimately, symptoms (biliary colic) develop in 10–25% of patients by 10 years. "Symptomatic" cholelithiasis usually means characteristic right upper quadrant or epigastric discomfort or pain (biliary colic). Occasional patients present with small intestinal obstruction due to "gallstone ileus" as the initial manifestation of cholelithiasis.

Treatment

Laparoscopic cholecystectomy is the treatment of choice for symptomatic gallbladder disease. The mini-mal trauma to the abdominal wall makes it possible for patients to go home within 2 days after the procedure and to return to work within 7 days (instead of weeks for those undergoing standard open cholecystectomy). In selected cases, the procedure may even be performed on an outpatient basis. This procedure is suitable in most patients, including those with acute cholecystitis. If problems are encountered, the surgery can be converted to a conventional open cholecystectomy. Bile duct injuries occur in 0.1% of cases done by experienced surgeons. Emerging data suggest that cholecystectomy may increase the risk of esophageal and proximal small intestinal adenocarcinoma because of increased duodenogastric reflux and changes in intestinal exposure to bile, respectively. A conservative approach to biliary colic is advised in pregnant patients, but for patients with repeated attacks of biliary colic or acute cholecystitis, cholecystectomy can be performed—even by the laparoscopic route—preferably in the second trimester. Enterolithotomy alone is considered adequate treatment in most patients with gallstone ileus.

Persistence of symptoms after removal of the gallbladder (postcholecystectomy syndrome) implies either mistaken diagnosis, functional bowel disorder, technical error, retained or recurrent common bile duct stone, or spasm of the sphincter of Oddi (see below).

Table 15–6. Diseases of the biliary tract.

	Clinical Features	Laboratory Features	Diagnosis	Treatment
Gallstones	Asymptomatic	Normal	Ultrasound	None
Gallstones	Biliary colic	Normal	Ultrasound	Laparoscopic cholecystectomy
Cholesterolosis of gallbladder	Usually asymptomatic	Normal	Oral cholecystography	None
Adenomyomatosis	May cause biliary colic	Normal	Oral cholecystography	Laparoscopic cholecystectomy if symptomatic
Porcelain gallbladder	Usually asymptomatic, high risk of gallbladder cancer	Normal	X-ray or CT	Laparoscopic cholecystectomy
Acute cholecystitis	Epigastric or right upper quadrant pain, nausea, vomiting, fever, Murphy's sign	Leukocytosis	Ultrasound, HIDA scan	Antibiotics, laparoscopic cholecystectomy
Chronic cholecystitis	Biliary colic, constant epigastric or right upper quadrant pain, nausea	Normal	Ultrasound (stones), oral cholecystography (nonfunctioning gallbladder)	Laparoscopic cholecystectomy
Choledocholithiasis	Asymptomatic or biliary colic, jaundice, fever; gallstone pancreatitis	Cholestatic liver function tests; leukocytosis and positive blood cultures in cholangitis; elevated amylase and lipase in pancreatitis	Ultrasound (dilated ducts), ERCP	Endoscopic sphincterotomy and stone extraction; antibiotics for cholangitis

ERCP = endoscopic retrograde cholangiopancreatography; HIDA = hepatic iminodiacetic acid.

Cheno- and ursodeoxycholic acids are bile salts that when given orally for up to 2 years dissolve some cholesterol stones and may be considered in selected patients who refuse cholecystectomy. The dose is 7 mg/kg/d of each or 8–13 mg/kg of ursodeoxycholic acid in divided doses daily. They are most effective in patients with a functioning gallbladder, as determined by gallbladder visualization on oral cholecystography, and multiple small "floating" gallstones (representing not more than 15% of patients with gallstones). In half of patients, gallstones recur within 5 years after treatment is stopped.

Lithotripsy in combination with bile salt therapy for single radiolucent stones less than 20 mm in diameter was an option in the past but is no longer generally employed in the USA.

Acalovschi M: Cholesterol gallstones: from epidemiology to prevention. Postgrad Med J 2001;77:221. [PMID: 11264482]

Freedman J et al: Association between cholecystectomy and adenocarcinoma of the esophagus. Gastroenterology 2001;121:548. [PMID: 11522738] (A population-based retrospective cohort study in Sweden suggesting that the risk of adenocarcinoma of the esophagus is increased (standardized incidence ratio 1.3, confidence interval 1.0–1.8) after cholecystectomy, presumably because of increased duodenogastric reflux.)

Johnson CD: ABC of the upper gastrointestinal tract. Upper abdominal pain: Gall bladder. BMJ 2001;323:1170. [PMID: 11711412] (Epidemiology, pathogenesis, symptoms, diagnosis, and management.)

Lagergren J et al: Intestinal cancer after cholecystectomy: Is bile involved in carcinogenesis? Gastroenterology 2001;121:542. [PMID: 11522737] (Another population-based retrospective cohort study in Sweden suggesting that the risk of adenocarcinoma of the proximal small bowel—and, to a lesser extent, the proximal colon—is increased after cholecystectomy.)

Ruhl CE et al: Association of diabetes, serum insulin, and C-peptide with gallbladder disease. Hepatology 2000;31:299. [PMID: 10655249] (In women without overt diabetes, serum insulin and C-peptide levels were independent risk factors for gallstone formation.)

Simon JA et al: Effect of estrogen plus progestin on risk for biliary tract surgery in postmenopausal women with coronary artery disease: The Heart and Estrogen/Progestin Replacement Study. Ann Intern Med 2001;135:493. [PMID: 11578152] (In this randomized, double-blind, placebo-controlled trial involving 2253 postmenopausal women, hormone replacement therapy resulted in a marginally significant 38% increase in the relative risk for biliary tract surgery (*P* = .05); the association became insignificant after adjustment for statin use.)

ACUTE CHOLECYSTITIS

ESSENTIALS OF DIAGNOSIS

- *Steady, severe pain and tenderness in the right hypochondrium or epigastrium.*
- *Nausea and vomiting.*
- *Fever and leukocytosis.*

General Considerations

Cholecystitis is associated with gallstones in over 90% of cases. It occurs when a stone becomes impacted in the cystic duct and inflammation develops behind the obstruction. Acalculous cholecystitis should be considered when unexplained fever or right upper quadrant pain occurs within 2–4 weeks of major surgery or in a critically ill patient who has had no oral intake for a prolonged period. Primarily as a result of ischemic changes secondary to distention, gangrene may develop, resulting in perforation. Although generalized peritonitis is possible, the leak usually remains localized and forms a chronic, well-circumscribed abscess cavity. Acute cholecystitis caused by infectious agents (eg, cytomegalovirus, cryptosporidiosis, or microsporidiosis) may occur in patients with AIDS.

Clinical Findings

A. SYMPTOMS AND SIGNS

The acute attack is often precipitated by a large or fatty meal and is characterized by the relatively sudden appearance of severe, steady pain which is localized to the epigastrium or right hypochondrium and which may gradually subside over a period of 12–18 hours. Vomiting occurs in about 75% of patients and in half of instances affords variable relief. Right upper quadrant abdominal tenderness is almost always present and is usually associated with muscle guarding and rebound pain. A palpable gallbladder is present in about 15% of cases. Jaundice is present in about 25% of cases and, when persistent or severe, suggests the possibility of choledocholithiasis. Jaundice also may result from compression of the common bile or hepatic duct by a cystic duct that is inflamed because of an impacted stone (Mirizzi's syndrome). Fever is usually present.

B. LABORATORY FINDINGS

The white blood cell count is usually high (12,000–15,000/μL). Total serum bilirubin values of 1–4 mg/dL may be seen even in the absence of common duct obstruction. Serum aminotransferase and alkaline phosphatase are often elevated—the former as high as 300 units/mL, or even higher when associated with ascending cholangitis. Serum amylase may also be moderately elevated.

C. IMAGING

Plain films of the abdomen may show radiopaque gallstones in 15% of cases. ^{99m}Tc hepatobiliary imaging (using iminodiacetic acid compounds), also known as the HIDA scan, is useful in demonstrating an obstructed cystic duct, which is the cause of acute cholecystitis in most patients. This test is reliable if the bilirubin is under 5 mg/dL (98% sensitivity and 81% specificity for acute cholecystitis). Right upper quadrant abdominal ultrasound may show the presence of gallstones but is not sensitive for acute cholecystitis (67% sensitivity, 82% specificity).

Differential Diagnosis

The disorders most likely to be confused with acute cholecystitis are perforated peptic ulcer, acute pancreatitis, appendicitis in a high-lying appendix, perforated colonic carcinoma or diverticulum of the hepatic flexure, liver abscess, hepatitis, and pneumonia with pleurisy on the right side. Definite localization of pain and tenderness in the right hypochondrium, with radiation around to the infrascapular area, strongly favors the diagnosis of acute cholecystitis. True cholecystitis without stones suggests the rare possibility of polyarteritis nodosa affecting the cystic artery.

Complications

A. Gangrene of the Gallbladder

Continuation or progression of right upper quadrant abdominal pain, tenderness, muscle guarding, fever, and leukocytosis after 24–48 hours suggests severe inflammation and possible gangrene of the gallbladder. Necrosis may occasionally develop without definite signs in the obese, diabetic, elderly, or immunosuppressed patient.

B. Cholangitis

Cholangitis classically presents with Charcot's triad, namely, fever and chills, right upper quadrant pain, and jaundice. Although 95% of patients who present with this picture will have common duct stones, only a minority of patients with acute cholecystitis have common duct stones that will present in this manner.

C. Chronic Cholecystitis and Other Complications

Chronic cholecystitis results from repeated episodes of acute cholecystitis or chronic irritation of the gallbladder wall by stones and is characterized pathologically by varying degrees of chronic inflammation of the gallbladder. Calculi are usually present. In about 4–5% of cases, the villi of the gallbladder undergo polypoid enlargement due to deposition of cholesterol that may be visible to the naked eye ("strawberry gallbladder," cholesterolosis). In other instances, adenomatous hyperplasia of all or part of the gallbladder wall may be so marked as to give the appearance of a myoma (pseudotumor). Hydrops of the gallbladder results when acute cholecystitis subsides but cystic duct obstruction persists, producing distention of the gallbladder with a clear mucoid fluid. Occasionally, a stone in the neck of the gallbladder may compress the bile duct and cause jaundice (Mirizzi's syndrome). Xanthogranulomatous cholecystitis is a rare variant of chronic cholecystitis characterized by grayish-yellow nodules or streaks, representing lipid-laden macrophages, in the wall of the gallbladder.

Cholelithiasis with chronic cholecystitis may be associated with acute exacerbations of gallbladder inflammation, common duct stone, fistulization to the bowel, pancreatitis, and, rarely, carcinoma of the gallbladder. Calcified (porcelain) gallbladder has generally been thought to have a high association with gallbladder carcinoma and to be an indication for cholecystectomy, though the risk of gallbladder cancer may be higher when calcification is mucosal rather than intramural.

Treatment

Acute cholecystitis will usually subside on a conservative regimen (withholding of oral feedings, intravenous alimentation, analgesics, and antibiotics). Meperidine may be preferable to morphine for pain because of less spasm of the sphincter of Oddi. Because of the high risk of recurrent attacks (up to 10% by 1 month and over 30% by 1 year), cholecystectomy—generally laparoscopically—should generally be performed within 2–3 days after hospitalization. If nonsurgical treatment has been elected, the patient (especially if diabetic or elderly) should be watched carefully for recurrent symptoms, evidence of gangrene of the gallbladder, or cholangitis. In high-risk patients, ultrasound-guided aspiration of the gallbladder or percutaneous cholecystostomy may postpone or even avoid the need for surgery. Cholecystectomy is mandatory when there is evidence of gangrene or perforation.

Surgical treatment of chronic cholecystitis is the same as for acute cholecystitis. If indicated, cholangiography can be performed during laparoscopic cholecystectomy. Choledocholithiasis can also be excluded by either pre- or postoperative ERCP or MRCP.

Prognosis

The overall mortality rate of cholecystectomy is less than 1%, but hepatobiliary tract surgery is a more formidable procedure in the elderly, in whom the mortality rate is 5–10%. A technically successful surgical procedure in an appropriately selected patient is generally followed by complete resolution of symptoms.

Chatziioannou SN et al: Hepatobiliary scintigraphy is superior to abdominal ultrasonography in suspected acute cholecystitis. Surgery 2000;127:609. [PMID: 10840354] (The accuracy rate of scintigraphy was 92% compared with 61% for ultrasonography.)

Chen PF et al: The clinical diagnosis of chronic acalculous cholecystitis. Surgery 2001;130:578. [PMID: 11602887] (Description of a group of patients with typical biliary colic, absence of stones or other gallbladder abnormalities on ultrasound, absence of other structural abnormalities of the gastrointestinal tract, a low gallbladder ejection fraction on cholecystokinin-stimulated HIDA scan, the finding of chronic cholecystitis on histologic examination of the gallbladder, and lasting symptomatic relief after laparoscopic cholecystectomy.)

McMahon AJ et al: Impact of laparoscopic cholecystectomy: a population-based study. Lancet 2000;356:1632. [PMID: 11089821] (In Scottish public hospitals, the introduction of laparoscopic cholecystectomy increased cholecystectomy rates and reduced hospital stay but had no effect on postoperative mortality.)

PRE- & POSTCHOLECYSTECTOMY SYNDROMES

Precholecystectomy

In a small group of patients (mostly women) with biliary colic, conventional radiographic studies of the upper gastrointestinal tract and gallbladder—including cholangiography—are unremarkable. However, emptying of the gallbladder is markedly reduced on gallbladder scintigraphy following injection of cholecystokinin. Cholecystectomy is curative. Anatomic and histologic examination of the operative specimen may reveal obstruction of the cystic duct because of fibrotic stenosis or adhesions and kinking. Additional diagnostic considerations are ampullary spasm and biliary dyskinesia (see below).

Postcholecystectomy

Following cholecystectomy, some patients complain of continuing symptoms, ie, right upper quadrant pain, flatulence, and fatty food intolerance. The persistence of symptoms in this group of patients suggests the possibility of an incorrect diagnosis prior to cholecystectomy, eg, esophagitis, pancreatitis, radiculopathy, or functional bowel disease. It is important to rule out the possibility of choledocholithiasis or common duct stricture as a cause of persistent symptoms in the postoperative period.

Pain has been associated with dilation of the cystic duct remnant, neuroma formation in the ductal wall, foreign body granuloma, or traction on the common duct by a long cystic duct. The clinical presentation of colicky pain, chills, fever, or jaundice should suggest biliary tract disease. Biliary colic associated with elevated liver tests or amylase suggests the possibility of spasm or stenosis of the sphincter of Oddi. Abdominal or endoscopic ultrasonography or retrograde cholangiography may be necessary to demonstrate or exclude biliary tract disease. Biliary manometry may be useful in documenting elevated baseline sphincter of Oddi pressures typical of sphincter dysfunction. Biliary scintigraphy shows promise as a screening test for sphincter dysfunction. In some such cases, treatment with calcium channel blockers, long-acting nitrates, or possibly injection of the sphincter with botulinum toxin may be beneficial. Endoscopic sphincterotomy is most likely to relieve symptoms when they are associated with elevated liver chemistry tests, a dilated common duct, or an elevated sphincter of Oddi pressure. In some cases, surgical sphincteroplasty or removal of the cystic duct remnant may be necessary.

Amaral J et al: Gallbladder muscle dysfunction in patients with chronic acalculous disease. Gastroenterology 2001;120:506. [PMID: 11159891] (Describes a group of patients with recurrent biliary colic, no stones in the gallbladder by ultrasound, impaired gallbladder contraction in response to intravenous cholecystokinin, impaired gallbladder muscle cell contraction in vitro in response to cholecystokinin, and resolution of symptoms after cholecystectomy.)

Toouli J et al: Sphincter of Oddi function and dysfunction. Can J Gastroenterol 2000;14:411. [PMID: 10851282] (Reviews the physiology of the sphincter of Oddi, the clinical syndromes associated with sphincter dysfunction, diagnosis, and treatment.)

CHOLEDOCHOLITHIASIS & CHOLANGITIS

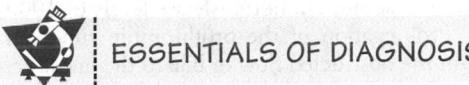

ESSENTIALS OF DIAGNOSIS

- *Often a history of biliary colic or jaundice.*
- *Sudden onset of severe right upper quadrant or epigastric pain, which may radiate to the right scapula or shoulder.*
- *Occasional patients present with painless jaundice.*
- *Nausea and vomiting.*
- *Fever, which may be followed by hypothermia and gram-negative shock, jaundice, and leukocytosis.*
- *Abdominal films may reveal gallstones.*

General Considerations

About 15% of patients with gallstones have choledocholithiasis (common bile duct stones). The percentage rises with age, and the frequency in elderly people with gallstones may be as high as 50%. Common duct stones usually originate in the gallbladder but may also form spontaneously in the common duct after cholecystectomy. The stones are frequently "silent" as no symptoms result unless there is obstruction.

Clinical Findings

A. SYMPTOMS AND SIGNS

A history suggestive of biliary colic or prior jaundice may be obtained. Biliary colic results from rapid increases in common bile duct pressure due to obstructed bile flow. The additional features that suggest the presence of a common duct stone are (1) frequently recurring attacks of right upper abdominal pain that is severe and persists for hours; (2) chills and fever associated with severe colic; and (3) a history of jaundice associated with episodes of abdominal pain. The combination of pain, fever (and chills), and jaundice represents **Charcot's triad** and denotes the classic picture of cholangitis. The presence of altered sensorium, lethargy, and septic shock connotes acute suppurative cholangitis and represents an endoscopic or surgical emergency.

Hepatomegaly may be present in calculous biliary obstruction, and tenderness is usually present in the right upper quadrant and epigastrium.

B. Laboratory Findings

Bilirubinuria and elevation of serum bilirubin are present if the common duct is obstructed; levels commonly fluctuate. Serum alkaline phosphatase elevation is especially suggestive of obstructive jaundice. Not uncommonly, serum amylase elevations are present because of secondary pancreatitis. On occasion, acute obstruction of the bile duct produces a transient striking increase in serum aminotransferase levels (> 1000 units/L). Prolongation of the prothrombin time can result from the obstructed flow of bile to the intestine. When extrahepatic obstruction persists for more than a few weeks, differentiation of obstruction from chronic cholestatic liver disease becomes progressively more difficult.

C. Imaging

Ultrasonography, CT scan, and radionuclide imaging may demonstrate dilated bile ducts and impaired bile flow. Endoscopic ultrasonography, helical CT, and MR cholangiography have been found to be accurate in demonstrating common duct stones and, if available, may be used in patients thought to be at low or intermediate risk for choledocholithiasis. Endoscopic retrograde cholangiopancreatography (ERCP) or percutaneous transhepatic cholangiography provides the most direct and accurate means of determining the cause, location, and extent of obstruction. If the likelihood that obstruction is caused by a stone is high, ERCP is the procedure of choice because it permits papillotomy or balloon dilation of the papilla with stone extraction or stent placement.

Differential Diagnosis

The most common cause of obstructive jaundice is common duct stone. Next in frequency is carcinoma of the pancreas, ampulla of Vater, or common duct. Extrinsic compression of the common duct may result from metastatic carcinoma (usually from the gastrointestinal tract or breast) involving porta hepatis lymph nodes or, rarely, from a large duodenal diverticulum. Gallbladder cancer extending into the common duct often presents as obstructive jaundice. Chronic cholestatic liver diseases (primarily biliary cirrhosis, sclerosing cholangitis, drug-induced) must be considered. Hepatocellular jaundice can usually be differentiated by the history, clinical findings, and liver tests, but liver biopsy is necessary on occasion. Recurrent pyogenic cholangitis should be considered in persons from Asia (and occasionally elsewhere), persons with intrahepatic biliary stones (particularly in the left ductal system), and those with recurrent cholangitis.

Complications

A. Biliary Cirrhosis

Common duct obstruction lasting longer than 30 days results in liver damage leading to cirrhosis. Hepatic failure with portal hypertension occurs in untreated cases.

B. Hypoprothrombinemia

Patients with obstructive jaundice or liver disease may bleed excessively as a result of prolonged prothrombin times. In contrast to hepatocellular dysfunction, hypoprothrombinemia due to obstructive jaundice will respond to 10 mg of parenteral vitamin K or water-soluble oral vitamin K (phytonadione, 5 mg) within 24–36 hours.

Treatment

Common duct stone in a patient with cholelithiasis and cholecystitis is usually treated by endoscopic papillotomy and stone extraction followed by laparoscopic cholecystectomy. For the poor-risk patient, however, cholecystectomy may be deferred because the risk of subsequent cholecystitis is low. ERCP should be performed before cholecystectomy in patients with gallstones and jaundice (serum total bilirubin > 2 mg/dL), a dilated common bile duct (> 7 mm), or stones in the bile duct seen on ultrasound or computed tomography. When biliary pancreatitis resolves rapidly, the stone usually passes into the intestine, and ERCP prior to cholecystectomy is not necessary if an intraoperative cholangiogram is done.

Choledocholithiasis discovered at laparoscopic cholecystectomy may be managed via laparoscopic removal or, if necessary, conversion to open surgery or by postoperative endoscopic sphincterotomy. In the postcholecystectomy patient with choledocholithiasis, endoscopic papillotomy with stone extraction is preferable to transabdominal surgery. Lithotripsy (endoscopic or external) or biliary stenting may be a therapeutic consideration for large stones. For the patient with a T tube and common duct stone, the stone may be extracted via the T tube (see below).

Urgent ERCP, sphincterotomy, and stone extraction are generally indicated for choledocholithiasis complicated by ascending cholangitis. Before ERCP, liver function should be evaluated thoroughly. Prothrombin time should be restored to normal by parenteral administration of vitamin K (see above). Nutrition should be restored by a high-carbohydrate, high-protein diet and vitamin supplementation. Ciprofloxacin, 250 mg intravenously every 12 hours, penetrates well into bile and is effective treatment for cholangitis. An alternative regimen in severely ill patients is mezlocillin, 3 g intravenously every 4 hours, plus either metronidazole or gentamicin (or both). The dose of metronidazole is 500 mg intravenously every 6 hours (if there has been no prior manipulation of the duct); the dose of gentamicin is 2 mg/kg intravenously as loading dose, plus 1.5 mg/kg every 8 hours adjusted for renal function. Aminoglycosides should not be given for more than a few days because the risk of aminoglycoside nephrotoxicity is increased in patients with cholestasis. Emergent decompression of the bile duct, generally by ERCP, is required for patients who are septic or fail to improve on antibiotics within 12–24 hours.

At cholecystectomy, operative cholangiography via the cystic duct should be considered. Operative findings of choledocholithiasis are palpable stones in the common duct, dilation or thickening of the wall of the common duct, and gallbladder stones small enough to pass through the cystic duct. If stones in the common duct are found, common duct exploration can be performed or a postoperative ERCP and sphincterotomy can be planned.

Following operative choledochostomy, a simple catheter or T tube is placed in the common duct for decompression. A properly placed tube should drain bile at the operating table and continuously thereafter; otherwise, it should be considered blocked or dislocated. The volume of bile drainage varies from 100 to 1000 mL daily (average, 200–400 mL). Above-average drainage may be due to obstruction at the ampulla (usually by edema).

Postoperative antibiotics are not administered routinely after biliary tract surgery. Cultures of the bile are always taken at operation. If biliary tract infection was present preoperatively or is apparent at operation, ampicillin (500 mg every 6 hours intravenously) with gentamicin (1.5 mg/kg every 8 hours) and metronidazole (500 mg every 6 hours) or ciprofloxacin (250 mg intravenously every 12 hours) or a third-generation cephalosporin (eg, cefoperazone, 1–2 g intravenous every 12 hours) is administered postoperatively until the results of sensitivity tests on culture specimens are available.

A T-tube cholangiogram should be done before the tube is removed, usually about 3 weeks after surgery. A small amount of bile frequently leaks from the tube site for a few days.

Binmoelle KF et al: Endoscopic management of bile duct stones. J. Clin Gastroenterol 2001;32.106. [PMID: 11205644] (Reviews the spectrum of techniques for stone removal and approaches to the management of choledocholithiasis in relation to the timing of cholecystectomy.)

Chak A et al: Effectiveness of ERCP in cholangitis: a community-based study. Gastrointest Endosc 2000;52:484. [PMID: 11023564] (Compared with other interventions, ERCP performed within 24 hours of admission shortens the severity-adjusted length of stay in patients with cholangitis.)

Eisen GM et al: An annotated algorithm for the evaluation of choledocholithiasis. Gastrointest Endosc 2001;53:864. [PMID: 11375619] (Practice guidelines.)

Hui CK et al: Acute cholangitis—predictive factors for emergency ERCP. Aliment Pharmacol Ther 2001;15:1633. [PMID: 11564004] (Among 142 consecutive patients with acute cholangitis, medical therapy failed and ERCP was required in 31 [22%]; predictive factors for failure of medical therapy were heart rate > 100/min, serum albumin < 3 g/dL, bilirubin > 50 μmol/L, and PT > 14 s on admission.)

Kim DI et al: Risk factors for recurrence of primary bile duct stones after endoscopic biliary sphincterotomy. Gastrointest

Endosc 2001;54:42. [PMID: 11427840] (The overall recurrence rate was 21% after 2 years; recurrence was associated with persistent dilation of the bile duct and location of the papilla in a diverticulum. Lower rates of recurrence (< 10%) have been reported in other studies.)

BILIARY STRICTURE

Benign biliary strictures are the result of surgical anastomosis or injury in about 95% of cases. The remainder are caused by blunt external injury to the abdomen, pancreatitis, erosion of the duct by a gallstone, or prior endoscopic sphincterotomy.

Signs of injury to the duct may or may not be recognized in the immediate postoperative period. If complete occlusion has occurred, jaundice will develop rapidly; more often, however, a tear has been accidentally made in the duct, and the earliest manifestation of injury may be excessive or prolonged loss of bile from the surgical drains. Bile leakage may predispose to localized infection, which in turn accentuates scar formation and the ultimate development of a fibrous stricture.

Cholangitis is the most common complication of stricture. Typically, the patient experiences episodes of pain, fever, chills, and jaundice within a few weeks to months after cholecystectomy. Physical findings may include jaundice during an attack of cholangitis and right upper quadrant abdominal tenderness.

Serum alkaline phosphatase is usually elevated. Hyperbilirubinemia is variable, fluctuating during exacerbations and usually remaining in the range of 5–10 mg/dL. Blood cultures may be positive during an episode of cholangitis. Endoscopic retrograde cholangiopancreatography or percutaneous transhepatic cholangiography can be valuable in demonstrating the stricture, permitting biopsy and cytologic specimens, and allowing dilation and stent placement, thereby avoiding surgical repair in some cases. Placement of multiple plastic stents may be more effective than placement of a single stent. Metal stents, which cannot be removed endoscopically, are generally avoided in benign strictures.

Differentiation from cholangiocarcinoma may require surgical exploration. Significant hepatocellular disease due to secondary biliary cirrhosis will inevitably occur if a biliary stricture is not treated. Operative treatment of a stricture frequently necessitates performance of an end-to-end ductal repair, choledochojejunostomy, or hepaticojejunostomy to reestablish bile flow into the intestine.

Bergman JJ et al: Long-term follow-up after biliary stent placement for postoperative bile duct stenosis. Gastrointest Endosc 2001;54:154. [PMID: 11474383] (In 74 patients with a postoperative bile duct stricture, placement of two 10F for a maximum of 12 months with stent exchange every 3 months was feasible in 80% and led to long-term resolution of the stricture in 52%.)

Lillemoe KD et al: Postoperative bile duct strictures: Management and outcome in the 1990s. Ann Surg 2000; 232:430.

[PMID: 10973393] (A majority of strictures occur from laparoscopic cholecystectomy. Surgical repair at a referral center led to a successful outcome in over 90% of cases.)

PRIMARY SCLEROSING CHOLANGITIS

Primary sclerosing cholangitis is an uncommon disease characterized by a diffuse inflammation of the biliary tract leading to fibrosis and strictures of the biliary system. The disease is most common in men aged 20–40 and is closely associated with ulcerative colitis, which is present in approximately two-thirds of patients with primary sclerosing cholangitis; however, only 1–4% of patients with ulcerative colitis develop clinically significant sclerosing cholangitis. As in ulcerative colitis, smoking is associated with a decreased risk of primary sclerosing cholangitis. Primary sclerosing cholangitis is associated with the histocompatible antigens HLA-B8 and -DR3 or -DR4, suggesting that genetic factors may play an etiologic role. Antineutrophil cytoplasmic antibodies (ANCA), with fluorescent staining characteristics and target antigens distinct from those found in patients with Wegener's granulomatosis or vasculitis, are found in 70% of patients. In patients with AIDS, sclerosing cholangitis may result from infections caused by CMV, cryptosporidium, or microsporum.

Clinically, primary sclerosing cholangitis presents as progressive obstructive jaundice, frequently associated with malaise, pruritus, anorexia, and indigestion. Some patients are diagnosed in the presymptomatic phase because of an elevated alkaline phosphatase level.

The diagnosis of primary sclerosing cholangitis is generally made by endoscopic retrograde cholangiography; magnetic resonance cholangiography is also a useful diagnostic test. Biliary obstruction by a stone or tumor should be excluded. The disease may be confined to small intrahepatic bile ducts, in which case ERCP is normal and the diagnosis is suggested by liver biopsy. Liver biopsy is also needed for staging, which is based on the degree of inflammation and fibrosis. In addition to ANCA, patients may have serum antinuclear, anticardiolipin, and antithyroperoxidase antibodies and rheumatoid factor. Occasional patients have clinical and histologic features of both sclerosing cholangitis and autoimmune hepatitis. Even more rarely, an association with chronic pancreatitis (sclerosing pancreaticocholangitis) is seen, and this entity is often responsive to corticosteroids. In general, the diagnosis of primary sclerosing cholangitis is difficult to make after biliary surgery or intrahepatic artery chemotherapy, which may result in bile duct injury. Primary sclerosing cholangitis must be distinguished from idiopathic adulthood ductopenia, a rare disorder affecting young to middle-aged adults who manifest cholestasis resulting from loss of interlobular and septal bile ducts yet who have a normal cholangiogram.

Cholangiocarcinoma may complicate the course of primary sclerosing cholangitis in at least 10% of cases and may be difficult to diagnose by cytologic examination or biopsy because of false-negative results. A serum CA 19-9 level > 100 units/mL is suggestive but not diagnostic of cholangiocarcinoma.

Treatment with corticosteroids and broad-spectrum antimicrobial agents has been employed with inconsistent and unpredictable results. Episodes of acute bacterial cholangitis may be treated with ciprofloxacin. Ursodeoxycholic acid in standard doses (10–15 mg/kg/d) may improve liver function test results but does not appear to alter the natural history. However, recent experience suggests that high-dose ursodeoxycholic acid (20 mg/kg/d) may reduce cholangiographic progression and liver fibrosis. Careful endoscopic evaluation of the biliary tree may permit balloon dilation of localized strictures. If there is a major stricture, short-term placement of a stent may relieve symptoms and improve biochemical abnormalities with sustained improvement after the stent is removed. However, long-term stenting may increase the rate of complications such as cholangitis. In patients without cirrhosis, surgical resection of a dominant bile duct stricture may lead to longer survival than endoscopic therapy by decreasing the subsequent risk of cholangiocarcinoma. In patients with ulcerative colitis, primary sclerosing cholangitis is an independent risk factor for the development of colorectal dysplasia and cancer, and strict adherence to a colonoscopic surveillance program is advisable. For patients with cirrhosis and clinical decompensation, liver transplantation is the procedure of choice.

Survival of patients with primary sclerosing cholangitis averages 10 years once symptoms appear. Adverse prognostic markers are older age, higher serum bilirubin and aspartate aminotransferase levels, lower albumin levels, and a history of variceal bleeding. Actuarial survival rates with liver transplantation are as high as 85% at 3 years, but rates are much lower once cholangiocarcinoma has developed. Following transplantation, patients have an increased risk of nonanastomotic biliary strictures and—in those with ulcerative colitis—colon cancer. Those patients who are unable to undergo liver transplantation will ultimately require high-quality palliative care (see Chapter 5).

Baluyut AR et al: Impact of endoscopic therapy on the survival of patients with primary sclerosing cholangitis. Gastrointest Endosc 2001;53:308. [PMID: 11231388] (Repeated balloon dilation of dominant strictures was associated with a 5-year survival rate of 83% compared with a rate of 65% predicted by the Mayo Clinic model.)

Kaya M et al: Balloon dilation compared to stenting of dominant strictures in primary sclerosing cholangitis. Am J. Gastroenterol 2001;96:1059. [PMID: 11316147] (A nonrandomized review of 71 cases showing no difference in relief of cholestasis but a higher rate of complications such as cholangitis with long-term stenting.)

Kim WR et al: A revised natural history model for primary sclerosing cholangitis. Mayo Clin Proc 2000;75:688. [PMID: 10907383] (Updated version of a model for predicting survival based on age, serum bilirubin, serum albumin, serum aspartate aminotransferase, and history of variceal bleeding.)

Mitchell SA et al: A preliminary trial of high-dose ursodeoxycholic acid in primary sclerosing cholangitis. Gastroenterology 2001;121:900. [PMID: 11606503] (A 2-year double-blind, placebo-controlled study showing that ursodeoxycholic acid, 20 mg/kg/d, led to significant improvement in liver biochemistry and a reduction in cholangiographic progression and liver fibrosis.)

CARCINOMA OF THE BILIARY TRACT

Carcinoma of the gallbladder occurs in approximately 2% of all people operated on for biliary tract disease. It is notoriously insidious, and the diagnosis is often made unexpectedly at surgery. Cholelithiasis (often large, symptomatic stones) is usually present. Other risk factors are chronic infection of the gallbladder with *Salmonella typhi*, gallbladder polyps over 1 cm in diameter, calcification of the gallbladder (porcelain gallbladder), and anomalous pancreaticobiliary ductal junction. Spread of the cancer—by direct extension into the liver or to the peritoneal surface—may be the initial manifestation. The TNM classification includes the following stages: Tis, carcinoma in situ; T1, invasion of mucosa (T1a) or muscle layer (T1b); T2, invasion of perimuscular connective tissue; T3, extension into serosa or into an adjacent organ; T4: invasion > 2 cm into liver or two or more adjacent organs; N1: metastasis in cystic duct, pericholedochal, or hilar nodes; N2: metastasis in peripancreatic head, periduodenal, periportal, celiac, or superior mesenteric nodes.

Carcinoma of the bile ducts (cholangiocarcinoma) accounts for 3% of all cancer deaths in the USA, and the incidence and mortality rate have increased dramatically in the past 2 decades. It affects both sexes equally but is more prevalent in individuals aged 50–70. Two-thirds arise at the confluence of the hepatic ducts (Klatskin tumors), and one-fourth arise in the distal extrahepatic bile duct; the remainder are intrahepatic. Staging is similar to that for carcinoma of the gallbladder. The frequency of carcinoma in persons with choledochal cysts has been reported to be over 14% at 20 years, and surgical excision is recommended. There is an increased incidence in patients with ulcerative colitis, especially those with primary sclerosing cholangitis. In southeast Asia, infection of the bile ducts with helminths *(Clonorchis sinensis, Opisthorchis viverrini, Fasciola hepatica)* is associated with chronic cholangitis and an increased risk of cholangiocarcinoma.

Clinical Findings

Progressive jaundice is the most common and usually the first sign of obstruction of the extrahepatic biliary system. Pain in the right upper abdomen with radiation into the back is usually present early in the course of gallbladder carcinoma, but this occurs later in the course of bile duct carcinoma. Anorexia and weight loss are common and often associated with fever and chills due to cholangitis. Rarely, hematemesis or melena results from erosion of tumor into a blood vessel (hemobilia). Fistula formation between the biliary system and adjacent organs may also occur. The course is usually one of rapid deterioration, with death occurring within a few months.

Physical examination reveals profound jaundice. A palpable gallbladder with obstructive jaundice usually is said to signify malignant disease (Courvoisier's law); however, this clinical generalization has been proved to be accurate only about 50% of the time. Hepatomegaly is usually present and is associated with liver tenderness. Ascites may occur with peritoneal implants. Pruritus and skin excoriations are common.

Laboratory examination reveals predominantly conjugated hyperbilirubinemia, with total serum bilirubin values ranging from 5 to 30 mg/dL. There is usually concomitant elevation of the alkaline phosphatase and serum cholesterol. AST is normal or minimally elevated. An elevated CA 19-9 level may help distinguish cholangiocarcinoma from a benign biliary stricture (in the absence of cholangitis).

Ultrasonography and CT may show a gallbladder mass in gallbladder carcinoma and intrahepatic mass or biliary dilation in carcinoma of the bile ducts. CT may also show involved regional lymph nodes. MRI with MRCP permits visualization of the biliary tree and detection of vascular invasion and obviates the need for angiography. Preliminary observations suggest that positron emission tomography (PET) can detect cholangiocarcinomas as small as 1 cm. The most helpful diagnostic studies before surgery are either percutaneous transhepatic or endoscopic retrograde cholangiography with biopsy and cytologic specimens, though false-negative biopsy and cytology results are common. Fine-needle aspiration of tumors under endoscopic ultrasonographic guidance and choledochoscopy also have potential roles in the diagnosis of cholangiocarcinoma.

Treatment

In young and fit patients, curative surgery may be attempted if the tumor is well localized. The 5-year survival rate for localized carcinoma of the gallbladder (stage 1, T1a, N0, M0) is as high as 80% with laparoscopic cholecystectomy but drops to 15%, even with a more extended open resection, if there is muscular invasion (T1b). If the tumor is unresectable at laparotomy, cholecystoduodenostomy or T-tube drainage of the common duct can be performed. Carcinoma of the bile ducts is curable by surgery in less than 10% of cases. Palliation can be achieved by placement of a self-expandable metal stent via the endoscopic or percutaneous transhepatic route. Plastic stents are less expensive but more prone to occlude than metal ones; they are suitable for patients expected to survive only a few months. Preliminary experience supports a palliative role for photodynamic therapy. Radiotherapy may relieve pain and contribute to biliary decompression.

There is limited response to chemotherapy such as with gemcitabine. In general, the prognosis is poor, with few patients surviving for more than 12 months after surgery. Although cholangiocarcinoma is generally considered to be a contraindication to liver transplantation because of rapid tumor recurrence, a 62% 5-year survival rate has been reported in patients with a single peripheral cholangiocarcinoma undergoing either transplantation or resection, with clear resection margins and no lymph node involvement.

For those patients whose disease progresses despite treatment, meticulous efforts at palliative care are essential (see Chapter 5).

Jarnagin WR et al: Staging, resectability, and outcome in 225 patients with hilar cholangiocarcinoma. Ann Surg 2001;234: 507. [PMID: 11573044] (Predictors of long-term survival following surgical resection are well-differentiated tumor histology, negative histologic margins, and concomitant partial hepatectomy.)

Patel T: Increasing incidence and mortality of primary intrahepatic cholangio-carcinoma in the United States. Hepatology 2001;33:1353. [PMID: 11391522] (Over the past 2 decades, incidence and mortality rate rose an estimated 9% annually. One- and 2-year survival rates following diagnosis are only 25% and 13%, respectively.)

Stephen AE et al: Carcinoma in the porcelain gallbladder: A relationship revisited. Surgery 2001;129:699. [PMID: 11391368] (A retrospective review of 25,900 resected gallbladders showing that the frequency of carcinoma in association with gallbladder calcification was lower than previously reported—7% in mucosal calcification and nil in those with diffuse intramural calcification.)

■ DISEASES OF THE PANCREAS

ACUTE PANCREATITIS

ESSENTIALS OF DIAGNOSIS

- *Abrupt onset of deep epigastric pain, often with radiation to the back.*
- *Nausea, vomiting, sweating, weakness.*
- *Abdominal tenderness and distention, fever.*
- *Leukocytosis, elevated serum amylase, elevated serum lipase.*
- *History of previous episodes, often related to alcohol intake.*

General Considerations

Acute pancreatitis is thought to result from "escape" of activated pancreatic enzymes from acinar cells into surrounding tissues. Most cases are related to biliary tract disease (a passed gallstone, usually < 5 mm in diameter) or heavy alcohol intake. The exact pathogenesis is not known but may include edema or obstruction of the ampulla of Vater, resulting in reflux of bile into pancreatic ducts, or direct injury to the acinar cells. Among the numerous other causes or associations are hypercalcemia, hyperlipidemias (chylomicronemia, hypertriglyceridemia, or both), abdominal trauma (including surgery), drugs (including azathioprine, mercaptopurine, asparaginase, pentamidine, didanosine, valproic acid, tetracyclines, estrogen, sulfonamides, thiazides, and possibly glucocorticoids), vasculitis, viral infections (eg, mumps), peritoneal dialysis, cardiopulmonary bypass, and ERCP. In patients with pancreas divisum, a congenital anomaly in which the dorsal and ventral pancreatic ducts fail to fuse, acute pancreatitis may result from stenosis of the minor papilla with obstruction to flow from the accessory pancreatic duct. Rarely, acute pancreatitis may be the presenting manifestation of a pancreatic or ampullary neoplasm. Apparently "idiopathic" acute pancreatitis is often caused by occult biliary microlithiasis.

Pathologic changes vary from acute edema and cellular infiltration to necrosis of the acinar cells, hemorrhage from necrotic blood vessels, and intra- and extrapancreatic fat necrosis. All or part of the pancreas may be involved.

Clinical Findings

A. SYMPTOMS AND SIGNS

Epigastric abdominal pain, generally abrupt in onset, is steady, boring, and severe and often made worse by walking and lying supine and better by sitting and leaning forward. The pain usually radiates into the back but may radiate to the right or left. Nausea and vomiting are usually present. Weakness, sweating, and anxiety are noted in severe attacks. There may be a history of alcohol intake or a heavy meal immediately preceding the attack, or a history of milder similar episodes or biliary colic in the past.

The abdomen is tender mainly in the upper abdomen, most often without guarding, rigidity, or rebound. The abdomen may be distended, and bowel sounds may be absent with associated paralytic ileus. Fever of 38.4–39 °C, tachycardia, hypotension (even true shock), pallor, and cool clammy skin are often present. Mild jaundice is common. Occasionally, an upper abdominal mass due to the inflamed pancreas or a pseudocyst may be palpated. Acute renal failure (usually prerenal) may occur early in the course of acute pancreatitis.

B. ASSESSMENT OF SEVERITY

Ranson's criteria are generally used in assessing the severity of acute alcoholic pancreatitis on presentation (pancreatitis due to other causes is assessed by similar criteria). When three or more of the following are present on admission, a severe course complicated by pancreatic necrosis can be predicted with a sensitivity of 60–80%.

1. Age over 55 years.
2. White blood cell count over 16,000/µL.
3. Blood glucose over 200 mg/dL.
4. Serum LDH over 350 units/L.
5. AST over 250 units/L.

Development of the following in the first 48 hours indicates a worsening prognosis:

1. Hematocrit drop of more than ten percentage points.
2. BUN rise greater than 5 mg/dL.
3. Arterial PO_2 of less than 60 mm Hg.
4. Serum calcium of less than 8 mg/dL.
5. Base deficit over 4 meq/L.
6. Estimated fluid sequestration of more than 6 L.

Mortality rates correlate with the number of criteria present:

Number of Criteria	Mortality Rate
0–2	1%
3–4	16%
5–6	40%
7–8	100%

The Acute Physiology and Chronic Health (APACHE) II scoring system may also be used to assess severity.

C. LABORATORY FINDINGS

Leukocytosis (10,000–30,000/µL), proteinuria, granular casts, glycosuria (10–20% of cases), hyperglycemia, and elevated serum bilirubin may be present. Blood urea nitrogen and serum alkaline phosphatase may be elevated and coagulation tests abnormal. Decrease in serum calcium may reflect saponification and correlates well with severity of disease. Levels lower than 7 mg/dL (when serum albumin is normal) are associated with tetany and an unfavorable prognosis. In patients with clear evidence of acute pancreatitis, a serum ALT level of more than 80 units/L suggests biliary pancreatitis.

Serum amylase and lipase are elevated, usually in excess of three times the upper limit of normal, within 24 hours in 90% of cases; their return to normal is variable depending on the severity of disease. Other tests that offer the possibility of simplicity, rapidity, ease of use, and low cost, including urinary trypsinogen activation peptide and carboxypeptidase B, are under study. In patients who develop ascites or left pleural effusions, fluid amylase content is high. An elevated C-reactive protein concentration after 48 hours suggests the development of pancreatic necrosis. Electrocardiography may show ST–T wave changes.

D. IMAGING

Plain radiographs of the abdomen may show gallstones, a "sentinel loop" (a segment of air-filled small intestine most commonly in the left upper quadrant), the "colon cutoff sign"—a gas-filled segment of transverse colon abruptly ending at the area of pancreatic inflammation—or linear focal atelectasis of the lower lobe of the lungs with or without pleural effusion. CT scan is useful in demonstrating an enlarged pancreas when the diagnosis of pancreatitis is uncertain, in detecting pseudocysts, and in differentiating pancreatitis from other possible intra-abdominal catastrophes. Dynamic intravenous contrast-enhanced CT is of particular value after the first 3 days of severe acute pancreatitis to identify areas of necrotizing pancreatitis, though the use of intravenous contrast may increase the risk of complications of pancreatitis and of renal failure and should be avoided when the serum creatinine level is greater than 1.5 mg/dL. The presence of a fluid collection in the pancreas correlates with an increased mortality rate. CT-guided needle aspiration of areas of necrotizing pancreatitis may disclose infection, usually by enteric organisms, which invariably leads to death unless surgical debridement is performed. The presence of gas bubbles on CT scan implies that infection by gas-forming organisms is present. Ultrasonography is less reliable, because the echoes are deflected by the gas-distended small intestine frequently associated with pancreatitis but is the initial imaging study required when pancreatitis is thought to be caused by gallstones. Endoscopic ultrasonography is useful in identifying occult biliary disease (eg, small stones, sludge, microlithiasis) in a majority of patients with apparently idiopathic acute pancreatitis.

Differential Diagnosis

Acute pancreatitis must be differentiated from an acutely perforated duodenal ulcer, acute cholecystitis, acute intestinal obstruction, leaking aortic aneurysm, renal colic, and acute mesenteric vascular insufficiency or thrombosis. Serum amylase may also be elevated in high intestinal obstruction, in mumps not involving the pancreas (salivary amylase), in ectopic pregnancy, after administration of narcotics, and after abdominal surgery. Serum lipase usually is normal in these conditions.

Complications

Intravascular volume depletion secondary to leakage of fluids in the pancreatic bed and ileus with fluid-filled loops of bowel may result in prerenal azotemia and even acute tubular necrosis without overt shock. This usually occurs within 24 hours of the onset of acute pancreatitis and lasts 8–9 days. Some patients require peritoneal dialysis or hemodialysis.

As mentioned above, sterile or infected necrotizing pancreatitis may complicate the course of 5–10% of cases and accounts for most of the deaths. The risk of infection does not correlate with the extent of necrosis. Pancreatic necrosis is often associated with fever, leukocytosis, and, in some cases, shock and is associated with organ failure (eg, pulmonary, renal, gastrointestinal bleeding) in 50% of cases. Because infected pancreatic necrosis is an absolute indication for operative treatment, fine-needle aspiration of necrotic tissue under CT guidance should be performed (if necessary, repeatedly) for Gram stain and culture.

A serious complication of acute pancreatitis is acute respiratory distress syndrome (ARDS); cardiac dysfunction may be superimposed. It usually occurs 3–7 days after the onset of pancreatitis in patients who have required large volumes of fluid and colloid to maintain blood pressure and urine output. Most patients with ARDS require assisted respiration with positive end-expiratory pressure.

Pancreatic abscess is a suppurative process characterized by rising fever, leukocytosis, and localized tenderness and epigastric mass usually 6 or more weeks into the course of acute pancreatitis. This may be associated with a left-sided pleural effusion or an enlarging spleen secondary to splenic vein thrombosis. In contrast to infected necrosis, the mortality rate is low following drainage.

Pseudocysts, encapsulated fluid collections with high enzyme content, commonly appear in pancreatitis when CT scans are used to monitor the evolution of an acute attack. Although the natural history of pseudocysts is still not well delineated, it appears that those less than 6 cm in diameter often resolve spontaneously. They most commonly are within or adjacent to the pancreas but can present anywhere (eg, mediastinal, retrorectal), by extension along anatomic planes. Pseudocysts are multiple in 14% of cases. Pseudocysts may become secondarily infected, necessitating drainage as for an abscess. Erosion of the inflammatory process into a blood vessel can result in a major hemorrhage into the cyst.

Pancreatic ascites may present after recovery from acute pancreatitis as a gradual increase in abdominal girth and persistent elevation of the serum amylase level in the absence of frank abdominal pain. Marked elevations in the ascitic protein (> 3 g/dL) and amylase (> 1000 units/L) concentrations are typical. The condition results from rupture of the pancreatic duct or drainage of a pseudocyst into the peritoneal cavity.

Rare complications of acute pancreatitis include hemorrhage caused by erosion of a blood vessel to form a pseudoaneurysm and colonic necrosis. Chronic pancreatitis develops in about 10% of cases. Permanent diabetes mellitus and exocrine pancreatic insufficiency occur uncommonly after a single acute episode.

Treatment

A. MANAGEMENT OF ACUTE DISEASE

In most patients, acute pancreatitis is a mild disease that subsides spontaneously within several days. The pancreatic rest program includes withholding food and liquids by mouth, bed rest, and, in patients with moderately severe pain or ileus and abdominal distention or vomiting, nasogastric suction. Pain is controlled with meperidine, up to 100–150 mg intramuscularly every 3–4 hours as necessary. In those with severe hepatic or renal dysfunction, the dose may need to be reduced. (Morphine has been thought to cause sphincter of Oddi spasm but is probably an acceptable alternative.) No fluid or foods should be given orally until the patient is largely free of pain and has bowel sounds. Clear liquids are then given, and gradual advancement to a regular low-fat diet is prescribed, guided by the patient's tolerance and by the absence of pain. Following recovery from acute biliary pancreatitis, laparoscopic cholecystectomy should be performed.

In more severe pancreatitis—particularly necrotizing pancreatitis—there may be considerable leakage of fluids, necessitating large amounts of intravenous fluids to maintain intravascular volume. Calcium gluconate must be given intravenously if there is evidence of hypocalcemia with tetany. Infusions of fresh frozen plasma or serum albumin may be necessary in patients with coagulopathy or hypoalbuminemia. With colloid solutions, there may be an increased risk of developing adult respiratory distress syndrome. If shock persists after adequate volume replacement (including packed red cells), pressors may be required. For the patient requiring a large volume of parenteral fluids, central venous pressure and blood gases should be monitored at regular intervals. Total parenteral nutrition (including lipids) should be considered in patients who have severe pancreatitis and ileus and will be without oral nutrition for at least 7–10 days. Enteral nutrition via a jejunal feeding tube is preferable in the absence of ileus. Imipenem (500 mg every 8 hours intravenously) or possibly cefuroxime (1.5 g intravenously three times daily, then 250 mg orally twice daily) administered to patients with sterile pancreatic necrosis may also reduce the risk of pancreatic infection. The role of intravenous somatostatin in severe acute pancreatitis is uncertain, but octreotide is thought to have no benefit. There is some evidence that the risk of pancreatitis after ERCP can be reduced by the administration of somatostatin or gabexate mesilate, a protease inhibitor. In preliminary trials, lexipafant, an antagonist of platelet-activating factor, was reported to reduce rates of multiple organ failure and mortality in patients with severe acute pancreatitis, but a subsequent larger trial failed to demonstrate benefit.

The patient with severe pancreatitis requires attention in an intensive care unit. Close follow-up of white blood count, hematocrit, serum electrolytes, serum calcium, serum creatinine, BUN, serum AST and LDH, and arterial blood gases is mandatory. Cultures of blood, urine, sputum, and pleural effusion (if present) and needle aspirations of areas of pancreatic necrosis (with CT guidance) should be obtained.

B. TREATMENT OF COMPLICATIONS AND FOLLOW-UP

A surgeon should be consulted in all cases of severe acute pancreatitis. If the diagnosis is in doubt and investigations indicate a strong possibility of a serious surgically correctable lesion (eg, perforated peptic ulcer), exploration is indicated. When acute pancreatitis is unexpectedly found on exploratory laparotomy, it is usually wise to close without intervention of any kind. If the pancreatitis appears mild and cholelithiasis is present, cholecystostomy or cholecystectomy may be justified. When severe pancreatitis results from choledocholithiasis—particularly if jaundice (serum total bilirubin > 5 mg/dL) or cholangitis is present—ERCP with endoscopic sphincterotomy and stone extraction is indicated. The role of MRCP in this setting is evolving; eventually, MRCP may be useful in selecting patients for therapeutic ERCP.

Operation may improve survival in patients with necrotizing pancreatitis and clinical deterioration with multiorgan failure or lack of resolution by 4–6 weeks. Surgery is always indicated for infected necrosis. The goal of surgery is to debride necrotic pancreas and surrounding tissue and establish adequate drainage. In selected cases, nonsurgical drainage of necrotizing pancreatitis under radiologic or endoscopic guidance may be feasible depending on local expertise. Peritoneal lavage has not been shown to improve survival in severe acute pancreatitis, in part because the risk of late septic complications is not reduced.

The development of a pancreatic abscess is an indication for prompt percutaneous or surgical drainage. Chronic pseudocysts require endoscopic, percutaneous catheter, or surgical drainage when infected or associated with persisting pain, pancreatitis, or common duct obstruction. For pancreatic infections, imipenem, 500 mg every 8 hours intravenously, is a good antibiotic because it achieves bactericidal levels in pancreatic tissue for most causative organisms.

Prognosis

The mortality rate for severe acute pancreatitis (more than three Ranson criteria) is high, especially when hepatic, cardiovascular, or renal impairment is present in association with pancreatic necrosis. Recurrences are common in alcoholic pancreatitis.

Abou-Assi S et al: Nutrition in acute pancreatitis. J Clin Gastroenterol 2001;32:203. [PMID: 11246344] (Enteral nutrition via a nasojejunal tube appears to be cheaper, safer, and more effective in reducing the systemic inflammatory response than total parenteral nutrition.)

Arguedas MR et al: Where do ERCP, endoscopic ultrasound, magnetic resonance cholangiography, and intraoperative cholangiography fit in the management of acute biliary pancreatitis? A decision analysis model. Am J Gastroenterol 2001;96:2892. [PMID: 11693323] (Intraoperative cholangiography at laparoscopic cholecystectomy is the most cost-effective strategy when the probability of common bile duct stones is < 7%; endoscopic ultrasound is most cost-effective when the probability is 7–45%; and ERCP is most cost-effective when the probability is > 45%.)

Ashley SW et al: Necrotizing pancreatitis: Contemporary analysis of 99 consecutive cases. Ann Surg 2001;234:572. [PMID: 11573050] (Overall mortality rate was 14%. Of 62 patients without infection, all but three were managed nonoperatively, with a mortality rate of 11%. Of 34 patients with infected necrosis, 31 underwent surgery and three underwent percutaneous drainage, with an overall mortality rate of 12%.)

Büchler MW et al: Acute necrotizing pancreatitis: Treatment strategy according to the status of infection. Ann Surg 2000;232:619. [PMID: 11066131] (Retrospective study suggesting that when infection is excluded, surgery can often be avoided in patients with pancreatic necrosis in whom imipenem is begun early in the course.)

Chang L et al: Preoperative versus postoperative endoscopic retrograde cholangiopancreatography in mild to moderate gallstone pancreatitis: A prospective randomized trial. Ann Surg 2000;231:82. [PMID: 10636106] (Selective postoperative ERCP and common duct stone extraction is associated with a shorter hospital stay and less cost than routine preoperative ERCP.)

Levy MJ et al: Idiopathic acute recurrent pancreatitis. Am J Gastroenterol 2001;96:2540. [PMID: 11569674] (Causes include biliary microlithiasis, sphincter of Oddi dysfunction, pancreas divisum with stenosis of the minor papilla, and uncommon congenital anomalies such as choledochocele and annular pancreas.)

Sakorafas GH et al: Etiology and pathogenesis of acute pancreatitis: current concepts. J Clin Gastroenterol 2000;30:343. [PMID: 10875461] (Detailed discussion of the differential diagnosis and pathogenesis of acute pancreatitis.)

CHRONIC PANCREATITIS

Chronic pancreatitis occurs most often in patients with alcoholism (70–80% of all cases). The risk of chronic pancreatitis increases with the duration and amount of alcohol consumed, but only 5–10% of heavy drinkers develop pancreatitis. Ethanol is thought to cause secretion of insoluble pancreatic proteins that calcify and occlude the pancreatic duct. Progressive fibrosis and destruction of functioning glandular tissue then occur, perhaps as a result of repeated episodes of necroinflammation and activation of pancreatic stellate cells. About 2% of patients with hyperparathyroidism develop pancreatitis. In tropical Africa and Asia, tropical pancreatitis, related in part to malnutrition, is the most common cause of chronic pancreatitis. A stricture, stone, or tumor obstructing the pancreas can lead to obstructive chronic pancreatitis. Rare cases of autoimmune chronic pancreatitis associated with hypergammaglobulinemia responsive to corticosteroids have been reported. About 10–20% of cases are idiopathic. Genetic factors may predispose to chronic pancreatitis in some of these cases. For example, a mutant trypsinogen gene for hereditary pancreatitis, transmitted as an autosomal dominant trait with variable penetrance, has been identified on chromosome 7. Furthermore, mutations of the cystic fibrosis transmembrane conductance regulator (CFTR) gene have been identified in as many as 50% of patients with idiopathic chronic pancreatitis and no other clinical features of cystic fibrosis. Mutations of the pancreatic secretory trypsin inhibitory gene (PSTI) have also been associated with idiopathic chronic pancreatitis. A useful mnemonic for the predisposing factors to chronic pancreatitis is TIGAR-O: toxic-metabolic, idiopathic, genetic; autoimmune, recurrent and severe acute pancreatitis, or obstructive.

In many cases, chronic pancreatitis is a self-perpetuating disease characterized by chronic pain or recurrent episodes of acute pancreatitis and ultimately by pancreatic exocrine or endocrine insufficiency. After many years, chronic pain may resolve spontaneously or as a result of surgery tailored to the cause of pain. Over 80% of adults develop diabetes 25 years after the clinical onset of chronic pancreatitis.

Clinical Findings

A. SYMPTOMS AND SIGNS

Persistent or recurrent episodes of epigastric and left upper quadrant pain with referral to the upper left lumbar region are typical. Anorexia, nausea, vomiting, constipation, flatulence, and weight loss are common. Abdominal signs during attacks consist chiefly of tenderness over the pancreas, mild muscle guarding, and paralytic ileus. Attacks may last only a few hours or as long as 2 weeks; pain may eventually be almost continuous. Steatorrhea (as indicated by bulky, foul, fatty stools) may occur late in the course.

B. LABORATORY FINDINGS

Serum amylase and lipase may be elevated during acute attacks; normal amylase does not exclude the diagnosis, however. Serum alkaline phosphatase and bilirubin may be elevated owing to compression of the common duct. Glycosuria may be present. Excess fecal fat may be demonstrated on chemical analysis of the stool; pancreatic insufficiency may be confirmed by response to therapy with pancreatic enzyme supplements, by a bentiromide (NBT-PABA) test or secretin stimulation test if available. Where available, detection of decreased fecal chymotrypsin or elastase levels may be used to diagnose pancreatic insufficiency, though the tests lack sensitivity and specificity. Vitamin B_{12} malabsorption is detectable in about 40% of patients, but clinical deficiency of vitamin B_{12} and fat-soluble vitamins is rare.

C. IMAGING

Plain films show calcifications due to pancreaticolithiasis in 30% of affected patients. CT may show calcifications not seen on plain films as well as ductal dilation and heterogeneity or atrophy of the gland. Endoscopic ultrasonography also can detect changes of chronic pancreatitis. Endoscopic retrograde cholangiopancreatography is the most sensitive imaging study for chronic pancreatitis and may show dilated ducts, intraductal stones, strictures, or pseudocyst, but the results may be normal in patients with so-called minimal change pancreatitis. Magnetic resonance cholangiopancreatography (MRCP) and endoscopic ultrasonography (with pancreatic tissue sampling) are promising alternatives to endoscopic retrograde cholangiopancreatography.

Complications

Opioid addiction is common. Other frequent complications include often brittle diabetes mellitus, pancreatic pseudocyst or abscess, cholestatic liver enzymes with or without jaundice, common bile duct stricture, steatorrhea, malnutrition, and peptic ulcer. Pancreatic cancer develops in 4% of patients after 20 years; the risk may relate to tobacco and alcohol use.

Treatment

Correctable coexistent biliary tract disease should be treated surgically.

A. MEDICAL MEASURES

A low-fat diet should be prescribed. Alcohol is forbidden because it frequently precipitates attacks. Narcotics should be avoided if possible. Steatorrhea is treated with pancreatic supplements that are selected on the basis of their high lipase activity. A total dose of 30,000 units of lipase in capsules is given before, during, and after meals (Table 15–7). Concurrent administration of H_2 receptor antagonists (eg, ranitidine, 150 mg twice daily), or a proton pump inhibitor (eg, omeprazole, 20–60 mg daily), or sodium bicarbonate, 650 mg before and after meals, decreases the inactivation of lipase by acid and may thereby further decrease steatorrhea. In selected cases of alcoholic pancreatitis and in cystic fibrosis, enteric-coated mi-

Table 15–7. Selected pancreatic enzyme preparations.[1]

Product	Enzyme Content Per Unit Dose		
	Lipase	Amylase	Protease
Conventional preparations			
Viokase	8000	30,000	30,000
Ilozyme	11,000	≥ 30,000	≥ 30,000
Cotazym	8000	30,000	30,000
Enteric-coated microencapsulated preparations			
Creon	8000	30,000	13,000
Creon 10	10,000	33,200	37,500
Creon 20	20,000	66,400	75,000
Pancrease	4500	20,000	25,000
Pancrease MT10	10,000	30,000	30,000
Pancrease MT16	16,000	48,000	48,000
Pancrease MT20	20,000	56,000	44,000
Pancrease MT25	25,000	75,000	75,000
Cotazym-S	5000	20,000	20,000
Ultrase MT12	12,000	39,000	39,000
Ultrase MT18	18,000	58,500	58,500

[1]Modified from *Drug Facts and Comparisons*, 2001.

croencapsulated preparations may offer an advantage. However, in patients with cystic fibrosis, high-dose pancreatic enzyme therapy has been associated with strictures of the ascending colon. Pain secondary to idiopathic chronic pancreatitis may be alleviated in some cases by the use of pancreatic enzymes (not enteric-coated) or octreotide, 200 μg subcutaneously three times daily. Associated diabetes should be treated (Chapter 27).

B. SURGICAL AND ENDOSCOPIC TREATMENT

Surgery may be indicated in chronic pancreatitis to drain persistent pseudocysts, treat other complications, or attempt to relieve pain. The objectives of surgical intervention are to eradicate biliary tract disease, ensure a free flow of bile into the duodenum, and eliminate obstruction of the pancreatic duct. Liver fibrosis may regress after biliary drainage. When obstruction of the duodenal end of the duct can be demonstrated by endoscopic retrograde cholangiopancreatography, dilation of the duct or resection of the tail of the pancreas with implantation of the distal end of the duct by pancreaticojejunostomy may be successful. When the pancreatic duct is diffusely dilated, anastomosis between the duct after it is split longitudinally and a defunctionalized limb of jejunum (modified Puestow procedure), in some cases combined with local resection of the head of the pancreas, is associated with relief of pain in 80% of cases. In advanced cases, subtotal or total pancreatectomy may be considered as a last resort but has variable efficacy and is associated with a high rate of pancreatic insufficiency and diabetes. Perioperative administration of somatostatin or octreotide may reduce the risk of postoperative pancreatic fistulas. Endoscopic or surgical drainage is indicated for symptomatic pseudocysts and, in many cases, those over 6 cm in diameter. Endoscopic ultrasound may facilitate selection of an optimal site for endoscopic drainage. Recent experience suggests that pancreatic ascites or pancreaticopleural fistulas due to a disrupted pancreatic duct can be managed by endoscopic placement of a stent across the disrupted duct. Fragmentation of stones in the pancreatic duct by lithotripsy and endoscopic removal of stones from the duct, pancreatic sphincterotomy, or pseudocyst drainage may relieve pain in selected patients. For patients with chronic pain and nondilated ducts, a percutaneous celiac plexus nerve block may be considered under either CT or endoscopic ultrasound guidance, with pain relief in approximately 50% of patients.

Prognosis

This is a serious disease and often leads to chronic disability. The prognosis is best in patients with recurrent acute pancreatitis caused by a remediable condition such as cholelithiasis, choledocholithiasis, stenosis of the sphincter of Oddi, or hyperparathyroidism. Medical management of the hyperlipidemias frequently associated with the condition may also prevent recurrent attacks of pancreatitis. In alcoholic pancreatitis, pain relief is most likely when a dilated pancreatic duct can be decompressed. In patients with disease not amenable to decompressive surgery, addiction to narcotics is a frequent outcome of treatment.

Etemad B et al: Chronic pancreatitis: Diagnosis, classification, and new genetic developments. Gastroenterology 2001;120: 682. [PMID: 11726846]

Gress F et al: Endoscopic ultrasound-guided celiac plexus block for managing abdominal pain associated with chronic pancreatitis: A prospective single center experience. Am J Gastroenterol 2001;96:409. [PMID: 11255521] (Significant pain relief occurred in 55% of patients.)

Lankisch MR et al: The effect of small amounts of alcohol on the clinical course of chronic pancreatitis. Mayo Clin Proc 2001;76:242. [PMID: 11243270] (Retrospective study suggesting that among patients with the onset of pancreatitis after age 35, even moderate alcohol consumption [< 50 g/d] leads to more frequent severe pain, calcification, and complications; larger amounts lead to earlier mortality.)

Lankisch PG: Natural course of chronic pancreatitis. Pancreatology 2001;1:3. (Although it has been claimed that pain decreases with increasing duration of disease, more than half of patients continue to have attacks of pain after 10 years. Further natural history studies are required.)

Malka D et al: Risk factors for diabetes mellitus in chronic pancreatitis. Gastroenterology 2000;119:1324. [PMID: 11054391] (The cumulative rate of diabetes was 83% 25 years after the clinical onset of chronic pancreatitis. Surgery did not increase the risk, though the risk at 5 years was higher in those who had undergone distal pancreatectomy compared with other operations.)

Noone PG et al: Cystic fibrosis gene mutations and pancreatic risk: relation to epithelial ion transport and trypsin inhibitor gene mutations. Gastroenterology 2001;121:1310. [PMID: 11729110] (By sequencing the *CFTR* gene, these authors identified *CFTR* gene mutations in 47% of patients with otherwise idiopathic chronic pancreatitis. The mechanism may involve decreased pancreatic bicarbonate secretion, but only 1:100 persons with such mutations develops chronic pancreatitis.)

CARCINOMA OF THE PANCREAS & THE PERIAMPULLARY AREA

 ESSENTIALS OF DIAGNOSIS

- *Obstructive jaundice (may be painless).*
- *Enlarged gallbladder (may be painful).*
- *Upper abdominal pain with radiation to back, weight loss, and thrombophlebitis are usually late manifestations.*

General Considerations

Carcinoma is the commonest neoplasm of the pancreas. About 75% are in the head and 25% in the body and tail of the organ. Carcinomas involving the head of the pancreas, the ampulla of Vater, the distal common bile duct, and the duodenum are considered together, because they are usually indistinguishable clinically; of these, carcinomas of the pancreas constitute over 90%. They comprise 2% of all cancers and 5% of cancer deaths. Risk features include age, obesity, tobacco use, prior abdominal radiation, and family history. About 7–8% of patients with pancreatic cancer have a family history of pancreatic cancer in a first-degree relative, compared with 0.6% of control subjects. Neuroendocrine tumors account for 2–5% of pancreatic neoplasms. Cystic neoplasms account for only 1% of pancreatic cancers, but they are important because they are often mistaken for pseudocysts. A cystic neoplasm should be suspected when a cystic lesion in the pancreas is found in the absence of a history of pancreatitis. Whereas serous cystadenomas are benign, mucinous cystadenomas, intraductal papillary mucinous tumors, and papillary cystic neoplasms are premalignant, though their prognoses are better than the prognosis of adenocarcinoma of the pancreas.

Clinical Findings

A. SYMPTOMS AND SIGNS

Pain is present in over 70% of cases and is often vague, diffuse, and located in the epigastrium or left upper quadrant when the lesion is in the tail. Radiation of pain into the back is common and sometimes predominates. Sitting up and leaning forward may afford some relief, and this usually indicates that the lesion has spread beyond the pancreas and is inoperable. Diarrhea, perhaps due to maldigestion, is an occasional early symptom. Migratory thrombophlebitis is a rare sign. Weight loss is a common but late finding and may be associated with depression. Occasionally a patient presents with acute pancreatitis in the absence of an alternative cause. Jaundice is usually due to biliary obstruction by a cancer in the pancreatic head. A palpable gallbladder is also indicative of obstruction by neoplasm (Courvoisier's law), but there are frequent exceptions. A hard, fixed, occasionally tender mass may be present.

B. LABORATORY FINDINGS

There may be mild anemia. Glycosuria, hyperglycemia, and impaired glucose tolerance or true diabetes mellitus are found in 10–20% of cases. The serum amylase or lipase level is occasionally elevated. Liver function tests may suggest obstructive jaundice. Steatorrhea in the absence of jaundice is uncommon. Occult blood in the stool is suggestive of carcinoma of the ampulla of Vater. CA 19-9, with a sensitivity of 70% and a specificity of 87%, has not proved sensitive enough for early detection; increased values are also found in acute and chronic pancreatitis and cholangitis. Point mutations in codon 12 of the K-*ras* oncogene are found in 70–100%, and inactivation of the tumor suppressor genes *P16* on chromosome 9, *P53* on chromosome 17, and *DCP4* on chromosome 18 are found in 95%, 50–70%, and 50% of pancreatic cancers, respectively.

C. IMAGING

With carcinoma of the head of the pancreas, the upper gastrointestinal series may show a widening of the duodenal loop, mucosal abnormalities in the duodenum ranging from edema to invasion or ulceration, or spasm or compression. Ultrasound is not reliable because of interference by intestinal gas. Dual-phase spiral CT and MRI detect a mass in over 80% of cases and are helpful in delineating the extent of the tumor and allowing for percutaneous fine-needle aspiration for cytologic studies and tumor markers. Preliminary experience suggests that positron emission tomography is also a sensitive technique for detecting pancreatic cancer and metastases. Selective celiac and superior mesenteric arteriography may demonstrate vessel invasion by tumor, a finding that would interdict attempts at surgical resection, but it is less widely used since the advent of dual-phase spiral CT. Endoscopic ultrasonography, if available, is useful for diagnosing pancreatic cancer and for demonstrating venous or gastric invasion. Endoscopic ultrasonography may also be used to guide fine-needle aspiration for tissue diagnosis. ERCP may clarify an ambiguous CT or MRI study by delineating the pancreatic duct system or confirming an ampullary or biliary neoplasm. MRCP appears to be at least as sensitive as ERCP in diagnosing pancreatic cancer. With obstruction of the splenic vein, splenomegaly or gastric varices are present, the latter delineated by endoscopy, endoscopic ultrasonography, or angiography.

Staging by the TNM classification includes the following definitions: T1: tumor limited to the pancreas (T1a if < 2 cm, T1b if > 2 cm); T2: extension into duodenum, bile duct, or peripancreatic tissues; T3: extension to stomach, spleen, colon, or adjacent large vessels.

Treatment

Abdominal exploration is usually necessary when cytologic diagnosis cannot be made or if resection is to be attempted, which includes about 30% of patients. In a patient with a localized mass in the head of the pancreas and without jaundice, laparoscopy may detect tiny peritoneal or liver metastases and thereby avoid resection in 4–13% of patients. Radical pancreaticoduodenal (Whipple) resection is indicated for lesions strictly limited to the head of the pancreas, periampullary zone, and duodenum (T1, N0, M0). Five-year survival rates are 20–25% in this group and as high as 40% in those with negative resection margins and without lymph node involvement. Adjuvant radiation therapy and fluorouracil-based chemotherapy or gemcitabine are of potential benefit. When resection is not feasible, cholecystojejunostomy or endoscopic stenting of the bile duct is performed to relieve jaundice. A gastrojejunostomy is also done if duodenal obstruction is expected to develop later; alternatively, endoscopic placement of a self-expandable duodenal stent may be feasible. Combined irradiation and chemotherapy may be used for palliation of unresectable cancer confined to the pancreas. Chemotherapy has been disappointing in metastatic pancreatic cancer, though improved response rates have been reported with gemcitabine. Celiac plexus nerve block or thoracoscopic splanchnicectomy may improve pain control.

Surgical resection is indicated for all mucinous cystic neoplasms, symptomatic serous cystadenomas, and cystic tumors that remain undefined after helical CT, endoscopic ultrasound, and diagnostic aspiration. Survival is higher than for adenocarcinoma. Endoscopic resection or ablation may be feasible for ampullary adenomas.

Prognosis

Carcinoma of the pancreas, especially in the body or tail, has a poor prognosis. Reported 5-year survival rates range from 2% to 5%. Lesions of the ampulla have a better prognosis, with reported 5-year survival rates of 20–40% after resection. In carefully selected patients, resection of cancer of the pancreatic head is feasible and results in reasonable survival. In persons with a family history of pancreatic cancer, screening with spiral CT and endoscopic ultrasonography should be considered beginning 10 years before the age at which pancreatic cancer was diagnosed in a family member.

For those patients whose disease progresses despite treatment, meticulous efforts at palliative care are essential (see Chapter 5).

Gunaratnam NT et al: A prospective study of EUS-guided celiac plexus neurolysis for pancreatic cancer pain. Gastrointest Endosc 2001;54:316. [PMID: 11522971] (Improvement in pain scores occurred in 45 of 58 [78%] patients.)

Kim MH et al: Tumors of the major duodenal papilla. Gastrointest Endosc 2001;54:609. [PMID: 11677478] (Reviews benign and malignant neoplasms and the spectrum of treatment approaches, including advanced endoscopic therapies.)

Michaud DS et al: Physical activity, obesity, height and the risk of pancreatic cancer. JAMA 2001;286:921. [PMID: 11509056] (In two prospective cohort studies, obesity [BMI $\geq$ 30 kg/m^2] was associated with an increased risk of pancreatic cancer, and physical activity decreased the risk.)

Sohn TA et al: Intraductal papillary mucinous neoplasms of the pancreas: An increasingly recognized clinicopathologic entity. Ann Surg 2001;234:313. [PMID: 11524584] (Description of 60 cases seen between 1987 and 2000; the 5-year survival rate after surgical resection was 57%, much higher than that for ductal adenocarcinoma.)

Sohn TA et al: Resected adenocarcinoma of the pancreas—616 patients: results, outcomes, and prognostic indicators. J Gastrointest Surg 2000;4:567. (Five-year survival was 17%, with a median survival of 17 months. Favorable prognostic factors on multivariate analysis were negative resection margins, tumor diameter < 3 cm, blood loss < 750 mL, well- or moderately differentiated tumor, and postoperative chemoradiation.)

Breast

16

Armando E. Giuliano, MD

See www.current-med.com/ch16.html

■ BENIGN BREAST DISORDERS

FIBROCYSTIC DISEASE

 ESSENTIALS OF DIAGNOSIS

- *Painful, often multiple, usually bilateral masses in the breast.*
- *Rapid fluctuation in the size of the masses is common.*
- *Frequently, pain occurs or increases and size increases during premenstrual phase of cycle.*
- *Most common age is 30–50. Rare in postmenopausal women not receiving hormonal replacement.*

General Considerations

This disorder is the most frequent lesion of the breast. It is common in women 30–50 years of age but rare in postmenopausal women who are not taking hormonal replacement medications. Estrogen hormone is considered a causative factor. Fibrocystic disease encompasses a wide variety of pathologic entities. These lesions are always associated with benign changes in the breast epithelium, some of which are found so commonly in normal breasts that they are probably variants of normal breast histology but have nonetheless been termed a "disease."

The microscopic findings of fibrocystic disease include cysts (gross and microscopic), papillomatosis, adenosis, fibrosis, and ductal epithelial hyperplasia. Although fibrocystic disease has generally been considered to increase the risk of subsequent breast cancer, only the variants in which proliferation (especially with atypia) of epithelial components is demonstrated represent true risk factors.

Clinical Findings

A. SYMPTOMS AND SIGNS

Fibrocystic disease may produce an asymptomatic lump in the breast that is discovered by accident, but pain or tenderness often calls attention to the mass. There may be discharge from the nipple. In many cases, discomfort occurs or is increased during the premenstrual phase of the cycle, at which time the cysts tend to enlarge. Fluctuation in size and rapid appearance or disappearance of a breast mass are common in cystic disease. Multiple or bilateral masses are common, and many patients will give a history of a transient lump in the breast or cyclic breast pain.

B. DIAGNOSTIC TESTS

Because a mass due to fibrocystic disease is frequently indistinguishable from carcinoma on the basis of clinical findings, suspicious lesions should be biopsied. Fine-needle aspiration cytology may be used, but if a suspicious mass that is nonmalignant on cytologic examination does not resolve over several months, it must be excised. Surgery should be conservative, since the primary objective is to exclude cancer. Occasionally, core needle biopsy will suffice. Simple mastectomy or extensive removal of breast tissue is rarely, if ever, indicated for mammary dysplasia.

Differential Diagnosis

Pain, fluctuation in size, and multiplicity of lesions are the features most helpful in differentiation from carcinoma. If a dominant mass is present, the diagnosis of cancer should be assumed until disproved by biopsy. Final diagnosis often depends on excisional biopsy. Mammography may be helpful, but the breast tissue in these young women is usually too radiodense to permit a worthwhile study. Sonography is useful in differentiating a cystic from a solid mass.

Treatment

When the diagnosis of fibrocystic disease has been established by previous biopsy or is likely because the history is classic, aspiration of a discrete mass suggestive of a cyst is indicated in order to alleviate pain and, more importantly, to confirm the cystic nature of the mass. The patient is reexamined at intervals thereafter. If no fluid is obtained or if fluid is bloody, if a mass persists after aspiration, or if at any time during follow-up a persistent lump is noted, biopsy is performed.

Breast pain associated with generalized fibrocystic disease is best treated by avoiding trauma and by wearing (night and day) a brassiere that gives good support and protection. Hormone therapy is not advisable, because it does not cure the condition and has undesirable side effects. Danazol (100–200 mg twice daily orally), a synthetic androgen, has been used for patients with severe pain. This treatment suppresses pituitary gonadotropins, but androgenic effects (acne, edema, hirsutism) usually make this treatment intolerable; in practice, it is rarely used.

The role of caffeine consumption in the development and treatment of fibrocystic disease is controversial. Some studies suggest that eliminating caffeine from the diet is associated with improvement. Many patients are aware of these studies and report relief of symptoms after giving up coffee, tea, and chocolate. Similarly, many women find vitamin E (400 IU daily) helpful. However, these observations remain anecdotal.

Prognosis

Exacerbations of pain, tenderness, and cyst formation may occur at any time until the menopause, when symptoms usually subside, except in patients receiving hormonal replacement therapy. The patient should be advised to examine her own breasts each month just after menstruation and to inform her physician if a mass appears. The risk of breast cancer in women with fibrocystic disease showing proliferative or atypical changes in the epithelium is higher than that of women in general. These women should be followed carefully with physical examinations and mammography.

Cady B et al: Evaluation of common breast problems: Guidance for primary care providers. CA Cancer J Clin 1998;48:49. [PMID: 9449933]

Fitzgibbons PL et al: Benign breast changes and the risk for subsequent breast cancer: an update of the 1985 consensus statement. Cancer Committee of the College of American Pathologists. Arch Pathol Lab Med 1998;122:1053. [PMID: 9870852] (A definition of the relative breast cancer risk associated with specific histologic abnormalities; includes data from recent case-control studies.)

Marchant DJ: Controversies in benign breast disease. Surg Oncol Clin N Am 1998;7:285. [PMID: 9537977]

Morrow M: The evaluation of common breast problems. Am Fam Physician 2000;61:2371. [PMID: 10794579]

FIBROADENOMA OF THE BREAST

This common benign neoplasm occurs most frequently in young women, usually within 20 years after puberty. It is somewhat more frequent and tends to occur at an earlier age in black women. Multiple tumors are found in 10–15% of patients.

The typical fibroadenoma is a round or ovoid, rubbery, discrete, relatively movable, nontender mass 1–5 cm in diameter. It is usually discovered accidentally. Clinical diagnosis in young patients is generally not difficult. In women over 30, cystic disease of the breast and carcinoma of the breast must be considered. Cysts can be identified by aspiration or ultrasonography. Fibroadenoma does not normally occur after the menopause, but may occasionally develop after administration of hormones.

No treatment is usually necessary if the diagnosis can be made by needle biopsy or cytologic examination. Excision with pathologic examination of the specimen is performed if the diagnosis is uncertain.

Phyllodes tumor is a fibroadenoma-like tumor with cellular stroma that grows rapidly. It may reach a large size and if inadequately excised will recur locally. The lesion can be benign or malignant. If benign, phyllodes tumor is treated by local excision with a margin of surrounding breast tissue. The treatment of malignant phyllodes tumor is more controversial, but complete removal of the tumor with a rim of normal tissue avoids recurrence. Since these tumors may be large, simple mastectomy is sometimes necessary. Lymph node dissection is not performed, since the sarcomatous portion of the tumor metastasizes to the lungs and not the lymph nodes.

Chilcote WA et al: Stereotactic breast biopsy: a less-invasive option. Cleve Clin J Med 1997;64:550. [PMID: 9385742]

Greenberg R et al: Management of breast fibroadenomas. J Gen Intern Med 1998;13:640. [PMID: 9754521] (Transformation of fibroadenoma is rare, and excision should be limited to fibroadenomas that fail to increase in size.)

Mangi AA et al: Surgical management of phyllodes tumors. Arch Surg 1999;134:487. [PMID: 10323420] (Phyllodes tumors mimic fibroadenomas clinically; 1-cm excision margins are recommended, or mastectomy for large lesions.)

NIPPLE DISCHARGE

In order of decreasing frequency, the following are the commonest causes of nipple discharge in the nonlactating breast: duct ectasia, intraductal papilloma, and carcinoma. The important characteristics of the discharge and some other factors to be evaluated by history and physical examination are as follows:

(1) Nature of discharge (serous, bloody, or other).

(2) Association with a mass.

(3) Unilateral or bilateral.

(4) Single or multiple duct discharge.

(5) Discharge is spontaneous (persistent or intermittent) or must be expressed.

(6) Discharge produced by pressure at a single site or by general pressure on the breast.

(7) Relation to menses.

(8) Premenopausal or postmenopausal.

(9) Patient taking contraceptive pills or estrogen.

Unilateral, spontaneous serous or serosanguineous discharge from a single duct is usually caused by an intraductal papilloma or, rarely, by an intraductal cancer. A mass may not be palpable. The involved duct may be identified by pressure at different sites around the nipple at the margin of the areola. Bloody discharge is suggestive of cancer but is more often caused by a benign papilloma in the duct. Cytologic examination may identify malignant cells, but negative findings do not rule out cancer, which is more likely in women over age 50. In any case, the involved duct—and a mass if present—should be excised. Ductography is of limited value since excision of the bloody duct system is indicated regardless of findings. Ductoscopy is being evaluated as a means of identifying intraductal lesions.

In premenopausal women, spontaneous multiple duct discharge, unilateral or bilateral, most marked just before menstruation, is often due to mammary dysplasia. Discharge may be green or brownish. Papillomatosis and ductal ectasia are usually seen on biopsy. If a mass is present, it should be removed.

Milky discharge from multiple ducts in the nonlactating breast occurs in certain endocrine syndromes, as a result of hyperprolactinemia. Serum prolactin levels should be obtained to search for a pituitary tumor. TSH helps exclude causative hypothyroidism. Numerous antipsychotic drugs and other drugs may also cause milky discharge that ceases on discontinuance of the medication.

Oral contraceptive agents or estrogen replacement therapy may cause clear, serous, or milky discharge from a single duct, but multiple duct discharge is more common. The discharge is more evident just before menstruation and disappears on stopping the medication. If it does not and is from a single duct, exploration should be considered.

Purulent discharge may originate in a subareolar abscess and require removal of the abscess and related lactiferous sinus.

When localization is not possible, no mass is palpable, and the discharge is nonbloody, the patient should be reexamined every 2 or 3 months for a year, and mammography should be done. Cytologic examination of nipple discharge for exfoliated cancer cells may rarely be helpful in diagnosis.

Jardines L: Management of nipple discharge. Am Surg 1996;62: 119. [PMID: 8554189]

FAT NECROSIS

Fat necrosis is a rare lesion of the breast but is of clinical importance because it produces a mass, often accompanied by skin or nipple retraction, that is indistinguishable from carcinoma. Trauma is presumed to be the cause, though only about half of patients give a history of injury. Ecchymosis is occasionally present. If untreated, the mass effect gradually disappears. The

safest course is to obtain a biopsy. Needle biopsy is often adequate, but frequently the entire mass must be excised, primarily to exclude carcinoma. Fat necrosis is common after segmental resection, radiation therapy, or flap reconstruction after mastectomy.

BREAST ABSCESS

During nursing, an area of redness, tenderness, and induration may develop in the breast. The organism most commonly found in these abscesses is *Staphylococcus aureus*. In the early stages, the infection can often be treated while nursing is continued from that breast by administering an antibiotic such as dicloxacillin or oxacillin, 250 mg four times daily for 7–10 days (see Puerperal Mastitis, Chapter 18). If the lesion progresses to form a localized mass with local and systemic signs of infection, surgical drainage is performed and nursing is discontinued.

A subareolar abscess may develop (rarely) in young or middle-aged women who are not lactating. These infections tend to recur after incision and drainage unless the area is explored during a quiescent interval, with excision of the involved lactiferous duct or ducts at the base of the nipple. Otherwise, infection in the breast is very rare unless the patient is lactating. In the nonlactating breast, inflammatory carcinoma is always considered. Thus, findings suggestive of abscess or cellulitis in the nonlactating breast are an indication for incision and biopsy of any indurated tissue. If the abscess can be percutaneously drained and completely resolves, the patient may be followed conservatively.

Schein M: Subareolar breast abscesses. Surgery 1996;120:902. [PMID: 8909529] (Highly successful nonoperative ultrasound-guided aspiration and antibiotic therapy of breast abscesses. This should probably be the first choice for treatment of small lesions.)

DISORDERS OF THE AUGMENTED BREAST

At least 4 million American women have had breast implants. Breast augmentation is performed by placing implants usually under the pectoralis muscle or, less desirably, in the subcutaneous tissue of the breast. Most implants are made of an outer silicone shell filled with a silicone gel, saline, or some combination of the two. About 15–25% of the patients develop capsule contraction or scarring around the implant, leading to a firmness and distortion of the breast that can be painful. Some require removal of the implant and capsule.

Implant rupture may occur in as many as 5–10% of women, and bleeding of gel through the capsule is noted even more commonly. While silicone gel may be an immunologic stimulant, there is no increase in autoimmune disorders in patients with such implants. The FDA has advised symptomatic women with ruptured implants to discuss possible surgical removal with their physicians. However, women who are asymptomatic and have no evidence of rupture of a silicone gel prosthesis should probably not undergo removal of the implant. Women with symptoms of autoimmune illnesses should address the possibility of removal.

Studies have failed to show any association between implants and an increased incidence of breast cancer. However, breast cancer may develop in a patient with a silicone gel prosthesis, as it does in women without them. Detection in patients with implants is made more difficult since mammography is less able to detect early lesions. However, local recurrence after breast reconstruction for cancer is usually cutaneous or subcutaneous and is easily palpated. If a cancer develops, it should be treated in the same manner as in women without implants. Such women should be offered the option of mastectomy or breast-conserving therapy, which may require removal or replacement of the implant. Radiotherapy of the augmented breast often results in marked capsular contracture. Adjuvant treatments should be given for the same indications as for women who have no implants.

Brinton LA et al: Breast implants and cancer. J Natl Cancer Inst 1997;89:1341. [PMID: 9308703] (No apparent biologic basis for implants increasing cancer risk or worsening prognosis.)

Gabriel SE et al: Complications leading to surgery after breast implantation. N Engl J Med 1997;336:677. [PMID: 9041097]

Gertzten PC: A formal risk assessment of silicone breast implants. Biomaterials 1999;20:1063. [PMID: 10378807] (Review of scientific evidence for safety of silicone breast implants.)

Nyren O et al: Risk of connective tissue disease and related disorders among women with breast implants: A nation-wide retrospective cohort study in Sweden. BMJ 1998;316:417. [PMID: 8190133].

■ CARCINOMA OF THE FEMALE BREAST

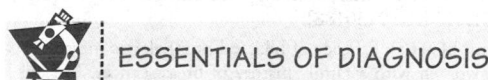

ESSENTIALS OF DIAGNOSIS

- *Risk factors include delayed childbearing, positive family history of breast cancer or genetic mutations (BRCA-1, BRCA-2), and personal history of breast cancer or some types of mammary dysplasia.*

- *Most women with breast cancer do not have identifiable risk factors.*

- *Early findings: Single, nontender, firm to hard mass with ill-defined margins; mammographic abnormalities and no palpable mass.*

- *Later findings: Skin or nipple retraction; axillary lymphadenopathy; breast enlargement, red-ness, edema, pain; fixation of mass to skin or chest wall.*

INCIDENCE & RISK FACTORS

Aside from skin cancer, the breast is the most common site of cancer in women, and cancer of the breast is second only to lung cancer as a cause of death from cancer among women. The probability of developing breast cancer increases throughout life. The mean and the median age of women with breast cancer is between 60 and 61 years.

There will be about 203,500 new cases of breast cancer and about 40,000 deaths from this disease in women in the USA in the year 2002. An additional 54,000 cases of ductal carcinoma in situ will be detected, principally by screening mammography. One out of every eight or nine American women will develop breast cancer during her lifetime. The incidence of breast cancer continues to increase, but mortality has stayed the same. Women whose mothers or sisters had breast cancer are three to four times more likely to develop the disease. Risk is further increased in patients whose mothers' or sisters' breast cancers occurred before menopause or was bilateral and in those with a family history of breast cancer in two or more first-degree relatives. However, there is no history of breast cancer among female relatives in over 75% of patients. Nulliparous women and women whose first full-term pregnancy was after age 35 have a 1.5 times higher incidence of breast cancer than multiparous women. Late menarche and artificial menopause are associated with a lower incidence, whereas early menarche (under age 12) and late natural menopause (after age 50) are associated with a slight increase in risk. Fibrocystic disease, when accompanied by proliferative changes, papillomatosis, or atypical epithelial hyperplasia, is associated with an increased incidence. A woman who has had cancer in one breast is at increased risk of developing cancer in the other breast. Such women develop a contralateral cancer at the rate of 1% or 2% per year. Women with cancer of the uterine corpus have a breast cancer risk significantly higher than that of the general population, and women with breast cancer have a comparably increased endometrial cancer risk. In the USA, breast cancer is more common in whites. The incidence of the disease among nonwhites (mostly blacks) is increasing, especially in younger women. In general, rates reported from developing countries are low, whereas rates are high in developed countries, with the notable exception of Japan. Some of the variability may be due to underreporting in the developing countries, but a real difference probably exists. Dietary factors, particularly increased fat consumption, may account for some differences in incidence. Oral contraceptives do not appear to increase the risk of breast cancer. There is evidence that administration of estrogens to postmenopausal women may result in a slightly increased risk of breast cancer, but only with higher, long-term doses of estrogens. Concomitant administration of progesterone and estrogen may markedly increase the incidence of breast cancer compared with the use of estrogen alone. Alcohol consumption increases the risk slightly. Some inherited breast cancers have been found to be associated with a gene on chromosome 17. This gene, *BRCA1*, is mutated in families with early-onset breast cancer and ovarian cancer. As many as 85% of women with *BRCA1* gene mutations will develop breast cancer in their lifetime. Other genes are associated with increased risk of breast and other cancers, such as *BRCA2*, ataxia-telangiectasia mutation, and *TP53*, the tumor suppressor gene. *TP53* mutations have been found in approximately 1% of breast cancers in women under 40 years of age. Genetic testing is now commercially available for women at high risk of breast cancer. Women with genetic mutations who develop breast cancer may be treated in the same way as women who do not have mutations (ie, lumpectomy). Such women with mutations often elect bilateral mastectomy as treatment. Problems associated with management of patients with identified mutations, their insurability, and potential social conflicts are anticipated. Some states have enacted legislation to prevent insurance companies from considering mutations as "preexisting conditions" preventing insurability.

Women at greater than normal risk of developing breast cancer (Table 16–1) should be identified by their physicians, taught the techniques of breast self-examination, and followed carefully. Those with an exceptional family history should be counseled and given the option of genetic testing. Some of these high-risk women may consider prophylactic mastectomy or tamoxifen.

The NSABP conducted the Breast Cancer Prevention Trial (BCPT), which studied the efficacy of tamoxifen as a preventive agent in women who had never had breast cancer but were at high risk for developing the disease. Women who received tamoxifen for 5 years had about a 50% reduction in noninvasive and invasive cancers compared with women taking placebo. However, women above the age of 50 who received the drug had an increased incidence of endometrial cancer and deep venous thrombosis. Unfortunately, no survival data will be produced from this trial. The estrogen replacement raloxifene, effective in preventing osteoporosis, may also prevent breast cancer. Several large studies to examine this hypothesis are under way.

Audrain J et al: Genetic counseling and testing for breast-ovarian cancer susceptibility: What do women want? J Clin Oncol 1998;16:133. [PMID: 9440734]

Beckhardt S for the American Society of Clinical Oncology. Statement of the American Society of Clinical Oncology: Genetic testing for cancer susceptibility. J Clin Oncol 1996; 14:1730.

[PMID: 8622094] (Summarizes the position of the American Society of Clinical Oncology on genetic testing for cancer susceptibility.)

Clemons M et al: Estrogen and the risk of breast cancer. N Engl J Med 2001;344:276. [PMID: 11172156]

Collaborative Group on Hormonal Factors in Breast Cancer (Radcliffe Infirmary, Oxford, England): Breast cancer and hormonal contraceptives: Collaborative reanalysis of individual data on 53,297 women with breast cancer and 100,239 women without breast cancer from 54 epidemiological studies. Lancet 1996;347:1713. [PMID: 8656904] (The relationship appears more complex than previously appreciated.)

Fisher B et al: Tamoxifen for prevention of breast cancer: Report of the National Surgical Adjuvant Breast and Bowel Project P-1 Study. J Natl Cancer Inst 1998; 90:1371. [PMID: 9747868] (This important study is the first to show that breast cancer can be prevented by a drug.)

Greely HT: Genetic testing for cancer susceptibility for creators of practice guidelines. Oncology (Huntingt) 1997;11(11A): 171. [PMID: 9430188]

Hartmann LC et al: Efficacy of bilateral prophylactic mastectomy in women with a family history of breast cancer. N Engl J Med 1999;340:77. [PMID: 9887158]

JAMA patient page: Breast cancer. JAMA 1999;281:772. [Cit ID: 99159816]

Kodish E et al: Genetic testing for cancer risk: How to reconcile the conflicts. JAMA 1998;279:179. [PMID:9438721]

Martin AM et al: Genetic and hormonal risk factors in breast cancer. J Natl Cancer Inst 2000;92:1126. [PMID: 10904085]

Meijers-Heijboer H et al: Breast cancer after prophylactic bilateral mastectomy in women with a BRCA1 or BRCA2 mutation. N Engl J Med 2001;345:159. [PMID: 11463009]

Pierce LJ et al: Effect of radiotherapy after breast-conserving treatment in women with breast cancer and germline BRCA1/2 mutations. J Clin Oncol 2000;18:3360. [PMID: 11013276]

Table 16–1. Factors associated with increased risk of breast cancer.[1]

Race	White
Age	Older
Family history	Breast cancer in mother, sister, or daughter (especially bilateral or premenopausal)
Genetics	*BRCA1* or *BRCA2* mutation
Previous medical history	Endometrial cancer Proliferative forms of fibrocystic disease Cancer in other breast
Menstrual history	Early menarche (under age 12) Late menopause (after age 50)
Pregnancy	Nulliparous or late first pregnancy

[1]Normal lifetime risk in white women = 1 in 8 or 9.

Schairer C et al: Menopausal estrogen and estrogen-progestin replacement therapy and breast cancer risk. JAMA 2000;283:485. [PMID: 10659874] (Estrogen-progestin hormone regimen increases breast cancer risk more than estrogen alone.)

EARLY DETECTION OF BREAST CANCER

Screening Programs

A number of mass screening programs consisting of physical and mammographic examination of the breasts of asymptomatic women have been conducted. Such programs frequently identify about ten cancers per 1000 women older than age 50 and about two cancers per 1000 women younger than age 50. About 80% of these women have negative axillary lymph nodes at the time of surgery, whereas only 50% of nonscreened women found in the course of usual medical practice have uninvolved axillary nodes. Detecting breast cancer before it has spread to the axillary nodes greatly increases the chance of survival, and about 85% of such women will survive at least 5 years.

Both physical examination and mammography are necessary for maximum yield in screening programs, since about 35–50% of early breast cancers can be discovered only by mammography and another 40% can be detected only by palpation. About one-third of the abnormalities detected on screening mammograms will be found to be malignant when biopsy is performed. Women 20–40 years of age should have a breast examination as part of routine medical care every 2–3 years. Women over age 40 should have yearly breast examinations. The sensitivity of mammography varies from approximately 60% to 90%. This sensitivity depends on several factors, including patient age (breast density), tumor size, location, and mammographic appearance. In young women with dense breasts, mammography is less sensitive than in older woman with fatty breasts, in whom mammography can detect at least 90% of malignancies. Smaller tumors, particularly those without calcifications, are more difficult to detect, especially in dense breasts. The lack of sensitivity and the low incidence of breast cancer in young women has led to questions concerning the value of mammography for screening in women 40–50 years of age. The specificity of mammography in women under 50 varies from about 30% to 40% for nonpalpable mammographic abnormalities to 85% to 90% for clinically evident malignancies.

Doubt exists about the beneficial effect of screening, especially in women under age 50. Questions such as the potential harmful effects of x-rays in a large population of young women and the general value of early detection were raised and largely ignored as various groups supported screening between ages 40 and 50. While the Health Insurance Plan Project study did show a beneficial effect of screening in such women, reducing breast cancer mortality 25% between 10 and 18 years after entry into the study, a Canadian trial demonstrated an unexplained shortening of survival from time of random assignment to death in the screening group. The small number of patients in this study experienced no beneficial effect, but the 95% confidence interval included a potential lifesaving effect as well as a potential harmful effect. A very large number of patients is necessary to show a beneficial effect of screening among patients age 40–49, where the incidence of breast cancer is low. In addition, the problems of crossover of patients in the control group with women undergoing physician examination and nonscreening mammograms, problems with mammography quality, and problems in recruitment, randomization, and compliance make the interpretation of such trials difficult. The beneficial effect of screening in women aged 50–69 is undisputed and has been confirmed by all clinical trials. The efficacy of screening in older women—those older than 70—is inconclusive and is difficult to determine because of the few women screened.

More recent studies showing a beneficial effect of screening young women and the recommendation of a Swedish consensus panel led the NCI to reconsider its position on screening mammography for women in their 40s. Two Swedish trials that had shown a 13% decrease in breast cancer mortality (not statistically significant) now showed a statistical advantage for screening women in their 40s, and a meta-analysis similarly revealed a statistical survival advantage for screened women with longer follow-up. In March 1997, the National Cancer Advisory Board recommended that women with average risk factors should have screening mammography every 1–2 years in their 40s and that women at higher risk should seek medical advice on when to begin screening. The American Cancer Society then recommended screening every year for asymptomatic women starting at age 40.

In 2001, a Danish review of the literature concluded that there is no survival advantage to screening mammography. This result has been questioned, and other studies continue to support the value of screening mammography.

Self-Examination

All women over age 20 should be advised to examine their breasts monthly. Premenopausal women should perform the examination 7–8 days after the menstrual period. The breasts should be inspected initially while standing before a mirror with the hands at the sides, overhead, and pressed firmly on the hips to contract the pectoralis muscles. Masses, asymmetry of breasts, and slight dimpling of the skin may become apparent as a result of these maneuvers. Next, in a supine position, each breast should be carefully palpated with the fingers of the opposite hand. Some women discover small breast lumps more readily when their skin is moist while bathing or showering. Physicians should instruct women in the technique of self-examination and advise them to report a mass or other abnormality.

Mammography

Mammography is the most useful technique for the detection of early breast cancer. Film screen mammography delivers less than 0.4 cGy to the mid breast per view and has largely replaced the older xeromammographic technique, which delivers more radiation.

Mammography is the only reliable means of detecting breast cancer before a mass can be palpated. Slowly growing cancers can be identified by mammography at least 2 years before reaching a size detectable by palpation.

Calcifications are the most easily recognized mammographic abnormality. The most common findings associated with carcinoma of the breast are clustered polymorphic microcalcifications. Such calcifications are usually at least five to eight in number, aggregated in one part of the breast and differing from each other in size and shape, often including branched or V- or Y-shaped configurations. There may be an associated mammographic mass density or, at times, only a mass density with no calcifications. Such a density usually has irregular or ill-defined borders and may lead to architectural distortion within the breast. A small mass or architectural distortion, particularly in a dense breast, may be subtle and difficult to detect.

Indications for mammography are as follows: (1) to screen at regular intervals women at high risk for developing breast cancer (see above); (2) to evaluate each breast when a diagnosis of potentially curable breast cancer has been made, and at yearly intervals thereafter; (3) to evaluate a questionable or ill-defined breast mass or other suspicious change in the breast; (4) to search for an occult breast cancer in a woman with metastatic disease in axillary nodes or elsewhere from an unknown primary; (5) to screen women prior to cosmetic operations or prior to biopsy of a mass, to examine for an unsuspected cancer; and (6) to follow those women with breast cancer who have been treated with breast-conserving surgery and radiation.

Patients with a dominant or suspicious mass must undergo biopsy despite mammographic findings. The mammogram should be obtained prior to biopsy so that other suspicious areas can be noted and the contralateral breast can be checked. Mammography is never a substitute for biopsy, because it may not reveal clinical cancer in a very dense breast, as may be seen in young women with mammary dysplasia, and may not reveal medullary cancers.

Communication and documentation between the patient, the referring physician, and the interpreting physician are critical for high-quality screening and diagnostic mammography. The patient should be informed about *how* she will receive timely results of her mammogram, that mammography does not "rule out" cancer, and that she should expect a correlative examination at the mammography facility if referred for a suspicious lesion. She should also be aware of the technique and need for breast compression and that this may be uncomfortable. The mammography facility should be informed *in writing* of abnormal physical examination findings. It is strongly recommended in the AHCPR Clinical Practice Guidelines that all mammography reports be communicated with the patient as well as the health care provider in writing. Additional phone communication about any abnormal findings should take place between the interpreting and referring physicians. MRI and PET may play a role in imaging atypical lesions but only after diagnostic mammography has been performed.

Alberg AJ et al: Epidemiology, prevention, and early detection of breast cancer. Curr Opin Oncol 1997;9:505. [PMID: 9370070]

Feig SA: Doubtful results in the Canadian national breast screening study. Breast Diseases 1996;6:354.

Gail M et al: Risk-based recommendations for mammographic screening for women in their forties. J Clin Oncol 1998;16:3105. [PMID: 9738582] (Recommendations are based on individual risk factors and empirical assumptions.)

Kopans DB: Updated results of the trials of screening mammography. Surg Oncol Clin N Am 1997;6:233. [PMID: 9115494]

Leitch AM et al: American Cancer Society guidelines for the early detection of breast cancer: Update 1997. CA Cancer J Clin 1997;47:150. [PMID: 9152172](Includes the most recent recommendations of the American Cancer Society, similar to but not identical with those of the National Cancer Institute.)

Nystrom L et al: Long-term effects of mammography screening: updated overview of the Swedish randomised trials. Lancet 2001;359:909. [PMID: 11918907] (Randomized study showing a 21% reduction in mortality among women screened by mammograms.)

Obdeijn IM et al: MR lesion detection in a breast cancer population. J Magn Reson Imaging 1996;6:849. [PMID: 8956127]

Olson O et al: Cochrane review on screening for breast cancer with mammography. Lancet 2001;358:1340. [PMID: 11684218] (Questions the value of screening mammography. An occasion for international controversy.)

Clinical Clues to Early Detection of Breast Cancer

A. SYMPTOMS AND SIGNS

The presenting complaint in about 70% of patients with breast cancer is a lump (usually painless) in the breast. About 90% of breast masses are discovered by the patient herself. Less frequent symptoms are breast pain; nipple discharge; erosion, retraction, enlargement, or itching of the nipple; and redness, generalized hardness, enlargement, or shrinking of the breast. Rarely, an axillary mass or swelling of the arm may be the first symptom. Back or bone pain, jaundice, or weight loss may be the result of systemic metastases, but these symptoms are rarely seen on initial presentation.

The relative frequency of carcinoma in various anatomic sites in the breast is shown in Figure 16–1.

Inspection of the breast is the first step in physical examination and should be carried out with the patient sitting, arms at sides and then overhead. Abnor-

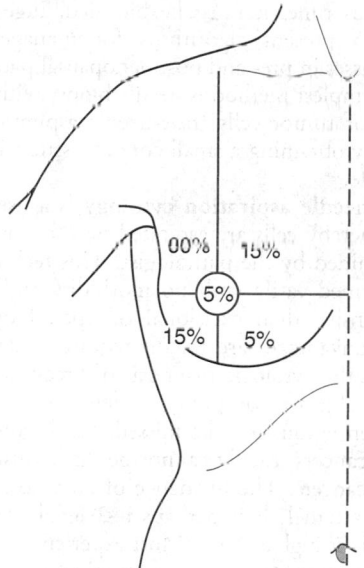

Figure 16-1. Frequency of breast carcinoma at various anatomic sites.

mal variations in breast size and contour, minimal nipple retraction, and slight edema, redness, or retraction of the skin can be identified. Asymmetry of the breasts and retraction or dimpling of the skin can often be accentuated by having the patient raise her arms overhead or press her hands on her hips in order to contract the pectoralis muscles. Axillary and supraclavicular areas should be thoroughly palpated for enlarged nodes with the patient sitting (Figure 16–2). Palpation of the breast for masses or other changes

should be performed with the patient both seated and supine with the arm abducted (Figure 16–3). Some authorities recommend palpation with a rotary motion of the examiner's fingers as well as a horizontal stripping motion.

Breast cancer usually consists of a nontender, firm or hard mass with poorly delineated margins (caused by local infiltration). Slight skin or nipple retraction is an important sign. Minimal asymmetry of the breast may be noted. Very small (1–2 mm) erosions of the nipple epithelium may be the only manifestation of Paget's carcinoma. Watery, serous, or bloody discharge from the nipple is an occasional early sign but is more often associated with benign disease.

A lesion smaller than 1 cm in diameter may be difficult or impossible for the examiner to feel and yet may be discovered by the patient. She should always be asked to demonstrate the location of the mass; if the physician fails to confirm the patient's suspicions, the examination should be repeated in 2–3 months, preferably 1–2 weeks after the onset of menses. During the premenstrual phase of the cycle, increased innocuous nodularity may suggest neoplasm or may obscure an underlying lesion. If there is any question regarding the nature of an abnormality under these circumstances, the patient should be asked to return after her period. Ultrasound is often valuable and mammography essential when an area is felt by the patient to be abnormal but the physician feels no mass.

Metastases tend to involve regional lymph nodes, which may be palpable. One or two movable, nontender, not particularly firm axillary lymph nodes 5 mm or less in diameter are frequently present and are generally of no significance. Firm or hard nodes larger than 1 cm are typical of metastases. Axillary nodes that are matted or fixed to skin or deep structures indicate advanced disease (at least stage III). Microscopic metastases are present in about 30% of patients with clinically negative nodes. On the other hand, if the examiner thinks that the axillary nodes are involved, that impression will be borne out by histologic section in

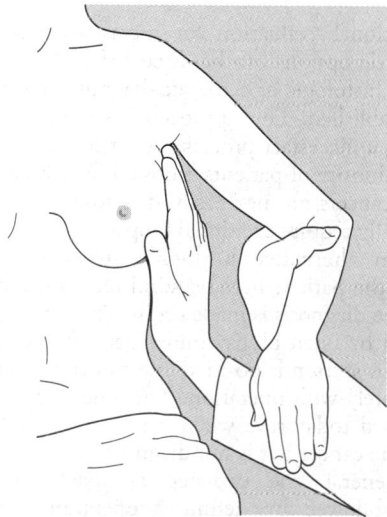

Figure 16–2. Palpation of axillary region for enlarged lymph nodes.

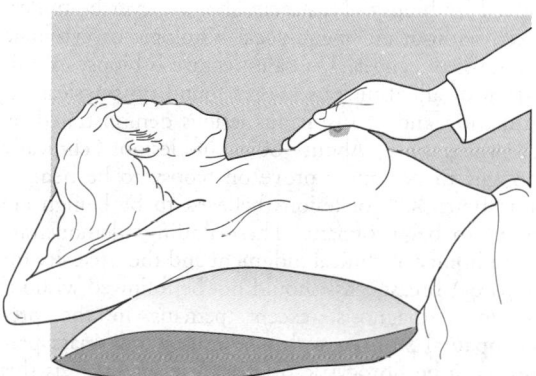

Figure 16–3. Palpation of breasts. Palpation is performed with the patient supine and arm abducted.

about 85% of cases. The incidence of positive axillary nodes increases with the size of the primary tumor. Noninvasive cancers do not metastasize.

In most cases no nodes are palpable in the supra-clavicular fossa. Firm or hard nodes of any size in this location or just beneath the clavicle are suggestive of metastatic cancer and should be biopsied. Ipsilateral supraclavicular or infraclavicular nodes containing cancer indicate that the tumor is in an advanced stage (stage IV). Edema of the ipsilateral arm, commonly caused by metastatic infiltration of regional lymphatics, is also a sign of advanced cancer.

B. Laboratory Findings

A consistently elevated sedimentation rate may be the result of disseminated cancer. Liver or bone metastases may be associated with elevation of serum alkaline phosphatase. Hypercalcemia is an occasional important finding in advanced cancer of the breast. Carcinoembryonic antigen (CEA) and CA 15-3 or CA 27–29 may be used as markers for recurrent breast cancer.

C. Imaging for Metastases

Chest x-ray may show pulmonary metastases. CT scanning of the liver and brain is of value only when metastases are suspected in these areas. Bone scans utilizing technetium Tc 99m-labeled phosphates or phosphonates are more sensitive than skeletal x-rays in detecting metastatic breast cancer. Bone scanning has not proved to be of clinical value as a routine preoperative test in the absence of symptoms, physical findings, or abnormal alkaline phosphatase or calcium levels. The frequency of abnormal findings on bone scan parallels the status of the axillary lymph nodes on pathologic examination. Positron emission tomography (PET) may prove to be an effective single scan for bone and soft tissue or visceral metastases in patients with symptoms or signs of metastatic disease.

D. Diagnostic Tests

1. Biopsy—The diagnosis of breast cancer depends ultimately upon examination of tissue or cells removed by biopsy. Treatment should never be undertaken without an unequivocal histologic or cytologic diagnosis of cancer. The safest course is biopsy examination of all suspicious masses found on physical examination and of suspicious lesions demonstrated by mammography. About 60% of lesions clinically thought to be cancer prove on biopsy to be benign, and about 30% of lesions believed to be benign are found to be malignant. These findings demonstrate the fallibility of clinical judgment and the necessity for biopsy. A breast mass should not be followed without histologic diagnosis, except perhaps in the premenopausal woman with a nonsuspicious mass presumed to be fibrocystic disease. A lesion such as this could be observed through one or two menstrual cycles. However, if the mass does not completely resolve

during this time, it must be biopsied. Figures 16–4 and 16–5 present algorithms for management of breast masses in pre- and postmenopausal patients.

The simplest method is needle biopsy, either by aspiration of tumor cells (fine-needle aspiration cytology) or by obtaining a small core of tissue with a hollow needle.

Fine-needle aspiration cytology is a useful technique whereby cells are aspirated with a small needle and examined by the pathologist. This technique can be performed easily with no morbidity and is much less expensive than excisional or open biopsy. The main disadvantages are that it requires a pathologist skilled in the cytologic diagnosis of breast cancer and that it is subject to sampling problems, particularly because deep lesions may be missed. Furthermore, noninvasive cancers usually cannot be distinguished from invasive cancers. The incidence of false-positive diagnoses is extremely low, perhaps 1–2%. The false-negative rate is as high as 10%. Most experienced clinicians would not leave a suspicious dominant mass in the breast even when fine-needle aspiration cytology is negative unless the clinical diagnosis, breast imaging studies, and cytologic studies were all in agreement.

Large-needle (core needle) biopsy removes a core of tissue with a large cutting needle. Hand-held biopsy devices make large-core needle biopsy of a palpable mass easy and cost-effective in the office with local anesthesia. As in the case of any needle biopsy, the main problem is sampling error due to improper positioning of the needle, giving rise to a false-negative test result.

Open biopsy under local anesthesia as a separate procedure prior to deciding upon definitive treatment is the most reliable means of diagnosis. Needle biopsy or aspiration, when positive, offers a more rapid approach with less expense and morbidity, but when nondiagnostic it must be followed by excisional biopsy.

Additional evaluation for metastatic disease and therapeutic options can be discussed with the patient after the histologic or cytologic diagnosis of cancer has been established. This approach has the advantage of avoiding unnecessary procedures, since cancer is found in the minority of patients biopsied for a breast lump. In situ cancers are not easily diagnosed cytologically and usually require excisional biopsy.

As an alternative in highly suspicious circumstances, the patient may be admitted to the hospital, where the diagnosis is made on frozen section of tissue obtained by open biopsy under general anesthesia. If the frozen section is positive, the surgeon can proceed immediately with operation. This one-step method is rarely used today save when cytologic study has suggested the cancer but is not diagnostic.

In general, the two-step approach—outpatient biopsy followed by definitive operation at a later date—is preferred in the diagnosis and treatment of breast cancer, because patients can be given time to

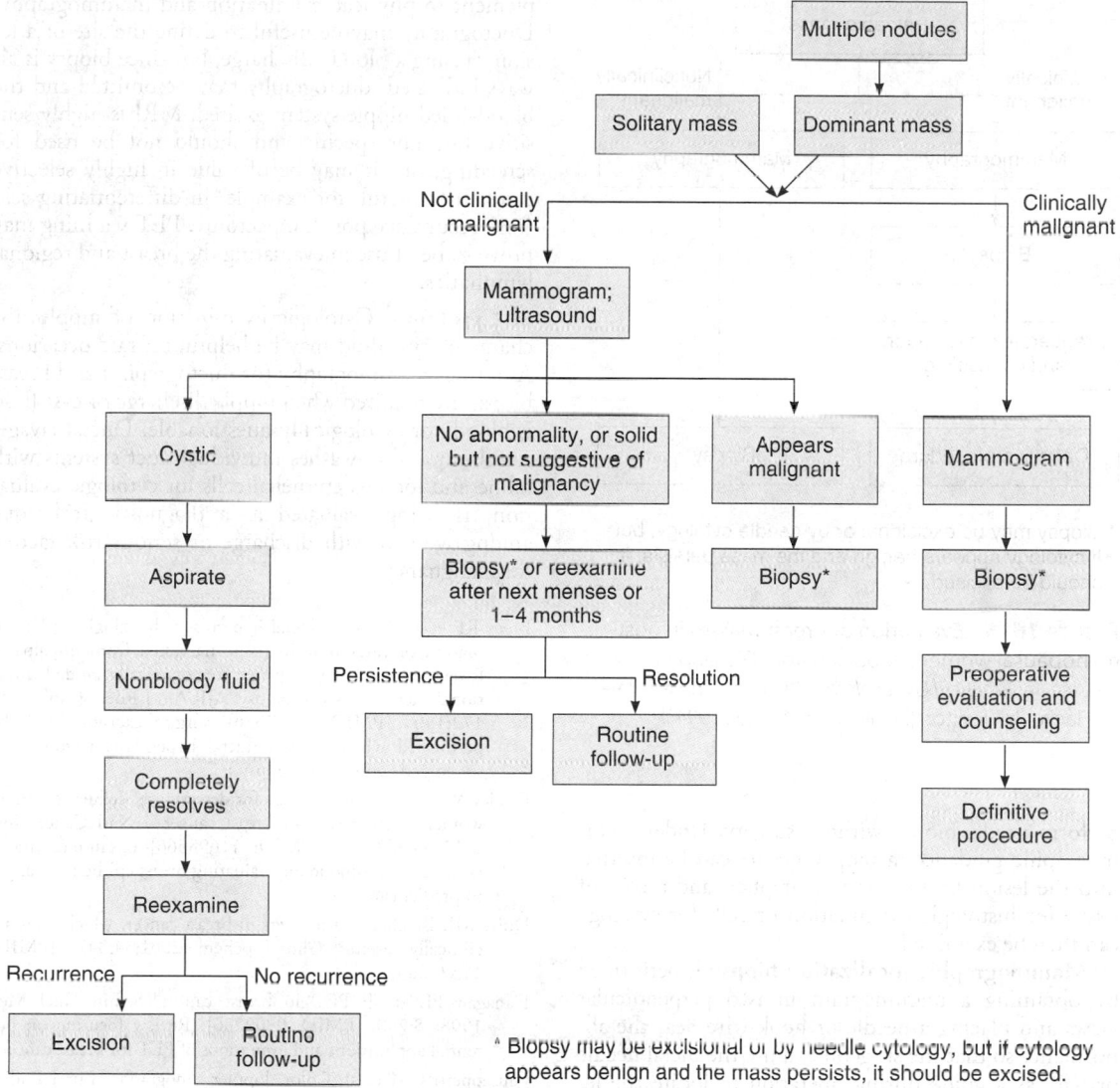

Figure 16–4. Evaluation of breast masses in premenopausal women. (Modified from Giuliano AE: Breast disease. In: *Practical Gynecologic Oncology*, 2nd ed. Berek JS, Hacker NF [editors]. Williams & Wilkins, 1994.)

adjust to the diagnosis of cancer, can consider alternative forms of therapy, and can seek a second opinion if they wish. There is no adverse effect from the short (1–2 weeks) delay of the two-step procedure, and this is the current recommendation of the National Cancer Institute.

2. Ultrasonography—Ultrasonography is performed chiefly to differentiate cystic from solid lesions. Though not diagnostic, ultrasound may reveal features highly suggestive of malignancy such as irregular margins on a new solid mass. Ultrasonography may show an irregular mass within a cyst in the rare case of intracystic carcinoma. If a tumor is palpable and feels like a cyst, an 18-gauge needle can be used to aspirate the

fluid and make the diagnosis of cyst. If a cyst is aspirated and the fluid is nonbloody, it does not have to be examined cytologically. If the mass does not recur, no further diagnostic test is necessary. Nonpalpable mammographic densities that appear benign should be investigated with ultrasound to determine whether the lesion is cystic or solid. These may even be needle-biopsied with ultrasound guidance.

3. Mammography—When a suspicious abnormality is identified by mammography alone and cannot be palpated by the clinician, the lesion should be biopsied by **computerized stereotactic guided core needle** technique. These units have been added to mammographic suites in order to localize abnormalities and

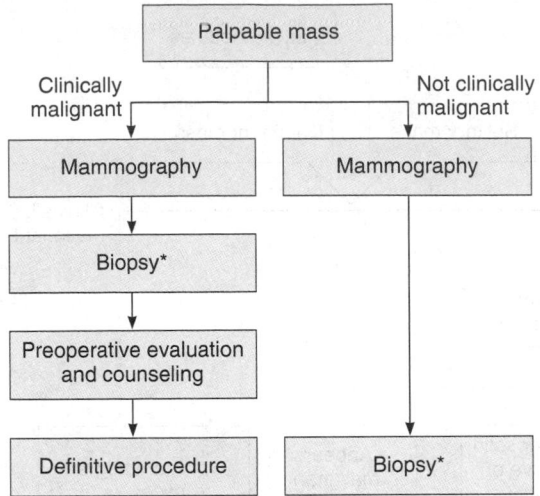

* Biopsy may be excisional or by needle cytology, but if cytology appears benign and the mass persists, it should be excised.

Figure 16–5. Evaluation of breast masses in post-menopausal women. (Modified from Giuliano AE: Breast disease. In: *Practical Gynecologic Oncology,* 2nd ed. Berek JS, Hacker NF [editors]. Williams & Wilkins, 1994.)

perform needle biopsy without surgery. Under mammographic guidance, a biopsy needle can be inserted into the lesion by the mammographer, and a core of tissue for histologic examination or cells for cytology can then be examined.

Mammographic localization biopsy is performed by obtaining a mammogram in two perpendicular views and placing a needle or hook-wire near the abnormality so that the surgeon can use the metal needle or wire as a guide during operation to locate the lesion. After mammography confirms the position of the needle in relation to the lesion, an incision is made and the subcutaneous tissue is dissected until the needle is identified. Using the films as a guide, the abnormality can then be localized and excised. It often happens that the abnormality cannot even be palpated through the incision—this is the case with microcalcifications—and thus it is essential to obtain a mammogram of the specimen to document that the lesion was excised. At that time, a second marker needle can further localize the lesion for the pathologist. Stereotactic core needle biopsies have proved equivalent to mammographic localization biopsies. Core biopsy is preferable to mammographic localization for accessible lesions.

4. Other imaging modalities—Other modalities of breast imaging have been investigated. Automated breast ultrasonography is useful in distinguishing cystic from solid lesions but should be used only as a sup-

plement to physical examination and mammography. Ductography may be useful to define the site of a lesion causing a bloody discharge, but since biopsy is always indicated, ductography may be omitted and the blood-filled nipple system excised. MRI is highly sensitive but not specific and should not be used for screening, but it may be of value in highly selective cases. It is useful, for example, in differentiating scar from recurrence post lumpectomy. PET scanning may prove to be of use in evaluating the breast and regional lymphatics.

5. Cytology—Cytologic examination of nipple discharge or cyst fluid may be helpful on rare occasions. As a rule, mammography (or ductography) and breast biopsy are required when nipple discharge or cyst fluid is bloody or cytologically questionable. Ductal lavage, a technique that washes individual duct systems with saline and loosens epithelial cells for cytologic evaluation, is being evaluated as a diagnostic technique among women with discharge or serious risk factors for malignancy.

Brem RF et al: Atypical ductal hyperplasia: histologic underestimation of carcinoma in tissue harvested from impalpable breast lesions using 11-gauge stereotactically guided directional vacuum-assisted biopsy. AJR Am J Roentgenol 1999; 172:1405. [PMID: 10227526] (Surgical excision should be performed when atypical ductal hyperplasia is found on stereotactic core breast biopsy.)

Dooley WC et al: Ductal lavage for detection of cellular atypia in women at high risk for breast cancer. J Natl Cancer Inst 2001;93:1624-32. [PMID: 11698566] (Examines ductal lavage as a technique for evaluating breast epithelial changes to predict cancer.)

Duffy MJ: Biochemical markers in breast cancer: which ones are clinically useful? Clin Biochem 2001;34:347. [PMID: 11522269]

Flanagan FL et al: PET in breast cancer. Semin Nucl Med 1998;28:290. [PMID: 9800236] (Review focusing on potential applications and limitations of PET for breast cancer.)

Giuseppetti GM et al: Color doppler sonography. Eur J Radiol 1998;27(Suppl 2):S254. [PMID: 9652531] (Doppler sonography may be a useful adjunct to mammography and sonography in the differential diagnosis of breast nodules.)

Olson J et al: Magnetic resonance imaging facilitates breast conservation for occult breast cancer. Ann Surg Oncol 2000; 7:411. [PMID: 10894136]

Shen K et al: Fiberoptic ductoscopy for patients with nipple discharge. Cancer 2000;89:1512. [PMID: 11013365]

Tartter PI et al: Factors associated with clear biopsy margins and clear re-excision margins in breast cancer specimens from candidates for breast conservation. J Am Coll Surg 1997; 185:268. [PMID: 9291405] (Clear margins facilitated by small tumor size and preoperative diagnosis by FNA.)

DIFFERENTIAL DIAGNOSIS

The lesions to be considered most often in the differential diagnosis of breast cancer are the following, in descending order of frequency: mammary dysplasia (cystic disease of the breast), fibroadenoma, intraductal papilloma, lipoma, and fat necrosis.

Table 16–2. TNM staging for breast cancer.[1]

Stage	T	N	M
0	Tis	N0	M0
I	T1	N0	M0
IIA	T0	N1	M0
	T1	N1	M0
	T2	N0	M0
IIB	T2	N1	M0
	T3	N0	M0
IIIA	T0	N2	M0
	T1	N2	M0
	T2	N2	M0
	T3	N1, N2	M0
IIIB	T4	Any N	M0
	Any T	N3	M0
IV	Any T	Any N	M1

Tumor Size (T)	
TX	Primary tumor cannot be assessed.
T0	No evidence of primary tumor.
Tis	Carcinoma in situ; intraductal carcinoma, lobular carcinoma in situ, or Paget's disease of the nipple with no tumor.
T1	Tumor 2 cm or less in greatest dimension.
T1mic	Microinvasion 0.1 cm or less in greatest dimension
T1a	Tumor more than 0.1 cm but not more than 0.5 cm in greatest dimension.
T1b	Tumor more than 0.5 cm but not more than 1 cm in greatest dimension.
T1c	Tumor more than 1 cm but not more than 2 cm in greatest dimension.
T2	Tumor more than 2 cm but not more than 5 cm in greatest dimension.
T3	Tumor more than 5 cm in greatest dimension.
T4	Tumor of any size with direct extension to (a) chest wall or (b) skin, only as described below.
T4a	Extension to chest wall.
T4b	Edema (including peau d'orange) or ulceration of the skin of the breast or satellite nodules confined to the same breast.
T4c	Both (T4a and T4b).
T4d	Inflammatory carcinoma (see text).

Regional Lymph Nodes (N)	
NX	Regional lymph nodes cannot be assessed (eg, previously removed).
N0	No regional lymph node metastasis.

(continued)

Regional Lymph Nodes (N) (cont.)	
N1	Metastasis to movable ipsilateral axillary lymph node(s).
N2	Metastasis to ipsilateral axillary lymph node(s) fixed to one another or to other structures.
N3	Metastasis to ipsilateral internal mammary lymph node(s).

Distant Metastases (M)	
MX	Presence of distant metastasis cannot be assessed.
M0	No distant metastasis
M1	Distant metastasis (includes metastasis to ipsilateral supraclavicular lymph node[s]).

[1]From: *AJCC Cancer Staging Manual,* 5th ed. Lippincott-Raven, 1997.

STAGING

Currently, the American Joint Committee on Cancer and the International Union Against Cancer have agreed on a TNM (tumor, regional lymph nodes, distant metastases) staging system for breast cancer. The use of this uniform TNM staging system will enhance communication between investigators and clinicians. Table 16–2 sets forth the TNM classification.

PATHOLOGIC TYPES

Numerous pathologic subtypes of breast cancer can be identified histologically (Table 16–3). These types are distinguished by the histologic appearance and growth pattern of the tumor. In general, breast cancer arises either from the epithelial lining of the large or intermediate-sized ducts (ductal) or from the epithelium of

Table 16–3. Histologic types of breast cancer.

Type	Frequency of Occurrence
Infiltrating ductal (not otherwise specified)	80–90%
Medullary	5–8%
Colloid (mucinous)	2–4%
Tubular	1–2%
Papillary	1–2%
Invasive lobular	6–8%
Noninvasive	4–6%
Intraductal	2–3%
Lobular in situ	2–3%
Rare cancers	< 1%
Juvenile (secretory)	
Adenoid cystic	
Epidermoid	
Sudoriferous	

the terminal ducts of the lobules (lobular). The cancer may be invasive or in situ. Most breast cancers arise from the intermediate ducts and are invasive (invasive ductal, infiltrating ductal), and most histologic types are merely subtypes of invasive ductal cancer with unusual growth patterns (colloid, medullary, scirrhous, etc). Ductal carcinoma that has not invaded the extraductal tissue is intraductal or in situ ductal. Lobular carcinoma may be either invasive or in situ.

Except for the in situ cancers, the histologic subtypes have only a slight bearing on prognosis when outcomes are compared after accurate staging. Various histologic parameters, such as invasion of blood vessels, tumor differentiation, invasion of breast lymphatics, and tumor necrosis have been examined, but they too seem to have little prognostic value.

The noninvasive cancers by definition are confined by the basement membrane of the ducts and lack the ability to spread. However, in patients whose biopsies show noninvasive intraductal cancer, associated invasive ductal cancers metastasize to lymph nodes in about 1–3% of cases. Lobular carcinoma in situ (LCIS) is a premalignant lesion that is not a true cancer but is a risk factor associated with subsequent development of invasive cancer in at least 20% of cases.

SPECIAL CLINICAL FORMS OF BREAST CANCER

Paget's Carcinoma

The basic lesion is usually an infiltrating ductal carcinoma, usually well differentiated, or a ductal carcinoma in situ (DCIS). The ducts of the nipple epithelium are infiltrated, but gross nipple changes are often minimal, and a tumor mass may not be palpable. The first symptom is often itching or burning of the nipple, with superficial erosion or ulceration. The diagnosis is established by biopsy of the erosion.

Paget's carcinoma is not common (about 1% of all breast cancers), but it is important because the nipple changes appear innocuous. These are frequently diagnosed and treated as dermatitis or bacterial infection, leading to delay in detection. When the lesion consists of nipple changes only, the incidence of axillary metastases is less than 5%, and the prognosis is excellent. When a breast mass is also present, the incidence of axillary metastases rises, with an associated marked decrease in prospects for cure by surgical or other treatment.

Inflammatory Carcinoma

This is the most malignant form of breast cancer and constitutes less than 3% of all cases. The clinical findings consist of a rapidly growing, sometimes painful mass that enlarges the breast. The overlying skin becomes erythematous, edematous, and warm. Often there is no distinct mass, since the tumor infiltrates the involved breast diffusely. The diagnosis should be made when the redness involves more than one-third of the skin over the breast and biopsy shows infiltrating carcinoma with invasion of the subdermal lymphatics. The inflammatory changes, often mistaken for an infection, are caused by carcinomatous invasion of the subdermal lymphatics, with resulting edema and hyperemia. If the physician suspects infection but the lesion does not respond rapidly (1–2 weeks) to antibiotics, biopsy is performed. Metastases tend to occur early and widely, and for this reason inflammatory carcinoma is rarely curable. Mastectomy is seldom indicated unless chemotherapy and radiation have resulted in clinical remission with no evidence of distant metastases. In these cases, residual disease in the breast may be eradicated. Radiation, hormone therapy, and chemotherapy are the measures most likely to be of value rather than operation.

Breast Cancer Occurring During Pregnancy or Lactation

Breast cancer complicates approximately one in 3000 pregnancies. The diagnosis is frequently delayed, because physiologic changes in the breast may obscure the lesion. This results in a tendency of both patients and physicians to misinterpret findings and to delay biopsy. When the cancer is confined to the breast, the 5-year survival rate after mastectomy is about 70%. Axillary metastases are already present in 60–70% of patients, and for them the 5-year survival rate after mastectomy is only 30–40%. Pregnancy (or lactation) is not a contraindication to operation, and treatment should be based on the stage of the disease as in the nonpregnant (or nonlactating) woman. Overall survival rates have improved, since cancers are now diagnosed in pregnant women earlier than in the past. Breast-conserving surgery may be performed—and radiation and chemotherapy given—even during the pregnancy.

Bilateral Breast Cancer

Clinically evident simultaneous bilateral breast cancer occurs in less than 1% of cases, but there is a 5–8% incidence of later occurrence of cancer in the second breast. Bilaterality occurs more often in familial breast cancer, in women under age 50, and when the tumor in the primary breast is lobular. The incidence of second breast cancers increases directly with the length of time the patient is alive after her first cancer—about 1% per year.

In patients with breast cancer, mammography should be performed before primary treatment and at regular intervals thereafter, to search for occult cancer in the opposite breast. Routine biopsy of the opposite breast is usually not warranted even for lobular cancer.

Noninvasive Cancer

Noninvasive cancer can occur within the ducts (ductal carcinoma in situ) or lobules (lobular carcinoma in situ). While ductal carcinoma in situ (DCIS) behaves as an early malignancy, lobular carcinoma in situ (LCIS) would perhaps better be called lobular neoplasia because it is not truly carcinoma. DCIS tends to be unilateral and most often progresses to invasive cancer if untreated. Approximately 40–60% of women who have DCIS treated with biopsy alone develop invasive cancer within the same breast. Lobular carcinoma in situ, however, appears to be a risk factor calling attention to the probability of developing invasive cancer in either breast. One in five women with lobular carcinoma in situ develop invasive cancer. This invasive cancer may occur in either breast regardless of the side of the original biopsy and is usually ductal.

The treatment of intraductal lesions is controversial. Ductal carcinoma can be treated with total mastectomy or by wide excision with or without radiation therapy. Lobular carcinoma in situ is well managed with observation, but patients unwilling to accept the increased risk of breast cancer may be offered bilateral total mastectomy. Another alternative is tamoxifen, which is effective in preventing invasive breast cancer from developing in both lobular cancer in situ and intraductal cancer in situ. Axillary metastases from in situ cancers should not occur unless there is an occult invasive cancer.

Fisher B et al: Tamoxifen in treatment of intraductal breast cancer: National Surgical Adjuvant Breast and Bowel Project B-24 randomised controlled trial. Lancet 1999;353:1993. [PMID: 10376613]

Fisher ER et al: Pathologic findings from the National Surgical Adjuvant Breast Project (NSABP) eight-year update of Protocol B-17: intraductal carcinoma. Cancer 1999;86:429. [PMID: 10430251] (Degree of comedo necrosis is sufficient for defining high and low risk for second ipsilateral breast tumor after lumpectomy; low-risk patients benefit from radiotherapy.)

Silverstein MJ et al: The influence of margin width on local control of ductal carcinoma in situ of the breast. N Engl J Med 1999;340:1455. [PMID: 10320383] (Patients with margins < 1 mm benefit from adjuvant radiotherapy; those with margins > 10 mm showed no benefit from postoperative radiotherapy.)

Turner R et al: Histopathologic validation of the sentinel node hypothesis for breast carcinoma. Ann Surg 1997;226:271. [PMID: 9339933]

Winchester DP et al: The diagnosis and management of ductal carcinoma in-situ of the breast. CA Cancer J Clin 2000; 50:184. [PMID: 10901741]

HORMONE RECEPTOR SITES

The presence or absence of estrogen and progesterone receptors in the cytoplasm of tumor cells is of paramount importance in managing patients with breast cancer. Patients whose primary tumors are receptor-positive have a more favorable course than those whose tumors are receptor-negative. Receptors are of value in determining adjuvant therapy and for treatment of advanced disease. Up to 60% of patients with metastatic breast cancer will respond to hormonal manipulation if their tumors contain estrogen receptors. Fewer than 5% of patients with metastatic, estrogen

receptor-negative tumors can be treated successfully in this fashion.

Receptor status is valuable not only in management of metastatic disease but also helps select patients for adjuvant therapy. Adjuvant hormonal therapy (tamoxifen) with receptor-positive tumors and adjuvant chemotherapy with receptor-negative tumors improve survival rates even in the absence of lymph node metastases (see Adjuvant Therapy, below).

Progesterone receptors may be a more sensitive indicator than estrogen receptors of patients who may respond to hormonal manipulation. Up to 80% of patients with metastatic progesterone receptor-positive tumors improve with hormonal manipulation. Receptors have no relationship to response to chemotherapy.

The estrogen, progesterone, and HER-2/neu receptor status and proliferative indices of the tumor should be determined at the time of initial biopsy. This is performed on paraffin-fixed tissue by immunohistochemistry. HER-2/neu assessment in breast cancer by immunohistochemistry is appropriate for patients with tumors that score 3+. Fluorescence in situ hybridization (FISH) is recommended for women with 2+ immunohistochemistry scores to more accurately assess HER-2/neu amplification and provide better prognostic information. Receptor status may change after hormonal therapy, radiotherapy, or chemotherapy.

Carmeci C et al: Analysis of estrogen receptor messenger RNA in breast carcinomas from archival specimens is predictive of tumor biology. Am J Pathol 1997;150:1563. [PMID: 9137083]

Kakar S et al: HER-2/neu assessment in breast cancer by immunohistochemistry and florescence in situ hybridization comparison of results and correlation with survival. Mol Diagn 2000;5:191. [PMID: 11070154]

Raabe NK et al: Hormone receptor measurements and survival in 1335 consecutive patients with primary invasive breast carcinoma. Int J Oncol 1998;12:1091. [PMID: 9538134] (Evaluation of relationship between ER and PR content to relapse and survival in patients without systemic adjuvant treatment.)

CURATIVE TREATMENT

Treatment may be curative or palliative. Curative treatment is advised for clinical stage I and stage II disease (Table 16–2). Patients with locally advanced (stage III) and even inflammatory tumors may be cured with multimodality therapy, but in most palliation is all that can be expected. Palliative treatment is appropriate for all patients with stage IV disease and for previously treated patients who develop distant metastases or who have unresectable local cancers.

The growth potential of tumors and host resistance factors vary widely from patient to patient and may be altered during the course of the disease. The doubling time of breast cancer cells ranges from several weeks in a rapidly growing lesion to a year in a slowly growing one. Assuming that the rate of doubling is constant and that the neoplasm originates in one cell, a carcinoma with a doubling time of 100 days may not reach clinically detectable size (1 cm) for about 8 years. Rapidly growing cancers have a much shorter preclinical course and a greater tendency to metastasize by the time a breast mass is discovered.

The long preclinical growth phase and the tendency of breast cancers to metastasize have led clinicians to believe that most breast cancer is a systemic disease at the time of diagnosis. Although it may be true that breast cancer cells are released from the tumor prior to diagnosis, variations in the host-tumor relationship prohibit the growth of disseminated disease in many patients. Clearly, not all breast cancer is systemic at the time of diagnosis. For this reason, a pessimistic attitude concerning the management of localized breast cancer is unwarranted, and many patients can be cured.

Controversy surrounds the timing of surgery with respect to the menstrual cycle. Some suggest that operation during the time of unopposed estrogen adversely affects survival, but most studies support no such effect. Several trials are currently examining this question.

Choice of Primary Therapy

The extent of disease and its biologic aggressiveness are the principal determinants of the outcome of primary therapy. Clinical and pathologic staging help in assessing extent of disease (Table 16–2), but each is to some extent imprecise. Other factors such as DNA flow cytometry, tumor grade, hormone receptor assays, and oncogene amplification may be of prognostic value but are not important in determining the type of local therapy. Since two-thirds of patients eventually manifest distant disease regardless of the form of primary therapy, there is a tendency to think of breast carcinoma as being systemic in most patients at the time of presentation.

Controversy surrounds the choice of primary therapy of stage I, II, and III breast carcinoma. A number of states require physicians to inform patients of alternative treatment methods in the management of breast cancer.

Breast-Conserving Therapy

Many nonrandomized trials, the Milan trial, and a large randomized trial conducted by the National Surgical Adjuvant Breast Project (NSABP) in the USA show that disease-free survival rates are similar for patients treated by partial mastectomy plus axillary dissection followed by radiation therapy and for those treated by modified radical mastectomy (total mastectomy plus axillary dissection). All patients whose axillary nodes contained tumor received adjuvant chemotherapy.

In the NSABP trial, patients were randomized to three treatment types: (1) "lumpectomy" (removal of the tumor with *confirmed* tumor-free margins) plus whole breast irradiation, (2) lumpectomy alone, and (3) total mastectomy. All patients underwent axillary

lymph node dissection, and some had tumors as large as 4 cm with (or without) palpable axillary lymph nodes. The lowest local recurrence rate was among patients treated with lumpectomy and postoperative irradiation; the highest—nearly 40% at 8 years of follow-up—was among patients treated with lumpectomy alone. However, no statistically significant differences were observed in overall or disease-free survival among the three treatment groups. This study shows that lumpectomy and axillary dissection with postoperative radiation therapy is as effective as modified radical mastectomy for the management of patients with stage I and stage II breast cancer.

The results of these and other trials have demonstrated that much less aggressive surgical treatment of the primary lesion than has previously been thought necessary gives equivalent therapeutic results and may preserve an acceptable cosmetic appearance.

Tumor size is a major consideration in determining the feasibility of breast conservation. The lumpectomy trial of the NSABP randomized patients with tumors as large as 4 cm. To achieve an acceptable cosmetic result, the patient must have a breast of sufficient size to enable excision of a 4 cm tumor without considerable deformity. Therefore, large size is only a relative contraindication. Subareolar tumors are also difficult to excise without deformity, but this location is not a contraindication to breast conservation. Clinically detectable multifocality is a relative contraindication to breast-conserving surgery, as is fixation to the chest wall or skin or involvement of the nipple or overlying skin. The patient and not the surgeon should be the judge of what is cosmetically acceptable.

Axillary dissection is valuable in preventing axillary recurrences, in staging cancer, and in planning therapy. Intraoperative lymphatic mapping and sentinel node dissection identify lymph nodes most likely to harbor metastases if they are present in the axillary nodes. Numerous studies have confirmed the validity of this technique. Ongoing trials are examining the replacement of formal axillary dissection with sentinel node dissection. Results to date suggest that sentinel node biopsy may replace axillary dissection for staging and treatment in histopathologically node-negative women. A trial by the American College of Surgeons Oncology Group is examining the role of sentinel node dissection without axillary dissection for node-positive women. Bone marrow biopsy with examination by immunocytochemistry to detect early metastases may be as sensitive a staging procedure as axillary dissection and may identify patients at high risk for disseminating disease.

Recommendations

Earlier consensus held that breast-conserving surgery with radiation was the preferred form of treatment for patients with early-stage breast cancer. Despite the numerous randomized trials showing no survival benefit of mastectomy over breast-conserving partial mastectomy and irradiation, breast-conserving surgery appears underutilized and mastectomy remains the more common treatment. About 25% of patients in the United States with stage I or stage II breast cancer are treated with breast-conserving surgery and radiation therapy, compared with 75% treated with mastectomy. Use of breast-conserving surgery and radiation therapy varies by region of the country, ranging from 15% in the South Central United States to 30% in the Pacific Region.

Modified radical mastectomy (total mastectomy plus axillary lymph node dissection) has been the standard therapy for most patients with breast cancer. This operation removes the entire breast, overlying skin, nipple, and areolar complex as well as the underlying pectoralis fascia with the axillary lymph nodes in continuity. The major advantage of modified radical mastectomy is that radiation therapy is usually not necessary. The disadvantage, of course, is the psychologic trauma associated with breast loss. Radical mastectomy, which removes the underlying pectoralis muscle, should be performed rarely if at all. Axillary node dissection is not indicated for noninfiltrating cancers, because nodal metastases are rarely present. At an international consensus conference in Philadelphia in April 2001, participants recommended sentinel node biopsy as an alternative to axillary dissection in selected patients with invasive cancer. Radiotherapy after partial mastectomy consists of 5–6 weeks of five daily fractions to a total dose of 5000–6000 cGy. Some radiotherapists use a boost dose. Current studies suggest that radiotherapy after mastectomy may improve survival.

Preoperatively, full discussion with the patient regarding the rationale for operation and various alternative forms of treatment is essential. Breast-conserving surgery and radiation should be offered whenever possible, since most patients would prefer to save the breast. Breast reconstruction should be discussed with patients who choose or require mastectomy, and the option of simultaneous mastectomy with immediate reconstruction added. Time spent preoperatively in educating the patient and her family about these matters is well spent.

Adjuvant Systemic Therapy

Following surgery and radiation therapy, chemotherapy or hormonal therapy is advocated for most patients with curable breast cancer. The objective of adjuvant systemic therapy is to eliminate the occult metastases responsible for late recurrences while they are microscopic and most vulnerable to anticancer agents. In addition, adjuvant chemotherapy may decrease local recurrence in patients treated with breast conservation, and adjuvant tamoxifen decreases contralateral breast cancer occurrence.

Numerous clinical trials with various adjuvant chemotherapeutic regimens have been completed. The most extensive clinical experience is with the CMF (cyclophosphamide, methotrexate, and fluorouracil) regimen. Cyclophosphamide can be given either orally, in a dose of 100 mg/m² daily for 14 days; or intravenously, in a dose of 600 mg/m² on days 1 and 8. Methotrexate is given intravenously, 40 mg/m² on days 1 and 8; and fluorouracil is given intravenously, 600 mg/m² on days 1 and 8. This cycle is repeated every 4 weeks. Some clinicians prefer to give the drugs on 1 day only every 3 weeks. There appears to be no obvious advantage except that patient compliance is assured when the cyclophosphamide is given intravenously. The regimen is continued for 6 months in patients with axillary metastases. Premenopausal women with positive axillary nodes benefit from adjuvant chemotherapy. The recurrence rate in premenopausal patients who received no adjuvant chemotherapy is more than 1.5 times that of those who received such therapy. No therapeutic effect with CMF has been shown in postmenopausal women with positive nodes, perhaps because therapy was modified so often in response to side effects that the total amount of drugs administered was less than planned. Other trials with different agents support the value of adjuvant chemotherapy in postmenopausal women. There are many forms of combination chemotherapy that are effective. Most are variations of CMF or AC (Adriamycin [doxorubicin] plus cyclophosphamide). The addition of taxanes (docetaxel, paclitaxel) to AC improved survival in node-positive women.

Selection of patients to receive chemotherapy must take into account common health problems in older women and the effects of chemotherapy on the patient's overall health. Tamoxifen can be given with few side effects even in the elderly. It appears to increase bone density and favorably affect lipid and lipoprotein profiles, which may explain the observed decreased mortality rate from coronary artery disease seen in patients taking tamoxifen.

The addition of hormonal therapy, usually with tamoxifen, may improve the results of adjuvant therapy. It also has been shown to enhance the beneficial effects of melphalan and fluorouracil in postmenopausal women whose tumors are estrogen receptor (ER)-positive. Tamoxifen alone in a dosage of 10 mg orally twice a day has long been the recommended treatment for postmenopausal women with ER-positive tumors. Finally, an NSABP trial showed that tamoxifen plus chemotherapy (Adriamycin [doxorubicin] plus cyclophosphamide [AC] or prednisone plus Adriamycin plus fluorouracil [PAF]) lowered recurrence rates more than tamoxifen alone in postmenopausal women with ER-positive tumors.

The length of time adjuvant therapy must be administered remains uncertain. Shorter treatment periods may be as effective as longer ones. For example, one study compared 6 versus 12 cycles of postoperative CMF and found 5-year disease-free survival rates to be comparable. One of the earliest adjuvant trials used a 6-day perioperative regimen of intravenous cyclophosphamide alone; follow-up at 15 years shows a 15% improvement in disease-free survival rates for treated patients, suggesting that short-term therapy may be effective. An NSABP study shows that 5 years of treatment with tamoxifen may be superior to 10 years.

Several studies of adjuvant therapy in node-negative women reveal a beneficial effect of adjuvant chemotherapy or tamoxifen in delaying recurrence and improving survival. A number of protocols, including CMF with leucovorin rescue as well as tamoxifen alone, have increased disease-free survival. The magnitude of this improvement is about one-third, ie, a group of women with an estimated 30% recurrence rate would have a 20% recurrence rate after adjuvant systemic therapy. Quality of life while receiving chemotherapy does not appear to be greatly altered.

An NIH consensus conference has reexamined the standards for adjuvant therapy of breast cancer. Since the last conference on this topic in 1990, the long-term advantage of systemic therapy has been further established. In the last 10 years, no new prognostic factors have been validated to aid in the selection of patients for adjuvant treatment. Its use should be based on the patient's age; on the size, histopathologic grade, and hormone receptor status of the breast tumor; and on the status of the regional lymph nodes. The value of HER-2/*neu*, *P53*, angiogenesis factors, and vascular invasion are being investigated but as yet are not proven prognostic factors. However, patients whose tumors overexpress HER-2/*neu* are being treated with trastuzumab even though studies evaluating this drug in the adjuvant setting have not been completed. The panel concluded that regardless of other factors, adjuvant systemic chemotherapy with drug combinations improves survival and should be used for most women who have potentially curable breast cancer. The use of anthracyclines is superior to combinations without anthracyclines. Tamoxifen should be used as a systemic agent in all women whose tumors are hormone receptor-positive—regardless of age, menopausal status, or other prognostic factors. HER-2-*neu* status should not affect the choice of agents or the use of hormone therapy. Ovarian ablation in premenopausal patients with estrogen receptor-positive tumors may produce a benefit similar to that of adjuvant systemic chemotherapy. Taxanes have demonstrated benefit in patients with metastatic cancer but have not yet proved to be of value in node-negative patients. Adjuvant systemic therapy should not be given to women who have small node-negative breast cancers with favorable histologic subtypes, such as mucinous or tubular carcinoma.

In practice, most medical oncologists are currently using systemic adjuvant therapy for patients with node-negative and node-positive breast cancer. Other prognostic factors being used to determine the patient's risks are tumor size, estrogen and progesterone receptor status, nuclear grade, histologic type, proliferative rate, and oncogene expression (Table 16–4). The assumption is made that all patients with node-negative aggressive tumors should receive adjuvant therapy

Table 16–4. Prognostic factors in node-negative breast cancer.

Prognostic Factor	Increased Recurrence	Decreased Recurrence
Size	T3, T2	T1, T0
Hormone receptors	Negative	Positive
DNA flow cytometry	Aneuploid	Diploid
Histologic grade	High	Low
Tumor labeling index	< 3%	> 3%
S phase fraction	> 5%	< 5%
Lymphatic or vascular invasion	Present	Absent
Cathepsin D	High	Low
HER-2/*neu* oncogene	High	Low
Epidermal growth factor receptor	High	Low

save those who have serious coexistent medical problems. Few patients cannot tolerate at least tamoxifen. The use of chemotherapy prior to resection of the primary tumor has also been examined. This "neoadjuvant" chemotherapy enables the assessment of in vivo chemosensitivity. A complete tumor response in vivo prior to operation appears to be associated with improvement in survival. Neoadjuvant chemotherapy also permits breast conservation by shrinking the primary tumor in women who would otherwise need mastectomy for local control.

Important questions remaining to be answered are the timing and duration of adjuvant chemotherapy, which chemotherapeutic agents should be applied for which subgroups of patients, how best to coordinate adjuvant chemotherapy with postoperative radiation therapy, the use of combinations of hormonal therapy and chemotherapy, and the value of prognostic factors other than hormone receptors in predicting response to adjuvant therapy. Adjuvant systemic therapy is not generally used in patients with small tumors and those with negative lymph nodes who have favorable tumor markers. A small disease-free survival benefit even in patients with small favorable tumors has been suggested. It appears that adjuvant systemic therapy benefits all breast cancer patients, but the clinician must decide if the benefits outweigh the risks, complications, and expense.

Abrams JS: Adjuvant therapy for breast cancer—results from the USA Consensus Conference. Breast Cancer 2001;8:298. [PMID: 11791121] (Results of the NCI Consensus Conference on adjuvant therapy for breast cancer.)

Adjuvant systemic therapy for women with node-negative breast cancer. The Steering Committee on Clinical Practice Guidelines for the Care and Treatment of Breast Cancer. Can Med Assoc J 1998;10:158. [PMID: 9484288]

Adjuvant systemic therapy for women with node-positive breast cancer. The Steering Committee on Clinical Practice Guidelines for the Care and Treatment of Breast Cancer. Can Med Assoc J 1998;10(Suppl):S52. [PMID: 9484279]

Adjuvant therapy for breast cancer. NIH Consensus Statement 2000 November 1 3;17:1–23.

Aebi S et al: Is chemotherapy alone adequate for young women with oestrogen-receptor-positive breast cancer? Lancet 2000;355:1869. [PMID: 10866443]

Borden EC et al: Biological therapies for breast carcinoma: concepts for improvements in survival. Semin Oncol 1999;26(4 Suppl 12):28. [PMID: 10482192] (Review of recent clinical and preclinical research in immune and cytotoxic cancer therapies.)

Braun S et al: Cytokeratin-positive cells in the bone marrow and survival of patients with stage I, II, or III breast cancer. N Engl J Med 2000;342:525. [PMID: 10684910] (Presence of occult metastatic cells in bone marrow indicates increased risk of relapse in breast cancer patients.)

Cady B et al: The surgeon's role in outcome in contemporary breast cancer. Surg Oncol Clin N Am 2000;9:119. [PMID: 10601528]

Favourable and unfavourable effects on long-term survival of radiotherapy for early breast cancer: an overview of the randomised trials. Early Breast Cancer Trialists' Collaborative Group. Lancet 2000;355:1757. [PMID: 10832826]

Fisher B et al: Findings from recent national surgical adjuvant breast and bowel project adjuvant studies in Stage I breast cancer. J Natl Cancer Inst Monogr 2001;30:62. [PMID: 11773294] (This article summarizes the NSABP randomized trials with adjuvant systemic therapy for early breast cancer.)

Giuliano AE et al: Sentinel lymphadenectomy in breast cancer. J Clin Oncol 1997;15:2345. [PMID: 9196149] (SLND with frozen section and immunohistochemical staining is minimally invasive and an accurate method of intraoperative axillary staging.)

Giuliano AE et al: Prospective observational study of sentinel lymphadenectomy without further axillary dissection in patients with sentinel node-negative breast cancer. J Clin Oncol 2000;18(13):2553. [PMID: 10893286] (This is the first trial using sentinel node biopsy instead of axillary node dissection in clinically node-negative patients.)

Goldhirsch A et al: Meeting Highlights: International consensus panel on the treatment of primary breast cancer. J Clin Oncol 2001;19:3817. [PMID: 11559719] (Results of an international consensus panel on adjuvant systemic therapy.)

Ingle JN: Current status of adjuvant endocrine therapy for breast cancer. Clin Cancer Res. 2001;7:4392. [PMID: 11916230] (This article summarizes the value of adjuvant hormonal therapy in breast cancer and emphasizes the use of third generation aromatase inhibitors.)

Jordan VC: Tamoxifen: A personal retrospective. Lancet Oncol 2000;1:43. [PMID: 11905688] (The development and use of tamoxifen and some of the newer SERMS.)

Keleher AJ et al: Multi-disciplinary management of breast cancer concurrent with pregnancy. J Am Coll Surg 2002;194:54. [PMID: 11800340]

Krag D et al: The sentinel node in breast cancer—a multicenter validation study. N Engl J Med 1998;339:941. [PMID: 9753708] (Sentinel node biopsy is predictive of axillary lymph node metastasis in breast cancer patients.)

Lazovich D et al. Breast conservation therapy in the United States following the 1990 National Institutes of Health Consensus Development Conference on the treatment of patients with early stage invasive breast carcinoma. Cancer 1999;86:628. [PMID: 10440690]

Margolese RG: Surgical considerations for invasive breast cancer. Surg Clin North Am 1999;79:1031. [PMID: 10572549] (Discussion of when breast-conserving surgery is and is not appropriate based on review of clinical data.)

Mehta K et al: Long-term outcome in patients with four or more positive lymph nodes treated with conservative surgery and radiation therapy. Int J Radiat Oncol Biol Phys 1996;35:679. [PMID: 8690633] (For patients with four or more positive axillary lymph nodes, breast conserving surgery, radiotherapy to the breast, and adjuvant systemic therapy yield reasonable long-term survival with a high rate of local regional control.)

Munster PN et al: Tamoxifen versus the aromatase inhibitors: News from San Antonio, 2001. Cancer Control 2001;8:478. [PMID: 11807416]

Ramirez AJ et al: Do patients with advanced breast cancer benefit from chemotherapy? Br J Cancer 1998;78:1488. [PMID: 9836482] (Advanced breast cancer patients benefit from six cycles of first-line palliative treatment; factors predicting treatment failure or negative treatment outcomes are identified.)

Touboul E et al: Local recurrences and distant metastases after breast-conserving surgery and radiation therapy for early stage breast cancer. Int J Radiat Oncol Biol Phys 1999;43:25. [PMID: 9989511] (Different factors predict local and metastatic recurrence.)

Zurrida S et al: Timing of breast cancer surgery in relation to the menstrual cycle: an update of developments. Crit Rev Oncol Hematol 2001;38:223. [PMID: 11369255] (This study shows the timing of surgery with respect to the menstrual cycle does affect prognosis.)

PALLIATIVE TREATMENT

This section covers palliative therapy of disseminated disease incurable by surgery (stage IV).

Radiotherapy

Palliative radiotherapy may be advised for locally advanced cancers with distant metastases in order to control ulceration, pain, and other manifestations in the breast and regional nodes. Irradiation of the breast and chest wall and the axillary, internal mammary, and supraclavicular nodes should be undertaken in an attempt to cure locally advanced and inoperable lesions when there is no evidence of distant metastases. A small number of patients in this group are cured in spite of extensive breast and regional node involvement. Neoadjuvant chemotherapy should be considered for such patients.

Palliative irradiation is of value also in the treatment of certain bone or soft tissue metastases to control pain or avoid fracture. Radiotherapy is especially useful in the treatment of isolated bony metastasis, chest wall recurrences, brain metastases, and acute spinal cord compression.

Hormone Therapy

Disseminated disease may shrink—or grow less rapidly—after endocrine therapy such as administration of hormones (eg, estrogens, androgens, progestins; see Table 16–5); ablation of the ovaries, adrenals, or pituitary; or administration of drugs that block hormone receptor sites (eg, antiestrogens) or drugs that block the synthesis of hormones (eg, aminoglutethimide). Hormonal manipulation is usually more successful in postmenopausal women even if they have received estrogen replacement therapy. If treatment is based on the presence of estrogen receptor protein in the primary tumor or metastases, however, the rate of response is nearly equal in premenopausal and postmenopausal women. A favorable response to hormonal manipulation occurs in about one-third of patients with metastatic breast cancer. Of those whose tumors contain estrogen receptors, the response is about 60% and perhaps as high as 80% for patients whose tumors contain progesterone receptors as well. Because only 5–10% of women whose tumors do not contain estrogen receptors respond, they should not receive hormonal therapy except in unusual circumstances, eg, in an older patient who cannot tolerate chemotherapy.

Since the quality of life during a remission induced by endocrine manipulation is usually superior to a remission following cytotoxic chemotherapy, it is usually best to try endocrine manipulation first in cases where the estrogen receptor status is unknown. When receptor status is unknown but the disease is progressing rapidly or involves visceral organs, however, endocrine therapy is rarely successful, and introducing it may waste valuable time.

In general, only one type of therapy should be given at a time unless it is necessary to irradiate a destructive lesion of weight-bearing bone while the patient is on another regimen. The regimen should be changed only if the disease is clearly progressing. This is especially important for patients with destructive bone metastases, since changes in the status of these lesions are difficult to determine radiographically. A plan of therapy that would simultaneously minimize toxicity and maximize benefits is often best achieved by hormonal manipulation.

The choice of endocrine therapy depends on the menopausal status of the patient. Women within 1 year of their last menstrual period are considered to be premenopausal, while women whose menstruation ceased more than a year ago are postmenopausal. If endocrine therapy is the initial choice, it is referred to as primary hormonal manipulation; subsequent endocrine treatment is called secondary or tertiary hormonal manipulation.

A. The Premenopausal Patient

1. Primary hormonal therapy—The potent antiestrogen tamoxifen is the endocrine treatment of choice in the premenopausal patient. Tamoxifen is usually given orally in a dose of 20 mg daily. There is no significant difference in survival or response between tamoxifen therapy and bilateral oophorectomy. Tamoxifen is by far the most common and preferred method of hormonal manipulation for both pre- and postmenopausal women. The average remission is about 12 months. Tamoxifen can be given with little morbidity and few side effects. Controversy continues about whether a response to tamoxifen is predictive of probable success with other forms of endocrine manipulation. A new tamoxifen analog, toremifene, appears as effective as tamoxifen as primary hormonal therapy.

Bilateral oophorectomy is less desirable than primary hormonal manipulation in premenopausal women because tamoxifen is so well tolerated. Oophorectomy can be achieved rapidly and safely by surgery, however, or, if the patient is a poor operative risk, by irradiation of the ovaries. Ovarian radiation therapy should be avoided in otherwise healthy patients because of the high rate of complications and the longer time necessary to achieve results. Chemical ovarian ablation using a GnRH analog can also be utilized. Oophorectomy presumably works by eliminating estrogens, progestins, and androgens, which stimulate growth of the tumor.

2. Secondary or tertiary hormonal therapy—Although patients who do not respond to tamoxifen or oophorectomy should be treated with cytotoxic drugs, those who respond and then relapse may subsequently respond to another form of endocrine treatment

Table 16–5. Agents commonly used for hormonal management of metastatic breast cancer.

Drug	Action	Usual Oral Dose	Major Side Effects
Tamoxifen (Nolvadex)	Antiestrogen	10 mg twice daily	Hot flushes, uterine bleeding, thrombophlebitis, rash
Diethylstilbestrol (DES)	Estrogen	5 mg three times daily	Fluid retention, uterine bleeding, thrombophlebitis, nausea
Megestrol acetate (Megace)	Progestin	40 mg four times daily	Fluid retention
Aminoglutethimide (Cytadren)[1]	Aromatase inhibitor	250 mg four times daily	Adrenal suppression, skin rashes, neurologic reactions

[1]Used with hydrocortisone.

(Table 16–5). The initial choice for secondary endocrine manipulation has not been clearly defined.

Patients who improve after oophorectomy but subsequently relapse should receive tamoxifen. If tamoxifen fails, aminoglutethimide or megestrol acetate should be considered. Aminoglutethimide is an inhibitor of adrenal hormone synthesis and, when combined with a corticosteroid, provides a therapeutically effective "medical adrenalectomy." Megestrol is a progestational agent. Both drugs cause less morbidity and mortality than surgical adrenalectomy; can be discontinued once the patient improves; and are not associated with the many problems of postsurgical hypoadrenalism, so that patients who require chemotherapy are more easily managed. Adrenalectomy or hypophysectomy induces regression in 30–50% of patients who have previously responded to oophorectomy. Pharmacologic hormonal manipulation has in large part replaced these invasive procedures. Toremifene is not likely to be of value in women whose tumors no longer respond to tamoxifen.

B. THE POSTMENOPAUSAL PATIENT

1. Primary hormonal therapy—Tamoxifen, 20 mg daily, is the initial therapy of choice for postmenopausal women with metastatic breast cancer amenable to endocrine manipulation. It has fewer side effects than diethylstilbestrol, the former therapy of choice, and is equally as effective. The main side effects of tamoxifen are nausea, vomiting, and skin rash. Rarely, it may induce hypercalcemia in patients with bony metastases.

2. Secondary or tertiary hormonal therapy—Postmenopausal patients who do not respond to tamoxifen should be given cytotoxic drugs such as cyclophosphamide, methotrexate, and fluorouracil (CMF) or Adriamycin (doxorubicin) and cyclophosphamide (AC). Postmenopausal women who respond initially to tamoxifen but later manifest progressive disease may be given diethylstilbestrol or megestrol acetate. Aromatase inhibitors (aminoglutethimide) have been available for the treatment of advanced breast cancer in postmenopausal women who fail tamoxifen treatment. Recent trials comparing an aromatase inhibitor, anastrazole, with tamoxifen suggest that the former is just as effective and has fewer side effects. Aromatase inhibitors may achieve the status of primary hormonal therapy in postmenopausal women. Clinical trials have proved the efficacy of anastrozole for such purposes. Anastrozole, easily administered in daily doses of 1 mg, has few side effects. Androgens have many toxicities and should rarely be used. As in premenopausal patients, neither hypophysectomy nor adrenalectomy is still being performed.

Chemotherapy

Cytotoxic drugs should be considered for the treatment of metastatic breast cancer (1) if visceral metastases are present (especially brain or lymphangitic pulmonary); (2) if hormonal treatment is unsuccessful or the disease has progressed after an initial response to hormonal manipulation; or (3) if the tumor is ER-negative. The most useful single chemotherapeutic agent to date is doxorubicin (Adriamycin), with a response rate of 40–50%. Single agents are rarely used but rather given in combination with other cytotoxic drugs.

Combination chemotherapy using multiple agents has proved to be more effective, with objectively observed favorable responses achieved in 60–80% of patients with stage IV disease. Various combinations of drugs have been used, and clinical trials are continuing in an effort to improve results and reduce undesirable side effects. Nausea and vomiting are well controlled with drugs that directly affect the central nervous system, such as ondansetron and granisetron. These drugs are selective antagonists of serotonin receptors in the central nervous system and block nausea caused by cytotoxic chemotherapy. Doxorubicin (40 mg/m^2 intravenously on day 1) and cyclophosphamide (200 mg/m^2 orally on days 3–6) produce an objective response in about 85% of patients so treated. Other chemotherapeutic regimens have consisted of various combinations of drugs, including cyclophosphamide, vincristine, methotrexate, fluorouracil, and taxanes with response rates ranging up to 60–70%. Prior adjuvant chemotherapy does not seem to alter response rates in patients who relapse. Growth factors such as erythropoietin (epoetin alfa), which stimulates red blood cell production and mimics the effect of erythropoietin, and filgrastim (granulocyte colony-stimulating factor; G-CSF), which stimulates proliferation and differentiation of hematopoietic cells, prevent life-threatening anemia and neutropenia seen commonly with high doses of chemotherapy. These agents greatly diminish the incidence of infections that may complicate the use of myelosuppressive chemotherapy.

Paclitaxel, given by intravenous infusion in a dose of 135–175 mg/m^2, has been shown to be very effective for patients with breast cancer. It is usually given after failure of combination chemotherapy for metastatic disease or relapse shortly after completion of adjuvant chemotherapy. Paclitaxel has response rates of 30–40% in patients with metastatic disease and is used as both a first-line agent and as an adjuvant systemic agent, usually in combination with doxorubicin.

Docetaxel is another taxane (like paclitaxel) that shows promise for treatment of patients with anthracycline-resistant tumors. Both agents are currently being used after treatment with anthracyclines in patients with advanced disease as well as in adjuvant and neoadjuvant settings. Trastuzumab is a monoclonal antibody that binds to HER-2/*neu* receptors on the cancer cell and has been shown to be highly effective in HER-2/*neu*-expressive cancers. It appears superior to doxorubicin alone or doxorubicin and cyclophosphamide.

High-dose chemotherapy and autologous bone marrow or stem cell transplantation have aroused widespread interest for the treatment of metastatic breast cancer. With this technique, the patient receives high doses of cytotoxic agents, eradicating the marrow, for which the patient subsequently undergoes autologous bone marrow or stem cell transplantation. Complete response rates are as high as 30–35%—considerably better than what can be achieved with conventional chemotherapy. Most randomized trials, however, comparing high-dose chemotherapy with stem cell support show no improvement in survival over conventional chemotherapy. A study purporting to show an advantage to high-dose chemotherapy in South Africa was found to be falsified and discredited. Enthusiasm for high-dose chemotherapy with stem cell support has waned, but additional studies continue. The technique is extremely costly, and the treatment itself is associated with a mortality rate of about 3–7%.

Malignant Pleural Effusion

This condition develops at some time in almost half of patients with metastatic breast cancer (see Chapter 9).

Burstein HJ et al: New cytotoxic agents and schedules for advanced breast cancer. Semin Oncol 2001;28:344. [PMID: 11398829] (Summarizes newer agents used in the treatment of metastatic breast cancer.)

Clarke M: Tamoxifen for early breast cancer: an overview of the randomised trials. Lancet 1998;351:1451. [Cit ID: 98266838] (Adjuvant tamoxifen yields significant improvement in 10-year survival rates in women with ER-positive tumors and in women with tumors of unknown ER status.)

Cristofanilli M et al: New horizons in treating metastatic disease. Clin Breast Cancer 2001;1:276. [PMID: 11899350]

Harris S: Radiotherapy for early and advanced breast cancer. Intl J Clin Pract 2001;55:609. [PMID: 11770358]

Johnston SR et al: Endocrine manipulation in advanced breast cancer: Recent advances with SERM therapies. Clin Cancer Res 2001;7(Suppl):4376s. [PMID: 11916228] (This article summarizes recent studies evaluating SERMS.)

Miles DW: Update on HER-2 as a target for cancer therapy: Herceptin in the clinical setting. Breast Cancer Res 2001;3:380. [PMID: 11737889] (This article reviews the use of trastuzumab as treatment for advanced breast cancer.)

Nabholtz JM et al: Third-generation aromatase inhibitors in the treatment of advanced breast cancer. Breast Cancer 2001;8:305-9. (This article describes the use of aromatase inhibitors in the treatment of advanced breast cancer in postmenopausal women and their superiority to tamoxifen.)

Pegram MD et al: Combination therapy with trastuzumab (Herceptin) and cisplatin for chemoresistant metastatic breast cancer: evidence for receptor-enhanced chemosensitivity. Semin Oncol 1999;26(4 Suppl 12):89. [PMID: 10482199] (The combination yielded higher response rates than either single agent alone.)

Stadtmauer EA et al: Conventional-dose chemotherapy compared with high-dose chemotherapy plus autologous hematopoietic stem-cell transplantation for metastatic breast cancer. N Engl J Med 2000;342:1069. [PMID: 10760307] (Randomized trial, high-dose chemotherapy given after induction of complete or partial remission with conventional-dose chemotherapy does not improve survival.)

PROGNOSIS

Stage of breast cancer is the most reliable indicator of prognosis (Table 16–6). Patients with disease localized to the breast and no evidence of regional spread after microscopic examination of the lymph nodes have by far the most favorable prognosis. Axillary lymph node status is the best-analyzed prognostic factor and correlates with survival at all tumor sizes. In addition, increased number of axillary nodes involved correlates directly with lower survival rates. Estrogen and progesterone receptors are prognostic variables because patients with hormone receptor-negative tumors and no evidence of metastases to the axillary lymph nodes have a much higher recurrence rate than do patients with hormone receptor-positive tumors and no regional metastases. The histologic subtype of breast cancer (eg, medullary, lobular, colloid) seems to have little significance in prognosis once these tumors are truly invasive. Flow cytometry of tumor cells to analyze DNA index and S-phase frequency aid in prognosis. Tumors with marked aneuploidy have a poor prognosis (Table 16–4). HER-2/*neu* oncogene amplification, epidermal growth factor receptors, and cathepsin D may have some prognostic value, but no markers are as significant as lymph node metastases in predicting outcome.

The mortality rate of breast cancer patients exceeds that of age-matched normal controls for nearly 20 years. Thereafter, the mortality rates are equal, though deaths that occur among breast cancer patients are often directly the result of tumor. Five-year statistics do not accurately reflect the final outcome of therapy.

When cancer is localized to the breast, with no evidence of regional spread after pathologic examination, the clinical cure rate with most accepted methods of therapy is 75–90%. Exceptions to this generalization may be related to the hormonal receptor content of the tumor, tumor size, host resistance, or associated illness. Patients with small mammographically de-

Table 16–6. Approximate survival (%) of patients with breast cancer by TNM stage.

TNM Stage	Five Years	Ten Years
0	95	90
I	85	70
IIA	70	50
IIB	60	40
IIIA	55	30
IIIB	30	20
IV	5–10	2
All	65	30

tected estrogen and progesterone receptor-positive tumors and no evidence of axillary spread probably have a 5-year survival rate greater than 90%. When the axillary lymph nodes are involved with tumor, the survival rate drops to 40–50% at 5 years and probably around 25% at 10 years. In general, breast cancer appears to be somewhat more malignant in younger than in older women, and this may be related to the fact that fewer younger women have ER-positive tumors.

For those patients whose disease progresses despite treatment, supportive group therapy may improve survival. As they approach the end of life, such patients will require meticulous efforts at palliative care (see Chapter 5).

Fitzgibbons PL et al: Prognostic factors in breast cancer. College of American Pathologists Consensus Statement 1999. Arch Pathol Lab Med 2000;124:966. [PMID: 10888772]

Younes M et al: Stratified multivariate analysis of prognostic markers in breast cancer; a preliminary report. Anticancer Res 1997;17:1383. [PMID: 9137503] (Discussion of a proposed integration of commonly used prognostic factors into prognostic scheme for use in making treatment decisions.)

FOLLOW-UP CARE

After primary therapy, patients with breast cancer should be followed for life for at least two reasons: to detect recurrences and to observe the opposite breast for a second primary carcinoma. Local and distant recurrences occur most frequently within the first 3 years. During this period, the patient should be examined every 6 months. Thereafter, examination is done annually. Special attention is paid to the remaining breast, because 10% of patients will develop a contralateral primary malignancy. The patient should examine her own breast monthly, and a mammogram should be obtained annually. In some cases, metastases are dormant for long periods and may appear 10–15 years or longer after removal of the primary tumor. Estrogen and progestational agents are rarely used for a patient free of disease after treatment of primary breast cancer, particularly if the tumor was hormone receptor-positive. Studies nevertheless have failed to show an adverse effect of hormonal agents in patients who are free of disease. Even pregnancy has not been clearly associated with shortened survival of patients rendered disease-free—yet most oncologists are reluctant to advise a young patient with breast cancer that she may become pregnant, and most are less than enthusiastic about prescribing hormone replacement therapy for the postmenopausal breast cancer patient. Estrogen replacement therapy may be prescribed for a woman with a history of breast cancer after discussion of the benefits and risks of such therapy for such conditions as osteoporosis and hot flushes. Raloxifene may prove to be appropriate replacement therapy to prevent osteoporosis after breast cancer, but as yet it has not been adequately studied.

Local Recurrence

The incidence of local recurrence correlates with tumor size, the presence and number of involved axillary nodes, the histologic type of tumor, the presence of skin edema or skin and fascia fixation with the primary, and the type of initial local (breast) therapy. About 8% of patients develop local recurrence on the chest wall after total mastectomy and axillary dissection. When the axillary nodes are not involved, the local recurrence rate is 5%, but the rate is as high as 25% when they are heavily involved. A similar difference in local recurrence rate was noted between small and large tumors. Factors affecting the rate of local recurrence in patients who have had partial mastectomies are not yet determined. Early studies show that factors such as multifocal cancer, in situ tumors, positive resection margins, chemotherapy, and radiotherapy are important.

Chest wall recurrences usually appear within the first 2 years but may occur as late as 15 or more years after mastectomy. Suspicious nodules and skin lesions should be biopsied. Local excision or localized radiotherapy may be feasible if an isolated nodule is present. If lesions are multiple or accompanied by evidence of regional involvement in the internal mammary or supraclavicular nodes, the disease is best managed by radiation treatment of the entire chest wall including the parasternal, supraclavicular, and axillary areas.

Local recurrence after mastectomy usually signals the presence of widespread disease and is an indication for bone scans, abdominal CT or liver ultrasound, posteroanterior and lateral chest x-rays, and other examinations as needed to search for evidence of metastases. Most patients with locally recurrent tumor will develop distant metastases within 2 years. When there is no evidence of metastases beyond the chest wall and regional nodes, irradiation for cure or complete local excision should be attempted. Patients with local recurrence may be cured with local resection and radiation. After partial mastectomy, local recurrence may not have as serious a prognostic significance as after mastectomy. However, those patients who do develop a breast recurrence have a worse prognosis than those who do not. It is speculated that the ability of a cancer to recur locally after radiotherapy is a sign of aggressiveness. Completion of the mastectomy should be done for local recurrence after partial mastectomy; some of these patients will survive for prolonged periods, especially if the breast recurrence is DCIS or more than 5 years after initial treatment. Systemic chemotherapy or hormonal treatment should be used for women who develop disseminated disease or those in whom local recurrence occurs.

Edema of the Arm

Significant edema of the arm occurs in about 10–30% of patients after radical mastectomy. It occurs more commonly if radiotherapy has been given or if there was postoperative infection. Partial mastectomy with radiation to the axillary lymph nodes is followed by chronic edema of the arm in 10–20% of patients. To avoid this complication, many authorities advocate axillary lymph node sampling rather than complete axillary dissection. However, since axillary dissection is a more accurate staging operation than axillary sampling, it is recommended that at least level I and II lymph nodes be removed, in combination with partial mastectomy. Sentinel lymph node dissection may offer accurate staging without the risk of lymphedema for node-negative patients. Judicious use of radiotherapy, with treatment fields carefully planned to spare the axilla as much as possible, can greatly diminish the incidence of edema, which will occur in only 5% of patients if no radiotherapy is given to the axilla after a partial mastectomy and lymph node dissection.

Late or secondary edema of the arm may develop years after treatment, as a result of axillary recurrence or of infection in the hand or arm, with obliteration of lymphatic channels. Infection in the arm or hand on the dissected side should be treated with antibiotics, rest, and elevation. When edema develops, careful examination of the axilla for recurrence should be done. If there is no sign of recurrence, the swollen extremity should be treated with rest and elevation. A mild diuretic may be helpful. If there is no improvement, a compressor pump decreases the swelling, and the patient is then fitted with an elastic glove or sleeve. Most patients are not bothered enough by mild edema to wear an uncomfortable glove or sleeve and will treat themselves with elevation alone. Benzopyrones have been reported to decrease lymphedema but are not approved for this use in the USA. Rarely, edema may be severe enough to interfere with use of the limb.

Breast Reconstruction

Breast reconstruction, with the implantation of a prosthesis, is usually feasible after standard or modified radical mastectomy. Reconstruction should be discussed with patients prior to mastectomy, because it offers an important psychologic focal point for recovery. Reconstruction is not an obstacle to the diagnosis of recurrent cancer. The most common breast reconstruction has been implantation of a silicone gel prosthesis in the subpectoral plane between the pectoralis minor and pectoralis major muscles. The FDA has placed a moratorium on the purely cosmetic use of silicone gel implants because of possible leakage of silicone and possible associated autoimmune phenomena. This remote possibility should not prevent the cancer patient from having a reconstruction, and breast cancer patients are exempt from the moratorium. Most plastic surgeons currently would place a saline-filled prosthesis rather than a silicone gel implant. Alternatively, autologous tissue can be used for reconstruction. Autologous tissue flaps are aesthetically superior to implant recon-

struction in most patients. They also have the advantage of not feeling like a foreign body to the patient. The most popular autologous technique currently is the trans-rectus abdominis muscle flap (TRAM flap), which is done by rotating the rectus abdominis muscle with attached fat and skin cephalad to make a breast mound. The free TRAM flap is done by completely removing the rectus with overlying fat and skin and using microvascular surgical techniques reconstructing the vascular supply on the chest wall. A latissimus dorsi flap can be swung from the back but offers less fullness than the TRAM flap and is therefore less acceptable cosmetically. Reconstruction may be performed immediately (at the time of initial mastectomy) or may be delayed until later, usually when the patient has completed adjuvant therapy.

Risks of Pregnancy

Data are insufficient to determine whether interruption of pregnancy improves the prognosis of patients who are discovered during pregnancy to have potentially curable breast cancer and who receive definitive treatment. Theoretically, the increasingly high levels of estrogen produced by the placenta as the pregnancy progresses could be detrimental to the patient with occult metastases of hormone-sensitive breast cancer. Moreover, occult metastases are present in most patients with positive axillary nodes, and treatment by adjuvant chemotherapy could be potentially harmful to the fetus, although chemotherapy has been given to pregnant women. Under these circumstances, interruption of early pregnancy seems reasonable, with progressively less rationale for the procedure as term approaches. The decision is affected by many factors, including the patient's desire to have the baby and the generally poor prognosis when axillary nodes are involved.

Equally important is the advice regarding future pregnancy (or abortion in case of pregnancy) to be given to women of child-bearing age who have had definitive treatment for breast cancer. Under these circumstances, one must assume that pregnancy will be harmful if occult metastases are present, though this has not been demonstrated. Patients whose tumors are ER-negative probably would not be affected by pregnancy. To date, no adverse effect of pregnancy on survival of pregnant women who have had breast cancer has been demonstrated, though most oncologists advise against it.

In patients with inoperable or metastatic cancer (stage IV disease), induced abortion is usually advisable because of the possible adverse effects of hormonal treatment, radiotherapy, or chemotherapy upon the fetus.

Herd-Smith A et al: Prognostic factors for lymphedema after primary treatment of breast carcinoma. Cancer 2001;92:1783. [PMID: 11745250] (The authors examine risk factors for the development of lymphedema after treatment for breast cancer. The use of postoperative radiotherapy and number of lymph nodes removed increase the risk of lymphedema.)

Loudon L et al: Lymphedema in women treated for breast cancer. Cancer Practice 2000;8:65. [PMID: 11898179] (This summary discusses the etiology, prevention, and treatment of lymphedema in breast cancer.)

Velentgas P et al: Pregnancy after breast carcinoma: outcomes and influence on mortality. Cancer 1999;85:2424. [PMID: 10357413] (Findings indicate that pregnancy after breast cancer diagnosis does not have adverse effect on survival.)

Williams JK et al: The effects of radiation after TRAM flap breast reconstruction. Plast Reconstr Surg 1997;100:1153. [PMID: 9326776]

■ CARCINOMA OF THE MALE BREAST

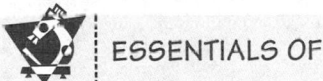

ESSENTIALS OF DIAGNOSIS

- A painless lump beneath the areola in a man usually over 50 years of age.
- Nipple discharge, retraction, or ulceration may be present.

General Considerations

Breast cancer in men is a rare disease; the incidence is only about 1% of that in women. The average age at occurrence is about 60—somewhat older than the commonest presenting age in women. The prognosis, even in stage I cases, is worse in men than in women. Blood-borne metastases are commonly present when the male patient appears for initial treatment. These metastases may be latent and may not become manifest for many years. As in women, hormonal influences are probably related to the development of male breast cancer. There is a high incidence of both breast cancer and gynecomastia in Bantu men, theoretically owing to failure of estrogen inactivation by a damaged liver by associated liver disease.

Clinical Findings

A painless lump, occasionally associated with nipple discharge, retraction, erosion, or ulceration, is the chief complaint. Examination usually shows a hard, ill-defined, nontender mass beneath the nipple or areola. Gynecomastia not uncommonly precedes or accompanies breast cancer in men. Nipple discharge is an uncommon presentation for breast cancer in men, as it is in women, but is an ominous finding associated with carcinoma in nearly 75% of cases.

Breast cancer staging is the same in men as in women. Gynecomastia and metastatic cancer from another site (eg, prostate) must be considered in the differential diagnosis. Biopsy settles the issue.

Treatment

Treatment consists of modified radical mastectomy in operable patients, who should be chosen by the same criteria as women with the disease. Irradiation is the first step in treating localized metastases in the skin, lymph nodes, or skeleton that are causing symptoms. Examination of the cancer for hormone receptor proteins may prove to be of value in predicting response to endocrine ablation. Adjuvant chemotherapy is used for the same indications as in breast cancer in women.

Since breast cancer in men is frequently a disseminated disease, endocrine therapy is of considerable importance in its management. Tamoxifen and castration are the main therapeutic resources for management of advanced breast cancer in men. Tamoxifen (20 mg daily) should be the initial treatment, though there is little experience. Castration in advanced breast cancer is a successful palliative measure and more beneficial than the same procedure in women. Objective evidence of regression may be seen in 60–70% of men who are castrated—approximately twice the proportion in women. The average duration of tumor growth remission is about 30 months, and life is prolonged. Bone is the most frequent site of metastases from breast cancer in men (as in women), and castration relieves bone pain in most patients so treated. The longer the interval between mastectomy and recurrence, the longer the tumor growth remission following castration. As in women, there is no correlation between the histologic type of the tumor and the likelihood of remission following castration.

Aminoglutethimide (250 mg orally four times a day) should replace adrenalectomy in men as it has in women. Corticosteroid therapy alone has been considered to be efficacious but probably has no value when compared with major endocrine ablation.

Estrogen therapy—5 mg of diethylstilbestrol three times daily orally—may be effective as secondary hormonal manipulation after medical adrenalectomy (with aminoglutethimide). Androgen therapy may exacerbate bone pain. Chemotherapy should be administered for the same indications and using the same dosage schedules as for women with metastatic disease.

Prognosis

The prognosis of breast cancer is poorer in men than in women. The crude 5- and 10-year survival rates for clinical stage I breast cancer in men are about 58% and 38%, respectively. For clinical stage II disease, the 5- and 10-year survival rates are approximately 38% and 10%. The survival rates for all stages at 5 and 10 years are 36% and 17%. For those patients whose disease progresses despite treatment, meticulous efforts at palliative care are essential (see Chapter 5).

Friedman LS et al: Mutation analysis of BRCA1 and BRCA2 in a male breast cancer population. Am J Hum Genet 1997; 60:313. [PMID: 9012404] (Reports BRCA genetic mutations in male breast cancer.)

Meijer-van Gelder ME et al: Clinical relevance of biologic factors in male breast cancer. Breast Cancer Res Treat 2001;68: 249. [PMID: 11727961]

Memon MA et al: Male breast cancer. Br J Surg 1997;84:433. [PMID: 9112887]

Pich A et al: Oncogenes and male breast carcinoma: c-erbB-2 and p53 coexpression predicts a poor survival. J Clin Oncol 2000;18:2948. [PMID: 10944127]

Wolpert N et al: Prevalence of BRCA1 and BRCA2 mutations in male breast cancer patients in Canada. Clin Breast Cancer 2000;1:57. [PMID: 11899391]

Gynecology

17

H. Trent MacKay, MD, MPH
See www.current-med.com/ch17.html

ABNORMAL PREMENOPAUSAL BLEEDING

Normal menstrual bleeding lasts an average of 4 days (range, 2–7 days), with a mean blood loss of 40 mL. Blood loss of over 80 mL per cycle is abnormal and frequently produces anemia. Excessive bleeding, often with the passage of clots, may occur at regular menstrual intervals (**menorrhagia**) or irregular intervals (**dysfunctional uterine bleeding**). When there are fewer than 21 days between the onset of bleeding episodes, the cycles are likely to be anovular. **Ovulation bleeding,** a single episode of spotting between regular menses, is quite common. Heavier or irregular intermenstrual bleeding warrants investigation.

Dysfunctional uterine bleeding is usually caused by overgrowth of endometrium due to estrogen stimulation without adequate progesterone to stabilize growth; this occurs in anovular cycles. Anovulation associated with high estrogen levels commonly occurs in teenagers, in women aged late 30s to late 40s, and in extremely obese women or those with polycystic ovary syndrome.

Clinical Findings

A. SYMPTOMS AND SIGNS

The diagnosis of the disorders underlying the bleeding usually depends upon the following: (1) A careful description of the duration and amount of flow, related pain, and relationship to the last menstrual period (LMP). The presence of blood clots or the degree of inconvenience caused by the bleeding may be more useful indicators. (2) A history of pertinent illnesses. (3) A history of all medications the patient has taken in the past month. (4) A careful pelvic examination to look for pregnancy, uterine myomas, adnexal masses, or infection.

B. LABORATORY STUDIES

Cervical smears should be obtained as needed for cytologic and culture studies. Blood studies should include a complete blood count, sedimentation rate, and glu-cose levels to rule out diabetes. Diabetes may occasionally initially present with abnormal bleeding. A test for pregnancy and studies of thyroid function and blood clotting should be considered in the clinical evaluation. Tests for ovulation in cyclic menorrhagia include basal body temperature records, serum progesterone measured 1 week before the expected onset of menses, and analysis of an endometrial biopsy specimen for secretory activity shortly before the onset of menstruation.

C. IMAGING

Ultrasound may be useful to evaluate endometrial thickness or to diagnose intrauterine or ectopic pregnancy or adnexal masses. Endovaginal ultrasound with saline infusion sonohysterography may be used to diagnose endometrial polyps or subserous myomas. MRI can definitively diagnose submucous myomas and adenomyosis.

D. CERVICAL BIOPSY AND ENDOMETRIAL CURETTAGE

Biopsy, curettage, or aspiration of the endometrium and curettage of the endocervix may be necessary to diagnose the cause of bleeding. These and other invasive gynecologic diagnostic procedures are described in Table 17–1. Polyps, endometrial hyperplasia, and submucous myomas are commonly identified in this way. If cancer of the cervix is suspected, colposcopically directed biopsies and endocervical curettage are indicated as first steps.

E. HYSTEROSCOPY

Hysteroscopy can visualize endometrial polyps, submucous myomas, and exophytic endometrial cancers. It is useful immediately before D&C.

Treatment

Premenopausal patients with abnormal uterine bleeding include those with submucous myomas, infection, early abortion, or pelvic neoplasms. The history, physical examination, and laboratory findings should identify such patients, who require definitive therapy depending upon the cause of the bleeding. A large group

Table 17–1. Common gynecologic diagnostic procedures.

Colposcopy

Visualization of cervical, vaginal, or vulvar epithelium under 5–50× magnification to identify abnormal areas requiring biopsy. Used to identify genital warts on males as well as females. An office procedure.

D&C

Dilation of the cervix and curettage of the entire endometrial cavity, using a metal curette or suction cannula and often using forceps for the removal of endometrial polyps. Performed to diagnose endometrial disease and to stop heavy bleeding. Can usually be done in the office under local anesthesia.

Endometrial biopsy

Removal of one or more areas of the endometrium by means of a curette or small aspiration device without cervical dilation. Less accurate diagnostically than D&C. An office procedure performed under local anesthesia.

Endocervical curettage

Removal of endocervical epithelium with a small curette for diagnosis of cervical dysplasia and cancer. An office procedure performed under local anesthesia.

Hysteroscopy

Visual examination of the uterine cavity with a small fiberoptic endoscope passed through the cervix. Biopsies, excision of myomas, and other procedures can be performed. Can be done in the office under local anesthesia or in the operating room under general anesthesia.

Hysterosalpingography

Injection of radiopaque dye through the cervix to visualize the uterine cavity and oviducts. Mainly used in investigation of infertility.

Laparoscopy

Visualization of the abdominal and pelvic cavity through a small fiberoptic endoscope passed through a subumbilical incision. Permits diagnosis, tubal sterilization, and treatment of many conditions previously requiring laparotomy. General anesthesia is usually used.

of patients remains, most of whom have dysfunctional uterine bleeding on a hormonal basis.

Dysfunctional uterine bleeding can usually be treated hormonally. Women over the age of 35 should have endometrial sampling to rule out endometrial hyperplasia or carcinoma prior to initiation of hormonal therapy. Progestins, which limit and stabilize endometrial growth, are generally effective. Office D&C is usually not necessary in women under age 40. Medroxyprogesterone acetate, 10 mg/d, or norethindrone acetate, 5 mg/d, should be given for 10–14 days starting on day 15 of the cycle, following which withdrawal bleeding (so-called medical curettage) will occur. The treatment is repeated for several cycles; it can be reinstituted if amenorrhea or dysfunctional bleeding recurs. In women who are bleeding actively, any of the combination oral contraceptives can be

given four times daily for one or 2 days followed by two pills daily through day 5 and then one pill daily through day 20; after withdrawal bleeding occurs, pills are taken in the usual dosage for three cycles. In cases of intractable heavy bleeding, danazol, 200 mg four times daily, is sometimes used to create an atrophic endometrium. Alternatively, a GnRH agonist such as depot leuprolide, 3.75 mg intramuscularly monthly, or nafarelin, 0.2–0.4 mg intranasally twice daily, can be used for up to 6 months to create a temporary cessation of menstruation by ovarian suppression.

In cases of heavy bleeding, intravenous conjugated estrogens, 25 mg every 4 hours for three or four doses, can be used, followed by oral conjugated estrogens, 2.5 mg daily, or ethinyl estradiol, 20 μg daily, for 3 weeks, with the addition of medroxyprogesterone acetate, 10 mg daily for the last 10 days of treatment, or a combination oral contraceptive daily for 3 weeks. This will thicken the endometrium and control the bleeding. If the abnormal bleeding is not controlled by hormonal treatment, a D&C is necessary to check for incomplete abortion, polyps, submucous myomas, or endometrial cancer.

Endometrial ablation through the hysteroscope with laser photocoagulation or electrocautery is an option; this technique is designed to reduce or prevent any future menstrual flow.

Nonsteroidal anti-inflammatory drugs such as naproxen or mefenamic acid in the usual anti-inflammatory doses will often reduce blood loss in menorrhagia—even that associated with an IUD.

Prolonged use of a progestin, as in a minipill, in injectable contraceptives, or in the therapy of endometriosis, can also lead to intermittent bleeding, sometimes severe. In this instance, the endometrium is atrophic and fragile. If bleeding occurs, it should be treated with estrogen as follows: ethinyl estradiol, 20 μg/d for 7 days, or conjugated estrogens, 1.25 mg/d for 7 days.

It is useful for the patient and the clinician to discuss stressful situations or life-styles that may contribute to anovulation and dysfunctional bleeding, such as prolonged emotional turmoil or excessive use of drugs or alcohol.

Cooper JM: Contemporary management of abnormal uterine bleeding. Obstet Gynecol Clin North Am 2000;27. (Entire volume.)

Farquhar CM et al: An evaluation of the risk factors for endometrial hyperplasia in premenopausal women with abnormal menstrual bleeding. Am J Obstet Gynecol 1999;181:525. [PMID: 10486458] (Risk factors included body weight ≥ 90 kg, age ≥ 45 years, infertility, family history of colon cancer, and nulliparity.)

Pasqualotto EB et al: Accuracy of preoperative diagnostic tools and outcome of hysteroscopic management of menstrual dysfunction. J Am Assoc Gynecol Laparosc 2000;7:201. [PMID: 10806263] (Reviews sensitivities of preoperative diagnostic tools for all intrauterine abnormalities. Sensitivities for myomas and polyps for transvaginal sonography were 74% and 39%, respectively; for saline-infusion sonography, 96% and 96%; for hysteroscopy, 100% and 99%; and for Pipelle endometrial biopsy, 24% and 10%.)

POSTMENOPAUSAL VAGINAL BLEEDING

Vaginal bleeding that occurs 6 months or more following cessation of menstrual function should be investigated. The most common causes are atrophic endometrium, endometrial proliferation or hyperplasia, endometrial or cervical cancer, and administration of estrogens without added progestin. Other causes include atrophic vaginitis, trauma, endometrial polyps, friction ulcers of the cervix associated with prolapse of the uterus, and blood dyscrasias. Uterine bleeding is usually painless, but pain will be present if the cervix is stenotic, if bleeding is severe and rapid, or if infection or torsion or extrusion of a tumor is present. The patient may report a single episode of spotting or profuse bleeding for days or months.

Diagnosis

The vulva and vagina should be inspected for areas of bleeding, ulcers, or neoplasms. A cytologic smear of the cervix and vaginal pool should be taken. If available, transvaginal sonography should be used to measure endometrial thickness. A measurement of 4 mm or less indicates a very low likelihood of hyperplasia or endometrial cancer. In 20 studies of a total of 4759 women with postmenopausal bleeding and an endometrial thickness of 4 mm or less, only 0.25% were found to have endometrial cancer. If the thickness is greater than 4 mm, endocervical curettage and endometrial aspiration should be performed, preferably in conjunction with hysteroscopy.

Treatment

Aspiration curettage (with polypectomy if indicated) will frequently be curative. Simple endometrial hyperplasia calls for cyclic progestin therapy (medroxyprogesterone acetate, 10 mg/d, or norethindrone acetate, 5 mg/d) for 21 days of each month for 3 months. A repeat D&C or endometrial biopsy should be performed, and if tissues are normal and estrogen replacement therapy is reinstituted, a progestin should be prescribed (as above) in a cyclic or continuous regimen. If endometrial hyperplasia with atypical cells or carcinoma of the endometrium is found, hysterectomy is necessary.

Gull B et al: Transvaginal ultrasonography in women with postmenopausal bleeding: is it always necessary to perform an endometrial biopsy? Am J Obstet Gynecol 2000;185:509. [PMID: 10739500] (In 163 women with postmenopausal bleeding and an endometrial thickness of ≤ 4 mm, only one woman had endometrial cancer. and that case was detected with cervical cytology.)

PREMENSTRUAL SYNDROME (Premenstrual Tension)

The premenstrual syndrome is a recurrent, variable cluster of troublesome physical and emotional symptoms that develop during the 7–14 days before the onset of menses and subside when menstruation occurs. The syndrome intermittently affects about one-third of all premenopausal women, primarily those 25–40 years of age. In about 10% of affected women, the syndrome may be severe. Although not every woman experiences all the symptoms or signs at one time, many describe bloating, breast pain, ankle swelling, a sense of increased weight, skin disorders, irritability, aggressiveness, depression, inability to concentrate, libido change, lethargy, and food cravings.

The pathogenesis of premenstrual syndrome is still uncertain. Psychosocial factors may play a role. Suppression of ovarian function with a GnRH agonist has been shown to diminish all symptoms during therapy. "Add-back therapy" to provide the hormones suppressed by the GnRH agonist with low-dose estrogen and progestin may allow extended use of a GnRH agonist. Suppression of ovulation with an oral contraceptive is sometimes helpful, but the patient often complains that she still has premenstrual syndrome.

Current treatment methods are mainly empirical. The clinician should provide the best support possible for the patient's emotional and physical distress. This includes the following:

(1) Careful evaluation of the patient, with understanding, explanation, and reassurance, is of first importance.

(2) Advise the patient to keep a daily diary of all symptoms for 2–3 months, to help in evaluating the timing and characteristics of the syndrome. If her symptoms occur throughout the month rather than in the 2 weeks before menses, she may be depressed or may have other emotional problems in addition to premenstrual syndrome.

(3) A diet emphasizing complex carbohydrates can be recommended. Foods high in sugar content and alcohol should be avoided to minimize reactive hypoglycemia. Use of caffeine should be minimized whenever tension and irritability predominate.

(4) Vitamin B_6, up to 100 mg/d, may be beneficial in the treatment of premenstrual symptoms and premenstrual depression. At this dosage level, neurologic side effects are rare.

(5) A program of regular conditioning exercise, such as jogging, has been found to decrease depression, anxiety, and fluid retention premenstrually in several studies.

(6) Serotonin reuptake inhibitors such as fluoxetine, 20 mg/d, are effective in relieving tension, irritability, and dysphoria with few side effects.

(7) Luteal phase administration of danazol, 200 mg/d on cycle days 14–28, is effective in reducing symptoms of mastalgia. Other symptoms are not affected by this low-dose therapy.

Freeman EW et al: Full- or half-cycle treatment of severe premenstrual syndrome with a serotonergic antidepressant. J Clin Psychopharmacol 1999;19:3. [PMID: 9934936] (The SSRI sertraline, 50–100 mg/d, in the luteal phase is as effective as full-cycle treatment for the relief of severe premenstrual symptoms.)

Kessel B: Premenstrual syndrome, Advances in diagnosis and treatment. Obstet Gynecol Clin North Am 2000;27:625 [PMID: 10958008] (Summary of current state of knowledge of PMS.)

Wyatt KM et al: Efficacy of vitamin B$_6$ in the treatment of premenstrual syndrome: systematic review. BMJ 1999;318: 1375. [PMID: 10334745] (Review of nine published randomized clinical trials shows an OR = 2.32 [95% CI, 1.95–2.54] compared with placebo for improvement in overall PMS symptoms and an OR = 1.69 [95% CI, 1.39–2.06] for improvement in PMS depressive symptoms with vitamin B$_6$, 50–100 mg/d.)

DYSMENORRHEA

1. Primary Dysmenorrhea

Primary dysmenorrhea is menstrual pain associated with ovular cycles in the absence of pathologic findings. The pain usually begins within 1–2 years after the menarche and may become more severe with time. The frequency of cases increases up to age 20 and then decreases with age and markedly with parity. Fifty to 75 percent of women are affected at some time, and 5–6% have incapacitating pain.

Primary dysmenorrhea is low, midline, wave-like, cramping pelvic pain often radiating to the back or inner thighs. Cramps may last for 1 or more days and may be associated with nausea, diarrhea, headache, and flushing. The pain is produced by uterine vasoconstriction, anoxia, and sustained contractions mediated by prostaglandins.

Clinical Findings

The pelvic examination is normal between menses; examination during menses may produce discomfort, but there are no pathologic findings.

Treatment

Nonsteroidal anti-inflammatory drugs (ibuprofen, ketoprofen, mefenamic acid, naproxen) are generally helpful. Drugs should be started at the onset of bleeding to avoid inadvertent drug use during early pregnancy. Medication should be continued on a regular basis for 2–3 days. Ovulation can be suppressed and dysmenorrhea usually prevented by oral contraceptives.

2. Secondary Dysmenorrhea

Secondary dysmenorrhea is menstrual pain for which an organic cause exists. It usually begins well after menarche, sometimes even as late as the third or fourth decade of life.

Clinical Findings

The history and physical examination commonly suggest endometriosis or pelvic inflammatory disease. Other causes may be submucous myoma, IUD use, cervical stenosis with obstruction, or blind uterine horn (rare).

Diagnosis

Laparoscopy is often needed to differentiate endometriosis from pelvic inflammatory disease. Submucous myomas can be detected most reliably by MRI but also by hysterogram, by hysteroscopy, or by passing a sound or curette over the uterine cavity during D&C. Cervical stenosis may result from induced abortion, creating crampy pain at the time of expected menses with no blood flow; this is easily cured by passing a sound into the uterine cavity after administering a paracervical block.

Treatment

A. SPECIFIC MEASURES

Periodic use of analgesics, including the nonsteroidal anti-inflammatory drugs given for primary dysmenorrhea, may be beneficial, and oral contraceptives may give relief, particularly in endometriosis. Danazol and GnRH agonists are effective in the treatment of endometriosis (see below).

B. SURGICAL MEASURES

If disability is marked or prolonged, laparoscopy or exploratory laparotomy is usually warranted. Definitive surgery depends upon the degree of disability and the findings at operation.

Coco AS: Primary dysmenorrhea. Am Fam Physician 1999;60: 489. [PMID: 10465224] (Epidemiology, etiology, diagnosis, and treatment.)

Wilson M et al: Dysmenorrhea. Clin Evidence 2001;6:1388. (Evidence-based summary of therapies for primary dysmenorrhea.)

VAGINITIS

Inflammation and infection of the vagina are common gynecologic problems, resulting from a variety of pathogens, allergic reactions to vaginal contraceptives or other products, or the friction of coitus. The normal vaginal pH is 4.5 or less, and lactobacillus is the predominant organism. At the time of the midcycle estrogen surge, clear, elastic, mucoid secretions from the cervical os are often profuse. In the luteal phase and during pregnancy, vaginal secretions are thicker, white, and sometimes adherent to the vaginal walls. These normal secretions can be confused with vaginitis by concerned women.

Clinical Findings

When the patient complains of vaginal irritation, pain, or unusual discharge, a careful history should be taken, noting the onset of the last menstrual period; recent sexual activity; use of contraceptives, tampons, or douches; and the presence of vaginal burning, pain, pruritus, or unusually profuse or malodorous discharge. The physical examination should include careful inspection of the vulva and speculum examination of the vagina and cervix. The cervix is cultured for gonococcus or chlamydia if applicable. A specimen of vaginal discharge is examined under the microscope in a drop of 0.9% saline solution to look for trichomonads or clue cells and in a drop of 10% potassium hydroxide to search for candida. The vaginal pH should be tested; it is frequently greater than 4.5 in infections due to trichomonads and bacterial vaginosis. A bimanual examination to look for evidence of pelvic infection should follow.

A. Candida albicans

Pregnancy, diabetes, and use of broad-spectrum antibiotics or corticosteroids predispose to candida infections. Heat, moisture, and occlusive clothing also contribute to the risk. Pruritus, vulvovaginal erythema, and a white curd-like discharge that is not malodorous are found. Microscopic examination with 10% potassium hydroxide reveals filaments and spores. Cultures with Nickerson's medium may be used if candida is suspected but not demonstrated.

B. Trichomonas vaginalis

This protozoal flagellate infects the vagina, Skene's ducts, and lower urinary tract in women and the lower genitourinary tract in men. It is transmitted through coitus. Pruritus and a malodorous frothy, yellow-green discharge occur, along with diffuse vaginal erythema and red macular lesions on the cervix in severe cases. Motile organisms with flagella are seen by microscopic examination of a wet mount with saline solution.

C. Bacterial Vaginosis

This condition is considered to be a polymicrobial disease which is not sexually transmitted. An overgrowth of gardnerella and other anaerobes is often associated with increased malodorous discharge without obvious vulvitis or vaginitis. The discharge is grayish and sometimes frothy, with a pH of 5.0–5.5. An amine-like ("fishy") odor is present if a drop of discharge is alkalinized with 10% potassium hydroxide. On wet mount in saline, epithelial cells are covered with bacteria to such an extent that cell borders are obscured (clue cells). Vaginal cultures are generally not useful in diagnosis.

D. Condylomata Acuminata (Genital Warts)

Warty growths on the vulva, perianal area, vaginal walls, or cervix are caused by various types of the human papillomavirus. They are sexually transmitted. Pregnancy and immunosuppression favor growth. Vulvar lesions may be obviously wart-like or may be diagnosed only after application of 4% acetic acid (vinegar) and colposcopy, when they appear whitish, with prominent papillae. Fissures may be present at the fourchette. Vaginal lesions may show diffuse hypertrophy or a cobblestone appearance. Cervical lesions may be visible only by colposcopy after pretreatment with 4% acetic acid. These lesions may be related to dysplasia and cervical cancer. Vulvar cancer is also currently considered to be associated with the human papillomavirus.

Treatment

A. Candida albicans

A variety of regimens are available to treat vulvovaginal candidiasis. The short-term cure rates are similar with all listed regimens.

1. Three-day regimens—Butoconazole (2% cream, 5 g), clotrimazole (two 100 mg vaginal tablets), terconazole (0.8% cream, 5 g, or 80 mg suppository), or miconazole (200 mg vaginal suppository) once daily.

2. Seven-day regimens—Clotrimazole (1% cream or 100 mg vaginal tablet), miconazole (2% cream, 5 g, or 100 mg vaginal suppository), or terconazole (0.4% cream, 5 g) once daily.

3. Single-dose regimens—Clotrimazole (500 mg tablet) or tioconazole ointment (6.5%, 5 g). Fluconazole, 150 mg orally in a single dose, is also effective.

4. Fourteen-day regimens—Nystatin (100,000 unit vaginal tablet once daily).

5. Recurrent vulvovaginitis—Ketoconazole, 100 mg orally once daily for up to 6 months.

B. Trichomonas vaginalis

Treatment of both partners simultaneously is recommended; metronidazole, 2 g as a single dose, is usually employed. In the case of treatment failure in the absence of reexposure, the patient should be re-treated with metronidazole, 500 mg twice a day for 7 days. If this is not effective in eradicating the organisms, metronidazole susceptibility testing can be arranged with the CDC at 404-639-8363.

C. Bacterial Vaginosis

The recommended regimens are metronidazole, 500 mg twice daily for 7 days; clindamycin vaginal cream

(2%, 5 g), once daily for 7 days; or metronidazole gel (0.75%, 5 g), twice daily for 5 days. Alternative regimens include metronidazole, 2 g orally as a single dose, or clindamycin, 300 mg orally twice daily for 7 days.

D. CONDYLOMATA ACUMINATA

Recommended treatments for vulvar warts include podophyllum resin 25% in tincture of benzoin (do not use during pregnancy or on bleeding lesions) or 80–90% trichloroacetic or bichloroacetic acid, carefully applied to avoid the surrounding skin. The pain of bi- or trichloroacetic acid application can be lessened by a sodium bicarbonate paste applied immediately after treatment. Podophyllum resin must be washed off after 2–4 hours. Freezing with liquid nitrogen or a cryoprobe and electrocautery are also effective. Patient-applied regimens include podofilox 0.5% solution or gel and imiquimod 5% cream. Vaginal warts may be treated with cryotherapy with liquid nitrogen, trichloroacetic acid, or podophyllum resin. Extensive warts may require treatment with CO_2 laser under local or general anesthesia. Interferon is not recommended for routine use because it is very expensive, associated with systemic side effects, and no more effective than other therapies. Routine examination of sex partners is not necessary for the management of genital warts since the risk of reinfection is probably minimal and curative therapy to prevent transmission is not available. However, partners may wish to be examined for detection and treatment of genital warts and other STDs.

Egan ME: Diagnosis of vaginitis. Am Fam Physician 2000; 62:1095. [PMID: 10997533] (General review.)

1998 Guidelines for treatment of sexually transmitted diseases. MMWR Recomm Rep 1998;47(RR-1):1. [PMID: 9461053]

1998 Guidelines for the treatment of sexually transmitted diseases. Clin Infect Dis 1999;28(Suppl 1). [PMID: 10028105–10028113] (Series of articles constituting the background information for the 1998 CDC STD Treatment Guidelines.)

CERVICITIS

Infection of the cervix must be distinguished from physiologic ectopy of columnar epithelium, which is common in young women. Mucopurulent cervicitis is characterized by a red edematous cervix with a purulent yellow discharge. The infection may result from a sexually transmitted pathogen such as *Neisseria gonorrhoeae*, chlamydia, or herpesvirus (which presents with vesicles and ulcers on the cervix during a primary herpetic infection), though in most cases none of these organisms can be isolated.

Mucopurulent cervicitis is an insensitive predictor of either gonorrheal or chlamydial infection and in addition has a low positive predictive value. Treatment should be based on microbiologic testing. Presumptive antibiotic treatment of mucopurulent cervicitis is not indicated unless there is a high prevalence of either *N*

gonorrhoeae or chlamydia in the population or if the patient is unlikely to return for treatment. (See Chapter 33 for discussion.) Three months after treatment, approximately 20% of women will have persistent or recurrent mucopus in the cervix, not explained by relapse or reinfection.

CERVICAL POLYPS

Cervical polyps commonly occur after menarche and are occasionally noted in postmenopausal women. The cause is not known, but inflammation may play an etiologic role. The principal symptoms are discharge and abnormal vaginal bleeding. However, abnormal bleeding should not be ascribed to a cervical polyp without sampling the endocervix and endometrium. The polyps are visible in the cervical os on speculum examination.

Cervical polyps must be differentiated from polypoid neoplastic disease of the endometrium, small submucous pedunculated myomas, and endometrial polyps. Cervical polyps rarely contain malignant foci.

Treatment

Cervical polyps can generally be removed in the office by avulsion with a uterine packing forceps or ring forceps. If the cervix is soft, patulous, or definitely dilated and the polyp is large, surgical D&C is required (especially if the pedicle is not readily visible). Because of the possibility of endometrial disease, cervical polypectomy should be accompanied by endometrial sampling, and all tissue removed should be submitted for microscopic examination.

Ozsaran AA et al: Endometrial hyperplasia co-existing with cervical polyps. Int J Obstet Gynecol 1999;66:185. [PMID: 10468348] (In a group of 210 women with cervical polyps, 19% with symptomatic polyps [discharge or bleeding] and 7.9% with asymptomatic polyps had endometrial hyperplasia on endometrial sampling.)

CYST & ABSCESS OF BARTHOLIN'S DUCT

Trauma or infection may involve Bartholin's duct, causing obstruction of the gland. Drainage of secretions is prevented, leading to pain, swelling, and abscess formation. The infection usually resolves and pain disappears, but stenosis of the duct outlet with distention often persists. Reinfection causes recurrent tenderness and further enlargement of the duct.

The principal symptoms are periodic painful swelling on either side of the introitus and dyspareunia. A fluctuant swelling 1–4 cm in diameter in the inferior portion of either labium minus is a sign of occlusion of Bartholin's duct. Tenderness is evidence of active infection.

Pus or secretions from the gland should be cultured for gonococci, chlamydiae, and other pathogens and treated accordingly (see Chapter 33); frequent warm soaks may be helpful. If an abscess develops, aspiration or incision and drainage are the simplest forms of therapy, but the problem may recur. Marsupialization, incision and drainage with the insertion of an indwelling Word catheter, or laser treatment will establish a new duct opening. An asymptomatic cyst does not require therapy.

EFFECTS OF EXPOSURE TO DIETHYLSTILBESTROL IN UTERO

Between 1947 and 1971, diethylstilbestrol (DES) was widely used in the USA for diabetic women during pregnancy and to treat threatened abortion. It is estimated that 2–3 million fetuses were exposed. A relationship between fetal DES exposure and clear cell carcinoma of the vagina was later discovered, and a number of other related anomalies have since been noted. In one-third of all exposed women, there are changes in the vagina (adenosis, septa), cervix (deformities and hypoplasia of the vaginal portion of the cervix), or uterus (T-shaped cavity).

At present, all exposed women are advised to have an initial colposcopic examination to outline vaginal and cervical areas of abnormal epithelium, followed by cytologic examination of the vagina (all four quadrants of the upper half of the vagina) and cervix at yearly intervals. Lugol's iodine stain of the vagina and cervix will also outline areas of metaplastic squamous epithelium.

Many women are not aware of having been exposed to DES. Therefore, in the age groups at risk (30–56 years), examiners should pay attention to structural changes of the vagina and cervix that may signal the possibility of DES exposure and indicate the need for follow-up.

The incidence of clear cell carcinoma is approximately one in 1000 exposed women, and the incidence of cervical and vaginal intraepithelial neoplasia (dysplasia and carcinoma in situ) is twice as high as in unexposed women. DES daughters have more difficulty conceiving and have an increased incidence of early abortion, ectopic pregnancy, and premature births. In addition, mothers treated with DES in pregnancy appear to have a small increase in the incidence of breast cancer, beginning 20 years after exposure.

Goldberg JM et al: Effect of diethylstilbestrol on reproductive function. Fertil Steril 1999;72:1. [PMID: 10418139] (Review of published literature on in utero diethylstilbestrol exposure and the effects on rates of fertility, ectopic pregnancy, spontaneous abortion, and live births.)

CERVICAL INTRAEPITHELIAL NEOPLASIA
(CIN; Dysplasia of the Cervix)

The squamocolumnar junction of the cervix is an area of active squamous cell proliferation. In childhood, this junction is located on the exposed vaginal portion of the cervix. At puberty, because of hormonal influence and possibly because of changes in the vaginal pH, the squamous margin begins to encroach on the single-layered, mucus-secreting epithelium, creating an area of metaplasia (transformation zone). Factors associated with coitus (see Prevention, below) may lead to cellular abnormalities, which over a period of time can result in the development of squamous cell dysplasia or cancer. There are varying degrees of dysplasia (Table 17–2), defined by the degree of cellular atypia; all types must be observed and treated if they persist or become more severe. At present, the malignant potential of a specific lesion cannot be predicted. Some lesions remain stable for long periods of time; some regress; and others advance.

Clinical Findings

There are no specific symptoms or signs of cervical intraepithelial neoplasia. The presumptive diagnosis is made by cytologic screening of an asymptomatic population with no grossly visible cervical changes. All visibly abnormal cervical lesions should be biopsied.

Diagnosis

A. CYTOLOGIC EXAMINATION (PAPANICOLAOU SMEAR)

Specimens should be taken from a nonmenstruating patient, spread on a single slide, and fixed or rinsed directly into preservative solution if a thin layer slide system (ThinPrep) is to be used. A specimen should be obtained from the squamocolumnar junction with a

Table 17–2. Classification systems for Papanicolaou smears.

Numerical	Dysplasia	CIN	Bethesda System
1	Benign	Benign	Normal
2	Benign with inflammation	Benign with Inflammation	Normal, ASC-US
3	Mild dysplasia	CIN I	Low-grade SIL
3	Moderate dysplasia	CIN II	
3	Severe dysplasia	CIN III	High-grade SIL
4	Carcinoma in situ		
5	Invasive cancer	Invasive cancer	Invasive cancer

CIN = cervical intraepithelial neoplasia; SIL = squamous intraepithelial lesion; ASC-US-atypical squamous cells of undetermined significance wooden or plastic spatula and from the endocervix with a cotton swab or nylon brush.

Cytologic reports from the laboratory may describe findings in one of several ways (see Table 17–2). While use of class I–IV is decreasing, the CIN classification continues to be used along with a description of abnormal cells, including evidence of human papillomavirus (HPV). The term "squamous intraepithelial lesions (SIL)," low-grade or high-grade, is increasingly used. Cytopathologists consider a Papanicolaou smear to be a medical consultation and will recommend further diagnostic procedures, treatment for infection, and comments on factors preventing adequate evaluation of the specimen. HPV testing of cytologic smears may be useful for triage of atypia (atypical squamous cells of unknown significance; ASCUS).

B. COLPOSCOPY

Viewing the cervix with 10–20× magnification allows for assessment of the size and margins of an abnormal transformation zone and determination of extension into the endocervical canal. The application of 3–5% acetic acid (vinegar) dissolves mucus, and the acid's desiccating action sharpens the contrast between normal and actively proliferating squamous epithelium. Abnormal changes include white patches and vascular atypia, which indicate areas of greatest cellular activity. Paint the cervix with Lugol's solution (strong iodine solution [Schiller's test]). Normal squamous epithelium will take the stain; nonstaining squamous epithelium should be biopsied. (The single-layered, mucus-secreting endocervical tissue will not stain either but can readily be distinguished by its darker pink, shinier appearance.)

C. BIOPSY

Colposcopically directed punch biopsy and endocervical curettage are office procedures. If colposcopic examination is not available, the normal-appearing cervix shedding atypical cells can be evaluated by endocervical curettage and multiple punch biopsies of nonstaining squamous epithelium or biopsies from each quadrant of the cervix.

Data from both cervical biopsy and endocervical curettage are important in deciding on treatment.

Prevention

Current data suggest that cervical infection with the human papillomavirus (HPV) is associated with a high percentage of all cervical dysplasias and cancers. There are over 60 recognized HPV subtypes, of which types 6 and 11 tend to cause mild dysplasia, while types 16, 18, 31, and others cause higher grade cellular changes.

Cervical cancer almost never occurs in virginal women; it is epidemiologically related to the number of sexual partners a woman has had and the number of other female partners a male partner has had. Use of the diaphragm or condom has a protective effect.

Long-term oral contraceptive users develop more dysplasias and cancers of the cervix than users of other forms of birth control, and smokers are also more at risk. Preventive measures include the following:

(1) Regular cytologic screening to detect abnormalities.

(2) Limiting the number of sexual partners.

(3) Using a diaphragm or condom for coitus.

(4) Stopping smoking.

Women with HIV infection appear to be at increased risk of the disease and of recurrent disease after treatment. Women with HIV infection should receive regular cytologic screening and should be followed closely after treatment for cervical intraepithelial neoplasia.

Because of the very low rate of abnormal Papanicolaou smears in women who have undergone hysterectomy for benign disease, routine screening is not justified in this population.

Treatment

Treatment varies depending on the degree and extent of cervical intraepithelial neoplasia. Biopsies should always precede treatment.

A. CAUTERIZATION OR CRYOSURGERY

The use of either hot cauterization or freezing (cryosurgery) is effective for noninvasive small lesions visible on the cervix without endocervical extension.

B. CO_2 LASER

This well-controlled method minimizes tissue destruction. It is colposcopically directed and requires special training. It may be used with large visible lesions. In current practice it involves the vaporization of the transformation zone on the cervix and the distal 5–7 mm of endocervical canal.

C. LOOP RESECTION

When the CIN is clearly visible in its entirety, a wire loop can be used for excisional biopsy. Cutting and hemostasis are effected with a low-voltage electrosurgical machine (Bovie). This office procedure with local anesthesia is quick and uncomplicated.

D. CONIZATION OF THE CERVIX

Conization is surgical removal of the entire transformation zone and endocervical canal. It should be reserved for cases of severe dysplasia or cancer in situ (CIN III), particularly those with endocervical extension. The procedure can be performed with the scalpel, the CO_2 laser, the needle electrode, or by large-loop excision.

E. FOLLOW-UP

Because recurrence is possible—especially in the first 2 years after treatment—and because the false-negative rate of a single cervical cytologic test is 20%, close follow-up is imperative. Vaginal cytologic examination should be repeated at 3-month intervals for at least 1 year.

Sawaya GF et al: Current practice. Current approaches to cervi-cal-cancer screening. N Engl J Med 2001;344:1603. [PMID: 11372013] (Summary of the current status of cervical can-cer screening.)

Sherman ME et al: Effects of age and human papilloma viral load on colposcopy triage: Data from the Randomized Atypical Squamous Cells of Undetermined Significance/Low-grade Squamous Intraepithelial Lesion Triage Study (ALTS). J Natl Cancer Inst 2002;94:102. [PMID: 11792748] (For women with ASC-US, HPV testing was highly sensitive for detecting CIN3 and cancer, and it was particularly useful in reducing referrals for colposcopy among older women.)

Stoler MH: New Bethesda terminology and evidence-based man-agement guidelines for cervical cytology findings. JAMA 2002;287:2140. [PMID: 11966390]

Wright TC Jr et al: 2001 Consensus Guidelines for the manage-ment of women with cervical cytological abnormalities. JAMA 2002,287.2120. [PMID: 11966387] (Women with ASC-US [atypical squamous cells of undetermined signifi-cance] should have 2 repeat cytology tests, immediate col-poscopy, or DNA testing for high-risk types of human papillomavirus (HPV). Most cases of ASC-H [atypical squamous cells, cannot exclude high-grade squamous in-traepithelial lesion {HSIL}], low-grade squamous intraep-ithelial lesion, HSIL, and atypical glandular cells should be referred for immediate colposcopic evaluation.)

CARCINOMA OF THE CERVIX

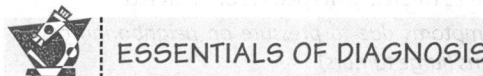

ESSENTIALS OF DIAGNOSIS

- *Abnormal uterine bleeding and vaginal discharge.*
- *Cervical lesion may be visible on inspection as a tumor or ulceration.*
- *Vaginal cytology usually positive; must be con-firmed by biopsy.*

General Considerations

Cancer appears first in the intraepithelial layers (the preinvasive stage, or carcinoma in situ). Preinvasive cancer (CIN III) is a common diagnosis in women 25–40 years of age and is etiologically related to infec-tion with the human papillomavirus. Two to 10 years are required for carcinoma to penetrate the basement membrane and invade the tissues. After invasion, death usually occurs within 3–5 years in untreated or unresponsive patients.

Clinical Findings

A. SYMPTOMS AND SIGNS

The most common signs are metrorrhagia, postcoital spotting, and cervical ulceration. Bloody or purulent,

odorous, nonpruritic discharge may appear after inva-sion. Bladder and rectal dysfunction or fistulas and pain are late symptoms.

B. CERVICAL BIOPSY AND ENDOCERVICAL CURETTAGE, OR CONIZATION

These procedures are necessary steps after a positive Papanicolaou smear to determine the extent and depth of invasion of the cancer. Even if the smear is positive, treatment is never justified until definitive di-agnosis has been established through biopsy.

C. "STAGING," OR ESTIMATE OF GROSS SPREAD OF CANCER OF THE CERVIX

The depth of penetration of the malignant cells be-yond the basement membrane is a reliable clinical guide to the extent of primary cancer within the cervix and the likelihood of metastases. It is customary to stage cancers of the cervix under anesthesia as shown in Table 17–3. Further assessment may be carried out by abdominal and pelvic CT scanning or MRI.

Complications

Metastases to regional lymph nodes occur with in-creasing frequency from stage I to stage IV. Paracervi-cal extension occurs in all directions from the cervix. The ureters are often obstructed lateral to the cervix, causing hydroureter and hydronephrosis and conse-quently impaired kidney function. Almost two-thirds of patients with untreated carcinoma of the cervix die of uremia when ureteral obstruction is bilateral. Pain in the back, in the distribution of the lumbosacral plexus, is often indicative of neurologic involvement. Gross edema of the legs may be indicative of vascular and lymphatic stasis due to tumor.

Vaginal fistulas to the rectum and urinary tract are severe late complications. Hemorrhage is the cause of death in 10–20% of patients with extensive invasive carcinoma.

Treatment

A. EMERGENCY MEASURES

Vaginal hemorrhage originates from gross ulceration and cavitation in stage II–IV cervical carcinoma. Liga-tion and suturing of the cervix are usually not feasible, but ligation of the uterine or hypogastric arteries may be lifesaving when other measures fail. Styptics such as Monsel's solution or acetone are effective, although delayed sloughing may result in further bleeding. Wet vaginal packing is helpful. Emergency irradiation usu-ally controls bleeding.

B. SPECIFIC MEASURES

1. Carcinoma in situ (stage 0)—In women who have completed childbearing, total hysterectomy is the treatment of choice. In women who wish to retain the

Table 17–3. FIGO staging
of cancer of the cervix.[1]

Preinvasive carcinoma	
Stage 0	Carcinoma in situ
Invasive carcinoma	
Stage I	Carcinoma strictly confined to the cervix.
IA	Invasive cancer diagnosed only by microscopy. All gross lesions, even with superficial invasion, are stage IB.
IA1	Measured invasion of stroma no greater than 3 mm in depth and no wider than 7 mm.
IA2	Measured invasion of stroma greater than 3 mm in depth and no greater than 5 mm in depth and no wider than 7 mm.
IB	Clinical lesions confined to the cervix or preclinical lesions greater than 1A.
IB1	Clinical lesions no greater than 4 cm.
IB2	Clinical lesions greater than 4 cm.
Stage II	Carcinoma extends beyond the cervix but has not extended to the pelvic wall. The carcinoma involves the vagina but not as far as the lower third.
IIA	No obvious parametrial involvement.
IIB	Obvious parametrial involvement.
Stage III	Carcinoma has extended either to the lower third of the vagina or to the pelvic sidewall. All cases of hydronephrosis.
IIIA	Involvement of lower third of vagina. No extension to pelvic sidewall.
IIIB	Extension onto the pelvic wall and/or hydronephrosis or nonfunctioning kidney.
Stage IV	Carcinoma extended beyond the true pelvis or clinically involving the mucosa of the bladder or rectum.
IVA	Spread of growth to adjacent organs.
IVB	Spread of growth to distant organs.

uterus, acceptable alternatives include cervical conization or ablation of the lesion with cryotherapy or laser. Close follow-up with Papanicolaou smears every 3 months for 1 year and every 6 months for another year is necessary after cryotherapy or laser.

2. Invasive carcinoma—Microinvasive carcinoma (stage IA) is treated with simple, extrafascial hysterectomy. Stage IB and stage IIA cancers may be treated with either radical hysterectomy or radiation therapy. Stage IIB and stage III and IV cancers must be treated with radiation therapy. Because radical surgery results in fewer long-term complications than irradiation and may allow preservation of ovarian function, it may be the preferred mode of therapy in younger women without contraindications to major surgery.

Prognosis

The overall 5-year relative survival rate for carcinoma of the cervix is 68% in white women and 55% in black women in the United States. Survival rates are inversely proportionate to the stage of cancer: stage 0, 99–100%; stage IA, > 95%; stage IB-IIA, 80–90%; stage IIB, 65%; stage III, 40%; stage IV, < 20%.

Canavan TP et al: Cervical cancer. Am Family Physician 2000; 61:1369. [PMID: 10735343] (Review article.)

Ferrante JM et al: Clinical and demographic predictors of late-stage cervical cancer. Arch Fam Med 2000;9:439. [PMID: 10810949] (Women who are elderly, uninsured, and unmarried are more likely to be diagnosed with late-stage cervical cancer. Cervical cancer screening programs should target these women.)

LEIOMYOMA OF THE UTERUS (Fibroid Tumor)

 ESSENTIALS OF DIAGNOSIS

- *Irregular enlargement of the uterus (may be asymptomatic).*
- *Heavy or irregular vaginal bleeding, dysmenorrhea.*
- *Acute and recurrent pelvic pain if the tumor becomes twisted on its pedicle or infarcted.*
- *Symptoms due to pressure on neighboring organs (large tumors).*

General Considerations

Uterine leiomyoma is the most common benign neoplasm of the female genital tract. It is a discrete, round, firm, often multiple uterine tumor composed of smooth muscle and connective tissue. The most convenient classification is by anatomic location: (1) intramural, (2) submucous, (3) subserous, (4) intraligamentous, (5) parasitic (ie, deriving its blood supply from an organ to which it becomes attached), and (6) cervical. A submucous myoma may become pedunculated and descend through the cervix into the vagina.

Clinical Findings

A. SYMPTOMS AND SIGNS

In nonpregnant women, myomas are frequently asymptomatic. However, they can cause urinary frequency, dysmenorrhea, heavy bleeding (often with anemia), or other complications due to the presence of an abdominal mass. Occasionally, degeneration occurs, causing intense pain. Infertility may be due to a myoma that significantly distorts the uterine cavity.

B. LABORATORY FINDINGS

Hemoglobin levels may be decreased as a result of blood loss, but in rare cases polycythemia is present, presumably as a result of the production of erythropoietin by the myomas.

C. IMAGING

Ultrasonography will confirm the presence of uterine myomas and can be used sequentially to monitor growth. When multiple subserous or pedunculated myomas are being followed, ultrasonography is important to exclude ovarian masses. MRI can delineate intramural and submucous myomas accurately. Hysterography or hysteroscopy can also confirm cervical or submucous myomas.

Differential Diagnosis

Irregular myomatous enlargement of the uterus must be differentiated from the similar but symmetric enlargement that may occur with pregnancy or adenomyosis (the presence of endometrial glands and stroma in the myometrium). Subserous myomas must be distinguished from ovarian tumors. Leiomyosarcoma is an unusual tumor occurring in 0.5% of women operated on for symptomatic myoma. It is very rare under the age of 40 and increases in incidence thereafter.

Treatment

A. EMERGENCY MEASURES

If the patient is markedly anemic as a result of long, heavy menstrual periods, preoperative treatment with depot medroxyprogesterone acetate, 150 mg intramuscularly every 28 days, or danazol, 400–800 mg orally daily, will slow or stop bleeding, and medical treatment of anemia can be given prior to surgery. Emergency surgery is required for acute torsion of a pedunculated myoma. The only emergency indication for myomectomy during pregnancy is torsion; abortion is not an inevitable result.

B. SPECIFIC MEASURES

Women who have small asymptomatic myomas should be examined at 6-month intervals. If necessary, elective myomectomy can be done to preserve the uterus. Myomas do not require surgery on an urgent basis unless they cause significant pressure on the ureters, bladder, or bowel or severe bleeding leading to anemia or unless they are undergoing rapid growth. Cervical myomas larger than 3–4 cm in diameter or pedunculated myomas that protrude through the cervix must be removed. Submucous myomas can be removed using a hysteroscope and laser or resection instruments.

Because the risk of surgical complications increases with the increasing size of the myoma, preoperative reduction of myoma size is desirable. GnRH analogs such as depot leuprolide, 3.75 mg intramuscularly monthly, or nafarelin, 0.2–0.4 mg intranasally twice a day, are used preoperatively for 3- to 4-month periods to induce reversible hypogonadism, which temporarily reduces the size of myomas, suppresses their further growth, and reduces surrounding vascularity.

C. SURGICAL MEASURES

Surgical measures available for the treatment of myoma are myomectomy and total or subtotal abdominal, vaginal, or laparoscopy-assisted vaginal hysterectomy. Myomectomy is the treatment of choice during the childbearing years. Recent developments include transcatheter bilateral uterine artery embolization and myolysis with cryotherapy or cauterization. While these approaches are promising, randomized clinical trials comparing these new methods with conventional therapy are needed.

Prognosis

Surgical therapy is curative. Future pregnancies are not endangered by myomectomy, although cesarean delivery may be necessary after wide dissection with entry into the uterine cavity.

Olive DL: New approaches to the management of fibroids. Obstet Gynecol Clin North Am 2000;27:669. [PMID: 10958011] (Summary of new approaches to therapy.)

CARCINOMA OF THE ENDOMETRIUM

Adenocarcinoma of the uterine corpus is the second most common cancer of the female genital tract. It occurs most often in women 50–70 years of age. Some patients will have taken unopposed estrogen in the past; their increased risk appears to persist for 10 or more years after stopping the drug. Obesity, nulliparity, diabetes, and polycystic ovaries with prolonged anovulation and the extended use of tamoxifen for the treatment of breast cancer are also risk factors.

Abnormal bleeding is the presenting sign in 80% of cases. Endometrial carcinoma may cause obstruction of the cervix with collection of pus (pyometra) or blood (hematometra) causing lower abdominal pain. However, pain generally occurs late in the disease, with metastases or infection.

Papanicolaou smears of the cervix occasionally show atypical endometrial cells but are an insensitive diagnostic tool. Endocervical and endometrial sampling is the only reliable means of diagnosis. Adequate specimens of each can usually be obtained during an office procedure performed following local anesthesia (paracervical block). Simultaneous hysteroscopy can be a valuable addition in order to localize polyps or other lesions within the uterine cavity. Vaginal ultrasonography may be used to determine the thickness of the endometrium as an indication of hypertrophy and possible neoplastic change.

Pathologic assessment is important in differentiating hyperplasias, which often can be treated with cyclic oral progestins.

Prevention

Prompt endometrial sampling for patients who report abnormal menstrual bleeding or postmenopausal uterine bleeding will reveal many incipient as well as clinical cases of endometrial cancer. In comparison with the use of unopposed estrogen for menopausal therapy, there is a relative risk of endometrial cancer of 0.3 among women using continuous combined regimens of estrogen and progestin. Younger women with chronic anovulation are at risk for endometrial hyperplasia and subsequent endometrial cancer. They can reduce the risk of hyperplasia almost completely with the use of oral contraceptives or cyclic progestin therapy.

Staging

Examination under anesthesia, endometrial and endocervical sampling, chest x-ray, intravenous urography, cystoscopy, sigmoidoscopy, transvaginal sonography, and MRI will help determine the extent of the disease and its appropriate treatment. The staging is based on the surgical and pathologic evaluation.

TREATMENT

Treatment consists of total hysterectomy and bilateral salpingo-oophorectomy. Peritoneal material for cytologic examination is routinely taken. Preliminary external irradiation or intracavitary radium therapy is indicated if the cancer is poorly differentiated or if the uterus is definitely enlarged in the absence of myomas. If invasion deep into the myometrium has occurred or if sampled preaortic lymph nodes are positive for tumor, postoperative irradiation is indicated.

Palliation of advanced or metastatic endometrial adenocarcinoma may be accomplished with large doses of progestins, eg, medroxyprogesterone, 400 mg intramuscularly weekly, or megestrol acetate, 80–160 mg daily orally.

Prognosis

With early diagnosis and treatment, the 5-year survival is 80–85%.

Hernandez E: Endometrial carcinoma: A primer for the generalist. Obstet Gynecol North Am 2001;28:743. [PMID: 11766149] (Summary of current diagnosis and treatment.)

CARCINOMA OF THE VULVA

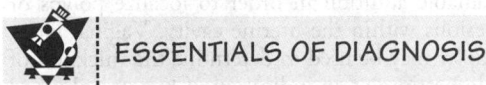

ESSENTIALS OF DIAGNOSIS

- *History of genital warts.*
- *History of prolonged vulvar irritation, with pruritus, local discomfort, or slight bloody discharge.*

- *Early lesions may suggest or include nonneoplastic epithelial disorders.*
- *Late lesions appear as a mass, an exophytic growth, or a firm, ulcerated area in the vulva.*
- *Biopsy is necessary to make the diagnosis.*

General Considerations

The vast majority of cancers of the vulva are squamous lesions that classically have occurred in women over 50 years of age. Several subtypes (particularly 16, 18, and 31) of the human papillomavirus have been identified in some but not all vulvar cancers. As with squamous cell lesions of the cervix, a grading system of vulvar intraepithelial neoplasia (VIN) from mild dysplasia to carcinoma in situ has been established.

Differential Diagnosis

Biopsy is essential for the diagnosis of vulvar cancer and should be performed with any localized atypical vulvar lesion, including white patches. Multiple skin-punch specimens can be taken in the office under local anesthesia, with care to include tissue from the edges of each lesion sampled.

Benign vulvar disorders that must be excluded in the diagnosis of carcinoma of the vulva include chronic granulomatous lesions (eg, lymphogranuloma venereum, syphilis), condylomas, hidradenoma, or neurofibroma. Lichen sclerosus and other associated leukoplakic changes in the skin should be biopsied. The likelihood that a superimposed vulvar cancer will develop in a woman with a nonneoplastic epithelial disorder (vulvar dystrophy) ranges from 1% to 5%.

Treatment

A. General Measures

Early diagnosis and treatment of irritative or other predisposing or contributing causes to carcinoma of the vulva should be pursued. A 7:3 combination of betamethasone and crotamiton is particularly effective for itching. After an initial response, fluorinated steroids should be replaced with hydrocortisone because of their skin atrophying effect. For lichen sclerosus, recommended treatment is clobetasol propionate cream 0.05% twice daily for 2–3 weeks, then once daily until symptoms resolve. Application one to three times a week can be used for long-term maintenance therapy.

B. Surgical Measures

In situ squamous cell carcinoma of the vulva and small, invasive basal cell carcinoma of the vulva should be excised with a wide margin. If the squamous carcinoma in situ is extensive or multicentric, laser therapy or superficial surgical removal of vulvar skin may be required. In this way, the clitoris and uninvolved portions of the vulva may be spared. Skin grafting may be necessary, but mutilating vulvectomy is avoided.

Invasive carcinoma confined to the vulva without evidence of spread to adjacent organs or to the regional lymph nodes will necessitate radical vulvectomy and inguinal lymphadenectomy if the patient is able to withstand surgery. Debilitated patients may be candidates for palliative irradiation only.

Prognosis

Basal cell carcinomas very seldom metastasize, and carcinoma in situ by definition has not metastasized. With adequate excision, the prognosis for both lesions is excellent. Patients with invasive vulvar squamous cell carcinoma 3 cm in diameter or less without inguinal lymph node metastases who can sustain radical surgery have about a 90% chance of a 5-year survival. If the lesion is greater than 3 cm and has metastasized, the likelihood of 5-year survival is less than 25%.

Nash JD et al: Vulvar cancer. Surg Oncol Clin N Am 1998; 7:335. [PMID: 9537980] (A review of surgical and medical treatment of vulvar cancer.)

Thomas E et al: Premalignant vulval disorders. Clin Evidence 2000;4:1115. (Topical clobetasol is the most effective treatment for lichen sclerosus and is associated with minimal side effects.)

ENDOMETRIOSIS

Endometriosis is an aberrant growth of endometrium outside the uterus, particularly in the dependent parts of the pelvis and in the ovaries and is a common cause of abnormal bleeding and secondary dysmenorrhea. Its causes, pathogenesis, and natural course are poorly understood. The prevalence in the USA is 2% among fertile women and three- to fourfold greater than that in the infertile. Depending on the location and extent of the endometrial implants, infertility, dyspareunia, or rectal pain with bleeding may result. Aching pain tends to be constant, beginning 2–7 days before the onset of menses, and becomes increasingly severe until flow slackens. Pelvic examination may disclose tender indurated nodules in the cul-de-sac, especially if the examination is done at the onset of menstruation.

Endometriosis must be distinguished from pelvic inflammatory disease, ovarian neoplasms, and uterine myomas. In general, only in salpingitis and endometriosis are the symptoms aggravated by menstruation. Bowel invasion by endometrial tissue may produce clinical findings, including blood in the stool, that must be distinguished from bowel neoplasm. Differentiation in these instances depends upon proctosigmoidoscopy and biopsy.

Ultrasound examination will often reveal complex fluid-filled masses that cannot be distinguished from neoplasms. MRI is more sensitive and specific than ultrasound, particularly in the diagnosis of adnexal masses. However, the clinical diagnosis of endometriosis is presumptive and usually confirmed by laparoscopy or laparotomy.

Treatment

A. MEDICAL TREATMENT

The goal of medical treatment is to preserve the fertility of women wanting future pregnancies, ameliorate symptoms, and simplify future surgery or make it unnecessary. Medications are designed to inhibit ovulation over 4–9 months and lower hormone levels, thus preventing cyclic stimulation of endometriotic implants and decreasing their size. The optimum duration of therapy is not clear, and the relative merits in terms of pregnancies, side effects, and long-term risks and benefits show insignificant differences when compared with each other, with surgery (including laser surgery), and, in mild cases, with placebo.

1. The GnRH analogs such as nafarelin nasal spray, 0.2–0.4 mg twice daily, or long-acting injectable leuprolide acetate, 3.75 mg intramuscularly monthly, used for 6 months, suppress ovulation. Side effects consisting of vasomotor symptoms and bone demineralization may be relieved by "add-back" therapy with norethindrone, 5–10 mg daily.

2. Danazol is used for 6–9 months in the lowest dose necessary to suppress menstruation, usually 200–400 mg twice daily. Side effects are androgenic and include decreased breast size, weight gain, acne, and hirsutism.

3. Any of the combination oral contraceptives may be given, one daily, without interruption, for 6–12 months. Breakthrough bleeding can be treated with conjugated estrogens, 1.25 mg daily for 1 week, or estradiol, 2 mg daily for 1 week.

4. Medroxyprogesterone acetate, 100 mg intramuscularly every 2 weeks for four doses; then 100 mg every 4 weeks; add oral estrogen or estradiol valerate, 30 mg intramuscularly, for breakthrough bleeding. Use for 6–9 months.

5. Low-dose oral contraceptives can also be given cyclically; prolonged suppression of ovulation will often inhibit further stimulation of residual endometriosis, especially if taken after one of the therapies mentioned above.

6. Analgesics, with or without codeine, may be needed during menses. Nonsteroidal anti-inflammatory drugs may be helpful.

B. SURGICAL MEASURES

The surgical treatment of moderately extensive endometriosis depends upon the patient's age and symptoms and her desire to preserve reproductive function. If the patient is under 35, resect the lesions, free adhesions, and suspend the uterus. At least 20% of patients so treated can become pregnant, although some must undergo surgery again if the disease progresses. If the patient is over 35 years old, is disabled by pain, and has involvement of both ovaries, bilateral salpingo-oophorectomy and hysterectomy will probably be necessary.

Foci of endometriosis can be treated at laparoscopy by bipolar coagulation or laser vaporization. Because pelvic endometriosis can take forms other than the classic powder burns and hemorrhagic cysts, a meticulous survey of the peritoneum is required.

Prognosis

The prognosis for reproductive function in early or moderately advanced endometriosis is good with conservative therapy. Bilateral ovariectomy is curative for patients with severe and extensive endometriosis with pain. Following hysterectomy and oophorectomy, estrogen replacement therapy is indicated.

Farquhar C: Endometriosis. Clin Evidence 2000;4:1058. (Danazol, DMPA, GnRH analogs, and oral contraceptives appear to be equally effective at reducing pain associated with endometriosis.)

Ling FW: Randomized controlled trial of depot leuprolide in patients with chronic pelvic pain and clinically suspected endometriosis. Pelvic Pain Study Group. Obstet Gynecol 1999;93:51. [PMID: 9916956] (Empiric use of depot leuprolide in women with chronic pelvic pain suspected of having endometriosis is a cost-effective approach to nonsurgical diagnosis and treatment.)

Olive DL et al: Treatment of endometriosis. N Engl J Med 2001; 345:266. [PMID: 11474666] (Summary of current treatment approaches.)

GENITAL PROLAPSE (CYSTOCELE, RECTOCELE, ENTEROCELE)

Cystocele, rectocele, and enterocele are vaginal hernias commonly seen in multiparous women. Cystocele is a hernia of the bladder wall into the vagina, causing a soft anterior fullness. Cystocele may be accompanied by urethrocele, which is not a hernia but a sagging of the urethra following its detachment from the pubic symphysis during childbirth. Rectocele is a herniation of the terminal rectum into the posterior vagina, causing a collapsible pouch-like fullness. Enterocele is a vaginal vault hernia containing small intestine, usually in the posterior vagina and resulting from a deepening of the pouch of Douglas. Enterocele may also accompany uterine prolapse or follow hysterectomy, when weakened vault supports or a deep unobliterated cul-de-sac containing intestine protrudes into the vagina. Two or all three types of hernia may occur in combination.

Supportive measures include a high-fiber diet. Weight reduction in obese patients and limitation of straining and lifting are helpful. Pessaries may reduce cystocele, rectocele, or enterocele temporarily and are helpful in women who do not wish surgery or are chronically ill.

The only cure for symptomatic cystocele, rectocele, or enterocele is corrective surgery. The prognosis following an uncomplicated procedure is good.

UTERINE PROLAPSE

Uterine prolapse most commonly occurs as a delayed result of childbirth injury to the pelvic floor (particularly the transverse cervical and uterosacral ligaments). Unrepaired obstetric lacerations of the levator musculature and perineal body augment the weakness. Attenuation of the pelvic structures with aging and congenital weakness can accelerate the development of prolapse.

In slight prolapse, the uterus descends only part way down the vagina; in moderate prolapse, the corpus descends to the introitus and the cervix protrudes slightly beyond; and in marked prolapse (procidentia), the entire cervix and uterus protrude beyond the introitus and the vagina is inverted. Inability to walk comfortably because of protrusion or discomfort from the presence of a vaginal mass is an indication that surgical treatment should be considered.

Treatment

The type of surgery depends upon the extent of prolapse and the patient's age and her desire for menstruation, pregnancy, and coitus. The simplest, most effective procedure is vaginal hysterectomy with appropriate repair of the cystocele and rectocele. If the patient desires pregnancy, a partial resection of the cervix with plication of the cardinal ligaments can be attempted. For elderly women who do not desire coitus, partial obliteration of the vagina is surgically simple and effective. Abdominal uterine suspension or ventrofixation will fail in the treatment of prolapse.

A well-fitted vaginal pessary (eg, inflatable doughnut type, Gellhorn pessary) may give relief if surgery is refused or contraindicated.

Poma PA: Nonsurgical management of genital prolapse. A review and recommendations for clinical practice J Reprod Med 2000;45:789. [PMID: 11077625] (Review article.)

PELVIC INFLAMMATORY DISEASE (PID; Salpingitis, Endometritis)

Pelvic inflammatory disease is a polymicrobial infection of the upper genital tract associated with the sexually transmitted organisms *N gonorrhoeae* and *C trachomatis* as well as endogenous organisms, including anaerobes, *H influenzae,* enteric gram-negative rods, and streptococci. It is most common in young, nulliparous, sexually active women with multiple partners. Other risk markers include nonwhite race, douching, and smoking. The use of oral contraceptives or barrier methods of contraception may provide significant protection.

Tuberculous salpingitis is rare in the USA but more common in developing countries; it is characterized by pelvic pain and irregular pelvic masses not responsive to antibiotic therapy. It is not sexually transmitted.

Clinical Findings

A. SYMPTOMS AND SIGNS

Patients with pelvic inflammatory disease may have lower abdominal pain, chills and fever, menstrual disturbances, purulent cervical discharge, and cervical and adnexal tenderness. Right upper quadrant pain (Fitz-Hugh and Curtis syndrome) may indicate an associated perihepatitis. However, diagnosis of PID is complicated by the fact that many women may have subtle or mild symptoms, not readily recognized as PID.

B. MINIMUM DIAGNOSTIC CRITERIA

Women with lower abdominal, adnexal, or cervical motion tenderness should be considered to have PID and be treated with antibiotics unless there is a competing diagnosis such as ectopic pregnancy or appendicitis.

C. ADDITIONAL CRITERIA

The following criteria may be used to enhance the specificity of the diagnosis: (1) oral temperature > 38.3 °C, (2) abnormal cervical or vaginal discharge with white cells on saline microscopy, (3) elevated erythrocyte sedimentation rate, (4) elevated C-reactive protein, and (5) laboratory documentation of cervical infection with *N gonorrhoeae* or *C trachomatis*. Endocervical culture should be performed routinely, but treatment should not be delayed while awaiting results.

D. DEFINITIVE CRITERIA

In selected cases where the diagnosis based on clinical or laboratory evidence is uncertain, the following criteria may be used: (1) histopathologic evidence of endometritis on endometrial biopsy, (2) transvaginal sonography or other imaging techniques showing thickened fluid-filled tubes with or without free pelvic fluid or tubo-ovarian complex, and (3) laparoscopic abnormalities consistent with PID.

Differential Diagnosis

Appendicitis, ectopic pregnancy, septic abortion, hemorrhagic or ruptured ovarian cysts or tumors, twisted ovarian cyst, degeneration of a myoma, and acute enteritis must be considered. Pelvic inflammatory disease is more likely to occur when there is a history of pelvic inflammatory disease, recent sexual contact, recent onset of menses, or an IUD in place or if the partner has a sexually transmitted disease. Acute pelvic inflammatory disease is highly unlikely when recent intercourse has not taken place or an IUD is not being used. A sensitive serum pregnancy test should be obtained to rule out ectopic pregnancy. Culdocentesis will differentiate hemoperitoneum (ruptured ectopic pregnancy or hemorrhagic cyst) from pelvic sepsis (salpingitis, ruptured pelvic abscess, or ruptured appendix). Pelvic and vaginal ultrasound is helpful in the differential diagnosis of ectopic pregnancy of over 6 weeks. Laparoscopy is often utilized to diagnose pelvic inflammatory disease, and it is imperative if the diagnosis is not certain or if the patient has not responded to antibiotic therapy after 48 hours. The appendix should be visualized at laparoscopy to rule out appendicitis. Cultures obtained at the time of laparoscopy are often specific and helpful.

Treatment

A. HOSPITALIZATION

Patients with acute pelvic inflammatory disease should be admitted for intravenous antibiotic therapy if (1) surgical emergencies such as appendicitis cannot be ruled out; (2) the patient has a tubo-ovarian abscess; (3) the patient is pregnant; (4) the patient is unable to follow or tolerate an outpatient regimen; (5) the patient has failed to respond clinically to outpatient therapy; (6) the patient has severe illness, nausea and vomiting, or high fever; or (7) the patient is immunodeficient (ie, has HIV infection with low CD4 counts, is taking immunosuppressive therapy, or has another immunosuppressing disease). In the past, many experts recommended that all patients with PID be hospitalized for bed rest and supervised treatment with parenteral antibiotics. Outpatient parenteral therapy is available in some settings and may be an acceptable alternative, though data are lacking on the efficacy of this approach. Patients with tubo-ovarian abscesses should have direct inpatient observation for at least 24 hours prior to switching to outpatient parenteral therapy.

B. ANTIBIOTICS

Early treatment with appropriate antibiotics effective against *N gonorrhoeae, C trachomatis,* and the endogenous organisms listed above is essential to prevent long-term sequelae. The sexual partner should be examined and treated appropriately.

Two inpatient regimens have been shown to be effective in the treatment of acute pelvic inflammatory disease: (1) Cefoxitin, 2 g intravenously every 6 hours, or cefotetan, 2 g every 12 hours, plus doxycycline, 100 mg intravenously or orally every 12 hours. This regimen is continued for at least 24 hours after the patient shows significant clinical improvement. Doxycycline, 100 mg twice daily, should be continued to complete a total of 14 days therapy. (2) Clindamycin, 900 mg intravenously every 8 hours, plus gentamicin intravenously in a loading dose of 2 mg/kg followed by 1.5 mg/kg every 8 hours. This regimen is continued for at least 24 hours after the patient shows significant clinical improvement and is followed by either clindamycin, 450 mg four times daily, or doxycycline, 100 mg twice daily, to complete a total of 14 days of therapy.

Limited data exist on other parenteral regimens. Three regimens providing broad-spectrum coverage have been investigated in at least one clinical trial: (1) ofloxacin, 400 mg intravenously every 12 hours, plus metronidazole, 500 mg intravenously every 8 hours; (2) ampicillin-sulbactam, 3 g intravenously every 6 hours, plus doxycycline, 100 mg intravenously or orally every 12 hours; and (3) ciprofloxacin, 200 mg intravenously every 12 hours, plus doxycycline, 100 mg intravenously or orally every 12 hours, plus metronidazole, 500 mg intravenously every 8 hours.

Two outpatient regimens are recommended: (1) ofloxacin, 400 mg orally twice daily for 14 days, plus metronidazole, 500 mg orally twice daily, for 14 days; and (2) either a single dose of cefoxitin, 2 g intramuscularly, with probenecid, 1 g orally, or ceftriaxone, 250 mg intramuscularly, plus doxycycline, 100 mg orally twice daily, for 14 days.

C. SURGICAL MEASURES

Tubo-ovarian abscesses may require surgical excision or transcutaneous or transvaginal aspiration. Unless rupture is suspected, institute high-dose antibiotic therapy in the hospital, and monitor therapy with ultrasound. In 70% of cases, antibiotics are effective; in 30%, there is inadequate response in 48–72 hours, and intervention is required. Unilateral adnexectomy is acceptable for unilateral abscess. Hysterectomy and bilateral salpingo-oophorectomy may be necessary for overwhelming infection or in cases of chronic disease with intractable pelvic pain.

Prognosis

In spite of treatment, one-fourth of women with acute disease develop long-term sequelae, including repeated episodes of infection, chronic pelvic pain, dyspareunia, ectopic pregnancy, or infertility. The risk of infertility increases with repeated episodes of salpingitis: it is estimated at 10% after the first episode, 25% after a second episode, and 50% after a third episode.

1998 guidelines for treatment of sexually transmitted diseases. MMWR Morb Mortal Wkly Rep 1998;47(RR-1):79. [PMID: 9461043]

Paavonen J: Pelvic inflammatory disease: From diagnosis to prevention. Dermatol Clin 1998;16:747. [PMID: 9891675] (Review of current approaches to diagnosis, management, and prevention.)

OVARIAN TUMORS

ESSENTIALS OF DIAGNOSIS

- *Vague gastrointestinal discomfort.*
- *Pelvic pressure and pain.*
- *Many cases of early-stage cancer are asymptomatic.*
- *Pelvic examination, CA 125, and ultrasound are mainstays of diagnosis.*

General Considerations

Ovarian tumors are common. Most are benign, but malignant ovarian tumors are the leading cause of death from reproductive tract cancer. The wide range of types and patterns of ovarian tumors is due to the complexity of ovarian embryology and differences in tissues of origin (Table 17–4).

In women with no family history of ovarian cancer, the lifetime risk is 1.6%, whereas a woman with one affected first-degree relative has a 5% lifetime risk. With two or more affected first-degree relatives, the risk is 7%. Approximately 3% of women with two or more affected first-degree relatives will have a hereditary ovarian cancer syndrome with a lifetime risk of 40%. Women with a *BRCA1* gene mutation have a 45% lifetime risk of ovarian cancer and those with a *BRAC2* mutation a 25% risk. These women should be screened annually with transvaginal sonography (TVS) and CA 125 testing, and prophylactic oophorectomy is recommended by age 35 or whenever childbearing is completed because of the high risk of disease. The benefits of such screening for women with one or no affected first-degree relatives are unproved, and the risks associated with unnecessary surgical procedures may outweigh the benefits in low-risk women.

Clinical Findings

A. SYMPTOMS AND SIGNS

Unfortunately, most women with both benign and malignant ovarian neoplasms are either asymptomatic or experience only mild nonspecific gastrointestinal symptoms or pelvic pressure. Women with early disease are typically detected on routine pelvic examination. Women with advanced malignant disease may experience abdominal pain and bloating, and a palpable abdominal mass with ascites is often present.

B. LABORATORY FINDINGS

An elevated serum CA 125 (> 35 units) indicates a greater likelihood that an ovarian tumor is malignant. CA 125 is elevated in 80% of women with epithelial ovarian cancer overall but in only 50% of women with early disease. Furthermore, serum CA 125 may be elevated in premenopausal women with benign disease such as endometriosis.

C. IMAGING STUDIES

TVS is useful for screening high-risk women but has inadequate sensitivity for screening low-risk women. Ultrasound is helpful in differentiating ovarian masses that are benign and likely to resolve spontaneously from those with malignant potential. Color Doppler imaging may further enhance the specificity of ultrasound diagnosis.

Table 17–4. Ovarian functional and neoplastic tumors.

Tumor	Incidence	Size	Consistency	Menstrual Irregularities	Endocrine Effects	Potential for Malignancy	Special Remarks
Follicle cysts	Rare in childhood; frequent in menstrual years; never in postmenopausal years.	< 6 cm, often bilateral.	Moderate	Occasional	Occasional anovulation with persistently proliferative endometrium	None	Often disappear after a 2-month regimen of oral contraceptives.
Corpus luteum cysts	Occasional, in menstrual years.	4–6 cm, unilateral.	Moderate	Occasional delayed period	Prolonged secretory phase	None	Functional cysts. Intraperitoneal bleeding occasionally.
Theca lutein cysts	Occurs with hydatidiform mole, choriocarcinoma; also with gonadotropin or clomiphene therapy.	To 4–5 cm, multiple, bilateral. (Ovaries may be ≥ 20 cm in diameter.)	Tense	Amenorrhea	hCG elevated as a result of trophoblastic proliferation	None	Functional cysts. Hematoperitoneum or torsion of ovary may occur. Surgery is to be avoided.
Inflammatory (tuboovarian abscess)	Concomitant with acute salpingitis.	To 15–20 cm, often bilateral.	Variable, painful	Menometrorrhagia	Anovulat on usual	None	Unilateral removal indicated if possible.
Endometriotic cysts	Never in preadolescent or postmenopausal years. Most common in women aged 20–40 years.	To 10–12 cm, occasionally bilateral.	Moderate to softened	Rare	None	Very rare	Associated pelvic endometriosis. Medical treatment or conservative surgery recommended.
Teratoid tumors: Benign teratomas (dermoid cysts)	Childhood to postmenopause.	< 15 cm; 15% are bilateral.	Moderate to softened	None	None	Rare	Torsion can occur. Partial oophorectomy recommended.
Malignant teratomas	< 1% of ovarian tumors. Usually in infants and young adults.	> 20 cm, unilateral.	Irregularly firm	None	Occasionally, hCG elevated	All	Unresponsive to any therapy.

(continued)

Table 17–4. Ovarian functional and neoplastic tumors. (continued)

Tumor	Incidence	Size	Consistency	Menstrual Irregularities	Endocrine Effects	Potential for Malignancy	Special Remarks
Cystadenoma, cyst-adenocarcinoma	Common in reproductive years.	Serous: < 25 cm, 33% bilateral; mucinous: up to 1 cm, 10% bilateral.	Moderate to softened	None	None	> 50% for serous, about 5% for mucinous	Peritoneal implants often occur with serous, rarely with mucinous. If mucinous tumor is ruptured, pseudomyxoma peritonei may occur.
Endometrioid carcinoma	15% of ovarian carcinomas.	Moderate, 13% bilateral.	Firm	None	None	All	Adenocarcinoma of endometrium coexists in 15–30% of cases.
Fibroma	< 5% of ovarian tumors.	Usually < 15 cm.	Very firm	None	None	Rare	Ascites in 20% (rarely, pleural fluid).
Arrhenoblastoma	Rare. Average age 30 years or more.	Often small (< 10 cm), unilateral.	Firm to softened	Amenorrhea	Androgens elevated	< 20%	Recurrences are moderately sensitive to irradiation.
Theca cell tumor (thecoma)	Uncommon.	< 10 cm, unilateral.	Firm	Occasional irregularity	Estrogens or androgens elevated	< 1%	
Granulosa cell tumor	Uncommon. Usually in prepubertal girls or women older than 50 years.	May be very small.	Firm to softened	Menometrorrhagia	Estrogens elevated	15–20%	Recurrences are moderately sensitive to irradiation.
Dysgerminoma	About 1–2% of ovarian tumors.	< 30 cm, bilateral in 33%.	Moderate to softened	None	...	All	Very radiosensitive.
Brenner tumor	About 1% of ovarian tumors.	< 30 cm, unilateral.	Firm	None	...	Very rare	> 50% occur in postmenopausal years.
Secondary ovarian tumors	10% of fatal malignant disease in women.	Varies; often bilateral.	Firm to softened	Occasional	Very rare (thyroid, adreno-cortical origin)	All	Bowel or breast metastases to ovary common.

Differential Diagnosis

Once an ovarian mass has been detected, it must be categorized as functional, benign neoplastic, or potentially malignant. Predictive factors include age, size of the mass, ultrasound configuration, CA 125 levels, the presence of symptoms, and whether the mass is unilateral or bilateral. In a premenopausal woman, an asymptomatic, mobile, unilateral, simple cystic mass less than 8–10 cm may be observed for 4–6 weeks. Most will resolve spontaneously. If the mass is larger or unchanged on repeat pelvic examination and TVS, surgical evaluation is required.

Most ovarian masses in postmenopausal women require surgical evaluation. However, a postmenopausal woman with an asymptomatic unilateral simple cyst less than 5 cm in diameter and a normal CA 125 level may be followed closely with TVS. All others require surgical evaluation.

Exploratory laparotomy has been the standard approach. Laparoscopy may be considered for a premenopausal woman with an ovarian mass small enough to be removed using a laparoscopic approach. If malignancy is suspected, preoperative workup should include chest x-ray, evaluation of liver and kidney function, and hematologic indices.

Treatment

If a malignant ovarian mass is suspected, surgical evaluation should be performed by a gynecologic oncologist. For benign neoplasms, tumor removal or unilateral oophorectomy is usually performed. For ovarian cancer in an early stage, the standard therapy is complete surgical staging followed by abdominal hysterectomy and bilateral salpingo-oophorectomy with omentectomy and selective lymphadenectomy. With more advanced disease, aggressive removal of all visible tumor improves survival. Except for women with low-grade ovarian cancer in an early stage, postoperative chemotherapy is indicated. Several chemotherapy regimens are effective, such as the combination of cisplatin or carboplatin with paclitaxel, with clinical response rates of up to 60–70%.

Prognosis

Unfortunately, approximately 75% of women with ovarian cancer are diagnosed with advanced disease after regional or distant metastases have become established. The overall 5-year survival is approximately 17% with distant metastases, 36% with local spread, and 89% with early disease.

Holschneider CH et al: Ovarian cancer: epidemiology, biology, and prognostic factors. Semin Surg Oncol 2000;19:3. [PMID: 10883018] (Review article.)

PERSISTENT ANOVULATION
(Polycystic Ovary Syndrome)

ESSENTIALS OF DIAGNOSIS

- Chronic anovulation.
- Infertility.
- Elevated plasma testosterone and LH values and a reversed FSH/LH ratio.
- Hirsutism (in 70% of patients).

General Considerations

Polycystic ovary syndrome is a common endocrine disorder affecting 2–5% of women of reproductive age. The primary lesion is unknown. These patients have a steady state of relatively high estrogen, androgen, and LH levels rather than the fluctuating condition seen in ovulating women. Increased levels of estrone come from obesity (conversion of ovarian and adrenal androgens to estrone in body fat) or from excessive levels of androgens seen in some women of normal weight. The high estrone levels are believed to cause suppression of pituitary FSH and a relative increase in LH. Constant LH stimulation of the ovary results in anovulation, multiple cysts, and theca cell hyperplasia with excess androgen output. The polycystic ovary has a thickened, pearly white capsule and may not be enlarged.

Women with Cushing's syndrome, congenital adrenal hyperplasia, and androgen-secreting adrenal tumors also tend to have high circulating androgen levels and anovulation with polycystic ovaries.

Clinical Findings

Polycystic ovary syndrome is manifested by hirsutism (70% of cases), obesity (40%), and virilization (20%). Fifty percent of patients have amenorrhea, 30% have abnormal uterine bleeding, and 20% have normal menstruation. Additionally, they show insulin resistance and hyperinsulinemia when infused with glucose, and these women are at increased risk of early-onset type 2 diabetes mellitus. The patients are generally infertile, although they may ovulate occasionally. They have an increased long-term risk of cancer of the breast and endometrium because of unopposed estrogen secretion.

Differential Diagnosis

Anovulation in the reproductive years may also be due to (1) premature menopause (high FSH and LH levels); (2) rapid weight loss, extreme physical exertion (normal FSH and LH levels for age), or obesity; (3) discontinuation of oral contraceptives (anovulation for 6 months or more occasionally occurs); (4) pituitary adenoma with elevated prolactin (galactorrhea may or may not be present); (5) hyper- or hypothyroidism. When amenorrhea has persisted for 6 months or more without a diagnosis, FSH, LH, prolactin, TSH, testosterone, and dehydroepiandrosterone sulfate (DHEAS) should be checked. A 10-day course of progestin (eg, medroxyprogesterone acetate, 10 mg/d) will cause withdrawal bleeding if estrogen levels are high. This will aid in the diagnosis and prevent endometrial hyperplasia. In long-term anovular patients over age 35, it is wise to search for an estrogen-stimulated cancer with mammography and endometrial aspiration.

Treatment

In obese patients with polycystic ovaries, weight reduction is often effective; a decrease in body fat will lower the conversion of androgens to estrone and thereby help to restore ovulation.

If the patient wishes to become pregnant, clomiphene or other drugs can be employed for ovulatory stimulation. (See Infertility, this chapter.) The addition of dexamethasone 0.5 mg at bedtime to a clomiphene regimen may increase the likelihood of ovulation by suppression of ACTH and circulating adrenal androgens. For women who are unresponsive to clomiphene, 3- to 6-month courses of the oral hypoglycemic agent metformin, 500 mg three times daily, may bring resumption of regular cycles and ovulation. This agent reduces the hyperinsulinemia and hyperandrogenemia seen with polycystic ovary syndrome.

If the patient does not desire pregnancy, medroxyprogesterone acetate, 10 mg/d for the first 10 days of each month, should be given. This will ensure regular shedding of the endometrium so that hyperplasia will not occur. If contraception is desired, a low-dose combination oral contraceptive can be used; this is also useful in controlling hirsutism, for which treatment must be continued for 6–12 months before results are seen.

Hirsutism may be managed with epilation and electrolysis. Dexamethasone, 0.5 mg each night, is helpful in women with excess adrenal androgen secretion. If hirsutism is severe, some patients will elect to have a hysterectomy and bilateral oophorectomy followed by estrogen replacement therapy. Spironolactone, an aldosterone antagonist, is also useful for hirsutism in doses of 25 mg three or four times daily.

Guzick DS (editor): Polycystic ovarian syndrome. Obstet Gynecol Clin North Am 2001;28:1. [PMID: 11292997–11293007] (State-of-the-art articles on pathogenesis, diagnosis, and treatment.)

Moghetti P et al: Metformin effects on clinical features, endocrine and metabolic profiles, and insulin sensitivity in polycystic ovarian syndrome: a randomized, double-blind, placebo-controlled 6-month trial, followed by open, long-term clinical evaluation. J Clin Endocrinol Metab 2000;85:139. [PMID: 10634377] (Metformin treatment of women with polycystic ovarian syndrome reduced hyperinsulinemia and hyperandrogenemia and in many patients produced sustained improvements in menstrual abnormalities and resumption of ovulation.)

PAINFUL INTERCOURSE (Dyspareunia)

Questions related to sexual functioning should be asked as part of the reproductive history. Two helpful questions are, "Are you sexually active?" and "Are you having any sexual difficulties at this time?"

During the pelvic examination, the patient should be placed in a half-sitting position and given a handheld mirror and then asked to point out the site of pain and describe the type of pain.

Etiology

A. Vulvovaginitis

Vulvovaginitis is inflammation or infection of the vagina. Areas of marked tenderness in the vulvar vestibule without visible inflammation occasionally show lesions resembling small condylomas on colposcopy (see Vaginitis, this chapter).

B. Vaginismus

Vaginismus is voluntary or involuntary contraction of muscles around the introitus. It results from fear, pain, sexual trauma, or having learned negative attitudes toward sex during childhood.

C. Remnants of the Hymen

The hymen is usually adequately stretched during initial intercourse, so that pain does not occur subsequently. In some women, the pain of initial intercourse may produce vaginismus. In others, a thin or thickened rim or partial rim of hymen remains after several episodes of intercourse, causing pain.

D. Insufficient Lubrication of the Vagina

See Vaginal Atrophy, this chapter.

E. Infection, Endometriosis, Tumors, or Other Pathologic Conditions

Pain occurring with deep thrusting during coitus is usually due to acute or chronic infection of the cervix, uterus, or adnexa; endometriosis; adnexal tumors; or adhesions resulting from prior pelvic disease or operation. Careful history taking and a pelvic examination will generally help in the differential diagnosis.

F. Vulvodynia

This is the most frequent cause of dyspareunia in premenopausal women. It is characterized by a sensation of burning along with other symptoms including pain, itching, stinging, irritation, and rawness. The discomfort may be constant or intermittent, focal or diffuse, and experienced as either deep or superficial. There are generally no physical findings except minimal erythema that may be associated with a subset of vulvodynia, vulvar vestibulitis.

Treatment

A. VULVOVAGINITIS

Lesions resembling warts on colposcopy or biopsy should be treated in the appropriate way (see Vaginitis). Irritation from spermicides may be a factor. The couple may be helped by a discussion of noncoital techniques to achieve orgasm until the infection subsides.

B. VAGINISMUS

Sexual counseling and education on anatomy and sexual functioning may be appropriate. The patient can be instructed in self-dilation, using a lubricated finger or test tubes of graduated sizes. Before coitus (with adequate lubrication) is attempted, the patient—and then her partner—should be able to easily and painlessly introduce two fingers into the vagina. Penetration should never be forced, and the woman should always be the one to control the depth of insertion during dilation or intercourse.

C. REMNANTS OF THE HYMEN

In rare situations, manual dilation of a remaining hymen under general anesthesia is necessary. Surgery should be avoided.

D. INSUFFICIENT LUBRICATION OF THE VAGINA

If inadequate sexual arousal is the cause, sexual counseling is helpful. Lubricants may be used during sexual foreplay. For women with low plasma estrogen levels, use of a lubricant during coitus is sometimes sufficient. If not, systemic hormone replacement therapy (see Menopausal Syndrome, this chapter) may be used and is preferable to estrogen vaginal cream. An alternative is the estradiol vaginal ring. The ring may be worn continuously and replaced every 3 months. Concomitant progestin therapy is not needed with the ring.

E. INFECTION, ENDOMETRIOSIS, TUMORS, OR OTHER PATHOLOGIC CONDITIONS

Medical treatment of acute cervicitis, endometritis, or salpingitis and temporary abstention from coitus usually relieve pain. Hormonal or surgical treatment of endometriosis may be helpful. Dyspareunia resulting from chronic pelvic inflammatory disease or any condition causing extensive adhesions or fixation of pelvic organs is difficult to treat without extirpative surgery. Couples can be advised to try coital positions that limit deep thrusting and to use manual and oral sexual techniques.

F. VULVODYNIA

Since the cause of vulvodynia is unknown, management is difficult. Few treatment approaches have been subjected to methodologically rigorous trials. Surgery, usually consisting of vestibulectomy, has reportedly been the most consistently successful approach. A variety of specific (antiviral or antifungal) and nonspecific (corticosteroid or anesthetic) agents have been tried with varying degrees of success. Pain control through behavioral therapy, biofeedback, or acupuncture has also been tried. No single approach has been consistently shown to be effective. Patients with continuous genital burning or pain may benefit from treatment with a tricyclic antidepressant such as amitriptyline in gradually increasing doses from 10 mg/d to 75–100 mg/d.

Davis GD et al: Clinical management of vulvodynia. Clin Obstet Gynecol 1999;42:221. [PMID: 10370843] (Diagnosis and treatment of vulvar pain syndromes.)

Masheb RM et al: Vulvodynia: an introduction and critical review of a chronic pain condition. Pain 2000;86:3. [PMID: 10779654] (Review article summarizing current knowledge of etiology, diagnosis, treatment, and psychosocial sequelae. The authors emphasize the need to approach vulvodynia from a multidimensional, chronic pain perspective.)

INFERTILITY

A couple is said to be infertile if pregnancy does not result after 1 year of normal sexual activity without contraceptives. About 25% of couples experience infertility at some point in their reproductive lives; the incidence of infertility increases with age. The male partner contributes to about 40% of cases of infertility, and a combination of factors is common.

Diagnostic Survey

During the initial interview, the clinician can present an overview of infertility and discuss a plan of study. Separate private consultations are then conducted, allowing appraisal of psychosexual adjustment without embarrassment or criticism. Pertinent details (eg, sexually transmitted disease or prior pregnancies) must be obtained. The ill effects of cigarettes, alcohol, and other recreational drugs on male fertility should be discussed. Prescription drugs that impair male potency should be discussed as well. The gynecologic history should include queries regarding the menstrual pattern. The present history includes use and types of contraceptives, douches, libido, sex techniques, frequency and success of coitus, and correlation of intercourse with time of ovulation. Family history includes repeated abortions and maternal DES use.

General physical and genital examinations are performed on both partners. Basic laboratory studies include complete blood count, urinalysis, cervical culture for chlamydia, serologic test for syphilis, rubella antibody determination, and thyroid function tests. Tay-Sachs screening should be offered if both parents are Jews and sickle cell screening if both parents are black.

The patient is instructed to chart her basal body temperature orally daily on arising and to record on a graph episodes of coitus and days of menstruation. Self-performed urine tests for the midcycle LH surge can be used to enhance temperature observations relating to ovulation. Couples should be advised that coitus resulting in conception occurs during the 6-day period ending with the day of ovulation.

The male partner is instructed to bring a complete ejaculate for analysis. Sexual abstinence for at least 3 days before the semen is obtained is emphasized. A clean, dry, wide-mouthed bottle for collection is preferred. Condoms should not be employed, as the protective powder or lubricant may be spermicidal. Semen should be examined within 1–2 hours after collection. Semen is considered normal with the following minimum values: volume, 3 mL; concentration, 20 million sperm per milliliter; motility, 50% after 2 hours; and normal forms, 60%. If the sperm count is abnormal, further evaluation includes a search for exposure to environmental and workplace toxins, alcohol or drug abuse, and hypogonadism.

A. First Testing Cycle

While the contribution of cervical factors to infertility is controversial, most gynecologists include a postcoital test in their workup. The test is scheduled for just before ovulation (eg, day 12 or 13 in an expected 28-day cycle). Preovulation timing can be enhanced by serial urinary LH tests. The patient is examined within 6 hours after coitus. The cervical mucus should be clear, elastic, and copious owing to the influence of the preovular estrogen surge. (The mucus is scantier and more viscid before and after ovulation.) A good spinnbarkeit (stretching to a fine thread 4 cm or more in length) is desirable. A small drop of cervical mucus should be obtained from within the cervical os and examined under the microscope. The presence of five or more active sperm per high-power field constitutes a satisfactory postcoital test. If no spermatozoa are found, the test should be repeated (assuming that active spermatozoa were present in the semen analysis). Sperm agglutination and sperm immobilization tests should be considered if the sperm are immotile or show ineffective tail motility.

The presence of more than three white blood cells per high-power field in the postcoital test suggests cervicitis in the woman or prostatitis in the man. When estrogen levels are normal, the cervical mucus dried on the slide will form a fern-like pattern when viewed with a low-power microscope. This type of mucus is necessary for normal sperm transport.

The serum progesterone level should be measured at the midpoint of the secretory phase (21st day); a level of 10–20 ng/mL confirms adequate luteal function.

B. Second Testing Cycle

Hysterosalpingography using an oil dye is performed within 3 days following the menstrual period. This x-ray study will demonstrate uterine abnormalities (septa, polyps, submucous myomas) and tubal ob-

struction. A repeat x-ray film 24 hours later will confirm tubal patency if there is wide pelvic dispersion of the dye. This test has been associated with an increased pregnancy rate by some observers. If the woman has had prior pelvic inflammation, one should give doxycycline, 100 mg twice daily, beginning immediately before and for 7 days after the x-ray study.

C. Further Testing

1. Gross deficiencies of sperm (number, motility, or appearance) require repeat analysis. Zona-free hamster egg penetration tests are available to evaluate the ability of human sperm to fertilize an egg.

2. Obvious obstruction of the uterine tubes requires assessment for microsurgery or in vitro fertilization.

3. Absent or infrequent ovulation requires additional laboratory evaluation. Elevated FSH and LH levels indicate ovarian failure causing premature menopause. Elevated LH levels in the presence of normal FSH levels confirm the presence of polycystic ovaries. Elevation of blood prolactin (PRL) levels suggests pituitary microadenoma.

4. Major histocompatibility antigen typing of both partners will confirm human leukocyte antigen-B locus homozygosity, which is found in greater than expected numbers among couples with unexplained infertility.

5. Ultrasound monitoring of folliculogenesis may reveal the occurrence of unruptured luteinized follicles.

6. Endometrial biopsy in the luteal phase associated with simultaneous serum progesterone levels will rule out luteal phase deficiency.

D. Laparoscopy

Approximately 25% of women whose basic evaluation is normal will have findings on laparoscopy explaining their infertility (eg, peritubal adhesions, endometriotic implants).

Treatment

A. Medical Measures

Fertility may be restored by appropriate treatment in many patients with endocrine imbalance, particularly those with hypo- or hyperthyroidism. Antibiotic treatment of cervicitis is of value. In women with abnormal postcoital tests and demonstrated antisperm antibodies causing sperm agglutination or immobilization, condom use for up to 6 months may result in lower antibody levels and improved pregnancy rates.

Women who engage in vigorous athletic training often have low sex hormone levels; fertility improves with reduced exercise and some weight gain.

B. Surgical Measures

Excision of ovarian tumors or ovarian foci of endometriosis can improve fertility. Microsurgical relief of tubal obstruction due to salpingitis or tubal ligation will reestablish fertility in a significant number of cases. In special instances of cornual or fimbrial block, the prognosis with newer surgical techniques has become much better. Peritubal adhesions or endometriotic implants often can be treated via laparoscopy or via laparotomy immediately following laparoscopic examination if prior consent has been obtained.

With varicocele in the male, sperm characteristics are often improved following surgical treatment.

C. INDUCTION OF OVULATION

1. Clomiphene citrate—Clomiphene citrate stimulates gonadotropin release, especially LH. Consequently, plasma estrone (E_1) and estradiol (E_2) also rise, reflecting ovarian follicle maturation. If E_2 rises sufficiently, an LH surge occurs to trigger ovulation.

After a normal menstrual period or induction of withdrawal bleeding with progestin, one should give 50 mg of clomiphene orally daily for 5 days. If ovulation does not occur, the dosage is increased to 100 mg orally daily for 5 days. If ovulation still does not occur, the course is repeated with 150 mg daily and then 200 mg daily for 5 days, with the addition of chorionic gonadotropin, 10,000 units intramuscularly, 7 days after clomiphene.

The rate of ovulation following this treatment is 90% in the absence of other infertility factors. The pregnancy rate is high. Twinning occurs in 5% of these patients, and three or more fetuses are found in rare instances (< 0.5% of cases). An increased incidence of congenital anomalies has not been reported. Painful ovarian cyst formation occurs in 8% of patients and may warrant discontinuation of therapy. Several recent studies have suggested a two- to threefold increased risk of ovarian cancer with the use of clomiphene for more than 1 year.

In the presence of increased androgen production (DHEA-S > 200 μg/dL), the addition of dexamethasone, 0.5 mg, or prednisone, 5 mg, at bedtime, improves the response to clomiphene. Dexamethasone should be discontinued after pregnancy is confirmed.

2. Bromocriptine—Bromocriptine is used only if PRL levels are elevated and there is no withdrawal bleeding following progesterone administration (otherwise, clomiphene is used). To minimize side effects (nausea, diarrhea, dizziness, headache, fatigue), bromocriptine should be taken with meals. The initial dosage is 2.5 mg once daily, increased to two or three times daily in increments of 1.25 mg. The drug is discontinued once pregnancy has occurred.

3. Human menopausal gonadotropins (hMG)—hMG or recombinant FSH is indicated in cases of hypogonadotropism and most other types of anovulation (exclusive of ovarian failure). Because of the complexities, laboratory tests, and expense associated with this treatment, these patients should be referred to a specialist.

4. Gonadotropin-releasing hormone (GnRH)—Hypothalamic amenorrhea unresponsive to clomi-phene will be reliably and successfully treated with subcutaneous pulsatile gonadotropin-releasing hormone (GnRH). Use of this substance will avoid the dangerous ovarian complications and the 25% incidence of multiple pregnancy associated with hMG, though the overall rate of ovulation and pregnancy is lower than when hMG is used.

D. TREATMENT OF ENDOMETRIOSIS

See above.

E. TREATMENT OF INADEQUATE TRANSPORT OF SPERM

Intrauterine insemination of concentrated washed sperm has been used to bypass a poor cervical environment associated with scant or hostile cervical mucus. The sperm must be handled by sterile methods, washed in sterile saline or tissue culture solutions, and centrifuged. A small amount of fluid (0.5 mL) containing the sperm is then instilled into the uterus.

F. ARTIFICIAL INSEMINATION IN AZOOSPERMIA

If azoospermia is present, artificial insemination by a donor usually results in pregnancy, assuming female function is normal. The use of frozen sperm is currently preferable to fresh sperm because the frozen specimen can be held pending cultures and blood test results for sexually transmitted diseases, including HIV infection.

G. ASSISTED REPRODUCTIVE TECHNOLOGIES

Couples who have failed to respond to traditional infertility treatments, including those with tubal disease, severe endometriosis, oligospermia, and immunologic or unexplained infertility, may benefit from in vitro fertilization (IVF), gamete intrafallopian transfer (GIFT), and zygote intrafallopian transfer (ZIFT). These techniques are complex and require a highly organized team of specialists. All of the procedures involve ovarian stimulation to produce multiple oocytes, oocyte retrieval by TVS-guided needle aspiration, and handling of the oocytes outside the body. With IVF, the eggs are fertilized in vitro and the embryos transferred to the uterine fundus. Extra embryos may be cryopreserved for subsequent cycles. The rate of live births per retrieval for 360 programs in the United States and Canada in 1998 was 29%. Age is an important determinant of success—for couples under the age of 35, the average rate of live birth was 32% per retrieval, while the rate for women over 40 was 8%. In 1998, 38% of pregnancies were multiple.

GIFT involves the placement of sperm and eggs in the uterine tube by laparoscopy or minilaparotomy and is more invasive than IVF. In 1998, for all age groups, the success rate for GIFT was 28%. GIFT is not appropriate for women with severe tubal diseases and is less successful than IVF with male factor infertility since fertilization cannot be documented. With ZIFT, fertilization occurs in vitro, and the early development of the embryo occurs in the uterine tube after transfer by laparoscopy or minilaparotomy. The average rate of live births per retrieval in 1998 was 30%.

A recent development is intracytoplasmic sperm injection (ICSI), which allows fertilization with a single sperm. This provides the opportunity for men with severe oligospermia or obstructive azoospermia to father children.

Prognosis

The prognosis for conception and normal pregnancy is good if minor (even multiple) disorders can be identified and treated; it is poor if the causes of infertility are severe, untreatable, or of prolonged duration (over 3 years).

It is important to remember that in the absence of identifiable causes of infertility, 60% of couples will achieve a pregnancy within 3 years. Couples with unexplained infertility who do not achieve pregnancy within 3 years should be offered ovulation induction or assisted reproductive technology. Also, offering appropriately timed information about adoption is considered part of a complete infertility regimen.

Assisted reproductive technology in the United States: 1998 results generated from the American Society for Reproductive Medicine/Society for Assisted Reproductive Technology Registry. Fertil Steril 2002;77:18. [PMID: 11779586]

Rosene-Montella K et al: Evaluation and management of infertility in women: the internist's role. Ann Intern Med 2000;132:973. [PMID: 10858181] (Review of the scope of infertility, the interventions used for its treatment, the medical complications of these interventions, the potential risks of fertility treatments, and important issues for preconceptual counseling.)

CONTRACEPTION

Voluntary control of childbearing benefits women, men, and the children born to them. Contraception should be available to all women and men of reproductive ages. Education about contraception and access to contraceptive pills or devices are especially important for sexually active teenagers and for women following childbirth or abortion.

1. Oral Contraceptives

Combined Oral Contraceptives

A. Efficacy and Methods of Use

Oral contraceptives have a theoretical failure rate of less than 0.5% if taken absolutely on schedule and a typical failure rate of 3%. Their primary mode of action is suppression of ovulation. The pills are initially started on the first or fifth day of the ovarian cycle and taken daily for 21 days, followed by 7 days of placebos or no medication, and this schedule is then continued for each cycle. If a pill is missed at any time, two pills should be taken the next day, and another method of contraception should be used for the rest of the cycle (eg, condoms or foam). A backup method should also be used during the first cycle if the pills are started later than the fifth day. Low-dose oral contraceptives are no longer contraindicated in women aged 35–50 who are nonsmokers and have no risk factors for cardiovascular disease.

B. Benefits of Oral Contraceptives

There are many noncontraceptive advantages to oral contraceptives. Menstrual flow is lighter, resultant anemia is less common, and dysmenorrhea is relieved for most women. Functional ovarian cysts generally disappear with oral contraceptive use, and new cysts do not occur. Pain with ovulation and postovulatory aching are relieved. The risk of ovarian and endometrial cancer is decreased. The risks of salpingitis and ectopic pregnancy may be diminished. Acne is usually improved. The frequency of developing myomas is lower in long-term users (> 4 years). There is a beneficial effect on bone mass.

C. Selection of an Oral Contraceptive

Any of the combination oral contraceptives containing less than 50 μg of estrogen are suitable for most women. There is some variation in potency of the various progestins in the pills, but there are essentially no clinically significant differences for most women among the progestins in the low-dose pills. Women who have acne or hirsutism may benefit from use of one of the pills containing the third-generation progestins, desogestrel or norgestimate, as they are the least androgenic. The low-dose oral contraceptives commonly used in the United States are listed in Table 17–5.

D. Drug Interactions

Several drugs interact with oral contraceptives to decrease their efficacy by causing induction of microsomal enzymes in the liver, by increasing sex hormone-binding globulin, and by other mechanisms. Some commonly prescribed drugs in this category are phenytoin, phenobarbital (and other barbiturates), primidone, carbamazepine, and rifampin. Women taking these drugs should use another means of contraception for maximum safety.

E. Contraindications and Adverse Effects

Oral contraceptives have been associated with many adverse effects; they are contraindicated in some situations and should be used with caution in others (Table 17–6).

1. Myocardial infarction—The risk of heart attack is higher with use of oral contraceptives, particularly with pills containing 50 μg of estrogen or more. Cigarette smoking, obesity, hypertension, diabetes, or hypercholesterolemia increases the risk. Young nonsmoking women have minimal increased risk. Smokers over age 40 and women with other cardiovascular risk factors should use other methods of birth control.

Table 17–5. Commonly used low-dose oral contraceptives.

Name	Type	Progestin	Estrogen (Ethinyl Estradiol)	Cost per Month[1]
Alesse	Combination	0.1 mg levonorgestrel	20 μg	$32.95
Cyclessa	Triphasic	0.1 mg desogestrel (days 1–7) 0.125 mg desogestrel (days 8–14) 0.15 mg desogestrel (days 15–21)	25 μg	$31.48
Mircette	Combination	0.5 mg desogestrel	20 μg	$31.48
Loestrin 1/20 Microgestin 1/20	Combination	1 mg norethindrone acetate	20 μg	$33.17 $28.66
Estrostep	Triphasic	1.0 mg norethindrone acetate (days 1–5)	20 μg	$33.17
		1.0 mg norethindrone acetate (days 6–12)	30 μg	
		1.0 mg norethindrone acetate (days 13–21)	35 μg	
Lo-Ovral Low-ogestrel	Combination	0.3 mg dl-norgestrel	30 μg	$34.04 $30.52
Nordette Levlen Levora	Combination	0.15 mg levonorgestrel	30 μg	$31.93 $34.33 $30.93
Norinyl 1/35 Ortho-Novum 1/35 Necon 1/35	Combination	1 mg norethindrone	35 μg	$29.61 $32.78 $27.65
Loestrin 1.5/30 Microgestin 1.5/30	Combination	1.5 mg norethindrone acetate	30 μg	$33.49 $28.94
Demulen 1/35 Zovia 1/35E	Combination	1 mg ethynodiol diacetate	35 μg	$33.31 $29.29
Brevicon Modicon Necon 0.5/35	Combination	0.5 mg norethindrone	35 μg	$27.63 $35.75 $30.15
Ovcon 35	Combination	0.4 mg norethindrone	35 μg	$31.76
Ortho-Cept Desogen	Combination	0.15 mg desogestrel	30 μg	$32.78 $28.53
Ortho-Cyclen	Combination	0.25 mg norgestimate	35 μg	$32.78
Ortho-Tricyclen	Triphasic	0.15 mg norgestimate (days 1–7) 0.215 mg norgestimate (days 8–14) 0.25 mg norgestimate (days 15–21)	35 μg	$32.46
Ortho-Novum 7/7/7	Triphasic	0.5 mg norethindrone (days 1–7) 0.75 mg norethindrone (days 8–14) 1 mg norethindrone (days 15–21)	35 μg	$32.78
Tri-Norinyl	Triphasic	0.5 mg norethindrone (days 1–7) 1 mg norethindrone (days 8–16) 0.5 mg norethindrone (days 17–21)	35 μg	$32.00
Triphasil Trivora	Triphasic	0.05 mg levonorgestrel (days 1–6) 0.0075 mg levonorgestrel (days 7–11) 0.125 mg levonorgestrel (days 12–21)	30 μg 40 μg 30 μg	$30.65 $27.49
Yasmin	Combination	3 mg drospirenone	30 μg	$28.19
Micronor Nor-QD	Progestin-only minipill	0.35 mg norethindrone to be taken continuously	(None)	$38.06 $36.92
Ovrette	Progestin-only minipill	0.075 mg dl-norgestrel to be taken continuously	(None)	$33.63

[1]Cost to pharmacist (average wholesale price, generic when possible) for quantity listed. Source: *Drug Topics Red Book,* March 2002; Vol. 21, No. 3.

Table 17–6. Contraindications to use of oral contraceptives.

Absolute contraindications
  Pregnancy
  Thrombophlebitis or thromboembolic disorders (past or present)
  Stroke or coronary artery disease (past or present)
  Cancer of the breast (known or suspected)
  Undiagnosed abnormal vaginal bleeding
  Estrogen-dependent cancer (known or suspected)
  Benign or malignant tumor of the liver (past or present)
Relative contraindications
  Age over 35 years and heavy cigarette smoking (> 15 cigarettes daily)
  Migraine or recurrent persistent severe headache
  Hypertension
  Cardiac or renal disease
  Diabetes
  Gallbladder disease
  Cholestasis during pregnancy
  Active hepatitis or infectious mononucleosis
  Sickle cell disease (S/S or S/C type)
  Surgery, fracture, or severe injury
  Lactation
  Significant psychologic depression

---

2. Thromboembolic disease—An increased rate of venous thromboembolism is found in oral contraceptive users, especially if the dose of estrogen is 50 μg or more. While the overall risk is very low (15 per 100,000 woman-years), several studies have reported a twofold increased risk in women using oral contraceptives containing the progestins gestodene (not available in the United States) or desogestrel compared with women using oral contraceptives with levonorgestrel and norethindrone. Women who develop thrombophlebitis should stop using this method, as should those at risk of thrombophlebitis because of surgery, fracture, serious injury, or immobilization.

3. Cerebrovascular disease—Overall, a small increased risk of hemorrhagic stroke and subarachnoid hemorrhage and a somewhat greater increased risk of thrombotic stroke has been found; smoking, hypertension, and age over 35 years are associated with increased risk. Women who develop warning symptoms such as severe headache, blurred or lost vision, or other transient neurologic disorders should stop using oral contraceptives.

4. Carcinoma—A relationship between long-term (3–4 years) oral contraceptive use and occurrence of cervical dysplasia and cancer has been found in various studies. A reanalysis of data from 54 studies of oral contraceptives and breast cancer indicated a small increase in the risk among current users (RR = 1.24), while women who had discontinued use 10 or more years previously had a slightly decreased risk (RR = 0.88). One study has suggested the possibility of an increased risk of breast cancer in women who have ever used oral contraceptives if they have first-degree relatives with breast cancer. Combination oral contraceptives reduce the risk of endometrial carcinoma by 40% after 2 years of use and 60% after 4 or more years of use. The risk of ovarian cancer is reduced by 30% with pill use for less than 4 years, by 60% with use for 5–11 years, and by 80% after 12 or more years. Rarely, oral contraceptives have been associated with the development of benign or malignant hepatic tumors; this may lead to rupture of the liver, hemorrhage, and death. The risk increases with higher dosage, longer duration of use, and older age.

5. Metabolic disorders—A decrease in glucose tolerance and an increase in triglyceride levels is seen in pill takers, and women with diabetes using this method should be carefully monitored.

6. Hypertension—Oral contraceptives may cause hypertension in some women; the risk is increased with longer duration of use and older age. Women who develop hypertension while using oral contraceptives should use other contraceptive methods. However, with regular blood pressure monitoring, nonsmoking women under the age of 40 with well-controlled mild hypertension may use oral contraceptives.

7. Headache—Migraine or other vascular headaches may occur or worsen with pill use. If severe or frequent headaches develop while using this method, it should be discontinued.

8. Amenorrhea—Postpill amenorrhea lasting a year or longer occurs occasionally, sometimes with galactorrhea. Prolactin levels should be checked; if elevated, a pituitary prolactinoma may be present.

9. Disorders of lactation—Combined oral contraceptives can impair the quantity and quality of breast milk. While it is preferable to avoid the use of combination oral contraceptives during lactation, the effects on milk quality are small and are not associated with developmental abnormalities in infants. Combination oral contraceptives should be started no earlier than 6 weeks postpartum to allow for establishment of lactation. Progestin-only pills, levonorgestrel implants, and depot medroxyprogesterone acetate are alternatives with no adverse effects on milk quality.

10. Other disorders—Depression may occur or be worsened with oral contraceptive use. Fluid retention may occur. Patients who had cholestatic jaundice during pregnancy may develop it while taking birth control pills.

F. MINOR SIDE EFFECTS

Nausea and dizziness may occur in the first few months of pill use. A weight gain of 2–5 lb commonly occurs. Spotting or breakthrough bleeding between menstrual periods may occur, especially if a pill is skipped or taken late; this may be helped by switching to a pill of slightly greater potency (see section C, above). Missed menstrual periods may occur, especially with low-dose pills. A pregnancy test should be performed if pills have been skipped or if two or more menstrual periods are missed. Depression, fatigue, and decreased libido can occur. Chloasma may occur, as in pregnancy, and is increased by exposure to sunlight.

Progestin Minipill

A. Efficacy and Methods of Use

Formulations containing 0.35 mg of norethindrone or 0.075 mg of norgestrel are available in the USA. Their efficacy is slightly lower than that of combined oral contraceptives, with failure rates of 1–4% being reported. The minipill is believed to prevent conception by causing thickening of the cervical mucus to make it hostile to sperm, alteration of ovum transport (which may account for the higher rate of ectopic pregnancy with these pills), and inhibition of implantation. Ovulation is inhibited inconsistently with this method. The minipill is begun on the first day of a menstrual cycle and then taken continuously for as long as contraception is desired.

B. Advantages

The low dose and absence of estrogen make the minipill safe during lactation; it may increase the flow of milk. It is often tried by women who want minimal doses of hormones and by patients who are over age 35. The minipill can be used by women with uterine myomas or sickle cell disease (S/S or S/C). Like the combined pill, the minipill decreases the likelihood of pelvic inflammatory disease by its effect on cervical mucus.

C. Complications and Contraindications

Minipill users often have bleeding irregularities (eg, prolonged flow, spotting, or amenorrhea); such patients may need monthly pregnancy tests. Ectopic pregnancies are more frequent, and complaints of abdominal pain should be investigated with this in mind. The absolute contraindications and many of the relative contraindications listed in Table 17–6 apply to the minipill. Exceptions are mentioned in section E, above. Minor side effects of combination oral contraceptives such as weight gain and mild headache may also occur with the minipill.

Beral V et al: Mortality associated with oral contraceptive use: 25 year follow up of cohort of 46,000 women from Royal College of General Practitioners' oral contraceptive study. BMJ 1999;318:96. [PMID: 9880284] (There was no difference in the overall rate of death among ever-users and never-users. Among current and recent [< 10 years] users, the relative risk of death from ovarian cancer was 0.2 [95% CI, 0.1–0.8], from cervical cancer, 2.5 [1.1–6.1], and from cerebrovascular disease, 1.9 [1.2–3.1].)

Grabrick DM et al: Risk of breast cancer with oral contraceptive use in women with a family history of breast cancer. JAMA 2000;284:1791. [PMID: 11025831] (A historical cohort study that suggests that women who have ever used an early formulation of oral contraceptives and who have a first-degree relative with breast cancer may be at increased risk for breast cancer [RR = 3.3, 95%, CI = 1.6–6.7]. Studies are

needed of women with a family history of breast cancer who have used low-dose oral contraceptives.)

2. Contraceptive Injections & Implants (Long-Acting Progestins)

The injectable progestin medroxyprogesterone acetate is approved for contraceptive use in the USA. There is extensive worldwide experience with this method over the past 3 decades. The medication is given as a deep intramuscular injection of 150 mg every 3 months and has a contraceptive efficacy of 99.7%. Common side effects include irregular bleeding, amenorrhea, weight gain, and headache. Bone mineral loss may occur. Users commonly have irregular bleeding initially and subsequently develop amenorrhea. Ovulation may be delayed after the last injection. Contraindications are similar to those for the minipill.

A monthly injectable containing both depot medroxyprogesterone acetate and an estrogen, estradiol cypionate (Lunelle), is available in the United States. It is highly effective, with a first-year pregnancy rate of 0.2% and a side effect profile similar to that of oral contraceptives.

The other available long-acting progestin is the Norplant system, a contraceptive implant containing levonorgestrel. The system consists of six small Silastic capsules that are inserted subcutaneously in the inner aspect of the upper arm. They release daily and provide highly effective contraception for 5 years. In the first year of use, Norplant is 99.8% effective. Contraceptive effectiveness drops slightly in succeeding years, but even in the fifth year it is more effective than the combination pill. The most common side effects include irregular bleeding and spotting, amenorrhea, headache, acne, and weight gain. Irregular bleeding is the most common reason for discontinuation. Hormone levels drop rapidly after removal of the implants, and there is no delay in the return of fertility. Contraindications are similar to those for the minipill. Insertion of the implants requires a minor surgical procedure under local anesthesia. Removal is also done under local anesthesia and may be more difficult than insertion. Removal may be facilitated by the "U" technique, involving use of a modified vasectomy clamp through a 4 mm incision parallel to the implants between implants three and four.

Kaunitz AM: Injectable long-acting contraceptives. Clin Obstet Gynecol 2001;44:73. [PMID: 11219248] (Review article.)

Kovalevsky G et al: Norplant and other Implantable Contraceptives. Clin Obstet Gynecol 2001;44:92. [PMID: 11219249] (Review article.)

3. Other Hormonal Methods

A transdermal contraceptive patch containing 150 µg norelgestromin and 20 µg ethinyl estradiol and measuring 20 cm^2 is available. The patch is applied to the lower abdomen, upper torso, or buttock once a week for 3 consecutive weeks, followed by 1 week without the patch. The mechanism of action, side effects, and efficacy are similar to those associated with oral contraceptives, though compliance may be better.

A contraceptive vaginal ring that measures 54 mm in diameter and releases 120 μg of etonogestrel and 15 μg of ethinyl estradiol daily is available. The ring is soft and flexible and is placed in the upper vagina for 3 weeks, removed, and replaced 1 week later. The efficacy, mechanism of action, and systemic side effects are similar to those associated with oral contraceptives. In addition, users may experience an increased incidence of vaginal discharge.

4. Intrauterine Devices (IUDs)

IUDs available in the United States include the Mirena (which releases levonorgestrel) and the copper-bearing TCu380A. The mechanism of action of IUDs is thought to involve either spermicidal or inhibitory effects on sperm capacitation and transport. IUDs are not abortifacients.

The Mirena is effective for 5 years and the TCu380A for 10 years. The hormone-containing IUDs have the advantage of reducing cramping and menstrual flow.

The IUD is an excellent contraceptive method for most women. The devices are highly effective, with failure rates similar to those achieved with surgical sterilization. Nulliparity is not a contraindication to IUD use. Women who are not in mutually monogamous relationships should use condoms for protection from STDs. The Mirena may have a protective effect against upper tract infection similar to that of the oral contraceptives.

Insertion

Insertion can be performed during or after the menses, at midcycle to prevent implantation, or later in the cycle if the patient has not become pregnant. Most clinicians wait for 6–8 weeks postpartum before inserting an IUD. When insertion is performed during lactation, there is greater risk of uterine perforation or embedding of the IUD. Insertion immediately following abortion is acceptable if there is no sepsis and if follow-up insertion a month later will not be possible; otherwise, it is wise to wait until 4 weeks postabortion.

Contraindications & Complications

Contraindications to use of IUDs are outlined in Table 17–7.

A. Pregnancy

A copper-containing IUD can be inserted within 5 days following a single episode of unprotected midcycle coitus as a postcoital contraceptive. An IUD

Table 17–7. Contraindications to IUD use.

Absolute contraindications
Pregnancy
Acute or subacute pelvic inflammatory disease or purulent cervicitis
Relative contraindications
History of pelvic inflammatory disease since the last pregnancy
Lack of available follow-up care
Menorrhagia or severe dysmenorrhea (copper IUD)
Cervical or uterine neoplasia
Abnormal size or shape of uterus, including myomas distorting cavity

should not be inserted into a pregnant uterus. If pregnancy occurs as an IUD failure, there is a greater chance of spontaneous abortion if the IUD is left in situ (50%) than if it is removed (25%). Spontaneous abortion with an IUD in place is associated with a high risk of severe sepsis, and death can occur rapidly. Women using an IUD who become pregnant should have the IUD removed if the string is visible. It can be removed at the time of abortion if this is desired. If the string is not visible and the patient wants to continue the pregnancy, she should be informed of the serious risk of sepsis and, occasionally, death with such pregnancies. She should be informed that any flu-like symptoms such as fever, myalgia, headache, or nausea warrant immediate medical attention for possible septic abortion.

Since the ratio of ectopic to intrauterine pregnancies is increased among IUD wearers, clinicians should search for adnexal masses in early pregnancy and should always check the products of conception for placental tissue following abortion.

B. Pelvic Infection

There is an increased risk of pelvic infection during the first month following insertion. The subsequent risk of pelvic infection appears to be primarily related to the risk of acquiring sexually transmitted infections. Infertility rates do not appear to be increased among women who have previously used the currently available IUDs. At the time of insertion, women with an increased risk of STDs should be screened for gonorrhea and chlamydiosis. Women with a history of recent or recurrent pelvic infection are not good candidates for IUD use.

C. Menorrhagia or Severe Dysmenorrhea

The copper IUD can cause heavier menstrual periods, bleeding between periods, and more cramping, so it is generally not suitable for women who already suffer from these problems. However, hormone-releasing IUDs can be tried in these cases, as they often cause decreased bleeding and cramping with menses. Nonsteroidal anti-inflammatory drugs are also helpful in decreasing bleeding and pain in IUD users.

D. COMPLETE OR PARTIAL EXPULSION

Spontaneous expulsion of the IUD occurs in 10–20% of cases during the first year of use. Any IUD should be removed if the body of the device can be seen or felt in the cervical os.

E. MISSING IUD STRINGS

If the transcervical tail cannot be seen, this may signify unnoticed expulsion, perforation of the uterus with abdominal migration of the IUD, or simply retraction of the string into the cervical canal or uterus owing to movement of the IUD or uterine growth with pregnancy. Once pregnancy is ruled out, one should probe for the IUD with a sterile sound or forceps designed for IUD removal, after administering a paracervical block. If the IUD cannot be detected, pelvic ultrasound will demonstrate the IUD if it is in the uterus. Alternatively, obtain anteroposterior and lateral x-rays of the pelvis with another IUD or a sound in the uterus as a marker, to confirm an extrauterine IUD. If the IUD is in the abdominal cavity, it should generally be removed by laparoscopy or laparotomy. Open-looped all-plastic IUDs such as the Lippes Loop can be left in the pelvis without danger, but ring-shaped IUDs may strangulate a loop of bowel and copper-bearing IUDs may cause tissue reaction and adhesions.

Perforations of the uterus are less likely if insertion is performed slowly, with meticulous care taken to follow directions applicable to each type of IUD.

Grimes DA: Intrauterine device and upper-genital-tract infection. Lancet 2000;356:1013. [PMID: 11041414] (Concern about pelvic infection has limited IUD use. However, most studies have used inappropriate comparison groups, have overdiagnosed pelvic inflammatory disease in IUD users, and have not controlled for the confounding effect of sexual behavior. Recent evidence suggests that IUDs are much safer than previously thought and are an appropriate contraceptive method for most women.)

5. Diaphragm & Cervical Cap

The diaphragm (with contraceptive jelly) is a safe and effective contraceptive method with features that make it acceptable to some women and not others. Failure rates range from 2% to 20%, depending on the motivation of the woman and the care with which the diaphragm is used. The advantages of this method are that it has no systemic side effects and gives significant protection against pelvic infection and cervical dysplasia as well as pregnancy. The disadvantages are that it must be inserted near the time of coitus and that pressure from the rim predisposes some women to cystitis after intercourse.

The cervical cap (with contraceptive jelly) is similar to the diaphragm but fits snugly over the cervix only (the diaphragm stretches from behind the cervix to behind the pubic symphysis). The cervical cap is more difficult to insert and remove than the diaphragm. The main advantages are that it can be used by women who cannot be fitted for a diaphragm because of a relaxed anterior vaginal wall or by women who have discomfort or develop repeated bladder infections with the diaphragm.

Because of the small risk of toxic shock syndrome, a cervical cap or diaphragm should not be left in the vagina for over 12–18 hours, nor should these devices be used during the menstrual period (see above).

6. Contraceptive Foam, Cream, Film, Sponge, Jelly, & Suppository

These products are available without prescription, are easy to use, and are fairly effective, with reported failure rates of 2–30%. All contain the spermicide nonoxynol-9, which also has some virucidal and bactericidal activity. Nonoxynol-9 does not appear to adversely affect the vaginal colonization of hydrogen peroxide-producing lactobacilli. Recent unpublished data suggest that nonoxynol-9 may not be protective against HIV infection, particularly in women who have frequent intercourse. The products have the advantages of being simple to use and easily available. Their disadvantage is a slightly higher failure rate than the diaphragm or condom.

Richardson BA et al: Use of nonoxynol-9 and changes in vaginal lactobacilli. J Infect Dis 1998;178:441. [PMID: 9697724] (A randomized controlled clinical trial demonstrated that daily use of nonoxynol-9 for 2 weeks reduced the likelihood of bacterial vaginosis.)

7. Condom

The male sheath of latex or animal membrane affords good protection against pregnancy—equivalent to that of a diaphragm and spermicidal jelly; latex (but not animal membrane) condoms also offer protection against sexually transmitted disease and cervical dysplasia. Men and women seeking protection against HIV transmission are advised to use a latex condom along with spermicide during vaginal or rectal intercourse. When a spermicide such as vaginal foam is used with the condom, the failure rate approaches that of oral contraceptives. Condoms coated with spermicide are available in the USA. The disadvantages of condoms are dulling of sensation and spillage of semen due to tearing, slipping, or leakage with detumescence of the penis.

A female condom made of polyurethane is available in the USA. The reported failure rates range from 5% to 21%; the efficacy is comparable to that of the diaphragm. This is the only female-controlled method that offers significant protection from both pregnancy and sexually transmitted diseases.

Rosen AD et al: Study of condom integrity after brief exposure to over-the-counter vaginal preparations. South Med J 1999;92:305. [PMID: 10094272] (Over-the-counter vaginal products that contain mineral oil or vegetable oil—as do some moisturizers, antipruritics, and antifungals—may weaken latex condoms and reduce their efficacy.)

8. Contraception Based on Awareness of Fertile Periods

There is renewed interest in methods to identify times of ovulation and avoidance of unprotected intercourse at that time as a means of family planning. These methods are most effective when the couple restricts intercourse to the postovular phase of the cycle or uses a barrier method at other times. Women benefit from learning to identify their fertile periods. Well-instructed, motivated couples may achieve low pregnancy rates with fertility awareness, but in many field trials, the pregnancy rates were as high as 20%.

"Symptothermal" Natural Family Planning

The basis for this approach is patient-observed increase in clear elastic cervical mucus, brief abdominal midcycle discomfort ("mittelschmerz"), and a sustained rise of the basal body temperature about 2 weeks after onset of menstruation. Unprotected intercourse is avoided from shortly after the menstrual period, when fertile mucus is first identified, until 48 hours after ovulation, as identified by a sustained rise in temperature and the disappearance of clear elastic mucus.

Calendar Method

After the length of the menstrual cycle has been observed for at least 8 months, the following calculations are made: (1) The first fertile day is determined by subtracting 18 days from the shortest cycle; (2) the last fertile day is determined by subtracting 11 days from the longest cycle. For example, if the observed cycles run from 24 to 28 days, the fertile period would extend from the sixth day of the cycle (24 minus 18) through the 17th day (28 minus 11). Day 1 of the cycle is the first day of menses.

Basal Body Temperature Method

This method indicates the safe time for intercourse after ovulation has passed. The temperature must be taken immediately upon awakening, before any activity. A slight drop in temperature often occurs 12–24 hours before ovulation, and a rise of about 0.4 °C occurs 1–2 days after ovulation. The elevated temperature continues throughout the remainder of the cycle. Data suggest that the risk of pregnancy increases starting 5 days prior to the day of ovulation, peaks on the day of ovulation, and then rapidly decreases to zero by the day after ovulation.

Frank-Herrmann P et al: Natural family planning with and without barrier method use in the fertile phase: efficacy in relation to sexual behavior: A German prospective long-term study. Adv Contracept 1997;13:179. [PMID: 9288336] (Among 758 couples using natural family planning with and without barrier methods, "perfect use" of the method resulted in failure rates under 1%.)

Wilcox AJ et al: Timing of sexual intercourse in relation to ovulation. N Engl J Med 1995;333:1517. [PMID: 7477165] (Among 221 women attempting conception, all pregnancies occurred with coitus during the 6-day period ending on the day of ovulation.)

9. Emergency Contraception

If unprotected intercourse occurs in midcycle and the woman is certain she has not inadvertently become pregnant earlier in the cycle, the following regimens are effective in preventing implantation. These methods should be started within 72 hours after unprotected coitus. (1) Levonorgestrel, 0.75 mg given in two doses 12 hours apart (available in the United States prepackaged as Plan B), has a 1% failure rate and is associated with less nausea and vomiting than the following combination regimen. (2) Ethinyl estradiol, 50 μg, with 0.5 mg norgestrel (available in the United States prepackaged as Preven), given in a regimen of two tablets initially followed by two tablets 12 hours later. A comparable regimen includes four pills 12 hours apart of Lo/Ovral, Nordette, or Levlen, or the same regimen with the yellow pills of Triphasil or Tri-Levlen. The failure rate is approximately 3%, and antinausea medication should be provided. (3) Ethinyl estradiol, 2.5 mg twice daily for 5 days. This regimen is as efficacious as the others but is associated with a higher likelihood of nausea, vomiting, and breast tenderness. Mifepristone, 10 mg as a single dose, has been shown to have the same failure rate as the levonorgestrel regimen, with minimal side effects, and appears to be effective given up to 120 hours after unprotected intercourse. It is not currently available at this dose in the United States.

IUD insertion within 5 days after one episode of unprotected midcycle coitus will also prevent pregnancy; copper-bearing IUDs have been tested for this purpose. The disadvantage of this method is possible infection, especially in rape cases; the advantage is ongoing contraceptive protection if this is desired in a patient for whom the IUD is a suitable choice.

Information on clinics or individual clinicians providing emergency contraception in the United States may be obtained by calling 1-888-668-2528.

Comparison of three single doses of mifepristone as emergency contraception: A randomized trial. Lancet 1999;353:697. [PMID: 10073511] (A single 10 mg dose of mifepristone was as effective as a 600 mg dose for emergency contraception.)

Piaggio G et al: Timing of emergency contraception with levonorgestrel or the Yuzpe regimen. Task Force on Postovulatory Methods of Fertility Regulation. Lancet 1999;353:721. [PMID: 10017517] (There is a linear relationship between efficacy and time from intercourse to treatment with both regimens. The pregnancy rate increased from 0.5% when treatment was given within 12 hours to 4.1% when given between 61 and 72 hours after intercourse.)

Randomized controlled trial of levonorgestrel versus the Yuzpe regimen of combined oral contraceptives for emergency contraception. Lancet 1998;352:428. [PMID: 9708750] (The levonorgestrel regimen was better tolerated and more effective than the current standard approach to hormonal emergency contraception.)

10. Abortion

Since the legalization of abortion in the USA in 1973, the related maternal mortality rate has fallen markedly, because illegal and self-induced abortions have been replaced by safer medical procedures. Abortions in the first trimester of pregnancy are performed by vacuum aspiration under local anesthesia. A similar technique, dilation and evacuation, is often used in the second trimester, with general or local anesthesia. Techniques utilizing intra amniotic instillation of hypertonic saline solution or prostaglandins are also occasionally used after 18 weeks from the LMP but are more difficult for the patient. Abortions are rarely performed after 20 weeks from the LMP. It is currently believed that fetal viability is established at about 24 weeks. Legal abortion has a mortality rate of 1:100,000. Rates of morbidity and mortality rise with length of gestation. Currently in the USA, 90% of abortions are performed before 12 weeks' gestation and only 3–4% after 17 weeks. If abortion is chosen, every effort should be made to encourage the patient to seek an early procedure.

Complications resulting from abortion include retained products of conception (often associated with infection and heavy bleeding) and unrecognized ectopic pregnancy. Immediate analysis of the removed tissue for placenta can exclude or corroborate the diagnosis of ectopic pregnancy. Women presenting with fever, bleeding, or abdominal pain after abortion should be examined; use of broad-spectrum antibiotics and reaspiration of the uterus are frequently necessary. Hospitalization is advisable if acute salpingitis requires intravenous administration of antibiotics. Complications following illegal abortion often need emergency care for hemorrhage, septic shock, or uterine perforation.

Rh immune globulin should be given to all Rh-negative women following abortion. Contraception should be thoroughly discussed and contraceptive supplies or pills provided at the time of abortion. In women with a past history of pelvic inflammatory disease, prophylactic antibiotics are indicated: A one-dose regimen is doxycycline, 200 mg orally 1 hour before the procedure, or aqueous penicillin G, 1 million units intravenously 30 minutes before. In the second trimester, use cefazolin, 1 g intravenously 30 minutes before the procedure. Many clinics prescribe tetracycline, 500 mg four times daily for 5 days after the procedure for all patients.

Long-term sequelae of repeated induced abortions have been studied, but as yet there is no consensus on whether there are increased rates of fetal loss or premature labor. It is felt that such adverse sequelae can be minimized by performing early abortion with minimal cervical dilation or by the use of osmotic dilators to induce gradual cervical dilation. One population-based study showed no evidence of an increased risk of breast cancer in women who had undergone an induced abortion.

An FDA-approved oral abortifacient, mifepristone (RU 486), 600 mg as a single dose followed in 36–48 hours by a prostaglandin vaginally or orally, is 95% successful in spontaneously terminating pregnancies of up to 9 weeks' duration with minimum complications. The drug acts as an antihormone to progesterone and glucocorticoids without producing adrenal insufficiency. Although not approved by the FDA for this indication, a combination of intramuscular methotrexate, 50 mg/m^2 of body surface area, followed 7 days later by vaginal misoprostol, 800 μg, was 98% successful in terminating pregnancy at 8 weeks or less. Minor side effects such as nausea, vomiting, and diarrhea are common with these regimens. There is a 5–10% incidence of hemorrhage or incomplete abortion requiring curettage, but there are no known long-term complications.

Grimes DA: A 26-year-old woman seeking an abortion. JAMA 1999;282:1169. [PMID: 10501121] (A thoughtful discussion of a number of aspects of induced abortion.)

Newhall EP et al: Abortion with mifepristone and misoprostol: regimens, efficacy, acceptability and future directions. Am J Obstet Gynecol 2000;183:S44. [PMID: 10944369] (Mifepristone 200 mg orally followed by misoprostol 800 mg vaginally appears to be as effective as the FDA-approved 600 mg regimen up to 9 weeks of gestation.)

11. Sterilization

In the USA, sterilization is the most popular method of birth control for couples who want no more children. Although sterilization is reversible in some instances, reversal surgery in both men and women is costly, complicated, and not always successful. Therefore, patients should be counseled carefully before sterilization and should view the procedure as final.

Vasectomy is a safe, simple procedure in which the vas deferens is severed and sealed through a scrotal incision under local anesthesia. Long-term follow-up studies on vasectomized men show no excess risk of cardiovascular disease. Several studies have shown a possible association with prostate cancer, but the evidence is weak and inconsistent.

Female sterilization is currently performed via laparoscopic bipolar electrocoagulation or plastic ring application on the uterine tubes or via minilaparotomy with Pomeroy tubal resection. The advantages of laparoscopy are minimal postoperative pain, small incisions, and rapid recovery. The advantages of minilaparotomy are that it can be performed with standard surgical instruments under local or general anesthesia. However, there is more postoperative pain and a longer recovery period. The cumulative 10-year failure rate for all methods combined is 1.85%, varying from

0.75% for postpartum partial salpingectomy and laparoscopic unipolar coagulation to 3.65% for spring clips; this fact should be discussed with women preoperatively. Some studies have found an increased risk of menstrual irregularities as a long-term complication of tubal ligation, but findings in different studies have been inconsistent.

Westoff C et al: Tubal sterilization: focus on the U.S. experience. Fertil Steril 2000;73:913. [PMID: 10785216] (Review article.)

RAPE

Rape, or sexual assault, is legally defined in different ways in various jurisdictions. Clinicians and emergency room personnel who deal with rape victims should be familiar with the laws pertaining to sexual assault in their own state. From a medical and psychologic viewpoint, it is essential that persons treating rape victims recognize the nonconsensual and violent nature of the crime. About 95% of reported rape victims are women. Penetration may be vaginal, anal, or oral and may be by the penis, hand, or a foreign object. The absence of genital injury does not imply consent by the victim. The assailant may be unknown to the victim or, more frequently, may be an acquaintance or even the spouse.

"Unlawful sexual intercourse," or statutory rape, is intercourse with a female before the age of majority even with her consent.

Rape represents an expression of anger, power, and sexuality on the part of the rapist. The rapist is usually a hostile man who uses sexual intercourse to terrorize and humiliate a woman. Women neither secretly want to be raped nor do they expect, encourage, or enjoy rape.

Rape involves severe physical injury in 5–10% of cases and is always a terrifying experience in which most victims fear for their lives. Consequently, all victims suffer some psychologic aftermath. Moreover, some rape victims may acquire sexually transmissible disease or become pregnant.

Because rape is a personal crisis, each patient will react differently. The rape trauma syndrome comprises two principal phases. (1) Immediate or acute: Shaking, sobbing, and restless activity may last from a few days to a few weeks. The patient may experience anger, guilt, or shame or may repress these emotions. Reactions vary depending on the victim's personality and the circumstances of the attack. (2) Late or chronic: Problems related to the attack may develop weeks or months later. The lifestyle and work patterns of the individual may change. Sleep disorders or phobias often develop. Loss of self-esteem can rarely lead to suicide.

Clinicians and emergency room personnel who deal with rape victims should work with community rape crisis centers whenever possible to provide ongoing support and counseling.

General Office Procedures

The clinician who first sees the alleged rape victim should be empathetic. Begin with a statement such as, "This is a terrible thing that has happened to you. I want to help."

(1) Secure written consent from the patient, guardian, or next of kin for gynecologic examination; and for photographs if they are likely to be useful as evidence. If police are to be notified, do so, and obtain advice on the preservation and transfer of evidence.

(2) Obtain and record the history in the patient's own words. The sequence of events, ie, the time, place, and circumstances, must be included. Note the date of the LMP, whether or not the woman is pregnant, and the time of the most recent coitus prior to the sexual assault. Note the details of the assault such as body cavities penetrated, use of foreign objects, and number of assailants.

Note whether the victim is calm, agitated, or confused (drugs or alcohol may be involved). Record whether the patient came directly to the hospital or whether she bathed or changed her clothing. Record findings but do not issue even a tentative diagnosis lest it be erroneous or incomplete.

(3) Have the patient disrobe while standing on a white sheet. Hair, dirt, and leaves; underclothing; and any torn or stained clothing should be kept as evidence. Scrape material from beneath fingernails and comb pubic hair for evidence. Place all evidence in separate clean paper bags or envelopes and label carefully.

(4) Examine the patient, noting any traumatized areas that should be photographed. Examine the body and genitals with a Wood light to identify semen, which fluoresces; positive areas should be swabbed with a premoistened swab and air-dried in order to identify acid phosphatase. Colposcopy can be used to identify small areas of trauma from forced entry especially at the posterior fourchette.

(5) Perform a pelvic examination, explaining all procedures and obtaining the patient's consent before proceeding gently with the examination. Use a narrow speculum lubricated with water only. Collect material with sterile cotton swabs from the vaginal walls and cervix and make two air-dried smears on clean glass slides. Wet and dry swabs of vaginal secretions should be collected and refrigerated for subsequent acid phosphatase and DNA evaluation. Swab the mouth (around molars and cheeks) and anus in the same way, if appropriate. Label all slides carefully. Collect secretions from the vagina, anus, or mouth with a premoistened cotton swab, place at once on a slide with a drop of saline, and cover with a coverslip. Look for motile or nonmotile sperm under high, dry magnification, and record the percentage of motile forms.

(6) Perform appropriate laboratory tests as follows. Culture the vagina, anus, or mouth (as appropriate) for *N gonorrhoeae* and chlamydia. Perform a Papanicolaou smear of the cervix, a wet mount for *T vaginalis*, a baseline pregnancy test, and VDRL test. A confidential test for HIV antibody can be obtained if desired by the patient and repeated in 2-4 months if initially negative. Repeat the pregnancy test if the next menses is missed, and repeat the VDRL test in 6 weeks. Obtain blood (10 mL without anticoagulant) and urine (100 mL) specimens if there is a history of forced ingestion or injection of drugs or alcohol.

(7) Transfer clearly labeled evidence, eg, laboratory specimens, directly to the clinical pathologist in charge or to the responsible laboratory technician, in the presence of witnesses (never via messenger), so that the rules of evidence will not be breached.

Treatment

(1) Give analgesics or sedatives if indicated.

(2) Administer tetanus toxoid if deep lacerations contain soil or dirt particles.

(3) Give ceftriaxone, 125 mg intramuscularly, to prevent gonorrhea. In addition, give metronidazole, 2 g as a single dose, and doxycycline, 100 mg twice daily for 7 days to treat chlamydial infection. Incubating syphilis will probably be prevented by these medications, but the VDRL test should be repeated 6 weeks after the assault.

(4) Prevent pregnancy by using one of the methods discussed under Postcoital Contraception, if necessary (this chapter).

(5) Vaccinate against hepatitis B.

(6) Consider HIV prophylaxis (see Chapter 31).

(7) Make sure the patient and her family and friends have a source of ongoing psychologic support.

Linden JA: Sexual assault. Emerg Med Clin North Am 1999; 17:685. [PMID: 10516847] (Review article.)

MENOPAUSAL SYNDROME

ESSENTIALS OF DIAGNOSIS

- *Cessation of menses due to aging or to bilateral oophorectomy.*
- *Elevation of FSH and LH levels.*
- *Hot flushes and night sweats (in 80% of women).*
- *Decreased vaginal lubrication; thinned vaginal mucosa with or without dyspareunia.*

General Considerations

The term "menopause" denotes the final cessation of menstruation, either as a normal part of aging or as the result of surgical removal of both ovaries. In a broader sense, as the term is commonly used, it denotes a 1- to 3-year period during which a woman adjusts to a diminishing and then absent menstrual flow and the physiologic changes that may be associated—hot flushes, night sweats, and vaginal dryness.

The average age at menopause in Western societies today is 51 years. Premature menopause is defined as ovarian failure and menstrual cessation before age 40; this often has a genetic or autoimmune basis. Surgical menopause due to bilateral oophorectomy is common and can cause more severe symptoms owing to the sudden rapid drop in sex hormone levels.

There is no objective evidence that cessation of ovarian function is associated with severe emotional disturbance or personality changes. However, mood changes toward depression and anxiety can occur at this time. Furthermore, the time of menopause often coincides with other major life changes, such as departure of children from the home, a midlife identity crisis, or divorce. These events, coupled with a sense of the loss of youth, may exacerbate the symptoms of menopause and cause psychologic distress.

Clinical Findings

A. SYMPTOMS AND SIGNS

1. Cessation of menstruation—Menstrual cycles generally become irregular as menopause approaches. Anovular cycles occur more often, with irregular cycle length and occasional menorrhagia. Menstrual flow usually diminishes in amount owing to decreased estrogen secretion, resulting in less abundant endometrial growth. Finally, cycles become longer, with missed periods or episodes of spotting only. When no bleeding has occurred for one year, the menopausal transition can be said to have occurred. Any bleeding after this time warrants investigation by endometrial curettage or aspiration to rule out endometrial cancer.

2. Hot flushes—Hot flushes (feelings of intense heat over the trunk and face, with flushing of the skin and sweating) occur in 80% of women as a result of the decrease in ovarian hormones. Hot flushes can begin before the cessation of menses. An increase in pulsatile release of gonadotropin-releasing hormone from the hypothalamus is believed to trigger the hot flushes by affecting the adjacent temperature-regulating area of the brain. Hot flushes are more severe in women who undergo surgical menopause. Flushing is more pronounced late in the day, during hot weather, after ingestion of hot foods or drinks, or during periods of tension. Occurring at night, they often cause sweating and insomnia and result in fatigue on the following day.

3. Vaginal atrophy—With decreased estrogen secretion, thinning of the vaginal mucosa and decreased vaginal lubrication occur and may lead to dyspareunia. The introitus decreases in diameter. Pelvic examination reveals pale, smooth vaginal mucosa and a small cervix and uterus. The ovaries are not normally palpable after the menopause. Continued sexual activity will help prevent tissue shrinkage.

4. Osteoporosis—Osteoporosis may occur as a late sequela of menopause.

B. LABORATORY FINDINGS

Serum FSH and LH levels are elevated. Vaginal cytologic examination will show a low estrogen effect with predominantly parabasal cells, indicating lack of epithelial maturation due to hypoestrinism.

Treatment

A. NATURAL MENOPAUSE

Education and support from health providers, midlife discussion groups, and reading material will help most women having difficulty adjusting to the menopause. Physiologic symptoms can be treated as follows:

1. Vasomotor symptoms—Oral conjugated estrogens, 0.3 mg or 0.625 mg; estradiol, 0.5 or 1 mg; or estrone sulfate, 0.625 mg; or estradiol can be given transdermally as skin patches that are changed once or twice weekly and secrete 0.05–0.1 mg of hormone daily. When either form of estrogen is used, add a progestin (medroxyprogesterone acetate) to prevent endometrial hyperplasia or cancer. The hormones can be given in several differing regimens. Give estrogen on days 1–25 of each calendar month, with 5–10 mg of medroxyprogesterone acetate added on days 14–25. Withhold hormones from day 26 until the end of the month, when the endometrium will be shed, producing a light, generally painless monthly period. Alternatively, give the estrogen along with 2.5 mg of medroxyprogesterone acetate daily, without stopping. This regimen causes some initial bleeding or spotting, but within a few months it produces an atrophic endometrium that will not bleed. If the patient has had a hysterectomy, a progestin need not be used. Explain to the patient that hot flushes will probably return if the hormone is discontinued. When women wish to stop hormone therapy, the dose should be tapered.

In women who cannot use estrogen, megestrol acetate, 20 mg twice daily, is effective in reducing the frequency of hot flushes. Clonidine given orally or transdermally, 100–150 μg daily, may also reduce the frequency of hot flushes, but its use is limited by side effects, including dry mouth, drowsiness, and hypotension.

2. Vaginal atrophy—This problem can be treated with hormone therapy as outlined above. Alternatively, an estradiol vaginal ring that can be left in place for 3 months and is suitable for long-term use provides effective relief of vaginal atrophy. There is mini-mal systemic absorption of estradiol with the ring, and progestin therapy to protect the endometrium is unnecessary. Short-term use of estrogen vaginal cream will relieve symptoms of atrophy, but because of variable absorption, therapy with either systemic hormone replacement or the vaginal ring is preferable. Testosterone propionate 1–2%, 0.5–1 g, in a vanishing cream base used in the same manner is also effective if estrogen is contraindicated. A bland lubricant such as unscented cold cream or water-soluble gel can be helpful at the time of coitus.

3. Osteoporosis—(See also discussion in Chapter 26.) Women should ingest at least 800 mg of calcium daily throughout life. Nonfat or low-fat milk products, calcium-fortified orange juice, green leafy vegetables, corn tortillas, and canned sardines or salmon consumed with the bones are good dietary sources. In addition, 1 g of elemental calcium should be taken as a daily supplement at the time of the menopause and thereafter; calcium supplements should be taken with meals to increase their absorption. Vitamin D, 400 units/d from food, sunlight, or supplements, is necessary to enhance calcium absorption. A daily program of energetic walking and exercise to strengthen the arms and upper body helps maintain bone mass.

Women most at risk for osteoporotic fractures should consider hormone replacement therapy. This includes Caucasian and Asian women, especially if they have a family history of osteoporosis; are thin, short, cigarette smokers, and physically inactive; or have had a low calcium intake in adult life.

B. ADVANTAGES AND RISKS OF HORMONE THERAPY

A number of observational studies have demonstrated a 35–50% decrease in the primary risk of cardiovascular disease with estrogen therapy and menopause. However, double-blinded randomized, controlled trials have shown no overall cardiovascular benefit with estrogen-progestin replacement therapy in a group of postmenopausal women with or without established coronary disease. Both in the Women's Health Initiative trial and the Heart and Estrogen/Progestin Replacement Study (HERS), the overall health risks (increased risk of coronary heart events, strokes, thromboembolic disease, breast cancers, gallstones) exceeded the benefits from the use of combination estrogen and progesterone. The trial of unopposed estrogen use in the Women's Health Initiative study is ongoing. Progestins counteract some but not all favorable effects of estrogen. Whether women who have been on long-term estrogen-progestin hormone replacement therapy (HRT) without complications should stop is unclear, but it seems prudent to do so, especially if they do not have menopausal symptoms. Definitive evidence of beneficial effects of HRT on cognitive function is lacking. Several studies have shown an increased risk of breast cancer in women taking estrogen-progestin therapy, while estrogen alone did not increase the risk. Endometrial cancer can occur if adequate progestin is not used. Estrogen may cause the growth of uterine myomas, which otherwise shrink after the menopause. (See also discussions of estrogen and progestin replacement therapy in Chapter 26.)

C. SURGICAL MENOPAUSE

The abrupt hormonal decrease resulting from oophorectomy generally results in severe vasomotor symptoms and rapid onset of dyspareunia and osteoporosis unless treated. Estrogen replacement is generally started immediately after surgery. Conjugated estrogens 1.25 mg, estrone sulfate 1.25 mg, or estradiol 2 mg is given for 25 days of each month. After age 45–50 years, this dose can be tapered to 0.625 mg of conjugated estrogens or equivalent.

Grady D et al: Cardiovascular disease outcomes during 6.8 years of hormone therapy: Heart and Estrogen/progestin Replacement Study follow-up (HERS II). JAMA 2002;288:49. [PMID: 12090862]

Grady D. A 60-year-old woman trying to discontinue hormone replacement therapy. JAMA 2002;287:2130. [PMID: 11966388]

Hulley S et al: Noncardiovascular disease outcomes during 6.8 years of hormone therapy: Heart and Estrogen/progestin Replacement Study follow-up (HERS II). JAMA 2002; 288:58. [PMID: 12090863]

Hulley S et al: Randomized trial of estrogen plus progestin for secondary prevention of coronary heart disease in postmenopausal women. Heart and Estrogen/Progestin Replacement Study (HERS) Research Group. JAMA 1998;280: 605. [PMID: 9718051] (A randomized secondary prevention trial of 2763 women with coronary disease found no significant difference between the placebo and hormone replacement therapy [HRT] group with respect to cardiovascular outcomes during an average of 4.1 years of follow-up despite beneficial lipid changes. There was a significant time trend, with more coronary heart disease events in the HRT group in year 1 and fewer in years 4 and 5.)

Manson JE et al: Clinical practice. Postmenopausal hormone replacement therapy. N Engl J Med 2001;345:34. [PMID: 11439947] (Review article covering current knowledge of risks and benefits; includes a useful decision tree for use of hormone replacement therapy.)

Mendelsohn ME et al: The protective effects of estrogen on the cardiovascular system. N Engl J Med 1999;340:1801. [PMID: 10362825] (Review article.)

Risks and benefits of estrogen plus progestin in healthy postmenopausal women: principal results From the Women's Health Initiative randomized controlled trial. JAMA 2002;288:321. [PMID: 12117397] (A randomized controlled primary prevention trial involving 16,608 postmenopausal women aged 50–79 years with an intact uterus who received conjugated estrogens 0.625 mg/d plus medroxyprogesterone acetate 2.5 mg/d versus placebo found that overall health risks exceeded benefits of treatment. Among those treated with estrogen-progestin, there were significantly more women with nonfatal myocardial infarction and coronary heart disease death; breast cancer, stroke, and pulmonary emboli. There were significantly fewer women with hip fracture and colorectal cancer. Absolute excess risks per 10,000 person-years attributable to estrogen plus progestin were seven more coronary deart disease events, eight more strokes, eight more pulmonary emboli, and eight more invasive breast cancers, while absolute risk reductions per 10,000 person-years were six fewer colorectal cancers and five fewer hip fractures.)

Schairer C et al: Menopausal estrogen and estrogen-progestin replacement therapy and breast cancer risk. JAMA 2000; 283:485. [PMID: 10659874] (In a cohort study of 46,355 postmenopausal women, the relative risk of breast cancer with estrogen and estrogen-progestin use for up to 4 years, compared with that of nonusers, was 1.2 [95% CI, 1.0–1.4] and 1.4 [1.1–1.8], respectively. The relative risk increased 0.01 for each year of estrogen use and 0.08 for each year of estrogen-progestin use.)

Obstetrics

18

William R. Crombleholme, MD
See www.current-med.com/ch18.html

DIAGNOSIS & DIFFERENTIAL DIAGNOSIS OF PREGNANCY

It is advantageous to diagnose pregnancy as promptly as possible when a sexually active woman misses a menstrual period or has symptoms suggestive of pregnancy. In the event of a desired pregnancy, prenatal care can begin early, and potentially harmful medications and activities such as drug and alcohol use, smoking, and occupational chemical exposure can be halted. In the event of an unwanted pregnancy, counseling about adoption or termination of the pregnancy can be provided at an early stage.

Pregnancy Tests

All urine or blood pregnancy tests rely on the detection of hCG produced by the placenta. hCG levels increase shortly after implantation, double approximately every 48 hours, reach a peak at 50–75 days, and fall to lower levels in the second and third trimesters. Laboratory and home pregnancy tests now use monoclonal antibodies specific for hCG. These tests are performed on serum or urine and are accurate at the time of the missed period or shortly after it.

Compared with intrauterine pregnancies, ectopic pregnancies may show lower levels of hCG that level off or fall in serial determinations. Quantitative assays of hCG repeated at 48- to 72-hour intervals are used in the diagnosis of ectopic pregnancy as well as in cases of molar pregnancy, threatened abortion, and missed abortion. Comparison of hCG levels between laboratories may be misleading in a given patient because different international standards may produce results that vary by as much as twofold.

Manifestations of Pregnancy

The following symptoms and signs are usually due to pregnancy, but none are diagnostic. A record of the time and frequency of coitus is helpful for diagnosing and dating a pregnancy.

A. SYMPTOMS

Amenorrhea, nausea and vomiting, breast tenderness and tingling, urinary frequency and urgency, "quickening" (perception of first movement noted at about the 18th week), weight gain.

B. SIGNS (IN WEEKS FROM LMP)

Breast changes (enlargement, vascular engorgement, colostrum), abdominal enlargement, cyanosis of vagina and cervical portio (about the seventh week), softening of the cervix (seventh week), softening of the cervicouterine junction (eighth week), generalized enlargement and diffuse softening of the corpus (after eighth week).

The uterine fundus is palpable above the pubic symphysis by 12–15 weeks from the LMP and reaches the umbilicus by 20–22 weeks. Fetal heart tones can be heard by doppler at 10–12 weeks of gestation and at 20 weeks with an ordinary fetoscope.

Differential Diagnosis

The nonpregnant uterus enlarged by myomas can be confused with the gravid uterus, but it is usually very firm and irregular. An ovarian tumor may be found midline, displacing the nonpregnant uterus to the side or posteriorly. Ultrasonography and a pregnancy test will provide accurate diagnosis in these circumstances.

ESSENTIALS OF PRENATAL CARE

The first prenatal visit should occur as early as possible after the diagnosis of pregnancy and should include the following.

History

Age, ethnic background, occupation. Onset of LMP and its normality, possible conception dates, bleeding after LMP, medical history, all prior pregnancies (duration, outcome, and complications), symptoms of present pregnancy. Use of drugs, alcohol, tobacco, caffeine, nutritional habits (Table 18–1). Family history of congenital anomalies and heritable diseases. History of childhood varicella. Prior STDs or risk factors for HIV infection.

Physical Examination

Height, weight, blood pressure, general physical examination. Abdominal and pelvic examination: (1) estimate uterine size or measure fundal height; (2) evaluate bony pelvis for symmetry and adequacy; (3) evaluate cervix for structural anatomy, infection, effacement, dilation; (4) detect fetal heart sounds by doppler device after 10 weeks or fetoscope after 18 weeks.

Laboratory Tests

Urinalysis, culture of a clean-voided midstream urine sample, complete blood count with red cell indices, serologic test for syphilis, rubella antibody titer, blood group, Rh type, atypical antibody screening, and HBsAg evaluation. Human immunodeficiency virus (HIV) screening should be offered to all pregnant women. Cervical cultures are usually obtained for *Neisseria gonorrhoeae* and chlamydia, along with a Pa-

Table 18–1. Common drugs that are teratogenic or fetotoxic.[1]

ACE inhibitors	Estrogens
Alcohol	Griseofulvin
Amantadine	Hypoglycemics, oral
Aminopterin	Isotretinoin
Androgens	Lithium
Anticonvulsants	Methotrexate
Aminoglutethimide	Misoprostol
Carbamazepine	NSAIDs (third trimester)
Ethotoin	Opioids (prolonged use)
Phenytoin	Progestins
Valproic acid	Radioiodine (antithyroid)
Aspirin and other	Reserpine
salicylates (third	Ribavirin
trimester)	Sulfonamides (third trimester)
Benzodiazepines	Tetracycline (third trimester)
Carbarsone	Thalidomide
(amebicide)	Tobacco smoking
Chloramphenicol	Trimethoprim (third trimester)
(third trimester)	Warfarin and other coumarin
Cyclophosphamide	anticoagulants
Diazoxide	
Diethylstilbestrol	
Disulfiram	
Ergotamine	

[1]Many other drugs are also contraindicated during pregnancy. Evaluate any drug for its need versus its potential adverse effects. Further information can be obtained from the manufacturer or from any of several teratogenic registries around the country.

panicolaou smear of the cervix. All black women should have sickle cell screening. Women of African, Asian, or Mediterranean ancestry with anemia or low MCV values should have hemoglobin electrophoresis performed to identify abnormal hemoglobins (Hb S, C, F, α-thalassemia, β-thalassemia). Tuberculosis skin testing is increasingly indicated for immigrant and inner city populations. Genetic counseling with the option of chorionic villus sampling or genetic amniocentesis should be offered to all women who will be 35 years of age or older at delivery and those who have had prior offspring with chromosomal abnormalities. Tay-Sachs blood screening is offered to Jewish women with Jewish partners. Screening for cystic fibrosis is offered based on the family history. Hepatitis C antibody screening should be offered only to those pregnant women who are at high risk of infection.

Pregnant women who work in medical-dental health care or the police and fire departments and those who are household contacts of a hepatitis B virus carrier or a hemodialysis patient and are HBsAg-negative at prenatal screening are at high risk of acquiring hepatitis B. They should be vaccinated during pregnancy.

Advice to Patients

A. PRENATAL VISITS

Prenatal care should begin early and maintain a schedule of regular prenatal visits: 0–28 weeks, every 4 weeks; 28–36 weeks, every 2 weeks; 36 weeks on, weekly.

B. DIET

1. Eat a balanced diet containing the major food groups.
2. Take prenatal vitamins with iron and folic acid.
3. Expect to gain 20–40 lb. Do not diet to lose weight during pregnancy.
4. Decrease caffeine intake to 0–1 cup of coffee, tea, or caffeinated cola daily.
5. Avoid eating raw or rare meat, and wash hands after handling raw meat.
6. Eat fresh fruits and vegetables and wash them before eating.

C. MEDICATIONS

Do not take medications unless prescribed or authorized by your provider.

D. ALCOHOL AND OTHER DRUGS

Abstain from alcohol, tobacco, and all recreational ("street") drugs. No safe level of alcohol intake has been established for pregnancy. Fetal effects are manifest in the **fetal alcohol syndrome,** which includes growth restriction, facial abnormalities, and serious central nervous system dysfunction. These effects are thought to result from direct toxicity of ethanol itself as well as of its metabolites such as acetaldehyde.

Characteristic findings include shortened palpebral fissures, low-set ears, midfacial hypoplasia, a smooth philtrum, a thin upper lip, microcephaly, mental retardation, and attention deficit disorder. Skeletal and cardiac abnormalities may also be seen.

Cigarette smoking results in fetal exposure to carbon monoxide and nicotine, and this is thought to eventuate in a number of adverse pregnancy outcomes. An increased risk of abruptio placentae, placenta previa, and premature rupture of the membranes is documented among women who smoke. Premature delivery occurs 20% more frequently among smoking pregnant women, and the birth weights of their infants are on average 200 g lower than infants of nonsmokers. Women who smoke should quit smoking or at least reduce the number of cigarettes smoked per day to as few as possible. Pregnant women should also avoid exposure to environmental smoke ("passive smoking").

Sometimes compounding the above effects on pregnancy outcome are the independent adverse effects of illicit drugs. Cocaine use in pregnancy is associated with an increased risk of premature rupture of membranes, preterm delivery, placental abruption, intrauterine growth restriction, neurobehavioral deficits, and sudden infant death syndrome. Similar adverse pregnancy effects are associated with amphetamine use, perhaps reflecting the vasoconstrictive potential of both amphetamines and cocaine. Adverse effects associated with opioid use include intrauterine growth restriction, prematurity, stillbirth, and fetal death.

E. X-Rays and Noxious Exposures

Avoid x-rays unless essential and approved by a physician. Inform your dentist and your providers that you are pregnant. Avoid chemical or radiation hazards. Avoid excessive heat in hot tubs or saunas. Avoid handling cat feces or cat litter. Wear gloves when gardening.

F. Rest and Activity

Obtain adequate rest each day. Abstain from strenuous physical work or activities, particularly when heavy lifting or weight bearing is required. Exercise regularly at a mild to moderate level. Avoid exhausting or hazardous exercises or new athletic training programs during pregnancy. Heart rate should be kept below 140 beats/min during exercise.

G. Birth Classes

Enroll with your partner in a childbirth preparation class well before your due date.

Tests & Procedures

A. Each Visit

Weight, blood pressure, fundal height, fetal heart rate, urine specimen for protein and glucose. Review patient's concerns about pregnancy, health, and nutrition.

B. 6–12 Weeks

Confirm uterine size and growth by pelvic examination. Document fetal heart tones (audible at 10–12 weeks of gestation by doppler). Transvaginal chorionic villus sampling (CVS) between 10 and 12 weeks when indicated.

C. 12–18 Weeks

Genetic counseling for women age 35 years or older at EDC and those with a family history of congenital anomalies or a previous child with a chromosomal abnormality, metabolic disease, or neural tube defect. Amniocentesis is performed as indicated and requested by the patient.

D. 12–24 Weeks

Fetal ultrasound examination to determine pregnancy dating and evaluate fetal anatomy. An earlier examination provides the most accurate dating, and a later examination demonstrates fetal anatomy in greater detail. The best compromise is at 18–20 weeks of gestation.

E. 16–20 Weeks

Maternal serum alpha-fetoprotein testing is offered to all women to screen for neural tube defects. In some states, such testing is mandatory. Serum α-fetoprotein is usually combined with measurement of estriol and hCG (triple screen) for the detection of fetal Down's syndrome.

F. 20–24 Weeks

Instruct patient in symptoms and signs of preterm labor and rupture of membranes.

G. 24 Weeks to Delivery

Ultrasound examination is performed as indicated. Typically, fetal size and growth are evaluated when fundal height is 3 cm less than or more than expected for gestational age. In multiple pregnancies, ultrasound should be performed every 4 weeks to evaluate for discordant growth.

H. 26–28 Weeks

Screening for gestational diabetes by a 50-g glucose load (Glucola) and a 1-hour post-Glucola blood glucose determination. Abnormal values should be followed up with a 3-hour glucose tolerance test (Table 18–3).

I. 28 Weeks

If initial antibody screen is negative, repeat antibody testing for Rh-negative patients, but result is not required before $Rh_o(D)$ immune globulin is administered.

J. 28–32 WEEKS

Repeat the complete blood count to evaluate for anemia of pregnancy.

K. 28 WEEKS TO DELIVERY

Determination of fetal position and presentation. Question the patient at each visit for symptoms or signs of preterm labor or rupture of membranes. Assess maternal perception of fetal movement at each visit. Antepartum fetal testing is performed as medically indicated.

L. 36 WEEKS TO DELIVERY

Repeat syphilis and HIV testing, cervical cultures for *N gonorrhoeae,* and *Chlamydia trachomatis* in at-risk patients. Discuss with the patient the indicators of onset of labor, admission to hospital, management of labor and delivery, and options for analgesia and anesthesia. Weekly cervical examinations are not necessary unless indicated to assess a specific clinical situation. Elective delivery (whether by induction or cesarean section) prior to 39 weeks of gestation requires confirmation of fetal lung maturity.

The CDC has approved two approaches—screening-based and risk factor-based—for management of group B streptococcal colonization in pregnancy: (1) In the **screening-based approach,** a single standard culture of the distal vagina and anorectum is collected at 35–37 weeks. No prophylaxis is needed if the screening culture is negative. Patients whose cultures are positive receive intrapartum penicillin prophylaxis with labor. Patients with risk factors such as a previous infant with invasive group B streptococcal disease, or group B streptococcal bacteriuria during the pregnancy, or delivery at less than 37 weeks of gestation also receive intrapartum prophylaxis. Patients whose cultures at 35–37 weeks were not done or whose results are not known receive prophylaxis only with the risk factors of intrapartum temperature greater than 38 °C or membrane rupture greater than 18 hours. (2) In the **risk factor approach,** no screening cultures are performed, and all patients with any of the risk factors noted above are treated.

The routine recommended regimen for prophylaxis is penicillin G, 5 million units intravenously as a loading dose and then 2.5 million units intravenously every 4 hours until delivery. In penicillin-allergic patients, clindamycin, 900 mg intravenously every 8 hours until delivery, is substituted.

M. 41 WEEKS AND BEYOND

Cervical examination to determine the probability of successful induction of labor. Based on this, induction of labor is undertaken if the cervix is favorable; if unfavorable, antepartum fetal testing is begun.

Haertsch M et al: What is recommended for healthy women during pregnancy? A comparison of seven prenatal clinical practice guideline documents. Birth 1999;26:24. [PMID: 10352052]

Koren G et al: Drugs in pregnancy. N Engl J Med 1998;338: 1128. [PMID: 9545362]

Schrag SJ et al: Group B streptococcal disease in the era of intrapartum antibiotic prophylaxis. N Engl J Med 2000;342:15. [PMID: 10620644]

NUTRITION IN PREGNANCY

Nutrition in pregnancy significantly affects maternal health and infant size and well-being. Pregnant women should have nutrition counseling early in prenatal care and access to supplementary food programs if necessary. Counseling should stress abstention from alcohol, smoking, and recreational drugs. Caffeine and artificial sweeteners should be used only in small amounts. "Empty calories" should be avoided, and the diet should contain the following foods: protein foods of animal and vegetable origin, milk and milk products, whole-grain cereals and breads, and fruits and vegetables—especially green leafy vegetables.

Weight gain in pregnancy should be 20–40 lb, which includes the added weight of the fetus, placenta, and amniotic fluid and of maternal reproductive tissues, fluid, blood, increased fat stores, and increased lean body mass. Maternal fat stores are a caloric reserve for pregnancy and lactation; weight restriction in pregnancy to avoid developing such fat stores may affect the development of other fetal and maternal tissues and is not advisable. Obese women can have normal infants with less weight gain (15–20 lb) but should be encouraged to eat high-quality foods. Normally, a pregnant woman gains 2–5 lb in the first trimester and slightly less than 1 lb/wk thereafter. She needs approximately an extra 200–300 kcal/d (depending on energy output) and 30 g/d of additional protein for a total protein intake of about 75 g/d. Appropriate caloric intake in pregnancy helps prevent the problems associated with low birth weight.

Rigid salt restriction is not necessary. While consumption of highly salted snack foods and prepared foods is not desirable, 2–3 g/d of sodium is permissible. The increased calcium needs of pregnancy (1200 mg/d) can be met with milk, milk products, green vegetables, soybean products, corn tortillas, and calcium carbonate supplements.

The increased need for iron and folic acid should be met from foods as well as vitamin and mineral supplements. (See section on anemia in pregnancy.) Megavitamins should not be taken in pregnancy, as they may result in fetal malformation or disturbed metabolism. However, a balanced prenatal supplement containing 30–60 mg of elemental iron, 0.5–0.8 mg of folate, and the recommended daily allowances of various vitamins and minerals is widely used in the USA and is probably beneficial to many women with marginal diets. There is evidence that periconceptional folic acid supplements can decrease the risk of neural tube defects in the fetus. For this reason, the United States Public Health Service recommends the consumption of 0.4

mg of folic acid per day for all pregnant women (and thus all women capable of becoming pregnant). Women with a prior pregnancy complicated by neural tube defect may require higher supplemental doses as determined by their providers. Lactovegetarians and ovolactovegetarians do well in pregnancy; vegetarian women who eat neither eggs nor milk products should have their diets assessed for adequate calories and protein and should take oral vitamin B_{12} supplements during pregnancy and lactation.

Institute of Medicine, National Academy of Sciences: *Nutrition During Pregnancy.* Part I, *Weight Gain;* Part II, *Nutrient Supplements.* National Academy Press, 1990.

Locksmith GJ et al: Preventing neural tube defects: The importance of periconceptional folic acid supplements. Obstet Gynecol 1998;91:1027. [PMID: 9611019]

TRAVEL & IMMUNIZATIONS DURING PREGNANCY

During an otherwise normal low-risk pregnancy, travel can be planned most safely between the 18th and 32nd weeks. Commercial flying in pressurized cabins does not pose a threat to the fetus. An aisle seat will allow frequent walks. Adequate fluids should be taken during the flight.

It is not advisable to travel to endemic areas of yellow fever in Africa or Latin America; similarly, it is inadvisable to travel to areas of Africa or Asia where chloroquine-resistant falciparum malaria is a hazard, since complications of malaria are more common in pregnancy.

Ideally, all immunizations should precede pregnancy. Live virus products are contraindicated (measles, rubella, yellow fever). Inactivated poliovaccine (Salk) can be used instead of the oral vaccine. Vaccines against pneumococcal pneumonia, meningococcal meningitis, and hepatitis A can be used as indicated. Influenza vaccine is indicated in all pregnant women who will be in their second or third trimester during "flu season."

Pooled immune globulin to prevent hepatitis A is safe and does not carry a risk of HIV transmission. Hepatitis A vaccine contains formalin-inactivated virus but can be given in pregnancy when needed. Chloroquine can be used for malaria prophylaxis in pregnancy, and proguanil is also safe.

Water should be purified by boiling, since iodine purification may provide more iodine than is safe during pregnancy.

Do not use prophylactic antibiotics or bismuth subsalicylate during pregnancy to prevent diarrhea. Use oral rehydration fluids, and treat bacterial diarrhea with erythromycin or ampicillin if necessary.

Prevention and control of influenza: Recommendations of the Advisory Committee on Immunization Practices (ACIP). Morb Mortal Wkly Rep 1999;48(RR-4):1. [PMID: 10366138]

Rose SR: Pregnancy and travel. Emerg Med Clin N Am 1997;15:93. [PMID: 9056572]

VOMITING OF PREGNANCY (Morning Sickness) & HYPEREMESIS GRAVIDARUM (Pernicious Vomiting of Pregnancy)

Morning or evening nausea and vomiting usually begins soon after the first missed period and ceases by the fifth month of gestation. Up to three-fourths of women complain of nausea and vomiting during early pregnancy, with the vast majority noting nausea throughout the day. This problem exerts no adverse effects on the pregnancy and does not presage other complications, though it is particularly common with multiple pregnancy and hydatidiform mole. The cause of vomiting during pregnancy is believed to be high estrogen levels.

Persistent, severe vomiting during pregnancy—hyperemesis gravidarum—can be disabling and require hospitalization. Dehydration, acidosis, and nutritional deficiencies may develop with protracted vomiting. Thyroid dysfunction can be associated with hyperemesis gravidarum, so it is advisable to determine TSH and free T_4 values in these patients.

Treatment

A. MILD NAUSEA AND VOMITING OF PREGNANCY

Reassurance and dietary advice are all that is required in most instances. Because of possible teratogenicity, drugs used during the first half of pregnancy should be restricted to those of major importance to life and health. Antiemetics, antihistamines, and antispasmodics are generally unnecessary to treat nausea of pregnancy. Vitamin B_6 (pyridoxine), 50–100 mg/d orally, is nontoxic and may be helpful in some patients.

B. HYPEREMESIS GRAVIDARUM

Hospitalize the patient in a private room at bed rest. Give nothing by mouth for 48 hours, and maintain hydration and electrolyte balance by giving appropriate parenteral fluids and vitamin supplements as indicated. Rarely, total parenteral nutrition may become necessary. As soon as possible, place the patient on a dry diet consisting of six small feedings daily plus clear liquids 1 hour after eating. Prochlorperazine rectal suppositories may be useful. After in-patient stabilization, the patient can be maintained at home even if she requires intravenous fluids in addition to her oral intake.

Lacroix R et al: Nausea and vomiting during pregnancy: A prospective study of its frequency, intensity, and patterns of change. Am J Obstet Gynecol 2000; 182:931. [PMID: 10764476]

Mazzotta P et al: A risk-benefit assessment of pharmacological and non-pharmacological treatments for nausea and vomiting of pregnancy. Drugs 2000;59:781. [PMID: 10804035]

SPONTANEOUS ABORTION

Abortion is defined as termination of gestation before the 20th week of pregnancy. About three-fourths of spontaneous abortions occur before the 16th week; of these, three-fourths occur before the eighth week. Almost 20% of all clinically recognized pregnancies terminate in spontaneous abortion.

More than 60% of spontaneous abortions result from chromosomal defects due to maternal or paternal factors; about 15% appear to be associated with maternal trauma, infections, dietary deficiencies, diabetes mellitus, hypothyroidism, or anatomic malformations. There is no reliable evidence that abortion may be induced by psychic stimuli such as severe fright, grief, anger, or anxiety. In about one-fourth of cases, the cause of abortion cannot be determined. There is no evidence that video display terminals or associated electromagnetic fields are related to an increased risk of spontaneous abortion.

It is important to distinguish women with a history of incompetent cervix from those with more typical early abortion and those with premature labor or rupture of the membranes. Characteristically, incompetent cervix presents as "silent" cervical dilation (ie, with minimal uterine contractions) between 16 and 28 weeks of gestation. Women with incompetent cervix often present with significant cervical dilation (2 cm or more) and minimal symptoms. When the cervix reaches 4 cm or more, active uterine contractions or rupture of the membranes may occur secondary to the degree of cervical dilation. This does not change the primary diagnosis. Factors that predispose to incompetent cervix are a history of incompetent cervix with a previous pregnancy; cervical conization or surgery; cervical injury; DES exposure; and anatomic abnormalities of the cervix. Prior to pregnancy or during the first trimester, there are no methods for determining whether the cervix will eventually be incompetent. After 14–16 weeks, ultrasound may be used to evaluate the internal anatomy of the lower uterine segment and cervix for the funneling and shortening abnormalities consistent with cervical incompetence.

Clinical Findings

A. SYMPTOMS AND SIGNS

1. Threatened abortion—Bleeding or cramping occurs, but the pregnancy continues. The cervix is not dilated.

2. Inevitable abortion—The cervix is dilated and the membranes may be ruptured, but passage of the products of conception has not occurred. Bleeding and cramping persist, and passage of the products of conception is considered inevitable.

3. Complete abortion—The fetus and placenta are completely expelled. Pain ceases, but spotting may persist.

4. Incomplete abortion—Some portion of the products of conception (usually placental) remain in the uterus. Only mild cramps are reported, but bleeding is persistent and often excessive.

5. Missed abortion—The pregnancy has ceased to develop, but the conceptus has not been expelled. Symptoms of pregnancy disappear. There is a brownish vaginal discharge but no free bleeding. Pain does not develop. The cervix is semifirm and slightly patulous; the uterus becomes smaller and irregularly softened; the adnexa are normal.

B. LABORATORY FINDINGS

Pregnancy tests show low or falling levels of hCG. A complete blood count should be obtained if bleeding is heavy. Determine Rh type, and give $Rh_o(D)$ immune globulin if the type is Rh-negative. All tissue recovered should be assessed by a pathologist and may be sent for genetic analysis in selected cases.

C. ULTRASONOGRAPHIC FINDINGS

The gestational sac can be identified at 5–6 weeks from the LMP, a fetal pole at 6 weeks, and fetal cardiac activity at 6–7 weeks. Serial observations are often required to evaluate changes in size of the embryo. A small, irregular sac without a fetal pole with accurate dating is diagnostic of an abnormal pregnancy.

Differential Diagnosis

The bleeding that occurs in abortion of a uterine pregnancy must be differentiated from the abnormal bleeding of an ectopic pregnancy and anovular bleeding in a nonpregnant woman. The passage of hydropic villi in the bloody discharge is diagnostic of hydatidiform mole.

Treatment

A. GENERAL MEASURES

1. Threatened abortion—Place the patient at bed rest for 24–48 hours followed by gradual resumption of usual activities, with abstinence from coitus and douching. Hormonal treatment is contraindicated. Antibiotics should be used only if there are signs of infection.

2. Missed or inevitable abortion—This calls for counseling regarding the fate of the pregnancy and planning for its elective termination at a time chosen by the patient and physician. Insertion of a laminaria to dilate the cervix followed by aspiration is the method of choice for a missed abortion. Prostaglandin vaginal suppositories are an effective alternative.

B. SURGICAL MEASURES

1. Incomplete abortion—Prompt removal of any products of conception remaining within the uterus is required to stop bleeding and prevent infection. Analgesia and a paracervical block are useful, followed by uterine exploration with ovum forceps or uterine aspiration.

2. Cerclage and restriction of activities—These are the treatment of choice for incompetent cervix. A variety of suture materials including a 5 mm Mersilene band can be used to create a purse-string type of stitch around the cervix, using either the McDonald or Shirodkar method. Cerclage should be undertaken with caution when there is advanced cervical dilation or when the membranes are prolapsed into the vagina. Rupture of the membranes and infection are specific contraindications to cerclage. Cervical cultures for *N gonorrhoeae,* chlamydia, and group B streptococci should be obtained before or at the time of cerclage.

Hurd WW et al: Expectant management versus elective curettage for the treatment of spontaneous abortion. Fertil Steril 1997;68:601. [PMID: 9341597]

Ness RB et al: Cocaine and tobacco use and the risk of spontaneous abortion. N Engl J Med 1999;340:333. [PMID: 9929522]

RECURRENT (HABITUAL) ABORTION

Recurrent abortion has been defined for years as the loss of three or more previable (< 500 g) pregnancies in succession. Recurrent abortion occurs in about 0.4–0.8% of all pregnancies. Abnormalities related to recurrent abortion can be identified in approximately half of the couples. If a woman has lost three previous pregnancies without identifiable cause, she still has a 70–80% chance of carrying a fetus to viability. If she has aborted four or five times, the likelihood of a successful pregnancy is 65–70%.

Recurrent abortion is a clinical rather than pathologic diagnosis. The clinical findings are similar to those observed in other types of abortion (see above).

Treatment

A. PRECONCEPTION THERAPY

Preconception therapy is aimed at detection of maternal or paternal defects that may contribute to abortion. A thorough general and gynecologic examination is essential. Polycystic ovaries should be ruled out. A random blood glucose test and thyroid function studies (including thyroid antibodies) should be done. Detection of lupus anticoagulant and other hemostatic abnormalities (proteins S and C and antithrombin III deficiency, hyperhomocysteinemia, anticardiolipin antibody, factor V Leiden mutation) and an antinuclear antibody test may be indicated. Endometrial tissue should be examined in the postovulation stage of the cycle to determine the adequacy of the response of the endometrium to hormones. The competency of the cervix must be determined and hysteroscopy or hys-

terography used to exclude submucous myomas and congenital anomalies. Chromosomal (karyotype) analysis of both partners rules out balanced translocations (found in 5% of infertile couples).

Studies have focused on the major histocompatibility complex (MHC) of chromosome 6, which carries HLA loci and other genes that may influence reproductive success. Some women demonstrate a lack of maternal antibody response to paternal lymphocytes, which is customarily found in normal women after successful childbearing. However, several randomized controlled trials have found no benefit of IGIV therapy for recurrent spontaneous abortion.

B. POSTCONCEPTION THERAPY

Provide early prenatal care and schedule frequent office visits. Complete bed rest is justified only for bleeding or pain. Empiric sex steroid hormone therapy is contraindicated.

Prognosis

The prognosis is excellent if the cause of abortion can be corrected.

Coumans AB et al: Haemostatic and metabolic abnormalities in women with unexplained recurrent abortion. Hum Reprod 1999;14:211. [PMID: 10374132]

Jablonowska B et al: Prevention of recurrent spontaneous abortion by intravenous immunoglobulin: A double-blind placebo-controlled study. Hum Reprod 1999;14:838. [PMID: 10221723]

Ridker PM et al: Factor V Leiden mutation as a risk factor for recurrent pregnancy loss. Ann Intern Med 1998;128(12 Part 1):1000. [PMID: 9625662]

ECTOPIC PREGNANCY

Any pregnancy arising from implantation of the ovum outside the cavity of the uterus is ectopic. Ectopic implantation occurs in about one out of 150 live births. About 98% of ectopic pregnancies are tubal. Other sites of ectopic implantation are the peritoneum or abdominal viscera, the ovary, and the cervix. Any condition that prevents or retards migration of the fertilized ovum to the uterus can predispose to an ectopic pregnancy, including a history of infertility, pelvic inflammatory disease, ruptured appendix, and prior tubal surgery. Combined intra- and extrauterine pregnancy (heterotopic) may occur rarely. In the USA, undiagnosed or undetected ectopic pregnancy is currently the most common cause of maternal death during the first trimester.

Clinical Findings

A. SYMPTOMS AND SIGNS

The cardinal symptoms and signs of tubal pregnancy are (1) amenorrhea or irregular bleeding and spotting, followed by (2) pelvic pain, and (3) pelvic (adnexal) mass formation. They may be acute or chronic.

1. Acute (40%)—Severe lower quadrant pain occurs in almost every case. It is sudden in onset, lancinating, intermittent, and does not radiate. Backache is present during attacks. Shock occurs in about 10%, often after pelvic examination. At least two-thirds of patients give a history of abnormal menstruation; many have been infertile.

2. Chronic (60%)—Blood leaks from the tubal ampulla over a period of days, and considerable blood may accumulate in the peritoneum. Slight but persistent vaginal spotting is reported, and a pelvic mass can be palpated. Abdominal distention and mild paralytic ileus are often present.

B. LABORATORY FINDINGS

Blood studies may show anemia and slight leukocytosis. Quantitative serum pregnancy tests will show levels generally lower than expected for normal pregnancies of the same duration. If pregnancy tests are followed over a few days, there may be a slow rise or a plateau rather than the near doubling every 2 days associated with normal early intrauterine pregnancy or the falling levels that occur with spontaneous abortion.

C. IMAGING

Ultrasonography can reliably demonstrate a gestational sac 6 weeks from the LMP and a fetal pole at 7 weeks if located in the uterus. An empty uterine cavity raises a strong suspicion of extrauterine pregnancy, which can occasionally be revealed by endovaginal ultrasound. Specified levels of serum hCG have been reliably correlated with ultrasound findings of an intrauterine pregnancy. For example, an hCG level of 6500 mU/mL with an empty uterine cavity by transabdominal ultrasound is virtually diagnostic of an ectopic pregnancy. Similarly, an hCG value of 2000 mU/mL or more can be indicative of an ectopic pregnancy if no products of conception are detected within the uterine cavity by transvaginal ultrasound.

D. SPECIAL EXAMINATIONS

With the advent of high-resolution transvaginal ultrasound, culdocentesis is rarely used in evaluation of possible ectopic pregnancy. Laparoscopy is the surgical procedure of choice both to confirm an ectopic pregnancy and in most cases to permit pelviscopic removal of the ectopic pregnancy without the need for exploratory laparotomy.

Differential Diagnosis

Clinical and laboratory findings suggestive or diagnostic of pregnancy will distinguish ectopic pregnancy from many acute abdominal illnesses such as acute appendicitis, acute pelvic inflammatory disease, ruptured corpus luteum cyst or ovarian follicle, and urinary calculi. Uterine enlargement with clinical findings similar to those found in ectopic pregnancy is also characteristic of an aborting uterine pregnancy or hydatidiform mole. Ectopic pregnancy should be suspected when

postabortal tissue examination fails to reveal placenta. Steps must be taken for immediate diagnosis, including prompt microscopic tissue examination, ultrasonography, and serial hCG titers every 48 hours. Patients must be warned of possible ectopic pregnancy problems and followed very closely.

Treatment

When a patient is unstable or when surgical therapy is planned, the patient is hospitalized with a diagnosis of ectopic pregnancy. Blood is typed and cross-matched. Ideally, diagnosis and operative treatment should precede frank rupture of the tube and intra-abdominal hemorrhage.

Surgical treatment is definitive. In a stable patient, diagnostic laparoscopy is the initial surgical procedure performed. Depending on the size of the ectopic pregnancy and whether or not it has ruptured, salpingostomy with removal of the ectopic or a partial or complete salpingectomy can usually be performed pelviscopically through the laparoscope. Clinical conditions permitting, patency of the contralateral tube can be established by injection of indigo carmine into the uterine cavity and flow through the contralateral tube confirmed visually by the surgeon.

In a stable patient, methotrexate (50 mg/m²)—given systemically as single or multiple doses—is acceptable medical therapy for early ectopic pregnancy. Favorable criteria are that the pregnancy should be less than 3.5 cm and unruptured, with no active bleeding.

Iron therapy for anemia may be necessary during convalescence. Give Rh₀(D) immune globulin (300 μg) to Rh-negative patients.

Prognosis

Repeat tubal pregnancy occurs in about 12% of cases. This should not be regarded as a contraindication to future pregnancy, but the patient requires careful observation and early ultrasound confirmation of an intrauterine pregnancy.

Buster J et al: Medical management of ectopic pregnancy. Clin Obstet Gynecol 1999;42:23. [PMID: 10073296]

Hajenius PJ et al: Interventions for tubal ectopic pregnancy. Cochrane Database Syst Rev 2000;(2):CD000324. [PMID: 10796710]

Kamwendo F et al: Epidemiology of ectopic pregnancy during a 28-year period and the role of pelvic inflammatory disease. Sex Transm Infect 2000;76:28. [PMID: 10817065]

PREECLAMPSIA-ECLAMPSIA

Preeclampsia-eclampsia can occur any time after 20 weeks of gestation and up to 6 weeks postpartum. It is a disease unique to pregnancy, with the only cure being delivery of the fetus and placenta. Approximately 7% of pregnant women in the United States develop preeclampsia-eclampsia. Primiparas are most frequently affected; however, the incidence of preeclampsia-eclampsia is increased with multiple pregnancies, chronic hypertension, diabetes, renal disease, collagen-vascular and autoimmune disorders, and gestational trophoblastic disease. Five percent of women with preeclampsia progress to eclampsia. Uncontrolled eclampsia is a significant cause of maternal death.

The basic cause of preeclampsia-eclampsia is not known. Epidemiologic studies suggest an immunologic cause for preeclampsia, since it occurs predominantly in women who have had minimal exposure to sperm (having used barrier methods of contraception) or have new consorts; in primigravidas; and in women both of whose parents have similar HLA antigens. Preeclampsia is an endothelial disorder resulting from poor placental perfusion, which releases a factor that injures the endothelium, causing activation of coagulation and an increased sensitivity to pressors. Before the syndrome becomes clinically manifest in the second half of pregnancy, there has been vasospasm in various small vessel beds, accounting for the pathologic changes in maternal organs and the placenta with consequent adverse effects on the fetus.

The use of diuretics, dietary restriction or enhancement, sodium restriction, aspirin, and vitamin-mineral supplements such as calcium has not been shown to be useful in clinical studies. The only cure is termination of the pregnancy at a time as favorable as possible for fetal survival.

Definition

Preeclampsia is defined as the presence of elevated blood pressure and proteinuria during pregnancy. Eclampsia occurs with the addition of seizures. The abnormalities of preeclampsia-eclampsia are defined as follows: (1) A sustained elevation of blood pressure of 140 mm Hg systolic or 90 mm Hg diastolic or more (in the absence of chronic hypertension) after 20 weeks of gestation. All abnormal blood pressure readings must be confirmed with two separate readings at least 6 hours apart. (2) Proteinuria of at least 0.3 g/24 h as determined by 24-hour urine collection.

Classically, the presence of three elements was required for the diagnosis of preeclampsia-eclampsia: hypertension, proteinuria, and edema. Clinically, however, there is a great deal of variation in presentation. Edema was difficult to objectively quantify and is no longer a required element. Hypertension occurs most frequently, but proteinuria may be the dominant abnormality at presentation. The absence of one component does not exclude the diagnosis of preeclampsia-eclampsia, and many women with the disorder are asymptomatic early. Diagnosis at an early stage thus requires careful attention to details and a high index of suspicion.

Clinical Findings

Clinically, the severity of preeclampsia-eclampsia can be measured with reference to the six major sites in which it exerts its effects: the central nervous system,

the kidneys, the liver, the hematologic and vascular systems, and the fetal-placental unit. By evaluating each of these areas for the presence of mild to moderate versus severe preeclampsia-eclampsia, the degree of involvement can be assessed, and an appropriate management plan can be formulated that is integrated with gestational age assessment (Table 18–2).

A. PREECLAMPSIA

1. **Mild to moderate**—Precise differentiation between mild and moderate preeclampsia-eclampsia is difficult because the abnormalities that define the disease are quite variable and fail to accurately predict progression to more severe disease. Symptoms are generally minimal or mild. With mild preeclampsia, patients usually have few complaints, and the diastolic blood pressure is less than 90–100 mm Hg. Edema is usually more pronounced with moderate disease, and diastolic blood pressures are in the range of 90–110 mm Hg. The platelet count is over 100,000/μL, antepartum fetal testing is reassuring, central nervous

Table 18–2. Indicators of mild to moderate versus severe preeclampsia-eclampsia.

Site	Indicator	Mild to Moderate	Severe
Central nervous system	Symptoms and signs	Hyperreflexia Headache	Seizures Blurred vision Scotomas Headache Clonus Irritability
Kidney	Proteinuria	0.3–5 g/24 h	> 5 g/24 h or catheterized urine with 4+ protein
	Urine output	> 20–30 mL/h	< 20–30 mL/h
Liver	AST, ALT, LDH	Normal	Elevated LFTs Epigastric pain Ruptured liver
Hematologic	Platelets Hemoglobin	> 100,000/μL Normal range	< 100,000/mL Elevated
Vascular	Blood pressure Retina	< 160/110 mm Hg Arteriolar spasm	> 160/110 mm Hg Retinal hemorrhages
Fetal-placental unit	Growth retardation Oligohydramnios Fetal distress	Absent May be present Absent	Present Present Present

AST, aspartate aminotransferase; ALT, alanine aminotransferase; LDH, lactate dehydrogenase; LFTs, liver function tests.

system irritability is minimal, epigastric pain is not present, and liver enzymes are not elevated.

2. Severe—Symptoms are more dramatic and persistent. The blood pressure is often quite high, with readings over 160/110 mm Hg. Thrombocytopenia (platelet counts < 100,000/μL) may be present and progress to disseminated intravascular coagulation. Severe epigastric pain may be present from hepatic subcapsular hemorrhage with significant stretch or rupture of the liver capsule. The HELLP syndrome (hemolysis, elevated liver enzymes, low platelets) is a form of severe preeclampsia.

B. ECLAMPSIA

The occurrence of seizures defines eclampsia. It is a manifestation of severe central nervous system involvement. The other abnormal findings of severe preeclampsia are also observed with eclampsia.

Differential Diagnosis

Preeclampsia-eclampsia can mimic and be confused with many other diseases, including chronic hypertension, chronic renal disease, primary seizure disorders, gallbladder and pancreatic disease, immune or thrombotic thrombocytopenic purpura, and hemolytic uremic syndrome. It must always be considered a possibility in any pregnant woman beyond 20 weeks of gestation. It is particularly difficult to diagnose when preexisting disease such as hypertension is present. Uric acid values can be quite helpful in such situations, since hyperuricemia is uncommon in pregnancy except with gout, renal failure, or preeclampsia-eclampsia.

Treatment

A. PREECLAMPSIA

Early recognition is the key to treatment. This requires careful attention to the details of prenatal care—especially subtle changes in blood pressure and weight. The objectives are to prolong pregnancy if possible, to allow fetal lung maturity while preventing progression to severe disease and eclampsia. The critical factors are the gestational age of the fetus, fetal pulmonary maturity status, and the severity of maternal disease. Preeclampsia-eclampsia at 36 weeks or more of gestation is managed by delivery regardless of how mild the disease is judged to be. Prior to 36 weeks, severe preeclampsia-eclampsia requires delivery except in unusual circumstances associated with extreme fetal prematurity, in which case prolongation of pregnancy may be attempted. Epigastric pain, thrombocytopenia, and visual disturbances are strong indications for delivery of the fetus. For mild to moderate preeclampsia-eclampsia, bed rest is the cornerstone of therapy. This increases central blood flow to the kidneys, heart, brain, liver, and placenta and may stabilize or even improve the degree of preeclampsia-eclampsia for a period of time.

Bed rest may be attempted at home or in the hospital. Prior to making this decision, the provider should evaluate the six sites of involvement listed in Table 18–2 and make an assessment about the severity of disease.

1. Home management—Home management with bed rest may be attempted for patients with mild preeclampsia and a stable home situation. This requires homemaking assistance, rapid access to the hospital, a reliable patient, and the ability to obtain frequent blood pressure readings. A home health nurse can often provide frequent home visits and assessment.

2. Hospital care—Hospitalization is required for women with moderate or severe preeclampsia or those with unreliable home situations. Regular assessment of blood pressure, reflexes, urine protein, and fetal heart tones and activity are required. A complete blood count, platelet count, and electrolyte panel including liver enzymes should be checked every 1 or 2 days. A 24-hour urine collection for creatinine clearance and total protein should be obtained on admission and repeated as indicated. Sedatives and opioids should be avoided because the fetal central nervous system depressant effects interfere with fetal testing. Magnesium sulfate is not used until the diagnosis of severe preeclampsia-eclampsia is made or until labor occurs.

Fetal evaluation should be obtained as part of the workup. If the patient is being admitted to the hospital, fetal testing must be performed on the same day to make certain that the fetus is safe. This may be done by fetal heart rate testing with nonstress or stress testing or by biophysical profile. A regular schedule of fetal surveillance must then be followed. Daily fetal kick counts can be recorded by the patient herself. Consideration should be given to amniocentesis to evaluate fetal lung maturity status if hospitalization occurs at 30–37 weeks of gestation. If immaturity is present, steroids (betamethasone 12 mg or dexamethasone 16 mg, two doses intramuscularly 12–24 hours apart) can be administered to the mother. Fetuses between 26 and 30 weeks of gestation can be presumed to be immature, and steroids should be given.

The method of delivery is determined by the maternal and fetal status. Cesarean section is reserved for the usual fetal indications.

B. ECLAMPSIA

1. Emergency care—If the patient is convulsing, she is turned on her side to prevent aspiration and to improve blood flow to the placenta. Fluid or food is aspirated from the glottis or trachea. The seizure may be stopped by giving an intravenous bolus of either magnesium sulfate, 4 g, or diazepam, 5–10 mg, over 4 minutes or until the seizure stops. A continuous intravenous infusion of magnesium sulfate is then started at a rate of 2–3 g/h unless the patient is known to have significantly reduced renal function. Magnesium blood levels are then checked every 4–6 hours and the infusion rate adjusted to maintain a therapeutic blood level (4–6 meq/L). Urine output is checked hourly and the patient assessed for signs of possible magnesium toxicity such as loss of deep tendon reflexes or decrease in respiratory rate and depth, which can be reversed with calcium gluconate.

2. General care—The occurrence of eclampsia necessitates delivery once the patient is stabilized. It is important, however, that assessment of the status of the patient and fetus take place first. Continuous fetal monitoring must be performed and blood typed and cross-matched quickly. A urinary catheter is inserted to monitor urine output, and blood is sent for complete blood count, platelets, liver enzymes, uric acid, creatinine or urea nitrogen, and electrolytes. If hypertension is present with diastolic values over 110 mm Hg, antihypertensive medications should be administered to reduce the diastolic blood pressure to 90–100 mm Hg. Lower blood pressures than this may induce placental insufficiency through reduced perfusion. Hydralazine given in 5- to 10-mg increments intravenously every 20 minutes is frequently used to lower blood pressure. Nifedipine, 10 mg sublingually or orally, or labetalol, 10–20 mg intravenously, both every 20 minutes, can also be used.

3. Delivery—Except in unusual circumstances, delivery is mandated once eclampsia has occurred. Vaginal delivery may be attempted if the patient has already been in active labor or the cervix is quite favorable *and* the patient is clinically stable. The rapidity with which delivery must be achieved depends on the fetal and maternal status following the seizure and the availability of laboratory data on the patient. Oxytocin may be used to induce or augment labor. Regional analgesia or anesthesia is acceptable. Cesarean section is used for the usual obstetric indications or when rapid delivery is necessary for maternal or fetal indications.

4. Postpartum—Magnesium sulfate infusion (2–3 g/h) should be continued until preeclampsia-eclampsia has begun to resolve postpartum. This may take 1–7 days. The most reliable indicator of this is the onset of diuresis with urine output of over 100–200 mL/h. When this occurs, magnesium sulfate can be discontinued. Late-onset preeclampsia-eclampsia can occur during the postpartum period. It is usually manifested by either hypertension or seizures. Treatment is the same as prior to delivery—ie, with magnesium sulfate—though other antiseizure medications can be used since the fetus is no longer present.

Chronic Hypertension in Pregnancy. ACOG Practice Bulletin, No. 29, 7/2001 in 2002 Compendium of Selected Publications. ACOG, Washington, DC, 2002:285.

Mattar F et al: Eclampsia. VIII. Risk factors for maternal morbidity. Am J Obstet Gynecol 2000;182:307. [PMID: 10694329]

Roberts JM: Preeclampsia: What we know and what we do not know. Semin Perinatol 2000;24: 24. [PMID: 10709854]

GESTATIONAL TROPHOBLASTIC NEOPLASIA (Hydatidiform Mole & Choriocarcinoma)

Gestational trophoblastic neoplasia is a spectrum of disease that includes hydatidiform mole, invasive mole, and choriocarcinoma. Partial moles generally show evidence of an embryo or gestational sac; are polypoid, slower-growing, and less symptomatic; and often present clinically as a missed abortion. Partial moles tend to follow a benign course, while complete moles have a greater tendency to become choriocarcinomas.

The highest rates of gestational trophoblastic neoplasia occur in some developing countries, with rates of 1:125 pregnancies in certain areas of Asia. In the USA, the frequency is 1:1500 pregnancies. Risk factors include low socioeconomic status, a history of mole, and age below 18 or above 40. Approximately 10% of women require further treatment after evacuation of the mole; 5% develop choriocarcinoma.

Clinical Findings

A. SYMPTOMS AND SIGNS

Excessive nausea and vomiting occur in over one-third of patients with hydatidiform mole. Uterine bleeding, beginning at 6–8 weeks, is observed in virtually all instances and is indicative of threatened or incomplete abortion. In about one-fifth of cases, the uterus is larger than would be expected in a normal pregnancy of the same duration. Intact or collapsed vesicles may be passed through the vagina. These grape-like clusters of enlarged villi are diagnostic. Bilaterally enlarged cystic ovaries are sometimes palpable. They are the result of ovarian hyperstimulation due to excess of hCG.

Preeclampsia-eclampsia, frequently of the fulminating type, may develop during the second trimester of pregnancy, but this is unusual.

Choriocarcinoma may be manifested by continued or recurrent uterine bleeding after evacuation of a mole or following delivery, abortion, or ectopic pregnancy. The presence of an ulcerative vaginal tumor, pelvic mass, or evidence of distant metastatic tumor may be the presenting observation. The diagnosis is established by pathologic examination of curettings or by biopsy.

B. LABORATORY FINDINGS

A serum hCG β-subunit value above 40,000 mU/mL or a urinary hCG value in excess of 100,000 units/24 h increases the likelihood of hydatidiform mole, though such values are occasionally seen with a normal pregnancy (eg, in multiple gestation).

C. IMAGING

Ultrasound has virtually replaced all other means of preoperative diagnosis of hydatidiform mole. The multiple echoes indicating edematous villi within the enlarged uterus and the absence of a fetus and placenta are pathognomonic. A preoperative chest film is indicated to rule out pulmonary metastases of trophoblast.

Treatment

A. Specific (Surgical) Measures

The uterus should be emptied as soon as the diagnosis of hydatidiform mole is established, preferably by suction. Ovarian cysts should not be resected nor ovaries removed; spontaneous regression of theca lutein cysts will occur with elimination of the mole.

If malignant tissue is discovered at surgery or during the follow-up examination, chemotherapy is indicated.

Thyrotoxicosis indistinguishable clinically from that of thyroid origin may occur. While hCG usually has minimal TSH-like activity, the very high hCG levels associated with moles result in the release of T_3 and T_4 and cause hyperthyroidism. Patients thyrotoxic on this basis should be stabilized with beta-blockers prior to induction of anesthesia for their surgical evacuation. Surgical removal of the mole promptly corrects the thyroid overactivity.

B. Follow-Up Measures

Effective contraception (preferably birth control pills) should be prescribed. Weekly quantitative hCG level measurements are initially required. Following successful surgical evacuation, moles show a progressive decline in hCG. After two negative weekly tests (< 5 mU/mL), the interval may be increased to monthly for 6 months and then to every 2 months for a total of 1 year. If levels plateau or begin to rise, the patient should be evaluated by repeat chest film and D&C before the initiation of chemotherapy.

C. Antitumor Chemotherapy:

For low-risk patients with a good prognosis, methotrexate, 0.4 mg/kg intramuscularly over a 5-day period, or dactinomycin, 10–12 μg/kg/d intravenously over a 5-day period, is used (see Table 40–3). Patients with a poor prognosis should be referred to a cancer center, where multiple-agent chemotherapy probably will be given. The side effects—anorexia, nausea and vomiting, stomatitis, rash, diarrhea, and bone marrow depression—usually are reversible in about 3 weeks and can be ameliorated by the administration of leucovorin (0.1 mg/kg). Repeated courses of methotrexate 2 weeks apart generally are required to destroy the trophoblast and maintain a zero chorionic gonadotropin titer, as indicated by β-hCG determination.

D. Supportive Measures

Oral contraceptives (if acceptable) or another reliable birth control method should be prescribed to avoid the hazard and confusion of elevated hCG from a new pregnancy. hCG levels should be negative for a year before pregnancy is again attempted. In the pregnancy following a mole, the hCG level should be checked 6 weeks postpartum.

Prognosis

Five years' survival after courses of chemotherapy, even when metastases have been demonstrated, can be expected in at least 85% of cases of choriocarcinoma.

Newlands ES et al: Recent advances in gestational trophoblastic disease. Hematol Oncol Clin North Am 1999;13:225. [PMID: 10080078]

Seckl MJ et al: Choriocarcinoma and partial hydatidiform moles. Lancet 2000;356:36. [PMID: 10892763]

THIRD-TRIMESTER BLEEDING

Five to 10 percent of women have vaginal bleeding in late pregnancy. The clinician must distinguish between placental causes (placenta previa, placental abruption, vasa previa) and nonplacental causes (infection, disorders of the lower genital tract, systemic disease). The approach to bleeding in late pregnancy should be conservative and expectant unless fetal distress or risk of maternal hemorrhage occurs.

The patient should be hospitalized and placed at bed rest with continuous fetal monitoring. A complete blood count (including platelets) should be obtained and two to four units of blood typed and crossmatched. Coagulation studies should be ordered as clinically indicated. Ultrasound examination should be performed to determine placental location. Speculum and digital pelvic examinations are done only after ultrasound study has ruled out placenta previa. Continuous electronic fetal monitoring is required to exclude fetal distress. While uterine contractions, pain, or tenderness often indicate associated abruptio placentae, an ultrasound negative for retroplacental clot does not exclude it.

If the patient is at less than 36 weeks of gestation, continued hospitalization and bed rest may be necessary, especially with placenta previa during the initial 7–10 days following vaginal bleeding. If the patient has close proximity to the hospital and immediate access, can be on strict bed rest, and has complete resolution of bleeding and uterine contractions, home management may be considered. She must be well instructed and counseled regarding the risks. Patients with vaginal bleeding at less than 36 weeks of gestation should also be considered for amniocentesis to test for fetal lung maturity. Steroid therapy (betamethasone 12 mg intramuscularly, two doses 12–24 hours apart) is indicated if fetal lung immaturity is present.

Towers CV et al: Is tocolysis safe in the management of third-trimester bleeding? Am J Obstet Gynecol 1999;180:1572. [PMID: 10368505]

MEDICAL CONDITIONS COMPLICATING PREGNANCY

Anemia

Plasma volume increases 50% during pregnancy, while red cell volume increases 25%, causing lower hemoglobin and hematocrit values, which are maximally changed around the 24th to 28th weeks. Anemia in pregnancy is often defined as a hemoglobin measurement below 10 g/dL or hematocrit below 30%. Anemia is very common in pregnancy, causing fatigue, anorexia, dyspnea, and edema. Prevention through optimal nutrition and iron and folic acid supplementation is desirable.

A. Iron Deficiency Anemia

Many women enter pregnancy with low iron stores resulting from heavy menstrual periods, previous pregnancies, breast feeding, or poor nutrition. It is difficult to meet the increased requirement for iron through diet, and anemia often develops unless iron supplements are given. Red cells may not become hypochromic and microcytic until the hematocrit has fallen significantly. When this occurs, a serum iron level below 40 μg/dL and a transferrin saturation less than 10% suggest iron deficiency anemia (see Chapter 13). Treatment consists of a diet containing iron-rich foods and 60 mg of elemental iron (eg, 300 mg of ferrous sulfate) three times a day with meals. Iron is best absorbed if taken with a source of vitamin C (raw fruits and vegetables, lightly cooked greens). All pregnant women should take daily iron supplements.

B. Folic Acid Deficiency Anemia

Folic acid deficiency anemia is the main cause of macrocytic anemia in pregnancy, since vitamin B_{12} deficiency anemia is rare in the childbearing years. The daily requirement of folic acid doubles from 0.4 mg to 0.8 mg in pregnancy. Twin pregnancies, infections, malabsorption, and use of anticonvulsant drugs such as phenytoin can precipitate folic acid deficiency. The anemia may first be seen in the puerperium owing to the increased need for folate during lactation.

The diagnosis is made by finding macrocytic red cells and hypersegmented neutrophils in a blood smear (see Chapter 13). However, blood smears in pregnancy may be difficult to interpret, since they frequently show iron deficiency changes as well. Because the deficiency is hard to diagnose and folate intake is inadequate in some socioeconomic groups, 0.8–1 mg of folic acid is given as a supplement in pregnancy; the dose in established deficiency is 1–5 mg/d.

Good sources of folate in food are leafy green vegetables, orange juice, peanuts, and beans. Cooking and storage of food destroy folic acid. Strict vegetarians who eat no eggs or milk products should take vitamin B_{12} supplements during pregnancy and lactation.

C. Sickle Cell Anemia

Women with sickle cell anemia are subject to serious complications in pregnancy. The anemia becomes more severe, and crises may occur more frequently. Complications include infections, bone pain, pulmonary infarction, congestive heart failure, and preeclampsia. There is an increased rate of spontaneous abortion and higher maternal and perinatal mortality rates. Intensive medical treatment may improve the outcome for mother and fetus. Frequent indicated transfusions of packed cells or leukocyte-poor washed red cells lower the level of hemoglobin S and elevate the level of hemoglobin A; this minimizes the severity of anemia and the risk of sickle cell crises.

Genetic counseling should be offered to patients with sickle cell disease or sickle trait. They may wish to undergo first-trimester chorionic villus biopsy or second-trimester amniocentesis to determine whether the abnormality has been passed on to the fetus. IUDs and oral contraceptives are relatively contraindicated, but progestin-only contraceptives may be used. Women with sickle cell trait alone usually have an uncomplicated gestation except for an increased risk of urinary tract infection. Sickle cell-hemoglobin C disease in pregnancy is similar to sickle cell anemia and is treated similarly.

Allen LH: Anemia and iron deficiency: Effects on pregnancy outcome. Am J Clin Nutr 2000;71(5 Suppl):1280S. [PMID: 10799402]

Mason E et al: Medical problems during pregnancy. Med Clin North Am 1998;82:249. [PMID: 9531925]

Lupus Anticoagulant-Anticardiolipin-Antiphospholipid Antibody Syndrome

The presence of antibodies to phospholipids and a variety of clinical symptoms, including vascular thromboses, thrombocytopenia, and recurrent pregnancy loss, characterize the lupus anticoagulant-anticardiolipin-antiphospholipid antibody syndrome. Many of these patients have SLE-like symptoms but do not meet specific diagnostic criteria for that disease. The lupus anticoagulant and anticardiolipin antibody may occur in these patients, and both may cause arterial and venous thromboses. Detection of these antiphospholipid antibodies may require a combination of laboratory tests. The lupus anticoagulant will prolong both the partial thromboplastin time (PTT) and the Russell viper venom time. The latter is a more sensitive predictor of disease. Such patients should also be screened for the presence of the factor V Leiden mutation. Anticardiolipin antibody may be detected with ELISA testing. Either antibody may cause false-positive serologic tests for syphilis.

This syndrome may require treatment with immunosuppressive or anticoagulant medications. In a small number of patients with recurrent pregnancy loss and a diagnosis of lupus anticoagulant syndrome, improved outcomes have been reported following treatment with either (1) daily high-dose prednisone (40 mg/d) and low-dose aspirin (81 mg) or (2) heparin anticoagulation (8000–20,000 units in two or three doses daily) and low-dose aspirin begun before or early in pregnancy and continued until the postpartum period. Although complications have been reported with both regimens, current opinion seems to favor the heparin and low-dose aspirin combination. The addition of monthly infusions of IGIV to this regimen did not improve outcomes in such patients.

Backos M et al: Pregnancy complications in women with recurrent miscarriage associated with antiphospholipid antibodies treated with low dose aspirin and heparin. Br J Obstet Gynecol 1999;106:102. [PMID: 10426674]

Branch DW et al: A multi-center placebo-controlled pilot study of intravenous immune globulin treatment of antiphospholipid syndrome during pregnancy, The Pregnancy Loss Study Group. Am J Obstet Gynecol 2000;182(1 Part 1): 122. [PMID: 10649166]

Asthma

The effect of pregnancy on asthma is unpredictable. About 50% of patients have no change, 25% improve, and 25% get worse. Management of acute and chronic asthma during pregnancy does not differ significantly from that of nonpregnant women. The goal is to maintain maternal PO_2 > 80 mm Hg to sustain normal fetal oxygenation (see Chapter 9).

Alexander S et al: Perinatal outcomes in women with asthma during pregnancy. Obstet Gynecol 1998;92:435. [PMID: 9721785] (A retrospective cohort study included 817 asthmatic women and 13,709 nonasthmatic women.)

The use of newer asthma and allergy medications during pregnancy. ACOG and ACAAI. Ann Allergy Asthma Immunol 2000;84:475. [PMID: 10830999]

AIDS During Pregnancy

Heterosexual acquisition (40%) and injecting drug use (41%) are the principal modes of HIV infection in women. In 15%, no risk factor is reported or identified. Asymptomatic infection is associated with a normal pregnancy rate and no increased risk of adverse pregnancy outcomes. There is no evidence that pregnancy causes AIDS progression.

Although some fetuses appear to acquire HIV infection antenatally by transplacental transmission, approximately two-thirds are infected close to or during the time of delivery. Zidovudine given to the mother antenatally (500 mg/d orally) and during labor (1 mg/kg/h intravenously) and then to the infant (2 mg/kg orally four times daily) for the first 6 weeks of life reduces the transmission rate from 25% to 8%. Pregnancy does not preclude the use of combinations of highly active antiretroviral therapy (HAART). HIV-positive pregnant women should be assessed by CD4 count, plasma RNA levels, and prior or current antiretroviral use. In general, pregnant HIV-positive women should receive at least zidovudine but also HAART as appropriate for their HIV disease status after counseling regarding the potential impact of therapy on the fetus and infant after delivery. The use of prophylactic elective cesarean section before the onset of labor or rupture of the membranes to prevent vertical transmission of HIV infection from mother to fetus has been shown to reduce the transmission rate to 2% in infants of mothers taking zidovudine. There is limited information on the impact of elective cesarean section on transmission rates in infants of mothers on HAART or with viral loads less than 1000 copies/mL. HIV-infected women should be advised not to breast-feed their infants.

ACOG committee opinion. Scheduled cesarean delivery and the prevention of vertical transmission of HIV infection. Number 219, August 1999. Committee on Obstetric Practice, American College of Obstetricians and Gynecologists. Int J Gynaecol Obstet 1999;66:305. [PMID: 10580685]

The mode of delivery and the risk of vertical transmission of human immunodeficiency virus type 1—a meta-analysis of 15 prospective cohort studies. The International Perinatal HIV Group. N Engl J Med 1999;340:977. [PMID: 10099139]

Public Health Service Task Force Recommendations for Use of Antiretroviral Drugs in Pregnant HIV-1 Infected Women for Maternal Health and Interventions to Reduce Perinatal HIV-1 Transmission in the United States (http://www.hivatis.org). (Provides antiretroviral treatment guidelines; perinatal prophylaxis guidelines.)

Diabetes Mellitus

Pregnancy is associated with increased tissue resistance to insulin, resulting in increased levels of blood insulin as well as glucose and triglycerides. These changes are due to placental lactogen and elevated circulating estrogens and progesterone. Although pregnancy does not appear to alter the long-term consequences of diabetes, retinopathy and nephropathy may first appear or become worse during pregnancy. The White classification of diabetes has been largely abandoned. The emphasis in classifying diabetes mellitus has shifted more to etiology. Type 1 diabetics often express particular HLA haplotypes and have anti-islet cell antibodies contributing to their insulin dependence and risk of ketoacidosis. Type 2 diabetics have minimal to no risk of ketoacidosis even though they may require insulin to control their blood glucose levels. Debate continues over whether gestational diabetics are women whose glucose intolerance is solely a function of their pregnant compared with their nonpregnant state. Alternatively, pregnancy may merely serve to unmask an underlying propensity for glucose intolerance, which will be evident even in the nonpregnant state at some time in the future if not in the immediate postpartum period. However, goals for glycemic control during pregnancy are the same whether the diagnosis is made before or during the pregnancy.

Prepregnancy counseling and evaluation of diabetic women should include a complete chemistry panel, HbA_{1c} determination, 24-hour urine collection for total protein and creatinine clearance, funduscopic examination, and an ECG. Any medical problems should be addressed, and HbA_{1c} levels of less than 8% should be achieved before pregnancy. Euglycemia should be established before conception and maintained during pregnancy with daily home glucose monitoring by the patient. A well-planned dietary program is a key component, with an intake of 1800–2200 kcal/d divided into three meals and three snacks. Insulin is given subcutaneously in a split-dose regimen with frequent dosage adjustments. Patients taking oral agents prior to pregnancy should be switched to insulin. However, limited information suggests that agents such as glyburide may be safe and effective in pregnancy. The use of continuous insulin pump therapy has been found to be very useful during pregnancy in women with type 1 diabetes mellitus.

Congenital anomalies result from hyperglycemia during the first 4–8 weeks of pregnancy. They occur in 4–10% of diabetic pregnancies (two to three times the rate in nondiabetic pregnancies). Euglycemia in the early weeks of pregnancy, when organogenesis is occurring, reduces the rate of anomalies to near-normal levels. Even so, because few women with diabetes begin a rigorous program to achieve euglycemia until well after they have become pregnant, congenital anomalies are the principal cause of perinatal fetal deaths in diabetic pregnancies. All women with diabetes should receive counseling about pregnancy and, when the decision has been made to start a family, should receive prepregnancy management by physicians experienced in diabetic pregnancies.

Fasting and preprandial glucose values are lower during pregnancy in both diabetic and nondiabetic women. Euglycemia is considered to be 60–80 mg/dL while fasting and 30–45 minutes before meals and < 120 mg/dL 2 hours after meals. This is the target for good diabetic control during pregnancy. Glycated hemoglobin levels help determine the quality of glucose control both before and during pregnancy.

While perinatal problems for mother and baby are decreased by fastidious diabetic control, the incidence of hydramnios, preeclampsia-eclampsia, infections, and prematurity is increased even in carefully managed diabetic pregnancies. Diabetes is an inherently unstable disease characterized by fluctuations of blood glucose levels, particularly late in pregnancy. The risk of fetal demise in the third trimester (stillbirth) and neonatal death increases with the level of hyperglycemia. Consequently, pregnant women with diabetes must receive regular antepartum fetal testing (nonstress testing, contraction stress testing, biophysical profile) during the third trimester. The timing of delivery is dictated by the quality of diabetic control, the presence or absence of medical complications, and fetal status. The goal is to reach 39 weeks (38 completed weeks) and then proceed with delivery. Confirmation of lung maturity is necessary only for delivery prior to 39 weeks. Cesarean sections are performed for obstetric indications.

Because 15% of patients with gestational diabetes require insulin during pregnancy and because the infants of gestational diabetics have some risks similar to those of infants of diabetic mothers (particularly macrosomia), screening of women for glucose intolerance has been recommended between the 24th and 28th weeks of pregnancy (Table 18–3). Patients with gestational diabetes should be evaluated 6–8 weeks postpartum by a 2-hour oral glucose tolerance test (75 g glucose load).

Diabetes and Pregnancy. ACOG Technical Bulletin No. 200, 2001. Compendium of Selected Publications, American College of Obstetricians and Gynecologists, Dec 2000:393.

Gabbe SG et al: Benefits, risks, costs and patient satisfaction associated with insulin pump therapy for the pregnancy complicated by type 1 diabetes mellitus. Am J Obstet Gynecol 2000;182:1283. [PMID: 10871440]

Langer O et al: A comparison of glyburide and insulin in women with gestational diabetes mellitus. N Engl J Med 2000; 343:1134. [PMID:11036118]

Metzger BE et al: Summary and recommendations of the Fourth International Workshop-Conference on Gestational Diabetes Mellitus. The Organizing Committee. Diabetes Care 1998;21(Suppl 2):B161. [PMID: 9704245]

Table 18–3. Screening and diagnostic criteria for gestational diabetes mellitus.

Screening for gestational diabetes mellitus
1. 50 g oral glucose load, administered between the 24th and 28th weeks, without regard to time of day or time of last meal. Recent recommendations suggest that universal blood glucose screening is appropriate for patients who are of Hispanic, African, Native American, South or East Asian, Pacific Island, or Indigenous Australian ancestry. Other patients who have no known diabetes in first-degree relatives, are under 25 years of age, have normal weight before pregnancy, and have no history of abnormal glucose metabolism or poor obstetric outcome do not require routine screening.
2. Venous plasma glucose measure 1 hour later.
3. Value of 130 mg/dL (7.2 mmol/L) or above in venous plasma indicates the need for a full diagnostic glucose tolerance test.

Diagnosis of gestational diabetes mellitus
1. 100 g oral glucose load, administered in the morning after overnight fast lasting at least 8 hours but not more than 14 hours, and following at least 3 days of unrestricted diet (> 150 g carbohydrate) and physical activity.
2. Venous plasma glucose is measured fasting and at 1, 2, and 3 hours. Subject should remain seated and should not smoke throughout the test.
3. Two or more of the following venous plasma concentrations must be equaled or exceeded for a diagnosis of gestational diabetes: fasting, 95 mg/dL (5.3 mmol/L); 1 hour, 180 mg/dL (10 mmol/L); 2 hours, 155 mg/dL (8.6 mmol/L); 3 hours, 140 mg/dL (7.8 mmol/L).

Heart Disease

Overall, 5% of maternal deaths are due to heart disease. Most heart disease complicating pregnancy in the USA is congenital heart disease. Normal pregnancy causes a faster pulse, an increase of cardiac output of more than 30%, and a rise in plasma volume greater than red cell mass with relative hemodilution. Vital capacity and oxygen consumption rise only slightly.

For practical purposes, the functional capacity of the heart is the best single measurement of cardiopulmonary status.

FUNCTIONAL CARDIAC ASSESSMENT

Class I — Ordinary physical activity causes no discomfort (perinatal mortality rate about 5%).

Class II — Ordinary activity causes discomfort and slight disability (perinatal mortality rate 10–15%).

Class III — Less than ordinary activity causes discomfort or disability; patient is barely compensated (perinatal mortality rate about 35%).

Class IV — Patient decompensated; any physical activity causes acute distress (perinatal mortality rate over 50%).

In general, patients with class I or class II functional disability (80% of pregnant women with heart disease) do well obstetrically, with four-fifths of maternal deaths due to heart disease occurring in women with class III or class IV disability. Congestive failure is the usual cause of death. Most deaths occur in the early puerperium. Pregnancy is contraindicated in Eisenmenger's complex, in primary pulmonary hypertension, in severe mitral stenosis with secondary pulmonary hypertension, and in Marfan's syndrome, in which the aorta is prone to dissection and rupture. In addition, pregnancy is poorly tolerated in patients with aortic stenosis, aortic coarctation, tetralogy of Fallot, and active rheumatic carditis.

Therapeutic abortion and elective sterilization should be offered to patients with significant cardiac disease. Cesarean section should be performed only for obstetric indications. Women with valvular heart disease, mitral valve prolapse associated with mitral insufficiency, or idiopathic hypertrophic subaortic stenosis should receive appropriate antibiotic prophylaxis against infective endocarditis during labor and delivery or termination of pregnancy.

Mendelson M: Congenital cardiac disease and pregnancy. Clin Perinatol 1997;24:467. [PMID: 9209813]

Sadler L et al: Pregnancy outcomes and cardiac complications in women with mechanical bioprosthetic and homograft valves. Br J Obstet Gynaecol 2000;107:245. [PMID: 10688509]

Peripartum Cardiomyopathy

Cardiac failure that develops during pregnancy or during the first 6 months postpartum in a woman without a history of heart disease and with no cause for heart failure other than pregnancy is termed peripartum cardiomyopathy. The incidence varies from 1:4000 to 1:1000. It is higher in Africa. It occurs more often in older women, those with twins, and in patients with pregnancy-induced hypertension. The cause of peripartum cardiomyopathy is unknown. In patients who continue to have symptoms and signs of disease for more than 6 months postpartum, the mortality rate is high, and subsequent pregnancy is especially dangerous.

Symptoms of peripartum cardiomyopathy are those of congestive heart failure. An ECG may reveal tachycardia and atrial or ventricular arrhythmias. Death may occur as a result of arrhythmia or embolism. Autopsy usually reveals an enlarged, dilated heart, and mural thrombi (the source of pulmonary and systemic emboli) are often found.

The treatment of peripartum cardiomyopathy is that of congestive cardiomyopathy (see Chapter 10). Patients with persistent cardiomegaly or mural thrombi shown by echocardiography require anticoagulant therapy. The long-term prognosis in these patients depends on whether cardiomegaly resolves within 6 months after the onset of symptoms. If it does not resolve, the 5-year mortality rate is 35%. If it does resolve, the mortality rate is still about 15%. If cardiomegaly does not resolve and another pregnancy intervenes, cardiomyopathy recurs in 50% of cases, with an almost 100% mortality rate.

Pearson GD et al: Peripartum cardiomyopathy: National Heart Lung and Blood Institute and Office of Rare Disease (National Institutes of Health) workshop recommendations and review. JAMA 2000;283:1183. [PMID: 10703781]

Herpes Genitalis
(See also Chapter 6.)

Infection of the lower genital tract by herpes simplex virus type 2 (HSV-2) is a common sexually transmitted disease of potential seriousness to pregnant women and their newborn infants. Although up to 20% of women in an obstetric practice may have antibodies to HSV-2, a history of the infection is unreliable and the incidence of neonatal infection is low (1:20,000–1:3000 live births). Most infected neonates are born to women with no symptoms, signs, or history of infection.

Women who have had *primary* herpes infection late in pregnancy are at high risk of shedding virus at delivery. Some authors suggest use of prophylactic acyclovir, 400 mg orally twice daily, to decrease the likelihood of active lesions at the time of labor and delivery.

Women with a history of *recurrent* genital herpes have a neonatal attack rate of 5% and should be followed by clinical observation and culture of any suspicious lesions. Since asymptomatic viral shedding is not predictable by antepartum cultures, current recommendations do not include routine cultures in individuals with a history of herpes without active disease. However, when labor begins, vulvar and cervical inspection and cultures should be performed, with prompt treatment of a newborn after a positive culture.

For treatment, see Chapter 32. The use of acyclovir in pregnancy is acceptable when there is significant fetal or neonatal risk.

Cesarean section is indicated at the time of labor if there are prodromal symptoms, active genital lesions, or a positive cervical culture obtained within the preceding week.

ACOG Practice Bulletin. Management of herpes in pregnancy. Number 8 October 1999, Clinical management guidelines for obstetrician-gynecologists. Int J Gynaecol Obstet 2000; 68:165. [PMID: 10717827]

Brocklehurst P et al: A randomised placebo controlled trial of suppressive acyclovir in late pregnancy in women with recurrent genital herpes infection. Br J Obstet Gynaecol 1998; 105:275. [PMID: 9532986]

Brown ZA et al: The acquisition of herpes simplex virus during pregnancy. N Engl J Med 1997;337:509. [PMID: 9262493]

Hensleigh PA et al: Genital herpes during pregnancy: Inability to distinguish primary and recurrent infections clinically. Obstet Gynecol 1997;89:891. [PMID: 9170460]

Hypertensive Disease

Hypertensive disease in women of childbearing age is usually essential hypertension, but secondary causes should be considered: coarctation of the aorta, pheochromocytoma, hyperaldosteronism, and renovascular and renal hypertension.

Preeclampsia is superimposed on 20% of pregnancies in hypertensive women and appears earlier, is more severe, and is more often associated with intrauterine growth retardation. It may be difficult to determine whether or not hypertension in a pregnant woman precedes or derives from the pregnancy if she is not examined until after the 20th week. Serum uric acid can help differentiate, since it is elevated with preeclampsia and normal in chronic hypertension unless the patient is receiving diuretics. If hypertension persists for 6–8 weeks postpartum, essential hypertension is likely.

Pregnant women with chronic hypertension require medication only if the diastolic pressure is sustained at or above 100 mm Hg. For initiation of treatment, methyldopa is still the drug of choice in a dosage of 250 mg orally twice daily and increase in divided doses as needed to as much as 3 g daily. The goal is to keep the diastolic pressure between 80 and 100 mm Hg.

If a hypertensive woman is being managed successfully by medical treatment when she registers for antenatal care, one may generally continue the antihypertensive medication. Diuretics may be continued in pregnancy. ACE inhibitors should be replaced with a drug of another class because of reports of fetal and neonatal renal failure with these compounds.

Use of antihypertensive medications in preeclampsia remains controversial. This should be attempted only with significant fetal prematurity, absence of fetal compromise, and close supervision of the patient.

Therapeutic abortion may be indicated in cases of severe hypertension during pregnancy. If pregnancy is allowed to continue, the risk to the fetus must be assessed periodically in anticipation of early delivery. An early second-trimester ultrasound examination will confirm the duration of pregnancy, and follow-up examinations after 28 weeks will evaluate intrauterine growth retardation.

Rey E et al: Report of the Canadian Hypertension Society Consensus Conference 3. Pharmacologic treatment of hypertensive disorders in pregnancy. Can Med Assoc J 1997; 157:1245. [PMID: 9361646]

Maternal Hepatitis B & C Carrier State

There are an estimated 200 million chronic carriers of hepatitis B virus worldwide. Among these people there is an increased incidence of chronic active hepatitis, cirrhosis, and hepatocellular carcinoma. The frequency of the hepatitis B carrier state varies from 1% in the USA and Western Europe to 35% in parts of Africa and Asia. All pregnant women should be screened for hepatitis B surface antigen (HBsAg). Transmission of the virus to the baby after delivery is likely if both surface antigen and e antigen are positive. Vertical transmission can be blocked by the immediate postdelivery administration to the newborn of 0.5 mL of hepatitis B immunoglobulin and hepatitis B vaccine intramuscularly. The vaccine dose is repeated at 1 and 6 months of age.

Hepatitis C virus infection is the most common chronic blood-borne infection in the United States. Risk factors for transmission include blood transfusion, injecting drug use, employment in patient care or clinical laboratory work, exposure to a sex partner or household member who has had a history of hepatitis, exposure to multiple sex partners, and low socioeconomic level. The average rate of HCV infection among infants born to HCV-positive, HIV-negative women is 5–6%. However, the average infection rate increases to 14% when mothers are coinfected with HCV and HIV. The principal factor associated with transmission is the presence of HCV RNA in the mother at the time of birth.

Recommendations for prevention and control of hepatitis C virus (HCV) infection and HCV-related chronic disease. MMWR Morb Mortal Wkly Rep 1998;47(RR-19):1. [PMID: 9790221]

Thomas DL et al: Perinatal transmission of hepatitis C virus from human immunodeficiency virus type 1-infected mothers. Women and Infants Transmission Study. J Infect Dis 1998; 177:1480. [PMID: 9607823]

Acute Fatty Liver of Pregnancy

Acute fatty liver of pregnancy is a disorder limited to the gravid state. It occurs in the third trimester of pregnancy and involves acute hepatic failure. The mortality rate has been reported to be as high as 85%, but with improved recognition and immediate delivery, the mortality range is 20–30%. The disorder is usually seen after the 35th week of gestation and is more common in primigravidas and those with twins. The incidence is about 1:14,000 deliveries.

The cause of acute fatty liver of pregnancy is not known. Pathologic findings are unique to the disorder, with fatty engorgement of hepatocytes. Clinical onset is gradual, with flu-like symptoms that progress to the development of abdominal pain, jaundice, encephalopathy, disseminated intravascular coagulation, and death. On examination, the patient shows signs of hepatic failure.

Laboratory findings show marked elevation of alkaline phosphatase but only moderate elevations of ALT and AST. Prothrombin time and bilirubin are also elevated. The white blood cell count is elevated, and the platelet count is depressed. Hypoglycemia may be extreme.

The differential diagnosis is that of fulminant hepatitis. However, liver aminotransferases for fulminant hepatitis are higher (> 1000 units/mL) than those for acute fatty liver of pregnancy (usually < 500 units/ mL). It is also important to review the appropriate history and perform the appropriate tests for toxins that cause liver failure. Preeclampsia may involve the liver but typically does not cause jaundice. The elevations in liver function tests in patients with preeclampsia usually do not reach the levels seen in patients with acute fatty liver of pregnancy.

Diagnosis of acute fatty liver of pregnancy mandates immediate delivery. Supportive care during labor includes administration of glucose, platelets, and fresh frozen plasma as needed. Vaginal delivery is preferred. Resolution of encephalopathy occurs over days, and supportive care with a low-protein diet is needed.

Recurrence rates for this liver disorder are unclear. Most authorities advise against subsequent pregnancy, but there have been reported cases of successful outcomes in later pregnancies.

Castro MA et al: Reversible peripartum liver failure: a new perspective on the diagnosis, treatment, and cause of acute fatty liver of pregnancy, based on 28 consecutive cases. Am J Obstet Gynecol 1999;181:389. [PMID: 10454689]

Seizure Disorders

Epileptic women contemplating pregnancy who have not had a seizure for 5 years should consider a pre-pregnancy trial of withdrawal from treatment. Those with recurrent epilepsy should use a single drug with blood level monitoring. Trimethadione and valproate are contraindicated during pregnancy; phenytoin and carbamazepine may be teratogenic in the first trimester and should not be used unless absolutely necessary. Newer antiepilepsy drugs have recently been introduced, but there is little information available on their safety in pregnancy and they should generally be avoided.

Phenobarbital is considered the drug of choice. Serum levels should be measured in each trimester and dosage adjustments made to keep serum levels in the low normal therapeutic range. Pregnant women taking phenobarbital and phenytoin should receive vitamin supplements, including folic acid and vitamin D, throughout pregnancy. Vitamin K, 10–20 mg/d, is administered during the last month to help prevent bleeding problems in the newborn, who is at risk of bleeding tendencies due to decreased levels of clotting factors. Such infants should receive an injection of vitamin K_1, 1 mg subcutaneously immediately after delivery, and should have clotting studies 2–4 hours later. Breast feeding is not contraindicated for infants of mothers taking antiseizure medications.

ACOG educational bulletin. Seizure disorders in pregnancy. Number 231, December 1996. Committee on Educational Bulletins of the American College of Obstetricians and Gynecologists. Int J Gynaecol Obstet 1997;56:279. [PMID: 9127164]

Syphilis, Gonorrhea, & *Chlamydia trachomatis* Infection (See also Chapters 33 and 34.)

These sexually transmitted diseases have significant consequences for mother and child. Untreated syphilis in pregnancy will cause late abortion, stillbirth, transplacental infection, and congenital syphilis. Gonorrhea will produce large-joint arthritis by hematogenous spread as well as ophthalmia neonatorum. Maternal chlamydial infections are largely asymptomatic but are manifested in the newborn by inclusion conjunctivitis and, at age 2–4 months, by pneumonia. The diagnosis of each can be reliably made by appropriate laboratory tests, which should be included in all prenatal care. The sexual partners of women with sexually transmitted diseases should be identified and treated also if that can be done.

Gene M et al: Syphilis in pregnancy. Sex Transm Infect 2000; 76:73. [PMID: 10858706]

Group B Streptococcal Infection

Group B streptococci frequently colonize the lower female genital tract, with an asymptomatic carriage rate in pregnancy of 5–30%. This rate depends on maternal age, gravidity, and geographic variation. Vaginal carriage is asymptomatic and intermittent, with spontaneous clearing in approximately 30% and recolonization in about 10% of women. Adverse perinatal outcomes associated with group B streptococcal colonization include urinary tract infection, intrauterine infection, premature rupture of membranes, preterm delivery, and postpartum endometritis.

Women with postpartum endometritis due to infection with group B streptococci, especially after cesarean section, develop fever, tachycardia, and abdominal distention, usually within 24 hours after delivery. Approximately 35% of these women are bacteremic.

Group B streptococcal infection is a common cause of neonatal sepsis. Transmission rates are high, yet the rate of neonatal sepsis is surprisingly low at less than 4:1000 live births. Unfortunately, the mortality rate associated with early-onset disease can be as high as 50% in premature infants and approaches 25% even in those at term. Moreover, these infections can contribute markedly to chronic morbidity, including mental retardation and neurologic disabilities. Late-onset disease develops through contact with hospital nursery personnel. Up to 45% of these health care workers can carry the bacteria on their skin and transmit the infection to newborns.

CDC recommendations for screening for and prophylaxis of group B streptococcal colonization are set forth in this chapter in the section on Tests and Procedures.

Brozanski BS et al: Effect of a screening-based prevention policy on prevalence of early-onset group B streptococcal sepsis. Obstet Gynecol 2000;95:496. [PMID: 10725479]

Varicella

Commonly known as chickenpox, varicella-zoster virus (VZV) infection has a fairly benign course when incurred during childhood but may result in serious illness in adults, particularly during pregnancy. Infection results in lifelong immunity. Approximately 95% of women born in the USA have VZV antibodies by the time they reach reproductive age. The incidence of VZV infection during pregnancy has been reported as up to 7:10,000.

The incubation period for this infection is 10–20 days. A primary infection follows and is characterized by a flu-like syndrome with malaise, fever, and development of a pruritic maculopapular rash on the trunk which becomes vesicular and then crusts. Pregnant women are prone to the development of VZV pneumonia, often a fulminant infection sometimes requiring respiratory support. After primary infection, the virus becomes latent, ascending to dorsal root ganglia. Subsequent reactivation can occur as zoster, often under circumstances of immunocompromise, though this is rare during pregnancy.

Two types of fetal infection have been documented. The first is congenital VZV syndrome, which typically occurs in 2–3% of fetuses exposed to primary VZV infection during the first trimester. Anomalies include limb and digit abnormalities, microphthalmos, and microcephaly.

Infection during the second and third trimesters is less threatening. Maternal IgG crosses the placenta, protecting the fetus. The only infants at risk for severe infection are those born after maternal viremia but before development of maternal protective antibody. Maternal infection manifesting 5 days before or after delivery is the time period arbitrarily determined to be most hazardous for transmission to the fetus.

Diagnosis is commonly made on clinical grounds. Laboratory verification of recent infection is made most often by antibody detection techniques, including ELISA, fluorescent antibody, and hemagglutination inhibition. Serum obtained by cordocentesis may be tested for VZV IgM to document fetal infection.

Varicella-zoster immune globulin (VZIG) has been shown to prevent or modify the symptoms of infection in some women. Treatment success depends on identification of susceptible women at or just following exposure. Women with a questionable or negative history of chickenpox should be checked for antibody, since the overwhelming majority will have been exposed previously. If the antibody is negative, VZIG (625 units intramuscularly) should be given within 96 hours after exposure. There are no known adverse effects of VZIG administration during pregnancy. Infants born within 5 days after onset of maternal infection should also receive VZIG (125 units).

Infected pregnant women should be closely observed and hospitalized at the earliest signs of pulmonary involvement. Intravenous acyclovir (10–15 mg/kg every 8 hours for 7–10 days) is recommended in the treatment of VZV pneumonia.

Chapman SJ: Varicella in pregnancy. Semin Perinatol 1998;22: 339. [PMID: 9738999]

Thyroid Disease

Thyrotoxicosis during pregnancy may result in fetal anomalies, late abortion, or preterm labor and fetal hyperthyroidism with goiter. Thyroid storm in late pregnancy or labor is a life-threatening emergency.

Radioactive isotope therapy must never be given during pregnancy. The thyroid inhibitor of choice is propylthiouracil, which acts to prevent further thyroxine formation by blocking iodination of tyrosine. There is a 2- to 3-week delay before the pretreatment hormone level begins to fall. The initial dose of propylthiouracil is 100–150 mg three times a day; the dose is lowered as the euthyroid state is approached. It is desirable to keep free T_4 in the high normal range during pregnancy. A maintenance dose of 100 mg/d minimizes the chance of fetal hypothyroidism and goiter.

Recurrent postpartum thyroiditis occurs 3–6 months after delivery. A hyperthyroid state of 1–3 months' duration is followed by hypothyroidism, sometimes misdiagnosed as depression. Thyroperoxidase antibodies and thyroglobulin antibodies are present. Recovery is spontaneous in over 90% of cases after 3–6 months.

Maternal hypothyroidism—even subclinical hypothyroidism manifested only by elevated levels of thyroid stimulating hormone (TSH)—may adversely affect subsequent neuropsychologic development of the child. Mothers with known or suspected hypothyroidism should have the TSH level measured at the first prenatal visit. Replacement therapy with levothyroxine should be adjusted to maintain levels of TSH in the normal range.

Lazarus JH et al: Thyroid disease in relation to pregnancy: A decade of change. Clin Endocrinol 2000;53:265. [PMID: 10971442]

Tuberculosis

The diagnosis of tuberculosis in pregnancy is made by history taking, physical examination, and skin testing, with special attention to women from ethnic groups with a high prevalence of the disease (such as women from southeast Asia). Chest films should not be obtained as a routine screening measure in pregnancy but should be used only in patients with a skin test conversion or with suggestive findings in the history and physical examination. Abdominal shielding must be used if a chest film is obtained.

If adequately treated, tuberculosis in pregnancy has an excellent prognosis. There is no increase in spontaneous abortion, fetal problems, or congenital anomalies.

Treatment is with isoniazid and ethambutol or isoniazid and rifampin (see Chapters 9 and 33). Because isoniazid therapy may result in vitamin B_6 deficiency, a supplement of 50 mg/d of vitamin B_6 should be given simultaneously. Streptomycin, ethionamide, and most other antituberculous drugs should be avoided in pregnancy.

Urinary Tract Infection

The urinary tract is especially vulnerable to infections during pregnancy because the altered secretions of steroid sex hormones and the pressure exerted by the gravid uterus upon the ureters and bladder cause hypotonia and congestion and predispose to urinary stasis. Labor and delivery and urinary retention postpartum also may initiate or aggravate infection. *Escherichia coli* is the offending organism in over two-thirds of cases.

From 2% to 8% of pregnant women have asymptomatic bacteriuria, which some believe to be associated with an increased risk of prematurity. It is estimated that 20–40% of these women will develop pyelonephritis during pregnancy if untreated.

A first-trimester urine culture is indicated in women with a history of recurrent or recent episodes of urinary tract infection. If the culture is positive,

treatment should be initiated as a prophylactic measure. Nitrofurantoin (100 mg twice daily), ampicillin (500 mg four times daily), and cephalexin (500 mg four times daily) are acceptable medications for 3–7 days. Sulfonamides should not be given in the third trimester because they interfere with bilirubin binding and thus impose a risk of neonatal hyperbilirubinemia and kernicterus. Fluoroquinolones are also contraindicated because of their potential teratogenic effects on fetal cartilage and bone. If bacteriuria returns, suppressive medication (one daily dose of an appropriate antibiotic) for the remainder of the pregnancy is indicated. Acute pyelonephritis requires hospitalization for intravenous administration of antibiotics until the patient is afebrile; this is followed by a full course of oral antibiotics.

Delzell JE Jr et al: Urinary tract infections during pregnancy. Am Fam Physician 2000;61:713. [PMID: 10695584]

SURGICAL COMPLICATIONS DURING PREGNANCY

Elective major surgery should be avoided during pregnancy. Normal uncomplicated pregnancy does not alter operative risk except as it may interfere with the diagnosis of abdominal disorders and increase the technical problems of intra-abdominal surgery. Abortion is not a serious hazard after operation unless peritoneal sepsis or other significant complications occur. During the first trimester, congenital anomalies may be induced in the developing fetus by hypoxia. Thus, the second trimester is usually the optimal time for operative procedures.

Appendicitis

Appendicitis occurs in about one of 1500 pregnancies. Diagnosis may be difficult, since the appendix is carried high and to the right, away from McBurney's point, as the uterus enlarges, and localization of pain does not always occur. Nausea, vomiting, fever, and leukocytosis occur regularly. Any right-sided abdominal pain associated with these symptoms should arouse suspicion. In at least 20% of obstetric patients, the diagnosis of appendicitis is not made until rupture occurs and peritonitis has become established. Such a delay may lead to premature labor or abortion. With early diagnosis and appendectomy, the prognosis is good for mother and baby.

Mourad J et al: Appendicitis in pregnancy: New information that contradicts long-held clinical beliefs. Am J Obstet Gynecol 2000;182:1027. [PMID: 10819817]

Carcinoma of the Breast

Cancer of the breast (see also Chapter 16) is diagnosed approximately once in 3500 pregnancies. Pregnancy may accelerate the growth of cancer of the breast, and delay in diagnosis affects the outcome of treatment.

Inflammatory carcinoma is an extremely virulent type of breast cancer that occurs most commonly during lactation. Prepregnancy mammography should be encouraged for women over age 35 who are anticipating a pregnancy.

Breast enlargement during pregnancy obscures parenchymal masses, and breast tissue hyperplasia decreases the accuracy of mammography. Any discrete mass should be evaluated by aspiration to verify its cystic structure, with fine-needle biopsy if it is solid. A definitive diagnosis may require excisional biopsy under local anesthesia. If breast biopsy confirms the diagnosis of cancer, surgery should be done regardless of the stage of the pregnancy. If spread to the regional glands has occurred, irradiation or chemotherapy should be considered. Under these circumstances, the alternatives are termination of an early pregnancy or delay of therapy for fetal maturation.

Choledocholithiasis, Cholecystitis, & Idiopathic Cholestasis of Pregnancy

Severe choledocholithiasis and cholecystitis are not uncommon during pregnancy. When they do occur, it is usually in late pregnancy or in the puerperium. About 90% of patients with cholecystitis have gallstones; 90% of stones will be visualized by ultrasonography. Symptomatic relief may be all that is required.

Conventional gallbladder surgery in pregnant women should be attempted only in complicated cases (eg, obstruction), because it may increase the perinatal mortality rate to about 15%. Cholecystostomy and lithotomy may be all that is feasible during advanced pregnancy, cholecystectomy being deferred until after delivery. On the other hand, withholding surgery may result in necrosis and perforation of the gallbladder and peritonitis. Cholangitis due to impacted common duct stone requires surgical removal of gallstones and establishment of biliary drainage. Endoscopic retrograde cholangiopancreatography and endoscopic retrograde sphincterotomy can be performed safely in pregnant women if precautions are taken to minimize exposure to radiation. In early to mid-second trimester, laparoscopic cholecystectomy can be performed with minimal maternal morbidity and no fetal mortality.

Idiopathic cholestasis of pregnancy is due to a hereditary metabolic (hepatic) deficiency aggravated by the high estrogen levels of pregnancy. It causes intrahepatic biliary obstruction of varying degrees. The rise in bile acids is sufficient in the third trimester to cause severe, intractable, generalized itching and sometimes clinical jaundice. There may be mild elevations in blood bilirubin and alkaline phosphatase levels. The fetus is also threatened by this condition. An increased incidence of preterm delivery has been reported as well as unexplained intrauterine fetal demise. For this reason, antenatal surveillance of the fetus is mandatory in patients with this diagnosis. Resins such as cholestyramine (4 g three times a day) absorb bile acids in the large bowel and relieve pruritus but are difficult to take and may cause constipation. Their use requires vitamin K supplementation. The disorder is relieved once the infant has been delivered, but it recurs in subsequent pregnancies and sometimes with the use of oral contraceptives.

Ovarian Tumors

The most common adnexal mass in early pregnancy is the corpus luteum, which may become cystic and enlarge to 6 cm in diameter. Any persistent mass over 6 cm should be evaluated by ultrasound examination; unilocular cysts are likely to be corpus luteum cysts, whereas septated or semisolid tumors are likely to be neoplasms. The incidence of malignancy in ovarian masses over 6 cm in diameter is 2.5%. Ovarian tumors may undergo torsion and cause abdominal pain and nausea and vomiting and must be differentiated from appendicitis, other bowel disease, and ectopic pregnancy. Patients with suspected ovarian cancer should be referred to a tertiary perinatal center to determine whether the pregnancy can progress to fetal viability or whether treatment should be instituted without delay.

PREVENTION OF HEMOLYTIC DISEASE OF THE NEWBORN (Erythroblastosis Fetalis)

The antibody anti-Rh_o(D) is responsible for most severe instances of hemolytic disease of the newborn (erythroblastosis fetalis). About 15% of whites and much lower proportions of blacks and Asians are Rh_o(D)-negative. If an Rh_o(D)-negative woman carries an Rh_o(D)-positive fetus, she may develop antibodies against Rh_o(D) when fetal red cells enter her circulation during small fetomaternal bleeding episodes in the early third trimester or during delivery, abortion, ectopic pregnancy, abruptio placentae, or other antepartum bleeding problems. This antibody, once produced, remains in the woman's circulation and poses the threat of hemolytic disease for subsequent Rh-positive fetuses.

Passive immunization against hemolytic disease of the newborn is achieved with Rh_o(D) immune globulin, a purified concentrate of antibodies against Rh_o(D) antigen. The Rh_o(D) immune globulin (one vial of 300 µg intramuscularly) is given to the mother within 72 hours after delivery (or spontaneous or induced abortion or ectopic pregnancy). The antibodies in the immune globulin destroy fetal Rh-positive cells so that the mother will not produce anti-Rh_o(D). During her next Rh-positive gestation, erythroblastosis will be prevented. An additional safety measure is the administration of the immune globulin at the 28th week of pregnancy. The passive antibody titer that results is too low to significantly affect an Rh-positive fetus. The maternal clearance of the globulin is slow enough that protection will continue for 12 weeks.

Hemolytic disease of varying degrees, from mild to serious, continues to occur in association with Rh subgroups (C, c, or E) or Kell, Kidd, and other factors. Therefore, the presence of atypical antibodies should be checked in the third trimester of all pregnancies.

ACOG practice bulletin. Prevention of Rh D alloimmunization. Number 4, May 1999. Clinical management guidelines for obstetrician-gynecologists. American College of Obstetrics and Gynecology. Int J Gynaecol Obstet 1999;66:63. [PMID: 10458556]

PREVENTION OF PRETERM (PREMATURE) LABOR

Preterm (premature) labor is labor that begins before the 37th week of pregnancy; it is responsible for 85% of neonatal illnesses and deaths. The onset of labor is a result of a complex sequence of biologic events involving regulatory factors that are still poorly understood. Significant risk factors for the onset of preterm labor are a past history of preterm delivery, premature rupture of the membranes, urinary tract infection, exposure to diethylstilbestrol, multiple gestation, and abdominal or cervical surgery. In high-risk women (prior preterm birth), ultrasound measurement of cervical length (< 25 mm) in the second trimester may also identify a significant risk.

Low rates of preterm delivery are associated with success in educating patients to identify regular, frequent uterine contractions and in alerting medical and nursing staff to evaluate these patients early and initiate treatment if cervical changes can be identified. Distinguishing true from false labor in patients with a history of previous preterm births can be facilitated by the use of fetal fibronectin measurement in cervicovaginal specimens. This ubiquitous protein can be released by several different stimuli. Its absence (< 50 ng/mL) in the face of uterine contractions in a patient with a previous preterm birth has a negative predictive value of 93–97% for delivery within 7–14 days. On the other hand, despite initial promising findings, several prospective randomized controlled trials have failed to demonstrate a benefit of home uterine activity monitoring in preventing preterm birth.

In more acute situations, intravenous magnesium sulfate is effective, as are intravenous beta-adrenergic drugs. Magnesium sulfate is given as a 4- or 6-g bolus followed by a continuous infusion of 2–3 g/h. The rate may be increased by 1 g/h every 1½–2 hours until contractions cease or a blood magnesium concentration of 6–8 mg/dL is reached. Magnesium levels are determined every 4–6 hours to monitor the therapeutic blood level. After contractions have ceased for 12–24 hours, magnesium can be stopped and the situation reassessed.

Uterine smooth muscle is largely under sympathetic nervous system control, and stimulation of β_2-adrenergic receptors relaxes the myometrium. Consequently, inhibition of uterine contractility often can be accomplished by the administration of beta-adrenergic drugs such as ritodrine or terbutaline. Alternatively, use of an oxytocin receptor antagonist might also be expected to inhibit uterine contractility. However, trials of one such antagonist, atosiban, have shown only minimal efficacy.

Ritodrine is no longer manufactured. Terbutaline can be given as an intravenous infusion starting at 2.5 μg/min and increased by 2.5 μg/min every 20 minutes until contractions cease or to a maximum dose of 20 μg/min. Terbutaline can also be administered as subcutaneous injections of 250 μg every 3 hours. Oral terbutaline therapy following parenteral treatment is often elected and consists of giving 2.5–5 mg every 2–4 hours. With terbutaline, a dose-related elevation of heart rate of 20–40 beats/min may occur. An increase of systolic blood pressure up to 10 mm Hg is likely, and the diastolic pressure may fall 10–15 mm Hg during the infusion. Nifedipine has also been used in doses of 10–20 mg orally every 4–6 hours. Blood pressure may fall with nifedipine, but cardiac output increases considerably. Transient elevation of blood glucose, insulin, and fatty acids together with slight reduction of serum potassium have been reported with beta-adrenergic drugs. Fetal tachycardia may be slight or absent. No drug-related perinatal deaths have been reported with beta-agonists. Maternal side effects requiring dose limitation are tachycardia (≥ 120 beats/min), palpitations, and nervousness. Fluids should be limited to 2500 mL/24 h. Serious side effects (pulmonary edema, chest pain with or without electrocardiographic changes) are often idiosyncratic, not dose-related, and warrant termination of therapy.

One must identify cases in which untimely delivery is the sole threat to the life or health of the infant. An effort should be made to eliminate (1) maternal conditions that compromise the intrauterine environment and make premature birth the lesser risk, eg, preeclampsia-eclampsia; (2) fetal conditions that either are helped by early delivery or render attempts to stop premature labor meaningless, eg, severe erythroblastosis fetalis; and (3) clinical situations in which it is likely that an attempt to stop labor will be futile, eg, ruptured membranes with chorioamnionitis, cervix fully effaced and dilated more than 3 cm, or strong labor in progress.

In pregnancies of less than 34 weeks' duration, betamethasone, 12 mg intramuscularly, or dexamethasone, 16 mg intramuscularly, repeated in 12–24 hours, is administered to hasten fetal lung maturation and permit delivery 48 hours after initial treatment when further prolongation of pregnancy is contraindicated.

ACOG practice bulletin. Assessment of risk factors for preterm birth. Clinical management guidelines for obstetrician-gynecologists. Number 31, October 2001. In: 2002 Compendium of Selected Publications, ACOG, Washington, DC, 2002:277.

Dyson D et al: Monitoring women at risk for preterm labor. N Engl J Med 1998;338:15. [PMID: 9414326]

Table 18–4. Drugs and substances that require a careful assessment of risk before they are prescribed for breast-feeding women.[1]

Category	Specific Drugs or Compounds	Management Plan and Rationale
Analgesic drugs	Meperidine, oxycodone	Use alternatives to meperidine and oxycodone. Breast-fed infants whose mothers were receiving meperidine had a higher risk of neurobehavioral depression than breast-fed infants whose mothers were receiving morphine. In breast-fed infants, the level of exposure to oxycodone may reach 10% of the therapeutic dose. For potent analgesia, morphine may be given cautiously. Acetaminophen and nonsteroidal anti-inflammatory drugs are safe.
Antiarthritis drugs	Gold salts, methotrexate, high-dose aspirin	Consider alternatives to gold therapy. Although the bioavailability of elemental gold is unknown, a small amount is excreted in breast milk for a prolonged period. Therefore, the total amount of elemental gold that an infant could ingest may be substantial. No toxicity has been reported. Consider alternatives to methotrexate therapy, although low-dose methotrexate therapy for breast-feeding women with rheumatic diseases had lower risks of adverse effects in their infants than did anticancer chemotherapy. High-dose aspirin should be used with caution, since there is a case report of metabolic acidosis in a breast-fed infant whose mother was receiving high-dose therapy. Although the risk seems small, the infant's condition should be monitored clinically if the mother is receiving long-term therapy with high-dose aspirin.
Anticoagulant drugs	Phenindione[2]	Use alternatives to phenindione. Currently available vitamin K antagonists such as warfarin and acenocoumarol are considered safe, as is heparin.
Antidepressant drugs and lithium	Fluoxetine, doxepin, lithium[2]	Use fluoxetine, doxepin, and lithium with caution. Although the concentrations of these drugs in breast milk are low, colic (with fluoxetine) and sedation (with doxepin) have been reported in exposed infants. Near-therapeutic plasma concentrations of lithium were reported in an infant exposed to the drug in utero and through breast-feeding. The incidence of these adverse events is unknown.
Antiepileptic drugs	Phenobarbital, ethosuximide, primidone	In breast-fed infants, the level of exposure to phenobarbital, ethosuximide, and primidone may exceed 10% of the weight-adjusted therapeutic dose. Consider alternatives such as carbamazepine, phenytoin, and valproic acid.
Antimicrobial drugs	Chloramphenicol, tetracycline	Use alternatives to chloramphenicol and tetracycline. Idiosyncratic aplastic anemia is a possibility among breast-fed infants whose mothers are receiving chloramphenicol. Although tetracycline-induced discoloration of the teeth of breast-fed infants has not been reported, the potential risk of this event needs to be clearly communicated to lactating women.
Anticancer drugs	All (eg, cyclophosphamide,[2] methotrexate,[2] doxorubicin[2])	Because of their potent pharmacologic effects, cytotoxic drugs should not be given to breast-feeding women.
Anxiolytic drugs	Diazepam, alprazolam	Avoid long-term use of diazepam and alprazolam in breast-feeding women. Intermittent use poses little risk to their infants, but regular use may result in the accumulation of the drug and its metabolites in the infants. Lethargy and poor weight gain have been reported in an infant exposed to diazepam in breast milk, and the withdrawal syndrome was reported in a breast-fed infant after the mother discontinued alprazolam.
Cardiovascular and antihypertensive drugs	Acebutolol, amiodarone, atenolol, nadolol, sotalol	The use of acebutolol, amiodarone, atenolol, nadolol, and sotalol by breast-feeding women may cause relatively high levels of exposure among their infants, and these agents should therefore be used with caution. The two β-adrenergic antagonists propranolol and labetalol are considered safe.

(continued)

Table 18–4. Drugs and substances that require a careful assessment of risk before they are prescribed for breast-feeding women. (continued)

Category	Specific Drugs or Compounds	Management Plan and Rationale
Endocrine drugs and hormones	Estrogens, bromocriptine[2]	Estrogens and bromocriptine may suppress milk production. Oral contraceptives containing little or no estrogen have smaller risk than formulations with higher concentrations of estrogen. Nevertheless, caution should be exercised in their use.
Immunosuppressive drugs	Cyclosporine,[2] azathioprine	Maternal plasma concentrations of cyclosporine and azathioprine should be monitored. In nine reported cases in breast-fed infants who were exposed to azathioprine in breast milk, no obvious adverse effects were noted.
Respiratory drugs	Theophylline	Theophylline should be used with caution. When the mother's doses are high, the levels of exposure in the infant may be substantial (ie, 20% of the therapeutic dose).
Radioactive compounds	All	Breast-feeding should be stopped for the length of the half-life of the radiolabeled compound used.
Drugs of abuse	All[1]	The use of drugs of abuse precludes breast-feeding; cocaine-induced toxicity has been reported among breast-fed infants whose mothers abused cocaine. Methadone, used for the treatment of addiction, is safe for infants of breast-feeding women, at doses of up to 80 mg per day. Buprenorphine may be a safer alternative to methadone.
Nonmedicinal substances	Ethanol, caffeine, nicotine	In order to avoid exposure of the infant to ethanol, the mother should not consume alcohol or should consume no more than one drink 2 to 3 hours before breast-feeding. The ingestion of moderate amounts of caffeine should be safe. Because of the effects of second-hand smoke and the fact that nicotine is excreted in breast milk, smoking is contraindicated in breast-feeding women.
Miscellaneous compounds	Iodides and iodine, ergotamine,[2] ergonovine	Use alternatives to iodine-containing antiseptic agents. Ergotamine and ergonovine may suppress prolactin secretion in breast-feeding women. However, the use of methylergonovine to stimulate uterine involution is considered safe in breast-feeding women.

[1]Data modified from Ito S: Drug therapy for breast-feeding women. N Engl J Med 2000;343:120. Drugs for which there is no information are not included, though a careful risk assessment is necessary before such drugs are prescribed.
[2]The use of this drug or these drugs by breast-feeding women is contraindicated according to the American Academy of Pediatrics.

Romero R et al: An oxytocin receptor antagonist (atosiban) in the treatment of preterm labor: A randomized double-blind, placebo-controlled trial with tocolytic rescue. Am J Obstet Gynecol 2000;182:1173. [PMID: 10819855]

LACTATION

Breast feeding should be encouraged by education throughout pregnancy and the puerperium. Mothers should be told the benefits of breast feeding—it is emotionally satisfying, promotes mother-infant bonding, is economical, and gives significant immunity to the infant. The period of amenorrhea associated with frequent and consistent breast feeding provides some (though not completely reliable) birth control until menstruation begins at 6–12 months postpartum or the intensity of breast feeding diminishes. If the mother must return to work, even a brief period of nursing is beneficial. Transfer of immunoglobulins in colostrum and breast milk protects the infant against many systemic and enteric infections. Macrophages and lymphocytes transferred to the infant from breast milk play an immunoprotective role. The intestinal flora of breast-fed infants inhibits the growth of pathogens. Breast-fed infants have fewer bacterial and viral infections, less severe diarrhea, and fewer allergy problems than bottle-fed infants and are less apt to be obese as children and in adult life.

Frequent breast feeding on an infant demand schedule enhances milk flow and successful breast feeding. Mothers breast feeding for the first time need help and encouragement from providers, nurses, and other nursing mothers. Milk supply can be increased by increased suckling and increased rest.

Nursing mothers should have a fluid intake of over 2 L/d. The United States RDA calls for 21 g of extra protein (over the 44 g/d baseline for an adult woman) and 550 extra kcal/d in the first 6 months of nursing. Calcium intake should be 1200 mg/d. Continuation of a prenatal vitamin and mineral supplement is wise. Strict vegetarians who eschew both milk and eggs should always take vitamin B_{12} supplements during pregnancy and lactation.

Effects of Drugs in a Nursing Mother

Drugs taken by a nursing mother may accumulate in milk and be transmitted to the infant (Table 18–4). The amount of drug entering the milk depends on the drug's lipid solubility, mechanism of transport, and degree of ionization.

Suppression of Lactation

A. MECHANICAL SUPPRESSION

The simplest and safest method of suppressing lactation after it has started is to gradually transfer the baby to a bottle or a cup over a 3-week period. Milk supply will decrease with decreased demand, and minimal discomfort ensues. If nursing must be stopped abruptly, the mother should avoid nipple stimulation, refrain from expressing milk, and use a snug brassiere. Ice packs and analgesics can be helpful. If suppression is desired before nursing has begun, use this same technique. Engorgement will gradually recede over a 2- to 3-day period.

B. HORMONAL SUPPRESSION

Oral and long-acting injections of hormonal preparations were used at one time to suppress lactation. Because of their questionable efficacy and particularly because of associated side effects such as thromboembolic episodes and hair growth, their use for this purpose has largely been abandoned in recent years. Simi-larly, lactation suppression with bromocriptine is to be avoided because of reports of severe hypertension, seizures, strokes, and myocardial infarctions associated with its use.

Ito S: Drug therapy for breast feeding women. N Engl J Med 2000;343:118. [PMID: 10891521]

Neifert MR: Clinical aspects of lactation. Promoting breastfeeding success. Clin Perinatol 1999;26:281. [PMID: 10394489]

PUERPERAL MASTITIS (See also Chapter 16.)

Postpartum mastitis occurs sporadically in nursing mothers shortly after they return home, or it may occur in epidemic form in the hospital. *Staphylococcus aureus* is usually the causative agent. Inflammation is generally unilateral, and women nursing for the first time are more often affected. Rarely, inflammatory carcinoma of the breast can be mistaken for puerperal mastitis.

Mastitis frequently begins within 3 months after delivery and may start with a sore or fissured nipple. There is obvious cellulitis in an area of breast tissue, with redness, tenderness, local warmth, and fever. Treatment consists of antibiotics effective against penicillin-resistant staphylococci (dicloxacillin or a cephalosporin, 500 mg orally every 6 hours for 5–7 days) and regular emptying of the breast by nursing followed by expression of any remaining milk by hand or with a mechanical suction device.

If the mother begins antibiotic therapy before suppuration begins, infection can usually be controlled in 24 hours. If delay is permitted, breast abscess can result. Incision and drainage are required for abscess formation. Despite puerperal mastitis, the baby usually thrives without prophylactic antimicrobial therapy.

Allergic & Immunologic Disorders 19

Jeffrey L. Kishiyama, MD, & Daniel C. Adelman, MD

See www.current-med.com/ch19.html

■ I. ALLERGIC DISEASES

Allergy is an immunologically mediated (antibody- or cellular-mediated) reaction to a foreign antigen (allergen) manifested by tissue inflammation and organ dysfunction. Atopic responses have a genetic basis, but the clinical expression of disease depends on both immunologic responsiveness and exposure to relevant antigens. Allergic hypersensitivity disorders may be local or systemic. Because the allergen is foreign (ie, environmental), the skin and respiratory tract are the organs most frequently involved in allergic disease. Allergic reactions may also localize to the vasculature, gastrointestinal tract, or other visceral organs. Anaphylaxis is the most extreme form of systemic allergy.

Immunologic Classification

Hypersensitivity diseases can be classified according to (1) the immunologic mechanism involved in pathogenesis, (2) the organ system affected, and (3) the nature and source of the allergen. An immunologic classification is preferred because it serves as a rational basis for diagnosis and treatment. The Gell and Coombs classification of the hypersensitivity diseases is as follows:

A. Type I—IgE-Mediated (Immediate) Hypersensitivity

IgE antibodies occupy receptor sites on mast cells. Within minutes after exposure to the allergen, a multivalent antigen links adjacent IgE molecules, activating and degranulating mast cells. Both preformed and newly generated mediators cause vasodilation, visceral smooth muscle contraction, mucus secretory gland stimulation, vascular permeability, and tissue inflammation. Arachidonic acid metabolites, cytokines, and other mediators induce a late-phase inflammatory response that appears several hours later. There are two clinical subgroups of IgE-mediated allergy: atopy and anaphylaxis.

1. Atopy—The term atopy is applied to a group of diseases (allergic rhinitis, allergic asthma, atopic dermatitis, and allergic gastroenteropathy) occurring in certain persons with an inherited tendency to develop antigen-specific IgE to multiple common organic environmental allergens. Aeroallergens such as pollens, mold spores, animal danders, and house dust mite antigen are common triggers for ocular, nasal, and pulmonary allergic disorders. The allergic origin of atopic dermatitis is less well understood, but it is clear that some patients' symptoms can be triggered by exposure to dust mite antigen and certain foods.

The allergic reaction is localized to a susceptible target organ, but more than one of these diseases may occur in an allergic individual. There is a strong familial tendency.

2. Anaphylaxis—Certain allergens—especially drugs, insect venoms, latex, and foods—may induce an IgE antibody response, causing a generalized release of mediators from mast cells and resulting in systemic anaphylaxis. This is characterized by (1) hypotension or shock from widespread vasodilation, (2) bronchospasm, (3) gastrointestinal and uterine muscle contraction, and (4) urticaria or angioedema (see Chapter 6). The condition is potentially fatal and can affect both nonatopic and atopic persons. Isolated urticaria and angioedema are cutaneous forms of anaphylaxis, are much more common, and have a better prognosis.

B. Type II—Antibody-Mediated (Cytotoxic) Hypersensitivity

Cytotoxic reactions involve the specific reaction of either IgG or IgM antibody to cell-bound antigens. This typically results in activation of the complement cascade and the destruction of the cell to which the antigen is bound. Examples of tissue injury by this mechanism include immune hemolytic anemia and Rh hemolytic disease in the newborn.

C. Type III—Immune Complex-Mediated Hypersensitivity

Antibodies of the IgG or IgM isotype can form complexes with the allergen, be deposited in tissues, and activate the complement cascade. With similar concentrations of both allergen and antibody, the Arthus reaction, a localized cutaneous and subcutaneous inflammatory response to injected allergen, occurs, as well as serum sickness, a systemic disease characterized by fever, arthralgias, and dermatitis.

D. Type IV—T Cell-Mediated Hypersensitivity (Delayed Hypersensitivity, Cell-Mediated Hypersensitivity)

The most common expression of T cell-mediated hypersensitivity is allergic contact dermatitis, in which the allergen causes dermal inflammation on direct contact with the skin. The reaction occurs after a latent period of 1–2 days from the time of contact. Hypersensitivity pneumonitis (extrinsic allergic alveolitis) is a pulmonary T cell-mediated hypersensitivity disease.

Immunopathophysiology

Atopic disorders are associated with tissue inflammation, characterized immunohistologically by infiltration with certain subsets of CD4 lymphocytes. This has generated interest in the T helper 1 (TH1)/T helper 2 (TH2) paradigm of allergic immunopathology. In this model, antigen-specific CD4 (T helper) cells develop into one of two lymphocyte subsets: TH1 or TH2. The terms TH1 and TH2 comprise the functional phenotype of the T helper cell. TH1 cells are characterized by the production of gamma interferon (IFN-γ). TH2 cells synthesize interleukin-4 (IL-4), interleukin-5 (IL-5), and interleukin-13 (IL-13). Since both IL-4 and IL-13 stimulate isotype switching with IgE synthesis and since IL-5 promotes eosinophil survival and function, these cytokines have been implicated in the generation of allergic inflammation. TH1 and TH2 phenotypes appear to be mutually exclusive. The development of a dominant TH2 response to an environmental allergen can cause IgE-mediated hypersensitivity disease. As the pathophysiology of these atopic diseases becomes better elucidated, novel therapies are being developed to modulate aberrant immunologic responses.

Upper & Lower Airway Connections

Up to 80% of patients with asthma suffer from rhinitis, and, conversely, 15% of patients with allergic rhinitis suffer from asthma. Furthermore, the immunopathophysiology of inflammation is similar in the upper and lower airways. Both airways are lined by pseudostratified columnar epithelium. In atopic states, these airways are characterized by edematous mucosa, hyperplasia of mucus-secreting goblet cells, numerous mast cells, infiltration with mononuclear cells, including TH2-type lymphocytes and eosinophils, and airway hyperresponsiveness. Only the lower airways contain bronchial smooth muscle, but the similarities in immunohistology otherwise suggests an overlap in the causes of and possible treatments for disease. Several clinical studies have demonstrated a measurable reduction in bronchial hyperreactivity after treatment of upper airway inflammation with topical nasal corticosteroids alone. Concomitant sinusitis can lead to a worsening of asthma in some patients, and sinobronchial reflexes have been identified in physiologic investigations. These observations suggest a coordinated approach to airways disease to optimize patient care in atopic individuals.

The Late-Phase Allergic Response

The immediate allergic response occurs after reexposure to allergen in previously sensitized individuals. Six to 12 hours following allergen exposure, a late-phase allergic response can cause a recrudescence of symptoms in anaphylaxis or allergic airways disease. Histologically, the late-phase allergic responses are characterized by infiltration with inflammatory cells, including mononuclear cells, basophils, and eosinophils. These cells release mediators that cause symptoms but also set the stage for chronic inflammation, persistence of disease, and the phenomenon of "priming" or heightened sensitivity to antigen. Increased nonspecific hyperresponsiveness to respiratory irritants can also be secondary to mediators released during the late phase. A rationale for using topical corticosteroids or allergen immunotherapy in the treatment of allergic rhinitis or allergic asthma is based on the observation that suppression of the late-phase reaction will decrease eosinophil activity, inhibit allergen-induced cytokine production and mediator release, and thereby inhibit proinflammatory responses and chronic symptoms.

■ ATOPIC DISEASE

Clinical manifestations resembling allergic hypersensitivity can also occur in the absence of an immunologic mechanism. Specific examples include nonallergic (intrinsic) asthma, which is triggered by the nonimmunologic effect of inhaled dusts and fumes, weather changes, viral respiratory infections, and stress rather than by aeroallergen-induced IgE-mediated mast cell degranulation; irritant dermatitis, which is the result of physical or chemical damage to skin rather than development of sensitized lymphocytes; and "anaphylactoid reactions" from nonimmunologic release of mast cell mediators. Therefore, the diagnosis of allergy requires answers to the following questions: (1) What is the nature of the disease? (2) Is the disease caused by an IgE-mediated mechanism? (3) What specific allergens are responsible?

The relevant history includes a survey of allergen exposure associated with home, work, hobbies, and habits as well as medications. Physical examination is most useful if performed during exposure. Demonstration of allergic hypersensitivity by in vivo or in vitro testing confirms clinical suspicions of allergic disease.

Specific-IgE Antibody Tests

Allergy tests reveal an immune response to a particular allergen. To maximize the positive predictive value of allergy testing, a positive test result must be correlated with the history before one can conclude that the allergen caused the illness. Patients selected for testing include those with moderate to severe disease, those who are potential candidates for allergen immunotherapy, and those with strong predisposing factors for atopic diatheses, eg, a strong family history of atopy or ongoing exposure to potential sources of allergen. Since the development of rhinitis precedes the presentation of asthma in over half of cases, early intervention may decrease the risk of more severe clinical allergic disease. Patients with a risk for allergic bronchopulmonary aspergillosis should be screened for sensitivity to aspergillus antigens. The type of immune response must be consistent with the nature of the disease. For example, IgE antibody causes allergic rhinitis but not delayed-type allergic contact dermatitis. IgE antibodies are detected by in vivo (skin tests) or in vitro methods.

A. Skin Tests

Epicutaneous or cutaneous allergen testing produces a localized pruritic wheal (induration) and flare (erythema) which is maximal at 15–20 minutes. It is used most commonly in the diagnosis of allergic respiratory disease (rhinitis and asthma) but also in suspected cases of food or drug allergy and hymenoptera (bee, wasp, hornet or yellow jacket) venom hypersensitivity. Allergen extracts are available for pollens, fungi, animal danders, and dust mites and are selected appropriately for the patient's geographic area.

Skin testing is preferred to in vitro methods (discussed below) because it detects the presence of IgE antibody in tissue and shows biologic activity. For most applications, in vivo skin testing is more sensitive, more specific, more rapid, and less expensive than in vitro radioallergosorbent (RAST) testing. Any drug with antihistamine effects (H_1 antagonists, tricyclic antidepressants, phenothiazines) must be withdrawn prior to testing. Appropriate controls with a negative diluent and a positive histamine response are mandatory for valid results and accurate interpretation. There is a remote risk of inducing a systemic reaction. To avoid this, most allergists perform epicutaneous (prick) testing first, followed by selected intradermal tests to allergens negative by prick testing. Intradermal skin testing techniques are often employed for diagnostic confirmation of hymenoptera (insect venom) or penicillin hypersensitivity, as this method increases sensitivity of the assay for detection of IgE-mediated anaphylaxis. Skin testing with hymenoptera venom or a drug is performed by serial titration, starting with diluted solutions. Special allergenic extracts can be prepared for other allergens (food or latex).

Skin testing for allergy to drugs is reliable for high-molecular-weight protein drugs (eg, heterologous serum, insulin) but not for low-molecular-weight compounds (most drugs), which must bind to larger proteins (haptens) to become immunogenic. With the exception of penicillin, in vivo skin testing for low-molecular-weight drugs is limited in sensitivity and availability. Penicillin testing is available because the immunochemistry has been delineated, identifying all haptenated molecules including the native drug and all immunogenic metabolites. The combination of skin testing with the major and minor metabolic determinants of penicillin is highly predictive of anaphylaxis. (The minor determinants are not available commercially, though they may be synthesized and are often available at specialized centers.) The negative predictive value of skin tests for IgE-mediated reactions to subsequently administered penicillin is good.

B. In Vitro Tests of IgE Antibody

IgE antibodies can be detected in serum by radioallergosorbent test (RAST) or enzyme-linked immunosorbent assay (ELISA). Protein allergens are covalently linked to the immunosorbent (solid) phase. After a patient's serum is allowed to incubate with the allergen-coated solid phase, the system is washed and a second incubation is performed utilizing labeled anti-IgE antibody (rabbit anti-human IgE). The allergen-specific IgE is quantified by comparing colorimetric changes or radioactive counts against a standard curve. Many of the usual atopic allergens are available commercially for RAST or ELISA testing.

In vitro tests detect allergen-specific antibody in serum. Since IgE-mediated allergy is caused by IgE antibodies bound to mast cells (not by circulating IgE), in vitro tests generally are less sensitive than skin tests for diagnostic use. They are not affected by antihistamine therapy but can give false-positive results in patients with high total serum IgE levels and false-negative results in patients treated with immunotherapy who have significant allergen-specific IgG antibodies. The test is significantly more expensive than skin testing, and results are not immediately available. The RAST or ELISA method is particularly useful for detecting IgE antibodies to certain occupational chemicals or potentially toxic allergens.

The total IgE level in serum is higher in atopic patients. Because there is considerable overlap, it is not a satisfactory diagnostic test for atopy.

ALLERGIC RHINITIS

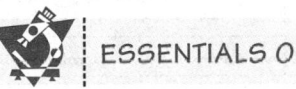

ESSENTIALS OF DIAGNOSIS

- *Presence of specific-IgE antibody to tested aeroallergens.*
- *Nasal pruritus, congestion, rhinorrhea, or paroxysms of sneezing, associated with lower respiratory symptoms (chronic cough, wheezing, chest*

tightness, or dyspnea); eye irritation and pruritus; or eczematous dermatitis.

• *Environmental allergen exposure.*

Clinical Findings

In addition to the symptoms listed above, the physical examination may reveal edematous or inflamed nasal mucosa. In severe cases, the affected mucosa may be pale, boggy, or blue-tinged from vascular engorgement and venous congestion.

Treatment

The three basic principles of allergy management are avoidance of the allergen, symptomatic pharmacologic therapy, and specific allergen immunotherapy.

A. AVOIDANCE THERAPY

Avoidance is the most effective treatment for any allergic condition. It cures the clinical manifestations but does not reduce the sensitivity to the allergen.

1. Pollens—Airborne allergens can travel significant distances, but concentrations are highest near their source. Pollen release occurs in the early morning, and airborne levels depend on temperature and wind velocity. Closing windows and remaining in air-conditioned environments can decrease exposure when pollen counts are high.

2. Animal danders—If the allergy is slight, the patient may benefit from merely keeping the animal out of the bedroom; usually, however, it is necessary to remove the animal from the home altogether. Hypersensitivity to animal dander can be exquisite, and passively transferred dander can accumulate to significant levels in "off-limits" areas. Washing or otherwise treating the fur of a live animal has not been proved to reduce allergenicity.

3. House dust and dust mites—The mattress and pillows should be encased in dust-proof material, and the bedroom floor should be uncarpeted. The room should be dusted frequently. Electronic air purifiers are of unproved effectiveness. Acaricides to eliminate dust mites are under investigation.

4. Mold spores—Out of doors, mold spores are unavoidable during certain seasons. Nevertheless, activities such as gardening and farming can be associated with acute high levels of exposure and should be avoided. Indoor mold contamination can be controlled by repairing leaks and cleaning mold buildup in sinks, shower curtains, pipes, etc.

B. DRUG THERAPY

Three classes of pharmacotherapy are useful for IgE-mediated diseases, based on (1) inhibition of release of mediators from mast cells, (2) inhibition of the action of mediators on their target cells, and (3) reversal of the vascular and inflammatory responses in the target tissues (Table 19–1).

1. Antihistamines—Of the numerous mediators released from mast cells by reaction of allergen with IgE antibody, histamine is the only one that can be effectively blocked by drugs. Antihistamine drugs are competitive inhibitors of the receptors. Those that inhibit H_1 receptors are used to treat IgE-mediated allergy. There are a number of such drugs, but the use of first-generation antihistamines (chlorpheniramine, brompheniramine, diphenhydramine, clemastine, hydroxyzine) may be limited by sedation and dry mucous membranes. Tolerance to soporific effects may develop with continued use. Rare complications include seizures and tachyarrhythmias. Second-generation nonsedating histamine H_1 receptor-blocking drugs, loratadine, fexofenadine, and desloratadine appear not to be associated with arrhythmias and, along with cetirizine, are now the drugs of choice. Cetirizine is mildly sedating, but the incidence of side effects is markedly lower than that of its parent compound, hydroxyzine. Azelastine is a topical antihistamine preparation that is applied intranasally to decrease its systemic side effects.

Antihistamine therapy is helpful in allergic rhinitis and in urticaria but not in all patients. It rarely allevi-

Table 19–1. Effectiveness of agents used in treatment of allergic disorders.

Drug Class	Sneezing	Pruritus	Rhinorrhea	Congestion	Inflammation	Onset of Action
Antihistamines	++++	++++	+++	+	–	Rapid
Sympathomimetics	–	–	+	++++	–	Rapid
Glucocorticoids	+++	+++	+++	++++	++++	Slow (days)
Cromolyn-nedocromil sodium	++	+	+	+	++	Slow (weeks)
Anticholinergics	–	–	++++	–	–	Rapid
Immunotherapy	++++	++++	++++	++++	++++	Slow (months)

ates symptoms of asthma, though it is not contraindicated when used to treat concomitant rhinitis or pruritus. The antipruritic effect of antihistamines may be a useful adjunct in treatment of eczematous diseases. Intramuscular or intravenous antihistamines are used in systemic anaphylaxis as adjunctive treatment only. They relieve cutaneous and gastrointestinal symptoms but have no effect on vascular collapse or airway obstruction.

2. Sympathomimetic drugs—Adrenergic agonists are used for both α-adrenergic (vasoconstricting) and β-adrenergic (bronchodilating) properties. Alpha-adrenergic agonists can be used orally (pseudoephedrine) or topically (phenylephrine, naphazoline, oxymetazoline) as nasal decongestants and (topically) as conjunctival vasoconstrictors. Daily use of topical preparations can lead to rapid development of rebound vasodilation (rhinitis medicamentosa). The main side effects of oral decongestants are insomnia, tremor, and tachycardia.

3. Glucocorticoids—These drugs have a therapeutic role in virtually all types of allergic diseases because of their anti-inflammatory action rather than by their immunosuppressive effects. Although effective, they do not modify the underlying disease. Their use in allergy requires close attention to toxicity. Steroids are available in oral, intramuscular, intravenous, intranasal, and bronchial inhalation forms; as eye drops; and in topical formulations for dermatologic use. Short-term systemic burst therapy is indicated for treatment of severe asthma, allergic contact dermatitis, marked allergic rhinitis, acute exacerbations of hypersensitivity pneumonitis, and allergic bronchopulmonary aspergillosis. Because of complications, including cataracts, corneal ulceration, keratitis, and glaucoma, steroid eye drops are most commonly prescribed by ophthalmologists.

Topical corticosteroid nasal spray is effective and probably safe for long-term use, but epistaxis can occur and nasal septal perforation is a complication. Flunisolide, fluticasone, beclomethasone, mometasone, budesonide, and triamcinolone are similarly efficacious, often requiring only a single daily dose after an initial period of therapy with multiple doses daily for 1 week. Long-term topical corticosteroid therapy for allergic rhinitis is an essential aspect of management of the inflammatory phase of the disease.

4. Cromolyn sodium and sodium nedocromil—Pretreatment with these drugs prevents the response to allergen by stabilizing the mast cell, though the specific molecular mechanisms of action are unknown. Although unrelated, they have similar effects and, because of poor bioavailability, are effective only when applied directly to the involved organ. Their action is short-lived, so that they must be given three or four times a day. Cromolyn is available as a bronchial inhaler, nasal spray, and ophthalmologic preparation;

nedocromil is available in metered-dose inhalers. Not all patients respond, but the drugs have very few side effects and wide margins of safety. A high-dose oral form of cromolyn has been released for use in treating systemic mastocytosis, but poor oral absorption limits its effectiveness.

5. Anticholinergic agents—Ipratropium bromide is effective as a nasal topical agent for use in rhinitis. Mucous membrane glandular secretion is under cholinergic control and can be inhibited by anticholinergic agents. First-generation antihistamines have systemic anticholinergic activity, but ipratropium is preferred as adjunctive treatment of allergic rhinitis or as primary treatment for many types of nonallergic rhinitis. Ipratropium does not alleviate sneezing, pruritus, or nasal congestion but can be useful for treatment of postnasal drip and rhinorrhea.

C. IMMUNOTHERAPY

Treatment of atopy—especially allergic rhinitis—by the repeated long-term injection of allergen has been shown in many controlled clinical trials to be an effective method for reducing or eliminating symptoms and signs of the allergic disorder.

1. Indications—This treatment is recommended for patients with severe allergic rhinitis who respond poorly to drug therapy and whose allergens are not avoidable. Immunotherapy is unequivocally effective in patients with allergic rhinitis and allergic conjunctivitis. In allergic asthma it has also shown proof of efficacy, but conflicting accounts are reported. The lower clinical response rates observed in asthma have been attributed to the multifactorial nature of the disease. There is no current evidence for an effect in atopic dermatitis. Food or drug hypersensitivity is treated by avoidance only, since immunotherapy is not available.

2. Immunologic effects—"Allergen immunotherapy" is preferable to "desensitization" because the immunologic basis for this treatment is unknown. Nevertheless, certain immunologic changes can be induced by these injections. Circulating levels of IgE antibodies specific to the injected allergens increase slightly during the first few months, then decrease, eventually to substantially lower levels than before treatment. Seasonal rises in IgE antibodies to pollens are blunted or eliminated. IgG blocking antibody is produced. Changes in regulatory T cells favoring suppression of IgE antibody production have been reported. There is some evidence that TH2 cytokine responses are shifted toward TH1 responses in peripheral blood mononuclear cells. Higher thresholds for release of inflammatory mediators and decreases in late phase allergic reactions may be related to the reduction in biologic sensitivity of end organ systems (eyes, nose, bronchi, skin).

3. Clinical effects—Most patients with allergic rhinitis caused by aeroallergens become more tolerant to natural pollen exposure during successive seasons while on immunotherapy. A small minority become completely asymptomatic, but most patients enjoy a significant decrease in symptoms and medication usage. Only high-dose injected immunotherapy has been demonstrated to be effective in double-blind, placebo-controlled trials. A beneficial response may persist after treatment is stopped. The clinical effects and immunologic responses are antigen-specific.

4. Procedure—A sterile aqueous solution of the allergen or allergens responsible for the patient's disease is administered by subcutaneous injection in increasing doses once or twice a week until a maintenance dose is reached, at which time the interval is advanced to every 4 weeks. The maintenance dose is typically one to ten thousand times the starting dose. Ascending doses are used to minimize the risk of systemic allergic reactions during initial stages of immunotherapy. Three to 5 years is a typical course of therapy. As of 2002, oral immunotherapy is experimental in the United States, and sublingual or low-dose immunotherapy is unconventional and of unproved efficacy.

5. Adverse effects—Reactions to treatment may be local or systemic. Localized immediate and late-phase skin reactions occur at injection sites. These are not harmful, but the dose must be adjusted to avoid excessively large or prolonged local reactions. Immediate systemic reactions or anaphylaxis are a potential problem with each injection and must be prevented by monitoring of dosage. The patient must remain at the treatment facility for at least 20 minutes after each injection so that drugs and equipment for treating anaphylaxis will be available if needed. No long-term adverse consequences of aqueous allergen extract immunotherapy are known to have occurred in immunocompetent individuals.

Abramson MJ et al: Allergen immunotherapy for asthma. Cochrane Database Syst Rev 2000;CD001186. [PMID: 10796617]

Barnes PJ: New directions in allergic diseases: mechanism-based anti-inflammatory therapies. J Allergy Clin Immunol 2000; 106:5. [PMID: 10887299]

Bousquet J, et al: WHO position paper. Allergen immunotherapy: Therapeutic vaccines for allergic diseases. Allergy 1998;S53:1. [PMID: 9860031] (A comprehensive review from a consensus meeting of American and European organizations.)

Bousquet J: Specific immunotherapy in asthma. Allergy 1999;54 Suppl 56:37. [PMID: 10532302]

Demoly P, Michel FB, Bousquet J: In vivo methods for study of allergy skin tests, techniques, and interpretation. In: *Allergy Principles and Practice*, 5th ed. Middleton E Jr et al (editors). Mosby, 1998.

Durham SR et al: Long-term clinical efficacy of grass-pollen immunotherapy. N Engl J Med 1999;341:468. [PMID: 10441602]

Munir AKM, et al: Exposure to indoor allergens in early infancy and sensitization. J Allergy Clin Immunol 1997;100:177. [PMID: 9275137] (Looks at threshold levels of allergen exposure for sensitization.)

ANAPHYLAXIS, URTICARIA, ANGIOEDEMA

 ESSENTIALS OF DIAGNOSIS

- *Urticaria is characterized by large, irregularly shaped pruritic, erythematous wheals.*
- *Angioedema is painless, deeper, subcutaneous swelling, often involving periorbital, circumoral, and facial regions.*
- *Anaphylaxis is a systemic reaction with cutaneous symptoms, associated with dyspnea, visceral edema, and hypotension.*
- *These disorders may be diagnosed clinically, especially in the context of allergen exposure; detection of specific IgE or elevated serum tryptase can confirm diagnosis.*

General Considerations

Certain allergens—especially drugs, insect venoms, and foods—may induce an IgE antibody response, causing a generalized release of mediators from mast cells and resulting in systemic anaphylaxis. This potentially fatal condition affects both nonatopic and atopic persons. Isolated urticaria and angioedema are more common cutaneous forms of anaphylaxis with a better prognosis.

Clinical Findings

A. SYMPTOMS AND SIGNS

The manifestations are (1) hypotension or shock from widespread vasodilation, (2) respiratory distress from bronchospasm or laryngeal edema, (3) gastrointestinal and uterine muscle contraction, and (4) urticaria and angioedema.

B. LABORATORY FINDINGS

In vivo allergy skin testing and in vitro RAST testing can detect allergen-specific IgE for a variety of foods, hymenoptera (bee, wasp, hornet, fire ant) venom, latex, and some medicines. Skin testing for food allergy is appropriate only if the patient has symptoms consistent with IgE-mediated allergy (eg, urticaria, angioedema, or anaphylaxis) within 2 hours after eating the suspect food.

Determination of serum tryptase can be used to identify recent anaphylactic reactions or other reactions due to systemic mast cell activation. Tryptase is a mast cell-derived neutral protease with a half-life of 60–90 minutes. Elevated tryptase levels have been associated with anaphylaxis, systemic mastocytosis, and non-IgE-mediated diseases characterized by mast cell degranulation ("anaphylactoid reactions"). Histamine is released during these disorders but has a very short serum half-life, making detection difficult even during symptomatic periods.

Treatment

A. TREATMENT OF ANAPHYLAXIS

At the first suspicion, aqueous epinephrine 1:1000 in a dose of 0.2–0.5 mL (0.2–0.5 mg) is injected subcutaneously or intramuscularly. Repeated injections can be given every 15–30 minutes when necessary. Rapid intravenous infusion of large volumes of fluids (saline, lactated Ringer's, plasma, colloid solutions, or plasma expanders) is essential to replace loss of intravascular plasma into tissues. Other vasopressor drugs (high-dose dopamine, norepinephrine, phenylephrine) may be necessary if the patient remains hypotensive despite epinephrine.

Airway obstruction may be caused by edema of the larynx and hypopharynx or by bronchospasm. The former is treated by maintenance of an airway with endotracheal intubation or trachcostomy. Bronchospasm responds to subcutaneous epinephrine or terbutaline. Inhalation of selective β$_2$-adrenergic agonists such as albuterol or terbutaline and intravenous administration of theophylline are effective for bronchospasm.

Antihistamines (H$_1$ and H$_2$ receptor antagonists) may be useful as adjuvant therapy for alleviating the cutaneous manifestations of urticaria or angioedema and pruritus and for the gastrointestinal and uterine smooth muscle spasms. Corticosteroids will not reverse respiratory obstruction or shock. Long-term combined oral antihistamine and prednisone therapy reduces the number and severity of attacks in patients with frequent life-threatening episodes of idiopathic anaphylaxis. Medical therapy does not reliably prevent true IgE-mediated hypersensitivity reactions.

There may be a clinical late-phase response in anaphylaxis, causing a recrudescence of symptoms hours (most commonly 6–12 hours) after exposure to the allergen. Since this may occur after subsidence of the immediate-phase response, all patients with anaphylaxis should be monitored for up to 24 hours.

Anaphylaxis in a patient being treated with β-adrenergic blocker drugs is a special problem because of refractoriness to epinephrine and selective β-adrenergic agonists. Higher doses of adrenergic drugs are required for the desired effect; glucagon in patients taking beta-blockers may be beneficial. Patients being treated with angiotensin-converting enzyme (ACE) inhibitors may suffer from more severe hypotension due to blockade of renin-angiotensin-dependent compensatory mechanisms.

B. TREATMENT OF URTICARIA AND ANGIOEDEMA

These disorders are discussed fully in Chapter 6.

C. VENOM IMMUNOTHERAPY

Patients with immediate hypersensitivity reactions to stinging insects and documented venom-specific IgE on allergy testing should receive venom immunotherapy for prevention of anaphylaxis. Untreated individuals have a 50–60% risk of anaphylactic response to subsequent stings. Venom immunotherapy is highly protective, affording 98% protection from life-threatening reactions on rechallenge.

Charous BL et al: Natural rubber latex allergy after 12 years: Recommendations and perspectives. J Allergy Clin Immunol 2002;109(1 Part 1):31. [PMID: 11799362

Kaplan AP: Diagnostic tests for urticaria and angioedema. Clin Allergy Immunol 2000;15:111. [PMID: 10943290]

Korenblat P et al: A retrospective study of epinephrine administration for anaphylaxis: how many doses are needed? Allergy Asthma Proc 1999;20:383. [PMID: 10624495]

Reisman RE: Insect stings. N Engl J Med 1994;331:523. [PMID: 8041420] (Venom immunotherapy is effective in decreasing the risk of anaphylactic reactions in people at risk to 2% after 3 years of therapy.)

DRUG ALLERGY

Clinical Findings

A. SYMPTOMS AND SIGNS

The development of symptoms and the nature of the reaction can suggest whether an immunologic process is responsible for symptoms. In previously sensitized individuals, immediate hypersensitivity is manifested by rapid development of urticaria, angioedema, or anaphylaxis. Delayed onset of urticaria accompanied by fever, arthralgias, and nephritis may indicate the development of an immune complex-mediated disorder. Many drugs can be associated with recognizable known toxicities, drug interactions, or idiosyncratic reactions that are not immune-mediated. These must be distinguished from true hypersensitivity reactions because the prognosis and management differs.

B. LABORATORY FINDINGS

1. Allergy testing—Allergy skin testing is available for a limited number of drugs, since patients may react to the native drug as well as any metabolite that covalently binds to native protein and becomes immunoreactive. Skin testing is available for patients with suspected immediate hypersensitivity to penicillin or beta-lactam antibiotics. The degree of cross-reactivity between the cephalosporin antibiotics and penicillins is uncertain. The incidence of IgE-mediated hypersensitivity appears to be less than 5%. There appears to be no allergic cross-reactivity between the monobactam antibiotics (aztreonam) and penicillin or other beta-lactam antibiotics. A high degree of cross-reactivity exists between penicillin and the carbapenem, imipenem, so this drug should be given to the penicillin-allergic patient with the same degree of caution as if the patient were to receive penicillin.

If the likelihood of immunologic reaction is low—based on the history and the assessment of likely offending agents—and if no allergy testing is available, judicious test dose challenges may be considered in a monitored setting. If the likelihood of IgE-mediated reaction is significant, these challenges are risky and rapid drug desensitization is indicated.

2. Provocation tests—Occasionally, direct allergen challenge of the target organ or tissue under controlled conditions is required for definitive diagnosis. Such challenges may be bronchial, nasal, conjunctival, oral, or cutaneous. A positive test confirms that the reaction can be caused by the test substance, but it does not prove that an immunologic mechanism is responsible.

a. Bronchoprovocation testing—Natural provocation field testing can be done by having the patient make serial determinations of peak expiratory flow rate (PEFR) using a portable peak flowmeter during periods of natural exposure to a suspected airborne allergen. Bronchoprovocation is not necessary in the routine diagnosis of allergic asthma, but it may be helpful in some cases of occupational asthma. Bronchial provocation with exercise or with inhalation of methacholine, histamine, or cold air can document the presence of nonspecific bronchial hyperactivity during the diagnostic workup for respiratory symptoms but does not detect allergic sensitivities.

b. Oral provocation—In most cases of suspected allergy to a food or drug, placebo-controlled oral challenge is the definitive test. To be considered a positive result, the reported clinical findings must be reproduced during provocation testing. A blinded provocation test may be preceded by an open challenge (no placebo control), which, if negative, negates the necessity for logistically difficult blinded challenge. Freeze-dried foods in large opaque capsules provide a sufficient dose of allergen for testing. This should not be done in patients with suspected food-induced anaphylaxis.

Treatment

Acute rapid desensitization for IgE allergy to certain drugs—especially penicillin and insulin—has been successful in many cases. This is accomplished by a course of oral or parenteral doses starting with extremely low doses (dilutions of 1×10^{-6} or 1×10^{-5} units) and increasing to the full dose over a period of hours. IgE-mediated reactivity diminishes during the course of this desensitization, creating a temporary drug-specific refractory state. During the refractory period, skin histamine responsiveness is maintained, and mast cells may be activated by other stimuli but the patient may receive the desired drug with a very low risk of anaphylaxis. Acute rapid desensitization may work through cellular mechanisms different from those involved in standard injection immunotherapy, and the refractory period is maintained only throughout the course of uninterrupted therapy.

Marshall GD Jr et al: Determining allergic versus nonallergic drug reactions. Clin Allergy Immunol 2000;15:217. [PMID:10943295]

Patterson R et al: Drug allergy and protocols for management of drug allergies. Allergy Proc 1994;15:239. [NLM Cit ID: 95137378]

Sampson HA, Ho DG: Relationship between food-specific IgE concentrations and the risk of positive food challenges in children and adolescents. J Allergy Clin Immunol 1997; 100:444. [NLM Cit ID: 97478240]

IMMUNE COMPLEX DISEASE
(Serum Sickness)

 ESSENTIALS OF DIAGNOSIS

- Fever, pruritus, and arthropathy.
- Reaction is delayed in onset, usually 7–10 days, when specific-IgG antibodies are generated against the allergen.
- Immune complexes found circulating in serum or deposited in affected tissues.

General Considerations

Serum sickness reactions occur when immune complexes are formed by the binding of antigens (eg, drugs, heterologous serum) to antibodies. Deposition of these complexes in tissues or in vascular endothelium can produce immune complex-mediated tissue injury by activation of complement, generation of anaphylatoxins, chemoattraction of polymorphonuclear leukocytes, and tissue injury. The commonly affected organs include skin (urticaria, vasculitis), joints (arthritis), and kidney (nephritis).

Clinical Findings

A. SYMPTOMS AND SIGNS

Constitutional symptoms, such as drug fever, are common.

B. LABORATORY FINDINGS

The specific IgG antibody may be present in sufficient quantity in serum to be detected by the precipitin-in-gel method. Detection of these precipitating antibodies by gel diffusion can be useful in the diagnosis of allergic bronchopulmonary aspergillosis or hypersensitivity pneumonitis. ELISA will detect antibodies present in lesser amounts.

Circulating antigen-nonspecific immune complexes can be detected in a variety of malignancies and in autoimmune, hypersensitivity, and infectious diseases. Immunohistochemical techniques can identify immune complexes or complement fragments deposited in tissue biopsy specimens. Depressed serum levels of C3, C4, or CH50 may be sought as nonspecific evidence of immune complex disease with consumption of soluble factors.

The erythrocyte sedimentation rate is increased, and other nonspecific laboratory findings may include elevated hepatic aminotransferases or reduced complement levels. Circulating immune complexes may be found, but current assays are limited in sensitivity. Evidence of nephritis may be found by observing red cell casts at urinalysis.

Treatment

This disease is self-limited, so treatment is usually conservative. Aspirin will relieve the arthralgias. Antihistamines and topical steroids will control the dermatitis. Corticosteroid therapy may be necessary for serious reactions—especially glomerulonephritis, neuropathy, and other manifestations of vasculitis.

PSEUDOALLERGIC REACTIONS

These reactions resemble immediate hypersensitivity reactions but are not mediated by allergen-IgE interaction. Instead, direct mast cell activation occurs. Examples of pseudoallergic or "anaphylactoid" reactions include the now rare "red man syndrome" from rapid infusion of vancomycin, direct mast cell activation by opioids, and radiocontrast reactions. In contrast to IgE-mediated reactions, these can often be prevented by prophylactic medical regimens.

Radiocontrast Media Reactions

Reactions to radiocontrast media do not appear to be mediated by IgE antibodies, yet clinically they are similar to anaphylaxis. If a patient has had an anaphylactoid reaction to conventional radiocontrast media, the risk for a second reaction upon reexposure may be as high as 30%. Patients with asthma or those being treated with β-adrenergic blocking medications may be at increased risk. The management of patients at risk for radiocontrast medium reactions includes use of the low-osmolality contrast preparations and prophylactic administration of prednisone (50 mg orally every 6 hours beginning 18 hours before the procedure) and diphenhydramine (25–50 mg intramuscularly 60 minutes before the procedure). The use of the lower-osmolality radiocontrast media in combination with the pretreatment regimen decreases the incidence of reactions to less than 1%.

■ II. CLINICAL IMMUNOLOGY

CELLS INVOLVED IN IMMUNITY

Development of T & B Lymphocytes

Thymus-derived cells (T lymphocytes) mediate cellular immune responses; bone marrow-derived cells (B lymphocytes) are involved in humoral immunity. Both T and B lymphocytes are derived from precursor or stem cells in the marrow. Precursors of T cells migrate to the thymus, where they develop some of the functional and cell surface characteristics of mature T cells. Through positive and negative selection, clones of autoreactive T cells are eliminated, and mature T cells migrate to the peripheral lymphoid tissues. There they enter the pool of long-lived lymphocytes that recirculate from the blood to the lymph.

B cell maturation proceeds in antigen-independent and antigen-dependent stages. Antigen-independent maturation includes development from precursor cells in the marrow through the naive B cell (a cell that has not been exposed to antigen previously) found in the peripheral lymphoid tissues. Antigen-dependent maturation occurs following the interaction of antigen with naive B cells. The final products of B cell development are circulating long-lived memory B cells and plasma cells found predominantly in primary follicles and germinal centers of the lymph nodes and spleen. Plasma cells are terminally differentiated B cells responsible for synthesis and secretion of immunoglobulin.

Subpopulations of T Cells

T lymphocytes are heterogeneous with respect to their cell surface features (Table 19–2) and functional characteristics. At least three subpopulations of T cells are now recognized.

A. Helper-Inducer T Cells

These cells help to amplify the production of antibody-forming cells from B lymphocytes after interaction with antigen. Helper (CD4) T cells also amplify the production of effector T cells that mediate cytotoxicity. Activated CD4 T cells regulate immune responses by two mechanisms: through cell-to-cell contact and through elaboration of soluble factors or cytokines. Two subsets of helper T cells can be identified on the basis of their pattern of cytokine production. The subsets are called type 1 T helper (TH1) cells, which produce interleukin (IL)-2 and gamma interferon; and type 2 T helper (TH2) cells, which produce interleukins-4, -5, and -6, among others. Both subsets produce IL-3 and GM-CSF. The TH1 subset of CD4 T cells provides cellular immune responses to intracellular pathogens and underlies the pathogenesis of delayed-type hypersensitivity.

TH2 helper T cells play a central role in immediate hypersensitivity and humoral immune responses, since IL-4 promotes IgE production and IL-5 is an eosinophil proliferation and differentiation factor (Table 19–3).

B. Cytotoxic or Killer T Cells

These cells are generated after mature T cells interact with certain foreign antigens. They are responsible for defense against intracellular pathogens (eg, viruses), tumor immunity, and organ graft rejection. Most

Table 19–2. Selected surface antigens on immune cells detected by monoclonal antibodies.

Cluster of Differentiation	Primary Cellular Distribution	Function
CD2	T cells, NK cells	Adhesion molecule
CD3	Pan-T cell marker	T cell receptor
CD4	T helper-inducer cells, macrophage	Binds to MHC class II
CD5	T cells, B cell subset	
CD7	T cells	
CD8	T cytotoxic-suppressor cells	Binds MHC class I
CD10	Immature B cells	CALLA; also found in ALL
CD11a CD11b CD11c	Leukocytes	Adhesion molecule
CD13/33	Granulocytes	Granulocyte marker
CD14	Monocytes	Monocyte marker
CD16/56	NK cells	NK cell markers; CD16 is low-affinity Fcγ receptor
CD19	Pan-B cell marker	Appears early in B cell maturation
CD20/21/22	B cell markers	Appear after CD19; CD21 is complement receptor (CR2)
CD23	Activated B cells, macrophages	Low-affinity Fcε receptor
CD25	Activated T, B cells and macrophages	IL-2 receptor; activation marker
CD28	T cells	Costimulatory receptor
CD34	Hematopoietic progenitor cells	"Stem cell" marker
CD38	Plasma cells	
CD45	Leukocytes	Panleukocyte marker
CD45RA/RO	T cells	CD45RA on "naive" T cells; CD45RO on "memory" T cells

killer T cells express the CD8 phenotype, though in certain circumstances CD4 T cells can be cytotoxic. Cytotoxic T cells may kill their target through osmotic lysis, by secretion of tumor necrosis factor (TNF), or by induction of apoptosis, ie, programmed cell death.

C. SUPPRESSOR T CELLS

Suppressor T cells are CD8 regulatory cells that modulate antibody formation and cellular immunity in an antigen-specific manner. It is unclear, however, whether suppressor T cells are a distinct T cell phenotype or if their inhibitory functions merely reflect the profile of the factors they secrete.

B Lymphocytes

The majority of B cells express both IgM and IgD on the surface and are derived from pre-B cells found mainly in the bone marrow. Pre-B cells contain intracytoplasmic IgM but do not express surface immunoglobulin.

B cells have been commonly identified by other surface markers in addition to immunoglobulins. These include the receptor for the Fc portion of immunoglobulins, B cell-specific antigens CD19 and CD20, and surface antigens coded for by the HLA-D genetic region in humans. All mature B cells bear surface immunoglobulin that is the antigen-specific receptor. The major role of B cells is differentiation to antibody-secreting plasma cells. However, B cells may also release cytokines and function as antigen-presenting cells.

Other Cells Involved in Immune Responses

A. MACROPHAGES

Macrophages are involved in the ingestion, processing, and presentation of antigens for interaction with lymphocytes. These CD14 cells play an important role in T and B lymphocyte cooperation in the induction of antibody responses. In addition, they are effector cells for certain types of tumor immunity.

Table 19–3. Major activities of selected cytokines.

Cytokine	Primary Biologic Activity
IL-1	Major source is activated macrophages. Enhances T and B cell activation. Endogenous pyrogen and major inflammatory mediator.
IL-2	Autocrine and paracrine T cell activation and growth factor.
IL-3	Multilineage hematopoietic growth factor.
IL-4	T and B cell growth factor. Induces IgE isotype switching; TH2 CD4 cell and mast cell growth factor.
IL-5	Promotes eosinophil growth and differentiation and IgA synthesis.
IL-6	B cell differentiation factor; acute phase reactant.
IL-7	Growth factor for very early B and T lymphocytes.
IL-8	Chemotactic factor for neutrophils, lymphocytes. Up-regulates adhesion molecule expression.
IL-10	Down-regulates cellular activation. Inhibits production of proinflammatory cytokines by monocytes and macrophages.
IL-12	Augments IFN-γ production, enhances TH1 CD4 response.
IL-13	Functions overlap with those of IL-4.
TNF	Overlaps with activity with IL-1 but has more antitumor activity. Mediates host response to gram-negative bacteria and systemic toxicity of LPS.
IFN-α, -β, −γ	Antiviral and antitumor activities. Activates macrophages. Enhances cytotoxic lymphocyte and NK activity.
GM-CSF	Growth factor for granulocytes, macrophages, and eosinophils. Activates neutrophil phagocytosis. Enhances eosinophil-mediated cytotoxicity. Promotes basophil histamine release.
TGF-β	Major regulatory factor, inhibiting leukocyte growth, proliferation and proinflammatory cytokines.

B. NK (NATURAL KILLER) CELLS

These lymphocytic cells, which are indirectly related to the T cell lineage, can kill a wide spectrum of target cells. They are recognized by the presence of specific surface antigens (CD16 or CD56) and Fc receptors. Many appear as large granular lymphocytes. Their role in host defense is probably the killing of virally infected cells and tumor cells in the absence of prior sensitization and without MHC restriction.

Cytokines

Many T cell functions are mediated by cytokines, humoral factors secreted by immunologically active cells. Cytokines are secreted when cells are activated by antigens or other cytokines. Table 19–3 lists some examples of cytokines and their functions. The cytokines can be functionally organized into groups according to their major activities: (1) those that promote and mediate natural immunity, such as IL-1, IL-6, interferon (IFN)-γ, and IL-8; (2) those that support allergic inflammation, such as IL-4, IL-5, and IL-13; (3) those controlling lymphocyte regulatory activity, such as IL-10, produced by the TH2 helper T cell, and IFN-γ and IL-12, which are produced by the TH1 T helper cell; and (4) those that act as hematopoietic growth factors (IL-3, IL-7, and GM-CSF). This complicated network of interacting cytokines functions to modulate and regulate cellular function in such a way that the host is able to survive in a hostile environment.

Favero J et al: Effector pathways regulating T cell activation. Biochem Pharmacol 1998;56:1539. [PMID: 9973174]

Kay AB: Allergy and allergic diseases. First of two parts. N Engl J Med 2001;344:30. [PMID: 11136958]

Kay AB: Allergy and allergic diseases. Second of two parts. N Engl J Med 2001 344:109. [PMID: 11150362] (Part 1 discusses the pathophysiology of allergic diseases and allergic inflammation, including the contribution of genetic and environmental factors and cellular mechanisms of disease. Part 2 discusses allergic diseases and their treatments.)

Romagnani S: T-cell subsets (Th1 versus Th2). Ann Allergy Asthma Immunol 2000;85:9. [PMID: 10923599]

Seaman WE: Natural killer cells and natural killer T cells. Arthritis Rheum 2000;43:1204. [PMID: 10857779]

Teyton L et al: Function and dysfunction of T cell receptor: structural studies. Immunol Res 2000;21:325. [PMID: 10852133]

TESTS FOR CELLULAR IMMUNITY

Leukocyte Immunophenotyping by Flow Cytometry

Utilizing fluorescent-labeled monoclonal antibodies directed against specific cell surface antigens, or clusters of differentiation (CD), leukocytes can be immunophenotyped and enumerated by flow cytometry. During lymphocyte development, different patterns of CD markers are expressed at various stages of maturation (Table 19–2). Flow cytometry segregates populations of leukocytes for analysis by cellular size and complexity. By these parameters, polymorphonuclear cells and monocytes can be enumerated and analyzed separately from peripheral blood lymphocyte populations.

In normal individuals, roughly 75% of circulating lymphocytes are T cells (CD3), two-thirds of which are CD4 T helper-inducer cells and one-third CD8 suppressor or cytotoxic T cells. CD19 B cells make up 7–24% of circulating lymphocytes, and the remainder are CD16/CD56 NK cells. Lymphocyte immunophenotyping can be utilized in suspected cases of immunodeficiency or lymphoproliferative syndromes or following organ transplantation.

Thymic hypoplasia (DiGeorge syndrome) is associated with a marked decrease in the number of T cells in the peripheral blood; the absence of B cells in the blood is a feature of X-linked agammaglobulinemia. Marked reductions of both T and B cells occur in severe combined immunodeficiency disease (SCID). Patients with AIDS have reduced numbers of T cells and reduced CD4:CD8 ratios.

Many hematologic neoplasms can express aberrant CD markers or lose characteristic phenotypic patterns. B cell lymphomas can express inappropriate maturational markers or even T cell- or granulocyte-associated clusters of differentiation. In lymphoproliferative diseases, the suspicious lymphocyte population may demonstrate a monoclonal pattern by bearing surface immunoglobulin of a single isotype (IgM, IgG or IgA) or a single immunoglobulin light chain (κ or λ). Immunophenotyping may be used in conjunction with histopathologic analysis of bone marrow biopsies and fine-needle aspirates from suspicious lymph nodes or peripheral blood. In poorly differentiated leukemias and lymphomas, it can also provide prognostic information and help optimize treatment regimens.

T Cell Antigen Receptors

The structure of T cell antigen receptors and the genes that encode these glycoproteins have been defined. The receptor structure is a complex of two molecules, one containing variable α/β or γ/δ chains and the other the monomorphic CD3 molecule. Genes encoding the β chain are homologous with immunoglobulin genes. Rearrangement of T cell receptor genes proceeds during T cell development to generate diversity for antigen recognition in a fashion similar to that of immunoglobulin genes in B cells. Lymphoid malignancies often feature chromosomal translocations that occur disproportionately in or near the T cell receptor genes. Identification of T cell receptor gene rearrangements have been used to distinguish clonal T cell leukemias and lymphomas from reactive processes.

Functional Testing of Cell-Mediated Immunity

A. Delayed Type Hypersensitivity Skin Testing

Cell-mediated immune function can be assessed qualitatively by evaluating skin reactivity following intradermal injection of a battery of recall antigens to which humans are frequently sensitized (ie, streptokinase, streptodornase, purified protein derivative, trichophyton, dermatophyton, mumps, tetanus, or candida). Intradermal injections of 0.1 mL of recommended test strengths are observed for maximal induration and erythema at 24 and 48 hours. A positive reaction varies in size with particular antigens but is generally 5–10 mm in diameter. Anergy or lack of skin reactivity to all of these substances indicates a depression of cell-mediated immunity. Delayed hypersensitivity skin tests depend on complex interactions of T cells, macrophages, and other immunoreactants; thus, failure to respond cannot identify the exact cellular defect.

Patch testing can be clinically indicated for the diagnosis of suspected allergic contact dermatitis. The patch test is performed by topical application of the suspected contactant allergen. A positive test at 48–72 hours consists of erythema, swelling, and papules. Concentrations of allergens for patch testing must be screened in nonallergic subjects to avoid false-positive irritant responses.

B. In Vitro Lymphocyte Proliferation After Stimulation With Mitogens or Antigens

T lymphocytes are transformed to blast cells upon short-term incubation with mitogens or recall antigens in vitro. Mitogens stimulate lymphocytes nonspecifically. Phytohemagglutinin (PHA), pokeweed mitogen (PWM), and concanavalin A (ConA) can all be used in clinical laboratory assays. T cell activation is determined quantitatively by following the cellular uptake and incorporation of [^{3}H]thymidine introduced into the culture medium. The uptake indicates T cell function and correlates well with other manifestations of cell-mediated immunity as measured by skin tests. These tests can detect abnormalities in T cells despite normal or slightly reduced cell counts, particularly following bone marrow transplantation or in congenital immunodeficiency diseases. Stimulation of recipients' lymphocytes or donor lymphocytes (the mixed lymphocyte reaction) is a critical test for determining histocompatibility, especially after renal and bone marrow transplantation.

Dutton RW et al: T cell memory. Annu Rev Immunol 1998;16:201. [PMID: 9597129]

Wulfing C et al: Visualizing the dynamics of T cell activation. Proc Natl Acad Sci U S A 1998; 95:6302. [PMID: 9600960]

IMMUNOGLOBULIN STRUCTURE & FUNCTION

Disorders of immune function are the cause of many human illnesses. The basic unit of all immunoglobulins consists of four polypeptide chains linked by disulfide bonds. There are two identical heavy chains and two identical light chains. Both heavy and light chains have a carboxyl terminal constant (C) region and an amino terminal variable (V) region. A hypervariable portion of the V regions of heavy and light chains folded together in a three-dimensional conformation forms the combining site, which is responsible for the specific interaction with antigen.

Antibodies contain one of five classes of heavy chains (γ, α, μ, δ, and ε) and one of two types of light chains (κ and λ). About 10 million different antibody specificities are thought to exist in a given individual.

Immunoglobulin Classes

A. IMMUNOGLOBULIN M (IgM)

The IgM molecule is found predominantly in the intravascular compartment and on the surface of B lymphocytes and does not normally cross the placenta. IgM antibody predominates in early, primary immune responses; carbohydrate antigens such as blood group antigens stimulate IgM.

B. IMMUNOGLOBULIN A (IgA)

IgA is present in blood and in relatively high concentrations in saliva, colostrum, tears, and secretions of the bronchi and gastrointestinal tract. Secretory IgA plays an important role in host defense against viral and bacterial infections by blocking transport of mi crobes across mucosa.

C. IMMUNOGLOBULIN G (IgG)

IgG comprises about 85% of total serum immunoglobulins and is distributed in the extracellular fluid; it is the only immunoglobulin that normally crosses the placenta. Antigen-bound IgG fixes complement via the Fc region of the constant chain. Immune effector cells express Fc receptors and complement receptors that facilitate phagocytosis and cytolysis. Immune complex activation of the classic complement pathway also generates soluble factors that chemoattract neutrophils, increase vascular permeability, and amplify the inflammatory response.

D. IMMUNOGLOBULIN E (IgE)

IgE is present in serum in very low concentrations as a single immunoglobulin unit with ε heavy chains. Fifty percent of patients with allergic diseases have increased serum IgE levels. The specific interaction between antigen and mast cell-bound IgE results in the release of histamine, leukotrienes, proteases, chemotactic factors, and cytokines. These mediators can produce bronchospasm, vasodilation, increased vascular permeability, smooth muscle contraction, and chemoattraction of other inflammatory and immune cells.

E. IMMUNOGLOBULIN D (IgD)

IgD is present in the serum in very low concentrations and is found on the surface of most B lymphocytes in association with IgM, where it probably serves as a receptor for antigen.

Tests for Immunoglobulins

In some diseases, increased serum immunoglobulins, especially monoclonal types, are critical for diagnosis. Chronic liver diseases, chronic infection, or idiopathic inflammatory states can cause polyclonal or oligoclonal increases in immunoglobulins which are incidental or of unknown significance. If immunodeficiency is suspected in the presence of recurrent bacterial infections, measurement of serum immunoglobulin levels provides an essential test of B cell and plasma cell function. In acquired immune deficiencies such as AIDS, paradoxical increases in immunoglobulins can occur.

Antibodies and immunoglobulins can be measured in three ways: (1) by quantitative and qualitative determinations of serum immunoglobulins; (2) by determination of isohemagglutinin and febrile agglutinin titers; and (3) by determination of antibody titers following immunization with tetanus toxoid, diphtheria toxoid, or pneumococcal polysaccharide vaccines. The first method tests for the presence of serum immunoglobulins but not for the functional adequacy of the immunoglobulins. The second tests for functional antibodies present in the serum of almost all individuals as a consequence of exposure to blood group antigens (ABO blood groups) or infection. The third method examines functional humoral immunity in the serum after intentional immunization.

Protein Electrophoresis & Immunoelectrophoresis

Serum protein electrophoresis is a test to measure semiquantitatively various proteins in serum or urine. Proteins are electrically separated on a strip of cellulose acetate on the basis of charge, into albumin, α_1, α_2, β, and γ globulins. This test is useful to screen for diseases with excess or deficiency of immunoglobulins.

Immunoelectrophoresis is used to identify the specific immunoglobulin class in a body fluid. Serum, for example, is separated electrophoretically and then reacted with appropriate antisera directed against IgG, IgA, or IgM. The resulting patterns allow identification of abnormal immunoglobulins such as myeloma (M) proteins. This method is also useful in differentiation of monoclonal from polyclonal increases in immunoglobulins. It is only semiquantitative and thus cannot be used to determine immunoglobulin levels precisely, eg, in Waldenström's macroglobulinemia.

A similar technique called immunofixation electrophoresis has to a large extent replaced immunoelectrophoresis. Serum proteins are separated electrophoretically in a gel and then immunoprecipitated in situ with monospecific antisera. This method has the advantages of more rapid results and slightly higher resolution of low levels of monoclonal immunoglobulin chains. If protein electrophoresis is normal despite suspicion of an M protein, immunoelectrophoresis or immunofixation electrophoresis of both serum and concentrated urine should be performed because of the greater sensitivity of these tests combined.

Quantitative Immunoglobulin Determinations

Quantitative determinations of total serum IgG, IgA, IgE, and IgM levels can be made rapidly and accurately by nephelometry. Nephelometry detects scattered light when specific antiserum immunoprecipitates soluble antigen. Antiserum is available for a variety of antigens, including all immunoglobulin isotypes. Measurement of serum IgD levels has no recognized clinical use, and antigen-specific IgE levels should be measured with more sensitive techniques such as in vitro radioallergosorbent testing (RAST) or in vivo allergy skin testing.

Functional Testing of Humoral Immunity

Laboratory evaluation of humoral function should include assessment of specific antibody responses. Isohemagglutinins are naturally occurring IgM antibodies against ABO blood groups and can be detected in most patients depending on blood type. Humoral responses can also be assessed by immunization with protein and carbohydrate antigens. This is most easily accomplished by measuring antitetanus, antidiphtheria, and antipneumococcal antibody titers before and 3–4 weeks after vaccination with diphtheria-tetanus (dT) and polyvalent pneumococcal vaccine. In this context, a fourfold increase in antibody titer is considered normal. In patients suspected to be suffering from humoral immunodeficiency, quantification of IgG subclasses may be appropriate, particularly when total IgG immunoglobulins are at the low end of the normal range.

Bengten E et al: Immunoglobulin isotypes: structure, function, and genetics. Curr Top Microbiol Immunol 2000;248:189. [PMID: 10793479] (A comprehensive review.)

Huston DP: The biology of the immune system. JAMA 1997;278:1804. [PMID: 9396641] (Provides a framework for understanding physiologic immune responses and the pathogenesis of immunologic disorders.)

Rose NR, Hamilton RG, Detrick B (editors): *Manual of Clinical Laboratory Immunology*, 6th ed. American Society for Microbiology, 2002. (General reference for diagnostic laboratory immunology.)

■ IMMUNODEFICIENCY DISORDERS

The primary immunologic deficiency diseases include congenital and acquired disorders of humoral immunity (B cell function) or cell-mediated immunity (T cell function). Most of these diseases are rare, and since they are genetically determined, are seen primarily in children. Several immunodeficiency disorders affect adults, and are discussed below. The WHO classification of immunodeficiency disorders

more often affecting adults is set forth in the accompanying box.

WHO CLASSIFICATION

- Primary Immunodeficiency Disorders:

  Selective IgA deficiency.

  Common variable immunodeficiency.

  X-linked agammaglobulinemia.

  Immunodeficiency with normal serum globulins or hyperimmunoglobulinemia.

  Immunodeficiency with thymoma.

- Secondary Immunodeficiency Disorders (for example, AIDS)

Buckley RH: Advances in immunology: primary immunodeficiency diseases due to defects in lymphocytes. N Engl J Med 2000;343:1313. [PMID: 11058677]

Sicherer SH et al: Primary immunodeficiency diseases in adults. JAMA 1998;279:58. [NLM Cit ID: 98084662]

SELECTIVE IMMUNOGLOBULIN A DEFICIENCY

Selective IgA deficiency is the most common primary immunodeficiency disorder and is characterized by the absence of serum IgA with normal levels of IgG and IgM; its prevalence is about 1:500 individuals. Most patients are asymptomatic because of compensatory increases in secreted IgG and IgM. Some affected patients have frequent and recurrent infections such as sinusitis, otitis, and bronchitis. Some cases of IgA deficiency may spontaneously remit. When IgG$_2$ subclass deficiency occurs in combination with IgA deficiency, affected patients are more susceptible to encapsulated bacteria and the degree of immune impairment can be more severe. Patients with a combined IgA and IgG subclass deficiency should be assessed for functional antibody responses to glycoprotein antigen immunization.

Atopic disease and autoimmune disorders can be associated with IgA deficiency. Occasionally, a sprue-like syndrome with steatorrhea has been associated with an isolated IgA deficit. Treatment with commercial immune globulin is ineffective, since IgA and IgM are present only in trace quantities in these preparations. Frequent infusions of plasma (containing IgA) or unwashed blood transfusions are hazardous, since anti-IgA antibodies may develop, resulting in systemic anaphylaxis or serum sickness.

Burrows PD et al: IgA deficiency. Adv Immunol 1997;65:245. [NLM Cit ID: 97381155]

COMMON VARIABLE IMMUNODEFICIENCY

 ESSENTIALS OF DIAGNOSIS

- *Defect in terminal differentiation of B cells, with absent plasma cells and deficient synthesis of secreted antibody.*
- *Frequent sinopulmonary infections secondary to humoral immune deficiency.*
- *Confirmation by evaluation of serum immunoglobulin levels and deficient functional antibody responses.*

General Considerations

The most common cause of panhypogammaglobulinemia in adults is common variable immunodeficiency, a heterogeneous immunodeficiency disorder clinically characterized by an increased incidence of recurrent infections, autoimmune phenomena, and neoplastic diseases. The onset generally is during adolescence or early adulthood but can occur at any age. The prevalence of common variable immunodeficiency is about 1:80,000 in the United States.

Clinical Findings

A. SYMPTOMS AND SIGNS

The pattern of immunoglobulin isotype deficiency is variable. Most patients present with significantly depressed IgG levels, but over time all antibody classes (IgG, IgA, and IgM) may be affected. Increased susceptibility to pyogenic infections is the hallmark of the disease. Virtually all patients suffer from recurrent sinusitis, with bronchitis, otitis, pharyngitis, and pneumonia also being common infections. Infections may be of prolonged duration or associated with unusual complications such as meningitis or sepsis.

Gastrointestinal disorders are commonly associated, and patients may develop a sprue-like syndrome, with diarrhea, steatorrhea, malabsorption, protein-losing enteropathy, and hepatosplenomegaly. Paradoxically, there is an increased incidence of autoimmune disease (20%), though patients may not display the usual serologic markers. Autoimmune cytopenias are most common, but also commonly seen are autoimmune endocrinopathies, seronegative rheumatic disease, and gastrointestinal disorders. Lymph nodes may be enlarged in these patients, yet biopsies show marked reduction in plasma cells. Noncaseating granulomas are frequently found in the spleen, liver, lungs, or skin. There is an increased propensity for the development of B cell neoplasms (50- to 400-fold increase risk of lymphoma), gastric carcinomas, and skin cancers.

B. LABORATORY FINDINGS

Diagnosis is confirmed in patients with recurrent infections by demonstration of functional or quantitative defects in antibody production. Serum IgG levels are usually less than 250 mg/dL; serum IgA and IgM levels are also subnormal. Decreased to absent functional antibody responses to protein antigen immunizations establish the diagnosis.

The cause of the panhypogammaglobulinemia in the majority of common variable immunodeficiency patients is an intrinsic B cell defect preventing terminal maturation into antibody-secreting plasma cells. In a small number, excessive suppressor T cell activity that inhibits B cells—or helper T cell activity inadequate to assist B cells to make antibody—has been identified. The absolute B cell count in the peripheral blood in most patients, despite the underlying cellular defect, is normal. A subset of these patients have concomitant T cell immunodeficiency with increased numbers of activated CD8 cells, splenomegaly, and decreased delayed-type hypersensitivity.

Treatment

Patients may be treated aggressively with antibiotics at the first sign of infection. Since antibody deficiency predisposes patients to high-risk pyogenic infections, antibiotic coverage should be sure to cover encapsulated bacteria. Only after the development of bronchiectasis or after sinus surgery do patients become significantly affected by more virulent organisms such as *Staphylococcus aureus* or *Pseudomonas aeruginosa*. Maintenance intravenous immune globulin (IGIV) therapy is indicated, with infusions of 300–500 mg/kg of IGIV given at about monthly intervals. Adjustment of dosage or of the infusion interval is made on the basis of clinical responses and steady state trough serum IgG levels. Such therapy is effective in decreasing the incidence of potentially life-threatening infections and increasing quality of life. The yearly cost of monthly infusions can be in excess of $20,000–$30,000.

Spickett GP et al: Common variable immunodeficiency: How many diseases? Immunol Today 1997;18:325. [NLM Cit ID: 97381556]

DISEASES OF IMMUNOGLOBULIN OVERPRODUCTION (Gammopathies)

The monoclonal gammopathies include those diseases in which there is a proliferation of a single clone of immunoglobulin-forming cells that produce a homogeneous heavy chain, light chain, or complete molecule. The amino acid sequence of the variable (V) regions is fixed, and only one type (κ or λ) of light chain is produced. Polyclonal gammopathies result from proliferation of many B cell clones, resulting in a diffuse increase of immunoglobulins.

Monoclonal Gammopathy of Uncertain Significance (MGUS)

This diagnosis is made upon finding a monoclonal spike on serum protein electrophoresis, confirmed by immunoelectrophoresis to be a homogeneous immunoglobulin (with either κ or λ chains). The incidence of MGUS increases with age and may approach 3% in persons 70 years of age or older. As many as one-third of individuals with apparently benign monoclonal gammopathies will develop lymphoid malignancies, amyloidosis, or multiple myeloma. No specific therapy is necessary, but close observation is required. Risk for the development of a malignant disorder is 33% at 20 years. Parameters that suggest a favorable prognosis include (1) concentration of homogeneous immunoglobulin less than 2 g/dL, (2) no increase in concentration of the immunoglobulin from the time of diagnosis, (3) no decrease in the concentration of normal immunoglobulins, (4) absence of a homogeneous light chain in the urine, and (5) normal hematocrit and serum albumin.

Multiple Myeloma (See also Chapter 13.)

This disease is characterized by the overproduction and spread of neoplastic plasma cells throughout the bone marrow. Myeloma cells sometimes express molecules of early B cell or myelomonocytic lineages. Rarely, extraosseous plasmacytomas may be found. Anemia, hypercalcemia, increased susceptibility to infection, and bone pain are frequent. Diagnosis depends upon the presence of the following: (1) radiographic findings of osteolytic lesions or diffuse osteoporosis, (2) the presence of a homogeneous serum immunoglobulin (myeloma protein) or a single type of light chain in the urine (Bence Jones proteinuria), and (3) finding of an abnormal plasma cell infiltrate in the bone marrow biopsy (see Chapter 13). The presence of over 20% bone marrow plasma cells reliably differentiates early myeloma from MGUS. There is an approximate correlation between the incidence of immunoglobulin type in myeloma and the normal serum concentration of the immunoglobulin involved.

Waldenström's Macroglobulinemia

In Waldenström's macroglobulinemia, there is proliferation of abnormal lymphoid cells that have morphologic features of both B cells and plasma cells. These cells secrete a homogeneous macroglobulin (IgM) detectable by immunoelectrophoresis. Monoclonal light chains are present in 10% of cases. Clinical manifestations depend upon the physicochemical characteristics of the macroglobulin. Raynaud's phenomenon and peripheral vascular occlusions are associated with cold-insoluble proteins (cryoglobulins). Retinal hemorrhages, visual impairment, and transient neurologic deficits are common with high-viscosity serum. Bleeding diatheses or hemolytic anemia can occur when the macroglobulin complexes with coagulation factors or binds to the surface of red blood cells.

Amyloidosis

Amyloidosis is a group of disorders manifested by impaired organ function caused by infiltration of tissues with insoluble protein fibrils. Different fibril composition can be correlated with the clinical syndromes.

In primary amyloidosis (AL), the protein fibrils are monoclonal immunoglobulin light chains, whereas secondary amyloid (AA) proteins are derived from acute phase reactant apolipoprotein precursors. Other types of amyloidosis may also be hereditary. Over 20 types of fibrils have been identified in amyloid deposits.

Symptoms and signs of amyloid infiltration are related to malfunction of the organ involved (eg, nephrotic syndrome and renal failure, cardiomyopathy and cardiac conduction defects, intestinal malabsorption and pseudo-obstruction, carpal tunnel syndrome, macroglossia, peripheral neuropathy, end-organ insufficiency of endocrine glands, respiratory failure, and capillary damage with ecchymosis). Such widespread deposition is typical of primary amyloidosis; secondary amyloidosis more often is confined to liver, spleen, and adrenals. Familial syndromes commonly cause infiltrative neuropathies. Amyloidosis due to deposition of β_2-microglobulin in carpal ligaments occurs in chronic hemodialysis patients.

The diagnosis of primary amyloidosis is based on clinical suspicion, protein electrophoresis, and microscopic examination of biopsy specimens. In patients with systemic disease, rectal or gingival biopsies show a sensitivity of about 80%, bone-marrow biopsy about 50%, and abdominal fat aspiration between 70% and 80%. Fine-needle biopsy of subcutaneous abdominal fat is a simple and reliable method for diagnosing systemic amyloidosis.

Treatment of localized amyloid tumors is by surgical excision. There is no effective treatment of systemic amyloidosis, and death usually occurs within 1–3 years. Care is generally supportive, though hemodialysis and immunosuppressive therapy may be useful. When concomitant multiple myeloma is found, it is treated in the standard fashion (Chapter 13). Secondary disease is usually approached by aggressively treating the predisposing disease, but remission of fibril deposition does not occur.

Heavy Chain Disease
(α, γ, μ)

These are rare disorders in which the abnormal serum and urine protein is a part of a homogeneous α, γ, or μ heavy chain. The clinical presentation is more typical of lymphoma than multiple myeloma, and there are no destructive bone lesions. Gamma chain disease presents as a lymphoproliferative disorder with autoimmune features. Alpha chain disease is frequently associated with severe diarrhea and infiltration of the lamina propria of the small intestine with abnormal plasma cells. Mu chain disease is associated with chronic lymphocytic leukemia.

Bataille R et al: Multiple myeloma. N Engl J Med 1997;36:1657. [PMID: 9171069]

Buxbaum J et al: Nonamyloidotic monoclonal immunoglobulin deposition disease. Light-chain, heavy-chain, and light- and heavy-chain deposition diseases. Hematol Oncol Clin North Am 1999;13:1235. [PMID: 10626147]

Falk RH et al: The systemic amyloidoses. N Engl J Med 1997;337:898. [PMID: 9302305]

Fermand JP et al: Heavy-chain diseases. Hematol Oncol Clin North Am 1999;13:1281. [PMID: 10626151]

Kambham et al: Heavy chain deposition disease: the disease spectrum. Am J Kidney Dis 1999;33:954. [PMID: 10213655]

Kyle RA: Clinical aspects of multiple myeloma and related disorders including amyloidosis. Pathol Biol (Paris) 1999; 47:148. [PMID: 10192881]

Samuels J et al: Familial Mediterranean fever at the millennium: Clinical spectrum, ancient mutations and a survey of 100 American referrals to the National Institutes of Health. Medicine 1998;77:268. [PMID: 9715731]

■ AUTOIMMUNITY

Autoimmune diseases cannot be explained by a solitary cause or mechanism. Small amounts of autoantibodies are normally produced and may have physiologic roles in cellular interactions. The major theories regarding the development of autoimmune disease are (1) release of normally sequestered antigens; (2) escape from anergy or defective apoptosis (programmed cell death) leading to abnormal autoreactive cellular clones; (3) shared antigens between the host and microorganisms, ie, "molecular mimicry"; and (4) defects in helper or suppressor T cell function. A genetic susceptibility is also a likely determinant of autoimmune disease. In nearly all autoimmune diseases, multiple mechanisms of autoimmunity are operative.

Cell-Mediated Autoimmunity

Certain autoimmune diseases are mediated by T cells that have become specifically immunized to autologous tissues. Cytotoxic or killer T cells generated by this aberrant immune response injure specific organs in the absence of serum autoantibodies. Diminished suppressor T cell activity or loss of clonal anergy results in disordered regulation of immune function and consequent autoreactivity. The immune damage in systemic (non-organ-specific) diseases such as systemic lupus erythematosus may be due to such a mechanism.

Antibody-Mediated Autoimmunity

Several autoimmune diseases have been shown to be caused by autoantibodies in the absence of cell-mediated autoimmunity. The autoimmune hemolytic anemias, idiopathic thrombocytopenia, and Goodpasture's syndrome appear to be mediated solely by autoantibodies directed against autologous cell membrane constituents. In these diseases, antibody attaches to cell membranes and fixes complement; the ensuing inflammatory reaction injures the cells.

Anti-receptor antibodies that compete with or mimic physiologic agonists for cellular receptors cause several diseases. In Graves' disease, antibodies are present that bind to thyroid cells' TSH receptors and thereby stimulate thyroid hormone production. In rare instances of type 1 diabetes mellitus, anti-insulin receptor antibodies cause insulin resistance in peripheral target tissues. Antibodies to acetylcholine receptors of the myoneural junction in myasthenia gravis block neuromuscular transmission and produce muscle weakness.

Immune Complex Disease

In this group of diseases (systemic lupus erythematosus, lupus nephritis, rheumatoid arthritis, some drug-induced hemolytic anemias, and thrombocytopenias), autologous tissues are injured as "innocent bystanders." Autoantibodies are not directed against cellular components of the target organ but rather against autologous or heterologous antigens in the serum. The resultant antigen-antibody complexes bind nonspecifically to autologous membranes (eg, glomerular basement membrane) and fix complement. Fixation and subsequent activation of complement components produce a local inflammatory response resulting in tissue injury.

AUTOIMMUNE DISEASES
(See also Chapter 20.)

The diagnosis and treatment of specific autoimmune diseases are described elsewhere in this book. Autoantibodies associated with certain autoimmune diseases may not be pathogenetic but are thought to be markers or by-products of the injury (eg, autoimmune thyroiditis and antithyroglobulin antibody). See Table 19–4 for autoantibody patterns in connective tissue diseases.

Table 19–4. Autoantibodies: Associations with connective tissue diseases.[1]

Suspected Disease State	Test	Primary Disease Association (Sensitivity, Specificity)	Other Disease Associations	Comments
CREST[2] syndrome	Anticentromere antibody	CREST (70–90%, high)	Scleroderma (10–15%), Raynaud's disease (10–30%).	Predictive value of a positive test is > 95% for scleroderma or related disease (CREST, Raynaud's). Diagnosis of CREST is made clinically.
Systemic lupus erythematosus (SLE)	Antinuclear antibody (ANA)	SLE (> 95%, low)	Rheumatoid arthritis (30–50%), discoid lupus, scleroderma (60%), drug-induced lupus (100%), Sjögren's syndrome (80%), miscellaneous inflammatory disorders.	Often used as a screening test; a negative test virtually excludes SLE; a positive test, while nonspecific, increases posttest probability of SLE. Titer does not correlate with disease activity.
	Anti-double-stranded-DNA (anti-ds-DNA)	SLE (60–70%, high)	Lupus nephritis, rarely rheumatoid arthritis, other connective tissue disease, usually in low titer.	Predictive value of a positive test is > 90% for SLE if present in high titer; a decreasing titer may correlate with worsening renal disease. Titer generally correlates with disease activity.
	Anti-Smith antibody (anti-Sm)	SLE (30–40%, high)		SLE-specific. A positive test substantially increases posttest probability of SLE. Test rarely indicated.
Mixed connective tissue disease (MCTD)	Anti-ribonucleoprotein antibody (RNP)	Scleroderma (20–30%, low), MCTD (95–100%, low)	SLE (30%), Sjögren's syndrome, rheumatoid arthritis (10%), discoid lupus (20–30%)	A negative test essentially excludes MCTD; a positive test in high titer, while nonspecific, increases posttest probability of MCTD.
Rheumatoid arthritis	Rheumatoid factor (RF)	Rheumatoid arthritis (50–90%)	Other rheumatic diseases, chronic infections, some malignancies, some healthy individuals, elderly patients.	Titer does not correlate with disease activity.
Scleroderma	Anti-Scl-70 antibody	Scleroderma (15–20%, low)		Predictive value of a positive test is > 95% for scleroderma.
Sjögren's syndrome	Anti-SS-A/Ro antibody	Sjögren's (60–70%, low)	SLE (30–40%), rheumatoid arthritis (10%), subacute cutaneous lupus, vasculitis.	Useful in counseling women of childbearing age with known connective tissue disease, since a positive test is associated with a small but real risk of neonatal SLE and congenital heart block.
Wegener's granulomatosis	Anti-neutrophil cytoplasmic antibody (ANCA)	Wegener's granulomatosis (systemic necrotizing vasculitis) (56–96%, high)	Crescentic glomerulonephritis or other systemic vasculitis (eg, polyarteritis nodosa).	Ability of this assay to reflect disease activity remains unclear.

[1]Modified, with permission, from Harvey AM et al (editors): *The Principles and Practice of Medicine,* 22nd ed. Appleton & Lange, 1988; White RH, Robbins DL: Clinical significance and interpretation of antinuclear antibodies. West J Med 1987;147:210; and Tan EM: Autoantibodies to nuclear antigens (ANA): Their immunobiology and medicine. Adv Immunol 1982;33:167.
[2]CREST = calcinosis, Raynaud's phenomenon, esophageal dysmotility, sclerodactyly, and telangiectasia.

TESTS FOR AUTOANTIBODIES ASSOCIATED WITH AUTOIMMUNE DISEASE

Agglutination Assays

Red cells are incubated with purified specific antigen (eg, thyroglobulin), which is adsorbed to the cell surface. The antigen-coated cells are suspended in the patient's serum, and antibody is detected by red cell agglutination. Antigen-coated latex particles are substituted for red cells in latex fixation tests.

Enzyme-Linked Immunosorbent Assays (ELISA)

Antibodies to various tissue antigens can be readily detected by these tests. Extracted and purified antigens are fixed to a plastic microtiter well or beads. The patient's serum is added, and excess proteins are removed by washing and centrifugation. Adherent immunoglobulin is then detected when a second antibody coupled to an enzyme (eg, alkaline phosphatase) is added. Finally, the enzyme's substrate is added; color forms and is measured in a spectrophotometer. This test can also be adapted for antigen detection by placing the antibody on the plastic surface. ELISA assays are very sensitive and less cumbersome than radioimmunoassay techniques.

Immunofluorescence Microscopy

This technique is most frequently used for detection of antinuclear antibody (ANA). Frozen sections of mouse liver or other substrates are cut and placed on glass slides or, alternatively, monolayers of cultured cell lines may be used. A patient's serum is placed over the sections and incubated. Fluorescein-conjugated rabbit anti-human immunoglobulin is then applied and washed. Antinuclear antibody specifically binds to the nucleus, and the fluorescein conjugate binds to the human antibody. Fluorescence of the cell nucleus on microscopy indicates a positive test.

Complement Fixation

Specific antigen, unknown serum, and complement are combined. Sheep red blood cells coated with anti-sheep cell antibody are added for 30 minutes at 37 °C. If antigen-specific antibody is present in the patient's serum, complement is bound and consumed, preventing lysis of sheep red cells.

Egner W: The use of laboratory tests in the diagnosis of SLE. J Clin Pathol 2000;53:424. [PMID: 10911799]

Fleisher TA et al: Introduction to diagnostic laboratory immunology. JAMA 1997;278:1823. [PMID: 9396643] (Reviews diagnostic laboratory assays.)

Moder KG et al: The current use and interpretation of rheumatologic tests. Adolesc Med 1998;9:25. [PMID: 10961249]

Winkelstein A et al: Immunohematologic disorders. JAMA 1997;278:1982. [PMID: 9396661] (Immune reactions can produce hemolytic anemia, thrombocytopenia, or neutropenia. Autoimmune phenomena and drug-induced reactions are the most common mechanisms.)

■ IMMUNOGENETICS & TRANSPLANTATION

GENETIC CONTROL OF THE IMMUNE RESPONSE

The ability to mount a specific immune response is under the direct control of genes for the major transplantation antigens (major histocompatibility complex; MHC). These MHC molecules play a critical role in the positive and negative selection of thymocytes during T cell development, the process of antigen presentation between immunocompetent cells, and transplantation rejection reactions to foreign tissue. In a rare immunodeficiency disorder, "bare lymphocyte syndrome," the surface expression of HLA molecules is deficient, leading to impaired immune defenses and recurrent infection.

In humans, this genetic region has been designated the **human leukocyte antigen (HLA)** complex because these antigens were first detected on peripheral blood lymphocytes. The complex includes antigens HLA-A, -B, -C, -DR, and others, each with many alleles. The HLA region has been localized to chromosome 6 and codes for over 200 genes. In nearly all instances, the HLA complex is inherited intact as two haplotypes (one from each parent), and within any particular family, therefore, the number of different combinations found is 25% (ie, siblings have a 1:4 chance of being HLA-identical). In contrast, the number of antigen combinations among unrelated individuals is enormous, resulting in probabilities of less than one in several thousand, depending upon the phenotype involved, of finding HLA-compatible individuals in a random donor pool. This is particularly important when compatible donors are needed for allosensitized patients requiring platelet transfusions or organ transplantation. Family members have the highest likelihood of being compatible donors, whereas compatibility between unrelated individuals has a low probability. HLA-A and -B typing or cross-matching is utilized for selection of compatible donors for platelet transfusions to allosensitized, thrombocytopenic recipients. Typing for these class I antigens as well as for HLA-D (class II) antigens is important in determining compatibility for organ transplantation. Typing for HLA markers is of value in studying associations between the HLA system and genetic control of disease susceptibility.

Klein J et al: The HLA system. First of two parts. N Engl J Med 2000;343:702. [PMID: 10974135]

Klein J et al: The HLA system. Second of two parts. N Engl J Med 2000;343:782. [PMID: 10984567]

VanBuskirk AM et al: Transplantation immunology. JAMA 1997;278:1993. [PMID: 9396662] (This review discusses the three forms of graft rejection, each of which is addressed at the level of histopathology, pathobiology, incidence, and clinical strategies.)

ASSOCIATIONS BETWEEN HLA ANTIGENS & SPECIFIC DISEASES

In humans, very striking associations are observed between particular HLA antigens and specific diseases. Some of these are listed in Table 19–5. In some diseases, the HLA molecule may be implicated in the pathogenesis. In others, the specific HLA allele may be linked to a gene determining immune responsiveness to a particular antigen.

The standard method for detecting HLA-A, -B, and -C antigens is that of lymphocyte microcytotoxicity. Lymphocytes isolated from peripheral blood or lymph nodes are added to each well of a typing tray filled with sera containing the appropriate cytotoxic alloantibody. When complement is added, cells to which antibody has been specifically bound will have complement activated at the cell surface, resulting in cell death or lysis. It is thus possible to type for all of the known HLA-A, -B, and -C specificities. An appreciable majority of typing serum samples are obtained from multiparous women since they form antibodies to fetal alloantigens.

Typing for the class II antigens HLA-DR and -DQ by serologic methods is technically more difficult. Antigens of the HLA-D, -DR, -DQ, and -DP series may also be detected by in vitro mixed lymphocyte culture (MLC). Lymphocytes of one individual (responder cells) will undergo proliferation upon encountering lymphocytes from another individual possessing foreign HLA-DR and -DQ antigens (stimulator cells). Lymphocyte proliferation can be readily measured by DNA incorporation of tritiated thymidine. Responders possessing matching -DR and -DQ antigens will remain nonreactive.

Increasingly, HLA class II typing is being performed by molecular technology. The DNA sequences for the HLA genes and their flanking sequences are known. Selected primers that amplify the gene of interest using the polymerase chain reaction (PCR) technique are known as sequence-specific primers. HLA typing by PCR provides better resolution than serologic identification because typing is done at the genetic level.

Apanius V et al: The nature of selection on the major histocompatibility complex. Crit Rev Immunol 1997;17:179. [PMID: 9094452] (A comprehensive review of evidence for differing hypotheses on the mechanisms of gene diversity and immune responses.)

Gonzalez S et al: Immunogenetics, HLA-B27 and spondyloarthropathies. Curr Opin Rheumatol 1999;11:257. [PMID: 10411379]

McCurdy D: Genetic susceptibility to the connective tissue diseases. Curr Opin Rheumatol 1999;11:399. [PMID: 10503661]

CLINICAL TRANSPLANTATION

Organ transplants are in widespread use. Limitations include the scarcity of donor organs and expense. Failure to achieve successful grafts is primarily due to histoincompatibility and lack of safe and effective immunosuppressive regimens to halt rejection. Avoiding transmission of infectious agents (eg, HIV, HBV, HCV, CMV) from donor to recipient requires extensive pretransplant serologic testing.

Kidney Transplantation

End-stage renal disease is the indication for kidney transplantation. Factors that determine outcome include antigenic disparity (ABO blood groups and major histocompatibility or HLA) between donor and recipient, the type of immunologic response mounted by the host, and the immunosuppressive regimen used to prevent graft rejection. Nonimmunologic factors that affect the risk of chronic rejection include age and race of recipient, donor age, length of time on dialysis, and coexisting hyperlipidemia, hypertension, or cytomegalovirus infection.

Kidneys from living related donors who are HLA-identical and also red cell ABO-matched grafts have 90% survival at 1 year; grafts from less well matched relatives and from living unrelated donors have lower rates. Antigens are matched for HLA-A, -B and -DR loci, with -DR compatibility most important for long-term graft survival. Grafts from cadaver donors with zero HLA mismatches have a half-life of 11.3 years. Those with six mismatches have a half-life of 6.8 years, compared with those from HLA-identical siblings, which have a half-life of 23.6 years.

Some donors are highly sensitized to HLA antigens from previous transfusions, ie, possess high panel reactive antibody levels. It may be difficult to find a suitable donor, since a positive cross-match by cytotoxicity testing is likely and would be a contraindication to transplant. Donor screening is performed in all cases to assess suitability, rule out hypertension or anatomic anomalies, and avoid transmission of hepatitis viruses, HIV, and other infectious agents. Owing to the scarcity of related donors, living unrelated donors may be used in certain circumstances. Pretreatment of recipients with blood transfusions from the donor appears to extend graft survival even longer.

Delayed allograft function can be due to hyperacute graft rejection, post ischemic acute tubular necrosis, cyclosporine toxicity, or obstructive nephropathy. If conservative measures do not improve function or patients are at high risk of allograft rejection, renal biopsy should be performed for definitive diagnostic purposes. Renal allograft rejection may be due to hyperacute rejection from binding of cytotoxic antibod-

Table 19-5. Association between the presence of various HLA markers and selected autoimmune diseases.[1]

Disease	Associated HLA Marker[2]	Relative Risk of Disease[3]
Ankylosing spondylitis	B27	87.4
Reactive arthropathy, including Reiter's syndrome	B27	37.0
Rheumatoid arthritis	DR4	4.2
Behçet's syndrome	B51	3.8
Systemic lupus erythematosus	DR3	5.8
Insulin-dependent (type 1) diabetes mellitus	DR3	3.3
	DQB1*0201	2.4
	DR4	6.4
	DQB1*0302	9.5
	DR2	0.19
	DRB*1501[4]	
	DRB*0101[4]	
	DQB1*0602[4]	0.15
Idiopathic Addison's disease	DR3	6.3
Graves' disease	DR3	3.7
Hashimoto's disease	DR11	3.2
Postpartum thyroiditis	DR4	5.3
Celiac disease	DR3	10.8
	DQB1*0201[4]	
	DQA1*0501[4]	
	DR7,11	6.0–10.00
	DR7, DQB1*0201[4]	
	DR11, DQA1*0501[4]	
Dermatitis herpetiformis	DR3	15.9
Sicca syndrome	DR3	9.7
Myasthenia gravis	DR3	2.5
	B8	3.4
Idiopathic membranous glomerulonephritis	DR3	12.0
Goodpasture's syndrome	DR2	15.9
Multiple sclerosis	DR2	4.1
	DRB1*1501[4]	
	DRB5*0101[4]	
	DQB1*0602[4]	
Pemphigus vulgaris (among Ashkenazi Jews)	DR4	14.4
Psoriasis vulgaris	Cw6	13.3
Birdshot retinochoroidopathy	A29	109.0

[1]Reproduced, with permission, from Klein J et al: The HLA system. First of two parts. N Engl J Med 2000;343:782.
[2]Symbols with asterisks indicate alleles, and symbols without asterisks indicate serologically defined antigens. For each disease, the marker or markers with the strongest associations are given. In many cases in which it is difficult to decide whether HLA-DR or DQ markers are responsible for association, both markers are given.
[3]The relative risk indicates the frequency of a disease in persons with the HLA marker as compared with persons without the marker. A positive association (ie, when the HLA marker is more frequent in persons with the disease than in those without it) is indicated by a relative risk of more than 1.0, a negative association by a relative risk of less than 1.0, and no association by a relative risk of 1.0.
[4]The risk has not been assessed separately for this allele.

ies and complement activation, acute rejection from cellular immune responses or chronic rejection. A form of interstitial nephritis secondary to polyomavirus infection is associated with aggressive immunosuppression.

Chronic allograft nephropathy is characterized by vasculopathy and immune-mediated graft obliteration. Previous acute rejection is strongly linked with later chronic rejection, and severity of those episodes has prognostic implications. Cyclosporine-induced nephrotoxicity and recurrent or de novo renal disease are also significant factors affecting long-term survival.

High-Dose Chemotherapy With Hematopoietic Progenitor Cell Transplantation

Transient myelosuppression after cancer chemotherapy is a well-established adverse effect of such treatments. For most regimens, it is rapidly reversible and requires no intervention. Some malignancies (eg, many leukemias, lymphomas, and chemotherapy-sensitive breast and small-cell lung carcinomas) may demonstrate a higher cure rate with higher-dose therapy; however, associated with this approach is an increase in hematologic toxicity. Administering the maximal tolerated chemotherapy dose and thus restoring all hematopoietic functions as rapidly as possible has led to evolution of the concept of hematopoietic progenitor cell (HPC) or "stem cell" transplant. HPC transplants have also expanded somewhat into the therapy of certain nonmalignant disorders of hematopoiesis and hematologic function; examples are aplastic anemia, sickle cell anemia, myelodysplasia, amyloidosis, and paroxysmal nocturnal hemoglobinuria.

The sources of HPC are the bone marrow, peripheral blood, and cord blood. They comprise less than 0.5–1% of all nucleated bone marrow cells. Recently, it has become common practice to harvest HPCs from the peripheral blood by apheresis. As the peripheral blood has approximately one-fortieth the number of circulating HPCs as the bone marrow, these cells must be "mobilized" by the administration of cytotoxic chemotherapy (with the harvest being performed during the recovery phase) or enriched by the administration of hematopoietic growth factors. The cells are frozen and administered at a later date.

Because syngeneic transplants between identical (monozygotic) twins are rare, the two predominant transplants are autologous, where the HPCs are harvested from and returned to the patient; or allogeneic, where the source is an HLA-matched donor, ideally a sibling. The goals of the two procedures—and their associated adverse effects—are frequently different. Allogeneic transplants are most commonly offered to patients with malignant and nonmalignant disorders involving the bone marrow. Chemotherapy is given to ablate the marrow, resulting in maximal suppression or eradication of the recipient's native immune system. The bone marrow is repopulated by infusion of donor cells containing not only HPCs but also functional donor T lymphocytes. These T cells can cause graft-versus-host disease, in which the recipient's tissues are recognized as nonself. While this is occasionally desirable, as in the "graft-versus-leukemia" effect, it is the cause of considerable morbidity and can be fatal. There are two separate phases of graft-versus-host disease: acute, secondary to cytokine-mediated cytotoxicity against the cells of the liver, the mucosa of the gastrointestinal tract, and skin; and chronic, characterized by fibrosis and collagen deposition and resembling autoimmune disease such as scleroderma. The incidence of graft-versus-host disease can be decreased by depleting the donor marrow of T cells, but this is associated with a higher incidence of graft failure and, in the case of leukemia, a higher relapse rate. Though only a few allogeneic peripheral HPC transplants have been reported, graft-versus-host disease in such cases does not appear to be as severe, though experience is still very limited.

Autologous HPC transplants are performed solely for the treatment of malignancies. In these cases the chemotherapy is intensively myelosuppressive though not necessarily myeloablative. One prominent exception is patients with chronic myelogenous leukemia in blast crisis, who receive their autologous HPC in an effort to return their disease to the chronic phase. Since patients usually have some residual immune function and are receiving their own HPC—and thus do not require posttransplant immunosuppression— the risk of opportunistic infections and immunosuppression-related neoplasia is markedly reduced.

The success rates of HPC transplantation depend mostly upon the underlying disease and the associated risk of relapse (in cases of leukemia), the level of matching between donor and recipient (and thus the likelihood of graft-versus-host disease), the age of the recipient (over age 30, the incidence increases), and the complications associated with conditioning (venoocclusive liver disease and infection). Overall, the survival rates at 1 year are about 60–70% in aplastic anemia and 40–75% in various forms of leukemia and other neoplasms such as non-Hodgkin's lymphomas; results in breast carcinoma are less well defined.

Bhatia V et al: Novel approaches to allogeneic stem cell therapy. Expert Opin Biol Ther 2001;1:3. [PMID: 11727545]

Champlin RE et al: Blood stem cells compared with bone marrow as a source of hematopoietic cells for allogeneic transplantation. IBMTR Histocompatibility and Stem Cell Sources Working Committee and the European Group for Blood and Marrow Transplantation (EBMT). Blood 2000;95: 3702. [PMID: 10845900]

Gyger M et al: Immunobiology of allogeneic peripheral blood mononuclear cells mobilized with granulocyte-colony stimulating factor. Bone Marrow Transplant 2000;26:1. [PMID: 10918400]

Hariharan S: Long-term kidney transplant survival. Am J Kidney Dis 2001;38(6 Suppl 6):S44. [PMID: 11729005]

Terasaki PI et al: High survival rates of kidney transplants from spousal and living unrelated donors. N Engl J Med

1995;333:333. [PMID: /609/48] (Excellent outcomes from use of spousal donors—equal to that of parental donors.)

MECHANISM OF ACTION OF IMMUNOSUPPRESSIVE DRUGS

The most frequently used immunosuppressive drugs and their modes of action are briefly summarized below.

Corticosteroids

This group of drugs has potent and direct anti-inflammatory effects on immunocompetent cells. Corticosteroids inhibit lymphocyte proliferation and cell-mediated immune responses more severely than they inhibit antibody responses. T helper cells, eosinophils, and monocytes are reduced in peripheral blood. Corticosteroids down-regulate cytokine gene expression through interference with transcription regulation. By inhibition of phospholipase A_2, synthesis of inflammatory arachidonic acid metabolites (prostaglandins and leukotrienes) is suppressed. Corticosteroids have been shown to block the activation of T cells by interleukin-1 (IL-1) derived from macrophages. They also inhibit the expression of class II histocompatibility antigens on the macrophage surface, thereby interfering with presentation of antigen to T cells. Cumulatively, these cellular changes result in reduced inflammatory responses.

Cytotoxic Drugs

The most frequently used cytotoxic drugs are the antimetabolites (see below) and cyclophosphamide. Cyclophosphamide is an alkylating agent that damages cells by cross-linking DNA. Although this cycle-specific drug is most effective in killing cells going through the mitotic cycle, it can also cause intermitotic cell injury and death. Cyclophosphamide can inhibit both T and B cell immunity as well as inflammation. Azathioprine and cyclophosphamide are effective inhibitors of the production of serum antibodies.

Antimetabolites

The most commonly used antimetabolites are methotrexate, an inhibitor of folic acid synthesis, and azathioprine, a structural analog of mercaptopurine, an antagonist of purine synthesis. Azathioprine is a phase-specific drug that kills rapidly replicating cells. It inhibits proliferation of both T and B cells as well as macrophages. Methotrexate inhibits rapidly proliferating cells in S phase and suppresses both cell-mediated and humoral immunity as well as inflammation. Without immunosuppression, the incidence of graft-versus-host disease after allogeneic HPC transplant is almost 100%; this can be reduced to 20–30% with immunosuppressive therapy, especially the combination of methotrexate and cyclosporine, in addition to corticosteroids. Cyclosporine prevents T cell activation, while methotrexate inhibits the function of T cells that are already activated.

Cyclosporine

This cyclic polypeptide derived from a fungus is used as an immunosuppressive drug in organ transplant recipients. Cyclosporine binds to cyclophilin, a cytoplasmic protein, thereby interfering with calcium-dependent events including secretion of interleukin-2 (IL-2) by T lymphocytes. Since IL-2 is necessary for T cell replication, this drug is a potent inhibitor of T cell proliferation and thereby inhibits T cell-mediated immune responses. Little effect has been shown on direct B cell immune responses or on inflammation. Its toxic effects are primarily on renal and, to a lesser extent, hepatic function. In addition to methotrexate, methylprednisolone has also been utilized with cyclosporine to treat graft-versus-host disease, though T cell-directed immunotoxins have not proved to be of any benefit. A recently developed microemulsion formulation offers improved oral bioavailability, safety, and efficacy.

Tacrolimus

This drug was developed for use in transplantation and is a macrolide with potent anti-T cell properties and a mode of action similar to that of cyclosporine. Like cyclosporine, tacrolimus inhibits IL-2 and interferon-γ production and T cell activation. It has been approved for use in kidney and liver transplantation as a primary immunosuppressive agent or as rescue therapy. Both cyclosporine and tacrolimus block the intracellular pathway of calcineurin dephosphorylation of nuclear transcription factors.

Tacrolimus is approximately 100 times more potent than cyclosporine. Rates of graft-versus-host disease are lower for tacrolimus-based regimens. Tacrolimus appears to be at least as effective as cyclosporine, possibly better as prophylaxis of acute rejection. The major toxicities include hyperglycemia, nephrotoxicity, and neurotoxicity.

Mycophenolate Mofetil

Mycophenolate mofetil is used primarily as an adjunctive agent in kidney transplantation. By blocking lymphocyte production of guanine nucleotides, it inhibits T and B lymphocyte proliferation. Its use in combination with cyclosporine or tacrolimus has led to a lower incidence of acute graft rejection, reducing the need for high-dose corticosteroids or OKT3 (muromonab-CD3).

Humanized Anti-Interleukin-2 Receptor Antibody

A humanized monoclonal antibody directed to the low-affinity IL-2 receptor is approved for use in kidney transplantation. This antibody, administered for 8 weeks following the transplant, when added to standard immunosuppressive therapy, results in a reduction of the incidence of acute graft rejection to about 25%. Although the incidence of acute rejection is not substantially lower than that of other combinations of immunosuppressive agents, there appears to be a lower incidence and severity of side effects compared with antilymphocyte alternatives.

Muromonab-CD3

A murine monoclonal antibody, muromonab-CD3, is directed against human CD3, the T cell receptor. Indicated for acute graft rejection refractory to corticosteroids, large doses of the drug purge T cells from the systemic circulation. The drug has numerous side effects related to the release of cytokines, including fever, myalgias, dyspnea, and aseptic meningitis, and has also been associated with increased susceptibility to cytomegalovirus infection. Most patients are limited to a single course of therapy since recurrent courses may be associated with posttransplant lymphoproliferative disease.

Tumor Necrosis Factor (TNF) Antagonists

Several approaches have been developed to mitigate the biologic effects of TNF, a cytokine produced by macrophages and other antigen-presenting cells. TNF activates gene expression of proinflammatory mediators, up-regulates adhesion molecule expression, stimulates neutrophil function, possesses antitumor and antiviral activity, and is an endogenous pyrogen. In addition to its proinflammatory properties, TNF has been associated with bone resorption and cartilage degradation and appears to play a central role in rheumatic joint disease. Two molecules have been designed to inhibit binding of TNF to its cellular receptor and thereby reduce its cellular and biologic effects. Etanercept is a dimeric construct—containing the soluble TNF receptor—joined to the Fc domain of a human IgG molecule. Infliximab is a chimeric antibody molecule containing a human Fc domain and a murine variable region. Both are disease-modifying drugs that have been shown to slow joint destruction and markedly decrease symptomatology in rheumatoid arthritis; etanercept may also be effective in ankylosing spondylitis. It must be administered by subcutaneous injection twice weekly; infliximab is given intravenously every 2 months.

IMMUNOMODULATING THERAPIES

Cytokine Therapy

The experimental and clinical applications of cytokines, as biologic response modifiers and therapeutic agents, have been greatly expanded in recent years. Some cytokines, such as tumor necrosis factor and interferon alfa, have direct antitumor activity. Other cytokines affect tumor immune responses by lymphokine-activated killer cells, tumor-infiltrating lymphocytes, and activated natural killer cells. Cytokines have been used to activate immune cells ex vivo prior to adoptive transfer or have been given concurrently with activated effector cells. Phase I and phase II trials of cellular adoptive therapy, with IL-2 activated killer cells, for the treatment of renal cell carcinoma and melanoma have demonstrated feasibility and regression of metastasis in some patients. Modest results, significant morbidity, and high cost have hampered widespread adoption of these techniques.

Interferon alfa is used in hairy cell leukemia, chronic myelogenous leukemia, Kaposi's sarcoma, and chronic active hepatitis B and C. Interferon beta is used for multiple sclerosis and interferon gamma for the treatment of chronic granulomatous disease. Constitutional symptoms are common with cytokine therapy, and in some instances the toxicity is considerable.

Intravenous Gamma Globulin

Immune globulin IV (IGIV) has numerous immunomodulatory and anti-inflammatory activities and is the standard of care for immunologically mediated disorders such as Kawasaki's syndrome and for antibody replacement in humoral immunodeficiency. When used in humoral immunodeficiency, serum IgG levels can become normal but the IGIV contains virtually no IgM and only traces of IgA.

Each lot of IGIV produced from donated serum contains millions of antibody specificities, reflecting the humoral immune repertoire from thousands of normal blood donors. Most current products undergo numerous purification and viral inactivation steps, including solvent-detergent treatment or pasteurization. The antibody reactivities can be directed against a wide range of foreign and self antigens. In addition to the above disorders, IGIV is effective in Guillain-Barré syndrome, immune-mediated neuropathies, idiopathic thrombocytopenic purpura, pediatric HIV infection, and after bone marrow transplantation. Many other potential indications have been supported only by anecdotal reports or uncontrolled trials.

Allison AC et al: Mycophenolate mofetil and its mechanisms of action. Immunopharmacology 2000;47:85. [PMID: 10878285]

Allison AC: Immunosuppressive drugs: the first 50 years and a glance forward. Immunopharmacology 2000;47:63. [PMID: 10878284]

Matsuda S et al: Mechanisms of action of cyclosporine. Immunopharmacology 200047:119. [PMID: 10878286]

Arthritis & Musculoskeletal Disorders

David B. Hellmann, MD, FACP, & John H. Stone, MD, MPH

See www.current-med.com/ch20.html

■ DIAGNOSIS & EVALUATION

Examination of the Patient

In the patient with arthritis, the two clinical clues most helpful for diagnosis are the joint pattern and the presence or absence of extra-articular manifestations. The joint pattern is defined by answering three questions: (1) Is inflammation present? (2) How many joints are involved? and (3) What joints are affected? Joint inflammation is manifested by redness, warmth, swelling, and morning stiffness of at least 30 minutes' duration. Both the number of affected joints and the specific sites of involvement help determine the differential diagnosis (Table 20–1). Some diseases—gout, for example—are characteristically monarticular, whereas other diseases, such as rheumatoid arthritis, are chiefly polyarticular. The location of joint involvement can also be distinctive. Only two diseases cause prominent involvement of the distal interphalangeal joint (DIP): osteoarthritis and psoriatic arthritis. Extra-articular manifestations such as fever, rash, nodules, or neuropathy help narrow the differential diagnosis (see Table 20–1).

Arthrocentesis & Examination of Joint Fluid

Synovial fluid examination (Table 20–2) may provide specific diagnostic information in joint disease. Contraindications to arthrocentesis include infection of the overlying skin, bleeding disorder, or inability of the patient to cooperate. For patients who are chronically anticoagulated with warfarin, joints can be aspirated if the INR is less 3.0. In such patients, use of a small-gauge needle (eg, 22F or 25F) and application of firm pressure to the aspiration site are prudent measures. Most large joints are easily aspirated (Figure 20–1).

A. TYPES OF STUDIES

1. Gross examination—If fluid is green or purulent, a Gram's stain is indicated. If bloody, a bleeding disorder, trauma, or traumatic tap is most likely.

2. Microscopic examination—Compensated polarized light microscopy identifies and distinguishes monosodium urate (gout) and calcium pyrophosphate (pseudogout) crystals.

3. Culture—Bacterial cultures as well as special studies for gonococci, tubercle bacilli, or fungi are ordered as appropriate.

B. INTERPRETATION

(See Table 20–2.) Although synovial fluid analysis is diagnostic in infectious or microcrystalline arthritis, there is considerable overlap in the cytologic and biochemical values obtained in these and other diseases (Table 20–3). These studies do make possible, however, a differentiation according to severity of inflammation. Inflammatory joint fluids have more than 3000 white blood cells per microliter, of which 50% or more are polymorphonuclear neutrophils (Table 20–2). Noninflammatory fluids have less than 3000/µL white cells and less than 25% polymorphonuclear neutrophils. Synovial fluid glucose and protein levels (Table 20–2) add little information.

■ DEGENERATIVE & CRYSTAL-INDUCED ARTHRITIS

DEGENERATIVE JOINT DISEASE (Osteoarthritis)

ESSENTIALS OF DIAGNOSIS

- *Commonly secondary to other articular disease.*
- *A degenerative disorder without systemic manifestations.*

  Pain relieved by rest, morning stiffness brief, articular inflammation minimal.
- *X-ray findings: narrowed joint space, osteophytes, increased density of subchondral bone, bony cysts.*

Table 20–1. Diagnostic value of the joint pattern.

Characteristic	Status	Representative Disease
Inflammation	Present	Rheumatoid arthritis, systemic lupus erythematosus, gout
	Absent	Osteoarthritis
Number of involved joints	Monarticular	Gout, trauma, septic arthritis, Lyme disease
	Oligoarticular (2–4 joints)	Reiter's disease, psoriatic arthritis, inflammatory bowel disease
	Polyarticular (≥ 5 joints)	Rheumatoid arthritis, systemic lupus erythematosus
Site of joint involvement	Distal interphalangeal	Osteoarthritis, psoriatic arthritis (not rheumatoid arthritis)
	Metacarpophalangeal, wrists	Rheumatoid arthritis, systemic lupus erythematosus (not osteoarthritis)
	First metatarsal phalangeal	Gout, osteoarthritis

General Considerations

Osteoarthritis is the most common form of joint disease, sparing no age, race, or geographic area. At least 20 million adults in the USA suffer from the effects of this condition at any one time, and 90% of all people will have radiographic features of osteoarthritis in weight-bearing joints by age 40. Symptomatic disease also increases with age.

This arthropathy is characterized by degeneration of cartilage and by hypertrophy of bone at the articular margins. Inflammation is usually minimal. Hereditary and mechanical factors may be involved in the pathogenesis.

Degenerative joint disease is divided into two types: (1) primary, which most commonly affects some or all of the following: the terminal interphalangeal joints (Heberden's nodes) and less commonly the proximal interphalangeal joints (Bouchard's nodes), the metacarpophalangeal and carpometacarpal joints of the thumb, the hip, the knee, the metatarsophalangeal joint of the big toe, and the cervical and lumbar spine; and (2) secondary, which may occur in any joint as a sequela to articular injury resulting from either intra-articular (including rheumatoid arthritis) or extra-articular causes. The injury may be acute, as in a fracture; or chronic, as that due to occupational overuse of a joint, metabolic disease (eg, hyperparathyroidism, hemochromatosis, ochronosis), or neurologic disorders (tabes dorsalis; see below). Obesity is a risk factor for knee osteoarthritis and probably for the hip. Recreational running does not increase the incidence of osteoarthritis, but participation in competitive contact sports does. Jobs requiring frequent bending and carrying increase the risk of knee osteoarthritis.

Pathologically, the articular cartilage is first roughened and finally worn away, and spur formation and lipping occur at the edge of the joint surface. The syn-

Table 20–2. Examination of joint fluid.

Measure	Normal	Group I (Noninflammatory)	Group II (Inflammatory)	Group III (Purulent)
Volume (mL) (knee)	< 3.5	Often > 3.5	Often > 3.5	Often > 3.5
Clarity	Transparent	Transparent	Translucent to opaque	Opaque
Color	Clear	Yellow	Yellow to opalescent	Yellow to green
WBC (per μL)	< 200	200–300	3000–50,000	> 50,000[1]
Polymorphonuclear leukocytes	< 25%	< 25%	50% or more	75% or more[1]
Culture	Negative	Negative	Negative	Usually positive
Glucose (mg/dL)	Nearly equal to serum	Nearly equal to serum	> 25, lower than serum	< 25, much lower than serum

[1]Counts are lower with infections caused by organisms of low virulence or if antibiotic therapy has been started.

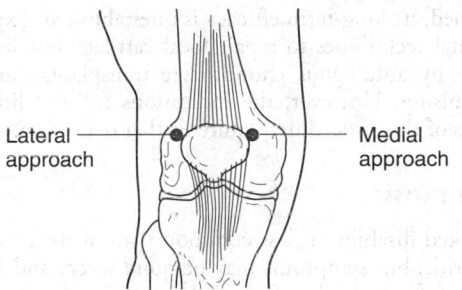

Figure 20–1. Aspiration of the knee joint. The knee joint—the most commonly aspirated joint—can be entered either medially or laterally. The patient should be supine, with the leg fully extended. Apply pressure on the side of the joint opposite to the puncture site to assist in directing the needle toward the bulging synovium. From the lateral approach, the needle (held parallel to the examining table) is directed medially, just beneath the patella, into the suprapatellar space. From the medial approach, the needle (held parallel to the examining table) is introduced between the patella and the medial condyle and advanced upward and laterally, beneath the patella and into the joint space. (Reproduced, with permission, from Nicoll D et al: *Pocket Guide to Diagnostic Tests* McGraw-Hill, 1997.)

ovial membrane becomes thickened, with hypertrophy of the villous processes; the joint cavity, however, never becomes totally obliterated, and the synovial membrane does not form adhesions. Inflammation is prominent only in occasional patients with acute interphalangeal joint involvement.

Clinical Findings

A. SYMPTOMS AND SIGNS

The onset is insidious. Initially, there is articular stiffness, seldom lasting more than 15 minutes; this develops later into pain on motion of the affected joint and is made worse by activity or weight bearing and relieved by rest. Deformity may be absent or minimal; however, bony enlargement of the interphalangeal joints is occasionally prominent, and flexion contracture or varus deformity of the knee is not unusual. There is no ankylosis, but limitation of motion of the affected joint or joints is common. Coarse crepitus may often be felt in the joint. Joint effusion and other articular signs of inflammation are mild. There are no systemic manifestations.

B. LABORATORY FINDINGS

Elevated sedimentation rate and other laboratory signs of inflammation are not present.

C. IMAGING

Radiographs may reveal narrowing of the joint space, sharpened articular margins, osteophyte formation and lipping of marginal bone, and thickened, dense subchondral bone. Bone cysts may also be present.

Differential Diagnosis

Because articular inflammation is minimal and systemic manifestations are absent, degenerative joint disease should seldom be confused with other arthritides. The distribution of joint involvement in the hands also helps distinguish osteoarthritis from rheumatoid arthritis. Osteoarthritis chiefly affects the distal and proximal interphalangeal joints and spares the wrist

Table 20–3. Differential diagnosis by joint fluid groups.[1]

Group 1 (Noninflammatory)	Group II (Inflammatory)	Group III (Purulent)	Hemorrhagic
Degenerative joint disease	Rheumatoid arthritis	Pyogenic bacterial infections	Hemophilia or other hemorrhagic diathesis
Trauma[2]	Acute crystal-induced synovitis		Trauma with or without fracture
Osteochondritis dissecans	(gout and pseudogout)		Neuropathic arthropathy
Osteochondromatosis	Reiter's syndrome		Pigmented villonodular synovitis
Neuropathic arthropathy[2]	Ankylosing spondylitis		Synovioma
Subsiding or early inflammation	Psoriatic arthritis		Hemangioma and other benign neoplasms
Hypertrophic osteoarthropathy[3]	Arthritis accompanying ulcerative colitis and regional enteritis		
Pigmented villonodular synovitis[2]	Rheumatic fever[3]		
	Systemic lupus erythematosus[3]		
	Progressive systemic sclerosis (scleroderma)[3]		
	Tuberculosis		
	Mycotic infections		

[1]Reproduced from Rodnan GP (editor): Primer on the rheumatic diseases, 7th ed. JAMA 1973;224(Suppl):662.
[2]May be hemorrhagic.
[3]Group I or II.

and metacarpophalangeal joints (except at the thumb); rheumatoid arthritis involves the wrists and metacarpophalangeal joints and spares the distal interphalangeal joints. Furthermore, the joint enlargement is bony-hard and cool in osteoarthritis but spongy and warm in rheumatoid arthritis. Skeletal symptoms due to degenerative changes in joints, especially in the spine, may cause coexistent metastatic neoplasia, osteoporosis, multiple myeloma, or other bone disease to be overlooked.

Prevention

Weight reduction in women reduces the risk of developing symptomatic knee osteoarthritis. Estrogen replacement therapy may reduce the risk of knee and hip osteoarthritis and maintaining normal vitamin D levels can reduce the occurrence and progression of osteoarthritis.

Treatment

A. GENERAL MEASURES

For patients with mild to moderate osteoarthritis of weight-bearing joints, a supervised walking program may result in clinical improvement of functional status without aggravating the joint pain. Weight loss can also improve the symptoms.

B. ANALGESIC AND ANTI-INFLAMMATORY DRUGS

NSAIDs (Table 5–6) are more effective (and more toxic) than acetaminophen for osteoarthritis of the knee or hip. Their superiority is most convincing in those with severe disease. Patients with mild disease should start with acetaminophen (2.6–4 g/d). Glucosamine and chondroitin sulfate also appear to be effective and safe. NSAIDs should be considered for patients who fail to respond to acetaminophen, chondroitin sulfate, and glucosamine. (See discussion of NSAID toxicity in the section on treatment of rheumatoid arthritis.) High doses of NSAIDs, as used in more inflammatory arthritides, are unnecessary.

For many patients, it is possible eventually to reduce the dosage or limit use of drugs to periods of exacerbation. For patients with knee osteoarthritis and effusion, intra-articular injection of triamcinolone (20–40 mg) may obviate the need for analgesics or NSAIDs but should not be repeated more than two or three times in a year. Intra-articular injections of sodium hyaluronate reduce symptoms moderately in some patients. Capsaicin cream 0.025% applied twice daily can also reduce knee pain without NSAIDs.

C. SURGICAL MEASURES

Total hip replacement provides excellent symptomatic and functional improvement when that joint is seriously afflicted, as indicated by severely restricted walking and pain at rest, particularly at night. Knee replacement is also effective. Although arthroscopic surgery for knee osteoarthritis is commonly per-

formed, its long-term efficacy is unestablished. Experimental techniques to repair focal cartilage loss in the knee by autologous chondrocyte transplantation are promising. However, the indications for and limitations of this procedure require further definition.

Prognosis

Marked disability is less common than in rheumatoid arthritis, but symptoms may be quite severe and limit activity considerably (especially with involvement of the hips, knees, and cervical spine).

Geba GP et al: Efficacy of rofecoxib, celecoxib, and acetaminophen in osteoarthritis of the knee. A randomized trial. JAMA 2002;287:64. [PMID: 11754710] (Rofecoxib 25 mg/d was more effective than acetaminophen 4000 mg/d, celecoxib 200 mg/d, or rofecoxib 12.5 mg/d in this 6-week trial.)

Pincus T et al: A randomized, double-blind, crossover clinical trial of diclofenac plus misoprostol versus acetaminophen in patients with osteoarthritis of the hip or knee. Arthritis Rheum 2001;44:1587. [PMID: 11465710] (Diclofenac plus misoprostol was more effective than acetaminophen, especially in patients with severe osteoarthritis.)

Reginster JY et al: Long-term effects of glucosamine sulphate on osteoarthritis progression: a randomised, placebo-controlled clinical trial. Lancet 2001;357:251. [PMID: 11214126] (Glucosamine-treated patients did not experience progression of x-ray damage whereas those on placebo did.)

CRYSTAL DEPOSITION ARTHRITIS

1. Gouty Arthritis

 ESSENTIALS OF DIAGNOSIS

- *Acute onset, typically nocturnal and usually monarticular, often involving the first metatarsophalangeal joint.*
- *Postinflammatory desquamation and pruritus.*
- *Hyperuricemia in most; identification of urate crystals in joint fluid or tophi is diagnostic.*
- *Dramatic therapeutic response to NSAIDs or colchicine.*
- *With chronicity, urate deposits in subcutaneous tissue, bone, cartilage, joints, and other tissues.*

General Considerations

Gout is a metabolic disease of heterogeneous nature, often familial, associated with abnormal amounts of urates in the body and characterized early by a recurring acute arthritis, usually monarticular, and later by chronic deforming arthritis. The associated hyperuricemia is due to overproduction or underexcretion of uric acid—sometimes both. The disease is especially common in Pacific islanders, eg, Filipinos and Samoans. It is rarely caused by a specifically determined genetic aberration (eg, Lesch-Nyhan syndrome). Secondary gout, which may have a heritable component, is related to acquired causes of hyperuricemia, eg, medication use (especially diuretics, cyclosporine, low-dose aspirin, and niacin), myeloproliferative disorders, multiple myeloma, hemoglobinopathies, chronic renal disease, hypothyroidism, psoriasis, sarcoidosis, and lead poisoning. Alcohol ingestion promotes hyperuricemia by increasing urate production and decreasing the renal excretion of uric acid. Finally, hospitalized patients frequently suffer attacks of gout because of changes in diet (eg, inability to take oral feedings following abdominal surgery) or medications that lead either to rapid reductions or increases in the serum urate level.

About 90% of patients with primary gout are men, usually over 30 years of age. In women the onset is typically postmenopausal. The characteristic lesion is the tophus, a nodular deposit of monosodium urate monohydrate crystals, with an associated foreign body reaction. These are found in cartilage, subcutaneous and periarticular tissues, tendon, bone, the kidneys, and elsewhere. Urates have been demonstrated in the synovial tissues (and fluid) during acute arthritis; indeed, the acute inflammation of gout is believed to be activated by the phagocytosis by polymorphonuclear cells of urate crystals with the ensuing release from the neutrophils of chemotactic and other substances capable of mediating inflammation. The precise relationship of hyperuricemia to gouty arthritis is still obscure, since chronic hyperuricemia is found in people who never develop gout or uric acid stones (Table 20–4). Rapid fluctuations in serum urate levels, either increasing or decreasing, are important factors in precipitating acute gout. The mechanism of the late, chronic stage of gouty arthritis is better understood. This is characterized pathologically by tophaceous invasion of the articular and periarticular tissues, with structural derangement and secondary degeneration (osteoarthritis).

Uric acid kidney stones are present in 5–10% of patients with gouty arthritis. Hyperuricemia correlates highly with the likelihood of developing stones, with the risk of stone formation reaching 50% in patients with a serum urate level above 13 mg/dL. Chronic urate nephropathy is caused by the deposition of monosodium urate crystals in the renal medulla and pyramids. Although progressive renal failure occurs in a substantial percentage of patients with chronic gout, the role of hyperuricemia in causing this outcome is controversial, because many patients with gout have numerous confounding risk factors for renal failure (eg, hypertension, alcohol use, lead exposure, and other risk factors for vascular disease).

Unless there is a rapid breakdown of cellular nucleic acid following aggressive treatment of leukemia or lymphoma, uric acid-lowering drugs need not be instituted until arthritis, renal calculi, or tophi become

Table 20–4. Origin of hyperuricemia.[1]

Primary hyperuricemia
  A. Increased production of purine:
    1. Idiopathic.
    2. Specific enzyme defects (eg, Lesch-Nyhan syndrome, glycogen storage diseases).
  B. Decreased renal clearance of uric acid (idiopathic).

Secondary hyperuricemia
  A. Increased catabolism and turnover of purine:
    1. Myeloproliferative disorders.
    2. Lymphoproliferative disorders.
    3. Carcinoma and sarcoma (disseminated).
    4. Chronic hemolytic anemias.
    5. Cytotoxic drugs.
    6. Psoriasis.
  B. Decreased renal clearance of uric acid:
    1. Intrinsic kidney disease.
    2. Functional impairment of tubular transport:
      a. Drug-induced (eg, thiazides, probenecid).
      b. Hyperlacticacidemia (eg, lactic acidosis, alcoholism).
      c. Hyperketoacidemia (eg, diabetic ketoacidosis, starvation).
      d. Diabetes insipidus (vasopressin-resistant).
      e. Bartter's syndrome.

[1]Modified from Rodnan GP: Gout and other crystalline forms of arthritis. Postgrad Med (Oct) 1975;58:6.

apparent. Asymptomatic hyperuricemia should not be treated.

Clinical Findings

A. SYMPTOMS AND SIGNS

The acute arthritis is characterized by its sudden onset, frequently nocturnal, either without apparent precipitating cause or following rapid fluctuations in serum urate levels, from alcohol excess or medication changes (see above). The metatarsophalangeal joint of the great toe is the most susceptible joint ("podagra"), although others, especially those of the feet, ankles, and knees, are commonly affected. Gouty attacks may develop in periarticular soft tissues such as the arch of the foot. Hips and shoulders are rarely involved in gout. More than one joint may occasionally be affected during the same attack; in such cases, the distribution of the arthritis is usually asymmetric. As the attack progresses, the pain becomes intense. The involved joints are swollen and exquisitely tender and the overlying skin tense, warm, and dusky red. Fever is common and may reach 39 °C. Local desquamation and pruritus during recovery from the acute arthritis are characteristic of gout but are not always present. Tophi may be found in the external ears, hands, feet, olecranon, and prepatellar bursas. They are usually seen only after several attacks of acute arthritis.

Asymptomatic periods of months or years commonly follow the initial acute attack. After years of recurrent severe monarthritis attacks of the lower extremities, gout can evolve into a chronic, deforming polyarthritis of upper and lower extremities that mimics rheumatoid arthritis.

B. LABORATORY FINDINGS

The serum uric acid is elevated (> 7.5 mg/dL) in 95% of patients who have serial measurements during the course of an attack. However, a single uric acid determination is normal in up to 25% of cases, so it does not exclude gout, especially in patients taking uricopenic drugs. During an acute attack, the erythrocyte sedimentation rate and white cell count are frequently elevated. Material aspirated from a tophus shows the typical crystals of sodium urate and confirms the diagnosis. Further confirmation is obtained by identification of sodium urate crystals by compensated polariscopic examination of wet smears prepared from joint fluid aspirates. Such crystals are negatively birefringent and needle-like and may be found free or in neutrophils.

C. IMAGING

Early in the disease, radiographs show no changes. Later, punched-out erosions with an overhanging rim of cortical bone ("rat bite") develop. When these are adjacent to a soft tissue tophus, they are diagnostic of gout.

Differential Diagnosis

Acute gout is often confused with cellulitis. Bacteriologic studies usually exclude acute pyogenic arthritis. Pseudogout is distinguished by the identification of calcium pyrophosphate crystals (strong positive birefringence) in the joint fluid, usually normal serum uric acid, the x-ray appearance of chondrocalcinosis, and the relative therapeutic ineffectiveness of colchicine.

Chronic tophaceous arthritis may rarely mimic chronic rheumatoid arthritis. In such cases, the diagnosis of gout is suggested by an earlier history of monarthritis and is established by the demonstration of urate crystals in a suspected tophus. Likewise, hips and shoulders are generally spared in tophaceous gout. Biopsy may be necessary to distinguish tophi from rheumatoid nodules. An x-ray appearance similar to that of gout may be found in rheumatoid arthritis, sarcoidosis, multiple myeloma, hyperparathyroidism, or Hand-Schüller-Christian disease. Chronic lead intoxication may result in attacks of gouty arthritis (saturnine gout); abdominal pain, peripheral neuropathy, renal insufficiency, and basophilic stippling of red cells are clues to the diagnosis.

Treatment

A. ACUTE ATTACK

The most common mistake in managing gout is starting drug treatment for the acute arthritis and the hyperuricemia simultaneously. Treatment must be separated by treating the acute arthritis first and hyperuricemia later, if at all. Sudden reduction of serum uric acid often precipitates further episodes of gouty arthritis.

1. Nonsteroidal anti-inflammatory drugs— NSAIDs (Table 5–6) have become the treatment of choice for acute gout. Traditionally, indomethacin has been the most frequently used agent, but all of the other newer NSAIDs are probably equally effective. Indomethacin is initiated at a dosage of 25–50 mg every 8 hours and continued until the symptoms have resolved (usually 5–10 days). Active peptic ulcer disease, impaired renal function, and a history of allergic reaction to NSAIDs are contraindications. For patients at high risk for upper gastrointestinal bleeding, a COX-2 inhibitor may be an appropriate first choice for management of an acute gout attack.

2. Colchicine—Colchicine is also effective for acute gout but is less favored, since 80% of treated patients develop significant abdominal cramping, diarrhea, nausea, or vomiting. Colchicine is thought to work by inhibiting chemotaxis and thereby interfering with the inflammatory response to urate crystals; thus, it is most effective when given in the first few hours after onset of symptoms. The dose is 0.5 or 0.6 mg by mouth every hour until pain is relieved or until nausea or diarrhea appears; the drug is then stopped. The usual total dose required is 4–6 mg and should not exceed 8 mg. Oral colchicine should not be used in patients with inflammatory bowel disease. For patients who cannot tolerate oral medications (eg, postoperative patients), colchicine can be administered intravenously. However, local pain, tissue damage from extravasation, and marrow suppression may occur. The initial dose is 2 mg in 20–50 mL of saline solution given through an intravenous catheter. Two additional doses of 1 mg each can be administered at 6-hour intervals. The total dose should not exceed 4 mg, and no additional colchicine should be given by mouth for 3 weeks. Dosages must be reduced by at least 50% in the presence of renal or hepatic disease or old age. Failure to adjust the dose of intravenous colchicine can cause the patient's death. Combined renal and hepatic disease contraindicates the use of intravenous colchicine.

3. Corticosteroids—Corticosteroids often give dramatic symptomatic relief in acute episodes of gout and will control most attacks. They are best reserved for patients unable to take oral NSAIDs. If the patient's gout is monarticular, intra-articular administration (eg, triamcinolone, 10–40 mg depending on the size of the joint) is most effective. For polyarticular gout, corticosteroids may be given intravenously (eg, methylprednisolone, 40 mg/d tapered off over 7 days) or orally (eg, prednisone, 40–60 mg/d tapered off over 7 days). Gouty and septic arthritis can coexist, albeit rarely. Therefore, joint aspiration and Gram stain of synovial fluid should be performed before corticosteroids are given.

4. Analgesics—At times the pain of an acute attack may require opioids. Aspirin should be avoided since it aggravates hyperuricemia (see below).

5. Bed rest—Bed rest is important in the management of the acute attack and should be continued for about 24 hours after the acute attack has subsided. Early ambulation may precipitate a recurrence.

B. MANAGEMENT BETWEEN ATTACKS

Treatment during symptom-free periods is intended to minimize urate deposition in tissues, which causes chronic tophaceous arthritis, and to reduce the frequency and severity of recurrences.

1. Diet—Potentially reversible causes of hyperuricemia are a high purine diet, obesity, frequent alcohol consumption, and use of certain medications (see below). Although dietary purines usually contribute only 1 mg/dL to the serum uric acid level, moderation in eating foods with high-purine content is advisable (Table 20–5). A high liquid intake and, more importantly, a daily urinary output of 2 L or more will aid urate excretion and minimize urate precipitation in the urinary tract.

2. Avoidance of hyperuricemic medications—Thiazide and loop diuretics inhibit renal excretion of uric acid and should be avoided in patients with gout. Similarly, low doses of aspirin (< 3 g daily) aggravate hyperuricemia, as does niacin.

Table 20–5. The purine content of foods.[1,2]

Low-purine foods
 Refined cereals and cereal products, cornflakes, white bread, pasta, flour, arrowroot, sago, tapioca, cakes
 Milk, milk products, and eggs
 Sugar, sweets, and gelatin
 Butter, polyunsaturated margarine, and all other fats
 Fruit, nuts, and peanut butter
 Lettuce, tomatoes, and green vegetables (except those listed below)
 Cream soups made with low-purine vegetables but without meat or meat stock
 Water, fruit juice, cordials, and carbonated drinks

High-purine foods
 All meats, including organ meats, and seafood
 Meat extracts and gravies
 Yeast and yeast extracts, beer, and other alcoholic beverages
 Beans, peas, lentils, oatmeal, spinach, asparagus, cauliflower, and mushrooms

[1]Reproduced, with permission, from Emmerson BT: The management of gout. N Engl J Med 1996;334:445.
[2]The purine content of a food reflects its nucleoprotein content and turnover. Foods containing many nuclei (eg, liver) have many purines, as do rapidly growing foods such as asparagus. The consumption of large amounts of a food containing a small concentration of purines may provide a greater purine load than consumption of a small amount of a food containing a large concentration of purines.

3. Colchicine—The decision to begin chronic pharmacologic treatment of gout should be based on an estimate of the likelihood of further attacks. Patients with a single episode of gout who are willing to lose weight and stop drinking alcohol are at low risk of another attack and therefore unlikely to benefit from chronic medical therapy. In contrast, older individuals with mild chronic renal failure who require diuretic use and have a history of multiple attacks of gout are more likely to benefit from pharmacologic treatment. In general, the higher the uric acid level and the more frequent the attacks, the more likely that chronic medical therapy will be beneficial.

There are two indications for daily colchicine administration: (1) It can be used to prevent future attacks. For the person who has mild hyperuricemia and occasional attacks of gouty arthritis, chronic colchicine prophylaxis may be all that is needed. The usual dose is 0.6 mg twice a day. Patients who have coexisting moderate renal insufficiency or heart failure should have the dose reduced to once a day in order to avoid the development of a peripheral neuromyopathy and myositis that can complicate the use of higher doses. (2) It is also used when uricosuric drugs or allopurinol (see below) are started, to suppress the acute attacks that can be precipitated by abrupt changes in the serum uric acid level.

4. Reduction of serum uric acid—Indications include frequent acute arthritis not controlled by colchicine prophylaxis, tophaceous deposits, or renal damage. Hyperuricemia with infrequent attacks of arthritis may not require treatment; asymptomatic hyperuricemia should not be treated. If instituted, the goal of medical treatment is to maintain the serum uric acid below 6 mg/dL, which should prevent crystallization of urate.

Two classes of agents may be used to lower the serum uric acid—the uricosuric drugs and allopurinol (neither is of value in the treatment of acute gout). The choice of one or the other depends on the result of a 24-hour urine uric acid determination. A value under 800 mg/d indicates undersecretion of uric acid, which is amenable to uricosuric agents if renal function is preserved. Patients with more than 800 mg of uric acid in a 24-hour urine collection are overproducers of uric acid who require allopurinol.

a. Uricosuric drugs—These drugs, by blocking tubular reabsorption of filtered urate and reducing the metabolic pool of urates, prevent the formation of new tophi and reduce the size of those already present. Furthermore, when administered concomitantly with colchicine, they may lessen the frequency of recurrences of acute gout. The indication for uricosuric treatment is the increasing frequency or severity of acute attacks. Uricosuric agents are ineffective in patients with renal insufficiency, with a serum creatinine of more than 2 mg/dL.

The following uricosuric drugs may be employed: (1) Probenecid, 0.5 g daily initially, with gradual increase to 1–2 g daily; or (2) sulfinpyrazone, 50–100 mg twice daily initially, with gradual increase to 200–400 mg twice daily. Hypersensitivity to either with fever and rash occurs in 5% of cases; gastrointestinal complaints are observed in 10%. Probenecid also inhibits the excretion of penicillin, indomethacin, dapsone, and acetazolamide.

Precautions with uricosuric drugs. It is important to maintain a daily urinary output of 2000 mL or more in order to minimize the precipitation of uric acid in the urinary tract. This can be further prevented by giving alkalinizing agents (eg, potassium citrate, 30–80 meq/d) to maintain a urine pH of above 6.0. Uricosuric drugs are best avoided in patients with a history of uric acid lithiasis. Aspirin in moderate doses antagonizes the action of uricosuric agents, but low doses (325 mg or less per day) do not; doses greater than 3 g daily are themselves uricosuric.

b. Allopurinol—The xanthine oxidase inhibitor allopurinol promptly lowers plasma urate and urinary uric acid concentrations and facilitates tophus mobilization. The drug is of special value in uric acid overproducers; in tophaceous gout; in patients unresponsive to the uricosuric regimen; and in gouty patients with uric acid renal stones. It should be used in low doses in patients with renal insufficiency and is not indicated in asymptomatic hyperuricemia. The most frequent adverse effect is the precipitation of an acute gouty attack. However, the commonest sign of hypersensitivity to allopurinol (occurring in 2% of cases) is a pruritic rash that may progress to toxic epidermal necrolysis. Vasculitis and hepatitis are other rare complications.

The daily dose is determined by the serum uric acid response. Initially, 100 mg/d of allopurinol is given for 1 week; the dose is increased if the serum uric acid is still high. A normal serum uric acid level is often obtained with a daily dose of 200–300 mg. Occasionally (and in selected cases) it may be helpful to continue the use of allopurinol with a uricosuric drug.

Allopurinol interacts with other drugs. The combined use of allopurinol and ampicillin causes a drug rash in 20% of patients. Allopurinol can increase the half-life of probenecid, while probenecid increases the excretion of allopurinol. Thus, a patient taking both drugs may need to use slightly higher than usual doses of allopurinol and lower doses of probenecid. Allopurinol potentiates the effect of azathioprine. If allopurinol cannot be avoided, the dose of azathioprine should be reduced by 75% before allopurinol is started.

C. CHRONIC TOPHACEOUS ARTHRITIS

Tophaceous deposits can be made to shrink and disappear altogether with allopurinol therapy. Resorption of extensive tophi may require maintaining a serum uric acid below 5 mg/dL, which may be achievable only with concomitant use of allopurinol and a uricosuric agent. Surgical excision of large tophi offers mechanical improvement in selected deformities.

D. GOUT IN THE TRANSPLANT PATIENT

Since many transplant patients have decreased renal function and require drugs that inhibit uric acid excretion (especially cyclosporine and diuretics), these patients commonly develop hyperuricemia and gout. Treating these patients is challenging: NSAIDs are usually contraindicated because of renal impairment; intravenous colchicine should be avoided for the same reason; and corticosteroids are already being used. Often the best approach for monarticular gout—after excluding infection—is injecting corticosteroids into the joint (see above). For polyarticular gout, increasing the dose of systemic corticosteroid may be the only alternative. Since transplant patients often have multiple attacks of gout, long-term relief requires lowering the serum uric acid with allopurinol. Renal impairment seen in many transplant patients would make uricosuric agents ineffective.

Prognosis

Without treatment, the acute attack may last from a few days to several weeks, but proper treatment quickly terminates the attack. The intervals between acute attacks vary up to years, but the asymptomatic periods often become shorter if the disease progresses. Chronic tophaceous arthritis occurs after repeated attacks of acute gout, but only after inadequate treatment. The younger the patient at the onset of disease, the greater the tendency to a progressive course. Destructive arthropathy is rarely seen in patients whose first attack is after age 50.

Patients with gout are said to have an increased incidence of hypertension, renal disease (eg, nephrosclerosis, interstitial nephritis, pyelonephritis), diabetes mellitus, hypertriglyceridemia, and atherosclerosis, although these relationships are anecdotal and not well studied.

Fam AG et al: Efficacy and safety of desensitization to allopurinol following cutaneous reactions. Arthritis Rheum 2001;44: 231. [PMID: 11212165] (Details a successful method for oral desensitization.)

Harris M et al: Effect of low dose daily aspirin on serum urate levels and urinary excretion in patients receiving probenecid for gouty arthritis. J Rheumatol 2000;27:2873. [PMID: 11128679] (Aspirin 325 mg/d does not raise serum uric acid or decrease urate excretion in patients taking probenecid.)

2. Chondrocalcinosis & Pseudogout (Calcium Pyrophosphate Dihydrate [CPPD] Deposition Disease)

The term chondrocalcinosis refers to the presence of calcium-containing salts in articular cartilage. It is most often first diagnosed radiologically. It may be familial and is commonly associated with a wide variety of metabolic disorders, eg, hemochromatosis, hyperparathyroidism, ochronosis, diabetes mellitus, hypothyroidism, Wilson's disease, and true gout.

Pseudogout, most often seen in persons age 60 or older, is characterized by acute, recurrent and rarely chronic arthritis involving large joints (most commonly the knees and the wrists) and is almost always accompanied by chondrocalcinosis of the affected joints. Other joints frequently affected by CPPD are the metacarpophalangeal joints, hips, shoulders, elbows, and ankles. Involvement of the distal interphalangeal and proximal interphalangeal joints is no more common in CPPD deposition disease than in other age-matched controls. Pseudogout, like gout, frequently develops 24–48 hours after major surgery. Identification of calcium pyrophosphate crystals in joint aspirates is diagnostic of pseudogout. With light microscopy, the rhomboid-shaped pseudogout crystals can usually be distinguished from the needle-shaped gout crystals. A red compensator is used for positive identification, since pseudogout crystals are blue when parallel and yellow when perpendicular to the axis of the compensator. Urate crystals give the exact opposite color pattern. X-ray examination shows not only calcification (usually symmetric) of cartilaginous structures but also signs of degenerative joint disease (osteoarthritis). Unlike gout, pseudogout is usually associated with normal serum urate levels and is not dramatically improved by colchicine.

Treatment of chondrocalcinosis is directed at the primary disease, if present. Some of the nonsteroidal anti inflammatory agents (salicylates, indomethacin, naproxen, and other drugs) are helpful in the treatment of acute episodes. Patients at increased risk for upper gastrointestinal bleeding may use a COX-2 inhibitor to treat acute attacks of pseudogout. Colchicine, 0.6 mg orally twice daily, appears to be more effective for prophylaxis than for acute attacks. Aspiration of the inflamed joint and intra-articular injection of triamcinolone, 10–40 mg, depending on the size of the joint, are also of value in resistant cases.

Rosenthal AK: Calcium crystal-associated arthritides. Curr Opin Rheumatol 1998;10:273. [PMID: 9608333] (Extra-articular and spinal calcium pyrophosphate dihydrate deposits occur; association between hypothyroidism and chondrocalcinosis is debated.)

■ PAIN SYNDROMES

NECK PAIN

ESSENTIALS OF DIAGNOSIS

- *Most chronic neck pain is caused by degenerative joint disease and responds to conservative approaches.*
- *Whiplash, the most common type of traumatic injury to the neck, responds to early mobilization.*
- *Serious erosive disease of joints in the neck that may lead to neurologic complications sometimes occurs in rheumatoid arthritis and occasionally in ankylosing spondylitis; the usual joint involved in these disorders is the atlantoaxial joint (C1–2).*

General Considerations

A large group of articular and extra-articular disorders are characterized by pain that may involve simultaneously the neck, shoulder girdle, and upper extremity. Diagnostic differentiation among these disorders may be difficult. Some of these entities and clinical syndromes represent primary disorders of the cervicobrachial region; others are local manifestations of systemic disease.

Clinical Findings

A. Symptoms and Signs

Neck pain may be limited to the posterior neck region or, depending upon the level of the symptomatic joint, may radiate segmentally to the occiput, anterior chest, shoulder girdle, arm, forearm, and hand. It may be intensified by active or passive neck motions. The general distribution of pain and paresthesias corresponds roughly to the involved dermatome in the upper extremity. Radiating pain in the upper extremity is often intensified by hyperextension of the neck and deviation of the head to the involved side. Limitation of cervical movements is the most common objective finding. Neurologic signs depend upon the extent of compression of nerve roots or the spinal cord. Compression of the spinal cord may cause long-tract involvement resulting in paraparesis or paraplegia.

B. Imaging

The radiographic findings depend on the cause of the pain; many plain x-rays are completely normal in patients who have suffered an acute cervical strain. Loss of the normal anterior convexity of the cervical curve (loss of cervical lordosis) is frequently seen but is a nonspecific result of paraspinal muscle spasm. In osteoarthritis, comparative reduction in height of the involved disk space is a frequent finding. The most common late x-ray finding is osteophyte formation anteriorly, adjacent to the disk; other late changes occur around the apophysial joint clefts, chiefly in the lower cervical spine.

Use of advanced imaging techniques is indicated in the patient who has severe pain of unknown cause that fails to respond to conservative therapy or in the patient who has evidence of myelopathy. MRI is more sensitive than CT in detecting disk disease, extradural compression, and intramedullary cord disease. CT is more sensitive for demonstration of fractures.

Differential Diagnosis & Treatment

The causes of neck pain include acute and chronic cervical strain or sprains, herniated nucleus pulposus, osteoarthritis, ankylosing spondylitis, rheumatoid arthritis, osteomyelitis, neoplasms, spinal stenosis, polymyalgia rheumatica, compression fractures, and functional disorders.

A. ACUTE OR CHRONIC CERVICAL MUSCULOTENDINOUS STRAIN

Cervical strain is generally caused by mechanical postural disorders, overexertion, or injury (eg, whiplash). Acute episodes are associated with pain, decreased cervical spine motion, and paraspinal muscle spasm, resulting in stiffness of the neck and loss of motion. Muscle trigger points can often be localized. After whiplash injury, patients often experience not only neck pain but also shoulder girdle discomfort and headache. Management includes a cervical collar, and administration of analgesics. Corticosteroid injection into cervical facet joints is ineffective. Gradual return to full activity is encouraged.

Patients with chronic symptoms often have few objective findings. Mechanical stress due to work or recreational activities is often implicated. Chronic pain, especially that radiating into the upper extremity, may require additional treatment such as bracing. Chronic pain in the zygapophysial joints resulting from whiplash injuries may benefit from percutaneous radiofrequency neurotomy.

B. HERNIATED NUCLEUS PULPOSUS

Rupture or prolapse of the nucleus pulposus of the cervical disks into the spinal canal causes pain that radiates to the arms at the level of C6–7. When intra-abdominal pressure is increased by coughing, sneezing, or other movements, symptoms are aggravated, and cervical muscle spasm may often occur. Neurologic abnormalities may include decreased reflexes of the deep tendons of the biceps and triceps and decreased sensation and muscle atrophy or weakness in the forearm or hand. Cervical traction, bed rest, and other conservative measures are usually successful. Radicular symptoms usually respond to conservative therapy, including NSAIDs, activity modification, intermittent cervical traction, and neck immobilization. Cervical epidural steroid injections may help those who fail. Surgery is indicated for unremitting pain and progressive weakness despite a full trial of conservative therapy and if a surgically correctable abnormality is identified by MRI or CT myelography. Surgical decompression achieves excellent results in 70–80% of such patients.

C. ARTHRITIC DISORDERS

Cervical spondylosis (degenerative arthritis) is a collective term describing degenerative changes that occur in the apophysial joints and intervertebral disk joints, with or without neurologic signs. Osteoarthritis of the articular facets is characterized by progressive thinning of the cartilage, subchondral osteoporosis, and osteophytic proliferation around the joint margins. Degeneration of cervical disks and joints may occur in adolescents but is more common after age 40. Degeneration is progressive and is marked by gradual narrowing of the disk space, as demonstrated by x-ray. Osteocartilaginous proliferation occurs around the margin of the vertebral body and gives rise to osteophytic ridges that may encroach upon the intervertebral foramina and spinal canal, causing compression of the neurovascular contents.

Osteoarthritis of the cervical spine is often asymptomatic but may cause diffuse neck pain, radicular pain, or myelopathy. Myelopathy develops insidiously and is manifested by numb, clumsy hands. Some patients also complain of unsteady walking, urinary frequency and urgency, or electrical shock sensations with neck flexion or extension (Lhermitte's sign). Weakness, sensory loss, and spasticity with exaggerated reflexes develop below the level of spinal cord compression. Motor neuron disease, multiple sclerosis, syringomyelia, spinal cord tumors, and tropical spastic paresis from HTLV-1 infection can mimic myelopathy from cervical arthritis. The mainstay of conservative therapy is immobilizing the cervical spine with a collar. With moderate to severe symptoms, surgical treatment is indicated.

Ankylosing spondylitis is discussed below. Atlantoaxial subluxation may occur in patients with rheumatoid arthritis, regardless of the severity of disease. Inflammation of the synovial structures resulting from erosion and laxity of the transverse ligament can lead to neurologic signs of spinal cord compression. Treatment may vary from use of a cervical collar or more rigid bracing to operative treatment, depending on the degree of subluxation and neurologic progression. Surgical treatment may involve stabilization of the cervical spine.

D. OTHER DISORDERS

Osteomyelitis and neoplasms are discussed below. Osteoporosis is discussed in Chapter 26.

Hardin J Jr: Pain and the cervical spine. Bull Rheum Dis 2001;50:1. [PMID: 11688257] (Most causes of neck pain not associated with neurologic symptoms or signs can be managed conservatively with physical therapy, particularly interrupted traction.)

Narayan P et al: Treatment of degenerative cervical disc disease. Neurol Clin 2001;19:217. [PMID: 11471766] (Indications for surgery in radiculopathy and myelopathy are reviewed.)

THORACIC OUTLET SYNDROMES

Thoracic outlet syndromes include those disorders that result in compression of the neurovascular structures supplying the upper extremity. Patients often have a history of trauma to the head and neck areas.

Symptoms and signs arise from intermittent or continuous pressure on elements of the brachial plexus and the subclavian or axillary vessels by a variety of anatomic structures of the shoulder girdle region. The neurovascular bundle can be compressed between the anterior or middle scalene muscles and a normal first thoracic rib or a cervical rib. Descent of the shoulder girdle may continue during adulthood and cause compression. Faulty posture, chronic illness, and occupation may be other predisposing factors. The components of the median nerve that encircle the axillary artery may cause compression and vascular symptoms. Sudden or repetitive strenuous physical activity may precipitate thrombosis of the axillary or subclavian vein.

Pain may radiate from the point of compression to the base of the neck, the axilla, the shoulder girdle region, arm, forearm, and hand. Paresthesias are frequently present and are commonly distributed to the volar aspect of the fourth and fifth digits. Sensory symptoms may be aggravated at night or by prolonged use of the extremities. Weakness and muscle atrophy are the principal motor abnormalities. Vascular symptoms consist of arterial ischemia characterized by pallor of the fingers on elevation of the extremity, sensitivity to cold, and, rarely, gangrene of the digits or venous obstruction marked by edema, cyanosis, and engorgement.

Deep reflexes are usually not altered. When the site of compression is between the upper rib and clavicle, partial obliteration of subclavian artery pulsation may be demonstrated by abduction of the arm to a right angle with the elbow simultaneously flexed and rotated externally at the shoulder so that the entire extremity lies in the coronal plane. Neck or arm position has no effect on the diminished pulse, which remains constant in the subclavian steal syndrome.

Chest x-ray will identify patients with cervical rib. MRI with the arms held in different positions is useful in identifying sites of impaired blood flow. Intra-arterial or venous obstruction is confirmed by angiography. Determinations of the conduction velocities of the ulnar and other peripheral nerves of the upper extremity may help to localize the site of their compression.

Thoracic outlet syndrome must be differentiated from osteoarthritis of the cervical spine, tumors of the cervical spinal cord or nerve roots, and periarthritis of the shoulder.

Treatment is directed toward relief of compression of the neurovascular bundle. Overhead pulley exercises are useful to improve posture. Shoulder bracing, although uncomfortable, provides a constant stimulus to improve posture. When lying down, the shoulder girdle should be bolstered by arranging pillows in an inverted "V" position.

Symptoms may disappear spontaneously or may be relieved by conservative treatment. Operative treatment is more likely to relieve the neurologic rather than the vascular component that causes symptoms.

LOW BACK PAIN

Low back pain is exceedingly common, experienced at some time by up to 80% of the population. The differential diagnosis is broad and includes muscular strain, primary spine disease (eg, disk herniation, degenerative arthritis), systemic diseases (eg, metastatic cancer), and regional diseases (eg, aortic aneurysm). A precise diagnosis cannot be made in the majority of cases. Even when anatomic defects—such as vertebral osteophytes or a narrowed disk space—are present, clinical disease cannot be assumed since such defects are common in asymptomatic patients. The majority of patients will improve in 1–4 weeks and need no evaluation beyond the initial history and physical examination. The diagnostic challenge is to identify those patients who require more extensive or urgent evaluation.

In practice, this means identifying those patients with pain caused by (1) infection, (2) cancer, (3) inflammatory back disease such as ankylosing spondylitis, (4) or nonrheumatologic conditions, especially leaking aortic aneurysm. Significant or progressive neurologic deficits also require identification. If there is no evidence of these problems, conservative therapy is called for.

1. Clinical Approach to Diagnosis

General History & Physical Examination

Low back pain is a final common pathway of many processes; the pain of vertebral osteomyelitis, for example, is not very different in quality and intensity from the pain due to back strain of the weekend gardener. Historical factors of importance include smoking, weight loss, age over 50, and cancer, all of which are risk factors for vertebral body metastasis. Osteomyelitis most frequently occurs in adults with a history of recurrent urinary tract infections and is especially common in diabetics.

Previous peptic ulcer disease suggests that a patient's back pain is due to a penetrating ulcer. A history of cardiac murmurs should raise concern about endocarditis, since back pain is a not uncommon manifestation. A history of renal stones might indicate another cause of referred back pain.

History of the Back Pain

Certain qualities of a patient's pain can indicate a specific diagnosis. Low back pain radiating down the buttock and below the knee suggests a herniated disk causing nerve root irritation. Other conditions—including sacroiliitis, facet joint degenerative arthritis, spinal stenosis, or irritation of the sciatic nerve from a wallet—can also cause this pattern.

The diagnosis of disk herniation is further suggested by physical examination (see below) and confirmed by imaging techniques. Disk herniation can be asymptomatic, so its presence does not invariably link it to the symptom.

Low back pain at night, unrelieved by rest or the supine position, should suggest the possibility of malignancy, either vertebral body metastasis (chiefly from prostate, breast, lung, multiple myeloma, or lymphoma) or a cauda equina tumor. Similar pain can also be caused by compression fractures (from osteoporosis or myeloma).

Symptoms of large or rapidly evolving neurologic deficits identify patients who need urgent evaluation for possible cauda equina tumor, epidural abscess, or, rarely, massive disk herniation. Even with a herniated disk and nerve root impingement, pain is the most prominent symptom; numbness and weakness are less commonly reported and when present are of the magnitude consistent with compression of a single nerve root. Thus, symptoms of bilateral leg weakness (from multiple lumbar nerve root compressions) or of saddle area anesthesia, bowel or bladder incontinence, or impotence (indicating multiple sacral nerve root compressions) indicate a cauda equina process.

Low back pain that worsens with rest and improves with activity is characteristic of ankylosing spondylitis or other seronegative spondyloarthropathies, especially when the onset is insidious and begins before age 40. Most degenerative back diseases produce precisely the opposite pattern, with rest alleviating and activity aggravating the pain.

Low back pain causing the patient to writhe occurs in renal colic but can also indicate a leaking aneurysm.

Low back pain associated with pseudoclaudication from lumbar spinal stenosis is discussed below.

Physical Examination of the Back

Although examination of the back usually does not suggest a specific cause, several physical findings should be sought because they do help identify those few patients who need more than just conservative management.

Neurologic examination of the lower extremities will detect the small deficits produced by disk disease and the large deficits complicating such problems as cauda equina tumors. A positive straight leg raising test indicates nerve root irritation. The examiner performs the test on the supine patient by passively raising the patient's leg. The test is positive if radicular pain is produced with the leg raised 60 degrees or less. The test has a specificity of 40% but is 95% sensitive in patients with herniation at the L4–5 or L5–S1 level (the sites of 95% of disk herniations). It can be falsely negative, especially in patients with herniation above the L4–5 level.

The crossed straight leg sign has a sensitivity of 25% but is 90% specific for disk herniation and is positive when raising the contralateral leg reproduces the sciatica.

Detailed examination of the sacral and lumbar nerve roots, especially L5 and S1, is essential for detecting neurologic deficits associated with back pain. Disk herniation produces deficits predictable for the site involved (Table 20–6). Deficits of multiple nerve roots suggest a cauda equina tumor, an epidural abscess, or some other important process that requires urgent evaluation and treatment.

Measurement of spinal motion in the patient with acute pain is rarely of diagnostic utility and usually simply confirms that pain limits motion. An exception to this general rule is that evidence of decreased range of motion in multiple regions of the spine (cervical, thoracic, and lumbar) indicates a diffuse spinal disease such as ankylosing spondylitis. But by the time the patient has such limits, the diagnosis is usually straightforward.

If back pain is not severe and does not itself limit motion, Schober's test of lumbar motion is helpful in early diagnosis of ankylosing spondylitis. To perform this test, two marks are made, one 10 cm above S1 and another 5 cm below. The patient then bends forward as far as possible, and the distance between the points is measured. Normally, the distance increases at least 5 cm. Anything less indicates reduced lumbar motion, which in the absence of severe pain is most commonly due to ankylosing spondylitis or other seronegative spondyloarthropathies.

Palpation of the spine usually does not yield diagnostic information. Point tenderness over a vertebral body is reported to suggest osteomyelitis, but this association is uncommon. A step-off noted between the spinous process of adjacent vertebral bodies may indicate spondylolisthesis, but the sensitivity of this finding is extremely low. Tenderness of the soft tissues overlying the greater trochanter of the hip is a manifestation of trochanteric bursitis.

Inspection of the spine is not often of value in identifying serious causes of low back pain. The classic posture of ankylosing spondylitis is a late finding. Scoliosis of mild degree is not associated with an increased risk of clinical back disease. Cutaneous neurofibromas can identify the very rare patient who has nerve root encasement.

Examination of the hips should be part of the complete examination. While hip arthritis usually produces groin pain, some patients have buttock or low back symptoms.

Table 20–6. Neurologic testing of lumbosacral nerve disorders.

Nerve Root	Motor	Reflex	Sensory Area
L4	Dorsiflexion of foot	Knee jerk	Medial calf
L5	Dorsiflexion of great toe	None	Medial fore-foot
S1	Eversion of foot	Ankle jerk	Lateral foot

Further Examination

If the history and physical examination do not suggest the presence of infection, cancer, inflammatory back disease, major neurologic deficits, or pain referred from abdominal or pelvic disease, further evaluation can be eliminated or deferred while conservative therapy is tried. The great majority of patients will spontaneously improve with conservative care over 1–4 weeks.

Regular radiographs of the lumbosacral spine give 20 times the radiation dose of a chest x-ray and provide limited, albeit important, information. Oblique films double the radiation dose and are not routinely needed. X-rays can provide evidence of vertebral body osteomyelitis, cancer, fractures, or ankylosing spondylitis. Degenerative changes in the lumbar spine are ubiquitous in patients over 40 and do not prove clinical disease. Plain x-rays have very low sensitivity or specificity for disk disease. Thus, plain x-rays are warranted promptly for patients suspected of having infection, cancer, fractures, or inflammation; selected other patients who fail to improve after 2–4 weeks of conservative therapy are also candidates. The Agency for Health Care Policy and Research guidelines for obtaining lumbar radiographs are summarized in Table 20–7.

MRI provides exquisite anatomic detail but is reserved for patients in whom the information would change therapy. It is needed urgently in any patient suspected of having an epidural mass or cauda equina tumor but not if a patient is felt to have a routine disk herniation, since most will improve over 4–6 weeks of conservative therapy. Noncontrast CT does not image cauda equina tumors or other intradural lesions, and if used instead of MRI it must include intrathecal contrast.

Radionuclide bone scanning has limited utility. It is most useful for early detection of vertebral body osteomyelitis or metastases. The bone scan is often normal in multiple myeloma because lytic lesions do not take up isotope.

2. Management

While any management plan must be individualized, key elements of most conservative treatments for back pain include analgesia and education. Analgesia can usually be provided with NSAIDs (Table 5–6), but severe pain may require opioids (Table 5–7). Rarely does the need for opioids extend beyond 1–2 weeks.

Limited evidence supports the use of "muscle relaxants" such as diazepam, cyclobenzaprine, carisoprodol, and methocarbamol. These drugs should be reserved for patients who fail NSAIDs and should also be limited to courses of 1–2 weeks. Their use should be avoided in older patients, who are at risk of falling. All patients should be taught how to protect the back in daily activities—ie, not to lift heavy objects, to use the legs rather than the back when lifting, to use a chair with arm rests, and to rise from bed by first rolling to one side and then using the arms to push to an upright position. Back manipulation for benign, mechanical low back pain appears safe and as effective as therapies provided by physicians.

Rest and back exercises, once thought to be cornerstones of conservative therapy, are now known to be ineffective for acute back pain. Two days of bed rest gives better results than 7 days. Indeed, no bed rest with continuation of ordinary activities as tolerated is superior to either 2 days of bed rest or back mobilizing exercises. The value of corsets or traction is dubious. Epidural corticosteroid injections can provide short-term relief of sciatica but do not improve functional status or reduce the need for surgery. Corticosteroid injections into facet joints are ineffective for chronic low back pain.

Surgical consultation is needed urgently for any patient with a large or evolving neurologic deficit. Surgery for disk disease is indicated when there is documentation of herniation by some imaging procedure, a consistent pain syndrome, and a consistent neurologic deficit that has failed to respond to 4–6 weeks of conservative therapy. Percutaneous lumbar discectomy, performed under local anesthesia, is a safe and effective (up to 75%) alternative to laminectomy. The percutaneous procedure is contraindicated in the presence of tumor, infection, spondylolisthesis, foraminal stenosis, loose disk fragments, or severe facet joint arthritis.

Complaints without objective findings suggest a psychologic role in symptom formation. Treatment includes reassurance and nonopioid analgesics.

LUMBAR SPINAL STENOSIS

Lumbar spinal stenosis may be congenital or (more commonly) acquired. Narrowing of the spinal canal most frequently results from enlarging osteophytes at the facet joints, hypertrophy of the ligamentum

Table 20–7. AHRQ criteria for lumbar radiographs in patients with acute low back pain.[1]

Possible fracture
  Major trauma
  Minor trauma in patients > 50 years
  Chronic steroid use
  Osteoporosis
  > 70 years
Possible tumor or infection
  > 50 years
  < 20 years
  History of cancer
  Constitutional symptoms
  Recent bacterial infection
  Intravenous drug use
  Immunosuppression
  Supine pain
  Nocturnal pain

[1] Agency for Healthcare Research and Quality (modified from JAMA 1997;277:1784.)

flavum, and protrusion or bulging of intervertebral disks. Exactly how spinal stenosis results in the pain syndromes described below is not defined, but is-chemia from compression of nutrient arterioles is one possible mechanism.

Since age is the greatest risk factor for spinal degen-erative changes, most patients with lumbar spinal stenosis are over 60 years old. Patients may present ei-ther with trouble walking or with back pain. Patients with gait disturbance notice the gradual onset of pain, weakness, or unsteadiness in both legs that is precipi-tated by walking or prolonged standing and relieved by sitting. The onset of symptoms with standing by it-self, the location of the maximal discomfort to the thighs, and the preservation of pedal pulses help dis-tinguish the "pseudoclaudication" of spinal stenosis from true claudication caused by vascular insuffi-ciency. In some patients, unsteadiness of gait is the most prominent complaint. Because the lumbar spinal canal volume increases with back flexion and decreases with extension, some patients observe that they have fewer symptoms walking uphill than down. When low back pain is the chief symptom, it is bilateral and often diffuse over the buttocks.

The back examination in patients with lumbar spinal stenosis is often unimpressive. Fewer than 10% have a positive straight leg raise sign, 25% have dimin-ished deep tendon reflexes, and 60% have slight proxi-mal weakness. Walking with the patient may reveal unsteadiness, though usually the patient's perception of gait disturbance is greater than that of any other ob-server. The diagnosis of spinal stenosis in a patient with symptoms is best confirmed by MRI. Weight loss and exercises aimed at reducing lumbar lordosis, which aggravates symptoms of spinal stenosis, can help. When disabling symptoms persist, decompres-sive laminectomy provides at least short-term relief in approximately 80%.

Andersson GB et al: A comparison of osteopathic spinal manipu-lation with standard care for patients with low back pain. N Engl J Med 1999;341:1426.[PMID: 10547405] (Osteo-pathic manual care and one or more standard medical thera-pies—analgesics, NSAIDs, physical therapy, ultrasound, and TENS units—had comparable outcomes at 12 weeks.)

Browning R et al: Cyclobenzaprine and back pain. A meta-analy-sis. Arch Intern Med 2001;161:1613. [PMID: 11434793] (Cyclobenzaprine is more effective than placebo, with effect greatest at 4 days.)

Cherkin DC et al: A comparison of physical therapy, chiropractic manipulation, and provision of an educational booklet for the treatment of patients with low back pain. N Engl J Med 1998;339:1021. [PMID: 9761803] (Chiropractic manipu-lation [$437] and physical therapy [$429] are more expen-sive and very slightly more effective than an education booklet [$153].)

Deyo RA et al: Low back pain. N Engl J Med 2001;344:363. [PMID: 11172169] (Comprehensive but concise review of the clinical features, imaging strategies, and treatment ap-proaches.)

JAMA patient page: low back pain. JAMA 1998;279:1846. [PMID: 9828721]

Vroomen PCAJ et al: Lack of effectiveness of bed rest for sciatica. N Engl J Med 1999;340:418. [PMID: 9971865]

FIBROMYALGIA

ESSENTIALS OF DIAGNOSIS

- Most frequent in women aged 20–50.
- Chronic widespread musculoskeletal pain syn-drome with multiple tender points.
- Fatigue, headaches, numbness common.
- Objective signs of inflammation absent; labora-tory studies normal.
- Partially responsive to exercise, tricyclic antide-pressants.

General Considerations

Fibromyalgia is one of the most common rheumatic syndromes in ambulatory general medicine affecting 3–10% of the general population. It shares many fea-tures with the chronic fatigue syndrome, namely, an increased frequency among women aged 20–50, ab-sence of objective findings, and absence of diagnostic laboratory tests. While many of the clinical features of the two conditions overlap, musculoskeletal pain pre-dominates in fibromyalgia whereas lassitude domi-nates the chronic fatigue syndrome.

The cause is unknown, but sleep disorders, depres-sion, viral infections, and aberrant perception of nor-mal stimuli have all been proposed. Fibromyalgia can be a rare complication of hypothyroidism, rheumatoid arthritis, or, in men, sleep apnea.

Clinical Findings

The patient complains of chronic aching pain and stiffness, frequently involving the entire body but with prominence of pain around the neck, shoulders, low back, and hips. Fatigue, sleep disorders, subjective numbness, chronic headaches, and irritable bowel symptoms are common. Even minor exertion aggra-vates pain and increases fatigue. Physical examination is normal except for "trigger points" of pain produced by palpation of various areas such as the trapezius, the medial fat pad of the knee, and the lateral epicondyle of the elbow.

Differential Diagnosis

Fibromyalgia is a diagnosis of exclusion. A detailed history and repeated physical examination can obviate the need for extensive laboratory testing. Rheumatoid arthritis and systemic lupus erythematosus present with objective physical findings or abnormalities on routine testing, including the erythrocyte sedimentation rate. Thyroid function tests are useful, since hypothyroidism can produce a secondary fibromyalgia syndrome. Polymyositis produces weakness rather than pain. The diagnosis of fibromyalgia probably should be made hesitantly in a patient over age 50 and should never be invoked to explain fever, weight loss, or any other objective signs. Polymyalgia rheumatica produces shoulder and girdle pain, is associated with anemia and an elevated sedimentation rate, and occurs after age 50. Hypophosphatemic states, such as oncogenic osteomalacia, should also be included in the differential diagnosis of musculoskeletal pain unassociated with physical findings. In contrast to fibromyalgia, oncogenic osteomalacia usually produces pain in only a few areas and is associated with a low serum phosphate level.

Treatment

Patient education is essential. Patients can be comforted that they have a diagnosable syndrome treatable by specific though imperfect therapies and that the course is not progressive. There is modest efficacy of amitriptyline, fluoxetine, chlorpromazine, or cyclobenzaprine. Amitriptyline is initiated at a dosage of 10 mg at bedtime and gradually increased to 40–50 mg depending on efficacy and toxicity. Exercise programs are also beneficial. NSAIDs are generally ineffective. Opioids and corticosteroids are ineffective and should not be used to treat fibromyalgia.

Prognosis

All patients have chronic symptoms. With treatment, however, many do eventually resume increased activities. Progressive or objective findings do not develop.

Bennett RM: Emerging concepts in the neurobiology of chronic pain: evidence of abnormal sensory processing in fibromyalgia. Mayo Clin Proc 1999;74:385.[PMID: 10221469] (Review of the neurobiology of chronic pain, with particular reference to fibromyalgia.)

Goldenberg DL: Fibromyalgia syndrome a decade later: what have we learned? Arch Intern Med 1999;159:777. [PMID: 10219923] (Acknowledges psychosocial factors in patients with fibromyalgia who seek medical care, compared with persons in the community who meet criteria for the syndrome who do not.)

Leventhal LJ: Management of fibromyalgia. Ann Intern Med 1999;131:850. [PMID: 10610631]

CARPAL TUNNEL SYNDROME

An entrapment neuropathy, carpal tunnel syndrome is a painful disorder caused by compression of the median nerve between the carpal ligament and other structures within the carpal tunnel. The contents of the tunnel can be increased by organic lesions such as synovitis of the tendon sheaths or carpal joints, recent or malhealed fractures, tumors, and occasionally congenital anomalies. Even though no anatomic lesion is apparent, flattening or even circumferential constriction of the median nerve may be observed during operative section of the ligament. The disorder may occur in pregnancy, is seen in individuals with a history of repetitive use of the hands, and may follow injuries of the wrists. There is a familial type of carpal tunnel syndrome in which no etiologic factor can be identified.

Carpal tunnel syndrome can also be a feature of many systemic diseases: rheumatoid arthritis and other rheumatic disorders (inflammatory tenosynovitis); myxedema, amyloidosis, sarcoidosis, and leukemia (tissue infiltration); acromegaly; and hyperparathyroidism.

Clinical Findings

Pain in the distribution of the median nerve, which may be burning and tingling (acroparesthesia), is the initial symptom. Aching pain may radiate proximally into the forearm and occasionally proximally to the shoulder and over the neck and chest. Pain is exacerbated by manual activity, particularly by extremes of volar flexion or dorsiflexion of the wrist. It is most bothersome at night. Impairment of sensation in the median nerve distribution may or may not be demonstrable. Subtle disparity between the affected and opposite sides can be shown by testing for two-point discrimination or by requiring the patient to identify different textures of cloth by rubbing them between the tips of the thumb and the index finger. Tinel's or Phalen's sign may be positive. (Tinel's sign is tingling or shock-like pain on volar wrist percussion; Phalen's sign, pain or paresthesia in the distribution of the median nerve when the patient flexes both wrists to 90 degrees with the dorsal aspects of the hands held in apposition for 60 seconds.) The carpal compression test, in which numbness and tingling are induced by the direct application of pressure over the carpal tunnel, may be more sensitive and specific than the Tinel and Phalen tests. Muscle weakness or atrophy, especially of the thenar eminence, appears later than sensory disturbances. Specific examinations include electromyography and determinations of segmental sensory and motor conduction delay. Sensory conduction delay is evident before motor delay.

Differential Diagnosis

This syndrome should be differentiated from other cervicobrachial pain syndromes, from compression syndromes of the median nerve in the forearm or arm, and from mononeuritis multiplex. When left-sided, it may be confused with angina pectoris.

Treatment

Treatment is directed toward relief of pressure on the median nerve. When a primary lesion is discovered, specific treatment should be given. When soft tissue swelling is a cause, elevation of the extremity may relieve symptoms. Splinting of the hand and forearm at night may be beneficial. Injection of corticosteroid by an experienced operator into the carpal tunnel can alleviate symptoms in some patients, particularly those with synovitis of the wrist.

Operative division of the volar carpal ligament gives lasting relief from pain, which usually subsides within a few days. The presence of muscle atrophy is a strong indication for surgery; ideally median nerve entrapment is treated before atrophy occurs. Muscle strength returns gradually, but complete recovery cannot be expected when atrophy is pronounced.

Atroshi I et al: Prevalence of carpal tunnel syndrome in a general population. JAMA 1999;282:153. [PMID: 10411196] (One in five symptomatic people had confirmation of the diagnosis by clinical examination and electrophysiologic testing.)

D'Arcy CA et al: Does this patient have carpal tunnel syndrome? JAMA 2000;283:3110. [PMID: 10865306] (Meta-analysis of studies evaluating the use of physical examination to diagnose carpal tunnel syndrome debunks the utility of several traditional findings. Hand symptom diagrams, hypalgesia, and thumb abduction weakness are helpful in diagnosis.)

Katz JN et al: Predictors of outcomes of carpal tunnel release. Arthritis Rheum 2001;44:1184. [PMID: 11352253] (Two-thirds were very satisfied with the long-term results of surgery. Consulting an attorney or having worse psychologic problems were predictors of less favorable outcomes.)

DUPUYTREN'S CONTRACTURE

This relatively common disorder is characterized by hyperplasia of the palmar fascia and related structures, with nodule formation and contracture of the palmar fascia. The cause is unknown, but the condition has a genetic predisposition and occurs primarily in white men over 50 years of age. The incidence is higher among alcoholics and patients with chronic systemic disorders (especially cirrhosis). It is also associated with systemic fibrosing syndrome, which includes Peyronie's disease, mediastinal and retroperitoneal fibrosis, and Riedel's struma. The onset may be acute, but slowly progressive chronic disease is more common.

Dupuytren's contracture manifests itself by nodular or cord-like thickening of one or both hands, with the fourth and fifth fingers most commonly affected. The patient may complain of tightness of the involved digits, with inability to satisfactorily extend the fingers, and on occasion there is tenderness. The resulting cosmetic problems may be unappealing, but in general the contracture is well tolerated since it exaggerates the normal position of function of the hand. Fasciitis involving other areas of the body may lead to plantar fibromatosis (10% of patients) or Peyronie's disease (1–2%).

If the palmar nodule is growing rapidly, injections of triamcinolone into the nodule may be of benefit. Surgical intervention is indicated in patients with significant flexion contractures, depending on the location, but recurrence is not uncommon.

REFLEX SYMPATHETIC DYSTROPHY

Reflex sympathetic dystrophy is a syndrome of pain and swelling of an extremity accompanied by signs of skin changes in the extremity (eg, skin atrophy, hyperhidrosis) and signs and symptoms of vasomotor instability. Complex regional pain syndrome may be a more appropriate name. Any extremity can be involved, but the disorder most commonly occurs in the hand and is associated with ipsilateral restricted shoulder motion (shoulder-hand syndrome). The swelling in reflex sympathetic dystrophy is diffuse ("catcher's mitt hand") and not restricted to joints. Pain is often described as burning in quality. The shoulder-hand variant of reflex sympathetic dystrophy sometimes complicates myocardial infarction or injuries to the neck or shoulder. Direct trauma to the hand or foot can also provoke this syndrome. Reflex sympathetic dystrophy may occur after a knee injury or after arthroscopic knee surgery. There are no systemic symptoms, and x-rays reveal severe generalized osteopenia. In the posttraumatic variant of reflex sympathetic dystrophy, this is known as Sudeck's atrophy. Bone scans also show increased uptake. Symptoms and findings are bilateral in some.

This syndrome should be differentiated from other cervicobrachial pain syndromes, rheumatoid arthritis, and scleroderma, among others.

In addition to addressing the underlying disorder, treatment is directed toward restoration of function. Physical therapy is the cornerstone of treatment. Patients who have restricted shoulder motion may benefit from the treatment described for scapulohumeral periarthritis. In resistant cases, prednisone, 30–40 mg/d for 2 weeks and then tapered over 2 weeks, may be effective. Stellate ganglion block can also be effective for reflex sympathetic dystrophy.

The prognosis depends in part upon the stage in which the lesions are encountered and the extent and severity of associated organic disease. Early treatment offers the best prognosis for recovery.

Kemler MA et al: Spinal cord stimulation in patients with chronic reflex sympathetic dystrophy. N Engl J Med 2000;343:618. [PMID: 10965008] (This invasive but safe modality is effective for relief of intractable pain without functional improvement.)

Schwartzman RJ: New treatments for reflex sympathetic dystrophy. N Engl J Med 2000;343:654. [PMID: 10979798] (Editorial summarizing clinical features and outlining nomenclature and new therapeutic approaches.)

Van Hilten BJ et al: Intrathecal baclofen for the treatment of dystonia in patients with reflex sympathetic dystrophy. N Engl J Med 2000;343:625. [PMID: 10965009]

BURSITIS

Inflammation of the synovium-like cellular membrane overlying bony prominences may be secondary to trauma, infection, or arthritic conditions such as gout, rheumatoid arthritis, or osteoarthritis. The most common locations are the subdeltoid, olecranon, ischial, trochanteric, semimembranous-gastrocnemius (Baker's cyst) and prepatellar bursae.

There are several ways to distinguish bursitis from arthritis. Bursitis is more likely than arthritis to begin abruptly and cause focal tenderness and swelling. Olecranon bursitis, for example, causes an oval swelling at the tip of the elbow, whereas elbow joint inflammation produces more diffuse swelling. Similarly, a patient with prepatellar bursitis has a small focus of swelling over the kneecap and no distention of the knee joint itself. Active and passive range of motion are usually much more limited in arthritis than in bursitis. A patient with trochanteric bursitis will have normal internal rotation of the hip, whereas a patient with hip arthritis will not. Bursitis caused by trauma responds to local heat, rest, immobilization, NSAIDs, and local corticosteroid injections.

Bursitis can result from infection. The two most common sites are the olecranon and prepatellar bursae. Acute swelling and redness at either of these two sites calls for aspiration to rule out infection. The absence of fever does not exclude infection; and one-third of those with septic olecranon bursitis are afebrile. A bursal fluid white blood cell count of greater than 1000/μL indicates inflammation from infection, rheumatoid arthritis, or gout. In septic bursitis, the white cell count averages over 50,000/μL. Most cases are caused by *Staphylococcus aureus;* the Gram stain is positive in two-thirds. Treatment involves antibiotics and repeated aspiration for tense effusions.

Chronic, stable olecranon bursa swelling unaccompanied by erythema or other signs of inflammation does not suggest infection and does not require aspiration. Aspiration of the olecranon bursa in rheumatoid arthritis and in gout runs the risk of creating a chronic drainage site. This risk can be reduced by using a small needle (25 gauge if possible) and pulling the skin over the bursa before introducing the needle. Applying a pressure bandage may also help prevent chronic drainage. Surgical removal of the bursa is indicated only for cases in which repeated infections occur. Repetitive minor trauma to the olecranon bursa should be eliminated by avoiding resting the elbow on a hard surface or by wearing an elbow pad.

A bursa can also become symptomatic when it ruptures. This is particularly true for Baker's cyst, whose rupture can cause calf pain and swelling that mimic thrombophlebitis. The ruptured cyst can be imaged with sonography, MRI, or arthrography. In most cases, none of these tests are necessary because Baker's cyst or the frequently associated knee effusion is detectable on physical examination. Often it is more important to exclude thrombophlebitis than it is to visualize Baker's cyst. Treatment of a ruptured cyst includes rest, leg elevation, and injection of triamcinolone, 20–40 mg into the knee (which communicates with the cyst). Rarely, Baker's cyst can compress vascular structures and cause leg edema and true thrombophlebitis.

SPORTS MEDICINE INJURIES

Musculoskeletal problems commonly occur as a result of both serious athletic pursuits and activities of daily living. For most such disorders, the diagnosis is made easily. Physical therapy is an increasingly important adjunct to the management of these disorders.

1. Rotator Cuff Disorders

A substantial majority of shoulder problems stem from disorders of the rotator cuff. The tendons of the rotator cuff form a musculotendinous unit near their insertions into the proximal humerus. As a result of years of cumulative irritation, attenuation of these tendons occurs. Among the relevant muscles, the supraspinatus is most often affected. Distinguishing between the various soft tissue disorders that cause shoulder pain is difficult. Rotator cuff tendinitis, subacromial bursitis, partial and complete rotator cuff tears, and calcific tendinitis frequently cause similar symptoms. In addition, these disorders often occur together, though precise distinction is frequently unimportant for purposes of therapy.

Clinical Findings

Patients usually present with nonspecific pain localized to the shoulder, often noticed more at night when lying on the affected side. Locking sensations occur with motion of the shoulder, particularly through abduction. Because of the shared innervation, symptoms are frequently referred down the proximal lateral arm. With rotator cuff tears, there may be an inability to abduct or flex the shoulder depending on the site of the tear.

The rotator cuff may be palpated just lateral to the head of the acromion. Maximum tenderness is usually noted over the supraspinatus insertion. The acromioclavicular joint may also be tender if there is accompanying degenerative arthritis in that joint. There may be prominent crepitus. Pain with range of motion is most pronounced between 60 and 120 degrees of abduction, the site of greatest impingement of the rotator cuff tissues between the humerus and coracoacromial arch.

For patients with partial rotator cuff tendon ruptures, the findings are identical to those of chronic tendinitis and bursitis. Patients with partial ruptures often demonstrate mild abduction weakness. With complete ruptures, weakness of abduction (and, to a lesser extent, flexion) is substantial, even though full range of motion may be maintained by the shoulder's accessory rotator muscles. Patients with complete tears usually have positive "drop" signs: inability to sustain passive abduction of the arm to 90 degrees.

Treatment

For most rotator cuff disorders, the central tenets of therapy are rest and abstention from inciting activities.

Temporary use of a sling is occasionally helpful in enforcing rest. NSAIDs and moist heat afford some symptomatic relief. For patients with symptoms persisting after 2 weeks of conservative management, injections of a corticosteroid preparation (eg, 1 mL of triamcinolone, 40 mg/mL) mixed with 2–3 mL of lidocaine hydrochloride (1–2%) may be useful. Tears or partial tears of the rotator cuff tendons that are believed to be chronic do not preclude a corticosteroid injection. Most patients obtain significant relief with one injection, but the procedure—along with continued rest—may be repeated after 2–3 weeks. Physical therapy is valuable for refractory cases—if the patient fails to maintain the shoulder's normal range of motion, stiffness and impaired function may ensue.

Aside from patients with complete rotator cuff tears, only those who fail to improve after months of conservative therapy are candidates for operation. Persistent symptoms may be a sign of complete tear, which may be diagnosed by MRI. Patients with symptoms that continue in the absence of a complete tear, however, sometimes require surgery to excise the inferolateral portion of the acromion, release obstructed soft tissue, and repair partial tendon tears. Depending on the degree of symptoms and functional status, complete tears may not always require surgical repair. Patients over 75 years of age rarely have symptoms or limitations that necessitate surgery. Moreover, surgical repairs are frequently less successful because of the attrition of the rotator cuff that occurs with aging.

2. Lateral & Medial Epicondylitis

These disorders are better known by their sports associations: "tennis elbow" and "golf elbow," respectively. Lateral epicondylitis is the more common of the two. The conditions are caused by overuse, and the pain results from minor tears in the tendons of the forearm's extensor and flexor muscles.

Clinical Findings

The patient presents with pain at the site of tendon insertion. Tasks that require grasping and squeezing, such as shaking hands or opening jars, are impaired and cause pain.

The diagnoses are easily confirmed on physical examination by elicitation of point tenderness over the involved site. The characteristic pain may also be reproduced by extension or flexion of the wrist against pressure. Clenching the fist and extending the wrist against the pressure of the examiner's palm is a useful maneuver for localizing lateral epicondylitis. Medial epicondylitis may be demonstrated by performing the same maneuver in flexion.

Treatment

The use of "counterforce" straps (bands worn distal to the elbow, over the bulk of the forearm musculature), intended to decrease the forces transmitted to the elbow during activity, are inadequate substitutes for rest. NSAIDs are effective in mild cases. Symptoms that persist after 2 weeks of conservative therapy usually respond to infiltration of triamcinolone 10–20 mg mixed with 1–2 mL of 1% lidocaine around the involved epicondyle. After the pain and tenderness have subsided, patients may begin a physical therapy program involving daily stretching of the flexor and extensor tendons. There are anecdotal reports of dramatic relief with operative treatment.

3. Patellofemoral Syndrome

Patellofemoral syndrome is among the most common causes of knee complaints in primary care medicine, particularly among adolescent and young adult patients. The syndrome frequently gives rise to the chief complaint of anterior knee pain. The belief that furrowing and roughening of the cartilage on the patella's posterior surface cause the syndrome (chondromalacia patellae) is erroneous. This finding is common, rarely leads to symptomatology, and requires no intervention. A variety of injuries or anatomic abnormalities predispose patients to irregular patellar movements, however, leading to the patellofemoral syndrome. Such predisposing conditions include imbalance of quadriceps strength, patella alta, recurrent patellar subluxation, direct trauma to the patella, and meniscal injuries. For most of these causes, the therapeutic approach is similar.

Clinical Findings

Patients frequently have difficulty localizing the source of their complaint but generally confirm that the pain is in the front of the knee, around or underneath the patella. Questions regarding specific precipitants of the pain may be useful in establishing the diagnosis. For example, because of the flexion load, patients have difficulty going up or down staircases. Another characteristic symptom is the positive "theater" sign: after remaining seated for a prolonged period, patients describe extreme discomfort with their first few steps after rising. The symptoms improve with further walking. Finally, patients with patellofemoral syndrome often complain of crepitus, joint locking, or sensations of joint instability, all of which lack anatomic explanations.

The physical examination is less useful than the history in establishing the diagnosis, but a significant number of patients have characteristic physical findings. In particular, when the knee is held in slight flexion, gentle pressure against the patella as the patient contracts the quadriceps muscles may reproduce the symptoms. In some cases, with the knee extended and the quadriceps relaxed, the typical pain may be reproduced by digital pressure under the medial or lateral border of the patella, with side-to-side movement of the bone. Inflammatory findings on examination are incompatible with the diagnosis of patellofemoral syndrome and suggest other disorders.

Treatment

Therapy includes avoidance of flexion loads and strengthening of the quadriceps. Referral to a physical therapist is helpful in educating the patient about home exercises. Many patients learn that the most effective therapy is bicycling, with the seat high enough to permit nearly full knee extension with each cycle. Although most cases respond to these interventions and even resolve altogether, some persist for years. Even in the latter, conservative therapy remains the rule; operation is rarely indicated.

4. Overuse Syndromes of the Knee

Runners—particularly those who overtrain, fail to stretch prior to running, or do not attain the proper level of conditioning before starting a running program—may develop a variety of painful overuse syndromes of the knee. Most of these conditions are forms of tendinitis or bursitis that can be diagnosed on examination. The most common conditions include anserine bursitis, the iliotibial band syndrome, and popliteal and patellar tendinitis.

Clinical Findings

Symptoms resulting from all of these conditions worsen as the patient continues to run and often require cessation of the activity. Anserine bursitis results in pain medial and inferior to the knee joint over the medial tibia. The iliotibial band syndrome and popliteal tenosynovitis may be difficult to differentiate, because the popliteus tendon inserts into the lateral femoral condyle underneath the iliotibial band. Both conditions result in pain on the lateral side of the knee. Patellar tendinitis, a cause of anterior knee discomfort, typically occurs at the tendon's insertion into the patella rather than at its more inferior insertion.

All of these diagnoses are confirmed by palpation at the relevant sites around the knee. None is associated with joint effusions or other signs of synovitis.

Treatment

Rest and abstention from the associated physical activities for a period of days to weeks are essential. Once the acute pain from these conditions has subsided, a program of gentle stretching (particularly prior to resuming exercise) may prevent recurrence. Corticosteroid with lidocaine injections may be useful when intense discomfort is present, but caution must be employed when injecting corticosteroids into the region of a tendon.

5. Medial Meniscus Injuries

Tears of the medial meniscus are the most common knee injuries encountered in primary care. Because the medial meniscus is firmly tethered to the underlying tibia, injuries to the medial meniscus occur ten times more commonly than injuries to the lateral meniscus. Both types of injury result from a twisting action exerted on the knee joint while the foot is in a weight-bearing position.

Clinical Findings

The injury is heralded by a tearing or popping sensation followed by severe pain. Occasionally, meniscal tears result from seemingly minor trauma. In contrast to ligamentous injuries, in which hemorrhage causes immediate swelling, effusions associated with meniscal injuries accumulate over hours and are typically worse on the day following the injury. Several days after resolution (full or partial), the patient may experience joint locking or instability, recurrent swelling with activity, and pain. The sensation of locking, which may result from mechanical blockage by a fragment of torn meniscus, more commonly results from "pseudolocking" caused by muscle spasm and swelling.

Joint effusion is usually present, frequently accompanied by a ballottable patella. Tenderness may be localized to the medial joint line, and range of motion in the knee may be restricted. In patients without an acutely painful, swollen knee, McMurray's test may suggest the diagnosis. This test is performed with the patient supine and the hip and knee in full flexion. The examiner has one hand on the involved knee and the other on the ipsilateral foot. As the foot is externally rotated, the examiner extends the patient's knee. The presence of a "snap" (palpable or audible) suggests a medial meniscus lesion. MRI is now the optimal test for confirming the diagnosis if plain films exclude other conditions.

Treatment

Initial management is conservative, with elevation of the joint and application of a compression dressing and ice. Weight bearing should be minimized for the first few days after the injury but may be resumed slowly thereafter. The patient should perform quadriceps-strengthening exercises under the instruction of a physical therapist. Surgery is reserved for patients with symptoms that recur upon resumption of normal activities or for patients with irreducible locking caused by mechanical problems.

6. Ankle Sprains

Ankle sprains are among the most common of all sports injuries. Most sprains involve the lateral ligament complex, particularly the anterior talofibular ligament. In more severe injuries, the calcaneofibular ligament may also be involved. If both of these ligaments are ruptured, the injury results in significant joint instability and is classified as a grade III (severe) sprain. (Grades I and II correspond to mild and moderate injuries, respectively.) This section reviews only the type of ankle sprain resulting from inversion (varus) injuries, which account for 85% of all sprains.

Clinical Findings

Varus sprains include a spectrum of severity, ranging from slight loss of function to injuries in which the swelling is prompt, the pain prominent, and weight-bearing impossible. A history of hearing a "pop" at the time of injury is frequently associated with the latter.

Hemorrhage resulting from torn ligaments and damaged peroneal muscle tendons may cause substantial ecchymosis. Tenderness is typically present at the site of injury, and the associated swelling may be considerable. Stability of the anterior talofibular and calcaneofibular ligaments should be assessed with the "anterior drawer" sign: With the foot held in slight plantar flexion, the examiner cups the patient's heel with one hand and the patient's shin with the other. The examiner then applies gentle anterior force in the plane of the patient's foot. Excessive anterior motion of the foot constitutes a positive test (grade III sprain). Plain radiographs exclude associated bony injury.

Treatment

Most ankle sprains—even grade III sprains—usually are treated identically. The acronym "RICE" (rest, ice, compression, elevation) applies more accurately to ankle sprains than to any other injury. Early application of a compression dressing is essential to control swelling and provide stability to the traumatized joint. Weight bearing should be minimal, with liberal use of crutches. Elevation of the ankle for several days hastens functional recovery by diminishing pain and swelling, and ice is also helpful (alternating 30 minutes on, 30 minutes off). The ice should be applied on top of the compression dressing and not against the skin both because close apposition of the dressing to the skin is critical to control swelling and because direct application of ice is uncomfortable and even deleterious to the skin. Referral to a physical therapist may expedite recovery. Patients should be informed that symptoms from lateral ankle sprains may take weeks or months to resolve, and that this period will be prolonged by premature attempts to bear weight on the injured ankle. Surgical repairs of ruptured lateral ligaments provide excellent outcomes but are usually necessary only in cases of chronically unstable joints.

7. Plantar Fasciitis

The most common cause of foot pain in outpatient medicine is plantar fasciitis, which results from constant strain on the plantar fascia at its insertion into the medial tubercle of the calcaneus. Although certain inflammatory disorders such as the seronegative spondyloarthropathies predispose patients to enthesopathies, the majority of cases occur in patients with no associated disease. Most occur as the result of excessive standing and improper footwear.

Clinical Findings

Patients with plantar fasciitis report severe pain on the bottoms of their feet in the morning—the first steps out of bed in particular—but the pain subsides after a few minutes of ambulation.

The diagnosis may be confirmed by palpation over the plantar fascia's insertion on the medial heel. Radiographs have no role in the diagnosis of this condition—heel spurs frequently exist in patients without plantar fasciitis, and most symptomatic patients do not have heel spurs.

Treatment

Treatment consists of imposing an interval of days without prolonged standing and the use of arch supports. Arch supports give relief by requiring the arches to bear more of the patient's weight, thus unloading the plantar enthesis. NSAIDs may provide some relief. In severe cases, a corticosteroid with lidocaine injection (small volume—no more than a total of 1.5 mL) directly into the most tender area on the sole of the foot is helpful. Rare patients require release of the plantar fascia from its attachment site at the os calcis.

Carette S: Adhesive capsulitis: research advances frozen in time? J Rheumatol 2000;27:1329. [PMID: 10852248] (Classic adhesive capsulitis is usually self-limited, but time to the conclusion of the "thawing" or recovery phase may be 2 or 3 years.)

Liu SH et al: Ankle sprains and other soft tissue injuries. Curr Opin Rheumatol 1999;11:132. [PMID: 10319217] (Review of the management of patients with residual ankle pain and lateral ankle instability.)

Solomon DH et al: Does this patient have a torn meniscus or ligament of the knee? Value of the physical examination. JAMA 2001;286:1610. [PMID: 11585485] (Synthesis of the history and several examination maneuvers are more accurate than any single maneuver.)

Speed CA et al: Calcific tendinitis of the shoulder. N Engl J Med 1999;340: 1582. [PMID: 10332023] (Concise review of the problem and an approach to therapy.)

Tandeter HB et al: Acute knee injuries: use of decision rules for selective radiograph ordering. Am Fam Phys 1999;60:2599. [PMID: 10605994] (Radiographs are principally useful for ruling out bone fractures.)

Thomee et al: Patello-femoral pain syndrome: a review of current issues. Sports Med 1999;28:245. [PMID: 10565551] (Thoughtful review of the problem of anterior knee pain, acknowledging the shortcomings of current explanations for pain in this region.)

■ AUTOIMMUNE DISEASES

The autoimmune disorders are a protean group of acquired diseases in which genetic factors appear to play a role. They have in common widespread immunologic and inflammatory alterations of connective tissue.

These illnesses share certain clinical features, and differentiation among them is often difficult because of this. Common findings include synovitis, pleuritis, myocarditis, endocarditis, pericarditis, peritonitis, vasculitis, myositis, skin rash, alterations of connective tissues, and nephritis. Laboratory tests may reveal Coombs-positive hemolytic anemia, thrombocytopenia, leukopenia, immunoglobulin excesses or deficiencies, antinuclear antibodies (which include antibodies to many nuclear constituents, including DNA and extractable nuclear antigen), rheumatoid factors, cryoglobulins, false-positive serologic tests for syphilis, elevated muscle enzymes, and alterations in serum complement.

Some of the laboratory alterations that occur in this group of diseases (eg, false-positive serologic tests for syphilis, rheumatoid factor) occur in asymptomatic individuals. These changes may also be demonstrated in certain asymptomatic relatives of patients with connective tissue diseases, in older persons, in patients using certain drugs, and in patients with chronic infectious diseases.

RHEUMATOID ARTHRITIS

ESSENTIALS OF DIAGNOSIS

- *Prodromal systemic symptoms of malaise, fever, weight loss, and morning stiffness.*
- *Onset usually insidious and in small joints; progression is centripetal and symmetric; deformities common.*
- *Radiographic findings: juxta-articular osteoporosis, joint erosions, and narrowing of the joint spaces.*
- *Rheumatoid factor usually present.*
- *Extra-articular manifestations: subcutaneous nodules, pleural effusion, pericarditis, lymphadenopathy, splenomegaly with leukopenia, and vasculitis.*

General Considerations

Rheumatoid arthritis is a chronic systemic inflammatory disease of unknown cause, chiefly affecting synovial membranes of multiple joints. The disease has a wide clinical spectrum with considerable variability in joint and extra-articular manifestations. The prevalence in the general population is 1–2%; female patients outnumber males almost 3:1. The usual age at onset is 20–40 years, although rheumatoid arthritis may begin at any age. Susceptibility to rheumatoid arthritis is genetically determined. Most patients have a class 2 human leukocyte antigen (HLA) with an identical five-

amino-acid sequence. Although rheumatoid arthritis was once considered to be a relatively benign disorder that could be kept in check by slowly adding layers of treatment, it is now known to be a disease with such a strong tendency to shorten life and cause severe disability that early and aggressive treatment—often with drugs used in combination—is preferred.

The pathologic findings in the joint include chronic synovitis with pannus formation. The pannus erodes cartilage, bone, ligaments, and tendons. In the acute phase, effusion and other manifestations of inflammation are common. In the late stage, organization may result in fibrous ankylosis; true bony ankylosis is rare. In both acute and chronic phases, inflammation of soft tissues around the joints may be prominent and is a significant factor in joint damage.

The microscopic findings most characteristic of rheumatoid arthritis are those of the subcutaneous nodule. This is a granuloma with a central zone of fibrinoid necrosis, a surrounding palisade of radially arranged elongated connective tissue cells, and a periphery of chronic granulation tissue. Pathologic alterations indistinguishable from those of the subcutaneous nodule are occasionally seen in the myocardium, pericardium, endocardium, heart valves, visceral pleura, lungs, sclera, dura mater, spleen, and larynx as well as in the synovial membrane, periarticular tissues, and tendons. Nonspecific pericarditis and pleuritis are found in 25–40% of patients at autopsy. Additional nonspecific lesions associated with rheumatoid arthritis include inflammation of small arteries, pulmonary fibrosis, mononuclear cell infiltration of skeletal muscle and perineurium, and hyperplasia of lymph nodes. Secondary amyloidosis may also be present.

Clinical Findings

A. SYMPTOMS AND SIGNS

The clinical manifestations of rheumatoid disease are highly variable. The onset of articular signs of inflammation is usually insidious, with prodromal symptoms of malaise, weight loss, and vague periarticular pain or stiffness. Less often, the onset is acute, apparently triggered by a stressful situation such as infection, surgery, trauma, emotional strain, or the postpartum period. There is characteristically symmetric joint swelling with associated stiffness, warmth, tenderness, and pain. Stiffness persisting for over 30 minutes is prominent in the morning and subsides during the day; its duration is a useful indicator of activity of disease. Stiffness may recur after daytime inactivity and may be much more severe after strenuous activity. Although any joint may be affected in rheumatoid arthritis, the proximal interphalangeal and metacarpophalangeal joints of the fingers as well as the wrists, knees, ankles, and toes are most often involved. Monarticular disease is occasionally seen early. Synovial cysts and rupture of tendons may occur. Entrapment syndromes are not unusual—particularly entrapment of the median nerve at the carpal tunnel of the wrist. Palmar erythema is noted occasionally, as are tiny hemorrhagic infarcts in the nail folds or finger pulps, which are signs of vasculitis. Twenty percent of patients have subcutaneous nodules, most commonly situated over bony prominences but also observed in the bursas and tendon sheaths; these occur in seropositive patients, as do most other extra-articular manifestations. A small number of patients have splenomegaly and lymph node enlargement. Low-grade fever, anorexia, weight loss, fatigue, and weakness often persist; chills are rare. After months or years, deformities may occur; the most common are ulnar deviation of the fingers, boutonnière deformity (hyperextension of the distal interphalangeal joint with flexion of the proximal interphalangeal joint), "swan-neck" deformity (flexion of the distal interphalangeal with extension of the proximal interphalangeal joint), and valgus deformity of the knee. Atrophy of skin or muscle is common. Dryness of the eyes, mouth, and other mucous membranes is found especially in advanced disease (see Sjögren's Syndrome). Other ocular manifestations include episcleritis and scleromalacia, the latter due to scleral nodules and capable of causing retinal detachment. Pericarditis and pleural disease, when present, are frequently silent clinically. Aortitis is a rare late complication that can result in aortic regurgitation or rupture and is usually associated with evidence of rheumatoid vasculitis elsewhere in the body.

B. Laboratory Findings

Serum protein abnormalities are often present. Rheumatoid factor, an IgM antibody directed against the Fc fragment of IgG, is present in the sera of more than 75% of patients. High titers of rheumatoid factor are commonly associated with severe rheumatoid disease. Titers may also be significantly elevated in a number of diverse conditions, including syphilis, sarcoidosis, infective endocarditis, tuberculosis, leprosy, and parasitic infections; in advanced age; and in asymptomatic relatives of patients with autoimmune diseases. Antinuclear antibodies are demonstrable in 20% of patients, though their titers are lower than in systemic lupus erythematosus.

During both the acute and chronic phases, the erythrocyte sedimentation rate and the gamma globulins (most commonly IgM and IgG) are typically elevated. A moderate hypochromic normocytic anemia is common. The white cell count is normal or slightly elevated, but leukopenia may occur, often in the presence of splenomegaly (eg, Felty's syndrome). The platelet count is often elevated, roughly in proportion to the severity of overall joint inflammation. Joint fluid examination is valuable, reflecting abnormalities that are associated with varying degrees of inflammation. (See Tables 20–1 and 20–2.)

C. Imaging

Of all the laboratory tests, x-ray changes are the most specific for rheumatoid arthritis. X-rays, however, are not sensitive in that most of those taken during the first 6 months are read as normal. The earliest changes occur in the wrists or feet and consist of soft tissue swelling and juxta-articular demineralization. Later, diagnostic changes of uniform joint space narrowing and erosions develop. The erosions are often first evident at the ulnar styloid and at the juxta-articular margin, where the bony surface is not protected by cartilage. Diagnostic changes also occur in the cervical spine, with C1–2 subluxation, but these changes usually take many years to develop.

Differential Diagnosis

The differentiation of rheumatoid arthritis from other diseases of connective tissue can be difficult. However, certain clinical features are helpful. Rheumatic fever is characterized by the migratory nature of the arthritis, an elevated antistreptolysin titer, and a more dramatic and prompt response to aspirin; carditis and erythema marginatum may occur in adults, but chorea and subcutaneous nodules virtually never do. Butterfly rash, discoid lupus erythematosus, photosensitivity, alopecia, high titer to anti-DNA, renal disease, and central nervous system abnormalities point to the diagnosis of systemic lupus erythematosus. Degenerative joint disease (osteoarthritis) is not associated with constitutional manifestations, and the joint pain is characteristically relieved by rest, in contrast to the morning stiffness of rheumatoid arthritis. Signs of articular inflammation, prominent in rheumatoid arthritis, are usually minimal in degenerative joint disease. Osteoarthritis—in contrast to rheumatoid arthritis—spares the wrist and the metacarpophalangeal joints. While in the early years gouty arthritis is almost always intermittent and monarticular, in later years it can become a chronic polyarticular process that mimics rheumatoid arthritis. Gouty tophi can at times resemble rheumatoid nodules. The early history of intermittent monarthritis and the presence of synovial urate crystals are distinctive features of gout. Septic arthritis can be distinguished by chills and fever, demonstration of the causative organism in joint fluid, and the frequent presence of a primary focus elsewhere, eg, gonococcal arthritis. Septic arthritis can complicate rheumatoid arthritis and should be considered whenever a patient with rheumatoid arthritis has one joint inflamed out of proportion to the rest. Chronic Lyme disease typically involves only one joint, most commonly the knee, and is associated with positive serologic tests (see Chapter 34). Human parvovirus B19 infection in adults can occasionally mimic rheumatoid arthritis. The mean age at onset is 35–37; arthralgias are much more prominent than arthritis; and rash—on the cheeks, torso, or extremities—is common. The patients are rheumatoid factor-negative, do not have erosions, and have IgM antibodies to human parvovirus B19 infection. Polymyalgia rheumatica occasionally causes polyarthritis in patients over age 50, but these patients remain rheumatoid factor-negative and have chiefly proximal muscle pain and stiffness. A variety of cancers produce paraneoplastic syndromes, including polyarthritis. One form is hypertrophic pulmonary osteoarthropathy most often produced by lung and gastrointestinal carcinomas, characterized by a rheumatoid-like arthritis associated with clubbing, periosteal new bone formation, and a negative rheumatoid factor. Diffuse swelling of the hands with palmar fasciitis has also been reported with a variety of cancers, especially ovarian carcinoma.

Treatment

A. BASIC PROGRAM (NONPHARMACOLOGIC MANAGEMENT)

The primary objectives in treating rheumatoid arthritis are reduction of inflammation and pain, preservation of function, and prevention of deformity. Patient satisfaction and the success of therapy depend on how effectively the clinician utilizes the nonpharmacologic measures outlined in the following paragraphs.

1. Education and emotional factors—The clinician should explain the disease, describe its fluctuations, and involve the patient in decisions about therapy. Education of the family is invaluable to the patient's long-term well-being.

2. Physical and occupational therapies—Physical and occupational therapists understand nonpharmacologic treatments of arthritis (described below) and can effectively teach them. The therapist can develop a program the patient can follow at home, with only periodic monitoring.

3. Systemic rest—The amount of systemic rest required depends upon the presence and severity of inflammation. Complete bed rest may be desirable in patients with profound systemic and articular inflammation, as can occur in rheumatoid arthritis, systemic lupus erythematosus, or psoriatic arthritis. With mild inflammation, 2 hours of rest each day may suffice. In general, rest should be continued until significant improvement is sustained for at least 2 weeks; thereafter, the program may be liberalized. However, the increase of physical activity must proceed gradually and with appropriate support for any involved weight-bearing joints.

4. Articular rest—Decrease of articular inflammation may be expedited by articular rest. Relaxation and stretching of the hip and knee muscles, to prevent flexion contractures, can be accomplished by having the patient lie in the prone position for 15 minutes several times daily. Sitting in a flexed position for prolonged periods is a poor form of joint rest. Appropriate adjustable supports provide rest for inflamed weight-bearing joints, relieve spasm, and may reduce deformities, soft tissue contracture, or instability of the ligaments. The supports must be removable to permit daily range of motion and exercise of the affected extremities (see below).

5. Exercise—Exercises are designed to preserve joint motion, muscular strength, and endurance. Initially, for inflammatory disease, passive range of motion and isometric exercises (such as straight leg raising) are best tolerated. The buoyancy of water permits maximum isotonic and isometric exercise with no more stress on joints than active range of motion exercises. Although ideal for arthritic patients, the cost of hydrotherapy often precludes its use. As tolerance for exercise increases and the activity of the disease subsides, progressive resistance exercises may be introduced. Patients should follow the general rule of eliminating any exercise that produces increased pain 1 hour after the exercise has ended.

6. Heat and cold—These are used primarily for their muscle-relaxing and analgesic effects. Radiant or moist heat is generally most satisfactory. The ambulatory patient will find warm tub baths convenient. Exercise may be better performed after exposure to heat. Some patients derive more relief of joint pain from local application of cold.

7. Assistive devices—Patients with significant hip or knee arthritis may benefit from having a raised toilet seat, a gripping bar, or a cane. Patients hold the cane in the hand opposite to the affected knee or hip, thus leaning away from the affected joint. Crutches or walkers may be needed for patients with more extensive disease.

8. Splints—Splints may provide joint rest, reduce pain, and prevent contracture, but certain principles should be adhered to.

    a. Night splints of the hands or wrists (or both) should maintain the extremity in the position of optimum function. The elbow and shoulder lose motion so rapidly that other local measures and corticosteroid injections are usually preferable to splints.

    b. The best "splint" for the hip is prone-lying for several hours a day on a firm bed. For the knee, prone-lying may suffice, but splints in maximum tolerated extension are frequently needed. Ankle splints are of the simple right-angle type.

    c. Splints should be applied for the shortest period needed, should be made of lightweight materials for comfort, and should be easily removable for range-of-motion exercises once or twice daily to prevent loss of motion.

    d. Corrective splints, such as those for overcoming knee flexion contractures, should be used under the guidance of a clinician familiar with their proper use.

    Note: Avoidance of prolonged sitting or knee pillows may decrease the need for splints.

9. Weight loss—For overweight patients, achieving ideal body weight will reduce the wear and tear placed on arthritic joints of the lower extremities.

B. NONSTEROIDAL ANTI-INFLAMMATORY DRUGS (NSAIDs)

The first drug used to treat rheumatoid arthritis is an NSAID. These agents have analgesic and anti-inflammatory effects but are believed not to be capable of preventing erosions or altering progression of the disease. A number of NSAIDs are available, including aspirin, ibuprofen, fenoprofen, naproxen, tolmetin, sulindac, meclofenamate sodium, piroxicam, flurbiprofen, diclofenac, oxaprozin, nabumetone, etodolac, ketoprofen, celecoxib, and rofecoxib.

NSAIDs work in arthritis by the same mechanism that causes side effects: inhibition of cyclooxygenase, the enzyme that converts arachidonic acid to prostaglandins. Although prostaglandins play important roles in promoting inflammation and pain, they also help maintain homeostasis in several organs—especially the stomach, where prostaglandin E serves as a local hormone responsible for gastric mucosal cytoprotection. The discovery that cyclooxygenase (COX) exists in two isomers—COX-1 (which is expressed continuously in many cells and is responsible for the salutary effects of prostaglandins) and COX-2 (which is induced by cytokines and expressed in inflammatory tissues)—was initially of little practical consequence since all traditional NSAIDs inhibit both isomers. However, selective COX-2 inhibitors (celecoxib and rofecoxib) are FDA-approved for the treatment of osteoarthritis. Celecoxib is also approved for rheumatoid arthritis. Compared with traditional NSAIDs, COX-2 inhibitors are just as effective for treating rheumatoid arthritis and less likely to cause clinically significant upper gastrointestinal events (eg, obstruction, perforation, hemorrhage, or ulceration). Rheumatoid arthritis patients taking rofecoxib for 9 months are about half as likely as those taking naproxen to develop important gastrointestinal complications Thus, 41 patients treated with rofecoxib rather than naproxen for 1 year would prevent one gastrointestinal event.

In terms of efficacy, all NSAIDs appear equivalent. Anecdotes more than data suggest that indomethacin is more effective than other NSAIDs for ankylosing spondylitis (see below). But for rheumatoid arthritis, no NSAID is convincingly more effective than another.

For traditional NSAIDs that inhibit both COX-1 and COX-2, gastrointestinal side effects, such as gastric ulceration, perforation, and gastrointestinal hemorrhage, are the most common serious side effects. The overall rate of bleeding with NSAID use is low (1:6000 users or less) but is increased by chronic use, concomitant corticosteroids or anticoagulants, the presence of rheumatoid arthritis, history of peptic ulcer disease or alcoholism, and age over 70. Approximately 25% of all hospitalizations and deaths from peptic ulcer disease result from traditional NSAID therapy. Some reports suggest that each year 1:1000 patients with rheumatoid arthritis will require hospitalization for NSAID-related gastrointestinal bleeding or perforation. Although all traditional NSAIDs can cause massive gastrointestinal bleeding, the risk may be higher with indomethacin and piroxicam, probably because these drugs preferentially inhibit COX-1 in the stomach.

There are two approaches to reducing the gastrointestinal toxicity of NSAIDs. One approach is to use a COX-2 inhibitor, either celecoxib (100–200 mg twice daily for rheumatoid arthritis or 100 mg twice daily for osteoarthritis) or rofecoxib (12.5–25 mg once daily for osteoarthritis). The other approach is to use a traditional NSAID and add either a proton pump inhibitor (eg, omeprazole 20 mg daily), famotidine 40 mg twice daily, or misoprostol. The expense of these medications dictates that their use should be reserved for patients with risk factors for NSAID-induced gastrointestinal toxicity (noted above). Carafate, antacids, and ranitidine either do not work or do not work as well as omeprazole. The efficacy of misoprostol is limited by its poor tolerance; 20% of patients cannot tolerate the diarrhea and bloating associated with full doses (200 μg four times daily). Giving smaller amounts of misoprostol (eg, 100 μg four times daily) or using less frequent dosing (eg, 200 μg twice daily) improves tolerance while reducing efficacy only modestly. Misoprostol is an abortifacient and is contraindicated in patients who are or might become pregnant.

NSAIDs can also affect the lower intestinal tract, causing perforation or aggravating inflammatory bowel disease.

Acute liver injury from NSAIDs is rare, occurring in about one out of every 25,000 patients using these agents. Having rheumatoid arthritis or taking sulindac may increase the risk. Minor transient increases in aminotransferase levels do not predict risk for NSAID-associated hepatotoxicity.

All of the NSAIDs, including aspirin, can produce renal toxicity, resulting in interstitial nephritis, nephrotic syndrome, reversible renal failure, and aggravation of baseline hypertension. Hyperkalemia due to hyporeninemic hypoaldosteronism may also be seen. The risk of renal toxicity is low but is increased by age over 60, a history of renal disease, congestive heart failure, ascites, and diuretic use. COX-2 inhibitors appear to cause as much renal toxicity as traditional NSAIDs.

All NSAIDs except the nonacetylated salicylates and the COX-2 inhibitors interfere with platelet function and prolong bleeding time. For all older NSAIDs except aspirin, the effect on bleeding time resolves as the drug is cleared. Aspirin irreversibly inhibits platelet function, so the bleeding time effect resolves only as new platelets are made. COX-2 inhibitors, which differ from other NSAIDs in not inhibiting platelet function, do not increase the risk of bleeding with surgical procedures as most NSAIDs do. Whether this lack of platelet inhibition with COX-2 inhibitors generally increases the risk of myocardial infarction or thrombosis is not yet clear. Patients who require low-dose aspirin but do not take it have a greater risk of developing a thrombotic event while taking a "coxib" than while taking a traditional NSAID. Whether combination therapy with low-dose aspirin and a coxib maintains the gastrointestinal advantage of selective COX-2 inhibitors is not yet known.

Although groups of patients with rheumatoid arthritis respond similarly to NSAIDs, individuals may respond differently—an NSAID that works for one patient may not work for another. Thus, if the first NSAID chosen is not effective after 2–3 weeks of use, another should be tried.

C. ADDITIONAL DRUGS

Disease-modifying antirheumatic drugs (DMARDs) should be started as soon as the diagnosis of rheumatoid disease is certain.

1. Methotrexate—Many now believe that methotrexate is the treatment of choice for patients with rheumatoid arthritis who fail to respond to NSAIDs. Methotrexate is generally well-tolerated and often produces a beneficial effect in 2–6 weeks—compared with the 2- to 6-month onset of action for drugs such as gold, penicillamine, and antimalarials. The usual initial dose is 7.5 mg of methotrexate orally once weekly. If the patient has tolerated methotrexate but has not responded in 1 month, the dose can be increased to 15 mg orally once per week. The maximal dose is approximately 20 mg/wk. The most frequent side effects are gastric irritation and stomatitis. If needed to minimize gastrointestinal toxicity, methotrexate can be administered by subcutaneous or intramuscular injection. A severe, potentially life-threatening interstitial pneumonitis occurs rarely and usually responds to cessation of the drug and institution of corticosteroids. Hepatotoxicity with fibrosis and cirrhosis is another important toxic effect of methotrexate that fortunately appears to be very rare, with a risk of approximately 1:1000 after 5 years of methotrexate therapy. Still, methotrexate is contraindicated in a patient with any form of chronic hepatitis. Diabetes, obesity, and renal disease appear to increase the risk of hepatotoxicity. Liver function tests should be monitored every 4–8 weeks, along with the CBC, serum creatinine, and serum albumin. Heavy alcohol use increases the hepatotoxicity, so patients should be advised not to drink. In a patient with no risk factors for hepatotoxicity, liver biopsy is not needed initially but is performed if aminotransferase levels are elevated, despite dosage reduction, in 6 out of 12 monthly determinations or if the serum albumin falls below normal. Cytopenia due to bone marrow suppression and infection are other important potential problems. The risk of developing cytopenia is much higher in patients with a serum creatinine of 2 mg/dL or higher. Side effects, including hepatotoxicity, may be reduced by prescribing either daily folate (1 mg) or weekly leucovorin calcium (2.5–5 mg taken 24 hours after the dose of methotrexate). To date, methotrexate has not been proved to increase the risk of malignancy. The combination of methotrexate and other folate antagonists, such as trimethoprim-sulfamethoxazole, should be used cautiously, since pancytopenia can result. Probenecid should also be avoided since it increases methotrexate drug levels and toxicity.

2. Tumor necrosis factor inhibitors—For years it has been hoped that biologic therapies with designer monoclonal antibodies and anticytokines would provide effective and more specific treatment for rheumatoid arthritis. Inhibitors of tumor necrosis factor (TNF) are at last fulfilling that hope and are now frequently added to the treatment of patients who have not responded adequately to methotrexate. TNF inhibitors work faster than methotrexate and may replace that drug as the remitting agent of first choice. TNF has been targeted because it is a cytokine that activates lymphocytes and leukocytes and is greatly increased in the synovial fluid of patients with rheumatoid arthritis. Two inhibitors of TNF have been released. The first is etanercept, a soluble recombinant TNF receptor:Fc fusion protein (administered at a dosage of 25 mg subcutaneously twice weekly). The second is infliximab, an anti-TNF antibody that is administered at a dosage of 3–10 mg/kg intravenously initially and then repeated after 2, 6, 10, and 14 weeks. Both drugs produce substantial improvement in over 60% of patients. Etanercept is usually very well tolerated. Minor irritation at injection sites is the most common side effect. Rarely, patients develop nonrecurrent leukopenia. Since TNF may play a physiologic role in combating infection, there has been concern that TNF inhibitors increase the risk of developing infections. Infliximab very likely multiplies fourfold the risk of tuberculosis. Screening for latent tuberculosis is now recommended before TNF blockers are initiated. Still, it is prudent to discontinue treatment with TNF blockers when a patient develops fever or other manifestations of a clinically important infection. Multiple sclerosis-like attacks have been reported rarely in patients taking TNF inhibitors, but the importance of this association has not yet been determined. Infliximab can rarely cause anaphylaxis and can induce anti-DNA antibodies. Concomitant use of methotrexate appears to enhance the clinical response to infliximab and to prevent development of neutralizing antibodies to the drug (which is a hybrid human-mouse antibody). Because both drugs cost more than $10,000 per year, many insurers do not cover their cost unless the patient has a definite diagnosis of rheumatoid arthritis and has failed methotrexate.

3. Antimalarials—Hydroxychloroquine sulfate is the antimalarial agent most often used against rheumatoid arthritis. It should be reserved for patients with mild disease, since only 25–50% will respond and in some of those cases only after 3–6 months of therapy. The advantage of hydroxychloroquine is its comparatively low toxicity. A dosage of 200–400 mg/d minimizes the likelihood of toxic reactions. The most important reaction, pigmentary retinitis causing visual loss, is fortunately rare when the dosage is kept low. Ophthalmologic examinations every 6–12 months are required when this drug is employed for long-term therapy. Other reactions include neuropathies and myopathies of both skeletal and cardiac muscle, which usually improve when the drug is withdrawn.

4. Corticosteroids—Corticosteroids usually produce an immediate and dramatic anti-inflammatory effect in rheumatoid arthritis, and they may be able to slow the rate of bony destruction. However, the problem of untoward reactions resulting from prolonged use greatly limits its long-term efficacy. Another disadvantage that might stem from the use of steroids lies in the tendency of the patient and the physician to neglect the less spectacular but proved benefits derived from general supportive treatment, physical therapy, and orthopedic measures.

Corticosteroids may be used on a short-term basis to tide patients over acute disabling episodes, to facilitate other treatment measures (eg, physical therapy), or to manage serious extra-articular manifestations (eg, pericarditis, perforating eye lesions). Corticosteroids may also be indicated for active and progressive disease that does not respond favorably to conservative management and when there are contraindications to or therapeutic failure of methotrexate, gold salts, or other disease-modifying agents.

No more than 10 mg of prednisone or equivalent per day is appropriate for articular disease. Many patients do reasonably well on 5–7.5 mg daily. (The use of 1 mg tablets is to be encouraged.) When the steroids are to be discontinued, they should be phased out gradually on a planned schedule appropriate to the duration of treatment. All patients receiving chronic corticosteroid therapy should take measures to prevent osteoporosis.

Intra-articular corticosteroids may be helpful if one or two joints are the chief source of difficulty. Intra-articular triamcinolone, 10–40 mg depending on the size of the joint to be injected, may be given for symptomatic relief, but no more often than four times a year.

5. Sulfasalazine—This drug has become established as a second-line agent for rheumatoid arthritis. Sulfasalazine is usually introduced at a dosage of 0.5 g twice daily and then increased each week by 0.5 g until the patient improves or the daily dose reaches 3 g. Side effects, particularly neutropenia and thrombocytopenia, occur in 10–25% and are serious in 2–5%. Sulfasalazine also causes hemolysis in patients with glucose-6-phosphate dehydrogenase (G6PD) deficiency. Patients taking sulfasalazine should have complete blood counts monitored every 2–4 weeks for the first 3 months, then every 3 months.

6. Leflunomide—Leflunomide, a pyrimidine synthesis inhibitor, is also FDA-approved for treatment of rheumatoid arthritis. Leflunomide is begun at a dosage of 100 mg/d for 3 days followed by a maintenance dosage of 20 mg daily. The most frequent side effects are diarrhea, rash, reversible alopecia, and hepatotoxicity. Some patients experience dramatic unexplained weight loss. The drug is carcinogenic, teratogenic, and has a half-life of 2 weeks. Thus, it is contraindicated in premenopausal women or in men who wish to father children.

7. Azathioprine—This agent, like methotrexate, is an antimetabolite that is effective for severe rheumatoid arthritis not responsive to gold or antimalarials. The usual initial dose is 1 mg/kg, gradually increased as needed to a maximum of 2.5–3 mg/kg. Its potential for severe toxicity, including immunosuppression complicated by opportunistic infection, restricts its use.

8. Minocycline—Minocycline is more effective than placebo for rheumatoid arthritis. It is reserved for early, mild cases, since its efficacy is modest, and it works better during the first year of rheumatoid arthritis. The mechanism of action is not clear, but tetracyclines do have anti-inflammatory properties, including the ability to inhibit destructive enzymes such as collagenase. The dosage of minocycline is 200 mg/d. Adverse effects are uncommon except for dizziness, which occurs in about 10%.

9. Gold salts and penicillamine—Gold and penicillamine are very rarely used. Careful monitoring for toxicity is essential with either of these agents.

10. Combination therapy—Combination therapy can be considered for patients who have failed to respond to individual agents. The combination of methotrexate, hydroxychloroquine, and sulfasalazine appears more effective than methotrexate alone. The combination of cyclosporine (2.5–5 mg/kg/d) plus methotrexate also appears more effective than methotrexate alone.

D. OTHER THERAPIES

Anakinra, a recombinant form of human IL-1 receptor antagonist, may be given to adult patients who have failed one or more DMARDs. Anakinra can be used alone or in combination with DMARDs other than TNF-blocking agents. This agent must be administered daily by subcutaneous injection. Since anakinra has been associated with an increased incidence of serious infection, it should be discontinued whenever suggestive symptoms develop.

The efficacy of removing rheumatoid factor by performing apheresis and passing the patient's plasma over a Prosorba column containing staphylococcal protein A (which binds rheumatoid factor) has been demonstrated in short-term studies.

Dietary modification, especially supplementation with n-3 fatty acids in doses of 2.5–3 g/d, has been helpful to some patients, as has oral administration of collagen from articular cartilage.

E. SURGICAL MEASURES

See below.

Course & Prognosis

Determining the best initial treatment is difficult because patients suspected of having rheumatoid arthritis can follow two widely divergent courses. Of all patients who present with polyarthritis that appears to be (but probably is not) rheumatoid arthritis, 50–75% experience remission within 2 years. These patients are often negative for rheumatoid factor, have good functional status even during disease activity, and are commonly seen in community practices but rarely in academic centers. Clearly, conservative therapy makes good sense for this patient population.

For patients whose joint symptoms persist beyond 2 years the outcome is not so favorable. Patients in this group die, on average, 10–15 years earlier than people without rheumatoid arthritis. In fact, for patients who have persistent symptoms and poor functional status, the mortality curve resembles that for stage IV Hodgkin's disease or triple-vessel coronary artery disease. The most common causes of death are infection, heart disease, respiratory failure, renal failure, and gastrointestinal disease. Factors that identify those at particular risk of early death include positive rheumatoid factor, poor functional status, more than 30 inflamed joints, and extra-articular manifestations (eg, rheumatoid lung disease). These patients, then, need aggressive therapy and probably need it early, since extensive bone damage can occur during the first 2 years.

Since some patients with polyarthritis will remit and others will sustain substantial damage within the first 2 years, a guidepost for early decisions about aggressive treatment is needed. Patients who have polyarthritis lasting more than 12 weeks are those at greatest risk of having persistent disease and are appropriate candidates for aggressive therapy. Although genetic risk factors for developing rheumatoid arthritis have been identified, it has not been possible in this way to consistently identify those patients needing aggressive therapy.

Bathon JM et al: A comparison of etanercept and methotrexate in patients with early rheumatoid arthritis. N Engl J Med 2000;343:1586. [PMID: 11096165] (Etanercept works faster.)

Catella-Lawson F et al: Cyclooxygenase inhibitors and the antiplatelet effects of aspirin. N Engl J Med 2001;345:1809. [PMID: 11752357] (Concomitantly administered ibuprofen—but not diclofenac, acetaminophen, or rofecoxib—antagonizes the antiplatelet effect of aspirin.)

del Rincón I et al: High incidence of cardiovascular events in a rheumatoid arthritis cohort not explained by traditional cardiac risk factors. Arthritis Rheum 2001;44:2737. [PMID: 11762933] (Study of 236 patients demonstrating a nearly fourfold greater risk of cardiovascular events in patients with rheumatoid arthritis.)

FitzGerald GA et al: The coxibs, selective inhibitors of cyclooxygenase-2. N Engl J Med 2001;345:433. [PMID: 11496855]

Huang JQ et al: Role of *Helicobacter pylori* infection and non-steroidal anti-inflammatory drugs in peptic-ulcer disease: a meta-analysis. Lancet 2002;359:14. [PMID: 11899181] (*H pylori* infection and NSAIDs interact synergistically to increase the risk of peptic ulcer.)

Keane J et al: Tuberculosis associated with infliximab, a tumor necrosis factor α neutralizing agent. N Engl J Med 2001;345:1098. [PMID: 11596589] (Tuberculosis is four times more common in rheumatoid arthritis patients taking infliximab. Extrapulmonary and disseminated tuberculosis are common.)

Lipsky PE et al: Infliximab and methotrexate in the treatment of rheumatoid arthritis. N Engl J Med 2000;343:1594. [PMID: 11096166] (The combination works well.)

Mukherjee D et al: Risk of cardiovascular events associated with selective COX-2 inhibitors. JAMA 2001;286:954. [PMID: 11509060] (Review of literature suggesting COX-2 inhibitors increase risk of myocardial infarction, coronary vascular disease. The validity of this concern is not yet established.)

van Everdingen AA et al: Low-dose prednisone therapy for patients with early active rheumatoid arthritis. Clinical efficacy, disease-modifying properties, and side effects. A randomized, double-blind, placebo-controlled clinical trial. Ann Intern Med 2002;136:1. [PMID: 11777359] (Prednisone 10 mg/d is effective but toxic.)

ADULT STILL'S DISEASE

Still's disease is considered a variant of rheumatoid arthritis in which high spiking fevers are much more prominent, especially at the outset, than arthritis. This syndrome also occurs in adults. Most adults are in their 20s or 30s, and onset after age 60 is rare. The fever is dramatic, often spiking to 40 °C, associated with sweats and chills, and then plunging to several degrees below normal. Many patients initially complain of sore throat. An evanescent salmon-colored nonpruritic rash, chiefly on the chest and abdomen, is a characteristic feature. However, the rash can easily be missed since it often appears only with the fever spike. Many patients also have lymphadenopathy and pericardial effusions. Joint symptoms are mild or absent in the beginning, but a destructive arthritis, especially of the wrists, may develop months later. Anemia and leukocytosis, with white blood counts sometimes exceeding 40,000/μL, are the rule. Although the diagnosis requires exclusion of other causes of fever, the diagnosis of adult Still's disease is strongly suggested by the fever pattern, sore throat, and the classic rash. About half of the patients respond to high-dose aspirin (eg, 1 g three times daily) or other NSAIDs, and half require prednisone, sometimes in doses greater than 60 mg/d. About one-third of patients have recurrent episodes.

Fautrel B et al: Corticosteroid sparing effect of low dose methotrexate treatment in adult Still's disease. J Rheumatol 1999;26:373. [PMID: 9972972] (Methotrexate is an effective second-line drug.)

SYSTEMIC LUPUS ERYTHEMATOSUS

 ESSENTIALS OF DIAGNOSIS

- *Occurs mainly in young women.*
- *Rash over areas exposed to sunlight.*

- *Joint symptoms in 90% of patients. Multiple system involvement.*
- *Depression of hemoglobin, white blood cells, platelets.*
- *Serologic findings: antinuclear antibody with high titer to native DNA.*

General Considerations

Systemic lupus erythematosus (SLE) is an inflammatory autoimmune disorder that may affect multiple organ systems. Many of its clinical manifestations are secondary to the trapping of antigen-antibody complexes in capillaries of visceral structures or to autoantibody-mediated destruction of host cells (eg, thrombocytopenia). The clinical course is marked by spontaneous remission and relapses. The severity may vary from a mild episodic disorder to a rapidly fulminant, life-threatening illness.

The prevalence of SLE is influenced by many factors, including gender, race, and genetic inheritance. About 85% of patients are women. Sex hormones appear to play some role, since most cases develop after menarche and before menopause. Among the patients who develop SLE during childhood or after the age of 50, the gender distribution is more equal. Race is also a factor, as SLE occurs in 1:1000 white women but in 1:250 black women. Familial occurrence of SLE has been repeatedly documented, and the disorder is concordant in 25–70% of identical twins. If a mother has SLE, her daughters' risk of developing the disease is 1:40 and her sons' risk is 1:250. Aggregation of serologic abnormalities (positive antinuclear antibody) is seen in asymptomatic family members, and the prevalence of other rheumatic diseases is increased among close relatives of patients. The importance of specific genes in SLE is emphasized by the high frequency of certain HLA haplotypes, especially DR2 and DR3, and null complement alleles.

Before making a diagnosis of SLE, it is imperative to ascertain that the condition has not been induced by a drug. A host of pharmacologic agents have been implicated as causing a lupus-like syndrome, but only a few cause the disorder with appreciable frequency (Table 20–8). Procainamide, hydralazine, and isoniazid are the best-studied drugs. While antinuclear antibody tests and other serologic findings become positive in many persons receiving these agents, clinical manifestations occur in only a few.

Four features of drug-induced lupus separate it from SLE: (1) the sex ratio is nearly equal; (2) nephritis and central nervous system features are not ordinarily present; (3) hypocomplementemia and antibodies to native DNA are absent; and (4) the clinical features and most laboratory abnormalities often revert toward normal when the offending drug is withdrawn.

Table 20–8. Drugs associated with lupus erythematosus.[1]

Definite association	
Chlorpromazine	Methyldopa
Hydralazine	Procainamide
Isoniazid	Quinidine
Possible association	
Beta-blockers	Methimazole
Captopril	Nitrofurantoin
Carbamazepine	Penicillamine
Cimetidine	Phenytoin
Ethosuximide	Propylthiouracil
Hydrazines	Sulfasalazine
Levodopa	Sulfonamides
Lithium	Trimethadione
Unlikely association	
Allopurinol	Penicillin
Chlorthalidone	Phenylbutazone
Gold salts	Reserpine
Griseofulvin	Streptomycin
Methysergide	Tetracyclines
Oral contraceptives	

[1]Modified and reproduced, with permission, from Hess EV, Mongey AB: Drug-related lupus. Bull Rheum Dis 1991;40:1.

The diagnosis of SLE should be suspected in patients having a multisystem disease with serologic positivity (eg, antinuclear antibody, false-positive serologic test for syphilis). Differential diagnosis includes rheumatoid arthritis, vasculitis, scleroderma, chronic active hepatitis, acute drug reactions, polyarteritis, and drug-induced lupus.

The diagnosis of SLE can be made with reasonable probability if 4 of the 11 criteria set forth in Table 20–9 are met. These criteria should be viewed as rough guidelines that do not supplant clinical judgment in the diagnosis of SLE.

Clinical Findings

A. Symptoms and Signs

The systemic features include fever, anorexia, malaise, and weight loss. Most patients have skin lesions at some time; the characteristic "butterfly" rash affects fewer than half of patients. Other cutaneous manifestations are discoid lupus, typical fingertip lesions, periungual erythema, nail fold infarcts, and splinter hemorrhages. Alopecia is common. Mucous membrane lesions tend to occur during periods of exacerbation. Raynaud's phenomenon, present in about 20% of patients, often antedates other features of the disease.

Joint symptoms, with or without active synovitis, occur in over 90% of patients and are often the earliest manifestation. The arthritis is seldom deforming; erosive changes are almost never noted on radiographs. Subcutaneous nodules are rare.

Table 20–9. Criteria for the classification of SLE.[1] (A patient is classified as having SLE if any four or more of eleven criteria are met.)

1. Malar rash
2. Discoid rash
3. Photosensitivity
4. Oral ulcers
5. Arthritis
6. Serositis
7. Renal disease
   a. > 0.5 g/d proteinuria, or—
   b. ≥ 3+ dipstick proteinuria, or—
   c. Cellular casts
8. Neurologic disease
   a. Seizures, or—
   b. Psychosis (without other cause)
9. Hematologic disorders
   a. Hemolytic anemia, or—
   b. Leukopenia (< 4000/mL), or—
   c. Lymphopenia (< 1500/mL), or—
   d. Thrombocytopenia (< 100,000/mL)
10. Immunologic abnormalities
    a. Positive LE cell preparation, or—
    b. Antibody to native DNA, or—
    c. Antibody to Sm, or—
    d. False-positive serologic test for syphilis
11. Positive antinuclear antibody (ANA)

[1]Modified and reproduced, with permission, from Tan EM et al: The 1982 revised criteria for the classification of systemic lupus erythematosus. Arthritis Rheum 1982;25:1271.

Ocular manifestations include conjunctivitis, photophobia, transient or permanent monocular blindness, and blurring of vision. Cotton-wool spots on the retina (cytoid bodies) represent degeneration of nerve fibers due to occlusion of retinal blood vessels.

Pleurisy, pleural effusion, bronchopneumonia, and pneumonitis are frequent. Restrictive lung disease is often demonstrated.

The pericardium is affected in the majority of patients. Cardiac failure may result from myocarditis and hypertension. Cardiac arrhythmias are common. Atypical verrucous endocarditis of Libman-Sacks is usually clinically silent but occasionally can produce acute or chronic valvular incompetence—most commonly mitral regurgitation—and can serve as a source of emboli.

Mesenteric vasculitis occasionally occurs in SLE and may closely resemble polyarteritis nodosa, including the presence of aneurysms in medium-sized blood vessels. Abdominal pain (particularly postprandial), ileus, peritonitis, and perforation may result.

Neurologic complications of SLE include psychosis, organic brain syndrome, seizures, peripheral and cranial neuropathies, transverse myelitis, and strokes. Severe depression and psychosis are sometimes exacerbated by the administration of large doses of corticosteroids.

Several forms of glomerulonephritis may occur, including mesangial, focal proliferative, diffuse proliferative, and membranous (see Chapter 22). Some patients may also have interstitial nephritis. With appropriate therapy, the survival rate even for patients with serious renal disease (proliferative glomerulonephritis) is favorable.

Other clinical features include arterial and venous thrombosis, lymphadenopathy, splenomegaly, Hashimoto's thyroiditis, hemolytic anemia, and thrombocytopenic purpura.

B. LABORATORY FINDINGS

(Tables 20–10, 20–11, and 19–4.) SLE is characterized by the production of many different autoantibodies, some of which produce specific laboratory abnormalities (eg, hemolytic anemia). Antinuclear antibody tests are sensitive but not specific for systemic lupus—ie, they are positive in virtually all patients with lupus but are positive also in many patients with nonlupus conditions such as rheumatoid arthritis, various forms of hepatitis, and interstitial lung disease. Antibodies to double-stranded DNA and to Sm are specific for systemic lupus but not sensitive, since they are present in only 60% and 30% of patients, respectively. Depressed serum complement—a finding suggestive of disease activity—often returns toward normal in remission. Anti-double-stranded DNA antibody levels also correlate with disease activity; anti-Sm levels do not.

Three types of antiphospholipid antibodies occur (Table 20–11). The first causes the biologic false-positive tests for syphilis; the second is the lupus anticoagulant, which despite its name is a risk factor for venous and arterial thrombosis and miscarriage. It is most commonly identified by prolongation of the activated partial thromboplastin time, an in vitro phenomenon related to antibody reacting to phospholipid in the test materials. Anticardiolipin antibodies are the third type of antiphospholipid antibodies. In many cases, the "anticardiolipin antibody" appears to be directed at a serum cofactor (β_2-glycoprotein-I) rather than at phospholipid itself. A primary **antiphospholipid antibody syndrome** is diagnosed in patients who have recurrent venous or arterial occlusions, recurrent fetal loss, or thrombocytopenia in the presence of antiphospholipid antibodies but without features of SLE. Livedo reticularis, skin ulcers, mental status changes, and mitral regurgitation are also noted.

Abnormality of urinary sediment is almost always found in association with renal lesions. Showers of red blood cells, with or without casts, and mild proteinuria are frequent during exacerbation of the disease; these usually abate with remission.

Treatment

Some patients with SLE have a benign form of the disease requiring only supportive care and need little or no medication. Emotional support, as described for

Table 20–10. Frequency (%) of autoantibodies in rheumatic diseases.

	ANA	Anti-Native DNA	Rheumatoid Factor	Anti-Sm	Anti-SS-A	Anti-SS-B	Anti-SCL-70	Anti-Centromere	Anti-Jo-1	ANCA
Rheumatoid arthritis	30–60	0–5	72–85	0	0–5	0–2	0	0	0	0
Systemic lupus erythematosus	95–100	60	20	10–25	15–20	5–20	0	0	0	0–1
Sjögren's syndrome	95	0	75	0	60–70	60–70	0	0	0	0
Diffuse scleroderma	80–95	0	25–33	0	0	0	33	1	0	0
Limited scleroderma (CREST syndrome)	80–95	0	25–33	0	0	0	20	50	0	0
Polymyositis/dermatomyositis	80–95	0	33	0	0	0	0	0	20–30	0
Wegener's granulomatosis	0–15	0	50	0	0	0	0	0	0	93–96[1]

ANA = antinuclear antibodies; ANCA = anti-neutrophil cytoplasmic antibody.
[1]Frequency for generalized, active disease.

rheumatoid arthritis, is especially important for patients with lupus. Patients with photosensitivity should be cautioned against sun exposure and should apply a protective lotion to the skin while out of doors. Skin lesions often respond to the local administration of corticosteroids. Minor joint symptoms can usually be alleviated by rest and NSAIDs. Every drug that may have precipitated the condition should be withdrawn if possible.

Antimalarials (hydroxychloroquine) may be helpful in treating lupus rashes or joint symptoms that do not

Table 20–11. Frequency of laboratory abnormalities in systemic lupus erythematosus.[1]

Anemia	60%
Leukopenia	45%
Thrombocytopenia	30%
Biologic false-positive tests for syphilis	25%
Lupus anticoagulant	7%
Anti-cardiolipin antibody	25%
Direct Coombs-positive	30%
Proteinuria	30%
Hematuria	30%
Hypocomplementemia	60%
ANA	95–100%
Anti-native DNA	50%
Anti-Sm	20%

[1]Modified and reproduced, with permission, from Hochberg MC et al: Systemic lupus erythematosus: A review of clinicolaboratory features and immunologic matches in 150 patients with emphasis on demographic subsets. Medicine 1985;64:285.

respond to NSAIDs. When these are used, the dose should not exceed 400 mg/d, and biannual monitoring for retinal changes is recommended. Drug-induced neuropathy and myopathy may be erroneously ascribed to the underlying disease.

Corticosteroids are required for the control of certain serious complications. These include thrombocytopenic purpura, hemolytic anemia, myocarditis, pericarditis, convulsions, and nephritis. Forty to 60 mg of prednisone is often needed initially; however, the lowest dose of corticosteroid that controls the condition should be employed. Central nervous system lupus may require higher doses of corticosteroids than are usually given; however, steroid psychosis may mimic lupus cerebritis, in which case reduced doses are appropriate. In lupus nephritis, sequential studies of serum complement and antibodies to DNA often permit early detection of disease exacerbation and thus prompt increase in corticosteroid therapy. Such studies also allow for lowering the dosage of the drugs and withdrawing them when they are no longer needed. Immunosuppressive agents such as cyclophosphamide, chlorambucil, and azathioprine are used in cases resistant to corticosteroids. The exact role of immunosuppressive agents is controversial. Cyclophosphamide improves renal survival. Overall patient survival, however, is no better than in the prednisone-treated group. Very close follow-up is needed to watch for potential side effects when immunosuppressants are employed; these agents should be given by physicians experienced in their use. The androgenic steroid danazol may be effective therapy for thrombocytopenia not responsive to corticosteroids. Dehydroepiandrosterone (DHEA) appears to have a therapeutic role comparable to that of the antimalarial agents in the treatment of SLE, but its side effects (particularly acne) may be troubling to some patients. Anticoagulation, most commonly with warfarin to achieve an INR > 3.0, is prescribed for patients who have antiphospholipid antibodies and clotting of the arterial or venous systems. Systemic steroids are not usually given for minor arthritis, skin rash, leukopenia, or the anemia associated with chronic disease. Positive serologic findings in asymptomatic patients are not an indication for treatment.

Course & Prognosis

The prognosis for patients with systemic lupus appears to be considerably better than older reports implied. From both community settings and university centers, 10-year survival rates exceeding 85% are routine. In most patients, the illness pursues a relapsing and remitting course. Corticosteroids, often needed in doses of 40 mg/d or more during severe flares, can usually be tapered to low doses (10–15 mg/d) during disease inactivity. However, there are some in whom the disease pursues a virulent course, leading to serious impairment of vital structures such as lung, heart, brain, or kidneys, and the disease may lead to death. With improved control of lupus activity and with increasing use of corticosteroids and immunosuppressive drugs, the mortality and morbidity patterns in lupus have changed. Infections—especially with opportunistic organisms—have become the leading cause of death, followed by active SLE, chiefly due to renal or central nervous system disease. Although such manifestations are more likely to be seen in the early phases of the illness, one must be alert to the possibility of their occurrence at any time. Accelerated atherosclerosis attributed, in part, to corticosteroid use, has been responsible for a rise in late deaths due to myocardial infarction. With more patients living longer, it has become evident that avascular necrosis of bone, affecting most commonly the hips and knees, is responsible for substantial morbidity. Still, it must be emphasized that the outlook for most patients with SLE has become increasingly favorable.

Gomez-Pacheco L et al: Serum anti-beta₂-glycoprotein I anticardiolipin antibodies during thrombosis in systemic lupus erythematosus patients. Am J Med 1999;106:417. [PMID: 99239750] (Beta₂-glycoprotein-I antibodies are strongly associated with thrombosis in SLE.)

Guidelines for referral and management of systemic lupus erythematosus in adults. American College of Rheumatology Ad Hoc Committee on Systemic Lupus Erythematosus Guidelines. Arthritis Rheum 1999;42:1785. [PMID: 10513791] (Useful algorithm for the diagnosis, referral, and treatment of SLE, with discussion of difficult clinical questions such as when to perform renal biopsy.)

Ho A et al: A decrease in complement is associated with increased renal and hematologic activity in patients with systemic lupus erythematosus. Arthritis Rheum 2001;44:2350. [PMID: 11665976] (Renal and hematologic flares depress complement levels; other types of flares do not.)

Illei GG et al: Combination therapy with pulse cyclophosphamide plus pulse methylprednisolone improves long-term renal outcome without adding toxicity in patients with lupus nephritis. Ann Intern Med 2001;135:248. [PMID: 11511139] (For lupus nephritis, combination therapy of pulse cyclophosphamide plus pulse methylprednisolone is better than pulse cyclophosphamide alone, which is better than pulse methylprednisolone alone.)

Wilson WA et al: International consensus statement on preliminary classification criteria for definite antiphospholipid syndrome: report of an international workshop. Arthritis Rheum 1999;42:1309. [PMID: 10403256] (Concise discussion of the clinical and laboratory criteria for the diagnosis of antiphospholipid syndrome.)

SYSTEMIC SCLEROSIS (Scleroderma; SSC)

 ESSENTIALS OF DIAGNOSIS

- Diffuse thickening of skin, with telangiectasia and areas of increased pigmentation and depigmentation.
- Raynaud's phenomenon in 90% of patients.
- Systemic features of dysphagia, hypomotility of gastrointestinal tract, pulmonary fibrosis, and cardiac and renal involvement.
- Positive test for antinuclear antibodies nearly universal.

General Considerations

Systemic sclerosis is a chronic disorder characterized by diffuse fibrosis of the skin and internal organs. The causes of systemic sclerosis are not known, but autoimmunity, fibroblast dysregulation, graft-versus-host disease from fetal lymphocytes retained in the maternal circulation, and occupational exposure to silica have been implicated. Symptoms usually appear in the third to fifth decades, and women are affected two to three times as frequently as men.

Two forms of systemic sclerosis are generally recognized: limited (80% of patients) and diffuse (20%). Two bedside clues help distinguish the two subsets. First, in the CREST syndrome, hardening of the skin (scleroderma) is limited to the face and hands, whereas in diffuse scleroderma the skin changes also involve the trunk and proximal extremities. Second, tendon friction rubs, especially frequent over the wrists, ankles, and knees, occur uniquely (but not universally) in diffuse scleroderma. Patients with CREST syndrome have a much better prognosis than those with diffuse disease, in large part because patients with limited disease do not develop renal failure or interstitial lung disease. Curiously, patients with limited disease are more liable to develop digital ischemia and pulmonary hypertension. Gastrointestinal and cardiac disease also tend to be more severe and more rapidly progressive in diffuse scleroderma.

Clinical Findings

A. SYMPTOMS AND SIGNS

Most frequently, the disease makes its appearance in the skin, although visceral involvement may precede cutaneous alteration. Polyarthralgia and Raynaud's phenomenon (present in 90% of patients) are early manifestations. Subcutaneous edema, fever, and malaise are common. With time the skin becomes thickened and hidebound, with loss of normal folds. Telangiectasia, pigmentation, and depigmentation are characteristic. Ulceration about the fingertips and subcutaneous calcification are seen. Dysphagia due to esophageal dysfunction is common and results from abnormalities in motility and later from fibrosis. Fibrosis and atrophy of the gastrointestinal tract cause hypomotility, and malabsorption results from bacterial overgrowth. Large-mouthed diverticula occur in the jejunum, ileum, and colon. Diffuse pulmonary fibrosis and pulmonary vascular disease are reflected in low diffusing capacity and decreased lung compliance. Cardiac abnormalities include pericarditis, heart block, myocardial fibrosis, and right heart failure secondary to pulmonary hypertension. Systemic sclerosis renal crisis, resulting from obstruction of smaller renal blood vessels, indicates a grave prognosis.

B. LABORATORY FINDINGS

Mild anemia is often present, and it is occasionally hemolytic because of mechanical damage to red cells from diseased small vessels. Elevation of the sedimentation rate is unusual. Proteinuria and cylindruria appear in association with renal involvement. Antinuclear antibody tests are nearly always positive, frequently in high titers (Tables 20–10 and 19–4). The scleroderma antibody (SCL-70) directed against topoisomerase III is found in one-third of patients with diffuse systemic sclerosis and in 20% of those with CREST syndrome; an anticentromere antibody is seen in 50% of those with CREST syndrome and in 1% of individuals with diffuse systemic sclerosis (Tables 20–10 and 19–4). Although present in only a minority of patients with diffuse systemic sclerosis, anti-Scl-70 antibodies may portend a poor prognosis, with a high likelihood of serious internal organ involvement (eg, interstitial lung disease). Anticentromere antibodies are highly specific for limited systemic sclerosis, but they also occur occasionally in overlap syndromes.

Differential Diagnosis

Several conditions classified as "localized" sclerosis may mimic systemic morphea and limited systemic sclerosis. These disorders are generally limited to the skin (typically in a localized fashion) and are associated with excellent prognoses. Linear scleroderma is occasionally associated with atrophy of underlying muscle and bone and may cause deformities that are both cosmetically and functionally disabling.

Eosinophilic fasciitis is a rare disorder presenting with skin changes that resemble diffuse systemic sclerosis. The inflammatory abnormalities, however, are limited to the fascia rather than the dermis and epidermis. Patients with eosinophilic fasciitis are further distinguished from those with systemic scleroderma by the presence of peripheral blood eosinophilia, the absence of Raynaud's phenomenon, the good response to prednisone, and an increased risk of developing aplastic anemia.

The eosinophilia-myalgia syndrome was first noted in patients who ingested tryptophan, an essential amino acid that was sold as an over-the-counter remedy for insomnia and premenstrual symptoms—until banned by the Food and Drug Administration. Weeks to months after beginning ingestion, affected patients developed a syndrome of severe generalized myalgias, and cutaneous abnormalities ranging from hives to generalized swelling and induration of the arms and legs. Peripheral eosinophilia (> 1000/μL) is characteristic. Other common clinical manifestations have included pulmonary symptoms, fever, myopathy, lymphadenopathy, and ascending polyneuropathy. Besides eosinophilia, laboratory features include mild elevations of aldolase with normal creatine kinase levels and, frequently, positive ANA tests. Full-thickness biopsies may reveal features of systemic sclerosis, evidence of fasciitis or myositis, or small vessel vasculitis. While some patients improve after discontinuing tryptophan, others progress and require corticosteroid therapy, which is not always effective. Deaths have been reported, especially from neurologic involvement. Patients presenting with systemic sclerosis or an eosinophilic fasciitis-like syndrome should be asked about tryptophan use.

Case reports once suggested that silicone breast implants can cause scleroderma or other rheumatic diseases, including SLE and undifferentiated autoimmune diseases, but population studies have failed to detect a link between silicone breast implants and any defined rheumatic disease.

Treatment

Treatment of systemic sclerosis is symptomatic and supportive. Severe Raynaud's syndrome may respond to calcium channel blockers, eg, long-acting nifedipine, 30–120 mg/d, or to losartan, 50 mg/d. Intravenous iloprost, a prostacyclin analog that causes vasodilation and platelet inhibition, is moderately effective in healing digital ulcers. Patients with esophageal disease should take medications in liquid or crushed form. Esophageal reflux can be reduced and scarring prevented by avoiding late-night meals, elevating the head of the bed, and using antacids and H_2 blockers. Proton pump inhibitors (eg, omeprazole,

20–40 mg/d) are the only drugs that achieve near-complete inhibition of gastric acid production, and they are remarkably effective for refractory esophagitis. Patients with delayed gastric emptying maintain their weight better if they eat small, frequent meals and remain upright for at least 2 hours after eating. Prokinetic drugs (eg, cisapride) infrequently produce a meaningful improvement in gastric emptying and are ineffective in promoting esophageal emptying. Octreotide, a somatostatin analog, has helped a few patients with bacterial overgrowth and pseudo-obstruction. Malabsorption due to bacterial overgrowth also responds to antibiotics, eg, tetracycline, 500 mg four times daily. The hypertensive crises associated with systemic sclerosis renal crisis must be treated early and aggressively (in the hospital) with angiotensin-converting enzyme inhibitors, eg, captopril, 37.5–75 mg/d in three divided doses. Prednisone has little or no role in the treatment of scleroderma. Cyclophosphamide, a drug with many important side effects, may improve severe interstitial lung disease.

The 9-year survival rate in scleroderma averages approximately 40%. The prognosis tends to be worse in those with diffuse scleroderma, in blacks, in males, and in older patients. In most cases, death results from renal, cardiac, or pulmonary failure. Those who do not develop severe internal organ involvement in the first 3 years do much better, with 72% surviving at least 9 years. Breast and lung cancer may be more common in patients with scleroderma.

LeRoy EC et al: Criteria for the classification of early systemic sclerosis. J Rheumatol 2001;28:1573. [PMID: 11469464] (Raynaud's phenomenon, defined as episodic, bilateral, di- or triphasic vascular reactions [pallor, cyanosis, suffusion] of the fingers, toes, ears or nose, is essential to the diagnosis of systemic sclerosis.)

Sule SD et al: Update on management of scleroderma. Bull Rheum Dis 2000;49:1. [PMID: 11286150] (No effective modifying agent of the underlying disease process currently exists for treatment of scleroderma.)

Wigley FM: When is scleroderma really scleroderma? J Rheumatol 2001;28:1471. [PMID: 11469447] (Three features should be present before the diagnosis of systemic sclerosis is made: tissue fibrosis; evidence of a vasculopathy—usually Raynaud's phenomenon or nailfold capillary abnormalities—and a specific autoantibody response.)

IDIOPATHIC INFLAMMATORY MYOPATHIES
(Polymyositis & Dermatomyositis)

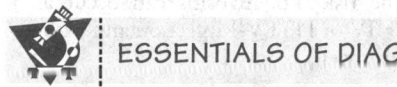

ESSENTIALS OF DIAGNOSIS

- *Bilateral proximal muscle weakness.*
- *Characteristic cutaneous manifestations in dermatomyositis (Gottron's papules, heliotrope rash).*
- *Diagnostic tests: elevated creatine kinase and other muscle enzymes, muscle biopsy, electromyography.*
- *Increased risk of malignancy, particularly in adult dermatomyositis.*
- *Inclusion body myositis can mimic polymyositis but is less responsive to treatment.*

General Considerations

Polymyositis and dermatomyositis are systemic disorders of unknown cause whose principal manifestation is muscle weakness. Although their clinical presentations (aside from the presence of certain skin findings in dermatomyositis, some of which are pathognomonic) and treatments are similar, the two diseases are pathologically quite distinct. They affect persons of any age group, but the peak incidence is in the fifth and sixth decades of life. Women are affected twice as commonly as men, and the diseases (particularly polymyositis) also occur more often among blacks than whites. There is an increased risk of malignancy, particularly in adult patients with dermatomyositis. Indeed, up to one patient in four with dermatomyositis has an occult malignancy. Malignancies may be evident at the time of presentation with the muscle disease but may not be detected until months afterward in some cases. Rare patients with dermatomyositis have skin disease without overt muscle involvement, a condition termed "dermatomyositis sine myositis."

Clinical Findings

A. SYMPTOMS AND SIGNS

Polymyositis may begin abruptly, but the usual presentation is one of gradual and progressive muscle weakness. The weakness chiefly involves proximal muscle groups of the upper and lower extremities as well as the neck. Leg weakness (eg, difficulty in rising from a chair or climbing stairs) typically precedes arm symptoms. In contrast to myasthenia gravis, polymyositis and dermatomyositis do not cause facial or ocular muscle weakness. Pain and tenderness of affected muscles occur in one-fourth of cases, but these are rarely the chief complaints. About one-fourth of patients have dysphagia. In contrast to scleroderma, which affects the smooth muscle of the lower esophagus and can cause a "sticking" sensation below the sternum, polymyositis or dermatomyositis involves the striated muscles of the upper pharynx and can make initiation of deglutition difficult. Muscle atrophy and contractures occur as late complications of advanced disease. Clinically significant myocarditis is uncommon even though there is often CK-MB elevation. Patients who are bed-bound from myositis should be screened for respiratory muscle weakness that can be severe enough to cause CO_2 retention and to require mechanical ventilation.

In dermatomyositis, the characteristic rash is dusky red and may appear in malar distribution mimicking the classic rash of SLE. Erythema also occurs over other areas of the face, neck, shoulders, and upper chest and back ("shawl sign"). Periorbital edema and a purplish (heliotrope) suffusion over the eyelids are typical signs. Periungual erythema, dilations of nailbed capillaries, and scaly patches over the dorsum of proximal interphalangeal and metacarpophalangeal joints (Gottron's sign) are highly suggestive.

A subset of patients with polymyositis and dermatomyositis develop the "antisynthetase syndrome," a group of findings including inflammatory arthritis, Raynaud's phenomenon, interstitial lung disease, and often severe muscle disease associated with certain autoantibodies (eg, anti-Jo1 antibodies).

B. LABORATORY FINDINGS

Measurement of serum levels of muscle enzymes, especially creatine kinase and aldolase, is most useful in diagnosis and in assessment of disease activity. Anemia is uncommon. The sedimentation rate is not appreciably elevated in half of the patients. Rheumatoid factor is found in a minority of patients. Antinuclear antibodies are present in many patients, and anti-Jo-1 antibodies are seen in the subset of patients who have associated interstitial lung disease (Tables 20–10 and 19–4). Chest radiographs are usually normal, though interstitial fibrosis is occasionally seen. Electromyographic abnormalities consisting of polyphasic potentials, fibrillations, and high-frequency action potentials are helpful in establishing the diagnosis. None of the studies are specific. The search for an occult malignancy should begin with a history and physical examination, supplemented with a complete blood count, comprehensive biochemical panel, serum protein electrophoresis, and urinalysis, and should include age and risk-appropriate cancer screening tests. If these evaluations are unrevealing, then a more invasive or extensive laboratory evaluation is probably not cost-effective. No matter how extensive the initial screening, some malignancies will not become evident for months after the initial presentation.

C. MUSCLE BIOPSY

Biopsy of clinically involved muscle is the only specific diagnostic test. The pathology findings in polymyositis and dermatomyositis are distinct. Although both include lymphoid inflammatory infiltrates, the findings in dermatomyositis are localized to perivascular regions and there is evidence of humoral and complement-mediated destruction of microvasculature associated with the muscle. In addition to its vascular orientation, the inflammatory infiltrate in dermatomyositis centers on the interfascicular septa and is located around, rather than in, muscle fascicles. In contrast, the pathology of polymyositis characteristically includes endomysial infiltration of the inflammatory infiltrate. Owing to the sometimes patchy distribution of pathologic abnormalities, however, false-negative biopsies sometimes occur in both disorders.

Differential Diagnosis

Muscle inflammation may occur as a component of SLE, systemic sclerosis, or Sjögren's syndrome. In those cases, associated findings usually permit the precise diagnosis of the primary condition.

Inclusion body myositis, because of its tendency to mimic polymyositis, is a common cause of "treatment-resistant polymyositis." In contrast to the epidemiologic features of polymyositis, however, the typical inclusion body myositis patient is white, male, and over the age of 50. The onset of inclusion body myositis is even more insidious than that of polymyositis or dermatomyositis (eg, occurring over years rather than months), and asymmetric distal motor weakness is common in inclusion body myositis. Inclusion body myositis is less likely to respond to therapy and is associated with characteristic pathologic findings evident on frozen section or electron microscopy.

Most endocrine diseases can be associated with proximal muscle weakness. This is particularly true for hyper- and hypothyroidism, and the latter is associated also with elevations of creatinine phosphokinase. Patients with polymyalgia rheumatica are over the age of 50 and—in contrast to patients with polymyositis—have pain but no objective weakness. Disorders of the peripheral and central nervous systems (eg, chronic inflammatory polyneuropathy, multiple sclerosis, myasthenia gravis, Eaton-Lambert disease and amyotrophic lateral sclerosis) can produce weakness but are distinguished by characteristic symptoms and neurologic signs and often by distinctive electromyographic abnormalities. Many drugs, including corticosteroids, alcohol, clofibrate, penicillamine, tryptophan, and hydroxychloroquine, can produce proximal muscle weakness. Chronic use of colchicine at doses as low as 0.6 mg twice a day in elderly patients with mild to moderate renal insufficiency can produce a mixed neuropathy-myopathy that mimics polymyositis. The weakness and muscle enzyme elevation reverse with cessation of the drug. HMG-CoA reductase inhibitors, which are frequently used to treat hypercholesterolemia, can cause myopathy and rhabdomyolysis. Although only about 0.1% of patients taking a statin drug alone develop myopathy, concomitant administration of other drugs (especially gemfibrozil, cyclosporine, niacin, and itraconazole) increases the risk. Polymyositis can occur as a complication of HIV or HTLV-I infection and with zidovudine therapy as well.

Treatment

Most patients respond to corticosteroids. Often a daily dose of 40–60 mg or more of prednisone is required initially. The dose is then adjusted downward according to the response of sequentially observed serum levels of muscle enzymes. Long-term use of steroids is often needed, and the disease may recur or reemerge when they are withdrawn. Patients with an associated neoplasm have a poor prognosis, although remission may follow treatment of the tumor; steroids may or may not be effective in these patients. In patients resistant or intolerant to corticosteroids, therapy with methotrexate or azathioprine may be helpful, but these agents should be used with caution in view of their adverse effects. Intravenous immune globulin has also been shown to be effective for dermatomyositis resistant to prednisone, but leukapheresis and plasma exchange are not.

Hilton-Jones D: Inflammatory muscle diseases. Curr Opin Neurol 2001;14.591. [PMID: 11562570] (Muscle enzyme elevations are usually lower in inclusion body myositis than in polymyositis and dermatomyositis.)

OVERLAP (OR MIXED) CONNECTIVE TISSUE DISEASE

Not infrequently, patients have features of more than one rheumatic disease. Special attention has been drawn to patients who have overlapping features of SLE, systemic sclerosis, and polymyositis. Initially, these patients were thought to have a distinct entity ("mixed connective tissue disease") defined by a specific autoantibody to ribonuclear protein (RNP). With time in many patients, the manifestations evolve to one predominant disease, such as scleroderma, and many patients with antibodies to RNP have clear-cut SLE. Therefore, "overlap connective tissue disease" is the preferred designation for patients having features of different rheumatic diseases.

SJÖGREN'S SYNDROME

 ESSENTIALS OF DIAGNOSIS

- Ninety percent of patients are women; the average age is 50 years.
- Dryness of eyes and dry mouth (sicca components) are the most common features; they occur alone or in association with rheumatoid arthritis or other connective tissue disease.
- Rheumatoid factor and other autoantibodies common.
- Increased incidence of lymphoma.

General Considerations

Sjögren's syndrome, an autoimmune disorder, is the result of chronic dysfunction of exocrine glands in many areas of the body. It is characterized by dryness of the eyes, mouth, and other areas covered by mucous membranes and is frequently associated with a rheumatic disease, most often rheumatoid arthritis. The disorder is predominantly a disease of women, in a ratio of 9:1, with greatest incidence between age 40 and 60 years.

Disorders with which Sjögren's syndrome is frequently associated include rheumatoid arthritis, SLE, primary biliary cirrhosis, scleroderma, polymyositis, Hashimoto's thyroiditis, polyarteritis, and interstitial pulmonary fibrosis. When Sjögren's syndrome occurs without rheumatoid arthritis, HLA-DR2 and -DR3 antigens are present with increased frequency.

Clinical Findings

A. SYMPTOMS AND SIGNS

Keratoconjunctivitis sicca results from inadequate tear production caused by lymphocyte and plasma cell infiltration of the lacrimal glands. Symptoms include burning, itching, ropy secretions, and impaired tear production during crying. Parotid enlargement, which may be chronic or relapsing, develops in one-third of patients. Dryness of the mouth (xerostomia) leads to difficulty in speaking and swallowing and to severe dental caries. There may be loss of taste and smell. Desiccation may involve the nose, throat, larynx, bronchi, vagina, and skin.

Systemic manifestations include dysphagia, pancreatitis, pleuritis, obstructive lung disease (in the absence of smoking), neuropsychiatric dysfunction, and vasculitis; they may be related to the associated diseases noted above. Renal tubular acidosis (type I, distal) occurs in 20% of patients. Chronic interstitial nephritis, which may result in impaired renal function, may be seen. A glomerular lesion is rarely observed but may occur secondary to associated cryoglobulinemia.

A spectrum of lymphoproliferation ranging from benign to malignant may be found. Malignant lymphomas and Waldenström's macroglobulinemia occur nearly 50 times more frequently than can be explained by chance alone in primary Sjögren's syndrome.

B. LABORATORY FINDINGS

Laboratory findings include mild anemia, leukopenia, and eosinophilia. Rheumatoid factor is found in 70% of patients. Heightened levels of gamma globulin, antinuclear antibodies, and antibodies against RNA, salivary gland, lacrimal duct, and thyroid may be noted. Antibodies against the cytoplasmic antigens SS-A and SS-B (also called Ro and La, respectively) are often present in Sjögren's syndrome (Tables 20–10 and 19–4). When SS-A antibodies are present, extraglandular manifestations of Sjögren's syndrome are far more common.

Useful ocular diagnostic tests include the Schirmer test, which measures the quantity of tears secreted. Lip biopsy, a simple procedure, is the only specific diagnostic technique and has minimal risk; if lymphoid foci are seen in accessory salivary glands, the diagnosis is confirmed. Biopsy of the parotid gland should be reserved for patients with atypical presentations such as unilateral gland enlargement.

Treatment & Prognosis

Treatment is symptomatic and supportive. Artificial tears applied frequently will relieve ocular symptoms and avert further desiccation. Sipping water frequently or using sugar-free gums and hard candies usually relieves dry mouth symptoms. Although they are FDA-approved for xerostomia, pilocarpine (5 mg four times daily) and the acetylcholine derivative cevimeline (30 mg three times daily) are rarely needed. The mouth should be kept well lubricated. Atropinic drugs and decongestants decrease salivary secretions and should be avoided. A program of oral hygiene is essential in order to preserve dentition. If there is an associated rheumatic disease, its treatment is not altered by the presence of Sjögren's syndrome.

The disease is usually benign and may be consistent with a normal life span; it is influenced mainly by the nature of the associated disease. The patients (3–10% of the total Sjögren's population) at greatest risk of developing lymphoma have severe dryness, marked parotid gland enlargement, splenomegaly, vasculitis, peripheral neuropathy, anemia, and mixed monoclonal cryoglobulinemia.

Carsons S: A review and update of Sjögren's syndrome: manifestations, diagnosis, and treatment. Am J Manag Care 2001; 7(14 Suppl):S433. [PMID: 11605978]

RHABDOMYOLYSIS

Defined strictly, rhabdomyolysis is necrosis of skeletal muscle and may be encountered in a wide variety of clinical settings, alone or in concert with other disorders of muscle. One of the latter is myopathy, or objective weakness of muscle; another is myalgia, or pain in the muscle. In some conditions, such as polymyositis, all three processes may coexist, as in a patient with proximal muscle weakness, pain, and an elevated creatine kinase (the biochemical indicator of skeletal muscle necrosis). The myopathies are dealt with elsewhere in this chapter, and myalgias are sufficiently nonspecific and widespread so that they need not be discussed separately—the exception being polymyalgia rheumatica. When the term "rhabdomyolysis" is employed without being otherwise defined, physicians ordinarily think of the syndrome of crush injury to muscle, associated with myoglobinuria, renal insufficiency, markedly elevated creatine kinase levels, and, frequently, multiorgan failure as a consequence of other complications of the trauma. Renal insufficiency in myoglobinuria is caused by tubular damage resulting from filtered myoglobin postinjury and is nearly always associated with hypovolemia. Experimental models of severe rhabdomyolysis in which blood volume and pressure are maintained ordinarily are not associated with acute tubular necrosis. From a practical point of view, however, many patients who suffer crush injuries are indeed volume-contracted, and oliguric renal failure is encountered routinely.

Vigorous fluid resuscitation, mannitol, and urine alkalinization are suggested early in the course, but it is not clear that the outcome is affected by these measures. On occasion, oliguric tubular necrosis may be converted to a nonoliguric variety, and—though the prognosis for recovery of renal function and mortality is the same—many clinicians believe it is easier to care for nonoliguric disease, since hyperkalemia and pulmonary edema are less important concerns.

In addition to crush injuries, prolonged immobility, particularly after drug overdose or intoxication and commonly associated with exposure hypothermia, may be associated with rhabdomyolysis. Often there is little evidence for muscle injury on external examination of these patients—and specifically, neither myalgia nor myopathy present. The clue to muscle necrosis in such individuals may be a urinary dipstick testing positive for blood in the absence of red cells in the sediment. This false-positive finding is due to myoglobinuria, which results in a positive reading for blood. Such an abnormality is investigated by serum creatine kinase determination. Other studies elevated in rhabdomyolysis include ALT and LDH—and once again, these studies may be obtained for other reasons, such as suspected liver disease or hemolysis. When disproportionately elevated, it is prudent to establish that they are not of muscle origin by confirming them with CK determination.

A number of other causes of rhabdomyolysis are encountered, and the statin group of drugs for treatment of hyperlipidemia are common offenders (see above). A simple intramuscular injection may cause some elevation of CK, and acute alcoholic intoxication is also culpable on rare occasions. For the most part, however, rhabdomyolysis is seen with concomitant myopathy, though the term rhabdomyolysis refers only to a test abnormality. Certain types of myopathies—notably the endocrine myopathies associated with hyperthyroidism and hypercortisolism—are not found with elevated muscle enzymes. The same is true of polymyalgia rheumatica, in fact not a myopathy. If these conditions are thought to be present but the CK is elevated, alternative explanations need to considered.

Holt SG et al: Pathogenesis and treatment of renal dysfunction in rhabdomyolysis. Intensive Care Med 2001;27:803. [PMID: 11430535] (Renal failure in rhabdomyolysis is due to vasoconstriction and oxidant injury to tubules as well as to tubular obstruction.)

Vanholder R et al: Rhabdomyolysis. J Am Soc Nephrol 2000; 1:1553. [PMID: 10906171] (Aggressive fluid administration is essential to preventing the acute renal failure of rhabdomyolysis. Up to 10–12 L of fluid may be administered in the first 24 hours.)

■ VASCULITIS SYNDROMES

The vasculitis syndromes are a heterogeneous group of disorders characterized by the pathologic features of inflammation and necrosis of blood vessels. The causes of most forms of vasculitis are not known. Infection is important in the pathogenesis of some forms of vasculitis. In polyarteritis nodosa, 10–30% of patients have evidence of hepatitis B or C. Most patients with mixed cryoglobulinemia are infected with hepatitis C. Infective endocarditis and syphilis can be associated with vasculitis, and cases of herpes zoster are in rare instances followed by central nervous system vasculitis. Drug reactions—especially to penicillins, sulfonamides, and allopurinol—can produce serum sickness associated with vasculitis. No common pathogenic link has been identified for these disorders, though the deposition of immune complexes in the vascular system occurs in many.

Although there are multiple forms of vasculitis, including primary and secondary forms, only the major vasculitides will be discussed here.

POLYARTERITIS NODOSA & MICROSCOPIC POLYANGIITIS

ESSENTIALS OF DIAGNOSIS

- Microscopic polyangiitis may involve small blood vessels (capillaries, arterioles, venules) as well as medium-sized vessels. Classic polyarteritis nodosa involves only medium-sized vessels, but substantial overlap occurs.
- Clinical findings depend on the arteries involved.
- Common symptoms of both disorders include fever and other constitutional symptoms, abdominal pain, livedo reticularis, mononeuritis multiplex, anemia, and an elevated sedimentation rate.
- Classic polyarteritis nodosa is often associated with hypertension but spares the lung.
- Ten to 30 percent of polyarteritis nodosa are associated with hepatitis B or C.
- Microscopic polyangiitis is frequently associated with antineutrophil cytoplasmic antibodies (ANCAs), pulmonary hemorrhage, and glomerulonephritis.

General Considerations

Polyarteritis nodosa was the first form of vasculitis recognized (in 1866). For many years, all forms of inflammatory vascular disease were termed "polyarteritis nodosa." In recent decades, numerous subtypes of vasculitis have been recognized, greatly narrowing the spectrum of vasculitis called polyarteritis nodosa. Currently, the term is reserved for a medium-sized necrotizing arteritis that has a predilection for involving peripheral nerves, mesenteric vessels (including renal arteries), heart, and brain but the capability of involving most organs. Microscopic polyangiitis, as its name implies, is the term given to nongranulomatous vasculitis involving small blood vessels. It is often associated with ANCAs that produce a p-ANCA pattern on immunofluorescence testing and are directed against myeloperoxidase, a constituent of neutrophil granules. Because microscopic polyangiitis may involve medium-sized as well as small blood vessels, its spectrum overlaps that of polyarteritis nodosa. Although the causes of polyarteritis and microscopic polyangiitis are not usually known, chronic hepatitis B or C causes 10–30% of cases of polyarteritis. In a minority of cases, microscopic polyangiitis appears to be induced by reactions to medications, particularly propylthiouracil, hydralazine, allopurinol, penicillamine, and sulfasalazine.

Clinical Findings

A. SYMPTOMS AND SIGNS

The clinical onset is usually insidious, with fever, malaise, weight loss, and other symptoms developing over weeks to months. Pain in the extremities is often a prominent early feature caused by arthralgia, myalgia (particularly affecting the calves), or neuropathy. The combination of mononeuritis multiplex (with the most common finding being foot-drop) and features of a systemic illness is one of the earliest specific clues to the presence of an underlying vasculitis. Polyarteritis and microscopic polyangiitis are among the forms of vasculitis most commonly associated with vasculitic neuropathy.

A wide variety of findings suggesting vasculitis of small blood vessels may develop in microscopic polyangiitis. These include palpable purpura and numerous other signs of cutaneous vasculitis; hematuria, proteinuria, and red blood cell casts in the urine; and pulmonary hemorrhage. The renal lesion is a segmental, necrotizing glomerulonephritis, often with localized intravascular coagulation. The pathologic findings in the lung are typically those of capillaritis.

In polyarteritis nodosa, the typical findings reflect the involvement of deeper, medium-sized blood vessels. Skin findings often include livedo reticularis, subcutaneous nodules, and skin ulcers. Digital gangrene is not an unusual occurrence. Involvement of the renal arteries leads to a renin-mediated hypertension (much less characteristic of vasculitides involving smaller blood vessels). For unclear reasons, classic polyarteritis nodosa seldom involves the lung.

Abdominal pain—particularly diffuse periumbilical pain precipitated by eating—is common to both polyarteritis nodosa and microscopic polyangiitis. Nausea and vomiting are frequently associated. Infarction compromises the function of major viscera and may lead to acalculous cholecystitis or appendicitis. Some patients present dramatically with an acute abdomen caused by mesenteric vasculitis and gut perforation or with hypotension resulting from rupture of a microaneurysm in the liver, kidney, or bowel.

Subclinical cardiac involvement is common in polyarteritis nodosa, and overt cardiac dysfunction occasionally occurs (eg, myocardial infarction secondary to coronary vasculitis, or myocarditis).

B. LABORATORY FINDINGS

The sedimentation rate is almost always elevated, often strikingly so. Most patients have a slight anemia, and leukocytosis is common. Three-fourths of patients with microscopic polyangiitis are ANCA-positive (usually with antibodies directed against myeloperoxidase, causing a p-ANCA pattern on immunofluorescence testing). Patients with classic polyarteritis nodosa are ANCA-negative. Serologic tests for hepatitis B or C are positive in 10–30% of patients with polyarteritis nodosa.

C. BIOPSY AND ANGIOGRAPHY

The diagnosis of both of these disorders requires confirmation with either a tissue biopsy or, in the case of polyarteritis nodosa, an angiogram. Biopsies of symptomatic sites (eg, nerve, muscle, lung, or kidney) have high sensitivities and specificities. The least invasive tests should usually be obtained first, but biopsy of an involved organ is essential. If performed by experienced physicians, tissue biopsies normally have high benefit-risk ratios because of the importance of establishing the diagnosis. Patients suspected of having polyarteritis nodosa—eg, on the basis of mesenteric ischemia or new-onset hypertension occurring in the setting of a systemic illness—may be diagnosed by the angiographic finding of aneurysmal dilations in the renal, mesenteric, or hepatic arteries. Angiography must be performed cautiously in patients with baseline renal dysfunction.

Treatment

For polyarteritis nodosa, corticosteroids in high doses (up to 60 mg of prednisone daily) may control fever and constitutional symptoms and heal vascular lesions. Pulse methylprednisolone (eg, 1 g intravenously daily for 3 days) may be necessary for patients who are critically ill at presentation. Immunosuppressive agents, especially cyclophosphamide, appear to improve the survival of patients when given with steroids. Some patients who have polyarteritis nodosa associated with viral hepatitis may respond to a short course of prednisone followed by antiviral treatment and plasmapheresis.

In microscopic polyangiitis, patients are more likely to require cyclophosphamide because of the urgency in treating pulmonary hemorrhage and glomerulonephritis. Cyclophosphamide may be administered either in an oral daily fashion or via intermittent (usually monthly) intravenous pulses.

Prognosis

Without treatment, the 5-year survival rate in these disorders is poor—on the order of 20%. With appropriate therapy, remissions are possible in many cases and the 5-year survival rate has improved to 60–90%. Poor prognostic factors are renal insufficiency, proteinuria, gastrointestinal ischemia, central nervous system disease, and cardiac involvement. Relapses following disease remissions may occur in both disorders—approximately 35% among patients with microscopic polyangiitis and perhaps less in those with idiopathic polyarteritis nodosa. For polyarteritis nodosa associated with hepatitis B or C, the likelihood of chronic disease may be higher.

Bonsib SM: Polyarteritis nodosa. Semin Diagn Pathol 2001; 18:14. [PMID: 11296989]

Jennette JC et al: Microscopic polyangiitis (microscopic polyarteritis). Semin Diagn Pathol 2001;18:3. [PMID: 11296991] (Microscopic polyangiitis is the most common cause for pulmonary-renal vasculitic syndromes—substantially more common than anti-glomerular basement membrane disease [Goodpasture's disease]).

POLYMYALGIA RHEUMATICA & GIANT CELL ARTERITIS

 ESSENTIALS OF DIAGNOSIS

- *Giant cell arteritis is characterized by headache, jaw claudication, polymyalgia rheumatica, visual abnormalities, and a markedly elevated ESR.*
- *The hallmark of polymyalgia rheumatica is pain and stiffness in shoulders and hips.*

General Considerations

Polymyalgia rheumatica and giant cell arteritis probably represent a spectrum of one disease: Both affect the same population (patients over the age of 50), show preference for the same HLA haplotypes, and show similar patterns of cytokines in blood and arteries. Polymyalgia rheumatica and giant cell arteritis also frequently coexist. Clinically, the important difference between the two conditions is that polymyalgia rheumatica alone does not cause blindness and responds to low-dose (10–20 mg/d) prednisone therapy, whereas giant cell arteritis can cause blindness and large artery complications and requires high-dose therapy (40–60 mg/d).

Clinical Findings

A. POLYMYALGIA RHEUMATICA

Polymyalgia rheumatica is a clinical diagnosis based on pain and stiffness of the shoulder and pelvic girdle areas, frequently in association with fever, malaise, and weight loss. It can occur in the absence of giant cell arteritis. Anemia and a markedly elevated sedimentation rate are almost always present. Because of the stiffness and pain in the shoulders, hips, and lower back, patients have trouble combing their hair, putting on a coat, or getting up out of a chair. In contrast to polymyositis, polymyalgia rheumatica does not cause muscular weakness. A few patients have joint swelling, particularly of the knees, wrists, and sternoclavicular joints. The differential diagnosis of malaise, anemia, and a markedly elevated sedimentation rate includes rheumatic diseases such as rheumatoid arthritis, other forms of vasculitis, multiple myeloma and other malignant disorders, and chronic infections such as bacterial endocarditis.

B. GIANT CELL ARTERITIS

Giant cell arteritis is a systemic panarteritis affecting medium-sized and large vessels in patients over the age of 50. The condition is also called temporal arteritis, since that artery is frequently involved, as are other extracranial branches of the carotid artery. About 50% of patients with giant cell arteritis also have polymyalgia rheumatica. The classic symptoms suggesting that a patient has arteritis are headache, scalp tenderness, visual symptoms, jaw claudication, or throat pain. The temporal artery is usually normal on physical examination but may be nodular, enlarged, tender, or pulseless. Blindness results from occlusive arteritis of the posterior ciliary branch of the ophthalmic artery. The ischemic optic neuropathy of giant cell arteritis may produce no funduscopic findings for the first 24–48 hours after the onset of blindness. Asymmetry of pulses in the arms, a murmur of aortic regurgitation, or bruits heard near the clavicle resulting from subclavian artery stenoses identify patients in whom giant cell arteritis has affected the aorta or its major branches. Large vessel involvement, particularly thoracic aortic aneurysms, occurs in approximately 15% of patients with giant cell arteritis, sometimes years after the diagnosis. Forty percent of patients with giant cell arteritis have nonclassic symptoms at presentation, chiefly respiratory tract problems (most frequently dry cough), mononeuritis multiplex (most frequently with painful paralysis of a shoulder), or fever of unknown origin. Giant cell arteritis accounts for 15% of all cases of fever of unknown origin in patients over the age of 65. The fever can be as high as 40 °C and is frequently associated with rigors and sweats. In contrast to patients with infection, patients with giant cell arteritis and fever almost always have a normal white blood count (before prednisone is started). Thus, in an older patient with fever of unknown origin, a very high erythrocyte sedimentation rate, and a normal white blood count, giant cell arteritis must be considered even in the absence of specific features such as headache or jaw claudication. In some cases, instead of having the well-known symptom of jaw claudication, patients complain of vague pain affecting other locations, including the tongue, nose, or ears. Indeed, unexplained head or neck pain in an older patient may signal the presence of giant cell arteritis.

C. LABORATORY FINDINGS

An elevated ESR, with a median result of about 65 mm/h, occurs in more than 90% of patients with polymyalgia rheumatica or giant cell arteritis. Other acute phase reactants such as C-reactive protein are also elevated. Interleukin-6 may be the most sensitive serologic indicator of disease activity yet described, but routine clinical testing for this cytokine is not widely available. Most patients also have a mild normochromic, normocytic anemia and thrombocytosis. The alkaline phosphatase (liver source) is elevated in 20% of patients with giant cell arteritis.

Treatment

A. POLYMYALGIA RHEUMATICA

Patients with isolated polymyalgia rheumatica are treated with prednisone, 10–20 mg/d. If the patient fails to experience a dramatic improvement within 72 hours, the diagnosis should be revisited. Within 1–2 months after beginning treatment, the patient's symptoms and laboratory abnormalities will resolve. The total duration of treatment varies considerably but ranges from 6 months to more than 2 years. Disease flares are common (50% or more) as prednisone is tapered.

B. GIANT CELL ARTERITIS

The urgency of early diagnosis and treatment in giant cell arteritis relates to the prevention of blindness. Once blindness develops, it is usually permanent. Therefore, when a patient has symptoms and findings suggestive of temporal arteritis, therapy with prednisone, 60 mg daily, is initiated immediately, and temporal artery biopsy is promptly obtained. Although it is prudent to obtain a temporal artery biopsy as soon as possible after instituting treatment, diagnostic findings of giant cell arteritis may still be present 2 weeks (or even considerably longer) after starting corticosteroids. Typically, a positive biopsy shows inflammatory infiltrate in the media and adventitia with lymphocytes, histiocytes, plasma cells, and giant cells. An adequate biopsy specimen (2 cm in length) is essential, because the disease may be segmental. Unilateral temporal artery biopsies are positive in approximately 80–85% of patients; bilateral biopsies add 10–15% to the yield. Prednisone should be continued in a dosage of 60 mg/d for 1–2 months before tapering. When only the symptoms of polymyalgia rheumatica are present, temporal artery biopsy is not necessary.

In adjusting the dosage of steroid, the erythrocyte sedimentation rate is a useful but not absolute guide to disease activity. A common error is treating the ESR rather than the patient. The ESR often rises slightly as the prednisone is tapered, even as the disease remains quiescent. Because elderly individuals often have baseline ESRs that are outside the "normal" range, mild ESR elevations should not be an occasion for renewed treatment with prednisone in patients who are asymptomatic. Thoracic aortic aneurysms occur 17 times more frequently in patients with giant cell arteritis than in normal individuals. The aneurysms can develop at any time but typically occur 7 years after the diagnosis of giant cell arteritis is made.

Evans JM et al: Polymyalgia rheumatica and giant cell arteritis. Rheum Dis Clin North Am 2000;26:493. [PMID: 10989509] (Interleukin-6 levels may be the most sensitive serologic marker of disease activity.)

Jover JA et al: Combined treatment of giant cell arteritis with methotrexate and prednisone. Ann Intern Med 2001; 134:106. [PMID: 11177313] (Methotrexate plus prednisone decreased risk of flare but not drug toxicity.)

Salvarani C et al: Giant cell arteritis with low erythrocyte sedimentation rate: frequency of occurrence in a population-based study. Arthritis Rheum 2001;45:140. [PMID: 11324777] (Eleven percent of patients with biopsy-proved temporal arteritis had sedimentation rates of < 50 mm/h at presentation. Five percent had sedimentation rates < 40 mm/h.)

Smetana GW et al: Does this patient have temporal arteritis? JAMA 2002;287:92. [PMID: 11754714] (Historical features that increased the likelihood of temporal arteritis were jaw claudication and diplopia. Physical examination findings that predicted the diagnosis were temporal artery nodularity, prominence, and tenderness.)

WEGENER'S GRANULOMATOSIS

ESSENTIALS OF DIAGNOSIS

- Originally defined by the triad of upper respiratory tract disease, lower respiratory disease, and glomerulonephritis.
- Suspect this diagnosis whenever mundane respiratory systems (eg, nasal congestion, sinusitis) are refractory to usual treatment.
- Pathology defined by the triad of small vessel vasculitis, granulomatous inflammation, and necrosis.
- c-ANCA relatively sensitive and specific.
- Renal disease often rapidly progressive without treatment.

General Considerations

Wegener's granulomatosis is a rare disorder (prevalence of three per 100,000) characterized by vasculitis of small arteries, arterioles, and capillaries, necrotizing granulomatous lesions of both upper and lower respiratory tract, and glomerulonephritis. Without treatment it is invariably fatal, most patients surviving less than a year after diagnosis. It occurs most commonly in the fourth and fifth decades of life and affects men and women with equal frequency.

Clinical Findings

A. SYMPTOMS AND SIGNS

The disorder usually develops over 4–12 months, with 90% of patients presenting with upper or lower respiratory tract symptoms or both. Upper respiratory tract symptoms can include nasal congestion, sinusitis, otitis media, mastoiditis, inflammation of the gums, or stridor due to subglottic stenosis. Since many of these symptoms are common, the underlying disease is not often suspected until the patient develops systemic symptoms or the original problem is refractory to treatment. The lung is affected initially in 40% and eventually in 80%, with symptoms including cough, dyspnea, and hemoptysis. Other early symptoms can include unilateral proptosis (from pseudotumor), red eye from scleritis, arthritis, purpura, and dysesthesia due to neuropathy. Renal involvement, which develops in three-fourths of the cases, may be subclinical until renal insufficiency is advanced. Fever, malaise, and weight loss are common.

Physical examination can be remarkable for congestion, crusting, ulceration, bleeding, and even perforation of the nasal mucosa. Destruction of the nasal cartilage with "saddle nose" deformity occurs late. Otitis media, proptosis, scleritis, episcleritis, and conjunctivitis are other common findings. Newly acquired hypertension, a frequent feature of polyarteritis, is rare in Wegener's granulomatosis.

Although limited forms of Wegener's granulomatosis have been described in which the kidney is spared initially, most untreated patients will develop renal disease. In such cases the urinary sediment invariably contains red cells, with or without white cells, and red cell casts. Renal biopsy discloses a segmental necrotizing glomerulonephritis with multiple crescents; this is characteristic but not diagnostic. Granulomas are observed in only 10% of renal biopsy specimens but are found much more commonly on lung biopsy.

B. LABORATORY FINDINGS

Most patients have slight anemia, mild leukocytosis, and an elevated erythrocyte sedimentation rate. Chest CT is more sensitive than chest radiography; lesions include infiltrates, nodules, masses, and cavities. Often the radiographs prompt concern about lung cancer. Hilar adenopathy is unusual in Wegener's granulomatosis; if present, sarcoidosis, tumor, or infection is more likely. Other common laboratory or radiographic abnormalities include hematuria, red blood cell casts, and sinus destruction.

Histologic features of Wegener's granulomatosis include vasculitis, granulomatous inflammation, geographic necrosis, and acute and chronic inflammation. The full range of pathologic changes are usually evident only on thoracoscopic lung biopsy. Nasal biopsies often do not show vasculitis but may show chronic inflammation and other changes which, interpreted by an experienced pathologist, can serve as convincing evidence of the diagnosis.

Serum tests for antineutrophil cytoplasmic antibodies (ANCA) help in the diagnosis of Wegener's granulomatosis and related forms of vasculitis (Tables 20–10 and 19–4). Several different types of ANCA are recognized. The cytoplasmic pattern of immunofluorescence (c-ANCA), caused by antibodies to proteinase-3, a constituent of neutrophil granules, has a high specificity (> 90%) for Wegener's granulomatosis. In the setting of active disease, the sensitivity of c-ANCA is also reasonably high (≥ 70%). Although ANCA testing may be very helpful when used properly, it does not eliminate the need in most cases for confirmation of the diagnosis by tissue biopsy. Furthermore, ANCA levels correlate erratically with disease activity, and changes in titer should not dictate changes in therapy in the absence of supporting clinical data. The perinuclear (p-ANCA) pattern is caused by antibodies to myeloperoxidase and is much less specific for Wegener's granulomatosis. Approximately 10–25% of patients with classic Wegener's granulomatosis have p-ANCA. Owing to involvement of the same types of blood vessels, similar patterns of organ involvement, and the possibility of failing to identify granulomatous pathology on tissue biopsies because of sampling error, Wegener's granulomatosis is often difficult to differentiate from microscopic polyangiitis.

Atypical patterns of ANCA—often mistaken for p-ANCA—occur frequently in patients with systemic lupus erythematosus and inflammatory bowel disease.

Treatment

It is essential that the diagnosis of Wegener's granulomatosis be made early, since treatment may be lifesaving. Early treatment is also crucial in preventing renal failure. While Wegener's granulomatosis may involve the sinuses or lung for months, once proteinuria or hematuria develops, progression to renal failure can be rapid (over several weeks). Remissions have been induced in up to 75% of patients treated with cyclophosphamide and prednisone, though half of these patients eventually suffer disease recurrences. The cyclophosphamide is best given daily by mouth; intermittent high-dose intravenous cyclophosphamide is less effective. Unfortunately, the traditional therapy of oral cyclophosphamide continued for 12 months after the patient achieves remission has resulted in severe toxicity, including a 2.4 times increased risk of all malignancies, a 33-fold increase in bladder cancer, and a 60% chance of ovarian failure. Methotrexate, 20–25 mg/wk, is a reasonable substitute for oral cyclophosphamide in patients who do not have immediately life-threatening disease. Another strategy to limit cyclophosphamide use is to employ the drug for about 3 months in order to induce remission and then switch to methotrexate. Trimethoprim-sulfamethoxazole (one double-strength tablet twice daily) is ineffective for life-threatening Wegener's disease; however, the drug may help maintain disease remissions. Trimethoprim-sulfamethoxazole and methotrexate are both folate antagonists; the combination can cause aplastic anemia and should be used with great care.

Hoffman GS et al: Antineutrophil cytoplasmic antibodies. Arthritis Rheum 1998;41:1521. [PMID: 9551084] (Although this article is now several years old, it remains the most lucid and comprehensive review of ANCA testing. All positive immunofluorescence assays should be followed up by specific enzyme immunoassays for antibodies to proteinase-3 and myeloperoxidase.)

Regan MJ et al: Treatment of Wegener's granulomatosis. Rheum Dis Clin North Am 2001;27:863. [PMID: 11723769] (After the diagnosis is made, remission is achieved by a high percentage of patients. Keeping patients in remission while avoiding the adverse effects commonly associated with conventional treatments for the disease is the greatest challenge.)

CRYOGLOBULINEMIA

Vasculitis secondary to cryoglobulinemia is uncommon but should be considered when patients present with palpable purpura and peripheral neuropathy. Abnormal liver function tests, abdominal pain, and pulmonary disease may also occur. The diagnosis is based on a compatible clinical picture and a positive serum test for cryoglobulins. Type I cryoglobulins (monoclonal proteins that lack rheumatoid factor activity) are more commonly seen in lymphoproliferative disease. (Type I cryoglobulins usually cause hyperviscosity syndromes rather than vasculitis.) The diseases most commonly associated with cryoglobulinemic vasculitis are hepatitis C and connective tissues diseases, especially Sjögren's syndrome. Type II (monoclonal antibody with rheumatoid factor activity) and type III (polyclonal antibody with rheumatoid factor activity) cryoglobulins cause vasculitis. Because 90% of cryoglobulinemia cases are associated with hepatitis C infections, the optimal approach to treatment is viral suppression with interferon alfa with or without ribavirin. Because immunosuppressive agents may facilitate viral replication, corticosteroids, cyclophosphamide, and other agents should be reserved for organ-threatening complications.

Lamprecht P et al: Cryoglobulinemic vasculitis. Arthritis Rheum 1999;42:2507. [PMID: 10615995]

HENOCH-SCHÖNLEIN PURPURA

Henoch-Schönlein purpura, the most common systemic vasculitis in children, occurs in adults as well. Typical features are palpable purpura, abdominal pain, arthritis, and hematuria. Pathologic features include leukocytoclastic vasculitis with IgA deposition. The cause is not known.

The purpuric skin lesions are typically located on the lower extremities but may also be seen on the hands, arms, trunk, and buttocks. Joint symptoms are present in the majority of patients, the knees and ankles being most commonly involved. Abdominal pain secondary to vasculitis of the intestinal tract is often associated with gastrointestinal bleeding. Hematuria signals the presence of a renal lesion that is usually reversible, although it occasionally may progress to renal insufficiency. Children tend to have more frequent and more serious gastrointestinal vasculitis, whereas adults more often suffer from renal disease. Biopsy of the kidney reveals segmental glomerulonephritis with crescents and mesangial deposition of IgA.

The disease is usually self-limited, lasting 1–6 weeks, and subsides without sequelae if renal involvement is not severe. Chronic courses with persistent or intermittent skin disease are more likely to occur in adults than in children. The efficacy of treatment is not well established.

Saulsbury FT: Henoch-Schönlein purpura. Curr Opin Rheumatol 2001;13:35. [PMID: 111489713] (This disorder is associated with preferential deposition of IgA1 in involved tissues. The reason for the exclusive involvement of IgA1 as opposed to IgA2 remains unclear.)

RELAPSING POLYCHONDRITIS

This is characterized by inflammatory destructive lesions of cartilaginous structures, principally the ears, nose, trachea, and larynx. It may be associated either with other immunologic disorders such as SLE, rheumatoid arthritis, or Hashimoto's thyroiditis or with cancers, especially multiple myeloma. The disease, which is usually episodic, affects males and females equally. The cartilage is painful, swollen, and tender during an attack and subsequently becomes atrophic, resulting in permanent deformity. Biopsy of the involved cartilage shows inflammation and chondrolysis. Noncartilaginous manifestations of the disease include fever, episcleritis, uveitis, deafness, aortic insufficiency, and rarely glomerulonephritis. In 85% of patients, a migratory, asymmetric, and seronegative arthropathy occurs, affecting both large and small joints and the costochondral junctions.

Prednisone, 0.5–1 mg/kg/d, is often effective. Dapsone (100–200 mg/d) may also be effective, sparing the need for chronic high-dose corticosteroid treatment. Involvement of the tracheobronchial tree, leading to tracheomalacia, may lead to difficult management issues.

Molina JF et al: Relapsing polychondritis. Baillieres Best Pract Res Clin Rheumatol 2000;14:97. [PMID: 10882216] (Corticosteroids remain the drugs of choice.)

BEHÇET'S SYNDROME

Named after the Turkish dermatologist who first described it, this disease of unknown cause is characterized by recurrent oral and genital ulcers, uveitis, seronegative arthritis, and central nervous system abnormalities. Other features include ulcerative skin lesions, erythema nodosum, thrombophlebitis, and vasculitis. Arthritis occurs in about two-thirds of patients, most commonly affecting the knees and ankles. Keratitis, retinal vasculitis, and anterior uveitis (often with hypopyon—pus in the anterior chamber) are observed. The ocular involvement is often fulminant and may result in blindness. Involvement of the central nervous system, which may mimic multiple sclerosis radiologically, often results in serious disability or death. Findings include cranial nerve palsies, convulsions, encephalitis, mental disturbances, and spinal cord lesions.

The clinical course may be chronic but is often characterized by remissions and exacerbations. Corticosteroids, azathioprine, chlorambucil, pentoxifylline, and cyclosporine have been used with beneficial results. Oral base corticosteroids may be of some help for oral ulcerations.

Direskeneli H: Behçet's disease: infectious aetiology, new autoantigens, and HLA-B51. Ann Rheum Dis 2001;60:996. [PMID: 11602462] (In case-control studies, the presence of the HLA-B51 allele is associated with an increased odds ratio of 1.5–16 for the diagnosis of Behçet's disease.)

Yazici H et al: Behçet disease. Curr Opin Rheumatol 2001;13:18. [PMID: 11148711] (Brain stem lesions are the most common type of parenchymal brain involvement, occurring in 51% of patients with central nervous system disease).

PRIMARY ANGIITIS OF THE CENTRAL NERVOUS SYSTEM

Primary angiitis of the central nervous system is a syndrome with several possible causes that produces small and medium-sized vasculitis limited to the brain and spinal cord. Biopsy-proved cases have predominated in men who present with a history of weeks to months of headaches, encephalopathy, and multifocal strokes. Systemic signs and symptoms are absent, and routine laboratory tests are usually normal. MRI of the brain is almost always abnormal, and the spinal fluid often reveals a mild lymphocytosis and a modest increase in protein level. Angiograms classically reveal a "string of beads" pattern produced by alternating segments of arterial narrowing and dilation. However, neither the MRI nor the angiogram appearance is specific for vasculitis. Many conditions, including vasospasm, can produce the same angiographic pattern as vasculitis. Definitive diagnosis requires a compatible clinical picture; exclusion of infection, neoplasm, or metabolic disorder or drug exposure (eg, cocaine) that can mimic primary angiitis of the central nervous system, and a positive brain biopsy. When a patient meeting the above criteria has a positive angiogram without a confirming biopsy, the diagnosis should be considered possible. Angiographically defined cases of central nervous system vasculopathy differ from biopsy-proved cases chiefly involving women who have had an abrupt onset of headaches and stroke (often in the absence of encephalopathy) with normal spinal fluid findings. Many patients who fit this clinical profile and have disease diagnosed by angiography (but not biopsy) probably have vasospasm rather than true vasculitis. Such cases may require shorter and less intensive courses of immunosuppression—or none at all—as opposed to those with biopsy-proved cases. The latter usually improve with prednisone therapy and may require cyclophosphamide.

Calabrese LH et al: Vasculitis in the central nervous system. Arthritis Rheum 1997;40:1189. [PMID:9214418] (The diagnostic and therapeutic approaches to possible central nervous system vasculitis have changed very little in the past several years. This review summarizes the logical strategies for work-up.)

■ SERONEGATIVE SPONDYLOARTHROPATHIES

The seronegative spondyloarthropathies are ankylosing spondylitis, psoriatic arthritis, Reiter's syndrome (also called reactive arthritis), and the arthritis associated with inflammatory bowel disease. These disorders are noted for onset usually before age 40, inflammatory arthritis of the spine or the large peripheral joints (or both), uveitis in a significant minority, the absence of autoantibodies in the serum, and a striking association with HLA-B27. Present in only 8% of normal whites and 3% of normal blacks, HLA-B27 is positive in 90% of patients with ankylosing spondylitis and 75% with Reiter's syndrome. HLA-B27 also occurs in 50% of the psoriatic and inflammatory bowel disease patients who have sacroiliitis. Patients with only peripheral arthritis in these latter two syndromes do not show an increase in HLA-B27.

That HLA-B27 itself (and not some other gene) confers susceptibility to these diseases has been demonstrated by experiments with transgenic rats. When the human HLA-B27 gene is expressed in rats, the animals develop a spinal and peripheral arthritis, psoriasiform nail and skin changes, and bowel inflammation. Thus, HLA-B27 is an important risk factor for the spondyloarthropathies. However, some patients with these disorders are HLA-B27-negative, and the great majority of HLA-B27-positive individuals do not develop spondyloarthropathies. The gene is therefore neither necessary nor sufficient to cause spondyloarthropathies.

Infection also appears to play a key role in some of the spondyloarthropathies, especially Reiter's syndrome, which characteristically develops days to weeks after bacterial dysentery or a nongonococcal sexually transmitted infection (see below). The interplay of susceptibility genes and environmental infections is demonstrated by the fact that the risk of developing Reiter's syndrome is 0.2% in the general population, 2% in the HLA-B27 individuals, and 20% in patients with HLA-B27 who become infected with salmonella, shigella, or enteric organisms. Despite these gains in our understanding of the importance of HLA-B27 and infection, the precise mechanism by which genes and infection cause spondyloarthropathy is not yet known.

ANKYLOSING SPONDYLITIS

 ESSENTIALS OF DIAGNOSIS

- *Chronic low backache in young adults.*
- *Progressive limitation of back motion and of chest expansion.*
- *Transient (50%) or permanent (25%) peripheral arthritis.*
- *Anterior uveitis in 20–25%.*
- *Diagnostic x-ray changes in sacroiliac joints.*
- *Accelerated erythrocyte sedimentation rate and negative serologic tests for rheumatoid factor. HLA-B27 usually positive.*

General Considerations

Ankylosing spondylitis is a chronic inflammatory disease of the joints of the axial skeleton, manifested clinically by pain and progressive stiffening of the spine. The age at onset is usually in the late teens or early 20s. The incidence is greater in males than in females, and symptoms are more prominent in men, with ascending involvement of the spine more likely to occur.

Clinical Findings

A. SYMPTOMS AND SIGNS

The onset is usually gradual, with intermittent bouts of back pain that may radiate down the thighs. As the disease advances, symptoms progress in a cephalad direction and back motion becomes limited, with the normal lumbar curve flattened and the thoracic curvature exaggerated. Chest expansion is often limited as a consequence of costovertebral joint involvement. Radicular symptoms due to cauda equina fibrosis may occur years after onset of the disease. In advanced cases, the entire spine becomes fused, allowing no motion in any direction. Transient acute arthritis of the peripheral joints occurs in about 50% of cases, and permanent changes in the peripheral joints—most commonly the hips, shoulders, and knees—are seen in about 25%.

Spondylitic heart disease, characterized chiefly by atrioventricular conduction defects and aortic insufficiency, occurs in 3–5% of patients with long-standing severe disease. Anterior uveitis is associated in as many as 25% of cases and may be a presenting feature. Pulmonary fibrosis of the upper lobes, with progression to cavitation and bronchiectasis mimicking tuberculosis, may occur, characteristically long after the onset of skeletal symptoms. Constitutional symptoms similar to those of rheumatoid arthritis are absent in most patients.

B. LABORATORY FINDINGS

The erythrocyte sedimentation rate is elevated in 85% of cases, but serologic tests for rheumatoid factor are characteristically negative. Anemia may be present but is often mild.

HLA-B27 is found in 90% of patients with ankylosing spondylitis. Because this antigen occurs in 8% of the normal population, it is not a specific diagnostic test.

C. IMAGING

The earliest radiographic changes are usually in the sacroiliac joints. In the first few months of the disease process, the sacroiliac changes may be detectable only by CT scanning. Later, erosion and sclerosis of these joints are evident on plain radiographs. Involvement of the apophysial joints of the spine, ossification of the annulus fibrosus, calcification of the anterior and lateral spinal ligaments, and squaring and generalized demineralization of the vertebral bodies may occur in more advanced stages. The term "bamboo spine" has been used to describe the late radiographic appearance of the spinal column.

Additional x-ray findings include periosteal new bone formation on the iliac crest, ischial tuberosities and calcanei, and alterations of the pubic symphysis and sternomanubrial joint similar to those of the sacroiliacs. Radiologic changes in peripheral joints, when present, tend to be asymmetric and lack the demineralization and erosions seen in rheumatoid arthritis.

Differential Diagnosis

In contrast to ankylosing spondylitis, rheumatoid arthritis predominantly affects multiple, small, peripheral joints of the hands and feet. Rheumatoid arthritis also spares the sacroiliac joints, has little effect on the rest of the spine except for C1–C2. Finally, rheumatoid arthritis is often associated with rheumatoid nodules and with rheumatoid factor, not with HLA-B27. The history and physical findings of ankylosing

spondylitis serve to distinguish this disorder from other causes of low back pain such as disk disease, osteoporosis, soft tissue trauma, and tumors. The single most valuable distinguishing radiologic sign of ankylosing spondylitis is the appearance of the sacroiliac joints, although a similar pattern may be seen in Reiter's syndrome and in the arthritis associated with inflammatory intestinal diseases and psoriasis. In ankylosing hyperostosis (diffuse idiopathic skeletal hyperostosis [DISH], Forestier's disease), there is exuberant osteophyte formation. The osteophytes are thicker and more anterior than the syndesmophytes of ankylosing spondylitis, and the sacroiliac joints are not affected. The x-ray appearance of the sacroiliac joints in spondylitis should be distinguished from that in osteitis condensans ilii.

Belanger TA et al: Diffuse idiopathic skeletal hyperostosis: musculoskeletal manifestations. J Am Acad Orthop Surg 2001;9: 258. [PMID:11476536] ("Flowing" osteophytes along the anterolateral margins of at least four contiguous vertebrae in the absence of spondyloarthropathy or degenerative spondylosis are diagnostic. There is often a delay in diagnosis of spinal fractures in these patients because they often have some back pain at baseline and because the degree of trauma required to cause fracture is low.)

Treatment

A. BASIC PROGRAM

The general principles of managing chronic arthritis (see above) apply equally well to ankylosing spondylitis. The importance of postural and breathing exercises should be stressed.

B. DRUG THERAPY

The nonsteroidal anti-inflammatory agents are employed in the treatment of this disorder. Of these, indomethacin appears to be the most effective, though it can be quite toxic. The dosage of indomethacin is usually 25–50 mg three times a day, but the smallest effective dose should be used. Indomethacin may produce a variety of untoward reactions, including headache, giddiness, nausea and vomiting, peptic ulcer, renal insufficiency, depression, and psychosis. Other NSAIDs are valuable alternatives and may be used as primary therapy. Sulfasalazine (1000 mg twice daily) is sometimes useful for the peripheral arthritis in patients with spondyloarthropathies but has little symptomatic effect on spinal and sacroiliac joint disease. Recent studies with tumor necrosis factor inhibitors demonstrate that these agents are highly effective in both the spinal and peripheral arthritis of ankylosing spondylitis. Either etanercept (25 mg subcutaneously twice a week) or infliximab (5 mg/kg every other month) is reasonable for patients whose symptoms are refractory to physical therapy and other interventions.

C. PHYSICAL THERAPY

See above.

Prognosis

Almost all patients have persistent symptoms over decades; rare individuals experience long-term remissions. The severity of disease varies greatly, with about 10% of patients having work disability after 10 years. Developing hip disease within the first 2 years of disease onset presages a worse prognosis.

Braun J et al: New treatment options in spondyloarthropathies: increasing evidence for significant efficacy of anti-tumor necrosis factor therapy. Curr Opin Rheumatol 2001;13: 245. [PMID: 11555723] (Specific tumor necrosis factor inhibition is an exciting new approach to treating severe spondyloarthropathies.)

Reveille JD et al: HLA-B27 and genetic predisposing factors in spondyloarthropathies. Curr Opin Rheumatol 2001;13: 265. [PMID: 11555726] (HLA-B27 contributes only 16–50% of the total genetic risk for ankylosing spondylitis, indicating clearly that other genes are involved.)

PSORIATIC ARTHRITIS

ESSENTIALS OF DIAGNOSIS

- *Psoriasis precedes onset of arthritis in 80% of cases.*
- *Arthritis usually asymmetric, with "sausage" appearance of fingers and toes; resembles rheumatoid arthritis; rheumatoid factor is negative.*
- *Sacroiliac joint involvement common; ankylosis of the sacroiliac joints may occur.*
- *X-ray findings: osteolysis; pencil-in-cup deformity; relative lack of osteoporosis; bony ankylosis; asymmetric sacroiliitis and atypical syndesmophytes.*

General Considerations

In 15–20% of patients with psoriasis, arthritis coexists. The patterns or subsets of arthritis that may accompany psoriasis include the following:

(1) Joint disease that resembles rheumatoid arthritis in which polyarthritis is symmetric. Usually, fewer joints are involved than in rheumatoid arthritis.

(2) An oligoarticular form that may lead to considerable destruction of the affected joints.

(3) A pattern of disease in which the distal interphalangeal joints are primarily affected. Early, this may be monarticular, and often the joint involvement is asymmetric. Pitting of the nails and onycholysis are frequently associated.

(4) A severe deforming arthritis (arthritis mutilans) in which osteolysis is marked.

(5) A spondylitic form in which sacroiliitis and spinal involvement predominate; 50% of these patients are HLA-B27-positive.

Clinical Findings

A. Symptoms and Signs

Although psoriasis usually precedes the onset of arthritis, arthritis precedes or occurs simultaneously with the skin disease in approximately 20% of cases. Arthritis is at least five times more common in patients with severe skin disease than in those with only mild skin findings. Occasionally, however, patients may have a single patch of psoriasis (typically hidden in the scalp, gluteal cleft, or umbilicus) and are unaware of its connection to the arthritis. Thus, a detailed search for cutaneous lesions is essential in patients with arthritis of new onset. Also, the psoriatic lesions may have cleared when arthritis appears—in such cases, the history is most useful in diagnosing previously unexplained cases of mono- or oligoarthritis. Nail pitting, a residue of previous psoriasis, is sometimes the only clue.

B. Laboratory Findings

Laboratory studies show an elevation of the sedimentation rate, but rheumatoid factor is not present. Uric acid levels may be high, reflecting the active turnover of skin affected by psoriasis. There is a correlation between the extent of psoriatic involvement and the level of uric acid, but gout is no more common than in patients without psoriasis. Desquamation of the skin may also reduce iron stores.

C. Imaging

Radiographic findings are most helpful in distinguishing the disease from other forms of arthritis. There are marginal erosions of bone and irregular destruction of joint and bone, which, in the phalanx, may give the appearance of a sharpened pencil. Fluffy periosteal new bone may be marked, especially at the insertion of muscles and ligaments into bone. Such changes will also be seen along the shafts of metacarpals, metatarsals, and phalanges. Paravertebral ossification occurs, which may be distinguished from ankylosing spondylitis by the absence of ossification in the anterior aspect of the spine.

Treatment

Treatment regimens are symptomatic. Nonsteroidal anti-inflammatory drugs are usually sufficient for mild cases. Corticosteroids are less effective in psoriatic arthritis than in other forms of inflammatory arthritis. In addition, they may exacerbate the skin disease during tapers. Antimalarials may also exacerbate psoriasis. In resistant cases, methotrexate may be helpful. For cases with disease that is refractory to methotrexate, etanercept or infliximab is usually effective for both arthritis and psoriatic skin disease. Successful treatment of the skin lesions (eg, by PUVA therapy) commonly—though not invariably—is accompanied by an improvement in peripheral articular symptoms.

Mease PJ et al: Etanercept in the treatment of psoriatic arthritis and psoriasis: a randomized trial. Lancet 2000;356:385. [PMID: 10972371] (In this 12-week trial with 60 patients, 87% taking etanercept improved versus 23% on placebo. Benefit was less for psoriasis itself.)

REITER'S SYNDROME
(Reactive Arthritis)

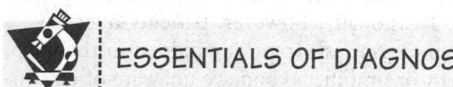

ESSENTIALS OF DIAGNOSIS

- *Fifty to 80 percent of patients are HLA-B27-positive.*
- *Oligoarthritis, conjunctivitis, urethritis, and mouth ulcers most common features.*
- *Usually follows dysentery or a sexually transmitted infection.*

General Considerations

Reiter's syndrome, also called "reactive arthritis," is a clinical tetrad of urethritis, conjunctivitis (or, less commonly, uveitis), mucocutaneous lesions, and aseptic arthritis. It occurs most commonly in young men, is associated with HLA-B27 in 80% of white patients and 50–60% of blacks, and often follows infection (see above).

Clinical Findings

A. SYMPTOMS AND SIGNS

Most cases of Reiter's syndrome develop within days or weeks after either a dysenteric infection (with shigella, salmonella, yersinia, campylobacter) or a sexually transmitted infection (with *Chlamydia trachomatis* or perhaps *Ureaplasma urealyticum*). Whether the inciting infection is sexually transmitted or dysenteric does not affect the subsequent manifestations but does influence the gender ratio: The ratio is 1:1 after enteric infections but 9:1 with male predominance after sexually transmitted infections.

Although affected joints are culture-negative, fragments of putative organisms have been identified by polymerase chain reaction studies on synovial fluid. The exact role of infection remains unclear.

The arthritis is most commonly asymmetric and frequently involves the large weight-bearing joints (chiefly the knee and ankle); sacroiliitis or ankylosing spondylitis is observed in at least 20% of patients, especially after frequent recurrences. Systemic symptoms including fever and weight loss are common at the onset of disease. The mucocutaneous lesions may in-

clude balanitis, stomatitis, and keratoderma blennorrhagicum, indistinguishable from pustular psoriasis. Involvement of the fingernails in Reiter's syndrome may also mimic psoriatic changes. Carditis and aortic regurgitation may occur. While most signs of the disease disappear within days or weeks, the arthritis may persist for several months or even years. Recurrences involving any combination of the clinical manifestations are common and are sometimes followed by permanent sequelae, especially in the joints.

B. IMAGING

X-ray signs of permanent or progressive joint disease may be seen in the sacroiliac as well as the peripheral joints.

Differential Diagnosis

Gonococcal arthritis can initially mimic Reiter's syndrome, but the marked improvement after 24–48 hours of antibiotic administration and the culture results distinguish the two disorders. Rheumatoid arthritis, ankylosing spondylitis, and psoriatic arthritis must also be considered.

The association of Reiter's syndrome and HIV has been debated, but evidence now indicates Reiter's syndrome is equally common in sexually active men regardless of HIV status.

Treatment

NSAIDs have been the mainstay of therapy. Antibiotics given at the time of a nongonococcal sexually transmitted infection reduce the chance that the individual will develop Reiter's syndrome. Tetracycline (250 mg four times daily) given for 3 months to patients with Reiter's syndrome associated with *C trachomatis* reduces the duration of symptoms. Tetracyclines have anti-inflammatory properties, so the response need not be attributed solely to an antimicrobial effect. Patients who fail NSAIDs and tetracycline may respond to sulfasalazine, 1000 mg twice daily. Anti-TNF agents (etanercept, infliximab) are reasonable therapies for patients with refractory disease.

Toivanen A et al: Reactive arthritis. Isr Med Assoc J 2001;3:681. [PMID: 11574987] (Relapsing, chronic cases are not uncommon. Early treatment of the precipitating infection may prevent the development of reactive arthritis).

ARTHRITIS & INFLAMMATORY INTESTINAL DISEASES

One-fifth of patients with inflammatory bowel disease have arthritis, making it second only to anemia as the most common extraintestinal manifestation. Arthritis complicates Crohn's disease somewhat more frequently than it does ulcerative colitis. In both diseases, two distinct forms of arthritis occur. The first is peripheral arthritis—usually a nondeforming asymmetric oligoarthritis of large joints—in which the activity of the joint disease parallels that of the bowel disease. The arthritis usually begins months to years after the bowel disease, but occasionally the joint symptoms develop earlier and may be prominent enough to cause the patient to overlook intestinal symptoms. The second form of arthritis is a spondylitis that is indistinguishable by symptoms or x-ray from ankylosing spondylitis and follows a course independent of the bowel disease. About 50% of these patients are HLA-B27-positive.

Controlling the intestinal inflammation usually eliminates the peripheral arthritis. The spondylitis often requires NSAIDs, which need to be used cautiously since these agents may activate the bowel disease in a few patients. Range-of-motion exercises as prescribed for ankylosing spondylitis can be helpful.

About two-thirds of patients with Whipple's disease experience arthralgia or arthritis, most often an episodic, large-joint polyarthritis. The arthritis usually precedes the gastrointestinal manifestations by years. In fact, the arthritis resolves as the diarrhea develops. Thus, Whipple's disease should be considered in the differential diagnosis of unexplained episodic arthritis.

■ INFECTIOUS ARTHRITIS*

NONGONOCOCCAL ACUTE BACTERIAL (SEPTIC) ARTHRITIS

ESSENTIALS OF DIAGNOSIS

- Sudden onset of acute arthritis, usually monarticular, most often in large weight-bearing joints and wrists.
- Previous joint damage or intravenous drug abuse common risk factors.
- Infection with causative organisms commonly found elsewhere in body.
- Joint effusions are usually large, with white blood counts commonly > 50,000/µL.

General Considerations

Nongonococcal acute bacterial arthritis is a disease of an abnormal host. The key risk factors are persistent bacteremia (eg, intravenous drug use, endocarditis) and damaged joints (eg, rheumatoid arthritis). *Staphylococcus aureus* is the most common cause of nongono-

coccal septic arthritis, followed by group A and group B streptococci. Gram-negative septic arthritis, once rare, has become more common, especially in intravenous drug abusers and in other immunocompromised hosts. *Escherichia coli* and *Pseudomonas aeruginosa* are the most common gram-negative isolates in adults.

The widespread use of arthroscopy and prosthetic joint surgery has also increased the frequency of septic arthritis. In the latter conditions, *Staphylococcus epidermidis* is the usual offending organism. Pathologic changes include varying degrees of acute inflammation, with synovitis, effusion, abscess formation in synovial or subchondral tissues, and, if treatment is not adequate, articular destruction.

Clinical Findings

A. SYMPTOMS AND SIGNS

The onset is usually sudden, with acute pain, swelling, and heat of one joint—most frequently the knee. Other commonly affected sites are the hip, wrist, shoulder, and ankle. Unusual sites, such as the sternoclavicular or sacroiliac joint, can be involved in intravenous drug abusers. Chills and fever are common but are absent in up to 20% of patients. Infection of the hip usually does not produce apparent swelling but results in groin pain greatly aggravated by walking.

B. LABORATORY FINDINGS

Blood cultures are positive in approximately 50% of patients. The leukocyte count of the synovial fluid exceeds 50,000 and often 100,000/µL, with 90% or more polymorphonuclear cells. Synovial fluid glucose is usually low. Gram stain of the synovial fluid is positive in 75% of staphylococcal infections and in 50% of gram-negative infections.

C. IMAGING

Radiographs are usually normal early in the disease, but evidence of demineralization may be present within days of onset. Bony erosions and narrowing of the joint space followed by osteomyelitis and periostitis may be seen within 2 weeks.

Differential Diagnosis

The septic course with chills and fever, the acute systemic reaction, the joint fluid findings, evidence of infection elsewhere in the body, and the evidence of response to appropriate antibiotics are diagnostic of bacterial arthritis. Gout and pseudogout are excluded by the failure to find crystals on synovial fluid analysis. Acute rheumatic fever and rheumatoid arthritis commonly involve many joints; Still's disease may mimic septic arthritis, but laboratory evidence of infection is absent. Pyogenic arthritis may be superimposed on other types of joint disease, notably rheumatoid arthri-

*Lyme disease is discussed in Chapter 34.

tis, and must be excluded (by joint fluid examination) in any apparent acute relapse of the primary disease, particularly when a joint has been needled or when one is more strikingly inflamed than the others.

Treatment

Prompt systemic antibiotic therapy of any septic arthritis should be based on the best clinical judgment of the causative organism and the results of smear and culture of joint fluid, blood, urine, or other specific sites of potential infection. If the organism cannot be determined clinically, treatment should be started with bactericidal antibiotics effective against staphylococci, pneumococci, and gram-negative organisms.

Frequent (even daily) local aspiration is indicated when synovial fluid rapidly reaccumulates and causes symptoms. Immediate surgical drainage is reserved for septic arthritis of the hip, because that site is inaccessible to repeated aspiration. For most other joints, surgical drainage is used only if medical therapy fails over 2–4 days to improve the fever and the synovial fluid volume, white blood count, and culture results. Pain can be relieved with local hot compresses and by immobilizing the joint with a splint or traction. Rest, immobilization, and elevation are used at the onset of treatment. Early active motion exercises within the limits of tolerance will hasten recovery.

Prognosis

With prompt antibiotic therapy and no serious underlying disease, functional recovery is usually good. Five to 10 percent of patients with an infected joint die, chiefly from respiratory complications of sepsis. The mortality rate is 30% for patients with polyarticular sepsis. Bony ankylosis and articular destruction commonly also occur if treatment is delayed or inadequate.

Ho G Jr: Bacterial arthritis. Curr Opin Rheumatol 2001;13:310. [PMID: 11555734]

GONOCOCCAL ARTHRITIS

ESSENTIALS OF DIAGNOSIS

- *Prodromal migratory polyarthralgias.*
- *Tenosynovitis most common sign.*
- *Purulent monarthritis in 50%.*
- *Characteristic skin rash.*
- *Most common in young women during menses or pregnancy.*
- *Symptoms of urethritis frequently absent.*
- *Dramatic response to antibiotics.*

General Considerations

In contrast to nongonococcal bacterial arthritis, gonococcal arthritis usually occurs in otherwise healthy individuals. Host factors, however, influence the expression of the disease: gonococcal arthritis is two to three times more common in women than in men, is especially common during menses and pregnancy, and is rare after age 40. Gonococcal arthritis is also common in male homosexuals, whose high incidence of asymptomatic gonococcal pharyngitis and proctitis predisposes them to disseminated gonococcal infection. Some of the signs of disseminated gonococcal infection may result from an immunologic reaction to nonviable fragments of the organism's cell wall; this may explain the frequent inability to culture organisms from skin and joint lesions. Recurrent disseminated gonococcal infection should prompt evaluation for a congenital deficiency of complement components, especially C7 and C8.

Clinical Findings

A. Symptoms and Signs

One to 4 days of migratory polyarthralgias involving the wrist, knee, ankle, or elbow is the most common initial course. Thereafter, two patterns emerge, one (60% of patients) characterized by tenosynovitis and the other (40%) by purulent monarthritis, most frequently involving the knee. Less than half of patients have fever, and less than one-fourth have any genitourinary symptoms. Most patients will have asymptomatic but highly characteristic skin lesions that usually consist of two to ten small necrotic pustules distributed over the extremities, especially the palms and soles.

B. Laboratory Findings

The peripheral blood leukocyte count averages about 10,000 cells/μL and is elevated in less than one-third of patients. The synovial fluid white blood cell count, however, is typically over 50,000 cells/μL. The synovial fluid Gram stain is positive in one-fourth of cases and culture in less than half. Positive blood cultures are seen in 40% of patients with tenosynovitis and virtually never in patients with suppurative arthritis. Urethral, throat, and rectal cultures should be done in all patients, since they are often positive in the absence of local symptoms. Culturing *Neisseria gonorrhoeae* is facilitated by rapid transport to the microbiology laboratory, inoculation on appropriate media, and incubation in carbon dioxide.

C. Imaging

Radiographs are usually normal or show only soft tissue swelling.

Differential Diagnosis

Reiter's syndrome can also produce acute monarthritis in a young person but is distinguished by negative cultures, sacroiliitis, and failure to respond to antibiotics. Lyme disease involving the knee is less acute, does not show positive cultures, and may be preceded by known tick exposure and characteristic rash. The synovial fluid analysis will exclude gout, pseudogout, and nongonococcal bacterial arthritis. Rheumatic fever and sarcoidosis can produce migratory tenosynovitis but have other distinguishing features. Infective endocarditis with septic arthritis can mimic disseminated gonococcal infection.

Treatment

In most cases, patients suspected of having gonococcal arthritis should be admitted to the hospital to confirm the diagnosis, to exclude endocarditis, and to start treatment. While outpatient treatment has been recommended in the past, the rapid rise in gonococci resistant to penicillin makes initial inpatient treatment advisable. Approximately 4–5% of all gonococcal isolates produce a β-lactamase that confers penicillin resistance. An additional 15–20% of gonococcal species have chromosomal mutations that result in relative resistance to penicillin. Therefore, the current recommendations for initial treatment of gonococcal arthritis are to give ceftriaxone, 1 g intravenously daily (or cefotaxime, 1 g intravenously every 8 hours; or ceftizoxime, 1 g intravenously every 8 hours; or spectinomycin, 2 g intramuscularly every 12 hours, for patients with beta-lactam allergy). Once improvement from parenteral antibiotics has been achieved for 24–48 hours, patients can be switched to oral cefixime, 400 mg orally twice daily, or ciprofloxacin, 500 mg orally twice daily, to complete a 7- to 10-day course.

Prognosis

Generally, gonococcal arthritis responds dramatically in 24–48 hours after initiation of antibiotics so that daily joint aspirations are rarely needed. Complete recovery is the rule.

RHEUMATIC MANIFESTATIONS OF HIV INFECTION

Infection with human immunodeficiency virus (HIV) has been associated with various rheumatic disorders, most commonly arthralgias or Reiter's syndrome. More rarely myositis, psoriatic arthritis, Sjögren's syndrome, or vasculitis occur (see Chapter 31). It is possible that these disorders stem directly from HIV infection itself or from the many other infections that occur in immunodeficient patients. The rheumatic syndromes may follow the diagnosis of AIDS or may precede it by several months. Thus, coexistent HIV infection must be considered in patients presenting with Reiter's syndrome. The lower extremity joints, especially the knees and ankles, are most commonly affected. Often, as in classic Reiter's syndrome,

Achilles tendon inflammation (enthesopathy) or knee periarthritis is a prominent and distinguishing feature. Many patients respond to NSAIDs, though a few are unresponsive and develop progressive deformities. Immunosuppressive agents must be employed with great caution in these patients.

Reveille JD: The changing spectrum of rheumatic disease in human immunodeficiency virus infection. Semin Arthritis Rheum 2000;30:147. [PMID: 1112428]

VIRAL ARTHRITIS

Arthritis may be a manifestation of many viral infections. It is generally mild and of short duration, terminating without lasting ill effects. Mumps arthritis may occur in the absence of parotitis. Rubella arthritis, which occurs more commonly in adults than in children, may appear immediately before, during, or soon after the disappearance of the rash. Its usual polyarticular and symmetric distribution mimics that of rheumatoid arthritis. However, the seronegative tests for rheumatoid factor and the rising rubella titers in convalescent serum help to confirm the diagnosis. Post-rubella vaccination arthritis may have its onset as long as 6 weeks following vaccination and occurs in all age groups. In adults, arthritis may follow infection with human parvovirus B19.

Transient polyarthritis may be associated with type B hepatitis and typically occurs before the onset of jaundice; it may occur in anicteric hepatitis as well. Urticaria or other types of skin rash may be present. Indeed, the clinical picture may be indistinguishable from that of serum sickness. Serum transaminase levels are elevated, and hepatitis B surface antigen is most often present. Serum complement levels are usually low during active arthritis and become normal after remission of arthritis. False-positive tests for rheumatoid factor, when present, disappear within several weeks. The arthritis is mild; it rarely lasts more than a few weeks and is self-limiting and without deformity. Hepatitis C infection may be associated with chronic polyarthralgia or polyarthritis that mimics rheumatoid arthritis.

Lovy MR: Rheumatic disorders associated with hepatitis C. Baillieres Best Pract Res Clin Rheumatol 2000;14:535. [PMID: 10985985]

■ INFECTIONS OF BONES

Direct microbial contamination of bones results from open fracture, surgical procedures, gunshot wounds, diagnostic needle aspirations, and therapeutic or self-administered drug injections.

Indirect or secondary infections are first noticed in other areas of the body and extend to bones by hematogenous routes.

ACUTE PYOGENIC OSTEOMYELITIS

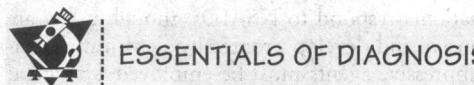

ESSENTIALS OF DIAGNOSIS

- *Fever and chills associated with pain and tenderness of involved bone.*
- *Aspiration of involved bone is usually diagnostic.*
- *Culture of blood or lesion tissue is essential for precise diagnosis.*
- *Radiographs early in the course are typically negative.*

General Considerations

Osteomyelitis is a serious infection that is often difficult to diagnose and treat. Infection of bone occurs as a consequence of (1) hematogenous dissemination of bacteria, (2) invasion from a contiguous focus of infection, and (3) skin breakdown in the setting of vascular insufficiency.

Clinical Findings

A. SYMPTOMS AND SIGNS

1. Hematogenous osteomyelitis—Osteomyelitis resulting from bacteremia is a disease associated with sickle cell disease, intravenous drug users, or the elderly. Patients with this form of osteomyelitis often present with sudden onset of high fever, chills, and pain and tenderness of the involved bone. The site of osteomyelitis and the causative organism depend on the host. Among patients with hemoglobinopathies such as sickle cell anemia, osteomyelitis is caused by salmonellae ten times as often as by other bacteria. Intravenous drug users develop osteomyelitis most commonly in the spine. Although in this setting *S aureus* is most common, gram-negative infections, especially *P aeruginosa* and serratia species, are also frequent pathogens. Rapid progression to epidural abscess causing fever, pain, and sensory and motor loss is not uncommon. In older patients with hematogenous osteomyelitis, the most common sites are the thoracic and lumbar vertebral bodies. Risk factors for these patients include diabetes, intravenous catheters, and indwelling urinary catheters. These patients often have more subtle presentations, with low-grade fever and gradually increasing bone pain.

2. Osteomyelitis from a contiguous focus of infection—Prosthetic joint replacement, decubitus ulcer, neurosurgery, and trauma most frequently cause soft tissue infections that can spread to bone. *S aureus* and *S epidermidis* are the most common organisms. Localized signs of inflammation are usually evident, but high fever and other signs of toxicity are usually absent.

3. Osteomyelitis associated with vascular insufficiency—Patients with diabetes and vascular insufficiency are susceptible to developing a very challenging form of osteomyelitis. The foot and ankle are the most commonly affected sites. Infection originates from an ulcer or other break in the skin that is usually still present when the patient presents but may appear disarmingly unimpressive. Bone pain is often absent or muted by the associated neuropathy. Fever is also commonly absent. One of the best bedside clues that the patient has osteomyelitis is the ability to easily advance a sterile probe through a skin ulcer to bone.

B. IMAGING AND LABORATORY FINDINGS

The plain film is the most readily available imaging procedure to establish the diagnosis of osteomyelitis, but it can be falsely negative early. Early radiographic findings may include soft tissue swelling, loss of tissue planes, and periarticular demineralization of bone. About 2 weeks after onset of symptoms, erosion of bone and alteration of cancellous bone appear, followed by periostitis.

MRI, CT, and nuclear medicine bone scanning are more sensitive than conventional radiography. MRI is believed to be the most sensitive and is particularly helpful in demonstrating the extent of soft tissue involvement. Radionuclide bone scanning is most valuable when osteomyelitis is suspected but no site is obvious.

Identifying the offending organism is a crucial step in selection of antibiotic therapy. Bone biopsy for culture is required except in those with hematogenous osteomyelitis, who have positive blood cultures. Cultures from overlying ulcers, wounds, or fistulas are unreliable.

Differential Diagnosis

Acute hematogenous osteomyelitis should be distinguished from suppurative arthritis, rheumatic fever, and cellulitis. More subacute forms must be differentiated from tuberculosis or mycotic infections of bone and Ewing's sarcoma or, in the case of vertebral osteomyelitis, from metastatic tumor. When osteomyelitis involves the vertebrae, it commonly traverses the disk—a finding not observed in tumor.

Complications

Inadequate treatment of bone infections results in chronicity of infection, and this possibility is increased by delaying diagnosis and treatment. Extension to adjacent bone or joints may complicate acute osteomyelitis. Recurrence of bone infections often results in anemia, a markedly elevated erythrocyte sedimentation rate, weight loss, weakness, and, rarely, amyloidosis or nephrotic syndrome. Pseudoepitheliomatous hyperplasia, squamous cell carcinoma, or fibrosarcoma may occasionally arise in persistently infected tissues.

Treatment

Most patients require both debridement of necrotic bone and prolonged administration of antibiotics. Patients with vertebral body osteomyelitis and epidural abscess require urgent neurosurgical decompression. Depending on the site and extent of debridement, surgical procedures to stabilize, fill in, cover, or revascularize may be needed. Traditionally, in adults, antibiotics have been administered parenterally for at least 4–6 weeks. Oral therapy with quinolones (eg, ciprofloxacin, 750 mg twice daily) for 6–8 weeks has been shown to be as effective as standard parenteral antibiotic therapy for chronic osteomyelitis in adults with susceptible organisms. When treating osteomyelitis caused by *S aureus,* quinolones are usually combined with rifampin, 300 mg twice daily.

Prognosis

If sterility of the lesion is achieved within 2–4 days, a good result can be expected in most cases if there is no compromise of the patient's immune system. However, progression of the disease to a chronic form may occur. It is especially common in the lower extremities and in patients in whom circulation is impaired (eg, diabetics).

Carek PJ et al: Diagnosis and management of osteomyelitis. Am Fam Physician 2001;63:2413. [PMID: 11430456]

Kothari NA et al: Imaging of musculoskeletal infections. Radiol Clin North Am 2001;39:653. [PMID: 11549164] (MRI is the study of choice for evaluation of the local extent of musculoskeletal infections).

MYCOTIC INFECTIONS OF BONES & JOINTS

Fungal infections of the skeletal system are usually secondary to a primary infection in another organ, frequently the lungs (see Chapter 36). Although skeletal lesions have a predilection for the cancellous portions of long bones and vertebral bodies, the predominant lesion—a granuloma with varying degrees of necrosis and abscess formation—does not produce a characteristic clinical picture.

Differentiation from other chronic focal infections depends upon culture studies of synovial fluid or tissue obtained from the local lesion. Serologic tests provide presumptive support of the diagnosis.

1. Candidiasis

Candidal osteomyelitis most commonly develops in debilitated, malnourished patients undergoing prolonged hospitalization for cancer, neutropenia, trauma, complicated abdominal surgical procedures, or intravenous drug use. Infected intravenous catheters frequently serve as a hematogenous source.

For susceptible candida species, fluconazole, 200 mg orally twice daily, is probably as effective as amphotericin B.

2. Coccidioidomycosis

Coccidioidomycosis of bones and joints is usually secondary to primary pulmonary infection. Arthralgia with periarticular swelling, especially in the knees and ankles, occurring as a nonspecific manifestation of systemic coccidioidomycosis, should be distinguished from actual bone or joint infection. Osseous lesions commonly occur in cancellous bone of the vertebrae or near the ends of long bones at tendinous insertions. These lesions are initially osteolytic and thus may mimic metastatic tumor or myeloma.

The precise diagnosis depends upon recovery of *Coccidioides immitis* from the lesion or histologic examination of tissue obtained by open biopsy. Rising titers of complement-fixing antibodies also provide evidence of the disseminated nature of the disease.

Itraconazole, 200 mg twice daily for 6–12 months, has become the treatment of choice for bone and joint coccidioidomycosis. Chronic infection is rarely cured with antifungal agents and may require operative excision of infected bone and soft tissue; amputation may be the only solution for stubbornly progressive infections. Immobilization of joints by plaster casts and avoidance of weight bearing provide benefit. Synovectomy, joint debridement, and arthrodesis are reserved for more advanced joint infections.

3. Histoplasmosis

Focal skeletal or joint involvement in histoplasmosis is rare and generally represents dissemination from a primary focus in the lungs. Skeletal lesions may be single or multiple and are not characteristic.

Muller RJ: A brief review of antifungal treatment for deep fungal infections. Oncology (Huntingt) 2001;15(11 Suppl 9):21. [PMID: 11757847]

Rogers TR: Optimal use of existing and new antifungal drugs. Curr Opin Crit Care 2001;7:238. [PMID: 11571420] (Some of the new liposomal amphotericin preparations may have less renal toxicity. Evidence for this is controversial.)

TUBERCULOSIS OF BONES & JOINTS

ESSENTIALS OF DIAGNOSIS

- *A disease of children, the elderly, or those with HIV infection.*
- *In most cases, a single site of bone or joint is infected.*
- *Spine—especially lower thoracic—or knee most common sites.*
- *Chest x-ray abnormal in less than half.*

General Considerations

Most tuberculous infections in the USA are caused by the human strain of *Mycobacterium tuberculosis* (see Chapter 9). Infection of the musculoskeletal system is caused by hematogenous spread from a primary lesion of the respiratory tract; it may occur shortly after primary infection or may be seen years later as a disease reactivation. Tuberculosis of the thoracic or lumbar spine (Pott's disease) usually occurs in the absence of extraspinal infection. It is a disease of children in developing nations and of the elderly in the United States. Tuberculosis of peripheral joints is almost always monarticular, with the knee the most common site. Extra-articular tuberculosis occurs in only 20%.

Clinical Findings

A. SYMPTOMS AND SIGNS

The onset of symptoms is generally insidious and not accompanied by general manifestations of fever, sweating, toxicity, or prostration. Pain may be mild at onset, is usually worse at night, and may be accompanied by stiffness. As the disease process progresses, limitation of joint motion becomes prominent because of muscle contractures and joint destruction. The knee is the most commonly involved peripheral joint. Symptoms of pulmonary tuberculosis may also be present.

Local findings during the early stages may be limited to tenderness, soft tissue swelling, joint effusion, and increase in skin temperature about the involved area. As the disease progresses without treatment, muscle atrophy and deformity become apparent. Abscess formation with spontaneous drainage externally leads to sinus formation. Progressive destruction of bone in the spine may cause a gibbus, especially in the thoracolumbar region.

B. LABORATORY FINDINGS

The precise diagnosis rests upon recovery of the acid-fast organism from joint fluid, pus, or tissue specimens. Biopsy of the bony lesion, synovium, or a regional lymph node may demonstrate the characteristic histopathologic picture of caseating necrosis and giant cells.

C. IMAGING

There is a latent period between the onset of symptoms and the initial positive radiographic finding. The earliest changes of tuberculous arthritis are those of soft tissue swelling and distention of the capsule by effusion. Subsequently, bone atrophy causes thinning of the trabecular pattern, narrowing of the cortex, and enlargement of the medullary canal. As joint disease progresses, destruction of cartilage, both in the spine and in peripheral joints, is manifested by narrowing of the joint cleft and focal erosion of the articular surface, especially at the margins. Where the lesion is limited to bone, especially in the cancellous portion of the metaphysis, radiography may demonstrate single or multilocular cysts surrounded by sclerotic bone. With spinal tuberculosis, CT scanning is helpful in demonstrating paraspinal soft tissue extensions of the infection (eg, psoas abscess, epidural extension).

Differential Diagnosis

Tuberculosis of the musculoskeletal system must be differentiated from all subacute and chronic infections, rheumatoid arthritis, gout, and, occasionally, osseous dysplasia. In the spine, metastatic tumor may be suggested.

Complications

Destruction of bones or joints may occur in a few weeks or months if adequate treatment is not provided. Deformity due to joint destruction, abscess formation with spread into adjacent soft tissues, and sinus formation are common. Paraplegia is the most serious complication of spinal tuberculosis. As healing of severe joint lesions takes place, spontaneous fibrous or bony ankylosis follows.

Treatment
(See also Chapter 33.)

A. GENERAL MEASURES

General care is especially important when prolonged recumbency is necessary; skillful nursing care must be provided.

B. CHEMOTHERAPY

Because of the rise of resistant organisms, the new recommendation for treating bony tuberculosis is to begin with four drugs: isoniazid, 300 mg/d; rifampin, 600 mg/d; pyrazinamide, 25 mg/kg/d; and ethambutol, 15 mg/kg/d. If the isolate is sensitive to isoniazid and rifampin, the ethambutol can be stopped, with the pyrazinamide maintained for 2 months. Isoniazid and rifampin are continued for a total of 6 months. Cure without need for surgical intervention may be effected in most cases, even with extensive disease.

C. SURGICAL MEASURES

In acute infections where synovitis is the predominant feature, treatment can be conservative, at least initially. Immobilization by splint or plaster, aspiration, and chemotherapy may suffice to control the infection. Synovectomy may be valuable for less acute hypertrophic lesions that involve tendon sheaths, bursae, or joints.

Turgut M: Spinal tuberculosis (Pott's disease): Its clinical presentation, surgical management, and outcome. A survey study on 694 patients. Neurosurg Rev 2001;24:8. [PMID: 11339471]

ARTHRITIS IN SARCOIDOSIS

The frequency of arthritis among patients with sarcoidosis is variously reported between 10% and 35%. It is usually acute in onset, but articular symptoms may appear insidiously and often antedate other manifestations of the disease. Knees and ankles are most commonly involved, but any joint may be affected. Distribution of joint involvement is usually polyarticular and symmetric. The arthritis is commonly self-limited, resolving after several weeks or months and rarely resulting in chronic arthritis, joint destruction, or significant deformity. Sarcoid arthropathy is often associated with erythema nodosum, but the diagnosis is contingent upon the demonstration of other extra-articular manifestations of sarcoidosis and, notably, biopsy evidence of noncaseating granulomas. In chronic arthritis, radiographs show typical changes in the bones of the extremities with intact cortex and cystic changes.

Treatment of arthritis in sarcoidosis is usually symptomatic and supportive. Colchicine may be of value. A short course of corticosteroids may be effective in patients with severe and progressive joint disease.

■ TUMORS & TUMOR-LIKE LESIONS OF BONE

 ESSENTIALS OF DIAGNOSIS

- Persistent pain, swelling, or tenderness of a skeletal part.
- Pathologic ("spontaneous") fractures.
- Suspicious areas of bony enlargement, deformity, radiodensity, or radiolucency on x-ray.
- Histologic evidence of bone neoplasm on biopsy specimen.

General Considerations

Primary tumors of bone are relatively uncommon in comparison with secondary or metastatic neoplasms. They are, however, of great clinical significance because some grow rapidly and metastasize widely.

Although tumors of bone have been categorized classically as primary or secondary, there is some disagreement about which tumors are primary to the skeleton. Tumors of mesenchymal origin that reflect skeletal tissues (eg, bone, cartilage, and connective tissue) and tumors developing in bones that are of hematopoietic, nerve, vascular, fat cell, and notochordal origin should be differentiated from secondary malignant tumors that involve bone by direct extension or hematogenous spread. Because of the great variety of bone tumors, it is difficult to establish a satisfactory simple classification of bone neoplasms.

Clinical Findings

Persistent skeletal pain and swelling, with or without limitation of motion of adjacent joints or spontaneous fracture, are indications for prompt clinical, radiographic, laboratory, and possibly biopsy examination. Radiographs may reveal the location and extent of the lesion and certain characteristics that may suggest the specific diagnosis. The so-called classic radiographic findings of certain tumors (eg, punched-out areas of the skull in multiple myeloma, "sun ray" appearance of osteogenic sarcoma, and "onion peel" effect of Ewing's sarcoma), although suggestive, are not pathognomonic. Even a bone tumor's histologic characteristics, considered in isolation, provide incomplete information about the nature of the disease. The age of the patient, the duration of complaints, the site of involvement and the number of bones involved, and the presence or absence of associated systemic disease—as well as the histologic characteristics—must all be considered for proper management.

The possibility of benign developmental skeletal abnormalities, metastatic neoplastic disease, infections (eg, osteomyelitis), posttraumatic bone lesions, or metabolic disease of bone must always be kept in mind. If bone tumors occur in or near the joints, they may be confused with the various types of arthritis, especially monarticular arthritis.

Specific Bone Tumors

Tumors arising from osteoblastic connective tissue include osteoid osteoma and osteosarcoma. Osteoid osteomas are benign tumors of children and adolescents that should be surgically removed. Osteosarcoma, the most common malignancy of bone, typically occurs in an adolescent who presents with pain or swelling in a bone or joint (especially in or around the knee). Since the symptoms often appear to begin following a sports-related injury, accurate diagnosis may be delayed. Osteosarcoma can also develop in patients with Paget's disease of bone, enchondromatosis, fibrous dysplasia, or hereditary multiple exostoses. Osteosarcomas are treated by resection and chemotherapy, with 5-year survival rates improving from 15% in 1965 to 60% at this time. Fibrosarcomas, which are derived from nonosteoblastic connective tissue, have a prognosis similar to that of the osteogenic sarcomas. Tumors derived from cartilage include enchondromas, chondromyxoid fibromas, and chondrosarcomas. Histologic examination is confirmatory in this group, and the prognosis with appropriate curettement or surgery is generally good.

Other bone tumors include giant cell tumors (osteoclastomas), chondroblastomas, and Ewing's sarcoma. Of these, chondroblastomas are almost always benign. About 50% of giant cell tumors are benign, while the rest may be frankly malignant or recur after excision. Ewing's sarcoma, which affects children, adolescents, and young adults, has a 50% mortality rate in spite of chemotherapy, irradiation, and surgery.

Treatment

Although prompt action is essential for optimal treatment of certain bone tumors, accurate diagnosis is required because of the great potential for harm that may result from temporization, radical or ablative operations, or unnecessary irradiation.

Arndt C et al: Common musculoskeletal tumors of childhood and adolescence. N Engl J Med 1999;341:342. [PMID: 10423470] (Review of rhabdomyosarcoma, osteosarcoma, and Ewing's sarcoma.)

NEUROGENIC ARTHROPATHY (Charcot's Joint)

Neurogenic arthropathy is joint destruction resulting from loss or diminution of proprioception, pain, and temperature perception. Although traditionally associated with tabes dorsalis, it is more frequently seen in diabetic neuropathy, syringomyelia, spinal cord injury, pernicious anemia, leprosy, and peripheral nerve injury. Prolonged administration of hydrocortisone by the intra-articular route may also cause Charcot's joint. As normal muscle tone and protective reflexes are lost, secondary degenerative joint disease ensues, resulting in an enlarged, boggy, painless joint with extensive cartilage erosion, osteophyte formation, and multiple loose joint bodies. Radiographic changes may be degenerative or hypertrophic in the same patient.

Treatment is directed against the primary disease; mechanical devices are used to assist in weight bearing and prevention of further trauma. In some instances, amputation becomes unavoidable.

Pinzur MS: Charcot's foot. Foot Ankle Clin 2000;5:897. [PMID: 11232475]

■ OTHER RHEUMATIC DISORDERS

RHEUMATIC MANIFESTATIONS OF CANCER

Rheumatologic syndromes may be the presenting manifestations for a variety of cancers. Dermatomyositis in adults, for example, is associated with cancer. Middle-aged or older patients with polyarthritis that mimics rheumatoid arthritis but is associated with new onset of clubbing and periosteal new bone formation should be suspected of having hypertrophic pulmonary osteoarthropathy, a disorder commonly associated with both malignant diseases (eg, lung and intrathoracic cancers) and nonmalignant ones (eg, cyanotic heart disease, cirrhosis, and lung abscess). Palmar fasciitis is characterized by bilateral palmar swelling and finger contraction and may be the first indication of cancer, particularly ovarian carcinoma. Palpable purpura due to leukocytoclastic vasculitis may be the presenting complaint in myeloproliferative disorders. Hairy cell leukemia can be associated with medium-sized vessel vasculitis such as polyarteritis nodosa. Acute leukemia can produce joint pains that are disproportionately severe in comparison to the minimal swelling and heat that are present. Leukemic arthritis complicates approximately 5% of cases. Rheumatic manifestations of myelodysplastic syndromes include cutaneous vasculitis, lupus-like syndromes, neuropathy, and episodic intense arthritis. Erythromelalgia, a painful warmth and redness of the extremities that (unlike Raynaud's) improves with cold exposure or with elevation of the extremity, is often associated with myeloproliferative diseases.

Abu-Shakra M et al: Cancer and autoimmunity: autoimmune and rheumatic features in patients with malignancies. Ann Rheum Dis 2001;60:433. [PMID: 11302861]

PALINDROMIC RHEUMATISM

Palindromic rheumatism is a disease of unknown cause characterized by frequent recurring attacks (at irregular intervals) of acutely inflamed joints. Periarticular pain with swelling and transient subcutaneous nodules may also occur. The attacks cease within several hours to several days. The knee and finger joints are most commonly affected, but any peripheral joint may be involved. Systemic manifestations other than fever do not occur. Although hundreds of attacks may take place over a period of years, there is no permanent articular damage. Laboratory findings are usually normal. Palindromic rheumatism must be distinguished from acute gouty arthritis and an atypical, acute onset of rheumatoid arthritis. In some patients, palindromic rheumatism is a prodrome of rheumatoid arthritis.

Symptomatic treatment with NSAIDs is usually all that is required during the attacks. Hydroxychloroquine may be of value in preventing recurrences.

AVASCULAR NECROSIS OF BONE

Avascular necrosis of bone is a complication of corticosteroid use, trauma, SLE, pancreatitis, alcoholism, gout, sickle cell disease, and infiltrative diseases (eg, Gaucher's disease). The most commonly affected sites are the proximal and distal femoral heads, leading to hip or knee pain. Many patients with hip disease actually first present with pain referred to the knee. Physical examination will reveal that it is internal rotation of the hip—not movement of the knee—that is painful. Other commonly affected sites include the ankle, shoulder, and elbow. Initially, radiographs are often normal; MRI, CT scan, and bone scan are all more sensitive techniques. Treatment involves avoidance of weight bearing on the affected joint for at least several weeks. The value of surgical core decompression is controversial. Unfortunately, the natural history of avascular necrosis is usually progression of the bony infarction to cortical collapse, resulting in significant joint dysfunction. Total hip replacement is the usual outcome for all patients who are candidates for that procedure.

Pavelka K: Osteonecrosis. Baillieres Best Pract Res Clin Rheumatol 2000;14:399. [PMID: 10925752]

■ SOME ORTHOPEDIC PROCEDURES FOR ARTHRITIC JOINTS

Synovectomy

This procedure attempts to eliminate inflammation at a joint by surgically removing as much of the synovium as possible. The procedure has been performed most commonly in patients with rheumatoid arthritis who, despite medical therapy, have a persistent pannus of inflamed synovium (usually around a wrist or a knee). Patients with degenerative diseases do not have marked synovial inflammation and are not candidates for this procedure.

Unfortunately, synovium can regrow. Even in patients with rheumatoid arthritis, the long-term benefits of synovectomy remain unproved.

Arthroplasty

Realigning arthritic joints (arthroplasty) generally does not work as well as complete joint replacement, but it can defer the need for joint replacement. The typical candidate is an adult under 50 years of age who has severe osteoarthritis of one compartment of the knee (typically the medial compartment). Excising a wedge of femur will realign the patient's knee so as to shift weight to the compartment with normal cartilage and thereby eliminate or reduce the patient's pain.

Tendon Rupture

This is a fairly common complication in rheumatoid arthritis and requires immediate orthopedic referral. The most common sites are the finger flexors and extensors, the patellar tendon, and the Achilles tendon.

Arthrodesis

Arthrodesis (fusion) is being used less now than formerly, but a chronically infected, painful joint may be an indication for this surgical procedure.

Total Joint Arthroplasty

In the last 3 decades, remarkable progress has been made in the replacement of severely damaged joints with prosthetic materials. Although many different joints can be replaced, the largest experience and greatest success have been with hip and knee replacement. Indication for total joint arthroplasty is severe pain (usually including pain at rest) accompanied by loss of function and severe destruction of the joint on x-ray. Age is also a consideration, as the durability of artificial joints beyond 10–15 years is limited with older surgical techniques and unproved with newer techniques. Thus, patients over 65 are less likely than younger ones to face the challenge of revision.

Whatever the patient's age, success of the replacement depends upon the amount of physical stress to which the prosthetic components are subjected. Vigorous impact activity, even with the most advanced biomaterials and design, will result in failure of the prosthesis with time. Revision operations are technically more difficult, and the results may not be as good as with the primary procedure. The patient, therefore, must understand the limitations of joint replacement and the consequences of unrestrained joint usage.

A. TOTAL HIP ARTHROPLASTY

Hip replacement was originally designed for use in patients over 65 years of age with severe osteoarthritis. In these patients—usually less active physically—the prosthesis not only functioned well but outlasted the patients. Severe arthritis that fails to respond to conservative measures remains the principal indication for hip arthroplasty. Hip arthroplasty may also be indicated in younger patients severely disabled by painful hip disease (eg, rheumatoid arthritis), since in such cases it can be assumed that stress on the prosthetic joint will not be great. Contraindications to the operation include active infection and neurotrophic joint disease. Obesity is a relative contraindication. Serious complications may occur in about 1% of patients and include thrombophlebitis, pulmonary embolization, infection, and dislocation of the joint. Extensive experience has now been accumulated, and the short-term results are highly successful in properly selected patients. The long-term success has been limited by loosening of the prosthesis, a complication seen in 30–50% of patients 10 years after replacement with "first generation" techniques. Although loosening and periprosthetic osteolysis were blamed on the cement, second-generation cementing techniques for prosthetic hips have proved more durable than cementless hips in one out of four cases.

B. TOTAL KNEE ARTHROPLASTY

The indications and contraindications for total knee arthroplasty are similar to those for hip arthroplasty. Results are slightly better in osteoarthritis patients than in those with rheumatoid arthritis. Complications are similar to those with hip arthroplasty. The failure rate of knee arthroplasty is slightly higher than that of hip arthroplasty.

Colwell CW Jr: Low molecular weight heparin prophylaxis in total knee arthroplasty: the answer. Clin Orthop 2001; 392:245. [PMID: 11716391] (The answer is, "Yes—use it!" Without prophylaxis, the rate of deep venous thromboses in these patients may be over 80%, with proximal extension in 20%.)

Huo MH et al: What's new in hip arthroplasty? J Bone Joint Surg Am 2001;83:1598. [PMID: 11679623] (The clinical efficacy and safety of total hip arthroplasty in older patients has been demonstrated provided that appropriate preoperative and perioperative medical support is provided.)

Fluid & Electrolyte Disorders

Masafumi Fukagawa, MD, PhD, Kiyoshi Kurokawa, MD, MACP, & Maxine A. Papadakis, MD

See www.current-med.com/ch21.html

APPROACH TO THE PATIENT

History & Physical Examination

Causes of changes in body fluid volume can usually be determined by the history and physical examination. **Volume overload** is manifested by an increase in weight and peripheral edema or ascites. Edema from local obstruction of venous return must be differentiated from systemic processes (congestive heart failure, cirrhosis, and nephrotic syndrome). A history of increased dietary sodium intake and use of medications that affect the renin-angiotensin system (angiotensin converting enzyme inhibitors, prostaglandin synthesis inhibitors, mineralocorticoids, calcium channel blockers) should be sought. **Volume depletion** is characterized by weight loss, excessive thirst, and dry mucous membranes. The term **dehydration,** pure water deficit, should be distinguished from volume depletion, in which both water and salt are lost. There may be resting tachycardia, orthostatic hypotension, or shock. Causes include vomiting or diarrhea, diuretic use, renal disease, diabetes mellitus or diabetes insipidus, inadequate oral intake associated with altered mental status, and excessive insensible losses from sweating or fever.

Further Evaluation

Treatment of fluid and electrolyte disorders is based on (1) assessment of total body water and its distribution, (2) serum electrolyte concentrations, (3) urine electrolyte concentrations, and (4) serum osmolality. Serial changes in body weight constitute the best way of knowing if there has been an acute change in body water balance.

A. BODY WATER

Table 21–1 shows the sex difference in total body water and the decrease in total body water that occurs with aging.

B. SERUM ELECTROLYTES

Table 21–2 shows the normal values for serum electrolytes.

C. EVALUATION OF URINE

Urinalysis provides information about underlying renal disorders. Samples also should be obtained for analysis of urine electrolyte abnormalities. An electrolyte concentration in urine is a useful indicator of renal handling of water and the electrolyte, ie, whether the kidney loses or preserves the electrolyte.

In addition to the total urine per day, a spot urine may be used. Simple concentration, or concentration per gram creatinine excretion, is usually sufficient for initial analysis. More precisely, fractional excretion is used. Fractional excretion (FE) of an electrolyte X is calculated using a random urine sample with simultaneously obtained serum samples for X and creatinine.

$$FEX(\%) = \frac{Urine\ X/Serum\ X}{Urine\ Cr/Serum\ Cr} \times 100$$

D. SERUM OSMOLALITY

Serum osmolality (normally 285–295 mosm/kg) can be calculated from the following formula:

$$Osmolality = 2\ (Na^+\ meq/L) + \frac{Glucose\ mg/dL}{18} + \frac{BUN\ mg/dL}{28}$$

(1 mosm of glucose equals 180 mg/L, and 1 mosm of urea nitrogen equals 28 mg/L.)

Solute concentration is usually expressed in terms of osmolality. The number of particles in solution (ie, osmolytes; either molecules or ions) determines the number of milliosmoles. Each particle has a unit value of 1, so if a substance ionizes, each ion contributes the same amount as a nonionizable molecule. More importantly, permeability of the particle across the cell membrane determines if it acts as a physiologically active osmolyte. Only impermeable particles contribute to tonicity, and it is tonicity, not osmolality, that stimulates both thirst and ADH release. Substances that easily permeate cell membranes (eg, urea, ethanol) are not

Table 21–1. Total body water (as percentage of body weight) in relation to age and sex.

Age	Male	Female
18–40	60%	50%
41–60	60–50%	50–40%
Over 60	50%	40%

effective osmolytes and therefore do not cause shifting of fluid in body fluid compartments. For example, glucose in solution is nonionizable. Therefore, 1 mmol of glucose has an osmole concentration of 1 mosm/kg H_2O. One millimole of NaCl, however, forms two ions in water (one Na^+ and one Cl^-) and has an osmole concentration of roughly 2 mosm/kg H_2O. "Osmoles per kilogram of water" is *osmolality;* "osmoles per liter of solution" is *osmolarity.* At the solute concentration of body fluids, the two measurements correspond so closely that they are interchangeable.

Clinical Implications

In many instances, electrolyte disorders are asymptomatic. However, patients may develop lethargy, weakness, confusion, delirium, and seizures, especially in the presence of an abnormal serum sodium concentration. Often these symptoms are mistaken for primary neurologic or metabolic disorders. Muscle weakness occurs in patients with severe hypokalemia, hyperkalemia, and hypophosphatemia; confusion, seizures, and coma may develop in those with severe hypercalcemia. Measurement of electrolytes (sodium, potassium, chloride, bicarbonate, calcium, magnesium, and phosphorus) is indicated for any patient with even vague neuromuscular symptoms.

Table 21–2. Normal values and mass conversion factors.[1]

	Normal Plasma Values	Mass Conversion
Na^+	135–145 meq/L	23 mg = 1 meq
K^+	3.5–5 meq/L	39 mg = 1 meq
Cl^-	98–107 meq/L	35 mg = 1 meq
HCO_3^-	22–28 meq/L	61 mg = 1 meq
Ca^{2+}	8.5–10.5 mg/dL	40 mg = 1 mmol
Phosphorus	2.5–4.5 mg/dL	31 mg = 1 mmol
Mg^{2+}	1.6–3 mg/dL	24 mg = 1 mmol
Osmolality	280–295 mosm/kg	...

[1]Modified and reproduced, with permission, from Cogan MG: *Fluid and Electrolytes: Physiology and Pathophysiology.* McGraw-Hill, 1991.

■ DISORDERS OF SODIUM CONCENTRATION

An abnormal serum sodium concentration does not necessarily imply abnormal sodium balance but rather abnormal water balance. Thus, most instances of abnormal sodium concentration are associated with abnormal serum osmolality. An abnormal sodium balance is often associated either with volume depletion or with edema formation.

HYPONATREMIA

Hyponatremia (defined as a serum sodium concentration less than 130 meq/L) is the most common electrolyte abnormality observed in a general hospitalized population, seen in about 2% of patients. The initial approach to its investigation is the determination of serum osmolality (Figure 21–1).

The Urine Sodium

Measurement of urine sodium helps distinguish renal from nonrenal causes of hyponatremia. Urine sodium exceeding 20 meq/L is consistent with renal salt wasting (diuretics, ACE inhibitors, mineralocorticoid deficiency, salt-losing nephropathy). Urine sodium less than 10 meq/L or fractional excretion of sodium less than 1% (unless diuretics have been given) implies avid sodium retention by the kidney to compensate for extrarenal fluid losses from vomiting, diarrhea, sweating, or third-spacing, as with ascites.

Isotonic Hyponatremia

In hyperlipidemia and hyperproteinemia, the marked increases in lipids (chylomicrons and triglycerides, but not cholesterol) and proteins (> 10 g/dL) occupy a disproportionately large portion of the plasma volume. Plasma osmolality remains normal because its measurement is unaffected by the lipids or proteins. A decreased volume of water results, so that the sodium concentration in total plasma volume is decreased. Because the sodium concentration in the plasma water is actually normal, hyperlipidemia and hyperproteinemia cause pseudohyponatremia. Most United States laboratories measure serum electrolytes using ion-specific electrodes and thus avoid misdiagnosis.

Hypotonic Hyponatremia

Hypotonic hyponatremia is true hyponatremia in a physiologic sense. Since the capacity of the kidney to excrete electrolyte-free water is potentially great—up to 20–30 L/d—in the presence of a normal GFR (100 L/d), electrolyte-free water intake must theoretically exceed 30 L/d for hyponatremia to develop.

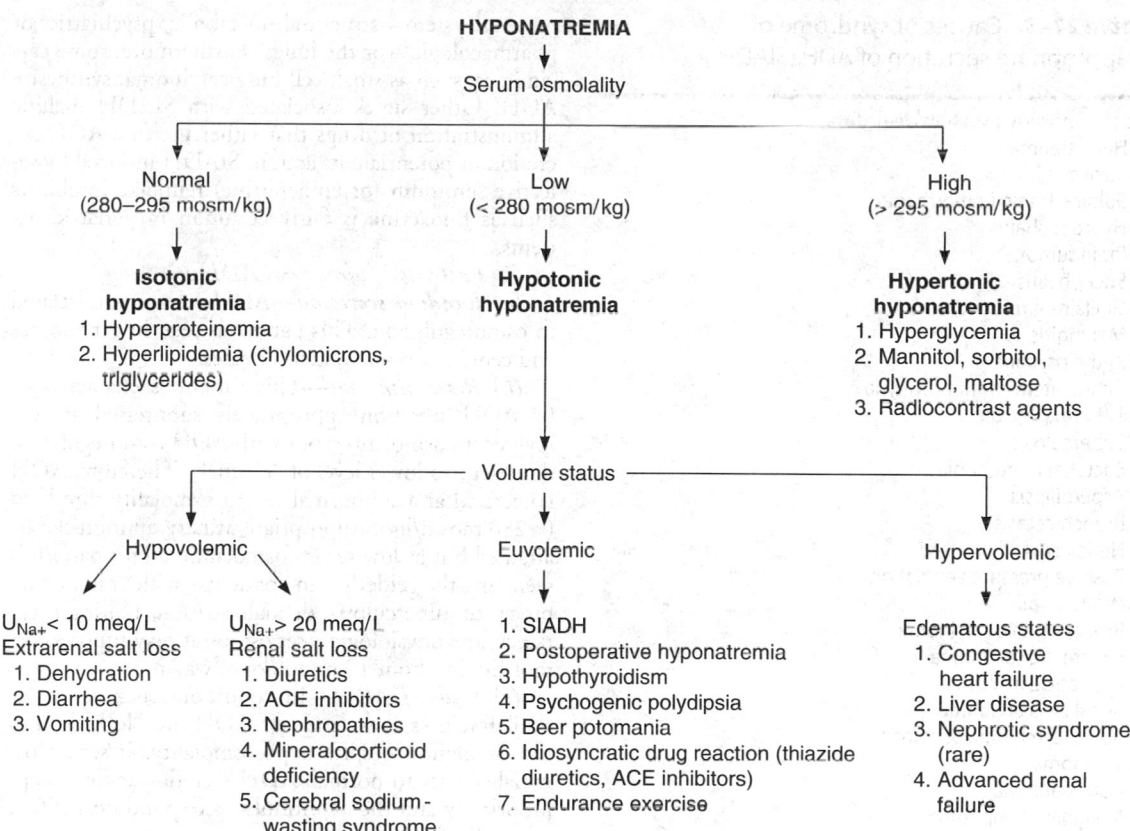

HYPONATREMIA

Serum osmolality

Normal
(280–295 mosm/kg)

Isotonic hyponatremia
1. Hyperproteinemia
2. Hyperlipidemia (chylomicrons, triglycerides)

Low
(< 280 mosm/kg)

Hypotonic hyponatremia

High
(> 295 mosm/kg)

Hypertonic hyponatremia
1. Hyperglycemia
2. Mannitol, sorbitol, glycerol, maltose
3. Radiocontrast agents

Volume status

Hypovolemic

U_{Na+}< 10 meq/L
Extrarenal salt loss
1. Dehydration
2. Diarrhea
3. Vomiting

U_{Na+}> 20 meq/L
Renal salt loss
1. Diuretics
2. ACE inhibitors
3. Nephropathies
4. Mineralocorticoid deficiency
5. Cerebral sodium - wasting syndrome

Euvolemic
1. SIADH
2. Postoperative hyponatremia
3. Hypothyroidism
4. Psychogenic polydipsia
5. Beer potomania
6. Idiosyncratic drug reaction (thiazide diuretics, ACE inhibitors)
7. Endurance exercise

Hypervolemic
Edematous states
1. Congestive heart failure
2. Liver disease
3. Nephrotic syndrome (rare)
4. Advanced renal failure

Figure 21–1. Evaluation of hyponatremia using serum osmolality and extracellular fluid volume status.

Instead, in hypotonic hyponatremia, retention of electrolyte-free water nearly always occurs because of impaired excretion (renal failure, inappropriate ADH excess, etc).

A. Hypovolemic Hypotonic Hyponatremia

Hyponatremia with decreased extracellular fluid volume occurs in the setting of renal or extrarenal volume loss (Figure 21–1). Total body sodium is decreased. To maintain intravascular volume, antidiuretic hormone (ADH) secretion increases, and free water is retained. The drive to replenish intravascular volume overrides the need to sustain normal osmolality; losses of salt and water are replaced by water alone. The combination of low fractional excretion of sodium (< 0.5%) and low fractional urea clearance (< 55%) is the best way to predict improvement with saline therapy. Hyponatremia has been shown to develop in patients with intracranial diseases through renal sodium wasting. Unlike those with SIADH, these patients are hypovolemic, though plasma levels of ADH are inappropriately high for the osmolality. Observations in patients with subarachnoid hemorrhage suggest that the cerebral salt-wasting syndrome is caused by increased secretion of brain natriuretic peptide with suppression of aldosterone secretion.

Treatment consists of replacement of lost volume with isotonic or half-normal (0.45%) saline or lactated Ringer's infusion. The rate of correction must be adjusted to prevent permanent cerebral damage (see below). Corticosteroids can be used empirically if hypocortisolism is considered in the differential diagnosis. See Adrenocortical Hypofunction in Chapter 26 for diagnosis (by means of the cosyntropin stimulation test) and treatment of hypocortisolism.

B. Euvolemic Hypotonic Hyponatremia

In this setting, determinations of urine osmolality (Figure 21–1) along with urine sodium are useful for appropriate diagnosis.

1. Clinical syndromes—

a. Syndrome of inappropriate ADH secretion (SIADH)—(Table 21–3.) Hypovolemia physiologically stimulates ADH secretion, so the diagnosis of SIADH is made only if the patient is euvolemic. In SIADH, increased ADH release occurs without osmolality-dependent or volume-dependent physiologic stimulation. Normal regulation of ADH release occurs from both the central nervous system and the chest via baroreceptors and neural input. It follows that the causes of SIADH are disorders affecting the central

Table 21–3. Causes of syndrome of inappropriate secretion of ADH (SIADH).

Central nervous system disorders
  Head trauma
  Stroke
  Subarachnoid hemorrhage
  Hydrocephalus
  Brain tumor
  Encephalitis
  Guillain-Barré syndrome
  Meningitis
  Acute psychosis
  Acute intermittent porphyria
Pulmonary lesions
  Tuberculosis
  Bacterial pneumonia
  Aspergillosis
  Bronchiectasis
  Neoplasms
  Positive pressure ventilation
Malignancies
  Bronchogenic carcinoma
  Pancreatic carcinoma
  Prostatic carcinoma
  Renal cell carcinoma
  Adenocarcinoma of colon
  Thymoma
  Osteosarcoma
  Malignant lymphoma
  Leukemia
Drugs
  Increased ADH production
    Antidepressants: tricyclics, monoamine oxidase
      inhibitors, SSRIs
    Antineoplastics: cyclophosphamide, vincristine
    Carbamazepine
    Methylenedioxymethamphetamine (MDMA; Ecstasy)
    Clofibrate
    Neuroleptics: thiothixene, thioridazine, fluphenazine,
      haloperidol, trifluoperazine
  Potentiated ADH action
    Carbamazepine
    Chlorpropamide, tolbutamide
    Cyclophosphamide
    NSAIDs
    Somatostatin and analogs
Others
  Postoperative
  Pain
  Stress
  AIDS
  Pregnancy (physiologic)
  Hypokalemia

nervous system—structural, metabolic, psychiatric, or pharmacologic—or the lungs. Furthermore, some carcinomas, such as small cell lung carcinoma, synthesize ADH. Other states associated with SIADH include administration of drugs that either increase ADH secretion or potentiate its action. SIADH induced by selective serotonin (or epinephrine) reuptake inhibitors such as fluoxetine is fairly common in geriatric patients.

(1) Patterns of abnormal ADH secretion—

*(a) Random secretion—*ADH release is unrelated to osmoregulation. This pattern is seen in carcinomas and central nervous system diseases.

*(b) Reset osmostat—*This variant is characterized by ADH secretion appropriately suppressed at very low serum osmolalities but with ADH osmoregulation downset to a lower level of "normal." Therefore, ADH is secreted at a subnormal serum osmolality threshold (< 280 mosm/kg). Appropriate urinary dilution can be attained but at low serum osmolalities. This pattern is seen in the elderly, in patients with pulmonary processes, tuberculosis, or malnutrition. During pregnancy, the physiologic reset osmostat may suppress osmolality by about 10 mmol/kg of water.

*(c) Leak of ADH—*In conditions such as basilar skull fractures, low levels of ADH are "leaked" into the circulation despite hypo-osmolality. If serum osmolality rises to normal, ADH secretion increases appropriately and then continues to respond normally if osmolality further increases.

*(2) Clinical features—*SIADH is characterized by (1) hyponatremia; (2) decreased osmolality (< 280 mosm/kg) with inappropriately increased urine osmolality (> 150 mosm/kg); (3) absence of cardiac, renal, or liver disease; (4) normal thyroid and adrenal function (see Chapter 26 for thyroid function tests and cosyntropin stimulation test); and (5) urine sodium usually over 20 meq/L. Natriuresis compensates for the slight increase in volume from ADH secretion. The mechanisms that regulate sodium excretion in response to increases in extracellular volume, such as suppression of the sympathetic nervous and renin-angiotensin systems and increased secretion of atrial natriuretic factor, are preserved and account for the increase in urinary sodium. The expansion of extracellular volume is not large enough to cause clinical hypervolemia, hypertension, or edema. Other changes frequently seen in SIADH include low blood urea nitrogen (BUN) (< 10 mg/dL) and hypouricemia (< 4 mg/dL), which are not only dilutional but result from increased urea and uric acid clearances in response to the volume-expanded state. A high BUN suggests a volume-contracted state, which excludes a diagnosis of SIADH.

b. Postoperative hyponatremia—Severe postoperative hyponatremia can develop in 2 days or less after elective surgery in healthy patients, especially premenopausal women. Most have received excessive postoperative hypotonic fluid in the setting of elevated

ADH levels related to pain of surgery with continuing excretion of hypertonic urine. Similar mechanisms have been suspected for hyponatremia after colonoscopy. Patients awake normally from general anesthesia but within 2 days develop nausea, headache, seizures, and even respiratory arrest. Serum sodium levels may be less than 110 meq/L. Premenopausal women who develop hyponatremic encephalopathy are about 25 times more likely than menopausal women to die or to suffer permanent brain damage, suggesting a hormonal role in the pathophysiology of this disorder. Hyponatremia may also result from direct absorption of hypotonic irrigating fluids through veins during endometrial ablation or transurethral prostate resection. These patients can be symptomatic intraoperatively, with tremulousness, hypothermia, or hypoxia, or upon awakening from anesthesia, with headache, nausea, and vomiting.

c. Hypothyroidism—Hyponatremia is not commonly caused by hypothyroidism, but it can occur on occasion with serum sodium levels as low as 105 meq/L. Water retention is the cause, probably both from inappropriately elevated ADH levels and from nonhormonal alterations in the handling of water by the kidneys.

d. Psychogenic polydipsia and beer potomania—Marked excess free water intake (generally > 10 L/d) may produce hyponatremia. Euvolemia is maintained through the renal excretion of sodium. Urine sodium is therefore generally elevated (> 20 meq/L), but unlike SIADH, levels of ADH are suppressed. Urine osmolality is appropriately low (< 300 mosm/kg) as the increased free water is excreted. Hyponatremia from bursts of ADH occurs in manic-depressive patients with excess free water intake. Psychogenic polydipsia is observed in patients with psychologic problems, and these patients frequently take drugs interfering with water excretion. Similarly, excessive intake of beer, which contains very small amounts of sodium (< 5 meq/L), can cause severe hyponatremia in cirrhotic patients, who have elevated ADH and often decreased GFR.

e. Idiosyncratic diuretic reaction—In addition to hyponatremia developing from volume contraction due to diuretic therapy (see above), a less common diuretic-induced hyponatremia can occur in euvolemic patients, typically from thiazides. This syndrome is most often seen in healthy older women (over 70 years of age) often after a few days of therapy. The mechanism for the hyponatremia appears to be a combination of excessive renal sodium loss and water retention.

f. Idiosyncratic ACE inhibitor reactions—ACE inhibitors can cause central polydipsia and increased antidiuretic hormone secretion, both of which result in severe, symptomatic hyponatremia. Patients given ACE inhibitors who develop polydipsia should have their serum Na+ levels checked.

g. Endurance exercise hyponatremia—Hyponatremia after endurance exercise (eg, triathlon events) may be caused by a combination of excessive fluid overload and continued ADH secretion. Reperfusion of the exercise-induced ischemic splanchnic bed causes delayed absorption of excessive quantities of hypotonic fluid ingested during exercise. Sustained elevation of ADH prevents water excretion in this setting. The retention of hypotonic fluid may be further exacerbated by NSAIDs frequently used by athletes.

2. Treatment—

a. Symptomatic hyponatremia—Symptomatic hyponatremia is usually seen in patients with serum sodium levels less than 120 meq/L. If there are central nervous system symptoms, hyponatremia should be rapidly treated at any level of serum sodium concentration.

(1) Rate and degree of correction—Central pontine myelinolysis may occur from osmotically induced demyelination due to overly rapid correction of serum sodium (an increase of more than 1 meq/L/h, or 25 meq/L within the first day of therapy). Hypoxic-anoxic episodes during hyponatremia may contribute to the demyelination. A reasonable approach is to increase the serum sodium concentration by no more than 1–2 meq/L/h and not more than 25–30 meq/L in the first 2 days; the rate should be reduced to 0.5–1 meq/L/h as soon as neurologic symptoms improve. The initial goal is to achieve a serum sodium concentration of 125–130 meq/L, guarding against overcorrection.

(2) Saline plus furosemide—Hypertonic (eg, 3%) saline with furosemide is indicated for symptomatic hyponatremic patients. If one administers 3% saline without a diuretic to a patient with SIADH, the serum sodium concentration increases temporarily, but euvolemic patients excrete the excess sodium. If one adds furosemide (0.5–1 mg/kg intravenously), however, the kidney cannot concentrate urine even in the presence of high levels of ADH. Infusion of 3% saline is accompanied by excretion of isotonic urine with a net loss of free water. The sodium concentration of 3% saline is 513 meq/L. In order to determine how much 3% saline to administer, a spot urinary Na+ is determined after a furosemide diuresis has begun. The excreted Na+ is replaced with 3% saline, empirically begun at 1–2 mL/kg/h and then adjusted based on urinary output and urinary sodium. For example, after administration of furosemide, urine volume may be 400 mL/h and sodium plus potassium excretion 100 meq/L. The excreted Na+ plus K+ is 40 meq/h, which is replaced with 78 mL/h of 3% saline (40 meq/h divided by 513 meq/L). Free water loss is about 1% of total body water. Therefore, an approximately 1% rise in plasma sodium concentration (1–1.5 meq/L/h) can be expected. Measurements of plasma sodium should be done approximately every 4 hours and the patient observed closely.

b. Asymptomatic hyponatremia—In asymptomatic hyponatremia, the correction rate of hyponatremia need be no more than 0.5 meq/L/h. No specific treatment is needed for patients with reset osmostats.

(1) Water restriction—Water intake should be restricted to 0.5–1 L/d. Gradual increase of serum sodium will occur over days.

(2) 0.9% saline—0.9% saline with furosemide may be used in asymptomatic patients whose serum sodium is less than 120 meq/L. Urinary sodium and potassium losses are replaced as above.

(3) Demeclocycline—Demeclocycline (300–600 mg twice daily) is useful for patients who cannot adhere to water restriction or need additional therapy; it inhibits the effect of ADH on the distal tubule. Onset of action may require 1 week, and concentrating may be permanently impaired. Therapy with demeclocycline in cirrhosis appears to increase the risk of renal failure.

(4) Fludrocortisone—Hyponatremia occurring as part of the cerebral salt-wasting syndrome can be treated with fludrocortisone.

(5) Selective vasopressin V2 antagonist—The renal effect of ADH on water excretion is mediated by the V2 receptor. Oral selective V2 antagonists have been in clinical trials and may be available for treatment of SIADH in the near future.

C. HYPERVOLEMIC HYPOTONIC HYPONATREMIA

Hyponatremia with increased extracellular fluid volume is seen when hyponatremia is accompanied by edema-associated disorders such as congestive heart failure, cirrhosis, nephrotic syndrome, and advanced renal disease (Figure 21–1). In congestive heart failure, total body sodium is increased, yet effective circulating volume is sensed as inadequate by baroreceptors. Increased ADH and aldosterone results, with retention of water and sodium.

The **urine sodium** concentration is generally less than 10 meq/L unless the patient has been taking diuretics.

Treatment

A. WATER RESTRICTION

The treatment of hyponatremia is that of the underlying condition (eg, improving cardiac output in congestive heart failure) and water restriction (to < 1–2 L of water daily).

B. DIURETICS

To hasten excretion of water and salt, use of diuretics may be indicated. Since diuretics may worsen hyponatremia, the patient must be cautioned not to increase free water intake.

C. HYPERTONIC (3%) SALINE

Hypertonic saline administration is dangerous in volume-overloaded states and is not routinely recommended. In patients with severe hyponatremia (serum sodium < 110 meq/L) and central nervous system symptoms, judicious administration of small amounts (100–200 mL) of 3% saline with diuretics may be necessary. Emergency dialysis should also be considered.

Hypertonic Hyponatremia

Hypertonic hyponatremia is most commonly seen with hyperglycemia. When blood glucose becomes acutely elevated, water is drawn from the cells to the extracellular space, diluting the serum sodium. The plasma sodium level falls 1.6 meq/L for every 100 mg/dL rise when the glucose concentration is between 200 and 400 mg/dL. If the glucose concentration is above 400 mg/dL, the plasma sodium concentration falls 4 meq/L for every 100 mg/dL rise in glucose. This dilutional hyponatremia is not pseudohyponatremia, since the sodium concentration does indeed fall. Infusion of hypertonic solutions containing osmotically active osmoles (eg, mannitol) may also cause hypertonic hyponatremia by drawing water to the extracellular space.

Hyponatremia in AIDS

Hyponatremia is seen in up to 50% of patients hospitalized for AIDS and in 20% of ambulatory AIDS patients, often associated with pneumonia and central nervous system processes. If hyponatremia is present at the time of hospital admission, it is just as likely to be due to hypovolemic gastrointestinal loss as to euvolemic SIADH. However, if hyponatremia develops after hospital admission, most patients have euvolemic SIADH. Infrequently, hypovolemic hyponatremia is due to adrenal insufficiency, isolated mineralocorticoid deficiency with hyporeninemic hypoaldosteronism, or an HIV-specific impairment in renal sodium conservation. Hyponatremia from adrenal insufficiency may coexist with hypokalemia—rather than hyperkalemia—if the patient also has diarrhea. Adrenal function can be tested with corticotropin stimulation to determine the adequacy of serum cortisol response (see Chapter 26). Patients with isolated hyporeninemic hypoaldosteronism have normal cortisol responses to corticotropin but have decreased serum aldosterone levels.

Adrogue HJ et al: Hyponatremia. N Engl J Med 2000;342:1581. [PMID: 10824078]

Bouman WP et al: Incidence of selective serotonin reuptake inhibitor (SSRI) induced hyponatremia due to the syndrome of inappropriate antidiuretic hormone (SIADH) secretion in the elderly. Int J Geriatr Psychiatry 1998;13:12. [PMID: 9489575]

Cadnapaphornchai MA et al: Pathogenesis and management of hyponatremia. Am J Med 2000;109:688. [PMID: 11099692]

Gross P: Correction of hyponatremia. Semin Nephrol 2001;21:269. [PMID: 11320492]

Hillier TA et al: Hyponatremia: Evaluating the correction factor for hyperglycemia. Am J Med 1999;106:399. [PMID: 10225241]

Kumar S et al: Sodium. Lancet 1998;352:220. [PMID: 9683227] (Up-to-date review of the pathogenesis of and practical treatment recommendations for sodium imbalance.)

Oster JR et al: Hyponatremia, hyposmolality, and hypotonicity: tables and fables. Arch Intern Med 1999;159:333. [PMID: 10030305] (An insightful review of the interpretation of hyponatremia.)

Palmer BF: Hyponatraemia in a neurosurgical patient: syndrome of inappropriate antidiuretic hormone secretion versus cerebral salt wasting. Nephrol Dial Transplant 2000;15:262. [PMID: 10648680]

Thaler SM et al: "Beer potomania" in non-beer drinkers: effect of low dietary solute intake. Am J Kidney Dis 1998;31:1028. [PMID: 9631849] (Low solute intake as a cause of free water excretion defect.)

HYPERNATREMIA

An intact thirst mechanism usually prevents hypernatremia (> 145 meq/L). Thus, whatever the underlying disorder (eg, dehydration, lactulose or mannitol therapy, central and nephrogenic diabetes insipidus), excess water loss can cause hypernatremia only when adequate water intake is not possible, as with unconscious patients.

Rarely, excessive sodium intake may cause hypernatremia. Hypernatremia in primary aldosteronism is mild and usually does not cause symptoms. Hypernatremia in the presence of salt and water overload is uncommon but has been reported in very ill patients in the course of therapy.

Clinical Findings

A. SYMPTOMS AND SIGNS

When dehydration exists, orthostatic hypotension and oliguria are typical findings. Hyperthermia, delirium, and coma may be seen with severe hyperosmolality.

B. LABORATORY FINDINGS

1. Urine osmolality > 400 mosm/kg—Renal water-conserving ability is functioning.

a. Nonrenal losses—Hypernatremia will develop if water ingestion fails to keep up with hypotonic losses from excessive sweating, exertional losses from the respiratory tract, or through stool water. Lactulose causes an osmotic diarrhea with loss of free water.

b. Renal losses—While diabetic hyperglycemia can cause pseudohyponatremia (see above), progressive volume depletion from the osmotic diuresis of glycosuria can result in true hypernatremia. Osmotic diuresis can occur with the use of mannitol or urea.

2. Urine osmolality < 250 mosm/kg—A dilute urine with osmolality less than 250 mosm/kg with hypernatremia is characteristic of central and nephrogenic diabetes insipidus. Nephrogenic diabetes insipidus, seen with lithium or demeclocycline therapy, after relief of prolonged urinary tract obstruction, or with interstitial nephritis, results from renal insensitivity to ADH. Hypercalcemia and hypokalemia may be contributing factors when present.

Treatment

Treatment of hypernatremia is directed toward correcting the cause of the fluid loss and replacing water and, as needed, electrolytes. In response to increases in plasma osmolality, brain cells synthesize solutes—or idiogenic osmoles—which increase osmotic flow of water back into the brain cells to regulate their volume. This begins 4–6 hours after dehydration and takes several days to reach a steady state. If hypernatremia is too rapidly corrected, the osmotic imbalance may cause water to preferentially enter brain cells, causing cerebral edema and potentially severe neurologic impairment. Fluid therapy should be administered over a 48-hour period, aiming for a decrease in serum sodium of 1 meq/L/h (1 mmol/L/h). Potassium and phosphate may be added as indicated by serum levels; other electrolytes are also monitored frequently.

A. CHOICE OF TYPE OF FLUID FOR REPLACEMENT

1. Hypernatremia with hypovolemia—Severe hypovolemia should be treated with isotonic (0.9%) saline to restore the volume deficit and to treat the hyperosmolality, since the osmolality of isotonic saline (308 mosm/kg) is often lower than that of the plasma. This should be followed by 0.45% saline to replace any remaining free water deficit. Milder volume deficit may be treated with 0.45% saline and 5% dextrose in water.

2. Hypernatremia with euvolemia—Water drinking or 5% dextrose and water intravenously will result in excretion of excess sodium in the urine. If GFR is decreased, diuretics will increase urinary sodium excretion but may impair renal concentrating ability, increasing the quantity of water that needs to be replaced.

3. Hypernatremia with hypervolemia—Treatment consists of providing water as 5% dextrose in water to reduce hyperosmolality, but this will expand vascular volume. Thus, loop diuretics such as furosemide (0.5–1 mg/kg) should be administered intravenously to remove the excess sodium. In severe renal insufficiency, hemodialysis may be necessary.

B. CALCULATION OF WATER DEFICIT

When calculating fluid replacement, both the deficit and the maintenance requirements should be added to each 24-hour replacement regimen.

1. Acute hypernatremia—In acute dehydration without much solute loss, free water loss is similar to the weight loss. Initially, 5% dextrose in water may be employed. As correction of water deficit progresses, therapy should continue with 0.45% saline with dextrose.

2. Chronic hypernatremia—Water deficit is calculated to restore normal osmolality for total body water. Total body water (TBW) (Table 21–1) correlates with muscle mass and therefore decreases with advancing age, cachexia, and dehydration and is lower in women than in men. Current TBW equals 0.4–0.6 of current body weight.

$$\frac{\text{Volume (in L)}}{\text{to be replaced}} = \text{Current TBW} \times \frac{[Na^+] - 140}{140}$$

Adrogue HJ et al: Hypernatremia. N Engl J Med 2000;342:1493. [PMID: 10816188]

Kahn T: Hypernatremia with edema. Arch Intern Med 1999; 159:93. [PMID: 9892337]

Kugler JP et al: Hyponatremia and hypernatremia in the elderly. Am Fam Physician 2000;61:3623. [PMID: 10892634]

■ DISORDERS OF POTASSIUM CONCENTRATION

HYPOKALEMIA

The total potassium content of the body is 50 meq/kg, more than 95% of which is intracellular. The plasma potassium concentration is maintained in a narrow range through two main regulating mechanisms: potassium shift between intracellular and extracellular compartments and modulation of renal potassium excretion. A deficit of 4–5 meq/kg occurs for each 1 meq/L decrement in serum potassium concentration below a level of 4 meq/L.

Clinical Findings

A. SYMPTOMS AND SIGNS

Muscular weakness, fatigue, and muscle cramps are frequent complaints in mild to moderate hypokalemia. Smooth muscle involvement may result in constipation or ileus. Flaccid paralysis, hyporeflexia, hypercapnia, tetany, and rhabdomyolysis may be seen with severe hypokalemia (< 2.5 meq/L).

B. LABORATORY FINDINGS

The ECG shows decreased amplitude and broadening of T waves, prominent U waves, premature ventricular contractions, and depressed ST segments. Hypokalemia also increases the likelihood of digitalis toxicity. Thus, in patients with heart disease, hypokalemia induced by certain drugs such as β_2-adrenergic agonists and diuretics may impose a substantial risk.

Pathophysiology & Diagnosis

Hypokalemia can occur as a result of shifting of potassium intracellularly from the extracellular space, extrarenal potassium loss (or insufficient potassium intake), or renal potassium loss (Table 21–4). Potassium uptake by the cell is stimulated by insulin in the presence of glucose. It is also facilitated by adrenergic beta-stimulation, whereas adrenergic alpha-stimulation blocks it. All of these effects are transient. Self-limited

Table 21–4. Causes of hypokalemia.

Decreased potassium intake
Potassium shift into the cell
  Increased postprandial secretion of insulin
  Alkalosis
  Trauma (via beta-adrenergic stimulation?)
  Periodic paralysis (hypokalemic)
Renal potassium loss
  Increased aldosterone (mineralocorticoid) effects
    Primary hyper-aldosteronism
    Secondary aldosteronism (dehydration, heart failure)
    Renovascular hypertension
    Malignant hypertension
    Ectopic ACTH-producing tumor
    Bartter's syndrome
    Cushing's syndrome
    Licorice (European)
    Renin-producing tumor
    Congenital abnormality of steroid metabolism (eg, adrenogenital syndrome, 17α-hydroxylase defect, apparent mineralocorticoid excess)
  Increased flow of distal nephron
    Diuretics (furosemide, thiazides)
    Salt-losing nephropathy
  Hypomagnesemia
    Unreabsorbable anion
    Carbenicillin, penicillin
  Renal tubular acidosis (type I or II)
    Fanconi's syndrome
    Interstitial nephritis
    Metabolic alkalosis (bicarbonaturia)
  Congenital defect of distal nephron
    Liddle's syndrome
Extrarenal potassium loss
  Vomiting, diarrhea, laxative abuse
  Villous adenoma, Zollinger-Ellison syndrome

hypokalemia occurs in 50–60% of trauma patients, perhaps related to enhanced release of epinephrine. Profound hypokalemia due to barium intoxication has been reported that may also be the result of transport of potassium into cells.

Aldosterone, which facilitates urinary potassium excretion through enhanced potassium secretion at the distal renal tubules, is the most important regulator of body potassium content. Urinary potassium concentration is low (< 20 meq/L) as a result of extrarenal fluid loss (eg, diarrhea, vomiting) and inappropriately high (> 40 meq/L) with urinary losses (eg, mineralocorticoid excess, Bartter's syndrome, Liddle's syndrome). Various genetic mutations that affect fluid and electrolyte metabolism, including disorders of potassium metabolism, have been reported recently (Table 21–5). Licorice-induced hypokalemia results from inhibition of 11β-hydroxysteroid dehydrogenase, which inactivates cortisol. Cortisol thus escapes degradation, binds to aldosterone receptors, and exerts aldosterone-like effects.

Table 21–5. Genetic disorders associated with electrolyte metabolism disturbances.

Disease	Site of Mutation
Potassium	
Hypokalemia	
Hypokalemic periodic paralysis	Dihydropyridine-sensitive skeletal muscle voltage-gated calcium channel
Bartter's syndrome	Na-K-2Cl cotransporter, K$^+$ channel (ROMK), or Cl$^-$ channel of thick ascending limb of Henle (hypofunction)
Liddle's syndrome	β or γ subunit of amiloride-sensitive Na$^+$ channel (hyperfunction)
Apparent mineralocorticoid excess	11β-Hydroxysteroid dehydrogenase (failure to inactivate cortisol)
Glucocorticoid-remediable hyperaldosteronism	Regulatory sequence of 11β-hydroxylase controls aldosterone synthase inappropriately
Hyperkalemia	
Hyperkalemic periodic paralysis	α subunit of calcium channel
Pseudohypoaldosteronism type I	β or γ subunit of amiloride-sensitive Na$^+$ channel (hypofunction)
Calcium	
Familial hypocalciuric hypercalcemia	Ca^{2+}-sensing protein (hypofunction)
Familial hypocalcemia	Ca^{2+}-sensing protein (hyperfunction)
Phosphate	
Hypophosphatemic rickets	*PEX* gene
Water	
X-linked (type I) nephrogenic diabetes insipidus	Vasopressin receptor

Recently, the transtubular K$^+$ concentration gradient (TTKG) has been used for simple and rapid reevaluation of net potassium secretion. TTKG is calculated as follows:

$$TTKG = \frac{Urine\ K^+ / Plasma\ K^+}{Urine\ osm / Plasma\ osm}$$

Hypokalemia with a TTKG > 4 suggests renal potassium loss with increased distal K$^+$ secretion. In such cases, plasma renin and aldosterone levels are helpful in differential diagnosis. The presence of nonabsorbed anions, including bicarbonate, also increases TTKG.

Treatment

The safest way to treat mild to moderate deficiency is with oral potassium, and all potassium formulations are easily absorbed. Dietary potassium is almost entirely coupled to phosphate—rather than chloride—and is therefore not effective in correcting potassium loss associated with chloride depletion, such as from diuretics or vomiting. In the setting of abnormal renal function and mild to moderate diuretic dosage, 20 meq/d of oral potassium is generally sufficient to prevent hypokalemia, but 40–100 meq/d over a period of days to weeks is needed to treat hypokalemia and fully replete potassium stores.

Intravenous potassium replacement is indicated for patients with severe hypokalemia and for those who cannot take oral supplementation. For severe deficiency, potassium may be given through a peripheral intravenous line in a concentration that should not exceed 40 meq/L at rates of up to 40 meq/L/h. Continuous electrocardiographic monitoring is indicated, and the serum potassium level should be checked every 3–6 hours.

Magnesium is an important cofactor for potassium uptake and for maintenance of intracellular potassium levels. Loop diuretics (eg, furosemide) cause substantial renal potassium and magnesium losses. Coexisting magnesium and potassium depletion can result in refractory hypokalemia despite potassium repletion if there is no magnesium repletion.

Cohn JN et al: New guidelines for potassium replacement in clinical practice. Arch Intern Med 2000;160:2429. [PMID: 10979053]

Gennari FJ: Hypokalemia. N Engl J Med 1998;339:451. [PMID: 9700180] (Comprehensive review.)

Halperin ML et al: Potassium. Lancet 1998;352:135. [PMID: 9672294] (Pathophysiologic review of potassium disorders.)

Rastegar A et al: Hypokalaemia and hyperkalaemia. Postgrad Med J 2001;77:759. [PMID: 11723313]

Scheinmann SJ et al: Genetic disorders of renal electrolyte transport. N Engl J Med 1999;340:1177. [PMID: 10202170] (A comprehensive review of the molecular pathogenesis of several genetic disorders, including Bartter's syndrome and Liddle's syndrome.)

Stewart OM: Mineralocorticoid hypertension. Lancet 1999;353:1341. [PMID: 10218547]

HYPERKALEMIA

Many cases of hyperkalemia are spurious or associated with acidosis (Table 21–6). The common practice of repeatedly clenching and unclenching a fist during venipuncture may raise the potassium concentration by 1–2 meq/L by causing acidosis and consequent potassium loss from cells.

Intracellular potassium shifts to the extracellular fluid in hyperkalemia associated with acidosis. Serum

Table 21–6. Causes of hyperkalemia.

Spurious
  Leakage from erythrocytes when separation of serum
    from clot is delayed (plasma K⁺ normal)
  Marked thrombocytosis or leukocytosis with release of K⁺
    (plasma K⁺ normal)
  Repeated fist clenching during phlebotomy, with release
    of K⁺ from forearm muscles
  Specimen drawn from arm with K⁺ infusion
Decreased excretion
  Renal failure, acute and chronic
  Renal secretory defects (may or may not have frank renal
    failure): renal transplant, interstitial nephritis, systemic
    lupus erythematosus, sickle cell disease, amyloidosis,
    obstructive uropathy
  Hyporeninemic hypoaldosteronism (often in diabetic
    patients with mild to moderate nephropathy) or selec-
    tive hypoaldosteronism (some patients with AIDS)
  Heparin (regardless of molecular size; suppresses
    aldosterone secretion)
  Drugs that inhibit potassium excretion (spironolactone,
    triamterene, ACE inhibitors, trimethoprim, NSAIDs, cy-
    closporine, tacrolimus)
Shift of K⁺ from within the cell
  Massive release of intracellular K⁺ in burns, rhabdomyoly-
    sis, hemolysis, severe infection, internal bleeding,
    vigorous exercise
  Metabolic acidosis (in the case of organic acid
    accumulation—eg, lactic acidosis—a shift of K⁺ does
    not occur since organic acid can easily move across the
    cell membrane)
  Hypertonicity (solvent drag)
  Insulin deficiency (metabolic acidosis may not be
    apparent)
  Hyperkalemic periodic paralysis
  Drugs: succinylcholine, arginine, digitalis toxicity, beta-
    adrenergic antagonists
  Alpha-adrenergic stimulation?
Excessive intake of K⁺

potassium concentration rises about 0.7 meq/L for every decrease of 0.1 pH unit during acidosis. Potassium movement out of cells occurs primarily in metabolic acidosis due to the accumulation of minerals such as NH_4Cl or HCl. The inability of the chloride anion to permeate the cell membrane results in the transcellular exchange of H⁺ for K⁺. Metabolic acidosis from organic acids (keto acids and lactic acid) does not induce hyperkalemia. Unlike the minerals, these organic acids easily permeate cell membranes and retard Na^+-K^+ ATPase. The hyperkalemia frequently observed in diabetic ketoacidosis is not due to the acidosis but to a combination of the hyperosmolality (the intracellular K⁺ concentration of the dehydrated cell increases and K⁺ diffuses extracellularly) and deficiencies of insulin, catecholamines, and aldosterone. In the absence of acidosis, serum potassium concentration

rises about 1 meq/L when there is a total body potassium excess of 1–4 meq/kg. However, the higher the serum potassium concentration, the smaller the excess necessary to raise the potassium levels further.

Trimethoprim is structurally related to amiloride and triamterene, and all three drugs inhibit renal potassium excretion through suppression of sodium channels in the distal nephron. Serum potassium levels rise progressively over 4–5 days in patients treated with standard or high-dose trimethoprim (combined with sulfamethoxazole or dapsone), especially if there is concurrent renal insufficiency. Over half of inpatients taking this drug have potassium levels over 5 meq/L, and 20% have marked hyperkalemia (> 5.5 meq/L). The potassium concentration returns to baseline after drug discontinuation.

In addition, it is of note that immunosuppressive drugs such as cyclosporine and tacrolimus can induce hyperkalemia in organ transplant recipients—and especially in kidney transplant patients. This is partly due to the suppression of basolateral Na^+-K^+ ATPase in principal cells.

Hyperkalemia is commonly seen in patients with AIDS and has been attributed to impaired renal excretion of potassium due to the use of pentamidine or trimethoprim-sulfamethoxazole or to hyporeninemic hypoaldosteronism. An abnormality in the redistribution between the intracellular and extracellular compartments may also play a role.

Clinical Findings

An elevated K⁺ concentration interferes with normal neuromuscular function to produce muscle weakness and, rarely, flaccid paralysis; abdominal distention and diarrhea may occur. Electrocardiography is not a sensitive method for detecting hyperkalemia, since nearly half of patients with a serum potassium level greater than 6.5 meq/L will not manifest electrocardiographic changes. Electrocardiographic changes in hyperkalemia include peaked T waves of increased amplitude, widening of the QRS, and biphasic QRS–T complexes. Inhibition of atrial depolarization despite normal conduction through usual pathways may occur. This sinoventricular rhythm resembles a junctional mechanism and occurs because of greater sensitivity of atrial myocytes to hyperkalemia than is the case for ventricular muscle cells. The heart rate may be slow; ventricular fibrillation and cardiac arrest are terminal events.

Treatment
(Table 21–7)

One first confirms that the elevated level of serum K⁺ is genuine. Potassium concentration can be measured in plasma rather than in serum to avoid leakage of potassium out of cells into the serum of the blood

Table 21–7. Treatment of hyperkalemia.[1]

EMERGENCY					
Modality	**Mechanism of Action**	**Onset**	**Duration**	**Prescription**	**K⁺ Removed From Body**
Calcium	Antagonizes cardiac conduction abnormalities	0–5 minutes	1 hour	Calcium gluconate 10%, 5–30 mL IV; or calcium chloride 5%, 5–30 mL IV	0
Bicarbonate	Distributes K⁺ into cells	15–30 minutes	1–2 hours	$NaHCO_3$, 44–88 meq (1–2 ampules) IV	0
Insulin	Distributes K⁺ into cells	15–60 minutes	4–6 hours	Regular insulin, 5–10 units IV, plus glucose 50%, 25 g (1 ampule) IV	0
Albuterol	Distributes K⁺ into cells	15–30 minutes	2–4 hours	Nebulized albuterol, 10–20 mg in 4 mL normal saline, inhaled over 10 minutes	0

NONEMERGENCY				
Modality	**Mechanism of Action**	**Duration of Treatment**	**Prescription**	**K⁺ Removed From Body**
Loop diuretic	↑ Renal K⁺ excretion	0.5–2 hours	Furosemide, 40–160 mg IV or orally with or without $NaHCO_3$, 0.5–3 meq/kg daily	Variable
Sodium polystyrene sulfonate (Kayexalate)	Ion exchange resin binds K⁺	1–3 hours	Oral: 15–30 g in 20% sorbitol (50–100 mL) Rectal: 50 g in 20% sorbitol	0.5–1 meq/g
Hemodialysis	Extracorporeal K⁺ removal	48 hours	Blood flow ≥ 200–300 mL/min. Dialysate [K⁺] ~ 0	200–300 meq
Peritoneal dialysis	Peritoneal K⁺ removal	48 hours	Fast exchange, 3–4 L/h	200–300 meq

[1]Modified and reproduced, with permission, from Cogan MG: *Fluid and Electrolytes: Physiology and Pathophysiology.* McGraw-Hill, 1991.

sample in the course of clotting, which may be observed in thrombocytosis.

Treatment consists of withholding potassium and giving cation exchange resins by mouth or enema. Sodium polystyrene sulfonate, 40–80 g/d in divided doses, is usually effective. Emergent treatment of hyperkalemia is indicated if cardiac toxicity or muscular paralysis is present or if the hyperkalemia is severe (serum potassium > 6.5–7 meq/L) even in the absence of electrocardiographic changes. Insulin plus 10–50% glucose (5–10 g of glucose per unit of insulin) may be employed to deposit K⁺ with glycogen in the liver. Calcium may be given intravenously as an antagonist ion—but not when digoxin toxicity is suspected, since calcium may augment the deleterious effects of digoxin on the heart. Transcellular shifts of potassium can also be mediated by β_2-adrenergic stimulation. Albuterol, a nebulized β_2 agonist, is effective in decreasing serum potassium in patients on hemodialysis. For such patients, one or two standard doses of nebulized albuterol can reduce serum K⁺ 0.5–1 meq/L within 30 minutes after administration, and this effect is sustained for at least 2 hours. Albuterol and insulin are probably equally efficacious in lowering potassium in uremic patients, and the hypokalemic effects of coadministration of the two drugs (with glucose) are additive and appear not to constitute a hazard. Sodium bicarbonate can be given intravenously as an emergency measure in severe hyperkalemia; the increase in blood pH results in a shift of K⁺ into cells. Hemodialysis or peritoneal dialysis may be required to remove K⁺ in the presence of protracted renal insufficiency. Therapy of the precipitating event proceeds concurrently.

Caramelo C et al: Hyperkalemia in patients infected with the human immunodeficiency virus: involvement of a systemic mechanism. Kidney Int 1999;56:198. [PMID: 10411693]

Charytan D et al: Indications for hospitalization of patients with hyperkalemia. Arch Intern Med 2000;160:1605. [PMID: 10847253]

Perazella MA: Drug-induced hyperkalemia: Old culprits and new offenders. Am J Med 2000;109:307. [PMID: 10996582]

Reardon LC et al: Hyperkalemia in outpatients using angiotensin-converting enzyme inhibitors. How much should we worry? Arch Intern Med 1998;158:26. [PMID: 9437375] (Serious hyperkalemia is uncommon in ACE-treated patients under 70 who have normal renal function.)

Schepkens H et al: Life-threatening hyperkalemia during combined therapy with angiotensin-converting enzyme inhibitors and spironolactone: An analysis of 25 cases. Am J Med 2001;110:438. [PMID: 11331054]

■ DISORDERS OF CALCIUM CONCENTRATION

Calcium constitutes about 2% of body weight, but only about 1% of the total body calcium is in solution in body fluid. In the plasma, only 50% of calcium is present as ionized calcium; the remainder forms a complex with protein—mostly albumin (40%)—or anions, including citrate, bicarbonate, and phosphate (10%). The normal total plasma (or serum) calcium concentration is 9–10.3 mg/dL. It is ionized calcium (normal: 4.7–5.3 mg/dL) which, under physiologic regulation, is necessary for muscle contraction and nerve function. Calcium-sensing protein, a receptor-like protein with the special function of detecting extracellular calcium ion concentrations, has been identified in parathyroid cells and in the kidney. Some diseases (eg, familial hypocalcemia and familial hypocalciuric hypercalcemia) associated with disturbed calcium metabolism are due to functional defects of this protein (Table 21–5).

HYPOCALCEMIA

Development of hypocalcemia implies insufficient action of PTH or active vitamin D. Important causes of hypocalcemia are listed in Table 21–8.

Table 21–8. Causes of hypocalcemia.

Decreased intake or absorption
  Malabsorption
  Small bowel bypass, short bowel
  Vitamin D deficit (decreased absorption, decreased production of 25-hydroxyvitamin D or 1,25-dihydroxy vitamin D)
Increased loss
  Alcoholism
  Chronic renal insufficiency
  Diuretic therapy
Endocrine disease
  Hypoparathyroidism (genetic, acquired; including hypo- and hypermagnesemia)
  Sepsis
  Pseudohypoparathyroidism
  Calcitonin secretion with medullary carcinoma of the thyroid
  Familial hypocalcemia
Physiologic causes
  Associated with decreased serum albumin[1]
  Decreased end-organ response to vitamin D
  Hyperphosphatemia
  Induced by aminoglycoside antibiotics, plicamycin, loop diuretics, foscarnet

[1]Calcium ion concentration is normal.

The most common cause of hypocalcemia is renal failure, in which decreased production of active vitamin D_3 and hyperphosphatemia both play a role. (See Chapter 22.) Some cases of primary hypoparathyroidism are due to mutation of calcium-sensing protein in which inappropriate suppression of PTH release leads to hypocalcemia. Hypocalcemia in pancreatitis is also a marker for severe disease (see Chapter 15).

Clinical Findings

A. SYMPTOMS AND SIGNS

Hypocalcemia increases excitation of nerve and muscle cells, primarily affecting the neuromuscular and cardiovascular systems. Extensive spasm of skeletal muscle causes cramps and tetany. Laryngospasm with stridor can obstruct the airway. Convulsions can occur as well as paresthesias of lips and extremities and abdominal pain. Chvostek's sign (contraction of the facial muscle in response to tapping the facial nerve anterior to the ear) and Trousseau's sign (carpal spasm occurring after occlusion of the brachial artery with a blood pressure cuff for 3 minutes) are usually readily elicited. Prolongation of the QT interval (due to lengthened ST segment) predisposes to the development of ventricular arrhythmias. In chronic hypoparathyroidism, cataracts and calcification of basal ganglia of the brain may appear. (See Hypoparathyroidism, Chapter 26.)

B. LABORATORY FINDINGS

Serum Ca^{2+} is low (< 9 mg/dL). The depressed level of serum Ca^{2+} must be correlated with the simultaneous concentration of serum albumin: When albumin is low, serum Ca^{2+} concentration is depressed in a ratio of 0.8–1 mg of Ca^{2+} to 1 g of albumin. Serum phosphate is usually elevated in hypoparathyroidism or end-stage renal failure, whereas it is suppressed in early stage renal failure or vitamin D deficiency. Serum Mg^{2+} is commonly low, and hypomagnesemia reduces both parathyroid hormone release and tissue responsiveness to parathyroid hormone, causing hypocalcemia. In respiratory alkalosis, total serum calcium is normal but ionized calcium is low. The ECG shows a prolonged QT interval.

Treatment*

A. SEVERE, SYMPTOMATIC HYPOCALCEMIA

In the presence of tetany, arrhythmias, or seizures, calcium gluconate 10% (10–20 mL) administered intravenously over 10–15 minutes is indicated. Because of the short duration of action, calcium infusion is usually required. Ten to 15 milligrams of calcium per kilogram body weight, or six to eight 10-mL vials of 10% calcium gluconate (558–744 mg of calcium), is added to 1 L of D_5W and infused over 4–6 hours. By monitoring the serum calcium level frequently (every 4–6 hours), the infusion rate is adjusted to maintain the serum calcium level at 7–8.5 mg/dL.

B. ASYMPTOMATIC HYPOCALCEMIA

Oral calcium (1–2 g) and vitamin D preparations (Table 26–10) are used. Calcium carbonate is well tolerated and less expensive than many other calcium tablets. The low serum Ca^{2+} associated with low serum albumin concentration does not require replacement therapy. If serum Mg^{2+} is low, therapy must include replacement of magnesium, which by itself usually will correct hypocalcemia.

Bushinsky DA et al: Calcium. Lancet 1998;352:306. [PMID: 9690425] (Pathophysiology, differential diagnosis, and treatment of hypocalcemia and hypercalcemia.)

HYPERCALCEMIA

Important causes of hypercalcemia are listed in Table 21–9. Primary hyperparathyroidism is the most common cause of hypercalcemia in ambulatory patients. Tumor production of PTH-related protein is the commonest paraneoplastic endocrine syndrome, accounting for most cases of hypercalcemia in inpatients. The neoplasm is clinically apparent in nearly all cases when the hypercalcemia is detected, and the prognosis is poor. Chronic hypercalcemia (over 6

*See also Chapter 26 for discussion of the treatment of hypoparathyroidism.

Table 21–9. Causes of hypercalcemia.

Increased Intake or absorption
Milk-alkali syndrome
Vitamin D or vitamin A excess
Endocrine disorders
Primary hyperparathyroidism (adenoma, hyperplasia, carcinoma)
Secondary hyperparathyroidism (renal insufficiency, malabsorption)
Acromegaly
Adrenal insufficiency
Neoplastic diseases
Tumors producing PTH-related proteins (ovary, kidney, lung)
Multiple myeloma (elaboration of osteoclast-activating factor)
Miscellaneous causes
Thiazide diuretic-induced
Sarcoidosis
Paget's disease of bone
Hypophosphatasia
Immobilization
Familial hypocalciuric hypercalcemia
Complications of renal transplantation
Iatrogenic

months) or some manifestation such as nephrolithiasis suggests a benign cause. Primary hyperparathyroidism and malignancy account for 90% of all cases of hypercalcemia.

Milk-alkali syndrome, which had become rare with the advent of nonabsorbable antacid therapy for ulcer disease, should be considered as a cause of hypercalcemia with the current popularity of calcium ingestion for osteoporosis prevention. In the milk-alkali syndrome, massive calcium and vitamin D ingestion can cause hypercalcemic nephropathy. Because of the decreased GFR, retention of the alkali in the calcium antacid occurs and causes metabolic alkalosis, which can be worsened by the vomiting associated with this disorder.

Hypercalcemia also causes nephrogenic diabetes insipidus. Development of polyuria is mediated through activation of calcium-sensing receptors in collecting ducts. Volume depletion further worsens hypercalcemia.

Clinical Findings

A. SYMPTOMS AND SIGNS

Symptoms of hypercalcemia irrespective of cause are constipation and polyuria. The focus of the history and physical examination should be on the duration of the process of hypercalcemia and evidence for a neoplasm. Symptoms usually occur if the serum calcium is above 12 mg/dL and tend to be more severe if hypercalcemia develops acutely.

Interestingly, polyuria is absent in hypercalcemia in familial hypocalciuric hypercalcemia, in which function of calcium-sensing protein is altered in the kidney as well. A variety of neurologic symptoms also are observed. Stupor, coma, and azotemia may develop in severe hypercalcemia. Ventricular extrasystoles and idioventricular rhythm occur and can be accentuated by digitalis.

B. LABORATORY FINDINGS

A significant elevation of serum Ca^{2+} is seen; the level must be interpreted in relation to the serum albumin level (see Hypocalcemia). The highest serum calcium levels (> 15 mg/dL) generally occur in malignancy. More than 200 mg/d of urinary calcium excretion suggests hypercalciuria; less than 100 mg/d, hypocalciuria. Hypercalciuric patients—such as those with malignancy or those receiving oral active vitamin D therapy—may easily develop hypercalcemia in case of volume depletion. Serum phosphate may or may not be low, depending on the cause.

The ECG shows a shortened QT interval. Measurements of PTH and PTH-related protein (PTHrP) help distinguish between malignancy-associated hypercalcemia (elevated PTHrP) and hyperparathyroidism (elevated PTH).

Treatment

Until the primary disease can be brought under control, renal excretion of calcium with resultant decrease in serum Ca^{2+} concentration is promoted. Excretion of Na^+ is accompanied by excretion of Ca^{2+}.

The tendency in hypercalcemia is toward volume depletion from nephrogenic diabetes insipidus. Therefore, establishing euvolemia and inducing natriuresis by giving saline with furosemide is the emergency treatment of choice. In dehydrated patients with normal cardiac and renal function, 0.45% saline or 0.9% saline can be given rapidly (250–500 mL/h). Intravenous furosemide (20–40 mg every 2 hours) prevents volume overload and enhances Ca^{2+} excretion. Thiazides can actually worsen hypercalcemia (as can furosemide if inadequate saline is given). In the treatment of hypercalcemia of malignancy, bisphosphonates are safe and effective in more than 95% of patients and are the mainstay of treatment. In emergency cases, dialysis with low or no calcium dialysate may be needed. See Chapter 40 for a discussion of the treatment of hypercalcemia of malignancy and Chapter 26 for a discussion of the treatment of hypercalcemia of hyperparathyroidism.

Body JJ: Current and future directions in medical therapy: hypercalcemia. Cancer 2000;88(12 Suppl):3054. [PMID: 10898351]

Strewler GL: The physiology of a parathyroid hormone-related protein. N Engl J Med 2000;342:177. [PMID: 10639544] (An updated review on the action of PTHrP.)

Ziegler R: Hypercalcemic crisis. J Am Soc Nephrol 2001;17:S39. [PMID: 11251025]

■ DISORDERS OF PHOSPHORUS CONCENTRATION

Phosphate is important in the body as a constituent of bone and is crucial in cellular energy transfer and metabolism. Phosphate occupies 1% of body weight, and 80% of it is combined with calcium in bones and teeth. Only 10% is incorporated into a variety of organic compounds, and 10% is combined with proteins, lipids, carbohydrates, and other compounds in muscle and blood. Organic phosphate is the principal intracellular anion. In plasma, phosphate is mainly present as inorganic phosphate, and this fraction is very small (< 0.2% of total phosphate). However, body phosphate metabolism is regulated through plasma inorganic phosphate. Important determinants of plasma inorganic phosphate concentration are its intestinal absorption, renal excretion, and shift between the intracellular and extracellular spaces. Intestinal absorption of phosphate is facilitated by active vitamin D. Parathyroid hormone stimulates phosphate release from bone and suppresses proximal tubular reabsorption of phosphate, leading to hypophosphatemia and to bone phosphate store depletion if hypersecretion continues. Renal proximal tubular reabsorption of phosphate is decreased by volume expansion, glucocorticoid administration, and proximal tubular dysfunction, such as occurs in Fanconi's syndrome due to myeloma or other diseases. Growth hormone, on the other hand, augments proximal tubular reabsorption of phosphate. Recently, additional phosphaturic hormones such as fibroblast growth factor 23 have been identified.

Cellular phosphate uptake is stimulated by various factors and conditions, including alkalemia, insulin, epinephrine, feeding, hungry bone syndrome, and accelerated cell proliferation.

Phosphorus metabolism and homeostasis are intimately related to calcium metabolism. See sections on metabolic bone disease in Chapter 26.

HYPOPHOSPHATEMIA

Hypophosphatemia may occur in the presence of normal phosphate stores. Serious depletion of body phosphate stores may exist with low, normal, or high concentrations of phosphorus in serum. Leading causes of hypophosphatemia are listed in Table 21–10.

In the presence of severe hypophosphatemia (1 mg/dL or less), affinity of hemoglobin for oxygen is increased through a decrease in the erythrocyte 2,3-diphosphoglycerate concentration. This impairs tissue

Table 21–10. Causes of hypophosphatemia.

Diminished supply or absorption
  Starvation
  Parenteral alimentation with inadequate phosphate
    content
  Malabsorption syndrome, small bowel bypass
  Absorption blocked by oral aluminum hydroxide or
    bicarbonate
  Vitamin D-deficient and vitamin D-resistant osteomalacia
Increased loss
  Phosphaturic drugs: theophylline, diuretics,
    bronchodilators, corticosteroids
  Hyperparathyroidism (primary or secondary)
  Hyperthyroidism
  Renal tubular defects permitting excessive phosphaturia
    (congenital, induced by monoclonal gammopathy,
    heavy metal poisoning), alcoholism
  Hypokalemic nephropathy
  Inadequately controlled diabetes mellitus
  Hypophosphatemic rickets
  Oncogenic osteomalacia
Intracellular shift of phosphorus
  Administration of glucose
  Anabolic steroids, estrogen, oral contraceptives, beta-
    adrenergic agonists, xanthine derivatives
  Respiratory alkalosis
  Salicylate poisoning
Electrolyte abnormalities
  Hypercalcemia
  Hypomagnesemia
  Metabolic alkalosis
Abnormal losses followed by inadequate repletion
  Diabetes mellitus with acidosis, particularly during
    aggressive therapy
  Recovery from starvation or prolonged catabolic state
  Chronic alcoholism, particularly during restoration of
    nutrition; associated with hypomagnesemia
  Recovery from severe burns

oxygenation and thus cell metabolism, which underlies the effects of hypophosphatemia such as muscle weakness or even rhabdomyolysis.

Severe hypophosphatemia is common and multifactorial in alcoholic patients. In acute alcohol withdrawal, increased plasma insulin and epinephrine along with respiratory alkalosis promote intracellular shift of phosphate. Vomiting, diarrhea, and poor dietary intake contribute to hypophosphatemia. Chronic alcohol use results in a decrease in the renal threshold of phosphate excretion. This renal tubular dysfunction reverses after a month of abstinence. Patients with chronic obstructive pulmonary disease and asthma commonly have hypophosphatemia, attributed to xanthine derivatives causing shifts of phosphate intracellularly and the phosphaturic effects of beta-adrenergic agonists, loop diuretics, xanthine derivatives, and corticosteroids.

Hypophosphatemia is a potent stimulator of 1α-hydroxylation of vitamin D in the kidney to form active vitamin D. However, in oncogenic osteomalacia, which accompanies various mesenchymal tumors, activation of vitamin D is suppressed in spite of hypophosphatemia. This suppression may be due to overproduction of phosphatonin, a poorly understood factor that stimulates phosphaturia.

Clinical Findings

A. SYMPTOMS AND SIGNS

Acute, severe hypophosphatemia (0.1–0.2 mg/dL) can lead to acute hemolytic anemia with increased erythrocyte fragility, increased susceptibility to infection from impaired chemotaxis of leukocytes, and platelet dysfunction with petechial hemorrhages. Rhabdomyolysis, encephalopathy (irritability, confusion, dysarthria, seizures, and coma), and heart failure are uncommon but serious manifestations.

Chronic severe depletion may be manifested by anorexia, pain in muscles and bones, and fractures.

B. LABORATORY FINDINGS

In addition to hypophosphatemia, evidence of anemia due to hemolysis may be present (eg, elevated serum lactate dehydrogenase). Rhabdomyolysis results in elevated serum creatine kinase (which contains mostly the MM fraction but also some MB fraction) and, in many cases, myoglobin in the urine. Other values vary according to the cause. Renal glycosuria and hypouricemia together with hypophosphatemia indicate Fanconi's syndrome. In chronic depletion, radiographs and biopsies of bones show changes resembling those of osteomalacia.

Treatment

Treatment is best directed toward prophylaxis by including phosphate in repletion and maintenance fluids. A rapid decline in calcium levels can occur with parenteral administration of phosphate; therefore, when possible, oral replacement of phosphate is preferable. For parenteral alimentation, 620 mg (20 mmol) of phosphorus is required for every 1000 nonprotein kcal to maintain phosphate balance and to ensure anabolic function. A daily ration for prolonged parenteral fluid maintenance is 620–1240 mg (20–40 mmol) of phosphorus. For asymptomatic hypophosphatemia (serum phosphorus 0.7–1 mg/dL), an infusion should provide 279–310 mg (9–10 mmol)/12 h until the serum phosphorus exceeds 1 mg/dL. Since the response to phosphate supplementation is not predictable, frequent monitoring of plasma and urine phosphate is necessary. A magnesium deficit often coexists and should be treated simultaneously. In administering phosphate-containing solutions, serum creatinine and calcium must be monitored to guard against hypocalcemia.

For oral use, phosphate salts are available in skim milk (approximately 1 g [33 mmol]/L). Tablets or capsules of mixtures of sodium and potassium phosphate may be given to provide 0.5–1 g (18–32 mmol) per day.

Contraindications to therapy with phosphate salts include hypoparathyroidism, renal insufficiency, tissue damage and necrosis, and hypercalcemia. When hyperglycemia due to any cause is treated, phosphate accompanies glucose into cells, and hypophosphatemia may ensue.

Barak V et al: Prevalence of hypophosphatemia in sepsis and infection: The role of cytokines. Am J Med 1998;104:40. [PMID: 9528718] (Hypophosphatemia observed in sepsis may be related to overproduction of cytokines.)

Miller DW et al: Hypophosphatemia in the emergency department therapeutics. Am J Emerg Med 2000;18:457. [PMID: 10919539]

Subramian R et al: Severe hypophosphatemia: Pathophysiologic implications, clinical presentations, and treatment. Medicine 2000;79:1. [PMID: 10670405]

HYPERPHOSPHATEMIA

Causes of hyperphosphatemia are given in Table 21–11. Growing children normally have serum phosphate levels higher than those of adults.

Clinical Findings

A. SYMPTOMS AND SIGNS

The clinical manifestations are those of the underlying disorders (eg, chronic renal failure, hypoparathyroidism). Hyperphosphatemia in chronic renal failure

Table 21–11. Causes of hyperphosphatemia.

Massive load of phosphate into the extracellular fluid
From outside the body
Hypervitaminosis D
Laxatives or enemas containing phosphate
Intravenous phosphate supplement
From inside the body
Rhabdomyolysis (especially if renal insufficiency coexists)
Cell destruction by chemotherapy of malignancy, particularly lymphoproliferative diseases
Metabolic acidosis (lactic acidosis, ketoacidosis)
Respiratory acidosis (phosphate incorporation into cells is disturbed)
Decreased excretion into urine
Renal failure (acute, chronic)
Hypoparathyroidism
Pseudohypoparathyroidism
Excessive growth hormone (acromegaly)
Pseudohyperphosphatemia
Multiple myeloma, hypertriglyceridemia, cell lysis

leads to secondary hyperparathyroidism and renal osteodystrophy.

B. LABORATORY FINDINGS

In addition to elevated phosphate, other blood chemistry values are those characteristic of the underlying disease.

Treatment

Treatment is that of the underlying disease and of associated hypocalcemia if present. In acute and chronic renal failure, dialysis will reduce serum phosphate. Absorption of phosphate can be reduced by administration of calcium carbonate, 0.5–1.5 g three times daily with meals (500 mg tablets). This approach is preferred to the traditional use of aluminum hydroxide because of concerns about aluminum toxicity. Another phosphate binder is sevelamer hydrochloride. Since this agent does not contain calcium or aluminum, it may be especially useful for patients with hypercalcemia or uremia.

Levin NW et al: Consequences of hyperphosphatemia and elevated levels of the calcium-phosphorus product in dialysis patients. Curr Opin Nephrol Hypertens 2001;10:563. [PMID: 11496047]

Slatopolsky EA et al: Renagel, a nonabsorbed calcium- and aluminum-free phosphate binder, lowers serum phosphorus and parathyroid hormone. Kidney Int 1999;55:299. [PMID: 9893140]

Weisinger JR et al: Magnesium and phosphorus. Lancet 1998; 352:391. [PMID: 9717944] (Review of the significance of abnormal levels of magnesium and phosphorus.)

■ DISORDERS OF MAGNESIUM CONCENTRATION

About 50% of total body magnesium exists in the insoluble state in bone. Only 5% is present as extracellular cation; the remaining 45% is contained in cells as intracellular cation. The normal plasma concentration is 1.5–2.5 meq/L, with about one-third bound to protein and two-thirds existing as free cation. Excretion of magnesium ion is via the kidney. Normally, about 3% of magnesium filtered by the glomerulus is excreted in urine.

Magnesium is an important activator ion, participating in the function of many enzymes involved in phosphate transfer reactions. Magnesium exerts physiologic effects on the nervous system resembling those of calcium. Magnesium acts directly upon the myoneural junction.

Altered concentration of Mg^{2+} in the plasma usually provokes an associated alteration of Ca^{2+}. Hypermagnesemia suppresses secretion of parathyroid hormone with consequent hypocalcemia. Severe and prolonged magnesium depletion impairs secretion of

PTH with consequent hypocalcemia. Hypomagnesemia may impair end-organ response to PTH as well.

HYPOMAGNESEMIA

Causes of hypomagnesemia are given in Table 21–12. Nearly half of hospitalized patients in whom serum electrolytes are ordered have unrecognized hypomagnesemia. Common causes include use of large volumes of intravenous fluids, diuretics, cisplatin in cancer patients (with concomitant hypokalemia), and administration of nephrotoxic agents such as aminoglycosides and amphotericin B.

Clinical Findings

A. SYMPTOMS AND SIGNS

Common symptoms are weakness, muscle cramps, and tremor. There is marked neuromuscular and central nervous system hyperirritability, with tremors, athetoid movements, jerking, nystagmus, and a positive Babinski response. There may be hypertension, tachycardia, and ventricular arrhythmias. Confusion and disorientation may be prominent features.

B. LABORATORY FINDINGS

Urinary excretion of magnesium exceeding 10–30 mg/d or a fractional excretion more than 2% indicates renal magnesium wasting. In calculating fractional excretion of magnesium, since only 30% is protein bound, it follows that 70% of circulating magnesium

Table 21–12. Causes of hypomagnesemia.

Diminished absorption or intake
  Malabsorption, chronic diarrhea, laxative abuse
  Prolonged gastrointestinal suction
  Small bowel bypass
  Malnutrition
  Alcoholism
  Total parenteral alimentation with inadequate Mg^{2+} content
Increased renal loss
  Diuretic therapy (loop diuretics, thiazide diuretics)
  Hyperaldosteronism, Gitelman's syndrome (Bartter's syndrome)
  Hyperparathyroidism, hyperthyroidism
  Hypercalcemia
  Volume expansion
  Tubulointerstitial diseases
  Transplant kidney
  Drugs (aminoglycoside, cisplatin, amphotericin B, pentamidine)
Others
  Diabetes mellitus
  Post parathyroidectomy (hungry bone syndrome)
  Respiratory alkalosis
  Pregnancy

is filtered by the glomerulus. In addition to hypomagnesemia, hypocalcemia and hypokalemia are often present. The ECG shows a prolonged QT interval, due to lengthening of the ST segment. Parathyroid hormone secretion is often suppressed (see Hypocalcemia, above).

Treatment

Treatment consists of the use of intravenous fluids containing magnesium as chloride or sulfate, 240–1200 mg/d (10–50 mmol/d) during the period of severe deficit, followed by 120 mg/d (5 mmol/d) for maintenance. Magnesium sulfate may also be given intramuscularly in a dosage of 200–800 mg/d (8–33 mmol/d) in four divided doses. Serum levels must be monitored and dosage adjusted to keep the concentration from rising above 2.5 mmol/L. K^+ and Ca^{2+} may be required as well. Magnesium oxide, 250–500 mg by mouth two to four times daily, is useful for repleting stores in those with chronic hypomagnesemia. Hypokalemia and hypocalcemia of hypomagnesemia do not recover without magnesium supplementation.

Argus ZS: Hypomagnesemia. J Am Soc Nephrol 1999;10:1616. [PMID: 10405219]

Dacey M: Hypomagnesemic disorders. Crit Care Clin 2001;17: 155. [PMID: 11219227]

HYPERMAGNESEMIA

Magnesium excess is almost always the result of renal insufficiency and the inability to excrete what has been taken in from food or drugs, especially antacids and laxatives.

Clinical Findings

A. SYMPTOMS AND SIGNS

Muscle weakness, decreased deep tendon reflexes, mental obtundation, and confusion are characteristic manifestations. Weakness—even flaccid paralysis—and hypotension are noted. There may be respiratory muscle paralysis or cardiac arrest.

B. LABORATORY FINDINGS

Serum Mg^{2+} is elevated. In the common setting of renal insufficiency, concentrations of BUN and of serum creatinine, phosphate, and uric acid are elevated; serum K^+ may be elevated. Serum Ca^{2+} is often low. The ECG shows increased PR interval, broadened QRS complexes, and peaked T waves, probably related to associated hyperkalemia.

Treatment

Treatment is directed toward alleviating renal insufficiency. Calcium acts as an antagonist to Mg^{2+} and may be given intravenously as calcium chloride, 500 mg or more at a rate of 100 mg (4.5 mmol)/min. Hemodialysis or peritoneal dialysis may be indicated.

Weisinger JR et al: Magnesium and phosphorus. Lancet 1998; 352:391. [PMID: 9717944] (Review of the significance of abnormal levels of magnesium and phosphorus.)

■ HYPEROSMOLAR DISORDERS & OSMOLAR GAPS

HYPEROSMOLALITY WITH TRANSIENT OR NO SIGNIFICANT SHIFT IN WATER

Urea and alcohol are two substances that readily cross cell membranes and can produce hyperosmolality. Because of its permeant nature, urea has little effect on the shift of water across the cell membrane. Alcohol quickly equilibrates between intracellular and extracellular water, adding 22 mosm/L for every 1000 mg/L. This measured hyperosmolality does not produce symptoms by itself because of the equilibrium described, but in any case of stupor or coma in which measured osmolality exceeds that calculated from values of serum Na^+ and glucose and BUN, ethanol intoxication should be considered as a possible explanation of the discrepancy (osmolar gap). Toxic alcohol ingestion, particularly methanol or ethylene glycol, also causes an osmolar gap characterized by anion gap metabolic acidosis (Chapter 39).

The combination of anion gap metabolic acidosis and an osmolar gap exceeding 10 mosm/kg is not specific for toxic alcohol ingestion. Nearly half of patients with alcoholic ketoacidosis or lactic acidosis have similar findings, caused in part by elevations of endogenous glycerol, acetone, and acetone metabolites.

Delaney MF et al: Diabetic ketoacidosis and hyperglycemic hyperosmolar nonketotic syndrome. Endocrinol Metab Clin North Am 2000;29:683. [PMID: 11149157]

Glaser OS: Utility of the serum osmol gap in the diagnosis of methanol or ethylene glycol ingestion. Ann Emerg Med 1996;27:343. [PMID: 8599495] (Limitations of the test.)

Magee MF et al: Management of decompensated diabetes. Diabetic ketoacidosis and hyperglycemic hyperosmolar syndrome. Crit Care Clin 2001;17:75. [PMID: 11219236]

HYPEROSMOLALITY ASSOCIATED WITH SIGNIFICANT SHIFTS IN WATER

Increased concentrations of solutes that do not readily enter cells produce a shift of water from the intracellular space to effect a true intracellular dehydration. Sodium and glucose are the solutes commonly involved. In these instances, the hyperosmolality does produce symptoms.

Clinical symptoms are mainly referred to the central nervous system. The severity of symptoms depends on the degree of hyperosmolality and rapidity of development. In acute hyperosmolality, symptoms of somnolence and confusion can appear when the osmolality exceeds 320–330 mosm/L, and coma, respiratory arrest, and death when it exceeds 340–350 mosm/L.

■ ACID-BASE DISORDERS

About 1 meq/L/kg/d of nonvolatile acid (H^+) is produced, together with volatile acid (CO_2), by whole body metabolism. Body fluid pH, however, remains relatively constant at about 7.40. This constancy of body fluid pH is achieved by removal of CO_2 and H^+ through lung and kidney, respectively.

In order to assess a patient's acid-base status, measurement of arterial pH, partial pressure of carbon dioxide (P_{CO_2}), and plasma bicarbonate (HCO_3^-) is needed. Blood gas analyzers directly measure pH and P_{CO_2}, and the HCO_3^- value is calculated from the Henderson-Hasselbalch equation:

$$pH = 6.1 + \log \frac{HCO_3^-}{0.3 \times P_{CO_2}}$$

The total venous CO_2 measurement is a more direct determination of HCO_3^-. Because of the dissociation characteristics of carbonic acid (H_2CO_3) at body pH, dissolved CO_2 is almost exclusively in the form of HCO_3^-, and for clinical purposes the total carbon dioxide content is equivalent ($\pm$ 3 meq/L) to the HCO_3^- concentration:

$$H^+ + HCO_3^- \leftrightarrow H_2CO_3 \leftrightarrow CO_2 + H_2O$$

If precise measurements of oxygenation are not needed or if oxygen saturation obtained from the pulse oximeter is adequate, venous blood gases generally provide useful information for assessment of acid-base balance and can be used interchangeably with arterial blood gases since the arteriovenous differences in pH and P_{CO_2} are small and relatively constant. Venous blood pH is usually 0.03–0.04 units lower than that of arterial blood, and venous blood P_{CO_2} is 7 or 8 mm Hg higher. Calculated HCO_3^- concentration in venous blood is at most 2 meq/L higher than that of arterial blood. An important exception to the rule of interchangeability between arterial and venous blood gases for determination of acid-base balance is during cardiopulmonary arrest. In this setting, arterial pH may be 7.41 and venous pH 7.15, and arterial blood P_{CO_2} can be 32 mm Hg with a venous blood P_{CO_2} of 74 mm Hg.

Types of Acid-Base Disorders

There are two types of acid-base disorders: respiratory and metabolic. Primary respiratory disorders affect blood acidity by causing changes in P_{CO_2}, and primary metabolic disorders are caused by disturbances in the

HCO_3^- concentration. The primary disturbances are usually accompanied by compensatory changes; however, even though these changes attenuate a pH shift from the normal value (7.40), they do not fully compensate for the primary acid-base disorders even if the disorders are chronic. Therefore, if the pH is less than 7.40, the primary process is acidosis (either respiratory or metabolic). If the pH is higher than 7.40, the primary process is either respiratory or metabolic alkalosis. The presence of one disorder with its appropriate compensatory change is a simple disorder.

Mixed Acid-Base Disorders

The presence of more than one simple disorder (not compensatory) is a mixed disorder. Double or triple disorders can coexist but not quadruple ones, since simultaneous respiratory acidosis and alkalosis are not possible.

Clinicians frequently find it difficult to decide if a mixed disorder is present. One useful scheme is to determine if the degree of compensation for the primary disorder is appropriate (Table 21–13). In respiratory disorders, if the magnitude of compensation in HCO_3^- level differs from that which is predicted, the patient has a mixed disorder. Therefore, superimposed metabolic acidosis will decrease HCO_3^- to lower than the predicted level, and a metabolic alkalosis will increase HCO_3^- over the predicted value. For example, a patient with chronic respiratory acidosis and PCO_2 of 60 mm Hg should have a HCO_3^- of 31 meq/L (assuming that normal HCO_3^- is 24 meq/L). If the HCO_3^- is 25 meq/L, a superimposed metabolic acidosis exists, and if the HCO_3^- is 45 meq/L, there is a superimposed metabolic alkalosis. Using data from Table 21–13, similar calculations can be made for primary metabolic disorders.

Furthermore, corrected bicarbonate ($cHCO_3^-$), calculated from measured HCO_3^- plus the increase in anion gap (see below), is useful to assess the superimposed metabolic alkalosis or normal anion gap metabolic acidosis. In increased anion gap acidosis, there

must be a mole for mole decrease in HCO_3^- as anion gap decreases. Therefore, an HCO_3^- value higher or lower than normal (24 meq/L) indicates the concomitant presence of metabolic alkalosis or normal anion gap acidosis, respectively.

STEP-BY-STEP ANALYSIS OF ACID-BASE STATUS

Step 1: Determine the primary (or main) disorder—whether it is metabolic or respiratory—from blood pH, HCO_3^-, and PCO_2 values.

Step 2: Determine the presence of mixed acid-base disorders by calculating the range of compensatory responses (Table 21–13).

Step 3: Calculate the anion gap (Table 21–15).

Step 4: Calculate the HCO_3^- concentration if the anion gap is increased (see above).

Step 5: Examine the patient to determine whether the clinical signs are compatible with the acid-base analysis thus obtained.

Gluck SL: Acid-base. Lancet 1998;352:474. [PMID: 9708770] (A clinical approach to diagnosis and management.)

Laski ME et al: Acid-base disorders in medicine. Dis Mon 1996;42(2):51. [PMID: 8631223]

RESPIRATORY ACIDOSIS

Respiratory acidosis results from decreased alveolar ventilation and subsequent hypercapnia. Pulmonary as well as nonpulmonary disorders can cause hypoventilation. The clinician must be mindful of readily reversible causes of respiratory acidosis, especially opioid-induced central nervous system depression.

Acute respiratory failure is associated with severe acidosis and only a small increase in the plasma bicar-

Table 21–13. Primary acid-base disorders and expected compensation.

Disorder	Primary Defect	Compensatory Response	Magnitude of Compensation
Respiratory acidosis Acute	↑PCO_2	↑HCO_3^-	↑HCO_3^- 1 meq/L per 10 mm Hg ↑PCO_2
Chronic	↑PCO_2	↑HCO_3^-	↑HCO_3^- 3.5 meq/L per 10 mm Hg ↑PCO_2
Respiratory alkalosis Acute	↓PCO_2	↓HCO_3^-	↓HCO_3^- 2 meq/L per 10 mm Hg ↓PCO_2
Chronic	↓PCO_2	↓HCO_3^-	↓HCO_3^- 5 meq/L per 10 mm Hg ↓PCO_2
Metabolic acidosis	↓PCO_2	↓PCO_2	↓PCO_2 1.3 mm Hg per 1 meq/L ↓HCO_3^-
Metabolic alkalosis	↑PCO_2	↑PCO_2	↑PCO_2 0.7 mm Hg per 1 meq/L ↑HCO_3^-

bonate. After 6–12 hours, the primary increase in P_{CO_2} evokes a renal compensatory response to generate more HCO_3^-, which tends to ameliorate the respiratory acidosis. This usually takes several days to complete.

Chronic respiratory acidosis is generally seen in patients with underlying lung disease, such as chronic obstructive disease. Urinary excretion of acid in the form of NH_4^+ and Cl^- ions results in the characteristic hypochloremia of chronic respiratory acidosis. When chronic respiratory acidosis is corrected suddenly, especially in patients who receive mechanical ventilation, there is a 2- to 3-day lag in renal bicarbonate excretion, resulting in posthypercapnic metabolic alkalosis.

Clinical Findings

A. SYMPTOMS AND SIGNS

With acute onset, there is somnolence and confusion, and myoclonus with asterixis may be seen. Coma from CO_2 narcosis ensues. Severe hypercapnia increases cerebral blood flow and cerebrospinal fluid pressure. Signs of increased intracranial pressure (papilledema, pseudotumor cerebri) may be seen.

B. LABORATORY FINDINGS

Arterial pH is low, and P_{CO_2} is increased. Serum HCO_3^- is elevated, but not enough to completely compensate for the hypercapnia. If the disorder is chronic, hypochloremia is seen.

Treatment

Since drug overdose is an important reversible cause of acute respiratory acidosis, administration of naloxone, 0.04–2 mg intravenously (see Chapter 39) is given to all such patients if no obvious cause for respiratory depression is present. In all forms of respiratory acidosis, treatment is directed at the underlying disorder to improve ventilation.

RESPIRATORY ALKALOSIS

Respiratory alkalosis, or hypocapnia, occurs when hyperventilation reduces the P_{CO_2}, which increases the pH. The most common cause of respiratory alkalosis is hyperventilation syndrome (Table 21–14), but bacterial septicemia and cirrhosis are other common causes. Symptoms in acute respiratory alkalosis are related to decreased cerebral blood flow induced by the disorder. Pregnancy is another cause of chronic respiratory alkalosis, probably from progesterone stimulation of the respiratory center, with an average P_{CO_2} of 30 mm Hg.

Determination of appropriate compensatory changes in the HCO_3^- is useful to sort out the presence of an associated metabolic disorder (see above under Mixed Acid-Base Disorders). As in respiratory acidosis, the changes in HCO_3^- values are greater if the respiratory alkalosis is chronic (Table 21–13). While serum HCO_3^- is frequently below 15 meq/L in

Table 21–14. Causes of respiratory alkalosis.[1]

Hypoxia
  Decreased inspired oxygen tension
  High altitude
  Ventilation/perfusion inequality
  Hypotension
  Severe anemia
CNS-mediated disorders
  Voluntary hyperventilation
    Anxiety-hyperventilation syndrome
  Neurologic disease
  Cerebrovascular accident (infarction, hemorrhage)
  Infection
  Trauma
  Tumor
  Pharmacologic and hormonal stimulation
    Salicylates
    Nicotine
    Xanthines
    Pregnancy (progesterone)
  Hepatic failure
  Gram-negative septicemia
  Recovery from metabolic acidosis
  Heat exposure
Pulmonary disease
  Interstitial lung disease
  Pneumonia
  Pulmonary embolism
  Pulmonary edema
Mechanical overventilation

[1]Adapted from Gennari FJ: Respiratory acidosis and alkalosis. In: *Maxwell and Kleeman's Clinical Disorders of Fluid and Electrolyte Metabolism*, 5th ed. Narins RG (editor). McGraw-Hill, 1994.

metabolic acidosis, it is unusual to see such a low level in respiratory alkalosis, and its presence would imply a superimposed (noncompensatory) metabolic acidosis.

Clinical Findings

A. SYMPTOMS AND SIGNS

In acute cases (hyperventilation), there is light-headedness, anxiety, paresthesias, numbness about the mouth, and a tingling sensation in the hands and feet. Tetany occurs in more severe alkalosis from a fall in ionized calcium. In chronic cases, findings are those of the responsible condition.

B. LABORATORY FINDINGS

Arterial blood pH is elevated, and P_{CO_2} is low. Serum bicarbonate is decreased in chronic respiratory alkalosis.

Treatment

Treatment is directed toward the underlying cause. In acute hyperventilation syndrome from anxiety, rebreathing into a paper bag will increase the P_{CO_2}. The processes are usually self-limited since muscle weakness caused by hyperventilation-induced alkalemia will suppress ventilation. Sedation may be necessary if the process persists. Rapid correction of chronic respiratory alkalosis may result in metabolic acidosis as PCO_2 is increased in the setting of previous compensatory decrease in HCO_3^-.

Laffey JG et al: Hypocapnia. N Engl J Med 2002;347:43. [PMID: 12097540]

METABOLIC ACIDOSIS

The hallmark of metabolic acidosis is decreased HCO_3^-, seen also in respiratory alkalosis (see above), but the pH distinguishes between the two disorders. Calculation of the anion gap is useful in determining the cause of the metabolic acidosis (Table 21–15). The anion gap represents the difference between readily measured anions and cations.

In plasma,

$$Na^+ + \frac{Unmeasured}{cations} = HCO_3^- + Cl^- + \frac{Unmeasured}{anions}$$

$$Anion\ gap = Na^+ - (HCO_3^- + Cl^-)$$

Table 21–15. Abnormal anion gap.[1]

Decreased (< 6 meq)
  Hypoalbuminemia (decreased unmeasured anion)
  Plasma cell dyscrasias
    Monoclonal protein (cationic paraprotein)
      (accompanied by chloride and bicarbonate)
  Bromide intoxication
Increased (>12 meq)
  Metabolic anion
    Diabetic ketoacidosis
    Alcoholic ketoacidosis
    Lactic acidosis
    Renal insufficiency (PO_4^{3-}, SO_4^{2-})
    Starvation
    Metabolic alkalosis (increased number of negative
      charges on protein)
  Drug or chemical anion
    Salicylate intoxication
    Sodium carbenicillin therapy
    Methanol (formic acid)
    Ethylene glycol (oxalic acid)
Normal (6–12 meq)
  Loss of HCO_3^-
  Diarrhea
  Recovery from diabetic ketoacidosis
  Pancreatic fluid loss ileostomy (unadapted)
  Carbonic anhydrase inhibitors
  Chloride retention
  Renal tubular acidosis
  Ileal loop bladder
  Administration of HCl equivalent or NH_4Cl
  Arginine and lysine in parenteral nutrition

[1]Reference ranges for anion gap may vary based on differing laboratory methods.

The major unmeasured cations are calcium (1 meq/L), magnesium (2 meq/L), gamma globulins, and potassium (4 meq/L). The major unmeasured anions are negatively charged albumin (2 meq/L per g/dL), phosphate (2 meq/L), sulfate (1 meq/L), lactate (1–2 meq/L), and other organic anions (3–4 meq/L). Traditionally, the normal anion gap has been 12 ± 4 meq/L. With the current generation of autoanalyzers, the reference range may be lower (6 ± 1 meq/L), primarily from an increase in Cl^- values. Despite its usefulness, the serum anion gap can be misleading. Nonacid-base disorders that may contribute to an error in anion gap interpretation include hypoalbuminemia (see below), antibiotic administration (eg, carbenicillin is an unmeasured anion; polymyxin is an unmeasured cation), hypernatremia, or hyponatremia.

Decreased Anion Gap

A decreased anion gap can occur because of a reduction in unmeasured anions or an increase in unmeasured cations.

A. DECREASED UNMEASURED ANIONS

If the sodium concentration remains normal but HCO_3^- and Cl^- increase, the anion gap will decrease. This is seen when there are decreased unmeasured anions, especially in hypoalbuminemia. For every 1 g/dL decline in serum albumin, a 2 meq/L decrease in anion gap will occur.

B. INCREASED UNMEASURED CATIONS

If the sodium concentration falls because of addition of unmeasured cations but HCO_3^- and Cl^- remain unchanged, the anion gap will decrease. This is seen in (1) severe hypercalcemia, hypermagnesemia, or hyperkalemia; (2) IgG myeloma, where the immunoglobulin is cationic in 70% of cases; and (3) lithium toxicity.

Jurado RL et al: Low anion gap. South Med J 1998;91:624. [PMID: 9671832] (Differential diagnosis of the low anion gap and the importance of this clue in the diagnosis of occult myeloma or intoxications.)

Increased Anion Gap Acidosis (Increased Unmeasured Anions)

The hallmark of this disorder is that metabolic acidosis (thus low HCO_3^-) is associated with normal serum Cl^-, so that the anion gap increases. Normochloremic metabolic acidosis generally results from addition to the blood of nonchloride acids such as lactate, acetoacetate, β-hydroxybutyrate, and exogenous toxins. An exception is uremia, with underexcretion of organic acids and anions.

A. LACTIC ACIDOSIS

Lactic acid is formed from pyruvate in anaerobic glycolysis. Therefore, most of the lactate is produced in tissues with high rates of glycolysis, such as gut (responsible for over 50% of lactate production), skeletal muscle, brain, skin, and erythrocytes. Normally, lactate levels remain low (1 meq/L) because of metabolism of lactate principally by the liver through gluconeogenesis or oxidation via the Krebs cycle. Furthermore, the kidneys metabolize about 30% of lactate.

In lactic acidosis, lactate levels are at least 4–5 meq/L but commonly 10–30 meq/L. The mortality rate exceeds 50%. There are two basic types of lactic acidosis, both associated with increased lactate production and decreased lactate utilization. Type A is characterized by hypoxia or decreased tissue perfusion, whereas in type B there is no clinical evidence of hypoxia. Type A (hypoxic) lactic acidosis is the more common type, resulting from poor tissue perfusion; cardiogenic, septic, or hemorrhagic shock; and carbon monoxide or cyanide poisoning. These conditions not only cause lactic acid production to increase peripherally but, more importantly, hepatic metabolism of lactate to decrease as liver perfusion declines. In addition, severe acidosis impairs the ability of the liver to extract the perfused lactate.

Type B lactic acidosis may be due to metabolic causes, such as diabetes, ketoacidosis, liver disease, renal failure, infection, leukemia, or lymphoma; or may occur as a result of toxicity from ethanol, methanol, salicylates, or isoniazid. AIDS without AIDS-related lymphoma is associated with type B lactic acidosis.

Idiopathic lactic acidosis, usually in debilitated patients, has an extremely high mortality rate. (For treatment of lactic acidosis, see below and Chapter 27.)

B. DIABETIC KETOACIDOSIS

This metabolic abnormality is characterized by hyperglycemia and metabolic acidosis (pH < 7.25 or plasma bicarbonate < 16 meq/L). Anion gap metabolic acidosis is the acid-base disturbance generally ascribed to diabetic ketoacidosis:

$$H + B^- + NaHCO_3 \leftrightarrow CO_2 + NaB + H_2O$$

where B^- is β-hydroxybutyrate or acetoacetate.

The anion gap should be calculated from the serum electrolytes as measured, since correction of the serum sodium for the dilutional effect of hyperglycemia will incorrectly exaggerate the anion gap. The increased anion gap is due to hyperketonemia (acetoacetate and β-hydroxybutyrate) and at times to an increase in serum lactate secondary to reduced tissue perfusion and increased anaerobic metabolism. If a rise in anion gap from normal is equal to a fall in HCO_3^-, a diagnosis of simple metabolic acidosis can be made. However, the presence of concurrent metabolic alkalosis or normal anion gap metabolic acidosis is suggested if the value of the measured HCO_3^- plus the increase in anion gap ($cHCO_3^-$) is higher or lower than the normal value for HCO_3^-, respectively.

During the recovery phase of diabetic ketoacidosis, anion gap acidosis can be transformed into hyper-chloremic non-anion gap acidosis. The mechanism for this is as follows: As GFR increases from NaCl therapy of diabetic ketoacidosis, the retention of Cl^- causes a mild decrease in the anion gap from dilution. More importantly, the increased GFR causes the urinary excretion of ketone salts (NaB), which are formed as bicarbonate is consumed:

$$HB + NaHCO_3^- \rightarrow NaB + H_2CO_3$$

The kidney reabsorbs ketone anions poorly but can compensate for the loss of anions (and therefore Na^+) by increasing the reabsorption of Cl^-. Conversely, even on presentation, patients with diabetic ketoacidosis and normal renal perfusion may have marked ketonuria, severe metabolic acidosis, and only a mildly increased anion gap. Again, the variable relationship between the rise in the anion gap and the fall in the HCO_3^- can occur with the urinary loss of Na^+ or K^+ salts of β-hydroxybutyrate, which will lower the anion gap without altering the H^+ excretion or the severity of the acidosis.

Since Ketostix reacts to acetoacetate, less to acetone, and not at all to the predominant keto acid, β-hydroxybutyrate, the test may become more positive even as the patient improves owing to the metabolism of hydroxybutyrate. Thus, the patient's clinical status and the reduction of the anion gap are better markers of improvement than monitoring the serum acetone test. Conversely, in the presence of concomitant lactic acidosis, a shift in the redox state can increase β-hydroxybutyrate and decrease the readily detectable acetoacetate, thus lowering the nitroprusside reaction.

C. ALCOHOLIC KETOACIDOSIS

This is a common disorder of chronically malnourished patients who consume large quantities of alcohol daily. Most of these patients have mixed acid-base disorders (10% have a triple acid-base disorder). While decreased HCO_3^- is usual, half the patients may have normal or alkalemic pH. The three types of metabolic acidosis seen in alcoholic ketoacidosis are the following: (1) Ketoacidosis due to β-hydroxybutyrate and acetoacetate excess. (2) Lactic acidosis: Alcohol metabolism increases the NADH:NAD ratio, causing increased production and decreased utilization of lactate. Accompanying thiamin deficiency, which inhibits pyruvate carboxylase, further enhances lactic acid production in many cases. Moderate to severe elevations of lactate (> 6 mmol/L) are seen with concomitant disorders such as sepsis, pancreatitis, or hypoglycemia. (3) Hyperchloremic acidosis from bicarbonate loss in the urine associated with ketonuria (see above). Metabolic alkalosis occurs from volume contraction and vomiting. Respiratory alkalosis results from alcohol withdrawal, pain, or associated disorders such as sepsis or liver disease. Half of the patients have either hypoglycemia or hyperglycemia. When serum glucose levels are greater than 250 mg/dL, the distinction from diabetic ketoacidosis is difficult. The diagnosis of alcoholic ketoacidosis is supported by absence of a diabetic history and by no evidence of glucose intolerance after initial therapy.

D. TOXINS

(See also Chapter 39.) Multiple toxins and drugs can increase the anion gap by increasing endogenous acid production. Examples include methanol (metabolized to formic acid), ethylene glycol (glycolic and oxalic acid), and salicylates (salicylic acid and lactic acid), which can cause a mixed disorder of metabolic acidosis with respiratory alkalosis.

E. UREMIC ACIDOSIS

At glomerular filtration rates below 20 mL/min, the inability to excrete H^+ with retention of acid anions such as PO_4^{3-} and SO_4^{2-} result in an increased anion gap acidosis, which rarely is severe. The unmeasured anions "replace" HCO_3^- (which is consumed as a buffer). Hyperchloremic normal anion gap acidosis may be seen in milder cases of renal insufficiency.

Normal Anion Gap Acidosis (Table 21–16)

The hallmark of this disorder is that the low HCO_3^- of metabolic acidosis is associated with hyperchloremia, so that the anion gap remains normal. The most common causes are gastrointestinal HCO_3^- loss and defects in renal acidification (renal tubular aci-

doses). The urinary anion gap can differentiate between these two common causes (see below).

A. GASTROINTESTINAL HCO_3^- LOSS

Bicarbonate is secreted in multiple areas in the gastrointestinal tract. Small bowel and pancreatic secretions contain large amounts of HCO_3. Therefore, massive diarrhea or pancreatic drainage can result in HCO_3^- loss because of increased HCO_3^- secretion and decreased absorption. Hyperchloremia occurs because the ileum and colon secrete HCO_3^- in a one-to-one exchange for Cl^- by countertransport. The resultant volume contraction causes further increased Cl^- retention by the kidney in the setting of decreased anion, HCO_3^-. Patients with ureterosigmoidostomies can develop hyperchloremic metabolic acidosis because the colon secretes HCO_3^- in the urine in exchange for Cl^-.

B. RENAL TUBULAR ACIDOSIS

In renal tubular acidosis, the defect is either inability to excrete H^+ (inadequate generation of new HCO_3^-) or inappropriate reabsorption of HCO_3^-. Four discrete types can be differentiated by the clinical setting, urinary pH, urinary anion gap (see below), and serum K^+ level. Since mutations of Cl^-/HCO_3^- exchanger and H^+-ATPase genes have been recently demonstrated in hereditary distal renal tubular acidosis, further classification depending upon molecular mechanisms may soon become possible.

1. Classic distal renal tubular acidosis (type I)— This disorder is characterized by hypokalemic hyper-

Table 21–16. Hyperchloremic, normal anion gap metabolic acidoses.[1]

	Renal Defect	Serum [K^+]	Distal H^+ Secretion: Urinary NH_4^+ Plus Minimal Urine pH	Titratable Acid	Urinary Anion Gap	Treatment
Gastrointestinal HCO_3^- loss	None	↓	< 5.5	↑↑	Negative	Na^+, K^+, and HCO_3^- as required
Renal tubular acidosis I. Classic distal	Distal H^+ secretion	↓	> 5.5	↓	Positive	$NaHCO_3$ (1–3 meq/kg/d)
II. Proximal secretion	Proximal H^+	↓	< 5.5	Normal	Positive	$NaHCO_3$ or $KHCO_3$ (10–15 meq/kg/d), thiazide
III. Glomerular insufficiency	NH_3 production	Normal	< 5.5	↓	Positive	$NaHCO_3$ (1–3 meq/kg/d)
IV. Hyporeninemic hypoaldosteronism	Distal Na^+ reabsorption, K^+ secretion, and H^+ secretion	↑	< 5.5	↓	Positive	Fludrocortisone (0.1–0.5 mg/d), dietary K^+ restriction, furosemide (40–160 mg/d), $NaHCO_3$ (1–3 meq/kg/d)

[1]Modified and reproduced, with permission, from Cogan MG: *Fluid and Electrolytes: Physiology and Pathophysiology.* McGraw-Hill, 1991.

chloremic metabolic acidosis and is due to selective deficiency in H^+ secretion in the distal nephron. Despite acidosis, urinary pH cannot be acidified and is above 5.5, which retards the binding of H^+ to phosphate ($H^+ + HPO_4^{2-} \rightarrow H_2PO_4$), and thus inhibits titratable acid excretion. Furthermore, urinary excretion of $NH_4^+Cl^-$ is decreased, and the urinary anion gap is positive (see below). Enhanced K^+ excretion occurs probably because there is less competition from H^+ in the distal nephron transport system. Furthermore, as a response to renal salt wasting, hyperaldosteronism occurs. Nephrocalcinosis and nephrolithiasis frequently accompany this disorder since chronic acidosis decreases tubular calcium reabsorption. The hypercalciuria, alkaline urine, and lowered level of urinary citrate cause calcium phosphate stones and nephrocalcinosis.

2. Proximal renal tubular acidosis (type II)—Proximal renal tubular acidosis is a hypokalemic hyperchloremic metabolic acidosis due to a selective defect in the proximal tubule's ability to adequately reabsorb filtered HCO_3^-. Carbonic anhydrase inhibitors (acetazolamide) can cause proximal renal tubular acidosis. About 90% of filtered HCO_3^- is absorbed by the proximal tubule. The distal nephron has a limited ability to absorb HCO_3^- but becomes overwhelmed and does not function adequately when there is increased delivery. Eventually, distal delivery of filtered HCO_3^- declines because the plasma HCO_3^- level has dropped as a result of progressive urinary HCO_3^- wastage. When the plasma HCO_3^- level drops to 15–18 meq/L, delivery of HCO_3^- drops to the point where the distal nephron is no longer overwhelmed and can regain function. At that point, bicarbonaturia disappears, and urinary pH can be acidic. Thiazide-induced volume contraction can be used to enhance proximal HCO_3^- reabsorption, leading to the decrease in distal HCO_3^- delivery and improvement of bicarbonaturia and renal acidification. The increased delivery of HCO_3^- to the distal nephron also increases K^+ secretion, and hypokalemia results if a patient is loaded with excess HCO_3^- and K^+ is not adequately supplemented. Proximal renal tubular acidosis often exists with other defects of absorption in the proximal tubule, resulting in glucosuria, aminoaciduria, phosphaturia, and uricaciduria. Causes include multiple myeloma with Fanconi's syndrome and nephrotoxic drugs.

3. Renal tubular acidosis of glomerular insufficiency (type III)—When GFR decreases to 20–30 mL/min, ability to generate adequate NH_3 is impaired, with subsequent decreased $NH_4^+Cl^-$ excretion. A normokalemic, hyperchloremic metabolic acidosis ensues. Further reduction in GFR results in increased anion gap acidosis of uremia (see above).

4. Hyporeninemic hypoaldosteronemic renal tubular acidosis (type IV)—Type IV is the only type characterized by hyperkalemic, hyperchloremic acidosis. The defect is aldosterone deficiency or antag-

onism, which impairs distal nephron Na^+ reabsorption and K^+ and H^+ excretion. Renal salt wasting is frequently present. Relative hypoaldosteronism from hyporeninemia is most commonly found in diabetic nephropathy, tubulointerstitial renal diseases, hypertensive nephrosclerosis, and AIDS. In patients with these disorders, caution must be taken when using drugs that can exacerbate the hyperkalemia, such as angiotensin-converting enzyme inhibitors (which will further reduce aldosterone levels), aldosterone receptor blockers such as spironolactone, and NSAIDs.

C. DILUTIONAL ACIDOSIS

Rapid dilution of plasma volume by 0.9% NaCl may cause a mild hyperchloremic acidosis.

D. RECOVERY FROM DIABETIC KETOACIDOSIS

See above.

E. POSTHYPOCAPNIA

In prolonged respiratory alkalosis, HCO_3^- decreases and Cl^- increases from decreased renal $NH_4^+Cl^-$ excretion. If the respiratory alkalosis is corrected quickly, P_{CO_2} will increase acutely but HCO_3^- will remain low until the kidneys can generate new HCO_3^-, which generally takes several days. In the meantime, the increased P_{CO_2} with low HCO_3^- causes metabolic acidosis.

F. HYPERALIMENTATION

Hyperalimentation fluids may contain amino acid solutions that acidify when metabolized, such as arginine hydrochloride and lysine hydrochloride.

Urinary Anion Gap to Assess Hyperchloremic Metabolic Acidosis

Increased renal $NH_4^+Cl^-$ excretion to enhance H^+ removal is a normal physiologic response to metabolic acidosis. NH_3 reacts with H^+ to form NH_4^+, which is accompanied by the anion Cl^- for excretion. The normal daily urinary excretion of NH_4Cl of about 30 meq can be increased up to 200 meq in response to acid load.

Urinary anion gap from a random urine sample ($[Na^+ + K^+] - Cl^-$) reflects the ability of the kidney to excrete NH_4Cl as in the following equation:

$$Na^+ + K^+ + NH_3^+ = Cl^- + 80$$

where 80 is the average value for the difference in the urinary anions and cations other than Na^+, K^+, NH_3^+, and Cl^-.

Therefore, urinary anion gap is equal to ($80 - NH_3^+$), and thus aids in the distinction between gastrointestinal and renal causes of hyperchloremic acidosis. If the cause of the metabolic acidosis is gastrointestinal HCO_3^- loss (diarrhea), renal acidification ability remains normal and NH_4Cl excretion increases in response to the acidosis. The urinary anion gap is negative (eg, −30 meq/L). If the cause is distal renal tubular acidosis, the urinary anion gap is positive (eg, +25 meq/L), since the basic lesion in the disorder is inability of the kidney to excrete H⁺ and thus inability to increase NH_4Cl excretion. Urinary pH may not as readily differentiate between the two causes. Despite acidosis, if volume depletion from diarrhea causes inadequate Na⁺ delivery to the distal nephron and therefore decreased exchange with H⁺, urinary pH may not be lower than 5.3. In the presence of this relatively high urine pH, however, H⁺ excretion continues due to buffering of NH_3 to NH_4^+, since the pK of this reaction is as high as 9.1. Potassium depletion, which can accompany diarrhea (and surreptitious laxative abuse), may also impair renal acidification. Thus, when volume depletion is present, the urinary anion gap is a better measurement of ability to acidify the urine than urinary pH.

Clinical Findings

A. SYMPTOMS AND SIGNS

Symptoms of metabolic acidosis are mainly those of the underlying disorder. Compensatory hyperventilation is an important clinical sign and may be misinterpreted as a primary respiratory disorder; when severe, Kussmaul respirations (deep, regular, sighing respirations) are seen.

B. LABORATORY FINDINGS

Blood pH, serum HCO_3^-, and PCO_2 are decreased. Anion gap may be normal (hyperchloremic) or increased (normochloremic). Hyperkalemia may be seen (see above).

Treatment

A. INCREASED ANION GAP ACIDOSIS

Treatment is aimed at the underlying disorder, such as insulin and fluid therapy for diabetes and appropriate volume resuscitation to restore tissue perfusion. The metabolism of lactate will produce HCO_3^- and increase pH. The use of supplemental HCO_3^- is indicated for treatment of hyperkalemia (Table 21–7) and some forms of normal anion gap acidosis but has been controversial for treatment of increased anion gap metabolic acidosis. Administration of large amounts of HCO_3^- may have deleterious effects, including hypernatremia and hyperosmolality. Furthermore, intracellular pH may decrease because administered HCO_3^- is converted to CO_2, which easily diffuses into cells. There, it combines with water to create additional hydrogen ions and worsening of intracellular acidosis. Theoretically, this could impair cellular function, but the clinical significance of this phenomenon is uncertain. In addition, alkali administration is known to stimulate phosphofructokinase activity, thus exacerbating lactic acidosis via enhanced lactate production. Ketogenesis is also augmented by alkali ther-

apy. In salicylate intoxication, however, alkali therapy must be started unless blood pH is already alkalinized by respiratory alkalosis, since the increment in pH converts salicylate to more impermeable salicylic acid and thus prevents central nervous system damage. In alcoholic ketoacidosis, thiamine should be given together with glucose to avoid the development of Wernicke's encephalopathy. The amount of HCO_3^- deficit can be calculated as follows:

$$\text{Amount of } HCO_3^- \text{ deficit} = 0.5 \times$$
$$\text{Body weight} \times (24 - HCO_3)$$

Half of the calculated deficit should be administered within the first 3–4 hours to avoid overcorrection and volume overload.

In methanol intoxication, ethanol has been used as a competitive substrate for alcohol dehydrogenase, which metabolizes methanol to formaldehyde. Recently, direct inhibition of alcohol dehydrogenase by fomepizole has been reported and may be used in near future.

B. NORMAL ANION GAP ACIDOSIS

(Table 21–16.) In distal renal tubular acidosis, supplementation of bicarbonate is necessary since acid accumulates systemically in this disorder. However, in proximal renal tubular acidosis, correction of low serum bicarbonate is sometimes hazardous and unnecessary except in severe cases. If the blood bicarbonate concentration is elevated in response to its administration, and the concentration in the glomerular filtrate exceeds the capacity of the proximal tubule to reabsorb it, a large quantity of bicarbonate is excreted into the urine accompanied by potassium, exacerbating hypokalemia. Thus, potassium should also be given when bicarbonate therapy is indicated in proximal renal tubular acidosis.

Adrogue HJ et al: Management of life threatening acid base disorders. (Part 1.) N Engl J Med 1998;338:26. [PMID: 9414329]

Adrogue HJ et al: Management of life-threatening acid-base disorders. Second of two parts. N Engl J Med 1998;338:107. [PMID: 9420343]

Batlle D et al: Hereditary distal renal tubular acidosis: new understandings. Annu Rev Med 2001;52:471. [PMID: 11160790]

Brent J et al: Fomepizole for the treatment of methanol poisoning. N Engl J Med 2001;344:424. [PMID: 11172179]

Galla JH: Metabolic alkalosis. J Am Soc Nephrol 2000;11:369. [PMID: 10665945]

Hood VL et al: Protection of acid base balance by pH regulation of acid production. N Engl J Med 1998;339:819. [PMID: 9738091] (Systemic pH regulates acid production in a negative feedback manner.)

Luft FC: Lactic acidosis update for critical care clinicians. J Am Soc Nephrol 2001;12:S15. [PMID: 11251027]

Salem MM et al: Gaps in the anion gap. Arch Intern Med 1992; 152:1625. [PMID: 1497396]

Smulders YM et al: Renal tubular acidosis: Pathophysiology and diagnosis. Arch Intern Med 1996;156:1629. [PMID: 8694660]

METABOLIC ALKALOSIS

Classification

Metabolic alkalosis is characterized by high HCO_3^-. The high HCO_3^- is seen also in chronic respiratory acidosis (see above), but pH differentiates the two disorders. It is useful to classify the causes of metabolic alkalosis into two groups based on "saline responsiveness" or urinary Cl^-, which are markers for volume status (Table 21–17). Saline-responsive metabolic alkalosis is a sign of extracellular volume contraction, and saline-unresponsive alkalosis implies a volume-expanded state. It is rare for a compensatory increase in PCO_2 to exceed 55 mm Hg. A higher value implies a superimposed respiratory acidosis.

A. SALINE-RESPONSIVE METABOLIC ALKALOSIS

Saline-responsive metabolic alkalosis is by far the more common disorder. It is characterized by normotensive extracellular volume contraction and hypokalemia. Less frequently, hypotension or orthostatic hypotension may be seen. In vomiting or nasogastric suction, for example, loss of acid (HCl) initiates the alkalosis, but volume contraction from loss of Cl^- sustains the alkalosis because the decline in GFR causes avid renal Na^+ and HCO_3^- reabsorption. Since there is Cl^- depletion from loss of HCl, NaCl, and KCl from the stomach, the available anion is HCO_3^-, whose reabsorption is increased proximally, and urine pH may remain acidic despite alkalemia (paradoxical aciduria). Renal Cl^- reabsorption (as well as Na^+) reabsorption is high, and the urinary Cl^- is therefore low (< 10–20 meq/L). In alkalosis, bicarbonaturia may force Na^+ excretion as the accompanying cation even if volume depletion is present. Therefore, urinary Cl^- is preferred to urinary Na^+ as a measure of extracellular volume. An exception to the usefulness of urinary Cl^- is in patients who have recently received diuretics. Their urine may contain high Na^+ and Cl^- despite extracellular volume contraction. If diuretics are discontinued, the urinary Cl^- will decrease.

Metabolic alkalosis is generally associated with hypokalemia. This is due partly to the direct effect of alkalosis per se on renal potassium excretion and partly to secondary hyperaldosteronism from volume depletion. Hypokalemia induced in this fashion further worsens the metabolic alkalosis by increasing bicarbonate reabsorption in the proximal tubule and hydrogen ion secretion in the distal tubule. Administration of KCl will correct the disorder. Repletion of KCl is important to reverse the disorder.

1. Contraction alkalosis—Diuretics can acutely decrease extracellular volume from urinary loss of NaCl and water. There is no associated bicarbonaturia, so that body HCO_3^- content remains normal. However, plasma HCO_3^- increases because of extracellular fluid contraction—the reverse of what occurs in dilutional acidosis.

2. Posthypercapnia alkalosis—In chronic respiratory acidosis, compensatory increases in HCO_3^- occur (Table 21–13). Hypercapnia also directly affects the proximal tubule to decrease NaCl reabsorption, which can cause extracellular volume depletion. If PCO_2 is corrected rapidly, as with mechanical ventilation,

Table 21–17. Metabolic alkalosis.[1]

Saline-Responsive ($U_{Cl} < 10$ meq/d)	Saline-Unresponsive ($U_{Cl} > 10$ meq/d)
Excessive body bicarbonate content	**Excessive body bicarbonate content**
Renal alkalosis	Renal alkalosis
Diuretic therapy	Normotensive
Poorly reabsorbable anion therapy:	Bartter's syndrome (renal salt wasting and secondary
carbenicillin, penicillin, sulfate, phosphate	hyperaldosteronism)
Posthypercapnia	Severe potassium depletion
Gastrointestinal alkalosis	Refeeding alkalosis
Loss of HCl from vomiting or nasogastric	Hypercalcemia and hypoparathyroidism
suction	Hypertensive
Intestinal alkalosis: chloride diarrhea	Endogenous mineralocorticoids
Exogenous alkali	Primary aldosteronism
$NaHCO_3$ (baking soda)	Hyperreninism
Sodium citrate, lactate, gluconate, acetate	Adrenal enzyme deficiency: 11- and 17-hydroxylase
Transfusions	Liddle's syndrome
Antacids	Exogenous mineralocorticoids
Normal body bicarbonate content	Licorice
"Contraction alkalosis"	

[1]Modified and reproduced, with permission, from Narins RG et al: Diagnostic strategies in disorders of fluid, electrolyte and acid-base homeostasis. Am J Med 1982;72:496.

metabolic alkalosis will ensue until adequate bicarbonaturia occurs. Hypovolemia will inhibit bicarbonaturia until Cl⁻ is repleted. Many patients with chronic respiratory acidosis receive diuretics, which further exacerbates the metabolic alkalosis.

B. Saline-Unresponsive Alkalosis

1. Hyperaldosteronism—Primary hyperaldosteronism causes expansion of extracellular volume with hypertension. Metabolic alkalosis with hypokalemia results from the renal mineralocorticoid effect. In an attempt to decrease extracellular volume, high levels of NaCl are excreted, and for that reason the urinary Cl is high (> 20 meq/L, often higher). Therapy with NaCl will only increase volume expansion and hypertension and will not treat the underlying problem of mineralocorticoid excess.

2. Alkali administration with decreased GFR—Despite large ingestions of HCO₃⁻, enhanced bicarbonaturia almost always prevents a patient with normal renal function from developing metabolic alkalosis. However, with renal insufficiency, urinary excretion of bicarbonate is inadequate. If large amounts of HCO₃⁻ or metabolizable salts of organic acids such as sodium lactate, sodium citrate, or sodium gluconate are consumed, as with intensive antacid therapy, metabolic alkalosis will occur. In milk-alkali syndrome, large and sustained ingestion of absorbable antacids and milk causes renal insufficiency from hypercalcemia. Decreased GFR prevents appropriate bicarbonaturia from the ingested alkali, and metabolic alkalosis occurs. Volume contraction from renal hypercalcemic effects further exacerbates the alkalosis.

Clinical Findings

A. Symptoms and Signs

There are no characteristic symptoms or signs. Orthostatic hypotension may be encountered. Weakness and hyporeflexia occur if serum K⁺ is markedly low. Tetany and neuromuscular irritability occur rarely.

B. Laboratory Findings

The arterial blood pH and bicarbonate are elevated. The arterial P_{CO_2} is increased. Serum potassium and chloride are decreased. There may be an increased anion gap.

Treatment

Mild alkalosis is generally well tolerated. Severe or symptomatic alkalosis (pH > 7.60) requires urgent treatment.

A. Saline-Responsive Metabolic Alkalosis

Therapy for saline-responsive metabolic alkalosis is aimed at correction of extracellular volume deficit. Depending on the degree of hypovolemia, adequate amounts of 0.9% NaCl and KCl should be administered. Discontinuation of diuretics and administration of H₂-blockers in patients whose alkalosis is due to nasogastric suction can be useful. If impaired pulmonary or cardiovascular status prohibits adequate volume repletion, acetazolamide, 250–500 mg intravenously every 4–6 hours, can be used. One must be alert to the possible development of hypokalemia, since potassium depletion can be induced by forced kaliuresis via bicarbonaturia. Administration of acid can be used as emergency therapy. HCl, 0.1 mol/L, is infused via a central vein (the solution is sclerosing). Dosage is calculated to decrease the HCO₃⁻ level by one-half over 2–4 hours, assuming a HCO₃⁻ volume of distribution (L) of 0.5 × body weight (kg). Patients with marked renal insufficiency may require dialysis.

B. Saline-Unresponsive Metabolic Alkalosis

Therapy for saline-unresponsive metabolic alkalosis includes surgical removal of a mineralocorticoid-producing tumor and blockage of aldosterone effect with an angiotensin-converting enzyme inhibitor or with spironolactone. Metabolic alkalosis in primary aldosteronism can be treated only with potassium repletion.

Table 21–18. Replacement guidelines for sweat and gastrointestinal fluid losses.

	Average Electrolyte Composition				Replacement Guidelines per Liter Lost				
	Na⁺ (meq/L)	K⁺ (meq/L)	Cl⁻ (meq/L)	HCO₃⁻ (meq/L)	0.9% saline (mL)	0.45% saline (mL)	D₅W (mL)	KCl (meq/L)	7.5% NaHCO₃ (45 meq HCO₃⁻/amp)
Sweat	30–50	5	50			500	500	5	
Gastric secretions	20	10	10			300	700	20	
Pancreatic juice	130	5	35	115		400	600	5	2 amps
Bile	145	5	100	25	600		400	5	0.5 amp
Duodenal fluid	60	15	100	10		1000		15	0.25 amp
Ileal fluid	100	10	60	60		600	400	10	1 amp
Colonic diarrhea	140[1]	10	85	60		1000		10	1 amp

[1]In the absence of diarrhea, colonic fluid Na⁺ levels are low (40 meq/L).

Adrogue HJ et al: Management of life threatening acid base disorders. (Part 2.) N Engl J Med 1998;338:107. [PMID: 98069970]

Khanna A et al: Metabolic alkalosis. Respir Care 2001;46:354. [PMID: 11262555]

■ FLUID MANAGEMENT

Most of those who require water and electrolyte intravenously are relatively normal people who cannot take orally what they require for maintenance. The range of tolerance for water and electrolytes (homeostatic limits) permits reasonable latitude in therapy provided normal renal function exists to accomplish the final regulation of volume and concentration.

An average adult whose entire intake is parenteral would require for maintenance 2500–3000 mL of 5% dextrose in 0.2% saline solution (34 meq Na^+ plus 34 meq Cl^-/L). To each liter, 30 meq of KCl could be added. In 3 L, the total chloride intake would be 192 meq, which is easily tolerated. Guidelines for gastrointestinal fluid losses are shown in Table 21–18.

In situations requiring maintenance or maintenance plus replacement of fluid and electrolyte by parenteral infusion, the total daily ration should be administered continuously over the 24-hour period in order to ensure the best utilization by the patient.

If parenteral fluids are the only source of water, electrolytes, and calories for longer than a week, more complex fluids containing amino acids, lipid, trace metals, and vitamins may be indicated. (See Total Parenteral Nutrition, Chapter 29.)

Kidney

22

Suzanne Watnick, MD, & Gail Morrison, MD

See www.current-med.com/ch22.html

■ APPROACH TO RENAL DISEASE

A patient will present with renal disease in one of two ways: discovered incidentally during a routine medical evaluation or with evidence of renal dysfunction such as hypertension, edema, nausea, and hematuria. The initial approach in both situations should be to assess the cause and severity of renal abnormalities. In all cases this evaluation includes (1) an estimation of disease duration, (2) a careful urinalysis, and (3) an assessment of the glomerular filtration rate (GFR). The history and physical examination, though equally important, are variable among renal syndromes—thus, specific symptoms and signs are discussed under each disease entity. Further diagnostic categorization is according to anatomic distribution: prerenal disease, postrenal disease, and intrinsic renal disease. Intrinsic renal disease can further be divided into glomerular, tubular, interstitial, and vascular abnormalities.

DISEASE DURATION

Renal disease may be acute or chronic. Acute renal failure is worsening of renal function over hours to days, resulting in the retention of nitrogenous wastes (such as urea nitrogen) and creatinine in the blood. Retention of these substances is called azotemia. Chronic renal failure results from an abnormal loss of renal function over months to years. Differentiating between the two is important for diagnosis, treatment, and outcome. Oliguria is unusual in chronic renal insufficiency. Anemia (from low renal erythropoietin production) is rare in the initial period of acute renal failure. Small kidneys are most consistent with chronic renal failure, whereas normal to large sizes can be seen with both.

URINALYSIS

A urinalysis has been likened to "a poor man's renal biopsy." The urine is collected in midstream or, if that is not feasible, by bladder catheterization. The urine should be examined within 1 hour after collection.

Urinalysis includes a dipstick examination followed by microscopic assessment if the dipstick has positive findings. The dipstick examination measures urinary specific gravity, pH, protein, hemoglobin, glucose, ketones, bilirubin, nitrites, and leukocyte esterase. Microscopy searches for all formed elements—crystals, cells, casts, and infecting organisms.

Various findings on the urinalysis are indicative of certain patterns of renal disease (Table 22–1). A bland urinary sediment is common, especially in chronic renal disease and prerenal and postrenal disorders. Red blood cells are misshapen during passage from the capillary through the glomerular basement membrane into the urinary space of Bowman's capsule. The presence of hematuria with dysmorphic red blood cells, red blood cell casts, and mild proteinuria is indicative of glomerulonephritis. Casts are composed of Tamm-Horsfall urinary mucoprotein in the shape of the nephron segment where they were formed. Heavy proteinuria and lipiduria are consistent with the nephrotic syndrome. Pigmented granular casts and renal tubular epithelial cells alone or in casts suggest acute tubular necrosis. White blood cells, including neutrophils and eosinophils, white blood cell casts, red blood cells, and small amounts of protein can be found in interstitial nephritis and pyelonephritis; Wright's stain can detect eosinophilia. Pyuria alone can indicate a urinary tract infection. Hematuria and proteinuria are discussed more thoroughly below.

Proteinuria

Proteinuria is defined as excessive protein excretion in the urine, generally > 150–160 mg/24 h in adults. Significant proteinuria is a sign of an underlying renal abnormality, usually glomerular in origin when greater than 1 g/d. It is typically accompanied by other clinical abnormalities—elevated BUN and serum creatinine levels, abnormal urinary sediment, or evidence of systemic illness (eg, fever, rash, vasculitis).

There are four primary reasons for development of proteinuria.

(1) Functional proteinuria is a benign process stemming from stressors such as acute illness, exercise,

Table 22–1. Significance of specific urinary casts.

Type	Significance
Hyaline casts	Concentrated urine, febrile disease, after strenuous exercise, in the course of diuretic therapy (not indicative of renal disease)
Red cell casts	Glomerulonephritis
White cell casts	Pyelonephritis, interstitial nephritis (indicative of infection or inflammation)
Renal tubular cell casts	Acute tubular necrosis, interstitial nephritis
Coarse, granular casts	Nonspecific; can represent acute tubular necrosis
Broad, waxy casts	Chronic renal failure (indicative of stasis in collecting tubule)

and "orthostatic proteinuria." The latter condition, generally found in people under age 30, results in the excretion of abnormal amounts of urinary protein, typically less than 1 g/d.

(2) Overload proteinuria can result from overproduction of circulating, filterable plasma proteins, such as Bence Jones proteins associated with multiple myeloma. Urinary protein electrophoresis will exhibit a discrete protein peak. Other examples of overload proteinuria include myoglobinuria in rhabdomyolysis and lysozymuria in certain leukemias.

(3) Glomerular proteinuria results from effacement of epithelial cell foot processes and altered glomerular permeability with an increased filtration fraction of normal plasma proteins. All glomerular diseases exhibit some degree of proteinuria. The urinary electrophoresis will have a pattern exhibiting a large albumin spike indicative of increased permeability of albumin across a damaged GBM.

(4) Tubular proteinuria occurs as a result of damaged reabsorption of normally filtered proteins in the proximal tubule, particularly β_2-microglobulin. Causes include acute tubular necrosis, toxic injury (lead, aminoglycosides), drug-induced interstitial nephritis, and hereditary metabolic disorders (Wilson's disease and Fanconi's syndrome).

Evaluation of proteinuria by urinary dipstick primarily detects albumin and intact globulins, while overlooking positively charged light chains of immunoglobulins. These proteins can be detected by the addition of sulfosalicylic acid to the urine specimen. The lack of precipitation indicates the absence of paraproteins.

The next step—and the most reliable way to quantify proteinuria—is a 24-hour urine collection. A finding of > 150 mg/24 h is abnormal, and > 3.5 g/24 h is consistent with nephrotic-range proteinuria. A simpler and less accurate method is to collect a random urine sample. The ratio of the urinary protein concentration to the urinary creatinine concentration ($U_{protein}/U_{creatinine}$) correlates with 24-hour urine protein collection (< 0.2 is normal and corresponds to excretion of less than 200 mg/d). If a patient has proteinuria with loss of renal function, renal biopsy may be indicated, particularly if the renal insufficiency is acute in onset. The clinical consequences of proteinuria are discussed in the section on the nephrotic syndrome.

In both diabetics and nondiabetics, therapy aimed at reducing proteinuria may also reduce progression of renal disease. ACE inhibitors are effective by lowering efferent arteriolar resistance out of proportion to afferent arteriolar resistance, thereby reducing glomerular capillary pressure and lowering urinary protein excretion. Other effects include alterations of glomerular mesangial proliferation. ACE inhibitors can be used in patients despite compromised GFR as long as significant hyperkalemia does not occur and serum creatinine rises less than 30%, stabilizing over 2 months. More recently, large randomized controlled trials (the RENAAL and IDNT studies) have also proved the benefit of angiotensin II receptor blockers in reducing proteinuria and preventing the progression of renal disease in diabetic nephropathy. The consequences of dietary restrictions in patients with proteinuria are discussed in the section on chronic renal failure.

Hematuria

Hematuria is significant if there are more than three to five red cells per high-power field. It is usually detected incidentally by the urine dipstick examination or by an episode of macroscopic hematuria. The diagnosis must be confirmed via microscopic examination, as false-positive dipstick tests can be caused by vitamin C, beets and rhubarb, bacteria, and myoglobin. Transient hematuria is common, but in patients under 40 it is less often of clinical significance.

Hematuria may be due to renal or extrarenal causes. Extrarenal causes are addressed in Chapter 23; the most worrisome of these are urologic malignancies. Renal causes account for approximately 10% of cases and are best considered anatomically as glomerular or nonglomerular. The most common extraglomerular sources include cysts, calculi, interstitial nephritis, and renal neoplasia. Glomerular causes include IgA nephropathy, thin GBM disease, postinfectious glomerulonephritis, membranoproliferative glomerulonephritis, and the systemic nephritic syndromes.

Currently, the United States Health Preventive Services Task Force does not recommend screening for hematuria. See Chapter 23 for evaluation of hematuria.

ESTIMATION OF GFR

The glomerular filtration rate (GFR) provides a useful index of overall renal function; however, patients with renal disease can actually have a normal or increased GFR. The GFR measures the amount of plasma ultrafiltered across the glomerular capillaries and correlates with the ability of the kidneys to filter fluids and various substances. Daily GFR in normal individuals is variable, with a range of 150–250 L/24 h or 100–120 mL/min/1.73 m^2 of body surface area. GFR can be measured indirectly by determining the renal clearance of plasma substances which are not bound to plasma proteins, are freely filterable across the glomerulus, and are neither secreted nor reabsorbed along the renal tubules.

The formula used to determine the renal clearance of a substance is

$$C = \frac{U \times \dot{V}}{P}$$

where C is the clearance, U and P are the urine and plasma concentrations of the substance (mg/dL), and $\dot{V}$ is the urine flow rate (mL/min). Inulin and creatinine clearance are used as markers of GFR. Inulin clearance following a continuous infusion is one of the most accurate methods for measurement of GFR. The cost and the complexity of the administration and analysis of inulin preclude its routine use. In clinical practice, the clearance rate of endogenous creatinine, the creatinine clearance (C_{cr}), is the usual means of estimating GFR.

Creatinine is a product of muscle metabolism produced at a relatively constant rate and cleared by renal excretion. It is freely filterable by the glomerulus and not reabsorbed by the renal tubules. With stable renal function, creatinine production and excretion are equal, thus, plasma creatinine concentrations remain constant. However, it is not a perfect indicator of GFR for the following reasons: (1) a small amount is normally eliminated by tubular secretion, and the fraction secreted progressively increases as GFR declines (overestimating GFR); (2) with severe renal failure, gut microorganisms degrade creatinine; (3) an individual's meat intake and muscle mass affect baseline plasma creatinine levels; (4) commonly used drugs such as cimetidine, probenecid, and trimethoprim reduce tubular secretion of creatinine, increasing the plasma creatinine concentration and falsely indicating renal dysfunction; and (5) the accuracy of the measurement necessitates a stable plasma creatinine concentration over a 24-hour period, so that during the development of and recovery from acute renal failure, the C_{cr} is a questionable value (see Table 22–2).

To measure creatinine clearance, collect a 24-hour urine sample and determine the plasma creatinine level on the same day. An incomplete or prolonged urine collection is a common source of error. One way of estimating the completeness of the collection is to calculate a 24-hour creatinine excretion; the amount should be constant:

$$U_{cr} \times V = 15 - 20 \text{ mg/kg for healthy young women}$$
$$U_{cr} \times V = 20 - 25 \text{ mg/kg for healthy young men}$$

The creatinine clearance is approximately 100 mL/min/1.73 m^2 in healthy young women and 120 mL/min/1.73 m^2 in healthy young men. The C_{cr} declines by 1 mL/min/yr after age 40 as part of the aging process.

Since urine collection may be difficult, creatinine clearance can be estimated from the formula of Cockcroft and Gault, which incorporates age, sex, and weight to estimate creatinine clearance from plasma creatinine levels without any urinary measurements:

$$C_{cr} = \frac{(140 - Age) \times Weight \text{ (kg)}}{P_{cr} \times 72}$$

For women, the estimated GFR is multiplied by 0.85 because muscle mass is less. This formula overestimates GFR in patients who are obese or edematous.

Urea is another index helpful in assessing renal function. It is synthesized mainly in the liver and is the end product of protein catabolism. Urea is freely filtered by the glomerulus, and about 30–70% is reabsorbed in the nephron. Unlike creatinine clearance, which overestimates GFR, urea clearance underestimates GFR. Urea reabsorption may be decreased in well-hydrated patients, whereas dehydration causes increased reabsorption, increasing blood urea nitrogen (BUN). A normal BUN:creatinine ratio is 10:1. With dehydration, the ratio can increase to 20:1 or higher.

Table 22–2. Conditions affecting serum creatinine independently of GFR.

Condition	Mechanism
Conditions causing elevation	
Ketoacidosis	Noncreatinine chromogen
Cephalothin, cefoxitin	Noncreatinine chromogen
Other drugs: aspirin, cimetidine, trimethoprim	Inhibition of tubular creatinine secretion
Conditions causing decrease	
Advanced age	Physiologic decrease in muscle mass
Cachexia	Pathologic decrease in muscle mass
Liver disease	Decreased hepatic creatine synthesis and cachexia

Other causes of increased BUN include increased catabolism (gastrointestinal bleeding, cell lysis, and steroid usage), increased dietary protein, and decreased renal perfusion (congestive heart failure, renal artery stenosis (Table 22–3). Reduced BUN is seen in liver disease and in the syndrome of inappropriate antidiuretic hormone secretion (SIADH).

As patients approach end-stage renal disease, a more accurate measure of GFR than creatinine clearance is the average of the creatinine and urea clearances. The creatinine clearance overestimates GFR, as mentioned above, while the urea clearance underestimates GFR.

IMAGING STUDIES

Radionuclide Studies

Radionuclide studies can measure renal function. ^{125}I-iothalamate gives a surprisingly accurate measurement of GFR. It is injected intravenously, excreted renally, and sampled from the venous circulation over time. Technetium diethylenetriamine pentaacetic acid (^{99m}Tc-DTPA) is freely filtered by the glomerulus and not reabsorbed and is used to estimate GFR. Technetium dimercaptosuccinate (^{99m}Tc-DMSA) is bound to the tubules and provides an assessment of functional renal mass. Radioiodinated (^{131}I) orthoiodohippurate is secreted into the renal tubules and assesses renal plasma flow (RPF). The indications for nuclear renography are to measure function and flow; to determine the contribution of each kidney to overall renal function; to demonstrate the presence or absence of functioning renal tissue in mass lesions; to detect obstruction; and to evaluate renovascular disease.

Poor flow along with poor function is consistent with acute tubular necrosis or end-stage renal disease. Decreased flow to one kidney suggests arterial occlusion of that kidney. To further investigate renal artery stenosis, the test is done both with and without captopril (see Chapter 11).

Table 22–3. Conditions affecting BUN independently of GFR.

Increased BUN
  Reduced effective circulating blood volume (prerenal
    azotemia)
  Catabolic states
  High-protein diets
  Gastrointestinal bleeding
  Glucocorticoids
  Tetracycline
Decreased BUN
  Liver disease
  Malnutrition
  Sickle cell anemia
  SIADH

Ultrasonography

Ultrasonography can identify the thickness and echogenicity of the renal cortex, medulla, pyramids, and a distended urinary collecting system. Kidney size can be determined; a kidney less than 9 cm in length indicates significant irreversible renal disease. A difference in size of more than 1.5 cm between the two kidneys is observed in unilateral renal disease. Renal ultrasound is also performed to search for hydronephrosis, characterize renal mass lesions, screen for autosomal dominant polycystic kidney disease, evaluate the perirenal space, localize the kidney for a percutaneous invasive procedure, and assess postvoiding bladder residual.

Intravenous Urography

The intravenous pyelogram (IVP) has been for many years the standard imaging procedure for evaluating the urinary tract since it provides an assessment of the kidneys, ureters, and bladder. The dye is filtered and secreted by the renal tubules in normal kidneys, resulting in a nephrogram formed by opacification of the renal parenchyma. The density of the nephrogram is dependent on the GFR. Filling of the pelvicaliceal system produces the pyelogram. The IVP can demonstrate differential function between the right and left kidneys by the rate of appearance of the nephrogram phase.

An IVP necessitates the injection of contrast and is relatively contraindicated in patients with an increased risk for developing acute renal failure (eg, diabetes mellitus with serum creatinine > 2 mg/dL, severe volume contraction, or prerenal azotemia), chronic renal failure with serum creatinine greater than 5 mg/dL, and multiple myeloma. IVP is performed to obtain a detailed view of the pelvicaliceal system, assess renal size and shape, detect and localize renal stones, and assess renal function. Helical computed tomography is replacing IVP for stone evaluation, and ultrasonography is replacing IVP to avoid dye administration.

Computed Tomography

Computed tomography (CT) is required for further investigation of abnormalities detected by ultrasound or IVP. Although the routine study requires radiographic contrast administration, no contrast is necessary if the reason for the study is to demonstrate hemorrhage or calcifications in the kidneys such as suspected stone disease. Since contrast is filtered by the glomeruli and concentrated in the tubules, there is enhancement of parenchymal tissue, making abnormalities such as cysts or neoplasms easily identified and allowing good visualization of renal vessels and ureters. CT is especially useful for evaluation of solid or cystic lesions in the kidney or the retroperitoneal space, particularly if the ultrasound results are suboptimal.

Magnetic Resonance Imaging (MRI)

MRI can easily distinguish renal cortex from medulla. Loss of corticomedullary function, which can be seen in a variety of disorders (glomerulonephritis, hydronephrosis, renal vascular occlusion, and renal failure) will be evident on MRI. Renal cysts seen on a CT scan can also be identified by MRI. For some solid lesions, MRI may be superior to CT scanning. MRI is indicated as an addition or alternative to CT for staging renal cell cancer and as a substitute for CT in the evaluation of a renal mass, especially for patients in whom contrast is contraindicated; in addition, the adrenals are well imaged.

Arteriography & Venography

Renal arteriography is useful in the evaluation of atherosclerotic or fibrodysplastic stenotic lesions, aneurysms, vasculitis, and renal mass lesions. Venography is useful to diagnose renal vein thrombosis, though CT and MRI are less invasive for this purpose.

RENAL BIOPSY

Indications for percutaneous needle biopsy include (1) unexplained acute renal failure or chronic renal insufficiency; (2) acute nephritic syndromes; (3) unexplained proteinuria and hematuria; (4) previously identified and treated lesions to plan future therapy; (5) systemic diseases associated with kidney dysfunction, such as systemic lupus erythematosus, Goodpasture's syndrome, and Wegener's granulomatosis, to confirm the extent of renal involvement and to guide management suspected transplant rejection, to differentiate it from other causes of acute renal failure and to guide treatment. Relative contraindications include a solitary or ectopic kidney (exception: transplant allografts), horseshoe kidney, uncorrected bleeding disorder, severe uncontrolled hypertension, renal infection, renal neoplasm, hydronephrosis, end-stage renal disease, congenital anomalies, multiple cysts, or an uncooperative patient. Prior to biopsy, patients should have well-controlled blood pressure, a hematocrit, platelet count, prothrombin time, partial thromboplastin time, and perhaps a bleeding time. After biopsy, hematuria occurs in nearly all patients. Fewer than 10% will have macroscopic hematuria. A patient with a postbiopsy hematocrit more than 3% lower than baseline should be closely monitored.

Percutaneous kidney biopsies are generally safe. One percent of patients will experience significant bleeding and 0.1% will require blood transfusions. The risks of nephrectomy and mortality are about 0.01–0.06%. When a percutaneous needle biopsy is technically not feasible and renal tissue is deemed clinically essential, a closed renal biopsy via interventional radiologic techniques or open renal biopsy under general anesthesia can be done.

Andreucci VE et al: Role of renal biopsy in the diagnosis and prognosis of acute renal failure. Kidney Int 1998;66 (Suppl):S91. [PMID: 9573582]

Grossfeld GD et al: Asymptomatic microscopic hematuria in adults: summary of the AUA best practice policy recommendations. Am Fam Physician 2001;63:1145. [PMID:11277551]

Manjunath G et al: Estimating the glomerular filtration rate. Postgraduate Med 2001;110:55. [PMID: 11787409]

Mucelli RP et al: Imaging techniques in acute renal failure. Kidney Int 1998;66(Suppl):S102. [PMID: 9573584]

Ruggenenti P et al: Cross sectional longitudinal study of spot morning urine protein:creatinine ratio, 24 hour urine protein excretion rate, glomerular filtration rate, and end stage renal failure in chronic renal disease in patients without diabetes. BMJ 1998;316:504. [PMID: 9501711] (Cross-sectional study of 177 nondiabetic outpatients with chronic renal disease. When compared with 24-hour urinary protein collection, the protein:creatinine ratio in a spot urine sample is a precise indicator of proteinuria.)

Wingo CS et al: Proteinuria: potential causes and approach to evaluation. Am J Med Sci 2000;320:188. [PMID: 11014373]

■ ACUTE RENAL FAILURE

 ESSENTIALS OF DIAGNOSIS

- *Sudden increase in BUN or serum creatinine.*
- *Oliguria often associated.*
- *Symptoms and signs depend on cause.*

General Considerations

Five percent of hospital admissions and 30% of ICU admissions have acute renal failure, and 25% of hospitalized patients will develop it. Acute renal failure is defined as a sudden decrease in renal function, resulting in an inability to maintain fluid and electrolyte balance and to excrete nitrogenous wastes. Serum creatinine is a convenient marker. In the absence of functioning kidneys, serum creatinine concentration will typically increase 1–1.5 mg/dL daily—although with certain conditions, such as rhabdomyolysis, serum creatinine can increase more rapidly.

Clinical Findings

A. SYMPTOMS AND SIGNS

The uremic milieu of acute renal failure can cause nonspecific symptoms. When present, they are often due to azotemia and the underlying cause of acute renal failure. Azotemia can cause nausea, vomiting, malaise, and altered sensorium. Hypertension is rare, but fluid homeostasis is often altered. Hypovolemia can cause prerenal failure, whereas hypervolemia can result from intrinsic renal failure or postrenal failure. Pericardial effusions can occur with azotemia, and a pericardial friction rub can be present. Effusions may result in cardiac tamponade. Arrhythmias occur especially with hyperkalemia. The pulmonary examination may show rales in the presence of hypervolemia. Acute renal failure can cause nonspecific diffuse abdominal pain and ileus as well as platelet dysfunction; thus, bleeding is more common in these patients. The neurologic examination reveals encephalopathic changes with asterixis and confusion; seizures may ensue.

B. LABORATORY FINDINGS

Elevated BUN and creatinine are present, though these elevations do not in themselves distinguish acute from chronic renal failure (Table 22–4). Hyperkalemia often occurs from impaired renal potassium excretion. The ECG can reveal peaked T waves, PR prolongation, and QRS widening. A long QT segment can occur with hypocalcemia. Anion gap metabolic acidosis (due to decreased organic acid clearance) is often noted. Hyperphosphatemia occurs when phosphorus cannot be secreted by damaged tubules either with or without increased cell catabolism. Hypocalcemia with metastatic calcium phosphate deposition may be observed when the product of calcium and phosphorus exceeds 70 mg/dL. Anemia can occur as a result of decreased erythropoietin production, and associated platelet dysfunction is typical.

Classification & Etiology

Acute renal failure can be divided into three categories: prerenal azotemia, intrinsic renal failure, and postrenal azotemia. Identifying the cause is the first step toward managing the patient. (See Table 22–4.)

A. PRERENAL AZOTEMIA

Prerenal azotemia is the most common cause of acute renal failure. It is due to renal hypoperfusion. This is an appropriate physiologic change. If it can be immediately reversed with restoration of renal blood flow, renal parenchymal damage does not occur. If hypoperfusion persists, ischemia can result, causing intrinsic renal failure.

Decreased renal perfusion can occur in one of three ways: a decrease in intravascular volume, a change in vascular resistance, or low cardiac output. Causes of volume depletion include hemorrhage, gastrointestinal losses, dehydration, excessive diuresis, extravascular space sequestration, pancreatitis, burns, trauma, and peritonitis.

Changes in vascular resistance can occur systemically with sepsis, anaphylaxis, anesthesia, and afterload-reducing drugs. ACE inhibitors prevent efferent renal arteriolar constriction out of proportion to the afferent arteriole; thus, GFR will decrease. NSAIDs prevent afferent arteriolar vasodilation by inhibiting prostaglandin-mediated signals. Thus, in cirrhosis and congestive heart failure, when prostaglandins are recruited to increase renal blood flow, NSAIDs will have particularly deleterious effects. Epinephrine, norepinephrine, high-dose dopamine, anesthetic agents, and cyclosporine also can cause renal vasoconstriction. Renal artery stenosis causes increased resistance and decreased perfusion.

Low cardiac output is a state of effective hypovolemia. This occurs in states of cardiogenic shock, congestive heart failure, pulmonary embolus, and peri-

Table 22–4. Classification and differential diagnosis of renal failure.

| | Prerenal Azotemia | Postrenal Azotemia | Intrinsic Renal Disease | | |
			Acute Tubular Necrosis (Oliguric or Polyuric)	Acute Glomerulonephritis	Acute Interstitial Nephritis
Etiology	Poor renal perfusion	Obstruction of the urinary tract	Ischemia, nephrotoxins	Poststreptococcal; collagen-vascular disease	Allergic reaction; drug reaction
Urinary indices Serum BUN:Cr ratio	> 20:1	> 20:1	< 20:1	> 20:1	< 20:1
U_{Na} (meq/L)	< 20	Variable	> 20	< 20	Variable
FE_{Na} (%)	< 1	Variable	> 1	< 1	< 1; > 1
Urine osmolality (mosm/kg)	> 500	< 400	250–300	Variable	Variable
Urinary sediment	Benign, or hyaline casts	Normal or red cells, white cells, or crystals	Granular casts, renal tubular casts	Dysmorphic red cells and red cell casts	White cells, white cell casts, with or without eosinophils

cardial tamponade. Arrhythmias and valvular disorders can also reduce cardiac output. In the ICU setting, positive-pressure ventilation will decrease venous return, also decreasing cardiac output.

When GFR falls acutely, it is important to determine whether acute renal failure is due to prerenal or intrinsic renal causes. The history and physical examination are important, and urinalysis can be helpful. The BUN:creatinine ratio will typically exceed 20:1 owing to increased urea reabsorption. Another useful index is the fractional excretion of sodium. With decreased GFR, the kidney will reabsorb salt and water avidly if there is no intrinsic tubular dysfunction. Thus, patients with prerenal failure should have a low fractional excretion percent of sodium (< 1%). The FE_{Na} is calculated as follows: Fractional excretion of Na^+ (FE_{Na}) = clearance of Na^+/GFR = Clearance of Na^+/creatinine clearance (C_{Cr}):

$$FE_{Na} = \frac{Urine_{sodium} / Plasma_{sodium}}{Urine_{creatinine} / Plasma_{creatinine}} \times 100\%$$

The causes of oliguric states are more accurately assessed with this formula than the causes of nonoliguric states because the kidneys do not avidly reabsorb water and sodium in nonoliguric states. (Oliguria is defined as urine output < 500 mL/d.) Diuretics can cause increased sodium excretion. Thus, if the FE_{Na} is high within 12–24 hours after diuretic administration, the cause of acute renal failure may not be accurately predicted. Acute renal failure due to glomerulonephritis can have a low FE_{Na} because sodium reabsorption and tubular function may not be compromised.

Treatment of prerenal azotemia depends entirely on its cause, but maintenance of euvolemia, attention to serum potassium, and avoidance of nephrotoxic drugs are the benchmarks of therapy. This involves careful assessment of volume status, drug usage, and cardiac function.

B. POSTRENAL AZOTEMIA

Postrenal azotemia is the least common cause of acute renal failure, accounting for approximately 5% of cases, but is perhaps the most important cause to detect because of its reversibility. It occurs when urinary flow from both kidneys is obstructed. Each nephron has an elevated intraluminal pressure, causing a decrease in GFR.

Causes include urethral obstruction, bladder dysfunction or obstruction, and obstruction of both ureters or renal pelvises. In men, benign prostatic hyperplasia is the most common cause. Patients taking anticholinergic drugs are particularly at risk. Bladder, prostate, and cervical cancers as well as retroperitoneal processes and neurogenic bladder can also cause obstruction. Less common causes are blood clots, bilateral ureteral stones, urethral stones or stricture, and bilateral papillary necrosis. In patients with a single

functioning kidney, obstruction of a solitary ureter can cause postrenal azotemia.

Patients may be anuric or polyuric and may complain of lower abdominal pain. Obstruction can be constant or intermittent and partial or complete. On examination, the patient may have an enlarged prostate, distended bladder, or a mass detected on pelvic examination.

Laboratory examination may initially reveal high urine osmolality, low urine sodium, high BUN:creatinine ratio, and low FE_{Na}. These indices are similar to a prerenal picture because extensive intrinsic renal damage has not occurred. After several days, the urine sodium increases as the kidneys fail and are unable to concentrate the urine—thus, isosthenuria is present. The urine sediment is generally benign.

Patients with acute renal failure and suspected postrenal azotemia should undergo bladder ultrasonography and bladder catheterization if hydroureter and hydronephrosis are present along with an enlarged bladder. These patients often undergo a postobstructive diuresis, and care should be taken to avoid dehydration. Rarely, the presence of obstruction is not seen via ultrasonography. For example, patients with retroperitoneal fibrosis from tumor or radiation may not show dilation of the urinary tract. If suspicion does exist, a CT scan or MRI can establish the diagnosis. Promptly treated obstruction with catheters or stents can result in complete reversal of the acute process.

C. INTRINSIC RENAL FAILURE

Intrinsic renal disorders account for half of all cases of acute renal failure. Intrinsic (or parenchymal) dysfunction is considered after prerenal and postrenal causes have been excluded. The sites of injury are the tubules, the interstitium, the vasculature, and the glomeruli.

ACUTE TUBULAR NECROSIS

 ESSENTIALS OF DIAGNOSIS

- *Acute renal insufficiency.*
- *$FE_{Na} > 1\%$.*
- *Urine sediment with pigmented granular casts and renal tubular epithelial cells.*

General Considerations

Acute renal failure due to tubular damage is termed acute tubular necrosis and accounts for 85% of intrinsic acute renal failure. The two major causes of acute tubular necrosis are ischemia and toxin exposure. Ischemia causes tubular damage from states of low perfusion and is often preceded by a state of prerenal azotemia. Ischemic acute renal failure is characterized not only by inadequate GFR but also by renal blood flow inadequate to maintain parenchymal cellular formation. This occurs in the setting of prolonged hypotension or hypoxemia such as dehydration, shock, and sepsis. Major surgical procedures can involve prolonged periods of hypoperfusion which are exacerbated by vasodilating anesthetic agents.

The other major cause of acute tubular necrosis is nephrotoxin exposure. Exogenous nephrotoxins more commonly cause damage than endogenous toxins.

A. Exogenous Nephrotoxins

Up to 25% of hospitalized patients receiving therapeutic levels of aminoglycosides sustain some degree of acute tubular necrosis. Nonoliguric renal failure typically occurs after 5–10 days of exposure. Predisposing factors include underlying renal damage, dehydration, and advanced age. Monitoring of peak and trough levels is important, but trough levels are more helpful in predicting renal toxicity. Gentamicin is the most and tobramycin the least nephrotoxic. Amphotericin B is typically nephrotoxic after a dose of 2–3 g. This causes severe vasoconstriction with distal tubular damage and can lead to distal renal tubular acidosis with hypokalemia and nephrogenic diabetes insipidus. Vancomycin, acyclovir, and several cephalosporins have been known to cause acute tubular necrosis.

Radiographic contrast media can be directly nephrotoxic. Contrast nephropathy is the third leading cause of new acute renal failure in hospitalized patients. It results from the synergistic combination of direct renal tubular epithelial cell toxicity and renal medullary ischemia. Predisposing factors include advanced age, preexisting renal disease (serum creatinine > 2 mg/dL), volume depletion, diabetic nephropathy, congestive heart failure, repeated doses of contrast, and recent exposure to other nephrotoxic agents, including NSAIDs and ACE inhibitors. The combination of diabetes mellitus and renal dysfunction poses the greatest risk for contrast nephropathy. Lower volumes of contrast are recommended in high-risk patients, though this has never been consistently demonstrated in trials. Toxicity usually occurs 24–48 hours after the radiocontrast study. Nonionic contrast media may be less toxic, but this has never been proved. Prevention should be the goal when using these agents. Patients should be hydrated with 1 L of 0.45% saline over 12 hours both before and after the contrast administration—cautiously to patients with preexisting cardiac dysfunction. Neither mannitol nor furosemide offers benefit over saline hydration. In a recent study, acetylcysteine given before and after contrast decreased the incidence of dye-induced nephrotoxicity. These results have not yet been validated. Other nephrotoxic agents should be avoided during the day before and after administration.

Cyclosporine toxicity is usually dose-dependent. It causes distal tubular dysfunction from severe vasoconstriction. Regular blood level monitoring is important to prevent nephrotoxicity. With patients who are taking cyclosporine for renal transplant rejection, kidney biopsy is often necessary to distinguish transplant rejection from cyclosporine toxicity. Renal function usually improves after reducing the dose or stopping the drug.

Other exogenous nephrotoxins include antineoplastics, such as cisplatin and organic solvents, and heavy metals such as mercury, cadmium, and arsenic.

B. Endogenous Nephrotoxins

Endogenous nephrotoxins include heme-containing products, uric acid, and paraproteins. Myoglobinuria as a consequence of rhabdomyolysis leads to acute tubular necrosis. Necrotic muscle releases large amounts of myoglobin, which is freely filtered across the glomerulus. The myoglobin is reabsorbed by the renal tubules, and direct damage can occur. Distal tubular obstruction from pigmented casts and intrarenal vasoconstriction can also cause damage. This type of renal failure occurs in the setting of crush injury, muscle necrosis from prolonged unconsciousness, seizures, cocaine, and alcohol abuse. Dehydration and acidosis predisposes to the development of myoglobinuric acute renal failure. Patients may complain of muscular pain and often have signs of muscle injury. Rhabdomyolysis of clinical importance commonly occurs with a serum creatine kinase > 20,000–50,000 IU/L. One study showed that 58% of patients with acute renal failure from rhabdomyolysis had CK levels > 16,000 IU/L. Only 11% of patients without renal failure had CK values > 16,000 IU/L. The globin moiety of myoglobin will cause the urine dipstick to read falsely positive for hemoglobin: the urine appears dark brown, but no red cells are present. With lysis of muscle cells, patients also become hyperkalemic, hyperphosphatemic, and hyperuricemic. The mainstay of treatment is hydration. Other adjunctive treatments include mannitol for free radical clearance and diuresis as well as alkalinization of the urine. These modalities have not been proved to change outcomes in human trials.

Hemoglobin can cause a similar form of acute renal tubular necrosis. Massive intravascular hemolysis is seen in transfusion reactions and in certain hemolytic anemias. Reversal of the underlying disorder and hydration are the mainstays of treatment.

Hyperuricemia can occur in the setting of rapid cell turnover and lysis. Chemotherapy for germ cell neoplasms and leukemia and lymphoma are the primary causes. Acute renal failure occurs with intratubular deposition of uric acid crystals; serum uric acid levels are often > 20 mg/dL and urine uric acid levels > 600 mg/24 h. A urine uric acid to urine creatinine ratio > 1.0 indicates risk for acute renal failure.

Bence Jones protein seen in conjunction with multiple myeloma can cause direct tubular toxicity and tubular obstruction. Other renal complications from multiple myeloma include hypercalcemia and proximal renal tubular acidosis.

Clinical Findings

A. SYMPTOMS AND SIGNS

See Acute Renal Failure, above.

B. LABORATORY FINDINGS

Urinalysis may show evidence of acute tubular damage. The urine may be brown. On microscopic examination, an active sediment may show pigmented granular casts or "muddy brown" casts. Renal tubular epithelial cells and epithelial cell casts are often present as well. Hyperkalemia and hyperphosphatemia are commonly encountered.

Treatment

Treatment is aimed at hastening recovery and avoiding complications. Preventive measures should be taken to avoid volume overload and hyperkalemia. Loop-blocking diuretics may be used in large doses (eg, furosemide in doses ranging from 20 mg to 160 mg orally or intravenously twice daily) to effect adequate diuresis, and may help convert oliguric to nonoliguric renal failure. Side effects of supranormal dosing include deafness. This is mainly due to peak furosemide levels and can be avoided by the use of a furosemide drip. A starting dose of 0.4–0.6 mg/kg/h is appropriate, increasing to a maximum of 1 mg/kg/h. A bolus of the hourly dose should be administered at the beginning of treatment. Intravenous thiazide diuretics can be used to augment urine output; chlorothiazide, 500 mg intravenously every 8–12 hours, is a reasonable choice. Nutritional support should maintain adequate intake while preventing excessive catabolism. Dietary protein restriction of 0.6 g/kg/d helps to prevent metabolic acidosis. Hypocalcemia and hyperphosphatemia can be improved with diet and phosphate-binding agents such as aluminum hydroxide (500 mg orally with meals) over the short term, calcium carbonate (500–1500 mg orally three times daily), calcium acetate, or sevelamer. Hypocalcemia should not be treated in patients with rhabdomyolysis unless they are symptomatic. Hypermagnesemia can occur because of reduced magnesium excretion by the renal tubules, so magnesium-containing antacids and laxatives should be avoided in these patients. Dosages must be adjusted according to the estimated degree of renal impairment for drugs eliminated by the kidney.

Indications for dialysis in acute renal failure from acute tubular necrosis or other intrinsic disorders are as follows: life-threatening electrolyte disturbances (such as hyperkalemia), volume overload unresponsive to diuresis, worsening acidosis, and uremic complications (eg, encephalopathy, pericarditis, and seizures). In gravely ill patients, less severe but worsening abnormalities may also be indications for dialytic support.

Course & Prognosis

The clinical course of acute tubular necrosis is often divided into three phases: initial injury, maintenance, and recovery. The maintenance phase is expressed as either oliguric (urine output < 500 mL/d) or nonoliguric. Nonoliguric acute tubular necrosis has a better outcome. Conversion from oliguric to nonoliguric states may be attempted but has not been shown to change the prognosis. Drugs such as dopamine and diuretics are sometimes used for this purpose but have not been shown to improve outcomes. "Renal dose" dopamine (1–3 μg/kg/min) can increase renal blood flow but can also potentiate arrhythmias and myocardial ischemia. Rarely, dopamine can cause a significant diuresis. If dopamine does not improve urinary output within a few hours, it should be discontinued. Average duration of this period is 1–3 weeks but may be several months. Cellular repair and removal of tubular debris occur during the maintenance phase. The recovery phase is heralded by diuresis. GFR begins to rise; BUN and serum creatinine fall.

The mortality rate from acute renal failure is 20–50% in medical illness and up to 70% in a surgical setting. Increased mortality is associated with advanced age, severe underlying disease, and multisystem organ failure. Leading causes of death are infections, fluid and electrolyte disturbances, and worsening of underlying disease. Mortality rates have not changed significantly over 20 years, making prevention of acute renal failure a high priority.

INTERSTITIAL NEPHRITIS

 ESSENTIALS OF DIAGNOSIS

- *Fever.*
- *Transient maculopapular rash.*
- *Acute renal insufficiency.*
- *Pyuria (including eosinophiluria), white blood cell casts, and hematuria.*

General Considerations

Acute interstitial nephritis accounts for 10–15% of cases of intrinsic renal failure. An interstitial inflammatory response with edema and possible tubular cell damage is the typical pathologic finding. Cell-mediated immune reactions prevail over humoral responses. T lymphocytes can cause direct cytotoxicity or release lymphokines that recruit monocytes and inflammatory cells.

Although drugs account for over 70% of cases, acute interstitial nephritis also occurs in infectious diseases or immunologic disorders or may be idiopathic. The most common drugs are penicillins and cephalosporins, sulfonamides and sulfonamide-containing diuretics, NSAIDs, rifampin, phenytoin, and allopurinol. Infectious causes include streptococcal infections, leptospirosis, CMV, histoplasmosis, and Rocky Mountain spotted fever. Immunologic entities are more commonly associated with glomerulonephritis, but systemic lupus erythematosus, Sjögren's syndrome, sarcoidosis, and cryoglobulinemia can cause interstitial nephritis.

Clinical Findings

Clinical features can include fever (> 80%), rash (25–50%), arthralgias, and peripheral blood eosinophilia (80%). The urine often contains red cells (95%), white cells, and white cell casts. Proteinuria can be a feature, particularly in NSAID-induced interstitial nephritis but is usually modest. Eosinophiluria can be detected by Wright's stain.

Treatment & Prognosis

Acute interstitial nephritis often carries a good prognosis. Recovery occurs over weeks to months, but acute dialytic therapy may be necessary in up to one-third of all patients before resolution. (See indications for dialysis, above.) Patients rarely progress to end-stage renal disease. Those with prolonged courses of oliguric failure and advanced age have a worse prognosis. Treatment consists of supportive measures and removal of the inciting agent. If renal failure persists after removal of the inciting agent, a short course of steroids can be given. Short-term, high dose methylprednisolone (0.5–1 g/d for 1–4 days) or prednisone (60 mg/d for 1–2 weeks) followed by a prednisone taper can be used in these more severe cases of drug-induced interstitial nephritis.

GLOMERULONEPHRITIS

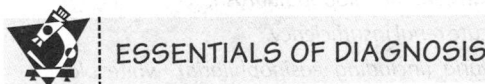

ESSENTIALS OF DIAGNOSIS

- *Hematuria, dysmorphic red cells, red cell casts, and mild proteinuria.*
- *Dependent edema and hypertension.*
- *Acute renal insufficiency.*

General Considerations

Acute glomerulonephritis is a relatively uncommon cause of acute renal failure, accounting for about 5% of cases of intrinsic renal failure. Pathologically, inflammatory glomerular lesions are seen. These include mesangioproliferative, focal and diffuse proliferative, and crescentic lesions. The larger the percentage of glomeruli involved and the more severe the lesion, the more likely it is that the patient will have a poor clinical outcome.

Categorization of acute glomerulonephritis can be done by serologic analysis. Markers include antineutrophil cytoplasmic antibodies (ANCA), anti-glomerular basement membrane (GBM) antibodies, and other immune markers of disease.

Immune complex deposition usually occurs when moderate antigen excess over antibody production occurs. Complexes formed with marked antigen excess tend to remain in the circulation. Antibody excess with large antigen-antibody aggregates usually results in phagocytosis and clearance of the precipitates by the mononuclear phagocytic system in the liver and spleen. Causes include IgA nephropathy (Berger's disease), peri- or postinfectious glomerulonephritis, lupus nephritis, cryoglobulinemic glomerulonephritis (often associated with hepatitis C virus), and membranoproliferative glomerulonephritis.

Anti-GBM-associated acute glomerulonephritis is either confined to the kidney or associated with pulmonary hemorrhage. The latter is termed Goodpasture's syndrome. Injury is related to autoantibodies aimed against type IV collagen in the glomerular basement membrane rather than to immune complex deposition.

Pauci-immune acute glomerulonephritis is a form of small-vessel vasculitis associated with ANCA, causing primary and secondary renal diseases that do not have direct immune complex deposition or antibody binding. Tissue injury is believed to be due to cell-mediated immune processes. An example is Wegener's granulomatosis, a systemic necrotizing vasculitis of small arteries and veins associated with intravascular and extravascular granuloma formation. In addition to glomerulonephritis, these patients can have upper airway, pulmonary, and skin manifestations of disease. Cytoplasmic ANCA (c-ANCA) is both specific (88%) and sensitive (95%) for this entity. Microscopic polyangiitis is another pauci-immune vasculitis causing acute glomerulonephritis. Perinuclear staining (p-ANCA) is the common pattern. ANCA-associated and anti-GBM-associated acute glomerulonephritis can evolve to crescentic glomerulonephritis and often have poor outcomes unless treatment is started early. Both are described more fully below.

Other vascular causes of acute glomerulonephritis include malignant hypertension and the thrombotic microangiopathies such as hemolytic-uremic syndrome (Chapter 11) and thrombotic thrombocytopenic purpura (Chapter 13).

Clinical Findings

A. SYMPTOMS AND SIGNS

Patients with acute glomerulonephritis are often hypertensive, edematous, and have an abnormal urinary sediment. The edema is found first in body parts with low tissue tension such as the periorbital and scrotal regions.

B. LABORATORY FINDINGS

Dipstick and microscopic evaluation will reveal evidence of hematuria, moderate proteinuria (usually < 2 g/d), and cellular elements such as red cells, red cell casts, and white cells. Red cell casts are specific for glomerulonephritis, and a detailed search is warranted. Twenty-four hour urine for protein excretion and creatinine clearance quantifies the amount of proteinuria and documents the degree of renal dysfunction. However, in cases of rapidly changing serum creatinine values, the urinary creatinine clearance is an unreliable marker of GFR. FE_{Na} is usually low unless renal dysfunction is marked.

Further tests include complement levels (C3, C4, CH50), ASO titer, anti-GBM antibody levels, ANCAs, ANA titers, cryoglobulin and hepatitis panels, C3 nephritic factor, renal ultrasound, and renal biopsy.

Treatment

Depending on the nature and severity of disease, treatment can consist of high-dose steroids and cytotoxic agents such as cyclophosphamide. Plasma exchange can be used in Goodpasture's disease. Treatment and prognosis for specific diseases are more fully discussed below.

Albright RC Jr: Acute renal failure: a practical update. Mayo Clin Proc 2001;76:67. [PMID:11155415]

Andreucci M et al: Edema and acute renal failure. Semin Nephrol 2001;21:251. [PMID: 11320489]

Hebert LA et al: The urgent call of albuminuria/proteinuria. Heeding its significance in early detection of kidney disease. Postgrad Med 2001;110:79. [PMID:11675984]

Holt SG et al: Pathogenesis and treatment of renal dysfunction in rhabdomyolysis. Intensive Care Med 2001;27:803. [PMID: 11430535]

Michel DM et al: Acute interstitial nephritis. J Am Soc Nephrol 1998;9:506. [PMID: 9513915]

Murphy SW et al: Contrast nephropathy. J Am Soc Nephrol 2000;11:177. [PMID: 10616853] (Review of causes and management of contrast nephropathy.)

Nissenson AR: Acute renal failure: Definition and pathogenesis. Kidney Int 1998;66(Suppl):S7. [PMID: 9573567] (Review of four main pathophysiologic mechanisms of acute renal failure.)

Perazella MA: COX-2 inhibitors and the kidney. Hosp Pract (Off Ed) 2001;36:43. [PMID:11263799]

Perazella MA: Crystal-induced acute renal failure. Am J Med 1999;106:459. [PMID: 10225250]

Vanholder R et al: Rhabdomyolysis. J Am Soc Nephrol 2000;11: 1553. [PMID: 10906171]

■ CHRONIC RENAL DISEASE

ESSENTIALS OF DIAGNOSIS

- *Progressive azotemia over months to years.*
- *Symptoms and signs of uremia when nearing end-stage disease.*
- *Hypertension in the majority.*
- *Isosthenuria and broad casts in urinary sediment are common.*
- *Bilateral small kidneys on ultrasound are diagnostic.*

General Considerations

Over 50% of cases of chronic renal failure are due to diabetes mellitus and hypertension. Glomerulonephritis, cystic diseases, and other urologic diseases account for another 20–25%, and nearly one-sixth of patients have unknown causes. The major causes of chronic renal failure are listed in Table 22–5.

Chronic renal disease is rarely reversible and leads to progressive decline in renal function. This occurs even after an inciting event has been removed. Reduction in renal mass leads to hypertrophy of the remaining nephrons with hyperfiltration, and the glomerular

Table 22–5. Major causes of chronic renal failure.

Glomerulopathies
  Primary glomerular diseases:
    1. Focal and segmental glomerulosclerosis
    2. Membranoproliferative glomerulonephritis
    3. IgA nephropathy
    4. Membranous nephropathy
  Secondary glomerular diseases:
    1. Diabetic nephropathy
    2. Amyloidosis
    3. Post infectious glomerulonephritis
    4. HIV-associated nephropathy
    5. Collagen vascular diseases
    6. Sickle cell nephropathy
    7. HIV-associated membranoproliferative glomerulonephritis
Tubulointerstitial nephritis
  Drug hypersensitivity
  Heavy metals
  Analgesic nephropathy
  Reflux/chronic pyelonephritis
  Idiopathic
Hereditary diseases
  Polycystic kidney disease
  Medullary cystic disease
  Alport's syndrome
Obstructive nephropathies
  Prostatic disease
  Nephrolithiasis
  Retroperitoneal fibrosis/tumor
  Congenital
Vascular diseases
  Hypertensive nephrosclerosis
  Renal artery stenosis

Table 22–6. Symptoms and signs of uremia.

Organ System	Symptoms	Signs
General	Fatigue, weakness	Sallow-appearing, chronically ill
Skin	Pruritus, easy bruisability	Pallor, ecchymoses, excoriations, edema, xerosis
ENT	Metallic taste in mouth, epistaxis	Urinous breath
Eye		Pale conjunctiva
Pulmonary	Shortness of breath	Rales, pleural effusion
Cardiovascular	Dyspnea on exertion, retrosternal pain on inspiration (pericarditis)	Hypertension, cardiomegaly, friction rub
Gastrointestinal	Anorexia, nausea, vomiting, hiccup	
Genitourinary	Nocturia, impotence	Isosthenuria
Neuromuscular	Restless legs, numbness and cramps in legs	
Neurologic	Generalized irritability and inability to concentrate, decreased libido	Stupor, asterixis, myoclonus, peripheral neuropathy

filtration rate in these nephrons are transiently at supranormal levels. These adaptations place a burden on the remaining nephrons and lead to progressive glomerular sclerosis and interstitial fibrosis, suggesting that hyperfiltration may worsen renal function. However, decreased renal mass in kidney donors is not associated with chronic renal failure.

Clinical Findings

A. SYMPTOMS AND SIGNS

The symptoms of chronic renal failure often develop slowly and are nonspecific (Table 22–6). Individuals can remain asymptomatic until renal failure is far-advanced (GFR < 10–15 mL/min). Manifestations include fatigue, weakness, and malaise. Gastrointestinal complaints such as anorexia, nausea, vomiting, a metallic taste in the mouth, and hiccups are common. Neurologic problems include irritability, difficulty in concentrating, insomnia, restless legs, and twitching. Pruritus is common and difficult to treat. As uremia progresses, decreased libido, menstrual irregularities, chest pain from pericarditis, and paresthesias can develop. Symptoms of drug toxicity—especially for drugs eliminated by the kidney—increase as renal clearance worsens. (See Table 22–7 for antimicrobial dosages.)

On physical examination, the patient appears chronically ill. Hypertension is common. The skin may be yellow, with signs of easy bruisability. Rarely seen in the dialysis era is uremic frost, a cutaneous re-

Table 22–7. Antimicrobial dosages in renal failure.[1]

	No Change	Moderate Reduction	Marked Reduction	Avoid
Aminoglycoside Amikacin			✓	
Gentamicin			✓	
Netilmicin			✓	
Tobramycin			✓	
Amphotericin B			✓	
Azithromycin	✓			
Cephalosporins First-generation: Cefadroxil			✓	
Cephradine			✓	
Cephalexin	✓			
Cephalothin		✓		
Cephapirin		✓		
Cefazolin			✓	

(continued)

Table 22–7. Antimicrobial dosages in renal failure.[1] (continued)

	No Change	Moderate Reduction	Marked Reduction	Avoid
Second-generation: Cefaclor	✓			
Cefonicid			✓	
Cefotetan			✓	
Cefoxitin			✓	
Cefuroxime			✓	
Third-generation: Cefoperazone	✓			
Cefotaxime			✓	
Ceftazidime			✓	
Ceftizoxime			✓	
Ceftriaxone	✓			
Chloramphenicol	✓			
Clarithromycin		✓		
Clindamycin	✓			
Erythromycin	✓			
Monobactams (aztreonam)			✓	
Nitrofurantoin				✓
Penicillins Amoxicillin		✓		
Ampicillin		✓		
Azlocillin			✓	
Carbenicillin	✓			
Dicloxacillin		✓		
Methicillin		✓		
Mezlocillin	✓			
Nafcillin	✓			
Penicillin G		✓		
Piperacillin			✓	
Ticarcillin			✓	
Quinolones Ciprofloxacin		✓		
Norfloxacin		✓		
Trimethoprim-sulfamethoxazole			✓	
Tetracyclines Doxycycline	✓			
Tetracycline				✓
Vancomycin			✓	

[1]GFR = < 10 mL/min

flection of end-stage renal disease. Uremic fetor is the characteristic fishy odor of the breath. Cardiopulmonary signs may include rales, cardiomegaly, edema, and a pericardial friction rub. Mental status can vary from decreased concentration to confusion, stupor, and coma. Myoclonus and asterixis are additional signs of uremic effects on the central nervous system.

The term "uremia" is used for this clinical syndrome, but the exact cause remains unknown. BUN and serum creatinine are believed to be markers for unknown toxins, with urea and parathyroid hormone believed to play a partial role in the syndrome.

In any patient with renal failure, it is important to identify and correct all possibly reversible causes. Urinary tract infections, obstruction, extracellular volume depletion, nephrotoxins, hypertension, and congestive heart failure should be excluded (Table 22–8). Any of the above can worsen underlying chronic renal failure.

B. LABORATORY FINDINGS

The diagnosis of renal failure is made by documenting elevations of the BUN and serum creatinine concentrations. Further evaluation is needed to differentiate between acute and chronic renal failure. Evidence of previously elevated BUN and creatinine, abnormal prior urinalyses, and stable but abnormal serum creatinine on successive days is most consistent with a chronic process. It is helpful to plot the inverse of serum creatinine ($1/S_{Cr}$) versus time if three or more prior measurements are available; this estimates time to end-stage renal disease (Figure 22–1). If the slope of the line acutely declines, new causes of renal failure

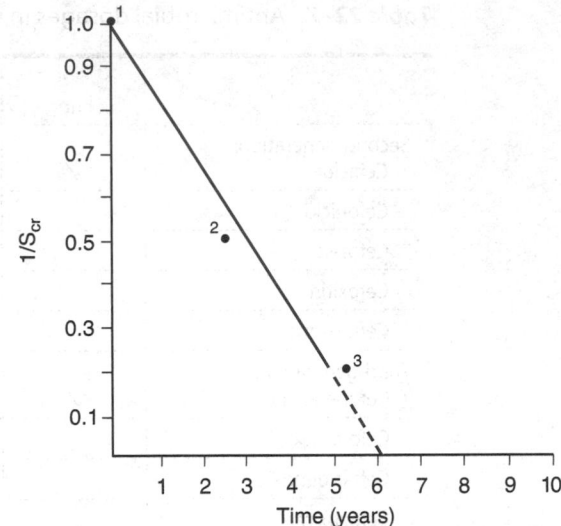

^{1} Value of serum creatinine level = 1.0 mg/dL
^{2} Value of serum creatinine level = 2.0 mg/dL
^{3} Value of serum creatinine level = 5.0 mg/dL

Figure 22–1. Decline in renal function plotted against time to end-stage renal disease. The solid line indicates the linear decline in renal function over time. The dotted line indicates the approximate time to end-stage renal disease.

should be excluded as outlined above. Anemia, metabolic acidosis, hyperphosphatemia, hypocalcemia, and hyperkalemia can occur with both acute and chronic renal failure. The urinalysis shows isosthenuria if tubular concentrating and diluting ability are impaired. The urinary sediment can show broad waxy casts as a result of dilated, hypertrophic nephrons.

C. IMAGING

The findings of small echogenic kidneys bilaterally (< 10 cm) by ultrasonography supports a diagnosis of chronic renal failure, though normal or even large kidneys can be seen with chronic renal failure caused by adult polycystic kidney disease, diabetic nephropathy, HIV-associated nephropathy, multiple myeloma, amyloidosis, and obstructive uropathy. Radiologic evidence of renal osteodystrophy is another helpful finding, since x-ray changes of secondary hyperparathyroidism do not appear unless parathyroid levels have been elevated for at least 1 year. Evidence of subperiosteal reabsorption along the radial sides of the digital bones of the hand confirms hyperparathyroidism.

Complications

A. HYPERKALEMIA

Potassium balance generally remains intact in chronic renal failure until the GFR is less than 10–20

Table 22–8. Reversible causes of renal failure.

Reversible Factors	Diagnostic Clues
Infection	Urine culture and sensitivity tests
Obstruction	Bladder catheterization, then renal ultrasound
Extracellular fluid volume depletion	Orthostatic blood pressure and pulse: ↓BP and ↑pulse upon sitting up from a supine position
Hypokalemia, hypercalcemia, and hyperuricemia (usually > 15 mg/dL)	Serum electrolytes, calcium, phosphate, uric acid
Nephrotoxic agents	Drug history
Pericarditis	Echocardiography, chest x-ray
Hypertension	Blood pressure, chest x-ray
Congestive heart failure	Physical examination, chest x-ray

mL/min. However, certain states pose an increased risk of hyperkalemia at higher GFRs. Endogenous causes include any type of cellular destruction such as hemolysis and trauma, the hyporeninemic hypoaldosteronism (type IV renal tubular acidosis, seen particularly in diabetes mellitus), and acidemic states (0.6 meq/L elevation in K^+ for each 0.1 unit decrease in pH). Exogenous causes include diet (eg, citrus fruits and salt substitutes containing potassium) and drugs that decrease K^+ secretion (amiloride, triamterene, spironolactone, NSAIDs, ACE inhibitors) or block cellular uptake (beta-blockers).

Treatment of acute hyperkalemia involves cardiac monitoring, intravenous calcium chloride or gluconate, insulin administration with glucose, bicarbonate, and an orally or rectally administered ion exchange resin (sodium polystyrene sulfonate). The resin exchanges sodium for potassium and can administer a significant sodium load to a patient (see Chapter 22). Chronic hyperkalemia is best treated with dietary potassium restriction and sodium polystyrene sulfonate when necessary. The usual dose is 15–30 g once a day in juice or sorbitol.

B. ACID-BASE DISORDERS

Damaged kidneys are unable to excrete the 1 meq/kg/d of acid generated by metabolism of dietary proteins. The resultant metabolic acidosis is primarily due to loss of renal mass. This limits production of ammonia (NH_3) and limits buffering of H^+ in the urine. (Other causes include decreased filtration of titratable acids such as sulfates and phosphates, decreased proximal tubular bicarbonate resorption, and decreased renal tubular hydrogen ion secretion.) Although patients with chronic renal failure are in positive hydrogen ion balance, the arterial blood pH is maintained at 7.33–7.37 and serum bicarbonate concentration rarely falls below 15 meq/L. The excess hydrogen ions are buffered by the large calcium carbonate and calcium phosphate stores in bone. This contributes to the renal osteodystrophy of chronic renal failure described below.

The serum bicarbonate level should be maintained at > 20 meq/L. Base supplements include sodium bicarbonate, calcium bicarbonate, and sodium citrate. Administration should begin with 20–30 mmol/d of alkali divided into two doses per day and titrated as needed.

C. CARDIOVASCULAR COMPLICATIONS

1. Hypertension—As renal failure progresses, hypertension due to salt and water retention usually develops. Hyperreninemic states and exogenous erythropoietin administration can also exacerbate hypertension. Hypertension is the most common complication of end-stage renal disease and must be meticulously controlled. Failure to do so can accelerate the progression of renal damage.

Control of hypertension can be achieved with salt and water restriction, weight loss if indicated, and pharmacologic therapy. The ability of the kidney to adjust to variations in sodium and water intake becomes limited as renal failure progresses. An elevated sodium chloride intake leads to congestive heart failure, edema, and hypertension, whereas low salt intake leads to volume contraction and hypotension. A mildly decreased salt diet (4–6 g/d) can be started, and salt intake should be reduced to 2 g/d if hypertension persists. Initial drug therapy can include ACE inhibitors or angiotensin II receptor blockers (if serum potassium and GFR permit), calcium channel-blocking agents, diuretics, and beta-blocking agents. The adjunctive drugs that are often needed (clonidine, hydralazine, minoxidil, etc) reflect the difficulty of achieving and maintaining hypertensive control in these patients.

2. Pericarditis—With uremia, pericarditis may develop. The cause is believed to be retention of metabolic toxins. Symptoms include chest pain and fever. Pulsus paradoxus can be present. A friction rub may be auscultated, but the lack of a rub does not rule out a significant pericardial effusion. Chest radiography will show an enlarged cardiac silhouette, and electrocardiography will show characteristic findings as explained in Chapter 10. Cardiac tamponade can occur; these patients have signs of poor cardiac output, with jugular venous distention and lungs clear to auscultation. Pericarditis is an absolute indication for initiation of hemodialysis.

3. Congestive heart failure—Patients with end-stage renal disease tend toward a high cardiac output. They often have extracellular fluid overload, shunting of blood through an arteriovenous fistula for dialysis, and anemia. In addition to hypertension, these abnormalities cause increased myocardial work and oxygen demand. Patients with chronic renal failure may also have accelerated rates of atherosclerosis. All of these factors contribute to left ventricular hypertrophy and dilation. Parathyroid hormone may also play a role in the pathogenesis of the cardiomyopathy of renal failure.

Water and salt intake should be controlled in patients who are oliguric or anuric. Diuretics are of value, though thiazides are ineffective when the GFR is less than 10–15 mL/min. Loop diuretics are commonly used, and higher doses are required as renal function declines. Digoxin should be used with caution since it is excreted by the kidney. The proved efficacy of ACE inhibitors in congestive heart failure holds true for patients with chronic renal failure. However, they are typically not used with a serum creatinine greater than 3 mg/dL without close supervision because of the risks of hyperkalemia and worsening renal function. Nonetheless, ACE inhibitors are being increasingly used with higher levels of stable serum creatinines. Along with angiotensin II receptor-blocking drugs, they have been shown to slow the progression to end-stage renal disease. (See above section regarding treatment of proteinuria.) Once a patient is on dialysis, these risks become less relevant. When an ACE inhibitor is initiated, patients should have serum creatinine and potassium checked within 2–7 days.

D. Hematologic Complications

1. Anemia—The anemia of chronic renal failure is characteristically normochromic and normocytic. It is due primarily to decreased erythropoietin production, which becomes clinically significant when GFR falls below 20–25 mL/min. Many patients are iron-deficient as well. Low-grade hemolysis and blood loss from platelet dysfunction or hemodialysis play an additional role.

Recombinant erythropoietin (epoetin alfa) is used in patients whose hematocrits are less than 30–35%. The effective dose can vary, and patients are started on 50 units/kg (3000–4000 units/dose) once or twice a week. It can be given intravenously (eg, in the hemodialysis patient) or subcutaneously (eg, in the peritoneal dialysis patient or one who has not yet started dialysis). Iron stores must be adequate to ensure response. Subcutaneous administration is preferable to intravenous administration because it requires a lower overall dose for the same effect. Iron supplementation is given at the minimum if the serum ferritin is less than 100 ng/mL or if iron saturation is < 20–25%. Oral therapy with ferrous sulfate, 325 mg once daily to three times daily, is adequate but not always well tolerated. Ferrous fumarate is the best-accepted formulation, and intravenous iron may be used in dialysis patients. The importance of observing trends in iron stores and hemoglobin levels cannot be overemphasized.

Hypertension is a complication of epoetin alfa therapy in about 20% of patients. It develops more abruptly in the patients with the lowest hematocrit values at initiation of therapy. Patients may require dosage adjustment or may have to be started on antihypertensive drugs. Hemoglobin levels should rise no more than 1 g/dL every 3–4 weeks.

2. Coagulopathy—The coagulopathy of chronic renal failure is mainly caused by platelet dysfunction. Platelet counts are only mildly decreased, but the bleeding time is prolonged. Platelets show abnormal adhesiveness and aggregation. Clinically, patients can have petechiae, purpura, and an increased tendency for bleeding during surgery.

Treatment is required only in patients who are symptomatic. Raising the hematocrit to 30% can reduce bleeding time in many patients. Desmopressin (25 μg intravenously every 8–12 hours for 2 doses) is effective and often used in preparation for surgery. It causes release of factor VIII bound to von Willebrand's factor from endothelial cells. Conjugated estrogens, 0.6 mg/kg diluted in 50 mL of 0.9% sodium chloride infused over 30–40 minutes daily, or 2.5–5 mg orally for 5–7 days, have an effect for several weeks. Dialysis improves the bleeding time but does not normalize it. Peritoneal dialysis is preferable to hemodialysis because

the latter requires heparin use to prevent clotting in the dialyzer. Cryoprecipitate (10–15 bags) is rarely used and lasts less than 24 hours.

E. Neurologic Complications

Uremic encephalopathy does not occur until GFR falls below 10–15 mL/min. Parathyroid hormone is believed to be one of the uremic toxins. Patients can develop markedly elevated intact PTH levels from tertiary hyperparathyroidism. When calcium levels exceed 12–15 mg/dL, mental status changes often follow. Symptoms begin with difficulty in concentrating and can progress to lethargy, confusion, and coma. Physical findings include nystagmus, weakness, asterixis, and hyperreflexia. These symptoms and signs may improve after initiation of dialysis.

Neuropathy is found in 65% of patients on or nearing dialysis but not until GFR is 10% of normal. Peripheral neuropathies manifest themselves as sensorimotor polyneuropathies (stocking and glove distribution) and isolated or multiple isolated mononeuropathies. Patients can have restless legs, loss of deep tendon reflexes, and distal pain. The earlier initiation of dialysis may prevent peripheral neuropathies, and the response to dialysis is variable. Other neuropathies result in impotence and autonomic dysfunction.

F. Disorders of Mineral Metabolism

The disorders of calcium, phosphorus, and bone are referred to as renal osteodystrophy. The most common disorder is osteitis fibrosa cystica—the bony changes of secondary hyperparathyroidism. As GFR decreases below 25% of normal, phosphorus excretion is impaired. Hyperphosphatemia leads to hypocalcemia, stimulating secretion of parathyroid hormone, which has a phosphaturic effect and normalizes serum phosphorus. This continuous process leads to markedly elevated parathyroid hormone levels and high bone turnover with osteoclastic bone resorption and subperiosteal lesions. Clinically, patients experience bony pain and proximal muscle weakness. Metastatic calcifications can occur. Radiographically, lesions are most prominent in the phalanges and lateral ends of the clavicles.

Osteomalacia is a form of renal osteodystrophy with low bone turnover. With worsening renal function, there is decreased renal conversion of 25-hydroxycholecalciferol to the 1,25-dihydroxy form. Gut absorption of calcium is diminished, leading to hypocalcemia and abnormal bone mineralization. Deposition of aluminum in bone can also lead to osteomalacia. Elevated aluminum levels are seen in patients after years of chronic aluminum hydroxide administration for phosphorus binding. This entity is seen with decreasing frequency because aluminum-based binders are used less in the chronic setting and water used for hemodialysis is now cleared of aluminum.

Both of the above entities can cause bony pain and proximal muscle weakness. Spontaneous bone fractures can occur which are slow to heal. When the calcium-phosphorus product (serum calcium [mg/dL] × serum phosphate [mg/dL]) is above 60–70, metastatic calcifications are commonly seen in blood vessels, soft tissues, lungs, and myocardium. Treatment should begin with dietary phosphorus restriction. Oral phosphorus binding agents such as calcium carbonate or calcium acetate act in the gut and are given in divided doses three or four times daily with meals. These should be titrated to a serum calcium of 10 mg/dL (preventing hypercalcemia) and serum phosphorus of 4.5 mg/dL. Aluminum hydroxide is another effective phosphorus binder but can cause osteomalacia and neurologic complications. It can be used in the acute setting; however, chronic use should be avoided. If aluminum levels are high, chelation with deferoxamine can be effective. Vitamin D or vitamin D analogs should be given with hyperparathyroidism (iPTH more than two to three times normal) if phosphorus levels are < 7 mg/dL and calcium < 11 mg/dL. Vitamin D suppresses PTH and increases serum calcium and phosphorus levels; both need to be followed closely to prevent hypercalcemia and hyperphosphatemia. If calcitriol is used, the dosage should be 0.25–0.5 μg daily or every other day initially.

G. ENDOCRINE DISORDERS

Circulating insulin levels are higher because of decreased renal insulin clearance. Glucose intolerance can occur in chronic renal failure when GFR is less than 10–20 mL/min. Primarily, this is due to peripheral insulin resistance. Fasting glucose levels are usually normal or only slightly elevated. Therefore, patients can be either hyperglycemic or hypoglycemic depending on the predominant disturbance. Most commonly, diabetic patients require decreased doses of hypoglycemic agents.

Decreased libido and impotence are common in chronic renal failure. Men have decreased testosterone levels; women are often anovulatory. Despite a high degree of infertility, pregnancy can occur—particularly in women who are well dialyzed and well nourished. Therefore, contraception is advisable for women who do not wish to become pregnant.

Thyroid, pituitary, and adrenal function are often normal despite abnormalities in thyroxine, growth hormone, aldosterone, and cortisol levels.

Treatment

A. DIETARY MANAGEMENT

Every patient with chronic renal failure should be evaluated by a renal nutritionist. Specific recommendations should be made concerning protein, salt, water, potassium, and phosphorus intake.

1. Protein restriction—Experimental models have shown that protein restriction slows the progression to end-stage renal disease; however, clinical trials have not consistently proved this. The Modification of Diet in Renal Disease (MDRD) Study was meant to clarify the issue, but the results were inconclusive. A subsequent meta-analysis of five clinical trials did show a significant benefit but did not control for certain effects such as ACE inhibitor therapy. Protein intake should not exceed 1 g/kg/d, and if protein restriction proves to be beneficial, it should not exceed 0.6 g/kg/d.

2. Salt and water restriction—In advanced renal failure, the kidney is unable to adapt to large changes in sodium intake. Intake greater than 3–4 g/d can lead to edema, hypertension, and congestive heart failure, whereas intake of less than 1 g/d can lead to volume depletion and hypotension. For the nondialysis patient approaching end-stage renal disease, 2 g/d of sodium is an initial recommendation. A daily intake of 1–2 L of fluid maintains water balance.

3. Potassium restriction—Restriction is needed once the GFR has fallen below 10–20 mL/min. Patients should receive detailed lists concerning potassium content of foods and should limit their intake to less than 60–70 meq/d. (Normal intake is about 100 meq/d.)

4. Phosphorus restriction—Phosphorus levels should be kept below 4.5 mg/dL. Foods rich in phosphorus such as cola beverages, eggs, dairy products, and meat should be limited. Renal failure patients with a GFR > 10–20 mL/min should restrict phosphorus intake to 5–10 mg/kg/d. Below this GFR, phosphorus binders are usually required. The treatment of hyperphosphatemia is discussed in the section on disorders of mineral metabolism.

5. Magnesium restriction—Magnesium is excreted primarily by the kidneys. Dangerous hypermagnesemia is rare unless the patient ingests medications high in magnesium or receives it parenterally. All magnesium-containing laxatives and antacids are relatively contraindicated in renal failure.

B. DIALYSIS

When conservative management of end-stage renal disease is inadequate, hemodialysis, peritoneal dialysis, and kidney transplantation are alternatives (see below). Indications for dialysis include the following: (1) uremic symptoms such as pericarditis, encephalopathy, or coagulopathy; (2) fluid overload unresponsive to diuresis; (3) refractory hyperkalemia; (4) severe metabolic acidosis (pH < 7.20); and (5) neurologic symptoms such as seizures or neuropathy. According to the Dialysis Outcomes Quality Initiative (DOQI) guidelines, dialysis should be started when a patient has a GFR of 10 mL/min or serum creatinine of 8 mg/dL. Diabetics should start when the GFR reaches 15 mL/min or serum creatinine is 6 mg/dL. Preparation for dialysis requires a team approach. Dietitians, social workers, psychiatrists, and transplant surgeons should be involved as well as primary care physicians and nephrologists. The patient and family need early counseling regarding the risks and benefits of therapy. The option of not starting therapy or withdrawing therapy should be discussed openly.

1. Hemodialysis—Hemodialysis requires a constant flow of blood along one side of a semipermeable membrane with a cleansing solution, or dialysate, along the other. Diffusion and convection allow the dialysate to remove unwanted substances from the blood while adding back needed components. Vascular access for hemodialysis can be accomplished by an arteriovenous fistula or prosthetic shunt. Indwelling catheters should be considered temporary measures. Native fistulas typically last longer than prosthetic shunts but require longer (6–8 weeks or more after surgical construction) before they can be used. Infection, thrombosis, and aneurysm formation are complications seen more often in shunts than fistulas. *Staphylococcus aureus* is the most common infecting agent.

Patients typically require hemodialysis three times a week. Sessions last 3–5 hours depending on patient size, type of dialyzer used, and other factors. Periodic measurement of dialysis adequacy should determine the duration of treatment. Home hemodialysis is an option that is becoming less popular because of the need for a trained helper, large equipment, and costs.

2. Peritoneal dialysis—With peritoneal dialysis, the peritoneal membrane is the "dialyzer." Fluids and solutes move across the capillary bed that lies between the visceral and parietal layers of the membrane into the dialysate. Dialysate enters the peritoneal cavity through a catheter. The most common kind of peritoneal dialysis is continuous ambulatory peritoneal dialysis (CAPD). Patients exchange the dialysate four to six times a day. Continuous cyclic peritoneal dialysis (CCPD) utilizes a cycler machine to automatically perform exchanges at night. The dialysate remains in the peritoneal cavity between exchanges. As with hemodialysis, actual peritoneal dialysis prescriptions are guided by adequacy measurements.

The percentage of dialysis patients using peritoneal dialysis has been decreasing over the past several years. Peritoneal dialysis permits greater patient autonomy; its continuous nature minimizes the symptomatic swings observed in hemodialysis patients; and poorly dialyzable compounds such as phosphates are better cleared, which permits less dietary restriction. The dialysate removes large amounts of albumin, and nutritional status must be closely watched.

The most common complication of peritoneal dialysis is peritonitis. Rates are as high as 0.8 episodes per patient year. The patient can experience nausea and vomiting, abdominal pain, diarrhea or constipation, and fever. The dialysate will be cloudy and contain > 100 white cells per microliter of which over 50% should be polymorphonuclear neutrophils. *S aureus* is the most common infecting organism.

The total costs of peritoneal dialysis and hemodialysis are approximately the same. Equipment expenses are less for peritoneal dialysis, but the costs of peritonitis are high. Patients treated with both modalities more often prefer peritoneal to hemodialysis.

Survival rates on dialysis depend on the underlying disease process. Five-year Kaplan-Meier survival rates vary from 21% for diabetics to 47% for patients with glomerulonephritis. Overall 5-year survival is currently estimated at 36%. Patients undergoing dialysis have an average life expectancy of 3–4 years, but survival for as long as 25 years is seen depending on the disease entity. Most studies have shown no survival advantage associated with either peritoneal dialysis or hemodialysis.

C. KIDNEY TRANSPLANTATION

Up to one-half of all patients with end-stage renal disease are suitable for transplantation. Age is becoming less of a barrier. Two-thirds of kidney transplants come from cadaveric donors; the remainder from living related or unrelated donors. Immunosuppressive drugs include corticosteroids, azathioprine, mycophenolate mofetil, tacrolimus, and cyclosporine. A patient with a cadaveric renal transplant typically requires stronger immunosuppression than patients with living related kidney transplants. However, this depends to a great extent on the degree of HLA-type matching. The 1- and 5-year kidney graft survival rates approximately 94% and 72%, respectively, for living related and living unrelated donor transplants and 89% and 58%, respectively, for cadaveric donor transplants. The average wait for a cadaveric transplant is 2–4 years. Aside from medication use, the life of a transplanted patient can return to nearly normal.

D. PROGNOSIS

Mortality is higher for patients on dialysis than for age-matched controls. Yearly mortality is 22.4 deaths per 100 patient years. The expected remaining lifetime for the age group 55–64 is 22 years, whereas that of the end-stage renal disease population is 5 years. The most common cause of death is cardiac dysfunction (48%). Other causes include infection (15%), cerebrovascular disease (6%), and malignancy (4%). Diabetes, age, a low serum albumin, lower socioeconomic status, and inadequate dialysis are all significant predictors of mortality.

For those who require dialysis to sustain life but elect not to undergo dialysis, death ensues within days to weeks. In general, patients develop uremia and lose consciousness prior to death. Arrhythmias can occur as a result of electrolyte imbalance. Volume overload and dyspnea can be managed by volume restriction and opioids as described in Chapter 5. Meticulous efforts at palliative care are essential.

Barrett BJ et al: Clinical practice guidelines for the management of anemia coexistent with chronic renal failure. J Am Soc Nephrol 1999;10(Suppl 13): S292. [PMID: 10425612]

Collins AJ et al: Cardiovascular disease in end-stage renal disease patients. Am J Kidney Dis 2001;38(4 Suppl 1):S26. [PMID:11576917]

Curtis JJ: End-stage renal disease patients: referral for transplantation. J Am Soc Nephrol 1998;9(12 Suppl):S137. [PMID: 11443761]

Drueke TB: Medical management of secondary hyperparathyroidism in uremia. Am J Med Sci 1999;317:383. [PMID: 10272838]

Fan SL et al: Bisphosphonates in renal osteodystrophy. Curr Opin Nephrol Hypertens 2001;10:581. [PMID: 11496050]

Gaede P et al: Intensified multifactorial intervention in patients with type 2 diabetes mellitus and microalbuminuria: the Steno type 2 randomised study. Lancet 1999;353:617. [PMID: 10030326] (Randomized trial demonstrating that intensified multifactorial treatment of risk factors in diabetic patients with microalbuminuria can slow the progression of nephropathy, retinopathy, and neuropathy.)

Mackenzie HS et al: Current strategies for retarding progression of renal disease. Am J Kidney Dis 1998;31:161. [PMID: 9428469] (A review of the mechanisms of renal disease progression and clinical trials to prevent disease progression, with a particular focus on protein restriction, ACE inhibitor use, antihypertensive therapy, and glycemic control.)

Mathur RV et al: Calciphylaxis. Postgrad Med J 2001;77:557. [PMID: 11524512]

McCarthy JR: A practical approach to the management of patients with chronic renal failure. Mayo Clin Proc 1999;74: 269. [PMID: 10089997] (Review of the predialysis care of patients with renal failure.)

Ramanathan V et al: Renal transplantation. Semin Nephrol 2001; 21:213. [PMID: 11245782]

Rao VK: Posttransplant medical complications. Surg Clin North Am 1998;78:113. [PMID: 9531939] (Medical, surgical, and psychosocial problems.)

Rostand S: Coronary heart disease in chronic renal insufficiency: some management considerations. J Am Soc Nephrol 2000; 11:1948. [PMID: 11004228]

Ruggenenti P et al: Progression, remission, regression of chronic renal diseases. Lancet 2001;357:1601. [PMID: 11377666]

Smogorzewski MJ: Central nervous dysfunction in uremia. Am J Kidney Dis 2001;38(4 Suppl 1):S122. [PMID: 11576937]

RENAL ARTERY STENOSIS

The two most common forms of renal artery stenosis are atherosclerotic ischemic renal disease and fibromuscular dysplasia. The prevalence of this condition has only been estimated by autopsy and angiographic studies. Approximately 5% of Americans with hypertension suffer from renal artery stenosis.

Atherosclerotic ischemic renal disease accounts for 67–95% of all cases of renal artery stenosis. It occurs most commonly in those over 45 years of age with a history of atherosclerotic disease. Other risk factors include renal insufficiency, diabetes mellitus, tobacco use, and hypertension.

Clues to diagnosis include refractory hypertension, new-onset hypertension in an older patient, pulmonary edema with poorly controlled blood pressure, and acute renal failure upon starting an angiotensin-converting enzyme inhibitor. In addition to hypertension, physical examination may reveal an audible abdominal bruit on the affected side. Laboratory values can show elevated BUN and serum creatinine levels in the setting of significant renal ischemia, and abdominal ultrasound discloses asymmetric kidney size when one renal artery is affected out of proportion to the other.

Three prevailing methods used for screening are doppler ultrasonography, captopril renography, and magnetic resonance angiography (MRA). Doppler ultrasonography is highly sensitive and specific (> 90% with an experienced ultrasonographer) and relatively inexpensive. However, this method is extremely operator- and patient-dependent. Measurements of blood flow must be made at the aorta and along each third of the renal artery in order to assess the disease. This test is a poor choice for patients who are obese, unable to lie supine, or have interfering bowel gas patterns.

Captopril renography capitalizes on the difference in renal perfusion with and without ACE inhibitors. A kidney distal to a significant stenosis requires high angiotensin II levels to maintain adequate perfusion. With an ACE inhibitor, perfusion is markedly diminished. The affected kidney enhances less, whereas the unaffected one enhances more in the setting of a captopril challenge. Sensitivity ranges from 75% to 100% and specificity from 60% to 90%. This procedure is not accurate in moderate to severe renal insufficiency.

MRA is an excellent but expensive way to screen for renal artery stenosis. Sensitivity is 99–100%. Specificity ranges from 71% to 96%. Turbulent blood flow can cause falsely positive results.

Renal angiography is the best procedure for diagnosis. CO_2 subtraction angiography can be used in place of dye when the risk of dye nephropathy exists— eg, in diabetic patients with renal insufficiency. Lesions are most commonly found in the proximal third or ostial region of the renal artery. The risk of atheroembolic phenomena after angiography is not trivial in this population, ranging from 5% to 10%.

Treatment is controversial. Options include medical management, angioplasty with or without stenting, and surgical bypass. Angioplasty might reduce the number of antihypertensive medications but does not significantly change outcome in comparison to patients medically managed. Stenting produces significantly better angioplastic results. However, blood pressure is equally improved, and serum creatinines are similar at 6 months of observation. Angioplasty is equally as effective as and safer than surgical revision.

Fibromuscular dysplasia primarily affects young women. Unexplained hypertension in a young woman is reason to screen for this disorder. The noninvasive tests mentioned above should be used for detection. This disorder has a characteristic "beads-on-a-string" appearance on angiography. Treatment with percutaneous transluminal angioplasty is often curative.

Block MJ: An evidence-based approach to diagnosing renovascular hypertension. Curr Cardiol Rep 2001;3:477. [PMID: 11602079]

Klassen PS et al: Diagnosis and management of renovascular hypertension. Cardiol Rev 2000;8:17. [PMID: 11174870]

Plouin P et al: Management of the patient with atherosclerotic renal artery stenosis. New information from randomized trials. Nephrol Dial Transplant 1999;14:1623. [PMID: 10435867]

Textor SC et al: Renal artery stenosis: a common, treatable cause of renal failure? Annu Rev Med 2001;52:421. [PMID: 112160787]

Zierler RE: Is duplex scanning the best screening test for renal artery stenosis? Semin Vasc Surg 2001;14:177. [PMID: 11561278]

■ GLOMERULONEPHROPATHIES

Abnormalities of glomerular function can be caused by damage to the major components of the glomerulus: the epithelium (podocytes), the basement membrane, the capillary endothelium, or the mesangium. The damage is often manifested as an inflammatory process. A specific histologic pattern of glomerular injury can be seen on renal biopsy, one of the most helpful techniques available for defining the cause of glomerular disease. Clinically, hematuria, proteinuria, hypertension, and a reduced GFR are typical findings of glomerular diseases presenting as *nephritic* syndromes; heavy proteinuria (> 3.5 g/24 h), hypoalbuminemia, hyperlipidemia, and edema are typical findings of glomerular diseases presenting as *nephrotic* syndromes.

Classification

Glomerular diseases generally can be classified into one of three major syndromes: nephritic syndrome, nephrotic syndrome, and asymptomatic renal disease. Specific glomerular diseases usually exhibit characteristics of one of the above syndromes, though some can have varying components of all three.

Glomerular diseases can also be classified according to whether they cause only renal abnormalities (primary renal disease) or whether the renal abnormalities result from a systemic disease (secondary renal disease).

NEPHRITIC SYNDROME

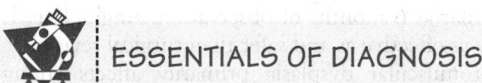

ESSENTIALS OF DIAGNOSIS

- Edema.
- Hypertension.
- Hematuria (with or without dysmorphic red cells, red blood cell casts).

General Considerations

Acute glomerulonephritis usually signifies an inflammatory process causing renal dysfunction over days to weeks that may or may not resolve. If the inflammatory process is severe, the glomerulonephritis may lead to a greater than 50% loss of nephron function over the course of just weeks to months. Such a process, called rapidly progressive acute glomerulonephritis, can cause permanent damage to glomeruli if not identified and treated rapidly. Prolonged inflammatory changes can result in chronic glomerulonephritis with persistent renal abnormalities that progress to end-stage renal disease.

Clinical Findings

A. SYMPTOMS AND SIGNS

Edema is first seen in regions of low tissue pressure such as the periorbital and scrotal areas. Hypertension, if present, is due to volume overload rather than vasoactive substances such as angiotensin II, whose levels are low.

B. LABORATORY FINDINGS

1. Serum chemistries—There are no serum chemistries characteristic of nephritic syndrome, but certain special tests are often performed depending on the history and the results of the preliminary evaluation. These include complement levels, antinuclear antibodies (ANA), cryoglobulins, hepatitis panels, ANCA, anti-GBM antibodies, ASO titers, and C3 nephritic factor. (See Figure 22–2.)

2. Urinalysis—The urinalysis shows red blood cells. These may be misshapen from traversing a damaged capillary membrane—so-called dysmorphic red blood cells. Red blood cell casts and moderate degrees of proteinuria are also characteristic of the urinary sediment. Placing the patient in a lordotic position for an hour increases sensitivity for finding red cell casts in the next urine specimen.

3. Biopsy—Renal biopsy should be considered if there are no other contraindications to biopsy (eg, bleeding disorders, thrombocytopenia, uncontrolled hypertension). Rapidly progressive glomerulonephritis is likely when over 50% of glomeruli contain crescents. The type of disease can be categorized according to the immunofluorescent pattern and appearance on electron microscopy (see Table 22–9).

Treatment

Treatment includes aggressive reduction of hypertension and fluid overload and specific therapeutic maneuvers aimed at the underlying cause. Salt and water restriction, diuretic therapy, and possibly dialysis are needed. The inflammatory glomerular injury may require corticosteroids and cytotoxic agents. (See specific diseases discussed below.)

POSTINFECTIOUS GLOMERULONEPHRITIS

Postinfectious glomerulonephritis is most often associated with poststreptococcal infection due to nephritogenic group A beta-hemolytic streptococci, especially

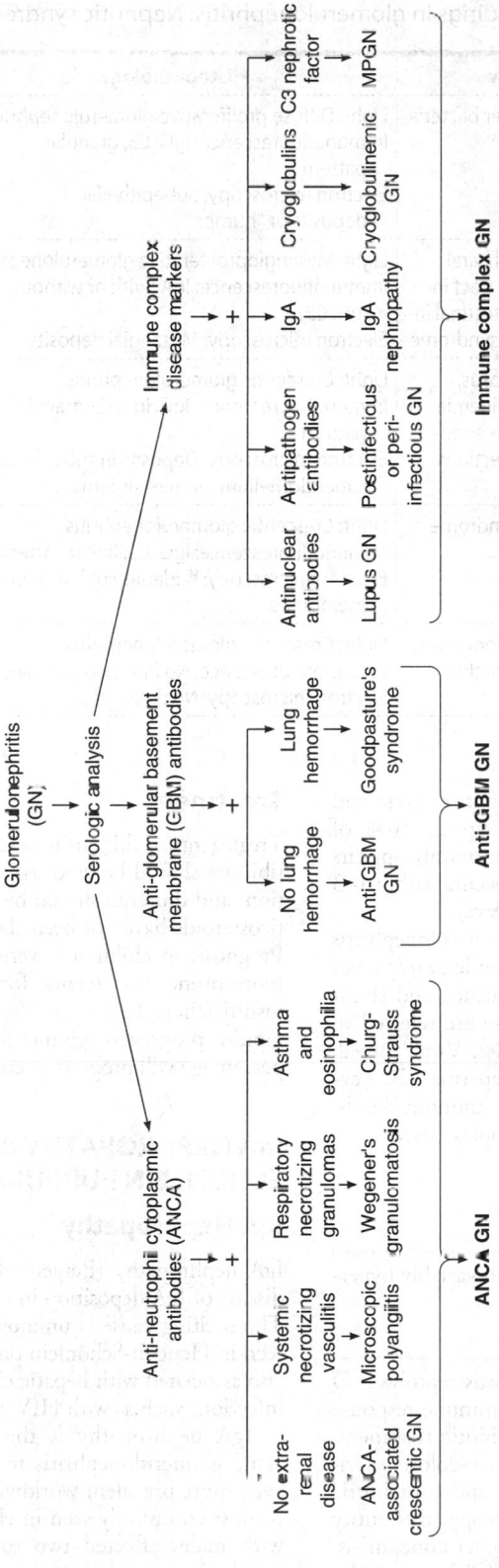

Figure 22–2. Serologic analysis of patients with glomerulonephritis. ANCA, anti-neutrophil cytoplasmic antibodies; GBM, glomerular basement membrane GN, glomerulonephritis; MPGN, membranoproliferative glomerulonephritis. (Reproduced, with permission, from Jennette JC, Falk RJ: *Primer on Kidney Diseases.* Academic Press, 1994.)

Table 22–9. Classification and findings in glomerulonephritis: Nephritic syndromes.

	Etiology	Histopathology	Pathogenesis
Acute (postinfectious) glomerulonephritis	Streptococci, other bacteria	Light: Diffuse proliferative glomerulonephritis Immunofluorescence: IgG; C3, granular pattern Electron microscopy: Subepithelial deposits or "humps"	Trapped immune complexes
IgA nephropathy (Berger's disease and Henoch-Schönlein purpura)	In association with viral upper respiratory tract infections; gastrointestinal infection or flu-like syndrome	Light: Mesangioproliferative glomerulonephritis Immunofluorescence: IgA (with or without IgG, C3) Electron microscopy: Mesangial deposits	Unknown
Rapidly progressive glomerulonephritis	Lupus erythematosus, mixed cryoglobulinemia, subacute infective endocarditis, shunt infections	Light: Crescentic glomerulonephritis Immunofluorescence: IgG, IgA; C3 granular pattern Electron microscopy: Deposits in subepithelium, subendothelium, or mesangium	Trapped immune complexes
	Goodpasture's syndrome or idiopathic	Light: Crescentic glomerulonephritis Immunofluorescence: IgG; C3, linear pattern Electron microscopy: Widening of basement membrane	Anti-GBM antibodies
	Wegener's granulomatosis, polyarteritis, idiopathic	Light: Crescentic glomerulonephritis Immunofluorescence: No immunoglobulins Electron microscopy: No deposits	Unknown

type 12. It can occur sporadically or in clusters and during epidemics can account for up to 10% of known streptococcal infections. It commonly appears after pharyngitis or impetigo. Onset occurs within 1–3 weeks after infection (average, 7–10 days).

Other causes of postinfectious glomerulonephritis include bacteremic states such as systemic *Staphylococcus aureus* infection. Infective endocarditis and shunt infections cause similar lesions. These are referred to as peri-infectious glomerulonephritides. Viral, fungal, and parasitic causes include hepatitis B, cytomegalovirus infection, infectious mononucleosis, coccidioidomycosis, malaria, and toxoplasmosis.

Clinical Findings

A. SYMPTOMS AND SIGNS

The patient is oliguric, edematous, and variably hypertensive.

B. LABORATORY FINDINGS

Serum complement levels are low; antistreptolysin O (ASO) titers can be high unless the immune response had been blunted with previous antibiotic treatment. Classically, the urine is described as cola-colored. Urinary red blood cells, red cell casts, and proteinuria under 3.5 g/d is present. On microscopy, this entity appears as a diffuse proliferative glomerulonephritis. Immunofluorescence shows IgG and C3 in a granular pattern in the mesangium and along the capillary basement membrane. Electron microscopy shows large, dense subepithelial deposits or "humps."

Treatment

Treatment for this entity is supportive. Appropriate antibiotics should be used. Antihypertensives, salt restriction, and diuretics should be employed if needed. Corticosteroids have not been shown to improve outcome. Prognosis in children is very favorable, but adults are more prone to crescentic formation and chronic renal insufficiency. Less than 5% of adults will develop a rapidly progressive glomerulonephritis, and a smaller percentage will progress to end-stage renal disease.

IgA NEPHROPATHY & HENOCH-SCHÖNLEIN PURPURA

IgA Nephropathy

IgA nephropathy (Berger's disease) is a primary renal disease of IgA deposition in the glomerular mesangium. The inciting cause is unknown, but the same lesion is seen in Henoch-Schönlein purpura. IgA nephropathy is also associated with hepatic cirrhosis, celiac disease, and infections such as with HIV and CMV.

IgA nephropathy is the most common form of acute glomerulonephritis in the United States and is even more prevalent worldwide, particularly in Asia. It is most commonly seen in children and young adults, with males affected two to three times more commonly than females.

An episode of gross hematuria is the commonest presenting complaint. Frequently this is associated with an upper respiratory infection (50%), gastrointestinal symptoms (10%), or a flu-like illness (15%). The urine becomes red or cola-colored 1–2 days after onset. In contrast to postinfectious glomerulonephritis, this feature has been called "synpharyngitic hematuria" since there is no significant latent period. Other findings include asymptomatic microscopic hematuria as an incidental finding and the nephrotic syndrome (see below). Approximately one-third of patients will experience a clinical remission. Forty to 50 percent of patients will have progressive renal insufficiency. The remainder will show chronic microscopic hematuria and a stable serum creatinine. The most unfavorable prognostic indicator is proteinuria > 1 g/d. Others include hypertension, persistent microscopic hematuria and proteinuria, glomerulosclerosis, and abnormal renal function.

The serum IgA level is increased in up to 50% of patients, and for that reason a normal serum IgA does not rule out the disease. Serum complement levels are usually normal, and renal biopsy is the standard for diagnosis. Glomeruli show a focal glomerulonephritis with diffuse mesangial IgA deposits and proliferation of mesangial cells. IgG and C3 can also be seen in the mesangium of all glomeruli. Skin biopsy often reveals granular deposits of IgA in dermal capillaries of affected patients.

In patients with significant proteinuria (> 1 g/d), ACE inhibitors or angiotensin II receptor-blocking drugs should be used to reduce proteinuria. The target blood pressure is < 130/80 mm Hg. In nephrotic patients, prior regimens suggested short courses of steroids, but this practice rarely prevented progression of disease. A recent regimen showed a 2% doubling of creatinine after 6 years in the treatment group versus a 21% doubling of creatinine in the control group. The regimen consisted of giving methylprednisolone, 1 g/d intravenously, for 3 days during months 1, 3, and 5, plus prednisone in a dosage of 0.5 mg/kg every other day for 6 months. This was aimed at patients with creatinine clearances > 70 mL/min. ACE inhibitors or angiotensin II receptor antagonists should also be considered as first-line therapy for the treatment of hypertension in this population.

Other treatments have included fish oil, with variable results in clinical trials. Recent studies that have shown a benefit also show that low doses (2–5g/d) are just as efficacious as high doses (9–12 g/d). There are very few side effects of long-term fish oil administration. Thus, many clinicians will use this as adjunctive therapy. Renal transplantation is an excellent option for patients with end-stage renal disease, but recurrent disease has been documented in 30% of patients 5–10 years posttransplant. Fortunately, recurrent disease rarely leads to failure of the allograft.

Henoch-Schönlein Purpura (Anaphylactoid Purpura)

This disease is a leukocytoclastic vasculitis of unknown cause. It is most common in children and has a male predominance. It classically presents with palpable purpura, arthralgias, and abdominal symptoms such as nausea, colic, and melena. Purpuric skin lesions are most often found on the lower extremities. Renal insufficiency is common with a nephritic presentation. The renal lesions are identical to those found in IgA nephropathy. Most patients will recover fully over several weeks.

Further details about Henoch-Schönlein purpura are provided in Chapter 20.

David JC et al: What is the difference between IgA nephropathy and Henoch-Schönlein purpura nephritis? Kidney Int 2001;59:823. [PMID:11231337]

Donadio JV Jr et al: The long term outcome of patients with IgA nephropathy treated with fish oil in a controlled trial. J Am Soc Nephrol 1999;10:1772. [PMID: 10446945] (Early and prolonged treatment with fish oil retards renal progression for high-risk patients with IgA nephropathy.)

Lang MM et al: Identifying poststreptococcal glomerulonephritis. Nurse Pract 2001;26:34. [PMID: 11521409]

Rostoker G: Schönlein-Henoch purpura in children and adults; diagnosis, pathophysiology and management. BioDrugs 2001;15:99. [PMID:11437679]

Saulsbury FT: Henoch Schönlein purpura. Curr Opin Rheumatol 2001;13:35. [PMID:11148713]

PAUCI-IMMUNE GLOMERULONEPHRITIS (ANCA-Associated)

Pauci-immune glomerular lesions are seen with Wegener's granulomatosis and microscopic polyangiitis. Both are small-vessel vasculirides. Wegener's granulomatosis also involves granulomatous inflammation of the respiratory tract with a necrotizing vasculitis of small and medium-sized vessels. Microscopic polyangiitis (polyarteritis) is similar to Wegener's granulomatosis without granulomatous inflammation, but both commonly exhibit a necrotizing glomerulonephritis. ANCA-associated glomerulonephritis can also present as a primary renal lesion. The pathogenesis of these entities is unknown, but more than 80% of pauci-immune glomerulonephritis is associated with antineutrophil cytoplasmic antibodies.

Clinical Findings

A. SYMPTOMS AND SIGNS

Patients can present with symptoms of a systemic inflammatory disease, including fever, malaise, and weight loss. In addition to hematuria and proteinuria from glomerular inflammation, some patients exhibit purpura from dermal capillary involvement and mononeuritis multiplex from nerve arteriolar involvement. Ninety percent of patients with Wegener's will have upper or lower respiratory tract symptoms with nodular lesions that can cavitate and bleed.

B. LABORATORY FINDINGS

Serologically, ANCA subtype analysis can be done. A cytoplasmic pattern (c-ANCA) is specific for antiproteinase 3 antibodies, while a perinuclear pattern (p-ANCA) is specific for antimyeloperoxidase antibodies. Over 90% of patients with Wegener's syndrome will have c-ANCA; the remainder can have a p-ANCA pattern. Microscopic angiitis will have either a p-ANCA or c-ANCA pattern about 80% of the time. Pathologically, the small vessels and glomeruli will lack immune deposits (pauci-immune); however, a cell-mediated immune response is often seen. Necrotizing lesions and crescents signify a rapidly progressive glomerulonephritis.

Treatment

Treatment should be instituted early if aggressive disease is suspected. High doses of corticosteroids (methylprednisolone, 1–2 g/d for 3 days, followed by prednisone, 1 mg/kg for 1 month, with a slow taper over the next 6 months) and cytotoxic agents (cyclophosphamide, 1.5–2 mg/kg orally for 3 months, tapered over 1 year) are recommended for controlling end-organ damage. Without treatment, prognosis is extremely poor, but with the above regimen complete remission can be achieved in about 75% of patients. The addition of plasmapheresis does not seem to improve outcomes. Prognosis depends mainly on the extent of glomerular involvement before treatment is started. ANCA levels can be followed to help determine the efficacy of treatment.

ANTI-GBM GLOMERULONEPHRITIS & GOODPASTURE'S SYNDROME

Goodpasture's syndrome is defined by the clinical constellation of glomerulonephritis and pulmonary hemorrhage; injury to both is mediated by antiglomerular basement membrane (anti-GBM) antibodies. Up to one-third of patients with anti-GBM glomerulonephritis have no evidence of lung injury. Anti-GBM-associated glomerulonephritis accounts for about 5% of patients with rapidly progressive acute glomerulonephritis. The incidence in males is approximately six times that in females, and the disease occurs most commonly in the second and third decades but has a wide range. It has been associated with influenza A infection, hydrocarbon solvent exposure, and HLA-DR2 and -B7 antigens.

Clinical Findings

A. Symptoms and Signs

The onset of disease is preceded by an upper respiratory tract infection in 20–60% of cases. Patients experience hemoptysis, dyspnea, and possible respiratory failure. Hypertension and edema are seen as components of the nephritic syndrome.

B. Laboratory Findings

Laboratory evaluation can show iron deficiency anemia, and complement levels are normal. Sputum contains hemosiderin-laden macrophages. Chest x-rays can show shifting pulmonary infiltrates due to pulmonary hemorrhage. The diffusion capacity of carbon monoxide is markedly increased. Diagnosis is confirmed by finding circulating anti-GBM antibodies, which are positive in over 90% of patients.

Treatment

The treatment of choice is a combination of plasma exchange therapy to remove circulating antibodies and administration of immunosuppressive drugs to prevent formation of new antibodies and control the inflammatory response. Steroids are given initially in pulse doses of prednisone or methylprednisolone, 1–2 g/d for 3 days, then 1 mg/kg/d. Cyclophosphamide is administered at a dosage of 2–3 mg/kg/d. Daily plasmapheresis is performed for up to 2 weeks. A poorer prognosis exists in patients with oliguria and a serum creatinine greater than 6–7 mg/dL. Anti-GBM antibody levels should decrease as the clinical course improves. A recently published retrospective review emphasized the importance of aggressive treatment.

CRYOGLOBULIN-ASSOCIATED GLOMERULONEPHRITIS

Essential (mixed) cryoglobulinemia is a disorder associated with cold-precipitable immunoglobulins (cryoglobulins). Glomerular disease results from the precipitation of cryoglobulins in glomerular capillaries. The cause is typically an underlying infection such as hepatitis B and C or other occult viral, bacterial, and fungal infections.

Patients exhibit necrotizing skin lesions in dependent areas, arthralgias, fever, and hepatosplenomegaly. Serum complement levels are depressed. Rapidly progressive glomerulonephritis is seen on pathologic examination with the presence of crescents.

Treatment consists of aggressively treating the underlying infection. Pulse steroids, plasma exchange, and cytotoxic agents can be used. Alfa-interferon has been shown to benefit patients with hepatitis C-related cryoglobulinemia.

Other important examples of glomerulonephritis include systemic lupus erythematosus and membranoproliferative glomerulonephritis. These are described below under the heading of diseases exhibiting manifestations of nephritic and nephrotic syndrome.

Cohen Tervaert JW et al: Novel therapies for anti-neutrophil cytoplasmic antibody-associated vasculitis. Curr Opin Nephrol Hypertens 2001;10:211. [PMID:11224696]

D'Amico G: Natural history of idiopathic IgA nephropathy: role of clinical and histological prognostic factors. Am J Kidney Dis 2000;36:227. [PMID: 10922300]

Gaskin G et al: Plasmapheresis in antineutrophil cytoplasmic antibody-associated systemic vasculitis. Ther Apher 2001;5:176. [PMID:11467753]

Hricik DE et al: Glomerulonephritis. N Engl J Med 1998;339: 888. [PMID: 9744974]

Jennett JC et al: Microscopic polyangiitis (microscopic polyarteritis). Semin Diagn Pathol 2001;18:3. [PMID:11296991]

Kaplan AA: Apheresis for renal disease. Ther Apher 2001;5:134. [PMID: 11354298]

Kluth DC et al: Antiglomerular basement membrane disease. J Am Soc Nephrol 1999;10:2446. [PMID: 10541306] (Review of the epidemiology, pathogenesis, and management of glomerular basement membrane disease.)

Levy JB et al: Long-term outcome of anti-glomerular basement membrane antibody disease treated with plasma exchange and immunosuppression. Ann Intern Med 2001;134:1033. [PMID: 11388816] (71 patients with anti-GBM antibody disease were treated with plasma exchange, prednisolone, and cyclophosphamide. Those with SCr of < 5.7 mg/dL experienced 95% renal survival at 1 year, whereas those who require dialysis with SCr > 5.7 mg/dL showed an 8% renal survival at 1 year.)

Nolin L et al: Management of IgA nephropathy: evidence-based recommendations. Kidney Int 1999;70(Suppl):S56. [PMID: 10369196] (Review of the evidence for the use of steroids, fish oils, and control of hypertension.)

Ritz E et al: Nephropathy in patients with type 2 diabetes mellitus. N Engl J Med 1999;341:1127. [PMID: 10511612] (Review of renal complications of diabetes with an emphasis on prevention and control of disease.)

Specks U: Diffuse alveolar hemorrhage syndromes. Curr Opin Rheumatol 2001;13:12. [PMID: 11148710]

NEPHROTIC SYNDROME

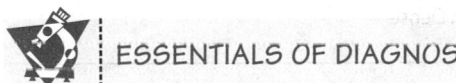

ESSENTIALS OF DIAGNOSIS

- Urine protein excretion > 3.5 g/1.73 m² per 24 hours.
- Hypoalbuminemia (albumin < 3 g/dL).
- Peripheral edema.

General Considerations

In adults, about one-third of patients with nephrotic syndrome have a systemic renal disease such as diabetes mellitus, amyloidosis, or systemic lupus erythematosus. With the current epidemic of type 2 diabetes mellitus, this proportion is slowly increasing. The remainder have idiopathic nephrotic syndrome. The four most common are minimal change disease, focal glomerular sclerosis, membranous nephropathy, and membranoproliferative glomerulonephritis.

Clinical Findings

A. SYMPTOMS AND SIGNS

Peripheral edema is a hallmark of the nephrotic syndrome, occurring when the serum albumin concentration is less than 3 g/dL. Edema is most likely due to sodium retention (from renal disease) rather than arterial underfilling from low plasma oncotic pressure. Initially this presents in the dependent areas of the body such as the lower extremities; however, such edema can become generalized. Patients can experience dyspnea due to pulmonary edema, pleural effusions, and diaphragmatic compromise with ascites. Complaints of abdominal fullness may also be present in patients with ascites.

Patients may show signs and symptoms of infection more frequently than the general population owing to loss of immunoglobulins and certain complement moieties in the urine.

B. LABORATORY FINDINGS

1. Urinalysis—Proteinuria occurs as a result of an alteration of the negative charge in the GBM. The screening test for proteinuria is the urinary dipstick analysis; however, one must bear in mind that this test indicates albumin only. The addition of sulfosalicylic acid to the urine sediment can detect the presence of abnormal paraproteins. Urine dipstick testing can detect as little as 15 mg/dL of protein, but the results must be interpreted along with the urine specific gravity. Trace protein seen on highly concentrated specimens may be insignificant, while trace protein on dilute specimens may indicate true renal disease.

Microscopically, the urinary sediment has relatively few cellular elements or casts. However, if marked hyperlipidemia is present, patients can have oval fat bodies in the urine. These represent lipid deposits in sloughed renal tubular epithelial cells. They appear as "grape clusters" under light microscopy and "Maltese crosses" under polarized light.

2. Blood chemistries—Characteristic blood chemistries include a decreased serum albumin (< 3 g/dL) and total serum protein < 6 g/dL. Hyperlipidemia occurs in over one-half of those with early nephrotic syndrome. As patients excrete larger amounts of protein per day, the frequency of hyperlipidemia increases. There is increased hepatic production of lipids (cholesterol and apolipoprotein B), owing to a fall in oncotic pressure. There is also decreased clearance of VLDLs, causing hypertriglyceridemia. Patients can also have an elevated erythrocyte sedimentation rate as a result of alterations in some plasma components such as increased levels of fibrinogen.

Other less common tests may be necessary depending on the patient's clinical presentation, including complement levels, serum and urine protein electrophoresis, ANA, and serologic tests for hepatitis. Patients may become deficient in vitamin D, zinc, and copper from loss of binding proteins in the urine.

3. Renal biopsy—Specific classification and findings are set forth in Table 22–10. Specimens are examined by light microscopy, with immunofluorescent stains, and by electron microscopy. Renal biopsy is often performed in adults with new-onset idiopathic nephrotic syndrome if one suspects a primary renal disease that may require drug therapy (eg, corticosteroids, cytotoxic agents). Significantly elevated creatinine levels may indicate irreversible renal disease mitigating the

Table 22–10. Classification and findings in glomerulonephritis: Nephrotic syndromes.

	Etiology	Histopathology	Pathogenesis
Minimal change disease (nil disease; lipoid nephrosis)	Associated with allergy, Hodgkin's disease, NSAIDs	Light: Normal (with or without mesangial proliferation) Immunofluorescence: No immunoglobulins Electron microscopy: Fusion foot processes	Unknown
Focal and segmental glomerulosclerosis	Associated with heroin abuse, HIV infection, reflux nephropathy, obesity	Light: Focal segmental sclerosis Immunofluorescence: IgM and C3 in sclerotic segments Electron microscopy: Fusion foot processes	Unknown
Membranous nephropathy	Associated with non-Hodgkin's lymphoma, carcinoma (gastrointestinal, renal, bronchogenic, thyroid), gold therapy, penicillamine, lupus erythematosus	Light: Thickened GBM and spikes Immunofluorescence: Granular IgG and C3 along capillary loops Electron microscopy: Dense deposits in subepithelial area	In situ immune complex formation
Membranoproliferative glomerulonephropathy	Type I associated with upper respiratory infection	Light: Increase mesangial cells and matrix with splitting of basement membrane Immunofluorescence: Granular C3, C1q, C4 with IgG and IgM Electron microscopy: Dense deposits in subendothelium	Unknown
	Type II	Light: Same as type I Immunofluorescence: C3 only Electron microscopy: Dense material in GBM	Unknown

need for renal biopsy. Disease due to amyloid or diabetes mellitus often does not need to be biopsied, since nephrotic range proteinuria in these diseases represents irreversible damage, although bone marrow transplant with high-dose chemotherapy can be considered in some patients with amyloid. The role of biopsy for other systemic renal diseases is debated. However, it can be useful for prognosis and treatment. An occasional unexpected diagnosis is made, such as membranous nephropathy due to lupus erythematosus without serologic evidence of that illness.

Management of Nephrotic Syndrome

A. Protein Loss

The daily total dietary protein intake should replace the daily urinary protein losses so as to avoid negative nitrogen balance. Protein malnutrition often occurs with urinary protein losses greater than 10 g/d. In the past, protein restriction was suggested for patients with renal insufficiency because experimental animal models had demonstrated a decrease in glomerulosclerosis among those animals fed low-protein diets. The largest human trial to date (the Modification of Diet in Renal Disease Study) did not show a significant benefit, but two recent meta-analyses have shown a mild renal benefit. For this reason, the Kidney Disease Outcomes Quality Initiative (K/DOQI) recommends

protein restriction to 0.6 g/kg/d in patients with a GFR < 25 mL/min prior to starting dialysis.

B. Edema

Dietary salt restriction is essential for managing edema; however, most patients also require diuretic therapy. Commonly used diuretics include thiazide and loop diuretics. Both are highly protein-bound. With hypoalbuminemia, diuretic delivery to the kidney is reduced, and patients often require large doses. The combination of loop and thiazide diuretics can potentiate the diuretic effect. This may be needed for patients with refractory fluid retention associated with pleural effusions and ascites.

C. Hyperlipidemia

Hypercholesterolemia and hypertriglyceridemia occur as outlined above. Dietary management in patients with nephrotic syndrome is of little value; however, dietary modification and exercise should be advocated. Aggressive pharmacologic treatment should be pursued. This is discussed in Chapter 27.

D. Hypercoagulable State

Patients with serum albumin less than 2 g/dL can become hypercoagulable. Nephrotic patients have urinary losses of antithrombin III, protein C, and protein S and increased platelet activation. Patients are prone to renal vein thrombosis and other venous thromboemboli, especially with membranous glomerulopathy. Anticoagulation therapy is warranted for at least 3–6 months in patients with evidence of thrombosis. Patients with renal vein thrombosis and recurrent thromboemboli require indefinite anticoagulation.

NEPHROTIC DISEASE IN PRIMARY RENAL DISORDERS

MINIMAL CHANGE DISEASE

Minimal change disease is most commonly seen in children but is occasionally present in adults. In patients over 40 with primary nephrotic syndrome, the incidence of minimal change disease is 20–25%, with equal distribution between men and women. In younger patients, there is a male predominance. Minimal change disease can be idiopathic but also occurs following viral upper respiratory infections, in association with tumors such as Hodgkin's disease, with drugs (gold and lithium), and with hypersensitivity reactions (especially to NSAIDs and bee stings).

Clinical Findings

A. SYMPTOMS AND SIGNS

Patients can exhibit the manifestations of nephrotic syndrome. They are more susceptible to infection, especially with gram-positive organisms, have a tendency toward thromboembolic events, develop severe hyperlipidemia, and experience protein malnutrition. Minimal change disease can rarely cause acute renal failure due to tubular changes and interstitial edema.

B. HISTOLOGIC FINDINGS

Glomeruli show no changes on light microscopy or immunofluorescence. On electron microscopy, there is a characteristic fusion of epithelial foot processes. A subgroup of patients also show mesangial cell proliferation. These people have more hematuria and hypertension and respond poorly to steroid treatment.

Treatment

Treatment is with prednisone, 1 mg/kg/d. In children the response is excellent, but about 10% of patients become steroid-resistant after 4–6 weeks. Adults often require longer therapy. It can take up to 16 weeks to achieve a response to steroids. Treatment should be continued for several weeks after complete remission of proteinuria. A significant number of patients will relapse and require further steroid treatment. Patients with frequent relapses and steroid resistance may need cyclophosphamide or chlorambucil to induce subsequent remissions. Progression to end-stage renal disease is rare. Complications most often arise from prolonged steroid use.

MEMBRANOUS NEPHROPATHY

Membranous nephropathy is the most common cause of primary nephrotic syndrome in adults. It is an immune-mediated disease characterized by immune complex deposition in the subepithelial portion of glomerular capillary walls. The antigens in primary disease are not known. Secondary disease is associated with infections such as hepatitis B, endocarditis, and syphilis; autoimmune disease such as systemic lupus erythematosus, mixed connective tissue disease, and thyroiditis; carcinoma; and certain drugs such as gold, penicillamine, and captopril. Membranous nephropathy occurs most commonly in adults in their fifth and sixth decades and almost always after age 30.

Clinical Findings

A. SYMPTOMS AND SIGNS

Patients exhibit the signs of nephrotic syndrome and have a higher incidence of renal vein thrombosis than most nephrotic patients. A higher incidence of occult neoplasms of lung, stomach, and colon are found in people over 50. The course of disease is variable, with about 50% of patients progressing to end-stage renal disease over 3–10 years. Poorer outcome is associated with concomitant tubulointerstitial fibrosis, male gender, elevated serum creatinine, hypertension, and heavy proteinuria (> 10 g/d).

B. LABORATORY FINDINGS

By light microscopy, capillary wall thickness is increased without inflammatory changes or cellular proliferation. When stained with silver methenamine, a "spike and dome" pattern may be observed owing to projections of excess basement membrane between the subepithelial deposits. Immunofluorescence shows IgG and C3 uniformly along capillary loops. Electron microscopy shows a discontinuous pattern of dense deposits along the subepithelial surface of the basement membrane.

Treatment

Treatment is controversial. After underlying causes are excluded, treatment should depend on the risk of renal disease progression. One algorithm is based on the degree of proteinuria. In patients with proteinuria < 4 g/d, the risk of progression is low. These individuals should be closely monitored with a low-salt diet, strict blood pressure control, and an ACE inhibitor for reduction of proteinuria. Patients with proteinuria of 4–8 g/d but normal renal function are at medium risk. They should follow the above suggestions and can elect immunosuppressive regimens with steroids and chlorambucil or cyclophosphamide for 6 months. Cyclosporine is a second choice. The highest-risk patients—those with > 8 g/d of proteinuria and possible renal dysfunction—might receive cyclosporine as a first-line immunosuppressant, though the choice of steroids with a cytotoxic agent is also reasonable. These treatments should be carefully chosen in consultation with a nephrologist. Patients with membranous nephropathy are excellent candidates for transplant.

FOCAL SEGMENTAL GLOMERULAR SCLEROSIS

This lesion can present as idiopathic disease or secondary to conditions such as heroin use, morbid obesity, and HIV infection. Clinically, patients show evidence of nephrotic syndrome, but they also have more nephritic features than membranous nephropathy or minimal change disease. Eighty percent of patients have microscopic hematuria at presentation, and many are hypertensive. Decreased renal function is present in 25–50% at time of diagnosis. Patients with focal segmental glomerular sclerosis and nephrotic syndrome typically progress to end-stage renal disease in 6–8 years.

Diagnosis requires renal biopsy. Light microscopy shows the lesions of focal segmental glomerular sclerosis. It is thought that these lesions occur first in the juxtamedullary glomeruli and are then seen in the superficial renal cortex. IgM and C3 are seen in the sclerotic lesions on immunofluorescence. Electron microscopy shows fusion of epithelial foot processes as seen in minimal change disease (Table 22–10).

Treatment is controversial, though supportive care for nephrotic patients is indicated. Longer courses of steroids are now being used because a higher percentage of patients are entering remissions. High-dose oral prednisone (1–1.5 mg/kg/d) for 2–3 months followed by a slow steroid taper can induce remission in over half of patients. Most patients achieve remission within 5–9 months. Other cytotoxic drug therapy can be considered but is disappointing (< 20% remission in most series).

DeSanto NG et al: Nephrotic edema. Semin Nephrol 2001;21: 262. [PMID: 11320491]

Geddes C et al: The treatment of idiopathic membranous nephropathy. Semin Nephrol 2000;20:299. [PMID: 10855940]

Khoshnoodi J et al: Congenital nephritic syndromes. Curr Opin Genet Dev 2001;11:322. [PMID: 11377970]

Madaio MP et al: The diagnosis of glomerular diseases: acute glomerulonephritis and the nephrotic syndrome. Arch Intern Med 2001;161:25. [PMID: 11146695]

Orth SR et al: The nephrotic syndrome. N Engl J Med 1998;338:1202. [PMID: 9554862] (Etiology, pathogenesis, and treatment.)

Ponticelli C et al: Can prolonged treatment improve the prognosis in adults with focal segmental glomerulosclerosis? Am J Kidney Dis 1999;34:618. [PMID: 10516340]

Schwarz A: New aspects of the treatment of nephrotic syndrome. J Am Soc Nephrol 2001;(12 Suppl)17:S44. [PMID: 11251031]

Whelton A: Renal and related cardiovascular effects of conventional and COX-2-specific NSAIDs and non-NSAID analgesics. Am J Ther 2000;7:63. [PMID: 11319575]

■ NEPHROTIC DISEASE FROM SYSTEMIC DISORDERS

AMYLOIDOSIS

Amyloidosis consists of extracellular deposition of the fibrous protein amyloid in one or more sites in the body. Primary amyloidosis may occur in the absence of systemic disease or associated with multiple myeloma; indeed, both are plasma cell dyscrasias. Secondary amyloidosis is due to a chronic inflammatory disease such as rheumatoid arthritis, inflammatory bowel disease, or chronic infection. The acute phase reactant serum amyloid A is synthesized in the liver and deposited in the tissues. Primary amyloidosis usually occurs in older age groups and displays a benign urinary sediment; the amyloid is derived from immunoglobulin light chain. The degree of proteinuria is not associated with the extent of renal lesions. Kidneys can be enlarged as a result of amyloid deposition. Pathologically, glomeruli are filled with amorphous deposits that stain positive with Congo red and show green birefringence.

Treatment options are few. Remissions can occur in secondary amyloidosis if the inciting agent is removed. Primary amyloidosis of the kidney progresses to end-stage renal disease in an average of 2–3 years. Five-year overall survival is less than 20%, with death occurring from end-stage renal disease and heart disease. The use of alkylating agents and corticosteroids—eg, melphalan and prednisone—can reduce proteinuria and improve renal function in a small percentage of patients. Melphalan and stem cell transplantation is associated with high toxicity (45% deaths) but induces remission in the remaining 80% of patients. Renal transplant is an option in patients with secondary amyloid.

DIABETIC NEPHROPATHY

Diabetic nephropathy is the most common cause of end-stage renal disease in the United States (about 4000 cases a year). Type 1 diabetes mellitus carries a 30–40% chance of nephropathy after 20 years, whereas Type 2 has a 15–20% chance after 20 years. With the current epidemic of type 2 diabetes mellitus, rates of diabetic nephropathy are projected to continue to increase over at least the next 2 decades. Patients at higher risk include males, African-Americans, and Native Americans.

Patients at risk for nephropathy progress to develop the nephrotic syndrome. Diabetic retinopathy is invariably present in these patients. Initial screening of diabetics should always include urine examination for microalbuminuria. Dipstick examination may not be sensitive enough; a 24-hour urine collection is the accepted standard measure. (An albumin excretion of > 30 mg/d is abnormal.) However, an early morning spot urine albumin or albumin-creatinine ratio is adequate. (More than 20–30 μg/L of albumin or 30 mg of albumin per gram of creatinine is considered abnormal.) In patients prone to nephropathy, microalbuminuria will develop within 10–15 years after onset of diabetes and progress over the next 3–7 years to overt proteinuria. During the onset of subclinical proteinuria, aggressive treatment is called for. Strict glycemic control and treatment of hypertension have been proved to slow progression of disease. In particular, ACE inhibitors and angiotensin II receptor antagonists lower the rate of progression to clinical proteinuria; angiotensin II receptor antagonists have been shown to slow progression to end-stage renal disease. They may reduce intraglomerular pressure as well as treat hypertension.

The most common lesion is diffuse glomerulosclerosis, but nodular glomerulosclerosis (Kimmelstiel-Wilson nodules) is pathognomonic for this entity. The kidneys in these patients are usually enlarged as a result of cellular hypertrophy and proliferation. At the onset of diabetic nephropathy, glomerular disease will cause an increase in GFR. As the nephropathy progresses, with the development of macroalbuminuria, the GFR returns to normal and continues to decrease.

Patients with diabetes are prone to other renal disease. These include papillary necrosis, chronic interstitial nephritis, and type IV renal tubular acidosis (hyporeninemic hypoaldosteronemic type). Patients are more susceptible to acute renal failure from contrast material and have a poor prognosis once dialysis is begun.

HIV-ASSOCIATED NEPHROPATHY

HIV-associated nephropathy can present as the nephrotic syndrome in patients with HIV infection. Most patients are young black men. In these patients, the more common mode of acquisition of HIV is through intravenous drug use.

Patients can have a nephrotic picture with normal complement levels. Light microscopy shows focal segmental glomerulosclerosis as described above. Lesions can be of the collapsing variety and often exhibit severe tubulointerstitial damage.

There is no effective treatment for HIV-associated nephropathy. Highly active antiretroviral therapy (HAART) for a prolonged course may be beneficial. Occasionally, corticosteroid treatment has been used with variable success at dosages of 1 mg/kg/d along with cyclosporine and ACE inhibitors.

■ DISEASES DEMONSTRATING NEPHRITIC & NEPHROTIC COMPONENTS

SYSTEMIC LUPUS ERYTHEMATOSUS

Systemic lupus erythematosus is a systemic autoimmune disease in which renal involvement is common. In various series, clinical renal involvement ranges from 35% to 90%.

Patients present with nephritic or nephrotic syndromes. All patients with systemic lupus erythematosus should have routine urinalyses to monitor for the appearance of hematuria or proteinuria. If urinary abnormalities are detected, renal biopsy is often performed. The type of glomerular injury depends on the site of immune complex deposition. Five patterns of renal histology are seen on biopsy: type I, normal; type II, mesangial proliferative; type III, focal and segmental proliferative; type IV, diffuse proliferative; and type V, membranous nephropathy.

Individuals with type I and type II patterns require no treatment. Transformation of these types to a more active lesion is usually accompanied by an increase in lupus serologic activity and evidence of deteriorating renal function (eg, rising serum creatinine, increasing proteinuria). Repeat biopsy to confirm the transformation in these patients is standard. Patients with extensive type III lesions and all type IV lesions should receive aggressive immunosuppressive therapy. Poorest prognostic features in patients with type IV lesions are an elevated serum creatinine, hematocrit < 26%, and black race. Indications for treatment of type V disease are unclear; however, if superimposed proliferative lesions exist, aggressive therapy should be instituted.

Corticosteroids are the mainstay of treatment (methylprednisolone 1 g intravenously daily for 3 days followed by prednisone, 60 mg orally daily for 4–6 weeks) but are associated with many side effects and may not prevent progression of chronic lesions. Cytotoxic agents such as cyclophosphamide are almost always added because they improve long-term renal survival in patients with aggressive type III and type IV nephritis. They are typically used for 18–24 months (eg, cyclophosphamide intravenously every month for six doses and then every 3 months for six doses). Ongoing trials of newer therapies include cyclosporine and mycophenolate mofetil. In a recent randomized study, patients receiving mycophenolate mofetil and prednisolone versus cyclophosphamide and prednisolone had the same rates of remission and relapse but had fewer side effects. The return of serologic measurements to normal can be useful in monitoring treatment. Markers include dsDNA antibodies, C3, C4, CH50, and serum creatinine. Urinary protein and sediment are also helpful markers. Systemic lupus erythematosus patients on dialysis have a favorable prospect for long-term survival. Patients with kidney transplants have recurrent renal disease in 8% of cases.

MEMBRANOPROLIFERATIVE GLOMERULONEPHRITIS

Membranoproliferative glomerulonephritis in its primary form is an idiopathic syndrome that can present with nephritic or nephrotic features. (The secondary form can be seen in the immune complex, paraprotein deposition, and thrombotic microangiopathic glomerulonephritides discussed above.) Most patients are under 30 years of age. At least two major subgroups are recognized: type I and type II.

Patients with type I membranoproliferative glomerulonephritis present with a history of recent upper respiratory tract infection about a third of the time. Patients typically have a nephrotic picture, and complement levels are low. Histologically, the GBM is thickened because of immune complex deposition and abnormal mesangial cell proliferation between the GBM and the endothelial cells. This gives a characteristic "splitting" appearance to the capillary wall. Immunofluorescence shows IgG, IgM, and granular deposits of C3, C1q, and C4 (Table 22–10).

Type II membranoproliferative glomerulonephritis often presents with a nephritic picture and is less common than type I. Light microscopy is similar to type I. Serologically, type II is associated with C3 nephritic factor, which is a circulating IgG antibody. EM shows a characteristic dense deposit of homogeneous material that replaces part of the glomerular basement membrane.

Treatment is controversial in this disorder. After ruling out secondary causes, it consists of steroid therapy (there is no standard dosage for adults) and antiplatelet drugs (aspirin, 500–975 mg/d, plus dipyridamole 225 mg/d). The rationale for antiplatelet therapy is that platelet consumption is increased in membranoproliferative glomerulonephritis and may play a role in glomerular injury. Fifty percent of patients used to progress to end-stage renal disease in 10 years; these rates may now be slightly lower with the introduction of more aggressive therapy. Less favorable prognostic findings include type II disease, early renal insufficiency, hypertension, and persistent nephrotic syndrome. Both types of membranoproliferative glomerulonephritis will recur after renal transplantation; however, type II recurs more commonly.

Cameron JS: Lupus nephritis. J Am Soc Nephrol 1999;10:413. [PMID: 10215343] (Review of etiology, pathogenesis and management.)

Chan TM et al: Efficacy of mycophenolate mofetil in patients with diffuse proliferative lupus nephritis. N Engl J Med 2000;343:1156. [PMID: 11036121] (Mycophenolate is an alternative to cyclophosphamide in treating diffuse proliferative lupus nephritis.)

Daghestani L et al: Renal manifestations of hepatitis C infection. Am J Med 1999;106:347. [PMID: 10190385] (Includes review of hepatitis C-associated renal disease, with or without cryoglobulinemia.)

Markowitz GS: Membranous glomerulopathy: emphasis on secondary forms and disease variants. Adv Anat Pathol 2001;8:119. [PMID: 11345236]

Rai A et al: Henoch-Schönlein purpura nephritis. J Am Soc Nephrol 1999;10:2637. [PMID: 10589705] (Pathogenesis and management.)

Rao TK: Acute renal failure syndromes in human immunodeficiency virus infection. Semin Nephrol 1998;18:378. [PMID: 9692351] (In-depth review of acute renal failure in patients with human immunodeficiency virus.)

Szczech LA: Renal diseases associated with human immunodeficiency virus infection: epidemiology, clinical course, and management. Clin Infect Dis 2001;33:115. [PMID: 11389504]

Zimmerman R et al: Advances in the treatment of lupus nephritis. Annu Rev Med 2001;52:63. [PMID: 11160768]

■ TUBULOINTERSTITIAL DISEASES

Tubulointerstitial disease may be acute or chronic. Acute disease is most commonly associated with toxins and ischemia. Interstitial edema, infiltration with polymorphonuclear neutrophils, and tubular cell necrosis can be seen. (See Acute Renal Failure, above, and Table 22–11.) Chronic disease is associated with insult from an acute factor or progressive insult without any obvious acute cause. Interstitial fibrosis and tubular atrophy are present, with a mononuclear cell predominance. The chronic disorders are described below.

Table 22–11. Causes of acute tubulointerstitial nephritis.

Drug reactions
Antibiotics
  Beta-lactam antibiotics: methicillin, penicillin, ampicillin, cephalosporins
  Ciprofloxacin
  Erythromycin
  Sulfonamides
  Tetracycline
  Vancomycin
  Trimethoprim-sulfamethoxazole
  Ethambutol
  Rifampin
Nonsteroidal anti-inflammatory drugs
Diuretics
  Thiazides
  Furosemide
Miscellaneous
  Allopurinol
  Cimetidine
  Phenytoin
Systemic Infections
  Bacteria
    Streptococcus
    Corynebacterium diphtheriae
    Legionella
  Viruses
    Epstein-Barr virus
  Others
    Mycoplasma
    Rickettsia rickettsii
    Leptospira icterohaemorrhagiae
    Toxoplasma
Idiopathic
  Tubulointerstitial nephritis-uveitis (TIN–U)

CHRONIC TUBULOINTERSTITIAL DISEASES

ESSENTIALS OF DIAGNOSIS

- *Kidney size: small and contracted.*
- *Decreased urinary concentrating ability.*
- *Hyperchloremic metabolic acidosis.*
- *Hyperkalemia.*
- *Reduced GFR.*

General Considerations

There are four main causes of chronic tubulointerstitial disease. Other causes include multiple myeloma and gout, which are discussed in the section on multisystem disease with variable kidney involvement.

A. OBSTRUCTIVE UROPATHY

The most common cause of chronic tubulointerstitial disease is prolonged obstruction of the urinary tract. In partial obstruction, urine output alternates between polyuria (due to vasopressin insensitivity) and oliguria (due to decreased GFR). Azotemia and hypertension (due to increased renin-angiotensin production) are usually present. The major causes are prostatic disease in men; bilateral ureteral calculi; carcinoma of the cervix, colon, and bladder; and involvement of the retroperitoneum with other tumors or fibrosis.

Abdominal, rectal, and genitourinary examinations are helpful. Urinalysis can show hematuria, pyuria, and bacteriuria but is often benign. Abdominal ultrasound may detect mass lesions, hydroureter, and hydronephrosis. CT scanning and MRI provide more detailed information.

B. VESICOURETERAL REFLUX

Reflux nephropathy is primarily a disorder of childhood and occurs when urine passes retrograde from the bladder to the kidneys during voiding. It is the second most common cause of chronic tubulointerstitial disease. It occurs as a result of an incompetent vesicoureteral sphincter. Urine can extravasate into the interstitium; an inflammatory response develops, and fibrosis occurs. The inflammatory response is due to either bacteria or the normal urinary components.

Patients present as adolescents or young adults with hypertension, renal insufficiency, and a history of urinary tract infections as a child. Focal glomerulosclerosis is often seen. This is a cause of substantial proteinuria, unusual in most tubular diseases. Renal ultrasound or IVP can show renal scarring and hydronephrosis. Although most damage occurs before age 5, progressive renal deterioration to end-stage renal disease continues as a result of the early insults.

C. ANALGESICS

Analgesic nephropathy is most commonly seen in patients who ingest large quantities of analgesic combinations. The drugs of concern are phenacetin, paracetamol, aspirin, and NSAIDs. Chronic ingestion of 1 g/d for 3 years is the typical amount needed for renal dysfunction. This disorder occurs most frequently in individuals who are using analgesics for chronic headaches, muscular pains, and arthritis. Most patients grossly underestimate their analgesic use.

Tubulointerstitial inflammation and papillary necrosis are seen on pathologic examination. Papillary tip and inner medullary concentrations of some analgesics are tenfold higher than in the renal cortex. Phenacetin—once a common cause of this disorder and now rarely available—is metabolized in the papillae by the prostaglandin hydroperoxidase pathway to reactive intermediates that bind covalently to interstitial cell macromolecules, causing necrosis. Aspirin and other NSAIDs may worsen the damage by decreasing medullary blood flow (via inhibition of prostaglandin synthesis) and decreasing glutathione levels (which are necessary for detoxification).

Patients can exhibit hematuria, mild proteinuria, polyuria (from tubular damage), anemia (from gastrointestinal bleeding) and sterile pyuria. As a result of papillary necrosis, sloughed papillae can be found in the urine. An IVP may be helpful for detecting these—contrast will fill the area of the sloughed papillae, leaving a "ring shadow" sign at the papillary tip.

D. HEAVY METALS

Environmental exposure to heavy metals—such as lead and cadmium—is seen less frequently now in the United States. Chronic lead exposure can lead to tubulointerstitial disease. Individuals at risk are those with occupational exposure (eg, among welders who work with lead-based paint) and drinkers of alcohol distilled in automobile radiators (moonshine users). Lead is filtered by the glomerulus and is transported across the proximal convoluted tubules, where it accumulates and causes cell damage. Fibrosed arterioles and cortical scarring also lead to damaged kidneys. Proximal tubular damage leads to decreased secretion of uric acid, resulting in hyperuricemia and saturnine gout. Patients commonly are hypertensive. Diagnosis is most reliably performed with a calcium disodium edetate (EDTA) chelation test. Urinary excretion of more than 600 mg of lead in 24 hours following 1 g of EDTA indicates excessive lead exposure.

Occupational exposure to cadmium also causes proximal tubular dysfunction. Hypercalciuria and nephrolithiasis can be seen. Other heavy metals that can cause tubulointerstitial disease include mercury and bismuth.

Clinical Findings

A. SYMPTOMS AND SIGNS

Polyuria is common because tubular damage leads to inability to concentrate the urine. Dehydration can also occur as a result of salt-wasting defect in some individuals.

B. LABORATORY FINDINGS

Patients are hyperkalemic because the distal tubules become aldosterone-resistant. A hyperchloremic renal tubular acidosis is characteristic. The cause of the renal tubular acidosis is threefold: (1) reduced ammonia production, (2) inability to acidify the distal tubules, and (3) proximal tubular bicarbonate wasting. The urinalysis is nonspecific, as opposed to that seen in acute interstitial nephritis. Proteinuria is typically less than 2 g/d (owing to inability of the proximal tubule to reabsorb freely filterable proteins); a few cells may be seen; and broad waxy casts are often present.

Treatment

Treatment depends first upon identifying the disorder responsible for renal dysfunction. The degree of interstitial fibrosis that has developed can help to predict recovery of renal function. Once there is evidence for loss of parenchyma (small shrunken kidneys or interstitial fibrosis on biopsy), nothing can prevent the progression toward end-stage renal disease. Treatment is then directed at medical management. Tubular dysfunction may require potassium and phosphorus restriction and sodium, calcium, or bicarbonate supplements.

If hydronephrosis is present, relief of obstruction should be accomplished promptly. Prolonged obstruction leads to further tubular damage—particularly in the distal nephron—which may be irreversible despite relief of obstruction. Neither surgical correction of reflux nor medical therapy with antibiotics can prevent deterioration toward end-stage renal disease once renal scarring has occurred.

Those suspected of having lead nephropathy should continue chelation therapy with EDTA if there is no evidence of irreversible renal damage (eg, renal scarring or small kidneys). Continued exposure should be avoided.

Treatment of analgesic nephropathy requires withdrawal of all analgesics. Stabilization or improvement of renal function may occur if significant interstitial fibrosis is not present. Hydration during exposure to analgesics may also have some beneficial effects.

De Broe ME et al: Analgesic nephropathy. N Engl J Med 1998;338:446. [PMID: 9459649]

Harris DC: Tubulointerstitial renal disease. Curr Opin Nephrol Hypertens 2001;10:303. [PMID:11342791]

Michel DM et al: Acute interstitial nephritis. J Am Soc Nephrol 1998;9:506. [PMID: 9513915] (Causes and management.)

Rastegar A et al: The clinical spectrum of tubulointerstitial nephritis. Kidney Int 1998;54:313. [PMID: 9690198]

■ CYSTIC DISEASES OF THE KIDNEY

Renal cysts are epithelium-lined cavities filled with fluid or semisolid material. They develop primarily from renal tubular elements. One or more simple cysts are found in 50% of individuals over the age of 50. They are rarely symptomatic and have little clinical significance. In contrast, generalized cystic diseases are associated with cysts scattered throughout the cortex and medulla of both kidneys and can progress to end-stage renal disease (Table 22–12).

SIMPLE OR SOLITARY CYSTS

Simple cysts account for 65–70% of all renal masses. They are generally found at the outer cortex and contain fluid that is consistent with an ultrafiltrate of plasma. Most are found incidentally on ultrasonographic examination. Simple cysts are typically asymptomatic but can become infected.

The main concern with simple cysts is to differentiate them from malignancy, abscess, or polycystic kidney disease. Renal cystic disease can develop in dialysis patients. These cysts have a potential for progression to malignancy. Ultrasound and CT scanning are the recommended procedures for evaluating these masses. Simple cysts must meet three sonographic criteria to be considered benign: (1) echo-free, (2) sharply demarcated mass with smooth walls, and (3) an enhanced back wall (indicating good transmission through the cyst). Complex cysts can have thick walls, calcifications, solid components, and mixed echogenicity. On CT scan, the simple cyst should have a smooth thin wall which is sharply demarcated. It should not enhance with contrast media. A renal cell carcinoma will enhance but typically is of lower density than the rest of the parenchyma. Arteriography can also be used to evaluate a mass preoperatively. A renal cell carcinoma is hypervascular in 80%, hypovascular in 15%, and avascular in 5% of cases.

If a cyst meets the criteria for being benign, periodic reevaluation is the standard of care. If the lesion is not consistent with a simple cyst, surgical exploration is recommended.

AUTOSOMAL DOMINANT POLYCYSTIC KIDNEY DISEASE

This disorder is among the most common hereditary disease in the United States, affecting 1:1000 to 1:400 individuals. Fifty percent of patients will have end-stage renal disease by age 60. The disease has variable penetrance but accounts for 10% of dialysis patients in the USA. At least two genes account for this disorder: *ADPKD1* on the short arm of chromosome 16 (86% of patients) and *ADPKD2* on chromosome 4.

Table 22–12. Clinical features of renal cystic disease.

	Simple Renal Cysts	Acquired Renal Cysts	Autosomal Dominant Polycystic Kidney Disease	Medullary Sponge Kidney	Medullary Cystic Kidney
Prevalence	Common	Dialysis patients	1:1000	1:5000	Rare
Inheritance	None	None	Autosomal dominant	None	Autosomal dominant
Age at onset	...	...	20–40	40–60	Adulthood
Kidney size	Normal	Small	Large	Normal	Small
Cyst location	Cortex and medulla	Cortex and medulla	Cortex and medulla	Collecting ducts	Corticomedullary junction
Hematuria	Occasional	Occasional	Common	Rare	Rare
Hypertension	None	Variable	Common	None	None
Associated complications	None	Adenocarcinoma in cysts	Urinary tract infections, renal stones, cerebral aneurysms 10–15%, hepatic cysts 40–60%	Renal stones, urinary tract infections	Polyuria, salt wasting
Renal failure	Never	Always	Frequently	Never	Always

Clinical Findings

Most patients present with abdominal or flank pain and microscopic or gross hematuria. A history of urinary tract infections and nephrolithiasis is common. A family history is positive in 75% of cases, and more than 50% of patients have hypertension (see below) that may antedate the clinical manifestations of the disease. Patients have large kidneys that may be palpable on abdominal examination. The combination of hypertension and an abdominal mass should suggest the disease. Forty to 50 percent have concurrent hepatic cysts, and pancreatic and splenic cysts occur also. Hemoglobin and hematocrit tend to be maintained as a result of erythropoietin production by the cysts. The urinalysis may show hematuria and mild proteinuria. Ultrasonography confirms the diagnosis—two or more cysts in patients under age 30, two or more cysts in each kidney in patients age 30–59, and four or more cysts in each kidney in patients age 60 or over are diagnostic for autosomal dominant polycystic kidney disease. If sonographic results are unclear, CT scan is recommended and highly sensitive.

Complications & Treatment

A. PAIN

Abdominal or flank pain is caused by infection, bleeding into cysts, and nephrolithiasis. Bed rest and analgesics are recommended. Cyst decompression can help with chronic pain.

B. HEMATURIA

Gross hematuria is most commonly due to rupture of a cyst into the renal pelvis, but it can also be caused by a renal stone or urinary tract infection. Hematuria typically resolves within 7 days with bed rest and hydration. Recurrent bleeding should suggest the possibility of underlying renal cell carcinoma, particularly in men over age 50.

C. RENAL INFECTION

Patients presenting with flank pain, fever, and leukocytosis should be suspected of having an infected renal cyst. Blood cultures may be positive, and urinalysis may be normal because the cyst does not communicate directly with the urinary tract. CT scans can be helpful because an infected cyst may have an increased wall thickness. Bacterial cyst infections are difficult to treat. Antibiotics with cystic penetration should be used, eg, fluoroquinolones, trimethoprim-sulfamethoxazole, and chloramphenicol. Treatment may require 2 weeks of parenteral therapy followed by long-term oral therapy.

D. NEPHROLITHIASIS

Up to 20% of patients have kidney stones, primarily calcium oxalate. Hydration (2–3 L/d) is recommended.

E. HYPERTENSION

Fifty percent of patients have hypertension at time of presentation, and most will develop it during the course of the disease. Cyst-induced ischemia appears to cause activation of the renin-angiotensin system, and cyst decompression can lower blood pressure temporarily. Hypertension should be treated aggressively, as this may prolong the time to end-stage renal disease. (Diuretics should be used cautiously since the effect on renal cyst formation is unknown.)

F. CEREBRAL ANEURYSMS

About 10–15% of these patients have arterial aneurysms in the circle of Willis. Screening arteriography is not recommended unless the patient has a family history of aneurysms or is undergoing elective surgery with a high risk of developing hypertension.

G. OTHER COMPLICATIONS

Vascular problems include mitral valve prolapse in up to 25% of patients, aortic aneurysms, and aortic valve abnormalities. Colonic diverticula are more common in this population.

Prognosis

No medical therapy has been shown to prevent the development of renal failure, though treatment of hypertension and a low-protein diet may slow the progression of disease.

MEDULLARY SPONGE KIDNEY

This disease is a relatively common and benign disorder that is present at birth and not usually diagnosed until the fourth or fifth decade. Kidneys have a marked irregular enlargement of the medullary and interpapillary collecting ducts. This is associated with medullary cysts that are diffuse, giving a "Swiss cheese" appearance in these regions.

Clinical Findings

Medullary sponge kidney presents with gross or microscopic hematuria, recurrent urinary tract infections, or nephrolithiasis. Common abnormalities are a decreased urinary concentrating ability and nephrocalcinosis; less common is incomplete type I distal renal tubular acidosis. The diagnosis is confirmed with intravenous pyelography, which shows striations in the papillary portions of the kidney produced by the accumulation of contrast in dilated collecting ducts.

Treatment

There is no known therapy. Adequate fluid intake (2 L/d) helps to prevent stone formation. If hypercalciuria is present, thiazide diuretics are recommended because they decrease calcium excretion. Alkali therapy is recommended if renal tubular acidosis is present.

Prognosis

Renal function is well maintained unless there are complications from recurrent urinary tract infections and nephrolithiasis.

JUVENILE NEPHRONOPHTHISIS-MEDULLARY CYSTIC DISEASE

This is a rare disorder associated with almost universal progression to end-stage renal disease. The childhood type—juvenile nephronophthisis—is an autosomal re-

cessive disorder; the type appearing in adulthood—medullary cystic disease—is autosomal dominant. Both types are manifested by multiple small renal cysts at the corticomedullary junction and medulla. The cortex becomes fibrotic, and as the disease progresses, interstitial inflammation and glomerular sclerosis appear.

Clinical Findings

Patients with both forms exhibit polyuria, pallor, and lethargy. Hypertension occurs at the later stages of disease. The juvenile form causes growth retardation and end-stage renal disease before age 20. Patients require large amounts of salt and water as a result of renal salt wasting. Ultrasound and CT scan show small, scarred kidneys, and an open renal biopsy may be necessary to recover tissue from the corticomedullary junction.

Treatment & Prognosis

There is no medical therapy that will prevent progression to renal failure. Adequate salt and water intake are essential to replenish renal losses.

Davis ID et al: Can progression of autosomal dominant or autosomal recessive polycystic kidney disease be prevented? Semin Nephrol 2001;21:430. [PMID: 10922300]

Hildebrandt F et al: New insights: nephronophthisis-medullary cystic kidney disease. Pediatr Nephrol 2001;16:168. [PMID: 11261687]

Hwang DY et al: Unilateral renal cystic disease in adults. Nephrol Dial Transplant 1999;14:1999. [PMID: 10462284] (Case reports and review emphasizing the lack of a genetic background or progressive renal failure in patients with unilateral renal cystic disease compared with those with autosomal dominant polycystic kidney disease.)

Peters DJ et al: Autosomal-dominant polycystic kidney disease: modification of disease progression. Lancet 2001;358:1439. [PMID: 11705510]

■ MULTISYSTEM DISEASES WITH VARIABLE KIDNEY INVOLVEMENT*

MULTIPLE MYELOMA

Multiple myeloma is a malignancy of plasma cells (see Chapter 13). Renal involvement occurs in about one-fourth of all patients. "Myeloma kidney" is the presence of light chain immunoglobulins (Bence Jones protein) in the urine causing renal toxicity. Bence Jones protein causes direct renal tubular toxicity and

---

*Other diseases with variable renal involvement described elsewhere in this chapter include systemic lupus erythematosus, diabetes mellitus, and the vasculitides such as Wegener's granulomatosis and Goodpasture's disease.

results in tubular obstruction by precipitating in the tubules. The earliest tubular damage results in Fanconi's syndrome (a type II proximal renal tubular acidosis). The proteinuria seen with multiple myeloma is primarily due to light chains which are not detected on urine dipstick, which mainly detects albumin. Patients with multiple myeloma can also develop glomerular amyloidosis; in these patients, dipstick protein determinations are positive. Hypercalcemia and hyperuricemia are frequently seen. Other conditions resulting in renal dysfunction include plasma cell infiltration of the renal parenchyma and a hyperviscosity syndrome compromising renal blood flow.

SICKLE CELL DISEASE

Renal dysfunction associated with sickle cell disease is most commonly due to sickling of red blood cells in the renal medulla because of low oxygen tension and hypertonicity. Congestion and stasis lead to hemorrhage, interstitial inflammation, and papillary infarcts. Clinically, hematuria is common. Damage to renal capillaries also leads to diminished concentrating ability. Isosthenuria (urine osmolality equal to that of serum) is routine, and patients can easily become dehydrated. Papillary necrosis occurs as well. These abnormalities are commonly encountered in sickle cell trait. Sickle cell glomerulopathy is less common but will inexorably progress to end-stage renal disease. Its primary clinical manifestation is proteinuria. Optimal treatment requires adequate hydration and control of the sickle cell disease.

TUBERCULOSIS

The classic renal manifestation of tuberculosis is the presence of microscopic pyuria with a sterile urine culture—or "sterile pyuria." More often, other bacteria are present in addition. Microscopic hematuria is often present with pyuria. Urine cultures may demonstrate tubercle bacilli, and cavitation of the renal parenchyma occurs. Adequate drug therapy can result in resolution of renal involvement.

GOUT & THE KIDNEY

The kidney is the primary organ for excretion of uric acid. Depending on the pH and uric acid concentration, deposition can occur in the tubules, the interstitium, or the urinary tract. The more alkaline pH of the interstitium causes urate salt deposition, whereas the acidic environment of the tubules and urinary tract causes uric acid crystal deposition at high concentrations.

Three disorders are commonly seen: (1) uric acid nephrolithiasis, (2) acute uric acid nephropathy, and (3) chronic urate nephropathy. Renal dysfunction with uric acid nephrolithiasis stems from obstructive nephropathy. Acute uric acid nephropathy presents similarly to acute tubulointerstitial nephritis with direct toxicity from uric acid crystals. Chronic nephropathy is caused by deposition of urate crystals in the alkaline medium of the interstitium; this can lead to fibrosis and atrophy.

Treatment between gouty attacks involves avoidance of food and drugs causing hyperuricemia, aggressive hydration, and pharmacotherapy aimed at reducing serum uric acid levels. These disorders are seen in both "overproducers" and "underexcretors" of uric acid. The latter situation may seem counterintuitive; however, these patients have hyperacidic urine, which explains the deposition of relatively insoluble uric acid crystals.

■ THE KIDNEY & AGING

Renal mass declines progressively after the fourth decade. The renal medulla is spared in comparison to the cortex. Renal blood flow decreases with a resultant increase in arteriolar resistance. This allows for an increased filtration fraction and a relative sparing of the glomerular filtration rate (GFR). After the age of 40, GFR declines at a rate of approximately 0.8 mL/min/1.73 m^2/yr (though some older patients show little or no change). Serum creatinine values remain relatively constant because of decreased muscle mass along with the decrease in GFR. GFR impairment is partially due to thickening of the glomerular basement membrane, leading to glomerulosclerosis.

Renal tubular changes include impaired sodium handling, decreased concentration and dilutional ability, and impaired acidification. Thus, older patients are more prone to volume overload, hypo- and hypernatremia, and acidosis. Decreased renin synthesis and 1α-hydroxylase activity is also observed. These abnormalities can result in hyperkalemia, hypocalcemia, and elevated parathyroid hormone activity.

More adverse drug reactions occur in older patients. Three main pharmacokinetic changes occur: (1) altered volume of distribution, (2) altered drug half-life, and (3) altered elimination. The latter two are directly related to impaired renal clearance of drug.

The average age of patients starting dialysis is 61; the average age of patients receiving dialysis is 65. Both are increasing steadily. Hemodialysis is the modality of choice for those with functional impairment. Peritoneal dialysis is tolerated much better in those with cardiovascular disease. Sudden fluid and electrolyte shifts can cause hypotension, ischemia, and arrhythmias.

Renal transplantation is being offered to older individuals more often as it seems to benefit even those over 65. The main complications in this population are infection and cardiovascular disease. A reduced steroid requirement with the introduction of steroid-sparing agents such as cyclosporine has diminished infection rates.

Bruno D et al: Genitourinary complications of sickle cell disease. J Urol 2001;166:803. [PMID: 11490223]

Kaplan AA: Therapeutic apheresis for the renal complications of multiple myeloma and the dysglobulinemias. Ther Apher 2001;5:171. [PMID: 11467752]

Kapoor M et al: Malignancy and renal disease. Crit Care Clin 2001;17:571. [PMID: 11525049]

Rodriguez-Puyol D: The aging kidney. Kidney Int 1998;54:2247. [PMID: 9853294]

Ruilope LM et al: Hyperuricemia and renal function. Curr Hypertens Rep 2001;3:197. [PMID: 11353569]

Urology

23

Marshall L. Stoller, MD, & Peter R. Carroll, MD, FACS
See www.current-med.com/ch23.html

■ UROLOGIC EVALUATION

HISTORY

Pain

Pain in the genitourinary tract is usually associated with distention of a hollow viscus (ureteral obstruction, urinary retention) or the capsule of an organ (acute prostatitis, acute pyelonephritis). Pain may be local or referred. Pain associated with malignancy is usually a late manifestation and indicative of advanced disease.

A. RENAL PAIN

Pain of renal origin is usually located in the ipsilateral costovertebral angle. It may radiate to the umbilicus and may be referred to the ipsilateral testicle in men or the labium in women. In infection, the pain is typically constant, whereas in obstruction it may come and go. Nausea and vomiting may result from reflex stimulation of the celiac ganglion. Patients with intraperitoneal pathology will typically lie motionless to avoid pain, while patients with renal disease will move about to try to find a more comfortable position.

B. URETERAL PAIN

Ureteral pain is usually acute and a result of obstruction. Distention of the ureter along with hyperperistalsis and spasm of the smooth muscle of the ureter may result in two different pain patterns. Distention may cause a constant dull ache, while the spasms result in colic. The site of obstruction is often predicted by the site of pain. Upper ureteral obstruction may result in pain referred to the scrotum in males or to the labium in females. Midureteral obstruction may cause pain in the lower quadrant and thus may be confused with appendicitis in right-sided ureteral obstruction or diverticulitis in left-sided ureteral obstruction. Lower ureteral obstruction may cause inflammation of the ureteral orifice and thus be associated with symptoms of vesical irritability.

C. VESICAL PAIN

Acute urinary retention results in severe suprapubic discomfort. Chronic urinary retention is usually painless despite tremendous vesical distention. Suprapubic pain not related to the act of micturition is rarely vesical in origin. Acute cystitis pain is usually referred to the distal urethra and is associated with micturition.

D. PROSTATIC PAIN

Prostatic pain is associated with inflammation and is located in the perineum. Pain radiates to the lumbosacral spine, inguinal canals, or lower extremities. Because of its location near the bladder neck, inflammatory processes of the prostate result in irritative voiding complaints.

E. PENILE PAIN

Pain in the flaccid penis is secondary to inflammatory processes caused by sexually transmitted diseases or paraphimosis, a condition of the uncircumcised male in which the retracted foreskin is trapped behind the glans penis, resulting in vascular congestion and painful swelling of the glans. Pain in the erect penis may be due to Peyronie's disease (fibrous plaque of the tunica albuginea, resulting in painful curvature of the erect penis) or to priapism (prolonged painful erection).

F. TESTICULAR PAIN

Acute conditions such as trauma, torsion of the testis or one of its appendices, or epididymo-orchitis cause acute pain within the scrotum with radiation to the ipsilateral groin. Chronic pain may persist for months following successful treatment of acute epididymitis. Chronic pain produced by a varicocele or hydrocele results in "heaviness" without radiation. Disorders of the kidney, retroperitoneal structures, or inguinal canal may result in pain referred to the testis.

Hematuria

Gross hematuria in adults is considered a sign of malignancy until proved otherwise.

The character of the hematuria may give a clue to the site of origin. **Initial hematuria,** the presence of blood at the beginning of the urinary stream that clears during the stream, implies an anterior (penile) urethral source. **Terminal hematuria,** the presence of blood at the end of the urinary stream, implies a bladder neck or prostatic urethral source. **Total hematuria,** the presence of blood throughout the urinary stream, implies a bladder or upper tract source.

Associated symptoms give clues to the cause. Hematuria associated with renal colic suggests ureteral stone, but the passage of blood clots from a bleeding tumor mimics this scenario. Irritative voiding symptoms in a young woman may suggest acute bacterial infection and associated hemorrhagic cystitis, yet the same picture in an older woman or in any male raises concerns about neoplasm. In any situation, if cultures are negative or symptoms persist after therapy, further evaluation is warranted. Absent other symptoms, gross hematuria may be more indicative of tumor, but staghorn calculi, glomerulonephropathies, and polycystic kidney disease are in the differential.

Irritative Voiding Symptoms

Urgency is the sudden desire to void. It is observed in inflammatory conditions such as cystitis or in hyperreflexic neuropathic conditions such as neurogenic bladders resulting from upper motor neuron lesions. **Dysuria** (painful urination) is usually associated with inflammation. The pain is typically referred to the tip of the penis in men or to the urethra in women. **Frequency** is the increased number of voids during the daytime, and **nocturia** is nocturnal frequency. Adults normally void five or six times a day and once at most during the nighttime hours. Increased numbers of voidings may result from increased urinary output or decreased functional bladder capacity. Diabetes mellitus, diabetes insipidus, excess fluid ingestion, and diuretics (including caffeine and alcohol) are a few of the causes of increased urinary output. Decreased functional bladder capacities may result from bladder outlet obstruction (increased residual urine volume results in a lower functional capacity), neurogenic bladder disorders (spasticity and reduced compliance), extrinsic bladder compression (uterine fibroids, radiation-induced fibrosis, pelvic neoplasms), or psychologic factors (anxiety).

Obstructive Voiding Symptoms

Hesitancy is a delay in the initiation of micturition. It results from the increased time required for the bladder to attain the high pressure necessary to exceed that of the urethra in the obstructed setting. **Decreased force of stream** results from the high resistance the bladder faces and is often associated with a decrease in caliber of the stream. **Intermittency** and **postvoid dribbling** are interruption of the urinary stream and the uncontrolled release of the terminal few drops of urine, respectively. Obstructive symptoms are most commonly due to benign prostatic hyperplasia, urethral stricture, or neurogenic bladder disorders. Pro-

static or urethral carcinoma and foreign body are other causes.

Incontinence

Urinary incontinence is the involuntary loss of urine. The history permits subclassification into one of four categories of incontinence. Such a distinction is necessary, as the workup and treatment vary with each of the categories. With **total incontinence,** patients lose urine at all times and in all positions. **Stress incontinence** is the loss of urine associated with activities that result in an increase in intra-abdominal pressure (coughing, sneezing, lifting, exercising). Uncontrolled loss of urine preceded by a strong urge to void is known as **urge incontinence.** Chronic urinary retention may result in **overflow incontinence.**

Systemic Manifestations

Fever when associated with other symptoms of a urinary tract infection (see below) helps to localize the site of infection. In women, high fevers occur in acute pyelonephritis. Fevers are not typical of uncomplicated cystitis. In men, a febrile urinary tract infection implies acute pyelonephritis, acute prostatitis, or acute epididymitis. Fever may also be seen associated with malignancy of the kidney, bladder, or testis.

Weight loss and malaise also may be associated with tumor or disease states associated with chronic renal failure.

Other Symptoms

Hematospermia, the presence of blood in the ejaculate, results from inflammation of the prostate or seminal vesicles. Blood in the initial portion of the ejaculate implicates the prostate, whereas terminal hematospermia implies a seminal vesicle origin. Workup should include urinalysis, digital rectal examination with prostate massage, and microscopic evaluation of the expressed prostatic secretions. More invasive procedures such as cystoscopy or transrectal ultrasound with prostate biopsy are reserved for patients with hematuria or abnormal rectal examinations, respectively. Persistent hematospermia warrants similar testing. The risk of malignancy with isolated hematospermia, normal urinalysis, and normal digital rectal examination is low.

Pneumaturia, the presence of gas in the urine, is usually secondary to a fistula between the bladder and the gastrointestinal tract. Diverticulitis is the most common cause, followed by colonic carcinoma, Crohn's disease, and radiation enteritis. The patient reports bubbles or particulate matter in the urine. On occasion, pneumaturia may be due to infection by gasproducing organisms.

Urethral discharge is the most common symptom of sexually transmitted diseases. Dysuria and urethral itching are seen in association with the discharge. A bloody urethral discharge, especially in an elderly patient, suggests urethral carcinoma.

Cloudy urine may be secondary to a urinary tract infection, yet in the absence of infection it can be a result of an alkaline urinary pH. Such conditions result in phosphate crystal precipitation. Chyluria, the presence of lymph in the urine, results from a fistula between the urinary tract and the lymphatic system. Filariasis, tuberculosis, and retroperitoneal tumors are some of the possible causes of this rare symptom.

PHYSICAL EXAMINATION

General Examination

The pallor of anemia and cachexia may be seen in malignancy. Gynecomastia occurs in testicular carcinomas or as a complication of hormonal therapy in prostatic cancer. Hypertension can be a result of renovascular disease or adrenal cancer.

Detailed Examination

A. KIDNEY

Because of the liver, the right kidney is lower than the left. The lower pole of the right kidney may be palpable in thin patients, yet the left kidney is usually not palpable unless abnormally enlarged. To palpate the kidney, one hand is placed posteriorly in the costovertebral angle to push the kidney anteriorly, while the second hand is placed anteriorly under the costal margin. With inspiration, the kidney may be palpated between the two hands.

Auscultation of the upper abdominal quadrants in hypertensive patients may reveal a systolic bruit associated with renal artery stenosis or an arteriovenous malformation; however, aortic bruits or transmitted heart murmurs may give similar findings.

Patients with flank pain should be tested for hyperesthesia of the overlying skin by pin testing, as this may be secondary to nerve root irritation and radiculitis rather than being of renal origin.

B. BLADDER

The normal adult bladder is not palpable unless filled with at least 150 mL of urine. Percussion is better than palpation in diagnosing the distended bladder. Dullness is appreciated over the full bladder and changes to tympany if the air-filled bowel is anterior to the bladder.

Bimanual examination under anesthesia is helpful in the evaluation of patients with suspected bladder neoplasms. In the male, the bladder is palpated between the abdominal wall and the rectum while in the female it is palpated between the abdominal wall and the vagina. This is the best means of assessing vesical mobility and thus resectability.

C. PENIS

The foreskin must be retracted in the uncircumcised male to permit inspection of the urethral meatus and glans. The position of the urethral meatus, the presence of urethral discharge, inflammation, penile tumor, and skin lesions must be noted. In **phimosis,** the foreskin cannot be retracted over the glans. In **paraphimosis,** the foreskin has been left retracted behind the glans, resulting in painful engorgement and edema of the glans. If not attended to, this may result in glandular ischemia. Congenital anomalies of position of the urethral meatus are called **hypospadias** when the meatus is located on the ventral aspect of the penis, scrotum, or perineum and **epispadias** when it is located on the dorsal aspect of the penis. A thick yellow urethral discharge is seen in gonococcal urethritis, whereas a thin clear or white discharge is noted in nongonococcal urethritis. Palpation of the dorsal penile shaft for plaques of Peyronie's disease and of the ventral surface for urethral tumors should be performed.

D. SCROTUM AND ITS CONTENTS

The most common referral to the urologist concerning the scrotum is for evaluation of a mass. It is important to determine whether the lesion resides within the testicle or is related to the epididymis or cord structures. The testes are palpated between the fingertips of both hands. Normal testes measure 4.5×2.5 cm and are rubbery in consistency. The epididymis rests posterolateral to the testis and varies in its degree of testicular attachment. Masses arising from within the testes are usually malignant; those from the epididymis and spermatic cord structures are usually benign. Transillumination will distinguish solid and cystic lesions.

The history and physical examination can make the diagnosis in the majority of cases. Tumors of the testis are usually painless, firm, solid lesions within the substance of the testis. These lesions do not transilluminate.

Acute epididymitis is an acute infectious process and is associated with painful enlargement of the epididymis. Fever and irritative voiding symptoms are common. In advanced states, the infection can spread to the testis, making the distinction between the epididymis and the testicle difficult on physical examination. The entire scrotal contents may be painful on palpation, yet relief may be offered to the supine patient by elevation of the scrotum above the pubic symphysis (Prehn's sign).

A **hydrocele** is a collection of fluid between the two layers of the tunica vaginalis. The diagnosis is readily made by transillumination. Evaluation of the testis is necessary, as approximately 10% of testicular tumors may have an associated hydrocele.

A **varicocele** is engorgement of the internal spermatic veins above the testis. These almost always occur on the left side as the left spermatic vein empties into the left renal vein while the right empties into the inferior vena cava. Varicoceles should diminish in size or disappear with the patient in the supine position. The sudden onset of a right varicocele should raise the question of a retroperitoneal malignancy resulting in obstruction of the right spermatic vein; a left varicocele suggests obstruction of the left renal vein, as in renal cell carcinoma.

Torsion of the testis typically occurs in the 10- to 20-year age group and presents with acute onset of pain and swelling within the testis. Examination reveals a painful testis that may have a "high lie" in relation to the other testis. The acute onset, lack of voiding symptoms, and the different age distribution may help distinguish it from epididymitis.

Torsion of the appendices of the testis or epididymis may be indistinguishable from torsion of the testis and affects a similar age group as torsion of the testis. On occasion a small palpable lump on the superior pole of the testis or epididymis is discernible that may appear blue when the skin is pulled tautly over it ("blue dot sign").

E. Rectal Examination in the Male

Inspection for anal pathology (fissures, warts, carcinoma, hemorrhoids) should be performed first. Upon insertion of the finger, anal tone can be estimated and a bulbocavernosus reflex can be elicited. As the anal and urinary sphincter derive from a common innervation, clues to neurogenic disorders may be obtained. The entire prostate is then examined, with attention being directed toward size and consistency. The normal prostate is approximately 4×4 cm and weighs 25 g. Normal consistency is that of the contracted thenar eminence with the thumb opposed to the little finger. Rubbery enlargement of the prostate is noted in benign prostatic hyperplasia. Induration may be perceived with carcinoma but also with chronic inflammation. The remainder of the rectum is then examined to exclude primary rectal disease.

F. Pelvic Examination in the Female

Examination of the introitus should include inspection for atrophic changes, ulcers, discharge, and warts. The urethral meatus can be inspected for caruncles and palpated for tumors or diverticula. Bimanual examination of the bladder, uterus, and adnexa should be performed with two fingers in the vagina and one hand on the abdomen, and attention is directed toward abnormal masses.

URINALYSIS

Collection of Specimens

In the male, a clean-catch urine is obtained in separate aliquots. Such a scheme may permit localization of disease. The first 5–10 mL is collected and represents the urethral specimen; a midstream specimen reflects conditions in the bladder and upper urinary tracts. If necessary, the prostate is then massaged and the expressed secretions collected. If no fluid is obtained, the next 2–3 mL of urine are collected, which reflects prostatic pathology. (See also Hematuria.)

Dipstick Urinalysis

A. pH

There is no role for dipstick urinalysis screening for urinary tract disorders in asymptomatic adults except for pregnant women. Urinary pH (range 5.0–9.0) may be helpful in the diagnosis and treatment of some urologic conditions. Alkaline urine in a patient with a urinary tract infection suggests the presence of a urea-splitting organism, most commonly *Proteus mirabilis,* though some strains of klebsiella, pseudomonas, providencia, and staphylococcus may also produce urease. Acidic urine in a patient with urolithiasis suggests uric acid or cystine stones. Failure to acidify the urine below a pH of 5.5 despite a metabolic acidosis suggests a distal renal tubular acidosis.

B. Protein

Dipsticks using bromphenol blue can detect protein in concentrations exceeding 10 mg/dL. It measures albumin and is not sensitive for the light chain of immunoglobulins (Bence Jones proteins). False-positive results are seen in urine containing numerous leukocytes or epithelial cells. (See Proteinuria in Chapter 22.)

C. Urobilinogen and Bilirubin

Urobilinogen is formed from the catabolism of conjugated bilirubin in the gut by bacteria, and the majority is cleared by the liver. Normally, only 1–4 mg of urobilinogen is excreted in the urine per day. Hemolytic processes or hepatocellular disease can lead to increased urinary levels, while complete biliary obstruction or broad-spectrum antibiotics that alter the gut bacterial flora may result in absent urinary urobilinogen. Unconjugated bilirubin is not filtered by the glomerulus, while only 1% of conjugated bilirubin is filtered. Normally no bilirubin is detected by urinary dipstick, since only concentrations greater than 0.4 mg/dL are detectable. Conditions manifesting elevated conjugated bilirubin in the serum will result in higher urinary levels. Ascorbic acid may cause false-negative results, while phenazopyridine may cause false-positive results.

D. Glucose and Ketones

Only small amounts of glucose are normally excreted in the urine, and these levels are below the sensitivity of the dipstick. Any positive finding requires evaluation for diabetes. The test is specific for glucose and does not cross-react with any other sugars. Ascorbic acid or elevated ketones may result in false-negative results.

Ketones are not normally found in the urine, but fasting, postexercise states, and pregnancy may result in elevated urinary ketones. Diabetics often demonstrate elevated urinary ketone levels prior to an elevation in serum levels. False-positive results occur in dehydration or in the presence of levodopa metabolites, mesna (sodium mercaptoethanesulfonate), and other sulfhydryl-containing compounds.

E. NITRITES

Normally, the urine does not contain nitrites. Many gram-negative bacteria can reduce nitrate to nitrite, which is thus an indicator of bacteriuria. However, the low sensitivity of the test requires clarification. Adequate numbers of bacteria must be present (10^5 organisms/mL), nitrates must be available in the urine, and the bacteria must be in contact with the urine for a sufficient time (usually 4 hours). Therefore, the first morning voided sample is preferable. False-negative results may be due to non-nitrate-reducing organisms, frequent urination, dilute or acidic urine (pH < 6.0), and the presence of urobilinogen. False-positive results are usually secondary to contaminated specimens, so that bacteria are indeed present in the sample yet not present in the urinary tract.

F. LEUKOCYTE ESTERASE

Leukocyte esterase is an enzyme produced by white cells. The dipstick detects leukocytes in the urine, which is thus suggestive but not diagnostic for bacteria. False-positive tests result from specimen contamination. False-negative tests result from high specific gravity, glycosuria, the presence of urobilinogen, and medications, including rifampin, phenazopyridine, and ascorbic acid.

G. BLOOD

The urinary dipstick for blood measures intact erythrocytes, free hemoglobin, and myoglobin. False-positive results in women may occur as a result of contamination at collection with menstrual blood. Concentrated urine may also cause a false-positive result, as patients normally excrete 1000 erythrocytes per milliliter of urine. Vigorous exercise and vitamins or foods associated with high oxidant levels may also give a false-positive result. High ascorbic acid levels may give a false-negative result.

Microscopic Urinalysis

A. LEUKOCYTES

The presence of more than five leukocytes per high-power field is considered significant pyuria. Leukocytes in the urine are indicative of injury to the urinary tract, which may or may not be due to infection. Other causes of pyuria include calculous disease, strictures, neoplasm, glomerulonephropathy, or interstitial cystitis. Leukocyte counts will vary by the state of hydration, method of collection, and degree of injury to the urinary tract.

B. ERYTHROCYTES

The presence of more than five erythrocytes per high-power field is considered significant and warrants further investigation. (See Evaluation of Hematuria, below.) The appearance of the red cells sometimes gives a clue to their origin within the urinary tract. Dysmorphic (irregularly shaped) cells have an uneven distribution of hemoglobin and cytoplasm, and usually indicate glomerular disease. Red cells that are round, with evenly distributed hemoglobin, suggest disease along the epithelial lining of the urinary tract. All patients with hematuria require further diagnostic workup (see below); morphology, though of interest, is not of sufficient accuracy to allow firm diagnostic conclusions.

C. EPITHELIAL CELLS

The presence of squamous epithelial cells in the urinary sediment is indicative of contamination and thus requires a repeat collection. Transitional epithelial cells are occasionally noted in normal urinary sediment, but if present in large numbers or clumps they cause concern about possible neoplasm. Cytologic examination may be necessary to confirm the finding.

D. BACTERIA AND YEASTS

The identification of organisms in an uncontaminated specimen implies infection, which must be confirmed by culture. The presence of several organisms per high-power field usually correlates with a culture count of 10^5 organisms per milliliter. Gram staining may further aid in characterizing the organism. *Candida albicans* is the most common yeast seen in the urine, and characteristic budding and clumps are typically observed.

E. CASTS

Casts are formed in the distal tubules and collecting ducts as a result of Tamm-Horsfall mucoprotein precipitation. They congregate near the edges of the coverslip and are detected best in a fresh specimen viewed under low power. If the urine is devoid of cells, hyaline casts are formed. Casts with entrapped red cells are indicative of glomerulonephritis or vasculitis. Leukocyte casts are suggestive of pyelonephritis. Epithelial casts in small numbers are normal, but in large numbers they suggest intrinsic renal disease. Granular casts result from degeneration of other cellular casts and also suggest intrinsic renal disease.

F. CRYSTALS

Uric acid, oxalate, and cystine crystals are more often precipitated in acid urine, while phosphate crystals are more commonly seen in alkaline urine. The presence of uric acid, phosphate, and oxalate crystals can be seen in normal patients as well as in stone-formers. Cystine crystals, with a characteristic hexagonal benzene ring shape, are seen only in patients with cystinuria and are thus pathologic.

Bove P et al: Reexamining the value of hematuria testing in patients with acute flank pain. J Urol 1999;162(3 Part 1):685. [PMID: 10458342] (Fourteen percent of patients presenting with ureterolithiasis had a negative dipstick for blood and fewer than two red cells per high-power field.)

■ EVALUATION OF HEMATURIA

If gross hematuria occurs, a description of the timing (initial, terminal, total) may give a clue to the localization of disease. Associated symptoms (ie, renal colic, irritative voiding symptoms, constitutional symptoms) should be investigated. Drug ingestion and associated medical problems may also provide diagnostic clues. Anticoagulants, analgesic abuse (papillary necrosis), cyclophosphamide (chemical cystitis), antibiotics (interstitial nephritis), diabetes mellitus, sickle cell trait or disease (papillary necrosis), a history of stone disease, or malignancy should all be investigated. The presence of hematuria in patients on anticoagulation therapy warrants a complete evaluation consisting of upper tract imaging, cystoscopy, and urine cytology.

Physical examination should emphasize signs of systemic disease (fever, rash, lymphadenopathy, abdominal or pelvic masses) as well as signs of medical renal disease (hypertension, volume overload). Urologic evaluation may demonstrate an enlarged prostate, flank mass, or urethral disease.

Initial laboratory investigations include a urinalysis and urine culture. Proteinuria and casts suggest renal origin. Irritative voiding symptoms, bacteriuria, and a positive urine culture in the female suggest urinary tract infection, but follow-up urinalysis is important after treatment to ensure resolution of the hematuria.

Further evaluation includes urinary cytology, upper tract imaging, and cystoscopy. Cytology especially assists in the diagnosis of bladder neoplasm, and three voided samples are recommended to maximize sensitivity. Upper tract imaging (usually abdominal and pelvic CT with and without contrast) may identify neoplasms of the kidney or ureter as well as identifying benign conditions such as urolithiasis, obstructive uropathy, papillary necrosis, medullary sponge kidney, or polycystic kidney disease. The role of ultrasonographic evaluation of the urinary tract for hematuria is unclear. While it may provide adequate information for the kidney, its sensitivity in detecting ureteral disease may be lower. In addition, its higher degree of operator dependence may further confound the issue. Cystoscopy can assess for bladder or urethral neoplasm, benign prostatic enlargement, and radiation or chemical cystitis. For gross hematuria, cystoscopy is ideally performed while the patient is actively bleeding to allow better localization (ie, lateralize to one side of the upper tracts, bladder, or urethra).

In patients with gross or microscopic hematuria, an upper tract source (kidneys and ureters) can be identified in 10% of cases. For upper tract sources, stone disease accounts for 40%, medical renal disease (medullary sponge kidney, glomerulonephritis, papillary necrosis) for 20%, renal cell carcinoma for 10%, and transitional cell carcinoma of the ureter or renal pelvis for 5%. In the absence of infection, gross hematuria from a lower tract source is most commonly from transitional cell carcinoma of the bladder. Microscopic hematuria in the male is most commonly from benign prostatic hyperplasia. In patients with negative evaluations, repeat evaluations are warranted to avoid a missed malignancy; however, the ideal frequency of such evaluations is not defined. Urinary cytology can be repeated in 3–6 months, and cystoscopy and upper tract imaging after a year.

Angulo JC et al: The value of comparative volumetric analysis of urinary and blood erythrocytes to localize the source of hematuria. J Urol 1999;162:119. [PMID: 10379753] (Red cells originating from the kidney and going through the glomerulus are smaller than those originating from other nonrenal sources of the genitourinary collecting system.)

Avidor Y et al: Clinical significance of gross hematuria and its evaluation in patients receiving anticoagulant and aspirin treatment. Urology 2000;55:22. [PMID: 10654888] (A complete urologic evaluation is required for patients with hematuria whether or not the patient is taking anticoagulants.)

■ GENITOURINARY TRACT INFECTIONS

Urinary tract infections are among the most common entities encountered in medical practice. In acute infections, a single pathogen is usually found, whereas two or more pathogens are often seen in chronic infections. Coliform bacteria are responsible for most nonnosocomial, uncomplicated urinary tract infections, with E coli being the most common. Such infections typically are sensitive to a wide variety of orally administered antibiotics and respond quickly. Nosocomial infections often are due to more resistant pathogens and may require parenteral antibiotics. Renal infections are of particular concern because if they are inadequately treated, loss of renal function may result. Previously, a colony count > 10^5/mL was considered the criterion for urinary tract infection. However, it is now recognized that up to 50% of women with symptomatic infections have lower counts. In addition, the presence of pyuria correlates poorly with the diagnosis of urinary tract infection, and thus urinalysis alone is not adequate for diagnosis. With respect to treatment, soft tissue infections (pyelonephritis, prostatitis) require intensive therapy for 1–2 weeks, while mucosal infections (cystitis) may require 1–3 days of therapy.

Classification & Pathogenesis

First infections—ie, first documented infections—in young women tend to be uncomplicated. **Unresolved bacteriuria** occurs when the urinary tract is never sterilized during therapy. This may result from bacterial resistance to therapy, noncompliance, mixed infections with organisms having different susceptibilities, renal insufficiency, or the rapid emergence of resistance from an initially sensitive organism. **Persistent bacteriuria** occurs when the urinary tract is initially sterilized during therapy but a persistent source of infection in contact with the urinary tract remains. This may result from infected stones, chronic pyelonephritis or prostatitis, vesicoenteric or vesicovaginal fistulas, obstructive uropathy, foreign bodies, or urethral diverticula. **Reinfections** occur when new infections with new pathogens occur following successful treatment.

Ascending infection from the urethra is the most common route. Women are particularly at risk for urinary tract infections because the female urethra is short and the vagina becomes colonized with bacteria. Sexual intercourse is a major precipitating factor in young women, and the use of diaphragms and spermicidal creams (alters normal vaginal bacterial flora) further increases the risk for cystitis. Pyelonephritis most commonly results from ascent of infection up the ureter. **Hematogenous spread** to the urinary tract is uncommon, the exceptions being tuberculosis and cortical renal abscesses. **Lymphogenous spread** is rare. **Direct extension** from other organs may occur, especially from intraperitoneal abscesses in inflammatory bowel disease or pelvic inflammatory disease.

Susceptibility Factors

A. Bacterial Virulence Factors

Over 90% of first infections are caused by *E coli*. While there are over 150 strains of *E coli*, most infections are caused by only five serogroups (O1, O4, O6, O18, and O75). It appears that strains implicated in infection have a higher degree of bacterial adherence, which is mediated by the bacterial fimbriae or pili. A relationship between the type of fimbriae and the type of infection exists. P-fimbriated strains of *E coli* are associated with pyelonephritis in normal urinary tracts, whereas strains without P fimbriae are associated with pyelonephritis only when vesicoureteral reflux is present.

B. Host Susceptibility Factors

1. Bladder and upper tract factors—Intrinsic defense mechanisms in the bladder include efficient emptying of the bladder with voiding, which decreases colony counts; a protective glycosaminoglycan layer, which interferes with bacterial adherence; and the antimicrobial properties of urine (high osmolality and extremes of pH). The presence of vesicoureteral reflux, diminished renal blood flow, or intrinsic renal disease may increase the likelihood of upper tract involvement.

2. Female-specific factors—The anatomically short female urethra facilitates the ascent of organisms from the introitus into the bladder. Women with recurrent urinary tract infections have more adhesin receptors on their genitourinary mucosa and therefore have more binding sites for pathogens. Women whose mucosal secretions lack fucosyltransferase activity ("nonsecretors") are more prone to urinary tract infections. The lack of this enzyme results in lack of expression of the A, B, and H blood group antigens that normally may mask some of the bacterial adhesin receptors, making these receptors more available for pathogen binding.

3. Male-specific factors—A higher incidence of urinary tract infections in the uncircumcised male in comparison to the circumcised male has been observed. The mucosal surface of the foreskin has a propensity for colonization with P-fimbriated bacteria in a fashion analogous to that of the female introitus. The prostate in normal males secretes zinc, which is a potent antibacterial agent and thus prevents ascending infection. Lower zinc levels are seen in prostatic secretions of men with bacterial prostatitis.

Prevention of Reinfections

Prophylactic antibiotic therapy is given to prevent recurrence after treatment of urinary tract infection.

Women who have more than three episodes of cystitis per year are considered candidates for prophylaxis. Prior to institution of therapy, a thorough urologic evaluation is warranted to exclude any anatomic abnormality (stones, reflux, fistula, etc). Only selected antimicrobial agents are effective in prophylaxis. To be successful, the agent must eliminate pathogenic bacteria from the fecal or introital reservoirs and not cause bacterial resistance. Single dosing at bedtime or at the time of intercourse is the recommended schedule. The three most commonly used agents for prophylaxis are trimethoprim-sulfamethoxazole (40 mg/200 mg), nitrofurantoin (100 mg), and cephalexin (250 mg).

Proceedings of the 5th International Symposium on Clinical Evaluation of Drug Efficacy in Urinary Tract Infection and of the Urinary Tract Infections Symposia of the Commission for Treatment of Urinary Tract Infection of the International Society of Chemotherapy. 29 June–3 July1997. Sydney, Australia. Int J Antimicrob Agents 1999;11:183. [PMID: 10465618]

Semeniuk H et al: Evaluation of the leukocyte esterase and nitrite urine dipstick screening tests for detection of bacteriuria in women with suspected uncomplicated urinary tract infections. J Clin Microbiol 1999;37:3051. [PMID: 10449505] (A urine dipstick screen for leukocyte esterase or nitrite may be negative in 19% of patients with significant bacteriuria.)

Talan DA et al: Comparison of ciprofloxacin (7 days) and trimethoprim-sulfamethoxazole (14 days) for acute uncomplicated pyelonephritis in women: a randomized trial. JAMA 2000;283:1583. [PMID: 10735395] (Uncomplicated pyelonephritis can be successfully treated with a 7-day course of oral antibiotics.)

ACUTE CYSTITIS

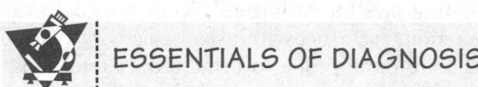

ESSENTIALS OF DIAGNOSIS

- Irritative voiding symptoms.
- Patient usually afebrile.
- Positive urine culture; blood cultures may also be positive.

General Considerations

Acute cystitis is an infection of the bladder most commonly due to the coliform bacteria (especially *E coli*) and occasionally gram-positive bacteria (enterococci). The route of infection is typically ascending from the urethra. Viral cystitis due to adenovirus is sometimes seen in children but is rare in adults.

Clinical Findings

A. SYMPTOMS AND SIGNS

Irritative voiding symptoms (frequency, urgency, dysuria) and suprapubic discomfort are common. Women may experience gross hematuria, and symptoms in women may often appear following sexual intercourse. Physical examination may elicit suprapubic tenderness, but examination is often unremarkable. Systemic toxicity is absent.

B. LABORATORY FINDINGS

Urinalysis shows pyuria and bacteriuria and varying degrees of hematuria. The degree of pyuria and bacteriuria does not necessarily correlate with the severity of symptoms. Urine culture is positive for the offending organism, but colony counts exceeding 10^5/mL are not essential for the diagnosis.

C. IMAGING

Follow-up imaging is warranted only if pyelonephritis, recurrent infections, or anatomic abnormalities are suspected.

Differential Diagnosis

In women, infectious processes such as vulvovaginitis and pelvic inflammatory disease can usually be distinguished by pelvic examination and urinalysis. In men, urethritis and prostatitis may be distinguished by

physical examination (urethral discharge or prostatic tenderness). Cystitis in men is rare and implies a pathologic process such as infected stones, prostatitis, or chronic urinary retention requiring further investigation.

Noninfectious causes of cystitis-like symptoms include pelvic irradiation, chemotherapy (cyclophosphamide), bladder carcinoma, interstitial cystitis, voiding dysfunction disorders, and psychosomatic disorders.

Treatment

Uncomplicated cystitis in women can be treated with short-term antimicrobial therapy, which consists of single-dose therapy or 1–3 days of therapy. Trimethoprim-sulfamethoxazole can be ineffective in significant numbers of patients because of the emergence of resistant organisms. Nitrofurantoin and fluoroquinolones are now the drugs of choice for uncomplicated cystitis (Table 23–1). Because uncomplicated cystitis is rare in men, elucidation of the underlying problem with appropriate investigations is warranted. Hot sitz baths or urinary analgesics (phenazopyridine, 200 mg orally three times daily) may provide symptomatic relief.

Prognosis

Infections typically respond rapidly to therapy, and failure to respond suggests resistance to the selected drug or anatomic abnormalities requiring further investigation.

Chew LD et al: Recurrent cystitis in nonpregnant women. West J Med 1999;170:274. [PMID: 10379218] (Continuous or postcoital antibiotic prophylaxis with nitrofurantoin, fluoroquinolones, or TMP-SMZ can reduce infection rates in women with recurrent cystitis.)

Gupta K et al: The prevalence of antimicrobial resistance among uropathogens causing acute uncomplicated cystitis in young women. Int J Antimicrob Agents 1999;11:305. [PMID: 10394988] (Increasing resistance to many antibiotics is noted. *E coli*, the most common species isolated, was resistant to ampicillin [25% of the time], tetracycline [24%], and TMP-SMZ [11%].)

Gupta K et al: Increasing prevalence of antimicrobial resistance among uropathogens causing acute uncomplicated cystitis in women. JAMA 1999;281:736. [PMID: 10052444] (Resistance of *E coli* in women with uncomplicated cystitis increased from 9% in 1992 to 18% in 1996 and from 8% to 16% among all isolates combined.)

ACUTE PYELONEPHRITIS

ESSENTIALS OF DIAGNOSIS

- Fever.
- Flank pain.

Table 23-1. Empirical therapy for urinary tract infections.

Diagnosis	Antibiotic	Route	Duration	Cost per Duration Noted[1]
Acute pyelonephritis	Ampicillin, 1 g every 6 hours, and gentamicin, 1 mg/kg every 8 hours	IV	21 days	$290.00 not including IV supplies
	Ciprofloxacin, 750 mg every 12 hours	Orally	21 days	$210.00
	Ofloxacin, 200–300 mg every 12 hours	Orally	21 days	$217.00
	Trimethoprim-sulfamethoxazole, 160/800 mg every 12 hours[2]	Orally	21 days	$46.00
Chronic pyelonephritis	Same as for acute pyelonephritis, but duration of therapy is 3–6 months			
Acute cystitis	Cephalexin, 250–500 mg every 6 hours	Orally	1–3 days	$15.00/3 days (500 mg)
	Ciprofloxacin, 250–500 mg every 12 hours	Orally	1–3 days	$30.00/3 days (500 mg)
	Nitrofurantoin (macrocrystals), 100 mg every 12 hours	Orally	7 days	$17.00
	Norfloxacin, 400 mg every 12 hours	Orally	1–3 days	$24.00/3 days
	Ofloxacin, 200 mg every 12 hours	Orally	1–3 days	$26.00/3 days
	Trimethoprim-sulfamethoxazole, 160/800 mg, two tablets[2]	Orally	Single dose	$2.00
Acute bacterial prostatitis	Same as for acute pyelonephritis		21 days	
Chronic bacterial prostatitis	Ciprofloxacin, 250–500 mg every 12 hours	Orally	1–3 months	$297.00/1 month (500 mg)
	Ofloxacin, 200–400 mg every 12 hours	Orally	1–3 months	$326.00/1 month (400 mg)
	Trimethoprim-sulfamethoxazole, 160/800 mg every 12 hours[2]	Orally	1–3 months	$65.00/1 month
Acute epididymitis Sexually transmitted	Ceftriaxone, 250 mg as single dose, plus: Doxycycline, 100 mg every 12 hours	IM Orally	10 days	$17.00/250 mg $8.00
Non-sexually transmitted	Same as for chronic bacterial prostatitis	Orally	3 weeks	

[1]Cost to pharmacist (average wholesale price, generic when possible) for quantity listed. Source: *Drug Topics Red Book,* March 2002; Vol. 21, No. 3.
[2]Increasing resistance noted (up to 20%).

- *Irritative voiding symptoms.*
- *Positive urine culture.*

General Considerations

Acute pyelonephritis is an infectious inflammatory disease involving the kidney parenchyma and renal pelvis. Gram-negative bacteria are the most common causative agents including *E coli*, proteus, klebsiella, enterobacter, and pseudomonas. Gram-positive bacte-ria are less commonly seen but include *Enterococcus faecalis* and *Staphylococcus aureus*. The infection usually ascends from the lower urinary tract—with the exception of *S aureus*, which usually is spread by a hematogenous route.

Clinical Findings

A. SYMPTOMS AND SIGNS

Symptoms include fever, flank pain, shaking chills, and irritative voiding symptoms (urgency, frequency, dysuria). Nausea and vomiting and diarrhea are not uncommon. Signs include fever and tachycardia. Costovertebral angle tenderness is usually pronounced.

B. LABORATORY FINDINGS

Complete blood count shows leukocytosis and a left shift. Urinalysis shows pyuria, bacteriuria, and varying degrees of hematuria. White cell casts may be seen. Urine culture demonstrates heavy growth of the offending agent, and blood culture may also be positive.

C. IMAGING

In complicated pyelonephritis, renal ultrasound may show hydronephrosis from a stone or other source of obstruction.

Differential Diagnosis

Acute intra-abdominal disease such as appendicitis, cholecystitis, pancreatitis, or diverticulitis must be distinguished from pyelonephritis. A normal urinalysis is usually seen in gastrointestinal disorders; however, on occasion, inflammation from adjacent bowel (appendicitis or diverticulitis) may result in hematuria or pyuria. Abnormal liver function tests or elevated amylase levels may assist in the differentiation. Lower lobe pneumonia is distinguishable by the abnormal chest radiograph.

In males, the main differential diagnosis for acute pyelonephritis includes acute epididymitis, acute prostatitis, and acute cystitis. Physical examination and the location of the pain should permit this distinction.

Complications

Sepsis with shock can occur with acute pyelonephritis. In diabetics, emphysematous pyelonephritis resulting from gas-producing organisms may be life-threatening if not adequately treated. Healthy adults usually recover complete renal function, yet if coexistent renal disease is present, scarring or chronic pyelonephritis may result. Inadequate therapy could result in abscess formation.

Treatment

Severe infections or complicating factors require hospital admission. Urine and blood cultures are obtained to identify the causative agent and to determine antimicrobial sensitivity. Intravenous ampicillin and an aminoglycoside are initiated prior to obtaining sensitivity results (Table 23–1). In the outpatient setting, quinolones or nitrofurantoin may be initiated (Table 23–1). Antibiotics are adjusted according to sensitivities. Fevers may persist for up to 72 hours; failure to respond warrants radiographic imaging (ultrasound) to exclude complicating factors that may require intervention. Catheter drainage may be necessary in the face of urinary retention and nephrostomy drainage if there is ureteral obstruction. In inpatients, intravenous antibiotics are maintained for 24 hours after the patient defervesces, and oral antibiotics are then given to complete a 7-day course of therapy. Follow-up urine cultures are mandatory several weeks following the completion of treatment.

Prognosis

With prompt diagnosis and appropriate treatment, acute pyelonephritis carries a good prognosis. Complicating factors, underlying renal disease, and increasing patient age may lead to a less favorable outcome.

Weidner W et al: Rational diagnostic steps in acute pyelonephritis with special reference to ultrasonography and computed tomography scan. Int J Antimicrob Agents 1999;11:257. [PMID: 10394980] (Ultrasonography is an excellent modality to rule out urinary tract obstruction. Patients who respond poorly to antibiotic therapy should have CT of the kidney with and without contrast.)

ACUTE BACTERIAL PROSTATITIS

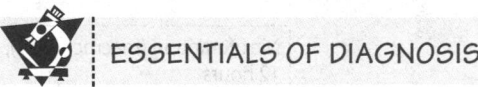 ESSENTIALS OF DIAGNOSIS

- *Fever.*
- *Irritative voiding symptoms.*
- *Perineal or suprapubic pain; exquisite tenderness common on rectal examination.*
- *Positive urine culture.*

General Considerations

Acute bacterial prostatitis is usually caused by gram-negative rods, especially *E coli* and pseudomonas species and less commonly by gram-positive organisms (eg, enterococcus). The most likely routes of infection include ascent up the urethra and reflux of infected urine into the prostatic ducts. Lymphatic and hematogenous routes are probably rare.

Clinical Findings

A. SYMPTOMS AND SIGNS

Perineal, sacral, or suprapubic pain, fever, and irritative voiding complaints are common. Varying degrees of obstructive symptoms may occur as the acutely inflamed prostate swells, which may lead to urinary retention. High fevers and a warm and often exquisitely tender prostate are detected on examination. Care should be taken in performing a gentle rectal examination, as vigorous manipulations may result in septicemia. Prostatic massage is contraindicated.

B. LABORATORY FINDINGS

Complete blood count shows leukocytosis and a left shift. Urinalysis shows pyuria, bacteriuria, and varying degrees of hematuria. Urine cultures will demonstrate the offending pathogen.

Differential Diagnosis

Acute pyelonephritis or acute epididymitis should be distinguishable by the location of pain as well as by physical examination. Acute diverticulitis is occasionally confused with acute prostatitis; however, the history and urinalysis should permit clear distinction. Urinary retention from benign or malignant prostatic enlargement is distinguishable by initial or follow-up rectal examination.

Treatment

Hospitalization may be required, and parenteral antibiotics (ampicillin and aminoglycoside) should be initiated until organism sensitivities are available (Table 23–1). After the patient is afebrile for 24–48 hours, oral antibiotics (quinolones) are used to complete 4–6 weeks of therapy. If urinary retention develops, urethral catheterization or instrumentation is contraindicated, and a percutaneous suprapubic tube is required. Follow-up urine culture and examination of prostatic secretions should be performed after the completion of therapy to ensure eradication.

Prognosis

With effective treatment, chronic bacterial prostatitis is rare.

CHRONIC BACTERIAL PROSTATITIS

ESSENTIALS OF DIAGNOSIS

- Irritative voiding symptoms.
- Perineal or suprapubic discomfort, often dull and poorly localized.
- Positive expressed prostatic secretions and culture.

General Considerations

Although chronic bacterial prostatitis may evolve from acute bacterial prostatitis, many men have no history of acute infection. Gram-negative rods are the most common etiologic agents, but only one gram-positive organism (enterococcus) is associated with chronic infection. Routes of infection are the same as discussed for acute infection.

Clinical Findings

A. SYMPTOMS AND SIGNS

Clinical manifestations are variable. Some patients are asymptomatic, but most have varying degrees of irritative voiding symptoms. Low back and perineal pain is not uncommon. Many patients report a history of urinary tract infections. Physical examination is often unremarkable, though the prostate may feel normal, boggy, or indurated.

B. LABORATORY FINDINGS

Urinalysis is normal unless a secondary cystitis is present. Expressed prostatic secretions demonstrate increased numbers of leukocytes (> 10/hpf), especially lipid laden macrophages. However, this finding is consistent with inflammation and is not diagnostic of bacterial prostatitis. Culture of the secretions or the post-prostatic massage urine specimen is necessary to make the diagnosis.

C. IMAGING

Imaging tests are not necessary, though pelvic radiographs or transrectal ultrasound may demonstrate prostatic calculi.

Differential Diagnosis

Chronic urethritis may mimic chronic prostatitis, though cultures of the fractionated urine may localize the source of infection. Cystitis may be secondary to prostatitis, but fractionated urine samples should localize the infection. Anal disease may share some of the symptoms of prostatitis, but physical examination should permit a distinction between the two.

Treatment

Few antimicrobial agents attain therapeutic intraprostatic levels in the absence of acute inflammation. Trimethoprim does diffuse into the prostate, and trimethoprim-sulfamethoxazole is associated with the best cure rates (Table 23–1). Other effective agents include carbenicillin, erythromycin, cephalexin, and the quinolones. The optimal duration of therapy remains controversial, ranging from 6 to 12 weeks. Symptomatic relief may be provided by anti-inflammatory agents (indomethacin, ibuprofen) and hot sitz baths.

Prognosis

Chronic bacterial prostatitis is difficult to cure, but its symptoms and tendency to cause recurrent urinary tract infections can be controlled by suppressive antibiotic therapy.

NONBACTERIAL PROSTATITIS

ESSENTIALS OF DIAGNOSIS

- Irritative voiding symptoms.
- Perineal or suprapubic discomfort, similar to that of chronic bacterial prostatitis.

• *Positive expressed prostatic secretions, but culture is negative.*

General Considerations

Nonbacterial prostatitis is the most common of the prostatitis syndromes, and its cause is unknown. Speculation implicates chlamydiae, mycoplasmas, ureaplasma, and viruses, but no substantial proof exists. In some cases, nonbacterial prostatitis may represent a noninfectious inflammatory disorder. Some investigators have postulated an autoimmune origin. Because the cause of nonbacterial prostatitis remains unknown, the diagnosis is usually one of exclusion.

Clinical Findings

A. SYMPTOMS AND SIGNS

The clinical presentation is identical to that of chronic bacterial prostatitis; however, no history of urinary tract infections is present.

B. LABORATORY FINDINGS

Increased numbers of leukocytes are seen on expressed prostatic secretions, but all cultures are negative.

Differential Diagnosis

The major distinction is from chronic bacterial prostatitis. The absence of a history of urinary tract infection and of positive cultures makes the distinction (Table 23–2). In older men with irritative voiding symptoms and negative cultures, the possibility of bladder cancer must be excluded. Urinary cytologic examination and cystoscopy are warranted.

Treatment

Because of the uncertainty regarding the etiology of nonbacterial prostatitis, a trial of antimicrobial therapy directed against ureaplasma, mycoplasma, or chlamydia is warranted. Erythromycin (250 mg orally four times daily) can be initiated for 14 days yet should only be continued (for 3–6 weeks) if a favorable clinical response ensues. Some symptomatic relief may be obtained with anti-inflammatory agents or sitz baths. Dietary restrictions are not necessary unless the patient relates a history of symptom exacerbation by certain substances such as alcohol, caffeine, and perhaps certain foods.

Prognosis

Annoying, recurrent symptoms are common, but serious sequelae have not been identified.

Litwin MS et al: The National Institutes of Health chronic prostatitis symptom index: development and validation of a new outcome measure. Chronic Prostatitis Collaborative Research Network. J Urol 1999;162:369. [PMID: 10411041]

Nickel JC et al: Research guidelines for chronic prostatitis: consensus report from the first National Institutes of Health International Prostatitis Collaborative Network. Urology 1999;54:229. [PMID: 10443716]

PROSTATODYNIA

Prostatodynia is a noninflammatory disorder that affects young and middle-aged men and has variable causes, including voiding dysfunction and pelvic floor musculature dysfunction. The term "prostatodynia" is a misnomer, as the prostate is actually normal.

Clinical Findings

A. SYMPTOMS AND SIGNS

Symptoms are the same as those seen with chronic prostatitis, yet there is no history of urinary tract infection. Additional symptoms may include hesitancy and interruption of flow. Patients may relate a lifelong history of voiding difficulty. Physical examination is unremarkable, but increased anal sphincter tone and periprostatic tenderness may be observed.

B. LABORATORY FINDINGS

Urinalysis is normal. Expressed prostatic secretions show normal numbers of leukocytes. Urodynamic

Table 23–2. Clinical characteristics of prostatitis and prostatodynia syndromes.

Findings	Acute Bacterial Prostatitis	Chronic Bacterial Prostatitis	Nonbacterial Prostatitis	Prostatodynia
Fever	+	–	–	–
Urinalysis	+	–	–	–
Expressed prostatic secretions	Contraindicated	+	+	–
Bacterial culture	+	+	–	–

testing may show signs of dysfunctional voiding (detrusor contraction without urethral relaxation, high urethral pressures, spasms of the urinary sphincter) and is indicated in patients failing empiric trials of alpha-blockers or anticholinergics.

Differential Diagnosis

Normal urinalysis will distinguish it from acute infectious processes. Examination of expressed prostatic secretions will distinguish this entity from prostatitis syndromes (Table 23–2).

Treatment

Bladder neck and urethral spasms can be treated by α-blocking agents (terazosin, 1–10 mg orally once a day; or doxazosin, 1–8 mg orally once a day). Pelvic floor muscle dysfunction may respond to diazepam and biofeedback techniques. Sitz baths may contribute to symptomatic relief.

Prognosis

Prognosis is variable depending upon the specific cause.

Lummus WE et al: Prostatitis. Emerg Med Clin North Am 2001; 19:691. [PMID: 11554282] (Reviews the etiology of prostatitis. Possible mechanism is reflux of urine into prostatic ducts.)

Nickel JC et al: Prevalence of prostatitis-like symptoms in a population based study using the National Institutes of Health chronic prostatitis symptom index. J Urol 2001;165:842. [PMID: 11176483] (Prostatitis-like symptoms are common among men aged 20–74.)

ACUTE EPIDIDYMITIS

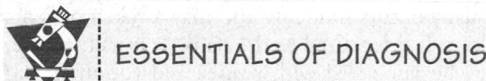

ESSENTIALS OF DIAGNOSIS

- *Fever.*
- *Irritative voiding symptoms.*
- *Painful enlargement of epididymis.*

General Considerations

Most cases of acute epididymitis are infectious and can be divided into one of two categories that have different age distributions and etiologic agents. Sexually transmitted forms typically occur in men under age 40, are associated with urethritis, and result from *C trachomatis* or *N gonorrhoeae*. Non-sexually transmitted forms typically occur in older men, are associated with urinary tract infections and prostatitis, and are caused by gram-negative rods. The route of infection is probably via the urethra to the ejaculatory duct and then down the vas deferens to the epididymis. Amiodarone has been associated with self-limited epididymitis.

Clinical Findings

A. Symptoms and Signs

Symptoms may follow acute physical strain (heavy lifting), trauma, or sexual activity. Associated symptoms of urethritis (pain at the tip of the penis and urethral discharge) or cystitis (irritative voiding symptoms) may occur. Pain develops in the scrotum and may radiate along the spermatic cord or to the flank. Fever and scrotal swelling are usually apparent. Early in the course, the epididymis may be distinguishable from the testis; however, later the two may appear as one enlarged, tender mass. The prostate may be tender on rectal examination.

B. Laboratory Findings

Complete blood count shows leukocytosis and a left shift. In the sexually transmitted variety, Gram staining of a smear of urethral discharge may be diagnostic of gram-negative intracellular diplococci (*N gonorrhoeae*). White cells without visible organisms on urethral smear represent nongonococcal urethritis, and *C trachomatis* is the most likely pathogen. In the nonsexually transmitted variety, urinalysis shows pyuria, bacteriuria, and varying degrees of hematuria. Urine cultures will demonstrate the offending pathogen.

C. Imaging

Scrotal ultrasound may aid in the diagnosis if examination is difficult because of the presence of a large hydrocele or because questions exist regarding the diagnosis.

Differential Diagnosis

Tumors generally cause painless enlargement of the testis. Urinalysis is negative, and examination reveals a normal epididymis. Scrotal ultrasound is helpful to define the pathology. Testicular torsion usually occurs in prepubertal males but is occasionally seen in young adults. Acute onset of symptoms and a negative urinalysis favor testicular torsion or torsion of one of the testicular or epididymal appendages. Prehn's sign (elevation of the scrotum above the pubic symphysis improves pain from epididymitis) may be helpful but is not reliable.

Treatment

Bed rest with scrotal elevation is important in the acute phase. Treatment is directed toward the identified pathogen (Table 23–1). The sexually transmitted variety is treated with 10–21 days of antibiotics, and the sexual partner must be treated as well. Non-sexually transmitted forms are treated for 21–28 days with appropriate antibiotics, at which time evaluation of the urinary tract is warranted to identify underlying disease.

Prognosis

Prompt treatment usually results in a favorable outcome. Delayed or inadequate treatment may result in epididymo-orchitis, decreased fertility, or abscess formation.

Barloon TJ et al: Diagnostic imaging of patients with acute scrotal pain. Am Fam Physician 1996;53:1734. [PMID: 8623698] (Doppler ultrasound can be useful in distinguishing between epididymitis [increased blood flow] and testicular torsion [decreased blood flow].)

Joly-Guillou ML et al: Practical recommendations for the drug treatment of bacterial infections of the male genital tract including urethritis, epididymitis and prostatitis. Drugs 1999;57:743. [PMID: 10353299] (Men less than 35 years of age usually have infections caused by sexually transmitted bacteria, while those over 35 usually have infections related to Enterobacteriaceae.)

■ URINARY STONE DISEASE

Urinary stone disease is exceeded in frequency as a urinary tract disorder only by infections and prostatic disease and is estimated to afflict 240,000–720,000 Americans per year. Men are more frequently affected by urolithiasis than women, with a ratio of 3:1. Initial presentation predominates in the third and fourth decades. The ratio of men to women approaches parity in the sixth and seventh decades.

Urinary calculi are polycrystalline aggregates composed of varying amounts of crystalloid and a small amount of organic matrix. Stone formation requires saturated urine that is dependent upon pH, ionic strength, solute concentration, and complexation. There are five major types of urinary stones: calcium oxalate, calcium phosphate, struvite, uric acid, and cystine. The most common types are composed of calcium, and for that reason most urinary stones (85%) are radiopaque. Uric acid stones can be radiolucent yet frequently are composed of a combination of uric acid and calcium oxalate and thus are radiopaque. Cystine stones frequently have a smooth-edged ground-glass appearance.

Geographic factors contribute to the development of stones. Areas of high humidity and elevated temperatures appear to be contributing factors, and the incidence of symptomatic ureteral stones is greatest during hot summer months.

Diet and fluid intake may be important factors in the development of urinary stones. Those afflicted with recurrent urinary stone disease are encouraged to maintain a diet restricted in sodium and protein intake. Sodium should be restricted to 100 meq/d. Increased sodium intake will increase sodium and calcium excretion and increase monosodium urate saturation (that can act as a nidus for stone growth), and increase the relative saturation of calcium phosphate, and a decrease in urinary citrate excretion. All of these factors encourage stone growth. Protein intake should be limited to 1 g/kg/d. An increased protein load can also increase calcium, oxalate, and uric acid excretion and can also decrease urinary citrate excretion. Carbohydrates and fats have not been proved to have any impact on urinary stone disease. Bran can significantly decrease urinary calcium by increasing bowel transit time and mechanically binding to calcium. Excess intake of oxalate and purines can increase the incidence of stones in predisposed individuals. Although a reduction in dietary calcium results in reduced urinary calcium, the concurrent increase in urinary oxalate may promote stone formation. Only type II absorptive hypercalciuric patients (see below) benefit from a low-calcium diet. Persons in sedentary occupations have a higher incidence of stones than manual laborers.

Genetic factors may contribute to urinary stone formation. Cystinuria is an autosomal recessive disorder. Homozygous individuals have markedly increased excretion of cystine and frequently have numerous recurrent episodes of urinary stones despite attempts to optimize medical treatment. Distal renal tubular acidosis may be transmitted as a hereditary trait, and urolithiasis occurs in up to 75% of patients affected with this disorder.

Clinical Findings

A. Symptoms and Signs

Obstructing urinary stones usually present with colic. Pain usually occurs suddenly and may awaken patients from sleep. It is localized to the flank, is usually severe, and may be associated with nausea and vomiting. Patients are constantly moving—in sharp contrast to those with an acute abdomen. The pain may occur episodically and may radiate anteriorly over the abdomen. As the stone progresses down the ureter, the pain may be referred into the ipsilateral testis or labium. If the stone becomes lodged at the ureterovesical junction, patients will complain of marked urinary urgency and frequency. Stone size does not correlate with the severity of the symptoms.

B. Metabolic Evaluation

Stone analysis should be performed on recovered stones. Controversy exists in deciding which patients need a thorough metabolic evaluation for stone disease. Uncomplicated first-time stone-formers should probably undergo blood screening for abnormalities of serum calcium, phosphate, electrolytes, and uric acid as a baseline.

More extensive evaluation is required in recurrent stone-formers or patients with a family history of stone disease. A 24-hour urine collection on a random diet should ascertain volume, urinary pH, and calcium, uric acid, oxalate, phosphate, and citrate excretion. A second collection on a restricted calcium (400 mg/d) and sodium (100 meq/d) diet is undertaken to subcategorize patients, if necessary. Serum PTH and calcium load tests can be performed at a third visit. A calcium load test is performed as follows: After a patient has been on a restricted calcium diet for at least 1 week, the patient is told to fast from 9 PM. The patient discards his early morning voided specimen (7 AM). While still fasting, the patient voids at 9 AM, which is the fasting sample. The patient then ingests 1 g of calcium gluconate, and all urine is collected from 9 AM to 1 PM, the calcium load sample. Table 23–3 demonstrates the diagnostic criteria for the hypercalciuric states. (See discussion below.)

C. LABORATORY FINDINGS

Urinalysis usually reveals microscopic or gross (≈ 10%) hematuria. However, the absence of microhematuria does not exclude urinary stones. Infection must be excluded, because the combination of infection and urinary tract obstruction requires prompt intervention as described below. Urinary pH is a valuable clue to the cause of the possible stone. Normal urine pH is 5.85. There is a normal postprandial urinary alkaline tide. Numerous dipstick measurements are valuable in the complete workup of a stone patient. Persistent urinary pH below 5.0 is suggestive of uric acid or cystine stones, both relatively radiolucent as seen on plain films of the abdomen. In contrast, a persistent pH above 7.5 is suggestive of a struvite infection stone, radiopaque on plain films.

D. IMAGING

A plain film of the abdomen and renal ultrasound examination will diagnose most stones. Spiral CT has emerged as a useful tool in evaluating flank pain with sensitivities for kidney stones in some trials exceeding those of ultrasound and intravenous urography. Stones suspected of being located at the ureterovesical junction can be imaged with abdominal ultrasonography with the aid of the acoustic window of a full bladder. Alternatively, transvaginal or transrectal ultrasonography will help identify calculi near the ureterovesical junction. When the diagnosis remains uncertain, intravenous urography is indicated.

Medical Treatment & Prevention

To reduce the recurrence rate of urinary stones, one must attempt to achieve a stone-free status. Small stone fragments may serve as a nidus for future stone development. Selected patients must be thoroughly evaluated to reduce stone recurrence rates. Uric acid stone-formers may have recurrences within months if appropriate therapy is not initiated. If no medical treatment is provided after surgical stone removal, stones will generally recur in 50% of patients within 5 years. Of greatest importance in reducing stone recurrence is an increased fluid intake. Absolute volumes are not established, but doubling previous fluid intake is recommended. Patients are encouraged to ingest fluids during meals, 2 hours after each meal (when the body is most dehydrated), and prior to going to sleep in the evening—enough to awaken the patient to void and to ingest additional fluids during the night. Increasing fluids only during daylight hours may not dilute a supersaturated urine overnight and thus initiate a new stone.

A. CALCIUM NEPHROLITHIASIS

1. Hypercalciuric—Hypercalciuric calcium nephrolithiasis (> 200 mg/24 h) can be caused by absorptive, resorptive, and renal disorders.

Absorptive hypercalciuria is secondary to increased absorption of calcium at the level of the small bowel, predominantly in the jejunum, and can be further subdivided into types I, II, and III. Type I absorptive hypercalciuria is independent of calcium intake. There is increased urinary calcium on a regular or even a calcium-restricted diet. Treatment is centered upon

Table 23–3. Diagnostic criteria of different types of hypercalciuria.

	Absorptive Type I	Absorptive Type II	Absorptive Type III	Resorptive	Renal
Serum					
Calcium	N	N	N	↑	N
Phosphorus	N	N	↓	↓	N
PTH	N	N	N	↑	↑
Vitamin D	N	N	↑	↑	↑
Urinary calcium					
Fasting	N	N	↑	↑	↑
Restricted	↑	N	↑	↑	↑
After calcium load	↑	↑	↑	↑	↑

Key: ↑ = elevated, ↓ = low, N = normal

decreasing bowel absorption of calcium. Cellulose phosphate, a chelating agent, is an effective form of therapy. An average dose is 10–15 g in three divided doses. It binds to the calcium and impedes small bowel absorption due to its increased bulk. Cellulose phosphate does not change the intestinal transport mechanism. It should be given with meals so it will be available to bind to the calcium. Taking this chelating agent prior to bedtime is ineffective. Postmenopausal women should be treated with caution. It is interesting, however, that there is no enhanced decline in bone density after long-term use. Inappropriate use without an initial metabolic evaluation (see above) may result in a negative calcium balance and a secondary parathyroid stimulation. Long-term use without follow-up metabolic surveillance may result in hypomagnesemia and secondary hyperoxaluria and recurrent calculi. Routine follow-up every 6–8 months will help encourage medical compliance and permit adjustments in medical therapy based upon repeat metabolic studies.

Thiazide therapy is an alternative to cellulose phosphate in the treatment of type I absorptive hypercalciuria. Thiazides decrease renal calcium excretion but have no impact on intestinal absorption. This therapy results in increased bone density of approximately 1% per year. Thiazides have limited long-term utility (< 5 years) as they lose their hypocalciuric effect with continued therapy.

Type II absorptive hypercalciuria is diet-dependent. Decreasing calcium intake by 50% (approximately 400 mg/d) will decrease the hypercalciuria to normal values (150–200 mg/24 h). There is no specific medical therapy.

Type III absorptive hypercalciuria is secondary to a renal phosphate leak. This results in increased vitamin D synthesis and secondarily increased small bowel absorption of calcium. This can be readily reversed by orthophosphates (0.5 g three times per day). Orthophosphates do not change intestinal absorption but rather inhibit vitamin D synthesis.

Resorptive hypercalciuria is secondary to hyperparathyroidism. Hypercalcemia, hypophosphatemia, hypercalciuria, and an elevated parathyroid hormone value are found. Appropriate surgical resection of the adenoma cures the disease and the urinary stones. Medical management is invariably a failure.

Renal hypercalciuria occurs when the renal tubules are unable to efficiently reabsorb filtered calcium, and hypercalciuria results. Spilling calcium in the urine results in secondary hyperparathyroidism. Serum calcium is normal. Thiazides are effective long-term therapy in patients with this disorder.

2. Hyperuricosuric—Hyperuricosuric calcium nephrolithiasis is secondary to dietary excesses or uric acid metabolic defects. Both disorders can be treated with purine dietary restrictions or allopurinol therapy (or both). In contrast to uric acid nephrolithiasis, patients with hyperuricosuric calcium stones will maintain a urinary pH greater than 5.5. Monosodium urates absorb inhibitors and promote heterogeneous nucleation. Hyperuricosuric calcium nephrolithiasis is probably secondary to epitaxy, or heterogeneous nucleation. In such situations, similar crystal structures (ie, uric acid and calcium oxalate) can grow together with the aid of a protein matrix infrastructure.

3. Hyperoxaluric—Hyperoxaluric calcium nephrolithiasis is usually due to primary intestinal disorders. Patients usually present with a history of chronic diarrhea frequently associated with inflammatory bowel disease or steatorrhea. Increased bowel fat combines with intraluminal calcium to form a soap-like product. Calcium is therefore unavailable to bind to oxalate, which is then freely and rapidly absorbed. A small increase in oxalate absorption will significantly increase stone formation. If the diarrhea or steatorrhea cannot be effectively curtailed, oral calcium supplements should be given with meals. It remains controversial whether excess ascorbic acid increases urinary oxalate levels. Emphasis on encouraging increased fluid intake is required for these patients as for all stone-formers.

4. Hypocitraturic—Hypocitraturic calcium nephrolithiasis may be secondary to chronic diarrhea, type I (distal) renal tubular acidosis, chronic hydrochlorothiazide treatment, and, in rare cases, is idiopathic. Any condition that results in metabolic acidosis (including prolonged fasting, hypomagnesemia, and hypokalemia) will decrease urinary citrate excretion, since it will be consumed by the citric acid cycle within the mitochondria of renal cells. Hypocitraturia is frequently associated with other forms of calcium stone formation. Citrate appears to bind to calcium in solution, thereby decreasing available calcium for stone formation. Potassium citrate supplements are usually effective. Urinary citrate is decreased in acidosis and is increased during alkalosis. The potassium will supplement the frequent hypokalemic states, and citrate will help to correct the acidosis. A typical dose is 20 meq three times a day (available in solution or in 5 and 10 meq tablets or in crystal formulations).

B. URIC ACID CALCULI

The average urinary pH is 5.85. Uric acid stone-formers frequently have urinary pH values less than 5.5. The pK of uric acid is 5.75, at which point half of the uric acid is ionized as a urate salt and is soluble, while the other half is insoluble. Increasing the pH above 6.5 dramatically increases solubility and can effectively dissolve large calculi. Potassium citrate is the most frequently used medication to increase urinary pH. It can be given in liquid preparation, as crystals that need to be taken with fluids, or as tablets (10 meq), two by mouth three or four times daily. Compliant urinary alkalinization may dissolve uric acid calculi at a rate of 1 cm of stone per month. Patients with uric acid calculi should be given Nitrazine pH paper with which to monitor the effectiveness of their urinary alkalinization. Other contributing factors include hyperuricemia, myeloproliferative disorders, malignancy with increased uric acid production, abrupt and dramatic weight loss, and uricosuric medications. If hyperuricemia is present, allopurinol (300 mg/d) may be given. Although pure uric acid stones are relatively radiolucent, most have some calcium components and can be visualized on plain abdominal radiographs. Renal ultrasonography is a helpful adjunct for appropriate diagnosis and long-term management.

C. Struvite Calculi

Struvite stones are synonymous with magnesium-ammonium-phosphate stones. They are commonly seen in women with recurrent urinary tract infections recalcitrant to appropriate antibiotics. They rarely form as ureteral stones without prior upper tract endourologic intervention. Frequently they are discovered as a large staghorn calculus forming a cast of the renal collecting system. These stones are radiodense. Urinary pH is high, usually above 7.0–7.5. These stones are formed secondary to urease-producing organisms, including proteus, pseudomonas, providencia, and, less commonly, klebsiella, staphylococci, and mycoplasma. An *E coli* urinary tract infection is not consistent with an infectious reservoir originating from a struvite calculus. These frequently large stones are relatively soft and amenable to percutaneous nephrolithotomy. Appropriate perioperative antibiotics are required. They can recur rapidly, and efforts should be taken to render the patient stone-free. Postoperative irrigation through nephrostomy tubes can eliminate small fragments. Acetohydroxamic acid is an effective urease inhibitor, but it is poorly tolerated by most patients because of its gastrointestinal toxicity.

D. Cystine Calculi

Cystine stones are a result of abnormal excretion of cystine, ornithine, lysine, and arginine. Cystine is the only amino acid that becomes insoluble in urine. These stones are particularly difficult to manage medically. Prevention is centered around increased fluid intake, alkalinization of the urine above pH 7.5 (monitored with Nitrazine pH paper), and a variety of medications including penicillamine and tiopronin.

Surgical Treatment

Forced intravenous fluids will not push stones down the ureter. Effective peristalsis directing a bolus of urine down the ureter requires opposing ureteral walls to approach each other and touch, which large dilated systems cannot do. In fact, diuresis is counterproductive and will exacerbate the pain. Associated fever may represent infection, a medical emergency requiring prompt drainage by a ureteral catheter or a percutaneous nephrostomy tube. Antibiotics alone are inadequate unless obstruction is released.

A. Ureteral Stones

Impediment to urine flow by ureteral stones usually occurs at three sites: (1) at the ureteropelvic junction,

(2) at the crossing of the ureter over the iliac vessels, and finally (3) as the ureter enters the bladder at the ureterovesical junction. Prediction of spontaneous stone passage is difficult. Stones less than 6 mm in diameter as seen on a plain abdominal radiograph will usually pass spontaneously. Conservative observation with appropriate pain medications is appropriate for the first 6 weeks. If spontaneous stone passage has failed, therapeutic intervention is required. Distal ureteral stones are best managed either with ureteroscopic stone extraction or in situ extracorporeal shock wave lithotripsy (ESWL). Ureteroscopic stone extraction involves placement of a small endoscope through the urethra and into the ureter. Under direct vision, basket extraction or fragmentation followed by extraction is performed. Complications during endoscopic retrieval increase as the duration of conservative observation increases beyond 6 weeks. Indications for earlier intervention include severe pain unresponsive to medications, fever, persistent nausea and vomiting requiring intravenous hydration, social requirements requiring return to work, or anticipated travel. Most upper tract stones that enter the bladder can exit the urethra with minimal discomfort.

In situ ESWL, an alternative, utilizes an external energy source that is focused upon the stone. This focused energy is additive, resulting in minimal tissue insult except at the focus where the stone is positioned with the aid of fluoroscopy or ultrasonography. This can be performed under anesthesia as an outpatient procedure and usually results in stone fragmentation. Most stone fragments will pass uneventfully within 2 weeks, but those that have not passed within 3 months are unlikely to pass without intervention. Women of childbearing age are best not treated with ESWL for a stone in the lower ureter, as the impact upon the ovary is unknown.

Proximal and midureteral stones—those above the inferior margin of the sacroiliac joint—can be treated with ESWL or ureteroscopy. ESWL is delivered directly to the stone (in situ), or the stones can be pushed back into the renal pelvis (via a retrograde ureteral catheter) to allow for a more capacious surrounding space and more efficient fragmentation. To help ensure adequate drainage after ESWL, a double J ureteral stent is frequently placed. Double J stents do not ensure passage of stone fragments after ESWL. Occasionally, stone fragments will obstruct the ureter after ESWL. Conservative management will usually result in spontaneous resolution with eventual passage of the stone fragments. If this is unsuccessful, adequate proximal drainage through a percutaneous nephrostomy tube will facilitate passage. In rare instances, ureteroscopic extraction will be required.

B. Renal Stones

Patients with renal calculi presenting without pain, urinary tract infections, or obstruction need not be treated. They should be followed with serial abdominal radiographs or renal ultrasonographic examinations. If calculi are growing or become symptomatic, intervention should be undertaken. Renal stones less than 3 cm in diameter are best treated with ESWL. Stones located in the inferior calix frequently result in suboptimal stone-free rates as measured at 3 months by x-ray. Such stones and others of larger diameter are best treated via percutaneous nephrolithotomy. Perioperative antibiotic coverage should be given on the basis of preoperative urine cultures.

Denton ER et al: Unenhanced helical CT for renal colic—is the radiation dose justifiable? Clin Radiol 1999;54:444. [PMID: 10437695] (Noncontrast CT avoids the risks of intravenous contrast associated with an intravenous pyelogram but exposes the patient to three times the radiation.)

Kosar A et al: Comparative study of long-term stone recurrence after extracorporeal shock wave lithotripsy and open stone surgery for kidney stones. Int J Urol 1999;6:125. [PMID: 10226822] (Stone burden is a key determinant of recurrent urinary stone disease after ESWL or open stone surgery.)

Larkin GL et al: Efficacy of ketorolac tromethamine versus meperidine in the ED treatment of acute renal colic. Am J Emerg Med 1999;17:6. [PMID: 9928687] (Ketorolac was more effective than meperidine in reducing renal colic.)

Pak CY et al: Adequacy of a single stone risk analysis in the medical evaluation of urolithiasis. J Urol 2001;165:378. [PMID: 11176377] (A single 24-hour urine collection is reproducible and adequate to assess for metabolic abnormalities for urinary stone disease.)

Parivar F et al: The influence of diet on urinary stone disease. J Urol 1996;155:432. [PMID: 8558629] (In an extensive literature review, dietary manipulation was beneficial in the prevention of recurrent urolithiasis in only a selected group of patients.)

■ URINARY INCONTINENCE

Urinary incontinence is most common in older patients. Its prevalence varies from 5% to 15% in the community to perhaps more than 50% in long-term care facilities. The normal urinary bladder can store relatively large volumes of urine at low pressures. Continence is dependent upon a compliant reservoir and sphincteric efficiency that has two components: the involuntary smooth muscle of the bladder neck and the voluntary skeletal muscle of the external sphincter. (See also discussion in Chapter 3.)

Classification

Urinary incontinence occurs when urine leaks involuntarily and can be classified into one of four categories.

A. Total Incontinence

With total incontinence, patients lose urine at all times and in all positions. This results when sphincteric efficiency is lost (previous surgery, nerve damage,

cancerous infiltration) or when an abnormal connection between the urinary tract and the skin exists that bypasses the urinary sphincter (vesicovaginal or ureterovaginal fistulas).

B. Stress Incontinence

Stress incontinence is the loss of urine associated with activities that result in an increase in intra-abdominal pressure (coughing, sneezing, lifting, exercising). Patients do not leak in the supine position. Laxity of the pelvic floor musculature—most commonly seen in the multiparous woman or in patients who have undergone pelvic surgery—results in urethral sphincteric insufficiency.

C. Urge Incontinence

The uncontrolled loss of urine that is preceded by a strong, unexpected urge to void is known as urge incontinence. It is unrelated to position or activity and is indicative of detrusor hyperreflexia or sphincter dysfunction. Inflammatory conditions or neurogenic disorders of the bladder are commonly associated with urge incontinence.

D. Overflow Incontinence

Chronic urinary retention may result in overflow incontinence. Incontinence results from the chronically distended bladder receiving an additional increment of urine, so that intravesical pressure just exceeds the outlet resistance, allowing a small amount of urine to dribble out.

Clinical Findings

A. Symptoms and Signs

The history is the most important step in the evaluation of urinary incontinence. It may be supplemented with a voiding diary prepared by the patient. Physical examination is important to exclude fistula for cases of total incontinence, neurologic abnormalities in cases of urge incontinence (spasticity, flaccidity, rectal sphincter tone), or the distended bladder in cases of overflow incontinence. Rectal examination will reveal the general function of the pelvic floor. Normal anal tone suggests an intact external sphincter. A tender levator ani suggests an overfacilitated pelvic floor. A lax sphincter suggests a lower motor neuron lesion. The bulbocavernosus reflex further confirms the integrity of the lower motor neurons. This reflex is confirmed by feeling an anal contraction in response to pressure on the glans penis or the clitoris.

B. Laboratory Findings

Urinalysis and urine culture are important to exclude urinary tract infection in cases of urge incontinence. Abnormal renal function may be detected in cases of overflow incontinence. Cystograms may demonstrate fistula sites. Lateral stress cystograms may show descensus of the bladder neck (descent of bladder neck more than 1.5 cm on straining view) in cases of stress incontinence. Those suspected of overflow incontinence can have postvoid residual urine volume assessed by urethral catheterization or ultrasonography.

C. SPECIAL TESTS

Urinary continence depends upon both bladder and sphincteric mechanisms; dysfunction of either component may result in incontinence. Urodynamic evaluation can assess both bladder and sphincteric function. Such testing is indicated in patients with moderate to severe incontinence, those suspected of having neurologic disease, and those with urge incontinence when infection and neoplasm have been excluded.

Bladder capacity, accommodation, sensation, voluntary control, contractility, and response to pharmacologic intervention can be assessed by cystometry. Cystometry is performed by filling the bladder with water or CO_2 and simultaneously recording intravesical pressure.

During filling, the normal bladder has the ability to maintain a low pressure. As volume increases, compliance increases. Normal sensation is first appreciated with volumes less than 150 mL. There is a strong sensation prior to micturition. Normal capacity in an adult bladder is 350–500 mL. Micturition is consciously initiated starting with pelvic floor relaxation followed by a sustained bladder contraction. Normal bladder function will empty the bladder completely. Uninhibited contractions during the normal filling phase are abnormal and are usually associated with a strong urge to void. Causes of decreased urinary capacity include incontinence, infections, interstitial cystitis, radiation damage, upper motor neuron lesions, and postoperative changes. Increased bladder capacity is seen with chronic urinary tract obstruction, lower motor neuron lesions, and sensory neuropathies.

Responses to routine medications during cystometry will help confirm a diagnosis and facilitate appropriate therapy. Lack of an appropriate detrusor contraction may be secondary to poor bladder muscle function or inadequate filling. Myogenic function can be assessed with bethanechol chloride, a parasympathomimetic drug. Lack of response to intravenous bethanechol suggests intrinsic muscle damage. In contrast, an exaggerated response is suggestive of a lower motor neuron lesion.

Sphincteric function assessment is necessary in the evaluation of urinary incontinence. More formal evaluation of the urinary sphincter may be performed using urethral profilometry, electromyography, or combined video studies.

Treatment

A. TOTAL INCONTINENCE

True incontinence is due to anatomic abnormalities, either congenital or acquired. Congenital defects, including bladder exstrophy, ectopic ureteral orifices, and urethral diverticula, and acquired lesions such as vesicovaginal fistulas require surgical correction. Sphincter injuries following prostatectomy may be managed by surgical reconstruction (bladder neck reconstruction), periurethral collagen injections, or placement of an artificial urinary sphincter.

B. STRESS INCONTINENCE

In patients with stress urinary incontinence, the bladder neck will descend below the midportion of the pubic symphysis when viewed on a lateral stress cystogram. Urodynamic investigations usually reveal a shortened functional urethral length, decreased urethral closure pressure, minimal augmentation of closure pressure with stress activities, decreased urethral pressure and length when assuming an upright position, and decreased closure pressure with bladder filling.

If hypoestrogenism of the vagina or urethra is discovered, topical estrogen creams applied locally are indicated. Surgical treatment is centered upon placing the bladder neck into an appropriate anatomic location, allowing increased intra-abdominal pressure to be transmitted to both the bladder and the bladder neck. These procedures also lengthen the urethra. Transvaginal sling suspension or suprapubic (culpocystourethropexy) approaches can pull the bladder neck into proper position. Surgery is usually corrective.

C. URGE INCONTINENCE

The etiology of urge urinary incontinence includes urethral or detrusor instability or a combination of these mechanisms. Treatment is medical rather than surgical. Effective agents include antispasmodic medication (oxybutinin, 5 mg orally three times daily), anticholinergic medication (propantheline 15 mg orally three times daily), or tricyclic antidepressants (imipramine, 25–75 mg orally at bedtime). Sacral nerve stimulation can be effective in treating refractory urinary urge incontinence.

D. OVERFLOW INCONTINENCE

Placement of a urethral catheter is both diagnostic and therapeutic in the acute setting. Further treatment must address the underlying disease. Men with benign prostatic hyperplasia can be treated with medical therapy, prostatectomy, or newer less invasive procedures (see below). Patients with urethral strictures can be treated with a direct internal urethrotomy or open urethroplasty. Neurogenic causes (external sphincteric spasticity) may be managed with intermittent catheterization regimens with or without pharmacotherapy.

Andersson KE: Drug therapy for urinary incontinence. Baillieres Best Pract Res Clin Obstet Gynaecol 2000;14:291. [PMID: 10897323] (Stress urinary incontinence rarely responds to pharmacologic therapy.)

Assessment and treatment of urinary incontinence. Scientific Committee of the First International Consultation on Incontinence. Lancet 2000;355:2153. [PMID: 2035843]

(Therapeutic algorithms are presented which are applicable in most health care systems.)

Butler RN et al: Urinary incontinence: keys to diagnosis of the older woman. 1. Geriatrics 1999;54:22, 29. [PMID: 10542858] (The topic of urinary incontinence should be addressed, especially in older patients.)

Jackson S et al: The effect of oestrogen supplementation on post-menopausal urinary stress incontinence: a double-blind placebo-controlled trial. Br J Obstet Gynaecol 1999;106: 711. [PMID: 10428529] (Estrogen supplementation is ineffective in treating postmenopausal stress urinary incontinence.)

JAMA patient page: Incontinence. JAMA 1998;280:2054. [PMID: 9863861]

Knapp PM Jr: Identifying and treating urinary incontinence: The crucial role of the primary care physician. Postgrad Med 1998;103:279. [PMID: 9553601] (General review.)

Parazzini F et al: Risk factors for urinary incontinence in women. Eur Urol 2000;37:637. [PMID: 10828661] (The incidence of urinary incontinence increases with age. The causes are varied.)

Schmidt RA et al: Sacral nerve stimulation for treatment of refractory urinary urge incontinence. Sacral Nerve Stimulation Study Group. J Urol 1999;162:352. [PMID: 10411037] (Sacral nerve stimulation is a treatment option for refractory urge urinary incontinence.)

INTERSTITIAL CYSTITIS

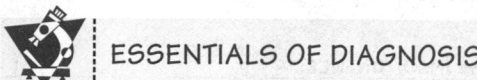

ESSENTIALS OF DIAGNOSIS

- *Pain with a full bladder or urinary urgency.*
- *Submucosal petechiae on cystoscopic examination.*
- *Diagnosis of exclusion.*

General Considerations

Interstitial cystitis is characterized by pain with bladder filling that is relieved by emptying and is often associated with urgency and frequency. This is a diagnosis of exclusion, and patients must have a negative urine culture and cytology and no other obvious cause such as radiation cystitis, chemical cystitis (cyclophosphamide), vaginitis, urethral diverticulum, or genital herpes.

Population-based studies have demonstrated a prevalence of between 18 and 40 per 100,000 people. Both sexes are involved, but the majority of patients are women, with a mean age of 40 years at onset. Patients with interstitial cystitis are more likely to report bladder problems in childhood, and there appears to be a higher prevalence in Jewish women. Up to 50% of patients may experience spontaneous remission of symptoms, with a mean duration of 8 months without treatment.

The etiology of interstitial cystitis is unknown, and it is most likely not a single disease but rather several diseases with similar symptomatology. Associated diseases include severe allergies, irritable bowel syndrome, or inflammatory bowel disease. Theories regarding the cause of interstitial cystitis include increased epithelial permeability, neurogenic causes (sensory nervous system abnormalities), and autoimmunity.

Clinical Findings

A. SYMPTOMS AND SIGNS

Pain with bladder filling that is relieved with urination or urgency, frequency, and nocturia are the most common symptoms. Exposures such as pelvic radiation or prior cyclophosphamide should be inquired about. Examination should exclude genital herpes, vaginitis, or a urethral diverticulum.

B. LABORATORY FINDINGS

Urinalysis and urine culture are obtained to exclude infectious causes. Urinary cytology is obtained to exclude bladder malignancy. Urodynamic testing assesses bladder sensation and compliance and excludes detrusor instability.

C. CYSTOSCOPY

The bladder is distended with fluid (hydrodistention) to detect glomerulations (submucosal hemorrhage), which must be present in at least three quadrants of the bladder. Biopsy should be performed to exclude other causes such as carcinoma, eosinophilic cystitis, and tuberculous cystitis. The presence of submucosal mast cells is not needed to make the diagnosis of interstitial cystitis.

Differential Diagnosis

Exposures to radiation or cyclophosphamide are obtained by the history. Bacterial cystitis, genital herpes, or vaginitis can be excluded by urinalysis, culture, and physical examination. A urethral diverticulum may be suspected if palpation of the urethra demonstrates an indurated mass that results in the expression of pus from the urethral meatus. Urethral carcinoma presents as a firm mass on palpation.

Treatment

There is no cure for interstitial cystitis, but most patients achieve symptomatic relief from one of several approaches, including hydrodistention, which is usually done as part of the diagnostic evaluation. Approximately 20–30% of patients will notice symptomatic improvement following this maneuver. Also of importance is the measurement of bladder capacity during hydrodistention, since patients with very small bladder capacities (< 200 mL) are unlikely to respond to medical therapy.

Amitriptyline is often used as first-line medical therapy in patients with interstitial cystitis. Both central and peripheral mechanisms may contribute to its activity. Nifedipine and other calcium channel blockers have also demonstrated some activity in patients with interstitial cystitis patients. Pentosan polysulfate sodium (Elmiron) is an oral synthetic sulfated polysaccharide that helps restore integrity to the epithelium of the bladder in a few patients.

The mainstay of therapy for interstitial cystitis is intravesical instillation of dimethyl sulfoxide (DMSO). Other agents, including heparin and BCG, are being investigated, with the latter achieving up to 60% response rates.

Other treatment modalities include transcutaneous electric nerve stimulation (TENS) and acupuncture. Surgical therapy for interstitial cystitis should only be considered as a last resort and may require cystourethrectomy with urinary diversion.

Hanno PM et al: The diagnosis of interstitial cystitis revisited: lessons learned from the National Institutes of Health Interstitial Cystitis Database study. J Urol 1999;161:553. [PMID: 99112653] (Initial criteria used to diagnose interstitial cystitis may be too restrictive.)

Jepsen JV et al: Long-term experience with pentosanpolysulfate in interstitial cystitis. Urology 1998;51:381. [PMID: 9510339] (Ninety-seven patients followed for up to 116 months demonstrated a response rate between 6% and 18%.)

Propert KJ et al: A prospective study of interstitial cystitis: results of longitudinal followup of the interstitial cystitis data base cohort. The Interstitial Cystitis Data Base Study Group. J Urol 2000;163:1434. [PMID: 10751852]. (Interstitial cystitis is a chronic disease.)

Sant GR et al: Interstitial cystitis. Curr Opin Urol 1999;9:297. [PMID: 10459464] (Interstitial cystitis is a common inflammatory condition of the bladder.)

■ MALE ERECTILE DYSFUNCTION & SEXUAL DYSFUNCTION

Erectile dysfunction is defined as the consistent inability to maintain an erect penis with sufficient rigidity to allow sexual intercourse. This condition is thought to affect 10 million American men, and its incidence is age-related. Approximately 25% of all men older than age 65 suffer from this disorder. Most cases of male erectile disorders have an organic rather than a psychogenic cause. Normal male erection is a neurovascular phenomenon relying on an intact autonomic and somatic nerve supply to the penis, smooth and striated musculature of the corpora cavernosa and pelvic floor, and arterial inflow supplied by the paired pudendal arteries. Erection is precipitated and maintained by an increase in arterial flow, active relaxation of the smooth muscle elements of the sinusoids within the corporal bodies of the penis, and an increase in venous resistance. Contraction of the bulbocavernosus and ischiocavernosus muscles results in further rigidity of the penis. The neurotransmitters that initiate the process have not been identified with certainty, though nitric oxide, vasoactive intestinal peptide, acetylcholine, and prostaglandins have all been postulated to initiate or contribute to male erection.

Male sexual dysfunction may be manifested in a variety of ways, and the history is critical to the proper classification and subsequent treatment. Androgens have a strong influence on the sexual desire of men. A **loss of libido** may indicate androgen deficiency on the basis of either hypothalamic, pituitary or testicular disease. Serum testosterone and gonadotropin levels may help localize the site of disease. **Loss of erections** may result from arterial, venous, neurogenic, or psychogenic causes. Concurrent medical problems may damage one or more of the mechanisms. In addition, many medications, especially antihypertensives, are associated with erectile dysfunction. Centrally acting sympatholytics (methyldopa, clonidine, reserpine) can result in loss of erection, while vasodilators, alphablockers, and diuretics rarely alter erections. Betablockers and spironolactone may result in loss of libido. It is important to determine whether the patient ever has any normal erections, such as early morning or during sleep. If normal erections do occur, an organic cause is unlikely. The gradual loss of erections over a period of time is more suggestive of an organic cause. The **loss of emission** (lack of antegrade seminal fluid during ejaculation) may result from several underlying disorders. **Retrograde ejaculation** may occur as a result of mechanical disruption of the bladder neck, especially following transurethral resection of the prostate or sympathetic denervation as a result of medications (alpha-blockers), diabetes mellitus, or radical pelvic or retroperitoneal surgery. Androgen deficiency may also result in lack of emission by decreasing the amount of prostatic and seminal vesicle secretions. If libido and erection are intact, the **loss of orgasm** is usually of psychologic origin. **Premature ejaculation** is usually an anxiety-related disorder and rarely has an organic cause. The history may elucidate the presence of a new partner, unreasonable expectations about performance, or emotional disorders.

Clinical Findings

A. SYMPTOMS AND SIGNS

Erectile dysfunction should be clearly distinguished from problems of ejaculation, libido, and orgasm. The degree of the dysfunction (whether chronic, occasional, or situational) as well as its timing should be noted. The history should include inquiries about hyperlipidemia, hypertension, neurologic disease, diabetes mellitus, renal failure, and adrenal and thyroid disorders. Trauma to the pelvis or pelvic or peripheral vascular surgery also identifies patients at increased risk of impotence. A complete recording of drug use should be made, since about 25% of all cases of sexual dysfunction may be drug-related. The use of alcohol, tobacco, and recreational drugs should be recorded as well, since each is associated with an increased risk of sexual dysfunction.

During the physical examination, secondary sexual characteristics should be assessed. Neurologic and peripheral vascular examination should be performed. Motor and sensory examination should be performed as well as palpation and quantification of lower extremity vascular pulsations. The genitalia should be examined, noting the presence of penile scarring or plaque formation (Peyronie's disease) and any abnormalities in size or consistency of either testicle. Examination of the prostate is essential.

B. LABORATORY FINDINGS

Laboratory evaluation is limited and should consist of a complete blood count, urinalysis, lipid profile, determination of serum testosterone, glucose, and prolactin. Patients with abnormalities of testosterone or prolactin require further evaluation with measurement of serum FSH and LH, and endocrinologic consultation is advised.

C. SPECIAL TESTS

Further testing is based on the patient's goals. Patients who will accept only noninvasive forms of therapy may be offered medical therapy or a vacuum constriction device, as described below. Most patients undergo further evaluation with direct injection of vasoactive substances into the penis. Such substances (prostaglandin E_1, papaverine, or a combination of drugs) will induce erections in men with intact vascular systems. Patients who respond with a rigid erection require no further vascular evaluation. However, organic and psychogenic impotence can be differentiated by use of nocturnal penile tumescence testing, where the frequency as well as the rigidity of erections are recorded by a simple device attached to the penis before sleep. Patients with psychogenic impotence will have nocturnal erections of adequate frequency and rigidity.

Additional vascular testing is indicated in patients who fail to achieve an erection with injection of vasoactive substances on serial attempts using increasing doses or combination of drugs and who would consider vascular reconstructive surgery. The diameter and flow in the cavernous arteries can be assessed using duplex ultrasound. Patients with poor arterial inflow in the absence of known peripheral vascular disease (as in patients who have sustained pelvic trauma) are candidates for pelvic arteriography before planned arterial reconstruction. Patients with normal arterial inflow should be suspected of suffering from venous leak. Further testing in this group would include cavernosometry (measurement of flow required to maintain erection) and cavernosography (contrast study of the penis to determine site and extent of venous leak).

Treatment

The vast majority of men suffering from erectile dysfunction can be managed successfully with one of the approaches outlined below. Men who do not suffer from organic dysfunction will probably benefit from behaviorally oriented sex therapy.

A. HORMONAL REPLACEMENT

Testosterone injections (200 mg intramuscularly every 3 weeks) or topical patches (2.5–6 mg/d) are offered to men with documented androgen deficiency who have undergone endocrinologic evaluation as described and in whom prostatic cancer has been excluded by PSA screening and digital rectal examination.

B. VACUUM CONSTRICTION DEVICE

The vacuum constriction device is a cylindric device that draws the penis into an erect state by inducing a vacuum within the cylinder. Once adequate tumescence has been achieved, a rubber constriction device or band is placed around the proximal penis to prevent loss of erection, and the cylinder is removed. Such devices are suitable for patients with venous disorders of the penis and those who fail to achieve an adequate erection with injection of vasoactive substances. Complications are rare.

C. VASOACTIVE THERAPY

Direct injection of vasoactive prostaglandins into the penis is an acceptable form of treatment for most men with impotence. These injections are performed using a tuberculin syringe. The base and lateral aspect of the penis is used as the injection site to avoid injury to the superficial blood supply located anteriorly. Complications are rare and include dizziness, local pain, fibrosis, and infection. A prolonged erection requiring aspiration of blood and injection of epinephrine and phenylephrine to achieve detumescence occurs very rarely. A mechanism of delivering vasoactive prostaglandins (alprostadil) via a urethral suppository has been developed, and results are good. Pellet sizes are 125, 250, 500, and 1000 μg.

Sildenafil (Viagra) inhibits phosphodiesterase 5—itself an inhibitor of erection—and allows cGMP to function unopposed. Ordinarily, nitric oxide-mediated release from parasympathetic nerves and endothelium generates this compound, and prolongation of its half-life results in sustained inflow of blood into the erect penis. Fifty milligrams taken 1 hour prior to anticipated sexual activity is recommended, with peak action at 2 hours. There is no effect on libido, nor is priapism a problem, but the additive effect on nitrates may lead to exaggerated cardiac preload reduction and hypotension. Thus, the drug is contraindicated in patients receiving nitroglycerin. All patients being evaluated for acute chest pain should be asked if they are taking sildenafil before administering nitroglycerin. Fixed atherosclerotic disease in the aortoiliac system is associated with diminished efficacy.

D. PENILE PROSTHESES

Prosthetic devices may be implanted directly into the paired corporal bodies. Such prostheses may be rigid, malleable, hinged, or inflatable. Each is manufactured in a variety of sizes and diameters. Inflatable models may result in a more cosmetic appearance but may be associated with a greater likelihood of mechanical failure.

E. VASCULAR RECONSTRUCTION

Patients with disorders of the arterial system are candidates for various forms of arterial reconstruction, including endarterectomy and balloon dilation for proximal arterial occlusion and arterial bypass procedures utilizing arterial (epigastric) or venous (deep dorsal vein) segments for distal occlusion. Patients with disorders of venous occlusion may be managed with ligation of certain veins (deep dorsal or emissary veins) or the crura of the corpora cavernosa. Experience with vascular reconstructive procedures is still limited, and many patients so treated still fail to achieve a rigid erection.

Goldstein I et al: Oral sildenafil in the treatment of erectile dysfunction. Sildenafil Study Group. N Engl J Med 1998; 338:1397. [PMID: 9580646] (Sildenafil is an effective, well-tolerated treatment for erectile dysfunction due to organic, psychogenic, and mixed causes.)

JAMA patient page: Sexual dysfunction. JAMA 1999;281:584. [PMID: 10022117]

Lue TF: Erectile dysfunction. N Engl J Med 2000;342:1802. [PMID: 10853004] (A complete review of the pathophysiology and treatment options for erectile dysfunction.)

Padma-Nathan H et al: Treatment of men with erectile dysfunction with transurethral alprostadil. Medicated Urethral System for Erection (MUSE) Study Group. N Engl J Med 1997;336:1. [PMID: 8970933] (Alprostadil was delivered transurethrally in a double-blind, placebo-controlled study of 1511 men who had chronic erectile dysfunction from various organic causes. Sixty-six percent of patients had erections sufficient for intercourse. The most common side effect was mild penile pain, which occurred in 11%.)

MALE INFERTILITY

Primary infertility affects 15–20% of married couples. Approximately one-third of cases result from male factors, one-third from female factors, and one-third from combined factors. It is thus critical to have simultaneous evaluation of the female partner. Clinical evaluation is warranted following 6 months of unprotected intercourse. Endocrinologic profiles and detailed semen analyses are the cornerstones of laboratory investigations after the history and physical examination. **Oligospermia** is the presence of less than 20 million sperm/mL of the ejaculate; **azoospermia** is the absence of sperm. As spermatogenesis takes approximately 74 days, it is thus important to review events from the past 3 months.

Clinical Findings

A. SYMPTOMS AND SIGNS

The history should include prior testicular insults (torsion, cryptorchism, trauma), infections (mumps orchitis, epididymitis), environmental factors (excessive heat, radiation, chemotherapy), medications (anabolic steroids, cimetidine, and spironolactone may affect spermatogenesis; phenytoin may lower FSH; sulfasalazine and nitrofurantoin affect sperm motility), and drugs (alcohol, marijuana). Sexual habits, frequency and timing of intercourse, use of lubricants, and each partner's previous fertility experiences are important. Loss of libido and headaches or visual disturbances may indicate a pituitary tumor. The past medical or surgical history may reveal thyroid or liver disease (abnormalities of spermatogenesis), diabetic neuropathy (retrograde ejaculation), radical pelvic or retroperitoneal surgery (absent seminal emission secondary to sympathetic nerve injury), or hernia repair (damage to the vas deferens or testicular blood supply).

Physical examination should pay particular attention to features of hypogonadism: underdeveloped secondary sexual characteristics, diminished male pattern hair distribution (axillary, body, facial, pubic), eunuchoid skeletal proportions (arm span 2 inches > height; upper to lower body ratio < 1.0), and gynecomastia. The scrotal contents should be carefully evaluated. Testicular size should be noted (normal size approximately 4.5 × 2.5 cm, volume 18 mL). Varicoceles should be looked for in the standing position and on occasion may only be appreciated with the Valsalva maneuver. The vas deferens, epididymis, and prostate should be palpated.

B. LABORATORY FINDINGS

Semen analysis should be performed after 72 hours of abstinence. The specimen should be analyzed within 1 hour after collection. Abnormal sperm concentrations are less than 20 million/mL. Normal semen volumes range between 1.5 and 5 mL (volumes < 1.5 mL may result in inadequate buffering of the vaginal acidity and may be due to retrograde ejaculation or androgen insufficiency). Normal sperm motility and morphology demonstrate 50–60% motile cells and more than 60% normal morphology. Abnormal motility may result from antisperm antibodies or infection. Abnormal morphology may result from a varicocele, infection, or exposure history.

Endocrinologic evaluation is warranted if sperm counts are low or if there is a clinical basis (from the history and physical examination) for suspecting an endocrinologic origin. Testing should include serum FSH, LH, and testosterone. Elevated FSH and LH and low testosterone (hypergonadotropic hypogonadism) are associated with primary testicular failure, which is usually irreversible. Low FSH and LH associated with low testosterone occur in secondary testicular failure (hypogonadotropic hypogonadism) and may be of hypothalamic or pituitary origin. Such defects may be correctable. In such cases, serum prolactin should be checked to exclude pituitary prolactinoma.

C. IMAGING

Scrotal ultrasound may detect a subclinical varicocele. Vasography may be required in patients with suspected ductal obstruction.

D. SPECIAL TESTS

Azoospermic patients should have postmasturbation urine samples centrifuged and analyzed for sperm to exclude retrograde ejaculation. Azoospermic patients and patients with ejaculate volumes less than 1 mL should have fructose levels determined on the ejaculate. Fructose is produced in the seminal vesicles and if absent in the ejaculate implies obstruction of the ejaculatory ducts.

Treatment

A. GENERAL MEASURES

Education with respect to the proper timing for intercourse in relation to the female's ovulatory cycle as well as the avoidance of spermicidal lubricants should be discussed. In cases of toxic exposure or medication-related factors, the offending agent should be removed. Patients with active genitourinary tract infections should be treated with appropriate antibiotics.

B. ENDOCRINE THERAPY

Hypogonadotropic hypogonadism may be treated with chorionic gonadotropin once primary pituitary disease has been excluded or treated. Dosage is usually 2000 IU intramuscularly three times a week. If sperm counts fail to rise after 12 months, FSH therapy should be initiated. Menotropins (Pergonal) is available as a premixed vial of 75 IU of FSH and 75 IU of LH. The usual dosage ranges from one-half to one vial intramuscularly three times per week.

C. RETROGRADE EJACULATION THERAPY

Oligospermic patients with retrograde ejaculation may benefit from alpha-adrenergic agonists (pseudoephedrine, 60 mg orally three times a day) or imipramine (25 mg orally three times a day). Medical failures may require the collection of postmasturbation urine for intrauterine insemination or electroejaculation in the case of absent emission.

D. VARICOCELE

Surgical approaches to varicoceles may be accomplished via a scrotal, inguinal, or laparoscopic approach. More recently, percutaneous venographic approaches have been developed, obviating the need for an anesthetic.

E. DUCTAL OBSTRUCTION

The level of obstruction must be delineated via a vasogram prior to operative treatment. Mechanical obstruction of the ejaculatory duct may be corrected by transurethral resection and unroofing of the ducts in the prostatic urethra. Obstruction of the vas deferens is best managed by a microsurgical approach, and a vasovasostomy or vasoepididymostomy may be required.

F. ASSISTED REPRODUCTIVE TECHNIQUES

Advances in reproductive technology may provide alternatives to patients who have failed other means of treating reduced sperm counts and motility. Such measures include intrauterine insemination, in vitro fertilization, and gamete intrafallopian transfer.

Bartoov B et al: Quantitative ultramorphological analysis of human sperm: fifteen years of experience in the diagnosis and management of male factor infertility. Arch Androl 1999;43:13. [PMID: 10445101] (The utility of quantitative ultramorphological sperm analysis in the diagnosis and treatment of male infertility is presented.)

McClure RD: Male infertility—realistic treatment options [editorial; comment]. J Urol 1999;161:1166. [PMID: 10081862]

■ BENIGN PROSTATIC HYPERPLASIA

ESSENTIALS OF DIAGNOSIS

- *Obstructive or irritative voiding symptoms.*
- *May have enlarged prostate on rectal examination.*
- *Absence of urinary tract infection, neurologic disorder, stricture disease, prostatic or bladder malignancy.*

General Considerations

Benign prostatic hyperplasia is the most common benign tumor in men, and its incidence is age-related. The prevalence of histologic benign prostatic hyperplasia in autopsy studies rises from approximately 20% in men aged 41–50 years, to 50% in men aged 51–60 and to over 90% in men over 80 years of age. Although clinical evidence of disease occurs less commonly, symptoms of prostatic obstruction are also age-related. At age 55, approximately 25% of men report obstructive voiding symptoms. At age 75 years, 50% of men report a decrease in the force and caliber of the urinary stream.

Risk factors for the development of benign prostatic hyperplasia are poorly understood. Some studies have suggested a genetic predisposition and some have noted racial differences. Approximately 50% of men under age 60 who undergo surgery for benign prostatic hyperplasia may have a heritable form of the disease. This form is most likely an autosomal dominant trait, and first-degree male relatives of such patients carry an increased relative-risk of approximately fourfold.

Etiology

The etiology is not completely understood, but the disorder seems to be multifactorial and under endocrine control. The prostate is composed of both stromal and epithelial elements, and each, either alone or in combination, can give rise to hyperplastic nodules and the symptoms associated with benign prostatic hyperplasia. Each element may be targeted in medical management schemes.

Laboratory and clinical studies have identified two factors necessary for the development of benign prostatic hyperplasia: dihydrotestosterone (DHT) and aging. Animal studies have demonstrated that the aging prostate becomes more sensitive to androgens. Prostatic growth in aging dogs appears to be related more to a decrease in cell death than to an increase in cell proliferation. Laboratory studies have suggested several theories in this area, including the following: (1) stromal-epithelial interactions (stroma cell may regulate growth of epithelial cell or other stromal cells via a paracrine or autocrine mechanism by secreting growth factors such as basic fibroblast growth factor or transforming growth factor-β); and (2) aging may result in stem cells undergoing a block in the maturation process, preventing them from entering into programmed cell death (apoptosis). The impact of aging in animal studies appears to be mediated via estrogen synergism. In canines, estrogens induce the androgen receptor; alter steroid metabolism, resulting in higher levels of intraprostatic DHT; inhibit cell death when given in the presence of androgens; and stimulate stroma collagen production.

Studies have demonstrated that benign prostatic hyperplasia is under endocrine control. Castration results in the regression of established disease and improvement in urinary symptoms. Administration of a luteinizing hormone-releasing hormone (LHRH) analog in men reversibly shrinks established benign prostatic hyperplasia, resulting in objective improvement in flow rate and subjective improvement in symptoms. Further investigations have demonstrated a positive correlation between levels of free testosterone and estrogen and the volume of the gland. The latter may suggest that the association between aging and benign prostatic hyperplasia might reflect increasing estrogen levels of aging, resulting in induction of the androgen receptor and thus sensitizing the prostate to free testosterone. However, no studies to date have been able to demonstrate elevated estrogen receptor levels in humans with the disease.

Pathology

Benign prostatic hyperplasia is truly a hyperplastic process, resulting from an increase in cell numbers. Microscopic evaluation reveals a nodular growth pattern consisting of varying amounts of stroma or epithelium. Stroma is composed of varying amounts of collagen and smooth muscle. The differential representation of various histologic components of benign prostatic hyperplasia in part explains the potential responsiveness to medical therapy. Thus, alpha-blocker therapy may result in excellent responses in patients with benign prostatic hyperplasia when there is a significant component of smooth muscle, while hyperplasia composed

predominantly of epithelium might respond better to 5α-reductase inhibitors. Patients with significant components of collagen in the stroma may not respond to either form of medical therapy. One cannot reliably predict responsiveness to specific therapy (see below).

As benign prostatic hyperplasia nodules in the transition zone enlarge, they compress the outer zones of the prostate, resulting in the formation of a "surgical capsule." This boundary separates the transition zone from the peripheral zone of the gland and serves as a cleavage plane for open enucleation of the prostate during simple prostatectomies.

Pathophysiology

One can relate the symptoms of benign prostatic hyperplasia either to the obstructive component of the prostate or to the secondary response of the bladder to the outlet resistance. The obstructive component can be subdivided into mechanical obstruction and dynamic obstruction.

As prostatic enlargement occurs, mechanical obstruction may result from intrusion into the urethral lumen or bladder neck, resulting in a higher bladder outlet resistance. Prostatic size on digital rectal examination (DRE) correlates poorly with symptoms.

The dynamic component of prostatic obstruction explains the variable nature of the symptoms. The prostatic stroma is composed of smooth muscle and collagen and is rich in adrenergic nerve supply. The level of autonomic stimulation thus sets a "tone" to the prostatic urethra. Alpha-blocker therapy decreases this tone, resulting in a decrease in outlet resistance.

The irritative voiding complaints (see below) of benign prostatic hyperplasia result from the secondary response of the bladder to the increased outlet resistance. Bladder outlet obstruction results in detrusor muscle hypertrophy and hyperplasia as well as collagen deposition. The latter is most likely responsible for a decrease in bladder compliance, but detrusor instability also occurs. On gross inspection, thickened detrusor muscle bundles are seen as trabeculation on cystoscopic examination. If left unchecked, mucosal herniation between detrusor muscle bundles ensues, resulting in diverticulum formation ("false" diverticula composed of mucosa and serosa only).

Clinical Findings

A. Symptoms

The symptoms of benign prostatic hyperplasia can be divided into obstructive and irritative complaints. Obstructive symptoms include hesitancy, decreased force and caliber of the stream, sensation of incomplete bladder emptying, double voiding (urinating a second time within 2 hours), straining to urinate, and postvoid dribbling. Irritative symptoms include urgency, frequency, and nocturia.

The American Urological Association (AUA) has developed a self-administered questionnaire that is reliable in identifying patients who need therapy and in monitoring the response to therapy. The AUA symptom index (Table 23–4) is perhaps the single most important tool used in the evaluation of patients with this disorder and should be calculated for all patients before starting therapy. The answers to seven questions quantitate the severity of obstructive or irritative complaints on a scale of 0–5. Thus, the score can range from 0 to 35, in increasing severity of symptoms.

A detailed history focusing on the urinary tract should be obtained to exclude other possible causes of symptoms such as prostate cancer or disorders unrelated to the prostate such as urinary tract infection, neurogenic bladder, or urethral stricture.

B. SIGNS

A physical examination, DRE, and a focused neurologic examination should be performed on all patients. The size and consistency of the prostate should be noted, but prostate size does not correlate with the severity of symptoms or the degree of obstruction. Benign prostatic hyperplasia usually results in a smooth, firm, elastic enlargement of the prostate. Induration, if detected, must alert the physician to the possibility of cancer, and further evaluation is needed (ie, PSA, transrectal ultrasound, and biopsy). Examination of the lower abdomen should be performed to assess for a distended bladder.

C. LABORATORY FINDINGS

Urinalysis should be done to exclude infection or hematuria, and serum creatinine should be measured to assess renal function. Renal insufficiency may be observed in 10% of patients with prostatism and if observed warrants upper tract imaging. Patients with renal insufficiency are at an increased risk of developing complications following operative treatment for benign prostatic hyperplasia. A serum PSA is considered optional, yet most physicians will include it in the initial evaluation. PSA certainly increases the ability to detect prostate cancer over DRE alone, yet because there is much overlap between levels seen in benign prostatic hyperplasia and prostate cancer, its use remains controversial (see below in the section on screening for prostate cancer).

D. IMAGING

Upper tract imaging (intravenous pyelogram or renal ultrasound) is only recommended in the presence of concomitant urinary tract disease or complications from benign prostatic hyperplasia (ie, hematuria, urinary tract infection, renal insufficiency, history of stone disease).

E. CYSTOSCOPY

Cystoscopy is not recommended to determine the need for treatment but may assist in determining the

Table 23–4. American Urological Association symptom index for benign prostatic hyperplasia.[1,2]

Questions to Be Answered	Not at all	Less Than One Time in Five	Less Than Half the Time	About Half the Time	More Than Half the Time	Almost Always
1. Over the past month, how often have you had a sensation of not emptying your bladder completely after you finish urinating?	0	1	2	3	4	5
2. Over the past month, how often have you had to urinate again less than 2 hours after you finished urinating?	0	1	2	3	4	5
3. Over the past month, how often have you found you stopped and started again several times when you urinated?	0	1	2	3	4	5
4. Over the past month, how often have you found it difficult to postpone urination?	0	1	2	3	4	5
5. Over the past month, how often have you had a weak urinary stream?	0	1	2	3	4	5
6. Over the past month, how often have you had to push or strain to begin urination?	0	1	2	3	4	5
7. Over the past month, how many times did you most typically get up to urinate from the time you went to bed at night until the time you got up in the morning?	0 (None)	1 (1 time)	2 (2 times)	3 (3 times)	4 (4 times)	5 (5 times)

[1]Sum of seven circled numbers equals the symptom score. See text for explanation.
[2]Reproduced, with permission, from Barry MJ et al: The American Urological Association symptoms index for benign prostatic hyperplasia. J Urol 1992;148:1549.

surgical approach in patients opting for invasive therapy.

F. ADDITIONAL TESTS

Cystometrograms and urodynamic profiles should be reserved for patients with suspected neurologic disease or those who have failed prostate surgery. Flow rates, postvoid residual urine determination, and pressure-flow studies are considered optional.

Differential Diagnosis

Other obstructive conditions of the lower urinary tract such as urethral stricture, bladder neck contracture, bladder stone, or carcinoma of the prostate must be considered when evaluating men with presumptive benign prostatic hyperplasia. A history of prior urethral instrumentation, urethritis, or trauma should be elucidated to exclude urethral stricture or bladder neck contracture. Hematuria and pain are commonly associated with bladder stones. Carcinoma of the prostate may be detected by abnormalities on the DRE or an elevated PSA (see below). A urinary tract infection can mimic the irritative symptoms of benign prostatic hyperplasia and can be readily identified by urinalysis and culture, however, a urinary tract infection can also be a complication of benign prostatic hyperplasia. Carcinoma of the bladder, especially carcinoma in situ, may also present with irritative voiding complaints; however, urinalysis usually shows evidence of hematuria. Patients with neurogenic bladder may also have many of the same signs and symptoms as those with benign prostatic hyperplasia; however, a history of neurologic disease, stroke, diabetes mellitus, or back injury may be obtained, and diminished perineal or lower extremity sensation or alterations in rectal sphincter tone or the bulbocavernosus reflex might be observed on examination. Simultaneous alterations in bowel function (constipation) might also alert one to the possibility of a neurologic disorder.

Treatment

Clinical practice guidelines exist for the evaluation and treatment of patients with benign prostatic hyperplasia (Figure 23–1). Following evaluation as outlined above, patients should be offered various forms of therapy for benign prostatic hyperplasia. Patients are advised to consult with their primary care physicians and make an educated decision on the basis of the relative efficacy and side effects of the treatment options (Table 23–5).

Patients with mild symptoms (scores 0–7) should be managed by watchful waiting only. Absolute surgical indications are refractory urinary retention (failing at least one attempt at catheter removal), large bladder diverticula, or any of the following sequelae of benign prostatic hyperplasia: recurrent urinary tract infection, recurrent gross hematuria, bladder stones, or renal insufficiency.

A. WATCHFUL WAITING

The risk of progression or complications is uncertain. However, in men with symptomatic disease, it is clear that progression is not inevitable and that some men undergo spontaneous improvement or resolution of their symptoms.

Retrospective studies on the natural history of benign prostatic hyperplasia are inherently subject to bias, relating in part to patient selection and also to the type and extent of follow-up. Very few prospective studies addressing the natural history have been reported. One small series demonstrated that approximately 10% of symptomatic men may progress to urinary retention while half of patients demonstrate marked improvement or resolution of symptoms. Recently, a large randomized study was reported comparing finasteride with placebo in men with moderate to severely symptomatic disease and enlarged prostates on DRE. Patients in the placebo arm demonstrated a 7% risk of developing urinary retention over 4 years.

Men with moderate or severe symptoms can be managed also in this fashion if they so choose. The optimal interval for follow-up is not defined, nor are the specific end points for intervention.

B. MEDICAL THERAPY

1. Alpha blockers—The human prostate and bladder base contains α_1 adrenoceptors, and the prostate will show a contractile response to such agonists. The contractile properties of the prostate and bladder neck seem to be mediated primarily by α_{1a} receptors. Alpha blockade has been shown to result in both objective and subjective degrees of improvement in the symptoms and signs of benign prostatic hyperplasia in some patients. Alpha-blockers can be classified according to their receptor selectivity as well as their half-life (Table 23–6).

The efficacies of phenoxybenzamine and prazosin are comparable with respect to symptomatic relief; however, the higher side effect profile of phenoxybenzamine, resulting from its lack of alpha-receptor specificity, precludes its use in benign prostatic hyperplasia patients. Dose titration is necessary with prazosin, with typical therapy starting at 1 mg orally at bedtime for 3 nights, then increasing to 1 mg orally twice daily and then titrating up to 2 mg orally twice daily if necessary. Little additional symptomatic improvement is observed at higher doses, and side effects increase. Typical side effects include orthostatic hypotension, dizziness, tiredness, retrograde ejaculation, rhinitis, and headache.

Long-acting alpha-blockers allow for once-a-day dosing, but dose titration is still necessary. Terazosin is started at a dosage of 1 mg orally daily for 3 days, increased to 2 mg orally daily for 11 days, then 5 mg orally daily. Additional dose escalation to 10 mg orally daily can be performed if necessary. Doxazosin is started at a dosage of 1 mg orally daily for 7 days, increased to 2 mg orally daily for 7 days, then 4 mg

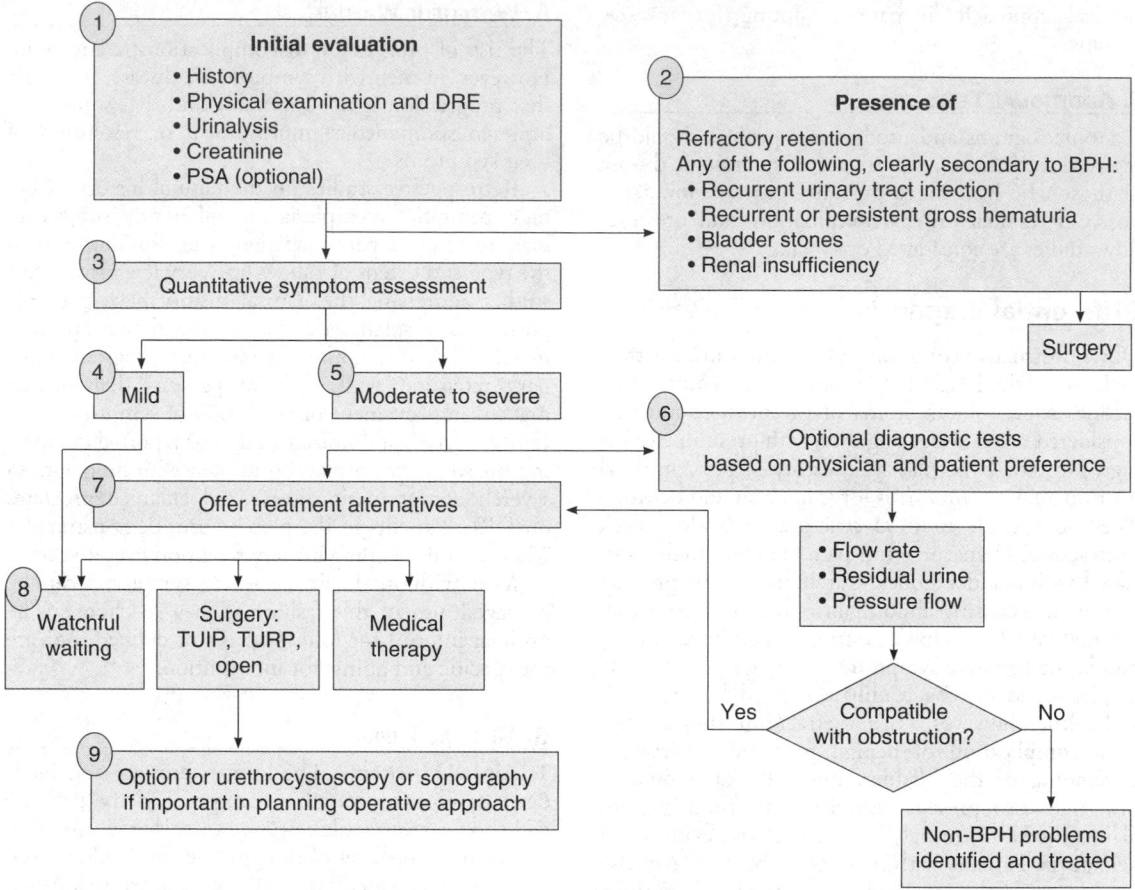

Figure 23–1. Benign prostatic hyperplasia decision diagram. (BPH, benign prostatic hyperplasia; DRE, digital rectal examination; TUIP, transurethral incision of the prostate; TURP, transurethral resection of the prostate.)

orally daily. Additional dose escalation to 8 mg orally daily can be performed if necessary. Side effects are similar to those described above for prazosin.

The most recent advance in alpha-blocker therapy has been the identification of subtypes of α_1 receptors. The α_{1a} receptors are those localized to the prostate and bladder neck, and selective blockade results in fewer systemic side effects (orthostatic hypotension, dizziness, tiredness, rhinitis, and headache), thus obviating the need for dose titration. Tamsulosin is started at a dosage of 0.4 mg orally daily and can be increased to 0.8 mg orally daily if necessary.

Several randomized, double-blind, placebo-controlled trials have been performed comparing terazosin, doxazosin, or tamsulosin with placebo. All agents have demonstrated safety and efficacy. Comparative trials between different alpha-blockers are ongoing.

2. 5α-Reductase inhibitors—Finasteride is a 5α-reductase inhibitor that blocks the conversion of testosterone to dihydrotestosterone. This drug impacts

upon the epithelial component of the prostate, resulting in reduction in size of the gland and improvement in symptoms. Six months of therapy are required for maximum effects on prostate size (20% reduction) and symptomatic improvement.

Several randomized, double-blind, placebo-controlled trials have been performed comparing finasteride with placebo. Efficacy, safety, and durability are well established. However, symptomatic improvement is seen only in men with enlarged prostates (> 40 mL). Side effects include decreased libido, decrease in volume of ejaculate, and impotence. Serum PSA is reduced by approximately 50% in patients receiving finasteride therapy. However, individual values may vary, thus complicating cancer detection.

A recent report suggests that finasteride therapy may decrease the incidence of urinary retention and the need for operative treatment in men with enlarged prostates and moderate to severe symptoms. However, optimal identification of appropriate patients for prophylactic therapy remains to be determined.

Table 23–5. Balance sheet for benign prostatic hyperplasia treatment outcomes.[1]

Outcome	TUIP	Open Surgery	TURP	Watchful Waiting	Alpha Blockers	Finasteride[2]
Chance for improvement[1]	78–83%	94–99.8%	75–96%	31–55%	59–86%	54–78%
Degree of symptom improvement (% reduction in symptom score)	73%	79%	85%	Unknown	51%	31%
Morbidity and complications[1]	2.2–33.3%	7–42.7%	5.2–30.7%	1–5%	2.9–43.3%	13.6–8.8%
Death within 30–90 days[1]	0.2–1.5%	1–4.6%	0.5–3.3%	0.8%	0.8%	0.8%
Total incontinence[1]	0.1–1.1%	0.3–0.7%	0.7–1.4%	2%	2%	2%
Need for operative treatment for surgical complications[1]	1.3–2.7%	0.6–14.1%	0.7–10.1%	0	0	0
Impotence[1]	3.9–24.5%	4.7–39.2%	3.3–34.8%	3%	3%	2.5–5.3%
Retrograde ejaculation	6–55%	36–95%	25–99%	0	4–11%	0
Loss of work in days	7–21	21–28	7–21	1	3.5	1.5
Hospital stay in days	1–3	5–10	3–5	0	0	0

TUIP = transurethral incision of the prostate; TURP = transurethral resection of the prostate
[1]90% confidence interval.
[2]Most of the data reviewed for finasteride is derived from three trials that have required an enlarged prostate for entry. The chance of improvement in men with symptoms yet minimally enlarged prostates may be much less, as noted from the VA Cooperative Trial.

3. Combination therapy—The first randomized, double-blind, placebo-controlled study investigating combination therapy of an alpha-blocker and a 5α-reductase inhibitor was recently reported. This was a four-arm Veterans Administration Cooperative Trial comparing placebo, finasteride alone, terazosin alone, and combination of finasteride and terazosin. Over 1200 patients participated, and significant decreases in symptom scores and increases in urinary flow rates were seen only in the arms containing terazosin. However, one must note that enlarged prostates were not an entry criterion, and in fact prostate size in this study was much smaller than in previous controlled trials using finasteride (32 versus 52 mL). Additional combination therapy trials are ongoing.

4. Phytotherapy—Phytotherapy is the use of plants or plant extracts for medicinal purposes. Its use in be-nign prostatic hyperplasia has been popular in Europe for years, and its use in the United States is growing as a result of patient-driven enthusiasm. Several plant extracts have been popularized, including the saw palmetto berry, the bark of *Pygeum africanum,* the roots of *Echinacea purpurea* and *Hypoxis rooperi,* pollen extract, and the leaves of the trembling poplar. The mechanisms of action of these agents are unknown, and their efficacy and safety have not been tested in multicenter, randomized, double-blind, placebo-controlled studies.

C. CONVENTIONAL SURGICAL THERAPY

1. Transurethral resection of the prostate (TURP)—Ninety-five percent of simple prostatectomies can be performed endoscopically. Most of these procedures are performed under a spinal anesthetic and require a 1- to 2-day hospital stay. Symptom scores and flow rate improvement are superior following TURP relative to any minimally invasive therapy; however, the length of the hospital stay is greater. Much controversy revolves around possible higher rates of morbidity and mortality associated with TURP in comparison with open surgery, but the higher rates observed in one study probably related to more significant comorbidities in the TURP patients compared with the patients who received open surgical treatment. Several other studies could not confirm the difference in mortality when controlling for age and comorbidities. The risks of TURP include retrograde ejaculation (75%), impotence (5–10%), and urinary incontinence (< 1%). Complications include bleeding, urethral stricture or bladder neck contrac-

Table 23–6. Alpha blockade for benign prostatic hyperplasia.

Agent	Action	Dose
Phenoxybenzamine	α_1 and α_2 blockade	5–10 mg twice daily
Prazosin	α_1 blockade	1–5 mg twice daily
Terazosin	α_1 blockade	1–10 mg daily
Doxazosin	α_1 blockade	1–8 mg daily
Tamsulosin	α_{1a} blockade	0.4 or 0.8 mg daily

ture, perforation of the prostate capsule with extravasation, and, if severe, transurethral resection syndrome, a hypervolemic, hyponatremic state resulting from absorption of the hypotonic irrigating solution. Clinical manifestations of the syndrome include nausea, vomiting, confusion, hypertension, bradycardia, and visual disturbances. The risk of transurethral resection syndrome increases with resection times over 90 minutes. Treatment includes diuresis and, in severe cases, hypertonic saline administration.

2. Transurethral incision of the prostate (TUIP)— Men with moderate to severe symptoms and small prostates often have posterior commissure hyperplasia or an "elevated bladder neck." These patients will often benefit from incision of the prostate. The procedure is more rapid and less morbid than TURP. Outcomes in well-selected patients are comparable, though a lower rate of retrograde ejaculation has been reported (25%). The technique involves two incisions using the Collins knife at the 5 and 7 o'clock positions. The incisions are started just distal to the ureteral orifices and extended outward to the verumontanum.

3. Open simple prostatectomy— When the prostate is too large to remove endoscopically, open enucleation is necessary. What size is "too large" depends upon the surgeon's experience with TURP. Glands over 100 g are usually considered for open enucleation. In addition to size, other relative indications for open prostatectomy include concomitant bladder diverticulum or bladder stone and whether dorsal lithotomy positioning is or is not possible.

Open prostatectomies can be performed with either a suprapubic or retropubic approach. Simple suprapubic prostatectomy is performed transvesically and is the operation of choice if there is concomitant bladder pathology. After the bladder is opened, a semicircular incision is made in the bladder mucosa distal to the trigone. The dissection plane is initiated sharply, and blunt dissection with the finger is then performed to deliver the adenoma. The apical dissection should be performed sharply to avoid injury to the distal sphincteric mechanism. After the adenoma is removed, hemostasis is attained with suture ligatures and both a urethral and a suprapubic catheter are inserted prior to closure.

In simple retropubic prostatectomy, the bladder is not entered but rather a transverse incision is made in the surgical capsule of the prostate and the adenoma is enucleated as described above. Only a urethral catheter is needed at the end of the case.

D. MINIMALLY INVASIVE THERAPY

1. Laser therapy— Many techniques of laser surgery for the prostate have been described. Two main energy sources of lasers have been utilized—neodymium: yttrium-aluminum-garnet (Nd:YAG) and holmium-YAG.

Several different coagulation necrosis techniques have been described. TULIP (transurethral laser-in-duced prostatectomy) is performed under transrectal ultrasound guidance. The instrument is placed in the urethra and transrectal ultrasound is used to direct the device as it is slowly pulled from the bladder neck to the apex. The depth of treatment is monitored with ultrasound.

Most urologists prefer to use visually directed laser techniques. Visual coagulative necrosis is performed under cystoscopic control, and the laser fiber is pulled through the prostate at several designated areas depending upon the size and configuration of the gland. Four-quadrant and sextant approaches have been described for lateral lobes, with additional treatments directed at enlarged median lobes. Coagulative techniques do not create an immediate visual defect in the prostatic urethra—tissue is sloughed over the course of several weeks up to 3 months following the procedure.

Visual contact ablative techniques take longer in the operating room because the fiber is placed in direct contact with the prostate tissue, which is vaporized. An immediate defect is obtained in the prostatic urethra, similar to that seen during TURP.

Interstitial laser therapy places fibers directly into the prostate, usually under cystoscopic control. At each puncture, the laser is fired, resulting in submucosal coagulative necrosis. Irritative voiding symptoms may be less in these patients as the urethral mucosa is spared and prostate tissue is resorbed by the body rather than sloughed.

Advantages to laser surgery include minimal blood loss, rare occurrence of transurethral resection syndrome, the ability to treat patients while on anticoagulation therapy, and outpatient surgery. Disadvantages are the lack of tissue for pathologic examination, the longer postoperative catheterization time, the more frequent irritative voiding complaints, and the expense of laser fibers and generators.

Large multicenter, randomized studies with long-term follow-up are needed in comparing laser prostate surgery with TURP and other forms of minimally invasive surgery.

2. Transurethral needle ablation of the prostate (TUNA)— This procedure uses a specially designed urethral catheter that is passed into the urethra. Interstitial radiofrequency needles are then deployed from the tip of the catheter, piercing the mucosa of the prostatic urethra. Radiofrequencies are then used to heat the tissue, resulting in coagulative necrosis. Bladder neck and median lobe enlargement are not well treated by TUNA. Subjective and objective improvement in voiding occurs. In randomized trials comparing TUNA to transurethral resection of the prostate (TURP), similar improvement was seen when comparing life scores, peak urinary flow rates, and postvoid residual urine.

3. Transurethral electrovaporization of the prostate— This technique uses the standard resectoscope but replaces a conventional loop with a variation of a grooved rollerball. High current densities result in heat vaporization of tissue, creating a cavity in the prostatic urethra. Because the device requires slower sweeping speeds over the prostatic urethra and the depth of vaporization is approximately one-third of a standard loop, this procedure usually takes longer than a standard TURP. Long-term comparative data are needed.

4. Hyperthermia—Microwave hyperthermia is most commonly delivered with a transurethral catheter. Some devices cool the urethral mucosa to decrease the risk of injury. However, if temperatures do not go above 45 °C, cooling is unnecessary. Symptom score and flow rate improvement are obtained, but (as with laser surgery) large randomized studies with long-term follow-up are needed to assess durability and cost-effectiveness.

5. High-intensity focused ultrasound (HIFU)—HIFU is another means of performing thermal tissue ablation. A specially designed dual-function ultrasound probe is placed in the rectum. This probe allows transrectal imaging of the prostate and also delivers short bursts of high-intensity focused ultrasound energy, which heats the prostate tissue and causes coagulative necrosis. Bladder neck and median lobe enlargement are not well treated by HIFU. Ongoing clinical trials demonstrate some improvement in symptom score and flow rate, but the durability of the response is not known.

6. Intraurethral stents—Intraurethral stents are placed endoscopically in the prostatic fossa to keep the prostatic urethra patent. They are usually covered by urothelium within 4–6 months following insertion. These devices are typically used for patients with limited life expectancies who are not deemed good surgical or anesthetic candidates; however, with the advent of other minimally invasive techniques requiring minimal anesthesia (conscious sedation, or prostatic blocks), their application has become more limited.

7. Transurethral balloon dilation of the prostate—Balloon dilation of the prostate is performed with specially designed catheters that permit dilation of the prostatic fossa alone or dilation of the prostatic fossa and bladder neck. The technique is most effective in small prostates (< 40 mL), and while it may result in improvement in symptom score and flow rates, the effects are transient. This technique is rarely used today.

Arai Y et al: Impact of interventional therapy for benign prostatic hyperplasia on quality of life and sexual function: a prospective study. J Urol 2000;164:1206. [PMID: 10992367] (Sexual desire and erectile function are intact after treatment for benign prostatic hyperplasia; retrograde ejaculation is a common finding postoperatively.)

Djavan B et al: Prospective randomized comparison of high energy transurethral microwave thermotherapy versus alpha-blocker treatment of patients with benign prostatic hyperplasia. J Urol 1999;161:139. [PMID: 10037386] (Alpha blockade resulted in rapid improvement in symptoms.

Transurethral microwave therapy was associated with superior outcomes at 12 weeks to 6 months.)

Fawzy A et al: Long-term (4 year) efficacy and tolerability of doxazosin for the treatment of concurrent benign prostatic hyperplasia and hypertension. Int J Urol 1999;6:346. [PMID: 10445304] (Doxazosin is well-tolerated and effective long-term therapy for concurrent benign prostatic hyperplasia and hypertension.)

Floratos DL et al: Long-term followup of randomized transurethral microwave thermotherapy versus transurethral prostatic resection study. J Urol 2001;165:1533. [PMID: 11342912]. (Transurethral microwave thermotherapy and transurethral prostatic resection alleviate lower urinary tract symptoms. The magnitude of the resection is greater with the resection technique.)

Medina JJ et al: Benign prostatic hyperplasia (the aging prostate). Med Clin North Am 1999;83:1213. [PMID: 10503061]

Wilde MI et al: Finasteride: an update of its use in the management of symptomatic benign prostatic hyperplasia. Drugs 1999;57:557. [PMID: 10235693] (Finasteride reduces disease progression and decreases the incidence of acute urinary retention. It is a therapeutic option for patients unable or unwilling to undergo more definitive operative management.)

■ MALIGNANT GENITOURINARY TRACT DISORDERS

PROSTATE CANCER

ESSENTIALS OF DIAGNOSIS

- *Prostatic induration on digital rectal examination or elevation of PSA.*
- *Most often asymptomatic.*
- *Rarely: systemic symptoms (weight loss, bone pain).*

General Considerations

Prostatic cancer is the most common cancer detected in American men and the second leading cause of cancer-related death. In the United States in 2001, over 198,000 new cases of prostate cancer were diagnosed, and about 31,500 deaths resulted. However, the clinical incidence of the disease does not match the prevalence noted at autopsy, where more than 40% of men over 50 years of age are found to have prostatic carcinoma. Most such occult cancers are small and contained within the prostate gland. Few are associated with regional or distant disease. The incidence of prostatic cancer increases with age. Whereas 30% of men age 60–69 will have the disease, autopsy incidence increases to 67% in men aged 80–89 years. Although the prevalence of prostatic cancer in autopsy specimens around the world varies little, the clinical incidence is considerably different (high in North America and European countries, intermediate in South America, and low in the Far East), suggesting that environmental or dietary differences among populations may be important for prostatic cancer growth. A 50-year-old American man has a lifetime risk of 40% for latent cancer, 9.5% for developing clinically apparent cancer, and a 2.9% risk of death due to prostatic cancer. Blacks, men with a family history of prostatic cancer or a history of high dietary fat intake, and perhaps men who have undergone vasectomy are at an increased risk of developing it.

Clinical Findings

A. Symptoms and Signs

Prostate cancer may be manifested as focal nodules or areas of induration within the prostate at the time of digital rectal examination. However, a large number of prostate cancers are associated with palpably normal prostates and are detected on the basis of elevations in serum prostate-specific antigen.

Rarely, patients present with signs of urinary retention (palpable bladder) or neurologic symptoms as a result of epidural metastases and cord compression. Obstructive voiding symptoms are most often due to benign prostatic hyperplasia, which occurs in the same age group. However, large or locally extensive prostatic cancers can cause obstructive voiding symptoms. Lymph node metastases can lead to lower extremity lymphedema. As the axial skeleton is the most common site of metastases, patients may present with back pain or pathologic fractures.

B. Laboratory Findings

1. Serum tumor markers—Prostate-specific antigen (PSA) is a glycoprotein produced only in the cytoplasm of benign and malignant prostate cells. The serum level correlates with the volume of both benign and malignant prostatic tissue. Measurement of PSA may be useful in detecting and staging prostatic cancer, monitoring response to treatment, and detecting recurrence before it becomes obvious clinically. As a first-line screening test, PSA will be elevated in approximately 10–15% of men self-referred for screening. Approximately 18–30% of men with intermediate degrees of elevation (4.1–10 ng/mL; normal < 4 ng/mL) will be found to have prostatic cancer. Between 50% and 70% of those with elevations greater than 10 ng/mL will have prostatic cancer. (See age-specific PSA reference ranges under Screening for Prostatic Cancer, below.) Patients with intermediate levels of PSA will usually have localized and therefore potentially curable cancers. However, it should be remembered that approximately 20% of patients who undergo radical prostatectomy for localized prostatic cancer will have normal levels of PSA.

In untreated patients with prostatic cancer, the level of PSA correlates with the volume and stage of the disease. Whereas most organ-confined cancers are associated with PSA levels less than 10 ng/mL, more advanced disease (seminal vesicle invasion, lymph node involvement, or occult distant metastases) is more common in patients with PSA levels in excess of 40 ng/mL. Approximately 98% of patients with metastatic prostatic cancer will have elevated PSA. However, there are occasional cancers which are localized despite substantial elevations in PSA. Therefore, treatment decisions in patients with untreated cancers cannot be made on the basis of PSA testing alone. A rising level of PSA after treatment is usually consistent with progressive disease whether it be locally recurrent or metastatic.

2. Miscellaneous laboratory testing—Patients in urinary retention or those with ureteral obstruction due to locally or regionally advanced prostatic cancers may present with elevations in serum urea nitrogen or creatinine. Patients with bony metastases may have elevations in alkaline phosphatase or hypercalcemia. Laboratory and clinical evidence of disseminated intravascular coagulation can occur in patients with advanced prostatic cancers.

3. Prostatic biopsy—Transrectal ultrasound-guided biopsy seems to be a better method for detection of prostatic cancer than finger-guided biopsy. The use of a spring-loaded, 18-gauge biopsy needle has allowed transrectal biopsy to be performed with little patient discomfort and low attendant morbidity. The specimen preserves glandular architecture and allows for accurate grading as described below. Transrectal ultrasound-guided biopsies are taken from the apex, mid portion, and base of the prostate in men who have an abnormal digital rectal examination or an elevated serum PSA. Systematic rather than only lesion-directed biopsies are usually performed. Patients with abnormalities of the seminal vesicles can have guided biopsies of these structures performed to allow for detection of local tumor invasion. Aspiration biopsies of the prostate, though accurate and associated with low morbidity, have been used rarely since the introduction of the spring-loaded biopsy device but should be considered in patients at an increased risk of bleeding.

C. Imaging

Modern transrectal ultrasound instrumentation provides high-definition images of the prostate. Transrectal ultrasonography has been used largely for the staging of prostatic carcinomas. In addition, transrectal ultrasound-guided—rather than digitally guided—biopsy of the prostate may be a more accurate way to investigate suspicious lesions. Most prostatic cancers are hypoechoic.

MRI of the prostate allows for evaluation of the prostatic lesion as well as regional lymph nodes. The positive predictive value for detection of both capsular penetration and seminal vesicle invasion is similar for both transrectal ultrasound and MRI. CT scanning plays little role in evaluation because of its inability to accurately identify or stage prostatic cancers.

Radionuclide bone scan is superior to conventional plain skeletal x-rays in detecting bony metastases. Most prostatic cancer metastases are multiple and are most commonly localized to the axial skeleton. Because of the high frequency of abnormal scans in patients in this age group resulting from degenerative joint disease, plain films are often useful in evaluating patients with indeterminate radionuclide findings. Intravenous urography and cystoscopy are not routinely used to evaluate patients with prostatic cancer.

Imaging can be tailored to the likelihood of advanced disease in newly diagnosed patients. Asymptomatic patients with well to moderately well differentiated cancers—thought to be localized to the prostate on digital rectal examination and transurethral ultrasound and associated with normal or only modest elevations of PSA (ie, < 10 ng/mL)— need no further evaluation.

Those with more advanced local lesions, symptoms of metastases (ie, bone pain), and elevations in PSA greater than 10 ng/mL should undergo radionuclide bone scan. Cross-sectional imaging of the prostate is usually indicated only in those patients in the latter group who have negative bone scans in an attempt to detect lymph node metastases. Patients found to have enlarged pelvic lymph nodes are candidates for fine-needle aspiration. Despite application of modern and sophisticated imaging, understaging of prostatic cancer occurs in at least 20% of patients.

Screening for Prostatic Cancer

The reported incidence of prostate cancer rose significantly in the United States when early detection techniques (PSA testing and transrectal ultrasound) became widely available. The goal of a screening effort should be to detect and effectively treat only those prostatic carcinomas most likely to cause morbidity or mortality if left untreated. Detection of latent, non-progressive cancers would expose patients to unnecessary treatment and its attendant complications and costs. Whether screening for prostatic cancer will result in a decrease in yearly mortality rates due to the disease is the subject of much current debate.

The screening tests currently available include digital rectal examination, PSA testing, and transrectal ultrasound. Depending on the patient population being evaluated, detection rates using digital rectal examination alone will vary from 1.5% to 7%. Unfortunately, most cancers detected in this way are advanced (stages T3 or greater). Transrectal ultrasound should not be used as a first-line screening tool because of its expense, its low specificity (and therefore high biopsy rate), and the fact that it increases the detection rate very little when compared with the combined use of digital rectal examination and PSA testing.

PSA testing will increase the detection rate of prostatic cancers compared with digital rectal examination. Approximately 2–2.5% of men older than age 50 will be found to have prostatic cancer using PSA testing compared with a rate of approximately 1.5% using digital rectal examination alone. PSA is not specific for cancer, and there is considerable overlap of values between men with benign prostatic hyperplasia and those with prostatic cancers. The sensitivity, specificity, and positive predictive value of PSA and digital rectal examination are listed in Table 23–7. PSA-detected cancers are more likely to be localized compared with those detected with digital rectal examination alone.

In order to improve the performance of PSA as a screening test, several investigators have developed alternative methods for its use. The serial measurement of PSA (PSA velocity) may increase specificity for cancer detection with little loss in sensitivity. A rate of change in PSA greater than 0.75 ng/mL per year is associated with an increased likelihood of cancer detection. In a patient with a normal digital rectal examination, an elevated PSA, and a normal transrectal ultrasound, the indications for prostate biopsy may be refined by calculating PSA density (serum PSA/volume of the prostate as measured by ultrasound). Patients with high PSA density are more likely to have disease in spite of a normal digital rectal examination and normal transrectal ultrasound. Some have found measurement of PSA transition zone density (the zone of the prostate that undergoes enlargement during development of benign prostatic hyperplasia) to be more predictive of the presence or absence of cancer than PSA density calculated using the entire prostate volume. As PSA concentration is directly related to patient age, establishment of age-specific reference ranges would increase specificity (fewer older men with benign prostatic hyperplasia would undergo evaluation) and increase sensitivity (more younger men with cancer would undergo evaluation). Age-specific

Table 23–7. Screening for prostatic cancer: Test performance.[1]

Test	Sensitivity	Specificity	Positive Predictive Value
Abnormal PSA (> 4 ng/mL)	0.67	0.97	0.43
Abnormal DRE	0.50	0.94	0.24
Abnormal PSA or DRE	0.84	0.92	0.28
Abnormal PSA and DRE	0.34	0.995	0.49

Key: DRE = digital rectal examination; PSA = prostate-specific antigen.
[1]Modified from Kramer BS et al: Prostate cancer screening: What we know and what we need to know. Ann Intern Med 1993; 119:914.

reference ranges have been established: men 40–49, < 2.5 ng/mL; men 50–59, < 3.5 ng/mL; men 60–69, < 4.5 ng/mL; men 70–79, < 6.5 ng/mL (based on a previously normal serum PSA of < 4 ng/mL). Black men have lower age-specific reference ranges (age 40–49, < 2 ng/mL; age 50–59, < 4 ng/mL; age 60–69, < 4.5 ng/mL; age 70–79, < 5.5 ng/mL). The most recent attempt at refining PSA has been the measurement of free serum and protein-bound levels (cancer patients have a lower percentage of free serum PSA). Numerous centers are analyzing this assay to define an optimal cutoff level. Generally, men with free fractions exceeding 25% are unlikely to have prostate cancer, whereas those with free fractions less than 10% have an approximately 50% chance of having prostate cancer. Early reports using cutoffs of 18–20% of free PSA resulted in 5–10% lost sensitivity for 15–40% gains in specificity. The frequency of PSA testing remains a matter of some debate. In men with a normal DRE and a PSA > 2.5 ng/mL, PSA testing should be performed yearly because approximately 50% of these patients convert to having a PSA > 4 ng/mL. It can be performed biennially in those with a normal DRE and serum PSA < 2.5 ng/mL. Conversion in this group is much less likely.

Pathology & Staging

The majority of prostatic cancers are adenocarcinomas. Most arise in the periphery of the prostate (peripheral zone), though a small percentage arise in the central (5–10%) and transition zones (20%) of the gland. Most pathologists employ the Gleason grading system whereby a "primary" grade is applied to the architectural pattern of cancerous glands occupying the largest area of the specimen and a "secondary" pattern is assigned to the next largest area of cancerous growth. Grading is based on architectural (rather than histologic) criteria, and five possible "grades" are possible. Adding the score of the primary and secondary patterns gives a Gleason score. Grade correlates well with tumor volume, stage, and prognosis. The TNM classification of the American Joint Cancer Committee for prostatic cancer is shown in Table 23–8.

The patterns of prostatic cancer progression have been well defined. The likelihood of both local invasion and metastases is greater in larger or less well differentiated cancers. Small and well-differentiated cancers (grades 1 and 2) are usually confined within the prostate, whereas large-volume (> 4 mL) or poorly differentiated (grades 4 and 5) cancers are more commonly locally extensive or metastatic to regional lymph nodes or bone. Penetration of the prostatic capsule by cancer is common and often occurs along perineural spaces. Seminal vesicle invasion is associated with a high likelihood of regional or distant disease. Lymphatic metastases are most often identified in the obturator lymph node chain. The axial skeleton, as mentioned previously, is the most common site of distant metastases.

Table 23–8. TNM staging system for prostate cancer.

T: Primary tumor	
Tx	Cannot be assessed
T0	No evidence of primary tumor
Tis	Carcinoma in situ (CIS)
T1a	Carcinoma in 5% or less of tissue resected; normal DRE
T1b	Carcinoma in more than 5% of tissue resected; normal DRE
T1c	Detected from elevated PSA alone; normal DRE
T2a	Tumor in one lobe
T2b	Tumor in both lobes
T3a	Extracapsular extension
T3b	Seminal vesicle involvement
T4	Adjacent organ involvement
N: Regional lymph nodes	
Nx	Cannot be assessed
N0	No regional lymph node metastasis
N1	Metastasis in one or more regional lymph nodes
M: Distant metastasis	
Mx	Cannot be assessed
M0	No distant metastasis
M1	Distant metastasis present

DRE = digital rectal examination; PSA = prostate-specific antigen.

Treatment

A. LOCALIZED DISEASE

What constitutes the optimal form of treatment for patients with clinically localized cancers remains controversial. Treatment decisions are at present made on the basis of tumor grade and stage and the age and health of the patient. Although selected patients may be candidates for surveillance based on age or health and the presence of small-volume or well-differentiated cancers, most patients with an anticipated survival in excess of 10 years should be considered for treatment. Both radiation therapy and radical prostatectomy allow for acceptable levels of local control. A randomized trial comparing watchful waiting and radical prostatectomy in men with clinically localized prostate cancer is currently under way in the United States (PIVOT: Prostate Cancer Intervention Versus Observation Trial). This trial will randomize 1000 patients and will run for 15 years. Patients need to be advised of all treatment options (including surveillance) along with their particular benefits, risks, and limitations.

B. RADICAL PROSTATECTOMY

In radical prostatectomy, the seminal vesicles, prostate, and ampullae of the vas deferens are removed. Refinements in technique have allowed maintenance of urinary continence in most patients and erectile function in selected patients. Local recurrence is uncommon after radical prostatectomy, and its incidence is related to pathologic stage. Organ-confined cancers rarely recur. However, cancers found to be locally extensive (capsular penetration, seminal vesicle invasion) are associated with higher local (10–25%) and distant (20–50%) relapse rates.

Ideal candidates for the procedure include healthy patients with stages T1 and T2 prostatic cancers. Patients with advanced local tumors (T3 and T4) and those with lymph node metastases are rarely candidates for this procedure.

Patients with positive surgical margins are at an increased risk for local and distant tumor relapse. Such patients are often considered candidates for adjuvant therapy (radiation for positive margins or androgen deprivation for lymph node metastases). Although adjuvant radiation seems to be associated with fewer local recurrences (0–5% with radiation versus 15–30% without), it has little or no impact on distant failure rates (30–35% with radiation versus 30–45% without).

C. Radiation Therapy

Radiation can be delivered by a variety of techniques including use of external beam radiotherapy and transperineal implantation of radioisotopes. Morbidity is limited, and the survival of patients with localized cancers (T1, T2, and selected T3) approaches 65% at 10 years. As with surgery, the likelihood of local failure correlates with technique and tumor stage. The likelihood of a positive prostatic biopsy more than 18 months after surgery varies between 20% and 60% in selected series. Patients with local recurrence are at an increased risk of cancer progression and cancer death compared with those who have negative biopsies. Ambiguous target definitions, inadequate radiation doses, and understaging of patients may be responsible for the failure noted in some series. Newer techniques of radiation (implantation, conformal therapy using three-dimensional reconstruction of CT-based tumor volumes, heavy particle, charged particle, and heavy charged particle) may improve local control rates. Three-dimensional conformal radiation delivers a higher dose because of improved targeting and appears to be associated with improved efficacy and a lower likelihood of adverse side effects compared with previous radiation techniques. As a result of improvements in imaging—most notably transrectal ultrasound—there has been a resurgence of interest in brachytherapy, the implantation of permanent or temporary radioactive sources (palladium, iodine, or iridium) into the prostate. Brachytherapy can be combined with external beam radiation in patients with higher-grade or higher-volume disease or as monotherapy in those with low-grade or low-volume malignancies.

D. Surveillance

A positive impact of localized prostatic cancer treatment with regard to survival has not been conclusively demonstrated. Surveillance alone may be an appropriate form of management for selected patients with prostatic cancer. However, many patients in such series are older and have very small and well-differentiated cancers. Even in such a selected population, cancer death rates approach 10%. In addition, end points for intervention in patients on surveillance regimens have not been defined.

E. Cryosurgery

Cryosurgery is a technique whereby liquid nitrogen is circulated through small hollow-core needles inserted into the prostate under ultrasound guidance. The freezing process results in tissue destruction. There has been a resurgence of interest in less invasive forms of therapy for localized prostate cancer as well as several recent technical innovations, including improved percutaneous techniques, expertise in transrectal ultrasound, improved cryotechnology, and better understanding of cryobiology. The positive biopsy rate after cryoablation ranges between 7% and 23%.

F. Locally and Regionally Advanced Disease

Prostatic cancers associated with minimal degrees of capsular penetration are candidates for standard irradiation or surgery. Those with locally extensive cancers, including those with seminal vesicle and bladder neck invasion, are at increased risk of both local and distant relapse despite conventional therapy. Currently, a variety of investigational regimens are being tested in an effort to improve local and distant relapse rates in such patients. Combination therapy (androgen deprivation combined with surgery or irradiation), newer forms of irradiation, and hormonal therapy alone are being tested in such patients. Neoadjuvant androgen deprivation therapy combined with external beam radiation therapy have demonstrated improved survival over external beam radiation therapy alone. Similarly, patients with lymph node metastases may benefit little from aggressive local therapy and are best treated with androgen deprivation, occasionally combined with local therapy.

G. Metastatic Disease

Since death due to prostatic carcinoma is almost invariably a result of failure to control metastatic disease, research has emphasized efforts to improve control of distant disease. It is well known that most prostatic carcinomas are hormone-dependent, and approximately 70–80% of men with metastatic prostatic carcinoma will respond to various forms of androgen deprivation. Testosterone, the major circulating androgen, is produced by Leydig cells in the testes (95%), with a smaller amount being produced by peripheral conversion of other steroids. Although 98% of serum testosterone is protein-bound, free testosterone enters prostate cells and is converted to dihydrotestosterone, the major intracellular androgen. Dihydrotestosterone binds a cytoplasmic receptor protein, and the complex moves to the cell nucleus,

Table 23–9. Androgen ablation for prostatic cancer.

Level	Agent	Dose	Sequelae
Pituitary, hypothalamus	Estrogens	1–3 mg daily	Gynecomastia, hot flushes, thromboembolic disease, erectile dysfunction
	LHRH agonists	Monthly or 3-monthly depot injection	Erectile dysfunction, hot flushes, gynecomastia, rarely anemia
Adrenal	Ketoconazole	400 mg three times daily	Adrenal insufficiency, nausea, rash, ataxia
	Aminoglutethimide	250 mg four times daily	Adrenal insufficiency, nausea, rash, ataxia
	Glucocorticoids	Prednisone: 20–40 mg daily	Gastrointestinal bleeding, fluid retention
Testis	Orchiectomy		Gynecomastia, hot flushes, erectile dysfunction
Prostate cell	Antiandrogens	Flutamide: 250 mg three times daily Bicalutamide: 50 mg daily	No erectile dysfunction when used alone; nausea, diarrhea

where it modulates transcription. Androgen deprivation may be induced at several levels along the pituitary-gonadal axis using a variety of methods or agents (Table 23–9). Use of LHRH agonists (leuprolide, goserelin)—drugs delivered in monthly or 3-monthly depot—has allowed induction of androgen deprivation without orchiectomy or administration of diethylstilbestrol. Presently, administration of LHRH agonists and orchiectomy are the most common forms of primary androgen blockade used. Because of its rapid onset of action, ketoconazole should be considered in patients with advanced prostatic cancer who present with spinal cord compression, bilateral ureteral obstruction, or disseminated intravascular coagulation. Although testosterone is the major circulating androgen, the adrenal gland secretes the androgens dehydroepiandrosterone, dehydroepiandrosterone sulfate, and androstenedione. Some investigators believe that suppressing both testicular and adrenal androgens will allow for a better initial and longer response than methods which inhibit production of only testicular androgens. Complete androgen blockade can be achieved by combining an antiandrogen with use of an LHRH agonist or orchiectomy. Nonsteroidal antiandrogen agents appear to act by competitively binding the receptor for dihydrotestosterone, the intracellular androgen responsible for prostatic cell growth and development. A meta-analysis of trials comparing the use of either an LHRH agonist or orchiectomy alone with the use of either in combination with an antiandrogen agent shows marginal (if any) benefit to the use of combination therapy. However, patients at risk of disease-related symptoms (bone pain, obstructive voiding symptoms) due to the initial elevation of serum testosterone that accompanies the use of an LHRH agonist should receive antiandrogens initially.

Barry MJ et al: Outcomes for men with clinically nonmetastatic prostate carcinoma managed with radical prostatectomy, external beam radiotherapy, or expectant management: a retrospective analysis. Cancer 2001;91:2302. [PMID: 11413519]. (Disease-specific mortality estimates were as follows: expectant management, 75%; radiotherapy, 67%; and radical prostatectomy cohort, 86%. Direct comparisons are difficult due to patient selection.)

Fowler JE Jr et al: Race and cause specific survival with prostate cancer: influence of clinical stage, Gleason score, age and treatment [see comments]. J Urol 2000; 163:137. [PMID: 10604331] (Localized prostate cancer is more lethal in black than in white men.)

JAMA patient page: Prostate cancer. JAMA 1998;280:1030. [PMID: 9749489]

Klutke JJ et al: Long-term results after antegrade collagen injection for stress urinary incontinence following radical retropubic prostatectomy. Urology 1999;53:974. [PMID: 10223492] (Collagen injection cured or improved 45% of patients with stress urinary incontinence after radical prostatectomy.)

Koppie TM et al: Patterns of treatment of patients with prostate cancer initially managed with surveillance: results from The CaPSURE database. Cancer of the Prostate Strategic Urological Research Endeavor. J Urol 2000;164:81. [PMID: 10840429] (Patients who elect watchful waiting after diagnosis of prostate cancer typically have lower serum PSAs and more favorable disease characteristics.)

Labrie F: Screening and early hormonal treatment of prostate cancer are accumulating strong evidence and support [see comments]. Prostate 2000;43:215. [PMID: 10797496] (Treatment for localized prostate cancer results in a marked decrease in the number of prostate cancer deaths.)

Oh WK et al: Management of hormone refractory prostate cancer: Current standards and future prospects. J Urol 1998; 160:1220. [PMID: 9751323]

Rietbergen JB et al: The changing pattern of prostate cancer at the time of diagnosis: characteristics of screen detected prostate cancer in a population based screening study. J Urol 1999; 161:1192. [PMID: 10081868]

Rodriguez RR et al: High dose rate brachytherapy in the treatment of prostate cancer. Hematol Oncol Clin North Am 1999;13:503. [PMID: 10432425]

Walsh PC: Treatment with finasteride preserves usefulness of prostate-specific antigen in the detection of prostate cancer: results of a randomized, double-blind, placebo-controlled clinical trial. J Urol 1999;161:350. [PMID: 10037436

BLADDER CANCER

ESSENTIALS OF DIAGNOSIS

- Irritative voiding symptoms.
- Gross or microscopic hematuria.
- Positive urinary cytology in most patients.
- Filling defect within bladder noted on imaging.

General Considerations

Bladder cancer is the second most common urologic cancer, occurs more commonly in men than women (2.7:1), and the mean age at diagnosis is 65 years. Cigarette smoking and exposure to industrial dyes or solvents are risk factors for the disease and account for approximately 60% and 15% of new cases, respectively.

Clinical Findings

A. SYMPTOMS AND SIGNS

Hematuria—gross or microscopic, chronic or intermittent—is the presenting symptom in 85–90% of patients with bladder cancer. Irritative voiding symptoms (urinary frequency and urgency) will occur in a small percentage of patients as a result of the location or size of the cancer. Most patients with bladder cancer will fail to have signs of the disease because of its superficial nature. Masses detected on bimanual examination may be present in patients with large-volume or deeply infiltrating cancers. Hepatomegaly or supraclavicular lymphadenopathy may be present in patients with metastatic disease, and lymphedema of the lower extremities may be present as a result of locally advanced cancers or metastases to pelvic lymph nodes.

B. LABORATORY FINDINGS

Urinalysis will reveal hematuria in the majority of cases. On occasion, it may be accompanied by pyuria. Azotemia may be present in a small number of cases associated with ureteral obstruction. Anemia may occasionally be due to chronic blood loss or to bone marrow metastases. Exfoliated cells from normal and abnormal urothelium can be readily detected in voided urine specimens. Cytology may be useful in detecting the disease at the time of initial presentation or to detect recurrence. Cytology is very sensitive in detecting cancers of higher grade and stage (80–90%) but less so in detecting superficial or well-differentiated lesions (50%). Sensitivity of detection using exfoliated cells may be enhanced by flow cytometry.

C. IMAGING

Bladder cancers may be detected using intravenous urography, ultrasound, CT, or MRI where filling defects within the bladder are noted. However, the presence of cancer is confirmed by cystoscopy and biopsy, so imaging is useful primarily for evaluating the upper urinary tract and in staging the more advanced lesions.

D. CYSTOURETHROSCOPY AND BIOPSY

The diagnosis and staging of bladder cancers is made by cystoscopy and transurethral resection. If cystoscopy—performed usually under local anesthesia—confirms the presence of bladder cancer, the patient is scheduled for transurethral resection under general or regional anesthesia. A careful bimanual examination is performed initially and at the end of the procedure, noting the size, position, and degree of fixation of a mass, if present. Any suspicious lesions are resected using electrocautery. Resection is carried down to the muscular elements of the bladder wall so as to allow complete staging. Random bladder and, on occasion, prostatic urethral biopsies are performed to detect occult disease elsewhere in the bladder and, therefore, identify patients at high risk of recurrence and progression.

Pathology & Selection of Treatment

Ninety-eight percent of primary bladder cancers are epithelial malignancies, with the majority being transitional cell carcinomas (90%). These latter cancers most often appear as papillary growths, but higher-grade lesions are often sessile and ulcerated. Grading is based on histologic appearance: size, pleomorphism, mitotic rate, and hyperchromatism. The frequency of recurrence and progression is strongly correlated with grade. Whereas progression may be noted in few grade I cancers (19–37%), it is common with poorly differentiated lesions (33–67%). Carcinoma in situ is recognizable as a flat, nonpapillary, anaplastic epithelium and may occur focally or diffusely, but it is most often found in association with papillary bladder cancers. Its presence identifies a patient at increased risk of recurrence and progression.

Adenocarcinomas and squamous cell cancers account for approximately 2% and 7% (respectively) of all bladder cancers detected in the USA. The latter is often associated with schistosomiasis, vesical calculi, or chronic catheter use.

Bladder cancer staging is based on the extent of bladder wall penetration and the presence of either regional or distant metastases. The TNM classification of the American Joint Cancer Committee for bladder cancer is shown in Table 23–10.

The natural history of bladder cancer is based on two separate but related processes: tumor recurrence and progression to higher stage disease. Both are related to tumor grade and stage. At initial presentation, approximately 50–80% of bladder cancers will be superficial: Ta, Tis, T1. Lymph node metastases and progression are uncommon in such patients when they are properly treated, and survival is excellent at 81%. Patients with superficial cancers (Ta, T1) are treated

Table 23–10. TNM staging system for bladder cancer.

T: Primary tumor

Tx	Cannot be assessed
T0	No evidence of primary tumor
Tis	Carcinoma in situ (CIS)
Ta	Noninvasive papillary carcinoma
T1	Invasion into lamina propria
T2a	Invasion into superficial layer of muscularis propria
T2b	Invasion into deep layer of muscularis propria
T3	Invasion through serosa into perivesical fat
T4a	Invasion into adjacent organs
T4b	Invasion into pelvic sidewall

N: Regional lymph nodes

Nx	Cannot be assessed
N0	No regional lymph node metastasis
N1	Metastasis in a single lymph node 2 cm or less
N2	Metastasis in a single lymph node > 2 cm and < 5 cm or multiple nodes none > 5 cm
N3	Metastasis in lymph node > 5 cm

M: Distant metastasis

Mx	Cannot be assessed
M0	No distant metastasis
M1	Distant metastasis present

with complete transurethral resection and the selective use of intravesical chemotherapy. The latter is used to prevent or delay recurrence. Patients who present with large, high-grade, recurrent Ta lesions, T1 cancers, and those with carcinoma in situ are good candidates for intravesical chemotherapy. Patients with more invasive (T2, T3) but still localized cancers are at risk of both nodal metastases and progression, and they require more aggressive surgery, irradiation, or the combination of chemotherapy and selective surgery or irradiation due to the much higher risk of progression compared to patients with lower-stage lesions. Patients with evidence of lymph node or distant metastases should undergo systemic chemotherapy initially.

Treatment

A. INTRAVESICAL CHEMOTHERAPY

Immuno- or chemotherapeutic agents can be delivered directly into the bladder by a urethral catheter. They can be used to eradicate existing disease or to reduce the likelihood of recurrence in those who have undergone complete transurethral resection. Such therapy is more effective in the latter situation. Most agents are administered weekly for 6–12 weeks. The use of maintenance therapy after the initial induction regimen may be beneficial. Efficacy may be increased by prolonging contact time to 2 hours. Common agents include thiotepa, mitomycin, doxorubicin, and BCG, the latter being the most effective agent when compared with the others. Side effects of intravesical chemotherapy include irritative voiding symptoms and hemorrhagic cystitis. Systemic effects are rare. Patients who develop symptoms from BCG may require antituberculous therapy.

B. SURGICAL TREATMENT

Although transurethral resection is the initial form of treatment for all bladder cancers as it is diagnostic, allows for proper staging, and will control superficial cancers, muscle infiltrating cancers will require more aggressive treatment. Partial cystectomy may be indicated in patients with solitary lesions and those with cancers in a bladder diverticulum. Radical cystectomy entails removal of the bladder, prostate, seminal vesicles, and surrounding fat and peritoneal attachments in men and in women also the uterus, cervix, urethra, anterior vaginal vault, and usually the ovaries. Bilateral pelvic lymph node dissection is performed simultaneously.

Urinary diversion can be performed using a conduit of small or large bowel. However, continent forms of diversion have been developed that avoid the necessity of an external appliance.

C. RADIOTHERAPY

External beam radiotherapy delivered in fractions over a 6- to 8-week period is generally well tolerated, but approximately 10–15% of patients will develop bladder, bowel, or rectal complications. Unfortunately, local recurrence is common after radiotherapy (30–70%). Increasingly, radiotherapy is being combined with systemic chemotherapy in an effort to improve local and distant relapse rates.

D. CHEMOTHERAPY

Fifteen percent of patients with newly diagnosed bladder cancer will present with metastatic disease, and 40% of those thought to have localized disease at the time of cystectomy or definitive radiotherapy will develop metastases usually within 2 years after the start of treatment. Cisplatin-based combination chemotherapy will result in partial or complete responses in 15–35% and 15–45% of patients, respectively.

Combination chemotherapy has been integrated into trials of surgery and radiotherapy. It has been used to decrease recurrence rates with either modality and in an attempt to preserve the bladder in those treated with radiation. Chemotherapy should be considered before surgery in those with bulky lesions or those suspected of having regional disease. Chemoradiation may be best suited for those with T2 or limited T3 disease without hydronephrosis. Alternatively, chemotherapy has been employed postoperatively in patients who have undergone cystectomy and have been found to be at high risk of recurrence. In current practice, adjuvant chemotherapy when indicated—ie, when the primary tumor invades perivesical fat or adjacent organs or when lymph nodes are found to have metastatic disease—is being offered mainly to patients being treated with radical cystectomy.

Carroll PR: Urothelial carcinoma: Cancers of the bladder, ureter and renal pelvis. In: *Smith's General Urology*, 15th ed. Tanagho EA, McAninch JW (editors). McGraw-Hill, 2000.

Kim HL et al: The current status of bladder preservation in the treatment of muscle invasive bladder cancer. J Urol 2000;164(3 Part 1):627. [PMID: 10953112] (Radical surgery is still the gold standard for muscle invasive bladder cancer. Bladder sparing protocols are being performed in select medical centers with dedicated multispecialty teams.)

Savage SJ et al: Laparoscopic radical nephroureterectomy. J Endourol 2000;14:859. [PMID: 11206620]. (Laparoscopic means are now routinely utilized to remove kidneys or ureters harboring transitional cell carcinomas.)

Smith JA Jr et al: Bladder cancer clinical guidelines panel summary report on the management of nonmuscle invasive bladder cancer (stages Ta, T1 and Tis). The American Urological Association. J Urol 1999;162:1697. [PMID: 10524909]

CANCERS OF THE URETER & RENAL PELVIS

Cancers of the renal pelvis and ureter are rare and occur more commonly in smokers, in those with Balkan nephropathy, in those exposed to Thorotrast (a contrast agent with radioactive thorium in use until the 1960s), or those with a long history of analgesic abuse. The majority are transitional cell carcinomas. Gross or microscopic hematuria occurs in most patients, and flank pain secondary to bleeding and obstruction occurs less commonly. Like primary bladder cancers, urinary cytology is often positive. The most common signs identified at the time of intravenous pyelography include an intraluminal filling defect, unilateral nonvisualization of the collecting system, and hydronephrosis. Ureteral and renal pelvic tumors must be differentiated from calculi, blood clots, papillary necrosis, or inflammatory or infectious lesions. On occasion, such lesions are accessible to direct biopsy, fulguration, or resection using a ureteroscope. Treatment is based on the site, size, depth of penetration, and number of tumors present. Most such cancers are excised with nephroureterectomy (renal pelvic and upper ureteral lesions) or segmental excision of the ureter (distal ureteral lesions). Endoscopic resection may be indicated in patients with limited renal function and in the management of focal, low-grade, upper tract cancers.

[Transitional Cell Cancer of Renal Pelvis and Ureter]
  http://www.cancer.gov/CancerInformation/ CancerType/transitionalcell

PRIMARY TUMORS OF THE KIDNEY

1. Renal Cell Carcinoma

ESSENTIALS OF DIAGNOSIS

- Gross or microscopic hematuria.
- Flank pain or mass in some patients.
- Systemic symptoms such as fever, weight loss may be prominent.
- Solid renal mass on imaging.

General Considerations

Renal cell carcinoma accounts for 2.3% of all adult cancers. In the United States in 2001, approximately 30,800 cases of renal cell carcinoma were diagnosed and 12,100 deaths resulted. Renal cell carcinoma has a peak incidence in the sixth decade of life and a male-to-female ratio of 2:1.

The cause is unknown. Cigarette smoking is the only significant environmental risk factor that has been identified. Familial settings for renal cell carcinoma have been identified (von Hippel-Lindau syndrome) as well as an association with dialysis-related acquired cystic disease, but sporadic tumors are far more common.

Renal cell carcinoma originates from the proximal tubule cells. Various cell types (clear, granular, spindle) and histologic patterns (acinar, papillary, solid) are observed. However, cell type and histologic pattern do not affect treatment. The TNM classification of the American Joint Cancer Committee for kidney cancer is shown in Table 23–11.

Clinical Findings

A. SYMPTOMS AND SIGNS

Historically, 60% of patients presented with gross or microscopic hematuria. Flank pain or an abdominal mass was detected in approximately 30% of cases. The triad of flank pain, hematuria, and mass was found in only 10–15% of patients and is often a sign of advanced disease. Symptoms of metastatic disease (cough, bone pain) occur in 20–30% of patients at presentation. Because of the more widespread use of ultrasound and CT scanning for diverse indications, renal tumors are being detected incidentally in patients with no urologic symptoms.

B. LABORATORY FINDINGS

Hematuria is present in 60% of patients. Paraneoplastic syndromes are not uncommon in renal cell carcinoma. Erythrocytosis from increased erythropoietin

Table 23–11. TNM staging system for kidney cancer.

T: Primary tumor	
Tx	Cannot be assessed
T0	No evidence of primary tumor
T1	Tumor ≤ 7 cm limited to kidney
T2	Tumor > 7 cm limited to kidney
T3a	Tumor invades adrenal gland or perinephric tissue
T3b	Tumor extends into renal vein or vena cava
T3c	Tumor extends into renal vein or vena cava above diaphragm
T4	Tumor invades outside of Gerota's fascia
N: Regional lymph nodes	
Nx	Cannot be assessed
N0	No regional lymph node metastasis
N1	Metastasis in a single lymph node
N2	Metastasis in multiple nodes
N3	Metastasis in lymph node > 5 cm
M: Distant metastasis	
Mx	Cannot be assessed
M0	No distant metastasis
M1	Distant metastasis present

production occurs in 5%, though anemia is far more common; hypercalcemia may be present in up to 10% of patients. Stauffer's syndrome is a reversible syndrome of hepatic dysfunction in the absence of metastatic disease.

C. IMAGING

Renal masses are often first detected by intravenous urography. Further evaluation requires ultrasound to determine whether it is solid or cystic. CT scanning is the most valuable imaging test for renal cell carcinoma. It confirms the character of the mass and further stages the lesion with respect to regional lymph nodes, renal vein, or hepatic involvement. It also gives valuable information on the contralateral kidney (function, bilaterality of neoplasm). Chest radiographs exclude pulmonary metastases, and bone scans should be performed for large tumors and in patients with bone pain or elevated alkaline phosphatase levels. MRI and duplex Doppler ultrasonography are excellent methods of assessing for the presence and extent of tumor thrombus within the renal vein or vena cava in selected patients.

Differential Diagnosis

Solid lesions of the kidney are renal cell carcinoma until proved otherwise. Other solid masses include angiomyolipomas (fat density usually visible by CT); transitional cell cancers of the renal pelvis (more centrally located, involvement of the collecting system,

positive urinary cytology reports); adrenal tumors (supero-anterior to the kidney) and oncocytomas (indistinguishable from renal cell carcinoma preoperatively); and renal abscesses.

Treatment & Prognosis

Radical nephrectomy is the primary treatment for localized renal cell carcinoma. Patients with a single kidney, bilateral lesions, or significant medical renal disease should be considered for partial nephrectomy. Patients with a normal contralateral kidney and good renal function but a small cancer may be good candidates for partial nephrectomy as well. The use of radiofrequency or cryosurgical ablation is being studied. Tumors confined to the renal capsule (T1–T2) demonstrate 5-year disease-free survivals of 90–100%. Tumors extending beyond the renal capsule (T3 or T4) and node-positive tumors have 50–60% and 0–15% 5-year disease-free survivals, respectively.

No effective chemotherapy is available for metastatic renal cell carcinoma. Vinblastine is the single most effective agent, with short-term partial response rates of 15%. Biologic response modifiers have received much attention, including alpha interferon and interleukin-2. Partial response rates of 15–20% and 15–35%, respectively, have been reported. Responders tend to have lower tumor burdens, metastatic disease confined to the lung, and a high performance status. Because of these low response rates, new investigations are ongoing with tumor vaccines and gene therapy. Nephrectomy is rarely considered in those with metastatic disease; such patients usually should be considered for palliative therapy. However, two randomized trials have shown a benefit to surgery followed by the use of systemic therapy—specifically, biologic response modifiers—compared with the use of systemic therapy alone.

One subgroup of metastatic patients has demonstrated long-term survival, namely, those with solitary resectable metastases. In this setting, radical nephrectomy with resection of the metastasis has resulted in 5-year disease-free survival rates of 15–30%.

Chan DY et al: Laparoscopic radical nephrectomy: cancer control for renal cell carcinoma. J Urol 2001;166:2095. [PMID: 11696714]. (Laparoscopic nephrectomy is an effective alternative option for the surgical management of renal cell carcinoma.)

Figlin RA: Renal cell carcinoma: management of advanced disease. J Urol 1999;161:381. [PMID: 9915408] (IL-2 can produce durable complete remissions.)

Flanigan RC et al: Nephrectomy followed by interferon alfa-2b compared with interferon alfa-2b alone for metastatic renal-cell cancer. N Engl J Med 2001;345:1655. [PMID: 11759643]. (This trial showed that patients with metastatic renal cell carcinoma who were managed with surgery followed by interferon survived longer than those receiving interferon alone.)

Javidan J et al: Prognostic significance of the 1997 TNM classification of renal cell carcinoma. J Urol 1999;162:1277. [PMID: 10492179]

Mickisch GH et al: Radical nephrectomy plus interferon-alfa-based immunotherapy compared with interferon alfa alone in metastatic renal-cell carcinoma: a randomised trial. Lancet 2001;358:966. [PMID: 11583750]. (Radical nephrectomy before interferon-based immunotherapy might improve survival in patients with metastatic renal cell carcinoma with a good performance status.)

2. Other Primary Tumors of the Kidney

Oncocytomas account for 3–5% of renal tumors and are indistinguishable from renal cell carcinoma by all imaging modalities. The biologic potential of these lesions is not well defined. These tumors are seen in other organs, including the adrenals, the salivary glands, and the thyroid and parathyroid glands.

Angiomyolipomas are rare benign tumors composed of fat, smooth muscle, and blood vessels. They are most commonly seen in patients with tuberous sclerosis (often multiple and bilateral) or in young to middle-aged women. CT scanning may identify the fat component, which is diagnostic for angiomyolipoma. Asymptomatic lesions less than 5 cm in diameter usually do not require intervention.

Dechet CB et al: Renal oncocytoma: multifocality, bilateralism, metachronous tumor development and coexistent renal cell carcinoma. J Urol 1999;162:40. [PMID: 10379735] (Oncocytomas are benign. Renal cell carcinoma may coexist in 10% of these tumors.)

SECONDARY TUMORS OF THE KIDNEY

The kidney is not an infrequent site for metastatic disease. Of the solid tumors, the lung is the most common (20%), followed by breast (10%), stomach (10%), and the contralateral kidney (10%). Lymphoma, both Hodgkin's and non-Hodgkin's, may also involve the kidney, though it tends to be a diffusely infiltrative process resulting in renal enlargement rather than a discrete mass.

PRIMARY TUMORS OF THE TESTIS

ESSENTIALS OF DIAGNOSIS

- *Commonest neoplasm in men aged 20–35.*
- *Typical presentation as a patient-identified painless nodule.*
- *Orchiectomy necessary for diagnosis.*

General Considerations

Malignant tumors of the testis are rare, with approximately two to three new cases per 100,000 males being reported in the United States each year. Ninety to 95 percent of all primary testicular tumors are germ cell tumors (seminoma and nonseminoma), while the remainder are nongerminal neoplasms (Leydig cell, Sertoli cell, gonadoblastoma). The lifetime probability of developing testicular cancer is 0.2% for an American white male. For the purposes of this review, we will only consider germ cell tumors. Survival in testicular cancer has improved dramatically in recent years as a result of the development and application of effective combination chemotherapy.

Testicular cancer is slightly more common on the right than on the left, which parallels the increased incidence of cryptorchism on the right side. One to 2 percent of primary testicular tumors are bilateral, and up to 50% of these men have a history of unilateral or bilateral cryptorchism. Primary bilateral testicular tumors may occur synchronously or asynchronously but tend to be of the same histology. Seminoma is the most common histologic finding in bilateral *primary* testicular tumors, while malignant lymphoma is the most common bilateral testicular tumor.

While the cause of testicular cancer is unknown, both congenital and acquired factors have been associated with tumor development. Approximately 5% of testicular tumors develop in a patient with a history of cryptorchism, with seminoma being the most common. However, 5–10% of these tumors occur in the contralateral, normally descended testis. The relative risk of development of malignancy is highest for the intra-abdominal testis (1:20) and lower for the inguinal testis (1:80). Placement of the cryptorchid testis into the scrotum (orchiopexy) does not alter the malignant potential of the cryptorchid testis; however, it does facilitate examination and tumor detection.

In animal models, exogenous estrogen administration during pregnancy has been associated with an increased relative risk for testicular tumors ranging from 2.8 to 5.3. Other acquired factors such as trauma and infection-related testicular atrophy have been associated with testicular tumors; however, a causal relationship has not been established.

Histopathology & Clinical Staging

From a treatment standpoint, testicular carcinoma can be divided into two major categories: (1) nonseminomas, which include embryonal cell carcinomas (20%), teratomas (5%), choriocarcinomas (< 1%), and mixed cell types (40%); and (2) seminomas (35%). In a commonly used staging system for nonseminoma germ cell tumors, a stage A lesion is confined to the testis; stage B demonstrates regional lymph node involvement in the retroperitoneum; and stage C indicates distant metastasis. For seminoma, the M.D. Anderson system is commonly used. In this system, a stage I lesion is confined to the testis, a stage II lesion has spread to the retroperitoneal lymph nodes, and a stage III lesion has supradiaphragmatic nodal or visceral involvement. The TNM classification of the American Joint Cancer Committee for testis cancer is shown in Table 23–12.

Table 23–12. TNM staging system for testicular cancer.

T: Primary tumor	
Tx	Cannot be assessed
T0	No evidence of primary tumor
Tis	Intratubular cancer (CIS)
T1	Limited to testis without vascular invasion
T2	Invades beyond tunica albuginea or into epididymis, or limited to testis with vascular invasion
T3	Invades spermatic cord
T4	Invades scrotum
N: Regional lymph nodes	
Nx	Cannot be assessed
N0	No regional lymph node metastasis
N1	Metastasis in a single lymph node 2 cm or less
N2	Metastasis in a single lymph node > 2 cm and < 5 cm or multiple nodes none > 5 cm
N3	Metastasis in lymph node > 5 cm
M: Distant metastasis	
Mx	Cannot be assessed
M0	No distant metastasis
M1	Distant metastasis present

Clinical Findings

A. SYMPTOMS AND SIGNS

The most common symptom of testicular cancer is painless enlargement of the testis. Sensations of heaviness are not unusual. Patients are usually the first to recognize an abnormality, yet the typical delay in seeking medical attention ranges from 3 to 6 months. Acute testicular pain resulting from intratesticular hemorrhage occurs in approximately 10% of cases. Ten percent of patients are asymptomatic at presentation, and 10% manifest symptoms relating to metastatic disease such as back pain (retroperitoneal metastases), cough (pulmonary metastases), or lower extremity edema (vena cava obstruction).

A testicular mass or diffuse enlargement of the testis is found in the majority of cases on physical examination. Secondary hydroceles may be present in 5–10% of cases. In advanced disease, supraclavicular adenopathy may be detected, and abdominal examination may palpate a retroperitoneal mass. Gynecomastia is seen in 5% of germ cell tumors.

B. LABORATORY FINDINGS

Several biochemical markers are important in the diagnosis and treatment of testicular carcinoma, including human chorionic gonadotropin (hCG), alphafetoprotein, and LDH. Alpha-fetoprotein is never elevated in seminomas, and while hCG is occasionally elevated in seminomas, levels tend to be lower than those seen in nonseminomas. LDH may be elevated in either type of tumor. Liver function tests may be elevated in the presence of hepatic metastases, and anemia may be present in advanced disease. In patients with advanced disease who will receive chemotherapy, renal function is assessed with a 24-hour urine creatinine clearance.

C. IMAGING

Scrotal ultrasound can readily determine whether the mass is intra- or extratesticular in origin. Once the diagnosis of testicular cancer has been established by inguinal orchiectomy, clinical staging of the disease is accomplished by chest, abdominal, and pelvic CT scanning.

Differential Diagnosis

An incorrect diagnosis is made at the initial examination in up to 25% of patients with testicular tumors. The differential diagnosis of scrotal masses has been discussed previously in this chapter. Scrotal ultrasonography should be performed if any uncertainty exists with respect to the diagnosis. Although most intratesticular masses are malignant, one benign lesion, an epidermoid cyst, may rarely been seen. Epidermoid cysts are usually very small benign nodules located just underneath the tunica albuginea; on occasion, however, they can be large.

Treatment

Inguinal exploration with early vascular control of the spermatic cord structures is the initial intervention to exclude neoplasm. If cancer cannot be excluded by examination of the testis, radical orchiectomy is warranted. Scrotal approaches and open testicular biopsies should be avoided. Further therapy is dependent upon the histology of the tumor as well as the clinical stage.

The 5-year disease-free survival rates for stage I and IIa (retroperitoneal disease < 10 cm in diameter) seminomas treated by radical orchiectomy and retroperitoneal irradiation are 98% and 92–94%, respectively. High-stage seminomas of stage IIb (> 10 cm retroperitoneal involvement) and stage III receive primary chemotherapy (etoposide and cisplatin or cisplatin, etoposide, and bleomycin). Ninety-five percent of patients with stage III disease will attain a complete response following orchiectomy and chemotherapy. Surgical resection of residual retroperitoneal masses is warranted only if the mass is larger than 3 cm in diameter, under which circumstances 40% will harbor residual carcinoma.

Up to 75% of stage A nonseminomas are cured by orchiectomy alone. Currently, such patients may be treated by modified retroperitoneal lymph node dissections designed to preserve the sympathetic innervation for ejaculation. Selected patients who meet specific criteria may be offered surveillance. These criteria are as follows: (1) tumor is confined within the tunica albuginea; (2) tumor does not demonstrate vascular invasion; (3) tumor markers normalize after orchiectomy; (4) radiographic imaging shows no evidence of disease (chest x-ray and CT); and (5) the patient is reliable. Patients most likely to experience relapse on a surveillance regimen include those with predominantly embryonal cancer and those with vascular or lymphatic invasion identified in the orchiectomy specimen. Surveillance should be considered an active process both by the physician and by the patient. Patients are followed monthly for the first 2 years and bimonthly in the third year. Tumor markers are obtained at each visit, and chest x-ray and CT scans are obtained every 3–4 months. Follow-up continues beyond the initial 3 years; however, the majority of relapses will occur within the first 8–10 months. With rare exceptions, patients who relapse can be cured by chemotherapy or surgery. The 5-year disease-free survival rate for patients with stage A disease ranges from 96% to 100%. For low-volume stage B disease, 90% 5-year disease-free survival is attainable.

Patients with bulky retroperitoneal disease (> 3 cm nodes) or metastatic nonseminomas are treated with primary cisplatin-based combination chemotherapy following orchiectomy (etoposide and cisplatin or cisplatin, etoposide, and bleomycin). If tumor markers normalize and a residual mass greater than 3 cm is apparent on imaging studies, resection of that mass is mandatory because 20% of the time it will harbor residual cancer and 40% of the time it will be teratoma. Even if patients have a complete response to chemotherapy, retroperitoneal lymphadenectomy is advocated by some as 10% of patients may harbor residual carcinoma and 10% may have teratoma in the retroperitoneum. If tumor markers fail to normalize following primary chemotherapy, salvage chemotherapy is required (cisplatin, etoposide, bleomycin, ifosfamide).

Prognosis

Patients with bulky retroperitoneal or disseminated disease treated with primary chemotherapy followed by surgery have a 5-year disease-free survival rate of 55–80%.

Heidenreich A et al: Organ-sparing surgery for malignant germ cell tumor of the testis. J Urol 2001;166:2161. [PMID: 11696727]. (Follow-up greater than 7 years revealed that organ-sparing surgery for bilateral testicular germ cell tumors had an excellent outcome.)

Sweeney CJ et al: Results and outcome of retroperitoneal lymph node dissection for clinical stage I embryonal carcinoma–predominant testis cancer. J Clin Oncol 2000;18:358. [PMID: 10637250] (Patients with clinical stage I embryonal carcinoma of the testis are at high risk for metastatic disease.)

SECONDARY TUMORS OF THE TESTIS

Secondary tumors of the testis are rare. Lymphoma is the most common testis tumor in a patient over the age of 50 and is the most common secondary neoplasm of the testis, accounting for 5% of all testicular tumors. It may be seen in three clinical settings: (1) as a late manifestation of widespread lymphoma; (2) as the initial presentation of clinically occult disease; and (3) as primary extranodal disease. Radical orchiectomy is indicated to make the diagnosis. Prognosis is related to the stage of disease.

Metastasis to the testis is rare. The most common primary site is the prostate, followed by the lung, gastrointestinal tract, melanoma, and kidney.

Nervous System

24

Michael J. Aminoff DSc, MD, FRCP
See www.current-med.com/ch24.html

HEADACHE

Headache is such a common complaint and can occur for so many different reasons that its proper evaluation may be difficult. Chronic headaches are commonly due to migraine, tension, or depression, but they may be related to intracranial lesions, head injury, cervical spondylosis, dental or ocular disease, temporomandibular joint dysfunction, sinusitis, hypertension, and a wide variety of general medical disorders. Although underlying structural lesions are not present in most patients presenting with headache, it is nevertheless important to bear this possibility in mind. About one-third of patients with brain tumors, for example, present with a primary complaint of headache.

The intensity, quality, and site of pain—and especially the duration of the headache and the presence of associated neurologic symptoms—may provide clues to the underlying cause. Migraine or tension headaches are often described as pulsating or throbbing; a sense of tightness or pressure is also common with tension headache. Sharp lancinating pain suggests a neuritic cause; ocular or periorbital icepick-like pains occur with migraine or cluster headache; and a dull or steady headache is typical of an intracranial mass lesion. Ocular or periocular pain suggests an ophthalmologic disorder; band-like pain is common with tension headaches; and lateralized headache is common with migraine or cluster headache. In patients with sinusitis, there may be tenderness of overlying skin and bone. With intracranial mass lesions, headache may be focal or generalized; in patients with trigeminal or glossopharyngeal neuralgia, the pain is localized to one of the divisions of the trigeminal nerve or to the pharynx and external auditory meatus, respectively.

Inquiry should be made of precipitating factors. Recent sinusitis or hay fever, dental surgery, head injury, or symptoms suggestive of a systemic viral infection may suggest the underlying cause. Migraine may be exacerbated by emotional stress, fatigue, foods containing nitrite or tyramine, or the menstrual period. Alcohol may precipitate cluster headache. Temporomandibular joint dysfunction causes headache or facial pain that comes on with chewing; trigeminal or glossopharyngeal neuralgia may also be precipitated by chewing, and masticatory claudication sometimes occurs with giant cell arteritis. Cough-induced headache occurs with structural lesions of the posterior fossa, but in many instances no specific cause can be found.

The timing of symptoms is important. Headaches are typically worse on awakening in patients with sinusitis or an intracranial mass. Cluster headaches tend to occur at the same time each day or night. Tension headaches are worse with stress or at the end of the day.

The onset of severe headache in a previously well patient is more likely than chronic headache to relate to an intracranial disorder such as subarachnoid hemorrhage or meningitis. The need for further investigation is determined by the initial clinical impression.

A progressive headache disorder, new onset of headache in middle or later life, headaches that disturb sleep or are related to exertion, and headaches that are associated with neurologic symptoms or a focal neurologic deficit usually require cranial MRI or CT scan to exclude an intracranial mass lesion. Signs of meningeal irritation and impairment of consciousness also indicate the need for further investigation (cranial CT scan or MRI and examination of the cerebrospinal fluid) to exclude subarachnoid hemorrhage or meningeal infection. The diagnosis and treatment of primary neurologic disorders associated with headache are considered separately under these disorders.

Tension Headache

Patients frequently complain of poor concentration and other vague nonspecific symptoms, in addition to constant daily headaches that are often vise-like or tight in quality and may be exacerbated by emotional stress, fatigue, noise, or glare. The headaches are usually generalized, may be most intense about the neck or back of the head, and are not associated with focal neurologic symptoms.

When treatment with simple analgesics is not effective, a trial of antimigrainous agents (see Migraine, below) is worthwhile. Techniques to induce relaxation are also useful and include massage, hot baths, and biofeedback. Exploration of underlying causes of chronic anxiety is often rewarding. Anecdotal reports of beneficial responses to local injection of botulinum toxin type A have been published.

Depression Headache

Depression headaches are frequently worse on arising in the morning and may be accompanied by other symptoms of depression. Headaches are occasionally the focus of a somatic delusional system. Antidepressant drugs are often helpful, as may be psychiatric consultation.

Migraine

Classic migrainous headache is a lateralized throbbing headache that occurs episodically following its onset in adolescence or early adult life. In many cases, however, the headaches do not conform to this pattern, although their associated features and response to antimigrainous preparations nevertheless suggest that they have a similar basis. In this broader sense, migrainous headaches may be lateralized or generalized, may be dull or throbbing, and are sometimes associated with anorexia, nausea, vomiting, photophobia, phonophobia, and blurring of vision. They usually build up gradually and may last for several hours or longer. They have been related to dilation and excessive pulsation of branches of the external carotid artery. Focal disturbances of neurologic function may precede or accompany the headaches and have been attributed to constriction of branches of the internal carotid artery. Visual disturbances occur quite commonly and may consist of field defects; of luminous visual hallucinations such as stars, sparks, unformed light flashes (photopsia), geometric patterns, or zigzags of light; or of some combination of field defects and luminous hallucinations (scintillating scotomas). Other focal disturbances such as aphasia or numbness, tingling, clumsiness, or weakness in a circumscribed distribution may also occur.

Patients often give a family history of migraine. Attacks may be triggered by emotional or physical stress, lack or excess of sleep, missed meals, specific foods (eg, chocolate), alcoholic beverages, menstruation, or use of oral contraceptives.

An uncommon variant is **basilar artery migraine,** in which blindness or visual disturbances throughout both visual fields are initially accompanied or followed by dysarthria, disequilibrium, tinnitus, and perioral and distal paresthesias and are sometimes followed by transient loss or impairment of consciousness or by a confusional state. This, in turn, is followed by a throbbing (usually occipital) headache, often with nausea and vomiting.

In **ophthalmoplegic migraine,** lateralized pain—often about the eye—is accompanied by nausea, vom-

iting, and diplopia due to transient external ophthalmoplegia. The ophthalmoplegia is due to third nerve palsy, sometimes with accompanying sixth nerve involvement, and may outlast the orbital pain by several days or even weeks. The ophthalmic division of the fifth nerve has also been affected in some patients. Ophthalmoplegic migraine is rare; more common causes of a painful ophthalmoplegia are internal carotid artery aneurysms and diabetes.

In rare instances, the neurologic or somatic disturbance accompanying typical migrainous headaches becomes the sole manifestation of an attack ("migraine equivalent"). Very rarely, the patient may be left with a permanent neurologic deficit following a migrainous attack.

The pathophysiology of migraine probably relates to the neurotransmitter serotonin. Headache may result from release of neuropeptides acting as neurotransmitters at trigeminal nerve branches, leading to an inflammatory process; another possible mechanism involves activation of the dorsal raphe nucleus.

Management of migraine consists of avoidance of any precipitating factors, together with prophylactic or symptomatic pharmacologic treatment if necessary.

During acute attacks, many patients find it helpful to rest in a quiet, darkened room until symptoms subside. A simple analgesic (eg, aspirin) taken right away often provides relief, but treatment with extracranial vasoconstrictors or other drugs is sometimes necessary. Cafergot, a combination of ergotamine tartrate (1 mg) and caffeine (100 mg), is often particularly helpful; one or two tablets are taken at the onset of headache or warning symptoms, followed by one tablet every 30 minutes, if necessary, up to six tablets per attack and ten tablets per week. Because of impaired absorption or vomiting during acute attacks, oral medication sometimes fails to help. Cafergot given rectally as suppositories (one-half to one suppository containing 2 mg of ergotamine); ergotamine tartrate given by inhalation (0.36 mg per puff; up to six puffs per attack) or sublingually (2 mg tablets; not more than three tablets per 24 hours); or dihydroergotamine mesylate (0.5–1 mg intravenously or 1–2 mg subcutaneously or intramuscularly) may be useful in such cases. Alternatively, prochlorperazine administered rectally (25 mg suppository) or intravenously (10 mg) may be prescribed. Ergotamine-containing preparations may affect the gravid uterus and thus should be avoided during pregnancy. Sumatriptan is a rapidly effective agent for aborting attacks when given subcutaneously by an autoinjection device. It has a high affinity for serotonin$_1$ receptors. It should probably be avoided in pregnancy. Sumatriptan can also be taken in a nasal form, but absorption is limited and a bitter aftertaste may be disturbing; an oral preparation is available but is poorly absorbed. Zolmitriptan, another selective serotonin$_1$ receptor agonist, has high bioavailability after oral administration and is also effective for the acute treatment of migraine. The optimal initial dose is 2.5 mg, and relief usually occurs within 1 hour. Intravenous propofol in subanesthetic doses may help in intractable cases.

Prophylactic treatment may be necessary if migrainous headaches occur more frequently than two or three times a month. Some of the more common drugs used for this purpose are listed in Table 24–1. Their mode of action is unclear and may involve both an effect on extracerebral vasculature and a cerebral effect, eg, by stabilizing serotonergic neurotransmission. Several drugs may have to be tried in turn before the headaches are brought under control. Once a drug has been found to help, it should be continued for several months. If the patient remains headache-free, the dose can then be tapered and the drug eventually withdrawn.

Calcium channel antagonist drugs may decrease the frequency of attacks after an interval of several weeks, but the severity and duration of attacks are not influenced. They should not be used with beta-blockers.

Cluster Headache (Migrainous Neuralgia)

Cluster headache affects predominantly middle-aged men. Its cause is unclear but may relate to a vascular headache disorder or a disturbance of serotonergic mechanisms. There is often no family history of headache or migraine. Episodes of severe unilateral periorbital pain occur daily for several weeks and are often accompanied by one or more of the following: ipsilateral nasal congestion, rhinorrhea, lacrimation, redness of the eye, and Horner's syndrome. Episodes

usually occur at night, awaken the patient, and last for less than 2 hours. Spontaneous remission then occurs, and the patient remains well for weeks or months before another bout of closely spaced attacks occurs. During a bout, many patients report that alcohol triggers an attack; others report that stress, glare, or ingestion of specific foods occasionally precipitates attacks. In occasional patients, typical attacks of pain and associated symptoms recur at intervals without remission. This variant has been referred to as chronic cluster headache.

Examination reveals no abnormality apart from Horner's syndrome that either occurs transiently during an attack or, in long-standing cases, remains as a residual deficit between attacks.

Treatment of an individual attack with oral drugs is generally unsatisfactory, but subcutaneous sumatriptan (6 mg) or dihydroergotamine (1–2 mg) or use of ergotamine tartrate aerosol or inhalation of 100% oxygen (7 L/min for 15 minutes) may be effective. Butorphanol tartrate, a synthetic opioid agonist-antagonist, may also be helpful when administered by nasal spray. The dose is 1 mg (one spray in one nostril), repeated after 60–90 minutes if necessary. Ergotamine tartrate is an effective prophylactic and can be given as rectal suppositories (0.5–1 mg at night or twice daily), by mouth (2 mg daily), or by subcutaneous injection (0.25 mg three times daily for 5 days per week). Various prophylactic agents that have been found to be effective in individual patients are propranolol, amitriptyline, valproate, cyproheptadine, lithium carbonate (monitored by plasma lithium determination), prednisone (20–40 mg

Table 24–1. Prophylactic treatment of migraine.

Drug	Usual Adult Daily Dose	Common Side Effects
Aspirin	650–1950 mg	Dyspepsia, gastrointestinal bleeding.
Propranolol	80–240 mg	Fatigue, lassitude, depression, insomnia, nausea, vomiting, constipation.
Amitriptyline	10–150 mg	Sedation, dry mouth, constipation, weight gain, blurred vision, edema, hypotension, urinary retention.
Imipramine	10–150 mg	Similar to those of amitriptyline (above).
Sertraline	50–200 mg	Anxiety, insomnia, sweating, tremor, gastrointestinal disturbances.
Fluoxetine	20–60 mg	Similar to those of sertraline (above).
Ergonovine maleate	0.6–2 mg	Nausea, vomiting, abdominal pain, diarrhea.
Cyproheptadine	12–20 mg	Sedation, dry mouth, epigastric discomfort, gastrointestinal disturbances.
Clonidine	0.2–0.6 mg	Dry mouth, drowsiness, sedation, headache, constipation.
Methysergide	4–8 mg	Nausea, vomiting, diarrhea, abdominal pain, cramps, weight gain, insomnia, edema, peripheral vasoconstriction. Retroperitoneal and pleuropulmonary fibrosis and fibrous thickening of cardiac valves may occur.
Verapamil[1]	80–160 mg	Headache, hypotension, flushing, edema, constipation. May aggravate atrioventricular nodal heart block and congestive heart failure.

[1]Other calcium channel antagonists (eg, nimodipine, nifedipine, and diltiazem) may also be used.

daily or on alternate days for 2 weeks, followed by gradual withdrawal), verapamil (240–480 mg daily), and methysergide (4–6 mg daily).

Giant Cell (Temporal or Cranial) Arteritis

The superficial temporal, vertebral, ophthalmic, and posterior ciliary arteries are often the most severely affected pathologically. Most patients are elderly. The major symptom is headache, often associated with or preceded by myalgia, malaise, anorexia, weight loss, and other nonspecific complaints. Loss of vision is the most feared manifestation and occurs quite commonly. Clinical examination often reveals tenderness of the scalp and over the temporal arteries. Further details, including approaches to treatment, are given in Chapter 20.

Posttraumatic Headache

A variety of nonspecific symptoms may follow closed head injury, regardless of whether consciousness is lost. Headache is often a conspicuous feature. Some authorities believe that psychologic factors may be important because there is no correlation of severity of the injury with neurologic signs.

The headache itself usually appears within a day or so following injury, may worsen over the ensuing weeks, and then gradually subsides. It is usually a constant dull ache, with superimposed throbbing that may be localized, lateralized, or generalized. It is sometimes accompanied by nausea, vomiting, or scintillating scotomas.

Disequilibrium, sometimes with a rotatory component, may also occur and is often enhanced by postural change or head movement. Impaired memory, poor concentration, emotional instability, and increased irritability are other common complaints and occasionally are the sole manifestations of the syndrome. The duration of symptoms relates in part to the severity of the original injury, but even trivial injuries are sometimes followed by symptoms that persist for months.

Special investigations are usually not helpful. The electroencephalogram may show minor nonspecific changes, while the electronystagmogram sometimes suggests either peripheral or central vestibulopathy. CT scans or MRI of the head usually show no abnormal findings.

Treatment is difficult, but optimistic encouragement and graduated rehabilitation, depending upon the occupational circumstances, are advised. Headaches often respond to simple analgesics, but severe headaches may necessitate treatment with amitriptyline, propranolol, or ergot derivatives.

Cough Headache

Severe head pain may be produced by coughing (and by straining, sneezing, and laughing) but, fortunately, usually lasts for only a few minutes or less. The pathophysiologic basis of the complaint is not known, and often there is no underlying structural lesion. However, intracranial lesions, usually in the posterior fossa (eg, Arnold-Chiari malformation), are present in about 10% of cases, and brain tumors or other space-occupying lesions may certainly present in this way. Accordingly, CT scanning or MRI should be undertaken in all patients and repeated annually for several years, since a small structural lesion may not show up initially.

The disorder is usually self-limited, although it may persist for several years. For unknown reasons, symptoms sometimes clear completely after lumbar puncture. Indomethacin (75–150 mg daily) may provide relief.

Headache Due to Intracranial Mass Lesions

Intracranial mass lesions of all types may cause headache owing to displacement of vascular structures. Posterior fossa tumors often cause occipital pain, and supratentorial lesions lead to bifrontal headache, but such findings are too inconsistent to be of value in attempts at localizing a pathologic process. The headaches are nonspecific in character and may vary in severity from mild to severe. They may be worsened by exertion or postural change and may be associated with nausea and vomiting, but this is true of migraine also. Headaches are also a feature of pseudotumor cerebri (see below). Signs of focal or diffuse cerebral dysfunction or of increased intracranial pressure will indicate the need for further investigation. Similarly, a progressive headache disorder or the new onset of headaches in middle or later life merits investigation if no cause is apparent.

Headache Due to Other Neurologic Causes

Cerebrovascular disease may be associated with headache, but the mechanism is unclear. Headache may occur with internal carotid artery occlusion or carotid dissection and after carotid endarterectomy. Diagnosis is facilitated by the clinical accompaniments and the circumstances in which the headache developed.

Acute severe headache accompanies subarachnoid hemorrhage and meningeal infections; accompanying signs of meningeal irritation and impairment of consciousness indicate the need for further investigations.

Dull or throbbing headache is a frequent sequela of lumbar puncture and may last for several days. It is aggravated by the erect posture and alleviated by recumbency. The exact mechanism is unclear, but it is commonly attributed to leakage of cerebrospinal fluid through the dural puncture site. Its incidence may be reduced if a small-diameter needle is used for the spinal tap, and perhaps also if the patient lies prone or supine after the procedure.

Goadsby PJ: Mechanisms and management of headache. J R Coll Physicians Lond 1999;33:228. [PMID: 10402569]

Gobel H et al: Botulinum toxin A in the treatment of headache syndromes and pericranial pain syndromes. Pain 2001; 91:195. [PMID: 11275374] (Review.)

Krusz JC et al: Intravenous propofol: unique effectiveness in treating intractable migraine. Headache 2000;40:224. [PMID: 10759925]

FACIAL PAIN

Trigeminal Neuralgia

Trigeminal neuralgia ("tic douloureux") is most common in middle and later life. It affects women more frequently than men. The disorder is characterized by momentary episodes of sudden lancinating facial pain that commonly arises near one side of the mouth and then shoots toward the ear, eye, or nostril on that side. The pain may be triggered or precipitated by such factors as touch, movement, drafts, and eating. Indeed, in order to lessen the likelihood of triggering further attacks, many patients try to hold the face still while talking. Spontaneous remissions for several months or longer may occur. As the disorder progresses, however, the episodes of pain become more frequent, remissions become shorter and less common, and a dull ache may persist between the episodes of stabbing pain. Symptoms remain confined to the distribution of the trigeminal nerve (usually the second or third division) on one side only.

The characteristic features of the pain in trigeminal neuralgia usually distinguish it from other causes of facial pain. Neurologic examination shows no abnormality except in a few patients in whom trigeminal neuralgia is symptomatic of some underlying lesion, such as multiple sclerosis or a brain stem neoplasm, in which case the finding will depend on the nature and site of the lesion. Similarly, CT scans and radiologic contrast studies are normal in patients with classic trigeminal neuralgia.

In a young patient presenting with trigeminal neuralgia, multiple sclerosis must be suspected even if there are no other neurologic signs. In such circumstances, findings on evoked potential testing and examination of cerebrospinal fluid may be corroborative. When the facial pain is due to a posterior fossa tumor, CT scanning and MRI generally reveal the lesion.

The drug most helpful for treatment of trigeminal neuralgia is carbamazepine, given in a dose of up to 1200 mg/d, with monitoring by serial blood counts and liver function tests. If carbamazepine is ineffective or cannot be tolerated, phenytoin should be tried. (Doses and side effects of these drugs are shown in Table 24–2.) Baclofen (10–20 mg three or four times daily) may also be helpful, either alone or in combination with carbamazepine or phenytoin. Gabapentin, another anticonvulsant agent, may also relieve pain, especially in patients refractory to conventional medical therapy and those with multiple sclerosis. Depending on response and tolerance, up to 2400 mg/d is given in divided doses.

In the past, alcohol injection of the affected nerve, rhizotomy, or tractotomy was recommended if pharmacologic treatment was unsuccessful. More recently, however, posterior fossa exploration has frequently revealed some structural cause for the neuralgia (despite normal findings on CT scans, MRI, or arteriograms), such as an anomalous artery or vein impinging on the trigeminal nerve root. In such cases, simple decompression and separation of the anomalous vessel from the nerve root produce lasting relief of symptoms. In elderly patients with a limited life expectancy, radiofrequency rhizotomy is sometimes preferred because it is easy to perform, has few complications, and provides symptomatic relief for a period of time. Gamma radiosurgery to the trigeminal root is another noninvasive approach that appears to be successful in 80% of patients, with essentially no side effects other than facial paresthesias in a few instances. Surgical exploration generally reveals no abnormality and is inappropriate in patients with trigeminal neuralgia due to multiple sclerosis.

Kondziolka DE et al: Stereotactic radiosurgery for the treatment of trigeminal neuralgia. Clin J Pain 2002;18;42. [PMID: 11803302] (Clinical study.)

Sindrup SH et al: Pharmacotherapy of trigeminal neuralgia. Clin J Pain 2002;18;22. [PMID: 11803299]

Atypical Facial Pain

Facial pain without the typical features of trigeminal neuralgia is generally a constant, often burning pain that may have a restricted distribution at its onset but soon spreads to the rest of the face on the affected side and sometimes involves the other side, the neck, or the back of the head as well. The disorder is especially common in middle-aged women, many of them emotionally depressed, but it is not clear whether depression is the cause of or a reaction to the pain. Simple analgesics should be given a trial, as should tricyclic antidepressants, carbamazepine, and phenytoin; the response is often disappointing. Opioid analgesics pose a danger of addiction in patients with this disorder. Attempts at surgical treatment are not indicated.

Glossopharyngeal Neuralgia

Glossopharyngeal neuralgia is an uncommon disorder in which pain similar in quality to that in trigeminal neuralgia occurs in the throat, about the tonsillar fossa, and sometimes deep in the ear and at the back of the tongue. The pain may be precipitated by swallowing, chewing, talking, or yawning and is sometimes accompanied by syncope. In most instances, no underlying structural abnormality is present; multiple sclerosis is sometimes responsible. Carbamazepine is the treatment of choice and should be tried (in daily

Table 24–2. Drug treatment for seizures.

Drug	Usual Adult Daily Dose	Minimum No. of Daily Doses	Time to Steady-State Drug Levels	Optimal Drug Level	Selected Side Effects and Idiosyncratic Reactions
Generalized tonic-clonic (grand mal) or partial (focal) seizures					
Phenytoin	200–400 mg	1	5–10 days	10–20 μg/mL	Nystagmus, ataxia, dysarthria, sedation, confusion, gingival hyperplasia, hirsutism, mega-loblastic anemia, blood dyscrasias, skin rashes, fever, systemic lupus erythematosus, lymphadenopathy, peripheral neuropathy, dyskinesias.
Carbamazepine	600–1200 mg	2–3	3–4 days	4–8 μg/mL	Nystagmus, dysarthria, diplo-pia, ataxia, drowsiness, nausea, blood dyscrasias, hepatotox-icity, hyponatremia. May exa-cerbate myoclonic seizures.
(extended-release formulation)		(2)			
Valproic acid	1500–2000 mg	3	2–4 days	50–100 μg/mL	Nausea, vomiting, diarrhea, drowsiness, alopecia, weight gain, hepatotoxicity, throm-bocytopenia, tremor.
Phenobarbital	100–200 mg	1	14–21 days	10–40 μg/mL	Drowsiness, nystagmus, ataxia, skin rashes, learning difficul-ties, hyperactivity.
Primidone	750–1500 mg	3	4–7 days	5–15 μg/mL	Sedation, nystagmus, ataxia, ver-tigo, nausea, skin rashes, mega-loblastic anemia, irritability.
Felbamate[1,2]	1200–3600 mg	3	4–5 days	?	Anorexia, nausea, vomiting, headache, insomnia, weight loss, dizziness, hepatotoxicity, aplastic anemia.
Gabapentin[2]	900–1800 mg	3	1 day	?	Sedation, fatigue, ataxia, nys-tagmus, weight loss.
Lamotrigine	100–500 mg	2	4–5 days	?	Sedation, skin rash, visual dis-turbances, dyspepsia, ataxia.
Topiramate[2]	200–400 mg	2	4 days	?	Somnolence, nausea, dyspepsia, irritability, dizziness, ataxia, nystagmus, diplopia, renal calculi, weight loss.
Oxcarbazepine[4]	900–1800 mg	2	2–3 days	?	As for carbamazepine.
Levetiracetam[2]	1000–3000 mg	2	2 days	?	Somnolence, ataxia, headache.
Zonisamide[2]	200–600 mg	1–2	10 days	?	Somnolence, ataxia, anorexia, nausea, vomiting, rach, confu-sion, renal calculi. Do not use in patients with sulfonamide al-lergy.
Tiagabine[3]	32–56 mg	2	2 days	?	Somnolence, anxiety, dizzi-ness, poor concentration, tremor, diarrhea.
Absence (petit mal) seizures					
Ethosuximide	100–1500 mg	2	5–10 days	40–100 μg/mL	Nausea, vomiting, anorexia, headache, lethargy, unsteadi-ness, blood dyscrasias, sys-temic lupus erythematosus, urticaria, pruritus.

(continued)

Table 24–2. Drug treatment for seizures. (continued)

Drug	Usual Adult Daily Dose	Minimum No. of Daily Doses	Time to Steady-State Drug Levels	Optimal Drug Level	Selected Side Effects and Idiosyncratic Reactions
Valproic acid	1500–2000 mg	3	2–4 days	50–100 µg/mL	See above.
Clonazepam	0.04–0.2 mg/kg	2	?	20–80 ng/mL	Drowsiness, ataxia, irritability, behavioral changes, exacerbation of tonic-clonic seizures.
Myoclonic seizures					
Valproic acid	1500–2000 mg	3	2–4 days	50–100 µg/mL	See above.
Clonazepam	0.04–0.2 mg/kg	2	?	20–80 ng/mL	See above.

[1]Not to be used as a first-line drug; when used, blood counts should be performed regularly (every 2–4 weeks). Should be used only in selected patients because of risk of aplastic anemia and hepatic failure.
[2]Approved as adjunctive therapy for partial and secondarily generalized seizures.
[3]Approved as adjunctive therapy for partial seizures.
[4]Approved as monotherapy for partial seizures.

doses up to 1200 mg) before any surgical procedures are considered. Microvascular decompression is generally preferred over destructive surgical procedures such as partial rhizotomy in medically refractory cases and is often effective without causing severe complications.

Minagar A et al: Glossopharyngeal neuralgia and MS. Neurology 2000;54:1368. [PMID: 10746612] (Clinical study.)

Postherpetic Neuralgia

Herpes zoster (shingles) is due to infection of the nervous system by varicella-zoster virus. About 15% of patients who develop shingles suffer from postherpetic neuralgia. This complication seems especially likely to occur in the elderly, when the rash is severe, and when the first division of the trigeminal nerve is affected. A history of shingles and the presence of cutaneous scarring resulting from shingles aid in the diagnosis. Severe pain with shingles correlates with the intensity of postherpetic symptoms.

The incidence of postherpetic neuralgia may be reduced by the treatment of shingles with oral acyclovir or famciclovir, but this is disputed; systemic corticosteroids do not help. Management of the established complication is essentially medical. If simple analgesics fail to help, a trial of a tricyclic drug (eg, amitriptyline, up to 100–150 mg/d) in conjunction with a phenothiazine (eg, perphenazine, 2–8 mg/d) is often effective. Other patients respond to carbamazepine (up to 1200 mg/d), phenytoin (300 mg/d), or gabapentin (up to 3600 mg/d). Topical application of capsaicin cream (eg, Zostrix, 0.025%) may also be helpful, perhaps because of depletion of pain-mediating peptides from peripheral sensory neurons.

Alper BS et al: Does treatment of acute herpes zoster prevent or shorten postherpetic neuralgia? J Fam Pract 2000;49:255. [PMID: 10735485] (Systematic literature review.)

Rice AS et al: Gabapentin in postherpetic neuralgia: a randomized, double blind, placebo controlled study. Pain 2001; 94;215. [PMID: 11690735] (Clinical trial.)

Facial Pain Due to Other Causes

Facial pain may be caused by temporomandibular joint dysfunction in patients with malocclusion, abnormal bite, or faulty dentures. There may be tenderness of the masticatory muscles, and an association between pain onset and jaw movement is sometimes noted. Treatment consists of correction of the underlying problem.

A relationship of facial pain to chewing or temperature changes may suggest a dental disturbance. The cause is sometimes not obvious, and diagnosis requires careful dental examination and x-rays. Pain on mastication may also occur in giant cell arteritis. Sinusitis and ear infections causing facial pain are usually recognized by the history of respiratory tract infection, fever, and, in some instances, aural discharge. There may be localized tenderness. Radiologic evidence of sinus infection or mastoiditis is confirmatory.

Glaucoma is an important ocular cause of facial pain, usually localized to the periorbital region.

On occasion, pain in the jaw may be the principal manifestation of angina pectoris. Precipitation by exertion and radiation to more typical areas establish the cardiac origin.

EPILEPSY

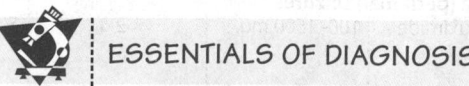 ESSENTIALS OF DIAGNOSIS

- *Recurrent seizures.*
- *Characteristic electroencephalographic changes accompany seizures.*

• *Mental status abnormalities or focal neurologic symptoms may persist for hours postictally.*

General Considerations

The term epilepsy denotes any disorder characterized by recurrent seizures. A seizure is a transient disturbance of cerebral function due to an abnormal paroxysmal neuronal discharge in the brain. Epilepsy is common, affecting approximately 0.5% of the population in the USA.

Etiology

Epilepsy has several causes. Its most likely cause in individual patients relates to the age at onset.

A. IDIOPATHIC OR CONSTITUTIONAL EPILEPSY

Seizures usually begin between 5 and 20 years of age but may start later in life. No specific cause can be identified, and there is no other neurologic abnormality.

B. SYMPTOMATIC EPILEPSY

There are many causes for recurrent seizures.

1. Pediatric age groups—Congenital abnormalities and perinatal injuries may result in seizures presenting in infancy or childhood.

2. Metabolic disorders—Withdrawal from alcohol or drugs is a common cause of recurrent seizures, and other metabolic disorders such as uremia and hypoglycemia or hyperglycemia may also be responsible.

3. Trauma—Trauma is an important cause of seizures at any age, but especially in young adults. Posttraumatic epilepsy is more likely to develop if the dura mater was penetrated and generally becomes manifest within 2 years following the injury. However, seizures developing in the first week after head injury do not necessarily imply that future attacks will occur. There is no clear evidence that prophylactic anticonvulsant drug treatment reduces the incidence of posttraumatic epilepsy.

4. Tumors and other space-occupying lesions—Neoplasms may lead to seizures at any age, but they are an especially important cause of seizures in middle and later life, when the incidence of neoplastic disease increases. The seizures are commonly the initial symptoms of the tumor and often are partial (focal) in character. They are most likely to occur with structural lesions involving the frontal, parietal, or temporal regions. Tumors must be excluded by appropriate imaging studies in all patients with onset of seizures after 30 years of age, focal seizures or signs, or a progressive seizure disorder.

5. Vascular diseases—Vascular diseases become increasingly frequent causes of seizures with advancing age and are the most common cause of seizures with onset at age 60 years or older.

6. Degenerative disorders—Alzheimer's disease and other degenerative disorders are a cause of seizures in later life.

7. Infectious diseases—Infectious diseases must be considered in all age groups as potentially reversible causes of seizures. Seizures may occur with an acute infective or inflammatory illness, such as bacterial meningitis or herpes encephalitis, or in patients with more long-standing or chronic disorders such as neurosyphilis or cerebral cysticercosis. In patients with AIDS, they may result from central nervous system toxoplasmosis, cryptococcal meningitis, secondary viral encephalitis, or other infective complications. Seizures are a common sequela of supratentorial brain abscess, developing most frequently in the first year after treatment.

Classification of Seizures

Seizures can be categorized in various ways, but the descriptive classification proposed by the International League Against Epilepsy is clinically the most useful. Seizures are divided into those that are generalized and those affecting only part of the brain (partial seizures).

A. PARTIAL SEIZURES

The initial clinical and electroencephalographic manifestations of partial seizures indicate that only a restricted part of one cerebral hemisphere has been activated. The ictal manifestations depend upon the area of the brain involved. Partial seizures are subdivided into simple seizures, in which consciousness is preserved, and complex seizures, in which it is impaired. Partial seizures of either type sometimes become secondarily generalized, leading to a tonic, clonic, or tonic-clonic attack.

1. Simple partial seizures—Simple seizures may be manifested by focal motor symptoms (convulsive jerking) or somatosensory symptoms (eg, paresthesias or tingling) that spread (or "march") to different parts of the limb or body depending upon their cortical representation. In other instances, special sensory symptoms (eg, light flashes or buzzing) indicate involvement of visual, auditory, olfactory, or gustatory regions of the brain, or there may be autonomic symptoms or signs (eg, abnormal epigastric sensations, sweating, flushing, pupillary dilation). The sole manifestations of some seizures are phenomena such as dysphasia, dysmnesic symptoms (eg, déjà vu, jamais vu), affective disturbances, illusions, or structured hallucinations, but such symptoms are usually accompanied by impairment of consciousness.

2. Complex partial seizures—Impaired consciousness may be preceded, accompanied, or followed by the psychic symptoms mentioned above, and automatisms may occur. Such seizures may also begin with some of the other simple symptoms mentioned above.

B. GENERALIZED SEIZURES

There are several different varieties of generalized seizures, as outlined below. In some circumstances, seizures cannot be classified because of incomplete information or because they do not fit into any category.

1. Absence (petit mal) seizures—These are characterized by impairment of consciousness, sometimes with mild clonic, tonic, or atonic components (ie, reduction or loss of postural tone), autonomic components (eg, enuresis), or accompanying automatisms. Onset and termination of attacks are abrupt. If attacks occur during conversation, the patient may miss a few words or may break off in mid sentence for a few seconds. The impairment of external awareness is so brief that the patient is unaware of it. Absence seizures almost always begin in childhood and frequently cease by the age of 20 years, although occasionally they are then replaced by other forms of generalized seizure. Electroencephalographically, such attacks are associated with bursts of bilaterally synchronous and symmetric 3-Hz spike-and-wave activity. A normal background in the electroencephalogram and normal or above-normal intelligence imply a good prognosis for the ultimate cessation of these seizures.

2. Atypical absences—There may be more marked changes in tone, or attacks may have a more gradual onset and termination than in typical absences.

3. Myoclonic seizures—Myoclonic seizures consist of single or multiple myoclonic jerks.

4. Tonic-clonic (grand mal) seizures—In these seizures, which are characterized by sudden loss of consciousness, the patient becomes rigid and falls to the ground, and respiration is arrested. This tonic phase, which usually lasts for less than a minute, is followed by a clonic phase in which there is jerking of the body musculature that may last for 2 or 3 minutes and is then followed by a stage of flaccid coma. During the seizure, the tongue or lips may be bitten, urinary or fecal incontinence may occur, and the patient may be injured. Immediately after the seizure, the patient may either recover consciousness, drift into sleep, have a further convulsion without recovery of consciousness between the attacks (**status epilepticus**), or after recovering consciousness have a further convulsion (**serial seizures**). In other cases, patients will behave in an abnormal fashion in the immediate postictal period, without subsequent awareness or memory of events (**postepileptic automatism**). Headache, disorientation, confusion, drowsiness, nausea, soreness of the muscles, or some combination of these symptoms commonly occurs postictally.

5. Tonic, clonic, or atonic seizures—Loss of consciousness may occur with either the tonic or clonic accompaniments described above, especially in children. Atonic seizures (**epileptic drop attacks**) have also been described.

Clinical Findings

A. SYMPTOMS AND SIGNS

Nonspecific changes such as headache, mood alterations, lethargy, and myoclonic jerking alert some patients to an impending seizure hours before it occurs. These prodromal symptoms are distinct from the aura which may precede a generalized seizure by a few seconds or minutes and which is itself a part of the attack, arising locally from a restricted region of the brain.

In most patients, seizures occur unpredictably at any time and without any relationship to posture or ongoing activities. Occasionally, however, they occur at a particular time (eg, during sleep) or in relation to external precipitants such as lack of sleep, missed meals, emotional stress, menstruation, alcohol ingestion (or alcohol withdrawal; see below), or use of certain drugs. Fever and nonspecific infections may also precipitate seizures in known epileptics. In a few patients, seizures are provoked by specific stimuli such as flashing lights or a flickering television set (**photosensitive epilepsy**), music, or reading.

Clinical examination between seizures shows no abnormality in patients with idiopathic epilepsy, but in the immediate postictal period, extensor plantar responses may be seen. The presence of lateralized or focal signs postictally suggests that seizures may have a focal origin. In patients with symptomatic epilepsy, the findings on examination will reflect the underlying cause.

B. IMAGING

MRI is indicated for patients with focal neurologic symptoms or signs, focal seizures, or electroencephalographic findings of a focal disturbance; some clinicians routinely order imaging studies for all patients with new-onset seizure disorders. Such studies should certainly be performed in patients with clinical evidence of a progressive disorder and in those presenting with new onset of seizures after the age of 20 years, because of the possibility of an underlying neoplasm. A chest radiograph should also be obtained in such patients, since the lungs are a common site for primary or secondary neoplasms.

C. LABORATORY AND OTHER STUDIES

Initial investigations should always include a full blood count, blood glucose determination, liver and renal function tests, and serologic tests for syphilis. The hematologic and biochemical screening tests are important both in excluding various causes of seizures and in providing a baseline for subsequent monitoring of long-term effects of treatment.

Electroencephalography may support the clinical diagnosis of epilepsy (by demonstrating paroxysmal abnormalities containing spikes or sharp waves), may provide a guide to prognosis, and may help classify the seizure disorder. Classification of the disorder is important for determining the most appropriate anticonvulsant drug with which to start treatment. For example, absence (petit mal) and complex partial seizures may be difficult to distinguish clinically, but the electroencephalographic findings and treatment of choice differ in these two conditions. Finally, by localizing the epileptogenic source, the electroencephalographic findings are important in evaluating candidates for surgical treatment.

Differential Diagnosis

The distinction between the various disorders likely to be confused with generalized seizures is usually made on the basis of the history. The importance of obtaining an eyewitness account of the attacks cannot be overemphasized.

A. DIFFERENTIAL DIAGNOSIS OF PARTIAL SEIZURES

1. Transient ischemic attacks—These attacks are distinguished from seizures by their longer duration, lack of spread, and symptomatology. Level of consciousness, which is unaltered, does not distinguish them. There is a loss of motor or sensory function (eg, weakness or numbness) with transient ischemic attacks, whereas positive symptomatology (eg, convulsive jerking or paresthesias) characterizes seizures.

2. Rage attacks—Rage attacks are usually situational and lead to goal-directed aggressive behavior.

3. Panic attacks—These may be hard to distinguish from simple or complex partial seizures unless there is evidence of psychopathologic disturbances between attacks and the attacks have a clear relationship to external circumstances.

B. DIFFERENTIAL DIAGNOSIS OF GENERALIZED SEIZURES

1. Syncope—Syncopal episodes usually occur in relation to postural change, emotional stress, instrumentation, pain, or straining. They are typically preceded by pallor, sweating, nausea, and malaise and lead to loss of consciousness accompanied by flaccidity; recovery occurs rapidly with recumbency, and there is no postictal headache or confusion. In some instances, however, motor accompaniments may simulate a seizure. Serum creatine kinase measured about 3 hours after the event is generally normal after syncopal episodes but markedly elevated after tonic-clonic seizures.

2. Cardiac dysrhythmias—Cerebral hypoperfusion due to a disturbance of cardiac rhythm should be suspected in patients with known cardiac or vascular disease or in elderly patients who present with episodic loss of consciousness. Prodromal symptoms are typically absent. A relationship of attacks to physical activity and the finding of a systolic murmur is suggestive of aortic stenosis. Repeated Holter monitoring may be necessary to establish the diagnosis; monitoring initi-

ated by the patient ("event monitor") may be valuable if the disturbances of consciousness are rare.

3. Brain stem ischemia—Loss of consciousness is preceded or accompanied by other brain stem signs. Basilar artery migraine and vertebrobasilar vascular disease are discussed elsewhere in this chapter.

4. Pseudoseizures—The term pseudoseizures is used to denote both hysterical conversion reactions and attacks due to malingering when these simulate epileptic seizures. Many patients with pseudoseizures also have true seizures or a family history of epilepsy. Although pseudoseizures tend to occur at times of emotional stress, this may also be the case with true seizures.

Clinically, the attacks superficially resemble tonic-clonic seizures, but there may be obvious preparation before pseudoseizures occur. Moreover, there is usually no tonic phase; instead, there is an asynchronous thrashing of the limbs, which increases if restraints are imposed and which rarely leads to injury. Consciousness may be normal or "lost," but in the latter context the occurrence of goal-directed behavior or of shouting, swearing, etc, indicates that it is feigned. Postictally, there are no changes in behavior or neurologic findings.

Laboratory studies may aid in recognition of pseudoseizures. There are no electrocerebral changes, whereas the electroencephalogram changes during organic seizures accompanied by loss of consciousness. The serum level of prolactin has been found to increase dramatically between 15 and 30 minutes after a tonic-clonic convulsion in most patients, whereas it is unchanged after a pseudoseizure.

Treatment

A. GENERAL MEASURES

For patients with recurrent seizures, drug treatment is prescribed with the goal of preventing further attacks and is usually continued until there have been no seizures for at least 3 years. Epileptic patients should be advised to avoid situations that could be dangerous or life-threatening if further seizures should occur. State legislation may require clinicians to report to the state department of public health any patients with seizures or other episodic disturbances of consciousness.

1. Choice of medication—The drug with which treatment is best initiated depends upon the type of seizures to be treated (Table 24–2). The dose of the selected drug is gradually increased until seizures are controlled or side effects prevent further increases. If seizures continue despite treatment at the maximal tolerated dose, a second drug is added and the dose increased depending on tolerance; the first drug is then gradually withdrawn. In treatment of partial and secondarily generalized tonic-clonic seizures, the success rate is higher with carbamazepine, phenytoin, or valproic acid than with phenobarbital or primidone. Gabapentin, topiramate, lamotrigine, oxcarbazepine, levetiracetam, and zonisamide are newer antiepileptic drugs that are effective for partial or secondarily generalized seizures. Felbamate is also effective for such seizures but, because it may cause aplastic anemia or fulminant hepatic failure, it should be used only in selected patients unresponsive to other measures. Tiagabine is another adjunctive agent for partial seizures. In most patients with seizures of a single type, satisfactory control can be achieved with a single anticonvulsant drug. Treatment with two drugs may further reduce seizure frequency or severity, but usually only at the cost of greater toxicity. Treatment with more than two drugs is almost always unhelpful unless the patient is having seizures of different types.

2. Monitoring—Monitoring serum drug levels has led to major advances in the management of seizure disorders. The same daily dose of a particular drug leads to markedly different blood concentrations in different patients, and this will affect the therapeutic response. In general, the dose of an antiepileptic agent is increased depending on the clinical response regardless of the serum drug level. The trough drug level is then measured to provide a reference point for the maximum tolerated dose. Dosing should not be based simply on serum levels because many patients require levels that exceed the therapeutic range ("toxic levels") but tolerate these without ill effect. Steady-state drug levels in the blood should be measured after treatment is initiated, dosage is changed, or another drug is added to the therapeutic regimen and when seizures are poorly controlled. Dose adjustments are then guided by the laboratory findings. The most common cause of a lower concentration of drug than expected for the prescribed dose is poor patient compliance. Compliance can be improved by limiting to a minimum the number of daily doses. Recurrent seizures or status epilepticus may result if drugs are taken erratically, and in some circumstances noncompliant patients may be better off without any medication.

All anticonvulsant drugs have side effects, and some of these are shown in Table 24–2. In most patients, a complete blood count should be performed at least annually because of the risk of anemia or blood dyscrasia. Treatment with certain drugs may require more frequent monitoring or use of additional screening tests. For example, periodic tests of hepatic function are necessary if valproic acid, carbamazepine, or felbamate is used, and serial blood counts are important with carbamazepine, ethosuximide, or felbamate.

3. Discontinuance of medication—Only when patients have been seizure-free for several (at least 3) years should withdrawal of medication be considered. Unfortunately, there is no way of predicting which patients can be managed successfully without treatment, although seizure recurrence is more likely in patients who initially failed to respond to therapy, those with seizures having focal features or of multiple types, and those with continuing electroencephalographic abnormalities. Dose reduction should be gradual over a period of weeks or months, and drugs should be withdrawn one at a time. If seizures recur, treatment is reinstituted with the same drugs used previously. Seizures are no more difficult to control after a recurrence than before.

4. Surgical treatment—Patients with surgically remediable epilepsy or seizures refractory to pharmacologic management may be candidates for operative treatment, which is best undertaken in specialized centers.

5. Vagal nerve stimulation—Treatment by chronic vagal nerve stimulation for adults and adolescents with medically refractory partial-onset seizures is approved in the USA and provides an alternative approach for patients who are not optimal candidates for surgical treatment. The mechanism of therapeutic action is unknown. Adverse effects consist mainly of transient hoarseness during stimulus delivery.

B. SPECIAL CIRCUMSTANCES

1. Solitary seizures—In patients who have had only one seizure, investigation as outlined above should exclude an underlying cause requiring specific treatment. An EEG should also be performed, preferably within 24 hours after the seizure, because the findings may influence management—especially when focal abnormalities are present. Prophylactic anticonvulsant drug treatment is generally not required unless further attacks occur or investigations reveal some underlying pathology that itself is untreatable. The risk of seizure recurrence varies in different series between about 30% and 70%. Epilepsy should not be diagnosed on the basis of a solitary seizure. If seizures occur in the context of transient, nonrecurrent systemic disorders such as acute cerebral anoxia, the diagnosis of epilepsy is inaccurate, and long-term prophylactic anticonvulsant drug treatment is unnecessary.

2. Alcohol withdrawal seizures—One or more generalized tonic-clonic seizures may occur within 48 hours or so of withdrawal from alcohol after a period of high or chronic intake. If the seizures have consistently focal features, the possibility of an associated structural abnormality, often traumatic in origin, must be considered. Head CT scan should be performed in patients with new onset of generalized seizures and whenever there are focal features associated with any seizures. Treatment with anticonvulsant drugs is generally not required for alcohol withdrawal seizures, since they are self-limited. Status epilepticus may rarely follow alcohol withdrawal and is managed along conventional lines (see below). Further attacks will not occur if the patient abstains from alcohol.

3. Tonic-clonic status epilepticus—Poor compliance with the anticonvulsant drug regimen is the most common cause; others include alcohol withdrawal, intracranial infection or neoplasms, metabolic disorders, and drug overdose. The mortality rate may be as high as 20%, and among survivors the incidence of neurologic and mental sequelae may be high. The prognosis relates to the length of time between onset of status epilepticus and the start of effective treatment.

Status epilepticus is a medical emergency. Initial management includes maintenance of the airway and 50% dextrose (25–50 mL) intravenously in case hypoglycemia is responsible. If seizures continue, 10 mg of diazepam is given intravenously over the course of 2 minutes, and the dose is repeated after 10 minutes if necessary. Alternatively, a 4 mg intravenous bolus of lorazepam, repeated once after 10 minutes if necessary, is given in place of diazepam. This is usually effective in halting seizures for a brief period but occasionally causes respiratory depression.

Regardless of the response to diazepam or lorazepam, phenytoin (18–20 mg/kg) is given intravenously at a rate of 50 mg/min; this provides initiation of long-term seizure control. The drug is best injected directly but can also be given in saline; it precipitates, however, if injected into glucose-containing solutions. Because arrhythmias may develop during rapid administration of phenytoin, electrocardiographic monitoring is prudent. Hypotension may complicate phenytoin administration, especially if diazepam has also been given. In the United States, injectable phenytoin has been replaced by fosphenytoin, which is rapidly and completely converted to phenytoin following intravenous administration. No dosing adjustments are necessary because fosphenytoin is expressed in terms of phenytoin equivalents (PE); fosphenytoin is less likely to cause reactions at the infusion site, can be given with all common intravenous solutions, and may be administered at a faster rate (150 mg PE/min). It is also more expensive.

If seizures continue, phenobarbital is then given in a loading dose of 10–20 mg/kg intravenously by slow or intermittent injection (50 mg/min). Respiratory depression and hypotension are common complications and should be anticipated; they may occur also with diazepam alone, though less commonly. If these measures fail, general anesthesia with ventilatory assistance and neuromuscular junction blockade may be required. Alternatively, intravenous midazolam may provide control of refractory status epilepticus; the suggested loading dose is 0.2 mg/kg, followed by 0.05–0.2 mg/kg/h.

After status epilepticus is controlled, an oral drug program for the long-term management of seizures is started, and investigations into the cause of the disorder are pursued.

4. Nonconvulsive status epilepticus—Absence (petit mal) and complex partial status epilepticus are characterized by fluctuating abnormal mental status, confusion, impaired responsiveness, and automatism. Electroencephalography is helpful both in establishing the diagnosis and in distinguishing the two varieties. Initial treatment with intravenous diazepam is usually helpful regardless of the type of status epilepticus, but phenytoin, phenobarbital, carbamazepine, and other drugs may also be needed to obtain and maintain control in complex partial status epilepticus.

Alldredge BK et al: A comparison of lorazepam, diazepam, and placebo for the treatment of out-of-hospital status epilepticus. N Engl J Med 2001;345:631. [PMID:11547716] (Clinical trial.)

Benbadis SR et al: Advances in the treatment of epilepsy. Am Fam Physician 2001;64:91. [PMID: 11456438] (Review.)

Brodie MJ et al: Management of epilepsy in adolescents and adults. Lancet 2000;356:323. [PMID: 11071202] (Review.)

Kwan P et al: Early identification of refractory epilepsy. N Engl J Med 2000;342:314. [PMID: 10660394] (Clinical study.)

Kwan P et al: The mechanisms of action of commonly used antiepileptic drugs. Pharmacol Ther 2001;90:21. [PMID: 11448723] (Review.)

Wiebe S et al: A randomized, controlled trial of surgery for temporal lobe epilepsy. N Engl J Med 2001;345:311. [PMID: 11484687] (Clinical trial.)

SYNCOPE & DYSAUTONOMIA

Dysautonomia may occur as a result of central or peripheral pathologic processes. It is manifested by a variety of symptoms that may occur in isolation or in various combinations and relate to abnormalities of blood pressure regulation, thermoregulatory sweating, gastrointestinal function, sphincter control, sexual function, respiration, and ocular function. Such symptoms include syncope, postural hypotension, paroxysmal hypertension, persistent tachycardia without other cause, facial flushing, hypo- or hyperhidrosis, vomiting, constipation, diarrhea, dysphagia, abdominal distention, disturbances of micturition or defecation, apneic episodes, and declining night vision.

Syncope is characterized by a transient loss of consciousness, usually accompanied by hypotension and bradycardia. It may occur in response to emotional stress, postural hypotension, vigorous exercise in a hot environment, obstructed venous return to the heart, acute pain or its anticipation, fluid loss, and a variety of other circumstances. A prodrome of malaise, nausea, headache, diaphoresis, pallor, visual disturbance, loss of postural tone, and a sense of weakness and impending loss of consciousness is followed by actual loss of consciousness. Although the patient is usually flaccid, some motor activity is not uncommon, and urinary (and, rarely, fecal) incontinence may also occur, thereby simulating a seizure. Recovery is rapid once the patient becomes recumbent, but headache, nausea, and fatigue are common postictally.

Evaluation of the Patient

Clinical evaluation is important to exclude reversible, nonneurologic causes of symptoms. Postural hypotension and syncope, for example, may relate to a reduced cardiac output (eg, from aortic stenosis or cardiomyopathy), paroxysmal cardiac dysrhythmias, volume depletion, various medications, and endocrine and metabolic disorders such as Addison's disease, hypo- or hyperthyroidism, pheochromocytoma, and carcinoid syndrome. Testing of autonomic function helps to establish the diagnosis of dysautonomia, to exclude other causes of symptoms, to assess the severity of involvement, and to guide prognostication. Such testing includes evaluating the cardiovascular response to the Valsalva maneuver, startle, mental stress, postural change, and deep respiration, and the sudomotor (sweating) responses to warming or a deep inspiratory gasp. Tilt-table testing may reproduce syncopal or presyncopal symptoms. Pharmacologic studies to evaluate the pupillary responses, radiologic studies of the bladder or gastrointestinal tract, uroflowmetry and urethral pressure profiles, and recording of nocturnal penile tumescence may also be necessary in selected cases. Further investigation depends on the presence of other associated neurologic abnormalities. In patients with a peripheral cause, work-up for peripheral neuropathy may be required as discussed below. For those with evidence of a central lesion, imaging studies will exclude a treatable structural cause.

Neurologic Causes

A. CENTRAL CAUSES

Disease at certain sites in the central nervous system, regardless of its nature, may lead to dysautonomic symptoms. Postural hypotension, which is usually the most troublesome and disabling symptom, may result from spinal cord transection and other myelopathies (eg, due to tumor or syringomyelia) above the T6 level or from brain stem lesions such as syringobulbia and posterior fossa tumors. Sphincter or sexual disturbances may result from cord lesions below T6. Certain primary degenerative disorders are responsible for dysautonomia occurring in isolation (**pure autonomic failure**) or in association with more widespread abnormalities (**multisystem atrophy** or **Shy-Drager syndrome**) that may include parkinsonian, pyramidal symptoms, and cerebellar deficits.

B. PERIPHERAL CAUSES

A pure autonomic neuropathy may occur acutely or subacutely after a viral infection or as a paraneoplastic disorder related usually to small cell lung cancer. Patients typically present with postural hypotension, impaired thermoregulatory sweating, xerostomia or xerophthalmia, abnormal gastrointestinal motility, dilated pupils, or acute urinary retention. Dysautonomia is often conspicuous in patients with Guillain-Barré syndrome, manifesting with marked hypotension or hypertension or cardiac arrhythmias that may have a fatal outcome. It may also occur with diabetic, uremic, amyloidotic, and various other metabolic or toxic neuropathies; in association with leprosy or Chagas' dis-

ease; and as a feature of certain hereditary neuropathies. Autonomic symptoms are prominent in the crises of hepatic porphyria. Patients with botulism or the Lambert-Eaton myasthenic syndrome may have constipation, urinary retention, and a sicca syndrome as a result of impaired cholinergic function.

Treatment

The most disabling symptom of dysautonomia is usually postural hypotension and syncope. Abrupt postural change, prolonged recumbency, and other precipitants should be avoided. Medications associated with postural hypotension should be discontinued or reduced in dose. Treatment may include wearing waist-high elastic hosiery, salt supplementation, sleeping in a semierect position (which minimizes the natriuresis and diuresis that occur during recumbency), and fludrocortisone (0.1–0.2 mg daily). Vasoconstrictor agents may be helpful and include midodrine (2.5–10 mg three times daily) and ephedrine (15–30 mg three times daily). Other agents that have been used occasionally or experimentally are dihydroergotamine, yohimbine, and clonidine; refractory cases may respond to erythropoietin (epoetin alfa) or desmopressin. Patients must be monitored for recumbent hypertension. Postprandial hypotension is helped by caffeine. There is no satisfactory treatment for disturbances of sweating, but an air-conditioned environment is helpful in avoiding extreme swings in body temperature.

Kaufmann H et al: Why do we faint? Muscle Nerve 2001;24:981. [PMID: 11439373] (Review.)

SENSORY DISTURBANCES

Patients may complain of either lost or abnormal sensations. The term "numbness" is often used by patients to denote loss of feeling, but the word also has other meanings and the patient's intention must be clarified. Abnormal spontaneous sensations are generally called paresthesias, and unpleasant or painful sensations produced by a stimulus that is usually painless are called dysesthesias.

Sensory symptoms may be due to disease located anywhere along the peripheral or central sensory pathways. The character, site, mode of onset, spread, and temporal profile of sensory symptoms must be established and any precipitating or relieving factors identified. These features—and the presence of any associated symptoms—help identify the origin of sensory disturbances, as do the physical signs as well. Sensory symptoms or signs may conform to the territory of individual peripheral nerves or nerve roots. Involvement of one side of the body—or of one limb in its entirety—suggests a central lesion. Distal involvement of all four extremities suggests polyneuropathy, a cervical cord or brain stem lesion, or—when symptoms are transient—a metabolic disturbance such as hyperventilation syndrome. Short-lived sensory complaints may be indicative of sensory seizures or cerebral ischemic phenomena as well as metabolic disturbances. In patients with cord lesions, there may be a transverse sensory level. "Dissociated sensory loss" is characterized by loss of some sensory modalities with preservation of others. Such findings may be encountered in patients with either peripheral or central disease and must therefore be interpreted in the clinical context in which they are found.

The absence of sensory signs in patients with sensory symptoms does not mean that symptoms have a nonorganic basis. Symptoms are often troublesome before signs of sensory dysfunction have had time to develop.

WEAKNESS & PARALYSIS

Loss of muscle power may result from central disease involving the upper or lower motor neurons; from peripheral disease involving the roots, plexus, or peripheral nerves; from disorders of neuromuscular transmission; or from primary disorders of muscle. The clinical findings help to localize the lesion and thus reduce the number of diagnostic possibilities.

Weakness due to upper motor neuron lesions is characterized by selective involvement of certain muscle groups and is associated with spasticity, increased tendon reflexes, and extensor plantar responses. The site of upper motor neuron (pyramidal) involvement may be indicated by the presence of other clinical signs or by the distribution of the motor deficit. Lower motor neuron lesions lead to muscle wasting as well as weakness, with flaccidity and loss of tendon reflexes, but no change in the plantar responses unless the neurons subserving them are directly involved. Fasciculations may be evident over affected muscles. In distinguishing between a root, plexus, or peripheral nerve lesion, the distribution of the motor deficit and of any sensory changes is of particular importance. In patients with disturbances of neuromuscular transmission, weakness is patchy in distribution, often fluctuates over short periods of time, and is not associated with sensory changes. In myopathic disorders, weakness is usually most marked proximally in the limbs, is not associated with sensory loss or sphincter disturbance, and is not accompanied by muscle wasting or loss of tendon reflexes—at least not until an advanced stage.

TRANSIENT ISCHEMIC ATTACKS

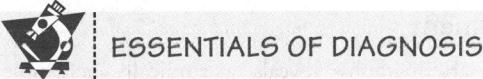

ESSENTIALS OF DIAGNOSIS

- Risk factors for vascular disease often present.
- Focal neurologic deficit of acute onset.
- Clinical deficit resolves completely within 24 hours.

General Considerations

Transient ischemic attacks are characterized by focal ischemic cerebral neurologic deficits that last for less than 24 hours (usually less than 1–2 hours). About 30% of patients with stroke have a history of transient ischemic attacks, and proper treatment of the attacks is an important means of prevention. The incidence of stroke does not relate to either the number or the duration of individual attacks but is increased in patients with hypertension or diabetes. The risk of stroke is highest in the month after a transient ischemic attack and progressively declines thereafter.

Etiology

An important cause of transient cerebral ischemia is embolization. In many patients with these attacks, a source is readily apparent in the heart or a major extracranial artery to the head, and emboli sometimes are visible in the retinal arteries. Moreover, an embolic phenomenon explains why separate attacks may affect different parts of the territory supplied by the same major vessel. Cardiac causes of embolic ischemic attacks include rheumatic heart disease, mitral valve disease, cardiac arrhythmia, infective endocarditis, atrial myxoma, and mural thrombi complicating myocardial infarction. Atrial septal defects and patent foramen ovale may permit emboli from the veins to reach the brain ("paradoxical emboli"). An ulcerated plaque on a major artery to the brain may serve as a source of emboli. In the anterior circulation, atherosclerotic changes occur most commonly in the region of the carotid bifurcation extracranially, and these changes may cause a bruit. In some patients with transient ischemic attacks or strokes, an acute or recent hemorrhage is found to have occurred into this atherosclerotic plaque, and this finding may have pathologic significance. Patients with AIDS have an increased risk of developing transient ischemic deficits or strokes.

Other (less common) abnormalities of blood vessels that may cause transient ischemic attacks include fibromuscular dysplasia, which affects particularly the cervical internal carotid artery; atherosclerosis of the aortic arch; inflammatory arterial disorders such as giant cell arteritis, systemic lupus erythematosus, polyarteritis, and granulomatous angiitis; and meningovascular syphilis. Hypotension may cause a reduction of cerebral blood flow if a major extracranial artery to the brain is markedly stenosed, but this is a rare cause of transient ischemic attack.

Hematologic causes of ischemic attacks include polycythemia, sickle cell disease, and hyperviscosity syndromes. Severe anemia may also lead to transient focal neurologic deficits in patients with preexisting cerebral arterial disease.

The **subclavian steal syndrome** may lead to transient vertebrobasilar ischemia. Symptoms develop when there is localized stenosis or occlusion of one subclavian artery proximal to the source of the vertebral artery, so that blood is "stolen" from this artery. A bruit in the supraclavicular fossa, unequal radial pulses, and a difference of 20 mm Hg or more between the systolic blood pressures in the arms should suggest the diagnosis in patients with vertebrobasilar transient ischemic attacks.

Clinical Findings

A. SYMPTOMS AND SIGNS

The symptoms of transient ischemic attacks vary markedly among patients; however, the symptoms in a given individual tend to be constant in type. Onset is abrupt and without warning, and recovery usually occurs rapidly, often within a few minutes.

If the ischemia is in the carotid territory, common symptoms are weakness and heaviness of the contralateral arm, leg, or face, singly or in any combination. Numbness or paresthesias may also occur either as the sole manifestation of the attack or in combination with the motor deficit. There may be slowness of movement, dysphasia, or monocular visual loss in the eye contralateral to affected limbs. During an attack, examination may reveal flaccid weakness with pyramidal distribution, sensory changes, hyperreflexia or an extensor plantar response on the affected side, dysphasia, or any combination of these findings. Subsequently, examination reveals no neurologic abnormality, but the presence of a carotid bruit or cardiac abnormality may provide a clue to the cause of symptoms.

Vertebrobasilar ischemic attacks may be characterized by vertigo, ataxia, diplopia, dysarthria, dimness or blurring of vision, perioral numbness and paresthesias, and weakness or sensory complaints on one, both, or alternating sides of the body. These symptoms may occur singly or in any combination. Drop attacks due to bilateral leg weakness, without headache or loss of consciousness, may occur, sometimes in relation to head movements.

The natural history of attacks is variable. Some patients will have a major stroke after only a few attacks, whereas others may have frequent attacks for weeks or months without having a stroke. Attacks may occur intermittently over a long period of time, or they may stop spontaneously. In general, carotid ischemic attacks are more liable than vertebrobasilar ischemic attacks to be followed by stroke. The stroke risk is greater in patients older than 60 years, in diabetics, or after TIAs that last longer than 10 minutes and with symptoms or signs of weakness, speech impairment, or gait disturbance. When stroke does occur, it is often during the first 48 hours after a TIA.

B. IMAGING

CT scan of the head will exclude the possibility of a small cerebral hemorrhage or a cerebral tumor masquerading as a transient ischemic attack. A number of noninvasive techniques, such as ultrasonography, have been developed for studying the cerebral circulation and imaging the major vessels to the head. Carotid duplex ultrasonography is useful for detecting significant stenosis of the internal carotid artery, but arteriography remains important for demonstrating the status of the cerebrovascular system. MR angiography may reveal stenotic lesions of large vessels but is less sensitive than conventional arteriography. Accordingly, if findings on CT scan are normal, if there is no cardiac source of embolization, and if age and general condition indicate that the patient is a good operative risk, bilateral carotid arteriography should be considered in the further evaluation of carotid ischemic attacks, although the ultrasound findings may help in selecting patients for study.

C. LABORATORY AND OTHER STUDIES

Clinical and laboratory evaluation must include assessment for hypertension, heart disease, hematologic disorders, diabetes mellitus, hyperlipidemia, and peripheral vascular disease. It should include complete blood count, fasting blood glucose and serum cholesterol and homocysteine determinations, serologic tests for syphilis, and an ECG and chest x-ray. Echocardiography with bubble contrast is performed if a cardiac source is likely, and blood cultures are obtained if endocarditis is suspected. Holter monitoring is indicated if a transient, paroxysmal disturbance of cardiac rhythm is suspected.

Differential Diagnosis

Focal seizures usually cause abnormal motor or sensory phenomena such as clonic limb movements, paresthesias, or tingling, rather than weakness or loss of feeling. Symptoms generally spread ("march") up the limb and may lead to a generalized tonic-clonic seizure.

Classic migraine is easily recognized by the visual premonitory symptoms, followed by nausea, headache, and photophobia, but less typical cases may be hard to distinguish. The patient's age and medical history (including family history) may be helpful in this regard. Patients with migraine commonly have a history of episodes since adolescence and report that other family members have a similar disorder.

Focal neurologic deficits may occur during periods of hypoglycemia in diabetic patients receiving insulin or oral hypoglycemic agent therapy.

Treatment

When arteriography reveals a surgically accessible high-grade stenosis (70–99% in luminal diameter) on the side appropriate to carotid ischemic attacks and there is relatively little atherosclerosis elsewhere in the cerebrovascular system, operative treatment (carotid thromboendarterectomy) reduces the risk of ipsilateral carotid stroke, especially when transient ischemic attacks are of recent onset (< 2 months). Surgery is not indicated for mild stenosis (< 30%); its benefits are unclear with severe stenosis plus diffuse intracranial atherosclerotic disease. See Chapter 12 for additional discussion.

In patients with carotid ischemic attacks who are poor operative candidates (and thus have not undergone arteriography) or who are found to have extensive vascular disease, medical treatment should be instituted. Similarly, patients with vertebrobasilar ischemic attacks are treated medically and are not subjected to arteriography unless there is clinical evidence of stenosis or occlusion in the carotid or subclavian arteries.

Medical treatment is aimed at preventing further attacks and stroke. Cigarette smoking should be stopped, and cardiac sources of embolization, hypertension, diabetes, hyperlipidemia, arteritis, or hematologic disorders should be treated appropriately.

A. EMBOLIZATION FROM THE HEART

If anticoagulants are indicated for the treatment of embolism from the heart, they should be started immediately, provided there is no contraindication to their use. There is no advantage in delay, and the common fear of causing hemorrhage into a previously infarcted area is misplaced, since there is a far greater risk of further embolism to the cerebral circulation if treatment is withheld. Treatment is initiated with intravenous heparin (in a loading dose of 5000–10,000 units of standard molecular weight heparin, and maintenance infusion of 1000–2000 units per hour depending on the partial thromboplastin time) while warfarin sodium is introduced in a daily dose of 5–15 mg orally, depending on the INR. Warfarin is more effective than aspirin in reducing the incidence of cardioembolic events, but when its use is contraindicated aspirin (325 mg daily) may be used in patients with nonrheumatic atrial fibrillation to reduce the risk of stroke.

B. EMBOLIZATION FROM THE CARDIOVASCULAR SYSTEM

In patients with presumed or angiographically verified atherosclerotic changes in the extracranial or intracranial cerebrovascular circulation, antithrombotic medication is prescribed. The evidence supporting a therapeutic role for aspirin to suppress platelet aggregation is convincing. Platelets adhere to and aggregate around an atherosclerotic plaque and release various substances including thromboxane A_2. Treatment with aspirin significantly reduces the frequency of transient ischemic attacks and the incidence of stroke or myocardial infarcts in high-risk patients. A daily dose of 325 mg is adequate; higher doses may provide added benefit but are associated with a higher incidence of gastrointestinal side effects. Dipyridamole is not as effective, and when added to aspirin does not offer any advantage over aspirin alone for stroke prevention. In patients intolerant of aspirin, ticlopidine (another platelet aggregation inhibitor) may be used in

a dose of 250 mg twice daily, but patients must be monitored closely for the development of neutropenia or agranulocytosis. Some physicians use anticoagulant drugs (eg, warfarin, with temporary heparinization until the dose of warfarin is adequate) unless they are medically contraindicated, continuing them for 3–6 months before they are tapered and ultimately replaced with aspirin, which is continued for another year. However, there is no convincing evidence that anticoagulant drugs are of value.

Surgical extracranial-intracranial arterial anastomosis is generally not helpful in patients with transient ischemic attacks associated with stenotic lesions of the distal internal carotid or the proximal middle cerebral arteries.

Johnston SC et al: Short-term prognosis after emergency department diagnosis of TIA. JAMA 2000;284:2901. [PMID: 11147987] (Clinical study.)

Kelly J et al: Transient ischaemic attacks: under-reported, over-diagnosed, under-treated. Age Ageing 2001;30:379. [PMID: 11709374] (Review.)

STROKE

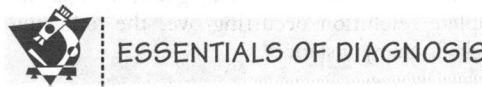 ESSENTIALS OF DIAGNOSIS

- Sudden onset of characteristic neurologic deficit.
- Patient often has history of hypertension, diabetes mellitus, valvular heart disease, or atherosclerosis.
- Distinctive neurologic signs reflect the region of the brain involved.

General Considerations

In the USA, stroke remains the third leading cause of death, despite a general decline in the incidence of stroke in the last 30 years. The precise reasons for this decline are uncertain, but increased awareness of risk factors (hypertension, diabetes, hyperlipidemia, cigarette smoking, cardiac disease, AIDS, recreational drug abuse, heavy alcohol consumption, family history of stroke) and improved prophylactic measures and surveillance of those at increased risk have been contributory. Elevation of the blood homocysteine level is also a risk factor for stroke, but it is unclear whether this risk is reduced by treatment to lower the level. A previous stroke makes individual patients more susceptible to further strokes.

For years, strokes have been subdivided pathologically into infarcts (thrombotic or embolic) and hemorrhages, and clinical criteria for distinguishing between these possibilities have been emphasized. However, it is often difficult to determine on clinical grounds the pathologic basis for stroke.

1. Lacunar Infarction

Lacunar infarcts are small lesions (usually < 5 mm in diameter) that occur in the distribution of short penetrating arterioles in the basal ganglia, pons, cerebellum, anterior limb of the internal capsule, and, less commonly, the deep cerebral white matter. Lacunar infarcts are associated with poorly controlled hypertension or diabetes and have been found in several clinical syndromes, including contralateral pure motor or pure sensory deficit, ipsilateral ataxia with crural paresis, and dysarthria with clumsiness of the hand. The neurologic deficit may progress over 24–36 hours before stabilizing.

Lacunar infarcts are sometimes visible on CT scans as small, punched-out, hypodense areas, but in other patients no abnormality is seen. In some instances, patients with a clinical syndrome suggestive of lacunar infarction are found on CT scanning to have a severe hemispheric infarct.

The prognosis for recovery from the deficit produced by a lacunar infarct is usually good, with partial or complete resolution occurring over the following 4–6 weeks in many instances.

2. Cerebral Infarction

Thrombotic or embolic occlusion of a major vessel leads to cerebral infarction. Causes include the disorders predisposing to transient ischemic attacks (see above) and atherosclerosis of cerebral arteries. The resulting deficit depends upon the particular vessel involved and the extent of any collateral circulation. Cerebral ischemia leads to release of excitatory and other neuropeptides that may augment calcium flux into neurons, thereby leading to cell death and increasing the neurologic deficit.

Clinical Findings

A. SYMPTOMS AND SIGNS

Onset is usually abrupt, and there may then be very little progression except that due to brain swelling. Clinical evaluation always includes examination of the heart and auscultation over the subclavian and carotid vessels to determine whether there are any bruits.

1. Obstruction of carotid circulation—Occlusion of the ophthalmic artery is probably symptomless in most cases because of the rich orbital collaterals, but its transient embolic obstruction leads to amaurosis fugax—sudden and brief loss of vision in one eye.

Occlusion of the anterior cerebral artery distal to its junction with the anterior communicating artery causes weakness and cortical sensory loss in the contralateral leg and sometimes mild weakness of the arm,

especially proximally. There may be a contralateral grasp reflex, paratonic rigidity, and abulia (lack of initiative) or frank confusion. Urinary incontinence is not uncommon, particularly if behavioral disturbances are conspicuous. Bilateral anterior cerebral infarction is especially likely to cause marked behavioral changes and memory disturbances. Unilateral anterior cerebral artery occlusion proximal to the junction with the anterior communicating artery is generally well tolerated because of the collateral supply from the other side.

Middle cerebral artery occlusion leads to contralateral hemiplegia, hemisensory loss, and homonymous hemianopia (ie, bilaterally symmetric loss of vision in half of the visual fields), with the eyes deviated to the side of the lesion. If the dominant hemisphere is involved, global aphasia is also present. It may be impossible to distinguish this clinically from occlusion of the internal carotid artery. With occlusion of either of these arteries, there may also be considerable swelling of the hemisphere, leading to drowsiness, stupor, and coma in extreme cases. Occlusions of different branches of the middle cerebral artery cause more limited findings. For example, involvement of the anterior main division leads to a predominantly expressive dysphasia and to contralateral paralysis and loss of sensations in the arm, the face, and, to a lesser extent, the leg. Posterior branch occlusion produces a receptive (Wernicke's) aphasia and a homonymous visual field defect. With involvement of the nondominant hemisphere, speech and comprehension are preserved, but there may be a confusional state, dressing apraxia, and constructional and spatial deficits.

2. Obstruction of vertebrobasilar circulation—Occlusion of the posterior cerebral artery may lead to a thalamic syndrome in which contralateral hemisensory disturbance occurs, followed by the development of spontaneous pain and hyperpathia. There is often a macular-sparing homonymous hemianopia and sometimes a mild, usually temporary, hemiparesis. Depending on the site of the lesion and the collateral circulation, the severity of these deficits varies and other deficits may also occur, including involuntary movements and alexia. Occlusion of the main artery beyond the origin of its penetrating branches may lead solely to a macular-sparing hemianopia.

Vertebral artery occlusion distally, below the origin of the anterior spinal and posterior inferior cerebellar arteries, may be clinically silent because the circulation is maintained by the other vertebral artery. If the remaining vertebral artery is congenitally small or severely atherosclerotic, however, a deficit similar to that of basilar artery occlusion is seen unless there is good collateral circulation from the anterior circulation through the circle of Willis. When the small paramedian arteries arising from the vertebral artery are occluded, contralateral hemiplegia and sensory deficit occur in association with an ipsilateral cranial nerve palsy at the level of the lesion. An obstruction of the posterior inferior cerebellar artery or an obstruction of the vertebral artery just before it branches to this vessel leads ipsilaterally to spinothalamic sensory loss involving the face, ninth and tenth cranial nerve lesions, limb ataxia and numbness, and Horner's syndrome, combined with contralateral spinothalamic sensory loss involving the limbs.

Occlusion of both vertebral arteries or the basilar artery leads to coma with pinpoint pupils, flaccid quadriplegia and sensory loss, and variable cranial nerve abnormalities. With partial basilar artery occlusion, there may be diplopia, visual loss, vertigo, dysarthria, ataxia, weakness or sensory disturbances in some or all of the limbs, and discrete cranial nerve palsies. In patients with hemiplegia of pontine origin, the eyes are often deviated to the paralyzed side, whereas in patients with a hemispheric lesion, the eyes commonly deviate from the hemiplegic side.

Occlusion of any of the major cerebellar arteries produces vertigo, nausea, vomiting, nystagmus, ipsilateral limb ataxia, and contralateral spinothalamic sensory loss in the limbs. If the superior cerebellar artery is involved, the contralateral spinothalamic loss also involves the face; with occlusion of the anterior inferior cerebellar artery, there is ipsilateral spinothalamic sensory loss involving the face, usually in conjunction with ipsilateral facial weakness and deafness. Massive cerebellar infarction may lead to coma, tonsillar herniation, and death.

3. Coma—Infarction in either the carotid or vertebrobasilar territory may lead to loss of consciousness. For example, an infarct involving one cerebral hemisphere may lead to such swelling that the function of the other hemisphere or the rostral brain stem is disturbed and coma results. Similarly, coma occurs with bilateral brain stem infarction when this involves the reticular formation, and it occurs with brain stem compression after cerebellar infarction.

B. IMAGING

Radiography of the chest may reveal cardiomegaly or valvular calcification; the presence of a neoplasm would suggest that the neurologic deficit is due to metastasis rather than stroke, or rarely to nonbacterial thrombotic endocarditis. A CT scan of the head (without contrast) is important in excluding cerebral hemorrhage, but it may not permit distinction between a cerebral infarct and tumor. CT scanning is preferable to MRI in the acute stage because it is quicker and because intracranial hemorrhage is not easily detected by MRI within the first 48 hours after a bleeding episode. In selected patients, carotid duplex studies, MRI and MR angiography, and conventional angiography may also be necessary. Diffusion-weighted MRI is more sensitive than standard MRI in detecting cerebral ischemia.

C. LABORATORY AND OTHER STUDIES

Investigations should include a complete blood count, sedimentation rate, blood glucose determination, and serologic tests for syphilis. Antiphospholipid antibodies (lupus anticoagulants and anticardiolipin antibodies) promote thrombosis and are associated with an increased incidence of stroke. Similarly, elevated serum cholesterol and lipids and serum homocysteine may indicate an increased risk of thrombotic stroke. Electrocardiography will help exclude a cardiac arrhythmia or recent myocardial infarction that might be serving as a source of embolization. Blood cultures should be performed if endocarditis is suspected, echocardiography if heart disease is suspected, and Holter monitoring if paroxysmal cardiac arrhythmia requires exclusion. Examination of the cerebrospinal fluid is not always necessary but may be helpful if there is diagnostic uncertainty; it should be delayed until after CT scanning.

Treatment

If the neurologic deficit progresses over the following minutes or hours, heparinization may be of value in limiting or arresting further deterioration. Since the signs of progressing stroke may be simulated by an intracerebral hematoma, the latter must be excluded by immediate CT scanning or angiography before the patient is heparinized.

Intravenous thrombolytic therapy with recombinant tissue plasminogen activator (0.9 mg/kg to a maximum of 90 mg, with 10% given as a bolus over 1 minute and the remainder over 1 hour) is effective in reducing the neurologic deficit in selected patients without CT evidence of intracranial hemorrhage when administered within 3 hours after onset of ischemic stroke, but later administration has not been proved effective or safe. Recent hemorrhage, increased risk of hemorrhage (eg, treatment with anticoagulants), arterial puncture at a noncompressible site, and systolic pressure above 185 mm Hg or diastolic pressure above 110 mm Hg are among the contraindications to this treatment. Early management of a completed stroke otherwise consists of attention to general supportive measures. During the acute stage, there may be marked brain swelling and edema, with symptoms and signs of increasing intracranial pressure, an increasing neurologic deficit, or herniation syndrome. Corticosteroids have been prescribed in an attempt to reduce vasogenic cerebral edema. Prednisone (up to 100 mg/d) or dexamethasone (16 mg/d) has been used, but the evidence that corticosteroids are of any benefit is conflicting. Dehydrating hyperosmolar agents have also been prescribed in efforts to reduce brain swelling, but there is little evidence of any lasting benefit. Likewise, clinical benefit from treatment with vasodilators such as papaverine is minimal. Neither hypercapnia nor hypocapnia has been shown to have any benefit. Barbiturates are known to decrease neuronal metabolism and energy requirements and have been reported to improve functional recovery in experimental stroke models; their use in humans, however, is experimental. Attempts to lower the blood pressure of hypertensive patients during the acute phase (ie, within 2 weeks) of a stroke should generally be avoided, as there is loss of cerebral autoregulation and lowering the blood pressure may further compromise ischemic areas. However, if the systolic pressure exceeds 200 mm Hg, it can be lowered with continuous monitoring to 170–200 mm Hg and then, after 2 weeks, the blood pressure reduced further to less than 140/90 mm Hg.

Anticoagulant drugs should be started when there is a cardiac source of embolization. Treatment is with intravenous heparin while warfarin is introduced. The target is an INR of 2–3 for the prothrombin time. If the CT scan shows no evidence of hemorrhage and the cerebrospinal fluid is clear, anticoagulant treatment may be started without delay. Some physicians prefer to wait for 2 or 3 days before initiating anticoagulant treatment; the CT scan is then repeated and anticoagulant therapy is initiated if it again shows no evidence of hemorrhagic transformation.

Physical therapy has an important role in the management of patients with impaired motor function. Passive movements at an early stage will help prevent contractures. As cooperation increases and some recovery begins, active movements will improve strength and coordination. In all cases, early mobilization and active rehabilitation are important. Occupational therapy may improve morale and motor skills, while speech therapy may be beneficial in patients with expressive dysphasia or dysarthria. When there is a severe and persisting motor deficit, a device such as a leg brace, toe spring, frame, or cane may help the patient move about, and the provision of other aids to daily living may improve the quality of life.

Prognosis

The prognosis for survival after cerebral infarction is better than after cerebral or subarachnoid hemorrhage. The only proved effective therapy for acute stroke requires initiation within 3 hours after stroke onset, and the prognosis therefore depends on the time that elapses before arrival at the hospital. Patients receiving such treatment with tissue plasminogen activator are at least 30% more likely to have minimal or no disability at 3 months than those not treated by this means. Loss of consciousness after a cerebral infarct implies a poorer prognosis than otherwise. The extent of the infarct governs the potential for rehabilitation. Patients who have had a cerebral infarct are at risk for further strokes and for myocardial infarcts. Statin therapy to lower serum lipid levels may reduce this risk. Antiplatelet therapy reduces the recurrence rate by 30% among patients without a cardiac cause for the stroke who are not candidates for carotid endarterectomy. Nevertheless, the cumulative risk of recurrence of noncardioembolic stroke is still 3–7% annually. A 2-year comparison did not show benefit of warfarin (INR 1.4–2.8) over aspirin (325 mg daily),

and higher doses of warfarin should be avoided as they lead to an increased incidence of major bleeding. Patients with massive strokes from which meaningful recovery is unlikely should receive palliative care (Chapter 5).

Albers GW et al: Intravenous tissue-type plasminogen activator for treatment of acute stroke: the Standard Treatment with Alteplase to Reverse Stroke (STARS) study. JAMA 2000;283:1145. [PMID: 10703776]

Callahan A: Cerebrovascular disease and statins: a potential addition to the therapeutic armamentarium from stroke prevention. Am J Cardiol 2001;88;33J. [PMID: 11595197] (Review.)

JAMA patient page: Stroke. JAMA 1999;281:1146. [PMID: 10188669]

Mohr JP et al: A comparison of warfarin and aspirin for the prevention of recurrent ischemic stroke. N Engl J Med 2001;345:1444. [PMID: 11794192] (Clinical trial.)

Powers WJ: Oral anticoagulant therapy for the prevention of stroke. N Engl J Med 2001;345:1493. [PMID: 11794201] (Review.)

Sacco RL: Identifying patient populations at high risk for stroke. Neurology 1998;51(3 Suppl 3):S27. [PMID: 9744829]

3. Intracerebral Hemorrhage

Spontaneous intracerebral hemorrhage in patients with no angiographic evidence of an associated vascular anomaly (eg, aneurysm or angioma) is usually due to hypertension. The pathologic basis for hemorrhage is probably the presence of microaneurysms that develop on perforating vessels of 100–300 μm in diameter in hypertensive patients. Hypertensive intracerebral hemorrhage occurs most frequently in the basal ganglia and less commonly in the pons, thalamus, cerebellum, and cerebral white matter. Hemorrhage may extend into the ventricular system or subarachnoid space, and signs of meningeal irritation are then found. Hemorrhages usually occur suddenly and without warning, often during activity.

In addition to its association with hypertension, nontraumatic intracerebral hemorrhage may occur with hematologic and bleeding disorders (eg, leukemia, thrombocytopenia, hemophilia, or disseminated intravascular coagulation), anticoagulant therapy, liver disease, cerebral amyloid angiopathy, and primary or secondary brain tumors. Bleeding is primarily into the subarachnoid space when it occurs from an intracranial aneurysm or arteriovenous malformation (see below), but it may be partly intraparenchymal as well. In some cases, no specific cause for cerebral hemorrhage can be identified.

Clinical Findings

A. SYMPTOMS AND SIGNS

With hemorrhage into the cerebral hemisphere, consciousness is initially lost or impaired in about one-half of patients. Vomiting occurs very frequently at the onset of bleeding, and headache is sometimes present. Focal symptoms and signs then develop, depending on the site of the hemorrhage. With hypertensive hemorrhage, there is generally a rapidly evolving neurologic deficit with hemiplegia or hemiparesis. A hemisensory disturbance is also present with more deeply placed lesions. With lesions of the putamen, loss of conjugate lateral gaze may be conspicuous. With thalamic hemorrhage, there may be a loss of upward gaze, downward or skew deviation of the eyes, lateral gaze palsies, and pupillary inequalities.

Cerebellar hemorrhage may present with sudden onset of nausea and vomiting, disequilibrium, headache, and loss of consciousness that may terminate fatally within 48 hours. Less commonly, the onset is gradual and the course episodic or slowly progressive—clinical features suggesting an expanding cerebellar lesion. In yet other cases, however, the onset and course are intermediate, and examination shows lateral conjugate gaze palsies to the side of the lesion; small reactive pupils; contralateral hemiplegia; peripheral facial weakness; ataxia of gait, limbs, or trunk; periodic respiration; or some combination of these findings.

B. IMAGING

CT scanning (without contrast) is important not only in confirming that hemorrhage has occurred but also in determining the size and site of the hematoma. It is superior to MRI for detecting intracranial hemorrhage of less than 48 hours duration. If the patient's condition permits further intervention, cerebral angiography may be undertaken thereafter to determine if an aneurysm or arteriovenous malformation is present (see below).

C. LABORATORY AND OTHER STUDIES

A complete blood count, platelet count, bleeding time, prothrombin and partial thromboplastin times, and liver and renal function tests may reveal a predisposing cause for the hemorrhage. Lumbar puncture is contraindicated because it may precipitate a herniation syndrome in patients with a large hematoma, and CT scanning is superior in detecting intracerebral hemorrhage.

Treatment

Neurologic management is generally conservative and supportive, regardless of whether the patient has a profound deficit with associated brain stem compression, in which case the prognosis is grim, or a more localized deficit not causing increased intracranial pressure or brain stem involvement. Decompression is helpful, however, when a superficial hematoma in cerebral white matter is exerting a mass effect and causing incipient herniation. In patients with cerebellar hemorrhage, prompt surgical evacuation of the hematoma is appropriate, because spontaneous unpredictable deterioration may otherwise lead to a fatal outcome and because operative treatment may lead to complete res-

olution of the clinical deficit. The treatment of underlying structural lesions or bleeding disorders depends upon their nature.

Hill MD et al: Rate of stroke recurrence in patients with primary intracerebral hemorrhage. Stroke 2000;31:123. [PMID: 10625726] (Clinical study.)

4. Subarachnoid Hemorrhage

Between 5% and 10% of strokes are due to subarachnoid hemorrhage. Although hemorrhage is usually from rupture of an aneurysm or arteriovenous malformation, no specific cause can be found in 20% of cases.

Clinical Findings

A. SYMPTOMS AND SIGNS

Subarachnoid hemorrhage has a characteristic clinical picture. Its onset is with sudden headache of a severity never experienced previously by the patient. This may be followed by nausea and vomiting and by a loss or impairment of consciousness that can either be transient or progress inexorably to deepening coma and death. If consciousness is regained, the patient is often confused and irritable and may show other symptoms of an altered mental status. Neurologic examination generally reveals nuchal rigidity and other signs of meningeal irritation, except in deeply comatose patients. A focal neurologic deficit is occasionally present and may suggest the site of the underlying lesion.

B. IMAGING

A CT scan should be performed immediately to confirm that hemorrhage has occurred and to search for clues regarding its source. It is preferable to MRI because it is faster and more sensitive in detecting hemorrhage in the first 24 hours. CT findings sometimes are normal in patients with suspected hemorrhage, and the cerebrospinal fluid must then be examined for the presence of blood or xanthochromia before the possibility of subarachnoid hemorrhage is discounted.

Cerebral arteriography may be undertaken to determine the source of bleeding; it is not performed unless or until the patient's condition has stabilized and is good enough so that operative treatment is feasible. In general, bilateral carotid and vertebral arteriography are necessary because aneurysms are often multiple, while arteriovenous malformations may be supplied from several sources. MR angiography may also permit these vascular anomalies to be visualized but is less sensitive than conventional arteriography.

Treatment

The measures outlined below in the section on stupor and coma are applied to comatose patients. Conscious patients are confined to bed, advised against any exertion or straining, treated symptomatically for headache and anxiety, and given laxatives or stool softeners. If there is severe hypertension, the blood pressure can be lowered gradually, but not below a diastolic level of 100 mm Hg. Phenytoin is generally prescribed routinely to prevent seizures. Further comment concerning the specific operative management of arteriovenous malformations and aneurysms follows.

Johnston SC et al: The burden, trends, and demographics of mortality from subarachnoid hemorrhage. Neurology 1998; 50:1413. [PMID: 9595997]

5. Intracranial Aneurysm

Saccular aneurysms ("berry" aneurysms) tend to occur at arterial bifurcations, are frequently multiple (20% of cases), and are usually asymptomatic. They may be associated with polycystic kidney disease and coarctation of the aorta. Risk factors for aneurysm formation include smoking, hypertension, and hypercholesterolemia. Most aneurysms are located on the anterior part of the circle of Willis—particularly on the anterior or posterior communicating arteries, at the bifurcation of the middle cerebral artery, and at the bifurcation of the internal carotid artery.

Clinical Findings

A. SYMPTOMS AND SIGNS

Aneurysms may cause a focal neurologic deficit by compressing adjacent structures. However, most are asymptomatic or produce only nonspecific symptoms until they rupture, at which time subarachnoid hemorrhage results. There is often a paucity of focal neurologic signs in patients with subarachnoid hemorrhage, but when present, such signs may relate either to a focal hematoma or to ischemia in the territory of the vessel with the ruptured aneurysm. Hemiplegia or other focal deficit sometimes occurs after a delay of 4–14 days and is due to focal arterial spasm in the vicinity of the ruptured aneurysm. This spasm is of uncertain, probably multifactorial, cause, but it sometimes leads to significant cerebral ischemia or infarction, and it may further aggravate any existing increase in intracranial pressure. Subacute hydrocephalus due to interference with the flow of cerebrospinal fluid may occur after 2 or more weeks, and this leads to a delayed clinical deterioration that is relieved by shunting.

In some patients, "warning leaks" of a small amount of blood from the aneurysm precede the major hemorrhage by a few hours or days. They lead to headaches, sometimes accompanied by nausea and neck stiffness, but the true cause of these symptoms is often not appreciated until massive hemorrhage occurs.

B. IMAGING

The CT scan generally confirms that subarachnoid hemorrhage has occurred, but occasionally it is normal.

Angiography (bilateral carotid and vertebral studies) generally indicates the size and site of the lesion, sometimes reveals multiple aneurysms, and may show arterial spasm. If subarachnoid hemorrhage is confirmed by lumbar puncture or CT scanning but arteriograms show no abnormality, the examination should be repeated after 2 weeks, because vasospasm may have prevented detection of an aneurysm during the initial study.

C. LABORATORY AND OTHER STUDIES

The cerebrospinal fluid is bloodstained. The electroencephalogram sometimes indicates the side or site of hemorrhage but frequently shows only a diffuse abnormality. Electrocardiographic evidence of arrhythmias or myocardial ischemia has been well described and probably relates to excessive sympathetic activity. Peripheral leukocytosis and transient glycosuria are also common findings.

Treatment

The major aim of treatment is to prevent further hemorrhages. Definitive treatment requires a surgical approach to the aneurysm and ideally consists of clipping of its base. Alternatively, endovascular treatment (coil embolization) by interventional radiologists may be undertaken and is sometimes feasible even for inoperable aneurysms. Otherwise, medical management as outlined above for subarachnoid hemorrhage is continued for about 6 weeks and is followed by gradual mobilization.

The risk of further hemorrhage is greatest within a few days of the first hemorrhage; approximately 20% of patients will have further bleeding within 2 weeks and 40% within 6 months. Attempts have been made to reduce this risk pharmacologically. Treatment with an antifibrinolytic agent such as aminocaproic acid during the first 14 days reduces the risk of recurrent hemorrhage but is associated with such an increase in cerebral ischemic complications that the mortality rate and the degree of disability among survivors are unchanged. Thus, early operation (ie, within about 2 days of hemorrhage) is preferred for good operative candidates.

Calcium channel-blocking agents have helped to reduce or reverse experimental vasospasm, and nimodipine has been shown to reduce, in neurologically normal patients, the incidence of ischemic deficits from arterial spasm without producing any side effects. The dose of nimodipine is 60 mg every 4 hours for 21 days. After surgical obliteration of any aneurysms, symptomatic vasospasm may also be treated by intravascular volume expansion, induced hypertension, or transluminal balloon angioplasty of involved intracranial vessels.

With regard to unruptured aneurysms, those that are symptomatic merit prompt treatment, either surgically or by endovascular coil embolization, whereas small asymptomatic ones discovered incidentally are often followed arteriographically and corrected surgically only if they increase in size to over 10 mm. The natural history of unruptured aneurysms is not clearly defined.

Connolly ES et al: Management of symptomatic and asymptomatic unruptured aneurysms. Neurosurg Clin North Am 1998;9:509. [PMID: 9668183] (Literature review.)

International Study of Unruptured Intracranial Aneurysms Investigators: Unruptured intracranial aneurysms: Risks of rupture and risks of surgical intervention. N Engl J Med 1998;339:1725. [PMID: 9867550] (Multicenter study.)

Johnston SC et al: Which unruptured cerebral aneurysms should be treated? A cost-utility analysis. Neurology 1999;52:1806. [PMID: 10371527] (Cost-utility analysis.)

Polin RS et al: Efficacy of transluminal angioplasty for the management of symptomatic cerebral vasospasm following aneurysmal subarachnoid hemorrhage. J Neurosurg 2000;92:284. [PMID: 10659016] (Clinical study.)

Wardlaw JM et al: The detection and management of unruptured intracranial aneurysms. Brain 2000;123:205. [PMID: 10648430] (Clinical review.)

6. Arteriovenous Malformations

Arteriovenous malformations are congenital vascular malformations that result from a localized maldevelopment of part of the primitive vascular plexus and consist of abnormal arteriovenous communications without intervening capillaries. They vary in size, ranging from massive lesions that are fed by multiple vessels and involve a large part of the brain to lesions so small that they are hard to identify at arteriography, surgery, or autopsy. In approximately 10% of cases, there is an associated arterial aneurysm, while 1–2% of patients presenting with aneurysms have associated arteriovenous malformations. Clinical presentation may relate to hemorrhage from the malformation or an associated aneurysm or may relate to cerebral ischemia due to diversion of blood by the anomalous arteriovenous shunt or due to venous stagnation. Regional maldevelopment of the brain, compression or distortion of adjacent cerebral tissue by enlarged anomalous vessels, and progressive gliosis due to mechanical and ischemic factors may also be contributory. In addition, communicating or obstructive hydrocephalus may occur and lead to symptoms.

Clinical Findings

A. Symptoms and Signs

1. Supratentorial lesions—Most cerebral arteriovenous malformations are supratentorial, usually lying in the territory of the middle cerebral artery. Initial symptoms consist of hemorrhage in 30–60% of cases, recurrent seizures in 20–40%, headache in 5–25%, and miscellaneous complaints (including focal deficits) in 10–15%. Up to 70% of arteriovenous malformations bleed at some point in their natural history, most commonly before the patient reaches the age of 40 years. This tendency to bleed is unrelated to the le-

sion site or to the patient's sex, but small arteriovenous malformations are more likely to bleed than large ones. Arteriovenous malformations that have bled once are more likely to bleed again. Hemorrhage is commonly intracerebral as well as into the subarachnoid space, and it has a fatal outcome in about 10% of cases. Focal or generalized seizures may accompany or follow hemorrhage, or they may be the initial presentation, especially with frontal or parietal arteriovenous malformations. Headaches are especially likely when the external carotid arteries are involved in the malformation. These sometimes simulate migraine but more commonly are nonspecific in character, with nothing about them to suggest an underlying structural lesion.

In patients presenting with subarachnoid hemorrhage, examination may reveal an abnormal mental status and signs of meningeal irritation. Additional findings may help to localize the lesion and sometimes indicate that intracranial pressure is increased. A cranial bruit always suggests the possibility of a cerebral arteriovenous malformation, but bruits may also be found with aneurysms, meningiomas, acquired arteriovenous fistulas, and arteriovenous malformations involving the scalp, calvarium, or orbit. Bruits are best heard over the ipsilateral eye or mastoid region and are of some help in lateralization but of no help in localization. Absence of a bruit in no way excludes the possibility of arteriovenous malformation.

2. Infratentorial lesions—Brain stem arteriovenous malformations are often clinically silent, but they may hemorrhage, cause obstructive hydrocephalus, or lead to progressive or relapsing brain stem deficits. Cerebellar arteriovenous malformations may also be clinically inconspicuous but sometimes lead to cerebellar hemorrhage.

B. Imaging

In patients presenting with suspected hemorrhage, CT scanning indicates whether subarachnoid or intracerebral bleeding has recently occurred, helps to localize its source, and may reveal the arteriovenous malformation. If the CT scan shows no evidence of bleeding but subarachnoid hemorrhage is diagnosed clinically, the cerebrospinal fluid should be examined.

When intracranial hemorrhage is confirmed but the source of hemorrhage is not evident on the CT scan, arteriography is necessary to exclude aneurysm or arteriovenous malformation. MR angiography is not sensitive enough for this purpose. Even if the findings on CT scan suggest arteriovenous malformation, arteriography is required to establish the nature of the lesion with certainty and to determine its anatomic features so that treatment can be planned. The examination must generally include bilateral opacification of the internal and external carotid arteries and the vertebral arteries. Arteriovenous malformations typically appear as a tangled vascular mass with distended tortuous afferent and efferent vessels, a rapid circulation time, and arteriovenous shunting. Findings on plain radiographs of the skull are often normal unless an intracerebral hematoma is present, in which case there may be changes suggestive of raised intracranial pressure and displacement of a calcified pineal gland.

In patients presenting without hemorrhage, CT scan or MRI usually reveals the underlying abnormality, and MRI frequently also shows evidence of old or recent hemorrhage that may have been asymptomatic. The nature and detailed anatomy of any focal lesion identified by these means is delineated by angiography, especially if operative treatment is under consideration.

C. LABORATORY AND OTHER STUDIES

Electroencephalography is usually indicated in patients presenting with seizures and may show consistently focal or lateralized abnormalities resulting from the underlying cerebral arteriovenous malformation. This should be followed by CT scanning.

Treatment

Surgical treatment to prevent further hemorrhage is justified in patients with arteriovenous malformations that have bled, provided that the lesion is accessible and the patient has a reasonable life expectancy. Surgical treatment is also appropriate if intracranial pressure is increased and to prevent further progression of a focal neurologic deficit. In patients presenting solely with seizures, anticonvulsant drug treatment is usually sufficient, and operative treatment is unnecessary unless there are further developments.

Definitive operative treatment consists of excision of the arteriovenous malformation if it is surgically accessible. Arteriovenous malformations that are inoperable because of their location are sometimes treated solely by embolization; although the risk of hemorrhage is not reduced, neurologic deficits may be stabilized or even reversed by this procedure. Two other techniques for the treatment of intracerebral arteriovenous malformations are injection of a vascular occlusive polymer through a flow-guided microcatheter and permanent occlusion of feeding vessels by positioning detachable balloon catheters in the desired sites and then inflating them with quickly solidifying contrast material. Stereotactic radiosurgery with the gamma knife is also useful in the management of inoperable cerebral arteriovenous malformations.

Al-Shahi R et al: A systematic review of the frequency and prognosis of arteriovenous malformations of the brain in adults. Brain 2001;124:1900. [PMID: 11571210] (Review.)

Ogilvy CS et al: AHA Scientific Statement: recommendations for the management of intracranial arteriovenous malformations. Stroke 2001;32:1458. [PMID: 11387517] (Practice guideline.)

7. Intracranial Venous Thrombosis

Intracranial venous thrombosis may occur in association with intracranial or maxillofacial infections, hypercoagulable states, polycythemia, sickle cell disease, and cyanotic congenital heart disease and in pregnancy or during the puerperium. It is characterized by headache, focal or generalized convulsions, drowsiness, confusion, increased intracranial pressure, and focal neurologic deficits—and sometimes by evidence of meningeal irritation. The diagnosis is confirmed by CT scanning and MRI, MR venography, or angiography.

Treatment includes anticonvulsant drugs if seizures have occurred and antiedema agents (eg, dexamethasone, 4 mg four times daily and continued as necessary) to reduce intracranial pressure. Anticoagulation with dose-adjusted intravenous heparin followed by oral anticoagulation for 6 months reduces morbidity and mortality of venous sinus thrombosis.

8. Spinal Cord Vascular Diseases
Infarction of the Spinal Cord

Infarction of the spinal cord is rare. It occurs only in the territory of the anterior spinal artery because this vessel, which supplies the anterior two-thirds of the cord, is itself supplied by only a limited number of feeders. Infarction usually results from interrupted flow in one or more of these feeders, eg, with aortic dissection, aortography, polyarteritis, or severe hypotension, or after surgical resection of the thoracic aorta. The paired posterior spinal arteries, by contrast, are supplied by numerous arteries at different levels of the cord.

Since the anterior spinal artery receives numerous feeders in the cervical region, infarcts almost always occur caudally. Clinical presentation is characterized by acute onset of flaccid, areflexive paraplegia that evolves after a few days or weeks into a spastic paraplegia with extensor plantar responses. There is an accompanying dissociated sensory loss, with impairment of appreciation of pain and temperature but preservation of sensations of vibration and position. Treatment is symptomatic.

Goodin DS: Neurological complications of aortic disease and surgery. In: *Neurology and General Medicine,* 3rd ed. Aminoff MJ (editor). Churchill Livingstone, 2001. (Clinical review.)

Epidural or Subdural Hemorrhage

Epidural or subdural hemorrhage may lead to sudden severe back pain followed by an acute compressive myelopathy necessitating urgent myelography and surgical evacuation. It may occur in patients with bleeding disorders or those who are taking anticoagulant drugs, sometimes following trauma or lumbar puncture. Epidural hemorrhage may also be related to a vascular malformation or tumor deposit.

Arteriovenous Malformation of the Spinal Cord

Arteriovenous malformations of the cord are congenital lesions that present with spinal subarachnoid hemorrhage or myeloradiculopathy. Since most of these malformations are located in the thoracolumbar region, they lead to motor and sensory disturbances in the legs and to sphincter disorders. Pain in the legs or back is often severe. Examination reveals an upper, lower, or mixed motor deficit in the legs; sensory deficits are also present and are usually extensive, although occasionally they are confined to radicular distribution. Cervical arteriovenous malformations lead also to symptoms and signs in the arms. Spinal MRI may not detect the arteriovenous malformation, and negative findings do not exclude the diagnosis. In general, the diagnosis is suggested at myelography (performed with the patient prone and supine) when serpiginous filling defects due to enlarged vessels are found. Selective spinal arteriography confirms the diagnosis. Most lesions are extramedullary, are posterior to the cord (lying either intra- or extradurally), and can easily be treated by ligation of feeding vessels and excision of the fistulous anomaly or by embolization procedures. Delay in treatment may lead to increased and irreversible disability or to death from recurrent subarachnoid hemorrhage.

INTRACRANIAL & SPINAL SPACE-OCCUPYING LESIONS

1. Primary Intracranial Tumors

ESSENTIALS OF DIAGNOSIS

- Generalized or focal disturbance of cerebral function, or both.
- Increased intracranial pressure in some patients.
- Neuroradiologic evidence of space-occupying lesion.

General Considerations

Half of all primary intracranial neoplasms (Table 24–3) are gliomas and the remainder meningiomas, pituitary adenomas, neurofibromas, and other tumors. Certain tumors, especially neurofibromas, hemangioblastomas, and retinoblastomas, may have a familial basis, and congenital factors bear on the development of craniopharyngiomas. Tumors may occur at any age, but certain gliomas show particular age predilections (Table 24–3).

Clinical Findings

A. SYMPTOMS AND SIGNS

Intracranial tumors may lead to a generalized disturbance of cerebral function and to symptoms and signs of increased intracranial pressure. In consequence, there may be personality changes, intellectual decline, emotional lability, seizures, headaches, nausea, and malaise. If the pressure is increased in a particular cranial compartment, brain tissue may herniate into a compartment with lower pressure. The most familiar syndrome is herniation of the temporal lobe uncus through the tentorial hiatus, which causes compression of the third cranial nerve, midbrain, and posterior cerebral artery. The earliest sign of this is ipsilateral pupillary dilation, followed by stupor, coma, decerebrate posturing, and respiratory arrest. Another important herniation syndrome consists of displacement of the cerebellar tonsils through the foramen magnum, which causes medullary compression leading to apnea, circulatory collapse, and death. Other herniation syndromes are less common and of less clear clinical importance.

Intracranial tumors also lead to focal deficits depending on their location.

1. Frontal lobe lesions—Tumors of the frontal lobe often lead to progressive intellectual decline, slowing of mental activity, personality changes, and contralateral grasp reflexes. They may lead to expressive aphasia if the posterior part of the left inferior frontal gyrus is involved. Anosmia may also occur as a consequence of pressure on the olfactory nerve. Precentral lesions may cause focal motor seizures or contralateral pyramidal deficits.

2. Temporal lobe lesions—Tumors of the uncinate region may be manifested by seizures with olfactory or gustatory hallucinations, motor phenomena such as licking or smacking of the lips, and some impairment of external awareness without actual loss of consciousness. Temporal lobe lesions also lead to depersonalization, emotional changes, behavioral disturbances, sensations of déjà vu or jamais vu, micropsia or macropsia (objects appear smaller or larger than they are), visual field defects (crossed upper quadrantanopia), and auditory illusions or hallucinations. Left-sided lesions may lead to dysnomia and receptive aphasia, while right-sided involvement sometimes disturbs the perception of musical notes and melodies.

3. Parietal lobe lesions—Tumors in this location characteristically cause contralateral disturbances of sensation and may cause sensory seizures, sensory loss or inattention, or some combination of these symptoms. The sensory loss is cortical in type and involves postural sensibility and tactile discrimination, so that the appreciation of shape, size, weight, and texture is impaired. Objects placed in the hand may not be recognized (astereognosis). Extensive parietal lobe lesions may produce contralateral hyperpathia and spontaneous pain (thalamic syndrome). Involvement of the optic radiation leads to a contralateral homonymous field defect that sometimes consists solely of lower quadrantanopia. Lesions of the left angular gyrus cause Gerstmann's syndrome (a combination of alexia, agraphia, acalculia, right-left confusion, and finger agnosia), whereas involvement of the left submarginal gyrus causes ideational apraxia. Anosognosia (the denial, neglect, or rejection of a paralyzed limb) is seen in patients with lesions of the nondominant (right)

Table 24–3. Primary intracranial tumors.

Tumor	Clinical Features	Treatment and Prognosis
Glioblastoma multiforme	Presents commonly with nonspecific complaints and increased intracranial pressure. As it grows, focal deficits develop.	Course is rapidly progressive, with poor prognosis. Total surgical removal is usually not possible. Radiation therapy and chemotherapy may prolong survival.
Astrocytoma	Presentation similar to glioblastoma multiforme but course more protracted, often over several years. Cerebellar astrocytoma may have a more benign course.	Prognosis is variable. By the time of diagnosis, total excision is usually impossible; tumor often is not radiosensitive. In cerebellar astrocytoma, total surgical removal is often possible.
Medulloblastoma	Seen most frequently in children. Generally arises from roof of fourth ventricle and leads to increased intracranial pressure accompanied by brainstem and cerebellar signs. May seed subarachnoid space.	Treatment consists of surgery combined with radiation therapy and chemotherapy.
Ependymoma	Glioma arising from the ependyma of a ventricle, especially the fourth ventricle; leads early to signs of increased intracranial pressure. Arises also from central canal of cord.	Tumor is not radiosensitive and is best treated surgically if possible.
Oligodendroglioma	Slow-growing. Usually arises in cerebral hemisphere in adults. Calcification may be visible on skull x-ray.	Treatment is surgical and usually successful.
Brain stem glioma	Presents during childhood with cranial nerve palsies and then with long tract signs in the limbs. Signs of increased intracranial pressure occur late.	Tumor is inoperable; treatment is by irradiation and shunt for increased intracranial pressure.
Cerebellar hemangioblastoma	Presents with dysequilibrium, ataxia of trunk or limbs, and signs of increased intracranial pressure. Sometimes familial. May be associated with retinal and spinal vascular lesions, polycythemia, and renal cell carcinoma.	Treatment is surgical.
Pineal tumor	Presents with increased intracranial pressure, sometimes associated with impaired upward gaze (Parinaud's syndrome) and other deficits indicative of midbrain lesion.	Ventricular decompression by shunting is followed by surgical approach to tumor; irradiation is indicated if tumor is malignant. Prognosis depends on histopathologic findings and extent of tumor.
Craniopharyngioma	Originates from remnants of Rathke's pouch above the sella, depressing the optic chiasm. May present at any age but usually in childhood, with endocrine dysfunction and bitemporal field defects.	Treatment is surgical, but total removal may not be possible.
Acoustic neurinoma	Ipsilateral hearing loss is most common initial symptom. Subsequent symptoms may include tinnitus, headache, vertigo, facial weakness or numbness, and long tract signs. (May be familial and bilateral when related to neurofibromatosis.) Most sensitive screening tests are MRI and brainstem auditory evoked potential.	Treatment is excision by translabyrinthine surgery, craniectomy, or a combined approach. Outcome is usually good.
Meningioma	Originates from the dura mater or arachnoid; compresses rather than invades adjacent neural structures. Increasingly common with advancing age. Tumor size varies greatly. Symptoms vary with tumor site—eg, unilateral exophthalmos (sphenoidal ridge); anosmia and optic nerve compression (olfactory groove). Tumor is usually benign and readily detected by CT scanning; may lead to calcification and bone erosion visible on plain x-rays of skull.	Treatment is surgical. Tumor may recur if removal is incomplete.
Primary cerebral lymphoma	Associated with AIDS and other immunodeficient states. Presentation may be with focal deficits or with disturbances of cognition and consciousness. May be indistinguishable from cerebral toxoplasmosis.	Treatment is by whole brain irradiation; chemotherapy may have an adjunctive role. Prognosis depends upon CD4 count at diagnosis.

hemisphere. Constructional apraxia and dressing apraxia may also occur with right-sided lesions.

4. Occipital lobe lesions—Tumors of the occipital lobe characteristically produce crossed homonymous hemianopia or a partial field defect. With left-sided or bilateral lesions, there may be visual agnosia both for objects and for colors, while irritative lesions on either side can cause unformed visual hallucinations. Bilateral occipital lobe involvement causes cortical blindness in which there is preservation of pupillary responses to light and lack of awareness of the defect by the patient. There may also be loss of color perception, prosopagnosia (inability to identify a familiar face), simultagnosia (inability to integrate and interpret a composite scene as opposed to its individual elements), and Balint's syndrome (failure to turn the eyes to a particular point in space, despite preservation of spontaneous and reflex eye movements). The denial of blindness or a field defect constitutes Anton's syndrome.

5. Brain stem and cerebellar lesions—Brain stem lesions lead to cranial nerve palsies, ataxia, incoordination, nystagmus, and pyramidal and sensory deficits in the limbs on one or both sides. Intrinsic brain stem tumors, such as gliomas, tend to produce an increase in intracranial pressure only late in their course. Cerebellar tumors produce marked ataxia of the trunk if the vermis cerebelli is involved and ipsilateral appendicular deficits (ataxia, incoordination and hypotonia of the limbs) if the cerebellar hemispheres are affected.

6. False localizing signs—Tumors may lead to neurologic signs other than by direct compression or infiltration, thereby leading to errors of clinical localization. These false localizing signs include third or sixth nerve palsy and bilateral extensor plantar responses produced by herniation syndromes, and an extensor plantar response occurring ipsilateral to a hemispheric tumor as a result of compression of the opposite cerebral peduncle against the tentorium.

B. IMAGING

CT scanning or MRI with gadolinium enhancement may detect the lesion and may also define its location, shape, and size; the extent to which normal anatomy is distorted; and the degree of any associated cerebral edema or mass effect. CT scanning is less helpful with tumors in the posterior fossa, but MRI is of particular value there. The characteristic appearance of meningiomas on CT scanning is virtually diagnostic; ie, a lesion in a typical site (parasagittal and sylvian regions, olfactory groove, sphenoidal ridge, tuberculum sellae) that appears as a homogeneous area of increased density in noncontrast CT scans and enhances uniformly with contrast.

Arteriography may show stretching or displacement of normal cerebral vessels by the tumor and the presence of tumor vascularity. The presence of an avascular mass is a nonspecific finding that could be due to tumor, hematoma, abscess, or any space-occupying lesion. In patients with normal hormone levels

and an intrasellar mass, angiography is necessary to distinguish with confidence between a pituitary adenoma and an arterial aneurysm.

C. LABORATORY AND OTHER STUDIES

The electroencephalogram provides supporting information concerning cerebral function and may show either a focal disturbance due to the neoplasm or a more diffuse change reflecting altered mental status. Lumbar puncture is rarely necessary; the findings are seldom diagnostic, and the procedure carries the risk of causing a herniation syndrome.

Treatment

Treatment depends on the type and site of the tumor (Table 24–3) and the condition of the patient. Complete surgical removal may be possible if the tumor is extra-axial (eg, meningioma, acoustic neuroma) or is not in a critical or inaccessible region of the brain (eg, cerebellar hemangioblastoma). Surgery also permits the diagnosis to be verified and may be beneficial in reducing intracranial pressure and relieving symptoms even if the neoplasm cannot be completely removed. Clinical deficits are sometimes due in part to obstructive hydrocephalus, in which case simple surgical shunting procedures often produce dramatic benefit. In patients with malignant gliomas, radiation therapy increases median survival rates regardless of any preceding surgery, and its combination with chemotherapy provides additional benefit. Indications for irradiation in the treatment of patients with other primary intracranial neoplasms depend upon tumor type and accessibility and the feasibility of complete surgical removal. Corticosteroids help reduce cerebral edema and are usually started before surgery. Herniation is treated with intravenous dexamethasone (10–20 mg as a bolus, followed by 4 mg every 6 hours) and intravenous mannitol (20% solution given in a dose of 1.5 g/kg over about 30 minutes). Anticonvulsants are also commonly administered in standard doses (Table 24–2). For those patients whose disease deteriorates despite treatment, palliative care is important (Chapter 5).

Akinwunmi J et al: Understanding cerebral tumours. Practitioner 2001;245:494. [PMID: 11436261] (Review.)

DeAngelis LM et al: Malignant glioma: who benefits from adjuvant chemotherapy. Ann Neurol 1998;44:691. [PMID: 10371527]

Hall WA: Targeted toxin therapy for malignant astrocytoma. Neurosurgery 2000;46:544. [PMID: 10719849] (Review.)

Pech IV et al: Chemotherapy for brain tumors. Oncology 1998; 12:537. [PMID: 9575527]

2. Metastatic Intracranial Tumors

Cerebral Metastases

Metastatic brain tumors present in the same way as other cerebral neoplasms, ie, with increased intracranial pressure, with focal or diffuse disturbance of cerebral function, or with both of these manifestations. Indeed, in patients with a single cerebral lesion, the metastatic nature of the lesion may only become evident on histopathologic examination. In other patients, there is evidence of widespread metastatic disease, or an isolated cerebral metastasis develops during treatment of the primary neoplasm.

The most common source of intracranial metastasis is carcinoma of the lung; other primary sites are the breast, kidney, and gastrointestinal tract. Most cerebral metastases are located supratentorially. Laboratory and radiologic studies used to evaluate patients with metastases are those described for primary neoplasms. They include MRI and CT scanning performed both with and without contrast material. Lumbar puncture is necessary only in patients with suspected carcinomatous meningitis (see below). In patients with verified cerebral metastasis from an unknown primary, investigation is guided by symptoms and signs. In women, mammography is indicated; in men under 50, germ cell origin is sought since both have therapeutic implications.

In patients with only a single cerebral metastasis who are otherwise well, it may be possible to remove the lesion and then treat with irradiation; the latter may also be selected as the sole treatment. In patients with multiple metastases or widespread systemic disease, the prognosis is poor, and treatment is palliative only.

Leptomeningeal Metastases (Carcinomatous Meningitis)

The neoplasms metastasizing most commonly to the leptomeninges are carcinoma of the breast, lymphomas, and leukemia. Leptomeningeal metastases lead to multifocal neurologic deficits, which may be associated with infiltration of cranial and spinal nerve roots, direct invasion of the brain or spinal cord, obstructive hydrocephalus, or some combination of these factors.

The diagnosis is confirmed by examination of the cerebrospinal fluid. Findings may include elevated cerebrospinal fluid pressure, pleocytosis, increased protein concentration, and decreased glucose concentration. Cytologic studies may indicate that malignant cells are present; if not, spinal tap should be repeated at least twice to obtain further samples for analysis.

CT scans showing contrast enhancement in the basal cisterns or showing hydrocephalus without any evidence of a mass lesion support the diagnosis. Gadolinium-enhanced MRI frequently shows enhancing foci in the leptomeninges. Myelography may show deposits on multiple nerve roots.

Treatment is by irradiation to symptomatic areas, combined with intrathecal methotrexate. The long-term prognosis is poor—only about 10% of patients survive for 1 year—and palliative care is therefore important (Chapter 5).

3. Intracranial Mass Lesions in AIDS Patients

AIDS patients may present with **primary cerebral lymphoma.** This leads to disturbances in cognition or consciousness, focal motor or sensory deficits, aphasia, seizures, and cranial neuropathies. Similar clinical disturbances may result from **cerebral toxoplasmosis,** which is also a common complication in patients with AIDS. Neither CT nor MRI findings distinguish these two disorders, and serologic tests for toxoplasmosis are unreliable in AIDS patients. Accordingly, for neurologically stable patients, a trial of treatment for toxoplasmosis with sulfadiazine (100 mg/kg/d up to 8 g/d in four divided doses) and pyrimethamine (75 mg/d for 3 days, then 25 mg/d) is recommended for 3 weeks; the imaging studies are then repeated, and if any lesion has improved, the regimen is continued indefinitely. If any lesion does not improve, cerebral biopsy is necessary. Primary cerebral lymphoma is treated with whole-brain irradiation.

Cryptococcal meningitis is also a commonly opportunistic infection in AIDS patients. Clinically, it may resemble cerebral toxoplasmosis or lymphoma, but cranial CT scans are usually normal. The diagnosis is made on the basis of cerebrospinal fluid studies, with positive India ink staining in 75–80% and cryptococcal antigen tests in 95% of cases. Treatment is with amphotericin B, sometimes accompanied by flucytosine, as set forth in Table 36–1.

Berger JR: AIDS and the nervous system. In: *Neurology and General Medicine,* 3rd ed. Aminoff MJ (editor). Churchill Livingstone, 2001. (Clinical review.)

Evaluation and management of intracranial mass lesions in AIDS. Report of the Quality Standards Subcommittee of the American Academy of Neurology. Neurology 1998;50:21. [PMID: 9443452]

4. Primary & Metastatic Spinal Tumors

Approximately 10% of spinal tumors are intramedullary. Ependymoma is the most common type of intramedullary tumor; the remainder are other types of glioma. Extramedullary tumors may be extradural or intradural in location. Among the primary extramedullary tumors, neurofibromas and meningiomas are relatively common, are benign, and may be intra- or extradural. Carcinomatous metastases, lymphomatous or leukemic deposits, and myeloma are usually extradural; in the case of metastases, the prostate, breast, lung, and kidney are common primary sites.

Tumors may lead to spinal cord dysfunction by direct compression, by ischemia secondary to arterial or venous obstruction, and, in the case of intramedullary lesions, by invasive infiltration.

Clinical Findings

A. SYMPTOMS AND SIGNS

Symptoms usually develop insidiously. Pain is often conspicuous with extradural lesions; is characteristically aggravated by coughing or straining; may be radicular, localized to the back, or felt diffusely in an extremity; and may be accompanied by motor deficits, paresthesias, or numbness, especially in the legs. When sphincter disturbances occur, they are usually particularly disabling. Pain, however, often precedes specific neurologic symptoms from epidural metastases.

Examination may reveal localized spinal tenderness. A segmental lower motor neuron deficit or dermatomal sensory changes (or both) are sometimes found at the level of the lesion, while an upper motor neuron deficit and sensory disturbance are found below it.

B. IMAGING

Findings on plain radiography of the spine may be normal but are commonly abnormal when there are metastatic deposits. CT myelography or MRI may be necessary to identify and localize the site of cord compression. The combination of known tumor elsewhere in the body, back pain, and either abnormal plain films of the spine or neurologic signs of cord compression is an indication to perform these studies on an urgent basis. Some clinicians proceed to myelography based solely on new back pain in a cancer patient. If a complete block is present at lumbar myelography, a cisternal myelogram is performed to determine the upper level of the block and to investigate the possibility of block higher in the cord.

C. LABORATORY FINDINGS

The cerebrospinal fluid removed at myelography is often xanthochromic and contains a greatly increased protein concentration with normal cell content and glucose concentration.

Treatment

Intramedullary tumors are treated by decompression and surgical excision (when feasible) and by irradiation. The prognosis depends upon the cause and severity of cord compression before it is relieved.

Treatment of epidural spinal metastases consists of irradiation, irrespective of cell type. Dexamethasone is also given in a high dosage (eg, 25 mg four times daily for 3 days, followed by rapid tapering of the dosage, depending on response) to reduce cord swelling and relieve pain. Surgical decompression is reserved for patients with tumors that are unresponsive to irradiation or have previously been irradiated and for cases in which there is some uncertainty about the diagnosis. The long-term outlook is poor, but radiation treatment may at least delay the onset of major disability.

5. Brain Abscess

Brain abscess presents as an intracranial space-occupying lesion and arises as a sequela of disease of the ear or nose, may be a complication of infection elsewhere in the body, or may result from infection introduced intracranially by trauma or surgical procedures. The most common infective organisms are streptococci, staphylococci, and anaerobes; mixed infections are not uncommon. Headache, drowsiness, inattention, confusion, and seizures are early symptoms, followed by signs of increasing intracranial pressure and then a focal neurologic deficit. There may be little or no systemic evidence of infection.

A CT scan of the head characteristically shows an area of contrast enhancement surrounding a low-density core. Similar abnormalities may be found in patients with metastatic neoplasms. MRI findings often permit earlier recognition of focal cerebritis or an abscess. Arteriography indicates the presence of a space-occupying lesion, which appears as an avascular mass with displacement of normal cerebral vessels, but this procedure provides no clue to the nature of the lesion. Examination of the cerebrospinal fluid does not help in diagnosis and may precipitate a herniation syndrome.

Treatment consists of intravenous antibiotics, combined with surgical drainage (aspiration or excision) if necessary to reduce the mass effect, or sometimes to establish the diagnosis. Abscesses smaller than 2 cm can often be cured medically. Broad-spectrum antibiotics are used if the infecting organism is unknown. A common regimen is penicillin G (2 million units every 2 hours intravenously) plus either chloramphenicol (1–2 g intravenously every 6 hours), metronidazole (750 mg intravenously every 6 hours), or both. Nafcillin is added if *Staphylococcus aureus* infection is suspected. Antimicrobial treatment is usually continued parenterally for 6–8 weeks, followed by orally for a further 2–3 weeks. The patient should be monitored by serial CT scans or MRI every 2 weeks and at deterioration. Dexamethasone (4–25 mg four times daily, depending on severity, followed by tapering of dose, depending on response) may reduce any associated edema, but intravenous mannitol is sometimes required.

Roos KL: Acute bacterial infections of the central nervous system. In: *Neurology and General Medicine,* 3rd ed. Aminoff MJ (editor). Churchill Livingstone, 2001.

NONMETASTATIC NEUROLOGIC COMPLICATIONS OF MALIGNANT DISEASE

A variety of nonmetastatic neurologic complications of malignant disease (Table 40–6) can be recognized:

(1) Metabolic encephalopathy due to electrolyte abnormalities, infections, drug overdose, or the failure

of some vital organ may be reflected by drowsiness, lethargy, restlessness, insomnia, agitation, confusion, stupor, or coma. The mental changes are usually associated with tremor, asterixis, and multifocal myoclonus. The electroencephalogram is generally diffusely slowed. Laboratory studies are necessary to detect the cause of the encephalopathy, which must then be treated appropriately.

(2) Immune suppression resulting from either the malignant disease or its treatment (eg, by chemotherapy) predisposes patients to brain abscess, progressive multifocal leukoencephalopathy, meningitis, herpes zoster infection, and other opportunistic infectious diseases. Moreover, an overt or occult cerebrospinal fluid fistula, as occurs with some tumors, may also increase the risk of infection. CT scanning aids in the early recognition of a brain abscess, but metastatic brain tumors may have a similar appearance. Examination of the cerebrospinal fluid is essential in the evaluation of patients with meningitis but is of no help in the diagnosis of brain abscess.

(3) Cerebrovascular disorders that cause neurologic complications in patients with systemic cancer include nonbacterial thrombotic endocarditis and septic embolization. Cerebral, subarachnoid, or subdural hemorrhages may occur in patients with myelogenous leukemia and may be found in association with metastatic tumors, especially malignant melanoma. Spinal subdural hemorrhage sometimes occurs after lumbar puncture in patients with marked thrombocytopenia.

Disseminated intravascular coagulation occurs most commonly in patients with acute promyelocytic leukemia or with some adenocarcinomas and is characterized by a fluctuating encephalopathy, often with associated seizures, that frequently progresses to coma or death. There may be few accompanying neurologic signs.

Venous sinus thrombosis, which usually presents with convulsions and headaches, may also occur in patients with leukemia or lymphoma. Examination commonly reveals papilledema and focal or diffuse neurologic signs. Anticonvulsants, anticoagulants, and drugs to lower the intracranial pressure may be of value.

(4) Paraneoplastic cerebellar degeneration occurs most commonly in association with carcinoma of the lung. Symptoms may precede those due to the neoplasm itself, which may be undetected for several months or even longer. Typically, there is a pancerebellar syndrome causing dysarthria, nystagmus, and ataxia of the trunk and limbs. The disorder probably has an autoimmune basis. Treatment is of the underlying malignant disease.

(5) Encephalopathy, characterized by impaired recent memory, disturbed affect, hallucinations, and seizures, occurs in some patients with carcinomas. The cerebrospinal fluid is often abnormal. EEGs may show diffuse slow-wave activity, especially over the temporal regions. Pathologic changes are most marked in the inferomedian portions of the temporal lobes. There is no specific treatment.

(6) Malignant disease may be associated with sensorimotor polyneuropathy and less commonly with pure sensory neuropathy (ie, dorsal root ganglionitis) or autonomic neuropathy. A subacute motor neuronopathy may be associated with lymphomas.

(7) Dermatomyositis or a myasthenic syndrome may be seen in patients with underlying carcinoma (see Chapter 20). The myasthenic syndrome may have an autoimmune basis and differs clinically from myasthenia gravis.

Posner JB: Paraneoplastic syndromes involving the nervous system. In: *Neurology and General Medicine,* 3rd ed. Aminoff MJ (editor). Churchill Livingstone, 2001.

PSEUDOTUMOR CEREBRI (Benign Intracranial Hypertension)

Symptoms of pseudotumor cerebri consist of headache, diplopia, and other visual disturbances due to papilledema and abducens nerve dysfunction. Examination reveals the papilledema and some enlargement of the blind spots, but patients otherwise look well. Investigations reveal no evidence of a space-occupying lesion, and the CT scan shows small or normal ventricles. Lumbar puncture confirms the presence of intracranial hypertension, but the cerebrospinal fluid is normal.

There are many causes of pseudotumor cerebri. Thrombosis of the transverse venous sinus as a noninfectious complication of otitis media or chronic mastoiditis is one cause, and sagittal sinus thrombosis may lead to a clinically similar picture. MR venography is helpful in screening for these disorders. Other causes include chronic pulmonary disease, endocrine disturbances such as hypoparathyroidism or Addison's disease, vitamin A toxicity, and the use of tetracycline or oral contraceptives. Cases have also followed withdrawal of corticosteroids after long-term use. In many instances, however, no specific cause can be found, and the disorder remits spontaneously after several months.

Untreated pseudotumor cerebri leads to secondary optic atrophy and permanent visual loss. Acetazolamide (250 mg orally three times daily) reduces formation of cerebrospinal fluid and can be used to start treatment. Oral corticosteroids (eg, prednisone, 60–80 mg daily) may also be necessary. Obese patients should be advised to lose weight. Repeated lumbar puncture to lower the intracranial pressure by removal of cerebrospinal fluid is effective, but pharmacologic approaches to treatment are now more satisfactory. Treatment is monitored by checking visual acuity and visual fields, funduscopic appearance, and pressure of the cerebrospinal fluid.

If medical treatment fails to control the intracranial pressure, surgical placement of a lumboperitoneal or other shunt—or subtemporal decompression or optic nerve sheath fenestration—should be undertaken to preserve vision.

In addition to the above measures, any specific cause of pseudotumor cerebri requires appropriate treatment. Thus, hormone therapy should be initiated if there is an underlying endocrine disturbance. Discontinuing the use of tetracycline, oral contraceptives, or vitamin A will allow for resolution of pseudotumor cerebri due to these agents. If corticosteroid withdrawal is responsible, the medication should be reintroduced and then tapered more gradually.

Kessler LA et al: Surgical treatment of benign intracranial hypertension—subtemporal decompression revisited. Surg Neurol 1998;50:73. [PMID: 9657496] (Clinical study.)

SELECTED NEUROCUTANEOUS DISEASES

Tuberous Sclerosis

Tuberous sclerosis may occur sporadically or on a familial basis with autosomal dominant inheritance. The responsible gene is located on the long arm of chromosome 9 in at least some cases. Its pathogenesis is unknown. Neurologic presentation is with seizures and progressive psychomotor retardation beginning in early childhood. The cutaneous abnormality, adenoma sebaceum, becomes manifest usually between 5 and 10 years of age and typically consists of reddened nodules on the face (cheeks, nasolabial folds, sides of the nose, and chin) and sometimes on the forehead and neck. Other typical cutaneous lesions include subungual fibromas, shagreen patches (leathery plaques of subepidermal fibrosis, situated usually on the trunk), and leaf-shaped hypopigmented spots. Associated abnormalities include retinal lesions and tumors, benign rhabdomyomas of the heart, lung cysts, benign tumors in the viscera, and bone cysts.

The disease is slowly progressive and leads to increasing mental deterioration. There is no specific treatment, but anticonvulsant drugs may help in controlling seizures.

Neurofibromatosis

Neurofibromatosis may occur either sporadically or on a familial basis with autosomal dominant inheritance. Two distinct forms are recognized: Type 1 (**Recklinghausen's disease**) is characterized by multiple hyperpigmented macules and neurofibromas and type 2 by **eighth nerve tumors,** often accompanied by other intracranial or intraspinal tumors. Among familial cases, the gene for type 1 is located on chromosome 17 and that for type 2 on chromosome 22.

Neurologic presentation is usually with symptoms and signs of tumor. Multiple neurofibromas characteristically are present and may involve spinal or cranial nerves, especially the eighth nerve. Examination of the superficial cutaneous nerves usually reveals palpable mobile nodules. In some cases, there is an associated marked overgrowth of subcutaneous tissues (plexiform neuromas), sometimes with an underlying bony abnormality. Associated cutaneous lesions include axillary freckling and patches of cutaneous pigmentation (café au lait spots). Malignant degeneration of neurofibromas occasionally occurs and may lead to peripheral sarcomas. Meningiomas, gliomas (especially optic nerve gliomas), bone cysts, pheochromocytomas, scoliosis, and obstructive hydrocephalus may also occur.

It may be possible to correct disfigurement by plastic surgery. Intraspinal or intracranial tumors and tumors of peripheral nerves should be treated surgically if they are producing symptoms.

Hirsch NP et al: Neurofibromatosis: clinical presentations and anaesthetic implications. Br J Anaesth 2001;86;555. [PMID: 11573632] (Review of etiology and clinical manifestations.)

Wolkenstein P et al: Quality-of-life impairment in neurofibromatosis type 1: a cross-sectional study of 128 cases. Arch Dermatol 2001;137:1421. [PMID: 11708944] (Clinical study.)

Sturge-Weber Syndrome

Sturge-Weber syndrome consists of a congenital, usually unilateral, cutaneous capillary angioma involving the upper face, leptomeningeal angiomatosis, and, in many patients, choroidal angioma. It has no sex predilection and usually occurs sporadically. The cutaneous angioma sometimes has a more extensive distribution over the head and neck and is often quite disfiguring, especially if there is associated overgrowth of connective tissue. Focal or generalized seizures are the usual neurologic presentation and may commence at any age. There may be contralateral homonymous hemianopia, hemiparesis and hemisensory disturbance, ipsilateral glaucoma, and mental subnormality. Skull x-rays taken after the first 2 years of life usually reveal gyriform ("tramline") intracranial calcification, especially in the parieto-occipital region, due to mineral deposition in the cortex beneath the intracranial angioma.

Treatment is aimed at controlling seizures pharmacologically. Ophthalmologic advice should be sought concerning the management of choroidal angioma and of increased intraocular pressure.

MOVEMENT DISORDERS

1. Benign Essential (Familial) Tremor

The cause of benign essential tremor is uncertain, but it is sometimes inherited in an autosomal dominant manner. Tremor may begin at any age and is enhanced by emotional stress. The tremor usually involves one or both hands, the head, or the hands and head, while the legs tend to be spared. Examination reveals no other abnormalities. Ingestion of a small quantity of alcohol commonly provides remarkable but short-lived relief by an unknown mechanism.

Although the tremor may become more conspicuous with time, it generally leads to little disability, and treatment is often unnecessary. Occasionally, it interferes with manual skills and leads to impairment of handwriting. Speech may also be affected if the laryngeal muscles are involved. In such circumstances, propranolol may be helpful but will need to be continued indefinitely in daily doses of 60–240 mg. However, intermittent therapy is sometimes useful in patients whose tremor becomes exacerbated in specific predictable situations. Primidone may be helpful when propranolol is ineffective, but patients with essential tremor are often very sensitive to it. They are therefore started on 50 mg daily, and the daily dose is increased by 50 mg every 2 weeks depending on the response; a maintenance dose of 125 mg three times daily is commonly effective. Occasional patients fail to respond to these measures but are helped by alprazolam (up to 3 mg daily in divided doses), clozapine (30–50 mg twice daily), or mirtazapine (15 or 30 mg at night).

Disabling tremor unresponsive to medical treatment may be helped by contralateral thalamotomy. Unilateral high-frequency thalamic stimulation is an alternative approach that is equally effective, is associated with only mild and transient side effects, and is therefore preferred. Bilateral thalamotomy has significant morbidity, whereas the risks of bilateral stimulation are appreciably lower.

Louis ED et al: Clinical subtypes of essential tremor. Arch Neurol 2000;57:1194. [PMID: 10927801] (Clinical study.)

Louis ED: Essential tremor. N Engl J Med 2001;345:887. [PMID:11565522] (Clinical review.)

Pact V et al: Mirtazapine treats resting tremor, essential tremor, and levodopa-induced dyskinesias. Neurology 1999;53:1154. [PMID: 10496290] (Clinical report.)

2. Parkinsonism

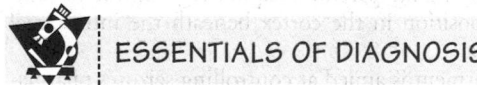 ESSENTIALS OF DIAGNOSIS

- *Any combination of tremor, rigidity, bradykinesia, progressive postural instability.*
- *Seborrhea of skin quite common.*
- *Mild intellectual deterioration may occur.*

General Considerations

Parkinsonism is a relatively common disorder that occurs in all ethnic groups, with an approximately equal sex distribution. The most common variety, idiopathic Parkinson's disease (paralysis agitans), begins most often between 45 and 65 years of age.

Etiology

Parkinsonism may rarely occur on a familial basis, and the parkinsonian phenotype may result from mutations of several different genes. Postencephalitic parkinsonism is becoming increasingly rare. Exposure to certain toxins (eg, manganese dust, carbon disulfide) and severe carbon monoxide poisoning may lead to parkinsonism. Typical parkinsonism has occurred in individuals who have taken 1-methyl-4-phenyl-1,2,5,6-tetrahydropyridine (MPTP) for recreational purposes. This compound is converted in the body to a neurotoxin that selectively destroys dopaminergic neurons in the substantia nigra. Reversible parkinsonism may develop in patients receiving neuroleptic drugs (see Chapter 25), reserpine, or metoclopramide. Only rarely is hemiparkinsonism the presenting feature of a progressive space-occupying lesion.

In idiopathic parkinsonism, dopamine depletion due to degeneration of the dopaminergic nigrostriatal system leads to an imbalance of dopamine and acetylcholine, which are neurotransmitters normally present in the corpus striatum. Treatment is directed at redressing this imbalance by blocking the effect of acetylcholine with anticholinergic drugs or by the administration of levodopa, the precursor of dopamine.

Clinical Findings

Tremor, rigidity, bradykinesia, and postural instability are the cardinal features of parkinsonism and may be present in any combination. There may also be a mild decline in intellectual function. The tremor of about four to six cycles per second is most conspicuous at rest, is enhanced by emotional stress, and is often less severe during voluntary activity. Although it may ultimately be present in all limbs, the tremor is commonly confined to one limb or to the limbs on one side for months or years before it becomes more generalized. In some patients, tremor is absent.

Rigidity (an increase in resistance to passive movement) is responsible for the characteristically flexed posture seen in many patients, but the most disabling symptoms of parkinsonism are due to bradykinesia, manifested as a slowness of voluntary movement and a reduction in automatic movements such as swinging of the arms while walking. Curiously, however, effective voluntary activity may briefly be regained during an emergency (eg, the patient is able to leap aside to avoid an oncoming motor vehicle).

Clinical diagnosis of the well-developed syndrome is usually simple. The patient has a relatively immobile face with widened palpebral fissures, infrequent blinking, and a certain fixity of facial expression. Seborrhea of the scalp and face is common. There is often mild blepharoclonus, and a tremor may be present about the mouth and lips. Repetitive tapping (about twice per second) over the bridge of the nose produces a sustained blink response (Myerson's sign). Other findings may include saliva drooling from the mouth, perhaps due to impairment of swallowing; soft and poorly modulated voice; a variable rest tremor and rigidity in some or all of the limbs; slowness of voluntary movements; impairment of fine or rapidly alternating movements; and micrographia. There is typically no muscle weakness (provided that sufficient time is allowed for power to be developed) and no alteration in the tendon reflexes or plantar responses. It is difficult for the patient to arise from a sitting position and begin walking. The gait itself is characterized by small shuffling steps and a loss of the normal automatic arm swing; there may be unsteadiness on turning, difficulty in stopping, and a tendency to fall.

Differential Diagnosis

Diagnostic problems may occur in mild cases, especially if tremor is minimal or absent. For example, mild hypokinesia or slight tremor is commonly attributed to old age. Depression, with its associated expressionless face, poorly modulated voice, and reduction in voluntary activity, can be difficult to distinguish from mild parkinsonism, especially since the two disorders may coexist; in some cases, a trial of antidepressant drug therapy is necessary. The family history, the character of the tremor, and lack of other neurologic signs should distinguish essential tremor from parkinsonism. Wilson's disease can be distinguished by its early age at onset, the presence of other abnormal movements, Kayser-Fleischer rings, and chronic hepatitis, and by increased concentrations of copper in the tissues. Huntington's disease presenting with rigidity and bradykinesia may be mistaken for parkinsonism unless the family history and accompanying dementia are recognized. In Shy-Drager syndrome, the clinical features of parkinsonism are accompanied by autonomic insufficiency (leading to postural hypotension, anhidrosis, disturbances of sphincter control, impotence, etc) and more widespread neurologic deficits (pyramidal, lower motor neuron, or cerebellar signs). In progressive supranuclear palsy, bradykinesia and rigidity are accompanied by a supranuclear disorder of eye movements, pseudobulbar palsy, and axial dystonia. Creutzfeldt-Jakob disease may be accompanied by features of parkinsonism, but dementia is usual, myoclonic jerking is common, ataxia and pyramidal signs may be conspicuous, and the electroencephalographic findings are usually characteristic. In cortical-basal ganglionic degeneration, parkinsonism is accompanied by conspicuous signs of cortical dysfunction (eg, apraxia, sensory inattention, dementia, aphasia).

Treatment

A. MEDICAL MEASURES

Drug treatment is not required early in the course of parkinsonism, but the nature of the disorder and the availability of medical treatment for use when necessary should be discussed with the patient.

1. Amantadine—Patients with mild symptoms but no disability may be helped by amantadine. This drug improves all of the clinical features of parkinsonism, but its mode of action is unclear. Side effects include restlessness, confusion, depression, skin rashes, edema, nausea, constipation, anorexia, postural hypotension, and disturbances of cardiac rhythm. However, these are relatively uncommon with the usual dose (100 mg twice daily).

2. Anticholinergic drugs—Anticholinergics are more helpful in alleviating tremor and rigidity than bradykinesia. Treatment is started with a small dose (Table 24–4) and gradually increased until benefit occurs or side effects limit further increments. If treatment is ineffective, the drug is gradually withdrawn and another preparation then tried.

Common side effects include dryness of the mouth, nausea, constipation, palpitations, cardiac arrhythmias, urinary retention, confusion, agitation, restlessness, drowsiness, mydriasis, increased intraocular pressure, and defective accommodation.

Anticholinergic drugs are contraindicated in patients with prostatic hypertrophy, narrow-angle glaucoma, or obstructive gastrointestinal disease and are often tolerated poorly by the elderly.

3. Levodopa—Levodopa, which is converted in the body to dopamine, improves all of the major features of parkinsonism, including bradykinesia, but does not stop progression of the disorder. The commonest early side effects of levodopa are nausea, vomiting, and hypotension, but cardiac arrhythmias may also occur. Dyskinesias, restlessness, confusion, and other behavioral changes tend to occur somewhat later and become more common with time. Levodopa-induced dyskinesias may take any conceivable form, including chorea, athetosis, dystonia, tremor, tics, and myoclonus. An even later complication is the "on-off

Table 24–4. Some anticholinergic antiparkinsonian drugs.[1]

Drug	Usual Daily Dose
Benztropine mesylate (Cogentin)	1–6 mg
Biperiden (Akineton)	2–12 mg
Orphenadrine (Disipal, Norflex)	150–400 mg
Procyclidine (Kemadrin)	7.5–30 mg
Trihexyphenidyl (Artane)	6–20 mg

[1]Modified, with permission, from Aminoff MJ: Pharmacologic management of parkinsonism and other movement disorders. In: *Basic & Clinical Pharmacology*, 8th ed. Katzung BG (editor). McGraw-Hill, 2001.

phenomenon," in which abrupt but transient fluctuations in the severity of parkinsonism occur unpredictably but frequently during the day. The "off" period of marked bradykinesia has been shown to relate in some instances to falling plasma levels of levodopa. During the "on" phase, dyskinesias are often conspicuous but mobility is increased.

Carbidopa, which inhibits the enzyme responsible for the breakdown of levodopa to dopamine, does not cross the blood-brain barrier. When levodopa is given in combination with carbidopa, the extracerebral breakdown of levodopa is diminished. This reduces the amount of levodopa required daily for beneficial effects, and it lowers the incidence of nausea, vomiting, hypotension, and cardiac irregularities. Such a combination does not prevent the development of the "on-off phenomenon," and the incidence of other side effects (dyskinesias or psychiatric complications) may actually be increased.

Sinemet, a commercially available preparation that contains carbidopa and levodopa in a fixed ratio (1:10 or 1:4), is generally used. Treatment is started with a small dose—eg, one tablet of Sinemet 25/100 (containing 25 mg of carbidopa and 100 mg of levodopa) three times daily—and gradually increased depending on the response. Sinemet CR is a controlled-release formulation (containing 25 or 50 mg of carbidopa and 100 or 200 mg of levodopa). It is sometimes helpful in reducing fluctuations in clinical response to treatment and in reducing the frequency with which medication must be taken. Response fluctuations are also reduced by keeping the daily intake of protein at the recommended minimum and taking the main protein meal as the last meal of the day.

The dyskinesias and behavioral side effects of levodopa are dose-related, but reduction in dose may eliminate any therapeutic benefit.

Levodopa therapy is contraindicated in patients with psychotic illness or narrow-angle glaucoma. It should not be given to patients taking monoamine oxidase A inhibitors or within 2 weeks of their withdrawal, because hypertensive crises may result. Levodopa should be used with care in patients with suspected malignant melanomas or with active peptic ulcers because of concerns that it may exacerbate these disorders.

4. Dopamine agonists—Dopamine agonists act directly on dopamine receptors, and their use in parkinsonism is associated with a lower incidence of the response fluctuations and dyskinesias that occur with long-term levodopa therapy. They were previously reserved for patients who had either become refractory to levodopa or developed the "on-off phenomenon." However, they are now best given either before the introduction of levodopa or with a low dose of Sinemet-25/100 (carbidopa 25 mg and levodopa 100 mg), one tablet three times daily when dopaminergic therapy is first introduced; the dose of Sinemet is kept constant, while the dose of the agonist is gradually increased.

Two widely used agonists are bromocriptine and pergolide, which are equally effective ergot derivatives. The initial dosage of bromocriptine is 1.25 mg twice daily; this is increased by 2.5 mg at 2-week intervals until benefit occurs or side effects limit further increments. The usual daily maintenance dose in patients with parkinsonism is between 10 and 30 mg. Pergolide is similarly started in a low dose (eg, 0.05 mg daily) and built up gradually depending on the response and tolerance.

Side effects include anorexia, nausea, vomiting, constipation, postural hypotension, digital vasospasm, cardiac arrhythmias, various dyskinesias and mental disturbances, headache, nasal congestion, erythromelalgia, and pulmonary infiltrates. Bromocriptine and pergolide are contraindicated in patients with a history of mental illness or recent myocardial infarction and are probably best avoided in those with peripheral vascular disease or peptic ulcers as bleeding from the latter has been reported.

Pramipexole and ropinirole are two newer dopamine agonists that are not ergot derivatives. It is not clear that they have any benefit over the older agents, except that ergot-related side effects are unlikely. They are effective in early Parkinson's disease as well as in advanced stages of the disease. In each case, the daily dose is built up gradually. Pramipexole is started at a dosage of 0.125 mg three times daily, and the dose is doubled after 1 week and again after another week; the daily dose is then increased by 0.75 mg at weekly intervals depending on response and tolerance. Most patients require between 0.5 and 1.5 mg three times daily. Ropinirole is begun in a dosage of 0.25 mg three times daily, and the total daily dose is increased at weekly intervals by 0.75 mg until the fourth week and by 1.5 mg thereafter. Most patients require between 2 and 8 mg three times daily for benefit. Adverse effects include fatigue, somnolence, nausea, peripheral edema, dyskinesias, confusion, and postural hypotension. Less commonly, an irresistible urge to sleep may occur, sometimes in inappropriate and hazardous circumstances.

5. Selegiline—Selegiline is a monoamine oxidase B inhibitor that is sometimes used as adjunctive treatment for parkinsonism in patients receiving levodopa. By inhibiting the metabolic breakdown of dopamine, selegiline has been used to improve fluctuations or declining response to levodopa. In general, however, the response to treatment with it has been disappointing. The drug is taken in a standard dose of 5 mg with breakfast and 5 mg with lunch. It may increase any adverse effects of levodopa.

There are reasons to believe that selegiline may arrest the progression of Parkinson's disease. Studies have failed to establish this conclusively, but this remains an important consideration for patients who are young or have mild disease.

6. COMT inhibitors—Catecholamine-O-methyltransferase inhibitors reduce the metabolism of levodopa to 3-O-methyldopa and thereby alter the plasma pharmacokinetics of levodopa, leading to more sustained plasma levels and more constant dopaminergic stimulation of the brain. Two such agents, tolcapone and entacapone, are currently available and may be used as an adjunct to levodopa-carbidopa in patients with response fluctuations or an otherwise inadequate response and who either have failed with other adjunctive therapies or are not candidates for such therapies. Treatment results in reduced response fluctuations, with a greater period of responsiveness to administered levodopa. Tolcapone is given in a dosage of 100 mg or 200 mg three times daily, and entacapone is given as 200 mg with each dose of Sinemet (levodopa-carbidopa). With either preparation, the dose of Sinemet taken concurrently may have to be reduced by up to one-third to avoid side effects such as dyskinesias, confusion, hypotension, and syncope. Diarrhea is sometimes troublesome. Because rare cases of fulminant hepatic failure have followed its use, tolcapone should be avoided in patients with preexisting liver disease. Serial liver function tests should be performed at 2-week intervals for the first year and at longer intervals thereafter in patients receiving the drug—as recommended by the manufacturer. Hepatotoxicity has not been reported with entacapone, and serial liver function tests are not required.

7. Atypical antipsychotics—Confusion and psychotic symptoms, which may be iatrogenic, often respond to atypical antipsychotic agents, which have few extrapyramidal side effects and do not block the effects of dopaminergic medication. Olanzapine, quetiapine, and risperidone may be tried, but the most effective of these agents is clozapine, a dibenzodiazepine derivative. Clozapine may rarely cause marrow suppression, and weekly blood counts are therefore necessary for patients taking it. The patient is started on 6.25 mg at bedtime and the dosage increased to 25–100 mg/d as needed. In low doses, it may also improve iatrogenic dyskinesias.

B. GENERAL MEASURES

Physical therapy or speech therapy helps many patients. The quality of life can often be improved by the provision of simple aids to daily living, eg, rails or banisters placed strategically about the home, special table cutlery with large handles, nonslip rubber table mats, and devices to amplify the voice.

C. SURGICAL MEASURES

Thalamotomy or pallidotomy may be helpful for patients who become unresponsive to medical treatment or have intolerable side effects from antiparkinsonian agents, especially if they have no evidence of diffuse vascular disease or significant cognitive decline. Surgery should generally be confined to one side because the morbidity is considerably greater after bilateral procedures. Surgical implantation of adrenal medullary or fetal substantia nigra tissue into the cau-

date nucleus has been reported to benefit some patients, but other investigators have failed to substantiate such claims or have found only modest benefits or major adverse effects, and the procedure is still being evaluated.

D. BRAIN STIMULATION

High-frequency thalamic stimulation is effective in suppressing the rest tremor of Parkinson's disease, and chronic bilateral stimulation of the subthalamic nuclei or globus pallidus internus may benefit all the major features of the disease. Electrical stimulation of the brain has the advantage of being reversible and of causing minimal or no damage to the brain, and its utility is being explored in several centers. There is no evidence that the natural history of Parkinson's disease is affected.

Deep-Brain Stimulation for Parkinson's Disease Study Group: Deep-brain stimulation of the subthalamic nucleus or the pars interna of the globus pallidus in Parkinson's disease. N Engl J Med 2001;345;956. [PMID 11575287] (Clinical study.)

Freed C et al: Transplantation of embryonic dopamine neurons for severe Parkinson's disease. N Engl J Med 2001;344;710. [PMID: 11236774] (Clinical trial.)

Miyasaki JM et al: Practice parameter: initiation of treatment for Parkinson's disease: an evidence-based review. Neurology 2002;58:11. [PMID 11781398]

Mouradian MM: Recent advances in the genetics and pathogenesis of Parkinson disease. Neurology 2002;58:179. [PMID 11805242] (Review.)

Olanow CW et al: An algorithm (decision tree) for the management of Parkinson's disease: Treatment guidelines. Neurology 1998;50(3 Suppl 3):S1. [PMID: 9524552]

Rascol O et al: A five-year study of the incidence of dyskinesia in patients with early Parkinson's disease who were treated with ropinirole or levodopa. N Engl J Med 2000;342:1484. [PMID: 10816186] (Clinical study.)

3. Huntington's Disease

ESSENTIALS OF DIAGNOSIS

- Gradual onset and progression of chorea and dementia.
- Family history of the disorder.
- Responsible gene identified on chromosome 4.

General Considerations

Huntington's disease is characterized by chorea and dementia. It is inherited in an autosomal dominant manner and occurs throughout the world, in all ethnic groups, with a prevalence rate of about 5 per 100,000. The gene responsible for the disease has been located on the short arm of chromosome No. 4. At 4p16.3

there is an expanded and unstable CAG trinucleotide repeat.

Clinical Findings

Clinical onset is usually between 30 and 50 years of age. The disease is progressive and usually leads to a fatal outcome within 15–20 years. The initial symptoms may consist of either abnormal movements or intellectual changes, but ultimately both occur. The earliest mental changes are often behavioral, with irritability, moodiness, antisocial behavior, or a psychiatric disturbance, but a more obvious dementia subsequently develops. The dyskinesia may initially be no more than an apparent fidgetiness or restlessness, but eventually choreiform movements and some dystonic posturing occur. Progressive rigidity and akinesia (rather than chorea) sometimes occur in association with dementia, especially in cases with childhood onset. CT scanning usually demonstrates cerebral atrophy and atrophy of the caudate nucleus in established cases. MRI and positron emission tomography (PET) have shown reduced glucose utilization in an anatomically normal caudate nucleus.

Chorea developing with no family history of choreoathetosis should not be attributed to Huntington's disease, at least not until other causes of chorea have been excluded clinically and by appropriate laboratory studies. In younger patients, self-limiting Sydenham's chorea develops after group A streptococcal infections on rare occasions. If a patient presents solely with progressive intellectual failure, it may not be possible to distinguish Huntington's disease from other causes of dementia unless there is a characteristic family history or a dyskinesia develops.

A clinically similar autosomal dominant disorder (**dentatorubral-pallidolysian atrophy**), manifested by chorea, dementia, ataxia, and myoclonic epilepsy, is uncommon except in persons of Japanese ancestry. It is due to a mutant gene mapping to 12p13.31. Treatment is as for Huntington's disease.

Treatment

There is no cure for Huntington's disease; progression cannot be halted; and treatment is purely symptomatic. The reported biochemical changes suggest a relative underactivity of neurons containing gamma-aminobutyric acid (GABA) and acetylcholine or a relative overactivity of dopaminergic neurons. Treatment with drugs blocking dopamine receptors, such as phenothiazines or haloperidol, may control the dyskinesia and any behavioral disturbances. Haloperidol treatment is usually begun with a dose of 1 mg once or twice daily, which is then increased every 3 or 4 days depending on the response. Tetrabenazine, a drug that depletes central monoamines, is widely used in Europe to treat dyskinesia but is not available in the USA. Reserpine is similar in its actions to tetrabenazine and may be helpful; the daily dose is built up gradually to

between 2 and 5 mg, depending on the response. Behavioral disturbances may respond to clozapine. Attempts to compensate for the relative GABA deficiency by enhancing central GABA activity or to compensate for the relative cholinergic underactivity by giving choline chloride have not been therapeutically helpful. High levels of somatostatin (a neuropeptide) have recently been reported in certain areas of the brain in patients with Huntington's disease, and the therapeutic response to cysteamine (a selective depleter of somatostatin in the brain) is currently under study. Neuroprotective strategies are also being explored.

Offspring should be offered genetic counseling. Genetic testing permits presymptomatic detection and definitive diagnosis of the disease.

Davies S et al: Huntington's disease. Mol Pathol 2001;54:409. [PMID 11724916] (Review of molecular pathology.)

Emerich DF: Neuroprotective possibilities for Huntington's disease. Expert Opin Biol Ther 2001;1:467. [PMID 11727519] (Review.)

4. Idiopathic Torsion Dystonia

 ESSENTIALS OF DIAGNOSIS

- *Dystonic movements and postures.*
- *Normal birth and developmental history. No other neurologic signs.*
- *Investigations (including CT scan or MRI) reveal no cause of dystonia.*

General Considerations

Idiopathic torsion dystonia may occur sporadically or on a hereditary basis, with autosomal dominant, autosomal recessive, and X-linked recessive modes of transmission. The responsible gene is located at 9q34 (and has been named *DYT1*) and involves a unique mutation consisting of a GAG deletion in the dominantly inherited disorder, and maps to the long arm of the X chromosome in the X-linked recessive form; the responsible gene in the autosomal recessive disorder is unknown. Other autosomal dominant forms have also been recognized, with different or unidentified genetic loci. Symptoms may begin in childhood or later and persist throughout life.

Clinical Findings

The disorder is characterized by the onset of abnormal movements and postures in a patient with a normal birth and developmental history, no relevant past medical illness, and no other neurologic signs. Investigations (including CT scan) reveal no cause for the abnormal movements. Dystonic movements of the head and neck may take the form of torticollis, blepharospasm, facial grimacing, or forced opening or closing of the mouth. The limbs may also adopt abnormal but characteristic postures. The age at onset influences both the clinical findings and the prognosis. With onset in childhood, there is usually a family history of the disorder, symptoms commonly commence in the legs, and progression is likely until there is severe disability from generalized dystonia. In contrast, when onset is later, a positive family history is unlikely, initial symptoms are often in the arms or axial structures, and severe disability does not usually occur, although generalized dystonia may ultimately develop in some patients. If all cases are considered together, about one-third of patients eventually become so severely disabled that they are confined to chair or bed, while another one-third are affected only mildly.

Before a diagnosis of idiopathic torsion dystonia is made, it is imperative to exclude other causes of dystonia. For example, perinatal anoxia, birth trauma, and kernicterus are common causes of dystonia, but abnormal movements usually then develop before the age of 5, the early development of the patient is usually abnormal, and a history of seizures is not unusual. Moreover, examination may reveal signs of mental retardation or pyramidal deficit in addition to the movement disorder. Dystonic posturing may also occur in Wilson's disease, Huntington's disease, or parkinsonism; as a sequela of encephalitis lethargica or previous neuroleptic drug therapy; and in certain other disorders. In these cases, diagnosis is based on the history and accompanying clinical manifestations.

Treatment

Idiopathic torsion dystonia usually responds poorly to drugs. Levodopa, diazepam, baclofen, carbamazepine, amantadine, or anticholinergic medication (in high dosage) is occasionally helpful; if not, a trial of treatment with phenothiazines or haloperidol may be worthwhile. In each case, the dose has to be individualized, depending on response and tolerance. However, the doses of these latter drugs that are required for benefit lead usually to mild parkinsonism. Stereotactic thalamotomy is sometimes helpful in patients with predominantly unilateral dystonia, especially when this involves the limbs.

A distinct variety of dominantly inherited dystonia, mapping to a genetic locus on chromosome 14q, is remarkably responsive to levodopa.

Bressman SB: Dystonia. Curr Opin Neurol 1998;11:363. [PMID: 9725083] (Review of recent advances.)

Ozelius LJ et al: The early-onset torsion dystonia gene (*DYT1*) encodes an ATP-binding protein. Nat Genet 1997;17:40. [PMID: 9288096] (Identification of gene.)

5. Focal Torsion Dystonia

A number of the dystonic manifestations that occur in idiopathic torsion dystonia may also occur as isolated phenomena. They are best regarded as focal dystonias that either occur as formes frustes of idiopathic torsion dystonia in patients with a positive family history or represent a focal manifestation of the adult-onset form of that disorder when there is no family history. Mapping of responsible genes to chromosome 8 (*DYT6*) and chromosome 18 (*DYT7*) has been reported in some instances of cervical or cranial dystonia. Medical treatment is generally unsatisfactory. A trial of the drugs used in idiopathic torsion dystonia is worthwhile, however, since a few patients do show some response. In addition, with restricted dystonias such as blepharospasm or torticollis, local injection of botulinum A toxin into the overactive muscles may produce worthwhile benefit for several weeks or months and can be repeated as needed.

Both blepharospasm and oromandibular dystonia may occur as an isolated focal dystonia. The former is characterized by spontaneous involuntary forced closure of the eyelids for a variable interval. Oromandibular dystonia is manifested by involuntary contraction of the muscles about the mouth causing, for example, involuntary opening or closing of the mouth, roving or protruding tongue movements, and retraction of the platysma.

Spasmodic torticollis, usually with onset between 25 and 50 years of age, is characterized by a tendency for the neck to twist to one side. This initially occurs episodically, but eventually the neck is held to the side. Spontaneous resolution may occur in the first year or so. The disorder is otherwise usually lifelong. Selective section of the spinal accessory nerve and the upper cervical nerve roots is sometimes helpful if medical treatment is unsuccessful. Local injection of botulinum A toxin provides benefit in most cases.

Writer's cramp is characterized by dystonic posturing of the hand and forearm when the hand is used for writing and sometimes when it is used for other tasks, eg, playing the piano, using a screwdriver or eating utensils. Drug treatment is usually unrewarding, and patients are often best advised to learn to use the other hand for activities requiring manual dexterity. Injections of botulinum A toxin are helpful in some instances.

6. Myoclonus

Occasional myoclonic jerks may occur in anyone, especially when drifting into sleep. General or multifocal myoclonus is common in patients with idiopathic epilepsy and is especially prominent in certain hereditary disorders characterized by seizures and progressive intellectual decline, such as the lipid storage diseases. It is also a feature of various rare degenerative disorders, notably Ramsay Hunt syndrome, and is common in subacute sclerosing panencephalitis and Creutzfeldt-Jakob disease. Generalized myoclonic jerking may accompany uremic and other metabolic encephalopathies, result from levodopa therapy, occur in alcohol or drug withdrawal states, or follow anoxic brain damage. It also occurs on a hereditary or sporadic basis as an isolated phenomenon in otherwise healthy subjects.

Segmental myoclonus is a rare manifestation of a focal spinal cord lesion. It may also be the clinical expression of **epilepsia partialis continua,** a disorder in which a repetitive focal epileptic discharge arises in the contralateral sensorimotor cortex, sometimes from an underlying structural lesion. An electroencephalogram is often helpful in clarifying the epileptic nature of the disorder, and CT or MRI scan may reveal the causal lesion.

Myoclonus may respond to certain anticonvulsant drugs, especially valproic acid, or to one of the benzodiazepines, particularly clonazepam (Table 24–2). It may also respond to piracetam (up to 16.8 g daily). Myoclonus following anoxic brain damage is often responsive to oxitriptan (5-hydroxytryptophan), an investigational agent that is the precursor of serotonin, and sometimes to clonazepam. Oxitriptan is given in gradually increasing doses up to 1–1.5 mg daily. In patients with segmental myoclonus, a localized lesion should be searched for and treated appropriately.

7. Wilson's Disease

In this metabolic disorder, abnormal movement and posture may occur with or without coexisting signs of liver involvement. It is discussed in Chapter 15.

8. Drug-Induced Abnormal Movements

Phenothiazines and butyrophenones may produce a wide variety of abnormal movements, including parkinsonism, akathisia (ie, motor restlessness), acute dystonia, chorea, and tardive dyskinesia. These complications are discussed in Chapter 25. Chorea may also develop in patients receiving levodopa, bromocriptine, anticholinergic drugs, phenytoin, carbamazepine, lithium, amphetamines, or oral contraceptives, and it resolves with withdrawal of the offending substance. Similarly, dystonia may be produced by levodopa, bromocriptine, lithium, metoclopramide, or carbamazepine; and parkinsonism by reserpine, tetrabenazine, and metoclopramide. Postural tremor may occur with a variety of drugs, including epinephrine, isoproterenol, theophylline, caffeine, lithium, thyroid hormone, tricyclic antidepressants, and valproic acid.

9. Gilles de la Tourette's Syndrome

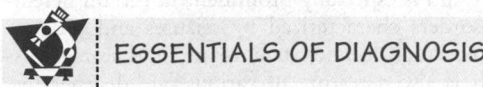 ESSENTIALS OF DIAGNOSIS

- Multiple motor and phonic tics.
- Symptoms begin before age 21 years.

- Tics occur frequently for at least 1 year.
- Tics vary in number, frequency, and nature over time.

Clinical Findings

Motor tics are the initial manifestation in 80% of cases and most commonly involve the face whereas in the remaining 20%, the initial symptoms are phonic tics; all patients ultimately develop a combination of different motor and phonic tics. These are noted first in childhood, generally between the ages of 2 and 15. Motor tics occur especially about the face, head, and shoulders (eg, sniffing, blinking, frowning, shoulder shrugging, head thrusting, etc). Phonic tics commonly consist of grunts, barks, hisses, throat-clearing, coughs, etc, but sometimes also of verbal utterances including coprolalia (obscene speech). There may also be echolalia (repetition of the speech of others), echopraxia (imitation of others' movements), and palilalia (repetition of words or phrases). Some tics may be self-mutilating in nature, such as nail-biting, hair-pulling, or biting of the lips or tongue. The disorder is chronic, but the course may be punctuated by relapses and remissions. Obsessive-compulsive behaviors are commonly associated and may be more disabling than the tics themselves.

Examination usually reveals no abnormalities other than the tics. In addition to obsessive-compulsive behavior disorders, psychiatric disturbances may occur because of the associated cosmetic and social embarrassment. Electroencephalography may show minor nonspecific abnormalities of no diagnostic relevance.

The diagnosis of the disorder is often delayed for years, the tics being interpreted as psychiatric illness or some other form of abnormal movement. Patients are thus often subjected to unnecessary treatment before the disorder is recognized. The tic-like character of the abnormal movements and the absence of other neurologic signs should differentiate this disorder from other movement disorders presenting in childhood. Wilson's disease, however, can simulate the condition and should be excluded.

Treatment

Treatment is symptomatic and may need to be continued indefinitely. Haloperidol is generally regarded as the drug of choice. It is started in a low daily dose (0.25 mg) that is gradually increased (by 0.25 mg every 4 or 5 days) until there is maximum benefit with a minimum of side effects or until side effects limit further increments. A total daily dose of between 2 and 8 mg is usually optimal, but higher doses are sometimes necessary. Treatment with clonazepam (in a dose that depends on response and tolerance) or clonidine (2–5 μg/kg/d) may also be helpful, and it seems sensible to begin with one of these drugs in order to avoid some of the long-term extrapyramidal side effects of haloperidol. Phenothiazines, such as fluphenazine (2–15 mg daily), have been used, but patients unresponsive to haloperidol are usually unresponsive to these as well.

Pimozide, an oral dopamine-blocking drug related to haloperidol, may be helpful in patients who cannot tolerate or have not responded to haloperidol. Treatment is started with 1 mg daily and the daily dose increased by 1–2 mg every 10 days; the average dose is between 7 and 16 mg daily.

Treatment with risperidone, calcium channel blockers, tetrabenazene, or clomipramine has yielded mixed results.

Jankovic J: Tourette's syndrome. N Engl J Med 2001;345;1184. [PMID 11642235] (Review.)

DEMENTIA

Dementia, the symptom complex of progressive global impairment of intellectual function, is a major medical, social, and economic problem that is worsening as the number of elderly people in the general population increases. It is discussed in Chapter 4, and the only point to be reiterated here is the importance of recognizing early any treatable or reversible causes of dementia, such as normal-pressure hydrocephalus, intracranial mass lesions, vascular disease, hypothyroidism, thiamin or vitamin B_{12} deficiency, Wilson's disease, hepatic or renal failure, neurosyphilis, and the chronic meningitides.

MULTIPLE SCLEROSIS

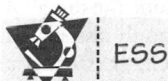

ESSENTIALS OF DIAGNOSIS

- Episodic neurologic symptoms.
- Patient usually under 55 years of age at onset.
- Single pathologic lesion cannot explain clinical findings.
- Multiple foci best visualized by MRI.

General Considerations

This common neurologic disorder, which probably has an autoimmune basis, has its greatest incidence in young adults. Epidemiologic studies indicate that multiple sclerosis is much more common in persons of western European lineage who live in temperate zones. No population with a high risk for multiple sclerosis exists between latitudes 40 °N and 40 °S. Genetic, dietary, and climatic factors cannot account for these differences. Nevertheless, a genetic susceptibility to the disease is likely, based on twin studies, familial cases, and an association with specific HLA antigens (HLA-DR2). Pathologically, focal—often perivenular—areas of demyelination with reactive gliosis are found scattered in the white matter of brain and spinal cord and in the optic nerves.

Clinical Findings

A. SYMPTOMS AND SIGNS

The common initial presentation is weakness, numbness, tingling, or unsteadiness in a limb; spastic paraparesis; retrobulbar neuritis; diplopia; disequilibrium; or a sphincter disturbance such as urinary urgency or hesitancy. Symptoms may disappear after a few days or weeks, although examination often reveals a residual deficit.

Several forms of the disease are recognized. In most patients, there is an interval of months or years after the initial episode before new symptoms develop or the original ones recur (relapsing-remitting disease). Eventually, however, relapses and usually incomplete remissions lead to increasing disability, with weakness, spasticity, and ataxia of the limbs, impaired vision, and urinary incontinence. The findings on examination at this stage commonly include optic atrophy, nystagmus, dysarthria, and pyramidal, sensory, or cerebellar deficits in some or all of the limbs. In some of these patients, the clinical course changes so that a steady deterioration occurs, unrelated to acute relapses (secondary progressive disease).

Less commonly, symptoms are steadily progressive from their onset, and disability develops at a relatively early stage (primary progressive disease). The diagnosis cannot be made with confidence unless the total clinical picture indicates involvement of different parts of the central nervous system at different times.

A number of factors (eg, infection, trauma) may precipitate or trigger exacerbations. Relapses are also more likely during the 2 or 3 months following pregnancy, possibly because of the increased demands and stresses that occur in the postpartum period.

B. IMAGING

MRI of the brain or cervical cord is often helpful in demonstrating the presence of a multiplicity of lesions. CT scans are less helpful.

In patients presenting with myelopathy alone and in whom there is no clinical or laboratory evidence of more widespread disease, myelography or MRI may be necessary to exclude a congenital or acquired surgically treatable lesion. The foramen magnum region must be visualized to exclude the possibility of Arnold-Chiari malformation, in which part of the cerebellum and the lower brain stem are displaced into the cervical canal and produce mixed pyramidal and cerebellar deficits in the limbs.

C. LABORATORY AND OTHER STUDIES

A definitive diagnosis can never be based solely on the laboratory findings. If there is clinical evidence of only a single lesion in the central nervous system, multiple sclerosis cannot properly be diagnosed unless it can be shown that other regions are affected subclinically. The electrocerebral responses evoked by monocular visual stimulation with a checkerboard pattern stimulus, by monaural click stimulation, and by electrical stimulation of a sensory or mixed peripheral nerve have been used to detect subclinical involvement of the visual, brain stem auditory, and somatosensory pathways, respectively. Other disorders may also be characterized by multifocal electrophysiologic abnormalities.

There may be mild lymphocytosis or a slightly increased protein concentration in the cerebrospinal fluid, especially soon after an acute relapse. Elevated IgG in cerebrospinal fluid and discrete bands of IgG (oligoclonal bands) are present in many patients. The presence of such bands is not specific, however, since they have been found in a variety of inflammatory neurologic disorders and occasionally in patients with vascular or neoplastic disorders of the nervous system.

D. DIAGNOSIS

Multiple sclerosis should not be diagnosed unless there is evidence that two or more different regions of the central white matter have been affected at different times. A diagnosis of clinically definite disease can be made in patients with a relapsing-remitting course and evidence on examination of at least two lesions involving different regions of the central white matter. The diagnosis is probable in patients with multifocal white matter disease but only one clinical attack, or with a history of at least two clinical attacks but signs of only a single lesion.

Treatment

At least partial recovery from acute exacerbations can reasonably be expected, but further relapses may occur without warning, and there is no means of preventing progression of the disorder. Some disability is likely to result eventually, but about half of all patients are without significant disability even 10 years after onset of symptoms.

Recovery from acute relapses may be hastened by treatment with corticosteroids, but the extent of recovery is unchanged. A high dose (eg, prednisone, 60 or 80 mg) is given daily for 1 week, after which medication is tapered over the following 2 or 3 weeks. Such a regimen is often preceded by methylprednisolone, 1 g intravenously for 3 days. Long-term treatment with steroids provides no benefit and does not prevent further relapses.

In patients with relapsing-remitting or secondary progressive disease, treatment with beta interferon or with daily subcutaneous administration of glatiramer acetate reduces the frequency of exacerbations. Several recent studies have suggested that immunosuppressive therapy with cyclophosphamide, azathioprine, methotrexate, cladribine, or mitoxantrone may help to arrest the course of secondary progressive multiple sclerosis. The evidence of benefit is incomplete, however. There

is little evidence that plasmapheresis enhances any beneficial effects of immunosuppression in multiple sclerosis. Intravenous immunoglobulins may reduce the clinical attack rate in relapsing-remitting disease, but the available studies are inadequate to permit treatment recommendations.

Treatment for spasticity (see below) and for neurogenic bladder may be needed in advanced cases. Excessive fatigue must be avoided, and patients should rest during periods of acute relapse.

Goodin DS et al: Disease modifying therapies in multiple sclerosis: subcommittee of the American Academy of Neurology and the MS Council for Clinical Practice Guidelines. Neurology 2002;58;169. [PMID 11805241] (Review.)

VITAMIN E DEFICIENCY

Vitamin E deficiency may produce a disorder somewhat similar to Friedreich's ataxia (see below). There is spinocerebellar degeneration involving particularly the posterior columns of the spinal cord and leading to limb ataxia, sensory loss, absent tendon reflexes, slurring of speech, and, in some cases, pigmentary retinal degeneration. The disorder may occur as a consequence of malabsorption or on a hereditary basis. Treatment is with alpha-tocopheryl acetate (eg, Aquasol E capsules or drops) as discussed in Chapter 29.

SPASTICITY

The term "spasticity" is commonly used for an upper motor neuron deficit, but it properly refers to a velocity-dependent increase in resistance to passive movement that affects different muscles to a different extent, is not uniform in degree throughout the range of a particular movement, and is commonly associated with other features of pyramidal deficit. It is often a major complication of stroke, cerebral or spinal injury, static perinatal encephalopathy, and multiple sclerosis.

Physical therapy with appropriate stretching programs is important during rehabilitation after the development of an upper motor neuron lesion and in subsequent management of the patient. The aim is to prevent joint and muscle contractures and perhaps to modulate spasticity.

Drug management is important also, but treatment may increase functional disability when increased extensor tone is providing additional support for patients with weak legs. Dantrolene weakens muscle contraction by interfering with the role of calcium. It is best avoided in patients with poor respiratory function or severe myocardial disease. Treatment is begun with 25 mg once daily, and the daily dose is built up by 25 mg increments every 3 days, depending on tolerance, to a maximum of 100 mg four times daily. Side effects include diarrhea, nausea, weakness, hepatic dysfunction (that may rarely be fatal, especially in women older than 35), drowsiness, light-headedness, and hallucinations.

Lioresal is an effective drug for treating spasticity of spinal origin and painful flexor (or extensor) spasms. The maximum recommended daily dose is 80 mg; treatment is started with a dose of 5 or 10 mg twice daily and then built up gradually. Side effects include gastrointestinal disturbances, lassitude, fatigue, sedation, unsteadiness, confusion, and hallucinations. Diazepam may modify spasticity by its action on spinal interneurons and perhaps also by influencing supraspinal centers, but effective doses often cause intolerable drowsiness and vary with different patients. Tizanidine, a centrally acting α_2-adrenergic agonist, is as effective as these other agents but is probably better tolerated. The daily dose is built up gradually, usually to 8 mg taken three times daily. Side effects include sedation, lassitude, hypotension, and dryness of the mouth.

Motor-point blocks by intramuscular phenol have been used to reduce spasticity selectively in one or a few important muscles and may permit return of function in patients with incomplete myelopathies. Intramuscular administration of botulinum toxin may also be helpful. Intrathecal injection of phenol or absolute alcohol may be helpful in more severe cases, but greater selectivity can be achieved by nerve root or peripheral nerve neurolysis. These procedures should not be undertaken until the spasticity syndrome is fully evolved, ie, only after about 1 year or so, and only if long-term drug treatment either has been unhelpful or carries a significant risk to the patient.

In patients with severe spasticity and limited use of the legs, a surgically implanted lioresal pump may provide significant relief and improve hygiene. A number of surgical procedures, eg, adductor or heel cord tenotomy, may also help in the management of spasticity and facilitate patient management. For example, obturator neurectomy is helpful in patients with marked adductor spasms that interfere with personal hygiene or cause gait disturbances. Posterior rhizotomy reduces spasticity, but its effect may be short-lived, whereas anterior rhizotomy produces permanent wasting and weakness in the muscles that are denervated.

Spasticity may be exacerbated by decubitus ulcers, urinary or other infections, and nociceptive stimuli.

Auff E et al: Clinical applications of botulinum toxin type A. Eur J Neurol 1999;6:Suppl 4. (Entire issue provides a review of clinical uses.)

MYELOPATHIES IN AIDS

A variety of myelopathies may occur in patients with AIDS. These are discussed in Chapter 31.

MYELOPATHY OF HUMAN T CELL LEUKEMIA VIRUS

Human T cell leukemia virus (HTLV-1), a human retrovirus, is transmitted by breast feeding, sexual contact, blood transfusion, and contaminated needles.

Most patients are asymptomatic, but after a variable latent period (may be as long as several years) a myelopathy develops in some instances. The MRI, electrophysiologic, and cerebrospinal fluid findings are similar to those of multiple sclerosis, but HTLV-1 antibodies are present in serum and spinal fluid. There is no specific treatment.

Engström JW: HTLV-I infection and the nervous system. In: *Neurology and General Medicine,* 3rd ed. Aminoff MJ (editor). Churchill Livingstone, 2001. (Clinical review.)

SUBACUTE COMBINED DEGENERATION OF THE SPINAL CORD

Subacute combined degeneration of the spinal cord is due to vitamin B_{12} deficiency, such as occurs in pernicious anemia. It is characterized by myelopathy with predominant pyramidal and posterior column deficits, sometimes in association with polyneuropathy, mental changes, or optic neuropathy. Megaloblastic anemia may also occur, but this does not parallel the neurologic disorder, and the former may be obscured if folic acid supplements have been taken. Treatment is with vitamin B_{12}. For pernicious anemia, a convenient therapeutic regimen is 100 mg cyanocobalamin intramuscularly daily for 1 week, then weekly for 1 month, and then monthly for the remainder of the patient's life.

WERNICKE'S ENCEPHALOPATHY

Wernicke's encephalopathy is characterized by confusion, ataxia, and nystagmus leading to ophthalmoplegia (lateral rectus muscle weakness, conjugate gaze palsies); peripheral neuropathy may also be present. It is due to thiamin deficiency and in the USA occurs most commonly in alcoholics. It may also occur in patients with AIDS. In suspected cases, thiamin (50 mg) is given intravenously immediately and then intramuscularly on a daily basis until a satisfactory diet can be ensured. Intravenous glucose given before thiamin may precipitate the syndrome or worsen the symptoms. The diagnosis is confirmed by the response in 1 or 2 days to treatment, which must not be delayed while laboratory confirmation is obtained.

Messing RO: Alcohol and the nervous system. In: *Neurology and General Medicine,* 3rd ed. Aminoff MJ (editor). Churchill Livingstone, 2001. (Clinical review.)

STUPOR & COMA

The patient who is stuporous is unresponsive except when subjected to repeated vigorous stimuli, while the comatose patient is unarousable and unable to respond to external events or inner needs, although reflex movements and posturing may be present.

Coma is a major complication of serious central nervous system disorders. It can result from seizures, hypothermia, metabolic disturbances, or structural lesions causing bilateral cerebral hemispheric dysfunction or a disturbance of the brain stem reticular activating system. A mass lesion involving one cerebral hemisphere may cause coma by compression of the brain stem.

Assessment & Emergency Measures

The diagnostic workup of the comatose patient must proceed concomitantly with management. Supportive therapy for respiration or blood pressure is initiated; in hypothermia, all vital signs may be absent, all such patients should be rewarmed before the prognosis is assessed.

The patient can be positioned on one side with the neck partly extended, dentures removed, and secretions cleared by suction; if necessary, the patency of the airways is maintained with an oropharyngeal airway. Blood is drawn for serum glucose, electrolyte, and calcium levels; arterial blood gases; liver and renal function tests; and toxicologic studies as indicated. Dextrose 50% (25 g), naloxone (0.4–1.2 mg), and thiamine (50 mg) are given intravenously.

Further details are then obtained from attendants of the patient's medical history, the circumstances surrounding the onset of coma, and the time course of subsequent events. Abrupt onset of coma suggests subarachnoid hemorrhage, brain stem stroke, or intracerebral hemorrhage, whereas a slower onset and progression occur with other structural or mass lesions. A metabolic cause is likely with a preceding intoxicated state or agitated delirium. On examination, attention is paid to the behavioral response to painful stimuli, the pupils and their response to light, the position of the eyes and their movement in response to passive movement of the head and ice-water caloric stimulation, and the respiratory pattern.

A. RESPONSE TO PAINFUL STIMULI

Purposive limb withdrawal from painful stimuli implies that sensory pathways from and motor pathways to the stimulated limb are functionally intact. Unilateral absence of responses despite application of stimuli to both sides of the body in turn implies a corticospinal lesion; bilateral absence of responsiveness suggests brain stem involvement, bilateral pyramidal tract lesions, or psychogenic unresponsiveness. Inappropriate responses may also occur. Decorticate posturing may occur with lesions of the internal capsule and rostral cerebral peduncle, decerebrate posturing with dysfunction or destruction of the midbrain and rostral pons, and decerebrate posturing in the arms accompanied by flaccidity or slight flexor responses in the legs in patients with extensive brain stem damage extending down to the pons at the trigeminal level.

B. OCULAR FINDINGS

1. Pupils—Hypothalamic disease processes may lead to unilateral Horner's syndrome, while bilateral diencephalic involvement or destructive pontine lesions may lead to small but reactive pupils. Ipsilateral pupillary dilation with no direct or consensual response to light occurs with compression of the third cranial nerve, eg, with uncal herniation. The pupils are slightly smaller than normal but responsive to light in many metabolic encephalopathies; however, they may be fixed and dilated following overdosage with atropine, scopolamine, or glutethimide, and pinpoint (but responsive) with opiates. Pupillary dilation for several hours following cardiopulmonary arrest implies a poor prognosis.

2. Eye movements—Conjugate deviation of the eyes to the side suggests the presence of an ipsilateral hemispheric lesion or a contralateral pontine lesion. A mesencephalic lesion leads to downward conjugate deviation. Dysconjugate ocular deviation in coma implies a structural brain stem lesion unless there was preexisting strabismus.

The oculomotor responses to passive head turning and to caloric stimulation relate to each other and provide complementary information. In response to brisk rotation of the head from side to side and to flexion and extension of the head, normally conscious patients with open eyes do not exhibit contraversive conjugate eye deviation (doll's-head eye response) unless there is voluntary visual fixation or bilateral frontal pathology. With cortical depression in lightly comatose patients, a brisk doll's-head eye response is seen. With brain stem lesions, this oculocephalic reflex becomes impaired or lost, depending on the site of the lesion. The oculovestibular reflex is tested by caloric stimulation using irrigation with ice water. In normal subjects, jerk nystagmus is elicited for about 2 or 3 minutes, with the slow component toward the irrigated ear. In unconscious patients with an intact brain stem, the fast component of the nystagmus disappears, so that the eyes tonically deviate toward the irrigated side for 2–3 minutes before returning to their original position. With impairment of brain stem function, the response becomes perverted and finally disappears. In metabolic coma, oculocephalic and oculovestibular reflex responses are preserved, at least initially.

C. RESPIRATORY PATTERNS

Diseases causing coma may lead to respiratory abnormalities. Cheyne-Stokes respiration may occur with bihemispheric or diencephalic disease or in metabolic disorders. Central neurogenic hyperventilation occurs with lesions of the brain stem tegmentum; apneustic breathing (in which there are prominent end-inspiratory pauses) suggests damage at the pontine level (eg, due to basilar artery occlusion); and atactic breathing (a completely irregular pattern of breathing with deep and shallow breaths occurring randomly) is associated with lesions of the lower pontine tegmentum and medulla.

1. Stupor & Coma Due to Structural Lesions

Supratentorial mass lesions tend to affect brain function in an orderly way. There may initially be signs of hemispheric dysfunction, such as hemiparesis. As coma develops and deepens, cerebral function becomes progressively disturbed, producing a predictable progression of neurologic signs that suggest rostrocaudal deterioration.

Thus, as a supratentorial mass lesion begins to impair the diencephalon, the patient becomes drowsy, then stuporous, and finally comatose. There may be Cheyne-Stokes respiration; small but reactive pupils; doll's-head eye responses with side-to-side head movements but sometimes an impairment of reflex upward gaze with brisk flexion of the head; tonic ipsilateral deviation of the eyes in response to vestibular stimulation with cold water; and initially a positive response to pain but subsequently only decorticate posturing. With further progression, midbrain failure occurs. Motor dysfunction progresses from decorticate to bilateral decerebrate posturing in response to painful stimuli; Cheyne-Stokes respiration is gradually replaced by sustained central hyperventilation; the pupils become middle-sized and fixed; and the oculocephalic and oculovestibular reflex responses become impaired, perverted, or lost. As the pons and then the medulla fail, the pupils remain unresponsive; oculovestibular responses are unobtainable; respiration is rapid and shallow; and painful stimuli may lead only to flexor responses in the legs. Finally, respiration becomes irregular and stops, the pupils often then dilating widely.

In contrast, a subtentorial (ie, brain stem) lesion may lead to an early, sometimes abrupt disturbance of consciousness without any orderly rostrocaudal progression of neurologic signs. Compressive lesions of the brain stem, especially cerebellar hemorrhage, may be clinically indistinguishable from intraparenchymal processes.

A structural lesion is suspected if the findings suggest focality. In such circumstances, a CT scan should be performed before, or instead of, a lumbar puncture in order to avoid any risk of cerebral herniation. Further management is of the causal lesion and is considered separately under the individual disorders.

2. Stupor & Coma Due to Metabolic Disturbances

Patients with a metabolic cause of coma generally have signs of patchy, diffuse, and symmetric neurologic involvement that cannot be explained by loss of function at any single level or in a sequential manner, although focal or lateralized deficits may occur in hypoglycemia. Moreover, pupillary reactivity is usually preserved, while other brain stem functions are often grossly impaired. Comatose patients with meningitis, encephalitis, or subarachnoid hemorrhage may also exhibit little in the way of focal neurologic signs, however, and clinical evidence of meningeal irritation is sometimes very subtle in comatose patients. Examination of the cerebrospinal fluid in such patients is essential to establish the correct diagnosis.

In patients with coma due to cerebral ischemia and hypoxia, the absence of pupillary light reflexes at the time of initial examination indicates that there is little chance of regaining independence; by contrast, preserved pupillary light responses, the development of spontaneous eye movements (roving, conjugate, or better), and extensor, flexor, or withdrawal responses to pain at this early stage imply a relatively good prognosis.

Treatment of metabolic encephalopathy is of the underlying disturbance and is considered in other chapters. If the cause of the encephalopathy is obscure, all drugs except essential ones may have to be withdrawn in case they are responsible for the altered mental status.

Feske SK: Coma and confusional states: Emergency diagnosis and management. Neurol Clin North Am 1998;16:237. [PMID: 9537961]

Young GB (editor): *Coma and Impaired Consciousness: A Clinical Perspective.* McGraw-Hill, 1998.

3. Brain Death

The definition of brain death is controversial, and diagnostic criteria have been published by many different professional organizations. In order to establish brain death, the irreversibly comatose patient must be shown to have lost all brain stem reflex responses, including the pupillary, corneal, oculovestibular, oculocephalic, oropharyngeal, and respiratory reflexes, and should have been in this condition for at least 6 hours. Spinal reflex movements do not exclude the diagnosis, but ongoing seizure activity or decerebrate or decorticate posturing is not consistent with brain death. The apnea test (presence or absence of spontaneous respiratory activity at a $PaCO_2$ of at least 60 mm Hg) serves to determine whether the patient is capable of respiratory activity.

Reversible coma simulating brain death may be seen with hypothermia (temperature < 32 °C) and overdosage with central nervous system depressant drugs, and these conditions must be excluded. Certain ancillary tests may assist the determination of brain death but are not essential. An isoelectric electroencephalogram, when the recording is made according to the recommendations of the American Electroencephalographic Society, is especially helpful in confirming the diagnosis. Alternatively, the demonstration of an absent cerebral circulation by intravenous radioisotope cerebral angiography or by four-vessel contrast cerebral angiography can be confirmatory.

Wijdicks EFM: Brain death worldwide. Neurology 2002,50.20. [PMID 11781400] (Review of diagnostic criteria in different countries.)

4. Persistent Vegetative State

Patients with severe bilateral hemispheric disease may show some improvement from an initially comatose state, so that, after a variable interval, they appear to be awake but lie motionless and without evidence of awareness or higher mental activity. This persistent vegetative state has been variously referred to as akinetic mutism, apallic state, or coma vigil. Most patients in this persistent vegetative state will die in months or years, but partial recovery has occasionally occurred and in rare instances has been sufficient to permit communication or even independent living.

5. Locked-In Syndrome (De-efferented State)

Acute destructive lesions (eg, infarction, hemorrhage, demyelination, encephalitis) involving the ventral pons and sparing the tegmentum may lead to a mute, quadriparetic but conscious state in which the patient is capable of blinking and of voluntary eye movement in the vertical plane, with preserved pupillary responses to light. Such a patient can mistakenly be regarded as comatose. Physicians should recognize that "locked-in" individuals are fully aware of their surroundings. The prognosis is variable, but recovery has occasionally been reported—in some cases including resumption of independent daily life, though this may take up to 2 or 3 years.

HEAD INJURY

Trauma is the most common cause of death in young people, and head injury accounts for almost half of these trauma-related deaths. The prognosis following head injury depends upon the site and severity of brain damage. Some guide to prognosis is provided by the mental status, since loss of consciousness for more than 1 or 2 minutes implies a worse prognosis than otherwise. Similarly, the degree of retrograde and posttraumatic amnesia provides an indication of the severity of injury and thus of the prognosis. Absence of skull fracture does not exclude the possibility of severe head injury. During the physical examination, special attention should be given to the level of consciousness and extent of any brain stem dysfunction.

Note: Patients who have lost consciousness for 2 minutes or more following head injury should be admitted to the hospital for observation, as should patients with focal neurologic deficits, lethargy, or skull fractures. If admission is declined, responsible family members should be given clear instructions about the need for, and manner of, checking on them at regular (hourly) intervals and for obtaining additional medical help if necessary.

Skull radiographs or CT scans may provide evidence of fractures. Because injury to the spine may have accompanied head trauma, cervical spine radiographs (especially in the lateral projection) should always be obtained in comatose patients and in patients with severe neck pain or a deficit possibly related to cord compression. CT scanning has an important role in demonstrating intracranial hemorrhage and may also provide evidence of cerebral edema and displacement of midline structures.

Cerebral Injuries

These are summarized in Table 24–5 along with comments about treatment. Increased intracranial pressure may result from ventilatory obstruction, abnormal

Table 24–5. Acute cerebral sequelae of head injury.

Sequelae	Clinical Features	Pathology
Concussion	Transient loss of consciousness with bradycardia, hypotension, and respiratory arrest for a few seconds followed by retrograde and posttraumatic amnesia. Occasionally followed by transient neurologic deficit.	Bruising on side of impact (coup injury) or contralaterally (contrecoup injury).
Cerebral contusion or laceration	Loss of consciousness longer than with concussion. May lead to death or severe residual neurologic deficit.	Cerebral contusion, edema, hemorrhage, and necrosis. May have subarachnoid bleeding.
Acute epidural hemorrhage	Headache, confusion, somnolence, seizures, and focal deficits occur several hours after injury and lead to coma, respiratory depression, and death unless treated by surgical evacuation.	Tear in meningeal artery, vein, or dural sinus, leading to hematoma visible on CT scan.
Acute subdural hemorrhage	Similar to epidural hemorrhage, but interval before onset of symptoms is longer. Treatment is by surgical evacuation.	Hematoma from tear in veins from cortex to superior sagittal sinus or from cerebral laceration, visible on CT scan.
Cerebral hemorrhage	Generally develops immediately after injury. Clinically resembles hypertensive hemorrhage. Surgical evacuation is sometimes helpful.	Hematoma, visible on CT scan.

neck position, seizures, dilutional hyponatremia, or cerebral edema; an intracranial hematoma requiring surgical evacuation may also be responsible. Other measures that may be necessary to reduce intracranial pressure include induced hyperventilation, intravenous mannitol infusion, and intravenous furosemide; corticosteroids provide no benefit in this context.

Scalp Injuries & Skull Fractures

Scalp lacerations and depressed or compound depressed skull fractures should be treated surgically as appropriate. Simple skull fractures require no specific treatment.

The clinical signs of basilar skull fracture include bruising about the orbit (raccoon sign), blood in the external auditory meatus (Battle's sign), and leakage of cerebrospinal fluid (which can be identified by its glucose content) from the ear or nose. Cranial nerve palsies (involving especially the first, second, third, fourth, fifth, seventh, and eighth nerves in any combination) may also occur. If there is any leakage of cerebrospinal fluid, conservative treatment, with elevation of the head, restriction of fluids, and administration of acetazolamide (250 mg four times daily), is often helpful; but if the leak continues for more than a few days, lumbar subarachnoid drainage may be necessary. Antibiotics are given if infection occurs, based on culture and sensitivity studies. Only very occasional patients require intracranial repair of the dural defect because of persistence of the leak or recurrent meningitis.

Late Complications of Head Injury

The relationship of chronic subdural hemorrhage to head injury is not always clear. In many elderly persons there is no history of trauma, but in other cases a head injury, often trivial, precedes the onset of symptoms by several weeks. The clinical presentation is usually with mental changes such as slowness, drowsiness, headache, confusion, memory disturbances, personality change, or even dementia. Focal neurologic deficits such as hemiparesis or hemisensory disturbance may also occur but are less common. CT scan is an important means of detecting the hematoma, which is sometimes bilateral. Treatment is by surgical evacuation to prevent cerebral compression and tentorial herniation. There is no clear evidence that prophylactic anticonvulsant therapy reduces the incidence of posttraumatic seizures.

Normal-pressure hydrocephalus may follow head injury, subarachnoid hemorrhage, or meningoencephalitis.

Other late complications of head injury include posttraumatic seizure disorder and posttraumatic headache.

Attia J et al: Prognosis in anoxic and traumatic coma. Crit Care Clin 1998;14:497. [PMID: 9700444] (Meta-analysis.)

Schierhout G et al: Prophylactic antiepileptic agents after head injury: A systematic review. J Neurol Neurosurg Psychiatry 1998;64:108. [PMID: 9436738] (Meta-analysis.)

SPINAL TRAUMA

While spinal cord damage may result from whiplash injury, severe injury usually relates to fracture-dislocation causing compression or angular deformity of the cord either cervically or in the lower thoracic and upper lumbar regions. Extreme hypotension following injury may also lead to cord infarction.

Total cord transection results in immediate flaccid paralysis and loss of sensation below the level of the lesion. Reflex activity is lost for a variable period, and there is urinary and fecal retention. As reflex function returns over the following days and weeks, spastic paraplegia or quadriplegia develops, with hyperreflexia and extensor plantar responses, but a flaccid atrophic (lower motor neuron) paralysis may be found depending on the segments of the cord that are affected. The bladder and bowels also regain some reflex function, permitting urine and feces to be expelled at intervals. As spasticity increases, flexor or extensor spasms (or both) of the legs become troublesome, especially if the patient develops bed sores or a urinary tract infection. Paraplegia with the legs in flexion or extension may eventually result.

With lesser degrees of injury, patients may be left with mild limb weakness, distal sensory disturbance, or both. Sphincter function may also be impaired, urinary urgency and urgency incontinence being especially common. More particularly, a unilateral cord lesion leads to an ipsilateral motor disturbance with accompanying impairment of proprioception and contralateral loss of pain and temperature appreciation below the lesion (Brown-Séquard's syndrome). A central cord syndrome may lead to a lower motor neuron deficit and loss of pain and temperature appreciation, with sparing of posterior column functions. A radicular deficit may occur at the level of the injury—or, if the cauda equina is involved, there may be evidence of disturbed function in several lumbosacral roots.

Treatment of the injury consists of immobilization and—if there is cord compression—decompressive laminectomy and fusion. Early treatment with high doses of corticosteroids (eg, methylprednisolone, 30 mg/kg by intravenous bolus, followed by 5.4 mg/kg/h for 23 hours) has been shown to improve neurologic recovery if commenced within 8 hours after injury. Treatment with G_{M1} ganglioside for 3 or 4 weeks is an experimental approach that has also been helpful. Anatomic realignment of the spinal cord by traction and other orthopedic procedures is also important. Subsequent care of the residual neurologic deficit—paraplegia or quadriplegia—requires treatment of spasticity and care of the skin, bladder, and bowels.

Yu D: A crash course in spinal cord injury. Postgrad Med 1998;104:109. [PMID: 9721582]

SYRINGOMYELIA

Destruction or degeneration of gray and white matter adjacent to the central canal of the cervical spinal cord leads to cavitation and accumulation of fluid within the spinal cord. The precise pathogenesis is unclear, but many cases are associated with Arnold-Chiari malformation, in which there is displacement of the cerebellar tonsils, medulla, and fourth ventricle into the spinal canal, sometimes with accompanying meningomyelocele. In such circumstances, the cord cavity connects with and may merely represent a dilated central canal. In other cases, the cause of cavitation is less clear. There is a characteristic clinical picture, with segmental atrophy and areflexia and loss of pain and temperature appreciation in a "cape" distribution owing to the destruction of fibers crossing in front of the central canal. Thoracic kyphoscoliosis is usually present. With progression, involvement of the long motor and sensory tracts occurs as well, so that a pyramidal and sensory deficit develops in the legs. Upward extension of the cavitation (syringobulbia) leads to dysfunction of the lower brain stem and thus to bulbar palsy, nystagmus, and sensory impairment over one or both sides of the face.

Syringomyelia, ie, cord cavitation, may also occur in association with an intramedullary tumor or following severe cord injury, and the cavity then does not communicate with the central canal.

In patients with Arnold-Chiari malformation, there are commonly skeletal abnormalities on plain x-rays of the skull and cervical spine. CT scans show caudal displacement of the fourth ventricle. MRI or positive contrast myelography may demonstrate the malformation itself. Focal cord enlargement is found at myelography or by MRI in patients with cavitation related to past injury or intramedullary neoplasms.

Treatment of Arnold-Chiari malformation with associated syringomyelia is by suboccipital craniectomy and upper cervical laminectomy, with the aim of decompressing the malformation at the foramen magnum. The cord cavity should be drained, and if necessary an outlet for the fourth ventricle can be made. In cavitation associated with intramedullary tumor, treatment is surgical, but radiation therapy may be necessary if complete removal is not possible. Posttraumatic syringomyelia is also treated surgically if it leads to increasing neurologic deficits or to intolerable pain.

Goel A et al: Surgery for syringomyelia: an analysis based on 163 surgical cases. Acta Neurochir (Wien) 2000;142:293. [PMID: 10819260] (Clinical study.)

MOTOR NEURON DISEASES

This group of disorders is characterized clinically by weakness and variable wasting of affected muscles, without accompanying sensory changes.

Motor neuron disease in adults generally commences between 30 and 60 years of age. There is degeneration of the anterior horn cells in the spinal cord, the motor nuclei of the lower cranial nerves, and the corticospinal and corticobulbar pathways. The disorder is usually sporadic, but familial cases may occur.

Classification

Five varieties have been distinguished on clinical grounds.

A. PROGRESSIVE BULBAR PALSY

Bulbar involvement predominates owing to disease processes affecting primarily the motor nuclei of the cranial nerves.

B. PSEUDOBULBAR PALSY

Bulbar involvement predominates in this variety also, but it is due to bilateral corticobulbar disease and thus reflects upper motor neuron dysfunction.

C. PROGRESSIVE SPINAL MUSCULAR ATROPHY

This is characterized primarily by a lower motor neuron deficit in the limbs due to degeneration of the anterior horn cells in the spinal cord.

D. PRIMARY LATERAL SCLEROSIS

There is a purely upper motor neuron deficit in the limbs.

E. AMYOTROPHIC LATERAL SCLEROSIS

A mixed upper and lower motor neuron deficit is found in the limbs. This disorder is sometimes associated with dementia or parkinsonism.

Clinical Findings

A. SYMPTOMS AND SIGNS

Difficulty in swallowing, chewing, coughing, breathing, and talking (dysarthria) occur with bulbar involvement. In progressive bulbar palsy, there is drooping of the palate, a depressed gag reflex, pooling of saliva in the pharynx, a weak cough, and a wasted, fasciculating tongue. In pseudobulbar palsy, the tongue is contracted and spastic and cannot be moved rapidly from side to side. Limb involvement is characterized by motor disturbances (weakness, stiffness, wasting, fasciculations) reflecting lower or upper motor neuron dysfunction; there are no objective changes on sensory examination, though there may be vague sensory complaints. The sphincters are generally spared.

The disorder is progressive, and amyotrophic lateral sclerosis is usually fatal within 3–5 years; death usually results from pulmonary infections. Patients with bulbar involvement generally have the poorest prognosis.

B. LABORATORY AND OTHER STUDIES

Electromyography may show changes of chronic partial denervation, with abnormal spontaneous activity in the resting muscle and a reduction in the number of motor units under voluntary control. In patients with suspected spinal muscular atrophy or amyotrophic lateral sclerosis, the diagnosis should not be made with confidence unless such changes are found in at least three extremities. Motor conduction velocity is usually normal but may be slightly reduced, and sensory conduction studies are also normal. Biopsy of a wasted muscle shows the histologic changes of denervation. The serum creatine kinase may be slightly elevated but never reaches the extremely high values seen in some of the muscular dystrophies. The cerebrospinal fluid is normal.

A familial form of amyotrophic lateral sclerosis has been described with autosomal dominant inheritance, related to mutations in the copper-zinc superoxide dismutase gene on the long arm of chromosome 21. X-linked bulbospinal neuronopathy is associated with an expanded trinucleotide repeat sequence on the androgen receptor gene and carries a more benign prognosis than other forms of motor neuron disease. There have been recent reports of juvenile spinal muscular atrophy due to hexosaminidase deficiency, with abnormal findings on rectal biopsy and reduced hexosaminidase A in serum and leukocytes. Pure motor syndromes resembling motor neuron disease may also occur in association with monoclonal gammopathy or multifocal motor neuropathies with conduction block. A motor neuronopathy may also develop in Hodgkin's disease and has a relatively benign prognosis.

Treatment

Riluzole, which reduces the presynaptic release of glutamate, may slow progression of amyotrophic lateral sclerosis. There is otherwise no specific treatment except in patients with gammopathy, in whom plasmapheresis and immunosuppression may lead to improvement. Therapeutic trials of various neurotrophic factors to slow disease progression have yielded generally disappointing results. Symptomatic and supportive measures may include prescription of anticholinergic drugs (such as trihexyphenidyl, amitriptyline, or atropine) if drooling is troublesome, braces or a walker to improve mobility, and physical therapy to prevent contractures. Spasticity may be helped by baclofen or diazepam. A semiliquid diet or nasogastric tube feeding may be needed if dysphagia is severe. Gastrostomy or cricopharyngomyotomy is sometimes resorted to in extreme cases of predominant bulbar involvement, and tracheostomy may be necessary if respiratory muscles are severely affected; however, in the terminal stages of these disorders, the aim of treatment should be to keep patients as comfortable as possible.

Benditt JO et al: Empowering the individual with ALS at the end-of-life: disease-specific advance care planning. Muscle Nerve 2001;24:1706. [PMID: 11745983] (Suggested advance care planning document.)

Miller RG: New approaches to therapy of amyotrophic lateral sclerosis. West J Med 1998;168:262. [PMID: 9584665]

Parton MJ et al: Motor neuron disease and its management. J R Coll Physicians Lond 1999;33:212. [PMID: 10402566] (Review.)

PERIPHERAL NEUROPATHIES

Peripheral neuropathies can be categorized on the basis of the structure primarily affected. The predominant pathologic feature may be axonal degeneration (axonal or neuronal neuropathies) or paranodal or segmental demyelination. The distinction may be possible on the basis of neurophysiologic findings. Motor and sensory conduction velocity can be measured in accessible segments of peripheral nerves. In axonal neuropathies, conduction velocity is normal or reduced only mildly and needle electromyography provides evidence of denervation in affected muscles. In demyelinating neuropathies, conduction may be slowed considerably in affected fibers, and in more severe cases, conduction is blocked completely, without accompanying electromyographic signs of denervation.

Nerves may be injured or compressed by neighboring anatomic structures at any point along their course. Common **mononeuropathies** of this sort are considered below. They lead to a sensory, motor, or mixed deficit that is restricted to the territory of the affected nerve. A similar clinical disturbance is produced by peripheral nerve tumors, but these are rare except in patients with Recklinghausen's disease. Multiple mononeuropathies suggest a patchy multifocal disease process such as vasculopathy (eg, diabetes, arteritis), an infiltrative process (eg, leprosy, sarcoidosis), radiation damage, or an immunologic disorder (eg, brachial plexopathy). Diffuse **polyneuropathies** lead to a symmetric sensory, motor, or mixed deficit, often most marked distally. They include the hereditary, metabolic, and toxic disorders; idiopathic inflammatory polyneuropathy (Guillain-Barré syndrome); and the peripheral neuropathies that may occur as a nonmetastatic complication of malignant diseases. Involvement of motor fibers leads to flaccid weakness that is most marked distally; dysfunction of sensory fibers causes impaired sensory perception. Tendon reflexes are depressed or absent. Paresthesias, pain, and muscle tenderness may also occur.

1. Polyneuropathies & Mononeuritis Multiplex

The cause of polyneuropathy or mononeuritis multiplex is suggested by the history, mode of onset, and predominant clinical manifestations. Laboratory workup includes a complete blood count and sedimentation rate, serum protein electrophoresis, determination of plasma urea and electrolytes, liver and thyroid function tests, tests for rheumatoid factor and antinuclear antibody, HBsAg determination, a serologic test for syphilis, fasting blood glucose level, urinary heavy metal levels, cerebrospinal fluid examination, and chest radiography. These tests should be ordered selectively, as guided by symptoms and signs. Measurement of nerve conduction velocity is important in confirming the peripheral nerve origin of symptoms and providing a means of following clinical changes, as well as indicating the likely disease process (ie, axonal or demyelinating neuropathy). Cutaneous nerve biopsy may help establish a precise diagnosis (eg, polyarteritis, amyloidosis). In about half of cases, no specific cause can be established; of these, slightly less than half are subsequently found to be heredofamilial.

Treatment is of the underlying cause, when feasible, and is discussed below under the individual disorders. Physical therapy helps prevent contractures, and splints can maintain a weak extremity in a position of useful function. Anesthetic extremities must be protected from injury. To guard against burns, patients should check the temperature of water and hot surfaces with a portion of skin having normal sensation, measure water temperature with a thermometer, and use cold water for washing or lower the temperature setting of their hot-water heaters. Shoes should be examined frequently during the day for grit or foreign objects in order to prevent pressure lesions.

Patients with polyneuropathies or mononeuritis multiplex are subject to additional nerve injury at pressure points and should therefore avoid such behavior as leaning on elbows or sitting with crossed legs for lengthy periods.

Neuropathic pain is sometimes troublesome and may respond to simple analgesics such as aspirin. Narcotics or narcotic substitutes may be necessary for severe hyperpathia or pain induced by minimal stimuli, but their use should be avoided as far as possible. The use of a frame or cradle to reduce contact with bedclothes may be helpful. Many patients experience episodic stabbing pains, which may respond to phenytoin, carbamazepine, gabapentin, or tricyclic antidepressants.

Symptoms of autonomic dysfunction are occasionally troublesome. Postural hypotension is often helped by wearing waist-high elastic stockings and sleeping in a semierect position at night. Fludrocortisone reduces postural hypotension, but doses as high as 1 mg/d are sometimes necessary in diabetics and may lead to recumbent hypertension. Midodrine, an alpha agonist, is sometimes helpful in a dose of 2.5–10 mg three times daily. Impotence and diarrhea are difficult to treat; a flaccid neuropathic bladder may respond to parasympathomimetic drugs such as bethanechol chloride, 10–50 mg three or four times daily.

Inherited Neuropathies

A. CHARCOT-MARIE-TOOTH DISEASE

Several distinct varieties of Charcot-Marie-Tooth disease can be recognized. There is usually an autosomal dominant mode of inheritance, but occasional cases occur on a sporadic, recessive, or X-linked basis. The responsible gene is commonly located on the short arm of chromosome 17 and less often shows linkage to chromosome 1 or the X chromosome. Clinical presentation may be with foot deformities or gait disturbances in childhood or early adult life. Slow progres-

sion leads to the typical features of polyneuropathy, with distal weakness and wasting that begin in the legs, a variable amount of distal sensory loss, and depressed or absent tendon reflexes. Tremor is a conspicuous feature in some instances. Electrodiagnostic studies show a marked reduction in motor and sensory conduction velocity (hereditary motor and sensory neuropathy [HMSN] type I).

In other instances (HMSN type II), motor conduction velocity is normal or only slightly reduced, sensory nerve action potentials may be absent, and signs of chronic partial denervation are found in affected muscles electromyographically. The predominant pathologic change is axonal loss rather than segmental demyelination.

A similar disorder may occur in patients with progressive distal spinal muscular atrophy, but there is no sensory loss; electrophysiologic investigation reveals that motor conduction velocity is normal or only slightly reduced, and nerve action potentials are normal.

B. DEJERINE-SOTTAS DISEASE (HMSN TYPE III)

Most cases are sporadic or autosomal recessive. The recessive form has its onset in infancy or childhood and leads to a progressive motor and sensory polyneuropathy with weakness, ataxia, sensory loss, and depressed or absent tendon reflexes. The peripheral nerves may be palpably enlarged and are characterized pathologically by segmental demyelination, Schwann cell hyperplasia, and thin myelin sheaths. Electrophysiologically, there is slowing of conduction, and sensory action potentials may be unrecordable.

C. FRIEDREICH'S ATAXIA

Patients generally present in childhood or early adult life with this autosomal recessive disorder, which has been related to an unstable mutation of the *X25* gene on chromosome 9q13–q21.1. The gait becomes atactic, the hands become clumsy, and other signs of cerebellar dysfunction develop accompanied by weakness of the legs and extensor plantar responses. Involvement of peripheral sensory fibers leads to sensory disturbances in the limbs and depressed tendon reflexes. There is bilateral pes cavus. Pathologically, there is a marked loss of cells in the posterior root ganglia and degeneration of peripheral sensory fibers. In the central nervous system, changes are conspicuous in the posterior and lateral columns of the cord. Electrophysiologically, conduction velocity in motor fibers is normal or only mildly reduced, but sensory action potentials are small or absent.

D. REFSUM'S DISEASE (HMSN TYPE IV)

This autosomal recessive disorder is due to a disturbance in phytanic acid metabolism. Clinically, pigmentary retinal degeneration is accompanied by progressive sensorimotor polyneuropathy and cerebellar signs. Auditory dysfunction, cardiomyopathy, and cutaneous manifestations may also occur. Motor and sensory conduction velocity is reduced, often markedly, and there may be electromyographic evidence of denervation in affected muscles. Dietary restriction of phytanic acid and its precursors may be helpful therapeutically.

E. PORPHYRIA

Peripheral nerve involvement may occur during acute attacks in both variegate porphyria and acute intermittent porphyria. Motor symptoms usually occur first, and weakness is often most marked proximally and in the upper limbs rather than the lower. Sensory symptoms and signs may be proximal or distal in distribution. Autonomic involvement is sometimes pronounced. The electrophysiologic findings are in keeping with the results of neuropathologic studies suggesting that the neuropathy is axonal in type. Hematin (4 mg/kg intravenously over 15 minutes once or twice daily) may lead to rapid improvement. A high-carbohydrate diet and, in severe cases, intravenous glucose or levulose may also be helpful. Propranolol (up to 100 mg every 4 hours) may control tachycardia and hypertension in acute attacks. Porphyria is discussed further in Chapter 40.

Neuropathies Associated With Systemic & Metabolic Disorders

A. DIABETES MELLITUS

In this disorder, involvement of the peripheral nervous system may lead to symmetric sensory or mixed polyneuropathy, asymmetric motor radiculoneuropathy or plexopathy (diabetic amyotrophy), thoracoabdominal radiculopathy, autonomic neuropathy, or isolated lesions of individual nerves. These may occur singly or in any combination and are discussed in Chapter 27.

B. UREMIA

Uremia may lead to a symmetric sensorimotor polyneuropathy that tends to affect the lower limbs more than the upper limbs and is more marked distally than proximally (Chapter 22). The diagnosis can be confirmed electrophysiologically, for motor and sensory conduction velocity is moderately reduced. The neuropathy improves both clinically and electrophysiologically with renal transplantation and to a lesser extent with chronic dialysis.

C. ALCOHOLISM AND NUTRITIONAL DEFICIENCY

Many alcoholics have an axonal distal sensorimotor polyneuropathy that is frequently accompanied by painful cramps, muscle tenderness, and painful paresthesias and is often more marked in the legs than in the arms. Symptoms of autonomic dysfunction may also be conspicuous. Motor and sensory conduction velocity may be slightly reduced, even in subclinical cases, but gross slowing of conduction is uncommon. A similar distal sensorimotor polyneuropathy is a well-recognized feature of beriberi (thiamin deficiency). In vitamin B_{12} deficiency, distal sensory polyneuropathy may develop but is usually overshadowed by central nervous system manifestations (eg, myelopathy, optic neuropathy, or intellectual changes).

D. PARAPROTEINEMIAS

A symmetric sensorimotor polyneuropathy that is gradual in onset, progressive in course, and often accompanied by pain and dysesthesias in the limbs may occur in patients (especially men) with multiple myeloma. The neuropathy is of the axonal type in classic lytic myeloma, but segmental demyelination (primary or secondary) and axonal loss may occur in sclerotic myeloma and lead to predominantly motor clinical manifestations. Both demyelinating and axonal neuropathies are also observed in patients with paraproteinemias without myeloma. A small fraction will develop myeloma if serially followed. The demyelinating neuropathy in these patients may be due to the monoclonal protein's reacting to a component of the nerve myelin. The neuropathy of classic multiple myeloma is poorly responsive to therapy. The polyneuropathy of benign monoclonal gammopathy may respond to immunosuppressant drugs and plasmapheresis.

Polyneuropathy may also occur in association with macroglobulinemia and cryoglobulinemia and sometimes responds to plasmapheresis. Entrapment neuropathy, such as carpal tunnel syndrome, is more common than polyneuropathy in patients with (nonhereditary) generalized amyloidosis. With polyneuropathy due to amyloidosis, sensory and autonomic symptoms are especially conspicuous, whereas distal wasting and weakness occur later; there is no specific treatment.

Neuropathies Associated With Infectious & Inflammatory Diseases

A. LEPROSY

Leprosy is an important cause of peripheral neuropathy in certain parts of the world. Sensory disturbances are mainly due to involvement of intracutaneous nerves. In tuberculoid leprosy, they develop at the same time and in the same distribution as the skin lesion but may be more extensive if nerve trunks lying beneath the lesion are also involved. In lepromatous leprosy, there is more extensive sensory loss, and this develops earlier and to a greater extent in the coolest regions of the body, such as the dorsal surfaces of the hands and feet, where the bacilli proliferate most actively. Motor deficits result from involvement of superficial nerves where their temperature is lowest, eg, the ulnar nerve in the region proximal to the olecranon groove, the median nerve as it emerges from beneath the forearm flexor muscle to run toward the carpal tunnel, the peroneal nerve at the head of the fibula, and the posterior tibial nerve in the lower part of the leg; patchy facial muscular weakness may also occur owing to involvement of the superficial branches of the seventh cranial nerve.

Motor disturbances in leprosy are suggestive of multiple mononeuropathy, whereas sensory changes resemble those of distal polyneuropathy. Examination, however, relates the distribution of sensory deficits to the temperature of the tissues; in the legs, for example, sparing frequently occurs between the toes and in the popliteal fossae, where the temperature is higher. Treatment is with antileprotic agents (see Chapter 33).

B. AIDS

A variety of neuropathies occur in HIV-infected patients (see Chapter 31). Patients with AIDS may develop a chronic symmetric sensorimotor axonal **polyneuropathy** associated usually with no abnormal cerebrospinal fluid findings. Treatment is symptomatic. AIDS patients may also develop progressive **polyradiculopathy** or radiculomyelopathy that leads to leg weakness and urinary retention; sensory loss is less conspicuous than in polyneuropathy. The cerebrospinal fluid may show mononuclear pleocytosis and increased protein and low glucose concentrations. Cytomegalovirus is responsible in at least some cases. The prognosis is generally poor, but some patients respond to intravenous ganciclovir (2.5 mg/kg every 8 hours for 10 days, then 7.5 mg/kg daily 5 days per week).

An inflammatory **demyelinating polyradiculoneuropathy** sometimes occurs in HIV-seropositive patients without AIDS and may follow an acute, subacute, or chronic course. Weakness is usually more conspicuous distally than proximally and tends to overshadow sensory symptoms. Tendon reflexes are depressed or absent. The cerebrospinal fluid shows an increased cell count and protein concentration. Treatment with plasmapheresis has helped some patients. Spontaneous improvement may also occur. Seropositive patients without AIDS may also develop a **mononeuropathy multiplex** that sometimes responds to treatment with plasmapheresis.

C. LYME BORRELIOSIS

The neurologic manifestations of Lyme disease include meningitis, meningoencephalitis, polyradiculoneuropathy, mononeuropathy multiplex, and cranial neuropathy. Serologic tests establish the underlying disorder. Treatment is as described in Chapter 34.

D. SARCOIDOSIS

Cranial nerve palsies (especially facial palsy), multiple mononeuropathy, and, less commonly, symmetric polyneuropathy may all occur, the latter sometimes preferentially affecting either motor or sensory fibers. Improvement may occur with use of corticosteroids.

E. POLYARTERITIS

Involvement of the vasa nervorum by the vasculitic process may result in infarction of the nerve. Clinically, one encounters an asymmetric sensorimotor polyneuropathy (mononeuritis multiplex) that pursues a waxing and waning course. Steroids and cytotoxic agents—especially cyclophosphamide—may be of benefit in severe cases.

F. RHEUMATOID ARTHRITIS

Compressive or entrapment neuropathies, ischemic neuropathies, mild distal sensory polyneuropathy, and severe progressive sensorimotor polyneuropathy can occur in rheumatoid arthritis.

Neuropathy Associated With Critical Illness

Patients in intensive care units with sepsis and multiorgan failure sometimes develop polyneuropathies. This may be manifested initially by unexpected difficulty in weaning patients from a mechanical ventilator and in more advanced cases by wasting and weakness of the extremities and loss of tendon reflexes. Sensory abnormalities are relatively inconspicuous. The neuropathy is axonal in type. Its pathogenesis is obscure, and treatment is supportive. The prognosis is good provided patients recover from the underlying critical illness.

Toxic Neuropathies

Axonal polyneuropathy may follow exposure to industrial agents or pesticides such as acrylamide, organophosphorus compounds, hexacarbon solvents, methyl bromide, and carbon disulfide; metals such as arsenic, thallium, mercury, and lead; and drugs such as phenytoin, perhexiline, isoniazid, nitrofurantoin, vincristine, and pyridoxine in high doses. Detailed occupational, environmental, and medical histories and recognition of clusters of cases are important in suggesting the diagnosis. Treatment is by preventing further exposure to the causal agent. Isoniazid neuropathy is prevented by pyridoxine supplementation.

Diphtheritic neuropathy results from a neurotoxin released by the causative organism and is common in many areas. Palatal weakness may develop 2–4 weeks after infection of the throat, and infection of the skin may similarly be followed by focal weakness of neighboring muscles. Disturbances of accommodation may occur about 4–5 weeks after infection and distal sensorimotor demyelinating polyneuropathy after 1–3 months.

Neuropathies Associated With Malignant Diseases (Table 40–6)

Both a sensorimotor and a purely sensory polyneuropathy may occur as a nonmetastatic complication of malignant diseases. The sensorimotor polyneuropathy may be mild and occur in the course of known malignant disease; or it may have an acute or subacute onset, lead to severe disability, and occur before there is any clinical evidence of the cancer, occasionally following a remitting course.

Acute Idiopathic Polyneuropathy (Guillain-Barré Syndrome)

This acute or subacute polyradiculoneuropathy sometimes follows infective illness, inoculations, or surgical procedures. There is an association with preceding *Campylobacter jejuni* enteritis. The disorder probably has an immunologic basis, but the precise mechanism is unclear. The main complaint is of weakness that varies widely in severity in different patients and often has a proximal emphasis and symmetric distribution. It usually begins in the legs, spreading to a variable extent but frequently involving the arms and often one or both sides of the face. The muscles of respiration or deglutition may also be affected. Sensory symptoms are usually less conspicuous than motor ones, but distal paresthesias and dysesthesias are common, and neuropathic or radicular pain is present in many patients. Autonomic disturbances are also common, may be severe, and are sometimes life-threatening; they include tachycardia, cardiac irregularities, hypotension or hypertension, facial flushing, abnormalities of sweating, pulmonary dysfunction, and impaired sphincter control.

The cerebrospinal fluid characteristically contains a high protein concentration with a normal cell content, but these changes may take 2 or 3 weeks to develop. Electrophysiologic studies may reveal marked abnormalities, which do not necessarily parallel the clinical disorder in their temporal course. Pathologic examination has shown primary demyelination or, less commonly, axonal degeneration.

When the diagnosis is made, the history and appropriate laboratory studies should exclude the possibility of porphyric, diphtheritic, or toxic (heavy metal, hexacarbon, organophosphate) neuropathies. Poliomyelitis, botulism, and tick paralysis must also be considered. The presence of pyramidal signs, a markedly asymmetric motor deficit, a sharp sensory level, or early sphincter involvement should suggest a focal cord lesion.

Most patients eventually make a good recovery, but this may take many months, and 10–20% patients of are left with persisting disability. Treatment with prednisone is ineffective and may prolong recovery time. Plasmapheresis is of value; it is best performed within the first few days of illness and is best reserved for clinically severe or rapidly progressive cases or those with ventilatory impairment. Intravenous immunoglobulin (400 mg/kg/d for 5 days) is also helpful and imposes less stress on the cardiovascular system than plasmapheresis. Patients should be admitted to intensive care units if their forced vital capacity is declining, and intubation is considered if the forced vital capacity reaches 15 mL/kg, dyspnea becomes evident, or the oxygen saturation declines. Respiratory toilet and chest physical therapy help prevent atelectasis. Marked hypotension may respond to volume replacement or pressor agents. Low-dose heparin to prevent pulmonary embolism should be considered.

Approximately 3% of patients with acute idiopathic polyneuropathy have one or more clinically similar relapses, sometimes several years after the initial illness. Plasma exchange therapy may produce improvement in chronic and relapsing inflammatory polyneuropathy.

Chronic Inflammatory Polyneuropathy

Chronic inflammatory demyelinating polyneuropathy, an acquired immunologically mediated disorder, is clinically similar to Guillain-Barré syndrome except that it has a relapsing or steadily progressive course over months or years. In the relapsing form, partial recovery may occur after some relapses, but in other instances there is no recovery between exacerbations. Although remission may occur spontaneously with time, the disorder frequently follows a progressive downhill course leading to severe functional disability.

Electrodiagnostic studies show marked slowing of motor and sensory conduction, and focal conduction block. Signs of partial denervation may also be present owing to secondary axonal degeneration. Nerve biopsy may show chronic perivascular inflammatory infiltrates in the endoneurium and epineurium, without accompanying evidence of vasculitis. However, a normal nerve biopsy result or the presence of nonspecific abnormalities does not exclude the diagnosis.

Corticosteroids may be effective in arresting or reversing the downhill course. Treatment is usually begun with prednisone, 60 mg daily, continued for 2–3 months or until a definite response has occurred. If no response has occurred despite 3 months of treatment, a higher dose may be tried. In responsive cases, the dose is gradually tapered, but most patients become corticosteroid-dependent, often requiring prednisone, 20 mg daily on alternate days, on a long term basis. Patients unresponsive to corticosteroids may benefit instead from treatment with a cytotoxic drug such as azathioprine. There are increasing anecdotal reports of short-term benefit with plasmapheresis; high-dose intravenous immunoglobulin treatment (eg, 400 mg/kg/d) may produce clinical improvement lasting for weeks to months.

Jensen PG et al: Management of painful diabetic neuropathy. Drugs Aging 2001;18;737. [PMID: 11735621] (Clinical review.)

Manji H: Neuropathy in HIV infection. Curr Opin Neurol 2000;13;589. [PMID: 11073368] (Review .)

Saperstein DS et al: Clinical spectrum of chronic acquired demyelinating polyneuropathies. Muscle Nerve 2001;24;311. [PMID: 11353415] (Clinical review.)

Wicklund MP et al: Paraproteinemic neuropathy. Curr Treat Options Neurol 2001;3;147. [PMID: 11180752] (Review.)

Winer JB: Guillain-Barré syndrome. Mol Pathol 2001;54;381. [PMID: 11724912] (Review.)

2. Mononeuropathies

An individual nerve may be injured along its course or may be compressed, angulated, or stretched by neighboring anatomic structures, especially at a point where it passes through a narrow space (entrapment neuropathy). The relative contributions of mechanical factors and ischemia to the local damage are not clear. With involvement of a sensory or mixed nerve, pain is commonly felt distal to the lesion. Symptoms never develop with some entrapment neuropathies, resolve rapidly and spontaneously in others, and become progressively more disabling and distressing in yet other cases. The precise neurologic deficit depends on the nerve involved. Percussion of the nerve at the site of the lesion may lead to paresthesias in its distal distribution.

Entrapment neuropathy may be the sole manifestation of subclinical polyneuropathy, and this must be borne in mind and excluded by nerve conduction studies. Such studies are also indispensable for the accurate localization of the focal lesion.

In patients with acute compression neuropathy such as may occur in intoxicated individuals, ("Saturday night palsy") no treatment is necessary. Complete recovery generally occurs, usually within 2 months, presumably because the underlying pathology is demyelination. However, axonal degeneration can occur in severe cases, and recovery then takes longer and may never be complete.

In chronic compressive or entrapment neuropathies, avoidance of aggravating factors and correction of any underlying systemic conditions are important. Local infiltration of the region about the nerve with corticosteroids may be of value; in addition, surgical decompression may help if there is a progressively increasing neurologic deficit or if electrodiagnostic studies show evidence of partial denervation in weak muscles.

Peripheral nerve tumors are uncommon, except in Recklinghausen's disease, but also give rise to mononeuropathy. This may be distinguishable from entrapment neuropathy only by noting the presence of a mass along the course of the nerve and by demonstrating the precise site of the lesion with appropriate electrophysiologic studies. Treatment of symptomatic lesions is by surgical removal if possible.

Carpal Tunnel Syndrome

See Chapter 20.

Pronator Teres or Anterior Interosseous Syndrome

The median nerve gives off its motor branch, the anterior interosseous nerve, below the elbow as it descends between the two heads of the pronator teres muscle. A lesion of either nerve may occur in this region, sometimes after trauma or owing to compression from, for example, a fibrous band. With anterior interosseous nerve involvement, there is no sensory loss, and weakness is confined to the pronator quadratus, flexor pollicis longus, and the flexor digitorum profundus to the second and third digits. Weakness is more widespread and sensory changes occur in an appropriate distribution when the median nerve itself is affected. The prognosis is variable. If improvement does not occur spontaneously, decompressive surgery may be helpful.

Ulnar Nerve Lesions

Ulnar nerve lesions are likely to occur in the elbow region as the nerve runs behind the medial epicondyle and descends into the cubital tunnel. In the condylar groove, the ulnar nerve is exposed to pressure or trauma. Moreover, any increase in the carrying angle of the elbow, whether congenital, degenerative, or traumatic, may cause excessive stretching of the nerve when the elbow is flexed. Ulnar nerve lesions may also result from thickening or distortion of the anatomic structures forming the cubital tunnel, and the resulting symptoms may also be aggravated by flexion of the elbow, because the tunnel is then narrowed by tightening of its roof or inward bulging of its floor. A severe lesion at either site causes sensory changes in the medial 1½ digits and along the medial border of the hand. There is weakness of the ulnar-innervated muscles in the forearm and hand. With a cubital tunnel lesion, however, there may be relative sparing of the flexor carpi ulnaris muscle. Electrophysiologic evaluation using nerve stimulation techniques allows more precise localization of the lesion.

If conservative measures are unsuccessful in relieving symptoms and preventing further progression, surgical treatment may be necessary. This consists of nerve transposition if the lesion is in the condylar groove, or a release procedure if it is in the cubital tunnel.

Ulnar nerve lesions may also develop at the wrist or in the palm of the hand, usually owing to repetitive trauma or to compression from ganglia or benign tumors. They can be subdivided depending upon their presumed site. Compressive lesions are treated surgically. If repetitive mechanical trauma is responsible, this is avoided by occupational adjustment or job retraining.

Radial Nerve Lesions

The radial nerve is particularly liable to compression or injury in the axilla (eg, by crutches or by pressure when the arm hangs over the back of a chair). This leads to weakness or paralysis of all the muscles supplied by the nerve, including the triceps. Sensory changes may also occur but are often surprisingly inconspicuous, being marked only in a small area on the back of the hand between the thumb and index finger. Injuries to the radial nerve in the spiral groove occur characteristically during deep sleep, as in intoxicated individuals (Saturday night palsy), and there is then sparing of the triceps muscle, which is supplied more proximally. The nerve may also be injured at or above the elbow; its purely motor posterior interosseous branch, supplying the extensors of the wrist and fingers, may be involved immediately below the elbow, but then there is sparing of the extensor carpi radialis longus, so that the wrist can still be extended. The superficial radial nerve may be compressed by handcuffs or a tight watch strap.

Femoral Neuropathy

The clinical features of femoral nerve palsy consist of weakness and wasting of the quadriceps muscle, with sensory impairment over the anteromedian aspect of the thigh and sometimes also of the leg to the medial malleolus, and a depressed or absent knee jerk. Isolated femoral neuropathy may occur in diabetics or from compression by retroperitoneal neoplasms or hematomas (eg, expanding aortic aneurysm). Femoral neuropathy may also result from pressure from the inguinal ligament when the thighs are markedly flexed and abducted, as in the lithotomy position.

Meralgia Paresthetica

The lateral femoral cutaneous nerve, a sensory nerve arising from the L2 and L3 roots, may be compressed or stretched in obese or diabetic patients and during pregnancy. The nerve usually runs under the outer portion of the inguinal ligament to reach the thigh, but the ligament sometimes splits to enclose it. Hyperextension of the hip or increased lumbar lordosis—such as occurs during pregnancy—leads to nerve compression by the posterior fascicle of the ligament. However, entrapment of the nerve at any point along its course may cause similar symptoms, and several other anatomic variations predispose the nerve to damage when it is stretched. Pain, paresthesia, or numbness occurs about the outer aspect of the thigh, usually unilaterally, and is sometimes relieved by sitting. Examination shows no abnormalities except in severe cases when cutaneous sensation is impaired in the affected area. Symptoms are usually mild and commonly settle spontaneously. Hydrocortisone injections medial to the anterosuperior iliac spine often relieve symptoms temporarily, while nerve decompression by transposition may provide more lasting relief.

Sciatic & Common Peroneal Nerve Palsies

Misplaced deep intramuscular injections are probably still the most common cause of sciatic nerve palsy. Trauma to the buttock, hip, or thigh may also be responsible. The resulting clinical deficit depends on whether the whole nerve has been affected or only certain fibers. In general, the peroneal fibers of the sciatic nerve are more susceptible to damage than those destined for the tibial nerve. A sciatic nerve lesion may therefore be difficult to distinguish from peroneal neuropathy unless there is electromyographic evidence of involvement of the short head of the biceps femoris muscle. The common peroneal nerve itself may be compressed or injured in the region of the head and neck of the fibula, eg, by sitting with crossed legs or wearing high boots. There is weakness of dorsiflexion and eversion of the foot, accompanied by numbness or blunted sensation of the anterolateral aspect of the calf and dorsum of the foot.

Tarsal Tunnel Syndrome

The tibial nerve, the other branch of the sciatic, supplies several muscles in the lower extremity, gives origin to the sural nerve, and then continues as the posterior tibial nerve to supply the plantar flexors of the foot and toes. It passes through the tarsal tunnel behind and below the medial malleolus, giving off calcaneal branches and the medial and lateral plantar nerves that supply small muscles of the foot and the skin on the plantar aspect of the foot and toes. Compression of the posterior tibial nerve or its branches between the bony floor and ligamentous roof of the tarsal tunnel leads to pain, paresthesias, and numbness over the bottom of the foot, especially at night, with sparing of the heel. Muscle weakness may be hard to recognize clinically. Compressive lesions of the individual plantar nerves may also occur more distally, with similar clinical features to those of the tarsal tunnel syndrome. Treatment is surgical decompression.

Aminoff MJ: *Electromyography in Clinical Practice: Clinical and Electrodiagnostic Aspects of Neuromuscular Disease*, 3rd ed. Churchill Livingstone, 1998.

Facial Neuropathy

An isolated facial palsy may occur in patients with HIV seropositivity, sarcoidosis, or Lyme disease (Chapter 34), but most often it is idiopathic (Bell's palsy).

3. Bell's Palsy

Bell's palsy is an idiopathic facial paresis of lower motor neuron type that has been attributed to an inflammatory reaction involving the facial nerve near the stylomastoid foramen or in the bony facial canal. Reactivation of herpes simplex virus has been postulated, but there is limited evidence to support that view.

The clinical features of Bell's palsy are characteristic. The facial paresis generally comes on abruptly, but it may worsen over the following day or so. Pain about the ear precedes or accompanies the weakness in many cases but usually lasts for only a few days. The face itself feels stiff and pulled to one side. There may be ipsilateral restriction of eye closure and difficulty with eating and fine facial movements. A disturbance of taste is common, owing to involvement of chorda tympani fibers, and hyperacusis due to involvement of fibers to the stapedius occurs occasionally.

The management of Bell's palsy is controversial. Approximately 60% of cases recover completely without

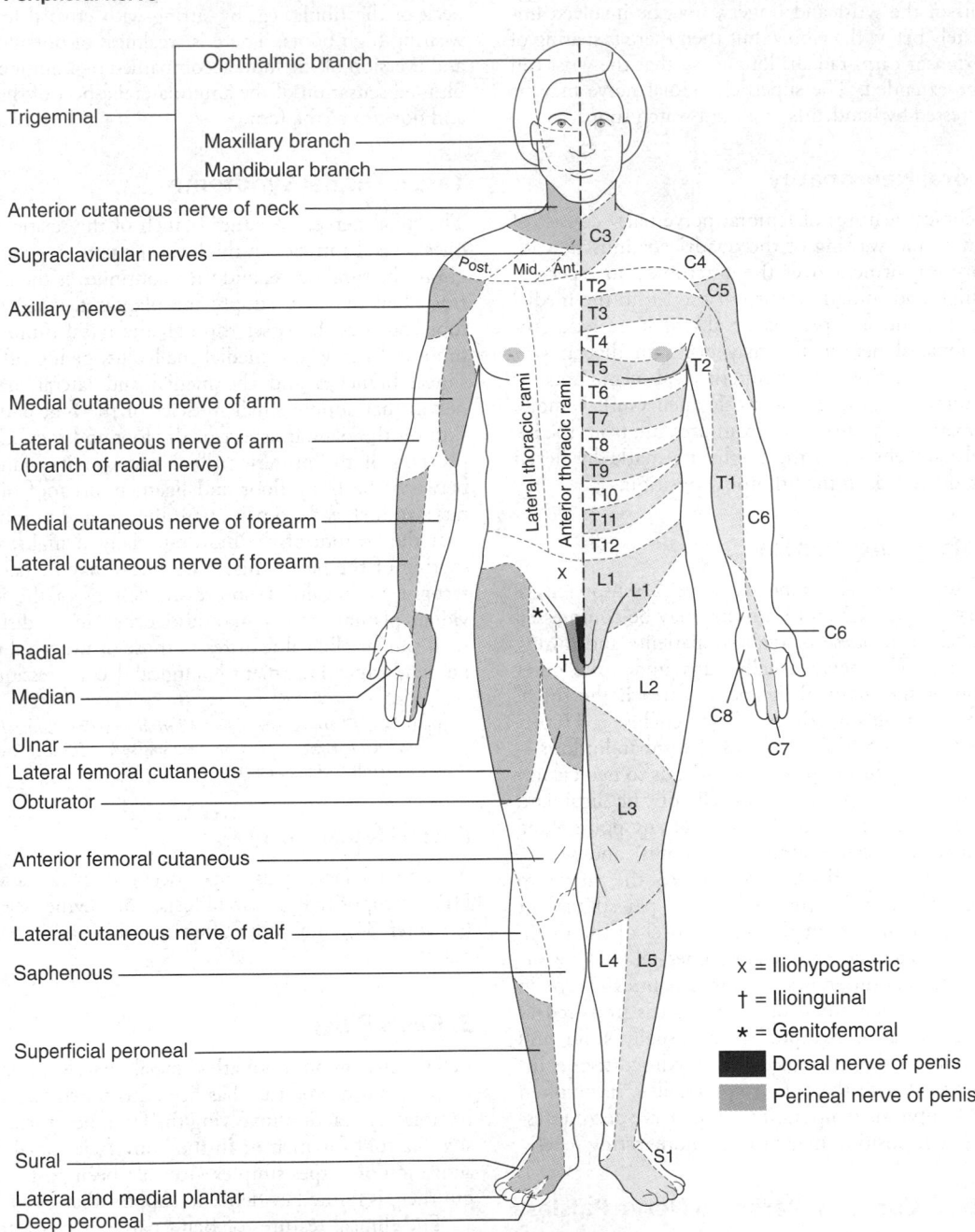

Peripheral nerve

Trigeminal
- Ophthalmic branch
- Maxillary branch
- Mandibular branch

Anterior cutaneous nerve of neck

Supraclavicular nerves

Axillary nerve

Medial cutaneous nerve of arm

Lateral cutaneous nerve of arm
(branch of radial nerve)

Medial cutaneous nerve of forearm

Lateral cutaneous nerve of forearm

Radial

Median

Ulnar

Lateral femoral cutaneous

Obturator

Anterior femoral cutaneous

Lateral cutaneous nerve of calf

Saphenous

Superficial peroneal

Sural

Lateral and medial plantar

Deep peroneal

Nerve root

Post. Mid. Ant.

Lateral thoracic rami

Anterior thoracic rami

C3
C4
C5
T2
T3
T4
T5
T6
T7
T8
T9
T10
T11
T12
L1
T2
T1
C6
C8
C7
L2
L3
L4 L5
S1

x = Iliohypogastric
† = Ilioinguinal
* = Genitofemoral
■ Dorsal nerve of penis
▨ Perineal nerve of penis

Figure 24–1. Cutaneous innervation. The segmental or radicular (root) distribution is shown on the left side of the body and the peripheral nerve distribution on the right side. **Above:** anterior view; **facing page:** posterior view. (Reproduced, with permission, from Simon RP, Aminoff MJ, Greenberg DA: *Clinical Neurology,* 4th ed. McGraw-Hill, 1999.)

Nerve root

Peripheral nerve

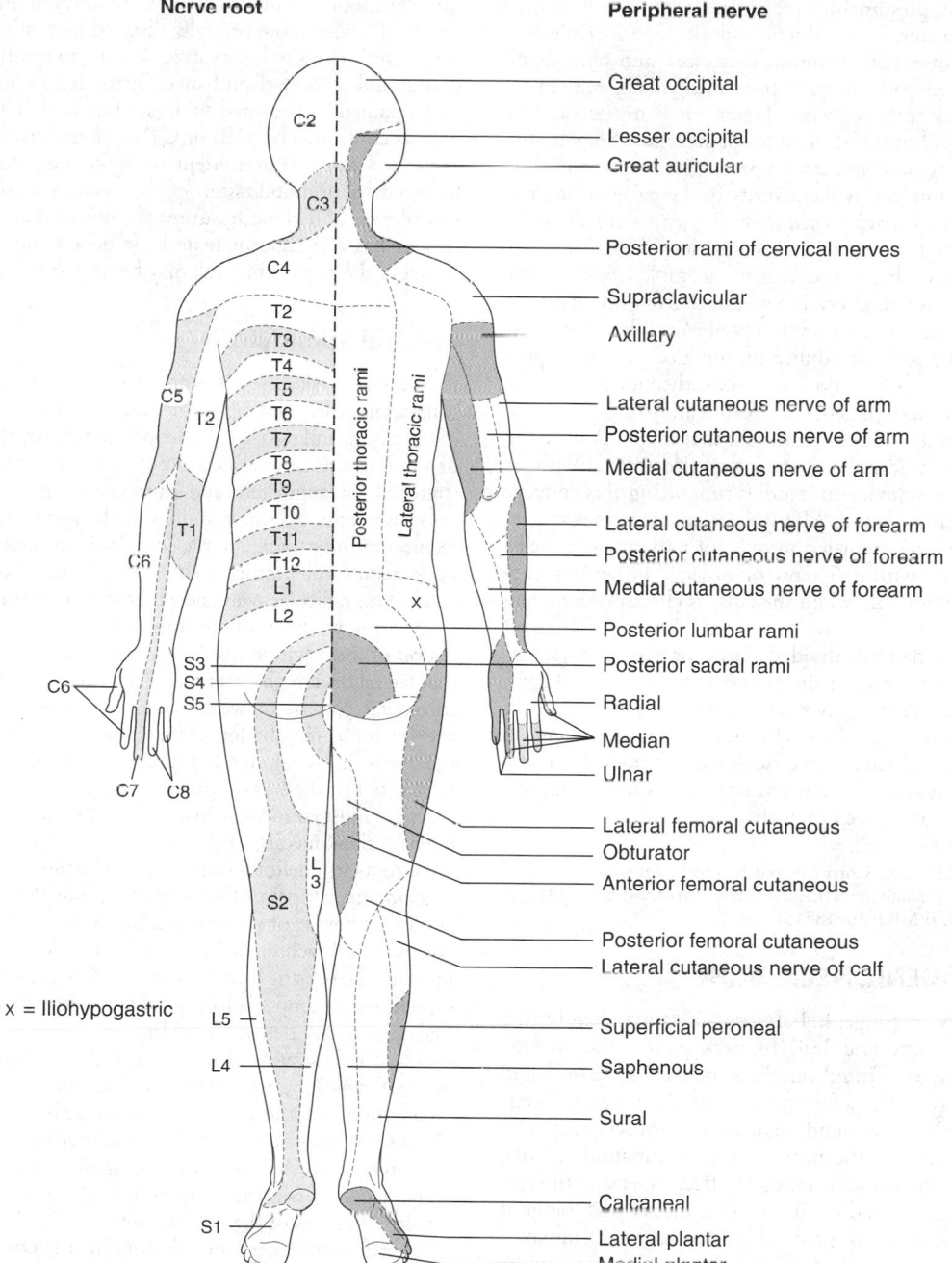

Great occipital

Lesser occipital

Great auricular

Posterior rami of cervical nerves

Supraclavicular

Axillary

Lateral cutaneous nerve of arm

Posterior cutaneous nerve of arm

Medial cutaneous nerve of arm

Lateral cutaneous nerve of forearm

Posterior cutaneous nerve of forearm

Medial cutaneous nerve of forearm

Posterior lumbar rami

Posterior sacral rami

Radial

Median

Ulnar

Lateral femoral cutaneous

Obturator

Anterior femoral cutaneous

Posterior femoral cutaneous

Lateral cutaneous nerve of calf

Superficial peroneal

Saphenous

Sural

Calcaneal

Lateral plantar

Medial plantar

x = Iliohypogastric

C2

C3

C4

T2
T3
T4
T5
T6
T7
T8
T9
T10
T11
T12
L1
L2

C5

T2

T1

C6

S3
S4
S5

C6

C7 C8

Posterior thoracic rami

Lateral thoracic rami

x

L
3

S2

L5

L4

S1

treatment, presumably because the lesion is so mild that it leads merely to conduction block. Considerable improvement occurs in most other cases, and only about 10% of all patients have permanent disfigurement or other long-term sequelae. Treatment is unnecessary in most cases but is indicated for patients in whom an unsatisfactory outcome can be predicted. The best clinical guide to progress is the severity of the palsy during the first few days after presentation. Patients with clinically complete palsy when first seen are less likely to make a full recovery than those with an incomplete one. A poor prognosis for recovery is also associated with advanced age, hyperacusis, and severe initial pain. Electromyography and nerve excitability or conduction studies provide a guide to prognosis but not early enough to aid in the selection of patients for treatment.

The only medical treatment that may influence the outcome is administration of corticosteroids with or without acyclovir, but studies supporting this concept have been criticized. Many clinicians nevertheless routinely prescribe corticosteroids for patients with Bell's palsy seen within 5 days of onset. The author prescribes them only when the palsy is clinically complete or there is severe pain. Treatment with prednisone, 60 or 80 mg daily in divided doses for 4 or 5 days, followed by tapering of the dose over the next 7–10 days, is a satisfactory regimen. It is helpful to protect the eye with lubricating drops (or lubricating ointment at night) and a patch if eye closure is not possible. There is no evidence that surgical procedures to decompress the facial nerve are of benefit.

Ramsey MJ et al: Corticosteroid treatment for idiopathic facial nerve paralysis: a meta-analysis. Laryngoscope 2000;110: 335. [PMID: 10718415]

DISCOGENIC NECK PAIN*

A variety of congenital abnormalities may involve the cervical spine and lead to neck pain; these include hemivertebrae, fused vertebrae, basilar impression, and instability of the atlantoaxial joint. Traumatic, degenerative, infective, and neoplastic disorders may also lead to pain in the neck. When rheumatoid arthritis involves the spine, it tends to affect especially the cervical region, leading to pain, stiffness, and reduced mobility; displacement of vertebrae or atlantoaxial subluxation may lead to cord compression that can be life-threatening if not treated by fixation. Further details are given in Chapter 20, and discussion here is restricted to disk disease.

Acute Cervical Disk Protrusion

Acute cervical disk protrusion leads to pain in the neck and radicular pain in the arm, exacerbated by head movement. With lateral herniation of the disk, motor, sensory, or reflex changes may be found in a radicular

*Low back pain is discussed in Chapter 20.

(usually C6 or C7) distribution on the affected side (Figure 24–1); with more centrally directed herniations, the spinal cord may also be involved, leading to spastic paraparesis and sensory disturbances in the legs, sometimes accompanied by impaired sphincter function. The diagnosis is confirmed by MRI or CT myelography. In mild cases, bed rest or intermittent neck traction may help, followed by immobilization of the neck in a collar for several weeks. If these measures are unsuccessful or the patient has a significant neurologic deficit, surgical removal of the protruding disk may be necessary.

Cervical Spondylosis

Cervical spondylosis results from chronic cervical disk degeneration, with herniation of disk material, secondary calcification, and associated osteophytic outgrowths. One or more of the cervical nerve roots may be compressed, stretched, or angulated; and myelopathy may also develop as a result of compression, vascular insufficiency, or recurrent minor trauma to the cord. Patients present with neck pain and restricted head movement, occipital headaches, radicular pain and other sensory disturbances in the arms, weakness of the arms or legs, or some combination of these symptoms. Examination generally reveals that lateral flexion and rotation of the neck are limited. A segmental pattern of weakness or dermatomal sensory loss (or both) may be found unilaterally or bilaterally in the upper limbs, and tendon reflexes mediated by the affected root or roots are depressed. The C5 and C6 nerve roots are most commonly involved, and examination frequently then reveals weakness of muscles supplied by these roots (eg, deltoids, supra- and infraspinatus, biceps, brachioradialis), pain or sensory loss about the shoulder and outer border of the arm and forearm, and depressed biceps and brachioradialis reflexes. Spastic paraparesis may also be present if there is an associated myelopathy, sometimes accompanied by posterior column or spinothalamic sensory deficits in the legs.

Plain radiographs of the cervical spine show osteophyte formation, narrowing of disk spaces, and encroachment on the intervertebral foramina, but such changes are common in middle-aged persons and may be unrelated to the presenting complaint. CT or MRI helps to confirm the diagnosis and exclude other structural causes of the myelopathy.

Restriction of neck movements by a cervical collar may relieve pain. Operative treatment may be necessary to prevent further progression if there is a significant neurologic deficit or if root pain is severe, persistent, and unresponsive to conservative measures.

BRACHIAL & LUMBAR PLEXUS LESIONS

Brachial Plexus Neuropathy

Brachial plexus neuropathy may be idiopathic, sometimes occurring in relationship to a number of different nonspecific illnesses or factors. In other instances, brachial plexus lesions follow trauma or result from congenital anomalies, neoplastic involvement, or injury by various physical agents. In rare instances, the disorder occurs on a familial basis.

Idiopathic brachial plexus neuropathy (neuralgic amyotrophy) characteristically begins with severe pain about the shoulder, followed within a few days by weakness, reflex changes, and sensory disturbances involving especially the C5 and C6 segments. Symptoms and signs are usually unilateral but may be bilateral. Wasting of affected muscles is sometimes profound. The disorder relates to disturbed function of cervical roots or part of the brachial plexus, but its precise cause is unknown. Recovery occurs over the ensuing months but may be incomplete. Treatment is purely symptomatic.

Cervical Rib Syndrome

Compression of the C8 and T1 roots or the lower trunk of the brachial plexus by a cervical rib or band arising from the seventh cervical vertebra leads to weakness and wasting of intrinsic hand muscles, especially those in the thenar eminence, accompanied by pain and numbness in the medial two fingers and the ulnar border of the hand and forearm. The subclavian artery may also be compressed, and this forms the basis of Adson's test for diagnosing the disorder; the radial pulse is diminished or obliterated on the affected side when the seated patient inhales deeply and turns the head to one side or the other. Electromyography, nerve conduction studies, and somatosensory evoked potential studies may help confirm the diagnosis. X-rays sometimes show the cervical rib or a large transverse process of the seventh cervical vertebra, but normal findings do not exclude the possibility of a cervical band. Treatment of the disorder is by surgical excision of the rib or band.

Lumbosacral Plexus Lesions

A lumbosacral plexus lesion may develop in association with diseases such as diabetes, cancer, or bleeding disorders or in relation to injury. It occasionally occurs as an isolated phenomenon similar to idiopathic brachial plexopathy, and pain and weakness then tend to be more conspicuous than sensory symptoms. The distribution of symptoms and signs depends on the level and pattern of neurologic involvement.

DISORDERS OF NEUROMUSCULAR TRANSMISSION

1. Myasthenia Gravis

ESSENTIALS OF DIAGNOSIS

- Fluctuating weakness of commonly used voluntary muscles, producing symptoms such as diplopia, ptosis, and difficulty in swallowing.
- Activity increases weakness of affected muscles.
- Short-acting anticholinesterases transiently improve the weakness.

General Considerations

Myasthenia gravis occurs at all ages, sometimes in association with a thymic tumor or thyrotoxicosis, as well as in rheumatoid arthritis and lupus erythematosus. It is commonest in young women with HLA-DR3; if thymoma is associated, older men are more commonly affected. Onset is usually insidious, but the disorder is sometimes unmasked by a coincidental infection that leads to exacerbation of symptoms. Exacerbations may also occur before the menstrual period and during or shortly after pregnancy. Symptoms are due to a variable degree of block of neuromuscular transmission caused by autoantibodies binding to acetylcholine receptors; these are found in most patients with the disease and have a primary role in reducing the number of functioning acetylcholine receptors. Additionally, cellular immune activity against the receptor is found. Clinically, this leads to weakness; initially powerful movements fatigue readily. The external ocular muscles and certain other cranial muscles, including the masticatory, facial, and pharyngeal muscles, are especially likely to be affected, and the respiratory and limb muscles may also be involved.

Clinical Findings

A. SYMPTOMS AND SIGNS

Patients present with ptosis, diplopia, difficulty in chewing or swallowing, respiratory difficulties, limb weakness, or some combination of these problems. Weakness may remain localized to a few muscle groups, especially the ocular muscles, or may become generalized. Symptoms often fluctuate in intensity during the day, and this diurnal variation is superimposed on a tendency to longer-term spontaneous relapses and remissions that may last for weeks. Nevertheless, the disorder follows a slowly progressive course and may have a fatal outcome owing to respiratory complications such as aspiration pneumonia.

Clinical examination confirms the weakness and fatigability of affected muscles. In most cases, the extraocular muscles are involved, and this leads to ocular palsies and ptosis, which are commonly asymmetric. Pupillary responses are normal. The bulbar and limb muscles are often weak, but the pattern of involvement is variable. Sustained activity of affected muscles increases the weakness, which improves after a brief rest. Sensation is normal, and there are usually no reflex changes.

The diagnosis can generally be confirmed by the response to a short-acting anticholinesterase. Edrophonium can be given intravenously in a dose of 10 mg (1 mL), 2 mg being given initially and the remaining 8 mg about 30 seconds later if the test dose is well tolerated; in myasthenic patients, there is an obvious improvement in strength of weak muscles lasting for about 5 minutes. Alternatively, 1.5 mg of neostigmine can be given intramuscularly, and the response then lasts for about 2 hours; atropine sulfate (0.6 mg) should be available to reverse muscarinic side effects.

B. Imaging

Lateral and anteroposterior x-rays of the chest and CT scans should be obtained to demonstrate a coexisting thymoma, but normal studies do not exclude this possibility.

C. Laboratory and Other Studies

Electrophysiologic demonstration of a decrementing muscle response to repetitive 2- or 3-Hz stimulation of motor nerves indicates a disturbance of neuromuscular transmission. Such an abnormality may even be detected in clinically strong muscles with certain provocative procedures. Needle electromyography of affected muscles shows a marked variation in configuration and size of individual motor unit potentials, and single-fiber electromyography reveals an increased jitter, or variability, in the time interval between two muscle fiber action potentials from the same motor unit.

Assay of serum for elevated levels of circulating acetylcholine receptor antibodies is another approach—increasingly used—to the laboratory diagnosis of myasthenia gravis and has a sensitivity of 80–90%.

Treatment

Medication such as aminoglycosides that may exacerbate myasthenia gravis should be avoided. Anticholinesterase drugs provide symptomatic benefit without influencing the course of the disease. Neostigmine, pyridostigmine, or both can be used, the dose being determined on an individual basis. The usual dose of neostigmine is 7.5–30 mg (average, 15 mg) taken four times daily; of pyridostigmine, 30–180 mg (average, 60 mg) four times daily. Overmedication may temporarily increase weakness, which is then unaffected or enhanced by intravenous edrophonium.

Thymectomy usually leads to symptomatic benefit or remission and should be considered in all patients younger than age 60, unless weakness is restricted to the extraocular muscles. If the disease is of recent onset and only slowly progressive, operation is sometimes delayed for a year or so, in the hope that spontaneous remission will occur.

Treatment with corticosteroids is indicated for patients who have responded poorly to anticholinesterase drugs and have already undergone thymectomy. It is introduced with the patient in the hospital, since weakness may initially be aggravated. Once weakness has stabilized after 2–3 weeks or any improvement is sustained, further management can be on an outpatient

basis. Alternate-day treatment is usually well tolerated, but if weakness is enhanced on the nontreatment day it may be necessary for medication to be taken daily. The dose of corticosteroids is determined on an individual basis, but an initial high daily dose (eg, prednisone, 60–100 mg) can gradually be tapered to a relatively low maintenance level as improvement occurs; total withdrawal is difficult, however. Treatment with azathioprine may also be effective. The usual dose is 2–3 mg/kg orally daily after a lower initial dose.

In patients with major disability in whom conventional treatment is either unhelpful or contraindicated, plasmapheresis or intravenous immunoglobulin therapy may be beneficial. It may also be useful for stabilizing patients before thymectomy and for managing acute crisis. Mycophenolate mofetil, an immunosuppressant, has also been used, and preliminary studies indicate that it may provide symptomatic benefit and allow the steroid dose to be reduced.

Palace J et al: Myasthenia gravis: diagnostic and management dilemmas. Curr Opin Neurol 2001;14:583. [PMID: 11562569] (Review of diagnostic tests and treatment.)

Vincent A et al: Myasthenia gravis. Lancet 2001;357:2122. [PMID:11445126] (Review.)

2. Myasthenic Syndrome (Lambert-Eaton Syndrome)

Myasthenic syndrome (Table 40–6) may be associated with small-cell carcinoma, sometimes developing before the tumor is diagnosed, and occasionally occurs with certain autoimmune diseases. There is defective release of acetylcholine in response to a nerve impulse, and this leads to weakness especially of the proximal muscles of the limbs. As is not the case in myasthenia gravis, however, power steadily increases with sustained contraction. The diagnosis can be confirmed electrophysiologically, because the muscle response to stimulation of its motor nerve increases remarkably if the nerve is stimulated repetitively at high rates, even in muscles that are not clinically weak.

Treatment with plasmapheresis and immunosuppressive drug therapy (prednisone and azathioprine) may lead to clinical and electrophysiologic improvement, in addition to therapy aimed at tumor when present. Prednisone is usually initiated in a daily dose of 60–80 mg and azathioprine in a daily dose of 2 mg/kg. Guanidine hydrochloride (25–50 mg/kg/d in divided doses) is occasionally helpful in seriously disabled patients, but adverse effects of the drug include marrow suppression. The response to treatment with anticholinesterase drugs such as pyridostigmine or neostigmine, either alone or in combination with guanidine, is variable.

3. Botulism

The toxin of *Clostridium botulinum* prevents the release of acetylcholine at neuromuscular junctions and autonomic synapses. Botulism occurs most commonly following the ingestion of contaminated home-canned food and should be suggested by the development of sudden, fluctuating, severe weakness in a previously healthy person. Symptoms begin within 72 hours following ingestion of the toxin and may progress for several days. Typically, there is diplopia, ptosis, facial weakness, dysphagia, and nasal speech, followed by respiratory difficulty and finally by weakness that appears last in the limbs. Blurring of vision (with unreactive dilated pupils) is characteristic, and there may be dryness of the mouth, constipation (paralytic ileus), and postural hypotension. Sensation is preserved, and the tendon reflexes are not affected unless the involved muscles are very weak. If the diagnosis is suspected, the local health authority should be notified and a sample of serum and contaminated food (if available) sent to be assayed for toxin. Support for the diagnosis may be obtained by electrophysiologic studies; with repetitive stimulation of motor nerves at fast rates, the muscle response increases in size progressively.

Patients should be hospitalized in case respiratory assistance becomes necessary. Treatment is with trivalent antitoxin, once it is established that the patient is not allergic to horse serum. Guanidine hydrochloride (25–50 mg/kg/d in divided doses) to facilitate release of acetylcholine from nerve endings sometimes helps to increase muscle strength. Anticholinesterase drugs are of no value. Respiratory assistance and other supportive measures should be provided as necessary. Further details are provided in Chapter 33.

4. Disorders Associated With Use of Aminoglycosides

Aminoglycoside antibiotics, eg, gentamicin, may produce a clinical disturbance similar to botulism by preventing the release of acetylcholine from nerve endings, but symptoms subside rapidly as the responsible drug is eliminated from the body. These antibiotics are particularly dangerous in patients with preexisting disturbances of neuromuscular transmission and are therefore best avoided in patients with myasthenia gravis.

MYOPATHIC DISORDERS

Muscular Dystrophies

These inherited myopathic disorders are characterized by progressive muscle weakness and wasting. They are subdivided by mode of inheritance, age at onset, and clinical features, as shown in Table 24–6. In the Duchenne type, pseudohypertrophy of muscles frequently occurs at some stage; intellectual retardation is common; and there may be skeletal deformities, muscle contractures, and cardiac involvement. The serum creatine kinase level is increased, especially in the Duchenne and Becker varieties, and mildly increased also in limb-girdle dystrophy. Electromyography may

help to confirm that weakness is myopathic rather than neurogenic. Similarly, histopathologic examination of a muscle biopsy specimen may help to confirm that weakness is due to a primary disorder of muscle and to distinguish between various muscle diseases.

A genetic defect on the short arm of the X chromosome has been identified in Duchenne dystrophy. The affected gene codes for the protein dystrophin, which is markedly reduced or absent from the muscle of patients with the disease. Dystrophin levels are generally normal in the Becker variety, but the protein is qualitatively altered.

Duchenne muscular dystrophy can now be recognized early in pregnancy in about 95% of women by genetic studies; in late pregnancy, DNA probes can be used on fetal tissue obtained for this purpose by amniocentesis. The genes causing some of the other muscular dystrophies are listed in Table 24–6.

There is no specific treatment for the muscular dystrophies, but it is important to encourage patients to lead as normal lives as possible. Prolonged bed rest must be avoided, as inactivity often leads to worsening of the underlying muscle disease. Physical therapy and orthopedic procedures may help to counteract deformities or contractures.

Cohn RD et al: Molecular basis of muscular dystrophies. Muscle Nerve 2000;23:1456. [PMID: 11003781] (Review.)

Myotonic Dystrophy

Myotonic dystrophy, a slowly progressive, dominantly inherited disorder, usually manifests itself in the third or fourth decade but occasionally appears early in childhood. The genetic defect has been localized to the long arm of chromosome 19. Myotonia leads to complaints of muscle stiffness and is evidenced by the marked delay that occurs before affected muscles can relax after a contraction. This can often be demonstrated clinically by delayed relaxation of the hand after sustained grip or by percussion of the belly of a muscle. In addition, there is weakness and wasting of the facial, sternocleidomastoid, and distal limb muscles. Associated clinical features include cataracts, frontal baldness, testicular atrophy, diabetes mellitus, cardiac abnormalities, and intellectual changes. Electromyographic sampling of affected muscles reveals myotonic discharges in addition to changes suggestive of myopathy.

Myotonia can be treated with phenytoin (100 mg three times daily), quinine sulfate (300–400 mg three times daily), or procainamide (0.5–1 g four times daily). More recently, tocainide and mexiletine have been used. Phenytoin is preferred, since the other drugs may have undesirable effects on cardiac conduction. Neither the weakness nor the course of the disorder is influenced by treatment.

Meola G: Clinical and genetic heterogeneity in myotonic dystrophies. Muscle Nerve 2000;23:1789. [PMID: 11102902] (Review.)

Table 24–6. The muscular dystrophies.

Disorder	Inheritance	Age at Onset (years)	Distribution	Prognosis	Genetic Locus
Duchenne type	X-linked recessive	1–5	Pelvic, then shoulder girdle; later, limb and respiratory muscles	Rapid progression. Death within about 15 years after onset.	Xp21
Becker's	X-linked recessive	5–25	Pelvic, then shoulder girdle	Slow progression. May have normal life span.	Xp21
Limb-girdle (Erb's)	Autosomal recessive (may be sporadic or dominant)	10–30	Pelvic or shoulder girdle initially, with later spread to the other	Variable severity and rate of progression. Possible severe disability in middle life.	Multiple
Facioscapulo-humeral	Autosomal dominant	Any age	Face and shoulder girdle initially; later, pelvic girdle and legs	Slow progression. Minor disability. Usually normal life span.	4q35
Emery-Dreifuss	X-linked recessive or autosomal dominant	5–10	Humeroperoneal or scapuloperoneal	Variable	Xq28, 1q11
Distal	Autosomal dominant or recessive	40–60	Onset distally in extremities; proximal involvement later	Slow progression.	2q13, 2p13
Ocular	Autosomal dominant (may be recessive)	Any age (usually 5–30)	External ocular muscles; may also be mild weakness of face, neck, and arms		
Oculopharyn-geal	Autosomal dominant	Any age	As in the ocular form but with dysphagia		14q11.2–q13

Myotonia Congenita

Myotonia congenita is commonly inherited as a dominant trait. The responsible gene may be on the long arm of chromosome 7. Generalized myotonia without weakness is usually present from birth, but symptoms may not appear until early childhood. Patients complain of muscle stiffness that is enhanced by cold and inactivity and relieved by exercise. Muscle hypertrophy, at times pronounced, is also a feature. A recessive form with later onset is associated with slight weakness and atrophy of distal muscles. Treatment with quinine sulfate, procainamide, tocainide, mexiletine, or phenytoin may help the myotonia, as in myotonic dystrophy.

Polymyositis & Dermatomyositis

See Chapter 20.

Inclusion Body Myositis

This disorder, of unknown cause, begins insidiously, usually after middle age, with progressive proximal weakness of first the lower and then the upper extremities. Distal weakness is usually mild. Serum creatine kinase levels may be normal or increased. The diagnosis is confirmed by muscle biopsy. In contrast to polymyositis, corticosteroid therapy is usually ineffective. The role of intravenous immunoglobulin therapy is unclear.

Dalakas MC et al: A controlled study of intravenous immunoglobulin combined with prednisone in the treatment of IBM. Neurology 2001;56;323. [PMID: 11171896] (Clinical trial.)

Mitochondrial Myopathies

The mitochondrial myopathies are a clinically diverse group of disorders that on pathologic examination of skeletal muscle with the modified Gomori stain show characteristic "ragged red fibers" containing accumulations of abnormal mitochondria. Patients may present with progressive external ophthalmoplegia or with limb weakness that is exacerbated or induced by activity. Other patients present with central neurologic dysfunction, eg, myoclonic epilepsy (myoclonic epilepsy, ragged red fiber syndrome, or MERRF), or the combination of myopathy, encephalopathy, lactic acidosis, and stroke-like episodes (MELAS). These disorders result from separate abnormalities of mitochondrial DNA. (See also Chapter 19.)

Myopathies Associated With Other Disorders

Myopathy may occur in association with chronic hypokalemia, any endocrinopathy, and in patients taking corticosteroids, chloroquine, colchicine, clofibrate, emetine, aminocaproic acid, lovastatin, bretylium tosylate, or drugs causing potassium depletion. Weakness is mainly proximal, and serum creatine kinase is typically normal, except in hypothyroidism and some of the toxic myopathies. Treatment is of the underlying cause. Myopathy also occurs with chronic alcoholism, whereas acute reversible muscle necrosis may occur shortly after acute alcohol intoxication. Inflammatory myopathy may occur in patients taking penicillamine; myotonia may be induced by clofibrate; and preexisting myotonia may be exacerbated or unmasked by depolarizing muscle relaxants (eg, suxamethonium), beta-blockers (eg, propranolol), fenoterol, ritodrine, and, possibly, certain diuretics.

PERIODIC PARALYSIS SYNDROME

Periodic paralysis may have a familial (dominant inheritance) basis. Episodes of flaccid weakness or paralysis occur, sometimes in association with abnormalities of the plasma potassium level. Strength is normal between attacks. The **hypokalemic** variety is characterized by attacks that tend to occur on awakening, after exercise, or after a heavy meal and may last for several days. Patients should avoid excessive exertion. A low-carbohydrate and low-salt diet may help prevent attacks, as may acetazolamide, 250–750 mg/d. An ongoing attack may be aborted by potassium chloride given orally or by intravenous drip, provided the ECG can be monitored and renal function is satisfactory. In young Asian men, it is commonly associated with hyperthyroidism; treatment of the endocrine disorder then prevents recurrences. In **hyperkalemic** periodic paralysis, attacks also tend to occur after exercise but usually last for less than an hour. They may be terminated by intravenous calcium gluconate (1–2 g) or by intravenous diuretics (furosemide, 20–40 mg), glucose, or glucose and insulin; daily acetazolamide or chlorothiazide may prevent recurrences. Genetic linkage studies suggest that many families with this disorder have a defect in the sodium channel gene on the long arm of chromosome 17. **Normokalemic** periodic paralysis is similar clinically to the hyperkalemic variety, but the plasma potassium level remains normal during attacks; treatment is with acetazolamide.

Ptacek L: The familial periodic paralyses and nondystrophic myotonias. Am J Med 1998;104:58. [PMID: 9688022]

Psychiatric Disorders

25

Stuart J. Eisendrath, MD, & Jonathan E. Lichtmacher, MD
See www.current-med.com/ch25.html

Psychiatric disorders are functional impairments that may result from disturbance of one or more of the following interrelated factors: (1) biologic function, (2) psychodynamic adaptation, (3) learned behavior, and (4) social and environmental conditions. Although the clinical situation at a given time determines which area of dysfunction will be emphasized, proper patient care requires an approach that adequately evaluates all factors.

Biologic Function

Psychiatric disorders of biologic origin may be secondary to identifiable physical illness or caused by biochemical disturbances of the brain. A wide variety of psychiatric disorders (eg, psychosis, depression, delirium, anxiety) as well as nonspecific symptoms are caused by organic brain disease or by derangement of cerebral metabolism resulting from illness, biochemical aberrations (usually neurotransmitter dysfunction), nutritional deficiencies, or toxic agents.

Neurotransmitter functions have been correlated with the major psychiatric disorders. Cholinergic deficiency is present in some dementias, and adrenergic imbalance is important in some psychoses. Serotonergic mechanisms are significantly involved in affective disorders, aggression, autism, and the anxiety disorders, particularly obsessive-compulsive disorders and panic disorder.

Psychodynamic Adaptations

Psychodynamic adaptation involves a healthy balancing of intrapsychic motivations. Psychodynamic maladaptation involves intrapsychic aberrations and is usually treated by a psychotherapeutic approach. There are many forms of psychotherapy: supportive, interpretive, cognitive, persuasive, educative, or some combination of these methods. Depth, duration, intensity, and frequency of sessions may vary.

Learned Behavior

Learned behavior is part of the pathogenetic mechanism in all psychiatric disorders. For example, in somatization disorder, the patient may have learned that being sick is the only way to get attention. Altering such positive reinforcement may be critical in producing a change in behavior. Personality disorders are examples of failure to learn to incorporate patterns of behavior acceptable in social surroundings.

Social & Environmental Conditions

Social and environmental factors have always been considered of vital importance in the mental balance of the individual. Without encounter with the environment, there can be no socially recognized illness: The exigencies of everyday life contribute both to the development of a stable personality and to the deviations from the norm. There is a constantly changing cultural mix of influences that determines which types of behavior will be tolerated or considered deviant. Cultural attitudes and fears play key roles in the perception of illness and acceptance of treatment.

Gabbard GO: A neurobiologically informed perspective on psychotherapy. Br J Psychiatry 2000;177:117. [PMID: 11026950]

Olfson M et al: Mental disorders and disability among patients in a primary care group practice. Am J Psychiatry 1997; 154:1734. [PMID: 9396954] (Mental disorders in a population of primary care patients are significantly associated with a decline in work, family, and social functioning.)

■ PSYCHIATRIC ASSESSMENT

Psychiatric diagnosis rests upon the established principles of a thorough history and examination. All of the forces contributing to the individual's life situation must be identified, and this can be done only if the examination includes the history; mental status; medical conditions (including drugs); and pertinent social, cultural, and environmental factors impinging on the individual.

The examination of a psychiatric patient must include a complete medical history and physical examination (with emphasis on the neurologic examination) as well as all necessary laboratory and other special studies. Physical illness may frequently present as psychiatric disease, and vice versa.

Interview

Every psychiatric history should cover the following points: (1) complaint, from the patient's viewpoint; (2) the present illness, or the evolution of the symptoms; (3) neurovegetative signs such as libido, appetite, and sleep; (4) previous disorders and the nature and extent of their treatment; (5) the family history—important for genetic aspects and family influences; (6) the personal history—childhood development, adolescent adjustment, level of education, and adult coping patterns; (7) current life functioning, with attention to vocational, social, educational, and avocational areas; and (8) present or past use of alcohol and other drugs.

It is often essential to obtain additional information from the family. Observing interactions of the patient with significant others in the context of a family interview may give important diagnostic information and may even underscore the nature of the problem and suggest a therapeutic approach.

The formal mental status examination should be particularly detailed when there is any evidence or high risk of cognitive dysfunction. The mental status examination includes the following: (1) Appearance: Note unusual modes of dress, use of makeup, etc. (2) Activity and behavior: Gait, gestures, coordination of bodily movements, etc. (3) Affect: Outward manifestation of emotions such as depression, anger, elation, fear, resentment, or lack of emotional response. (4) Mood: The patient's report of feelings and observable emotional manifestations. (5) Speech: Coherence, spontaneity, articulation, hesitancy in answering, and duration of response. (6) Content of thought: Associations, preoccupations, obsessions, depersonalization, delusions, hallucinations, paranoid ideation, anger, fear, or unusual experiences; suicidal and homicidal ideation. (7) Thought process: Loose associations, flight of ideas, thought blocking, tangentiality, circumstantiality, perseveration, racing thought. (8) Cognition: (a) orientation to person, place, time, and circumstances; (b) remote and recent memory and recall; (c) calculations, digit retention (six forward is normal), serial sevens or threes; (d) general fund of knowledge (presidents, states, distances, events); (e) abstracting ability, often tested with common proverbs or with analogies and differences (eg, "How are a lie and a mistake the same, and how are they different?"); (f) ability to identify by naming, reading, and writing specified test names and objects; (g) ideomotor function, which combines understanding and the ability to perform a task (eg, "Show me how to throw a ball"); (h) ability to reproduce geometric constructions (eg, parallelogram, intersecting squares); and (i) right-left differentiation. (9) Judgment regarding commonsense problems such as what to do when one runs out of medicine. (10) Insight into the nature and extent of the current difficulty and its ramifications in the patient's daily life.

Formal cognitive screens can quantify impairments and point to the need for further evaluation. The Mini-Mental State Examination produces a numerical score with up to 30 points given for correct answers to questions (likely organic < 27 points) (Figure 25–1). Specific cognitive assessment must be performed, since many patients are able to cover a deficit in routine conversation.

Special Diagnostic Aids

Many tests and evaluation procedures are available that can be used to support and clarify initial diagnostic impressions.

A. PSYCHOLOGIC TESTING

Testing by a psychologist may measure intelligence and cognitive functioning; provide information about personality, feelings, psychodynamics, and psychopathology; and differentiate psychic problems from organic ones. The place of such tests is similar to that of other tests in medicine—helpful in diagnostic problems but may be an unnecessary expense.

1. Objective tests—These tests provide quantitative evaluation compared to standard norms.

a. Intelligence tests—The test most frequently used is the Wechsler Adult Intelligence Scale–Revised (WAIS-R). Intelligence tests often reveal more than IQ. The results, given expert interpretation, can quantify intellectual deterioration that has occurred.

b. Minnesota Multiphasic Personality Inventory (MMPI-2)—The MMPI-2 is an empirically based test of personality assessment. The patient's scores are interpreted in comparison with data about others with the same response pattern to assess psychopathologic changes.

c. Screening instruments—These tests include the Beck Depression Inventory, which quantifies degrees of dysphoria; and the Mental Health Screener (Prime MD), which is a broad measure of the patient's concerns and assists with differential diagnosis.

d. Neuropsychologic assessment—Such an assessment is made when an organic deficit is present but information on anatomic location and extent of dysfunction is required.

2. Projective tests—These tests are unstructured, so that the patient is forced to respond in ways that reflect fantasies and individual modes of adaptation. They are particularly useful in identifying psychotic disorders and unconscious motivations.

a. Rorschach Psychodiagnostics—This test utilizes ten inkblots to provide important information on psychodynamic themes and aberrations.

b. Thematic Apperception Test (TAT)—This test uses 20 pictures of people in different situations to assess areas of interpersonal conflicts.

COMPLETE IF INDICATED CLINICALLY
(Ask general question and then ask specific questions to the right.)

Orientation *(Score 1 for each correct. max = 10)*

Where are you? Name this place (building or hospital)
 What floor are you on now?
 What state are you in?
 What country are you in?
 (If not in a country, score correct if city is correct.)
 What city are you in (or near) now?

What is the date today? What year is it?
 What season is it?
 What month is it?
 What is the day of the week?
 What is the date today?

Registration *(Score 1 for each object correctly repeated. max = 3)*

 Name three objects (ball, flag, and tree) and have patient repeat them.
(Say objects at about 1 word per second. If patient misses object, ask patient to repeat them after you until he/she learns them. Stop at 6 repeats.)

Attention and calculation *(Score 1 for each correct to 65. max = 5)*

 Subtract 7s from 100 in a serial fashion to 65
(Alternatively, ask serial 3s from 20 or spell WORLD backwards.)

Recall *(Score 1 for each object recalled. max = 3)*

 Do you recall the names of the three objects?

Language *(max = 8)*

 Ask the patient to provide names of a watch and pen as you show them to him/her
  (Score 1 for each object correct. max = 2)
 Repeat "No ifs, ands, or buts."
  (Only one trial. Score 1 if correct. max = 1)
 Give the patient a piece of plain blank paper and say, "Take the paper in your right hand
  (1), fold it in half (2), and put it on the floor (3)."
  (Score 1 for each part done correctly. max = 3)
 Ask the patient to read and perform the following task written on paper: "Close your eyes."
  (Score 1 if patient closes eyes. max = 1)
 Ask the patient to write a sentence on a piece of paper.
  (Score total of 1 if sentence has a subject, object and verb. max = 1)

Construction

 Ask patient to copy the two interlocking pentagons.
  *(Score total of 1, if all 10 angles are present and the two angles intersect.
  Ignore tremor and rotation. max = 1)*

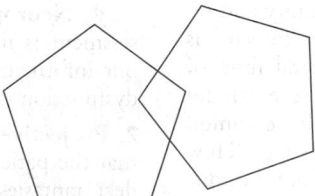

Total Score *(Maximum = 30)*

Figure 25–1. MINI-MENTAL STATE EXAM. (Adapted from Folstein MF et al: Mini-mental state: A practical method for grading the cognitive state of patients for the clinician. J Psychiatr Res 1975;12:189.)

B. NEUROLOGIC EVALUATION

Consultation is often necessary and may include specialized tests. Brain imaging is useful for detecting structural abnormalities in the patient who presents with a nondefinitive history and examination (eg, dissociative episodes, unusual psychotic episodes not explained by drug abuse, or an acute change in mental status). MRI is particularly useful in delineating lesions and identifying demyelinating and degenerative diseases (eg, Huntington's disease). Electroencephalography is particularly useful for the diagnosis of seizure disorders and in differentiating delirium from depression or dementia. Typically, delirium is associated with generalized electroencephalographic slowing, while depression and dementia do not have this change. Single photon emission computed tomography (SPECT) is a gamma imaging technology like PET, and both provide tomographic images of brain activity. SPECT is cheaper but has the disadvantages of lower image resolution and lower quantification of regional brain activity.

Formulation of the Diagnosis

A psychiatric diagnosis must be based upon positive evidence accumulated by the above techniques. It must not be based simply on the exclusion of organic findings.

A thorough psychiatric evaluation has therapeutic as well as diagnostic value and should be expressed in ways best understood by the patient, family, and other clinicians.

Crum RM et al: Population-based norms for the Mini-Mental State Examination by age and educational level. JAMA 1993;269:2386. [PMID: 8479064] (Older or less well educated subjects may score somewhat lower but still may be normal.)

Spitzer RL et al: Validation and utility of a self-report version of Prime-MD: the PHQ primary care study. JAMA 1999; 282:1737. [PMID: 10568646] (This increasingly popular test is self-administered and is an excellent screen for common mental health problems.)

Wells KP et al: Impact of disseminating quality improvement programs for depression in managed primary care. JAMA 2000;283:212. [PMID: 10634337] (Quality improvement programs that improved opportunities for depression treatment appeared to improve outcomes and employment retention.)

■ TREATMENT APPROACHES

The approaches to treatment of psychiatric patients are, in a broad sense, similar to those in other branches of medicine. For example, the internist treating a patient with heart disease uses not only **medical** measures such as drugs and pacemakers but also **psychologic** techniques to change attitudes and behaviors, **social** and **environmental** manipulation to mitigate deleterious influences, and **behavioral** techniques to change behavior patterns.

Regardless of the methods employed, treatment must be directed toward an objective, ie, it must be **goal-oriented.** This usually involves (1) obtaining active cooperation on the part of the patient; (2) establishing reasonable goals and modifying the goal if failure occurs; (3) emphasizing positive behavior (goals) instead of symptom behavior (problems); (4) delineating the method; and (5) setting a time frame (which can be modified later).

The clinician must resist pressures for instantaneous results. In almost all cases, psychiatric treatment involves the active participation of the significant people in the patient's life. Time must be spent with the patient, but the frequency and duration of appointments are highly variable and should be adjusted to meet both the patient's psychologic needs and financial restrictions. Adherence (collaboration) is the end product of many factors, the most important being clear communication, attention to cost, and simple dosage regimens when drugs are prescribed. The clinician can unwittingly promote chronic illness by prescribing medication inappropriately. The patient may come to believe that problems respond only to medication, and the more drugs prescribed, the stronger the misconception becomes.

Psychiatric Consultation

All clinicians are in an excellent position to meet their patients' emotional needs in an organized and competent way, referring to psychiatrists for consultation or for ongoing treatment of patients whose problems are considered beyond the expertise of the referring clinician. The most pressing problems involve evaluation of suicidal or assaultive potential and diagnostic differentiation in mood disorders and psychoses. Psychiatric problems associated with unusual psychopharmacologic therapy and with medications used in other branches of medicine may require pharmacologic consultation. When a psychiatric referral is made, it should be conducted like any other referral: in an open manner, with full explanation of the problem to the patient.

Hospitalization

Hospital care may be indicated when patients are too sick to care for themselves or when they present serious threats to themselves or others; when observation and diagnostic procedures are necessary; or when specific kinds of treatment such as complex medication trials or a hospital environment ("milieu therapy") are required. Symptoms calling for hospitalization include self-neglect, violent or bizarre behavior, suicidal risk, paranoid ideation or delusions, marked intellectual impairment, and poor judgment. The trend over recent years has been to admit patients to hospitals and treat them aggressively with the expectation of prompt discharge to the next appropriate level of care—day hospital, halfway house, outpatient therapy, etc. The decision to propose involuntary hospitalization should be taken only after weighing the potential benefits to the patient and the community against the individual's loss of autonomy.

The disadvantages of psychiatric hospitalization include decreased self-confidence as a result of needing hospitalization; the stigma of being a "psychiatric patient"; possible increased dependency and regression; and the expense. Generally, there is no advantage to prolonged hospital stays for most psychiatric disorders. Partial hospitalization or "day" programs are providing many of the benefits of hospitalization without some of the disadvantages; in these programs, the patient attends daytime treatment but sleeps at home.

Bateman A et al: Effectiveness of partial hospitalization in the treatment of borderline personality disorder: a randomized controlled trial. Am J Psychiatry 1999;156:1563. [PMID: 10518167] (Psychotherapy in a structured day program can improve mood symptoms, decrease self-destructive behaviors, and reduce inpatient days.)

■ COMMON PSYCHIATRIC DISORDERS

STRESS & ADJUSTMENT DISORDERS (Situational Disorders)

ESSENTIALS OF DIAGNOSIS

- Anxiety or depression clearly secondary to an identifiable stress.
- Subsequent symptoms of anxiety or depression commonly elicited by similar stress of lesser magnitude.
- Alcohol and other drugs are commonly used in self-treatment.

General Considerations

Stress exists when the adaptive capacity of the individual is overwhelmed by events. The event may be an insignificant one objectively considered, and even favorable changes (eg, promotion and transfer) requiring adaptive behavior can produce stress. For each individual, stress is subjectively defined, and the response to stress is a function of each person's personality and physiologic endowment.

Classification & Clinical Findings

Opinion differs about what events are most apt to produce stress reactions. The causes of stress are different at different ages—eg, in young adulthood, the

sources of stress are found in the marriage or parent-child relationship, the employment relationship, and the struggle to achieve financial stability; in the middle years, the focus shifts to changing spousal relationships, problems with aging parents, and problems associated with having young adult offspring who themselves are encountering stressful situations; in old age, the principal concerns are apt to be retirement, loss of physical capacity, major personal losses, and thoughts of death.

An individual may react to stress by becoming anxious or depressed, by developing a physical symptom, by running away, having a drink, starting an affair, or in limitless other ways. Common subjective responses are fear (of repetition of the stress-inducing event), rage (at frustration), guilt (over aggressive impulses), and shame (over helplessness). Acute and reactivated stress may be manifested by restlessness, irritability, fatigue, increased startle reaction, and a feeling of tension. Inability to concentrate, sleep disturbances (insomnia, bad dreams), and somatic preoccupations often lead to self-medication, most commonly with alcohol or other central nervous system depressants. Maladaptive behavior in response to stress is called adjustment disorder, with the major symptom specified (eg, "adjustment disorder with depressed mood").

Posttraumatic stress disorder (included among the anxiety disorders in *DSM-IV*) is a syndrome characterized by "reexperiencing" a traumatic event (eg, rape, severe burns, military combat), along with decreased responsiveness and avoidance of current events associated with the trauma. Patients experience physiologic hyperarousal, which includes startle reactions, intrusive thoughts, illusions, overgeneralized associations, sleep problems, nightmares, dreams about the precipitating event, impulsivity, difficulties in concentration, and hyperalertness. The symptoms may be precipitated or exacerbated by events that are a reminder of the original stress. Symptoms frequently arise after a long latency period (eg, child abuse can result in later-onset posttraumatic stress syndrome). The sooner the symptoms arise after the initial trauma and the sooner therapy is initiated, the better the prognosis. The therapeutic approach is to facilitate the normal recovery that was blocked at the time of the trauma. Therapy at that time should be brief and simple (catharsis and working through of the traumatic experience), expecting quick recovery and promoting a sense of mastery over the traumatic event.

Treatment initiated later, when symptoms have crystallized, includes programs for cessation of alcohol and other drug abuse, group and individual psychotherapy, and improved social support systems.

Differential Diagnosis

Adjustment disorders must be distinguished from anxiety disorders, affective disorders, and personality disorders exacerbated by stress and from somatic disorders with psychic overlay.

Treatment

A. BEHAVIORAL

Stress reduction techniques include immediate symptom reduction (eg, rebreathing in a bag for hyperventilation) or early recognition and removal from a stress source before full-blown symptoms appear. It is often helpful for the patient to keep a daily log of stress precipitators, responses, and alleviators. Relaxation and exercise techniques are also helpful in reducing the reaction to stressful events.

B. SOCIAL

The stress reactions of life crisis problems are—more than any other category—a function of psychosocial upheaval, and patients frequently present with somatic symptoms. While it is not easy for the patient to make necessary changes (or they would have been made long ago), it is important for the therapist to establish the framework of the problem, since the patient's denial system may obscure the issues. Clarifying the problem allows the patient to begin viewing it within the proper context and facilitates the sometimes difficult decisions the patient eventually must make (eg, change of job or relocation of adult dependent offspring).

C. PSYCHOLOGIC

Prolonged in-depth psychotherapy is seldom necessary in cases of isolated stress response or adjustment disorder. Supportive psychotherapy (see above) with an emphasis on the here and now and strengthening of existing defenses is a helpful approach so that time and the patient's own resiliency can restore the previous level of function. Posttraumatic stress syndromes respond to early catharsis and dynamic psychotherapy oriented toward acceptance of the event, with the expectation of quick recovery and return to the previous level of function. Marital problems are a major area of concern, and it is important that the clinician have available a dependable referral source when marriage counseling is indicated. In posttraumatic stress disorder, group psychotherapy and individual counseling are both helpful.

D. MEDICAL

Judicious use of sedatives (eg, lorazepam, 1–2 mg orally daily) for a limited time and as part of an overall treatment plan can provide relief from acute anxiety symptoms. Problems arise when the situation becomes chronic through inappropriate treatment or when the treatment approach supports the development of chronicity (see Sedative-Hypnotic Drugs, below).

In posttraumatic stress disorder, antidepressant drugs—particularly selective serotonin reuptake inhibitors (SSRIs)—in full dosage are helpful in ameliorating depression, panic attacks, sleep disruption, and startle responses. Sertraline is FDA-approved for this purpose. Beta-blockers (eg, propranolol, 80–160 mg daily) may be used to lessen the peripheral symptoms of anxiety (eg, tremors, palpitations). Antiseizure medications such as carbamazepine (400–800 mg daily) will often mitigate impulsivity and difficulty with anger management. Benzodiazepines such as clonazepam (1–4 mg daily) will reduce anxiety and panic attacks when used in adequate dosage, but dependency problems are a concern, particularly when the patient has had such problems in the past.

Prognosis

Return to satisfactory function after a short period is part of the clinical picture of this syndrome. Resolution may be delayed if others' responses to the patient's difficulties are thoughtlessly harmful or if the secondary gains outweigh the advantages of recovery. The longer the symptoms persist, the worse the prognosis.

Ladwig KH et al: Long acting psychotraumatic properties of a cardiac arrest experience. Am J Psychiatry 1999;156:912. [PMID: 10360132] (Cardiac patients with PTSD symptoms are at high risk for emotional disability.)

Stein MB et al: Posttraumatic stress disorder in the primary medical care setting. Gen Hosp Psychiatry 2000;224:261. [PMID: 10889283] (Such patients are frequently encountered in primary care.)

ANXIETY DISORDERS & DISSOCIATIVE DISORDERS

 ESSENTIALS OF DIAGNOSIS

- Overt anxiety or an overt manifestation of a defense mechanism (such as a phobia), or both.
- Not limited to an adjustment disorder.
- Somatic symptoms referable to the autonomic nervous system or to a specific organ system (eg, dyspnea, palpitations, paresthesias).
- Not a result of physical disorders, psychiatric conditions (eg, schizophrenia), or drug abuse (eg, cocaine).

General Considerations

Stress, fear, and anxiety all tend to be interactive. The principal components of anxiety are **psychologic** (tension, fears, difficulty in concentration, apprehension) and **somatic** (tachycardia, hyperventilation, palpitations, tremor, sweating). Other organ systems (eg, gastrointestinal) may be involved in multiple system complaints. Fatigue and sleep disturbances are common. Sympathomimetic symptoms of anxiety are both a response to a central nervous system state and a reinforcement of further anxiety. Anxiety can become self-generating, since the symptoms reinforce the reaction, causing it to spiral. This is often the case when the anxiety is an epiphenomenon of other medical or psychiatric disorders.

Anxiety may be free-floating, resulting in acute anxiety attacks, occasionally becoming chronic. When one or several defense mechanisms (see above) are functioning, the consequences are well-known problems such as phobias, conversion reactions, dissociative states, obsessions, and compulsions. Lack of structure is frequently a contributing factor, as noted in those people who have "Sunday neuroses." They do well during the week with a planned work schedule but cannot tolerate the unstructured weekend. Planned-time activities tend to bind anxiety, and many people have increased difficulties when this is lost, as in retirement.

Some believe that various manifestations of anxiety are not a result of unconscious conflicts but are "habits"—persistent patterns of nonadaptive behavior acquired by learning. The "habits," being nonadaptive, are unsatisfactory ways of dealing with life's problems—hence the resultant anxiety. Help is sought only when the anxiety becomes too painful. Exogenous factors such as stimulants (eg, caffeine, cocaine) must be considered as a contributing factor.

Clinical Findings

A. GENERALIZED ANXIETY DISORDER

This is the most common of the clinically significant anxiety disorders. Initial manifestations appear at age 20–35 years, and there is a slight predominance in women. The anxiety symptoms of apprehension, worry, irritability, difficulty in concentrating, insomnia, and somatic complaints are present more days than not for at least 6 months. Manifestations include cardiac (eg, tachycardia, increased blood pressure), gastrointestinal (eg, increased acidity, nausea, epigastric pain), and neurologic (eg, headache, near-syncope) systems. The focus of the anxiety may be a number of everyday activities.

B. PANIC DISORDER

This is characterized by short-lived, recurrent, unpredictable episodes of intense anxiety accompanied by marked physiologic manifestations. Agoraphobia may be present. Distressing symptoms and signs such as dyspnea, tachycardia, palpitations, headaches, dizziness, paresthesias, choking, smothering feelings, nausea, and bloating are associated with feelings of impending doom (alarm response). Recurrent sleep panic attacks (not nightmares) occur in about 30% of panic disorders. Anticipatory anxiety develops in all these patients and further constricts their daily lives. Panic disorder tends to be familial, with onset usually under age 25; it affects 3–5% of the population, and the female-to-male ratio is 2:1. The premenstrual period is one of heightened vulnerability. Patients frequently undergo emergency medical evaluations (eg, for "heart attacks" or "hypoglycemia") before the correct diagnosis is made. Gastrointestinal symptoms are especially common, occurring in about one-third of cases. Myocardial infarction, pheochromocytoma, hyperthyroidism, and various recreational drug reactions can mimic panic disorder. Mitral valve prolapse may be present but is not usually a significant factor. Patients who have recurrent panic disorder often become **demoralized, hypochondriacal, agoraphobic,** and **depressed.** These individuals are at increased risk for major depression and the suicide attempts associated with that disorder. Alcohol abuse (about 20%) results from self-treatment and is not infrequently combined with dependence on sedatives. Some patients have atypical panic attacks associated with seizure-like symptoms that often include psychosensory phenomena (a history of stimulant abuse often emerges). About 25% of panic disorder patients also have obsessive-compulsive disorder.

C. OBSESSIVE-COMPULSIVE DISORDER (OCD)

In the obsessive-compulsive reaction, the irrational idea or the impulse persistently intrudes into awareness. Obsessions (constantly recurring thoughts such as fears of exposure to germs) and compulsions (repetitive actions such as washing the hands many times) are recognized by the individual as absurd and are resisted, but anxiety is alleviated only by ritualistic performance of the action or by deliberate contemplation of the intruding idea or emotion. The primary underlying concern of the patient is not to lose control. Many patients do not mention the symptoms and must be asked about them. These patients are usually predictable, orderly, conscientious, and intelligent—traits that are seen in many compulsive behaviors such as food binging and purging and compulsive running. There is an overlapping of obsessive-compulsive disorder and other behaviors ("OCD spectrum"), including tics, trichotillomania (hair pulling), onychophagia (nail biting), hypochondriasis, Tourette's syndrome, and eating disorders (see Chapter 29). The 2–3% incidence of OCD in the general population is much higher than was previously recognized. In addition, there is a high comorbidity of OCD and major depression; two-thirds of OCD patients will develop major depression during their lifetime. Male:female ratios are similar, with the highest rates occurring in the young, divorced, separated, and unemployed (all high stress categories). Neurologic abnormalities of fine motor coordination and involuntary movements are common. Under extreme stress, these patients sometimes exhibit paranoid and delusional behaviors, often associated with depression, and can mimic schizophrenia.

D. PHOBIC DISORDER

Phobic ideation can be considered a mechanism of "displacement" in which patients transfer feelings of anxiety from their true object to one that can be avoided. However, since phobias are ineffective defense mechanisms, there tends to be an increase in their scope, intensity, and number. Social phobias are global or specific; in the former, all social situations are poorly tolerated, while the latter group includes performance anxiety or well-delineated phobias. Agoraphobia (fear of open places and public areas) is frequently associated with severe panic attacks. Patients often develop the agoraphobia in early adult life, making a normal lifestyle difficult.

E. DISSOCIATIVE DISORDER

Fugue (the sudden, unexpected travel away from one's home with inability to recall one's past), amnesia, somnambulism, dissociative identity disorder (multiple personality disorder), and depersonalization are all dissociative states. The reaction is precipitated by emotional crisis. The symptom produces anxiety reduction and a temporary solution of the crisis. Mechanisms include repression and isolation as well as particularly limited concentration as seen in hypnotic states. Dissociative symptoms are similar in many ways to symptoms seen in patients with temporal lobe dysfunction.

Treatment

In all cases, underlying medical disorders must be ruled out (eg, cardiovascular, endocrine, respiratory, and neurologic disorders and substance-related syndromes, both intoxication and withdrawal states). These and other disorders can coexist with panic disorder.

A. MEDICAL

1. Generalized anxiety—Benzodiazepines are the anxiolytics of choice in the acute management of generalized anxiety (Table 25–1). They are almost immediately effective. Antidepressants can be efficacious for the long-term treatment of generalized anxiety disorder, panic disorder, social phobia, and obsessive-compulsive disorder.

All of the benzodiazepines may be given orally, and several are available in parenteral formulations. Benzodiazepines such as lorazepam are absorbed rapidly

Table 25–1. Commonly used antianxiety and hypnotic agents.

Drug	Usual Daily Oral Dose	Usual Daily Maximum Dose	Cost for 30 Days' Treatment Based on Maximum Dosage[1]
Benzodiazepines (used for anxiety)			
Alprazolam (Xanax)[7]	0.5 mg	4 mg	$118.80
Chlordiazepoxide (Librium)[3]	10–20 mg	100 mg	$40.80
Clonazepam (Klonopin)[3]	1–2 mg	10 mg	$177.00
Clorazepate (Tranxene)[3]	15–30 mg	60 mg	$260.40
Diazepam (Valium)[3]	5–15 mg	30 mg	$27.90
Lorazepam (Ativan)[2]	2–4 mg	4 mg	$76.80
Oxazepam (Serax)[2]	10–30 mg	60 mg	$95.40
Benzodiazepines (used for sleep)			
Estazolam (Prosom)[2]	1 mg	2 mg	$29.70
Flurazepam (Dalmane)[3]	15 mg	30 mg	$10.50
Midazolam (Versed IV)[4]	5 mg IV		$1.56/dose
Quazepam (Doral)[3]	7.5 mg	15 mg	$92.70
Temazepam (Restoril)[2]	15 mg	30 mg	$24.30
Triazolam (Halcion)[5]	0.125 mg	0.25 mg	$20.25
Miscellaneous (used for anxiety)			
Buspirone (Buspar)[2]	10–30 mg	60 mg	$218.10
Phenobarbital[3]	15–30 mg	90 mg	$3.60
Miscellaneous (used for sleep)			
Chloral hydrate (Noctec)[2]	500 mg	1000 mg	$36.00
Hydroxyzine (Vistaril)[2]	50 mg	100 mg	$13.20
Zolpidem (Ambien)[5]	5–10 mg	10 mg	$76.50
Zaleplon (Sonata)[6]	5–10 mg	10 mg	$70.50

[1]Cost to pharmacist (average wholesale price, generic when possible) for quantity listed. Source: *Drug Topics Red Book,* March 2002; Vol. 23, No. 3.
[2]Intermediate physical half-life (10–20 hours).
[3]Long physical half-life (> 20 hours).
[4]Intravenously for procedures.
[5]Short physical half-life (1–5 hours).
[6]Short physical half-life (about 1 hour).

when given intramuscularly. In psychiatric disorders, the benzodiazepines are usually given orally; in controlled medical environments (eg, the ICU), where the rapid onset of respiratory depression can be assessed, they are often given intravenously. Onset of action is a function of the rate of absorption (related to lipophilic property) and varies, with diazepam and clorazepate being the most rapidly absorbed. This characteristic, along with high lipid solubility, may explain the popularity of diazepam. In the average case of anxiety, diazepam, 5–10 mg orally every 6–8 hours as needed, is a reasonable starting regimen.

The duration of action of the benzodiazepines varies as a function of the active metabolites they produce. Benzodiazepines such as lorazepam do not produce active metabolites and have intermediate half-lives of 10–20 hours, characteristics useful in treating elderly patients. Ultra-short-acting agents such as triazolam have half lives of 1–3 hours and may lead to rebound withdrawal anxiety. Longer-acting benzodiazepines such as flurazepam and diazepam produce active metabolites, have half-lives of 20–120 hours, and should be avoided in the elderly. Since people vary widely in their response and since the drugs are long-lasting, one must individualize the dosage. Once this is established, an adequate dose early in the course of symptom development will obviate the need for "pill popping," which contributes to dependency problems. Panic disorder does not usually respond to benzodiazepines other than clonazepam and alprazolam. Those high-potency benzodiazepines and the antidepressants are most commonly used for panic disorder. Notably, alprazolam has a relatively short half-life and over time can lead to interdose rebound anxiety.

Whether the indications for benzodiazepines are anxiety or insomnia, the drugs should be used judiciously. The longer-acting benzodiazepines are used for the treatment of alcohol withdrawal and anxiety symptoms; the intermediate drugs are useful as sedatives for insomnia (eg, lorazepam), while short-acting agents (eg, midazolam) are used for medical procedures such as endoscopy.

The side effects of all the benzodiazepine antianxiety agents are mainly behavioral and depend on patient reaction and dosage. As the dosage exceeds the levels necessary for sedation, the side effects include disinhibition, ataxia, dysarthria, nystagmus, and errors of commission. (The patient should be told not to operate machinery until he is well stabilized without side effects.)

Paradoxical agitation, anxiety, psychosis, confusion, mood lability, and anterograde amnesia have been reported, particularly with the shorter-acting benzodiazepines. These agents produce cumulative clinical effects with repeated dosage (especially if the patient has not had time to metabolize the previous dose); additive effects when given with other classes of sedatives or alcohol (many apparently "accidental" deaths are the result of concomitant use of sedatives and alcohol); and residual effects after termination of treatment (particularly in the case of drugs that undergo slow biotransformation).

Overdosage results in respiratory depression, hypotension, shock syndrome, coma, and death. Flumazenil, a benzodiazepine antagonist, is effective in overdosage. Overdosage (see Chapter 39) and withdrawal states are medical emergencies. Serious side effects of chronic excessive dosage are development of tolerance, resulting in increasing dose requirements, and physiologic dependence, resulting in withdrawal symptoms similar in appearance to alcohol and barbiturate withdrawal (withdrawal effects must be distinguished from reemergent anxiety). Abrupt withdrawal of sedative drugs may cause serious and even fatal convulsive seizures. Psychosis, delirium, and autonomic dysfunction have also been described. Both duration of action and duration of exposure are major factors. Common withdrawal symptoms after low to moderate daily use of benzodiazepines are classified as **somatic** (disturbed sleep, tremor, nausea, muscle aches), **psychologic** (anxiety, poor concentration, irritability, mild depression), or **perceptual** (poor coordination, mild paranoia, mild confusion). The presentation of symptoms will vary depending on the half-life of the drug. There are no significant side effects on organ systems other than the brain, and the drugs are safe in most medical conditions. Benzodiazepine interactions with other drugs are listed in Table 25–2.

Antidepressants are the first-line medications for sustained treatment of generalized anxiety, having the advantage of not causing serious physiologic dependency problems. At initiation of treatment, antidepressants can themselves be anxiogenic—thus, an initial dose, in conjunction with short-term treatment with a benzodiazepine, is often indicated. Venlafaxine (a sustained-release serotonin and norepinephrine reuptake inhibitor, is FDA-approved for the treatment of generalized anxiety disorder in usual antidepressant doses (75–225 mg). Initial daily dosing should start low (37.5–75 mg) and be tapered upward as needed. Similarly, buspirone,

Table 25–2. Benzodiazepine interactions with other drugs.

Drug	Effects
Antacids	Decreased absorption of benzodiazepines
Cimetidine	Increased half-life of diazepam and triazolam
Contraceptives	Increased levels of diazepam and triazolam
Digoxin	Alprazolam and diazepam raise digoxin level
Disulfiram	Increased duration of action of sedatives
Isoniazid	Increased plasma diazepam
Levodopa	Inhibition of antiparkinsonism effect
Propoxyphene	Impaired clearance of diazepam
Rifampin	Decreased plasma diazepam
Warfarin	Decreased prothrombin time

sometimes used as an augmenting agent in the treatment of agitated depression and compulsive behaviors, is also effective for generalized anxiety. Buspirone is usually given in a dosage of 15–60 mg/d in three divided doses. Higher doses tend to be counterproductive and produce gastrointestinal symptoms and dizziness. There is a 2- to 4-week delay before antidepressants and buspirone take effect, and patients require education regarding this lag. Sleep is sometimes negatively effected. Beta-blockers such as propranolol may help reduce peripheral somatic symptoms. Ethanol is the most frequently self-administered drug and should be interdicted. The highly addicting drugs with a narrow margin of safety such as glutethimide, ethchlorvynol, methprylon, meprobamate, and the barbiturates (with the exception of phenobarbital) should be avoided. Phenobarbital, in addition to its anticonvulsant properties, is a reasonably safe and very cheap sedative but has the disadvantage of causing hepatic microsomal enzyme stimulation (not the case with benzodiazepines), which markedly reduces its usefulness if any other relevant medications are being used by the patient.

2. Panic attacks—Panic attacks may be treated in several ways. A sublingual dose of lorazepam (0.5–2 mg) or alprazolam (0.5–1 mg) is often effective for urgent treatment. For sustained treatment, serotonin-selective reuptake inhibitors (SSRIs) are the initial drugs of choice (adequate blood levels will require dosages similar to those used in the treatment of depression). For example, sertraline starting at 25 mg/d and increased after 1 week to 50 mg/d may be effective. Lithium may be used to augment the antidepressant drugs. Because of initial agitation in response to antidepressants, doses should start low and be very gradually increased. High-potency benzodiazepines may be used for symptomatic treatment as the antidepressant dose is titrated upward. Clonazepam (1–6 mg/d orally) and alprazolam (0.5–6 mg/d orally) are effective alternatives to antidepressants. Both drugs may produce marked withdrawal if stopped abruptly and should always be tapered. Because of chronicity of the disorders and the problem of dependency with benzodiazepine drugs, it is generally desirable to use antidepressant drugs as the principal pharmacologic approach. Antidepressants have been used in conjunction with beta-blockers in resistant cases. Propranolol (40–160 mg/d orally) can mute the peripheral symptoms of anxiety without significantly affecting motor and cognitive performance. They block symptoms mediated by sympathetic stimulation (eg, palpitations, tremulousness) but not nonadrenergic symptoms (eg, diarrhea, muscle tension). Contrary to current belief, they usually do not cause depression as a side effect and can be used cautiously in patients with depression. Valproate has been found to be as effective in panic disorder as the antidepressants and is another useful alternative.

3. Phobic disorder—Phobic disorder may be part of the panic disorder and is treated within that framework. Global social phobias may be treated with SSRIs,

such as paroxetine, sertraline, and fluvoxamine, or MAO inhibitors in the same dosage as used for depression. Gabapentin, an anticonvulsant with anxiolytic properties, may be an alternative to antidepressants in the treatment of social phobia in a dosage of 900–3600 mg/d. Specific phobias such as performance anxiety may respond to moderate doses of beta-blockers, such as propranolol, 20–40 mg 1 hour prior to exposure. A sustained effect is often not obtained with drugs alone; a combination of drugs, behavioral techniques, and cognitive psychotherapy is most effective. If there is any indication of seizure-like phenomena, carbamazepine or valproic acid should be considered.

4. Obsessive-compulsive disorders—Obsessive-compulsive disorders respond to serotonergic drugs in about 60% of cases and usually require a longer response time than for depression (up to 12 weeks). Clomipramine has proved effective in doses equivalent to those used for depression. Fluoxetine (an SSRI drug) has been widely used in this disorder but in doses higher than those used in depression (up to 60–80 mg/d). The other SSRI drugs such as sertraline, paroxetine, and fluvoxamine are being used with comparable efficacy, each with its own side effect profile. Buspirone in doses of 15–60 mg/d appears to be effective primarily as an antiobsessional augmenting agent for the SSRI drugs. Psychosurgery has a limited place in selected cases of severe unremitting obsessive-compulsive disorder. The stereotactic techniques now being used, including modified cingulotomy, are great improvements over the crude methods of the past.

B. BEHAVIORAL

Behavioral approaches are widely used in various anxiety disorders, often in conjunction with medication. Any of the behavioral techniques (see above) can be used beneficially in altering the contingencies (precipitating factors or rewards) supporting any anxiety-provoking behavior. Relaxation techniques can sometimes be helpful in reducing anxiety. Desensitization, by exposing the patient to graded doses of a phobic object or situation, is an effective technique and one that the patient can practice outside the therapy session. Emotive imagery, wherein the patient imagines the anxiety-provoking situation while at the same time learning to relax, helps to decrease the anxiety when the patient faces the real-life situation. Physiologic symptoms in panic attacks respond well to relaxation training.

C. PSYCHOLOGIC

Cognitive approaches have been effective in treatment of panic disorders, phobias, and obsessive-compulsive disorder when erroneous beliefs need correction. The combination of medical and cognitive therapy is more effective than either alone. Group therapy is the treatment of choice when the anxiety is clearly a function of the patient's difficulties in dealing with others, and if these other people are part of the family it is appropriate to include them and initiate family or couples therapy.

D. SOCIAL

Peer support groups for panic disorder and agoraphobia have been particularly helpful. Social modification may require measures such as family counseling to aid acceptance of the patient's symptoms and avoid counterproductive behavior in behavioral training. Any help in maintaining the social structure is anxiety-alleviating, and work, school, and social activities should be maintained. School and vocational counseling may be provided by professionals, who often need help from the clinician in defining the patient's limitations.

Prognosis

Anxiety disorders are usually of long standing and may be quite difficult to treat. All can be relieved to varying degrees with medications and behavioral techniques. The prognosis is much better if one can break the commonly observed anxiety-panic-phobia-depression cycle with a combination of the therapeutic interventions discussed above.

Brady K et al: Efficacy and safety of sertraline treatment of posttraumatic stress disorder. JAMA 2000;283:1837. [PMID: 10770145] (Suggests that sertraline is safe and effective.)

Hohagen F: Cognitive-behavioral therapy and integrated approaches in the treatment of obsessive-compulsive disorder. CNS Spectrums 1999;5:35. (Cognitive-behavioral therapy and SSRIs can be used together or independently in the treatment of obsessive-compulsive disorder. Further research may refine their application in subtypes of the disorder.)

JAMA patient page: Obsessive-compulsive disorder. JAMA 1998;280:1806. [PMID: 9842960]

Pande AC et al: Treatment of social phobia with gabapentin: a placebo controlled study. J Clin Psychopharmacol 1999;19:341. [PMID: 10440462] (Gabapentin may have efficacy in the treatment of social phobia.)

Pohl RB et al: Sertraline in the treatment of panic disorder: A double-blind multicenter trial. Am J Psychiatry 1998;155:1189. [PMID: 9734541] (Effective and well tolerated.)

Stein MB et al: Paroxetine treatment of generalized social phobia (social anxiety disorder). JAMA 1998;280:708. [PMID: 9728642] (Symptoms and disability were substantially reduced.)

SOMATOFORM DISORDERS (Abnormal Illness Behaviors)

ESSENTIALS OF DIAGNOSIS

- *Physical symptoms may involve one or more organ systems and are not intentional.*
- *Subjective complaints exceed objective findings.*
- *Correlations of symptom development and psychosocial stresses.*
- *Combination of biogenetic and developmental patterns.*

General Considerations

A major source of diagnostic confusion in medicine has been to assume cause-and-effect relationships when parallel conditions exist. This problem is particularly vexing in situations where the individual exhibits psychosocial distress that could well be secondary to a chronic illness but has been assumed to be primary and causative. An example is the person with a chronic bowel disease who becomes querulous and demanding. Is this behavior a result of problems of coping with a chronic disease, or is it a personality pattern that causes the gastrointestinal problem?

Vulnerability in one or more organ systems and exposure to family members with somatization problems play a major role in the development of particular symptoms, and the "functional" versus "organic" dichotomy is a hindrance to good treatment. Clinicians should suspect psychiatric disorders in a number of conditions. For example, 45% of patients complaining of palpitations had lifetime psychiatric diagnoses including generalized anxiety, depression, panic, and somatization disorders. Similarly, 33–44% of patients who undergo coronary angiography for chest pain but have negative results have been found to have panic disorder.

In any patient presenting with a condition judged to be somatoform, depression must be considered in the diagnosis.

Clinical Findings

A. CONVERSION DISORDER

"Conversion" (formerly "hysterical conversion") of psychic conflict into physical symptoms in parts of the body innervated by the sensorimotor system (eg, paralysis, aphonia) is a disorder that is more common in individuals from lower socioeconomic classes and certain cultures. The defense mechanisms utilized in this condition are repression (a barring from consciousness) and isolation (a splitting of the affect from the idea). The somatic manifestation that takes the place of anxiety is typically paralysis, and in some instances the organ dysfunction may have symbolic meaning (eg, arm paralysis in marked anger). Pseudoepileptic ("hysterical") seizures are often difficult to differentiate from intoxication states or panic attacks. Retention of consciousness, random flailing with asynchronous movements of the right and left sides, and resistance to having the nose and mouth pinched closed during the attack all point toward a pseudoepileptic event. Electroencephalography, particularly in a video-EEG assessment unit, during the attack is the most helpful diagnostic aid in excluding genuine seizure states. Serum prolactin levels rise abruptly in the postictal state only in true epilepsy. La belle indifférence (a lack of affect) is not a significant characteristic, as commonly believed. Important criteria in diagnosis include a history of conversion or somatization disorder, modeling the symptom after someone else who had a similar presentation, a serious precipitating emotional event, associated psychopathology (eg, depression, schizophrenia, personality disorders), a temporal correlation between the precipitating event and the symptom, and a temporary "solving of the problem" by the conversion. It is important to identify physical disorders with unusual presentations (eg, multiple sclerosis).

B. SOMATIZATION DISORDER (BRIQUET'S SYNDROME, HYSTERIA)

This is characterized by multiple physical complaints referable to several organ systems. Anxiety, panic disorder, and depression are often present, and **major depression** is an important consideration in the differential diagnosis. There is a significant relationship (20%) to a lifetime history of panic-agoraphobia-depression. It usually occurs before age 30 and is ten times more common in women. Polysurgery is often a feature of the history. Preoccupation with medical and surgical therapy becomes a lifestyle that excludes most other activities. The symptoms are a reflection of maladaptive coping techniques and reactivity of the particular organ system. There is often evidence of long-standing somatic symptoms (particularly dysmenorrhea, a lump in the throat, vomiting, shortness of breath, burning in the sex organs, painful extremities, and amnesia), often with a history of similar organ system involvement in other family members. Multiple symptoms that constantly change and inability of more than three doctors to make a diagnosis are strong clues to the problem.

C. PAIN DISORDER ASSOCIATED WITH PSYCHOLOGIC FACTORS (FORMERLY SOMATOFORM PAIN DISORDER)

This involves a long history of complaints of severe pain not consonant with anatomic and clinical signs. This diagnosis must not be one of exclusion and should be made only after extended evaluation has established a clear correlation of psychogenic factors with exacerbations and remissions of complaints.

D. HYPOCHONDRIASIS

This is a fear of disease and preoccupation with the body, with perceptual amplification and heightened responsiveness. A process of social learning is usually involved, frequently with a role model who was a member of the family and may be a part of the underlying psychodynamic causation. It is common in panic disorders.

E. FACTITIOUS DISORDERS

These disorders, in which symptom production is intentional, are not somatoform conditions in that symptoms are produced consciously, in contrast to the unconscious process of the above conditions. They are characterized by self-induced symptoms or false physical and laboratory findings for the purpose of deceiving clinicians or other hospital personnel. The deceptions may involve self-mutilation, fever, hemorrhage, hypoglycemia, seizures, and an almost endless variety of manifestations—often presented in an exaggerated and dramatic fashion (Munchausen syndrome). "Munchausen by proxy" is the term used when a parent creates an illness in a child so the adult (usually the mother) can maintain a relationship with clinicians. The duplicity may be either simple or extremely complex and difficult to recognize. The patients are frequently connected in some way with the health professions; they are often migratory; and there is no apparent external motivation other than achieving the patient role.

Complications

A poor doctor-patient relationship, with iatrogenic disorders and "doctor shopping," tends to exacerbate the problem. Sedative and analgesic dependency is the most common iatrogenic complication.

Treatment

A. MEDICAL

Medical support with careful attention to building a therapeutic doctor-patient relationship is the mainstay of treatment. It must be accepted that the patient's distress is real. Every problem not found to have an organic basis is not necessarily a mental disease. Diligent attempts should be made to relate symptoms to adverse developments in the patient's life. It may be useful to have the patient keep a meticulous diary, paying particular attention to various pertinent factors evident in the history. Regular, frequent, short appointments that are not symptom-contingent may be helpful. Drugs (frequently abused) should not be prescribed to replace appointments. One doctor should be the primary clinician, and consultants should be used mainly for evaluation. An empathic, realistic, optimistic approach must be maintained in the face of the expected ups and downs. Ongoing reevaluation is necessary, since somatization can coexist with a concurrent physical illness.

B. PSYCHOLOGIC

Psychologic approaches can be used by the primary clinician when it is clear that the patient is ready to make some changes in lifestyle in order to achieve symptomatic relief. This is often best approached on a here-and-now basis and oriented toward pragmatic changes rather than an exploration of early experiences that the patient frequently fails to relate to current distress. Group therapy with other individuals who have similar problems is sometimes of value to improve coping, allow ventilation, and focus on interpersonal adjustment. Hypnosis or lorazepam interviews used early are helpful in resolving conversion disorders. If the primary clinician has been working with the patient on psychologic problems related to the physical illness, the groundwork is often laid for successful psychiatric referral.

For patients who have been identified as having a factitious disorder, early psychiatric consultation is indicated. There are two main treatment strategies for these patients. One consists of a conjoint confrontation of the patient by both the primary clinician and the psychiatrist. The patient's disorder is portrayed as a cry for help, and psychiatric treatment is recommended. The second approach avoids direct confrontation and attempts to provide a face-saving way to relinquish the symptom without overt disclosure of the disorder's origin. Techniques such as biofeedback and self-hypnosis may foster recovery using this strategy. Another face-saving approach is to utilize a double bind with the patient. For example, the patient is told there are two possible diagnoses: (1) an organic disease that should respond to the next medical intervention (usually modest and noninvasive), or (2) factitious disorder for which the patient will need psychiatric treatment. Given these options, many patients will choose to recover and not have to admit the origin of their problem.

C. BEHAVIORAL

Behavioral therapy is probably best exemplified by biofeedback techniques. In biofeedback, the particular abnormality (eg, increased peristalsis) must be recognized and monitored by the patient and therapist (eg, by an electronic stethoscope to amplify the sounds). This is immediate feedback, and after learning to recognize it the patient can then learn to identify any change thus produced (eg, a decrease in bowel sounds) and so become a conscious originator of the feedback instead of a passive recipient. Relief of the symptom operantly conditions the patient to utilize the maneuver that relieves symptoms (eg, relaxation causing a decrease in bowel sounds). With emphasis on this type of learning, the patient is able to identify symptoms early and initiate the countermaneuvers, thus decreasing the symptomatic problem. Migrainoid and tension headaches have been particularly responsive to biofeedback methods.

D. SOCIAL

Social endeavors include family, work, and other interpersonal activity. Family members should come for some appointments with the patient so they can learn how best to live with the patient. This is particularly important in treatment of somatization and pain disorders. Peer support groups provide a climate for encouraging the patient to accept and live with the problem. Ongoing communication with the employer may be necessary to encourage long-term continued interest in the employee. Employers can become just as discouraged as clinicians in dealing with employees who have chronic problems.

Prognosis

The prognosis is much better if the primary clinician is able to intervene early before the situation has deteriorated. After the problem has crystallized into chronicity, it is very difficult to effect change.

Eisendrath SJ: Factitious physical disorders. West J Med 1994; 160:177. [PMID: 8169474]

Eisendrath SJ et al: Somatization disorders: Effective management in primary care. J Musculoskel Med 1997;4:47. (The successful physician-patient relationship is the main "medicine" for this population.)

Noyes R et al: Fluvoxamine for somatoform disorders: an open trial. Gen Hosp Psychiatry 1998;20:339. [PMID: 9862258] (Modest benefits in the treatment of patients with somatoform disorders may warrant further study.)

CHRONIC PAIN DISORDERS

 ESSENTIALS OF DIAGNOSIS

- *Chronic complaints of pain.*
- *Symptoms frequently exceed signs.*
- *Minimal relief with standard treatment.*
- *History of having seen many clinicians.*
- *Frequent use of several nonspecific medications.*

General Considerations

A problem in the management of pain is the lack of distinction between acute and chronic pain syndromes. Most clinicians are adept at dealing with acute pain problems but have difficulty handling the patient with a chronic pain disorder. This type of patient frequently takes too many medications, stays in bed a great deal, has seen many clinicians, has lost skills, and experiences little joy in either work or play. All relationships suffer (including those with clinicians), and life becomes a constant search for succor. The search results in complex clinician-patient relationships that usually include many drug trials, particularly sedatives, with adverse consequences (eg, irritability, depressed mood) related to long-term use. Treatment failures provoke angry responses and depression from both the patient and the clinician, and the pain syndrome is exacerbated. When frustration becomes too great, a new clinician is found, and the cycle is repeated. The longer the existence of the pain disorder, the more important become the psychologic factors of anxiety and depression. As with all other conditions, it is counterproductive to speculate about whether the pain is "real." It is real to the patient, and acceptance of the problem must precede a mutual endeavor to alleviate the disturbance.

Clinical Findings

Components of the chronic pain syndrome consist of anatomic changes, chronic anxiety and depression, anger, and changed lifestyle. Usually, the anatomic problem is irreversible, since it has already been subjected to many interventions with increasingly unsatisfactory results. An algorithm for assessing chronic pain and differentiating it from other psychiatric conditions is illustrated in Figure 25–2.

Chronic anxiety and depression produce heightened irritability and overreaction to stimuli. A marked decrease in pain threshold is apparent. This pattern develops into a hypochondriacal preoccupation with the body and a constant need for reassurance. The pressure on the clinician becomes wearing and often leads to covert rejection devices, such as not being available or making referrals to other clinicians. This is perceived by the patient, who then intensifies the effort to find help, and the typical cycle is repeated. Anxiety and depression are seldom discussed, almost as if there is a tacit agreement not to deal with these issues.

Changes in lifestyle involve some of the pain behaviors. These usually take the form of a family script in which the patient accepts the role of being sick, and this role then becomes the focus of most family inter-actions and may become important in maintaining the family, so that neither the patient nor the family wants the patient's role to change. Demands for attention and efforts to control the behavior of others revolve around the central issue of control of other people (including clinicians). Cultural factors frequently play a role in the behavior of the patient and how the significant people around the patient cope with the problem. Some cultures encourage demonstrative behavior, while others value the stoic role.

Another secondary gain that frequently maintains the patient in the sick role is financial compensation or other benefits ("green poultice"). Frequently, such systems are structured so that they reinforce the maintenance of sickness and discourage any attempts to give up the role. Clinicians unwittingly reinforce this role because of the very nature of the practice of medicine, which is to respond to complaints of illness. Helpful suggestions from the clinician are often met

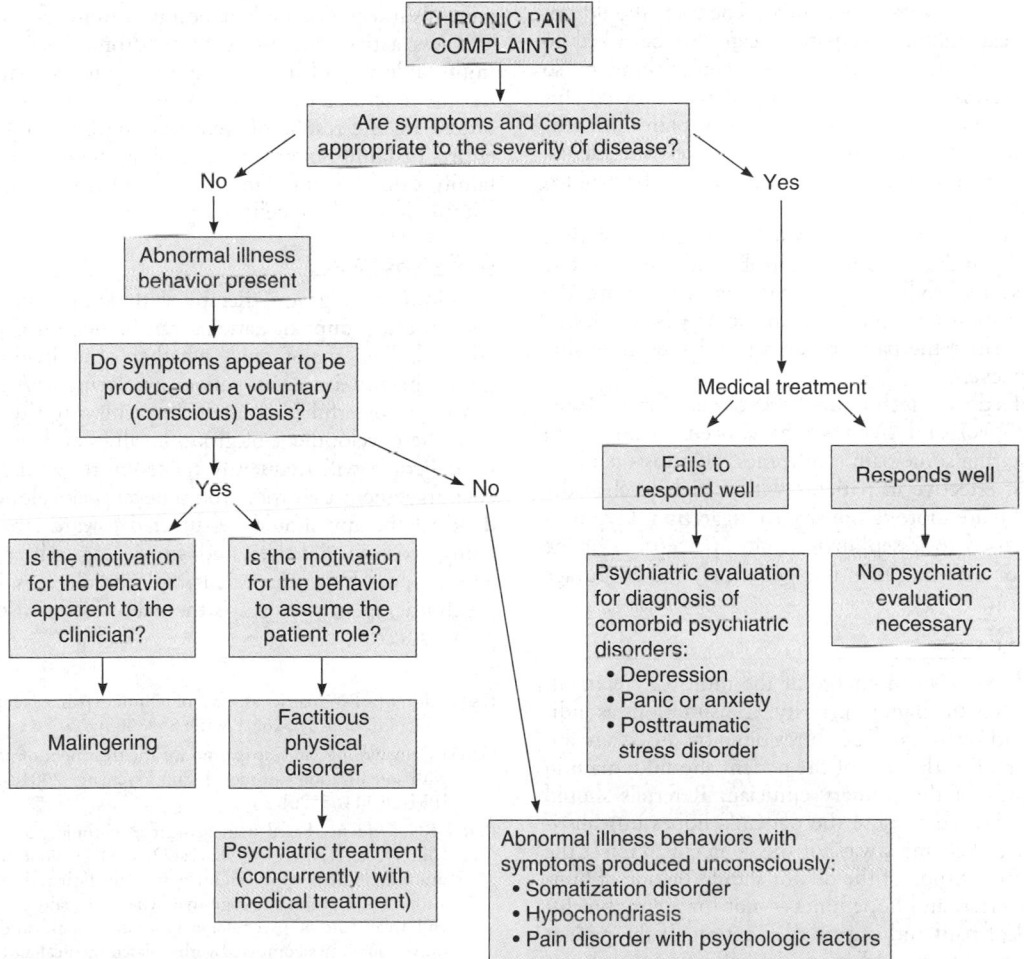

Figure 25–2. Algorithm for assessing psychiatric component of chronic pain. (Modified and reproduced, with permission, from Eisendrath SJ: Psychiatric aspects of chronic pain. Neurology 1995;45 [Suppl 9]:S20.)

with responses like, "Yes, but. . . ." Medications then become the principal approach, and drug dependency problems may develop.

Treatment

A. BEHAVIORAL

The cornerstone of a unified approach to chronic pain syndromes is a comprehensive behavioral program. This is necessary to identify and eliminate pain reinforcers, to decrease drug use, and to use effectively those positive reinforcers that shift the focus from the pain. It is critical that the patient be made a partner in the effort to alleviate pain. The clinician must shift from the idea of biomedical cure to ongoing care of the patient. The patient should agree to discuss the pain only with the clinician and not with family members; this tends to stabilize the patient's personal life, since the family is usually tired of the subject. At the beginning of treatment, the patient should be assigned self-help tasks graded up to maximal activity, as a means of positive reinforcement. The tasks should not exceed capability. The patient can also be asked to keep a self-rating chart to log accomplishments, so that progress can be measured and remembered. Instruct the patient to record degrees of pain on a self-rating scale in relation to various situations and mental attitudes so that similar circumstances can be avoided or modified.

Avoid positive reinforcers for pain such as marked sympathy and attention to pain. Emphasize a positive response to productive activities, which remove the focus of attention from the pain. Activity is also desensitizing, since the patient learns to tolerate increasing activity levels.

Biofeedback techniques (see Somatoform Disorders, above) and hypnosis have been successful in ameliorating some pain syndromes. Hypnosis tends to be most effective in patients with a high level of denial, who are more responsive to suggestion. Hypnosis can be used to lessen anxiety, alter perception of the length of time that pain is experienced, and encourage relaxation.

B. MEDICAL

A *single clinician* in charge of the multiple treatment approach is the highest priority. Consultations as indicated and technical procedures done by others are appropriate, but the care of the patient should remain in the hands of the primary clinician. Referrals should not be allowed to raise the patient's hopes unrealistically or to become a way for the clinician to reject the case. The attitude of the doctor should be one of honesty, interest, and hopefulness—not for a cure but for control of pain and improved function. If the patient manifests narcotic addiction, detoxification may be an early treatment goal.

If analgesics or sedatives are prescribed, they should not be given on an "as-needed" schedule (see Chapter 1). A fixed schedule lessens the conditioning effects of these drugs. Tricyclic antidepressants (eg, nortriptyline) and venlafaxine in doses up to those used in depression may be helpful, particularly in neuropathic pain syndromes. In other conditions, their effects on pain may be less clear, but ameliorating depression is usually important nonetheless. Gabapentin, an anticonvulsant with possible applications in the treatment of mood and anxiety disorders, has been shown to be useful in postherpetic and diabetic neuropathy and somatoform disorders.

In addition to medications, a variety of alternative strategies may be offered, including physical therapy and acupuncture.

C. SOCIAL

Involvement of family members and other significant persons in the patient's life should be an early priority. The best efforts of both patient and therapists can be unwittingly sabotaged by other persons who may feel that they are "helping" the patient. They frequently tend to reinforce the negative aspects of the chronic pain disorder. The patient becomes more dependent and less active, and the pain syndrome becomes an immutable way of life. The more destructive pain behaviors described by many experts in chronic pain disorders are the results of well-meaning but misguided efforts of family members. Ongoing therapy with the family can be helpful in the early identification and elimination of these behavior patterns.

D. PSYCHOLOGIC

In addition to group therapy with family members and others, groups of patients can be helpful if properly led. The major goal, whether of individual or group therapy, is to gain patient involvement. A group can be a powerful instrument for achieving this goal, with the development of group loyalties and cooperation. People will frequently make efforts with group encouragement that they would never make alone. Individual therapy should be directed toward strengthening existing defenses and improving self-esteem. The rapport between patient and clinician, as in all psychotherapeutic efforts, is the major factor in therapeutic success.

Eisendrath SJ: Psychiatric aspects of chronic pain. Neurology 1995;45(Suppl 9):S26. [PMID: 8538883]

Garcia-Campayo J et al: Gabapentin for the treatment of patients with somatization disorder. J Clin Psychiatry 2001;62:474. [PMID: 11465526]

Reiter RC: Evidence-based management of chronic pelvic pain. Clin Obstet Gynecol 1998;41:422. [PMID: 9646974] (A multidisciplinary approach integrating medical and socioenvironmental problems, cognitive behavioral pain strategies, and treatment of psychologic morbidity significantly improves outcomes compared with isolated medical and surgical interventions.)

Rowbotham M et al: Gabapentin for the treatment of postherpetic neuralgia. JAMA 1998;280:1837. [PMID: 9846778] (Gabapentin is effective in the treatment of pain and sleep interference in this population.)

PSYCHOSEXUAL DISORDERS

The stages of sexual activity include **excitement** (arousal), **orgasm,** and **resolution.** The precipitating excitement or arousal is psychologically determined. Arousal response leading to plateau is a physiologic and psychologic phenomenon of vasocongestion, a parasympathetic reaction causing erection in men and labial-clitoral congestion in women. The orgasmic response includes emission in men and clonic contractions of the analogous striated perineal muscles of both men and women. Resolution is a gradual return to normal physiologic status.

While the arousal stimuli—vasocongestive and orgasmic responses—constitute a single response in a well-adjusted person, they can be considered as separate stages that can produce different syndromes responding to different treatment procedures.

Clinical Findings

There are three major groups of sexual disorders.

A. PARAPHILIAS (SEXUAL AROUSAL DISORDERS)

In these conditions, formerly called "deviations" or "variations," the excitement stage of sexual activity is associated with sexual objects or orientations different from those usually associated with adult sexual stimulation. The stimulus may be a woman's shoe, a child, animals, instruments of torture, or incidents of aggression. The pattern of sexual stimulation is usually one that has early psychologic roots. Poor experiences with sexual activity frequently reinforce this pattern over time.

Exhibitionism is the impulsive behavior of exposing the genitalia to unsuspecting strangers in order to achieve sexual excitation. It is a childhood sexual behavior carried into adult life.

Transvestism consists of recurrent cross-dressing behavior in a heterosexual man for the purpose of sexual excitation. Such fetishistic behavior can be part of masturbation foreplay. Transvestism in homosexuality and transsexualism is not for the purpose of sexual excitement but is a function of the homosexual preference or gender disorder.

Voyeurism involves the achievement of sexual arousal by watching the activities of an unsuspecting person, usually in various stages of undress or sexual activity. In both exhibitionism and voyeurism, excitation leads to masturbation as a replacement for sexual activity.

Pedophilia is the use of a child of either sex to achieve sexual arousal and, in many cases, gratification. Contact is frequently oral, with either participant being dominant, but pedophilia includes intercourse of any type. Adults of both sexes engage in this behavior, but because of social and cultural factors it is more commonly identified with men. The pedophile has difficulty in adult sexual relationships, and men who perform this act are frequently impotent.

Incest involves a sexual relationship with a person in the immediate family, most frequently a child. In many ways it is similar to pedophilia (intrafamilial pedophilia). Incestuous feelings are fairly common, but cultural mores are usually sufficiently strong to act as a barrier to the expression of sexual feelings.

Sexual sadism is the attainment of sexual arousal by inflicting pain upon the sexual object. Much sexual activity has aggressive components (eg, biting, scratching). However, forced sexual acquiescence (eg, rape) is considered to be primarily an act of aggression.

Sexual masochism is the achievement of erotic pleasure by being humiliated, enslaved, physically bound, and restrained. It is life-threatening, since neck binding or partial asphyxiation usually forms part of the ritual. It is estimated that bondage is responsible for about 1000 accidental deaths a year in men (the practice is much less common in women).

Necrophilia is sexual intercourse with a dead body or the use of parts of a dead body for sexual excitation, often with masturbation.

B. GENDER IDENTITY DISORDER

Core gender identity reflects a biologic self-image—the conviction that "I am a boy" or "I am a girl" that is usually well developed by age 3 or 4. Gender dysphoria refers to the development of a sexual identity that is the opposite of the biologic one.

Transsexualism is an attempt to deny and reverse biologic sex by maintaining sexual identity with the opposite gender. Transsexuals do not alternate between gender roles; rather, they assume a fixed role of attitudes, feelings, fantasies, and choices consonant with those of the opposite sex, all of which clearly date back to early development. For example, male transsexuals in early childhood behave, talk, and fantasize as if they were girls. They do not grow out of feminine patterns; they do not work in professions traditionally considered to be masculine; and they have no interest in their own penises either as evidence of maleness or as organs for erotic behavior. The desire for sex change starts early and may culminate in assumption of a feminine lifestyle, hormonal treatment, and use of surgical procedures, eg, castration and vaginoplasty.

C. PSYCHOSEXUAL DYSFUNCTION

This category includes a large group of vasocongestive and orgasmic disorders. Often, they involve problems of sexual adaptation, education, and technique that are often initially discussed with, diagnosed by, and treated by the primary care provider.

There are two conditions common in men: erectile dysfunction and ejaculation disturbances.

Erectile dysfunction (impotence) is inability to achieve or maintain an erection firm enough for satisfactory intercourse; patients sometimes use the term to mean premature ejaculation. Careful questioning is necessary, since causes of this vasocongestive disorder can be psychologic, physiologic, or both. The majority are pathophysiologic and, to varying degrees, treatable.

After onset of the problem, a history of occasional erections—especially nocturnal penile tumescence, which may be evaluated by a simple monitoring device, or a sleep study in the sleep laboratory—is usually evidence that the dysfunction is psychologic in origin, with the caveat that decreased nocturnal penile tumescence occurs in some depressed patients. **Psychologic erectile dysfunction** is caused by interpersonal or intrapsychic factors (eg, marital disharmony, depression). **Organic factors** are discussed in Chapter 23.

Ejaculation disturbances include premature ejaculation, inability to ejaculate, and retrograde ejaculation. (One may ejaculate even though impotent.) Ejaculation is usually connected with orgasm, and ejaculatory control is an acquired behavior that is minimal in adolescence and increases with experience. Pathogenic factors are those that interfere with learning control, most frequently sexual ignorance. Intrapsychic factors (anxiety, guilt, depression) and interpersonal maladaptation (marital problems, unresponsiveness of mate, power struggles) are also common. Organic causes include interference with sympathetic nerve distribution (often due to surgery or trauma) and the effects of pharmacologic agents (eg, SSRIs or sympatholytics).

In women, the two most common forms of sexual dysfunction are vaginismus and frigidity.

Vaginismus is a conditioned response in which a spasm of the perineal muscles occurs if there is any stimulation of the area. The desire is to avoid penetration. Sexual responsiveness and vasocongestion may be present, and orgasm can result from clitoral stimulation.

Frigidity is a complex condition in which there is a general lack of sexual responsiveness. The woman has difficulty in experiencing erotic sensation and does not have the vasocongestive response. Sexual activity varies from active avoidance of sex to an occasional orgasm. Orgasmic dysfunction—in which a woman has a vasocongestive response but varying degrees of difficulty in reaching orgasm—is sometimes differentiated from frigidity. Causes for the dysfunctions include poor sexual techniques, early traumatic sexual experiences, interpersonal disharmony (marital struggles, use of sex as a means of control), and intrapsychic problems (anxiety, fear, guilt). Organic causes include any conditions that might cause pain in intercourse, pelvic pathology, mechanical obstruction, and neurologic deficits.

Disorders of sexual desire consist of diminished or absent libido in either sex and may be a function of organic or psychologic difficulties (eg, anxiety, phobic avoidance). Any chronic illness can sap desire. Hormonal disorders, including hypogonadism or use of antiandrogen compounds such as cyproterone acetate, and chronic renal failure contribute to deterioration in sexual activity. Though menopause may lead to diminution of sexual desire in some women, the relationship between menopause and libido is complicated and may be influenced by sociocultural factors. Alcohol, sedatives, narcotics, marijuana, and some medications may affect sexual drive and performance.

Treatment

A. Paraphilias and Gender Identity Disorders

1. Psychologic—Sexual arousal disorders involving variant sexual activity (paraphilia), particularly those of a more superficial nature (eg, voyeurism) and those of recent onset, are responsive to psychotherapy in a moderate percentage of cases. The prognosis is much better if the motivation comes from the individual rather than the legal system; unfortunately, however, judicial intervention is frequently the only stimulus to treatment, because the condition persists and is reinforced until conflict with the law occurs. Therapies frequently focus on barriers to normal arousal response; the expectation is that the variant behavior will decrease as normal behavior increases.

2. Behavioral—Aversive and operant conditioning techniques have been tried frequently in gender role disorders but have only occasionally been successful. In some cases, the sexual arousal disorders improve with modeling, role-playing, and conditioning procedures. Emotive imagery is occasionally helpful in lessening anxiety in fetish problems.

3. Social—Although they do not produce a change in sexual arousal patterns or gender role, self-help groups have facilitated adjustment to an often hostile society. Attention to the family is particularly important in helping persons in such groups to accept their situation and alleviate their guilt about the role they think they had in creating the problem.

4. Medical—Medroxyprogesterone acetate, a suppressor of libidinal drive, is used to mute disruptive sexual behavior in men of all ages. Onset of action is usually within 3 weeks, and the effects are generally reversible. Fluoxetine or other SSRIs may reduce some of the compulsive sexual behaviors including the paraphilias. Although some transsexuals are treated with genital reconstructive surgery, many others are screened out by trial periods of living as females prior to operation.

B. Psychosexual Dysfunction

1. Medical—Identification of a contributory reversible cause is most important. Even if the condition is not reversible, identification of the specific cause helps the patient to accept the condition. Marital disharmony, with its exacerbating effects, may thus be avoided. Of all the sexual dysfunctions, erectile dysfunction is the condition most likely to have an organic basis. Sildenafil citrate is an effective oral agent for the treatment of penile erectile dysfunction in the recommended dose of 25–100 mg 1 hour prior to intercourse. Sildenafil is effective for SSRI-induced erectile dysfunction in men and in some cases for SSRI-associated sexual dysfunction in women. Use of the medication in conjunction with any nitrates, particularly in individuals with coronary artery disease, can have significant hypotensive effects leading to death in some cases. The medication, which does not appear to impact sexual desire, should be used only once a day. Because of their common effect in delaying ejaculation, the SSRIs have been effective in premature ejaculation.

2. Behavioral—Syndromes resulting from conditioned responses have been treated by conditioning techniques, with excellent results. Vaginismus responds well to desensitization with graduated Hegar dilators along with relaxation techniques. Masters and Johnson have used behavioral approaches in all of the sexual dysfunctions, with concomitant supportive psychotherapy and with improvement of the communication patterns of the couple.

3. Psychologic—The use of psychotherapy by itself is best suited for those cases in which interpersonal difficulties or intrapsychic problems predominate. Anxiety and guilt about parental injunctions against sex may contribute to sexual dysfunction. Even in these cases, however, a combined behavioral-psychologic approach usually produces results most quickly.

4. Social—The proximity of other people (eg, a mother-in-law) in a household is frequently an inhibiting factor in sexual relationships. In such cases, some social engineering may alleviate the problem.

Boyce EG et al: Sildenafil citrate, a therapeutic update. Clin Ther 2001;23:2. [PMID: 11219477]

JAMA patient page: Sexual abuse. JAMA 1998;280:1888. [PMID: 9846750]

JAMA patient page: Sexual dysfunction. JAMA 1999;281:584. [PMID: 1022117]

Reilly DR et al: Protocols for the use of cyproterone, medroxyprogesterone, and leuprolide in the treatment of paraphilia. Can J Psychiatry 2000;45:559. [PMID: 10986575] (Complications associated with each drug can be detected early and avoided.)

Speckens AE et al: Psychosexual functioning of partners of men with presumed nonorganic erectile dysfunction: Cause or consequence of the disorder? Arch Sex Behav 1995;24:157. [PMID: 7794106] (Relationship problems, female psychosexual dysfunction, and the possible effect of relatively high levels of female sexual interest may contribute to the onset, exacerbation, and maintenance of erectile dysfunction.)

PERSONALITY DISORDERS

 ESSENTIALS OF DIAGNOSIS

- Long history dating back to childhood.
- Recurrent maladaptive behavior.
- Low self-esteem and lack of confidence.
- Minimal introspective ability with a tendency to blame others for all problems.
- Major difficulties with interpersonal relationships or society.
- Depression with anxiety when maladaptive behavior fails.

General Considerations

Personality—a hypothetical construct—is the result of a genetic substrate and the prolonged interaction of an individual with personal drives and with outside influences (parent-child interactions, peer influences, random events). The sum of the effects produces the enduring and unique patterns of behavior that are adopted in order to cope with the environment and which characterize one as an individual. The personality structure, or character, is an integral part of self-image and is important to one's sense of personal identity.

The classification of subtypes depends upon the predominant symptoms and their severity. The most severe disorders—those that bring the patient into greatest conflict with society—tend to be classified as antisocial (psychopathic) or borderline.

Personality disorders can be considered a matrix for some of the more severe psychiatric problems (eg, schizotypal, relating to schizophrenia; avoidance types, relating to some anxiety disorders).

Classification & Clinical Findings

See Table 25–3.

Differential Diagnosis

Patients with personality disorders tend to show anxiety and depression when pathologic coping mechanisms fail, and their symptoms can be similar to those occurring with anxiety disorders. Occasionally, the more severe cases may decompensate into psychosis under stress and mimic other psychotic disorders.

Treatment

A. SOCIAL

Social and therapeutic environments such as day hospitals, halfway houses, and self-help communities utilize peer pressures to modify the self-destructive behavior. The patient with a personality disorder often has failed to profit from experience, and difficulties with authority impair the learning experience. The use of peer relationships and the repetition possible in a structured setting of a helpful community enhance the behavioral treatment opportunities and increase learning. When problems are detected early, both the school and the home can serve as foci of intensified social pressure to change the behavior, particularly with the use of behavioral techniques.

B. BEHAVIORAL

The behavioral techniques used are principally operant conditioning and aversive conditioning. The former simply emphasizes the recognition of acceptable behavior and its reinforcement with praise or other tangible rewards. Aversive responses usually mean punishment, though this can range from a mild rebuke to some specific punitive responses such as depri-

Table 25–3. Personality disorders: Classification and clinical findings.

Personality Disorder	Clinical Findings
Paranoid	Defensive, oversensitive, secretive, suspicious, hyperalert, with limited emotional response.
Schizoid	Shy, introverted, withdrawn, avoids close relationships.
Obsessive-compulsive	Perfectionist, egocentric, indecisive, with rigid thought patterns and need for control.
Histrionic (hysterical)	Dependent, immature, seductive, egocentric, vain, emotionally labile.
Schizotypal	Superstitious, socially isolated, suspicious, with limited interpersonal ability, eccentric behaviors, and odd speech.
Narcissistic	Exhibitionist, grandiose, preoccupied with power, lacks interest in others, with excessive demands for attention.
Avoidant	Fears rejection, hyperreacts to rejection and failure, with poor social endeavors and low self-esteem.
Dependent	Passive, overaccepting, unable to make decisions, lacks confidence, with poor self-esteem.
Antisocial	Selfish, callous, promiscuous, impulsive, unable to learn from experience, has legal problems.
Borderline	Impulsive; has unstable and intense interpersonal relationships; is suffused with anger, fear, and guilt; lacks self-control and self-fulfillment; has identity problems and affective instability; is suicidal (a serious problem—up to 80% of hospitalized borderline patients make an attempt at some time during treatment, and the incidence of completed suicide is as high as 5%); aggressive behavior, feelings of emptiness, and occasional psychotic decompensation. This group has a high drug abuse rate, which plays a role in symptomatology. There is extensive overlap with other diagnostic categories, particularly mood disorders and posttraumatic stress disorder.

vation of privileges. Extinction plays a role in that an attempt is made not to respond to inappropriate behavior, and the lack of response eventually causes the person to abandon that type of behavior. Pouting and tantrums, for example, diminish quickly when such behavior elicits no reaction. Dialectical behavioral therapy is a program of individual and group therapy specifically designed for patients with chronic suicidality and borderline personality disorder. It adapts a cognitive-behavioral model to address self-awareness, interpersonal functioning, affective lability, and reactions to stress.

C. PSYCHOLOGIC

Psychologic intervention is best conducted in group settings. Group therapy is helpful when specific interpersonal behavior needs to be improved (eg, schizoid and inadequate types, in which involvement with people is markedly impaired). This mode of treatment also has a place with so-called acting-out patients, ie, those who frequently act in an impulsive and inappropriate way. The peer pressure in the group tends to impose restraints on rash behavior. The group also quickly identifies the patient's types of behavior and helps to improve the validity of the patient's self-assessment, so that the antecedents of the unacceptable behavior can be effectively handled, thus decreasing its frequency. Individual therapy should initially be supportive, ie, helping the patient to restabilize and mobilize defenses. If the individual has the ability to observe his or her own behavior, a longer-term and more introspective therapy may be warranted. The therapist must be able to handle countertransference feelings (which are frequently negative), maintain appropriate boundaries in the relationship (no physical contacts, however well-meaning), and refrain from premature confrontations and interpretations.

D. MEDICAL

Hospitalization is rarely indicated except in the case of serious suicidal danger. In most cases, treatment can be accomplished in the day treatment center or self-help community. Antipsychotics may be required for short periods in conditions that have temporarily decompensated into transient psychoses (eg, haloperidol, 2–5 mg orally every 3–4 hours until the patient has quieted down and is regaining contact with reality). Olanzapine (2.5–10 mg/d) or risperidone (0.5–2 mg/d) may be given with lorazepam (1–2 mg orally every 4 hours as needed). In most cases, these drugs are required only for several days and can be discontinued after the patient has regained a previously established level of adjustment. Carbamazepine, 400–800 mg orally daily in divided doses, decreases the severity of behavioral dyscontrol. Antidepressants have improved anxiety, depression, and sensitivity to rejection in some borderline patients. Selective serotonin reuptake inhibitors (SSRIs) may have a role in reducing aggressive behavior in impulsive aggressive patients.

Prognosis

Antisocial and borderline categories generally have a guarded prognosis. Those patients with poor outcomes are more likely to have a history of parental abuse and a family history of mood disorder, whereas persons with mild schizoid or passive-aggressive tendencies have a better prognosis with appropriate treatment.

Hueston WJ et al: Personality disorder traits: prevalence and effects on health status in primary care patients. Int J Psychiatry Med 1999;29:63. [PMID: 10376233] (Patients with borderline, dependent, schizoid, and schizotypal traits are common in primary care settings and are more likely to show depressive symptoms on screening.)

Schultz S et al. Olanzapine safety and efficacy in patients with borderline personality disorder and comorbid dysthymia. Biol Psychiatry 1999;46:1429. [PMID: 10578457] (Low-dose olanzapine improved symptoms of psychosis, mood, and anxiety in patients with borderline personality disorder.)

Simpson EB et al: Use of dialectical behavior therapy in a partial hospitalization program for women with borderline personality disorder. Psychiatr Serv 1998;49:669. [PMID: 9603574]

SCHIZOPHRENIC & OTHER PSYCHOTIC DISORDERS

ESSENTIALS OF DIAGNOSIS

- *Social withdrawal, usually slowly progressive, often with deterioration in personal care.*
- *Loss of ego boundaries, with inability to perceive oneself as a separate entity.*
- *Loose thought associations, often with slowed thinking or overinclusive and rapid shifting from topic to topic.*
- *Autistic absorption in inner thoughts and frequent sexual or religious preoccupations.*
- *Auditory hallucinations, often of a derogatory nature.*
- *Delusions, frequently of a grandiose or persecutory nature.*
- *Symptoms of at least 6 months' duration.*

Frequent additional signs:

- *Flat affect and rapidly alternating mood shifts irrespective of circumstances.*
- *Hypersensitivity to environmental stimuli, with a feeling of enhanced sensory awareness.*
- *Variability or changeable behavior incongruent with the external environment.*
- *Concrete thinking with inability to abstract; inappropriate symbolism.*
- *Impaired concentration worsened by hallucinations and delusions.*
- *Depersonalization, wherein one behaves like a detached observer of one's own actions.*

General Considerations

The schizophrenic disorders are a group of syndromes manifested by massive disruption of thinking, mood, and overall behavior as well as poor filtering of stimuli. The characterization and nomenclature of the disorders are quite arbitrary and are influenced by sociocultural factors and schools of psychiatric thought.

It is currently believed that the schizophrenic disorders are of multifactorial cause, with genetic, environmental, and neurotransmitter pathophysiologic components. At present, there is no laboratory method for confirmation of a diagnosis of schizophrenia. There may or may not be a history of a major disruption in the individual's life (failure, loss, physical illness) before gross psychotic deterioration is evident.

"Other psychotic disorders" are conditions that are similar to schizophrenic disorders in their acute symptoms but have a less pervasive influence over the long term. The individual usually attains higher levels of functioning. The acute psychotic episodes tend to be less disruptive of the person's lifestyle, with a fairly quick return to previous levels of functioning.

Classification

A. SCHIZOPHRENIC DISORDERS

Schizophrenic disorders are subdivided on the basis of certain prominent phenomena that are frequently present. **Disorganized (hebephrenic) schizophrenia** is characterized by marked incoherence and an incongruous or silly affect. **Catatonic schizophrenia** is distinguished by a marked psychomotor disturbance of either excitement (purposeless and stereotyped) or rigidity with mutism. Infrequently, there may be rapid alternation between excitement and stupor (see under catatonic syndrome, below). **Paranoid schizophrenia** includes marked persecutory or grandiose delusions often consonant with hallucinations of similar content and with less marked disorganization of speech and behavior. **Undifferentiated schizophrenia** denotes a category in which symptoms are not specific enough to warrant inclusion of the illness in the other subtypes. **Residual schizophrenia** is a classification that includes persons who have clearly had an episode warranting a diagnosis of schizophrenia but who at present have no overt psychotic symptoms, though they show milder signs such as social withdrawal, flat affect, and eccentric behaviors.

B. DELUSIONAL DISORDERS

Delusional disorders are psychoses in which the predominant symptoms are persistent, nonbizarre delusions with minimal impairment of daily functioning. (The schizophrenic disorders show significant impairment.) Intellectual and occupational activities are little affected, whereas social and marital functioning tend to be markedly involved. Hallucinations are not usually present. Common delusional themes include paranoid delusions of persecution, delusions of being related to or loved by a well-known person, and delusions that one's partner is unfaithful.

C. SCHIZOAFFECTIVE DISORDERS

Schizoaffective disorders are those cases that fail to fit comfortably either in the schizophrenic or in the affective categories. They are usually cases with affective symptoms that precede or develop concurrently with psychotic manifestations.

D. SCHIZOPHRENIFORM DISORDERS

Schizophreniform disorders are similar in their symptoms to schizophrenic disorders except that the duration of prodromal, acute, and residual symptoms is less than 6 months but more than 1 week.

E. BRIEF PSYCHOTIC DISORDERS

These disorders last less than 1 week. They are the result of psychologic stress. The shorter duration is significant and correlates with a more acute onset and resolution as well as a much better prognosis.

F. LATE LIFE PSYCHOSIS

Brain abnormalities occur in 40% of patients who develop psychotic symptoms after age 60. The psychotic symptoms are typical, and there are other findings such as low IQ scores and diminished cognitive function.

G. ATYPICAL PSYCHOSES

This group includes a wide range of conditions with psychotic symptomatology. The cause is often not clear, but later events (eg, new symptoms) may clarify the diagnosis. The most common example is chronic psychosis developing either during periods of heavy abuse of drugs or at some time after the drug use has ceased. Other conditions include temporal lobe dysfunction, HIV infection, and a number of the conditions noted in the differential diagnosis (see below). They often have a good premorbid history, a precipitous onset, and an episodic course with symptom-free intervals.

Clinical Findings

The symptoms and signs of schizophrenia vary markedly among individuals as well as in the same person at different times. The patient's **appearance** may be bizarre, though the usual finding is a mild to moderate unkempt blandness. **Motor activity** is generally reduced, though extremes ranging from catatonic stupor to frenzied excitement occur. **Social behavior** is characterized by marked withdrawal coupled with disturbed interpersonal relationships and a reduced ability to experience pleasure. Dependency and a poor self-image are common. **Verbal utterances** are variable, the language being concrete yet symbolic, with unassociated rambling statements (at times interspersed with mutism) during an acute episode. Neologisms (made-up words or phrases), echolalia (repetition of words spoken by others), and verbigeration (repetition of senseless words or phrases) are occasionally present. **Affect** is usually flattened, with occasional inappropriateness. **Depression** is present in almost all cases but may be less apparent during the acute psychotic episode and more obvious during recovery. Depression is sometimes confused with akinetic side effects of antipsychotic drugs. It is also related to **boredom,** which increases symptoms and decreases the response to treatment. Work is generally unavailable and time unfilled, providing opportunities for counterproductive activities such as drug abuse, withdrawal, and increased psychotic symptoms.

Thought content may vary from a paucity of ideas to a rich complex of delusional fantasy with archaic thinking. One frequently notes after a period of conversation that little if any information has actually been conveyed. Incoming stimuli produce varied responses. In some cases a simple question may trigger explosive outbursts, whereas at other times there may be no overt response whatsoever (catatonia). When paranoid ideation is present, the patient is often irritable and less cooperative. **Delusions** (false beliefs) are characteristic of paranoid thinking, and they usually take the form of a preoccupation with the supposedly threatening behavior exhibited by other individuals. This ideation may cause the patient to adopt active countermeasures such as locking doors and windows, taking up weapons, covering the ceiling with aluminum foil to counteract radar waves, and other bizarre efforts. Somatic delusions revolve around issues of bodily decay or infestation. **Perceptual distortions** usually include auditory hallucinations—visual hallucinations are more commonly associated with organic mental states—and may include illusions (distortions of reality) such as figures changing in size or lights varying in intensity. Cenesthetic hallucinations (eg, a burning sensation in the brain, feeling blood flowing in blood vessels) occasionally occur. Lack of humor, feelings of dread, depersonalization (a feeling of being apart from the self), and fears of annihilation may be present. Any of the above symptoms generate higher anxiety levels, with heightened arousal and occasional panic and suicidal ideation, as the individual fails to cope.

Schizophrenic symptoms have been classified into positive and negative categories. Positive symptoms include hallucinations, delusions, and formal thought disorders. These symptoms appear to be related to increased (D_2) dopaminergic activity in the mesolimbic region. Negative symptoms include diminished sociability, restricted affect, and poverty of speech and appear to be related to decreased dopaminergic activity in the mesocortical system.

Ventricular enlargement and cortical atrophy, as seen on the CT scan, have been correlated with a chronic course, severe cognitive impairment, and nonresponsiveness to neuroleptic medications. Decreased frontal lobe activity on positron emission tomography has been associated with negative symptoms.

The development of the acute episode in schizophrenia frequently is the end product of a gradual decompensation. Frustration and anxiety appear early, followed by depression and alienation, along with decreased effectiveness in day-to-day coping. This often leads to feelings of panic and increasing disorganization, with loss of the ability to test and evaluate the reality of perceptions. The stage of so-called psychotic resolution includes delusions, autistic preoccupations, and psychotic insight, with acceptance of the decompensated state. The process is frequently complicated by the use of caffeine, alcohol, and other recreational drugs. Life expectancy of schizophrenics is as much as 20% shorter than that of cohorts in the general population (usually because of a higher mortality rate in younger people).

Polydipsia may produce water intoxication with hyponatremia—characterized by symptoms of confusion, lethargy, psychosis, seizures, and occasionally death—in any psychiatric disorder, but most commonly in schizophrenia. These problems exacerbate the schizophrenic symptoms. Possible pathogenetic factors include a hypothalamic defect, inappropriate ADH secretion, neuroleptic medications (anticholinergic effects, stimulation of hypothalamic thirst center, effect on ADH), smoking (nicotine and SIADH), psychotic thought processes (delusions), and other medications (eg, diuretics, antidepressants, lithium, alcohol). Other causes of polydipsia must be ruled out (eg, diabetes mellitus, diabetes insipidus, renal disease).

Differential Diagnosis

One should not hesitate to reconsider the diagnosis of schizophrenia in any person who has received that diagnosis in the past, particularly when the clinical course has been atypical. A number of these patients have been found to actually have atypical episodic affective disorders that have responded well to lithium. Manic episodes often mimic schizophrenia. Furthermore, many individuals have been diagnosed as schizophrenic because of inadequacies in psychiatric nomenclature. Thus, persons with brief reactive psychoses, obsessive-compulsive disorder, paranoid disorders, and schizophreniform disorders were often inappropriately diagnosed as having schizophrenia.

Psychotic depressions, psychotic organic mental states, and any illness with psychotic ideation tend to be confused with schizophrenia, partly because of the regrettable tendency to use the terms interchangeably. Adolescent phases of growth and counterculture behaviors constitute another area of diagnostic confusion. It is particularly important to avoid a misdiagnosis in these groups, because of the long-term implications arising from having such a serious diagnosis made in a formative stage of life.

Medical disorders such as thyroid dysfunction, adrenal and pituitary disorders, reactions to toxic materials (eg, mercury, PCBs), and almost all of the organic mental states in the early stages must be ruled out. Postpartum psychosis is discussed under Mood Disorders. Complex partial seizures, especially when psychosensory phenomena are present, are an important differential consideration. Toxic drug states arising from prescription, over-the-counter, and street drugs

may mimic all of the psychotic disorders. The chronic use of amphetamines, cocaine, and other stimulants frequently produces a psychosis that is almost identical to the acute paranoid schizophrenic episode. The presence of formication and stereotypy suggests the possibility of stimulant abuse. Phencyclidine (see below), a very common street drug, may cause a reaction that is difficult to distinguish from other psychotic disorders. Cerebellar signs, excessive salivation, dilated pupils, and increased deep tendon reflexes should alert the clinician to the possibility of a toxic psychosis. Industrial chemical toxicity (both organic and metallic), degenerative disorders, and metabolic deficiencies must be considered in the differential diagnosis.

Catatonic syndrome, frequently assumed to exist solely as a component of schizophrenic disorders, is actually the end product of a number of illnesses, including various organic conditions. Neoplasms, viral and bacterial encephalopathies, central nervous system hemorrhage, metabolic derangements such as diabetic ketoacidosis, sedative withdrawal, and hepatic and renal malfunction have all been implicated. It is particularly important to realize that drug toxicity (eg, overdoses of antipsychotic medications such as fluphenazine or haloperidol) can cause catatonic syndrome, which may be misdiagnosed as a catatonic schizophrenic disorder and inappropriately treated with more antipsychotic medication.

Treatment

A. MEDICAL

Hospitalization is often necessary, particularly when the patient's behavior shows gross disorganization. The presence of competent family members lessens the need for hospitalization, and each case should be judged individually. The major considerations are to prevent self-inflicted harm or harm to others and to provide the patient's basic needs. A full medical evaluation and CT scan or MRI should be considered in first episodes of schizophreniform disorder and other psychotic episodes of unknown cause.

Antipsychotic medications (see below) are the treatment of choice. They block the response to stimulation. The relapse rate can be reduced by 50% with proper maintenance neuroleptic therapy. Long-acting, injectable depot neuroleptics are used in noncompliant patients or nonresponders to oral medication.

Antipsychotic drugs include the "typical" neuroleptics: **phenothiazines, thioxanthenes** (both similar in structure), **butyrophenones, dihydroindolones, dibenzoxazepines,** and **benzisoxazoles;** and the newer "atypical" neuroleptics: clozapine, risperidone, olanzapine, quetiapine, and ziprasidone (Table 25–4). Generally, increasing milligram potency of the typical neuroleptics is associated with decreasing anticholinergic and adrenergic side effects and increasing extrapyramidal symptoms (Table 25–5). For example, chlorpromazine has lower potency and more severe anticholinergic and adrenergic side effects. The in-

Table 25–4. Commonly used antipsychotics.

Drug	Usual Daily Oral Dose	Usual Daily Maximum Dose[1]	Cost per Unit	Cost for 30 Days' Treatment Based on Maximum Dosage[2]
Phenothiazines				
Chlorpromazine (Thorazine; others)	100–400 mg	1 g	$0.95/200 mg	$142.50
Thioridazine (Mellaril)	100–400 mg	600 mg	$0.95/200 mg	$85.50
Mesoridazine (Serentil)	50–200 mg	400 mg	$1.39/100 mg	$166.80
Perphenazine (Trilafon)[3]	16–32 mg	64 mg	$1.08/16 mg	$129.60
Trifluoperazine (Stelazine)	5–15 mg	60 mg	$1.52/10 mg	$273.60
Fluphenazine (Permitil, Prolixin)[3]	2–10 mg	60 mg	$1.15/10 mg	$207.00
Thioxanthenes				
Thiothixene (Navane)[3]	5–10 mg	80 mg	$0.65/10 mg	$156.00
Dihydroindolone				
Molindone (Moban)	30–100 mg	225 mg	$3.44/50 mg	$464.40
Dibenzoxazepine				
Loxapine (Loxitane)	20–60 mg	200 mg	$2.18/50 mg	$261.60
Dibenzodiazepine				
Clozapine (Clozaril)	300–450 mg	900 mg	$3.33/100 mg	$899.10
Butyrophenone				
Haloperidol (Haldol)	2–5 mg	60 mg	$1.16/20 mg	$104.40
Benzisoxazole				
Risperidone[4] (Risperdal)	2–6 mg	10 mg	$4.64/2 mg	$696.00
Thienbenzodiazepine				
Olanzapine (Zyprexa)	5–10 mg	10 mg	$10.50/10 mg	$315.10
Dibenzothiazepine				
Quetiapine (Seroquel)	200–400 mg	800 mg	$5.06/200 mg	$607.20

[1]Can be higher in some cases.
[2]Cost to pharmacist (average wholesale price, generic when possible) for quantity listed. Source: *Drug Topics Red Book,* March 2002; Vol. 21, No. 3.
[3]Indicates piperazine structure.
[4]For risperidone, daily doses above 6 mg increase the risk of extrapyramidal syndrome. Risperidone 6 mg is approximately equivalent to haloperidol 20 mg.

creased anticholinergic effect of chlorpromazine, however, lowers the risk of extrapyramidal symptoms.

The phenothiazines comprise the bulk of the currently used typical neuroleptic drugs. The only butyrophenone commonly used in psychiatry is haloperidol, which is totally different in structure but very similar in action and side effects to the piperazine phenothiazines such as fluphenazine, perphenazine, and trifluoperazine. These drugs and haloperidol (dopamine [D_2] receptor blockers) have high potency, a paucity of autonomic side effects, and act to markedly lower arousal levels. Molindone and loxapine, while less potent, are similar in action, side effects, and safety to the piperazine phenothiazines.

The first "atypical" (novel) antipsychotic drug developed, clozapine, a dibenzodiazepine derivative, has dopamine (D_4) receptor-blocking activity as well as central serotonergic, histaminergic, and alpha-noradrenergic receptor-blocking activity. It is effective in the treatment of about 30% of psychoses resistant to other neuroleptic drugs. It is associated with a 1% risk

of agranulocytosis, which requires weekly white blood cell count monitoring for the first 6 months followed by monitoring every other week. Weekly monitoring for 1 month after discontinuation of the medication is recommended. Risperidone is an antipsychotic that blocks some serotonin receptors (5-HT_2) and dopamine receptors (D_2). Risperidone causes fewer extrapyramidal side effects than the typical antipsychotics at doses less than 6 mg. It appears to be as effective as haloperidol and possibly as effective as clozapine in treatment-resistant patients without requiring weekly white cell counts. Risperidone-induced hyperprolactinemia, even on low doses, has been reported, and that effect is thought to be more common with risperidone than with other atypical antipsychotics.

Olanzapine is a potent blocker of muscarinic, anticholinergic, 5-HT_2, and dopamine D_1, D_2, and D_4 receptors. High doses of olanzapine (12.5–17.5 mg daily) appear to be more effective than lower doses. The drug appears to be more effective than haloperidol in the treatment of negative symptoms. It has,

Table 25–5. Relative potency and side effects of antipsychotics.

Drug	Chlorpromazine Potency Ratio	Anticholinergic Effects	Extrapyramidal Effects
Phenothiazines			
Chlorpromazine	1:1	4	1
Thioridazine	1:1	4	1
Mesoridazine	1:2	3	2
Perphenazine	1:10	2	3
Trifluoperazine	1:20	1	4
Fluphenazine	1:50	1	4
Thioxanthene			
Thiothixene	1:20	1	4
Dihydroindolone			
Molindone	1:10	2	3
Dibenzoxazepine			
Loxapine	1:10	2	3
Butyrophenone			
Haloperidol	1:50	1	4
Dibenzodiazepine			
Clozapine	1:1	4	—
Benzisoxazole			
Risperidone	1:50	1	1
Thienbenzodi-azepine			
Olanzapine	1:20	1	1
Dibenzothiazepine			
Quetiapine	1:1	1	—
Benzisothiazolyl piperazine			
Ziprasidone	1:1	1	1

Key: 4 = strong effect; 1 = weak effect

however, been associated with more elevated serum alanine aminotransferase than those taking haloperidol. It is associated with a much lower incidence of dystonic reaction than haloperidol and is perhaps less likely to induce tardive dyskinesia. Its most common side effects include somnolence, agitation, nervousness, headache, insomnia, dizziness, and significant weight gain. Multiple case reports have linked olanzapine and clozapine to new-onset type-2 diabetes. Further investigation to clarify the risk, risk factors, and pathophysiology is needed.

Quetiapine is a neuroleptic with greater 5-HT$_2$ relative to D$_2$ receptor blockade as well as a relatively high affinity for α_1- and α_2-adrenergic receptors. It appears to be as efficacious as haloperidol in treating positive and negative symptoms of schizophrenia, with less extrapyramidal side effects even at high doses. More common side effects include somnolence, dizziness, and postural hypotension. Because of an association with lens changes seen in patients on long-term treatment, an eye examination to detect cataract for-

mation is recommended at initiation of treatment and then at 6-month intervals during treatment.

Ziprasidone, the newest atypical neuroleptic available in the United States, has both anti-dopamine receptor and anti-serotonin receptor antagonist effects, with good efficacy for both positive and negative symptoms of schizophrenia. Ziprasidone is not associated with significant weight gain, hyperlipidemia, or new-onset diabetes and offers a good alternative for some patients. It has been implicated in QTc interval delay of > 500 ms in some patients, though in several cases of overdose there were no incidents of torsade de pointes or sudden death. Patients taking ziprasidone should be screened for cardiac risk factors. A pretreatment ECG is indicated for patients at risk of cardiac sequelae (including patients taking other medications that might prolong the QTc interval).

None of the antipsychotics produce true physical dependency, and they have wide safety margins between therapeutic and toxic effects. All decrease adrenergic responses. Despite higher costs, atypical neuroleptics are often considered preferable to traditional antipsychotics because they are thought to be associated with reduced extrapyramidal symptoms and a lesser risk of tardive dyskinesia.

Clinical Indications

The antipsychotics are used to treat all forms of the schizophrenias as well as psychotic ideation in organic brain psychoses, delirium and dementia, drug-induced psychoses, psychotic depression, and mania. They are also effective in Tourette's disorder. They quickly lower the arousal (activity) level and, perhaps indirectly, gradually improve socialization and thinking. The improvement rate is about 80%. Patients whose behavioral symptoms worsen with use of antipsychotic drugs may have an undiagnosed organic condition such as anticholinergic toxicity.

Symptoms that are ameliorated by these drugs include hyperactivity, hostility, aggression, delusions, hallucinations, irritability, and poor sleep. Individuals with acute psychosis and good premorbid function respond quite well. The most common cause of failure in the treatment of acute psychosis is inadequate dosage, and the most common cause of relapse is noncompliance.

Though typical antipsychotics are efficacious in the treatment of so-called positive symptoms of schizophrenia such as hallucinations and delusions, atypical antipsychotics are thought to have efficacy in reducing both positive symptoms and negative symptoms such as withdrawal, psychomotor retardation, and poor interpersonal relationships. Antidepressant drugs may be used in conjunction with neuroleptics if significant depression is present. Resistant cases may require concomitant use of lithium, carbamazepine, or valproic acid. The addition of a benzodiazepine drug to the neuroleptic regimen may prove helpful in treating the agitated or catatonic psychotic patient who has not responded to neuroleptics alone—lorazepam, 1–2 mg orally, can produce a rapid resolution of catatonic symptoms and may allow maintenance with a lower neuroleptic dose. ECT has also been effective in treating catatonia.

Dosage Forms & Patterns

The dosage range is quite broad. For example, risperidone, 0.5–1 mg orally at bedtime, may be sufficient for the elderly person with mild dementia, whereas up to 6 mg/d may be used in a young patient with acute schizophrenia. For quick response, one may start with an atypical antipsychotic in combination with a benzodiazepine (eg, risperidone oral solution, 2 mg, or olanzapine, 10 mg orally, and lorazepam, 2 mg orally, every 2–4 hours as needed). In an acutely distressed, psychotic patient one might use haloperidol, 10 mg intramuscularly, which is absorbed rapidly and achieves an initial tenfold plasma level advantage over equal oral doses. Psychomotor agitation, racing thoughts, and general arousal are quickly reduced. The dose can be repeated every 3–4 hours; when the patient is less symptomatic, oral doses can replace parenteral administration in most cases.

Various factors play a role in the absorption of oral medications. Of particular importance are previous gastrointestinal surgery and concomitant administration of other drugs. There are racial differences in metabolizing the neuroleptic drugs—eg, many Asians require only about half the usual dosage. Bioavailability is influenced by other factors such as smoking or hepatic microsomal enzyme stimulation with alcohol or barbiturates and enzyme-altering drugs such as carbamazepine or methylphenidate. Neuroleptic plasma drug level determinations are not currently of major clinical assistance.

Divided daily doses are not necessary after a maintenance dose has been established, and most patients can then be maintained on a single daily dose, usually taken at bedtime. This is particularly appropriate in a case where the sedative effect of the drug is desired for nighttime sleep, and undesirable sedative effects can be avoided during the day. Risperidone is an exception, being given twice daily. First-episode patients especially should be tapered off medications after about 6 months of stability and carefully monitored; their rate of relapse is lower than that of multiple-episode patients.

Psychiatric patients—particularly paranoid individuals—often neglect to take their medication. In these cases and in nonresponders to oral medication, the enanthate and decanoate (the latter is slightly longer-lasting and has fewer extrapyramidal side effects) forms of fluphenazine or the decanoate form of haloperidol may be given by deep subcutaneous injection or intramuscularly to achieve an effect that will usually last 7–28 days. A patient who cannot be depended on to take oral medication (or who overdoses on minimal provocation) will generally agree to come to the clinician's office for a "shot." The usual dose of the fluphenazine long-acting preparations is 25 mg every 2 weeks. Dosage and frequency of administration vary from about 100 mg weekly to 12.5 mg monthly. Use the smallest effective amount as infrequently as possible. A monthly injection of 25 mg of fluphenazine decanoate is equivalent to about 15–20 mg of oral fluphenazine daily. Concomitant use of a benzodiazepine (eg, lorazepam, 2 mg orally twice daily) may permit reduction of the required dosage of oral or parenteral antipsychotic drug.

Intravenous haloperidol, the neuroleptic most commonly used by this route, is often used in critical care units in the management of agitated, delirious patients. Intravenous haloperidol should be given no faster than 1 mg/min to reduce cardiovascular side effects, such as torsades de pointes, and is associated with a lower risk of extrapyramidal side effects.

Side Effects

For both typical and atypical neuroleptic agents, a range of side effects are reported. The most common anticholinergic side effects include dry mouth (which can lead to ingestion of caloric liquids and weight gain or hyponatremia), blurred near vision, urinary retention (particularly in elderly men with enlarged prostates), delayed gastric emptying, esophageal reflux, ileus, delirium, and precipitation of acute glaucoma in patients with narrow anterior chamber angles. Other autonomic effects include orthostatic hypotension and sexual dysfunction—problems in achieving erection, ejaculation (including retrograde ejaculation), and orgasm in men (approximately 50% of cases) and women (approximately 30%). Delay in achieving orgasm is often a factor in medication noncompliance. Electrocardiographic changes occur frequently, but clinically significant arrhythmias are much less common. Elderly patients and those with preexisting cardiac disease are at greater risk. The most frequently seen electrocardiographic changes include diminution of the T wave amplitude, appearance of prominent U waves, depression of the ST segment, and prolongation of the QT interval. Thioridazine has been given an FDA warning for dose-related QTc delay and risk of fatal cardiac arrhythmias. As noted above, ziprasidone can produce QTc prolongation. An ECG prior to treatment in some patients may be indicated. In some critical care patients, torsade de pointes has been associated with the use of high-dose intravenous haloperidol (usually > 30 mg/24 h).

Associations have been suggested between the atypical neuroleptics and new-onset diabetes, hyperlipidemia, QTc prolongation, and weight gain (Table 25–6). Neuroleptic medications in general may have metabolic and endocrine effects, including weight gain, hyperglycemia, infrequent temperature irregularities (particularly in hot weather), and water intoxication, that may be due to inappropriate antidiuretic hormone secretion. Lactation and menstrual irregularities are common (antipsychotic drugs should be avoided, if possible, in breast cancer patients because of potential trophic effects of elevated prolactin levels on the breast). Both antipsychotic and antidepressant drugs inhibit sperm motility. Bone marrow depression and cholestatic jaundice occur rarely; these are hypersensitivity reactions, and they usually appear in the first 2 months of treatment. They subside on discontinuance of the drug. There is cross-sensitivity among all of the phenothiazines, and a drug from a different group should be used when allergic reactions occur.

Clozapine is associated with a 1.6% risk of **agranulocytosis** (higher in persons of Ashkenazi Jewish ancestry), and its use must be strictly monitored with weekly blood counts during the first 6 months of treatment, with monitoring every other week monitoring thereafter. Discontinuation of the medication requires weekly monitoring of the white blood cell count for 1 month. Clozapine lowers the seizure threshold and has many side effects, including sedation, hypotension, increased liver enzyme levels, hypersalivation, respiratory arrest, weight gain, and changes in both the ECG and the EEG.

Photosensitivity, retinopathy, and hyperpigmentation are associated with use of fairly high dosages of chlorpromazine and thioridazine. The appearance of particulate melanin deposits in the lens of the eye is related to the total dose given, and patients on long-term medication should have periodic eye examinations. Teratogenicity has not been causally related to these drugs, but prudence is indicated particularly in the first trimester of pregnancy. The seizure threshold is lowered, but it is safe to use these medications in epileptics controlled by anticonvulsants.

The **neuroleptic malignant syndrome (NMS)** is a catatonia-like state manifested by extrapyramidal signs, blood pressure changes, altered consciousness, and hyperpyrexia; it is an uncommon but serious complication of neuroleptic treatment. Muscle rigidity, involun-

Table 25–6. Adverse factors associated with atypical antipsychotics.[1]

	Weight Gain	Hyperlipidemia	New–Onset Diabetes	QTc Prolongation[2]
Clozapine	++++	+++	++	+/–
Olanzapine	++++	++	+++	+/–
Risperidone	++	–	–	+
Quetiapine	+/–	++	no data	++
Ziprasidone	–	–	no data	+++

[1]Compiled with assistance from Luriko Ajari, PharmD, BCPP, Pharmacy Director, Langley Porter Psychiatric Institute, University of California, San Francisco.
[2]QTc prolongation is a side effect of many medications and suggests a possible risk for arrhythmia. Among atypical neuroleptics, only ziprasidone carries a special warning regarding the risk of QTc prolongation.

tary movements, confusion, dysarthria, and dysphagia are accompanied by pallor, cardiovascular instability, fever, pulmonary congestion, and diaphoresis and may result in stupor, coma, and death. The cause may be related to a number of factors, including poor dosage control of neuroleptic medication, affective illness, decreased serum iron, dehydration, and increased sensitivity of dopamine receptor sites. Lithium in combination with a neuroleptic drug may increase vulnerability, which is already increased in patients with an affective disorder. In most cases, the symptoms develop within the first 2 weeks of antipsychotic drug treatment. The syndrome may occur with small doses of the drugs. Intramuscular administration is a risk factor. Elevated creatine kinase and leukocytosis with a shift to the left are present early in about half of cases. Treatment includes controlling fever and providing fluid support. Dopamine agonists such as bromocriptine, 2.5–10 mg orally three times a day, and amantadine, 100–200 mg orally twice a day, have also been useful. Dantrolene, 50 mg intravenously as needed, is used to alleviate rigidity (do not exceed 10 mg/kg/d). There is ongoing controversy about the efficacy of these three agents as well as the use of calcium channel blockers and benzodiazepines. Electroconvulsive therapy has been used effectively in resistant cases. Clozapine has been used with relative safety and fair success as an antipsychotic drug for patients who have had NMS. The syndrome must be differentiated from acute lethal catatonia, malignant hyperthermia, neurotoxic syndromes (including AIDS), and a variety of other conditions such as viral encephalitis, Wilson's disease, central anticholinergic syndrome, and hypertonic states (eg, tetany, strychnine poisoning).

Akathisia is the most common (about 20%) so-called **extrapyramidal symptom.** It usually occurs early in treatment (but may persist after neuroleptics are discontinued) and is frequently mistaken for anxiety or exacerbation of psychosis. It is characterized by a subjective desire to be in constant motion followed by an inability to sit or stand still and consequent pacing. It may include suicidality or feelings of fright, rage, terror, or sexual torment. Insomnia is often present. In all cases, reevaluate the dosage requirement or the type of neuroleptic drug. One should inquire also about cigarette smoking, which in women has been associated with an increased incidence of akathisia. Antiparkinsonism drugs such as trihexyphenidyl, 2–5 mg orally three times daily, or benztropine mesylate, 1–2 mg twice daily, may be helpful. In resistant cases, symptoms may be alleviated by propranolol, 30–80 mg/d orally; diazepam, 5 mg three times daily; or amantadine, 100 mg orally three times daily.

Acute dystonias usually occur early, though a late (tardive) occurrence is reported in patients (mostly men after several years of therapy) who previously had early severe dystonic reactions and a mood disorder (see below). Younger patients are at higher risk for acute dystonias. The most common signs are bizarre muscle spasms of the head, neck, and tongue. Fre-

quently present are torticollis, oculogyric crises, swallowing or chewing difficulties, and masseter spasms. Laryngospasm is particularly dangerous. Back, arm, or leg muscle spasms are occasionally reported. Diphenhydramine, 50 mg intramuscularly, is effective for the acute crisis; one should then give benztropine mesylate, 2 mg orally twice daily, for several weeks, and then discontinue gradually, since few of the extrapyramidal symptoms require long-term use of the antiparkinsonism drugs (all of which are about equally efficacious—though trihexyphenidyl tends to be mildly stimulating and benztropine mildly sedating).

Drug-induced parkinsonism is indistinguishable from idiopathic parkinsonism, but it is reversible, occurs later in treatment than the preceding extrapyramidal symptoms, and in some cases appears after neuroleptic withdrawal. The condition includes the typical signs of apathy and reduction of facial and arm movements (akinesia, which can mimic depression), festinating gait, rigidity, loss of postural reflexes, and pill-rolling tremor. AIDS patients seem particularly vulnerable to extrapyramidal side effects. High-potency neuroleptics often require antiparkinsonism drugs (Table 24–5). The neuroleptic dosage should be reduced, and immediate relief can be achieved with antiparkinsonism drugs in the same dosages as above. After 4–6 weeks, these antiparkinsonism drugs can often be discontinued with no recurrent symptoms. In any of the extrapyramidal symptoms, amantadine, 100–400 mg daily, may be used instead of the antiparkinsonism drugs. Neuroleptic-induced catatonia is similar to catatonic stupor with rigidity, drooling, urinary incontinence, and cogwheeling. It usually responds slowly to withdrawal of the offending medication and use of antiparkinsonism agents.

Tardive dyskinesia is a syndrome of abnormal involuntary stereotyped movements of the face, mouth, tongue, trunk, and limbs that may occur after months or (usually) years of treatment with neuroleptic agents. The syndrome affects 20–35% of patients who have undergone long-term neuroleptic therapy. Predisposing factors include older age, many years of treatment, cigarette smoking, and diabetes mellitus. Pineal calcification is higher in this condition by a margin of 3:1. There are no known differences among any of the antipsychotic drugs in the development of this syndrome, though the atypical antipsychotics appear to offer lower risk.

Early manifestations include fine worm-like movements of the tongue at rest, difficulty in sticking out the tongue, facial tics, increased blink frequency, or jaw movements of recent onset. Later manifestations may include bucco-linguo-masticatory movements, lip smacking, chewing motions, mouth opening and closing, disturbed gag reflex, puffing of the cheeks, disrupted speech, respiratory distress, or choreoathetoid movements of the extremities (the last being more prevalent in younger patients). The symptoms do not necessarily worsen and in rare cases may lessen even though neuroleptic drugs are continued. The dyskinesias do not occur during sleep and can be voluntarily suppressed for short periods. Stress and movements in other parts of the body will often aggravate the condition.

Early signs of dyskinesia must be differentiated from those reversible signs produced by ill-fitting dentures or nonneuroleptic drugs such as levodopa, tricyclic antidepressants (TCAs), antiparkinsonism agents, anticonvulsants, and antihistamines. Other neurologic conditions such as Huntington's chorea can be differentiated by history and examination.

The emphasis should be on prevention. Use the least amount of neuroleptic drug necessary to mute the psychotic symptoms. Detect early manifestations of dyskinesias. When these occur, stop anticholinergic drugs and gradually discontinue neuroleptic drugs. Weight loss and cachexia sometimes appear on withdrawal of neuroleptics. In an indeterminate number of cases, the dyskinesias will remit. Keep the patient off the drugs until reemergent psychotic symptoms dictate their resumption, at which point they are restarted in low doses and gradually increased until there is clinical improvement. If neuroleptic drugs are restarted, clozapine and olanzapine appear to offer less risk of recurrence. The use of adjunctive agents such as benzodiazepines or lithium may help directly or indirectly by allowing control of psychotic symptoms with a low dosage of neuroleptics. If the dyskinesic syndrome recurs and it is necessary to continue neuroleptic drugs to control psychotic symptoms, informed consent should be obtained. Benzodiazepines, buspirone (in doses of 15–60 mg/d), phosphatidylcholine, clonidine, calcium channel blockers, vitamin E, and propranolol all have had limited usefulness in treating the dyskinetic side effects.

B. SOCIAL

Environmental considerations are most important in the individual with a chronic illness, who usually has a history of repeated hospitalizations, a continued low level of functioning, and symptoms that never completely remit. Family rejection and work failure are common. In these cases, board and care homes staffed by personnel experienced in caring for psychiatric patients are most important. There is frequently an inverse relationship between stability of the living situation and the amounts of required antipsychotic drugs, since the most salutary environment is one that reduces stimuli. Nonresidential self-help groups such as Recovery, Inc., should be utilized whenever possible. They provide a setting for sharing, learning, and mutual support and are frequently the only social involvement with which this type of patient is comfortable. Vocational rehabilitation and work agencies (eg, Goodwill Industries, Inc.) provide assessment, training, and job opportunities at a level commensurate with the person's clinical condition.

C. PSYCHOLOGIC

The need for psychotherapy varies markedly depending on the patient's current status and history. In a person with a single psychotic episode and a previously good level of adjustment, supportive psychotherapy may help the patient reintegrate the experience, gain some insight into antecedent problems, and become a more self-observant individual who can recognize early signs of stress. Insight-oriented psychotherapy is often counterproductive in this type of disorder. Early research suggests that cognitive behavioral therapy—in conjunction with medication management, may have some efficacy in the treatment of symptoms of schizophrenia. Family therapy should be given concomitantly to help alleviate the patient's stress and to assist relatives in coping with the patient.

D. BEHAVIORAL

Behavioral techniques (see above) are most frequently used in therapeutic settings such as day treatment centers, but there is no reason why they cannot be incorporated into family situations or any therapeutic setting. Many behavioral techniques are used unwittingly (eg, positive reinforcement—whether it be a word of praise or an approving nod—after some positive behavior), and with some careful thought this approach can be a powerful instrument for helping a person learn behaviors that will facilitate social acceptance. Music from portable cassette players with earphones is one of many ways to divert the patient's attention from auditory hallucinations.

Prognosis

In any psychosis in the large majority of patients, the prognosis is excellent for alleviation of positive symptoms such as hallucinations or delusions treated with medication. Negative symptoms such as diminished affect and sociability are much more difficult to treat but appear responsive to atypical antipsychotics. Unavailability of structured work situations and lack of family therapy are two other reasons why the prognosis is so guarded in such a large percentage of schizophrenic patients. Psychosis connected with a history of serious drug abuse has a guarded prognosis because of the central nervous system damage, usually from the drugs themselves and associated medical illnesses.

Andersson C et al: Emerging roles for novel antipsychotic medications in the treatment of schizophrenia. Psychiatr Clin North Am 1998;21:151. [PMID: 9551495] (Superior efficacy and more benign side effect profile of atypical antipsychotics provide a rationale for their use as first-line treatment.)

Eisendrath SJ, Chamberlain J: Psychiatry in the critical care unit. In: *Current Diagnosis and Treatment in Critical Care,* 2nd ed. Bongard FS, Sue DY (editors). Appleton & Lange, 2002.

Glassman AH et al: Antipsychotic drugs: prolonged QTc interval, torsade de pointes, and sudden death. Am J Psychiatry 2001;158:1774. [PMID: 11691681]

Rector NA et al: Cognitive behavioral therapy for schizophrenia: an empirical review. J Nerv Ment Dis 2001;189:278. [PMID: 11379970]

MOOD DISORDERS
(Depression & Mania)

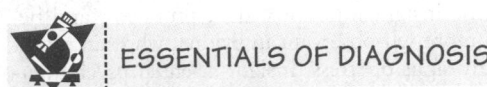 ESSENTIALS OF DIAGNOSIS

Present in most depressions:

- *Lowered mood, varying from mild sadness to intense feelings of guilt, worthlessness, and hopelessness.*
- *Difficulty in thinking, including inability to concentrate, ruminations, and lack of decisiveness.*
- *Loss of interest, with diminished involvement in work and recreation.*
- *Somatic complaints such as headache; disrupted, lessened, or excessive sleep; loss of energy; change in appetite; decreased sexual drive.*
- *Anxiety.*

Present in some severe depressions:

- *Psychomotor retardation or agitation.*
- *Delusions of a hypochondriacal or persecutory nature.*
- *Withdrawal from activities.*
- *Physical symptoms of major severity, eg, anorexia, insomnia, reduced sexual drive, weight loss, and various somatic complaints.*
- *Suicidal ideation.*

Present in mania:

- *Mood ranging from euphoria to irritability.*
- *Sleep disruption.*
- *Hyperactivity.*
- *Racing thoughts.*
- *Grandiosity.*
- *Variable psychotic symptoms.*

General Considerations

Depression is extremely common, with up to 30% of primary care patients having depressive symptoms. Depression may be the final expression of (1) genetic factors (neurotransmitter dysfunction), (2) developmental problems (personality defects, childhood events), or (3) psychosocial stresses (divorce, unemployment). It frequently presents in the form of somatic complaints with negative medical workups. Although sadness and grief are normal responses to loss, depression is not. Patients experiencing normal grief tend to produce sympathy and sadness in the clinician caregiver; depression often produces frustration and irritation in the clinician. Grief is usually accompanied by intact self-esteem, whereas depression is marked by a sense of guilt and worthlessness.

Mania is often combined with depression and may occur alone, together with mania in a mixed episode, or in cyclic fashion with depression.

Clinical Findings

In general, there are four major types of depressions, with similar symptoms in each group.

A. Adjustment Disorder With Depressed Mood

Depression may occur in reaction to some identifiable stressor or adverse life situation, usually loss of a person by death (grief reaction), divorce, etc; financial reversal (crisis); or loss of an established role, such as being needed. Anger is frequently associated with the loss, and this in turn often produces a feeling of guilt. The disorder occurs within 3 months of the stressor and causes significant impairment in social or occupational functioning. The symptoms range from mild sadness, anxiety, irritability, worry, lack of concentration, discouragement, and somatic complaints to the more severe symptoms of the next group.

B. Depressive Disorders

The subclassifications include major depressive disorder and dysthymia.

1. Major depressive disorder—A major depressive disorder (eg, "endogenous" unipolar disorder, melancholia) consists of at least one episode of serious mood depression that occurs at any time of life. Many consider a physiologic or metabolic aberration to be causative. Complaints vary widely but most frequently include a loss of interest and pleasure (anhedonia), withdrawal from activities, and feelings of guilt. Also included are inability to concentrate, some cognitive dysfunction, anxiety, chronic fatigue, feelings of worthlessness, somatic complaints (unidentifiable somatic complaints frequently indicate depression), loss of sexual drive, and thoughts of death. Diurnal variation with improvement as the day progresses is common. Vegetative signs that frequently occur are insomnia, anorexia with weight loss, and constipation. Occasionally, severe agitation and psychotic ideation (paranoid thinking, somatic delusions) are present. These symptoms are more common in postmenopausal depression (involutional melancholia). Paranoid symptoms may range from general suspiciousness to ideas of reference with delusions. The somatic delusions frequently revolve around feelings of impending annihilation or hypochondriacal beliefs (eg, that the body is rotting away with cancer). Hallucinations are uncommon.

Subcategories include **major depression with atypical features** characterized by hypersomnia, overeating, lethargy, and rejection sensitivity. **Major depression with a seasonal onset (seasonal affective disorder)** is a dysfunction of circadian rhythms that occurs more commonly in the winter months and is believed to be due to decreased exposure to full-spectrum light. Common symptoms include carbohydrate craving, lethargy, hyperphagia, and hypersomnia. **Major depression with postpartum onset** usually occurs 2 weeks to 6 months postpartum.

Most women (up to 80%) experience some mild letdown of mood in the postpartum period. For some of these (10–15%), the symptoms are more severe and similar to those usually seen in serious depression, with an increased emphasis on concerns related to the baby (obsessive thoughts about harming it or inability to care for it). When psychotic symptoms occur, there is frequently associated sleep deprivation, volatility of behavior, and manic-like symptoms. Postpartum psychosis is much less common (< 2%), often occurs within the first 2 weeks, and requires early and aggressive management. Biologic vulnerability with hormonal changes and psychosocial stressors all play a role. The chances of a second episode are about 25% and may be reduced with prophylactic treatment.

2. Dysthymia—Dysthymia is a chronic depressive disturbance. Sadness, loss of interest, and withdrawal from activities over a period of 2 or more years with a relatively persistent course is necessary for this diagnosis. Generally, the symptoms are milder but longer-lasting than those in a major depressive episode.

3. Premenstrual dysphoric disorder—Depressive symptoms during the late luteal phase of the menstrual cycles may occur throughout the year.

C. BIPOLAR DISORDERS

Bipolar disorders consist of episodic mood shifts into mania, major depression, hypomania, and mixed mood states. The ability of bipolar disorder to mimic aspects of many other Axis I disorders and a high comorbidity with substance abuse can make the initial diagnosis of bipolar disorder difficult.

1. Mania—A manic episode is a mood change characterized by elation with hyperactivity, overinvolvement in life activities, increased irritability, flight of ideas, easy distractibility, and little need for sleep. The overenthusiastic quality of the mood and the expansive behavior initially attract others, but the irritability, mood lability with swings into depression, aggressive behavior, and grandiosity usually lead to marked interpersonal difficulties. Activities may occur that are later regretted, eg, excessive spending, resignation from a job, a hasty marriage, sexual acting out, and exhibitionistic behavior, with alienation of friends and family. Atypical manic episodes can include gross delusions, paranoid ideation of severe proportions, and auditory hallucinations usually related to some grandiose perception. The episodes begin abruptly (sometimes precipitated by life stresses) and may last from several days to months. Spring and summer tend to be the peak periods. Generally, the manic episodes are of shorter duration than the depressive episodes. In almost all cases, the manic episode is part of a broader bipolar (manic-depressive) disorder. Patients with four or more discrete episodes of

a mood disturbance in 1 year are called "rapid cyclers." (Substance abuse, particularly cocaine, can mimic rapid cycling.) These patients have a higher incidence of hypothyroidism. Manic patients differ from schizophrenics in that the former use more effective interpersonal maneuvers, are more sensitive to the social maneuvers of others, and are more able to utilize weakness and vulnerability in others to their own advantage. Creativity has been positively correlated with mood disorders, but the best work done is between episodes of mania and depression.

2. Cyclothymic disorders—These are chronic mood disturbances with episodes of depression and hypomania. The symptoms must have at least a 2-year duration and are milder than those that occur in depressive or manic episodes. Occasionally, the symptoms will escalate into a full-blown manic or depressive episode, in which case reclassification as bipolar I or bipolar II disorder would be warranted.

D. MOOD DISORDERS SECONDARY TO ILLNESS AND DRUGS

Any illness, severe or mild, can cause significant depression. Conditions such as rheumatoid arthritis, multiple sclerosis, and chronic heart disease are particularly likely to be associated with depression, as are other chronic illnesses. Hormonal variations clearly play a role in some depressions. Varying degrees of depression occur at various times in schizophrenic disorders, central nervous system disease, and organic mental states. **Alcohol dependency** frequently coexists with serious depression.

The classic model of drug-induced depression occurs with the use of reserpine, both in a clinical and a neurochemical sense. Corticosteroids and oral contraceptives are commonly associated with affective changes. Antihypertensive medications such as methyldopa, guanethidine, and clonidine have been associated with the development of depressive syndromes, as have digitalis and antiparkinsonism drugs (eg, levodopa). It is unusual for beta-blockers to produce depression when given for short periods, such as in the treatment of performance anxiety. Sustained use of beta-blockers for medical conditions such as hypertension may produce depression in some patients, though the literature is unclear on this subject. It is also unclear whether non-lipid-soluble beta-blockers are less likely to be associated with depression than lipid-soluble ones. Infrequently, disulfiram and anticholinesterase drugs may be associated with symptoms of depression. All stimulant use results in a depressive syndrome when the drug is withdrawn. Alcohol, sedatives, opiates, and most of the psychedelic drugs are depressants and, paradoxically, are often used in self-treatment of depression.

Differential Diagnosis

Since depression may be a part of any illness—either reactively or as a secondary symptom—careful attention must be given to personal life adjustment problems and the role of medications (eg, reserpine, corticosteroids, levodopa). Schizophrenia, partial complex seizures, organic brain syndromes, panic disorders, and anxiety disorders must be differentiated. Subtle thyroid dysfunction must be ruled out.

Complications

The longer the depression continues, the more crystallized it becomes—particularly when there is an element of secondary reinforcement. The most important complication is suicide, which often includes some elements of aggression. Suicide rates in the general population vary from 9 per 100,000 in Spain to 20 per 100,000 in the USA to 58 per 100,000 in Hungary. In individuals with depression, the lifetime risk rises to 10–15%. Men tend toward successful suicide, particularly in older age groups, whereas women make more attempts with lower mortality rates. An increased suicide rate is being observed in the younger population, ages 15–35. Patients with cancer, respiratory illnesses, AIDS, and those being maintained on hemodialysis have higher suicide rates. Alcohol is a significant factor in many suicide attempts.

There are four major groups of people who make suicide attempts:

(1) Those who are overwhelmed by problems in living (the despair of ordinary people). By far the greatest number fall into this category. There is often great ambivalence; they don't really want to die, but they don't want to go on as before either. These may be impulsive or aggressive acts not associated with significant depression.

(2) Those who are clearly attempting to control others. This is the blatant attempt in the vicinity of a significant other person in order to hurt or control that person.

(3) Those with severe depressions (high-risk group). This group includes both exogenous conditions (eg, AIDS, whose victims have a suicide rate over 30 times that of the general population) and endogenous conditions (eg, panic disorders). It also includes those who may not be diagnosed as having depression but who are overwhelmed by a serious stressful situation (eg, the man charged with child molestation who hangs himself in his cell). Anxiety, panic, and fear are major findings in suicidal behavior. A patient may seem to make a dramatic improvement, but the lifting of depression may be due to the patient's decision to commit suicide.

(4) Those with psychotic illness (high-risk group). These individuals tend not to verbalize their concerns, are unpredictable, and are often successful but comprise a small percentage of the total. (Suicide is ten times more prevalent in schizophrenics than in the general population, and jumping from bridges is more common. In one study of 100 jumpers, 47% were schizophrenic.)

The immediate goal of psychiatric evaluation is to assess the current suicidal risk and the need for hospitalization versus outpatient management. The intent is less likely to be truly suicidal, for example, if small amounts of poison or drugs were ingested or scratching of wrists was superficial; if the act was performed in the vicinity of others or with early notification of others; or if the attempt was arranged so that early detection would be anticipated. Alcohol, hopelessness, delusional thoughts, and complete or nearly complete loss of interest in life or ability to experience pleasure are all positively correlated with suicide attempts. Other risk factors are previous attempts, a family history of suicide, medical or psychiatric illness (eg, anxiety, depression, psychosis), male sex, older age, contemplation of violent methods, a humiliating social stressor, and drug use (including long-term sedative or alcohol use), which contributes to impulsiveness or mood swings. Successful treatment of the patient at risk for suicide cannot be achieved if the patient continues to abuse drugs.

The patient's current mood status is best evaluated by direct evaluation of plans and concerns about the future, personal reactions to the attempt, and thoughts about the reactions of others. The patient's immediate resources should be assessed—people who can be significantly involved (most important), family support, job situation, financial resources, etc.

If hospitalization is not indicated (eg, gestures, impulsive attempts; see above), the clinician must formulate and institute a treatment plan or make an adequate referral. Medication should be dispensed in small amounts to at-risk patients. Although tricyclics and SSRIs are associated with an equal incidence of suicide attempts, the risk of successful suicide is higher with tricyclic overdose. Guns and drugs should be removed from the patient's household. Driving should be interdicted until the patient improves. The problem is often worsened by the long-term complications of the suicide attempt, eg, brain damage due to hypoxia; peripheral neuropathies caused by staying for long periods in one position, causing nerve compressions; and medical or surgical problems such as esophageal strictures and tendon dysfunctions.

The reasons for self-mutilation, most commonly wrist cutting (but also autocastration, autoamputation, and autoenucleation, which are associated with psychoses), may be very different from the reasons for a suicide attempt. The initial treatment plan, however, should presume suicidal ideation, and conservative treatment should be initiated.

Sleep disturbances in the depressions are discussed below.

Treatment of Depression

A. MEDICAL

Depression associated with reactive disorders usually does not call for drug therapy and can be managed by psychotherapy and the passage of time. In severe cases—particularly when vegetative signs are significant and symptoms have persisted for more than a few weeks—antidepressant drug therapy is often effective. Drug therapy is also suggested by a family history of major depression in first-degree relatives or a past history of prior episodes.

The antidepressant drugs may be conveniently classified into three groups: (1) the newer antidepressants, including the serotonin-selective reuptake inhibitors (SSRIs) and bupropion, venlafaxine, nefazodone, and mirtazapine; (2) the tricyclic antidepressants (TCAs) and clinically similar drugs; and (3) the monoamine oxidase (MAO) inhibitors. These groups are described in greater detail below. Electroconvulsive therapy is effective in all types of depression (particularly involutional melancholia) and will also rapidly resolve a manic episode. It is also very effective for postpartum depression. Megavitamin treatment, acupuncture, and electrosleep are of unproved usefulness for any psychiatric condition.

Hospitalization is necessary if suicide is a major consideration or if complex treatment modalities are required.

Drug selection is influenced by the history of previous responses if that information is available. If a relative has responded to a particular drug, this suggests that the patient may respond similarly. If no background information is available, a drug such as desipramine, starting with 50 mg and gradually increasing to 150 mg daily, or sertraline, 50 mg daily, can be selected and a *full trial* instituted. The medication trial should be monitored every 1–2 weeks until week 6. If successful, the medication should be continued for 6–12 months at the full therapeutic dose before tapering is considered. Antidepressants should be continued indefinitely at full dosage in individuals with more than two episodes after age 40 or one episode after age 50. If the response is inadequate despite a diagnosis supported by review and adequate drug levels, a drug from a different group (eg, fluoxetine) should be substituted and given a trial. If the second drug fails, augmentation with lithium (eg, 600–900 mg/d) or thyroid medication (eg, liothyronine, 25 μg/d) should be considered. Dysthymia is also treated in this way. The Agency for Health Care Policy and Research has produced clinical practice guidelines that outline one algorithm of treatment decisions (Figure 25–3).

Psychotic depression can be treated with a combination of an antipsychotic such as perphenazine (used initially) and an antidepressant such as an SSRI at their usual doses.

Major depression with atypical features or seasonal onset can be treated with an MAO inhibitor or an SSRI with good results.

Stimulants such as dextroamphetamine (5–30 mg/d) and methylphenidate (10–45 mg/d) have enjoyed a resurgence of interest for the short-term treatment of depression in medically ill and geriatric patients. Their 50–60% efficacy rate is slightly below that of other agents. The stimulants are notable for rapid onset of action (hours) and a paucity of side effects (tachycardia, agitation) in most patients. They are usually given in two divided doses early in the day (eg, 7 AM and noon) so as to avoid interfering with sleep. These agents may also be useful as adjunctive agents in refractory depression.

Caution: Depressed patients may have suicidal thoughts, and the amount of drug dispensed should be appropriately controlled. The older tricyclics have a narrow therapeutic index, and one advantage of the newer drugs is their wider margin of safety. In all cases of pharmacologic management of depressed states, caution is indicated until the risk of suicide is considered minimal.

1. SSRIs and atypical antidepressants—The chief advantages of these agents are that they do not generally cause significant cardiovascular or anticholinergic side effects, as do the tricyclic agents. The serotonin selective reuptake inhibitors (SSRIs) include fluoxetine, sertraline, paroxetine, fluvoxamine, and citalopram. The atypical antidepressants are bupropion, which appears to exert its effect through the dopamine neurotransmitter system; venlafaxine, which inhibits the reuptake of both serotonin and norepinephrine; nefazodone, which blocks the reuptake of serotonin but also inhibits the $5-HT_2$ postsynaptic receptors; and mirtazapine, which selectively blocks presynaptic α_2-adrenergic receptors and enhances both noradrenergic and serotonergic transmission. All of these antidepressants are effective in the treatment of depression, both typical and atypical. The SSRI drugs have been effective in the treatment of panic attacks, bulimia, and obsessive-compulsive disorders, while bupropion may have some particular effectiveness in the treatment of rapid-cycling bipolar disorder. They do not seem to be as clearly effective in some pain syndromes as the tricyclics, though venlafaxine may have some efficacy in the treatment of neuropathic pain.

Most of the drugs in this group tend to be activating and are given in the morning so as not to interfere with sleep. Some patients, however, may have sedation, requiring that the drug be given at bedtime. This reaction occurs most commonly with paroxetine, fluvoxamine, and mirtazapine. The SSRIs can be given in once-daily dosage. Bupropion is usually given in two divided doses daily. Nefazodone and venlafaxine are usually given twice daily. Bupropion and venlafaxine are available in extended-release formulations. There is usually some delay in response; fluoxetine, for example, requires 2–6 weeks to act in depression, 4–8 weeks to be effective in panic disorder, and 6–12 weeks in treatment of obsessive-compulsive disorder. The starting dose (10–20 mg) is the usual daily dose for depression, while obsessive-compulsive disorder may require up to 80 mg daily. Some patients, particularly the elderly, may tolerate and benefit from as little as 10 mg/d or every other day. The other SSRIs (sertraline, paroxetine, and fluvoxamine) have shorter

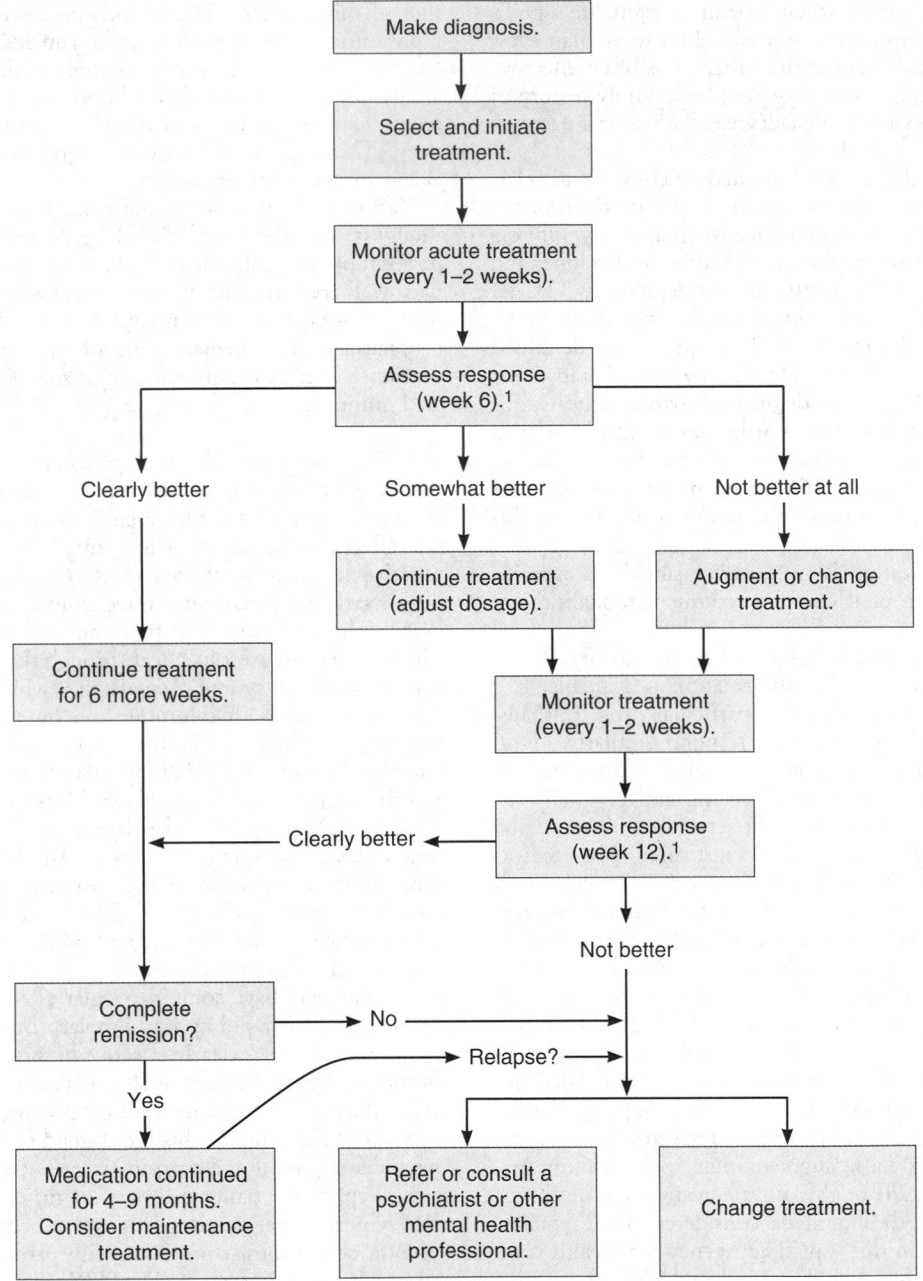

Figure 25–3. Overview of treatment for depression. (Reproduced, with permission, from Agency for Health Care Policy and Research: *Depression in Primary Care.* Vol. 2: *Treatment of Major Depression.* United States Department of Health and Human Services, 1993.)

half-lives and a lesser effect on hepatic enzymes, which reduces their impact on the metabolism of other drugs (thus not increasing significantly the serum concentrations of other drugs as much as fluoxetine). The shorter half-lives also allow for more rapid clearing if adverse side effects appear. Venlafaxine appears to be more effective with doses greater than 200 mg/d, although some individuals respond at 75 mg/d.

The side effects common to all of these drugs are headache, nausea, tinnitus, insomnia, and nervousness. Akathisia has been common with the SSRIs; other extrapyramidal symptoms (eg, dystonias) have occurred infrequently but particularly in withdrawal states. Sexual side effects of erectile dysfunction, retrograde ejaculation, and dysorgasmia are very common with the SSRIs. Antidotes to SSRI-induced sexual dysfunction are occasionally helpful. Sildenafil, 25–50 mg 2 hours prior to sexual activity, can improve erectile dysfunction in some patients. Cyproheptadine, 4 mg orally prior to sexual activity, may be helpful in countering drug-induced anorgasmia. Adjunctive bupropion (75–150 mg daily) may also help with restoring erectile function. Because of early research with bulimic patients, bupropion has been burdened with an unwarranted reputation for causing seizures. The SSRIs are strong serotonin uptake blockers and may in high dosage or in combination with MAO inhibitors, including the antiparkinsonian drug selegiline, cause a "serotonin syndrome." This syndrome is manifested by rigidity, hyperthermia, autonomic instability, myoclonus, confusion, delirium, and coma. This syndrome can be a particularly troublesome problem in the elderly. Several cases of angina have been reported in association with SSRIs. Early research raised the possibility that SSRIs might induce vasospasm in the presence of coronary artery disease. However, current research indicates that SSRIs are safer agents to use than tricyclic antidepressants in patients with cardiac disease.

Withdrawal syndromes have been reported for the SSRIs and venlafaxine. These include dysphoric mood, agitation, and a flu-like state. These medications should be discontinued gradually over a period of weeks or months to reduce the risk of withdrawal phenomena.

Research indicates that fluoxetine, fluvoxamine, paroxetine, sertraline, and venlafaxine in customary antidepressant doses do not appear to increase the risk of major fetal malformation when used during pregnancy. Postpartum developmental effects are thought to be minimal, but this question has not been well studied. The decision to use SSRIs and other psychotropic agents during pregnancy must be based on a risk-benefit analysis for each individual.

Venlafaxine is reported to be well tolerated without significant anticholinergic or cardiovascular side effects. Nausea, nervousness, and profuse sweating appear to be the major side effects. Venlafaxine appears to have few drug-drug interactions. It does require monitoring of blood pressure because some individuals develop a dose-related hypertension. Nefazodone appears to lack the anticholinergic effects of the TCAs and the agitation sometimes induced by SSRIs. Nefazodone should not be give with terfenadine, astemizole, or cisapride. Because nefazodone inhibits the liver's cytochrome P450 3A4 isoenzymes, concurrent use of these medications can lead to serious QT prolongation, ventricular tachycardia, or death. Through the same mechanism of enzyme inhibition, nefazodone can elevate cyclosporine levels sixfold to tenfold. Nefazodone has been given an FDA warning because it has been implicated in liver failure in rare cases. Pretreatment and ongoing monitoring of liver enzymes are indicated.

Mirtazapine is thought to enhance central noradrenergic and serotonergic activity with minimal sexual side effects as compared with the SSRIs. Its action as a potent antagonist of histaminergic receptors may make it a useful agent for patients with depression and insomnia. Its most common adverse side effects include somnolence, increased appetite, weight gain, lipid abnormalities, and dizziness. There have been reports of agranulocytosis in two of 2796 patients. Although it is metabolized by P450 isoenzymes, it is not an inhibitor of this system. It is given in a single dose at bedtime starting at 15 mg and increasing in 15 mg increments every week or every other week up to 45 mg.

2. Tricyclic antidepressants and clinically similar drugs—These drugs were the mainstay of drug therapy for depression for many years. They have also been effective in panic disorders, pain syndromes, and anxiety states. Specific ones have been effective in obsessive-compulsive disorder (clomipramine), enuresis (imipramine), psychotic depression (amoxapine), and reduction of craving in cocaine withdrawal (desipramine).

The tricyclics are characterized more by their similarities than by their differences. There is a lag in clinical response for up to several weeks, partly as a result of side effects that prevent rapid increase in dosage and partly because of their neurotransmitter effects. They tend to affect both serotonin and norepinephrine reuptake; some drugs act mainly on the former and others principally on the latter neurotransmitter system. Individuals receiving the same dosages vary markedly in therapeutic drug levels achieved (elderly patients require smaller doses), and determination of plasma drug levels is helpful when clinical response has been disappointing. Nortriptyline is usually effective when plasma levels are between 50 and 150 ng/mL; imipramine at plasma levels of 200–250 ng/mL; and desipramine at plasma levels of 100–250 ng/mL. High blood levels are not more effective than moderate levels and may be counterproductive (eg, delirium, seizures). Patients with gastrointestinal side effects benefit from plasma level monitoring to assess absorption of the drug. Most of the tricyclics can be given in a single dose at bedtime, starting at fairly low doses (eg, nortriptyline 25 mg orally) and increasing by 25 mg every several days as tolerated until the therapeutic response is achieved (eg, nortriptyline, 100–150 mg) or to maximum dose if necessary (eg, nortriptyline, 150 mg). The most common cause of treatment failure is an inadequate trial. A full trial consists of giving maximum daily dosage for at least 6 weeks. To reach maximum dosage, the trial encompasses a total of about 8 weeks. Because of marked anticholinergic and sedating side effects, clomipramine is started at a low dose (25 mg/d orally) and increased slowly in divided doses up to 100 mg/d, held at that level for several days, and then gradually increased as necessary up to 250 mg/d. Any of the TCA-like drugs should be started at very low doses (eg, 10–25 mg/d) and increased slowly in the treatment of panic disorder.

The tricyclic antidepressants have anticholinergic side effects to varying degrees (amitriptyline 100 mg is equivalent to atropine 5 mg). One must be particularly wary of the effect in elderly men with prostatic hyperplasia. The anticholinergic effects also predispose to other medical problems such as heat stroke or dental problems from xerostomia. Orthostatic hypotension is fairly common, may not remit with time, and may predispose to falls and hip fractures in the elderly. Cardiac effects of the TCAs are functions of the anticholinergic effect, direct myocardial depression (quinidine-like effect), and interference with adrenergic neurons. These factors may produce altered rate, rhythm, and contractility, particularly in patients with preexisting cardiac disease, such as bundle-branch or bifascicular block. Electrocardiographic changes range from benign ST segment and T wave changes and sinus tachycardia to a variety of complex and serious arrhythmias, the latter requiring a change in medication. Because TCAs have class I antiarrhythmic effects, they should be used with caution in patients with ischemic heart disease, arrhythmias, or conduction disturbances. SSRIs or the atypical antidepressants may be better initial choices for this population. TCAs lower the seizure threshold so this is of particular concern in patients with a propensity for seizures (eg, previous head injury, alcohol withdrawal). Loss of libido and erectile, ejaculatory, and orgasmic dysfunction are fairly common and can compromise compliance. Trazodone rarely causes priapism, which requires treatment within 12 hours (epinephrine 1:1000 injected into the corpus cavernosum). Delirium, agitation, and mania are infrequent complications. Sudden discontinuation of some of these drugs can produce "cholinergic rebound," manifested by headaches and nausea with abdominal cramps. Overdoses of the tricyclic compounds are often serious because of the narrow therapeutic index and quinidine-like effects (see Chapter 39).

3. Monoamine oxidase inhibitors—The MAO inhibitors are now generally used as third-line drugs for depression (after a failure of SSRIs, TCAs, or the atypical antidepressants) because of the dietary and other restrictions required (see below and Table 25–7).

Table 25–7. Principal dietary restrictions in MAOI use.

1. Cheese, except cream cheese and cottage cheese and fresh yogurt
2. Fermented or aged meats such as bologna, salami
3. Broad bean pods such as Chinese bean pods
4. Liver of all types
5. Meat and yeast extracts
6. Red wine, sherry, vermouth, cognac, beer, ale
7. Soy sauce, shrimp paste, sauerkraut

They should be considered third-line drugs for refractory panic disorder and depression.

MAO inhibitors are administered in gradual stepwise dosage and may be given in the morning or evening, depending upon their effect on sleep. They tend to take effect in a fairly low dosage range (Table 25–8). Blood levels are not congruent with therapeutic response.

The MAO inhibitors commonly cause symptoms of orthostatic hypotension (which may persist) and sympathomimetic effects of tachycardia, sweating, and tremor. Nausea, insomnia (often associated with intense afternoon drowsiness), and sexual dysfunction are common. Trazodone, 25–75 mg orally at bedtime, may ameliorate the MAO-induced insomnia. Central nervous system effects include agitation and toxic psychoses. Dietary limitations (Table 25–7) and abstinence from drug products containing phenylpropanolamine, phenylephrine, meperidine, dextromethorphan, and pseudoephedrine are mandatory for MAO-A type inhibitors (those marketed for treatment of depression), since the reduction of available monoamine oxidase leaves the patient vulnerable to exogenous amines (eg, tyramine in foodstuffs).

Treatment for a resultant hypertensive crisis has been the same as for pheochromocytoma (see Chapter 26), but there have been reports of success with nifedipine, 10 mg chewed and placed under the tongue, normalizing blood pressure in 1–5 minutes. The restrictions on the proscribed foodstuffs and sympathomimetic drugs are in effect during treatment and for 2–3 weeks after cessation of therapy. Termination of therapy with MAO inhibitors may be associated with anxiety, agitation, cognitive slowing, and headache. Very gradual withdrawal and short-term benzodiazepine therapy will ameliorate symptoms.

4. Switching and combination therapy—If the therapeutic response has been poor after an adequate trial with the chosen drug, one should reassess the diagnosis. Assuming that the trial has been adequate and the diagnosis is correct, a trial with a drug from another group is appropriate. In switching from one group to another, an adequate "washout time" must be allowed. This is critical in certain situations—eg, in switching from an MAO inhibitor to a tricyclic, allow 2–3 weeks between stopping one drug and starting another; in switching from an SSRI to an MAO inhibitor, allow 4–5 weeks. In switching within groups—eg, from one tricyclic to another (amitriptyline to desipramine, etc)—no washout time is needed, and one can rapidly decrease the dosage of one drug while increasing the other. Combining two antidepressants requires caution and is usually reserved for refractory patients after psychiatric consultation.

However, in any of the three groups, one can augment the antidepressant drug if the therapeutic response has been less than satisfactory. Psychiatric consultation may be helpful in selecting the augmenting agent. Lithium and thyroid hormone (eg, 25 μg daily of liothyronine) are the most commonly used aug-

Table 25–8. Commonly used antidepressants.

Drug	Usual Daily Oral Dose (mg)	Usual Daily Maximum Dose (mg)	Sedative Effects[1]	Anticho-llnergic Effects[1]	Cost per Unit	Cost for 30 Days' Treatment Based on Maximum Dosage[2]
SSRIs AND OTHER NEW COMPOUNDS						
Fluoxetine (Prozac, Sarafem)	5–40	80	< 1	< 1	$2.67/20 mg	$320.40
Fluvoxamine (Luvox)	100–300	300	1	< 1	$2.64/100 mg	$237.60
Nefazodone (Serzone)	300–600	600	2	< 1	$1.52/200 mg	$136.80
Paroxetine (Paxil)	20–30	50	1	1	$2.71/20 mg	$203.25
Sertraline (Zoloft)	50–150	200	< 1	< 1	$2.52/100 mg	$151.20
Venlafaxine (Effexor)	150–225	375	1	< 1	$1.55/75 mg	$232.50
Venlafaxine XR (Effexor)	150–225	225	1	< 1	$2.62/75 mg	$235.80
Mirtazapine (Remeron)	15–45	45	4	2	$2.86/30 mg	$87.30
Citalopram (Celexa)	20	40	< 1	1	$2.34/40 mg	$70.20
TRICYCLIC AND CLINICALLY SIMILAR COMPOUNDS						
Amitriptyline (Elavil)	150–250	300	4	4	$0.31/150 mg	$18.60
Amoxapine (Asendin)	150–200	400	2	2	$1.67/100 mg	$200.40
Clomipramine (Anafranil)	100	250	3	3	$1.40/75 mg	$126.00
Desipramine (Norpramin)	100–250	300	1	1	$1.00/100 mg	$90.00
Doxepin (Sinequan)	150–200	300	4	3	$1.00/100 mg	$90.00
Imipramine (Tofranil)	150–200	300	3	3	$0.69/50 mg	$24.20
Maprotiline (Ludiomil)	100–200	300	4	2	$0.93/75 mg	$111.60
Nortriptyline (Aventyl, Pamelor)	100–150	150	2	2	$1.46/50 mg	$131.40
Protriptyline (Vivactil)	15–40	60	1	3	$0.64/10 mg	$115.20
Trazodone (Desyrel)	100–300	400	4	< 1	$0.73/100 mg	$87.60
Trimipramine (Surmontil)	75–200	200	4	4	$2.24/100 mg	$134.40
Bupropion (Wellbutrin)	300[3]	450[3]		< 1	$0.96/100 mg	$129.60
Bupropion SR (Wellbutrin SR)	300	400[4]		< 1	$1.64/100 mg $1.76/150 mg	$196.80 $105.60
MONOAMINE OXIDASE INHIBITORS						
Phenelzine (Nardil)	45–60	90	...	...	$0.53/15 mg	$95.40
Tranylcypromine (Parnate)	20–30	50	...	...	$0.61/10 mg	$91.50

[1]**Key:** 4 = strong effect; 1 = weak effect
[2]Cost to pharmacist (average wholesale price, generic when possible) for quantity listed. Source: *Drug Topics Red Book,* March 2002; Vol. 23, No. 3.
[3]No single dose should exceed 150 mg.
[4]200 mg twice daily.

menting agents. Lithium is an excellent augmentation agent for the 25–40% of depressed patients who fail to respond to an adequate trial of an antidepressant. One-half of these patients will respond to the addition of lithium (600–900 mg/d) with an enhanced antidepressant effect. An empirical trial of liothyronine, 25 μg, may produce effects within a week in certain patients irrespective of whether or not thyroid function is normal at baseline.

5. Maintenance and tapering—When clinical relief of symptoms is obtained, medication is continued for 12 months in the effective maintenance dosage, which is the dosage required in the acute stage. The full dosage should be continued indefinitely when the individual has a first episode before age 20 or after age 50; is over age 40 with two episodes; or has had three episodes at any age. Major depression should often be considered as a chronic disease. If the medication is

Table 25–9. Antidepressant drug interactions with other drugs.

Drug	Effects
Tricyclic and other non-MAOI antidepressants	
Antacids	Decreased absorption of antidepressants.
Anticoagulants	Increased hypoprothrombinemic effect.
Cimetidine	Increased antidepressant blood levels and psychosis.
Clonidine	Decreased antihypertensive effect.
Digitalis	Increased incidence of heart block.
Disulfiram	Increased antidepressant blood levels.
Guanethidine	Decreased antihypertensive effect.
Haloperidol	Increased clomipramine levels.
Insulin	Decreased blood sugar.
Lithium	Increased lithium levels with fluoxetine.
Methyldopa	Decreased antihypertensive effect.
Other anticholinergic drugs	Marked anticholinergic responses.
Phenytoin	Increased blood levels.
Procainamide	Decreased ventricular conduction.
Procarbazine	Hypertensive crisis.
Propranolol	Increased hypotension.
Quinidine	Decreased ventricular conduction.
Rauwolfia derivatives	Increased stimulation.
Sedatives	Increased sedation.
Sympathomimetic drugs	Increased pressor effect.
Terfenadine	Torsade de pointes
Monoamine oxidase inhibitors	
Antihistamines	Increased sedation.
Belladonna-like drugs	Increased blood pressure.
Dextromethorphan	Same as meperidine.
Guanethidine	Decreased blood pressure.
Insulin	Decreased blood sugar.
Levodopa	Increased blood pressure.
Meperidine	Increased agitation, seizures, coma, death.
Methyldopa	Decreased blood pressure.
Pseudoephedrine	Hypertensive crisis (increased blood pressure).
Reserpine	Increased blood pressure and temperature.
Succinylcholine	Increased neuromuscular blockade.
Sulfonylureas	Decreased blood sugar.
Sympathomimetic drugs	Increased blood pressure.

being tapered, it should be done gradually over several months, monitoring closely for relapse.

6. Drug interactions—Interactions with other drugs are listed in Table 25–9.

7. Electroconvulsive therapy (ECT)—ECT causes a generalized central nervous system seizure (peripheral convulsion is not necessary) by means of electric current. The key objective is to exceed the seizure threshold, which can be accomplished by a variety of means. Electrical stimulation is more reliable and simpler than the use of chemical convulsants. The mechanism of action is not known, but it is thought to involve major neurotransmitter responses at the cell membrane. Current insufficient to cause a seizure produces no therapeutic benefit.

Electroconvulsive therapy is the most effective (about 70–85%) treatment of severe depression, particularly the delusions and agitation commonly seen with depression in the involutional period. It is indicated when medical conditions preclude the use of antidepressants or in cases of nonresponsiveness to these medications. Comparative controlled studies of electroconvulsive therapy in severe depression show that it is more effective than chemotherapy. It is also effective in the manic disorders and psychoses during pregnancy (when drugs may be contraindicated). It has not been shown to be helpful in chronic schizophrenic disorders, and it is generally not used in acute schizophrenic episodes unless drugs are not effective and it is urgent that the psychosis be controlled (eg, a catatonic stupor complicating an acute medical condition).

The most common side effects are memory disturbance and headache. Memory loss or confusion is usually related to number and frequency of electroconvulsive therapy treatments and proper oxygenation during treatment. Some memory loss is occasionally permanent, but most memory faculties return to full capacity within several weeks. There have been reports that lithium administration concurrent with electroconvulsive therapy resulted in greater memory loss. Before anesthesia was used, spinal compression fractures and severe anticipatory anxiety were common.

Increased intracranial pressure is a serious contraindication. Other problems such as cardiac disorders, aortic aneurysms, bronchopulmonary disease, and venous thrombosis are relative contraindications and must be evaluated in light of the severity of the medical problem versus the need for electroconvulsive therapy. Serious complications arising from electroconvulsive therapy occur in less than one in 1000 cases. Most of these problems are cardiovascular or respiratory in nature (eg, aspiration of gastric contents). Poor patient understanding and lack of acceptance of the technique by the public are the biggest obstacles to the use of electroconvulsive therapy.

8. Phototherapy—Phototherapy is used in major depression with seasonal onset. It consists of exposure (at a 3-foot distance) to a light source of 2500 lux for 2 hours daily. Light visors are an adaptation that provides greater mobility and an adjustable light intensity. The price of these full-spectrum light sources range between $300 and $400. The dosage varies, with some patients requiring morning and night exposure. One effect is alteration of biorhythm through melatonin mechanisms.

9. Experimental treatments—In preliminary studies, transcranial magnetic stimulation has appeared to be effective in nonpsychotic depression. Vagal nerve stimulation has shown promise in extremely refractory cases.

B. PSYCHOLOGIC

It is seldom possible to engage an individual in penetrating psychotherapeutic endeavors during the acute stage of a severe depression. While medications may be taking effect, a supportive approach to strengthen existing defenses and appropriate consideration of the patient's continuing need to function at work, to engage in recreational activities, etc, are necessary as the severity of the depression lessens. If the patient is not seriously depressed, it is often quite appropriate to initiate intensive psychotherapeutic efforts, since flux periods are a good time to effect change. A catharsis of repressed anger and guilt may be beneficial. Therapy during or just after the acute stage may focus on coping techniques, with some practice of alternative choices. When lack of self-confidence and identity problems are factors in the depression, individual psychotherapy can be oriented to ways of improving self-esteem, increasing assertiveness, and lessening dependency. Interpersonal psychotherapy for depression has shown efficacy in the treatment of acute depression, helping patients master interpersonal stresses and develop new coping strategies. Cognitive psychotherapy addresses patients' patterns of negative thoughts, called cognitive distortions, that lead to feelings of depression and anxiety. Treatment usually includes homework assignments such as keeping a journal of cognitive distortions and of positive responses to them. As previously noted, numerous studies have shown that the combination of drug therapy plus interpersonal psychotherapy or cognitive psychotherapy is more effective than either modality alone. It is usually helpful to involve the spouse or other significant family members early in treatment.

C. SOCIAL

Flexible use of appropriate social services can be of major importance in the treatment of depression. Since alcohol is often associated with depression, early involvement in alcohol treatment programs such as Alcoholics Anonymous can be important to future success (see Alcohol Dependency and Abuse, below). The structuring of daily activities during severe depression is often quite difficult for the patient, and loneliness is often a major factor. The help of family, employer, or friends is often necessary to mobilize the patient who experiences no joy in daily activities and tends to remain uninvolved and to deteriorate. Insis-

tence on sharing activities will help involve the patient in simple but important daily functions. In some severe cases, the use of day treatment centers or support groups of a specific type (eg, mastectomy groups) is indicated. It is not unusual for a patient to have multiple legal, financial, and vocational problems requiring legal and vocational assistance.

D. BEHAVIORAL

When depression is a function of self-defeating coping techniques such as passivity, the role-playing approach can be useful. Behavioral techniques, including desensitization, may be used in problems such as phobias where depression is a by-product. When depression is a regularly used interpersonal style, behavioral counseling to family members or others can help in extinguishing the behavior in the patient.

Treatment of Mania

Acute manic or hypomanic symptoms will respond to lithium therapy after several days of treatment, but it is common to use neuroleptic drugs or high-potency benzodiazepines (eg, clonazepam) to immediately treat the excited or psychotic manic stage. Some schizoaffective disorders and some cases of so-called schizophrenia are probably atypical bipolar affective disorder, for which lithium treatment may be effective.

A. NEUROLEPTICS

Acute manic symptoms of agitation and psychosis may be initially treated with the atypical antipsychotic olanzapine, 5–20 mg orally in conjunction with a benzodiazepine if indicated. Alternatively, haloperidol, 5–10 mg orally or intramuscularly every 2–3 hours until symptoms subside, may be used. The dosage of olanzapine or haloperidol is gradually reduced after lithium or another mood stabilizer is started (see below).

B. CLONAZEPAM

Clonazepam can be an alternative or adjunct to a neuroleptic in controlling acute behavioral symptoms. Clonazepam has the advantage of causing no extrapyramidal side effects. Although 1–2 mg orally every 4–6 hours may be effective, up to 16 mg/d may be necessary.

C. LITHIUM

As a prophylactic drug for bipolar affective disorder, lithium significantly decreases the frequency and severity of both manic and depressive attacks in about 70% of patients. A positive response is more predictable if the patient has a low frequency of episodes (no more than two per year with intervals free of psychopathology). A positive response occurs more frequently in individuals who have blood relatives with a diagnosis of manic or hypomanic attacks. Patients who swing rapidly back and forth between manic and depressive attacks (at least four cycles per year) usually respond poorly to lithium prophylaxis initially, but some improve with continued long-term treatment.

Carbamazepine (see below) has been used with success in this group.

In addition to its use in manic states, lithium is sometimes useful in the prophylaxis of recurrent unipolar depressions (perhaps undiagnosed bipolar disorder). Lithium may ameliorate nonspecific aggressive behaviors and dyscontrol syndromes. The dosages are the same as used in bipolar disorder. Most patients with bipolar disease can be managed long-term with lithium alone, though some will require continued or intermittent use of a neuroleptic, antidepressant, or carbamazepine. An excellent resource for information pertaining to lithium is the Information Centers, Madison Institute of Medicine, 7617 Mineral Point Road, Suite 300, Madison, WI 53717-1914.

Before treatment, the clinical workup should include a medical history and physical examination; complete blood count; T_4, TSH, blood urea nitrogen, serum creatinine, and serum electrolyte determinations; urinalysis; and electrocardiography in patients over age 45 or with a history of cardiac disease.

1. **Dosage**—Lithium carbonate is generally prescribed in the 300 mg unit. In a small minority of patients, a slow release form or units of different dosage may be required. Lithium citrate is available as a syrup. The dosage is that required to maintain blood levels in the therapeutic range. For acute attacks, this ranges from 1 to 1.5 meq/L. Although there is controversy about the optimal chronic maintenance dose, many clinicians reduce the acute level to 0.6–1 meq/L in order to reduce side effects. The dose required to meet this need will vary in different individuals. For acute mania, doses of 1200–1800 mg/d are generally recommended. Augmentation of antidepressants is usually achieved with one-half of these doses. Once-a-day dosage is acceptable, but most patients have less nausea when they take the drug in divided doses with meals.

Lithium is readily absorbed, with peak serum levels occurring within 1–3 hours and complete absorption in 8 hours. Half of the total body lithium is excreted in 18–24 hours (95% in the urine). Blood for lithium levels should be drawn 12 hours after the last dose. Serum levels should be measured 5–7 days after initiation of treatment and changes in dose. For maintenance treatment, lithium levels should be monitored initially every 1–2 months but may be measured every 6–12 months in stable, long-term patients. Levels should be monitored more closely when there is any condition that causes volume depletion (eg, diarrhea; dehydration; use of diuretics).

2. **Side effects**—Mild gastrointestinal symptoms (take lithium with food), fine tremors (treat with propranolol, 20–60 mg/d orally, only if persistent), slight muscle weakness, and some degree of somnolence are early side effects that are usually transient. Moderate polyuria (reduced renal responsiveness to antidiuretic hormone) and polydipsia (associated with increased plasma renin concentration) are often present. Potassium administration can blunt this effect, as may once-daily dosing of lithium. Weight gain (often a result of calories in fluids taken for polydipsia) and leukocytosis not due to infection are fairly common.

Other side effects include goiter (3%; often euthyroid), hypothyroidism (10%; concomitant administration of lithium and iodide or lithium and carbamazepine enhances the hypothyroid and goitrogenic effect of either drug), changes in the glucose tolerance test toward a diabetes-like curve, nephrogenic diabetes insipidus (usually resolving about 8 weeks after cessation of lithium therapy), nephrotic syndrome, edema, folate deficiency, and pseudotumor cerebri (ophthalmoscopy is indicated if there are complaints of headache or blurred vision). A metallic taste, hair loss, and Raynaud's phenomenon have been reported in a few cases. Thyroid and kidney function should be checked at 3- to 4-month intervals. Most of these side effects subside when lithium is discontinued; when residual side effects exist, they are usually not serious. Most clinicians treat lithium-induced hypothyroidism (more common in women) with thyroid hormone while continuing lithium therapy. Hypercalcemia and elevated parathyroid hormone levels occur in some patients. Electrocardiographic abnormalities (principally T wave flattening or inversion) may occur during lithium administration but are not of major clinical significance. Sinoatrial block may occur, particularly in the elderly. It is important that other drugs which prolong intraventricular conduction, such as tricyclics, be used with caution in conjunction with lithium. Lithium impairs ventilatory function in patients with airway obstruction. Lithium alone does not have a significant effect on sexual function, but when combined with benzodiazepines (clonazepam in most symptomatic patients) it causes sexual dysfunction in about 50% of men. Lithium may precipitate or exacerbate psoriasis in some patients.

Patients receiving long-term lithium therapy may have cogwheel rigidity and, occasionally, other extrapyramidal signs. Lithium potentiates the parkinsonian effects of haloperidol. Long-term lithium therapy has also been associated with a relative lowering of the level of memory and perceptual processing (affecting compliance in some cases). Some impairment of attention and emotional reactivity has also been noted. Lithium-induced delirium with therapeutic lithium levels is an infrequent complication usually occurring in the elderly and may persist for several days after serum levels have become negligible. Encephalopathy has occurred in patients receiving combined lithium and neuroleptic therapy and in those who have cerebrovascular disease, thus requiring careful evaluation of patients who develop neurotoxic signs at subtoxic blood levels.

Some reports have suggested that the long-term use of lithium may have adverse effects on renal function (with interstitial fibrosis or tubular atrophy). A rise in serum creatinine levels is an indication for in-depth evaluation of renal function. Incontinence has been reported in women, apparently related to changes in bladder cholinergic-adrenergic balance.

Lithium exposure in early pregnancy increases the frequency of congenital anomalies, especially Ebstein's and other major cardiovascular anomalies. As with any woman taking psychotropic medications who has a planned or unplanned pregnancy, the decision to make a change in medication is complex and requires informed consent regarding the relative risks to the patient and fetus. Recent prospective studies suggest that the risk imposed by lithium in pregnancy may be overemphasized. Indeed, the risk of untreated bipolar disorder carries its own risks for pregnancy. Formula feeding should be considered in mothers using lithium, since concentration in breast milk is one-third to one-half that in serum.

Frank toxicity usually occurs at blood lithium levels above 2 meq/L. Because sodium and lithium are reabsorbed at the same loci in the proximal renal tubules, any sodium loss (diarrhea, use of diuretics, or excessive perspiration) results in increased lithium levels. Symptoms and signs include vomiting and diarrhea, the latter exacerbating the problem since more sodium is lost and more lithium is absorbed. Other symptoms and signs, some of which may not be reversible, include tremors, marked muscle weakness, confusion, dysarthria, vertigo, choreoathetosis, ataxia, hyperreflexia, rigidity, lack of coordination, myoclonus, seizures, opisthotonos, and coma. Toxicity is more severe in the elderly, who should be maintained on slightly lower serum levels. Lithium overdosage may be accidental or intentional or may occur as a result of poor monitoring.

Patients with massive ingestions of lithium or blood lithium levels above 2.5 meq/L should be treated with induced emesis and gastric lavage. If renal function is normal, osmotic and saline diuresis increases renal lithium clearance. Urinary alkalinization is also helpful, since sodium bicarbonate decreases lithium reabsorption in the proximal tubule, as does acetazolamide as well. Aminophylline potentiates the diuretic effect by increasing the clearance of lithium. Drugs affecting the distal loop have no effect on lithium reabsorption. Blood lithium levels above 2.5 meq/L (confirmed by cerebrospinal fluid lithium levels) should be considered an indication for hemodialysis.

Compliance with lithium therapy is adversely affected by the loss of some hypomanic experiences valued by the patient. These include social extroversion and a sense of heightened enjoyment in many activities such as sex and business dealings, often with increased productivity in the latter.

3. Drug interactions—Patients receiving lithium should use diuretics with caution and only under close medical supervision. The thiazide diuretics cause increased lithium reabsorption from the proximal renal

Table 25–10. Lithium interactions with other drugs.

Drug	Effects
ACE inhibitors	↑ Lithium levels
Fluoxetine	↑ Lithium levels
Ibuprofen	↑ Lithium levels
Indomethacin	↑ Lithium levels
Methyldopa	Rigidity, mutism, fascicular twitching
Osmotic diuretics (urea, mannitol)	↑ Lithium excretion
Phenylbutazone	↑ Lithium levels
Potassium-sparing diuretics (spironolactone, amiloride, triamterene)	↑ Lithium levels
Sodium bicarbonate	↑ Lithium excretion
Succinylcholine	↑ Duration of action of succinylcholine
Theophylline, aminophylline	↑ Lithium excretion
Thiazide diuretics	↑ Lithium levels
Valproic acid	↓ Lithium levels

tubules, resulting in increased serum lithium levels (Table 25–10), and adjustment of lithium intake must be made to compensate for this. Reduce lithium dosage by 25–40% when the patient is receiving 50 mg of hydrochlorothiazide daily. Potassium-sparing diuretics (spironolactone, amiloride, triamterene) may also increase serum lithium levels and require careful monitoring of lithium levels. Loop diuretics (furosemide, ethacrynic acid, bumetanide) do not appear to alter serum lithium levels. Concurrent use of lithium and ACE inhibitors requires a 50–75% reduction in lithium intake to achieve therapeutic lithium levels.

D. VALPROIC ACID

Valproic acid (divalproex) is an antiseizure drug whose activity is at least partially related to GABA neurotransmission. It is gaining favor as a first-line treatment for mania because it has a broader index of safety than lithium. This issue is particularly important in AIDS or other medically ill patients prone to dehydration or malabsorption with wide swings in serum lithium levels. Valproic acid has also been utilized effectively in panic disorder and migraine headache. Treatment is often started at a dose of 750 mg/d orally in divided doses, and dosage is then titrated to achieve therapeutic serum levels. Oral loading in acutely manic bipolar patients in an inpatient setting (initiated at a dosage of 20 mg/kg/d) can safely achieve serum therapeutic levels in 2–3 days. Concomitant use of aspirin, carbamazepine, warfarin, or phenytoin may affect serum levels. Gastrointestinal symptoms are the main side effects. Liver function tests and complete blood counts should be monitored, and teratogenic effects are a concern.

E. CARBAMAZEPINE

Carbamazepine, an antiseizure drug that stabilizes the activity of cell membranes, has been used with increasing frequency in the treatment of bipolar patients who cannot be satisfactorily treated with lithium (nonresponsive, excessive side effects, or rapid cycling). It is often effective at 800–1600 mg/d orally. It has also been used in the treatment of resistant depressions, alcohol withdrawal, and hallucinations (in conjunction with neuroleptics) and in patients with behavioral dyscontrol or panic attacks. It suppresses some phases of kindling (see Stimulants) and has been used to treat residual symptoms in previous stimulant abusers (eg, posttraumatic stress disorder with impulse control problems). Dose-related side effects include sedation and ataxia. Dosages start at 400–600 mg orally daily and are increased slowly to therapeutic levels. Skin rashes and a mild reduction in white count are common. SIADH occurs rarely. Nonsteroidal anti-inflammatory drugs (except aspirin); the antibiotics erythromycin and isoniazid; the calcium channel blockers verapamil and diltiazem (but not nifedipine); fluoxetine, propoxyphene, and cimetidine all increase carbamazepine levels. Carbamazepine can be effective in conjunction with lithium, though there have been reports of reversible neurotoxicity with the combination. Carbamazepine stimulates hepatic microsomal enzymes and so tends to decrease levels of haloperidol and oral contraceptives. It also lowers T_4, free T_4, and T_3 levels. Cases of fetal malformation (particularly spina bifida) have been reported along with growth deficiency and developmental delay. Liver tests and complete blood counts should be monitored in patients taking carbamazepine. Oxcarbazepine, a derivative of carbamazepine, does not appear to induce its own metabolism and is associated with fewer drug interactions and a lower risk of hepatotoxicity than carbamazepine, though it may impose a higher risk of hyponatremia. FDA-approved for partial seizures, oxcarbazepine may have efficacy as a mood stabilizer.

F. CALCIUM CHANNEL BLOCKERS

Calcium channel blockers (eg, verapamil) have been used in bipolar states that have failed to respond to lithium, carbamazepine, or valproic acid. This has come about with the realization that a number of drugs used in psychiatry (eg, lithium, antidepressants, neuroleptics, and carbamazepine) have calcium channel-blocking activity. There is also preliminary evidence that these drugs may be useful in the treatment of tardive dyskinesia and panic attacks. Verapamil may be safer than lithium or carbamazepine during pregnancy, though it decreases uterine contractility and must be discontinued before delivery.

G. NEWER ANTICONVULSANTS

Lamotrigine, which has a primary indication for adjunctive treatment of partial seizures, may have some efficacy in the treatment of bipolar disorder. It is thought to inhibit neuronal sodium channels and the release of excitatory amino acids, glutamate and aspartate. Two double-blind studies support its efficacy in the treatment of bipolar depression as adjunctive therapy or as monotherapy. One double-blind study suggests that it may have efficacy as maintenance monotherapy for patients with rapid-cycling bipolar disorder. Its metabolism is inhibited by coadministration of valproic acid, doubling its half-life, and accelerated by hepatic enzyme-inducing agents such as carbamazepine. More frequent mild side effects include headache, dizziness, nausea, and diplopia. Rash occurring in 10% of patients is an indication for immediate cessation of dosing since lamotrigine has been associated with Stevens-Johnson syndrome (1:1000) and, rarely, toxic epidermal necrolysis. Dosing starts at 25–50 mg/d and is titrated upward slowly to decrease the likelihood of rash. A slower titration is indicated for patients taking valproic acid. Topiramate, which has been labeled for use as an anticonvulsant, has been found efficacious in the adjunctive treatment of bipolar disorder in a series of open-label studies. It has the unique feature of promoting weight loss as a side effect. Other common side effects include somnolence, difficulty with memory, dizziness, and anxiety.

Prognosis

Reactive depressions are usually time-limited, and the prognosis with treatment is good if a pathologic pattern of adjustment does not intervene. Major affective disorders frequently respond well to a full trial of drug treatment.

Mania and bipolar disorder have a good prognosis with adequate treatment.

Glass RM: Treating depression as a recurrent or chronic disease. JAMA 1999;281:83. [PMID: 9892456] (Current thinking regarding major depression requires a long-term view of the illness, just as with other chronic medical problems.)

JAMA patient page: Depression. JAMA 1998;279:1760. [PMID: 9624033]

Kulin NA et al: Pregnancy outcome following maternal use of the new selective serotonin reuptake inhibitors: A prospective controlled multicenter study. JAMA 1998;279:609. [PMID: 9486756] (Prospective multicenter controlled study suggests that fluvoxamine, paroxetine, and sertraline at recommended doses do not increase teratogenic risk.)

Reynolds CF et al: Nortriptyline and interpersonal psychotherapy as maintenance therapies for recurrent major depression: A randomized controlled trial in patients older than 59 years. JAMA 1999;281:39. [PMID: 9892449] (In geriatric patients, maintenance treatment with nortriptyline or interpersonal therapy is effective in preventing recurrence. Combining both treatments appears to be the optimal strategy.)

Roose SP et al: Comparison of paroxetine and nortriptyline in depressed patients with ischemic heart disease. JAMA 1998;

279:287. [PMID: 9450712] (Paroxetine had a significantly lower risk of adverse cardiac events.)

Young LT et al: Double-blind comparison of addition of second mood stabilizer versus an anti-depressant to an initial mood stabilizer for treatment of patients with bipolar depression. Am J Psychiatry 2000;157:124. [PMID: 10618026] (Both treatments are effective, but paroxetine was better tolerated than the second mood-stabilizer.)

SLEEP DISORDERS

Sleep consists of two distinct states as shown by electroencephalographic studies: REM (rapid eye movement) sleep, also called dream sleep, D state sleep, paradoxic sleep; and NREM (non-REM) sleep, also called S stage sleep, which is divided into stages 1, 2, 3, and 4 recognizable by different electroencephalographic patterns. Stages 3 and 4 are "delta" sleep. Dreaming occurs mostly in REM and to a lesser extent in NREM sleep.

Sleep is a cyclic phenomenon, with four or five REM periods during the night accounting for about one-fourth of the total night's sleep (1½–2 hours). The first REM period occurs about 80–120 minutes after onset of sleep and lasts about 10 minutes. Later REM periods are longer (15–40 minutes) and occur mostly in the last several hours of sleep. Most stage 4 (deepest) sleep occurs in the first several hours.

Age-related changes in normal sleep include an unchanging percentage of REM sleep and a marked decrease in stage 3 and stage 4 sleep, with an increase in wakeful periods during the night. These normal changes, early bedtimes, and daytime naps play a role in the increased complaints of insomnia in older people. Variations in sleep patterns may be due to circumstances (eg, "jet lag") or to idiosyncratic patterns ("night owls") in persons who perhaps because of different "biologic rhythms" habitually go to bed late and sleep late in the morning. Creativity and rapidity of response to unfamiliar situations are impaired by loss of sleep. There are also rare individuals who have chronic difficulty in adapting to a 24-hour sleep-wake cycle (desynchronization sleep disorder), which can be resynchronized by altering exposure to light.

The three major sleep disorders are discussed below.

1. Dyssomnias (Insomnia)

Classification & Clinical Findings

Patients may complain of difficulty getting to sleep or staying asleep, intermittent wakefulness during the night, early morning awakening, or combinations of any of these. Transient episodes are usually of little significance. Stress, caffeine, physical discomfort, daytime napping, and early bedtimes are common factors.

Psychiatric disorders are often associated with persistent insomnia. **Depression** is usually associated with fragmented sleep, decreased total sleep time, earlier onset of REM sleep, a shift of REM activity to the first half of the night, and a loss of slow wave sleep—all of which are nonspecific findings. In **manic disorders,** sleeplessness is a cardinal feature and an important early sign of impending mania in bipolar cases. Total sleep time is decreased, with shortened REM latency and increased REM activity. Sleep-related panic attacks occur in the transition from stage 2 to stage 3 sleep in some patients with a longer REM latency in the sleep pattern preceding the attacks.

Abuse of alcohol may cause or be secondary to the sleep disturbance. There is a tendency to use alcohol as a means of getting to sleep without realizing that it disrupts the normal sleep cycle. Acute alcohol intake produces a decreased sleep latency with reduced REM sleep during the first half of the night. REM sleep is increased in the second half of the night, with an increase in total amount of slow wave sleep (stages 3 and 4). Vivid dreams and frequent awakenings are common. Chronic alcohol abuse increases stage 1 and decreases REM sleep (most drugs delay or block REM sleep), with symptoms persisting for many months after the individual has stopped drinking. Acute alcohol or other sedative withdrawal causes delayed onset of sleep and REM rebound with intermittent awakening during the night.

Heavy smoking (more than a pack a day) causes difficulty falling asleep—apparently independently of the often associated increase in coffee drinking. Excess intake near bedtime of caffeine, cocaine, and other stimulants (eg, OTC cold remedies) causes decreased total sleep time—mostly NREM sleep—with some increased sleep latency.

Sedative-hypnotics—specifically, the benzodiazepines, which are the prescription drugs of choice to promote sleep—tend to increase total sleep time, decrease sleep latency, and decrease nocturnal awakening, with variable effects on NREM sleep. Withdrawal causes just the opposite effects and results in continued use of the drug for the purpose of preventing withdrawal symptoms. Antidepressants decrease REM sleep (with marked rebound on withdrawal in the form of nightmares) and have varying effects on NREM sleep. The effect on REM sleep correlates with reports that REM sleep deprivation produces improvement in some depressions.

Persistent insomnias are also related to a wide variety of medical conditions, particularly delirium, pain, respiratory distress syndromes, uremia, asthma, and thyroid disorders. Adequate analgesia and proper treatment of medical disorders will reduce symptoms and decrease the need for sedatives.

Treatment

In general, there are two broad classes of treatment for insomnia, and the two may be combined: psychologic (cognitive-behavioral) and pharmacologic. In situations of acute distress, such as a grief reaction, pharmacologic measures may be most appropriate. With primary insomnia, however, initial efforts should be psychologically based. This is particularly true in the elderly to avoid the potential adverse reactions of medications. The elderly population is at risk for complaints of insomnia because sleep becomes lighter and more easily disrupted with aging. Medical disorders that become more common with age may also predispose to insomnia.

A. PSYCHOLOGIC

Psychologic strategies should include educating the patient regarding good sleep hygiene: (1) Go to bed only when sleepy. (2) Use the bed and bedroom only for sleeping and sex. (3) If still awake after 20 minutes, leave the bedroom and only return when sleepy. (4) Get up at the same time every morning regardless of the amount of sleep during the night. (5) Discontinue caffeine and nicotine, at least in the evening if not completely. (6) Establish a daily exercise regimen. (7) Avoid alcohol as it may disrupt continuity of sleep. (8) Limit fluids in the evening. (9) Learn and practice relaxation techniques.

The clinician should also discuss any myths or misconceptions about sleep that the patient may hold.

B. MEDICAL

When the above measures are insufficient, medications may be useful. Pharmacologic measures currently rely primarily on safe hypnotic medications that are difficult to overdose with. Lorazepam (0.5 mg nightly), temazepam (7.5–15 mg nightly), zolpidem (5–10 mg nightly), and zaleplon (5–10 mg nightly) are often effective for the elderly population and can be given in larger doses—twice what is prescribed for the elderly—in younger patients. It is important to note that short-acting agents like triazolam or zolpidem may lead to amnestic episodes if used on a daily ongoing basis. Longer-acting agents such as flurazepam (half-life of > 48 hours) may accumulate in the elderly and lead to cognitive slowing, ataxia, falls, and somnolence. In general, it is appropriate to use medications for short courses of 1–2 weeks. The medications described above have largely replaced barbiturates as hypnotic agents because of their greater safety in overdose and their lesser hepatic enzyme induction effects. Antihistamines such as diphenhydramine (25 mg nightly) or hydroxyzine (25 mg nightly) may also be useful for sleep, as they produce no pharmacologic dependency; their anticholinergic effects may, however, produce confusion or urinary symptoms in the elderly. Trazodone, an atypical antidepressant, is a non-habit-forming, effective sleep medication in lower than antidepressant doses (25–150 mg at bedtime). Priapism is a rare side effect requiring emergent treatment.

Triazolam has achieved popularity as a hypnotic drug because of its very short duration of action. Because it has been associated with dependency, transient psychotic reactions, anterograde amnesia, and re-

bound anxiety, it has been removed from the market in several European countries. If used, it must be prescribed only for short periods of time.

2. Hypersomnias (Disorders of Excessive Sleepiness)

The hypersomnias are a more severe problem than insomnia.

Classification & Clinical Findings

A. SLEEP APNEA

This disorder is characterized by cessation of breathing for at least 30 episodes (each lasting about 10 seconds) during the night. There are two types: obstructive and central. (See Chapter 9.)

B. NARCOLEPSY

Narcolepsy consists of a tetrad of symptoms: (1) Sudden, brief (about 15 minutes) sleep attacks that may occur during any type of activity; (2) cataplexy—sudden loss of muscle tone involving specific small muscle groups or generalized muscle weakness that may cause the person to slump to the floor, unable to move, often associated with emotional reactions and sometimes confused with seizure disorder; (3) sleep paralysis—a generalized flaccidity of muscles with full consciousness in the transition zone between sleep and waking; and (4) hypnagogic hallucinations, visual or auditory, which may precede sleep or occur during the sleep attack. The attacks are characterized by an abrupt transition into REM sleep—a necessary criterion for diagnosis. The disorder begins in early adult life, affects both sexes equally, and usually levels off in severity at about 30 years of age.

REM sleep behavior disorder, characterized by motor dyscontrol and often violent dreams during REM sleep, may be related to narcolepsy.

C. KLEINE-LEVIN SYNDROME

This syndrome, which occurs mostly in young men, is characterized by hypersomnic attacks three or four times a year lasting up to 2 days, with hyperphagia, hypersexuality, irritability, and confusion on awakening. It has often been associated with antecedent neurologic insults. It usually remits after age 40.

D. NOCTURNAL MYOCLONUS

Periodic lower leg movements occur during sleep with subsequent daytime sleepiness, anxiety, depression, and cognitive impairment.

Treatment

Narcolepsy can be managed by daily administration of a stimulant such as dextroamphetamine sulfate, 10 mg in the morning, with increased dosage as necessary. Modafinil is a schedule IV medication FDA-approved for treating the excessive daytime fatigue of narcolepsy. Usual dosing is 200 mg each morning. Its mechanism of action is unknown, yet it is thought to be less of an abuse risk than stimulants that are primarily dopaminergic. Common side effects include headache and anxiety; however, Modafinil appears to be generally well tolerated. Modafinil may reduce the efficacy of cyclosporine, oral contraceptives, and other medications by inducing their hepatic metabolism. Imipramine, 75–100 mg daily, has been effective in treatment of cataplexy but not narcolepsy.

Nocturnal myoclonus and REM sleep behavior disorder can be treated with clonazepam with variable results. There is no treatment for Kleine-Levin syndrome.

Treatment of sleep apnea is discussed in Chapter 9.

3. Parasomnias (Abnormal Behaviors During Sleep)

These disorders are fairly common in children and less so in adults.

Classification & Clinical Findings

A. Sleep Terror

Sleep terror (pavor nocturnus) is an abrupt, terrifying arousal from sleep, usually in preadolescent boys though it may occur in adults as well. It is distinct from sleep panic attacks. Symptoms are fear, sweating, tachycardia, and confusion for several minutes, with amnesia for the event.

B. Nightmares

Nightmares occur during REM sleep; sleep terrors in stage 3 or stage 4 sleep.

C. Sleepwalking

Sleepwalking (somnambulism) includes ambulation or other intricate behaviors while still asleep, with amnesia for the event. It affects mostly children aged 6–12 years, and episodes occur during stage 3 or stage 4 sleep in the first third of the night and in REM sleep in the later sleep hours. Sleepwalking in elderly people may be a feature of dementia. Idiosyncratic reactions to drugs (eg, marijuana, alcohol) and medical conditions (eg, partial complex seizures) may be causative factors in adults.

D. Enuresis

Enuresis is involuntary micturition during sleep in a person who usually has voluntary control. Like other parasomnias, it is more common in children, usually in the 3–4 hours after bedtime, but is not limited to a specific stage of sleep. Confusion during the episode and amnesia for the event are common.

Treatment

Treatment for sleep terrors is with benzodiazepines (eg, diazepam, 5–20 mg at bedtime), since it will sup-

press stage 3 and stage 4 sleep. Somnambulism responds to the same treatment for the same reason, but simple safety measures should not be neglected. Enuresis may respond to imipramine, 50–100 mg at bedtime, though desmopressin nasal spray (an antidiuretic hormone preparation) has increasingly become the treatment of choice for nocturnal enuresis. Behavioral approaches (eg, bells that ring when the pad gets wet) have also been successful.

JAMA patient page: Insomnia. JAMA 1999;281:1056. [PMID: 1086442]

Morin CM et al: Behavioral and pharmacological therapies for late-life insomnia; a randomized controlled trial. JAMA 1999;281:991. [PMID: 10086433] (Behavioral treatment for late-life insomnia may have more sustained efficacy than pharmacotherapy, though both are effective.)

Simon GE et al: Prevalence, burden and treatment of insomnia in primary care. Am J Psychiatry 1997;154:1417. [PMID: 9326825] (Insomnia among primary care patients is associated with broad functional impairment comparable to that found with other psychiatric and medical conditions.)

DISORDERS OF AGGRESSION

Acts performed with the deliberate intent of causing physical harm to persons or property have a wide variety of causative features. Aggression and violence are symptoms rather than diseases, and most frequently they are not associated with an underlying medical condition. Clinicians are unable to predict dangerous behavior with greater than chance accuracy. In terms of demographic characteristics, the perpetrator of an act of aggression is often a male under age 25, a member of a socioeconomically deprived group, and a resident of an inner city area. Depression, schizophrenia, personality disorders, mania, paranoia, temporal lobe dysfunction, and organic mental states may be associated. Anabolic steroid usage by athletes has been associated with increased tendencies toward violent behavior.

In the USA, a significant proportion of all violent deaths are alcohol-related. The ingestion of even small amounts of alcohol can result in pathologic intoxication that resembles an acute organic mental condition. Amphetamines, crack cocaine, and other stimulants are frequently associated with aggressive behavior. Phencyclidine is a drug commonly associated with violent behavior that is occasionally of a bizarre nature, partly due to lowering of the pain threshold. Impulse control disorders are characterized by physical abuse, usually of the aggressor's domestic partner or children, pathologic intoxication, impulsive sexual activities, and reckless driving.

Domestic violence and rape are much more widespread than heretofore recognized. Awareness of the problem is to some degree due to increasing recognition of the rights of women and the understanding by women that they do not have to accept abuse. Acceptance of this kind of aggression inevitably leads to more, with the ultimate aggression being murder—20–50% of murders in the USA occur within the family. Police are called in more domestic disputes than all other criminal incidents combined. Children living in such family situations frequently become victims of abuse.

Features of individuals who have been subjected to chronic physical or sexual abuse are as follows: trouble expressing anger, staying angry longer, general passivity in relationships, feeling "marked for life" with an accompanying feeling of deserving to be victimized, lack of trust, and dissociation of affect from experiences. They are prone to express their psychologic distress with somatization symptoms, often pain complaints. They may also have symptoms related to posttraumatic stress, as discussed above. The clinician should be suspicious about the origin of any injuries not fully explained, particularly if such incidents recur.

Treatment

A. Psychologic

Management of any violent individual includes appropriate psychologic maneuvers. Move slowly, talk slowly with clarity and reassurance, and evaluate the situation. Strive to create a setting that is minimally disturbing and eliminate people or things threatening to the violent individual. Do not threaten or abuse and do not touch or crowd the person. Allow no weapons in the area (an increasing problem in hospital emergency rooms). Proximity to a door is comforting to both the patient and the examiner. Use a negotiator the violent person can relate to comfortably. Food and drink are helpful in defusing the situation (as are cigarettes for those who smoke). Honesty is important. Make no false promises, bolster the patient's self-esteem, and continue to engage the subject verbally until the situation is under control. This type of individual does better with strong external controls to replace the lack of inner controls over the long term. Close probationary supervision and judicially mandated restrictions can be most helpful. There should be a major effort to help the individual avoid drug use (eg, Alcoholics Anonymous). Victims of abuse are essentially treated as any victim of trauma and, not infrequently, have evidence of posttraumatic stress disorder.

B. Pharmacologic

Pharmacologic means are often necessary whether or not psychologic approaches have been successful. This is particularly true in the agitated or psychotic patient. The drug of choice in psychotic aggressive states is haloperidol, 5–10 mg intramuscularly every hour until symptoms are alleviated. Benzodiazepine sedatives (eg, diazepam, 5 mg orally or intravenously every several hours) can be used for mild to moderate agitation, but an antipsychotic drug is preferred for management of the seriously violent and psychotic patient. Chronic aggressive states, particularly in retardation and brain damage (rule out causative organic conditions and medications such as anticholinergic drugs in amounts sufficient to cause confusion), have been ameliorated

with propranolol, 40–240 mg/d orally, or pindolol, 5 mg twice daily orally (pindolol causes less bradycardia and hypotension). Carbamazepine and valproic acid are effective in the treatment of aggression and explosive disorders, particularly when associated with known or suspected brain lesions. Lithium and SSRIs are also effective for some intermittent explosive outbursts. Buspirone (10–45 mg/d orally) is helpful for aggression, particularly in mentally retarded patients.

C. Physical

Physical management is necessary if psychologic and pharmacologic means are not sufficient. It requires the active and visible presence of an adequate number of personnel (five or six) to reinforce the idea that the situation is under control despite the patient's lack of inner controls. Such an approach often precludes the need for actual physical restraint. When adequate personnel are not available, however, two people shielded by a mattress (single-bed size) can usually corner and subdue the patient without injury to anyone. Seclusion rooms and restraints should be used only when necessary (ambulatory restraints are an alternative), and the patient must then be observed at frequent intervals. Design of corridors and seclusion rooms is important. Narrow corridors, small spaces, and crowded areas exacerbate the potential for violence in an anxious patient.

D. Other

The treatment of victims (eg, battered women) is challenging and often complicated by their reluctance to leave the situation. Reasons for staying vary, but common themes include the fear of more violence because of leaving; the hope that the situation may ameliorate (in spite of steady worsening); and the financial aspects of the situation, which are seldom to the woman's advantage. Concerns for the children often finally compel the woman to seek help. An early step is to get the woman into a therapeutic situation that provides the support of others in similar straits. Al-Anon is frequently a valuable asset and quite appropriate when alcohol is a factor. The group can support the victim while she gathers strength to consider alternatives without being paralyzed by fear. Many cities now offer temporary emergency centers and counseling. Use the available resources, attend to any medical or psychiatric problems, and maintain a compassionate interest. Some states now require physicians to report injuries caused by abuse to police authorities.

Abbott J et al: Domestic violence against women: Incidence and prevalence in an emergency department population. JAMA 1995;273:1763. [PMID: 776770] (The incidence of acute domestic violence among the 418 women with a current male partner was 11.7%.)

Kyriacou DN et al: Risk factors for injury to women from domestic violence against women. N Engl J Med 1999;341:1892. [PMID: 10601509]

Rodriguez MA et al: Patient attitudes about mandatory reporting of domestic violence: Implications for health care professionals. West J Med 1998;169:337. [PMID: 9866430] (Mandatory reporting may pose a threat to the safety of abused women.)

■ SUBSTANCE USE DISORDERS (DRUG DEPENDENCY, DRUG ABUSE)

The term "drug dependency" is used in a broad sense here to include both addictions and habituations. It involves the triad of compulsive drug use referred to as drug addiction, which includes (1) a **psychologic dependence** or craving and the behavior involved included in procurement of the drug; (2) **physiologic dependence,** with withdrawal symptoms on discontinuance of the drug; and (3) **tolerance,** ie, the need to increase the dose to obtain the desired effects. Drug dependency is a function of the amount of drug used and the duration of usage. The amount needed to produce dependency varies with the nature of the drug and the idiosyncratic nature of the user. The frequency of use is usually daily, and the duration is inevitably greater than 2–3 weeks. Polydrug abuse is very common. Transgenerational continuity of drug abuse is also common.

There is accumulating evidence that an impairment syndrome exists in many former (and current) drug users. It is believed that drug use produces damaged neurotransmitter receptor sites and that the consequent imbalance produces symptoms that may mimic other psychiatric illnesses. **"Kindling"**—repeated stimulation of the brain—renders the individual more susceptible to focal brain activity with minimal stimulation. Stimulants and depressants can produce kindling, leading to relatively spontaneous effects no longer dependent on the original stimulus. These effects may be manifested as mood swings, panic, psychosis, and occasionally overt seizure activity. The imbalance also results in personal nonproductivity: frequent job changes, marital problems, and generally erratic behavior. Patients with posttraumatic stress disorder frequently have treated themselves with a variety of drugs. Chronic abusers of a wide variety of drugs exhibit cerebral atrophy on CT scans, a finding that may relate to the above symptoms. Early recognition is important, mainly to establish realistic treatment programs that are chiefly symptom-directed.

The clinician faces three problems with substance abuse: (1) the prescribing of substances such as sedatives, stimulants, or narcotics that might produce dependency; (2) the treatment of individuals who have already abused drugs, most commonly alcohol; and (3) the detection of illicit drug use in patients presenting with psychiatric symptoms. The usefulness of urinalysis for detection of drugs varies markedly with different drugs and under different circumstances (pharmacokinetics is a major factor). Water-soluble drugs (eg, alcohol, stimulants, opioids) are eliminated in a day or so. Lipophilic substances (eg, barbiturates, tetrahydrocannabinol) appear in the urine over longer periods of time: several days in most cases, 1–2 months in chronic marijuana users. Sedative drug determinations are quite variable, amount of drug and duration of use being important determinants. False-positives can be a problem related to ingestion of some legitimate drugs (eg, phenytoin for barbiturates, phenylpropanolamine for amphetamines, chlorpromazine for opioids) and some foods (eg, poppy seeds for opioids, coca leaf tea for cocaine). Manipulations can alter the legitimacy of the testing. Dilution, either in vivo or in vitro, can be detected by checking urine specific gravity. Addition of ammonia, vinegar, or salt may invalidate the test, but odor and pH determinations are simple. Hair analysis can determine drug use over longer periods, particularly sequential drug taking patterns. The sensitivity and reliability of such tests are considered good, and the method may be complementary to urinalysis.

Denning P: Strategies for implementation of harm reduction in treatment settings. J Psychoactive Drugs 2001;33:23. [PMID: 11332997] (Harm reduction involves a range of interventions, including abstinence, and emphasizes a collaborative model of care that is not punitive.)

Hughes JR et al: Recent advances in the pharmacotherapy of smoking. JAMA 1999;281:72. [PMID: 9892454] (Pharmacotherapy can be effective and should be made available to patients.)

Phillips DP et al: An increase in the number of deaths in the United States in the first week of the month—an association with substance abuse and other causes of death. N Engl J Med 1999; 341:93. [PMID: 10395634]

ALCOHOL DEPENDENCY & ABUSE (Alcoholism)

 ESSENTIALS OF DIAGNOSIS

Major criteria:

- *Physiologic dependence as manifested by evidence of withdrawal when intake is interrupted.*
- *Tolerance to the effects of alcohol.*
- *Evidence of alcohol-associated illnesses, such as alcoholic liver disease, cerebellar degeneration.*
- *Continued drinking despite strong medical and social contraindications and life disruptions.*
- *Impairment in social and occupational functioning.*
- *Depression.*
- *Blackouts.*

Other signs:

- *Alcohol stigmas: alcohol odor on breath, alcoholic facies, flushed face, scleral injection, tremor, ecchymoses, peripheral neuropathy.*
- *Surreptitious drinking.*
- *Unexplained work absences.*
- *Frequent accidents, falls, or injuries of vague origin; in smokers, cigarette burns on hands or chest.*
- *Laboratory tests (elevated values of liver function tests, mean corpuscular volume, serum uric acid and triglycerides).*

General Considerations

Alcoholism is a syndrome consisting of two phases: problem drinking and alcohol addiction. Problem drinking is the repetitive use of alcohol, often to alleviate anxiety or solve other emotional problems. Alcohol addiction is a true addiction similar to that which occurs following the repeated use of other sedative-hypnotics. Alcohol and other drug abuse patients have a much higher prevalence of lifetime psychiatric disorders. While male-to-female ratios in alcoholic treatment agencies remain at 4:1, there is evidence that the rates are converging. Women delay seeking help, and when they do they tend to seek it in medical or mental health settings. Adoption and twin studies indicate some genetic influence. Ethnic distinctions are important—eg, 40% of Japanese have aldehyde dehydrogenase deficiency and are more susceptible to the effects of alcohol. Depression is often present and should be evaluated carefully. The majority of suicides and intrafamily homicides involve alcohol, and alcohol is a major factor in rapes and other assaults also.

There are several screening instruments that may help identify alcoholism. One of the most useful is the CAGE questionnaire (Table 1–10).

Clinical Findings

A. ACUTE INTOXICATION

The signs of alcoholic intoxication are the same as those of overdosage with any other central nervous system depressant: drowsiness, errors of commission, psychomotor dysfunction, disinhibition, dysarthria, ataxia, and nystagmus. For a 70-kg person, an ounce of whiskey, a 4- to 6-oz glass of wine, or a 12-oz bottle of beer (roughly 15, 11, and 13 grams of alcohol, respectively) may raise the level of alcohol in the blood by 25 mg/dL. For a 50-kg person, the blood alcohol level would rise even higher (35 mg/dL) with the same consumption. Blood alcohol levels below 50 mg/dL rarely cause significant motor dysfunction. Intoxication as manifested by ataxia, dysarthria, and nausea and vomiting indicates a blood level above 150

mg/dL, and lethal blood levels range from 350 to 900 mg/dL. In severe cases, overdosage is marked by respiratory depression, stupor, seizures, shock syndrome, coma, and death. Serious overdoses are frequently due to a combination of alcohol with other sedatives.

B. WITHDRAWAL

There is a wide spectrum of manifestations of alcoholic withdrawal, ranging from anxiety, decreased cognition, and tremulousness through increasing irritability and hyperreactivity to full-blown **delirium tremens.** Symptoms of mild withdrawal, including tremor, elevated vital signs, and anxiety, begin within about 8 hours after the last drink and usually have passed by day 3. Generalized seizures occur within the first 24–38 hours and are more prevalent in persons who have a history of withdrawal syndromes. Delirium tremens is an acute organic psychosis that is usually manifest within 24–72 hours after the last drink (but may occur up to 7–10 days later). It is characterized by mental confusion, tremor, sensory hyperacuity, visual hallucinations (often of snakes, bugs, etc), autonomic hyperactivity, diaphoresis, dehydration, electrolyte disturbances (hypokalemia, hypomagnesemia), seizures, and cardiovascular abnormalities. The acute withdrawal syndrome is often completely unexpected and occurs when the patient has been hospitalized for some unrelated problem and presents as a diagnostic problem. Suspect alcohol withdrawal in every unexplained delirium. The mortality rate from delirium tremens has steadily decreased with early diagnosis and improved treatment.

In addition to the immediate withdrawal symptoms, there is evidence of persistent longer-term ones, including sleep disturbances, anxiety, depression, excitability, fatigue, and emotional volatility. These symptoms may persist for 3–12 months, and in some cases they become chronic.

C. ALCOHOLIC (ORGANIC) HALLUCINOSIS

This syndrome occurs either during heavy drinking or on withdrawal and is characterized by a paranoid psychosis without the tremulousness, confusion, and clouded sensorium seen in withdrawal syndromes. The patient appears normal except for the auditory hallucinations, which are frequently persecutory and may cause the patient to behave aggressively and in a paranoid fashion.

D. CHRONIC ALCOHOLIC BRAIN SYNDROMES

These encephalopathies are characterized by increasing erratic behavior, memory and recall problems, and emotional instability—the usual signs of organic brain injury due to any cause. Wernicke-Korsakoff syndrome due to thiamin deficiency may develop with a series of episodes. Wernicke's encephalopathy consists of the triad of confusion, ataxia, and ophthalmoplegia (typically sixth nerve). Early recognition and treatment with thiamine can minimize damage. One of the possible sequelae is Korsakoff's psychosis, characterized by both anterograde and retrograde amnesia, with confabulation early in the course. Early recognition and treatment of the alcoholic with intravenous thiamine and B complex vitamins can minimize damage.

Differential Diagnosis

The differential diagnosis of problem drinking is essentially between primary alcoholism (when no other major psychiatric diagnosis exists) and secondary alcoholism, when alcohol is used as self-medication for major underlying psychiatric problems such as schizophrenia or affective disorder. The differentiation is important, since the latter group requires treatment for the specific psychiatric problem.

The differential diagnosis of alcohol withdrawal includes other sedative withdrawals and other causes of delirium. Acute alcoholic hallucinosis must be differentiated from other acute paranoid states such as amphetamine psychosis or paranoid schizophrenia. An accurate history is the most important differentiating factor. The history and laboratory test results (elevated liver function tests, increased mean corpuscular volume, increased serum uric acid and triglycerides, decreased serum potassium and magnesium) are the most important features in differentiating chronic organic brain syndromes due to alcohol from those due to other causes. The form of the brain syndrome is of little help—eg, chronic brain syndromes from lupus erythematosus may be associated with confabulation similar to that resulting from long-standing alcoholism.

Complications

The medical, economic, and psychosocial problems of alcoholism are staggering. The central and peripheral nervous system complications include chronic brain syndromes, cerebellar degeneration, cardiomyopathy, and peripheral neuropathies. Direct effects on the liver include cirrhosis, esophageal varices, and eventual hepatic failure. Indirect effects include protein abnormalities, coagulation defects, hormone deficiencies, and an increased incidence of liver neoplasms.

Fetal alcohol syndrome includes one or more of the following developmental defects in the offspring of alcoholic women: (1) low birth weight and small size with failure to catch up in size or weight; (2) mental retardation, with an average IQ in the 60s; and (3) a variety of birth defects, with a large percentage of facial and cardiac abnormalities. The fetuses are very quiet in utero, and there is an increased frequency of breech presentations. There is a higher incidence of delayed postnatal growth and behavior development. The risk is appreciably higher the more alcohol ingested by the mother each day. Cigarette and marijuana smoking as well as cocaine use can produce similar effects on the fetus.

Treatment of Problem Drinking

A. PSYCHOLOGIC

The most important consideration for the clinician is to suspect the problem early and take a nonjudgmental attitude, though this does not mean a passive one. The problem of **denial** must be faced, preferably with significant family members at the first meeting. This means dealing from the beginning with any enabling behavior of the spouse or other significant people. Enabling behavior allows the alcoholic to avoid facing the consequences of his or her behavior.

There must be an emphasis on the things that can be done. This approach emphasizes the fact that the clinician cares and strikes a positive and hopeful note early in treatment. Valuable time should not be wasted trying to find out why the patient drinks; come to grips early with the immediate problem of how to stop the drinking. Total abstinence (not "controlled drinking") should be the goal.

B. SOCIAL

Get the patient into Alcoholics Anonymous (AA) and the spouse into Al-Anon. Success is usually proportionate to the utilization of AA, religious counseling, and other resources. The patient should be seen frequently for short periods and charged an appropriate fee.

Do not underestimate the importance of religion, particularly since the alcoholic is often a dependent person who needs a great deal of support. Early enlistment of the help of a concerned religious adviser can often provide the turning point for a personal conversion to sobriety.

One of the most important considerations is the patient's job—fear of losing a job is one of the most powerful motivations for giving up drink. The business community has become painfully aware of the problem, with the result that about 70% of the Fortune 500 companies offer programs to their employees to help with the problem of alcoholism. In the latter case, some specific recommendations to employers can be offered: (1) Avoid placement in jobs where the alcoholic must be alone, eg, as a traveling buyer or sales executive. (2) Use supervision but not surveillance. (3) Keep competition with others to a minimum. (4) Avoid positions that require quick decision making on important matters (high stress situations).

C. MEDICAL

Hospitalization is not usually necessary. It is sometimes used to dramatize a situation and force the patient to face the problem of alcoholism, but generally it should be used on medical indications.

Because of the many medical complications of alcoholism, a complete physical examination with appropriate laboratory tests is mandatory, with special attention to the liver and nervous system. Two tests that may provide clues to an alcohol problem are γ-glutamyl transpeptidase measurement (levels above 30 units/L are suggestive of heavy drinking) and mean corpuscular volume (> 95 fL in men and > 100 fL in women). If both are elevated, a serious drinking problem is likely. Use of other recreational drugs with alcohol skews and negates the significance of these tests. HDL cholesterol elevations combined with elevated γ-glutamyl transpeptidase concentrations also can help to identify heavy drinkers.

Use of sedatives as a replacement for alcohol is not desirable. The usual result is concomitant use of sedatives and alcohol and worsening of the problem. Lithium is not helpful in the treatment of alcoholism.

Disulfiram (250–500 mg/d orally) has been used for many years as an aversive drug to discourage alcohol use. Disulfiram inhibits alcohol dehydrogenase, causing toxic reactions when alcohol is consumed. The results have generally been of limited effectiveness and depend on the motivation of the individual to be compliant.

Naltrexone, an opiate antagonist, in a dosage of 50 mg daily, has been helpful in lowering relapse rates over the 3–6 months after cessation of drinking, apparently by lessening the pleasurable effects of alcohol. One study suggests that naltrexone is most efficacious when given during periods of drinking in combination with therapy that supports abstinence but accepts the fact that relapses occur. Naltrexone is FDA-approved for maintenance therapy. Studies indicate that it reduces alcohol craving when used as part of a comprehensive treatment program.

A double-blind study suggests that ondansetron, a selective 5-HT$_3$ receptor blocker, effectively reduces alcohol consumption and increases abstinence in patients with early-onset (under age 26) alcoholism. A dose of 4 μg/kg twice daily is the most efficacious among a range of doses tested. The study suggests an underlying serotonergic abnormality in the early-onset subtype. Early-onset alcoholism is associated with a family history of alcoholism, more severe disease course, and psychiatric comorbidity. Any pharmacologic intervention should be accompanied by psychosocial treatment.

D. BEHAVIORAL

Conditioning approaches have been used in some settings in the treatment of alcoholism, most commonly as a type of aversion therapy. For example, the patient is given a drink of whiskey and then a shot of apomorphine, and proceeds to vomit. In this way a strong association is built up between the vomiting and the drinking. Although this kind of treatment has been successful in some cases, many people do not sustain the learned aversive response.

Treatment of Hallucinosis & Withdrawal

A. MEDICAL

1. Alcoholic hallucinosis—Alcoholic hallucinosis, which can occur either during or on cessation of a prolonged drinking period, is not a typical withdrawal syndrome and is handled differently. Since the symptoms are primarily those of a psychosis in the presence of a clear sensorium, they are handled like any other psychosis: hospitalization (when indicated) and adequate amounts of antipsychotic drugs. Haloperidol, 5 mg orally twice a day for the first day or so, usually ameliorates symptoms quickly, and the drug can be decreased and discontinued over several days as the patient improves. It then becomes necessary to deal with the chronic alcohol abuse, which has been discussed.

2. Withdrawal symptoms—The onset of withdrawal symptoms is usually 8–12 hours and the peak intensity of symptoms is 48–72 hours after alcohol consumption is stopped. Providing adequate central nervous system depressants (eg, benzodiazepines) is important to counteract the excitability resulting from sudden cessation of alcohol intake. The choice of a specific sedative is less important than using adequate doses to bring the patient to a level of moderate sedation, and this will vary from person to person. Mild dependency requires "drying out." In some instances for outpatients, a short course of tapering benzodiazepines—eg, 20 mg of diazepam initially, decreasing by 5 mg daily—may be a useful adjunct. In moderate to severe withdrawal, hospitalize the patient and use diazepam orally in a dosage of 5–10 mg hourly depending on the clinical need as judged by withdrawal symptoms, including nausea, tremor, autonomic hyperactivity, agitation; tactile, visual, and auditory hallucinations; and disorientation. This type of symptom-driven medication regimen for withdrawal appears to reduce total benzodiazepine usage over fixed-dose schedules. Antipsychotic drugs should not be used. Monitoring of vital signs and fluid and electrolyte levels is essential for the severely ill patient.

In very severe withdrawal, intravenous administration is necessary. After stabilization, the amount of diazepam required to maintain a sedated state may be given orally every 8–12 hours. If restlessness, tremulousness, and other signs of withdrawal persist, the dosage is increased until moderate sedation occurs. The dosage is then gradually reduced by 20% every 24 hours until withdrawal is complete. This usually requires a week or so of treatment. Clonidine, 5 μg/kg orally every 2 hours, or the patch formulation of appropriate dosage strength, suppresses cardiovascular signs of withdrawal and has some anxiolytic effect. Carbamazepine, 400–800 mg daily orally, compares favorably with benzodiazepines for alcohol withdrawal.

Atenolol, as an adjunct to benzodiazepines, can reduce symptoms of alcohol withdrawal. The daily oral atenolol dose is 100 mg when the heart rate is above 80 beats per minute and 50 mg for a heart rate between 50 and 80 beats per minute. Atenolol should not be used when bradycardia is present.

Meticulous examination for other medical problems is necessary. Alcoholic hypoglycemia can occur with low blood alcohol levels (see Chapter 27). Alcoholics commonly have liver disease and associated clotting problems and are also prone to injury—and the combination all too frequently leads to undiagnosed subdural hematoma.

Phenytoin does not appear to be useful in managing alcohol withdrawal seizures per se. Sedating doses of benzodiazepines are effective in treating alcohol withdrawal seizures. Thus, other anticonvulsants are not usually needed unless there is a preexisting seizure disorder.

A general diet should be given, and vitamins in high doses: thiamine, 50 mg intravenously initially, then intramuscularly on a daily basis; pyridoxine, 100 mg/d; folic acid, 1 mg/d; and ascorbic acid, 100 mg twice a day. Intravenous glucose solutions should not be given prior to thiamine for fear of precipitation of Wernicke's syndrome. Thiamine is necessary as a ketolase enzyme cofactor. Concurrent administration is satisfactory, and hydration should be meticulously assessed on an ongoing basis.

Chronic brain syndromes secondary to a long history of alcohol intake are not clearly responsive to thiamine and vitamin replenishment. Attention to the social and environmental care of this type of patient is paramount.

B. Psychologic and Behavioral

The comments in the section on problem drinking apply here also; these methods of treatment become the primary consideration after successful treatment of withdrawal or alcoholic hallucinosis. Psychologic and social measures should be initiated in the hospital shortly before discharge. This increases the possibility of continued posthospitalization treatment.

Adams WL et al: Screening for problem drinking in older primary care patients. JAMA 1996;276:1964. [PMID: 89711065] (The CAGE survey and other questions can identify alcohol abuse in elderly populations.)

Cornelius JR et al: Fluoxetine in depressed alcoholics. Arch Gen Psychiatry 1997;54:700. [PMID: 9283504] (In patients with major depression and alcohol dependence, fluoxetine reduces symptoms and alcohol consumption.)

JAMA patient page: Alcohol. JAMA 1999;281:1352. [PMID: 10208153]

Johnson BA: Ondansetron for reduction of drinking among biologically predisposed alcoholic patients. JAMA 2000;284:963. [PMID: 10944641] (Ondansetron may reduce consumption in some patients with early-onset alcoholism.)

Sinclair JD: Evidence about the use of naltrexone and for different ways of using it in the treatment of alcoholism. Alcohol Alcohol 2001;36:2. [PMID: 11139409]

See also Substance Abuse references in Chapter 1.

OTHER DRUG & SUBSTANCE DEPENDENCIES

Opioids

The terms "opioids" and "narcotics" are used interchangeably and include a group of drugs with actions that mimic those of morphine. The group includes natural derivatives of opium (opiates), synthetic surrogates (opioids), and a number of polypeptides, some of which have been discovered to be natural neurotransmitters. The principal narcotic of abuse is heroin (metabolized to morphine), which is not used as a legitimate medication. The other common narcotics are prescription drugs and differ in milligram potency, duration of action, and agonist and antagonist capabilities (see Chapter 1). All of the narcotic analgesics can be reversed by the narcotic antagonist naloxone.

The clinical symptoms and signs of mild narcotic intoxication include changes in mood, with feelings of euphoria; drowsiness; nausea with occasional emesis; needle tracks; and miosis. The incidence of snorting and inhaling heroin ("smoking") is increasing, particularly among cocaine users. This coincides with a decrease in the availability of methaqualone (no longer marketed) and other sedatives used to temper the cocaine "high" (see discussion of cocaine under Stimulants, below). Overdosage causes respiratory depression, peripheral vasodilation, pinpoint pupils, pulmonary edema, coma, and death.

Dependency is a major concern when continued use of narcotics occurs, though withdrawal causes only moderate morbidity (similar in severity to a bout of "flu"). Addicted patients sometimes consider themselves more addicted than they really are and may not require a withdrawal program. Grades of withdrawal are categorized from 0 to 4: grade 0 includes craving and anxiety; grade 1, yawning, lacrimation, rhinorrhea, and perspiration; grade 2, previous symptoms plus mydriasis, piloerection, anorexia, tremors, and hot and cold flashes with generalized aching; grades 3 and 4, increased intensity of previous symptoms and signs, with increased temperature, blood pressure, pulse, and respiratory rate and depth. In withdrawal from the most severe addiction, vomiting, diarrhea, weight loss, hemoconcentration, and spontaneous ejaculation or orgasm commonly occur. Complications of heroin administration include infections (eg, pneumonia, septic emboli, hepatitis, and HIV infection from using nonsterile needles), traumatic insults (eg, arterial spasm due to drug injection, gangrene), and pulmonary edema.

Treatment for overdosage (or suspected overdosage) is naloxone, 2 mg intravenously. If an overdose has been taken, the results are dramatic and occur within 2 minutes. Since the duration of action of naloxone is much shorter than that of the narcotics, the patient must be under close observation. Hospitalization, supportive care, repeated naloxone administration, and observation for withdrawal from other drugs should be maintained for as long as necessary.

Treatment for withdrawal begins if grade 2 signs develop. If a withdrawal program is necessary, use methadone, 10 mg orally (use parenteral administration if the patient is vomiting), and observe. If signs (piloerection, mydriasis, cardiovascular changes) persist for more than 4–6 hours, give another 10 mg; continue to administer methadone at 4- to 6-hour intervals until signs are not present (rarely more than 40 mg of methadone in 24 hours). Divide the total amount of drug required over the first 24-hour period by 2 and give that amount every 12 hours. Each day, reduce the total 24-hour dose by 5–10 mg. Thus, a moderately addicted patient initially requiring 30–40 mg of methadone could be withdrawn over a 4- to 8-day period. Clonidine, 0.1 mg several times daily over a 10- to 14-day period, is both an alternative and an adjunct to methadone detoxification; it is not necessary to taper the dose. Clonidine is helpful in alleviating cardiovascular symptoms but does not significantly relieve anxiety, insomnia, or generalized aching. There is a protracted abstinence syndrome of metabolic, respiratory, and blood pressure changes over a period of 3–6 months.

Alternative strategies for the treatment of opioid withdrawal include rapid and ultrarapid detoxification techniques. In rapid detoxification, withdrawal is precipitated by opioid antagonists followed by naltrexone maintenance. Ultrarapid detoxification precipitates withdrawal with opioid antagonists under general anesthesia in a hospital. The impact of rapid detoxification on relapse rates, compared to more traditional methods, is not known at this time. The research literature on these techniques is limited.

Methadone maintenance programs are of some value in chronic recidivism. Under carefully controlled supervision, the narcotic addict is maintained on fairly high doses of methadone (40–120 mg/d) that satisfy craving and block the effects of heroin to a great degree.

Narcotic antagonists (eg, naltrexone) can also be used successfully for treatment of the patient who has been free of opioids for 7–10 days. Naltrexone blocks the narcotic "high" of heroin when 50 mg is given orally every 24 hours initially for several days and then 100 mg is given every 48–72 hours. Liver disorders are a major contraindication. Compliance tends to be poor, partly because of the dysphoria that can persist long after opioid discontinuance.

Sedatives (Anxiolytics)

See Anxiety Disorders, this chapter.

Psychedelics

About 6000 species of plants have psychoactive properties. All of the common psychedelics (LSD, mescaline, psilocybin, dimethyltryptamine, and other derivatives of phenylalanine and tryptophan) can produce similar behavioral and physiologic effects. An initial feeling of tension is followed by emotional release such as crying or laughing (1–2 hours). Later, perceptual distortions occur, with visual illusions and hallucinations, and occasionally there is fear of ego disintegration (2–3 hours). Major changes in time sense and mood lability then occur (3–4 hours). A feeling of detachment and a sense of destiny and control occur (4–6 hours). Of course, reactions vary among individuals, and some of the drugs produce markedly different time frames. Occasionally, the acute episode is terrifying (a "bad trip") which may include panic, depression, confusion, or psychotic symptoms. Preexisting emotional problems, the attitude of the user, and the setting where the drug is used affect the experience.

Treatment of the acute episode primarily involves protection of the individual from erratic behavior that may lead to injury or death. A structured environment is usually sufficient until the drug is metabolized. In severe cases, antipsychotic drugs with minimal side effects (eg, haloperidol, 5 mg intramuscularly) may be given every several hours until the individual has regained control. In cases where "flashbacks" occur (mental imagery from a "bad trip" that is later triggered by mild stimuli such as marijuana, alcohol, or psychic trauma), a short course of an antipsychotic drug—(eg, olanzapine, 5–10 mg/d, or risperidone, 2 mg/d, initially, and up to 20 mg/d and 6 mg/d, respectively—is usually sufficient. Lorazepam, 1–2 mg orally or intramuscularly every 2 hours as needed for acute agitation, maybe a useful adjunct. An occasional patient may have "flashbacks" for much longer periods and require small doses of neuroleptic drugs over the longer term.

Phencyclidine

Phencyclidine (PCP, angel dust, peace pill, hog), developed as an anesthetic agent, first appeared as a street drug deceptively sold as tetrahydrocannabinol (THC). Because it is simple to produce and mimics to some degree the traditional psychedelic drugs, PCP has become a common deceptive substitute for LSD, THC, and mescaline. It is available in crystals, capsules, and tablets to be inhaled, injected, swallowed, or smoked (it is commonly sprinkled on marijuana).

Absorption after smoking is rapid, with onset of symptoms in several minutes and peak symptoms in 15–30 minutes. Mild intoxication produces euphoria accompanied by a feeling of numbness. Moderate intoxication (5–10 mg) results in disorientation, detachment from surroundings, distortion of body image, combativeness, unusual feats of strength (partly due to its anesthetic activity), and loss of ability to integrate sensory input, especially touch and proprioception. Physical symptoms include dizziness, ataxia, dysarthria, nystagmus, retracted upper eyelid with blank stare, hyperreflexia, and tachycardia. There are increases in blood pressure, respiration, muscle tone, and urine production. Usage in the first trimester of pregnancy is associated with an increase in spontaneous abortion and congenital defects. Severe intoxication (20 mg or more) produces an increase in degree of moderate symptoms, with the addition of seizures, deepening coma, hypertensive crisis, and severe psychotic ideation. The drug is particularly long-lasting (several days to several weeks) owing to high lipid solubility, gastroenteric recycling, and the production of active metabolites. Overdosage may be fatal, with the major causes of death being hypertensive crisis, respiratory arrest, and convulsions. Acute rhabdomyolysis has been reported and can result in myoglobinuric renal failure.

Differential diagnosis involves the whole spectrum of street drugs, since in some ways phencyclidine mimics sedatives, psychedelics, and marijuana in its effects. Blood and urine testing can detect the acute problem.

Treatment is discussed in Chapter 39.

Marijuana

Cannabis sativa, a hemp plant, is the source of marijuana. The parts of the plant vary in potency. The resinous exudate of the flowering tops of the female plant (hashish, charas) is the most potent, followed by the dried leaves and flowering shoots of the female plant (bhang) and the resinous mass from small leaves of inflorescence (ganja). The least potent parts are the lower branches and the leaves of the female plant and all parts of the male plant. Mercury may be a contaminant in marijuana grown in volcanic soil. The drug is usually inhaled by smoking. Effects occur in 10–20 minutes and last 2–3 hours. "Joints" of good quality contain about 500 mg of marijuana (which contains approximately 5–15 mg of tetrahydrocannabinol with a half-life of 7 days). Marijuana soaked in formaldehyde and dried ("AMP") has produced unusual effects, including autonomic discharge and severe though transient cognitive impairment.

With moderate dosage, marijuana produces two phases: mild euphoria followed by sleepiness. In the acute state, the user has an altered time perception, less inhibited emotions, psychomotor problems, impaired immediate memory, and conjunctival injection. High doses produce transient psychotomimetic effects. No specific treatment is necessary except in the case of the occasional "bad trip," in which case the person is treated in the same way as for psychedelic usage. Marijuana frequently aggravates existing mental illness and adversely affects motor performance.

Studies of long-term effects have conclusively shown abnormalities in the pulmonary tree. Laryngitis and rhinitis are related to prolonged use, along with chronic obstructive pulmonary disease. Electrocardiographic abnormalities are common, but no long-term cardiac disease has been linked to marijuana use. Chronic usage has resulted in depression of plasma testosterone levels and reduced sperm counts. Abnormal menstruation and failure to ovulate have occurred in some women. Cognitive impairments are probable, though studies are not conclusive. Health care utilization for a variety of health problems is increased in chronic marijuana smokers. Sudden withdrawal produces insomnia, nausea, myalgia, and irritability. Psychologic effects of chronic marijuana usage are still unclear. Urine testing is reliable if samples are carefully collected and tested. Detection periods span 4–6 days in acute users and 20–50 days in chronic users.

Stimulants: Amphetamines & Cocaine

Stimulant abuse is quite common, either alone or in combination with abuse of other drugs. The **amphetamines,** including Methedrine ("speed")—one variant is a smokable form called "ice," which gives an intense and fairly long-lasting high—methylphenidate, and phenmetrazine, are under prescription control, but street availability remains high. Moderate usage of any of the stimulants produces hyperactivity, a sense of enhanced physical and mental capacity, and sympathomimetic effects. The clinical picture of acute stimulant intoxication includes sweating, tachycardia, elevated blood pressure, mydriasis, hyperactivity, and an acute brain syndrome with confusion and disorientation. Tolerance develops quickly and, as the dosage is increased, hypervigilance, paranoid ideation (with delusions of parasitosis), stereotypy, bruxism, tactile hallucinations of insect infestation, and full-blown psychoses occur, often with persecutory ideation and aggressive responses. Stimulant withdrawal is characterized by depression with symptoms of hyperphagia and hypersomnia.

People who have used stimulants chronically (eg, anorexigenics) occasionally become sensitized (**"kindling"**) to future use of stimulants. In these individuals, even small amounts of mild stimulants such as caffeine can cause symptoms of paranoia and auditory hallucinations.

Cocaine is a stimulant. It is a product of the coca plant. The derivatives include seeds, leaves, coca paste, cocaine hydrochloride, and the free base of cocaine. Coca paste is a crude extract that contains 40–80% cocaine sulfate and other impurities. Cocaine hydrochloride is the salt and the most commonly used form. Free base, a purer (and stronger) derivative called "crack," is prepared by simple extraction from cocaine hydrochloride.

There are various modes of use. Coca leaf chewing involves toasting the leaves and chewing with alkaline material (eg, the ash of other burned leaves) to enhance buccal absorption. One achieves a mild high, with onset in 5–10 minutes and lasting for about an hour. Intranasal use is simply snorting cocaine through a straw. Absorption is slowed somewhat by vasoconstriction (which may eventually cause tissue necrosis and septal perforation); the onset of action is in 2–3 minutes, with a moderate high (euphoria, excitement, increased energy) lasting about 30 minutes. The purity of the cocaine is a major determinant of the high. Intravenous use of cocaine hydrochloride or "freebase" is effective in 30 seconds and produces a short-lasting, fairly intense high of about 15 minutes' duration. The combined use of cocaine and ethanol results in the metabolic production of cocaethylene by the liver. This substance produces more intense and long-lasting cocaine-like effects. Smoking freebase (volatilized cocaine because of the lower boiling point) acts in seconds and results in an intense high lasting several minutes. The intensity of the reaction is related to the marked lipid solubility of the freebase form and produces by far the most severe medical and psychiatric symptoms.

Cardiovascular collapse, arrhythmias, myocardial infarction, and transient ischemic attacks have been reported. Seizures, strokes, migraine symptoms, hyperthermia, and lung damage may occur, and there are several obstetric complications, including spontaneous abortion, abruptio placentae, teratogenic effects, delayed fetal growth, and prematurity. Cocaine can cause anxiety, mood swings, and delirium, and chronic use can cause the same problems as other stimulants (see above).

Clinicians should be alert to cocaine use in patients presenting with unexplained nasal bleeding, headaches, fatigue, insomnia, anxiety, depression, and chronic hoarseness. Sudden withdrawal of the drug is not life-threatening but usually produces craving, sleep disturbances, hyperphagia, lassitude, and severe depression (sometimes with suicidal ideation) lasting days to weeks.

Treatment is imprecise and difficult. Since the high is related to blockage of dopamine reuptake, the dopamine agonist bromocriptine, 1.5 mg orally three times a day, alleviates some of the symptoms of craving associated with acute cocaine withdrawal. Other dopamine agonists such as apomorphine, levodopa, and amantadine are under study for this purpose. Carbamazepine may be a useful adjunct in treating symptoms of alcohol withdrawal, and desipramine in moderate doses has been useful in helping maintain abstinence in the early stages of treatment. Treatment of psychosis is the same as that of any psychosis: antipsychotic drugs in dosages sufficient to alleviate the symptoms. Any medical symptoms (eg, hyperthermia, seizures, hypertension) are treated specifically. These approaches should be used in conjunction with a structured program, most often based on the Alcoholics Anonymous model. Hospitalization may be required if self-harm or violence toward others is a perceived threat (usually indicated by paranoid delusions).

Caffeine

Caffeine, along with nicotine and alcohol, is one of the most commonly used drugs worldwide. About 10 billion pounds of coffee (the richest source of caffeine) are consumed yearly throughout the world. Tea, cocoa, and cola drinks also contribute to an intake of caffeine that is often astoundingly high in a large number of people. Low to moderate doses (30–200 mg/d) tend to improve some aspects of performance (eg, vigilance). The approximate content of caffeine in a (180 mL) cup of beverage is as follows: brewed coffee, 80–140 mg; instant coffee, 60–100 mg; decaffeinated coffee, 1–6 mg; black leaf tea, 30–80 mg; tea bags, 25–75 mg; instant tea, 30–60 mg; cocoa, 10–50 mg; and 12-oz cola drinks, 30–65 mg. A 2-oz chocolate candy bar has about 20 mg. Some herbal teas (eg, "morning thunder") contain caffeine. Caffeine-containing analgesics usually contain approximately 30 mg per unit. Symptoms of caffeinism (usually associated with ingestion of over 500 mg/d) include anxiety, agitation, restlessness, insomnia, a feeling of being "wired," and somatic symptoms referable to the heart and gastrointestinal tract. It is common for a case of caffeinism to present as an anxiety disorder. It is also common for caffeine and other stimulants to precipitate severe symptoms in

compensated schizophrenic and manic-depressive patients. Chronically depressed patients often use caffeine drinks as self-medication. This diagnostic clue may help distinguish some major affective disorders. Withdrawal from caffeine (> 250 mg/d) can produce headaches, irritability, lethargy, and occasional nausea.

Miscellaneous Drugs, Solvents

The principal OTC drugs of concern have been phenylpropanolamine and an assortment of antihistaminic agents, frequently in combination with a mild analgesic promoted as cold remedies (eg, Dristan, Triaminic). Appetite suppressant combinations of phenylpropanolamine and caffeine were also heavily marketed as "stay-awake" drugs. Practically all of the so-called sleep aids are now antihistamines. Scopolamine and bromides have generally been removed from OTC products.

The major problem in the use of all these drugs related to phenylpropanolamine, which had all the side effects of any stimulant, including precipitation of anxiety states, increased pressor effect, auditory and visual hallucinations, paranoid ideation, and occasionally delirium. Aggressiveness and some loss of impulse control were reported, as well as sleep disturbances even with small doses. Medications containing phenylpropanolamine have been removed from sale due to an FDA ban.

Antihistamines usually produce some central nervous system depression—thus their use as OTC sedatives. Drowsiness may be a problem. The mixture of antihistamines with alcohol usually exacerbates the central nervous system effects.

The abuse of laxatives sometimes can lead to electrolyte disturbances that may contribute to the manifestations of a delirium. The greatest use of laxatives tends to be in the elderly and in those with eating disorders, both of whom are the most vulnerable to physiologic changes.

Anabolic steroids are being abused by people who wish to increase muscle mass for cosmetic reasons or for greater strength. In addition to the medical problems, the practice is associated with significant mood swings, aggressiveness, and paranoid delusions. Alcohol and stimulant use is higher in these individuals. Withdrawal symptoms of steroid dependency include fatigue, depressed mood, restlessness, and insomnia.

Amyl nitrite has been used in recent years as an "orgasm expander." The changes in time perception, "rush," and mild euphoria caused by the drug prompted its nonmedical use, and popular lore concerning the effects of inhalation just prior to orgasm has led to increased use. Subjective effects last from 5 seconds to 15 minutes. Tolerance develops readily, but there are no known withdrawal symptoms. Abstinence for several days reestablishes the previous level of responsiveness. Long-term effects may include damage to the immune system and respiratory difficulties.

Sniffing of solvents and inhaling of gases (including aerosols) produce a form of inebriation similar to that of the volatile anesthetics. Agents include gasoline, toluene, petroleum ether, lighter fluids, cleaning fluids, paint thinners, and solvents that are present in many household products (eg, nail polish, typewriter correction fluid). Typical intoxication states include euphoria, slurred speech, hallucinations, and confusion, and with high doses, acute manifestations are unconsciousness and cardiorespiratory depression or failure; chronic exposure produces a variety of symptoms related to the liver, kidney, bone marrow, or heart. Lead encephalopathy can be associated with sniffing leaded gasoline. In addition, studies of workers chronically exposed to jet fuel showed significant increases in neurasthenic symptoms, including fatigue, anxiety, mood changes, memory difficulties, and somatic complaints. These same problems have been noted in long-term solvent abuse.

The so-called designer drugs are synthetic substitutes for commonly used recreational drugs and are produced in small, clandestine laboratories. The most common designer drugs have been methyl analogues of fentanyl and have been used as heroin substitutes. MDMA (methylenedioxymethamphetamine), an amphetamine derivative sometimes called "ecstasy," is also a designer drug with high abuse potential and neurotoxicity. Often not detected by standard toxicology screens, these substances can present a vexing problem for clinicians faced with symptoms from a totally unknown cause.

Harder S et al: Concentration-effect relationship of delta-9-tetrahydrocannabinol and prediction of psychotropic effects after smoking marijuana. Int J Clin Pharmacol Ther 1997; 35:155. [PMID: 9112136] (Smoking marijuana can lead to a plateau THC blood level that persists for 150 minutes after the last joint.)

National Consensus Development Panel on Effective Medical Treatment of Opiate Addiction: Effective medical treatment of opiate addiction. JAMA 1998;280:1936. [PMID: 9851480] (Patients with opiate dependence should have access to methadone hydrochloride maintenance therapy.)

O'Connor PG et al: Rapid and ultrarapid opioid detoxification techniques. JAMA 1998;279:229. [PMID: 9438745]

■ DELIRIUM, DEMENTIA, & OTHER COGNITIVE DISORDERS (Formerly: Organic Brain Syndrome [OBS])

ESSENTIALS OF DIAGNOSIS

- Transient or permanent brain dysfunction.
- Cognitive impairment to varying degrees: may include impaired recall and recent memory, inability to focus attention, random psychomotor activity such as stereotypy, and problems in perceptual processing, often with psychotic ideation.
- Emotional disorders frequently present: depression, anxiety, irritability.
- Behavioral disturbances may include problems of impulse control, sexual acting-out, attention deficits, aggression, and exhibitionism.

General Considerations

The organic problem may be a primary brain disease or a secondary manifestation of some general disorder. All of the cognitive disorders show some degree of impaired thinking depending on the site of involvement, the rate of onset and progression, and the duration of the underlying brain lesion. Emotional disturbances (eg, depression) are often present as significant comorbidities. The behavioral disturbances tend to be more common with chronicity, more directly related to the underlying personality or central nervous system vulnerability to drug side effects, and not necessarily correlated with cognitive dysfunction.

The causes of cognitive disorders are listed in Table 25–11.

Clinical Findings

The manifestations are many and varied and include problems with orientation, short or fluctuating attention span, loss of recent memory and recall, impaired judgment, emotional lability, lack of initiative, impaired impulse control, inability to reason through problems, depression (worse in mild to moderate types), confabulation (not limited to alcohol organic brain syndrome), constriction of intellectual functions, visual and auditory hallucinations, and delusions. Physical findings will naturally vary according to the cause. The EEG usually shows generalized slowing in delirium.

A. DELIRIUM

Delirium (acute confusional state) is a transient global disorder of attention, with clouding of consciousness, usually a result of systemic problems (eg, drugs, hypoxemia). Onset is usually rapid. The mental status fluctuates (impairment is usually least in the morning), with varying inability to concentrate, maintain attention, and sustain purposeful behavior. ("Sundowning"—mild to moderate delirium at night—is more common in patients with preexisting dementia and may be precipitated by hospitalization, drugs, and sensory deprivation.) There is a marked deficit of short-term memory and recall. Anxiety and irritability are common. Amnesia is retrograde (impaired recall of past memories) and anterograde (inability to recall events after the onset of the delirium). Orientation problems follow the inability to retain information. Perceptual disturbances (often visual hallucinations) and psychomotor restlessness with

Table 25–11. Etiology of delirium and other cognitive disorders

Disorder	Possible Causes
Intoxication	Alcohol, sedatives, bromides, analgesics (eg, pentazocine), psychedelic drugs, stimulants, and household solvents.
Drug withdrawal	Withdrawal from alcohol, sedative-hypnotics, corticosteroids
Long-term effects of alcohol	Wernicke-Korsakoff syndrome
Infections	Septicemia; meningitis and encephalitis due to bacterial, viral, fungal, parasitic, or tuberculous organisms or to central nervous system syphilis; acute and chronic infections due to the entire range of microbiologic pathogens.
Endocrine disorders	Thyrotoxicosis, hypothyroidism, adrenocortical dysfunction (including Addison's disease and Cushing's syndrome), pheochromocytoma, insulinoma, hypoglycemia, hyperparathyroidism, hypoparathyroidism, panhypopituitarism, diabetic ketoacidosis.
Respiratory disorders	Hypoxia, hypercapnia.
Metabolic disturbances	Fluid and electrolyte disturbances (especially hyponatremia, hypomagnesemia, and hypercalcemia), acid-base disorders, hepatic disease (hepatic encephalopathy), renal failure, porphyria.
Nutritional deficiencies	Deficiency of vitamin B_1 (beriberi), vitamin B_{12} (pernicious anemia), folic acid, nicotinic acid (pellagra); protein-calorie malnutrition.
Trauma	Subdural hematoma, subarachnoid hemorrhage, intracerebral bleeding, concussion syndrome.
Cardiovascular disorders	Myocardial infarctions, cardiac arrhythmias, cerebrovascular spasms, hypertensive encephalopathy, hemorrhages, embolisms, and occlusions indirectly cause decreased cognitive function.
Neoplasms	Primary or metastatic lesions of the central nervous system, cancer-induced hypercalcemia.
Seizure disorders	Ictal, interictal, and postictal dysfunction.
Collagen-vascular and immunologic disorders	Autoimmune disorders, including systemic lupus erythematosus, Sjögren's syndrome, and AIDS.
Degenerative diseases	Alzheimer's disease, Pick's disease, multiple sclerosis, parkinsonism, Huntington's chorea, normal pressure hydrocephalus.
Medications	Anticholinergic drugs, antidepressants, H_2-blocking agents, digoxin, salicylates (chronic use), and a wide variety of other OTC and prescribed drugs.

insomnia are common. Autonomic changes include tachycardia, dilated pupils, and sweating. The average duration is about 1 week, with full recovery in most cases. Delirium can coexist with dementia.

B. DEMENTIA

(See also Chapter 3.) Dementia is characterized by chronicity and deterioration of selective mental functions. Onset is insidious over months to years in most cases. Dementia is usually progressive, more common in the elderly, and rarely reversible even if underlying disease can be corrected. Dementia can be classified as cortical or subcortical.

There are three types of cortical dementia: (1) primary degenerative dementia (eg, Alzheimer's), accounting for about 50–60% of cases; (2) atherosclerotic (multi-infarct) dementia, 15–20% of cases (this figure is probably low because of the tendency to overuse the di-

agnosis of Alzheimer's dementia); and (3) mixtures of the first two types or dementia due to miscellaneous causes, 15–20% of cases (see also Chapter 3). Examples of primary degenerative dementia are Alzheimer's dementia (most common) and Pick, Creutzfeldt-Jakob, and Huntington dementias (less common).

In all types, loss of impulse control (sexual and language) is common. The tenuous level of functioning makes the individual most susceptible to minor physical and psychologic stresses. The course depends on the underlying cause, and the general trend is steady deterioration.

HIV infection can produce a primary neurogenic disorder (partially due to neuronal loss) and secondary effects due to opportunistic infections, neoplasias, or the effects of drug therapy. At present there has been a reduction in dementia symptoms in both early and late stages, perhaps due to earlier use of zidovudine.

The general trend is variable, and patients require ongoing monitoring of neuropsychiatric status.

Pseudodementia is a term applied to depressed patients who appear to be demented. These patients are often identifiable by their tendency to complain about memory problems vociferously rather than try to cover them up. They usually say they can't complete cognitive tasks but with encouragement can often do so.

C. AMNESTIC SYNDROME

This is a memory disturbance without delirium or dementia. It is usually associated with thiamin deficiency and chronic alcohol use (eg, Korsakoff's syndrome). There is an impairment in the ability to learn new information or recall previously learned information.

D. SUBSTANCE-INDUCED HALLUCINOSIS

This condition is characterized by persistent or recurrent hallucinations (usually auditory) without the other symptoms usually found in delirium or dementia. Alcohol or hallucinogens are often the cause. There does not have to be any other mental disorder, and there may be complete spontaneous resolution.

E. PERSONALITY CHANGES DUE TO A GENERAL MEDICAL CONDITION (FORMERLY ORGANIC PERSONALITY SYNDROME)

This syndrome is characterized by emotional lability and loss of impulse control along with a general change in personality. Cognitive functions are preserved. Social inappropriateness is common. Loss of interest and lack of concern with the consequences of one's actions are often present. The course depends on the underlying cause (eg, frontal lobe contusion may resolve completely).

Differential Diagnosis

The differential diagnosis consists mainly of schizophrenia and the other psychoses, which are sometimes confused with cognitive disorders which are often accompanied by psychotic symptoms.

Complications

Chronicity may result from delayed correction of the defect, eg, subdural hematoma, low-pressure hydrocephalus. Accidents secondary to impulsive behavior and poor judgment are a major consideration. Secondary depression and impulsive behavior not infrequently lead to suicide attempts. Drugs—particularly sedatives—may worsen thinking abilities and contribute to the overall problems.

Treatment

(See also Chapter 3.)

A. MEDICAL

Delirium should be considered a syndrome of acute brain dysfunction analogous to acute renal failure. The first aim of treatment is to identify and correct the etiologic medical problem. Evaluation should consist of a comprehensive physical examination including a search for neurologic abnormalities, infection, or hypoxia. Routine laboratory tests may include serum electrolytes, serum glucose, BUN, serum creatinine, liver function tests, thyroid function tests, arterial blood gases, complete blood count, serum calcium, phosphorus, magnesium, vitamin B_{12}, folate, blood cultures, urinalysis, and cerebrospinal fluid analysis. Discontinue drugs that may be contributing to the problem (eg, analgesics, corticosteroids, cimetidine, lidocaine, anticholinergic drugs, central nervous system depressants, mefloquine). Do not overlook any possibility of reversible organic disease. Electroencephalography, CT, MRI, PET, and SPECT evaluations may be helpful in diagnosis. Ideally, the patient should be monitored without further medications while the evaluation is carried out. There are, however, two indications for medication in delirious states: behavioral control (eg, pulling out lines) and subjective distress (eg, pronounced fear due to hallucinations). If these indications are present, medications may be employed. If there is any hint of alcohol or substance withdrawal (the most common cause of delirium in the general hospital), a benzodiazepine such as lorazepam (1–2 mg every hour) can be given parenterally. If there is little likelihood of withdrawal syndrome, haloperidol is often used in doses of 1–10 mg every hour. Given intravenously, it appears to impose slight risk of extrapyramidal side effects. In addition to the medication, a pleasant, comfortable, nonthreatening, and physically safe environment with adequate nursing or attendant services should be provided. Once the underlying condition has been identified and treated, adjunctive medications can be tapered.

Treatment of dementia syndrome usually involves symptomatic management with one exception. Since there is a cholinergic deficiency in Alzheimer's disease, research has focused on drugs to increase cholinergic activity by inhibiting cholinesterase. Tacrine (tetrahydroaminoacridine; THA) is the first reversible cholinesterase inhibitor approved by the FDA for the treatment of cognitive deficits associated with Alzheimer's disease. Studies suggest that tacrine (80–160 mg/d in four divided doses) may improve cognition in 25–42% of patients, with higher doses producing better effects. There was, however, no functional improvement in the subjects. Serum ALT levels increase in half of patients, requiring hepatic monitoring. Most levels return to normal when the drug is discontinued. Three newer FDA-approved cholinesterase inhibitors are donepezil (5–10 mg at night), rivastigmine (3–6 mg twice daily), and galantamine (8–12 mg twice daily, adjusted for renal and hepatic impairment). They are thought to be efficacious in the short-term preservation of cognitive function and activities of daily living in mild to moderate dementia and, unlike tacrine, are not thought to be hepatotoxic. Gastrointestinal side effects are common but may be least frequent with donepezil. Further research continues to clarify the long-term efficacy of these medications on cognition and behavior. None of the cholinesterase inhibitors to date are thought to slow disease progression.

Aggressiveness and rage states in central nervous system disease can be reduced with lipophilic beta-blockers (eg, propranolol, metoprolol) in moderate doses. Since the serotonergic system has been implicated in arousal conditions, drugs that affect serotonin have been found to be of some benefit in aggression and agitation. Included in this group are lithium, trazodone, buspirone, and clonazepam. Dopamine blockers (eg, the neuroleptic drugs such as haloperidol) have been used for many years to attenuate aggression. Atypical neuroleptics appear to have a role. There are also recent reports of reduced agitation in Alzheimer's disease from carbamazepine, 100–400 mg/d orally (with slow increase as needed). Emotional lability in some cases responds to small doses of imipramine (25 mg orally one to three times per day) or fluoxetine (5–20 mg/d orally); and depression, which often occurs early in the course of Alzheimer's dementia, responds to the usual doses of antidepressant drugs, preferably those with the least anticholinergic side effects (eg, SSRIs and MAO inhibitors).

Cerebral vasodilators were originally used on the assumption that cerebral arteriosclerosis and ischemia were the principal causes of the dementias. Although there is a slight reduction of blood flow in primary degenerative dementia (probably as a result of the basic disorder), there is no evidence that this is a major factor in this group of disorders or that vasodilators are of value. Ergotoxine alkaloids (ergoloid mesylates: Hydergine, others) have been studied with mixed results; improvement in ambulatory self-care and depressed mood has been noted, but there has been no improvement of cognitive functioning on any standardized tests. Hyperbaric oxygen treatment has not produced significant improvement. Stimulant drugs (eg, methylphenidate) do not change cognitive function but can improve affect and mood, which helps the caretakers cope with the problem.

Failing sensory functions should be supported as necessary, with hearing aids, cataract surgery, etc.

B. SOCIAL

Substitute home care, board and care, or convalescent home care may be most useful when the family is unable to care for the patient. The setting should include familiar people and objects, lights at night, and a simple schedule. Counseling may help the family to cope with problems and may help keep the patient at home as long as possible. Information about local groups can be obtained from the Alzheimer's Disease and Related Disorders Association, 70 East Lake Street, Suite 600, Chicago, IL 60601. Volunteer services, including homemakers, visiting nurses, and adult protective services, may be helpful in maintaining the patient at home.

C. BEHAVIORAL

Behavioral techniques include operant responses that can be used to induce positive behaviors, eg, paying attention to the patient who is trying to communicate appropriately, and extinction by ignoring inappropriate responses. Alzheimer's patients can learn skills and retain them but do not recall the circumstances in which they were learned.

D. PSYCHOLOGIC

Formal psychologic therapies are not usually helpful and may make things worse by taxing the patient's limited cognitive resources.

Prognosis

The prognosis is good for recovery of mental functioning in delirium when the underlying condition is reversible. For most dementia syndromes, the prognosis is for gradual deterioration, though new drug treatments may prove helpful.

Delagarza VW: New drugs for Alzheimer's disease. Am Fam Physician 1998;58:1175. [PMID: 9787282]

Gruetzner H: *Alzheimer's: A Complete Guide for Families and Loved Ones.* Wiley, 1997. (An excellent guide for family caregivers.)

JAMA patient page: Alzheimer disease. JAMA 1998;280:674. [PMID: 9718065]

Rogers SL: Perspective in the management of Alzheimer's disease: Clinical profile of donepezil. Dement Geriatr Cogn Disord 1998;9:29. [PMID: 9853200]

■ GERIATRIC PSYCHIATRIC DISORDERS (See Also Chapter 4.)

There are three basic factors in the process of aging: biologic, sociologic, and psychologic.

The complex **biologic** changes depend on inherited characteristics (the best chance of long life is to have long-lived parents), nutrition, declining sensory functions such as hearing or vision, disease, trauma, and lifestyle. A definite correlation between hearing loss and paranoid ideation exists in the elderly. (See Dementia, above.) As a person ages, relatively minor disorders or combinations of disorders may cause deficits in cognition and affective response. Hypochondriasis is frequently a mechanism of compensating for decreased function (eg, preoccupation with bowel function).

The **sociologic** factors derive from stresses connected with occupation, family, and community. Any or all of these areas may be disrupted in a general phenomenon of "disengagement" and lack of intimacy that older people experience as friends die, the children move away, and the surroundings become less familiar. Retirement commonly precipitates a major disruption in a well-established life structure. This is particularly stressful in the person whose compulsive devotion to a job has inhibited the development of other interests, so that sudden loss of this outlet leaves a void that is not easily filled. New duties, such as caring for a spouse with dementia, may also lead to depression.

The **psychologic** withdrawal of the elderly person is frequently related to a loss of self-esteem, which is based on the economic insecurity of older age with its congruent loss of independence, the recognition of decreasing physical and mental ability, loneliness, and the fear of approaching death. The process of aging is often poorly accepted, and the real or imagined loss of physical attractiveness may have a traumatic impact that the plastic surgeon can only soften for a time. In a culture that stresses physical and sexual attractiveness, it is difficult for some people to accept the change.

Clinical Findings & Complications

The most common psychiatric syndrome in the elderly is dementia of varying degrees. Psychotic ideation (usually paranoid) may coexist with dementia. Frequently, in milder cases, the individual is aware of the deficiency in cognition and becomes depressed about actual or threatened loss of function. Depression may then amplify the apparent cognitive decline.

Overt depression, often presenting as a somatic complaint, is often related to life changes (80% of people over age 65 have some kind of medical problem). Alcoholism is present in approximately 15% of older patients presenting with psychiatric symptoms. The incidence of suicide is higher in elderly people—loneliness, age, and medical problems being directly related. Deprivation of full-spectrum light may be a factor in some patients (eg, nursing home residents). Anxiety, often associated with organic illness, heightens preexisting confusion in the patient with cognitive dysfunction.

Abuse of the elderly—both physical neglect (passive) and physical injury (active)—demands early recognition. Bruises, welts, fractures, and debilitation should alert the clinician. The battered elderly are probably just as numerous as battered children, but less reported, and require the same diligence in clinician recognition.

Polypharmacy (with both prescription and OTC drugs) is a major cause of accidents (often with resultant hip fracture) and illness in the elderly. Cognitive impairment increases as the number of drugs used increases; sedatives and anticholinergic drugs are the major culprits (eg, overuse in sleep problems). The increased and varied complaints are often an attempt to compensate and divert attention from decreased mental function.

Treatment

A. SOCIAL

Socialization, a structured schedule of activities, familiar surroundings, continued achievement, and avoidance of loneliness (probably the most important factor) are some of the major considerations in prevention and amelioration of the psychiatric problems of old age. The patient can be supported in the primary environment by various agencies that can help avoid a premature change of habits. For patients with disabilities that make it difficult to cope with the problems of living alone, homemaker services can assist in continuing the day-to-day activities of the household; visiting nurses can administer medications and monitor the physical condition of the patient; and geriatric social groups can help maintain socialization and human contacts. In the hospital or nursing home, attention to the kinds of people placed in the same room is most important (mix active and inactive patients).

B. MEDICAL

Treatment of any reversible components of a dementia syndrome is obviously the major medical consideration. One commonly overlooked factor is self-medication, frequently with nonprescription drugs or herbal remedies that further impair the patient's already precarious functioning. Common culprits are antihistamines and anticholinergic drugs, sometimes mixed with ethanol abuse.

Any signs of psychosis, such as paranoid ideation, agitation, and delusions, respond very well to *small doses* of antipsychotics. Risperidone, 0.5–1 mg orally daily, or olanzapine, 2.5–5 mg orally once a day, will usually decrease psychotic ideation markedly.

Do not use drugs that cause significant orthostatic hypotension (resulting in dizziness, falls, fractures).

Antidepressants (in one-third to one-half the doses given to young adults) are used when indicated for depression. Occasionally, a stimulant in small doses (eg, methylphenidate, 5–30 mg orally usually given in two doses at 7 AM and noon) can be used to treat apathy. The stimulant may help increase the patient's energy for social involvement and help the patient to maintain life activities.

The appropriate use of wine and beer for mild sedative effects is quite rewarding in the hospital and other care facilities as well as at home.

C. BEHAVIORAL

The impaired cognitive abilities of the geriatric patient necessitate simple behavioral techniques. Positive responses to appropriate behavior encourage the patient to repeat desirable kinds of behavior, and frequent repetition offsets to some degree the defects in recent memory and recall. It also results in participation—a most important element, since there is a tendency in the older population to withdraw, thus increasing isolation and functional decline.

One must be careful not to reinforce and encourage obstreperous behavior by responding to it; in this way, extinction or at least gradual reduction of inappropriate behavior will occur. At the same time, the obstreperous behavior often represents a nondirective response to frustration and inability to function, and a structured program of activity is necessary.

D. PSYCHOLOGIC

Patients may require help in adjusting to changing roles and commitments and in finding new goals and viewpoints. The older person steadily loses an important commodity—the future—and may attempt to compensate by preoccupation with the past. Involvement with the present and psychotherapy on a here-and-now basis can help make the adjustment easier.

Grossman F: A review of anticonvulsants in treating agitated demented elderly patients. Pharmacotherapy 1998;18:600. [PMID: 9620110] (Divalproex sodium and carbamazepine are effective and well tolerated.)

Verma SD et al: Management of the agitated elderly patient in nursing homes: The role of the atypical antipsychotics. J Clin Psychiatry 1998;59(Suppl 19):50. [PMID: 0947052] (Although behavioral interventions are often effective, the newer antipsychotics appear to impose a lesser risk of tardive dyskinesia and extrapyramidal side effects.)

■ PSYCHIATRIC PROBLEMS ASSOCIATED WITH HOSPITALIZATION & MEDICAL & SURGICAL DISORDERS

Diagnostic Categories

A. ACUTE PROBLEMS

1. Delirium with psychotic features secondary to the medical or surgical problem, or compounded by effect of treatment.
2. Acute anxiety, often related to ignorance and fear of the immediate problem as well as uncertainty about the future.
3. Anxiety as an intrinsic aspect of the medical problem (eg, hyperthyroidism).
4. Denial of illness, which may present during acute or intermediate phases of illness.

B. INTERMEDIATE PROBLEMS

1. Depression as a function of the illness or acceptance of the illness, often associated with realistic or fantasied hopelessness about the future.
2. Behavioral problems, often related to denial of illness and, in extreme cases, causing the patient to leave the hospital against medical advice.

C. RECUPERATIVE PROBLEMS

1. Decreasing cooperation as the patient sees improvement and compliance is not compelled.
2. Readjustment problems with family, job, and society.

General Considerations

A. ACUTE PROBLEMS

1. **"Intensive care unit psychosis"**—The stressful ICU environment may be a cause of delirium. Critical care unit factors include sleep deprivation, increased arousal, mechanical ventilation, and social isolation. Other causes include those common to delirium and require vigorous investigation (see Delirium, above).

2. **Pre- and postsurgical anxiety states**—Such problems are common and commonly ignored. Presurgical anxiety is very common and is principally a fear of death (many surgical patients make out their wills). Patients may be fearful of anesthesia (improved by the preoperative anesthesia interview), the mysterious operating room, and the disease processes that might be uncovered by the surgeon. Such fears frequently cause people to delay examinations that might result in earlier surgery and a greater chance of cure.

The opposite of this is **surgery proneness,** the quest for surgery to escape from overwhelming life stresses. Polysurgery patients are not easily categorized. Dynamic motivations include narcissism, societal pressures (eg, breast implants), unconscious guilt, a masochistic need to suffer, an attempt to deal with another family member's illness, and somatoform disorders and body dysmorphic disorder (an obsession that a body part is disfigured). More apparent reasons may include an attempt to get relief from pain and a lifestyle that has become almost exclusively medically oriented, with all of the risks entailed in such an endeavor.

Postsurgical anxiety states are usually related to pain, procedures, and loss of body image. Acute pain problems are quite different from chronic pain disorders (see Chronic Pain Disorders, above); the former are readily handled with adequate analgesic medication (see Chapter 1). Alterations in body image, as with amputations, ostomies, and mastectomies, often raise concerns about relationships with others.

3. **Iatrogenic problems**—These usually pertain to medications, complications of diagnostic and treatment procedures, and impersonal and unsympathetic staff behavior. Polypharmacy is often a factor. Patients with unsolved diagnostic problems are at higher risk. They are desirous of relief, and the quest engenders more diagnostic procedures with a higher incidence of complications. The upset patient and family may be very demanding. Excessive demands usually result from anxiety. Such behavior is best handled with calm and measured responses.

B. INTERMEDIATE PROBLEMS

1. Prolonged hospitalization—Prolonged hospitalization presents unique problems in certain hospital services, eg, burn units, orthopedic services, and tuberculosis wards. The acute problems of the severely burned patient are discussed in Chapter 38. The problems often are behavioral difficulties related to length of hospitalization and necessary procedures. For example, in burn units, pain is a major problem in addition to anxiety about procedures. Disputes with staff are common and often concern pain medication or ward privileges. Some patients regress to infantile behavior and dependency. Staff members must agree about their approach to the patient in order to ensure the smooth functioning of the unit.

Denial of illness may present in the patient with acute myocardial infarction. Intervention by an authority figure (eg, immediate work supervisor) may help the patient accept treatment and eventually abandon the defense of denial.

2. Depression—Depression frequently occurs during this period. Therapeutic drugs (eg, corticosteroids) may be a factor. Depression can contribute to irritability and overt anger. Severe depression can lead to anorexia, which further complicates healing and metabolic balance. It is during this period that the issue of disfigurement arises—relief at survival gives way to concern about future function and appearance.

C. RECUPERATIVE PROBLEMS

1. Anxiety—Anxiety about return to the posthospital environment can cause regression to a dependent position. Complications increase, and staff forbearance again is tested. Anxiety occurring at this stage usually is handled more easily than previous behavior problems.

2. Posthospital adjustment—Adjustment difficulties after discharge are related to the severity of the deficits and the use of outpatient facilities (eg, physical therapy, rehabilitation programs, psychiatric outpatient treatment). Some patients may experience posttraumatic stress symptoms (eg, from traumatic injuries or even from necessary medical treatments). Lack of appropriate follow-up can contribute to depression in the patient, who may feel that he or she is making poor progress and may have thoughts of "giving up." Reintegration into work, educational, and social endeavors may be slow. Life is simply much more difficult when one is disfigured, disabled, or disfranchised.

Clinical Findings

The symptoms that occur in these patients are similar to those discussed in previous sections of this chapter, eg, delirium, stress and adjustment disorders, anxiety, and depression. Behavior problems may include lack of cooperation, increased complaints, demands for medication, sexual approaches to nurses, threats to leave the hospital, and actual signing out against medical recommendations. The underlying personality structure of the individual is a major factor in coping styles (eg, the compulsive individual increases indecision, the hysterical individual increases dramatic behavior).

Differential Diagnosis

Delirium and dementia (including cases associated with HIV infection and drug abuse) must always be ruled out, since they often present with symptoms resembling anxiety, depression, or psychosis. Personality disorders existing prior to hospitalization often underlie the various behavior problems, but particularly the management problems.

Complications

Prolongation of hospitalization causes increased expense, deterioration of patient-staff relationships, and increased probabilities of iatrogenic and legal problems. The possibility of increasing posthospital treatment problems is enhanced.

Treatment

A. MEDICAL

The most important consideration by far is to have one clinician in charge, a clinician whom the patient trusts and who is able to oversee multiple treatment approaches (see Somatoform Disorders, above). In acute problems, attention must be paid to metabolic imbalance, alcohol withdrawal, and previous drug use—prescribed, recreational, or OTC. Adequate sleep and analgesia are important in the prevention of delirium.

Most clinicians are attuned to the early detection of the surgery-prone patient. Plastic and orthopedic surgeons are at particular risk. Appropriate consultations may help detect some problems and mitigate future ones.

Postsurgical anxiety states can be alleviated by personal attention from the surgeon. Anxiety is not so effectively lessened by ancillary medical personnel, whom the patient perceives as lesser authorities, until after the physician has reassured the patient. Inappropriate use of "as needed" analgesia places an unfair burden on the nurse. "Patient-controlled analgesia" can improve pain control, decrease anxiety, and minimize side effects (see Chapter 1).

Depression should be recognized early. If severe, it may be treated by antidepressant medications (see Antidepressant Drugs, above). High levels of anxiety can be lowered with judicious use of anxiolytic agents. Unnecessary medications tend to reinforce the patient's impression that there must be a serious illness or medication would not be required.

B. PSYCHOLOGIC

Prepare the patient and family for what is to come. This includes the types of units where the patient will be quartered, the procedures that will be performed, and any disfigurements that will result from surgery. Repetition improves understanding. The nursing staff can be helpful, since patients frequently confide a lack of understanding to a nurse but are reluctant to do so to the physician.

Denial of illness is frequently a block to acceptance of treatment. This too should be handled with family members present (to help the patient face the reality of the situation) in a series of short interviews (for reinforcement). Dependency problems resulting from long hospitalization are best handled by focusing on the changes to come as the patient makes the transition to the outside world. Key figures are teachers, vocational counselors, and physical therapists. Challenges should be realistic and practical and handled in small steps.

Depression is usually related to the loss of familiar hospital supports, and the outpatient therapists and counselors help to lessen the impact of the loss. Some of the impact can be alleviated by anticipating, with the patient and family, the signal features of the common depression to help prevent the patient from assuming a permanent sick role (invalidism).

Suicide is always a concern when a patient is faced with despair. An honest, compassionate, and supportive approach will help sustain the patient during this trying period.

C. BEHAVIORAL

Prior desensitization can significantly allay anxiety about medical procedures. A "dry run" can be done to reinforce the oral description. Cooperation during acute problem periods can be enhanced by the use of appropriate reinforcers such as a favorite nurse or helpful family member. People who are positive reinforcers are even more helpful during the intermediate phases when the patient becomes resistant to the seemingly endless procedures (eg, debridement of burned areas).

Specific situations (eg, psychologic dependency on the respirator) can be corrected by weaning with appropriate reinforcers (eg, watching a favorite movie on a videorecorder when disconnected from the ventilator). Behavioral approaches should be employed in a positive and optimistic way for maximal reinforcement.

Relaxation techniques and attentional distraction can be used to block side effects of a necessary treatment (eg, nausea in cancer chemotherapy).

D. SOCIAL

A change in environment requires adaptation. Because of the illness, admission and hospitalization may be more easily handled than discharge. Reintegration into society can be difficult. In some cases, the family is a negative influence. A predischarge evaluation must be made to determine whether the family will be able to cope with the physical or mental changes in the patient. Working with the family while the patient is in the acute stage may presage a successful transition later on.

Development of a new social life can be facilitated by various self-help organizations (eg, the stoma club). Sharing problems with others in similar circumstances eases the return to a social life which may be quite different from that prior to the illness.

Prognosis

The prognosis is good in all patients who have reversible medical and surgical conditions. It is guarded when there is serious functional loss that impairs vocational, educational, or societal possibilities—especially in the case of progressive and ultimately life-threatening illness.

Herrmann C et al: Diagnostic groups and depressed mood as predictors of 22-month mortality in medical inpatients. Psychosom Med 1998;60:570. [PMID: 9773760] (Depressed mood was an independent risk factor associated with an odds ratio of 3.2 in predicting 22-month survival.)

Nemeroff CB et al: Depression and cardiac disease. Depress Anxiety 1998;(8 Suppl 1):71. [PMID: 9809217] (Depression is a major risk factor for increased mortality of coronary artery disease but is often underdiagnosed and undertreated.)

Endocrinology

26

Paul A. Fitzgerald, MD

See www.current-med.com/ch26.html

Hormones exert their effects by interacting with receptors on the cell surface (catecholamines and peptide hormones) or inside the cell (thyroid and steroid hormones). Endocrine disorders result from an excess or deficiency of hormonal effects.

■ COMMON PRESENTATIONS IN ENDOCRINOLOGY

Obesity

Genetics is the most important determinant for obesity. In a given environment, up to 80% of human obesity is due to genetic factors. Several novel hormones appear to act upon brain receptors to regulate appetite and metabolism, thereby determining an individual's predisposition to obesity.

Leptin is a hormone secreted by subcutaneous adipose tissue in response to fat storage or overfeeding. Leptin binds to brain (α-melanocortin receptors and influences the secretion of neuropeptides, inhibiting neuropeptide Y and agouti-related peptide. It thereby promotes satiety and increases the body's metabolic rate. Leptin is also required for gonadotropin secretion. During starvation, reduced leptin secretion results in a lower metabolic rate and a reduction in gonadotropin secretion. Congenital leptin deficiency accounts for 1–2% of early-onset morbid obesity.

Ghrelin is a 28-amino-acid hormone that is secreted by the empty stomach; it stimulates appetite.

Alpha-melanocyte-stimulating hormone (α-MSH) is a neuropeptide that regulates the hypothalamic control of food intake. Defects in the α-MSH (melanocortin 4) receptor are present in up to 5% of morbidly obese patients.

Familial partial lipodystrophy (Dunnigan-Kobberling syndrome) is an autosomal dominant disorder caused by missense mutations in the lamin A/C gene. Beginning at puberty, affected patients develop atrophy of subcutaneous fat in the extremities but obese proximal thighs, trunk, and face (type I) or absence of subcutaneous fat everywhere but in the face, which is

very fat (type II). Patients may have muscle hypertrophy. Affected patients, especially women, are at risk for metabolic complications associated with insulin resistance, including glucose intolerance, diabetes mellitus, hypertriglyceridemia, low HDL cholesterol, and atherosclerosis.

Obesity is associated with mental retardation in several genetic syndromes expressing multiple congenital anomalies: eg, Prader-Willi syndrome (hypotonia, hypogonadism), Laurence Moon-Bardet-Biedl syndrome (polydactyly, renal anomalies, retinitis pigmentosa, hypogonadism), Cohen's syndrome (microcephaly, hypotonia, short stature, ocular anomalies, neutropenia), and Biemond syndrome (diabetes mellitus, polydactyly, coloboma, facial anomalies, hypogonadism).

Several endocrine disorders do cause obesity. Cushing's syndrome causes central obesity (due to intraperitoneal fat) with relatively thin extremities; such patients usually have plethoric, rounded (moon) facies along with prominent supraclavicular and dorsocervical fat pads (buffalo humps). Alcoholism causes hypercortisolism and a similar syndrome. Hypothyroidism occasionally causes mild weight gain due to edema and fat accumulation. Hyperthyroidism may cause mild weight gain due to hyperphagia. Pancreatic insulinomas secrete excessive amounts of insulin, causing hypoglycemia and compensatory overeating. Growth hormone deficiency usually causes obesity in both children and adults.

Insulin or thiazolidinedione therapy for type 2 diabetes usually worsens obesity.

Menopause is associated with a decrease in the resting metabolic rate, which increases body weight. Weight gain is greatest in the perimenopausal period. Hormone replacement therapy causes negligible weight gain. Obesity may be associated with other disorders as part of several recognized syndromes. Syndrome X (the cluster of obesity, diabetes, and hypertension) has a 50% hereditary component. Polycystic ovary syndrome refers to the combination of obesity with anovulation, amenorrhea, cystic ovaries, and hirsutism. Hypothalamic lesions can cause massive obesity and are often associated with headache, lethargy,

1067

depression, diabetes insipidus, and hypopituitarism. Congenital obesity may be due to various uncommon syndromes of hypothalamic obesity and hypogonadotropic hypogonadism.

Bowles L et al: Leptin: of mice and men? J Clin Pathol 2001;54:1. [PMID: 11271782] (Review article on leptin and its role in human energy metabolism.)

Ruhl CE et al: Leptin concentrations in the United States: relations with demographic and anthropometric measures. Am J Clin Nutr 2001;74:295. [PMID: 11522551] (Leptin concentrations from a large representative sample of the United States population correlated with anthropometric measurements.)

Wardlaw SL: Clinical review 127: Obesity as a neuroendocrine disease: lessons to be learned from proopiomelanocortin and melanocortin receptor mutations in mice and men. J Clin Endocrinol Metab 2001;86:1442. [PMID: 11297566]

Unintended Weight Loss

Uncontrolled diabetes mellitus may be associated with weight loss, polyphagia, polydipsia, and polyuria. Anorexia and nausea may be seen with diabetic ketoacidosis and with adrenal insufficiency (due either to pituitary ACTH deficiency or to Addison's disease). Patients with severe diabetes insipidus may also lose weight. Patients with hyperthyroidism typically lose weight despite increased appetite; some patients with hypothyroidism lose weight because of diminished appetite. About 15% of patients with pheochromocytoma lose over 10% of their basal weight. Some patients with Cushing's syndrome lose weight as a result of muscle wasting.

A great variety of nonendocrine conditions enter into the differential diagnosis of unintended weight loss (see Chapter 1). Anorexia is frequently a side effect of medications or radiation therapy and is also seen with azotemia, AIDS, and many gastrointestinal conditions. Malignancies typically produce diminished appetite and cachexia. Tuberculosis may cause weight loss even when occult. Chronic respiratory insufficiency is often associated with weight loss. Psychiatric illnesses producing diminished appetite include depressed or agitated affective disorder, catatonia, and anorexia nervosa.

Abnormal Skin Pigmentation

Increased skin pigmentation can be caused by excessive ACTH secretion in Addison's disease and can occur after bilateral adrenalectomy for Cushing's disease (Nelson's syndrome). Pigmentation can be generalized or may be localized to palmar creases, extensor joint surfaces, tongue, nails, belt or bra lines, freckles, or new scars.

Pigmentation of the upper lip, forehead, or malar eminences, known as **chloasma** can be caused by pregnancy ("mask of pregnancy"), oral contraceptives, or estrogen replacement therapy.

Acanthosis nigricans presents as velvety brown thickened skin of the neck and axillae. It may be asso-

ciated with syndromes of severe insulin resistance type A (ovarian dysfunction and hirsutism) or type B (autoimmune). It may also be familial or associated with obesity, acromegaly, or thyroid disease. Acanthosis presenting after age 40 is often a sign of an underlying malignancy.

Pretibial areas of pigmentation are common in diabetes ("diabetic shin spots") as a result of minor trauma or following necrobiosis lipoidica diabeticorum.

Prominent lentigines can be a sign of Carney's complex, an autosomal dominant condition associated with atrial myxomas, schwannomas, and endocrine overactivity (eg, tumors of the thyroid, gonads, or pigmented adrenal nodular hyperplasia). Similar skin pigmentation is seen in Peutz-Jeghers syndrome with an increased risk of intestinal polyposis, adenocarcinoma, breast cancer, and tumors of the gonads and thyroid.

Diffuse hyperpigmentation is seen in POEMS syndrome (polyneuropathy, organomegaly, endocrinopathy, monoclonal gammopathy, skin changes); adrenal insufficiency, hypoparathyroidism, diabetes, osteosclerotic bone lesions, or thiamin deficiency may occur.

Gray-brown ("bronze") hyperpigmentation is caused by hemochromatosis, which can cause endocrine deficiencies such as diabetes mellitus. An orange skin discoloration is characteristic of jaundice and carotenodermia (caused by ingestion of large amounts of carotene in vegetables, seaweed, or vitamin preparations).

Patchy hypopigmentation can be due to vitiligo, a condition sometimes associated with Addison's disease and with other endocrine deficiencies as part of the polyglandular autoimmune syndrome. Hypopigmentation can also be a manifestation of cobalamin deficiency, trisomy 13, and various dermatologic conditions.

Patients undergoing chronic hemodialysis frequently become hyperpigmented, and hypopigmentation has also been reported. Other causes of hyperpigmentation include sprue, malnutrition, HIV infection, and porphyria. Hyperpigmentation may be caused by certain drugs: amiodarone, arsenic, bleomycin, busulfan, clofazimine, hydroxychloroquine, chlorpromazine, doxorubicin (nail beds), imipramine, methimazole, minocycline, niacin, primaquine, propylthiouracil, topical tretinoin, and zidovudine (nails).

Stratakis CA et al: Carney complex, Peutz-Jeghers syndrome, Cowden disease, and Bannayan-Zonana syndrome share cutaneous and endocrine manifestations, but not genetic loci. J Clin Endocrinol Metab 1998;83:2972. [PMID: 9709978]

Gynecomastia

Gynecomastia is a glandular enlargement of the male breast that may be tender and is often asymmetric or unilateral. It must be distinguished from tumors and from the fatty breast enlargement of obesity.

Pubertal gynecomastia is common and is characterized by tender discoid enlargement of breast tissue 2–3 cm in diameter beneath the areola; the swelling usually subsides spontaneously within a year. Gynecomastia develops in about 50% of athletes who abuse androgens and anabolic steroids. Gynecomastia is also common among elderly men, particularly when there is associated weight gain. Gynecomastia can be the first sign of a serious disorder. Patients with Peutz-Jeghers syndrome are prone to development of gynecomastia caused by testicular tumors.

The causes of gynecomastia are multiple and diverse (Table 26–1).

Laboratory investigation of unclear cases should include the following:

(1) A chest x-ray to search for metastatic or bronchogenic carcinoma.

Table 26–1. Causes of gynecomastia.

Idiopathic	Androgens
	Bicalutamide
Physiologic causes	Busulfan
Neonatal period	Chorionic gonadotropin
Puberty	Cimetidine
Aging	Clomiphene
Obesity	Cyclophosphamide
	Diazepam
Endocrine diseases	Diethylstilbestrol
Androgen resistance	Digitalis preparations
syndromes	Estrogens (oral or topical)
Aromatase excess syndrome	Ethionamide
(sporadic or familial)	Finasteride
Diabetic lymphocytic	Flutamide
mastitis	Goserelin (Zoladex)
Hyperprolactinemia	HAART (Highly active anti-
	retroviral therapy)
Hyperthyroidism	Haloperidol
Klinefelter's syndrome	Hydroxyzine
Male hypogonadism	Isoniazid
Partial 17-ketosteroid	Ketoconazole
reductase deficiency	Leuprolide
	Marijuana
Systemic diseases	Meprobamate
Chronic liver disease	Methadone
Chronic renal disease	Methyldopa
Neurologic disorders	Metoclopramide
Refeeding after starvation	Molindone
Spinal cord injury	Nilutamide
	Omeprazole
Neoplasms	Opioids
Adrenal tumors	Penicillamine
Bronchogenic carcinoma	Phenothiazines
Carcinoma of the breast	Progestins
Testicular tumors	Protease inhibitors
Hepatocellular carcinoma	Reserpine
(rare)	Risperidone
	Somatropin (growth
Drugs (partial list)	hormone)
Alcohol	Spironolactone
Alkylating agents	Testosterone
Amiodarone	Thioridazine
Anabolic steroids	Tricyclic antidepressants

(2) Measurements of plasma levels of prolactin (see Hyperprolactinemia) and the beta subunit of human chorionic gonadotropin (β-hCG). Detectable levels implicate a testicular tumor (germ cell or Sertoli cell) or other malignancy (usually lung or liver). Detectable low levels of serum β-hCG (< 5 mU/mL) may be reported in men with primary hypogonadism and high serum LH levels if the assay for β-hCG cross-reacts with LH.

(3) Measurements of plasma testosterone and luteinizing hormone (LH) are valuable in the diagnosis of primary or secondary hypogonadism. A low testosterone and high LH are seen in primary hypogonadism. High testosterone levels *plus* high LH levels characterize partial androgen resistance.

(4) Other tests: Serum estradiol is determined but is usually normal; increased levels may result from testicular tumors, increased β-hCG, liver disease, obesity, adrenal tumors (rare), or true hermaphroditism (rare). Many estrogens and substances with estrogenic activity are not detected by estradiol assays. Serum TSH (sensitive) and free thyroxine levels are also determined. A karyotype (for Klinefelter's syndrome) is obtained in men with persistent gynecomastia without obvious cause.

(5) Needle biopsy with cytologic examination may be performed on suspicious areas of male breast enlargement (especially when unilateral or asymmetric) to distinguish gynecomastia from tumor or mastitis.

The treatment of gynecomastia is that of the underlying condition. Idiopathic and pubertal gynecomastia tends to occur in boys who are taller and heavier than average; gynecomastia often resolves spontaneously within 1–2 years. Drug-induced gynecomastia resolves after the offending drug is removed. Painful gynecomastia may be treated with tamoxifen (an antiestrogen), 10 mg orally twice daily; discomfort improves, and some degree of reduction in breast size occurs in over 50%. Recurrence of gynecomastia occurs in about 28% of men after tamoxifen is stopped. Danazol, 400 mg orally daily, produces some improvement in gynecomastia in 40%; relapses are uncommon after stopping it. Danazol can cause hepatic dysfunction, so liver enzymes must be monitored. Since both tamoxifen and danazol can produce adverse reactions, it is prudent to treat gynecomastia only when it becomes a troubling and continuing problem for the patient. Surgical correction is reserved for persistent or severe gynecomastia, since results are often disappointing. Endoscopically assisted transaxillary liposuction and subcutaneous mastectomy may produce acceptable results.

Amory JK et al: Klinefelter's syndrome. Lancet 2000;356:333. [PMID: 11071204] (Klinefelter syndrome affects one in 500 male patients, with gynecomastia and other variable manifestations.)

Manfredi R et al: Gynecomastia associated with highly active antiretroviral therapy. Ann Pharmacother 2001;35:438. [PMID: 11302408] (Treatment with nucleoside analogs with or without protease inhibitors can cause gynecomastia.)

Ting AC et al: Comparison of tamoxifen with danazol in the management of idiopathic gynecomastia. Am Surg 2000;66: 38. [PMID: 10651345]

Galactorrhea

Lactation that occurs in the absence of nursing is termed galactorrhea. A small amount of breast milk can be expressed from the nipple in many parous women and is not cause for concern. Normal breast milk may be various colors besides white. Galactorrhea requires evaluation when it occurs in significant amounts or in nulliparous women or when it is associated with amenorrhea, headache, visual field abnormalities, or other symptoms implying systemic illness.

Evaluation begins with serum prolactin measurement; a persistently elevated level should prompt further investigation to determine its cause (Table 26–4). MRI of the pituitary and hypothalamus is done for nonpregnant patients with serum prolactin levels over 200 mg/dL, those with headaches or visual field defects, and women with persistently elevated prolactin levels with no discernible cause. Treatment is directed at correcting the cause of the elevated prolactin. Galactorrhea due to antipsychotic drugs may resolve if the neuroleptic is changed to clozapine, an atypical antipsychotic. Galactorrhea may occur in the absence of elevated serum prolactin levels (idiopathic). Whatever the cause, galactorrhea can be reduced with cabergoline or bromocriptine administration.

Pena KS et al: Evaluation and treatment of galactorrhea. Am Fam Physician 2001;63:1763. [PMID: 11352287] (Review of the evaluation and treatment of galactorrhea.)

Erectile Dysfunction & Diminished Libido in Men

Erectile dysfunction is a frequent problem. Psychogenic factors as well as endocrine, vascular, or neurologic abnormalities may be important. Hypogonadism of whatever origin (Table 26–14) is associated with lack of libido and erectile dysfunction. These can also be the first clinical manifestations of a hyperprolactinemic disorder (Table 26–4). Other endocrine causes include hyperthyroidism, Addison's disease, and acromegaly. Impotence in diabetes may be related to inadequate penile blood flow or autonomic neuropathy. Vascular disease is a frequent factor in impotence in elderly men. Vascular claudication of the legs along with related impotence is known as **Leriche's syndrome.**

Many pharmacologic agents are known to cause varying degrees of impotence (Table 26–2). Selective serotonin reuptake inhibitors (SSRIs, eg, fluoxetine) cause reduced libido. SSRIs and clomipramine cause delayed ejaculation.

Evaluation and treatment of erectile dysfunction are covered in Chapter 23.

Table 26–2. Drugs causing erectile dysfunction.

Alcohol	Leuprolide
Amphetamines	Marijuana
Antihistamines	Methadone
Barbiturates	Methyldopa
Beta-blockers	Metoclopramide
Butyrophenones	Monoamine oxidase inhibitors
Carbamazepine	Opioids
Cimetidine	Phenothiazines
Clonidine	Sedatives
Cocaine	Spironolactone
	SSRIs
Guanethidine	Thiazides
Ketoconazole	Tricyclic antidepressants

Cryptorchism

One or both testes may be absent from the scrotum at birth in about 20% of premature males and in 3–6% at full term. Cryptorchism is found in 1–2% of males after 1 year of age but must be distinguished from retractile testes, which require no treatment. Cryptorchism should be corrected before age 18–24 months in an attempt to reduce the risk of infertility, which occurs in up to 75% of men with bilateral cryptorchism and in 50% with unilateral cryptorchism. It is not clear, however, whether early orchiopexy improves ultimate fertility. Many patients have underlying hypogonadism.

The ultimate incidence of significant testicular neoplasia is about 0.002% in normal males, 0.06% in cryptorchid males, and up to 5% in patients with intra-abdominal testes.

If the testes are not palpable, ultrasound or MRI can be used to locate them. Alternatively, human chorionic gonadotropin, 1500 units intramuscularly daily for 3 days, causes a significant rise in testosterone if the testes are present.

Orchiopexy decreases the risk of neoplasia when performed before 10 years of age. Orchiectomy after puberty is an option for intra-abdominal testes.

Rogers E et al: The role of orchiectomy in the management of postpubertal cryptorchidism. J Urol 1998;159:851. [PMID: 9474167] (Sixty-two percent of undescended testes were palpable. Diminished spermatogenesis was related to age and the severity of the maldescent; only 2% had normal spermatogenesis. Carcinoma in situ was present in 4% and torsion of the undescended testis in 2%.)

Vinardi S et al: Testicular function in men treated in childhood for undescended testes. J Pediatr Surg 2001;36:385. [PMID: 11172441] (Approximately 10% of young men treated in childhood for cryptorchism have reduced testicular volume and semen quality.)

Bone Pain & Pathologic Fractures

Onset of pathologic fractures at an early age is seen in osteogenesis imperfecta (blue scleras may be present).

Painful bowing of the bones and pseudofractures suggest rickets or osteomalacia. Hyperparathyroidism or malignancy is suspected in patients with bone pain and hypercalcemia. Back pain or pathologic fractures in hypogonadal men and women implicate osteoporosis; such pain may be relieved with calcitonin. In cases of osteopenia of unknown cause, hyperthyroidism and Cushing's syndrome should also be considered. Bone pain may occur also as a result of primary or metastatic tumors, multiple myeloma, and Paget's disease; such pain may be relieved with bisphosphonates such as pamidronate or alendronate. Treatment is that of the underlying disorder.

Muscle Cramps & Tetany

Muscle cramps are usually caused by sports or occupational muscle injury. Nocturnal leg cramps are commonly idiopathic but are seen in diabetes mellitus, Parkinson's disease, central nervous system or spinal cord lesions, peripheral neuropathy, hemodialysis, peripheral vascular disease, and cisplatin or vincristine. Various other drugs can cause myalgias that patients describe as cramps (eg, cimetidine, cholestyramine). Alkalosis due to any cause (eg, severe vomiting or hyperventilation) may decrease ionized calcium and cause muscle cramping and paresthesias. Leg cramps during walking may be due to vascular insufficiency, hyperthyroidism, or hypothyroidism.

McArdle's disease is caused by muscle phosphorylase deficiency; patients present with muscle fatigue, cramping, and high serum CK levels; vitamin B_6 (pyridoxine) supplementation reduces muscle cramps. Carnitine palmitoyltransferase II deficiency is a genetic disorder of lipid metabolism; patients present with myalgia, cramping, myoglobinuria, and elevated serum CK levels. Other conditions that may cause muscle cramping include stiff man syndrome (abdominal and back cramping), Brody's disease, phosphoglycerate kinase deficiency (myoglobinuria), muscle phosphofructokinase deficiency (Tarui's disease), and neuromyotonia (Isaac's syndrome).

Diffuse, recurrent, or severe muscle cramping requires evaluation for hypocalcemia (Table 21–8). Treatment of hypocalcemia is discussed in Chapter 21. Magnesium deficiency must be considered in tetany unresponsive to calcium.

For patients with recurrent, severe, or prolonged muscle cramping, gabapentin, 600–1200 mg/d orally, appears to be effective. Adverse effects of gabapentin may include leukopenia and central nervous system toxicities. Quinine, long used to prevent nocturnal muscle cramps, can cause arrhythmias, dizziness, hemolytic-uremic syndrome, and agranulocytosis. Leg cramps, usually nocturnal, affect 45% of women during pregnancy; oral calcium may reduce their frequency. Exertional claudication caused by vascular insufficiency may be treated with oral pentoxifylline, cilostazol, angioplasty, or arterial bypass.

Recurrent cervicofacial and laryngeal dystonias, as well as hand cramps, have been successfully treated with injections of botulinum toxin.

Serrao M et al: Gabapentin treatment for muscle cramps: an open label trial. Clin Neuropharmacol 2000;23:45. [PMID: 10682230]

Mental Changes

Disturbances of mentation may be important indications of underlying endocrine disorders. Nervousness and excitability are characteristic of the menopause and hyperthyroidism. Adult cretinism is the result of prolonged hypothyroidism in infancy. In adults, hypothyroidism is accompanied by mental slowness, depression, and lethargy. Occasionally it may be manifested by delusional psychosis ("myxedema madness"). Pheochromocytoma may cause anxiety, confusion, or psychosis. Prolonged hypocalcemia from untreated hypoparathyroidism may be associated with intellectual deterioration. Hypoglycemia of any origin may cause confusion, abnormal speech, and behavioral or personality changes as well as sudden loss of consciousness, somnolence and prolonged lethargy, or coma. Frank psychosis can occur but is rare. Mild hypercalcemia causes fatigue and emotional irritability. Severe hypercalcemia can cause confusion, psychosis, and coma. Confusion may occur in hypopituitarism or Addison's disease. Confusion, lethargy, and nausea may be the presenting symptoms of hyponatremia. Insomnia, mood changes, anxiety, and psychosis can be associated with Cushing's syndrome. Rapid changes in glucocorticoid status (either a sudden increase or a sudden decrease) may be associated with acute psychosis. Porphyria may cause affective and thought disorders, particularly during acute attacks.

Mental changes may result from vitamin deficiencies caused by malnutrition, malabsorption, and other conditions. Deficiency in vitamin B_1 (thiamin) is usually seen in alcoholism and can cause Korsakoff's syndrome with typical memory loss and confabulation. Deficiency in vitamin B_2 (riboflavin) may cause personality deterioration and occurs commonly with psychotropic and antimalarial drugs and with diabetes and other diseases. Vitamin B_3 (niacin) deficiency is seen with poor nutrition, alcoholism, mercaptopurine toxicity, and malignant carcinoid syndrome and can cause irritability, dementia, dermatitis, and diarrhea. Vitamin B_6 (pyridoxine) deficiency is frequently seen in alcoholics or during treatment with isoniazid or levodopa and can cause irritability, depression, and neuropathy. Deficiency of vitamin B_{12} (cobalamin) is caused by deficiency in gastric intrinsic factor and may be seen at any age; however, it is more common in the elderly, affecting about 10% of people over age 70 years. Vitamin B_{12} deficiency may cause depression, irritability, paranoia, confusion, and dementia. It is usually associated with other neurologic symptoms such as paresthesias and leg weakness. Mental changes may occur in the absence of megaloblastic anemia.

■ DISEASES OF THE HYPOTHALAMUS & PITUITARY GLAND

Anterior pituitary gland function is controlled by regulating hormones produced by the hypothalamus and by direct feedback inhibition. The **posterior pituitary** receives antidiuretic hormone and oxytocin from the hypothalamus, secreting them under central nervous system control (Table 26–3). Hypothalamic hormones generally stimulate the anterior pituitary except for dopamine, which inhibits the pituitary from spontaneously secreting prolactin.

HYPOPITUITARISM

ESSENTIALS OF DIAGNOSIS

- *Sexual dysfunction; weakness; easy fatigability; lack of resistance to stress, cold, and fasting; axillary and pubic hair loss.*
- *Low blood pressure; pituitary tumors may cause visual field defects.*
- *Low free thyroxine; deficient cortisol response to cosyntropin.*
- *Low serum testosterone (men); amenorrhea; serum prolactin may be elevated; FSH and LH are low or low normal.*
- *MRI may reveal a pituitary or hypothalamic lesion.*

Table 26–3. Pituitary hormones.

Anterior pituitary
Growth hormone (GH)[1]
Prolactin (PRL)
Adrenocorticotropic hormone (ACTH)
Thyroid-stimulating hormone (TSH)
Luteinizing hormone (LH)[2]
Follicle-stimulating hormone (FSH)
Posterior pituitary
Arginine vasopressin (AVP)[3]
Oxytocin

[1]GH closely resembles human placental lactogen (hPL).
[2]LH closely resembles human chorionic gonadotropin (hCG).
[3]AVP is identical with antidiuretic hormone (ADH).

General Considerations

Hypopituitarism can be caused by either hypothalamic or pituitary dysfunction. Patients with hypopituitarism may have single or multiple hormonal deficiencies. When one hormonal deficiency is discovered, others must be sought.

Mass lesions causing hypopituitarism include pituitary adenomas, granulomas, Rathke's cleft cysts, apoplexy, metastatic carcinomas, aneurysms, and brain tumors such as craniopharyngioma, meningioma, germinoma, glioma, chondrosarcoma, and chordoma of the clivus. Langerhans cell histiocytosis usually presents in youth with diabetes insipidus or hypopituitarism; MRI may reveal a mass lesion, thickening of the pituitary stalk, or no visible abnormality. Osteolytic bone lesions are noted on skeletal x-rays. Autoimmune hypophysitis, postpartum pituitary necrosis (Sheehan's syndrome), eclampsia-preeclampsia, sickle cell disease, and African trypanosomiasis are rare causes.

A pituitary tumor may be part of the syndrome of multiple endocrine neoplasia (type 1), with tumors of the parathyroid glands and pancreatic islets.

Hypopituitarism without mass lesions may be idiopathic or may be caused by trauma, cranial radiation, surgery, encephalitis, hemochromatosis, autoimmunity, or stroke. It may also occur after coronary artery bypass grafting. Pituitary hormone deficiencies may be congenital and caused by a *POU1F1* gene mutation. GnRH agonist therapy for prostate cancer causes hypogonadotropic hypogonadism. Long-term intrathecal administration of opioids causes hypogonadotropic hypogonadism in the overwhelming majority of patients; GH deficiency and secondary adrenal insufficiency each occur in about 15% of such patients.

Clinical Findings

Manifestations of hypopituitarism vary depending upon which specific hormones are lacking and whether their deficiency is partial or complete.

A. SYMPTOMS AND SIGNS

Gonadotropin deficiency includes loss of luteinizing hormone (LH) and follicle-stimulating hormone (FSH), which causes hypogonadism and infertility. Patients with isolated gonadotropin deficiency may present as delayed adolescence. (See also discussion of primary amenorrhea.) Congenital gonadotropin deficiency may be associated with micropenis, cryptorchism, or a decreased sense of smell (from hypoplasia of the olfactory bulbs) in Kallmann's syndrome. In males with X-linked adrenal hypoplasia, gonadotropin deficiency and azoospermia may present in adolescence or adulthood; primary adrenal insufficiency usually presents in childhood, but mild cases may remain undiagnosed until adulthood. In acquired gonadotropin deficiency, both men and women lose axillary, pubic, and body hair gradually, particularly if they are also hypoadrenal. Men may note diminished beard growth. Libido is diminished. Women have amenorrhea; men note decreased erections. Most patients are infertile. (See section on secondary amenorrhea.)

Thyroid-stimulating hormone (TSH) deficiency causes hypothyroidism with manifestations such as fatigue, weakness, weight change, and hyperlipidemia. (See Hypothyroidism and Myxedema.)

Adrenocorticotropic hormone (ACTH) deficiency results in diminished cortisol secretion (see Adrenocortical Hypofunction). Symptoms include weakness, fatigue, weight loss, and hypotension. Adrenal mineralocorticoid secretion continues, so manifestations of adrenal insufficiency in hypopituitarism are usually less striking than in bilateral adrenal gland destruction (Addison's disease).

Growth hormone (GH) deficiency in adulthood tends to cause mild to moderate obesity, asthenia, reduced cardiac output, and feelings of social isolation.

Panhypopituitarism is the absence of all anterior pituitary hormones. Besides the manifestations noted above, patients with long-standing hypopituitarism tend to have dry, pale, finely textured skin. The face has fine wrinkles and an apathetic countenance.

B. Laboratory Findings

The fasting blood glucose may be low. Hyponatremia is often present. Hyperkalemia usually does not occur, since aldosterone production is not affected.

The free T_4 level is low, and TSH is not elevated. Plasma levels of sex steroids (testosterone and estradiol) are low or low normal, as are the serum gonadotropins as well. Elevated prolactin levels are found in patients with prolactinomas, acromegaly, and hypothalamic disease.

In secondary hypoadrenalism, administration of cosyntropin (synthetic $ACTH_{1-24}$), 0.25 mg (intramuscularly or intravenously) usually causes serum cortisol to rise to less than 20 μg/dL by 30–60 minutes after the injection. A low-dose cosyntropin test (0.001 mg intravenously) is slightly more sensitive in detecting subtle ACTH-cortisol insufficiency. A baseline ACTH level is low or normal in secondary hypoadrenalism, distinguishing it from primary adrenal disease.

Patients with a normal cosyntropin test but with clinically suspected pituitary-adrenal insufficiency may have a metyrapone stimulation test: Metyrapone, 1.5 g orally, is administered at 11 PM; serum is collected at 8 AM for 11-deoxycortisol and cortisol determinations. Patients with hypoadrenalism usually have an 11-deoxycortisol concentration under 7 μg/dL in the presence of a cortisol suppressed to less than 5 μg/dL. The metyrapone test must be performed in the absence of replacement glucocorticoid. Side effects include frequent nausea and occasional vomiting.

The diagnosis of growth hormone (GH) deficiency is made difficult by the pulsatile nature of GH secretion and individual variability. GH deficiency is present in 96% of patients with three or four other pituitary hormone deficiencies. The insulin hypoglycemia

test, long considered the "gold standard," is actually somewhat unreliable, cumbersome, and uncomfortable; it is contraindicated in the elderly, in patients with cardiovascular or cerebrovascular disease, and in patients with any history of seizures, an abnormal EEG, or recent brain surgery. Instead, the arginine/GHRH stimulation test may be used. GH deficiency is diagnosed if the maximum stimulated serum GH concentration is less than 5 mg/mL (polyclonal radioimmunoassay) or less than 2.5 mg/mL (immunochemiluminescent assay). Serum IGF-1 levels are in the normal range in about 50% of adults with GH deficiency. However, very low levels of IGF-1 (< 84 μg/L) are indicative of GH deficiency except in conditions that naturally suppress serum IGF-1 (eg, malnutrition, prolonged fasting, oral estrogen, hypothyroidism, uncontrolled diabetes mellitus, liver failure). In GH deficiency, exercise-stimulated serum GH levels usually fail to rise and remain at < 5 ng/mL; however, by age 40 years, most normal adults have lost their GH response to exercise.

C. Imaging

MRI provides the best visualization of parasellar lesions. In hemochromatosis, MRI shows a very hypointense anterior lobe on T1-weighted images, which is surrounded by hyperintense cerebrospinal fluid on T2-weighted images. The posterior pituitary usually has a high-intensity signal on sagittal MRI that is lacking in central diabetes insipidus.

Differential Diagnosis

Reversible hypogonadotropic hypogonadism may occur with serious illness, malnutrition, or anorexia nervosa. The clinical situation, presence of normal sex hair, and normal adrenal and thyroid function allow ready distinction from hypopituitarism. Patients receiving chronic intrathecal infusion of opioids usually develop hypogonadotropic hypogonadism; GH deficiency and secondary adrenal insufficiency each occur in 15% of such patients. Reversible secondary adrenal insufficiency may persist for many months following high-dose glucocorticoid therapy.

Severe illness causes functional suppression of TSH and thyroxine. Hyperthyroxinemia reversibly suppresses TSH. Bexarotene, used to treat cutaneous T cell lymphoma, suppresses TSH secretion, resulting in reversible central hypothyroidism. Glucocorticoids or megestrol treatment reversibly suppresses endogenous ACTH and cortisol secretion.

Serum IGF-1 may be low in patients with malnutrition, liver disease, hypothyroidism, or uncontrolled diabetes mellitus.

Complications

Patients with destructive lesions (eg, tumors) may develop complications related to them or to surgery or radiation therapy. Among patients with craniopharyngiomas, diabetes insipidus is found in 16% preoperatively and in 60% postoperatively. Hyponatremia may present abruptly during the first 2 weeks following pituitary surgery. Visual field impairment may occur. Hypothalamic damage may result in morbid obesity as well as cognitive and emotional problems. Conventional radiation therapy results in an increased incidence of small vessel ischemic strokes and second tumors.

Patients with untreated hypoadrenalism and a stressful illness may become febrile and die in shock and coma.

Adults with growth hormone deficiency have experienced an increased cardiovascular morbidity. Rarely, acute hemorrhage may occur in large pituitary tumors, manifested by rapid loss of vision, headache, and evidence of acute pituitary failure (pituitary apoplexy) requiring emergency decompression of the sella.

Treatment

Transsphenoidal removal of pituitary tumors will sometimes reverse hypopituitarism. Postoperative hyponatremia often occurs; serum sodium must be checked frequently for 2 weeks after pituitary surgery. Hypogonadism due to prolactin excess usually resolves during treatment with dopamine agonists. Endocrine substitution therapy must be used before, during, and often permanently after such procedures.

GH-secreting tumors may respond to octreotide (see section on acromegaly). Radiation therapy with x-ray, gamma knife, or heavy particles may be necessary but increases the likelihood of hypopituitarism.

The mainstay of substitution therapy for pituitary insufficiency remains lifetime hormone replacement.

A. CORTICOSTEROIDS

Give hydrocortisone tablets, 15–25 mg/d orally in divided doses. Most patients do well with 15 mg in the morning and 5–10 mg in the late afternoon. Some patients feel better taking prednisone, 3–7.5 mg/d, or dexamethasone, 0.25 mg/d. A mineralocorticoid is rarely needed. Additional hydrocortisone must be given during states of stress, eg, during infection, trauma, or surgical procedures. For mild illness, corticosteroid doses are doubled or tripled. For trauma or surgical stress, hydrocortisone is given in doses of 50 mg intramuscularly or intravenously every 6 hours and then reduced to normal doses as the stress subsides.

Patients with secondary adrenal insufficiency due to treatment with glucocorticoids at supraphysiologic doses require their usual daily dose of glucocorticoid during surgery and acute illness; supplemental hydrocortisone is not usually required.

B. THYROID

Levothyroxine is given to correct hypothyroidism only after the patient is assessed for cortisol deficiency or is already receiving glucocorticoids. (See Hypothy-

roidism.) The usual maintenance dose is 0.125 mg daily (range, 0.05–0.3 mg daily).

C. SEX HORMONES

Androgen replacement is discussed in the section on male hypogonadism. Estrogen replacement is discussed in the section on female hypogonadism.

To improve spermatogenesis, chorionic gonadotropin (equivalent to luteinizing hormone) may be given at a dosage of 2000–3000 units intramuscularly three times weekly and testosterone replacement is discontinued. The dose of hCG is adjusted to normalize serum testosterone levels. After 6–12 months of hCG treatment, if the sperm count remains low, hCG injections are continued along with injections of FSH: follitropin beta (synthetic recombinant FSH) or urofollitropins (urine-derived FSH). An alternative for patients with an intact pituitary (eg, Kallmann's syndrome) is the use of leuprolide (GnRH analog) by intermittent subcutaneous infusion. With either treatment, testicular volumes double within 5–12 months, and spermatogenesis occurs in most cases. With the help of intracytoplasmic sperm injection for some cases, the total pregnancy success rate is about 70%. Clomiphene, 25–50 mg orally daily, can sometimes stimulate a man's own pituitary gonadotropins (when his pituitary is intact), thereby increasing testosterone and sperm production.

For fertility induction in females, ovulation may be induced with clomiphene, 50 mg daily for 5 days every 2 months. Follitropins and chorionic gonadotropin can induce multiple births and should be used only by those experienced with their administration. (See Chapter 17.)

D. HUMAN GROWTH HORMONE

hGH (somatotropin) is synthesized by recombinant DNA techniques. Symptomatic adults with severe growth hormone deficiency may be treated with subcutaneous somatotropin injection starting at a dosage of about 0.2 mg (0.6 IU) three times weekly or daily. The dosage of somatropin is increased every 2–4 weeks by increments of 0.1 mg (0.3 IU) until side effects occur or a sufficient salutary response is achieved. A sustained-release injectable suspension of growth hormone has been developed (somatropin depot). It can be given once monthly and is therefore more convenient than standard hGH preparations; however, its safety and dosing in adults remain to be established. If the desired effects (eg, improved energy and mentation, reduction in visceral adiposity) are not seen within 3–6 months at maximum tolerated dosage, somatropin is discontinued.

Oral estrogen replacement reduces hepatic IGF-1 production. Therefore, prior to commencing somatropin therapy, oral estrogen is changed to a transdermal estradiol system.

Side effects of somatotropin therapy may include peripheral edema, hand stiffness, arthralgias, myalgias, headache, pseudotumor cerebri, gynecomastia, carpal tunnel syndrome, tarsal tunnel syndrome, hypertension, and proliferative retinopathy. Side effects are more common in older patients, those with greater weight and higher BMI, and those with adult-onset GH deficiency. Such symptoms usually remit promptly after a sufficient reduction in dosage. Excessive doses of somatotropin could cause acromegaly; patients receiving chronic therapy require careful clinical monitoring. Serum IGF-1 levels may be helpful.

GH levels normally decline with aging. However, available data do not support the use of hGH to reverse normal aging. GH should not be administered during critical illness.

GH therapy appears to benefit some patients with Crohn's disease. It also improves phosphate retention in hypophosphatemic rickets.

E. OTHER DRUGS

Cabergoline, bromocriptine, or quinagolide may reverse the hypogonadism seen in hyperprolactinomas. (See Disorders of Prolactin Secretion.) Intravenous pamidronate may improve bone pain in Langerhans-cell histiocytosis.

Prognosis

The prognosis depends on the primary cause. Hypopituitarism resulting from a pituitary tumor may be reversible with bromocriptine, cabergoline, or quinagolide or with careful selective resection of the tumor. Spontaneous recovery from hypopituitarism associated with pituitary stalk enlargement has been reported. Patients can also recover from functional hypopituitarism, eg, hypogonadism due to starvation or severe illness, suppression of ACTH by glucocorticoids, or suppression of TSH by hyperthyroidism.

Abs R et al: Endocrine consequences of long-term intrathecal administration of opioids. J Clin Endocrinol Metab 2000;85: 2215. [PMID: 10852454]

Miller KK et al: Androgen deficiency in women with hypopituitarism. J Clin Endocrinol Metab 2001;86:561. [PMID: 11158090] (Women with hypopituitarism have markedly decreased serum levels of testosterone, free testosterone, androstenedione, and DHEAS.)

Tomlinson JW et al: Association between premature mortality and hypopituitarism. West Midlands Prospective Hypopituitary Study Group. Lancet 2001;357:425. [PMID: 11273062] (Patients with hypopituitarism had increased mortality rates compared with the general population in this large prospective study. Excess mortality was attributable mostly to vascular and respiratory disease. The following were independent risk factors for death: female sex, craniopharyngioma, and untreated gonadotropin deficiency.)

Vahl N et al: Continuation of growth hormone (GH) replacement in GH-deficient patients during transition from childhood to adulthood: a two-year placebo-controlled study. J Clin Endocrinol Metab 2000;85:1874. [PMID: 10843168] (Patients with childhood-onset GH deficiency whose GH was stopped at adulthood experienced a significant decline in muscle mass compared with those in whom GH therapy was continued.)

DIABETES INSIPIDUS

ESSENTIALS OF DIAGNOSIS

- Polyuria (2–20 L/d); polydipsia.
- Urine specific gravity usually < 1.006 during ad libitum fluid intake.
- Vasopressin reduces urine output (except in nephrogenic diabetes insipidus).

General Considerations

Diabetes insipidus is an uncommon disease characterized by an increase in thirst and the passage of large quantities of urine of low specific gravity. The urine is otherwise normal. It is caused by a deficiency of or resistance to vasopressin.

The causes may be classified as follows:

A. DEFICIENCY OF VASOPRESSIN

Primary diabetes insipidus (without an identifiable organic lesion noted on MRI of the pituitary and hypothalamus) may be familial, occurring as a dominant trait, or sporadic ("idiopathic"). **Secondary diabetes insipidus** is due to damage to the hypothalamus or pituitary stalk by tumor, anoxic encephalopathy, surgical or accidental trauma, infection (eg, encephalitis, tuberculosis, syphilis), sarcoidosis, or multifocal Langerhans cell (eosinophilic) granulomatosis ("histiocytosis X"). Metastases to the pituitary are more likely to cause diabetes insipidus (33%) than are pituitary adenomas (1%).

Vasopressinase-induced diabetes insipidus may be seen in the last trimester of pregnancy and in the puerperium; it is often associated with oligohydramnios, preeclampsia, or hepatic dysfunction. A circulating enzyme destroys native vasopressin; however, synthetic desmopressin is unaffected. The condition usually responds to desmopressin therapy (see below) and subsides spontaneously.

B. "NEPHROGENIC" DIABETES INSIPIDUS

This disorder is due to a defect in the kidney tubules that interferes with water reabsorption. The polyuria is unresponsive to vasopressin. These patients have normal secretion of vasopressin. Congenital nephrogenic diabetes insipidus is present from birth and is due to defective expression of renal vasopressin V2 receptors or vasopressin-sensitive water channels. It occurs as a familial X-linked trait; adults often have hyperuricemia as well.

Acquired forms of vasopressin-resistant diabetes insipidus are usually less severe and are seen in pyelonephritis, renal amyloidosis, myeloma, potassium depletion, Sjögren's syndrome, sickle cell anemia, or chronic hypercalcemia. The disorder may occur also as a glucocorticoid effect or as an acute side effect of diuretics. Certain drugs (eg, demeclocycline, lithium, foscarnet, or methicillin) may induce nephrogenic diabetes insipidus. The recovery from acute tubular necrosis may also be associated with transient nephrogenic diabetes insipidus.

Clinical Findings

A. SYMPTOMS AND SIGNS

The symptoms of the disease are intense thirst, especially with a craving for ice water, and polyuria, the volume of ingested fluid varying from 2 L to 20 L daily, with correspondingly large urine volumes. Partial diabetes insipidus presents with less intense symptoms and should be suspected in patients with unremitting enuresis. Diabetes insipidus may present with hypernatremia and dehydration, especially after hypothalamic damage due to shock or anoxia.

B. LABORATORY FINDINGS

Evaluation for diabetes insipidus should include a 24-hour urine collection for volume, glucose, and creatinine and serum for glucose, urea nitrogen, calcium, uric acid, potassium, and sodium.

The diagnosis of diabetes insipidus as a cause of polyuria or hypernatremia requires mostly clinical judgment. There is no single diagnostic laboratory test. Hyperuricemia implicates central diabetes insipidus, since reduced stimulation of the renal V1 receptor causes reduced urate clearance.

If the clinical situation implicates central diabetes insipidus (and no other causes for polyuria are present; see Differential Diagnosis, below), a supervised "vasopressin challenge test" may be given: Desmopressin acetate is given in an initial dose of 0.05–0.1 mL (5–10 μg) intranasally (or 1 μg subcutaneously or intravenously), with measurement of urine volume for 12 hours prior to and 12 hours after administration. Serum sodium must be obtained immediately in the event of symptoms of hyponatremia. The dosage of desmopressin is doubled if the response is marginal. Patients with central diabetes insipidus notice a distinct reduction in thirst and polyuria; serum sodium stays normal except in some salt-losing conditions.

When nephrogenic diabetes insipidus is a diagnostic consideration, measurement of serum vasopressin is done during modest fluid restriction; typically, the vasopressin level is high.

In nonfamilial central diabetes insipidus, MRI of the pituitary and hypothalamus and of the skull is done to look for mass lesions. Absence of a posterior pituitary "bright spot" on T1-weighted MRI is suggestive of central diabetes insipidus.

Differential Diagnosis of Polyuria

Central diabetes insipidus must be distinguished from polyuria caused by Cushing's syndrome or glucocorticoid treatment, lithium, and the nocturnal polyuria of Parkinson's disease. It must also be distinguished from the excessive fluid intake seen in psychogenic polydipsia, central nervous system sarcoidosis, and intravenous fluid administration.

Central diabetes insipidus is distinguished from diabetes mellitus by checking the urine for glucose. It must also be distinguished from nephrogenic diabetes insipidus (see above).

Complications

If water is not readily available, the excessive output of urine will lead to severe dehydration. Patients with an impaired thirst mechanism are very prone to hypernatremia, particularly since they usually also have impaired mentation and forget to take their desmopressin. All the complications of the primary disease may eventually become evident. In patients who are receiving desmopressin acetate therapy, there is a danger of induced water intoxication.

Treatment

A. DESMOPRESSIN

Desmopressin acetate is the treatment of choice for central diabetes insipidus. It is also useful in diabetes insipidus associated with pregnancy or the puerperium, since desmopressin is resistant to degradation by the circulating vasopressinase. It is usually given intranasally (100 μg/mL solution) every 12–24 hours as needed for thirst and polyuria. It may be administered via metered-dose nasal inhaler containing 0.1 mL/spray or via a plastic calibrated tube. Patients are started with 0.05–0.1 mL every 12–24 hours, and the dose is then individualized according to response.

Desmopressin is also available as a parenteral preparation containing 4 μg/mL. For central diabetes insipidus, it is given intravenously, intramuscularly, or subcutaneously in doses of 1–4 μg every 12–24 hours as needed to treat thirst or hypernatremia.

Desmopressin is also available as an oral preparation (0.1 or 0.2 mg tablets) which are given in a starting dose of 0.05 mg twice daily and increased to a maximum of 0.4 mg every 8 hours, if required. Oral desmopressin is particularly useful for patients with sinusitis from the nasal preparation. Mild increases in hepatic enzymes are common, so the drug is not given to patients with liver disease. Gastrointestinal symptoms and asthenia may occur.

Adverse reactions to desmopressin have included nasal irritation, occasional agitation, and erythromelalgia. Hyponatremia is uncommon if minimum effective doses are used and the patient allows thirst to occur periodically.

B. OTHER MEASURES

Mild cases require no treatment other than adequate fluid intake. Reduction of aggravating factors (eg, glucocorticoids, which directly increase renal free water clearance) will improve polyuria. Both central and nephrogenic diabetes insipidus respond partially to hydrochlorothiazide, 50–100 mg/d (with potassium supplement or amiloride). Nephrogenic diabetes insipidus may respond to combined treatments of indomethacin-hydrochlorothiazide, indomethacin-desmopressin, or indomethacin-amiloride. Indomethacin, 50 mg every 8 hours, is effective acutely.

Psychotherapy is required for most patients with compulsive water drinking. Thioridazine and lithium are best avoided if drug therapy is needed, since they cause polyuria.

Prognosis

Central diabetes insipidus appearing after pituitary surgery usually remits after days to weeks but may be permanent if the upper pituitary stalk is cut.

Central diabetes insipidus is made transiently worse by glucocorticoids in the high doses frequently given perioperatively.

Chronic diabetes insipidus is more an inconvenience than a dire medical condition. Treatment with desmopressin allows normal sleep and activity. Hypernatremia can occur, especially when the thirst center is damaged, but diabetes insipidus itself does not reduce life expectancy, and the prognosis is that of the underlying disorder.

Kaltsas GA et al: Hypothalamo-pituitary abnormalities in adult patients with Langerhans cell histiocytosis: clinical, endocrinological, and radiological features and response to treatment. J Clin Endocrinol Metab 2000;85:1370. [PMID: 10770168] (In Langerhans cell histiocytosis, granulomatous lesions are found in multiple sites. Patients with diabetes insipidus often have only subtle thickening of the pituitary stalk on MRI. Most develop deficiencies in anterior pituitary hormones. Radiation therapy does not reverse hormone deficiencies. Patients eventually develop extrapituitary lesions detectable on skeletal x-ray surveys more readily than bone scans.)

Maghnie M et al: Central diabetes insipidus in children and young adults. N Engl J Med 2000;343:998. [PMID: 11018166] (Of 79 patients with central diabetes insipidus, 61% developed anterior pituitary hormone deficiencies; 52% were idiopathic, 23% due to tumor, 15% due to Langerhans histiocytosis, 6% familial, and 6% due to trauma or autoimmunity.)

ACROMEGALY & GIGANTISM

ESSENTIALS OF DIAGNOSIS

- *Excessive growth of hands (increased glove and ring size), feet (increased shoe width), jaw (protrusion of lower jaw), and internal organs; or gigantism before closure of epiphyses.*
- *Coarsening facial features; deeper voice.*
- *Amenorrhea, headaches, visual field loss, sweating, weakness.*
- *Soft, doughy, sweaty handshake.*
- *Serum GH not suppressed following oral glucose.*
- *Elevated insulin-like growth factor 1 (IGF-1).*
- *Imaging: Terminal phalangeal "tufting" on radiographs. CT or MRI demonstration of pituitary tumor in 90%.*

General Considerations

Growth hormone exerts much of its growth-promoting effects through the release of IGF-1 produced in the liver and other tissues.

Acromegaly is nearly always caused by a pituitary adenoma. These tumors may be locally invasive, particularly into the cavernous sinus. Fewer than 1% are malignant. Most are macroadenomas (over 1 cm in diameter). Acromegaly is usually sporadic but may rarely be familial. The disease may be associated with endocrine tumors of the parathyroids or pancreas (multiple endocrine neoplasia type 1). Acromegaly may also be seen in McCune-Albright syndrome and as part of Carney's complex (atrial myxoma, acoustic neuroma, and spotty skin pigmentation). Acromegaly is rarely caused by ectopic GHRH or GH secreted by a lymphoma, hypothalamic tumor, bronchial carcinoid, or pancreatic tumor.

Clinical Findings

A. Symptoms and Signs

Excessive growth hormone causes tall stature and gigantism if it occurs before closure of epiphyses. Afterward, acromegaly develops. The term "acromegaly," meaning extremity enlargement, seriously understates the manifestations. The hands enlarge and a doughy, moist handshake is characteristic. The fingers widen, causing patients to enlarge their rings. Carpal tunnel syndrome is common. The feet also grow, particularly in width. Facial features coarsen since the bones and sinuses of the skull enlarge; hat size increases. The mandible becomes more prominent, causing prognathism and malocclusion. Tooth spacing widens.

Macroglossia occurs, as does hypertrophy of pharyngeal and laryngeal tissue; this causes a deep, coarse voice and sometimes makes intubation difficult. Obstructive sleep apnea may occur. A goiter may be noted. Hypertension (50%) and cardiomegaly are common; cardiovascular morbidity is increased. Weight gain is typical, particularly of muscle and bone. Insulin resistance is usually present and frequently causes diabetes mellitus (30%). Arthralgias and degenerative arthritis occur. Overgrowth of vertebral bone can cause spinal stenosis. Colon polyps are common, especially in patients with skin papillomas. The skin may also manifest hyperhidrosis, thickening, cystic acne, and areas of acanthosis nigricans.

GH-secreting pituitary tumors usually cause some degree of hypogonadism, either by cosecretion of prolactin or by direct pressure upon normal pituitary tissue. Decreased libido and impotence are common, as are irregular menses or amenorrhea. Secondary hypothyroidism sometimes occurs; hypoadrenalism is unusual. Headaches are frequent. Temporal hemianopia may occur as a result of the optic chiasm being impinged by a suprasellar growth of the tumor.

B. LABORATORY FINDINGS

After an overnight fast, a fasting serum specimen is obtained and assayed for prolactin (cosecreted by many GH-secreting tumors), IGF-1 (increased to over five times normal in most acromegalics), glucose (diabetes is common in acromegaly), liver enzymes and BUN, serum inorganic phosphorus (frequently elevated), serum free thyroxine, and TSH (secondary hypothyroidism is common in acromegaly; primary hypothyroidism may increase prolactin; hyperthyroidism may occur as a result of excess TSH). Serum calcium is determined to screen for hyperparathyroidism.

Glucose syrup (75 g) is then administered orally, and serum GH is measured 60 minutes afterward; acromegaly is excluded if the serum GH is less than 1 µg/L (IRMA or chemiluminescent assays) or less than 2 µg/L (older radioimmunoassays) after glucose syrup, and if the IGF-1 is normal.

C. IMAGING

MRI shows a pituitary tumor in 90% of acromegalics. MRI is generally superior to CT scanning, especially in the postoperative setting. X-rays of the skull may show an enlarged sella and thickened skull. X-rays may also show tufting of the terminal phalanges of the fingers and toes. A lateral view of the foot shows increased thickness of the heel pad.

Differential Diagnosis

Active acromegaly must be distinguished from familial coarse features, large hands and feet, and isolated prognathism and from inactive ("burned-out") acromegaly in which there has been a spontaneous remission due to infarction of the pituitary adenoma. GH-induced gigantism must be differentiated from familial tall stature and from aromatase deficiency. (See Osteoporosis.)

Misleadingly high serum GH levels can be caused by exercise or eating just prior to the test, acute illness or agitation, hepatic or renal failure, malnourishment, diabetes mellitus or concurrent treatment with estrogens, beta-blockers, or clonidine.

Complications

Complications include hypopituitarism, hypertension, glucose intolerance or frank diabetes mellitus, cardiac enlargement, and cardiac failure. Carpal tunnel syndrome may cause thumb weakness and thenar atrophy. Arthritis of hips, knees, and spine can be trouble-

some. Cord compression may be seen. Visual field defects may be severe and progressive. Acute loss of vision or cranial nerve palsy may occur if the tumor undergoes spontaneous hemorrhage and necrosis (pituitary apoplexy).

Treatment

Endoscopic transnsasal, transsphenoidal pituitary microsurgery removes the adenoma while preserving anterior pituitary function in most patients. Growth hormone levels fall immediately; diaphoresis and carpal tunnel syndrome often improve within a day after surgery. Transsphenoidal surgery is usually well tolerated, but complications occur in about 10%, including infection, cerebrospinal fluid leak, and hypopituitarism. Hyponatremia can occur 4–13 days postoperatively and is manifested by nausea, vomiting, headache, malaise, or seizure. Dietary salt supplements for 2 weeks postoperatively may prevent this complication.

Patients who fail to have a clinical or biochemical remission after surgery are treated with a dopamine agonist. This treatment is most successful for tumors that secrete both PRL and GH. About one-third of such tumors shrink by more than 50% with cabergoline given in dosages of 1–1.75 mg/wk orally.

Somatostatin analogs may be used to treat patients who have persistent acromegaly despite pituitary surgery: Octreotide and lanreotide are somatostatin analogs that are given by subcutaneous injection. Short-acting octreotide acetate in doses of 50 µg injected subcutaneously three times daily. Responders who tolerate the drug are switched to long-acting octreotide acetate injectable suspension in a dosage of 20 mg intragluteally per month. The dosage may be adjusted—up to a maximum of 40 mg monthly—to maintain the serum GH between 1 ng and 2.5 ng/mL, keeping IGF-1 levels normal. Lanreotide SR (not available in USA) is given by subcutaneous injection at a dosage of 30 mg every 7–14 days. Lanreotide Autogel (not available in USA) is a newer formulation that is administered by deep subcutaneous injection in doses of 60–120 mg every 28 days; this preparation is better-tolerated than lanreotide SR. All somatostatin analogs are expensive and must be continued indefinitely or until other treatment has been effective. Somatostatin analogs are fairly equivalent in effectiveness, suppressing GH to < 5 ng/mL in 60% of treated patients within 3–6 months. Headache often improves, but tumor shrinkage is usually marginal. Side effects are experienced by about one-third of patients and include injection site pain, loose acholic stools, abdominal discomfort, or cholelithiasis.

Pegvisomant (not available in USA) is a GH receptor antagonist. A series of 160 acromegalic patients were treated with pegvisomant 20 mg subcutaneously daily for 6–18 months. Serum IGF-1 levels fell to normal in over 90% of patients. Pegvisomant was well tolerated. GH levels rose, but only two patients were noted to have progressive growth of their pituitary tumors.

Pituitary irradiation is suggested for patients who are not cured by surgical and medical therapy. Stereotactic radiosurgery is the preferred modality.

Prognosis

Patients with untreated or persistent acromegaly tend to have premature cardiovascular disease and progressive acromegalic symptoms. Transsphenoidal pituitary surgery is successful in 80–90% of patients with tumors less than 2 cm in diameter and GH levels less than 50 ng/mL. Postoperatively, normal pituitary function is usually preserved. Soft tissue swelling regresses but bone enlargement is permanent. Hypertension frequently persists despite successful surgery. Conventional radiation therapy (alone) produces a remission in about 40% by 2 years and 75% by 5 years after treatment. Gamma knife radiation reduces GH levels an average of 77%, with 20% having a full remission after 12 months. Heavy particle pituitary radiation produces a remission in about 70% by 2 years and 80% by 5 years. Radiation therapy eventually produces some degree of hypopituitarism in most patients. Conventional radiation therapy may cause some degree of organic brain syndrome and predisposes to small strokes. Growth hormone levels over 5 ng/mL and rising usually indicate a recurrent tumor.

Caron P et al: Efficacy of the new long-acting formulation of lanreotide (lanreotide Autogel) in the management of acromegaly. J Clin Endocrinol Metab 2002;87:99. [PMID: 11788630] (Compared with standard lanreotide, lanreotide Autogel was just as effective and better tolerated.)

Colao A et al: Long-term effects of depot long-acting somatostatin analog octreotide on hormone levels and tumor mass in acromegaly. J Clin Endocrinol Metab 2001;86:2779. [PMID: 11397887] (Therapy with depot long-acting octreotide was effective in 36 patients with acromegaly. Over 1–2 years of therapy, clinical improvement was noted in all, GH hypersecretion was controlled in 69%, and IGF-1 levels were normal in 61%. Tumor shrinkage was noted in 12 of 15 patients treated de novo.)

Kreutzer J et al: Surgical management of GH-secreting pituitary adenomas: an outcome study using modern remission criteria. J Clin Endocrinol Metab 2001;86:4072. [PMID: 11549628] (A retrospective study of 57 patients treated with transsphenoidal surgery for GH-secreting pituitary adenomas showed the procedure to be safe, effective, and often definitive. Surgical remission was achieved in approximately 70% of patients followed for an average of 3 years. There were no perioperative deaths or serious morbidity. Permanent complications were seen in only three patients—one with diabetes insipidus, two with nasal septal perforations.)

van der Lely AJ et al: Long term treatment of acromegaly with pegvisomant, a growth hormone receptor antagonist. Lancet 2001;358:1754. [PMID: 11734231] (Pegvisomant 20 mg was given by subcutaneous injection daily to 160 patients with acromegaly. Pegvisomant was effective and well tolerated. Two patients had progressive enlargement of their pituitary tumors. Two other patients had increases in liver aminotransferases during therapy.)

HYPERPROLACTINEMIA

 ESSENTIALS OF DIAGNOSIS

- Women: Menstrual cycle disturbances (oligomenorrhea, amenorrhea); galactorrhea; infertility.
- Men: Hypogonadism; decreased libido and erectile dysfunction; infertility.
- Elevated serum prolactin.
- CT scan or MRI often demonstrates pituitary adenoma.

Normal Physiology

Prolactin's main role is to induce lactation. Serum prolactin levels increase during pregnancy from a normal (follicular phase) level of less than 20 ng/mL to as high as 600 ng/mL by the time of delivery. Under the combined effect of prolactin, increased estrogen, and progesterone, breast development takes place, with eventual formation of milk in the acini. Estrogens inhibit the actual secretion of milk. After parturition, the sudden withdrawal of estrogen caused by expulsion of the placenta results in the onset of lactation. During the puerperal period, suckling constitutes a powerful stimulus for the continued production of prolactin as well as oxytocin. Lactation will cease if prolactin secretion is interrupted by prolactin-lowering drugs or by pituitary destruction. Prolactin is an unusual hormone in terms of control of secretion in that it is under mainly inhibitory control. Thus, section of the pituitary stalk will result in marked increases in prolactin secretion. Prolactin inhibitory factor (PIF) is dopamine.

Prolactin circulates in different forms. Normally, the predominant form is "little prolactin" (molecular mass 23 kDa), with lesser amounts of "big prolactin" (50–60 kDa) and even lesser amounts of "macroprolactin" (150–170 kDa). Macroprolactin is relatively inactive but has a long serum half-life. Some individuals have normal pituitaries that preferentially secrete more macroprolactin; they account for about 10% of patients determined to have hyperprolactinemia. Elevated serum prolactin can be caused by numerous conditions (Table 26–4).

General Considerations

Prolactin-secreting pituitary tumors are more common in women than in men and are usually sporadic but may rarely be familial as part of multiple endocrine neoplasia (MEN 1). Most are microadenomas (< 1 cm in diameter) which do not grow even with pregnancy or oral contraceptives. However, some are

Table 26–4. Causes of hyperprolactinemia.

Physiologic Causes	Pharmacologic Causes	Pathologic Causes
Exercise	Amoxapine	Acromegaly
Idiopathic	Amphetamines	Chronic chest wall stimulation (postthoracotomy,
Macroprolactinemia	Anesthetic agents	postmastectomy, herpes zoster, breast
("big prolactin")	Butyrophenones	problems, nipple rings, etc)
Pregnancy	Cimetidine and rantidine (not famotidine	Cirrhosis
Puerperium	or nizatidine)	Hypothalamic disease
Sleep (REM phase)	Estrogens	Hypothyroidism
Stress (trauma, surgery)	Hydroxyzine	Multiple sclerosis
Suckling	Methyldopa	Optic neuromyelitis
	Metoclopramide	Pituitary stalk section
	Narcotics	Prolactin-secreting tumors
	Nicotine	Pseudocyesis (false pregnancy)
	Phenothiazines	Renal failure (especially with zinc deficiency)
	Protease inhibitors	Spinal cord lesions
	Progestins	Systemic lupus erythematosus
	Reserpine	
	Risperidone	
	Selective serotonin reuptake inhibitors	
	Tricyclic antidepressants	
	Verapamil	

quite large and can spread into the cavernous sinuses and suprasellar areas; rarely, they may erode the floor of the sella to invade the sinuses.

Clinical Findings

A. SYMPTOMS AND SIGNS

Hyperprolactinemia due to any cause may result in hypogonadotropic hypogonadism. Men usually have erectile dysfunction and diminished libido; gynecomastia sometimes occurs, but never with galactorrhea. Women may note oligomenorrhea or amenorrhea, though some women continue to menstruate normally; galactorrhea is common. Of women with secondary amenorrhea and galactorrhea, about 70% have hyperprolactinemia. Untreated hypogonadism ultimately increases the risk for developing osteoporosis.

Pituitary prolactinomas may cosecrete growth hormone and cause acromegaly (see above). Large tumors may cause headaches, visual symptoms, and pituitary insufficiency.

B. LABORATORY FINDINGS

Patients found to have hyperprolactinemia are evaluated for conditions known to cause it, particularly pregnancy (serum hCG), hypothyroidism (serum free thyroxine and TSH), renal failure (BUN and serum creatinine), and cirrhosis (clinical evaluation and serum bilirubin and liver enzymes). A serum calcium is obtained to screen for hyperparathyroidism. Patients are assessed for hypogonadism. An assay for macroprolactinemia should be considered for patients with hyperprolactinemia who are relatively asymptomatic and

have no apparent cause for hyperprolactinemia. Screening for macroprolactinemia may be done with gel filtration chromatography or polyethylene glycol gel precipitation. Patients having pituitary macroadenomas (> 3 cm in diameter) should have prolactin measured on serial dilutions of serum, since IRMA assays may otherwise report falsely low titers, the "high-dose hook effect."

C. IMAGING

When hyperprolactinemia persists without obvious cause, MRI of the pituitary and hypothalamus is indicated. Small prolactinomas may thus be demonstrated, but clear differentiation from normal variants is not always possible.

Differential Diagnosis

The differential diagnosis of prolactinoma should include acromegaly, since pituitary tumors often cosecrete prolactin and growth hormone. However, the most common causes of hyperprolactinemia are pregnancy and suckling. High prolactin levels are also commonly seen in conditions such as hypothyroidism, cirrhosis, renal failure, systemic lupus erythematosus, and hypothalamic disease. Chronic nipple stimulation, nipple piercing, augmentation mammoplasty, and mastectomy may stimulate prolactin secretion. Hyperprolactinemia may also be idiopathic or associated with secretion of macroprolactin, a relatively inactive "big prolactin." Many drugs cause hyperprolactinemia, particularly psychotropic agents, cimetidine, tricyclic antidepressants, and oral contraceptives.

(See Table 26–4.) Increased pituitary size is a normal variant in young women.

Treatment

Medications known to increase prolactin should be stopped if possible. Hyperprolactinemia due to hypothyroidism is corrected by thyroxine. Patients with hyperprolactinemia not induced by drugs, hypothyroidism, or pregnancy should be examined by pituitary MRI. Women with microprolactinomas who have amenorrhea or are desirous of contraception may safely take oral contraceptives or estrogen replacement—there is minimal risk of stimulating enlargement of the adenoma. Since estrogens or testosterone treatment can stimulate the growth of macroprolactinomas, they should not be used by patients with large pituitary adenomas unless in full remission with dopamine agonist medication or surgery.

A. DOPAMINE AGONISTS

Dopamine agonists are the initial treatment of choice for patients with macroprolactinomas and those with hyperprolactinemia desiring restoration of normal sexual function and fertility. Of the ergot-derived dopamine agonists, cabergoline is usually the best tolerated and is prescribed beginning with a dosage of 0.25 mg orally once weekly for 1 week, then 0.25 mg twice weekly for the next week, then 0.5 mg twice weekly. Further dosage increases may be required monthly, based upon serum prolactin levels, up to a maximum of 1.5 mg twice weekly. Alternative drugs include bromocriptine (1.25–20 mg/d orally) and pergolide (0.125–2 mg/d orally). Women who experience nausea with oral preparations may find relief with deep vaginal insertion of cabergoline or bromocriptine tablets; vaginal irritation sometimes occurs. Quinagolide (Norprolac; not available in USA) is a non-ergot-derived dopamine agonist for patients intolerant or resistant to ergot-derived medications; the starting dosage is 0.075 mg/d orally, increasing as needed and tolerated to a maximum of 0.6 mg/d.

Dopamine agonists are given at bedtime to minimize side effects of fatigue, nausea, dizziness, and orthostatic hypotension. These symptoms usually improve with dosage reduction and continued use. Erythromelalgia is rare. A variety of psychiatric side effects may be seen which are not dose-related and may take weeks to resolve once the dopamine agonist is discontinued.

With dopamine agonist treatment, 90% of patients with prolactinomas experience a fall in serum prolactin to 10% or less of pretreatment levels; about 80% of treated patients achieve a normal serum prolactin level. Shrinkage of a pituitary adenoma occurs early, but maximum effect may take up to a year. Nearly half—even massive tumors—shrink more than 50%. Discontinuing therapy after months or years usually results in reappearance of hyperprolactinemia and galactorrhea-amenorrhea, but a few patients with microadenomas remain in remission. Since fertility is

usually promptly restored with dopamine agonists, many pregnancies have resulted, with no evidence of teratogenicity. Women with microadenomas may have treatment safely withdrawn during pregnancy. Macroadenomas may enlarge significantly during pregnancy; if therapy is withdrawn, patients must be followed clinically and with computer-assisted visual field perimetry.

B. SURGICAL TREATMENT

Transsphenoidal pituitary surgery may be urgently required for large tumors undergoing apoplexy or those severely compromising visual fields. It is also used electively for patients who do not tolerate or respond to dopamine agonists. Craniotomy is rarely indicated, since even large tumors can usually be decompressed via the transsphenoidal approach.

C. RADIATION THERAPY

Radiation therapy is reserved for patients with macroadenomas that are growing despite treatment with dopamine agonists. Conventional radiation therapy is most commonly used, but it must be given over 5 weeks and carries a high risk of eventual hypopituitarism. Other possible side effects include some degree of memory impairment and an increased long-term risk of second tumors and small vessel ischemic strokes. After radiation therapy, patients are advised to take low-dose aspirin to reduce their stroke risk. A single gamma knife treatment may be preferable for certain patients whose optic chiasm is clear of tumor, since it is generally safer and more convenient.

Pinzone JJ et al: Primary medical therapy of micro- and macroprolactinomas in men. J Clin Endocrinol Metab 2000;85:3053. [PMID: 10999785] (Of 46 men referred for prolactinomas, 74% had macroadenomas over 1 cm in diameter. Treatment with dopamine agonists such as bromocriptine or cabergoline achieved normal serum PRL levels in 83% of microadenomas and 79% of macroadenomas.)

Vallette-Kasic S et al: Macroprolactinemia revisited: a study on 106 patients. J Clin Endocrinol Metab 2002;87:581. [PMID: 11836289] (A French study of 1106 patients with hyperprolactinemia discovered that 10% had macroprolactinemia as determined by serum prolactin chromatography. Patients with macroprolactinemia had serum prolactin levels ranging between 20 μg/L and 663 μg/L, exceeding 100 μg/L in 8.5% of patients. Some symptoms of hyperprolactinemia were present despite preserved fertility. Pituitary MRI was normal in 78%. Prolactin levels returned to normal in 47% of patients receiving dopaminergic therapy.)

■ DISEASES OF THE THYROID GLAND

An adult's thyroid gland normally weighs about 15–20 g. Embryologic defects may result in a rare lingual thyroid, retrosternal thyroid, or agenesis of one or both lobes.

Thyroid-stimulating hormone (TSH, thyrotropin) is secreted by the pituitary and stimulates several steps of thyroid hormone production: trapping of iodine, peroxidase linking of iodine to tyrosine, coupling of monoiodotyrosine or diiodotyrosine to form T_3 (triiodothyronine) or T_4 (thyroxine), and release of T_3 and T_4. The thyroid secretes mostly T_4 and very little T_3. About 90% of circulating T_3, the most active thyroid hormone, is derived from peripheral deiodination of T_4. Circulating thyroid hormones have a direct feedback inhibition effect upon the pituitary thyrotroph cells, desensitizing them from the stimulatory effect of hypothalamic thyrotropin-releasing hormone (TRH).

Over 99% of circulating thyroid hormones are bound to serum proteins, mostly thyroid-binding globulin (TBG). Only free hormone enters cells, binding to nuclear hormone receptors, which regulate DNA control of oxidative processes throughout the body.

The thyroid tests discussed in the following section are ordinarily very helpful in the evaluation of thyroid disorders. However, many conditions and drugs alter serum thyroxine levels without affecting clinical status (Table 26–5). Furthermore, a serum thyroxine determination is not sufficiently sensitive to detect mild degrees of hypo- or hyperthyroidism. Therefore, other tests may be used, but all are imperfect.

TESTS OF THYROID FUNCTION (Table 26–6)

The tests most widely used in clinical practice are serum immunoassays for TSH and "free" thyroxine (FT_4). Assays for FT_4 have largely supplanted measurements of total thyroxine (T_4), resin T_3 uptake (RT_3U), and free thyroxine index (FT_4I).

1. Serum Thyroid Tests

Thyroid-Stimulating Hormone (TSH) Immunoassay

TSH levels as low as 0.01 mU/L can be detected by ultrasensitive "third-generation" assays. In order to diagnose hyperthyroidism, an assay sensitive to at least 0.1 mU/L (sensitive "second-generation" assay) should be employed. Owing to discrepancies between different TSH assay methods, it is prudent to recheck unexpected results with a different assay.

TSH levels are **decreased** in patients with primary hyperthyroidism (eg, Graves' disease, toxic multin-

Table 26–5. Factors falsely altering serum thyroxine measurements without affecting clinical status.[1,2]

Factors Increasing T₄	Factors Decreasing T₄
Laboratory error	Laboratory error
AIDS (increased thyroid-binding globulin)	Severe illness (eg, chronic renal failure, major surgery, caloric
Autoimmunity	deprivation)
Acute illness (eg, viral hepatitis, chronic active hepatitis;	Acute psychiatric problems
primary biliary cirrhosis; acute intermittent porphyria;	Cirrhosis
AIDS)	Nephrotic syndrome
High-estrogen states (may also increase total T₃)	Hereditary TBG deficiency
Oral estrogen-containing contraceptives	Drugs
Pregnancy	Androgens
Estrogen replacement therapy	Asparaginase
Tamoxifen	Carbamazepine
Acute psychiatric problems	Chloral hydrate
Hyperemesis gravidarum and morning sickness (may	Fenclofenac
also increase T₃)	Fluorouracil
Familial thyroid-binding abnormalities	Glucocorticoids
Generalized resistance to thyroid hormone	Halofenate (lowers triglycerides and uric acid; not marketed in
Drugs	USA)
Amiodarone	Mitotane
Amphetamines	Nicotinic acid
Clofibrate	Phenobarbital
Heparin (dialysis method)	Phenylbutazone
Heroin	Phenytoin (T₄ may be as low as 2 µg/dL)
Levothyroxine (T₄) replacement therapy	Salicylates (large doses)
Methadone (may also increase T₃)	Sertraline
Perphenazine	Triiodothyronine (T₃) therapy

[1]Reproduced, with permission, from Fitzgerald PA: *Handbook of Clinical Endocrinology,* 2nd ed. McGraw-Hill 1992.
[2]Symptomatic hyperthyroidism or hypothyroidism may also be present incidentally.

Table 26 6. Appropriate use of thyroid tests.

Purpose	Test	Comment
Screening	Serum TSH (sensitive assay)	Most sensitive test for primary hypothyroidism and hyperthyroidism
	Free T_4	Excellent test
For hypothyroidism	Serum TSH	High in primary and low in secondary hypothyroidism
	Antithyroglobulin and antithyroid peroxidase antibodies	Elevated in Hashimoto's thyroiditis
For hyperthyroidism	Serum TSH (sensitive assay)	Suppressed except in TSH-secreting pituitary tumor or hyperplasia (rare)
	T_3 (RIA)	Elevated
	^{123}I uptake and scan	Increased diffuse versus "hot" areas
	Antithyroglobulin and antimicrosomal antibodies	Elevated in Graves' disease
	TSH receptor antibody (TSH-R Ab [stim])	Usually positive in Graves' disease
For nodules	Fine-needle aspiration (FNA)	Best diagnostic method for thyroid cancer
	^{123}I uptake and scan	Cancer is usually "cold." Less reliable than FNA.
	^{99m}Tc scan	Vascular versus avascular
	Ultrasonography	Solid versus cystic. Pure cysts are usually not malignant.

odular goiter, toxic nodule, subacute thyroiditis, or release of stored hormone in Hashimoto's thyroiditis). TSH levels may also be suppressed in some clinically euthyroid individuals with autonomous thyroid secretion (eg, euthyroid Graves' ophthalmopathy). TSH can also be suppressed by thyroid hormone administration in either excessive or adequate replacement amounts. TSH is also frequently low during severe nonthyroidal illness; distinction from hypopituitarism can usually be made clinically.

Dopamine and dopamine agonists (levodopa, bromocriptine) can cause suppression of TSH and may cause true secondary hypothyroidism during prolonged administration. Other conditions associated with decreased TSH include pregnancy (especially with morning sickness), hCG-secreting trophoblastic tumors, acute psychiatric illness (1% incidence), and acute administration of glucocorticoids. Certain drugs cause mild suppression of TSH without clinical hyperthyroidism; these include nonsteroidal anti-inflammatory agents, amphetamine, octreotide, opioids, and certain calcium channel blockers (especially nifedipine; also verapamil, but not diltiazem).

In clinically euthyroid persons age 60 or older, the TSH is very low (≤ 0.1 mU/L) in 3% and mildly low (0.1–0.4 mU/L) in 9%. The chance of developing atrial fibrillation is higher with very low TSH (2.8% yearly) than with normal TSH (1.1% yearly). Asymptomatic patients with very low TSH are followed closely but not treated unless they develop atrial fibrillation or other manifestations of hyperthyroidism.

TSH levels are **elevated** in primary hypothyroidism, either clinical or subclinical. TSH may also be elevated or inappropriately normal in the very rare cases of hyperthyroidism due to pituitary neoplastic or nonneoplastic inappropriate secretion of thyrotropin. Autoimmune disease may also falsely elevate serum TSH levels by interfering with the assay. TSH may be transiently elevated during recovery from nonthyroidal illness and in about 14% of patients with acute psychiatric admissions; the TSH returns to normal in the great majority of these patients. TSH may be increased by dopamine antagonists (eg, metoclopramide), phenothiazines, and atypical antipsychotics. TSH may be mildly elevated in some individuals, especially elderly women (10% incidence). Such patients with normal T_4 levels must be carefully evaluated for subtle signs of hypothyroidism (eg, fatigue, depression, hyperlipidemia). About 18% later become definitely hypothyroid.

Free Thyroxine Immunoassay (FT₄)

FT_4 is a direct measurement of the serum concentration of free (unbound) thyroxine. FT_4 represents only about 0.025% of the serum concentration of the total T_4. It is the only metabolically active fraction of T_4 that freely enters cells to produce its effects.

When performed properly, this assay is superior to the total T_4 assay and free thyroxine index, since it is not affected by variations in protein binding. It is the procedure of choice for following the thyroid's changing secretion of T_4 during treatment for hyperthyroidism. Serum FT_4 levels may be suppressed in patients with severe nonthyroid illness. In patients receiving heparin, measured levels of FT_4 may be falsely high, particularly when a dialysis assay is used. Serum FT_4 levels rise transiently in acute nonthyroidal illness, when thyroid-binding protein frequently falls.

T_4 Immunoassay

This test measures the total serum concentration of thyroxine (bound and free). An increased serum T_4 confirms a clinical diagnosis of hyperthyroidism, while a decreased serum T_4 confirms a clinical diagnosis of hypothyroidism. It is affected by altered states of thyroxine binding (see Table 26–5). Therefore, this test is usually run with a resin T_3 uptake to provide a free thyroxine index (see below).

Resin T_3 (or T_4) Uptake

This is an indirect inverse test of serum thyroid-binding proteins (TBP)—ie, it is high when thyroid-binding proteins are low. The assay involves adding labeled T_3 or T_4 to the serum sample; it competes with the patient's thyroxine for binding to TBP. This mixture is then added to a thyroid hormone-binding resin. The resin is then assayed for its uptake of the label. A high resin uptake indicates that the patient's serum contains relatively low amounts of TBP or high levels of thyroxine.

This test corrects a total serum thyroxine measurement for the effect of increased or decreased binding, creating a free thyroxine index (see below). A low resin uptake (high TBP) is seen with estrogen therapy, pregnancy, acute hepatitis, genetic TBP increase, and hypothyroidism. A low resin uptake with low TBP may be seen in severe illness. A high resin uptake (low TBP) is seen with hyperthyroidism and with chronic liver disease, nephrotic syndrome, anabolic steroid administration, and high-dose glucocorticoid administration.

Free Thyroxine Index (FTI)

The product of T_4 and resin T_3 uptake ($T_4 \times T_3$ uptake) helps correct for abnormalities of thyroxine binding. A good free T_4 assay is more accurate.

The FTI, when calculated using the RT_3U, may be elevated in euthyroid patients with familial dysalbuminemic hyperthyroxinemia. This is a benign autosomal dominant trait in which an abnormal albumin molecule binds T_4 with much greater affinity than T_3. The RT_3U is not decreased (failing to compensate for the increased binding, as it would for TBG excess), because the T_3 used in the RT_3U assay is not significantly affected. Serum levels of free thyroxine and TSH are normal.

T_3

This test is of value in the diagnosis of thyrotoxicosis with normal T_4 values (T_3 thyrotoxicosis). It is not useful for the diagnosis of hypothyroidism.

Free T_3

This test measures the very tiny amount of T_3 that circulates unbound. It is useful in looking for hyperthyroidism in women who are pregnant or taking oral estrogen.

2. Thyroid Radioactive Iodine Uptake & Scan

Radioiodine (^{123}I or ^{131}I) Uptake of Thyroid Gland

A. ELEVATED

Graves' disease, dietary iodine deficiency, toxic nodular goiter, pregnancy, early Hashimoto's thyroiditis, some thyroid enzyme deficiencies, nephrotic syndrome, recovery from subacute thyroiditis, recovery from thyroid hormone suppression.

B. LOW

Administration of iodides or iodine in any form (drugs, radiology contrast dyes, etc), antithyroid drugs, subacute thyroiditis, thyroid hormone administration, thyroid gland damage (from thyroiditis, surgery, or radioiodine), hypopituitarism, ectopic functioning thyroid tissue, azotemia, severe (high-turnover) Graves' disease, heart failure, and some thyroid enzyme abnormalities.

Radioiodine (RAI) Scans

A rectilinear scan over the neck may be obtained after radioiodine administration, thereby obtaining a life-sized picture of thyroid uptake. RAI scans are useful also for detecting metastatic thyroid cancer. (See Thyroid Cancer.) Following administration of a treatment dose of ^{131}I for thyroid cancer, a whole body scan is useful for detecting metastases.

3. Other Thyroid Tests

Thyroid Antibodies

Antibodies against several thyroid constituents (thyroglobulin and thyroperoxidase) are most commonly found in Hashimoto's thyroiditis and Graves' disease. Antithyroid antibodies are found in about 5–10% of normal subjects. There is an increasing incidence with age. About 20% of hospitalized patients have detectable antithyroid antibodies. In the latter, the titers tend to be low, and they increase with age. TSH receptor antibody (TSH-R Ab [stim]) titers are elevated in approximately 80% of patients with Graves' disease. These titers—and those of antithyroglobulin and antithyroperoxidase antibodies—often decrease during pregnancy and during treatment of Graves' disease with antithyroid drugs. TSH-R Ab [stim] titers have been used with variable results to predict the rate of relapse of Graves' disease after chronic thiourea therapy.

Serum Thyroglobulin

The level of serum thyroglobulin rises in autoimmune thyroid disease, thyroid injury or inflammation, and thyroid cancer. Levels are of little value in diagnosing or distinguishing among these conditions, but they provide a useful marker in thyroid cancer to indicate recurrence of disease and the need for further studies and therapy. Serum thyroglobulin is to be distinguished from serum thyroid binding globulin (see above).

Calcitonin Assay

This test is elevated in medullary thyroid carcinoma, azotemia, hypercalcemia, pernicious anemia, thyroiditis, and pregnancy. High levels are also seen in many other malignancies such as carcinomas of the lung (45%), pancreas, breast (38%), and colon (24%).

Ultrasound

Ultrasound may be used to guide fine-needle aspiration biopsy of clinically suspicious thyroid nodules and nodes. In patients with established thyroid malignancy, ultrasound of the neck is useful for surveillance, localization, and quantitation of residual or recurrent tumor. Small nonpalpable nodules are detected in half of "normal" thyroids and are rarely malignant.

Fine-Needle Thyroid Biopsy

Aspiration of thyroid tissue with a fine needle (25-gauge) is helpful in the diagnosis of thyroid disorders, especially nodular lesions. This technique has become the preferred approach to the diagnosis of thyroid masses. (See Nodular Thyroid.)

4. Effect of Nonthyroidal Illness & Drugs Upon Thyroid Function Tests

Many factors affect thyroid function tests, causing misleading laboratory evidence of hypothyroidism or hyperthyroidism in patients who are clinically euthyroid. (See Table 26–5.)

Serum thyroxine is frequently low in patients with severe illness, caloric deprivation, or major surgery who have accelerated peripheral metabolism of serum T_4 to reverse T_3 (rT_3). Furthermore, in most patients who are critically ill, there is a circulating inhibitor of thyroid hormone binding to serum thyroid binding proteins. This causes the resin uptake of thyroid hormone (RT_3U) to be misleadingly low, causing the computed free thyroxine index to be very low. The presence of a very low serum T_4 in severe nonthyroidal illness indicates a poor prognosis.

Direct assays of free thyroxine often show low levels of FT_4 in severe illness. Since studies of giving replacement thyroxine to such patients have shown no improvement in survival, they are considered "euthyroid." Serum TSH tends to be suppressed in severe nonthyroidal illness, making the diagnosis of concurrent primary hypothyroidism quite difficult, although the presence of a goiter suggests the diagnosis.

The clinician must decide whether such severely ill patients (with a low serum T_4 but nonelevated TSH) might have hypothyroidism due to pituitary insufficiency. Patients without symptoms of prior brain lesion or hypopituitarism are very unlikely to suddenly develop hypopituitarism during an unrelated illness. Patients with diabetes insipidus, hypopituitarism, or other signs of a central nervous system lesion may have thyroxine given empirically. Patients receiving prolonged dopamine infusions may develop true secondary hypothyroidism due to direct dopamine suppression of TSH-secreting cells.

Dayan CM: Interpretation of thyroid function tests. Lancet 2001;357:619. [PMID: 11558500] (Important pitfalls occur when interpreting thyroid function tests. If assays for TSH, free T_3, and free T_4 are all done, their patterns along with clinical information allow the proper diagnosis to be made in most cases.)

Despres N et al: Antibody interference in thyroid assays: a potential for clinical misinformation. Clin Chem 1998;44:440. [PMID: 9510847]

Isojarvi JI et al: Thyroid function in men taking carbamazepine, oxcarbazepine, or valproate for epilepsy. Epilepsia 2001;42: 930. [PMID: 11488894] (Serum T_4 and free T_4 levels fell below the reference normal range in 45% of men taking carbamazepine, in 24% of men taking oxcarbazepine, and in none of the men taking valproate. Serum levels of T_3 and TSH remained normal in all patients on each drug.)

THYROID NODULES & MULTINODULAR GOITER

 ESSENTIALS OF DIAGNOSIS

- *Single or multiple thyroid nodules are commonly found with careful thyroid examinations.*
- *Thyroid function tests mandatory.*
- *Thyroid biopsy for single or dominant nodules or for a history of prior head-neck radiation.*
- *Ultrasound examination sometimes useful for biopsy and follow-up.*
- *Clinical follow-up required.*

General Considerations

Palpable enlargement of the thyroid (goiter) may be diffuse or nodular and is detectable in 4% of North American adults. The incidence of goiter is higher in iodine-deficient geographic areas (see Endemic Goiter, below). The presence of a goiter warrants further testing and follow-up. Most patients with goiter are euthyroid, but there is a high incidence of hypothyroidism or hyperthyroidism. Diffuse and multinodular goiters are ordinarily benign and may be caused by numerous conditions, eg, benign multinodular goiter, iodine deficiency, pregnancy (in areas of iodine deficiency), Graves' disease, Hashimoto's thyroiditis, subacute thyroiditis, or infections. A solitary thyroid nodule is most often a benign adenoma, colloid nodule, or cyst but may sometimes be a primary thyroid malignancy or (less frequently) a metastatic neoplasm. The risk of a palpable nodule being malignant is higher among patients with a history of head-neck radiation, a family history of thyroid cancer, or a personal history of another malignancy. The risk of malignancy is higher if a thyroid nodule is large, adherent to the trachea or strap muscles, or associated with lymphadenopathy.

The thyroid is best examined in a well-lighted room. The seated patient is given water to drink and the anterior neck is observed during swallowing. The thyroid moves upward during swallowing and may be visible in a thin neck; enlargement or asymmetry of the thyroid may be noted. Palpation of the thyroid is best done from behind a seated patient using the second and third fingers of both hands. As the patient swallows water, thyroid nodules may be perceived moving beneath the fingers. The location of any nodules should be noted, along with their size, firmness, and tenderness. The neck should be examined for lymphadenopathy. Enlarged thyroids should be auscultated for bruits.

Clinical Evaluation (Table 26–7)

A. SYMPTOMS AND SIGNS

Most small thyroid nodules are asymptomatic and are discovered incidentally on routine neck inspection or palpation; some are discovered as an incidental finding during radiological imaging of the neck. Graves' disease, toxic multinodular goiter, hyperfunctioning nodules, and subacute thyroiditis can cause hyperthyroidism. Hashimoto's thyroiditis may cause goiter and hypothyroidism.

A thyroid nodule or multinodular goiter can grow to become visible and of concern to the patient. Particularly large nodular goiters can become a cosmetic embarrassment. Nodules can grow large enough to cause discomfort, hoarseness, or dysphagia. Retrosternal large multinodular goiters can cause dyspnea due to tracheal compression.

B. LABORATORY FINDINGS

Thyroid nodules are an indication for thyroid function testing. Serum determinations for TSH (sensitive assay) and free thyroxine (FT_4) are preferred. Tests for antithyroperoxidase antibodies and antithyroglobulin antibodies may also be helpful. Very high antibody levels are found in Hashimoto's thyroiditis. However, thyroiditis frequently coexists with malignancy, so a suspicious nodule should be biopsied.

Fine-needle aspiration (FNA) biopsy is the best way to assess a nodule for malignancy. A 25-gauge

Table 26–7. Clinical evaluation of thyroid nodules.[1]

Clinical Evidence	Low Index of Suspicion	High Index of Suspicion
History	Family history of goiter; residence in area of endemic goiter	Previous therapeutic radiation of head, neck, or chest; hoarseness
Physical characteristics	Older women; soft nodule; multinodular goiter	Young adults, men; solitary, firm nodule; vocal cord paralysis; enlarged lymph nodes; distant metastatic lesions
Serum factors	High titer of antithyroid antibody; hypothyroidism; hyperthyroidism	
Fine-needle aspiration biopsy	Colloid nodule or adenoma	Papillary carcinoma, follicular neoplasm, medullary or anaplastic carcinoma
Scanning techniques Uptake of [123]I Ultrasonogram Roentgenogram	"Hot" nodule Cystic lesion Shell-like calcification	"Cold" nodule Solid lesion Punctate calcification
Thyroxine therapy	Regression after 0.05–0.1 mg/d for 6 months or more	Increase in size

[1]Clinically suspicious nodules should be evaluated with fine-needle aspiration biopsy.

needle is used to biopsy suspicious nodules. The needle is attached to a syringe and special syringe holder. The biopsy is done without local anesthesia. The success rate of FNA biopsy is increased by ultrasound guidance. Care must be taken to avoid bloody dilution of the specimens. Material obtained is placed on a slide; a thin smear is obtained by laying a second slide over the material and then drawing the slides apart. One slide is air-dried while the other is preserved in 95% alcohol. Two or more biopsies may be obtained. Reading by an experienced cytopathologist is mandatory.

In one review of thyroid biopsies, about 70% were benign, 10% follicular neoplasm (suspicious), 5% malignant, and 15% nondiagnostic. About 20–40% of patients with "suspicious" cytology harbor a malignancy, with the risk being higher in young patients and those with nodules that are fixed or over 3 cm in diameter. Most such patients undergo thyroid surgery. However, a subgroup of elderly patients with "suspicious" cytology (nodules < 4 cm in diameter) have a malignancy rate of just 5%; such patients may elect to be followed every 6 months with palpation and ultrasound.

Cystic nodules yielding serous fluid are usually benign, but fluid should be submitted for cytology. Cystic nodules yielding bloody fluid have a higher chance of being malignant. Repeat FNA biopsy is done if the cytology is nondiagnostic (eg, diluted with blood or hypocellular) and the lesion remains palpable.

C. IMAGING STUDIES

Neck ultrasound should be performed on most patients with thyroid nodules, since it frequently adds important information. Ultrasound is more accurate than palpation in measuring the size of a nodule and can help determine whether a palpable nodule is part of a multinodular goiter, thus having less chance of being malignant. Ultrasound is also helpful in following thyroid nodules. The detection of calcification increases the risk of a nodule's being malignant. Ultrasound-guided fine-needle aspiration biopsy is helpful in obtaining representative and adequate specimens, especially from complex thyroid nodules. Ultrasonography is generally preferred over CT and MRI because of its accuracy, ease of use, and lower cost.

Radioactive iodine (RAI; ^{123}I or ^{131}I) scans have limited utility in the evaluation of thyroid nodules. Hypofunctioning (cold) nodules have a somewhat increased risk of being malignant, but most are benign. Hyperfunctioning (hot) nodules are ordinarily benign but may sometimes be malignant. RAI scanning and uptake are helpful if a patient is found to have evidence of hyperthyroidism. (See Hyperthyroidism, below.)

Treatment

All thyroid nodules, including those with benign cytology, need to be followed by regular periodic palpation and rebiopsied if growth occurs. Patients with elevated levels of serum TSH are treated with thyroxine replacement. Otherwise, for small nodules, thyroxine is not required. For larger nodules (> 2 cm), if TSH levels are elevated or normal, "suppression" with levothyroxine sodium (0.05–0.1 mg daily) can be considered. Levothyroxine should not be administered if the baseline TSH is low, since that is an indication of autonomous thyroid secretion, such that levothyroxine treatment will be ineffective and liable to cause clinical thyrotoxicosis. Long-term levothyroxine suppression of TSH tends to keep nodules from enlarging, but only a few will actually shrink. Additional nodules develop in fewer treated patients. Suppressive levothyroxine therapy is most suitable for younger patients. All patients require regular careful clinical evaluation and thyroid palpation or ultrasound examinations. Levothyroxine suppression therapy should usually not be given to patients with certain cardiovascular problems since it may increase the risk for angina and arrhythmia. Levothyroxine suppression causes a small loss of bone density in many postmenopausal women not taking estrogen replacement; estrogen appears protective in this regard. Patients at risk for osteoporosis are advised to have periodic bone density testing.

A. SOLITARY THYROID NODULES

Palpable solitary thyroid nodules call for fine-needle aspiration biopsy (see above). A solitary thyroid nodule in a patient with a remote history of radiation therapy to the head or neck (or exposure to nuclear fallout) is considered at high risk of malignancy and the nodule is resected. Cystic nodules can be managed by removal of fluid for cytologic examination, which may deflate the cyst. However, cysts tend to recur, requiring repeated aspirations. Solitary nodules in a patient with hyperthyroidism are an indication for radioactive iodine scan, which generally distinguishes toxic adenoma from Graves' disease. However, Graves' disease may occasionally be unilateral owing to agenesis of the contralateral lobe, so additional studies with antithyroid antibodies may be helpful. A "hot" nodule is usually benign but is resected to cure the hyperthyroidism.

B. MULTINODULAR GOITERS

A thyroid containing multiple nodules is likely to be a benign multinodular goiter. Nevertheless, fine-needle aspiration biopsy is performed on any nodule that is growing or is particularly dominant or hard. Large retrosternal goiters rarely harbor a malignancy but can be followed by CT scan or MRI. Continued growth or compressive symptoms are reasons for surgical excision. Patients found to be hyperthyroid may have a radioactive iodine scan and uptake for additional evaluation, especially if ^{131}I is a therapeutic consideration.

C. NONPALPABLE THYROID NODULES

Nonpalpable small thyroid nodules are detected in about 50% of scans of the neck (MRI, CT, ultrasound) done for other reasons. In one series, only 2% of such thyroids were found to have significant malignancy after surgical resection. Therefore, ultrasound-guided FNA biopsy is considered only for patients with nonpalpable nodules over 1.5 cm in diameter and for those with a history of head-neck irradiation. For incidentally discovered thyroid nodules of borderline concern, follow-up thyroid ultrasound in 3 months may be helpful; growing lesions may be biopsied or resected.

Microscopic "micropapillary" carcinoma is a variant of normal, being found in 24% of thyroidectomies performed for benign thyroid disease when 2 mm sections were carefully examined. It thus appears that the overwhelming majority of these microscopic foci never become clinically significant. The surgical pathology report of such a tiny papillary carcinoma that is otherwise benign does not justify aggressive follow-up or treatment because a cancer diagnosis is unwarranted and harmful. All that may be required is yearly follow-up with palpation of the neck and mild TSH suppression by thyroxine.

Prognosis

The great majority of thyroid nodules are benign. Benign thyroid nodules tend to persist or grow slowly, but they may involute. Only about 1% of benign nodules increase in diameter with follow-up. Conversion to a malignant nodule is rare. The prognosis for patients with thyroid nodules that prove to be malignant is determined by the histologic type and other factors (see below). Overall, differentiated thyroid carcinoma has an excellent prognosis, but metastases do occur. Multinodular goiters tend to persist or grow slowly, even in iodine-deficient areas where iodine repletion usually does not shrink established goiters. Patients with small incidentally discovered nonpalpable thyroid nodules are at very low risk for malignancy, and even those that are malignant have a minor effect on morbidity and mortality.

Braga M et al: Efficacy of ultrasound-guided fine-needle aspiration biopsy in the diagnosis of complex thyroid nodules. J Clin Endocrinol Metab 2001;86:4089. [PMID: 11549630] (Ultrasound-guided fine-needle aspiration is helpful in obtaining a satisfactory specimen from complex thyroid nodules.)

Gharib H et al: Thyroxine suppressive therapy in patients with nodular thyroid disease. Ann Intern Med 1998;128:386. [PMID: 9490600] (Patients with cytologically benign nodules are best followed without thyroxine suppression. Nodules that increase in size should be rebiopsied or resected.)

Marqusee E et al: Usefulness of ultrasonography in the management of nodular thyroid disease. Ann Intern Med 2000; 133:696. [PMID: 11074902] (Ultrasonography is an important adjunct to the physical examination of the thyroid gland. In this retrospective study of 223 patients with suspected nodular thyroid disease, ultrasonography changed the clinical management in 63%.)

Poller DN et al: Fine-needle aspiration of the thyroid. Cancer 2000;90:239. [PMID: 10966565] ("Indeterminate" fine-needle aspirates had a 15% risk of malignancy whereas "suspicious" aspirates had a 42% risk of malignancy.)

THYROID CANCER (Table 26–8)

ESSENTIALS OF DIAGNOSIS

- Painless swelling in region of thyroid.
- Thyroid function tests usually normal.
- Past history of irradiation to head and neck region may be present.
- Positive thyroid needle aspiration.

Table 26–8. Some characteristics of thyroid cancer.

	Papillary	Follicular	Medullary	Anaplastic
Incidence	Most common	Common	Uncommon	Uncommon
Average age	42	50	50	57
Females	70%	72%	56%	56%
Deaths due to thyroid cancer	6%	24%	33%	98%
Invasion:				
Juxtanodal	+++++	+	++++++	+++
Blood vessels	+	+++	+++	+++++
Distant sites	+	+++	++	++++
Resemblance to normal thyroid	+	+++	+	±
^{123}I uptake	+	++++	0	0
Degree of malignancy	+	++ to +++	+ to ++++	++++++++

General Considerations

The incidence of papillary and follicular (differentiated) thyroid carcinomas increases with age. The female:male ratio is 3:1. About 13% of persons in the USA are found to have microscopic thyroid cancer at autopsy. However, thyroid cancer is diagnosed in only about 40 per million population. Clearly, most thyroid cancers remain microscopic and indolent. Those cancers that do become aggressive often have mutations in the *P53* tumor suppressor gene or the *ras* and *gsp* oncogenes.

Papillary carcinoma is the most common thyroid malignancy. Pure papillary or mixed papillary-follicular carcinoma represents about 76% of all thyroid cancers. It usually presents as a single nodule, but it can arise out of a multinodular goiter. Patients who have had external x-ray treatments to the neck or head during childhood have an increased lifelong risk. Similarly, childhood exposure to radioactive isotopes of iodine in nuclear fallout (eg, after the Chernobyl accident) carries a high risk for later development of papillary thyroid cancer. It may also be familial (3%) or associated with Cowden's disease (multiple hamartomas of the skin and mucous membranes with a high incidence of breast cancer) or adenomatous polyposis coli.

Generally speaking, papillary carcinoma is the least aggressive thyroid malignancy. However, the tumor spreads via lymphatics within the thyroid, becoming multifocal in 60% and involving both lobes in 30%. About 80% of patients have microscopic metastases to cervical lymph nodes; palpable lymph node involvement is present in 15% of adults and 60% of youths. Unlike other forms of cancer, patients with papillary thyroid cancer who have palpable lymph node metastases do not have a particularly increased mortality rate; however their risk of local recurrence is increased.

Occult metastases to the lung occur in 10–15% of differentiated thyroid cancer; such lung metastases may be first noted on the whole-body scan following ^{131}I therapy. About 70% of small lung metastases resolve following ^{131}I therapy; however, larger pulmonary metastases have only a 10% remission rate.

Chronic low-grade papillary carcinoma can sometimes undergo a late anaplastic transformation into an aggressive carcinoma.

Follicular carcinoma accounts for about 16% of thyroid malignancies and is generally more aggressive than papillary carcinoma. Rarely, some follicular carcinomas secrete enough thyroxine to cause thyrotoxicosis if the tumor load becomes significant. Metastases commonly are found in neck nodes, bone, and lungs. Most follicular thyroid carcinomas avidly absorb iodine, making possible diagnostic scanning and treatment with ^{131}I after total thyroidectomy. Certain follicular histopathologic features are associated with a high risk of metastasis and recurrence: poorly differentiated and Hürthle cell (oncocytic) variants. The latter variants do not take up radioiodine.

Medullary thyroid carcinoma represents about 4% of thyroid cancers. About one-third are sporadic; one-third are familial; and one-third are associated with multiple endocrine neoplasia (MEN) type 2. Therefore, discovery of a medullary thyroid carcinoma makes family surveillance advisable. It arises from parafollicular thyroid cells that can secrete calcitonin, prostaglandins, serotonin, ACTH, corticotropin-releasing hormone (CRH), and other peptides. These peptides can cause symptoms and can be used as tumor markers. Early local metastases are usually present, usually to adjacent muscle and trachea as well as to local and mediastinal lymph nodes. Eventually, late metastases may appear in the bones, lungs, adrenals, or liver. This tumor does not concentrate iodine.

Anaplastic thyroid carcinoma represents about 1% of thyroid cancers. It usually presents in an older patient as a rapidly enlarging mass in a multinodular goiter. It is the most aggressive thyroid carcinoma and metastasizes early to surrounding nodes and distant sites. Local pressure symptoms include dysphagia or vocal cord paralysis. This tumor does not concentrate iodine.

Other thyroid malignancies together represent about 3% of thyroid cancers. Lymphoma of the thyroid is more common in older women. It usually presents as a rapidly enlarging, painful mass arising out of a multinodular or diffuse goiter affected by autoimmune thyroiditis, with which it may be confused microscopically. About 20% of cases have concomitant hypothyroidism. Thyroid lymphomas are most commonly B cell lymphomas (50%) or mucosa-associated lymphoid tissue (MALT; 23%); other types include follicular, small lymphocytic, and Burkitt's lymphoma and Hodgkin's disease. Thyroidectomy is rarely required. Metastatic cancers may sometimes involve the thyroid, particularly bronchogenic, breast, and renal carcinomas and malignant melanoma.

Clinical Findings

A. Symptoms and Signs

Thyroid carcinoma usually presents as a palpable, firm, nontender nodule in the thyroid. About 3% of thyroid malignancies present with a metastasis, usually to local lymph nodes but sometimes to distant sites such as bone or lung. Metastatic functioning differentiated thyroid carcinoma can sometimes secrete enough thyroid hormone to produce thyrotoxicosis.

Medullary thyroid carcinoma frequently causes flushing and diarrhea (30%), fatigue, and other symptoms; about 5% develop Cushing's syndrome from secretion of ACTH or CRH. Signs of pressure or invasion of surrounding tissues are present in anaplastic or long-standing tumors with recurrent laryngeal nerve palsy or fixation of nodule to neighboring structures.

B. Laboratory Findings

(Fine-needle aspiration is discussed above in the section on nodular thyroid.) Thyroid function tests are generally normal unless there is concomitant thyroiditis. Follicular carcinoma may secrete enough thyroxine to suppress TSH and cause clinical hyperthyroidism.

Serum thyroglobulin is high in most metastatic papillary and follicular tumors, making this a useful marker for recurrent or metastatic disease. Caution must be exercised for the following reasons: (1) Circulating antithyroglobulin antibodies can cause erroneous thyroglobulin determinations. (2) Thyroglobulin levels may be misleadingly elevated in thyroiditis, which often coexists with carcinoma. (3) Certain thyroglobulin assays falsely report the continued presence of thyroglobulin after total thyroidectomy and tumor resection, causing undue concern about possible metastases. Therefore, unexpected thyroglobulin levels should prompt a repeat assay in another reference laboratory.

A promising development is the use of reverse transcriptase polymerase chain reaction (RT-PCR) assay for the detection of thyroglobulin messenger RNA in peripheral blood. In patients who have had a thyroidectomy for differentiated thyroid cancer, analysis of peripheral blood by RT-PCR for thyroglobulin mRNA is very sensitive for the presence of residual normal thyroid or metastatic disease even in patients taking TSH-suppressive doses of thyroxine replacement.

Serum calcitonin levels are frequently elevated in medullary thyroid carcinoma, making this a marker for metastatic disease. However, serum calcitonin may be elevated in many other conditions such as thyroiditis, pregnancy, azotemia, hypercalcemia, and other malignancies, including pheochromocytomas, carcinoid tumors, and carcinomas of the lung, pancreas, breast, and colon.

Serum carcinoembryonic antigen (CEA) levels are usually elevated with medullary carcinoma, making this a useful second marker; however, it is not specific for this carcinoma.

Serum determinations for calcitonin and CEA should be obtained before surgery for medullary carcinoma, then periodically in postoperative follow-up. Calcitonin levels remain elevated in patients with persistent tumor but also in some patients with apparent cure. Therefore, rising levels of calcitonin or CEA are the best indication for recurrence.

Since up to two-thirds of medullary thyroid carcinoma cases are familial or MEN 2 (both autosomal dominant), siblings and children of patients with medullary carcinoma are advised to have genetic testing to detect *RET* proto-oncogene mutations. Mutation analysis of exons 10, 11, 13, and 14 detects 95% of the mutations causing MEN 2a and 90% of the mutations causing familial medullary thyroid carcinoma. (See Multiple Endocrine Neoplasia, below.)

C. IMAGING

Radioiodine (^{131}I or ^{123}I) whole-body scanning is typically performed about 2–4 months following surgery for differentiated thyroid carcinoma. Thyroid cancer tissue is generally not as avid for radioiodine as is normal thyroid tissue, which competes for radioiodine. About 65% of metastases are detectable by radioiodine scanning, but only after optimal preparation: Patients should ideally have had total or near-total thyroidectomy. Intravenous iodinated contrast must be avoided for at least 2 months before scanning. Patients must follow a low-iodine diet for at least 2 weeks before scanning. Patients are allowed to become hypothyroid; high levels of endogenous TSH are required to stimulate the uptake of radioiodine into metastases. Prior to scanning, serum TSH is assayed to confirm that it is elevated; serum hCG is assayed to screen for pregnancy in all women of reproductive age; serum thyroglobulin and antithyroglobulin antibody titers are also determined.

The radioisotope ^{131}I is generally available and most commonly used for scanning. However, ^{131}I given in scanning doses of 3 mCi (111 MBq) appears to reduce the effectiveness of radioiodine therapy by impairing the ability of the remnant tissue to take up subsequent therapeutic doses of ^{131}I (the "stunning" phenomenon). Lower scanning doses of 1 mCi (37 MBq) of ^{131}I are less likely to interfere with radioiodine therapy. The radioisotope ^{123}I has the advantage of a shorter half-life, allowing quicker dissipation of background radiation and next-day scanning. The lower-energy gamma radiation of ^{123}I also allows for single photon emission computed tomography (SPECT) to better localize metastases; the lack of beta emission from ^{123}I scanning avoids "stunning" the tumor, which might otherwise reduce the effectiveness of subsequent ^{131}I therapy.

Thyrotropin-stimulated Tg and radioiodine scanning may be useful for some patients who have no anti-Tg antibodies and a very low risk of metastatic thyroid cancer or who refuse thyroid hormone withdrawal because of the discomforts of hypothyroidism.

Thyrotropin alfa injections can stimulate uptake of ^{131}I by thyroid cancer or residual thyroid. The dosage is 0.9 mg intragluteally (not intravenously) every 24 hours for two doses or every 72 hours for three doses. Radioiodine is administered 24 hours after the final thyrotropin injection; 72 hours after the final injection, a whole-body scan is obtained and blood is drawn for serum thyroglobulin determination. Side effects of thyrotropin injections include nausea (11%) and headache (7%). Hyperthyroidism can occur in patients with significant metastases or residual normal thyroid. Thyrotropin has caused neurologic deterioration in 7% of patients with central nervous system metastases. The combination of thyrotropin-stimulated scan and thyroglobulin (Tg) level detects a thyroid remnant or cancer with a sensitivity of 94% (three injections) or 84% (two injections). The presence of anti-Tg antibodies renders the serum Tg determination uninterpretable. Thyrotropin injections do not stimulate radioiodine uptake sufficiently to allow ^{131}I ablative therapy of thyroid cancer.

Ultrasound of the neck is useful in determining the size and location of the malignancy as well as neck metastases. Bone and soft tissue metastases that take up radioiodine may be demonstrable on radioisotope scans. Chest x-ray or CT may demonstrate metastases. However, iodinated contrast greatly reduces the effectiveness of radioiodine scanning and therapy. Medullary carcinoma in the thyroid, nodes, and liver may calcify, but lung metastases rarely do so. Metastases may be detected with positron emission tomography (PET) scanning and MRI.

Differential Diagnosis

Lymphocytic thyroiditis, multinodular goiter, and colloid nodules can be distinguished from malignancies by FNA biopsy. However, FNA cannot distinguish benign follicular adenoma from follicular carcinoma. Overall, in such "suspicious" cases, the risk of malignancy is about 20%—higher in fixed lesions over 4 cm in diameter. The risk of malignancy is 5% for nodules in elderly patients with lesions under 4 cm in diameter having "suspicious" cytology.

Neuroendocrine carcinomas may metastasize to the thyroid and be confused with medullary thyroid carcinoma.

False-positive ^{131}I scans are common with normal residual thyroid tissue and have been reported with Zenker's diverticulum, struma ovarii, pleuropericardial cyst, gastric pull-up, and ^{131}I-contaminated bodily secretions. False-negative ^{131}I scans are common in early metastatic differentiated thyroid carcinoma but occur also in more advanced disease, including 14% of bone metastases.

Complications

The complications vary with the type of carcinoma. Differentiated thyroid carcinomas may have local or distant metastases. One-third of medullary carcinomas may secrete serotonin and prostaglandins, producing flushing and diarrhea, and may be complicated by the coexistence of pheochromocytomas or hyperparathyroidism. The complications of radical neck surgery often include permanent hypoparathyroidism and, less commonly, vocal cord palsy; permanent hypothyroidism is expected and should always be treated adequately.

Treatment of Differentiated Thyroid Carcinoma

A. SURGICAL TREATMENT

Surgical removal is the treatment of choice for thyroid carcinomas. Neck ultrasound is useful both preoperatively and in follow-up. Highly skilled surgeons can perform near-total thyroidectomies with a less than 1% rate of serious complications (hypoparathyroidism or recurrent laryngeal nerve damage). Other series have reported up to an 11% incidence of permanent hypoparathyroidism after total thyroidectomy.

Following thyroidectomy, patients should be hospitalized as inpatients until it is determined that they have safely recovered from surgery. This requires at least an overnight hospital admission, since late bleeding, airway problems, and tetany can occur. Ambulatory thyroidectomy is potentially dangerous and should not be done.

The incidence of hypoparathyroidism may be reduced if accidentally resected parathyroids are immediately autotransplanted into the neck muscles. The advantage of near-total thyroidectomy for differentiated thyroid carcinoma is that multicentric foci of carcinoma are more apt to be resected and there is then less normal thyroid tissue to compete with cancer for ^{131}I administered later for scans or treatment. Subtotal thyroidectomy is acceptable for adults under age 45 who have a single small tumor (≤ 1 cm in diameter). Neck muscle dissections are usually avoided for differentiated thyroid carcinoma. Thyroxine is prescribed in doses of 0.05–0.1 mg/d immediately postoperatively. The dosage is adjusted to keep the serum TSH slightly suppressed during long-term follow-up of differentiated thyroid carcinoma.

About 2–4 months after surgery, a whole-body ^{131}I scan is performed: Thyroxine is stopped for 6 weeks prior to the scan, thereby causing hypothyroidism; TSH then rises and stimulates iodide uptake and thyroglobulin release from residual tumor or normal thyroid. Iodine-containing foods and contrast media are avoided.

Metastases to the brain are best treated surgically, since treatment with radiation or radioactive iodide is ineffective. Patients with bulky recurrent tumor in the neck region also benefit from surgery.

B. MEDICAL TREATMENT

Patients who have had a thyroidectomy for differentiated thyroid cancer must take thyroid hormone replacement for life. Patients need to be followed regularly for recurrent or metastatic disease. Serum TSH levels must be monitored, and thyroxine must be given in doses that are adequate to keep serum TSH levels mildly suppressed without causing thyrotoxicosis.

C. RADIOIODINE

Patients must be prepared for ^{131}I therapy by stopping thyroid hormone replacement for 2–3 weeks, thereby inducing hypothyroidism and increasing TSH, which then stimulates tumor cells to take up iodine. Patients must follow a low iodine diet for 2 weeks before ^{131}I therapy. Just before therapy, serum is obtained for measurement of TSH (to make certain it is elevated), thyroglobulin, and hCG (in all reproductive-age women). Pregnant women may not receive radioiodine therapy; women are advised to avoid pregnancy for at least 4 months following ^{131}I therapy.

Sodium iodide I 131, 30–50 mCi, is administered orally to patients with an original papillary or follicular carcinoma ≥ 1.5 cm in diameter and also to patients having persistent radioiodine uptake in the thyroid bed following near-total thyroidectomy. Patients with extrathyroidal uptake from metastatic disease are given larger doses of about 150 mCi orally in the hospital. Another whole-body scan several days after ^{131}I treatment will sometimes detect metastases not visible on pretreatment scans.

About 35% of patients with metastatic differentiated thyroid carcinoma have poor uptake of radioiodine into metastases. Lithium inhibits the release of ^{131}I from differentiated thyroid cancer, while ^{131}I uptake is unaffected. Lithium thereby increases the absorbed radiation dose by augmenting the accumulation and retention of ^{131}I by metastases. Lithium is potentially useful for improving the efficacy of ^{131}I for treating metastases with relatively poor radioiodine uptake. Lithium carbonate, 300 mg orally once to three times daily (10 mg/kg daily). is taken beginning 7 days before ^{131}I therapy and continued for 5–7 days after. Serum lithium levels are measured every 1 or 2 days to achieve a therapeutic serum lithium concentration.

^{131}I ablation in doses over 100 mCi can cause gastritis, temporary oligospermia, sialadenitis, and xerostomia. Sialadenitis and xerostomia may be prevented by treatment with amifostine, 500 mg/m^2 intravenously before high-dose radioiodine. Cumulative doses of ^{131}I over 500 mCi can cause infertility, pancytopenia (4%), and leukemia (0.3%). The kidneys excrete radioiodine. In order to reduce the risk of radiation-induced side effects, patients receiving dialysis for renal failure require a dosage reduction to only 20% of the usual dose of ^{131}I.

D. EXTERNAL RADIATION THERAPY

External radiation may be delivered to bone metastases. Brain metastases do not usually respond to ^{131}I and are best resected or treated with gamma knife radiation therapy.

E. SURVEILLANCE

Patients with differentiated thyroid carcinoma are followed clinically with neck palpation, physical examination, and chest x-ray and observed for thyrotoxicosis that might indicate functioning metastases. About 6–12 months after their postoperative scan, patients usually receive another ^{131}I whole body scan and serum thyroglobulin measurement while hypothyroid (see above); these have a combined sensitivity of 95% for metastases. Serum thyroglobulin in a patient receiving thyroxine has a lower sensitivity of 62%. Regular neck ultrasound is advisable as an adjunct to the physical examination since neck palpation often does not detect local metastases. Patients who need particularly close surveillance include those with prior known metastases and those who have persistent elevation in serum thyroglobulin or who have detectable levels of antithyroglobulin antibodies.

Thallium-201 (^{201}Tl) scans may be useful for detecting metastatic differentiated thyroid carcinoma when ^{131}I scan is normal but serum thyroglobulin is elevated. MRI or ultrasound is useful in distinguishing recurrent thyroid tumor from postoperative changes.

Positron emission tomography whole-body scanning using ^{18}F-deoxyglucose (FDG-PET) is a sensitive method for detecting thyroid cancer metastases—particularly those that are not revealed on radioiodine scanning.

Patients with papillary carcinoma should have at least two consecutively negative scans before they are considered in remission. Patients with radioiodine uptake restricted to the thyroid bed need not have repeated $_{131}$I therapies. Further scans may be required for patients with more aggressive follicular carcinomas, prior metastases, rising serum thyroglobulin, or other evidence of metastases.

Treatment of Other Thyroid Malignancies

Patients with anaplastic thyroid carcinoma are treated with local resection and radiation. Thyroid lymphomas are best treated with external radiation therapy; chemotherapy is added for extensive lymphoma.

Medullary thyroid carcinoma is treated surgically; repeated neck dissections are often required over time. Patients found to have *RET* proto-oncogene mutations are advised to have a prophylactic total thyroidectomy, ideally at age 6 years. This cancer does not take up ^{131}I.

Anaplastic thyroid carcinoma is also treated surgically. It does not take up ^{131}I.

Patients with MALT lymphomas have a low risk of recurrence after simple thyroidectomy. Patients with other types of systemic lymphomas involving the thyroid are usually treated with chemotherapy.

Prognosis

The prognosis for differentiated (papillary and follicular) thyroid carcinoma is generally excellent, particularly for adults under age 45 years. The following characteristics imply a worse prognosis: older age, male sex, bone or brain metastases, large pulmonary metastases, and lack of ^{131}I uptake into metastases. Certain papillary histologic types are associated with a higher risk of recurrence: tall cell, columnar cell, and diffuse sclerosing types. Staging and survival rates are presented in Table 26–9. Brain metastases are detected in 1%; they reduce median survival to 12 months, but their prognosis is improved by surgical resection. Patients with follicular carcinoma have a cancer mortality rate that is 3.4 times higher than patients with papillary carcinoma. The Hürthle cell variant of follicular carcinoma is more aggressive. Patients with primary tumors over 1 cm in diameter who undergo limited thyroid surgery (subtotal thyroidectomy or lobectomy) have a 2.2-fold increased mortality over those having total or near-total thyroidectomies. Pa-

Table 26–9. Pathologic tumor-node-metastasis (pTNM) staging and survival rates for adults with appropriately treated differentiated (papillary and follicular) thyroid carcinoma based upon patient age, primary tumor size and invasiveness (T), lymph node involvement (N), and distant metastases (M).[1]

	Description	Five-Year Survival	Ten-Year Survival
Stage 1	Under 45: Any T, any N, no M; Over 45: T ≤1 cm, no N, no M	99%	98%
Stage 2	Under 45: Any T, any N, any M; Over 45: T >1 cm limited to thyroid, no N, no M	99%	85%
Stage 3	Over 45: T beyond thyroid capsule, no N, no M; or any T, regional N, no M	95%	70%
Stage 4	Over 45: Any T, any N, any M	80%	61%

[1]From Alsanea O et al: Surgery 2000;128:1043, Loh KC et al: J Endocrinol Metab 1997;82:3553, and Hay ID: Endocrinol Metabol Clin North Am 1990;19:545.
Note: Patients having a relatively worse prognosis include those with follicular thyroid carcinoma and those with familial differentiated thyroid carcinoma.

tients who have not received ^{131}I ablation have mortality rates that are increased twofold by 10 years and threefold by 25 years (over those who have received ablation). The risk of cancer recurrence is twofold higher in men than in women and 1.7-fold higher in multifocal than in unifocal tumors.

Medullary thyroid carcinoma has a variable prognosis. Patients with sporadic disease usually have lymph node involvement at the time of diagnosis, whereas distal metastases may not be noted for years; the 5-year survival is 82% and the 10-year survival rate is 69%. Familial cases or those associated with MEN 2a tend to be less aggressive; the 10-year survival rate is higher, in part due to earlier detection. Women with medullary thyroid carcinoma who are under age 40 also have a better prognosis. A better prognosis is also obtained in patients undergoing total thyroidectomy and neck dissection; radiation therapy reduces recurrence in patients with metastases to neck nodes. The mortality rate is increased 4.5-fold when primary or metastatic tumor tissue stains heavily for myelomonocytic antigen M-1. Conversely, tumors with heavy immunoperoxidase staining for calcitonin are associated with prolonged survival even in the presence of significant metastases.

Anaplastic thyroid carcinoma has a 1-year survival rate of about 10%, and a 5-year survival rate of about 5%. Patients with fully localized tumors on MRI have a better prognosis.

Patients with localized lymphoma have nearly 100% 5-year survival. Those with disease outside the thyroid have a 63% 5-year survival. However, the prognosis is better for those with the mucosa-associated lymphoid tissue (MALT) type. Patients presenting with stridor, pain, laryngeal nerve palsy or mediastinal extension tend to fare worse.

Alzahrani AS et al: [123]I isotope as a diagnostic agent in the follow-up of patients with differentiated thyroid cancer: comparison with post ^{131}I therapy whole body scanning. J Clin Endocrinol Metab 2001;86:5294. [PMID: 11701695] (^{123}I has advantages over ^{131}I as an isotope for scanning for metastatic differentiated thyroid cancer.)

Hundahl SA et al: Initial results from a prospective cohort study of 5583 cases of thyroid carcinoma treated in the United States during 1996. U.S. and German Thyroid Cancer Study Group. Cancer 2000;89:202. [PMID: 10897019] (The relative frequency of thyroid cancer histologic types in this study were papillary, 81%; follicular, 10%; Hurthle cell, 3.6%; familial medullary, 0.5%; sporadic medullary, 2.7%; and anaplastic, 1.7%. Postoperatively, residual tumor was detectable in 11%. Complications occurred most often in patients undergoing total thyroidectomy combined with lymph node dissection. Complications included hypocalcemia [10%] and recurrent laryngeal nerve injury [1.3%]. Thirty-day mortality was 0.3%.)

Kebebew E et al: Total thyroidectomy or thyroid lobectomy in patients with low-risk differentiated thyroid cancer: surgical decision analysis of a controversy using a mathematical model. World J Surg 2000;24:1295. [PMID: 11038197] (Total thyroidectomy is generally the preferred surgery for low-risk differentiated thyroid cancer, except for surgeons having a relatively high complication rate for this procedure.)

Koong SS et al: Lithium as a potential adjuvant to ^{131}I therapy of metastatic, well differentiated thyroid carcinoma. J Clin Endocrinol Metab 1999;84:912. [PMID: 10084570]

Mazzaferri EL et al: Current approaches to primary therapy for papillary and follicular thyroid cancer. J Clin Endocrinol Metab 2001;86:1447. [PMID: 11297567]

Mazzaferri EL, Kloos RT: Clinical review 128: Current approaches to primary therapy for papillary and follicular thyroid cancer. J Clin Endocrinol Metab 2001;86:1447. [PMID: 11297567]

Muros MA et al: Utility of fluorine-18-fluorodeoxyglucose positron emission tomography (FDG-PET) in differentiated thyroid carcinoma with negative radioiodine tomography and elevated serum thyroglobulin levels. Am J Surg 2000;179:457. [PMID: 11004330] (FDG-PET may detect metastases of thyroid cancer in patients with negative scans using ^{131}I and [201]Tl.)

Thieblemont C et al: Primary thyroid lymphoma is a heterogeneous disease. J Clin Endocrinol Metab. 2002;87:105. [PMID: 11788631]

Vitale G et al: Current approaches and perspectives in the therapy of medullary thyroid carcinoma. Cancer 2001;91:1797. [PMID: 11335906] (Surgery is the only curative therapy for medullary thyroid carcinoma.)

ENDEMIC GOITER

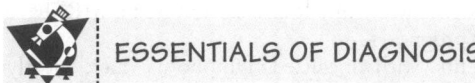

ESSENTIALS OF DIAGNOSIS

- *Common in regions of the world with low-iodine diets.*
- *High rate of congenital hypothyroidism and cretinism.*
- *Goiters may become multinodular and grow to great size.*
- *Most adults with endemic goiter are found to be euthyroid; however, some are hypothyroid or hyperthyroid.*
- *Impaired cognition and hearing may be subtle or severe in congenital hypothyroidism.*

General Considerations

Approximately 5% of the world's population have goiters. Of these, about 75% are in persons dwelling in areas of iodine deficiency. Such areas are found in 115 countries, mostly in developing areas but also in Europe.

In Pescopagano, Italy, 60% of adults have goiters. Hyperthyroidism (present or past) occurred in 2.9%; hypothyroidism was overt in 0.2% and subclinical in 3.8%. The incidence of thyroid cancer was less than 0.1%. Up to 0.5% of iodine-deficient populations have full-blown cretinism, with less severe manifestations of congenital hypothyroidism being even more common (eg, isolated deafness, short stature, or impaired mentation). Intelligence quotients in iodine-deficient adults are an average of 13 points lower than expected. Although iodine deficiency is the most common cause of endemic goiter, certain foods (eg, sorghum, millet, maize, cassava), mineral deficiencies (selenium, iron) and water pollutants can themselves cause goiter or aggravate a goiter proclivity caused by iodine deficiency. Pregnancy is associated with an increase in size of thyroid nodules and the emergence of new nodules. Some individuals are particularly susceptible to goiter owing to congenital partial defects in thyroid enzyme activity.

Clinical Findings

A. SYMPTOMS AND SIGNS

Endemic goiters may become multinodular and very large. Growth often occurs during pregnancy and may cause compressive symptoms.

Substernal goiters are usually asymptomatic but can cause tracheal compression, respiratory distress and failure, dysphagia, superior vena cava syndrome, gastrointestinal bleeding from esophageal varices, pal-

sies of the phrenic or recurrent laryngeal nerves, or Horner's syndrome. Cerebral ischemia and stroke can result from arterial compression or thyrocervical steal syndrome. Substernal goiters can rarely cause pleural or pericardial effusions. The incidence of significant malignancy is less than 1%.

Some patients with endemic goiter may become hypothyroid. Others may become thyrotoxic as the goiter grows and becomes more autonomous, especially if iodine is added to the diet.

B. LABORATORY FINDINGS

The serum thyroxine is usually normal. Serum TSH is generally normal. TSH falls in the presence of hyperthyroidism if a multinodular goiter has become autonomous in the presence of sufficient amounts of iodine for thyroid hormone synthesis. TSH rises with hypothyroidism. Thyroid radioactive iodine uptake is usually elevated, but it may be normal if iodine intake has improved. Serum levels of antithyroid antibodies are usually either undetectable or in low titers. Serum thyroglobulin is often elevated.

Differential Diagnosis

Endemic goiter must be distinguished from all other forms of nodular goiter that may coexist in an endemic region (see above).

Prevention

Iodine supplementation was started in Switzerland in 1922, initially by adding 5 mg of potassium iodide per kilogram of salt, with later increases to the current level of 20 mg/kg salt. Iodized salt has greatly reduced the incidence of endemic goiter. Unfortunately, many iodine-deficient countries have inadequate programs for iodine supplementation. The minimum dietary requirement for iodine is about 50 μg daily, with optimal iodine intake being 150–300 μg daily. Iodine sufficiency is assessed by measurement of urinary iodide excretion, the target being more than 10 μg/dL.

Initiating iodine supplementation in a geographic area causes an increased frequency of hyperthyroidism in the first year, followed by greatly reduced rates of toxic nodular goiter and Graves' disease thereafter.

Treatment

The addition of potassium iodide to table salt greatly reduces the prevalence of endemic goiter and cretinism but is less effective in shrinking established goiter. Dietary iodine supplementation increases the risk of autoimmune thyroid dysfunction which may result in hypothyroidism or thyrotoxicosis. Excessive iodine intake may increase the risk of goiter. Thyroxine supplementation can shrink goiters and reduce the risk of further goiter growth, but such treatment likewise carries a risk of inducing hyperthyroidism in individuals with autonomous multinodular goiters; therefore, thyroxine suppression should not be started in patients with suppressed TSH levels.

Adults with large multinodular goiter may require thyroidectomy for cosmesis, compressive symptoms, or thyrotoxicosis. Following partial thyroidectomy in iodine-deficient geographic areas, there is a high goiter recurrence rate, so total thyroidectomy is preferred when surgery is indicated. Certain patients may be treated with ^{131}I for large compressive goiters. Such patients may rarely develop Graves' disease 3–10 months after treatment.

Aghini-Lombardi F et al: The spectrum of thyroid disorders in an iodine-deficient community: The Pescopagano survey. J Clin Endocrinol Metab 1999;84:561. [PMID: 10022416]

Kahaly GJ et al: Iodide induces thyroid autoimmunity in patients with endemic goitre: a randomised, double-blind, placebo-controlled trial. Eur J Endocrinol 1998;139:290. [PMID: 9758438] (In 62 patients with endemic goiter, thyroxine [0.125 mg/d] caused an average decrease in thyroid volume from 32 mL to 17 mL. Iodine [0.5 mg/d] caused an average decrease in thyroid volume from 33 mL to 21 mL, but was associated with the development of antithyroid antibodies in 19%; hypothyroidism developed in 13% and hyperthyroidism in 6%. Thyroid dysfunction remitted when iodine supplementation was withdrawn.)

Wesche MFT et al: A randomized trial comparing levothyroxine with radioactive iodine in the treatment of sporadic nontoxic goiter. J Clin Endocrinol Metab 2001;86:998. [PMID: 11238476] (^{131}I therapy is more effective and better tolerated than levothyroxine treatment in patients with sporadic nontoxic goiter. Suppressive levothyroxine treatment results in significant bone loss.)

Zhao J et al: Endemic goiter associated with high iodine intake. Am J Public Health 2000;90:1633. [PMID: 11030003] (Goiter has been associated with excessive iodine in drinking water.)

HYPOTHYROIDISM & MYXEDEMA

ESSENTIALS OF DIAGNOSIS

- *Weakness, fatigue, cold intolerance, constipation, weight change, depression, menorrhagia, hoarseness.*
- *Dry skin, bradycardia, delayed return of deep tendon reflexes.*
- *Anemia, hyponatremia.*
- *T_4 and radioiodine uptake usually low.*
- *TSH elevated in primary hypothyroidism.*

General Considerations

Thyroid hormone deficiency may affect virtually all body functions. The degree of severity ranges from mild and unrecognized hypothyroid states to striking myxedema. The fluid retention seen in myxedema is caused by the interstitial accumulation of hydrophilic mucopolysaccharides, which leads to lymphedema. Hyponatremia is due to impaired renal tubular sodium reabsorption due to reductions in Na^+-K^+ ATPase. Cellular proteins are also affected in myxedema.

Hypothyroidism may be due to primary disease of the thyroid gland itself or lack of pituitary TSH. Florid hypothyroidism, ie, myxedema and cretinism, is readily recognized on clinical grounds alone, but mild hypothyroidism often escapes detection without screening (ie, serum TSH). Maternal hypothyroidism during pregnancy results in offspring with IQ scores that are an average 7 points lower than those of euthyroid mothers.

Goiter is frequently noted when hypothyroidism is due to Hashimoto's thyroiditis, iodide deficiency, genetic thyroid enzyme defects, drug goitrogens (lithium, iodide, propylthiouracil or methimazole, phenylbutazone, sulfonamides, amiodarone, interferon-alfa, interleukin-2), food goitrogens in iodide-deficient areas (eg, turnips, cassavas), or, rarely, peripheral resistance to thyroid hormone or infiltrating diseases (eg, cancer, sarcoidosis). A hypothyroid phase occurs in subacute (de Quervain's) viral thyroiditis following initial hyperthyroidism.

Goiter is usually absent when hypothyroidism is due to: deficient pituitary TSH secretion, or destruction of the gland by surgery, external radiation, or [131]I. Patients who have received central nervous system radiation for leukemia have a 15% chance of developing hypothyroidism years later. Patients with primary pulmonary hypertension have a 22% incidence of hypothyroidism.

Amiodarone, because of its high iodine content, causes clinically significant hypothyroidism in about 8% of patients. The T_4 level is normal or low, and the TSH is elevated, usually over 20 ng/dL. Another 17% of patients develop milder elevations of TSH and are asymptomatic. Low-dose amiodarone is less likely to cause hypothyroidism. Cardiac patients with amiodarone-induced symptomatic hypothyroidism are treated with just enough thyroxine to relieve symptoms. Patients with a high iodine intake from other sources may also develop hypothyroidism, especially if they have underlying lymphocytic thyroiditis.

Interferon-alfa treatment induces thyroid dysfunction (usually hypothyroidism, sometimes hyperthyroidism) in 6%. Spontaneous resolution occurs in over half of cases once interferon-alfa is discontinued.

Clinical Findings

These may vary from the rather rare full-blown myxedema to mild states of hypothyroidism, which are far more common.

A. SYMPTOMS AND SIGNS

1. Early—Frequent symptoms are fatigue, lethargy, weakness, arthralgias or myalgias, muscle cramps, cold intolerance, constipation, dry skin, headache, and menorrhagia. Physical findings may be few or absent. Features may include thin, brittle nails, thinning of hair, and pallor, with poor turgor of the mucosa. Delayed return of deep tendon reflexes is often noted.

2. Late—The symptoms are variable but may include slow speech, absence of sweating, constipation, peripheral edema, pallor, hoarseness, decreased sense of taste and smell, muscle cramps, aches and pains, dyspnea, weight changes (usually gain, but weight loss is not rare), and diminished auditory acuity. Some women have amenorrhea; others have menorrhagia. Galactorrhea may also be present. Physical findings may include goiter, puffiness of the face and eyelids, typical carotenemic skin color, thinning of the outer halves of the eyebrows, thickening of the tongue, hard pitting edema, and effusions into the pleural, peritoneal, and pericardial cavities, as well as into joints. Cardiac enlargement ("myxedema heart") is often due to pericardial effusion. The heart rate is slow; the blood pressure is more often normal than low, and reversible diastolic hypertension may be found. Hypothermia may be present. Pituitary enlargement due to hyperplasia of TSH-secreting cells, which is reversible following thyroid therapy, may be seen in long-standing hypothyroidism. Hypothyroidism rarely causes true obesity.

B. LABORATORY FINDINGS

The FT_4 may be low or low normal. TSH is increased with primary hypothyroidism but is low or normal with pituitary insufficiency. Other laboratory abnormalities may often be seen: increased serum cholesterol, liver enzymes, and creatine kinase; increased serum prolactin; hyponatremia, hypoglycemia, and anemia (with normal or increased mean corpuscular volume). Titers of antibodies against thyroperoxidase and thyroglobulin are high in patients with Hashimoto's thyroiditis. Serum T_3 is not a good test for hypothyroidism.

Differential Diagnosis

Hypothyroidism must be considered in states of asthenia, unexplained menstrual disorders, myalgias, constipation, weight change, hyperlipidemia, and anemia. Myxedema enters into the differential diagnosis of unexplained heart failure that does not respond to digitalis or diuretics, and unexplained ascites. The protein content of myxedematous effusions is high. The thick tongue may be confused with that seen in primary amyloidosis. Pernicious anemia may be suggested by the pallor and the macrocytic anemia sometimes seen in myxedema; the two disorders may even coexist. Some cases of depression, primary psychosis and structural diseases of the brain have been confused with myxedema. The pituitary is often quite enlarged in primary hypothyroidism due to reversible hyperplasia of TSH-secreting cells; the concomitant hyperprolactinemia seen in hypothyroidism can lead to the mistaken diagnosis of a pituitary adenoma.

A number of factors can lower serum T_4 levels without causing true hypothyroidism (Table 26–5).

Complications

Complications are mostly cardiac in nature, occurring as a result of advanced coronary artery disease and congestive failure, which may be precipitated by too vigorous thyroid therapy. There is an increased susceptibility to infection. Megacolon has been described in long-standing hypothyroidism. Organic psychoses with paranoid delusions may occur ("myxedema madness"). Rarely, adrenal crisis may be precipitated by thyroid therapy. Hypothyroidism is a rare cause of infertility, which may respond to thyroid medication. Pregnancy in a woman with untreated hypothyroidism often results in miscarriage. On the other hand, if the hypothyroidism is due to autoimmune disease, it may improve during pregnancy. Sellar enlargement and even well-defined TSH-secreting tumors may develop in untreated cases. These tumors decrease in size after replacement therapy is instituted.

A rare complication of severe hypothyroidism is deep stupor, at times progressing to **myxedema coma,** with severe hypothermia, hypoventilation, hyponatremia, hypoxia, hypercapnia, and hypotension. Convulsions and abnormal central nervous system signs may occur. Myxedema coma is often induced by an underlying infection; cardiac, respiratory, or central nervous system illness; cold exposure; or drug use. It is most often seen in elderly women. The mortality rate is high. Myxedematous patients are unusually sensitive to opiates and may die from average doses.

Refractory hyponatremia is often seen in severe myxedema. Inappropriate secretion of antidiuretic hormone has been observed in some patients, but a defect in distal tubular reabsorption of sodium and water has been demonstrated in many others.

Treatment

Levothyroxine (thyroxine, T_4) is the treatment of choice. It is partially converted in the body to T_3, the more active thyroid hormone. In patients taking a certain daily dose of levothyroxine, significant increases in serum T_4 levels are seen within 1–2 weeks, and near-maximum levels are seen within 3–4 weeks. It is best taken in the morning with water, avoiding concomitant intake of foods and drugs that may interfere with its absorption (see below). Brand preparations of levothyroxine in the USA appear to be bioequivalent to each other and certain generics. Before therapy with thyroid hormone is commenced, the hypothyroid patient requires at least a clinical assessment for adrenal insufficiency, which would require concurrent treatment.

A. ROUTINE INITIATION OF TREATMENT

Patients without coronary insufficiency who are under age 60 years may receive starting doses of levothyroxine, 50–100 μg daily orally. Women who are pregnant and significantly hypothyroid may begin therapy with levothyroxine at doses of 100–150 μg orally daily. Patients with coronary disease or those who are over age 60 are treated with smaller initial doses of levothyroxine, 25–50 μg daily. The dose can be increased by 25 μg every 1–3 weeks until the patient is euthyroid.

B. MYXEDEMA

Patients with severe hypothyroidism require larger initial doses of levothyroxine, particularly since myxedema itself can interfere with the intestinal absorption of thyroxine.

Myxedema coma is a medical emergency with a high mortality rate. It is caused by hypothyroidism but usually precipitated by an acute illness or trauma. Patients have the manifestations of hypothyroidism as well as impaired mentation. Hyponatremia and hypoglycemia are often present. Levothyroxine sodium 400 μg is given intravenously as a loading dose, followed by 100 μg intravenously daily. The hypothermic patient is warmed only with blankets, since faster warming can precipitate cardiovascular collapse. Patients with hypercapnia require intubation and assisted mechanical ventilation. Infections must be detected and treated aggressively. Patients suspected of having concomitant adrenal insufficiency are treated with hydrocortisone, 100 mg intravenously, followed by 25–50 mg every 8 hours.

C. MAINTENANCE

It is important to stress to the patient that levothyroxine therapy must be continued for life and that regular periodic dosage reassessments will be required. Most patients ultimately require 100–250 μg daily. Women with hypothyroidism require increased doses of thyroxine during pregnancy or therapy with estrogen. There is no standardized optimal dose of levothyroxine, so each patient's dose must be based upon careful clinical assessment. Although serum TSH levels can be helpful in determining optimal dosing, it is important not to rely entirely on this test.

Elevated serum TSH levels usually indicate underreplacement with levothyroxine. However, before increasing the T_4 dosage, it is wise to question the patient about compliance and the presence of angina and to consider the following: A high TSH in a patient receiving standard replacement doses of T_4 may indicate malabsorption of levothyroxine due to concurrent administration with binding substances, particularly iron preparations, sucralfate, aluminum hydroxide antacids, calcium supplements, or soy milk. Bile acid-binding resins such as cholestyramine can bind T_4 and impair its absorption even when administered 5 hours before the thyroxine. Malabsorption of T_4 can also occur in short bowel syndrome; therapy with medium chain triglyceride oil may improve absorption. Impaired absorption of T_4 can also be caused by diarrhea of any cause or malabsorption due to sprue, regional enteritis, liver disease, or pancreatic exocrine insufficiency.

Serum TSH may be elevated transiently in acute psychiatric illness and during recovery from nonthyroidal illness. Autoimmune disease can cause false elevations of TSH by interfering with the assay. A high TSH can also be caused by thyrotropin-secreting pituitary tumors.

Suppressed serum TSH levels < 0.1 mU/L (using a sensitive assay) may indicate overreplacement with levothyroxine; if such a patient has manifestations of hyperthyroidism, the dosage is reduced. However, patients with suppressed serum TSH levels may exhibit no symptoms of hyperthyroidism. For such patients, it is important to determine whether hypopituitarism or severe nonthyroidal illness is present, which can result in low serum TSH levels without hyperthyroidism. TSH can also be suppressed by certain medications, such as nonsteroidal anti-inflammatory agents, opioids, nifedipine, verapamil, and acute administration of glucocorticoids. Absent such conditions, a clinically euthyroid patient with a low serum TSH should be given a lower dosage of levothyroxine unless symptoms of hypothyroidism develop.

Some hypothyroid patients treated with levothyroxine complain of hypothyroid type symptoms despite having normal or suppressed levels of TSH and normal levels of free T_4. Such patients require careful assessment for other concurrent illnesses such as adrenal insufficiency, hypogonadism, anemia, or depression. If such conditions are ruled out or treated and hypothyroid type symptoms persist despite normal or low TSH levels, a serum T_3 level (free T_3 in women receiving oral estrogens) may help make the difficult decision about whether to increase the levothyroxine dose. If the T_3 level is low or low normal, such a patient may benefit from a careful increase in thyroxine dosage; if a definite clinical benefit is achieved, the higher dose is continued. However, long-term surveillance for atrial arrhythmias and for osteoporosis is recommended for such patients, though such complications are uncommon in those who are clinically euthyroid. The malaise felt by some hypothyroid patients despite apparent optimal replacement therapy with T_4 may be due to an abnormally low ratio of T_3/T_4 levels in certain tissues. In one small study, the addition of triiodothyronine, 12.5 μg daily, to the levothyroxine regimen caused an improvement in cognition, mood, and physical symptoms in some patients.

Prognosis

With early treatment, striking transformations take place both in appearance and mental function. Return to a normal state is usually the rule, but relapses will occur if treatment is interrupted. The patient may rarely die from the complications of myxedema coma. On the whole, response to thyroid treatment is most satisfactory. Hypothyroidism caused by interferon-alfa resolves within 17 months of stopping the drug in 50% of patients. Chronic maintenance therapy with unduly large doses of thyroid hormone may lead to subtle but important side effects (eg, bone demineralization) and is to be avoided.

Arafah BM: Increased need for thyroxine in women with hypothyroidism during estrogen therapy. N Engl J Med 2001;344:1743. [PMID: 11396440]

Behnia M et al: Management of myxedematous respiratory failure: review of ventilation and weaning principles. Am J Med Sci 2000;320:368. [PMID: 11149548] (Respiratory failure in myxedema is a complex medical emergency that may require prolonged ventilator assistance.)

Bunevicius R et al: Effects of thyroxine as compared with thyroxine plus triiodothyronine in patients with hypothyroidism. N Engl J Med 1999;340:424. [PMID: 9971866]

Cooper DS: Clinical practice. Subclinical hypothyroidism. N Engl J Med 2001;345:260. [PMID: 11474665]

Dong BJ et al: Bioequivalence of generic and brand-name levothyroxine products in the treatment of hypothyroidism. JAMA 1997;277:1205. [PMID: 9103344]

Helfand M et al: Clinical guideline, part 2. Screening for thyroid disease: an update. American College of Physicians. Ann Intern Med 1998;129:144. [PMID: 9669977] (Screening with serum TSH can detect symptomatic but unsuspected overt thyroid dysfunction. The highest yield is among women over age 50, in whom one in 71 was found to have symptomatic hypothyroidism that could benefit from treatment.)

Loh KC: Amiodarone-induced thyroid disorders: a clinical review. Postgrad Med J 2000;76:133. [PMID: 10684321]

Wall CR: Myxedema coma: diagnosis and treatment. Am Fam Physician 2000;62:2485. [PMID: 11130234]

HYPERTHYROIDISM (Thyrotoxicosis)

 ESSENTIALS OF DIAGNOSIS

- Sweating, weight loss or gain, anxiety, loose stools, heat intolerance, irritability, fatigue, weakness, menstrual irregularity.
- Tachycardia; warm, moist skin; stare; tremor.
- In Graves' disease: goiter (often with bruit); ophthalmopathy.
- Suppressed TSH in primary hyperthyroidism; increased T_4, free T_4, and free T_4 index.

General Considerations

The term "thyrotoxicosis" refers to the clinical manifestations associated with serum levels of thyroxine or triiodothyronine that are excessive for the individual.

The various causes include the following:

(1) By far the most common form of thyrotoxicosis is that associated with diffuse enlargement of the thyroid, hyperactivity of the gland, and the presence of antibodies against different fractions of the thyroid gland. This autoimmune thyroid disorder is called **Graves' disease** (Basedow's disease). It is much more common in women than in men (8:1), and its onset is usually between the ages of 20 and 40. It may be accompanied by infiltrative ophthalmopathy (Graves' exophthalmos) and, less commonly, by infiltrative dermopathy (pretibial myxedema). It may also be associated with other systemic autoimmune disorders such as pernicious anemia, myasthenia gravis, diabetes mellitus, etc. It has a familial tendency, and histocompatibility studies have shown an association with group HLA-B8 and HLA-DR3. The pathogenesis of the hyperthyroidism of Graves' disease involves the formation of autoantibodies that bind to the TSH receptor in thyroid cell membranes and stimulate the gland to hyperfunction. TSH receptor antibodies (TSH-R Ab [stim]) are demonstrable in the plasma of about 80% of patients with Graves' disease. Other antibodies such as ANA are generated in Graves' disease, with antithyroperoxidase or antithyroglobulin antibodies being increased in most patients. Patients with Graves' disease have an increased risk for developing Addison's disease, alopecia areata, celiac disease, diabetes mellitus type 1, myasthenia gravis, and hypokalemic periodic paralysis.

(2) Autonomous toxic adenomas of the thyroid may be single (Plummer's disease) or multiple (toxic multinodular goiter). These adenomas are not accompanied by infiltrative ophthalmopathy or dermopathy. Antithyroid antibodies are usually not present in the plasma, and tests for TSH-R Ab [stim] are negative.

(3) Subacute thyroiditis (thought to be due to viral infection) is characterized by a moderately enlarged, tender thyroid. If the gland is nontender, the disorder is called "silent thyroiditis." Hyperthyroidism is followed by hypothyroidism. During thyrotoxicosis, thyroid radioiodine uptake is low. A similar problem is seen with interleukin-2 therapy and after neck surgery for hyperparathyroidism.

(4) Jodbasedow disease, or iodine-induced hyperthyroidism, may occur in patients with multinodular goiters after intake of large amounts of iodine in the diet or in the form of radiographic contrast materials or drugs, especially amiodarone.

(5) Thyrotoxicosis factitia is due to ingestion of excessive amounts of exogenous thyroid hormone. Isolated epidemics of thyrotoxicosis have been caused by consumption of ground beef contaminated with bovine thyroid gland.

(6) Struma ovarii—Thyroid tissue is contained in about 3% of ovarian dermoid tumors and teratomas. This thyroid tissue may autonomously secrete thyroid hormone due to a toxic nodule or in concert with the woman's thyroid gland in Graves' disease or toxic multinodular goiter.

(7) TSH hypersecretion by the pituitary may be caused by a tumor and is a rare cause of hyperthyroidism. Serum TSH is elevated or normal (determined by a sensitive TSH assay) in the presence of

true thyrotoxicosis. No ophthalmopathy is present. Antithyroid antibodies and TSH-R Ab [stim] are usually normal. TSH hypersecretion may be caused by a pituitary adenoma, in which case it is known as "neoplastic inappropriate secretion of thyrotropin." The tumor may present as a mass lesion following treatment of hyperthyroidism. The pituitary adenoma is usually removed by transsphenoidal surgery; larger tumors may require radiation therapy; treatment with a somatostatin analog (octreotide, lanreotide) is also usually effective. Hyperthyroidism is treated symptomatically with propranolol.

This condition may also be due to pituitary hyperplasia, in which case it is known as "nonneoplastic inappropriate secretion of thyrotropin." Pituitary hyperplasia may be detected on MRI scan as pituitary enlargement without a discrete adenoma being visible. This condition appears to be due to a diminished feedback effect of T_4 upon the pituitary. It may be familial, but it can also be caused by prolonged untreated hypothyroidism, especially in youth. Hyperthyroid symptoms are treated with propranolol. Definitive treatment is with radioactive iodine or thyroid surgery.

(8) Hashimoto's thyroiditis may cause transient hyperthyroidism during the initial destructive phase. It may occur transiently postpartum. This is also seen in some patients receiving interferon-alfa, interferon-beta, and interleukin-2.

(9) Pregnancy and trophoblastic tumors—Although hCG generally has a low affinity for the thyroid's TSH receptors, very high serum levels of hCG may cause sufficient receptor activation to cause thyrotoxicosis. Mild gestational hyperthyroidism may occur during the first 4 months of pregnancy, when hCG levels are very high. Pregnant women are more likely to have thyrotoxicosis and hyperemesis gravidarum if they have high serum levels of asialo-hCG, a subfraction of hCG with greater affinity for TSH receptors.

Thyrotoxicosis may also be caused by the high serum levels of hCG seen in molar pregnancy, choriocarcinoma, and testicular malignancies.

(10) Metastatic functioning thyroid carcinoma is a rare cause of thyrotoxicosis.

(11) Amiodarone-induced thyrotoxicosis—Amiodarone is used to treat cardiac arrhythmias. The drug is concentrated in thyroid, adipose tissue, heart, and skeletal muscle and is 38% iodine by weight; its elimination half-life can be as long as 100 days. Amiodarone causes symptomatic hyperthyroidism in about 3% of patients in the USA; the incidence is higher in Europe and in iodine-deficient geographic areas. Hyperthyroidism can occur 4 months to 3 years after initiation of amiodarone and may develop many months after amiodarone has been discontinued. Thyrotoxicosis may cause angina or a relapse of the cardiac arrhythmia. Since high levels of T_4 and free T_4 are normally seen in patients taking amiodarone, suppressed TSH (sensitive assay) must be present along with a greatly elevated T_4 (> 20 μg/dL) or T_3 (> 200 ng/dL). (**Note:** *Hypo*thyroidism occurs in an additional 6% of patients receiving amiodarone after 2–39 weeks of therapy.) Amiodarone-induced thyrotoxicosis can occur by various mechanisms:

Type I amiodarone-induced thyrotoxicosis is caused by active elaboration of excessive thyroid hormone and may occur by either of two mechanisms: (a) Free iodine may cause toxic multinodular goiter in iodine-deficient patients with preexisting autonomous thyroid nodules (jodbasedow phenomenon). This is infrequently encountered in iodine-sufficient countries such as the USA. Thyroid radioiodine uptake ranges from low to high. (b) Excessive free iodine can trigger an immunologic attack on the thyroid; this may cause Graves' disease, commonly with diffuse thyroid enlargement and antithyroid peroxidase antibodies (70%). The presence of proptosis, thyroid-stimulating immunoglobulin (TSI), or thyrotropin-binding inhibitory immunoglobulin (TBII) is diagnostic. Thyroid radioiodine uptake is almost always negligible in the USA; however, up to 80% of such patients in Europe have detectable or normal radioiodine uptake.

Treatment of type I amiodarone-induced thyrotoxicosis usually requires a prolonged course of methimazole. After two doses of methimazole, iopanoic acid or sodium ipodate may be added to the regimen to further block conversion of T_4 to T_3; the recommended dosage for each is 500 mg orally twice daily for 3 days, followed by 500 mg once daily until thyrotoxicosis is resolved. Beta blockers may be required. Withdrawal of amiodarone does not have a significant therapeutic effect for several months. Therapy with ^{131}I may be successful in some patients with adequate radioiodine uptake. Thyroidectomy is reserved for resistant cases.

Type II amiodarone-induced thyrotoxicosis is caused by destructive thyroiditis, which releases stored thyroid hormone from damaged cells; hyperthyroidism can last 1–3 months and may be followed by hypothyroidism. Thyroid radioiodine uptake is very low. Serum levels of interleukin 6 (IL-6) are usually quite elevated. Treatment consists of prednisone plus either iopanoic acid or ipodate sodium (see above). Beta-blockers may be required. Withdrawal of amiodarone is not usually necessary. Since the condition is transient, thyroidectomy is rarely required.

Patients are likely to have Type I amiodarone-induced thyrotoxicosis if they have a pretreatment history of multinodular goiter or autoimmune thyroid disease, if they have proptosis, or if they have elevated serum levels of antithyroid antibodies or TSI. A thyroid radioiodine uptake is not usually obtained in the USA but may be useful elsewhere. It may be necessary to obtain a thyroid ultrasound with color flow Doppler sonography (CFDS). Ultrasound can usually detect thyroid nodularity characteristic of toxic multinodular goiter. In Graves' disease blood flow is normal or increased, whereas in destructive thyroiditis blood flow is decreased. In practice, the accuracy of this test may depend upon the proficiency of the ultrasonographer.

Patients in atrial fibrillation usually require anticoagulation with warfarin; close monitoring of the INR is required, since both methimazole and hyperthyroidism potentiate the hypoprothrombinemia of anticoagulants. Hyperthyroidism increases the catabolism of vitamin K-dependent clotting factors, and methimazole potentiates anti-vitamin K activity. Changing thyroid levels also modify the coagulation profile.

Clinical Findings

A. SYMPTOMS AND SIGNS

Thyrotoxicosis due to any cause produces many different manifestations of variable intensity among different individuals. Patients may complain of nervousness, restlessness, heat intolerance, increased sweating, fatigue, weakness, muscle cramps, frequent bowel movements, or weight change (usually loss). There may be palpitations or angina pectoris. Women frequently report menstrual irregularities.

Hypokalemic periodic paralysis occurs in about 15% of Asian or Native American men with thyrotoxicosis. It usually presents abruptly with paralysis (and few thyrotoxic symptoms), often after intravenous dextrose, oral carbohydrate, or vigorous exercise. Attacks last 7–72 hours.

Signs of thyrotoxicosis may include stare and lid lag, tachycardia or atrial fibrillation, fine resting finger tremors, moist warm skin, hyperreflexia, fine hair, onycholysis, and (rarely) heart failure. Chronic thyrotoxicosis may cause osteoporosis. At times there may be clubbing and swelling of the fingers (acropachy). Graves' disease usually presents with additional findings of goiter (often with a bruit).

Ophthalmopathy is clinically apparent in 20–40% of patients with Graves' disease and usually consists of chemosis, conjunctivitis, and mild proptosis. More severe lymphocytic infiltration of the eye muscles occurs in 5–10% and may produce exophthalmos and sometimes diplopia due to extraocular muscle entrapment. The optic nerve may be compressed in severe cases. Corneal drying may occur with inadequate lid closure. Eye changes may sometimes be asymmetric or unilateral. The severity of the eye disease is not closely correlated with the severity of the thyrotoxicosis. Some patients with Graves' ophthalmopathy are clinically euthyroid.

Diplopia can also be caused by coexistent ocular **myasthenia gravis,** which is more common in Graves' disease and is usually mild, often with selective eye involvement. Acetylcholinesterase receptor antibody (AchRAb) levels are elevated in only 36% of such patients, and a thymoma is present in 9%.

Graves' dermopathy (myxedema) occurs in about 3% of patients with Graves' disease, usually in the pretibial region. Glycosaminoglycan accumulation and lymphoid infiltration occur in affected skin, which becomes erythematous with a thickened, rough texture.

B. LABORATORY DIAGNOSIS

Serum T_3, T_4, thyroid resin uptake, and free thyroxine are usually all increased. Sometimes the T_4 level may be normal but the serum T_3 is elevated. A reliable sensitive TSH assay is the best test for thyrotoxicosis; it is suppressed except in the very rare cases of pituitary inappropriate secretion of thyrotropin. Other laboratory abnormalities may include hypercalcemia, increased alkaline phosphatase, anemia, and decreased granulocytes.

TSH receptor antibody (TSH-R Ab [stim]) levels are usually high (80%). Second-generation TSH-R Ab assays using human recombinant TSH-R are about 99% sensitive for Graves' disease. Antithyroglobulin or antimicrosomal antibodies are usually elevated in Graves' disease. Serum ANA and anti-double-stranded DNA antibodies are also usually elevated without any evidence of lupus erythematosus or other collagen-vascular disease.

Patients with subacute thyroiditis often have an increased erythrocyte sedimentation rate.

Thyroid radioactive iodine uptake and scan is usually performed on patients with an established diagnosis of thyrotoxicosis. A high radioactive iodine uptake is seen in Graves' disease and toxic nodular goiter but can be seen in other conditions as well. A low radioactive iodine uptake is characteristic of subacute thyroiditis but can also be seen in other conditions. (For conditions affecting radioactive iodine uptake, see section on tests of thyroid function.)

C. IMAGING

MRI of the orbits is the imaging method of choice to visualize Graves' ophthalmopathy affecting the extraocular muscles. CT scanning and ultrasound can also be used. Imaging is required only in severe cases or in euthyroid exophthalmos that must be distinguished from orbital tumors or other disorders.

Differential Diagnosis

True thyrotoxicosis must be distinguished from those conditions elevating serum thyroxine without affecting clinical status (Table 26–5).

Hyperthyroidism may be confused with anxiety neurosis or mania, but in the latter the thyroid is not enlarged and thyroid function tests are usually normal. Problems of diagnosis occur in patients with acute psychiatric disorders, about 30% of whom have hyperthyroxinemia without thyrotoxicosis. The TSH is not suppressed, distinguishing psychiatric disorder from true hyperthyroidism. T_4 levels return to normal gradually.

Exogenous thyroid administration will present the same laboratory features as thyroiditis. A rare pituitary tumor may produce the picture of thyrotoxicosis with high levels of TSH.

Some states of hypermetabolism without thyrotoxicosis—notably severe anemia, leukemia, polycythemia, and cancer—rarely cause confusion. Pheochromocytoma is often associated with hypermetabolism, tachycardia, weight loss, and profuse sweating. Acromegaly may also produce tachycardia, sweating, and thyroid enlargement. Appropriate laboratory tests will easily distinguish these entities.

Cardiac disease (eg, atrial fibrillation, angina) refractory to treatment suggests the possibility of underlying ("apathetic") hyperthyroidism. Other causes of ophthalmoplegia (eg, myasthenia gravis) and exophthalmos (eg, orbital tumor, pseudotumor) must be considered. Thyrotoxicosis must also be considered in the differential diagnosis of muscle weakness and osteoporosis. Diabetes mellitus and Addison's disease may coexist with thyrotoxicosis.

Complications

Cardiac complications of thyrotoxicosis include atrial fibrillation with a ventricular response that is difficult to control. Episodes of periodic paralysis induced by exercise or heavy carbohydrate ingestion and accompanied by hypokalemia may complicate thyrotoxicosis in Asian or Native American men. Hypercalcemia, osteoporosis, and nephrocalcinosis may occur. Decreased libido, impotence, decreased sperm count, and gynecomastia may be noted in men with hyperthyroidism.

Patients who have "subclinical hyperthyroidism" (suppressed TSH but normal free T_4 and clinically euthyroid) generally do well without treatment. No accelerated bone loss has been noted.

Treatment

The methods used to treat thyrotoxicosis will vary according to the cause and severity of the hyperthyroidism, the patient's age, the clinical situation, and the desires of the patient.

A. Graves' Disease

The treatment of Graves' disease involves a choice of methods rather than a method of choice:

1. **Propranolol**—Propranolol is generally used for symptomatic relief until the hyperthyroidism is resolved. It effectively relieves the tachycardia, tremor, diaphoresis, and anxiety that occur with hyperthyroidism due to any cause. It is the initial treatment of choice for thyroid storm. The periodic paralysis seen in association with thyrotoxicosis is also effectively treated with beta blockade. It has no effect on thyroid hormone secretion. Treatment is usually begun with 10 mg orally and increased progressively until an adequate response is achieved, usually 20 mg four times daily. Doses as high as 80 mg four times daily are occasionally required. Propranolol is available in a long-acting formulation that provides more consistent relief.

2. **Thiourea drugs**—Methimazole or propylthiouracil is generally used for young adults or patients with mild thyrotoxicosis, small goiters, or fear of isotopes. Aged patients usually respond particularly well. These drugs are also useful for preparing hyperthyroid patients for surgery and elderly patients for radioactive iodide treatment. The drugs do not permanently damage the thyroid and are associated with a lower chance of posttreatment hypothyroidism (compared with radioactive iodide or surgery). Unfortunately, there is a high rate of recurrent hyperthyroidism (about 50%) after a year or more of therapy. A greater likelihood of long-term remission is seen in patients with small goiters or mild hyperthyroidism. Patients whose thyroperoxidase and thyroglobulin antibodies remain high after 2 years of therapy have been reported to have only a 10% rate of relapse.

Agranulocytosis is an uncommon but serious complication of thiourea therapy, being reported in about 0.1% of patients taking methimazole and about 0.4% of patients taking propylthiouracil. Patients are warned that if they develop a sore throat or febrile illness, they should stop the drug while a white blood count is rechecked. The agranulocytosis is generally reversible; recovery is not improved by filgrastim (G-CSF). Periodic surveillance of the white blood count during treatment has been advocated by some clinicians, but onset is generally abrupt.

Other side effects common to thiourea drugs include pruritus, allergic dermatitis, nausea, and dyspepsia. Antihistamines may control mild pruritus without discontinuation of the drug. Since the two thiourea drugs are similar, patients who have had a major allergic reaction from one should not be given the other.

Primary hypothyroidism may occur. The patient may become clinically hypothyroid for 2 weeks or more before TSH levels rise, having been suppressed by the preceding hyperthyroidism. Therefore, the patient's changing thyroid status is best followed clinically and with serum levels of free thyroxine. Rapid growth of the goiter usually occurs if the patient is allowed to develop prolonged hypothyroidism; the goiter may sometimes become massive but usually regresses rapidly with thyroid hormone replacement.

a. Methimazole—Methimazole has the advantage of requiring less frequent dosing and fewer pills than propylthiouracil, making treatment more convenient. Patients treated with methimazole (compared with those taking propylthiouracil) have a lower risk of developing fulminant hepatic necrosis; methimazole therapy is also less likely to cause ^{131}I treatment failure. Rare complications peculiar to methimazole include serum sickness, cholestatic jaundice, loss of taste, alopecia, nephrotic syndrome, and hypoglycemia. Methimazole is given orally in initial doses of 30–60 mg once daily. The dosage is usually reduced as manifestations of hyperthyroidism resolve and as the free thyroxine level becomes normal.

b. Propylthiouracil—Propylthiouracil has been considered the drug of choice during breast feeding or pregnancy, possibly causing fewer problems in the newborn. Rare complications peculiar to propylthio-uracil include arthritis, lupus erythematosus, aplastic anemia, thrombocytopenia, and hypoprothrombine-mia. Acute hepatitis occurs rarely and is treated with prednisone but may progress to liver failure. Propylthiouracil is given orally in initial doses of 300–600 mg daily in four divided doses. The dosage and frequency of administration are generally reduced as symptoms of hyperthyroidism resolve and the free thyroxine level becomes normal. During pregnancy, the dose is kept below 200 mg/d in order to avoid goitrous hypothyroidism in the infant.

3. Iodinated contrast agents—These agents provide effective temporary treatment for thyrotoxicosis of any cause. Iopanoic acid (Telepaque) or ipodate sodium (Bilivist, Oragrafin) is given orally in a dosage of 500 mg twice daily for 3 days, then 500 mg once daily. These agents inhibit peripheral 5′-monodeiodination of thyroxine, thereby blocking its conversion to active triiodothyronine (T_3). Within 24 hours, serum T_3 levels fall an average of 62%. For patients with Graves' disease, methimazole is begun first in order to block iodine organification; the next day, ipodate sodium or iopanoic acid may be added. The iodinated contrast agents are particularly useful for patients who are very symptomatically thyrotoxic (see Thyroid Storm, below). They offer a therapeutic option for patients with thyroxine overdosage, subacute thyroiditis, and amiodarone-induced thyrotoxicosis and for those intolerant to thioureas and for newborns with thyrotoxicosis (due to maternal Graves' disease). Treatment periods of 8 months or more are possible, but efficacy tends to wane with time. In Graves' disease, thyroid radioiodine uptake may be suppressed during treatment but returns to pretreatment uptake by 7 days after discontinuation of the drug, allowing ^{131}I treatment.

4. Radioactive iodine (^{131}I)—The administration of radioiodine is an excellent method of destroying over-active thyroid tissue (either diffuse or toxic nodular goiter). The radioiodine damages the cells that concentrate it. Patients have no apparent risk of subsequent thyroid cancer, leukemia, or other malignancies. Children born to parents previously treated with ^{131}I show normal rates of congenital abnormalities.

Since fetal radiation is harmful, *radioactive iodine should not be given to pregnant women.* It is prudent to obtain a sensitive pregnancy test (serum β-hCG) on all women of reproductive age prior to ^{131}I therapy.

Most patients may receive ^{131}I while being symptomatically treated with just propranolol, which is then reduced in dosage as hyperthyroxinemia resolves. However, some patients (those with coronary diseases, the elderly, or those with severe hyperthyroidism) are usually rendered euthyroid with a thiouracil drug (see above) while the dosage of propranolol is reduced. Treatment with methimazole is discontinued for 1 week prior to ^{131}I therapy. Since pretreatment with propylthiouracil causes the risk of ^{131}I treatment failure to increase from 3% (without pretreatment) to 23%, the thiourea is

stopped for 2 weeks (if possible) before ^{131}I treatment and a somewhat higher dose of ^{131}I is administered.

Following ^{131}I treatment for hyperthyroidism, Graves' ophthalmopathy appears or worsens in 15% and improves in none, whereas during treatment with methimazole, ophthalmopathy worsens in 3% and improves in 2%. Among patients receiving 3 months of prednisone following ^{131}I treatment, preexistent ophthalmopathy worsens in none and improves in 67%.

Smoking increases the risk of having a flare in ophthalmopathy following ^{131}I treatment and also reduces the effectiveness of prednisone treatment. Therefore, patients who smoke are strongly encouraged to quit prior to ^{131}I treatment.

Free T_4 levels may sometimes drop within 2 months after starting ^{131}I treatment but then rise again to thyrotoxic levels, at which time thyroid radioiodine uptake is low. This phenomenon is caused by a release of stored thyroid hormone from injured thyroid cells and does not indicate a treatment failure. In fact, serum free T_4 then falls abruptly to hypothyroid levels.

There is a high incidence of hypothyroidism several years after ^{131}I even when small doses are given. However, hypothyroidism also occurs quite frequently years after surgical or medical treatment of Graves' disease, and eventual hypothyroidism may be part of the natural history of this condition. Lifelong clinical follow-up is mandatory, with measurements of free T_4 and TSH when indicated.

5. Thyroid surgery—Thyroid surgery for Graves' disease and toxic nodular goiter has been performed less frequently as radioiodine treatment has become more widely accepted. Surgery is usually preferred for pregnant women whose thyrotoxicosis is not controlled with low doses of thioureas, for patients with particularly large goiters, and whenever there is a significant chance of malignancy.

Patients are ordinarily rendered euthyroid with a thiourea drug or ipodate preoperatively. Propranolol is given until the T_3 is normal preoperatively. Thyroid vascularity is reduced by preoperative treatment with either ipodate sodium or iopanoic acid (500 mg twice daily for 3 days) or iodine (eg, Lugol's solution, 2 or 3 drops orally daily for several days). If a patient undergoes surgery while thyrotoxic, larger doses of propranolol are given perioperatively to reduce the likelihood of thyroid crisis.

Morbidity includes possible damage to the recurrent laryngeal nerve, with resultant vocal cord paralysis. Hypoparathyroidism also occurs, which means that calcium levels must be checked postoperatively. These complications are unusual (< 1%) when the surgery is performed by a competent, experienced neck surgeon. Thyroid surgery should be performed as an inpatient, with at least an overnight observational period.

B. TOXIC SOLITARY THYROID NODULES

Hyperthyroidism caused by a single hyperfunctioning thyroid nodule may be treated symptomatically with propranolol as in Graves' disease. Definitive treatment is with surgery or radioactive iodine. For patients under age 40, surgery is usually recommended; patients are made euthyroid with a thiourea preoperatively and given several days of iodine, ipodate sodium, or iopanoic acid before surgery as in Graves' disease (see above). Transient postoperative hypothyroidism resolves spontaneously. Permanent hypothyroidism occurs in about 14% of patients by 6 years after surgery. Patients over age 40 with a toxic solitary nodule are offered radioactive iodine. Permanent hypothyroidism occurs in about one-third of patients by 8 years after radioactive iodine. The nodule remains palpable in half and may grow in 10% of patients after radioactive iodine.

C. Toxic Multinodular Goiter

Hyperthyroidism caused by a toxic multinodular goiter may also be treated symptomatically with propranolol as in Graves' disease. This disorder usually affects older individuals, so radioactive iodine is ordinarily selected over surgery as definitive treatment. Thioureas do reverse hyperthyroidism, but there is a 95% recurrence rate after they are stopped. Older patients who are quite thyrotoxic are rendered nearly euthyroid with methimazole, which is stopped at least 3 days before radioactive iodine treatment. Meanwhile, the patient follows a low-iodine diet; this is done to enhance the thyroid gland's uptake of radioactive iodine, which may be relatively low in this condition (compared to Graves' disease). Relatively high doses of radioactive iodine are usually required; recurrent thyrotoxicosis and hypothyroidism are common, so patients must be followed closely. Surgery is generally reserved for pressure symptoms or cosmetic indications. Patients are prepared for surgery as in Graves' disease (see above).

D. Subacute Thyroiditis

Patients with hyperthyroidism due to subacute thyroiditis are treated symptomatically with propranolol. Ipodate sodium or iopanoic acid, 500 mg orally daily, promptly corrects elevated T_3 levels and is continued for 15–60 days until the serum FT_4 level normalizes. The condition subsides spontaneously within weeks to months. Thioureas are ineffective, since thyroid hormone production is actually low in this condition. Radioactive iodine is ineffective, since the thyroid's iodine uptake is low. Since periods of hypothyroidism may occur following the initial inflammatory episode, patients should have close clinical follow-up, with serum free thyroxine measurement when necessary. Prompt treatment of the transient hypothyroidism may reduce the incidence of recurrent thyroiditis. Pain can usually be managed with aspirin or other nonsteroidal anti-inflammatory agents.

E. Hashimoto's Thyroiditis

Rarely, patients develop hyperthyroidism as a result of release of stored thyroid hormone during severe Hashimoto's thyroiditis. The thyroperoxidase or thyroglobulin antibodies are usually high, but radioiodine uptake is low, thus distinguishing it from Graves' disease. This is especially common in postpartum women, in whom it may be transient. Treatment is with propranolol. Patients are followed carefully for the development of hypothyroidism and treated according to their thyroid status.

F. Treatment of Complications

1. Graves' ophthalmopathy—The risk of having a "flare" of ophthalmopathy following ^{131}I treatment for hyperthyroidism is about 6% for nonsmokers and 23% for smokers. For progressive exophthalmos, prednisone must be given promptly in doses of 40–60 mg/d, with dosage reduction over several weeks. Higher initial prednisone doses of 80–120 mg/d are used when there is optic nerve compression. Prednisone alleviates eye symptoms in 64% of nonsmokers, but only 14% of smokers respond well. Another treatment is low-dose radiation therapy (cumulative dose 20 Gy to each orbit over 2 weeks) to the extraocular muscles, avoiding the cornea and lens. Intravenous immune globulin (IGIV) is reportedly comparable to prednisone in effectiveness in doses of 1 g/kg for 2 consecutive days and repeated every 3 weeks for 3–4 months. For severe cases, orbital decompression surgery may save vision, though diplopia often persists postoperatively. General eye protective measures include wearing glasses to protect the protruding eye and taping the lids shut during sleep if corneal drying is a problem. Methylcellulose drops and gels ("artificial tears") may also help. Tarsorrhaphy or canthoplasty can frequently help protect the cornea and provide improved appearance. Hypothyroidism and hyperthyroidism must be treated promptly.

2. Cardiac complications—

a. Sinus tachycardia or heart pounding is usually present in thyrotoxicosis. Treatment consists of treating the thyrotoxicosis. A beta-blocker (as described above) such as propranolol is used in the interim unless there is an associated cardiomyopathy.

b. Atrial fibrillation is commonly seen in thyrotoxicosis and may be the presenting manifestation. Electrical cardioversion is unlikely to convert atrial fibrillation to normal sinus rhythm while the patient is thyrotoxic. Spontaneous conversion to normal sinus rhythm tends to occur with achievement of euthyroidism, but that likelihood decreases with age. Hyperthyroidism must be treated (see above). Other drugs may be required:

(1) Digoxin is used to slow a fast ventricular response to thyrotoxic atrial fibrillation; it must be used in larger than normal doses because of increased clearance and an increased number of cardiac sodium transport units requiring inhibition. Digoxin doses are reduced as hyperthyroidism is corrected.

(2) Beta-blockers may also reduce the ventricular rate, but they must be used with caution—particularly

in patients with cardiomegaly or signs of heart failure—since their negative inotropic effect may precipitate congestive heart failure. Therefore, an initial trial of a short-duration beta-blocker should be considered, such as esmolol intravenously. If a beta-blocker is used, doses of digoxin must be reduced.

(3) Anticoagulation is indicated to prevent arterial thromboembolism in thyrotoxicosis-induced atrial fibrillation in the following situations: left atrial enlargement on echocardiogram, global left ventricular dysfunction, recent congestive heart failure, hypertension, recurrent atrial fibrillation, or a history of previous thromboembolism. The doses of warfarin required in thyrotoxicosis are smaller than normal because of an accelerated plasma clearance of vitamin K-dependent clotting factors. Higher warfarin doses are usually required as hyperthyroidism subsides.

c. Heart failure due to thyrotoxicosis may be caused by extreme tachycardia, cardiomyopathy, or both. Very aggressive treatment of the hyperthyroidism is required in either case (see Thyroid Crisis, below). The tachycardia from atrial fibrillation is treated with digoxin as above. Intravenous furosemide is typically required. If tachycardia appears to be the main cause of the failure, beta-blockers are administered cautiously as described above.

Thyrotoxic dilated cardiomyopathy is caused by a direct toxic effect of prolonged excess thyroid hormone upon the heart and may occur at any age. Beta-blockers and calcium channel blockers are avoided. Emergency treatment may include afterload reduction, diuretics, digoxin, and other inotropic agents while the patient is being rendered euthyroid.

d. Apathetic hyperthyroidism may present with angina pectoris. Treatment is directed at reversing the hyperthyroidism as well as providing standard antianginal therapy. Coronary angioplasty or bypass grafting can often be avoided by prompt diagnosis and treatment.

3. Thyroid crisis or "storm"—This disorder, rarely seen today, is an extreme form of thyrotoxicosis that may occur with stressful illness, thyroid surgery, or radioactive iodine administration and is manifested by marked delirium, severe tachycardia, vomiting, diarrhea, dehydration, and, in many cases, very high fever. The mortality rate is high.

A thiourea drug is given (eg, propylthiouracil, 150–250 mg every 6 hours; or methimazole, 15–25 mg every 6 hours). Iodide is given 1 hour later as Lugol's solution (10 drops three times daily orally) or as sodium iodide (1 g intravenously slowly). Ipodate sodium (500 mg/d orally) can be helpful if begun 1 hour after the first dose of thiourea. Propranolol is given (cautiously in the presence of heart failure; see above) in a dosage of 0.5–2 mg intravenously every 4 hours or 20–120 mg orally every 6 hours. Hydrocortisone is usually given in doses of 50 mg every 6 hours, with rapid dosage reduction as the clinical situation improves. Aspirin is avoided since it displaces T_4 from

thyroid-binding globulin, raising free T_4 serum levels. Definitive treatment with ^{131}I or surgery is delayed until the patient is euthyroid.

4. Hyperthyroidism and pregnancy—The prevalence of hyperthyroidism in pregnancy—most commonly due to Graves' disease—is about 0.2%. Struma ovarii is rare. Diagnosis may be difficult, since normal pregnancy may be accompanied by tachycardia, warm skin, heat intolerance, increased sweating, and a palpable thyroid. Laboratory tests are helpful: The free T_4 is clearly elevated, while the TSH is suppressed. However, apparent lack of full TSH suppression can be seen due to misidentification of hCG as TSH in certain assays. Although the total T_4 is elevated in most pregnant women, values over 20 μg/dL are encountered only in hyperthyroidism. The T_3 resin uptake, which is low in normal pregnancy because of high TBG concentration, is normal or high in thyrotoxic subjects. Pregnancy can have a beneficial effect upon the thyrotoxicosis of Graves' disease, with decreasing antibody titers and decreasing free T_4 levels as the pregnancy advances. However, there is an increased risk of thyroid storm, preeclampsia-eclampsia, congestive heart failure, premature delivery, and abruptio placentae. Newborns have an increased risk of intrauterine growth retardation, prematurity, and transient thyrotoxicosis from transplacental transfer of TSH-R Ab [stim]. Pregnant women with hyperthyroidism are treated with methimazole or propylthiouracil in the smallest dose possible, permitting mild hyperthyroidism to occur since it is usually well tolerated. The drug does cross the placenta and rarely may induce TSH hypersecretion and fetal goiter. Thyroid hormone administration to the mother does not prevent hypothyroidism in the fetus, since T_4 and T_3 do not freely cross the placenta. Fetal hypothyroidism is rare if the mother's hyperthyroidism is controlled with small daily doses of propylthiouracil (50–150 mg/d) or methimazole (5–15 mg/d). Thyroidectomy is reserved for women who are allergic or resistant to antithyroid drugs (usually due to noncompliance) or who have very large goiters.

During lactation, women treated with propylthiouracil secrete very little of it into breast milk. Methimazole is secreted in higher concentrations in breast milk. However, the use of either propylthiouracil or methimazole during breast feeding does not significantly affect the infant's thyroid hormone levels. No adverse reactions to these drugs (eg, rash, hepatic dysfunction, leukopenia) have been reported in breast-fed infants. Recommended doses are 20 mg or less daily for methimazole and 450 mg or less daily for propylthiouracil. It is recommended that the medication be taken just after breast feeding.

5. Graves' dermopathy—An uncommon complication of Graves' disease, dermopathy is an abnormal thickening of the skin due to deposition of glycosaminoglycans. It is known as "pretibial myxedema" since it usually occurs in the anterior lower leg, sometimes also including the dorsum of the foot. Treatment involves application of a topical glucocorticoid (eg, fluocinolone) with nocturnal plastic occlusive dressings.

6. Thyrotoxic hypokalemic periodic paralysis—Asian or Native American men presenting with sudden symmetric flaccid paralysis, hypokalemia, and hypophosphatemia must always be suspected of having thyrotoxicosis, especially since classic signs of thyrotoxicosis may be lacking. Therapy with oral propranolol, 3 mg/kg, normalizes the serum potassium and phosphate levels and reverses the paralysis within 2–3 hours. No intravenous potassium or phosphate is ordinarily required. Intravenous dextrose and oral carbohydrate aggravate the condition and are to be avoided. Therapy is continued with propranolol, 60–80 mg every 8 hours (or sustained-action propranolol daily at equivalent daily dosage), along with a thiourea drug such as methimazole to treat the hyperthyroidism.

Prognosis

Graves' disease may rarely subside spontaneously and may even result in spontaneous hypothyroidism. However, it usually progresses. The ocular, cardiac, and psychologic complications often are more serious than the chronic wasting of tissues and may become irreversible even after treatment. Permanent hypoparathyroidism and vocal cord palsy are risks of surgical thyroidectomy. Recurrences are common following thiourea therapy but also occur after low-dose ^{131}I therapy or subtotal thyroidectomy. With adequate treatment and long-term follow-up, the results are usually good. However, despite treatment for their hyperthyroidism, women experience an increased long-term risk of death from thyroid disease, cardiovascular disease, stroke, and fracture of the femur. Posttreatment hypothyroidism is common. It may occur within a few months or up to several years after radioactive iodine therapy or subtotal thyroidectomy. Malignant exophthalmos has a poor prognosis unless treated aggressively.

Bartalena L et al: Cigarette smoking and treatment outcomes in Graves ophthalmopathy. Ann Intern Med 1998;129:632. [PMID: 9786811] (Smokers with thyroid-associated ophthalmopathy are more likely to have a flare in eye disease after ^{131}I treatment for hyperthyroidism and are less likely to respond to prednisone.)

Chopra IJ et al: Use of oral cholecystographic agents in the treatment of amiodarone-induced hyperthyroidism. J Clin Endocrinol Metab 2001;86:4707. [PMID: 11600529] (Patients with type II amiodarone-induced hyperthyroidism were treated with oral cholecystographic agents [OCAs] sodium ipodate [Oragrafin] or sodium tyropanoate [Telepaque]; amiodarone was discontinued; additionally, all patients received either methimazole or PTU. OCAs were safe and effective treatment for this condition.)

Daniels GH: Amiodarone-induced thyrotoxicosis. J Clin Endocrinol Metab 2001;86:3. [PMID: 11231968]

Klein I et al: Thyroid hormone and the cardiovascular system. N Engl J Med 2001;344:501. [PMID: 11172193] (Review article.)

Lin SH et al: Propranolol rapidly reverses paralysis, hypokalemia, and hypophosphatemia in thyrotoxic periodic paralysis. Am J Kidney Dis 2001;37:620. [PMID: 11228188]

Magsino CH Jr, et al: Thyrotoxic periodic paralysis. South Med J 2000;93:996. [PMID: 11147484] (Review article.)

Marcocci C et al: Comparison of the effectiveness and tolerability of intravenous or oral glucocorticoids associated with orbital radiotherapy in the management of severe Graves' ophthalmopathy: results of a prospective, single-blind, randomized study. J Clin Endocrinol Metab 2001;86:3562. [PMID: 11502779] (Intravenous glucocorticoid therapy is superior to oral therapy in the management of Graves' ophthalmopathy with orbital radiotherapy.)

Masiukiewicz US et al: Hyperthyroidism in pregnancy: diagnosis and treatment. Thyroid 1999;9:647. [PMID: 10447008]

Weetman AP: Graves' disease. N Engl J Med 2000;343:1236. [PMID: 11071676] (Review article.)

THYROIDITIS

 ESSENTIALS OF DIAGNOSIS

- *Swelling of thyroid gland, often causing pressure symptoms in acute and subacute forms; painless enlargement in chronic form.*
- *Thyroid function tests variable.*
- *Serum antithyroid antibody tests often positive.*

General Considerations

Thyroiditis may be classified as follows: (1) chronic lymphocytic ("Hashimoto's") thyroiditis due to autoimmunity, (2) subacute thyroiditis, (3) suppurative thyroiditis, and (4) Riedel's thyroiditis.

Clinical Findings

A. SYMPTOMS AND SIGNS

1. Hashimoto's thyroiditis—Hashimoto's thyroiditis—also called chronic lymphocytic thyroiditis—is the most common form of thyroiditis and probably the most common thyroid disorder in the USA. It tends to be familial and is six times more common in women than in men. Its frequency is increased by dietary iodine supplementation. Certain drugs (amiodarone, alpha interferon, interleukin-2, granulocyte-colony stimulating factor) frequently induce thyroid autoantibodies.

The thyroid gland is usually diffusely enlarged, firm, and finely nodular. One thyroid lobe may be asymmetrically enlarged, raising concerns about neoplasm. Although patients may complain of neck tightness, pain and tenderness are not usually present. About 10% of cases are atrophic, the gland being fibrotic, particularly in elderly women.

Thyroiditis often progresses to hypothyroidism, which is usually permanent, remitting in fewer than 5% of cases. Uncommonly, thyroiditis causes acute destruction of thyroid tissue and release of stored thyroid hormone, causing thyrotoxicosis. Rarely, a hypofunctioning gland may become hyperfunctioning with the onset of coexistent Graves' disease.

Systemic manifestations of Hashimoto's thyroiditis are mostly related to ambient levels of thyroid hormone. However, depression and chronic fatigue are more common in such patients, even after correction of hypothyroidism. About one-third of patients with Hashimoto's thyroiditis have mild dry mouth (xerostomia) or dry eyes (keratoconjunctivitis sicca) of an autoimmune nature related to Sjögren's syndrome. It may be associated with myasthenia gravis, which is usually of mild severity, mainly affecting the extraocular muscles and having a relatively low incidence of detectable acetylcholinesterase receptor antibodies or thymic disease.

Hashimoto's thyroiditis is sometimes associated with adrenal insufficiency (Schmidt's syndrome) and other endocrine deficiencies as part of polyglandular autoimmunity. Thyroiditis is also more common in patients with other autoimmune conditions, such as inflammatory bowel disease, or celiac disease (10%). Women with gonadal dysgenesis (Turner's syndrome) have a 15% incidence of significant thyroid dysfunction by age 40 years. Thyroiditis is also commonly seen in patients with hepatitis C.

Patients with clinically evident disease usually have increased circulating levels of antithyroid peroxidase (95%) or antithyroglobulin (60%) antibodies.

Subclinical thyroiditis is very common, and in autopsy series about 40% of women and 20% of men exhibit focal thyroiditis. Mildly elevated serum titers of antithyroid antibodies are found in 13% of women and 3% of men. However, only 1% of the population has antibody titers greater than 1:6400.

Postpartum thyroiditis is a form of autoimmune thyroiditis occurring soon after parturition and accompanied by transient hyperthyroidism followed by hypothyroidism; recovery of normal function occurs in most cases.

2. Subacute thyroiditis—This fairly common disorder—also called de Quervain's thyroiditis, granulomatous thyroiditis, and giant cell thyroiditis—is an acute, usually painful enlargement of the thyroid gland, with dysphagia. The pain may radiate to the ears. If there is no pain, it is called "silent thyroiditis." The manifestations may persist for weeks or months and may be associated with signs of thyrotoxicosis and malaise. Young and middle-aged women are most commonly affected. Viral infection has been suggested as the cause. The erythrocyte sedimentation rate is markedly elevated, and antithyroid antibodies are low, which helps differentiate this form of thyroiditis from others. Radioactive iodine uptake is low, distinguishing this disorder from Graves' disease. Aspiration biopsy is usually not required but shows characteristic giant multinucleated cells.

3. Suppurative thyroiditis—Suppurative thyroiditis is a rare disorder causing severe pain, tenderness, redness, and fluctuation in the region of the thyroid gland. It is caused by pyogenic organisms, usually in the course of systemic infection.

4. Riedel's thyroiditis—Riedel's thyroiditis is also called invasive fibrous thyroiditis, Riedel's struma, woody thyroiditis, ligneous thyroiditis, and invasive thyroiditis. It usually causes hypothyroidism and may cause hypoparathyroidism as well. It is the rarest form of thyroiditis and is found most frequently in middle-aged or elderly women. Enlargement is often asymmetric; the gland is stony hard and adherent to the neck structures, causing signs of compression and invasion, including dysphagia, dyspnea, pain, and hoarseness. It is usually a manifestation of a multifocal systemic fibrosis syndrome, with anterior neck symptoms predominating. Related conditions include retroperitoneal fibrosis, fibrosing mediastinitis, sclerosing cervicitis, subretinal fibrosis, and biliary tract sclerosis. It responds to therapy with tamoxifen (see Treatment, below).

B. LABORATORY FINDINGS

The T_4 and T_3 resin uptake are usually markedly elevated in acute and subacute thyroiditis and normal or low in the chronic forms. Radioiodine uptake is characteristically very low in the initial, hyperthyroid phase of subacute thyroiditis; it may be high with an uneven scan in chronic thyroiditis, with enlargement of the gland, and low in Riedel's struma. Thyroid autoantibodies are most commonly demonstrable in Hashimoto's thyroiditis but are also found in the other types. The serum TSH level is elevated if thyroid hormone is not elaborated in adequate amounts by the thyroid gland.

Complications

In the suppurative forms of thyroiditis, any of the complications of infection may occur; the subacute and chronic forms of the disease are complicated by the effects of pressure on the neck structures: dyspnea and, in Riedel's struma, vocal cord palsy. Hashimoto's thyroiditis may lead to hypothyroidism or transient thyrotoxicosis. Perimenopausal women with high serum levels of antithyroperoxidase antibodies have a higher relative risk of depression independently of ambient thyroid hormone levels. Graves' disease may sometimes develop. Carcinoma or lymphoma may be associated with chronic thyroiditis and must be considered in the diagnosis of uneven painless enlargements that continue in spite of treatment. Hashimoto's thyroiditis may be associated with Addison's disease, hypoparathyroidism, diabetes, pernicious anemia, biliary cirrhosis, vitiligo, and other autoimmune conditions.

Differential Diagnosis

Thyroiditis must be considered in the differential diagnosis of all types of goiters, especially if enlargement is rapid. The very low radioiodine uptake in subacute thyroiditis with elevated T_4 and T_3 are helpful. Chronic thyroiditis, especially if the enlargement is uneven and if there is pressure on surrounding structures, may resemble carcinoma, and both disorders may be present in the same gland. The subacute and suppurative forms of thyroiditis may resemble any infectious process in or near the neck structures. Thyroid autoantibody tests have been of help in the diagnosis of chronic lymphocytic (Hashimoto's) thyroiditis, but the tests are not specific and may also be positive in patients with goiters, carcinoma, and thyrotoxicosis—though the titers are usually higher in Hashimoto's thyroiditis. Biopsy may be required for diagnosis.

Treatment

A. Suppurative Thyroiditis

Treatment is with antibiotics and with surgical drainage when fluctuation is marked.

B. Subacute Thyroiditis:

All treatment is empirical and must be continued for several weeks. Recurrence is common. The drug of choice is aspirin, which relieves pain and inflammation. Thyrotoxic symptoms are treated with propranolol, 10–40 mg every 6 hours. Iodinated contrast agents cause a prompt fall in serum T_3 levels and a dramatic improvement in thyrotoxic symptoms. Sodium ipodate (Oragrafin, Bilivist) or iopanoic acid (Telepaque) is given orally in doses of 500 mg daily until serum free T_4 levels return to normal. Transient hypothyroidism is treated with thyroxine (0.05–0.1 mg/d) if symptomatic.

C. Hashimoto's Thyroiditis

Levothyroxine should be given in the usual doses (0.05–0.2 mg daily) if hypothyroidism or large goiter is present. In one study, selenium selenite (200 μg daily orally for 3 months) reduced the serum levels of antithyroperoxidase antibodies by 49% versus a 10% reduction in the placebo arm. If the thyroid gland is only minimally enlarged and the patient is euthyroid (with normal TSH levels), regular observation is in order, since hypothyroidism may develop subsequently—often years later. (See Hypothyroidism section.)

D. Riedel's Struma

The treatment of choice for invasive fibrous thyroiditis, like that of its related conditions, is tamoxifen, 10 mg orally twice daily. Tamoxifen can induce partial to complete remissions in most patients within 3–6 months. Tamoxifen treatment must be continued for years. Its mode of action appears to be unrelated to its antiestrogen activity. Short-term glucocorticoid treatment may be added for partial alleviation of pain and compression symptoms. Surgical decompression usually fails to permanently alleviate compression symptoms; such surgery is difficult due to dense fibrous adhesions, making surgical complications more likely.

Prognosis

The course of this group of diseases is quite variable. Spontaneous remissions and exacerbations are common in the subacute form, and therapy is nonspecific. The disease process may smolder for months. Hashimoto's thyroiditis is occasionally associated with other autoimmune disorders (diabetes mellitus, Addison's disease, pernicious anemia, etc). In general, however, patients with Hashimoto's thyroiditis have an excellent prognosis, since the condition either remains stable for years or progresses slowly to hypothyroidism, which is easily treated. Women with postpartum thyroiditis usually regain normal thyroid function.

Few J et al: Riedel's thyroiditis: treatment with tamoxifen. Surgery 1996;120:993. [PMID: 8957485]

Schuppert F et al: Patients treated with interferon-alpha, interferon-beta, and interleukin-2 have a different thyroid autoantibody pattern than patients suffering from endogenous autoimmune thyroid disease. Thyroid 1997;7:837. [PMID: 9459625]

Slatosky J et al: Thyroiditis: differential diagnosis and management. Am Fam Physician 2000;61:1047. [PMID: 10706157]

■ THE PARATHYROIDS

The main physiologic effects of parathyroid hormone are as follows: (1) It increases the osteoclastic activity in bone, with increased delivery of calcium and phosphorus to the circulation; (2) it increases the renal tubular reabsorption of calcium in the glomerular filtrate; (3) it inhibits the net absorption of phosphate and bicarbonate by the renal tubule; and (4) it stimulates the synthesis of 1,25-dihydroxycholecalciferol by the kidney. All of these steps result in a net increase in the amount of serum ionized calcium. Serum calcium is largely bound to albumin. Therefore, ionized calcium should be determined, or the serum calcium level should be corrected for serum albumin level as follows:

$$\text{"Corrected" serum Ca}^{2+} = \text{Serum Ca}^{2+} \text{ mg/dL} + (0.8 \times [4.0 - \text{Albumin g/dL}])$$

HYPOPARATHYROIDISM & PSEUDOHYPOPARATHYROIDISM

ESSENTIALS OF DIAGNOSIS

- *Tetany, carpopedal spasms, tingling of lips and hands, muscle and abdominal cramps, psychologic changes.*

- Positive Chvostek's sign and Trousseau's phenomenon; defective nails and teeth; cataracts.
- Serum calcium low; serum phosphate high; alkaline phosphatase normal; urine calcium excretion reduced.
- Serum magnesium may be low.

General Considerations

Hypoparathyroidism is most commonly seen following thyroidectomy, when it is usually transient but may be permanent. It may also occur after surgical removal of a parathyroid adenoma for primary hyperparathyroidism due to suppression of the remaining normal parathyroids and accelerated remineralization of the skeleton (hungry bone syndrome).

Hypoparathyroidism may also be seen in DiGeorge's syndrome, along with congenital cardiac and facial anomalies; hypocalcemia usually presents with tetany in infancy, but some cases are not detected until adulthood. Parathyroid deficiency may also be the result of damage from heavy metals such as copper (Wilson's disease) or iron (hemochromatosis, transfusion hemosiderosis), granulomas, sporadic autoimmunity, Riedel's thyroiditis, tumors, or infection.

Functional hypoparathyroidism may also occur as a result of magnesium deficiency (malabsorption, chronic alcoholism), which prevents the secretion of PTH. Correction of hypomagnesemia results in rapid disappearance of the condition. Hypoparathyroidism may rarely occur after neck irradiation.

Polyglandular autoimmunity type I (PGA-1) is also known as autoimmune polyendocrinopathy-candidiasis-ectodermal dystrophy (APECED). PGA-1 presents in childhood with at least two of the following manifestations: candidiasis, hypoparathyroidism, Addison's disease. Patients may also develop cataracts, uveitis, alopecia, vitiligo, or autoimmune thyroid disease.

Fat malabsorption occurs in 20% of patients with PGA-1 and may present as weight loss, diarrhea, or malabsorption of vitamin D, a fat-soluble vitamin used to treat the hypoparathyroidism. The fat malabsorption may be due to a deficiency in the jejunal enteroendocrine cells that produce cholecystokinin, causing a reduction in bile acid secretion.

Pseudohypoparathyroidism is a group of diseases characterized by hypocalcemia due to renal resistance to parathyroid hormone. There are several subtypes caused by different mutations involving the parathyroid hormone receptor or its G protein or adenylyl cyclase. PTH levels are high and the PTH receptors in bone are typically not involved, such that bony changes of hyperparathyroidism may be evident. Various phenotypic abnormalities may be associated—classically, short stature, round face, obesity, short fourth metacarpals, ectopic bone formation, and mental retardation. Patients without hypocalcemia but sharing the phenotypic abnormalities are said to have "pseudopseudohypoparathyroidism."

Clinical Findings

A. Symptoms and Signs

Acute hypoparathyroidism causes tetany, with muscle cramps, irritability, carpopedal spasm, and convulsions; tingling of the circumoral area, hands, and feet is almost always present. Symptoms of the chronic disease are lethargy, personality changes, anxiety state, blurring of vision due to cataracts, parkinsonism, and mental retardation.

Chvostek's sign (facial muscle contraction on tapping the facial nerve in front of the ear) is positive, and Trousseau's phenomenon (carpal spasm after application of a cuff) is present. Cataracts may occur; the nails may be thin and brittle; the skin is dry and scaly, at times with fungus infection (candidiasis), and there may be loss of hair (eyebrows); deep tendon reflexes may be hyperactive. Papilledema and elevated cerebrospinal fluid pressure are occasionally seen. Teeth may be defective if the onset of the disease occurs in childhood.

B. Laboratory Findings

Serum calcium is low, serum phosphate high, urinary calcium low, and alkaline phosphatase normal. Parathyroid hormone levels are low. Serum magnesium should be determined since hypomagnesemia frequently accompanies hypocalcemia and may exacerbate symptoms and decrease parathyroid function.

C. Imaging

Radiographs or CT scans of the skull may show basal ganglia calcifications; the bones may be denser than normal. Cutaneous calcification may occur.

D. Other Examinations

Slitlamp examination may show early posterior lenticular cataract formation. The ECG shows prolonged QT intervals and T wave abnormalities.

Complications

Acute tetany with stridor, especially if associated with vocal cord palsy, may lead to respiratory obstruction requiring tracheostomy. The complications of chronic hypoparathyroidism depend largely upon the duration of the disease. There may be associated autoimmunity causing sprue syndrome, pernicious anemia, or Addison's disease. In long-standing cases, cataract formation and calcification of the basal ganglia are seen. Occasionally, parkinsonian symptoms or choreoathetosis develops. Ossification of the paravertebral ligaments may occur with nerve root compression; surgical decompression may be required. Seizures are common in untreated patients. Overtreatment with vitamin D and calcium may produce nephrocalcinosis and impairment of renal function.

Differential Diagnosis

The symptoms of hypocalcemic tetany may be confused with paresthesias, muscle cramps, or tetany due to respiratory alkalosis, in which the serum calcium is normal. In fact, hyperventilation tends to accentuate hypocalcemic symptoms. Chronic hypocalcemia can cause heart failure and be confused with myocardial infarction and ischemic cardiomyopathy.

At times hypoparathyroidism is misdiagnosed as idiopathic epilepsy, choreoathetosis, or brain tumor (on the basis of brain calcifications, convulsions, choked disks) or, more rarely, as "asthma" (on the basis of stridor and dyspnea). Hypocalcemia is frequently seen in patients with hypoalbuminemia; serum levels of ionized calcium are normal.

Hypocalcemia may also be due to malabsorption of calcium, magnesium, or vitamin D; patients do not always have diarrhea. It may also be caused by certain drugs such as loop diuretics, plicamycin, phenytoin, alendronate, and foscarnet. In addition, hypocalcemia may be seen in cases of rapid intravascular volume expansion or due to chelation from transfusions of large volumes of citrated blood. Hypocalcemia is also frequently seen following parathyroidectomy for hyperparathyroidism. It is also observed in patients with acute pancreatitis. Some patients with certain osteoblastic metastatic carcinomas (especially breast, prostate) may develop hypocalcemia instead of the expected hypercalcemia. Hypocalcemia with hyperphosphatemia (simulating hypoparathyroidism) is seen in azotemia but may also be caused by large doses of intravenous, oral, or rectal phosphate preparations and by chemotherapy of responsive lymphomas or leukemias.

Hypocalcemia with hypercalciuria may be due to a familial syndrome involving a mutation in the calcium-sensing receptor; such patients have levels of serum PTH that are in the normal range, distinguishing it from hypoparathyroidism. It is transmitted as an autosomal dominant. Such patients are hypercalciuric; treatment with calcium and vitamin D may cause nephrocalcinosis.

Treatment

A. EMERGENCY TREATMENT FOR ACUTE ATTACK (HYPOPARATHYROID TETANY)

This usually occurs after surgery and requires immediate treatment.

1. Be sure an adequate airway is present.

2. Intravenous calcium gluconate—Calcium gluconate, 10–20 mL of 10% solution intravenously, may be given *slowly* until tetany ceases. Ten to 50 mL of 10% calcium gluconate may be added to 1 L of 5% glucose in water or saline and administered by slow intravenous drip. The rate should be so adjusted that the serum calcium is maintained between 8 and 9 mg/dL.

3. Oral calcium—Calcium salts should be given orally as soon as possible to supply 1–2 g of calcium daily. Liquid calcium carbonate (Titralac Plus), 500 mg/5 mL, may be especially useful. The dosage is 1–3 g calcium daily. Calcium citrate contains 21% calcium, but a higher proportion is absorbed with less gastrointestinal intolerance.

4. Vitamin D preparations—(Table 26–10.) Therapy should be started as soon as oral calcium is begun. The treatment of choice for chronic hypoparathyroidism is vitamin D_2 (ergocalciferol). The usual dose ranges from 25,000 to 150,000 units/d. It is a slow-acting preparation, and if toxicity develops, hypercalcemia—treatable with hydration and prednisone—may persist for weeks after it is discontinued. Ergocalciferol usually gives a more stable serum calcium level than do the shorter-acting preparations.

The active metabolite of vitamin D, 1,25-dihydroxycholecalciferol (calcitriol), has a very rapid onset of action, and if toxicity develops it is not long-lasting. It is of great use in the treatment of acute hypocalcemia in doses ranging from 0.25 to 4 µg/d. Despite its high cost, calcitriol is being used with increasing frequency for the treatment of chronic hypocalcemia. Therapy is commenced at a dosage of 0.25 µg orally

Table 26–10. Vitamin D preparations used in the treatment of hypoparathyroidism.[1]

	Potency	How Supplied	Daily Dose (Range)	Time Required for Hypercalcemia to Subside
Ergocalciferol (ergosterol, vitamin D_2)	40,000 USP units/mg	Capsules of 25,000 and 50,000 units; solution, 8000 units/mL	25,000–200,000 units	6–18 weeks
Dihydrotachysterol (Hytakerol)	120,000 USP units/mg	Tablets of 0.125, 0.2, and 0.4 mg	0.2–1 mg	1–3 weeks
Calcifediol (Calderol)	...	Capsules of 20 and 50 µg	20–200 µg	3–6 weeks
Calcitriol (Rocaltrol)	...	Capsules of 0.25 and 0.5 µg	0.25–4 µg	½–2 weeks

[1]Reproduced, with permission, from Greenspan FS, Baxter JD (editors): *Basic & Clinical Endocrinology,* 4th ed. McGraw-Hill 1994.

each morning with upward dosage titration to near-normocalcemia. Ultimately, doses of 0.5–2 μg/d are usually required.

Calcifediol (25-hydroxyvitamin D₃) is another option for treatment which has an intermediate onset and duration of action; the usual starting dose is 20 μg/d orally.

Dihydrotachysterol is faster in onset of action and is three times more potent than ergocalciferol. The usual daily maintenance dose is 0.125–1 mg/d. It is more expensive than vitamin D₂.

5. Magnesium—If hypomagnesemia is present (chronic alcoholism, malnutrition, renal loss, drugs such as cisplatin, etc), it must be corrected in order to treat the resulting hypocalcemia. Acutely, MgSO₄ is given intravenously, 1–2 g every 6 hours. Chronic magnesium replacement may be given as magnesium oxide tablets (600 mg), one or two per day, or as a combined magnesium and calcium preparation (Dolomite, others).

6. Transplantation of cryopreserved parathyroid tissue removed during prior surgery—Transplantation restores normocalcemia in about 23%.

B. MAINTENANCE TREATMENT

The goal should be to maintain the serum calcium in a slightly low but asymptomatic range (8–8.6 mg/dL). This will minimize the hypercalciuria that would otherwise occur and provides a margin of safety against overdosage and hypercalcemia, which may produce permanent damage to renal function. Calcium supplementation (1–2 g/d) is continued, and a vitamin D preparation (see above) is given. Monitoring of serum calcium at regular intervals (at least every 3 months) is mandatory. One should also monitor urine calcium with "spot" urine determinations and keep the level below 30 mg/dL if possible. Hypercalciuria may respond to oral hydrochlorothiazide, usually given with a potassium supplement.

Caution: Phenothiazine drugs should be administered with caution to hypocalcemic patients, since they may precipitate extrapyramidal symptoms. Furosemide should be avoided, since it may worsen hypocalcemia.

Prognosis

The outlook is good if the diagnosis is made promptly and treatment instituted. Any dental changes, cataracts, and brain calcifications are permanent. Periodic blood chemical evaluation is required, since changes in calcium levels may call for modification of the treatment schedule. Hypercalcemia that develops in patients with seemingly stable, treated hypoparathyroidism may be a presenting

Caccitolo JA et al: The current role of parathyroid cryopreservation and autotransplantation in parathyroid surgery: An institutional experience. Surgery 1997;122:1062. [PMID: 9426420]

Callies F et al: Management of hypoparathyroidism during pregnancy—report of twelve cases. Eur J Endocrinol 1998;139:284. [PMID: 9758437] (Hypoparathyroid women were treated during pregnancy with calcitriol 0.25 μg/d up to 3.25 μg/d, with a requirement for the higher doses as the pregnancies progressed.)

Högenauer C et al: Malabsorption due to cholecystokinin deficiency in a patient with autoimmune polyglandular syndrome type I. N Engl J Med 2001;344:270. [PMID: 11172154]

Marx SJ: Hyperparathyroid and hypoparathyroid disorders. N Engl J Med 2000;343:1863. [PMID: 11117980] (Review article.)

Thakker RV: Genetic developments in hypoparathyroidism. Lancet 2001;357:974. [PMID: 11293637] (A review of molecular genetic studies of hypoparathyroidism.)

HYPERPARATHYROIDISM

 ESSENTIALS OF DIAGNOSIS

- *Patients frequently asymptomatic, detected by screening.*
- *Renal stones, polyuria, hypertension, constipation, fatigue, mental changes.*
- *Bone pain; rarely, cystic lesions and pathologic fractures.*
- *Serum and urine calcium elevated; urine phosphate high with low to normal serum phosphate; alkaline phosphatase normal to elevated.*
- *Elevated parathyroid hormone.*

General Considerations

Primary hyperparathyroidism is an increasingly recognized disorder, present in up to 0.1% of adult patients examined. It can be seen at any age but is more frequent in persons over the age of 50 and is three times more common in women than in men.

The disease is caused by hypersecretion of parathyroid hormone, usually by a parathyroid adenoma, and less commonly by hyperplasia or carcinoma (rare). However, when hyperparathyroidism presents before age 30, there is a higher incidence of multiglandular disease (36%) and carcinoma (5%). The size of the parathyroid adenoma correlates with the serum parathyroid hormone level.

Parathyroid adenomas or hyperplasia can be familial (about 5%) and may be part of multiple endocrine neoplasia types 1, 2a, and 2b. (See Table 26–16.)

Hyperparathyroidism causes excessive excretion of calcium and phosphate by the kidneys. Parathyroid hormone stimulates renal tubular reabsorption of calcium; however, hyperparathyroidism causes hypercalcemia and an increase in calcium in the glomerular filtrate that overwhelms tubular reabsorption capacity, resulting in hypercalciuria. At least 5% of renal stones are associated with this disease. Diffuse parenchymal calcification (nephrocalcinosis) is seen less commonly. Chronic bone resorption induced by excessive PTH in the circulation may produce diffuse demineralization, pathologic fractures, or cystic bone lesions throughout the skeleton ("osteitis fibrosa cystica").

In chronic renal failure, hyperphosphatemia and decreased renal production of $1,25(OH)_2D_3$ initially produce a decrease in ionized calcium. The parathyroid glands are stimulated (secondary hyperparathyroidism) and may enlarge, becoming autonomous (tertiary hyperparathyroidism). The bone disease seen in this setting is known as "renal osteodystrophy." Diabetics seem somewhat less prone to develop this syndrome. Hypercalcemia often occurs after renal transplant but usually subsides spontaneously.

Parathyroid carcinoma is an unusual cause of hyperparathyroidism but is more common in patients with severe hypercalcemia.

Clinical Findings

A. SYMPTOMS AND SIGNS

Hypercalcemia is frequently discovered accidentally by routine chemistry panels. Most patients are asymptomatic. Parathyroid adenomas are usually so small and deeply located in the neck that they are almost never palpable; when a mass is palpated, it usually turns out to be an incidental thyroid nodule.

Although many patients with mild hypercalcemia offer no complaints, symptomatic patients are said to have problems with "bones, stones, abdominal groans, psychic moans, with fatigue overtones." The manifestations are more formally categorized as follows:

1. Skeletal manifestations— Hyperparathyroidism causes a loss of cortical bone and a gain of trabecular bone. Bone mineral concentration tends to be decreased in the distal radius and in the midshaft of the femur but not in the femoral neck. Similarly, bone mineral is decreased in vertebral posterior processes but increased in the vertebral bodies. Significant bone demineralization is uncommon in mild hyperparathyroidism, but osteitis fibrosa cystica may present as pathologic fractures or as "brown tumors" or cysts of the jaw. More commonly, patients have bone pain and arthralgias.

2. Urinary tract manifestations—Polyuria and polydipsia may be present and are due to hypercalcemia-induced nephrogenic diabetes insipidus. Calcium-containing kidney stones are reported in about 18% of those with newly discovered primary hyperparathyroidism. Nephrocalcinosis and renal failure can occur.

3. Manifestations of hypercalcemia—Mild hypercalcemia is often asymptomatic. In more severe cases, thirst, anorexia, nausea, and vomiting are present. Constipation, fatigue, anemia, weight loss, and hyper-

tension are commonly found. Pancreatitis occurs in 3%. Some patients present primarily with neuromuscular disorders such as muscle weakness, easy fatigibility, or paresthesias. Depression, intellectual weariness, and increased sleep requirement are common. Pruritus and psychosis or even coma may accompany severe hypercalcemia. Calcium may precipitate in the corneas ("band keratopathy") or soft tissue (calciphylaxis). Pancreatitis can occur.

B. LABORATORY FINDINGS

The hallmark of primary hyperparathyroidism is hypercalcemia (serum calcium > 10.5 mg/dL when corrected for serum albumin; see above). In hyperproteinemic states, the total serum calcium may be elevated but the ionized fraction is normal, whereas in primary hyperparathyroidism the ionized calcium is almost always elevated. The serum phosphate is often low (< 2.5 mg/dL). The urine calcium excretion may be high or normal (averaging 250 mg/g creatinine) but it is usually low for the degree of hypercalcemia. There is an excessive loss of phosphate in the urine in the presence of low (25% of cases) to low normal serum phosphate. (In secondary hyperparathyroidism due to renal failure, the serum phosphate is high.) The alkaline phosphatase is elevated only if bone disease is present. The plasma chloride and uric acid levels may be elevated. Elevated levels of parathyroid hormone confirm the diagnosis. The best immunoassay recognizes the intact molecule at two different sites—the amino terminal and the carboxyl terminal ends—with two different antibodies. This assay, known as immunoradiometric assay (IRMA), is specific and sensitive, making it easier to distinguish primary hyperparathyroidism from other causes of hypercalcemia.

C. IMAGING

Localizing preoperative imaging may allow a limited surgery and is especially important for patients with prior neck surgery. Performing two different types of studies reduces the chance of false positives. Since the gland or glands affected are rarely larger than 1.5 cm in diameter (and usually *much* smaller), preoperative imaging techniques are often unsuccessful. Imaging techniques include ultrasonography, CT, MRI, and Tc-99m MIBI studies. The accuracy of a given technique depends upon the available equipment and technical personnel. It is advisable to attempt preoperative localization with Tc-99m sestamibi/Tc-pertechnetate subtraction scintigraphy; this scan's sensitivity is 87%. Neck ultrasound may also be performed with a sensitivity of 80%. The sensitivity of combining both tests is 94%—but only about 55% in patients with multiglandular disease. Three-dimensional scintigraphic imaging techniques can help localize ectopic glands. Tc-99m MIBI specificity is over 95%, but false-positive scans can occur. Incidental small benign thyroid nodules are discovered incidentally in nearly half of patients with hyperparathyroidism who have imaging with ultrasound or MRI.

Bone x-rays are usually normal and not required to make the diagnosis of hyperparathyroidism. There may be demineralization, subperiosteal resorption of bone (especially in the radial aspects of the fingers), or loss of the lamina dura of the teeth. There may be cysts throughout the skeleton, mottling of the skull ("salt-and-pepper appearance"), or pathologic fractures. Articular cartilage calcification (chondrocalcinosis) is sometimes found.

Patients with renal osteodystrophy may have ectopic calcifications around joints or in soft tissue. Such patients may exhibit x-ray changes of osteopenia, osteitis fibrosa, or osteosclerosis, alone or in combination. Osteosclerosis of the vertebral bodies is known as "rugger jersey spine."

Complications

Pathologic fractures are more common in patients with hyperparathyroidism than in the general population. Urinary tract infection due to stone and obstruction may lead to renal failure and uremia. If the serum calcium level rises rapidly, clouding of sensorium, renal failure, and rapid precipitation of calcium throughout the soft tissues may occur. Peptic ulcer and pancreatitis may be intractable before surgery. Insulinomas or gastrinomas may be associated, as well as pituitary tumors (multiple endocrine neoplasia type 1). Pseudogout may complicate hyperparathyroidism both before and after surgical removal of tumors. Hypercalcemia during gestation produces neonatal hypocalcemia.

In secondary hyperparathyroidism due to renal failure, high serum calcium and phosphate levels may cause disseminated calcification in the skin, soft tissues, and arteries (calciphylaxis); this can result in painful ischemic necrosis of skin and gangrene, cardiac arrhythmias, and respiratory failure. The actual serum levels of calcium and phosphate have not correlated well with calciphylaxis, but a calcium (mg/dL) × phosphate (mg/dL) product over 70 is usually present.

Differential Diagnosis

(1) *Artifact*—A report of hypercalcemia may be due to laboratory error or excess tourniquet time and should always be repeated. Hypercalcemia may be due to high serum protein concentrations; serum calcium should be corrected for albumin (see above). It may also be seen with dehydration.

(2) *Hypercalcemia of malignancy*—Many malignant tumors (breast, lung, pancreas, uterus, hypernephroma, etc) can produce hypercalcemia. In some cases (breast carcinoma especially), bony metastases are present. In others, no metastases to bone can be demonstrated. Most of these tumors secrete parathyroid hormone-related protein (PTHrP), which has tertiary structural homologies to PTH and causes bone resorption and hypercalcemia similar to those of parathyroid hormone. The clinical features of the hypercalcemia of cancer can closely simulate hyperparathyroidism. Serum phosphate is often low, but the plasma level of PTH by IRMA is *low*. Serum PTHrP may be elevated.

Multiple myeloma is a common cause of hypercalcemia in the older population. Many other hematologic cancers such as monocytic leukemia, T cell leukemia and lymphoma, Burkitt's lymphoma, etc, have also been associated with hypercalcemia. Multiple myeloma causes renal dysfunction; resultant increased levels of carboxyl terminal PTH may cause it to be confused with hyperparathyroidism if a carboxyl terminal PTH assay is used. Serum protein and urine electrophoresis and bone marrow biopsy establish the diagnosis.

(3) *Sarcoidosis and other granulomatous disorders*—Macrophages and perhaps other cells present in granulomatous tissue have the ability to synthesize 1,25-dihydroxycholecalciferol. Hypercalcemia has been reported in patients with tuberculosis, sarcoidosis, berylliosis, histoplasmosis, coccidioidomycosis, leprosy, and even foreign-body granuloma. Increased intestinal calcium absorption and hypercalciuria are more common than hypercalcemia. Serum levels of 1,25-dihydroxycholecalciferol are elevated. Therapy with ketoconazole improves the hypercalcemia while treatment is directed at the underlying disorder.

(4) *Calcium or vitamin D ingestion*—Ingestion of large amounts of calcium (usually as an antacid) or vitamin D can cause hypercalcemia, which is reversible following its cessation. If it persists, the possibility of associated hyperparathyroidism should be strongly considered.

In vitamin D intoxication, patients may take large amounts of vitamin D for unclear reasons, so a check of all medications is important. Hypercalcemia may persist for several weeks. Serum levels of 25-hydroxycholecalciferol are helpful to confirm the diagnosis. A brief course of glucocorticoid therapy may be necessary if hypercalcemia is severe.

(5) *Familial hypocalciuric hypercalcemia*—This benign condition can be easily mistaken for mild hyperparathyroidism. It is an autosomal dominant inherited disorder characterized by hypocalciuria (usually < 50 mg/24 h), variable hypermagnesemia, and normal or minimally elevated levels of PTH. These patients do not normalize their hypercalcemia after subtotal parathyroid removal and should not be subjected to surgery. The condition has an excellent prognosis and is easily diagnosed with family history and urinary calcium clearance determination.

(6) *Adrenal insufficiency*—Hypercalcemia is common in untreated Addison's disease. This is partly due to disinhibition of calcium uptake by the renal tubule and gut. Additionally, Addison's disease can cause dehydration and hyperproteinemia, resulting in higher levels of nonionized calcium.

(7) *Hyperthyroidism*—Increased bone turnover is a feature of thyrotoxicosis. Mild hypercalcemia may also be present.

(8) Other causes—Other causes of hypercalcemia are shown in Table 21–9. Modest hypercalcemia is also occasionally seen in patients taking thiazide diuretics or lithium; such patients may have an inappropriately nonsuppressed PTH level in the face of hypercalcemia. Prolonged immobilization at bed rest may also cause hypercalcemia, especially in adolescents and patients with extensive Paget's disease of bone. Hypercalcemia is noted in up to one-third of acutely ill patients being treated in intensive care units, particularly patients with acute renal failure. Serum PTH levels are usually slightly elevated, consistent with mild hyperparathyroidism.

Treatment

A. Surgical Measures

Parathyroidectomy is recommended for patients with symptomatic hyperparathyroidism, kidney stones, or bone disease. Seemingly asymptomatic patients may be surgical candidates for other reasons such as (1) serum calcium 1 mg/dL above the upper limit of normal with urine calcium excretion > 50 mg/24 h; (2) urine calcium excretion over 400 mg/24 h; (3) cortical bone density ≥ 2 SD below normal; (4) relative youth (under age 50–60 years); (5) difficulty ensuring medical follow-up; or (6) pregnancy. Removal of a parathyroid adenoma usually results in cure. During pregnancy, parathyroidectomy is performed in the second trimester. If a parathyroid adenoma is identified preoperatively, limited neck exploration is usually sufficient to find and excise it. Without preoperative localization, bilateral neck exploration is usually advisable. Parathyroid glands are not uncommonly supernumerary (five or more) or ectopic (eg, intrathyroidal, carotid sheath, mediastinum). An intraoperative "quick" serum PTH determination is advisable to document the removal of the correct gland.

Parathyroid hyperplasia, commonly seen with chronic renal failure, is best treated with subtotal parathyroidectomy; three and one-half glands are usually removed, and a metal clip is left to mark the location of residual parathyroid tissue.

Complications: Serum PTH levels fall below normal in 70% of patients within hours after successful surgery, commonly causing hypocalcemic paresthesias or even tetany. Hypocalcemia tends to occur the evening after surgery or on the next day. Therefore, frequent postoperative monitoring of serum ionized calcium (or serum calcium plus albumin) is advisable beginning the evening after surgery. Once hypercalcemia has resolved, liquid or chewable calcium carbonate is given orally to reduce the likelihood of hypocalcemia. Symptomatic hypocalcemia is treated with larger doses of calcium; calcitriol (0.25–1 μg daily orally) may be added, with the dosage depending upon symptom severity. Magnesium salts are sometimes required postoperatively, since adequate magnesium is required for functional recovery of the remaining suppressed parathyroid glands.

In about 12% of patients having successful parathyroid surgery, PTH levels rise above normal (while serum calcium is normal or low) by 1 week postoperatively. This secondary hyperparathyroidism is probably due to "hungry bones" and is treated with calcium and vitamin D preparations. Such therapy is usually needed only for 3–6 months but is required chronically by some patients.

Hyperthyroidism commonly occurs immediately following parathyroid surgery. It is caused by release of stored thyroid hormone during surgical manipulation of the thyroid. Short-term treatment with propranolol may be required for several days.

B. Medical Measures

Hypercalcemia is treated with a large fluid intake unless contraindicated. Severe hypercalcemia requires hospitalization and intensive hydration with intravenous saline. (See Chapter 21.)

Bisphosphonates are potent inhibitors of bone resorption and can temporarily treat the hypercalcemia of hyperparathyroidism, malignancy, or immobilization. They may relieve bone pain as with patients with metastatic breast or prostate cancer. Pamidronate in doses of 30–90 mg (in 0.9% saline) is administered intravenously over 2–4 hours. Zoledronate 2–4 mg is administered intravenously over 15 minutes; it is quite effective but also quite expensive. These drugs cause a gradual decline in serum calcium over several days that may last for weeks to months. Other bisphosphonates such as alendronate may be effective orally, but their long-term use for chronic hyperparathyroidism has not been studied. Such bisphosphonates are used generally for patients with severe hyperparathyroidism in preparation for surgery.

Patients with parathyroid carcinoma are treated with surgical resections. Severe hypercalcemia may respond to the above measures and also to mithramycin. A calcium receptor agonist (R-568, calcimimetic) may also be effective.

Patients with mild, asymptomatic hyperparathyroidism are often followed closely medically. Such patients are advised to keep active, avoid immobilization, and drink adequate fluids. They need to avoid thiazide diuretics, large doses of vitamins D and A, and calcium-containing antacids or supplements. Serum calcium and albumin are checked about twice yearly, renal function and urine calcium once yearly, and bone density (of the distal radius) every 2 years.

Estrogen replacement is given to postmenopausal women. Digitalis preparations are avoided, since patients with hypercalcemia are sensitive to its toxic effects. Propranolol may be useful for preventing the adverse cardiac effects of hypercalcemia. Glucocorticoid therapy is ineffective for treating hypercalcemia in hyperparathyroidism.

Renal osteodystrophy is caused by secondary hyperthyroidism during renal failure; it may be prevented by avoiding hyperphosphatemia. Calcium acetate is given with meals to bind phosphate. Calcitriol, given orally or intravenously after dialysis, suppresses parathyroid hyperplasia of renal failure. New vitamin D analogs (eg, paricalcitol) suppress parathyroid hormone secretion but cause less hypercalcemia compared with calcitriol (see References; see also Chapter 22).

Prognosis

Completely asymptomatic patients with mild hypercalcemia may be followed and treated medically without compromising survival. There can be unexplained exacerbations and partial remissions. Surgical removal of sporadic parathyroid adenomas generally results in a permanent cure. Patients with MEN 1 undergoing subtotal parathyroidectomy may experience long remissions, but hyperparathyroidism usually recurs.

Spontaneous cure due to necrosis of the tumor has been reported but is exceedingly rare. The bones, in spite of severe cyst formation, deformity, and fracture, will heal if a parathyroid tumor is successfully removed. The presence of pancreatitis increases the mortality rate. Acute pancreatitis usually resolves with correction of hypercalcemia, whereas subacute or chronic pancreatitis tends to persist. Significant renal damage may progress even after removal of an adenoma. Parathyroid carcinoma tends to invade local structures and may sometimes metastasize; repeat surgical resections and radiation therapy can prolong life. Aggressive surgical and medical management of parathyroid carcinoma can result in an 85% 5-year survival rate and a 57% 10-year survival rate.

Irvin GL 3rd et al: Management changes in primary hyperparathyroidism. JAMA 2000;284:934. [PMID: 10944618] (Review article.)

Kort KC et al: Hyperparathyroidism and pregnancy. Am J Surg 1999;177:66. [PMID: 10037311]

Mandal AK et al: Secondary hyperparathyroidism is an expected consequence of parathyroidectomy for primary hyperparathyroidism: a prospective study. Surgery 1998;124:1021. [PMID: 9854578]

Marx SJ: Hyperparathyroid and hypoparathyroid disorders. N Engl J Med 2000;343:1863. [PMID: 11117980] (Review article.)

Shane E: Clinical review 122: Parathyroid carcinoma. J Clin Endocrinol Metab 2001;86:485. [PMID: 11157996] (Review article.)

Talpos GB et al: Randomized trial of parathyroidectomy in mild asymptomatic primary hyperparathyroidism: patient description and effects on the SF-36 health survey. Surgery 2000;128:1013. [PMID: 11114637] (Fifty-three asymptomatic patients with mild hyperparathyroidism were randomized to surgical therapy or observation. Patients undergoing parathyroidectomy reported improved function on two of the nine domains of the SF-36 health survey.)

Udelsman R et al: One hundred consecutive minimally invasive parathyroid explorations. Ann Surg 2000;232:331. [PMID: 10973383] (Most patients with hyperparathyroidism have a single adenoma. Minimally invasive parathyroidectomy requires a high-quality sestamibi scan using single-photon emission computed tomography [SPECT] to best localize the enlarged gland in three dimensions. Under cervical block anesthesia, patients undergo a limited neck exploration and parathyroidectomy; an intraoperative parathyroid

hormone assay is used to confirm the success of the resection.)

■ METABOLIC BONE DISEASE

The term "metabolic bone disease" denotes those conditions producing diffusely decreased bone density (osteopenia) and diminished bone strength. It is categorized by histologic appearance: osteoporosis (common; bone matrix and mineral both decreased) and osteomalacia (unusual; bone matrix intact, mineral decreased).

OSTEOPOROSIS

ESSENTIALS OF DIAGNOSIS

- Asymptomatic to severe backache from vertebral fractures.
- Spontaneous fractures often discovered incidentally on radiography; loss of height.
- Serum parathyroid hormone, 25(OH)D$_2$, calcium, phosphorus, and alkaline phosphatase usually normal.
- Demineralization, especially of spine, hip, and pelvis.

General Considerations

Osteoporosis is the most common metabolic bone disease and is estimated to cause 1.5 million fractures annually in the USA—mainly of the spine. The morbidity and indirect mortality rates are very high. Since the usual form of the disease is clinically evident in middle life and beyond and since women are more frequently affected than men, it is often referred to as "postmenopausal" osteoporosis. It is characterized by a decrease in the amount of bone present to a level below which it is capable of maintaining the structural integrity of the skeleton. The rate of bone formation is often normal, whereas the rate of bone resorption is increased. There is a greater loss of trabecular bone than compact bone, accounting for the primary features of the disease, ie, crush fractures of vertebrae, fractures of the neck of the femur, and fractures of the distal end of the radius. Whatever bone is present is normally mineralized.

Osteogenesis imperfecta (see Chapter 20) is caused by a major mutation in the gene encoding for type I collagen, the major collagen constituent of bone. This causes severe osteoporosis. Spontaneous fractures occur in utero or during childhood. Less severe mutations in the type I collagen gene are common, resulting in collagen disarray and predisposing to hypogonadal (eg, menopausal), or idiopathic osteoporosis.

Etiology

The causes of osteoporosis are listed in Table 26–11.

Clinical Findings

A. SYMPTOMS AND SIGNS

Osteoporosis is usually asymptomatic until fractures occur. It may present as backache of varying degrees of severity or as a spontaneous fracture or collapse of a vertebra. Loss of height is common. Once osteoporosis is identified, a carefully directed history and physical examination must be performed to determine its cause (see Table 26–11).

B. LABORATORY FINDINGS

Serum calcium, phosphate, and PTH are normal. The alkaline phosphatase is usually normal but may be slightly elevated, especially following a fracture. Once osteoporosis is identified, further testing for thyrotoxicosis, hypogonadism, and vitamin D deficiency may be required.

C. IMAGING

The principal areas of demineralization are the spine and pelvis, especially in the femoral neck and head; demineralization is less marked in the skull and extremities. Compression of vertebrae is common. Bone densitometry permits screening for osteopenia in high-risk individuals and allows assessment of response to therapy. CT densitometry of vertebrae is highly accurate and reproducible. Dual energy x-ray absorptiometry (DEXA) can determine the density of any bone, is quite accurate, and delivers negligible radiation.

Differential Diagnosis

Osteoporosis has many causes (Table 26–11). Additionally, osteopenia and fractures can be caused by osteomalacia (see below) and bone marrow neoplasia such as myeloma or metastatic bone disease. These conditions coexist in many patients.

Treatment

A. SPECIFIC MEASURES

Several treatment options are available, so a regimen is tailored to each patient.

1. **Sex hormones**—Women with hypogonadism should be considered for replacement estrogen (see Hormone Replacement Therapy) or raloxifene (see below). Men with hypogonadism are treated with testosterone (see Male Hypogonadism).

2. **Bisphosphonates**—These agents work similarly, inhibiting osteoclast-induced bone resorption. To ensure intestinal absorption, bisphosphonates must be taken in the morning with at least 8 oz of plain water at least 30 minutes before consumption of anything else. The patient must remain upright after taking alendronate to reduce the risk of esophagitis. Alendronate is excreted in the urine. However, no dosage adjustments are required for patients with creatinine clearances above 35 mL/min. There has been little experience giving alendronate to patients with severe renal insufficiency; if given, the dose would need to be

Table 26–11. Etiologic classification of osteoporosis.[1,2]

Hormone deficiency	**Genetic disorders**
Estrogen (women)	Aromatase deficiency
Androgen (men)	Type I collagen mutations
Hormone excess	Osteogenesis imperfecta
Cushing's syndrome or glucocorticoid	Idiopathic juvenile and adult osteoporosis
administration	Ehlers-Danlos syndrome
Thyrotoxicosis	Marfan's syndrome
Hyperparathyroidism	Homocystinuria
Immobilization and microgravity	**Miscellaneous**
Tobacco	Anorexia nervosa
Alcoholism	Protein-calorie malnutrition
Malignancy, especially multiple myeloma	Vitamin C deficiency
Medications	Copper deficiency
Excessive vitamin D intake	Liver disease
Excessive vitamin A intake	Rheumatoid arthritis
Heparin therapy	Uncontrolled diabetes mellitus
	Systemic mastocytosis

[1]Modified, with permission, from Fitzgerald PA: *Handbook of Clinical Endocrinology*, 2nd ed. McGraw-Hill, 1992.
[2]See Table 26–12 for causes of osteomalacia.

greatly reduced and serum phosphate levels monitored.

Alendronate, 10 mg/d orally, has proved effective for increasing bone density and reducing fracture risk; esophagitis can occur, especially in patients with hiatal hernia. Gastritis, anorexia, and weight loss are common side effects. Alendronate 70 mg orally once weekly appears to be as effective as daily dosing and is more convenient and possibly better-tolerated. An alternative oral bisphosphonate is risedronate. 5 mg orally daily. It must also be taken in the morning at least 30 minutes before eating, but it is associated with a lower incidence of gastrointestinal side-effects than daily alendronate. All patients should receive some supplementation with oral calcium (given with the evening meal) and vitamin D. Pamidronate is a parenteral bisphosphonate that can be given in doses of 60 mg by slow intravenous infusion in normal saline solution every 3 months for patients with osteoporosis who cannot tolerate the oral bisphosphonate preparations. Zoledronate is a recently developed third-generation bisphosphonate and a potent osteoclast inhibitor. It can be given every 3–4 months in doses of 2–4 mg intravenously over 15 minutes. It is very expensive.

Bisphosphonates have been effective in preventing corticosteroid-induced osteoporosis.

3. Selective estrogen receptor modulators (SERMs)—Raloxifene, 60 mg/d orally, can be used by postmenopausal women in place of estrogen for prevention of osteoporosis. Bone density increases about 1% over 2 years in postmenopausal women versus 2% increases with estrogen replacement. Raloxifene produces a reduction in LDL cholesterol but not the rise in HDL cholesterol seen with estrogen. It has no direct effect on coronary plaque. Unlike estrogen, raloxifene does not reduce hot flushes; in fact, it often intensifies them. It does not relieve vaginal dryness. Unlike estrogen, raloxifene does not cause endometrial hyperplasia, uterine bleeding, or cancer, nor does it cause breast soreness. The risk of breast cancer is reduced 76% in women taking raloxifene for 3 years. Since it is a potential teratogen, it is contraindicated in premenopausal women.

Raloxifene increases the risk for thromboembolism and should not be used by women with such a history. Leg cramps can also occur.

4. Calcitonin—A nasal spray of calcitonin-salmon (Miacalcin) is available that contains 2200 units/mL in 2 mL metered-dose bottles. The usual dose is one puff (0.09 mL, 200 IU) once daily, alternating nostrils. Nasal administration causes significantly less nausea and flushing than the parenteral route. However, nasal symptoms such as rhinitis and epistaxis occur commonly; other less common adverse reactions include flu-like symptoms, allergy, arthralgias, back pain, and headache. Five years of therapy increases bone 2–3% and reduces the number of new vertebral fractures. Both nasal and parenteral calcitonin have analgesic effects on bone pain; reduction of pain may be noted within 2–4 weeks after commencing therapy.

5. Calcium and vitamin D—Adequate oral intakes of calcium and vitamin D are required throughout life in order to maintain peak bone mass and reduce the risk of subsequent osteoporosis and osteomalacia. Supplements are recommended for patients at high risk for osteoporosis (see above) and for those with established osteoporosis. Other possible benefits are that the risk of breast cancer is reduced by vitamin D and that calcium supplements may reduce the risk of colon cancer. Calcium supplementation may be given as calcium citrate (0.4–0.7 g elemental calcium per day) or calcium carbonate (1–1.5 g elemental calcium per day). Vitamin D_2 is given in doses of 400–1000 IU daily.

Precautions: Patients who are taking glucocorticoids and thiazide diuretics may develop hypercalcemia when given oral calcium supplements. Calcium salts are given with meals in order to reduce the risk of calcium oxalate nephrolithiasis. Patients with renal failure who take calcium carbonate supplements experience a higher risk of calciphylaxis.

B. GENERAL MEASURES

For prevention and treatment of osteoporosis, the diet should be adequate in protein, total calories, calcium, and vitamin D. Pharmacologic glucocorticoid doses should be reduced or discontinued if possible. Thiazides may be useful if hypercalciuria is present. High-impact physical activity (eg, jogging) significantly increases bone density in men and women. Stair-climbing increases bone density in women. Patients who cannot exercise vigorously should be encouraged to engage in other exercise regularly, thereby increasing strength and reducing the risk of falling. Weight training is also helpful to increase muscle strength as well as bone density. Measures should be taken to avoid falls at home (eg, adequate lighting, handrails on stairs, handholds in bathrooms). Patients who have weakness or balance problems must use a cane or a walker; rolling walkers should have a brake mechanism. Balance exercises (eg, tai chi) can reduce the risk of falls. Patients should be kept active; bedridden patients should be given active or passive exercises. The spine may be adequately supported (though braces or corsets are usually not well tolerated), but rigid or excessive immobilization must be avoided. Alcohol and smoking should be avoided.

Prognosis

The prognosis is good for preventing postmenopausal osteoporosis if estrogen therapy or raloxifene is started early and maintained for years. Bisphosphonates can reverse osteoporosis and decrease fracture risk.

Altkorn D et al: Treatment of postmenopausal osteoporosis. JAMA 2001;285;1415. [PMID: 11255400]

Cauley JA et al: Effects of hormone replacement therapy on clinical fractures and height loss: The Heart and Estrogen/Progestin Replacement Study (HERS). Am J Med 2001;110: 442. [PMID: 11331055] (Secondary analysis of data from the HERS trial—a secondary prevention trial of estrogen and progestin replacement on cardiovascular disease—failed to show a beneficial effect of hormone replacement on clinical fracture risk.)

Cummings SR et al: The effect of raloxifene on risk of breast cancer in postmenopausal women: the results from the MORE randomized trial. Multiple Outcomes of Raloxifene Evaluation. JAMA 1999;281:2189. [PMID: 10376531] (Among 5129 postmenopausal women taking raloxifene versus 2576 women taking placebo, the incidence of breast cancer was reduced 76% in the raloxifene group during a median follow-up of 40 months. However, women taking raloxifene experienced a threefold increase in venous thromboembolic disorders.)

Greenspan SL et al: The effect of thyroid hormone on skeletal integrity. Ann Intern Med 1999;130:750. [PMID: 10357695] (Diminished bone density may occur in patients who have had hyperthyroidism or who use thyroid hormone to suppress TSH because of thyroid cancer or thyroid nodules. The effect is most notable in postmenopausal women. Such patients require assessment of cortical bone density in the hip or forearm. However, thyroid hormone replacement for hypothyroidism has negligible effect on bone density.)

Neer RM et al: Effect of parathyroid hormone (1–34) on fractures and bone mineral density in postmenopausal women with osteoporosis. N Engl J Med 2001;344:1434. [PMID: 11346808] (Postmenopausal women with vertebral compression fractures were randomized to receive once-daily subcutaneous injections of parathyroid hormone or placebo. Parathyroid hormone treatment decreased the risk of vertebral and nonvertebral fractures and increased vertebral, femoral, and total-body bone mineral density.)

Reid IR et al: Effect of pravastatin on frequency of fracture in the LIPID study: secondary analysis of a randomized controlled trial. Long-term Intervention with Pravastatin in Ischaemic Disease. Lancet 2001;357:509. [PMID: 11229669] (Secondary analysis of data from a large trial of pravastatin in patients with ischemic heart disease showed no effect of pravastatin on fracture risk.)

Villareal DT et al: Bone mineral density response to estrogen replacement in frail elderly women: a randomized controlled trial. JAMA 2001;286:815. [PMID: 11497535] (Compared with placebo, 9 months of hormone replacement therapy with estrogen significantly increased bone mineral density of the lumbar spine and hip in elderly women.)

OSTEOMALACIA

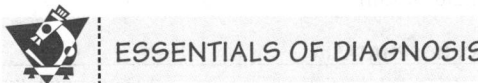

ESSENTIALS OF DIAGNOSIS

- *Painful proximal muscle weakness (especially pelvic girdle); bone pain and tenderness.*
- *Decreased bone density from diminished mineralization of osteoid.*
- *Laboratory abnormalities may include increases in alkaline phosphatase, decreased 25-hydroxy-*

vitamin D, or hypocalcemia, hypocalciuria, hypophosphatemia, secondary hyperparathyroidism.

- *Classic radiologic features may be present.*

General Considerations

Defective mineralization of the growing skeleton in childhood causes permanent bone deformities (rickets). Defective skeletal mineralization in adults is known as osteomalacia.

Osteomalacia is commonly caused by a deficiency in vitamin D, which is a hormone with a complex set of actions and mechanism of synthesis. Ergocalciferol (vitamin D_2) is derived from plants and is used in most pharmaceutical preparations of vitamin D. Cholecalciferol (vitamin D_3) is synthesized in the skin, under the influence of ultraviolet radiation, from 7-dehydrocholesterol. Both vitamin D_2 and vitamin D_3 are used to fortify foods and have equivalent potency. Two sequential hydroxylations are necessary for full biologic activity: The first one takes place in the liver—to 25-hydroxycholecalciferol (25[OH]D_3)—and the second one in the kidney, resulting in the formation of the most potent biologic metabolite of vitamin D, 1,25-dihydroxycholecalciferol (1,25[OH]$_2D_3$). The main action of vitamin D is to increase the absorption of calcium and phosphate from the intestine. However, vitamin D appears to have other systemic effects, since 1,25(OH)$_2$D receptors are also found in other tissues, including the parathyroids, bones, kidneys, skin, brain, pituitary, activated lymphocytes, and various tumors.

Etiology
(Table 26–12)

Osteomalacia is a common disorder and is caused by any condition that results in inadequate calcium or phosphate mineralization of bone osteoid.

A. VITAMIN D DEFICIENCY AND RESISTANCE

Vitamin D deficiency impairs the intestinal absorption of calcium and is the most common cause of osteomalacia. Borderline vitamin D deficiency (serum 25[OH]D < 50 nmol/L or < 20 ng/mL) was found in 24.3% of postmenopausal women from 25 countries in the MORE study. The incidence varied: < 1% in Southeast Asia, 29.3% in the USA, and 36% in Italy. Severe vitamin D deficiency (serum 25[OH]D < 25 nmol/L or < 10 ng/mL) was found in 4.1% of these women; 3.5% in the USA, and 12.5% in Italy. Vitamin D deficiency is particularly common in the institutionalized elderly, with the in-

Table 26–12. Causes of osteomalacia.[1,2]

Vitamin disorders
Decreased availability of vitamin D
Insufficient sunlight exposure
Nutritional deficiency of vitamin D
Malabsorption
Nephrotic syndrome
Vitamin D-dependent rickets type I
Liver disease
Chronic renal failure
Phenytoin, carbamazepine, or barbiturate therapy
Dietary calcium deficiency
Phosphate deficiency
Decreased intestinal absorption
Nutritional deficiency of phosphorus
Malabsorption
Phosphate-binding antacid therapy
Increased renal loss
X-linked hypophosphatemic rickets
Tumoral hypophosphatemic osteomalacia
Association with other disorders, including paraprotein-emias, glycogen storage diseases, neurofibromatosis, Wilson's disease, and Fanconi's syndrome
Disorders of bone matrix
Hypophosphatasia
Fibrogenesis imperfecta
Axial osteomalacia
Inhibitors of mineralization
Aluminum
Bisphosphonates

[1]Modified, with permission, from Fitzgerald PA: *Handbook of Clinical Endocrinology*, 2nd ed. McGraw-Hill, 1992.
[2]See Table 26–11 for causes of osteoporosis.

cidence exceeding 60% in some groups not receiving vitamin D supplementation. Deficiency of vitamin D may arise from insufficient sun exposure, malnutrition, or malabsorption (due to pancreatic insufficiency, cholestatic liver disease, sprue, inflammatory bowel disease, jejunoileal bypass, Billroth type II gastrectomy, etc). Cholestyramine binds bile acids necessary for vitamin D absorption. Patients with severe nephrotic syndrome lose large amounts of vitamin D-binding protein in the urine and may also develop osteomalacia.

Vitamin D-dependent rickets type I is caused by a rare autosomal recessive defect in renal synthesis of $1,25(OH)_2D$. It presents in childhood with rickets; adults develop osteomalacia unless treated with oral calcitriol in doses of 0.5–1 μg daily. Vitamin D-dependent rickets type II (now better known as hereditary $1,25[OH]_2D$-resistant rickets) is caused by a genetic defect in the $1,25(OH)_2D$ receptor. It presents in childhood with rickets and alopecia. Adults respond variably to oral calcitriol in very large doses (2–6 μg daily).

Anticonvulsants (eg, phenytoin, carbamazepine, valproate, phenobarbital) inhibit the hepatic production of $25(OH)D$ and sometimes cause osteomalacia. Phenytoin can also directly inhibit bone mineralization. Serum levels of $1,25(OH)_2D$ are usually normal.

B. DEFICIENT CALCIUM INTAKE

Rickets and osteomalacia continue to be common problems in many tropical countries despite adequate exposure to sunlight. A nutritional deficiency of calcium can occur in any severely malnourished patient. Some degree of calcium deficiency is common in the elderly, since intestinal calcium absorption declines with age. Ingestion of excessive wheat bran also causes calcium malabsorption.

C. PHOSPHATE DEFICIENCY

Phosphatonin is a circulating peptide that inhibits sodium-dependent phosphate transport in the renal tubule; high levels of this peptide cause excessive phosphaturia, resulting in hypophosphatemia. X-linked hypophosphatemic rickets is associated with high levels of phosphatonin, probably caused by familial or sporadic mutations in PHEX endopeptidase, which fails to cleave phosphatonin. Oncogenic osteomalacia is caused by excessive production of phosphatonin by a wide variety of soft tissue tumors (87% benign). The condition is characterized by hypophosphatemia, excessive phosphaturia, reduced serum $1,25(OH)_2D$ concentrations, and osteomalacia. Excessive renal phosphate losses are also seen in proximal renal tubular acidosis and Fanconi's syndrome. Some cases of hyperphosphaturia are idiopathic.

Other causes of hypophosphatemic osteomalacia include poor nutrition, alcoholism, or chelation of phosphate in the gut by aluminum hydroxide antacids, calcium acetate (Phos-Lo), or sevelamer hydrochloride (Renagel).

D. ALUMINUM TOXICITY

Bone mineralization is inhibited by aluminum. Osteomalacia may occur in patients receiving chronic renal hemodialysis with tap water dialysate or from aluminum-containing antacids used to reduce phosphate levels. Patients being maintained on long-term total parenteral nutrition may develop osteomalacia if the casein hydrolysate used for amino acids contains high levels of aluminum.

E. HYPOPHOSPHATASIA

Osteomalacia results from an autosomal recessive deficiency of bone alkaline phosphatase, which usually inactivates pyrophosphate; pyrophosphate inhibits bone mineralization. It may present in childhood as rickets or in adulthood as a propensity to fracture—due to osteomalacia. Patients have low serum levels of alkaline phosphatase and high urinary excretion of phosphoethanolamine.

F. Fibrogenesis Imperfecta Ossium

This rare condition sporadically affects middle-aged patients, who present with progressive bone pain and pathologic fractures. Bones have a dense "fishnet" appearance on x-ray. MRI of unfractured bone shows low signal intensity on both T1- and T2-weighted imaging. Serum alkaline phosphatase levels are elevated. Some patients have a monoclonal gammopathy, indicating a possible plasma cell dyscrasia causing an impairment in osteoblast function and collagen disarray. Remission has been reported after repeated courses of melphalan, corticosteroids, and vitamin D analog over 3 years.

Clinical Findings

The clinical manifestations of defective bone mineralization depend on the age at onset and the severity. In adults, osteomalacia is typically asymptomatic at first. Eventually, bone pain occurs, along with muscle weakness due to calcium deficiency. Fractures may occur with little or no trauma.

Diagnostic Tests

Serum is obtained for calcium, albumin, phosphate, alkaline phosphatase, parathyroid hormone. and 25-hydroxyvitamin D ($25[OH]D_3$) determinations. Bone densitometry helps document the degree of osteopenia. X-rays may show diagnostic features.

In one series of biopsy-proved osteomalacia, alkaline phosphatase was elevated in 94%; the calcium or phosphorus was low in 47%; $25(OH)D_3$ was low in 29%; pseudofractures were seen in 18%; and urinary calcium was low in 18%. $1,25(OH)_2D_3$ may be low even when $25(OH)D_2$ levels are normal.

Bone biopsy is not usually necessary but is diagnostic of osteomalacia if there is significant unmineralized osteoid.

Differential Diagnosis

Osteomalacia usually can be distinguished from osteoporosis by the relative absence of biochemical abnormalities in the latter. Phosphate deficiency must be distinguished from hypophosphatemia seen in hyperparathyroidism.

Prevention & Treatment

Prevention of vitamin D deficiency may be achieved with adequate sunlight exposure and vitamin D supplements. In the USA, the current recommended daily allowance (RDA) of vitamin D is at least 10 μg (400 IU) daily. However, in sunlight-deprived individuals (eg, veiled women, confined patients, or residents of higher latitudes during winter), the RDA should be 1000 IU daily. Patients receiving chronic phenytoin therapy may be treated prophylactically with vitamin D, 50,000 IU orally every 2–4 weeks.

Vitamin D deficiency is treated with ergocalciferol (D_2), 50,000 IU orally once or twice weekly for 6–12 months, followed by at least 1000 IU daily. Ergocalciferol has a long duration of action and may also be given orally every 2 months in doses of 50,000 IU. In patients with intestinal malabsorption, oral doses of 25,000–100,000 IU of vitamin D_2 daily may be required. Some patients with steatorrhea respond better to oral 25(OH)D (calcifediol), 50–100 μg daily. All patients receive supplemental oral calcium salts (eg, calcium citrate or calcium carbonate), which are given with meals. Recommended doses of calcium are as follows: calcium citrate (eg, Citracal), 0.4–0.6 g elemental calcium per day; or calcium carbonate (eg, OsCal, Tums), 1–1.5 g elemental calcium per day.

In hypophosphatemic osteomalacia, nutritional deficiencies are corrected, aluminum-containing antacids are discontinued, and patients with renal tubular acidosis are given bicarbonate therapy. In patients with sporadic adult-onset hypophosphatemia, hyperphosphaturia, and low serum $1,25(OH)_2D$ levels, a search is conducted for occult tumors that may be resected; whole-body MRI scanning may be required.

For those with X-linked or idiopathic hypophosphatemia and hyperphosphaturia, oral phosphate supplements must be given chronically; calcitriol, 0.25–0.5 μg/d, is given also to improve the impaired calcium absorption caused by the oral phosphate. Human recombinant growth hormone reduces phosphaturia and may be added to the above regimen.

Basha B et al: Osteomalacia due to vitamin D depletion: a neglected consequence of intestinal malabsorption. Am J Med 2000;108:296. [PMID: 11014722]

Kumar R: Tumor-induced osteomalacia and the regulation of phosphate homeostasis. Bone 2000;27:333. [PMID: 10962341]

Lips P et al: A global study of vitamin D status and parathyroid function in postmenopausal women with osteoporosis: baseline data from the Multiple Outcomes of Raloxifene Evaluation (MORE) clinical trial. J Clin Endocrinol Metab 2001;86:1212. [PMID: 11832511]

PAGET'S DISEASE OF BONE (Osteitis Deformans)

ESSENTIALS OF DIAGNOSIS

- *Often asymptomatic.*
- *Bone pain may be the first symptom.*
- *Kyphosis, bowed tibias, large head, deafness, and frequent fractures that vary with location of process.*

- Serum calcium and phosphate normal; alkaline phosphatase elevated; urinary hydroxyproline elevated.
- Dense, expanded bones on x-ray.

General Considerations

Paget's disease of bone is a common condition manifested by one or more bony lesions having high bone turnover and disorganized osteoid formation. Involved bones become vascular, weak, and deformed. Paget's disease is present in 1–2% of the population of the United States, with a higher prevalence in the elderly and in the Northeast. It is usually discovered incidentally during radiology imaging or due to incidentally discovered elevations in serum alkaline phosphatase. Only 27% of affected individuals are symptomatic at the time of diagnosis. Familial Paget's disease is unusual but is generally more severe than sporadic cases. A rare form occurs in young people.

Clinical Findings

A. Symptoms and Signs

Paget's disease is usually diagnosed in patients over 40 years of age and often mild and asymptomatic. It can involve just one bone (monostotic) or multiple bones (polyostotic), particularly the skull, femur, tibia, pelvis, and humerus. Pain is the usual first symptom. The bones become soft, leading to bowed tibias, kyphosis, and frequent fractures with slight trauma. If the skull is involved, the patient may report headaches and an increased hat size. Deafness may occur. Increased vascularity over the involved bones causes increased warmth.

B. Laboratory Findings

Serum calcium and phosphorus are normal, but serum alkaline phosphatase is markedly elevated. Urinary hydroxyproline is also elevated in active disease. Serum calcium may be elevated, particularly if the patient is at bed rest.

C. Imaging

On radiographs the involved bones are expanded and denser than normal. Multiple fissure fractures may be seen in the long bones. The initial lesion may be destructive and radiolucent, especially in the skull ("osteoporosis circumscripta"). Technetium pyrophosphate bone scans are helpful in delineating activity of bone lesions even before any radiologic changes are apparent.

Differential Diagnosis

Paget's disease must be differentiated from primary bone lesions such as osteogenic sarcoma, multiple myeloma, and fibrous dysplasia and from secondary bone lesions such as metastatic carcinoma and osteitis fibrosa cystica. Fibrogenesis imperfecta ossium is a rare symmetric disorder that can mimic the features of Paget's disease; alkaline phosphate is likewise elevated. If serum calcium is elevated, hyperparathyroidism may be present in some patients as well.

Complications

Fractures are frequent and occur with minimal trauma. If immobilization takes place and there is an excessive calcium intake, hypercalcemia and kidney stones may develop. Vertebral collapse may lead to spinal cord compression. Osteosarcoma may develop in long-standing lesions. Sarcomatous change is suggested by marked increase in bone pain, sudden rise in alkaline phosphatase, and appearance of a new lytic lesion. The increased vascularity may give rise to high-output cardiac failure. Arthritis frequently develops in joints adjacent to involved bone.

Extensive skull involvement may cause cranial nerve palsies from impingement of the neural foramina. Ischemic neurologic events may occur as a result of a vascular "steal" phenomenon. Involvement of the auditory region frequently causes hearing loss (mixed sensorineural and conductive) and occasionally tinnitus or vertigo.

Treatment

Asymptomatic patients require no treatment except for those with extensive skull involvement, in whom prophylactic treatment may prevent deafness and stroke.

A. Bisphosphonates

Bisphosphonates have become the treatment of choice for Paget's disease. The oral compounds should all be taken with 8 oz of plain water only. Bisphosphonates are usually given cyclically. Therapy is given until a therapeutic response occurs, as evidenced by normalization of the serum alkaline phosphatase. Patients are then given a break from therapy for about 3 months or until the serum alkaline phosphatase becomes elevated again; another cycle is then commenced.

1. Tiludronate, 400 mg orally daily for 3 months, is very effective in reducing the activity of bone lesions. It should not be taken within 2 hours of meals, aspirin, indomethacin, calcium, magnesium, or aluminum-containing antacids. Esophagitis is uncommon, so recumbency after dosing is not restricted, and it may be taken in the evening as well as during the day. The most common side effects have been gastrointestinal, including abdominal pain in 13% and nausea in 9%.

2. Alendronate, 20–40 mg orally daily (or 70 mg orally once weekly) for 3-month cycles, is also effective. It must be taken in the morning, at least one-half to 1 hour before breakfast. Its main side effect is esophagitis, so recumbency after dosing is prohibited, and the drug is contraindicated in patients with a history of esophagitis, esophageal stricture, dysphagia, hiatal hernia, or achalasia.

3. Risedronate, 30 mg orally daily for 3-month cycles, has been effective in normalizing alkaline phosphatase and eliminating bone pain in the majority of patients. It has been generally well tolerated, but arthralgias and gastrointestinal side effects do occur.

4. Etidronate disodium is given in doses of 5 mg/kg orally daily for 90–180 days. In severe disease, 10 mg/kg daily may be used for 90 days, with a rest period before another course is given. Etidronate can aggravate bone pain, particularly in the femur. It is much less effective than the other bisphosphonates.

5. Pamidronate, 60–120 mg intravenously over 2–4 hours, may produce improvements lasting several months. Alkaline phosphatase may continue to drop for 6 months after treatment. (See Treatment of Hypercalcemia.)

B. NASAL CALCITONIN-SALMON

Miacalcin, 200 IU/unit dose spray, is administered as one spray daily, alternating nostrils. It is just as effective as the parenteral preparation and is associated with fewer side effects. Nasal irritation may occur, as may occasional epistaxis. Calcitonin has been used for many years to treat Paget's disease. However, its use has declined dramatically with the introduction of more potent bisphosphonates.

Prognosis

The prognosis in general is good, but sarcomatous changes (in 1–3%) can alter the prognosis unfavorably. In general, the prognosis is worse the earlier in life the disease starts. Fractures usually heal well. In the severe forms, marked deformity, intractable pain, and cardiac failure are found. These complications should become rare with prompt bisphosphonate treatment.

Altman RD et al: Prevalence of pelvic Paget's disease of bone in the United States. J Bone Min Res 2000;15:461. [PMID: 10750560] (Paget's disease of bone is present in 1–2% of adults in the United States. The prevalence is highest in the Northeast [1.5%] and lowest in the South [0.3%]. The highest prevalence is among 65- to 75-year-old people [2.3%]. The condition is slightly more common in men, with near-equal racial distribution.)

Drake WM et al: Consensus statement on the modern therapy of Paget's disease of bone from a Western Osteoporosis Alliance symposium. Biannual Foothills Meeting on Osteoporosis, Calgary, Alberta, Canada, September 9–10, 2000. Clin Ther 2001;23:620. [PMID: 11354395]

Lombardi A: Treatment of Paget's disease of bone with alendronate. Bone 1999;24:59S. [PMID: 10321931] (The majority of patients with Paget's disease, treated with oral alendronate 40 mg/d, normalize their serum alkaline phosphatase within 6 months. The majority of those patients are likely to maintain biochemical remission for several years.)

Melton LJ 3rd et al: Fracture risk among patients with Paget's disease: a population-based cohort study. J Bone Miner Res 2000;15:2123. [PMID: 11092393] (Patients with Paget's disease had an increased risk of vertebral fractures.)

■ DISEASES OF THE ADRENAL CORTEX

ADRENAL CORTEX PHYSIOLOGY

Aldosterone is the major mineralocorticoid secreted by the zona glomerulosa, the outer layer of the adrenal cortex. It stimulates the renal tubule to reabsorb sodium and excrete potassium, thereby protecting against hypovolemia and hyperkalemia.

Aldosterone secretion is stimulated by hypovolemia in an indirect way. Hypovolemia causes the renal juxtaglomerular cells to secrete renin; renin stimulates the peripheral conversion of angiotensin I to angiotensin II; angiotensin II then causes aldosterone secretion. Hyperkalemia directly stimulates aldosterone secretion. Secretion is inhibited by atrial natriuretic factor and by dopamine.

Cortisol is the major glucocorticoid secreted by the middle zona fasciculata and the inner zona reticularis of the adrenal cortex.

Cortisol counters insulin effects, tending to cause hyperglycemia by inhibiting insulin secretion and by increasing hepatic gluconeogenesis, substrate being provided by the increased amino acids made available by cortisol's inhibition of protein synthesis in muscles.

Cortisol is secreted in a diurnal pattern, being highest upon awakening and lowest at bedtime. Cortisol production normally increases during exercise, making more glucose and fatty acids available for energy. Cortisol is also secreted in response to acute trauma, infection, and other stresses; it dampens defense mechanisms, helping prevent their dangerous overactivity. It inhibits the production or action of many mediators of inflammation and immunity such as interleukin-6 (IL-6), lymphokines, prostaglandins, and histamine. Cortisol is required for production of angiotensin II, thereby helping maintain adequate vascular tone.

Glucocorticoids increase renal free water clearance. They lower serum calcium by inhibiting calcium uptake by the renal tubule and gut and by redistributing calcium intracellularly.

Androgens are produced in the adrenal cortex, mostly by the inner zona fasciculata. The adrenal cortex's fetal zone atrophies after birth, but the adrenal continues to make large amounts of dehydroepiandrosterone sulfate (DHEAS) and dehydroepiandrosterone (DHEA), which have no known significance during adult life, having minimal androgenic activity; but they continue to be the adrenals' most abundantly secreted steroids. DHEAS secretion declines steadily with age. There are individual differences in secretion, and—for unknown reasons—there is a positive correlation between DHEAS levels and longevity.

Testosterone and androstenedione are the major functional androgens secreted by the adrenal. Their secretion causes adrenarche, which precedes gonadal androgen secretion and stimulates the first sexual hair of puberty.

ACUTE ADRENOCORTICAL INSUFFICIENCY
(Adrenal Crisis)

ESSENTIALS OF DIAGNOSIS

- *Weakness, abdominal pain, fever, confusion, nausea, vomiting, and diarrhea.*
- *Low blood pressure, dehydration; skin pigmentation may be increased.*
- *Serum potassium high, sodium low, blood urea nitrogen high.*
- *Cosyntropin (ACTH$_{1-24}$) unable to stimulate a normal increase in serum cortisol.*

General Considerations

Acute adrenal insufficiency is an emergency caused by insufficient cortisol. Crisis may occur in the course of chronic treated insufficiency, or it may be the presenting manifestation of adrenal insufficiency. Acute adrenal crisis is more commonly seen in primary adrenal insufficiency (Addison's disease) than in disorders of the pituitary gland causing secondary adrenocortical hypofunction.

Adrenal crisis may occur in the following situations: (1) Following stress, eg, trauma, surgery, infection, or prolonged fasting in a patient with latent insufficiency. (2) Following sudden withdrawal of adrenocortical hormone in a patient with chronic insufficiency or in a patient with temporary insufficiency due to suppression by exogenous glucocorticoids or megestrol. (3) Following bilateral adrenalectomy or removal of a functioning adrenal tumor that had suppressed the other adrenal. (4) Following sudden destruction of the pituitary gland (pituitary necrosis), or when thyroid is given to a patient with hypoadrenalism. (5) Following injury to both adrenals by trauma, hemorrhage, anticoagulant therapy, thrombosis, infection, or, rarely, metastatic carcinoma.

Clinical Findings

A. SYMPTOMS AND SIGNS

The patient complains of headache, lassitude, nausea and vomiting, abdominal pain, and often diarrhea.

Confusion or coma may be present. Fever may be 40.6 °C or more. The blood pressure is low. Patients with preexisting type-1 diabetes may present with recurrent hypoglycemia and reduced insulin requirements. Other signs may include cyanosis, dehydration, skin hyperpigmentation, and sparse axillary hair (if hypogonadism is also present). Meningococcemia may be associated with purpura and adrenal insufficiency secondary to adrenal infarction (Waterhouse-Friderichsen syndrome).

B. LABORATORY FINDINGS

The eosinophil count may be high. Hyponatremia or hyperkalemia (or both) are usually present. Hypoglycemia is frequent. Hypercalcemia may be present. Blood, sputum, or urine culture may be positive if bacterial infection is the precipitating cause of the crisis.

The diagnosis is made by a simplified cosyntropin stimulation test, which is performed as follows: (1) Synthetic ACTH$_{1-24}$ (cosyntropin), 0.25 mg, is given parenterally. (2) Serum is obtained for cortisol between 30 and 60 minutes after cosyntropin is administered. Normally, serum cortisol rises to at least 20 µg/dL. For patients receiving glucocorticoid treatment, hydrocortisone must not be given for at least 8 hours before the test. Other glucocorticoids (eg, prednisone, dexamethasone) do not interfere with specific assays for cortisol.

Plasma ACTH is markedly elevated if the patient has primary adrenal disease (generally > 200 pg/mL).

Differential Diagnosis

Acute adrenal insufficiency must be distinguished from other causes of shock (eg, septic, hemorrhagic, cardiogenic). Hyperkalemia is also seen with gastrointestinal bleeding, rhabdomyolysis, hyperkalemic paralysis, and certain drugs (eg, ACE inhibitors, spironolactone). Hyponatremia is seen in many other conditions (eg, hypothyroidism, diuretic use, heart failure, cirrhosis, vomiting, diarrhea, severe illness, or major surgery). It must also be distinguished from an acute abdomen where neutrophilia is the rule, whereas eosinophilia and lymphocytosis are characteristic of adrenal insufficiency.

Treatment

A. ACUTE PHASE

If the diagnosis is suspected, draw a blood sample for cortisol determination and treat with hydrocortisone, 100–300 mg intravenously, and saline *immediately*, without waiting for the results. Thereafter, give hydrocortisone phosphate or hydrocortisone sodium succinate, 100 mg intravenously immediately, and continue intravenous infusions of 50–100 mg every 6 hours for the first day. Give the same amount every 8 hours on the second day and then adjust the dosage in view of the clinical picture.

Since bacterial infection frequently precipitates acute adrenal crisis, broad-spectrum antibiotics should be administered empirically while waiting for the results of initial cultures. Hypoglycemia should be vigorously treated while serum electrolytes, blood urea nitrogen, and creatinine are monitored.

B. CONVALESCENT PHASE

When the patient is able to take food by mouth, give oral hydrocortisone, 10–20 mg every 6 hours, and reduce dosage to maintenance levels as needed. Most patients ultimately require hydrocortisone twice daily (AM, 10–20 mg; PM, 5–10 mg). Mineralocorticoid therapy is not needed when large amounts of hydrocortisone are being given, but as the dose is reduced it is usually necessary to add fludrocortisone acetate, 0.05–0.2 mg daily. Some patients never require fludrocortisone or become edematous at doses of more than 0.05 mg once or twice weekly. Once the crisis has passed, the patient must be investigated to assess the degree of permanent adrenal insufficiency and to establish the cause if possible.

Prognosis

Rapid treatment will usually be life-saving. However, acute adrenal insufficiency is frequently unrecognized and untreated since its manifestations mimic more common conditions; lack of treatment leads to shock that is unresponsive to volume replacement and vasopressors, resulting in death.

CHRONIC ADRENOCORTICAL INSUFFICIENCY (Addison's Disease)

ESSENTIALS OF DIAGNOSIS

- *Weakness, easy fatigability, anorexia, weight loss; nausea and vomiting, diarrhea; abdominal pain, muscle and joint pains; amenorrhea.*
- *Sparse axillary hair; increased skin pigmentation, especially of creases, pressure areas, and nipples.*
- *Hypotension, small heart.*
- *Serum sodium may be low; potassium, calcium, and urea nitrogen may be elevated; neutropenia, mild anemia, eosinophilia, and relative lymphocytosis may be present.*
- *Plasma cortisol levels are low or fail to rise after administration of corticotropin.*
- *Plasma ACTH level elevated.*

General Considerations

Addison's disease is an uncommon disorder caused by destruction or dysfunction of the adrenal cortices. It is characterized by chronic deficiency of cortisol, aldosterone, and adrenal androgens and causes skin pigmentation that can be subtle or strikingly dark. Volume and sodium depletion and potassium excess eventually occur in primary adrenal failure. In contrast, if chronic adrenal insufficiency is secondary to pituitary failure (atrophy, necrosis, tumor), mineralocorticoid production (controlled by the renin angiotensin system) persists and hyperkalemia is not present. Furthermore, if ACTH is not elevated, skin pigmentary changes are not encountered.

Etiology

(1) Autoimmune destruction of the adrenals is the most common cause of Addison's disease in the USA (accounting for about 80% of spontaneous cases). It may occur alone or as part of a polyglandular autoimmune (PGA) syndrome. Type 1 PGA is also known as autoimmune polyendocrinopathy-candidiasis-ectodermal dystrophy (APCED) syndrome and is caused by a defect in T cell-mediated immunity inherited as an autosomal recessive trait. It usually presents in early childhood with mucocutaneous candidiasis, followed by hypoparathyroidism and dystrophy of the teeth and nails; Addison's disease usually appears by age 15 years. Partial or late expression of the syndrome is common. A varied spectrum of associated diseases may be seen in adulthood, including hypogonadism, hypothyroidism, pernicious anemia, alopecia, vitiligo, hepatitis, malabsorption, and Sjögren's syndrome.

Type 2 PGA usually presents in adulthood with autoimmune adrenal insufficiency (no hypoparathyroidism) that is HLA-related. It is associated with autoimmune thyroid disease (usually hypothyroidism, sometimes hyperthyroidism), vitiligo, type 1 diabetes, alopecia areata, or celiac sprue. Autoimmune Addison's disease can also be associated with primary ovarian failure (40% of women before age 50), testicular failure (5%), and pernicious anemia (4%). The combination of Addison's disease and hypothyroidism is known as Schmidt's syndrome.

(2) Tuberculosis was formerly a leading cause of Addison's disease. The association is now relatively rare in the USA but common where tuberculosis is more prevalent.

(3) Bilateral adrenal hemorrhage may occur during sepsis, heparin-associated thrombocytopenia or anticoagulation, or with antiphospholipid antibody syndrome. It may occur in association with major surgery or trauma, presenting about 1 week later with pain, fever, and shock. It may also occur spontaneously.

(4) Adrenoleukodystrophy is an X-linked peroxisomal disorder causing accumulation of very long chain fatty acids in the adrenal cortex, testes, brain, and spinal cord. It may present at any age and accounts for

one-third of cases of Addison's disease in boys. Aldosterone deficiency occurs in 9%. Hypogonadism is common. Psychiatric symptoms often include mania, psychosis, or cognitive impairment. Neurologic deterioration may be severe or mild (particularly in heterozygote women), mimics symptoms of multiple sclerosis, and can occur years after the onset of adrenal insufficiency.

(5) Rare causes of adrenal insufficiency include lymphoma, metastatic carcinoma, coccidioidomycosis, histoplasmosis, cytomegalovirus infection (more frequent in patients with AIDS), syphilitic gummas, scleroderma, amyloid disease, and hemochromatosis.

Familial glucocorticoid deficiency is caused by a mutation in the gene encoding the adrenal ACTH receptor. Triple A (Allgrove's) syndrome is characterized by variable expression of the following: adrenal ACTH resistance with cortisol deficiency, achalasia, alacrima, nasal voice, and neuromuscular disease of varying severity (hyperreflexia to spastic paraplegia). Cortisol deficiency usually presents in infancy but may not occur until the third decade of life. Congenital adrenal hypoplasia causes adrenal insufficiency due to absence of the adrenal cortex; patients may also have hypogonadotropic hypogonadism, myopathy, and high-frequency hearing loss.

Patients with hereditary defects in adrenal enzymes for cortisol synthesis develop **congenital adrenal hyperplasia** due to ACTH stimulation. The most common enzyme defect is P450c21 (21-hydroxylase). Patients with severely defective P450c21 enzymes manifest deficiency of mineralocorticoids (salt wasting) in addition to deficient cortisol and excessive androgens. Women with milder enzyme defects have adequate cortisol but develop hirsutism in adolescence or adulthood and are said to have "late-onset" congenital adrenal hyperplasia. (See Hirsutism section.)

(6) Isolated hypoaldosteronism can be caused by various conditions. Hyporeninemic hypoaldosteronism can be caused by renal tubular acidosis type IV and is commonly seen with diabetic nephropathy, hypertensive nephrosclerosis, tubulointerstitial diseases, and AIDS; patients present with hyperkalemia, hyperchloremia, and metabolic acidosis (see Chapter 21). Hyperreninemic hypoaldosteronism can be seen in patients with myotonic dystrophy, aldosterone synthase deficiency, and congenital adrenal hyperplasia. Some patients with congenital adrenal hyperplasia (CYP17 deficiency) may present in adulthood with hyperkalemia, hypertension, and hypogonadism; cortisol deficiency is also usually present but may not be clinically evident.

Clinical Findings

A. SYMPTOMS AND SIGNS

The symptoms may include weakness and fatigability, weight loss, myalgias, arthralgias, fever, anorexia, nausea and vomiting, anxiety, and mental irritability.

Some of these symptoms may be due to high serum levels of IL-6. Pigmentary changes consist of diffuse tanning over nonexposed as well as exposed parts or multiple freckles; hyperpigmentation is especially prominent over the knuckles, elbows, knees, and posterior neck and in palmar creases and nail beds. Nipples and areolas tend to darken. The skin in pressure areas such as the belt or brassiere lines and the buttocks also darkens. New scars are pigmented. Some patients have associated vitiligo (10%). Emotional changes are common. Hypoglycemia, when present, may worsen the patient's weakness and mental functioning, rarely leading to coma. Manifestations of other autoimmune disease (see above) may be present. Patients tend to be hypotensive and orthostatic; about 90% have systolic blood pressures under 110 mm Hg; blood pressure over 130 mm Hg is rare. Other findings may include a small heart, hyperplasia of lymphoid tissues, and scant axillary and pubic hair (especially in women).

Patients with adult-onset adrenoleukodystrophy may present with neuropsychiatric symptoms, sometimes without adrenal insufficiency.

B. LABORATORY FINDINGS

The white count usually shows moderate neutropenia, lymphocytosis, and a total eosinophil count over 300/μL. Among patients with *chronic* Addison's disease, the serum sodium is usually low (90%) while the potassium is elevated (65%). Patients with diarrhea may not be hyperkalemic. Fasting blood glucose may be low. Hypercalcemia may be present. Young men with idiopathic Addison's disease are screened for adrenoleukodystrophy by determining plasma very long chain fatty acid levels; affected patients have high levels.

Low plasma cortisol (< 5 mg/dL) at 8 AM is diagnostic, especially if accompanied by simultaneous elevation of the plasma ACTH level (usually > 200 pg/mL). The cosyntropin stimulation test is performed as described above. Antiadrenal antibodies are found in the serum in about 50% of cases of autoimmune Addison's disease. Antibodies to thyroid (45%) and other tissues may be present.

Elevated plasma renin activity indicates the presence of depleted intravascular volume and the need for higher doses of fludrocortisone replacement.

C. IMAGING

When Addison's disease is not clearly autoimmune, a chest x-ray is obtained to look for tuberculosis, fungal infection, or cancer as possible causes. CT scan of the abdomen will show small noncalcified adrenals in autoimmune Addison's disease. The adrenals are enlarged in about 85% of cases due to metastatic or granulomatous disease. Calcification is noted in about 50% of cases of tuberculous Addison's disease but is also seen with hemorrhage, fungal infection, pheochromocytoma, and melanoma.

Differential Diagnosis

Addison's disease should be considered in any patient with hypotension or hyperkalemia. Unexplained weight loss, weakness, and anorexia may be mistaken for occult cancer. Nausea, vomiting, diarrhea, and abdominal pain may be misdiagnosed as intrinsic gastrointestinal disease. The hyperpigmentation may be confused with that due to ethnic or racial factors. Weight loss may simulate anorexia nervosa. The neurologic manifestations of Allgrove's syndrome and adrenoleukodystrophy (especially in women) often mimic multiple sclerosis. Hemochromatosis also enters the differential diagnosis of skin hyperpigmentation, but it should be remembered that it may truly be a cause of Addison's disease as well as diabetes mellitus and hypoparathyroidism. Serum ferritin is increased in most cases of hemochromatosis and is a useful screening test. About 17% of patients with AIDS have symptoms of cortisol resistance. AIDS can also cause frank adrenal insufficiency.

Complications

Any of the complications of the underlying disease (eg, tuberculosis) are more likely to occur, and the patient is susceptible to intercurrent infections that may precipitate crisis. Associated autoimmune diseases are common (see above).

Treatment

A. SPECIFIC THERAPY

Replacement therapy should include a combination of glucocorticoids and mineralocorticoids. In mild cases, hydrocortisone alone may be adequate.

1. Hydrocortisone is the drug of choice. Most addisonian patients are well maintained on 15–25 mg of hydrocortisone orally daily in two divided doses, two-thirds in the morning and one-third in the late afternoon or early evening. Some patients respond better to prednisone in a dosage of about 2–3 mg in the morning and 1–2 mg in the evening. Adjustments in dosage are made according to the clinical response. A proper dose usually results in a normal differential white count. Many patients, however, do not obtain sufficient salt-retaining effect and require fludrocortisone supplementation or extra dietary salt.

2. Fludrocortisone acetate has a potent sodium-retaining effect. The dosage is 0.05–0.3 mg orally daily or every other day. In the presence of postural hypotension, hyponatremia, or hyperkalemia, the dosage is increased. Similarly, in patients with fatigue, elevated plasma renin activity indicates the need for a higher replacement dose of fludrocortisone. If edema, hypokalemia, or hypertension ensues, the dose is decreased.

3. Dehydroepiandrosterone (DHEA) is given to some women with adrenal insufficiency. Women taking DHEA 50 mg orally each morning have experienced an improvement in their overall sense of well-being, mood, and sexuality. Since over-the-counter preparations of DHEA have variable potencies, it is best to have the pharmacy formulate this with pharmaceutical-grade DHEA.

B. GENERAL MEASURES

Treat all infections immediately and vigorously, and raise the dose of hydrocortisone appropriately. The dose of glucocorticoid should also be raised in case of trauma, surgery, stressful diagnostic procedures, or other forms of stress. The maximum hydrocortisone dose for severe stress is 50 mg intravenously or intramuscularly every 6 hours. Lower doses, oral or parenteral, are used for lesser stress. The dose is reduced back to normal as the stress subsides. Patients are advised to wear a medical alert bracelet or medal reading, "Adrenal insufficiency—takes hydrocortisone."

For patients with adrenoleukodystrophy, therapy with "Lorenzo's oil" normalizes serum very long-chain fatty acid concentrations but is ineffective clinically. Neurologic manifestations may improve following hematopoietic stem cell transplantation from normal donors.

Prognosis

Patients with Addison's disease can expect a normal life expectancy if their adrenal insufficiency is diagnosed and treated with appropriate replacement doses of glucocorticoids and (if required) mineralocorticoids. However, associated conditions can pose additional health risks. For example, patients with adrenoleukodystrophy or Allgrove syndrome may suffer from neurologic disease. Patients with adrenal tuberculosis may have a serious systemic infection that requires treatment. Adrenal crisis can occur in patients who stop their medication or who experience stress such as infection, trauma, or surgery without appropriately higher doses of glucocorticoids. Patients who take excessive doses of glucocorticoid replacement can develop Cushing's syndrome, which imposes its own risks. Many patients with treated Addison's disease complain of chronic low grade fatigue. Such fatigue may be due to epinephrine deficiency, which can result from adrenal destruction. Fatigue may also be an indication of suboptimal dosing of medication, electrolyte imbalance, or concurrent problems such as hypothyroidism or diabetes mellitus. However, most patients with Addison's disease are able to live fully active lives.

Arlt W et al: Dehydroepiandrosterone replacement in women with adrenal insufficiency. N Engl J Med 1999;341:1013. [PMID: 10502590] (DHEA raised initially low serum concentrations of DHEA, androstenedione, and testosterone to normal, and serum concentrations of sex hormone-binding globulin, cholesterol, and HDL cholesterol decreased. See editorial on page 1073.)

Huebner A et al: ACTH resistance syndromes. J Pediatr Endocrinol Metab 1999;12(Suppl 1):277. [PMID: 10698592] (Inherited ACTH insensitivity syndromes comprise a group of rare diseases manifested by cortisol deficiency alone or associated with other problems. Familial glucocorticoid deficiency is usually caused by mutations in the *MC2-R* gene encoding the adrenal ACTH receptor. Triple A syndrome is an autosomal dominant condition with variable phenotypic expression; a mutation on chromosome 12q13 has been implicated.)

Hunt PJ et al: Improvement in mood and fatigue after dehydroepiandrosterone replacement in Addison's disease in a randomized, double blind trial. J Clin Endocrinol Metab 2000;85:4650. [PMID: 11134123] (DHEA treatment improved some aspects of psychologic function in patients with Addison's disease.)

Ten S et al: Clinical review 130: Addison's disease 2001. J Clin Endocrinol Metab 2001;86:2909. [PMID: 11443143]

Vella A et al: Adrenal hemorrhage: a 25-year experience at the Mayo Clinic. Mayo Clin Proc 2001;76:161. [PMID: 11213304] (A review of 141 patients with adrenal insufficiency due to bilateral adrenal hemorrhage, which was diagnosed at autopsy in 48%. Adrenal hemorrhage most commonly occurred during sepsis and predisposed to the patient's death. It may be discovered as incidental adrenal masses. Adrenal hemorrhage also commonly occurs due to heparin-associated thrombocytopenia and antiphospholipid-antibody syndrome. It may occur postoperatively or spontaneously, presenting as abdominal pain and shock. It may also present during anticoagulant therapy or following trauma.)

CUSHING'S SYNDROME (Hypercortisolism)

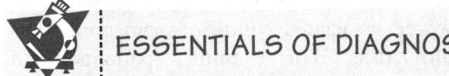

ESSENTIALS OF DIAGNOSIS

- *Central obesity, muscle wasting, thin skin, easy bruisability, psychologic changes, hirsutism, purple striae.*
- *Osteoporosis, hypertension, poor wound healing.*
- *Hyperglycemia, glycosuria, leukocytosis, lymphocytopenia, hypokalemia.*
- *Elevated serum cortisol and urinary free cortisol. Lack of normal suppression by dexamethasone.*

General Considerations

The term Cushing's "syndrome" refers to the manifestations of excessive corticosteroids, commonly due to supraphysiologic doses of glucocorticoid drugs and rarely due to spontaneous production of excessive corticosteroids by the adrenal cortex. Cases of spontaneous Cushing's syndrome are rare (2.6 new cases yearly per million population) and have several possible causes:

(1) About 43% are due to Cushing's "disease," by which is meant the manifestations of hypercortisolism due to ACTH hypersecretion by the pituitary. It is usually caused by a benign pituitary adenoma that is typically very small (< 5 mm). It is at least three times more frequent in women than men.

(2) About 10% are due to nonpituitary neoplasms (eg, small-cell lung carcinoma), which produce excessive amounts of ectopic ACTH. Hypokalemia and hyperpigmentation are commonly found in this group.

(3) About 15% are due to ACTH from a source that cannot be initially located.

(4) About 32% are due to excessive autonomous secretion of cortisol by the adrenals—independently of ACTH, serum levels of which are usually low. Most such cases are due to a unilateral adrenal tumor: benign adrenal adenomas are generally small and produce mostly cortisol; adrenal carcinomas are usually large when discovered and can produce excessive cortisol as well as androgens, with resultant hirsutism and virilization. ACTH-independent macronodular adrenal hyperplasia can also produce hypercortisolism due to the adrenal cortex cells' abnormal stimulation by hormones such as catecholamines, arginine vasopressin, serotonin, hCG/LH, or gastric inhibitory polypeptide; in the latter case, hypercortisolism may be intermittent and food-dependent and serum ACTH may not be completely suppressed. Pigmented bilateral adrenal macronodular adrenal hyperplasia is a rare cause of Cushing's syndrome in children and young adults; it may be an isolated condition or part of the Carney complex.

Clinical Findings

A. Symptoms and Signs

Patients with Cushing's syndrome usually have central obesity with a plethoric "moon face," "buffalo hump," supraclavicular fat pads, protuberant abdomen, and thin extremities; oligomenorrhea or amenorrhea (or impotence in the male); weakness, backache, headache; hypertension; osteoporosis; avascular bone necrosis; and acne and superficial skin infections. Patients may have thirst and polyuria (with or without glycosuria), renal calculi, glaucoma, purple striae (especially around the thighs, breasts, and abdomen), and easy bruisability. Wound healing is impaired. Mental symptoms may range from diminished ability to concentrate to increased lability of mood to frank psychosis. Patients are susceptible to opportunistic infections.

B. Laboratory Findings

Glucose tolerance is impaired as a result of insulin resistance. Polyuria is present as a result of increased free water clearance; diabetes mellitus with glycosuria may worsen it. Patients with Cushing's syndrome often have leukocytosis with relative granulocytosis and lymphopenia. Hypokalemia (but not hypernatremia) may be present, particularly in cases of ectopic ACTH secretion.

Tests for Hypercortisolism

The easiest screening test for hypercortisolism involves giving dexamethasone, 1 mg orally, at 11 PM and collecting serum for cortisol determination at about 8 AM the next morning; a cortisol level under 5 μg/dL (fluorometric assay) or under 2 μg/dL (HPLC assay) excludes Cushing's syndrome with 98% certainty. Other patients require further investigation, which includes a 24-hour urine collection for free cortisol and creatinine. An abnormally high 24-hour urine free cortisol (or free cortisol to creatinine ratio of > 95 μg cortisol/g creatinine) helps confirm hypercortisolism. A misleadingly high urine free cortisol excretion occurs with high fluid intake.

In cases of blatant Cushing's syndrome, no further confirmation of hypercortisolism is necessary. In less certain cases, a suppression test can also be done by giving dexamethasone, 0.5 mg orally every 6 hours for 48 hours; urine is collected on the second day. Urine free cortisol over 20 μg/d or urine 17-hydroxycorticosteroid over 4.5 mg/d also helps confirm hypercortisolism.

A midnight serum cortisol level > 7.5 μg/dL is indicative of Cushing's syndrome and distinguishes it from other conditions associated with a high urine free cortisol (pseudo-Cushing states; see Differential Diagnosis, below). Requirements for this test include being in the same time zone for at least 3 days, being without food for at least 3 hours, and having an indwelling intravenous line established in advance for the blood draw.

Certain drugs such as phenytoin, phenobarbital, and primidone accelerate the metabolism of dexamethasone, in that way causing a "false-positive" dexamethasone suppression test. Estrogens—during pregnancy or as oral contraceptives or estrogen replacement therapy—may also cause lack of dexamethasone suppressibility. In pregnancy, urine free cortisol is increased, while 17-hydroxycorticosteroids remain normal and diurnal variability of serum cortisol is normal.

Finding the Cause of Hypercortisolism

Once hypercortisolism is confirmed, a baseline plasma ACTH is obtained. It must be collected properly on ice and processed quickly by a laboratory with a reliable, sensitive assay. A level of ACTH below the normal range (about 20 pg/mL) indicates a probable adrenal tumor, whereas higher levels are produced by pituitary or ectopic tumors.

Localizing Techniques

In ACTH-dependent Cushing's syndrome, MRI of the pituitary can demonstrate a pituitary adenoma in about 50% of cases. Premature cerebral atrophy is often noted. When the pituitary MRI is normal or shows a tiny irregularity that may be incidental, selective inferior petrosal venous sampling for ACTH is performed (with CRH stimulation) where available to confirm a pituitary ACTH source, distinguishing it from an occult nonpituitary tumor secreting ACTH.

Two tests that are not useful for distinguishing the source of ACTH in Cushing's syndrome are the high-dose dexamethasone suppression test and the corticotropin releasing hormone (CRH) test.

Location of ectopic sources of ACTH is done with CT scan of the chest and abdomen, with special attention to the lungs (for carcinoid or small-cell carcinomas), the thymus, the pancreas, and the adrenals. Chest masses are frequently due to opportunistic infections, so biopsy is done to confirm the pathologic diagnosis prior to resection.

In non-ACTH-dependent Cushing's syndrome, a CT scan of the adrenals can localize the adrenal tumor in most cases.

Differential Diagnosis

Alcoholic patients can have hypercortisolism and many clinical manifestations of Cushing's syndrome. Depressed patients also have hypercortisolism that can be nearly impossible to distinguish biochemically from Cushing's syndrome but without clinical signs of Cushing's syndrome. Some adolescents develop violaceous striae on the abdomen, back, and breasts; these are known as "striae distensae" and are not indicative of Cushing's syndrome. Cushing's syndrome can be misdiagnosed as anorexia nervosa (and vice versa) owing to the muscle wasting and extraordinarily high urine free cortisol levels found in anorexia. Patients with severe obesity frequently have an abnormal dexamethasone suppression test, but the urine free cortisol is usually normal, as is diurnal variation of serum cortisol. Patients with familial cortisol resistance have hyperandrogenism, hypertension, and hypercortisolism without actual Cushing's syndrome. Patients with familial partial lipodystrophy type I develop central obesity and a moon facies, along with thin extremities due to atrophy of subcutaneous fat. However, their muscles are strong and may be hypertrophic, distinguishing this condition from Cushing's syndrome. Patients receiving antiretroviral therapy for HIV-1 infection frequently develop partial lipodystrophy with thin extremities and central obesity with a dorsocervical fat pad ("buffalo hump") that may mimic Cushing's syndrome.

Complications

Cushing's syndrome, if untreated, produces serious morbidity and even death. The patient may suffer from any of the complications of hypertension or of diabetes. Susceptibility to infections is increased. Compression fractures of the osteoporotic spine and aseptic necrosis of the femoral head may cause marked disability. Nephrolithiasis and psychosis may occur. Following bilateral adrenalectomy for Cushing's disease, a pituitary adenoma may enlarge progressively, causing local destruction (eg, visual field impairment) and hyperpigmentation; this complication is known as Nelson's syndrome.

Treatment

Cushing's disease is best treated by selective transsphenoidal resection of the pituitary adenoma, after which the rest of the pituitary usually returns to normal function; however, the normal corticotrophs are suppressed and require 6–36 months to recover normal function. Hydrocortisone replacement therapy is necessary in the meantime. Patients who fail to have a remission (or who have a recurrence) can be treated by bilateral laparoscopic adrenalectomy. Alternatively, stereotactic pituitary radiosurgery (gamma knife) induces normalization of urine free cortisol in two-thirds of patients within 12 months. Conventional radiation therapy results in a 23% cure rate. Patients who are not surgical candidates may be given a trial of ketoconazole in doses of about 200 mg every 6 hours; liver enzymes must be monitored for progressive elevation.

Adrenal neoplasms secreting cortisol are resected laparoscopically. The contralateral adrenal is suppressed, so postoperative hydrocortisone replacement is required until recovery occurs. Metastatic adrenal carcinomas may be treated with mitotane; ketoconazole or metyrapone can help suppress hypercortisolism in unresectable adrenal carcinoma.

Ectopic ACTH-secreting tumors should be surgically resected. If that cannot be done, medical treatment with ketoconazole or metyrapone (or both) may at least suppress the hypercortisolism; however, metyrapone may exacerbate female virilization. The somatostatin analog octreotide, given parenterally, suppresses ACTH secretion in about one-third of such cases.

Prognosis

Patients with Cushing's syndrome from a benign adrenal adenoma experience a 5-year survival of 95% and a 10-year survival of 90%, following a successful adrenalectomy. Patients with Cushing's disease from a pituitary adenoma experience a similar survival if their pituitary surgery is successful. However, transsphenoidal surgery incurs a failure rate of about 10–20%, often due to the adenoma's ectopic position or invasion of the cavernous sinus. Those patients who have a complete remission after transsphenoidal surgery have about a 15–20% chance of recurrence over the next 10 years. Patients with failed pituitary surgery may require pituitary radiation therapy, which has its own morbidity. Bilateral adrenalectomy is often complicated by infection; recurrence of hypercortisolism may occur as a result of growth of an adrenal remnant stimulated by high levels of ACTH. The prognosis for patients with ectopic ACTH-producing tumors is dependent upon the aggressiveness and stage of the particular tumor. Patients with ACTH of unknown source have a 5-year survival rate of 65% and a 10-year survival rate of 55%. Patients with adrenal carcinoma have a median survival of 7 months.

Boscaro M et al: The diagnosis of Cushing's syndrome: atypical presentations and laboratory shortcomings. Arch Intern Med 2001;161:1780 [PMID:11074733] (A review of atypical clinical presentations and laboratory findings in patients with Cushing's syndrome.)

Colao A et al: Inferior petrosal sinus sampling in the differential diagnosis of Cushing's syndrome: results of an Italian multicenter study. Eur J Endocrinol 2001;144:499. [PMID: 11331216] (Use of inferior petrosal sinus sampling improves the accuracy of imaging techniques in the evaluation of patients with ACTH-dependent Cushing's syndrome.)

Forget H et al: Cognitive decline in patients with Cushing's syndrome. J Int Neuropsychol Soc 2000;6:20. [PMID: 10761364] (Glucocorticoid receptors are found throughout the brain, particularly in the hippocampus; patients with Cushing's syndrome were found to have deficits in processing of visual and spatial information, reasoning, concept formation, memory, and attention.)

Kirk LF et al: Cushing's disease: clinical manifestations and diagnostic evaluation. Am Fam Physician 2000;62:1119 & 1133. [PMID: 10997535]

Lindholm J et al: Incidence and late prognosis of Cushing's syndrome: a population-based study. J Clin Endocrinol Metab 2001;86:117. [PMID: 11231987] (A population-based study of all patients with Cushing's syndrome in Denmark over an 11-year period. Standard mortality ratio was 3.68 for patients with nonmalignant disease, with most deaths occurring in the year following diagnosis.)

Papanicolaou DA et al: A single midnight serum cortisol measurement distinguishes Cushing's syndrome from pseudo-Cushing states. J Clin Endocrinol Metab 1998;83:1163. [PMID: 9543134]

HIRSUTISM & VIRILIZATION

 ESSENTIALS OF DIAGNOSIS

- *Menstrual disorders, hirsutism, acne.*
- *Virilization may occur: increased muscularity, androgenic alopecia, deepening of the voice, enlargement of the clitoris.*
- *Occasionally a palpable pelvic tumor.*
- *Urinary 17-ketosteroids and serum DHEAS and androstenedione elevated in adrenal disorders, variable in others.*
- *Serum testosterone often elevated.*

General Considerations

Major androgens include testosterone, androstenedione, and dehydroepiandrosterone sulfate (DHEAS).

In women, circulating testosterone is derived from direct ovarian secretion (60%) and from peripheral conversion from androstenedione (40%). Androstenedione is secreted in about equal amounts by the adrenals and ovaries. DHEAS is secreted exclusively by the adrenals.

Testosterone is the most potent androgen, but 98% circulates in a bound state: About 65% is strongly bound to sex hormone-binding globulin (SHBG), while 33% is weakly bound to albumin. Only free testosterone and a portion of the weakly bound testosterone can enter target cells to exert androgenic effect. Assays have therefore been devised to measure "total," "free," or "free and weakly bound" testosterone.

Testosterone is converted in the skin to dihydrotestosterone, which actually stimulates the hair follicle. Dihydrotestosterone is metabolized to androstanediol glucuronide, which can be measured and is elevated in most cases of hirsutism.

Etiology

Hirsutism may be caused by the following disorders:

(1) Idiopathic or familial—Most women with hirsutism or androgenic alopecia have no detectable hyperandrogenism. Patients often have a strong familial predisposition to hirsutism that may be considered normal in the context of their genetic background. Such patients may have elevated serum levels of androstanediol glucuronide, a metabolite of dihydrotestosterone that is produced by skin in cosmetically unacceptable amounts.

(2) Polycystic ovary syndrome (hyperthecosis, Stein-Leventhal syndrome)—This is a common functional disorder of the ovaries which accounts for at least half the cases of clinical hirsutism. Patients frequently have amenorrhea or oligomenorrhea with anovulation and obesity. The serum LH:FSH ratio is often greater than 2.0. Both adrenal and ovarian androgen hypersecretion are commonly present. Insulin resistance and obesity are common; fasting insulin levels are elevated in 70%. Diabetes mellitus is present in about 13%. Women frequently regain normal menstrual cycles with aging.

(3) Steroidogenic enzyme defects—Baby girls with "classic" 21-hydroxylase deficiency have ambiguous genitalia and may become virilized unless treated with corticosteroid replacement; about half of such patients have clinically evident mineralocorticoid deficiency (salt-wasting) as well.

About 2% of patients with adult-onset hirsutism have been found to have a partial defect in adrenal 21-hydroxylase, whose phenotypic expression is delayed until adolescence or adulthood; such patients do not have salt wasting.

Some rare patients with hyperandrogenism and hypertension have 11-hydroxylase deficiency. This is distinguished from cortisol resistance by high cortisol levels in the latter and by high 11-deoxycortisol levels in the former.

Patients with an XY karyotype and a deficiency in 17β-hydroxysteroid dehydrogenase 3 or a deficiency in 5α-reductase-2 may present as phenotypic girls who develop virilization at puberty.

(4) Ovarian tumors are very uncommon causes of hirsutism (0.8%) and include arrhenoblastomas, Sertoli-Leydig cell tumors, dysgerminomas, and hilar cell tumors.

(5) Adrenal carcinoma is a rare cause of hyperandrogenism that can be quite virilizing.

(6) Other rare causes of hirsutism include acromegaly and ACTH-induced Cushing's syndrome. Maternal virilization during pregnancy may occur as a result of a luteoma of pregnancy, hyperreactio luteinalis, or polycystic ovaries. In postmenopausal women, diffuse stromal Leydig cell hyperplasia is a rare cause of hyperandrogenism. Pharmacologic causes include minoxidil, cyclosporine, phenytoin, anabolic steroids, diazoxide, and certain progestins.

Clinical Findings

A. Symptoms and Signs

Modest androgen excess from any source increases sexual hair (chin, upper lip, abdomen, and chest) and increases sebaceous gland activity, producing acne. Menstrual irregularities, anovulation, and amenorrhea are common. If androgen excess is pronounced, defeminization (decrease in breast size, loss of feminine adipose tissue) and virilization (frontal balding, muscularity, clitoromegaly, and deepening of the voice) occurs. Virilization implies the presence of an androgen-producing neoplasm.

Hypertension may be seen in rare patients with Cushing's syndrome, adrenal 11-hydroxylase deficiency, or cortisol resistance syndrome.

A pelvic examination may disclose clitoromegaly or ovarian enlargement that may be cystic or neoplastic.

B. Laboratory Testing and Imaging

Serum androgen testing is mainly useful to screen for rare occult adrenal or ovarian neoplasms. Some general guidelines are presented here, though exceptions are common:

Serum is assayed for total testosterone and free testosterone. Certain assays for free testosterone are not reliable, including the free androgen index, the analog free testosterone assay, and the electrochemical luminescence assay. It is best to specify the assay desired, eg, free testosterone by equilibrium dialysis, calculated free testosterone, or non-sex hormone-bound testosterone assay.

A serum testosterone level greater than 200 ng/dL or free testosterone greater than 40 ng/dL indicates the need for pelvic examination and ultrasound. If that is negative, an adrenal CT scan is performed.

A serum androstenedione greater than 1000 ng/dL also implicates an ovarian or adrenal neoplasm.

Patients with milder elevations of serum testosterone or androstenedione usually are treated with an oral contraceptive.

Patients with very elevated serum DHEAS (> 700 μg/dL) have an adrenal source of androgen. This usually is due to adrenal hyperplasia and rarely to adrenal carcinoma. An adrenal CT scan is performed.

No firm guidelines exist as to which patients (if any) with hyperandrogenism should be screened for "late-onset" 21-hydroxylase deficiency. The evaluation requires levels of serum 17-hydroxyprogesterone to be drawn at baseline and at 30–60 minutes after the intramuscular injection of 0.25 mg of cosyntropin (ACTH$_{1-24}$). Patients with congenital adrenal hyperplasia will usually have a baseline 17-hydroxyprogesterone over 300 ng/dL or a stimulated level over 1000 ng/dL. The diagnosis, once made, is interesting academically but not helpful to the patient since glucocorticoid treatment is not particularly more effective in this condition than are other treatment modalities (see below).

Patients with any clinical signs of Cushing's syndrome should receive a screening test. (See Cushing's Syndrome.)

Serum levels of FSH and LH are elevated if amenorrhea is due to ovarian failure. An LH:FSH ratio greater than 2.0 is common in patients with polycystic ovary syndrome. On abdominal ultrasound, about 33% of normal young women have polycystic ovaries, so the appearance of ovarian cysts on ultrasound is not helpful diagnostically.

Virilizing tumors of the ovary can usually be detected by pelvic ultrasound or MRI. However, small virilizing ovarian tumors may not be detectable on imaging studies; selective venous sampling for testosterone may be employed for diagnosis in such patients.

Treatment

Any underlying cause of hyperandrogenism must be detected and treated if possible. Postmenopausal women with severe hyperandrogenism should undergo laparoscopic bilateral oophorectomy (if CT scan of the adrenals and ovaries is normal), since small hilar cell tumors of the ovary may not be visible on scans. Any drugs causing hirsutism are stopped. Treatment options for other cases include the following:

(1) Spironolactone may be taken in doses of 50–100 mg twice daily on days 5–25 of the menstrual cycle or daily if used concomitantly with an oral contraceptive. Hyperkalemia or hyponatremia is uncommon.

(2) Cyproterone acetate is a potent antiandrogen with progestational activity. A dose of 2 mg is effective. An oral contraceptive is usually prescribed also. Cyproterone is not available in the USA. It is available elsewhere as the progestin element in an oral contraceptive (Diane-35: ethinyl estradiol 35 μg with cyproterone acetate 2 mg). Side effects may include fatigue, nausea, or depression.

(3) Finasteride inhibits 5α-reductase, the enzyme that converts testosterone to active dihydrotestosterone in the skin. Given as 5 mg doses orally daily, it provides modest reduction in hirsutism over 6 months—comparable to results achieved with spironolactone. Finasteride is ineffective for androgenic alopecia in women. Side effects are rare.

(4) Flutamide, 250 mg/d, inhibits androgen reception uptake and also suppresses serum androgen. Used with an oral contraceptive, it appears to be more effective than spironolactone in improving hirsutism, acne, and male pattern baldness. Hepatotoxicity has been reported but is rare.

(5) Oral contraceptives stimulate menses, if desired, but are less effective for hirsutism. Contraceptives with low-androgenic progestins (desogestrel, gestodene) may be tried.

(6) Metformin, 500–1000 mg twice daily, in women with polycystic ovary syndrome and amenorrhea tends to restore normal menses and reduce hirsutism. It is contraindicated in renal disease. Gastrointestinal side effects are usually tolerable. Metformin can be taken by nondiabetics without causing hypoglycemia.

(7) Local treatment by shaving or depilatories, waxing, electrolysis, or bleaching should be encouraged. Laser therapy is an effective treatment for facial hirsutism, particularly for women with dark hair and light skin; complications include skin hypopigmentation (rare) and hyperpigmentation, which occurs in 20% but which usually resolves.

Women with androgenic alopecia may be effectively treated with topical minoxidil 2% solution applied chronically twice daily to a dry scalp. Hypertrichosis is an unwanted side effect of topical minoxidil, occurring in 3–5% of treated women; it may affect the forehead, cheeks, upper lip, or chin. Hypertrichosis resolves within 1–6 months after the drug is stopped.

Note: Antiandrogen treatments must be given only to nonpregnant women. Women must be counseled to take oral contraceptives, when indicated, and avoid pregnancy, since use during pregnancy causes malformations and pseudohermaphroditism in male infants.

Azziz R et al: Troglitazone improves ovulation and hirsutism in the polycystic ovary syndrome: a multicenter, double blind, placebo-controlled trial. J Clin Endocrinol Metab 2001;86: 1626. [PMID: 11297595] (In patients with polycystic ovary syndrome, the insulin-sensitizing agent troglitazone was statistically significantly more effective than placebo in treating hirsutism. Troglitazone has been withdrawn from the United States market, but pioglitazone and rosiglitazone are similar drugs that are available.)

Farquhar C et al: Spironolactone versus placebo or in combination with steroids for hirsutism and/or acne (Cochrane Review). Cochrane Database Syst Rev 2001;4:CD000194. [PMID: 11687072] (This review of clinical trial data concluded that 6 months of treatment with 100 mg of spironolactone daily compared with placebo was associated with a statistically significant subjective and objective reduction in hirsutism.)

Ibanez L et al: Treatment of hirsutism, hyperandrogenism, oligomenorrhea, dyslipidemia, and hyperinsulinism in nonobese, adolescent girls: effect of flutamide. J Clin Endocrinol Metab 2000;85:3251. [PMID: 10999817] (Flutamide is an antiandrogen that is widely used for the treatment of prostate cancer. Flutamide 250 mg/d, a relatively low dose, was administered to 18 young hirsute women for 18 months with marked reduction in hirsutism, serum testosterone, androstenedione, triglycerides, and LDL cholesterol. It was tolerated well.)

Price VH: Treatment of hair loss. N Engl J Med 1999;341:964. [PMID: 10498493]

Tartagni M et al: Comparison of Diane 35 and Diane 35 plus finasteride in the treatment of hirsutism. Fertil Steril 2000;73:718. [PMID: 10731531] (Diane 35 is an oral contraceptive with 35 µg ethinyl estradiol and 2 mg cyproterone acetate, an anti-androgen progestin. Combining this treatment with finasteride 5 mg/d for 2 weeks monthly led to rapid improvement in hirsutism.)

PRIMARY HYPERALDOSTERONISM

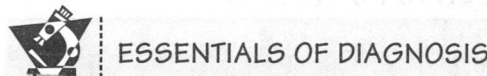

ESSENTIALS OF DIAGNOSIS

- *Hypertension, polyuria, polydipsia, muscular weakness.*
- *Hypokalemia, alkalosis.*
- *Elevated plasma and urine aldosterone levels and low plasma renin level.*

General Considerations

Classic hyperaldosteronism (with hypokalemia) accounts for about 0.7% of cases of hypertension; milder hyperaldosteronism is more frequent. The disorder is more common in women. Primary hyperaldosteronism may be due to unilateral adrenocortical adenoma (Conn's syndrome, 73%) or bilateral cortical hyperplasia (27%), which may be glucocorticoid-suppressible due to an autosomal dominant genetic defect allowing ACTH stimulation of aldosterone production.

Clinical Findings

A. SYMPTOMS AND SIGNS

Hypertension, muscular weakness (at times with paralysis simulating periodic paralysis), paresthesias with frank tetany, headache, polyuria, and polydipsia are the main complaints. Hypertension is typically moderate. Some patients have only diastolic hypertension, without other symptoms and signs. Malignant hypertension is rare. Edema is rarely seen in primary hyperaldosteronism.

B. LABORATORY FINDINGS

For a patient to be properly tested for hyperaldosteronism, all antihypertensive medications must be discontinued. Calcium channel blockers can normalize aldosterone secretion, thus interfering with the diagnosis. The patient must have a high sodium intake (> 120 meq/d) during the entire evaluation period; serum potassium is low. A 24-hour urine collection is assayed for aldosterone, free cortisol, and creatinine. A low plasma renin activity (< 5 µg/dL) with 24-hour urine aldosterone over 20 µg indicates hyperaldosteronism. A urine aldosterone of less than 20 µg/24 h is seen with rare adrenal or gonadal enzyme defects in the activity of 17α-hydroxylase (associated with ambiguous genitalia or primary amenorrhea) or 11β-hydroxylase (associated with virilization).

Once hyperaldosteronism is diagnosed, plasma is assayed for 18-hydroxycorticosterone; a level over 85 µg/dL is seen with adrenal neoplasms, whereas levels under 85 µg/dL are nondiagnostic. Additionally, plasma can be assayed for aldosterone at 8 AM while the patient is supine after overnight recumbency and again after 4 hours upright. Patients with an adrenal adenoma usually have a baseline plasma aldosterone greater than 20 µg/dL which does not rise. Patients with hyperplasia typically have a baseline plasma aldosterone less than 20 µg/dL which rises during upright posture. Exceptions occur.

C. IMAGING

If biochemical testing implicates an adrenal aldosterone-secreting adenoma, a thin-section CT scan of the adrenals is obtained. A discrete adrenal adenoma (> 1 cm in diameter with normal contralateral adrenal) is found is 60–80% of such patients. However, about 20% of such "adenomas" are found to be hyperplasia at surgery. Therefore, it is prudent to supplement CT localization with either adrenal vein catheterization for aldosterone or a dexamethasone-suppressed adrenal scan using ^{131}I-labeled 6β-iodomethyl-19-norcholesterol.

Differential Diagnosis

The differential diagnosis of hyperaldosteronism includes other causes of hypokalemia (see Chapter 21) in patients with essential hypertension. For example, many hypertensive patients taking diuretics develop hypokalemia even while taking potassium-sparing diuretics or potassium supplements. Chronic depletion of intravascular volume stimulates renin secretion and secondary hyperaldosteronism. Thus, it is important to discontinue diuretics and ensure adequate hydration and sodium intake when assessing a patient for primary hyperaldosteronism (see above).

Excessive ingestion of real licorice (black and derived from anise) may produce hypertension and hypokalemia caused by a derivative of its glycyrrhizinic acid inhibiting 11β-hydroxysteroid dehydrogenase, thereby enhancing cortisol's mineralocorticoid effect.

Oral contraceptives may increase aldosterone secretion in some patients. Renal vascular disease can cause severe hypertension with hypokalemia; plasma renin activity is high, distinguishing it from primary hyperaldosteronism.

Excessive adrenal secretion of other corticosteroids (besides aldosterone) may also cause hypertension with hypokalemia. This occurs with certain congenital adrenal enzyme disorders such as P450c11 deficiency (increased deoxycorticosterone with virilization and deficient cortisol) or P450c17 deficiency (increased deoxycorticosterone, corticosterone, and progesterone but deficient estradiol and testosterone). Primary cortisol resistance can cause hypertension and hypokalemia; renin and aldosterone are suppressed, while plasma levels of cortisol, ACTH, and deoxycorticosterone are high. Liddle's syndrome is an autosomal dominant cause of hypertension and hypokalemia resulting from excessive sodium absorption from the renal tubule; renin and aldosterone levels are low. Thyrotoxicosis and familial periodic paralysis may also present with hypokalemia. Hyperaldosteronism may rarely be due to a malignant ovarian tumor.

Treatment

Conn's syndrome (unilateral adrenal adenoma secreting aldosterone) is treated by laparoscopic adrenalectomy, though lifelong spironolactone therapy is an option. Bilateral adrenal hyperplasia is best treated with spironolactone; bilateral adrenalectomy corrects the hypokalemia but not the hypertension and should *not* be performed. Antihypertensive agents may also be necessary. Hyperplasia sometimes responds well to dexamethasone suppression.

Complications

All of the complications of chronic hypertension are encountered in primary hyperaldosteronism. Progressive renal damage is less reversible than hypertension. Following unilateral adrenalectomy for Conn's syndrome, suppression of the contralateral adrenal may result in temporary postoperative hypoaldosteronism, characterized by hyperkalemia and hypotension.

Prognosis

The hypertension is reversible in about two-thirds of cases but persists or returns in spite of surgery in the remainder. The prognosis is much improved by early diagnosis and treatment. Only 2% of aldosterone-secreting adrenal tumors are malignant.

The low renin levels found in this condition (and in about 25% of cases of essential hypertension) also confer a relatively good prognosis.

Brown MJ et al: Calcium-channel blockade can mask the diagnosis of Conn's syndrome. Postgrad Med J 1999;75:235. [PMID: 10715768]

Ganguly A: Primary aldosteronism. N Engl J Med 1998;339: 1828. [PMID: 9854120]

Harper R et al: Accuracy of CT scanning and adrenal vein sampling in the pre-operative localization of aldosterone-secreting adrenal adenomas. QJM 1999;92:643. [PMID: 10542304]

Sawka AM et al: Primary aldosteronism: factors associated with normalization of blood pressure after surgery. Ann Intern Med 2001;135:258. [PMID: 11511140] (A retrospective cohort study of patients who underwent adrenalectomy for primary hyperaldosteronism showed that postoperative resolution of hypertension was associated with a lack of familial hypertension and the use of two or fewer antihypertensive agents.)

Thakkar RB et al: Primary aldosteronism: a practical approach to diagnosis and treatment. J Clin Hypertens (Greenwich) 2001;3:189. [PMID: 11416708]

■ DISEASES OF THE ADRENAL MEDULLA

PHEOCHROMOCYTOMA

ESSENTIALS OF DIAGNOSIS

- *"Attacks" of headache, perspiration, palpitations.*
- *Hypertension, frequently sustained but often paroxysmal, especially during surgery or delivery.*
- *Attacks of nausea, abdominal pain, chest pain, weakness, dyspnea, tremor, visual disturbance.*
- *Anxiety, tremor, weight loss, or heat intolerance.*
- *Elevated urinary catecholamines or their metabolites. Normal serum T_4 and TSH.*

General Considerations

Pheochromocytomas are rare, being found in less than 0.3% of hypertensive individuals. The incidence is higher in patients with moderate to severe hypertension. About two new cases per million population are diagnosed annually. However, in autopsy cases, the incidence of pheochromocytoma is 250–1300 cases per million, indicating that most cases are not detected during life. The hypertension is caused by excessive plasma levels of norepinephrine or neuropeptide Y. Patients have disease characterized by paroxysmal or sustained hypertension due to a tumor located in either or both adrenals or anywhere along the sympathetic nervous chain, and rarely in such aberrant locations as the thorax, bladder, or brain. Primary extra-adrenal pheochromocytomas are known as "paragangliomas." Pheochromocytomas are characterized by a rough "rule of tens": About 10% of cases are not associated with hypertension; 10% are extra-adrenal, and of those about 10% are extra-abdominal (paraganglioma); 10% occur in children; most tumors are sporadic, with only 10–15% familial; in about 10%, the tumor involves both adrenal glands (bilateral adrenal tumors tend to occur more frequently in familial cases); and about 10% have metastatic disease noted around the time of diagnosis. Initially occult metastases are later discovered in another 5%.

Familial pheochromocytomas are usually bilateral (70%) and may be associated with the following: calcitonin-secreting medullary thyroid carcinoma and hyperparathyroidism (multiple endocrine neoplasia type 2); medullary thyroid carcinoma and the syndrome of multiple mucosal neuromas (multiple endocrine neoplasia type 2b); neurofibromatosis (Recklinghausen's disease; and islet cell tumors (rare).

Pheochromocytomas develop in about 20% of patients with von Hippel-Lindau disease (hemangiomas of the retina, cerebellum, brainstem, and spinal cord; pancreatic cysts; renal cysts, adenomas and carcinomas); inheritance is autosomal dominant.

Clinical Findings

A. SYMPTOMS AND SIGNS

Pheochromocytoma typically causes attacks of severe headache (80%), perspiration (70%), and palpitations (60%); other symptoms may include anxiety (50%), a sense of impending doom, or tremor (40%). Vasomotor changes during an attack cause mottled cyanosis and facial pallor; as the attack subsides, facial flushing may occur as a result of reflex vasodilation. Other findings may include tachycardia, precordial or abdominal pain, vomiting, increasing nervousness and irritability, increased appetite, and loss of weight. Anginal attacks may occur. Physical findings usually include hypertension (90%), which may be sustained (20%), sustained with paroxysms (50%), or paroxysmal only (25%). There may be cardiac enlargement; postural tachycardia (change of more than 20 beats/min) and postural hypotension; and mild elevation of basal body temperature. Retinal hemorrhage or cerebrovascular hemorrhage occurs occasionally.

The manifestations of pheochromocytoma are quite varied. Some patients are normotensive and asymptomatic. Besides the above symptoms, some patients can present with psychosis or confusion, seizures, hyperglycemia, bradycardia, hypotension, constipation, paresthesias, or Raynaud's phenomenon. Other patients may have pulmonary edema and heart failure due to cardiomyopathy. Epinephrine secretion may cause episodic tachyarrhythmias, hypotension, or syncope. Other patients may be entirely asymptomatic despite high serum levels of catecholamines. Some patients present with abdominal discomfort due to a pheochromocytoma presenting as a large abdominal mass.

Besides catecholamines and their metabolites, pheochromocytomas secrete a wide range of other peptides that can sometimes cause Cushing's syndrome (ACTH), erythrocytosis (erythropoietin), or hypercalcemia (parathyroid-related peptide; PTHrP). Serum chromogranin A is elevated in 90% and can serve as a tumor marker.

B. LABORATORY FINDINGS

Hypermetabolism is present; thyroid function tests are normal, including serum T_4, free T_4, T_3, and TSH. Hyperglycemia is present in about 35% but is usually mild. Leukocytosis is common. The erythrocyte sedimentation rate is sometimes elevated. Plasma renin activity may be increased by catecholamines.

C. SPECIAL TESTS

1. Assay of urinary catecholamines (total and fractionated), metanephrines, and creatinine detects most pheochromocytomas, especially when samples are obtained during or immediately following an episodic attack. A 24-hour urine specimen is usually obtained, although an overnight or shorter collection may be used: patients with pheochromocytomas generally have more that 2.2 µg of total metanephrine per milligram of creatinine, and more than 135 µg total catecholamines per gram creatinine. Urinary assay for total metanephrines is about 97% sensitive for detecting functioning pheochromocytomas. Urinary assay for vanillylmandelic acid (VMA) is about 89% sensitive and is not usually required.

Testing for catecholamines and metanephrines should be done using high-performance liquid chromatography with electrochemical detection (HPLC-ECD); this minimizes false test results. Nevertheless, some drugs and foods can interfere with certain assays, and stresses can also cause misleading elevations in catecholamine excretion (Table 26–13). About 10% of hypertensive patients have a misleadingly elevated level of one or more tests.

2. Direct assay of epinephrine and norepinephrine in blood and urine during or following an attack is a sensitive test for pheochromocytoma associated with paroxysmal hypertension. High epinephrine levels favor tumor localization within the adrenal gland. Proper, quiet collection of plasma specimens is essential.

3. Imaging should not replace biochemical testing since incidental adrenal adenomas are common (2–4% of scans) and can be misleading. CT scanning of the abdomen is performed using thin sections through the adrenals. Glucagon should not be used during scanning, since it can provoke hypertensive crisis; similarly, intravenous contrast can precipitate hypertensive crisis, particularly in patients whose hypertension is uncontrolled. MRI scanning has the advantage of not requiring intravenous contrast dye; its lack of radiation makes it the imaging of choice during pregnancy. On T2-weighted MRI, adrenal tumors that are hyperintense relative to liver have an in-

Table 26–13. Factors potientially causing misleading catecholamine or metanephrine results: High pressure liquid chromatography with electrochemical detection (HPLC-ECD).

Drugs	Foods	Conditions
Acetaminophen[2]	Bananas[1]	Amyotrophic lateral
Aldomet[2]	Caffeine[1]	sclerosis[1]
Amphetamines[1]	Coffee[2]	Brain lesions[1]
Bronchodilators[1]	Peppers[2]	Carcinoid[1]
Buspirone[2]		Eclampsia[1]
Captopril[2]		Emotion, severe[1]
Cocaine[1]		Exercise, vigorous[1]
Cimetidine[2]		Guillain-Barré
Codeine[2]		syndrome[1]
Decongestants[1]		Hypoglycemia[1]
Ephedrine[1]		Lead poisoning[1]
Fenfluramine[3]		Myocardial infarct,
Isoproterenol[1]		acute[1]
Levodopa[2]		Pain, severe[1]
Labetalol[1,2]		Porphyria, acute[1]
Mandelamine[2]		Psychosis, acute[1]
Metoclopramide[2]		Quadriplegia[1]
Nitroglycerin[1]		Renal failure[3]
Viloxazine[2]		

[1]Increases catecholamine excretion.
[2]May cause confounding peaks on HPLC chromatograms.
[3]Decreases catecholamine excretion.

creased likelihood of being pheochromocytomas. Both CT and MRI scanning have a sensitivity of about 90% for adrenal pheochromocytoma and a sensitivity of 95% for adrenal tumors over 0.5 cm in diameter. However, scanning is less sensitive for detecting recurrent tumors, metastases, and extra-adrenal paragangliomas. If no adrenal tumor is found, the scan is extended to include the entire abdomen, pelvis, and chest. A whole body ^{123}I mIBG scan can localize tumors with a sensitivity of 85% and a specificity of 99%. It is less sensitive for MEN 2a- or MEN 2b-related pheochromocytomas. Somatostatin receptor imaging using ^{111}In-octreotide is quite sensitive for head and neck paragangliomas and metastatic pheochromocytomas; it is less useful (25% sensitivity) for detecting primary pheochromocytomas.

4. Pharmacologic provocative and suppressive tests that evaluate the rise or fall in blood pressure are usually not required or recommended.

5. Patients or relatives suspected of having von Hippel-Lindau disease may have DNA analysis of the *VHL* gene performed (83% sensitivity). Patients or relatives suspected of having MEN 2a or 2b may have genetic testing for mutation of the *RET* proto-oncogene.

Differential Diagnosis

Tachycardia, tremor, palpitation, and hypermetabolism may give rise to confusion with thyrotoxicosis.

Pheochromocytoma may also be misdiagnosed as essential hypertension, myocarditis, glomerulonephritis or other renal lesions, toxemia of pregnancy, eclampsia, and psychoneurosis (anxiety attack). It can sometimes be mistaken for an acute abdomen.

Other conditions that have manifestations similar to those of pheochromocytoma include acute intermittent porphyria, hypogonadal vascular instability (hot flushes), cocaine or amphetamine use, clonidine withdrawal, hypertensive crisis caused by foods containing tyramine (eg, cheeses) in patients taking MAO inhibitor antidepressants, labile hypertension, and unstable angina. Patients with erythromelalgia can have hypertensive crises; their episodic painful flushing and leg swelling is relieved by cold, distinguishing this condition from pheochromocytoma. Pheochromocytomas can cause chest pain and electrocardiographic changes that mimic acute cardiac ischemia. Renal artery stenosis can cause severe hypertension and may coexist with pheochromocytoma.

False-positive testing for catecholamines and metabolites occurs in about 10% of hypertensives, but levels are usually less than 50% above normal and typically normalize with repeat testing.

Complications

All of the complications of severe hypertension may be encountered. Additionally, a catecholamine-induced cardiomyopathy may develop. Sudden death may occur due to cardiac arrhythmia. Hypertensive crises with sudden blindness or cerebrovascular accidents are not uncommon. Paroxysms may be precipitated by sudden movement, by manipulation during or after pregnancy, by emotional stress or trauma, or during surgical removal of the tumor. Decongestant medications, fluoxetine, and other SSRIs may induce hypertensive paroxysms. Cardiomyopathy may develop. Occasionally, the initial manifestation of pheochromocytoma may be hypotension or even shock.

After removal of the tumor, a state of severe hypotension and shock (resistant to epinephrine and norepinephrine) may ensue with precipitation of renal failure or myocardial infarction. Hypotension and shock may occur from spontaneous infarction or hemorrhage of the tumor.

On rare occasions, a patient dies as a result of the complications of diagnostic tests or during surgery.

Treatment

Laparoscopic removal of the tumor or tumors is the treatment of choice. Very large and invasive tumors are treated with open laparotomy. Preoperative administration of α-adrenergic blocking drugs has made pheochromocytoma surgery a great deal safer in recent years. Phenoxybenzamine is given initially in a dosage of 10 mg orally every 12 hours, increasing gradually—

about every 3 days—until hypertension is controlled. The usual maintenance dose is 40–120 mg daily. Optimal alpha blockade is achieved when supine arterial pressure is below 160/90 mm Hg and standing arterial pressure is above 80/45 mm Hg. Calcium channel blockers can also be effective and are better-tolerated than alpha-blockers.

After appropriate antihypertensive therapy, the beta-blocker propranolol (10–40 mg four times daily) can be employed to control tachycardia and other arrhythmias. Maintain blood pressure control for a minimum of 4–7 days or until optimal cardiac status is established. Monitor the ECG until it becomes stable. (It may take a week or even months to correct electrocardiographic changes in patients with catecholamine myocarditis, and it may be prudent to defer surgery until then in such cases.) Patients must be very closely monitored during surgery in order to promptly detect sudden changes in blood pressure or cardiac arrhythmias.

Hypertensive crisis can be managed initially with sublingual administration of nifedipine 10 mg (pierced capsule). Intraoperative severe hypertension is managed with continuous intravenous nicardipine (a short-acting calcium channel blocker), 2–6 μg/kg/ min; or nitroprusside, 0.5–10 μg/kg/min. Prolonged nitroprusside administration can cause cyanide toxicity. Tachyarrhythmia is treated with intravenous atenolol (1 mg boluses), esmolol, or lidocaine.

Autotransfusion of 1–2 units of blood at 12 hours preoperatively plus generous intraoperative volume replacement reduces the risk of postresection hypotension caused by desensitization of the vascular α_1 receptors. Shock may therefore occur following removal of the pheochromocytoma. It is treated with intravenous saline or colloid and high doses of intravenous norepinephrine. Intravenous 5% dextrose is infused postoperatively to prevent hypoglycemia.

Since there may be multiple or metastatic tumors, it is essential to recheck urinary catecholamine levels postoperatively (1–2 weeks after surgery). Thereafter, blood pressure and symptoms must be rechecked regularly; urinary catecholamines and metanephrines are rechecked postoperatively and if hypertension or symptoms recur or if metastases are evident.

For inoperable or metastatic tumors, metyrosine may be added to reduce catecholamine synthesis. Metyrosine is a competitive blocker in the synthesis of catecholamines that is also useful; the initial dosage is 250 mg four times daily, increased daily by increments of 250–500 mg to a maximum of 4 g/d. Metyrosine causes central nervous system side effects and crystalluria; hydration must be ensured. Metastatic pheochromocytomas may be treated with combination chemotherapy (eg, cyclophosphamide, vincristine, and dacarbazine) or with high doses of ^{131}I MIBG.

Prognosis

The prognosis depends upon how early the diagnosis is made. The malignancy of a pheochromocytoma cannot be determined by histologic examination. A tumor is considered malignant if metastases are present; this may take many years to become clinically evident. Therefore, lifetime surveillance is required. If the tumor is successfully removed before irreparable damage to the cardiovascular system has occurred, a complete cure is usually achieved. Complete cure (or improvement) may follow removal of a tumor that has been present for many years. In about 25%, hypertension persists or returns in spite of successful surgery. Although this may be essential hypertension, biochemical reevaluation is then required, looking for a second or metastatic pheochromocytoma.

Before the advent of blocking agents, the surgical mortality rate was as high as 30%, but this has rapidly decreased. A team approach—endocrinologist, anesthesiologist, and surgeon—is critically important. With optimal management, the surgical mortality rate is less than 3%.

Patients with metastatic pheochromocytoma have a 50% 5-year survival rate; however, prolonged survival does occur.

Mukherjee JJ et al: Treatment of metastatic carcinoid tumours, phaeochromocytoma, paraganglioma and medullary carcinoma of the thyroid with ^{131}I-meta-iodobenzylguanidine [^{131}I-mIBG]. Clin Endocrinol (Oxf) 2001;55:47. [PMID: 11453952] (Retrospective analysis of patients with metastatic neuroendocrine tumors treated with ^{131}I-mIBG showed symptomatic and hormonal improvement and moderate tumor stabilization with minimal adverse effects.)

Pacak K et al: Recent advances in genetics, diagnosis, localization, and treatment of pheochromocytoma. Ann Intern Med 2001;134:315. [PMID: 11182843]

Plouin PF et al: Factors associated with perioperative morbidity and mortality in patients with pheochromocytoma: analysis of 165 operations at a single center. J Clin Endocrinol Metab 2001;86:1477. [PMID: 11297571] (Retrospective review of patients undergoing surgery for pheochromocytoma showed a mortality rate of 2.4% and a morbidity rate of 23.6%. Spleen damage occurred with open laparotomy but not with laparoscopic adrenalectomy. Complications were more common in the setting of high preoperative systolic blood pressure, high urinary metanephrine excretion, and repeat operations.)

van der Harst E et al: [123]I metaiodobenzylguanidine and ^{111}In octreotide uptake in benign and malignant pheochromocytomas. J Clin Endocrinol Metab 2001;86:685. [PMID: 11158032]

van der Harst E et al: Proliferative index in phaeochromocytomas: does it predict the occurrence of metastases? J Pathol 2000;191:175. [PMID: 10861578] (Proliferative activity of pheochromocytomas was determined by MIB-1 immunostaining. A proliferative index > 2.5% was present in no benign pheochromocytomas and in 50% of pheochromocytomas with metastases. Other features associated with malignancy include extra-adrenal location, nonfamilial occurrence, and large size.)

Witteles RM et al: Sensitivity of diagnostic and localization tests for pheochromocytoma in clinical practice. Arch Intern Med 2000;160:2521. [PMID: 10979065]

■ PANCREATIC & DUODENAL NEUROENDOCRINE TUMORS*

ISLET CELL TUMORS

ESSENTIALS OF DIAGNOSIS

- Half the tumors are nonsecretory, and patients present with weight loss, abdominal pain, or jaundice.
- Secretory tumors cause a variety of manifestations depending upon the hormones secreted.

General Considerations

The pancreatic islets are composed of several types of cells, each with distinct chemical and microscopic features: the A cells (20%) secrete glucagon, the B cells (70%) secrete insulin, and the D cells (5%) secrete somatostatin or gastrin. F cells secrete "pancreatic polypeptide." Each type of cell may give rise to benign or malignant neoplasms that may be multiple and usually present with a clinical syndrome related to hypersecretion of a native or ectopic hormonal product. The endocrine diagnosis of a particular pancreatic islet neoplasm depends upon first suspecting it from its clinical manifestations. Many tumors secrete two or more different hormones.

Insulinomas are usually (about 82%) benign and secrete excessive amounts of insulin (as well as proinsulin and C-peptide), which causes hypoglycemia. The tumors may be multiple, especially in familial MEN 1—about 12% of cases (see Chapter 27).

Gastrinomas secrete excessive quantities of the hormone gastrin (as well as "big" gastrin), which stimulates the stomach to hypersecrete acid and thereby causing peptic ulceration (Zollinger-Ellison syndrome). Most gastrinomas are benign, but a minority are malignant and metastasize to the liver. Gastrinomas are typically found in the duodenum (49%), pancreas (24%), or lymph nodes (11%). Patients may present with abdominal pain (75%), diarrhea (73%), heartburn (44%), bleeding (25%), or weight loss (17%). Endoscopy usually discovers prominent gastric folds (94%). Sporadic Zollinger-Ellison syndrome is rarely suspected at the onset of symptoms; typically, there is a 5-year delay in diagnosis. About 22% of pa-

tients have multiple endocrine neoplasia type 1 (MEN 1). Patients with MEN 1 usually present at a younger age; hyperparathyroidism may occur from 14 years preceding the Zollinger-Ellison diagnosis to 38 years afterward. (See Multiple Endocrine Neoplasia, below.) Therapy with proton pump inhibitors is usually effective. Surgery is not usually employed because of the low cure rates, particularly in patients with MEN 1. Note that serum gastrin levels tend to be high in any patient who is taking a proton pump inhibitor; hypercalcemia also stimulates gastrin release.

The 5-, 10- and 20-year survival rates with MEN 1 are 94%, 75%, and 58%, respectively, while the survival rates for sporadic Zollinger-Ellison syndrome are 62%, 50%, and 31%, respectively. (See Chapter 14.)

Glucagonomas are usually malignant; weight loss and liver metastases are ordinarily present by the time of diagnosis. They usually secrete other hormones besides glucagon, often gastrin. Other initial symptoms often include diarrhea, nausea, peptic ulcer, or necrolytic migratory erythema. About 35% of patients ultimately develop diabetes. The median survival is 2.8 years after diagnosis.

Somatostatinomas are very rare and are associated with weight loss, diabetes mellitus, malabsorption, and hypochlorhydria.

Other rare tumors secrete excessive amounts of **vasoactive intestinal polypeptide (VIP)**, a substance that causes profuse watery diarrhea (Verner-Morrison syndrome). Treatment with octreotide improves the symptoms but does not halt tumor growth. Symptomatic improvement with calcitonin treatment has also been reported.

Islet cell tumors can secrete ectopic hormones in addition to native hormones, often in combinations producing a variety of clinical syndromes. They may secrete ACTH, producing Cushing's syndrome. Secretion of serotonin can produce an atypical carcinoid syndrome manifested by pain, diarrhea, and weight loss; skin flushing occurs in only 39%. Pancreatic carcinoid tumors grow slowly but usually metastasize to local and distant sites, particularly to other endocrine organs.

Islet cell tumors may be part of the syndrome of multiple endocrine adenomatosis type I (with pituitary and parathyroid adenomas).

Localization of noninsulinoma pancreatic islet cell tumors and their metastases is best done with somatostatin receptor scintigraphy (SRS); SRS detects about 75% of noninsulinomas. CT and MRI are also useful. Insulinomas can usually be located preoperatively by endoscopic ultrasonography. For insulinomas, preoperative localization studies are less successful and have the following sensitivities: ultrasonography 25%, computed tomography 25%, endoscopic ultrasonography 27%, transhepatic portal vein sampling 40%, arteriography 45%, intraoperative palpation 55%, intraoperative pancreatic ultrasound 75%. Nearly all insulinomas can be successfully located at surgery by intraoperative palpation and ultrasound. An abdomi-

*Diabetes mellitus and hyperglycemia are discussed in Chapter 27.

nal CT scan is usually obtained, but extensive preoperative localization procedures, especially with invasive methods, are not required. Tumors may be located in the pancreatic head or neck (57%), body (15%), or tail (19%) or in the duodenum (9%).

Direct resection of the tumor (or tumors), which often spreads locally, is the primary form of therapy for all types of islet cell neoplasm except Zollinger-Ellison syndrome, where use of a proton pump inhibitor, eg, omeprazole or lansoprazole, is the therapy of choice. Insulinomas are resected. However, in MEN 1, insulinomas are rarely cured, so surgery is reserved for dominant masses in such cases. Palliation of functioning malignant disease often requires both antihormonal and anticancer chemotherapy. The use of streptozocin, doxorubicin, and asparaginase, especially for malignant insulinoma, has produced some encouraging results, though these drugs are quite toxic. The hypoglycemia of insulinoma may be counteracted by verapamil or diazoxide. Octreotide, a somatostatin analog, is now used in the therapy of noninsulinoma islet cell tumor.

The prognosis in these neoplasms is variable. The surgical complication rate is about 40%, with patients commonly developing fistulas and infections. Extensive pancreatic resection may cause diabetes mellitus. The overall 5-year survival is higher with functional tumors (77%) than with nonfunctional ones (55%) and higher with benign tumors (91%) than with malignant ones (55%).

Arnold R et al: Treatment of neuroendocrine GEP tumours with somatostatin analogues: a review. Digestion 2000;62:84. [PMID: 10940693] (Current somatostatin analogs are not indicated for gastrinomas, since Zollinger-Ellison syndrome is best treated by proton pump inhibitors. They are ineffective for insulinomas. They cause limited stabilization of tumor growth in 50% of other pancreatic neuroendocrine tumors.)

Berger AC et al: Prognostic value of initial fasting serum gastrin levels in patients with Zollinger-Ellison syndrome. J Clin Oncol 2001;19:3051. [PMID: 11408501] (In patients with sporadic Zollinger-Ellison syndrome, higher initial fasting serum gastrin levels were associated with larger primary tumor size, greater likelihood of lymph node and liver metastases, and consequent reduced survival. Patients with Zollinger-Ellison syndrome due to MEN 1 have a better prognosis than do patients with sporadic Zollinger-Ellison syndrome. Higher serum gastrin levels are not associated with reduced survival in patients having gastrinomas due to MEN 1.)

Boukhman MP et al: Localization of insulinomas. Arch Surg 1999;134:818. [PMID: 10443803]

Chun J et al: Pancreatic endocrine tumors. Curr Opin Oncol 2001;13:52. [PMID: 11148686]

Norton JA et al: Surgery to cure the Zollinger-Ellison syndrome. N Engl J Med 1999; 341:635. [PMID: 10460814] (The surgical findings are presented for 151 patients with Zollinger-Ellison syndrome who underwent laparotomy. The 10-year recurrence rate was 34% for patients with sporadic gastrinoma and 100% for those with MEN 1. The overall 10-year survival was 94%.)

■ DISEASES OF THE TESTES

MALE HYPOGONADISM

ESSENTIALS OF DIAGNOSIS

- Diminished libido and erections.
- Decreased growth of body hair.
- Testes may be small or normal in size. Serum testosterone is usually decreased.
- Serum gonadotropins (LH and FSH) are decreased in hypogonadotropic hypogonadism; they are increased in testicular failure (hypergonadotropic hypogonadism).

General Considerations

Male hypogonadism is caused by deficient testosterone secretion by the testes. It may be classified according to whether it is due to (1) insufficient gonadotropin secretion by the pituitary (hypogonadotropic) or (2) pathology in the testes themselves (hypergonadotropic) (see Table 26–14). The evaluation for hypogonadism begins with a serum testosterone or free testosterone measurement. A low serum testosterone is evaluated with serum LH and FSH levels. Patients with low gonadotropins are further evaluated for other pituitary abnormalities, including hyperprolactinemia.

Etiology

A. HYPOGONADOTROPIC HYPOGONADISM

A deficiency in FSH and LH may be isolated or associated with other pituitary hormonal abnormalities. (See Hypopituitarism.) Patients must be evaluated for signs of Cushing's syndrome or adrenal insufficiency, growth hormone excess or deficiency, and thyroid hormone excess or deficiency.

Acquired hypogonadotropic hypogonadism may be due to pituitary or hypothalamic factors but may be idiopathic. Hyperprolactinemia (Table 26–4) may also induce hypogonadism.

Men receiving GnRH agonist therapy for prostate cancer develop hypogonadotropic hypogonadism that can persist following cessation of therapy.

B. HYPERGONADOTROPIC HYPOGONADISM

A failure in testicular secretion of testosterone causes a rise in LH. If testicular Sertoli cell function is deficient, FSH will be elevated. Conditions that can cause

Table 26–14. Causes of male hypogonadism.

Hypogonadotropic (Low or Normal LH)	Hypergonadotropic (High LH)
Alcohol	Antitumor chemotherapy
Chronic illness	Bilateral anorchia
Congenital syndromes	Idiopathic
Constitutional delay	Klinefelter's syndrome
Cushing's syndrome	Leprosy
Drugs	Lymphoma
Estrogen-secreting tumors (testicular, adrenal)	Male climacteric
	Mumps
GnRH agonist (leuprolide)	Myotonic dystrophy
Hemochromatosis	Noonan's syndrome
Hypopituitarism	Orchitis
Hypothyroidism	Radiation therapy
Idiopathic	Sertoli cell-only syndrome
Kallmann's syndrome	Testicular trauma
Ketoconazole	Tuberculosis
17-Ketosteroid reductase deficiency	Uremia
Malnourishment	
Marijuana	
Obesity (BMI > 40)	
Prader-Willi syndrome	
Prior androgens	
Spironolactone	

testicular failure include viral infection (eg, mumps), irradiation, cancer chemotherapy, autoimmunity, myotonic dystrophy, uremia, XY gonadal dysgenesis, partial 17-ketosteroid reductase deficiency, Klinefelter's syndrome, and male climacteric.

Klinefelter's syndrome (seminiferous tubule dysgenesis) is a common cause of male hypogonadism that is due to the expression of an abnormal karyotype, classically 47,XXY. Other forms are common, eg, 46,XY/47,XXY mosaicism, 48,XXYY, 48,XXXY, or 46,XX males.

The manifestations of Klinefelter's syndrome are variable. Testes feel normal during childhood, but during adolescence they usually become firm, fibrotic, small, and nontender to palpation. Although puberty occurs at the normal time, the degree of virilization is variable. About 85% have some gynecomastia at puberty.

Other common findings include tall stature and abnormal body proportions that are unusual for hypogonadal men (height greater than arm span; crownpubis length greater than pubis-floor). Patients with multiple X or Y chromosomes are more apt to have mental deficiency and other abnormalities such as clinodactyly or synostosis. They may also exhibit problems with coordination and social skills. Other problems include a higher incidence of breast cancer, chronic pulmonary disease, varicosities of the legs, and

diabetes mellitus (8%); impaired glucose tolerance occurs in an additional 19%.

Most men (about 95%) have azoospermia, but men with 46,XY/47,XXY mosaicism may be fertile. The diagnosis is confirmed by karyotyping or by determining the presence of RNA for X-inactive-specific transcriptase (XIST) in peripheral blood leukocytes by PCR.

The serum testosterone is low, and FSH and LH are elevated. Sometimes the serum testosterone is normal, but serum free testosterone is usually low.

All causes of gynecomastia (Table 26–1) must be differentiated from Klinefelter's syndrome.

C. Androgen Insensitivity

Partial resistance to testosterone is a rare condition in which phenotypic males have variable degrees of apparent hypogonadism, gynecomastia, hypospadias, cryptorchism, and gynecomastia. Serum testosterone levels are normal.

Clinical Findings

A. Symptoms and Signs

Hypogonadism that is congenital or acquired during childhood presents as delayed puberty. Men with acquired hypogonadism have variable manifestations. Most men experience decreased libido. Others complain of erectile dysfunction, hot sweats, fatigue, or depression. Their presenting complaint may also be infertility, gynecomastia, headache, fracture, or other symptoms related to the cause or result of the hypogonadism. The patient's history often gives a clue to the cause (Table 26–14).

Physical signs associated with hypogonadism may include decreased body, axillary, beard, or pubic hair; such diminished sexual hair growth is not reliably present except after years of severe hypogonadism. Men who develop hypogonadism tend to lose muscle mass and gain weight due to an increase in subcutaneous fat. Examination should include measurements of arm span and height. Testicular size should be assessed with an orchidometer (normal volume is about 10–25 mL; normal length is usually over 6 cm). Testicular size may decrease but usually remains within the normal range in men with postpubertal hypogonadotropic hypogonadism, but it may be diminished with testicular injury or Klinefelter's syndrome. The testes must also be carefully palpated for masses, since Leydig cell tumors may secrete estrogen and present with hypogonadism. The testicles must be carefully examined for evidence of trauma, infiltrative lesions (eg, lymphoma), or ongoing infection (eg, leprosy, tuberculosis).

B. Laboratory Findings

The hemoglobin and hematocrit may be slightly below the male range due to hypogonadism.

To evaluate a man for hypogonadism, the morning serum total testosterone concentration is determined.

Normal ranges for serum testosterone have been derived from nonfasting morning blood specimens, which tend to be the highest of the day. Later in the day, serum testosterone levels can be 25–50% lower. Therefore, a serum testosterone drawn fasting or late in the day may be misleadingly below the "normal range." Serum testosterone levels in men are highest at age 20–30 years and slightly lower at age 30–40 years; testosterone falls gradually but progressively after age 40 years. Elderly men have higher levels of SHBG, with consequently lower levels of free testosterone. The electrochemical luminescence assay for measuring serum total testosterone suffers interference in hyperlipidemic patients.

Serum free testosterone levels are low in hypogonadism. Different assay methodologies for free testosterone are in use. Assays employing equilibrium dialysis, calculated free testosterone, and non SHBG-bound testosterone are reasonably accurate. However, the free androgen index, direct radioimmunoassay, and analog free testosterone assays are inaccurate.

In patients with low or borderline-low serum testosterone levels, serum LH and FSH should be measured. LH and FSH tend to be high in patients with hypergonadotropic hypogonadism but low or inappropriately normal in men with hypogonadotropic hypogonadism. Bone densitometry may be reduced in long-standing male hypogonadism.

1. Hypogonadotropic hypogonadism—Men with hypogonadotropic hypogonadism have low serum testosterone levels without a compensatory increase in gonadotropins. A serum prolactin determination is obtained but may be elevated for many reasons (Table 26–4). Men with gynecomastia may be screened for partial 17-ketosteroid reductase deficiency with serum determinations for androstenedione and estrone, which are elevated in this condition. X-linked congenital adrenal hypoplasia is a rare condition in which a *DAX-1* gene mutation causes hypogonadotropic hypogonadism and azoospermia, which usually present in adolescence; the associated primary adrenal insufficiency usually presents in childhood, but it may remain undiagnosed into adulthood. The serum estradiol level may be elevated in patients with cirrhosis and in rare cases of estrogen-secreting tumors (testicular Leydig cell tumor or adrenal carcinoma). Men with no discernible definite cause for hypogonadotropic hypogonadism should be screened for hemochromatosis and have an MRI of the pituitary and hypothalamic region to look for a tumor or other lesion. (See Hypopituitarism.)

2. Hypergonadotropic hypogonadism—Men with hypergonadotropic hypogonadism have low serum testosterone levels with a compensatory increase in gonadotropins. Klinefelter's syndrome can be confirmed by karyotyping or by measurement of leukocyte X-inactive-specific transcriptase (XIST). Testicular biopsy is usually reserved for younger patients in whom the reason for primary hypogonadism is unclear.

Treatment

Testosterone replacement is ordinarily commenced once the diagnosis of hypogonadism is confirmed and the cause determined. It is prudent to screen older men for prostate cancer before testosterone therapy is begun. Testosterone helps reverse sexual dysfunction and muscle atrophy. Men with Klinefelter's syndrome have a reduced risk of developing verbal fluency problems if testosterone therapy is begun at the time of normal puberty. Hypogonadism is usually treated with parenteral testosterone (enanthate or cypionate). The usual dose is about 300 mg intramuscularly every 3 weeks or 200 mg every 2 weeks. The preparation is oil-based and is usually given in the gluteal area. The dose is adjusted according to the patient's response. Oral androgen preparations include methyltestosterone and fluoxymesterone. These oral preparations have rarely caused liver tumors or peliosis hepatis with long-term use. Cholestatic jaundice occurs in 1–2% but usually remits after the medication is discontinued. The oral androgens are not as effective as parenteral testosterone.

Testosterone transdermal systems (skin patches) are available in two formulations for application to nongenital skin. The testosterone may be mixed with the adhesive (eg, Testoderm II, 5 mg/d) with a new patch applied daily to a different site; this system leaves a sticky residue but causes little skin irritation. A different patch uses testosterone in a reservoir system applied to skin (eg, Androderm); this system adheres more tightly to the skin but may cause more skin irritation. Both produce reliable serum levels of testosterone which are somewhat lower that those achieved with injections. The patch systems also suffer from being rather inconvenient and expensive.

Topical 1% testosterone gel is commercially available as Androgel (2.5 g and 5 g packets). The starting dose is 5 g (50 mg testosterone) applied once daily to clean, dry skin of the shoulders, upper arms, or abdomen. The skin serves as a reservoir that slowly releases about 10% of the testosterone into the blood; serum testosterone levels reach a steady state in 1–3 days. The gel should not be applied to the genitals. The entire contents of a packet are squeezed onto the palm and then immediately applied. The hands should be washed and the application site allowed to dry for 3–5 minutes before dressing. A shirt must be worn during contact with women or children to prevent transfer of testosterone to them. The serum testosterone level should be determined about 14 days after starting therapy; if the level remains below normal or the clinical response is inadequate, the dose may be increased to 7.5 g or 10 g.

Side effects of any testosterone therapy may include acne, gynecomastia, aggravation of sleep apnea, and reduced HDL levels.

Men with hypogonadism due to endocrine therapy for prostate cancer usually develop severe hot flushes. Symptomatic relief can be obtained with the progestational agent megestrol acetate, 20 mg orally twice daily; the dose can be progressively reduced in some men. Megestrol has some glucocorticoid-like activity and tends to increase appetite and cause weight gain. Hyperglycemia and hypertriglyceridemia may occur, so the dosage should be kept minimal.

Men with mosaic Klinefelter's syndrome (eg, 46XY/47XXY) may be fertile. However men with nonmosaic Klinefelter's syndrome (eg, 47XXY) are usually azoospermic; fertility may be achieved by testicular sperm retrieval and in vitro intracytoplasmic sperm injection (ICSI) into an ovum.

Men with hypogonadotropic hypogonadism must receive further evaluation and specific treatment (see Hypopituitarism).

Prognosis of Hypogonadism

If hypogonadism is due to a pituitary lesion, the prognosis is that of the primary disease (eg, tumor, necrosis). The prognosis for restoration of virility is good if testosterone is given.

Basaria S et al: Hypogonadism and androgen replacement therapy in elderly men. Am J Med 2001;110:563. [PMID: 11343670]

Daniell HW et al: Hypogonadism following prostate-bed radiation therapy for prostate carcinoma. Cancer 2001;91:1889. [PMID: 11346871] (To investigate the possibility of testicular damage from radiation therapy, men with prostate carcinoma treated with external beam radiation therapy to the prostate bed were compared with men treated by radical prostatectomy. Hypogonadism was significantly more common among men treated with external beam radiation than radical prostatectomy.)

Howell SJ et al: Randomized placebo-controlled trial of testosterone replacement in men with mild Leydig cell insufficiency following cytotoxic chemotherapy. Clin Endocrinol (Oxf) 2001;55:315. [PMID: 11589674] (Treatment of young men with mild testosterone deficiency has not been well studied. This trial randomized 35 young men with mild hypogonadism secondary to cytotoxic chemotherapy to 12 months of transdermal testosterone or placebo. No significant changes were noted in bone mineral density, body composition, blood lipids, or quality of life.)

Mantovani G et al: Hypogonadotropic hypogonadism as a presenting feature of late-onset X-linked adrenal hypoplasia congenita. J Clin Endocrinol Metab 2002;87:44. [PMID: 11788621]

Seidman SN et al: Testosterone replacement therapy for hypogonadal men with major depressive disorder: a randomized, placebo-controlled clinical trial. J Clin Psychiatry 2001;62: 406. [PMID: 11465516]. (Men with hypogonadism and major depressive disorder did not show improvement in measures of depression with transdermal testosterone therapy. A small improvement was noted in sexual function.)

TESTICULAR TUMORS IN ADULTS
(See also Chapter 23.)

About 95% of testicular tumors are germ cell tumors (seminomas or nonseminomas). They may produce (as serum markers) hCG and alpha-fetoprotein. Seminomas do not produce alpha-fetoprotein, but about 5–10% produce some hCG; nonseminomas, on the other hand, produce increased serum levels of one or both of these markers in about 90% of cases. Men with liver disease may have misleadingly high levels of alpha-fetoprotein. Most germ cell tumors are sensitive to cisplatin-based chemotherapy. Sperm banking is advised.

About 5% of testicular tumors are Leydig or Sertoli cell tumors. Leydig cell tumors tend to produce estrogen (75%) and cause gynecomastia and impotence on that basis; they may sometimes produce androgens that can cause pseudoprecocious puberty in boys. Sertoli cell tumors may also produce estrogen (30%) with feminization; gynecomastia may be due to hCG secretion (25%).

Some testicular tumors may be small and nonpalpable yet may secrete sufficient amounts of hCG or estrogen to cause gynecomastia or impotence. Testicular ultrasound may help reveal small tumors.

After unilateral orchiectomy for testicular cancer, an elevated FSH level prior to further treatment indicates a patient at higher risk for cancer in the remaining testis.

Chaganti RS et al: Genetics and biology of adult human male germ cell tumors. Cancer Res 2000;60:1475. [PMID: 10749107] (Most testicular germ cell tumors are very sensitive to cisplatin-based chemotherapy.)

Dearnaley D et al: Regular review: Managing testicular cancer. BMJ 2001;322:1583. [PMID: 11431302]

Nichols CR: Testicular cancer. Curr Probl Cancer 1998;22:187. [PMID: 9743088] (A comprehensive review.)

■ AMENORRHEA & MENOPAUSE (See also Chapter 17.)

PRIMARY AMENORRHEA

Menarche ordinarily occurs between ages 11 and 15 years (average in USA: 12.7 years). The failure of any menses to appear is termed primary amenorrhea, and evaluation is commenced (1) at age 14 if neither menarche nor breast development has occurred or if height is in the lowest 3%, or (2) at age 16 if menarche has not occurred.

Etiology

The causes of primary amenorrhea include the following:

A. HYPOTHALAMIC-PITUITARY CAUSES (WITH LOW-NORMAL FSH)

A genetic deficiency of GnRH and gonadotropins may be isolated or associated with other pituitary deficiencies or diminished olfaction (Kallmann's syndrome). Hypothalamic lesions, particularly craniopharyngioma, may be present. Pituitary tumors may be nonsecreting or may secrete prolactin or growth hormone. Cushing's syndrome may be caused by glucocorticoid treatment, a cortisol-secreting adrenal tumor, or an ACTH secreting pituitary tumor. Hypothyroidism can delay adolescence. Head trauma or encephalitis can cause gonadotropin deficiency. Primary amenorrhea may also be caused by constitutional delay of adolescence, organic illness, vigorous exercise (eg, ballet dancing, running), stressful life events, dieting, or anorexia nervosa; however, these conditions should not be assumed to account for amenorrhea without a full physical and endocrinologic evaluation. (See section on hypopituitarism.)

B. HYPERANDROGENISM (WITH LOW-NORMAL FSH)

Excess testosterone may be secreted by adrenal tumors or by adrenal hyperplasia caused by steroidogenic enzyme defects such as P450c21 deficiency (salt-wasting) or P450c11 deficiency (hypertension). Ovarian tumors or polycystic ovaries may also secrete excess testosterone. Androgenic steroids may also cause this syndrome.

C. OVARIAN CAUSES (WITH HIGH FSH)

Gonadal dysgenesis (Turner's syndrome and variants; see below) is a frequent cause of primary amenorrhea. Ovarian failure due to autoimmunity is a common cause. Rare deficiencies in certain ovarian steroidogenic enzymes are causes of primary hypogonadism without virilization: 3β-hydroxysteroid dehydrogenase deficiency (adrenal insufficiency with low serum 17-hydroxyprogesterone) and P450c17 deficiency (hypertension and hypokalemia with high serum 17-hydroxyprogesterone). A whole-body deficiency in P450arom activity produces female hypogonadism associated with polycystic ovaries, tall stature, osteoporosis, and virilization.

D. PSEUDOHERMAPHRODITISM (WITH HIGH LH)

An enzymatic defect in testosterone synthesis may present as a sexually immature phenotypic girl with primary amenorrhea. Complete androgen resistance (testicular feminization) presents as a phenotypic young woman without sexual hair but with normal breast development and primary amenorrhea. In both cases, the uterus is absent and testes are intra-abdominal or cryptorchid. Intra-abdominal testes are surgically resected. Such patients are treated as normal but infertile, hypogonadal women.

E. UTERINE CAUSES (WITH NORMAL FSH)

Congenital absence or malformation of the uterus may be responsible for primary amenorrhea, as may an unresponsive or atrophic endometrium. An imperforate hymen is occasionally the reason for the absence of visible menses.

F. PREGNANCY (WITH HIGH hCG)

Pregnancy may be the cause of primary amenorrhea even when the patient denies ever having had sexual intercourse.

Clinical Findings

A. SYMPTOMS AND SIGNS

Patients with primary amenorrhea require a thorough history and physical examination to look for signs of the conditions noted above. Headaches or visual field abnormalities implicate a hypothalamic or pituitary tumor. Signs of pregnancy may be present. Blood pressure abnormalities, acne, and hirsutism should be noted. Short stature may be seen with an associated growth hormone or thyroid hormone deficiency. Short stature with manifestations of gonadal dysgenesis indicates Turner's syndrome (see below). Olfaction testing screens for Kallmann's syndrome. Obesity and short stature may be signs of Cushing's syndrome. Tall stature may be due to eunuchoidism or gigantism. Hirsutism or virilization suggests excessive testosterone.

An external pelvic examination plus a rectal examination should be performed to assess hymenal patency and the presence of a uterus.

B. LABORATORY FINDINGS

The initial endocrine evaluation should include serum determinations of FSH, LH, PRL, testosterone, TSH, free T_4, and hCG (pregnancy test). Patients who are virilized or hypertensive require serum electrolyte determinations and further hormonal evaluation. Girls with low-normal FSH and LH—especially those with high PRL levels—are evaluated by MRI of the hypothalamus and pituitary. Girls who have a normal uterus and high FSH without the classic features of Turner's syndrome may require a karyotype to diagnose X chromosome mosaicism.

Treatment

Treatment of primary amenorrhea is directed at the underlying cause. Girls with permanent hypogonadism are treated with estrogen replacement therapy (see below).

SECONDARY AMENORRHEA & MENOPAUSE

Secondary amenorrhea is defined as absence of menses for 3 consecutive months in women who have passed menarche. Menopause is defined as the terminal episode of naturally occurring menses; it is a retrospective diagnosis, usually made after 6 months of amenorrhea.

Etiology

The causes of secondary amenorrhea include the following:

A. PREGNANCY (HIGH hCG)

Pregnancy is the most common cause for secondary amenorrhea in women of childbearing age. The differential diagnosis includes rare ectopic secretion of hCG by a choriocarcinoma or bronchogenic carcinoma.

B. HYPOTHALAMIC-PITUITARY CAUSES (WITH LOW-NORMAL FSH)

The hypothalamus must release gonadotropin-releasing hormone (GnRH) in a pulsatile manner in order for the pituitary to secrete gonadotropins. GnRH pulses occurring more than once per hour favor LH secretion, while less frequent pulses favor FSH secretion. In normal ovulatory cycles, GnRH pulses in the follicular phase are rapid and favor LH synthesis and ovulation; ovarian luteal progesterone is then secreted that slows GnRH pulses, causing FSH secretion during the luteal phase. Most women with hypothalamic amenorrhea have a persistently low frequency of GnRH pulses.

Secondary "hypothalamic" amenorrhea may be caused by stressful life events such as school examinations or leaving home. Such women usually have a history of normal sexual development and irregular menses since menarche. Amenorrhea may also be the result of strict dieting, vigorous exercise, organic illness, or anorexia nervosa. Intrathecal infusion of opioids causes amenorrhea in most women. These conditions should not be assumed to account for amenorrhea without a full physical and endocrinologic evaluation. Young women in whom the results of evaluation and progestin withdrawal test are normal have noncyclic secretion of gonadotropins resulting in anovulation. Such women typically recover spontaneously but should have regular evaluations and a progestin withdrawal test about every 3 months to detect loss of estrogen effect.

Prolactin elevation due to any cause (see section on hyperprolactinemia) may cause amenorrhea. Pituitary tumors or other lesions may cause hypopituitarism. Glucocorticoid excess of any cause suppresses gonadotropins.

C. HYPERANDROGENISM (WITH LOW-NORMAL FSH)

Elevated serum levels of testosterone can cause hirsutism, virilization, and amenorrhea. In polycystic ovarian syndrome, GnRH pulses are persistently rapid, favoring LH synthesis with excessive androgen secretion; reduced FSH secretion impairs follicular maturation. Progesterone administration can slow the GnRH pulses, thus favoring FSH secretion that induces follicular maturation. Rare causes include adrenal P450c21 deficiency, ovarian or adrenal malignancies, ectopic ACTH secretion by a malignancy, and Cushing's disease. Anabolic steroids also cause amenorrhea.

D. UTERINE CAUSES (WITH NORMAL FSH)

Infection of the uterus commonly occurs following delivery or D&C but may occur spontaneously. Endometritis due to tuberculosis or schistosomiasis should be suspected in endemic areas. Endometrial scarring may result, causing amenorrhea (Asherman's syndrome). Such women typically continue to have monthly premenstrual symptoms. The vaginal estrogen effect is normal. Diagnosis and treatment is best done by direct hysteroscopic inspection of the endometrium and lysis of adhesions. A small Foley catheter is left in the uterus for 1 week while antibiotics are given. The catheter is then replaced by an IUD for about 2 months. Cyclic estrogen and progestin is given to build up the endometrial lining. After such treatment, menses usually resume and fertility is possible, but spontaneous abortions and other pregnancy complications occur commonly.

E. PREMATURE OVARIAN FAILURE (HIGH FSH)

This refers to primary hypogonadism that occurs before age 40. This affects about 1% of women. About 30% of such cases are due to autoimmunity against the ovary. About 8% of cases are due to X chromosome mosaicism. Other causes include surgical bilateral oophorectomy, radiation therapy for pelvic malignancy, and chemotherapy. Women who have undergone hysterectomy are prone to premature ovarian failure even though the ovaries were left intact. Myotonic dystrophy, galactosemia, and mumps oophoritis are additional causes. Other cases may be familial or idiopathic. Ovarian failure is usually irreversible. Treatment consists of estrogen replacement therapy plus a progestin if the uterus is present.

F. MENOPAUSE (HIGH FSH)

"Climacteric" is defined as the period of natural physiologic decline in ovarian function, generally occurring over about 10 years. By about age 40, the remaining ovarian follicles are those that are the least sensitive to gonadotropins. Increasing titers of FSH are required to stimulate estradiol secretion. Estradiol levels may actually rise during early climacteric. Frequent anovulation tends to cause menometrorrhagia (dysfunctional uterine bleeding). Fertility declines progressively. Psychologic symptoms may include depression and irritability. Women may experience fatigue, insomnia, headache, diminished libido, or rheumatologic symptoms. Vasomotor instability (hot flushes) are experienced by 80% of women, lasting seconds to many minutes. Hot flushes may be most severe at night or may be triggered by emotional stress; they must be distinguished from panic attacks. Some women continue to menstruate for many months despite symptoms of estrogen deficiency. Estrogen supplementation provides symptomatic relief.

The normal age for menopause in the USA ranges between 48 and 55 years, with an average of about 51.5 years. Serum estradiol levels fall and the remaining estrogen after menopause is estrone, derived mainly from peripheral aromatization of adrenal androstenedione. Such peripheral production of estrone is enhanced by obesity and liver disease. Individual differences in estrone levels partly explain why the symptoms noted above may be minimal in some women but severe in others. The acute symptoms of estrogen deficiency noted above tend to decline in severity within several years after menopause. However, about 35% of women have symptoms for more than 5 years. The late manifestations of estrogen deficiency include urogenital atrophy with vaginal dryness and dyspareunia; dysuria, frequency, and incontinence may occur. Increased bone osteoclastic activity increases the risk for osteoporosis and fractures. The skin becomes more wrinkled. Increases in the LDL:HDL cholesterol ratio cause an increased risk for arteriosclerosis.

Clinical Findings

A. SYMPTOMS AND SIGNS

All women with amenorrhea require a complete history and physical examination. Nausea and breast engorgement are typical signs of early pregnancy. Hot flushes are common in ovarian failure. Headache or visual field abnormalities are seen with pituitary or hypothalamic tumors. Complaints of thirst and polyuria require evaluation; diabetes insipidus implicates a hypothalamic lesion. Goiter may be due to hyperthyroidism. Weight loss, diarrhea, or skin darkening may indicate adrenal insufficiency. Weight loss with a distorted body image implicates anorexia nervosa. The breasts are examined carefully for galactorrhea, a common sign of hyperprolactinemia. Hirsutism or virilization may be a sign of hyperandrogenism. Manifestations of hypercortisolism (eg, weakness, psychiatric changes, hypertension, central obesity, hirsutism, thin skin, ecchymoses) may indicate alcoholism or Cushing's syndrome. Signs of acromegaly or gigantism may also indicate a pituitary tumor. Signs of systemic illness (eg, cirrhosis, renal failure) should be appreciated. Various drugs may elevate prolactin and cause amenorrhea (see section on hyperprolactinemia). Needle tracks may indicate heroin or amphetamine abuse.

A careful pelvic examination is always required to check for uterine or adnexal enlargement and to obtain a Papanicolaou smear and a vaginal smear for assessment of estrogen effect. Various life stresses, vigorous exercise, and "crash" dieting all predispose to amenorrhea; however, such factors should not be assumed to account for amenorrhea without a complete workup to screen for other causes.

B. LABORATORY FINDINGS

Since pregnancy is the most common cause of amenorrhea, women of childbearing age are immediately screened with a serum or urine hCG (pregnancy test). An elevated hCG overwhelmingly indicates pregnancy; false-positive testing may occur very rarely with ectopic hCG secretion (eg, choriocarcinoma or bronchogenic carcinoma). Women without an elevated hCG receive further laboratory evaluation including serum PRL, FSH, LH, TSH, and plasma potassium. Hyperprolactinemia or hypopituitarism (without obvious cause; see section on hypopituitarism) should prompt an MRI study of the pituitary region. Routine testing for renal and hepatic function (eg, BUN, serum creatinine, bilirubin, alkaline phosphatase, and ALT) is also performed. A serum testosterone level is obtained in hirsute or virilized women. Patients with manifestations of hypercortisolism receive a 1 mg overnight dexamethasone suppression test for initial screening (see section on Cushing's syndrome). Nonpregnant women without any laboratory abnormality may receive a 10-day course of a progestin (eg, medroxyprogesterone acetate, 10 mg/d); absence of withdrawal menses typically indicates a lack of estrogen or a uterine abnormality.

Treatment

Treatment of secondary amenorrhea is directed at the cause. Therapy of hypogonadism generally consists of hormone replacement therapy (see below). The doses of estrogen required for symptomatic relief from vasomotor symptoms are sometimes higher than typical physiologic replacement doses. If estrogen replacement therapy is declined or contraindicated, partial symptomatic relief from hot flushes may sometimes be afforded by progestins or phytoestrogens. Slow, deep breathing can also ameliorate hot flushes. Tamoxifen and raloxifene offer bone protection but aggravate hot flushes. Treatment or prevention of postmenopausal osteoporosis with bisphosphonates such as alendronate (see section on osteoporosis) is another therapeutic option.

Estrogen Replacement Therapy

The goals of estrogen replacement therapy are several: (1) to replace adequate estrogen to prevent osteoporosis; (2) to restore menses when the patient wants this for psychologic reasons; (3) to reduce manifestations of estrogen deficiency such as hot flushes, mood changes, vaginal dryness, urinary incontinence, and skin wrinkling; and (4) to improve the serum lipid profile, reducing the risk of cardiovascular disease.

Estrogen replacement therapy should begin with the onset of hypogonadism. However, it is not necessary to treat all cases, especially temporary amenorrhea or irregular menses. Patients who have normal menses after a short course of medroxyprogesterone acetate (see above) may have menses induced every 1–3 months in this manner.

Oral estrogen preparations include conjugated equine estrogens (0.3, 0.625, 0.9, 1.25, and 2.5 mg), ethinyl estradiol (20 and 50 μg), estradiol (0.5, 1, and 2 mg), estropipate (0.625, 1.25, and 2.5 mg), an plant-derived estrogen (eg, Estratab, 0.3, 0.625, and 2.5 mg); and synthetic estrogens (eg, Cenestin 0.625 mg and 0.9 mg).

Oral estrogen plus progestin preparations: Conjugated estrogens with medroxyprogesterone acetate (Prempro 0.625/2.5 or 0.625/5); estradiol with norgestimate (Ortho-Prefest, sequences of 1 mg estradiol daily for 3 days followed by a single tablet containing 1 mg estradiol combined with 0.09 mg norgestimate daily for 3 days. The 3-day sequences are repeated continuously during treatment.)

Estradiol transdermal systems (skin patches): Estradiol can be delivered systemically with different transdermal systems:

(1) Transdermal systems with estradiol mixed with adhesive: These systems tend to cause minimal skin irritation. Available preparations include the following: Climara (0.05 mg/d or 0.1 mg/d), replaced weekly; Fempatch (0.025 mg/d), replaced weekly; Alora (0.05 mg/d, 0.075 mg/d, or 0.1 mg/d), replaced twice weekly; Vivelle (0.0375 mg/d, 0.05 mg/d, 0.075 mg/d, or 0.1 mg/d), replaced twice weekly.

(2) Transdermal systems with estradiol in a drug reservoir: These systems cause significant skin irritation in some women. Available preparations include Estraderm (0.05 mg/d, or 0.1 mg/d), replaced twice weekly.

(3) Transdermal systems with estradiol (E) and norethindrone acetate (NA) mixed with adhesive: Available preparations include Combipatch (0.05 mg/d E & 0.14 mg/d NA, or 0.05 mg/d E & 0.25 mg/d NA), replaced twice weekly.

Intramuscular estrogen preparations include estradiol cypionate in oil (5 mg/mL; 1–5 mL every 3–4 weeks) and estradiol valerate (10, 20, and 40 mg/mL; 10–20 mg every 3–4 weeks). These preparations are rarely required.

Progestins: For a woman with an intact uterus, a progestin may be added to estrogen replacement in order to transform proliferative into secretory endometrium and to reduce the risk of endometrial carcinoma, which is otherwise increased by prolonged exposure to unopposed estrogen. Progestins also counter the increased risk of ovarian cancer caused by unopposed estrogen replacement. Progestins given on a daily or monthly cycled regimen appear to increase the risk of breast cancer more than estrogens alone. Progestins commonly increase the density of breast tissue, reducing the sensitivity of screening mammograms. Theoretically, less frequent administration of progestins (eg, for 10–14 days every 3–4 months) should reduce the adverse effects while causing the endometrium to slough any cells that might be undergoing early malignant transformation. Progestins may cause moodiness, particularly in women with a history of premenstrual dysphoric disorder. Cycled progestins may trigger migraines in certain women. Many other adverse reactions have been reported, including breast tenderness, alopecia, and fluid retention. Contraindications to the use of progestins include thromboembolic disorders, liver disease, breast cancer, and pregnancy. The type of progestin preparation, its dosage, and the timing of administration may be tailored to the given situation.

Micronized progesterone (Prometrium, 100 mg capsules) is an oral formulation of natural progesterone. Preliminary studies indicate that it may be associated with fewer adverse effects on quality of life than other progestins. It also appears to have a less deleterious effect on plasma lipids than other progestins. Micronized progesterone 100 mg/d may be administered with estrogen. Alternatively, estrogen may be given daily, with micronized progesterone (100–200 mg) added for 10–12 days of the month. If the estrogen is being cycled, micronized progesterone 200 mg/d may be given for the last 10 days of the estrogen cycle. It may cause drowsiness, in which case it is taken in the evening.

Medroxyprogesterone acetate (Provera, Cycrin, 2.5, 5, and 10 mg scored tabs) is the progestin that is in widest use. A dosage of 2.5–5 mg/d may be administered along with estrogen. If the estrogen is being cycled, medroxyprogesterone acetate 5 mg/d is given for the last 10 days of the estrogen cycle. Alternatively, estrogen may be given daily, with medroxyprogesterone acetate 5 mg/d added for 10–12 days of the month.

Topical progesterone (20–50 mg/d) may reduce hot flushes in women who are intolerant to oral hormone replacement therapy. It may be applied to the upper arms, thighs, or inner wrists daily. It may be compounded as micronized progesterone 250 mg/mL in a transdermal gel. Its effects upon the breast and endometrium are unknown.

Potential benefits of hormone replacement therapy: Women receiving long-term estrogen replacement therapy experience a significant reduction in overall mortality, mainly due to fewer cardiovascular deaths. A "healthy user" effect accounts for much of this observation. However, estrogen replacement does improve lipoprotein parameters in most women. Serum levels of atherogenic lipoprotein(a) are reduced by estrogen replacement with or without daily or cycled progestins. Improvement in serum HDL cholesterol is greatest with unopposed estrogen but is also seen with the addition of a progestin. However, in the HERS study, women with established coronary disease who received conjugated estrogens plus progestin were not protected from further coronary events. Similarly, women with cerebrovascular events were not protected from stroke by estrogen replacement.

Estrogen replacement improves or eliminates postmenopausal hot flushes and diaphoretic episodes. Vaginal moisture is improved. Libido is enhanced in some women. Perimenopause-related depression is improved by unopposed estrogen replacement; the addition of a progestin may negate this effect. Estrogen therapy may enhance verbal memory but does not protect against Alzheimer's disease. Estrogen replacement reduces bone loss and the risk of osteoporotic fractures. Women receiving estrogen replacement therapy experience a lower mortality rate from lung and colon cancers. In women with type 2 diabetes, unopposed estrogen replacement improves glycemic control. Estrogen replacement does not prevent facial skin wrinkling; however, it may improve facial skin moisture and thickness, reducing seborrhea and atrophy.

Potential risks of hormone replacement therapy: Women with an intact uterus who receive unopposed estrogens have a high risk of experiencing dysfunctional uterine bleeding. Continued abnormal bleeding necessitates a pelvic examination; endometrial biopsy may be required. Women receiving unopposed estrogen (conjugated estrogens, 0.625 mg/d or more) have a risk of endometrial carcinoma that is ten times greater than the risk in untreated patients. However, unopposed estrogen replacement at lower doses (eg, conjugated estrogens, 0.3 mg/d) does not appear to cause such an increased risk. Progestins, when added to estrogen replacement in either a continuous or cycled mode, greatly reduce the risk of endometrial cancer—but may have their own adverse effects (see below).

Long-term estrogen replacement therapy appears to increase the risk of breast cancer. The relative risk of breast cancer for women taking estrogen is 1.2, and the relative risk for women taking estrogen-progestin is 1.4. This increased risk for breast cancer appears to be confined to relatively thin women with a BMI < 24.4. Ironically, women receiving estrogen replacement experience a reduced mortality from breast cancer, possibly due to earlier detection. The Iowa Women's Health Study reported an increase in breast cancer with estrogen replacement only in women consuming more than 1 oz of alcohol weekly. No accelerated risk of breast cancer has been seen in users of estrogen replacement therapy who have benign breast disease or a family history of breast cancer.

Women receiving long-term unopposed estrogen appear to experience an increase in mortality from ovarian cancer. The annual age-adjusted ovarian cancer death rates for women who had taken estrogen replacement for ≥ 10 years were: 64:100,000 for baseline users, 38:100,000 for former users, and 26:100,000 for women who had never taken estrogen. Women taking combined estrogen-progestin replacement do not experience this risk of ovarian cancer.

Women receiving combined estrogen-progestin replacement experience an increased risk of developing asthma. Elderly women experience an increased risk of urinary incontinence. Some women complain of estrogen-induced edema or mastalgia. Estrogen replacement has been reported to lower the seizure threshold in some women with epilepsy. Untreated large pituitary prolactinomas may enlarge if exposed to estrogen.

There is an increased risk of venous thrombosis with oral estrogens. Oral estrogen therapy may cause hypertriglyceridemia, particularly in women with preexistent hyperlipidemia, which may rarely result in pancreatitis. Oral estrogens also reduce the effectiveness of growth hormone replacement. Using transdermal estrogen rather than oral estrogen replacement may avert the latter problems.

Androgen replacement: Women who have undergone a bilateral oophorectomy almost invariably have low serum androgens. Women with panhypopituitarism tend to have particularly low androgen levels. However, after natural menopause, the ovaries and adrenals continue to secrete testosterone, such that postmenopausal women are not always androgen-deficient. Androgen deficiency contributes to hot flushes, loss of libido and sexual hair, muscle atrophy, and osteoporosis. Selected women may be treated with low dose methyltestosterone, which is available in combination with conjugated estrogens (eg, Estratest). Tablets contain either 1.25 mg conjugated estrogens with 2.5 mg methyltestosterone or 0.625 mg conjugated estrogens with 1.25 mg methyltestosterone. Estratest is usually started at the lowest strength every 2 days, alternating days with standard estrogen replacement (see above). It should be given cyclically at the lowest dose that controls symptoms. At small doses, side effects of androgens are usually minimal but may include nausea, polycythemia, emotional changes, paresthesias, electrolyte disturbances, and potentiation of anticoagulant therapy. Reduction in HDL cholesterol may negate the beneficial effect on cardiovascular mortality conferred by estrogen replacement therapy. Cholestatic jaundice and elevation of liver enzymes occur rarely. Hepatocellular neoplasms and peliosis hepatis, rare complications of oral androgens at higher doses, have not been reported with lower doses. Side effects of excess androgen treatment include hirsutism and virilization. Androgens should not be given to women with liver disease or during pregnancy or breast feeding.

Selective estrogen receptor modulators (SERMs) (eg, raloxifene; Evista) are an alternative to estrogen replacement for hypogonadal women at risk for osteoporosis who prefer not to take estrogens because of their contraindications (eg, breast or uterine cancer) or side effects. Raloxifene does not reduce hot flushes, vaginal dryness, skin wrinkling, or breast atrophy; it does not improve cognition. However, in doses of 60 mg/d orally, it inhibits bone loss without stimulating effects upon the breasts or endometrium. Since raloxifene may slightly increase the risk of venous thromboembolism, it should not be used by women at prolonged bed rest or by those prone to thrombosis. In contrast with the use of estrogen replacement therapy, concomitant progesterone therapy is not needed, and raloxifene does not increase the risk of development of breast cancer. Tibolone (Livial) is a SERM whose metabolites have mixed estrogenic, progestogenic, and weak androgenic activity. It is comparable to hormone replacement therapy for the treatment of climacteric-related complaints. It does not appear to significantly stimulate proliferation of breast or endometrial tissue. It depresses both serum triglycerides and HDL cholesterol. Long-term studies are lacking. It is not available in the USA.

Phytoestrogens are substances found in plants (legumes) which bind to estrogen receptors. Isoflavones are phytoestrogens which bind weakly to estrogen receptor α but have over 80% of estrogen's affinity for estrogen receptor β. Soy and red clover isoflavones are selective estrogen receptor modulators, which act as estrogen on bone, brain, and vasculature but have no stimulatory effects upon the uterus or breast. Daily intake of 60 g of isolated soy protein reduces hot flushing by about 45% within 12 weeks. Isoflavones also improve the plasma lipid profile and inhibit the development of coronary atherosclerosis in male monkeys. In a study of female oophorectomized monkeys, soy phytoestrogens significantly inhibited carotid atherosclerosis, but the effect on coronary atherosclerosis was not statistically significant. In climacteric premenopausal women, soy supplementation does not appear to affect the menstrual cycle. Genistein, a flavone found in soy, has been proposed to account for the low incidence of breast cancer in Asian women. Genistein has a pronounced antiproliferative effect upon breast cancer cells in nude mice.

Binder EF et al: Effects of hormone replacement therapy on serum lipids in elderly women. A randomized, placebo-controlled trial. Ann Intern Med 2001;134:754. [PMID: 11329233] (In women aged 75 years or older, hormone replacement therapy improved lipoprotein profiles.)

Clemons M et al: Estrogen and the risk of breast cancer. N Engl J Med 2001;344:276. [PMID: 11172156] (In postmenopausal women, the relative risk [RR] of breast cancer among those receiving estrogen alone is 1.2, while those receiving combined estrogen-progestin replacement have a RR of 1.4. However, overall mortality is reduced among women receiving such hormone replacement therapy. Breast cancer risk is highest among postmenopausal women with mammographic breast density in the highest quartile [RR = 6], bone density in the highest quartile [RR = 3.1], or a family history of breast cancer [RR = 2.6]. Caution must be used when prescribing estrogen to this group of women.)

Gajdos C et al: Breast cancer diagnosed during hormone replacement therapy. Obstet Gynecol 2000;95:513. [PMID: 10725482] (Women taking hormone replacement therapy have an increased incidence of breast cancer but ironically have decreased breast cancer mortality. Their more favorable breast cancer survival may be due to earlier detection.)

Grady D et al: Postmenopausal hormones and incontinence: the Heart and Estrogen/Progestin Replacement Study. The HERS Research Group. Obstet Gynecol 2001;97:116. [PMID: 11152919] (Estrogen replacement aggravates incontinence in elderly women.)

Grodstein F et al: Postmenopausal hormone use and risk for colorectal cancer and adenoma. Ann Intern Med 1998;128:705. [PMID: 9556463] (A Nurses' Health Study with 59,002 participants determined that women currently receiving estrogen replacement have a reduced risk of colorectal cancer; relative risk = 0.65.)

Hulley S et al: Randomized trial of estrogen plus progestin for secondary prevention of coronary heart disease in postmenopausal women. Heart and Estrogen/Progestin Replacement Study (HERS) Research Group. JAMA 1998;280:605. [PMID: 9718051] (In postmenopausal women with established coronary disease, hormone replacement therapy with estrogen plus progestin did not alter the expected incidence of coronary events over 5 years.)

Lando JF et al: Hormone replacement therapy and breast cancer risk in a nationally representative cohort. Am J Prev Med 1999;17:176. [PMID: 10987632] (An analysis of data from the NHANES I Epidemiologic Follow-up Study. Subjects were interviewed repeatedly over 22 years for a total of 73,253 person-years of follow-up. There was no significant association between hormone replacement therapy and breast cancer in this study; relative risk = 0.8.)

LeBlanc ES et al: Hormone replacement therapy and cognition: systematic review and meta-analysis. JAMA 2001;285:1489. [PMID: 11255426] (Meta-analysis of trials examining the effect of hormone replacement on cognition showed a decreased risk of dementia in patients receiving hormone replacement; most trials had important methodologic limitations.)

Leonetti HB et al: Transdermal progesterone cream for vasomotor symptoms and postmenopausal bone loss. Obstet Gynecol 1999;94:225. [PMID: 10432132] (In a prospective, double-blinded, placebo-controlled study of 102 postmenopausal women, treatment with topical progesterone cream [20 mg/d] improved vasomotor symptoms in 83% while only 19% of the placebo-treated group noted such an improvement. Topical progesterone afforded no protective effect on bone density.)

Manson JE et al: Clinical practice. Postmenopausal hormone-replacement therapy. N Engl J Med 2001;345:34. [PMID: 11439947] (Review of the issues surrounding postmenopausal hormone-replacement therapy.)

Marshall JC et al: Hypothalamic dysfunction. Mol Cell Endocrinol 2001;183:29. [PMID: 11604221] (A review of the pathophysiology of hypothalamic amenorrhea.)

Rodriguez C et al: Estrogen replacement therapy and ovarian cancer mortality in a large prospective study of US women. JAMA 2001;285:1460. [PMID: 11255422] (The American Cancer Society's Cancer Prevention Study II, a prospective study of 211,581 postmenopausal women with mortality follow-up from 1982 to 1996. Annual age-adjusted ovarian cancer death rates for women who had taken estrogen replacement for ≥ 10 years were: 64:100,000 for baseline users, 38:100,000 for former users, and 26:100,000 for women who had never taken estrogen. Some increased risk persisted for up to 29 years after cessation of use.)

Ross RK et al: Effect of hormone replacement therapy on breast cancer risk: estrogen versus estrogen plus progestin. J Natl Cancer Inst 2000;94:328. [PMID: 10675382] (Postmenopausal women may receive unopposed estrogen replacement therapy [ERT]; progesterone may be added to estrogen as continuous combined replacement therapy [CCRT] or as sequential estrogen plus progestin therapy [SEPRT]. A case-control study of Los Angeles women reports relative risks [RR] for developing breast cancer: ERT = 1.06; CCRT = 1.24; SEPRT = 1.38. In hormone replacement therapy, the addition of a progestin appears to increase the risk of breast cancer. The difference between CCRT and SEPRT was not statistically significant.)

Schairer C et al: Menopausal estrogen and estrogen-progestin replacement therapy and breast cancer risk. JAMA 2000;283:485. [PMID: 10659874] (The National Cancer Institute reviewed the incidence of breast cancer among 46,355 postmenopausal women. Among women with a BMI ≤ 24.4, the relative risks of breast cancer for women taking hormone replacement with estrogen-only or estrogen-progestin were 1.2 and 1.4, respectively. The risk of breast cancer was not increased among heavier women on either replacement regimen.)

Seshadri S et al: Postmenopausal estrogen replacement therapy and the risk of Alzheimer disease. Arch Neurol 2001;58:435. [PMID: 11255447] (A large population-based nested case-control study involving more than 100,000 patients showed no decreased risk of Alzheimer's disease among women taking estrogen replacement therapy.)

Viscoli CM et al: A clinical trial of estrogen-replacement therapy after ischemic stroke. N Engl J Med 2001;345:1243.

[PMID: 11680444] (A randomized, double-blind, placebo controlled trial of estrogen therapy for women who recently suffered ischemic stroke or transient ischemic attack. Estradiol failed to reduce mortality or recurrence of stroke.)

TURNER'S SYNDROME
(Gonadal Dysgenesis)

Turner's syndrome is a chromosomal disorder associated with primary hypogonadism, short stature, and other phenotypic anomalies. It is a common cause of primary amenorrhea and early ovarian failure. Patients with the classic syndrome lack one of the two X chromosomes and have a 45,XO karyotype.

Typical Turner's Syndrome
(45,XO Gonadal Dysgenesis)

Features of Turner's syndrome (Table 26–15) are variable and may be subtle in girls with mosaicism. Typical manifestations in adulthood include short stature, hypogonadism, webbed neck, high-arched palate, wide-spaced nipples, hypertension, and renal abnormalities. 45,XO is the most common major chromosomal abnormality in humans. Less than 3% of these zygotes survive to term, with the incidence of Turner's syndrome being about 1:10,000 female newborns.

Girls with Turner's syndrome may be diagnosed at birth, since they tend to be small and may exhibit severe lymphedema. Evaluation for childhood short stature often leads to the diagnosis. Growth hormone and somatomedin levels are normal. Hypogonadism presents as "delayed adolescence" (80%) or early ovarian failure (20%); FSH and LH are high, making a diagnosis of primary hypogonadism. A blood karyotype showing 45,XO (or X chromosome abnormalities or mosaicism) establishes the diagnosis.

Treatment of short stature with daily injections of growth hormone (0.1 unit/kg/d) plus an androgen (eg, oxandrolone) for at least 4 years before epiphysial fusion increases final height by a mean of about 10.3 cm over the mean predicted height of 144.2 cm. Such growth hormone treatment rarely causes pseudotumor cerebri. After age 12, estrogen therapy is begun with low doses of conjugated estrogens (0.3 mg) or ethinyl estradiol (5 μg) given on days 1–21 per month. When growth stops, hormone replacement therapy is begun with estrogen and progestin (see below).

Women with Turner's syndrome have a reduced life expectancy due in part to their increased risk for diabetes mellitus (types 1 and 2), hypertension, dyslipidemia, and osteoporosis. Diagnostic vigilance and aggressive treatment of these conditions reduces the risk of ischemic heart disease, stroke, and fracture. Patients are prone to keloid formation after surgery or ear piercing. Yearly ocular examinations and periodic thyroid evaluations are recommended. It is advisable to evaluate patients for cardiac, aortic, and renal abnormalities.

Table 26–15. Manifestations of Turner's syndrome.

Short stature
Distinctive facial features
  Ptosis
  Micrognathia
  Low-set ears
  Epicanthal folds
Sexual infantilism due to gonadal dysgenesis with primary
  amenorrhea (80%)
Early ovarian failure with secondary amenorrhea (20%)
Webbed neck (40%)
Low hairline
High-arched palate
Cubitus valgus
Short fourth metacarpals (50%)
Lymphedema of hands and feet (30%)
Hypoplastic widely spaced nipples
Hyperconvex nails
Pigmented nevi
Keloid formation (eg, surgical scars or after ear piercing)
Recurrent otitis media
Renal abnormalities (60%)
  Horseshoe kidney
  Hydronephrosis
Hypertension (idiopathic or due to coarctation or renal
  disease)
Gastrointestinal bleeding from intestinal telangiectases
  (rare)
Impaired space-form recognition, direction sense, and
  mathematical reasoning
Cardiovasular anomalies
  Coarctation of the aorta (10–20%)
  Aortic stenosis
  Bicuspid aortic valve
  Aortic dissection due to coarctation and cystic medial
    necrosis of aorta
Associated conditions
  Obesity
  Diabetes mellitus (types 1 and 2)
  Dyslipidemia
  Hyperuricemia
  Hashimoto's thyroiditis
  Achlorhydria
  Cataracts, corneal opacities
  Neuroblastoma (1%)
  Rheumatoid arthritis
  Inflammatory bowel disease

Turner's Syndrome Variants

A. 46,X (ABNORMAL X) KARYOTYPE

An abnormality or deletion of certain genes on the short arm of the X chromosome causes short stature and other signs of Turner's syndrome; some gonadal function and even fertility is possible. Transmission of Turner's syndrome from mother to daughter can occur. There may be an increased risk of trisomy 21 in the conceptuses of women with Turner's syndrome.

Abnormalities or deletions of other genes located on both the long and short arms of the X chromosome can produce gonadal dysgenesis with few other somatic features.

B. 45,XO/46,XX MOSAICISM

This karyotype results in a modified form of Turner's syndrome. Such girls tend to be taller and may have more gonadal function and fewer other manifestations of Turner's syndrome.

C. OTHER VARIANTS

45,XO/46,XY mosaicism can produce some manifestations of Turner's syndrome. Patients may have ambiguous genitalia or male infertility with an otherwise normal phenotype.

Gravholt C et al: Morbidity in Turner's syndrome. J Clin Epidemiol 1998;51:147. [PM ID: 9474075]

Landin-Wilhelmsen K et al: Cardiac malformations and hypertension, but not metabolic risk factors, are common in Turner syndrome. J Clin Endocrinol Metab 2001;86:4166. [PMID: 11549644] (Cardiac malformations were found in 17% of patients with Turner's syndrome. Systolic hypertension, obesity, and inactivity were more common among these patients than in age-matched controls.)

Saenger P et al: Recommendations for the diagnosis and management of Turner syndrome. J Clin Endocrinol Metab 2001;86:3061. [PMID: 11443168] (Overview.)

■ MULTIPLE ENDOCRINE NEOPLASIA

Several syndromes with multiple gland involvement have been described (Table 26–16).

MEN 1
(Wermer's Syndrome)

The most common multiglandular syndrome is multiple endocrine neoplasia type 1 (MEN 1). Biochemical testing identifies affected individuals by age 14–18 years, but the syndrome usually becomes clinically manifest in the fourth decade. **Hyperparathyroidism** occurs in over 80% of patients; it presents with hypercalcemia and usually involves hyperplasia or adenomas of several parathyroid glands. **Pancreatic islet cell tumors** occur in about 75% of patients; gastrinomas are the most common tumor and can result in gastric hyperacidity (Zollinger-Ellison syndrome) with peptic ulcer disease or diarrhea. Islet cell tumors may also secrete insulin, somatostatin, or glucagon. **Pituitary adenomas** occur in about 60% and may secrete prolactin, growth hormone, or ACTH but are usually nonfunctional; such tumors may produce local pressure effects and hypopituitarism. About 37% of these patients have adrenal cortical adenomas or hyperplasia—bilateral in about half. They are generally benign and nonfunctional. In one series, one out of 12 such patients developed a feminizing adrenal carcinoma. These adrenal lesions are pituitary-independent.

Tumors of the pituitary gland, the parathyroid gland, and the pancreatic islets may occur in the same patient, though not necessarily at the same time. Some individuals in the same family express the abnormality as children, whereas in others the clinical manifestations may not appear until late in adult life. The clinical manifestations of MEN 1 are extremely variable, since the glandular tumors may secrete a variety of different hormones.

The kindreds expressing MEN 1 have been shown to harbor a gene mutation on the long arm of chromosome 11 (11q13), which causes phenotypic expres-

Table 26–16. Multiple endocrine neoplasia (MEN) syndromes: Incidence of tumor types.[1]

Tumor Type	MEN 1 (Wermer's Syndrome)	MEN 2a (Sipple's Syndrome)	MEN 2b
Parathyroid	>80%	50%	Rare
Pancreatic	75%		
Pituitary	60%		
Medullary thyroid carcinoma		>50%	80%
Pheochromocytoma		20%	60%
Mucosal and gastrointestinal ganglioneuromas		Rare	>90%
Lipoma	Occasional		
Adrenocortical adenoma	Occasional		
Carcinoid	Occasional		
Thyroid adenoma	Occasional		

[1]Modified from Fitzgerald PA (editor): *Handbook of Clinical Endocrinology,* 2nd ed. McGraw-Hill 1992.

sion as a dominant trait. Genetic linkage analysis can be used to determine which other family members will express this syndrome, permitting informed genetic counseling and avoiding unnecessary testing for unaffected individuals.

The differential diagnosis of MEN 1 includes sporadic or familial tumors of the pituitary, parathyroids, or pancreatic islets. Hypercalcemia (from any cause) may cause gastrointestinal symptoms and increased gastrin levels, simulating a gastrinoma. Treatment of gastrointestinal symptoms with H_2 blockers or metoclopramide causes hyperprolactinemia, simulating a pituitary prolactinoma.

Surgical treatment of hyperparathyroidism in MEN 1 can induce prolonged remissions, but relapse is typical. Aggressive parathyroid resection can cause permanent hypoparathyroidism. Medical treatment of hyperparathyroidism with bisphosphonates (eg, alendronate) is thus an important option.

MEN 2a
(Sipple's Syndrome)

A separate disorder of multiglandular hypersecretion of hormones is multiple endocrine neoplasia type 2a. It too is inherited as an autosomal dominant trait. In MEN 2a, patients may have **medullary thyroid carcinoma** (> 90%); hyperparathyroidism (20–50%), due to hyperplasia or multiple adenomas in over 70% of cases; **pheochromocytomas** (20–35%), which are often bilateral; or **Hirschsprung's disease.** The medullary thyroid carcinoma is of mild to moderate aggressiveness and generally occurs in the third or fourth decade in the familial syndrome and in the sixth decade in sporadic cases.

Siblings or children of patients with MEN 2a should have genetic testing to determine if they have a mutation of the *RET* proto-oncogene on chromosome 10q11-2; this identifies about 95% of affected individuals. Each kindred has a certain *RET* codon mutation that correlates with the particular variation in the MEN 2 syndrome, such as the age of onset and aggressiveness of medullary thyroid cancer. The specific mutation as well as case histories of family members should guide the timing for prophylactic thyroidectomy. Before any surgical procedure, MEN 2 carriers should be screened for pheochromocytoma. There is incomplete penetrance, and about 30% of those with such mutations never manifest endocrine tumors.

Patients may be screened with a serum calcitonin drawn after 3 days of omeprazole, 20 mg orally twice daily; calcitonin levels rise in the presence of medullary thyroid carcinoma to levels above 80 pg/mL in women or above 190 pg/mL in men.

MEN 2b

Patients with MEN 2b have a syndrome characterized by mucosal neuromas (> 90% with bumpy lips, enlarged tongue, Marfan-like habitus), pheochromocy-

tomas (60%), and medullary thyroid carcinoma (80%), which can be quite aggressive. Patients also have intestinal abnormalities (75%), skeletal abnormalities (87%), and delayed puberty (43%). The medullary thyroid carcinoma is aggressive and tends to present in the third to fourth decades. Prophylactic thyroidectomy is advisable for patients with mucosal neuromas and family members with the syndrome or *RET* proto-oncogene mutations after screening for pheochromocytoma.

Brandi ML et al: Guidelines for diagnosis and therapy of MEN type 1 and type 2. J Clin Endocrinol Metab 2001;86:5658. [PMID: 11739416] (A review and international consensus statement.)

Erdoğgan MF et al: Omeprazole:calcitonin stimulation test for the diagnosis, follow-up, and family screening in medullary thyroid carcinoma. J Clin Endocrinol Metab 1997;82:897. [PMID: 9062503]

■ CLINICAL USE OF GLUCOCORTICOIDS

Mechanisms of Action

Cortisol is a steroid hormone that is normally secreted by the adrenal cortex in response to ACTH. It exerts its action by binding to nuclear receptors which then act upon chromatin to regulate gene expression, producing effects throughout the body.

Table 26–17. Systemic versus topical activity of corticosteroids.
(Hydrocortisone = 1 in potency.)

	Systemic Activity	Topical Activity
Prednisone	4–5	1–2
Fluprednisolone	8–10	10
Triamcinolone	5	1
Triamcinolone acetonide	5	40
Dexamethasone	30–120	10
Betamethasone	30	5–10
Betamethasone valerate	...	50–150
Methylprednisolone	5	5
Fluocinolone acetonide	...	40–100
Flurandrenolone acetonide	...	20–50
Fluorometholone	1–2	40
Deflazocort	3–4	...

Relative Potencies

Hydrocortisone and cortisone acetate, like cortisol, have mineralocorticoid effects that become excessive at higher doses. Other synthetic glucocorticoids such as prednisone, dexamethasone, and deflazacort (an oxazoline derivative of prednisolone) have minimal mineralocorticoid activity. The relative potencies relative to hydrocortisone are listed in Table 26–17. Anticonvulsant drugs (eg, phenytoin, carbamazepine, phenobarbital) accelerate the metabolism of glucocorticoids other than hydrocortisone, making them significantly less potent. Megestrol, a synthetic progestin, has slight glucocorticoid activity that becomes significant when administered in high doses for appetite stimulation.

Adverse Effects

Prolonged treatment with systemic glucocorticoids causes a variety of adverse effects that can be life-threatening. Patients should be thoroughly informed of the major possible side effects of treatment such as insomnia, personality change, weight gain, muscle weakness, polyuria, kidney stones, diabetes mellitus, sex hormone suppression, occasional amenorrhea in women, candidiasis and opportunistic infections, osteoporosis with fractures, or aseptic necrosis of bones, particularly of the hips, which may become manifest many months after even brief treatment (see section on Cushing's syndrome). Alendronate, 5–10 mg orally daily, prevents the development of osteoporosis among patients receiving prolonged courses of glucocorticoids. For convenience, alendronate 70 mg orally may be taken once weekly. For patients who are unable to tolerate oral bisphosphonates (due to esophagitis, hiatal hernia, or gastritis), periodic intravenous infusions of pamidronate 60–90 mg or zoledronate 2–4 mg should also be effective. It is wise to follow an organized treatment plan such as the one outlined in Table 26–18.

Adachi JD et al: Two-year effects of alendronate on bone mineral density and vertebral fracture in patients receiving glucocorticoids: a randomized, double-blind, placebo-controlled ex-

---

Table 26–18. Management of patients receiving systemic glucocorticoids.[1]

- Do not administer glucocorticoids unless absolutely indicated or more conservative measures have failed.
- Keep dosage and duration of administration to the minimum required for adequate treatment.
- Screen for tuberculosis before treatment with a PPD test or chest x-ray.
- Screen for diabetes mellitus before treatment and at each physician visit. Train the patient to test urine weekly for glucose.
- Screen for hypertension before treatment and at each physician visit.
- Screen for glaucoma and cataracts before treatment, 3 months into treatment, and then at least yearly.
- Prepare the patient and family for possible adverse effects on mood, memory, and cognitive function. Inform them about other possible side effects, particularly weight gain, osteoporosis, and aseptic necrosis of bone.
- Institute a vigorous physical exercise and isometric regimen tailored to each patient's disabilities.
- Administer calcium (1 g elemental calcium) and vitamin D₃, 400–800 IU orally daily. Check spot morning urines, and alter dosage to keep urine calcium concentration below 30 mg/dL. If the patient is receiving thiazide diuretics, check for hypercalcemia, and administer only 500 mg elemental calcium daily. Consider a bisphosphonate such as alendronate (5–10 mg orally daily or 70 mg orally weekly) or periodic intravenous infusions of pamidronate or zoledronate.
- Avoid prolonged bed rest that will accelerate muscle weakness and bone mineral loss. Ambulate early after fractures.
- Treat hypogonadism in women or men.
- Avoid elective surgery, if possible. Vitamin A in a daily dose of 20,000 units orally for 1 week may improve wound healing, but it is not prescribed in pregnancy.
- Avoid activities that could cause falls or other trauma.
- Watch for fungal or yeast infections of skin, nails, mouth, vagina, and rectum, and treat appropriately.
- Ulcer prophylaxis: Administer oral glucocorticoids with meals. If administered with nonsteroidals, consider prophylaxis with omeprazole, 20–40 mg/d. Glucocorticoids alone do not need prophylaxis with H₂ blockers or omeprazole. Avoid large doses of antacids containing aluminum hydroxide (many popular brands); aluminum hydroxide binds phosphate and may cause a hypophosphatemic osteomalacia that can compound glucocorticoid osteoporosis.
- Treat infections aggressively. Consider unusual pathogens.
- Weigh daily. Use dietary measures to avoid obesity and optimize nutrition.
- Measure height frequently. This serves to document the degree of axial spine demineralization and compression.
- Treat edema as indicated.
- Monitor plasma potassium for hypokalemia. Treat as indicated.
- Obtain bone densitometry before treatment and then periodically. Treat osteoporosis.
- Council to avoid smoking and excessive ethanol consumption.
- With dosage reduction, watch for signs of adrenal insufficiency or glucocorticoid withdrawal syndrome.

[1]Modified and reproduced, with permission, from Fitzgerald PA: *Handbook of Clinical Endocrinology,* 2nd ed. McGraw-Hill, 1992.

tension trial. Arthritis Rheum 2001;44:202. [PMID: 11212161] (Glucocorticoid-induced osteoporosis can be prevented and treated with alendronate, a bisphosphonate. New vertebral fractures developed in 0.7% of patients treated with alendronate compared with 6.8% of patients taking placebo.)

Gonnelli S et al: Prevention of corticosteroid-induced osteoporosis with alendronate in sarcoid patients. Calcif Tissue Int 1997;61:382. [PMID: 9351879] (Alendronate, 5 mg/d orally, prevented bone loss in patients receiving prednisone over 12 months.)

Nasser SM et al: Lesson of the week: Depot corticosteroid treatment for hay fever causing avascular necrosis of both hips. BMJ 2001;322:1589. [PMID: 11431303]

Recommendations for the prevention and treatment of glucocorticoid-induced osteoporosis: 2001 update. American College of Rheumatology Ad Hoc Committee on Glucocorticoid-Induced Osteoporosis. Arthritis Rheum 2001;44:1496 [PMID: 11465699]

Diabetes Mellitus & Hypoglycemia 27

Umesh Masharani, MB, BS; MRCP(UK), & John H. Karam, MD
See www.current-med.com/ch27.html

■ DIABETES MELLITUS

ESSENTIALS OF DIAGNOSIS

Type 1 diabetes:

- *Polyuria, polydipsia, and weight loss associated with random plasma glucose ≥ 200 mg/dL.*
- *Plasma glucose of 126 mg/dL or higher after an overnight fast, documented on more than one occasion.*
- *Ketonemia, ketonuria, or both.*

Type 2 diabetes:

- *Most patients are over 40 years of age and obese.*
- *Polyuria and polydipsia. Ketonuria and weight loss generally are uncommon at time of diagnosis. Candidal vaginitis in women may be an initial manifestation. Many patients have few or no symptoms.*
- *Plasma glucose of 126 mg/dL or higher after an overnight fast on more than one occasion. After 75 g oral glucose, diagnostic values are 200 mg/dL or more 2 hours after the oral glucose.*
- *Hypertension, dyslipidemia, and atherosclerosis are often associated.*

Classification & Pathogenesis
(Table 27–1)

Diabetes mellitus is a syndrome with disordered metabolism and inappropriate hyperglycemia due to either a deficiency of insulin secretion or to a combination of insulin resistance and inadequate insulin secretion to compensate. An international committee

of experts in the field has recommended use of the terms "type 1 and type 2 diabetes," with arabic numerals being used rather than roman numerals, since the numeral II can be confused with the number 11. Type 1 diabetes is due to pancreatic islet B cell destruction predominantly by an autoimmune process, and these patients are prone to ketoacidosis. Type 2 diabetes is the more prevalent form and results from insulin resistance with a defect in compensatory insulin secretion.

A. TYPE 1 DIABETES MELLITUS

This form of diabetes is immune-mediated in over 90% of cases and idiopathic in less than 10%. The rate of pancreatic B cell destruction is quite variable, being rapid in some individuals and slow in others. Type 1 diabetes is usually associated with ketosis in its untreated state. It occurs most commonly in juveniles, with the highest incidence worldwide among the 10- to 14-year-old group, but occasionally occurs in adults, especially the nonobese and those who are elderly when hyperglycemia first appears. It is a catabolic disorder in which circulating insulin is virtually absent, plasma glucagon is elevated, and the pancreatic B cells fail to respond to all insulinogenic stimuli. Exogenous insulin is therefore required to reverse the catabolic state, prevent ketosis, reduce the hyperglucagonemia, and reduce blood glucose.

The highest incidence of immune-mediated type 1 diabetes is in Scandinavia and northern Europe, where the yearly incidence per 100,000 youngsters 14 years of age or less is as high as 37 in Finland, 27 in Sweden, 22 in Norway, and 19 in the United Kingdom. The incidence of type 1 diabetes generally decreases across the rest of Europe to 10 in Greece and 8 in France. Surprisingly, the island of Sardinia has as high an incidence as Finland (37) even though in the rest of Italy, including the island of Sicily, it is only 10 per 100,000 per year. The United States averages 15 per 100,000, with higher incidences in states more densely populated with persons of Scandinavian descent such as Minnesota. The lowest incidence of type 1 diabetes worldwide was found to be less than 1 per 100,000 per year in China and parts of South America.

Table 27–1. Clinical classification of common diabetes mellitus syndromes.

Type	Ketosis	Islet Cell Antibodies	HLA Association	Treatment
Type 1				
(A) Immune-mediated	Present	Present at onset	Positive	Eucaloric healthy diet and preprandial rapid-acting insulin, plus basal insulin replacement with intermediate-acting or long-acting insulin
(B) Idiopathic	Present	Absent	Absent	
Type 2				
(A) Nonobese	Absent	Absent	Negative	(1) Eucaloric diet alone (2) Diet plus insulin or oral agents
(B) Obese	Absent	Absent	Negative	(1) Weight reduction (2) Hypocaloric diet, plus oral agents or insulin

Certain human leukocyte antigens (HLA) are strongly associated with the development of type 1 diabetes. About 95% of type 1 patients possess either HLA-DR3 or HLA-DR4, compared with 45–50% of Caucasian controls. HLA-DQ genes are even more specific markers of type 1 susceptibility, since a particular variety (*HLA-DQB1*0302*) is found in the DR4 patients with type 1, while a "protective" gene (*HLA-DQB1*0602*) is often present in the DR4 controls. In addition, circulating islet cell antibodies have been detected in as many as 85% of patients tested in the first few weeks of their diabetes, and when sensitive immunoassays are used, the majority of these patients also have detectable anti-insulin antibodies prior to receiving insulin therapy. Most islet cell antibodies are directed against glutamic acid decarboxylase, an enzyme localized within pancreatic B cells. Immunoassays for this marker of type 1 diabetes facilitate screening of siblings of affected children as well as adults with atypical features of type 2 for an autoimmune cause of their diabetes.

Certain unrecognized patients with a milder expression of type 1 diabetes initially retain enough B cell function to avoid ketosis but later in life develop increasing dependency on insulin therapy as their B cell mass diminishes. Islet cell antibody surveys among northern Europeans indicate 15% of "type 2" patients may actually have this mild form of type 1 diabetes.

1. Immune-mediated type 1 diabetes mellitus— Immune-mediated type 1 diabetes is felt to result from an infectious or toxic insult to persons whose immune system is genetically predisposed to develop a vigorous autoimmune response either against altered pancreatic B cell antigens or against molecules of the B cell resembling the viral protein (molecular mimicry). Extrinsic factors that affect B cell function include damage caused by viruses such as mumps or coxsackie B4 virus, by toxic chemical agents, or by destructive cytotoxins and antibodies released from sensitized immunocytes. Specific HLA immune response genes are believed to predispose patients to a destructive autoimmune response against their own islet cells (autoaggression) which is mediated primarily by cytotoxic T cells. Amelioration of hyperglycemia in patients given an immunosuppressive agent (eg, cyclosporine) shortly after onset of type 1 diabetes lends further support to the pathogenetic role of autoimmunity.

2. Idiopathic type 1 diabetes mellitus—Fewer than 10% of subjects have no evidence of pancreatic B cell autoimmunity to explain their insulinopenia and ketoacidosis. This subgroup has been classified as "idiopathic type 1 diabetes" and designated as "type 1B." Although only a minority of patients with type 1 diabetes fall into this group, most of these are of Asian or African origin.

B. TYPE 2 DIABETES

This represents a heterogeneous group comprising milder forms of diabetes that occur predominantly in adults but occasionally in juveniles. More than 90% of all diabetics in the USA are included under this classification. Circulating endogenous insulin is sufficient to prevent ketoacidosis but is inadequate to prevent hyperglycemia in the face of increased needs owing to tissue insensitivity. In most cases of this type of diabetes, the cause is unknown.

Tissue insensitivity to insulin has been noted in most type 2 patients irrespective of weight and has been attributed to several interrelated factors. These include a putative (and as yet undefined) genetic factor, which is aggravated in time by additional enhancers of insulin resistance such as aging, a sedentary lifestyle, and abdominal-visceral obesity. In addition, there is an accompanying deficiency in the response of pancreatic B cells to glucose. Both the tissue resistance to insulin and the impaired B cell response to glucose appear to be further aggravated by increased hyperglycemia, and both defects are ameliorated by treatment that reduces the hyperglycemia toward normal. Most epidemiologic data indicate strong genetic influences, since in monozygotic twins over 40 years of age, concordance develops in over 70% of cases within a year whenever one twin develops type 2 diabetes. Attempts to identify genetic markers for type 2 have as yet been unsuccessful, though linkage to a gene on chromosome 2 encoding a cysteine protease, *calpain-10,* has been reported in a Mexican-American population. However, its association with other ethnic populations and any role it plays in the pathogenesis of type 2 diabetes remain to be clarified.

Two subgroups of patients are currently distinguished by the absence or presence of obesity. The degree and prevalence of obesity varies among different racial groups. While obesity is apparent in no more than 30% of Chinese and Japanese patients with type 2, it is found in 60–70% of North Americans, Europeans, or Africans with type 2 and approaches 100% of patients with type 2 among Pima Indians or Pacific Islanders from Nauru or Samoa.

Nonobese type 2 patients generally show an absent or blunted early phase of insulin release in response to glucose; however, it can be elicited in response to other insulinogenic stimuli such as acute intravenous administration of sulfonylureas, glucagon, or arginine.

Although insulin resistance may be detected with special tests, it does not seem to be clinically relevant to the treatment of most nonobese type 2 patients, who generally respond to appropriate therapeutic supplements of insulin in the absence of rare associated conditions such as lipoatrophy or acanthosis nigricans.

Among this heterogeneous subgroup of patients with nonobese type 2 diabetes, the majority are idiopathic. However, with increasing frequency, a variety of etiologic genetic abnormalities have been documented in a subset of these patients who have recently been reclassified within a group designated "other specific types." (See Table 27–2.)

Table 27–2. Other specific types of diabetes mellitus.

Genetic defects of pancreatic B cell function
   MODY 1 (HNF-4α); rare
   MODY 2 (glucokinase); less rare
   MODY 3 (HNF-1α); accounts for two-thirds of all MODY
   MODY 4 (IPF-1); very rare
   MODY 5 (HNF-1β); very rare
   MODY 6 (neuroD1); very rare
   Mitochondrial DNA
Genetic defects in insulin action
   Type A insulin resistance
   Leprechaunism
   Rabson-Mendenhall syndrome
   Lipoatrophic diabetes
Diseases of the exocrine pancreas
Endocrinopathies
Drug- or chemical-induced diabetes
Other genetic syndromes (Down's, Klinefelter's,
   Turners, others) sometimes associated with diabetes

C. OTHER SPECIFIC TYPES OF DIABETES MELLITUS

1. Maturity-onset diabetes of the young (MODY)—This subgroup is a relatively rare monogenic disorder characterized by non-insulin-dependent diabetes with autosomal dominant inheritance and an age at onset of 25 years or younger. Patients are nonobese, and their hyperglycemia is due to impaired glucose-induced secretion of insulin. Six types of MODY have been described. Except for MODY 2, in which a glucokinase gene is defective, all other types involve mutations of a nuclear transcription factor that regulates islet gene expression.

MODY 2 is quite mild, associated with only slight fasting hyperglycemia and few if any microvascular diabetic complications. It generally responds well to hygienic measures or low doses of oral hypoglycemic agents. MODY 3—the most common form—accounts for two-thirds of all MODY cases. It can progress similarly to type 2 diabetes as regards vascular complications and a subsequent need for supplemental or intensive insulin therapy.

2. Diabetes due to mutant insulins—This is a very rare subtype of nonobese type 2 diabetes, with no more than ten families having been described. Since affected individuals were heterozygous and possessed one normal insulin gene, diabetes was mild, did not appear until middle age, and showed autosomal dominant genetic transmission. There is generally no evidence of clinical insulin resistance and these patients respond well to standard therapy.

3. Diabetes due to mutant insulin receptors—Defects in one of their insulin receptor gene have been found in more than 40 people with diabetes, and most have extreme insulin resistance associated with acanthosis nigricans. In very rare instances when both insulin receptor genes are abnormal, newborns present with a leprechaun-like phenotype and seldom live through infancy.

4. Diabetes mellitus associated with a mutation of mitochondrial DNA—Since sperm do not contain mitochondria, only the mother transmits mitochondrial genes to her offspring. Diabetes due to a mutation of mitochondrial DNA that impairs the transfer of leucine or lysine into mitochondrial proteins has been described. Most patients have a mild form of diabetes that responds to oral hypoglycemic agents, some a nonimmune form of type 1 diabetes. Two-thirds of patients with this subtype of diabetes have a hearing loss, and a smaller proportion (15%) had a syndrome of myopathy, encephalopathy, lactic acidosis, and stroke-like episodes (MELAS).

5. Obese type 2 patients—This most common form of diabetes is secondary to extrapancreatic factors that produce insensitivity to endogenous insulin. When an associated defect of insulin production prevents adequate compensation for this insulin resistance, nonketotic mild diabetes occurs. The primary problem is a "target organ" disorder resulting in ineffective insulin action that can secondarily influence pancreatic B cell function. Hyperplasia of pancreatic B cells is often present and probably accounts for the fasting hyperinsulinism and exaggerated insulin and proinsulin responses to glucose and other stimuli seen in the milder forms of this disorder. In more severe cases, especially after several years' duration of diabetes, failure of B cell secretion may result. Chronic deposition of amyloid in the islets may combine with inherited genetic defects to progressively impair B cell function. Obesity is generally associated with abdominal distribution of fat, producing an abnormally high waist-to-hip ratio. This "visceral" obesity, due to accumulation of fat in the omental and mesenteric regions, correlates with insulin resistance; subcutaneous abdominal fat seems to have less of an association with insulin insensitivity. Exercise may affect the deposition of visceral fat as suggested by CT scans of Japanese wrestlers, whose extreme obesity is predominantly subcutaneous. Their daily vigorous exercise program prevents accumulation of visceral fat, and they have normal serum lipids and euglycemia despite daily intakes of 5000–7000 kcal and development of massive subcutaneous obesity.

A major cause of the observed resistance to insulin in target tissues of obese patients is believed to be a postreceptor defect in insulin action, resulting in a reduced ability to clear nutrients from the circulation after meals. The resulting hyperinsulinism can further enhance insulin resistance by down-regulation of insulin receptors. Moreover, when hyperglycemia develops, hexosamines accumulate in muscle and fat tissue to further inhibit glucose transport. This contributes to further defects in postreceptor insulin action, thereby aggravating hyperglycemia.

When exercise increases blood flow to muscle as well as increasing muscle mass, and when overfeeding is corrected so that storage depots become less saturated, the cycle is interrupted. There is improvement in insulin sensitivity, which is further restored toward normal by a reduction of both the hyperinsulinism and the hyperglycemia.

Several **adipokines,** secreted by fat cells, can affect insulin action in obesity. Two of these, **leptin** and **adiponectin,** seem to increase sensitivity to insulin, presumably by increasing hepatic responsiveness. Two others—**tumor necrosis factor-α,** which inactivates insulin receptors, and the newly discovered peptide **resistin**—interfere with insulin action on glucose metabolism and have been reported to be elevated in obese animal models. Mutations or abnormal levels of these adipokines may contribute to the development of insulin resistance in human obesity.

Epidemiologic Considerations

An estimated 16 million people in the USA are known to have diabetes, of which 1.4 million have type 1 diabetes and approximately 14.5 million have type 2 dia-

betes. The remainder, numbered only in the thousands, comprise a third group that was designated as "other specific types" by the American Diabetes Association (Table 27–2). These other types include disorders for which causes are known. Among these are the rare monogenic defects of either B cell function or of insulin action, primary diseases of the exocrine pancreas, endocrinopathies, and drug-induced diabetes.

Insulin Resistance Syndrome (Syndrome X)

In obese patients with type 2 diabetes, the association of **hyperglycemia, hyperinsulinemia, dyslipidemia,** and **hypertension,** which leads to coronary artery disease and stroke, may result from a genetic defect producing insulin resistance, with the latter being exaggerated by obesity. It has been proposed that insulin resistance predisposes to hyperglycemia, which results in hyperinsulinemia, which may or may not be of sufficient magnitude to correct the hyperglycemia; and that this excessive insulin level then contributes to increased VLDL production in the liver, leading to hypertriglyceridemia and to increased sodium retention by renal tubules, thus inducing hypertension. Moreover, high insulin levels can stimulate endothelial proliferation—by virtue of insulin's action on growth factor receptors—to initiate atherosclerosis. While these associations have long been well known, the mechanism for their interrelationship remains speculative and an invitation to experimental investigation. Some question the role of hyperinsulinism in hypertension, since they often coexist in Caucasians but not in blacks or Pima Indians. Moreover, patients with hyperinsulinism due to insulinoma are not hypertensive, and there is no fall in blood pressure after surgical removal of the insulinoma restores normal insulin levels. The main value of grouping these disorders as a syndrome, however, is to remind clinicians that the therapeutic goals are not only to correct hyperglycemia but also to manage the elevated blood pressure and dyslipidemia that result in increased cerebrovascular and cardiac morbidity and mortality in these patients. Clinicians aware of this syndrome are more cautious in prescribing therapies that correct hypertension but may raise lipids (diuretics, beta-blockers) or that correct hyperlipidemia but increase insulin resistance, with aggravation of diabetes (niacin). Finally, the use of long-acting insulins and sulfonylureas that promote sustained hyperinsulinism may have to be moderated, with insulin-sparing drugs such as metformin or a thiazolidinedione being preferable, if the hypothesis behind the insulin-resistance syndrome is ever substantiated.

Plasminogen activator-inhibitor 1 (PAI-1), produced by omental and visceral adipocytes, is elevated in the plasma of these patients. This contributes to the reduced fibrinolysis and higher risk for atherothrombosis in this syndrome.

Clinical Findings

The principal clinical features of the two major types of diabetes mellitus are listed for comparison in Table 27–3.

Patients with type 1 diabetes present with a characteristic symptom complex. An absolute deficiency of insulin results in accumulation of circulating glucose and fatty acids, with consequent hyperosmolality and hyperketonemia.

Patients with type 2 diabetes may or may not present with characteristic features. The presence of obesity or a strongly positive family history for mild diabetes suggests a high risk for the development of type 2 diabetes.

A. SYMPTOMS AND SIGNS

1. Type 1 diabetes—Increased urination is a consequence of osmotic diuresis secondary to sustained hyperglycemia. This results in a loss of glucose as well as free water and electrolytes in the urine. Thirst is a consequence of the hyperosmolar state, as is blurred vision, which often develops as the lenses and retinas are exposed to hyperosmolar fluids.

Weight loss despite normal or increased appetite is a common feature of type 1 when it develops subacutely. The weight loss is initially due to depletion of water, glycogen, and triglycerides; thereafter, reduced muscle mass occurs as amino acids are diverted to form glucose and ketone bodies.

Lowered plasma volume produces symptoms of postural hypotension. Total body potassium loss and the general catabolism of muscle protein contribute to the weakness.

Paresthesias may be present at the time of diagnosis, particularly when the onset is subacute. They reflect a temporary dysfunction of peripheral sensory nerves, which clears as insulin replacement restores glycemic levels closer to normal, suggesting neurotoxicity from sustained hyperglycemia.

Table 27–3. Clinical features of diabetes at diagnosis.

	Type 1 Diabetes	Type 2 Diabetes
Polyuria and thirst	++	+
Weakness or fatigue	++	+
Polyphagia with weight loss	++	−
Recurrent blurred vision	+	++
Vulvovaginitis or pruritus	+	++
Peripheral neuropathy	+	++
Nocturnal enuresis	++	−
Often asymptomatic	−	++

When absolute insulin deficiency is of acute onset, the above symptoms develop abruptly. Ketoacidosis exacerbates the dehydration and hyperosmolality by producing anorexia and nausea and vomiting, interfering with oral fluid replacement.

The patient's level of consciousness can vary depending on the degree of hyperosmolality. When insulin deficiency develops relatively slowly and sufficient water intake is maintained, patients remain relatively alert and physical findings may be minimal. When vomiting occurs in response to worsening ketoacidosis, dehydration progresses and compensatory mechanisms become inadequate to keep serum osmolality below 320–330 mosm/L. Under these circumstances, stupor or even coma may occur. The fruity breath odor of acetone further suggests the diagnosis of diabetic ketoacidosis.

Hypotension in the recumbent position is a serious prognostic sign. Loss of subcutaneous fat and muscle wasting are features of more slowly developing insulin deficiency. In occasional patients with slow, insidious onset of insulin deficiency, subcutaneous fat may be considerably depleted. An enlarged liver, eruptive xanthomas on the flexor surface of the limbs and on the buttocks, and lipemia retinalis indicate that chronic insulin deficiency has resulted in chylomicronemia, with circulating triglycerides elevated usually to over 2000 mg/dL.

2. Type 2 diabetes—While many patients with type 2 diabetes present with increased urination and thirst, many others have an insidious onset of hyperglycemia and are asymptomatic initially. This is particularly true in obese patients, whose diabetes may be detected only after glycosuria or hyperglycemia is noted during routine laboratory studies. Occasionally, type 2 patients may present with evidence of neuropathic or cardiovascular complications because of occult disease present for some time prior to diagnosis. Chronic skin infections are common. Generalized pruritus and symptoms of vaginitis are frequently the initial complaints of women. Diabetes should be suspected in women with chronic candidal vulvovaginitis as well as in those who have delivered large babies (> 9 lb, or 4.1 kg) or have had polyhydramnios, preeclampsia, or unexplained fetal losses.

Obese diabetics may have any variety of fat distribution; however, diabetes seems to be more often associated in both men and women with localization of fat deposits on the upper segment of the body (particularly the abdomen, chest, neck, and face) and relatively less fat on the appendages, which may be quite muscular. Standardized tables of waist-to-hip ratio indicate that ratios of "greater than 0.9" in men and "greater than 0.8" in women are associated with an increased risk of diabetes in obese subjects. Mild hypertension is often present in obese diabetics.

B. LABORATORY FINDINGS

1. Urinalysis—

a. Glucosuria—A specific and convenient method to detect glucosuria is the paper strip impregnated with glucose oxidase and a chromogen system (Clinistix, Diastix), which is sensitive to as little as 0.1% glucose in urine. Diastix can be directly applied to the urinary stream, and differing color responses of the indicator strip reflect glucose concentration.

A normal renal threshold for glucose as well as reliable bladder emptying is essential for interpretation.

b. Ketonuria—Qualitative detection of ketone bodies can be accomplished by nitroprusside tests (Acetest or Ketostix). Although these tests do not detect β-hydroxybutyric acid, which lacks a ketone group, the semiquantitative estimation of ketonuria thus obtained is nonetheless usually adequate for clinical purposes.

2. Blood testing procedures—

a. Glucose tolerance test—

(1) Methodology and normal fasting glucose— Plasma or serum from venous blood samples has the advantage over whole blood of providing values for glucose that are independent of hematocrit and that reflect the glucose concentration to which body tissues are exposed. For these reasons, and because plasma and serum are more readily measured on automated equipment, they are used in most laboratories. If serum is used or if plasma is collected from tubes that lack an agent to block glucose metabolism (such as fluoride), samples should be refrigerated and separated within 1 hour after collection.

(2) Criteria for laboratory confirmation of diabetes mellitus—If the fasting plasma glucose level is 126 mg/dL or higher on more than one occasion, further evaluation of the patient with a glucose challenge is unnecessary. However, when fasting plasma glucose is less than 126 mg/dL in suspected cases, a standardized oral glucose tolerance test may be done (Table 27–4).

Table 27–4. The Diabetes Expert Committee criteria for evaluating the standard oral glucose tolerance test.[1]

	Normal Glucose Tolerance	Impaired Glucose Tolerance	Diabetes Mellitus[2]
Fasting plasma glucose (mg/dL)	< 110	110–125	≥ 126
Two hours after glucose load (mg/dL)	< 140	≥ 140 but < 200	≥ 200

[1]Give 75 g of glucose dissolved in 300 mL of water after an overnight fast in subjects who have been receiving at least 150–200 g of carbohydrate daily for 3 days before the test.
[2]A fasting plasma glucose ≥ 126 mg/dL is diagnostic of diabetes if confirmed on a subsequent day.

For proper evaluation of the test, the subjects should be normally active and free from acute illness. Medications that may impair glucose tolerance include diuretics, contraceptive drugs, glucocorticoids, niacin, and phenytoin.

Because of difficulties in interpreting oral glucose tolerance tests and the lack of standards related to aging, these tests are being replaced by documentation of fasting hyperglycemia.

Since fasting plasma glucose is known to increase with aging, clinicians should be more tolerant of slight abnormalities of fasting glucose values in older people (over 70 years of age) and not deprive patients of occasional sugar-containing snacks when symptoms are not evident. However, an occasional elderly patient may benefit from the diagnosis of mild diabetes in that macular edema may be detected earlier and laser treatment initiated before vision deteriorates permanently.

b. Glycated hemoglobin (hemoglobin A$_1$) measurements—Glycated hemoglobin is abnormally high in diabetics with chronic hyperglycemia and reflects their metabolic control. It is produced by nonenzymatic condensation of glucose molecules with free amino groups on the globin component of hemoglobin. The higher the prevailing ambient levels of blood glucose, the higher will be the level of glycated hemoglobin.

The major form of glycohemoglobin is termed hemoglobin A$_{1c}$, which normally comprises only 4–6% of the total hemoglobin. The remaining glycohemoglobins (2–4% of the total) consist of phosphorylated glucose or fructose and are termed hemoglobin A$_{1a}$ and hemoglobin A$_{1b}$. Some laboratories measure the sum of these three glycohemoglobins and report it as hemoglobin A$_1$, but more laboratories are converting to the more intricate but highly specific HbA$_{1c}$ assay. There are now monoclonal immunoassays for measuring HbA$_{1c}$. Machines based on this technology can be used in clinicians' offices. They use capillary blood and give a result in about 9 minutes, allowing immediate feedback to the patient regarding their glycemic control.

Since glycohemoglobins circulate within red blood cells whose life span lasts up to 120 days, they generally reflect the state of glycemia over the preceding 8–12 weeks, thereby providing an improved method of assessing diabetic control. Measurements should be made in patients with either type of diabetes mellitus at 3- to 4-month intervals so that adjustments in therapy can be made if glycohemoglobin is either subnormal or if it is more than 2% above the upper limits of normal for a particular laboratory. In patients monitoring their own blood glucose levels, glycohemoglobin values provide a valuable check on the accuracy of monitoring. In patients who do not monitor their own blood glucose levels, glycohemoglobin values are essential for adjusting therapy. Use of glycohemoglobin for screening is controversial. Sensitivity in detecting known diabetes cases by hemoglobin A_{1c} measurements is only 85%, indicating that diabetes cannot be excluded by a normal value. On the other hand, elevated hemoglobin A_{1c} assays are fairly specific (91%) in identifying the presence of diabetes.

Occasionally, fluctuations in hemoglobin A_1 are due to an acutely generated, reversible, intermediary (aldimine-linked) product that can falsely elevate glycohemoglobins when measured with "short-cut" chromatographic methods. This can be eliminated by using specific HPLC methods that detect HbA_{1c} or by dialysis of the hemolysate before chromatography. When hemoglobin variants are present, such as negatively charged hemoglobin F, acetylated hemoglobin from high-dose aspirin therapy, or carbamoylated hemoglobin produced by the complexing of urea with hemoglobin in uremia, falsely high "hemoglobin A_1" values are obtained with commonly used chromatographic methods. In the presence of positively charged hemoglobin variants such as hemoglobin S or C, or when the life span of red blood cells is reduced by increased hemolysis or hemorrhage, falsely low values for "hemoglobin A_1" result.

Serum fructosamine is formed by nonenzymatic glycosylation of serum proteins (predominantly albumin). Since serum albumin has a much shorter half-life than hemoglobin, serum fructosamine generally reflects the state of glycemic control for only the preceding 2 weeks. Reductions in serum albumin (eg, nephrotic state or hepatic disease) will lower the serum fructosamine value. When abnormal hemoglobins or hemolytic states affect the interpretation of glycohemoglobin or when a narrower time frame is required, such as for ascertaining glycemic control at the time of conception in a diabetic woman who has recently become pregnant, serum fructosamine assays offer some advantage. Normal values vary in relation to the serum albumin concentration and are 1.5–2.4 mmol/L when the serum albumin level is 5 g/dL.

c. Self-monitoring of blood glucose—Capillary blood glucose measurements performed by patients themselves, as outpatients, are extremely useful. In type 1 patients in whom "tight" metabolic control is attempted, they are indispensable. A portable battery-operated glucometer provides a digital readout of the intensity of color developed when glucose oxidase paper strips are exposed to a drop of capillary blood for up to 45 seconds. A large number of blood glucose meters are now available. All are accurate, but they vary with regard to speed, convenience, size of blood samples required, and cost. Popular models include those manufactured by LifeScan (One Touch), Bayer Corporation (Glucometer Elite, DEX), Roche Diagnostics (Accu-Chek), Abbott Laboratories (ExacTech, Precision), and Home Diagnostics (Prestige). One Touch Ultra, for example, requires only 0.3 mL of blood and gives a result in 5 seconds—and illustrates how there has been continued progress in this technologic area. Various glucometers appeal to a particular consumer need and

are relatively inexpensive, ranging from $50.00 to $100.00 each. The more expensive models compute blood glucose averages and can be attached to printers for data records and graph production. Test strips remain a major expense, costing 50–75 cents apiece. In self-monitoring of blood glucose, patients must prick their finger with a 28-gauge lancet (Monolet, Ames Co.), which can be facilitated by a small plastic trigger device such as an Autolet (Ames Co.), SoftClix (Boehringer-Mannheim), or Penlet (Lifescan, Inc.). When used for multiple patients, as in a clinic, physician's office, or hospital ward, disposable finger-rest platforms are required to avoid inadvertent transmission of blood-borne viral diseases. Some meters such as the FreeStyle (Therasense) have been approved for measuring glucose in blood samples obtained at alternative sites such as the forearm and thigh. There is, however, a 5- to 20-minute lag in the glucose response on the arm with respect to the glucose response on the finger. Forearm blood glucose measurements could therefore result in a delay in detection of rapidly developing hypoglycemia.

The accuracy of data obtained by glucose monitoring requires education of the patient in sampling and measuring procedures as well as in proper calibration of the instruments. Bedside glucose monitoring in a hospital setting requires rigorous quality control programs and certification of personnel to avoid errors.

Noninvasive glucose monitoring is a subject of intensive research interest, and a prototype, the GlucoWatch, has been approved by the FDA. It utilizes reverse iontophoresis to measure interstitial glucose values with acceptable accuracy. Because of a lag period of 15–20 minutes, it records measurements only three times an hour. Sweating can result in skipped readings, which causes problems in warm humid climates. Further experience is needed to evaluate its clinical value.

3. Lipoprotein abnormalities in diabetes—Circulating lipoproteins are just as dependent on insulin as is the plasma glucose. In type 1 diabetes, moderately deficient control of hyperglycemia is associated with only a slight elevation of LDL cholesterol and serum triglycerides and little if any change in HDL cholesterol. Once the hyperglycemia is corrected, lipoprotein levels are generally normal. However, in obese patients with type 2 diabetes, a distinct "diabetic dyslipidemia" is characteristic of the insulin resistance syndrome. Its features are a high serum triglyceride level (300–400 mg/dL), a low HDL-cholesterol (less than 30 mg/dL), and a qualitative change in LDL particles, producing a smaller dense particle whose membrane carries supranormal amounts of free cholesterol. These smaller dense LDL particles are more susceptible to oxidation, which renders them more atherogenic. Since a low HDL-cholesterol is a major feature predisposing to macrovascular disease, the term "dyslipidemia" has preempted the term "hyperlipidemia," which mainly denoted the elevated triglycerides. Measures designed to correct the obesity and hyperglycemia, such as exercise, diet, and hypoglycemic therapy, are the treatment of choice for diabetic dyslipidemia, and in occasional patients in whom normal weight was achieved, all features of the lipoprotein abnormalities cleared. Since primary disorders of lipid metabolism may coexist with diabetes, persistence of lipid abnormalities after restoration of normal weight and blood glucose should prompt a diagnostic workup and possible pharmacotherapy of the lipid disorder. Chapter 28 discusses these matters in detail.

Differential Diagnosis

A. HYPERGLYCEMIA SECONDARY TO OTHER CAUSES

(Table 27–5.) Secondary hyperglycemia has been associated with various disorders of insulin target tissues (liver, muscle, and adipose tissue).

Other secondary causes of carbohydrate intolerance include endocrine disorders—often specific endocrine tumors—associated with excess production of growth hormone, glucocorticoids, catecholamines, glucagon, or somatostatin. In the first four situations, peripheral responsiveness to insulin is impaired. With excess of glucocorticoids, catecholamines, or glucagon, increased hepatic output of glucose is a contributory factor; in the case of catecholamines, decreased insulin release is an additional factor in producing carbohydrate intolerance, and with excess somatostatin production it is the major factor.

A rare syndrome of extreme insulin resistance associated with acanthosis nigricans afflicts either young women with androgenic features as well as insulin receptor mutations or older people, mostly women, in whom a circulating immunoglobulin binds to insulin receptors and reduces their affinity to insulin.

Table 27–5. Secondary causes of hyperglycemia.

Hyperglycemia due to tissue insensitivity to insulin
  Hormonal tumors (acromegaly, Cushing's syndrome, glucagonoma, pheochromocytoma)
  Pharmacologic agents (glucocorticoids, sympathomimetic drugs, niacin)
  Liver disease (cirrhosis, hemochromatosis)
  Muscle disorders (myotonic dystrophy)
  Adipose tissue disorders (lipodystrophy, truncal obesity)
  Insulin receptor disorders (acanthosis nigricans syndromes, leprechaunism)
Hyperglycemia due to reduced insulin secretion
  Hormonal tumors (somatostatinoma, pheochromocytoma)
  Pancreatic disorders (pancreatitis, hemosiderosis, hemochromatosis)
  Pharmacologic agents (thiazide diuretics, phenytoin, pentamidine)

Medications such as diuretics, phenytoin, niacin, and high-dose glucocorticoids can produce hyperglycemia that is reversible once the drugs are discontinued or when diuretic-induced hypokalemia is corrected. Chronic pancreatitis or subtotal pancreatectomy reduces the number of functioning B cells and can result in a metabolic derangement very similar to that of genetic type 1 diabetes except that a concomitant reduction in pancreatic A cells may reduce glucagon secretion so that relatively lower doses of insulin replacement are needed. Insulin-dependent diabetes is occasionally associated with Addison's disease and autoimmune thyroiditis (**Schmidt's syndrome,** or **polyglandular failure syndrome**). This occurs more commonly in women and represents an autoimmune disorder in which there are circulating antibodies to adrenocortical and thyroid tissue, thyroglobulin, and gastric parietal cells.

B. NONDIABETIC GLYCOSURIA

Nondiabetic glycosuria (renal glycosuria) is a benign, asymptomatic condition wherein glucose appears in the urine despite a normal amount of glucose in the blood, either basally or during a glucose tolerance test. Its cause may vary from an autosomally transmitted genetic disorder to one associated with dysfunction of the proximal renal tubule (Fanconi's syndrome, chronic renal failure), or it may merely be a consequence of the increased load of glucose presented to the tubules by the elevated glomerular filtration rate during pregnancy. As many as 50% of pregnant women normally have demonstrable sugar in the urine, especially during the third and fourth months. This sugar is practically always glucose except during the late weeks of pregnancy, when lactose may be present.

Goals of Treatment of Diabetes

Diabetes mellitus requires ongoing medical care as well as patient and family education both to prevent acute illness and to reduce the risk of long-term complications. The Diabetes Control and Complications Trial of type 1 diabetes and the United Kingdom Prospective Diabetes Study of type 2 diabetes (see below) both indicate that the therapeutic objective is to restore known metabolic derangements toward normal in order to prevent and delay progression of diabetic complications.

Treatment Regimens

A. DIET

A well-balanced, nutritious diet remains a fundamental element of therapy. However, in more than half of cases, diabetic patients fail to follow their diet. In prescribing a diet, it is important to relate dietary objectives to the type of diabetes. In obese patients with mild hyperglycemia, the major goal of diet therapy is weight reduction by caloric restriction. Thus, there is less need for exchange lists, emphasis on timing of meals, or periodic snacks, all of which are so essential in the treatment of insulin-requiring nonobese diabetics. This type of patient represents the most frequent challenge for the clinician. Weight reduction is an elusive goal that can only be achieved by close supervision and education of the obese patient. See Chapter 29 for dietary management of obesity.

1. Revised ADA recommendations—The American Diabetes Association releases an annual position statement on medical nutrition therapy that replaced the calculated ADA diet formula of the past with suggestions for an individually tailored dietary prescription based on metabolic, nutritional, and life-style requirements. They contend that the concept of one diet for "diabetes" and the prescription of an "ADA diet" no longer can apply to both major types of diabetes. In their recommendations for persons with type 2 diabetes, the 55–60% carbohydrate content of previous diets has been reduced considerably because of the tendency of high carbohydrate intake to cause hyperglycemia, hypertriglyceridemia, and a lowered HDL-cholesterol. In obese type 2 patients, glucose and lipid goals join weight loss as the focus of therapy. These patients are advised to limit their carbohydrate content by substituting noncholesterologenic monounsaturated oils such as olive oil, rapeseed (canola) oil, or the oils in nuts and avocados. This maneuver is also indicated in type 1 patients on intensive insulin regimens in whom near-normoglycemic control is less achievable on higher carbohydrate diets. They should be taught "carbohydrate counting" so they can administer 1 unit of regular insulin or insulin lispro for each 10 or 15 g of carbohydrate eaten at a meal. In these patients, the ratio of carbohydrate to fat will vary among individuals in relation to their glycemic responses, insulin regimens, and exercise pattern.

The current recommendations for both types of diabetes continue to limit cholesterol to 300 mg daily and advise a daily protein intake of 10–20% of total calories. They suggest that saturated fat be no higher than 8–9% of total calories with a similar proportion of polyunsaturated fat and that the remainder of caloric needs be made up of an individualized ratio of monounsaturated fat and of carbohydrate containing 20–35 g of dietary fiber. Poultry, veal, and fish continue to be recommended as a substitute for red meats for keeping saturated fat content low. The present ADA position statement proffers no evidence that reducing protein intake below 10% of intake (about 0.8 g/kg/d) is of any benefit in patients with nephropathy and renal impairment, and doing so may be detrimental.

Exchange lists for meal planning can be obtained from the American Diabetes Association and its affiliate associations or from the American Dietetic Association, 216 W. Jackson Blvd., Chicago, IL 60606 (312-899-0040). Their Internet address is http://www.eatright.org.

2. Dietary fiber—Plant components such as cellulose, gum, and pectin are indigestible by humans and are termed dietary "fiber." Insoluble fibers such as cellulose or hemicellulose, as found in bran, tend to increase intestinal transit and may have beneficial effects on colonic function. In contrast, soluble fibers such as gums and pectins, as found in beans, oatmeal, or apple skin, tend to retard nutrient absorption rates so that glucose absorption is slower and hyperglycemia may be slightly diminished. Although its recommendations do not include insoluble fiber supplements such as added bran, the ADA recommends food such as oatmeal, cereals, and beans with relatively high soluble fiber content as staple components of the diet in diabetics. High soluble fiber content in the diet may also have a favorable effect on blood cholesterol levels.

3. Artificial sweeteners—Aspartame (NutraSweet) has proved to be a popular sweetener for diabetic patients. It consists of two amino acids (aspartic acid and phenylalanine) that combine to produce a nutritive sweetener 180 times as sweet as sucrose. A major limitation is that it cannot be used in baking or cooking because of its lability to heat.

The nonnutritive sweetener saccharin continues to be available in certain foods and beverages despite warnings by the FDA about its potential long-term carcinogenicity to the bladder. The latest position statement of the ADA concludes that all nonnutritive sweeteners that have been approved by the FDA (such as aspartame and saccharin) are safe for consumption by all people with diabetes. Two other nonnutritive sweeteners have been approved by the FDA as safe for general use: sucralose (Splenda) and acesulfame potassium (Sunett, Sweet One, DiabetiSweet). These are both highly stable and, in contrast to aspartame, can be used in cooking and baking.

Nutritive sweeteners such as sorbitol and fructose have increased in popularity. Except for acute diarrhea induced by ingestion of large amounts of sorbitol-containing foods, their relative risk has yet to be established. Fructose represents a "natural" sugar substance that is a highly effective sweetener which induces only slight increases in plasma glucose levels. However, because of potential adverse effects of large amounts of fructose (up to 20% of total calories) on raising serum cholesterol and LDL-cholesterol, the ADA feels it may have no overall advantage as a sweetening agent in the diabetic diet. This does not preclude, however, ingestion of fructose-containing fruits and vegetables or fructose-sweetened foods in moderation.

B. ORAL DRUGS FOR TREATING HYPERGLYCEMIA

(Tables 27–6, 27–7, and 27–8.) The drugs for treating type 2 diabetes fall into three categories: (1) Drugs that primarily stimulate insulin secretion: Sulfonylureas remain the most widely prescribed drugs for treating hyperglycemia. The meglitinide analog repaglinide and the D-phenylalanine derivative nateglinide also bind the sulfonylurea receptor and

Table 27–6. Oral antidiabetic drugs that stimulate insulin secretion.

Drug	Tablet Size	Daily Dose	Duration of Action	Cost per Unit	Cost for 30 Days' Treatment Based on Maximum Dosage[1]
Sulfonylureas					
Tolbutamide (Orinase)	250 and 500 mg	0.5–2 g in 2 or 3 divided doses	6–12 hours	$0.28/500 mg	$33.60
Tolazamide (Tolinase)	100, 250, and 500 mg	0.1–1 g as single dose or in 2 divided doses	Up to 24 hours	$0.26/250 mg	$31.20
Acetohexamide (Dymelor)[2]	250 and 500 mg	0.25–1.5 g as single dose or in 2 divided doses	8–24 hours	$0.42/500 mg	$37.80
Chlorpropamide (Diabinese)[2]	100 and 250 mg	0.1–0.5 g as single dose	24–72 hours	$0.61/250 mg	$36.60
Glyburide					
(Diaβeta, Micronase)	1.25, 2.5, and 5 mg	1.25–20 mg as single dose or in 2 divided doses	Up to 24 hours	$0.78/5 mg	$93.60
(Glynase)	1.5, 3, and 6 mg	1.5–18 mg as single dose or in 2 divided doses	Up to 24 hours	$1.07/6 mg	$96.30
Glipizide					
(Glucotrol)	5 and 10 mg	2.5–40 mg as single dose or in 2 divided doses on an empty stomach	6–12 hours	$0.59/10 mg	$70.80
(Glucotrol XL)	5 and 10 mg	Up to 20 or 30 mg daily as a single dose	Up to 24 hours	$0.75/10 mg	$67.50
Glimeperide (Amaryl)	1, 2, and 4 mg	1–4 mg as single dose	Up to 24 hours	$0.87/4 mg	$26.10
Meglitinide analogs					
Repaglinide (Prandin)	0.5, 1, and 2 mg	4 mg in two divided doses given 15 minutes before breakfast and dinner	3 hours	$0.93/2 mg	$55.80
D-Phenylalanine derivative					
Nateglinide (Starlix)	60 mg and 120 mg	60 mg or 120 mg 3 times a day before meals	1.5 hours	$0.96/60 mg; $1.00/120 mg	$90.00

[1]Cost to pharmacist (average wholesale price, generic when possible) for maximum dosage listed. Source: *Drug Topics Red Book,* March 2002; Vol. 21, No. 3.

[2]There has been a decline in use of these formulations. In the case of chlorpropamide, the decline is due to its numerous side effects (see text).

stimulate insulin secretion. (2) Drugs that alter insulin action: Metformin works primarily in the liver. The thiazolidinediones appear to have their main effect on skeletal muscle and adipose tissue. (3) Drugs that principally affect absorption of glucose: The α-glucosidase inhibitors acarbose and miglitol are such currently available drugs.

1. Sulfonylureas—The mechanism of action of the sulfonylureas when they are acutely administered is due to their insulinotropic effect on pancreatic B cells. Sulfonylureas specifically bind to a receptor that closes an ATP-sensitive potassium channel of the pancreatic B cell, thereby depolarizing the cell membrane. This results in an influx of extracellular calcium through voltage-gated calcium channels, which causes insulin granules to move toward the cell surface, facilitating exocytosis.

Sulfonylureas are presently not indicated in the juvenile type ketosis-prone insulin-dependent diabetic,

Table 27–7. Oral antidiabetic drugs that are insulin-sparing.

Drug	Tablet Size	Daily Dose	Duration of Action	Cost per Unit	Cost for 30 Days' Treatment Based on Maximum Dosage[1]
Biguanides					
Metformin (Glucophage)	500, 850, 1000 mg	1–2.5 g. One tablet with meals 2 or 3 times daily	7–12 hours	$1.20/850 mg	$108.00
Extended-release metformin (Glucophage XR)	500 mg	500–2000 mg once a day	Up to 24 hours	$0.69/500 mg	$82.80
Thiazolidinediones					
Rosiglitazone (Avandia)	2, 4, 8 mg	4–8 mg daily (can be divided)	Up to 24 hours	$4.74/8 mg	$142.20
Pioglitazone (Actos)	15, 30, 45 mg	15–45 mg daily	Up to 24 hours	$4.74/30 mg	$142.20
Alpha-glucosidase inhibitors					
Acarbose (Precose)	50 and 100 mg	75–300 mg in 3 divided doses with first bite of food	4 hours	$0.74/100 mg	$66.60
Miglitol (Glyset)	25, 50, and 100 mg	75–300 mg in 3 divided doses with first bite of food	4 hours	$0.76/100 mg	$68.40

[1]Cost to pharmacist (average wholesale price, generic when possible) for maximum dosage listed. Source: *Drug Topics Red Book,* March 2002; Vol. 21, No. 3.

since these drugs seem to depend on functioning pancreatic B cells. There is little, if any, potentiation of insulin effectiveness on long-term glycemic control when sulfonylureas are added in type 1 patients, which argues against any substantial extrapancreatic effect of sulfonylureas.

The sulfonylureas seem most appropriate for use in nonobese mild type 2 diabetic patients. In this group, acute administration of sulfonylureas improves the early phase of insulin release that is refractory to acute glucose stimulation. In obese mild diabetics and others with peripheral insensitivity to levels of circulating insulin, primary emphasis should be on weight reduction. When hyperglycemia in obese diabetics has been more severe, with consequent impairment of pancreatic B cell function, sulfonylureas may improve glycemic control until concurrent measures such as diet, exercise, and weight reduction can sustain the improvement without the need for oral drugs. Sulfonylureas are generally contraindicated in patients

Table 27–8. Combination oral antidiabetic drugs.

Drug	Tablet Size	Daily Dose	Duration of Action	Cost per Unit	Cost for 30 Days' Treatment Based on Maximum Dosage[1]
Glyburide/metformin (Glucovance)	1.25 mg/250 mg 2.5 mg/500 mg 5 mg/500 mg	Maximum daily dose of 20 mg glyburide/ 2000 mg metformin	See individual drugs[2]	$0.86/5/ 500 mg	$103.20

[1]Cost to pharmacist (average wholesale price, generic when possible) for maximum dosage listed. Source: *Drug Topics Red Book,* March 2002; Vol. 21, No. 3.
[2]Glyburide, Table 27–6; metformin, Table 27–7.

with hepatic or renal impairment. Idiosyncratic reactions are rare, with skin rashes or hematologic toxicity (leukopenia, thrombocytopenia) occurring in less than 0.1% of users.

a. First-generation sulfonylureas (tolbutamide, tolazamide, acetohexamide, chlorpropamide)— **Tolbutamide** is supplied as 500 mg tablets. It is rapidly oxidized in the liver to inactive metabolites, and its approximate duration of effect is relatively short (6–10 hours). Tolbutamide is probably best administered in divided doses (eg, 500 mg before each meal and at bedtime); however, some patients require only one or two tablets daily with a maximum dose of 3000 mg/d. Because of its short duration of action, which is independent of renal function, tolbutamide is probably the safest sulfonylurea to use if liver function is normal. Prolonged hypoglycemia has been reported rarely with tolbutamide, mostly in patients receiving certain antibacterial sulfonamides (sulfisoxazole), phenylbutazone for arthralgias, or the oral azole antifungal drugs to treat candidiasis. These drugs apparently compete with tolbutamide for oxidative enzyme systems in the liver, resulting in maintenance of high levels of unmetabolized, active sulfonylurea in the circulation.

Tolazamide is supplied in tablets of 100, 250, and 500 mg. It has a longer duration of action than tolbutamide, lasting up to 20 hours, with maximal hypoglycemic effect occurring between the fourth and fourteenth hours. It is often effective, as are other longer-acting sulfonylureas also, when tolbutamide fails to correct prebreakfast hyperglycemia. Tolazamide is metabolized to several compounds that retain hypoglycemic effects. If more than 500 mg/d is required, the dose should be divided and given twice daily. Doses larger than 1000 mg daily do not improve the degree of glycemic control.

Acetohexamide and chlorpropamide are now rarely used. Chlorpropamide has a prolonged biologic effect, and severe hypoglycemia can occur especially in the elderly as their renal clearance declines with aging. Its other side effects include alcohol-induced flushing and hyponatremia due its effect on vasopresssin secretion and action.

b. Second-generation sulfonylureas—Glyburide, glipizide, and glimeperide are 100–200 times more potent than tolbutamide. These drugs should be used with caution in patients with cardiovascular disease or in elderly patients, in whom prolonged hypoglycemia would be especially dangerous.

Glyburide is available in 1.25, 2.5, and 5 mg tablets. The usual starting dose is 2.5 mg/d, and the average maintenance dose is 5–10 mg/d given as a single morning dose; maintenance doses higher than 20 mg/d are not recommended. Some reports suggest that 10 mg is a maximum daily therapeutic dose, with 15–20 mg having no additional benefit in poor responders and doses over 20 mg actually worsening hyperglycemia. Glyburide is metabolized in the liver into

products with hypoglycemic activity, which probably explains why assays specific for the unmetabolized compound suggest a plasma half-life of only 1–2 hours, yet the biologic effects of glyburide are clearly persistent 24 hours after a single morning dose in diabetic patients. Glyburide is unique among sulfonylureas in that it not only binds to the pancreatic B cell membrane sulfonylurea receptor but also becomes sequestered within the B cell. This may also contribute to its prolonged biologic effect despite its relatively short circulating half-life. A "Press Tab" formulation of "micronized" glyburide—easy to divide in half with slight pressure if necessary—is available in tablet sizes of 1.5 mg, 3 mg, and 6 mg.

Glyburide has few adverse effects other than its potential for causing hypoglycemia, which at times can be prolonged. Flushing has rarely been reported after ethanol ingestion. It does not cause water retention, as chlorpropamide does, but rather slightly enhances free water clearance. Glyburide is absolutely contraindicated in the presence of hepatic impairment and should not be used in patients with renal insufficiency, in elderly patients, or in those who would be put at serious risk from an episode of hypoglycemia.

Glipizide is available in 5 and 10 mg tablets. For maximum effect in reducing postprandial hyperglycemia, this agent should be ingested 30 minutes before meals, since rapid absorption is delayed when the drug is taken with food. The recommended starting dose is 5 mg/d with up to 15 mg/d given as a single daily dose before breakfast. When higher daily doses are required, they should be divided and given before meals. The maximum dose recommended by the manufacturer is 40 mg/d, though doses above 10–15 mg probably provide little additional benefit in poor responders and may even be *less* effective than smaller doses.

At least 90% of glipizide is metabolized in the liver to inactive products, and 10% is excreted unchanged in the urine. Glipizide therapy is therefore contraindicated in patients with hepatic or renal impairment, who would be at high risk for hypoglycemia, but because of its lower potency and shorter duration of action it is preferable to glyburide in elderly patients. Glipizide has also been marketed as Glucotrol-XL in 5 mg and 10 mg tablets. It provides extended release during transit through the gastrointestinal tract with greater effectiveness in lowering prebreakfast hyperglycemia than the shorter-duration immediate-release standard glipizide tablets. However, this formulation appears to have sacrificed its lower propensity for severe hypoglycemia compared with longer-acting glyburide without showing any demonstrable therapeutic advantages over glyburide.

Glimeperide is given once daily as monotherapy or in combination with insulin to lower blood glucose in diabetes patients who cannot control their glucose level through diet and exercise. Glimeperide achieves blood glucose lowering with the lowest dose of any sulfonylurea compound and this tends to increase its cost-effectiveness. A single daily dose of 1 mg/d has been shown to be effective, and the maximal recommended dose is 8 mg. It has a long duration of action with a pharmacodynamic half-life of 5 hours, allowing once-daily administration, which improves compliance. It is completely metabolized by the liver to relatively inactive metabolic products.

2. Meglitinide analogs—Repaglinide is structurally similar to glyburide but lacks the sulfonic acid-urea moiety. It acts by binding to the sulfonylurea receptor and closing the ATP-sensitive potassium channel. It is rapidly absorbed from the intestine and then undergoes complete metabolism in the liver to inactive biliary products, giving it a plasma half-life of less than 1 hour. The drug therefore causes a brief but rapid pulse of insulin. The starting dose is 0.5 mg three times a day 15 minutes before each meal. The dose can be titrated to a maximal daily dose of 16 mg. Like the sulfonylureas, repaglinide can be used in combination with metformin. Hypoglycemia is the main side effect. In clinical trials, when the drug was compared with a long-duration sulfonlyurea (glyburide), there was a trend toward less hypoglycemia. Like the sulfonylureas also, repaglinide causes weight gain. Metabolism is by cytochrome P450 3A4 isoenzyme, and other drugs that induce or inhibit this isoenzyme may increase or inhibit (respectively) the metabolism of repaglinide. The drug may be useful in patients with renal impairment or in the elderly. It remains to be shown that this drug has significant advantages over short-acting sulfonylureas.

3. D-Phenylalanine derivative—Nateglinide stimulates insulin secretion by binding to the sulfonylurea receptor and closing the ATP-sensitive potassium channel. This compound is rapidly absorbed from the intestine, reaching peak plasma levels within 1 hour. It is metabolized in the liver and has a plasma half-life of about 1.5 hours. Like repaglinide, it causes a brief rapid pulse of insulin, and when given before a meal it reduces the postprandial rise in blood glucose. The drug is available as 60 mg and 120 mg tablets. The 60 mg dose is used in patients who have mild elevations in HbA_{1c}. For most patients, the recommended starting and maintenance dose is 120 mg three times a day before meals. Like the other insulin secretagogues, its main side effects are hypoglycemia and weight gain. This drug has been approved for use either alone or in combination with metformin.

4. Metformin—Metformin (1,1-dimethylbiguanide hydrochloride) was introduced in France in 1957 as an oral agent for therapy of type 2 diabetes, either alone or in conjunction with sulfonylureas. In 1995 it became available in the United States.

a. Clinical pharmacology—The exact mechanism of action of metformin remains unclear. It reduces both the fasting level of blood glucose and the degree of postprandial hyperglycemia in patients with type 2 diabetes but has no effect on fasting blood glu-

cose in normal subjects. Metformin is particularly effective in reducing hepatic gluconeogenesis by interfering with lactate oxidation and uptake by the liver. Other proposed mechanisms include a slowing down of gastrointestinal absorption of glucose and increased glucose uptake by skeletal muscle, which have been reported in some but not all clinical studies. Because of its very high concentration in intestinal cells after oral administration, metformin increases glucose to lactate turnover, which may account for a reduction in hyperglycemia.

Metformin has a half-life of 1½–3 hours, is not bound to plasma proteins, and is not metabolized in humans, being excreted unchanged by the kidneys.

b. Indications and dosage—Metformin may be used as an adjunct to diet for the control of hyperglycemia and its associated symptomatology in patients with type 2 diabetes, particularly those who are obese or are not responding optimally to maximal doses of sulfonylureas. A side benefit of metformin therapy is its tendency to improve both fasting and postprandial hyperglycemia and hypertriglyceridemia in obese diabetics without the weight gain associated with insulin or sulfonylurea therapy. Metformin is not indicated for patients with type 1 diabetes and is contraindicated in diabetics with serum creatinine levels of 1.5 mg/dL or higher, hepatic insufficiency, alcoholism, or a propensity to develop tissue hypoxia.

Metformin is dispensed as 500 mg, 850 mg, and 1000 mg tablets. A 500 mg extended-release preparation is also available. Although the maximal dosage is 2.55 g, little benefit is seen above a total dose of 2000 mg. It is important to begin with a low dose and increase the dosage very gradually in divided doses—taken with meals—to reduce minor gastrointestinal upsets. A common schedule would be one 500 mg tablet three times a day with meals or one 850 mg or 1000 mg tablet twice daily at breakfast and dinner. One to four tablets of the extended-release preparation can be given once a day.

c. Adverse reactions—The most frequent side effects of metformin are gastrointestinal symptoms (anorexia, nausea, vomiting, abdominal discomfort, diarrhea), which occur in up to 20% of patients. These effects are dose-related, tend to occur at onset of therapy, and often are transient. However, in 3–5% of patients, therapy may have to be discontinued because of persistent diarrheal discomfort.

Hypoglycemia does not occur with therapeutic doses of metformin, which permits its description as a "euglycemic" or "antihyperglycemic" drug rather than an oral hypoglycemic agent. Dermatologic or hematologic toxicity is rare.

Lactic acidosis (see below) has been reported as a side effect but is uncommon with metformin in contrast to phenformin. While therapeutic doses of metformin reduce lactate uptake by the liver, serum lactate levels rise only minimally if at all, since other organs such as the kidney can remove the slight excess.

However, if tissue hypoxia occurs, the metformin-treated patient is at higher risk for lactic acidosis due to compromised lactate removal. Similarly, when renal function deteriorates, affecting not only lactate removal by the kidney but also metformin excretion, plasma levels of metformin rise far above the therapeutic range and block hepatic uptake enough to provoke lactic acidosis without associated increases in lactic acid production. Almost all reported cases have involved subjects with associated risk factors that should have contraindicated its use (renal, hepatic, or cardiorespiratory insufficiency, alcoholism, advanced age). Acute renal failure can occur rarely in certain patients receiving radiocontrast agents. Metformin therapy should therefore be temporarily halted on the day of the test and for 2 days following injection of radiocontrast agents to avoid potential lactic acidosis if renal failure occurs.

5. Thiazolidinediones—Drugs of this newer class of antihyperglycemic agents sensitize peripheral tissues to insulin. They bind a nuclear receptor called peroxisome proliferator-activated receptor gamma (PPAR-γ) and affect the expression of a number of genes and regulate the release of the adipokines—resistin and adiponectin—from adipocytes. Adiponectin secretion is stimulated, which sensitizes tissues to the effects of insulin; and resistin secretion is inhibited, which reduces insulin resistance. Observed effects of thiazolidinediones include increased glucose transporter expression (GLUT 1 and GLUT 4), decreased free fatty acid levels, decreased hepatic glucose output, and increased differentiation of preadipocytes into adipocytes. Like the biguanides, this class of drugs does not cause hypoglycemia.

Troglitazone was the first drug in this class to go into widespread clinical use. Unfortunately, about 1.9% of patients taking this drug developed elevations in liver enzymes greater than three times normal, which resolved when the drug was stopped. Liver failure, however, occurred if the drug was continued—at least 90 cases have been reported, and 63 of these patients have died. The drug has therefore been withdrawn from clinical use.

Two other drugs in the same class are available for clinical use: Rosiglitazone and pioglitazone. Both are effective as monotherapy and in combination with sulfonylureas or metformin. However, at present, only pioglitazone is approved by the FDA for use in combination with insulin. This is because in two clinical trials with 611 type 2 diabetic patients over a 26-week period, rosiglitazone in combination with insulin caused more congestive heart failure and other cardiovascular events than did insulin alone. Fluid retention has been invoked as the reason for this adverse effect of rosiglitazone when combined with insulin. When used as monotherapy, these drugs lower HbA$_{1c}$ by about 1 or 2 percentage points. When used in combination with insulin, they can result in a 30–50% reduction in insulin dosage, and some patients can come off insulin completely. The combination of a thiazolidinedione and metformin has the advantage of not causing hypoglycemia. Patients inadequately managed on sulfonylureas can do well on a combination of sulfonylurea and rosiglitazone or pioglitazone. About 25% of patients in clinical trials fail to respond to these drugs, presumably because they are significantly insulinopenic.

Rosiglitazone therapy is associated with increases in total cholesterol, LDL cholesterol (15%), and HDL cholesterol (10%). There is reduction in free fatty acids of about 8–15%. The changes in triglycerides were generally not different from placebo. The increase in the LDL cholesterol need not necessarily be detrimental—studies with troglitazone showed that there is a shift from the atherogenic small dense LDL particles to larger, less dense LDL particles. Pioglitazone in clinical trials lowered triglycerides (9%) and increased HDL cholesterol (15%) but did not cause a consistent change in total cholesterol and LDL cholesterol levels. There have not been any direct comparisons of rosiglitazone and pioglitazone, and the purported differences in the lipid profiles may simply reflect differences in the clinical study design rather than real differences in the drugs. Anemia occurs in 4% of patients treated with these drugs, but this effect may be due to a dilutional effect of increased plasma volume rather than a reduction in red cell mass. Weight gain occurs especially when the drug is combined with a sulfonylurea or insulin. Several studies suggest that thiazolidinediones cause a decrease in intra-abdominal fat mass but do not affect total body fat or body weight. It is believed that this class of drugs might increase proliferation of subcutaneous preadipocytes, thereby increasing target cell responsiveness to insulin. This would make the drugs of particular benefit for patients with syndrome X.

The dosage of rosiglitazone is 4–8 mg daily and of pioglitazone 15–45 mg daily, and the drugs do not have to be taken with food. Rosiglitazone is primarily metabolized by the CYP 2C8 isoenzyme and unlike troglitazone does not appear to affect CYP 3A4 isoenzyme and has no significant clinical effect on oral contraceptives. Pioglitazone is metabolized by CYP 2C8 and CYP 3A4. The pharmacokinetics of coadministration of pioglitazone and oral contraceptives has not been evaluated.

These two agents have so far not (unlike troglitazone) caused drug-induced hepatotoxicity. The FDA has, however, recommended that patients should not initiate drug therapy if the ALT is 2.5 times greater than the upper limit of normal. Obviously, caution should be used in initiation of therapy in patients with even mild ALT elevations. Liver function tests should be performed once every 2 months for the first year and periodically thereafter.

The thiazolidinediones have only recently become clinically available, and obviously it will take some time before their long-term safety is established.

6. Alpha-glucosidase inhibitors—This family of drugs competitively inhibits the alpha-glucosidase enzymes in the gut which digest dietary starch and sucrose. Two of these drugs—acarbose and miglitol—are available for clinical use. Both are potent inhibitors of glucoamylase, α-amylase, and sucrase but have less effect on isomaltase and hardly any on trehalase and lactase. A fundamental difference between acarbose and miglitol is in their absorption. Acarbose has the molecular mass and structural features of a tetrasaccharide, and very little (about 2%) crosses the microvillar membrane. Miglitol, however, has a structural similarity with glucose and is absorbable. Both drugs delay the absorption of carbohydrate and lower postprandial glycemic excursion.

a. Acarbose—Acarbose binds 1000 times more avidly to the intestinal disaccharidases than do products of carbohydrate digestion or sucrose. In diabetic patients, acarbose reduces postprandial hyperglycemia by 30–50%, and its overall effect is to lower the HbA_{1c} by 0.5–1%. The principal adverse effect, seen in 20–30% of patients, is flatulence. This is caused by undigested carbohydrate reaching the lower bowel, where gases are produced by bacterial flora. In 3% of cases, troublesome diarrhea occurs. This gastrointestinal discomfort tends to discourage excessive carbohydrate consumption and promotes improved compliance of type 2 patients with their diet prescriptions. The recommended starting dose of acarbose is 25 mg once or twice daily. This can be titrated upward slowly over 1 or 2 months to a maximum dosage of 100 mg three times a day. The more slowly the dose is raised, the less the bowel discomfort. For maximal benefit on postprandial hyperglycemia, acarbose should be given with the first mouthful of food ingested. When acarbose is given alone, there is no risk of hypoglycemia. However if combined with insulin or sulfonylureas, it might increase the risk of hypoglycemia from these agents. A slight rise in hepatic aminotransferases has been noted in clinical trials with acarbose (5% versus 2% in placebo controls, and particularly with doses > 300 mg/d). The levels generally return to normal on stopping the drug.

In the UKPDS, approximately 2000 patients on diet, sulfonylurea, metformin, or insulin therapy were randomized to acarbose or placebo therapy. By 3 years, 60% of the patients had discontinued the drug, mostly because of gastrointestinal symptoms. If one looked only at the 40% who remained on the drug, they had an 0.5% lower HbA_{1c} compared with placebo.

b. Miglitol—Miglitol is similar to acarbose in terms of its clinical effects. It is indicated for use in diet- or sulfonylurea-treated patients with type 2 diabetes. Therapy is initiated at the lowest effective dosage of 25 mg three times a day. The usual maintenance dose is 50 mg three times a day, though some patients may benefit from increasing the dose to 100 mg three times a day. Gastrointestinal side effects occur as with acarbose. The drug is not metabolized and is excreted unchanged by the kidney. Theoretically, absorbable α-glucosidase inhibitors could induce a deficiency of one or more of the α-glucosidases involved in cellular glycogen metabolism and biosynthesis of glycoproteins. This does not occur in practice because, unlike the intestinal mucosa, which sees a high concentration of the drug, the blood level is 200-fold to 1000-fold lower than the concentration needed to inhibit intracellular α-glucosidases. Miglitol should not be used in renal failure, when its clearance would be impaired.

7. Drug combinations—A glyburide and metformin combination (Glucovance) is available in dose forms of 1.25 mg/250 mg, 2.5 mg/500 mg, and 5 mg/500 mg. This combination, however, limits the clinician's ability to optimally adjust dosage of the individual drugs and for that reason is of questionable merit.

8. Safety of the oral hypoglycemic agents—The recently published United Kingdom Prospective Diabetes Study of type 2 diabetes (see below) has put to rest previous concerns regarding the safety of sulfonylureas. It did not confirm any cardiovascular hazard among over 1500 patients treated intensively with sulfonylureas for over 10 years, compared with a comparable number who received either insulin or diet therapy. Analysis of a subgroup of obese patients receiving metformin also showed no hazard and even a slight reduction in cardiovascular deaths compared with conventional therapy.

The currently available thiazolidinediones have not to date exhibited the idiosyncratic hepatotoxicity seen with troglitazone. Lactic acidosis from metformin (see above) is quite rare and probably not a major problem with its use in the absence of major risk factors such as impaired renal or hepatic disease or conditions predisposing to hypoxia.

C. INSULIN

Insulin is indicated for type 1 diabetes as well as for type 2 diabetic patients with insulinopenia whose hyperglycemia does not respond to diet therapy either alone or combined with oral hypoglycemic drugs.

With the development of highly purified human insulin preparations, immunogenicity has been markedly reduced, thereby decreasing the incidence of therapeutic complications such as insulin allergy, immune insulin resistance, and localized lipoatrophy at the injection site. However, the problem of achieving optimal insulin delivery remains unsolved with the present state of technology. It has not been possible to reproduce the physiologic patterns of intraportal insulin secretion with subcutaneous injections of soluble or longer-acting insulin suspensions. Even so, with the help of appropriate modifications of diet and exercise and careful monitoring of capillary blood glucose levels at home, it has often been possible to achieve acceptable control of blood glucose by using various mixtures of short- and longer-acting insulins injected at least twice daily or portable insulin infusion pumps.

1. Characteristics of available insulin preparations—Commercial insulin preparations differ with respect to the animal species from which they are obtained, their purity and solubility, and the time of onset and duration of their biologic action. As many as 17 different formulations of insulin are available in the USA.

a. Species of insulin—Human insulin is produced by recombinant DNA techniques (biosynthetic human insulin) as Humulin (Eli Lilly) and as Novolin (Novo Nordisk). It is dispensed as either regular (R), NPH (N), lente (L), or ultralente (U) formulations (see Table 27–9). Three analogs of human insulin—two rapidly acting (insulin lispro, insulin aspart) and one very long-acting (insulin glargine)—are now available for clinical use (see below). A limited supply of monospecies pork insulin (Iletin II) remains available for use in certain patients who may benefit from the slightly more prolonged and sustained effect of animal insulin compared with human insulin. The cost of human insulin is slightly less than the cost of purified pork insulin.

b. Purity of insulin—"Purified" insulin is defined by FDA regulations as the degree of purity wherein proinsulin contamination is less than 10 ppm, whether extracted from animal pancreas or produced from biosynthetic proinsulin. All human insulin and pork insulin products of Novo Nordisk and Eli Lilly presently available contain less than 10 ppm of proinsulin and are labeled as "purified." These purified insulins seem to preserve their potency quite well, so that refrigeration is recommended but not crucial. During travel, reserve supplies of insulin can thus be readily transported for weeks without losing potency if protected from extremes of heat or cold.

c. Concentration of insulin—At present, insulins are available in a concentration of 100 units/mL (U100), and all are dispensed in 10 mL vials. With the popularity of "low-dose" (0.5 or 0.3 mL) disposable insulin syringes, U100 can be measured with acceptable accuracy in doses as low as 1–2 units. For use in rare cases of severe insulin resistance in which large quantities of insulin are required, U500 regular human insulin (Humulin R) is available from Eli Lilly.

2. Insulin preparations—(Table 27–9.) Four principal types of insulins are available: (1) ultra-short-acting, with very rapid onset and short duration; (2) short-acting, with rapid onset of action; (3) intermediate-acting; and (4) long-acting, with slow onset of action (Table 27–9 and Figure 27–1). Ultra-short-acting and short-acting insulins are dispensed as clear solutions at neutral pH and contain small amounts of zinc to improve their stability and shelf life. All other commercial insulins have been modified to provide prolonged action and are dispensed as turbid suspensions at neutral pH with either protamine in phosphate buffer (NPH insulin) or varying concentrations of zinc in acetate buffer (ultralente and lente insulins). These suspensions of insulin are designed for subcutaneous administration only, while the short-acting and ultra-short-acting insulins can also be given intravenously.

a. Ultra-short-acting insulin—Insulin lispro (Humalog) is an insulin analog, produced by recombinant technology, wherein two amino acids near the carboxyl terminal of the B chain have been reversed in position: proline at position B28 has been moved to B29 and lysine has been moved from B29 to B28. Insulin aspart (Novolog) is a single substitution of proline by aspartic acid at position B28. These changes result in these two analogs having less tendency to form hexamers, in contrast to human insulin. When injected subcutaneously, the analogs quickly dissociate into monomers and are absorbed very rapidly, reaching peak serum values in as soon as 1 hour—in contrast to regular human insulin, whose hexamers require considerably more time to dissociate and become absorbed. The amino acid changes in these analogs do not interfere with their binding to the insulin receptor, with the circulating half-life, or with their immunogenicity, which are all identical with those of human regular insulin.

Clinical trials have demonstrated that the optimal times of preprandial subcutaneous injection of comparable doses of the ultrashort-acting insulin and analogs and of regular human insulin are 20 minutes and 60 minutes, respectively, before the meal. While this ultrarapid onset of action has been welcomed as a great convenience by diabetic patients who object to waiting as long as 60 minutes after injecting regular human insulin before they can begin their meal, patients must be taught to ingest adequate absorbable carbohydrate early in the meal to avoid hypoglycemia during the meal. Another desirable feature of insulin lispro is that its duration of action remains at about 4 hours irrespective of dosage. This contrasts with regular insulin, whose duration of action is prolonged when larger doses are used.

b. Short-acting insulin—Regular insulin is a short-acting soluble crystalline zinc insulin whose effect appears within 30 minutes after subcutaneous injection and lasts 5–7 hours when usual quantities are administered. Intravenous infusions of regular insulin are particularly useful in the treatment of diabetic ketoacidosis and during the perioperative management of insulin-requiring diabetics. When intravenous insulin is needed for hyperglycemic emergencies, insulin lispro has no advantage over regular human insulin, which is instantly converted to the monomeric form when given intravenously and which is 30–40% less costly than insulin lispro. Regular insulin is indicated when the subcutaneous insulin requirement is changing rapidly, such as after surgery or during acute infections—although the ultrashort-acting analogs may be preferable in these situations.

Table 27–9. Some insulin preparations available in the USA.[1,2]

Preparation	Species Source	Concentration	Cost[2]
Ultra-short-acting insulins			
Insulin lispro (Humalog, Lilly)	Human analog (recombinant)	U100	$50.09
Insulin aspart (Novolog, Novo Nordisk)	Human analog (recombinant)	U100	$50.09
Short-acting insulins "Purified"[3]			
Regular Novolin (Novo Nordisk)[4]	Human	U100	$26.56
Regular Humulin (Lilly)	Human	U100, U500 20 mL	$26.56 $191.09
Regular Iletin II (Lilly)	Pork	U100	$47.98
Velosulin (Novo Nordisk)[5]	Human	U100	$39.00
Intermediate-acting insulins "Purified"[3]			
Lente Humulin (Lilly)	Human	U100	$26.56
Lente Iletin II (Lilly)	Pork	U100	$47.98
Lente (Novo Nordisk) Novolin	Human	U100	$26.56
NPH Humulin (Lilly)	Human	U100	$26.56
NPH Iletin II (Lilly)	Pork	U100	$47.98
NPH (Novo Nordisk) Novolin	Human	U100	$26.56
Premixed insulins % NPH/% regular			
Novolin 70/30 (Novo Nordisk)	Human	U100	$26.56
Humulin 70/30 and 50/50 (Lilly)	Human	U100	$26.56
% NPL/% insulin lispro			
Humalog Mix 75/25 (Lilly)	Human analog (recombinant)	U100 (insulin pen, prefilled syringes, 5×3 mL cartridges)	Pen $100.80 Vial $50.09
Long-acting insulins "Purified"[3]			
Ultralente Humulin (Lilly)	Human	U100	$26.56
Insulin glargine (Lantus, Aventis)	Human analog (recombinant)	U100	$46.99[6]

[1]Modified and reproduced, with permission, from Katzung BG (editor): *Basic and Clinical Pharmacology*, 8th ed. McGraw-Hill, 2001.
[2]All of these agents (except insulin lispro and U500) are available without a prescription. Cost to pharmacist (average wholesale price, generic when possible) for 10 mL-vial unless otherwise specified. Source: *Drug Topics Red Book*, March 2002; Vol. 21, No. 3. Wholesale prices for all human preparations (except insulin lispro and U500) are similar.
[3]Less than 10 ppm proinsulin.
[4]Novo Nordisk human insulins are termed Novolin R, L, and N.
[5]Velosulin contains phosphate buffer, which favors its use to prevent insulin aggregation in pump tubing but precludes its being mixed with lente insulin. It is the only FDA-approved insulin for pump use.
[6]Personal communication and per Bergen Brunswick customer service information.

Aggregation of insulin solutions that cause clogging of tubing in insulin infusion pumps appears to be reduced by use of phosphate-buffered insulins. Novo Nordisk's Velosulin human insulin is a buffered regular insulin approved by the FDA for use in insulin pumps. The ultra-short-acting insulins are also com-

monly used in pumps. In a double-blind crossover study comparing insulin lispro with regular insulin in insulin pumps, subjects while using insulin lispro had lower HbA$_{1c}$ values and improved postprandial glucose control with the same frequency of hypoglycemia. Insulin aspart has been approved by the

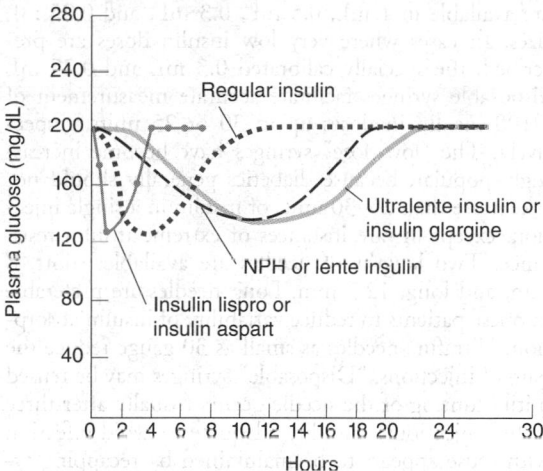

Figure 27–1. Extent and duration of action of various insulins (in a fasting diabetic). Duration is extended considerably when the dose of a given formulation increases above average therapeutic doses (except for insulin lispro).

FDA for use in insulin pumps. The concern remains that in the event of pump failure, users of the ultra-short-acting insulins will have more rapid onset of hyperglycemia and ketosis.

c. Intermediate-acting insulins—Lente insulin is a mixture of 30% semilente (an amorphous precipitate of insulin with zinc ions) with 70% ultralente insulin (an insoluble crystal of zinc and insulin). Its onset of action is delayed for up to 2 hours (Figure 27–1), and because its duration of action often is less than 24 hours (with a range of 18–24 hours), most patients require at least two injections daily to maintain a sustained insulin effect. Lente insulin has its peak effect in most patients between 8 and 12 hours, but individual variations in peak response time must be considered when interpreting unusual or unexpected patterns of glycemic responses in individual patients. While lente insulin is the most widely used of the lente series, particularly in conjunction with regular insulin, there has recently been a resurgence of use of ultralente in combination with multiple injections of rapid-acting insulin (regular insulin or insulin lispro) as a means of attempting optimal control in type 1 patients.

NPH (neutral protamine Hagedorn or isophane) insulin is an intermediate-acting insulin whose onset of action is delayed by combining two parts soluble crystalline zinc insulin with 1 part protamine zinc insulin. This produces equivalent amounts of insulin and protamine, so that neither is present in an uncomplexed form ("isophane").

The onset and duration of action of NPH insulin are comparable to those of lente insulin (Figure 27–1);

it is usually mixed with regular insulin and given at least twice daily for insulin replacement in type 1 patients. Occasional vials of NPH insulin have tended to show unusual clumping of their contents or "frosting" of the container, with considerable loss of bioactivity. This instability is rare and occurs less frequently if NPH human insulin is refrigerated when not in use and if bottles are discarded after 1 month of use.

d. Long acting insulins—Humulin ultralente is a crystalline insulin whose duration of action is less than that of the previously available beef ultralente. It is generally recommended that the daily dose be split into two equal doses given 12 hours apart. Its peak is less than that of NPH insulin, and it is often used to provide basal coverage while the short-acting insulins are used to cover the glucose rise associated with meals.

Insulin glargine is an insulin analog in which the asparagine at position 21 of the A chain of the human insulin molecule is replaced by glycine and two arginines are added to the carboxyl terminal of the B chain. The arginines raise the isoelectric point of the molecule closer to neutral, making it more soluble in an acidic environment. In contrast, human insulin has an isoelectric point of pH 5.4. Insulin glargine is a clear insulin which, when injected into the neutral pH environment of the subcutaneous tissue, forms microprecipitates that slowly release the insulin into the circulation. It lasts for about 24 hours without any pronounced peaks and is given once a day to provide basal coverage. This insulin cannot be mixed with the other human insulins because of its acidic pH. When this insulin was given as a single injection at bedtime to type 1 patients, fasting hyperglycemia was better controlled when compared with bedtime NPH insulin. The clinical trials also suggest that there may be less nocturnal hypoglycemia with this insulin when compared with NPH insulin.

In one clinical trial involving type 2 patients, insulin glargine was associated with a slightly higher progression of retinopathy when compared with NPH insulin. The frequency was 7.5% with the analog and 2.7% with the NPH. This finding, however, was not seen in other clinical trials with this analog. Insulin glargine does have a sixfold greater affinity for IgF 1 receptor compared with the human insulin. There has also been a report that insulin glargine had increased mitogenicity compared with human insulin in a human osteosarcoma cell line. The significance of these observations is not yet clear.

e. Mixtures of insulin—Since intermediate insulins require several hours to reach adequate therapeutic levels, their use in type 1 patients requires supplements of regular or lispro insulin preprandially. It is well established that insulin mixtures containing increased proportions of lente to regular insulins may retard the rapid action of admixed regular insulin. The excess zinc in lente insulin binds the soluble insulin and partially blunts its action, particularly when a relatively small proportion of regular insulin is mixed with lente (eg, 1 part regular to 1½ or more parts lente). NPH preparations do not contain excess protamine and so do not delay absorption of admixed regular insulin. They are therefore preferable to lente when mixtures of intermediate and regular insulins are prescribed. For convenience, regular and NPH insulin may be mixed together in the same syringe and injected subcutaneously in split dosage before breakfast and supper. It is recommended that the regular insulin be withdrawn first, then the NPH insulin. No attempt should be made to mix the insulins in the syringe, and the injection is preferably given immediately after loading the syringe. Stable premixed insulins (70% NPH and 30% regular or 50% of each) are available as a convenience to patients who have difficulty mixing insulin because of visual problems or impairment of manual dexterity.

With increasing use of ultra-short-acting insulin lispro as a popular and convenient preprandial insulin, it has become evident that combination with a more sustained insulin is essential to maintain postabsorptive glycemic control. It has been demonstrated that insulin lispro can be acutely mixed with either NPH or ultralente insulin without affecting its rapid absorption. There are no data on mixing insulin aspart with lente or ultralente insulins. Premixed preparations of lispro and NPH insulins are unstable because of exchange of insulin lispro with the human insulin in the protamine complex. Consequently, the soluble component becomes over time a mixture of regular and insulin lispro at varying ratios. In an attempt to remedy this, an intermediate insulin composed of isophane complexes of protamine with insulin lispro was developed called NPL (neutral protamine lispro). This insulin has the same duration of action as NPH insulin. Premixed combinations of NPL and insulin lispro (eg, 75:25, 50:50, and 25:75 of NPL:insulin lispro) have been tested. The 75% NPL:25% insulin lispro mixture (Humalog Mix 75/25) is available for clinical use. This new mixture has a more rapid onset of glucose-lowering activity compared with the 70% NPH:30% regular human insulin mixture, and it can therefore be given within 15 minutes of starting a meal. It remains to be shown that this new mixture has any other clinical advantage over the usual 70% NPH:30% regular mixture.

Since insulin lispro resists hexamer formation at pharmacologic concentrations, it appears to resist precipitation by high concentrations of zinc and thus cannot be used to make a lente or ultralente formulation. However, this lack of precipitation by zinc allows it to be mixed with any of the lente series—in contrast to regular insulin, which tends to be precipitated by the excess zinc in the lente series when mixed prior to injection.

3. Methods of insulin administration—

a. Insulin syringes and needles—Plastic disposable syringes with half-inch ultrafine needles attached are available in 1 mL, 0.5 mL, 0.3 mL, and 0.25 mL sizes. In cases where very low insulin doses are prescribed, the specially calibrated 0.3 mL and 0.25 mL disposable syringes facilitate accurate measurement of U100 insulin in doses up to 30 or 25 units, respectively. The "low-dose" syringes have become increasingly popular, because diabetics generally should not take more than 25–30 units of insulin in a single injection, except in rare instances of extreme insulin resistance. Two lengths of needles are available: short, 8 mm, and long, 12.7 mm. Long needles are preferable in obese patients to reduce variability of insulin absorption. Ultrafine needles as small as 30 gauge reduce the pain of injections. "Disposable" syringes may be reused until blunting of the needle occurs (usually after three to five injections). Sterility adequate to avoid infection with reuse appears to be maintained by recapping syringes between uses. Cleansing the needle with alcohol may not be desirable since it can dissolve the silicone coating and can increase the pain of skin puncturing.

b. Site of injection—Any part of the body covered by loose skin can be used, such as the abdomen, thighs, upper arms, flanks, and upper buttocks. Preparation with alcohol is no longer required prior to injection as long as the skin is clean. Rotation of sites continues to be recommended to avoid delayed absorption when fibrosis or lipohypertrophy occurs from repeated use of a single site. However, considerable variability of absorption rates from different sites, particularly with exercise, may contribute to the instability of glycemic control in certain type 1 patients if injection sites are rotated too frequently in different areas of the body. Consequently, it is best to limit injection sites to a single region of the body and rotate sites within that region. The abdomen is recommended for subcutaneous injections, since regular insulin has been shown to absorb more rapidly from there than from other subcutaneous sites.

c. Insulin delivery systems—In the United States, MiniMed, Disetronic, and Animas insulin infusion pumps are available for subcutaneous delivery of insulin. These pumps are small (about the size of a pager) and very easy to program. They offer many features, including the ability to set a number of different basal rates throughout the 24 hours and to adjust the time over which bolus doses are given. They also are able to detect pressure build-up if the catheter is kinked. Improvements have also been made in the infusion sets. The catheter connecting the insulin reservoir to the subcutaneous cannula can be disconnected, allowing the patient to remove the pump temporarily (eg, for bathing). The great advantage of continuous subcutaneous insulin infusion (CSII) is that it allows for establishment of a basal profile tailored to the patient. The patient therefore is able to eat with less regard to timing because the basal insulin infusion should maintain constant blood glucose between meals.

CSII therapy is appropriate for patients who are motivated, mechanically inclined, educated about diabetes (diet, insulin action, treatment of hypo- and hyperglycemia), and willing to monitor their blood glucose four to six times a day. Known complications of CSII include ketoacidosis, which can occur when insulin delivery is interrupted, and skin infections. Another disadvantage is its cost and the time demanded of physicians and staff in initiating therapy.

Standard methods of insulin administration with multiple subcutaneous injections of soluble, rapid-acting insulin before meals and injections of long-acting insulin or intermediate-acting insulin to maintain basal levels are therefore widely used for intensive insulin therapy. These regimens usually provide acceptable glycemic control if frequent self-monitoring of blood glucose is practiced.

To facilitate these multiple injection regimens, portable pen-sized injectors are available which contain cartridges of U100 regular human insulin and retractable needles (NovoPen, NovolinPen, Insuject). Cartridges of insulin lispro (Humalog) are available as well as disposable pens containing insulin lispro, NPH, 70/30 mixtures, and Humalog Mix 75/25. These injectors eliminate the need for carrying an insulin bottle and syringes during the day to provide multiple injections of insulin.

A novel method for delivering preprandial insulin by inhalation has been reported. A 12-week study in type 1 patients showed that inhaled insulin is as efficacious as subcutaneously delivered insulin without additional side effects. Patients required 300–400 units of insulin a day, since only 10% of the inhaled insulin is bioavailable. Studies are in progress to determine whether adequate glycemic control can be sustained with inhaled insulin and whether long-term use affects pulmonary tissues.

D. Insulin-Like Growth Factor-1 (IGF-1) Therapy

In patients with severe insulin resistance who respond poorly to insulin, the use of IGF-1 has been advocated. IGF-1 is a 70-amino-acid peptide which is homologous to human proinsulin. An intravenous bolus of 13 nmol produces hypoglycemia in humans similar to a bolus of 1 nmol of insulin. Several patients with severe insulin resistance due to insulin receptor mutations have responded to IGF-1 but not to insulin, suggesting that the hypoglycemic action of IGF-1 is via its own receptor and not by cross-reacting with the receptor for insulin. Although its use in some cases of severe insulin resistance has been advocated, IGF-1 may promote tumor growth, and there are serious questions about its safety in other than short-term use.

E. Aspirin Therapy

A dose of 81–325 mg of enteric-coated aspirin given once daily has been shown to effectively inhibit thromboxane synthesis by platelets and reduce the risk of diabetic atherothrombosis without increasing risks of either vitreous or gastrointestinal hemorrhage. Since diabetic patients have up to a fourfold increase in risk of dying from cardiovascular disease, the use of low-dose enteric-coated aspirin is recommended in diabetic adults with evident macrovascular disease or in those with increased cardiovascular risk factors. Contraindications for aspirin therapy are patients with aspirin allergy, bleeding tendency, recent gastrointestinal bleeding, or active hepatic disease.

General Considerations in Treatment of Diabetes

Insulin-treated patients with diabetes can have a full and satisfying life. However, "free" diets and unrestricted activity are still not advised. Until new methods of insulin replacement are developed that provide more normal patterns of insulin delivery in response to metabolic demands, multiple feedings with carbohydrate counting will continue to be recommended, and certain occupations potentially hazardous to the patient or others will continue to be prohibited because of risks due to hypoglycemia. The American Diabetic Association can act as a patient advocate in case of employment questions.

Exercise increases the effectiveness of insulin, and moderate exercise is an excellent means of improving utilization of fat and carbohydrate in diabetic patients. A judicious balance of the size and frequency of meals with moderate regular exercise can often stabilize the insulin dosage in diabetics who tend to slip out of control easily. Strenuous exercise can precipitate hypoglycemia in an unprepared patient, and diabetics must therefore be taught to reduce their insulin dosage in anticipation of strenuous activity or to take supplemental carbohydrate. Injection of insulin into a site farthest away from the muscles most involved in exercise may help ameliorate exercise-induced hypoglycemia, since insulin injected in the proximity of exercising muscle may be more rapidly mobilized.

All diabetic patients must receive adequate instruction on personal hygiene, especially with regard to care of the feet (see Box 27–1), skin, and teeth. All infections (especially pyogenic ones) provoke the release of high levels of insulin antagonists such as catecholamines or glucagon and thus bring about a marked increase in insulin requirements. Supplemental regular insulin is often required to correct hyperglycemia during infection.

Clinical Trials in Type 1 Diabetes:

A. Diabetes Prevention Trial-1 (DPT-1)

This NIH-sponsored multicenter study was designed to determine whether the development of type 1 diabetes could be prevented or delayed by immune intervention therapy. Daily low-dose insulin injections were administered for up to 8 years in first-degree relatives of type 1 diabetics who were selected as being at high risk for development of type 1 diabetes because

INSTRUCTIONS IN THE CARE OF THE FEET
FOR PERSONS WITH DIABETES MELLITUS OR VASCULAR DISTURBANCES

Hygiene of the Feet

(1) Wash feet daily with mild soap and lukewarm water. Dry thoroughly between the toes by pressure. Do not rub vigorously, as this is apt to break the delicate skin.

(2) When feet are thoroughly dry, rub well with vegetable oil to keep them soft, prevent excess friction, remove scales, and prevent dryness. Care must be taken to prevent foot tenderness.

(3) If the feet become too soft and tender, rub them with alcohol about once a week.

(4) When rubbing the feet, always rub upward from the tips of the toes. If varicose veins are present, massage the feet very gently; never massage the legs.

(5) If the toenails are brittle and dry, soften them by soaking for one-half hour each night in lukewarm water containing 1 tbsp of powdered sodium borate (borax) per quart. Follow this by rubbing around the nails with vegetable oil. Clean around the nails with an orangewood stick. If the nails become too long, file them with an emery board. File them straight across and no shorter than the underlying soft tissues of the toe. Never cut the corners of the nails. (The podiatrist should be informed if a patient has diabetes.)

(6) Wear low-heeled shoes of soft leather that fit the shape of the feet correctly. The shoes should have wide toes that will cause no pressure, fit close in the arch, and grip the heels snugly. Wear new shoes one-half hour only on the first day and increase by 1 hour each day following. Wear thick, warm, loose stockings.

Treatment of Corns & Calluses

(1) Corns and calluses are due to friction and pressure, most often from improperly fitted shoes and stockings. Wear shoes that fit properly and cause no friction or pressure.

(2) To remove excess calluses or corns, soak the feet in lukewarm (not hot) water, using a mild soap, for about 10 minutes and then rub off the excess tissue with a towel or file. Do not tear it off. Under no circumstances must the skin become irritated.

(3) Do not cut corns or calluses. If they need attention it is safer to see a podiatrist.

(4) Prevent callus formation under the ball of the foot (a) by exercise, such as curling and stretching the toes several times a day; (b) by finishing each step on the toes and not on the ball of the foot; and (c) by wearing shoes that are not too short and that do not have high heels.

Aids in Treatment of Impaired Circulation (Cold Feet)

(1) Never use tobacco in any form. Tobacco contracts blood vessels and so reduces circulation.

(2) Keep warm. Wear warm stockings and other clothing. Cold contracts blood vessels and reduces circulation.

(3) Do not wear circular garters, which compress blood vessels and reduce blood flow.

(4) Do not sit with the legs crossed. This may compress the leg arteries and shut off the blood supply to the feet.

(5) If the weight of the bedclothes is uncomfortable, place a pillow under the covers at the foot of the bed.

(6) Do not apply any medication to the feet without directions from a physician. Some medicines are too strong for feet with poor circulation.

(7) Do not apply heat in the form of hot water, hot water bottles, or heating pads without a physician's consent. Even moderate heat can injure the skin if circulation is poor.

(8) If the feet are moist or the patient has a tendency to develop athlete's foot, a prophylactic dusting powder should be used on the feet and in shoes and stockings daily. Change shoes and stockings at least daily or oftener.

Treatment of Abrasions of the Skin

(1) Proper first-aid treatment is of the utmost importance even in apparently minor injuries. Consult a physician immediately for any redness, blistering, pain, or swelling. Any break in the skin may become ulcerous or gangrenous unless properly treated by a physician.

(2) Dermatophytosis (athlete's foot), which begins with peeling and itching between the toes or discoloration or thickening of the toenails, should be treated immediately by a physician or podiatrist.

(3) Avoid strong irritating antiseptics such as tincture of iodine.

(4) As soon as possible after any injury, cover the area with sterile gauze, which may be purchased at drugstores. Only fine paper tape or cellulose tape should be used on the skin if adhesive retention of the gauze is required.

(5) Elevate and, as much as possible until recovery, avoid using the foot.

of detectable islet cell antibodies and reduced early-insulin release. Unfortunately, this immune intervention failed to affect the onset of type 1 diabetes in this cohort as compared with an untreated randomized group. Although this trial has been discontinued, a related study is still in progress using oral insulin in lower-risk first-degree relatives who have islet cell antibodies but whose early-insulin release remains intact.

B. The Diabetes Control and Complications Trial (DCCT)

A long-term therapeutic study involving 1441 type 1 patients reported that "near" normalization of blood glucose resulted in a delay in the onset and a major slowing of the progression of established microvascular and neuropathic complications of diabetes during an up to 10-year follow-up.

Multiple insulin injections (66%) or insulin pumps (34%) were used in the intensively treated group who were trained to modify their therapy depending on frequent glucose monitoring. The conventionally treated groups used no more than two insulin injections, and clinical well-being was the goal with no attempt to modify management based on HbA_{1c} or their glucose results.

In one-half of the subjects, a mean hemoglobin A_{1c} of 7.2% (normal: < 6%) and a mean blood glucose of 155 mg/dL was achieved using intensive therapy, while in the conventionally treated group, HbA_{1c} averaged 8.9% with an average blood glucose of 225 mg/dL. Over the study period, which averaged 7 years, there was an approximately 60% reduction in risk between the two groups in regard to diabetic retinopathy, nephropathy, and neuropathy.

Intensively treated patients had a threefold greater risk of serious hypoglycemia as well as a greater tendency toward weight gain. However, there were no deaths definitely attributable to hypoglycemia in any subjects in the DCCT study, and no evidence of posthypoglycemic cognitive damage was detected.

Reinterpretation of the published data from the DCCT trial suggests that "moderate" glycemic control (HbA_{1c} no higher than 2% above the upper limits of normal) rather than "tight" control was just as beneficial in reducing complications while producing fewer episodes of severe hypoglycemia. This implies that adjusting therapeutic glycemic goals a bit higher than those of the DCCT should retain the benefits of intensive insulin therapy at a somewhat lower risk.

The general consensus of the American Diabetes Association is that intensive insulin therapy associated with comprehensive self-management training should become standard therapy in type 1 patients after the age of puberty. Exceptions include those with advanced renal disease and the elderly, since, in these groups, the detrimental risks of hypoglycemia outweigh the benefits of tight glycemic control.

While patients with type 2 were not studied in the DCCT, the eye, kidney, and nerve abnormalities are quite similar in both types of diabetes, and it is likely that similar underlying mechanisms apply. Several important differences, however, must be considered. Since type 2 patients are generally from an older population with a high incidence of macrovascular disease, an episode of severe hypoglycemia entails much greater risk than it would in younger type 1 patients of the DCCT. Moreover, weight gain may be much greater in obese type 2 patients in whom intensive insulin therapy is attempted. These risks take on greater relevance in older type 2 patients who have a relatively lower prevalence of microangiopathy than type 1 patients and in whom prevention of microvascular disease over the long term is much less likely to influence morbidity and mortality because of the much more ominous consequences of their macrovascular disease.

To address these issues raised by the DCCT findings as well as a previous concern that sulfonylureas may *increase* cardiovascular deaths, as reported in 1970 by the University Group Diabetes Program, randomized clinical trials of intensive therapy have been conducted in patients with type 2 diabetes—as summarized in the following paragraphs.

Clinical Trials in Type 2 Diabetes

A. The Diabetes Prevention Program (DPP)

This is a randomized clinical trial in 3234 overweight men and women aged 25–85 years who showed impaired glucose tolerance. Preliminary results indicate that intervention with a low-fat diet and 150 minutes of moderate exercise (equivalent to a brisk walk) per week reduces the risk of progression to type 2 diabetes by 58% as compared with a matched control group.

Another arm of this trial demonstrated that use of 850 mg of metformin twice daily reduced the risk of developing type 2 diabetes by 31%, but this intervention was relatively ineffective in those who were either less obese or in the older age group.

With the demonstration that intervention can be successful in preventing progression to diabetes in these subjects, a recommendation has been made to change the terminology from the less comprehensible "impaired glucose tolerance" to "prediabetes." The latter is a term which the public can better understand and thus respond by implementing healthier diet and exercise habits.

B. The Veterans Administration Cooperative Study

This investigation involved 153 obese men who were moderately insulin-resistant and who were followed for only 27 months. Intensive insulin treatment resulted in mean HbA_{1c} differences from conventional insulin treatment (7.2% versus 9.5%) that were comparable to those reported from the Kumamoto Study. However, a difference in cardiovascular outcome in this study has prompted some concern. While conventional insulin therapy resulted in 26 total cardiovascular events, there were 35 total cardiovascular events in the intensively treated group. This difference in the relatively small population was not statistically significant, but when the total events were broken down to *major* events (myocardial infarction, stroke, cardiovascular death, congestive heart failure, or amputation), the 18 major events in the group treated intensively with insulin was reported to be statistically greater ($P = .04$) than the ten major events occurring with conventional treatment. While this difference may be a chance consequence of studying too few patients for too short a time, it raises the possibility that insulin-resistant patients with visceral obesity and long-standing type 2 diabetes may develop a greater risk of serious cardiovascular mishap when intensively treated with high doses of insulin. At the end of the study, 64% of the intensively treated group were either receiving (1) an average of 113 units of insulin per day when only two injections per day were used or (2) a mean dosage of 133 units per day when multiple injections were used. Unfortunately, the UKPDS (see below), which did not discern any effect of intensive therapy on cardiovascular outcomes, does not resolve the concern generated by the Veterans Administration Study since their patient population consisted of newly diagnosed diabetic patients in whom the obese subgroup seemed to be less insulin-resistant, requiring a median insulin dose for intensive therapy of only 60 units per day by the 12th year of the study.

C. The United Kingdom Prospective Diabetes Study (UKPDS)

This study began in 1977 as a multicenter clinical trial designed to establish, in type 2 diabetic patients, whether the risk of macrovascular or microvascular complications could be reduced by intensive blood glucose control with oral hypoglycemic agents or insulin and whether any particular therapy was of advantage. Newly diagnosed type 2 diabetic patients aged 25–65 years were recruited between 1977 and 1991, and a total of 3867 were studied over 10 years. The median age at baseline was 54 years; 44% were overweight (> 120% over ideal weight); and baseline HbA_{1c} was 9.1%. Therapies were randomized to include a control group on diet alone and separate groups intensively treated with either insulin, chlorpropamide, glyburide, or glipizide. Metformin was included as a randomization option in a subgroup of 342 overweight patients, and much later in the study an additional subgroup of both normal weight and overweight patients who were responding unsatisfactorily to sulfonylurea therapy were randomized to either continue on their sulfonylurea therapy alone or to have metformin combined with it.

In 1987, an additional modification was made to evaluate whether tight control of blood pressure with stepwise antihypertensive therapy would prevent macrovascular and microvascular complications in 758 hypertensive patients among this UKPDS population compared with 390 of them whose blood pressure was treated less intensively. The tight control group was randomly assigned to treatment with either an an-giotensin-converting enzyme (ACE) inhibitor (captopril) or a beta-blocker (atenolol). Both drugs were stepped up to maximum dosages of 100 mg/d and then, if blood pressure remained higher than the target level of < 150/85 mm Hg, more drugs were added in the following stepwise sequence: a diuretic, slow-release nifedipine, methyldopa, and prazosin—until the target level of tight control was achieved. In the control group, hypertension was conventionally treated to achieve target levels < 180/105 mm Hg, but these patients were not prescribed either ACE inhibitors or beta-blockers.

Intensive glycemic therapy in the entire group of 3897 newly diagnosed type 2 diabetic patients followed over 10 years showed the following: Intensive treatment with either sulfonylureas, metformin, combinations of those two, or insulin achieved mean HbA_{1c} levels of 7%. This level of glycemic control decreases the risk of microvascular complications (retinopathy and nephropathy) in comparison with conventional therapy (mostly diet alone), which achieved mean levels of HbA_{1c} of 7.9%. Weight gain occurred in intensively treated patients except when metformin was used as monotherapy. No cardiovascular benefit and no adverse cardiovascular outcomes were noted regardless of the therapeutic agent. Hypoglycemic reactions occurred in the intensive treatment groups, but only one death from hypoglycemia was documented during 27,000 patient-years of intensive therapy.

When therapeutic subgroups were analyzed, some unexpected and paradoxical results were noted. Among the obese patients, intensive treatment with insulin or sulfonylureas did not reduce microvascular complications compared with diet therapy alone. This was in contrast to the significant benefit of intensive therapy with these drugs in the total group. Furthermore, intensive therapy with metformin was more beneficial in obese persons than diet alone as regards less myocardial infarctions, strokes, and diabetes-related deaths, but there was no significant reduction by metformin of diabetic microvascular complications as compared with the diet group. Moreover, in the subgroup of obese and nonobese patients in whom metformin was added to sulfonylurea failures, rather than showing a benefit, there was a 96% *increase* in diabetes-related deaths compared with the matched cohort of patients with unsatisfactory glycemic control on sulfonylureas who remained on their sulfonylurea therapy. Chlorpropamide also came out poorly on subgroup analysis in that those receiving it as intensive therapy did less well as regards progression to retinopathy than those conventionally treated with diet.

Intensive antihypertensive therapy to a mean of 144/82 mm Hg had beneficial effects on microvascular disease as well as on all diabetes-related end points, including virtually all cardiovascular outcomes, in comparison with looser control at a mean of 154/87 mm Hg. In fact, the advantage of reducing hypertension by this amount was substantially more impressive than the benefit accrued by improving the degree of glycemic control from a mean HbA_{1c} of 7.9% to 7%. More than half of the patients needed two or more drugs for adequate therapy of their hypertension, and there was no demonstrable advantage of ACE-inhibitor therapy over therapy with beta-blockers with regard to diabetes end points. Use of a calcium channel blocker added to both treatment groups appeared to be safe over the long term in this diabetic population despite some controversy in the recent literature about its safety in diabetics.

Implications of the UKPDS

It appears that glycemic control to levels of HbA_{1c} to 7% shows benefit in reducing total diabetes end points, including a 25% reduction in microvascular disease as compared with HbA_{1c} levels of 7.9%. This reassures those who have questioned whether the value of intensive therapy, so convincingly shown by the DCCT in type 1 diabetes, can safely be extrapolated to older patients with type 2 diabetes. It also argues against the concept of a "threshold" of glycemic control since in this group there was a benefit from this modest reduction of HbA_{1c} below 7.9% whereas in the DCCT a threshold was suggested in that further benefit was less apparent at HbA_{1c} levels below 8%.

Because of the complexity of the overall design in which many of the original therapy groups received additional medications to achieve glycemic goals but remained assigned to their group, statistical analysis may have been compromised by these multiple crossovers. For instance, in the diet group that was used as a control for all the drug treatment groups, only 58% of their total "patient-years" were actually drug-free while the remainder consisted of nonintensive therapy with various hypoglycemic drug regimens to avoid unacceptable hyperglycemia. This probably partly explains why the mean HbA_{1c} for this group was only 7.9% on "diet alone" therapy for over 10 years. In view of these crossovers within treatment groups, caution is suggested regarding several subgroup analyses that are controversial. These include the implication that metformin was superior to insulin or sulfonylureas in reducing diabetes-related end points in obese patients compared with diet therapy even though all three treatment groups achieved the same degree of glycemic control. Conversely, the finding of excess mortality in the subgroup of patients receiving combination therapy with metformin and sulfonylureas need not necessarily preclude this combination in patients doing poorly on sulfonylureas alone, though it certainly indicates a need for clarification of this important question.

Probably the most striking implication of the UKPDS is the benefit to the *hypertensive* type 2 diabetic patient of intensive control of blood pressure. Of interest was the observation that there was no demonstrable advantage of ACE inhibitor therapy on outcome despite a number of short-term reports in smaller populations implying that these drugs have special efficacy in reducing glomerular pressure beyond their general antihypertensive effects. Moreover, slow-release nifedipine showed no evidence of cardiac toxicity in this study despite some previous reports claiming that calcium channel blockers may be hazardous in patients with diabetes. Finally, the greater benefit in diabetes end points from antihypertensive than from antihyperglycemic treatments may be that the difference between the mean blood pressures achieved (144/82 mm Hg versus 154/87 mm Hg) is therapeutically more influential than the slight difference in HbA_{1c} (7% versus 7.9%). Greater hyperglycemia in the control group would most likely have rectified this discrepancy in outcomes. At present, the American Diabetes Association recommends vigorous treatment of both hyperglycemia and hypertension when they occur with an expectation that reductions in microvascular and cardiovascular outcomes will be additive.

Steps in the Management of the Diabetic Patient

A. DIAGNOSTIC EXAMINATION

Any features of the clinical picture that suggest end-organ insensitivity to insulin, such as visceral obesity, must be identified. The family history should document not only the incidence of diabetes in other members of the family but also the age at onset, whether it was associated with obesity, and whether insulin was required. Other factors that increase cardiac risk, such as smoking history, presence of hypertension or hyperlipidemia, or oral contraceptive pill use, should be recorded.

Laboratory diagnosis should document fasting plasma glucose levels above 126 mg/dL or postprandial values consistently above 200 mg/dL and whether ketonuria accompanies the glycosuria. A glycohemoglobin measurement is useful for assessing the effectiveness of future therapy. Some flexibility of clinical judgment is appropriate when diagnosing diabetes mellitus in the elderly patient with borderline hyperglycemia.

Baseline values include fasting plasma triglycerides, total cholesterol and HDL cholesterol, electrocardiography, renal function studies, peripheral pulses, and neurologic, podiatric, and ophthalmologic examinations to help guide future assessments.

B. PATIENT EDUCATION (SELF-MANAGEMENT TRAINING)

Since diabetes is a lifelong disorder, education of the patient and the family is probably the most important obligation of the clinician who provides initial care. The best persons to manage a disease that is affected so markedly by daily fluctuations in environmental stress, exercise, diet, and infections are the patients themselves and their families. The "teaching curriculum" should include explanations by the physician or nurse of the nature of diabetes and its potential acute and chronic hazards and how they can be recognized early and prevented or treated. The importance of regular tests for glucose on capillary blood specimens should be stressed and instructions on proper testing and recording of data provided. Moreover, patients should be provided with algorithms they can use to adjust the timing and quantity of their insulin dose, food, and exercise in response to recorded blood glucose values for optimal blood glucose control. The targets for blood glucose control should be elevated appropriately in elderly patients since they have the greatest risk if subjected to hypoglycemia and the least long-term benefit from more rigid glycemic control. Advice on personal hygiene, including detailed instructions on foot care, as well as individual instruction on diet and specific hypoglycemic therapy, should be provided. Patients should be told about community agencies, such as Diabetes Association chapters, that can serve as a continuing source of instruction. Finally, vigorous efforts should be made to persuade new diabetics who smoke to give up the habit, since large vessel peripheral vascular disease and debilitating retinopathy are less common in nonsmoking diabetic patients.

C. SELF-MONITORING OF BLOOD GLUCOSE

Monitoring of blood glucose by patients has allowed greater flexibility in management while achieving improved glycemic control.

Self-monitoring of blood glucose is particularly useful in brittle diabetics, those attempting "ideal" glycemic control such as during pregnancy, patients who have little or no early warning of hypoglycemic attacks, and those with impaired gastric emptying from diabetic neuropathy or altered renal thresholds for glucose. Self-monitoring of blood glucose is recommended for all diabetic patients and especially for those on insulin therapy. The expert consensus on self-monitoring is that its proper use is to develop a database as an aid in making day-to-day informal decisions about therapy as well as to determine when emergency situations arise. It is particularly valuable as an educational and training tool to enhance understanding of diabetes by patients and their families. The usefulness of self-monitoring depends on the accuracy of the results obtained. Patients must be taught proper techniques, cautioned to calibrate instruments properly despite the expense of strips, to keep proper records, and, particularly, *how to respond to unacceptably high or low blood glucose levels with appropriate therapeutic maneuvers.* Self-monitoring has proved to be an effective and safe clinical tool that can improve glycemic control in compliant patients.

D. INITIAL THERAPY

Treatment must be individualized on the basis of the type of diabetes and specific needs of each patient.

However, certain general principles of management can be outlined for hyperglycemic states of different types.

1. The obese type 2 patient—The most common type of diabetic patient is obese, is non-insulin-dependent, and has hyperglycemia because of insensitivity to normal or elevated circulating levels of insulin.

a. Weight reduction—Treatment is directed toward achieving weight reduction, and prescribing a diet is only one means to this end. Behavior modification to achieve adherence to the diet, as well as increased physical activity to expend energy, is also required. Cure can be achieved by reducing adipose stores, with consequent restoration of tissue sensitivity to insulin, but weight reduction is hard to achieve and even more difficult to maintain with our current therapies. The presence of diabetes with its added risk factors may motivate the obese diabetic to greater efforts to lose weight. (See also Chapter 29.)

b. Hypoglycemic agents—Neither insulin nor sulfonylureas are indicated for long-term use in the obese patient with mild diabetes. The weight reduction program can be upset by real or imagined hypoglycemic reactions when insulin therapy or sulfonylureas are used and weight gain is a frequent complication. Monotherapy with alpha-glucosidase inhibitors or metformin may be useful in the obese patient with mild diabetes if pharmacotherapy is required since they are not associated with weight gain or drug-induced hypoglycemia.

If metformin therapy (combined with a weight reduction regimen) is inadequate to control symptoms of hyperglycemia (eg, nocturia, blurred vision, or candidal vulvovaginitis), a sulfonylurea should be added. If this combination of metformin and sulfonylurea is ineffective in achieving appropriate glycemic control, addition of a thiazolidinedione should be considered. Insulin therapy should be instituted if the combination of these three drugs fails to restore euglycemia. Generally, the sulfonylurea is discontinued when insulin therapy is instituted but the patient can stay on the metformin and the thiazolidinedione. Weight-reducing interventions should continue and may allow for simplification of this regimen in the future.

2. The nonobese patient—In the nonobese diabetic, mild to severe hyperglycemia is usually due to refractoriness of B cells to glucose stimulation. Treatment depends on whether insulinopenia is mild (type 2 or mild type 1 in partial remission) or severe, with ketoacidosis.

a. Diet therapy—If hyperglycemia is mild, normal metabolic control can occasionally be restored by means of multiple feedings of a diet limited in simple sugars and with a caloric content sufficient to maintain ideal weight. Restriction of saturated fats and cholesterol is also strongly advised.

b. Oral hypoglycemic agents—When diet therapy in nonketotic type 2 patients is not sufficient to correct hyperglycemia, a trial of sulfonylureas is often successful in reducing the glycohemoglobin concentration below 9.5%. Once the dosage of one of the more potent sulfonylureas reaches the upper recommended limit in a compliant patient without maintaining fasting blood glucose below 140 mg/dL during the day, combination therapy with metformin (up to 850 mg two or three times daily) and sulfonylureas should be tried. This has been effective in up to 50% of sulfonylurea failures. If the sulfonylurea and metformin combination fails to keep the fasting blood glucose below 140 mg/dL, a thiazolidinedione can be added. When the patient fails the combination of these three drugs, insulin therapy is indicated.

c. Treatment of type 1 diabetes with insulin— The patient requiring insulin therapy should be initially regulated under conditions of optimal diet and normal daily activities. Traditional once- or twice daily insulin regimens are usually ineffective in type 1 patients without residual endogenous insulin. In these patients, information and counseling based on the findings of the DCCT (see above) should be provided about the advantages of taking multiple injections of insulin in conjunction with self blood glucose monitoring. If near-normalization of blood glucose is attempted, at least three or four measurements of capillary blood glucose are required daily to avoid frequent hypoglycemic reactions.

(1) Intensive insulin therapy—In most type 1 diabetes cases, conventional split doses of insulin mixtures cannot maintain near normalization of blood glucose without hypoglycemia, particularly at night, and multiple injections of insulin are usually required. Small doses of regular insulin injected three times a day before meals with one injection of NPH at bedtime is a commonly used regimen. The advent of pen injectors has made such multiple-injection regimens more convenient. The dose of regular insulin prior to a meal should be selected so that each 10–15 g of carbohydrate is covered by 1 unit of regular insulin. With current availability of nutritional labeling, the counting of nutrient carbohydrates should be taught to all patients receiving intensive insulin therapy.

The ultra-short-acting insulin analogs have been advocated as a safer and much more convenient alternative to regular human insulin for preprandial use in regimens of intensive insulin therapy. In a study comparing regular insulin with insulin lispro, daily insulin doses and hemoglobin A_{1c} levels were similar, but insulin lispro improved postprandial control, reduced hypoglycemic episodes, and improved patient convenience compared with regular insulin. However, because of their relatively short duration (no more than 3–4 hours), the ultra-short-acting insulin analogs need to be combined with intermediate-acting or longer-acting insulin to provide basal coverage and avoid hyperglycemia prior to the next meal. In addition to carbohydrate content of the meal, the effect of simultaneous fat ingestion must also be considered a factor in determining the ultra-fast-acting insulin dosage required to control the glycemic increment during and just after the meal. With low-carbohydrate content and high-fat intake, there is an increased risk of hypoglycemia from insulin lispro within 2 hours after the meal. Table 27–10 illustrates some regimens that might be appropriate for a 70-kg person with type 1 diabetes eating meals providing standard carbohydrate intake and moderate to low fat content.

Since ultra-short-acting insulins reach peak serum levels so quickly after subcutaneous administration, smaller doses are generally required compared with regular human insulin. Multiple injections of NPH

Table 27–10. Examples of intensive insulin regimens using insulin lispro or insulin aspart and ultralente, NPH, or insulin glargine in a 70 kg man with type 1 diabetes.[1,2,3]

	Pre-Breakfast	Pre-Lunch	Pre-Dinner	At Bedtime
Insulin lispro or aspart	5 units	4 units	6 units	—
Ultralente insulin	8 units	—	8 units	—
		OR		
Insulin lispro or aspart	5 units	4 units	6 units	—
NPH insulin	3 units	3 units	2 units	8–14 units
Insulin lispro or aspart	5 units	4 units	6 units	—
Insulin glargine	—	—	—	15–16 units

[1]Assumes that patient is consuming approximately 75 g carbohydrate at breakfast, 60 g at lunch and 90 g at dinner.
[2]The dose of insulin lispro or insulin aspart can be raised by 1 or 2 units if extra carbohydrate (15–30 g) is ingested or if premeal blood glucose is > 170 mg/dL. Insulin lispro or insulin aspart can be mixed in the same syringe with ultralente or NPH insulin.
[3]Insulin glargine cannot be mixed with any of the available insulins and must be given as a separate injection.

insulin (or twice-daily ultralente insulin) can be mixed in the same syringe as the insulin lispro or insulin aspart.

Occasional patients do not accept multiple injections of insulin and prefer continuous subcutaneous infusions with portable open-loop insulin pumps, which require subcutaneous needle insertion only every 48 hours.

(3) Management of early morning hyperglycemia in type 1—(Table 27–11.) One of the more difficult therapeutic problems in managing patients with type 1 is determining the proper adjustment of insulin dose when the prebreakfast blood glucose level is high.

(a) Somogyi effect—Patients with type 1 may develop nocturnal hypoglycemia, which may in turn stimulate a surge of counterregulatory hormones (Somogyi effect) to produce high blood glucose levels by 7:00 AM. Reducing inappropriately high doses of administered insulin improves morning hyperglycemia.

(b) Dawn phenomenon—The dawn phenomenon is present in as many as 75% of type 1 patients and occurs in most type 2 and normal subjects as well. It is characterized by reduced tissue sensitivity to insulin developing between 5:00 AM and 8:00 AM. This phenomenon may be evoked by spikes of growth hormone released hours before, at the onset of sleep. When the dawn phenomenon occurs alone, it may produce only mild hyperglycemia in the early morning, but when it is associated with the Somogyi effect or the waning phenomenon (or both), the hyperglycemia may be more severe.

(c) Waning of circulating insulin levels—The most common cause of prebreakfast hyperglycemia is probably the waning of circulating insulin levels. This would suggest that more rather than less intermediate-acting insulin should be given in the evening.

Table 27–11 shows that diagnosis of the cause of prebreakfast hyperglycemia can be facilitated by self-monitoring of blood glucose at 3:00 AM in addition to the usual bedtime and 7:00 AM measurements. This is required for only a few nights until the diagnosis is established and appropriate adjustment of bedtime insulin dose or nighttime feeding is achieved.

(d) Therapy of prebreakfast hyperglycemia—When a particular pattern emerges from monitoring blood glucose levels overnight, appropriate therapeutic measures can be taken. The Somogyi effect can be treated by eliminating the dose of intermediate insulin at dinnertime and giving it at a lower dosage at bedtime or by supplying more food at bedtime. When the dawn phenomenon alone is present, the dosage of intermediate insulin can be divided between dinnertime and bedtime, or when insulin pumps are used, the basal infusion rate can be increased (eg, from 0.8 unit/h to 1 unit/h from 6:00 AM until breakfast). With waning insulin levels, either increasing the evening dose or shifting it from dinnertime to bedtime, or both, can be effective. A bedtime dose of either insulin glargine or of NPH insulin made from pork insulin provides more sustained overnight insulin levels than human NPH or human ultralente insulin and may be effective in managing refractory prebreakfast hyperglycemia. If this fails, insulin pump therapy may be required.

d. Treatment of type 2 diabetes with insulin—When the combination of metformin, sulfonylurea, and a thiazolidinedione fails and type 2 patients require insulin, various insulin regimens may be effective. Although a single morning injection of insulin is not recommended in type 1 diabetes, in some patients with type 2 diabetes enough residual insulin secretion persists to allow a single morning injection of 25–30 units of NPH or lente insulin to replace their deficient insulin secretion. If prebreakfast hyperglycemia persists on this regimen or if hypoglycemia occurs before dinner, a number of alternatives are available. A convenient regimen includes split doses of a fixed 70:30 mixture of NPH:regular insulin, which can be started as 20 units before breakfast and 15 units before dinner

Table 27–11. Prebreakfast hyperglycemia: Classification by blood glucose and insulin levels.

	Blood Glucose (mg/dL)			Free Immunoreactive Insulin (μU/mL)		
	10:00 PM	3:00 AM	7:00 AM	10:00 PM	3:00 AM	7:00 AM
Somogyi effect	90	40	200	High	Slightly high	Normal
Dawn phenomenon	110	110	150	Normal	Normal	Normal
Waning of insulin dose plus dawn phenomenon	110	190	220	Normal	Low	Low
Waning of insulin dose plus dawn phenomenon plus Somogyi effect	110	40	380	High	Normal	Low

and increased appropriately depending on target blood glucoses at 7:00 AM and 5:00 PM. A 75:25 mixture of NPL:insulin lispro can also be used in the same manner. When more than 50 units a day are required without achieving proper control, these patients may benefit from three or four injection regimens as described for type 1 in Table 27–10.

e. Acceptable levels of glycemic control—See above for a discussion of the Diabetes Control and Complications Trial (DCCT) and the United Kingdom Prospective Diabetes Study (UKPDS) and their implications for diabetes therapy. A reasonable aim of therapy is to approach normal glycemic excursions without provoking severe or frequent hypoglycemia. What has been considered "acceptable" control includes blood glucose levels of 90–130 mg/dL before meals and after an overnight fast, and levels no higher than 180 mg/dL 1 hour after meals and 150 mg/dL 2 hours after meals. Glycohemoglobin levels should be no higher than 2% above the upper limit of the normal range for any particular laboratory. It should be emphasized that the value of blood pressure control was as great as or greater than glycemic control in type 2 patients as regards microvascular as well as macrovascular complications.

Complications of Insulin Therapy

A. HYPOGLYCEMIA

Hypoglycemic reactions, the most common complication of insulin therapy, may result from delay in taking a meal or unusual physical exertion. With more type 1 patients attempting "tight" control, this complication has become even more frequent. In older diabetics, in those taking only longer-acting insulins, and often in those attempting to maintain euglycemia on infusion pumps, autonomic counterregulatory responses are less readily elicited during hypoglycemia, and central nervous system dysfunction may occur, ie, mental confusion, bizarre behavior, and ultimately coma. Even focal neurologic deficits mimicking stroke may be observed. More rapid development of hypoglycemia from the effects of regular insulin causes signs of autonomic hyperactivity, both sympathetic (tachycardia, palpitations, sweating, tremulousness) and parasympathetic (nausea, hunger), that may progress to coma and convulsions. Except for sweating, most of the sympathetic symptoms of hypoglycemia are blunted in patients receiving beta-blocking agents for angina or hypertension. Though not absolutely contraindicated, these drugs must be used with caution in insulin-requiring diabetics, and, β_1-selective blocking agents are preferred.

1. Altered awareness of hypoglycemia—Since autonomic responses correlate strongly with "awareness" of hypoglycemia, many poorly controlled diabetics—whose nervous systems have adapted to chronic hyperglycemia—may trigger adrenergic alarms at levels of blood glucose above the usual hypoglycemic range. Conversely, type 1 patients overtreated with insulin may be unaware of critically low levels of blood glucose because of an adaptive blunting of their alarm systems owing to repeated episodes of hypoglycemia. This has been shown to be reversible if higher average blood glucose levels are maintained in these patients to avoid recurrent hypoglycemia over a period of several weeks.

As evidenced by results of the DCCT, the risk of frequent severe hypoglycemic episodes is greatly increased when "normalization" of the blood glucose is attempted with presently available methods of insulin delivery, and this is independent of the species of insulin used. "Near normalization" is therefore a safer target for therapy to avoid hypoglycemic unawareness.

2. Lack of glucagon response in type 1—For unexplained reasons, patients with type 1 lose their glucagon responses to hypoglycemia (but not to amino acids in protein-containing meals) within a year or so after developing diabetes. These patients then rely predominantly on the sympathetic nervous system to counterregulate hypoglycemia and are at special risk in later years when aging, autonomic neuropathy, or frequent hypoglycemic episodes blunt their sympathetic responses.

3. Prevention and treatment of hypoglycemia—Because of the potential danger of insulin-induced reactions, the diabetic patient should carry packets of table sugar or a candy roll at all times for use at the onset of hypoglycemic symptoms. Tablets containing 3 g of glucose are available (dextrosol). The educated patient soon learns to take the amount of glucose needed and avoids the excess that may occur with eating candy or drinking orange juice, causing very high hyperglycemia. An ampule of glucagon (1 mg) should be provided to every diabetic receiving insulin therapy, and family or friends should be instructed how to inject it intramuscularly in the event that the patient is unconscious or refuses food. An identification MedicAlert bracelet, necklace, or card in the wallet or purse should be carried by every diabetic receiving hypoglycemic drug therapy. The telephone number for the MedicAlert Foundation International in Turlock, California, is 800-ID-ALERT.

All of the manifestations of hypoglycemia are rapidly relieved by glucose administration. If more severe hypoglycemia has produced unconsciousness or stupor, the treatment is 50 mL of 50% glucose solution by rapid intravenous infusion. If intravenous therapy is not available, 1 mg of glucagon injected intramuscularly will usually restore the patient to consciousness within 15 minutes to permit ingestion of sugar. If the patient is stuporous and glucagon is not available, small amounts of honey or syrup can be inserted within the buccal pouch, but, in general, oral feeding is contraindicated in unconscious patients.

Rectal administration of syrup or honey (30 mL per 500 mL of warm water) has been effective.

B. IMMUNOPATHOLOGY OF INSULIN THERAPY

At least five molecular classes of insulin antibodies are produced during the course of insulin therapy in diabetes, including IgA, IgD, IgE, IgG, and IgM. With the increased therapeutic use of purified pork and especially human insulin, the various immunopathologic syndromes such as insulin allergy, immune insulin resistance, and lipoatrophy have become quite rare since the titers and avidity of these induced antibodies are generally quite low. However, in parts of the world where less purified forms of beef insulin are still used, these disorders remain a clinical concern among some insulin-treated patients.

1. Insulin allergy—Insulin allergy, or immediate-type hypersensitivity, is a rare condition in which local or systemic urticaria is due to histamine release from tissue mast cells sensitized by adherence of anti-insulin IgE antibodies. In severe cases, anaphylaxis results. When only human insulin has been used from the onset of insulin therapy, insulin allergy is exceedingly rare. Antihistamines, corticosteroids, and even desensitization may be required, especially for systemic hypersensitivity. There have been case reports of successful use of insulin lispro in those rare patients who have a generalized allergy to human insulin or insulin resistance due to a high titer of insulin antibodies.

2. Immune insulin resistance—Most insulin-treated patients develop a low titer of circulating IgG anti-insulin antibodies that neutralize to a small extent the action of insulin. However, under rare circumstances, in some type 2 diabetic patients, principally those with some degree of tissue insensitivity to insulin (such as in the obese) and with a history of interrupted exposure to therapy with beef insulin, a high titer of circulating IgG anti-insulin antibodies may develop. This results in extremely high insulin requirements—often more than 200 units daily. This is often a self-limited condition and may clear spontaneously after several months. However, with advances in insulin purification and the use of human insulins, this syndrome has essentially disappeared in all industrialized countries.

C. LIPODYSTROPHY AT INJECTION SITES

Atrophy of subcutaneous fatty tissue leading to disfiguring excavations and depressed areas may rarely occur at the site of injection. This complication results from an immune reaction, and it has become rarer with the development of pure insulin preparations. Injection of these preparations directly into the atrophic area often results in restoration of normal contours. Lipohypertrophy, on the other hand, is a consequence of the pharmacologic effects of insulin being deposited in the same location repeatedly. It can occur with purified insulins and is best treated with localized liposuction of the hypertrophic areas by an experienced plastic surgeon. Rotation of injection sites will prevent lipohypertrophy. There is a case report of a patient who had intractable lipohypertrophy with human insulin but no longer had the problem when he switched to insulin lispro.

Chronic Complications of Diabetes

Late clinical manifestations of diabetes mellitus include a number of pathologic changes that involve small and large blood vessels, cranial and peripheral nerves, the skin, and the lens of the eye. These lesions lead to hypertension, renal failure, blindness, autonomic and peripheral neuropathy, amputations of the lower extremities, myocardial infarction, and cerebrovascular accidents. These late manifestations correlate with the duration of the diabetic state subsequent to the onset of puberty. In type 1 diabetes, up to 40% of patients develop end-stage renal disease, compared with less than 20% of patients with type 2 diabetes. As regards proliferative retinopathy, it ultimately develops in both types of diabetes but has a slightly higher prevalence in type 1 patients (25% after 15 years' duration). In patients with type 1 diabetes, complications from end-stage renal disease are a major cause of death, whereas patients with type 2 diabetes are more likely to have macrovascular diseases leading to myocardial infarction and stroke as the main causes of death. Cigarette use adds significantly to the risk of both microvascular and macrovascular complications in diabetic patients.

A. OCULAR COMPLICATIONS

1. Diabetic cataracts—Premature cataracts occur in diabetic patients and seem to correlate with both the duration of diabetes and the severity of chronic hyperglycemia. Nonenzymatic glycosylation of lens protein is twice as high in diabetic patients as in age-matched nondiabetic persons and may contribute to the premature occurrence of cataracts.

2. Diabetic retinopathy—Three main categories exist: background, or "simple," retinopathy, consisting of microaneurysms, hemorrhages, exudates, and retinal edema; preproliferative retinopathy with arteriolar ischemia manifested as cotton-wool spots (small infarcted areas of retina); and proliferative, or "malignant," retinopathy, consisting of newly formed vessels. Proliferative retinopathy is a leading cause of blindness in the USA, particularly since it increases the risk of retinal detachment. Vision-threatening retinopathy virtually never appears in type 1 patients in the first 3–5 years of diabetes or before puberty. Up to 20% of patients with type 2 diabetes have retinopathy at the time of diagnosis. Annual consultation with an ophthalmologist should be arranged for patients who have had type 1 diabetes for more than 3–5 years and for all patients with type 2 diabetes, because many were probably diabetic for an extensive period of time before diagnosis. Patients with any macular edema, severe nonproliferative retinopathy, or any proliferative retinopathy require the care of an ophthalmologist. Extensive "scatter" xenon or argon photocoagulation and focal treatment of new vessels reduce severe visual loss in those cases in which proliferative retinopathy is associated with recent vitreous hemorrhages or in which extensive new vessels are located on or near the optic disk. Macular edema, which is more common than proliferative retinopathy in patients with type 2 diabetes (up to 20% prevalence), has a guarded prognosis, but it has also responded to scatter therapy with improvement in visual acuity if detected early. Avoiding tobacco use and correction of associated hypertension are important therapeutic measures in the management of diabetic retinopathy. There is no contraindication to using aspirin in patients with proliferative retinopathy.

3. Glaucoma—Glaucoma occurs in approximately 6% of persons with diabetes. It is responsive to the usual therapy for open-angle disease. Neovascularization of the iris in diabetics can predispose to closed-angle glaucoma, but this is relatively uncommon except after cataract extraction, when growth of new vessels has been known to progress rapidly, involving the angle of the iris and obstructing outflow.

B. DIABETIC NEPHROPATHY

As many as 4000 cases of end-stage renal disease occur each year among diabetic people in the United States. This is about one-third of all patients being treated for end-stage renal disease and represents a considerable national health expense.

The cumulative incidence of nephropathy differs between the two major types of diabetes. Patients with type 1 diabetes have a 30–40% chance of having nephropathy after 20 years—in contrast to the much lower frequency in type 2 diabetes patients, in whom only about 15–20% develop clinical renal disease. However, since there are many more individuals affected with type 2 diabetes, end-stage renal disease is much more prevalent in type 2 than in type 1 diabetes in the United States and especially throughout the rest of the world. Improved glycemic control and more effective therapeutic measures to correct hypertension—and with the beneficial effects of angiotensin-converting enzyme inhibitors—can reduce the development of end-stage renal disease among diabetics.

Diabetic nephropathy is initially manifested by proteinuria; subsequently, as kidney function declines, urea and creatinine accumulate in the blood.

1. Microalbuminuria—Sensitive radioimmunoassay methods of detecting small amounts of urinary albumin have permitted detection of microgram concentrations—in contrast to the less sensitive dipstick strips, whose minimal detection limit is 0.3–0.5%. Conventional 24-hour urine collections, in addition to being inconvenient for patients, also show wide variability of albumin excretion, since several factors such as sustained erect posture, dietary protein, and exercise tend to increase albumin excretion rates. For

these reasons, a timed overnight urine collection or albumin-creatinine ratio in an early morning spot urine collected upon awakening is preferable. Normal subjects excrete less than 15 μg/min during overnight urine collections; values of 20 μg/min or higher are considered to represent abnormal microalbuminuria. In the early morning spot urine, a ratio of albumin (μg/L) to creatinine (mg/L) of < 30 μg/mg creatinine is normal, and a ratio of 30–300 μg/mg creatinine suggests abnormal microalbuminuria. At least two of three timed overnight or early morning spot urine collections over a 3- to 6-month period should be abnormal before a diagnosis of microalbuminuria is justified.

Subsequent renal failure can be predicted by persistent urinary albumin excretion rates exceeding 30 μg/min. Increased microalbuminuria correlates with increased levels of blood pressure and increased LDL cholesterol, and this may explain why increased proteinuria in diabetic patients is associated with an increase in cardiovascular deaths even in the absence of renal failure. Glycemic control as well as a low-protein diet (0.8 g/kg/d) may reduce both the hyperfiltration and the elevated microalbuminuria in patients in the early stages of diabetes and those with incipient diabetic nephropathy. Antihypertensive therapy also decreases microalbuminuria. Evidence from some studies—but not the UKPDS—supports a specific role for ACE inhibitors in reducing intraglomerular pressure in addition to their lowering of systemic hypertension. An ACE inhibitor (captopril, 50 mg twice daily) in normotensive diabetics impedes progression to proteinuria and prevents the increase in albumin excretion rate. Since microalbuminuria has been shown to correlate with elevated *nocturnal* systolic blood pressure, it is possible that "normotensive" diabetic patients with microalbuminuria have slightly elevated systolic blood pressure during sleep which is lowered during antihypertensive therapy. This action may contribute to the reported efficacy of ACE inhibitor drugs in reducing microalbuminuria in "normotensive" patients.

2. Progressive diabetic nephropathy—Progressive diabetic nephropathy consists of proteinuria of varying severity occasionally leading to nephrotic syndrome with hypoalbuminemia, edema, and an increase in circulating betalipoproteins as well as progressive azotemia. In contrast to all other renal disorders, the proteinuria associated with diabetic nephropathy does not diminish with progressive renal failure (patients continue to excrete 10–11 g daily as creatinine clearance diminishes). As renal failure progresses, there is an elevation in the renal threshold at which glycosuria appears.

Hypertension develops with progressive renal involvement, and coronary and cerebral atherosclerosis seems to be accelerated. Approximately two-thirds of adult patients with diabetes have hypertension. Once diabetic nephropathy has progressed to the stage of hypertension, proteinuria, or early renal failure, glycemic control is not beneficial in influencing its course. In this circumstance, antihypertensive medications, including ACE inhibitors, and restriction of dietary protein to 0.8 g/kg body weight per day are recommended. ACE inhibitors have been shown to protect against deterioration in renal function in type 1 diabetic patients with clinical nephropathy. This beneficial effect appears to be due to improved glomerular hemodynamics that cannot be explained only by the antihypertensive action of these drugs. Captopril (25 mg three times daily) has shown a 50% reduction in the risk of the combined end points of death, dialysis and transplantation in type 1 subjects with diabetic nephropathy and clinical proteinuria. During initiation of ACE-inhibitor therapy, an increment in serum creatinine greater than 2 mg/dL due to a rapid fall in intraglomerular pressure—or the occurrence of persistent hyperkalemia (above 6 meq/L) due to hyporeninemic hypoaldosteronism—is an indication to stop this medication.

Dialysis has been of limited value in the long-term treatment of renal failure due to diabetic nephropathy. At present, experience in renal transplantation—especially from related donors—is more promising and is the treatment of choice in cases where there are no contraindications such as severe cardiovascular disease.

C. GANGRENE OF THE FEET

The incidence of gangrene of the feet in diabetics is 20 times the incidence in matched controls. The factors responsible for its development are ischemia, peripheral neuropathy, and secondary infection. Occlusive vascular disease involves both microangiopathy and atherosclerosis of large and medium-sized arteries. Cigarette smoking should be avoided, and prevention of foot disease should be emphasized, since treatment is difficult once ulceration and gangrene have developed. Patients should be examined with a 10-g Semmes-Weinstein monofilament to ensure that protective sensation is intact. If it is not, cushioned socks, athletic shoes, and special foot care are needed since insensitive feet are at high risk for development of neuropathic ulcers. Patients should be instructed to inspect their feet daily for reddened areas, blisters, abrasions, or lacerations (see Instructions in the Care of the Feet). Clinicians should inspect the feet at each visit and instruct patients as necessary on filing calluses with an emery board, cutting toenails straight across, not walking barefoot, and avoiding tight shoes. When an uncomplicated neuropathic ulcer is present and blood flow is not impaired, consultation with a podiatrist or orthopedist is recommended. Cholesterol-lowering agents are useful as adjunctive therapy when early ischemic signs are detected. If blood supply is diminished or absent, patients with foot ulcers should be referred to an appropriate specialist (vascular or orthopedic surgeon). When chronic foot ulcers are refractory to standard debridement and antibiotics,

platelet-derived growth factor (Regranex) should be considered for local application. To Special custombuilt shoes are usually required to redistribute weight evenly over an insensitive foot when it has been deformed by surgery or asymptomatic fractures (Charcot's joint). Amputation of the lower extremities is sometimes required, but appropriate prophylactic foot care has greatly reduced its frequency.

Nonselective beta-blockers are relatively contraindicated in patients with ischemic foot ulcers, because these drugs may potentially reduce peripheral blood flow.

D. DIABETIC NEUROPATHY

Peripheral and autonomic neuropathy, the two most common chronic complications of diabetes, are poorly understood.

1. Peripheral neuropathy—

a. Distal symmetric polyneuropathy—This is the most common form of diabetic peripheral neuropathy where loss of function appears in a stockingglove pattern and is due to an axonal neuropathic process. Sensory involvement usually occurs first and is generally bilateral, symmetric, and associated with dulled perception of vibration, pain, and temperature, particularly in the lower extremities. At times, discomfort of the lower extremities can be incapacitating. Both motor and sensory nerve conduction are delayed in peripheral nerves, and ankle jerks may be absent. In most cases, motor weakness is mild and confined to the most distal intrinsic muscles of the hands and feet. Long-term complications of diabetic polyneuropathy include insensitivity of the feet, leading to repeated "silent" trauma that predisposes to neuropathic plantar ulcers or deformities of the feet secondary to multiple "silent" fractures (Charcot's joint).

b. Isolated peripheral neuropathy—Involvement of the distribution of only one nerve ("mononeuropathy"), or of several nerves ("mononeuropathy multiplex") is characterized by sudden onset with subsequent recovery of all or most of the function. This neuropathology has been attributed to vascular ischemia or traumatic damage. Femoral and cranial nerves are commonly involved, and motor abnormalities predominate. These can result in sudden onset of diplopia due to ophthalmoplegia or in acute pain and weakness of thigh muscles (diabetic amyotrophy). Spontaneous resolution of these ischemic neuropathies generally occurs in 6–12 weeks. In more severe cases with extensive atrophy of limb musculature, this disorder has been termed "malignant cachexia" and mimics the end stages of advanced neoplasia, particularly when depression produces anorexia and weight loss. With this more severe manifestation of diabetic amyotrophy, recovery of muscle function may only be partial.

c. Painful diabetic neuropathy—Hypersensitivity to light touch and occasionally severe "burning" pain, particularly at night, can become physically and emotionally disabling. Amitriptyline, 25–75 mg at bedtime, has been recommended for pain associated with diabetic neuropathy. Dramatic relief has often resulted within 48–72 hours. This rapid response is in contrast to the 2 or 3 weeks required for an antidepressive effect. Patients often attribute benefit to their having a full night's sleep after amitriptyline compared to many previously sleepless nights occasioned by neuropathic pain. Mild to moderate morning drowsiness is a side effect that generally improves with time or can be lessened by giving the medication several hours before bedtime. This drug should not be continued if improvement has not occurred after 5 days of therapy. Desipramine in doses of 25–150 mg/d seems to have the same efficacy as amitriptyline. Gabapentin (900–1800 mg/d in three divided doses) has also been shown to be effective in the treatment of painful neuropathy and should be tried if the tricyclic drugs prove ineffective. There has also been interest in use of the antiarrhythmic drug mexiletine for this purpose in doses of up to 10 mg/kg/d. Capsaicin, a topical irritant, has been found to be effective in reducing local nerve pain; it is dispensed as a cream (Zostrix 0.025%, Zostrix-HP 0.075%) to be rubbed into the skin over the painful region two to four times daily. Gloves should be used for application since hand contamination could result in discomfort if the cream comes in contact with eyes or sensitive areas such as the genitalia.

2. Autonomic neuropathy—With autonomic neuropathy, there is evidence of postural hypotension, decreased cardiovascular response to Valsalva's maneuver, gastroparesis, alternating bouts of diarrhea (particularly nocturnal) and constipation, inability to empty the bladder, and impotence. Gastroparesis should be considered in insulin-dependent diabetic patients who develop unexpected fluctuations and variability in their blood glucose levels after meals. Impotence due to neuropathy differs from psychogenic impotence in that the latter may be intermittent (erections occur under special circumstances), whereas diabetic impotence is usually persistent; aortoiliac occlusive disease may contribute to this problem.

a. Management of autonomic neuropathy— There is no consistently effective treatment for diabetic autonomic neuropathy. Metoclopramide has been of some help in treating diabetic gastroparesis over the short term, but its effectiveness seems to diminish over time. It is a dopamine antagonist that has central antiemetic effects as well as a cholinergic action to facilitate gastric emptying. It can be given intravenously (10 mg three or four times a day, 30 minutes before meals and at bedtime) or orally (20 mg of liquid metoclopramide) before breakfast and dinner. Drowsiness, restlessness, fatigue, and lassitude are common adverse effects. Tardive dyskinesia and extrapyramidal effects also occur. Because it has caused

life-threatening cardiac arrhythmias, including 80 deaths, cisapride has been withdrawn from use in the United States. Erythromycin appears to bind to motilin receptors in the stomach and has been found to improve gastric emptying in doses of 250 mg three times daily. Diarrhea associated with autonomic neuropathy has occasionally responded to broad-spectrum antibiotic therapy, though it often undergoes spontaneous remission. Refractory diabetic diarrhea is often associated with impaired sphincter control and fecal incontinence. Therapy with loperamide, 4–8 mg daily, or diphenoxylate with atropine, two tablets up to four times a day, may provide relief. In more severe cases, tincture of paregoric or codeine (60 mg tablets) may be required to reduce the frequency of diarrhea and improve the consistency of the stools. Clonidine has been reported to lessen diabetic diarrhea, but its tendency to lower blood pressure in these patients who already have autonomic neuropathy and some orthostatic hypotension often limits its usefulness. Constipation usually responds to stimulant laxatives such as senna. Bethanechol in doses of 10–50 mg three times a day has occasionally improved emptying of the atonic urinary bladder. Catheter decompression of the distended bladder has been reported to improve its function, and considerable benefit has been reported after surgical severing of the internal vesicle sphincter. Mineralocorticoid therapy with fludrocortisone, 0.2–0.3 mg/d, and elastic stockings or pressure suits have reportedly been of some help in patients with orthostatic hypotension occurring as a result of loss of postural reflexes.

b. Management of erectile dysfunction—There are medical, mechanical, and surgical treatments available for treatment of erectile dysfunction. Penile erection depends on relaxation of the smooth muscle in the arteries of the corpus cavernosum, and this is mediated by nitric oxide-induced cyclic 3′,5′-guanosine monophosphate (cGMP) formation. Sildenafil (Viagra) is a selective inhibitor of cGMP-specific phosphodiesterase type 5. In response to sexual stimulation, there is local release of nitric oxide and cGMP production, and sildenafil, by inhibiting the breakdown of cGMP, improves the ability to attain and maintain an erection. The recommended dose for most patients is one 50 mg tablet taken approximately 1 hour before sexual activity. The peak effect is at 1.5–2 hours, with some effect persisting for 4 hours. Patients with diabetes mellitus using sildenafil reported 50–60% improvement in erectile function. The maximum recommended dose is 100 mg. In clinical trials, only a few adverse effects have been reported—transient mild headache, flushing, dyspepsia, and some altered color vision, particularly with the 100 mg dose. There was no priapism or increase in libido. Because of sildenafil's potentiation of the hypotensive effects of nitrates, its use is contraindicated in patients who are concurrently using organic nitrates in any form. Following its approval and release, a number of deaths have resulted from its use in men with active cardiovascular disease. The FDA has mandated a warning label change in the package insert, advising caution for men who have suffered a heart attack, stroke, or life-threatening arrhythmia within the previous 6 months; men who have resting hypotension or hypertension; and men who have a history of cardiac failure or have unstable angina.

Intracorporeal injection of vasoactive drugs causes penile engorgement and erection. Drugs most commonly used include papaverine alone, papaverine with phentolamine, and alprostadil (prostaglandin E_1). Alprostadil injections are relatively painless, but careful instruction is essential to prevent local trauma, priapism, and fibrosis. Intraurethral pellets of alprostadil avoid the problem of injection of the drug.

External vacuum therapy (Erec-Aid System) is a nonsurgical treatment consisting of a suction chamber operated by a hand pump that creates a vacuum around the penis. This draws blood into the penis to produce an erection which is maintained by a specially designed tension ring inserted around the base of the penis and which can be kept in place for up to 20–30 minutes. While this method is generally effective, its cumbersome nature limits its appeal.

In view of the recent development of nonsurgical approaches to therapy of erectile dysfunction, resort to surgical implants of penile prostheses is becoming less common.

E. Skin and Mucous Membrane Complications

Chronic pyogenic infections of the skin may occur, especially in poorly controlled diabetic patients. Eruptive xanthomas can result from hypertriglyceridemia, associated with poor glycemic control. An unusual lesion termed **necrobiosis lipoidica diabeticorum** is usually located over the anterior surfaces of the legs or the dorsal surfaces of the ankles. They are oval or irregularly shaped plaques with demarcated borders and a glistening yellow surface and occur in women two to four times more frequently than in men.

"Shin spots" are not uncommon in adult diabetics. They are brownish, rounded, painless atrophic lesions of the skin in the pretibial area. Candidal infection can produce erythema and edema of intertriginous areas below the breasts, in the axillas, and between the fingers. It causes vulvovaginitis in most chronically uncontrolled diabetic women with persistent glucosuria and is a frequent cause of pruritus.

While antifungal creams containing miconazole or clotrimazole offer immediate relief of vulvovaginitis, recurrence is frequent unless glucosuria is reduced.

F. Special Situations

1. Insulin replacement during surgery—It is likely that target glucose levels between 100 and 250 mg/dL are adequate in most patients to avoid postoperative infections or wound dehiscence, though this view is based on clinical observations rather than conclusive evidence. All diabetic patients should have serum electrolytes measured preoperatively so that abnormalities can be corrected prior to surgery. During major surgery and in the immediate recovery period in patients with type 1 diabetes, 5% dextrose in physiologic saline containing 20 meq of potassium chloride should be infused intravenously at a rate of 100–200 mL/h with regular human insulin (25 units/250 mL 0.9% saline) infused into the intravenous tubing at a rate of 1–3 units/h. The patient's blood glucose should be monitored every hour initially and the rates of insulin or dextrose adjusted to maintain blood glucose values between 120 and 190 mg/dL (although levels up to 250 mg/dL may be acceptable).

Most patients with type 2 diabetes, whether or not they are receiving insulin therapy, should be treated with insulin during major surgery. In these patients, 10 units of regular human insulin added to 1000 mL of a D_5W solution containing 20 meq of potassium chloride and infused at a rate of 100 mL/h (1 unit/h) is generally adequate to regulate glycemia during surgery. The patient's glucose should be monitored hourly to prevent extremes of hyper- or hypoglycemia. If blood glucose values remain above 250 mg/dL at 1–2 hours, an infusion concentration of 15 units/L can be substituted.

Type 2 patients facing minor surgical procedures not requiring general anesthesia who have previously been controlled on oral agents or diet alone do not generally require insulin infusions. Glucose-containing solutions should be avoided during surgery in these patients, and blood glucose levels should be monitored every 4 hours. Regular human insulin or insulin lispro should be administered subcutaneously if needed to maintain blood glucose below 250 mg/dL (see Chapter 2).

2. Pregnancy and the diabetic patient—Several features distinguish the management of diabetics during pregnancy from the general therapy of diabetes. These include the following: (1) Oral hypoglycemic agents are contraindicated. (2) Weight reduction is not advised, since fetal nutrition can be adversely affected. (3) Intensive insulin therapy with frequent self-monitoring of blood glucose is generally recommended to improve the likelihood of having healthy normal babies. Every effort should be made, utilizing multiple injections of insulin or a continuous infusion of insulin by pump, to maintain near-normalization of fasting and preprandial blood glucose values while avoiding hypoglycemia. Glycohemoglobin should be maintained in the normal range.

Since many diabetic pregnancies persist beyond the expected term—or because the infants are usually large and hydramnios may be present—it has been suggested that pregnancy be terminated early (at 37–38 weeks), especially if glycemic control during pregnancy has been inadequate (eg, glycohemoglobin > 10%). There is a present trend away from elective cesarean section and toward induction of labor.

See Chapter 18 for further details.

Prognosis

The Diabetes Control and Complications Trial (DCCT) showed that the previously poor prognosis for as many as 40% of patients with type 1 diabetes is markedly improved by optimal care. DCCT participants were generally young and highly motivated and were cared for in academic centers by skilled diabetes educators and endocrinologists who were able to provide more attention and services than are usually available. Improved training of primary care providers may be beneficial.

For type 2 diabetes, the UKPDS documented a reduction in microvascular disease with glycemic control, though this was not apparent in the obese subgroup. Cardiovascular outcomes were not improved by glycemic control, though among hypertensive patients antihypertensive therapy showed benefit in reducing the number of adverse cardiovascular complications as well as in reducing the occurrence of microvascular disease. In those with visceral obesity, its successful management remains a major challenge in the attempt to achieve appropriate control of hyperglycemia, hypertension, and dyslipidemia. Once safe and effective methods are devised to prevent or manage obesity, the prognosis of type 2 diabetes with its high cardiovascular risks should improve considerably.

In addition to poorly understood genetic factors relating to differences in individual susceptibility to development of long-term complications of hyperglycemia, it is clear that in both types of diabetes, the diabetic patient's intelligence, motivation, and awareness of the potential complications of the disease contribute significantly to the ultimate outcome.

Internet Addresses

[American Association of Diabetes Educators]
http://www.aadenet.org/
[American Diabetes Association]
http://www.diabetesnet.com/ada.html
[American Dietetic Association]
http://www.eatright.org
[Juvenile Diabetes Foundation]
http://www.jdf.org/index.html

Classification, Pathophysiology, & Diagnosis of Diabetes Mellitus

Stumvoll M et al: Clinical features of insulin resistance and beta cell dysfunction and the relationship to type 2 diabetes. Clin Lab Med 2001;21:31. [PMID: 11211936] (This comprehensive review of the pathophysiology of type 2 diabetes emphasizes the presence of both insulin resistance and a defect in insulin secretion in most patients with this syndrome. While genetic factors could explain either or both of these abnormalities, the author indicates how acquired causes contribute to both defects and might even be primarily responsible. Until specific genes are identified, the relative influence of inheritance and environment on the etiology of type 2 diabetes remains to be clarified.)

Atkinson MA et al: Type 1 diabetes: new perspectives on disease pathogenesis and treatment. Lancet 2001;358:221. [PMID: 11476858] (This authoritative overview updates recent knowledge of the HLA genes that provide protection against or susceptibility to the development of type 1 diabetes and discusses the controversy over whether environmental factors play a role in pathogenesis of this complex disorder. It also cites the current dilemma presented by attempts to design prevention trials with current prophylactic agents that are not without some risk to the subjects. To justify their use, patient selection is delayed until B cell destruction has progressed to the brink of onset of type 1 diabetes, which consequently reduces the likelihood of a successful intervention.)

Report of the expert committee on the diagnosis and classification of diabetes mellitus. Diabetes Care 2001;24(Suppl 1):S5. (This revision of the previous 1997 therapeutic classification drops the terms "insulin-dependent" and "non-insulin dependent diabetes mellitus" and the acronyms IDDM and NIDDM. It provides an etiologic classification for a number of disorders of carbohydrate metabolism, including those whose genetic mechanisms are known, such as the forms of maturity-onset diabetes of the young, mitochondrial mutations of the pancreatic B cells, mutations of the insulin receptor, and other specific types of diabetes.)

Wajchenberg BL: Subcutaneous and visceral adipose tissue: their relation to the metabolic syndrome. Endocr Rev 2000;21:697. [PMID: 11133069] (This comprehensive review details techniques to measure visceral abdominal fat and discusses its correlation with gender, hormones, energy balance, and the metabolic profile. The ratio of visceral to subcutaneous fat in the abdomen as measured with computed tomography is a predictor of insulin resistance, elevated serum triglycerides, coronary artery disease, and diabetes. Differences in the endocrine regulation of abdominal visceral fat in comparison with fat from other areas are described.)

Therapy of Diabetes Mellitus

Abraira C et al: Intensive insulin therapy in patients with type 2 diabetes: implications of the veterans affairs (VA CSDM) feasibility trial. Am Heart J 1999;138: S360. [PMID: 10539798] (This preliminary study at five VAMCs in 153 men with type 2 diabetes in whom standard pharmacologic therapy had failed raised concern that intensive insulin therapy over 27 months was accompanied by a borderline significant excess in nonfatal cardiovascular events as the glycemic control became closer to normal. Because of the small sample size and the relatively short duration of the study, the authors feel that a longer expanded trial is needed before this unexpected conclusion can be accepted.)

American Diabetes Association: Clinical practice recommendations. Diabetes Care 2002;25(Suppl 1):S1. (A detailed compendium of all the current position statements of the ADA regarding screening, diagnostic procedures, and standards of medical care for treating the acute and chronic complications of type 1 and type 2 diabetes.)

American Diabetes Association: Diabetes mellitus and exercise. (Position statement) Diabetes Care 2002;25 (Suppl 1):S64. (Discussion on how to evaluate a patient with diabetes who wants to start an exercise program. There is also a discussion on the effects of exercise on metabolic control in both type 1 and type 2 diabetes.)

Cusi K et al: Metformin: A review of its metabolic effects. Diabetes Rev 1998;6:89. (A very comprehensive review that includes 471 references related to the pharmacology of metformin and its clinical efficacy when given alone or with other hypoglycemic drugs. The authors, who have extensive experience with this drug, conclude that metformin is an effective therapeutic agent in type 2 diabetes and relatively safe in the absence of impaired renal function or conditions predisposing to hypotension or hypoxia.)

Day C: Thiazolidinediones: a new class of antidiabetic drugs. Diabet Med 1999;16:179 [PMID: 10227562] (A review of the pharmacology of the thiazolidinediones and summary of the clinical studies using troglitazone.)

Effect of intensive blood-glucose control with metformin on complications in overweight patients with type 2 diabetes (UKPDS 34). UK Prospective Diabetes Study (UKPDS) Group. Lancet 1998;352:854. [PMID: 9742977] (Seven hundred and fifty-three obese newly diagnosed type 2 patients were randomized into groups receiving intensive therapy with metformin [n = 342], chlorpropamide [n = 265], glibenclamide [n = 277], or insulin [n = 409], and compared over a median duration of 10.7 years to a group receiving conventional therapy primarily with diet alone [n = 411]. In contrast to the results in the overall study population [see UKPDS 33 below], intensive therapy in these subgroups of obese patients did not reduce microvascular complications no matter what drug was used, as compared with conventional treatment with diet. A paradoxical finding was that metformin monotherapy reduced the risk for diabetes-related death and all-cause mortality compared with diet alone, but in a subgroup of 537 nonobese and obese patients responding poorly to sulfonylurea drugs alone, addition of metformin in half the group showed an increased risk of diabetes-related death compared with those staying on sulfonylureas alone. Since weight gain was less when type 2 obese patients received monotherapy with metformin and since hypoglycemia was uncommon, metformin was recommended as the first choice for drug therapy in obese type 2 patients.)

Efficacy of atenolol and captopril in reducing risk of macrovascular and microvascular complications in type 2 diabetes: UKPDS 39. UK Prospective Diabetes Study Group. BMJ 1998;317:713. [PMID: 9732338] (This analysis indicates that atenolol was just as effective as the ACE inhibitor captopril in reducing macrovascular and microvascular end points in hypertensive type 2 diabetes. Captopril had no specific beneficial effect regarding diabetic renal complications, suggesting that blood pressure reduction in itself may be more important than the medication used.)

Hebel G et al: Hypoglycemia: Pathophysiology and treatment. Endocrinol Metab Clin North Am 2000;29:725. [PMID: 11149159] (This review discusses in detail causation, pathophysiologic consequences, and treatment of the hypoglycemia associated with hypoglycemic therapy in patients with type 1 and type 2 diabetes mellitus.)

Intensive blood-glucose control with sulphonylureas or insulin compared with conventional treatment and risk of complications in patients with type 2 diabetes (UKPDS 33). UK Prospective Diabetes Study (UKPDS) Group. Lancet 1998;352:837. [PMID: 9742976] (Intensive glycemic control over a 10-year period in 3867 newly diagnosed type 2 patients with either sulfonylureas or insulin decreased the risk of microvascular complications but not macrovascular disease. All intensive treatment with these drugs increased the risk of hypoglycemia and weight gain. There were no adverse effects on cardiovascular outcomes.)

Owens DR et al. Insulins today and beyond. Lancet 2001;358:739. [PMID: 11551598] (A review of the pharmacokinetics, clinical benefits, and safety issues of the currently available insulin analogs. The authors also review the data on other analogs that are in development.)

Tight blood pressure control and risk of macrovascular and microvascular complications in type 2 diabetes: UKPDS 38. UK Prospective Diabetes Study Group. BMJ 1998;317: 703. [PMID: 9732337] (In this long-term study of 1148 hypertensive type 2 diabetic patients studied for a mean of 8.4 years, tight blood pressure control [mean of 144/82 mm Hg] reduced the risk of deaths related to diabetes as well as reducing microvascular complications related to diabetes such as progression of diabetic retinopathy and deterioration in visual acuity compared with less tight control with a mean blood pressure of 154/87 mm Hg. Intensive antihypertensive therapy was initially done with either atenolol or captopril, but stepwise addition of diuretics, long-acting nifedipine, and other drugs was needed to achieve target levels. At least 29% of the patients required three drugs to achieve tight control of blood pressure.)

Chronic Complications of Diabetes Mellitus

Aiello LP et al: Diabetic retinopathy. Diabetes Care 1998;21:143. [PMID: 9538986] (Screening strategies for comprehensive eye examinations in diabetic patients, lists outcomes of specific clinical therapies for retinopathy, and gives recommendations for treatment of the various stages of diabetic retinopathy. The American Diabetes Association based its 1998 statement upon evidence reviewed in this publication.)

American Diabetes Association Position Statement: Diabetes nephropathy. Diabetes Care 2002;25(Suppl 1):S85. (Reviews the natural history of diabetic nephropathy, discusses techniques to screen for microalbuminuria, and outlines therapy, including improved glycemic control, and aggressive antihypertensive treatment.)

American Diabetes Association Position Statement: Preventive foot care in people with diabetes. Diabetes Care 2002; 25(Suppl 1):S69. (An update on the foot examination in patients with diabetes and recommendations regarding prevention and management of high-risk foot problems.)

Dejgaard A: Pathophysiology and treatment of diabetic neuropathy. Diabetic Med 1998;15:97. [PMID: 9507909] (A comprehensive overview of pathogenesis and management of the wide range of subclinical and clinical syndromes comprising diabetic neuropathy. It reflects clinical experience as well as a careful review of numerous clinical trials regarding outcome of various pharmacotherapies with special attention to the use of local anesthetic agents in treating painful diabetic neuropathy.)

Lipshultz LI et al: Treatment of erectile dysfunction in men with diabetes. JAMA 1999;281:465. [PMID: 9952210] (All available therapeutic options are discussed, including a useful critical commentary reviewing the promising results of clinical trials with sildenafil [Viagra] while emphasizing the selection criteria needed to minimize cardiovascular complications.)

■ DIABETIC COMA

Coma may be due to a variety of causes not directly related to diabetes. Certain causes directly related to diabetes require differentiation: (1) Hypoglycemic coma resulting from excessive doses of insulin or oral hypoglycemic agents. (2) Hyperglycemic coma associated with either severe insulin deficiency (diabetic ketoacidosis) or mild to moderate insulin deficiency (hyperglycemic hyperosmolar state). (3) Lactic acidosis associated with diabetes, particularly in diabetics stricken with severe infections or with cardiovascular collapse.

DIABETIC KETOACIDOSIS

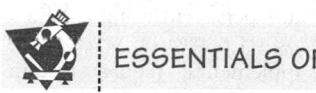 ESSENTIALS OF DIAGNOSIS

- *Hyperglycemia > 250 mg/dL.*
- *Acidosis with blood pH < 7.3.*
- *Serum bicarbonate < 15 meq/L.*
- *Serum positive for ketones.*

General Considerations

Diabetic ketoacidosis may be the initial manifestation of type 1 diabetes or may result from increased insulin requirements in type 1 diabetes patients during the course of infection, trauma, myocardial infarction, or surgery. It is a life-threatening medical emergency with a mortality rate just under 5% in individuals under 40 years of age, but with a more serious prognosis in the elderly, who have mortality rates over 20%. The National Data Group report an annual incidence of five to eight episodes of diabetic ketoacidosis per 1000 diabetic subjects. Type 2 diabetics may develop ketoacidosis under severe stress such as sepsis or trauma. Diabetic ketoacidosis has been found to be one of the more common serious complications of insulin pump therapy, occurring in approximately one per 80 patient-months of treatment. Many patients who monitor capillary blood glucose regularly ignore urine ketone measurements, which would signal the possibility of insulin leakage or pump failure before serious illness develops. Poor compliance is one of the most common causes of diabetic ketoacidosis, particularly when episodes are recurrent.

Clinical Findings

A. SYMPTOMS AND SIGNS

The appearance of diabetic ketoacidotic coma is usually preceded by a day or more of polyuria and polydipsia associated with marked fatigue, nausea and vomiting, and, finally, mental stupor that can progress to coma. On physical examination, evidence of dehydration in a stuporous patient with rapid deep breathing and a "fruity" breath odor of acetone would strongly suggest the diagnosis. Hypotension with tachycardia indicates profound fluid and electrolyte depletion, and mild hypothermia is usually present. Abdominal pain and even tenderness may be present in the absence of abdominal disease. Conversely, cholecystitis or pancreatitis may occur with minimal symptoms and signs.

B. LABORATORY FINDINGS

(Table 27–12.) Glycosuria of 4+ and strong ketonuria with hyperglycemia, ketonemia, low arterial blood pH, and low plasma bicarbonate are typical of diabetic ketoacidosis. Serum potassium is often elevated despite total body potassium depletion resulting from protracted polyuria or vomiting. Elevation of serum amylase is common but often represents salivary as well as pancreatic amylase. Thus, in this setting, an elevated serum amylase is not specific for acute pancreatitis. Azotemia may be a better indicator of renal status than serum creatinine, since multichannel chemical analysis of serum creatinine (SMA-6) is

Table 27–12. Laboratory diagnosis of coma in diabetic patients.

	Urine		Plasma		
	Glucose	Acetone	Glucose	Bicarbonate	Acetone
Related to diabetes					
Hypoglycemia	0[1]	0 or +	Low	Normal	0
Diabetic ketoacidosis	++++	++++	High	Low	++++
Nonketotic hyperglycemic coma	++++	0	High	Normal or slightly low	0
Lactic acidosis	0 or +	0 or +	Normal or low or high	Low	0 or +
Unrelated to diabetes					
Alcohol or other toxic drugs	0 or +	0 or +	May be low	Normal or low[2]	0 or +
Cerebrovascular accident or head trauma	+ or 0	0	Often high	Normal	0
Uremia	0 or +	0	High or normal	Low	0 or +

[1]Leftover urine in bladder might still contain glucose from earlier hyperglycemia.
[2]Alcohol can elevate plasma lactate as well as keto acids to reduce pH.

falsely elevated by nonspecific chromogenicity of keto acids and glucose. Most laboratories, however, now routinely eliminate this interference. Leukocytosis as high as 25,000/μL with a left shift may occur with or without associated infection. The presence of an elevated or even a normal temperature would suggest the presence of an infection, since patients with diabetic ketoacidosis are generally hypothermic if uninfected.

Complications

The two major metabolic aberrations of diabetic ketoacidosis are hyperglycemia and ketoacidemia, both due to insulin lack associated with hyperglucagonemia as well as elevated levels of other stress hormones such as catecholamines, cortisol, and growth hormone.

A. Hyperglycemia

Hyperglycemia results from increased hepatic production of glucose as well as diminished glucose uptake by peripheral tissues. Hepatic glucose output is a consequence of increased gluconeogenesis resulting from insulinopenia as well as from an associated hyperglucagonemia. When serum hyperosmolality exceeds 320–330 mosm/L, central nervous system depression or coma may ensue. Coma in a diabetic patient with a lower osmolality should prompt a search for cause of coma other than hyperosmolality.

B. Ketoacidemia

Ketoacidemia represents the effect of insulin lack at multiple enzyme loci. Insulin lack associated with elevated levels of growth hormone, catecholamines, and glucagon contributes to an increase in lipolysis from adipose tissue and in hepatic ketogenesis. In addition, there is evidence that reduced ketolysis by insulin-deficient peripheral tissues contributes to the ketoacidemia. The only true "keto" acid present is acetoacetic acid, which, along with its by-product acetone, is measured by nitroprusside reagents (Acetest and Ketostix). The sensitivity for acetone, however, is poor, requiring over 10 mmol, which is seldom reached in the plasma of ketoacidotic subjects—although this detectable concentration is readily achieved in urine. Thus, in the plasma of ketotic patients, only acetoacetate is measured by these reagents. The more prevalent β-hydroxybutyric acid has no ketone group and is therefore not detected by conventional nitroprusside tests. This takes on special importance in the presence of circulatory collapse during diabetic ketoacidosis, wherein an increase in lactic acid can shift the redox state to increase β-hydroxybutyric acid at the expense of the readily detectable acetoacetic acid. Bedside diagnostic reagents would then be unreliable, suggesting no ketonemia in cases where β-hydroxybutyric acid is a major factor in producing the acidosis.

Treatment

A. Prevention

Education of diabetic patients to recognize the early symptoms and signs of ketoacidosis has done a great deal to prevent severe acidosis. Urine ketones should be measured in patients with signs of infection or in insulin pump-treated patients when capillary blood glucose is unexpectedly and persistently high. When heavy ketonuria and glycosuria persist on several successive examinations, supplemental regular insulin should be administered and liquid foods such as lightly salted tomato juice and broth should be ingested to replenish fluids and electrolytes. The patient should be instructed to contact the physician if ketonuria persists, and especially if vomiting develops or if appropriate adjustment of the infusion rate on an insulin pump does not correct the hyperglycemia and ketonuria. In juvenile-onset diabetics, particularly in the teen years, recurrent episodes of severe ketoacidosis often indicate poor compliance with the insulin regimen, and these patients will require intensive family counseling.

B. Emergency Measures

If ketosis is severe, the patient should be placed in the hospital for correction of the hyperosmolality as well as the ketoacidemia. An intensive care unit or, at the least, a step-down unit is preferable for more severe cases.

1. Therapeutic flow sheet—One of the most important steps in initiating therapy is to start a flow sheet listing vital signs and the time sequence of diagnostic laboratory values in relation to therapeutic maneuvers. Indices of the metabolic defects include urine glucose and ketones as well as arterial pH, plasma glucose, acetone, bicarbonate, serum urea nitrogen, and electrolytes. Serum osmolality should be measured or estimated and tabulated during the course of therapy.

A convenient method of estimating effective serum osmolality is as follows (normal values in humans are 280–300 mosm/kg):

$$\text{mosm/kg} = 2[\text{Na}^+] + \frac{\text{Glucose (mg/dL)}}{18}$$

These calculated estimates are usually 10–20 mosm/kg lower than values measured by standard cryoscopic techniques in patients with diabetic coma. Urea is freely permeable across cell membranes and therefore not included in calculations of effective serum osmolality. One physician should be responsible for maintaining this therapeutic flow sheet and prescribing therapy. An indwelling urinary catheter is required in all comatose patients but should be avoided if possible in a fully cooperative diabetic because of the risk of introducing bladder infection.

Fluid intake and output should be recorded. Gastric intubation is recommended in the comatose patient to correct the commonly associated gastric dilatation that may lead to vomiting and aspiration. The patient should not receive sedatives or narcotics.

2. Insulin replacement—Only regular insulin should be used initially in all cases of severe ketoacidosis, and it should be given immediately after the diagnosis is established. Regular insulin can be given in a loading dose of 0.1 unit/kg as an intravenous bolus followed by 0.1 unit/kg/h, continuously infused or given hourly as an intramuscular injection; this is sufficient to replace the insulin deficit in most patients. Replacement of insulin deficiency helps correct the acidosis by reducing the flux of fatty acids to the liver, reducing ketone production by the liver, and also improving removal of ketones from the blood. Insulin treatment reduces the hyperosmolality by reducing the hyperglycemia. It accomplishes this by increasing removal of glucose through peripheral utilization as well as by decreasing production of glucose by the liver. This latter effect is accomplished by direct inhibition of gluconeogenesis and glycogenolysis, as well as by lowered amino acid flux from muscle to liver and reduced hyperglucagonemia.

The insulin dose should be "piggy-backed" into the fluid line so the rate of fluid replacement can be changed without altering the insulin delivery rate. For optimal effects, continuous low-dose insulin infusions should always be preceded by a rapid intravenous loading dose of regular insulin, 0.1 unit/kg, to prime the tissue insulin receptors. If the plasma glucose level fails to fall at least 10% in the first hour, a repeat loading dose is recommended. The availability of bedside glucometers and of laboratory instruments for rapid and accurate glucose analysis (Beckman or Yellow Springs glucose analyzer) has contributed much to achieving optimal insulin replacement. Rarely, a patient with immune insulin resistance is encountered, and this requires doubling the insulin dose every 2–4 hours if hyperglycemia does not improve after the first two doses of insulin.

3. Fluid and electrolyte replacement—In most patients, the fluid deficit is 4–5 L. Initially, 0.9% saline solution is the solution of choice to help reexpand the contracted vascular volume and should be started in the emergency room as soon as the diagnosis is established. The use of sodium bicarbonate has been questioned since clinical benefit was not demonstrated in one prospective randomized trial and because of the following potentially harmful consequences: (1) hypokalemia from rapid potassium shifts into cells; (2) tissue hypoxia from reduced dissociation of oxygen from hemoglobin when acidosis is rapidly reversed; (3) cerebral acidosis resulting from a reduction of cerebrospinal fluid pH; and (4) a worsening of hyperosmolality. However, these concerns are relatively less important in certain clinical settings. When the pH is

7.1 or higher, the use of sodium bicarbonate is contraindicated. However, when the arterial pH is 6.9–7.0, the current consensus statement of the American Diabetes Association suggests adding one ampule of 7.5% sodium bicarbonate (44 meq/L) to 200 mL of sterile water and administering it intravenously at a rate of 200 mL/h. If the pH is below 6.9, two ampules of sodium bicarbonate (88 meq) in 400 mL of sterile water given at the same rate of 200 mL/h is recommended. For each ampule of sodium bicarbonate added, 15 meq/L of potassium chloride should be added to the infusate as long as the serum potassium does not exceed 5.5 meq/L. *Once the pH reaches 7.1, no further bicarbonate should be given, since it aggravates rebound metabolic alkalosis as ketones are metabolized.* Alkalosis causes potassium shifts that increase the risk of cardiac arrhythmias. In the first hour, at least 1 L of 0.9% saline should be infused, and fluid should be given thereafter at a rate of 300–500 mL/h with careful monitoring of serum potassium. Failure to give enough volume replacement (at least 3–4 L in 8 hours) to restore normal perfusion is one of the most serious therapeutic shortcomings affecting satisfactory recovery. Likewise, excessive fluid replacement (more than 5 L in 8 hours) may contribute to acute respiratory distress syndrome or cerebral edema. When blood glucose falls to 250 mg/dL or less, 5% glucose solutions should be used to maintain blood glucose between 200 and 300 mg/dL while insulin therapy is continued in order to clear the ketonemia. Glucose administration has the dual advantage of preventing hypoglycemia and furthermore of reducing the likelihood of cerebral edema, which could result from too rapid a decline in hyperglycemia.

During therapy, **hyperchloremic acidosis** develops because of the considerable loss of keto acids in the urine during the initial phase of treatment. A portion of the bicarbonate deficit is replaced with chloride ions infused in large amounts as saline to correct the dehydration. Thus, in most patients, as the ketoacidosis clears during insulin replacement, they show a hyperchloremic, low bicarbonate pattern with a normal anion gap. This is a relatively benign condition that reverses itself over the subsequent 12–24 hours once intravenous saline is no longer being administered.

4. Potassium and phosphate replacement—Total body potassium loss from polyuria as well as from vomiting may be as high as several hundred milliequivalents. However, because of shifts from cells due to the acidosis, serum potassium is usually normal or high until after the first few hours of treatment, when acidosis improves and serum potassium returns into cells. Potassium in doses of 20–30 meq/h should be infused within 2–3 hours after beginning therapy, or sooner if initial serum potassium is inappropriately low. Potassium replacement should be deferred if serum potassium fails to respond to initial therapy and remains above 5 meq/L, as in cases of renal insufficiency.

Foods high in potassium content can be prescribed when the patient has recovered sufficiently to take food orally. (Tomato juice and grapefruit juice contain 14 meq of potassium per 240 mL and a medium-sized banana 10 meq.)

Phosphate replacement is seldom required in treating diabetic ketoacidosis. A significant therapeutic benefit of routine phosphate replacement has not been documented in several randomized trials. However, if severe hypophosphatemia of less than 0.35 mmol/L (< 1 mg/dL) develops during insulin therapy, a small amount of phosphate can be replaced as the potassium salt. Hypophosphatemia of this severity is detrimental to membranes of skeletal muscle and may lyse red blood cells. The potassium need is several times that of phosphate and should be replaced separately, since replacing phosphorus ions too rapidly (while meeting potassium requirements) can precipitate serum calcium in the tissues and induce tetany.

Treatment of severe hypophosphatemia helps to restore the buffering capacity of the plasma, thereby facilitating renal excretion of hydrogen; and it corrects the impaired oxygen dissociation from hemoglobin by regenerating 2,3-diphosphoglycerate. To minimize the risk of inducing tetany from an overload of phosphate replacement, an average deficit of 40–50 mmol phosphate in adults with diabetic ketoacidosis should be replaced by intravenous infusion at a rate not to exceed 3 mmol/h.

A stock solution available from Abbott Laboratories provides a mixture of 1.12 g KH_2PO_4 and 1.18 g K_2HPO_4 in a 5 mL single-dose vial representing 22 meq potassium and 15 mmol phosphate (27 meq). Five milliliters of this stock solution in 2 L of either 0.45% saline or 5% dextrose in water, infused at 400 mL/h, will replace the phosphate at the optimal rate of 3 mmol/h and will provide 4.4 meq of potassium per hour. If serum phosphate remains below 0.35 mmol/L (1 mg/dL), a repeat 5-hour infusion of potassium phosphate at a rate of 3 mmol/h would be reasonable.

5. Treatment of associated infection—Antibiotics are prescribed as indicated. Cholecystitis and pyelonephritis may be particularly severe in these patients.

Prognosis

The frequency of deaths due to diabetic ketoacidosis has been dramatically reduced by improved therapy of young diabetics, but this complication remains a significant risk in the aged and in patients in profound coma in whom treatment has been delayed. Acute myocardial infarction and infarction of the bowel following prolonged hypotension worsen the outlook. A serious prognostic sign is renal failure, and prior kidney dysfunction worsens the prognosis considerably because the kidney plays a key role in compensating for massive pH and electrolyte abnormalities. Cerebral edema has been reported to occur rarely as metabolic deficits return to normal. This is best prevented by avoiding sudden reversal of marked hyperglycemia. Maintaining glycemic levels of 200–300 mg/dL for the initial 24 hours after correction of severe hyperglycemia reduces this risk.

Kitabchi AE et al: Management of hyperglycemic crises in patients with diabetes. Diabetes Care 2001;24:131. [PMID: 11194218] (This detailed technical review of hyperglycemic emergencies reflects the extensive clinical experience of the authors, who were selected by the American Diabetes Association to provide the basis for a consensus report. It updates the pathogenesis, clinical features, and therapeutic recommendations for these critical diabetic emergencies. Criteria are given for classifying diabetic ketoacidosis as mild, moderate, or severe as a basis for prognosis and for directing therapy, such as deciding whether or not to administer bicarbonate.)

HYPERGLYCEMIC HYPEROSMOLAR STATE

 ESSENTIALS OF DIAGNOSIS

- *Hyperglycemia > 600 mg/dL.*
- *Serum osmolality > 310 mosm/kg.*
- *No acidosis; blood pH above 7.3.*
- *Serum bicarbonate > 15 meq/L.*
- *Normal anion gap (< 14 meq/L).*

General Considerations

This second most common form of hyperglycemic coma is characterized by severe hyperglycemia in the absence of significant ketosis, with hyperosmolality and dehydration. It occurs in patients with mild or occult diabetes, and most patients are at least middle-aged to elderly. Accurate figures are not available as to its true incidence, but from data on hospital discharges it is rarer than diabetic ketoacidosis even in older age groups. Lethargy and confusion develop as serum osmolality exceeds 310 mosm/kg, and coma can occur if osmolality exceeds 320–330 mosm/kg. A committee of the American Diabetes Association has recommended replacing the previous name of this disorder (hyperglycemic, hyperosmolar, nonketotic coma) with the consensus term hyperglycemic hyperosmolar state. Underlying renal insufficiency or congestive heart failure is common, and the presence of either worsens the prognosis. A precipitating event such as infection, myocardial infarction, stroke, or recent operation is often present. Certain drugs such as phenytoin, diazoxide, glucocorticoids, and diuretics have been implicated in its pathogenesis, as have procedures associated with glucose loading such as peritoneal dialysis.

Pathogenesis

A partial or relative insulin deficiency may initiate the syndrome by reducing glucose utilization of muscle, fat, and liver while inducing hyperglucagonemia and increasing hepatic glucose output. With massive glycosuria, obligatory water loss ensues. If a patient is unable to maintain adequate fluid intake because of an associated acute or chronic illness or has suffered excessive fluid loss, marked dehydration results. As plasma volume contracts, renal insufficiency develops, and the resultant limitation of renal glucose loss leads to increasingly higher blood glucose concentrations. Severe hyperosmolality develops that causes mental confusion and finally coma. It is not clear why ketosis is virtually absent under these conditions of insulin insufficiency, although reduced levels of growth hormone may be a factor, along with portal vein insulin concentrations sufficient to restrain ketogenesis.

Clinical Findings

A. SYMPTOMS AND SIGNS

Onset may be insidious over a period of days or weeks, with weakness, polyuria, and polydipsia. The lack of features of ketoacidosis may retard recognition of the syndrome and delay therapy until dehydration becomes more profound than in ketoacidosis. Reduced intake of fluid is not an uncommon historical feature, due to either inappropriate lack of thirst, nausea, or inaccessibility of fluids to elderly, bedridden patients. Lethargy and confusion develop, progressing to convulsions and deep coma. Physical examination confirms the presence of profound dehydration in a lethargic or comatose patient without Kussmaul respirations.

B. LABORATORY FINDINGS

Severe hyperglycemia is present, with blood glucose values ranging from 600 to 2400 mg/dL. In mild cases, where dehydration is less severe, dilutional hyponatremia as well as urinary sodium losses may reduce serum sodium to 120–125 meq/L, which protects to some extent against extreme hyperosmolality. However, as dehydration progresses, serum sodium can exceed 140 meq/L, producing serum osmolality readings of 330–440 mosm/kg. Ketosis and acidosis are usually absent or mild. Prerenal azotemia is the rule, with serum urea nitrogen elevations over 100 mg/dL being typical.

Treatment

A. SALINE

Fluid replacement is of paramount importance in treating nonketotic hyperglycemic coma. The onset of hyperosmolarity is more insidious in elderly people without ketosis than in younger individuals with high serum ketone levels, which provide earlier indicators of severe illness (vomiting, rapid deep breathing, acetone odor, etc). Consequently, diagnosis and treatment are often delayed until fluid deficit has reached levels of 6–10 L.

If hypovolemia is present as evidenced by hypotension and oliguria, fluid therapy should be initiated with isotonic 0.9% saline. In all other cases, hypotonic (0.45%) saline appears to be preferable as the initial replacement solution because the body fluids of these patients are markedly hyperosmolar. As much as 4–6 L of fluid may be required in the first 8–10 hours. Careful monitoring of the patient is required for proper sodium and water replacement. Once blood glucose reaches 250 mg/dL, fluid replacement should include 5% dextrose in either water, 0.45% saline solution, or 0.9% saline solution. The rate of dextrose infusion should be adjusted to maintain glycemic levels of 250–300 mg/dL in order to reduce the risk of cerebral edema. An important end point of fluid therapy is to restore urine output to 50 mL/h or more.

B. INSULIN

Less insulin may be required to reduce the hyperglycemia in nonketotic patients as compared to those with diabetic ketoacidotic coma. In fact, fluid replacement alone can reduce hyperglycemia considerably by correcting the hypovolemia, which then increases both glomerular filtration and renal excretion of glucose. An initial dose of only 15 units intravenously and 15 units subcutaneously of regular insulin is usually quite effective, and in most cases subsequent doses need not be greater than 10–20 units subcutaneously every 4 hours.

C. POTASSIUM

With the absence of acidosis, there may be no initial hyperkalemia unless associated renal failure is present. This results in less severe total potassium depletion than in diabetic ketoacidosis, and less potassium replacement is therefore needed. However, because initial serum potassium is usually not elevated and because it declines rapidly as a result of insulin's effect on driving potassium intracellularly, it has been recommended that potassium replacement be initiated earlier than in ketotic patients, assuming that no renal insufficiency or oliguria is present. Potassium chloride (10 meq/L) can be added to the initial bottle of fluids administered if the patient's serum potassium is not elevated.

D. PHOSPHATE

If severe hypophosphatemia (serum phosphate < 1 mg/dL [< 0.35 mmol/L]) develops during insulin therapy, phosphate replacement can be given as described for ketoacidotic patients (at 3 mmol/h).

Prognosis

The overall mortality rate of hyperglycemic, hyperosmolar, nonketotic coma is more than ten times that of diabetic ketoacidosis, chiefly because of its higher incidence in older patients, who may have compromised cardiovascular systems or associated major illnesses and whose dehydration is often excessive because of delays in recognition and treatment. (When patients are matched for age, the prognoses of these two hyperglycemic emergencies are reasonably comparable.) When prompt therapy is instituted, the mortality rate can be reduced from nearly 50% to that related to the severity of coexistent disorders.

Hyperglycemic crises in patients with diabetes mellitus. Diabetes Care 2001;24:154. [PMID:11221603] (This consensus statement provides the most current appraisal of the nomenclature, classification, and clinical features of these life-threatening hyperglycemic emergencies. The term "hyperglycemic, hyperosmolar state" has been chosen to replace the previously-used term "hyperglycemic, hyperosmolar, nonketotic coma." Differences between the pathogenesis and clinical manifestations of these hyperglycemic crises are contrasted, and a consensus as to their treatment is presented.)

Trence DL et al: Hyperglycemic crisis in diabetes mellitus type 2. Endocrinol Metab Clin North Am 2001;30:817. [PMID: 11727401] (The hyperglycemic hyperosmolar state is characterized as to its clinical presentation and treatment. Includes a detailed list of specific precipitating factors, including infections, coexisting illnesses, medications, and endocrine causes.)

LACTIC ACIDOSIS
(See also Metformin & Other Biguanides.)

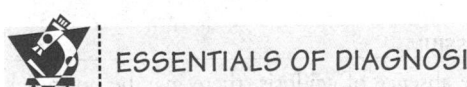 ESSENTIALS OF DIAGNOSIS

- *Severe acidosis with hyperventilation.*
- *Blood pH below 7.30.*
- *Serum bicarbonate < 15 meq/L.*
- *Anion gap > 15 meq/L.*
- *Absent serum ketones.*
- *Serum lactate > 5 mmol/L.*

General Considerations

Lactic acidosis is characterized by accumulation of excess lactic acid in the blood. Normally, the principal sources of this acid are the erythrocytes (which lack enzymes for aerobic oxidation), skeletal muscle, skin, and brain. Conversion of lactic acid to glucose and its oxidation principally by the liver but also by the kidneys represent the chief pathways for its removal. Overproduction of lactic acid (tissue hypoxia), deficient removal (hepatic failure), or both (circulatory collapse) can cause accumulation. Lactic acidosis is not uncommon in any severely ill patient suffering from cardiac decompensation, respiratory or hepatic failure, septicemia, or infarction of bowel or extremities. With the discontinuance of phenformin therapy in the USA, lactic acidosis in patients with diabetes mellitus has become uncommon but occasionally occurs in metformin-treated patients (see above) and it still must be considered in the acidotic diabetic, especially if the patient is seriously ill.

Clinical Findings

A. SYMPTOMS AND SIGNS

The main clinical feature of lactic acidosis is marked hyperventilation. When lactic acidosis is secondary to tissue hypoxia or vascular collapse, the clinical presentation is variable, being that of the prevailing catastrophic illness. However, in the idiopathic, or spontaneous, variety, the onset is rapid (usually over a few hours), blood pressure is normal, peripheral circulation is good, and there is no cyanosis.

B. LABORATORY FINDINGS

Plasma bicarbonate and blood pH are quite low, indicating the presence of severe metabolic acidosis. Ketones are usually absent from plasma and urine or at least not prominent. The first clue may be a high anion gap (serum sodium minus the sum of chloride and bicarbonate anions [in meq/L] should be no greater than 15). A higher value indicates the existence of an abnormal compartment of anions. If this cannot be clinically explained by an excess of keto acids (diabetes), inorganic acids (uremia), or anions from drug overdosage (salicylates, methyl alcohol, ethylene glycol), then lactic acidosis is probably the correct diagnosis. (See Chapter 21 also.) In the absence of azotemia, hyperphosphatemia may be a clue to the presence of lactic acidosis for reasons that are not clear. The diagnosis is confirmed by demonstrating, in a sample of blood that is promptly chilled and separated, a plasma lactic acid concentration of 5 mmol/L or higher (values as high as 30 mmol/L have been reported). Normal plasma values average 1 mmol/L, with a normal lactate/pyruvate ratio of 10:1. This ratio is greatly exceeded in lactic acidosis.*

Treatment

Aggressive treatment of the precipitating cause of lactic acidosis is the main component of therapy, such as ensuring adequate oxygenation and vascular perfusion

---

*In collecting samples, it is essential to rapidly chill and separate the blood in order to remove red cells, whose continued glycolysis at room temperature is a common source of error in reports of high plasma lactate. Frozen plasma remains stable for subsequent assay.

of tissues. Empirical antibiotic coverage for sepsis should be given after culture samples are obtained in any patient in whom the cause of the lactic acidosis is not apparent.

Alkalinization with intravenous sodium bicarbonate to keep the pH above 7.2 has been recommended by some in the emergency treatment of lactic acidosis; as much as 2000 meq in 24 hours has been used. However, there is no evidence that the mortality rate is favorably affected by administering bicarbonate, and its use remains controversial. Hemodialysis may be useful in cases where large sodium loads are poorly tolerated.

Prognosis

The mortality rate of spontaneous lactic acidosis is high. The prognosis in most cases is that of the primary disorder that produced the lactic acidosis.

Chan NN et al: Metformin-associated lactic acidosis: a rare or very rare clinical entity? Diabet Med 1999;16:273. [PMID: 10220200] (Analysis of over 170 reported cases of metformin-associated lactic acidosis found it to be 20 times less common than that associated with phenformin. They concluded that if recommended therapeutic guidelines are adhered to, metformin use appears to be safe and the case fatality rate is no higher than that seen in sulfonylurea-induced hypoglycemia.)

Forsythe SM et al: Sodium bicarbonate for the treatment of lactic acidosis. Chest 2000;117:260. [PMID: 10631227] (This perspective focuses on the treatment of lactic acidosis and presents evidence from an extensive literature search—as well as from the authors' extensive experience—that the use of sodium bicarbonate cannot be condoned for treating patients with lactic acidosis.)

■ THE HYPOGLYCEMIC STATES

Spontaneous hypoglycemia in adults is of two principal types: fasting and postprandial. Symptoms begin at plasma glucose levels in the range of 60 mg/dL and impairment of brain function at approximately 50 mg/dL. Fasting hypoglycemia is often subacute or chronic and usually presents with neuroglycopenia as its principal manifestation; postprandial hypoglycemia is relatively acute and is often heralded by symptoms of neurogenic autonomic discharge (sweating, palpitations, anxiety, tremulousness).

Differential Diagnosis
(Table 27–13)

Fasting hypoglycemia may occur in certain endocrine disorders, such as hypopituitarism, Addison's disease, or myxedema; in disorders related to liver malfunction, such as acute alcoholism or liver failure; and in instances of renal failure, particularly in patients requiring dialysis. These conditions are usually obvious,

Table 27–13. Common causes of hypoglycemia in adults.[1]

Fasting hypoglycemia
Hyperinsulinism
Pancreatic B cell tumor
Surreptitious administration of insulin or sulfonylureas
Extrapancreatic tumors
Postprandial (reactive) hypoglycemia
Early hypoglycemia (alimentary)
Postgastrectomy
Functional (increased vagal tone)
Late hypoglycemia (occult diabetes)
Delayed insulin release due to B cell dysfunction
Counterregulatory deficiency
Idiopathic
Alcohol-related hypoglycemia
Immunopathologic hypoglycemia
Idiopathic anti-insulin antibodies (which release their bound insulin)
Antibodies to insulin receptors (which act as agonists)
Pentamidine-induced hypoglycemia

[1]In the absence of clinically obvious endocrine, renal, or hepatic disorders and exclusive of diabetes treated with hypoglycemic agents.

with hypoglycemia being only a secondary feature. When fasting hypoglycemia is a primary manifestation developing in adults without apparent endocrine disorders or inborn metabolic diseases from childhood, the principal diagnostic possibilities include (1) hyperinsulinism, due to either pancreatic B cell tumors or surreptitious administration of insulin (or sulfonylureas); and (2) hypoglycemia due to non-insulin-producing extrapancreatic tumors.

Postprandial (reactive) hypoglycemia may be classified as early (within 2–3 hours after a meal) or late (3–5 hours after eating). Early, or alimentary, hypoglycemia occurs when there is a rapid discharge of ingested carbohydrate into the small bowel followed by rapid glucose absorption and hyperinsulinism. It may be seen after gastrointestinal surgery and is particularly associated with the dumping syndrome after gastrectomy. In some cases, it is functional and may represent overactivity of the parasympathetic nervous system mediated via the vagus nerve. Rarely, it results from defective counterregulatory responses such as deficiencies of growth hormone, glucagon, cortisol, or autonomic responses.

Alcohol-related hypoglycemia is due to hepatic glycogen depletion combined with alcohol-mediated inhibition of gluconeogenesis. It is most common in malnourished alcohol abusers but can occur in anyone who is unable to ingest food after an acute alcoholic episode followed by gastritis and vomiting.

Immunopathologic hypoglycemia is an extremely rare condition in which anti-insulin antibodies or antibodies to insulin receptors develop spontaneously. In the former case, the mechanism appears to relate to increasing dissociation of insulin from circulating pools of bound insulin. When antibodies to insulin receptors are found, most patients do not have hypoglycemia but rather severe insulin-resistant diabetes and acanthosis nigricans. However, during the course of the disease in these patients, certain anti-insulin receptor antibodies with agonist activity mimicking insulin action may develop, producing severe hypoglycemia.

Factitious hypoglycemia is self-induced hypoglycemia due to surreptitious administration of insulin or sulfonylureas.

HYPOGLYCEMIA DUE TO PANCREATIC B CELL TUMORS

Fasting hypoglycemia in an otherwise healthy, well-nourished adult is rare, and is most commonly due to an adenoma of the islets of Langerhans. Ninety percent of such tumors are single and benign, but multiple adenomas can occur as well as malignant tumors with functional metastases. B cell hyperplasia as a cause of fasting hypoglycemia is rare but has been documented in adults. Adenomas may be familial, and multiple adenomas have been found in conjunction with tumors of the parathyroids and pituitary (multiple endocrine neoplasia type 1 [MEN 1]).

Clinical Findings

A. SYMPTOMS AND SIGNS

The most important prerequisite to diagnosing an insulinoma is simply to consider it, particularly in relatively healthy-appearing persons who have fasting hypoglycemia associated with some degree of central nervous system dysfunction such as confusion or abnormal behavior. A delay in diagnosis can result in unnecessary treatment for psychomotor epilepsy or psychiatric disorders and may cause irreversible brain damage. In long-standing cases, obesity can result as a consequence of overeating to relieve symptoms.

Whipple's triad is characteristic of hypoglycemia regardless of the cause. It consists of (1) a history of hypoglycemic symptoms, (2) an associated fasting blood glucose of 40 mg/dL or less, and (3) immediate recovery upon administration of glucose. The hypoglycemic symptoms in insulinoma often develop in the early morning or after missing a meal. Occasionally, they occur after exercise. They typically begin with evidence of central nervous system glucose lack and can include blurred vision or diplopia, headache, feelings of detachment, slurred speech, and weakness. Personality and mental changes vary from anxiety to psychotic behavior, and neurologic deterioration can result in convulsions or coma. Sweating and palpitations may not occur.

Hypoglycemic unawareness is very common in patients with insulinoma. They adapt to chronic hypoglycemia by increasing their efficiency in transporting glucose across the blood-brain barrier, which masks awareness that their blood glucose is approaching critically low levels. Counterregulatory hormonal responses as well as neurogenic symptoms such as tremor, sweating, and palpitations are therefore blunted during hypoglycemia. If lack of these warning symptoms prevents recognition of the need to eat to correct the problem, patients can lapse into severe hypoglycemic coma. However, symptoms and normal hormone responses during experimental insulin-induced hypoglycemia have been shown to be restored after successful surgical removal of the insulinoma. Presumably with return of euglycemia, adaptive effects on glucose transport into the brain are corrected and thresholds of counterregulatory responses and neurogenic autonomic symptoms are therefore restored to normal.

B. LABORATORY FINDINGS

B cell adenomas do not reduce secretion in the presence of hypoglycemia, and the critical diagnostic test is to demonstrate inappropriately elevated serum insulin levels at a time when hypoglycemia is present. A reliable serum insulin level of 6 μU/mL or more in the presence of blood glucose values below 40 mg/dL is diagnostic of inappropriate hyperinsulinism. Other causes of hyperinsulinemic hypoglycemia must be considered, including factitious administration of insulin or sulfonylureas. An elevated circulating proinsulin level (above 0.2 ng/mL) in the presence of fasting hypoglycemia is characteristic of most B cell adenomas and does not occur in factitious hyperinsulinism.

In patients with epigastric distress, a history of renal stones, or menstrual or erectile dysfunction, a serum calcium, gastrin, or prolactin level may be useful in screening for MEN-1 associated with insulinoma.

C. DIAGNOSTIC TESTS

1. Prolonged fasting—Prolonged fasting under hospital supervision until hypoglycemia is documented is probably the most dependable means of establishing the diagnosis, especially in men. In 30% of patients with insulinoma, the blood glucose levels often drop below 40 mg/dL after an overnight fast, but some patients require up to 72 hours to develop symptomatic hypoglycemia. However, the term "72-hour fast" is actually a misnomer in most cases since the fast should be immediately terminated as soon as symptoms appear and laboratory confirmation of hypoglycemia is available. In normal male subjects, the blood glucose does not fall below 55–60 mg/dL during a 3-day fast. In contrast, in normal premenopausal women who have fasted for only 24 hours, the plasma glucose may fall normally to such an extent that it can reach values as low as 35 mg/dL. In these cases, however, the women are not symptomatic, presumably owing to the development of sufficient ketonemia to supply energy needs to the brain. Insulinoma patients, on the other hand, become symptomatic when plasma glucose drops to subnormal levels, since inappropriate insulin secretion restricts ketone formation. Moreover, the demonstration of a nonsuppressed insulin level (≥ 6 µU/mL) in the presence of hypoglycemia suggests the diagnosis of insulinoma. If hypoglycemia does not develop in a male patient after fasting for up to 72 hours—and particularly when this prolonged fast is terminated with a period of moderate exercise—insulinoma must be considered an unlikely diagnosis. A suggested protocol for the supervised fast is shown in Table 27–14.

2. Proinsulin determinations—In contrast to normal subjects, whose proinsulin concentration is less than 20% of the total immunoreactive insulin, most patients with insulinoma have elevated levels of proinsulin representing 30–90% of total immunoreactive insulin. While absolute proinsulin measurements may be elevated in other conditions besides insulinoma (such as in insulin-resistant states), an increased percentage of proinsulin-like components in relation to total insulin immunoreactivity is more specific for insulinoma. However, since this assay of the "percent proinsulin" requires laborious methodology to separate serum protein components, its usefulness is limited. Absolute proinsulin levels are more readily measured, and their specificity increases as plasma glucose falls during a supervised fast. If the laboratory diagnosis is not evident using insulin levels, it may be helpful to find that serum proinsulin fails to suppress below 0.2 ng/mL in the presence of hypoglycemia.

Table 27–14. Suggested hospital protocol for supervised fast in diagnosis of insulinoma.[1]

(1) Obtain baseline serum glucose, insulin, and C-peptide measurements at onset of fast and initiate reliable intravenous access with normal saline.

(2) Permit only calorie-free and caffeine-free fluids and encourage activity.

(3) Measure all voided urine for acetone.

(4) Obtain capillary glucose measurements with a reflectance meter every 4 hours until values < 60 mg/dL are obtained. Then increase the frequency of fingersticks to each hour, and when capillary glucose value is < 49 mg/dL send a venous blood sample to the laboratory for serum glucose, insulin, proinsulin, and C-peptide measurements. Check frequently for manifestations of neuroglycopenia.

(5) If symptoms of hypoglycemia occur or if a laboratory value of serum glucose is < 45 mg/dL, conclude the fast with a final blood sample for serum glucose, insulin, C-peptide, and sulfonylurea measurements. Intravenous glucose should then be administered (40–50 mL of 50% dextrose in water over 3–5 minutes through the intravenous access line) and adminster calorie-containing liquids and food.

[1]Adapted, with permission, from Service FJ: Hypoglycemic disorders. N Engl J Med 1995;332:1144.

3. Stimulation tests—Stimulation with pancreatic B cell secretagogues such as tolbutamide, glucagon, or leucine is generally not needed in most cases if basal insulin is found to be nonsuppressible and therefore inappropriately elevated during fasting hypoglycemia.

Intravenous glucagon (1 mg over 1 minute) can be useful in patients with "borderline" fasting inappropriate hyperinsulinism. A serum insulin rise above baseline of 200 µU/mL or more at 5 and 10 minutes strongly suggests insulinoma, although poorly differentiated tumors may not respond. Glucagon has the advantage over tolbutamide of correcting rather than provoking hypoglycemia during stimulation testing and is diagnostic in 60–70% of patients with insulinoma. False-negative results can occur if the tumor is poorly differentiated and agranular.

D. PREOPERATIVE LOCALIZATION OF B CELL TUMORS

Radiographic and arteriographic techniques are seldom helpful in localizing insulinomas preoperatively owing to the small size of most of these tumors (averaging 1.5 cm in diameter in one large series). These methods are often positive only when the tumor is large enough to be easily visualized or palpated intraoperatively.

Currently, there is a growing consensus among experts in this field that present techniques for preoperative localization are of limited usefulness and should be replaced by careful intraoperative ultrasonography and palpation by a surgeon experienced in insulinoma surgery. This approach has a success rate of over 90% in recent surveys and is the sole localizing approach relied upon by many centers, though a CT scan or MRI can be useful to screen for hepatic metastases from a malignant islet cell tumor.

When the insulinoma is not found at the initial surgery, three localization methods are available prior to reoperation. (1) The least invasive is a kinetic MRI with multiple imaging during gadolinium injection, but its accuracy for small tumors is no better than 40%. (2) Percutaneous transhepatic pancreatic vein catheterization with insulin assay can also be useful for localizing small insulinomas with about 70% reliability. However, this technique is not widely available, is invasive and expensive, and is associated with considerable discomfort and some risk to the patient. (3) A more acceptable and currently favored modification correlates imaging from selective arteriography of segments of the pancreas with simultaneous hepatic vein sampling for insulin during a bolus of intra-arterial calcium delivered selectively to these same pancreatic segments. Calcium has been found to be a secretagogue only for insulinomas and not for normal islet tissue, so that a rise in hepatic insulin concentration indicates segmental localization of an insulinoma. Furthermore, this technique may provide data which are particularly helpful when multiple insulinomas are suspected, as in patients with coexisting pituitary or parathyroid adenomas or in rare instances of pancreatic hyperplasia due to nesidioblastosis.

Treatment

A. SURGICAL MEASURES

It is imperative that the surgeon be convinced that the diagnosis of insulinoma has been unequivocally made by clinical and laboratory findings. Only then should surgery be considered, as there is no justification for exploratory operation—just as there is none for the use of current localization techniques as a preoperative diagnostic tool. Resection by a surgeon with previous experience in removing pancreatic B cell tumors is the treatment of choice. In patients with a single benign adenoma 90–95% have a successful cure at the first surgical attempt when intraoperative ultrasound is used by a skilled surgeon. Blood glucose should be monitored throughout surgery, and 10% dextrose in water should be infused at a rate of 100 mL/h or faster. In cases where the diagnosis has been established but no adenoma is located after careful palpation and use of intraoperative ultrasound, it is no longer advisable to blindly resect the body and tail of the pancreas, since a nonpalpable tumor missed by ultrasound is most likely embedded within the fleshy head of the pancreas that is left behind with subtotal resections. Most surgeons prefer to close the incision and schedule a selective arterial calcium stimulation with hepatic venous sampling to locate the tumor site prior to a repeat operation. Laparoscopy using ultrasound and enucleation has been successful with a single tumor of the body or tail of the pancreas, but open surgery remains necessary for tumors in the head of the pancreas.

B. DIET AND MEDICAL THERAPY

In patients with inoperable functioning islet cell carcinoma and in approximately 5–10% of MEN-1 cases when subtotal removal of the pancreas has failed to produce cure, reliance on frequent feedings is necessary. Since most tumors are not responsive to glucose, carbohydrate feedings every 2–3 hours are usually effective in preventing hypoglycemia, although obesity may become a problem. Glucagon should be available for emergency use as indicated in the discussion of treatment of diabetes, but its beneficial effect may be diminished by a concomitant stimulation of insulin release from the tumor. Diazoxide, 300–600 mg daily orally, has been useful with thiazide diuretic therapy to control sodium retention. When patients are unable to tolerate diazoxide because of gastrointestinal upset, hirsutism, or edema, the calcium channel blocker verapamil may be beneficial in view of its inhibitory effect on insulin release from insulinoma cells. Octreotide, a potent long-acting synthetic octapeptide analog of somatostatin, has been used to inhibit release of hormones from a number of endocrine tumors. A dose of 50 μg of octreotide injected subcutaneously twice daily has been tried in cases where surgery failed to remove the source of hyperinsulinism. However, its effectiveness is limited since its affinity for somatostatin receptors of the pancreatic B cell is very much less than for those of the anterior pituitary somatotrophs for which it was originally designed as treatment for acromegaly. When hypoglycemia persists after attempted surgical removal of the insulinoma and if diazoxide or verapamil is poorly tolerated or ineffective, multiple small feedings may be the only recourse until more selective somatostatin receptor agonists are available. Streptozocin can decrease insulin secretion in islet cell carcinomas, and effective doses have been delivered via selective arterial catheter so that the undue renal toxicity that characterized early experience is less of a problem.

Prognosis

When insulinoma is diagnosed early and cured surgically, complete recovery is likely, although brain damage following prolonged severe hypoglycemia is not reversible. A significant increase in survival rate has been shown in streptozocin-treated patients with islet cell carcinoma, with reduction in tumor mass as well as decreased hyperinsulinism.

Boukhman MP et al: Localization of insulinomas. Arch Surg 1999;134:818. [PMID: 10443803] (Surgical treatment of 58 insulinoma patients showed that extensive preoperative radiologic localization did not generally improve surgical outcome and that it was not cost-effective. Careful palpation with intraoperative ultrasonography was superior for tumor localization and led to successful operations for single benign tumors in 96% of patients.)

Grant CS: Surgical aspects of hyperinsulinemic hypoglycermia. Endocrinol Metab Clin North Am 1999;28:533. [PMID: 10500930] (A comprehensive review of the Mayo Clinic experience in 132 consecutive patients in whom 88% had a single tumor with an average size of 1.5 cm and in whom intraoperative ultrasound surpassed all other techniques for tumor localization, with a sensitivity of 96%.)

Hirshberg B et al: Forty-eight-hour fast: the diagnostic test for insulinoma. J Clin Endocrinol Metab 2000;85:3222. [PMID: 10999812] (In 127 patients with insulinoma at the National Institutes of Health, 94.5% developed hypoglycemia below 40 mg/dL accompanied by neuroglycopenic symptoms by 48 hours. Thus, the authors contend that 48 hours of a supervised fast is generally sufficient to provoke hypoglycemia in patients with insulinoma. They also found that 90% of insulinoma patients failed to suppress their proinsulin levels below 0.2 ng/mL during hypoglycemia provoked by a fast.)

HYPOGLYCEMIA DUE TO EXTRAPANCREATIC TUMORS

These rare causes of hypoglycemia include mesenchymal tumors such as retroperitoneal sarcomas, hepatocellular carcinomas, adrenocortical carcinomas, and miscellaneous epithelial type tumors. The tumors are frequently large and readily palpated or visualized on CT scans or MRI.

The expression and release of an incompletely processed insulin-like growth factor-2 (IGF-2) has provided the best explanation for the clinical manifestations of hypoglycemia in these cases. A larger immature form of the IGF-2 molecule is released which binds to a carrier protein but not to an acid-labile component of serum which inactivates normal IGF-2. This immature IGF-2 complex therefore remains active and binds to insulin receptors in muscle to promote glucose transport and to insulin receptors in liver and kidney to reduce glucose output. It also binds to receptors for IGF-1 in the pancreatic B cell to inhibit insulin secretion. Serum levels of IGF-2 may be increased but often are "normal" in quantity, despite the presence of the immature, higher-molecular-weight form of IGF-2, which can only be detected by special laboratory techniques. Laboratory diagnosis depends upon documenting fasting hypoglycemia associated with undetectable serum insulin levels.

The prognosis for these tumors is generally poor, and surgical removal should be attempted when feasible. Dietary management of the hypoglycemia is the mainstay of medical treatment, since diazoxide is usually ineffective.

Le Roith D: Tumor-induced hypoglycemia. N Engl J Med 1999;341:757. [PMID: 10471466] (An abnormal incompletely processed insulin-like growth factor-2 [IGF-2], with a high molecular weight, appears to explain many, but not all, cases of hypoglycemia secondary to extrapancreatic tumors.)

POSTPRANDIAL HYPOGLYCEMIA (Reactive Hypoglycemia)

Postgastrectomy Alimentary Hypoglycemia

Reactive hypoglycemia following gastrectomy is a consequence of hyperinsulinism resulting from rapid gastric emptying of ingested food. Symptoms result from adrenergic hyperactivity in response to the hypoglycemia. Treatment consists of more frequent feedings with smaller portions of less rapidly assimilated carbohydrate combined with more slowly absorbed fat and protein.

Functional Alimentary Hypoglycemia

This syndrome is classified as functional when no postsurgical explanation exists for the presence of early alimentary type reactive hypoglycemia. It is most often associated with chronic fatigue, anxiety, irritability, weakness, poor concentration, decreased libido, headaches, hunger after meals, and tremulousness. However, most patients with these symptoms do not have hypoglycemia after a mixed meal. (See Chronic Fatigue Syndrome in Chapter 1.)

Indiscriminate use and overinterpretation of glucose tolerance tests have led to an unfortunate tendency to overdiagnose functional hypoglycemia. As many as one-third or more of normal subjects have hypoglycemia reaching nadirs as low as 40–50 mg/dL with or without symptoms during a 4-hour glucose tolerance test. Accordingly, to increase diagnostic reli-

ability, hypoglycemia should preferably be documented during a spontaneous symptomatic episode accompanying routine daily activity, with clinical improvement following feeding. Oral glucose tolerance tests are overly sensitive and mixed meals are relatively insensitive in detecting postprandial reactive hypoglycemia. It has been shown that a high-carbohydrate breakfast has proved useful in differentiating persons with postprandial reactive hypoglycemia from normal controls. The test resulted in reactive hypoglycemia to levels below 59 mg/dL in 47% of 38 subjects, in contrast to only 2.2% of the 43 controls. This test was found to be much more sensitive than a standard mixed meal, which was also given to these two groups.

In patients with documented postprandial hypoglycemia on a functional basis, there is no harm and occasional benefit in reducing the proportion of carbohydrate in the diet while increasing the frequency and reducing the size of meals. Support and mild sedation should be the mainstays of therapy, with dietary manipulation only an adjunct.

Late Hypoglycemia (Occult Diabetes)

This condition is characterized by a delay in early insulin release from pancreatic B cells, resulting in initial exaggeration of hyperglycemia during a glucose tolerance test. In response to this hyperglycemia, an exaggerated insulin release produces a late hypoglycemia 4–5 hours after ingestion of glucose. These patients are usually quite different from those with early hypoglycemia occurring 2–3 hours after glucose ingestion, often being obese and frequently having a family history of diabetes mellitus.

In obese patients, treatment is directed at weight reduction to achieve ideal weight. Like all patients with postprandial hypoglycemia, regardless of cause, these patients often respond to reduced carbohydrate intake with multiple, spaced, small feedings. They should be considered potential diabetics and advised to have periodic medical evaluations.

Service FJ: Diagnostic approach to adults with hypoglycemic disorders. Endocrinol Metab Clin North Am 1999;28:519. [PMID: 10500929] (Reviews hypoglycemia—its clinical presentation and the diagnostic steps needed to confirm its etiology.)

ALCOHOL-RELATED HYPOGLYCEMIA

Fasting Hypoglycemia After Ethanol

During the postabsorptive state, normal plasma glucose is maintained by hepatic glucose output derived from both glycogenolysis and gluconeogenesis. With prolonged starvation, glycogen reserves become depleted within 18–24 hours and hepatic glucose output becomes totally dependent on gluconeogenesis. Under these circumstances, a blood concentration of ethanol as low as 45 mg/dL can induce profound hypoglycemia by blocking gluconeogenesis. Neuroglycopenia in a patient whose breath smells of alcohol may be mistaken for alcoholic stupor. Prevention consists of adequate food intake during ethanol ingestion. Therapy consists of glucose administration to replenish glycogen stores until gluconeogenesis resumes.

Postethanol Reactive Hypoglycemia

When sugar-containing soft drinks are used as mixers to dilute alcohol in beverages (gin and tonic, rum and cola), there seems to be a greater insulin release than when the soft drink alone is ingested and a tendency for more of a late hypoglycemic overswing to occur 3–4 hours later. Prevention would consist of avoiding sugar mixers while ingesting alcohol and ensuring supplementary food intake to provide sustained absorption.

FACTITIOUS HYPOGLYCEMIA

Factitious hypoglycemia may be difficult to document. A suspicion of self-induced hypoglycemia is supported when the patient is associated with the health professions or has access to insulin or sulfonylurea drugs taken by a diabetic member of the family. The triad of hypoglycemia, high immunoreactive insulin, and suppressed plasma C peptide immunoreactivity is pathognomonic of exogenous insulin administration. Demonstration of circulating insulin antibodies supports this diagnosis in suspected cases. When sulfonylureas are suspected as a cause of factitious hypoglycemia, a plasma level of these drugs to detect their presence may be required to distinguish laboratory findings from those of insulinoma. Unfortunately, the newer sulfonylurea, glimeperide, and other insulinotropic hypoglycemic drugs like repaglinide and nateglinide are not detected in the standard assays for sulfonylureas.

IMMUNOPATHOLOGIC HYPOGLYCEMIA

This rare cause of hypoglycemia, documented in isolated case reports, may occur as two distinct disorders: one associated with spontaneous development of circulating anti-insulin antibodies and another associated with antibodies to insulin receptors, in which the antibodies apparently have agonist capabilities. This latter disorder is extremely rare, having been documented in no more than five cases. However, development of anti-insulin antibodies has been reported in over 200 patients most of whom were being treated with methimazole for thyrotoxicosis. In western countries, 23 cases have been reported and include patients with a lupus-like syndrome or with various paraproteinemias. The hypoglycemia occurs 3–4 hours after meals following an initial postprandial hyperglycemic phase that is due to the antibodies interfering with the exit of insulin from the plasma to reach its target tissues. Later, after most of the meal is absorbed, inappropriate high levels of insulin dissociate from this antibody-bound compartment, resulting in hypoglycemia.

Redmon JB et al: Autoimmune hypoglycemia. Endocrinol Metab Clin North Am 1999;28:603. [PMID: 10500933] (A comprehensive review of this rare syndrome of hypoglycemia caused by the interaction of endogenous antibodies with insulin or the insulin receptor. Clinical manifestations, diagnosis, and therapy are discussed.)

PENTAMIDINE-INDUCED HYPOGLYCEMIA

With the increased prevalence of pulmonary infection by *Pneumocystis carinii* in patients with acquired immune deficiency syndrome, pentamidine given intravenously or by aerosol is being used more frequently and in 10–20% of patients produces symptomatic hypoglycemia, particularly when administered intravenously. This apparently is due to lytic destruction of pancreatic B cells, causing acute hyperinsulinemia and hypoglycemia, followed later by insulinopenia and hyperglycemia which occasionally is persistent. Intravenous glucose should be administered during intravenous pentamidine administration and for the period immediately following to prevent or ameliorate hypoglycemic symptoms. Following a complete course of therapy with pentamidine, fasting blood glucose or a subsequent glycohemoglobin should be monitored to assess the extent of pancreatic B cell recovery or residual damage.

Lipid Abnormalities

28

Robert B. Baron, MD, MS

See www.current-med.com/ch28.html

For patients with known cardiovascular disease (secondary prevention), cholesterol lowering leads to a reduction in total mortality in men and women and in middle-aged patients and older patients. Among patients without cardiovascular disease (primary prevention), the data are less conclusive, with heart disease mortality and all-cause mortality differing among studies. Nonetheless, treatment algorithms have been designed to assist clinicians in selecting patients for cholesterol-lowering therapy based on their lipid levels and their overall risk of developing cardiovascular disease.

LIPIDS & LIPOPROTEINS

The two main lipids in blood are cholesterol and triglyceride. They are carried in lipoproteins, globular particles that also contain proteins known as apoproteins. Cholesterol is an essential element of all animal cell membranes and forms the backbone of steroid hormones and bile acids; triglycerides are important in transferring energy from food into cells. Why lipids are deposited into the walls of large and medium-sized arteries—an event with potentially lethal consequences—is not known.

Lipoproteins are usually classified on the basis of density, which is determined by the amounts of triglyceride (which makes them less dense) and apoproteins (which makes them more dense). The least dense particles, known as chylomicrons, are normally found in the blood only after fat-containing foods have been eaten. They rise as a creamy layer when nonfasting serum is allowed to stand. The other lipoproteins are suspended in serum and must be separated using a centrifuge. The densest (and smallest) family of particles consists mainly of apoproteins and cholesterol and are called high-density lipoproteins (HDL). Somewhat less dense are the low-density lipoproteins (LDL). Least dense are the large, very-low-density lipoproteins (VLDL), consisting mainly of triglyceride. In fasting serum, most of the cholesterol is carried on LDL particles and is therefore referred to as LDL cholesterol; most of the triglyceride is found in VLDL particles. Specific apoproteins are associated with each lipoprotein class.

Chylomicrons are made in the gut and travel via the portal vein into the liver and via the thoracic duct into the circulation. They are normally completely metabolized, transferring energy from food into muscle and fat cells. The liver manufactures VLDL particles from its own stores of fat and carbohydrate. VLDL particles transfer triglyceride to cells; after losing enough, they eventually become LDL particles, which provide cholesterol for cellular needs. Excess LDL particles are taken up by the liver, and the cholesterol they contain is then excreted into the bile. HDL particles are made in the liver and intestine and appear to facilitate the transfer of apoproteins among lipoproteins. They also participate in reverse cholesterol transport, either by transferring cholesterol into other lipoproteins or directly into the liver.

LIPOPROTEINS & ATHEROGENESIS

The plaques in the arterial walls of patients with atherosclerosis contain large amounts of cholesterol. The higher the level of LDL cholesterol, the greater the risk of atherosclerotic heart disease; conversely, the higher the HDL cholesterol, the lower the risk of coronary heart disease (CHD). This is true in men and women, in different racial and ethnic groups, and at all ages up to age 75. Because most cholesterol in serum is LDL, high total cholesterol levels are also associated with an increased risk of CHD. Middle-aged men whose serum cholesterol levels are in the highest quintile for age (above about 230 mg/dL) have a risk of coronary death before age 65 of about 10%; men in the lowest quintile (below about 170 mg/dL) have a 3% risk. Death from CHD before age 65 is less common in women, with equivalent risks one-third those of men. In men, each 10 mg/dL increase in cholesterol (or LDL cholesterol) increases the risk of CHD by about 10%; each 5 mg/dL increase in HDL reduces the risk by about 10%. The effect of HDL cholesterol is greater in women, whereas the effects of total and LDL cholesterol are smaller. All of these relationships diminish with age.

The exact mechanism by which LDL particles result in the formation of atherosclerotic plaques—or the means whereby HDL particles protect against their formation—is not known. The model of LDL carrying cholesterol into the walls of arteries with HDL removing it is simple but not established. The natural oxidation of LDL particles may be particularly atherogenic. Receptors on the surface of macrophages within atherosclerotic plaques bind and accumulate oxidized LDL. The formation of antibodies to oxidized LDL may also be important in plaque formation. The size of the LDL molecule may also influence atherogenesis; at the same LDL concentrations, individuals with large numbers of smaller particles appear to be at higher risk for CHD.

The relationship of VLDL cholesterol to atherogenesis is less certain. The number, or size, or subtype of VLDL particles—in addition to the total amount in serum—may be important. In addition, HDL and VLDL levels are inversely related. Patients with a high VLDL level are likely to have a low HDL level and thus be at increased risk for CHD for that reason alone.

There are several genetic disorders that provide insight into the pathogenesis of lipid-related diseases. Most important—but rare in the homozygous state (about one per million)—is a condition in which the cell-surface receptors for the LDL molecule are absent or defective, **familial hypercholesterolemia,** resulting in unregulated synthesis of LDL. Patients with two abnormal genes (homozygotes) have extremely high levels—up to eight times normal—and present with atherosclerotic disease in childhood. Homozygotes may require liver transplantation to correct their severe lipid abnormalities. Those with one defective gene (heterozygotes) have LDL concentrations twice normal; persons with this condition may develop CHD in their 30s or 40s.

Another rare condition is caused by an abnormality of lipoprotein lipase, the enzyme that enables peripheral tissues to take up triglyceride from chylomicrons and VLDL particles. Patients with this condition, one cause of **familial hyperchylomicronemia,** have marked hypertriglyceridemia with recurrent pancreatitis and hepatosplenomegaly in childhood.

Numerous other genetic abnormalities of lipid metabolism are named for the abnormality noted when serum is electrophoresed (eg, dysbetalipoproteinemia) or from combinations of lipid abnormalities in families (eg, familial combined hyperlipidemia). Thus, family members of patients with severe lipid disorders are appropriately studied. Other patients have abnormalities in the production of apoproteins, such as increased apoprotein B and its affiliated lipoproteins, LDL and VLDL; reduced apoprotein AII and its affiliated particle; or excess lipoprotein(a). Other mutations occur in lipoprotein lipase and in the gene encoding for cholesterol efflux regulatory protein.

Genest J: Genetics and prevention: a new look at high-density lipoprotein cholesterol. Cardiol Rev 2002;10:61. [PMID: 11790271] (Some mutations causing high-density lipoprotein deficiency are associated with premature coronary artery disease, others paradoxically, may be associated with longevity.)

Gotto AM Jr: High-density lipoprotein cholesterol: an updated view. Curr Opin Pharmacol 2001;1:109. [PMID: 11714083] (ATP-binding-cassette A1 gene has been identified as an important genetic defect of this lipid fraction.)

Kawakami A et al: Remnant lipoproteins and atherogenesis. Ann N Y Acad Sci 2001;947:366. [PMID: 11795292] (Describes a simple immunoseparation method to separate remnant lipoproteins and the cellular mechanisms by which they contribute to atherogenesis.)

Kita T et al: Role of oxidized LDL in atherosclerosis. Ann N Y Acad Sci 2001;947:199. [PMID: 11795267] (Discusses the significance of oxidized LDL and its receptors, LOX-1 and SR-PSOX.)

Lamarche B et al: A prospective, population-based study of low density lipoprotein particle size as a risk factor for ischemic heart disease in men. Can J Cardiol 2001;17:859. [PMID: 11521128] (Supports the hypothesis that small, dense LDL particles may be associated with an increased risk of IHD. Also suggests that information on LDL diameter may improve the ability to predict IHD risk.)

Marcil M et al: Mutations in the *ABC1* gene in familial HDL deficiency with defective cholesterol efflux. Lancet 1999;354:1341. [PMID: 10533863] (A major cause of familial HDL deficiency.)

Miwa K et al: Lipoprotein(a) is a risk factor for occurrence of acute myocardial infarction in patients with coronary vasospasm. J Am Coll Cardiol 2000;35:1200. [PMID: 10758961] (Suggests that Lp[a] may play an important role in the genesis of thrombotic coronary occlusion and the occurrence of acute myocardial infarction subsequent to spasm.)

Neil HA et al: Extent of underdiagnosis of familial hypercholesterolaemia in routine practice: prospective registry study. BMJ 2000;321:148. [PMID: 10894692]

Packard CJ et al: Lipoprotein-associated phospholipase A2 as an independent predictor of coronary heart disease. West of Scotland Coronary Prevention Study Group. N Engl J Med 2000;343:1148. [PMID: 11036120] (Lipoprotein-associated platelet-activating factor acetylhydrolase was associated with doubling of the risk for a coronary event.)

Saku K et al: Hyperinsulinemic hypoalphalipoproteinemia as a new indicator for coronary heart disease. J Am Coll Cardiol 1999;34:1443. [PMID: 10551691] (A more potent indicator for coronary heart disease than either insulin resistance or low serum HDL-C levels alone.)

Shlipak MG et al: Estrogen and progestin, lipoprotein(a), and the risk of recurrent coronary heart disease events after menopause. JAMA 2000;283:1845. [PMID: 10770146] (Lp[a] is an independent risk factor and is lowered by treatment with estrogen and progestin.)

Wittrup HH et al: Lipoprotein lipase mutations, plasma lipids and lipoproteins, and risk of ischemic heart disease. A meta-analysis. Circulation 1999;99:2901. [PMID: 10359734] (Certain lipoprotein lipase mutations have an increased risk of ischemic heart disease; others are associated with reduced risk.)

LIPID FRACTIONS & THE RISK OF CORONARY HEART DISEASE

In fasting serum, cholesterol is carried primarily on three different lipoproteins—the VLDL, LDL, and HDL molecules. Total cholesterol equals the sum of these three components:

$$\text{Total cholesterol} = \text{HDL cholesterol} + \text{VLDL cholesterol} + \text{LDL cholesterol}$$

Most clinical laboratories measure the total cholesterol, the total triglycerides, and the amount of cholesterol found in the HDL fraction, which is easily precipitated from serum. Most triglyceride is found in VLDL particles, which contain five times as much triglyceride by weight as cholesterol. The amount of cholesterol found in the VLDL fraction can be estimated by dividing the triglyceride by 5:

$$\text{VLDL cholesterol} = \frac{\text{Triglycerides}}{5}$$

Because the triglyceride level is used as a proxy for the amount of VLDL, this formula only works in fasting samples. Furthermore, it only works when the triglyceride level is less than 400–500 mg/dL. At higher triglyceride levels, LDL and VLDL cholesterol levels can be determined after ultracentrifugation or by direct chemical measurement.

The total cholesterol is reasonably stable over time; however, measurements of HDL and especially triglycerides may vary considerably because of analytic error in the laboratory and biologic variation in a patient's lipid level. Thus, the LDL should always be estimated as the mean of at least two determinations; if those two estimates differ by more than 10%, a third lipid profile is obtained and is estimated as follows:

$$\text{LDL cholesterol} = \text{Total cholesterol} - \text{HDL cholesterol} - \frac{\text{Triglycerides}}{5}$$

When using SI units, the formula becomes:

$$\text{LDL cholesterol} \atop \text{(mmol/L)} = \text{cholesterol} \atop \text{(mmol/L)} - \text{cholesterol} \atop \text{(mmol/L)} - \frac{\text{Triglycerides}}{2.2}$$

Understanding the relationships of the different lipid fractions leads to a more accurate understanding of a patient's lipid-related coronary risk than the total cholesterol. Two persons with the same total cholesterol of 275 mg/dL may have very different lipid profiles. One may have an HDL cholesterol of 110 mg/dL with a triglyceride of 150 mg/dL, giving an estimated LDL cholesterol of 135 mg/dL; the other may have an HDL cholesterol of 25 mg/dL with a triglyceride of 200 mg/dL and an LDL cholesterol of 210 mg/dL. The second would have more than a tenfold higher CHD risk than the first, assuming no differences in other factors. Because of high HDL cholesterol levels in women, many with apparently high total cholesterol levels have favorable lipid profiles. Thus, evaluation of the lipid fractions is essential before therapy is initiated.

Some authorities use the ratio of the total to HDL cholesterol as an indicator of lipid-related coronary risk: the lower this ratio is, the better. (In the example above, the first person would have a ratio of $275 \div 110 = 2.5$, while the second would have a much less favorable ratio of $275 \div 25 = 11$.) The ratio may obscure important information (a total cholesterol of 300 mg/dL and an HDL of 60 mg/dL results in the same ratio of 5 as a total cholesterol of 150 mg/dL with an HDL of 30 mg/dL). Moreover, errors in the measurement of HDL cholesterol are common in many laboratories, and the total cholesterol-to-HDL cholesterol ratio magnifies their importance.

There is no true "normal" range for serum lipids. In Western populations, cholesterol values are about 20% higher than in Asian populations and exceed 300 mg/dL in nearly 5% of adults. About 10% of adults have LDL cholesterol levels above 200 mg/dL. Total and LDL cholesterol levels tend to rise with age in persons who are otherwise in good health.

Declines are seen in acute illness, and lipid studies in such patients are of little value with the exception of the serum triglyceride level in a patient with pancreatitis. Cholesterol levels (even when expressed as an age-matched percentile rank, such as the highest 20%) do not remain constant over time, especially from childhood through adolescence and young adulthood. Thus, children and young adults with relatively high cholesterol may have lower levels later in life, whereas those with low cholesterol may show increases.

THERAPEUTIC EFFECTS OF LOWERING CHOLESTEROL

Most studies of the effect of cholesterol lowering have distinguished between primary and secondary prevention. The important distinction is that primary prevention trials enroll healthy subjects who have relatively low rates of coronary disease but in whom other causes of morbidity and mortality are proportionately more common. Secondary prevention trials, on the other hand, follow patients who have a high rate of subsequent coronary disease; other causes of mortality are relatively less important.

Reducing cholesterol levels in healthy middle-aged men without CHD (primary prevention) reduces their risk in proportion to the reduction in LDL cholesterol and the increase in HDL cholesterol. Treated patients have statistically significant and clinically important reductions in the rates of myocardial infarctions, new cases of angina, and need for coronary artery bypass procedures. The West of Scotland Study showed a 31% decrease in myocardial infarctions in middle-aged men treated with pravastatin compared with placebo. The AFCAPS/TexCAPS study showed similar results with lovastatin. As with any primary prevention interventions, large numbers of healthy patients need to be treated to prevent a single event. The numbers of patients needed to treat (NNT) to prevent a nonfatal myocardial infarction or a coronary artery disease death in these two studies were 46 and 50, respectively.

Primary prevention studies have found a less consistent effect on total mortality. Although the West of Scotland study found a 20% decrease in total mortality, tending toward statistical significance, the AF-CAPS/TexCAPS study with lovastatin showed no difference in total mortality.

In patients with CHD, the benefits of cholesterol-lowering are more clear. Three major studies with statins have shown significant reductions in cardiovascular events, cardiovascular deaths, and all-cause mortality in men and women with coronary artery disease. The numbers of patients needed to treat (NNT) to prevent a nonfatal myocardial infarction or a coronary artery disease death in these three studies were between 12 and 34. Aggressive cholesterol lowering with these agents causes regression of atherosclerotic plaques in some patients, reduces the progression of atherosclerosis in saphenous vein grafts, and can slow or reverse carotid artery atherosclerosis. Meta-analysis suggests that this latter effect results in a significant decrease in strokes. Results with other classes of medications have been less consistent. For example, gemfi-brozil treatment subjects had fewer cardiovascular events, but there was no benefit in all-cause mortality when compared with placebo.

The disparities in results between primary and secondary prevention studies highlight several important points. The benefits and adverse effects of cholesterol lowering appear to be specific to each type of drug; the clinician cannot assume that the effects will generalize to other classes of medication. Second, the net benefits from cholesterol lowering depend upon the underlying risk of CHD and of other disease. In patients with atherosclerosis, morbidity and mortality rates associated with CHD are high, and measures that reduce it are more likely to be beneficial even if they have no effect—or even slightly harmful effects—on other diseases. Third, the full effects of cholesterol lowering in women and in older and younger men are uncertain.

Flaker GC et al: Pravastatin prevents clinical events in revascularized patients with average cholesterol concentrations. Cholesterol and Recurrent Events CARE Investigators. J Am Coll Cardiol 1999;34:106. [PMID: 10399998] (Lipid lowering with a statin reduced clinical events in revascularized postinfarction patients with average cholesterol levels.)

Gotto AM Jr et al: Relation between baseline and on-treatment lipid parameters and first acute major coronary events in the Air Force/Texas Coronary Atherosclerosis Prevention Study (AFCAPS/TexCAPS). Circulation 2000;101:477. [PMID: 20129878]

Jacobson TA: "The lower the better" in hypercholesterolemia therapy: a reliable clinical guideline? Ann Intern Med 2000;133:549. [PMID: 11015169]

Muldoon MF et al: Cholesterol reduction and non-illness mortality: meta-analysis of randomised clinical trials. BMJ 2001;322:11. [PMID: 11141142] (Nonillness mortality is not increased by cholesterol-lowering treatments; a modest increase may occur with dietary interventions and nonstatin drugs.)

Oliver MF: Cholesterol and strokes: Cholesterol-lowering is indicated for strokes due to carotid atheroma. BMJ 2000;320:459. [PMID: 10678841] (Meta-analyses of the coronary prevention trials show reduction in risk of stroke by about 30% without reducing mortality.)

Pedersen TR et al: Follow-up study of patients randomized in the Scandinavian simvastatin survival study (4S) of cholesterol lowering. Am J Cardiol 2000;86:257. [PMID: 10922429] (Eight-year follow-up continues to demonstrate a survival benefit.)

Ridker PM et al: Measurement of C-reactive protein for the targeting of statin therapy in the primary prevention of acute coronary events. N Engl J Med 2001;344:1959. [PMID: 11430324] (Shows that in subjects with lower than average lipids and a high C-reactive protein level, pravastatin prevented CHD events [NNT 43].)

Rubins HB et al: Gemfibrozil for the secondary prevention of coronary heart disease in men with low levels of high-density lipoprotein cholesterol. Veterans Affairs High-Density Lipoprotein Cholesterol Intervention Trial Study Group. N Engl J Med. 1999;341:410. [PMID: 10438259] (Gemfi-brozil therapy resulted in significant risk reduction of major cardiovascular events in patients with coronary disease whose primary lipid abnormality with low HDL cholesterol level but there was no effect on all-cause mortality.)

SECONDARY CONDITIONS THAT AFFECT LIPID METABOLISM

Several factors, including drugs, can influence serum lipids (Table 28–1). These are important for two reasons: abnormal lipid levels (or changes in lipid levels) may be the presenting sign of some of these conditions, and correction of the underlying condition may obviate the need to treat an apparent lipid disorder. Diabetes and alcohol use, in particular, are commonly associated with high triglyceride levels that decline with improvements in glycemic control or reduction in alcohol use, respectively. Thus, secondary causes of high blood lipids should be considered in each patient with a lipid disorder before lipid-lowering therapy is started. In most instances, special testing is not needed: a history and physical examination are sufficient. However, screening for hypothyroidism in patients with hyperlipidemia is cost-effective.

CLINICAL PRESENTATIONS

Most patients with high cholesterol levels have no specific symptoms or signs. The vast majority of patients with lipid abnormalities are detected by the laboratory, either as part of the workup of a patient with cardiovascular disease or as part of a preventive screening strategy. Extremely high levels of chylomicrons or VLDL particles (triglyceride level above 1000 mg/dL) result in the formation of **eruptive xanthomas** (red-yellow papules, especially on the buttocks). High LDL concentrations result in **tendinous xanthomas** on certain tendons (Achilles, patella, back of the hand). Such xanthomas usually indicate one of the underlying genetic hyperlipidemias. **Lipemia retinalis** (cream-colored blood vessels in the fundus) is seen with extremely high triglyceride levels (above 2000 mg/dL).

Table 28–1. Secondary causes of lipid abnormalities.

Cause	Associated Lipid Abnormality
Obesity	Increased triglycerides, decreased HDL cholesterol
Sedentary lifestyle	Decreased HDL cholesterol
Diabetes mellitus	Increased triglycerides, increased total cholesterol
Alcohol use	Increased triglycerides, increased HDL cholesterol
Hypothyroidism	Increased total cholesterol
Hyperthyroidism	Decreased total cholesterol
Nephrotic syndrome	Increased total cholesterol
Chronic renal insufficiency	Increased total cholesterol, increased triglycerides
Hepatic disease (cirrhosis)	Decreased total cholesterol
Obstructive liver disease	Increased total cholesterol
Malignancy	Decreased total cholesterol
Cushing's disease (or steroid use)	Increased total cholesterol
Oral contraceptives	Increased triglycerides, increased total cholesterol
Diuretics[1]	Increased total cholesterol, increased triglycerides
Beta-blockers[1,2]	Increased total cholesterol, decreased HDL

[1]Short-term effects only

[2]Beta-blockers with intrinsic sympathomimetic activity, such as pindolol and acebutolol, do not affect lipid levels.

SCREENING FOR HIGH BLOOD CHOLESTEROL

All patients with CHD or CHD risk equivalents (other clinical forms of atherosclerosis such as peripheral artery disease, abdominal aortic aneurysm, and symptomatic carotid artery disease; patients with diabetes mellitus; and patients with multiple risk factors that confer a greater than 20% 10-year risk for developing CHD) should be screened for elevated lipids. The only exceptions are patients in whom lipid lowering is not indicated or desirable for other reasons. Patients who already have evidence of atherosclerosis are the group at highest risk of suffering additional manifestations in the near term and thus have the most to gain from reduction of blood lipids. Additional risk reduction measures for atherosclerosis are discussed in Chapter 10; lipid lowering should be just one aspect of a program to reduce the progression and effects of the disease.

Given the high prevalence of lipid abnormalities in patients with cardiovascular disease, a complete lipid profile (total cholesterol, HDL cholesterol, and triglyceride levels) after an overnight fast should be obtained as a screening test. Those whose estimated

LDL cholesterol level is high should have at least one repeat measurement. Specific treatments for high LDL cholesterol levels are discussed below. The goal of therapy should be to reduce the LDL cholesterol to below 100 mg/dL, but any reduction in LDL is better than no reduction. Even treatment of only mildly elevated LDL cholesterol is clinically useful. Individuals with LDL cholesterol levels < 175 mg/dL have a 25% reduction in fatal CHD and recurrent myocardial infarctions when the LDL is lowered to 100 mg/dL.

The best screening and treatment strategy for adults who do not have atherosclerotic cardiovascular disease is not clear. Several algorithms have been developed to guide the clinician in treatment decisions, but management decisions are individualized.

Although the National Cholesterol Education Program (NCEP) recommends screening of all adults aged 20 or older for high blood cholesterol, both the American College of Physicians and the United States Preventive Services Task Force suggest beginning at age 35 in men and age 45 in women unless there is a striking family history or physical findings to suggest a genetic disorder. This strategy focuses cholesterol screening on those at most immediate risk of coronary artery disease and increases the cost effectiveness of cholesterol screening.

Individuals without cardiovascular disease can then be stratified according to risk factors as defined by the NCEP. Those with two or more risk factors are considered to be at intermediate risk of coronary artery disease, and those with less than two are at low risk. These include age and gender (men aged 45 or older, women aged 55 or older); a family history of premature CHD (myocardial infarction or sudden cardiac death before age 55 in a first-degree male relative or before age 65 in a first-degree female relative); hypertension (whether treated or not); current cigarette smoking (ten or more cigarettes per day); and low HDL cholesterol (< 35 mg/dL). Because HDL cholesterol is protective against CHD, a risk factor is subtracted if the level is greater than 60 mg/dL. Patients with two or more risk factors are then further stratified by evaluating their 10-year risk of developing CHD using Framingham projections of 10-year risk (Table 28–2).

Several strategies for obtaining the initial cholesterol measurement have been proposed, including (1) measuring total cholesterol alone, (2) measuring total cholesterol and HDL cholesterol, or (3) measuring LDL and HDL cholesterol. Each is acceptable, but treatment decisions are based on the LDL and HDL cholesterol levels. Measurement of the total cholesterol alone is the least expensive strategy and is adequate for low-risk individuals; those with total cholesterol greater than 200 mg/dL should then be reevaluated with a fasting LDL and HDL cholesterol measurement. Measurement of the total cholesterol and HDL cholesterol allows for better characterization of the risk factor profile but also requires reevaluation if the total cholesterol is greater than 200 mg/dL. Initial measure-

Table 28–2. Framingham 10-year coronary heart disease risk projections. Calculate the number of points for each risk factor. Sum the total risk score and estimate the 10-year risk.[1]

MEN			WOMEN	
Age	**Points**		**Age**	**Points**
20–34	–9		20–34	–7
35–39	–4		35–39	–3
40–44	0		40–44	0
45–49	3		45–49	3
50–54	6		50–54	6
55–59	8		55–59	8
60–64	10		60–64	10
65–69	11		65–69	12
70–74	12		70–74	14
75–79	13		75–79	16

MEN

Total Cholesterol	**Points**				
	Age 20–39	Age 40–49	Age 50–59	Age 60–69	Age 70–79
< 160	0	0	0	0	0
160–199	4	3	2	1	0
200–239	7	5	3	1	0
240–279	9	6	4	2	1
≥ 280	11	8	5	3	1

WOMEN

Total Cholesterol	**Points**				
	Age 20–39	Age 40–49	Age 50–59	Age 60–69	Age 70–79
< 160	0	0	0	0	0
160–199	4	3	2	1	1
200–239	8	6	4	2	1
240–279	11	8	5	3	2
≥ 280	13	10	7	4	2

MEN

Age	**Points**				
	20–39	40–49	50–59	60–69	70–79
Nonsmoker	0	0	0	0	0
Smoker	8	5	3	1	1

WOMEN

Age	**Points**				
	20–39	40–49	50–59	60–69	70–79
Nonsmoker	0	0	0	0	0
Smoker	9	7	4	2	1

HDL (mg/dL)	Points		HDL (mg/dL)	Points
≥ 60	–1		≥ 60	–1
50–59	0		50–59	0
40–49	1		40–49	1
< 40	2		< 40	2

Systolic BP (mm Hg)	Points if Untreated	Points if Treated	Systolic BP (mm Hg)	Points if Untreated	Points if Treated
< 120	0	0	< 120	0	0
120–129	0	1	120–129	1	3
130–139	1	2	130–139	2	4
140–159	1	2	140–159	3	5
≥ 160	2	3	≥ 160	4	6

(*continued*)

Table 28–2. Framingham 10-year coronary heart disease risk projections. Calculate the number of points for each risk factor. Sum the total risk score and estimate the 10-year risk.[1] (continued)

MEN			WOMEN		
Point Total	**10-Year Risk %**		**Point Total**	**10-Year Risk %**	
< 0	< 1		< 9	< 1	
0	1		9	1	
1	1		10	1	
2	1		11	1	
3	1		12	1	
4	1		13	2	
5	2		14	2	
6	2		15	3	
7	3		16	4	
8	4		17	5	
9	5		18	6	
10	6		19	8	
11	8		20	11	
12	10		21	14	
13	12		22	17	
14	16	Ten–Year risk	23	22	Ten–Year risk
15	20		24	27	
16	25		≥ 25	≥ 30	
≥ 17	≥ 30	%			%

[1]Reproduced, with permission, from Executive Summary of the third Report of The National Cholesterol Education Program (NCEP) Expert Panel on Detection, Evaluation, And Treatment of High Blood cholesterol In Adults (Adult Treatment Panel III). JAMA 2001;285:2486. http://www.nhlbi.nih.gov/guidelines/cholesterol/index.htm

ment of the LDL and HDL cholesterol is least likely to lead to patient misinformation and misclassification and is the strategy recommended by the NCEP.

Treatment decisions are based upon the LDL cholesterol and the patient's risk factor profile (including the HDL cholesterol level). Patients in the intermediate risk group (two or more risk factors) are selected for diet therapy (therapeutic lifestyle changes) if LDL cholesterol is greater than 130 mg/dL. If the 10-year risk of CHD is < 10%, drug treatment is recommended if LDL is > 160 mg/dL; if the 10-year CHD risk is between 10% and 20%, drug treatment is recommended if LDL is > 130 mg/dL. Low-risk individuals are selected for diet therapy if LDL cholesterol is greater than 160 mg/dL and for drug therapy if it is greater than 190 mg/dL.

Screening in Women

The foregoing screening and treatment guidelines, based largely on LDL cholesterol levels, are designed for both men and women. Yet observational studies suggest that a low HDL cholesterol is a more important risk factor for CHD in women than a high LDL cholesterol. Meta-analysis of studies including women with known heart disease, however, has found that medications which primarily lower LDL cholesterol do prevent recurrent myocardial infarctions in women. There is insufficient evidence to be certain of a similar effect from LDL-lowering therapy in women

without evidence of CHD. Although most experts recommend application of the same primary prevention guidelines for women as for men, clinicians should be aware of the uncertainty in this area.

Screening in Older Patients

Meta-analysis of evidence relating cholesterol to CHD in the elderly suggests that cholesterol is not a risk factor for CHD for persons over age 75. Clinical trials have rarely included such individuals. Although the NCEP recommends continuing treatment in the elderly, many clinicians will prefer to stop screening and treatment in patients age 75 or older who do not have CHD. In patients age 75 or older who have CHD, LDL-lowering therapy can be continued as recommended for younger patients with the disease. Decisions to discontinue therapy should be based on overall functional status and life expectancy, comorbidities, and patient preference and should be made in context with overall therapeutic goals and end-of-life decisions.

Ansell BJ: Developing a clinical strategy for cholesterol management in an era of unanswered questions. Am J Cardiol 2001;16;88(4 Suppl):25F. [PMID: 11529484] (Addresses unanswered questions about treatment, including the appropriate intensity of lipid-lowering therapy, the role of HDL cholesterol and triglycerides, and optimal treatment strategies for women, the elderly, and patients with diabetes.)

Atkins D et al: Lipid screening in women. J Am Med Womens Assoc 2000;55:234. [PMID: 10935359] (Screening beginning in middle age identified most women at high enough risk to merit drug therapy or more intensive individual lifestyle interventions.)

Avins AL et al: Improving the prediction of coronary heart disease to aid in the management of high cholesterol levels. What a difference a decade makes. JAMA 1998;279:445. [PMID: 9466637] (Placing greater emphasis on age as a risk factor for CHD improves the ability to discriminate between higher and lower risks.)

Beckett N et al: Is it advantageous to lower cholesterol in the elderly hypertensive? Cardiovasc Drugs Ther 2000;14:397. [PMID: 10999646] (Further trials are required before routinely suggesting it is advantageous to lower cholesterol in an elderly hypertensive patient without preexisting evidence of CHD.)

Brown WV: What are the priorities for managing cholesterol effectively? Am J Cardiol 2001;88(4 Suppl):21F. [PMID: 11520483] (LDL-C remains the primary target for treatment.)

Clearfield M et al: Air Force/Texas Coronary Atherosclerosis Prevention Study (AFCAPS/TexCAPS): efficacy and tolerability of long-term treatment with lovastatin in women. J Womens Health Gend Based Med 2001;10:971. [PMID: 11788107] (Insufficient evidence for a treatment group difference among women—seven of 499 first events in those receiving lovastatin versus 13 of 498 in those receiving placebo.)

Cui Y et al: Non-high-density lipoprotein cholesterol level as a predictor of cardiovascular disease mortality. Arch Intern Med 2001;161:1413. [PMID: 11386890] (Non-HDL cholesterol level is a somewhat better predictor of cardiovascular disease mortality than LDL level. Screening for it may be useful for risk assessment.)

D'Agostino RB et al: Validation of the Framingham coronary heart disease prediction scores: Results of a multiple ethnic groups investigation. JAMA 2001;286:180. [PMID: 11448281] (Framingham scores worked well in all ethnic groups.)

Deedwania PC: Hypercholesterolemia. Is lipid-lowering worthwhile for older patients? Geriatrics 2000;55:22. [PMID: 10826262] (Older persons benefit from lipid-lowering therapy as much as younger patients do.)

Executive Summery of the Third report of the National Cholesterol Education Program (NCEP) Expert Panel on Detection, Evaluation, and Treatment of High Blood Cholesterol in Adults (Adult Treatment Panel III). JAMA 2001; 285:2486. [PMID: 11368702] (Recommends a more aggressive approach, including a target of LDL < 100 mg/dL; using Framingham risk scores; and defining a more important role for treatment of triglycerides.)

Grover SA et al: Cost-effectiveness of treating hyperlipidemia in the presence of diabetes: who should be treated? Circulation 2000;102:722. [PMID: 10942738] (Diabetes identifies men and women in whom lipid therapy is effective and cost-effective even in the absence of other risk factors or known cardiovascular disease.)

Hunt D et al: Benefits of pravastatin on cardiovascular events and mortality in older patients with coronary heart disease are equal to or exceed those seen in younger patients: Results from the LIPID trial. Ann Intern Med 2001;134:931. [PMID: 11352694] (In older patients with CHD and average or moderately elevated cholesterol levels, pravastatin reduced the risk for all cardiovascular events and all-cause mortality.)

Newman TB et al: Cholesterol screening in children and adolescents. Pediatrics 2000;105:637. [PMID: 10699121]. (The evidence does not support routine screening for lipid abnormalities in children and adolescents.)

Pignone M et al: Use of lipid lowering drugs for primary prevention of coronary heart disease: meta-analysis of randomized trials. BMJ 2000;321:983. [PMID: 11039962] (Meta-analysis suggests that in patients with no history of coronary artery disease, lipid-lowering drugs decrease the risk for such events [NNT 69] but not coronary artery disease mortality or all-cause mortality.)

Rauoof MA et al: Measurement of plasma lipids in patients admitted with acute myocardial infarction or unstable angina pectoris. Am J Cardiol 2001;88:165. [PMID: 11448415] (Cholesterol and triglycerides within the first 24 hours after admission were significantly lower than corresponding values at 6 weeks. Early in-hospital lipid measurements can lead to underestimation of the lipid risk in these patients.)

Simons LA et al: Cholesterol and other lipids predict coronary heart disease and ischaemic stroke in the elderly, but only in those below 70 years. Atherosclerosis 2001;159:201. [PMID: 11689222] (Total cholesterol, LDL cholesterol, serum apo-B, total cholesterol/HDL cholesterol and apo-B/apo-A1 were most significant predictors of CHD in subgroup of 60–69 years.)

TREATMENT OF HIGH-LDL CHOLESTEROL (Table 28–3)

Reduction of LDL cholesterol is just one part of a program to reduce the risk of cardiovascular disease. Other measures—including smoking cessation, hypertension control, and aspirin—are also of central importance. Less well studied but of potential value is raising the HDL cholesterol level. Quitting smoking reduces the effect of other cardiovascular risk factors (such as a high cholesterol level); it may also increase the HDL cholesterol level. Exercise (and weight loss) may reduce the LDL cholesterol and increase the HDL. Modest alcohol use (1–2 ounces a day) also raises HDL levels and appears to have a salutary effect on CHD rates. While the clinician may not wish to recommend alcohol use to patients, its use in moderation need not be discouraged.

DIET THERAPY

Studies of nonhospitalized adults have reported only modest cholesterol-lowering benefits of dietary therapy, typically in the range of a 5–10% decrease in LDL cholesterol, with even less in the long term. The effect of diet therapy, however, varies considerably among individuals, as some patients will have striking reductions in LDL cholesterol—up to a 25–30% decrease—while others will have clinically important increases. Thus, the results of diet therapy should be assessed about 4 weeks after initiation.

Cholesterol-lowering diets may also have a variable effect on lipid fractions. Diets very low in total fat or in saturated fat may lower HDL cholesterol as much as LDL cholesterol. It is not known how these diet-induced changes affect coronary risk.

Table 28–3. LDL goals and treatment cutpoints: recommendations of the NCEP Adult Treatment Panel III Report.[1]

Risk Category	LDL Goal (mg/dL)	LDL at Which to Initiate Lifestyle Changes (mg/dL)	LDL Level at Which to Consider Drug Changes (mg/dL)
CHD or CHD risk equivalents	< 100	≥ 100	≥ 130
≥ 2 risk factors	< 130	≥ 130	10-year risk 10–20%: ≥ 130 10-year risk <10%: ≥ 160
0–1 risk factors	< 160	≥ 160	≥ 190

[1]Reproduced, with permission, from Executive Summary of The Third Report of The National Cholesterol Education Program (NCEP) Expert Panel on Detection, Evaluation, And Treatment of High Blood Cholesterol In Adults (Adult Treatment Panel III). JAMA 2001;285:2486. http://www.nhlbi.nih.gov/guidelines/cholesterol/index.htm

Several nutritional approaches to diet therapy are available. Most Americans currently eat 35–40% of calories as fat, of which 15% is saturated fat. Dietary cholesterol intake averages 400 mg/d. A cholesterol-lowering diet recommends reducing total fat to 25–30% and saturated fat to less than 7% of calories. Dietary cholesterol should be limited to less than 200 mg/d. These diets replace fat, particularly saturated fat, with carbohydrate. In most instances, this approach will also result in fewer total calories consumed and will facilitate weight loss in overweight patients. Other diet plans, including the Dean Ornish Diet, the Pritikin Diet, and most vegetarian diets, restrict fat even further. Low-fat, high-carbohydrate diets may, however, result in reductions in HDL cholesterol.

An alternative strategy is the "Mediterranean diet," which maintains total fat at approximately 35–40% of total calories but replaces saturated fat with monounsaturated fat such as that found in canola oil and in olives, peanuts, avocados, and their oils. This diet is equally effective at lowering LDL cholesterol but is less likely to lead to reductions in HDL cholesterol. This diet is less likely to lead to weight loss. Thus, a traditional low-fat approach is still preferred for patients with lipid disorders who are overweight.

Other dietary changes may also result in beneficial changes in blood lipids. Soluble fiber, such as that found in oat bran or psyllium, may reduce LDL cholesterol by 5–10%. Garlic, soy protein, vitamin C, pecans, and plant sterols may also result in reduction of LDL cholesterol. Because oxidation of LDL cholesterol as a potential initiating event in atherogenesis, diets rich in antioxidant vitamins, found primarily in fruits and vegetables, may be helpful (see Chapter 29).

Anderson JW et al: Cholesterol-lowering effects of psyllium intake adjunctive to diet therapy in men and women with hypercholesterolemia: meta-analysis of 8 controlled trials. Am J Clin Nutr 2000;71:472. [PMID: 10648260] (Psyllium lowers total and LDL-cholesterol concentrations in subjects consuming a low-fat diet.)

Berglund L et al: HDL-subpopulation patterns in response to reductions in dietary total and saturated fat intakes in healthy subjects. Am J Clin Nutr 1999;70:992. [PMID: 10584043] (A reduction in dietary total and saturated fat decreased both large—HDL(2) and HDL(2b)—and small, dense HDL subpopulations.)

Bunyard LB et al: Dietary intake and changes in lipoprotein lipids in obese, postmenopausal women placed on an American Heart Association Step 1 Diet. J Am Diet Assoc 2002;102:52. [PMID: 11794502] (The only dietary change predicting decreases in HDL concentrations was an increase in the percentage of energy from simple sugar.)

de Lorgeril M et al: Mediterranean diet, traditional risk factors and the rate of cardiovascular complications after myocardial infarction: Final report of the Lyon Diet Heart Study. Circulation 1999;99:779. [PMID: 9989963] (The protective effect of the Mediterranean diet was maintained up to 4 years.)

Denke MA et al: Individual cholesterol variation in response to a margarine- or butter-based diet. A study in families. JAMA 2000;284:2740. [PMID: 1055179] (Replacing butter with margarine results in an average 11% reduction in LDL-cholesterol levels in adults. The response varied among individuals; in some individuals, LDL levels increased.)

Harper CR et al: The fats of life: The role of omega-3 fatty acids in the prevention of coronary heart disease. Arch Intern Med 2001;161:2185. [PMID: 11575974] (Omega-3 fatty acids may have a role in the prevention of CHD.)

Maki KC et al: Lipid responses to plant-sterol-enriched reduced-fat spreads incorporated into a National Cholesterol Education Program Step I diet. Am J Clin Nutr 2001;74:33. [PMID: 11451715] (Subjects in the low- and high-sterol groups had total cholesterol values that were 5.2% and 6.6% lower, and LDL-cholesterol values that were 7.6% and 8.1% lower. Apolipoprotein B values and ratios of total to HDL cholesterol were also lower.)

Morgan WA et al: Pecans lower low-density lipoprotein cholesterol in people with normal lipid levels. J Am Diet Assoc 2000;100:312. [PMID: 10719404]

Schaefer EJ: Lipoproteins, nutrition, and heart disease. Am J Clin Nutr 2002;75:191. [PMID: 11815309] (Restricting saturated fat and cholesterol and increasing the intake of essential fatty acids, especially n-3 fatty acids, reduces CHD risk.)

Stampfer MJ et al: Primary prevention of coronary heart disease in women through diet and lifestyle. N Engl J Med 2000;343:16. [PMID: 10882764] (Women who adhered to all guidelines involving diet, exercise and abstinence from smoking had a very low risk of CHD.)

Stevinson C et al: Garlic for treating hypercholesterolemia. A meta-analysis of randomized clinical trials. Ann Intern Med 2000;133:420. [PMID: 10975959] (A meta-analysis suggesting that garlic is modestly superior to placebo in reducing total cholesterol levels.)

Yu-Poth S et al: Effects of the National Cholesterol Education Program's Step I and Step II dietary intervention programs on cardiovascular disease risk factors: a meta-analysis. Am J Clin Nutr 1999;69:632. [PMID: 10197564] (Plasma total cholesterol, LDL cholesterol, triacylglycerol, and TC:HDL cholesterol decreased by 10%, 12%, 8%, and 10%, respectively, in Step I intervention studies, and by 13%, 16%, 8%, and 7%, respectively, in Step II studies. HDL cholesterol decreased by 7% in response to Step II but not to Step I diets.)

Pharmacologic Therapy

All patients whose risk from CHD is considered high enough to warrant pharmacologic therapy of an elevated LDL cholesterol should be given aspirin prophylaxis at a dose of 81–325 mg/d unless there are contraindications such as aspirin sensitivity, bleeding diatheses, or active peptic ulcer disease. The benefit of aspirin in reducing the risk of CHD is equivalent to that of cholesterol lowering. Other CHD risk factors, such as hypertension and smoking, should also be controlled.

If the decision to treat a patient with an LDL-lowering drug is made, a goal for treatment is set. For patients with CHD or CHD risk equivalents, the goal is LDL < 100 mg/dL. For patients with two or more risk factors the goal is LDL < 130 mg/dL. For those with zero or one risk factor the goal is LDL < 160 mg/dL. In each instance, the therapeutic goal is approached slowly, watching for side effects and encouraging continued adherence to nonpharmacologic therapies. Combinations of drugs may be necessary. Once the goal is reached, the lipid profile should be monitored periodically (every 6–12 months), with consideration given to periodic reductions in drug dose. With the exception of niacin (available generically for a few dollars per month), lipid-lowering agents are expensive and may need to be given for decades. Thus, their cost-effectiveness is generally low, especially in primary prevention.

A. NIACIN (NICOTINIC ACID)

Niacin was the first lipid-lowering agent that was associated with a reduction in total mortality. Long-term follow-up of a secondary prevention trial of middle-aged men with previous myocardial infarction disclosed that about half of those who had been previously treated with niacin had died, compared with nearly 60% of the placebo group. This favorable effect on mortality was not seen during the trial itself, though there was a reduction in the incidence of recurrent coronary events.

Niacin reduces the production of VLDL particles, with secondary reduction in LDL and increases in

HDL cholesterol levels. The average effect of full-dose niacin therapy, 3–4.5 g/d, is a 15–25% reduction in LDL cholesterol and a 25–35% increase in HDL cholesterol. Full doses are required to obtain the LDL effect, but the HDL effect is observed at lower doses, eg, 1 g/d. Niacin will also reduce triglycerides by half and will lower lipoprotein(a) (Lp[a]) levels and will increase plasma homocysteine levels. Thus, its effect on blood lipids and CHD risk is nearly optimal. Unfortunately, intolerance to niacin is common; only 50–60% of patients tolerate full doses. Niacin causes a prostaglandin-mediated flushing that patients may describe as hot flashes or pruritus. This problem can be decreased by pretreatment with aspirin (81–325 mg/d) or other nonsteroidal anti-inflammatory agents. Flushing may also be decreased by initiating niacin therapy with a very small dose, eg, 100 mg with the evening meal. The dose can be doubled each week until 1.5 g/d is tolerated. After rechecking blood lipids, the dose is divided and increased until the goal of 3–4.5 g/d is reached. Extended-release niacin is also available and may be better tolerated by some patients. It is not known whether routine monitoring of liver enzymes results in early detection and thus reduced severity of this side effect. Niacin can also exacerbate gout and peptic ulcer disease. Although niacin may increase blood sugar in some patients, clinical trials have shown that niacin can be safely used in diabetics.

B. BILE ACID-BINDING RESINS (CHOLESTYRAMINE, COLESTIPOL)

Treatment with these agents reduces the incidence of coronary events in middle-aged men by about 20%, with no significant effect on total mortality. The resins work by binding bile acids in the intestine. The resultant reduction in the enterohepatic circulation causes the liver to increase its production of bile acids, using hepatic cholesterol to do so. Thus, hepatic LDL receptor activity increases, with a decline in plasma LDL levels. The triglyceride level tends to increase slightly in some patients treated with bile acid-binding resins; they should be used with caution in those with elevated triglycerides and probably not at all in patients who have triglyceride levels above 500 mg/dL. The clinician can anticipate a reduction of 15–25% in the LDL cholesterol level, with insignificant effects on the HDL level.

The usual dose of cholestyramine is 12–36 g of resin per day in divided doses with meals, mixed in water or, more palatably, juice. Doses of colestipol are 20% higher (the packets each contain 5 g of resin).

These agents often cause gastrointestinal symptoms, such as constipation and gas. They may interfere with the absorption of fat-soluble vitamins (thereby complicating the management of patients receiving warfarin) and may bind other drugs in the intestine. Concurrent use of psyllium may ameliorate the gastrointestinal side effects.

C. HMG-CoA REDUCTASE INHIBITORS (LOVASTATIN, PRAVASTATIN, SIMVASTATIN, FLUVASTATIN, ATORVASTATIN)

These agents work by inhibiting the rate-limiting enzyme in the formation of cholesterol. They reduce myocardial infarctions and total mortality in secondary prevention, as well as in middle-aged men free of CHD. A meta-analysis has demonstrated significant reduction in risk of stroke. Cholesterol synthesis in the liver is reduced, with a compensatory increase in hepatic LDL receptors (presumably so that the liver can take more of the cholesterol that it needs from the blood), and a reduction in the circulating LDL cholesterol level by up to 35%. There are also modest increases in HDL levels and decreases in triglyceride levels.

Doses are as follows: lovastatin, 10–80 mg/d; pravastatin, 10–40 mg/d; simvastatin, 5–40 mg/d; fluvastatin, 20–40 mg/d; and atorvastatin, 10–80 mg/d. These agents are usually given once a day in the evening (most cholesterol synthesis takes place overnight); at the high end of the dose ranges, twice-a-day dosing may be used. Side effects include myositis, whose incidence may be higher in patients concurrently taking fibrates or niacin. Manufacturers recommend monitoring liver and muscle enzymes. Several agents (notably erythromycin, cyclosporine, and azole antifungals) reduce the metabolism of these agents.

D. FIBRIC ACID DERIVATIVES (GEMFIBROZIL, FENOFIBRATE, CLOFIBRATE)

Gemfibrozil reduced CHD rates in hypercholesterolemic middle-aged men free of coronary disease in the Helsinki Heart Study. The effect was only observed among those who also had lower HDL cholesterol levels and high triglyceride levels. In a recent VA study, gemfibrozil was also shown to reduce cardiovascular events in men with existing CHD whose primary lipid abnormality was a low HDL-cholesterol. There was no effect on all-cause mortality.

The fibrates reduce the synthesis and increase the breakdown of VLDL particles, with secondary effects on LDL and HDL levels. They reduce LDL levels by about 10–15% and triglyceride levels by about 40% and raise HDL levels by about 15–20%. The usual dose of gemfibrozil is 600 mg once or twice a day. Side effects include cholelithiasis, hepatitis, and myositis. The incidence of the latter two conditions may be higher among patients also taking other lipid-lowering agents. In the largest clinical trial that used clofibrate, there were significantly more deaths—especially due to cancer—in the treatment group; it should not be used.

E. PROBUCOL

The effects of probucol on CHD—and its long-term safety—are not known. It does reduce the deposition of LDL into xanthomas in humans (and into atherosclerotic plaques in rabbits). The mechanism of action of probucol is not clear. It apparently reduces the amount of oxidized LDL (it was originally used as an industrial antioxidant). Probucol reduces LDL levels by 10–15% but has the potentially important adverse effect of lowering HDL levels by up to 10%. Probucol, if used at all, should be reserved for patients with a clear genetic disorder who have failed other therapies.

Initial Selection of Medication

At present there are no absolute guidelines for selection of available lipid-modifying medications in particular patients. Nonetheless, clinical trials provide guidance (Table 28–4). For most patients who require a lipid-modifying medication, an HMG-CoA reductase inhibitor is preferred. Although niacin will also have beneficial effects on lipids in both men and women with CHD, there is less evidence demonstrating the desired effects on CHD and all-cause mortality. While estrogen also has beneficial effects on lipids in postmenopausal women, it probably should not be used to treat lipid disorders (see Chapter 26). Resins are the only lipid-modifying medication considered safe in pregnancy.

Combinations of lipid-modifying medications may be more cost-effective than high doses of a single medication (usually an HMG-CoA reductase inhibitor) and may have beneficial effects on lipids. Low-dose niacin (0.5–1 g/d), for example, will substantially increase the HDL cholesterol when added to an HMG-CoA reductase inhibitor. Combinations, however, may increase the risk of severe complications of drug therapy. The combination of gemfibrozil and HMG-CoA reductase inhibitors increases the risk of myopathy more than either drug alone.

Albert MA et al: Effect of statin therapy on C-reactive protein levels. JAMA 2001:286:64. [PMID: 11434828] (Pravastatin reduced C-reactive protein levels independent of LDL effect.)

Choice of lipid-regulating drugs. Med Lett Drugs Ther 2001;43:43. [PMID: 11378632] (Maximum doses of atorvastatin decrease cholesterol the most. When both LDL and HDL are low in patients with established CHD, gemfibrozil lowers the incidence of CHD events.)

Cummings SR et al: Do statins prevent both cardiovascular disease and fracture? JAMA 2000;283:3255. [PMID: 10866875] (Editorial suggesting that recommendations to prescribe statins to prevent fractures must await results of further clinical trials.)

Elam MB et al: Effect of niacin on lipid and lipoprotein levels and glycemic control in patients with diabetes and peripheral arterial disease: the ADMIT study: A randomized trial. Arterial Disease Multiple Intervention Trial. JAMA 2000; 284:1263. [PMID: 10979113] (Niacin can be safely used and may be considered as an alternative to statin drugs or fibrates for patients who do not tolerate or fail to sufficiently correct hypertriglyceridemia or low HDL cholesterol levels with these agents.)

Garg R et al: Niacin treatment increases plasma homocyst(e)ine levels. Am Heart J 1999;138:1082. [PMID: 10577438]

Table 28–4. Effects of selected lipid-modifying drugs.

	Liqid-Modifying Effects			Initial Daily Dose	Maximum Daily Dose	Cost for 30 Days' Treatment With Dose Listed[1]
Drug	LDL	HDL	Triglyceride			
Atorvastatin (Lipitor)	−25 to −40%	+5 to −10%	↓↓	10 mg once	80 mg once	$101.20 (20 mg once)
Cholestyramine (Questran, others)	−15 to −25%	+5%	±	4 g bid	24 g divided	$83.61 (8 g divided)
Colestipol (Colestid)	−15 to −25%	+5%	±	5 g bid	30 g divided	$113.16 (10 g divided)
Fluvastatin (Lescol)	−20 to −30%	+5 to −10%	↓	20 mg once	40 mg once	$44.39 (20 mg once)
Gemfibrozil (Lopid)	−10 to −15%	+15 to −20%	↓↓	600 mg once	1200 mg divided	$74.80 (600 mg bid)
Lovastatin (Mevacor)	−25 to −40%	+5 to −10%	↓	10 mg once	80 mg divided	$71.10 (20 mg once)
Niacin	−15 to −25%	+25 to −35%	↓↓	100 mg once	3–4.5 g divided	$7.20 (1.5 g bid)
Pravastatin (Pravachol)	−25 to −40%	+5 to −10%	↓	20 mg once	40 mg once	$83.43 (20 mg once)
Simvastatin (Zocor)	−25 to −40%	+5 to −10%	↓↓	5 mg once	80 mg once	$75.60 (10 mg once)

[1]Cost to pharmacist (average wholesale price, generic when possible) for quantity listed. Source: *Drug Topics Red Book,* March 2002; Vol. 21, No. 3.
± = variable, if any.

Guyton JR et al: Extended-release niacin vs gemfibrozil for the treatment of low levels of high-density lipoprotein cholesterol. Niaspan-Gemfibrozil Study Group. Arch Intern Med 2000;24;160:1177. [PMID: 10789612] (High doses of extended-release niacin provided up to 2-fold greater HDL-C increases, decreases in lipoprotein(a), improvements in lipoprotein cholesterol ratios, and lower fibrinogen levels compared with gemfibrozil. Gemfibrozil gave a greater triglyceride reduction but also increased the low-density lipoprotein cholesterol level, which did not occur with Niaspan.)

Jacobson TA: Combination lipid-altering therapy: an emerging treatment paradigm for the 21st century. Curr Atheroscler Rep 2001;3:373. [PMID: 11487448] (Regimens involving statins with niacin, fibric-acid derivatives, or bile acid resins allow drugs to be given at lower doses, resulting in a lower risk of adverse events.)

Muldoon MF et al: Effects of lovastatin on cognitive function and psychological well-being. Am J Med 2000;108:538. [PMID: 10806282] (Treatment of hypercholesterolemia with lovastatin did not cause psychologic distress or substantially alter cognitive function.)

Ray JG et al: Use of statins and the subsequent development of deep vein thrombosis. Arch Intern Med 2001;161:1405. [PMID: 11386889] (Among individuals aged 65 years or older, statins were associated with a 22% relative risk reduction in the risk of DVT. A randomized clinical trial is needed to evaluate the efficacy of statins for primary and secondary prevention.)

Rubins HB et al: Gemfibrozil for the secondary prevention of coronary heart disease in men with low levels of high-den-sity lipoprotein cholesterol. Veterans Affairs High-Density Lipoprotein Cholesterol Intervention Trial Study Group. N Engl J Med 1999;341:410. [PMID: 10438259] (Significant reduction in the risk of major cardiovascular events in patients with coronary disease whose primary lipid abnormality was a low HDL cholesterol level; no effect on all-cause mortality.)

Schwartz GG et al: Atorvastatin for acute coronary syndromes. JAMA 2001;285:533. [PMID: 11476650] (Atorvastatin 80 mg started within 96 hours after admission was associated with a lower incidence of ischemic events in the following 16 weeks. Patients were lost to follow-up in the atorvastatin group.)

Secondary prevention by raising HDL cholesterol and reducing triglycerides in patients with coronary artery disease: the Bezafibrate Infarction Prevention (BIP) study. Circulation 2000;102:21. [PMID: 10880410] (No significant reduction in nonfatal myocardial infarction or sudden death.)

Waters DD et al: What is the role of intensive cholesterol lowering in the treatment of acute coronary syndromes? Am J Cardiol 2001;88(7 Suppl 2):7. [PMID: 11595193] (Intensive cholesterol lowering influences several mechanisms related to the pathogenesis of acute coronary syndromes.)

HIGH BLOOD TRIGLYCERIDES

Patients with very high levels of serum triglycerides are at risk of pancreatitis. The pathophysiology is not certain, since some patients with very high levels never develop pancreatitis. Most patients with congenital abnormalities in triglyceride metabolism present in childhood; hypertriglyceridemia-induced pancreatitis first presenting in adults is more commonly due to an acquired problem in lipid metabolism.

Although there are no clear triglyceride levels that predict pancreatitis, most clinicians are uncomfortable with fasting levels above 500 mg/dL. The risk of pancreatitis may be more related to the triglyceride level following consumption of a fatty meal. Because postprandial increases in triglyceride are inevitable if fat-containing foods are eaten, fasting triglyceride levels in persons prone to pancreatitis should be kept well below that level.

The primary therapy for high triglyceride levels is dietary, avoiding alcohol and fatty foods and restricting calories. Control of secondary causes of high triglyceride levels (see Table 28–1) may also be helpful. In patients with fasting triglycerides ≥ 500 mg/dL despite adequate dietary compliance—and certainly in those with a previous episode of pancreatitis—therapy with a triglyceride-lowering drug (eg, niacin, a fibric acid derivative, or an HMG-CoA reductase inhibitor) is indicated.

Whether patients with elevated triglycerides (> 150 mg/dL) should be treated to prevent CHD is not known. Meta-analysis of 17 observational studies suggests that after adjustment for other risk factors, elevated triglycerides increased CHD risk in men by 14% and in women by 37%. Triglyceride-rich lipoproteins (partially degraded VLDL, commonly called remnant lipoproteins) have been found in human atheromas, and elevated triglycerides are associated with small dense LDL in most instances. Elevated triglycerides are also an important feature of the **metabolic syndrome,** found in an estimated 25% of Americans—defined by three or more of the following five abnormalities: waist circumference > 102 cm in me or > 88 cm in women; serum triglycerides level of at least 150 mg/dL; HDL level of < 40 mg/dL in men or < 50 mg/dL in women; blood pressure of at least 130/85 mm Hg; and serum glucose level of at least 110 mg/dL. Other data, however, suggest that triglyceride measurements do not improve discrimination between those with and without CHD events, and clinical trial data are not available to support the routine treatment of high triglycerides in all patients.)

The recent NCEP Adult Treatment Panel III (ATP III) report, however, recommends an aggressive approach to triglyceride management. For those with borderline levels (150–199 mg/dL), emphasis is placed on calorie restriction and exercise. For patients with high triglycerides (> 200 mg/dL), the non-HDL cholesterol should be measured (total cholesterol – HDL cholesterol). The ATP III report recommends that non-HDL cholesterol should be treated with diet and medications to result in levels 30 mg/dL higher than the LDL goal. The ATP III report does not differentiate between primary and secondary prevention. A reasonable approach might be to use this approach for patients with CHD and risk equivalents for that disease but not for lower-risk patients.

Austin MA et al: Hypertriglyceridemia as a cardiovascular risk factor. Am J Cardiol 1998;81(4A):7B. [PMID: 9526807] (Meta-analysis of 17 studies of relation of plasma triglyceride levels and the risk of incident cardiovascular disease. After adjustment for high-density lipoprotein cholesterol and other risk factors, the risks were 14% in men and 37% in women and remained statistically significant.)

Avins AL et al: Do triglycerides provide meaningful information about heart disease risk? Arch Intern Med 2000;160:1937. [PMID: 10888968] (Reanalysis of data suggests that triglyceride measurements did not improve discrimination between those with and without CHD events in men; evidence does not support the routine measurement of serum triglycerides for assessing risk.)

Ford ES et al: Prevalence of the metabolic syndrome among US adults: findings from the third National Health and Nutrition Examination Survey. JAMA 2002;287:356. [PMID: 11790215] (The age-adjusted prevalence of the metabolic syndrome was 23.7% in the United States. Mexican-Americans had the highest age-adjusted prevalence, 31.9%).

Malloy MJ et al: A risk factor for atherosclerosis: triglyceride-rich lipoproteins. Adv Intern Med 2001;47:111. [PMID: 11795072] (Meta-analysis has established increased triglycerides as an independent risk factor for heart disease. The finding of triglyceride-rich lipoproteins in human atheromata provides pathophysiologic evidence for a direct role in atherogenesis. Hypertriglyceridemia also may underlie the phenomenon of small dense LDL in most instances.)

Miller M: Current perspectives on the management of hypertriglyceridemia. Am Heart J 2000;140:232. [PMID: 10925336] (Few data establishing that triglyceride reduction improves cardiovascular event rate.)

Stein EA et al: Comparison of statins in hypertriglyceridemia. Am J Cardiol 1998;81:66B. [PMID: 9526817] (All statins are effective in decreasing triglyceride levels, but only in hypertriglyceridemic patients. The more effective the statin is in decreasing LDL cholesterol, the more effective it will also be in decreasing triglyceride levels.)

Nutrition

Robert B. Baron, MD, MS

See www.current-med.com/ch29.html

29

■ NUTRITIONAL REQUIREMENTS

Approximately 40 nutrients are required by the human body. Nutrients are essential if they cannot be synthesized by the body and if a deficiency causes recognizable abnormalities that disappear when the deficit is corrected. Required nutrients include the essential amino acids, water-soluble vitamins, fat-soluble vitamins, minerals, and the essential fatty acids. The body also requires an adequate energy substrate, a small amount of metabolizable carbohydrate, indigestible carbohydrate (fiber), additional nitrogen, and water.

Nutritional requirements have been most commonly expressed by recommended dietary allowances (RDAs). Published and periodically reviewed by the Food and Nutrition Board of the National Academy of Sciences, the RDAs were initially designed to meet the known nutritional needs of practically all healthy persons. RDAs have been established for energy and protein; the water-soluble vitamins thiamin, riboflavin, niacin, vitamin B_6, folic acid, vitamin B_{12}, and vitamin C; the fat soluble vitamins A, D, and K; and the minerals calcium, phosphorus, magnesium, iron, zinc, iodine, and selenium (Table 29–1).

Recently, the Food and Nutrition Board has developed a broader approach to defining nutritional adequacy. Known as dietary reference intakes (DRIs), these new guidelines go beyond the prevention of classic nutritional deficiency diseases and address the role of nutrients and other food components in long-term health and the reduction of risk of chronic diseases. The DRIs consist of four reference intakes: the RDA, the estimated average requirement (EAR), the tolerable upper intake level (UL), and the adequate intake (AI). The RDA remains the dietary intake that is sufficient to meet the nutritional requirements of nearly all individuals in an age- and gender-specific group. RDAs are intended as goals for individuals. The EAR is the intake value that is estimated to meet the requirements of 50% of individuals in an age- and gender-specific group. The UL is the maximum level of daily nutrient intake that is unlikely to pose health risks to most individuals. The AI is determined when insufficient data are available to establish the EAR and RDA for a given nutrient. It is based on fewer data and more expert opinion but is also intended as goals for individuals. DRIs are divided into seven nutrient groups: (1) calcium, vitamin D, phosphorus, magnesium and fluoride; (2) folate and other B vitamins; (3) antioxidants (eg, vitamins C and E and selenium); (4) macronutrients (eg, protein, fat, carbohydrates); (5) trace elements (eg, iron and zinc); (6) electrolytes and water; and (7) other food components (eg, fiber, phytoestrogens).

ENERGY

The body requires energy to support normal functions and physical activity, growth, and repair of damaged tissues. Energy is provided by oxidation of dietary protein, fat, carbohydrate, and alcohol. Oxidation of 1 g of each provides 4 kcal of energy from protein and carbohydrate, 9 kcal from fat, and 7 kcal from alcohol.

In healthy adults, energy expenditure is primarily determined by three factors: basal energy expenditure (BEE), thermic effect of food (TEF), and physical activity.

The BEE is the amount of energy required to maintain basic physiologic functions. It is measured while the subject is resting in a warm room, not having eaten for 12 hours. In healthy persons, the BEE (in kcal/24 h) can be estimated by the Harris-Benedict equation, which will correctly predict measured BEE in 90% + 10% of healthy subjects. In clinical practice, patients rarely meet the strict criteria for BEE measurement. Instead, energy expenditure is measured in individuals at rest without food for 2 hours. This measurement, the resting energy expenditure (REE), is about 10% greater than BEE.

TEF is the amount of energy expended during and following the ingestion of food. TEF averages approximately 10% of the BEE.

Physical activity has a major impact on energy expenditure. The average energy expenditure per hour by adults engaged in typical activities is shown in Table 29–2.

Table 29–1. Recommended daily dietary allowances for adults (revised 1989).[1]

Category	Age (years) or Condition	Weight (kg)	Weight (lb)	Height (cm)	Height (in)	Protein (g)	Fat-Soluble Vitamins Vitamin A (mg RE)	Vitamin D (mg)	Vitamin E (mg α-TE)	Vitamin K (mg)	Water-Soluble Vitamins Vitamin C (mg)	Thiamine (mg)	Riboflavin (mg)	Niacin (mg)	Vitamin B6 (mg)	Folate (µg)	Vitamin B12 (µg)	Minerals Calcium (mg)	Phosphorus (mg)	Magnesium (mg)	Iron (mg)	Zinc (mg)	Iodine (µg)	Selenium (µg)
Males	15–18	66	145	176	69	59	1000	10	10	65	60	1.5	1.8	20	2.0	200	2.0	1200	1200	400	12	15	150	50
	19–24	72	160	177	70	58	1000	10	10	70	60	1.5	1.7	19	2.0	200	2.0	1200	1200	350	10	15	150	70
	25–50	79	174	176	70	63	1000	5	10	80	60	1.5	1.7	19	2.0	200	2.0	800	800	350	10	15	150	70
	51+	77	170	173	68	63	1000	5	10	80	60	1.2	1.4	15	2.0	200	2.0	800	800	350	10	15	150	70
Females	15–18	55	120	163	64	44	800	10	8	55	60	1.1	1.3	15	1.5	160	2.0	1200	1200	300	15	12	150	50
	19–24	58	128	164	65	46	800	10	8	60	60	1.1	1.3	15	1.6	180	2.0	1200	1200	280	15	12	150	55
	25–50	63	138	163	64	50	800	5	8	65	60	1.1	1.3	15	1.6	180	2.0	800	800	280	15	12	150	55
	51+	65	143	160	63	50	800	5	8	65	60	1.0	1.2	13	1.6	180	2.0	800	800	280	10	12	150	55
Pregnant						60	800	10	10	65	70	1.5	1.6	17	2.2	400[2]	2.2	1200	1200	320	30	15	175	65
Lactating	1st 6 months					65	1300	10	12	65	95	1.6	1.8	20	2.1	280	2.6	1200	1200	355	15	19	200	75
	2nd 6 months					62	1300	10	11	65	95	1.6	1.7	20	2.1	260	2.6	1200	1200	340	15	19	200	75

[1]From: National Research Council: Recommended Dietary Allowances, 10th ed. National Academy of Sciences, 1989.
[2]CDC recommendation is 800 µg.

Table 29–2. Average energy kilocalories expended per hour by adults at selected weights engaged in various activities.[1]

Activity	54 kg (120 lb)	64 kg (140 lb)	73 kg (160 lb)	82 kg (180 lb)	91 kg (200 lb)	100 kg (220 lb)
Sleeping: Reclining	50	58	69	78	86	99
Very light: Sitting	73	83	103	115	127	150
Light: Walking on level, shopping, light housekeeping	143	166	200	225	250	290
Moderate: Cycling, dancing, skiing, tennis	226	262	307	345	382	430
Heavy: Walking uphill, shoveling, swimming, playing basketball or football	440	512	598	670	746	840

Note: Range of rate of expenditure of calories per minute of activity (for a 70-kg man or a 58-kg woman): Sleeping, 0.9–1.2; very light, 1.5–2.5; light, 2–4.9; moderate, 5–7.4; heavy, 6–12.
[1]Data from McArdle WD, Katch FI, Katch VL: *Exercise Physiology: Energy, Nutrition and Human Performance.* Lea & Febiger, 1981.

Daily recommended energy intakes for healthy individuals are shown in Table 29–3.

PROTEIN

Protein is required for growth and for maintenance of body structure and function. Although the nutritional requirement is commonly stated in grams of protein, the true requirement is for nine **essential amino acids** plus additional nitrogen for protein synthesis. The essential amino acids are leucine, isoleucine, lysine, methionine, phenylalanine, threonine, tryptophan, valine, and histidine.

Adequate protein must be consumed each day to replace essential amino acids lost through protein turnover. On a protein-free diet, the average male loses 3.8 g of nitrogen per day—equivalent to 24 g of protein. Allowing for differences in protein quality and utilization and for individual variability, the RDA for protein is 56 g/d for men and 45 g/d for women.

Protein and energy requirements are closely related. Diets that provide insufficient energy will require additional protein to maintain nitrogen equilibrium.

CARBOHYDRATE

As long as adequate energy and protein are provided in the diet, there is no specific requirement for dietary carbohydrate. A small amount of carbohydrate—approximately 100 g/d—is necessary to prevent ketosis. In practice, however, most dietary energy should be provided by carbohydrate. The average American diet contains 45% of calories as carbohydrate. Current recommendations are to increase carbohydrate intakes to 55–60% of total calories in the diet.

Dietary carbohydrates include simple sugars, complex carbohydrates (starches), and indigestible carbohydrates (dietary fiber). Although simple sugars and starches provide equal amounts of calories, the bulk of

Table 29–3. Median heights and weights and recommended energy expenditure (REE).[1]

Category	Age (years)	Weight (kg)	Weight (lb)	Height (cm)	Height (in)	REE (kcal/d)	Average Energy Allowance[2] (kcal) Multiples of REE	Average Energy Allowance[2] (kcal) Per kg	Average Energy Allowance[2] (kcal) Per Day[3]
Males	19–24	72	160	177	70	1780	1.67	40	2900
	25–50	79	174	176	70	1800	1.60	37	2900
	51+	77	170	173	68	1530	1.50	30	2300
Females	19–24	58	128	164	65	1350	1.60	38	2200
	25–50	63	138	163	64	1380	1.55	36	2200
	51+	65	143	160	63	1280	1.50	30	1900

[1]Modified from: National Research Council: *Recommended Dietary Allowances,* 10th ed. National Academy of Sciences, 1989.
[2]In the range of light to moderate activity, the coefficient of variation is ± 20%.
[3]Figure is rounded.

dietary carbohydrates should be derived from starches. Simple sugars—particularly sucrose—are concentrated sources of calories without other sources of essential nutrients. Sucrose consumption is also thought to be an important factor in the development of tooth decay. Starches, when unrefined, provide carbohydrate calories and vitamins, minerals, and dietary fiber.

Dietary fiber is that portion of plant foods that cannot be digested by the human intestine. Fiber increases the bulk of the stool and facilitates excretion. Diets high in dietary fiber are associated with a lower incidence of digestive and cardiovascular diseases. The more insoluble fibers, such as those found in wheat bran, have the greatest effect on colonic function. Soluble fibers such as those found in legumes, oats, and fruit result in lower blood sugar levels in diabetics and lower blood cholesterol.

FAT

Dietary fat is the most concentrated source of food energy. Like energy from dietary carbohydrate, energy derived from fat can support protein synthesis. Dietary fat also provides the essential fatty acid linoleic acid. Other than the need for adequate quantities of linoleic acid, there is no specific requirement for dietary fat as long as the diet provides adequate nutrients oxidizable for energy. Although the average American diet contains 35–40% of calories as fat, most current recommendations are to limit dietary fat to 30% or less of total calories. Diets containing as little as 5–10% of total calories as fat appear to be safe and well tolerated.

Dietary fats are composed chiefly of fatty acids and dietary cholesterol. Fatty acids contain either no double bonds (saturated), one double bond (monounsaturated), or more than one double bond (polyunsaturated). Current recommendations are to decrease total fat and replace saturated fats with monounsaturated fatty acids and complex carbohydrates. Saturated fatty acids are associated with increased serum cholesterol, while polyunsaturated and monounsaturated fatty acids lower serum cholesterol. Saturated fats are solid at room temperature and in general are derived from animal foods; unsaturated fats are liquid at room temperature and in general are derived from plant foods.

The polyunsaturated fatty acid **linoleic acid** is an essential nutrient, required by the body for the synthesis of arachidonic acid, the major precursor of prostaglandins. Deficiency of linoleic acid results in dermatitis, hair loss, and impaired wound healing. For individuals with average energy requirements, approximately 5 g of linoleic acid per day—1–2% of total calories—is required to prevent essential fatty acid deficiency.

Cholesterol is a major constituent of cell membranes. It is synthesized by the body and is not an essential nutrient. Diets that contain large amounts of cholesterol partially inhibit endogenous cholesterol synthesis but result in a net increase in serum cholesterol concentrations because of suppression of synthesis of low-density lipoprotein receptors. Average American diets contain approximately 450 mg/d of cholesterol, but 300 mg or less per day is recommended.

VITAMINS

Vitamins are a heterogeneous group of organic molecules required by the body for a variety of essential metabolic functions. They are grouped as **water-soluble vitamins:** thiamin, riboflavin, niacin, vitamin B$_6$ (pyridoxine), vitamin B$_{12}$ (cobalamin), folate, pantothenic acid, biotin, and vitamin C (ascorbic acid); and **fat-soluble vitamins:** A, D, E, and K. Disorders of vitamin metabolism are discussed below.

MINERALS

The body also requires a number of inorganic minerals, commonly grouped as the **major minerals** calcium, magnesium, and phosphorus; the **electrolytes** sodium, potassium, and chloride; and the **trace elements** iron, zinc, copper, manganese, molybdenum, fluoride, iodine, cobalt, chromium, and selenium. Important characteristics of major minerals and electrolytes are summarized in Table 29–4.

DRUG-NUTRIENT INTERACTIONS

Many medications affect nutritional requirements. A variety of drugs induce nutrient deficiencies by appetite suppression, intestinal malabsorption, and alterations in nutrient metabolism or excretion. The effects of selected drugs on nutrient absorption and metabolism are summarized in Table 29–5.

DIETARY RECOMMENDATIONS

Prior to 1980, the emphasis in diet planning was to ensure that the RDAs were met by diets containing a wide variety of foods. The most important tool used for this purpose was *The Four Food Groups,* published by the United States Department of Agriculture (USDA). According to this model, two servings per day from both the milk group and the meat group and four servings per day from both the fruit and vegetable group and the cereal group would meet the minimal nutritional requirements for most individuals. This model, however, did not guarantee that selected foods were of high quality. The effects of food processing on the nutrient density of food, the balance of macronutrients, and the character of macronutrients (simple versus complex carbohydrate; saturated versus unsaturated fat) are omitted.

In the last 2 decades, numerous authorities have published dietary recommendations that address these issues. Although attention has been directed to the differences between these reports, most agree on the basic principles of eating a wide variety of foods; increasing

Table 29–4. Essential macrominerals: Summary of major characteristics.[1]

Elements	Functions	Deficiency Disease or Symptoms	Toxicity Disease or Symptoms[2]
Calcium	Constituent of bones, teeth; regulation of nerve, muscle function.	Children: rickets. Adults: osteomalacia. May contribute to osteoporosis.	Occurs with excess absorption due to hypervitaminosis D or hypercalcemia due to hyperparathyroidism or other causes of hypercalcemia.
Phosphorus	Constituent of bones, teeth, ATP, phosphorylated metabolic intermediates. Nucleic acids.	Children: rickets. Adults: osteomalacia.	Low serum Ca^{2+}:P_i ratio stimulates secondary hyperparathyroidism; may lead to bone loss.
Sodium	Principal cation in extracellular fluid. Regulates plasma volume, acid-base balance, nerve and muscle function, Na^+-K^+ ATPase.	Unknown on normal diet, secondary to injury or illness.	Hypertension (in susceptible individuals).
Potassium	Principal cation in intracellular fluid; nerve and muscle function, Na^+-K^+ ATPase.	Occurs secondary to illness, injury, or diuretic therapy; muscular weakness, paralysis, mental confusion.	Cardiac arrest, small bowel ulcers.
Chloride	Fluid and electrolyte balance; gastric fluid.	Infants fed salt-free formula. Secondary to vomiting, diuretic therapy, renal disease.	Cardiac arrest, small bowel ulcers.
Magnesium	Constituent of bones, teeth; enzyme cofactor (kinases, etc).	Secondary to malabsorption or diarrhea, alcoholism.	Depressed deep tendon reflexes and respiration.

[1]Modified from Murray RK et al: *Harper's Biochemistry*, 25th ed. Appleton & Lange, 1998.
[2]Excess mineral intake produces toxic symptoms. Unless otherwise specified, symptoms include nonspecific nausea, diarrhea, and irritability.

the consumption of foods containing complex carbohydrates; reducing the intake of sugar, fat (particularly saturated fat), cholesterol, salt, and alcohol; maintaining an ideal body weight, and being physically active each day.

A nutrition education guide, the "Food Guide Pyramid" (Figure 29–1), has been published by the USDA to guide food choices. The Pyramid emphasizes consumption of bread, cereal, rice, and pasta (six to eleven servings); vegetables (three to five servings); and fruit (two to four servings). It places lesser emphasis on milk, yogurt, and cheese (two or three servings) and meat, poultry, fish, dry beans, eggs, and nuts (two or three servings); and recommends that fats, oils, and sweets be used sparingly. "Food guide pyramids" have also been developed recently for use with older individuals and with children.

Bazzano LA et al: Legume consumption and risk of coronary heart disease in US men and women. NHANES I Epidemiologic Follow-up Study. Arch Intern Med 2001;161:2573. [PMID: 11718588] (Legume consumption four times per week compared with less than once per week was associated with a 22% lower risk of coronary heart disease and an 11% lower risk of cardiovascular disease.)

Bryant RJ et al: The new dietary reference intakes for calcium: implications for osteoporosis. J Am Coll Nutr 1999;18(5 Suppl):406S. [PMID: 10511321] (The new Dietary Reference Intakes [DRI] recommend calcium intakes for adults of 1000–1200 mg/d. Most people do not consume these amounts of calcium.)

Center for Nutrition Policy and Promotion. *Nutrition and Your Health: Dietary Guidelines for Americans*, 5th ed. USDA, 2000. (www.nutrition.gov/) (Dietary Guidelines have been published by the USDA every 5 years since 1980. The current edition provides ten guidelines clustered into three groups: aim for fitness, build a healthy base, choose sensibly.)

Feskanich D et al: Vitamin A intake and hip fractures among postmenopausal women. JAMA 2002;287:47. [PMID: 11754708] (Women in the highest quintile of total vitamin A intake had a 48% elevated relative risk of hip fracture compared with women in the lowest quintile of intake. Long-term intake of a diet high in retinol may promote the development of osteoporotic hip fractures in women.)

Freeland-Graves J et al: Position of the American Dietetic Association: total diet approach to communicating food and nutrition information. J Am Diet Assoc 2002;102:100. [PMID: 11794489] (Messages to the public about diet should emphasize the total diet, or overall pattern of food eaten, rather than any one food or meal. The value of a food should be determined within the context of the total diet because classifying foods as "good" or "bad" may foster unhealthy eating behaviors.)

Fung TT et al: Dietary patterns and the risk of coronary heart disease in women. Arch Intern Med 2001;161:1857. [PMID: 11493127] (A prudent dietary pattern—higher intakes of fruits, vegetables, legumes, fish, poultry, and whole grains—was compared with a Western pattern of red and processed

Table 29–5. Effect of drugs on nutrient absorption and metabolism.

Drug	Effect
Analgesics and anti-inflammatories	
Salicylates	Decrease serum ascorbic acid; increase urinary loss of ascorbic acid, potassium, and amino acids.
Sulfasalazine	Impairs folate absorption and antagonizes folate supplementation.
Antacids	
Aluminum antacids	Decrease absorption of phosphate and vitamin A.
H_2 blockers	Decrease iron and vitamin B_{12} absorption.
Octreotide acetate	Hypo- and hyperglycemia; decreases fat and carotene absorption.
Anticonvulsants	
Phenobarbital	Decreases serum folate; increases vitamin D and vitamin K turnover and may cause deficiency.
Phenytoin	Decreases serum folate; increases vitamin D and vitamin K turnover and may cause deficiency.
Primidone	Decreases serum folate and vitamins B_6 and B_{12}; decreases calcium absorption; increases vitamin D and vitamin K turnover and may cause anxiety.
Antimicrobials	
Neomycin	Binds bile acids. Decreases absorption of fat and carotene; of vitamins A, D, K, and B_{12}; and of potassium, sodium, calcium, and nitrogen.
Amphotericin B	Decreases serum magnesium and potassium.
Aminosalicylic acid	Increases absorption of folate, vitamin B_{12}, iron, cholesterol, and fat.
Chloramphenicol	Increases need for vitamins B_2, B_6, B_{12}; increases serum iron.
Penicillin	Hypokalemia; renal potassium wasting.
Tetracycline	Calcium, iron, magnesium inhibit drug absorption; decreases vitamin K synthesis.
Cycloserine	May decrease absorption of calcium, magnesium; may decrease serum folate and vitamins B_6 and B_{12}; decreases protein synthesis.
Isoniazid	Vitamin B_6 antagonist; may cause deficiency.
Sulfonamide	Decreases absorption of folate; decreases serum folate, iron.
Nitrofurantoin	Decreases serum folate.
Pyrimethamine	Decreases serum B_{12} and folate.
Antimitotics	
Methotrexate	Decreases activation of folate.
Colchicine	Decreases absorption of vitamin B_{12}, carotene, fat, sodium, potassium, cholesterol, lactose, nitrogen.
Cathartics	
Phenolphthalein	Malabsorption, hypokalemia; deficiency of vitamin D, calcium.
Mineral oil	Malabsorption; decreased absorption of vitamins A, D, K.
Diuretics	Some cause hypokalemia, hypomagnesemia; may increase urinary excretion of vitamins B_1 and B_6; calcium, magnesium, potassium.
Hypocholesterolemics	
Cholestyramine	Binds bile acids; decreases absorption of fat, carotene; vitamins A, D, K, and B_{12}; folate, iron.
Clofibrate	Decreases absorption of carotene, vitamin B_{12}, iron, glucose.
Hypotensives	
Hydralazine	Vitamin B_6 deficiency.
Captopril	May cause hyponatremia, hyperkalemia; decreases taste acuity.
Oral contraceptives	Vitamin B_6, folate deficiency; may increase the need for other nutrients.

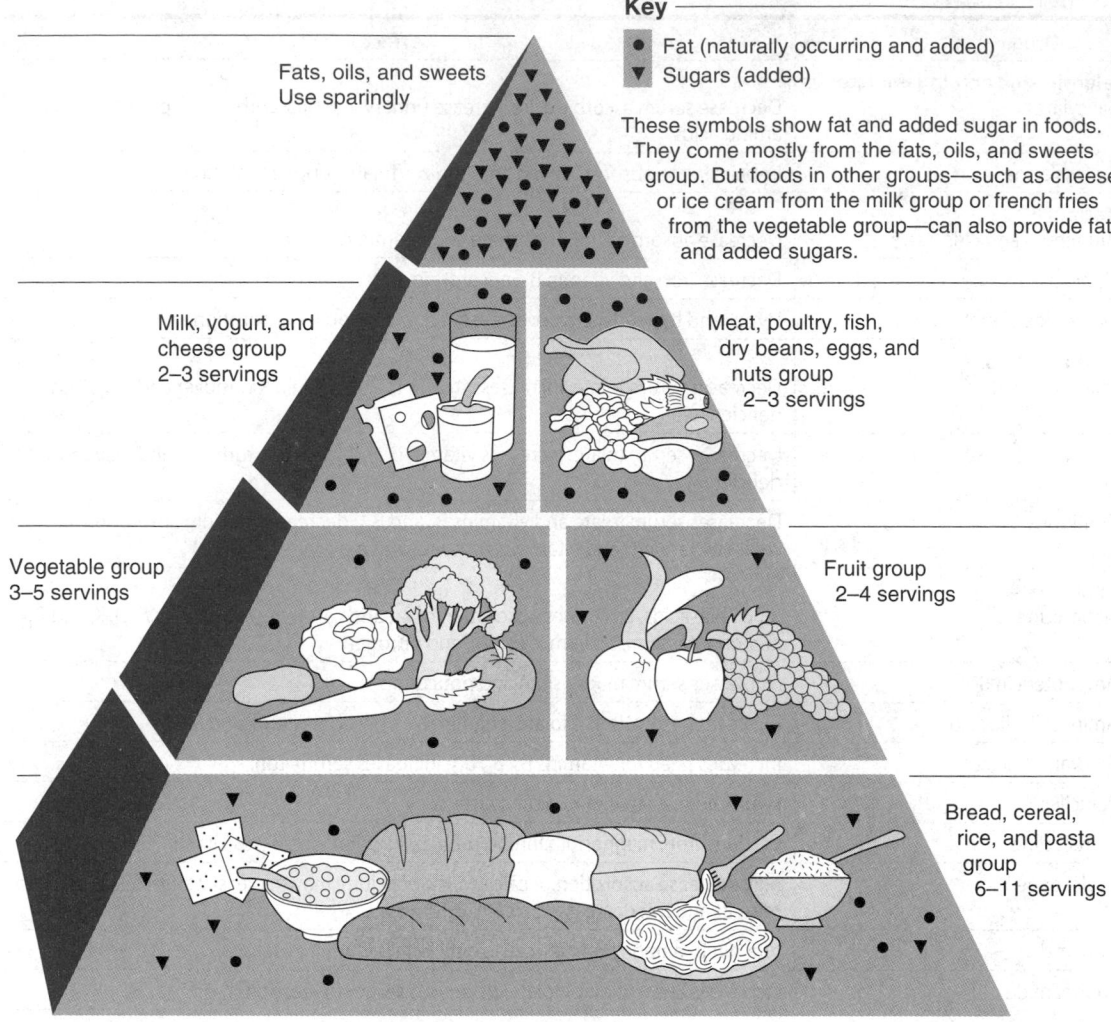

Key
- ● Fat (naturally occurring and added)
- ▼ Sugars (added)

These symbols show fat and added sugar in foods. They come mostly from the fats, oils, and sweets group. But foods in other groups—such as cheese or ice cream from the milk group or french fries from the vegetable group—can also provide fat and added sugars.

Fats, oils, and sweets
Use sparingly

Milk, yogurt, and cheese group
2–3 servings

Meat, poultry, fish, dry beans, eggs, and nuts group
2–3 servings

Vegetable group
3–5 servings

Fruit group
2–4 servings

Bread, cereal, rice, and pasta group
6–11 servings

Looking at the Pieces of the Pyramid
The Food Guide Pyramid emphasizes foods from the five major food groups shown in the three lower sections of the Pyramid. Each of these food groups provides some, but not all, of the nutrients you need. Foods in one group can't replace those in another. No one of these major food groups is more important than another—for good health, you need them all.

Figure 29–1. The Food Guide Pyramid. A guide to daily food choices.

meats, sweets and desserts, french fries, and refined grains. The top quintile of the prudent diet group had 36% less coronary heart disease events than the Western profile.)

Honein MA et al: Impact of folic acid fortification of the US food supply on the occurrence of neural tube defects. JAMA 2001;285:2981. [PMID: 11410096] (A 19% reduction in neural tube defects occurred following folic acid fortification in the United States.)

Joshipura KJ et al: The effect of fruit and vegetable intake on risk for coronary heart disease. Ann Intern Med 2001;134:1106. [PMID: 11412050] (Persons in the highest quintile of fruit and vegetable intake had a 20% reduction in risk of coronary heart disease. Green leafy vegetables and vitamin C-rich fruits and vegetables contributed most.)

Kant AK: Consumption of energy-dense, nutrient-poor foods by adult Americans: nutritional and health implications. The third National Health and Nutrition Examination Survey, 1988–1994. Am J Clin Nutr 2000;72:929. [PMID: 11010933] (Energy-dense, nutrient-poor foods are consumed at the expense of nutrient-dense foods, resulting in increased risk of high energy intake, marginal micronutrient intake, poor compliance with nutrient- and food group-related dietary guidance, and low serum concentrations of vitamins and carotenoids.)

Liu S et al: Intake of vegetables rich in carotenoids and risk of coronary heart disease in men: The Physicians' Health Study. Int J Epidemiol 2001;30:130. [PMID: 11171873] (Men eating two and one-half servings of vegetables per day had a relative risk of 0.77 of developing coronary heart disease compared with men eating one serving per day.)

Millward DJ: Optimal intakes of protein in the human diet. Proc Nutr Soc 1999;58:403. [PMID: 10466184] (Risks of high

What Counts as One Serving?

The amount of food that counts as one serving is listed below. If you eat a larger portion, count it as more than one serving. For example, a dinner portion of spaghetti would count as two or three servings of pasta.

Be sure to eat at least the lowest number of servings from the five major food groups listed below. You need them for the vitamins, minerals, carbohydrates, and protein they provide. Just try to pick the lowest fat choices from the food groups. No specific serving size is given for the fats, oils, and sweets group because the message is USE SPARINGLY.

Food groups

Milk, yogurt, and cheese

| 1 cup of milk or yogurt | 1½ ounces of natural cheese | 2 ounces of processed cheese |

Meat, poultry, fish, dry beans, eggs, and nuts

| 2–3 ounces of cooked lean meat, poultry, or fish | ½ cup of cooked dry beans, 1 egg, or 2 tablespoons of peanut butter count as 1 ounce of lean meat |

Vegetable

| 1 cup of raw leafy vegetables | ½ cup of other vegetables, cooked or chopped raw | ¾ cup of vegetable juice |

Fruit

| 1 medium apple, banana, orange | ½ cup of chopped, cooked, or canned fruit | ¾ cup of fruit juice |

Bread, cereal, rice, and pasta

| 1 slice of bread | 1 ounce of ready-to-eat cereal | ½ cup of cooked cereal, rice, or pasta |

How many servings do you need each day?

	Many women, older adults	Children, teenage girls, active women, most men	Teen-age boys, active men
Calorie level[1]	About 1600	About 2200	About 2800
Bread group servings	6	9	11
Vegetable group servings	3	4	5
Fruit group servings	2	3	4
Milk group servings	2–3[2]	2–3[2]	2–3[2]
Meat group servings	2, for a total of 5 ounces	2, for a total of 6 ounces	3, for a total of 7 ounces
Total fat (grams)	53	73	93

[1] These are the calorie levels if you choose low-fat, lean foods from the five major groups and use foods from the fats, oils, and sweets group sparingly.

[2] Women who are pregnant or breast feeding, teenagers, and young adults to age 24 need three servings.

Figure 29–1. (continued)

---

intakes of protein in adults may be overestimated. There is evidence to support raising the safe upper limit to more than the current value of 1.5 g/kg/d.)

Monsen ER: Dietary reference intakes for the antioxidant nutrients: vitamin C, vitamin E, selenium, and carotenoids. J Am Diet Assoc 2000;100:637. [PMID: 10863565]

Russell RM: The aging process as a modifier of metabolism. Am J Clin Nutr 2000;72(2 Suppl):529S. [PMID: 10919955] (The aging gastrointestinal tract is less efficient in absorbing vitamin B₁₂, vitamin D, and calcium. The new dietary reference intakes concluded that the recommended dietary allowances [RDAs] should be 1200 mg and 15 μg for calcium and vitamin D, respectively, for persons over the age of 70 years. The new RDAs for riboflavin, niacin, thiamin, folate, vitamin B₆, and vitamin B₁₂ are the same for those over age 70 as for those aged 51–70 years.)

Smith Warner SA et al: Intake of fruits and vegetables and risk of breast cancer: A pooled analysis of cohort studies JAMA 2001;285:769. [PMID: 11176915] (No protective associations were observed for green leafy vegetables, 8 botanical groups, and 17 specific fruits and vegetables. There were weak, nonsignificant associations for total fruit intake [RR = 0.93], total vegetables [RR = 0.96], and total fruits and vegetables [RR = 0.93]).

Suitor CW et al: Dietary folate equivalents: interpretation and application. J Am Diet Assoc 2000;100:88. [PMID: 10646010] (Dietary requirements for folate are expressed in dietary folate equivalents [DFEs]. DFEs account for the differences in absorption of naturally occurring food folate and the more bioavailable synthetic folic acid.)

Trumbo P et al: Dietary reference intakes: vitamin A, vitamin K, arsenic, boron, chromium, copper, iodine, iron, manganese, molybdenum, nickel, silicon, vanadium, and zinc. J Am Diet Assoc 2001;101:294. [PMID: 11269606]

Yates AA et al: Dietary Reference Intakes: The new basis for recommendations for calcium and related nutrients, B vitamins, and choline. J Am Diet Assoc 1998;98:699. [PMID: 9627630]

■ ASSESSMENT OF NUTRITIONAL STATUS

No single biochemical test or clinical technique is sufficiently accurate to serve as a reliable test for malnutrition. Techniques of nutritional assessment utilize a combination of methods, including evaluation of dietary intake, anthropometric measurements, clinical examination, and laboratory tests.

DIETARY HISTORY

Patients undergoing a history and physical examination should be asked questions to help identify those high-risk patients who require further evaluation for malnutrition. Of particular importance are the regularity and availability of meals; who does the shopping and food preparation; recent changes in appetite, intake, or body weight; use of special diets or dietary supplements; use of alcohol, drugs, or medications; food preferences and food allergies; and the presence of illnesses affecting nutritional intakes, losses, or requirements. Elderly and adolescent patients, pregnant or lactating women, and the poor and socially isolated are at particular risk for nutritional problems.

Further quantification of dietary intake can be performed using a variety of techniques. **Twenty-four-hour diet recalls** provide rough estimates of nutrient intakes. Patients are asked to describe their dietary intake over the preceding day, including snacks, beverages, and alcohol. Problems with this technique include poor patient recall, difficulties in estimating serving sizes, and the inaccuracy associated with generalizing from a single day's intake. More accurate information can be obtained by asking patients to complete a **3- to 5-day diet record.** Nutrient composition can then be analyzed with the aid of standard handbooks or computer software. Although prospective and less likely to be invalidated by memory lapses, omissions are still common, and the usual difficulties in estimating serving sizes persist.

CLINICAL EXAMINATION

A nutritionally focused physical examination should be performed on each patient at risk for nutritional problems. The examination targets body weight, muscle wasting, fat stores, volume status, and signs of micronutrient deficiencies (Table 29–6).

Evaluation of body weight is particularly useful. Body weight in relation to height can be assessed as the **relative weight** (the current weight/desirable weight × 100) or as the **body mass index** weight (in kilograms)/height (in meters)^2 (Table 29–7). In adult patients, however, a recent change in body weight is usually a better index of undernutrition than a low relative weight or a low body mass index. This change is best expressed as a percentage of usual weight lost per unit of time. A weight loss of 10% or more of usual weight within a period of 1–2 months is generally considered to be predictive of a poor clinical outcome.

Evaluation of body composition—particularly fat stores and skeletal muscle—can be performed by visual inspection or, more quantitatively, by using **anthropometric measurements.** The most commonly used are the triceps skin fold, and mid arm muscle circumference. Because of variations in measurement, they have limited clinical utility.

A number of more sophisticated techniques are available for assessment of body composition. Most have little role in patient care. These include bioelectrical impedance, dual energy x-ray absorptiometry, air-displacement plethysmography, hydrodensitometry, spectroscopy and mass spectrometry, neutron activation analysis, and MRI and body line scanners.

LABORATORY TESTS

Serum albumin is the most important laboratory test for the diagnosis of protein-calorie undernutrition. Most patients with severe protein depletion will have low serum albumin levels. Many nonnutritional conditions can also reduce serum albumin—particularly liver disease and severe illness in general. Other serum proteins with shorter half-lives (such as transferrin, transthyretin, prealbumin) may reflect short-term changes in nutritional status but suffer from similar shortcomings.

Tests of cellular immunity are also abnormal in many patients with protein-calorie undernutrition. Measurements of the **total lymphocyte count** and **delayed hypersensitivity reactions** to common skin test antigens are nonspecific; abnormalities may be due to nonnutritional factors.

Despite their poor specificity, these tests are useful prognostically. Patients with abnormal nutritional assessment parameters have a markedly increased risk of poor clinical outcomes.

Despite the use of a nutritionally focused history, physical examination, and laboratory tests, it is often difficult to confirm a diagnosis of malnutrition. Monitoring dietary intakes with **calorie counts** during hospitalization may be necessary.

Ahmad A et al: An evaluation of resting energy expenditure in hospitalized, severely underweight patients. Nutrition 1999;15:384. [PMID: 10355852] (Commonly employed formulas routinely underestimate the energy needs of severely underweight [< 50 kg] patients. An empirical calculation using 30–32 kcal/kg can be used when direct measurements are unavailable.)

Baxter JP: Problems of nutritional assessment in the acute setting. Proc Nutr Soc 1999;58:39. [PMID: 10343338] (Twenty to 50 percent of hospitalized patients suffer from nutritional

Table 29–6. Clinical signs that may be due to nutrient deficiency.

Clinical Sign	Nutrient Deficiency	Clinical Sign	Nutrient Deficiency
Hair		**Neck**	
Transverse depigmentation	Protein, copper	Goiter	Iodine
Easily pluckable	Protein	**Chest**	
Sparse and thin	Protein, zinc, biotin	Thoracic rosary	Vitamin D
Skin		**Heart**	
Dry, scaling	Zinc, vitamin A, essential fatty acids	High-output failure	Thiamin
		Decreased output	Protein-calorie
Flaky paint dermatitis	Protein, niacin, riboflavin	**Abdomen**	
Follicular hyperkeratosis	Vitamins A and C	Hepatosplenomegaly	Protein-calorie
Perifollicular petechiae	Vitamin C	Distention	Protein-calorie
Petechiae, purpura	Vitamins C and K	Diarrhea	Niacin, folate, vitamin B$_{12}$
Pigmentation, desquamation	Niacin	**Extremities**	
		Muscle tenderness, pain	Thiamin, vitamin C
Nasolabial seborrhea	Niacin, riboflavin, pyridoxine	Muscle wasting	Protein-calorie
Pallor	Iron, folate, vitamin B$_{12}$, copper	Edema	Protein, thiamin
		Bone tenderness	Vitamin C, vitamin D, calcium, phosphorus
Scrotal/vulvar dermatoses	Riboflavin		
Subcutaneous fat loss	Calories	**Neurologic**	
Nails		Hyporeflexia	Thiamin
Spooning	Iron	Decreased position and vibratory sense	Vitamin B$_{12}$, thiamin
Transverse lines, ridging	Protein-calorie		
Head		Paresthesias	Vitamin B$_{12}$, thiamin, niacin
Temporal muscle wasting	Protein-calorie	Confabulation, disorientation	Thiamin
Parotid enlargement	Protein		
Eyes		Dementia	Niacin
Night blindness	Vitamin A, zinc	Ophthalmoplegia	Thiamin, phosphorus
Corneal vascularization	Riboflavin	Tetany	Calcium, magnesium
Xerosis, Bitot's spots, keratomalacia	Vitamin A	**Other**	
		Delayed wound healing	Zinc, protein-calorie, vitamin C
Conjunctival inflammation	Riboflavin		
Mouth			
Glossitis (scarlet, raw)	Niacin, pyridoxine, riboflavin, vitamin B$_{12}$, folate		
Bleeding gums	Vitamin C, riboflavin		
Cheilosis, angular stomatitis	Riboflavin		
Atrophic lingual papillae	Niacin, iron, riboflavin, folate, vitamin B$_{12}$		
Hypogeusia	Zinc, vitamin A		
Tongue fissuring	Niacin		

depletion, and there is failure to recognize its existence and significance. More emphasis must be placed in clinical medicine on identifying subjects who are at high risk of developing disease-related malnutrition.)

Carney DE et al: Arch Surg 2002;137:42. Current concepts in nutritional assessment. [PMID: 11772213] (Review of nutritional assessment of surgical patients.)

Elia M et al: New techniques in nutritional assessment: body composition methods. Proc Nutr Soc 1999;58:33. [PMID: 10343337] (Several new techniques are improving the reproducibility and validity of body composition measurements.)

Niyongabo T et al: Comparison of methods for assessing nutritional status in HIV-infected adults. Nutrition 1999;15:740. [PMID: 10501285] (Subjective global assessment of nutritional status can serve as a basis for prescribing artificial nutrition, but assessment of body weight loss detects malnutrition at an earlier stage.)

Omran ML et al: Assessment of protein energy malnutrition in older persons, Part I: History, examination, body composition, and screening tools. Nutrition 2000;16:50. [PMID: 10674236] (The goal of nutrition assessment is to promote disease-free, active, and successful aging.)

Omran ML et al: Assessment of protein energy malnutrition in older persons, Part II: Laboratory evaluation. Nutrition 2000;16:131. [PMID: 10696638] (Biochemical measurements are a useful part of nutritional assessment in the elderly.)

Seidel S et al: Assessment of commercial laboratories performing hair mineral analysis. JAMA 2001;285.67. [PMID: 11150111] (Hair mineral analysis is unreliable and should not be used to assess nutritional status or suspected environmental exposures.)

Vellas B et al: Nutrition assessment in the elderly. Curr Opin Clin Nutr Metab Care 2001;4:5. [PMID: 11122552] (Review of assessment of nutritional status in the elderly.)

Table 29–7. Body mass index chart.

	BODY MASS INDEX																
	19	20	21	22	23	24	25	26	27	28	29	30	31	32	33	34	35
Height (inches)	Body weight (pounds)																
58	91	96	100	105	110	115	119	124	129	134	138	143	148	153	158	162	167
59	94	99	104	109	114	119	124	128	133	138	143	148	153	158	163	168	173
60	97	102	107	112	118	123	128	133	138	143	148	153	158	163	168	174	179
61	100	106	111	116	122	127	132	137	143	148	153	158	164	169	174	180	185
62	104	109	115	120	126	131	136	142	147	153	158	164	169	175	180	186	191
63	107	113	118	124	130	135	141	146	152	158	163	169	175	180	186	191	197
64	110	116	122	128	134	140	145	151	157	163	169	174	180	186	192	197	204
65	114	120	126	132	138	144	150	156	162	168	174	180	186	192	198	204	210
66	118	124	130	136	142	148	155	161	167	173	179	186	192	198	204	210	216
67	121	127	134	140	146	153	159	166	172	178	185	191	198	204	211	217	223
68	125	131	138	144	151	158	164	171	177	184	190	197	203	210	216	223	230
69	128	135	142	149	155	162	169	176	182	189	196	203	209	216	223	230	236
70	132	149	146	153	160	167	174	181	188	195	202	209	216	222	229	236	243
71	136	143	150	157	165	172	179	186	193	200	208	215	222	229	236	243	250
72	140	157	154	162	169	177	184	191	199	206	213	221	228	235	242	250	258
73	144	151	159	166	174	182	189	197	204	212	219	227	235	242	250	257	265
74	148	155	163	171	179	186	194	202	210	218	225	233	241	249	256	264	272
75	152	160	168	176	184	192	200	208	216	224	232	240	248	256	264	272	279
76	156	164	172	180	189	197	205	213	221	230	238	246	254	263	271	279	287

To use this table, find the appropriate height in the left-hand column. Move across to a given weight. The number at the top of the column is the BMI at that height and weight. Pounds have been rounded off. A normal BMI is 18.5–24.9. Overweight is defined as a BMI of 25–29.9. Class I obesity is 30–34.9; class II obesity is a BMI of 35–39.9; and class III (extreme) obesity is a BMI of > 40.

■ NUTRITIONAL DISORDERS

PROTEIN-ENERGY MALNUTRITION

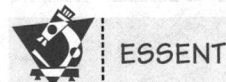

ESSENTIALS OF DIAGNOSIS

- *History of decreased intake of energy or protein, increased nutrient losses, or increased nutrient requirements.*
- *Manifestations range from weight loss and growth failure to distinct syndromes, kwashiorkor, and marasmus.*
- *In severe cases, virtually all organ systems affected.*
- *Protein loss correlates with weight loss. Thirty-five to 40 percent total body weight loss is usually fatal.*

General Considerations

Protein-energy malnutrition occurs as a result of a relative or absolute deficiency of energy and protein. It may be primary, due to inadequate food intake, or secondary, as a result of other illness. For most developing nations, primary protein-energy malnutrition remains among the most significant health problems. Protein-energy malnutrition has been described as two distinct syndromes. **Kwashiorkor,** caused by a deficiency of protein in the presence of adequate energy, is typically seen in weaning infants at the birth of a sibling in areas where foods containing protein are insufficiently abundant. **Marasmus,** caused by combined protein and energy deficiency, is most commonly seen where adequate quantities of food are not available.

In industrialized societies, protein-energy malnutrition is most often secondary to other diseases. **Kwashiorkor-like secondary protein-energy malnutrition** occurs primarily in association with hypermetabolic acute illnesses such as trauma, burns, and sepsis. **Marasmus-like secondary protein-energy malnutrition** typically results from chronic diseases such as COPD, congestive heart failure, cancer, or AIDS.

These syndromes have been estimated to be present in at least 20% of hospitalized patients. A substantially greater number of patients have risk factors that could result in these syndromes. In both syndromes, protein-energy malnutrition is caused either by decreased intake of energy and protein, increased nutrient losses, or increased nutrient requirements dictated by the underlying illness. For example, diminished oral intake may result from poor dentition or various gastrointestinal disorders. Loss of nutrients results from malabsorption and diarrhea as well as from glycosuria. Nutrient requirements are increased by fever, surgery, neoplasia, and burns.

Pathophysiology

Protein-energy malnutrition affects every organ system. The most obvious results are loss of body weight, adipose stores, and skeletal muscle mass. Weight losses of 5–10% are usually tolerated without loss of physiologic function; losses of 35–40% of body weight usually result in death. Loss of protein from skeletal muscle and internal organs is usually proportionate to weight loss. Protein mass is lost from the liver, gastrointestinal tract, kidneys, and heart.

As protein-energy malnutrition progresses, organ dysfunction develops. Hepatic synthesis of serum proteins decreases, and depressed levels of circulating proteins are observed. Cardiac output and contractility are decreased, and the ECG may show decreased voltage and a rightward axis shift. Autopsies of patients who die with severe undernutrition show myofibrillar atrophy and interstitial edema of the heart.

Respiratory function is affected primarily by weakness and atrophy of the muscles of respiration. Vital capacity and tidal volume are depressed, and mucociliary clearance is abnormal. The gastrointestinal tract is affected by mucosal atrophy and loss of villi of small intestine, resulting in malabsorption. Intestinal disaccharidase deficiency and mild pancreatic insufficiency also occur.

Changes in immunologic function are among the most important changes seen in protein-calorie undernutrition. T lymphocyte number and function are depressed. Changes in B cell function are more variable. Impaired complement activity, granulocyte function, and anatomic barriers to infection are noted, and wound healing is poor.

Clinical Findings

The clinical manifestations of protein-energy malnutrition range from mild growth retardation and weight loss to a number of distinct clinical syndromes. Children in the developing world manifest marasmus and kwashiorkor. In secondary protein-energy malnutrition as seen in industrialized nations, clinical manifestations are affected by the degree of protein and energy deficiency, the underlying illness that resulted in the deficiency, and the patient's nutritional status prior to illness.

In marasmus-like secondary protein-energy malnutrition, most patients typically develop progressive wasting that begins with weight loss and proceeds to more severe cachexia. In the most severe form of this disorder, virtually all body fat stores disappear and muscle mass decreases, most noticeably in the temporalis and interosseus muscles. Laboratory studies may be unremarkable—serum albumin, for example, may be normal or slightly decreased, rarely decreasing to < 2.8 g/dL. In contrast, owing to its rapidity of onset, kwashiorkor-like secondary protein-energy malnutrition may develop in patients with normal subcutaneous fat and muscle mass or, if the patient is obese, in patients with excess fat and muscle. The serum protein level, however, typically declines and the serum albumin is often < 2.8 g/dL. Dependent edema, ascites, or anasarca may develop. As with primary protein-energy malnutrition, combinations of the marasmus-like and kwashiorkor-like syndromes can occur simultaneously, typically in patients with progressive chronic disease who develop a superimposed acute illness.

Treatment

The treatment of severe protein-energy malnutrition is a slow process requiring great care. Initial efforts should be directed at correcting fluid and electrolyte abnormalities and infections. Of particular concern are depletion of potassium, magnesium, and calcium and acid-base abnormalities. The second phase of treatment is directed at repletion of protein, energy, and micronutrients. Treatment is started with modest quantities of protein and calories calculated according to the patient's actual body weight. Adult patients are given 1 g of protein and 30 kcal per kilogram. Concomitant administration of vitamins and minerals is obligatory. Either the enteral or parenteral route can be used, although the former is preferable. Enteral fat and lactose are withheld initially. Patients with less severe protein-calorie undernutrition can be given calories and protein simultaneously with the correction of fluid and electrolyte abnormalities. Similar quantities of protein and calories are recommended for initial treatment.

Patients treated for protein-energy malnutrition require close follow-up. In adults, both calories and protein are advanced as tolerated, adults to 1.5 g/kg/d of protein and 40 kcal/kg/d of calories.

Patients who are refed too rapidly may develop a number of untoward clinical sequelae. During refeeding, circulating potassium, magnesium, phosphorus, and glucose move intracellularly and can result in low serum levels of each. The administration of water and sodium with carbohydrate refeeding can overload hearts with depressed cardiac function and result in congestive heart failure. Enteral refeeding can lead to malabsorption and diarrhea due to abnormalities in the gastrointestinal tract.

Refeeding edema is a benign condition to be differentiated from congestive heart failure. Changes in renal sodium reabsorption and poor skin and blood vessel integrity result in the development of dependent edema without other signs of heart disease. Treatment includes reassurance, elevation of the dependent area, and modest sodium restriction. Diuretics are usually ineffective, may aggravate electrolyte deficiencies, and should not be used.

The prevention and early detection of protein-energy malnutrition in hospitalized patients require awareness of its risk factors and early symptoms and signs. Patients at risk require formal assessment of nutritional status and close observation of dietary intake, body weight, and nutritional requirements during the hospital stay.

Akner G et al: Treatment of protein-energy malnutrition in chronic nonmalignant disorders. Am J Clin Nutr 2001;74: 6. [PMID: 11451713] (Available treatment studies indicate that dietary supplements, either alone or in combination with hormonal treatment, may have benefit in patients with protein-energy malnutrition. In COPD, nutritional treatment may improve respiratory function. Nutritional therapy of elderly women after hip fractures may speed up the rehabilitation process. When administered to elderly patients with multiple disorders, diet therapy may improve functional capacity.)

Chandra RK: Nutrition and immunology: from the clinic to cellular biology and back again. Proc Nutr Soc 1999;58:681. [PMID: 10604203] (The interactions between nutrition and the immune system are of clinical, practical, and public health importance.)

Corish CA: Protein-energy undernutrition in hospital in-patients. Br J Nutr 2000;83:575. [PMID: 10911765] (To allow evidence-based practice, definitions of undernutrition and nutritional risk and cut-off values for the nutritional variables measured must first be agreed upon. Outcome measures that allow clear comparisons between groups and treatments must be used in studies assessing the effects of nutritional interventions.)

Herselman M et al: Protein-energy malnutrition as a risk factor for increased morbidity in long-term hemodialysis patients. J Ren Nutr 2000;10:7. [PMID: 10672628] (Protein-energy malnutrition contributes to morbidity in hemodialysis patients, possibly via an effect on the immune system and infection.)

Koretz RL: Does nutritional intervention in protein-energy malnutrition improve morbidity or mortality? J Ren Nutr 1999;9:119. [PMID: 10431028] (There is still need for large randomized controlled trials to establish or refute the efficacy of nutritional support in renal disease.)

Sullivan DH et al: Protein-energy undernutrition among elderly hospitalized patients: a prospective study. JAMA 1999;281: 2013. [PMID: 10359390] (Many hospitalized elderly patients were maintained on nutrient intakes far less than their estimated maintenance energy requirements, which may contribute to an increased risk of mortality.)

Thomas DR et al: Malnutrition in subacute care. Am J Clin Nutr 2002;75:308. [PMID: 11597412] (Ninety-one percent of subjects admitted to subacute care were either malnourished or at risk of malnutrition.)

OBESITY

ESSENTIALS OF DIAGNOSIS

- Excess adipose tissue, resulting in body mass index > 30.
- Upper body obesity (abdomen and flank) of greater health consequence than lower body obesity (buttocks and thighs).
- Associated with multiple metabolic and structural disorders, including diabetes mellitus, hypertension, and hyperlipidemia.

General Considerations

Obesity is one of the most common disorders in medical practice and among the most frustrating and difficult to manage. Little progress has been made in treatment, yet major changes have occurred in our understanding of its causes and its implications for health.

Definition & Measurement

Obesity is defined as an excess of adipose tissue. Accurate quantification of body fat requires sophisticated techniques not usually available in clinical practice. Physical examination is usually sufficient to detect excess body fat. Two methods commonly used for more quantitative evaluation are relative weight (RW) and body mass index (BMI).

Relative weight (RW) is the measured body weight divided by the "desirable weight" × 100. Desirable weight is defined as the midpoint value recommended for a given height in the weight tables published by the United States government (Table 29–7). There is controversy over which table best reflects the relationship between body weight and health. Weight tables published every few years since 1983 have varied significantly in their recommendations.

Because the RW does not differentiate between excess fat or excess muscle, the **body mass index (BMI)** can be used to more accurately reflect the presence of excess adipose tissue. The BMI is calculated by dividing measured body weight in kilograms by the height in meters squared.

The National Institutes of Health define a normal BMI as 18.5–24.9. Overweight is defined as BMI = 25–29.9. Class I obesity is 30–34.9, class II obesity is 35–39.9, and class III (extreme) obesity is BMI > 40. Other factors besides total weight, however, are also important. Upper body obesity (excess fat around the waist and flank) is a greater health hazard than lower body obesity (fat in the thighs and buttocks). Obese patients with increased abdominal circumference

(> 102 cm in men and 88 cm in women) or with high waist-hip ratios (> 1.0 in men; > 0.85 in women) have a greater risk of diabetes mellitus, stroke, coronary artery disease, and early death than equally obese patients with lower ratios. Further differentiation of the location of excess fat suggests that visceral fat within the abdominal cavity is more hazardous to health than subcutaneous fat around the abdomen.

The National Health and Nutrition Exam Survey III (NHANES III) found that 59.4% of men and 49.9% of women are overweight and that 19.9% of men and 25.1% of women are obese. Blacks—particularly black women—are more apt to be obese than whites, and the poor are more obese than the rich regardless of race.

Health Consequences of Obesity

Obesity is associated with significant increases in both morbidity and mortality. A great many disorders occur with greater frequency in obese people. The most important and common of these are hypertension, type II diabetes mellitus, hyperlipidemia, coronary artery disease, degenerative joint disease, and psychosocial disability. Certain cancers (colon, rectum, and prostate in men; uterus, biliary tract, breast, and ovary in women), thromboembolic disorders, digestive tract diseases (gallstones, reflux esophagitis), and skin disorders are also more prevalent in the obese. Surgical and obstetric risks are greater. Obese patients also have a greater risk of pulmonary functional impairment, endocrine abnormalities, proteinuria, and increased hemoglobin concentration.

In young and middle-aged adults, mortality from all causes and mortality from cardiovascular disease increase in proportion to the degree of obesity. The relative risk associated with obesity, however, decreases with age, and weight is no longer a risk factor in adults over age 75.

Etiology

Until recently, obesity was considered to be the direct result of a sedentary lifestyle plus chronic ingestion of excess calories. Although these factors are undoubtedly the principal cause in some cases, there is now evidence for strong genetic influences on the development of obesity. Adopted children demonstrate a close relationship between their body mass index and that of their biologic parents. No such relationship is found between the children and their adoptive parents. Twin studies also demonstrate substantial genetic influences on body mass index with little influence from the childhood environment. As much as 40–70% of obesity may be explained by genetic influences.

Genetic determinants of some types of obesity have now been established. Five genes affecting control of appetite have been identified in mice. Mutations of each gene result in obesity, and each has a human ho-

molog. One gene codes for a protein expressed by adipose tissue—leptin—and another for the leptin receptor in the brain. The other three genes affect brain pathways downstream from the leptin receptor. Numerous other candidate genes for human obesity have been identified. Only a very small number of humans, however, have been found with similar single gene mutations. Most human obesity undoubtedly develops from the interactions of multiple genes, environmental factors, and behavior.

Medical Evaluation of the Obese Patient

Historical information should be obtained about age at onset, recent weight changes, family history of obesity, occupational history, eating and exercise behavior, cigarette and alcohol use, previous weight loss experience, and psychosocial factors. Particular attention should be directed at use of laxatives, diuretics, hormones, nutritional supplements, and over-the-counter medications.

Physical examination should assess the degree and distribution of body fat, overall nutritional status, and signs of secondary causes of obesity.

Less than 1% of obese patients have an identifiable secondary cause of obesity. Hypothyroidism and Cushing's syndrome are important examples that can usually be diagnosed by physical examination in patients with unexplained recent weight gain. Such patients require further endocrinologic evaluation, including serum TSH determination and dexamethasone suppression testing (see Chapter 26).

All obese patients should be assessed for medical consequences of their obesity. Fasting levels of glucose, cholesterol, and triglycerides should be measured.

Treatment

Using conventional techniques, only 20% of patients will lose 20 lb and maintain the loss for over 2 years; 5% will maintain a 40-lb loss. Continued close provider-patient contact appears to be more important for success of treatment than the specific features of any given treatment regimen. Careful patient selection will improve success rates and lessen frustration of both patients and therapists. Only sufficiently motivated patients should enter treatment programs. Specific attempts to identify motivated patients—eg, requesting a 3-day diet record—are often useful.

Most successful programs employ a multidisciplinary approach to weight loss, with hypocaloric diets, behavior modification to change eating behavior, aerobic exercise, and social support. Emphasis must be on *maintenance* of weight loss.

Dietary instructions incorporate the same principles that apply to healthy people who are not obese, ie, a low-fat, high-complex carbohydrate, high-fiber diet. This is achieved by emphasizing intake of a wide variety of predominantly "unprocessed" foods. Special attention is usually paid to limiting foods that provide large amounts of calories without other nutrients, ie, fat, sucrose, and alcohol. There is no special advantage to diets that restrict carbohydrates, advocate large amounts of protein or fats, or recommend ingestion of foods one at a time.

Long-term changes in eating behavior are required to maintain weight loss. Although formal **behavior modification** programs are available to which patients can be referred, the clinician caring for obese patients can teach a number of useful behavioral techniques. The most important technique is to emphasize planning and record keeping. Patients can be taught to plan menus and exercise sessions and to record their actual behavior. Record keeping not only aids in behavioral change; the availability of records also helps the provider to make specific suggestions for problem solving. Patients can be taught to recognize "eating cues" (emotional, situational, etc) and how to avoid or control them. Reward systems and refundable financial contracts are also useful for many patients.

Exercise offers a number of advantages to patients trying to lose weight and keep it off. Aerobic exercise directly increases the daily energy expenditure and is particularly useful for long-term weight maintenance. Exercise will also preserve lean body mass and partially prevent the decrease in basal energy expenditure seen with semistarvation.

Social support is essential for a successful weight loss program. Continued close contact with the therapist and involvement of the family and peer group are useful techniques for reinforcing behavioral change and preventing social isolation.

Patients with severe obesity may require more aggressive treatment regimens. **Very low calorie diets** (≤ 800 kcal/d) result in rapid weight loss and marked improvement in obesity-related metabolic complications. Patients are commonly maintained on such programs for 4–6 months and lose an average of 2–4 lb per week. Long-term weight maintenance is less predictable and requires concurrent behavior modification and exercise. Side effects such as fatigue, orthostatic hypotension, cold intolerance, and fluid and electrolyte disorders are observed in proportion to the degree of calorie reduction and require regular supervision by a physician. Other less common complications include gout, gallbladder disease, and cardiac arrhythmias. Although weight loss is more rapidly achieved with very low-calorie diets as compared with traditional diets, long-term outcomes are equivalent.

Medications for the treatment of obesity are available both over the counter and with prescription. Medications can be classified as catecholaminergic or serotonergic. Catecholaminergic medications include amphetamines (with high abuse potential); the non-amphetamine schedule IV appetite suppressants phentermine, diethylpropion, and mazindol. The September 1997 withdrawal from the market of fenfluramine and dexfenfluramine has made true serotonergic appetite medications unavailable. The SSRI antidepressants, eg, fluoxetine and sertraline, also have serotonergic activity but are not approved by the FDA for weight loss.

Two newer medications are approved for weight loss: sibutramine and orlistat. Sibutramine blocks uptake of both serotonin and norepinephrine in the central nervous system. Orlistat reduces fat absorption in the gastrointestinal tract.

Considerable controversy exists as to the appropriate use of medications for obesity. The 1998 NIH clinical obesity guidelines state that obesity drugs may be used as part of a comprehensive weight loss program for patients with BMI > 30 or those with BMI > 27 with obesity-related risk factors. Nonetheless, use of medications has decreased markedly in the United States since the withdrawal from the market in 1997 of dexfenfluramine and fenfluramine after multiple reports of medication-associated valvular heart disease. Although recent studies have estimated the risk of valvular heart disease to be substantially less than the 30% prevalence first reported, this experience has led to considerable caution in the use of anorectic medications.

Several medications remain available for treatment of obesity. Older catecholaminergic medications (eg, phentermine, diethylpropion, mazindol) are approved for short-term use only and have limited utility. **Sibutramine,** typically at doses of 10 mg/d, results in average weight losses of 3–5 kg more than placebo in studies extending over 6–12 months. Sibutramine also appears to improve 1-year outcomes in patients on very low-calorie diets. Side effects include dry mouth, anorexia, constipation, insomnia, and dizziness. In some patients (< 5%), sibutramine may substantially increase blood pressure.

Orlistat is the first approved medication for obesity that works in the gastrointestinal tract rather than the central nervous system. By inhibiting intestinal lipase, orlistat reduces fat absorption. As expected, orlistat may result in diarrhea, gas, and cramping and perhaps also reduced absorption of fat-soluble vitamins. In randomized trials with up to 2 years of follow-up, orlistat has resulted in 2–4 kg greater weight loss than placebo. The recommended dose of orlistat is 120 mg three times daily with meals.

Despite FDA approval of sibutramine and orlistat and NIH guidelines supporting their use, long-term clinical benefits have not been demonstrated. Although these medications result in some additional weight loss at the end of 1- and 2-year clinical trials and, in some studies, improved obesity-related metabolic parameters, the impact of these medications on obesity-related clinical outcomes is unknown.

Although surgery is the last resort for treatment of obesity, large numbers of patients have had bariatric surgery. In the United States, gastric operations are considered the procedures of choice. Most popular are the vertical banded gastroplasty (VBG) and roux-en-Y gastric bypass (GBP). In some centers, these procedures can be done laparoscopically. Both operations lead to substantial amounts of weight loss—close to 50% of initial body weight in some studies. Direct comparisons of the two operations suggest that GBP is the more effective procedure. Complications occur in up to 50% of subjects undergoing both operations and include peritonitis due to anastomotic leak, abdominal wall hernias, staple line disruption, gallstones, neuropathy, marginal ulcers, stomal stenosis, wound infections, thromboembolic disease, and various nutritional deficiencies and gastrointestinal symptoms. Within 30 day operative mortality rates are nil to 1%. NIH consensus panel recommendations are to limit obesity surgery to patients with BMIs over 40, or over 35 if obesity-related comorbidities are present. Many third-party payers now cover obesity surgery.

Apfelbaum M et al: Long-term maintenance of weight loss after a very-low calorie diet: a randomized blinded trial of the efficacy and tolerability of sibutramine. Am J Med 1999;106: 179. [PMID: 10230747] (Seventy-five percent of subjects treated with sibutramine maintained 100% of the weight loss achieved with a very-low-calorie diet, compared with 42% in the placebo group.)

Blanck HM et al: Use of nonprescription weight loss products: results from a multistate survey. JAMA 2001;286:930. [PMID: 11509057] (A random-digit telephone survey conducted in five states showed that use of nonprescription weight loss products is common, including use by 28.4% of obese women.)

Chen Y et al: Obesity may increase the incidence of asthma in women but not in men: longitudinal observations from the Canadian national population health surveys. Am J Epidemiol 2002;155:191. [PMID: 1182124] (Obesity was an important predictor of asthma in women but not in men.)

Davidoff R et al: Echocardiographic examination of women previously treated with fenfluramine: Long-term follow-up of a randomized, double blind placebo-controlled trial. Arch Intern Med. 2001;161:1429. [PMID: 11386892] (In a 4.9-year follow-up of subjects randomly assigned to receive 3 months of fenfluramine or placebo as part of a smoking cessation randomized controlled trial, there were no differences in aortic or mitral regurgitation or in other echocardiographic or clinical abnormalities between groups.)

Davidson MH et al: Weight control and risk factor reduction in obese subjects treated for 2 years with orlistat: A randomized controlled trial. JAMA 1999;281:235. [PMID: 9918478] (After 2 years of treatment, orlistat 120 mg three times per day resulted in modest weight loss compared with placebo.)

Executive summary of the clinical guidelines on the identification, evaluation, and treatment of overweight and obesity in adults. Arch Intern Med 1998;158:1855. [PMID: 9759681] (Comprehensive evidence-based review of diagnosis and treatment of obesity from the NIH.)

Glazer G: Long-term pharmacotherapy of obesity 2000. A review of safety and efficacy. Arch Intern Med 2001;161:1814. [PMID: 11493122] (Weight loss attributable to medications—in excess of placebo—was 7.9 kg for phentermine resin, 4.3 kg for sibutramine, 3.4 kg for orlistat, and 1.5 kg for diethylpropion.)

Hauptman J et al: Orlistat in the long-term treatment of obesity in primary care settings. Arch Fam Med 2000;9:160. [PMID: 10693734] (Orlistat was associated with a 4-kg greater weight loss than placebo.)

Heymsfield SB et al: Recombinant leptin for weight loss in obese and lean adults: a randomized, controlled, dose-escalation trial. JAMA 1999;282:1568. [PMID: 10546697] (Leptin injections induced weight loss in some obese subjects with elevated endogenous serum leptin concentrations.)

Jakicic JM et al: Effects of intermittent exercise and use of home exercise equipment on adherence, weight loss, and fitness in overweight women: a randomized trial. JAMA 1999;282: 1554. [PMID: 10546695] (A dose-response relationship exists between amount of exercise and long-term weight loss in overweight adult women.)

Mantzoros CS: The role of leptin in human obesity and disease: a review of current evidence. Ann Intern Med 1999;130:671. [PMID: 11527094] (Review of leptin physiology and potential for therapeutic use.)

McMahon FG et al: Efficacy and safety of sibutramine in obese white and African American patients with hypertension: a 1-year, double-blind, placebo-controlled, multicenter trial. Arch Intern Med 2000;160:2185. [PMID: 10904462] (Among patients receiving sibutramine, 40.1% lost 5% and 13.4% lost 10% or more of body weight compared with 8.7% and 4.3% of patients in the placebo group [P < .05]. The most common adverse event resulting in discontinuation among patients receiving sibutramine was hypertension [5.3% of patients receiving sibutramine versus 1.4% of patients receiving placebo].)

Michaud DS et al: Physical activity, obesity, height, and the risk of pancreatic cancer. JAMA 2001;286:921. [PMID: 11509056] (Two large prospective cohort studies reporting 10–20 years of follow-up. In both, obesity significantly increased the risk of pancreatic cancer.)

Mokdad AH et al: The continuing epidemics of obesity and diabetes in the United States. JAMA 2001;286:1195. [PMID: 11559264] (Prevalence of obesity [BMI = 30] is 19.8%; diabetes is 7.3%. Twenty-seven percent of adults do not engage in any physical activity, and another 28.2% are not regularly active. Twenty-four percent of adults consume five servings of fruits and vegetables per day. Of obese individuals who had seen a health care professional, 42.8% had been advised to lose weight.)

Nguyen NT et al: Laparoscopic roux-en-Y gastric bypass for super/super obesity. Obes Surg 1999;9:403. [PMID: 10484302] (Roux-en-Y gastric bypass is increasingly done using a laparoscopic technique.)

Rossner S et al: Weight loss, weight maintenance, and improved cardiovascular risk factors after 2 years treatment with orlistat for obesity. European Orlistat Study Group. Obes Res 2000;8:49. [PMID: 10678259] (Orlistat-treated patients lost more weight than placebo-treated patients [6.6% versus 9.7% of initial weight] and regained less weight at 2-year follow-up.)

Smith IG et al: Randomized placebo-controlled trial of long-term treatment with sibutramine in mild to moderate obesity. J Fam Pract 2001;50:505. [PMID: 11407998] (Sibutramine [15 mg/d] resulted in 5 kg more weight loss than placebo at 1 year in obese patients.)

Stevens J et al: The effect of age on the association between body-mass index and mortality. N Engl J Med 1998;338:1. [PMID: 9414324] (Analysis of body weight and mortality. Although excess body weight increases the risk of death in adults, the risk is less than previously estimated and is no longer a factor in adults after age 75.)

Strauss RS et al: Epidemic increase in childhood overweight 1986–1998. JAMA 2001;286:2845. [PMID: 11735760] (Between 1986 and 1998, overweight increased significantly among African-American, Hispanic, and white children. By 1998, 21.5% of African-American children, 21.8% of Hispanic children, and 12.3% of white children were overweight. The increase was greatest among minorities and southerners.)

Wadden TA et al: Effects of sibutramine plus orlistat in obese women following 1 year of treatment by sibutramine alone: a placebo-controlled trial. Obes Res 2000;8:431. [PMID: 11011909] (The addition of orlistat to sibutramine did not induce further weight loss as compared with treatment with sibutramine alone.)

Wei M et al: Relationship between low cardiorespiratory fitness and mortality in normal-weight, overweight, and obese men. JAMA 1999;282:1547. [PMID: 10546694] (Fitness was an independent predictor of outcomes in obese subjects.)

Weissman NJ et al: Natural history of valvular regurgitation 1 year after discontinuation of dexfenfluramine therapy: A randomized double-blind placebo-controlled trial. Ann Intern Med 2001;134:267. [PMID: 11182836] (After dexfenfluramine is taken for 2 months and stopped, development or progression of regurgitation is unlikely.)

Wirth A et al: Long-term weight loss with sibutramine. A randomized controlled trial. JAMA 2001;286:1331. [PMID: 11560538] (Reporting a 48-week randomized controlled trial of 15 mg of sibutramine continuously, 15 mg sibutramine intermittently [weeks 1–12, 19–30, 37–48] or placebo. The results were 7.9 kg, 7.8 kg, and 3.8 kg of weight lost in the three groups, respectively.)

■ EATING DISORDERS

ANOREXIA NERVOSA

ESSENTIALS OF DIAGNOSIS

- *Disturbance of body image and intense fear of becoming fat.*
- *Weight loss leading to body weight 15% below expected.*
- *In females, absence of three consecutive menstrual cycles.*

General Considerations

Anorexia nervosa begins in the years between adolescence and young adulthood. Ninety percent of patients are females, most from the middle and upper socioeconomic strata. The diagnosis is based on weight loss leading to body weight 15% below expected, a distorted body image, fear of weight gain or of loss of control over food intake, and, in females, the absence of at least three consecutive menstrual cycles. Other medical or psychiatric illnesses that can account for anorexia and weight loss must be excluded.

The prevalence of anorexia nervosa is greater than previously suggested. In Rochester, Minnesota, for example, the prevalence per 100,000 population is estimated to be 270 for females and 22 for males. Many other adolescent girls have features of the disorder without the severe weight loss.

The cause of anorexia nervosa is not known. Although multiple endocrinologic abnormalities exist in these patients, most authorities believe they are secondary to malnutrition and not primary disorders. Most authors favor a primary psychiatric origin, but no hypothesis explains all cases. The patient characteristically comes from a family whose members are highly goal- and achievement-oriented. Interpersonal relationships may be inadequate or destructive. The parents are usually overly directive and concerned with slimness and physical fitness, and much of the family conversation centers around dietary matters. One theory holds that the patient's refusal to eat is an attempt to regain control of her body in defiance of parental control. The patient's unwillingness to inhabit an "adult body" may also represent a rejection of adult responsibilities and the implications of adult interpersonal relationships. Patients are commonly perfectionistic in behavior and exhibit obsessional personality characteristics. Marked depression or anxiety may be present.

Clinical Findings

A. Symptoms and Signs

Patients with anorexia nervosa may exhibit severe emaciation and may complain of cold intolerance or constipation. Amenorrhea is almost always present. Bradycardia, hypotension, and hypothermia may be present in severe cases. Examination demonstrates loss of body fat, dry and scaly skin, and increased lanugo body hair. Parotid enlargement and edema may also occur.

B. Laboratory Findings

Laboratory findings are variable but may include anemia, leukopenia, electrolyte abnormalities, and elevations of BUN and serum creatinine. Serum cholesterol levels are often increased. Endocrine abnormalities include depressed levels of luteinizing and follicle-stimulating hormones and impaired response of LH to luteinizing hormone-releasing hormone.

Diagnosis & Differential Diagnosis

The diagnosis can be difficult, since many common social and cultural factors promote and maintain anorexic behavior. The diagnosis depends upon identification of the common behavioral features and exclusion of medical disorders that would account for weight loss.

Behavioral features required for the diagnosis include intense fear of becoming obese, disturbance of body image, weight loss of at least 15%, and refusal to exceed a minimal normal weight.

The differential diagnosis includes endocrine and metabolic disorders such as panhypopituitarism, Addison's disease, hyperthyroidism, and diabetes mellitus; gastrointestinal disorders such as Crohn's disease and celiac sprue; chronic infections and cancers such as tuberculosis and lymphoma; and rare central nervous system disorders such as hypothalamic tumors.

Treatment

The goal of treatment is restoration of normal body weight and resolution of psychologic difficulties. Hospitalization may be necessary. Treatment programs conducted by experienced teams are successful in about two-thirds of cases, restoring normal weight and menstruation. One-half continue to experience difficulties with eating behavior and psychiatric problems. Occasional patients with anorexia develop obesity after treatment. Two to 6% of patients die from the complications of the disorder or commit suicide.

Various treatment methods have been used without clear evidence of superiority of one over another. Supportive care by physicians and nurses is probably the most important feature of therapy. Structured behavioral therapy, intensive psychotherapy, and family therapy may be tried. A variety of medications including tricyclic antidepressants, selective serotonin reuptake inhibitors, and lithium carbonate are effective in some cases. Patients with severe malnutrition must be hemodynamically stabilized and may require enteral or parenteral feeding. Forced feedings should be reserved for life-threatening situations, since the goal of treatment is to reestablish normal eating behavior.

American Dietetic Association: Position of the American Dietetic Association: Nutrition intervention in the treatment of anorexia nervosa, bulimia nervosa, and binge eating. http://www.eatright.org/adap0701.html. (Nutrition education and interventions should be integrated into the team treatment of patients with anorexia nervosa and other eating disorders.)

Becker AE et al: Eating disorders. N Engl J Med 1999;340:1092. [PMID: 10194240] (Pharmacologic agents are often useful as adjuncts to psychotherapy for bulimia nervosa or binge-eating disorder; in anorexia nervosa, medication is generally reserved for patients with concurrent psychiatric illness.)

Brown JM et al: Medical complications occurring in adolescents with anorexia nervosa. West J Med 2000;172:189. [PMID: 10734811]

Hetherington MM: Eating disorders: diagnosis, etiology and prevention. Nutrition 2000;16:547. [PMID: 10906551]

Kreipe RE et al: Eating disorders in adolescents and young adults. Obstet Gynecol Clin North Am 2000;27:101. [PMID: 10693185] (Eating disorders frequently result in gynecologic disorders.)

Polivy J et al: Causes of eating disorders. Annu Rev Psychol 2002;53:187. [PMID: 11752484] (Review of recent research on development of eating disorders, including sociocultural factors [eg, media and peer influences], family factors [eg, involvement and criticism], negative affect, low self-esteem, and body dissatisfaction.)

Practice guideline for the treatment of patients with eating disorders (revision). American Psychiatric Association Work Group on Eating Disorders. Am J Psychiatry 2000; 157(Suppl 1):1. [PMID: 10642782]

Walsh JM et al: Detection, evaluation, and treatment of eating disorders: the role of the primary care physician. J Gen Intern Med 2000; 15:577. [PMID: 10940151] (Primary care
providers have an important role in detecting and managing eating disorders.)

BULIMIA NERVOSA

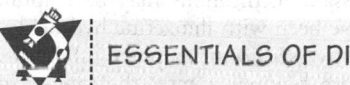 **ESSENTIALS OF DIAGNOSIS**

- *Uncontrolled episodes of binge eating at least twice weekly for 3 months.*
- *Recurrent inappropriate compensation to prevent weight gain such as self-induced vomiting, laxatives, diuretics, fasting, or excessive exercise.*
- *Overconcern with weight and body shape.*

General Considerations

Bulimia nervosa is the episodic uncontrolled ingestion of large quantities of food followed by recurrent inappropriate compensatory behavior in order to prevent weight gain such as self-induced vomiting, diuretic or cathartic use, or strict dieting or vigorous exercise.

Like anorexia nervosa, bulimia nervosa is predominantly a disorder of young, white middle- and upper-class women. It is more difficult to detect than anorexia, and some studies have estimated that the prevalence may be as high as 19% in college-age women.

Clinical Findings

Patients with bulimia nervosa typically consume large quantities of easily ingested high-calorie foods, usually in secrecy. Some patients may have several such episodes a day for a few days; others report regular and persistent patterns of binge eating. Binging is usually followed by vomiting, cathartics, or diuretics and is usually accompanied by feelings of guilt or depression. Periods of binging may be followed by intervals of self-imposed starvation. Body weights may fluctuate but generally are within 20% of desirable weights.

Some patients with bulimia nervosa also have a cryptic form of anorexia nervosa with significant weight loss and amenorrhea. Family and psychologic issues are generally similar to those encountered among patients with anorexia nervosa. Bulimics, however, have a higher incidence of premorbid obesity, greater use of cathartics and diuretics, and more impulsive or antisocial behavior. Menstruation is usually preserved.

Medical complications are numerous. Gastric dilatation and pancreatitis have been reported after binges. Vomiting can result in poor dentition, pharyngitis, esophagitis, aspiration, and electrolyte abnormalities. Cathartic and diuretic abuse also cause electrolyte abnormalities or dehydration. Constipation and hemorrhoids are common.

Treatment

Treatment of bulimia nervosa and bulimarexia requires supportive care and psychotherapy. Individual, group, family, and behavioral therapy have all been utilized. Antidepressant medications may be helpful. The best results have been with fluoxetine hydrochloride and other selective serotonin reuptake inhibitors. Although death from bulimia is rare, the long-term psychiatric prognosis in severe bulimia is worse than that in anorexia nervosa.

Bulik CM et al: Predictors of 1-year treatment outcome in bulimia nervosa. Compr Psychiatry 1998;39:206. [PMID: 9675505] (A history of obesity, the presence of depression, and several personality factors were predictive of poor treatment outcomes.)

Fitzgibbon ML et al: Binge eating disorder and bulimia nervosa: differences in the quality and quantity of binge eating episodes. Int J Eat Disord 2000;27:238. [PMID: 2012578] (Patients with binge eating disorder have as many binges as patients with bulimia nervosa, but patients with binge eating disorder do not purge and are more likely to be obese.)

Walsh BT et al: Fluoxetine for bulimia nervosa following poor response to psychotherapy. Am J Psychiatry 2000;157:1332-4. [PMID: 10910801] (Bulimic patients with a poor response to psychotherapy randomized to fluoxetine had significantly fewer binge eating and purging episodes than patients taking placebo.)

Wells LA et al: Bulimia nervosa: an update and treatment recommendations. Curr Opin Pediatr 2001;13:591. [PMID: 11753113] (Treatment should be comprehensive, individualized, and multifaceted. Many patients respond well to the use of an antidepressant, and cognitive-behavioral therapy is a useful approach for many patients. Combining these two treatments seems to be a good strategy.)

■ DISORDERS OF VITAMIN METABOLISM

Deficiencies of single vitamins are less often encountered than those of multiple vitamins. Although any cause of protein-calorie undernutrition can result in concurrent vitamin deficiency, most deficiencies are associated with malabsorption, alcoholism, medications, hemodialysis, total parenteral nutrition, food faddism, or inborn errors of metabolism.

Vitamin deficiency syndromes develop gradually. Symptoms are commonly nonspecific, and the physical examination is rarely helpful in early diagnosis. Most characteristic physical findings are seen late in the course of the syndrome. Other characteristic physical findings, such as glossitis and cheilosis, are seen with deficiencies of many B vitamins. Such abnormalities suggest the presence of a nutritional deficiency but do not indicate which nutrient is deficient.

Despite the relative ease of meeting the recommended daily allowances with a mixed diet, many adults in the USA take vitamin supplements. In fact, syndromes of vitamin excess may be more common than deficiency syndromes, particularly those due to excess of vitamins A, D, and B_6. Most claims for significant health benefits of such supplements, particularly those taken in megadoses, remain unsubstantiated.

Some vitamins can be used efficaciously as drugs. Derivatives of vitamin A are used to treat cystic acne and, more recently, skin wrinkles. Niacin is an effective medication for hyperlipidemia. Vitamin-responsive inborn errors of metabolism also commonly require pharmacologic doses of vitamins.

THIAMIN (B_1)

The primary role of thiamin is as precursor of thiamin pyrophosphate, a coenzyme required for several important biochemical reactions necessary for carbohydrate oxidation. Thiamin is also thought to have an independent role in nerve conduction in peripheral nerves. The recommended daily allowances of thiamin are listed in Table 29–1. There is no known toxicity of thiamin.

Thiamin Deficiency

A. CLINICAL FINDINGS

Most thiamin deficiency in the USA is due to alcoholism. Chronic alcoholics may have poor dietary intakes of thiamin and impaired thiamin absorption, metabolism, and storage. Thiamin deficiency is also associated with malabsorption, dialysis, and other causes of chronic protein-calorie undernutrition. Thiamin deficiency can be precipitated in patients with marginal thiamin status with intravenous dextrose solutions.

Early manifestations of thiamin deficiency include anorexia, muscle cramps, paresthesias, and irritability. Advanced deficiency affects chiefly the cardiovascular system ("wet beriberi") or the nervous system ("dry beriberi"). Wet beriberi occurs in thiamin deficiency accompanied by severe physical exertion and high carbohydrate intakes. Dry beriberi occurs in thiamin deficiency accompanied by inactivity and low-calorie intake.

Wet beriberi is characterized by marked peripheral vasodilation resulting in high-output heart failure with dyspnea, tachycardia, cardiomegaly, and pulmonary and peripheral edema, with warm extremities mimicking cellulitis.

Dry beriberi involves both the peripheral and the central nervous systems. Peripheral nerve involvement is typically a symmetric motor and sensory neuropathy with pain, paresthesias, and loss of reflexes. The legs are affected more than the arms. Central nervous system involvement results in Wernicke-Korsakoff syndrome. Wernicke's encephalopathy consists of nystagmus progressing to ophthalmoplegia, truncal ataxia, and confusion. Korsakoff's syndrome includes amnesia, confabulation, and impaired learning.

B. DIAGNOSIS

A variety of biochemical tests are available to assess thiamin deficiency. In most instances, however, the clinical response to empirical thiamine therapy is used to support a diagnosis of thiamin deficiency. The most commonly used and widely available biochemical tests are measurement of erythrocyte transketolase activity and urinary thiamin excretion. A transketolase activity coefficient greater than 15–20% suggests thiamin deficiency.

C. TREATMENT

Thiamin deficiency is treated with large parenteral doses of thiamine. Fifty to 100 mg/d is administered for the first few days, followed by daily oral doses of 5–10 mg/d. All patients should simultaneously receive therapeutic doses of other water-soluble vitamins. Although treatment results in complete resolution in one-half of patients (one-fourth immediately and another one-fourth over days), the other half obtain only partial resolution or no benefit.

Jamieson CP et al: The thiamin, riboflavin and pyridoxine status of patients on emergency admission to hospital. Clin Nutr 1999;18:87. [PMID: 10459067] (Almost half [49.2%] of patients were deficient in one or more vitamin.)

Ozawa H et al: Severe metabolic acidosis and heart failure due to thiamine deficiency. Nutrition 2001;17:351. [PMID: 11369178] (Case report of a male patient with severe metabolic acidosis and heart failure caused by deficiency.)

Shin RK et al: Wernicke encephalopathy. Arch Neurol 2000;57:405. [PMID: 10714669]

RIBOFLAVIN (B₂)

Riboflavin—as the coenzymes flavin mononucleotide and flavin adenine dinucleotide—participates in a variety of important oxidation-reduction reactions and is an essential component of a number of other enzymes. The recommended daily allowances of riboflavin are listed in Table 29–1. There is no known toxicity of riboflavin.

Riboflavin Deficiency

A. CLINICAL FINDINGS

Riboflavin deficiency almost always occurs in combination with deficiencies of other vitamins. Dietary inadequacy, interactions with a variety of medications, alcoholism, and other causes of protein-calorie undernutrition are the most common causes of riboflavin deficiency.

Manifestations of riboflavin deficiency include cheilosis, angular stomatitis, glossitis, seborrheic dermatitis, weakness, corneal vascularization, and anemia.

B. DIAGNOSIS

Riboflavin deficiency is usually treated empirically when the diagnosis is suspected. Deficiency can be confirmed by measuring the riboflavin-dependent enzyme erythrocyte glutathione reductase. Activity coefficients greater than 1.2–1.3 are suggestive of riboflavin deficiency. Urinary riboflavin excretion and serum levels of plasma and red cell flavins can also be measured.

C. TREATMENT

Riboflavin deficiency is easily treated with foods such as meat, fish, and dairy products or with oral preparations of the vitamin. Administration of 5–15 mg/d until clinical findings are resolved is usually adequate. Riboflavin can also be given parenterally, but it is poorly soluble in aqueous solutions.

Riboflavin Toxicity

There is no known toxicity of riboflavin.

Madigan SM et al: Riboflavin and vitamin B-6 intakes and status and biochemical response to riboflavin supplementation in free-living elderly people. Am J Clin Nutr 1998;68:389. [PMID: 9701198] (Almost half [49%] percent of elderly subjects were found to be deficient in riboflavin.)

Powers HJ: Current knowledge concerning optimum nutritional status of riboflavin, niacin and pyridoxine. Proc Nutr Soc 1999;58:435. [PMID: 10466188] (No single biochemical marker is wholly satisfactory as a marker of optimum nutritional status for these vitamins.)

NIACIN

Niacin is a generic term for nicotinic acid and other derivatives with similar nutritional activity. Unlike most other vitamins, niacin can be synthesized from the amino acid tryptophan. Niacin is an essential component of the coenzymes nicotinamide adenine dinucleotide (NAD) and nicotinamide adenine dinucleotide phosphate (NADP), which are involved in many oxidation-reduction reactions. The recommended daily allowances of niacin are listed in Table 29–1; major food sources are protein foods containing tryptophan and numerous cereals, vegetables, and dairy products.

Niacin in the form of nicotinic acid is used therapeutically for the treatment of hypercholesterolemia and hypertriglyceridemia. Daily doses of 3–6 g can result in significant reductions in levels of low-density lipoproteins (LDL) and very-low-density lipoproteins (VLDL) and in elevation of high-density lipoproteins (HDL). Niacinamide (the form of niacin usually used to treat niacin deficiency) does not exhibit the lipid-lowering effects of nicotinic acid.

Niacin Deficiency

A. CLINICAL FINDINGS

Historically, niacin deficiency occurred when corn, which is relatively deficient in both tryptophan and niacin, was the major source of calories. Currently, niacin deficiency is more commonly due to alcoholism and nutrient-drug interactions. Niacin deficiency can also occur in inborn errors of metabolism.

As with other B vitamins, the early manifestations of niacin deficiency are nonspecific. Common complaints include anorexia, weakness, irritability, mouth soreness, glossitis, stomatitis, and weight loss. More advanced deficiency results in the classic triad of pellagra: dermatitis, diarrhea, and dementia. The dermatitis is symmetric, involving sun-exposed areas. Skin lesions are dark, dry, and scaling. The dementia begins with insomnia, irritability, and apathy and progresses to confusion, memory loss, hallucinations, and psychosis. The diarrhea can be severe and may result in malabsorption due to atrophy of the intestinal villi. Advanced pellagra can result in death.

B. DIAGNOSIS

In advanced cases, the diagnosis of pellagra can be made on clinical grounds. In early deficiency, diagnosis requires a high index of suspicion and attempts at confirmation of niacin deficiency. Niacin metabolites, particularly *N*-methylnicotinamide, can be measured in the urine. Low levels suggest niacin deficiency but may also be found in patients with generalized undernutrition. Serum and red cell levels of NAD and NADP are also low but are similarly nonspecific.

C. TREATMENT

Niacin deficiency can be effectively treated with oral niacin, usually given as nicotinamide. Doses ranging from 10 to 150 mg/d have been used without difficulty.

Niacin Toxicity

At the high doses of niacin used to treat hyperlipidemia, side effects are common. These include cutaneous flushing (partially prevented by pretreatment with aspirin, 325 mg/d) and gastric irritation. Elevation of liver enzymes, hyperglycemia, and gout are less common untoward effects.

Kertesz SG: Pellagra in 2 homeless men. Mayo Clinic Proc 2001;76:315. [PMID: 11243279]

Knopp RH: Evaluating niacin in its various forms. Am J Cardiol 2000;86(12A):51L. [PMID: 11374857] (Immediate-release and extended-release niacin [Niaspan] are essentially equivalent with respect to their efficacy in reducing triglycerides and increasing high-density lipoprotein cholesterol, but there are fewer side effects and better compliance associated with the latter form.)

VITAMIN B$_6$ (Pyridoxine)

Vitamin B$_6$ (pyridoxine) is actually a group of closely related substances involved in intermediary metabolism. These include pyridoxine itself, pyridoxal, pyridoxamine, and their 5-phosphate esters. As the major coenzyme involved in the metabolism of amino acids, pyridoxal 5-phosphate is the most important. Pyridoxal phosphate is also required for the synthesis of heme. The recommended daily allowances of vitamin B$_6$ are listed in Table 29–1.

Vitamin B$_6$ Deficiency

A. CLINICAL FINDINGS

Vitamin B$_6$ deficiency most commonly occurs as a result of interactions with medications—especially isoniazid, cycloserine, penicillamine, and oral contraceptives—or of alcoholism. A number of inborn errors of metabolism and other pyridoxine-responsive syndromes, particularly pyridoxine-responsive anemia, are not clearly due to vitamin deficiency but commonly respond to high doses of the vitamin.

Vitamin B$_6$ deficiency results in a clinical syndrome similar to that seen with deficiencies of other B vitamins, including mouth soreness, glossitis, cheilosis, weakness, and irritability. Severe deficiency can result in peripheral neuropathy, anemia, and seizures.

B. DIAGNOSIS

The diagnosis of vitamin B$_6$ deficiency can be confirmed by measurement of pyridoxal phosphate in blood. Normal levels are greater than 50 ng/mL.

C. TREATMENT

Vitamin B$_6$ deficiency can be effectively treated with oral vitamin B$_6$ supplements. Doses of 10–20 mg/d are usually adequate, though some patients taking medications that interfere with pyridoxine metabolism may need doses as high as 100 mg/d. Inborn errors of metabolism and the pyridoxine-responsive syndromes often require up to 600 mg/d.

Vitamin B$_6$ should be routinely prescribed for patients receiving medications (such as isoniazid) that interfere with pyridoxine metabolism to prevent vitamin B$_6$ deficiency. This is particularly true for elderly patients, the urban poor, and alcoholics, who are more likely to have diets marginally adequate in vitamin B$_6$.

Vitamin B$_6$ Toxicity

A sensory neuropathy, at times irreversible, occurs in patients receiving large doses of vitamin B$_6$. Although most patients have taken 2 g or more per day, some patients have taken only 200 mg/d.

Lerner V et al: Vitamin B(6) in the treatment of tardive dyskinesia: a double-blind, placebo-controlled, crossover study. Am J Psychiatry 2001;158:1511. [PMID: 11532741] (Small randomized controlled trial showing benefit of vitamin B6 for symptoms of tardive dyskinesia.)

VITAMIN B$_{12}$ & FOLATE

Vitamin B$_{12}$ (cobalamin) and folate are discussed in Chapter 13. The recommended daily allowances of vitamin B$_{12}$ and folate are listed in Table 29–1. Vitamin B$_{12}$ is abundant in meat and dairy products; fresh fruits and vegetables supply ample folic acid.

Baik HW et al: Vitamin B$_{12}$ deficiency in the elderly. Annu Rev Nutr 1999;19:357. [PMID: 10448529] (Vitamin B$_{12}$ deficiency may be present in up to 10–15% of individuals over age 60.)

Bailey LB et al: Folate metabolism and requirements. J Nutr 1999;129:779. [PMID: 10203550] (The Recommended Dietary Allowance [RDA] for adults is 400 μg/d of dietary folate equivalents [DFE]; for lactating and pregnant women, the RDAs include an additional 100 μg/d and 200 μg/d, respectively, of DFE.)

Honein MA et al: Impact of folic acid fortification of the US food supply on the occurrence of neural tube defects. JAMA 2001;285:2981. [PMID: 11410096] (A 19% reduction in neural tube defects occurred in the United States following mandatory folic acid fortification.)

Quinlivan EP et al: Importance of both folic acid and vitamin B12 in reduction of risk of vascular disease. Lancet 2002;359:227. [PMID: 11812560] (A fortification policy based on folic acid and vitamin B12—rather than folic acid alone—is likely to be much more effective at lowering of homocysteine concentrations, with potential benefits for reduction of risk of vascular disease.)

Schnyder G et al: Decreased rate of coronary restenosis after lowering of plasma homocysteine levels. N Engl J Med 2001;345:1593. [PMID: 11757505] (Randomized controlled trial of folic acid, vitamin B12, and pyridoxine or placebo after successful coronary angioplasty. The rate of restenosis and revascularization was significantly lower in patients assigned to folate treatment.)

Snow CF: Laboratory diagnosis of vitamin B12 and folate deficiency: a guide for the primary care physician. Arch Intern Med 1999;159:1289. [PMID: 10386505] (New diagnostic tests have led to greater recognition of vitamin B12 deficiency and folate deficiency.)

Tice JA et al: Cost-effectiveness of vitamin therapy to lower plasma homocysteine levels for the prevention of coronary heart disease: effect of grain fortification and beyond. JAMA 2001;286:936. [PMID: 11509058] (Diets including grains enriched with folic acid or vitamin therapy with folic acid and cyanocobalamin are cost-effective to prevent coronary heart disease.)

VITAMIN C (Ascorbic Acid)

Vitamin C is a potent antioxidant involved in many oxidation-reduction reactions and is also required for the synthesis of collagen. It increases the absorption of nonheme iron and is involved in tyrosine metabolism, wound healing, and drug metabolism. With the exception of collagen synthesis, the mechanism of action for these functions is poorly understood. The recommended daily allowances of vitamin C are listed in Table 29–1; major food sources are fresh fruits and vegetables.

Vitamin C Deficiency

A. CLINICAL FINDINGS

Most cases of vitamin C deficiency seen in the USA are due to dietary inadequacy in the urban poor, the elderly, and chronic alcoholics. Patients with chronic illnesses such as cancer and chronic renal failure and individuals who smoke cigarettes are also at risk.

Early manifestations of vitamin C deficiency are nonspecific and include malaise and weakness. In more advanced stages, the typical features of scurvy develop. Manifestations include perifollicular hemorrhages, perifollicular hyperkeratotic papules, petechiae and purpura, splinter hemorrhages, bleeding gums, hemarthroses, and subperiosteal hemorrhages. Periodontal signs do not occur in edentulous patients. Anemia is common, and wound healing is impaired. The late stages of scurvy are characterized by edema, oliguria, neuropathy, intracerebral hemorrhage, and death.

B. DIAGNOSIS

The diagnosis of advanced scurvy can be made clinically on the basis of the skin lesions in the proper clinical situation. Atraumatic hemarthrosis is also highly suggestive. The diagnosis can be confirmed with decreased plasma ascorbic acid levels, typically below 0.1 mg/dL.

C. TREATMENT

Adult scurvy can be treated with 300–1000 mg of ascorbic acid per day. Improvement typically occurs within days. Some studies have suggested that high intakes of vitamin C are associated with a decreased risk of cancer. Vitamin C may also protect against coronary heart disease by modifying blood cholesterol levels and preventing LDL-cholesterol from oxidation. A decrease in all-cause and coronary heart disease mortality in individuals with high intakes (approximately 300–400 mg/d) has been reported.

Vitamin C Toxicity

Very large doses of vitamin C can cause gastric irritation, flatulence, or diarrhea. Oxalate kidney stones are of theoretic concern because ascorbic acid is metabolized to oxalate, but stone formation has not been frequently reported. Vitamin C can also confound common diagnostic tests by causing false-negative tests for fecal occult blood and both false-negative and false-positive tests for urine glucose.

Johnston CS et al: People with marginal vitamin C status are at high risk of developing vitamin C deficiency. J Am Diet Assoc 1999;99:854. [PMID: 10405686]

Khaw KT et al: Relation between plasma ascorbic acid and mortality in men and women in EPIC-Norfolk prospective study: a prospective population study. European Prospective Investigation into Cancer and Nutrition. Lancet 2001;357:657. [PMID: 11247548] (Plasma ascorbic acid concentration was inversely related to mortality from all-causes, and from cardiovascular disease, and from ischemic heart disease in men and women.)

Levine M et al: Criteria and recommendations for vitamin C intake. JAMA 1999;281:1415. [PMID: 10217058] (New evidence suggests the RDA for vitamin C, currently 60 mg/d, should be raised to 120 mg/d.)

Loria CM et al: Vitamin C status and mortality in US adults. Am J Clin Nutr 2000;72:139. [PMID: 10871572] (Men identified to be in the lowest quartile of serum vitamin C levels in NHANES II were found to have an all-cause mortality relative risk of 1.57 after 12–16 years follow-up compared with men in the highest quartile.)

VITAMIN A

Vitamin A (retinol) is a high-molecular-weight alcohol either ingested preformed or synthesized from plant carotenoids, particularly β-carotene. Isomers and derivatives of retinol are commonly called retinoids. Vitamin A is essential for normal retinal function and plays an important but still not fully understood role in cell growth and differentiation, particularly of epithelial cells. Vitamin A is also necessary for normal wound healing. The recommended daily allowances of vitamin A are listed in Table 29–1; the principal food sources are highly pigmented vegetables.

Because of its role in cell differentiation, vitamin A has been postulated to have a role in cancer prevention. The role of retinoids for chemoprevention of cancer is under intense investigation. The provitamin β-carotene may play an even more important role in prevention of cancer and heart disease by virtue of its antioxidant activity.

Vitamin A Deficiency

A. CLINICAL FINDINGS

Vitamin A deficiency is one of the most common vitamin deficiency syndromes, particularly in developing countries. In many such regions, it is the most common cause of blindness. In the USA, vitamin A deficiency is usually due to fat malabsorption syndromes or mineral oil laxative abuse and occurs most commonly in the elderly and urban poor.

Night blindness is the earliest symptom. Dryness of the conjunctiva (xerosis) and the development of small white patches on the conjunctiva (Bitot's spots) are early signs. Ulceration and necrosis of the cornea (keratomalacia), perforation, endophthalmitis, and blindness are late manifestations. Xerosis and hyperkeratinization of the skin and loss of taste may also occur.

B. DIAGNOSIS

Abnormalities of dark adaptation are strongly suggestive of vitamin A deficiency. Serum levels below the normal range of 30–65 mg/dL are commonly seen in advanced deficiency.

C. TREATMENT

Night blindness, poor wound healing, and other signs of early deficiency can be effectively treated with 30,000 IU of vitamin A daily for 1 week. Advanced deficiency with corneal damage calls for administration of 20,000 units/kg for at least 5 days. The potential antioxidant effects of β-carotene can be achieved with supplements of 25,000–50,000 IU of β-carotene.

Vitamin A Toxicity

Excess intake of β-carotenes (hypercarotenosis) results in staining of the skin a yellow-orange color but is otherwise benign. Skin changes are most marked on the palms and soles, while the scleras remain white, clearly distinguishing hypercarotenosis from jaundice.

Excessive vitamin A (hypervitaminosis A), on the other hand, can be quite toxic. Chronic toxicity usually occurs after ingestion of daily doses of over 50,000 units/d for more than 3 months. Early manifestations include dry, scaly skin, hair loss, mouth sores, painful hyperostoses, anorexia, and vomiting. More serious findings include hypercalcemia; increased intracranial pressure, with papilledema, headaches, and decreased cognition; and hepatomegaly, occasionally progressing to cirrhosis. Acute toxicity can result from ingestion of massive doses of vitamin A, such as in drug overdoses or consumption of polar bear liver. Manifestations include nausea, vomiting, abdominal pain, headache, papilledema, and lethargy.

The diagnosis can be confirmed by elevations of serum vitamin A levels. The only treatment is withdrawal of vitamin A from the diet. Most symptoms and signs improve rapidly.

Dawson MI: The importance of vitamin A in nutrition. Curr Pharm Des 2000;6:311. [PMID: 10637381] (Observational studies on vitamin A use and cancer prevention have produced mixed results.)

Feskanich D et al: Vitamin A intake and hip fractures among postmenopausal women. JAMA 2002;287:47. [PMID: 11754708] (Women in the highest quintile of total vitamin A intake had a 48% increased risk of hip fracture compared with women in the lowest quintile of intake. Beta-carotene did not contribute significantly to fracture risk.)

VITAMIN D

Vitamin D is discussed in Chapter 26. The recommended daily allowances of vitamin D are listed in Table 29–1; a major food source is fortified milk, but sunlight on the skin is a prime resource as well.

LeBoff MS et al: Occult vitamin D deficiency in postmenopausal US women with acute hip fracture. JAMA 1999;281:1505. [PMID: 10227320] (Postmenopausal community-living women who presented with hip fracture showed occult vitamin D deficiency.)

VITAMIN E

Vitamin E activity is derived from at least eight naturally occurring tocopherols, the most potent of which is α-tocopherol. Although the exact function and mechanism of action of vitamin E in humans are unclear, it is commonly thought to function as an antioxidant, protecting cell membranes and other cellular structures from attack by free radicals. Dietary selenium and other antioxidants work in conjunction with vitamin E and may partially spare its requirement and reverse signs of vitamin E deficiency in animals. The recommended daily allowances of vitamin E are listed in Table 29–1; the major food source is vegetable seed oil.

Vitamin E, like β-carotene and vitamin C, may also play a role in protection against cancer, coronary heart disease, Alzheimer's disease, and cataracts through its antioxidant function.

Vitamin E Deficiency

A. CLINICAL FINDINGS

Clinical deficiency of vitamin E is most commonly due to severe malabsorption, the genetic disorder abetalipoproteinemia, or, in children with chronic cholestatic liver disease, biliary atresia or cystic fibrosis. Manifestations of deficiency include areflexia, disturbances of gait, decreased proprioception and vibration, and ophthalmoplegia.

B. DIAGNOSIS

Plasma vitamin E levels can be measured; normal levels are 0.5–0.7 mg/dL or higher. Since vitamin E is normally transported in lipoproteins, the serum level should be interpreted in relation to circulating lipids.

C. TREATMENT

The optimum therapeutic dose of vitamin E has not been clearly defined. Large doses, often administered parenterally, can be used to improve the neurologic complications seen in abetalipoproteinemia and cholestatic liver disease. The potential antioxidant benefits of vitamin E can be achieved with supplements of 100–400 units/d.

Vitamin E Toxicity

Vitamin E is the least toxic of the fat-soluble vitamins. Large doses, 20–80 times the recommended daily requirement, have been taken for extended periods of time without apparent harm, although nausea, flatulence, and diarrhea have been reported. Large doses of vitamin E can increase the vitamin K requirement and can result in bleeding in patients taking oral anticoagulants.

de Gaetano G: Low-dose aspirin and vitamin E in people at cardiovascular risk: a randomised trial in general practice. Collaborative Group of the Primary Prevention Project. Lancet 2001;357:89. [PMID: 11197445] (A randomized controlled trial of low-dose aspirin and vitamin E in the prevention of cardiovascular events. Vitamin E showed no effect on any prespecified end point.)

Grundman M: Vitamin E and Alzheimer disease: the basis for additional clinical trials. Am J Clin Nutr 2000;71:630S. [PMID: 10681271] (A placebo-controlled clinical trial indicated that vitamin E may slow functional deterioration leading to nursing home placement.)

Willett WC et al: Clinical practice. What vitamins should I be taking, doctor? N Engl J Med 2001;345:1819. [PMID: 11752359] (Authors recommend daily multivitamins for most adults and especially women who may become pregnant, individuals who consume alcohol, the elderly, vegans, and the urban poor. The authors also recommend vitamin E 400 IU per day for middle-aged and older Americans at increased risk for coronary heart disease.)

Yusuf S et al: Vitamin E supplementation and cardiovascular events in high-risk patients. The Heart Outcomes Prevention Evaluation Study Investigators. N Engl J Med 2000;342:154. [PMID: 10639540] (Vitamin E supplementation for 4.5 years in men and women at high risk for coronary artery disease events had no effect on coronary artery disease outcomes or all-cause mortality.)

VITAMIN K

Vitamin K is discussed in Chapter 13. The recommended daily allowances of vitamin K are listed in Table 29–1. It is synthesized by intestinal bacteria.

Booth SL et al: Vitamin K: a practical guide to the dietary management of patients on warfarin. Nutr Rev 1999;57(9 Part 1):288. [PMID: 10568341] (A constant dietary intake of vitamin K that meets current dietary recommendations of 65–80 mg/day is the most acceptable practice for patients on warfarin therapy.)

Rashid M et al: Prevalence of vitamin K deficiency in cystic fibrosis. Am J Clin Nutr 1999;70:378. [PMID: 10479200] (Vitamin K deficiency is common in unsupplemented patients with cystic fibrosis and pancreatic insufficiency. Routine supplementation should be considered in all of these patients.)

■ DIET THERAPY

Specific therapeutic diets can be designed to facilitate the medical management of most common illnesses. In most cases, consultation with a registered dietitian is necessary in order to design and implement major dietary changes. Physicians should be familiar with the indications for special diets and their basic composition to facilitate patient referrals and to maximize patient compliance. Diet therapy is a difficult process, and not all patients are able to cooperate fully. Requesting the patient to record dietary intake for 3–5 days may provide useful insight into the patient's motivation.

Therapeutic diets can be divided into three groups: (1) diets that alter the consistency of food; (2) diets that restrict or otherwise modify dietary components; and (3) diets that supplement dietary components.

DIETS THAT ALTER CONSISTENCY

Clear Liquid Diet

This diet provides adequate water, 500–1000 kcal as simple sugar, and some electrolytes. It is fiber-free and requires minimal digestion or intestinal motility.

A clear liquid diet is useful for patients with resolving postoperative ileus, acute gastroenteritis, partial intestinal obstruction, and as preparation for diagnostic gastrointestinal procedures. It is commonly used as the first diet for patients who have been taking nothing by mouth for long periods. Because of the low calorie and minimal protein content of the clear liquid diet, it is used only for short periods.

Full Liquid Diet

The full liquid diet provides adequate water and can be designed to provide adequate calories and protein. Vitamins and minerals—especially folic acid, iron, and vitamin B_6—may be inadequate and should be provided in the form of supplements. Dairy products, soups, eggs, and soft cereals are used to supplement clear liquids. Commercial oral supplements can also be incorporated into the diet or used alone.

This diet is low in residue and can be used in many instances instead of the clear liquid diet described above—especially in patients with difficulty in chewing or swallowing, with partial obstructions, or in preparation for some diagnostic procedures. Full liquid diets are commonly used following clear liquid diets to advance diets in patients who have been taking nothing by mouth for long periods.

Soft Diets

Soft diets are designed for patients unable to chew or swallow hard or coarse food. Tender foods are used, and most raw fruits and vegetables and coarse breads and cereals are eliminated. Soft diets are commonly used to assist in progression from full liquid diets to regular diets in postoperative patients, in patients who are too weak or those whose dentition is too poor to handle a general diet, in head and neck surgical patients, in patients with esophageal strictures, and in other patients who have difficulty with chewing or swallowing.

The soft diet can be designed to meet all nutritional requirements.

DIETS THAT RESTRICT NUTRIENTS

Diets can be designed to restrict (or eliminate) virtually any nutrient or food component. The most commonly used restricted diets are those that limit sodium, fat, and protein. Other restrictive diets include gluten restriction in sprue, potassium and phosphate reduction in renal insufficiency, and various elimination diets for food allergies.

Sodium-Restricted Diets

Low-sodium diets are useful in the management of hypertension and in conditions in which sodium retention and edema are prominent features, particularly congestive heart failure, chronic liver disease, and chronic renal failure. Sodium restriction is beneficial with or without diuretic therapy. When used in conjunction with diuretics, sodium restriction allows lower dosage of the diuretic medication and may prevent side effects. Potassium excretion, in particular, is directly related to distal renal tubule sodium delivery, and sodium restriction will decrease diuretic-related potassium losses.

Typical American diets contain a minimum of 4–6 g (175–260 meq) of sodium per day. A no-added-salt diet contains approximately 3 g of sodium (132 meq) per day. Further restriction can be achieved with sodium diets 2 g or 1 g per day. Diets with more severe restriction are poorly accepted by patients and are rarely used.

Dietary sodium includes sodium naturally occurring in foods, sodium added during food processing, and sodium added by the consumer during cooking and at the table. About a third of current dietary intake is derived from each. Diets that allow 2000 mg of sodium daily are easiest to design and implement. Such diets generally eliminate added salt, most processed foods, and selected foods with particularly high sodium content. Patients who follow such diets for 2–3 months lose their craving for salty foods and can often continue to restrict their sodium intake indefinitely. Many patients with mild hypertension will achieve significant reductions in blood pressure (approximately 5 mm Hg diastolic) with this degree of sodium restriction. Other patients require more severe sodium restriction (approximately 1000 mg of sodium per day) for reduction in blood pressure.

Diets allowing 1000 mg of sodium require further restriction of commonly eaten foods. Special "low-sodium" products are now available to facilitate such diets. These diets are difficult for most people to follow and are generally reserved for hospitalized patients and highly motivated outpatients—most commonly those with severe liver disease and ascites.

Fat-Restricted Diets

Traditional fat-restricted diets are useful in the treatment of fat malabsorption syndromes. Such diets will improve the symptoms of diarrhea with steatorrhea independently of the primary physiologic abnormality by limiting the quantity of fatty acids that reach the colon. The degree of fat restriction necessary to control symptoms must be individualized. Patients with severe malabsorption can be limited to 40–60 g of fat per day. Diets containing 60–80 g of fat per day can be designed for patients with less severe abnormalities.

In general, fat-restricted diets require broiling, baking, or boiling meat and fish; discarding the skin of poultry and fish and using those foods as the main protein source; using nonfat dairy products; and avoiding desserts, sauces, and gravies.

Low-Cholesterol, Low-Saturated-Fat Diets

Fat-restricted diets that specifically restrict saturated fats and dietary cholesterol are the mainstay of dietary treatment of hyperlipidemia (see Chapter 28). Similar diets are recommended also for diabetes (Chapter 27) and for the prevention of coronary artery disease (Chapter 10). Current recommendations for the prevention of cancer by dietary modification also include fat restriction.

The aim of these diets is to restrict total fat to 30% of calories and to achieve a normal body weight by caloric restriction. Saturated fat is restricted to 10% of calories and dietary cholesterol to 300 mg/d. Saturated fat can be replaced either with complex carbohydrates or, if energy balance permits, with monounsaturated fats. Saturated fat, total fat, and dietary cholesterol can be restricted further, but studies suggest that more extreme restriction offers little further advantage in overall modification of serum lipids.

Protein-Restricted Diets

Protein-restricted diets are most commonly used in patients with hepatic encephalopathy due to chronic liver disease and in patients with renal failure to slow the progression of early disease and to decrease symptoms of uremia in more severe disease. Patients with selected inborn errors of amino acid metabolism and other abnormalities resulting in hyperammonemia also require restriction of protein or of specific amino acids.

Protein restriction is intended to limit the production of nitrogenous waste products. Energy intake must be adequate to facilitate the efficient use of dietary protein. Proteins must be of high biologic value and be provided in sufficient quantity to meet minimal requirements. For most patients, the diet should contain at least 0.6 g/kg/d of protein. Patients with encephalopathy who fail to respond to this degree of restriction are unlikely to respond to more severe restriction.

DIETS THAT SUPPLEMENT NUTRIENTS

High-Fiber Diet

Dietary fiber is a diverse group of plant constituents that are resistant to digestion by the human digestive tract. Typical American diets contain about 5–10 g of dietary fiber per day. Epidemiologic evidence has suggested that populations consuming greater quantities of fiber have a lower incidence of certain gastrointestinal disorders, including diverticulitis and colon cancer. Most authorities currently recommend higher intakes of dietary fiber for health maintenance.

Diets high in dietary fiber (20–35 g/d) are also commonly used in management of a variety of gastrointestinal disorders, particularly irritable bowel syndrome and recurrent diverticulitis. Diets high in fiber may also be useful to reduce blood sugar in patients with diabetes and to reduce cholesterol levels in patients with hypercholesterolemia. Such diets include greater intakes of fresh fruits and vegetables, whole grains, legumes and seeds, and bran products. For some patients, the addition of psyllium seed (2 tsp per day) or natural bran (½ cup per day) may be preferable.

High-Potassium Diets

Potassium-supplemented diets are used most commonly to compensate for potassium losses caused by diuretics. Although potassium losses can be partially prevented by using lower doses of diuretics, concurrent sodium restriction, and potassium-sparing diuretics, some patients require additional potassium to prevent hypokalemia. High-potassium diets may also have a direct antihypertensive effect. Typical American diets contain about 3 g (80 meq) of potassium per day. High-potassium diets commonly contain 4.5–7 g (120–180 meq) of potassium per day.

Most fruits, vegetables, and their juices contain high concentrations of potassium (see Chapter 21). Supplemental potassium can also be provided with potassium-containing salt substitutes (up to 20 meq in ¼ tsp) or as potassium chloride in solution or capsules, but this is rarely necessary if the above measures are followed to prevent potassium losses and supplement dietary potassium.

High-Calcium Diets

Additional intakes of dietary calcium have recently been recommended for the prevention of postmenopausal osteoporosis, the prevention and treatment of hypertension, and the prevention of colon cancer. Although the evidence in each case is preliminary, authorities recommend intakes of 1 g of calcium per day for most adults and 1.5 g/d for postmenopausal women. Average American daily intakes are approximately 700 mg/d.

Low-fat and nonfat dairy products are the mainstay of supplemental calcium intakes. Patients with lactose intolerance who cannot tolerate liquid dairy products may be able to tolerate nonliquid products such as cheese and yogurt. Leafy green vegetables and canned fish with bones also contain high concentrations of calcium, although the latter is also very high in sodium.

Alberts DS et al: Lack of effect of a high fiber cereal supplement on the recurrence of colorectal adenomas. N Engl J Med 2000;342:1156. [PMID: 10770980] (A randomized trial in which treating 1429 men and women with wheat bran fiber [13.5 g/d] did not demonstrate a reduction in recurrent colorectal adenomas.)

American Diabetes Association position statement: evidence-based nutrition principles and recommendations for the treatment and prevention of diabetes and related complications. J Am Diet Assoc 2002;102:109. [PMID: 11794490] (Medical nutrition therapy for people with diabetes should be individualized, with consideration given to the individual's usual food and eating habits, metabolic profile, treatment goals, and desired outcomes.)

Borghi L et al: Comparison of two diets for the prevention of recurrent stones in idiopathic hypercalciuria. N Engl J Med 2002;346:77. [PMID: 11784873] (Randomized controlled trial comparing a diet containing a normal amount of calcium but reduced animal protein and salt versus a traditional low-calcium diet. At 5 years, 12 of the 60 men on the normal-calcium, low-animal-protein, low-salt diet versus 23 of the 60 men on the low-calcium diet had had relapses—a 51% reduction in risk.)

Chandalia M et al: Beneficial effects of high dietary fiber intake in patients with type 2 diabetes mellitus. N Engl J Med 2000;342:1392. [PMID: 10805824] (A diet high in soluble fiber improves glycemic control and cholesterol levels in patients with type 2 diabetes mellitus.)

Haynes RB et al: Nutritionally complete prepared meal plan to reduce cardiovascular risk factors: a randomized clinical trial. J

Am Diet Assoc 1999;99:1077. [PMID: 10491676] (A nutritionally complete prepackaged meal plan offers greater improvements in lipids, blood sugars, homocysteine, and weight loss than usual care diet therapy.)

Hu FB et al: Diet, lifestyle, and the risk of type 2 diabetes mellitus in women. N Engl J Med 2001;345:790. [PMID: 11556298] (Ninety-one percent of the new cases of diabetes in this cohort could be attributed to habits and forms of behavior that did not conform to a low-risk pattern. A low-risk lifestyle pattern included BMI less than 25; a diet high in fiber and polyunsaturated fat and low in trans fat and glycemic load; moderate to vigorous physical activity for at least half an hour per day; no current smoking; and at least half a drink of an alcoholic beverage per day.)

Kasiske BL et al: A meta-analysis of the effects of dietary protein restriction on the rate of decline in renal function. Am J Kidney Dis 1998;31:954. [PMID: 9631839] (Meta-analysis of 13 trials demonstrates that protein restriction retards only somewhat the rate of renal function decline.)

Kopple JD: The National Kidney Foundation K/DOQI clinical practice guidelines for dietary protein intake for chronic dialysis patients. Am J Kidney Dis 2001;38(4 Suppl 1):S68. [PMID: 11576926] (Guidelines recommend a dietary protein intake of 1.2 g protein/kg body weight/d for clinically stable maintenance hemodialysis patients and 1.2–1.3 g protein/kg/d for clinically stable chronic peritoneal dialysis patients.)

Maki KC et al: Lipid responses to plant-sterol-enriched reduced-fat spreads incorporated into a National Cholesterol Education Program Step I diet. Am J Clin Nutr 2001;74:33. [PMID: 11451715] (A 5-week randomized controlled trial of a control reduced-fat spread or a reduced-fat spread enriched with plant sterol esters. Subjects in the low- and high-sterol groups had total cholesterol values that were 5.2% and 6.6% lower and LDL-cholesterol values that were 7.6% and 8.1% lower. Apolipoprotein B values and ratios of total to HDL cholesterol were also lower.)

Position of the American Dietetic Association: Medical nutrition therapy and pharmacotherapy. J Am Diet Assoc 1999;99:227. [PMID: 9972195] (Medical nutrition therapy and lifestyle counseling are integral components of the medical treatment of many conditions for which medications are also required.)

Sacks FM et al: Effects on blood pressure of reduced dietary sodium and the dietary approaches to stop hypertension (DASH) diet. N Engl J Med 2001;344:3. [PMID: 11136953] (Reconfirmation that the DASH diet reduces blood pressure, –5.9/2.9 mm Hg. A low-sodium diet [65 mmol/d] also reduced blood pressure, – 6.7/3.5 mm Hg. When the DASH diet and a low-sodium diet were used together, blood pressure was reduced by 8.9/4.5 mm Hg.)

Schatzkin A et al: Lack of effect of a low-fat, high fiber diet on the recurrence of colorectal adenoma. N Engl J Med 2000; 342:1149. [PMID: 10770979] (A randomized trial of 2079 men and women treated with a low-fat, high-fiber diet did not result in a decrease in recurrent colorectal adenomas.)

Sheils JF et al: The estimated costs and savings of medical nutrition therapy: the Medicare population. J Am Diet Assoc 1999;99:428. [PMID: 10207394] (After an initial period of implementation, coverage for medical nutrition therapy can result in a net reduction in health services utilization and costs for at least some populations. In the case of persons aged 55 years and older, the savings in utilization of hospital and other services will exceed the cost of providing the medical nutrition therapy benefit.)

Tuomilehto J et al: Prevention of type 2 diabetes mellitus by changes in lifestyle among subjects with impaired glucose tolerance. N Engl J Med 2001;344:1343. [PMID: 11333990] (Randomized controlled trial of 522 men and women with impaired glucose tolerance. The intervention arm received counseling to reduce weight, reduce total and saturated fat, increase fiber, and increase physical activity. At the end of 4 years, the incidence of diabetes was 58% less in the intervention group.)

■ NUTRITIONAL SUPPORT

Nutritional support is the provision of nutrients to patients who cannot meet their nutritional requirements by eating standard diets. Nutrients may be delivered enterally, using oral nutritional supplements, nasogastric and nasoduodenal feeding tubes, and tube enterostomies; or parenterally, using lines or catheters placed in peripheral or central veins, respectively. Current nutritional support techniques permit adequate nutrient delivery to virtually any patient. Nutrition support should only be utilized, however, if it is likely to improve the patient's clinical outcome. The financial costs and risks of side effects must be balanced against the potential advantages of improved nutritional status in each clinical situation.

INDICATIONS FOR NUTRITIONAL SUPPORT

The precise indications for nutritional support remain controversial. Most authorities agree that nutritional support is indicated for at least four groups of adult patients: (1) those with inadequate bowel syndromes; (2) those with severe prolonged hypercatabolic states (eg, due to extensive burns, multiple trauma, mechanical ventilation); (3) those requiring prolonged therapeutic bowel rest; and (4) those with severe protein-calorie undernutrition with a treatable disease who have sustained a loss of over 25% of body weight.

It has been difficult to prove the efficacy of nutritional support in the treatment of most other conditions. In most cases it has not been possible to show a clear advantage of treatment by means of nutritional support over treatment without such support.

The American Society for Parenteral and Enteral Nutrition (ASPEN) has published recommendations for the rational use of nutritional support. The recommendations emphasize the need to individualize the decision to begin nutritional support, weighing the risks and costs against the benefits to each patient. They also reinforce the need to identify high-risk malnourished patients by nutritional assessment.

NUTRITIONAL SUPPORT METHODS

Selection of the most appropriate nutritional support method involves consideration of gastrointestinal function, the anticipated duration of nutritional support, and the ability of each method to meet the patient's nutritional requirements. The method chosen should meet the patient's nutritional needs with the lowest risk and lowest cost possible. For most patients, enteral feeding is safer and cheaper and offers significant physiologic advantages. An algorithm for selection of the most appropriate nutritional support method is presented in Figure 29–2.

Prior to initiating specialized enteral nutritional support, efforts should be made to supplement food intake. Attention to patient preferences, timing of meals and diagnostic procedures and use of medications, and the use of foods brought to the hospital by family and friends can often increase oral intake. Patients unable to eat enough at regular mealtimes to meet nutritional requirements can be given **oral supplements** as snacks or to replace low-calorie beverages. Oral supplements of differing nutritional composition are available for the purpose of individualizing the diet in accordance with specific clinical requirements (see below). Fiber and lactose content, caloric density, protein level, and amino acid profiles can all be modified as necessary.

Patients unable to take adequate oral nutrients who have functioning gastrointestinal tracts and who meet the criteria for nutritional support are candidates for **tube feedings.** Small-bore feeding tubes are placed via the nose into the stomach or duodenum. Patients able to sit up in bed who can protect their airways can be fed into the stomach. Because of the increased risk of aspiration, patients who cannot adequately protect their airways should be fed nasoduodenally. Feeding tubes can usually be passed into the duodenum by leaving an extra length of tubing in the stomach and placing the patient in the right decubitus position. Metoclopramide, 10 mg intravenously, can be given 20 minutes prior to insertion and continued every 6 hours thereafter to facilitate passage through the pylorus. Occasionally patients will require fluoroscopic or endoscopic guidance to insert the tube distal to the pylorus. Placement of nasogastric and, particularly, nasoduodenal tubes should be confirmed radiographically before delivery of feeding solutions.

Feeding tubes can also be placed directly into the gastrointestinal tract using **tube enterostomies.** Most tube enterostomies are placed in patients who require long-term enteral nutritional support. Gastrostomies have the advantage of allowing bolus feedings, while jejunostomies require continuous infusions. Gastrostomies—like nasogastric feeding—should only be used in patients at low risk for aspiration. Gastrostomies can also be placed percutaneously with the aid of endoscopy. These tubes can then be advanced to jejunostomies. Tube enterostomies can also be placed surgically.

Patients who require nutritional support but whose gastrointestinal tracts are nonfunctional should receive **parenteral nutritional support.** Most patients receive parenteral feedings via a central vein—most commonly the subclavian vein. Peripheral veins can be used in some patients, but because of the high osmolality of parenteral solutions this is rarely tolerated for more than a few weeks.

Peripheral vein nutritional support is most commonly used in patients with nonfunctioning gastrointestinal tracts who require immediate support but whose clinical status is expected to improve within 1–2 weeks, allowing enteral feeding. Peripheral vein nutritional support is administered via standard intravenous lines. Solutions should always include lipid and dextrose in combination with amino acids to provide adequate nonprotein calories. Serious side effects are infrequent, but there is a high incidence of phlebitis and infiltration of intravenous lines.

Central vein nutritional support is delivered via intravenous catheters placed percutaneously using aseptic technique. Proper placement in the superior vena cava is documented radiographically before the

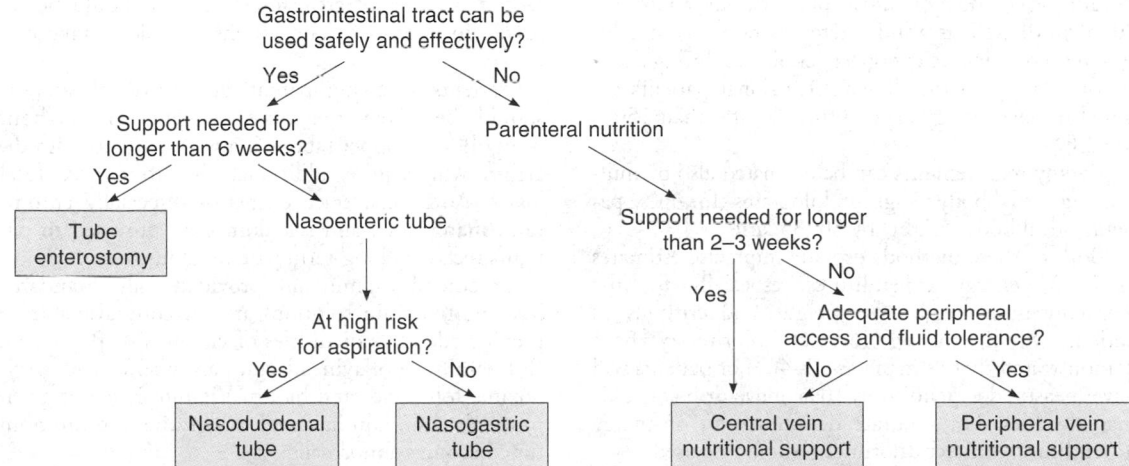

Figure 29–2. Nutritional support method decision tree.

solution is infused. Catheters must be carefully maintained by experienced nursing personnel and used solely for nutritional support to prevent infection and other catheter-related complications.

NUTRITIONAL REQUIREMENTS

Each patient's nutritional requirements should be determined independently of the method of nutritional support. In most situations, solutions of equal nutrient value can be designed for delivery via enteral and parenteral routes, but differences in absorption must be considered. A complete nutritional support solution must contain water, energy, amino acids, electrolytes, vitamins, minerals, and essential fatty acids.

Water

For most patients, water requirements can be calculated by allowing 1500 mL for the first 20 kg of body weight plus 20 mL for every kilogram over 20. Additional losses should be replaced as they occur. For average-sized adult patients, fluid needs are about 30–35 mL/kg, or approximately 1 mL/kcal of energy required (see below).

Energy

Energy requirements can be estimated by one of three methods: (1) by using standard equations to calculate resting energy expenditure (REE) plus additional calories for activity and illness; (2) by applying a simple calculation based on calories per kilogram of body weight; or (3) by measuring energy expenditure with indirect calorimetry.

Resting energy expenditure (REE) can be calculated by the **Harris-Benedict equation:** for men, REE = 666 + (13.7 × weight in kg) + (5 × height in cm) − (6.8 × age in years). For women, REE = 655 + (9.5 × weight in kg) + (1.8 × height in cm) − (4.7 × age). For undernourished patients, actual body weight should be used; and for obese patients, ideal body weight should be used. For most patients, an additional 20–50% of REE is administered as nonprotein calories to accommodate energy expenditures during activity or relating to the illness. Occasional patients are noted to have energy expenditures greater than 150% of REE.

Energy requirements can be estimated also by multiplying actual body weight in kilograms (for obese patients, ideal body weight) by 30–35 kcal.

Both of these methods provide imprecise estimates of actual energy expenditures, especially for the markedly underweight, overweight, and critically ill patient. Studies using indirect calorimetry have demonstrated that as many as 30–40% of patients will have measured expenditures 10% above or below estimated values. For accurate determination of energy expenditure, indirect calorimetry should be used.

Protein

Protein and energy requirements are closely related. If adequate calories are provided, most patients can be given 0.8–1.2 g of protein per kilogram per day. Patients undergoing moderate to severe stress should receive up to 1.5 g/kg/d. As in the case of energy requirements, actual weights should be used for normal and underweight patients and ideal weights for patients with significant obesity.

Patients who are receiving protein without adequate calories will catabolize protein for energy rather than utilizing it for protein synthesis. Thus, when energy intake is low, excess protein is needed for nitrogen balance. If both energy and protein intakes are low, extra energy will have a more significant positive effect on nitrogen balance than extra protein.

Electrolytes & Minerals

Requirements for sodium, potassium, and chloride vary widely. Most patients require 45–145 meq/d of each. The actual requirement in individual patients will depend on the patient's cardiovascular, renal, endocrine, and gastrointestinal status as well as measurements of serum concentration.

Patients receiving enteral nutritional support should receive adequate vitamins and minerals according to the recommended daily allowances (Table 29–1). Most premixed enteral solutions provide adequate vitamins and minerals as long as adequate calories are administered.

Patients receiving parenteral nutritional support require smaller amounts of minerals: calcium, 10–15 meq/d; phosphorus, 15–20 meq per 1000 nonprotein calories; and magnesium, 16–24 meq/d. Most patients receiving nutritional support do not require supplemental iron because body stores are adequate. Iron nutrition should be monitored closely by following the hemoglobin concentration, MCV, and iron studies. Parenteral administration of iron is associated with a number of adverse effects and should be reserved for iron-deficient patients unable to take oral iron.

Patients receiving parenteral nutritional support should be given the trace elements zinc (about 5 mg/d) and copper (about 2 mg/d). Patients with diarrhea will require additional zinc to replace fecal losses. Additional trace elements—especially chromium, manganese, and selenium—are provided to patients receiving long-term parenteral nutrition.

Parenteral vitamins are provided daily. Standardized multivitamin solutions are currently available to provide adequate quantities of vitamins A, B_{12}, C, D, E, thiamin, riboflavin, niacin, pantothenic acid, pyridoxine, folic acid, and biotin. Vitamin K is not given routinely but administered when the prothrombin time becomes abnormal.

Essential Fatty Acids

Patients receiving nutritional support should be given 2–4% of their total calories as linoleic acid to prevent essential fatty acid deficiency. Most prepared enteral solutions contain adequate linoleic acid. Patients receiving parenteral nutrition should be given at least 250 mL of a 20% intravenous fat (emulsified soybean or safflower oil) about two or three times a week. Intravenous fat can also be used as an energy source in place of dextrose.

ENTERAL NUTRITIONAL SUPPORT SOLUTIONS

Most patients who require enteral nutritional support can be given commercially prepared enteral solutions (Table 29–8). Nutritionally complete solutions have been designed to provide adequate proportions of water, energy, protein, and micronutrients. Nutritionally incomplete solutions are also available to provide specific macronutrients (eg, protein, carbohydrate, and fat) to supplement complete solutions for patients with unusual requirements or to design solutions that are not available commercially.

Nutritionally complete solutions are characterized as follows: (1) by osmolality (isotonic or hypertonic), (2) by lactose content (present or absent), (3) by the molecular form of the protein component (intact proteins; peptides or amino acids), (4) by the quantity of protein and calories provided, and (5) by fiber content (present or absent). For most patients, isotonic solutions containing no lactose or fiber are preferable. Such solutions generally contain moderate amounts of fat and intact protein. Most commercial isotonic solutions contain 1000 kcal and about 37–45 g of protein per liter.

Solutions containing hydrolyzed proteins or crystalline amino acids and with no significant fat content are called elemental solutions, since macronutrients are provided in their most "elemental" form. These solutions have been designed for patients with malabsorption, particularly pancreatic insufficiency and limited fat absorption. Elemental diets are extremely hypertonic and often result in more severe diarrhea. Their use should be limited to patients who cannot tolerate isotonic solutions.

Although formulas have been designed for specific clinical situations—solutions containing primarily essential amino acids (for renal failure), medium-chain triglycerides (for fat malabsorption), more fat (for respiratory failure and CO_2 retention), and more branched-chain amino acids (for hepatic encephalopathy and severe trauma)—they have not been shown to be superior to standard formulas for most patients.

Enteral solutions should be administered via continuous infusion, preferably with an infusion pump. Isotonic feedings should be started at full strength at

Table 29–8. Enteral solutions.

Complete

Blenderized (eg, Compleat Regular, Compleat Modified,[1] Vitaneed[1])

Whole protein, lactose-containing (eg, Mentene, Carnation and Delmark Instant Breakfast, Forta Shake)

Whole protein, lactose-free, low-residue:
  1 kcal/mL (eg, Ensure, Isocal, Osmolite, Nutren 1.0,[1] Nutrilan, Isolan,[1] Sustacal, Resource)
  1.5 kcal/mL (eg, Ensure Plus, Sustacal HC, Comply, Nutren 1.5, Resource Plus)
  2 kcal/mL (eg, Isocal HCN, Magnacal, TwoCal HN)
  High-nitrogen: > 15% total calories from protein (eg, Ensure HN, Attain,[1] Osmolite HN,[1] Replete, Entrition HN,[1] Isolan,[1] Isocal HN,[1] Sustacal HC, Isosource HN,[1] Ultralan)

Whole protein, lactose-free, high-residue:
  1 kcal/mL (eg, Jevity,[1] Profiber,[1] Nutren 1.0 with fiber,[1] Fiberian,[1] Sustacal with fiber, Ultracal,[1] Ensure with fiber, Fibersource)

Chemically defined peptide- or amino acid-based (eg, Accupep HPF, Criticare HN, Peptamen,[1] Reabfin, Vital HN, AlitraQ, Tolerex, Vivonex TEN)

"Disease-specific" formulas

Renal failure: with essential amino acids (eg, Amin-Aid, Travasorb Renal, Aminess)

Malabsorption: with medium-chain triglycerides (eg, Portagen,[1] Travasorb MCT)

Respiratory failure: with > 50% calories from fat (eg, Pulmocare, NutriVent)

Hepatic encephalopathy: with high amounts of branched-chain amino acids (eg, Hepatic-Acid II, Travasorb Hepatic)

Incomplete (modular)

Protein (eg, Nutrisource Protein, Promed, Propac)

Carbohydrate (eg, Nutrisource Carbohydrate, Polycose, Sumacal)

Fat (eg, MCT Oil, Microlipid, Nutrisource Lipid)

Vitamins (eg, Nutrisource Vitamins)

Minerals (eg, Nutrisource Minerals)

[1]Isotonic.

about 25–33% of the estimated final infusion rate. Feedings can be advanced by similar amounts every 12 hours as tolerated. Hypertonic feedings should be started at half strength. The strength and the rate can then be advanced every 6 hours as tolerated.

COMPLICATIONS OF ENTERAL NUTRITIONAL SUPPORT

Minor complications of tube feedings occur in 10–15% of patients. Gastrointestinal complications include diarrhea (most common), inadequate gastric emptying, emesis, esophagitis, and occasionally gastrointestinal bleeding. Diarrhea associated with tube feeding may be due to intolerance to the osmotic load or to one of the macronutrients (eg, fat, lactose) in the solution. Patients being fed in this way may also have diarrhea from other causes (as side effect of antibiotics or other drugs; associated with infection, etc), and these possibilities should always be investigated in appropriate circumstances.

Mechanical complications of tube feedings are potentially the most serious. Of particular importance is aspiration. All patients receiving nasogastric tube feedings are at risk for this life-threatening complication. Limiting nasogastric feedings to those patients who can adequately protect their airway and careful monitoring of patients being fed by tube should limit these serious complications to 1–2% of cases. Minor mechanical complications are common and include tube obstruction and dislodgment.

Metabolic complications during enteral nutritional support are common but in most cases easily managed. The most important problem is hypernatremic dehydration, most commonly seen in elderly patients given excessive protein intake who are unable to respond to thirst. Abnormalities of potassium, glucose, and acid-base balance may also occur.

PARENTERAL NUTRITIONAL SUPPORT SOLUTIONS

Parenteral nutritional support solutions can be designed to deliver adequate nutrients to virtually any patient. The basic parenteral solution is composed of dextrose, amino acids, and water. Electrolytes, minerals, trace elements, vitamins, and medications can also be added. Most commercial solutions contain the monohydrate form of dextrose that provides 3.4 kcal/g. Crystalline amino acids are available in a variety of concentrations, so that a broad range of solutions can be made up that will contain specific amounts of dextrose and amino acids as required.

Typical solutions for central vein nutritional support contain 25–35% dextrose and 2.75–6% amino acids depending upon the patient's estimated nutrient and water requirements. These solutions typically have osmolalities in excess of 1800 mosm/L and require infusion into a central vein. A typical formula for patients without organ failure is shown in Table 29–9.

Solutions with lower osmolalities can also be designed for infusion into peripheral veins. Typical solutions for peripheral infusion contain 5–10% dextrose and 2.75–4.25% amino acids. These solutions have osmolalities between 800 and 1200 mosm/L and result in a high incidence of thrombophlebitis and line infiltration. These solutions will provide adequate protein for most patients but inadequate energy. Additional energy must be provided in the form of emulsified soybean or safflower oil. Such intravenous fat solutions are currently available in 10% and 25% solutions providing 1.1 and 2.2 kcal/mL, respectively. Intravenous fat solutions are isosmotic and well tolerated by peripheral veins. Typical patients are given 200–500 mL of a

Table 29–9. Typical solution (for stable patients without organ failure).

Dextrose (3.4 kcal/g)	25%
Amino acids (4 kcal/g)	6%
Na^+	50 meq/L
K^+	40 meq/L
Ca^{2+}	5 meq/L
Mg^{2+}	8 meq/L
Cl^-	60 meq/L
P	12 meg/L
Acetate	Balance
MVI-12 (vitamins)	10 mL/d
MTE (trace elements)	5 mL/d
Fat emulsion 20%	250 mL 5 times a week
Typical rate	Day 1: 30 mL/h
	Day 2: 60 mL/h
By day 2, solution provides:	Calories: 1925 kcal total
	Protein: 86 g
	Fat: 19% of total kcal
	Fluid: 1690 mL

20% solution each day. As much as 60% of total calories can be administered in this manner.

Intravenous fat can also be provided to patients receiving central vein nutritional support. In this instance, dextrose concentrations should be decreased to provide a fixed concentration of energy. Intravenous fat has been shown to be equivalent to intravenous dextrose in providing energy to spare protein. Intravenous fat is associated with less glucose intolerance, less production of carbon dioxide, and less fatty infiltration of the liver and has been increasingly utilized in patients with hyperglycemia, respiratory failure, and liver disease. Intravenous fat has also been increasingly used in patients with large estimated energy requirements. Recent studies suggest that the maximum glucose utilization rate is approximately 5–7 mg/min/kg. Patients who require additional calories can be given them as fat to prevent excess administration of dextrose. Intravenous fat can also be used to prevent essential fatty acid deficiency. The optimal ratio of carbohydrate and fat in parenteral nutritional support has not been determined.

Infusion of parenteral solutions should be started slowly to prevent hyperglycemia and other metabolic complications. Typical solutions are given initially at a rate of 50 mL/h and advanced by about the same amount every 24 hours until the desired final rate is reached.

COMPLICATIONS OF PARENTERAL NUTRITIONAL SUPPORT

Complications of central vein nutritional support occur in up to 50% of patients. Although most are minor and easily managed, about 5% of patients will develop significant complications. Complications of central vein nutritional support can be divided into catheter-related complications and metabolic complications.

Catheter-related complications can occur during insertion or while the catheter is in place. Pneumothorax, hemothorax, arterial laceration, air emboli, and brachial plexus injury can occur during catheter placement. The incidence of these complications is inversely related to the experience of the physician performing the procedure but will occur in at least 1–2% of cases even in major medical centers. Each catheter placement should be documented by chest radiograph prior to initiation of nutritional support.

Catheter thrombosis and catheter-related sepsis are the most important complications of indwelling catheters. Patients with indwelling central vein catheters who develop fever without an apparent source should have their lines changed over a wire or removed immediately, the tip quantitatively cultured, and antibiotics begun empirically. Quantitative tip cultures and blood cultures will help guide further antibiotic therapy. Catheter-related sepsis occurs in 2–3% of patients even if maximal efforts are made to prevent infection.

Metabolic complications of central vein nutritional support occur in over 50% of patients (Table 29–10). Most are minor and easily managed, and termination of support is seldom necessary.

PATIENT MONITORING DURING NUTRITIONAL SUPPORT

Every patient receiving enteral or parenteral nutritional support should be followed closely. Formal nutritional support teams composed of a physician, a nurse, a dietitian, and a pharmacist have been shown to decrease the rate of complications.

Patients should be monitored both for the adequacy of treatment and to prevent complications or detect them early when they occur. Because estimates of nutritional requirements are imprecise, frequent reassessment is necessary. Daily intakes should be recorded and compared with estimated requirements. Body weight, hydration status, and overall clinical status should be followed. Patients who do not appear to be responding as anticipated can be evaluated for nitrogen balance by means of the following equation:

$$\text{Nitrogen balance} = \frac{\dfrac{24\text{-hour protein}}{\text{intake (g)}}}{6.25} - \left(\dfrac{25\text{-hour urinary}}{\text{nitrogen (g)}} + 4\right)$$

Patients with positive nitrogen balances can be continued on their current regimens; patients with negative balances should receive moderate increases in calorie and protein intake and then be reassessed.

Monitoring for metabolic complications includes daily measurements of electrolytes; serum glucose,

Table 29–10. Metabolic complications of parenteral nutritional support.

Complication	Common Causes	Possible Solutions
Hyperglycemia	Too rapid infusion of dextrose, "stress," glucocorticoids	Decrease glucose infusion. Insulin. Replacement of dextrose with fat.
Hyperosmolar nonketotic dehydration	Severe, undetected hyperglycemia	Insulin, hydration, potassium
Hyperchloremic metabolic acidosis	High chloride administration	Decrease chloride
Azotemia	Excessive protein administration	Decrease amino acid concentration
Hyperphosphatemia, hypokalemia, hypomagnesemia	Extracellular to intracellular shifting with refeeding	Increase solution concentration
Liver enzyme abnormalities	Lipid trapping in hepatocytes, fatty liver	Decrease dextrose
Acalculous cholecystitis	Biliary stasis	Oral fat
Zinc deficiency	Diarrhea, small bowel fistulas	Increase concentration
Copper deficiency	Biliary fistulas	Increase concentration

phosphorus, magnesium, calcium, and creatinine; and BUN until the patient is stabilized. Once the patient is stabilized, electrolytes, phosphorus, calcium, magnesium, and glucose should be obtained at least twice weekly. Red blood cell folate, zinc, and copper should be checked at least once a month.

Barrera R et al: Outcome of direct percutaneous endoscopic jejunostomy tube placement for nutritional support in critically ill, mechanically ventilated patients. Crit Care 2001; 16:178. [PMID: 11815903] (Direct percutaneous endoscopic jejunostomy placement is a safe and reliable procedure for critically ill mechanically ventilated patients. With this procedure, all patients can meet their nutritional requirements and eliminate the need for TPN.)

Beattie AH et al: A randomised controlled trial evaluating the use of enteral nutritional supplements postoperatively in malnourished surgical patients. Gut 2000;46:813. [PMID: 10807893] (Oral nutritional supplements reduced weight loss and the need for antibiotics in postoperative patients with evidence of malnutrition.)

Deitch EA et al: Prevention of multiple organ failure. Surg Clin North Am 1999;79:1471. [PMID: 10625989] (Despite lack of clinical trial evidence, early nutritional support may be useful in preventing multiple organ failure in high risk patients.)

Ferreira IM et al: Nutritional support for individuals with COPD: a meta-analysis. Chest 2000;117:672. [PMID: 10712990] (Nutritional support had no effect on improving anthropometric measures, lung function, or functional exercise capacity among patients with stable COPD.)

Finck C: How to provide nutritional support. Nutrition 2000;16:155. [PMID: 10696646]

Hasselgren PO: Burns and metabolism. J Am Coll Surg 1999;188:98. [PMID: 10024150]

Heyland DK et al: Should immunonutrition become routine in critically ill patients? A systematic review of the evidence. JAMA 2001;286:944. [PMID: 11509059] (Overall, no difference in mortality was noted among patients fed enterally with formulas containing immuno-modulating nutrients. Arginine-containing formulas, however, led to a decrease in infectious complications and a trend toward lower mortality.)

Heyland DK: Nutritional support in the critically ill patient. A critical review of the evidence. Crit Care Clin 1998;14:423. [PMID: 9700440]

Jensen GL: Hypoenergetic nutrition support in hospitalized obese patients: A simplified method for clinical application. J Parenter Enteral Nutr 1997;21:366. [PMID: 9406137] (Hypocaloric feedings can be used in obese patients who require nutritional support.)

Kearns PJ et al: The incidence of ventilator-associated pneumonia and success in nutrient delivery with gastric versus small intestinal feeding: a randomized clinical trial. Crit Care Med 2000;28:1742. [PMID: 10890612] (No difference in the incidence of pneumonia among ventilated patients receiving small-intestinal versus gastric feeding.)

Klein GL: Metabolic bone disease of total parenteral nutrition. Nutrition 1998;14:149. [PMID: 9437701] (The true incidence of parenteral nutrition-related metabolic bone disease remains unknown.)

Klein S et al: Nutrition support in clinical practice: A review of published data and recommendations for future research directions. National Institute of Health, American Society for Parenteral and Enteral Nutrition, and the American Society for Clinical Nutrition. J Parenter Enteral Nutr 1997; 21:133. [PMID: 9280194] (Extensive panel report on nutrition assessment, nutrition support in gastrointestinal diseases, nutrition support in wasting diseases, nutrition support in critically ill patients, and perioperative nutrition support.)

Mahesh C et al: Extended indications for enteral nutritional support. Nutrition 2000;16:129. [PMID: 10696637] (Enteral nutrition can be given to many patients who otherwise would have received parenteral nutrition.)

Mathus-Vliegen LM et al: Percutaneous endoscopic gastrostomy and gastrojejunostomy: a critical reappraisal of patient selection, tube function and the feasibility of nutritional support during extended follow-up. Gastrointest Endosc 1999;50: 746. [PMID: 10570331] (Clinical outcomes in 286 patients referred for percutaneous endoscopic gastrostomy.)

Rudberg MA et al: Effectiveness of feeding tubes in nursing home residents with swallowing disorders. JPEN J Parenter Enteral Nutr 2000;24:97. [PMID: 10772189] (Tube feeding can be life-prolonging, but the gain is not substantial.)

Wilmore DW: Nutrition and metabolic support in the 21st century. JPEN J Parenter Enteral Nutr 2000;24:1. [PMID: 10638464] (Recommends greater use of the enteral route for nutrient delivery, reductions in exogenous calories, utilization of nutrients for their pharmacologic effects, use of growth factors to enhance nutrient efficacy, and institution of nutritional supplementation before elective surgery.)

Zaloga GP: Early enteral nutritional support improves outcome: hypothesis or fact? Crit Care Med 1999;27:259. [PMID: 10075044]

General Problems in Infectious Diseases

30

Richard A. Jacobs, MD, PhD

See www.current-med.com/ch30.html

Most infections are confined to specific organ systems. In a book such as this—arranged principally by organ system—many of the important infectious disease entities are discussed in chapters dealing with specific anatomic areas. In this chapter are discussed some important general problems related to infectious diseases that are not covered elsewhere.

FEVER OF UNKNOWN ORIGIN (FUO)

To fulfill the original criteria for FUO as set forth in 1961, a patient must have an illness of at least 3 weeks' duration, fever over 38.3 °C on several occasions, and must remain undiagnosed after 1 week of study in the hospital. The intervals specified are arbitrary ones intended to exclude patients with protracted but self-limited viral illnesses and to allow time for the usual radiographic, serologic, and cultural studies to be performed. Because of concerns over costs of hospitalization and the availability of most screening tests on an outpatient basis, the criterion requiring 1 week of hospitalization has been modified to accept patients who remain undiagnosed after three outpatient visits or 3 days of hospitalization.

Over the ensuing decades, several additional categories of FUO have been added: (1) Nosocomial FUO refers to the hospitalized patient with fever of 38.3 °C or higher on several occasions, due to a process not present or incubating at the time of admission, in whom initial cultures are negative and the diagnosis remains unknown after 3 days of investigation (see Nosocomial Infections, below). (2) Neutropenic FUO includes patients with fever of 38.3 °C or higher on several occasions with less than 500 neutrophils per milliliter in whom initial cultures are negative and the diagnosis remains uncertain after 3 days (see Chapter 4 and Infections in the Immunocompromised Patient, below). (3) HIV-associated FUO refers to HIV-positive patients with fever of 38.3 °C or higher who have been febrile for 4 weeks or more as an outpatient or 3 days as an inpatient, in whom the diagnosis remains uncertain after 3 days of investigation with at least 2 days for cultures to incubate (see Chapter 31). Al-

though not usually considered a separate group, FUO in solid organ transplant recipients is a common scenario with a unique differential diagnosis and is discussed below.

For a general discussion of fever, see the section on fever and hyperthermia in Chapter 1.

Etiologic Considerations

Certain general principles about FUO should be kept in mind in the diagnostic approach to these patients.

A. COMMON CAUSES

Most cases represent unusual manifestations of common diseases and not rare or exotic diseases—ie, tuberculosis, endocarditis, gallbladder disease, and HIV (primary infection or opportunistic infection) are more common causes of FUO than Whipple's disease or familial Mediterranean fever.

B. AGE OF PATIENT

In adults, infections (25–40% of cases) and cancer (25–40% of cases) account for the majority of FUOs. In children, infections are the most common cause of FUO (30–50% of cases) and cancer a rare cause (5–10% of cases). Autoimmune disorders occur with equal frequency in adults and children (10–20% of cases), but the diseases differ. Juvenile rheumatoid arthritis is particularly common in children, whereas systemic lupus erythematosus, Wegener's granulomatosis, and polyarteritis nodosa are more common in adults. Adult Still's disease, giant cell arteritis, and polymyalgia rheumatica occur exclusively in adults.

C. DURATION OF FEVER

The cause of FUO changes dramatically in patients who have been febrile for a prolonged period of time—ie, 6 months or longer. Infection, cancer, and autoimmune disorders combined account for only 20% of FUOs in these patients. Instead, other entities such as granulomatous diseases (granulomatous hepatitis, Crohn's disease, ulcerative colitis) and factitious fever become important causes. Up to 27% of patients who say they have been febrile for 6 months or longer actually have no true fever or underlying disease. Instead, the usual normal circadian variation in temperature (temperature 1–2 °C higher in the afternoon than in the morning) is interpreted as abnormal. Patients with episodic or recurrent fever (ie, those who meet the classic criteria for FUO but have fever-free periods of 2 weeks or longer) are similar to patients with prolonged fever. Infection, malignancy, and autoimmune disorders account for only 20–25% of such fevers, whereas various miscellaneous diseases (Crohn's disease, familial Mediterranean fever, allergic alveolitis) account for another 25%. Approximately 50% remain undiagnosed but have a benign course with eventual resolution of symptoms.

D. Immunologic Status

In the neutropenic patient, fungal infections and occult bacterial infection are important and common causes of FUO. In the patient taking immunosuppressive medications (particularly organ transplant patients), cytomegalovirus infections are a frequent cause of fever, as are fungal infections, nocardiosis, *Pneumocystis carinii* pneumonia, and mycobacterial infections.

E. Classification of Causes of FUO

Most patients with FUO will fit into one of five categories.

1. Infection—Both systemic and localized infections can cause FUO. Tuberculosis and endocarditis are the most common systemic infections, but mycoses, viral diseases (particularly infection with Epstein-Barr virus and cytomegalovirus), toxoplasmosis, brucellosis, Q fever, cat-scratch disease, salmonellosis, malaria, and many other less common infections have been implicated. Primary infection with human immunodeficiency virus (HIV) or opportunistic infections associated with the acquired immunodeficiency syndrome (AIDS)—particularly mycobacterial infections—can also present as FUO. The most common form of localized infection causing FUO is an occult abscess. Liver, spleen, kidney, brain, and bone are organs in which abscess may be difficult to find. A collection of pus may form in the peritoneal cavity or in the subdiaphragmatic, subhepatic, paracolic, or other areas. Cholangitis, osteomyelitis, urinary tract infection, dental abscess, or a collection of pus in a paranasal sinus may cause prolonged fever.

2. Neoplasms—Many cancers can present as FUO. The most common are lymphoma (both Hodgkin's and non-Hodgkin's) and leukemia. Other diseases of lymph nodes, such as angioimmunoblastic lymphoma and Castleman's disease, can also cause FUO. Primary and metastatic tumors of the liver also are frequently associated with fever, as are renal cell carcinomas. Atrial myxoma is an often forgotten neoplasm that can result in fever. Chronic lymphocytic leukemia and multiple myeloma are rarely associated with fever, and the presence of fever in patients with these diseases should prompt a careful search for infection.

3. Autoimmune disorders—Still's disease, systemic lupus erythematosus, cryoglobulinemia, and polyarteritis nodosa are the most common autoimmune causes of FUO. Giant cell arteritis and polymyalgia rheumatica are seen almost exclusively in patients over 50 years of age and are nearly always associated with an elevated erythrocyte sedimentation rate (> 40 mm/h).

4. Miscellaneous causes—Many other diseases have been associated with FUO but less commonly than the foregoing types of illness. Examples include hyperthyroidism, thyroiditis, sarcoidosis, Whipple's disease, familial Mediterranean fever, recurrent pulmonary emboli, alcoholic hepatitis, drug fever, factitious fever, and others.

5. Undiagnosed FUO—Despite extensive evaluation, in 10–15% of patients the diagnosis remains elusive. In about three-fourths of these patients, the fever abates spontaneously and the clinician never knows the cause; in the remainder, more classic manifestations of the underlying disease appear over time, and the diagnosis then becomes obvious.

Approach to Diagnosis of FUO

Because the evaluation of a patient with FUO is so costly and time-consuming, it is imperative to document the presence of fever. This is done most reliably by observing the patient while the temperature is being taken to make certain that fever is not factitious (self-induced). Associated findings that usually accompany fever include tachycardia, chills, and piloerection. A thorough history—including family, occupational, social (sexual practices, use of intravenous drugs), dietary (unpasteurized products, raw meat), exposures (animals, chemicals), and travel histories—may give clues to the underlying diagnosis. Detailed and repeated physical examination may reveal subtle, evanescent clinical findings that are the key to diagnosis.

In addition to routine laboratory studies, blood cultures should always be obtained, preferably when the patient has been off antibiotics for several days, and should be held by the laboratory for 2 weeks to detect slow-growing organisms. Cultures on special media should be requested if legionella, bartonella, or nutritionally deficient streptococci are considered possible pathogens. "Screening tests" with immunologic or microbiologic serologies ("febrile agglutinins") are of low yield and should not be done. Specific serologic tests are helpful if the history or physical examination suggests a specific diagnosis. A single elevated titer rarely allows one to make a diagnosis of infection; instead, one must demonstrate a fourfold rise or fall in titer to confirm a specific infectious cause. Because infection is the most common cause of FUO, other body fluids are usually cultured, ie, urine, sputum, stool, cerebrospinal fluid, and morning gastric aspirates (if one suspects tuberculosis). Direct examination of blood smears may establish a diagnosis of malaria or relapsing fever (borrelia).

All patients with FUO should have a chest radiograph. Other studies such as sinus films, upper gastrointestinal series with small bowel follow-through, barium enema, proctosigmoidoscopy, and evaluation of gallbladder function are low-yield when performed as screening tests and should be reserved for patients who have symptoms, signs, or a history that suggest disease in these body regions. CT scan of the abdomen and pelvis is also frequently performed and can be quite useful in evaluating patients with FUO. It is particularly useful for looking at the liver, spleen, and retroperitoneum. When the CT scan is positive, the findings are usually confirmed and often lead to a specific diagnosis. It is important to realize that a negative CT scan is not quite as useful; even with a negative CT scan, more invasive procedures such as biopsy or exploratory laparotomy may lead to the diagnosis. The role of MRI in the investigation of FUO has not been evaluated. In general, however, MRI is better than CT for detecting lesions of the nervous system. Ultrasound is very sensitive for detecting lesions of the kidney, pancreas, and biliary tree. Echocardiography should be used if one is considering endocarditis or atrial myxoma. Transesophageal echocardiography is more sensitive than surface echocardiography for detecting valvular lesions, but even a negative transesophageal study does not exclude endocarditis (10% false-negative rate). The usefulness of radionuclide studies has not been extensively studied in FUO. Theoretically, a gallium scan would be more helpful than an indium-labeled white blood cell scan, because gallium is useful for detecting infection and neoplasm whereas the indium scan is useful only for detecting infection. Indium-labeled immunoglobulin is another radionuclide study that may prove to be useful in detecting infection and neoplasm and can be used in the neutropenic patient. It is not sensitive for lesions of the liver, kidney, and heart because of high background activity. Although not extensively studied, positron emission tomography (PET scan) may prove useful in diagnosis. In general, radionuclide scans are plagued by high rates of false-positive and false-negative results that are not useful when used as screening tests and, if used at all, should be limited to those patients whose history or examination suggests local inflammation or infection.

Invasive procedures are often required for diagnosis. Any abnormal finding should be aggressively evaluated: headache calls for lumbar puncture to rule out meningitis; skin from an area of rash should be biopsied to look for cutaneous manifestations of collagen vascular disease or infection; and enlarged lymph nodes should be aspirated or biopsied and examined for cytologic features to rule out neoplasm and sent for culture. Bone marrow aspiration with biopsy is a relatively low-yield procedure (except in HIV-positive patients, in whom mycobacterial infection is a common cause of FUO and bone marrow biopsy a high-yield

procedure), but the risk is low and the procedure should be done if other less invasive tests have not yielded a diagnosis. Liver biopsy will yield a specific diagnosis in 10–15% of patients with FUO. One should consider this procedure in any patient with abnormal liver function tests even if the liver is normal in size on physical examination. The role of exploratory laparotomy is debatable. Studies on the usefulness of laparotomy in the diagnosis of FUO have not been done since the advent of CT scanning and MRI. One should consider laparotomy or laparoscopy in the deteriorating patient if the diagnosis is elusive despite extensive evaluation.

Therapeutic Trials

Therapeutic trials are indicated if a diagnosis is strongly suspected—eg, it is reasonable to give antituberculous drugs if one suspects tuberculosis, or tetracycline if brucellosis is suspected. However, if there is no clinical response in several weeks, it is imperative to stop therapy and reevaluate the situation. In the seriously ill or rapidly deteriorating patient, empirical therapy is often given. Antituberculosis medications (particularly in the elderly or foreign-born) and broad-spectrum antibiotics are reasonable in this setting.

Empirical use of corticosteroids should be discouraged; these agents can suppress fever if given in high enough doses, but they can also exacerbate many infections, and infection remains a leading cause of FUO. Suppression of fever with low doses of nonsteroidal anti-inflammatory agents (eg, naproxen, 250 mg twice daily) has been reported to be specific for fever associated with malignancy, but published data are limited.

Davies GR et al: Fever of unknown origin. Clin Med 2001;1:177. [PMID: 11446608] (Diagnosis, etiology, and outcomes.)

INFECTIONS IN THE IMMUNOCOMPROMISED PATIENT

A description of the cellular basis of immune response, the role of various host responses in maintaining health, and the methods used for detection of deficiencies in the immune system can be found in Chapter 19.

Compromised hosts are individuals who have one or more defects in their natural defense mechanisms that put them at an increased risk of developing infections. Not only is the risk of infection greater in these individuals, but once infection develops it is often severe, rapidly progressive, and can be life-threatening. In addition, microorganisms that are not usually pathogens in the noncompromised patient may cause serious disease in the compromised patient. Individuals are most commonly compromised because of dysfunction of their immune system (granulocytopenia, T and B cell deficiency, hypogammaglobulinemia), but the presence of coexisting illness can also predispose to infection.

Granulocytopenia is common following bone marrow transplantation—as a result of myelosuppressive chemotherapy—and in acute leukemias. The risk of infection begins to increase when the absolute granulocyte count falls below 1000/μL, with a dramatic increase in frequency and severity when the granulocyte count falls below 100/μL. The granulocytopenic patient is particularly susceptible to infections with gram-negative enteric organisms, pseudomonas, gram-positive cocci (particularly *Staphylococcus aureus* and *Staphylococcus epidermidis*), candida, aspergillus, and other fungi that have recently emerged as pathogens such as trichosporon, scedosporium, fusarium, and pseudallescheria.

Defects in humoral immunity are often congenital, though hypogammaglobulinemia can occur in multiple myeloma and chronic lymphocytic leukemia. Patients with defects in humoral immunity lack opsonizing antibodies and are at particular risk of infection with encapsulated organisms such as *Haemophilus influenzae* and *Streptococcus pneumoniae*.

Patients with cellular immune deficiency encompass a large and rather heterogeneous group that includes patients with HIV infection (see Chapter 31), those with lymphoreticular malignancies such as Hodgkin's disease (which is associated with dysfunction of cellular immunity), and patients receiving immunosuppressive medications such as corticosteroids, cyclosporine, azathioprine, and other cytotoxic drugs. This latter group—immunosuppressed as a result of medications—includes transplant patients, many solid tumor patients receiving therapy, and patients receiving prolonged high-dose corticosteroid treatment (for asthma, temporal arteritis, systemic lupus, etc). Patients with cellular immune dysfunction are susceptible to infections by a large number of organisms, particularly ones that replicate intracellularly. Examples include bacteria such as listeria, legionella, salmonella, and mycobacterium; viruses such as herpes simplex, varicella, and cytomegalovirus; fungi such as cryptococcus, coccidioides, histoplasma, and pneumocystis; and protozoa such as toxoplasma.

Patients who are functionally or anatomically asplenic fail to clear organisms from the bloodstream and are at an increased risk of overwhelming bacteremia with encapsulated bacteria (primarily *S pneumoniae* but also *H influenzae* and *Neisseria meningitidis*).

Finally, a large group of patients who are not classically immunodeficient are at increased risk of infection because of debilitating injury (eg, burns or severe trauma), invasive procedures (eg, hyperalimentation lines, Foley catheters, dialysis catheters), central nervous system dysfunction (which predisposes to aspiration pneumonia and decubitus ulcers), the presence of obstructing lesions (eg, pneumonia due to an obstructed bronchus, pyelonephritis due to nephrolithiasis, cholangitis secondary to cholelithiasis), and use of broad-spectrum antibiotics.

Despite the generalizations made above about the relationship between type of immunosuppression and likely pathogen, it is important to remember that any pathogen can occur in any immunosuppressed patient at any time. Thus, a systematic evaluation to identify a specific organism is required.

Organisms not usually considered pathogens in the noncompromised patient may cause serious life-threatening infection in the compromised patient (eg, *S epidermidis, Corynebacterium jeikeium, Propionibacterium acnes,* bacillus species). Therefore, one must interpret culture results with caution and not disregard isolates as mere contaminants. A contaminating organism in the immunocompetent patient may be a pathogen in the immunocompromised one.

Approach to Diagnosis

Not all fevers are due to infection. Transplant rejection, organ ischemia and necrosis, thrombophlebitis, and lymphoma may all present as fever and must be considered in the differential diagnosis.

Because infections in the immunocompromised patient can be rapidly progressive and life-threatening, diagnostic procedures must be done promptly, and empirical therapy is often instituted before a specific diagnostic agent has been isolated:

(1) Routine evaluation includes complete blood count with differential, chest x-ray, and blood cultures; urine and sputum cultures should be obtained if indicated clinically or radiographically. Any focal complaints (localized pain, headache, rash) should prompt a thorough evaluation and cultures appropriate to the site.

(2) Because the types of organisms causing infection are so varied in the immunosuppressed patient, if a source of infection is identified every effort should be made to obtain specimens that may lead to a specific microbial diagnosis.

(3) Patients who remain febrile without an obvious source should be evaluated for viral infection (cytomegalovirus blood cultures or antigen test), abscesses (which usually occur near previous operative sites), systemic candidiasis that involves the liver or spleen, or aspergillosis. Serologic evaluation may be helpful if toxoplasmosis is a possible pathogen.

(4) Consider special diagnostic procedures. The cause of pulmonary infiltrates can be easily determined with simple techniques in some situations—eg, induced sputum yields a diagnosis of pneumocystis pneumonia in 50–80% of AIDS patients with this infection. In other situations, more invasive procedures may be required (bronchoalveolar lavage, transbronchial biopsy, or even open lung biopsy). Other procedures such as skin, liver, or bone marrow biopsy may be helpful in establishing a diagnosis.

(5) In patients who have undergone solid organ transplants, immediate postoperative infections often involve the transplanted organ. Following lung transplantation, pneumonia and mediastinitis are particularly common; following liver transplantation, intra-abdominal abscess, cholangitis, and peritonitis are common; following renal transplantation, urinary tract infections, perinephric abscesses, and infected lymphoceles can occur. In contrast to solid organ transplants, in bone marrow transplant patients the source of fever cannot be found in 60–70% of patients.

(6) The time of occurrence of infection, particularly following solid organ transplantation, can be helpful in determining the infectious origin. Most infections that occur in the first 2–4 weeks posttransplant are related to the operative procedure and to hospitalization itself (wound infection, intravenous catheter infection, urinary tract infection from a Foley catheter) or are related to the transplanted organ (see paragraph [5], above). Infections that occur between the first and sixth months are often related to immunosuppression. During this period, reactivation of viruses occurs, and herpes simplex, varicella-zoster, and CMV infections are quite common. Opportunistic infections with fungi (candida, aspergillus, cryptococcus, pneumocystis, and others), *Listeria monocytogenes,* nocardia, and toxoplasma are also common. After 6 months, when immunosuppression has been reduced to maintenance levels, common infections that are found in any population occur.

Prevention of Infection

There is great interest in preventing infection with prophylactic antimicrobial regimens, but there is no uniformity of opinion about what the optimal drugs or dosage regimens should be.

Trimethoprim-sulfamethoxazole (TMP-SMZ), one double-strength tablet three times a week, one double-strength tablet twice daily on weekends, or one single-strength tablet daily for 3–6 months, is frequently used to prevent pneumocystis infections in transplant patients. It may also decrease the incidence of bacterial pneumonia, urinary tract infections, nocardia infections, and toxoplasmosis. In patients allergic to trimethoprim-sulfamethoxazole, aerosolized pentamidine is used in a dosage of 300 mg once a month. Dapsone, 50 mg daily or 100 mg three times weekly, can also be used. (G6PD levels should be determined before therapy is instituted.) Acyclovir has been shown to be effective in preventing herpes simplex infections in bone marrow and solid organ transplant recipients and is given to seropositive patient who are not receiving acyclovir or ganciclovir for CMV prophylaxis. The usual dose is 200 mg orally three times daily for 4 weeks (bone marrow transplants) to 12 weeks (other solid organ transplants).

Prevention of CMV is more difficult, and no uniformly accepted approach has been adopted. Prevention strategies often depend on the serologic status of the donor and recipient and the organ transplanted, which determines the level of immunosuppression after transplant. In solid organ transplants (liver, kidney, heart, lung), the greatest risk of developing CMV disease is in seronegative patients who receive organs from seropositive donors. These high-risk patients usually receive ganciclovir, 2.5–5 mg/kg intravenously twice daily, during hospitalization (usually about 10 days) and then are placed on a regimen of oral ganciclovir, 1 g three times daily, for 3 months. Other solid organ transplant recipients (seropositive recipients) are at lower risk for developing CMV disease and usually receive intravenous ganciclovir while in the hospital followed by either high-dose oral acyclovir at a dosage of 800 mg four times daily or oral ganciclovir for 3 months. Both ganciclovir and acyclovir prevent herpesvirus reactivation. Because immunosuppression is increased during periods of rejection, patients treated for rejection usually receive intravenous ganciclovir during rejection therapy.

Recipients of bone marrow transplants are more severely immunosuppressed than recipients of solid organ transplants, are at greater risk for developing serious CMV infection, and thus usually receive more aggressive prophylaxis. Two approaches have been used: universal prophylaxis or preemptive therapy. In the former, all at-risk patients (seropositive patients or seronegative patients with seropositive donors) received 5 mg/kg of intravenous ganciclovir every 12 hours for a week, followed by 5 mg/kg once daily for 5 days each week to day 100. Although effective in preventing infection and disease, this method is costly and associated with significant toxicity and is therefore being used less frequently. Alternatively, patients can be followed without specific therapy and have blood sampled weekly for the presence of CMV. If CMV is detected by an antigenemia assay, preemptive therapy with ganciclovir is given (5 mg/kg intravenously twice daily for 7–14 days, followed by 5 mg/kg daily for 5 days each week for the first 100 days after transplantation). This approach is effective but does miss a small number of patients who subsequently develop CMV disease. Other preventive strategies include use of CMV-negative or leukocyte-depleted blood products for CMV-seronegative recipients.

Routine decontamination of the gastrointestinal tract to prevent bacteremia in the neutropenic patient is not recommended. Prophylactic administration of antibiotics in the afebrile, asymptomatic neutropenic patient is controversial, though many centers have adopted this strategy. Rates of bacteremia are decreased, but overall mortality is not affected and emergence of resistant organisms is a common problem. Use of intravenous immunoglobulin is reserved for the small number of patients with severe hypogammaglobulinemia following bone marrow transplantation and should not be routinely administered to all transplant patients.

Prophylaxis with antifungal agents to prevent invasive mold infections (primarily aspergillus) is routinely used, but the optimal agent, dose, and duration have not been standardized. Moderate-dose (0.5 mg/kg/d) and low-dose (0.1–0.25 mg/kg/d) amphotericin B, liposomal preparations of amphotericin B, aerosolized amphotericin B, and itraconazole (capsules and solution) have all been used with varying success in the neutropenic patient. In solid organ transplant recipients, the risk of invasive fungal infection varies considerably (1–2% in liver, pancreas, and kidney transplants and 6–8% in heart and lung transplants). Whether universal prophylaxis or careful observation with preemptive therapy is the best approach has not been determined. Although fluconazole is effective in preventing yeast infections, emergence of resistant strains of *Candida krusei,* other candida species, and molds (fusarium, aspergillus, mucor) has raised concerns about its routine use as a prophylactic agent.

Hand washing is the simplest and most effective means of decreasing nosocomial infections in *all* patients, especially the compromised host. Invasive devices such as central and peripheral lines and Foley catheters are a potential source of infection. The need for these devices should be continually assessed and their use discontinued at the earliest possible time.

Approach to Treatment

In addition to providing antimicrobial therapy, it is important to improve host defenses whenever possible, correct electrolyte imbalances, and maintain adequate nutrition. Because immunosuppression is often the reason for infection, it is important to decrease immunosuppressive medications even in organ transplant patients. Reduction or discontinuation of immunosuppressive medication may jeopardize the viability of the transplanted organ, but in life-threatening infections it is necessary as an adjunct to effective antimicrobial therapy. Hematopoietic growth factors (granulocyte and granulocyte-macrophage colony-stimulating factors) stimulate proliferation of bone marrow stem cells, resulting in an increase in peripheral leukocytes. These agents shorten the period of neutropenia and have been associated with fewer infections. Use of growth factors in patients with prolonged neutropenia (> 7 days) is an effective means of reversing immunosuppression.

Antimicrobial drug therapy should be rationally based on culture results (see Chapter 37). Therapy should be specific for isolated pathogens, and bactericidal agents should be used. Combinations of antimicrobials are often required to provide synergy, to prevent resistance, or to serve as broad-spectrum coverage of multiple pathogens (since infections in these patients are often polymicrobial).

Empirical therapy is often instituted at the earliest sign of infection in the immunosuppressed patient because prompt therapy favorably affects outcome. The antibiotic or combination of antibiotics used depends on the type of immunocompromise and the site of infection. For example, in the febrile neutropenic patient, one is concerned primarily about bacterial and fungal infections. Often in this patient population an algorithmic approach to therapy is used, with initial treatment directed at gram-positive and gram-negative organisms. If the patient fails to respond, broader-spectrum antibiotics and antifungal drugs are added. Although a number of different agents can be used, choices should be based on local microbiologic trends. One example would be to initiate therapy with levofloxacin, 500 mg orally or intravenously daily, when the absolute neutrophil count falls below 500/μL. If fever develops, cultures should be obtained; vancomycin, 10–15 mg/kg every 12 hours, is given (to cover methicillin-resistant *S aureus, S epidermidis,* and enterococcus), and amphotericin B, 0.3 mg/kg/d, is added. If after 48–72 hours fever continues, broader-spectrum antibiotics can be added sequentially—eg, to better cover acinetobacter, citrobacter, and pseudomonas, levofloxacin may be switched to cefipime, 2 g every 8 hours intravenously; with continued fever, imipenem, 500 mg every 6 hours with or without tobramycin, 1.8 mg/kg every 8 hours, may be used in place of cefipime, and amphotericin B may be increased to 0.6–1 mg/kg/d. Regardless of whether the patient becomes afebrile, therapy is continued until resolution of neutropenia. Failure to continue antibiotics through the period of neutropenia is associated with a high incidence of relapse that can be associated with septic shock. Patients with fever and neutropenia who are at low risk for developing complications (neutropenia expected to persist for less than 10 days, no comorbid complications requiring hospitalization, and cancer adequately treated) can be treated with oral antibiotic regimens (ciprofloxacin, 750 mg every 12 hours, plus amoxicillin-clavulanic acid, 500 mg every 8 hours). In the organ transplant patient with interstitial infiltrates, one is concerned mainly about pneumocystis or legionella species, so that empirical treatment with a macrolide and trimethoprim-sulfamethoxazole would be reasonable. If the patient fails to respond to empirical treatment, one must often decide between empirical addition of more antimicrobial agents or undertaking invasive procedures (see above) to make a specific diagnosis. By making a specific diagnosis, therapy can be specific and polypharmacy with multiple potentially toxic agents avoided.

Alexander SW et al: Current considerations in the management of fever and neutropenia. Curr Clin Top Infect Dis 1999; 19:160. [PMID: 10472485]

Guidelines for preventing opportunistic infections among hematopoietic stem cell transplant recipients. Recommendations of CDC, the Infectious Disease Society of America, and the American Society of Blood and Marrow Transplantation. MMWR Recomm Rep 2000;49(RR-10):1. [PMID: 11718124] (Comprehensive policy statement.)

Management of herpesvirus infections following transplantation. A report from the British Society of Antimicrobial Chemotherapy Working Party on Antiviral Therapy. J Antimicrob Chemother 2000;45:729. [PMID: 10837424]

Pizzo PA: Fever in immunocompromised patients. N Engl J Med 1999;341:893. [PMID: 10486422] (Review of etiology diagnosis and therapy in immunocompromised patients.)

Singh N: Invasive mycoses in organ transplant recipients: controversies in prophylaxis and management. J Antimicrob Chemother 2000;45:749. [PMID: 10837425]

Singh N: Presumptive therapy versus universal prophylaxis with ganciclovir for cytomegalovirus in solid organ transplant recipients. Clin Infect Dis 2001;32742. [PMID: 11229841] (Risks and benefits of these two approaches to prevention.)

NOSOCOMIAL INFECTIONS

Nosocomial infections are by definition those acquired during the course of hospitalization. In the USA, approximately 5% of patients who enter the hospital free of infection acquire a nosocomial infection resulting in prolongation of the hospital stay, increase in cost of care, significant morbidity, and a 5% mortality rate. Although most fevers that develop during the course of hospitalization are due to infections, about 25% of patients will have fever of noninfectious origin. Causes include drug fever, nonspecific postoperative fevers (atelectasis, tissue damage or necrosis), hematoma, pancreatitis, pulmonary embolus, myocardial infarction, and ischemic bowel disease. The most common infections are urinary tract infections, usually associated with Foley catheters or urologic procedures; bloodstream infections, most commonly from indwelling catheters but also from secondary sites such as surgical wounds, abscesses, pneumonia, the genitourinary tract, and the gastrointestinal tract; pneumonia in intubated patients or those with altered levels of consciousness; surgical wound infections; and *C difficile* colitis.

Some general principles are helpful in preventing, diagnosing, and treating nosocomial infections:

(1) Many infections are a direct result of the use of invasive devices for monitoring or therapy such as intravenous catheters (for hyperalimentation, fluids and electrolytes, medication, dialysis, hemodynamic monitoring, etc), Foley catheters, shunts, surgical drains, catheters placed by interventional radiology for drainage, nasogastric tubes and orotracheal or nasotracheal tubes for ventilatory support. To prevent infections associated with these devices, they should be removed as soon as is medically possible.

(2) Patients who develop nosocomial infections are often critically ill (in the intensive care unit), have been hospitalized for extended periods, and have received several courses of antibiotic therapy with agents that have a broad spectrum of activity. As a result, nosocomial infections are often caused by organisms that are multidrug resistant and are different from those encountered in community-acquired infections. Examples of nosocomial pathogens are *S aureus* and *S epidermidis* (a frequent cause of prosthetic device infection) that may be resistant to nafcillin and cephalosporins

and require vancomycin for therapy; *Enterococcus faecium* that is resistant to ampicillin and vancomycin (vancomycin-resistant enterococcus, or VRE); gram-negative infections caused by pseudomonas, citrobacter, enterobacter, acinetobacter, and stenotrophomonas, which may be sensitive only to fluoroquinolones, carbapenems, aminoglycosides, or trimethoprim-sulfamethoxazole. When choosing antibiotics to treat the seriously ill patient with a nosocomial infection, one must consider the previous antimicrobial the patient has received as well as the "local ecology" (ie, nosocomial pathogens for a given institution). It is often necessary to institute therapy with drugs such as vancomycin and a carbapenem (or aminoglycoside or a fluoroquinolone) until a specific agent is isolated and sensitivities are known, at which time the least toxic and most cost-effective drug can be used.

(3) Because widespread use of antimicrobial drugs contributes to the selection of drug-resistant organisms that cause nosocomial infections, every effort should be made to limit the use of antibiotics to treat documented infections. All too often, unreliable or uninterpretable specimens are obtained for culture that result in unnecessary use of antibiotics. The best example of this principle is the diagnosis of line-related or bloodstream infection in the febrile patient in the intensive care unit. Blood cultures from unidentified sites, a single blood culture from any site, or a blood culture through an existing line will often be positive for *S epidermidis* and will result in therapy with vancomycin. The likelihood that such a culture represents a true bacteremia is 10–20%. Unless two separate venipuncture cultures are obtained (*do not* sample through catheters), interpretation of results is impossible and unnecessary therapy is given. It has been estimated that every such "pseudobacteremia" increases laboratory costs, antibiotic use, and length of stay and increases costs of hospitalization by about $4500. To avoid unnecessary use of antibiotics, thoughtful consideration of culture results is mandatory. A positive wound culture without signs of inflammation or infection, a positive sputum culture without pulmonary infiltrates on chest x-ray, or a positive urine culture in a catheterized patient without signs or symptoms of pyelonephritis are all likely to represent colonization, not infection, and would not require antimicrobial therapy.

Prevention is of paramount importance in controlling nosocomial infections. The concept of universal precautions emphasizes that all patients should be treated as though they have a potential blood-borne transmissible disease, and thus all body secretions should be handled with care to prevent spread of disease. Almost all hospitals have implemented body substance isolation, which requires use of gloves whenever a health care worker anticipates contact with blood or other body secretions. The use of gloves is intended to prevent contamination of the hands of health care workers with infected secretions and subsequent spread of infection to other patients by direct contact. Hand washing is the easiest and most effective means of preventing nosocomial infections and should be done routinely even when gloves are utilized. Foley catheters, intravenous lines, hemodynamic monitoring devices, hyperalimentation lines, and similar invasive devices should be used only when critical to patient care and, when used, should be discontinued at the earliest possible time. Peripheral intravenous lines should be replaced every 3 days and arterial lines every 4 days. Lines in the central venous circulation (including those placed peripherally) can be left in indefinitely and are changed or removed when they are clinically suspected of being infected, when they are nonfunctional, or when they are no longer needed. Silver alloy-impregnated Foley catheters reduce the incidence of catheter-associated bacteriuria, and antibiotic-impregnated (minocycline plus rifampin or chlorhexidine plus silver sulfadiazine) venous catheters reduce line infections and bacteremia. Whether the increased cost of these devices justifies their routine use should be determined by individual institutions based on local infection rates. Selective decontamination of the digestive tract with nonabsorbable antibiotics to prevent nosocomial pneumonia is widely used in Europe, but the therapeutic efficacy of this expensive intervention is controversial. Attentive nursing care (positioning to prevent decubitus ulcers, wound care, elevating the head during tube feedings to prevent aspiration) is critical in preventing nosocomial infections. In addition, careful monitoring of high-risk areas (intensive care units, neonatal units, surgical floors, hemodialysis and transplant units, etc) by skilled personnel—hospital epidemiologists—to detect increases in infection rates early is a key factor in prevention of these types of infections.

Several highly efficacious vaccines have been approved by the FDA that add to our armamentarium for prevention of certain nosocomial infections. Hepatitis A, hepatitis B, and the varicella vaccine should be considered in the appropriate setting. (See section below on Immunization Against Infectious Diseases.)

Gerberding JL et al: Emerging nosocomial infections and antimicrobial resistance. Curr Clin Top Infect Dis 1999;19:83. [PMID: 10472481]

Kollef MH et al: Antibiotic resistance in the intensive care unit. Ann Intern Med 2001;134:298. [PMID: 11182841] (Reviews different strategies for reducing resistance.)

INFECTIONS OF THE CENTRAL NERVOUS SYSTEM

Infections of the central nervous system can be caused by almost any infectious agent, including bacteria, mycobacteria, fungi, spirochetes, protozoa, helminths, and viruses. Certain symptoms and signs are common to all types of central nervous system infection: headache, fever, sensorial disturbances, neck and back stiffness, positive Kernig and Brudzinski signs, and cerebrospinal fluid abnormalities. Although it is rare for all of these manifestations to be present in any one individual, the presence of even one of them should suggest the possibility of a central nervous system infection.

Central nervous system infection constitutes a *medical emergency*. Immediate diagnostic steps must be instituted to establish the specific cause. Normally, these include the history, physical examination, blood count, blood culture, lumbar puncture followed by careful study and culture of the cerebrospinal fluid, and a chest film. The fluid must be examined for cell count, glucose, and protein, and a smear must be stained for bacteria (and acid-fast organisms when appropriate) and cultured for pyogenic organisms and for mycobacteria and fungi when indicated. Latex agglutination tests can detect antigens of encapsulated organisms (*S pneumoniae, H influenzae, N meningitidis,* and *Cryptococcus neoformans*) but are rarely used except for detection of cryptococcus. Polymerase chain reaction (PCR) testing of cerebrospinal fluid has been employed to detect bacteria (*S pneumoniae, H influenzae, N meningitidis, Mycobacterium tuberculosis, Borrelia burgdorferi,* and *Tropheryma whippelii*) and viruses (herpes simplex, varicella-zoster, cytomegalovirus, Epstein-Barr virus, and enteroviruses) in patients with meningitis. The greatest experience is with PCR for herpes simplex, and the test is very sensitive (greater than 95%) and specific. Tests to detect the other organisms are generally more sensitive than culture, but the real value is the rapidity with which results are available, ie, hours compared with days or weeks. At present, with the exception of PCR for herpes simplex, these tests are performed only in reference laboratories. Although it is difficult to prove with existing clinical data that early antibiotic therapy improves outcome in bacterial meningitis, prompt therapy is still recommended.

Since performing a lumbar puncture in the presence of a space-occupying lesion (brain abscess, subdural hematoma, subdural abscess) can result in brain stem herniation and death, a CT scan is performed prior to lumbar puncture if a space-occupying lesion is suspected on the basis of papilledema, coma, seizures, or focal neurologic findings. If delays are encountered in obtaining a CT scan and bacterial meningitis is suspected, blood cultures should be drawn and antibiotics should be administered even before cerebrospinal fluid is obtained for culture to avoid unnecessary delays in treatment (Table 30–1). Animal studies suggest that antibiotics given within 4 hours before obtaining cerebrospinal fluid will not affect culture results.

Etiologic Classification

Central nervous system infections can be divided into several categories that usually can be readily distinguished from each other by cerebrospinal fluid exami-

Table 30–1. Initial antimicrobial therapy for purulent meningitis of unknown cause.

Age Group	Common Microorganisms	Standard Therapy
18–50 years	S pneumoniae,[1] N meningitidis	Cefotaxime or ceftriaxone[2]
Over 50 years	S pneumoniae,[1] N meningitidis, L monocytogenes, gram-negative bacilli	Ampicillin,[3] cefotaxime, or ceftriaxone[2]
Impaired cellular immunity	L monocytogenes, gram-negative bacilli, S pneumoniae	Ampicillin[3] plus ceftazidime[4]
Postsurgical or posttraumatic	S aureus, S pneumoniae,[1] gram-negative bacilli	Vancomycin[5] plus ceftazidime[4]

[1]In areas where penicillin-resistant pneumococcus is prevalent, vancomycin, 10–15 mg/kg every 6 hours, should be included in the regimen.
[2]The usual dose of cefotaxime is 2 g every 6 hours and that of ceftriaxone is 2 g every 12 hours. If the organism is sensitive to penicillin, 3–4 million units IV every 4 hours is given.
[3]The dose of ampicillin is usually 2 g IV every 4 hours.
[4]Ceftazidime is given in a dose of 50–100 mg/kg every 8 hours up to 2 g every 8 hours.
[5]The dose of vancomycin is 10–15 mg/kg every 6 hours.

nation as the first step toward etiologic diagnosis (Table 30–2).

A. PURULENT MENINGITIS

Patients with bacterial meningitis usually present acutely within hours or 1–2 days after onset of symptoms. The organisms responsible depend primarily on the age of the patient as summarized in Table 30–1. The diagnosis is usually based on the Gram-stained smear (positive in 60–80%) or culture (positive in over 90%).

B. CHRONIC MENINGITIS

Patients with chronic meningitis present less acutely with a history of symptoms lasting weeks to months.

The most common pathogens are *Mycobacterium tuberculosis*, atypical mycobacteria, fungi (cryptococcus, coccidioides, histoplasma), and spirochetes (*Treponema pallidum*, the agent of meningovascular syphilis; and *Borrelia burgdorferi*, the agent of Lyme disease). The diagnosis is made by culture or in some cases by serologic tests (cryptococcosis, coccidioidomycosis, syphilis, Lyme disease).

C. ASEPTIC MENINGITIS

Aseptic meningitis—a much more benign and self-limited syndrome than purulent meningitis—is caused principally by viruses, especially mumps virus and the enterovirus group (including coxsackieviruses

Table 30–2. Typical cerebrospinal fluid findings in various central nervous system diseases.

Diagnosis	Cells/μL	Glucose (mg/dL)	Protein (mg/dL)	Opening Pressure
Normal	0–5 lymphocytes	45–85[1]	15–45	70–180 mm H$_2$O
Purulent meningitis (bacterial)[2] community-acquired	200–20,000 polymorphonuclear neutrophils	Low (< 45)	High (> 50)	Markedly elevated
Granulomatous meningitis (mycobacterial, fungal)[3]	100–1000, mostly lymphocytes[3]	Low (< 45)	High (> 50)	Moderately elevated
Spirochetal meningitis	100–1000, mostly lymphocytes[3]	Normal	Moderately high (> 50)	Normal to slightly elevated
Aseptic meningitis, viral or meningoencephalitis[4]	25–2000, mostly lymphocytes[3]	Normal or low	High (> 50)	Slightly elevated
"Neighborhood reaction"[5]	Variably increased	Normal	Normal or high	Variable

[1]Cerebrospinal fluid glucose must be considered in relation to blood glucose level. Normally, cerebrospinal fluid glucose is 20–30 mg/dL lower than blood glucose, or 50–70% of the normal value of blood glucose.
[2]Organisms in smear or culture of cerebrospinal fluid; counterimmunoelectrophoresis or latex agglutination may be diagnostic.
[3]Polymorphonuclear neutrophils may predominate early.
[4]Viral isolation from cerebrospinal fluid early; antibody titer rise in paired specimens of serum; PCR for herpesvirus.
[5]May occur in mastoiditis, brain abscess, epidural abscess, sinusitis, septic thrombus, brain tumor. Cerebrospinal fluid culture results usually negative.

and echoviruses). Infectious mononucleosis may be accompanied by aseptic meningitis. Leptospiral infection is usually placed in the aseptic group because of the lymphocytic cellular response and its relatively benign course. This type of meningitis also occurs during secondary syphilis and stage 2 Lyme disease.

D. ENCEPHALITIS

Encephalitis (due to herpesviruses, arboviruses, rabies virus, flaviviruses [West Nile encephalitis, Japanese encephalitis], and many other viruses) produces disturbances of the sensorium, seizures, and many other manifestations. Patients present more acutely and are more ill than patients with aseptic meningitis. Cerebrospinal fluid may be entirely normal or may show some lymphocytes.

E. PARTIALLY TREATED BACTERIAL MENINGITIS

Previous effective antibiotic therapy given for 12–24 hours will decrease the rate of positive Gram stain results by 20% and culture by 30–40% but will have little effect on cell count, protein, or glucose. Occasionally, previous antibiotic therapy will change a predominantly polymorphonuclear response to a lymphocytic pleocytosis, and some of the cerebrospinal fluid findings may be similar to those seen in aseptic meningitis.

F. NEIGHBORHOOD REACTION

As noted in Table 30–2, this term denotes a purulent infectious process in close proximity to the central nervous system that spills some of the products of the inflammatory process—white blood cells or protein—into the cerebrospinal fluid. Such an infection might be a brain abscess, osteomyelitis of the vertebrae, epidural abscess, subdural empyema, or bacterial sinusitis or mastoiditis.

G. NONINFECTIOUS MENINGEAL IRRITATION

Meningismus, presenting with the classic signs of meningeal irritation with totally normal cerebrospinal fluid findings, may occur in the presence of other infections such as pneumonia and shigellosis. Carcinomatous meningitis, sarcoidosis, systemic lupus erythematosus, chemical meningitis, and certain drugs—NSAIDs, muromonab-CD3 (OKT3), trimethoprim-sulfamethoxazole, and others—can also produce symptoms and signs of meningeal irritation with associated cerebrospinal fluid pleocytosis, increased protein, and low or normal glucose.

H. BRAIN ABSCESS

Brain abscess presents as a space-occupying lesion; symptoms may include vomiting, fever, change of mental status, or focal neurologic manifestations. If brain abscess is suspected, a CT scan should be performed. If a CT scan reveals an abscess, lumbar puncture should *not* to be performed since results rarely provide clinically useful information and herniation can occur. The bacteriology of brain abscess is usually polymicrobial and includes *S aureus,* gram-negative bacilli, streptococci, and anaerobes (including anaerobic streptococci and prevotella species).

I. AMEBIC MENINGOENCEPHALITIS

These infections are caused by free-living amebas and present as two distinct syndromes. The diagnosis is confirmed by culture or identification of the organism in cerebrospinal fluid or on biopsy specimens. No effective therapy is available.

1. Primary amebic meningoencephalitis is caused by *Naegleria fowleri* and is an acute fulminant disease characterized by signs of meningeal irritation that rapidly progresses to encephalitis and death. Anecdotal reports of cure of primary amebic meningoencephalitis have been reported with intravenous and intraventricular administration of amphotericin B.

2. Granulomatous amebic encephalitis is caused by acanthamoeba species. It is an indolent disease characterized by headache, nausea, vomiting, cranial neuropathies, seizures, and hemiparesis.

Treatment

Treatment consists of supportive care and specific antimicrobial therapy directed at the causative organism. Increased intracranial pressure due to brain edema often requires therapeutic attention. Hyperventilation, mannitol (25–50 g as a bolus intravenous infusion), and even drainage of cerebrospinal fluid by repeated lumbar punctures or by placement of ventricular catheters have been employed to control cerebral edema and increased intracranial pressure. Dexamethasone (4 mg every 4–6 hours) may also decrease cerebral edema. In the case of purulent meningitis, proper antimicrobial treatment is imperative. Since the identity of the causative microorganism may remain unknown or doubtful for a few days, initial antibiotic treatment as set forth in Table 30–1 should be directed against the microorganisms most common for each age group.

The duration of therapy for bacterial meningitis varies depending upon the etiologic agent: *H influenzae* 7 days; *N meningitidis* 7 days; *S pneumoniae* 10–14 days; *L monocytogenes* 14–21 days; gram-negative bacilli 21 days.

Although dexamethasone therapy is standard in infants and children with meningitis, prospective controlled studies have not been performed in adults. Nonetheless, because adverse effects are minimal and some benefit may occur, some clinicians have recommended dexamethasone, 0.15 mg/kg intravenously every 6 hours for 2–4 days, especially in patients with high bacterial loads (ie, positive Gram stain), increased intracranial pressure, or altered mental status.

Therapy of brain abscess consists of drainage (excision or aspiration) in addition to 3–4 weeks of systemic antibiotics directed against organisms isolated. A regimen often used includes metronidazole, 500 mg intravenously or orally every 8 hours, plus ceftizoxime, 2 g intravenously every 8 hours, or ceftriaxone, 2 g every 12 hours. In cases where abscesses are less than 2 cm in size, there are multiple abscesses that cannot be drained, or if an abscess is located in an area where significant neurologic sequelae would result from drainage, antibiotics for 6–8 weeks without drainage can be employed.

Therapy of other types of meningitis is discussed elsewhere in this book (fungal meningitis, Chapter 36; syphilis and Lyme borreliosis, Chapter 33; tuberculous meningitis, Chapter 34; herpes encephalitis, Chapter 32).

Attia J et al: The rational clinical examination. Does this adult patient have acute meningitis? JAMA 1999;282:175. [PMID: 10411200] (Reliability of signs and symptoms in making diagnosis.)

Calfee DP et al: Brain abscess. Semin Neurol 2000;20:353. [PMID: 11051259] (Emphasizes changes in etiology due to immunocompromised patients and reviews diagnosis and therapy.)

Hussein AS et al: Acute bacterial meningitis in adults. A 12-year review. Medicine (Baltimore) 2000;79:360. [PMID: 11144034] (Review of 100 patients.)

ANIMAL & HUMAN BITE WOUNDS

It is estimated that about 900 new dog bite injuries require emergency department attention each day and that about 1% of emergency room visits in urban areas are for treatment of animal and human bites. Dog bites occur most commonly in the summer months. Biting animals are usually known by their victims, and most biting incidents are provoked (ie, bites occur while playing with the animal or after surprising the animal or waking it abruptly from sleep). Failure to elicit a history of provocation is important, because an unprovoked attack raises the possibility that the animal is rabid. Human bites are usually inflicted by children while playing or fighting; in adults, bites are associated with alcohol use and closed-fist injuries that occur during fights.

The animal inflicting the bite, the location of the bite, and the type of injury inflicted are all important determinants of whether these injuries become infected. Cat bites are more likely to become infected than human bites—between 30% and 50% of all cat bites subsequently become infected. Infections following human bites are variable: Those inflicted by children rarely become infected, because they are superficial; and bites by adults become infected in 15–30% of cases, with a particularly high rate of infection in closed-fist injuries. Dog bites, for unclear reasons, become infected only 5% of the time. Bites of the head, face, and neck are less likely to become infected than bites on the extremities. Puncture wounds become infected more frequently than lacerations, probably because the latter are easier to irrigate and debride.

The bacteriology of bite infections depends upon the biting animal and when the infection occurs after the biting incident. Early infections (within 24 hours after the bite) following dog and cat bites are most frequently caused by *Pasteurella multocida*. These infections are characterized by rapid onset and progression, fevers, chills, cellulitis, and local adenopathy. Early infections following human bites are usually caused by mixed aerobic and anaerobic mouth flora and can produce a rapidly progressive necrotizing infection. Late infections (longer than 24 hours after the bite) are caused mainly by staphylococci, streptococci, and anaerobes (fusobacterium, bacteroides, prevotella), but innumerable organisms have been implicated in these infections. *Capnocytophaga canimorsus* (formerly called a DF2 organism), a gram-negative organism that is part of canine oral flora; *Eikenella corrodens,* another gram-negative organism that can be part of human mouth flora; haemophilus species, pseudomonas species, and other gram-negative organisms—all have been implicated in bite infections.

There have been no documented cases of HIV transmission by human bites.

Treatment

A. LOCAL CARE

Vigorous cleansing and irrigation of the wound as well as debridement of necrotic material are the most important factors in decreasing the incidence of infections. X-rays should be obtained to look for fractures and the presence of foreign bodies. Careful examination to assess the extent of the injury (tendon laceration, joint space penetration) is critical to appropriate care.

B. SUTURING

If wounds require closure for cosmetic or mechanical reasons, suturing can be done. However, one should never suture a wound that is already infected, and wounds of the hand should generally not be sutured since a closed-space infection of the hand can result in loss of function.

C. PROPHYLACTIC ANTIBIOTICS

Prophylaxis is indicated in high-risk bites, eg, cat bites in any location (dicloxacillin, 0.5 g orally four times a day for 3–5 days) and hand bites by any animal or by humans (penicillin V, 0.5 g orally four times a day for 3–5 days). Although dicloxacillin and penicillin have been most extensively studied for prophylaxis, there is concern about their use because of their narrow spectrum of activity. Based on the microbiology of bite wounds noted above, other agents that have not been adequately studied but that have broader spectrums of activity may be even more effective as prophylactic agents. Examples include cefuroxime, amoxicillin-clavulanic acid, and, in the penicillin-allergic patient, clindamycin plus a fluoroquinolone. Immunocompromised patients and especially individuals without functional spleens are at risk for developing overwhelming bacteremia and sepsis following animal bites and should also receive prophylaxis.

D. ANTIBIOTICS

For wounds that are infected, antibiotics are clearly indicated. How they are given (orally or intravenously) and the need for hospitalization are individualized clinical decisions. In general, *P multocida* is best treated with penicillin or a tetracycline. Other active agents include second- and third-generation cephalosporins, fluoroquinolones, or azithromycin and clarithromycin. Response to therapy is slow, and therapy should be continued for at least 2–3 weeks. Human bites frequently require admission to the hospital and intravenous therapy with a β-lactam plus a β-lactamase inhibitor combination (Unasyn, Timentin, Zosyn), a second-generation cephalosporin with anaerobic activity (cefoxitin, cefotetan, cefmetazole), or, in the penicillin-allergic patient, clindamycin plus a fluoroquinolone. Because the bacteriology of these infections is so variable, one should always culture infected wounds and adjust therapy appropriately, especially if the patient is not responding to initial empirical treatment.

E. TETANUS AND RABIES

All patients must be evaluated for the need for tetanus (see Chapter 33) and rabies (see Chapter 32) prophylaxis.

Goldstein EJ: Current concepts on animal bites: bacteriology and therapy. Curr Clin Top Infect Dis 1999;19:99. [PMID: 10472482]

Talan DA et al: Bacteriologic analysis of infected dog and cat bites. N Engl J Med 1999;340:85. [PMID: 9887159] (Prospective analysis of bacteriology with discussion of therapy.)

SEXUALLY TRANSMITTED DISEASES

Some infectious diseases are transmitted most commonly—or most efficiently—by sexual contact. Most of the infectious agents that cause sexually transmitted diseases are fairly easily inactivated when exposed to a harsh environment. They are thus particularly suited to transmission by contact with mucous membranes. They may be bacteria (eg, gonococci), spirochetes (syphilis), chlamydiae (nongonococcal urethritis, cervicitis), viruses (eg, herpes simplex, hepatitis B virus, cytomegalovirus, HIV), or protozoa (eg, trichomonas). In most infections caused by these agents, early lesions occur on genitalia or other sexually exposed mucous membranes; however, wide dissemination may occur, and involvement of nongenital tissues and organs may mimic many noninfectious disorders. All sexually transmitted diseases have subclinical or latent phases that play an important role in long-term persistence of the infection or in its transmission from infected (but largely asymptomatic) persons to other contacts. Laboratory examinations are of particular importance in the diagnosis of such asymptomatic patients. Simultaneous infection by several different agents is common, and any person with a sexually transmitted disease should be tested for syphilis. If the test is negative, a repeat study should be done in 3 months, since seroconversion can be delayed.

For each patient, there are one or more sexual contacts who require diagnosis and treatment. As a rule, sexual partners should be treated simultaneously to avoid prompt reinfection. The commonest sexually transmitted diseases are gonorrhea,* syphilis,* condyloma acuminatum, chlamydial genital infections, herpesvirus genital infections, trichomonas vaginitis, chancroid,* granuloma inguinale,* scabies, louse infestation, and bacterial vaginosis (among lesbians). However, shigellosis,* hepatitis A, B, and C,* amebiasis,* giardiasis, cryptosporidiosis, salmonellosis,* and campylobacteriosis may also be transmitted by sexual (oral-anal) contact, especially in homosexual males. Homosexual contact is the most prevalent method of transmission of HIV and AIDS,* though bidirectional heterosexual transmission can also occur (see Chapter 31).

The risk of developing a sexually transmitted disease following a sexual assault has not been extensively studied. Victims of assault have a high baseline rate of infection (*N gonorrhoeae* 6%, *C trachomatis* 10%, *T vaginalis* 15%, and bacterial vaginosis 34%), and the risk of acquiring infection as a result of the assault is significant but is lower than the preexisting rate (*N gonorrhoeae* 6–12%, *C trachomatis* 4–17%, *T vaginalis* 12%, syphilis 0.5–3%, and bacterial vaginosis 19%). Victims should be evaluated within 24 hours after the assault, and cultures for *N gonorrhoeae*, *C trachomatis* (if culture is not available, nonculture tests, such as nucleic acid amplification tests, are acceptable), and herpes simplex virus should be obtained and vaginal secretions examined for trichomonas and bacterial vaginosis. In addition, a blood sample should be obtained for immediate serologic testing for syphilis, hepatitis B, and HIV. Follow-up examination for sexually transmitted disease should be repeated at 2 weeks, since concentrations of infecting organisms may not have been sufficient to produce a positive culture at the time of initial examination. Follow-up serologic testing for syphilis should be performed in 6, 12, and 24 weeks if the initial tests are negative. RNA testing for HIV should be done at 2 and 4 weeks if initial serologic tests are negative. Prophylactic antibiotics should be given if the assailant is known to be infected. The usefulness of presumptive therapy is controversial, some feeling that all patients should receive it and others that it should be limited to those in whom follow-up cannot be ensured or that it should be given only to those who request it. If therapy is given, a reasonable regimen would be hepatitis B vaccination (without hepatitis B immune globulin, the first dose given at the initial evaluation and follow-up doses at 1–2 months and 4–6 months) and one dose of ceftriaxone, 125 mg intramuscularly, plus metron-

*Reportable to public health authorities.

idazole, 2 g orally as a single dose, plus doxycycline, 100 mg orally twice daily for 7 days, or azithromycin, 1 g orally as a single dose. If the patient is pregnant, azithromycin should be used instead of doxycycline, and metronidazole should be given only after the first trimester.

Although seroconversion to HIV has been reported following sexual assault when this was the only known risk, the risk of acquiring HIV is felt to be low. The likelihood of HIV transmission from anal or vaginal receptive intercourse when the source is known to be HIV positive is 1–3 per 1000. Because prophylactic antiretroviral therapy has not been studied in this setting, firm recommendations cannot be made and the decision to institute therapy should be individualized. Because of the time-dependent nature of postexposure prophylaxis, if therapy is given it should be as soon as possible after the assault and certainly within 72 hours.

Bamberger JD et al: Post-exposure prophylaxis for human immunodeficiency virus (HIV) infection following sexual assault. Am J Med 1999;106:323-326. [PMID: 10190382] (Discussion of risk of infection and the risks and benefits of therapy with specific regimens.)

1998 guidelines for treatment of sexually transmitted diseases. Centers for Disease Control and Prevention. MMWR Recomm Rep 1998;47(RR-1):1. [PMID: 9461053]

INFECTIONS IN DRUG USERS

The use of parenterally administered recreational drugs has increased enormously in recent years. There are now an estimated 300,000 or more intravenous drug users in the USA, mostly in or near large urban centers. Consequently, clinicians and hospitals serving such urban and suburban populations must deal with many problems—including infections—related to drug abuse.

Common Infections That Occur With Greater Frequency in Drug Users

(1) **Skin infections** are associated with poor hygiene and use of nonsterile technique when injecting drugs. *S aureus* and oral flora (streptococci, eikenella, fusobacterium, peptostreptococcus) are the most common organisms, with enteric gram-negatives less common and seen in those who inject into the groin. Cellulitis and subcutaneous abscesses occur most commonly, particularly in association with subcutaneous ("skin-popping") or intramuscular injections and the use of cocaine and heroin mixtures (probably due to ischemia). Myositis and necrotizing fasciitis occur infrequently but are life-threatening. Wound botulism in association with brown heroin use has also been reported.

(2) **Hepatitis** is very common among habitual drug users and is transmissible both by the parenteral (hepatitis B, C, and D virus) and by the fecal-oral route (hepatitis A). Multiple episodes of hepatitis with different agents can occur.

(3) **Aspiration pneumonia** and its complications (lung abscess, empyema, brain abscess) result from altered consciousness associated with drug use. Mixed aerobic and anaerobic mouth flora are usually involved.

(4) **Tuberculosis** also occurs in drug users, and infection with HIV has fostered the spread of tuberculosis in this population. Morbidity and mortality rates are increased in HIV-infected individuals with tuberculosis. Tuberculosis should be suspected in those who have classic radiographic findings and in those with infiltrates who do not respond to antibiotics.

(5) **Pulmonary septic emboli** may originate from venous thrombi or right-sided endocarditis.

(6) **Sexually transmitted diseases** are not directly related to drug use, but the practice of exchanging sex for drugs has resulted in an increased frequency of sexually transmitted diseases. Syphilis, gonorrhea, and chancroid are the most common.

(7) **AIDS** has a high incidence among intravenous drug users and their sexual contacts and the offspring of infected women (see Chapter 31).

(8) **Infective endocarditis** (see below). A number of complications of endocarditis can occur, including splenic abscesses, central nervous system infections (meningitis, brain abscess, subdural empyema, epidural abscess), and endophthalmitis.

(9) **Other vascular infections** include septic thrombophlebitis and mycotic aneurysms. Mycotic aneurysms resulting from direct trauma to a vessel with secondary infection most commonly occur in femoral arteries and less commonly in arteries of the neck. Aneurysms resulting from hematogenous spread of organisms frequently involve intracerebral vessels and are seen in association with endocarditis.

Infections Rare in USA

A. TETANUS

In the 1950s and 1960s, tetanus was commonly seen in drug users, especially in unimmunized women who injected drugs subcutaneously ("skin-popping"). Increased tetanus immunization among drug users has resulted in a decline in this disease, though cases are still reported.

B. MALARIA

Needle transmission occurs from intravenous drug users who acquired the infection in malaria-endemic areas outside the USA.

C. MELIOIDOSIS

This chronic pulmonary infection caused by *Pseudomonas pseudomallei* is occasionally seen in debilitated drug users.

Osteomyelitis & Septic Arthritis

Osteomyelitis involving vertebral bodies, sternoclavicular joints, the pubic symphysis, the sacroiliac joints, and other sites usually results from hematogenous distribution of injected organisms or septic venous thrombi. Pain and fever precede radiographic changes, sometimes by several weeks. While staphylococci—often methicillin-resistant—are common organisms, serratia, pseudomonas, candida, and other pathogens rarely encountered in spontaneous bone or joint disease are found in intravenous drug users.

Infective Endocarditis

The organisms that cause infective endocarditis in those who use drugs intravenously are most commonly *S aureus,* candida (especially *Candida parapsilosis*), *Enterococcus faecalis,* other streptococci, and gram-negative bacteria (especially pseudomonas and *Serratia marcescens*).

Involvement of the right side of the heart is somewhat more frequent than involvement of the left side, and infection of more than one valve is not infrequent. Right-sided involvement, especially in the absence of murmurs, is often suggested by the presence of septic pulmonary emboli. The diagnosis must be established by blood culture. Therapy, including empirical treatment, is discussed in Chapter 33.

Approach to the Patient

A common and difficult clinical problem is management of the parenteral drug user who presents with fever. In general, after obtaining appropriate cultures (blood, urine, and sputum if the chest x-ray is abnormal), empirical therapy is begun. If the chest x-ray is suggestive of a community-acquired pneumonia (consolidation), therapy for outpatient pneumonia is begun with a second- or third-generation cephalosporin (many would add azithromycin or doxycycline to this regimen). If the chest x-ray is suggestive of septic emboli (nodular infiltrates), therapy for presumed endocarditis is initiated, usually with a combination of nafcillin and gentamicin. Ampicillin should be added if enterococci are a consideration. If the chest x-ray is normal and no focal site of infection can be found, endocarditis is presumed. While awaiting the results of blood cultures, empirical treatment with nafcillin and gentamicin (with or without ampicillin) is started. If blood cultures are positive for organisms that frequently cause endocarditis in drug users (see above), endocarditis is presumed to be present and treated accordingly. If blood cultures are positive for an organism that is an unusual cause of endocarditis, evaluation for an occult source of infection should go forward. In this setting, a transesophageal echocardiogram may be quite helpful since it is 90% sensitive in detecting vegetations and a negative study is strong evidence against endocarditis. If blood cultures are negative and the patient responds to antibiotics, therapy should be continued for 7–14 days (oral therapy can be given once an initial response has occurred). In every patient, careful examination for an occult source of infection (genitourinary, dental, sinus, gallbladder, etc) should be done.

Levine DP, Brown PD: Infections in injection drug users. In: *Principles and Practice of Infectious Diseases,* 5th ed. Mandell GL, Bennett JR, Dolin R (editors). Churchill Livingstone, 2000.

Murphy EL et al: Risk factors for skin and soft-tissue abscesses among injection drug users: a case-control study. Clin Infect Dis 2001;33:35. [PMID: 11389492]

ACUTE INFECTIOUS DIARRHEA

Diarrheal syndromes are arbitrarily divided into acute (those lasting less than 2 weeks) and chronic diseases and are said to be mild if there are three or fewer stools per day, moderate if there are four or more stools in association with local symptoms (abdominal cramps, nausea, tenesmus), and severe if there are four or more stools per day with systemic symptoms (fevers, chills, dehydration). Acute diarrhea can be caused by a number of different factors, including emotional stress, food intolerance, inorganic agents (eg, sodium nitrite), organic substances (eg, mushrooms, shellfish), drugs, and infectious agents (including viruses, bacteria, and protozoa). From a diagnostic and therapeutic standpoint, it is helpful to classify infectious diarrhea into syndromes that produce inflammatory or bloody diarrhea and those that are noninflammatory, nonbloody, or watery. In general, the term "inflammatory diarrhea" suggests colonic involvement by invasive bacteria or parasites or toxin production that affects the large bowel. Clinically, patients present with frequent bloody, small-volume stools, often associated with fever, abdominal cramps, tenesmus, and fecal urgency. Common causes of this syndrome include shigella, salmonella, campylobacter, yersinia, invasive strains of *E coli,* *E coli* O157:H7, *Entamoeba histolytica,* and *Clostridium difficile.* Tests for fecal leukocytes are frequently positive, and definitive etiologic diagnosis requires stool culture. Noninflammatory diarrhea is generally a milder disease and is caused by viruses or toxins that affect the small intestine and interfere with salt and water balance, resulting in large-volume watery diarrhea, often with nausea, vomiting, and cramps. Common causes of this syndrome include viruses (eg, rotavirus, Norwalk virus, enteric adenoviruses, astrovirus, coronavirus), vibrios *(V cholerae, V parahaemolyticus, V vulnificus),* enterotoxin-producing *E coli, Giardia lamblia,* cryptosporidia, and agents that can cause food-borne gastroenteritis.

The term "food poisoning" denotes diseases caused by toxins present in consumed foods. When the incubation period is short (1–6 hours after consumption), the toxin is usually preformed and present in the contaminated food. Vomiting is usually a major complaint, and fever is usually absent. Examples include intoxication from *S aureus* or *Bacillus cereus,* and toxin can be detected in the food. When the incubation period is longer—between 8 and 16 hours—the organism is present in the food and produces toxin after being ingested. Vomiting is less prominent, abdominal cramps are frequent, and fever is often absent. The best example of this disease is that due to *Clostridium perfringens*. Toxin can be detected in food or stool specimens.

The inflammatory and noninflammatory diarrheas discussed above can also be transmitted by food and water and usually have incubation periods between 12 and 72 hours. Cyclospora, cryptosporidia, and isospora are protozoans capable of causing disease in both immunocompetent and immunocompromised patients. Characteristics of disease include profuse watery diarrhea that is prolonged but usually self-limited (1–2 weeks) in the immunocompetent patient but can be chronic in the compromised host. Epidemiologic features may be helpful in determining etiology. Recent hospitalization or antibiotic use suggests *C difficile;* recent foreign travel suggests salmonella, shigella, campylobacter, *E coli,* or *V cholerae;* undercooked hamburger suggests *E coli,* especially O157:H7; fried rice consumption is associated with *B cereus* toxin. Prominent features of some of these causes of diarrhea are listed in Table 30–3.

Treatment usually consists of replacement of fluids and electrolytes and, very rarely, management of hypovolemic shock and respiratory compromise. In mild diarrhea, increasing ingestion of juices and clear soups is adequate. In more severe cases of dehydration (postural lightheadedness, decreased urination), oral glucose-based rehydration solutions can be used (Ceralyte, Pedialyte). In general, most cases of acute gastroenteritis are self-limited and do not require therapy other than supportive measures. When symptoms persist beyond 3–4 days, initial presentation is accompanied by fever or bloody diarrhea, or the patient is immunocompromised, cultures of stool are usually obtained. Symptoms have often resolved by the time cultures are completed. In this case, even if a pathogen is isolated, therapy is not needed (except for shigella, since the infecting dose is so small that therapy to eradicate organisms from the stool is indicated for epidemiologic reasons). If symptoms persist and a pathogen is isolated, it is reasonable to institute specific treatment even though therapy has not been conclusively shown to alter the natural history of disease for most pathogens. Exceptions include gastroenteritis due to salmonella (where therapy may prolong the carrier state and increase the relapse rate), infections with *E coli* O157:H7 (antibiotic therapy does not ameliorate symptoms and may increase the risk of developing hemolytic-uremic syndrome), and campylobacter infections (early therapy shortens the course of disease). Several studies examining the effect of antibiotic therapy on domestically acquired diarrhea have suggested that ciprofloxacin, 500 mg every 12 hours for 5 days, is effective in shortening the course of illness compared with placebo. Because of concerns about selecting for resistant organisms (especially campylobacter, where increasing resistance to fluoroquinolones has been documented and erythromycin is the drug of choice) coupled with the fact that most infectious diarrhea is self-limited, routine use of antibiotics for all patients with diarrhea is not recommended. Antibiotics should be considered in patients with evidence of invasive disease (white cells in stool, dysentery), with symptoms 3–4 days or more in duration, with multiple stools (eight to ten or more per day) and in those with impaired immune responses. Antimotility drugs may relieve cramping and decrease diarrhea in mild cases. Their use should be limited to patients without fever and without dysentery (bloody stools), and they should be used in low doses.

Therapeutic recommendations for specific agents can be found elsewhere in this book.

Aranda-Michel J et al: Acute diarrhea: a practical review. Am J Med 1999;106:670. [PMID: 10378626] (Review of causes with discussion of who should receive cultures and be treated.)

Guerrant RL et al: Practice guidelines for the management of infectious diarrhea. Clin Infect Dis 2001;32:331. [PMID: 11170940]

TRAVELER'S DIARRHEA

Whenever a person travels from one country to another—particularly if the change involves a marked difference in climate, social conditions, or sanitation standards and facilities—diarrhea is likely to develop within 2–10 days. There may be up to ten or even more loose stools per day, often accompanied by abdominal cramps, nausea, occasionally vomiting, and rarely fever. The stools do not usually contain mucus or blood, and aside from weakness and dehydration there are no systemic manifestations of infection. The illness usually subsides spontaneously within 1–5 days, although 10% remain symptomatic for a week or longer, and in 2% symptoms persist for longer than a month.

Bacteria cause 80% of cases of traveler's diarrhea, with enterotoxigenic *E coli,* shigella species, and *Campylobacter jejuni* being the most common pathogens. Less common causative agents include aeromonas, salmonella, noncholera vibrios, *Entamoeba histolytica,* and *Giardia lamblia.* Contributory causes may at times include unusual food and drink, change in living habits, occasional viral infections (adenoviruses or rotaviruses), and change in bowel flora. In patients with fever and bloody diarrhea, stool culture may be indicated, but in most cases cultures are reserved for those who do not respond to antibiotics. Chronic watery diarrhea may be due to amebiasis or giardiasis or, rarely, tropical sprue.

For most individuals, the affliction is short-lived, and symptomatic therapy with opioids or loperamide is all that is required provided the patient is not systemically ill (fever ≥ 39 °C) and does not have dysentery (bloody stools), in which case antimotility agents should be avoided. Packages of oral rehydration salts to treat dehydration are available over the counter in the USA (Infalyte, Pedialyte, others) and in many foreign countries. Avoidance of fresh foods and water sources that are likely to be contaminated is recommended for travelers to developing countries, where infectious diarrheal illnesses are endemic. Prophylaxis

Table 30–3. Acute bacterial diarrheas and "food poisoning."

Organism	Incubation Period (hours)	Vomiting	Diarrhea	Fever	Microbiology	Pathogenesis	Clinical Features and Treatment
Staphylococcus	1–8, rarely up to 18	+++	+	−	Staphylococci grow in meats and in dairy and bakery products and produce enterotoxin.	Enterotoxin acts on receptors in gut that transmit impulses to medullary centers.	Abrupt onset, intense vomiting for up to 24 hours, regular recovery in 24–48 hours. Occurs in persons eating the same food. No treatment usually necessary except to restore fluids and electrolytes.
Bacillus cereus	1–8, rarely up to 18	+++	+	−	Reheated fried rice causes vomiting or diarrhea.	Enterotoxins formed in food or in gut from growth of B cereus.	After 1–6 hours, mainly vomiting. After 8–16 hours, mainly diarrhea. Both self-limited to less than 1 day.
Clostridium perfringens	8–16	±	+++	−	Clostridia grow in rewarmed meat dishes and produce an enterotoxin.	Enterotoxin produced in food and in gut causes hypersecretion in small intestine.	Abrupt onset of profuse diarrhea; vomiting occasionally. Recovery usual without treatment in 1–4 days. Many clostridia in cultures of food and feces of patients.
Clostridium botulinum	24–96	±	Rare	−	Clostridia grow in anaerobic foods and produce toxin.	Toxin absorbed from gut blocks acetylcholine at neuromuscular junction.	Diplopia, dysphagia, dysphonia, respiratory embarrassment. Treatment requires clear airway, ventilation, and intravenous polyvalent antitoxin (see text). Toxin present in food and serum. Mortality rate high.
Clostridium difficile	?	−	+++	+	Associated with antimicrobial drugs, eg, clindamycin.	Enterotoxin causes epithelial necrosis in colon; pseudomembranous colitis.	Especially after abdominal surgery, abrupt bloody diarrhea and fever. Toxin in stool. Oral vancomycin or metronidazole useful in therapy.
Escherichia coli (some strains)	24–72	±	+	−	Organisms grow in gut and produce toxin. May also invade superficial epithelium.	Enterotoxin causes hypersecretion in small intestine.	Usually abrupt onset of diarrhea; vomiting rare. A serious infection in neonates. In adults, "traveler's diarrhea" is usually self-limited to 1–3 days and does respond to a fluoroquinolone.
Vibrio parahaemolyticus	6–96	+	+	±	Organisms grow in seafood and in gut and produce toxin or invade.	Hypersecretion in small intestine; stools may be bloody.	Abrupt onset of diarrhea in groups consuming the same food, especially crabs and other seafood. Recovery is usually complete in 1–3 days. Food and stool cultures are positive.
Vibrio cholerae (mild cases)	24–72	+	+++	−	Organisms grow in gut and produce toxin.	Enterotoxin causes hypersecretion in small intestine. Infective dose: 10^7–10^9 organisms.	Abrupt onset of liquid diarrhea in endemic area. Needs prompt replacement of fluids and electrolytes intravenously or orally. Tetracyclines shorten excretion of vibrios. Stool cultures positive.

(continued)

Table 30–3. Acute bacterial diarrheas and "food poisoning." (continued)

Organism	Incubation Period (hours)	Vomiting	Diarrhea	Fever	Microbiology	Pathogenesis	Clinical Features and Treatment
Campylobacter jejuni	2–10 days	–	+++	+	Organisms grow in jejunum and ileum.	Invasion and enterotoxin production uncertain.	Fever, diarrhea; PMNs and fresh blood in stool, especially in children. Usually self-limited. Special media needed for culture at 43 °C. Give a fluoroquinolone in severe cases with invasion. Recovery in 5–8 days is usual.
Shigella species (mild cases)	24–72	±	+	+	Organisms grow in superficial gut epithelium and gut lumen and produce toxin.	Organisms invade epithelial cells; blood, mucus, and PMNs in stools. Infective dose: 10^2–10^3 organisms	Abrupt onset of diarrhea, often with blood and pus in stools, cramps, tenesmus, and lethargy. Stool cultures are positive. Therapy depends on sensitivity testing, but the fluoroquinolones are most effective. Do not give opioids. Often mild and self-limited.
Salmonella species	8–48	±	+	+	Organisms grow in gut. Do not produce toxin.	Superficial infection of gut, little invasion. Infective dose: 10^5 organisms.	Gradual or abrupt onset of diarrhea and low-grade fever. No antimicrobials unless systemic dissemination is suspected, in which case give a fluoroquinolone. Stool cultures are positive. Prolonged carriage is common.
Yersinia enterocolitica	?	±	+	+	Fecal-oral transmission (occasionally). Food-borne. In pets.	Gastroenteritis or mesenteric adenitis. Occasional bacteremia. Enterotoxin produced.	Severe abdominal pain, diarrhea, fever. PMNs and blood in stool; polyarthritis, erythema nocosum in children. If severe, give tetracycline or gentamicin. Keep stool at 4 °C before culture.

is recommended for those with significant underlying disease (inflammatory bowel disease, AIDS, diabetes, heart disease in the elderly, conditions requiring immunosuppressive medications) and for those whose full activity status during the trip is so essential that even short periods of diarrhea would be unacceptable. Prophylaxis is started upon entry into the destination country and is continued for 1 or 2 days after leaving. For stays of more than 3 weeks, prophylaxis is not recommended because of the cost and increased toxicity. For prophylaxis, bismuth subsalicylate is effective but turns the tongue and the stools black and can interfere with doxycycline absorption, which may be needed for malaria prophylaxis. Numerous antimicrobial regimens for once-daily prophylaxis also are effective, such as norfloxacin 400 mg, ciprofloxacin 500 mg, ofloxacin 300 mg, or trimethoprim-sulfamethoxazole 160/800 mg. Because not all travelers will have diarrhea and because most episodes are brief and self-limited, an alternative approach that is currently recommended is to provide the traveler with a supply of antimicrobials to be taken if significant diarrhea occurs during the trip. Loperamide (4 mg loading dose, then 2 mg after each loose stool to a maximum of 16 mg/d) with a single dose of ciprofloxacin (750 mg), levofloxacin (500 mg), or ofloxacin (300 mg) cures most cases of traveler's diarrhea. If diarrhea is severe, associated with fever or bloody stools, or persists despite single-dose ciprofloxacin treatment, then 3–5 days of ciprofloxacin 500 mg twice daily, levofloxacin 500 mg once daily, norfloxacin 400 mg twice daily, or ofloxacin 300 mg twice daily can be given. Trimethoprim-sulfamethoxazole 160/800 mg twice daily can be used as an alternative, but resistance is common in many areas.

Ansdell VE et al: Prevention and empiric treatment of traveler's diarrhea. Med Clin North Am 1999;83:945. [PMID: 10453258] (Comprehensive review of epidemiology, prevention and therapy.)

Guerrant RL et al: Practice guidelines for the management of infectious diarrhea. Clin Infect Dis 2001;32:331. [PMID: 11170940]

Passaro DJ et al: Advances in prevention and management of traveler's diarrhea. Curr Clin Top Infect Dis 1998;18:217. [PMID: 9779357] (Review of causes, prevention, and therapy.)

■ ACTIVE IMMUNIZATION AGAINST INFECTIOUS DISEASES

RECOMMENDED IMMUNIZATION OF INFANTS, CHILDREN, & ADOLESCENTS

Every individual—child or adult—should maintain an adequate defense against infectious disease by immunization. The recommended schedules and dosages change often, so that one should always consult the manufacturer's package inserts.

The schedule for active immunizations in children is presented in Table 30–4. Of note is the recommendation that all adolescents should see a health care provider at age 11–12. The objective is to ensure vaccination of those who have not received varicella or hepatitis B vaccine; to make certain that a second dose of measles-mumps-rubella (MMR) has been given as well as a booster for tetanus and diphtheria (Td); and to provide immunizations (influenza and pneumococcal vaccines) that may be indicated for certain high-risk individuals.

RECOMMENDED IMMUNIZATION OF ADULTS

Several vaccines are recommended for adults depending upon the individual's previous vaccination status and the risks of exposure to certain diseases.

Tetanus-Diphtheria Toxoid

Everyone should receive a primary series of immunizations against tetanus and diphtheria once (Table 30–4). Adults who have not previously been immunized should receive two doses of Td 1–2 months apart, followed by a booster dose 6–12 months later. Adults partially immunized in childhood with DTP need only a total of three doses of tetanus and diphtheria toxoid (ie, if one dose was given in childhood, give two doses of Td; if two doses were given, only one dose of Td is needed to complete primary immunization). The traditional recommendation has been to give booster doses of Td every 10 years throughout life. An alternative approach emphasizes ensuring that all adults receive primary immunization and recommending a single midlife (age 50 years) booster dose of Td to those who have received the full pediatric immunization, including the booster in the teenage years. If booster doses are given too frequently, an Arthus reaction as well as severe local pain and swelling can occur. An acellular pertussis vaccine, which is highly immunogenic but associated with far fewer adverse effects than the whole cell vaccine, is now included with tetanus-diphtheria toxoid for use in childhood immunization (DTaP). Preliminary data suggest that the acellular vaccine is well tolerated in adolescents and adults, but large-scale trials have not been performed. Even though adolescents and adults with waning immunity may be reservoirs for *B pertussis*—making immunization attractive—because of lack of data, routine immunization of this population with the acellular vaccine is not presently recommended.

For tetanus prophylaxis in wound management see Chapter 33.

Measles

Adults born before 1957 are considered immune to measles. Adults born in 1957 or later who lack documentation of immunization after age 1 or who do not have a physician-documented history or laboratory evidence of previous infection should receive at least one dose of vaccine. Persons born between 1963 and 1967—a period when inactivated measles vaccine was the only product available—should also receive one dose of live attenuated vaccine. Persons vaccinated before their first birthday should also receive a single dose of vaccine. Because most adults do not have detailed information about childhood immunization or illnesses, a practical approach is to administer a single dose of MMR to all healthy adults born after 1956. Because outbreaks of measles have occurred in young adults who have received a single dose of measles vaccine, revaccination is recommended, particularly before going to college, entering a health care profession, or embarking on foreign travel to areas where measles is endemic. Even though birth before 1957 implies immunity, unvaccinated health care workers (especially women of childbearing age) who do not have a history of measles or laboratory evidence of immunity should be vaccinated. Entrants to colleges and universities and employees of health care institutions who have not previously been vaccinated should receive two doses of vaccine at least 1 month apart. Revaccination of an immune person is not associated with adverse effects—if the vaccination status is unknown and an indication for vaccination exists, it can be safely done. Vaccination of susceptible adults within 72 hours after exposure to an active case of measles is protective.

About 5–15% of unimmunized individuals will develop fever and about 5% a mild rash 5–12 days after vaccination. Fever and rash are self-limiting, lasting only 2–3 days. Local swelling and induration are particularly common in individuals previously vaccinated with inactivated vaccine. Pregnant women and immunosuppressed persons should not be vaccinated (with the exception of asymptomatic HIV-infected individuals who are not severely immunosuppressed [CD4 count < 200/µL], who should be vaccinated if susceptible). Recent data suggest that MMR vaccine can be safely given to patients with a history of egg allergy even when severe. A single 0.5 mL dose can be given without prior skin testing or desensitization as long as postvaccination observation for 90 minutes is possible.

Rubella

The major purpose of rubella vaccination is to prevent transmission to the fetus. Immunization is recommended for all adults but particularly for women of childbearing age who have not previously been immunized. Although persons born before 1957 are considered immune, this is not an acceptable criterion of immunity for women who could become pregnant. Thus, premenopausal women born before 1957 who might become pregnant should be vaccinated. In addition, both male and female hospital workers who may

be exposed to patients with rubella or who might have contact with pregnant patients should be immunized. A single immunization is given. MMR trivalent vaccine is recommended, but if immunity to one or more of the components can be demonstrated, monovalent or bivalent vaccines can be used. Because of the expense of serologic testing to identify susceptible individuals and because revaccination of immune individuals is not associated with adverse effects, routine serologic testing is not required prior to vaccination.

Adverse effects are usually mild. Up to 40% of unvaccinated adults (usually women) experience joint pain. Joint symptoms begin 1–3 weeks after vaccination and are self-limited, lasting 3–10 days. Frank arthritis is rare. Although vaccination of pregnant women is *not* recommended, available data suggest that with the RA27/3 vaccine strain (the one presently available), the congenital rubella syndrome does not occur in the offspring of those inadvertently vaccinated during pregnancy or within 3 months before conception. Persons immunosuppressed by virtue of disease or medication should not receive vaccine. HIV infection is an exception—vaccine should be given to asymptomatic individuals who do not have evidence of severe immunosuppression (CD5 count < 200/µL) and may be considered in symptomatic patients. Since the vaccine contains trace amounts of neomycin, a history of anaphylaxis to this agent is a contraindication to vaccine use.

Mumps

Mumps vaccine is recommended for all adults thought to be susceptible. Persons born before 1957 are considered to be naturally immune and do not require vaccination. Those born in 1957 or later should be considered susceptible unless they can document infection, prove vaccination, or have laboratory evidence of immunity. Vaccination in those already immune is not associated with an increased incidence of adverse effects.

Mumps vaccine is generally safe. It should not be given to those who are immunosuppressed (except HIV-infected individuals) or who have a history of anaphylaxis to neomycin.

Influenza

Influenza vaccination is recommended yearly. Those at greatest risk for severe complications of influenza should have priority in vaccination programs: (1) Adults and children with chronic cardiopulmonary disease, including children with asthma. (2) Residents of nursing homes and other chronic care facilities. (3) Healthy adults 50 years of age or older. (4) Adults and children who have required either regular medical follow-up or hospitalization in the last year for chronic metabolic disorders (including diabetes) or renal disease, those with hemoglobinopathies, and those receiving immunosuppressive drugs. (5) Children and

Table 30–4. Recommended childhood immunization schedule[*]—United States, 2002.

Vaccine	Birth	1 mo	2 mos	4 mos	6 mos	12 mos	15 mos	18 mos	24 mos	4–6 yrs	11–12 yrs	13–18 yrs
				Range of recommended ages				Catch-up vaccination		Preadolescent assessment		
Hepatitis B[1]	Hep B #1 only if mother HBsAg (*)									Hep B series		
		Hep B #2			Hep B #3							
Diphtheria, Tetanus, Pertussis[2]			DTaP	DTaP	DTaP		DTaP			DTaP	Td	
Haemophilus influenzae Type b[3]			Hib	Hib	Hib	Hib						
Inactivated Polio[4]			IPV	IPV		IPV				IPV		
Measles, Mumps, Rubella[5]						MMR #1				MMR #2	MMR #2	
Varicella[6]						Varicella					Varicella	
Pneumococcal[7]			PCV	PCV	PCV	PCV				PCV	PPV	
Hepatitis A[8]										Hepatitis A series		
Influenza[9]										Influenza (yearly)		

Vaccines below this line are for selected populations

[*]Indicates the recommended ages for routine administration of currently licensed childhood vaccines, as of December 1, 2001, for children through age 18 years. Any dose not given at the recommended age should be given at any subsequent visit when indicated and feasible. ▨ Indicates age groups that warrant special effort to administer those vaccines not given previously. Additional vaccines may be licensed and recommended during the year. Licensed combination vaccines may be used whenever any components of the combination are indicated and the vaccine's other components are not contraindicated. Providers should consult the manufacturers' package inserts for detailed recommendations.

[1]**Hepatitis B vaccine (Hep B).** All infants should receive the first dose of hepatitis B vaccine soon after birth and before hospital discharge; the first dose also may be given by age 2 months if the infant's mother is HBsAg-negative. Only monovalent hepatitis B vaccine can be used for the birth dose. Monovalent or combination vaccine containing Hep B may be used to complete the series; 4 doses of vaccine may be administered if combination vaccine is used. The second dose should be given at least 4 weeks after the first dose except for Hib-containing vaccine, which cannot be administered before age 6 weeks. The third dose should be given at least 16 weeks after the first dose and at least 8 weeks after the second dose. The last dose in the vaccination series (third or fourth dose) should not be administered before age 6 months. *Infants born to HBsAg-positive mothers* should receive hepatitis B vaccine and 0.5 mL hepatitis B immune globulin (HBIG) at separate sites within 12 hours of birth. The second dose is recommended at age 1–2 months and the vaccination series should be completed (third or fourth dose) at age 6 months. *Infants born to mothers whose HBsAg status is unknown* should receive the first dose of the hepatitis B vaccine series within 12 hours of birth. Maternal blood should be drawn at the time of delivery to determine the mother's HBsAg status; if the HBsAg test is positive, the infant should receive HBIG as soon as possible (no later than age 1 week).

[2]**Diphtheria and tetanus toxoids and acellular pertussis vaccine (DTaP).** The fourth dose of DTaP may be administered as early as age 12 months provided that 6 months have elapsed since the third dose and the child is unlikely to return at age 15–18 months.
Tetanus and diphtheria toxoids (Td) is recommended at age 11–12 years if at least 5 years have elapsed since the last dose of tetanus and diphtheria toxoid-containing vaccine. Subsequent routine Td boosters are recommended every 10 years.

[3]**Haemophilus influenzae type b (Hib) conjugate vaccine.** Three Hib conjugate vaccines are licensed for infant use. If PRP-OMP (PedvaxHIB® or ComVax® [Merck]) is administered at age 2 and 4 months, a dose at age 6 months is not required. DTaP/Hib combination products should not be used for primary immunization in infants at age 2, 4 or 6 months but can be used as boosters following any Hib vaccine.

[4]**Inactivated poliovirus vaccine (IPV).** An all-IPV schedule is recommended for routine childhood poliovirus vaccination in the United States. All children should receive 4 doses of IPV at age 2, 4, and 6–18 months, and 4–6 years.

[5]**Measles, mumps, and rubella vaccine (MMR).** The second dose of MMR is recommended routinely at age 4–6 years but may be administered during any visit provided at least 4 weeks have elapsed since the first dose and that both doses are administered beginning at or after age 12 months. Those who have not previously received the second dose should complete the schedule by the visit at age 11–12 years.

[6]**Varicella vaccine.** Varicella vaccine is recommended at any visit, at or after age 12 months for susceptible children (i.e., those who lack a reliable history of chickenpox). Susceptible persons aged ≥ 13 years should receive 2 doses given at least 4 weeks apart.

Table 30–4. Recommended childhood immunization schedule*—United States, 2002. (continued)

[7]**Pneumococcal vaccine.** The heptavalent **pneumococcal conjugate vaccine (PCV)** is recommended for all children aged 2–23 months and for certain children aged 24–59 months. **Pneumococcal polysaccharide vaccine** (PPV) is recommended in addition to PCV for certain high-risk groups. See *MMWR* 2000;49(No. RR-9):1–37.

[8]**Hepatitis A vaccine.** Hepatitis A vaccine is recommended for use in selected states and regions, and for certain high-risk groups. Consult local public health authority and *MMWR* 1999;48(No. RR-12):1–37.

[9]**Influenza vaccine.** Influenza vaccine is recommended annually for children aged ≥ 6 months with certain risk factors (including but not limited to asthma, cardiac disease, sickle cell disease, HIV, and diabetes; see *MMWR* 2001;50[No. RR-4]:1–44), and can be administered to all others wishing to obtain immunity. Children aged ≤ 12 years should receive vaccine in a dosage appropriate for their age (0.25 mL if 6–35 months or 0.5 mL if ≥ 3 years). Children aged ≤ 8 years who are receiving influenza vaccine for the first time should receive 2 doses separated by at least 4 weeks.

Additional information about vaccines, vaccine supply, and contraindications for immunization is available at http://www.cdc.gov/nip or at the National Immunization hotline, 800-232-2522 (English), or 800-232-0233 (Spanish). Copies of the schedule can be obtained at http://www.cdc.gov/nip/recs/child-schedule.htm. Approved by the **Advisory Committee of Immunization Practices** (http://www.cdc.gov/nip/acip), the **American Academy of Pediatrics** (http://www.aap.org), and the **American Academy of Family Physicians** (http://www.aafp.org).

teenagers (age 6 months to 18 years) who are on long-term aspirin therapy and would be at increased risk for developing Reye's syndrome following influenza. (6) Women who will be in the second or third trimester of pregnancy during the influenza season. Certain high-risk groups of patients (the elderly, persons with AIDS, transplant patients) may have a poor antibody response to vaccine, but there is no reason not to vaccinate them. Concern that vaccination of HIV-positive patients may result in a brief (2- to 4-week) period of increased HIV viremia and viral replication has been raised. The data are conflicting and the clinical significance is probably minimal, as progression of disease after vaccination has not been observed. Thus, the potential benefit of vaccination of HIV-positive individuals outweighs any theoretic risks. In an attempt to prevent disease in high-risk patients, vaccination is advised for household members and health care providers who have contact with these high-risk patients. Vaccination is recommended also for otherwise healthy adults who provide essential community services and for any individual who wants to decrease the risk of becoming ill with influenza.

Local reactions (erythema and tenderness) at the site of injection are common, but fevers, chills, and malaise (which last in any case only 2–3 days) are rare. Like measles, mumps, and yellow fever vaccines, influenza vaccine is prepared using embryonated chicken eggs, and persons with a history of anaphylaxis to eggs should not be vaccinated. The risk of Guillain-Barré syndrome is not increased following vaccination. Influenza vaccination may be associated with multiple false-positive serologic tests to HIV, HTLV-1, and hepatitis C. Seropositivity is self-limited, lasting 2–5 months.

Preliminary data suggest that a trivalent live attenuated influenza vaccine administered as a single-dose intranasal spray is effective in preventing disease. The product may be available for the next influenza season. Two neuraminidase inhibitors (zanamivir and os-

eltamivir) are approved for therapy of influenza A and B, and oseltamivir is approved for prophylaxis. The dose is 75 mg/d, and the duration of treatment depends on the clinical setting. Amantadine and rimantadine are also approved for prophylaxis, but these agents are active only against influenza A.

Pneumococcal Pneumonia

Pneumococcal vaccine contains purified polysaccharide from 23 of the most common strains of *S pneumoniae*, which cause 90% of bacteremic episodes in the USA. Antibody response following vaccination is dependent upon the patient's immune status and the presence of concomitant disease. Healthy adults have an excellent antibody response, as do patients who are postsplenectomy and those with sickle cell disease. Elderly individuals and those with chronic diseases (diabetes mellitus, alcoholic cirrhosis, chronic obstructive pulmonary disease, lupus erythematosus, rheumatoid arthritis) have increased antibody levels following vaccination but to a lesser extent than young healthy adults. Patients with Hodgkin's disease respond to vaccination if it is given before splenectomy, radiation, or chemotherapy, whereas patients with leukemia, lymphoma, and HIV infection respond poorly.

Although the efficacy of pneumococcal vaccine has been questioned, most postlicensure studies indicate that vaccination is about 60–70% effective in preventing bacteremic disease in immunocompetent persons. It is 50% effective in patients with underlying diseases (not severely immunocompromised) and even less effective in immunocompromised patients (only 10% effective) largely because of inability to mount an antibody response in this population of patients. It is presently recommended for patients at increased risk for developing severe pneumococcal disease, especially asplenic patients and those with sickle cell disease. It is also recommended for adults who are at increased risk of developing pneumococcal disease, including those with chronic illnesses (eg, cardiopulmonary disease, alcoholism, cirrhosis, cerebrospinal fluid leaks), those who are immunocompromised (eg, patients with Hodgkin's disease, lymphoma, chronic lymphocytic leukemia, multiple myeloma, chronic renal failure, nephrotic syndrome, organ transplant recipients receiving immunosuppressive therapy, including long-term systemic steroids, and asymptomatic or symptomatic HIV infection), and those taking immunosuppressive medications. Although not currently recommended for smokers and black adults, some feel that these groups should be routinely immunized because of their increased risk of developing invasive disease. In addition, it is recommended for all individuals over 65 years of age. Whether 65 is the appropriate age to vaccinate healthy adults is unclear. Antibody response declines with age, and some have suggested routine immunization at age 50 similar to the recommendation for tetanus (see above). A single dose of vaccine usually confers lifelong immunity. Revaccination every 5 years is recommended, regardless of age, in those at highest risk of fatal pneumococcal infection (eg, functionally or anatomically asplenic patients), those known to have a rapid decline in antibody titers (eg, those with nephrotic syndrome or renal failure, HIV infection, leukemia, lymphoma, multiple myeloma, those taking immunosuppressive medications, transplant patients), and those 65 years of age if they received the vaccine 5 years or more previously and were under age 65 at the time of primary vaccination. Elderly individuals with unknown vaccination status should be immunized once. Revaccination should also be considered for high-risk individuals previously immunized with the older 14-valent vaccine. Since immunocompetent patients respond best to the vaccine, it should be given 2 weeks before splenectomy or before starting chemotherapy if that can be anticipated.

A protein-conjugated heptavalent pneumococcal vaccine approved for use in children under 2 years of age has not been studied in adults.

Mild reactions (erythema and tenderness) to pneumococcal vaccine occur in up to 50% of recipients, but systemic reactions are uncommon. Similarly, revaccination at least 5 years after initial vaccination is associated with mild self-limited local reactions but not systemic reactions.

Hepatitis B

Recombinant hepatitis B vaccine is given intramuscularly in the deltoid (gluteal injection often results in deposition of vaccine in fat rather than muscle, with fewer serologic conversions) on three separate occasions: the first two doses 1 month apart and the last dose 5 months after the second one. It is recommended for all individuals at increased risk of developing hepatitis B for social reasons (intravenous drug users, male homosexuals), family reasons (household and sexual contacts of hepatitis B carriers), or occupational reasons (those with frequent exposure to blood

and blood products, hemodialysis patients and staff, house officers, medical students, morticians). For immunosuppressed patients, those being maintained on hemodialysis, and chronic alcoholics, seroresponse to standard doses of vaccine is low, and for that reason preparations delivering a higher vaccine dose (40 μg/mL) have become available. In addition to higher vaccine doses, these patients may require more frequent immunizations, and some experts have recommended annual screening to determine whether booster doses are needed. Although most often used for preexposure prophylaxis, the vaccine is also given as postexposure prophylaxis along with hepatitis B immunoglobulin following needle stick injury or mucous membrane exposure to blood from an individual who is HBsAg-positive. It is also given along with hepatitis B immunoglobulin to infants of mothers who are HBsAg-positive (Table 30–4). Immunity wanes with time, but periodic serologic monitoring is not recommended, and routine administration of booster doses is not necessary. Adverse reactions are minor and limited to local soreness.

Following vaccination, 90–95% of healthy young individuals develop protective antibodies. A number of factors decrease serologic response, including increasing age over 30, renal failure, HIV infection, diabetes, chronic liver disease, obesity, and smoking. Postvaccination serologic testing is not routinely done. It is reserved for those whose clinical management would be influenced by their immune status (eg, health care workers, infants born to HBsAg-positive mothers, dialysis patients), and those who may have an impaired response. Those who do not respond should receive a second three-dose vaccine series with serologic testing 1–2 months after completion. Those who fail to respond are unlikely to respond to further vaccination even with a different recombinant vaccine and should be considered susceptible; if exposed, they should receive hepatitis B immune globulin.

Varicella

A live attenuated varicella virus vaccine is currently recommended as part of routine childhood immunization (Table 30–4). Although only 10% of adults remain susceptible, varicella in adolescents and adults is a more severe disease. Only about 2% of all cases of varicella occur in adults, but almost 50% of all deaths are in the adult population. Thus, susceptible adolescents and adults should be immunized, with special emphasis on certain high-risk groups, ie, health care workers; susceptible household contacts of immunosuppressed individuals; persons who live or work in environments where transmission can occur, eg, teachers in day care centers or elementary schools, residents and workers in institutional settings such as the military and correctional institutions, college students; nonpregnant women of childbearing age; and international travelers. The role of the present vaccine in postexposure prophylaxis has not been widely studied, but several reports from Japan and the United States suggest that it is 90% effective in preventing varicella in an outbreak situation, particularly when given within 3–5 days after exposure. The Advisory Committee on Immunization Practices (ACIP) now recommends vaccination in susceptible persons following exposure. The vaccine is very immunogenic. Seroconversion occurs in 95% of children after a single dose. In adolescents (older than 12 years of age) and adults, seroconversion is seen in 78% after one dose and 99% after two doses. For this reason, two doses given 4–8 weeks apart are recommended in persons 12 years of age and older. The duration of immunity is not known but is probably 10 years. Although the vaccine is very effective in preventing disease, breakthrough infections do occur—but are much milder than in unvaccinated individuals (usually less than 50 lesions, with milder systemic symptoms). Although the vaccine is very safe, adverse reactions can occur as late as 4–6 weeks after vaccination. Tenderness and erythema at the injection site are seen in 25%, fever in 10–15%, a localized maculopapular or vesicular rash in 5%, and a smaller percentage develop a diffuse rash, usually with five or fewer vesicular lesions. Spread of virus from vaccinees to susceptible individuals is possible, but the risk of such transmission even to immunocompromised patients is small and disease, when it develops, is mild and treatable with acyclovir. Nonetheless, the vaccine, being a live attenuated virus, should not be given to immunocompromised individuals, including HIV-positive children and adults, or pregnant women. The vaccine is contraindicated in persons allergic to neomycin. For theoretic reasons, it is recommended that following vaccination salicylates should be avoided for 6 weeks (to prevent Reye's syndrome). Several unresolved issues remain, including the need for booster doses, whether universal childhood vaccination will shift the incidence of disease to adolescence or adulthood with the possibility of more severe disease, and whether vaccination might prevent development of herpes zoster.

Hepatitis A

Two inactivated hepatitis A vaccines (Havrix, VAQTA) are approved for use in the USA. They are indicated for individuals 2 years of age or older who are at an increased risk of developing hepatitis A. Potential vaccinees include travelers (including military personnel) to areas where hepatitis is endemic (Africa, Asia, Central and South America, Mexico, parts of the Caribbean); certain populations that experience episodic hepatitis A outbreaks (such as indigenous Alaskans, certain American Indian reservations, certain religious communities and certain states where the risk of hepatitis A is high among children); certain high-risk groups such as employees of day care centers, caretakers for developmentally impaired institutionalized individuals, and laboratory workers who handle live hepatitis A virus or work closely with nonhuman

primates; men who have sex with men; illicit drug users; persons who receive clotting factor concentrates; and those with chronic liver disease, particularly hepatitis B and hepatitis C. Vaccine has been used as a means of controlling spread of disease during outbreaks in communities with high rates of infection. The role of hepatitis A vaccine in controlling outbreaks in day care centers, hospitals, and institutions for the disabled has not been investigated, and immune globulin is used in those settings. A single intramuscular injection in adults elicits antibodies in 54–62% of individuals at 2 weeks and 96% by 1 month. The different formulations come in different strengths, and dosage depends on the age of the vaccinee and the preparation used (see package insert). In general, two doses are required, the second given 6–18 months after the first. The duration of immunity is not known but may be lifelong, and at present repeat vaccination is not recommended. Adverse effects are minimal and consist mainly of soreness at the injection site. If vaccine is not available, temporary passive immunity may be induced by the intramuscular injection of immune globulin, 0.02 mL/kg every 2–3 months or 0.1 mL/kg every 6 months. Protection with immune globulin is recommended for persons traveling to all parts of the world where sanitation is poor and the risk of exposure to hepatitis A is high because of contaminated food and water supplies and contact with infected persons. Preparation of immunoglobulin from plasma involves steps that inactivate HIV, thus making immunoglobulin preparations incapable of transmitting HIV infection.

Combined Hepatitis A & B Vaccine

A combined hepatitis A and B vaccine is approved for use in individuals 18 years of age and older. The components are identical to individual vaccines that have been used in the United States for many years. It is highly immunogenic and effective and should be used in individuals who have an indication for both hepatitis A and B vaccination such as patients with chronic liver disease, intravenous drug users, men who have sex with men, and individuals with clotting disorders who require frequent use of blood products. The product is safe, and adverse effects are similar to what is seen with the individual components.

RECOMMENDED IMMUNIZATIONS FOR TRAVELERS

Individuals traveling to other countries frequently require immunizations in addition to those listed above and may benefit from chemoprophylaxis against various diseases. Every traveler must fulfill the immunization requirements of the health authorities of different countries. These are listed in *Health Information for International Travel,* published by the Centers for Disease Control. An updated version is published yearly and is available from the Superintendent of Documents, United States Government Printing Office, Washington, DC 20402, or on the Internet: http://www.cdc.gov/nip/home.html.

When individuals request information and vaccinations for travel from a physician, their entire immunization history should be reviewed and updated, including those immunizations listed above that are not specifically required for travel.

Various vaccines can be given simultaneously at different sites. Some, such as cholera, plague, and typhoid vaccine, which cause significant discomfort, are best given at different times. In general, live attenuated vaccines (measles, mumps, rubella, yellow fever, and oral typhoid vaccine) should not be given to immunosuppressed individuals or household members of immunosuppressed people or to pregnant women. Immunoglobulin should not be given for 3 months before or at least 2 weeks after live virus vaccines, because it may attenuate the antibody response.

Chemoprophylaxis of malaria is discussed in Chapter 35.

Cholera

Because the incidence of cholera among travelers is very low and because the vaccine is only marginally effective, the World Health Organization does not routinely require immunization even for persons traveling to and from endemic areas. Although no country officially requires cholera vaccination, some local authorities may still require documentation of vaccination.

Cholera vaccine contains a suspension of killed vibrios, including prevalent antigenic types. Two injections are given intramuscularly 2–6 weeks apart, followed by booster injections every 6 months during periods of possible exposure. Protection depends largely on booster doses. An inactivated oral vaccine appears to be more effective than the parenteral vaccine but is not available in the USA. A live attenuated oral vaccine is being investigated. The WHO certificate is valid for 6 months only.

Hepatitis B

Persons traveling to and spending more than 6 months in endemic areas of HBV infection who will have close contact with the local population should be considered for vaccination. Short-term travelers to areas of moderate or high endemic infection (Southeast Asia, China, most of the Middle East, Haiti, the Dominican Republic, and most of Africa) who will be in contact with potentially infected body secretions of residents should be vaccinated. Vaccination should begin at least 6 months before travel to allow for completion of the series.

Hepatitis A

As indicated above, susceptible individuals traveling to areas of high or intermediate endemicity for hepatitis

A (eg, all areas except Canada, western Europe, Japan, Australia, and New Zealand) should be vaccinated. The vaccine should be given at least 4 weeks prior to travel, as protective antibodies develop in 96% of vaccinees by that time. If given 2 weeks before travel, up to 45% will not have protective antibodies, and if the person is traveling to a high-risk area, intramuscular immune globulin (0.02 mL/kg) should be administered at a separate site.

Meningococcal Meningitis

If travel is contemplated to an area where meningococcal meningitis is epidemic (Nepal, sub-Saharan Africa, the "meningitis belt" from Senegal in the west to Ethiopia in the east, northern India) or highly endemic, polysaccharide vaccines from types A, C, W-135, and Y may be indicated. (Saudi Arabia requires immunization for pilgrims to Mecca.) Follow the manufacturer's dosage recommendations. The vaccine is also recommended for persons with anatomic or functional asplenia and those with terminal complement deficiencies. College freshmen living in dormitories are at a modest increased risk for developing meningococcal infections. Vaccination will decrease but not eliminate the risk of disease and should be offered to those who want to decrease the risk of developing infection. Although the need for revaccination has not been determined, antibody levels decline over 2–3 years, and revaccination is reasonable in 3–5 years if risk continues.

Plague

Plague vaccine is a suspension of killed plague bacilli that is given intramuscularly. Three injections are given—the second, 4 weeks after the initial injection; and the third, 5 months after the second. The risk of acquiring plague is so low that routine vaccination is not recommended. Vaccination is reserved for travelers who will have exposure to rodents or rabbits in rural areas where plague is endemic (some areas in South America, Southeast Asia, occasionally others). For continuing exposures, booster doses at intervals of 1–2 years are recommended.

Poliomyelitis

Adult travelers to tropical or developing countries who have not previously been immunized against poliomyelitis should receive a primary series of three doses of inactivated enhanced-potency poliovaccine (IPV), as follows: two doses of 0.5 mL subcutaneously 4–8 weeks apart and then a third dose 6–12 months after the second dose. If more than 8 weeks will elapse before travel, three doses of IPV can be given 4 weeks apart. If 4–8 weeks will elapse before travel, two doses are given 4 weeks apart, and if less than 4 weeks will elapse, a single dose is given. Vaccination can be completed upon return if continued or future exposure to polio is anticipated. Travelers who have previously been fully immunized with OPV or IPV should receive a one-time booster dose with IPV. Data do not indicate the need for more than one adult booster. Live attenuated poliovaccine is no longer recommended because of the risk of vaccine-associated disease.

Rabies

For travelers to areas where rabies is common in domestic animals (eg, India, Asia, Mexico), preexposure prophylaxis with human diploid cell vaccine (HDCV), rabies vaccine adsorbed (RVA), or purified chick embryo cell culture (PCEC) vaccine should be considered. It usually consists of two intramuscular (deltoid area) injections of 1 mL given 1 week apart with a booster dose 2–3 weeks later. Alternatively, two intradermal injections of 0.1 mL of human diploid cell vaccine are given 1 week apart, with a booster dose given 2–3 weeks later. Chloroquine can blunt the immunologic response to rabies vaccine. If malaria prophylaxis with chloroquine is required, vaccination should be given intramuscularly (*not* intradermally) to ensure adequate antibody response. There are no data on the interaction between mefloquine and rabies vaccine. It would seem reasonable to administer rabies vaccine intramuscularly if mefloquine is to be given until further studies are done.

Typhoid

Typhoid vaccination is recommended for travelers to developing countries (especially Latin America, Africa, and Asia) who will have prolonged exposure to contaminated food and water. Three preparations of approximately equal efficacy (50–75% effective) are available: (1) a heat-phenol-inactivated vaccine for parenteral use; (2) an oral live-attenuated Ty21a vaccine supplied as enteric-coated capsules; and (3) a Vi capsular polysaccharide (Vi CPS) vaccine for parenteral use. The phenol-inactivated preparation that has been historically used is associated with the most side effects and is not recommended unless the other preparations are not available. The Ty21a vaccine is given as one capsule every other day for four doses. The capsules must be refrigerated and taken with cool liquids (37 °C or less) at least 1 hour before meals. All four doses must be taken for maximum protection. Adverse effects are minimal and consist primarily of gastrointestinal upset. The Vi CPS vaccine is given as a single intramuscular injection. Adverse effects consist mainly of local irritation at the site of injection, but fever and headache have been reported. If continued or repeated exposures are anticipated, booster doses are recommended. A booster dose of the heat-inactivated vaccine is recommended every 3 years. Boosters of the Vi CPS are given every 2 years. The optimal booster dose of the Ty21a is not known, but the manufacturer recommends repeating the four-dose series every 5 years. The live attenuated vaccine should not be used in immunosuppressed patients, including those with HIV infection.

Yellow Fever

The live attenuated yellow fever virus vaccine is administered once subcutaneously. Although the risk of yellow fever is low for most conventional travelers, a number of countries require vaccination for all visitors and others require it for travelers to or from endemic areas (mainly equatorial Africa and parts of South and Central America). The WHO certificate requires registration of the manufacturer and the batch number of the vaccine. Vaccination is available in the USA only at approved centers. (Contact the local health department for available resources.) Reimmunization is recommended at 10-year intervals if continued risk exists.

Because it is a live attenuated vaccine prepared in embryonated eggs, the yellow fever vaccine should not be given to immunosuppressed individuals or those with a history of anaphylaxis to eggs. Pregnancy is a relative contraindication to vaccination.

Although not proved to be causally related, between 1996 and 2001, seven cases of fever, jaundice, and multiple organ system failure following yellow fever vaccination were reported. Until further data are available, vaccination is still recommended but should be limited to those traveling to areas reporting yellow fever activity or to the yellow fever endemic area. (Current information about the vaccine and yellow fever activity can be found at http://www.cdc.gov/travel/yfever.htm)

Japanese B Encephalitis

This is a mosquito-borne viral encephalitis that affects primarily children and older adults (65 years and older) and usually occurs from May to September. It is the leading cause of encephalitis in Asia. Because the risk of infection is low and because adverse effects of the vaccine can be serious, not all travelers to Asia should be vaccinated. Vaccine should be given to travelers to endemic areas who will be staying at least 30 days and who are traveling during the transmission season, particularly if they are visiting rural areas. Travelers who spend less than 30 days in the region should be considered for vaccination if they intend to visit areas of epidemic transmission or if extensive outdoor activities are planned in rural rice-growing areas. The recommended primary immunization schedule is 1 mL of vaccine administered subcutaneously on days 0, 7, and 30. If time constraints are compelling, the last dose can be given on day 14. The last dose should be given at least 10 days before embarkation because adverse effects in the form of urticaria and angioedema have been described, occurring from minutes up to 10 days after vaccination. Following vaccination, patients should be observed for 30 minutes and advised of the possibility of delayed reactions of angioedema and urticaria. In addition, local reactions have been reported in 20% of vaccinees and systemic reactions (fever, chills, malaise, headache) in 10%.

Reid KC et al: Immunizations: Recommendations for practice. Mayo Clin Proc 1999;74:377. [PMID: 10221468] (Summary of indications for common adult immunizations.)

Ryan ET et al: Health advice and immunizations for travelers. N Engl J Med 2000;342:1716. [PMID: 10841875]

Vaccine recommendations—challenges and controversies. Infect Dis Clin North Am 2001;15(1). (Entire March 2001 issue devoted to immunizations, including routine, travel, in pregnancy, and in immunocompromised patients.)

Virk A: Medical advice for international travelers. Mayo Clinic Proc 2001;76:831. [PMID: 11499824] (Overview of general advice and specific vaccine recommendations.)

HYPERSENSITIVITY TESTS & DESENSITIZATION

One should test for hypersensitivity before injecting antitoxin, materials derived from animal sources, or drugs (eg, penicillin) to which a patient has had a severe reaction in the past. If the test described below is negative, desensitization is not necessary, and a full dose of the material may be given. If the test is positive, alternative drugs should be strongly considered. If that is not feasible, desensitization is necessary.

Intradermal Test for Hypersensitivity

Penicillin is the drug that most frequently serves as an indication for sensitivity testing and desensitization. A clinical history of penicillin allergy has a positive predictive value of only 15%. In determining whether allergy testing should be performed, the nature of the allergy should be determined. Immunoglobulin G-mediated delayed reactions such as erythematous or maculopapular skin rash, serum sickness (rash and arthritis), and pruritus should be distinguished from immediate-type immunoglobulin E-mediated reactions such as urticaria, angioedema, and anaphylaxis. Only patients with the latter history who require penicillin or a cephalosporin should undergo hypersensitivity testing. Skin testing requires two preparations: PPL (penicilloyl-polylysine) and a minor determinant mixture. Several points should be emphasized in performing and interpreting these tests. Whenever possible, both PPL and a minor determinant should be used, since 85% of skin test reactors are positive to PPL but 15% react only to the minor determinant mixture. In addition, if penicillin G is used instead of the minor determinant mixture, some allergic patients will be missed. About 25% of individuals who react to minor determinant mixture may not react to penicillin G, and such patients may still have an anaphylactic or accelerated reaction to penicillin. A pinprick test is performed with each solution at different sites by placing a small drop of solution on the skin and making small indentations of the skin with a needle. If there is no reaction within 10 minutes, 0.01–0.02 mL is injected intradermally, raising a small bleb. Development of a wheal greater than 5 mm in diameter is considered a positive test and an indication for desensitization. Even if the test is negative, about 1–2% of patients will have an immediate or accelerated reaction, but an anaphylactic reaction is exceedingly rare. Thus, if the test is negative, the drug can be administered with relative safety, but the first dose should be medically supervised and the patient observed for 1 hour (serious reactions after 1 hour are rare).

Patients with a history of allergy to penicillin are also at an increased risk of having a reaction to cephalosporins. A common approach to these patients is to assess the severity of the reaction. If an IgE-mediated reaction can be excluded by history, a cephalosporin can be administered. When the history justifies concern about an immediate type reaction, penicillin skin testing should be performed. If the test is negative, a cephalosporin can be given. If the test is positive, cephalosporin desensitization should be performed.

Desensitization

A. PRECAUTIONS

1. The desensitization procedure is not innocuous—deaths from anaphylaxis have been reported. If extreme hypersensitivity is suspected, it is advisable to use an alternative structurally unrelated drug and to reserve desensitization for situations when treatment cannot be withheld and no alternative drug is available.

2. An antihistaminic drug (25–50 mg of hydroxyzine or diphenhydramine intramuscularly or orally) should be administered before desensitization is begun in order to lessen any reaction that occurs.

3. Desensitization should be conducted in an intensive care unit where cardiac monitoring and emergency endotracheal intubation can be performed.

4. Epinephrine, 1 mL of 1:1000 solution, must be ready for immediate administration.

B. DESENSITIZATION METHOD

Several methods of desensitization have been described for penicillin, including use of both oral and intravenous preparations. All methods start with very small doses of drug and gradually increase the dose until therapeutic doses are achieved. For penicillin, 1 unit of drug is given intravenously and the patient observed for 15–30 minutes. If there is no reaction, some recommend doubling the dose while others recommend increasing it tenfold every 15–30 minutes until a dosage of 2 million units is reached; then give the remainder of the desired dose.

For recommendations on skin testing and desensitization for other preparations (botulism antitoxin, diphtheria antitoxin, etc), one should consult the manufacturer's package inserts.

Treatment of Reactions

A. MILD REACTIONS

If a mild reaction occurs, drop back to the next lower dose and continue with desensitization. If a severe reaction occurs, administer epinephrine (see below) and discontinue the drug unless treatment is urgently needed. If desensitization is imperative, continue slowly, increasing the dosage of the drug more gradually.

B. SEVERE REACTIONS

If bronchospasm occurs, epinephrine, 0.3–0.5 mL of 1:1000 dilution, should be given subcutaneously every 10–20 minutes. The following can also be given if symptoms persist: inhaled metaproterenol (0.3 mL of a 5% solution in 2.5 mL of saline), intravenous aminophylline (0.3–0.9 mL/kg/h maintenance after a 6 mg/kg loading dose over 30 minutes), or corticosteroids (250 mg of hydrocortisone or 50 mg of methylprednisolone intravenously every 6 hours for two to four doses). Hypotension should be treated with intravenous fluids (saline or colloid), epinephrine (1 mL of 1:1000 dilution in 500 mL of D_5W intravenously at a rate of 0.5–5 μg/min), and antihistamines (25–50 mg of hydroxyzine or diphenhydramine intramuscularly or orally every 6–8 hours as needed). Cutaneous reactions, manifested as urticaria or angioedema, respond to epinephrine subcutaneously and antihistamines in the doses set forth above.

Kelkar PS et al: Cephalosporin allergy. N Engl J Med 2001;345:804. (State of the art review.) [PMID: 11556301]

1998 guidelines for treatment of sexually transmitted diseases. Centers for Disease Control and Prevention. MMWR Recomm Rep 1998;47(RR-1):1. [PMID: 9461053] (Section on oral or intravenous desensitization to penicillin in patients with positive skin tests.)

Salkind AR et al: The rational clinical examination. Is this patient allergic to penicillin? An evidence-based analysis of the likelihood of penicillin allergy. JAMA 2001.288:2998. [PMID: 11368703] (A review of the value of skin testing, the role of the history, and cross-reactions with other drugs.)

HIV Infection

31

Harry Hollander, MD & Mitchell H. Katz, MD
See www.current-med.com/ch31.html

ESSENTIALS OF DIAGNOSIS

- *Risk factors: sexual contact with an infected person, parenteral exposure to infected blood by transfusion or needle sharing, perinatal exposure.*
- *Prominent systemic complaints such as sweats, diarrhea, weight loss, and wasting.*
- *Opportunistic infections due to diminished cellular immunity—often life-threatening.*
- *Aggressive cancers, particularly Kaposi's sarcoma and extranodal lymphoma.*
- *Neurologic manifestations, including dementia, aseptic meningitis, and neuropathy.*

General Considerations

When AIDS was first recognized in the USA in 1981, cases were identified by finding severe opportunistic infections such as pneumocystis pneumonia that indicated profound defects in cellular immunity in the absence of other causes of immunodeficiency. When the syndrome was found to be caused by the human immunodeficiency virus (HIV), it became obvious that severe opportunistic infections and unusual neoplasms were at one end of a spectrum of disease, while healthy seropositive individuals were at the other end.

The Centers for Disease Control and Prevention AIDS case definition (Table 31–1) includes opportunistic infections and malignancies that rarely occur in the absence of severe immunodeficiency (eg, pneumocystis pneumonia, central nervous system lymphoma). It also classifies persons as having AIDS if they have positive HIV serology and certain infections and malignancies that can occur in immunocompetent hosts but which are more common among persons infected with HIV (pulmonary tuberculosis, invasive cervical cancer). Several nonspecific conditions, including dementia and wasting (documented weight loss)—in the presence of a positive HIV serology—are considered AIDS. The definition includes criteria for both definitive and presumptive diagnoses of certain infections and malignancies. Finally, persons with positive HIV serology who have ever had a CD4 lymphocyte count below 200 cells/μL or a CD4 lymphocyte percentage below 14% are considered to have AIDS. Inclusion of persons with low CD4 counts as AIDS cases reflects the recognition that immunodeficiency is the defining characteristic of AIDS. The choice of a cutoff point at 200 cells/μL is supported by several cohort studies showing that over 80% of persons with counts below this level will develop AIDS within 3 years in the absence of effective antiretroviral therapy. The 1993 definition was also expanded to include persons with positive HIV serology and pulmonary tuberculosis, recurrent pneumonia, and invasive cervical cancer. Dramatic increases in the efficacy of antiretroviral treatments—especially those regimens that include protease inhibitors or nonnucleoside reverse transcriptase inhibitors—have improved the prognosis of persons with HIV/AIDS. One consequence is that fewer persons with HIV ever develop an infection or malignancy or have a low enough CD4 count to classify them as having AIDS, which means that the CDC definition has become a less useful measure of the impact of HIV/AIDS in the United States. Conversely, persons who had been diagnosed with AIDS based on a serious opportunistic infection, malignancy, or immunodeficiency may now be markedly healthier, with high CD4 counts, due to the use of highly active antiretroviral therapy. Therefore, the Social Security Administration as well as most social service agencies focus on functional assessment for determining eligibility for benefits rather than the simple presence or absence of an AIDS-defined illness.

Clinicians with limited experience in HIV/AIDS need to educate themselves about disease manifestations and treatment. Resources are available to help clinicians care for HIV-infected persons. Clinicians should call their state medical associations for a list of local resources.

Extra efforts should be made to obtain specialty consultation for patients failing their current regi-

Table 31–1. CDC AIDS case definition for surveillance of adults and adolescents.

Definitive AIDS diagnoses (with or without laboratory evidence of HIV infection)
1. Candidiasis of the esophagus, trachea, bronchi, or lungs.
2. Cryptococcosis, extrapulmonary.
3. Cryptosporidiosis with diarrhea persisting > 1 month.
4. Cytomegalovirus disease of an organ other than liver, spleen, or lymph nodes.
5. Herpes simplex virus infection causing a mucocutaneous ulcer that persists longer than 1 month; or bronchitis, pneumonitis, or esophagitis of any duration.
6. Kaposi's sarcoma in a patient < 60 years of age.
7. Lymphoma of the brain (primary) in a patient < 60 years of age.
8. *Mycobacterium avium* complex or *Mycobacterium kansasii* disease, disseminated (at a site other than or in addition to lungs, skin, or cervical or hilar lymph nodes).
9. *Pneumocystis carinii* pneumonia.
10. Progressive multifocal leukoencephalopathy.
11. Toxoplasmosis of the brain.

Definitive AIDS diagnoses (with laboratory evidence of HIV infection)
1. Coccidioidomycosis, disseminated (at a site other than or in addition to lungs or cervical or hilar lymph nodes).
2. HIV encephalopathy.
3. Histoplasmosis, disseminated (at a site other than or in addition to lungs or cervical or hilar lymph nodes).
4. Isosporiasis with diarrhea persisting > 1 month.
5. Kaposi's sarcoma at any age.
6. Lymphoma of the brain (primary) at any age.
7. Other non-Hodgkin's lymphoma of B cell or unknown immunologic phenotype.
8. Any mycobacterial disease caused by mycobacteria other than *Mycobacterium tuberculosis,* disseminated (at a site other than or in addition to lungs, skin, or cervical or hilar lymph nodes).
9. Disease caused by extrapulmonary *M tuberculosis.*
10. Salmonella (nontyphoid) septicemia, recurrent.
11. HIV wasting syndrome.
12. CD4 lymphocyte count below 200 cells/μL or a CD4 lymphocyte percentage below 14%.
13. Pulmonary tuberculosis.
14. Recurrent pneumonia.
15. Invasive cervical cancer.

Presumptive AIDS diagnoses (with laboratory evidence of HIV infection)
1. Candidiasis of esophagus: (a) recent onset of retrosternal pain on swallowing; and (b) oral candidiasis.
2. Cytomegalovirus retinitis. A characteristic appearance on serial ophthalmoscopic examinations.
3. Mycobacteriosis. Specimen from stool or normally sterile body fluids or tissue from a site other than lungs, skin, or cervical or hilar lymph nodes, showing acid-fast bacilli of a species not identified by culture.
4. Kaposi's sarcoma. Erythematous or violaceous plaque-like lesion on skin or mucous membrane.
5. *Pneumocystis carinii* pneumonia: (a) a history of dyspnea on exertion or nonproductive cough of recent onset (within the past 3 months); and (b) chest x-ray evidence of diffuse bilateral interstitial infiltrates or gallium scan evidence of diffuse bilateral pulmonary disease; and (c) arterial blood gas analysis showing an arterial oxygen partial pressure of < 70 mm Hg or a low respiratory diffusing capacity of < 80% of predicted values or an increase in the alveolar-arterial oxygen tension gradient; and (d) no evidence of a bacterial pneumonia.
6. Toxoplasmosis of the brain: (a) recent onset of a focal neurologic abnormality consistent with intracranial disease or a reduced level of consciousness; and (b) brain imaging evidence of a lesion having a mass effect or the radiographic appearance of which is enhanced by injection of contrast medium; and (c) serum antibody to toxoplasmosis or successful response to therapy for toxoplasmosis.
7. Recurrent pneumonia: (a) more than one episode in a 1-year period; and (b) acute pneumonia (new symptoms, signs, or radiologic evidence not present earlier) diagnosed on clinical or radiologic grounds by the patient's physician.
8. Pulmonary tuberculosis: (a) apical or miliary infiltrates and (b) radiographic and clinical response to antituberculous therapy.

mens, intolerant of standard antiviral drugs, those in need of systemic chemotherapy, and those with complicated opportunistic infections, particularly when invasive procedures or experimental therapies are needed. In many cases, a single consultation with follow-up to the primary care clinician will provide the needed expertise while ensuring continuity in care.

Epidemiology

The modes of transmission of HIV are similar to those of hepatitis B, in particular with respect to sexual, parenteral, and vertical transmission. Although certain sexual practices (eg, receptive anal intercourse) are significantly riskier than other sexual practices (eg, oral sex), it is difficult to quantify per-contact risks. The reason is that studies of sexual transmission of HIV show that most people at risk for HIV infection engage in a variety of sexual practices and have sex with multiple persons, only some of whom may actually be HIV-infected. Thus, it is difficult to determine which practice with which person actually resulted in HIV transmission.

Nonetheless, the best available estimates indicate that the risk of HIV transmission with receptive anal intercourse is between 1:100 and 1:30, with insertive anal intercourse 1:1000, with receptive vaginal intercourse 1:1000, with insertive vaginal intercourse 1:10,000, and with receptive fellatio with ejaculation 1:1000. The per-contact risk of HIV transmission with other behaviors, including receptive fellatio without ejaculation, insertive fellatio, and cunnilingus, are not known.

All per-contact risk estimates assume that the source is HIV-infected. If the HIV status of the source is unknown, the risk of transmission is the risk of transmission multiplied by the probability that the source is HIV-infected. This would vary by risk practices, age, and geographic area. A number of cofactors are known to increase the risk of HIV transmission during a given encounter, including the presence of ulcerative or inflammatory sexually transmitted diseases, trauma, menses, and lack of male circumcision.

The risk of acquiring HIV infection from a needlestick with infected blood is approximately 1:300. Factors known to increase the risk of transmission include depth of penetration, hollow bore needles, visible blood on the needle, and advanced stage of disease in the source. The risk of HIV transmission from a mucosal splash with infected blood is unknown but is assumed to be significantly lower.

The risk of acquiring HIV infection from illicit drug use with sharing of needles from an HIV-infected source is estimated to be 1:150. Use of clean needles markedly decreases the chance of HIV transmission but does not eliminate it if other drug paraphernalia are shared (eg, cookers).

When blood transfusion from an HIV-infected donor occurs, the risk of transmission is 95%. Fortunately, since 1985, blood donor screening using the HIV enzyme-linked immunosorbent assay (ELISA) has been universally practiced in the USA. Also, persons who have recently engaged in unsafe behaviors (eg, sex with a person at risk for HIV, injection drug use) are not allowed to donate. This eliminates donations from persons who are HIV-infected but have not yet developed antibodies (ie, persons in the "window" period). In recent years, HIV antigen and viral load testing have been added to the screening of blood to further lower the chance of HIV transmission. With these precautions, the chance of HIV transmission with receipt of blood transfusion is about 1:1,000,000.

In the absence of perinatal HIV prophylaxis, between 13% and 40% of children born to HIV-infected mothers contract HIV infection. The risk is higher with vaginal than with cesarean delivery, higher among mothers with high viral loads, and higher among those who breast feed their children. The risk can be decreased by administering antiretroviral treatment to the mother during pregnancy and to the infant immediately after birth (see below).

HIV has not been shown to be transmitted by respiratory droplet spread, by vectors such as mosquitoes, or by casual nonsexual contact.

Current estimates are that about 700,000 Americans are infected with HIV. Estimates of the number of people who have developed AIDS in the 1990s have been scaled down from prior estimates, based on recent AIDS incidence data. In 2000, there were 315,000 persons in the USA living with AIDS. Fifty-one percent of those are gay or bisexual men; 28% are heterosexual injection drug users; and 18% are heterosexual noninjection drug users. Women account for 24% of cases.

The rapid increase of AIDS cases among women is of great concern. In 1985, women represented only 7% of new AIDS cases; in 2000, women represented 24% of new cases. Intravenous drug use and heterosexual contact with an infected partner are the two major risk factors for women.

In general, the progression of HIV-related illness is similar in men and women. However, there are some important differences. Women appear later than men for medical care. They are at risk for gynecologic complications of HIV, including recurrent candidal vaginitis, pelvic inflammatory disease, and cervical dysplasia. Violence directed against women, pregnancy, and frequent occurrence of drug use and poverty all complicate the treatment of HIV-infected women. Although "safer sex" campaigns dramatically decreased the rates of seroconversions among gay men living in metropolitan areas in the United States by the mid 1980s, there is concern that relapse to unsafe sexual practices will result in an increase in the number of new seroconversions. Several studies have reported recent increases in the rates of unsafe sexual behaviors and sexually transmitted diseases among gay men in several large cities in the United States and in western Europe. The higher rates of unsafe sex appear to be related to decreased concern about acquiring HIV due to the availability of highly active antiretroviral treatment. Fatigue with following safe sex recommendations also appears be playing a role in the increased unsafe sex rates.

There are an estimated 10 million persons infected worldwide. In Central and East Africa in some urban areas, as many as one-third of sexually active adults are infected. HIV infection began to spread in Asia in the late 1980s. The most common mode of transmission is bidirectional heterosexual spread. The reason for the greater risk for transmission with heterosexual intercourse in Africa and Asia than in the United States may relate to cofactors such as general health status, the presence of genital ulcers, the number of sexual partners, and different HIV serotypes.

Increases in unsafe sex and rectal gonorrhea among men who have sex with men—San Francisco, California, 1994–1997. MMWR Recomm Rep 1999;48:45. [PMID: 9935141] (Increases in the incidence of rectal gonorrhea parallel decreased condom use and increased unsafe sex among men who have sex with men in San Francisco.)

Kleinman SH et al: The risks of transfusion-transmitted infection. Baillieres Best Pract Clin Haematol 2000;13:631. [PMID: 11102281] (Modeling of risk of HIV from transfusion of blood products.)

Vittinghoff E: Per-contact risk of human immunodeficiency virus transmission between male sexual partners. Am J Epidemiol 1999;150:306. [PMID: 10430236] (Detailed study of per-contact risk of transmission among men who have sex with men.)

Wade NA et al: Abbreviated regimens of zidovudine prophylaxis and perinatal transmission of the human immunodeficiency virus. N Engl J Med 1998;339:1409. [PMID: 9811915] (Zidovudine prophylaxis decreased the rate of perinatal transmission of HIV even if begun intrapartum or in the first 48 hours of life of the infant.)

Etiology

HIV, like other retroviruses, depends upon a unique enzyme, reverse transcriptase (RNA-directed DNA-polymerase), to replicate within host cells. The other major pathogenic human retrovirus, HTLV-I, is associated with lymphoma, while HIV is not directly oncogenic. The HIV genomes contain genes for three basic structural proteins and at least five other regulatory proteins; *gag* codes for group antigen proteins, *pol* codes for polymerase, and *env* codes for the external envelope protein. The greatest variability in strains of HIV occurs in the viral envelope. Since neutralizing activity is found in antibodies directed against the envelope, this variability presents problems for vaccine development.

In addition to the classic AIDS virus (HIV-1), a group of related viruses, HIV-2, have been isolated in West African patients. HIV-2 has the same genetic organization as HIV-1, but there are significant differences in the envelope glycoproteins. Some infected individuals exhibit AIDS-like illnesses, but most West Africans infected with HIV-2 are currently asymptomatic. HIV-2 has been found in several people in the USA. Thus, this variant may be less pathogenic or have a longer period of latency preceding disease. Cases have been documented in which AIDS-like illnesses have occurred in the absence of HIV infection or other known infectious causes of immunodeficiency.

Pathogenesis

The hallmark of symptomatic HIV infection is immunodeficiency caused by continuing viral replication. The virus can infect all cells expressing the T4 (CD4) antigen, which HIV uses to attach to the cell. Chemokine receptors (CCR5 and CXCR4) are important for virus import, and individuals with CCR5 deletions are less likely to become infected, and, once infected, the disease is more likely to progress slowly. Once it enters a cell, HIV can replicate and cause cell fusion or death. A latent state is also established, with integration of the HIV genome into the cell's genome. The cell principally infected is the CD4 (helper-inducer) lymphocyte, which directs many other cells in the immune network. With increasing duration of infection, the number of CD4 lymphocytes falls. Some of the immunologic defects, however, are explained not by *quantitative* abnormalities of lymphocyte subsets but by *qualitative* defects in CD4 responsiveness induced by HIV.

Other cells in the immune network that are infected by HIV include B lymphocytes and macrophages. The defect in B cells is mainly due to disordered CD4 lymphocyte function. These direct and indirect effects can lead to generalized hypergammaglobulinemia and can also depress B cell responses to new antigen challenges. Because of these defects, the immunodeficiency of HIV is mixed. Elements of humoral and cellular immunodeficiency are present, especially in children. Macrophages act as a reservoir for HIV and serve to disseminate it to other organ systems (eg, the central nervous system).

Apart from the immunologic effects of HIV, the virus can also directly cause a variety of neurologic effects. Neuropathology largely results from the release of cytokines and other neurotoxins by infected macrophages. Other factors such as coexistent CMV infection may also be important. Perturbations of excitatory neurotransmitters and calcium flux may contribute to neurologic dysfunction. Direct HIV infection of renal tubular cells and gastrointestinal epithelium may contribute to these organ system manifestations of infection.

Pathophysiology

Clinically, the syndromes caused by HIV infection are usually explicable by one of three known mechanisms.

A. IMMUNODEFICIENCY

Immunodeficiency is a direct result of the effects of HIV upon immune cells. A spectrum of infections and neoplasms is seen, as in other congenital or acquired immunodeficiency states. Two remarkable features of HIV immunodeficiency are the low incidence of certain infections such as listeriosis and aspergillosis and the frequent occurrence of certain neoplasms such as lymphoma or Kaposi's sarcoma. This latter complication has been seen primarily in gay or bisexual men, and its incidence has steadily declined through the first 10 years of the epidemic. Evidence now strongly suggests that a herpesvirus (KSHV or HHV-8) is the cause of Kaposi's sarcoma.

B. AUTOIMMUNITY

Autoimmunity can occur as a result of disordered cellular immune function or B lymphocyte dysfunction. Examples of both lymphocytic infiltration of organs (eg, lymphocytic interstitial pneumonitis) and autoantibody production (eg, immunologic thrombocytopenia) occur. These phenomena may be the only clinically apparent disease or may coexist with obvious immunodeficiency.

C. NEUROLOGIC, RENAL, AND GASTROINTESTINAL DYSFUNCTION

See discussion in Pathogenesis, above.

Clinical Findings

The complications of HIV-related infections and neoplasms affect virtually every organ. The general approach to the HIV-infected person with symptoms is to evaluate the organ systems involved, aiming to diagnose treatable conditions rapidly. As can be seen in Figure 31–1, the CD4 lymphocyte count provides very important prognostic information. Certain infections may occur at any CD4 count, while others rarely occur unless the CD4 lymphocyte count has dropped below a certain level. For example, a patient with a CD4 count of 600 cells/μL, cough, and fever may

have a bacterial pneumonia but would be very unlikely to have pneumocystis pneumonia.

A. SYMPTOMS AND SIGNS

Many individuals with HIV infection remain asymptomatic for years even without antiretroviral therapy, with a mean time of approximately 10 years between exposure and development of AIDS. When symptoms occur, they may be remarkably protean and nonspecific. Since virtually all the findings may be seen with other diseases, a combination of complaints is more suggestive of HIV infection than any one symptom.

Physical examination may be entirely normal. Abnormal findings range from completely nonspecific to highly specific for HIV infection. Those that are predictive of HIV infection include hairy leukoplakia of the tongue, disseminated Kaposi's sarcoma, and cutaneous bacillary angiomatosis.

1. Systemic complaints—Fever, night sweats, and weight loss are common symptoms in HIV-infected patients and may occur without a complicating opportunistic infection. Patients with persistent **fever** and no localizing symptoms should nonetheless be carefully examined, and evaluated with a chest radiograph (pneumocystis pneumonia can present without respiratory symptoms), bacterial blood cultures if the fever

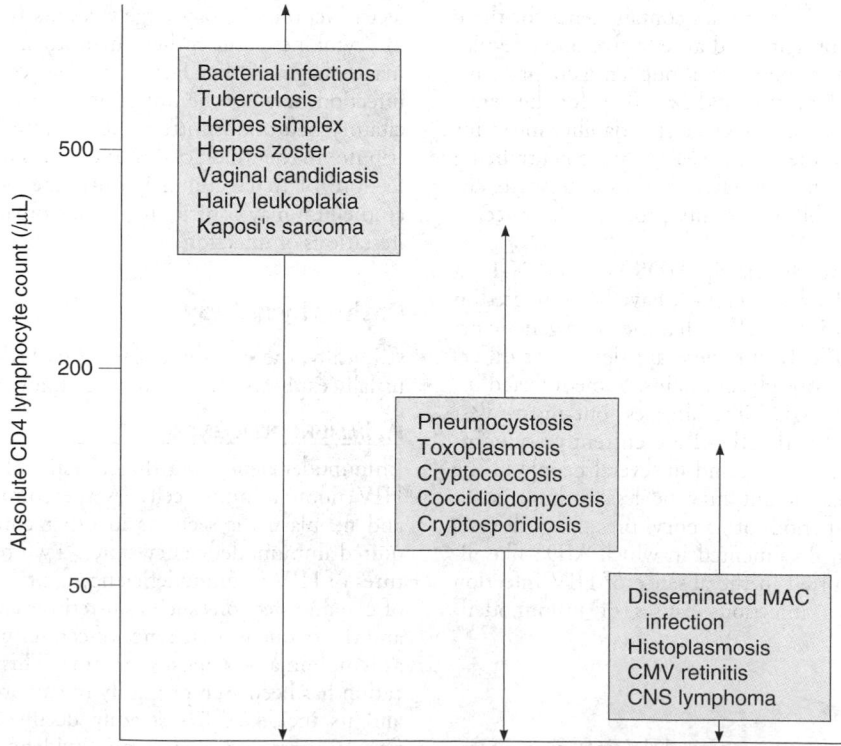

Figure 31–1. Relationship of CD4 count to development of opportunistic infections.

is greater than 38.5 °C, serum cryptococcal antigen, and mycobacterial cultures of the blood. Sinus CT scans or sinus radiographs should be considered to evaluate occult sinusitis. If these studies are normal, patients should be observed closely. Antipyretics are useful to prevent dehydration.

Weight loss is a particularly distressing complication of long-standing HIV infection. Patients typically have disproportionate loss of muscle mass, with maintenance or less substantial loss of fat stores. The mechanism of HIV-related weight loss is not completely understood but appears to be multifactorial.

AIDS patients frequently suffer from anorexia, nausea, and vomiting, all of which contribute to weight loss by decreasing caloric intake. In some cases, these symptoms are secondary to a specific infection, such as viral hepatitis. In other cases, however, evaluation of the symptoms yields no specific pathogen, and it is assumed to be due to a primary effect of HIV. Malabsorption also plays a role in decreased caloric intake. Patients may suffer diarrhea from infections with bacterial, viral, or parasitic agents.

Exacerbating the decrease in caloric intake, many AIDS patients have an increased metabolic rate. This increased rate has been shown to exist even among asymptomatic HIV-infected persons, but it accelerates with disease progression and secondary infection. AIDS patients with secondary infections also have decreased protein synthesis, which makes maintaining muscle mass difficult.

Several strategies have been developed to slow AIDS wasting. Food supplementation with high-calorie drinks may enable patients with not much appetite to maintain their intake. Selected patients with otherwise good functional status and weight loss due to unrelenting nausea, vomiting, or diarrhea may benefit from total parenteral nutrition. It should be noted, however, that TPN is more likely to increase fat stores than to reverse the muscle wasting process.

Two pharmacologic approaches for increasing appetite and weight gain are the progestational agent megestrol acetate (80 mg four times a day) and the antiemetic agent dronabinol (2.5–5 mg three times a day). Side effects from megestrol acetate are rare, but thromboembolic phenomena, edema, nausea, vomiting, and rash have been reported. Euphoria, dizziness, paranoia, and somnolence and even nausea and vomiting have been reported in 3–10% of patients using dronabinol. Dronabinol contains only one of the active ingredients in smoked marijuana, and many patients report better relief of nausea and improvement of appetite with smoking marijuana. Several states allow physicians to recommend the use of smoked marijuana to their patients. However, it is still illegal in the United States to sell marijuana. Thus, a physician's recommendation may at best decrease the chance that patients will be prosecuted for use of marijuana. Unfortunately, neither megestrol acetate or dronabinol increases lean body mass.

Two regimens that have resulted in increases in lean body mass are growth hormone and anabolic steroids. Growth hormone at a dose of 0.1 mg/kg/d subcutaneously for 12 weeks has resulted in modest increases in lean body mass; its cost is approximately $150 per day. Anabolic steroids also increase lean body mass among HIV-infected patients. They seem to work best for patients who are able to do weight training. The most commonly used regimens are testosterone enanthate or testosterone cypionate (100–200 mg intramuscularly every 2–4 weeks). Testosterone patches (4–6 mg/d) applied to the shaved scrotum and a testosterone gel that can be applied directly to the skin are also available. A transdermal delivery system (2.5 mg/d) is also available that can be applied to nonhairy parts of the body. Unfortunately, the patches tend to fall off, and the transdermal system often causes a local skin reaction. The anabolic steroid oxandrolone (15–20 mg orally in two to four divided doses) has also been found to increase lean body mass.

Nausea leading to weight loss is sometimes due to esophageal candidiasis. Patients with oral candidiasis and nausea should be empirically treated with an oral antifungal agent. Patients with weight loss due to nausea of unclear origin may benefit from use of antiemetics prior to meals (prochlorperazine, 10 mg three times daily; metoclopramide, 10 mg three times daily; or ondansetron, 8 mg three times daily). Effective fever control decreases the metabolic rate and may slow the pace of weight loss. Dronabinol (5 mg three times daily) can also be used to increase appetite. Depression and adrenal insufficiency are two potentially treatable causes of weight loss.

2. Sinopulmonary disease—

a. Pneumocystis pneumonia—(See also discussions in Chapter 36.) Pneumocystis pneumonia is the most common opportunistic infection associated with AIDS. Pneumocystis pneumonia may be difficult to diagnose because the symptoms—fever, cough, and shortness of breath—are nonspecific. Furthermore, the severity of symptoms ranges from fever and no respiratory symptoms through mild cough or dyspnea to frank respiratory distress.

Hypoxemia may be severe, with a P_{O_2} less than 60 mm Hg. The cornerstone of diagnosis is the chest radiograph. Diffuse or perihilar infiltrates are most characteristic, but only two-thirds of patients with pneumocystis pneumonia have this finding. Normal chest radiographs are seen in 5–10% of patients with pneumocystis pneumonia, while the remainder have atypical infiltrates. Apical infiltrates are commonly seen among patients with pneumocystis pneumonia who have been receiving aerosolized pentamidine prophylaxis. Large pleural effusions are uncommon with pneumocystis pneumonia; their presence suggests bacterial pneumonia, other infections such as tuberculosis, or pleural Kaposi's sarcoma.

Definitive diagnosis can be obtained in 50–80% of cases by Wright-Giemsa stain of induced sputum. Sputum induction is performed by having patients inhale an aerosolized solution of 3% saline produced by an ultrasonic nebulizer. Patients should not eat for at least 8 hours and should not use toothpaste or mouthwash prior to the procedure since they can interfere with test interpretation. The next step for patients with negative sputum examinations still suspected of having pneumocystis pneumonia should be bronchoalveolar lavage. This technique establishes the diagnosis in over 95% of cases.

In patients with symptoms suggestive of pneumocystis pneumonia but with negative or atypical chest radiographs and negative sputum examinations, other diagnostic tests may provide additional information in deciding whether to proceed to bronchoalveolar lavage. Elevation of serum lactate dehydrogenase occurs in 95% of cases of pneumocystis pneumonia, but the specificity of this finding is at best 75%. Either a normal diffusing capacity of carbon monoxide ($D_L CO$) or a high-resolution CT scan of the chest that demonstrates no interstitial lung disease makes the diagnosis of pneumocystis pneumonia very unlikely. In addition, a CD4 count above 250 cells/μL within 2 months prior to evaluation of respiratory symptoms makes a diagnosis of pneumocystis pneumonia unlikely; only 1–5% of cases occur above this CD4 count level (Figure 31–1). This is true even if the patient previously had a CD4 count lower than 200 cells/μL but has had an increase with antiretroviral therapy.

Pneumothoraces are common in HIV-infected patients with a history of pneumocystis pneumonia, especially if they have received aerosolized pentamidine treatment. Because patients may have a pneumothorax as their presenting symptom of recurrent pneumocystis pneumonia, such patients who have not had therapy for pneumocystis pneumonia in the preceding 3 months may need evaluation for pneumocystis. Pneumothoraces in HIV-infected individuals should be treated initially in the same fashion as in other patients. Unfortunately, they frequently recur with clamping or removal of the chest tube. Sclerosis with bleomycin or talc is the treatment of choice for recurrent pneumothoraces, but it is not uniformly successful even when multiple treatments are performed. If sclerosis fails, thoracoscopic stapling or thoracotomy may be required.

b. Other infectious pulmonary diseases— Other infectious causes of pulmonary disease in AIDS patients include bacterial, mycobacterial, and viral pneumonias. Community-acquired pneumonia is the most common cause of pulmonary disease in HIV-infected persons. An increased incidence of pneumococcal pneumonia with septicemia and *Haemophilus influenzae* pneumonia has been reported. *Pseudomonas aeruginosa* is an important respiratory pathogen in advanced disease. The incidence of infection with *Mycobacterium tuberculosis* has markedly increased in metropolitan areas because of HIV infection as well as homelessness. Tuberculosis occurs in an estimated 4% of persons who have AIDS. It is thought to result mainly from reactivation of prior infection; apical infiltrates and disseminated disease occur more commonly than among immunocompetent hosts. Although a PPD test should be performed on all HIV-infected persons in whom a diagnosis of tuberculosis is being considered, the lower the CD4 cell count, the greater the likelihood of anergy. Because "anergy" skin test panels do not accurately classify those patients who are infected with tuberculosis but unreactive to the PPD, they are not recommended. Treatment of HIV-infected persons with active tuberculosis is similar to treatment of HIV-uninfected tubercular individuals (see Chapter 9). However, rifampin should not be given to patients receiving indinavir, nelfinavir, amprenavir, lopinavir, or delavirdine. In these cases, rifabutin may be substituted, but it may require dosing modifications depending upon the antiretroviral regimen. Multidrug-resistant tuberculosis is a major problem in several metropolitan areas. Noncompliance with prescribed antituberculous drugs is a major risk factor. Several of the reported outbreaks appear to implicate nosocomial spread. The emergence of drug resistance makes it essential that antibiotic sensitivities be performed on all positive cultures. Drug therapy should be individualized. Patients with multidrug-resistant *M tuberculosis* infection should receive at least three drugs to which their organism is sensitive. Atypical mycobacteria can cause pulmonary disease in AIDS patients with or without preexisting lung disease and responds variably to treatment. Making a distinction between *M tuberculosis* and atypical mycobacteria requires culture of sputum specimens. If culture of the sputum produces acid-fast bacilli, definitive identification may take several weeks using traditional techniques. DNA probes allow for presumptive identification usually within days of a positive culture. While awaiting definitive diagnosis, clinicians should err on the side of treating patients as if they have *M tuberculosis* infection. In cases where the risk of atypical mycobacteria is very high (eg, a person without risk for tuberculosis exposure with a CD4 count under 50 cells/μL—see Figure 31–1), clinicians may wait for definitive diagnosis if the person is smear-negative for acid-fast bacilli, clinically stable, and not living in a communal setting. Isolation of cytomegalovirus from bronchoalveolar lavage fluid occurs commonly in AIDS patients but does not establish a definitive diagnosis. Diagnosis of cytomegalovirus pneumonia requires biopsy; response to treatment is poor. Histoplasmosis, coccidioidomycosis, and cryptococcal disease should also be considered in the differential diagnosis of unexplained pulmonary infiltrates.

c. Noninfectious pulmonary diseases—Noninfectious causes of lung disease include Kaposi's sarcoma, non-Hodgkin's lymphoma, and interstitial pneumonitis. In patients with known Kaposi's sarcoma, pulmonary involvement complicates the course in approximately one-third of cases. However, pulmonary involvement is rarely the presenting manifestation of Kaposi's sarcoma. Non-Hodgkin's lymphoma may involve the lung as the sole site of disease but more commonly involves other organs as well, especially the brain, liver, and gastrointestinal tract. Both of these processes may show nodular or diffuse parenchymal involvement, pleural effusions, and mediastinal adenopathy on chest radiographs.

Nonspecific interstitial pneumonitis may mimic pneumocystis pneumonia. Pulmonary involvement by HIV may result in a lymphocytic interstitial pneumonitis seen in lung biopsies. Whether this pathologic pattern represents direct HIV infection or is an autoimmune response to infection is unclear. It has a variable clinical course. Typically, these patients present with several months of mild cough and dyspnea; chest radiographs show interstitial infiltrates. Many patients with this entity undergo transbronchial biopsies in an attempt to diagnose pneumocystis pneumonia. Instead, the tissue shows interstitial inflammation ranging from an intense lymphocytic infiltration (consistent with lymphoid interstitial pneumonitis) to a mild mononuclear inflammation. Corticosteroids may be helpful in some cases.

d. Sinusitis—Chronic sinusitis can be a frustrating problem for HIV-infected patients. Symptoms include sinus congestion and discharge, headache, and fever. Some patients may have radiographic evidence of sinus disease on sinus CT scan or sinus x-ray in the absence of significant symptoms. Nonsmoking patients with purulent drainage should be treated with amoxicillin (500 mg orally three times a day). Patients who smoke should be treated with amoxicillin-potassium clavulanate (500 mg orally three times a day) to cover *H influenzae*. Prolonged treatment (3–6 weeks) with an antibiotic and guaifenesin (600 mg orally twice daily) to decrease sinus congestion may be required. For patients not responding to amoxicillin-potassium clavulanate, ciprofloxacin should be tried (500 mg orally twice a day). Some patients may require referral to an otolaryngologist for sinus drainage.

3. Central nervous system disease—Central nervous system disease in HIV-infected patients can be divided into intracerebral space-occupying lesions, encephalopathy, meningitis, and spinal cord processes. Many of these complications have declined markedly in prevalence in the era of highly active antiretroviral therapy.

a. Toxoplasmosis—Toxoplasmosis is the most common space-occupying lesion in HIV-infected patients. Patients may present with headache, focal neurologic deficits, seizures, or altered mental status. The diagnosis is usually made presumptively based on the characteristic appearance of cerebral imaging studies in an individual known to be seropositive for toxoplasma. Typically, toxoplasmosis appears as multiple contrast-enhancing lesions on CT scan. Lesions tend to be peripheral, with a predilection for the basal ganglia.

Single lesions are atypical of toxoplasmosis. When a single lesion has been detected by CT scanning, MRI scanning—because of its greater sensitivity—may reveal multiple lesions. If a patient has a single lesion on MRI and is neurologically stable, clinicians may pursue a 2-week empirical trial of toxoplasmosis therapy. A repeat scan should be performed at 2 weeks. If the lesion has not diminished in size, biopsy of the lesion should be performed. Since many HIV-infected patients will have detectable titers, a positive toxoplasma serologic test does not confirm the diagnosis. Conversely, as many as 15% of patients with toxoplasmosis have negative titers by enzyme immunoassay or immunofluorescence assays. Polymerase chain reaction assays of cerebrospinal fluid are useful adjunctive tests.

b. Central nervous system lymphoma—Primary non-Hodgkin's lymphoma is the second most common space-occupying lesion in HIV-infected patients. Symptoms are similar to those with toxoplasmosis. While imaging techniques cannot distinguish these two diseases with certainty, lymphoma more often is solitary. Other less common lesions should be suspected if there is preceding bacteremia, positive tuberculin test, fungemia, or intravenous drug use. These include bacterial abscesses, cryptococcomas, tuberculomas, and nocardia lesions.

Because techniques for stereotactic brain biopsy have improved, this procedure plays an increasing role in diagnosing cerebral lesions. Biopsy should be strongly considered if lesions are solitary or do not respond to toxoplasmosis treatment, especially if they are easily accessible. Diagnosis of lymphoma is important because many patients benefit from treatment (radiation therapy). In the future, it may be possible to avoid brain biopsy by utilizing PCR assay of cerebrospinal fluid for Epstein-Barr virus DNA, which is present in 90% of cases.

c. AIDS dementia complex—The diagnosis of AIDS dementia complex (HIV-associated cognitive-motor complex) is one of exclusion based on a brain imaging study and on spinal fluid analysis that excludes other pathogens. Neuropsychiatric testing is helpful in distinguishing patients with dementia from those with depression. Patients with AIDS dementia complex typically have difficulty with cognitive tasks and exhibit diminished motor speed. Patients may first notice a deterioration in their handwriting. The manifestations of dementia may wax and wane, with persons exhibiting periods of lucidity and confusion over the course of a day. Although the mechanism by which HIV causes neurologic dysfunction is not completely understood, many patients improve with effective antiretroviral treatment. Metabolic abnormalities may also cause changes in mental status: hypoglycemia, hyponatremia, hypoxia, and drug overdose are important considerations in this population. Other less common infectious causes of encephalopathy include progressive multifocal leukoencephalopathy (discussed below), cytomegalovirus, syphilis, and herpes simplex encephalitis.

d. Cryptococcal meningitis—Cryptococcal meningitis typically presents with fever and headache. Less than 20% of patients have meningismus. Diagnosis is based on a positive latex agglutination test (CRAG) or positive culture of spinal fluid for cryptococcus. Seventy to ninety percent of patients with cryptococcal meningitis have a positive serum CRAG. Thus, a negative serum CRAG test makes a diagnosis of cryptococcal meningitis unlikely and can be useful in the initial evaluation of a patient with headache, fever, and normal mental status. HIV meningitis, characterized by lymphocytic pleocytosis of the spinal fluid with negative culture, is common early in HIV infection and may mimic cryptococcal meningitis in its clinical presentation.

e. HIV myelopathy—Spinal cord function may also be impaired in HIV-infected individuals. HIV myelopathy presents with leg weakness and incontinence. Spastic paraparesis and sensory ataxia are seen on neurologic examination. Myelopathy is usually a late manifestation of HIV disease, and most patients will have concomitant HIV encephalopathy. Pathologic evaluation of the spinal cord reveals vacuolation of white matter. Because HIV myelopathy is a diagnosis of exclusion, symptoms suggestive of myelopathy should be evaluated by lumbar puncture to rule out cytomegalovirus polyradiculopathy (described below) and an MRI or CT scan to exclude epidural lymphoma.

f. Progressive multifocal leukoencephalopathy (PML)—PML is a viral infection of the white matter of the brain seen in patients with very advanced HIV infection. It typically results in focal neurologic deficits such as aphasia, hemiparesis, and cortical blindness. Imaging studies are strongly suggestive of the diagnosis if they show nonenhancing white matter lesions without mass effect. Extensive lesions may be difficult to differentiate from the changes caused by HIV. Several patients have stabilized or improved after the institution of combination antiretroviral therapy or cidofovir.

4. Peripheral nervous system—Peripheral nervous system syndromes include inflammatory polyneuropathies, sensory neuropathies, and mononeuropathies.

An inflammatory demyelinating polyneuropathy similar to Guillain-Barré syndrome occurs in HIV-infected patients, usually prior to frank immunodeficiency. The syndrome in many cases improves with plasmapheresis, supporting an autoimmune basis of the disease. Cytomegalovirus can cause an ascending polyradiculopathy characterized by lower extremity weakness and a neutrophilic pleocytosis on spinal fluid

analysis with a negative bacterial culture. Transverse myelitis can be seen with herpes zoster or cytomegalovirus.

Peripheral neuropathy is common among HIV-infected persons. Patients typically complain of numbness, tingling, and pain in the lower extremities. Symptoms are disproportionate to findings on gross sensory and motor evaluation. The most common cause is prior antiretroviral therapy with stavudine or didanosine. Patients who report these symptoms should be switched to an alternative agent if possible. Caution should be used when administering these agents to patients with a history of peripheral neuropathy. Unfortunately, drug-induced neuropathy is not always reversed when the offending agent is discontinued. Patients with advanced disease may also develop peripheral neuropathy even if they have never taken antiretroviral therapy. Evaluation should rule out other causes of sensory neuropathy such as alcoholism, thyroid disease, vitamin B_{12} deficiency, and syphilis.

Treatment of peripheral neuropathy is aimed at symptomatic relief. Patients should be initially treated with gabapentin (start at 300 mg at bedtime and increase to 300–900 mg orally three times a day). Although many clinicians initiate a trial of amitriptyline (10–25 mg orally at bedtime), responses to this agent are uncommon. A randomized study of recombinant nerve growth factor administered subcutaneously has shown that individuals with moderate to severe neuropathy tended to experience some reduction of pain. However, this therapy is currently unavailable.

5. Rheumatologic manifestations—Arthritis, involving single or multiple joints, with or without effusion, has been commonly noted in HIV-infected patients. Involvement of large joints is most common. While the cause of HIV-related arthritis is unknown, most patients will respond to nonsteroidal anti-inflammatory agents. Patients with a sizable effusion, especially if the joint is warm or erythematous, should have the joint tapped, followed by culture of the fluid to rule out suppurative arthritis as well as fungal and mycobacterial disease.

Several rheumatologic syndromes, including reactive arthritis (Reiter's syndrome), psoriatic arthritis, sicca syndrome, and systemic lupus erythematosus, have been reported in HIV-infected patients (Chapter 19). However, it is unclear if the prevalence is greater than in the general population.

6. Myopathy—Myopathies are increasingly noted in HIV-infected patients. Proximal muscle weakness is typical, and patients may have varying degrees of muscle tenderness. The most important clinical distinction is between myopathy due to the primary effect of HIV and that due to zidovudine. Patients with symptomatic myopathy, especially with creatine kinase levels greater than 1000 units/L, should have their dose of zidovudine decreased or stopped and be considered for alternative antiviral therapy. A muscle biopsy can distinguish HIV myopathy from zidovudine myopathy and should be considered in patients for whom continuation of zidovudine is essential.

7. Retinitis—Complaints of visual changes must be evaluated immediately in HIV-infected patients. Cytomegalovirus retinitis, characterized by perivascular hemorrhages and fluffy exudates, is the most common retinal infection in AIDS patients and can be rapidly progressive. In contrast, cotton wool spots, which are also common in HIV-infected people, are benign, remit spontaneously, and appear as small indistinct white spots without exudation or hemorrhage. This distinction may be difficult at times for the nonspecialist, and patients with visual changes should be seen by an ophthalmologist. Other rare retinal processes include other herpesvirus infections or toxoplasmosis.

8. Oral lesions—The findings of oral candidiasis and hairy leukoplakia are significant for several reasons. First, these lesions are highly suggestive of HIV infection. Second, several studies have indicated that patients with these lesions have a high rate of progression to AIDS even with statistical adjustment for CD4 count.

Hairy leukoplakia is caused by the Epstein-Barr virus. The lesion is not usually troubling to patients and sometimes regresses spontaneously. Hairy leukoplakia is commonly seen as a white lesion on the lateral aspect of the tongue. It may be flat or slightly raised, is usually corrugated, and has vertical parallel lines with fine or thick ("hairy") projections. Oral candidiasis can be bothersome to patients, many of whom report an unpleasant taste or mouth dryness. There are two types of oral candidiasis: pseudomembranous (removable white plaques) and erythematous (red friable plaques). Treatment is with topical agents such as clotrimazole 10 mg troches (one troche four or five times a day). Patients with candidiasis that does not respond to topical antifungals can be treated with fluconazole (50–100 mg orally once a day for 3–7 days). Chronic suppression of oral candidiasis with fluconazole has been associated with development of candidiasis resistant to all available azoles and thus should be avoided except in frequently recurring cases.

Angular cheilitis—fissures at the sides of the mouth—is usually due to candida as well and can be treated topically with ketoconazole cream (2%) twice a day.

Gingival disease is common in HIV-infected patients and is thought to be due to an overgrowth of microorganisms. It usually responds to professional dental cleaning and chlorhexidine rinses. Some HIV-infected patients will develop a particularly aggressive gingivitis or periodontitis; these patients should be started on antibiotics that cover anaerobic oral flora (eg, metronidazole, 250 mg four times a day for 4 or 5 days) and referred to oral surgeons with experience with these entities.

Aphthous ulcers are painful and may interfere with eating. They can be treated with fluocinonide (0.05% ointment mixed 1:1 with plain Orabase and applied six times a day to the ulcer). For lesions that are difficult to reach, patients should use dexamethasone swishes (0.5 mg in 5 mL elixir three times a day). The pain of the ulcers can be relieved with use of an anesthetic spray (10% lidocaine). For patients with refractory ulcers, thalidomide, starting at a dose of 50 mg orally daily and increasing to 100–200 mg daily, has proved useful. It should only be administered to patients at zero risk of procreation. The most common side effects are sedation and peripheral neuropathy. Other lesions seen in the mouths of HIV-infected patients include Kaposi's sarcoma (usually on the hard palate), and warts.

9. Gastrointestinal manifestations—

a. Candidal esophagitis—(See also discussion in Chapter 14.) Esophageal candidiasis is a common AIDS infection. In a patient with characteristic symptoms, empirical antifungal treatment is begun with fluconazole (200 mg daily for 10–14 days). Further evaluation to identify other causes of esophagitis (herpes simplex, cytomegalovirus) is reserved for patients who do not improve with treatment.

b. Hepatic disease—Autopsy studies have demonstrated that the liver is a frequent site of infections and neoplasms in HIV-infected patients. However, many of these infections are not clinically symptomatic. Clinicians may note elevations of alkaline phosphatase and aminotransferases on routine chemistry panels. Mycobacterial disease, cytomegalovirus, hepatitis B virus, hepatitis C virus, and lymphoma cause liver disease and can present with varying degrees of nausea, vomiting, and right upper quadrant abdominal pain. Sulfonamides, imidazole drugs, antituberculous medications, pentamidine, clarithromycin, and didanosine (ddI) have also been associated with hepatitis. HIV-infected patients with chronic active hepatitis may have less severe bouts of hepatitis because of the concomitant immunodeficiency. Percutaneous liver biopsy may be helpful in diagnosing liver disease, but frequently the cause can be determined by other tests (eg, blood culture, biopsy of a more accessible site). Moreover, because the majority of hepatic infections do not respond well to treatment (eg, *M avium* complex), liver biopsy should be reserved for people with persistent symptoms and laboratory abnormalities in whom no other cause for illness can be determined.

c. Biliary disease—Cholecystitis presents with manifestations similar to those seen in immunocompetent hosts but is more likely to be acalculous. Sclerosing cholangitis and papillary stenosis have also been increasingly reported in HIV-infected patients. Typically, the syndrome presents with severe nausea, vomiting, and right upper quadrant pain. Liver function tests generally show alkaline phosphatase elevations disproportionate to elevation of the aminotransferases. Although dilated ducts can be seen on ultrasound, the diagnosis is made by endoscopic retrograde cholangiopancreatography, which reveals intraluminal irregularities of the proximal intrahepatic ducts with "pruning" of the terminal ductal branches. Stenosis of the distal common bile duct at the papilla is commonly seen with this syndrome. Cytomegalovirus, cryptosporidium, and microsporidia are thought to play inciting roles in this syndrome. Initial reports of symptomatic improvement with performance of sphincterotomies were encouraging, but many patients had recurrence of symptoms.

d. Enterocolitis—Enterocolitis is a common problem in HIV-infected individuals. Organisms known to cause enterocolitis include bacteria (campylobacter, salmonella, shigella), viruses (cytomegalovirus, adenovirus), and protozoans (cryptosporidium, *Entamoeba histolytica,* giardia, isospora, Microsporida). HIV itself may cause enterocolitis. Several of the organisms causing enterocolitis in HIV-infected individuals also cause diarrhea in immunocompetent hosts. However, HIV-infected patients tend to have more severe and more chronic symptoms, including high fevers and severe abdominal pain that can mimic acute abdominal catastrophes. Bacteremia and concomitant biliary involvement are also more common with enterocolitis in HIV-infected patients. Relapses of enterocolitis following adequate therapy have been reported with both salmonella and shigella infections.

Because of the wide range of agents known to cause enterocolitis, a stool culture and multiple stool examinations for ova and parasites (including modified acid-fast staining for cryptosporidium) should be performed. Those patients who have cryptosporidium in one stool with improvement in symptoms in less than 1 month should not be considered to have AIDS, as cryptosporidium is a cause of self-limited diarrhea in HIV-negative hosts. More commonly, HIV-infected patients with cryptosporidium have persistent enterocolitis with profuse watery diarrhea.

To date, no consistently effective treatments have been developed for cryptosporidium infection. The most effective treatment of cryptosporidiosis is to improve immune function through the use of effective antiretroviral treatment. The diarrhea can be treated symptomatically with diphenoxylate with atropine (one or two tablets orally three or four times a day). Those who do not respond may be given paregoric with bismuth (5–10 mL orally three or four times a day). Octreotide in escalating doses (starting at 0.05 mg subcutaneously every 8 hours for 48 hours) has been found to ameliorate symptoms in approximately 40% of patients with cryptosporidial or idiopathic HIV-associated diarrhea.

Patients with a negative stool examination and persistent symptoms should be evaluated with colonoscopy and biopsy. Patients whose symptoms last longer than 1 month with no identified cause of diarrhea are considered to have a presumptive diagnosis of AIDS enteropathy. A primary effect of the HIV on the colonic epithelium may be the cause. Patients may respond to institution of effective antiretroviral treatment. Upper endoscopy with small bowel biopsy is not recommended as a routine part of the evaluation. Many patients who undergo upper endoscopy have nonspecific abnormalities, but these rarely reflect treatable diseases.

e. Other disorders—Two other important gastrointestinal abnormalities in HIV-infected patients are gastropathy and malabsorption. It has been documented that some HIV-infected patients do not produce normal levels of stomach acid and therefore are unable to absorb drugs such as itraconazole that require an acid medium. This decreased acid production may explain, in part, the susceptibility of HIV-infected patients to campylobacter, salmonella, and shigella, all of which are sensitive to acid concentration. There is no evidence that *Helicobacter pylori* is more common in HIV-infected persons.

A malabsorption syndrome occurs commonly in HIV-infected patients. It can be due to infection of the small bowel with *M avium* complex, cryptosporidium, or microsporidia. In other cases, biopsy of the small bowel reveals no pathogens but histologic changes consistent with Whipple's disease.

10. Endocrinologic manifestations—The adrenal gland is the most commonly afflicted endocrine gland in patients with AIDS. Abnormalities demonstrated on autopsy include infection (especially with cytomegalovirus and *M avium* complex), infiltration with Kaposi's sarcoma, and injury from hemorrhage and presumed autoimmunity. The prevalence of clinically significant adrenal insufficiency is low. Patients with suggestive symptoms should undergo a cosyntropin stimulation test.

While frank deficiency of cortisol is rare, an isolated defect in mineralocorticoid metabolism may lead to salt wasting and hyperkalemia. Such patients should be treated with fludrocortisone (0.1–0.2 mg daily).

AIDS patients appear to have abnormalities of thyroid function tests different from those of patients with other chronic diseases. AIDS patients have been shown to have high levels of triiodothyronine (T_3), thyroxine (T_4), and thyroid-binding globulin and low levels of reverse triiodothyronine (rT_3). The causes and clinical significance of these abnormalities are unknown.

11. Skin manifestations—HIV-infected patients commonly develop skin manifestations that can be grouped into viral, bacterial, fungal, neoplastic, and nonspecific dermatitides.

Herpes simplex infections occur more frequently, tend to be more severe, and are more likely to disseminate in AIDS patients than in immunocompetent hosts. Because of the risk of progressive local disease, all herpes simplex attacks should be treated with acyclovir (400 mg orally three times a day for 7 days), famciclovir (500 mg orally twice daily for 7 days), or valacyclovir (500 mg orally twice daily for 7 days). To avoid the complications of attacks, many clinicians recommend suppressive therapy for HIV-infected patients with a history of recurrent herpes. Options for suppressive therapy include acyclovir (400 mg orally twice daily), famciclovir (250 mg orally twice daily), and valacyclovir (500 mg orally daily).

Herpes zoster is a common manifestation of HIV infection. As with herpes simplex infections, patients with zoster should be treated with acyclovir to prevent dissemination (800 mg orally four or five times per day for 7 days). Alternatively, famciclovir (500 mg orally three times a day) or valacyclovir (500 mg three times a day) may be used. Vesicular lesions should be cultured if there is any question about their origin, since herpes simplex responds to much lower doses of acyclovir. Disseminated zoster and cases with ocular involvement should be treated with intravenous (10 mg/kg every 8 hours for 7–10 days) rather than oral acyclovir.

Molluscum contagiosum is seen in HIV-infected patients, as in other immunocompromised patients. Lesions have a propensity for spreading widely over the patient's skin and should be treated with topical liquid nitrogen.

Staphylococcus is the most common bacterial cause of skin disease in HIV-infected patients; it usually presents as **folliculitis, superficial abscesses (furuncles),** or **bullous impetigo.** Because dissemination with sepsis has been reported, attempts should be made to treat these lesions aggressively. Folliculitis is initially treated with topical clindamycin or mupirocin, and patients may benefit from regular washing with an antibacterial soap such as chlorhexidine. Intranasal mupirocin has been used successfully for staphylococcal decolonization in other settings. In HIV-infected patients with recurrent staphylococcal infections, weekly intranasal mupirocin should be considered in addition to topical care and systemic antibiotics. Abscesses often require incision and drainage. Patients may need antistaphylococcal antibiotics such as dicloxacillin, 250–500 mg orally four times daily, or erythromycin, 250 mg orally four times daily (with rifampin, 600 mg orally daily for 10 days for nasal staphylococcal decolonization), for severe folliculitis.

Bacillary angiomatosis is a well-described entity in HIV-infected patients. It is caused by two closely related organisms: *Bartonella henselae* and *Bartonella quintana.* The epidemiology of *B henselae* infection suggests zoonotic transmission from young cats. *B quintana* may be harbored by fleas. The most common manifestation is raised, reddish, highly vascular skin lesions that can mimic the lesions of Kaposi's sarcoma. Fever is a common manifestation of this infection; involvement of bone, lymph nodes, and liver has also been reported. The infection responds to doxycycline, 100 mg orally twice daily; or erythromycin, 250 mg orally four times daily. Therapy is continued for at least 14 days, and patients who are seriously ill

with visceral involvement may require months of therapy.

The majority of **fungal rashes** afflicting AIDS patients are due to dermatophytes and candida. These are particularly common in the inguinal region but may occur anywhere on the body. Fungal rashes generally respond well to topical clotrimazole (1% twice a day) or ketoconazole (2% twice a day).

Kaposi's sarcoma lesions are red or purple, flat or raised papules that generally do not blanch. Since they may be confused with lesions of bacillary angiomatosis, biopsy for definitive diagnosis should be performed. Individual lesions can be treated with radiation or with intralesional injection of vinblastine, 0.01–0.02 mg in 0.1 mL of saline. Other dermatologic malignancies seen disproportionately among HIV-infected persons include basal cell and squamous cell carcinomas.

Seborrheic dermatitis is more common in HIV-infected patients. Scrapings of seborrhea have revealed *Malassezia furfur (Pityrosporum ovale),* implying that the seborrhea is caused by this fungus. Consistent with the isolation of this fungus is the clinical finding that seborrhea responds well to topical clotrimazole (1% cream) as well as hydrocortisone (1% cream).

Xerosis presents in HIV-infected patients with severe pruritus. The patient may have no rash, or nonspecific excoriations from scratching. Treatment is with emollients (eg, absorption base cream) and antipruritic lotions (eg, camphor 9.5% and menthol 0.5%).

Psoriasis can be very severe in HIV-infected patients. Phototherapy and etretinate (0.25–9.75 mg/kg/d orally in divided doses) may be used for recalcitrant cases in consultation with a dermatologist. Because of the underlying immunodeficiency, methotrexate should be avoided.

12. HIV-related malignancies—Four cancers are currently included in the CDC classification of AIDS: Kaposi's sarcoma, non-Hodgkin's lymphoma, primary lymphoma of the brain, and invasive cervical carcinoma. Epidemiologic studies have shown that between 1973 and 1987 among single men in San Francisco, the risk of Kaposi's sarcoma increased more than 5000-fold and the risk of non-Hodgkin's lymphoma more than tenfold. The increase in incidence of malignancies is probably a function of impaired cell-mediated immunity.

Kaposi's sarcoma is still the most common HIV-related malignancy. Kaposi's lesions may appear anywhere; careful examination of the eyelids, conjunctiva, pinnae, palate, and toe webs is mandatory to locate potentially occult lesions. In light-skinned individuals, Kaposi's lesions usually appear as purplish, non-blanching lesions that can be papular or nodular. In dark-skinned individuals, the lesions may appear more brown. In the mouth, lesions are most often palatal papules, though exophytic lesions of the tongue and gingivae may also be seen. Kaposi's lesions may be confused with other vascular lesions such as angiomas and pyogenic granulomas. About 40% of patients with dermatologic Kaposi's sarcoma will develop visceral disease (eg, gastrointestinal, pulmonary). Rapidly progressive dermatologic or visceral disease is best treated with systemic chemotherapy. Liposomally encapsulated doxorubicin given intravenously every 3 weeks has a response rate of approximately 70%. Alpha interferon (10 million units subcutaneously three times a week) also has activity against Kaposi's sarcoma. However, symptoms such as malaise and anorexia limit the utility of this therapy. Bulky lesions of the lower extremities accompanied by lymphedema are a common presentation of Kaposi's sarcoma. Radiation and conservative measures (eg, leg elevation, elastic stockings) may be helpful.

Non-Hodgkin's lymphoma in HIV-infected persons tends to be very aggressive. The malignancies are usually of B cell origin and characterized as diffuse large-cell tumors. Over 70% of the malignancies are extranodal.

The prognosis of patients with systemic non-Hodgkin's lymphoma depends primarily on the degree of immunodeficiency at the time of diagnosis. Patients with high CD4 counts do markedly better than those diagnosed at a late stage of illness. Patients with primary central nervous system lymphoma are treated with radiation. Response to treatment is good, but prior to the availability of highly active antiretroviral treatment, most patients died within a few months after diagnosis due to their underlying disease. Systemic disease is treated with chemotherapy. Common regimens are CHOP (cyclophosphamide, doxorubicin, vincristine, and prednisone) and modified M-BACOD (methotrexate, bleomycin, doxorubicin, cyclophosphamide, vincristine, and dexamethasone). Granulocyte colony-stimulating factor (G-CSF; filgrastim) is used to maintain white blood counts with this latter regimen. Intrathecal chemotherapy is administered to prevent or treat meningeal involvement.

Although **Hodgkin's disease** is not included as part of the CDC definition of AIDS, studies have found that HIV infection is associated with a fivefold increase in the incidence of Hodgkin's disease. HIV-infected persons with Hodgkin's disease are more likely to have mixed cellularity and lymphocyte depletion subtypes of Hodgkin's disease and to present at an advanced stage of disease.

Anal dysplasia and squamous cell carcinoma have been noted in HIV-infected homosexual men. These lesions have been strongly correlated with previous infection by human papillomavirus (HPV). While many of the infected men report a history of anal warts or have visible warts, a significant percentage have silent papillomavirus infection. Cytologic (using Papanicolaou smears) and papillomavirus DNA studies can easily be performed on specimens obtained by anal swab. The growing frequency of these problems and the risk of progression from dysplasia to cancer in immunocompromised patients suggest that annual anal swabs for cytologic examination should be done in all HIV-infected persons who have engaged in receptive anal intercourse. An anal Pap smear is performed by rotating a moistened Dacron swab about 2 cm into the anal canal. The swab is immediately inserted into a cytology bottle.

HPV also appears to play a causative role in **cervical dysplasia and neoplasia.** The incidence and clinical course of cervical disease in HIV-infected women are discussed below.

13. Gynecologic manifestations—Vaginal candidiasis, cervical dysplasia and neoplasia, and pelvic inflammatory disease are more common in HIV-infected women than in uninfected women. These manifestations also tend to be more severe when they occur in association with HIV infection. Therefore, HIV-infected women need frequent gynecologic care. Vaginal candidiasis may be treated with topical agents (see Chapter 36). However, HIV-infected women with recurrent or severe vaginal candidiasis may need systemic therapy.

The incidence of cervical dysplasia in HIV-infected women is 40%. Because of this finding, HIV-infected women should have Papanicolaou smears every 6 months (as opposed to the AHRQ Guideline recommendation for every 12 months). Some clinicians recommend routine colposcopy or cervicography because cervical intraepithelial neoplasia has occurred in women with negative Papanicolaou smears. Cone biopsy is indicated in cases of serious cervical dysplasia.

Cervical neoplasia appears to be more aggressive among HIV-infected women. Most HIV-infected women with cervical cancer die of that disease rather than of AIDS. Because of its frequency and severity, cervical neoplasia was added to the CDC definition of AIDS in 1993.

While pelvic inflammatory disease appears to be more common in HIV-infected women, the bacteriology of this condition appears to be the same as among HIV-uninfected women. At present, HIV-infected women with pelvic inflammatory disease should be treated with the same regimens as uninfected women (see Chapter 17). However, inpatient therapy is generally recommended.

14. Inflammatory reactions—With initiation of highly active antiretroviral treatment, some patients experience inflammatory reactions based on immune reconstitution. Inflammatory reactions usually involve unusual presentations of opportunistic infections. For example, patients with cytomegalovirus retinitis have developed vitreitis after being treated with highly active antiretroviral treatment. *M avium* can present as focal lymphadenitis or granulomatous masses in patients receiving highly active antiretroviral treatment. Tuberculosis may paradoxically worsen. PML and cryptococcal meningitis may also behave atypically. Clinicians should be alert to new complications in patients with recovering immune function.

B. LABORATORY FINDINGS

Specific tests for HIV include antibody and antigen detection (Table 31–2). Screening serology is done by enzyme-linked immunosorbent assay (ELISA). Positive specimens are then confirmed by a different method (eg, Western blot). The sensitivity of screening serologic tests is greater than 99.5%. The specificity of positive results by two different techniques approaches 100% even in low-risk populations. False-positive screening tests may occur as normal biologic variants or in association with recent influenza vaccination or other disease states, such as connective tissue disease. These are usually detected by negative confirmatory tests. Molecular biology techniques (polymerase chain reaction) show a small incidence of individuals (< 1%) who are infected with HIV for up to 36 months without generating an antibody response. However, 95% of persons will develop antibodies detectable by screening serologic tests within 6 weeks after infection.

Nonspecific laboratory findings with HIV infection may include anemia, leukopenia (particularly lymphopenia) and thrombocytopenia in any combination, elevation of the erythrocyte sedimentation rate, polyclonal hypergammaglobulinemia, and hypocholesterolemia. Cutaneous anergy is common.

Several laboratory markers are available to provide prognostic information and guide therapy decisions (Table 31–2). The most widely used marker is the absolute CD4 lymphocyte count. As counts decrease, the risk of serious opportunistic infection over the subsequent 3–5 years increases (Figure 31–1).

There are many limitations to using the CD4 count, including diurnal variation, depression with intercurrent illness, and intra- and interlaboratory variability. Therefore, the trend is more important than a single determination. The frequency of performance of counts depends on the patient's health status. Patients whose CD4 counts are substantially above the threshold for initiation of antiviral therapy (350 cells/μL) should have counts performed every 6 months. Those who have counts near or below 350 cells/μL should have counts performed every 3 months. This is necessary for evaluating the efficacy of antiviral therapy and for initiating *P carinii* prophylactic therapy when the CD4 count drops below 200 cells/μL. Some studies suggest that the percentage of CD4 lymphocytes is a more reliable indicator of prognosis than the absolute counts because the percentage does not depend on calculating a manual differential. While the CD4 count measures immune dysfunction, it does not provide a measure of how actively HIV is replicating in the body. HIV viral load tests (discussed below) assess the level of viral replication and provide useful prognostic information which is independent of the information provided by CD4 counts.

DeSimone JA et al: Inflammatory reactions in HIV-1-infected persons after initiation of highly active antiretroviral therapy. Ann Intern Med 2000;133:447. [PMID: 10975963] (Describes the clinical characteristics and therapeutic man-

Table 31–2. Laboratory findings with HIV infection.

Test	Significance
HIV enzyme-linked immunosorbent assay (ELISA)	Screening test for HIV infection. 50% of ELISA tests are positive within 22 days after HIV transmission; 95% are positive within 6 weeks after transmission. Sensitivity > 99.9%; to avoid false-positive results, repeatedly reactive results must be confirmed with Western blot.
Western blot	Confirmatory test for HIV. Specificity when combined with ELISA > 99.99%. Indeterminate results with early HIV infection, HIV-2 infection, autoimmune disease, pregnancy, and recent tetanus toxoid administration.
CBC	Anemia, neutropenia, and thrombocytopenia common with advanced HIV infection.
Absolute CD4 lymphocyte count	Most widely used predictor of HIV progression. Risk of progression to an AIDS opportunistic infection or malignancy is high with CD4 < 200 cells/μL.
CD4 lymphocyte percentage	Percentage may be more reliable than the CD4 count. Risk of progression to an AIDS opportunistic infection or malignancy is high with percentage < 20%.
HIV viral load tests	These tests measure the amount of actively replicating HIV virus. Correlate with disease progression and response to antiretroviral drugs. Treatment is recommended for HIV-infected patients with > 30,000 viral copies by branched-chain DNA or > 55,000 viral copies by PCR testing. Best tests available for diagnosis of acute HIV infection; however, false positives are common, especially when the viral load is low.
β_2-Microglobulin	Cell surface protein indicative of macrophage-monocyte stimulation. Levels > 3.5 mg/dL associated with rapid progression of disease. Not useful with intravenous drug users.
p24 antigen	Indicates active HIV replication. Tends to be positive prior to seroconversion and with advanced disease.

agement of patients who have inflammatory presentations of opportunistic infections and malignancies following introduction of highly active antiretroviral treatment.)

Grabar S et al: Clinical outcome of patients with HIV-1 infection according to immunologic and virologic response after 6 months of highly active antiretroviral therapy. Ann Intern Med 2000;133:401. [PMID: 10975957] (Immunologic and virologic response are independent predictors of response to highly active antiretroviral treatment.)

Grinspoon S et al: Effects of testosterone and progressive resistance training in eugonadal men with AIDS wasting. A randomized, controlled trial. Ann Intern Med 2000;133:348. [PMID: 10979879] (Both testosterone and resistance training increased muscle mass; testosterone therapy also resulted in increased HDL levels.)

Kovacs JA et al: New insights into the transmission, diagnosis, and drug treatment of *Pneumocystis carinii* pneumonia. JAMA 2001;286:2450. [PMID: 11712941] (Review of recent advances in understanding of this important opportunistic infection.)

Little RF et al: HIV-associated non-Hodgkin lymphoma: incidence, presentation, and prognosis. JAMA 2001;285:1880. [PMID: 11308402] (Management of this entity in the era of highly active antiretroviral therapy.)

Differential Diagnosis

HIV infection may mimic a variety of other medical illnesses. Specific differential diagnosis depends upon the mode of presentation. In patients presenting with constitutional symptoms such as weight loss and fevers, differential considerations include cancer, chronic infections such as tuberculosis and endocarditis, and endocrinologic diseases such as hyperthyroidism. When pulmonary processes dominate the presentation, acute and chronic lung infections must be considered as well as other causes of diffuse interstitial pulmonary infiltrates. When neurologic disease is the mode of presentation, conditions that cause mental status changes or neuropathy—eg, alcoholism, liver disease, renal dysfunction, thyroid disease, and vitamin deficiency—should be considered. If a patient presents with headache and a cerebrospinal fluid pleocytosis, other causes of chronic meningitis enter the differential. When diarrhea is a prominent complaint, infectious enterocolitis, antibiotic-associated colitis, inflammatory bowel disease, and malabsorptive symptoms must be considered.

Prevention

A. PRIMARY PREVENTION

Until vaccination is a reality, prevention of HIV infection will depend upon effective precautions regarding sexual practices and intravenous drug use, use of perinatal HIV prophylaxis, screening of blood products, and infection control practices in the health care setting. Primary care clinicians should routinely obtain a sexual history and provide risk factor assessment of their patients and, when appropriate, screening for HIV infection with pre- and posttest counseling. Pretest counseling should include review of risk factors for HIV infection, discussion of safe sex and safe nee-dle use, and the meaning of a positive test. Posttest counseling should include a review of the importance of safe sex and needle use practices. For persons who test positive, information on available medical and mental health services should be provided as well as guidance for contacting sexual or needle-sharing partners. It is the duty of clinicians to counsel HIV-negative patients on how to avoid exposure to HIV. Patients should be counseled not to exchange bodily fluids unless they are in a long-term mutually monogamous relationship with someone who has tested HIV antibody-negative and has not engaged in unsafe sex, injection drug use, or other HIV risk behaviors for at least 6 months prior to or at any time since the negative test.

Only latex condoms should be used, along with a water-soluble lubricant. Although nonoxynol-9, a spermicide, kills HIV, it is not recommended because in some patients it may cause genital ulcers that could facilitate HIV transmission. Patients should be counseled that condoms are not 100% effective. They should be made familiar with the use of condoms, including, specifically, the advice that condoms must be used every time; that space should be left at the tip of the condom as a receptacle for semen; that intercourse with a condom should not be attempted if the penis is only partially erect; that men should hold on to the base of the condom when withdrawing the penis to prevent slippage; and that condoms should not be reused. Although anal intercourse remains the sexual practice at highest risk of transmitting HIV, seroconversions have been documented with vaginal and oral intercourse as well. Therefore, condoms should be used when engaging in these activities. Women as well as men should understand how to use condoms so as to be sure that their partners are using them correctly.

Persons using intravenous drugs should be cautioned never to exchange needles or other drug paraphernalia. When sterile needles are not available, bleach does appear to inactivate HIV and should be used to clean needles.

Current efforts to screen blood and blood products have lowered the risk of HIV transmission with transfusion of a unit of blood to 1:1,000,000.

In the hospital, concerns about nosocomial infection have led to the recommendation for universal body fluid precautions. This involves the rigorous use of gloves when handling any body fluid and the addition of gown, mask, and goggles for procedures that may result in splash or droplet spread as well as the use of specially designed needles with sheath devices to decrease the risk of needle sticks. Reports of transmission of drug-resistant tuberculosis in health care settings also have had infection control implications. All patients with cough in outpatient settings should be encouraged to wear masks. Hospitalized HIV-infected patients with cough should be placed in respiratory isolation until tuberculosis can be excluded by chest x-ray and sputum smear examination.

Primate model data have suggested that development of a protective vaccine may be possible, but clinical trials in humans using gp120 or its precursor gp160 have shown development of neutralizing antibodies to laboratory but not field isolates of HIV and may not be protective of infection. Many scientists have abandoned the quest for a fully protective HIV vaccine and are focusing on developing a vaccine that would reduce the chances of HIV transmission given a particular exposure.

B. SECONDARY PREVENTION

In the era prior to the development of highly effective antiretroviral treatment, cohort studies of individuals with documented dates of seroconversion demonstrate that approximately 50% of untreated seropositive persons develop AIDS within 10 years. Recent improvements in treatment would be expected to substantially improve this prognosis. Too few persons have been treated with these regimens prior to the development of AIDS to provide good data on progression of disease with these new regimens. Nevertheless, decreases in the incidence of AIDS reflecting successful treatment of HIV and successful HIV prevention efforts have been reported in the United States and western Europe.

There is substantial evidence that medical intervention with antiretroviral and prophylactic regimens can prevent opportunistic infections and improve survival. Prophylaxis and early intervention prevent several infectious diseases, including tuberculosis and syphilis, which are transmissible to others. Recommendations are listed in Table 31–3.

Because of the increased occurrence of tuberculosis among HIV-infected patients, all such individuals should undergo PPD testing. Although anergy is common among AIDS patients, the likelihood of a false-negative result is much lower when the test is done early in infection. Those with positive tests (defined for HIV-infected patients as > 5 mm of induration) need a chest x-ray. Patients with an infiltrate in any location, especially if accompanied by mediastinal adenopathy, should have sputum sent for acid-fast staining. Patients with a positive PPD but negative evaluations for active disease should receive isoniazid (300 mg daily) with pyridoxine (50 mg daily) for 9 months to a year. An alternative regimen of rifampin plus pyrazinamide for 2 months is no longer recommended because of the high associated incidence of hepatotoxicity. Recent analysis suggests also that HIV-infected individuals at high risk for tuberculosis should receive a course of isoniazid prophylaxis regardless of the PPD status. This may include homeless individuals and injection drug users.

HIV-infected patients are at increased risk of reactivation of syphilis and progression to tertiary syphilis despite standard treatment. Because the only widely available tests for syphilis are serologic and because HIV-infected individuals are known to have disordered antibody production, there is concern about the inter-

Table 31–3. Health care maintenance of HIV-infected individuals.

For all HIV-infected individuals:
CD4 counts every 3–6 months
Viral load tests every 3–6 months and 1 month following a change in therapy
PPD
INH for those with positive PPD and normal chest x-ray
RPR or VDRL
Toxoplasma IgG serology
Cytomegalovirus IgG serology
Pneumococcal vaccine
Influenza vaccine in season
Hepatitis B vaccine for those who are HBsAb-negative
Haemophilus influenzae b vaccination
Papanicolaou smears every 6 months for women
Consider anal swabs for cytologic evaluation yearly for men with history of receptive anal intercourse

For HIV-infected individuals with CD4 < 500 cells/μL:
Antiretroviral therapy (see Figure 31–2)

For HIV-infected individuals with CD4 < 200 cells/μL:
P carinii prophylaxis (see Table 31–6)

For HIV-infected individuals with CD4 < 75 cells/μL:
M avium complex prophylaxis

For HIV-infected individuals with CD4 < 50 cells/mL:
Consider CMV prophylaxis

pretation of these titers. This concern has been fueled by a report of an HIV-infected patient with secondary syphilis and negative syphilis serologic testing. Furthermore, HIV-infected individuals may lose FTA-ABS reactivity after treatment for syphilis, particularly if they have low CD4 counts. Thus, in this population, a nonreactive treponemal test does not rule out a past history of syphilis. In addition, persistence of treponemes in the spinal fluid after one dose of benzathine penicillin has been demonstrated in HIV-infected patients with primary and secondary syphilis. Therefore, the CDC has recommended an aggressive diagnostic approach to HIV-infected patients with reactive RPR or VDRL tests of greater than 1 year or unknown duration. All such patients should have a lumbar puncture with cerebrospinal fluid cell count and CSF-VDRL. Those with a normal cerebrospinal fluid evaluation are treated as having late latent syphilis (benzathine penicillin G, 2.4 million units intramuscularly weekly for 3 weeks) with follow-up titers. Those with a pleocytosis or a positive CSF-VDRL test are treated as having neurosyphilis (aqueous penicillin G, 2–4 million units intravenously every 4 hours; or procaine penicillin G, 2.4 million units intramuscularly daily, with probenecid, 500 mg four times daily, for 10 days). Some clinicians take a less aggressive approach to patients who have low titers (less than 1:8), a history of having been treated for syphilis, and a normal neurologic examination. Close follow-up of titers is mandatory if such a course is taken. For a more detailed discussion of this topic, see Chapter 34.

The efficacy of pneumococcal vaccine is debated, but since it is safe, HIV-infected individuals should receive it. Patients without evidence of hepatitis B antigen or surface antibody should receive hepatitis B vaccination. Live vaccines, such as yellow fever vaccine, should be avoided. Measles vaccination, while a live virus vaccine, appears relatively safe when administered to HIV-infected individuals and should be given if the patient has never had measles or been adequately vaccinated.

HIV-infected individuals should be counseled with regard to safe sex. Because of the risk of transmission, they should be warned to use condoms with sexual intercourse, including oral intercourse. Partners of HIV-infected women should use latex barriers such as dental dams (available at dental supply stores) to prevent direct oral contact with vaginal secretions. Substance abuse treatment should be recommended for persons who are using recreational drugs. They should be warned to avoid consuming raw meat or eggs to avoid infections with toxoplasma, campylobacter, and salmonella. HIV-infected patients should wash their hands thoroughly after cleaning cat litter or should forgo this household chore to avoid possible exposure to toxoplasmosis. To reduce the likelihood of infection with bartonella species, patients should avoid activities that might result in cat scratches or bites. Although there is not yet sufficient evidence on which to base a recommendation that HIV-infected persons not drink tap water to prevent infection with cryptosporidiosis, many clinicians recommend that HIV-infected persons—especially those with low CD4 counts—drink bottled water. Because of the emotional impact of HIV infection and subsequent illness, many patients will benefit from supportive counseling.

C. HIV RISK FOR HEALTH CARE PROFESSIONALS

Epidemiologic studies show that needle sticks occur commonly among health care professionals, especially among surgeons performing invasive procedures, inexperienced hospital house staff, and medical students. Efforts to reduce needle sticks should focus on avoiding recapping needles and use of safety needles whenever doing invasive procedures under controlled circumstances. The risk of HIV transmission from a needle stick with blood from an HIV-infected patient is about 1:300. The risk is higher with deep punctures, large inocula, and source patients with high viral loads. The risk from mucous membrane contact is too low to quantitate.

Health care professionals who sustain needle sticks should be counseled and offered HIV testing as soon as possible. HIV testing is done to establish a negative baseline for worker's compensation claims in case there is a subsequent conversion. Follow-up testing is usually performed at 6 weeks, 3 months, and 6 months.

A case-control study by the Centers for Disease Control and Prevention indicates that administration of zidovudine following a needle stick decreases the rate of HIV seroconversion by 79%. Therefore, providers should be offered therapy with Combivir (zidovudine 300 mg plus lamivudine 150 mg orally twice daily). Providers who have exposures to persons who are likely to have antiretroviral drug resistance (eg, persons receiving therapy who have detectable viral loads) should have their therapy individualized, using at least two drugs to which the source is unlikely to be resistant. Some clinicians recommend triple combination regimens, including a protease inhibitor for all occupational exposures, because of uncertainty about drug resistance. Others save these more aggressive regimens for the higher-risk exposures listed above. Since reports have noted hepatotoxicity due to nevirapine in this setting, this agent should be avoided. Therapy should be started as soon as possible after exposure and continued for 4 weeks. Unfortunately, there have been documented cases of seroconversion following potential parenteral exposure to HIV despite prompt use of zidovudine prophylaxis. Counseling of the provider should include "safe sex" guidelines.

D. POSTEXPOSURE PROPHYLAXIS FOR SEXUAL AND DRUG USE EXPOSURES TO HIV

Following publication of a case-control study indicating that antiretroviral therapy decreased the odds of seroconversion among health care workers who had occupational exposure, some experts have recommended offering antiretroviral therapy following potential exposure to HIV through sexual activity or drug use. While there are no efficacy data to support this practice, there are similarities between the immune response following transcutaneous and transmucosal exposures. The goal of postexposure prophylaxis is to reduce or prevent local viral replication prior to dissemination such that the infection can be aborted.

The choice of antiretroviral agents and the duration of treatment is the same as that for exposures that occur through the occupational route (see above). In contrast to those with occupational exposures, some individuals may present very late after exposure. Because the likelihood of success declines with length of time from HIV exposure, it is not recommended that treatment be offered after 72 hours. In addition, because the psychosocial issues involved with postexposure prophylaxis for sexual and drug use exposures are complex, it should be offered only in the context of prevention counseling. Counseling should focus on how to prevent future exposures.

E. PREVENTING PERINATAL TRANSMISSION OF HIV

A multicenter trial showed that when zidovudine is administered to women during pregnancy, labor, and delivery and to their newborns, the rate of HIV transmission is decreased by two-thirds. An observational trial demonstrated that zidovudine treatment is almost as effective when begun during labor or when administered only to the infant, as long as treatment is begun within 48 hours after birth. Nonetheless, treatment begun by at least the second trimester is still recommended. Many women are currently being offered combination antiretroviral treatment to further lower the risk of transmission. The availability of treatment makes it essential that all women who are pregnant or considering pregnancy be offered HIV counseling and testing. Many obstetricians recommend combination antiretroviral treatment, especially if zidovudine resistance is suspected. HIV-infected women receiving antiretroviral therapy in whom pregnancy is recognized during the first trimester should be counseled about the benefits and potential risks to the fetus of treatment during the first trimester. Since healthy mothers make healthy babies, continuation of therapy should be strongly considered. Because about half of fetal infections in non-breast-feeding women occur shortly before or during the birth process, antiretroviral therapy should be administered whenever a woman initiates perinatal care even if she did not begin therapy in the second trimester. Breast feeding is thought to increase the rate of transmission by 10–20% and should be avoided.

Katz MH et al: The care of persons with recent sexual exposure to HIV. Ann Intern Med 1998;128:306. [PMID: 9471935] (Information on the data supporting postexposure treatment, the indications for its use, the treatment regimen, and counseling recommendations.)

Osborn EH et al: Occupational exposures to body fluids among medical students: A seven-year longitudinal study. Ann Intern Med 1999;130:45. [PMID: 9890850]

Public Health Service guidelines for the management of health-care worker exposures to HIV and recommendations for postexposure prophylaxis. MMWR Recomm Rep 1998;47(RR-7):1. [PMID: 9603630] (Recommendations for treatment of occupational exposure to HIV.)

Public Health Service Task Force recommendations for the use of antiretroviral drugs in pregnant women infected with HIV-1 for maternal health and for reducing perinatal HIV-1 transmission in the United States. MMWR Recomm Rep 1998;48(RR-2):1. [PMID: 9461044] (Preclinical and clinical data regarding the use of a variety of antiretroviral regimens during pregnancy.)

Treatment

Treatment for HIV infection can be divided into four categories: therapy for opportunistic infections and malignancies, antiretroviral treatment, hematopoietic stimulating factors, and prophylaxis of opportunistic infections.

Experimental treatment regimens for HIV infection are constantly changing. Clinicians may obtain up-to-date information on experimental treatments by calling the AIDS Clinical Trials Information Service (ACTIS), 800-TRIALS-A (English and Spanish); the National AIDS Hot Line, 800-342-AIDS (English), 800-344-SIDA (Spanish), and 800-AIDS-TTY (hearing-impaired).

A. THERAPY FOR OPPORTUNISTIC INFECTIONS AND MALIGNANCIES

Treatment of common HIV infections and malignancies is detailed in Table 31–4. In the era prior to the use of highly active antiretroviral treatment (HAART), patients required lifelong treatment for many infections, including cytomegalovirus retinitis, toxoplasmosis, and cryptococcal meningitis. However, among patients who have a good response to HAART, maintenance therapy for some opportunistic infections can be terminated. For example, in consultation with an ophthalmologist, maintenance treatment for CMV infection can be discontinued in persons with durable suppression of viral load on HAART who have a CD4 count > 100–150 cells/µL. Similar results have been observed in patients with *M avium* complex bacteremia.

The emergence of resistance is more common for some infections of HIV-infected people (eg, acyclovir-resistant herpes simplex) than among immunocompetent individuals. In addition, HIV-infected patients have an increased incidence of side effects to standard drugs such as trimethoprim-sulfamethoxazole.

Treating patients with repeated episodes of the same opportunistic infection can pose difficult therapeutic challenges. For example, patients with second or third episodes of pneumocystis pneumonia may have developed allergic reactions to standard treatments with a prior episode. Fortunately, there are several alternatives available for the treatment of pneumocystis infection. Trimethoprim with dapsone—and primaquine and clindamycin—are two combinations that often are tolerated in patients with a prior allergic reaction to trimethoprim-sulfamethoxazole and intravenous pentamidine. On the positive side, patients who develop second episodes of pneumocystis pneumonia while taking prophylaxis tend to have milder courses.

Well-established alternative regimens now also exist for most AIDS-related opportunistic infections: amphotericin B or fluconazole for cryptococcal meningitis; ganciclovir, cidofovir, or foscarnet for cytomegalovirus infection; and sulfadiazine or clindamycin with pyrimethamine for toxoplasmosis.

Corticosteroids. Although conceptually it would seem that corticosteroid therapy should be avoided in HIV-infected patients, steroid use has been shown to improve the course of patients with moderate to severe pneumocystosis (oxygen saturation < 90%, PO_2 < 65 mm Hg) when administered within 72 hours after diagnosis. The mechanism of action is presumed to be a decrease in alveolar inflammation.

B. ANTIRETROVIRAL THERAPY

The availability of agents that alone and in combination suppress HIV replication (Table 31–5) has had a profound impact on the natural history of HIV infection. Patients who achieve excellent suppression of HIV generally have stabilization or improvement of their clinical course which results from partial immunologic reconstitution and a subsequent decrease in complications of immunosuppression. The best time to initiate antiretroviral treatment remains controversial. The recognition of continuous viral replica-

Table 31-4. Treatment of AIDS-related opportunistic infections and malignancies.[1]

Infection or Malignancy	Treatment	Complications
P carinii infection[2]	Trimethoprim-sulfamethoxazole, 15 mg/kg/d (based on trimethoprim component) orally or IV for 14–21 days.	Nausea, neutropenia, anemia, hepatitis, drug rash, Stevens-Johnson syndrome.
	Pentamidine, 3–4 mg/kg/d IV for 14–21 days.	Hypotension, hypoglycemia, anemia, neutropenia, pancreatitis, hepatitis.
	Trimethoprim, 15 mg/kg/d orally, with dapsone, 100 mg/d orally, for 14–21 days.[3]	Nausea, rash, hemolytic anemia in G6PD-deficient patients. Methemoglobinemia (weekly levels should be < 10% of total hemoglobin).
	Primaquine, 15–30 mg/d orally, and clindamycin, 600 mg every 8 hours orally, for 14–21 days.	Hemolytic anemia in G6PD-deficient patients. Methemoglobinemia, neutropenia, colitis.
	Atovaquone, 750 mg orally 3 times daily for 14–21 days.	Rash, elevated aminotransferases, anemia, neutropenia.
	Trimetrexate, 45 mg/m[2] IV for 21 days (given with leucovorin calcium) if intolerant of all other regimens.	Leukopenia, rash, mucositis.
M avium complex infection	Clarithromycin, 500 mg orally twice daily with ethambutol, 15 mg/kg/d orally (maximum, 1 g). May also add:	Clarithromycin: hepatitis, nausea, diarrhea; ethambutol: hepatitis, optic neuritis.
	Rifabutin, 300 mg orally daily.	Rash, hepatitis, uveitis.
Toxoplasmosis	Pyrimethamine, 100–200 mg orally as loading dose, followed by 50–75 mg/d, combined with sulfadiazine, 4–6 g orally daily in 4 divided doses, and folinic acid, 10 mg daily for 4–8 weeks; then pyrimethamine, 25–50 mg/d, with clindamycin, 2 g/d, and folinic acid, 5 mg/d, until clinical and radiographic resolution is achieved.	Leukopenia, rash.
Lymphoma	Combination chemotherapy (eg, modified CHOP,[4] M-BACOD,[4] with or without G-CSF[5] or GM-CSF[5]). Central nervous system disease: radiation treatment with dexamethasone for edema.	Nausea, vomiting, anemia, leukopenia, cardiac toxicity (with doxorubicin).
Cryptococcal meningitis	Amphotericin B, 0.6 mg/kg/d IV, with or without flucytosine, 100 mg/kg/d orally in 4 divided doses for 2 weeks, followed by:	Fever, anemia, hypokalemia, and azotemia.
	Fluconazole, 400 mg orally daily for 6 weeks, then 200 mg orally daily.	Hepatitis.
Cytomegalovirus infection	Ganciclovir, 10 mg/kg/d IV in 2 divided doses for 10 days, followed by 6 mg/kg 5 days a week indefinitely. (Decrease dose for renal impairment.) May use ganciclovir as maintenance therapy (1 g orally with fatty foods 3 times a day).	Neutropenia (especially when used concurrently with zidovudine).
	Foscarnet, 60 mg/kg IV every 8 hours for 10–14 days (induction), followed by 90 mg/kg once daily. (Adjust for changes in renal function.)	Nausea, hypokalemia, hypocalcemia, hyperphosphatemia, azotemia.

(continued)

Table 31–4. Treatment of AIDS-related opportunistic infections and malignancies.[1] (continued)

Infection or Malignancy	Treatment	Complications
Esophageal candidiasis or recurrent vaginal candidiasis	Fluconazole, 100–200 mg daily for 10–14 days.	Hepatitis, development of imidazole resistance.
	Ketoconazole, 200 mg orally twice daily for 10–14 days.	Hepatitis, adrenal insufficiency.
Herpes simplex infection	Acyclovir, 200 mg 5 times daily for 7–10 days; or acyclovir, 5 mg/kg IV every 8 hours for severe cases.	Resistant herpes simplex with chronic therapy.
	Famciclovir, 500 mg orally twice daily for 7 days.	Nausea
	Valacyclovir, 500 mg orally twice daily for 7 days	Nausea
	Foscarnet, 40 mg/kg IV every 8 hours, for acyclovir-resistant cases. (Adjust for changes in renal function.)	See above.
Herpes zoster	Acyclovir, 800 mg orally 4 or 5 times daily for 7 days. Intravenous therapy at 10 mg/kg every 8 hours for ocular involvement, disseminated disease.	See above.
	Famciclovir, 500 mg orally 3 times daily for 7 days.	Nausea.
	Valacyclovir, 500 mg orally 3 times daily for 7 days.	Nausea
	Foscarnet, 40 mg/kg IV every 8 hours for acyclovir-resistant cases. (Adjust for changes in renal function.)	See above.
Kaposi's sarcoma Limited cutaneous disease	Observation, intralesional vinblastine.	Inflammation, pain at site of injection.
Extensive or aggressive cutaneous disease	Systemic chemotherapy (eg, alternating weekly vinca alkaloids). Alpha interferon (for patients with CD4 > 200 cells/μL and no constitutional symptoms). Radiation (amelioration of edema).	Bone marrow suppression, peripheral neuritis, flu-like syndrome.
Visceral disease (eg, pulmonary)	Combination chemotherapy (eg, daunorubicin, bleomycin, vinblastine).	Bone marrow suppression, cardiac toxicity, fever.

[1]For treatment of *Mycobacterium tuberculosis* infection, see Chapter 9.
[2]For moderate to severe *P carinii* infection (oxygen saturation < 90%), corticosteroids should be given with specific treatment. The dose of prednisone is 40 mg twice daily for 5 days, then 40 mg daily for 5 days, and then 20 mg daily until therapy is complete.
[3]When considering use of dapsone, check G6PD level in African-American patients and those of Mediterranean origin.
[4]CHOP = cyclophosphamide, doxorubicin (hydroxydaunomycin), vincristine (Oncovin), and prednisone. Modified M-BACOD = methotrexate, bleomycin, doxorubicin, (Adriamycin), cyclophosphamide, vincristine (Oncovin), and dexamethasone.
[5]G-CSF = granulocyte colony stimulating factor (filgrastim); GM-CSF = granulocyte-macrophage colony stimulating factor (sargramostim).

tion during early HIV infection and the considerable risk of disease progression in individuals with even low levels of circulating HIV RNA gave impetus to the concept of treating the majority of infected individuals with antiretroviral therapy even if the CD4 lymphocyte count was normal. The rationale for hitting the virus "early and hard" was based on the hope that such a strategy might eradicate HIV infection. Even if HIV could not be eradicated, it was thought that this strategy would preserve immune function over time. With greater experience, it is clear that HAART does not eradicate HIV. While these regimens are generally successful in maintaining immune function, the development of severe drug side effects—especially lipodystro-

Table 31–5. Antiretroviral therapy.

Drug	Dose	Common Side Effects	Monitoring	Cost[1]	Cost/Month
Nucleoside analogs					
Zidovudine (AZT) (Retrovir)	500–600 mg orally daily in three divided doses	Anemia, neutropenia, nausea, malaise, headache, insomnia, myopathy	Complete blood count and differential (every 3 months once stable)	$1.96/100 mg	$354.60
Didanosine (ddI) (Videx)	125–200 mg orally twice daily (for pill formulation)	Peripheral neuropathy, pancreatitis, dry mouth, hepatitis	CBC and differential, aminotransferases, K^+, amylase, triglycerides, bimonthly neurologic questionnaire for neuropathy	$3.16/150 mg; $5.27/250 mg powder	$189.60; $316.10
Zalcitabine (ddC) (Hivid)	0.375–0.75 mg orally 3 times daily	Peripheral neuropathy, aphthous ulcers, hepatitis	Monthly neurologic questionnaire for neuropathy, aminotransferases	$2.73/0.75 mg	$245.70
Stavudine (d4T) (Zerit)	40 mg orally twice daily	Peripheral neuropathy, hepatitis, pancreatitis	Monthly neurologic questionnaire for neuropathy, aminotransferases, amylase	$5.30/40 mg	$318.04
Lamivudine (3TC) (Epivir)	150 mg orally twice daily	Rash, peripheral neuropathy	No additional monitoring	$5.06/150 mg	$303.40
Abacavir (Ziagen)	300 mg orally twice daily	Rash, fever—if occur, rechallenge may be fatal	No special monitoring	$6.80/300 mg	$407.70
Nucleotide analog					
Tenofovir	300 mg orally once daily	Gastrointestinal distress	Renal function	$13.60/300 mg	$408.00
Protease inhibitors					
Saquinavir soft gel (Fortovase)	1200 mg three times daily	Gastrointestinal distress, headache	Bimonthly aminotransferases, cholesterol, triglycerides	$1.34/200 mg	$720.96
Ritonavir (Norvir)	600 mg orally twice daily or 100–400 mg orally twice daily in combination with other protease inhibitors	Gastrointestinal distress, peripheral paresthesias	Bimonthly aminotransferases, CK, uric acid, triglycerides	$2.14/100 mg	$771.54
Indinavir (Crixivan)	800 mg orally three times daily	Kidney stones	Bimonthly aminotransferases, bilirubin level, cholesterol, triglycerides	$2.90/400 mg	$523.35
Nelfinavir (Viracept)	750 mg orally three times daily	Diarrhea	Cholesterol, triglycerides	$2.52/250 mg	$680.99

Protease inhibitors (cont.)			
Amprenavir (Agenerase)	1200 mg orally twice daily	Gastrointestinal, rash	Cholesterol, triglycerides	$1.47/150 mg	$706.12
Lopinavir/ritonavir (Kaletra)	400 mg/100 mg orally twice daily	Diarrhea	Cholesterol, triglycerides, every other month aminotransferases	$3.91/133 mg (lopinavir)	$703.50
Nonnucleoside reverse transcriptase inhibitors (NNRTIs)			
Nevirapine (Viramune)	200 mg orally daily for 2 weeks, then 200 mg orally twice daily	Rash	No additional monitoring	$5.60/200 mg	$336.08
Delavirdine (Rescriptor)	400 mg orally three times daily	Rash	No additional monitoring	$1.76/200 mg	$316.35
Efavirenz (Sustiva)	600 mg orally daily	Neurologic disturbances	No additional monitoring	$14.39/600 mg	$431.65

[1]Cost to pharmacist (average wholesale price, generic when possible) for quantity listed. Source: *Drug Topics Red Book,* March 2002; Vol. 21, No. 3.

phy and other metabolic complications—has significantly qualified enthusiasm for these regimens. Current recommendations are to initiate treatment for HIV-infected patients with CD4 cells < 350/μL or viral load > 30,000 copies/mL by branched-chain DNA or 55,000 copies/mL by PCR testing.

Once a decision to initiate therapy has been made, several important principles should guide therapy. First, since HIV develops drug resistance to antiretroviral agents, a major goal of therapy should be total suppression of viral replication as measured by the serum viral load, which has been shown to correlate with antiviral effect in other compartments. To achieve this and maintain virologic control over time, aggressive combination therapy is essential, and partially suppressive combinations such as dual nucleoside therapy should be avoided. Similarly, if toxicity develops, it is preferable to interrupt the entire regimen rather than reduce individual doses. The current standard is to use at least three agents simultaneously. Since the number of drugs and potential combinations is finite and the development of drug resistance may severely compromise the efficacy of treatment, patients must be able to adhere to these regimens. Patients should be counseled that if they think they will miss many doses of treatment, it would be preferable to defer starting therapy until they are able to adhere to the regimen. Adherence can be promoted through the use of medication boxes with compartments (eg, Medisets), supportive counseling, or daily supervision of therapy. Therefore, decisions to withhold treatment should not be based upon a patient's circumstances (eg, active drug use or housing status) alone. Often, a trial intervention such as offering pneumocystis pneumonia prophylaxis may be helpful in determining the likelihood of adherence to a more complex antiretroviral regimen.

Monitoring of antiretroviral therapy has two goals. Laboratory evaluation for toxicity depends upon the specific drugs in the combination but generally should be done approximately every 2–3 months once a patient is on a stable regimen. The second aspect of monitoring is to regularly measure objective markers of efficacy. The CD4 cell count and HIV viral load should be repeated 1–2 months after the initiation or change of antiretroviral regimen and every 3–4 months thereafter in clinically stable patients. Reasons for changing antiretroviral regimens include intolerable adverse reactions, rising or persistently high viral loads, the clinical progression of disease, and continued immunologic deterioration as reflected by a declining CD4 cell count. Although a rebound in HIV viral load is cited as an indication to change therapy, exact parameters have not been established, and many patients appear to have continued clinical benefit in the face of rising viral load measurements. When therapy is modified, clinicians should attempt to start at least two agents to which an individual has not been exposed. Conversely, there is a risk to stopping a single medication because of the possibility of its causing a side effect if the remaining regimen contains too few medications to prevent rapid development of resistance.

The roles of genotypic and phenotypic drug resistance assays are still being debated. Resistance testing is recommended for patients who are experiencing treatment failure (persistent or rising viral load despite adherence to an efficacious regimen). It is also recommended for guiding therapy in HIV-infected women who are pregnant. Resistance testing can also be considered when starting HAART in newly infected individuals living in areas where transmission of drug-resistant HIV is common. Of the two methods of resistance testing available, genotypic testing is more easily performed and less expensive. The presence of certain genetic mutations confers resistance to particular agents. Although phenotypic testing would appear to be more relevant than genotypic testing since it offers the promise of determining how a patient's virus actually responds to different agents, it is not well-standardized and is expensive.

Both methods of resistance testing are limited by the fact that they may measure resistance in only some of the viral strains present in an individual. Resistance results may also be misleading if a patient is not taking antiretroviral medications at the time of testing. Thus, resistance results must be viewed cumulatively—ie, if resistance is reported to an agent on one test, it should be presumed to be present thereafter even if subsequent tests do not give the same result.

Although the ideal combination of drugs has not yet been defined, possible choices can be better understood after a review of the available agents. These drugs can be grouped into three major categories: nucleoside and nucleotide analogs, protease inhibitors, and nonnucleoside reverse transcriptase inhibitors.

1. Nucleoside and nucleotide analogs—

a. Zidovudine—Zidovudine (azidothymidine; AZT) was the first approved antiviral drug for HIV infection and remains an important agent. It is administered at a dose of 300 mg orally twice daily. A combination of zidovudine 300 mg and lamivudine 150 mg (Combivir) allows more convenient dosing of medication for individuals taking both of these agents. The cost of zidovudine (at a dose of 600 mg/d) is approximately $270 a month. Higher doses of zidovudine (1000–2000 mg/d) have been shown to be of possible benefit in individuals with HIV-associated dementia. Side effects seen with zidovudine are listed in Table 31–5. Approximately 40% of patients experience subjective side effects which usually remit within 6 weeks. The common dose-limiting side effects are anemia and neutropenia, which can be exacerbated by other drugs such as ganciclovir that cause bone marrow suppression. Anemia is usually mild, indolent in course, and characterized by macrocytosis. It is unresponsive to vitamin B_{12} or folate supplementation. A minority of patients have the more rapid onset of red cell aplasia. Bone marrow toxicity is generally reversible with cessation of the drug. Erythropoietin (epoetin alfa), at a starting dose of 8000 units subcutaneously three times a week, and G-CSF (filgrastim), at a dose of 300 μg subcutaneously one to three times a week, can ameliorate these side effects in situations where alternatives to zidovudine therapy are limited. Long-term zidovudine administration may also be complicated by myopathy, with wasting and weakness usually most prominent in the gluteus and quadriceps muscles.

In monitoring patients receiving zidovudine, complete blood counts—with platelet and differential counts—should be done monthly for the first 2 months of therapy and then every 3 months. Creatine phosphokinase levels should be checked every 6 months. Zidovudine can be taken concomitantly with other medicines except probenecid, which prolongs the serum half-life of zidovudine. Long-term administration of zidovudine with ganciclovir can pose a difficult problem. Only 15% of patients tolerate this combination without significant hematologic toxicity. One approach to neutropenia is to add G-CSF (filgrastim) to the regimen; another is to substitute another agent for zidovudine.

b. Didanosine (ddI)—This agent also proved to have significant antiviral activity in early monotherapy trials and now is incorporated into combination regimens. Didanosine is available in three formulations: enteric-coated capsule, pill, and powder. Patients must take the medication on an empty stomach (1 hour before or 2–3 hours after meals). Indinavir and didanosine should be taken at least 1 hour apart.

For adults weighing at least 60 kg, the most convenient dosing is with the enteric-coated capsule (400 mg orally daily). Twice-daily dosing of didanosine with tablets or powder is by weight. For adults weighing < 60 kg, dosing is 125 mg (tablets) or 167 mg (powder) twice a day; for adults weighing ≥ 60 kg, 200 mg (tablets) or 250 mg (powder) twice a day. To ensure adequate buffering agent, the pills should be taken two at a time and thoroughly chewed or dissolved in water. Diarrhea (due to the buffering agent used) is more common with the powder.

Unlike zidovudine, didanosine does not cause anemia but may cause neutropenia. It has also been associated with pancreatitis. The incidence of pancreatitis with didanosine is 5–10%—of fatal pancreatitis, less than 0.4%. Patients with a history of pancreatitis, as well as those taking other medications associated with pancreatitis (including trimethoprim-sulfamethoxazole and intravenous pentamidine) are at higher risk of this complication. Patients should be warned to use alcohol judiciously while taking didanosine. Clinicians should also teach patients to watch for the symptoms of pancreatitis and to stop treatment if they develop abdominal pain, nausea, or vomiting while taking didanosine until it can be determined if they have pancreatitis. Other common side effects with didanosine include a dose-related, reversible, painful peripheral neuropathy which occurs in about 15% of patients, and dry mouth. Fulminant hepatic failure and electrolyte abnormalities, including hypokalemia, hypocalcemia, and hypomagnesemia, have been reported in patients taking didanosine.

c. Stavudine—Stavudine (d4T) has shown good activity as an antiretroviral drug. Side effects noted are peripheral neuropathy and, rarely, hepatitis. Pancreatitis has been reported in patients taking stavudine, but it is unclear if the drug was the cause of the pancreatitis. The dose is 40 mg orally twice daily for individuals weighing more than 70 kg.

d. Lamivudine—Lamivudine (3TC) is a safe and well-tolerated agent that has shown great promise when used in combination with zidovudine or stavudine. This combination results in more sustained suppression of viral replication and increase in CD4 cell counts than other combinations of nucleoside drugs studied to date. The dose of lamivudine is 150 mg orally twice daily. There are no significant side effects with this agent.

e. Abacavir—A daily dose of 300 mg orally twice daily results in potent antiretroviral activity, and the drug has pharmacokinetic features that allow twice-daily dosing. Abacavir retains activity against some HIV strains that have become resistant to other nucleoside drugs. Abacavir may be combined with two other nucleoside analogs instead of a protease inhibitor or NNRTI. In fact, abacavir is formulated with zidovudine and lamivudine in a single pill (Trizivir, one tablet orally twice daily). The main toxicity of abacavir is a hypersensitivity syndrome in about 5% of patients, characterized by a flu-like syndrome with rash and fever that worsens with successive doses; individuals who develop this syndrome *should not* be rechallenged with this agent.

f. Zalcitabine—Zalcitabine (ddC) is thought to be one of the least effective antiretroviral agents and is therefore not commonly used. Its advantages are that it is inexpensive, easy to administer, and has no known hematologic side effects. The usual dosage of zalcitabine is approximately 0.005–0.01 mg/kg orally every 8 hours. This drug is formulated in 0.375 mg and 0.75 mg tablets.

Zalcitabine, like didanosine, may cause peripheral neuropathy. It is also associated with aphthous ulcers, rash, and rare cases of pancreatitis.

g. Tenofovir— Tenofovir is the only licensed nucleotide analog. It is given as a single daily oral dose of 300 mg and is generally well tolerated.

2. Protease inhibitors—Six protease inhibitors—indinavir, nelfinavir, ritonavir, amprenavir, saquinavir, and lopinavir (in combination with ritonavir)—have been approved for use. Protease inhibitors have been shown to potently suppress HIV replication in vitro and in vivo and are always administered as part of a combination regimen, using either one or two agents from this class. If only one protease inhibitor is chosen as part of a regimen, possible choices include indinavir, amprenavir or nelfinavir.

All the protease inhibitors—to differing degrees—are metabolized by the cytochrome P450 system, and each can inhibit and induce various P450 isoenzymes. Therefore, drug interactions are common and difficult to predict. Clinicians should consult the product inserts before prescribing protease inhibitors with other medications. Drugs such as rifabutin that are known to induce the P450 system should be avoided.

The fact that the protease inhibitors are dependent on metabolism through the cytochrome P450 system has led to some innovative dosing strategies. In particular, ritonavir dramatically inhibits the hepatic clearance of saquinavir, thereby enhancing its antiviral effect; the combination has demonstrated potent suppression of HIV. When the drugs are used together, the doses are reduced to 400 mg of ritonavir twice daily and 400–600 mg of saquinavir (soft gel) twice daily. The only additional toxicity observed with this combination has been elevation of hepatic aminotransferases. Thus, liver enzymes should be regularly monitored, especially in patients who have underlying liver disease. Similar strategies combine ritonavir with either indinavir or nelfinavir, allowing twice-daily dosing of these protease inhibitors.

When any protease inhibitor is used incorrectly, drug resistance develops rapidly. Protease inhibitors should never be used alone, and they should not be dose-escalated.

Protease inhibitors have been linked to a constellation of metabolic abnormalities. These abnormalities include elevated cholesterol levels, elevated triglyceride levels, insulin resistance, diabetes mellitus, and changes in body fat composition (eg, abdominal obesity, skeletal wasting). The lipid abnormalities and body habitus changes are referred to as lipodystrophy. Its prevalence is known to be increased among persons treated with protease inhibitors, but it has been seen also in HIV-infected persons who have never been treated with these agents. The changes in body habitus are particularly disturbing to patients who are trying to maintain a positive body image. Of the different manifestations of lipodystrophy, the dyslipidemias that occur are of particular concern because of the likelihood that increased levels of cholesterol and triglycerides will result in increased prevalence of heart disease. All patients taking protease inhibitors or NNRTIs should have a fasting cholesterol, LDL, and triglyceride level performed every 3–6 months. Until there is longer follow-up of HIV-infected persons with elevated cholesterol levels, treatment decisions should be the same as those for uninfected persons (see Chapter 28). HIV-infected persons who do not respond to dietary interventions should be started on pravastatin (20 mg daily orally) or atorvastatin (10 mg daily orally). Lovastatin and simvastatin should be avoided because of their interactions with protease inhibitors. Patients with fasting serum triglyceride levels > 1000 mg/dL who do not respond to dietary intervention should be treated with gemfibrozil (600 mg twice daily prior to the morning and evening meals).

a. Indinavir—The standard dose of indinavir is 800 mg orally three times a day. Twice-daily dosing of indinavir is less effective and should not be used except in combination with ritonavir or nelfinavir. It is recommended that indinavir be taken without food but with water 1 hour before or 2 hours after a meal. Nausea and headache are common complaints with this drug. Indinavir crystals are present in the urine in approximately 40% of patients; this results in clinically apparent nephrolithiasis in about 15% of patients receiving indinavir. Lower urinary tract symptoms and acute renal failure have been rarely reported. Patients taking this drug should be instructed to drink at least 48 ounces of fluid a day to ensure adequate hydration in an attempt to avoid these complications, but if stones occur repeatedly, an alternative protease inhibitor may be needed. Mild indirect hyperbilirubinemia is also commonly observed in patients taking indinavir, but this does not portend more serious hepatotoxicity and is not an indication to discontinue the drug.

b. Nelfinavir—This agent appears to have slightly less potent antiviral activity than either indinavir or ritonavir but has shown short-term benefit in combination regimens. The dose of nelfinavir is 750 mg orally three times daily or 1250 mg orally twice daily. Diarrhea is a side effect in 25% of patients taking nelfinavir, and this symptom may be controlled in the majority of patients with over-the-counter antidiarrheal agents.

c. Ritonavir—Use of this potent protease inhibitor has been limited by its inhibition of the cytochrome P450 pathway causing a large number of drug-drug interactions and by its frequent side effects of fatigue, nausea, and paresthesias when the full dose of 600 mg orally twice daily is given. One of the major benefits of ritonavir is that it increases the bioavailability of other protease inhibitors (eg, saquinavir, lopinavir).

d. Saquinavir—As a single agent, in its original capsule formulation, saquinavir had limited bioavailability, which greatly curtailed its antiviral activity. A new soft-gel capsule formulation of saquinavir with greater bioavailability (Fortovase) is available. The dose of the soft gel formulation is 1200 mg three times a day with food. The most common side effects with saquinavir are diarrhea, nausea, dyspepsia, and abdominal pain. Soft-gel capsules of saquinavir do not require refrigeration if the capsules are kept at room temperature and used within 30 days.

e. Amprenavir—Amprenavir has efficacy and side effects similar to those of other protease inhibitors. Common side effects are nausea, vomiting, diarrhea, rash, and perioral paresthesia. The dose is 1200 mg orally twice daily. This requires that the patient take 16 capsules a day.

f. Lopinavir—This protease inhibitor appears to have less cross-resistance with other protease inhibitors. It is formulated with a low dose of ritonavir to maximize the bioavailability of lopinavir. It has been shown to be as effective as nelfinavir when used in combination with stavudine and lamivudine. The usual dose is 400 mg lopinavir with 100 mg of nelfinavir (three capsules) orally twice daily with food. When given along with efavirenz or nevirapine, a higher dose (533 mg/133 mg—four capsules) is needed. The most common side effect is diarrhea.

3. Nonnucleoside reverse transcriptase inhibitors (NNTRIs)—These agents inhibit reverse transcriptase at a site different from that of the nucleoside and nucleotide agents described above. All three have shown antiviral activity as measured by HIV viral load and CD4 responses. The major advantage of the NNRTIs is that two of them (nevirapine and efavirenz) have potencies comparable to that of protease inhibitors—with less toxicity. In particular, they do not appear to cause lipodystrophy; patients with lipodystrophy who are switched from a protease inhibitor to an NNRTI may have improvement in their symptoms. The resistance patterns of the NNRTIs are distinct from those of the protease inhibitors, so their use still leaves open the option for future protease inhibitor use.

The NNRTIs can be used with protease inhibitors in patients who are difficult to suppress on simpler regimens or when it is difficult to identify at least two agents to which the patient is not resistant. Because these agents may cause alterations in the clearance of protease inhibitors, dose modifications may be necessary when these two classes of medications are administered concomitantly. Resistance to one drug in this class uniformly predicts resistance to other drugs in the class. There is no therapeutic reason for using more than one NNRTI at the same time.

a. Nevirapine—The target dose of nevirapine is 200 mg orally twice daily, but it is initiated at a dose of 200 mg once a day to decrease the incidence of rash, which is as high as 40% when full doses are begun immediately. If rash develops while the patient is taking 200 mg a day, the dose should not be increased until the rash resolves. Patients with mild rash can continue to be treated with nevirapine. Diphenhydramine (25–50 mg orally three or four times daily) may provide symptomatic relief.

b. Efavirenz—The major advantage of this agent is that can be given once daily in a single dose (600 mg orally). The side effects are neurologic, with patients reporting symptoms ranging from lack of concentration and strange dreams to delusions and mania. Fortunately, the neurologic side effects of efavirenz subside over time, usually within a month.

c. Delavirdine—Of the three available NNRTIs, delavirdine is least used. It does not appear to be as potent as nevirapine or efavirenz. The dosage is 400 mg orally three times a day, which makes it less conve-

nient for patients than the other two medications in this class. As with nevirapine, the major side effect with delavirdine is rash, but the incidence of rash is lower with delavirdine.

4. Novel agents—

a. Hydroxyurea—This drug has no direct activity against HIV but potentiates the effect of several dideoxynucleosides, particularly didanosine, by decreasing clearance of the active compound. When hydroxyurea (at a dosage of 500 mg orally twice a day) is combined with didanosine, it can result in a short-term decrease of HIV viral load by greater than 1.5 log, an effect comparable to that seen with dual nucleoside regimens. Unfortunately, studies combining hydroxyurea with didanosine have not demonstrated retarded progression of disease. Because of its cytotoxic effect, patients treated with hydroxyurea tend to have less of a CD4 response to therapy than with other regimens; the clinical importance of this observation is unknown. The major toxicities of hydroxyurea are hematologic, with neutropenia being a dose-limiting toxicity about 8% of the time, and drug-induced hepatitis. The incidence of nucleoside-induced neuropathies is also higher in hydroxyurea-treated patients.

b. Peptide T20—Peptide T20 is the first drug in the new class of fusion inhibitors, which block the entry of HIV into cells. These drugs have antiviral activity even in heavily pretreated individuals. Other entry inhibitors are being developed, including inhibitors of chemokine receptors.

5. Constructing regimens—There is now little debate about the necessity for combining drugs to achieve long-term suppression of HIV and its associated clinical benefit. Only combinations of drugs have been able to decrease HIV viral load by 2–3 logs and allow suppression of HIV RNA to below the threshold of detection for longer than 4 years in some individuals. However, the ideal regimens for initial and second-line therapy have not yet been defined, so clinicians and their patients face difficult decisions in selecting therapy.

Several general principles should guide the choice of combinations. First, it is desirable to prescribe combinations that have demonstrated clinical benefit; since these data do not exist for many combinations, it is reassuring to know that the combination under consideration has shown beneficial effects upon HIV viral load levels in short-term studies. Second, to the extent possible, agents to which the patient has not been exposed are preferable to drugs for which resistance mutations may have already occurred. Third, toxicities should ideally be nonoverlapping. Fourth, an individual's relative contraindications to a given drug or drugs should be considered. Fifth, the regimen should not include agents that are either virologically antagonistic or incompatible in terms of drug-drug interactions. Sixth, compatible dosing schedules—prescribing medications that can be taken at the same time—improve adherence to treatment. Finally, highly complex therapeutic regimens should be reserved for individuals who are capable of adhering to the rigorous demands of taking multiple medications and having this therapy closely monitored. Conversely, simplified regimens that deliver the lowest number of pills given at the longest possible dosing intervals are desirable for patients who have difficulty taking multiple medications.

Possible ways of incorporating nonnucleoside agents and protease inhibitors into combinations are displayed in Figure 31–2. A number of points about the "nucleoside backbone" of regimens have become clearer. First, the dual nucleoside combinations with most activity probably include zidovudine plus lamivudine, zidovudine plus didanosine, stavudine plus didanosine, and stavudine plus lamivudine. In these pairings, both agents are given in full doses. The combination of stavudine plus didanosine does not seem to lead to syn-

ergistic development of neuropathy despite both drugs' predilection to cause this side effect. Also notable is the fact that the addition of lamivudine to didanosine does not appear to result in the same level of viral suppression as when lamivudine is combined with zidovudine or stavudine. Finally, the nucleoside pair of zidovudine and stavudine are antagonistic and should never be used together. This results from stavudine inhibiting the phosphorylation of zidovudine to its active metabolite.

In choosing which third agent to include in an initial antiretroviral regimen, ease of administration, minimization of side effects, and future treatment options should all be considered. For example, for patients for whom it is important to minimize the number of pills, a regimen of lamivudine/zidovudine (Combivir) and nevirapine offers a simple three-drug regimen (two pills twice a day). Another advantage of this regimen is that it reserves protease inhibitors for future use. Some persons who develop resistance to nelfinavir may still have sensitivity to indinavir and ri-

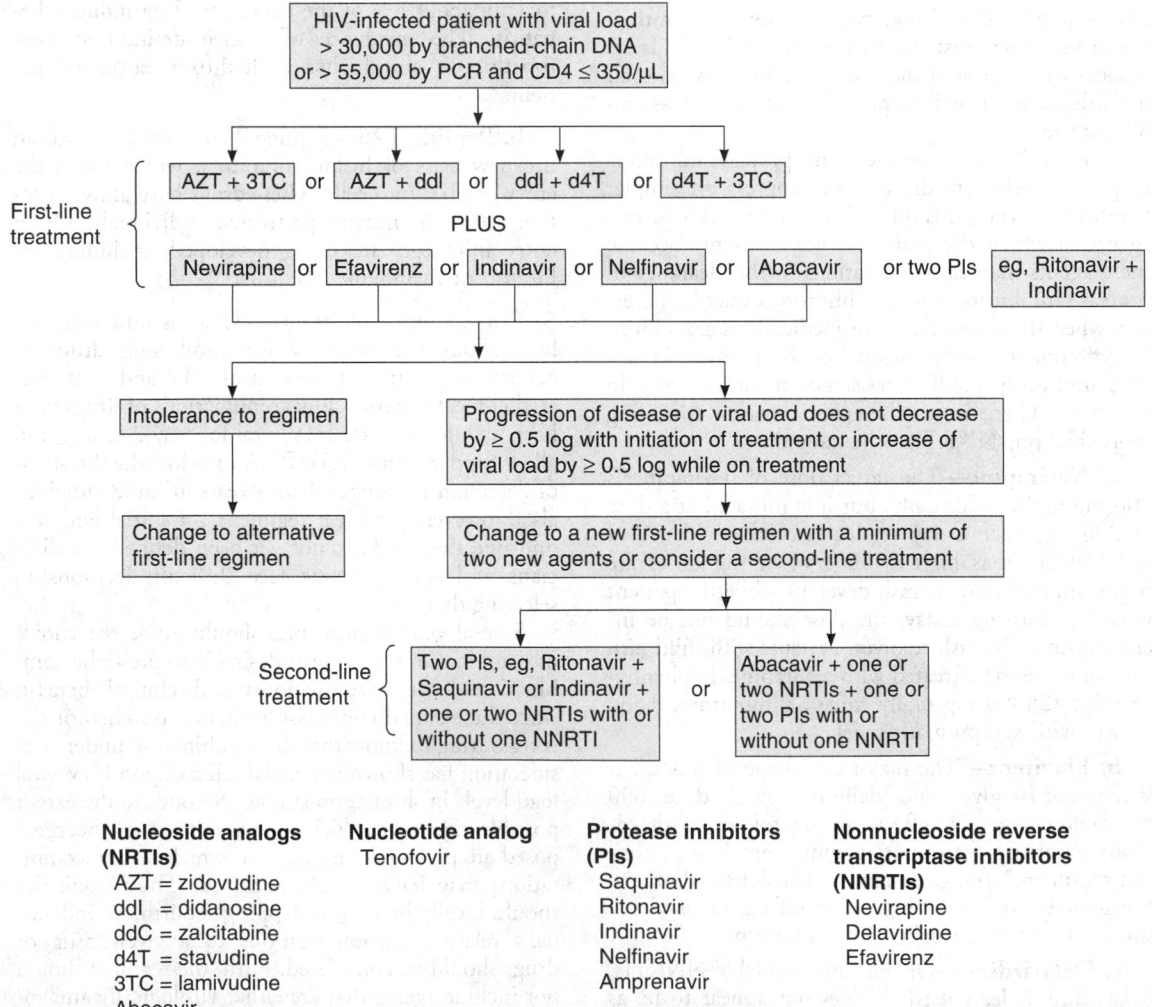

Figure 31–2. Approach to antiretroviral therapy.

tonavir. For this reason, many clinicians favor the use of nelfinavir as the initial protease inhibitor. Some clinicians advocate using two protease inhibitors simultaneously, particularly for patients with high viral loads (> 100,000/mL). The concern is that patients with particularly high viral loads are more likely to develop resistant virus on more conventional regimens. In addition to ritonavir-saquinavir, other combinations tried have included ritonavir-indinavir and indinavir-nelfinavir, with dosing of each agent reduced by roughly 50% of the usual recommended dose.

For some patients who have been heavily treated with antiretroviral agents it may be difficult to design second-line regimens when they are showing evidence of progression of disease on their existing regimen. In designing second-line regimens (sometimes called salvage regimens—a term that some patients may find offensive), the goal is to identify agents to which the patient is not resistant. This can be quite complicated because of cross resistance within types of agents. For example, the resistance patterns of ritonavir and indinavir are overlapping, and patients with virus resistant to these agents are unlikely to respond to nelfinavir or saquinavir even though they have never received treatment with these agents. Similarly, the resistance patterns of nevirapine and delavirdine are overlapping.

In addition to taking a careful history of what antiretroviral agents a patient has taken and for how long, genotypic and phenotypic resistance testing can provide useful information in designing second-line regimens. Interpretation of resistance testing often requires expert consultation.

Some clinicians have advocated the use of megadose highly active antiretroviral (HAART) regimens—regimens with six or more agents—for patients who have progressed on standard regimens. Although their use in some patients has resulted in virologic improvement, these regimens are difficult to adhere to, side effects are common, and they are expensive.

Whatever regimen is chosen, patients should be coached in ways to improve adherence. This should include taking medicines on an established schedule (eg, first thing in the morning), keeping a medication diary, and keeping medications in a variety of places the patient is likely to be (eg, car, workplace). For certain populations (eg, unstably housed individuals), specially tailored programs that include drug dispensing are needed.

For some patients, it is impossible to construct a tolerable regimen that fully suppresses HIV. In such cases, clinicians and patients should consider their goals. Patients maintained on effective antiretroviral agents often benefit from these regimens (eg, higher CD4 counts, fewer opportunistic infections) even if their virus is detectable. In some cases, patients appear to benefit from a drug holiday during which patients are taken off all medications. Patients often immediately feel better because of the absence of drug side effects. Structured treatment interruptions are being studied with two major goals: (1) to lessen side effects through decreased cumulative exposure to the medica-

tions, and (2) to stimulate an immunologic response by allowing low levels of viral replication. There is hope that achieving the first goal will result in a decreased long-term complication rate from therapy, but at present treatment interruption should be viewed as an experimental strategy. Patients should be monitored very closely during drug holidays, since viral rebound and CD4 decline can occur rapidly.

C. HEMATOPOIETIC STIMULATING FACTORS

Epoetin alfa (erythropoietin) is approved for use in HIV-infected patients with anemia, including those with anemia secondary to zidovudine use. It has been shown to decrease the need for blood transfusions. The drug is expensive, and a low endogenous erythropoietin level (less than 500 mU/mL) should be demonstrated before starting therapy. The starting dose is 8000 units subcutaneously three times a week. The target hematocrit is 35–40%. The dose may be increased by 12,000 units every 4–6 weeks as needed to a maximum dose of 48,000 units per week. Hypertension is the most common side effect.

Human granulocyte colony-stimulating factor (G-CSF [filgrastim]) and granulocyte-macrophage colony-stimulating factor (GM-CSF [sargramostim]) have been shown to increase the neutrophil counts of HIV-infected patients. G-CSF is preferred because of the theoretical concern of GM-CSF-stimulating HIV replication in infected monocytes. In patients receiving cytotoxic chemotherapy for lymphoma or Kaposi's sarcoma, daily subcutaneous doses of G-CSF at approximately 5 μg/kg (a 300 μg or 480 μg vial, depending upon weight) are given beginning 5–7 days after chemotherapy until the neutrophil count has rebounded to above 1000/μL. G-CSF may also have a role in ameliorating neutropenia caused by other drugs such as zidovudine or ganciclovir, when other therapeutic alternatives are not possible. Since the cost of this therapy is approximately $150 per vial, dosage should be closely monitored and minimized, aiming for a neutrophil count of 1000/μL. When the drug is used for indications other than cytotoxic chemotherapy, one or two doses at 5 μg/kg per week is usually sufficient.

D. PROPHYLAXIS OF OPPORTUNISTIC INFECTIONS

In general, decisions about prophylaxis of opportunistic infections are based on the CD4 count, other evidence of severe immune suppression (eg, oral candidiasis), and a history of having had the infection in the past. In the era prior to HAART, patients started on prophylactic regimens were maintained on them indefinitely. However, studies have shown that in patients with robust improvements in immune function—as measured by increases in CD4 counts above the levels that are used to initiate treatment—prophylactic regimens can safely be discontinued.

Primary prophylaxis for pneumocystis pneumonia should be offered to patients with CD4 counts below 200 cells/μL, a CD4 lymphocyte percentage below

14%, or weight loss or oral candidiasis. Patients with a history of pneumocystis pneumonia should receive secondary prophylaxis until they have had a durable virologic response to HAART for at least 3–6 months and maintain a CD4 count of > 250 cells/μL.

Three regimens for prophylaxis are trimethoprim-sulfamethoxazole, aerosolized pentamidine, and dapsone (see Table 31–6). Trimethoprim-sulfamethoxazole is inexpensive and widely available. In two studies comparing once-daily double-strength trimethoprim-sulfamethoxazole with aerosolized pentamidine for primary and secondary prophylaxis of pneumocystis pneumonia, patients randomized to trimethoprim-sulfamethoxazole were significantly less likely to develop pneumocystis pneumonia. Patients who receive trimethoprim-sulfamethoxazole are also less likely to develop bacterial infections (eg, pneumonia, sinusitis) than persons who receive pentamidine—another reason to use trimethoprim-sulfamethoxazole instead of aerosolized pentamidine. There is a higher incidence of side effects with trimethoprim-sulfamethoxazole (primarily fever, rash, and nausea and vomiting) than with aerosolized pentamidine. Nonetheless, trimethoprim-sulfamethoxazole (one double-strength tablet three times a week to once daily) should be considered the prophylactic agent of choice if tolerated. Patients who develop mild rashes on this regimen may be treated with diphenhydramine (25–50 mg every 4 hours). However, clinicians and patients must watch carefully for signs of Stevens-Johnson syndrome. Some clinicians are also using desensitization regimens to overcome allergic reactions. Reports suggest that desensitization may be successful in 40% of cases. Aerosolized pentamidine has the advantage of minimal systemic side effects. Its disadvantages are expense (approximately $160 per monthly treatment) and decreased effectiveness in the apical and peripheral areas of the lung. Cases of extrapulmonary pneumocystis infections in patients receiving aerosolized pentamidine have also been reported.

Aerosolized pentamidine may also increase the incidence of pneumothorax in patients with a history of pneumocystis infection.

Dapsone appears to be an effective prophylactic agent with minimal side effects. As with trimethoprim-sulfamethoxazole, it is inexpensive and widely available and may be used in patients with an allergic reaction to trimethoprim-sulfamethoxazole. Before prescribing dapsone, clinicians should document that the patient is not G6PD-deficient. Such patients are at high risk of developing hemolytic anemia with dapsone therapy. Patients taking dapsone concomitantly with didanosine should take the dapsone at least 2 hours prior to the didanosine. Dapsone is not absorbed well in the neutral pH stomach environment created by the didanosine buffering agent. Finally, atovaquone may be an option for individuals intolerant of other systemic therapies, but it appears to be less effective.

Patients who develop pneumocystis infection on a particular prophylactic regimen should be switched to a different one or should receive a combination regimen (eg, aerosolized pentamidine plus trimethoprim-sulfamethoxazole).

Prophylaxis against M avium complex infection should be given to patients whose CD4 counts fall below 75–100 cells/μL. Clarithromycin (500 mg orally twice daily) and azithromycin (1200 mg orally weekly) have both been shown to decrease the incidence of disseminated disease by approximately 75%, with a low rate of breakthrough of resistant disease. The latter regimen is generally preferred on the basis of ease of compliance and cost. Adding rifabutin increases the toxicity of the regimen but does not significantly increase its efficacy and is therefore not recommended. As sole therapy, rifabutin (300 mg orally daily) is less effective and more toxic than clarithromycin or azithromycin. Clinicians should make certain that patients do not have active M tuberculosis infection by examination of a chest radiograph prior to starting rifabutin because of concern about the development of resistance to rifabutin with cross-resistance to rifampin. Similarly, before initiating prophylaxis, clinicians should establish with a blood culture that the patient does not have disseminated M avium complex infection. Common side effects of both azithromycin and clarithromycin are nausea and diar-

Table 31–6. *Pneumocystis carinii* prophylaxis.

Drug	Dose	Side Effects	Limitations
Trimethoprim-sulfamethoxazole	One double-strength tablet 3 times a week to one tablet daily	Rash, neutropenia, hepatitis, Stevens-Johnson syndrome	Hypersensitivity reaction is common but, if mild, it may be possible to treat through.
Dapsone	50–100 mg daily or 100 mg 2 or 3 times per week	Anemia, nausea, methemoglobinemia, hemolytic anemia	Efficacy not established. G6PD level should be checked prior to therapy. Check methemoglobin level at 1 month.
Aerosolized pentamidine	300 mg monthly	Bronchospasm (pretreat with bronchodilators); rare reports of pancreatitis	Apical P carinii pneumonia, extrapulmonary P carinii infections, pneumothorax.

rhea. Two common side effects with rifabutin are rash and hepatic dysfunction. Rifabutin may induce hepatic enzymes, thereby decreasing the activity of some drugs metabolized by the liver.

Prophylaxis against *M avium* complex infection may be discontinued among patients whose CD4 counts go above 100 cells/μL in response to HAART.

Prophylaxis against *M tuberculosis* infection—isoniazid 300 mg daily plus pyridoxine 50 mg orally daily for 9 months to a year—should be given to all HIV-infected patients with positive PPD reactions (defined for HIV-infected patients as > 5 mm of induration).

Toxoplasmosis prophylaxis is desirable in patients with positive IgG toxoplasma serology. Trimethoprim-sulfamethoxazole (one double-strength tablet daily) offers good protection against toxoplasmosis, as does a combination of pyrimethamine, 25 mg orally once a week, plus dapsone, 100 mg orally daily.

Cytomegalovirus infection is also common in late HIV disease. Oral ganciclovir has been approved for CMV prophylaxis among HIV-infected persons with CD4 counts below 50 cells/μL. However, because the drug causes neutropenia, it is not widely used. Clinicians should consider performing serum CMV IgG antibody testing. Persons who are CMV IgG-negative are not at risk for development of CMV disease. Importantly, patients who are CMV IgG-negative should receive CMV-negative blood if they require a transfusion. Because over 99% of gay men are positive for CMV IgG, it is appropriate to reserve testing for heterosexuals with HIV.

Cryptococcosis, candidiasis, and endemic fungal diseases are also candidates for prophylaxis. One prophylactic trial showed a decreased incidence of cryptococcal disease with the use of fluconazole, 200 mg orally daily, but the treated group had no benefit in terms of mortality. Fluconazole (200 mg orally once a week) was found to prevent oral and vaginal candidiasis in women with CD4 counts below 300 cells/μL. In areas of the world where histoplasmosis and coccidioidomycosis are endemic and are frequent complications of HIV infection, prophylactic use of fluconazole or itraconazole may prove to be useful prophylactic strategies. However, the problem of identifying individuals at highest risk makes the targeting of prophylaxis difficult.

Since individuals with advanced HIV infection are susceptible to a number of opportunistic pathogens, the use of agents with activity against more than one pathogen is preferable. It has been shown, for example, that trimethoprim-sulfamethoxazole confers some protection against toxoplasmosis in individuals receiving this drug for pneumocystis prophylaxis. Similarly, clarithromycin and rifabutin may offer protection against development of cryptosporidiosis.

Course & Prognosis

With improvements in therapy, patients are living longer after the diagnosis of AIDS. This has resulted in dramatic decreases in AIDS deaths nationally. In 1999 in the USA there were 16,273 deaths due to AIDS, compared with 50,610 deaths in 1995. It remains to be seen whether the decreases in number of deaths can be sustained over the long term. Maintaining access to quality care and treatment is one key element. Unfortunately, studies continue to show less access to treatment for some underserved groups, especially blacks, the homeless, and injecting drug users. Another key element in sustaining lower mortality is developing new treatments for patients who have been heavily treated with existing agents. Despite new therapeutic options, people continue to die from HIV infection. For patients whose disease progresses even though they are receiving appropriate treatment, meticulous palliative care must be provided (see Chapter 4), with attention to pain control, spiritual needs, and family (biologic and chosen) dynamics.

Albrecht MA et al: Nelfinavir, efavirenz, or both after the failure of nucleoside treatment of HIV infection. N Engl J Med 2001;345;398. [PMID: 11496850] (Triple therapy with efavirenz was superior to triple therapy with nelfinavir; quadruple therapy including both had the best antiviral outcome.)

Bamberger JD et al: Helping the urban poor stay with antiretroviral HIV drug therapy. Am J Pub Health 2000:90:699. [PMID: 10800416] (A creative approach to assisting homeless, mentally ill, and substance-abusing patients adhere to antiretroviral regimens.)

Dube M et al: Preliminary guidelines for the evaluation and management of dyslipidemia in adults infected with human immunodeficiency virus and receiving antiretroviral therapy. Clin Infect Dis 2000;31;1216. [PMID: 11073755] (Consensus guidelines on management of lipid abnormalities in patients receiving highly active antiretroviral treatment.)

El-Sadr WM et al: Discontinuation of prophylaxis for *Mycobacterium avium* complex disease in HIV infected patients who have a response to antiretroviral therapy. N Engl J Med 2000;342:1085. [PMID: 10766581] (MAC prophylaxis can be discontinued among patients whose CD4 count has increased to > 100 cells/μL in response to HAART.)

Fauci AS et al: Guidelines for the use of antiretroviral agents in HIV-infected adults and adolescents. February 2001. Available at: www.hivatis.org. (Updated consensus guidelines on the use of antiretroviral medication.)

Gulick RM et al: Simultaneous versus sequential initiation of therapy with indinavir, zidovudine, and lamivudine for HIV-1 infection: 100-week follow-up. JAMA 1998;280:35. [PMID: 9660361] (Sustained viral suppression for 2 years in the majority of people who adhered to this regimen.)

Hirsch MS et al: Antiretroviral drug resistance testing in adult HIV-1 infection. JAMA 2000;283:2417. [PMID: 10815085] (Consensus recommendations on the use of drug resistance testing.)

Jacobson MA et al: Altered natural history of AIDS-related opportunistic infections in the era of potent combination antiretroviral therapy. AIDS 1998;12(Suppl A):S157. [PMID: 9632998] (Interesting review of newer manifestations of CMV, tuberculosis and other infections.)

Kovacs JA et al: Prophylaxis against opportunistic infections in patients with human immunodeficiency virus infection. N Engl J Med 2000;342:1416. [PMID: 10805828] (Review of strategies for prevention of opportunistic infections in HIV-infected persons, with consideration of immune reconstitution with HAART.)

Ledergerber B et al. AIDS-related opportunistic illnesses occurring after initiation of potent antiretroviral therapy: the Swiss HIV Cohort Study. JAMA 1999;282:2220. [PMID: 10605973] (Low rates of opportunistic infections among persons with undetectable viral loads after 6 months of HAART.)

Leoung GS et al: Trimethoprim-sulfamethoxazole (TMP-SMZ) dose escalation versus direct rechallenge for *Pneumocystis carinii* pneumonia prophylaxis in human immunodeficiency virus-infected patients with previous adverse reaction to TMP-SMZ. J Infect Dis 2001;184;992. [PMID: 11574913] (Dose escalation enabled 75% of those with prior mild to moderate reactions to continue prophylaxis with this agent.)

Staszewski S et al: Efavirenz plus zidovudine and lamivudine, efavirenz plus indinavir, and indinavir plus zidovudine and lamivudine in the treatment of HIV-1 infection in adults. N Engl J Med 1999;341:1865. [PMID: 10601505] (The combination of efavirenz, zidovudine, and lamivudine had greater antiviral activity and was better tolerated than the combination of indinavir, zidovudine, and lamivudine.)

Staszewski S et al: Abacavir-lamivudine-zidovudine vs indinavir-lamivudine-zidovudine in antiretroviral-naive HIV-infected adults: A randomized equivalence trial. JAMA 2001;285;1155. [PMID 11231744] (Both regimens had equivalent outcomes over the period of follow-up in previously untreated patients.)

Vincent I et al: Modalities of palliative care in hospitalized patients with advanced AIDS. AIDS Care 2000;12:211. [PMID: 10827862] (Advocates an integrated approach for palliative care of persons with AIDS.)

Whitcup SM et al: Discontinuation of anticytomegalovirus therapy in patients with HIV infection and cytomegalovirus retinitis. JAMA 1999;282:1633. [PMID: 10553789] (Maintenance therapy for CMV retinitis was safely stopped for patients with CD4 counts > 150 cells/μL who were being treated with HAART.)

Youle M et al: Two year outcome of a multidrug regimen in patients who did not respond to a protease inhibitor regimen. J AIDS 2002:29;58. [PMID: 11782591] (Small study showing success of salvage "mega-HAART" regimens in some patients.)

Zolopa AR et al: HIV-1 genotypic resistance patterns predict response to saquinavir-ritonavir therapy in patients in whom previous protease inhibitor therapy had failed. Ann Intern Med 1999;131:813. [PMID: 10610625] (Clinical features plus genotypic data were much better at predicting virologic response than clinical features alone.)

Infectious Diseases: Viral & Rickettsial

32

Wayne X. Shandera, MD, & Samuel Shelburne III, MD
See www.current-med.com/ch32.html

▮ I. VIRAL DISEASES

This section discusses viral diseases caused by herpesviruses, those preventable by vaccines, and others causing distinct syndromes. Rickettsial illnesses and Kawasaki syndrome are also included. Disorders caused by hepatotropic viruses (Chapter 15), papillomaviruses (Chapter 6), and human immunodeficiency virus (Chapters 17 and 31) are dealt with elsewhere.

Clinical Diagnosis

Some viral illnesses present with typical syndromes (measles, mumps, chickenpox). In others, the clinical picture suggests any of a number of viruses. For example, aseptic meningitis can be caused by the mumps virus, lymphocytic choriomeningitis virus, and several enteroviruses, among others. Symptoms of respiratory disease with many viruses are indistinguishable. Some viral diseases have a characteristic rash, though in most the rash associated with viral syndromes is not pathognomonic.

Identification of a virus is useful for confirmation of atypical cases, help with outbreak investigation, elucidation of confusing syndromes, and increasingly to support the need for specific antiviral therapy. The frequency with which certain pathogens cause certain diseases allows for educated guesses, eg, respiratory syncytial virus (RSV) for bronchiolitis or parainfluenza virus for croup. Instances where rapid diagnosis assists in patient management are noted.

Laboratory Diagnosis

Several techniques are used for diagnosis. Identification may be by stain (the nonspecific Tzanck smear for herpesviruses), cell culture (coxsackievirus in suckling mice), immunologic detection (seroconversion with arboviruses, rabies virus on skin biopsy, detection of secretory IgA), or molecular techniques such as polymerase chain reaction (for herpes simplex virus) or antigen assays (for cytomegalovirus). Isolation of virus

from a normally sterile site (cerebrospinal fluid, lung) or from a lesion (vesicles) in an immunocompetent individual is diagnostically significant. Isolation from nonsterile sites (nasopharynx, stool) may represent a carrier state, and seroconversion and pathologic change are needed to establish a diagnosis.

A. MICROSCOPIC METHODS

Microscopic techniques are used to examine cells, body fluids, or biopsy material in search of virus or cytopathic changes specific for one virus or a group of viruses (eg, multinucleated giant cells at the base of herpes lesions, rotavirus structures on electron micrographs of diarrheal stools).

Immunofluorescent methods, often with monoclonal antibodies, can rapidly identify some antigens (rabies, varicella, herpes simplex, respiratory syncytial virus) in desquamated or scraped cells.

B. IMMUNOLOGIC STUDIES OF SERA

Specific antibodies to viruses rise during the course of illness, though the rise and persistence of titer depend on both the virus and the host response. A fourfold or greater rise in antibody titer during illness is considered evidence of disease.

Single determinations are seldom helpful, and laboratories require paired sera (acute and convalescent, typically 2–3 weeks apart). Antigenic detection is used for certain viruses (HBsAg, CMV, HIV) and detects viral presence independently of disease duration or host response. Quantification of viral antigen titer is useful in the management of HIV disease and is becoming a standard of care for other chronic viral infections (eg, hepatitis C virus).

C. MOLECULAR TECHNIQUES

Molecular technology has provided techniques such as PCR and nucleic acid probes that have proved useful in the identification of new pathogens (eg, HCV and Kaposi's sarcoma herpesvirus) as well as for the management of patients in whom quantification of viral activity, as with immunologic techniques, assists in following the course of clinical illness or the response to therapy. Results vary among laboratories.

Treatment

The armamentarium of antiviral therapy has expanded greatly with the advent of the HIV outbreak (Table 31–5), though for many viruses there remains no definitive antiviral therapy.

The mainstay of controlling viral diseases is vaccination. Currently available live vaccines include those against measles, mumps, rubella, poliovirus (Sabin vaccine), yellow fever, and varicella. The inactivated vaccines protect against the agents implicated in poliovirus (Salk vaccine), hepatitis A, hepatitis B, influenza A and B, rabies, respiratory syncytial virus (RSV), and Japanese B encephalitis. Passive immunoprophylaxis remains important in prevention of hepatitis A and B, RSV infection, and, among the immunosuppressed, varicella.

Reusser P: Antiviral therapy: current options and challenges. Schweiz Med Wochenschr 2000;130:101. [PMID: 10780051]

HUMAN HERPESVIRUSES

These viruses cause a wide spectrum of human disease. Eight identified human herpesviruses include herpes simplex virus (HSV) type 1, HSV type 2, varicella-zoster virus (type 3), Epstein-Barr (EB)-infectious mononucleosis virus (type 4), and cytomegalovirus (CMV) (type 5). A sixth type (HHV-6) has been identified as a causative agent of roseola (exanthema subitum), and a seventh (HHV-7) is also serologically associated with roseola. Another herpesvirus (HHV-8) is linked with Kaposi's sarcoma (see Chapter 31).

Subclinical primary infection with the herpesviruses is more common than clinically manifest illness. Each persists in a latent state for the remainder of the host's life. With HSV and VZV, virus remains latent in sensory ganglia, and upon reactivation lesions appear in the distal sensory nerve distribution. As a result of disease-, drug-, or radiation-induced immunosuppression, virus reactivation may lead to widespread lesions in affected organs such as the viscera or the central nervous system. Severe or fatal illness may occur in infants and the immunodeficient. Herpesviruses can transform cells in tissue culture. Associations with malignancies include EBV with Burkitt's lymphoma and nasopharyngeal carcinoma and HHV-8 with body cavity lymphoma and Kaposi's sarcoma.

1. Herpesviruses 1 & 2

ESSENTIALS OF DIAGNOSIS

- Spectrum of illness from stomatitis and urogenital lesions to facial nerve paralysis (Bell's palsy) and encephalitis.

- Variable intervals between exposure and clinical disease, since HSV causes both primary (which may be subclinical) and reactivation disease.

- Successful management with acyclovir or related acyclic compounds (valacyclovir, famciclovir).

General Considerations

Herpesviruses 1 and 2 affect primarily the oral and genital areas, respectively. Seroprevalence to both agents increases with age and, for HSV-2, with sexual activity. Disease is typically a manifestation of reactivation, and the triggers for clinical reactivation are not well understood.

Clinical Findings

A. MUCOCUTANEOUS DISEASE

Herpes simplex type 1 (HSV-1) mucocutaneous disease largely involves the mouth and oral cavity ("herpes labialis"), although HSV-1 is increasingly recognized to cause urogenital infections. Vesicles form moist ulcers after several days and if untreated epithelialize over 1–2 weeks. Primary infection may be asymptomatic. Recurrences are usually milder, involve fewer lesions, tend to be labial, heal faster, and are induced by stress, fever, infection, sunlight, chemotherapy (eg, fludarabine), or other undetermined factors.

Herpes simplex type 2 lesions largely involve the genital tract. Virus remains latent in presacral ganglia. Typical lesions are multiple, painful, small, grouped, and vesicular. A manifestation of primary infection, predominantly in women, may be aseptic meningitis. Urinary retention may occur. Asymptomatic shedding is common, especially following primary infection or symptomatic recurrences, and appears to be responsible for transmission.

Diagnosis is usually made clinically, but viral cultures of vesicular fluid or direct fluorescent antibody staining of scraped lesions may confirm the diagnosis. HSV can be identified in serum using PCR, and its presence correlates with clinical reactivation. The presence of intranuclear inclusions and multinucleated giant cells on a Tzanck preparation is supportive of a diagnosis of herpes viral infection.

B. OCULAR DISEASE

HSV can cause keratitis, blepharitis, and keratoconjunctivitis. Keratitis is usually unilateral, is suggested by impaired visual acuity, and is diagnosed by branching (dendritic) ulcers that stain with fluorescein. It may be difficult to differentiate HSV conjunctivitis clinically from adenoviral conjunctivitis in the acute stage. Recurrences are frequent.

C. NEONATAL AND CONGENITAL INFECTION

Both herpesviruses can infect the fetus and induce congenital malformations (organomegaly, bleeding, central nervous system abnormalities). Neonatal transmission at the time of delivery is a more common mode of vertical spread. Such transmission is most common during acute disease in the mother but also occurs with subclinical shedding at the time of delivery (even without a history of symptomatic genital herpes).

D. ENCEPHALITIS AND RECURRENT MENINGITIS

Herpes simplex encephalitis presents with nonspecific symptoms: a flu-like prodrome, followed by headache, fever, behavioral and speech disturbances, and seizures that may be focal or generalized. A distinguishing feature is a propensity to involve the temporal lobe, with mass effect on imaging studies and temporal lobe seizure foci on EEGs. Cerebrospinal fluid white cell pleocytosis is common, with roughly equal numbers of red cells.

HSV DNA polymerase chain reaction (PCR) in the cerebrospinal fluid is a rapid and sensitive and specific tool for early diagnosis. Untreated disease and presentation with coma carry a high mortality rate, with many survivors suffering neurologic sequelae. HSV-2 has also been implicated as a major cause of benign recurrent lymphocytic meningitis (Mollaret's).

E. DISSEMINATED INFECTION

Disseminated HSV infection occurs in the setting of immunosuppression, either primary or iatrogenic, including steroid usage, or rarely with pregnancy. Skin lesions are not always present.

F. BELL'S PALSY

An association between HSV-1 and Bell's palsy has been established.

G. ESOPHAGITIS

Esophagitis from HSV-1 in AIDS and other immunocompromised patients is diagnosed by endoscopic biopsy and cultures. CMV esophagitis is distinguished by the size and depth of the lesion (smaller and deeper for HSV).

H. ERYTHEMA MULTIFORME

Herpes simplex viruses remain, with drugs, the leading association with erythema multiforme and with the more severe, mucosally involved Stevens-Johnson syndrome.

Treatment & Prevention

Drugs that inhibit replication of herpesvirus 1 and 2 include trifluridine (for keratitis), acyclovir and related compounds (for urogenital, encephalitic, or disseminated disease, and foscarnet (for resistant strains in the immunocompromised) (Table 32–1).

A. MUCOCUTANEOUS DISEASE

While treatment in immunocompetent patients is often not necessary, immunocompromised patients are treated with oral or topical acyclic derivatives, with intravenous acyclovir reserved for severe or recalcitrant disease. Lesions heal faster with topical penciclovir than with topical acyclovir. Oral agents are generally superior to topical ones and include (for primary infection) acyclovir, 200 mg five times a day; valacyclovir, 1000 mg twice daily; or famciclovir, 250 mg three times daily. Reactivation disease is treated with half the dose of the oral agents used against primary infection.

Acyclovir-resistant isolates associated with mucocutaneous lesions in the HIV-positive population are treated with foscarnet (phosphonoformic acid), 40–60 mg/kg intravenously every 8 hours, adjusting for renal function. The acyclic nucleoside analog cidofovir is used against HSV and CMV in rare cases of infection resistant to both acyclovir and foscarnet.

Acyclovir and related compounds are effective in secondary prevention. Patients with recurrent genital infections may be placed on maintenance acyclovir at a dosage of 400 mg twice a day. Prophylaxis for herpes labialis and mucocutaneous HSV infections may be especially useful for patients exposed to ultraviolet radiation such as during skiing or sailing trips when topical sun-blocking agents cannot be used or for wrestlers at risk for herpes gladiatorum. Famciclovir (250 mg twice daily or 500 mg once daily) and valacyclovir (500 mg twice daily or 1 g once daily) are more costly alternatives for preventing recurrent disease whose advantages include higher serum levels and less frequent administration. AIDS patients with a history of mucocutaneous disease should receive lifelong suppressive therapy.

B. KERATITIS

Ophthalmic trifluridine, vidarabine, and acyclovir given as drops for 10 days (without corticosteroids) are the available alternatives. Acyclovir at a dosage of 800 mg/d orally decreases recurrence rates.

C. NEONATAL DISEASE

Acyclovir intravenously is effective for disseminated lesions in neonatal disease. The dosage is 20 mg/kg intravenously every 8 hours for 14–21 days. The use of maternal antenatal suppressive therapy is not well established, but if undertaken it should be done with acyclovir or valacyclovir because of possible teratogenicity with famciclovir. The use of maternal antisuppressive therapy with acyclovir at 800 mg/d orally decreases the need for cesarean section with recurrent genital herpes.

D. ENCEPHALITIS

Because of the need for rapid treatment and the difficulties associated with brain biopsy, patients with suspected HSV encephalitis are given intravenous acy-

Table 32–1. Agents for viral infections.[1]

Drug	Dosing	Spectrum	Renal Clearance/ Hemodialysis	CNS/CSF Penetration	Toxicities
Acyclovir	200–800 mg orally five times daily; 250–500 mg/m² IV every 8 hours for 7 days	HSV	Yes/Yes	Yes	Neurotoxic reactions, reversible renal dysfunction, local reactions
Amantadine	100 mg orally twice daily (100 mg/d in elderly) for 10 days	Influenza A	Yes/No	Yes	Confusion, gastrointestinal symptoms
Cidofovir	5 mg/kg IV weekly for 2 weeks, then every other week	CMV	Yes/NA	NA	Neutropenia, renal failure, ocular hypotonia
Famciclovir	500 mg orally 3 times daily	VZV, ?HSV	Yes/NA	NA	NA
Foscarnet	20 mg/kg IV bolus, then 120 mg/kg IV every 8 hours for 2 weeks; maintain with 60 mg/kg/d IV for 5 days each week	CMV, HSV resistant to acyclovir, VZV, HIV-1	Yes/Yes	Variable	Nephrotoxicity, genital ulcerations, calcium disturbances
Ganciclovir	5 mg/kg IV bolus every 12 hours for 14–21 days; maintain with 3.75 mg/kg/d IV for 5 days each week	CMV	Yes/Yes	Yes	Neutropenia, thrombocytopenia, CNS side effects
Idoxuridine	Topical, 0.1% every 1–2 hours for 3–5 days	HSV keratitis	—	—	Local reactions
Interferon alfa-2b	3–5 million IU SC 3 times weekly to daily. Intralesionally: 1 million IU per 0.1 mL in up to 5 warts 3 times weekly for 3 weeks	HBV, HCV, papillomavirus	Yes/Yes	—	Influenza-like syndrome, myelosuppression, neurotoxicity
Interferon alfa-n3	0.05 mL/wart biweekly up to 8 weeks	HPV	NA/NA	NA	Local reactions
	3 mU IV 3 times per week	?HCV	NA/NA	NA	Influenza-like syndrome, myelosuppression, neurotoxicity
Lamivudine (3TC)	12 mg/kg/d	HIV-1, ?HIV-2, HBV	Yes/NA	Yes	Skin rash, headache, insomnia
Oseltamivir	75 mg twice daily for 5 days beginning 48 hours after onset of symptoms	Influenza A and B	Yes/NA	NA	Few
Penciclovir	Topical, 1% cream every 2 hours for 4 days	HSV	No/No	No	Local reactions
Palivizumab	15 mg/kg IM every month in RSV season	RSV	No/No	No	Upper respiratory infection symptoms
Ribavirin	Aerosol: 1.1 g/d as 20 mg/mL dilution over 12–18 hours for 3–7 days (See text for Lassa fever doses.)	RSV, severe influenza A or B, Lassa fever	Yes/No	Yes	Wheezing

(continued)

Table 32–1. Agents for viral infections. (continued)

Drug	Dosing	Spectrum	Renal Clearance/ Hemodialysis	CNS/CSF Penetration	Toxicities
Rimantadine	100 mg orally twice daily	Influenza A	Yes/No	Yes	Same as amantadine, but less severe
Trifluridine	Topical, 1% drops every 2 hours to 9 drops/d	HSV keratitis	—	—	Local reactions
Valacyclovir	1 g orally 3 times daily for 7 days for VZV; 500 mg twice daily for HSV	VZV, ?HSV	Yes/Poorly	NA	Thrombotic thrombocytopenic purpura or hemolytic uremic syndrome in AIDS
Valganciclovir	900 mg orally twice daily for 3 weeks; 900 mg daily as maintenance	CMV	Yes/Yes	Yes	See Ganciclovir
Vidarabine	15 mg/kg/d IV for 10 days	HSV, VZV	Yes/Yes	Yes	Teratogenic, megaloblastosis, neurotoxicity
Zanamivir	2–5 mg inhalations twice daily for 5 days	Influenza A and B	Yes/NA	NA	Few

[1]Agents used exclusively in the management of HIV infection and AIDS are found in Chapter 31.

clovir (10 mg/kg every 8 hours for 10 days or more, adjusting for renal impairment), starting upon suspicion of diagnosis, and stopping if another diagnosis is established. If the PCR is negative and clinical suspicion remains high in the absence of a biopsy, treatment should be continued for 10 days because of the relatively nontoxic nature of acyclovir.

E. DISSEMINATED DISEASE

Disseminated disease responds best to parenteral acyclovir (see the preceding paragraph for dosages) when treatment is initiated early.

F. BELL'S PALSY

The efficacy of treating Bell's palsy with acyclovir or steroids has not been established.

G. ESOPHAGITIS

Patients with esophagitis should receive either intravenous acyclovir at a dosage of 5–10 mg/kg every 8 hours or oral acyclovir, 400 mg five times daily. AIDS patients are maintained on acyclovir at a dosage of 400 mg three to five times daily.

H. ERYTHEMA MULTIFORME

Acyclovir may decrease the recurrence rate of HSV-associated erythema multiforme.

Prevention

Recurrent mucocutaneous disease is most effectively treated with acyclovir as outlined above; recurrent genital disease also requires use of barrier precautions during sexual activity. Preventing spread to hospital staff and other patients from cases with mucocuta-

neous, disseminated, or genital disease requires isolation and the use of hand washing and gloving-gowning precautions. Staff with active lesions (eg, whitlows) should not have contact with patients.

Chowsidow O et al: Famciclovir vs. aciclovir in immunocompetent patients with recurrent genital herpes infections: a parallel-groups, randomized, double-blind clinical trial. Br J Dermatol 2001;144:818. [PMID: 11298543]

Kimberlin DW et al: Safety and efficacy of high-dose intravenous acyclovir in the management of neonatal herpes simplex virus infections. Pediatrics 2001;108:230. [PMID: 11483782]

Mann JR et al: Effect of condoms on reducing the transmission of herpes simplex virus type 2 from men to women. JAMA 2001;285:3100. [PMID: 11427138] (Transmission can be reduced with condoms.)

Sauerbrei A et al: Virological diagnosis of herpes simplex encephalitis. J Clin Virol 2000;17:31. [PMID: 10814936] (PCR is needed for diagnosis early in the disease before antibodies become apparent.)

Whitley RJ et al: Herpes simplex virus infections. Lancet 2001;357:1513. [PMID: 11377626] (Epidemiology and pathophysiology.)

2. Varicella (Chickenpox) & Herpes Zoster (Shingles)

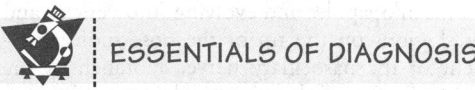

ESSENTIALS OF DIAGNOSIS

- *Exposure 14–21 days before onset.*
- *Fever and malaise just before or with eruption.*

• *Rash: pruritic, centrifugal, papular, changing to vesicular ("dewdrops on a rose petal"), pustular, and finally crusting.*

General Considerations

Varicella-zoster virus is human herpesvirus 3. Disease manifestations are either chickenpox (varicella) or shingles (its reactivation). Chickenpox is highly contagious and is generally a disease of childhood, with spread by inhalation of infective droplets or contact with lesions after 10–20 days (average, 14–15 days).

Clinical Findings

A. VARICELLA

1. Symptoms and signs—(Table 32–2.) Fever and malaise are mild in children and more marked in adults. Vesicular lesions, quickly rupturing to form small ulcers, may appear first in the oropharynx. The pruritic rash evolves centrifugally, beginning prominently on the face, scalp, and trunk, but to a lesser extent involving the extremities. Maculopapules change in a few hours to vesicles that become pustular and eventually form crusts. New lesions may erupt for 1–5 days, so that all stages of the eruption are generally present simultaneously. The crusts slough in 7–14 days. The vesicles and pustules are superficial and elliptical, with slightly serrated borders.

After the primary infection, the virus remains dormant in nervous tissue. Reactivation later in life is manifested as herpes zoster (see below). Widespread dissemination can occur in the immunosuppressed, sometimes in the absence of cutaneous lesions.

2. Laboratory findings—Diagnosis is usually made clinically, with confirmation by direct immunofluorescent antibody (DFA) staining or PCR of scrapings from lesions. Multinucleated giant cells are usually apparent on a Tzanck smear of material from the vesicle bases. Leukopenia is often present.

B. HERPES ZOSTER

Pain is often severe and may precede the appearance of rash. Lesions follow any nerve root distribution, with thoracic and lumbar roots commonest, and cervical or trigeminal involvement is typical. In most cases a single unilateral dermatome is involved. The occurrence of zoster does not correlate with progression to AIDS in HIV-infected patients, but recurrent and in particular multidermatomal zoster indicates a poorer prognosis in established AIDS.

Skin lesions resemble those of chickenpox, developing as maculopapules and evolving into vesicles and pustules. Lesions on the tip of the nose indicate involvement of the nasociliary nerve, a branch of the ophthalmic division of the trigeminal nerve; this nerve also serves the cornea. Facial palsy, lesions of the external ear with or without tympanic membrane involve-ment, vertigo and tinnitus, and deafness signify geniculate ganglion involvement (Ramsay Hunt syndrome). In either, treatment is indicated (see below).

Complications

A. VARICELLA

Interstitial pneumonia is more common in adults than in children and may result in ARDS. After healing, numerous densely calcified lesions are seen throughout the lung fields on chest x-rays. Ischemic strokes have been recognized in the wake of acute varicella and may be due to an associated vasculitis. Hepatitis is suggested by aminotransferase elevations and occurs in a small percentage of varicella-zoster patients. Encephalitis is infrequent (1:1000) and is characterized by ataxia and nystagmus and may be life-threatening. Cerebellar ataxia occurs among younger people at a lower frequency than encephalitis (1:4000).

Secondary bacterial infections, particularly with group A beta-hemolytic streptococci, are common; cellulitis, erysipelas, epiglottitis, osteomyelitis, scarlet fever, and, rarely, meningitis have been observed. Pitted scars are frequent sequelae.

Reye's syndrome (fatty liver with encephalopathy) also complicates varicella (and other viral infections, especially influenza B), usually in childhood, and has been associated with aspirin therapy (see Influenza, below). The many manifestations of VZV infection that occur in HIV infection include multifocal encephalitis, ventriculitis, myeloradiculitis, and arteritis.

When contracted during the first or second trimesters of pregnancy, varicella carries a small risk of congenital malformations, including cicatricial lesions of an extremity, growth retardation, microphthalmia, cataracts, chorioretinitis, deafness, and cerebrocortical atrophy. If a mother develops varicella within 5 days after delivery, the newborn is at risk of disseminated disease and should receive varicella-zoster immune globulin (VZIG). (See below for dosage.)

VZV is a major etiologic agent of Bell's palsy in patients lacking antibodies to HSV.

B. HERPES ZOSTER

In immunosuppressed and HIV-infected patients, herpes zoster may produce skin lesions beyond the dermatome, visceral lesions, and encephalitis. Postherpetic neuralgia occurs in 60–70% of zoster patients over age 60.

Prevention

Patients with active varicella or zoster are separated from seronegative patients. Respiratory isolation is needed in varicella pneumonia. Health care workers should be screened for varicella and vaccinated if seronegative. Health care workers should stay away from work when active vesicles are present, typically from the tenth day after onset through the twenty-first day. Varicella-zoster immune globulin (VZIG) is ef-

Table 32–2. Diagnostic features of some acute exanthems.

Disease	Prodromal Signs and Symptoms	Nature of Eruption	Other Diagnostic Features	Laboratory Tests
Eczema herpeticum	None.	Vesiculopustular lesions in area of eczema.		Herpes simplex virus isolated in cell culture. Multinucleate giant cells in smear of lesion.
Varicella (chicken-pox)	0–1 day of fever, anorexia, head-ache.	Rapid evolution of macules to papules, vesicles, crusts; all stages simultaneously present; lesions superficial, distribution centripetal.	Lesions on scalp and mucous mem-branes.	Specialized complement fixa-tion and virus neutralization in cell culture. Fluorescent antibody test of smear of le-sions.
Infectious mono-nucleosis (EBV)	Fever, adenopathy, sore throat.	Maculopapular rash resembling rubella, rarely papulovesicular.	Splenomegaly, tonsillar exudate.	Atypical lymphocytes in blood smears; heterophil agglutina-tion. Monospot test.
Exanthema subitum (HHV-6, 7; roseola)	3–4 days of high fever.	As fever falls by crisis, pink macu-lopapules appear on chest and trunk; fade in 1–3 days.		White blood count low.
Measles (rubeola)	3–4 days of fever, coryza, conjunc-tivitis, and cough.	Maculopapular, brick-red; begins on head and neck; spreads down-ward and outward, in 5–6 days rash brownish, desquamating. See atypical measles.	Koplik's spots on buccal mucosa.	White blood count low. Virus isolation in cell culture. Anti-body tests by hemagglutina-tion inhibition or neutraliza-tion.
Atypical measles	Same as measles.	Maculopapular centripetal rash, becoming confluent.	History of mea-sles vaccination.	Measles antibody present in past, with titer rise during illness.
Rubella	Little or no pro-drome.	Maculopapular, pink; begins on head and neck, spreads down-ward, fades in 3 days. No desqua-mation.	Lymphadenop-athy, postauricu-lar or occipital.	White blood count normal or low. Serologic tests for immu-nity and definitive diagnosis (hemagglutination inhi-bition).
Erythema in-fectiosum (parvo-virus B19)	None. Usually in epidemics.	Red, flushed cheeks; circumoral pallor; maculopapules on extremi-ties.	"Slapped face" ap-pearance.	White blood count normal.
Enterovirus infections	1–2 days of fever, malaise.	Maculopapular rash resembling rubella, rarely papulovesicular or petechial.	Aseptic meningitis.	Virus isolation from stool or cerebrospinal fluid; comple-ment fixation titer rise.
Typhus	3–4 days of fever, chills, severe headaches.	Maculopapules, petechiae, initial distribution centrifugal (trunk to extremities).	Endemic area, lice.	Complement fixation.
Rocky Moun-tain spotted fever	3–4 days of fever, vomiting.	Maculopapules, petechiae, initial distribution centripetal (extremi-ties to trunk, including palms).	History of tick bite.	Complement fixation.
Ehrlichiosis	Headache, malaise.	Rash in one-third, similiar to Rocky Mountain spotted fever.	Pancytopenia, elevated liver function tests.	Polymerase chain reaction, immunofluorescent antibody.
Scarlet fever	One-half to 2 days of malaise, sore throat, fever, vomiting.	Generalized, punctate, red; prominent on neck, in axillae, groin, skinfolds; circumoral pallor; fine desquamation involves hands and feet.	Strawberry tongue, exudative tonsillitis.	Group A beta-hemolytic streptococci in cultures from throat; antistreptolysin O titer rise.

(continued)

Table 32–2. Diagnostic features of some acute exanthems. (continued)

Disease	Prodromal Signs and Symptoms	Nature of Eruption	Other Diagnostic Features	Laboratory Tests
Meningo-coccemia	Hours of fever, vomiting.	Maculopapules, petechiae, purpura.	Meningeal signs, toxicity, shock.	Cultures of blood, cerebrospinal fluid. High white blood count.
Kawasaki disease	Fever, adenopathy, conjunctivitis.	Cracked lips, strawberry tongue, maculopapular polymorphous rash, peeling skin on fingers and toes.	Edema of extremities. Angiitis of coronary arteries.	Thrombocytosis, electrocardiographic changes.

fective in preventing chickenpox in exposed susceptible—particularly immunosuppressed—individuals. These include (1) susceptible persons receiving immunosuppressive therapy; (2) persons with congenital cellular immunodeficiency; (3) persons with an acquired immunodeficiency, including AIDS; (4) some adults, in particular pregnant females, considering the exposure history and the likelihood of previous chickenpox; (5) newborns; and (6) premature infants of low birth weight.

A. VARICELLA

A live attenuated vaccine is recommended for administration to all children over 12 months of age who have not had chickenpox. Patients with impaired cellular immunity should not be immunized, although the vaccine appears to be safe and effective when given to asymptomatic or mildly symptomatic HIV-infected children. Susceptible household contacts should also be vaccinated, assuming they are neither immunocompromised nor have had previous varicella. Under such conditions, the vaccine is 85% effective in preventing illness and 95% effective in preventing serious disease. Children receiving the vaccine should not take aspirin for at least 6 weeks, because of the possibility of Reye's syndrome. Adults should receive a second dose of the vaccine, typically 1–2 months after the first dose.

Varicella-zoster immune globulin (VZIG) is effective in preventing chickenpox in exposed susceptible, particularly immunosuppressed, individuals. It is given by intramuscular injection in a dosage of 12.5 units/kg up to a maximum of 625 units, with a repeat dose in 3 weeks if a high-risk patient remains exposed. VZIG has no place in therapy of established disease. Further information may be obtained by calling the Centers for Disease Control and Prevention's Immunization Information Hotline (800-232-2522). Because VZIG appears to bind the varicella vaccine, the two should not be given concomitantly.

B. ZOSTER

There is no effective prevention; whether the vaccine will serve that function is currently under investigation.

Treatment

A. GENERAL MEASURES

Patients should be isolated until primary crusts have disappeared and kept at bed rest until afebrile. Hospitalized patients with VZV infections should be isolated, and caregivers should wear gowns, gloves, and masks when in contact with them. The skin needs to be kept clean. Pruritus can be relieved with oral antihistamines, topical calamine lotion, and colloidal oatmeal baths. As an antipyretic, acetaminophen is used.

B. ANTIVIRAL THERAPY

For the infrequent varicella infection where antiviral therapy is indicated, the mainstay of therapy is acyclovir and its derivatives (valacyclovir and famciclovir are approved only for the immunocompetent). These agents are effective in reducing the severity and shortening the duration of chickenpox and zoster both in adults and in children. Acyclovir, if given in the first 72 hours of zoster, may reduce postherpetic pain. Valacyclovir, 1000 mg three times daily, and famciclovir, 500 mg three times daily, reduce pain and heal lesions faster than acyclovir, 800 mg five times daily. Data on the use of corticosteroids are conflicting, and their use is not routinely recommended. Otherwise healthy adults may benefit from a tapering course of prednisone over 21 days.

In immunocompromised patients, in pregnant women during the third trimester, and in patients with extracutaneous disease (encephalitis, pneumonitis), antiviral therapy with high-dose acyclovir (30 mg/kg/d in three divided doses intravenously for at least 7 days) should be started once the diagnosis is suspected. Acyclovir-resistant varicella has been observed in AIDS patients receiving chronic acyclovir therapy. Foscarnet may be used for acyclovir-resistant virus; however, resistance to foscarnet has also been observed.

C. TREATMENT OF COMPLICATIONS

The most troublesome issue with VZV infection is postherpetic neuralgia, especially in older patients. Initial treatment with antivirals and possibly steroids may reduce its incidence and severity. Once established, pain may respond to tricyclic antidepressants, lidocaine patches, gabapentin, or analgesics. Secondary bacterial infections of lesions are managed with antibiotics providing coverage for staphylococci.

Prognosis

The total duration of varicella from onset of symptoms to disappearance of crusts rarely exceeds 2 weeks. Fatalities are rare except in immunosuppressed patients.

Zoster resolves in 2–6 weeks. Antibodies persist longer and at higher levels than with primary varicella.

Kleinschmidt-Demasters BK et al: Varicella-Zoster virus infections of the nervous system: clinical and pathologic correlates. Arch Pathol Lab Med 2001;125:770. [PMID: 11371229]

Omrod D et al: Valaciclovir: a review of its use in the management of herpes zoster Drugs 2000;59:1317. [PMID: 10882165]

Schmader K: Herpes zoster in older adults. Clin Infect Dis 2001;32:1481. [PMID: 11317250]

Tyring S et al: A randomized, double-blind trial of famciclovir versus acyclovir for the treatment of localized dermatomal herpes zoster in immunocompromised patients. Cancer Invest 200119:13. [PMID: 11291551] (Famciclovir shown to be equivalent to acyclovir in efficacy and safety in immunocompromised patients.)

Vessey SJ et al: Childhood vaccination against varicella: persistence of antibody, duration of protection, and vaccine efficacy. J Pediatr 2001;139:297. [PMID: 11487760]

3. EBV & Infectious Mononucleosis

ESSENTIALS OF DIAGNOSIS

- *Malaise, fever, and sore throat, occasionally with exudate.*
- *Lymphadenopathy, splenomegaly and, occasionally, a maculopapular rash.*
- *Positive heterophil agglutination test (Monospot).*
- *"Atypical" large lymphocytes in blood smear; lymphocytosis.*
- *Possible complications: hepatitis, myocarditis, neuropathy, encephalitis, airway obstruction secondary to lymph node enlargement, anti-i hemolytic anemia, thrombocytopenia.*

General Considerations

Infectious mononucleosis is an acute infectious disease usually due to the Epstein-Barr (EB) virus (human herpesvirus 4). It is universal in distribution and may be seen at any age but usually occurs in the United States in persons between the ages of 10 and 35, either sporadically or in epidemic distribution. In the developing world, acute infections occur at much younger ages and tend to be less symptomatic. Rare cases have been reported in the elderly, usually without the full complex of symptoms. Its mode of transmission is probably by saliva. The incubation period is probably several weeks.

Clinical Findings

A. SYMPTOMS AND SIGNS

Symptoms are varied but typically include fever, sore throat, and toxic symptoms (malaise, anorexia, and myalgia) in the early phase of the illness. Physical findings include lymphadenopathy (discrete, nonsuppurative, slightly painful, especially along the posterior cervical chain), and splenomegaly (in about one-half). A maculopapular or occasionally petechial rash occurs in fewer than 15% of cases unless ampicillin has been given (when rash may be seen in > 90%). Exudative pharyngitis, tonsillitis, or gingivitis may occur and soft palatal petechiae may be noted.

Other manifestations of infectious mononucleosis include hepatitis, nervous system involvement with mononeuropathies and occasionally aseptic meningitis, encephalitis, or Guillain-Barré syndrome; hepatitis; renal failure from interstitial nephritis; pulmonary involvement with dyspnea and cough (in severe forms, "pseudocroup"); and myocarditis with tachycardia and arrhythmias. Airway obstruction from lymph node enlargement is a common indication for hospitalization or close observation.

B. LABORATORY FINDINGS

Initially, there is a granulocytopenia followed within 1 week by a lymphocytic leukocytosis. Many lymphocytes are larger than normal mature lymphocytes, stain more darkly, and frequently show vacuolated, foamy cytoplasm and dark chromatin in the nucleus. Hemolytic anemia, usually secondary to anti-i antibodies, is occasionally encountered, as is thrombocytopenia (at times marked).

Heterophil (sheep cell agglutination) antibody tests and the correlated mononucleosis spot (Monospot) test usually become positive in infectious mononucleosis within 4 weeks after onset of illness. Titer rises in antibodies directed at several EB virus antigens can be detected. During acute illness there is a rise and fall in IgM antibody to EB virus capsid antigen (VCA) and a rise in IgG antibody to VCA, which persists for life. Antibodies to EB virus nuclear antigen (EBNA) appear at 3–4 weeks after onset and also persist. A false-positive VDRL or RPR test occurs in 10% of cases. PCR for EBV DNA is useful in immunocompromised patients, who may not mount a typical antibody response.

Hepatic aminotransferases and bilirubin are commonly elevated. In aseptic meningitis, the cerebrospinal fluid may show increased opening pressure, lymphocytosis with abnormal morphology, and increased protein.

Differential Diagnosis

CMV infection, toxoplasmosis, acute HIV infection, and rubella may be indistinguishable from infectious mononucleosis due to EB virus, but exudative pharyngitis is usually absent and the heterophil antibody and Monospot tests are negative. With acute HIV infection, a rash is often seen. Mycoplasmal infection may also present primarily with pharyngitis, though lower respiratory symptoms usually predominate. A hypersensitivity syndrome induced by carbamazepine may mimic infectious mononucleosis.

The differential diagnosis of acute exudative pharyngitis includes diphtheria, gonococcal and streptococcal infections, and infections with adenovirus and herpes simplex. Head and neck soft tissue infections (pharyngeal and tonsillar abscesses) may occasionally be mistaken for the lymphadenopathy of mononucleosis.

Complications

Secondary bacterial throat infection can occur and is often streptococcal. Splenic rupture is a rare but dramatic complication, and a history of preceding trauma can be elicited in half of the cases. Pericarditis and myocarditis are also rare complications, although nonspecific electrocardiographic changes are seen in about 5% of all patients. Neurologic involvement—including transverse myelitis, encephalitis, and Guillain-Barré syndrome—is infrequent.

Treatment

A. General Measures

Given that over 95% of patients recover without specific antiviral therapy, treatment is largely symptomatic. Acyclovir has been shown to decrease viral shedding but does not have verified clinical benefit. There have been efforts to sensitize the virus to nucleoside analogs, but more studies in this area are needed. Symptomatic relief can be achieved by the administration of acetaminophen or other nonsteroidal anti-inflammatory agents and warm saline throat irrigations or gargles three or four times daily. The use of corticosteroids, while widespread, is not recommended in uncomplicated cases. Their use is reserved for impending airway obstruction from enlarged lymph nodes, hemolytic anemia, and severe thrombocytopenia. Their value in impending splenic rupture, pericarditis, myocarditis, and nervous system involvement is less well defined. If a throat culture grows beta-hemolytic streptococci, a 10-day course of penicillin or erythromycin is indicated. Ampicillin and amoxicillin are avoided because of the frequent association with rash in the presence of acute EBV infection.

B. Treatment of Complications

Hepatitis, myocarditis, and encephalitis are treated symptomatically. Rupture of the spleen requires emergency splenectomy; this complication is best avoided. It is most often caused by deep palpation of the spleen or vigorous activity.

Prognosis

In uncomplicated cases, fever disappears in 10 days and lymphadenopathy and splenomegaly in 4 weeks. The debility sometimes lingers for 2–3 months.

Death is uncommon; when it does occur it is usually due to splenic rupture, hypersplenic phenomena (severe hemolytic anemia, thrombocytopenic purpura), or encephalitis.

See references at end of next section.

4. Other EBV Syndromes

EBV viral antigens have been found in over 90% of patients with African Burkitt's lymphoma or nasopharyngeal carcinoma. A causative role for EBV has been postulated with both neoplasms. Chronic EBV infection is associated with X-linked lymphoproliferative syndrome (Duncan's disease). EBV-induced lymphoproliferation gives rise to B cell lymphomas among immunodeficient patients, such as the HIV-infected or after transplantation ("posttransplant lymphoproliferative disorder"). Immunologically privileged areas such as the central nervous system are particularly susceptible. The prophylactic use of EBV-specific cytotoxic T cell lymphocytes may prevent the development of EBV-associated lymphoproliferative disease.

EBV has also been associated with leiomyomas in children with AIDS and with nasal T cell lymphomas. There is no evidence that chronic fatigue syndrome is caused by chronic EBV infection. Oral hairy leukoplakia is discussed in Chapter 8.

EBV has been tentatively implicated in the pathogenesis of Hodgkin's disease but also in that of a variety of solid tumors and several medical syndromes, including systemic lupus erythematosus, encephalitis, rheumatoid arthritis, and Sjögren's syndrome.

Antinori A et al: Epstein-Barr virus in monitoring the response to therapy of AIDS-related primary central nervous system lymphoma. Ann Neurol 1999;45:259. [PMID: 9989631] (Mean EBV-DNA in cerebrospinal fluid may be useful in predicting response to therapy.)

Chien Y-C et al: Serologic markers of Epstein-Barr virus infection and nasopharyngeal carcinoma in Taiwanese men. N Engl J Med 2001; 345:1877. [PMID: 11756578] (IgA antibodies against EBV capsid antigen and neutralizing antibodies against EBV DNAse were predictive of nasopharyngeal carcinoma.)

Dehee A et al. Quantification of Epstein-Barr virus load in peripheral blood of human immunodeficiency virus-infected patients using real-time PCR. J Med Virol 2001;65:543. [PMID: 11596092]

Godshall SE et al: Infectious mononucleosis. Complexities of a common syndrome. Postgrad Med 2000;107:175. [PMID: 10887454]

Kimura H et al. Clinical and virologic characteristics of chronic active Epstein-Barr virus infection. Blood 2001;98:280. [PMID: 11435294] (A new clinical syndrome from Japan in which one half show chromosomal abnormalities.)

Preiksaitis JK et al. Diagnosis and management of posttransplant lymphoproliferative disorder in solid-organ transplant recipients. Clin Infect Dis 2001;33S1:S38-46. [PMID: 11389521]

5. Cytomegalovirus Disease

Most cytomegalovirus (CMV) infections are asymptomatic, with the virus remaining latent. The virus can be isolated from a variety of tissues under nonpathogenic conditions including up to 25% of salivary glands and 10% of uterine crevices. Nevertheless, the cells of latency are unknown. Seroprevalence increases with age and with the number of sexual partners. Detectable antibody is present in the serum of most homosexual men. Transmission is sexual, congenital, through blood products or transplantation, and person-to-person (eg, day care centers). Severe disease occurs primarily in the immunocompromised, especially AIDS and transplant patients.

Clinical Findings

A. CLASSIFICATION

There are three recognizable clinical syndromes.

1. Perinatal disease and CMV inclusion disease— This neonatal syndrome is acquired in utero and seen in 10% of newborns born to mothers with primary CMV infection during pregnancy. It is characterized by jaundice, hepatosplenomegaly, thrombocytopenia, periventricular central nervous system calcifications, mental retardation, motor disability, and purpura. Neonatally acquired disease is often asymptomatic, but neurologic deficits may ensue later in life.

2. Acute acquired CMV infection—This syndrome, akin to EBV-associated infectious mononucleosis, is characterized by fever, malaise, myalgias and arthralgias (but rarely exudative pharyngitis or cervical lymphadenopathy), splenomegaly, atypical lymphocytes, and abnormal liver function tests. Typically, leukopenia is followed by leukocytosis. Heterophil antibody is absent. Transmission occurs by sexual contact, in breast milk, via respiratory droplets among nursery or day care center attendants, and by transfusions of blood. Complications include mucosal gastrointestinal damage, encephalitis, Guillain-Barré syndrome, pericarditis, and myocarditis.

3. Disease in immunocompromised hosts—Tissue and bone marrow transplant patients are mainly at risk in the first 100 days after allograft transplantation. HIV-infected patients may have numerous manifestations. CMV is itself immunosuppressive and may worsen pneumocystis pneumonia. CMV may contribute to transplanted organ dysfunction.

a. CMV retinitis—Retinitis occurs primarily in AIDS patients with significant immunosuppression (CD4 count less than 50 cells/μL). Ophthalmologic documentation of neovascular, proliferative lesions ("pizza-pie" retinopathy) is required for diagnosis. With HAART, the frequency of retinitis is reduced, CD4 counts are less predictive, and active disease may be reversible.

b. Gastrointestinal and hepatobiliary CMV— Serious gastrointestinal CMV disease occurs in AIDS and after organ transplantation, cancer chemotherapy, or steroid therapy. Esophagitis presents with odynophagia; small bowel disease may mimic inflammatory bowel disease or may present as ulceration or perforation. Colonic CMV disease causes diarrhea, hematochezia, abdominal pain, fever, and weight loss. CMV has been identified, often with other pathogens, in up to 15% of patients with AIDS cholangiopathy. Diagnosis is by mucosal biopsy showing characteristic CMV histopathologic findings of intranuclear ("owl's eye") and intracytoplasmic inclusions.

c. Pulmonary CMV—CMV pneumonitis occurs in transplant recipients and in AIDS patients and is associated with a high mortality. In AIDS patients, the significant morbidity and mortality appears to be diminished by the use of highly active antiretroviral therapy (HAART). CMV seronegative blood products should be used in seronegative recipients of seronegative transplants. High-titer CMV immunoglobulins may be effective in preventing CMV pneumonia in seronegative recipients.

d. Neurologic CMV— Neurologic syndromes associated with CMV include polyradiculopathy, transverse myelitis, and encephalitis. The encephalitis has a subacute onset in patients with advanced AIDS and is usually associated with disseminated CMV infection. CMV can be isolated in the cerebrospinal fluid in cases of transverse myelitis or disseminated disease.

B. LABORATORY FINDINGS

Virus isolation is most useful when combined with the pathologic findings. Cultures alone are of little use in diagnosing AIDS-related CMV infections, but when positive have been associated with a risk of progressive retinitis. The acute mononucleosis-like syndrome is associated with lymphocytosis, often 2 weeks after the fever, but absolute leukopenia may also be noted. Serologic tests are useful primarily in seroepidemiologic studies and occasionally in confirming acute infection (with IgM) in nonimmunosuppressed patients. Antigen detection in blood components, urine, or cerebrospinal fluid by virus technology (including the PCR technique) should be interpreted in the context of clinical and pathologic findings but are increasingly being used to guide both treatment and prevention of CMV disease.

Prevention

No vaccine is currently available. Strategies for prevention of CMV disease in transplant recipients include antiviral agents and CMV immune globulin. The risk for CMV disease is proportionate to the intensity of immunosuppression, which depends in part on the organ being transplanted. PCR and antigen assays increase the ability to detect CMV disease prior to clinical disease. Oral ganciclovir is being replaced by oral valganciclovir in prevention of CMV disease because of its greater bioavailability. The optimum system for monitoring and preventing CMV disease among transplant patients remains to be elucidated. HAART is effective in preventing CMV infections in HIV-infected patients.

Treatment

Four antiviral agents with efficacy against CMV infections are ganciclovir, 5 mg/kg intravenously every 12 hours for 14–21 days; valganciclovir, 900 mg/kg twice daily; foscarnet, loading with 20 mg/kg intravenously, followed by 60 mg/kg every 8 hours over weeks; and cidofovir, 5 mg/kg intravenously, every week for 2 weeks. A daily maintenance regimen using both ganciclovir (3.75 mg/kg intravenously) and foscarnet (60 mg/kg intravenously), each over 1 hour, has been shown to be safe and effective in inhibiting CMV replication. Cidofovir is given only every 2 weeks, 375 mg intravenously, for maintenance. Oral valganciclovir (900 mg daily) is replacing oral ganciclovir for maintenance. Dosage adjustments of all medications are needed for renal impairment. In addition, a sustained-release ganciclovir implant has been shown to control disease in the implanted eye (but not elsewhere) more effectively than intravenous ganciclovir. Again, the role of HAART in reducing the need for CMV antivirals is primary. Fomivirsen is an intravitreal agent active against CMV strains that are resistant to ganciclovir, foscarnet, and cidofovir.

Drago F et al: Cytomegalovirus infection in normal and immunocompromised humans. A review. Dermatology 2000; 200:189. [PMID: 10828625]

Jouan M et al: Discontinuation of maintenance therapy for cytomegalovirus retinitis in HIV-infected patients receiving highly active antiretroviral therapy. AIDS 2001;15:23. [PMID: 11192865] (HAART can be safely stopped when CD4 counts are above 75 cells/μL.)

Kulkarni A et al: Molecular-based strategies for assessment of CMV infection and disease in immunosuppressed transplant recipients. Clin Microbiol Infect 2001;7:179. [PMID: 11422239]

Paya CV: Prevention of cytomegalovirus disease in recipients of solid-organ transplants. Clin Infect Dis 2001;32:596. [PMID: 11181123]

Perry CM et al: Fomivirsen. Drugs 1999;57:375. [PMID: 10193689]

van der Bij W et al: Management of cytomegalovirus infection and disease after solid-organ transplantation. Clin Infect Dis 2001;33(Suppl 1):S32. [PMID: 11389520]

Whitley RJ et al: Guidelines for the treatment of CMV diseases in patients with AIDS in the era of potent antiretroviral therapy. Arch Intern Med 1998;158:957. [PMID: 9588429]

6. Human Herpesviruses 6, 7, 8

Human herpesvirus 6 (HHV-6) is a B cell lymphotropic virus that is the principal cause of exanthema subitum (roseola infantum, sixth disease). Primary HHV-6 infection occurs most commonly in children under 2 years of age and is the most common cause of infantile febrile seizures. HHV-6 in adults is associated with immunocompromised states such as HIV and lymphoma. It is associated with graft rejection and bone marrow suppression in transplant patients and with encephalitis and pneumonitis in AIDS; it is mentioned as a factor in the etiology of multiple sclerosis.

Two variants (A and B) of HHV-6 have been identified. HHV6B is the predominant strain found in both normal and immunocompromised hosts. There are in-vitro data suggesting susceptibility to ganciclovir and foscarnet but not acyclovir, though this may not correlate in vivo.

HHV-7 is a T cell lymphotropic virus that has also been serologically associated with roseola. Infection with HHV-7 appears to be synergistic with CMV in renal transplant recipients. The membrane glycoprotein CD4 is involved in HHV-7 recognition, and an antagonistic interaction between HHV-7 and HIV is established. HHV-7 may invade the central nervous system in children.

HHV-8 is associated with Kaposi's sarcoma in AIDS patients. It has also been implicated in multicentric Castleman's disease and body-cavity lymphomas. See Chapter 31 for pathogenesis and management.

Caserta MT et al: Human herpesvirus 6. Clin Infect Dis 2001;33:829. [PMID: 11512088]

Emery VC: Human herpesviruses 6 and 7 in solid organ transplant recipients. Clin Infect Dis 2001;32:1357. [PMID: 11303272]

Leach CT: Human herpesvirus-6 and -7 infections in children: agents of roseola and other syndromes. Curr Opin Pediatr 2000;12:269. [PMID: 10836165]

Soldan SS et al: Elevated serum and cerebrospinal fluid levels of soluble human herpesvirus type 6 cellular receptor, membrane cofactor protein, in patients with multiple sclerosis. Ann Neurol 2001;50:486. [PMID: 11603380] (The receptor for HHV-6, CD46, is increased in patients with multiple sclerosis.)

MAJOR VACCINE-PREVENTABLE VIRAL INFECTIONS

1. Measles

ESSENTIALS OF DIAGNOSIS

- Exposure 10–14 days before onset in an unvaccinated patient.
- Prodrome of fever, coryza, cough, conjunctivitis, malaise, irritability, photophobia, Koplik's spots.

- *Rash: brick-red, irregular, maculopapular; onset 3–4 days after onset of prodrome; begins on the face and proceeds "downward and outward," affecting the palms and soles last.*
- *Leukopenia.*

General Considerations

Measles is an acute systemic paramyxoviral infection transmitted by inhalation of infective droplets. This virus tropic for monocytes is a major worldwide cause of pediatric morbidity and mortality, with an estimated 1 million deaths annually. Illness confers permanent immunity. Communicability is greatest during the preeruptive and catarrhal stages but continues as long as the rash remains. The largest recent outbreak in the Americas was in São Paolo, Brazil, with over 42,000 cases among largely unvaccinated young adults. This and other sporadic recent outbreaks of the disease in adults, adolescents, and unvaccinated preschool children in dense urban areas emphasize the need for specific recommendations concerning prevention (see below).

In the United States, in view of the preponderance of imported cases and the low number of geographically dispersed cases whose isolates fail to show a recurrent strain, measles is no longer considered endemic.

Clinical Findings

A. SYMPTOMS AND SIGNS

(Table 32–2.) Fever is often as high as 40–40.6 °C. It persists through the prodrome and early rash (about 5–7 days). Malaise may be marked. Coryza (nasal obstruction, sneezing, and sore throat) resembles that seen with upper respiratory infections. Cough is persistent and nonproductive. Conjunctivitis manifests as redness, swelling, photophobia, and discharge.

Koplik's spots are pathognomonic of measles. They appear about 2 days before the rash and last 1–4 days as tiny "table salt crystals" on the dull red mucous membranes of the cheeks and often on inner conjunctival folds and vaginal mucous membranes. Other findings include pharyngeal erythema, a yellowish exudate on the tonsils, coating of the tongue in the center with a red tip and margins, moderate generalized lymphadenopathy, and, in occasional cases, splenomegaly.

The rash usually appears first on the face and behind the ears 4 days after the onset of symptoms. The initial lesions are pinhead-sized papules which coalesce to form a brick-red, irregular, blotchy maculopapular rash. In severe cases, the rash may coalesce to form a nearly uniform erythema on some body areas. The rash next appears on the trunk, followed by the extremities, including the palms and soles. It fades in order of appearance. Hyperpigmentation remains in fair-skinned individuals and severe cases. Slight desquamation may follow.

Atypical measles is a syndrome occurring in adults who received inactivated measles vaccine (available 1963–1967) or who received live measles vaccine before age 12 months and as a result developed hypersensitivity rather than protective immunity. When infected later with wild measles virus, such individuals may develop a potentially fatal illness with high fever, unusual rashes (papular, hemorrhagic) without Koplik's spots, headache, arthralgias, hepatitis, and interstitial or nodular infiltrates, occasionally with pleural effusions.

Measles may occur in HIV-infected individuals in an uncharacteristic fashion, with higher rates of pneumonitis and higher mortality. Vaccine failure rates, both primary and secondary, are higher in HIV-infected children. The frequent difficulty in establishing a diagnosis suggests that measles may be more prevalent in epidemics than heretofore recognized.

B. LABORATORY FINDINGS

Leukopenia is usually present unless secondary bacterial complications exist. A lymphocyte count under 2000/μL is a poor prognostic sign. Proteinuria is often observed. Although technically difficult, virus can be cultured from nasopharyngeal washings and from blood. A fourfold rise in serum hemagglutination inhibition antibody supports the diagnosis. Fluorescent antibody staining of respiratory or urinary epithelial cells can also confirm the diagnosis.

Differential Diagnosis

Measles is easily recognizable from the clinical picture but may be mistaken for other exanthematous infections (see Table 32–2).

Complications

A. CENTRAL NERVOUS SYSTEM COMPLICATIONS

Encephalitis occurs in approximately 0.05–0.1% of cases. Its onset is usually 3–7 days after the rash. Vomiting, convulsions, coma, and a variety of severe neurologic symptoms and signs may develop. Treatment is symptomatic and supportive. Virus is usually not found in the central nervous system, though demyelination is prominent. There is an appreciable mortality rate (10–20%), and many patients are left with neurologic morbidity.

A similar form, "inclusion body encephalitis," is also reported to occur after measles vaccination but is associated with isolation of the measles virus.

Subacute sclerosing panencephalitis (SSPE) is a very late central nervous system complication, the measles virus acting as a "slow virus" to produce degenerative central nervous system disease years after the initial infection. SSPE is rare (1:100,000 cases of measles) and occurs more often when measles develops early in life, among males, and in persons living in rural environments.

An acute progressive encephalitis (subacute measles encephalitis), characterized by seizures, neurologic deficits, and often progressive stupor and death, can occur among immunosuppressed patients; measles virus opportunistically invades the central nervous system. Treatment is supportive, withholding immunosuppressive chemotherapy when feasible. Interferon and ribavirin have been variably successful.

B. RESPIRATORY TRACT DISEASE

Early in the course of the disease, bronchopneumonia or bronchiolitis due to the measles virus may occur in up to 5% and result in serious respiratory difficulties. Pneumonia occurring with or without an evanescent rash is seen in atypical measles.

C. SECONDARY BACTERIAL INFECTIONS

Immediately following measles, secondary bacterial infection, particularly cervical adenitis, otitis media, and pneumonia, occurs in about 15% of patients.

D. IMMUNE REACTIVITY

Measles produces temporary anergy to the tuberculin skin test.

E. GASTROENTERITIS

Diarrhea and protein-losing enteropathy (prodromal rectal Koplik spots may be seen) are significant complications when measles affects malnourished children.

Prevention

In the United States, it is recommended that children receive their first vaccine dose at 12–15 months and a second at age 4–6 years prior to entry into school (see Table 30–4).

Students beyond high school and medical staff starting employment must have the above vaccination schedule documented or must have serologic evidence of immunity if they were born after 1956. For individuals born before 1957, herd immunity can be assumed. Health care workers should be screened and vaccinated if necessary regardless of date of birth.

Outbreak control in the USA is similar. If outbreaks are occurring in preschool children under 1 year of age, initial vaccination may be given at 6 months, with repeat at 15 months. When outbreaks take place in day care centers, K–12 institutions, or colleges and universities, revaccination is probably indicated for all, in particular for students and their siblings born after 1956 who do not have documentation of immunity as defined above. Susceptible personnel who have been exposed should be isolated from patient contact from the fifth to the 21st day after exposure regardless of whether they have been vaccinated or have received immune globulin. If they develop measles, they should be isolated from patient contact until 7 days after the rash develops.

Ancillary control measures used in the developing world include "catch-up days"—when all children regardless of immunization history are vaccinated—maintenance and follow up of immunization histories ("catch-up, keep-up, and follow-up"), surveillance of acute cases, and confirmation of whether isolates from cases are imported or outbreak-associated.

When susceptible individuals are exposed to measles, the live virus vaccine can prevent disease if given within 5 days of exposure. This is rarely feasible in a household. Later, immune globulin (0.25 mL/kg [0.11 mL/lb] body weight) can be injected intramuscularly for prevention or modification of clinical illness if given within 6 days after exposure. This must be followed by active immunization with live measles vaccine 3 months later. Vaccination of all immunocompetent persons born after 1956 who travel to the developing world is important.

Pregnant women and the immunosuppressed should *not* receive this vaccine. There are two exceptions: asymptomatic HIV-infected patients, who have not shown adverse effects from measles vaccination; and HIV-infected children, in whom exposure to vaccines improves survival after measles. In the developing world, the use of "high-titer" vaccine is associated with a higher delayed mortality rate. Immune globulin should be considered for postexposure prophylaxis in any HIV-infected person exposed to measles.

Severe allergic reactions to the measles, mumps, and rubella (MMR) vaccine are rare, though fever and rash appear to occur slightly more often among female recipients.

Treatment

A. GENERAL MEASURES

The patient should be isolated for the week following onset of rash and kept at bed rest until afebrile. Treatment is symptomatic as needed. Vitamin A, 400,000 units/d orally (the beneficial effects of which include maintenance of gastrointestinal and respiratory epithelial mucosa and perhaps immune enhancement), reduces pediatric morbidity and mortality rates.

B. TREATMENT OF COMPLICATIONS

Secondary bacterial infections are treated with appropriate antimicrobial drugs. Pneumonia is managed with antibacterial antibiotics when clinical signs suggest sepsis or significant pulmonary findings. Postmeasles encephalitis, including SSPE, can only be managed symptomatically.

Prognosis

The mortality rate of measles in infants was 0.6% in a recent outbreak in California; the mortality rate may be as high as 10% in developing nations. Deaths in the USA are due principally to encephalitis (15% mortality rate) and secondary bacterial pneumonia. Deaths in the developing world are mainly related to diarrhea and protein-losing enteropathy.

Ceyhan M et al: Immunogenicity and efficacy of one dose MMR vaccine at 12 months of age as compared to monovalent measles vaccination at 9 months followed by MMR revaccination at 15 months of age. Vaccine 2001;19:4473. [PMID: 11483273] (The former regimen was associated with a significantly higher seroconversion rate.)

Gans H et al: Immune response to measles and mumps vaccination of infants at 6, 9, and 12 months. J Infect Dis 2001;184:817. [PMID: 11528592] (In this Stanford study, cellular immune responses of 6-month-olds were equivalent to those of older infants.)

Hung KL et al: Post-infectious encephalomyelitis: etiologic and diagnostic trends. J Child Neurol 2000;15:666. [PMID: 1106308] (More recent cases of postinfectious encephalomyelitis are caused by respiratory pathogens, EBV, and mycoplasma and not the traditional exanthematous diseases.)

Kaye JA et al: Mumps, measles, and rubella vaccine and the incidence of autism recorded by general practitioners: a time trend analysis. BMJ 2001;322:460. [PMID: 11222420] (Although the incidence of autisms increased sevenfold, the MMR vaccination rates remained stable and high throughout, suggesting that there is no significant association between the use of MMR vaccine and rising autism rates.)

Measles, rubella, and congenital rubella syndrome—United States and Mexico, 1997–1999. MMWR Morb Mortal Wkly Rep 2000;49:1048. [PMID: 11105768]

Okoko BJ et al: Influence of placental malaria infection and maternal hypergammaglobulinaemia on materno-faetal transfer of measles and tetanus antibodies in a rural west Africa population. J Health Popul Nutr 2001;19:59. [PMID: 11503348] (These two factors significantly impaired measles antibody production.)

Paunio M et al: Measles history and atopic diseases: a population-based cross-sectional study. JAMA 2000;283:343. [PMID: 10647796] (Despite theories that communicable diseases in childhood protect against atopic disease, this study shows an increased rate of atopy among Finnish children with a history of measles.)

Salama P et al: Malnutrition, measles, mortality, and the humanitarian response during a famine in Ethiopia. JAMA 2001;286:563. [PMID: 11476658] (Measles with or without wasting was responsible for 22% of deaths in children under age 5.)

2. Mumps

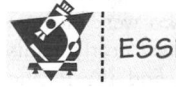

ESSENTIALS OF DIAGNOSIS

- Exposure 14–21 days before onset.
- Painful, swollen salivary glands, usually parotid.
- Frequent involvement of other tissues, including testes, pancreas, and meninges, in unvaccinated individuals.

General Considerations

Mumps is a paramyxoviral disease spread by respiratory droplets that usually produces inflammation of the salivary glands and, less commonly, orchitis, asep-

tic meningitis, pancreatitis, and oophoritis. Most patients are children, and the incidence is highest in spring. The incubation period is 14–21 days (average, 18 days). Infectivity occurs via saliva and urine and precedes the symptoms by about 1 day and is maximal for 3 days but may last a week.

Clinical Findings

A. SYMPTOMS AND SIGNS

Parotid tenderness and overlying facial edema are the most common physical findings. Occasionally, swelling in one gland subsides completely before the other parotid or salivary glands become involved. Swelling and tenderness of the submaxillary and sublingual glands are variable. The orifice of Stensen's duct may be red and swollen.

Fever and malaise are variable and are often minimal in young children. High fever usually accompanies meningitis or orchitis. Neck stiffness, headache, and lethargy suggest meningitis. Testicular swelling and tenderness (unilateral in 75%) denote orchitis. Orchitis, which develops typically 7–10 days after the onset of parotitis, occurs in about 25–40% of postpubertal men, but sterility is rare. Upper abdominal pain, nausea, and vomiting suggest pancreatitis. Mumps is the leading cause of pancreatitis in children. Lower abdominal pain and ovarian enlargement suggest oophoritis, but the diagnosis may be difficult to make. Pain and swelling of one or both (75%) of the parotid or other salivary glands occur, usually in succession 1–3 days apart. Occasionally, one gland subsides completely (usually in 7 days or less) before others become involved.

B. LABORATORY FINDINGS

Relative lymphocytosis may be present. Serum amylase is commonly elevated with or without pancreatitis because of salivary gland involvement. Lymphocytic pleocytosis (and normal to low glucose) of the cerebrospinal fluid is present in meningitis, which may be asymptomatic. The diagnosis of mumps is confirmed by isolating the virus from saliva or cerebrospinal fluid or demonstrating a fourfold rise in complement-fixing antibodies in paired sera.

Differential Diagnosis

Swelling of the parotid gland may be due to calculi in the parotid ducts or to a reaction to iodides. Other causes include starch ingestion, sarcoidosis, cirrhosis, diabetes, bulimia, and Sjögren's syndrome. Parotitis may also be produced by pyogenic organisms (eg, *Staphylococcus aureus*), particularly in debilitated individuals, drug reaction (phenothiazines, propylthiouracil), and other viruses (influenza A, parainfluenza, EBV infection, coxsackieviruses). Swelling of the parotid gland must be differentiated from inflammation of the lymph nodes located more posteriorly and inferiorly than the parotid gland.

Complications

Other manifestations of the disease are less common than inflammation of the salivary glands. These usually follow the parotitis but may precede it or occur without salivary gland involvement and include meningitis (30%), orchitis (on rare occasion leads to priapism or testicular infarction), pancreatitis, oophoritis, thyroiditis, neuritis, hepatitis, myocarditis, thrombocytopenia, migratory arthralgias, and nephritis. Mumps has also been associated with cases of endocardial fibroelastosis.

Rare neurologic complications include encephalitis, Guillain-Barré syndrome, cerebellar ataxia, and transverse myelitis. Encephalitis is associated with cerebral edema, serious neurologic manifestations, and sometimes death. Deafness develops rarely from eighth nerve neuritis.

Prevention

Mumps live virus vaccine is safe and highly effective. It is recommended for routine immunization for children over age 1 year, either alone or in combination with other virus vaccines (eg, with measles and rubella—in MMR vaccine). Reactions are reviewed in the measles section. It should not be given to pregnant women or to immunocompromised individuals, though the vaccine has been given to asymptomatic HIV-infected individuals without adverse sequelae. Its use has markedly decreased the incidence of mumps in the United States. The mumps skin test is less reliable in determining immunity than are serum neutralization titers.

Treatment

A. GENERAL MEASURES

The patient should be isolated until swelling subsides and kept at bed rest during the febrile period. Treatment is symptomatic as needed.

B. MANAGEMENT OF COMPLICATIONS

1. Meningitis—The treatment of aseptic meningitis is purely symptomatic. The management of encephalitis requires attention to cerebral edema, the airway, and vital functions.

2. Orchitis—The scrotum should be suspended in a suspensory or toweling "bridge" and ice bags applied. Incision of the tunica may be necessary in severe cases. Codeine or meperidine may be given as necessary for pain. Pain can also be relieved by injection of the spermatic cord at the external inguinal ring with 10–20 mL of 1% procaine solution. The merit of hydrocortisone sodium succinate (100 mg intravenously, followed by 20 mg orally every 6 hours for 2 or 3 days) to reduce the inflammatory reaction is not firmly established.

3. Pancreatitis—Symptomatic treatment is provided by emphasis on parenteral hydration.

Prognosis

The entire course of mumps rarely exceeds 2 weeks. Fatalities (usually from encephalitis) are rare.

Galazka AM et al: Mumps and mumps vaccine: a global review. Bull WHO 1999;77:3. [PMID: 10063655]

Iizuka M et al: No evidence of persistent mumps virus infection in inflammatory bowel disease. Gut 2001;48;637. [PMID: 11302960]

Patja A et al: Serious adverse events after MMR vaccination during a 14-year prospective follow-up. Pediatr Infect Dis 2000;19:1127. [PMID: 11144371] (Serious events related to MMR vaccination are rare and outweighed greatly by the risk of natural diseases.)

3. Poliomyelitis

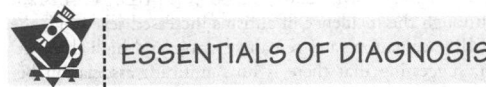

ESSENTIALS OF DIAGNOSIS

- *Muscle weakness, headache, stiff neck, fever, nausea and vomiting, sore throat.*
- *Lower motor neuron lesion (flaccid paralysis) with decreased deep tendon reflexes and muscle wasting.*
- *Cerebrospinal fluid shows excess leukocytes, with lymphocytic predominance; count is rarely more than 500/μL.*

General Considerations

Poliomyelitis virus, an enterovirus, is present in throat washings and stools. Infection is most commonly acquired by the fecal-oral route. Since the introduction of an effective vaccine, poliomyelitis has become a rare disease in developed areas of the world, and globally, between 1988 and 2000, the number of cases decreased by 85%. Among 133 cases reported in the United States between 1980 and 1994, six were imported and 125 (94%) were vaccine-associated (two were indeterminate). Wild poliovirus disease has been nearly eradicated from the Western hemisphere, and the Pacific Rim, Europe, and Central Asia appear to be polio-free. Polio remains endemic in Pakistan, India, and Southeast Asia, part of the Middle East (in particular Iraq), and Central and Western Africa. Three antigenically distinct types of poliomyelitis virus are recognized, with no cross-immunity between them. The incubation period is 5–35 days (usually 7–14 days). Disease with type 2 (of the three types) in particular is on the verge of extinction. Infectivity is maximal during the first week, but virus is excreted in stools for several weeks.

Several cases of polio reported in late 2000 from the Dominican Republic and Haiti were probably due to reversion to virulence of a strain isolated in an area where economic conditions necessitated the use of oral vaccines. Otherwise, polio appears to have been eradicated from the Western Hemisphere.

Clinical Findings

A. SYMPTOMS AND SIGNS

At least 95% of infections are asymptomatic, but in those who become ill the following manifestations are seen.

1. Minor illness (abortive poliomyelitis)—The symptoms are fever, headache, vomiting, diarrhea, constipation, and sore throat.

2. Nonparalytic poliomyelitis—In addition to the above symptoms, signs of meningeal irritation and muscle spasm occur in the absence of frank paralysis.

3. Paralytic poliomyelitis—Paralytic poliomyelitis represents 0.1% of all poliomyelitis cases (the incidence is higher when infections are acquired later in life). Paralysis may occur at any time during the febrile period. Tremors, muscle weakness, constipation, and ileus may appear. Paralytic poliomyelitis is divided into two forms, which may coexist: (1) **spinal poliomyelitis,** with involvement of the muscles innervated by the spinal nerves; and (2) **bulbar poliomyelitis,** with weakness of the muscles supplied by the cranial nerves (especially nerves IX and X) and of the respiratory and vasomotor centers.

In spinal poliomyelitis, paralysis of the shoulder girdle often precedes intercostal and diaphragmatic paralysis, which leads to diminished chest expansion and decreased vital capacity.

In bulbar poliomyelitis, symptoms include diplopia (uncommonly), facial weakness, dysphagia, dysphonia, nasal voice, weakness of the sternocleidomastoid and trapezius muscles, difficulty in chewing, inability to swallow or expel saliva, and regurgitation of fluids through the nose. The most life-threatening aspect of bulbar poliomyelitis is respiratory paralysis. Lethargy or coma may be due to hypoxia, most often from hypoventilation. Alterations in blood pressure and heart rate may occur. Convulsions are rare.

B. LABORATORY FINDINGS

The peripheral white blood cell count may be normal or mildly elevated. Cerebrospinal fluid pressure and protein are normal or slightly increased. Glucose is not decreased. White blood cells usually number fewer than 500/μL and are principally lymphocytes after the first 24 hours. Cerebrospinal fluid is normal in 5% of patients. The virus may be recovered from throat washings (early) and stools (early and late). Neutralizing and complement-fixing antibodies appear during the first or second week of illness.

Differential Diagnosis

Nonparalytic poliomyelitis is similar to other forms of enteroviral meningitis; the distinction is made serologically. Acute inflammatory polyneuritis (Guillain-Barré) and tick paralysis may initially resemble poliomyelitis. In Guillain-Barré syndrome (see Chapter 24), the weakness is more symmetric and ascending in most cases, but the Miller-Fisher variant is quite similar to bulbar polio. The cerebrospinal fluid usually has a high protein content but normal cell count in Guillain-Barré syndrome.

Complications

Urinary tract infection, atelectasis, pneumonia, myocarditis, and pulmonary edema may occur. Respiratory failure may be a result of paralysis of respiratory muscles, airway obstruction from involvement of cranial nerve nuclei, or lesions of the respiratory center.

Prevention

Given the above data regarding the epidemiologic distribution of poliomyelitis and the continued concern about vaccine-associated disease with the oral live vaccine, recommendations for prevention of poliomyelitis have been modified. Current recommendations in the USA are to provide the inactive (Salk) parenteral vaccination for all four doses (at ages 2, 4, and 6–18 months and 4–6 years). Oral vaccines are alternatively used for outbreak control, for travel to endemic areas within the ensuing month, and in protection of children whose parents do not accept the recommended number of immunizations. Oral vaccines, however, are being completely replaced by inactivated poliovirus vaccine for routine use in the developed world. The limited advantages of oral vaccination are the ease of administration, the effective local gastrointestinal and circulating immunity, and herd immunity.

Routine immunization of adults in the United States is not recommended because of the low incidence of the disease. Exceptions include adults exposed to poliomyelitis or planning to travel to endemic areas who have not received polio immunization within the past decade. They should be given inactivated poliomyelitis vaccine (Salk). Immunodeficient or immunosuppressed individuals and members of their households should also be given inactivated vaccines.

In the developing world, the interval between OPV doses should probably be longer than 1 month (because of interference from enteric pathogens). Intramuscular injections should be routinely avoided during the month following oral poliomyelitis vaccination to prevent provocation paralysis. Ancillary useful control measures in polio-endemic countries include national immunization days (mass campaigns in which all children are vaccinated twice, 4–6 weeks apart, regardless of vaccine history); cross-border vaccination activities; surveillance for "acute flaccid paralysis," an indicator for poliomyelitis; and aggressive outbreak responses and intensified immunization activities in countries recently affected by armed conflicts.

The recent outbreak in Hispaniola is a reminder of the need to maintain high levels of immunization coverage even in the absence of overt disease, the risks associated with oral vaccination, and the importance of continued surveillance for disease.

Treatment

Strict bed rest in the first few days of illness reduces the rate of paralysis. Cranial nerve involvement must be vigilantly sought. Comfortable but rotating positions should be maintained in a "polio bed": (firm mattress, footboard, sponge rubber pads or rolls, sandbags, and light splints). Fecal impaction and urinary retention (especially with paraplegia) are managed appropriately. In cases of respiratory weakness or paralysis, intensive care is needed.

Prognosis

During the febrile period, paralysis may develop or progress. Mild weakness of small muscles is more likely to regress than is severe weakness of large muscles. Bulbar poliomyelitis carries a mortality rate of up to 50%. New muscle weakness may develop and progress slowly years after recovery from acute paralytic poliomyelitis. This entity, postpoliomyelitis syndrome, presents with signs of chronic and new denervation, is not infectious in origin, and is associated with increasing dysfunction of surviving motor neurons. Series that report increased incidences of multiple sclerosis or other motor neuron diseases among poliomyelitis survivors need be evaluated in light of what is known about the postpoliomyelitis syndrome.

Caceres VM et al: Sabin monovalent oral polio vaccines: review of past experiences and their potential use after polio eradication. Clin Infect Dis 2001;33:531. [PMID: 11462191] (Vaccine-associated polio occurred most often with type 3 poliovirus.)

Fine PE et al: Transmissibility and persistence of oral polio vaccine viruses: implications for the global poliomyelitis eradication initiative. Am J Epidemiol 1999;150:1001. [PMID: 1056861] (Concern about the theoretical persistence of the oral poliomyelitis virus.)

Hull HF et al: Progress towards global polio eradication. Vaccine 2001;19:4378. [PMID:11483262] (The major locales where wild poliovirus transmission continues to occur are sub-Saharan Africa and South Asia.)

Prevention of poliomyelitis: recommendations for use of only inactivated poliovirus vaccine for routine vaccination. Committee on Infectious Diseases. American Academy of Pediatrics. Pediatrics 1999;108:1404. [PMID: 1058599]

Sutter RW et al: Poliomyelitis eradication: progress, challenges for the end game, and preparation for the post-eradication era. Infect Dis Clin North Am 2001;15:41. [PMID: 11301822]

4. Rubella

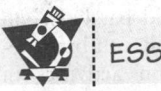

ESSENTIALS OF DIAGNOSIS

- *Exposure 14–21 days before onset.*
- *Arthralgia, particularly in young women.*

- *No prodrome in children, mild prodrome in adults; mild symptoms (fever, malaise, coryza) coinciding with eruption.*
- *Posterior cervical and postauricular lymphadenopathy 5–10 days before rash.*
- *Fine maculopapular rash of 3 days' duration; face to trunk to extremities.*
- *Leukopenia, thrombocytopenia.*

General Considerations

Rubella is a systemic disease caused by a togavirus transmitted by inhalation of infective droplets. It is only moderately communicable. One attack usually confers permanent immunity. The incubation period is 14–21 days (average, 16 days). The disease is transmissible from 1 week before the rash appears until 15 days afterward.

The clinical picture of rubella is difficult to distinguish from other viral illnesses such as infectious mononucleosis, echovirus infections, and coxsackievirus infections, though arthritis is more prominent in rubella. Definitive diagnosis can be made only by isolating the virus or serologically.

In the United States, rubella and congenital rubella syndrome are on the verge of elimination, though an outbreak of 83 cases of rubella occurred in 1999 in Nebraska, largely among Latin-Americans working in a meat-packing plant.

The principal importance of rubella lies in its devastating effects on the fetus in utero, producing teratogenic effects and a continuing congenital infection. Congenital rubella syndrome continues to occur in parts of the developing world at rates equivalent to those reported from the industrialized world during the prevaccine era. More than 100,000 cases occur annually in the developing world.

Clinical Findings
(Table 32–2)

A. SYMPTOMS AND SIGNS

Fever and malaise, usually mild, accompanied by tender suboccipital adenitis, may precede the eruption by 1 week. Mild coryza may be present. Polyarthritis occurs in about 25% of adult cases. These symptoms usually subside within 7 days but may persist for weeks.

Early posterior cervical and postauricular lymphadenopathy is very common. Erythema of the palate and throat, sometimes patchy, may be noted. A fine, pink maculopapular rash appears on the face, trunk, and extremities in rapid progression (2–3 days) and fades quickly, usually lasting 1 day in each area. Rubella without rash may be at least as common as the exanthematous disease. Diagnosis, when suspected because of epidemiologic evidence of the disease in the community, requires serologic confirmation.

B. Laboratory Findings

Leukopenia may be present early and may be followed by an increase in plasma cells. Virus isolation and serologic tests of immunity (rubella virus hemagglutination inhibition and fluorescent antibody tests) are available. Definitive diagnosis is based on a fourfold or greater rise in antibody titers.

Complications

A. Exposure During Pregnancy

Rubella antibodies are sought for at the beginning of pregnancy, since fetal infection during the first trimester leads to congenital rubella in at least 80% of fetuses.

When a pregnant woman is exposed to a possible case of rubella, an immediate hemagglutination-inhibiting rubella antibody level should be obtained; there is no reason for concern in positive tests. If no antibodies are found, clinical and serologic follow-up is essential. Confirmation of rubella in the expectant mother raises the question of therapeutic abortion, an alternative to be considered in the light of personal, religious, legal, and other factors. The risk to the fetus is highest for maternal infection in the first trimester but continues into the second trimester.

B. Congenital Rubella

An infant acquiring the infection in utero may be normal at birth but probably—half in a series of nearly 70 pregnant women with rubella in Mexico—will manifest a wide variety of manifestations, including early-onset cataracts, microphthalmia, and glaucoma, hearing deficits, psychomotor retardation, congenital heart defects, organomegaly, and maculopapular rash. Viral excretion in the throat and urine persists for many months despite high antibody levels. The diagnosis is confirmed by isolation of the virus. A specific test for IgM rubella antibody is useful for diagnosis in the newborn. Treatment is directed toward the many anomalies.

C. Postinfectious Encephalopathy

In 1:6000 cases, postinfectious encephalopathy develops 1–6 days after the rash; the virus cannot always be isolated. The mortality rate is 20%, but residual deficits are rare among the recovered. The mechanism is unknown.

Prevention

Live attenuated rubella virus vaccine should be given to all infants and to susceptible girls before the menarche. When women are immunized, they should not be pregnant, and the absence of antibodies should be established. (In the USA, about 80% of 20-year-old women are immune to rubella.) Postpartum administration to susceptible female hospital employees is recommended, though many hospitals fail to comply. While it is recommended that birth control be prac-

ticed for at least 3 months after vaccine administration, there are no reports of congenital rubella syndrome after rubella immunization, and inadvertent immunization of a pregnant woman is not considered an indication for therapeutic abortion. Arthritis is more marked after rubella vaccination than in native disease and appears to be immunologically mediated. The association between chronic arthropathies and rubella vaccination is controversial. MMR may be given in conjunction with DPT boosters as adequate serologic responses are documented.

Treatment

Acetaminophen provides symptomatic relief. Encephalitis and non-life-threatening thrombocytopenia should be treated symptomatically.

Prognosis

Rubella is a mild illness and rarely lasts more than 3–4 days. Congenital rubella, on the other hand, has a high mortality rate, and the associated congenital defects are largely permanent.

Barlow WE et al: The risk of seizures after receipt of whole-cell pertussis or measles, mumps, and rubella vaccine. N Engl J Med 2001;345:656. [PMID: 11547719] (Long-term adverse consequences are rare.)

Dykewicz CA et al: Rubella seropositivity in the United States, 1988–1994. Clin Infect Dis 2001;33:1279. [PMID: 11565065] (The lowest seropositivity was detected for those born in the early 1970s.)

Libman MD et al: Rubella susceptibility predicts measles susceptibility: implications for postpartum immunization. Clin Infect Dis 2000;31:1501. [PMID: 11096023] (7.6% of the rubella-susceptible were measles-susceptible, while the converse was only 0.8%.)

Plotkin SA: Rubella eradication. Vaccine 2001;19:3311. [PMID: 11348695] (Combining rubella and measles eradication strategies is advocated.)

Semerikov VV et al: Rubella in the Russian Federation: epidemiological factors and control measures to prevent the congenital rubella syndrome. Epidemiol Infect 2000;125:359. [PMID: 11117959] (Congenital rubella syndrome accounted for 15% of birth defects, and the incidence is 3.5 per 1000 live births in the Perm area of Russia.)

OTHER NEUROTROPIC VIRUSES

1. Rabies

 ESSENTIALS OF DIAGNOSIS

- *History of animal bite.*
- *Paresthesia, hydrophobia, rage alternating with calm.*
- *Convulsions, paralysis, thick tenacious saliva.*

General Considerations

Rabies is a viral (rhabdovirus) encephalitis transmitted by infected saliva that gains entry into the body by an animal bite or an open wound. Cases in the United States are rare but probably underreported. Bats, skunks, foxes, and raccoons are widely infected. Biting species that cause rabies in the United States and are geographically determined include raccoons in the East and New England; skunks in the Midwest, Southwest, and California; coyotes in Texas; foxes in the Southwest, New England, and Alaska. Dogs and cats are infected in developing countries (including the Mexican border). Ten out of 20 Americans with rabies acquired the disease abroad during the 1980s. Rodents and lagomorphs (eg, rabbits) are unlikely to have rabies. The virus gains entry into the salivary glands of dogs 5–7 days before their death from rabies, thus limiting their period of infectivity.

The incubation period may range from 10 days to many years but is usually 3–7 weeks. The interval is dependent in part on distance of the wound from the central nervous system. The virus travels in the nerves to the brain, multiplies there, and then migrates along the efferent nerves to the salivary glands.

Rabies is almost uniformly fatal, with four documented surviving cases; all received postexposure prophylaxis. The most common clinical problem confronting the physician is the management of a patient bitten by an animal (see Prevention).

Clinical Findings

A. Symptoms and Signs

There is usually a history of animal bite, though bat bites may not be remembered. The prodromal syndrome consists of pain at the site of the bite in association with fever, malaise, nausea, and vomiting. The skin is sensitive to changes of temperature, especially air currents. About 10 days later, the central nervous system stage begins, which may be either encephalitic ("furious") or paralytic ("dumb"). The encephalitic form produces the classic rabies manifestations of delirium alternating with periods of calm, when attempts at drinking cause extremely painful laryngeal spasms (hydrophobia). In the less common paralytic form, an acute ascending paralysis resembling Guillain-Barré syndrome predominates with relative sparing of higher cortical functions initially. Both forms progress relentlessly to coma, autonomic nervous system dysfunction, and death despite intensive support.

B. Laboratory Findings

Biting animals who are apparently well should be kept under observation for 7–10 days. Sick or dead animals should be examined for rabies. A wild animal, if captured, should be sacrificed and the head shipped on ice to the nearest laboratory qualified to examine the brain for evidence of rabies virus; the diagnosis is made by the fluorescent antibody technique. When the animal cannot be examined, skunks, bats, coyotes, foxes, and raccoons should be presumed to be rabid.

Fluorescent antibody testing of skin biopsy material from the posterior neck (where hair follicles are highly innervated) has a sensitivity of 60–80%.

Reverse transcriptase PCR and nucleic acid sequence-based amplification of the cerebrospinal fluid or saliva are being advocated as definitive diagnostic assays.

Prevention

Since rabies is almost always fatal, prevention is the only reasonable approach, and all exposures must be evaluated individually. Immunization of household dogs and cats and active immunization of persons with significant animal exposure (eg, veterinarians) are important. The most important common decisions, however, concern animal bites.

In the developing world, education, surveillance, and animal (particularly dog) vaccination programs are preferred over mass destruction of dogs, which is followed typically by invasion of susceptible feral animals into urban areas.

A. Local Treatment of Animal Bites and Scratches

Thorough cleansing, debridement, and repeated flushing of wounds with soap and water are important. If rabies immune globulin or antiserum is to be used, a portion should be infiltrated locally around the wound (see below) and the remainder given intramuscularly. Wounds caused by animal bites should not be sutured.

B. Postexposure Immunization

Therapy is indicated when the disease is seriously under consideration. Medical decisions should be based on recommendations of the USPHS Advisory Committee but also on circumstances of the bite, including the extent and location of the wound, the biting animal, history of prior vaccination, and the local endemicity of rabies. Consultation is available from state and local health departments. Postexposure treatment includes both passive antibody and vaccination.

The optimal form of passive immunization is rabies immune globulin (20 IU/kg). As much as possible of the full dose should be infiltrated around the wound, with any remaining injected intramuscularly at a site distant from the wound. If immune globulin (human) is not available, equine rabies antiserum (20–40 IU/kg) can be used after appropriate tests for horse serum sensitivity. An inactivated human diploid cell rabies vaccine (HDCV) is given as five injections of 1 mL intramuscularly (in the deltoid rather than the gluteal muscle) on days 0, 3, 7, 14, and 28 after exposure.

Several cell culture vaccines are available and are preferable to embryonated tissue vaccine (eg, duck embryo vaccine; DEV) because of better antigenic response and fewer systemic reactions. HDCV availability and cost limit its use in the developing world.

Rabies immune globulin and rabies vaccine (human diploid cell vaccine) should never be given in the same syringe or at the same site. Allergic reactions to the vaccine are rare, though local reactions (pruritus, erythema, tenderness) occur in about 25% and mild systemic reactions (headaches, myalgias, nausea) in about 20% of recipients. The vaccine is commercially available or can be obtained through health departments. For patients who previously received pre- or postexposure vaccine, rabies immune globulin should not be given; vaccine, 1 mL in the deltoid, should be given twice (on days 0 and 3).

In other countries, the less costly inactivated duck embryo vaccine or mouse brain vaccine may be available, but the method of administration is more complex, the rate of allergic reactions—including ascending paralysis—is higher, and the efficacy is less.

C. PREEXPOSURE IMMUNIZATION

Preexposure prophylaxis with three injections of diploid cell vaccine intramuscularly (1 mL on days 0, 7, and 21 or 28) or intradermally (0.1 mL on days 0, 7, and 28, over the deltoid) is recommended for persons at high risk of exposure: veterinarians (who should have rabies antibody titers checked every 2 years and be boosted with 1 mL intramuscularly or 0.1 mL intradermally if seronegative), animal handlers, Peace Corps workers, and travelers to remote areas (rabies immune globulin is in short supply worldwide). An intradermal route is available for preexposure prophylaxis only. Immunosuppressive illness and agents including corticosteroids as well as antimalarials—in particular chloroquine—may diminish the antibody response.

Treatment

This very severe illness with an almost universally fatal outcome requires intensive care with attention to the airway, maintenance of oxygenation, and control of seizures. Universal precautions are essential.

Prognosis

Once the symptoms have appeared, death almost inevitably occurs after 7 days, usually from respiratory failure.

Compendium of animal rabies prevention and control, 2001. National Association of State Public Health Veterinarians, Inc. MMWR Recomm Rep 2001;50(RR-8):1. [PMID: 11400959]

Moran GJ et al: Appropriateness of rabies postexposure prophylaxis treatment for animal exposures. Emergency ID Net Study Group. JAMA 2000;284:1001. [PMID: 10944646] (The use of rabies postexposure prophylaxis is often inappropriate, and the authors urge review of guidelines and consultation with public health officials in questionable cases.)

Plotkin SA: Rabies. Clin Infect Dis 2000;30:4. [PMID: 10619725] (Review and discussion of bat-related issues and detailed discussion of prophylaxis recommendations.)

Weiner HR: Diagnosis and prevention of rabies. Compr Ther 2001;27:60. [PMID: 11280857]

2. Arbovirus Encephalitides

ESSENTIALS OF DIAGNOSIS

- *Fever, malaise, stiff neck, sore throat, and nausea and vomiting, progressing to stupor, coma, and convulsions.*
- *Signs of an upper motor neuron lesion (exaggerated deep tendon reflexes, absent superficial reflexes, pathologic reflexes, spastic paralysis).*
- *Cerebrospinal fluid protein and opening pressure often increased, with lymphocytic pleocytosis.*

General Considerations

The arboviruses are arthropod-borne agents that produce clinical manifestations in humans. The mosquito-borne agents include three alphaviruses (causing Western, Eastern, and Venezuelan equine encephalitis), five flaviviruses (causing St. Louis and Japanese B encephalitis, dengue, yellow fever, and the West Nile agent; bunyaviruses (the California serogroup of viruses [in particular California encephalitis caused by the Lacrosse agent]); and some causes of viral hemorrhagic fever (Rift Valley fever). The tick-borne causes of encephalitis include the flavivirus Powassan (northeastern United States and Canada), and tick-borne encephalitides of Europe. Agents associated with viral hemorrhagic fever are discussed below, and only those viruses causing primarily encephalitis in the United States will be discussed here.

A new arboviral disease, West Nile encephalitis, in the USA was identified in 1999. Initial United States cases were largely in the New York City area, and presentations were similar to that of St. Louis encephalitis. Human infections are now documented along the Atlantic seaboard and in states as far West as Texas and Nebraska. The disease caused outbreaks in France in the early 1960s and in Romania in 1996, with occasional fatalities. West Nile encephalitis in the United States is distinctive because cases tend not to manifest a rash but do show relative lymphocytopenia.

The leading causes of arbovirus encephalitis in the USA are St. Louis and California encephalitis. Agent-specific reservoirs (typically small mammals or birds) are responsible for maintaining the encephalitis-producing viruses in nature; horses serve as sentinels for infection with the equine agents, though birds maintain the life cycle. Eleven North Americans died of

Japanese B encephalitis between 1981 and 1992, largely military personnel stationed in Asia.

Clinical Findings

A. SYMPTOMS AND SIGNS

The symptoms of arboviral encephalitis are fever, malaise, sore throat, nausea and vomiting, lethargy, stupor, coma, and convulsions. Signs include stiff neck, meningeal irritation, tremors, convulsions, cranial nerve palsies, paralysis of extremities, exaggerated deep tendon reflexes, absent superficial reflexes, and pathologic reflexes. With West Nile encephalitis, there are reports that a roseolar or maculopapular rash may occur in half of cases and that generalized lymphadenopathy is common.

While asymptomatic seroconversion is common, when frank encephalitis develops the outcome is age-dependent. St. Louis and West Nile encephalitides occur largely in adults, with residual damage principally in older patients. The other encephalitis-causing agents cause morbidity chiefly among children.

B. LABORATORY FINDINGS

The white blood cell count is variable. Cerebrospinal fluid pressure and protein content are often increased. Cerebrospinal fluid glucose is normal, though lymphocytic pleocytosis may be present (polymorphonuclear cells may predominate early). The virus may sometimes be isolated from blood or, rarely, from cerebrospinal fluid. PCR assays are available to assist with diagnosis. Serologic tests of blood or cerebrospinal fluid may be diagnostic in specific types of encephalitis (by demonstrating virus-specific IgM or a fourfold or greater change in complement-fixing or neutralizing antibodies). CT or MRI of the brain showing basal ganglial or thalamic involvement may be useful in excluding the temporal lobe lesions of herpesvirus or other space-occupying processes.

For West Nile encephalitis, IgM capture ELISAs on cerebrospinal fluid and serum samples are positive after the viremia (which ends with the fourth day of illness). Definitive diagnosis requires demonstration of a fourfold or greater rise in antibody titer. Nucleic acid amplification tests and direct viral isolation techniques are under development. MRI is reported to be especially sensitive for detecting meningeal enhancement.

Differential Diagnosis

Mild forms of encephalitis must be differentiated from aseptic meningitis, lymphocytic choriomeningitis, and nonparalytic poliomyelitis.

Severe forms of arbovirus encephalitides (Table 32–2) are to be differentiated from other causes of viral encephalitis (herpes simplex virus, mumps virus, poliovirus or other enteroviruses, HIV), encephalitis accompanying exanthematous diseases of childhood (measles, varicella, infectious mononucleosis, rubella), encephalitis following vaccination (a demyelinating type following rabies, measles, pertussis), toxic encephalitis (from drugs, poisons, or bacterial toxins such as *Shigella dysenteriae* type 1), Reye's syndrome, and severe forms of stroke, brain tumors, brain abscess, autoimmune processes such as lupus cerebritis, and intoxications.

Complications

Bronchial pneumonia, urinary retention and infection, and decubitus ulcers may occur. Late sequelae are mental deterioration, parkinsonism, and epilepsy.

Prevention

Effective measures include mosquito control (repellents, protective clothing, insecticides). A vaccine against Japanese B encephalitis is recommended for summer travelers to rural areas of East Asia.

Treatment

Although specific antiviral therapy is not available for most causative entities, vigorous supportive measures can be helpful. Such measures include reduction of intracranial pressure (mannitol) and monitoring of intraventricular pressure. The efficacy of corticosteroids in these infections is not established. Preliminary evidence that ribavirin was useful in West Nile encephalitis has not been substantiated.

Reducing the likelihood of contact between mosquitoes and humans is the best means of controlling infection. The use of DEET is discussed at http://ace.orst.edu./info/nptn or 800-858-7378.

Prognosis

The prognosis is always guarded, especially in younger children. Sequelae may become apparent late in the course of what appears to be a successful recovery. The prognosis is generally better for Western equine than for Eastern equine or St. Louis encephalitis. The case fatality rate for the original 78 patients with West Nile encephalitis from the New York City area was 12%.

Balkhy HH et al: Severe La Crosse encephalitis with significant neurologic sequelae. Pediatr Infect Dis J 2000;19:77. [PMID: 10643856] (A description of six cases with severe disease, requiring ICU care and causing neurologic sequelae.)

Kalita J et al: Comparison of CT scan and MRI findings in the diagnosis of Japanese encephalitis. J Neurol Sci 2000;174:3. [PMID: 10704974] (MRI is more sensitive than CT, and thalamic involvement is common in Japanese encephalitis.)

Marfin AA et al: West Nile encephalitis: an emerging disease in the United States. Clin Infect Dis 2001;33:1713. [PMID: 11595987] (During 2001 over 45 cases were reported from states ranging from Massachusetts to Louisiana, with most cases in New York and Florida. The early isolates all showed a high degree of homology.)

Outbreak of Powassan encephalitis—Maine, Vermont, 1999–2001. MMWR Morb Mortal Wkly Rep 2001;50:761. [PMID: 11787585] (Report of four cases.)

Wasay MN et al: St Louis encephalitis: a review of 11 cases in a 1995 Dallas, Texas, epidemic. Arch Neurol 2000;57:114. [PMID: 10634457] (Substantia nigra involvement may be more common with St. Louis encephalitis; HIV may be a risk factor.)

3. Lymphocytic Choriomeningitis

ESSENTIALS OF DIAGNOSIS

- *"Influenza-like" prodrome of fever, chills, malaise, and cough, followed by meningitis with associated stiff neck.*
- *Aseptic meningitis with positive Kernig's sign, headache, nausea, vomiting, and lethargy.*
- *Cerebrospinal fluid: slight increase of protein, lymphocytic pleocytosis (500–3000/μL); low glucose in 25% of patients.*
- *Complement-fixing antibodies within 2 weeks.*

General Considerations

Lymphocytic choriomeningitis is an arenaviral infection of the central nervous system. The main reservoir of infection is the infected house mouse, though other reservoirs include guinea pigs, monkeys, dogs, swine, and even pet hamsters. The virus is shed by the infected animal via oronasal secretions, urine, and feces, with transmission to humans probably through exposure to animal droppings via contaminated food and dust. The virus is not spread person-to-person, though vertical transmission occurs and lymphocytic choriomeningitis is considered a fetal teratogen. The incubation period is 8–13 days to the appearance of systemic manifestations and 15–21 days to the appearance of meningeal symptoms. CD4 cells may be involved in pathogenesis. Lymphocytic choriomeningitis is considered a model of cell-mediated immunity in vaccine development.

Outbreaks have occurred among persons with rodent exposure. Complications of clinical disease are rare.

This disease is principally confined to the eastern seaboard and northeastern states of the USA, and serologic evidence of infection is increased among women, the elderly, and members of lower socioeconomic groups.

Clinical Findings

A. SYMPTOMS AND SIGNS

Symptoms are biphasic. The prodromal illness is characterized by fever, chills, headache, myalgia, cough, and vomiting, the meningeal phase by headache, nausea and vomiting, and lethargy. Signs of pneumonia are occasionally present during the prodromal phase.

During the meningeal phase there may be neck and back stiffness with a positive Kernig sign. Obstructive hydrocephalus is a rare complication. Arthralgias can develop late.

The prodrome may terminate in complete recovery, or meningeal symptoms may appear after a few days of remission. Chorioretinitis also appears to be a sequela of lymphocytic choriomeningitis.

B. LABORATORY FINDINGS

Leukocytosis or leukopenia and thrombocytopenia may be present. Cerebrospinal fluid lymphocytic pleocytosis (total count is often 500–3000/μL) may occur, with slight increase in protein and normal to low glucose in at least 25%. Complement-fixing antibodies appear during or after the second week. The virus may be recovered from the blood and cerebrospinal fluid by mouse inoculation. A PCR technique for the detection of lymphocytic choriomeningitis virus in the cerebrospinal fluid has been described.

Differential Diagnosis

The influenza-like prodrome and latent period help distinguish this from other aseptic meningitides, and bacterial and granulomatous meningitis. A history of exposure to mice or other potential vectors is an important diagnostic clue.

Treatment

Treatment is supportive as for encephalitis or aseptic meningitis. The membrane protein alpha-dystroglycan interacts with lymphocytic choriomeningitis and Lassa fever virus (both arenaviruses), and this interaction provides a potential avenue for future interventions.

Prognosis

Fatalities are rare. The illness usually lasts 1–2 weeks, though convalescence may be prolonged.

Barton LL et al: Congenital lymphocytic choriomeningitis virus infection: decade of rediscovery. Clin Infect Dis 2001;33:370. [PMID: 11438904]. (This review emphasizes the teratogenicity of the pathogen.)

4. Prion Disease

Several neurologic diseases can be caused by communicable agents with slow replication and long latent intervals in the host. Such agents have been called *pro*teinaceous *i*nfectious particles, or "prions," and are resistant to most procedures that modify nucleic acid. The transmissible agents induce conversion of a normal brain protein (PrP^C) to an abnormal isoform (PrP^{Sc}), a process that appears to be both genetically determined and in need of the infectious agent. The accumulated abnormal isoform proteins are associated with disease, though the pathogenesis of spongiform changes and the accumulation in some cases of amyloid plaque are poorly understood. A variety of animal diseases exhibit these properties, including visna and scrapie in sheep and goats, chronic wasting disease of mule deer, and transmissible encephalopathy of mink. The agents or related agents that cause human disease are discussed here.

Kuru and **Creutzfeldt-Jakob disease** are transmissible in brain or eye tissue to primates, including humans. After an incubation period measured in years, disease ensues characterized by an inexorably progressive downhill course. Kuru—once prevalent in central New Guinea but no longer seen since abandonment of cannibalism—was characterized by cerebellar ataxia, tremors, dysarthria, and emotional lability.

The four forms of Creutzfeldt-Jakob disease are sporadic (classic, cCJD) (80–85%), familial (15%), iatrogenic (< 1%), and a new variant (vCJD), described below. There are no definitive risk factors for cCJD, which occurs worldwide with an incidence of 1 per million. Patients with cCJD usually present in the sixth or seventh decade with dementia progressive over several months, myoclonic fasciculations, ataxia, and somnolence. The characteristic electroencephalographic pattern shows paroxysms with high voltages and slow waves. MRI typically shows bilateral areas of increased signal intensity, predominantly in the caudate and putamen. Assays of the cerebrospinal fluid for 14-3-3 protein and neuron-specific enolase may help with the diagnosis. Familial cases are inherited in an autosomal dominant pattern with variable penetrance. Iatrogenic cases have occurred in patients who receive tissue such as cadaveric growth hormone and dural grafts from the central nervous systems of patients with Creutzfeldt-Jakob disease.

There is no specific treatment, and the only known means of prevention is avoidance of contamination by affected brain tissue, electrodes, or neurosurgical tools or by transplants of cornea, dura, or cadaveric growth hormone from infected donors. Disinfection of equipment requires autoclaving at 15 psi for 1 hour, and disinfection of contaminated surfaces requires 5% hypochlorite or 0.1-N sodium hydroxide solution.

New variant Creutzfeldt-Jakob disease (vCJD) was originally described in a small outbreak from Britain and since then increasingly from other countries in Western Europe. The patients are younger, the duration is longer, the clinical symptomatology is unique (psychiatric symptoms and cerebellar signs are more common), and the electroencephalographic findings are not typical of cCJD. The disease probably results from ingestion of beefsteak from livestock infected with **bovine spongiform encephalopathy (BSE)** ("mad cow disease").

Other prion diseases include fatal familial insomnia (rarely sporadic) and Gerstmann-Ströaussler-Scheinker disease (with dementia and spastic paraparesis).

Aksamit AJ Jr et al: Quantitation of 14-3-3 and neuron-specific enolase proteins in CSF in Creutzfeldt-Jakob disease. Neurology 2001;57:728. [PMID: 11524493] (Both assays are relatively sensitive and specific for the diagnosis of Creutzfeldt-Jakob disease.)

Coulthart MB et al: Variant Creutzfeldt-Jakob disease: a summary of current scientific knowledge in relation to public health. CMAJ. 2001;165:51. [PMID: 11468957]

Johnson RT et al: Medical progress: Creutzfeldt-Jakob disease and related transmissible spongiform encephalopathies. N Engl J Med 1998;339:1994. [PMID: 9869672] (Review by leading investigators, outlining the differences between sporadic and familial Creutzfeldt-Jakob disease and between that disease and bovine spongiform encephalopathy.)

MacKnight C: Clinical implications of bovine spongiform encephalopathy. Clin Infect Dis 2001;32:1726. [PMID: 11360215] (Discusses the likely impact on humans).

Worrall BB et al: Amyotrophy in prion disease. Arch Neurol 2000;57:33. [PMID: 10634430] (Amyotrophy was noted in 50 patients with clinically or biochemically proved prion disease, emphasizing the need to assess lower motor neuron function and spinal cord pathology in cases of Creutzfeldt-Jakob disease.)

5. Progressive Multifocal Leukoencephalopathy

Progressive multifocal leukoencephalopathy is a demyelinating central nervous system disorder with a propensity for affliction of immunosuppressed adults, especially AIDS patients. The cause is JC virus (JCV), a papovavirus that targets myelinating oligodendrocytes of the central nervous system. PCR of the cerebrospinal fluid for JCV is used for diagnosis in patients with compatible clinical and radiologic findings. Highly active antiretroviral therapy (HAART) for HIV infection is effective in improving survival as well as the clinical and radiographic features associated with this disease. The use of cidofovir, while becoming more widespread, is not routinely recommended at present.

Antonori A et al: Epidemiology and prognosis of AIDS-associated progressive multifocal leukoencephalopathy in the HAART era. J Neurovirol 2001;7:323. [PMID: 11517411] (Increased longevity in patients receiving HAART.)

Segarra-Newnham M et al: Use of cidofovir in progressive multifocal leukoencephalopathy. Ann Pharmacother 2001;35:741. [PMID: 11408993]

6. Human T Cell Lymphotropic Virus (HTLV)

Retroviruses include both the lympholytic HIV agents and the lymphotropic oncoviruses, human T cell leukemia viruses types 1 and 2 (HTLV-1 and -2). The isolation of HTLV-1 from a young man with T cell lymphoma established an association of the virus with adult T cell lymphoma/leukemia (ATL)—an association that has been confirmed from endemic areas throughout the world, including the Caribbean, southern Japan, sub-Saharan Africa (where over 10% of the population of Gabon and Cameroon are seropositive), Latin America, and the southeastern

United States (where seroprevalence is most common among intravenous drug users).

The lifetime risk of developing ATL among the seropositive is estimated to be 3% among women and 7% among men, with an incubation period of at least 15 years. HTLV-1 is oncogenic primarily through the simultaneous induction of both interleukin-2 and interleukin-2 receptor.

Common clinical features of ATL include diffuse lymphadenopathy, maculopapular skin lesions that may evolve into erythroderma, organomegaly, lytic bone lesions, and hypercalcemia.

There is a predisposition to opportunistic infections such as *Pneumocystis carinii* pneumonia and cryptococcal meningitis. A large percentage of patients are infected with *Strongyloides stercoralis*. Diagnosis requires identification of HTLV-1 antibodies. Confirmatory demonstration of monoclonal proviral DNA integration in tumor cells is helpful.

HTLV-1 also causes HTLV-associated myelopathy (HAM; tropical spastic paraparesis). It is characterized by progressive motor weakness, especially of the lower extremities, with spastic paraparesis or paraplegia with hyperreflexia. Sensory disturbances and urinary incontinence may also be seen. The disease may resemble multiple sclerosis but does not remit. Cranial nerve abnormalities are rare, and cognitive function is usually preserved. HAM develops in less than 1% of HTLV-1 seropositive individuals.

HTLV-2 was initially implicated in hairy cell leukemia, but this association has not been confirmed. HTLV-2 seropositivity is common in some American populations, especially intravenous drug users. It infects primarily CD8 cells, whereas HTLV-1 infects primarily CD4 cells. The role of HTLV-2 in disease is under investigation.

Management of ATL is similar to that for non-Hodgkin's lymphoma and includes combination chemotherapy and radiation of particular sites (weight-bearing bony lesions, paraspinal masses, intracerebral lesions). HTLV-associated myelopathy is treated with a variety of immune-modulating agents without consistent results. Antiretrovirals have not shown clear benefit for ATL- or HTLV-associated myelopathy.

Screening of the blood supply for HTLV-1 is required in the United States, since transfusion is a recognized mode of transmission along with sexual contact and vertical transfer. There is significant cross-reactivity between HTLV-1 and HTLV-2 on serologic studies, but PCR can differentiate the two.

Gotuzzo E et al: Human T-cell lymphotropic virus-1 in Latin America. Infect Dis Clin North Am 2000;14:211. [PMID: 10738680] (The role of screening blood donors in controlling the spread of HTLV-1.)

Merle H et al: A description of human T-lymphotropic virus type 1-related chronic interstitial keratitis in 20 patients. Am J Ophthalmol 2001;131:305. [PMID: 11239861] (New manifestations of HTLV-1 infection in the eye.)

Sonoda S et al: Ancient HTLV type 1 provirus DNA of Andean mummy. AIDS Res Hum Retroviruses 2000;1:1753. [PMID: 11080822] (Data supporting the theory that HTLV-1 was carried with ancient Mongoloids to the Andes in the pre Columbian era.)

OTHER SYSTEMIC VIRAL DISEASES

1. Hemorrhagic Fevers

This is a diverse group of illnesses resulting from several diverse viral infections (flaviviruses, alphaviruses, arenaviruses, bunyaviruses, and filoviruses) and immunologic responses to them. The common clinical features include high fever, leukopenia, altered mental status, and a hemorrhagic diathesis. Marked toxicity and death may occur. Modes of transmission are similarly diverse, and these viruses may be tick-borne (eg, tick-borne encephalitis, eastern Europe; Omsk hemorrhagic fever, Russia; Kyasanur Forest hemorrhagic fever, India); mosquito-borne (eg, Chikungunya hemorrhagic fever, yellow fever, dengue, and o'nyong-nyong fever); or zoonotic (often derived from rodents, eg, hemorrhagic fever with renal failure secondary to Hantaan virus infection, Junin hemorrhagic fever, Argentina; Machupo hemorrhagic fever, Bolivia; Lassa hemorrhagic fever, West Africa; the Puumala virus, Scandinavia). The zoonotic group also includes Marburg hemorrhagic fever and possibly Ebola hemorrhagic fever in central Africa. Lassa fever is associated with rodent contact or consumption. Dengue, yellow fever, and hantaviruses are discussed below.

The Nipah virus in Malaysia is a zoonotic paramyxovirus that does not cause hemorrhagic fever but instead causes a primarily encephalitic infection in most cases associated with a history of contact with pigs.

Persons who present with symptoms compatible with those of hemorrhagic fever and who have traveled from a possible endemic area should be isolated for diagnosis and symptomatic treatment. Diagnosis may be made by growing the virus from blood obtained early in the disease or by showing a significant specific four-fold or greater rise in antibody titer. Isolation is particularly important because some of these infections, such as Ebola virus, are highly transmissible and carry a mortality rate of 50–90%.

For most of these entities, no specific treatment is available. Lassa fever and hemorrhagic fever with renal failure can be effectively treated with intravenous ribavirin if started promptly: 33 mg/kg as loading dose, followed by 16 mg/kg every 6 hours for 4 days and then 8 mg/kg every 8 hours for 3 days (see Chapter 37). It is important to differentiate hemorrhagic fever from differently treated entities such as meningococcemia or other septicemias, Rocky Mountain spotted fever, dengue, and malaria. The likelihood of hemorrhagic fevers among travelers remains low.

Enria DA et al: Rodent-borne emerging viral zoonosis. Hemorrhagic fevers and hantavirus infections in South America. Infect Dis Clin North Am 2000;14:167. [PMID: 10738678]

Outbreak of Ebola hemorrhagic fever Uganda, August 2000–January 2001. MMWR Morb Mortal Wkly Rep 2001;50:73. [PMID: 11686289]

Paton NI et al: Outbreak of Nipah-virus infection among abattoir workers in Singapore. Lancet 1999;354:1253. [PMID: 10520634] (Nipah virus is a highly fatal zoonotic infection related to Hendra viruses of Australia. Pigs are the animal source, requiring slaughter for containment.)

2. Dengue

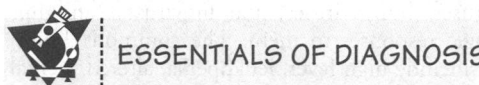

ESSENTIALS OF DIAGNOSIS

- *Exposure 7–10 days before onset.*
- *Sudden onset of high fever, chills, severe aching, headache, sore throat, prostration, and depression.*
- *Biphasic fever curve: initial phase, 3–7 days; remission, few hours to 2 days; second phase, 1–2 days.*
- *The rash is biphasic: first evanescent, followed by maculopapular, scarlatiniform, morbilliform, or petechial changes from extremities to torso.*
- *Leukopenia and thrombocytopenia in the hemorrhagic form.*

General Considerations

Dengue is a viral (togavirus, flavivirus) disease transmitted by the bite of the aedes mosquito. It may be caused by one of several serotypes widely distributed between latitudes 25 °N and 25 °S (eg, Thailand, India, Philippines; Caribbean, including Puerto Rico and Cuba; Central America and the northern half of South America; Africa). It occurs only in the active mosquito season (warm weather). The incubation period is 3–15 days (usually 7–10 days). Transmission occurred in the USA in southern Texas and nearby Mexican border towns in 1986 and 1999. A high level of suspicion is warranted in the southern United States since a new vector, the Asian tiger mosquito, *Aedes albopictus,* was admitted through imported tires into Texas in the 1980s.

Clinical Findings

A. SYMPTOMS AND SIGNS

Dengue is usually a nonspecific, self-limited, febrile illness, but its presentation may range from asymptomatic infection to severe hemorrhage (**dengue hemorrhagic fever**) and sudden fatal shock (**dengue shock syndrome**). Severe dengue begins with a sudden onset of high fever, chills, and severe aching ("breakbone")

of the head, back, and extremities, accompanied by sore throat, prostration, and depression. There may be conjunctival redness and flushing or blotching of the skin. The initial febrile phase lasts 3–7 days, typically but not inevitably followed by a remission of a few hours to 2 days.

The rash appears in 80% of cases during the remission or during the second febrile phase, which lasts 1–2 days and is accompanied by similar but usually milder symptoms than in the first phase. The rash may be scarlatiniform, morbilliform, maculopapular, or petechial, appearing first on the dorsum of the hands and feet and spreading to the arms, legs, trunk, and neck but rarely to the face. The rash lasts 2 hours to several days and may be followed by desquamation.

Petechial rashes and gastrointestinal hemorrhages occur with dengue hemorrhagic fever, caused by strains of many subtypes in Asia and increasingly in the Caribbean, Mexico, and Central America, typically as an anamnestic response, most often to serotype 2, and less often to serotypes 3, 4, and 1 (in decreasing order of frequency). Some dengue virus envelope glycoproteins are homologous with segments of clotting factors, including plasminogen, and thus the hemorrhagic fever may represent an autoimmune reaction. The early expression of the antigen CD69 on peripheral blood lymphocytes correlates in children with the development of dengue hemorrhagic fever. A subset of patients progress to dengue shock syndrome, in which a capillary leak process is prominent.

Before the rash of dengue appears, it is difficult to distinguish from malaria, yellow fever, or influenza; the rash makes dengue far more likely. A positive tourniquet test should alert one to the possible development of hemorrhagic fever.

B. LABORATORY FINDINGS

Leukopenia is characteristic. Thrombocytopenia occurs in the hemorrhagic form of the disease and appears to correlate with early CD69 expression on peripheral lymphocytes. Virus may be recovered from the blood during the acute phase. Several commercial rapid serologic assays are available.

Complications

Depression, pneumonia, bone marrow failure, iritis, orchitis, and oophoritis are unusual complications. Dengue shock syndrome occurs among a small subset of patients with severe dengue hemorrhagic fever, and children appear to be at particular risk.

Prevention

Available prophylactic measures include control of mosquitoes by screening and insect repellents, particularly during early morning and late afternoon exposures. An effective vaccine has been developed but is not produced commercially.

Treatment

Treatment entails the appropriate use of volume and pressors, acetaminophen rather than aspirin for analgesia, and the gradual restoration of activity during prolonged convalescence. Monitoring patients with platelet counts is useful in anticipating the complications of dengue hemorrhagic fever or shock syndrome.

Prognosis

Fatalities are rare, though convalescence tends to be slow.

Gill J et al: Dengue surveillance in Florida, 1997–98. Emerg Infect Dis 2000;6:30. [PMID: 10653566] (Proximity to endemic areas and the presence of the competent mosquito vector suggest that there is underrecognition and underreporting—18 cases in this 1-year surveillance—in Florida.)

Jacobs M: Dengue: emergence as a global public health problem and prospects for control. Trans R Soc Trop Med Hyg 2000;94:7. [PMID: 10748886] (There are an estimated 20 million infections annually, and several hundred thousand with hemorrhagic fever.)

Solomon T et al: Dengue and other emerging flaviviruses. J Infect 2991;42;104. [PMID: 11531316] (A reminder that mosquitoes are global vectors for the transmission of these viruses, although in cool environments ticks may be the transmitting agents.)

Solomon T et al: Neurological manifestations of dengue infection. Lancet 2000;355:1053. [PMID: 10744091] (Reduced consciousness and convulsions are the most common manifestations, and in this series of twenty-one cases, nine presented with encephalitis and six had neurologic sequelae on discharge.)

Underdiagnosis of dengue—Laredo, Texas, 1999. MMWR Morb Mortal Wkly Rep 2001;50:57. [PMID: 11243446] (Half of the 325 dengue cases were recognized only through heightened public health surveillance activities.)

3. Hantaviruses

Hantaviruses are rodent-borne RNA viruses with several distinct serotypes. These differ in rodent hosts, geographic distribution, and degree of pathogenicity for humans. They cause two major clinical syndromes: hemorrhagic fever (discussed above) and the hantavirus pulmonary syndrome. The ubiquitousness of hantaviruses is becoming recognized, with descriptions of infections from North and South America and additional infections from Europe and Asia. The Hantaan serotype viruses cause severe hemorrhagic fever with renal syndrome and are found primarily in Korea, China, and eastern Russia. The Seoul viruses produce a less severe form and are found primarily in Korea and China. The Puumala and Dobrava viruses are found in Scandinavia and Europe and are associated with a milder form of the syndrome.

The Sin Nombre (Muerto Canyon, Four Corners) virus is one of the viruses responsible for the **hantavirus pulmonary syndrome,** most cases of which have been seen in the southwestern United States. Approximately 300 cases have been reported from 31 states since 1993. Outbreaks are currently being reported from Central and South America. Hantavirus pulmonary syndrome begins as a nonspecific febrile illness followed by rapid progression to a shock-like state, associated with increased pulmonary vascular permeability and ARDS. Hematologic features include thrombocytopenia, hemoconcentration, and leukocytosis. Recently, it is recognized that clinical similarities—namely, renal involvement—exist between the New World hantaviruses and Old World counterparts.

Diagnosis can be made serologically, with the vast majority having both IgM and IgG antibodies at the time of presentation; by immunohistochemical staining; or by PCR amplification of viral tissue DNA. Since infection is thought to occur by inhalation of rodent wastes, prevention is aimed toward eradication of rodents in houses and avoidance of exposure to rodent excreta in rural settings.

No treatment has been established as definitely effective for hantavirus pulmonary syndrome. Intravenous ribavirin has been used with some success in hemorrhagic fever with renal syndrome, and studies are currently ongoing for its use in hantavirus pulmonary syndrome.

Bharadwaj M et al: Humoral immune responses in the hantavirus cardiopulmonary syndrome. J Infect Dis 2000;182:43. [PMID: 10882580] (Neutralizing antibody responses correlate inversely with severity of disease.)

Enria DA et al: Rodent-borne emerging viral zoonosis. Hemorrhagic fevers and hantavirus infections in South America. Infect Dis Clin North Am 2000;14:167. [PMID: 10738678]

Hantavirus pulmonary syndrome due to Andes virus in Temuco, Chile: clinical experience with 16 adults. Chest 2001;120: 548. [PMID: 11502657]

Hjelle B et al: Outbreak of hantavirus infection in the Four Corners region of the United States in the wake of the 1997–1998 El Nino–southern oscillation. J Infect Dis 2000;181: 1569. [PMID: 10823755] (Increasing prevalence correlated with increased rainfall and indoor exposure to deer mice.)

Padula PJ et al: Genetic diversity, distribution, and serological features of hantavirus infection in five countries in South America. J Clin Microbiol 2000;38:3029. [PMID: 10921972] (Eighty-seven cases are now reported from Argentina, Bolivia, Chile, Paraguay, and Uruguay.)

4. Yellow Fever

 ESSENTIALS OF DIAGNOSIS

- *Endemic area exposure (tropical South and Central America, Africa, but not Asia).*
- *Sudden onset of severe headache, aching in legs, and tachycardia.*
- *Brief (1 day) remission, followed by bradycardia, hypotension, jaundice, hemorrhagic tendency.*

• *Proteinuria, leukopenia, bilirubinemia, bilirubin-uria.*

General Considerations

Yellow fever is a zoonotic viral (group B arbovirus, to-gavirus) infection transmitted by the *Aedes* and jungle mosquitoes. It is endemic only in Africa and South America (tropical or subtropical), but epidemics have extended far into the temperate zone during warm seasons. Its role in thwarting economic development in tropical areas is devastating.

The mosquito transmits the infection by first biting an individual having the disease and then biting a susceptible individual after the virus has multiplied within the mosquito's body. The incubation period in humans is 3–6 days. Adults and children are equally susceptible, though attack rates are highest among adult males because of their work habits.

Clinical Findings

A. SYMPTOMS AND SIGNS

1. Mild form—Symptoms are malaise, headache, fever, retro-orbital pain, nausea, vomiting, and photophobia. Bradycardia may be present.

2. Severe form—About 15% of those infected with yellow fever develop severe illness. Initial symptoms are similar to the mild form, but a brief remission after about 3 days of acute illness is followed by a toxic phase manifested by fever and bradycardia (Faget's sign), hypotension, jaundice, hemorrhage (gastrointestinal, nasal, oral), and delirium that may progress to coma.

B. LABORATORY FINDINGS

Leukopenia occurs, although it may not be present at the onset. Proteinuria is present, sometimes as high as 5–6 g/L, and disappears completely with recovery. Abnormal liver function tests are seen, and prothrombin time may be elevated. Serologic diagnosis may be established by showing fourfold or greater increases in hemagglutination inhibition, complement fixation, or neutralizing antibodies. An IgM capture enzyme immunoassay (EIA) is a rapid, specific diagnostic aid.

Differential Diagnosis

It may be difficult to distinguish yellow fever from hepatitis, malaria, leptospirosis, dengue, and other hemorrhagic fevers on clinical evidence alone. Serologic confirmation is often needed.

Prevention

Transmission is prevented through mosquito control. Live virus vaccine is highly effective, safe, and should be provided for immunocompetent adults living in or traveling to endemic areas. Pregnant women should not be immunized and should defer travel to endemic areas (see Chapter 30). Eradication is difficult because of the sylvatic cycle, with forest rodents serving as a reservoir. (See Chapter 30.)

Treatment

No specific antiviral therapy is available. Treatment is directed toward symptomatic relief and management of complications.

Prognosis

The mortality rate is high in the severe form, with death occurring most commonly between the sixth and the tenth days. In survivors, the temperature returns to normal by the seventh or eighth day. The prognosis in any individual case is guarded at the onset, since sudden changes for the worse are common. Intractable hiccups, copious black vomitus, melena, and anuria are unfavorable signs. Convalescence is prolonged, including 1–2 weeks of asthenia.

Martin M et al: Fever and multisystem organ failure associated with 17D-204 yellow fever vaccination: a report of four cases. Lancet. 2001;358:98. [PMID: 11463410] (Rare reports suggest a relationship between vaccine receipt and the development of fever, hepatitis and multiorgan failure.)

Tomori O: Impact of yellow fever on the developing world. Adv Virus Res 1999;53:5. [PMID: 10582093]

Update on yellow fever in the Americas. Epidemiol Bull 2000;21:13. [PMID: 10909207]

5. Colorado Tick Fever

ESSENTIALS OF DIAGNOSIS

- *Onset 1–19 days (average, 4 days) following tick bite.*
- *Fever, chills, myalgia, headache, prostration.*
- *Leukopenia.*
- *Second attack of fever after remission lasting 2–3 days.*

General Considerations

Colorado tick fever is an acute coltivirus infection transmitted by *Dermacentor andersoni* bites. The disease is limited to the western USA and Canada and is most prevalent during the tick season (March to November). The incubation period is 3–6 days.

Clinical Findings

A. SYMPTOMS AND SIGNS

The onset of fever (to 38.9–40.6 °C) is abrupt, sometimes with chills. Severe myalgia, headache, photophobia, anorexia, nausea and vomiting, and generalized weakness are prominent symptoms. Physical findings are limited to an occasional faint rash. Fever continues for 3 days, followed by a remission of 1–3 days and then by a full recrudescence lasting 2–4 days. In an occasional case there may be three bouts of fever.

The differential diagnosis includes influenza, Rocky Mountain spotted fever, numerous other viral infections, and, in the right setting, relapsing fevers.

B. LABORATORY FINDINGS

Leukopenia (2000–3000/µL) with a shift to the left occurs. Viremia may be demonstrated by inoculation of blood into mice or by fluorescent antibody staining of the patient's red cells (with adsorbed virus). Complement-fixing antibodies appear during the third week of disease. A reverse transcriptase PCR assay is used to detect viremia.

Complications

Aseptic meningitis, encephalitis, and hemorrhagic fever occur rarely. Malaise may ensue, but fatalities are very rare.

Treatment

No specific treatment is available. Aspirin or another nonsteroidal anti-inflammatory agent such as codeine or hydrocodone may be given for pain.

Prognosis

The disease is usually self-limited and benign.

Attoui H et al: Serologic and molecular diagnosis of Colorado tick fever viral infections. Am J Trop Med Hyg 1998;59:763. [PMID: 9840594]

COMMON VIRAL RESPIRATORY INFECTIONS

Infections of the respiratory tract are perhaps the most common human ailments. Specific associations of some groups of viruses with certain disease syndromes have been established. In young infants and in the elderly, or in persons with impaired respiratory tract reserve, bacterial superinfection increases morbidity and mortality.

Croup, epiglottitis, and the common cold are discussed in Chapter 8.

Muether PS et al: Variant effect of first- and second-generation antihistamines as clues to their mechanism of action on the sneeze reflex in the common cold. Clin Infect Dis 2001; 33:1483. [PMID: 11588693] (Second generation antihistamines were less effective in blocking sneezing in the common cold.)

Seemungal T et al: Respiratory viruses, symptoms, and inflammatory markers in acute exacerbations and stable chronic obstructive pulmonary disease. Am J Respir Crit Care Med 2001;164:1618. [PMID: 11719299]

1. Respiratory Syncytial Virus

Respiratory syncytial virus (RSV) causes annual outbreaks of pneumonia, bronchiolitis, and tracheobronchitis, with the majority of cases occurring in the very young. Premature infants with bronchopulmonary dysplasia are at highest risk. Incomplete immunity commonly leads to reinfection manifested typically as an upper respiratory tract infection and tracheobronchitis in older children or adults. Serious pulmonary RSV infections have been described in elderly and immunocompromised adults. Outbreaks with a high mortality rate in bone marrow transplant and pediatric liver transplant patients are reported.

Annual epidemics occur in winter and spring. The average incubation period is 5 days. Inoculation may occur through the nose or the eyes.

In bronchiolitis, proliferation and necrosis of bronchiolar epithelium develop, producing obstruction from sloughed epithelium and increased mucus secretion. Signs include low-grade fever, tachypnea, and wheezes. Hyperinflated lungs, decreased gas exchange, and increased work of breathing are present. Otitis media is a frequent complication often with concomitant S pneumoniae infection.

RSV is the only respiratory pathogen that produces its most serious illness at a time when specific maternal antibody is invariably present. This—combined with the observation that infants who received a particular past live RSV vaccine had more severe disease—suggests an immune-mediated component to the disease.

Rapid diagnosis may be made by viral antigen identification of nasal washings using an ELISA or immunofluorescent assay. Culture of nasopharyngeal secretions remains the standard of diagnosis.

Treatment consists of hydration, humidification of inspired air, and ventilatory support as needed. While bronchodilating agents, ribavirin, and corticosteroids are widely used, evidence supporting their effectiveness in populations not at high risk is lacking. Pregnant women should avoid ribavirin exposure—and indeed, patients with upper respiratory RSV infections probably do not need ribavirin. Hyperimmune RSV immunoglobulin G (1500 mg/kg) is effective in combination with ribavirin in the management of RSV infections among immunocompromised adults; its role in the treatment of children with lower respiratory tract infections remains under study.

Given the high morbidity in certain infant subgroups, efforts have been made to develop preventive agents. At present, RSV immune globulin is being replaced with palivizumab, a monoclonal RSV antibody. The FDA recommends the administration of palivizumab prophylactically to infants with high-risk factors such as prematurity, bronchopulmonary dysplasia, and congenital heart disease. The search for an effective vaccine is ongoing. Because nosocomial RSV infections disseminate rapidly, prevention in hospitals entails rapid diagnosis, hand washing, and perhaps passive immunization.

Hall CB: Respiratory syncytial virus and parainfluenza virus. N Engl J Med 2001;344:1917. [PMID: 11419430]

Panitch HB: Bronchiolitis in infants. Curr Opin Pediatr 2001;13:256. [PMID: 11389361] (Therapeutic options.)

Randolph AT et al: Ribavirin for respiratory syncytial virus infection of the lower respiratory tract. Cochrane Database Syst Rev 2000;CD000181. [PMID: 10796503] (Ribavirin may reduce the length of ventilator support and the number of days of hospitalization.)

Sorrentino M et al: Effectiveness of palivizumab: evaluation of outcomes from the 1998 to 1999 respiratory syncytial virus season. The Palivizumab Outcomes Study Group. Pediatr Infect Dis J 2000;19:1068. [PMID: 11099087] (Recipients of palivizumab had a low admission rate [2.3%] for RSV infections.)

Walsh EE et al: Respiratory syncytial and other virus infection in persons with chronic cardiopulmonary disease. Am J Respir Crit Care Med 1999;160:791. [PMID: 10471598] (Respiratory syncytial virus aggravated the pulmonary status during the winter among patients with cardiopulmonary disease.)

2. Influenza

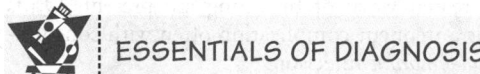

ESSENTIALS OF DIAGNOSIS

- Cases usually in epidemic pattern, not sporadic.
- Abrupt onset with fever, chills, malaise, cough, coryza, and muscle aches.
- Aching, fever, and prostration out of proportion to catarrhal symptoms.
- Leukopenia.

General Considerations

Influenza (an orthomyxovirus) is transmitted by the respiratory route. In contrast to RSV and rhinoviruses, transmission occurs by droplet nuclei rather than fomites or large particle aerosols. Although sporadic cases occur, epidemics and pandemics appear at varying intervals, usually in the fall or winter. Antigenic types A and B produce clinically indistinguishable infections, whereas type C is usually a minor illness. New epidemic strains may evolve from reassortment, through pig vectors, between avian and human strains. Pandemics—associated with higher mortality—typically are associated with type A infections in which significant genetic recombination of the virus (antigenic shift) has taken place. The incubation period is 1–4 days.

A small number of human cases of a new strain of avian influenza A (H5N1) were reported from Hong Kong in December 1997. Surveillance suggested that the highest risk for disease occurred among those with poultry exposure, though person-to-person transmission was not fully excluded. A massive poultry slaughter ensued based on these findings. The continued surveillance for future potentially pandemic strains is an important aspect of influenza control.

It is difficult to diagnose influenza in the absence of an epidemic. The disease resembles many other mild febrile illnesses but is almost always accompanied by a cough. Influenza A (H3N2) has been the dominating strain for three consecutive seasons (1997–1999), but for the 2000–2001 season the dominating strain was H1N1.

Clinical Findings

A. Symptoms and Signs

The onset is usually abrupt, with fever, chills, malaise, muscular aching, substernal soreness, headache, nasal stuffiness, and occasionally nausea. Fever lasts 1–7 days (usually 3–5). Coryza, nonproductive cough, and sore throat are present. Signs include mild pharyngeal injection, flushed face, and conjunctival redness.

B. Laboratory Findings

Leukopenia is common. Proteinuria may be present. The virus may be isolated from the throat washings by inoculation of embryonated eggs or cell cultures. Complement-fixing and hemagglutination-inhibiting antibodies appear during the second week.

Complications

Influenza causes necrosis of the respiratory epithelium, which predisposes to secondary bacterial infections. The interactions between bacteria and influenza are bidirectional, with bacterial enzymes (eg, proteases, trypsin-like compounds, streptokinase, plasminogen) activating influenza viruses. Frequent complications are acute sinusitis, otitis media, purulent bronchitis, and pneumonia. The elderly and the chronically ill are at high risk for complications. Rhabdomyolysis is a rare complication.

Pneumonia is commonly due to bacterial infection with pneumococci or, less often, staphylococci or haemophilus or, on occasion, the influenza virus itself. Pericarditis, myocarditis, and thrombophlebitis sometimes occur.

Reye's syndrome (fatty liver with encephalopathy) is a rare and severe complication of influenza and other viral diseases (eg, varicella), particularly in young children. It consists of rapidly progressive hepatic failure and encephalopathy, and there is a 30% fatality rate. The pathogenesis is unknown, but the syndrome is associated with aspirin use in such viral infections. Hypoglycemia, elevation of serum aminotransferases and blood ammonia, prolonged prothrombin time, and change in mental status all occur within 2–3 weeks after onset of the viral infection. Histologically, the periphery of liver lobules shows striking fatty infiltration and glycogen depletion. Treatment is supportive and directed toward the management of cerebral edema.

Prevention

Trivalent influenza virus vaccine provides partial immunity (about 85% efficacy) for a few months to 1 year. The vaccine's antigenic configuration changes yearly and is based on prevalent strains of the preceding year. Vaccination in October or November each year is recommended for persons over 50 (a substantial portion of the older population suffer from at least one chronic medical condition), children (over 6 months of age) and teenagers receiving chronic aspirin therapy, nursing home residents, patients with chronic lung or heart disease or other debilitating illnesses (including pregnant women during the second and third trimesters), and health care workers. The vaccine is contraindicated in persons with hypersensitivity to chicken eggs or other components of the vaccine, persons with an acute febrile illness, or thrombocytopenia. Concomitant warfarin or corticosteroid therapy is not a contraindication. Side effects are infrequent and include tenderness, redness, or induration at the site of the injection and, rarely, myalgias or fever.

Adequate immunity is achieved about 2 weeks after vaccination. In healthy subjects, the antibody level remains sufficiently high throughout the season. Levels wane quickly, however, in elderly nursing home patients. Therefore, the vaccine should not be administered too early in the influenza season. The vaccination effectively reduces both morbidity (preventing 35–60% of hospital admissions in the elderly) and mortality (preventing 35–80% of hospital deaths). A live attenuated vaccine has been widely used among Russian adults.

HIV-infected persons can be safely vaccinated, and concerns about activating replication of the HIV virus by the immunogen appear to be exaggerated and may be less severe than the increase in HIV viral load associated with a full influenza infection. Vaccination is less effective when CD4 counts are less than 100/μL. False-positive assays with HIV, HTLV-1, and HCV are reported in the wake of influenza vaccination.

Chemoprophylaxis for epidemiologically or virologically confirmed influenza A with amantadine hydrochloride, 200 mg/d orally in two divided doses (100 mg/d in the elderly, who are susceptible to central nervous system side effects), or rimantadine (200 mg/d in two divided doses) will markedly reduce the attack rate among exposed unvaccinated individuals if begun immediately and continued for 10 days. Amantadine or rimantadine may also be used during an outbreak while waiting for immunity to develop following vaccination. While the widespread use of antiviral agents as chemoprophylaxis is not usually recommended, recent data suggest that oseltamivir in a dosage of 75 mg daily lowers the contact rate among household contacts of influenza cases.

Treatment

Many patients with influenza prefer to rest in bed. Analgesics and a cough mixture may be used. Amantadine or rimantadine, in the same doses as are used for prophylaxis, appreciably decrease the duration of symptoms and signs. Rimantadine is preferred in patients with renal failure. The clinical significance of resistance to antiviral agents is controversial. Ribavirin (1.1 g/d, diluted to 20 mg/mL and delivered as particulate aerosol with oxygen over 12–18 hours a day for 3–7 days; [Table 32–1]) helps severely ill patients with influenza A or B. The new neuraminidase inhibitors, either inhaled zanamivir (two 5-mg inhalations twice daily for 5 days) or oral oseltamivir (75 mg twice daily for 5 days), are equally helpful in the treatment of influenza but are more costly. These agents are given only to patients over age 12 and only when symptoms are present for under 48 hours.

Antibacterial antibiotics should be reserved for treatment of bacterial complications. Acetaminophen rather than aspirin should be used for fever in children.

Prognosis

The duration of the uncomplicated illness is 1–7 days, and the prognosis is excellent. Purulent bronchitis and bronchiectasis may result in chronic pulmonary disease and fibrosis that persist throughout life. Most fatalities are due to bacterial pneumonia. Influenzal pneumonia has a high mortality rate among pregnant women and persons with a history of rheumatic heart disease. In recent epidemics, the mortality rate has been low except in debilitated individuals.

If the fever persists for more than 4 days with productive cough and white cell count over 10,000/μL, secondary bacterial infection should be suspected. Pneumococcal pneumonia is the most common such infection, and staphylococcal pneumonia is the most serious.

Bridges CB et al: Prevention and control of influenza. Recommendations of the Advisory Committee on Immunization Practices (ACIP). MMWR Recomm Rep 2001;50(RR-4):1. [PMID: 11334444] (The optimal period for immunization is extended through November.)

Couch RB: Influenza: prospects for control. Ann Intern Med 2000;133:992. [PMID: 11119401] (An overview of current preventive and treatment options and new developments.)

Demicheli V et al: Prevention and early treatment of influenza in healthy adults. Vaccine 2000;18:057. [PMID: 10590322] (The authors, reviewing as members of the Cochrane Collaboration, find that routine vaccination of healthy adults aged 15–64 is not warranted.)

Laver G et al: The origin and control of pandemic influenza. Science 2001;293:1776. [PMID: 11546857] (Two articles and two reviews in this issue [No. 5536] of Science discuss the molecular basis for the sudden emergence of Spanish flu and avian flu.)

Mossad SB: Underused options for preventing and treating influenza. Cleve Clin J Med 1999;66:19. [PMID: 9926627] (Influenza vaccine is the most effective preventive measure but is greatly underused.)

Neuzil KM et al: Influenza vaccine: issues and opportunities. Infect Dis Clin North Am 2001;15:123, ix. [PMID: 11301811]

Sandhu SK et al: Influenza in the older adult. Indications for the use of vaccine and antiviral therapy. Geriatrics 2001;54:43. [PMID: 11196338].

Welliver R et al: Effectiveness of oseltamivir in preventing influenza in household contacts: a randomized controlled trial. JAMA 2001;285:748. [PMID: 11176912] (Randomized controlled trial showing that oseltamivir, 75 mg daily for 7 days, was effective preventive therapy among household contacts aged 12 or over.)

ADENOVIRUS INFECTIONS

Adenoviruses (there are over 40 antigenic types) produce a variety of clinical syndromes. These infections are usually self-limited or clinically inapparent and most common among infants, young children, and military recruits. Outbreaks in liver, bone marrow, and renal transplant recipients have been reported, and dissemination may occur. The incubation period is 4–9 days. Adenoviruses, although a common cause of human disease, have also received particular recognition through their role in gene therapy.

Clinical syndromes of adenovirus infection, often overlapping, include the following:

(1) The common cold (see Chapter 8) is characterized by rhinitis, pharyngitis, and mild malaise without fever.

(2) Nonstreptococcal exudative pharyngitis is characterized by fever lasting 2–12 days and accompanied by malaise and myalgia. Sore throat is often manifested by diffuse injection, a patchy exudate, and cervical lymphadenopathy. Cough is sometimes accompanied by rales and x-ray evidence of pneumonitis. Conjunctivitis is often present.

(3) Lower respiratory tract infection may occur, including bronchiolitis, suggested by cough and rales, or pneumonia (type 3 and type 7 commonly cause acute respiratory disease and pneumonia).

(4) Pharyngoconjunctival fever is manifested by fever and malaise, conjunctivitis (often unilateral), and mild pharyngitis.

(5) Epidemic keratoconjunctivitis (transmissible person-to-person) occurs in adults and is manifested by unilateral conjunctival redness, pain, tearing, and an enlarged preauricular lymph node. Keratitis may lead to subepithelial opacities (especially with types 8, 19, or 37).

(6) Acute hemorrhagic cystitis is a disorder of children often associated with adenovirus type 11.

(7) Sexually transmitted genitourinary ulcers and urethritis may be caused by types 2, 8, and 37 in particular.

(8) Adenoviruses also cause acute gastroenteritis (types 40, 41), leading to intussusception, and are rarely associated with encephalitis and pericarditis.

Infected liver transplant recipients tend to develop hepatitis (type 5 adenovirus), whereas bone marrow and renal transplant recipients tend to develop pneumonia or hemorrhagic cystitis. Ribavirin is used in immunocompromised individuals with little success.

Vaccines are not available for general use. Live oral vaccines containing attenuated type 4 and type 7 are used in military personnel.

Treatment is symptomatic, though there is increasing interest in the use of cidofovir, especially in the immunocompromised.

Echavarria M et al: Prediction of severe disseminated adenovirus infection by serum PCR. Lancet 2001;358:384. [PMID: 11502321] (PCR assays are used to predict the development of severe disease.)

La Rosa AM: Adenovirus infections in adult recipients of blood and marrow transplants. Clin Infect Dis 2001;32:871. [PMID: 11247710] (Review of 85 cases at M.D. Anderson with 26% mortality and no response to ribavarin.)

OTHER EXANTHEMATOUS VIRAL INFECTIONS

1. Parvovirus Infections

Parvovirus B19 causes several syndromes. In children, an exanthematous illness ("fifth disease," erythema infectiosum) is characterized by fiery red "slapped cheek," circumoral pallor, and a subsequent lacy, maculopapular, evanescent truncal rash. Malaise, headache, and pruritus occur, but little fever. In immunosuppressed patients, including those with HIV infection, or post transplantation, or with hematologic conditions such as sickle cell disease, anemia due to red cell hypoplasia occurs as a consequence of binding to erythrocyte P antigen (globoside). Middle-aged persons (especially women) develop a symmetric polyarthritis that mimics lupus erythematosus and rheumatoid arthritis, preferentially involving the proximal interphalangeal joints of the hands and the wrists and knees. Arthralgias are uncommon in children. Rashes, especially facial, are uncommon in adults. Hepatitis may occur. In pregnancy, fetal loss and hydrops fetalis have been reported. An association with Henoch-Schönlein purpura has also been noted.

The diagnosis is clinical (Table 32–2) but may be confirmed by an elevated titer of IgM anti-parvovirus antibodies in serum. Scarlet fever is the most similar disorder. Arthritis with hypocomplementemia is a common complication in some outbreaks. Increasing attention is being directed toward the role of parvovirus in causing hydrops fetalis and fetal demise. Uncommon complications of infection include encephalitis, chronic hemolytic anemia, thrombotic thrombocytopenic purpuric syndrome, acute postinfectious glomerulonephritis, and hepatitis.

Treatment in healthy persons is symptomatic. NSAIDs can be used to treat arthralgias and transfusions to treat transient aplastic crises. In immunosuppressed patients, intravenous immunoglobulin aids in treatment.

Screening of donated blood could potentially prevent transfusion-related infection. Several nosocomial outbreaks have been documented, and hospital infection control personnel should administer standard containment guidelines, including hand washing after patient exposure and avoiding contact with pregnant women.

The prognosis is generally excellent in immunocompetent individuals. In immunosuppressed patients, persistent anemia may require continued transfusions and periodic evaluations. Remission of parvovirus infection in AIDS patients may occur with HAART.

Brennand JE et al: Human parvovirus B19 in pregnancy. Hosp Med 2000 (Feb);61:93. [PMID: 10748785]

Kerr JR: Pathogenesis of human parvovirus B19 in rheumatic disease. Ann Rheum Dis 2000;59:672. [PMID: 10976079]

Scroggie DA et al: Parvovirus arthropathy outbreak in southwestern United States. J Rheumatol 2000;27:2444. [PMID: 11036842] (Slightly over half of the patients showed an acute symmetric arthritis, the remainder migratory.)

Tolfvenstam T et al: Frequency of parvovirus B19 infection in intrauterine fetal death. Lancet 2001;357:1494. [PMID: 11377602]

2. Poxvirus Infections

Among the nine poxviruses causing disease in humans, the following are clinically important.

(1) **Variola:** Smallpox was a highly contagious disease characterized by severe headache, fever, and prostration and accompanied by a centrifugal rash developing in order of progression from macules to papules to vesicles to pustules. An international consensus among the scientific community in the 1990s resulted in a recommendation to destroy the virus since elimination of the disease had been achieved. As long as this recommendation is not implemented, there remains a risk of unauthorized access to the remaining samples and potential misuse for military or terrorist purposes, resulting in exposure of a large unvaccinated civilian population.

In the wake of the September 11, 2001 terrorism incidents, there exists a growing concern about the potential use of smallpox and other agents as biologic weapons. Most physicians in practice today have never seen a case of smallpox. The disseminated lesions of smallpox in the past were often confused with those of varicella, though the synchronous progression in smallpox readily distinguishes these lesions from those of varicella, wherein lesions of several stages are usually present simultaneously.

(2) **Molluscum contagiosum** may be transmitted sexually or by other close contact. It is manifested by pearly, raised, umbilicated skin nodules sparing the palms and soles. Marked and persistent lesions in AIDS patients appear to respond readily to combination antiretroviral therapy. The many anecdotal agents reported to hasten resolution include cimetidine and CO_2 laser therapy combined with natural interferon-beta gel. One percent imiquimod cream appeared to be effective in curing molluscum lesions.

(3) **Vaccinia:** Vaccination with vaccinia was responsible in part for smallpox eradication. Civilian vaccination is indicated only for laboratory workers who must handle virus. Vaccination is still practiced among some military forces but is not required for any international travel; it is effective in prevention of monkeypox (see below). Any form of immunosuppression is an absolute contraindication to smallpox vaccination. Eczema (or a history of it) in a patient or family member, other forms of dermatitis, and burns also contraindicate vaccination. While there is no current public indication for the therapeutic use of smallpox vaccine, if smallpox is used as a biologic weapon in the future, this recommendation may change. Efforts are under way to expand the availability of vaccine stores by use of dilution techniques of existing stocks.

(4) **Orf** (contagious pustular dermatitis or ecthyma contagiosa) and **paravaccinia** (milkers' nodules) are occupational diseases acquired by contact with sheep and cattle, respectively.

(5) **Monkeypox,** first identified in 1970, is enzootic in the rain forests of equatorial Africa and presents in humans with a syndrome similar to smallpox; case fatalities are about 3% (to 11% among the unvaccinated), and secondary attack rates, which are hard to determine because of diagnostic confusion with varicella in older series, appear to be about 10%. Primary prevention entails the use of vaccinia immunization, a procedure accompanied by a risk of dissemination in HIV-infected persons—a real concern considering the coincident areas of endemicity of HIV-1 and monkeypox.

Henderson DA: Countering the posteradication threat of smallpox and polio. Clin Infect Dis 2002;34:79. [PMID: 11731949]

Heymann DL et al: Re-emergence of monkeypox in Africa: a review of the past six years. Br Med Bull 1998;54:693. [PMID: 10326294] (The authors postulate that the termination of vaccinia vaccination after smallpox elimination may have increased the number of susceptibles and allowed this outbreak to emerge.)

VIRUSES & GASTROENTERITIS

Viruses are responsible for probably 30–40% of cases of infectious diarrhea in the USA, and rotaviruses are a leading worldwide cause of dehydrating gastroenteritis in young children. The agents that can cause disease include group B rotaviruses, Norwalk agent (which causes epidemics of vomiting and diarrhea and is often transmitted by food—especially shellfish—and water), and other caliciviruses, astroviruses, and enteric adenoviruses.

Rotaviruses (G1–G4 and G9 are the most common serotypes) are a major cause of diarrheal morbidity worldwide (due to dehydration) and can also cause infections in adults exposed to infected infants and are ubiquitous in the environment of an outbreak. (Secondary rates are between 16% and 30%.) The disease is usually mild, and cases also occur among travelers, in epidemic fashion, and after waterborne exposure. Sensitive and specific immunoassays to detect viral RNA in fecal specimens are available. Treatment is symptomatic, with fluid and electrolyte replacement.

The **Norwalk virus** was first identified using electron microscopy on infectious stool infiltrate derived from an outbreak of gastroenteritis at a school in Norwalk, Ohio. This virus and the related **Norwalk-like caliciviruses** are responsible for over 40% of cases of group-related and institutional outbreaks of diarrhea.

Norwalk virus is also often responsible for military outbreaks. While transmission is usually fecal-oral, airborne transmission is also documented. Infections appear to be more common during cold weather intervals. Symptoms include, in particular, nausea and vomiting. While a developed ELISA can detect the agent in stool samples and PCR assays are becoming increasingly available, the use of such assays remains restricted to the research laboratory. Treatment is largely symptomatic.

Atmar RL et al: Diagnosis of noncultivatable gastroenteritis viruses, the human caliciviruses. Clin Microbiol Rev 2001;14:15. [PMID: 11148001] (A review of the current status of diagnostic antigen and antibody assays.)

Dennehy PH et al: Rotavirus vaccine and intussusception. Where do we go from here? Infect Dis Clin North Am 2001;15:189, x.

Estes MK et al: Norwalk virus vaccines: challenges and progress. J Infect Dis 2000;181(Suppl 2):S367. [PMID: 10804150] (These viruses are excellent models for the study of human mucosal immunity.)

Kapikian AZ: The discovery of the 27-nm Norwalk virus: an historic perspective. J Infect Dis 2000;181(Suppl 2):S295. [PMID: 10804141] (This is one of the smaller viruses discovered; its size, indistinct morphology, and low concentration all complicated the original isolation.)

Kombo LA et al: Intussusception, infection, and immunization: summary of a workshop on rotavirus. Pediatrics 2001;108:E37. [PMID: 11483847] (Withdrawal of the rotavirus vaccine because of the association with intussusception has global public health implications.)

Lundgren O et al: Role of the enteric nervous system in the fluid and electrolyte secretion of rotavirus diarrhea. Science 2000;287:491. [PMID: 10642552]

Murphy TV et al: Intussusception among infants given an oral rotavirus vaccine. N Engl J Med 2001;344:564. [PMID: 11207352].

Weijer C: The future of research into rotavirus vaccine. BMJ 2000;321:525. [PMID: 10968800]

VIRUSES THAT PRODUCE SEVERAL SYNDROMES

1. Coxsackievirus Infections

Coxsackievirus infections cause several clinical syndromes. As with other enteroviruses, infections are most common during the summer. Two groups, A and B, are defined either serologically or by mouse bioassay. There are more than 50 serotypes.

Clinical Findings

A. SYMPTOMS AND SIGNS

The clinical syndromes associated with coxsackievirus infection may be described briefly as follows:

1. Summer grippe (A and B)—A febrile illness, principally of children, lasting 1–4 days. Minor symptoms and respiratory tract infection are often present.

2. Herpangina (A2–6, 10)—Sudden onset of fever, which may be as high as 40.6 °C, sometimes with febrile convulsions; headache, myalgia, vomiting; and sore throat, characterized early by petechiae or papules on the soft palate that become shallow ulcers in about 3 days and then heal.

3. Epidemic pleurodynia (Bornholm disease) (B1–5)—Pleuritic pain is prominent, and tenderness, hyperesthesia, and muscle swelling are present over the area of diaphragmatic attachment. Other findings include headache, sore throat, malaise, and nausea. Orchitis and aseptic meningitis are uncommon manifestations.

4. Aseptic meningitis (A and B) and other neurologic syndromes—Fever, headache, nausea, vomiting, stiff neck, drowsiness, and cerebrospinal fluid lymphocytosis without chemical abnormalities may occur, and pediatric clusters of group B meningitis are reported. Focal encephalitis, transverse myelitis, and acute flaccid paralysis are reported with coxsackievirus group A and a disseminated encephalitis after group B infection.

5. Acute nonspecific pericarditis (B types)—Sudden onset of anterior chest pain, often worse with inspiration and in the supine position, is typical. Fever, myalgia, headache, and pericardial friction rub appear early; evidence for pericardial effusion on imaging studies is often present, and the occasional patient has a paradoxic pulse. Electrocardiographic evidence of pericarditis is often present. Relapses may occur.

6. Myocarditis (B1–5)—Heart failure in the neonatal period secondary to in utero myocarditis and over 20% of adult cases of myocarditis and dilated cardiomyopathy are possibly associated with group B infections.

7. Hand, foot, and mouth disease (A5, 10, 16)—Sometimes epidemic and characterized by stomatitis and a vesicular rash on hands and feet. Enterovirus 71 is also a causative agent.

8. Hepatitis (B1)—Fulminant neonatal hepatitis with thrombocytopenia and coagulopathy occur rarely.

9. Type 1 diabetes mellitus (B types)—An association purportedly exists between coxsackievirus B infections and subsequent development of type 1 diabetes mellitus.

10. Glomerulopathy and tubular injury—Renal damage was recently reported with several group B infections.

B. LABORATORY FINDINGS

Routine laboratory studies show no characteristic abnormalities. Neutralizing antibodies appear during convalescence. The virus may be isolated from throat washings or stools inoculated into suckling mice.

Treatment & Prognosis

Treatment is symptomatic. With the exception of myocarditis, pericarditis, perhaps diabetes, and rare illnesses such as pancreatitis or polio-like syndrome, the syndromes caused by coxsackieviruses are benign and self-limited. There are anecdotal reports of success with intravenous immunoglobulin in severe disease.

Chaves SS et al: Coxsackie virus A24 infection presenting as acute flaccid paralysis. Lancet 2001;357:605. [PMID: 11558489]

Hoi-shan Chan S et al: Ventricular aneurysm complicating neonatal coxsackie B4 myocarditis. Pediatr Cardiol 2001;22:247. [PMID: 11343155]

2. Echovirus Infections

Echoviruses are enteroviruses that produce several clinical syndromes, particularly in children. Infection is most common during summer.

Over 30 serotypes have been demonstrated. Most cause aseptic meningitis, which may be associated with a rubelliform rash. Type 30 outbreaks have been reported from Japan, France, Germany, and Canada (Saskatchewan) while an increased number of type 13 cases occurred in the United States recently. Diseases associated with echoviruses range from common respiratory diseases and epidemic diarrhea (including type 22) to myocarditis, a hemorrhagic obstetric syndrome, keratoconjunctivitis, leukocytoclastic vasculitis, and neonatal as well as adult cases of encephalitis and sepsis to myocarditis, encephalitis, and septic shock.

As with other enterovirus infections, diagnosis is best established by correlation of clinical, epidemiologic, and laboratory evidence. Cytopathic effects are produced in tissue culture after recovery of virus from throat washings, blood, or cerebrospinal fluid. PCR of the cerebrospinal fluid may be diagnostic. Fourfold or greater rises in antibody titer signify systemic infection.

Treatment is usually symptomatic, and the prognosis is excellent, though there are reports of mild paralysis after central nervous system infection. Hand washing is an effective control measure in outbreaks of aseptic meningitis.

Starlin R et al: Acute flaccid paralysis syndrome associated with echovirus 19, managed with pleconaril and intravenous immunoglobulin. Clin Infect Dis 2001;33:730. [PMID: 11477532]

3. Enteroviruses 70 & 71

Several clinical syndromes are being described in association with newer enteroviruses. The most common of these are **enterovirus 70,** associated with **acute hemorrhagic conjunctivitis,** a ubiquitous agent first identified in 1969 and responsible for abrupt bilateral eye discharge and occasional systemic symptoms, but in most cases subconjunctival hemorrhage; and **enterovirus 71,** associated with **hand, foot, and mouth disease** as well as a form of **epidemic encephalitis,** most recently in children from East and Southeast Asia. Diagnosis of both entities is facilitated by the clinical and epidemiologic findings with the isolation of the suspect agent from either conjunctival scraping for enterovirus 70 or vesicle swabs, body secretions, or cerebrospinal fluid for enterovirus 71.

Treatment of both entities remains largely symptomatic, though there are increasing reports of the successful use of pleconaril, an agent available in some countries but not the United States. The major complication associated with enterovirus 70 is the development in a small percentage of cases of an acute neurologic illness with motor paralysis akin to poliomyelitis.

Enterovirus 72 is another term for hepatitis A virus (see Chapter 15).

Buxbaum S et al: Enterovirus infections in Germany: comparative evaluation of different laboratory diagnostic methods. Infection 2001;29:138. [PMID: 11440383] (Viral isolation or PCR was superior to serologies for diagnosis.)

Robart HA et al: Treatment of potentially life-threatening enterovirus infections with pleconaril. Clin Infect Dis 2001;32:228. [PMID: 11170912]

■ II. RICKETTSIAL DISEASES

The rickettsioses are febrile exanthematous diseases caused by rickettsiae, small gram-negative obligate intracellular bacteria. In arthropods, rickettsiae grow in the gut lining, often without harming the host. Human infection results from either an arthropod bite or contamination with its feces. In humans, rickettsiae grow principally in endothelial cells of small blood vessels, producing vasculitis, cell necrosis, thrombosis of vessels, skin rashes, and organ dysfunctions.

Different rickettsiae and their vectors are endemic in different parts of the world, but two or more types may coexist in the same geographic area. New organisms are identified regularly. A summary of epidemiologic features is given in Table 32–3. The clinical picture is variable but usually includes a prodromal stage followed by fever, rash, and prostration. Isolation of rickettsiae from the patient is difficult and potentially hazardous to laboratory workers. Diagnosis is usually based on clinical examination and epidemiologic evidence. Laboratory diagnosis relies on the development of specific antibodies detected by complement fixation (for diagnosis), immunofluorescence, or hemagglutination (for species identification) tests. Other newer

Table 32–3. Rickettsial diseases.

Disease	Rickettsial Pathogen	Geographic Areas of Prevalence	Insect Vector	Mammalian Reservoir
Typhus group				
Epidemic (louse-borne) typhus	*Rickettsia prowazekii*	South America, Africa, Asia, North America	Louse	Humans, flying squirrels
California flea rickettsiosis	*Rickettsia felis*	Southern California, Texas	Flea	Cats, opossums
Endemic (murine) typhus	*Rickettsia typhi*	Worldwide; small foci (USA: southeastern Gulf Coast)	Flea	Rodents
Scrub typhus	*Orientia tsutsugamushi*	Southeast Asia, Japan, Australia	Mite[1]	Rodents
Spotted fever group				
Rocky Mountain spotted fever	*Rickettsia rickettsii*	Western Hemisphere; USA (especially mid-Atlantic coast region)	Tick[1]	Rodents, dogs
Boutonneuse fever, Kenya tick typhus, South African tick fever, Indian tick typhus	*Rickettsia conorii*	Africa, India, Mediterranean regions	Tick[1]	Rodents, dogs
Queensland tick typhus	*Rickettsia australis*	Australia	Tick[1]	Rodents, marsupials
North Asian tick typhus	*Rickettsia sibirica*	Siberia, Mongolia	Tick[1]	Rodents
Rickettsialpox	*Rickettsia akari*	USA, Korea, former USSR	Mite[1]	Mice
RMSF-like	*Rickettsia canada*	North America	Tick[1]	Rodents
Other				
Ehrlichiosis				
Human monocytic	*Ehrlichia chaffeensis*	Southeastern USA	Tick[1]	Dogs
granulocytic	Organisms related to *Ehrlichia phago-cytophila*, *Ehrlichia equi*	Northeastern USA	Tick[1]	Rodents, deer, sheep
Q fever	*Coxiella burnetii*	Worldwide	None[2]	Cattle, sheep, goats

[1]Also serve as arthropod reservoir by maintaining rickettsiae through transovarian transmission.
[2]Human infection results from inhalation of dust.

means of isolation are the centrifugation shell-vial technique and PCR.

Prevention & Treatment

Preventive measures are directed at control of the vector, and avoidance of exposure by use of repellents and protective clothing. A search of body surfaces should be conducted after potential exposure and the vector (louse, tick, or mite) gently removed. Many patients do not recall exposure to a vector.

Rickettsiae can be inhibited by tetracyclines or chloramphenicol. All early infections respond to treatment with these drugs. Dosage schedules are listed below.

Parola P et al: Ticks and tickborne bacterial diseases in humans: An emerging infectious threat. Clin Infect Dis 2001;32:897. [PMID: 11247714]

TYPHUS GROUP

1. Epidemic Louse-Borne Typhus

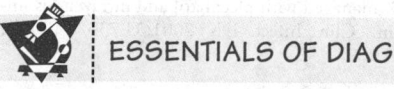

ESSENTIALS OF DIAGNOSIS

- *Prodrome of headache, then chills and fever.*
- *Severe, intractable headaches, prostration, persisting high fever.*

- Macular rash appearing on the fourth to seventh days on the trunk and in the axillae, spreading to the rest of the body but sparing the face, palms, and soles.
- Diagnosis confirmed by specific antibodies using complement fixation, microagglutination, or immunofluorescence.

General Considerations

Epidemic louse-borne typhus is due to infection with *Rickettsia prowazekii*, a parasite of the body louse that ultimately kills the louse. Transmission is favored by crowded living conditions, famine, war, or any circumstances that predispose to heavy infestation with lice. When the louse sucks the blood of a person infected with *R prowazekii*, the organism becomes established in the gut of the louse and grows there. When the louse is transmitted to another person (through contact or clothing) and has a blood meal, it defecates simultaneously, and the infected feces are rubbed into the itching bite wound. Dry, infectious louse feces may also enter the respiratory tract.

In a person who recovers from clinical or subclinical typhus infection, *R prowazekii* may survive in lymphoid tissues. Years later, there may be a recrudescence of disease (Brill's disease) without exposure to infected lice.

Mild and atypical cases of *R prowazekii* have rarely occurred in the USA after contact with flying squirrels or their ectoparasites or decades following exposure (eg, among concentration camp victims of World War II). Cases can be acquired by travel to pockets of infection (eg, central and northeastern Africa).

Clinical Findings

A. SYMPTOMS AND SIGNS

(Table 32–3.) Prodromal malaise, cough, headache, backache, arthralgia, and chest pain begin after an incubation period of 10–14 days, followed by an abrupt onset of chills, high fever, and prostration, with flu-like symptoms progressing to delirium and stupor. The headache is severe, the fever prolonged.

Other findings consist of conjunctivitis, hearing loss from neuropathy of the eighth cranial nerve, flushed facies, rales at the lung bases, and often splenomegaly. A macular rash (that may become confluent) appears first in the axillas and then over the trunk, spreading to the extremities but rarely involving the face, palms, or soles. In severely ill patients, the rash becomes hemorrhagic, and hypotension becomes marked. There may be renal insufficiency, stupor, and delirium. In spontaneous recovery, improvement begins 13–16 days after onset with rapid drop of fever.

B. LABORATORY FINDINGS

The white blood cell count is variable. Proteinuria and hematuria commonly occur. Serum obtained 5–12 days after onset of symptoms usually shows specific antibodies for *R prowazekii* antigens as demonstrated by complement fixation, microagglutination, or immunofluorescence. In primary rickettsial infection, early antibodies are IgM; in recrudescence (Brill's disease), early antibodies are predominantly IgG.

C. IMAGING

Radiographs of the chest may show patchy consolidation.

Differential Diagnosis

The prodromal symptoms and the early febrile stage are not specific enough to permit diagnosis in nonepidemic situations. The rash is usually sufficiently distinctive for diagnosis, but it may be absent in up to 10% of cases or may be difficult to observe in dark-skinned persons. A variety of other acute febrile diseases should be considered, including typhoid fever, meningococcemia, and measles.

Brill's disease (recrudescent epidemic typhus) has a more gradual onset than primary *R prowazekii* infection, fever and rash are of shorter duration, and the disease is milder and rarely fatal.

Complications

Pneumonia, thromboses, vasculitis with major vessel obstruction and gangrene, circulatory collapse, myocarditis, and uremia may occur.

Prevention

Prevention consists of louse control with insecticides, particularly by applying chemicals to clothing or treating it with heat, and frequent bathing. A deloused and bathed typhus patient is not infectious. The disease is not transmitted from person to person. Patients are infective for the lice during the febrile period and perhaps 2–3 days after the fever returns to normal. Infected lice pass rickettsiae in their feces within 2–6 days after the blood meal and can be infective earlier if crushed. Rickettsiae remain viable in a dead louse for weeks.

Immunization with vaccines consisting of inactivated egg-grown *R prowazekii* gives some protection to laboratory personnel, physicians, or field workers who are exposed to the parasite. This vaccine is not currently commercially available in the USA or Canada. An improved cell culture vaccine is being developed.

Treatment

Treatment consists of either tetracycline (25 mg/kg/d in four divided doses) or chloramphenicol (50–100 mg/kg/d in four divided doses) for 4–10 days.

Prognosis

The prognosis depends greatly upon age and immunization status. In children under age 10, the disease is usually mild. The mortality rate is 10% in the second and third decades but in the past reached 60% in the sixth decade. Effective vaccination can convert a potentially serious disease into a mild one.

Andersson JO et al: A century of typhus, lice and Rickettsia. Res Microbiol 2000;151:143. [PMID: 10865960]

Massung RF et al: Epidemic typhus meningitis in the southwestern United States. Clin Infect Dis 2001;32:979. [PMID: 11247722] (Describes the use of PCR to diagnose epidemic typhus in a patient in Texas.)

Raoult D et al: The body louse as a vector of reemerging human diseases. Clin Infect Dis 1999;29:888. [PMID: 10589908] (A description of pathogens and epidemics associated with the body louse, *Pediculus humanus humanus*.)

Raoult D et al: Outbreak of epidemic typhus associated with trench fever in Burundi. Lancet 1998;352:353. [PMID: 9717922] (A massive outbreak occurred at high altitudes in refugee camps of east Africa.)

2. Endemic Flea-Borne Typhus (Murine Typhus)

Rickettsia typhi, a ubiquitous pathogen, is transmitted from rat to rat through the rat flea. Humans usually acquire the infection in an urban or suburban setting when bitten by an infected flea, which releases infected feces while sucking blood. Rare cases in the developed world follow travel, usually to Southeast Asia. A second causative agent, *R felis*, has been linked to the cat flea and opossum exposures. Most cases in the USA are reported from southern Texas and California.

Endemic typhus resembles recrudescent epidemic typhus in that it has a gradual onset, less severe symptoms, and a shorter duration of illness than epidemic typhus (7–10 days versus 14–21 days). The presentation is nonspecific, including fever, headache, and chills. The rash is maculopapular and concentrated on the trunk and fades fairly rapidly. Fatalities are rare (less than 1%) and limited to the elderly.

The most common entity in the differential diagnosis is Rocky Mountain spotted fever, usually occurring after a rural exposure and with a different rash (centrifugal, versus centripetal for endemic typhus). Serologic confirmation may be necessary for differentiation, with complement-fixing or immunofluorescent antibodies detectable within 15 days after onset, with specific *R typhi* antigens.

Preventive measures are directed at control of rats and ectoparasites (rat fleas) with insecticides, rat poisons, and rat-proofing of buildings. Antibiotic treatment with tetracycline (25–50 mg/kg/d in four divided doses) or chloramphenicol (50–75 mg/kg/d in four divided doses) is indicated through 3 full days of defervescence.

Whiteford SF et al: Clinical, laboratory, and epidemiologic features of murine typhus in 97 Texas children. Arch Pediatr Adolesc Med 2001;155:396. [PMID: 11231808] (Classic triad of fever, rash, and headache seen in only half of patients, with gastrointestinal symptoms prominent.)

3. Scrub Typhus (Tsutsugamushi Fever)

 ESSENTIALS OF DIAGNOSIS

- *Exposure to mites in endemic area of Southeast Asia, the western Pacific (including Korea), and Australia.*
- *Black eschar at site of bite, with regional and generalized lymphadenopathy.*
- *Conjunctivitis and a short-lived macular rash.*
- *Frequent pneumonitis, encephalitis, and cardiac failure.*

General Considerations

Scrub typhus is caused by *Orientia tsutsugamushi*, which is principally a parasite of rodents transmitted by mites in the endemic areas listed above. The mites live on vegetation but complete their maturation cycle by biting humans who come in contact with infested vegetation. Vertical transmission occurs, and blood transfusions may transmit the pathogen. Serosurveys from Bangkok show prevalences over 20% for blood donors and nearly 60% for febrile malaria clinic patients. Rare occupational transmission via inhalation is documented among laboratory workers.

Clinical Findings

A. SYMPTOMS AND SIGNS

After a 1- to 3-week incubation period, malaise, chills, severe headache, and backache develop. At the site of the bite, a papule evolves into a flat black eschar. The regional lymph nodes are enlarged and tender, and there may be generalized adenopathy. Fever rises gradually, and a macular rash appears primarily on the trunk after a week of fever and may be fleeting or may last a week. The patient may become obtunded. During the second or third week, pneumonitis, myocarditis and cardiac failure, and encephalitis or meningitis, acute abdominal pain, granulomatous hepatitis, or acute renal failure may develop. In the gastrointestinal tract, there may appear superficial mucosal hemorrhage, multiple erosions, or ulcers. An attack confers prolonged immunity against homologous strains and transient immunity against heterologous strains. Heterologous strains produce mild disease if infection occurs within a year after the first episode.

B. LABORATORY FINDINGS

Blood obtained during the first few days of illness may permit isolation of the rickettsial organism by mouse inoculation. Fluorescein-labeled antirickettsial assays or commercial dot-blot ELISA dipstick assays are convenient means of establishing the diagnosis, though PCR may be the most sensitive test.

Differential Diagnosis

Leptospirosis, typhoid, dengue, malaria, and other rickettsial infections should be considered. Scrub typhus is a recognized cause of obscure tropical fevers, especially in children. When the rash is fleeting and the eschar not evident, laboratory results are required for diagnosis, including a conventional indirect fluorescent assay or a more sensitive rapid immunochromatographic flow assay that is under development. Upper tract endoscopy may help with gastrointestinal lesions.

Prevention

Repeated application of long-acting miticides can make endemic areas safe. Insect repellents on clothing and skin provide some protection. For short exposure, chemoprophylaxis with doxycycline (200 mg weekly) can prevent the disease but permits infection. No effective vaccines are available.

Treatment & Prognosis

Without treatment, fever subsides spontaneously after 2 weeks, but the mortality rate may be 10–30%. Treatment for 3 days with doxycycline, 100 mg twice daily, or for 7 days with chloramphenicol, 25 mg/kg/d in four divided doses, virtually eliminates deaths and relapses, though chloramphenicol- and tetracycline-resistant strains have been reported from Southeast Asia, and azithromycin may become the drug of choice for children, pregnant women, and patients with refractory disease. HIV infection does not appear to influence the severity of scrub typhus.

Choi YH et al: Scrub typhus: radiological and clinical findings. Clin Radiol 2000;55:140. [PMID: 10657161] (The most common clinical findings are fever, headache, and rash; the most common radiologic manifestation is a reticulonodular infiltrate.)

Moron CG et al: Identification of the target cells of *Orientia tsutsugamushi* in human cases of scrub typhus. Mod Pathol 2001;14:752. [PMID: 11504834] (The cardiac endothelia and myocytes were the targets in three patients examined postmortem).

Seong SY et al: *Orientia tsutsugamushi* infection: overview and immune responses. Microbes Infect 2001;3:11. [PMID: 11226850]

SPOTTED FEVERS

1. Rocky Mountain Spotted Fever

ESSENTIALS OF DIAGNOSIS

- *Exposure to tick bite in endemic area.*
- *An influenza-like prodrome followed by chills, fever, severe headache, myalgias, restlessness,*

and prostration; occasionally, delirium and coma.

- *Red macular rash appears between the second and sixth days of fever, first on the wrists and ankles and then spreading centrally; it may become petechial.*
- *Serial serologic examinations by indirect fluorescent antibody (IFA) confirm the diagnosis retrospectively.*

General Considerations

Despite its name, most cases occur outside the Rocky Mountain area, with cases in the United States concentrated along the Middle and Southern Atlantic seaboard and in the central Mississippi valley. The causative agent, *R rickettsii*, is transmitted to humans by the bite of ticks, including the wood tick, *Dermacentor andersoni*, in the western USA and by the bite of the dog tick, *Dermacentor variabilis*, in the eastern USA. Other hard ticks transmit the organism in the southern USA and in Central and South America and are responsible for transmitting it among rodents, dogs, porcupines, and other animals. Most human cases occur in late spring and summer. In the USA, most cases occur in the eastern third of the country, with about 1000 reported per year, primarily from April through September, and with a higher incidence among children and men.

Clinical Findings

A. Symptoms and Signs

Two to 14 days (mean, 7 days) after the bite of an infectious tick, symptoms begin with fever, chills, headache, nausea and vomiting, myalgias, restlessness, insomnia, and irritability. Cough and pneumonitis may develop. Delirium, lethargy, seizures, stupor, and coma may appear. The face is flushed and the conjunctiva injected. The rash (faint macules that progress to maculopapules and then petechiae) appears between days 2 and 6 of fever, first on the wrists and ankles, spreading centrally to the arms, legs, and trunk for 2–3 days; involvement of the palms and soles is characteristic. About 10% of cases occur without rash or with minimal rash. In some cases there is splenomegaly, hepatomegaly, jaundice, myocarditis, or uremia; acute respiratory distress syndrome (ARDS) is of greatest concern. About 3–5 % of reported cases in the USA during recent years have been fatal.

B. Laboratory Findings

Thrombocytopenia, hyponatremia, elevated aminotransferases, and hyperbilirubinemia are common. Cerebrospinal fluid may show hypoglycorrhachia and mild pleocytosis. Disseminated intravascular coagulation is observed in severe cases. Diagnosis during the acute phase of the illness can be made by immunohistologic demonstration of *R rickettsiae* in skin biopsy specimens, but this must be performed as soon as skin lesions become apparent to achieve maximum sensitivity. Isolation of the organism using the shell vial technique is available in some laboratories but is hazardous.

Serologic studies confirm the diagnosis, but the majority of patients do not mount an antibody response until the second week of illness. Indirect fluorescent antibody (IFA) is most commonly used. There is no longer any role for the Weil-Felix test.

Differential Diagnosis

The early symptoms and signs of Rocky Mountain spotted fever resemble those of many other infections. The rash may be confused with that of measles, typhoid, and ehrlichiosis, or—most importantly—meningococcemia. Blood cultures and cerebrospinal fluid examination establish the latter.

Prevention

Protective clothing, tick-repellent chemicals, and the removal of ticks at frequent intervals are helpful measures. Prophylactic therapy after a tick bite is not currently recommended.

Treatment & Prognosis

Doxycycline (200 mg/d) either orally or intravenously is the drug of choice. Chloramphenicol (50 mg/kg/d in four divided doses) is reserved for pregnant women. Patients usually defervesce within 48–72 hours. Mild cases in low-risk individuals may be observed without treatment.

The mortality rate for Rocky Mountain spotted fever varies strikingly with age. In the untreated elderly, it may be 70%, but it is usually less than 20% in children. Other risk factors for a fatal outcome include advanced age, atypical clinical features (absence of headache, no history of tick attachment, gastrointestinal symptoms), and a delay in initiation of appropriate antibiotic therapy. The usual cause of death is pneumonitis with respiratory or cardiac failure. Sequelae, more common than formerly recognized, may include seizures, encephalopathy, peripheral neuropathy, paraparesis, bowel and bladder incontinence, cerebellar and vestibular dysfunction, hearing loss, and motor deficits.

Gayle A et al: Tick-borne diseases. Am Fam Physician 2001;64:461 [PMID: 11515835] (A review of infectious diseases transmitted by ticks.)

Holman RC et al: Analysis of risk factors for fatal Rocky Mountain spotted fever: evidence for superiority of tetracyclines for therapy. J Infect Dis 2001;184:1437. [PMID: 11709786]

Thorner AR et al: Rocky Mountain spotted fever. Clin Infect Dis 1998;27:1353. [PMID: 9868640]

2. Rickettsialpox

Rickettsia akari is a parasite of mice, transmitted by mites *(Allodermanyssus sanguineus)*. Rickettsialpox occurs in humans where crowded conditions and mouse-infested housing allow transmission of the pathogen to humans. Pathologic findings include dermal edema, subepidermal vesicles, and at times a lymphocytic vasculitis. The incubation period is 7–12 days. Onset is sudden, with chills, fever, headache, photophobia, and disseminated aches and pains. The primary lesion is a painless red papule that vesiculates and forms a black eschar. Two to 4 days after onset of symptoms, a widespread papular eruption appears that becomes vesicular and forms crusts that are shed in about 10 days. Early lesions may resemble those of chickenpox (typically vesicular versus papulovesicular in rickettsialpox).

Leukopenia and a rise in antibody titer to rickettsial antigen with complement fixation or indirect fluorescent assays using a conjugated antirickettsial globulin can identify antigen in punch biopsies of skin lesions.

Treatment includes tetracycline, 15 mg/kg/d orally in four divided doses for 3–5 days.

Even without treatment, the disease is fairly mild and self-limited, treatment only hastening resolution. Control requires the elimination of mice from human habitations and insecticide applications to suppress the mite vectors.

Comer JA et al: Serologic evidence of rickettsialpox infection among intravenous drug users in inner-city Baltimore, Maryland. Am J Trop Med Hyg 1999;60:894. [PMID: 10403316] (Out of 631 patients, 112 [16%] showed a positive IFA against R akari.)

3. Tick Typhus

The term "tick typhus" denotes a variety of spotted rickettsial fevers. They are often named by geography, eg, Israel tick fever, Kenya tick fever, Mediterranean spotted fever, Queensland tick typhus, Flinders Island spotted fever; or morphology, eg, boutonneuse fever. These illnesses are transmitted by tick vectors of the rickettsial agents *R conorii, R australis, R japonica, R africae,* and *R sibirica.* Dogs and wild animals may serve as reservoirs. The pathogens usually produce a black spot (tâche noire) at the site of the tick bite that may be useful in diagnosis, though spotless boutonneuse fever occurs. Rarely, papulovesicular lesions may resemble rickettsialpox. Endothelial injury produces perivascular edema and dermal necrosis. Regional adenopathy, disseminated lesions, and focal hepatic necrosis may occur. The disease occurs among travelers, with occasional cases recorded among returnees from Africa in particular. Diagnosis is clinical, with serologic or PCR confirmation. Prevention entails protective clothing, repellents, and inspection for and removal of ticks. Treatment is with the following drugs given for 7–10 days: tetracycline (25–50 mg/kg/d in four divided doses), chloramphenicol (50–75 mg/kg/d in four divided doses), or ciprofloxacin (500 mg twice daily).

Cohen J et al: Mediterranean spotted fever in pregnancy. Scand J Infect Dis 1999;31:202. [PMID: 10447334] (The combination of erythromycin and rifampin was effective therapy.)

Parola P et al: Ticks and tickborne bacterial diseases in humans: an emerging infectious threat. Clin Infect Dis 2001;32:897. [PMID: 11247714]

OTHER RICKETTSIAL & RICKETTSIAL-LIKE DISEASES

1. Ehrlichiosis

Ehrlichiosis presents two clinical entities: human monocytic ehrlichiosis and human granulocytic ehrlichiosis. Human monocytic ehrlichiosis is caused by *Ehrlichia chaffeensis* and by the closely related agents *E equi* and *E canis*. Human granulocytic ehrlichiosis is caused by *E phagocytophilia*. *E sennetsu* is the etiologic agent of sennetsu fever, which appears to be confined to western Japan.

Ehrlichiae are small tick-borne gram-negative obligate intracellular bacteria. The major nonhuman hosts include mice, dogs, and horses. Ehrlichiae grow as microcolonies in phagosomes of hematopoietic cells and form characteristic inclusions seen with Giemsa's stain. Human monocytic ehrlichiosis is seen primarily in the Southeast, mid-Atlantic, and South Central states of the USA, though serologic evidence now documents a much more global endemicity (Israel, Japan, Mexico). Its major vector is the Lone Star tick *(Amblyomma americanus)*. Clinical disease ranges from mild to life-threatening. Typically, after about a 9-day incubation period and a prodrome consisting of malaise, rigors, and nausea, patients develop worsening fever and headache; a pleomorphic rash may occur. Leukopenia and absolute lymphopenia as well as thrombocytopenia occur often. Serious sequelae include acute respiratory failure and ARDS, encephalopathy, and acute renal failure, which may mimic thrombotic thrombocytopenic purpura. An indirect fluorescent antibody assay is available through CDC and requires acute and convalescent sera. A PCR assay applied to whole blood samples is a rapid diagnostic tool, if available.

Human granulocytic ehrlichiosis has a geographic area of distribution similar to that for Lyme disease, though the geographic boundaries are as yet not fully determined and seroconversion with clinically consistent cases are now reported from Israel and Europe also. The vectors are ticks of the *Ixodes* genus, and deer and possibly horses appear to be major nonhuman reservoirs. The incidence peaks in summer, but cases are seen year-round in warmer areas where ticks remain viable. The symptoms are similar to those seen with human monocytic ehrlichiosis. Coinfection with Lyme disease may occur, though patients with granulocytic ehrlichiosis appear to be older and sicker than those with acute Lyme disease.

Diagnosis is made by the history of tick exposure followed by a clinical illness with the characteristic symptoms and signs. Further laboratory evaluation is similar to that described for human monocytic ehrlichiosis.

Treatment for both forms of ehrlichiosis is with doxycycline, 200 mg orally or intravenously for at least 7 days or until 3 days of defervescence. Treatment should not be withheld while awaiting confirmatory serology when suspicion is high.

Bakker JS et al: Human granulocytic ehrlichiosis. Clin Infect Dis 2000;31:554. [PMID: 10987720]

Buller RS et al: *Ehrlichia ewingii*, a newly recognized agent of human ehrlichiosis. N Engl J Med 1999;15:148. [PMID: 10403852] (Reporting four patients from Missouri between 1996 and 1998, all with tick exposure, all of whom responded to doxycycline.)

Horowitz HW et al: Antimicrobial susceptibility of *Ehrlichia phagocytophila*. Antimicrob Agents Chemother 2001; 45:786. [PMID: 11181361] (Quinolones and rifampin may be acceptable alternatives to tetracyclines.)

McQuiston JH et al: The human ehrlichioses in the United States. Emerg Infect Dis 1999;5:635. [PMID: 10511519]

2. Q Fever

 **ESSENTIALS OF DIAGNOSIS**

- *Exposure to sheep, goats, cattle, or their products is common; some infections are laboratory-acquired.*
- *An acute or chronic febrile illness with severe headache, cough, prostration, and abdominal pain.*
- *Extensive pneumonitis, hepatitis, or encephalopathy; rarely endocarditis.*

General Considerations

Coxiella burnetii is unique among rickettsiae in that it is usually transmitted to humans not by arthropods but by inhalation or ingestion. It is distributed worldwide with few exceptions. Coxiella infections occur mostly in cattle, sheep, and goats, in which they cause mild or subclinical disease. Transmission by cows and goats is principally through the milk and placenta and by sheep through feces, placenta, and milk. Dry feces and milk, dust contaminated with them, and the tissues of these animals contain large numbers of infectious organisms that are spread by the airborne route. Inhalation of contaminated dust and of droplets from infected animal tissues is the main source of human infection. Outbreaks have been described in association with parturient cats. There is an occupational risk for animal handlers, slaughterhouse workers, veterinarians, and laboratory workers.

The route of acquisition appears to determine the main clinical syndrome. Endocarditis is an uncommon but serious form of coxiella infection and has been linked with immunocompromising conditions, urban residence, and raw milk ingestion. Coxiella is resistant to heat and drying, perhaps because the organism forms endospore-like structures. Thus, it survives in dust, on the fleece of infected animals, or in inadequately pasteurized milk. Spread from one human to another does not seem to occur even in the presence of florid pneumonitis, but maternal-fetal infection can occur.

Clinical Findings

A. SYMPTOMS AND SIGNS

After an incubation period of 1–3 weeks, a febrile illness develops with headache, prostration, and muscle pains, occasionally with a nonproductive cough. Physical signs of pneumonitis may occur. Granulomatous hepatitis is often present. A severe manifestation of chronic coxiella infection (and an occasional complication of acute coxiella infection) is endocarditis, usually of the aortic valve. It is found mainly in the setting of preexisting valve disease or immunosuppression and is typically characterized by large vegetations. Uncommon manifestations of coxiella infection include myocarditis, encephalitis, hemolytic anemia, orchitis, acute renal failure, and mediastinal lymphadenopathy. The clinical course may be acute or chronic and relapsing.

B. LABORATORY FINDINGS

Laboratory examination during the acute phase shows elevated liver function tests, occasionally leukocytosis, and a diagnostic rise in complement-fixing antibodies. Antibodies to phospholipids and antibody against phase 2 antigens have been reported.

In Q fever endocarditis, there is an IgG titer of 1:200 or more by complement fixation or indirect immunofluorescence with IgA or IgG antibodies against phase 1 antigen of *C burnetii*. Isolation of *C burnetii* is possible using the shell-vial technique. A serum ELISA is also available.

C. IMAGING

Radiographs of the chest show patchy pulmonary infiltrates, often more prominent than the physical signs would suggest.

Differential Diagnosis

Viral, mycoplasmal, and bacterial pneumonias; viral hepatitis; brucellosis; tuberculosis; psittacosis; and other animal-borne diseases must be considered. The history of exposure to animals or animal dusts or tissues (eg, in slaughterhouses) should lead to appropri-

ate specific serologic tests. Unexplained fevers with negative blood cultures in association with embolic or cardiac disease should make one consider Q fever, especially in immunocompromised patients.

Prevention

Prevention is based on detection of the infection in livestock, reduction of contact with infected animals or dusts contaminated by them, special care when working with animal tissues, and effective pasteurization of milk. A vaccine of formalin-inactivated phase 1 coxiella is being developed for persons at high risk of infection and appears to be protective. A vaccine is available in some countries for persons with high-risk exposures.

Treatment & Prognosis

Treatment with tetracycline (25 mg/kg/d in four divided doses) or doxycycline (100 mg twice daily) can suppress symptoms and shorten the clinical course but does not always eradicate the infection. Treatment should continue through 3 full days of defervescence. Even in untreated patients, the mortality rate is usually low, except when endocarditis develops (see below).

Treatment of endocarditis consists of protracted—often for years—antibiotic therapy with doxycycline (200 mg/d) and one of several alternatives, including trimethoprim-sulfamethoxazole (320/1600 mg/d), rifampin (900 mg/d), fluoroquinolones, or hydroxychloroquine. Potential interactions of antibiotics (rifampin, quinolones) with warfarin anticoagulation need be considered. Heart valves often need replacement, since the mainstays of antibiotic therapy (chloramphenicol, tetracycline) for rickettsial organisms are bacteriostatic. The combination of hydroxychloroquine and doxycycline appears to be the most effective regimen for treating endocarditis and may result in shorter dosing schedules. This combination should also be used even when there is a potential for developing endocarditis (because of the presence of valve prostheses or valve dysfunction.)

Domingo P et al: Acute Q fever in adult patients: report on 63 sporadic cases in an urban area. Clin Infect Dis 1999;29:874. [PMID: 10589906] (Doxycycline was the preferred agent in this outbreak from Barcelona.)

Fenollar F et al: Risk factors and prevention of Q fever endocarditis. Clin Infect Dis 2001;33:312. [PMID: 11438895] (The risk for developing endocarditis among patients with acute Q fever with valve defects was estimated at an astounding 39%.)

Hutson B et al: Vaccination of cattle workers at risk of Q fever on the north coast of New South Wales. Aust Fam Physician 2000;29:708. [PMID: 10914459] (Over 27% of cattle workers were seropositive for *Coxiella burnetii*, confirming the need for vaccination of certain occupational groups.)

Raoult D et al: Q fever 1985–1998. Clinical and epidemiologic features of 1,383 infections. Medicine (Baltimore) 2000;79:109. [PMID: 10771709] (Younger patients tend to develop hepatitis with Q fever. Older and immunocompromised patients more often have pneumonia or endocarditis. Myocarditis or meningoencephalitis is a poor prognostic sign.)

Voloudaki AE et al: Q fever pneumonia: CT findings. Radiology 2000;215:880. [PMID: 10831714] (The most common manifestation was multilobar airspace consolidation.)

■ KAWASAKI SYNDROME

Kawasaki syndrome is a worldwide multisystemic disease initially described by Tomisaku Kawasaki in 1967. It is also known as the "mucocutaneous lymph node syndrome." It occurs mainly in children under 10 but occasionally in adults, at times in epidemic fashion. Asian children are at higher risk. The epidemiology suggests an infectious origin, though no agent has been identified. While disease is probably not mediated by a bacterial toxin, a staphylococcal toxin may serve as a "superantigen" that interacts with T cells. IgA plasma cell infiltration is noted in the visceral organs, lungs, and coronary arteries of Kawasaki syndrome patients.

The disease is characterized by fever and four of the following for at least 5 days: bilateral nonexudative conjunctivitis, mucous membrane changes of at least one type (injected pharynx, cracked lips, strawberry tongue); extremity changes of at least one type (edema, desquamation, erythema); a polymorphous rash; and cervical lymphadenopathy greater than 1.5 cm.

A major complication is arteritis of the coronary vessels, occurring in about 25% of untreated cases and on occasion causing myocardial infarction. Noninvasive diagnosis can be made with magnetic resonance angiography or transthoracic ultrasound. Factors associated with the development of coronary artery aneurysms are leukocytosis and elevated C-reactive protein. Arteritis of extremity vessels and peripheral gangrene are also reported. Cerebrospinal fluid pleocytosis is reported in one-third of cases. The cause of these complications is also unknown. Differentiation from disseminated adenovirus infection is important and may be facilitated in the future with rapid adenovirus assays.

Management is with aspirin (80–100 mg/kg/d in divided doses with subsequent tapering) and intravenous immune globulin in high doses. Plasmapheresis may be useful in the up to 10% of cases that are unresponsive to immune globulin. Corticosteroids are used by some in refractory disease. Their role in increasing the likelihood of the development of coronary aneurysms is controversial. Warfarin is indicated for the management of coronary artery aneurysms larger than 6.5 mm in diameter. Regular follow-up by a cardiologist is recommended for patients with coronary artery disease or aneurysms. Success is reported with interventional catheter treatment, including stent implantation in patients with long-term cardiac complications. Percutaneous transluminal coronary angioplasty is successfully used in young children.

Johnson RM et al: Kawasaki-like syndromes associated with HIV infection. Clin Infect Dis 2001;32:1628. [PMID: 11340536] (Two case reports.)

Leung DY et al: The many faces of Kawasaki syndrome. Hosp Pract (Off Ed) 2000;35:77. [PMID: 10645991]

Lloyd AJ: Kawasaki disease: is it caused by an infectious agent? Br J Biomed Sci 2001;58:122. [PMID: 11440204]

Mason WH et al: Kawasaki syndrome. Clin Infect Dis 1999;28:169. [PMID: 10064222] (An excellent review including guidelines for management of coronary artery complications.)

Nasr I et al: Kawasaki disease: an update. Clin Exp Dermatol 2001;26:6. [PMID: 11260168]

33

Infectious Diseases: Bacterial & Chlamydial

Henry F. Chambers, MD

See www.current-med.com/ch33.html

■ INFECTIONS CAUSED BY GRAM-POSITIVE BACTERIA

STREPTOCOCCAL INFECTIONS

1. Pharyngitis

ESSENTIALS OF DIAGNOSIS

- Abrupt onset of sore throat, fever, malaise, nausea, and headache.
- Throat red and edematous, with or without exudate; cervical nodes tender.
- Diagnosis confirmed by culture of throat.

General Considerations

Group A beta-hemolytic streptococci *(Streptococcus pyogenes)* are the most common bacterial cause of exudative pharyngitis. Transmission is by droplets of infected secretions. Group A streptococci producing erythrogenic toxin may cause scarlet fever rashes in susceptible persons.

Clinical Findings

A. SYMPTOMS AND SIGNS

"Strep throat" is characterized by a sudden onset of fever, sore throat, pain on swallowing, tender cervical adenopathy, malaise, and nausea. The pharynx, soft palate, and tonsils are red and edematous. There may be a purulent exudate. The rash of scarlet fever is diffusely erythematous, resembling a sunburn, with superimposed fine red papules, and is most intense in the groin and axillas. It blanches on pressure, may become petechial, and fades in 2–5 days, leaving a fine desquamation. In scarlet fever, the face is flushed, with circumoral pallor; and the tongue is coated, with enlarged red papillae (strawberry tongue).

B. LABORATORY FINDINGS

Leukocytosis with neutrophil predominance is common. Throat culture onto a single blood agar plate has a sensitivity of 80–90%. Currently available rapid diagnostic tests, which are based on detection of streptococcal antigen, are slightly less sensitive than culture.

Complications

Suppurative complications include sinusitis, otitis media, mastoiditis, peritonsillar abscess, and suppuration of cervical lymph nodes, among others.

Nonsuppurative complications are rheumatic fever and glomerulonephritis. Rheumatic fever may follow recurrent episodes of pharyngitis beginning 1–4 weeks after the onset of symptoms. Glomerulonephritis follows a single infection with a nephritogenic strain of streptococcus group A (eg, types 4, 12, 2, 49, and 60), more commonly on the skin than in the throat, and begins 1–3 weeks after the onset of the infection.

Differential Diagnosis

Streptococcal sore throat resembles (and cannot be reliably distinguished clinically from) pharyngitis caused by adenoviruses, Epstein-Barr virus, *Arcanobacterium haemolyticus* (which also may cause a rash), and other agents. Pharyngitis and lymphadenopathy are common findings in primary HIV infection. Generalized lymphadenopathy, splenomegaly, atypical lymphocytosis, and a positive serologic test (eg, Monospot) distinguish mononucleosis from streptococcal pharyngitis. Diphtheria is characterized by a pseudomembrane; candidiasis shows white patches of exudate and less erythema; and necrotizing ulcerative gingivostomatitis (Vincent's fusospirochetal disease) presents with shallow ulcers in the mouth. Retropharyngeal abscess or bacterial epiglottitis should be considered when odynophagia and difficulty in handling secretions are present and when the severity of symptoms is disproportionate to findings on examination of the pharynx.

Treatment

Antimicrobial therapy has a minimal effect on resolution of symptoms. Because its main purpose is prevention of complications, therapy may be withheld pending results of culture. Because throat culture (especially if a single plate is used) and rapid detection methods may be falsely negative in 30% or more of cases, when clinical suspicion is high (eg, presence of exudative pharyngitis, tender adenopathy, high fever, and absence of cough and rhinorrhea) and the risk of therapy is low (eg, no drug allergy), antimicrobial therapy may be given without laboratory evaluation.

A. BENZATHINE PENICILLIN G

Benzathine penicillin G, 1.2 million units intramuscularly as a single dose, is optimal therapy.

B. PENICILLIN VK

Penicillin VK, 500 mg orally four times a day (or amoxicillin, 750 mg orally twice daily), is effective, but compliance may be poor after the patient becomes asymptomatic in 2–4 days.

C. MACROLIDES

Erythromycin, 500 mg orally four times a day, or azithromycin, 500 mg once daily for 3 days, are alternatives for the penicillin-allergic patient. Macrolides are less effective than penicillins. The prevalence of macrolide resistance among strains of group A streptococci is on the order of 25–40%. Therefore, macrolides are considered second-line agents because of the risk of treatment failure. Macrolide-resistant strains almost always are susceptible to clindamycin, which is an alternative for serious infections. A 10-day course of 300 mg three times a day orally should be effective.

Prevention of Recurrent Rheumatic Fever

Effectively controlling rheumatic fever depends upon identification and treatment of primary streptococcal infection and secondary prevention of recurrences. Patients who have had rheumatic fever should be treated with a continuous course of antimicrobial prophylaxis for at least 5 years. Effective regimens are erythromycin, 250 mg orally twice daily, or penicillin G, 500 mg orally daily.

Kuhn S et al: Evaluation of the Strep A OIA assay versus culture methods: ability to detect different quantities of group A Streptococcus. Diagn Microbiol Infect Dis 1999;34:275. [PMID: 10459477]

Kurtz B et al: Importance of inoculum size and sampling effect in rapid antigen detection for diagnosis of *Streptococcus pyogenes* pharyngitis. J Clin Microbiol 2000;38:279. [PMID: 10618101] (Evaluation of effect of inoculum on sensitivity and specificity of antigen detection versus culture for diagnosis of group A streptococcal pharyngitis.)

2. Streptococcal Skin Infections

Beta-hemolytic streptococci are not normal skin flora. Streptococcal skin infections usually result from colonization of normal skin by contact with other infected individuals or by preceding streptococcal respiratory infection.

Clinical Findings

A. SYMPTOMS AND SIGNS

Impetigo is a focal, vesicular, pustular lesion with a thick, amber-colored crust that has a "stuck-on" appearance.

Erysipelas is a painful superficial cellulitis that frequently involves the face. It is well demarcated from the surrounding normal skin. Erysipelas also affects skin with impaired lymphatic drainage, such as edematous lower extremities or wounds.

B. LABORATORY FINDINGS

Cultures obtained from a wound or pustule are likely to grow group A streptococci. Blood cultures are occasionally positive.

Treatment

Parenteral antibiotics are indicated for patients with facial erysipelas or evidence of systemic infection. Penicillin, 2 million units intravenously every 4 hours, is the drug of choice.

Cutaneous infections caused by staphylococci may at times be difficult to differentiate from streptococcal infections. Coinfection also occurs. Therefore, initial therapy for severely ill patients or those who have risk factors for staphylococcal infection (eg, intravenous drug use, wound infection, diabetes) should include an agent—such as nafcillin, 1.5 g intravenously every 6 hours—that also is active against *Staphylococcus aureus*. In the patient with minor penicillin allergy, cefazolin, 500 mg intravenously or intramuscularly every 8 hours, may be used. In the patient with a serious penicillin allergy (ie, anaphylaxis), vancomycin, 1000 mg intravenously every 12 hours, should be used.

Patients who do not require parenteral therapy may be treated with amoxicillin, 750 mg twice daily for 7–10 days. As mentioned for treatment of pharyngitis, relatively high prevalence of resistance among strains makes macrolides a less attractive alternative for penicillin-allergic patients. A first-generation oral cephalosporin, eg, cephalexin, 500 mg four times daily, or clindamycin, 300 mg orally three times daily, is an alternative to amoxicillin.

Carapetis JR et al: Epidemiology and prevention of group A streptococcal infections: acute respiratory tract infections, skin infections, and their sequelae at the close of the twentieth century. Clin Infect Dis 1999;28:205. [PMID: 10064227]

3. Other Group A Streptococcal Infections

Arthritis, pneumonia, empyema, endocarditis, and necrotizing fasciitis are relatively uncommon infections that may be caused by group A streptococci. A toxic shock-like syndrome also occurs.

Arthritis generally occurs in association with cellulitis. In addition to intravenous therapy with penicillin G, 2 million units every 4 hours (or cefazolin or vancomycin in doses recommended above for penicillin-allergic patients), frequent percutaneous needle aspiration should be performed to remove joint effusions. Open surgical drainage may be necessary when percutaneous drainage is difficult to achieve—eg, when the hip or shoulder is infected.

Pneumonia and **empyema** often are characterized by extensive tissue destruction and an aggressive, rapidly progressive clinical course associated with significant morbidity and mortality rates. High-dose penicillin and chest tube drainage are indicated for treatment of empyema. Vancomycin is an acceptable substitute in penicillin-allergic patients.

Group A streptococci can cause **endocarditis.** This complication should be suspected when bacteremia accompanies pneumonia, particularly if the patient abuses parenteral drugs. The tricuspid valve is most commonly involved. A patient with suspected endocarditis should be treated with 4 million units of penicillin G every 4 hours for 4 weeks. Vancomycin, 1000 mg every 12 hours, is recommended for persons allergic to penicillin.

Necrotizing fasciitis is a rapidly spreading infection involving the fascia of deep muscle. The clinical findings at presentation may be those of severe cellulitis, but the presence of systemic toxicity and severe pain, which may be followed by anesthesia of the involved area due to destruction of nerves as infection advances through the fascial planes, are important clues to the diagnosis. Surgical exploration is mandatory when the diagnosis is suspected. Early and extensive debridement is essential for survival.

Any streptococcal infection—and necrotizing fasciitis in particular—can be associated with **streptococcal toxic shock syndrome,** characterized by invasion of skin or soft tissues, acute respiratory distress syndrome, and renal failure. The very young, the elderly, and those with underlying medical conditions are at particularly high risk for invasive disease. Bacteremia, which is uncommon in staphylococcal toxic shock syndrome, occurs in the majority of cases. Skin rash and desquamation may not be present. Mortality rates up to 80% have been reported for patients with the full-blown syndrome. The syndrome is due to elaboration of pyrogenic erythrotoxin (which also causes **scarlet fever**), a superantigen that stimulates massive release of inflammatory cytokines felt to mediate the shock. Clindamycin—but not penicillin—inhibits toxin production.

Penicillin remains the drug of choice for treatment of serious streptococcal infections. Some authorities recommend adding clindamycin (600 mg every 8 hours intravenously) to the regimen for invasive disease, especially in the presence of shock. An uncontrolled observational study has suggested a possible survival benefit from administration of intravenous immune globulin for streptococcal toxic shock syndrome. Two dosage regimens were tested with no apparent differences in outcome: 450 mg/kg once daily for 5 days or a single dose of 2 g/kg with a repeat dose at 48 hours if the patient remained unstable. The presumed therapeutic benefit (which needs to be confirmed in a well-designed clinical trial) may be due to specific antibody to streptococcal exotoxins in immune globulin preparations.

Outbreaks of invasive disease have been associated with colonization by invasive clones that can be transmitted to close contacts who, though asymptomatic, may be a reservoir for disease. Tracing contacts of patients with invasive disease is controversial.

Kaul R et al: Intravenous immunoglobulin therapy for streptococcal toxic shock syndrome—a comparative observational study. The Canadian Streptococcal Study Group. Clin Infect Dis 1999;28:800. [PMID: 10825042]

Stevens DL: Streptococcal toxic shock syndrome associated with necrotizing fasciitis. Annu Rev Med 2000;51:271. [PMID: 10774464]

4. Non-Group A Streptococcal Infections

Non-group A streptococci produce a spectrum of disease similar to that of group A streptococci. Some non-group A streptococci are β-hemolytic (eg, groups B, C, and G). The treatment of infections caused by these strains is the same as for group A streptococci.

Group B streptococci are an important cause of sepsis, bacteremia, and meningitis in the neonate. This organism, which is part of the normal vaginal flora, may cause septic abortion, endometritis, or peripartum infections and, less commonly, cellulitis, bacteremia, and endocarditis in adults. Treatment of infections caused by group B streptococci is with either penicillin or vancomycin in doses recommended for group A streptococci. Because of in vitro synergism, some recommend the addition of low-dose gentamicin, 1 mg/kg every 8 hours.

Viridans streptococci, which are nonhemolytic or α-hemolytic (ie, producing a green zone of hemolysis on blood agar), are part of the normal oral flora. Although these strains may produce focal pyogenic infection, they are most notable as the leading cause of native valve endocarditis (see below).

Group D streptococci include *Streptococcus bovis* and the enterococci. *S bovis* is a cause of endocarditis in association with bowel neoplasia or cirrhosis and is treated like viridans streptococci.

Cabellos C et al: Streptococcal meningitis in adult patients: current epidemiology and clinical spectrum. Clin Infect Dis 1999;28:1104. [PMID: 10452643]

Perovic O et al: Invasive group B streptococcal disease in non-pregnant adults. Eur J Clin Microbiol Infect Dis 1999;18:362. [PMID: 10421045]

ENTEROCOCCAL INFECTIONS

Two species, *Enterococcus faecalis* and *Enterococcus faecium,* are responsible for most human enterococcal infections. Enterococci cause wound infections, urinary tract infections, and endocarditis. Except for serious infections such as meningitis, endocarditis, bacteremia in the immunocompromised host, and osteomyelitis, most enterococcal infections can still be treated with penicillin, 3 million units every 4 hours; ampicillin (which is slightly more active than penicillin in vitro), 2 g every 6 hours; or vancomycin, 1 g every 12 hours. Because these antibiotics are not bactericidal for enterococci, gentamicin in a dose of 1 mg/kg every 8 hours is added for treatment of endocarditis or other serious infection.

Resistance to vancomycin, penicillin, and gentamicin is common among enterococcal isolates, especially *E faecium;* it is essential to determine antimicrobial susceptibility of clinical isolates. Infection control measures that may be indicated to limit their spread include isolation, strict adherence to barrier precautions, and avoidance of overuse of vancomycin and gentamicin. Optimal therapy for infection caused by vancomycin- and gentamicin-resistant strains is not known. Quinupristin/dalfopristin and linezolid are FDA-approved for treatment of infections caused by vancomycin-resistant strains of enterococci. Quinupristin/dalfopristin is not active against strains of *Enterococcus faecalis* and should be used only for infections caused by *E faecium.* The dose is 7.5 mg/kg intravenously every 8–12 hours. Infusion-related events, including phlebitis and irritation at the infusion site (often requiring infusion via a central line), and an arthralgia-myalgia syndrome are relatively common side effects. Quinupristin/dalfopristin has important drug interactions with midazolam, nifedipine, and cyclosporine because it is an inhibitor of cytochrome P450 enzyme 3A4, which metabolizes these drugs. The reported microbiologic success rate is approximately 70% overall. Linezolid, an oxazolidinone, is active against both *E faecalis* and *E faecium.* The dose is 600 mg twice daily, and both intravenous and oral preparations are available. The overall microbiologic cure rate is approximately 85%. The drug is well tolerated, with hematologic abnormalities as the principal toxicity.

Chien JW et al: Use of linezolid, an oxazolidinone, in the treatment of multidrug-resistant gram-positive bacterial infections. Clin Infect Dis 2000;30:146. [PMID: 10619743]

Diekema DI et al: Oxazolidinones: a review. Drugs 2000;59:7. [PMID: 10718097]

Murray BE: Vancomycin-resistant enterococcal infections. N Engl J Med 2000;342:710. [PMID: 10706902]

PNEUMOCOCCAL INFECTIONS

1. Pneumococcal Pneumonia

 ESSENTIALS OF DIAGNOSIS

- Productive cough, fever, rigors, dyspnea, early pleuritic chest pain.
- Consolidating lobar pneumonia on chest x-ray.
- Lancet-shaped gram-positive diplococci on Gram stain of sputum.

General Considerations

The pneumococcus is the most common cause of community-acquired pyogenic bacterial pneumonia. Alcoholism, HIV infection, sickle cell disease, splenectomy, and hematologic disorders are predisposing factors. The mortality rate remains high in the setting of advanced age, multilobar disease, severe hypoxemia, extrapulmonary complications, and bacteremia.

Clinical Findings

A. SYMPTOMS AND SIGNS

The patient presents with high fever, productive cough, occasionally hemoptysis, and pleuritic chest pain. Rigors occur within the first few hours of infection but are uncommon thereafter. Bronchial breath sounds are an early sign.

B. LABORATORY FINDINGS

Pneumococcal pneumonia classically is a lobar pneumonia with radiographic findings of consolidation and occasionally effusion. However, differentiating pneumococcal from other bacterial pneumonias is not possible radiographically or clinically because of significant overlap in presentations. Diagnosis requires isolation of the organism in culture, although the Gram stain appearance of sputum can be highly suggestive. Gram stain should be performed on sputum of hospitalized patients, and sputum and blood cultures should be obtained prior to initiation of antimicrobial therapy. A good-quality sputum sample (less than 10 epithelial cells and more than 25 polymorphonuclear leukocytes per high-power field) shows gram-positive diplococci in 80–90% of cases. Sputum culture alone is less sensitive than Gram's stain, and false positives are common as well. Blood cultures are positive in up to 25% of selected cases and much more commonly so in HIV-positive patients.

Complications

Parapneumonic (sympathetic) effusion is common and may cause recurrence or persistence of fever.

These sterile fluid accumulations need no specific therapy. Empyema occurs in 5% or less of cases and is differentiated from sympathetic effusion by the presence of organisms on Gram-stained fluid or positive pleural fluid cultures.

Pneumococcal pericarditis is a rare complication that can cause tamponade. Pneumococcal arthritis also is uncommon. Pneumococcal endocarditis usually involves the aortic valve and often occurs in association with meningitis and pneumonia. Early heart failure and multiple embolic events are typical.

Treatment

A. SPECIFIC MEASURES

Initial antimicrobial therapy of pneumonia is empirical (see Chapter 9 for specific recommendations) pending isolation and identification of the causative agent. Once the pneumonia is determined to be caused by *S pneumoniae,* any of several antimicrobial agents may be used depending on the clinical setting, community patterns of penicillin resistance, and susceptibility of the particular isolate. Uncomplicated pneumococcal pneumonia (ie, arterial $PO_2 > 60$ mm Hg, no coexisting medical problems, and single-lobe disease without signs of extrapulmonary infection) caused by penicillin-susceptible strains of pneumococcus may be treated on an outpatient basis with amoxicillin, 750 mg twice daily for 7–10 days. For penicillin-allergic patients, alternatives are azithromycin, one 500 mg dose on the first day and 250 mg for the next 4 days; clarithromycin, 500 mg twice daily for 10 days; or doxycycline, 200 mg twice daily for 10 days. Patients should be followed for clinical response (eg, less cough, defervescence within 2–3 days) because pneumococci may be resistant to penicillin or any of the second-line agents. Lack of clinical response may indicate infection with a resistant strain, and hospitalization should be considered.

Parenteral therapy is generally recommended for the hospitalized patient at least until there has been clinical improvement. Aqueous penicillin G, 2 million units intravenously every 4 hours, is effective for strains that are not highly penicillin-resistant (ie, MIC > 1 μg/mL). A low-dose regimen of procaine penicillin, 600,000 units intramuscularly every 12 hours, can be used for pneumonia caused by penicillin-sensitive strains (MIC < 0.1 μg/mL). For penicillin-allergic patients without a history of immediate hypersensitivity reaction, ceftriaxone, 1 g intravenously every 24 hours, may be used. For serious penicillin allergy of infection caused by a highly penicillin-resistant strain, vancomycin, 1 g every 12 hours, is effective. Alternatively, a fluoroquinolone (eg, levofloxacin, 500 mg, or a comparable dose of any one of several newer fluoroquinolones now on the market, orally or intravenously) can be used. The total duration of therapy is not well defined, though a duration of 10–14 days is standard.

B. TREATMENT OF COMPLICATIONS

Pleural effusions developing after initiation of antimicrobial therapy usually are sterile, and thoracentesis need not be performed if the patient is otherwise improving. Thoracentesis is indicated for an effusion present prior to initiation of therapy and in the patient who has not responded to antibiotics after 3–4 days. Chest tube drainage may be required if pneumococci are identified by culture or Gram stain, especially if aspiration of the fluid is difficult.

Echocardiography should be done if pericardial effusion is suspected. Patients with pericardial effusion who are responding to therapy and have no signs of tamponade may be followed and treated with indomethacin, 50 mg three times daily, for pain. In patients with increasing effusion, unsatisfactory clinical response, or evidence of tamponade, pericardiocentesis will determine if the pericardial space is infected. Infected fluid must be drained either percutaneously (by tube placement or needle aspiration), by placement of a pericardial window, or by pericardiectomy. Pericardiectomy eventually may be required to prevent or treat constrictive pericarditis, a common sequela of bacterial pericarditis.

Endocarditis should be treated with 24 million units of penicillin G intravenously (or vancomycin, 30 mg/kg/d, for penicillin-allergic patients or for infections caused by penicillin-resistant strains) daily for 3–4 weeks. Mild heart failure may respond to medical therapy, but moderate to severe heart failure is an indication for prosthetic valve implantation, as are systemic emboli or large friable vegetations as determined by echocardiography.

C. PENICILLIN-RESISTANT PNEUMOCOCCI

The prevalence of penicillin-resistant pneumococci (MIC > 0.1 μg/mL) in the United States is increasing, accounting for 10–15% of bloodstream isolates in some regions. All blood and cerebrospinal fluid isolates should be tested for resistance to penicillin. The 1 μg oxacillin disk diffusion assay is an easily performed, reliable screen for resistance. Pneumonia caused by intermediately resistant strains (penicillin MIC > 0.1 μg/mL but ≤ 1 μg/mL) generally will respond to high-dose penicillin therapy. High-dose penicillin is likely to be effective for infections other than meningitis caused by highly penicillin-resistant strains (MIC > 1 μg/mL). However, ceftriaxone, 1 g once daily, or vancomycin, 1 g every 12 hours, results in a more favorable ratio between serum drug concentration and MIC and may be preferred, especially for immunocompromised patients. Fluoroquinolones with enhanced gram-positive activity (eg, levofloxacin 500 mg once daily, moxifloxacin 400 mg once daily, or gatifloxacin 400 mg once daily) are effective oral alternatives. Penicillin-resistant strains of pneumococci often are resistant to multiple antibiotics, including macrolides, trimethoprim-sulfamethoxazole, and chloramphenicol, and susceptibility to these agents must be documented prior to their use.

Pallares R: Treatment of pneumococcal pneumonia. Semin Respir Infect 1999;14:276. [PMID: 10501315]

Schneider RF et al: Pneumococcal infections in HIV-infected adults. Semin Respir Infect 1999;14:237. [PMID: 10501311] (This entire issue is devoted to pneumococcal infections. Four of the best articles address epidemiology, vaccination, clinical pathogenesis, and pathophysiology of the disease.)

2. Pneumococcal Meningitis

ESSENTIALS OF DIAGNOSIS

- Fever, headache, altered mental status.
- Meningismus.
- Gram-positive diplococci on Gram stain of cerebrospinal fluid; counterimmunoelectrophoresis may be positive in partially treated cases.

General Considerations

Streptococcus pneumoniae is the most common cause of meningitis in adults and the second most common cause of meningitis in children over the age of 6 years. Head trauma, cerebrospinal fluid leaks, and sinusitis may precede it.

Clinical Findings

A. SYMPTOMS AND SIGNS

The onset is rapid, with fever, headache, and altered mentation. Pneumonia may be present. Compared with meningitis caused by the meningococcus, pneumococcal meningitis lacks a rash, and focal neurologic deficits, cranial nerve palsies, and obtundation are more prominent features.

B. LABORATORY FINDINGS

The cerebrospinal fluid typically has more than 1000 white blood cells per microliter, over 60% of which are polymorphonuclear leukocytes; the glucose concentration is less than 40 mg/dL, or less than 50% of the simultaneous serum concentration; the protein usually exceeds 150 mg/dL. Not all cases of meningitis will have these typical findings, and alterations in cerebrospinal fluid cell counts and chemistries may be surprisingly minimal, overlapping with those of aseptic meningitis.

Gram stain of cerebrospinal fluid shows gram-positive cocci in 80–90% of cases, and in untreated cases blood or cerebrospinal fluid cultures are almost always positive. Tests such as counterimmunoelectrophoresis or latex agglutination to detect pneumococcal antigens in cerebrospinal fluid are less sensitive than culture and Gram stain. Antigen detection tests may occasionally be helpful in establishing the diagnosis in the patient who has been partially treated and in whom cultures and stains are negative.

Treatment

Antibiotics should be given as soon as the diagnosis of meningitis is suspected. If lumbar puncture must be delayed (eg, while awaiting results of an imaging study to exclude a mass lesion), ceftriaxone, 4 g, is given intravenously after blood cultures (positive in 50% of cases) have been obtained. If gram-positive diplococci are present on the Gram stain, then vancomycin, 45 mg/kg/d intravenously in three divided doses, should be administered in addition to ceftriaxone until the isolate is confirmed not to be penicillin-resistant. Once susceptibility to penicillin has been confirmed, penicillin, 24 million units daily in six divided doses, ceftriaxone, 4 g/d, or chloramphenicol, 6 g/d in four divided doses, is continued for 10–14 days in documented cases.

The best therapy for penicillin-resistant strains is not known. Penicillin-resistant strains often are cross-resistant to the third-generation cephalosporins as well as other antibiotics. Susceptibility testing is essential to proper management of this infection. Treatment failures have been reported with ceftriaxone or cefotaxime for meningitis caused by strains with penicillin MICs ≥ 2 μg/mL. If the MIC of ceftriaxone or cefotaxime is ≤ 0.5 μg/mL, single-drug therapy with either of these cephalosporins is likely to be effective. If the MIC is ≥ 1 μg/mL, treatment with a combination of ceftriaxone, 2 g every 12 hours, plus vancomycin, 45 mg/kg/d in three divided doses, is recommended. If a patient with a penicillin-resistant organism has not responded clinically to therapy with a third-generation cephalosporin, repeat lumbar puncture is indicated to assess the bacteriologic response.

The role of steroids in adjunctive therapy of meningitis in the adult remains controversial. Dexamethasone, 0.15 mg/kg intravenously every 6 hours, may be given when coma, focal deficits, or other signs of increased intracranial pressure are present.

Peltola H: Prophylaxis of bacterial meningitis. Infect Dis Clin North Am 1999;13:685. [PMID: 10470562]

Quagliarello VJ et al: Treatment of bacterial meningitis. N Engl J Med 1997;336:708. [PMID: 9041103]

Saaez-Llorens X et al: Antimicrobial and anti-inflammatory treatment of bacterial meningitis. Infect Dis Clin North Am 1999;13:619. [PMID: 10470558]

STAPHYLOCOCCUS AUREUS INFECTIONS

1. Skin & Soft Tissue Infections

ESSENTIALS OF DIAGNOSIS

- Localized erythema with induration.
- Tendency toward abscess formation.
- Folliculitis commonly observed.

- *Gram stain of pus with gram-positive cocci in clusters; cultures usually positive.*

General Considerations

Most staphylococci found on cultures of normal skin belong to the *Staphylococcus epidermidis* group. *Staphylococcus aureus* is not normal skin flora. *S aureus* tends to cause more localized skin infections than streptococci, and abscess formation is common.

Clinical Findings

A. SYMPTOMS AND SIGNS

S aureus skin infections may begin around one or more hair follicles, causing folliculitis. These infections may localize to form boils (or furuncles) or spread to adjacent skin and deeper subcutaneous tissue (ie, a carbuncle). Myositis or fasciitis may occur, often in association with a deep wound or other inoculation or injection.

B. LABORATORY FINDINGS

Cultures of the wound or abscess material will almost always yield the organism. In patients with other systemic signs of infection, blood cultures should be obtained because of potential endocarditis, osteomyelitis, or metastatic seeding of other sites.

Treatment

Proper drainage of abscess fluid or other focal infections is the mainstay of therapy. Drainage may be all that is needed for cutaneous abscess. Antibiotic therapy alone is unlikely to be effective if collections of infected material are undrained.

For uncomplicated skin infections, oral therapy is satisfactory. An oral penicillinase-resistant penicillin or cephalosporin, such as dicloxacillin or cephalexin, 500 mg four times a day for 7–10 days, is the drug of choice. Erythromycin, 500 mg four times a day, may be used in the penicillin-allergic patient, although the prevalence of erythromycin-resistant strains (40–60%) makes this regimen less attractive empirically.

For more complicated infections with extensive cutaneous or deep tissue involvement or fever, parenteral therapy is indicated initially. A penicillinase-resistant penicillin such as nafcillin or oxacillin in a dosage of 1.5 g every 6 hours intravenously is the drug of choice. In allergic patients without a serious reaction, cefazolin, 0.5–1 g intravenously or intramuscularly every 8 hours, can be used. In patients with a serious allergy to β-lactam antibiotics or if the strain is methicillin-resistant, vancomycin, 1000 mg intravenously every 12 hours, is the drug of choice.

2. Osteomyelitis

S aureus is the cause of approximately 60% of all cases of osteomyelitis. Osteomyelitis may be caused by direct inoculation, eg, from an open fracture or as a result of surgery; by extension from a contiguous focus of infection or open wound; or, more commonly, by hematogenous spread. Long bones and vertebrae are the usual sites. Epidural abscess with or without bone involvement is a common complication of vertebral osteomyelitis and should be suspected if fever and severe back or neck pain are accompanied by radicular pain or neurologic symptoms or signs indicative of spinal cord compression (eg, incontinence, extremity weakness, pathologic reflexes).

Clinical Findings

A. SYMPTOMS AND SIGNS

The infection may be acute, with abrupt development of local symptoms and systemic toxicity; or indolent, with insidious onset of vague pain over the site of infection, progressing to local tenderness. Fever is absent in one-third or more of cases. Abscess formation is a late and unusual manifestation. Draining sinus tracts occur in chronic infections or infections of foreign body implants.

B. LABORATORY FINDINGS

The diagnosis is established by isolation of *S aureus* from the blood, bone, or a contiguous focus of a patient with signs and symptoms of focal bone infection. Blood culture will be positive in approximately 60% of untreated cases of staphylococcal osteomyelitis. Bone biopsy and culture should be considered if blood cultures are sterile.

C. IMAGING

Bone scan and gallium scan, each with a sensitivity of approximately 95% and a specificity of 60–70%, are useful in identifying or confirming the site of bone infection. Plain bone films early in the course of infection are often normal but will become abnormal in most cases even with effective therapy. Spinal infection (unlike malignancy) traverses the disk space to involve the contiguous vertebral body. CT is more sensitive than plain films and can be useful in localizing associated abscesses. MRI is somewhat less sensitive than bone scan but has a specificity of 90%. MRI is indicated when epidural abscess is suspected in association with vertebral osteomyelitis.

Treatment

Prolonged therapy is required to cure staphylococcal osteomyelitis. Durations of 4–6 weeks or longer are recommended. Although oral regimens can be effective, parenteral regimens are advised during the acute phase of the infection for patients with systemic toxicity. Nafcillin or oxacillin, 9–12 g/d in six divided doses, is the drug of choice. Cefazolin, 1 g every 6–8 hours, also is effective. Vancomycin, 1 g every 12 hours, may be used for the penicillin-allergic patient.

Oral regimens are dicloxacillin or cephalexin, 1 g every 6 hours. Addition to the regimen of rifampin 300 mg twice daily probably prevents late relapse and should be strongly considered. For example, an oral regimen of ciprofloxacin 750 mg plus rifampin 300 mg twice daily improved outcome in implant related staphylococcal infections, which are very prone to relapse.

Herwaldt LA: Control of methicillin-resistant Staphylococcus aureus in the hospital setting. Am J Med 1999;106(Suppl 5A):11S. [PMID: 10388059]

Zimmerli W et al: Role of rifampin for treatment of orthopedic implant-related staphylococcal infections: A randomized controlled trial. Foreign-Body Infection Study Group. JAMA 1998;279:1537. [PMID: 9605897]

3. Staphylococcal Bacteremia

S aureus readily invades the bloodstream and infects sites distant from the primary site of infection, which may be relatively minor or even inapparent. Though commonly arising from skin lesions or intravenous lines, whenever S aureus is recovered from blood cultures, the possibility of endocarditis, osteomyelitis, or other metastatic deep infection must be considered. The appropriate duration of therapy for uncomplicated bacteremia arising from a removable source (eg, intravenous device) or drainable focus (eg, skin abscess) has not been well defined, but a 10- to 14-day course of therapy appears to be the minimum. However, approximately 5% or more of patients still relapse, usually with endocarditis or osteomyelitis, even if treated for 2 weeks.

Nafcillin or oxacillin, 1.5 g intravenously every 4–6 hours, cefazolin, 500–1000 mg every 8 hours, or vancomycin, 1000 mg every 12 hours, is recommended for uncomplicated staphylococcal bacteremia. Vancomycin should be reserved for patients with serious penicillin allergy or with infections caused by methicillin-resistant strains because of data suggesting that it is less active than β-lactam antibiotics. Longer courses of either parenteral or oral therapy may be considered for patients (eg, those with diabetes, immunocompromised persons) at risk for late complications from bacteremia and for those in whom endocarditis is suspected. Transesophageal echocardiography (TEE) is a sensitive and cost-effective method for excluding underlying endocarditis. The test should be considered for patients for whom the pretest probability of endocarditis is 5% or higher—and perhaps for all patients with unexplained S aureus bacteremia.

Treatment failures have been reported with the isolation of intermediate-resistant strains in foreign body infections, in association with prolonged or repeated courses of vancomycin therapy, and in patients with chronic renal failure. These strains have also been resistant to methicillin and numerous other antibiotics, severely limiting therapeutic options. An antistaphylococcal penicillin in combination with vancomycin may be synergistic in vitro against vancomycin-resistant strains and is an option for infections that do not respond to vancomycin alone. Cases of vancomycin treatment failures in which the staphylococcal isolate exhibits a vancomycin MIC $\geq$ 4 µg/mL should be reported to CDC to help track this potentially serious and emerging problem.

Rosen AB et al: Cost-effectiveness of transesophageal echocardiography to determine the duration of therapy for intravascular catheter-associated Staphylococcus aureus bacteremia. Ann Intern Med 1999;130:810. [PMID: 10366370]

Smith TL et al: Emergence of vancomycin resistance in Staphylococcus aureus. N Engl J Med 1999;340:493. [PMID: 10021469]

4. Toxic Shock Syndrome

Strains of staphylococci may produce toxins that can cause three important entities: "scalded skin syndrome" in children, toxic shock syndrome in adults, and enterotoxin food poisoning. Toxic shock syndrome is characterized by abrupt onset of high fever, vomiting, and watery diarrhea. Sore throat, myalgias, and headache are common. Hypotension with renal and cardiac failure is an ominous sign in severe cases. A diffuse macular erythematous rash and nonpurulent conjunctivitis are common, and desquamation, especially of palms and soles, is typical during recovery. Fatality rates may be as high as 15%. Although toxic shock syndrome has occurred in men, most cases (90% or more) have been reported in women of childbearing age. Of these, symptoms begin in nearly all patients within 5 days of the onset of a menstrual period in women who have used tampons. The syndrome is possible in any patient with a focus of toxin-producing S aureus. Nonmenstrual cases of toxic shock syndrome are now about as common as menstrual cases. Organisms from various sites, including the nasopharynx, bones, vagina, or rectum or from wounds, have all been associated with the illness. Toxic shock syndrome is most often caused by toxic shock syndrome toxin-1 (TSST-1). Nonmenstrual cases of toxic shock syndrome are frequently caused by strains that do not produce TSST-1. Blood cultures are negative, because symptoms are due to the effects of the toxin and not to the invasive properties of the organism.

Important aspects of treatment include rapid rehydration, antistaphylococcal drugs, management of renal or cardiac failure, and removal of sources of toxin, eg, removal of tampon, drainage of abscess. Intravenous immune globulin has been suggested as being effective in ameliorating toxicity (see section on streptococcal toxic shock syndrome), but confirmatory clinical data are lacking.

5. Infections Caused by Coagulase-Negative Staphylococci

Coagulase-negative staphylococci are an important cause of infections of intravascular and prosthetic devices and of wound infection following cardiothoracic surgery. Rarely, these organisms cause infections such as osteomyelitis and endocarditis in the absence of a prosthesis. More than 20 species have been identified, but most human infections are caused by *Staphylococcus epidermidis, S haemolyticus, S hominis, S warnerii, S saprophyticus, S saccharolyticus,* and *S cohnii.* These common nosocomial pathogens are less virulent than *S aureus,* and infections caused by them tend to be more indolent.

Because coagulase-negative staphylococci are normal inhabitants of human skin, it can be difficult to distinguish infection from contamination, the latter perhaps accounting for three-fourths of blood culture isolates. Infection is more likely if the patient has a foreign body (eg, sternal wires, prosthetic joint, prosthetic cardiac valve, pacemaker, intracranial pressure monitor, cerebrospinal fluid shunt, peritoneal dialysis catheter) or an intravascular device in place. Purulent or serosanguineous drainage, erythema, pain, or tenderness at the site of the foreign body or device suggests infection. Instability and pain are signs of prosthetic joint infection. Fever, a new murmur, instability of the prosthesis, or signs of systemic embolization are evidence of prosthetic valve infection. Immunosuppression and recent antimicrobial therapy also are risk factors for infection.

Infection is also more likely if the same strain is consistently isolated from two or more blood cultures (particularly if samples were obtained at different times) and from the foreign body site. Contamination is more likely when a single blood culture is positive or if more than one strain is isolated from blood cultures. The antimicrobial susceptibility pattern and speciation is commonly used to determine whether one or more strains have been isolated. More sophisticated typing methods, eg, pulse-field gel electrophoresis of restriction enzyme digested chromosomal DNA, may be required to identify distinct strains.

Whenever possible, the intravascular device or foreign body suspected of being infected by coagulase-negative staphylococci should be removed. However, removal and replacement of some devices (eg, prosthetic joint, prosthetic valve, cerebrospinal fluid shunt) can be a difficult or risky procedure, and it may sometimes be preferable to treat with antibiotics alone with the understanding that the probability of cure is reduced and that surgical management may eventually be necessary.

Coagulase-negative staphylococci are commonly resistant to methicillin and multiple other antibiotics. For patients with normal renal function, vancomycin, 1 g intravenously every 12 hours, is the treatment of choice for suspected or confirmed infection caused by these organisms until susceptibility to penicillinase-resistant penicillins or other agents has been confirmed. Duration of therapy has not been established for relatively uncomplicated infections, such as those secondary to intravenous devices, which may be eliminated by simply removing the infected device.

Infection involving bone or a prosthetic valve should be treated for 6 weeks. A combination regimen of vancomycin plus rifampin, 300 mg orally twice daily, and gentamicin, 1 mg/kg intravenously every 8 hours, is recommended for treatment of prosthetic valve endocarditis caused by methicillin-resistant strains.

Diekema DJ et al: Survey of infections due to Staphylococcus species: frequency of occurrence and antimicrobial susceptibility of isolates collected in the United States, Canada, Latin America, Europe, and the Western Pacific region for the SENTRY Antimicrobial Surveillance Program, 1997–1999. Clin Infect Dis 2001;32(Suppl 2):S114. [PMID: 11320452]

Sharma M et al: Molecular analysis of coagulase-negative Staphylococcus isolates from blood cultures: prevalence of genotypic variation and polyclonal bacteremia. Clin Infect Dis 2001;33:1317. [PMID: 11565071]

CLOSTRIDIAL DISEASES

1. Clostridial Myonecrosis (Gas Gangrene)

ESSENTIALS OF DIAGNOSIS

- Sudden onset of pain and edema in an area of wound contamination.
- Prostration and systemic toxicity.
- Brown to blood-tinged watery exudate, with skin discoloration of surrounding area.
- Gas in the tissue by palpation or x-ray.
- Gram-positive rods in culture or smear of exudate.

General Considerations

Gas gangrene or clostridial myonecrosis is produced by entry of one of several clostridia (*Clostridium perfringens, Clostridium ramosum, Clostridium bifermentans, Clostridium histolyticum, Clostridium novyi,* etc) into devitalized tissues. Toxins produced under anaerobic conditions result in shock, hemolysis, and myonecrosis.

Clinical Findings

A. SYMPTOMS AND SIGNS

The onset of gas gangrene is usually sudden, with rapidly increasing pain in the affected area, fall in blood pressure, and tachycardia. Fever is present but is not proportionate to the severity of the infection. In the last stages of the disease, severe prostration, stupor, delirium, and coma occur.

The wound becomes swollen, and the surrounding skin is pale. There is a foul-smelling brown, blood-tinged serous discharge. As the disease advances, the surrounding tissue changes from pale to dusky and finally becomes deeply discolored, with coalescent, red, fluid-filled vesicles. Gas may be palpable in the tissues.

B. LABORATORY FINDINGS

Gas gangrene is a clinical diagnosis, and empirical therapy is indicated whenever the diagnosis is suspected. Radiographic studies may show gas within the soft tissues, but this finding is not specific because other organisms may produce gas. The smear typically shows a remarkable absence of neutrophils and the presence of gram-positive rods. Anaerobic culture confirms the diagnosis.

Differential Diagnosis

Other types of infection can cause gas formation in the tissue, eg, enterobacter, escherichia, and mixed anaerobic infections including bacteroides and peptostreptococci. Clostridia may produce serious puerperal infection with hemolysis.

Treatment

Penicillin, 2 million units every 3 hours intravenously, is effective. Other agents (eg, tetracycline, clindamycin, metronidazole, chloramphenicol, cefoxitin) are active against clostridium species in vitro and probably in vivo as well. Adequate surgical debridement and exposure of infected areas is essential, with radical surgical excision often necessary. Hyperbaric oxygen therapy has been used, but clinical data supporting its efficacy is are not rigorously assessed. If hyperbaric oxygen therapy is used, it must be in conjunction with administration of an appropriate antibiotic and surgical debridement.

Petit L et al: *Clostridium perfringens:* toxinotype and genotype. Trends Microbiol 1999;7:104. [PMID: 10203838]

2. Tetanus

ESSENTIALS OF DIAGNOSIS

- *History of wound and possible contamination.*
- *Jaw stiffness followed by spasms of jaw muscles (trismus).*
- *Stiffness of the neck and other muscles, dysphagia, irritability, hyperreflexia.*
- *Finally, painful convulsions precipitated by minimal stimuli.*

General Considerations

Tetanus is caused by the neurotoxin tetanospasmin, elaborated by *Clostridium tetani.* Spores of this organism are ubiquitous in soil. When introduced into a wound, spores may germinate. The vegetative bacteria produce the toxin tetanospasmin, a zinc metalloprotease that cleaves synaptobrevin, a protein essential for neurotransmitter release. Tetanospasmin interferes with neurotransmission at spinal synapses of inhibitory neurons. As a result, minor stimuli result in uncontrolled spasms, and reflexes are exaggerated. The incubation period is 5 days to 15 weeks, with the average being 8–12 days.

Most cases occur in unvaccinated individuals. Persons at risk are the elderly, migrant workers, newborns, and injection drug users, who may acquire the disease through subcutaneous injections. While puncture wounds are recognized as particularly prone to causing tetanus, any wound, including decubiti, where dead tissue and anaerobic conditions are present may become colonized and infected by *C tetani.*

Clinical Findings

A. SYMPTOMS AND SIGNS

The first symptom may be pain and tingling at the site of inoculation, followed by spasticity of the muscles nearby. Stiffness of the jaw, neck stiffness, dysphagia, and irritability are other early signs. Hyperreflexia develops later, with spasms of the jaw muscles (trismus) or facial muscles and rigidity and spasm of the muscles of the abdomen, neck, and back. Painful tonic convulsions precipitated by minor stimuli are common. Spasms of the glottis and respiratory muscles may cause acute asphyxia. The patient is awake and alert throughout the illness. The sensory examination is normal. The temperature is normal or only slightly elevated.

B. LABORATORY FINDINGS

The diagnosis of tetanus is made clinically.

Differential Diagnosis

Tetanus must be differentiated from various acute central nervous system infections such as meningitis. Trismus may occasionally develop with the use of phenothiazines. Strychnine poisoning should also be considered.

Complications

Airway obstruction is common. Urinary retention and constipation may result from spasm of the sphincters. Respiratory arrest and cardiac failure are late, life-threatening events.

Prevention

Tetanus is completely preventable by active immunization. Immunizations for children include tetanus toxoid, usually as DTP (see Table 30–4 for schedule). For primary immunization of adults, tetanus toxoid is administered as two doses 4–6 weeks apart, with a third dose 6–12 months later. Booster doses are given every 10 years or at the time of major injury if it occurs more than 5 years after a dose.

Passive immunization should be used in nonimmunized individuals and those whose immunization status is uncertain whenever a wound is contaminated or likely to have devitalized tissue. Tetanus immune globulin, 250 units, is given intramuscularly. Active immunization with tetanus toxoid should be started concurrently. Table 33–1 provides a guide to prophylactic management.

Treatment

A. SPECIFIC MEASURES

Tetanus immune globulin, 5000 units, is administered intramuscularly. Tetanus does not produce natural immunity, and a full course of immunization with tetanus toxoid should be administered once the patient has recovered.

B. GENERAL MEASURES

Minimal stimuli can provoke spasms, so the patient should be placed at bed rest and monitored under the quietest conditions possible. Sedation, paralysis with curare-like agents, and mechanical ventilation are often necessary to control tetanic spasms. Penicillin, 20 million units daily, is given to all patients—even those with mild illness—to eradicate toxin-producing organisms.

Prognosis

High mortality rates are associated with a short incubation period, early onset of convulsions, and delay in

Table 33–1. Guide to tetanus prophylaxis in wound management.[1]

History of Absorbed Tetanus Toxoid	Clean, Minor Wounds		All Other Wounds[2]	
	Td[3]	TIG[4]	Td[3]	TIG[4]
Unknown or < 3 doses	Yes	No	Yes	Yes
3 or more doses	No[5]	No	No[6]	No

[1]From the Centers for Disease Control and Prevention. Recommended childhood immunization schedule—United States, 2002. JAMA 2002;287:707.
[2]Such as, but not limited to, wounds contaminated with dirt, feces, soil, saliva, etc; puncture wounds; avulsions; and wounds resulting from missiles, crushing, burns, and frostbite.
[3]Tetanus toxoid and diphtheria toxoid, adult form. Use only this preparation (Td-adult) in children older than 6 years.
[4]Tetanus immune globulin.
[5]Yes if more than 10 years have elapsed since last dose.
[6]Yes if more than 5 years have elapsed since last dose. (More frequent boosters are not needed and can enhance side effects.)

treatment. Contaminated lesions about the head and face are more dangerous than wounds on other parts of the body. The overall mortality rate historically is about 40%, but this can be considerably reduced with ventilator management as described.

Hsu SS et al: Tetanus in the emergency department: a current review. J Emerg Med 2001;20:357. [PMID: 11348815]

Botulism

 ESSENTIALS OF DIAGNOSIS

- *History of recent ingestion of home-canned or smoked foods or of injection drug use and demonstration of toxin in serum or food.*
- *Sudden onset of diplopia, dry mouth, dysphagia, dysphonia, and muscle weakness progressing to respiratory paralysis.*
- *Pupils are fixed and dilated in most cases.*

General Considerations

Botulism is a paralytic disease caused by botulinum toxin, which is produced by *Clostridium botulinum*, a ubiquitous, strictly anaerobic, spore-forming bacillus found in soil. Four toxin types—A, B, E, and F—cause human disease. Botulinum toxin is a zinc metalloprotease that inhibits release of acetylcholine at the neuromuscular junction by cleaving a specific component of the synaptic vesicle membrane docking and fusion complex.. Clinically, early nervous system involvement leads to respiratory paralysis and death in untreated cases. Botulinum toxin is extremely potent and is classified by the Centers for Disease Control and Prevention as a high-priority agent because of its potential for use as an agent of bioterrorism. Naturally occurring botulism occurs in one of three forms: foodborne botulism, infant botulism, or wound botulism. Food-borne botulism is caused by ingestion of preformed toxin present in canned, smoked, or vacuum-packed foods such as home-canned vegetables, smoked meats, and vacuum-packed fish. Commercial foods have also been associated with outbreaks of botulism. Infant botulism and wound botulism, are caused by organisms present in the gut or wound that elaborate toxin in vivo.

Clinical Findings

A. SYMPTOMS AND SIGNS

Twelve to 36 hours after ingestion of the toxin, visual disturbances appear, particularly diplopia and loss of accommodation. Ptosis, cranial nerve palsies with impairment of extraocular muscles, and fixed dilated pupils are characteristic signs. The sensory examination is normal. Other symptoms are dry mouth, dysphonia, and dysphonia. Nausea and vomiting may be present, particularly with type E toxin. The sensorium remains clear and the temperature normal. Respiratory paralysis may lead to death unless mechanical assistance is provided.

B. Laboratory Findings

Toxin in patients' serum and in suspected foods may be shown by mouse inoculation and identified with specific antiserum.

Differential Diagnosis

Cranial nerve involvement suggests vertebrobasilar insufficiency, the C. Miller Fisher variant of Guillain-Barré syndrome, myasthenia gravis, or any basilar meningitis, infectious or carcinomatous. Intestinal obstruction or other types of food poisoning are considered when nausea and vomiting are present.

Treatment

If botulism is suspected, the physician should contact the state health authorities or the Centers for Disease Control and Prevention for advice and help with procurement of botulinus antitoxin and for assistance in obtaining assays for toxin in serum, stool, or food. During off hours, the CDC provides assistance via a recorded message at 404-639-2206.

Respiratory failure is managed with intubation and mechanical ventilation. Parenteral fluids or alimentation should be given while swallowing difficulty persists.

The removal of unabsorbed toxin from the gut may be attempted. Any remnants of suspected foods should be assayed for toxin. Persons who might have eaten the suspected food must be located and observed.

Pellizzari R et al: Tetanus and botulinum neurotoxins: mechanism of action and therapeutic uses. Philos Trans R Soc London B Biol Sci 1999;354:259. [PMID: 10212474]

Shapiro RL et al: Botulism in the United States: A clinical and epidemiologic review. Ann Intern Med 1998;129:221. [PMID: 9696731]

ANTHRAX

ESSENTIALS OF DIAGNOSIS

- Appropriate epidemiologic setting, eg, exposure to animals or animal hides, or potential exposure resulting from an act of bioterrorism.
- A cutaneous black eschar, typically painless and on exposed areas of the skin, with marked surrounding edema and vesicles.

- Nonspecific flu-like symptoms that rapidly progress to extreme dyspnea and shock in association with mediastinal widening and pleural effusions on chest x-ray.

General Considerations.

The death of a Florida photo editor from inhalational anthrax acquired from a letter deliberately contaminated with spores of *Bacillus anthracis* thrust this extremely rare infection into the public awareness. Between September 18 and November 21 of 2001, there were 13 cases of cutaneous anthrax and 11 cases of inhalational anthrax in association with known or presumed exposure to anthrax spores in contaminated mail.

Naturally occurring anthrax is a disease of sheep, cattle, horses, goats, and swine. *B anthracis* is a gram-positive spore-forming aerobic rod. Spores—not vegetative bacteria—are the infectious form of the organism. These are transmitted to humans from contaminated animals, animal products, or soil by inoculation of broken skin or mucous membranes; by inhalation of aerosolized spores; or, rarely, by ingestion resulting in cutaneous, inhalational, or gastrointestinal forms of anthrax, respectively. The spores germinate into vegetative bacteria that multiply locally in cutaneous and gastrointestinal anthrax but may also disseminate to cause systemic infection. Spores entering the lungs are ingested by macrophages and carried via lymphatics to regional lymph nodes, where they germinate. The bacteria rapidly multiply within the lymphatics, causing a hemorrhagic lymphadenitis. Invasion of the bloodstream leads to overwhelming sepsis, killing the host. Virulence is determined by two plasmids, pXO1 and pXO2, which carry, respectively, genes for two toxins, lethal toxin and edema toxin; and genes for capsule production. Loss of either plasmid attenuates strain virulence. Edema toxin impairs neutrophil function and probably is responsible for the striking edema present in cutaneous anthrax. Lethal factor is thought to mediate the shock syndrome. The capsule allows the bacteria to evade host immune defenses.

Clinical Findings

A. Symptoms and Signs

1. Cutaneous anthrax—Onset occurs within 2 weeks after exposure to spores. Clinical data indicate no latency period for cutaneous disease. The initial lesion is an erythematous papule, often on an exposed area of skin, that vesiculates and then ulcerates and undergoes necrosis, ultimately progressing to a purple to black eschar. The eschar typically is painless; pain indicates secondary staphylococcal or streptococcal infection. The surrounding area is edematous and vesicular but not purulent. Regional adenopathy, fever, malaise, headache, and nausea and vomiting may be present. The infection is self-limited in most cases, but hematogenous spread with sepsis or meningitis may occur.

2. Inhalational anthrax—Onset of illness, which occurs in two stages, begins on average 10 days after exposure, although a longer incubation period of up to 6 weeks can occur. Nonspecific viral-like symptoms such as fever, malaise, headache, dyspnea, cough, and congestion of the nose, throat, and larynx are characteristic of the initial stage. Anterior chest pain is an early symptom of mediastinitis. Within hours to a few days, the patient progresses to the fulminant stage of infection in which signs and symptoms of overwhelming sepsis predominate. Delirium, obtundation, or findings of meningeal irritation suggest an accompanying hemorrhagic meningitis.

3. Gastrointestinal anthrax—This form has not been reported in the United States. Symptoms begin 2–5 days after ingestion of meat contaminated with anthrax spores. Fever, diffuse abdominal pain, rebound abdominal tenderness, vomiting, constipation, and diarrhea occur. Because the primary lesion is ulcerative, emesis is blood-tinged or coffee-grounds and stool may be blood-tinged or melenic. Bowel perforation can occur. The oropharyngeal form of the disease is characterized by local lymphadenopathy, cervical edema, dysphagia, and upper respiratory tract obstruction.

B. LABORATORY FINDINGS

Laboratory findings are nonspecific. The white blood cell count initially may be normal or modestly elevated, with polymorphonuclear predominance and an increase in early forms. Pleural fluid from patients with inhalational anthrax is typically hemorrhagic with a relative paucity of white cells. Cerebrospinal fluid from meningitis cases is also hemorrhagic. Gram stain of fluid from a cutaneous lesion, pleural fluid, cerebrospinal fluid, unspun blood, or blood culture may show the characteristic boxcar-shaped encapsulated rods in chains.

The diagnosis is established by isolation of the organism from culture of the skin lesion (or fluid expressed from it), blood, or pleural fluid—or cerebrospinal fluid in cases of meningitis. In the absence of prior antimicrobial therapy, cultures are invariably positive. Cultures obtained after initiation of antimicrobial therapy may be negative. If anthrax is suspected on clinical or epidemiologic grounds, immunohistochemical tests (eg, to detect capsular antigen), polymerase chain reaction assays, and serologic tests (useful for documenting past cutaneous infection) are available through the CDC and should be utilized to establish the diagnosis. Any suspected case of anthrax should be immediately reported to CDC so that a complete investigation can be conducted.

C. IMAGING STUDIES

The chest x-ray is the most sensitive test for inhalational disease, being abnormal (though the findings can be subtle) initially in every case of bioterrorism-associated disease. Mediastinal widening due to hemorrhagic lymphadenitis, a hallmark feature of the disease, was present in 70% of the bioterrorism-related cases. Pleural effusions were present initially or occurred over the course of illness in all cases, and approximately three-fourths had pulmonary infiltrates or signs of consolidation.

Differential Diagnosis

Cutaneous anthrax, despite its characteristic appearance, can be confused with a variety of other also uncommon or rare conditions such as ecthyma gangrenosum, rat-bite fever, ulceroglandular tularemia, plague, glanders, rickettsialpox, orf (parapoxvirus infection), or cutaneous mycobacterial infection. Inhalational anthrax must be differentiated from mediastinitis due to other bacterial causes, fibrous mediastinitis due to histoplasmosis, coccidioidomycosis, atypical or viral pneumonia, silicosis, sarcoidosis, and other causes of mediastinal widening (eg, superior vena cava syndrome or ruptured aortic aneurysm). Gastrointestinal anthrax shares clinical features with a variety of common intra-abdominal disorders, including bowel obstruction, perforated viscus, peritonitis, gastroenteritis, and peptic ulcer disease.

Treatment

Strains of *B anthracis* (including the strain isolated in the bioterrorism cases) are susceptible in vitro to penicillin, amoxicillin, chloramphenicol, clindamycin, imipenem, doxycycline, ciprofloxacin (as well as other fluoroquinolones), macrolides, rifampin, and vancomycin. Susceptibility to cephalosporins is variable. *B anthracis* may express beta-lactamases that confer resistance to cephalosporins and penicillins. For this reason, penicillin or amoxicillin is no longer recommended for use as a single agent in treatment of disseminated disease. Based on results of animal experiments and because of concern for engineered drug resistance in strains of *B anthracis* used in bioterrorism or weaponized, ciprofloxacin is considered the drug of choice (Table 33–2) for treatment and for prophylaxis following exposure to anthrax spores. Other fluoroquinolones with activity against gram-positive bacteria (eg, levofloxacin, gatifloxacin, moxifloxacin), though they have not been formally tested, are likely to be just as effective. Doxycycline is an alternative first-line agent. Combination therapy with at least one additional agent is recommended for inhalational or disseminated disease and in cutaneous infection involving the face, head, and neck or associated with extensive local edema or systemic signs of infection, eg, fever, tachycardia, elevated white blood cell count. Anecdotally, four of the six survivors of the recent in-

Table 33–2. Antimicrobial agents for treatment of or for prophylaxis against anthrax.

First-line agents and recommended doses
  Ciprofloxacin, 500 mg twice daily orally or 400 mg every 12 hours intravenously
  Doxycycline, 100 mg every 12 hours orally or intravenously
Second-line agents and recommended doses
  Amoxicillin, 500 mg three times daily orally
  Penicillin G, 2 mU every 4 hours intravenously
Alternative agents with in vitro activity and suggested doses
  Rifampin, 10 mg/kg/d orally or intravenously
  Clindamycin, 450–600 mg every 8 hours orally or intravenously
  Clarithromycin, 500 mg twice daily
  Erythromycin, 500 mg every 6 hours intravenously
  Vancomycin, 1 g every 12 hours intravenously
  Imipenem, 500 mg every 6 hours intravenously
  Vancomycin, 1 g every 12 hours intravenously

---

halational cases were treated with combinations that included both a fluoroquinolone and rifampin. Single-drug therapy is recommended for prophylaxis following exposure to spores.

The required duration of therapy is poorly defined. In naturally occurring disease, treatment for 7–10 days for cutaneous disease and for at least 2 weeks following clinical response for disseminated, inhalational, or gastrointestinal infection have been standard recommendations. Because of concern about relapse from latent spores acquired by inhalation of aerosol in bioterrorism-associated cases, the initial recommendation was treatment for 60 days. For postal workers receiving prophylaxis for exposure to contaminated mail, CDC has since set forth two new options: (1) antibiotics for 100 days (fearing that even with 60 days of treatment late relapses might occur) or (2) vaccination with an investigative agent (three doses administered over a 1-month period) in conjunction with 40 days of antibiotic administration to cover the time required for a protective antibody response to develop. As to the effectiveness of any of these options, there are as yet no data on which to base a recommendation for any one over another.

There is also an FDA-approved vaccine for persons at high risk of exposure to anthrax spores. The vaccine is cell-free antigen prepared from an attenuated strain of *B anthracis*. Multiple injections over 18 months and an annual booster dose are required to achieve and maintain protection. Existing supplies have been reserved for vaccination of military personnel.

The prognosis in cutaneous infection is excellent. Death is unlikely if the infection has remained localized, and lesions heal without complications in most cases. The reported mortality rate for gastrointestinal and inhalational infections is up to 85%. Recent experience with bioterrorism-associated inhalational cases in which six of eleven victims have survived suggest a somewhat better outcome with modern supportive care and antibiotics provided that treatment is initiated before the patient has progressed to the fulminant stage of disease. No cases of anthrax have occurred among the several thousand individuals receiving antimicrobial prophylaxis following exposure to spores.

[CDC Web site: Anthrax and Other Bioterrorism-Related Issues] http://www.bt.cdc.gov/

Borio L et al: Death due to bioterrorism-related inhalational anthrax: report of 2 patients. JAMA 2001;286:2554. [PMID: 11722269]

Bush LM et al: Index case of fatal inhalational anthrax due to bioterrorism in the United States. N Engl J Med 2001;345:1607. [PMID: 11704685]

Dixon TC et al: Anthrax. N Engl J Med 1999;341:815. [PMID: 10477781]

Inglesby TV et al: Anthrax as a biological weapon: medical and public health management. Working Group on Civilian Biodefense. JAMA 1999;281:1735. [PMID: 10328075]

Jernigan JA et al: Bioterrorism-related inhalational anthrax: the first 10 cases reported in the United States. Emerg Infect Dis 2001;7:933. [PMID: 11747719]

Mayer TA et al: Clinical presentation of inhalational anthrax following bioterrorism exposure: report of 2 surviving patients. JAMA 2001;286:2549. [PMID: 11722268]

Roche KJ et al: Images in clinical medicine. Cutaneous anthrax infection. N Engl J Med 2001;345:1611. [PMID: 11704684]

DIPHTHERIA

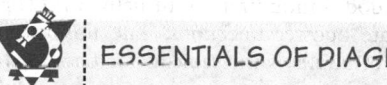 **ESSENTIALS OF DIAGNOSIS**

- Tenacious gray membrane at portal of entry in pharynx.
- Sore throat, nasal discharge, hoarseness, malaise, fever.
- Myocarditis, neuropathy.
- Culture confirms the diagnosis.

General Considerations

Diphtheria is an acute infection, caused by *Corynebacterium diphtheriae*, that usually attacks the respiratory tract but may involve any mucous membrane or skin wound. The organism is spread chiefly by respiratory secretions. Exotoxin produced by the organism is responsible for myocarditis and neuropathy. This exotoxin inhibits elongation factor, which is required for protein synthesis.

Clinical Findings

A. SYMPTOMS AND SIGNS

Nasal, laryngeal, pharyngeal, and cutaneous forms of diphtheria occur. Nasal infection produces few symptoms other than a nasal discharge. Laryngeal infection may lead to upper airway and bronchial obstruction. In pharyngeal diphtheria, the most common form, a tenacious gray membrane covers the tonsils and pharynx. Mild sore throat, fever, and malaise are followed by toxemia and prostration.

Myocarditis and neuropathy are the most common and most serious complications. Myocarditis causes cardiac arrhythmias, heart block, and heart failure. The neuropathy usually involves the cranial nerves first, producing diplopia, slurred speech, and difficulty in swallowing.

B. Laboratory Findings

The diagnosis is made clinically but can be confirmed by culture of the organism.

Differential Diagnosis

Diphtheria must be differentiated from streptococcal pharyngitis, infectious mononucleosis, adenovirus or herpes simplex infection, Vincent's angina, pharyngitis due to *Arcanobacterium haemolyticum,* and candidiasis. A presumptive diagnosis of diphtheria must be made on clinical grounds without waiting for laboratory verification, since emergency treatment is needed.

Prevention

Active immunization with diphtheria toxoid is part of routine childhood immunization (usually as DTP) with appropriate booster injections. The immunization schedule for adults is the same as for tetanus. In order to avoid major allergic reactions, only the "adult type" toxoid (Td) should be used.

Susceptible persons exposed to diphtheria should receive a booster dose of diphtheria toxoid plus active immunization if not previously immunized, as well as a course of penicillin or erythromycin.

Treatment

Antitoxin, which is prepared from horse serum, must be given in all cases when diphtheria is suspected. For mild early pharyngeal or laryngeal disease, the dose is 20,000–40,000 units; for moderate nasopharyngeal disease, 40,000–60,000 units; for severe, extensive, or late (3 days or more) disease, 80,000–100,000 units. Diphtheria equine antitoxin can be obtained from the Centers for Disease Control and Prevention.

Removal of membrane by direct laryngoscopy or bronchoscopy may be necessary to prevent or alleviate airway obstruction.

Either penicillin, 250 mg orally four times daily, or erythromycin, 500 mg orally four times daily, for 14 days is effective therapy, though erythromycin is slightly more effective in eliminating the carrier state. Azithromycin or clarithromycin is quite likely to be as effective as erythromycin. The patient should be isolated until three consecutive cultures at the completion of therapy have documented elimination of the organism from the oropharynx. Contacts to a case should receive erythromycin, 500 mg four times daily for 7 days, to eradicate carriage.

LISTERIOSIS

Listeria monocytogenes is a motile, gram-positive rod that is a facultative intracellular organism capable of invading several cell types. Most cases of infection caused by *L monocytogenes* are sporadic, but outbreaks have been traced to eating contaminated food, especially unpasteurized dairy products. Five types of infection are recognized:

(1) Infection during pregnancy, usually in the last trimester, is a mild febrile illness without an apparent primary focus. This is a relatively benign disease for both mother and fetus that may resolve without specific therapy.

(2) Granulomatosis infantisepticum is a neonatal infection acquired in utero and characterized by disseminated abscesses and granulomas and by a high mortality rate.

(3) Bacteremia with or without sepsis syndrome is an infection of neonates or immunocompromised adults. The presentation is that of a febrile illness without a recognized source.

(4) Meningitis caused by *L monocytogenes* affects infants under 2 months of age and adults, ranking third and fourth, respectively, among the common causes of bacterial meningitis. Adults with meningitis are usually immunocompromised, and cases have been associated with HIV infection. Cerebrospinal fluid shows a *neutrophilic* pleocytosis.

(5) Finally, focal infections, including adenitis, brain abscess, endocarditis, osteomyelitis, and arthritis, occur rarely.

Therapy of infections caused by listeria is controversial with respect both to the most effective agent and the duration of treatment. The drug of choice is probably ampicillin, 8–12 g/d intravenously in four to six divided doses (the higher dose being recommended in cases of meningitis). It has relatively good penetration into cerebrospinal fluid, and the response to ampicillin seems to be better than that to penicillin, erythromycin, or chloramphenicol. Gentamicin is synergistic with ampicillin against listeria in vitro and in animal models, and the use of combination therapy may for that reason be considered during the first few days of treatment to enhance eradication of organisms. Mortality and morbidity rates still are high, and relapse does occur, perhaps related to poor penetration of ampicillin into cells where organisms reside. Anecdotal clinical data indicating efficacy of trimethoprim-sulfamethoxazole and its excellent cellular and cerebrospinal fluid penetration into cells and into the cerebrospinal fluid support its use for therapy of listeriosis. The dose is 10–20 mg/kg/d of the trimethoprim component. Therapy should be administered for at least 2–3 weeks. Longer durations—between 3 and 6 weeks—have been recommended for treatment of meningitis, especially in severely immunocompromised patients.

Charpentier E et al: Antibiotic resistance in *Listeria* spp Antimicrob Agents Chemother 1999;43:2103. [PMID: 10471548]

Silver HM: Listeriosis during pregnancy Obstet Gynecol Surv 1998;53:737. [PMID: 9870235]

■ INFECTIVE ENDOCARDITIS

ESSENTIALS OF DIAGNOSIS

- Preexisting organic heart lesion.
- Fever.
- New or changing heart murmur.
- Evidence of systemic emboli.
- Positive blood culture.
- Evidence of vegetation on echocardiography.

General Considerations

Important factors that determine the clinical presentation are (1) the nature of the infecting organism; (2) which valve or valves are infected; and (3) the route of infection, since endocarditis in intravenous drug users and infections acquired during open heart surgery have special features.

More virulent organisms—*Staphylococcus aureus* in particular—tend to produce a more rapidly progressive and destructive infection. Patients are more likely to present with acute febrile illnesses, early embolization, and acute valvular regurgitation and myocardial abscess formation. Still, these organisms can produce a more gradual illness, and more indolent organisms can occasionally cause the acute presentation. Viridans strains of streptococci, enterococci, and a variety of other gram-positive and gram-negative bacilli, yeasts, and fungi tend to cause a more subacute picture. Systemic and peripheral manifestations may predominate. Acute deterioration due to valve perforations or large emboli may occur at any time.

Most patients who develop infective endocarditis have underlying cardiac disease, though this is not the case with intravenous drug users and hospital-acquired infections. Abnormal valves or endocardial changes due to jet flow effects in congenital lesions (most commonly ventricular septal defect, tetralogy of Fallot, coarctation of the aorta, or patent ductus arteriosus) provide a nidus for infection during bacteremic episodes. Predisposing valvular abnormalities include rheumatic involvement of any valve, bicuspid aortic valves, calcific or sclerotic aortic valves, hypertrophic subaortic stenosis, and mitral valve prolapse. In the past, rheumatic disease was the commonest predisposing condition; this is no longer the case in developed countries. Regurgitation lesions are more susceptible than stenotic ones.

The initiating event in infective endocarditis is colonization of the valve by bacteria during a transient or persistent bacteremia. Transient bacteremia is common during dental, upper respiratory, urologic, and lower gastrointestinal diagnostic and surgical procedures. It is less common during upper gastrointestinal and gynecologic procedures, though a high incidence has been reported during suction abortion.

Approximately 90% of cases of native valve endocarditis are due to viridans streptococci (60%), *S aureus* (20%), and enterococci (5–10%). Gram-negative organisms and fungi account for a small percentage.

The microbiology of native valve endocarditis in intravenous drug users differs from that of other patients. *S aureus* accounts for 60% or more of all cases and for 80–90% of cases in which the tricuspid valve is infected. Enterococci and streptococci comprise the balance in about equal proportions. Gram-negative aerobic bacilli, fungi, and unusual organisms that rarely infect others may cause endocarditis in intravenous drug users.

The microbiology of prosthetic valve endocarditis also is distinctive. Early infections (ie, those occurring within 2 months after valve implantation) are commonly caused by staphylococci—both coagulase-positive and coagulase-negative—gram-negative organisms, and fungi. Late prosthetic valve endocarditis resembles native valve endocarditis, with the majority of infections caused by streptococci, though coagulase-negative staphylococci still cause a significant proportion of cases.

Clinical Findings

A. Symptoms and Signs

Most patients present with a febrile illness that has lasted several days to 2 weeks. Nonspecific symptoms are common. Cough, dyspnea, arthralgias or arthritis, diarrhea, and abdominal or flank pain may occur as a result of embolization or immunologically mediated phenomena. The initial symptoms or signs of endocarditis may be caused by arterial emboli or cardiac damage.

Most patients are febrile, though older individuals may be euthermic. In the majority of cases of endocarditis, heart murmurs are stable, and although a changing murmur is significant diagnostically, it is the exception rather than the rule. The characteristic peripheral lesions—petechiae (on the palate or conjunctiva or beneath the fingernails); subungual ("splinter") hemorrhages; Osler nodes (painful, violaceous raised lesions of the fingers, toes, or feet); Janeway lesions (painless erythematous lesions of the palms or soles); and Roth spots (exudative lesions in the retina)—occur in 20–25% of patients, if that. Pallor and splenomegaly are other helpful signs.

In acute endocarditis, leukocytosis is common; in subacute cases, anemia of chronic disease and a normal white count are the rule. Hematuria and proteinuria as well as renal dysfunction may result from emboli or immunologically mediated glomerulonephritis.

B. DIAGNOSTIC STUDIES

Blood culture is the most important procedure for diagnosis; the current recommendation for maximizing the yield is to obtain three sets of blood cultures at least 1 hour apart before starting antibiotics. Even then, a small number of infected patients (up to 5% of cases) will be culture-negative, which is usually attributable to administration of antimicrobials prior to obtaining cultures. If antimicrobial therapy has been administered prior to cultures and the patient is clinically stable, it is reasonable to withhold further antimicrobial therapy for 2–3 days so that appropriate cultures can be obtained. These cases may also be due to a fungus (50% of patients with fungal endocarditis have negative blood cultures), organisms that require special media for growth (eg, legionella, bartonella, nutritionally deficient streptococci), organisms that do not grow on artificial media (agents of Q fever, psittacosis), or organisms that are slow-growing and may require several weeks of incubation (eg, brucella, anaerobes, certain haemophilus species, *Actinobacillus actinomycetemcomitans, Cardiobacterium hominis, Eikenella corrodens,* and kingella).

The chest x-ray may show evidence for the underlying cardiac abnormality and, in right-sided endocarditis, pulmonary infiltrates. The ECG is nondiagnostic. Changing conduction abnormalities suggest myocardial abscess formation.

Echocardiography is useful in diagnosis and may provide adjunctive information about the specific valve or valves that are infected. The sensitivity of transthoracic echocardiography is between 55% and 65%; therefore, it cannot reliably rule out endocarditis but may confirm a clinical suspicion. Transesophageal echocardiography is 90% sensitive in detecting vegetations and is particularly useful for identifying valve ring abscesses as well as pulmonary and prosthetic valve endocarditis.

Clinical criteria (commonly referred to as the Duke criteria) for the diagnosis of endocarditis have been proposed. Major criteria include (1) two positive blood cultures for a microorganism that typically causes infective endocarditis; and (2) evidence of endocardial involvement documented by echocardiography (definite vegetation, myocardial abscess, or new partial dehiscence of a prosthetic valve) or development of a new regurgitant murmur. Minor criteria include (1) the presence of a predisposing condition; (2) fever ≥ 38 °C; (3) embolic disease; (4) immunologic phenomena (glomerulonephritis, Osler nodes, Roth spots, rheumatoid factor); (5) positive blood cultures not meeting the major criteria; and (6) a positive echocardiogram not meeting the major criteria. A definite diagnosis can be made with 80% accuracy if two major criteria, one major criterion and three minor criteria, or five minor criteria are fulfilled. If none of these criteria are met and either an alternative explanation for illness is identified or the patient has defervesced within 4 days, endocarditis is highly unlikely.

Complications

The clinical course of infective endocarditis is determined by the degree of damage to the heart, by the site of infection (right- versus left-sided, aortic versus mitral valve), by the presence of metastatic foci of infection, by whether embolization from the site of infection occurs, and by immunologically mediated processes. Destruction of infected heart valves is especially common and precipitous with *S aureus* and often enterococci but can occur with any organism. The resulting regurgitation can be mild or severe and can progress even after bacteriologic cure. The infection can also extend into the myocardium, resulting in abscesses leading to conduction disturbances, and can also involve the wall of the aorta, creating sinus of Valsalva aneurysms.

Peripheral embolization can occur with any organism. The most catastrophic are cerebral and myocardial embolizations, with resulting infarctions. The spleen and kidneys are also common sites. Peripheral emboli may initiate metastatic infections or may become established in vessel walls, leading to mycotic aneurysms. Right-sided endocarditis, which usually involves the tricuspid valve, often leads to septic pulmonary emboli, causing infarction and lung abscesses.

Prevention

Some cases of endocarditis occur after dental procedures or operations involving the upper respiratory, genitourinary, or intestinal tract. Prophylactic antibiotics are given to patients with predisposing congenital or valvular anomalies who are to have any of these procedures (Tables 33–3 and 33–4). Current recommendations are given in Table 33–5.

Treatment

Empirical regimens for endocarditis while culture results are pending should include agents active against staphylococci, streptococci, and enterococci. Nafcillin or oxacillin, 1.5 g every 4 hours, plus penicillin, 2–3 million units every 4 hours (or ampicillin, 1.5 g every 4 hours), plus gentamicin, 1 mg/kg every 8 hours, is such a regimen. Vancomycin, 15 mg/kg every 12 hours, may be used instead of the penicillins in the penicillin-allergic patient or if infection by methicillin-resistant staphylococci is suspected.

A. VIRIDANS STREPTOCOCCI

For penicillin-susceptible viridans streptococcal endocarditis (ie, MIC ≤ 0.1 μg/mL), penicillin G, 2–3 mil-

Table 33–3. Cardiac lesions for which bacterial endocarditis prophylaxis is or is not recommended.[1,2]

Endocarditis prophylaxis recommended

1. High risk category

   Prosthetic cardiac valves, including bioprosthetic and homograft valves

   Previous bacterial endocarditis, even in the absence of heart disease

   Complex cyanotic congenital heart disease (eg, single ventricle states, transposition of the great arteries, tetralogy of Fallot)

   Surgically constructed systemic pulmonary shunts or conduits

2. Moderate-risk category

   Most congenital cardiac malformations (other than those listed above and below)

   Rheumatic and other acquired valvular dysfunction, even after valvular surgery

   Hypertrophic cardiomyopathy

   Mitral valve prolapse with valvular regurgitation[3,4]

- -

Endocarditis prophylaxis not recommended[5]

Isolated secundum septal defect

Surgical repair of atrial septal defect, ventricular septal defect, or patent ductus arteriosus (without residua beyond 6 months)

Previous coronary artery bypass graft surgery

Mitral valve prolapse without valvular regurgitation[6]

Physiologic, functional, or innocent heart murmurs

Previous Kawasaki disease without valvular dysfunction

Previous rheumatic fever without valvular dysfunction

Cardiac pacemakers (intravascular and epicardial) and implanted defibrillators

---

[1]Modified and reproduced, with permission, from Dajani AS et al: Prevention of bacterial endocarditis. Recommendations by the American Heart Association. JAMA 1997;277:1794. Copyright © 1997 by American Medical Association.

[2]This table lists selected conditions and is not meant to be all-inclusive.

[3]Mitral regurgitation determined by the presence of a murmur or by echo-Doppler.

[4]Men older than 45 without a consistent systolic murmur may warrant prophylaxis even in the absence of resting regurgitation.

[5]Negligible risk category—no greater than in the general population.

[6]Individuals who have a mitral valve prolapse associated with thickening or redundancy of the valve leaflets may be at increased risk for bacterial endocarditis.

lion units intravenously every 4 hours for 4 weeks, is recommended. The duration of therapy can be shortened to 2 weeks if gentamicin, 1 mg/kg every 8 hours, is used with penicillin. Ceftriaxone, 2 g once daily intravenously or intramuscularly for 4 weeks, is also effective therapy for penicillin-susceptible strains and is a convenient regimen for home therapy. For the penicillin-allergic patient, vancomycin, 15 mg/kg every 12 hours for 4 weeks should be used. The 2-week regimen is not recommended for patients with symptoms of more than 3 months' duration or patients with complications such as myocardial abscess or extracardiac infection. Prosthetic valve endocarditis should be treated with a 6-week course of penicillin with at least 2 weeks of gentamicin.

Viridans streptococci relatively resistant to penicillin (ie, MIC > 0.1 μg/mL but ≤ 0.5 μg/mL) should be treated for 4 weeks. Penicillin G, 3 million units intravenously every 4 hours is combined with gentamicin, 1 mg/kg every 8 hours for the first 2 weeks. In the patient with IgE-mediated allergy to penicillin, vancomycin alone, 15 mg/kg every 12 hours for 4 weeks, should be administered.

Viridans streptococci with an MIC > 0.5 μg/mL and nutritionally deficient streptococci should be treated like enterococci (see below).

B. OTHER STREPTOCOCCI

Endocarditis caused by *Streptococcus pneumoniae*, *Streptococcus pyogenes* (group A streptococcus), or groups B, C, and G streptococci is unusual. Large studies to determine efficacy of antibiotic regimens have not been published. *S pneumoniae* sensitive to penicillin (MIC < 0.1 μg/mL) can be treated with penicillin alone, 2–3 million units every 4 hours for 4–6 weeks. Strains resistant to penicillin (MIC > 0.1 μg/mL) are being reported with increasing frequency, and optimal therapy is not known, though vancomycin should be effective based on in vitro data. Group A streptococcal infection can be treated with penicillin, ceftriaxone, or vancomycin for 4–6 weeks. Groups B, C, and G streptococci tend to be more resistant to penicillin than group A streptococci, and some have recommended adding gentamicin, 1 mg/kg every 8 hours, to penicillin for the first 2 weeks of a 4- to 6-week course.

C. ENTEROCOCCI

For enterococcal endocarditis, the relapse rate is unacceptably high when penicillin is used alone; either streptomycin or gentamicin must be included in the regimen. Because aminoglycoside resistance occurs in enterococci, susceptibility should be documented. Gentamicin is the aminoglycoside of choice, because streptomycin resistance is more common than gentamicin resistance and the nephrotoxicity of gentamicin is generally more easily managed than the vestibular toxicity of streptomycin. Ampicillin, 2 g intravenously every 4 hours, or penicillin G, 3–4 million units every 4 hours (or, in the penicillin-allergic patient, vancomycin, 15 mg/kg every 12 hours), plus gentamicin, 1 mg/kg every 8 hours, is recommended. Standard practice is to continue this regimen for 4–6 weeks (the longer duration recommended for patients with symptoms for more than 3 months, relapse, or prosthetic valve endocarditis), though a recent retrospective

Table 33–4. Procedures for which bacterial endocarditis prophylaxis is or is not recommended.[1,2]

Endocarditis prophylaxis recommended[3]	Endocarditis prophylaxis not recommended

1. Dental
    Dental extractions
    Periodontal procedures
    Dental implant placement or reimplantation
    Endodontic (root canal) instrumentation or surgery
      only beyond the apex
    Subgingival placement of antibiotic fibers or strips
    Initial placement of orthodontic bands but not
      brackets
    Intraligamentary local anesthetic injections
    Prophylactic cleaning of teeth or implants where
      bleeding is anticipated
2. Respiratory tract
    Tonsillectomy, adenoidectomy
    Surgical operations that involve intestinal or
      respiratory mucosa
    Bronchoscopy with a rigid bronchoscope
3. Gastrointestinal tract[4]
    Sclerotherapy for esophageal varices
    Esophageal stricture dilation
    Endoscopic retrograde cholangiography with biliary
      obstruction
    Biliary tract surgery
    Surgical operations that involve intestinal mucosa
4. Genitourinary tract
    Prostatic surgery
    Cystoscopy
    Urethral dilation
	1. Dental
	    Restorative dentistry (filling cavities, operative and
	      prosthodontic) with or without retraction cord[5]
	    Local anesthetic injections (nonintraligamentary)
	    Intracanal endodontic treatment; post placement
	      and buildup
	    Placement of rubber dams, removable prostho-
	      dontic, or orthodontic appliances
	    Postoperative suture removal
	    Taking of oral impression
	    Fluoride treatments
	    Orthodontic appliance adjustment
	2. Respiratory tract
	    Endotracheal intubation
	    Bronchoscopy with a flexible bronchoscope, with
	      or without biopsy[6]
	    Tympanostomy (insertion)
	3. Gastrointestinal tract
	    Transesophageal echocardiography[6]
	    Endoscopy with or without gastrointestinal biopsy[6]
	4. Genitourinary tract
	    Vaginal hysterectomy[6]
	    Vaginal delivery[6]
	    Cesarean section
	    In the absence of infection: urethral catheteri-
	      zation, uterine dilation and curettage,
	      therapeutic abortion, sterilization procedures,
	      insertion or removal of intrauterine devices
	5. Other
	    Cardiac catheterization, including balloon angio-
	      plasty; implanting cardiac pacemakers or defib-
	      rillators and coronary stents; incision or biopsy
	      of surgically scrubbed skin; circumcision

[1]Reproduced, with permission, from Dajani AS et al: Prevention of bacterial endocarditis. Recommendation by the American Heart Association. JAMA 1997;277:1794. Copyright © 1997 by American Medical Association.
[2]This table lists selected procedures but is not meant to be all-inclusive.
[3]Recommended for individuals with high- and moderate-risk cardiac conditions (Table 33–3).
[4]Prophylaxis is recommended for high-risk patients, optional for moderate-risk patients.
[5]Clinical judgment may indicate antibiotic use in selected circumstances that may create significant bleeding.
[6]Prophylaxis is optional for high-risk patients.

study of native valve enterococcal endocarditis suggests that less than 4 weeks of aminoglycoside may be sufficient. Experience is more extensive with penicillin and ampicillin than with vancomycin for therapy of enterococcal endocarditis, and penicillin and ampicillin are superior to vancomycin in in vitro studies. Thus, whenever possible, either ampicillin or penicillin should be used. If endocarditis is caused by an organism that demonstrates high-level resistance to aminoglycosides (ie, not inhibited by 500 μg/mL of gentamicin), then the addition of an aminoglycoside will not be beneficial. Therapy with high doses of penicillin (eg, 6 g/d) administered as a continuous infusion, is recommended for 8–12 weeks, but the re-

lapse rate may be as high as 50%. Surgery may be the only option in such situations.

D. Staphylococci

For methicillin-susceptible *S aureus,* nafcillin or oxacillin, 1.5 g every 4 hours for 4–6 weeks, is the preferred therapy. For penicillin-allergic patients, cefazolin, 2 g intravenously every 8 hours, or vancomycin, 15 mg/kg every 12 hours, may be used. For methicillin-resistant strains, vancomycin is the only agent of proved effectiveness. Aminoglycoside combination regimens may be useful in shortening the duration of bacteremia. Their maximum benefit is achieved at low doses (1 mg/kg every 8 hours) and in the first 3–

Table 33–5. Endocarditis prophylaxis.[1,2]

DENTAL, RESPIRATORY, OR ESOPHAGEAL PROCEDURES		
Oral	Amoxicillin	2 g 1 hour before procedure
Penicillin allergy	Clindamycin	600 mg 1 hour before procedure
	or	
	Cephalexin or cefadroxil[3]	2 g 1 hour before procedure
	or	
	Azithromycin or clarithromycin	500 mg 1 hour before procedure
Parenteral	Ampicillin	2 g IM or IV 30 minutes before procedure
Penicillin allergy	Clindamycin	600 mg IV 1 hour before procedure
	or	
	Cefazolin[3]	1 g IM or IV 30 minutes before procedure
GASTROINTESTINAL (EXCEPT ESOPHAGEAL) OR GENITOURINARY PROCEDURES		
High-risk patient (Table 33–3)	Ampicillin plus gentamicin	Ampicillin, 2 g IM or IV, plus gentamicin, 1.5 mg/kg (not to exceed 120 mg) 30 minutes before procedure; 6 hours later, ampicillin, 1 g IM or IV, or amoxicillin, 1 g orally
Penicillin allergy	Vancomycin plus gentamicin	Vancomycin, 1 g IV over 1–2 hours, plus gentamicin, 1.5 mg/kg (not to exceed 120 mg) IV or IM; complete infusion or injection 30 minutes before procedure
Moderate-risk patient	Amoxicillin or ampicillin	Amoxicillin, 2 g orally 1 hour before procedure, or ampicillin, 2 g IM or IV 30 minutes before starting procedure
Penicillin allergy	Vancomycin	Vancomycin, 1 g IV over 1–2 hours; complete infusion 30 minutes before procedure

[1]Modified and reproduced, with permission, from Dajani AS et al: Prevention of bacterial endocarditis. Recommendations by the American Heart Association. JAMA 1997;277:1794. Copyright © 1997 by American Medical Association.
[2]Viridans streptococci are the most common cause of endocarditis occurring after dental or upper respiratory procedures; enterococci are the most common cause after gastrointestinal or genitourinary procedures.
[3]Cephalosporins should not be used in individuals with immediate type hypersensitivity reactions to penicillin.

5 days of therapy, and they should not be continued beyond the early phase of therapy. For treatment of tricuspid valve endocarditis (with or without pulmonary involvement) in the injection drug user who does not have serious extrapulmonary sites of infection, the total duration of therapy can be shortened from 4 weeks to 2 weeks if an aminoglycoside is added to an antistaphylococcal drug for the entire 2 weeks of therapy. The effect of rifampin with antistaphylococcal drugs is variable, and its routine use is not recommended.

Because coagulase-negative staphylococci—a common cause of prosthetic valve endocarditis—are routinely resistant to methicillin, β-lactam antibiotics should not be used for this infection until the isolate is known to be susceptible. A combination of vancomycin for 6 weeks, rifampin, 300 mg every 8 hours for 6 weeks, and gentamicin, 1 mg/kg every 8 hours for the first 2 weeks, is the regimen of choice. If the organism is sensitive to methicillin, either nafcillin or oxacillin or cefazolin can be used in combination with rifampin and gentamicin. Combination therapy with nafcillin or oxacillin (vancomycin for methicillin-resistant strains or patients allergic to β-lactams), rifampin, and gentamicin is also recom-

mended for treatment of *S aureus* prosthetic valve infection.

E. HACEK ORGANISMS

HACEK organisms *(Haemophilus aphrophilus, Haemophilus parainfluenzae, Actinobacillus actinomycetemcomitans, Cardiobacterium hominis, Eikenella corrodens, and Kingella kingae)* are slow-growing, fastidious gram-negative coccobacilli or bacilli that are normal oral flora and cause about 5–10% of all cases of endocarditis. These organisms can produce β-lactamase, and thus the treatment of choice is ceftriaxone (or some other third-generation cephalosporin), 2 g once daily for 4 weeks. Prosthetic valve endocarditis should be treated for 6 weeks. In the penicillin-allergic patient, experience is limited, but trimethoprim-sulfamethoxazole, quinolones, and aztreonam have in vitro activity and should be considered; desensitization may be preferable.

F. ROLE OF SURGERY

While most cases can be successfully treated medically, operative management is sometimes required. Valvular regurgitation resulting in acute heart failure that does not resolve promptly after institution of medical therapy is an indication for valve replacement even if active infection is present, especially if the aortic valve is involved. Infections that do not respond to appropriate antimicrobial therapy after 7–10 days (ie, persistent fevers, positive blood cultures despite therapy) are more likely to be eradicated if the valve is replaced. Surgery is nearly always required for fungal endocarditis and is more often necessary with gram-negative bacilli. Surgery is also indicated when the infection involves the sinus of Valsalva or produces septal abscesses. Recurrent infection with the same organism often indicates that surgery is necessary, especially with infected prosthetic valves. Continuing embolization presents a difficult problem when the infection is otherwise responding but may be an indication for surgery. Embolization after bacteriologic cure, however, does not necessarily imply recurrence of endocarditis.

G. ROLE OF ANTICOAGULATION

Anticoagulation is contraindicated in native valve endocarditis because it imposes a greatly increased risk of intracerebral hemorrhage. The role of anticoagulant therapy during active prosthetic valve endocarditis is more controversial. Reversal of anticoagulation may result in thrombosis of the mechanical prosthesis, particularly in the mitral position. On the other hand, anticoagulation during active prosthetic valve endocarditis caused by *S aureus* has been associated with fatal intracerebral hemorrhage. Therefore, anticoagulation perhaps should be stopped during the septic phase of *S aureus* prosthetic valve endocarditis. Indications for anticoagulation following prosthetic valve implantation for endocarditis are the same as for patients with prosthetic valves without endocarditis (eg, nonporcine mechanical valves and valves in the mitral position).

Response to Therapy

If infection is caused by viridans streptococci, enterococci, or coagulase-negative staphylococci, defervescence occurs in 3–4 days on average, whereas if infection is caused by *Staphylococcus aureus* or *Pseudomonas aeruginosa,* patients may remain febrile for 9–12 days. If fevers persist, blood cultures should be obtained to ensure adequacy of therapy. Other causes of persistent fever are myocardial or metastatic abscess, sterile embolization, superimposed nosocomial infection, and drug reaction. Careful posttreatment monitoring is critical. Most relapses occur within 1–2 months after completion of therapy. Obtaining one or two blood cultures during this period allows for early detection of recurrent infection.

Bayer AS et al: Diagnosis and management of infective endocarditis and its complications. Circulation 1998;98:2936. [PMID: 9860802]

Dajani AS et al: Prevention of bacterial endocarditis: Recommendations by the American Heart Association. JAMA 1997;277:1794. [PMID: 9178793]

Olaison L et al: Enterococcal endocarditis in Sweden, 1995–1999: can shorter therapy with aminoglycosides be used? Clin Infect Dis 2002 34:159. [PMID: 11740702]

■ INFECTIONS CAUSED BY GRAM-NEGATIVE BACTERIA

BORDETELLA PERTUSSIS INFECTION (Whooping Cough)

 ESSENTIALS OF DIAGNOSIS

- *Predominantly in infants under age 2 years. Adults are an important reservoir of infection.*
- *Two-week prodromal catarrhal stage of malaise, cough, coryza, and anorexia.*
- *Paroxysmal cough ending in a high-pitched inspiratory "whoop."*
- *Absolute lymphocytosis, often striking; culture confirms diagnosis.*

General Considerations

Pertussis is an acute infection of the respiratory tract caused by *Bordetella pertussis* that is transmitted by respiratory droplets. The incubation period is 7–17 days. Half of all cases occur before age 2 years. Neither immunization nor disease confers lasting immunity to pertussis. Consequently, adults are an important reservoir of the disease.

Clinical Findings

The symptoms of classic pertussis last about 6 weeks and are divided into three consecutive stages. The catarrhal stage is characterized by its insidious onset, with lacrimation, sneezing, and coryza, anorexia and malaise, and a hacking night cough that tends to become diurnal. The paroxysmal stage is characterized by bursts of rapid, consecutive coughs followed by a deep, high-pitched inspiration (whoop). The convalescent stage usually begins 4 weeks after onset of the illness with a decrease in the frequency and severity of paroxysms of cough. The diagnosis often is not considered in adults, who may not have a typical presentation. Cough persisting more than 2 weeks is suggestive of pertussis. Infection may also be asymptomatic.

The white blood cell count is usually 15,000–20,000/μL (rarely, as high as 50,000/μL or more), 60–80% of which are lymphocytes. The diagnosis is established by isolating the organism from nasopharyngeal culture. A special medium (eg, Bordet-Gengou agar) must be requested.

Prevention

Active immunization with pertussis vaccine is recommended for all infants, usually combined with diphtheria and tetanus toxoids (DTP). Infants and susceptible adults with significant exposure to pertussis should receive prophylaxis with erythromycin (40 mg/kg/d, up to 2 g/d, for 10 days). Booster doses of pertussis vaccine have not been recommended after age 6 except to control outbreaks. Recognition of adults as an important reservoir of infection and development of an effective acellular vaccine with fewer side effects than the whole cell vaccine undoubtedly will prompt a reevaluation of the current recommendations for vaccination of adults.

Treatment

Erythromycin, 500 mg four times a day orally for 10 days, shortens the duration of carriage. It also may diminish the severity of coughing paroxysms. Although clinical data are limited, azithromycin, 500 mg orally for 3 days, or clarithromycin, 500 mg orally twice daily for 7 days, is probably as effective as erythromycin and likely to be better tolerated.

Cherry JD: Epidemiological, clinical, and laboratory aspects of pertussis in adults. Clin Infect Dis 1999;28(Suppl 2):S112. [PMID: 10447028] (Illustrates the atypical presentation in adults and emphasizes that pertussis is not exclusively a childhood disease.)

Hewlett EL: A commentary on the pathogenesis of pertussis. Clin Infect Dis 1999;28(Suppl 2):S94. [PMID: 10447025]

OTHER BORDETELLA INFECTIONS

Bordetella bronchiseptica is a pleomorphic gram-negative coccobacillus that commonly causes kennel cough in dogs. It has been reported as a cause of upper and lower respiratory infection in humans, principally HIV-infected patients. Infection has been associated with contact with dogs and cats, suggesting animal-to-human transmission. Treatment of *B bronchiseptica* infection should be guided by results of in vitro susceptibility tests.

Dworkin MS et al: *Bordetella bronchiseptica* infection in human immunodeficiency virus-infected patients. Clin Infect Dis 1999;28:1095. [PMID: 10452641]

MENINGOCOCCAL MENINGITIS

 ESSENTIALS OF DIAGNOSIS

- *Fever, headache, vomiting, confusion, delirium, convulsions.*
- *Petechial rash of skin and mucous membranes in many.*
- *Neck and back stiffness with positive Kernig and Brudzinski signs is characteristic.*
- *Purulent spinal fluid with gram-negative intracellular and extracellular diplococci.*
- *Culture of cerebrospinal fluid, blood, or petechial aspiration confirms the diagnosis.*

General Considerations

Meningococcal meningitis is caused by *Neisseria meningitidis* of groups A, B, C, Y, W-135, and others. Meningitis due to serogroup A is uncommon in the United States. Serogroup B generally causes sporadic cases. The frequency of outbreaks of meningitis caused by group C meningococcus has increased in recent years, and this serotype is the most common cause of epidemic disease in the United States. Up to 40% of persons are nasopharyngeal carriers of meningococci, but relatively few develop disease. Infection is transmitted by droplets. The clinical illness may take the form of meningococcemia (a fulminant form of septicemia without meningitis), meningococcemia with meningitis, or predominantly meningitis. Chronic recurrent meningococcemia with fever, rash, and arthritis can occur, particular in those with terminal complement deficiencies.

Clinical Findings

A. SYMPTOMS AND SIGNS

High fever, chills, and headache; back, abdominal, and extremity pains; and nausea and vomiting are typical. In severe cases, rapidly developing confusion, delirium, seizures, and coma occur.

On examination, nuchal and back rigidity are typical, with positive Kernig and Brudzinski signs. (Kernig's sign is pain in the hamstrings upon extension of the knee with the hip at 90-degree flexion; Brudzinski's sign is flexion of the knee in response to flexion of the neck.) A petechial rash often first appearing in the lower extremities and at pressure points is found in most cases. Petechiae may vary from pinhead-sized to large ecchymoses or even areas of skin gangrene that may later slough if the patient survives.

B. LABORATORY FINDINGS

Lumbar puncture typically reveals a cloudy or purulent cerebrospinal fluid, with elevated pressure, increased protein, and decreased glucose content. The fluid usually contains more than 1000 cells/μL, with polymorphonuclear cells predominating and containing gram-negative intracellular diplococci. The absence of organisms in a Gram-stained smear of the cerebrospinal fluid sediment does not rule out the diagnosis. The capsular polysaccharide can often be demonstrated in cerebrospinal fluid or urine by latex agglutination; this is especially useful in partially treated patients, though sensitivity is only 60–80%.

The organism is usually demonstrated by smear or culture of the cerebrospinal fluid, oropharynx, blood, or aspirated petechiae.

Disseminated intravascular coagulation is an important complication of meningococcal infection. Prothrombin time and partial thromboplastin time are prolonged, fibrin dimers are elevated, fibrinogen is low, and the platelet count is depressed.

Differential Diagnosis

Meningococcal meningitis must be differentiated from other bacterial and viral meningitides. In small infants and in the elderly, the presentation may be atypical, without fever or stiff neck.

Rickettsial or echovirus infection and, rarely, other bacterial infections (eg, staphylococcal infections, scarlet fever) may also produce a petechial rash.

Prevention

Effective polysaccharide vaccines for groups A, C, Y, and W-135 are available. A and C vaccine has reduced the incidence of infections with these meningococcus groups in military recruits. The vaccines are effective for control of epidemics in civilian populations. The Advisory Committee on Immunization Practices now recommends immunization with a single dose of polyvalent vaccine (active against meningococcal groups A, C, Y, and W-135) for college freshmen—particularly those living in dormitories, who have been shown to have a modestly increased risk of invasive meningococcal disease.

Outbreaks in closed populations are best controlled by eliminating nasopharyngeal carriage of meningococci. Rifampin is the drug of choice; in a dosage of 600 mg twice a day for 2 days. A single 500 mg oral dose of ciprofloxacin or one intramuscular 250 mg dose of ceftriaxone in adults is also effective.

Household members exposed to a person with meningococcal meningitis are at increased risk and should be given rifampin prophylaxis as outlined above. Day care center contacts are treated in the same manner. School and work contacts need not be treated. Hospital contacts need not be treated unless intense exposure has occurred (eg, mouth-to-mouth resuscitation).

Accidentally discovered carriers without known close contact with meningococcal disease do not require prophylactic antimicrobials.

Treatment

Blood cultures must be obtained and intravenous antimicrobial therapy started immediately. This may be done prior to lumbar puncture in patients in whom the diagnosis is not straightforward and for those in whom MR or CT imaging is indicated to exclude mass lesions. Aqueous penicillin G is the antibiotic of choice (24 million units/24 h) in divided doses every 4 hours. In penicillin-allergic patients or those in whom

Haemophilus influenzae or gram-negative meningitis is a consideration, ceftriaxone, 4 g intravenously once a day, should be used. Chloramphenicol, 1 g every 6 hours, is an alternative in the severely penicillin- or cephalosporin-allergic patient.

Treatment should be continued in full doses by the intravenous route until the patient is afebrile for 5 days. Shorter courses—as few as 4 days if ceftriaxone is used—are also effective.

Obtundation or deterioration in mental status may result from cerebral edema and increased intracranial pressure. In critically ill patients with evidence of increased intracranial pressure, administration of dexamethasone (0.6 mg/kg/d in four divided doses) may help.

Heparinization is of theoretic value in disseminated intravascular coagulation and bleeding, but it does not influence prognosis.

Harrison LH et al: Risk of meningococcal infection in college students. JAMA 1999;281:1906. [PMID: 10349894]

Peltola H: Prophylaxis of bacterial meningitis. Infect Dis Clin North Am 1999;13:685. [PMID: 10470562]

Schuchat A et al: Bacterial meningitis in the United States in 1995. Active Surveillance Team. N Engl J Med 1997;337:970. [PMID: 9395430] (Incidence of *H influenzae* meningitis in adults is falling because of vaccination of children.)

INFECTIONS CAUSED BY HAEMOPHILUS SPECIES

Haemophilus influenzae and other haemophilus species may cause sinusitis, otitis, bronchitis, epiglottitis, pneumonitis, cellulitis, arthritis, meningitis, and endocarditis. **Pneumonia** is one of the more common infections of adults caused by *H influenzae* type b. Nontypeable strains are responsible for most disease in adults. The presentation is that of a typical bacterial pneumonia, with purulent sputum containing a predominance of gram-negative, pleomorphic rods. Alcoholism, smoking, chronic lung disease, advanced age, and HIV infection are important risk factors. Haemophilus species frequently colonize the upper respiratory tract. Consequently, in the absence of positive pleural fluid or blood cultures, distinguishing pneumonia from colonization or from bacterial bronchitis is difficult. Pneumonia from haemophilus species probably is overdiagnosed for this reason.

Beta-lactamase-producing strains are less common in adults than in children. For most adult patients with sinusitis, otitis, or respiratory tract infection, oral amoxicillin, 750 mg twice daily for 10–14 days, is adequate. For beta-lactamase-producing strains, use of the fixed drug combination of amoxicillin 875 mg with clavulanate 125 mg is indicated. For the penicillin-allergic patient, cefuroxime axetil, 250 mg twice daily, or trimethoprim-sulfamethoxazole, 800/160 mg orally twice daily, for 10 days is effective. Azithromycin and clarithromycin are less effective third-line agents.

In the more seriously ill patient (eg, the toxic patient with multilobar pneumonia), use of a second- or third-generation cephalosporin—cefuroxime, 750 mg every 8 hours, or ceftriaxone, 1 g/d—is advisable pending determination of whether the infecting strain is a β-lactamase producer. Trimethoprim-sulfamethoxazole, administered based on a dose of 10 mg/kg/d of trimethoprim, can be used for the penicillin-allergic patient. A 10- to 14-day course of therapy is adequate for most cases.

Epiglottitis, which occasionally occurs in adults, is characterized by an abrupt onset of high fever, drooling, and inability to handle secretions. The patient often has a severe sore throat despite an unimpressive examination of the pharynx. This is a clue to the diagnosis. Stridor and respiratory distress result from laryngeal obstruction. The diagnosis is best made by direct visualization of the cherry-red, swollen epiglottis at laryngoscopy. Because laryngoscopy may provoke laryngospasm and obstruction, especially in children, it should be performed in an intensive care unit or similar setting, and only at a time when intubation can be performed promptly. Cefuroxime, 1.5 g every 8 hours for 7–10 days, or ceftriaxone, 1 g every 24 hours for 7–10 days, is the drug of choice. Trimethoprim-sulfamethoxazole (see above for dosage) or chloramphenicol, 4 g/d, may be used in the patient with serious penicillin allergy.

Meningitis, rare in adults, becomes a consideration in the patient who has meningitis associated with sinusitis or otitis. Initial therapy of suspected *H influenzae* meningitis should be with ceftriaxone, 4 g/d in one or two divided doses, until the strain is proved not to produce β-lactamase. Chloramphenicol, 100 mg/kg/d in four divided doses, can be used if the patient has a serious, life-threatening allergy to β-lactam antibiotics. Traditionally, meningitis has been treated for 10–14 days. Dexamethasone, 0.15 mg/kg intravenously every 6 hours, is a valuable adjunctive agent in treatment of meningitis in infants and children, resulting in reduction in long-term sequelae, principally hearing loss. The role of steroids in adult meningitis is less clear.

INFECTIONS CAUSED BY *MORAXELLA CATARRHALIS*

Moraxella catarrhalis is a gram-negative aerobic coccus that is morphologically and biochemically similar to neisseria. This organism causes sinusitis, bronchitis, and pneumonia. Bacteremia and meningitis have also been reported in immunocompromised patients. The organism frequently colonizes the respiratory tract, and differentiation of colonization from infection can be difficult. If *M catarrhalis* is the predominant isolate, therapy should be directed against it. *M catarrhalis* typically produces β-lactamase and therefore is usually resistant to ampicillin and amoxicillin. It is susceptible to amoxicillin-clavulanate, ampicillin-sulbactam, trimethoprim-sulfamethoxazole, ciprofloxacin, and

second- and third-generation cephalosporins. Treatment is similar to that for haemophilus infections.

McGregor K et al: *Moraxella catarrhalis:* clinical significance, antimicrobial susceptibility and BRO beta-lactamases. Eur J Clin Microbiol Infect Dis 1998;17:219. [PMID: 9707304]

Niroumand M et al: Airway infection. Infect Dis Clin North Am 1998;12:671. [PMID: 9779384] (Reviews common causes of upper airway infection in adults, including moraxella.)

LEGIONNAIRE'S DISEASE

ESSENTIALS OF DIAGNOSIS

- *Patients are often immunocompromised, smokers, or have chronic lung disease.*
- *Scant sputum production, pleuritic chest pain, toxic appearance.*
- *Chest x-ray shows focal patchy infiltrates or consolidation.*
- *Gram's stain of sputum shows polymorphonuclear leukocytes and no organisms.*

General Considerations

Legionella infection ranks among the three or four most common causes of community-acquired pneumonia. The diagnosis must be considered whenever the etiology of a pneumonia is in question. Legionnaire's disease is more common in immunocompromised persons, in smokers, and in those with chronic lung disease. Outbreaks of legionellosis have been associated with contaminated water sources, such as shower heads and faucets in patient rooms and air conditioning cooling towers.

Clinical Findings

A. SYMPTOMS AND SIGNS

Legionnaire's disease is one of the atypical pneumonias, so called because a Gram-stained smear of sputum does not show organisms. However, many features of Legionnaire's disease are more like typical pneumonia, with high fevers, a "toxic" appearance of the patient, pleurisy, and purulent sputum (without predominant or identifiable organisms). Classically, this pneumonia is caused by *Legionella pneumophila,* though other species can cause disease that is clinically indistinguishable.

B. LABORATORY FINDINGS

Culture onto charcoal-yeast extract agar or similar enriched medium is the most sensitive method (80–90% sensitivity) for diagnosis of legionellosis and permits identification of infections caused by species and serotypes other than *L pneumophila* serotype 1. Dieterle's silver staining of tissue, pleural fluid, or other infected material is also a reliable method for detecting legionella species. Direct fluorescent antibody stains and serologic testing are less sensitive because these will detect only infection caused by *L pneumophila* serotype 1. In addition, making a serologic diagnosis requires that the host respond with sufficient specific antibody production. Urinary antigen tests, which are targeted for detection of *L pneumophila* serotype 1, are also less sensitive than culture.

Treatment

Erythromycin, 1 g every 6 hours intravenously, followed by 500 mg orally four times daily for 14–21 days, has been the preferred regimen for treatment of legionellosis. Alternative agents with excellent in vitro activity against legionella that are more easily administered and better tolerated than erythromycin are levofloxacin (500 mg once daily orally or intravenously), azithromycin (500 mg then 250 mg once daily, orally or intravenously), and clarithromycin (500 mg orally twice daily)—all administered for 10–14 days. Retrospective data indicate that azithromycin may be effective as a 5-day regimen. All indications are that these agents are just as effective as erythromycin and perhaps in some cases more effective and are now preferred to erythromycin. A 21-day course of treatment and combination therapy (eg, addition of rifampin 300 mg twice daily or macrolide-fluoroquinolone) have been recommended for legionellosis in the immunocompromised patient, but data supporting improved outcomes for combination regimens are lacking. Tetracyclines and trimethoprim-sulfamethoxazole also appear to be effective. Their use for documented infection has been limited, however, and they are best reserved for the patient who cannot be treated with either a macrolide or a fluoroquinolone.

File TM Jr et al: The role of atypical pathogens: *Mycoplasma pneumoniae, Chlamydia pneumoniae,* and *Legionella pneumophila* in respiratory infection. Infect Dis Clin North Am 1998;12:569. [PMID: 9779379]

Stout JE et al: Legionellosis. N Engl J Med 1997:682. [PMID: 9278466] (Epidemiology, pathogenesis, diagnosis, and treatment.)

Waterer GW et al: Legionella and community-acquired pneumonia: a review of current diagnostic tests from a clinician's viewpoint. Am J Med 2001;110:41. [PMID: 11152864]

GRAM-NEGATIVE BACTEREMIA & SEPSIS

There are numerous episodes of gram-negative sepsis in hospitals every year. Patients with rapidly fatal underlying diseases (neutropenic patients or those immunosuppressed by virtue of an underlying disease or medication) have a mortality rate of 40–60%; patients with ultimately fatal underlying diseases (diseases likely to be fatal in 5 years, such as solid tumors, severe liver disease, and aplastic anemia) have a mortality rate of 15–20%; and patients with no underlying disease have a low mortality rate—5% or less. Gram-negative bacteremia can originate in a number of sites, the most common being the genitourinary system, hepatobiliary tract, gastrointestinal tract, and lungs. Less common sources include intravenous lines, infusion fluids, surgical wounds, surgical drains, and decubitus ulcers.

Clinical Findings

A. SYMPTOMS AND SIGNS

Most patients have fevers and chills, often with an abrupt onset. However, 15% of patients are hypothermic (temperature ≤ 36.4 °C) at the onset of sepsis, and 5% of patients never develop a temperature above 37.5 °C. Hyperventilation with respiratory alkalosis and changes in mental status are important early manifestations. Hypotension and shock, which occur in 20–50% of patients, are unfavorable prognostic signs.

B. LABORATORY FINDINGS

Neutropenia or neutrophilia, often with increased numbers of immature forms of polymorphonuclear leukocytes, is the most common laboratory abnormality in septic patients. Thrombocytopenia occurs in 50% of patients, laboratory evidence of coagulation abnormalities in 10%, and frank DIC in 2–3%. Both clinical manifestations and the laboratory abnormalities are nonspecific and insensitive, which accounts for the relatively low rate of blood culture positivity (approximately 20–40%) in patients with suspected gram-negative sepsis. If possible, three blood cultures from separate sites should be obtained in rapid succession before starting antimicrobial therapy. The chance of recovering the organism from the blood of the septic patient with bacteremia in at least one of the three blood cultures is greater than 95%. The false-negative rate for a single culture of 5–10 mL of blood is 30%. This may be reduced to a 5–10% false-negative rate (albeit with a slight false-positive rate due to isolation of contaminants) if a single volume of 30 mL is inoculated into several blood culture bottles. Because blood cultures may be falsely negative, if the patient with presumed septic shock, negative blood cultures, and no other good explanation for the clinical course responds to antimicrobials, therapy should be continued for 10–14 days.

Treatment

Several factors are important in the management of patients with sepsis.

A. REMOVAL OF PREDISPOSING FACTORS

This usually means decreasing or stopping immunosuppressive medications and in certain circumstances (eg, documented positive blood cultures) giving granulocyte colony-stimulating factor (filgrastim; G-CSF) to the neutropenic patient.

B. IDENTIFYING THE SOURCE OF BACTEREMIA

A search for the source of bacteremia should be made. By simply finding the source and either removing it (intravenous line) or draining it (abscess), it is possible to transform what might be a fatal disease into one that is easily treatable.

C. SUPPORTIVE MEASURES

The use of fluids and pressors for maintaining blood pressure is discussed in Chapter 11; management of disseminated intravascular coagulation is discussed in Chapter 13.

D. ANTIBIOTICS

Antibiotics should be given as soon as the diagnosis of sepsis is seriously considered, since delays in therapy have been associated with increased mortality rates. In general, bactericidal antibiotics should be used and should be given intravenously to ensure therapeutic serum levels. Penetration of antibiotics into the site of primary infection is critical for successful therapy—ie, if the infection originates in the central nervous system, antibiotics that penetrate the blood-brain barrier should be used—eg, penicillin, ampicillin, chloramphenicol, and third-generation cephalosporins but not first-generation cephalosporins or aminoglycosides, which penetrate poorly. Sepsis caused by gram-positive organisms cannot be differentiated on clinical grounds from that due to gram-negative bacteria. Therefore, initial therapy should include antibiotics active against both types of organisms.

The number of antibiotics necessary to treat sepsis remains controversial and depends upon the underlying disease. Table 37–2 provides a guide for empirical therapy. Most authorities believe that for patients with rapidly fatal underlying diseases, a synergistic combination of antibiotics, including an aminoglycoside, should be used. For patients with nonfatal and ultimately fatal underlying diseases and who are not in shock, a single-drug regimen with any of several broad-spectrum antibiotics (eg, a third-generation cephalosporin, ticarcillin-clavulanate, imipenem) is adequate. Therapy can be altered once results of culture and sensitivity are known.

E. CORTICOSTEROIDS

There is no role for corticosteroids in the therapy of sepsis or septic shock.

F. ADJUNCTIVE THERAPY

Expanded knowledge of the pathophysiology of sepsis and septic shock and recognition that cytokines play a critical role have led to novel approaches to reduce morbidity and mortality associated with sepsis. Strategies include blocking the effects of endotoxin with anti-endotoxin monoclonal antibodies; blockade of

TNFα, a potent cytokine mediator of septic shock, with anti-TNF monoclonal antibody or soluble TNF receptor; use of IL-1 receptor antagonists to inhibit the proinflammatory effects of IL-1 binding to its receptor; and blocking platelet or thrombin activation. Results of clinical trials with these agents so far have been largely disappointing, with no significant improvement in overall survival. In 2001, however, a large study of recombinant human activated protein C (drotrecogin alfa) showed a significant mortality reduction in septic patients. This drug has been approved for clinical use but should be used cautiously because of the risk of bleeding. Patients enrolled in this study were considered to have an infectious cause of severe sepsis (defined as three or more signs of systemic inflammation—eg, fever or hypothermia, tachycardia, tachypnea—plus sepsis-induced dysfunction of at least one organ system) of less than 24 hours' duration. Patients who had platelet counts less than 30,000/μL, conditions associated with an increased risk of bleeding (eg, recent trauma, surgery, or bleeding episode; anticoagulation), or hypercoagulable state were excluded. These criteria should be followed when selecting candidates for treatment with drotrecogin alfa (activated). The agent is administered intravenously by constant infusion at a dosage of 24 μg/kg/h for 96 hours.

Bernard GR et al: Efficacy and safety of recombinant human activated protein C for severe sepsis. N Engl J Med 2001;344: 699. [PMID: 11236773] (Generically named drotrecogin alfa, this factor reduces mortality but may be associated with an increased risk of bleeding.)

Opal SM et al: Clinical gram-positive sepsis: does it fundamentally differ from gram-negative bacterial sepsis? Crit Care Med 1999;27:1608. [PMID: 10470773]

Wheeler AW et al: Current concepts: Treating patients with severe sepsis. N Engl J Med 1999;340:207. [PMID: 9895401]

SALMONELLOSIS

Salmonellosis includes infection by any of approximately 2000 serotypes of salmonellae. The taxonomy of salmonella species has been confusing. All salmonella serotypes are considered members of a single species, *S enterica*. Human infections are caused almost exclusively by *S enterica* subsp *enterica*, of which three serotypes—typhi, typhimurium, and choleraesuis—are predominantly isolated. Three clinical patterns of infection are recognized: (1) enteric fever, the best example of which is typhoid fever, due to serotype typhi; (2) acute enterocolitis, caused by serotype typhimurium, among others; and (3) the "septicemic" type, characterized by bacteremia and focal lesions, exemplified by infection with serotype choleraesuis. All types are transmitted by ingestion of the organism, usually from contaminated food or drink.

1. Enteric Fever (Typhoid Fever)

ESSENTIALS OF DIAGNOSIS

- Gradual onset of malaise, headache, sore throat, cough, and either diarrhea or constipation.
- Rose spots, relative bradycardia, splenomegaly, and abdominal distention and tenderness.
- Slow (stepladder) rise of fever to maximum and then slow return to normal.
- Leukopenia; blood, stool, and urine culture positive for salmonella.

General Considerations

Enteric fever is a clinical syndrome characterized by constitutional and gastrointestinal symptoms and by headache. It can be caused by any salmonella species. The term "typhoid fever" applies when serotype typhi is the cause of enteric fever accompanied by bacteremia. Infection is transmitted by consumption of contaminated food or drink. The incubation period is 5–14 days. Salmonella is an intracellular pathogen. Infection begins when organisms breach the mucosal epithelium of the intestines by transcytosis, an organism-mediated transport process through the cell via an endocytic vesicle. Having crossed the epithelial barrier, organisms invade and replicate in macrophages in Peyer's patches, mesenteric lymph nodes, and the spleen. Serotypes other than typhi usually do not cause invasive disease, presumably because they lack the necessary human-specific virulence factors. Bacteremia occurs, and the infection then localizes principally in the lymphoid tissue of the small intestine (particularly within 60 cm of the ileocecal valve). Peyer's patches become inflamed and may ulcerate, with involvement greatest during the third week of disease. The organism may disseminate to the lungs, gallbladder, kidneys, or central nervous system.

Clinical Findings

A. SYMPTOMS AND SIGNS

During the prodromal stage, there is increasing malaise, headache, cough, and sore throat, often with abdominal pain and constipation, while the fever ascends in a stepwise fashion. After about 7–10 days, the fever reaches a plateau and the patient is much more ill, appearing exhausted and often prostrated. There may be marked constipation, especially early, or "pea soup" diarrhea; marked abdominal distention occurs as well. If there are no complications, the patient's condition will gradually improve over 7–10 days.

However, relapse may occur for up to 2 weeks after defervescence.

During the early prodrome, physical findings are few. Later, splenomegaly, abdominal distention and tenderness, relative bradycardia, dicrotic pulse, and occasionally meningismus appear. The rash (rose spots) commonly appears during the second week of disease. The individual spot, found principally on the trunk, is a pink papule 2–3 mm in diameter that fades on pressure. It disappears in 3–4 days.

B. LABORATORY FINDINGS

Typhoid fever is best diagnosed by isolation of the organism from blood culture, which is positive in the first week of illness in 80% of patients who have not taken antimicrobials. The rate of blood culture positivity declines thereafter, but one-fourth or more of patients still have positive blood cultures in the third week. Cultures of bone marrow occasionally are positive when blood cultures are not. Stool culture is not reliable because it may be positive in gastroenteritis without typhoid fever.

Differential Diagnosis

Enteric fever must be distinguished from other gastrointestinal illnesses and from other infections that have few localizing findings. Examples include tuberculosis, infective endocarditis, brucellosis, lymphoma, and Q fever. Often there is a history of recent travel to endemic areas, and viral hepatitis, malaria, or amebiasis may be in the differential diagnosis as well.

Complications

Complications occur in about 30% of untreated cases and account for 75% of all deaths. Intestinal hemorrhage, manifested by a sudden drop in temperature and signs of shock followed by dark or fresh blood in the stool, or intestinal perforation, accompanied by abdominal pain and tenderness, is most likely to occur during the third week. Less frequent complications are urinary retention, pneumonia, thrombophlebitis, myocarditis, psychosis, cholecystitis, nephritis, osteomyelitis, and meningitis.

Prevention

Immunization is not always effective but should be provided for household contacts of a typhoid carrier, for travelers to endemic areas, and during epidemic outbreaks. A multiple-dose oral vaccine and a single-dose parenteral vaccine are available. Their efficacies are similar, but oral vaccine causes fewer side effects. Boosters, when indicated, should be given every 5 years and 3 years for oral and parenteral preparations, respectively.

Adequate waste disposal and protection of food and water supplies from contamination are important public health measures to prevent salmonellosis. Carriers must not be permitted to work as food handlers.

Treatment

A. SPECIFIC MEASURES

Ampicillin, chloramphenicol, and trimethoprim-sulfamethoxazole may be effective. All can be given orally or intravenously depending on the patient's condition. Because many salmonella strains are resistant to ampicillin and chloramphenicol, trimethoprim-sulfamethoxazole has been the agent of choice for treatment of salmonella infections. Resistance to trimethoprim-sulfamethoxazole now appears to be on the rise. Salmonellae remain susceptible to ceftriaxone and fluoroquinolones, though resistance to the latter is now appearing in anecdotal reports. The dose of ceftriaxone is 2 g orally once daily. The dose of ciprofloxacin is 750 mg orally twice daily. Fluoroquinolones are contraindicated in children and pregnant women. The recommended duration of therapy traditionally has been 2 weeks, but 5–10 days may be sufficient.

B. TREATMENT OF CARRIERS

Chemotherapy often is unsuccessful in eradicating the carrier state. While treatment of carriage with ampicillin, trimethoprim-sulfamethoxazole, or chloramphenicol may be successful, one recent study suggests that ciprofloxacin, 750 mg twice a day for 4 weeks, is highly effective. Cholecystectomy may also achieve this goal.

Prognosis

The mortality rate of typhoid fever is about 2% in treated cases. Elderly or debilitated persons are likely to do poorly.

With complications, the prognosis is poor. Relapses occur in up to 15% of cases. A residual carrier state frequently persists in spite of chemotherapy.

Akalin HE: Quinolones in the treatment of typhoid fever. Drugs 1999;58(Suppl 2):52. [PMID: 10553706] (The strengths and weaknesses of quinolones as therapy for infectious diarrhea.)

Chandel DS et al: Drug-resistant *Salmonella enterica* serotype paratyphi A in India. Emerg Infect Dis 2000;6:420. [PMID: 1090598]

Hakanen A et al: Increasing fluoroquinolone resistance in salmonella serotypes in Finland during 1995–1997. J Antimicrob Chemother 1999;43:145. [PMID: 10381114]

2. Salmonella Gastroenteritis

By far the most common form of salmonellosis is acute enterocolitis. Numerous salmonella serotypes may cause enterocolitis. The incubation period is 8–48 hours after ingestion of contaminated food or liquid.

Symptoms and signs consist of fever (often with chills), nausea and vomiting, cramping abdominal pain, and diarrhea, which may be grossly bloody, lasting 3–5 days. Differentiation must be made from viral gastroenteritis, food poisoning, shigellosis, amebic dysentery, acute ulcerative colitis, and acute surgical abdominal conditions. The diagnosis is made by culturing the organism from the stool.

The disease is usually self-limited, but bacteremia with localization in joints or bones may occur, especially in patients with sickle cell disease.

Treatment of uncomplicated enterocolitis is symptomatic only. Malnourished or severely ill patients, those with sickle cell disease, and those with suspected bacteremia should be treated for 3–5 days with trimethoprim-sulfamethoxazole (one double-strength tablet twice a day), ampicillin (100 mg/kg intravenously or orally), or ciprofloxacin (750 mg twice a day).

3. Salmonella Bacteremia

Salmonella infection may be manifested by prolonged or recurrent fevers accompanied by bacteremia and local infection in bone, joints, pleura, pericardium, lungs, or other sites. Mycotic abdominal aortic aneurysms may also be a complication. Serotypes other than typhi usually are isolated. This complication tends to occur in immunocompromised persons and is seen in HIV-infected individuals, who typically have bacteremia without an obvious source. Treatment is the same as for typhoid fever, plus drainage of any abscesses. In HIV-infected patients, relapse is common, and lifelong suppressive therapy may be needed. Ciprofloxacin, 750 mg twice a day, is effective both for therapy of acute infection and for suppression of recurrence.

SHIGELLOSIS

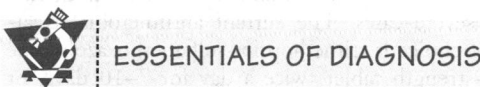

ESSENTIALS OF DIAGNOSIS

- *Diarrhea, often with blood and mucus.*
- *Crampy abdominal pain and systemic toxicity.*
- *White blood cells in stools; organism isolated on stool culture.*

General Considerations

Shigella dysentery is a common disease, often self-limited and mild but occasionally serious. *Shigella sonnei* is the leading cause in the USA, followed by *Shigella flexneri*. *Shigella dysenteriae* causes the most serious form of the illness. Shigellae are invasive organisms: The infective dose is 10^2–10^3 organisms. Recently, there has been a rise in strains resistant to multiple antibiotics.

Clinical Findings

A. SYMPTOMS AND SIGNS

The illness usually starts abruptly, with diarrhea, lower abdominal cramps, and tenesmus. The diarrheal stool often is mixed with blood and mucus. Systemic symptoms are fever, chills, anorexia and malaise, and headache. The patient becomes progressively weaker and more dehydrated. The abdomen is tender. Sigmoidoscopic examination reveals an inflamed, engorged mucosa with punctate, sometimes large areas of ulceration.

B. LABORATORY FINDINGS

The stool shows many leukocytes and red cells. Stool culture is positive for shigellae in most cases, but blood cultures grow the organism in less than 5% of cases.

Differential Diagnosis

Bacillary dysentery must be distinguished from salmonella enterocolitis and from disease due to enterotoxigenic *E coli*, campylobacter, and *Y enterocolitica*. Amebic dysentery may be similar clinically and is diagnosed by finding amebas in the fresh stool specimen. Ulcerative colitis in the adolescent and adult is an important cause of bloody diarrhea.

Complications

Temporary disaccharidase deficiency may follow the diarrhea. Reactive arthritis is an uncommon complication, usually occurring in HLA-B27 individuals infected by shigella.

Treatment

Treatment of dehydration and hypotension is lifesaving in severe cases. The current antimicrobial treatment of choice is trimethoprim-sulfamethoxazole, one double-strength tablet twice a day for 7–10 days, or ciprofloxacin (contraindicated in pregnancy), 750 mg twice daily for 7–10 days, a fluoroquinolone (ciprofloxacin, 750 mg twice daily, or levofloxacin, 500 mg once daily) for 3 days. Fluoroquinolones are contraindicated in pregnancy. Shigellae resistant to ampicillin are common, but if the isolate is susceptible, a dose of 500 mg four times a day is also effective. Amoxicillin, which is less effective, should not be used.

GASTROENTERITIS CAUSED BY *ESCHERICHIA COLI*

Escherichia coli causes gastroenteritis by a variety of mechanisms. Enterotoxigenic *E coli* (ETEC) elaborates either a heat-stable or heat-labile toxin that mediates the disease. ETEC is an important cause of traveler's diarrhea. Enteroinvasive *E coli* (EIEC) differs from other *E coli* bowel pathogens in that these strains invade cells, causing bloody diarrhea and dysentery similar to infection with shigella species. EIEC is uncommon in the United States. Neither ETEC nor EIEC strains are routinely isolated and identified from stool cultures because there is no selective medium. Antimicrobial therapy directed against salmonella and shigella shortens the clinical course, but the disease is self-limited.

Enterohemorrhagic *E coli* (EHEC) produces two shiga-like toxins that mediate the clinical manifestations, which include an asymptomatic carriage stage, nonbloody diarrhea, hemorrhagic colitis, hemolytic-uremic syndrome, and thrombotic thrombocytopenic purpura. Although there are several serotypes of EHEC, O157:H7 is responsible for most cases in the United States. *E coli* O157:H7 has been responsible for several outbreaks of diarrhea and hemolytic-uremic syndrome related to consumption of undercooked hamburger and unpasteurized apple juice. Elderly individuals and young children are most severely affected, with hemolytic-uremic syndrome being more common in the latter group. *E coli* O157:H7 is not identified by routine stool cultures. Isolation requires identification of sorbitol-negative colonies of *E coli* on sorbitol-MacConkey agar followed by serologic testing to confirm the serotype. Antimicrobial therapy does not alter the course of the disease, and may increase the risk of hemolytic-uremic syndrome. Treatment is primarily supportive. Hemolytic-uremic syndrome or thrombotic thrombocytopenic purpura occurring in association with a diarrheal illness suggests the diagnosis and should prompt evaluation for EHEC. Confirmed infections should be reported to public health officials.

Besser RE et al: *Escherichia coli* O157:H7 gastroenteritis and the hemolytic uremic syndrome: an emerging infectious disease. Annu Rev Med 1999;50:355. [PMID: 10073283]

Karch H et al: Epidemiology and diagnosis of Shiga toxin-producing *Escherichia coli* infections. Diagnostic Microbiol Infect Dis 1999;34:229. [PMID: 10403103]

Wong CS et al: The risk of the hemolytic-uremic syndrome after antibiotic treatment of *Escherichia coli* O157:H7 infections. N Engl J Med 2000;342:1930. [PMID: 10874060]

CHOLERA

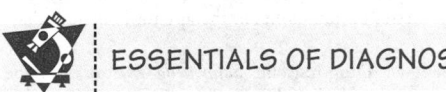

ESSENTIALS OF DIAGNOSIS

- *Voluminous diarrhea.*
- *Stool is liquid, gray, turbid, and without fecal odor, blood, or pus ("rice water stool").*
- *Rapid development of marked dehydration.*
- *History of travel in endemic area or contact with infected person.*
- *Positive stool cultures and agglutination of vibrios with specific sera.*

General Considerations

Cholera is an acute diarrheal illness caused by certain serotypes of *Vibrio cholerae*. The disease is toxin-mediated, and fever is unusual. The toxin activates adenylyl cyclase in intestinal epithelial cells of the small intestines, producing hypersecretion of water and chloride ion and a massive diarrhea of up to 15 L per day. Death results from profound hypovolemia.

Cholera occurs in epidemics under conditions of crowding, war, and famine (eg, in refugee camps) and where sanitation is inadequate. Infection is acquired by ingestion of contaminated food or water. Cholera was rarely seen in the United States until 1991, when epidemic cholera returned to the Western Hemisphere, originating as an outbreak in coastal cities of Peru. The epidemic spread to involve several countries in South and Central America as well as Mexico, and cases have been imported into the United States. Cholera should be considered in the differential diagnosis of severe watery diarrhea, especially in those who have traveled to affected countries.

Clinical Findings

Cholera is characterized by a sudden onset of severe, frequent watery diarrhea (up to 1 L per hour). The liquid stool is gray, turbid, and without fecal odor, blood, or pus ("rice water stool"). Dehydration and hypotension develop rapidly. Stool cultures are positive, and agglutination of vibrios with specific sera can be demonstrated.

Prevention

A vaccine is available that confers short-lived, limited protection and may be required for entry into or reentry after travel to some countries. It is administered in two doses 1–4 weeks apart. A booster dose every 6 months is recommended for persons remaining in areas where cholera is a hazard.

Vaccination programs are expensive and not particularly effective in managing outbreaks of cholera. When outbreaks occur, efforts should be directed toward establishing clean water and food sources and proper waste disposal.

Treatment

Treatment is by replacement of fluids. In mild or moderate illness, oral rehydration usually is adequate. A simple oral replacement fluid can be made from 1 teaspoon of table salt and 4 heaping teaspoons of sugar added to 1 L of water. Intravenous fluids are indicated for persons in shock or those with other signs of severe hypovolemia and those who cannot take adequate fluids orally. Lactated Ringer's infusion is satisfactory.

Antimicrobial therapy will shorten the course of illness. Several antimicrobials are active against V cholerae, including tetracycline, ampicillin, chloramphenicol, trimethoprim-sulfamethoxazole, and fluoroquinolones. Multiple antibiotic resistance does occur, so susceptibility testing, if available, is advisable.

Guerrant RL et al: How intestinal bacteria cause disease. J Infect Dis 1999;179(Suppl 2):S331. [PMID: 10081504]

INFECTIONS CAUSED BY OTHER VIBRIO SPECIES

Vibrios other than *Vibrio cholerae* that cause human disease are *Vibrio parahaemolyticus*, *Vibrio vulnificus*, and *Vibrio alginolyticus*. All are halophilic marine organisms. Infection is acquired by exposure to organisms in contaminated, undercooked, or raw crustaceans or shellfish and warm (> 20 °C) ocean waters and estuaries. Infections are more common during the summer months from regions along the Atlantic coast and the Gulf of Mexico in the United States and from tropical waters around the world. Oysters are implicated in up to 90% of food-related cases. *V parahaemolyticus* causes an acute watery diarrhea with crampy abdominal pain and fever, typically occurring within 24 hours after ingestion of contaminated shellfish. The disease is self-limited, and antimicrobial therapy is usually not necessary. *V parahaemolyticus* may also cause cellulitis and sepsis, though these findings are more characteristic of *V vulnificus* infection.

V vulnificus and *V alginolyticus*—neither of which is associated with diarrheal illness—are important causes of cellulitis and primary bacteremia, which may follow ingestion of contaminated shellfish or exposure to sea water. Cellulitis with or without sepsis may be accompanied by bulla formation and necrosis with extensive soft tissue destruction, at times requiring debridement and amputation. The infection can be rapidly progressive and is particularly severe in immunocompromised individuals—especially those with cirrhosis—with death rates as high as 50%. Patients with chronic liver disease and those who are immunocompromised should be cautioned to avoid eating raw oysters.

Tetracycline at a dose of 500 mg four times a day for 7–10 days is the drug of choice for treatment of suspected or documented primary bacteremia or cellulitis caused by vibrio species. *V vulnificus* is susceptible in vitro to penicillin, ampicillin, cephalosporins, chloramphenicol, aminoglycosides, and fluoroquinolones, and these agents may also be effective. *V parahaemolyticus* and *V alginolyticus* produce β-lactamase and therefore are resistant to penicillin and ampicillin, but susceptibilities otherwise are similar to those listed for *V vulnificus*.

INFECTIONS CAUSED BY CAMPYLOBACTER SPECIES

Campylobacters are microaerophilic, motile, gram-negative rods. Two species infect humans: *Campylobacter jejuni*, an important cause of diarrheal disease; and *Campylobacter fetus* subsp *fetus*, which typically causes systemic infection and not diarrhea. Dairy cattle and poultry are an important reservoir for campylobacters. Outbreaks of enteritis have been associated with consumption of raw milk. Campylobacter gastroenteritis is associated with fever, abdominal pain, and diarrhea characterized by loose, watery, or bloody stools. The differential diagnosis includes shigellosis, salmonella gastroenteritis, and enteritis caused by *Yersinia enterocolitica* or invasive *Escherichia coli*. The disease is self-limited, but its duration can be shortened with antimicrobial therapy. Both erythromycin, 250–500 mg four times daily for 5–7 days, and ciprofloxacin, 500 mg twice daily for 3–5 days, are effective regimens. Pending identification of the causative agent of suspected bacterial gastroenteritis, ciprofloxacin is a rational choice for empirical therapy because all of the common bacterial pathogens are susceptible.

C fetus causes systemic infections that can be fatal, including primary bacteremia, endocarditis, meningitis, and focal abscesses. It infrequently causes gastroenteritis. Patients infected with *C fetus* are often elderly, debilitated, or immunocompromised. Closely related species, collectively termed campylobacter-like organisms, cause bacteremia in HIV-infected individuals. Systemic infections respond to therapy with gentamicin, chloramphenicol, ceftriaxone, or ciprofloxacin. Ceftriaxone or chloramphenicol should be used to treat infections of the central nervous system because of their ability to penetrate the blood-brain barrier.

BRUCELLOSIS

ESSENTIALS OF DIAGNOSIS

- *Insidious onset: easy fatigability, headache, arthralgia, anorexia, sweating, irritability.*
- *History of animal exposure, ingestion of unpasteurized milk or cheese.*
- *Intermittent fever, especially at night, which may become chronic and undulant.*
- *Cervical and axillary lymphadenopathy; hepatosplenomegaly.*
- *Lymphocytosis, positive blood culture, elevated agglutination titer.*

General Considerations

The infection is transmitted from animals to humans. *Brucella abortus* (cattle), *Brucella suis* (hogs), and *Brucella melitensis* (goats) are the main agents. Transmission to humans occurs by contact with infected meat (slaughterhouse workers), placentae of infected animals (farmers, veterinarians), or ingestion of infected unpasteurized milk or cheese. The incubation period varies from a few days to several weeks. The disorder may become chronic. In the USA, brucellosis is very rare except in the midwestern states (from *B suis*) and in visitors or immigrants from countries where brucel-

losis is endemic (eg, Mexico, Spain, South American countries).

Clinical Findings

A. SYMPTOMS AND SIGNS

The onset may be acute, with fever, chills, and sweats, but typically is insidious. It may be weeks before the patient seeks medical care for weakness, weight loss, low-grade fevers, sweats, and exhaustion upon minimal activity. Symptoms also include headache, abdominal or back pains with anorexia and constipation, and arthralgia. Epididymitis occurs in 10% of cases in men. The chronic form may assume an undulant nature, with periods of normal temperature between acute attacks; symptoms may persist for years, either continuously or intermittently.

Physical findings are minimal. Half of cases have peripheral lymph node enlargement and splenomegaly; hepatomegaly is less common.

B. LABORATORY FINDINGS

Early in the course of infection, the organism can be recovered from the blood, cerebrospinal fluid, urine, and bone marrow. Because the organism is slow-growing, cultures should be incubated for 21 days before being read as negative. Cultures are more likely to be negative in chronic cases. The diagnosis often is made by serologic testing. Rising serologic titers or an absolute agglutination titer of greater than 1:100 supports the diagnosis.

Differential Diagnosis

Brucellosis must be differentiated from any other acute febrile disease, especially influenza, tularemia, Q fever, mononucleosis, and enteric fever. In its chronic form it resembles Hodgkin's disease, tuberculosis, HIV infection, malaria, and disseminated fungal infections such as histoplasmosis and coccidioidomycosis.

Complications

The most frequent complications are bone and joint lesions such as spondylitis and suppurative arthritis (usually of a single joint), endocarditis, and meningoencephalitis. Less common complications are pneumonitis with pleural effusion, hepatitis, and cholecystitis.

Treatment

Single-drug regimens are not recommended because the relapse rate may be as high as 50%. Combination regimens of two or three drugs are more effective. Either (1) doxycycline plus rifampin or streptomycin (or both) *or* (2) trimethoprim-sulfamethoxazole plus rifampin or streptomycin (or both) is effective in doses as follows for 21 days: doxycycline, 100–200 mg/d in divided doses; trimethoprim 320 mg/d plus sulfamethoxazole 1600 mg/d in divided doses; rifampin, 600–1200 mg/d; and streptomycin, 500 mg intramuscularly twice a day. Longer courses of therapy (eg, several months) may be required to cure relapses, osteomyelitis, or meningitis.

Yagupsky P: Detection of brucellae in blood cultures. J Clin Microbiol 1999;37:3437. [PMID: 10523530]

TULAREMIA

ESSENTIALS OF DIAGNOSIS

- *Fever, headache, nausea, and prostration.*
- *Papule progressing to ulcer at site of inoculation.*
- *Enlarged regional lymph nodes.*
- *History of contact with rabbits, other rodents, and biting arthropods (eg, ticks in summer) in endemic area.*
- *Serologic tests or culture of ulcer, lymph node aspirate, or blood confirm the diagnosis.*

General Considerations

Tularemia is an infection of wild rodents—particularly rabbits and muskrats—with *Francisella (Pasteurella) tularensis.* Humans usually acquire the infection by contact with animal tissues (eg, trapping muskrats, skinning rabbits) or from ticks. Investigation of an outbreak of pneumonic tularemia on Martha's Vineyard in Massachusetts implicated lawn-mowing and brush-cutting as risk factors for infection, underscoring the potential for probable aerosol transmission of the organism. *F tularensis* has been classified as a high-priority agent for potential bioterrorism use because of its virulence and relative ease of dissemination. Infection in humans often produces a local lesion and widespread organ involvement but may be entirely asymptomatic. The incubation period is 2–10 days.

Clinical Findings

A. Symptoms and Signs

Fever, headache, and nausea begin suddenly, and a local lesion—a papule at the site of inoculation—develops and soon ulcerates. Regional lymph nodes may become enlarged and tender and may suppurate. The local lesion may be on the skin of an extremity or in the eye. Pneumonia may develop from hematogenous spread of the organism or may be primary after inhalation of infected aerosols, which are responsible for human-to-human transmission. Following ingestion of infected meat or water, an enteric form may be manifested by gastrointestinal symptoms, stupor, and delirium. In any type of involvement, the spleen may be enlarged and tender and there may be nonspecific rashes, myalgias, and prostration.

B. Laboratory Findings

Culturing the organism from blood or infected tissue requires special media. For this reason and because cultures of *F tularensis* may be hazardous to laboratory personnel, the diagnosis is usually made serologically. A positive agglutination test (> 1:80) develops in the second week after infection and may persist for several years.

Differential Diagnosis

Tularemia must be differentiated from rickettsial and meningococcal infections, cat-scratch disease, infectious mononucleosis, and various bacterial and fungal diseases.

Complications

Hematogenous spread may produce meningitis, perisplenitis, pericarditis, pneumonia, and osteomyelitis.

Treatment

Streptomycin, 0.5 g intramuscularly every 6–8 hours, together with tetracycline 0.5 g orally every 6 hours, is administered until 4–5 days after the patient becomes afebrile. Chloramphenicol may be substituted for tetracycline in the same dosage.

Feldman KA et al: An outbreak of primary pneumonic tularemia on Martha's Vineyard. N Engl J Med 2001;345:1601. [PMID: 11757506]

PLAGUE

ESSENTIALS OF DIAGNOSIS

- *History of exposure to rodents in endemic area.*
- *Sudden onset of high fever, malaise, muscular pains, and prostration.*
- *Axillary or inguinal lymphadenitis (bubo).*
- *Bacteremia, sepsis, and pneumonitis may occur.*

• *Positive smear and culture from bubo and positive blood culture.*

General Considerations

Plague is an infection of wild rodents with *Yersinia pestis,* a small bipolar-staining gram-negative rod. Plague is endemic in California, Arizona, Nevada, and New Mexico. It is transmitted among rodents and to humans by the bites of fleas or from contact with infected animals. If a plague victim develops pneumonia, the infection can be transmitted by droplets to other individuals. The incubation period is 2–10 days.

Because of its extreme virulence, its potential for dissemination and person-to-person transmission, and efforts to develop the organism as an agent of biowarfare, plague bacillus is considered a high-priority agent for bioterrorism.

Following the flea bite, the organisms spread through the lymphatics to the lymph nodes, which become greatly enlarged (bubo). They may then reach the bloodstream to involve all organs. When pneumonia or meningitis develops, the outcome is often fatal.

Clinical Findings

A. SYMPTOMS AND SIGNS

The onset is sudden, with high fever, malaise, tachycardia, intense headache, and severe myalgias. The patient appears profoundly ill. Delirium may ensue. If pneumonia develops, tachypnea, productive cough, blood-tinged sputum, and cyanosis also occur. Signs of meningitis may develop. A pustule or ulcer at the site of inoculation and signs of lymphangitis may be observed. Axillary, inguinal, or cervical lymph nodes become enlarged and tender and may eventually suppurate and drain. With hematogenous spread, the patient may rapidly become toxic and comatose, with purpuric spots (black plague) appearing on the skin.

Primary plague pneumonia is a fulminant pneumonitis with bloody, frothy sputum and sepsis. It is usually fatal unless treatment is started within a few hours after onset.

B. LABORATORY FINDINGS

The plague bacillus may be found in smears from aspirates of buboes examined with Gram's stain. Cultures from bubo aspirate or pus and blood are positive but may grow slowly. In convalescing patients, an antibody titer rise may be demonstrated by agglutination tests.

Differential Diagnosis

The lymphadenitis of plague is most commonly mistaken for the lymphadenitis accompanying staphylococcal or streptococcal infections of an extremity, sexually transmitted diseases such as lymphogranuloma venereum or syphilis, and tularemia. The systemic manifestations resemble those of enteric or rickettsial fevers, malaria, or influenza. The pneumonia resembles other bacterial pneumonias, and the meningitis is similar to those caused by other bacteria.

Prevention

Drug prophylaxis may provide temporary protection for persons exposed to the risk of plague infection, particularly by the respiratory route. Tetracycline hydrochloride, 500 mg orally once or twice daily for 5 days, is effective.

Plague vaccines—both live and killed—have been used for many years, but their efficacy is not clearly established.

Treatment

Therapy should be started immediately once plague is suspected. Either streptomycin (the agent with which there is greatest experience), 1 g every 12 hours intravenously, or gentamicin, administered as a 2 mg/kg loading dose, then 1.7 mg/kg every 8 hours intravenously, is effective. Alternatively, doxycycline, 100 mg orally or intravenously, may be used. The duration of therapy is 10 days. Patients with plague pneumonia should be placed in strict respiratory isolation.

Galimand M: Brief report: Multidrug resistance in *Yersinia pestis* mediated by a transferable plasmid. N Engl J Med 1999;340:677. [PMID: 9278464]

Koornhof HJ et al: Yersiniosis. II: The pathogenesis of Yersinia infections. Eur J Clin Microbiol Infect Dis 1999;18:87. [PMID: 10219573]

GONOCOCCAL INFECTIONS

 ESSENTIALS OF DIAGNOSIS

• *Purulent and profuse urethral discharge, especially in men, with dysuria, yielding positive smear.*

• *Epididymitis, prostatitis, periurethral inflammation, proctitis in men.*

• *Cervicitis in women with purulent discharge, or asymptomatic, yielding positive culture; vaginitis, salpingitis, proctitis also occur.*

• *Fever, rash, tenosynovitis, and arthritis with disseminated disease.*

• *Gram-negative intracellular diplococci seen in a smear or cultured from any site, particularly the urethra, cervix, pharynx, and rectum.*

General Considerations

Gonorrhea is caused by *Neisseria gonorrhoeae,* a gram-negative diplococcus typically found inside polymorphonuclear cells. It is most commonly transmitted during sexual activity and has its greatest incidence in the 15- to 29-year-old age group. The incubation period is usually 2–8 days.

Anatomic Classification

A. Urethritis and Cervicitis

In men, there is initially burning on urination and a serous or milky discharge. One to 3 days later, the urethral pain is more pronounced and the discharge becomes yellow, creamy, and profuse, sometimes blood-tinged. The disorder may regress and become chronic or progress to involve the prostate, epididymis, and periurethral glands with acute, painful inflammation. Chronic infection leads to prostatitis and urethral strictures. Rectal infection is common in homosexual men. Atypical sites of primary infection (eg, the pharynx) must always be considered. Asymptomatic infection is common and occurs in both sexes.

Gonococcal infection in women often becomes symptomatic during menses. Women may have dysuria, urinary frequency, and urgency, with a purulent urethral discharge. Vaginitis and cervicitis with inflammation of Bartholin's glands are common. Infection may be asymptomatic, with only slightly increased vaginal discharge and moderate cervicitis on examination. Infection may remain as a chronic cervicitis—an important reservoir of gonococci. It may progress to involve the uterus and tubes with acute and chronic salpingitis and with ultimate scarring of tubes and sterility. In pelvic inflammatory disease, anaerobes and chlamydiae often accompany gonococci. Rectal infection may result from spread of the organism from the genital tract or from anal coitus.

Gram stain of urethral discharge in men, especially during the first week after onset, typically shows gram-negative diplococci in polymorphonuclear leukocytes. Gram stain is less often positive in women. Culture has been the gold standard for diagnosis, particularly when the Gram stain is negative. A ligase chain reaction (LCR) assay that detects both *N gonorrhoeae* and *Chlamydia trachomatis* in cervical and urethral swab specimens and urine permits more rapid diagnosis of gonococcal infection. LCR also has improved sensitivity (approximately 90–95% for urine and > 95% for swab) and high specificity (≥ 99%) compared with culture of swab specimens (overall sensitivity of approximately 80%). This test is likely to replace culture, particularly for screening, because of the convenience of obtaining a urine sample compared with swab and because it detects *C trachomatis* coinfection. Identification of *N gonorrhoeae* from rectal or pharyngeal sites and in joint fluid still requires culture.

B. Disseminated Disease

Systemic complications follow the dissemination of gonococci from the primary site via the bloodstream. Gonococcal bacteremia is associated with intermittent fever, arthralgia, and skin lesions ranging from maculopapular to pustular or hemorrhagic, which tend to be few in number and peripherally located. Rarely, gonococcal endocarditis or meningitis develops. Arthritis and tenosynovitis are common complications, particularly involving the knees, ankles, and wrists. One or occasionally a few joints usually are involved. Gonococci can be isolated from less than half of patients with gonococcal arthritis.

C. Conjunctivitis

The most common form of eye involvement is direct inoculation of gonococci into the conjunctival sac. In adults, this occurs by autoinoculation of a person with genital infection. The purulent conjunctivitis may rapidly progress to panophthalmitis and loss of the eye unless treated promptly. A single 1-g dose of ceftriaxone is effective.

Differential Diagnosis

Gonococcal urethritis or cervicitis must be differentiated from nongonococcal urethritis; cervicitis or vaginitis due to *Chlamydia trachomatis, Gardnerella vaginalis,* trichomonas, candida, and many other agents associated with sexually transmitted diseases; pelvic inflammatory disease, arthritis, proctitis, and skin lesions. Often, several such agents coexist in a patient. Reiter's disease (urethritis, conjunctivitis, arthritis) may mimic gonorrhea or coexist with it.

Prevention

Prevention is based on education, mechanical or chemical prophylaxis, and early diagnosis and treatment. The condom, if properly used, can reduce the risk of infection. Effective drugs taken in therapeutic doses within 24 hours of exposure can abort an infection.

Treatment

Therapy typically is administered before antimicrobial susceptibilities are known. The choice of which regimen to use should be based on the prevalence of penicillin-resistant organisms. Recent data indicate a nationwide distribution of penicillin- and tetracycline-resistant gonococci. Consequently, penicillin should no longer be considered first-line therapy. All sexual partners should be treated.

A. Uncomplicated Gonorrhea

For urethritis or cervicitis, either ceftriaxone, 125 mg intramuscularly, or cefixime, 400 mg orally as a single dose, is the treatment of choice. Fluoroquinolones are no longer recommended as first-line agents because of concerns about emerging resistance. A single oral dose of ciprofloxacin 500 mg, ofloxacin 400 mg, or levofloxacin 250 mg is also effective. Spectinomycin, 1 g intramuscularly once, may be used for the penicillin-allergic patient. Amoxicillin is no longer recommended owing to the prevalence of penicillin-resistant strains of gonococci. Anal gonorrhea in women responds to the same drugs, but in males ceftriaxone is most effective. Pharyngeal gonorrhea responds to ceftriaxone in the same dosage or to trimethoprim-sulfamethoxazole, nine regular-strength tablets orally daily for 5 days. Since coexistent chlamydial infection is common, one should give doxycycline, 100 mg twice daily orally for 7 days, or a single 1 g oral dose of azithromycin, concurrently.

B. TREATMENT OF OTHER INFECTIONS

Salpingitis, prostatitis, bacteremia, arthritis, and other complications due to susceptible strains in adults should be treated with penicillin G, 10 million units intravenously daily, for 5 days. Ceftriaxone, 1 g intravenously daily for 5 days, or an oral fluoroquinolone (ciprofloxacin, 500 mg twice daily, or levofloxacin, 500 mg once daily) for 5 days also are effective. Endocarditis should be treated with ceftriaxone, 1 g every 12 hours intravenously, for at least 3 weeks. Postgonococcal urethritis and cervicitis, which is usually caused by chlamydia, is treated with a regimen of erythromycin, doxycycline, or azithromycin as described above. Serologic tests for syphilis should also be obtained.

Pelvic inflammatory disease requires cefoxitin, 2 g parenterally every 6 hours, or cefotetan, 2 g intravenously every 12 hours. Clindamycin, 900 mg intravenously every 8 hours, plus gentamicin, administered as a 2 mg/kg loading dose followed by 1.5 mg/kg every 8 hours, is also effective. Cefoxitin, 2 g intramuscularly, plus probenecid, 1 g orally as a single dose, followed by a 14-day oral regimen of doxycycline, 100 mg twice a day, is an effective outpatient regimen. Concurrent treatment for chlamydial infection also is indicated. Alternative drug choices exist.

Woodward C et al: Drug treatment of common STDs: Part I. Herpes, syphilis, urethritis, chlamydia and gonorrhea. Am Fam Physician 1999;60:1387. [PMID: 10537386]

CHANCROID

Chancroid is a sexually transmitted disease caused by the short gram-negative bacillus *Haemophilus ducreyi*. The incubation period is 3–5 days. The initial lesion at the site of inoculation is a vesicopustule that breaks down to form a painful, soft ulcer with a necrotic base, surrounding erythema, and undermined edges. Multiple lesions—started by autoinoculation—and inguinal adenitis often develop. The adenitis is usually unilateral and consists of tender, matted nodes of moderate size with overlying erythema. These may become fluctuant and rupture spontaneously. With lymph node involvement, fever, chills, and malaise may develop. Balanitis and phimosis are frequent complications in men. Women may have no external signs of infection. The diagnosis is established by culturing a swab of the lesion onto special medium.

Chancroid must be differentiated from other genital ulcers. The chancre of syphilis, by contrast, is clean and painless, with a hard base. Mixed sexually transmitted disease is very common (including syphilis, herpes simplex, and HIV infection), as is infection of the ulcer with fusiforms, spirochetes, and other organisms.

A single dose of either azithromycin, 1 g orally, or ceftriaxone, 250 mg intramuscularly, is effective treatment. Effective multiple-dose regimens are amoxicillin-potassium clavulanate (500/125 mg) three times a day orally for 7 days; erythromycin, 500 mg orally four times a day for 7 days; or ciprofloxacin, 500 mg orally twice a day for 3 days.

GRANULOMA INGUINALE

Granuloma inguinale is a chronic, relapsing granulomatous anogenital infection due to *Calymmatobacterium (Donovania) granulomatis*. The pathognomonic cell, found in tissue scrapings or secretions, is large (25–90 μm) and contains intracytoplasmic cysts filled with bodies (Donovan bodies) that stain deeply with Wright's stain.

The incubation period is 8 days to 12 weeks. The onset is insidious. The lesions occur on the skin or mucous membranes of the genitalia or perineal area. They are relatively painless infiltrated nodules that soon slough. A shallow, sharply demarcated ulcer forms, with a beefy-red friable base of granulation tissue. The lesion spreads by contiguity. The advancing border has a characteristic rolled edge of granulation tissue. Large ulcerations may advance onto the lower abdomen and thighs. Scar formation and healing may occur along one border while the opposite border advances.

Superinfection with spirochete-fusiform organisms is common. The ulcer then becomes purulent, painful, foul-smelling, and extremely difficult to treat.

Several therapies are available. Because of the indolent nature of the disease, duration of therapy tends to be relatively long. Erythromycin or tetracycline, 500 mg four times a day for 21 days, is effective. Ampicillin, 500 mg four times a day, also is effective, but up to 12 weeks of therapy may be necessary.

Since other sexually transmitted diseases frequently coexist, cultures for these and a serologic test for syphilis must be performed.

National guideline for the management of donovanosis (granuloma inguinale). Clinical Effectiveness Group (Association of Genitourinary Medicine and the Medical Society for the Study of Venereal Diseases). Sex Transm Infect 1999;75(Suppl 1):S38. [PMID: 10616381]

BARTONELLA SPECIES

A revised classification of the α_2 subdivision of proteobacteria has grouped the species previously known as rochalimaea as members of the bartonellae based on ribosomal RNA. These organisms (which include *B quintana, B henselae, B vinsonii,* and *B elizabethae*) are responsible for a wide variety of clinical syndromes. **Bacillary angiomatosis,** an important manifestation of bartonellosis, is discussed in Chapter 31.

Trench fever is a self-limited, louse-borne relapsing febrile disease caused by *B quintana.* The disease has occurred epidemically in louse-infested troops and civilians during wars and endemically in residents of scattered geographic areas (eg, Central America). An urban equivalent of trench fever has been described among the homeless. Humans acquire infection when infected lice feces enter sites of skin breakdown. Onset of symptoms is abrupt and fever lasts 3–5 days, with relapses. The patient complains of weakness and severe pain behind the eyes and typically in the back and legs. Lymphadenopathy, splenomegaly, and a transient maculopapular rash may appear. Subclinical infection is frequent, and a carrier state is recognized. The differential diagnosis includes other febrile, self-limited states such as dengue, leptospirosis, malaria, relapsing fever, and typhus. Recovery occurs regularly even in the absence of treatment.

Brouqui P et al: Chronic *Bartonella quintana* bacteremia in homeless patients. N Engl J Med 1999;340:184. [PMID: 9895398]

Raoult D et al: The body louse as a vector of reemerging human diseases. Clin Infect Dis 1999;29:888. [PMID: 10589908]

Cat-scratch disease is an acute infection of children and young adults caused by *Bartonella henselae.* It is transmitted from cats to humans as the result of a scratch or bite. Within a few days, one-third of patients will develop a papule or ulcer at the inoculation site. One to 3 weeks later, fever, headache, and malaise occur. The regional lymph nodes become enlarged, often tender, and may suppurate. Lymphadenopathy from cat scratches must be differentiated from that due to neoplasm, tuberculosis, lymphogranuloma venereum, and bacterial lymphadenitis. The diagnosis is usually made clinically. Special cultures for bartonella, serology, or excisional biopsy, though rarely necessary, confirm the diagnosis. The biopsy reveals necrotizing lymphadenitis and is itself not specific for cat-scratch disease. Cat-scratch disease is usually self-limited, requiring no specific therapy. Encephalitis occurs rarely.

Disseminated forms of the disease—bacillary angiomatosis and peliosis hepatis—occur in HIV-infected persons. Clinically, the lesions are vasculoproliferative and histopathologically distinct from those of cat-scratch disease. *Bartonella quintana,* the agent of trench fever, can also cause bacillary angiomatosis as well as culture-negative endocarditis. Bacillary angiomatosis and endocarditis respond to treatment with a macrolide or tetracycline administered in standard doses for 4–8 weeks. Relapse may occur.

Koehler JE et al. Molecular epidemiology of bartonella infections in patients with bacillary angiomatosis-peliosis. N Engl J Med 1997;337:1876. [PMID: 9407154] (*Bartonella henselae* associated with peliosis hepatis and cat and flea exposure, *B quintana* associated with homelessness and lice.)

Robson JM et al: Cat-scratch disease with paravertebral mass and osteomyelitis. Clin Infect Dis 1999;28:274. [PMID: 10064243]

ANAEROBIC INFECTIONS

Anaerobic bacteria make up the majority of normal human flora. Prominent members of the normal microbial flora of the mouth (anaerobic spirochetes, prevotella, fusobacteria), the skin (anaerobic diphtheroids), the large bowel (bacteroides, anaerobic streptococci, clostridia), and the female tract (bacteroides, anaerobic streptococci, fusobacteria) may produce disease when displaced from their normal sites into tissues or closed body spaces.

Certain characteristics are suggestive of anaerobic infections: (1) They are polymicrobial. (2) Abscess formation is the rule. (3) Pus and infected tissue often are malodorous. (4) Septic thrombophlebitis and metastatic infection are frequent and may require incision and drainage. Many important anaerobes except *Bacteroides fragilis* are highly sensitive to penicillin G. Diminished blood supply that favors proliferation of anaerobes because of reduced tissue oxygenation interferes with the delivery of antimicrobials to the site of anaerobic infection. (5) Bacteriologic examination may yield negative results or only inconsequential aerobes unless rigorous culture conditions are used.

Important types of infections that are most commonly caused by anaerobic organisms are listed below. Treatment of all these infections consists of surgical exploration and judicious excision in conjunction with administration of antimicrobial drugs.

Upper Respiratory Tract

Prevotella melaninogenica (formerly *Bacteroides melaninogenicus*) and anaerobic spirochetes are commonly involved in periodontal infections. These organisms, fusobacteria, and peptostreptococci may cause chronic sinusitis, peritonsillar abscess, chronic otitis media, and mastoiditis. Hygiene, drainage, and surgical debridement are as important in treatment as antimicrobials. Oral anaerobic organisms have been uniformly susceptible to penicillin, but there has been a recent trend of increasing penicillin resistance, usually due to β-lactamase production. Penicillin, 1–2 million units intravenously every 4 hours (if parenteral therapy is required) or 0.5 g orally four times daily for less severe infections or clindamycin can be used (600 mg intravenously every 8 hours or 300 mg orally every 6 hours). Duration of therapy depends upon clinical response; antimicrobial treatment is continued for a few days after signs and symptoms of infection have resolved. Indolent, established infections (eg, mastoiditis or osteomyelitis) may require prolonged courses of therapy, eg, 4–6 weeks or longer.

Chest Infections

Usually in the setting of poor oral hygiene and periodontal disease, aspiration of saliva (which contains 10^8 anaerobic organisms per milliliter in addition to aerobes) may lead to necrotizing pneumonia, lung abscess, and empyema. While polymicrobial infection is the rule, anaerobes—particularly *P melaninogenica,* fusobacteria, and peptostreptococci—are common etiologic agents. Most pulmonary infections respond to antimicrobial therapy alone. Percutaneous chest tube or surgical drainage is indicated for empyema.

Penicillin has long been considered the drug of choice for treatment of anaerobic lung infections, but penicillin-resistant *B fragilis* and *P melaninogenica* are isolated in up to 25% of cases and have been associated with clinical failures. Clindamycin, 600 mg intravenously once, followed by 300 mg orally every 6–8 hours, is the treatment of choice for these infections. Penicillin, 2 million units intravenously every 4 hours, followed by amoxicillin, 500 mg every 8 hours orally, is a reasonable alternative. These infections respond slowly. A duration of 3–4 weeks or more of antimicrobial therapy is typical. The second-generation cephalosporins cefoxitin, cefotetan, and cefmetazole are active in vitro against anaerobes, including those that are penicillin-resistant.

Central Nervous System

Anaerobes are a common cause of brain abscess, subdural empyema, or septic central nervous system thrombophlebitis. The organisms reach the central nervous system by direct extension from sinusitis, otitis, or mastoiditis or by hematogenous spread from chronic lung infections. Antimicrobial therapy—eg, penicillin, 20 million units intravenously, in combination with metronidazole, 750 mg intravenously, every 8 hours—is an important adjunct to surgical drainage. Duration of therapy is 6–8 weeks. Some small multiple brain abscesses can be treated with antibiotics alone without surgical drainage. Alternatively, septic internal thrombophlebitis (Lemierre's syndrome) originates from mouth anaerobes and may cause septic pulmonary embolization.

Intra-Abdominal Infections

In the colon there are up to 10^{11} anaerobes per gram of content—predominantly *B fragilis*, clostridia, and peptostreptococci. These organisms play a central role in most intra-abdominal abscesses following trauma to the colon, diverticulitis, appendicitis, or perirectal abscess and may also participate in hepatic abscess and cholecystitis, often in association with aerobic coliform bacteria. The gallbladder wall may be infected with clostridia as well. The bacteriology includes anaerobes as well as enteric gram-negative rods and on occasion enterococci. Therapy should be directed both against anaerobes and gram-negative aerobes. Multiple antibiotics may be required. Antibiotics reliably active against *B fragilis* include metronidazole, chloramphenicol, imipenem, ampicillin-sulbactam, and ticarcillin-clavulanic acid. Cefoxitin, cefotetan, and clindamycin are active against 80–90% of strains, but most third-generation cephalosporins have poor activity, inhibiting only 50% of isolates. Non-fragilis species of bacteroides may be less susceptible to the cephalosporins.

Table 33–6 summarizes the antibiotic regimens for management of moderate to moderately severe infections (eg, patient hemodynamically stable, good surgical drainage possible or established, low APACHE score, no multiple organ failure) and severe infections (eg, major peritoneal soilage, large or multiple abscesses, patient hemodynamically unstable), particularly if drug-resistant organisms are suspected. An effective oral regimen for patients able to take oral medications is presented also.

Female Genital Tract & Pelvic Infections

The normal flora of the vagina and cervix includes several species of bacteroides, peptostreptococci, group B streptococci, lactobacilli, coliform bacteria, and, occasionally, spirochetes and clostridia. These organisms commonly cause genital tract infections and may disseminate from there.

While salpingitis is commonly caused by gonococci and chlamydiae, tubo-ovarian and pelvic abscesses are associated with anaerobes in a majority of cases. Postpartum infections may be caused by aerobic streptococci or staphylococci, but anaerobes are often found, and the most severe cases of postpartum or postabortion sepsis are associated with clostridia and bacteroides. These have a high mortality rate, and treat-

Table 33–6. Treatment of anaerobic intra-abdominal infections.

Oral therapy
  Ciprofloxacin, 750 mg twice daily, plus metronidazole, 500 mg three times daily
Intravenous therapy
  Moderate to moderately severe infections:
    Ticarcillin/clavulanate, 3 g/0.1 g every 6 hours
      or—
    Cefotetan, 2 g every 12 hours
      or—
    Clindamycin, 600 mg every 8 hours, or metronidazole, 500 mg every 8 hours, plus gentamicin, 5 mg/kg/d
  Severe infections:
    Imipenem, 0.5 g every 6–8 hours, or ceftriaxone, 1 g every 24 hours, plus either clindamycin, 600 mg every 8 hours, or metronidazole, 500 mg every 8 hours

ment requires both antimicrobials directed against anaerobes and coliforms (see above) and abscess drainage or early hysterectomy.

Bacteremia & Endocarditis

Anaerobic bacteremia usually originates from the gastrointestinal tract, the oropharynx, decubitus ulcers, or the female genital tract. Endocarditis due to anaerobic and microaerophilic streptococci and bacteroides originates from the same sites. Most cases of anaerobic or microaerophilic streptococcal endocarditis can be effectively treated with 12–20 million units of penicillin G daily for 4–6 weeks, but optimal therapy of other types of anaerobic bacterial endocarditis must rely on laboratory guidance. Anaerobic corynebacteria (propionibacterium), clostridia, and bacteroides occasionally cause endocarditis.

Skin & Soft Tissue Infections

Anaerobic infections in the skin and soft tissue usually follow trauma, inadequate blood supply, or surgery and are commonest in areas that are contaminated by oral or fecal flora. There may be progressive tissue necrosis and a putrid odor.

Several terms, such as bacterial synergistic gangrene, synergistic necrotizing cellulitis, necrotizing fasciitis, and nonclostridial crepitant cellulitis, have been used to classify these infections. Although there are some differences in microbiology among them, their differentiation on clinical grounds alone is difficult. All are mixed infections caused by aerobic and anaerobic organisms and require aggressive surgical debridement of necrotic tissue for cure. Surgical consultation is obligatory to assist in diagnosis and treatment.

Broad-spectrum antibiotics active against both anaerobes and gram-positive and gram-negative aerobes (eg, vancomycin plus metronidazole plus gentamicin or tobramycin) should be instituted empirically and modified by culture results (Table 37–2). They are given for about a week after progressive tissue destruction has been controlled and the margins of the wound remain free of inflammation.

Olsen I et al: A primer on anaerobic bacteria and anaerobic infections for the uninitiated. Infection 1999;27:159. [PMID: 10378125]

■ ACTINOMYCOSIS

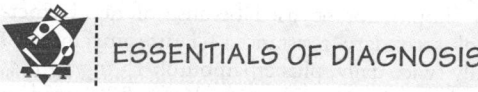

ESSENTIALS OF DIAGNOSIS

- *History of recent dental infection or abdominal trauma.*

- *Chronic pneumonia or indolent intra-abdominal or cervicofacial abscess.*
- *Sinus tract formation.*

General Considerations

Actinomyces israelii and other species of actinomyces occur in the normal flora of the mouth and tonsillar crypts. They are anaerobic, gram-positive, branching filamentous bacteria (1 µm in diameter) that may fragment into bacillary forms. When introduced into traumatized tissue and associated with other anaerobic bacteria, these actinomycetes become pathogens.

The most common site of infection is the cervicofacial area (about 60% of cases). Infection typically follows extraction of a tooth or other trauma. Lesions may develop in the gastrointestinal tract or lungs following ingestion or aspiration of the organism from its endogenous source in the mouth.

Clinical Findings

A. SYMPTOMS AND SIGNS

1. Cervicofacial actinomycosis—Cervicofacial actinomycosis develops slowly. The area becomes markedly indurated, and the overlying skin becomes reddish or cyanotic. Abscesses eventually draining to the surface persist for long periods. Sulfur granules—masses of filamentous organisms—may be found in the pus. There is usually little pain unless there is secondary infection. Trismus indicates that the muscles of mastication are involved. Radiography may reveal bony involvement.

2. Thoracic actinomycosis—Thoracic involvement begins with fever, cough, and sputum production with night sweats and weight loss. Pleuritic pain may be present. Multiple sinuses may extend through the chest wall, to the heart, or into the abdominal cavity. Ribs may be involved. Radiography shows areas of consolidation and in many cases pleural effusion. Cervicofacial or thoracic disease may occasionally result in central nervous system complications, most commonly brain abscess or meningitis.

3. Abdominal actinomycosis—Abdominal actinomycosis usually causes pain in the ileocecal region, spiking fever and chills, vomiting, and weight loss and may be confused with Crohn's disease. Irregular abdominal masses may be palpated. Pelvic inflammatory disease caused by actinomycetes has been associated with prolonged use of an intrauterine contraceptive device. Sinuses draining to the exterior may develop. CT scanning reveals an inflammatory mass that may extend to involve bone.

B. LABORATORY FINDINGS

The anaerobic, gram-positive organism may be demonstrated as a granule or as scattered branching gram-positive filaments in the pus. Anaerobic culture is necessary to distinguish actinomyces from nocardia because specific therapy differs for the two infections.

Treatment

Penicillin G is the drug of choice. Ten to 20 million units are given via a parenteral route for 2–4 weeks, followed by oral penicillin V, 500 mg four times daily.

Sulfonamides such as sulfamethoxazole may be an alternative regimen at a total daily dosage of 2–4 g. Response to therapy is slow. Therapy should be continued for weeks to months after clinical manifestations have disappeared in order to ensure cure. Surgical procedures such as drainage and resection may be beneficial.

With penicillin and surgery, the prognosis is good. The difficulties of diagnosis, however, may permit extensive destruction of tissue before the diagnosis is identified and therapy is started.

Lippes J: Pelvic actinomycosis: a review and preliminary look at prevalence. Am J Obstet Gynecol 1999;180(2 Part 1):265. [PMID: 9988785]

Zitsch RP 3rd et al: Actinomycosis: a potential complication of head and neck surgery. Am J Otolaryngol 1999;20:260. [PMID: 10442782]

■ NOCARDIOSIS

Nocardia asteroides, an aerobic filamentous soil bacterium, causes pulmonary and systemic nocardiosis. Bronchopulmonary abnormalities (eg, alveolar proteinosis) predispose to colonization, but infection is unusual unless the patient is also receiving systemic corticosteroids or is otherwise immunosuppressed.

Pulmonary involvement usually begins with malaise, loss of weight, fever, and night sweats. Cough and production of purulent sputum are the chief complaints. Radiography may show infiltrates accompanied by pleural effusion. The lesions may penetrate to the exterior through the chest wall, invading the ribs.

Dissemination may involve any organ. Brain abscesses and subcutaneous nodules are most frequent. Dissemination is seen exclusively in immunocompromised patients.

N asteroides is usually found as delicate, branching, gram-positive filaments. It may be weakly acid-fast, occasionally causing diagnostic confusion with tuberculosis. Identification is made by culture.

Therapy is initiated with intravenous trimethoprim-sulfamethoxazole administered at a dosage of 5–10 mg/kg/d (trimethoprim) and continued with oral trimethoprim-sulfamethoxazole, one double-strength tablet twice a day. Surgical procedures such as drainage and resection may be needed as adjunctive therapy.

Response may be slow, and therapy must be continued for at least 6 months. The prognosis in systemic nocardiosis is poor when diagnosis and therapy are delayed.

Nocardia brasiliensis typically causes a digital lesion—resembling herpetic whitlow—and ascending lymphangitis in normal hosts. Antimicrobial treatment is as for *N asteroides* infection, and the prognosis is excellent.

Case records of the Massachusetts General Hospital. Weekly clinicopathological exercises. Case 11-1999. A 60-year-old woman with epidural and paraspinal masses. N Engl J Med 1999;340:1188. [PMID: 10202171]

■ INFECTIONS CAUSED BY MYCOBACTERIA

NONTUBERCULOUS ATYPICAL MYCOBACTERIAL DISEASES

About 10% of mycobacterial infections seen in clinical practice are caused not by *Mycobacterium tuberculosis* but by atypical mycobacteria. Atypical mycobacterial infections are among the most common opportunistic infections in advanced HIV disease. These organisms have distinctive laboratory characteristics, occur ubiquitously in the environment, are not communicable from person to person, and are often strikingly resistant to antituberculous drugs.

Disseminated *Mycobacterium avium* Infection

Mycobacterium avium complex (MAC) produces asymptomatic colonization or a wide spectrum of diseases, including coin lesions, bronchitis in patients with chronic lung disease, and invasive pulmonary disease that is often cavitary and occurs in patients with underlying lung disease. MAC is a common cause of disseminated disease in the late stages of HIV infection, when the CD4 cell count is less than 50–100/μL. Persistent fever and weight loss are the most common symptoms. The organism can usually be cultured from multiple sites, including blood, liver, lymph node, or bone marrow. Blood culture is the preferred means of establishing the diagnosis and has a sensitivity of 98%.

Agents with proved activity against MAC in humans are rifabutin, azithromycin, clarithromycin, and ethambutol. Amikacin and ciprofloxacin have activity in vitro, but clinical data are lacking. Single-agent therapy should not be used because of rapid emergence of secondary resistance. Clarithromycin, 500 mg orally twice daily, plus ethambutol, 15 mg/kg/d as a single dose, with or without rifabutin, 300 mg/d, is the treatment of choice. Azithromycin, 500 mg once daily, may be used instead of clarithromycin. Too few data are available to permit specific recommendations about second-line regimens for patients intolerant of macrolides or those who have disease caused by macrolide-resistant organisms. However, a combination of two or more active agents should be used. The recommendation has been lifelong therapy for disseminated infection for patients with AIDS. It is not known whether immune reconstitution in patients receiving highly active antiretroviral therapy (HAART) whose CD4 counts exceed 100–200/μL is sufficient to permit discontinuation of therapy without relapse. This decision should be made on an individual basis.

Several clinical trials have now shown that antimicrobial prophylaxis of MAC prevents disseminated disease and prolongs survival. It is the standard of care to offer prophylaxis against MAC to all HIV-infected patients with CD4 counts ≤ 50/μL. Primary prophylaxis for MAC infection can be stopped in patients who have responded to HIV protease inhibitor antiretroviral combination therapy with elevation of CD4 counts above 100 cells/μL for 3–6 months. Single-drug regimens of clarithromycin, 500 mg twice daily, azithromycin, 1200 mg once weekly, or rifabutin, 300 mg once daily, have been shown to be effective. Clarithromycin and azithromycin are more effective and better tolerated than rifabutin, and for that reason a macrolide is preferred over rifabutin. Patients who develop disseminated disease while receiving macrolide prophylaxis may have macrolide-resistant organisms, a factor to consider when pondering treatment options. Which regimen to use is not established, but most authorities recommend addition of rifabutin and ethambutol. Whether to continue the macrolide if the isolate is resistant in vitro is controversial.

Pulmonary Infections

MAC causes a chronic, slowly progressive pulmonary infection resembling tuberculosis in immunocompetent patients, who typically have underlying pulmonary disease.

Treatment of immunocompetent patients with pulmonary infection is almost completely empirical and based almost entirely on anecdotal data. A combination of agents should be used. Rifampin, 600 mg once daily, plus ethambutol, 15–25 mg/kg/d, plus streptomycin, 1 g intramuscularly three to five times a week for the first 4–6 months, have been used. The role of rifabutin, fluoroquinolones, and the macrolides is not known, but based upon their excellent efficacy in immunocompromised AIDS patients, they may actually be more effective than the relatively weak agents traditionally used in immunocompetent patients. Clarithromycin is a very potent drug in the treatment of MAC in AIDS patients. Based on this, inclusion of clarithromycin in the initial treatment regimen of immunocompetent patients should be strongly considered. Therapy is continued for a total of 18–24 months.

Mycobacterium kansasii can produce clinical disease resembling tuberculosis, but the illness progresses more slowly. Most such infections occur in patients with preexisting lung disease, though 40% of patients have no known pulmonary disease. Microbiologically, *M kansasii* is similar to *M tuberculosis* and is sensitive to the same drugs except pyrazinamide, to which it is resistant. Therapy with isoniazid, ethambutol, and rifampin for 2 years (or 1 year after sputum conversion) has been highly successful.

Less common causes of pulmonary disease include *Mycobacterium xenopi*, *Mycobacterium szulgai*, and *Mycobacterium gordonae*. These organisms have variable sensitivities, and treatment is based on results of sensitivity tests. *Mycobacterium fortuitum* and *Mycobacterium chelonei* also can cause pneumonia.

Lymphadenitis

Most cases of lymphadenitis (scrofula) in adults are caused by *Mycobacterium tuberculosis* and can be a manifestation of disseminated disease. In children, the majority of cases are due to nontuberculous mycobacterial species, with *Mycobacterium scrofulaceum* and MAC being the most common. *Mycobacterium kansasii*, *Mycobacterium bovis*, *Mycobacterium chelonei*, and *Mycobacterium fortuitum* are less commonly observed. Unlike disease caused by *M tuberculosis*, which requires systemic therapy for 6 months, infection with nontuberculous mycobacteria can be successfully treated by surgical excision without antituberculous therapy.

Skin & Soft Tissue Infections

Skin and soft tissue infections such as abscesses, septic arthritis, and osteomyelitis can result from direct inoculation or hematogenous dissemination or may occur as a complication of surgery.

M chelonei and *M fortuitum* are frequent causes of this type of infection. Most cases occur in the extremities and initially present as nodules. Ulceration with abscess formation often follows. The organisms are resistant to the usual antituberculous drugs but may be sensitive to a variety of antibiotics, including erythromycin, doxycycline, amikacin, cefoxitin, sulfonamides, imipenem, and ciprofloxacin. Therapy includes surgical debridement along with drug therapy. Initially, parenteral drugs are given for several weeks, and this is followed by an oral regimen to which the organism is sensitive. The duration of therapy is variable but usually continues for several months after the soft tissue lesions have healed.

Mycobacterium marinum infection ("swimming pool granuloma") presents as a nodular skin lesion following exposure to nonchlorinated water. The lesions respond to therapy with doxycycline, minocycline, or trimethoprim-sulfamethoxazole.

Mycobacterium ulcerans infection (Buruli ulcer) is seen mainly in Africa and Australia and produces a large ulcerative lesion. Therapy consists of surgical excision and skin grafting.

Diagnosis and treatment of disease caused by nontuberculous mycobacteria. Medical Section of the American Lung Association. Am J Respir Crit Care Med 1997;156(2 Part 2):S1. [PMID: 9279284]

French AL et al: Nontuberculous mycobacterial infections. Med Clin North Am 1997;81:361. [PMID: 9093233]

Horsburgh Jr CR: The pathophysiology of disseminated *Mycobacterium avium* complex disease in AIDS. J Infect Dis 1999;179(Suppl 3):S461. [PMID: 10099120]

Kovacs J et al: Prophylaxis against opportunistic infection in patients with human immunodeficiency virus infection. N Engl J Med 2000;342:1416. [PMID: 10805828]

MYCOBACTERIUM TUBERCULOSIS INFECTIONS

Tuberculosis is discussed in Chapter 9. Further information and expert consultation can be obtained from the Francis J. Curry National Tuberculosis Center at the Web site http://www.nationaltbcenter.edu or, by phone, 415-502-4600, or fax, 415-502-4620.

TUBERCULOUS MENINGITIS

ESSENTIALS OF DIAGNOSIS

- Gradual onset of listlessness, irritability, and anorexia.
- Headache, vomiting, and seizures common.
- Cranial nerve abnormalities typical.
- Tuberculosis focus may be evident elsewhere.
- Cerebrospinal fluid shows several hundred lymphocytes, low glucose, and high protein.

General Considerations

Tuberculous meningitis is caused by rupture of a meningeal tuberculoma resulting from earlier hematogenous seeding of tubercle bacillus from a pulmonary focus, or it may be a consequence of miliary spread.

Clinical Findings

A. SYMPTOMS AND SIGNS

The onset is usually gradual, with listlessness, irritability, anorexia, and fever, followed by headache, vomiting, convulsions, and coma. In older patients, headache and behavioral changes are prominent early symptoms. Nuchal rigidity and cranial nerve palsies occur as the meningitis progresses. Evidence of active tuberculosis elsewhere or a history of prior tuberculosis is present in up to 75% of patients.

B. LABORATORY FINDINGS

The spinal fluid is frequently yellowish, with increased pressure, 100–500 cells/μL (predominantly lymphocytes, though neutrophils may be present early during infection), increased protein, and decreased glucose. Acid-fast stains of cerebrospinal fluid usually are negative, and cultures also may be negative in 15–25% of cases. Chest x-ray often reveals abnormalities compatible with tuberculosis but may be normal.

Differential Diagnosis

Tuberculous meningitis may be confused with any other type of meningitis, but the gradual onset, the predominantly lymphocytic pleocytosis of the spinal fluid, and evidence of tuberculosis elsewhere often point to the diagnosis. The tuberculin skin test is usually positive, though in a significant proportion of patients it is negative. Fungal and other granulomatous meningitides, syphilis, and carcinomatous meningitis are in the differential diagnosis.

Complications

Complications of tuberculous meningitis include chronic brain syndrome, seizure disorders, cranial nerve palsies, stroke, and obstructive hydrocephalus. These result from inflammatory exudate primarily involving the basilar meninges and arteries.

Treatment

Presumptive diagnosis followed by early, empirical antituberculous therapy is essential for survival and to minimize sequelae. Even if cultures are not positive, a full course of therapy is warranted if the clinical setting is suggestive of tuberculous meningitis.

Regimens that are effective for pulmonary tuberculosis are effective also for tuberculous meningitis (Table 9–14). Rifampin, isoniazid, and pyrazinamide all penetrate into cerebrospinal fluid well. The penetration of ethambutol is more variable, but therapeutic concentrations can be achieved, and the drug has been successfully used for meningitis. Aminoglycosides penetrate less well. Regimens that do not include both isoniazid and rifampin may be effective but are less reliable and generally must be given for longer periods.

Some authorities recommend the addition of corticosteroids for patients with focal deficits or altered mental status. Dexamethasone, 0.15 mg/kg four times daily for 1–2 weeks, then discontinued in a tapering regimen over 4 weeks, may be used.

LEPROSY

ESSENTIALS OF DIAGNOSIS

- Pale, anesthetic macular—or nodular and erythematous—skin lesions.
- Superficial nerve thickening with associated anesthesia.

- *History of residence in endemic area in child-hood.*
- *Acid-fast bacilli in skin lesions or nasal scrapings, or characteristic histologic nerve changes.*

General Considerations

Leprosy is a chronic infectious disease caused by the acid-fast rod *Mycobacterium leprae*. The mode of transmission probably is respiratory and involves prolonged exposure in childhood. The disease is endemic in tropical and subtropical Asia, Africa, Central and South America and the Pacific regions, and southern USA.

Clinical Findings

A. SYMPTOMS AND SIGNS

The onset is insidious. The lesions involve the cooler body tissues: skin, superficial nerves, nose, pharynx, larynx, eyes, and testicles. Skin lesions may occur as pale, anesthetic macular lesions 1–10 cm in diameter; discrete erythematous, infiltrated nodules 1–5 cm in diameter; or a diffuse skin infiltration. Neurologic disturbances are manifested by nerve infiltration and thickening, with resultant anesthesia, neuritis, and paresthesia. Bilateral ulnar neuropathy is highly suggestive. In untreated cases, disfigurement due to the skin infiltration and nerve involvement may be extreme, leading to trophic ulcers, bone resorption, and loss of digits.

The disease is divided clinically and by laboratory tests into two distinct types: lepromatous and tuberculoid. The lepromatous type occurs in persons with defective cellular immunity. The course is progressive and malignant, with nodular skin lesions; slow, symmetric nerve involvement; abundant acid-fast bacilli in the skin lesions; and a negative lepromin skin test. In the tuberculoid type, cellular immunity is intact and the course is more benign and less progressive, with macular skin lesions, severe asymmetric nerve involvement of sudden onset with few bacilli present in the lesions, and a positive lepromin skin test. Intermediate ("borderline") cases are frequent. Eye involvement (keratitis and iridocyclitis), nasal ulcers, epistaxis, anemia, and lymphadenopathy may occur.

B. LABORATORY FINDINGS

Laboratory confirmation of leprosy requires the demonstration of acid-fast bacilli in a skin biopsy. Biopsy of skin or of a thickened involved nerve also gives a typical histologic picture. *M leprae* does not grow in artificial media.

Differential Diagnosis

The skin lesions of leprosy often resemble those of lupus erythematosus, sarcoidosis, syphilis, erythema nodosum, erythema multiforme, cutaneous tuberculosis, and vitiligo.

Complications

Renal failure and hepatomegaly from secondary amyloidosis may occur with long-standing disease.

Treatment

Combination therapy is recommended for treatment of all types of leprosy. Single-drug treatment is accompanied by emergence of resistance, and primary resistance to dapsone also occurs. For borderline and lepromatous cases, a three-drug regimen such as dapsone, 50–100 mg/d, clofazimine, 50 mg/d, and rifampin, 10 mg/kg/d (up to 600 mg/d), all given orally, should be used. The triple drug combination should be administered for a minimum of 2–3 years and, ideally, until all biopsies are negative for acid-fast bacilli. For indeterminate and tuberculoid leprosy, the dapsone-rifampin combination is recommended for 6–12 months, often followed by a course of dapsone alone for 2 or more years.

Two reactional states—erythema nodosum leprosum and reversal reactions—may occur as a consequence of therapy. The reversal reaction, typical of borderline lepromatous leprosy, probably results from enhanced host immunity. Skin lesions and nerves become swollen and tender, but systemic manifestations are not seen. Erythema nodosum leprosum, typical of lepromatous leprosy, is a consequence of immune injury from antigen-antibody complex deposition in skin and other tissues; in addition to skin and nerve manifestations, fever and systemic involvement may be seen. Prednisone, 60 mg/d, or thalidomide, 300 mg/d (in the nonpregnant patient only), is effective for erythema nodosum leprosum. Improvement is expected within a few days after initiating prednisone, and thereafter the dose may be tapered over several weeks to avoid recurrence. Thalidomide is also tapered over several weeks to a 100 mg bedtime dose. Erythema nodosum leprosum is usually confined to the first year of therapy, and prednisone or thalidomide can be discontinued. Thalidomide is ineffective for reversal reactions, and prednisone, 60 mg/d, is indicated. Reversal reactions tend to recur, and the dose of prednisone should be slowly tapered over weeks to months. Therapy for leprosy should not be discontinued during treatment of reactional states.

Jacobson RR et al: Leprosy. Lancet 1999;353:655. [PMID: 10030346]

■ INFECTIONS CAUSED BY CHLAMYDIAE

Chlamydiae are a large group of obligate intracellular parasites closely related to gram-negative bacteria. They are assigned to three species—*Chlamydia tra-*

chomatis, Chlamydia psittaci, and *Chlamydia pneumoniae*—on the basis of intracellular inclusions, sulfonamide susceptibility, antigenic composition, and disease production. *C trachomatis* causes many different human infections involving the eye (trachoma, inclusion conjunctivitis), the genital tract (lymphogranuloma venereum, nongonococcal urethritis, cervicitis, salpingitis), or the respiratory tract (pneumonitis). *C psittaci* causes psittacosis in humans and many animal diseases. *Chlamydia pneumoniae* has recently been recognized as a cause of respiratory tract infections.

CHLAMYDIA TRACHOMATIS INFECTIONS

1. Lymphogranuloma Venereum

 ESSENTIALS OF DIAGNOSIS

- Evanescent primary genital lesion.
- Lymph node enlargement, softening, and suppuration, with draining sinuses.
- Proctitis and rectal stricture in women or homosexual men.
- Positive complement fixation test.

General Considerations

Lymphogranuloma venereum is an acute and chronic sexually transmitted disease caused by *Chlamydia trachomatis* types L1–L3. After the genital lesion disappears, the infection spreads to lymph channels and lymph nodes of the genital and rectal areas. The disease is acquired during intercourse or through contact with contaminated exudate from active lesions. The incubation period is 5–21 days. Inapparent infections and latent disease are not uncommon.

Clinical Findings

A. SYMPTOMS AND SIGNS

In men, the initial vesicular or ulcerative lesion (on the external genitalia) is evanescent and often goes unnoticed. Inguinal buboes appear 1–4 weeks after exposure, are often bilateral, and have a tendency to fuse, soften, and break down to form multiple draining sinuses, with extensive scarring. In women, the genital lymph drainage is to the perirectal glands. Early anorectal manifestations are proctitis with tenesmus and bloody purulent discharge; late manifestations are chronic cicatrizing inflammation of the rectal and perirectal tissue. These changes lead to obstipation and rectal stricture and, occasionally, rectovaginal and perianal fistulas. They are also seen in homosexual men.

B. LABORATORY FINDINGS

The complement fixation test may be positive, but cross-reaction with other chlamydiae occurs. Although a positive reaction may reflect remote infection, high titers usually indicate active disease. Specific immunofluorescence tests for IgM are more specific for acute infection.

Differential Diagnosis

The early lesion of lymphogranuloma venereum must be differentiated from the lesions of syphilis, genital herpes, and chancroid; lymph node involvement must be distinguished from that due to tularemia, tuberculosis, plague, neoplasm, or pyogenic infection; rectal stricture must be distinguished from that due to neoplasm and ulcerative colitis.

Treatment

The antibiotic of choice is tetracycline (contraindicated in pregnancy), 0.25–0.5 g orally four times daily, or doxycycline, 0.1 g twice daily for 21 days. Erythromycin, 500 mg four times a day, or trimethoprim-sulfamethoxazole, 160/800 mg twice a day for 21 days, also is effective.

2. Chlamydial Urethritis & Cervicitis

Chlamydia trachomatis immunotypes D–K are isolated in about 50% of cases of nongonococcal urethritis and cervicitis by appropriate techniques. In other cases, *Ureaplasma urealyticum* can be grown as a possible etiologic agent. *C trachomatis* is an important cause of postgonococcal urethritis. Co-infection with gonococci and chlamydiae is common, and postgonococcal (ie, chlamydial) urethritis may persist after successful treatment of the gonococcal component. Occasionally, epididymitis, prostatitis, or proctitis is caused by chlamydial infection.

Females infected with chlamydia may be asymptomatic or may have signs and symptoms of cervicitis, salpingitis, or pelvic inflammatory disease. Chlamydia is probably the leading cause of infertility in females in the United States.

The diagnosis of chlamydial infection has been clinical because *C trachomatis* is difficult and expensive to culture. The urethral or cervical discharge tends to be less painful, less purulent, and watery in chlamydial versus gonococcal infection. A patient with urethritis or cervicitis and absence of gram-negative diplococci on Gram stain and of *N gonorrhoeae* on culture is assumed to have chlamydial infection. Direct immunofluorescence assay, enzyme-linked immunoassay, and a DNA probe test, although less sensitive than culture, are sometimes used to confirm the diagnosis and for screening. The ligase chain reaction (LCR) test for *C trachomatis* has superior sensitivity compared with all other methods (eg, sensitivity of 60–70% for DNA probe versus 90–95% for LCR). LCR also has excellent specificity, approaching 100%, and it can be performed on urine. For these reasons, LCR will likely replace all other methods for diagnosis of chlamydial urethritis and cervicitis.

Therapy often must be given presumptively. Sexual partners of infected patients should also be treated. Effective treatment regimens are tetracycline or erythromycin, 500 mg four times a day, or doxycycline, 100 mg twice daily, for 7 days. Trimethoprim-sulfamethoxazole, 160/800 mg twice a day, is acceptable but may be less effective than tetracyclines or erythromycin. Erythromycin is the drug of choice in the pregnant patient. A single 1 g dose of azithromycin is effective for uncomplicated urethritis and cervicitis and has the advantage of improved patient compliance and minimal toxicity.

Cohen CR et al: Pathogenesis of chlamydia induced pelvic inflammatory disease. Sex Transm Infect 1999;75:21. [PMID: 10338337]

CHLAMYDIA PSITTACI & PSITTACOSIS (Ornithosis)

 ESSENTIALS OF DIAGNOSIS

- Fever, chills, and cough; headache common.
- Atypical pneumonia with slightly delayed appearance of signs of pneumonitis.
- Contact with infected bird (psittacine, pigeons, many others) 7–15 days previously.
- Isolation of chlamydiae or rising titer of complement-fixing antibodies.

General Considerations

Psittacosis is acquired from contact with birds (parrots, parakeets, pigeons, chickens, ducks, and many others), which may or may not be ill. The history may be difficult to obtain if the patient acquired infection from an illegally imported bird.

Clinical Findings

The onset is usually rapid, with fever, chills, myalgia, dry cough, and headache. Signs include temperature-pulse dissociation, dullness to percussion, and rales. Pulmonary findings may be absent early. Dyspnea and cyanosis may occur later. Endocarditis, which is culture-negative, may occur. The radiographic findings in typical psittacosis are those of atypical pneumonia, which tends to be interstitial and diffuse in appearance, though consolidation can occur. Psittacosis is indistinguishable from other bacterial or viral pneumonias by radiography.

The organism is rarely isolated from cultures. The diagnosis is usually made serologically; antibodies appear during the second week and can be demonstrated by complement fixation or immunofluorescence. Antibody response may be suppressed by early chemotherapy.

Differential Diagnosis

The illness is indistinguishable from viral, mycoplasmal, or other atypical pneumonias except for the history of contact with birds. Psittacosis is in the differential diagnosis of culture-negative endocarditis.

Treatment

Treatment consists of giving tetracycline, 0.5 g orally every 6 hours or 0.5 g intravenously every 12 hours, for 14–21 days. Erythromycin may be effective as well.

CHLAMYDIA PNEUMONIAE

Chlamydia pneumoniae causes pneumonia and bronchitis and has been associated seroepidemiologically with coronary artery disease. The clinical presentation of pneumonia is that of an atypical pneumonia. The organism accounts for approximately 10% of community-acquired pneumonias, ranking second to mycoplasma as an agent of atypical pneumonia. Its role in coronary artery disease remains to be defined, but *C zpneumoniae* has been detected in up to 50% of coronary atheromatous lesions.

Like *C psittaci*, strains of *C pneumoniae* are resistant to sulfonamides. Erythromycin or tetracycline, 500 mg four times a day for 10–14 days, appears to be effective therapy. Some of the newer fluoroquinolones, such as levofloxacin or trovafloxacin, are active in vitro against *C pneumoniae* and probably are effective clinically. The oral dose of levofloxacin is 500 mg once a day for 10–14 days.

Gurfinkel EP et al: Emerging role of antibiotics in atherosclerosis. Am Heart J 1999;138(5 Part 2):S537. [PMID: 10539868]

Mattila KJ et al: Role of infection as a risk factor for atherosclerosis, myocardial infarction, and stroke. Clin Infect Dis 1998;26:719. [PMID: 9524851] (Infections are being linked to atherosclerosis and thrombosis. *Chlamydia pneumoniae* is associated with coronary heart disease.)

Shor A et al: *Chlamydia pneumoniae* and atherosclerosis. JAMA 1999;282:2071. [PMID: 10591391]

Stamm WE: *Chlamydia trachomatis* infections: progress and problems. J Infect Dis 1999;179(Suppl 2):S380. [PMID: 10081511]

Infectious Diseases: Spirochetal

Richard A. Jacobs, MD, PhD
See www.current-med.com/ch34.html

■ SYPHILIS

NATURAL HISTORY & PRINCIPLES OF DIAGNOSIS & TREATMENT

Syphilis is a complex infectious disease caused by *Treponema pallidum,* a spirochete capable of infecting almost any organ or tissue in the body and causing protean clinical manifestations (Table 34–1). Transmission occurs most frequently during sexual contact, through minor skin or mucosal lesions; sites of inoculation are usually genital but may be extragenital. The risk of developing syphilis after unprotected sex with an individual with early syphilis is approximately 30–50%. The organism is extremely sensitive to heat and drying but can survive for days in fluids; therefore, it can be transmitted in blood from infected persons. Syphilis can be transferred via the placenta from mother to fetus after the tenth week of pregnancy (congenital syphilis).

The immunologic response to infection is complex, but it provides the basis for most clinical diagnoses. The infection induces the synthesis of a number of antibodies, some of which react specifically with pathogenic treponemes and some with components of normal tissues (see below). If the disease is untreated, sufficient defenses develop to produce a relative resistance to reinfection; however, in most cases these immune reactions fail to eradicate existing infection and may contribute to tissue destruction in the late stages. Patients treated early in the disease are fully susceptible to reinfection.

The natural history of acquired syphilis is generally divided into two major clinical stages: early (infectious) syphilis and late syphilis. The two stages are separated by a symptom-free latent phase during the first part of which (early latency) the infectious stage is liable to recur. Infectious syphilis includes the primary lesions (chancre and regional lymphadenopathy); the secondary lesions (commonly involving skin and mucous membranes, occasionally bone, central nervous system, or liver); relapsing lesions during early latency;

and congenital lesions. The hallmark of these lesions is an abundance of spirochetes; tissue reaction is usually minimal. Late syphilis consists of so-called benign (gummatous) lesions involving skin, bones, and viscera; cardiovascular disease (principally aortitis); and a variety of central nervous system and ocular syndromes. These forms of syphilis are not contagious. The lesions contain few demonstrable spirochetes, but tissue reactivity (vasculitis, necrosis) is severe and suggestive of hypersensitivity phenomena.

As a result of intensive public health efforts during and after World War II, there was a reduction in the incidence of infectious syphilis. With the marked increase in all sexually transmitted diseases since the 1970s, there has been a rise in the number of reported cases of syphilis. In the early 1980s, the incidence of infectious syphilis increased, with a particularly high rate among homosexual men. In the mid 1980s, there was a slight decrease in the incidence of syphilis, chiefly as a result of changes in sexual practices in response to the AIDS epidemic. Between 1985 and 1990, there was again a dramatic increase in infectious syphilis, with 50,223 cases of primary and secondary syphilis reported in 1990. This increase was broad-based, affecting both men and women in inner city urban and rural areas, particularly in the southern regions of the United States. Although adolescent and young adult blacks were primarily affected, increases were seen in other ethnic groups also, as well as adults over 60. Limited access to health care, decreases in health department clinical services, increased use of illicit drugs (especially "crack cocaine"), the exchange of sex for drugs or money to buy drugs, and the difficulty of contact tracing when multiple sexual partners are involved all contributed to the dramatic increase. Concomitantly with the increase in acquired syphilis, there has also been an increase in congenital syphilis, particularly in urban areas. In response to this increase in infectious syphilis in 1998, the United States Congress allocated funds for a syphilis elimination program. This included intensive syphilis control programs targeting high-risk populations—women of childbearing age, sexually active teens, drug users, inmates of penal institutions, persons with multiple sex-

Table 34–1. Stages of syphilis and common clinical manifestations.

Primary syphilis
  Genital ulcer: painless ulcer with clean base and firm
    indurated borders
  Regional lymphadenopathy
Secondary syphilis
  Skin and mucous membranes
    Rash: diffuse (including palms and soles), macular,
      papular, pustular, and combinations
    Condylomata lata
    Mucous patches: painless, silvery ulcerations of mucous
      membrane with surrounding erythema
  Generalized lymphadenopathy
  Constitutional symptoms
    Fever, usually low-grade
    Malaise
    Anorexia
    Arthralgias and myalgias
  Central nervous system
    Asymptomatic
    Symptomatic
    Headache
    Meningitis
    Cranial neuropathies (II–VIII)
  Ocular
    Iritis
    Iridocyclitis
  Other
    Renal: glomerulonephritis, nephrotic syndrome
    Liver: hepatitis
    Bone and joint: arthritis, periostitis
Late syphilis
  Late benign (gummatous): granulomatous lesion usually
    involving skin, mucous membranes and bones, but any
    organ can be involved
  Cardiovascular
    Aortic insufficiency
    Coronary ostial stenosis
    Aortic aneurysm
  Neurosyphilis
    Asymptomatic
    Meningovascular
      Seizures
      Hemiparesis or hemiplegia
    Tabes dorsalis
      Impaired proprioception and vibratory sensation
      Argyll Robertson pupil
      Shooting pains
      Ataxia
      Romberg's sign
      Urinary and fecal incontinence
      Charcot joint
      Cranial nerve involvement (II–VIII)
    General paresis
      Personality changes
      Hyperactive reflexes
      Argyll Robertson pupil
      Decreased memory
      Slurred speech
      Optic atrophy

ual partners or those who have sex with prostitutes—and emphasizing screening, early treatment, contact tracing, and condom use. This effort has been successful as evidenced by a 5.4% decrease in the number of primary and secondary cases reported in 1999 (6657 cases) compared with 1998 (7035 cases). Most cases are still reported from the South, with blacks and Hispanics being disproportionately affected. In addition, small urban outbreaks are still being reported, chiefly among men having sex with men.

Laboratory Diagnosis

Since the infectious agent of syphilis cannot be cultured in vitro, diagnostic measures must rely mainly on serologic testing, microscopic detection of *T pallidum* in lesions, and other examinations (biopsies, lumbar puncture, x-rays) for evidence of tissue damage.

A. SEROLOGIC TESTS FOR SYPHILIS

(Table 34–2.) There are two general categories of serologic tests for syphilis: (1) Nontreponemal tests detect antibodies to lipoidal antigens present in either the host or in *T pallidum*. The original antigens employed to measure these nonspecific antibodies (reagin) were crude extracts of beef heart or liver and resulted in significant numbers of false-positive reactions. The cardiolipin-cholesterol-lecithin preparation presently used is much purer and gives fewer false-positive reactions. (2) Treponemal tests employ live or killed *T pallidum* as antigen to detect antibodies specific for pathogenic treponemes.

1. Nontreponemal antigen tests—The most commonly used nontreponemal antigen tests are the VDRL and RPR, which measure the ability of heated serum to flocculate a suspension of cardiolipin-cholesterol-lecithin. The flocculation tests are inexpensive, rapid, and easy to perform and are therefore used primarily for routine screening. Quantitative expression of the reactivity of the serum, based upon titration of dilutions of serum, is valuable in establishing the diagnosis and in evaluating the efficacy of treatment.

The VDRL test (the nontreponemal test in widest use) generally becomes positive 4–6 weeks after infection, or 1–3 weeks after the appearance of a primary

Table 34–2. Percentage of patients with positive serologic tests for syphilis.[1]

Test	Stage		
	Primary	Secondary	Tertiary
VDRL[2]	70–75%	99%	75%
FTA-ABS[3]	85–95%	100%	98%

[1]Based on untreated cases.
[2]VDRL = Venereal Disease Research Laboratory test.
[3]FTA-ABS = Fluorescent treponemal antibody absorption test.

lesion; it is almost invariably positive in the secondary stage. The VDRL titer is usually high (> 1:32) in secondary syphilis and tends to be lower (< 1:4) or even negative in late forms of syphilis. These serologic tests are not highly specific and must be closely correlated with other clinical and laboratory findings. The tests are positive in patients with non-sexually transmitted treponematoses (see below). More importantly, "false-positive" serologic reactions are frequently encountered in a wide variety of nontreponemal states, including connective tissue diseases, infectious mononucleosis, malaria, febrile diseases, leprosy, intravenous drug use, infective endocarditis, old age, hepatitis C viral infection, and pregnancy. False-positive tests also occur more commonly in HIV-seropositive patients (4%) than in HIV-seronegative patients (0.8%). False-positive reactions are usually of low titer and transient and may be distinguished from true positives by specific treponemal antibody tests. False-negative results can be seen when very high antibody titers are present (the prozone phenomenon). If syphilis is strongly suspected and the nontreponemal test is negative, the laboratory should be instructed to dilute the specimen to detect a positive reaction. The rapid plasma reagin (RPR) test is a simple, rapid, and reliable substitute for the traditional VDRL test. RPR titers are often higher than VDRL titers and thus are not comparable.

Nontreponemal antibody titers are used to assess adequacy of therapy. The time required for the VDRL or RPR to become negative depends on the stage of the disease, the height of the initial titer, and whether the infection is an initial or repeat episode. In general, individuals with repeat infections, higher initial titers, and more advanced stages of disease at the time of treatment have a slower seroconversion rate and are more likely to remain serofast (ie, titers do not become negative). Older data derived from more intensive treatment regimens than are presently used indicate that in primary and secondary syphilis, the VDRL usually decreases fourfold by 3 months and eightfold by 6 months. Furthermore, seronegativity was seen in 97% of those with primary syphilis and 76% of those with secondary syphilis at 2 years. More recent data based on currently recommended treatment regimens (see below) suggest that decreases in titer may be slower—ie, in primary and secondary syphilis it may take 6 months to see a fourfold decrease in titer and 12 months to see an eightfold drop. In patients with early latent syphilis, response is even slower, with a fourfold drop in titer taking 12–24 months. Seronegativity was seen in 72% of patients with primary syphilis and only 56% of those with secondary syphilis after 3 years. Additional studies support a slower decline in titers with currently recommended treatment regimens.

2. Treponemal antibody tests—The fluorescent treponemal antibody absorption (FTA-ABS) test measures antibodies capable of reacting with killed *T pallidum* after absorption of the patient's serum with extracts of nonpathogenic treponemes. The FTA-ABS test is of value principally in determining whether a positive nontreponemal antigen test is "false-positive" or is indicative of syphilis. Because of its great sensitivity, particularly in the late stages of the disease, the FTA-ABS test is also of value when there is clinical evidence of syphilis but the nontreponemal serologic test for syphilis is negative. The test is positive in most patients with primary syphilis and in virtually all with secondary syphilis. Like nontreponemal antigen tests, the specific treponemal antibody test may revert to negative with adequate therapy. This is seen almost exclusively in initial infections in individuals with primary syphilis. In one study, 11% of individuals with a first episode of primary syphilis were seronegative by the FTA-ABS test at 1 year posttreatment, and 24% were negative by 3 years. Immunologic status may also affect antibody titers. Seven percent of asymptomatic HIV-infected patients became seronegative after treatment, as opposed to 38% of symptomatic HIV-infected individuals. The long-held belief that a positive FTA-ABS persists indefinitely is clearly not valid, and this test therefore cannot be used as a reliable marker of previous infection. False-positive FTA-ABS tests occur rarely in systemic lupus erythematosus and in other disorders associated with increased levels of gamma globulins. It is noteworthy that Lyme disease may cause a false-positive FTA-ABS test but rarely causes a false-positive reaginic test. The *T pallidum* hemagglutination (TPHA) test and the passive particle agglutination test (TPPA) are comparable in specificity and sensitivity to the FTA-ABS. The TPPA test, because of ease of performance, has supplanted the FTA-ABS test as the means of confirming the diagnosis of syphilis.

Investigational tests such as direct antigen detection, Western immunoblot, ELISA (CAPTIA Syph G, CAPTIA Syph M), latex agglutination (Syphilis Fast), and PCR are under study as diagnostic tools. They have shown promise in clinical trials, and the increased sensitivity (ELISA) and specificity (Western blot) of these tests make them attractive. However, because of limited clinical evaluation in field trials they have not yet supplanted the more traditional methods of diagnosis.

Final decisions about the significance of the results of serologic tests for syphilis must be based upon a total clinical appraisal.

B. MICROSCOPIC EXAMINATION

In infectious syphilis, *T pallidum* may be shown by darkfield microscopic examination of fresh exudate from lesions or material aspirated from regional lymph nodes. The darkfield examination requires considerable experience and care in the proper collection of specimens and in the identification of pathogenic spirochetes by observing characteristic features of morphology and motility. Repeated examinations may be necessary. Spirochetes usually are not found in late syphilitic lesions by this technique.

An immunofluorescent staining technique for demonstrating *T pallidum* in dried smears of fluid taken from early syphilitic lesions is available. Slides are fixed and treated with fluorescein labeled antitreponemal antibody that has been preabsorbed with nonpathogenic treponemes. The slides are then examined for fluorescing spirochetes in an ultraviolet microscope. Because of its simplicity and convenience to clinicians (slides can be mailed), this technique has replaced darkfield microscopy in most health departments and medical center laboratories.

C. SPINAL FLUID EXAMINATION

Cerebrospinal fluid findings in neurosyphilis are variable. In "classic" cases there is an elevation of total protein, lymphocytic pleocytosis, and a positive cerebrospinal fluid reagin test (VDRL). However, cerebrospinal fluid may be completely normal in neurosyphilis, and the VDRL may be negative. In one study, 25% of patients with primary or secondary syphilis in whom *T pallidum* was isolated from cerebrospinal fluid had a normal cerebrospinal fluid examination. In later stages of syphilis, normal cerebrospinal fluid analysis in the presence of infection can occur, but it is unusual. Because false-positive reagin tests rarely occur in the cerebrospinal fluid, a positive test confirms the presence of neurosyphilis. Because the cerebrospinal fluid VDRL may be negative in 30–70% of cases of neurosyphilis, *a negative test does not exclude neurosyphilis.* The use of cerebrospinal fluid FTA-ABS in the diagnosis of neurosyphilis is controversial. Some feel that it is more sensitive than the VDRL, but this is not accepted uniformly, and a high serum titer of FTA-ABS may result in a positive cerebrospinal fluid titer in the absence of neurosyphilis. However, the test is believed to be highly sensitive, and a negative cerebrospinal fluid FTA-ABS is strong evidence against the diagnosis of neurosyphilis. Other treponemal antibody tests likewise are not reliable in making the diagnosis of neurosyphilis, although a negative test is helpful in excluding the diagnosis.

Cerebrospinal fluid examination is recommended depending on the clinical manifestations and the stage of disease, as discussed below. Asymptomatic neurosyphilis (ie, positive cerebrospinal fluid findings without symptoms) requires prolonged penicillin treatment as given for symptomatic neurosyphilis. Adequate treatment is indicated by gradual decrease in cerebrospinal fluid cell count, protein concentration, and VDRL titer. Rarely, serologic tests of cerebrospinal fluid may remain positive for years after adequate treatment of neurosyphilis even though all other parameters have returned to normal.

Treatment

A. SPECIFIC MEASURES

1. Penicillin—Penicillin, as benzathine penicillin G or aqueous procaine penicillin G, is the drug of choice for all forms of syphilis and other spirochetal infections. Effective tissue levels must be maintained for several days or weeks because of the spirochete's long generation time (about 30 hours). Penicillin is highly effective in early infections and variably effective in the late stages. The principal contraindication is hypersensitivity to the penicillins. The recommended treatment schedules are included below in the discussion of the various forms of syphilis.

2. Other antibiotic therapy—Oral tetracyclines are effective in the treatment of syphilis for patients who are sensitive to penicillin. Tetracycline, 500 mg orally four times daily for 14 days, or doxycycline, 100 mg orally twice daily for 14 days, is given for infectious syphilis. In syphilis of more than 1 year's duration or of unknown duration, treatment is continued for 28 days in the same doses.

Although azithromycin, 500 mg daily for 10 days (total dose 5 g) or 500 mg on alternate days for 11 days (total dose 3 g), has been shown in one study to be effective for infectious syphilis, large numbers of patients have not been treated, and long-term follow-up data to identify failures are lacking. Thus, although this therapy may be effective, it is not currently recommended.

Human clinical trials using ceftriaxone for infectious syphilis are limited, and this agent is therefore not officially recommended at present. However, based on animal data and pharmacologic predictions, some have suggested that ceftriaxone in multiple-dose regimens (1 g intravenously or intramuscularly once a day for 7–14 days, or 2 g intravenously once daily for 10 days for neurosyphilis) may be efficacious against infectious syphilis. Single-dose ceftriaxone therapy is not effective for established syphilis.

B. LOCAL MEASURES (MUCOCUTANEOUS LESIONS)

Local treatment is usually not necessary. No local antiseptics or other chemicals should be applied to a suspected syphilitic lesion until specimens for microscopy have been obtained.

C. PUBLIC HEALTH MEASURES

Patients with infectious syphilis must abstain from sexual activity until rendered noninfectious by antibiotic therapy. All cases of syphilis must be reported to the appropriate public health agency for assistance in identifying and treating contacts. In addition, all patients with syphilis should have an HIV test at the time of diagnosis. In areas of high HIV prevalence, a repeat HIV test should be performed in 3 months if the initial test was negative.

D. EMPIRICAL POSTEXPOSURE TREATMENT

Patients who have been exposed to infectious syphilis within the preceding 3 months may be infected but seronegative and thus should be treated as for early syphilis. Persons exposed more than 90 days previously should be treated based on serologic results. If their partners are unavailable for testing or unreliable for follow-up, empirical therapy is indicated. Others at high risk either for infection (ie, those with other sexually transmitted diseases and those infected with HIV) or its consequences (ie, pregnant women) should undergo serologic tests for syphilis. The present recommended therapy for gonorrhea (ceftriaxone or cefixime) may not be effective in treating incubating syphilis. Therefore, patients with gonorrhea and a known exposure to syphilis should be treated with separate regimens effective against both diseases.

Complications of Specific Therapy

The Jarisch-Herxheimer reaction is ascribed to the sudden massive destruction of spirochetes by drugs and release of toxic products and is manifested by fever and aggravation of the existing clinical picture. It is most likely to occur in early syphilis. Treatment should not be discontinued unless the symptoms become severe or threaten to be fatal or unless syphilitic laryngitis, auditory neuritis, or labyrinthitis is present, where the reaction may cause irreversible damage.

The reaction may be prevented or modified by simultaneous administration of antipyretics or corticosteroids, though no proved method of prevention exists. It usually begins within the first 24 hours and subsides spontaneously within the next 24 hours of penicillin treatment.

Follow-Up Care

Because treatment failures can occur and reinfection is always a possibility, patients treated for syphilis should be followed clinically and serologically. Response to therapy is difficult to assess, and no definite criteria exist for cure in patients with primary or secondary syphilis. In primary and secondary syphilis, failure of nontreponemal antibody titers to decrease fourfold by 6 months may identify a group at high risk of treatment failure. Optimal management of these patients is unclear, but close clinical and serologic follow-up is indicated. If titers fail to decrease fourfold by 6 months, an HIV test should be repeated (all patients with syphilis should have an HIV test at the time of diagnosis); a lumbar puncture should be considered; and, if careful follow-up cannot be ensured (3-month intervals for HIV-positive individuals and 6-month intervals for HIV-negative patients), treatment should be repeated with 2.4 million units of benzathine penicillin intramuscularly weekly for 3 weeks. If symptoms or signs persist or recur after initial therapy or there is a fourfold or greater increase in nontreponemal titers, the patient has either failed therapy or has been reinfected. In those individuals, an HIV test should be performed, a lumbar puncture done (unless reinfection is a certainty), and re-treatment given as indicated above. In patients with latent syphilis, nontreponemal serologic tests should be repeated at 6, 12, and 24 months. If titers increase fourfold or if initially high titers (≥ 1:32) fail to decrease fourfold by 12–24

months—or if symptoms or signs consistent with syphilis develop—an HIV test and lumbar puncture should be performed and re-treatment given according to the stage of the disease.

Prevention

Avoidance of sexual contact is the only completely reliable method of prophylaxis but is an impractical public health measure for obvious reasons.

A. MECHANICAL

The standard latex condom is effective but protects covered parts only. The exposed parts should be washed with soap and water as soon after contact as possible. This applies to both sexes.

B. ANTIBIOTIC

If there is known exposure to infectious syphilis, abortive penicillin therapy may be used. Give 2.4 million units of procaine penicillin G intramuscularly. Treatment of gonococcal (and chlamydial) infection with tetracyclines and ceftriaxone is probably effective against incubating syphilis in most cases. However, other antimicrobial agents (eg, spectinomycin, quinolones) may be ineffective in aborting preclinical syphilis. Azithromycin administered as a single 1 g dose is also effective as preventive therapy in individuals exposed to infected partners. Because of concerns about treating incubating syphilis with nonpenicillin regimens, patients treated for gonorrhea should have a serologic test for syphilis 3–6 months after treatment.

Course & Prognosis
(See Table 34–3.)

The lesions associated with primary and secondary syphilis are self-limiting and resolve with few or no residua. Late syphilis may be highly destructive and permanently disabling and may lead to death. In broad terms, if no treatment is given, about one-third of people infected with syphilis will undergo spontaneous cure, about one-third will remain in the latent phase throughout life, and about one-third will develop serious late lesions.

CLINICAL STAGES OF SYPHILIS

1. Primary Syphilis

 ESSENTIALS OF DIAGNOSIS

- *History of sexual contact (often unreliable).*
- *Painless ulcer on genitalia, perianal area, rectum, pharynx, tongue, lip, or elsewhere 2–6 weeks after exposure.*
- *Nontender enlargement of regional lymph nodes.*

Table 34–3. Natural course of untreated syphilis.

Stage of Disease	Likelihood of Developing Clinical Manifestations	Comment
Latent	24%	90% of relapses occur in first year after infection.
Late		
Benign (gummatous)	15%	Many patients have more than one late manifestation.
Cardiovascular	10%	Seen only in those who develop syphilis after 15 years of age. Pathologic findings more common, ie, 50–80%.
Neurosyphilis	6.5%	Asymptomatic neurosyphilis has been reported in 8–40%.

- *Fluid expressed from lesion contains T pallidum by immunofluorescence or darkfield microscopy.*
- *Serologic test for syphilis often positive.*

General Considerations

This is the stage of invasion and may pass unrecognized. The typical lesion is the chancre at the site or sites of inoculation, most frequently located on the penis, labia, cervix, or anorectal region. Anorectal lesions are especially common among men who have sex with men. The primary lesion occurs occasionally in the oropharynx (lip, tongue, or tonsil) and rarely on the breast or finger. The chancre starts as a small erosion 10–90 days (average, 3–4 weeks) after inoculation that rapidly develops into a painless superficial ulcer with a clean base and firm, indurated margins, associated with enlargement of regional lymph nodes, which are rubbery, discrete, and nontender. Bacterial infection of the chancre may occur and may lead to pain. Healing occurs without treatment, but a scar may form, especially with secondary bacterial infection.

Laboratory Findings

The serologic test for syphilis is usually positive 1–2 weeks after the primary lesion is noted; rising titers are especially significant when there is a history of previous infection. Immunofluorescence or darkfield microscopy shows treponemes in at least 95% of chancres. Cerebrospinal fluid pleocytosis has been reported in 10–20% of patients with primary syphilis.

Differential Diagnosis

The syphilitic chancre may be confused with chancroid, lymphogranuloma venereum, genital herpes, or neoplasm. Any lesion on the genitalia should be considered a possible primary syphilitic lesion.

Treatment

Benzathine penicillin G, 2.4 million units intramuscularly in the gluteal area, is given once. For the nonpregnant penicillin-allergic patient, doxycycline, 100 mg orally twice daily for 2 weeks, or tetracycline, 500 mg orally four times a day for 2 weeks, can be used. There is more clinical experience with tetracycline, but compliance is probably better with doxycycline. Erythromycin, 500 mg orally four times a day for 2 weeks, can be used, but this regimen is generally considered less effective than others, and careful follow-up is mandatory in individuals treated with erythromycin.

2. Secondary Syphilis

ESSENTIALS OF DIAGNOSIS

- *Generalized maculopapular skin rash.*
- *Mucous membrane lesions, including patches and ulcers.*
- *Weeping papules (condylomas) in moist skin areas.*
- *Generalized nontender lymphadenopathy.*
- *Fever.*
- *Meningitis, hepatitis, osteitis, arthritis, iritis.*
- *Many treponemes in scrapings of mucous membrane or skin lesions by immunofluorescence or darkfield microscopy.*
- *Serologic tests for syphilis always positive.*

General Considerations & Treatment

The secondary stage of syphilis usually appears a few weeks (or up to 6 months) after development of the chancre, when sufficient dissemination of *T pallidum* has occurred to produce systemic signs (fever, lymphadenopathy) or infectious lesions at sites distant from the site of inoculation. The most common manifestations are skin and mucosal lesions. The skin lesions are nonpruritic, macular, papular, pustular, or follicular (or combinations of any of these types), though the maculopapular rash is the most common. The skin lesions usually are generalized; involvement of the palms and soles is especially suspicious. Annular lesions simulating ringworm are observed in blacks. Mucous membrane lesions range from ulcers and papules of the lips, mouth, throat, genitalia, and anus ("mucous patches") to a diffuse redness of the pharynx. Both skin and mucous membrane lesions are highly infectious at this stage. Specific lesions—**condylomata lata**—are fused, weeping papules on the moist areas of the skin and mucous membranes.

Meningeal (aseptic meningitis or acute basilar meningitis), hepatic, renal, bone, and joint invasion may occur, with resulting cranial nerve palsies, jaundice, nephrotic syndrome, and periostitis. Alopecia (moth-eaten appearance) and uveitis may also occur.

All serologic tests for syphilis are positive in almost all cases. The cutaneous and mucous membrane lesions often show *T pallidum* on darkfield microscopic examination. A transient cerebrospinal fluid pleocytosis is seen in 30–70% of patients with secondary syphilis, though only 5% have positive serologic cerebrospinal fluid reactions. There may be evidence of hepatitis or nephritis (immune complex type). Circulating immune complexes exist in the blood and are deposited in blood vessel walls.

Skin lesions may be confused with the infectious exanthems, pityriasis rosea, and drug eruptions. Visceral lesions may suggest nephritis or hepatitis due to other causes. The diffusely red throat may mimic other forms of pharyngitis.

Treatment is as for primary syphilis unless central nervous system or ocular disease is present, in which case treatment is as for neurosyphilis (see below). Isolation of the patient is important.

3. Relapsing Syphilis (Early Latent Syphilis)

The essentials of diagnosis are the same as in secondary syphilis.

The lesions of secondary syphilis heal spontaneously, but secondary syphilis may relapse if undiagnosed or inadequately treated. These relapses may include any of the findings noted under secondary syphilis: skin and mucous membrane, neurologic, ocular, bone, or visceral. Unlike the usual asymptomatic neurologic involvement of secondary syphilis, neurologic relapses may be fulminating, leading to death. Relapse is almost always accompanied by a rising titer in quantitative serologic tests; indeed, a rising titer may be the first or only evidence of relapse. About 90% of relapses occur during the first year after infection.

Treatment is as for primary syphilis unless central nervous system disease is present.

4. Late Latent ("Hidden") Syphilis

ESSENTIALS OF DIAGNOSIS

- No physical signs.
- History of syphilis with inadequate treatment.
- Positive serologic tests for syphilis.

General Considerations & Treatment

Latent syphilis is the clinically quiescent phase during the interval after disappearance of secondary lesions and before the appearance of tertiary symptoms. Early latency is defined as the first year after infection, during which time most infectious lesions recur ("relapsing syphilis"); after the first year, the patient is said to be in the late latent phase. Transmission to the fetus, however, can probably occur in any phase. There are (by definition) no clinical manifestations during the latent phase, and the only significant laboratory findings are positive serologic tests. A diagnosis of latent syphilis is justified only when the cerebrospinal fluid is entirely negative, x-ray and physical examination shows no evidence of cardiovascular involvement, and false-positive tests for syphilis have been ruled out. The latent phase may last from months to a lifetime.

It is important to differentiate latent syphilis from a false-positive serologic test for syphilis, which can be due to the many causes listed above.

Treatment is with benzathine penicillin G, 2.4 million units three times at 7-day intervals (total dose, 7.2 million units). In the penicillin-allergic patient, give tetracycline, 0.5 g orally four times a day for 28 days, or doxycycline, 100 mg orally twice daily for 28 days. If there is evidence of cerebrospinal fluid involvement, treat as for neurosyphilis. Only a small percentage of serologic tests will be appreciably altered by treatment with penicillin. The treatment of this stage of the disease is intended to prevent the late sequelae.

5. Late (Tertiary) Syphilis

ESSENTIALS OF DIAGNOSIS

- Infiltrative tumors of skin, bones, liver (gummas).
- Aortitis, aneurysms, aortic regurgitation.
- Central nervous system disorders, including meningovascular and degenerative changes,

paresthesias, shooting pains, abnormal reflexes, dementia, or psychosis.

General Considerations

This stage may occur at any time after secondary syphilis, even after years of latency, and is seen in about one-third of untreated patients (Table 34–3). Late lesions probably represent, at least in part, a delayed hypersensitivity reaction of the tissue to the organism and are usually divided into two types: (1) a localized gummatous reaction, with a relatively rapid onset and generally prompt response to therapy ("benign late syphilis"); and (2) diffuse inflammation of a more insidious onset that characteristically involves the central nervous system and large arteries, is often fatal if untreated, and is at best arrested by treatment. Gummas may involve any area or organ of the body but most often the skin or long bones. Cardiovascular disease is usually manifested by aortic aneurysm, aortic regurgitation, or aortitis. Various forms of diffuse or localized central nervous system involvement may occur.

Late syphilis must be differentiated from neoplasms of the skin, liver, lung, stomach, or brain; other forms of meningitis; and primary neurologic lesions.

Although almost any tissue and organ may be involved in late syphilis, the following are the most common types of involvement.

Skin

Cutaneous lesions of late syphilis are of two varieties: (1) multiple nodular lesions that eventually ulcerate (lues maligna) or resolve by forming atrophic, pigmented scars; and (2) solitary gummas that start as painless subcutaneous nodules, then enlarge, attach to the overlying skin, and eventually ulcerate.

Mucous Membranes

Late lesions of the mucous membranes are nodular gummas or leukoplakia, highly destructive to the involved tissue.

Skeletal System

Bone lesions are destructive, causing periostitis, osteitis, and arthritis with little or no associated redness or swelling but often marked myalgia and myositis of the neighboring muscles. The pain is especially severe at night.

Eyes

Late ocular lesions are gummatous iritis, chorioretinitis, optic atrophy, and cranial nerve palsies, in addition to the lesions of central nervous system syphilis.

Respiratory System

Respiratory involvement by late syphilis is caused by gummatous infiltrates into the larynx, trachea, and pulmonary parenchyma, producing discrete pulmonary densities. There may be hoarseness, respiratory distress, and wheezing secondary to the gummatous lesion itself or to subsequent stenosis occurring with healing.

Gastrointestinal System

Gummas involving the liver produce the usually benign, asymptomatic hepar lobatum. A picture resembling Laennec's cirrhosis is occasionally produced by liver involvement. Gastric involvement can consist of diffuse infiltration into the stomach wall or focal lesions that endoscopically and microscopically can be confused with lymphoma or carcinoma. Epigastric pain, early satiety, regurgitation, belching, and weight loss are common symptoms.

Cardiovascular System

Cardiovascular lesions (10–15% of late syphilitic lesions) are often progressive, disabling, and life-threatening. Central nervous system lesions are often present also. Involvement usually starts as an arteritis in the supracardiac portion of the aorta and progresses to cause one or more of the following: (1) narrowing of the coronary ostia, with resulting decreased coronary circulation, angina, and acute myocardial infarction; (2) scarring of the aortic valves, producing aortic regurgitation with its water-hammer pulse, aortic diastolic murmur, frequent aortic systolic murmur, cardiac hypertrophy, and eventually congestive heart failure, and (3) weakness of the wall of the aorta, with saccular aneurysm formation and associated pressure symptoms of dysphagia, hoarseness, brassy cough, back pain (vertebral erosion), and occasionally rupture of the aneurysm. Recurrent respiratory infections are common as a result of pressure on the trachea and bronchi.

Treatment of tertiary syphilis (excluding neurosyphilis; see below) is as for latent syphilis. Reversal of positive serologic tests does not usually occur. A second course of penicillin therapy may be given if necessary. There is no known method for reliable eradication of the treponeme from humans in the late stages of syphilis. Viable spirochetes are occasionally found in the eyes, in cerebrospinal fluid, and elsewhere in patients with "adequately" treated syphilis, but claims for their capacity to cause progressive disease are speculative.

Neurosyphilis

Neurosyphilis (15–20% of late syphilitic lesions; often present with cardiovascular syphilis) is also a progressive, disabling, and life-threatening complication. It develops more commonly in men than in women and in whites than in blacks.

A. Classification

There are four clinical types.

1. Asymptomatic neurosyphilis—This form is characterized by spinal fluid abnormalities (positive spinal fluid serology, increased cell count, occasionally increased protein) without symptoms or signs of neurologic involvement.

2. Meningovascular syphilis—This form is characterized by meningeal involvement or changes in the vascular structures of the brain (or both), producing symptoms of chronic meningitis (headache, irritability); cranial nerve palsies (basilar meningitis); unequal reflexes; irregular pupils with poor light and accommodation reflexes; and, when large vessels are involved, cerebrovascular accidents. The cerebrospinal fluid shows increased cells (100–1000/µL), elevated protein, and usually a positive serologic test for syphilis. The symptoms of acute meningitis are rare in late syphilis.

3. Tabes dorsalis—This form is a chronic progressive degeneration of the parenchyma of the posterior columns of the spinal cord and of the posterior sensory ganglia and nerve roots. The symptoms and signs are impairment of proprioception and vibration sense, Argyll Robertson pupils (which react poorly to light but well to accommodation), and muscular hypotonia and hyporeflexia. Impairment of proprioception results in a wide-based gait and inability to walk in the dark. Paresthesias, analgesia, or sharp recurrent pains in the muscles of the leg ("shooting" or "lightning" pains) may occur. Crises are also common in tabes: gastric crises, consisting of sharp abdominal pains with nausea and vomiting (simulating an acute abdomen); laryngeal crises, with paroxysmal cough and dyspnea; urethral crises, with painful bladder spasms; and rectal and anal crises. Crises may begin suddenly, last for hours to days, and cease abruptly. Neurogenic bladder with overflow incontinence is also seen. Painless trophic ulcers may develop over pressure points on the feet. Joint damage may occur as a result of lack of sensory innervation (Charcot joint). The cerebrospinal fluid may have a normal or increased cell count (3–200/µL), elevated protein, and variable results of serologic tests.

4. General paresis—This is generalized involvement of the cerebral cortex with insidious onset of symptoms. There is usually a decrease in concentrating power, memory loss, dysarthria, tremor of the fingers and lips, irritability, and mild headaches. Most striking is the change of personality; the patient becomes slovenly, irresponsible, confused, and psychotic. The cerebrospinal fluid findings resemble those of tabes dorsalis. Combinations of the various forms of neurosyphilis (especially tabes and paresis) are not uncommon.

B. Special Considerations in Treatment of Neurosyphilis

It is most important to prevent neurosyphilis by prompt diagnosis, adequate treatment, and follow-up of early syphilis. Indications for lumbar puncture vary depending upon the stage of the disease and the host's immune status. In early syphilis (primary and secondary syphilis and early latent syphilis of less than 1 year's duration), invasion of the central nervous system by *T pallidum* with cerebrospinal fluid abnormalities occur commonly, but neurosyphilis rarely develops in patients who have received the standard therapy outlined above. Thus, unless clinical symptoms and signs of neurosyphilis or ophthalmologic involvement (uveitis, neuroretinitis, optic neuritis, iritis) is present, a lumbar puncture in early syphilis is not recommended as part of the routine evaluation. In latent syphilis, the decision to perform a lumbar puncture should be individualized. Routine lumbar puncture for all patients is not indicated since the yield is low and findings rarely influence therapeutic decisions. Cerebrospinal fluid evaluation is recommended, however, in the later stages of syphilis if neurologic or ophthalmologic symptoms and signs are present; if therapy other than with penicillin is to be given; if the patient is HIV-positive (see next section); if there is evidence of treatment failure (see discussion above); if there is evidence of active tertiary syphilis (aortitis, iritis, optic atrophy, the presence of a gumma, etc); or if the serum nontreponemal antibody titer is ≥ 1:32. In the presence of definite cerebrospinal fluid or neurologic abnormalities, one should treat for neurosyphilis. The pretreatment clinical and laboratory evaluation should include neurologic, ocular, cardiovascular, psychiatric, and cerebrospinal fluid examinations.

The regimen of 2.4 million units of benzathine penicillin intramuscularly weekly for three consecutive weeks results in low to undetectable cerebrospinal fluid levels of penicillin, and treatment failures have been described when this regimen has been used to treat neurosyphilis. For these reasons, present recommendations for the therapy of neurosyphilis employ higher doses of short-acting penicillin in order to achieve better penetration and higher levels of drug in the cerebrospinal fluid. Recommended regimens include 3–4 million units of aqueous crystalline penicillin G intravenously every 4 hours for 10–14 days. Alternatively, 2.4 million units of procaine penicillin can be given intramuscularly once daily along with 500 mg of probenecid orally four times daily, both for 10–14 days. Because of concerns about slowly dividing organisms that may persist, many experts recommend subsequent administration of 2.4 million units of benzathine penicillin intramuscularly once weekly for 3 weeks as additional therapy. Alternative therapy to penicillin has not been established for treatment of neurosyphilis. Chloramphenicol (2 g daily for 30 days), doxycycline (200 mg twice daily for 21 days), and ceftriaxone (1 g daily for 14 days) have all been shown to achieve treponemicidal levels in the cerebrospinal fluid, but clinical experience is limited, and failures have been reported. Thus, patients with a history of penicillin allergy should be skin-tested, desensitized, and treated with penicillin.

All patients should have spinal fluid examinations at 6-month intervals until the cell count is normal. Response may be gauged by clinical improvement and reversal of cerebrospinal fluid changes. A second course of penicillin therapy may be given if the cell count has not decreased at 6 months or is not normal at 2 years. Not infrequently, there is progression of neurologic symptoms and signs despite high and prolonged doses of penicillin. It has been postulated that these treatment failures are related to the unexplained persistence of viable *T pallidum* in central nervous system or ocular lesions in at least some cases.

6. Syphilis in HIV-Infected Patients

Because syphilis has variable clinical manifestations and an unpredictable course, evaluation of case reports of unusual clinical or laboratory manifestations of syphilis in HIV-infected patients is difficult. Although unusual serologic responses have been reported in HIV-positive patients, including high titers of nontreponemal tests, delayed appearance of positive titers, and false-negative tests, most HIV-positive patients respond serologically in somewhat the same way as noninfected patients. Thus, interpretation of serologic tests should be the same for HIV-positive and HIV-negative individuals. Some recommend that all HIV-positive men be screened twice a year by RPR or VDRL to identify latent disease and to appropriately stage individuals. By establishing a serologic history, unnecessary lumbar punctures required for latent syphilis of unknown duration can be avoided. Because of concerns about false-negative serologic tests or a delayed immunologic response, if the diagnosis of syphilis is suggested on clinical grounds but reagin tests are negative, alternative tests should be performed. These tests include darkfield examination of lesions and direct fluorescent antibody staining for *T pallidum* of lesion exudate or biopsy specimens.

The diagnosis of neurosyphilis in HIV-infected patients is complicated by the fact that cerebrospinal fluid abnormalities are frequently seen and may be due to neurosyphilis or HIV infection itself. The significance of these abnormalities is unknown, and similar abnormalities are frequently seen in non-HIV-infected patients with primary or secondary syphilis. Despite occasional reports of HIV-infected patients who progress to develop neurosyphilis despite appropriate therapy for early disease, the vast majority of HIV-infected patients with primary or secondary syphilis respond appropriately to currently recommended regimens. Thus, although some recommend a cerebrospinal fluid examination for all HIV-positive patients with syphilis, such testing is probably not needed in those with early disease. In contrast, a lumbar puncture should be performed in HIV-positive patients if they have late latent syphilis or syphilis of unknown duration; if neurologic signs are present; or if they have failed therapy. As discussed above, the same criteria for failure apply to HIV-positive and HIV-

negative patients, and re-treatment regimens are the same.

Treatment of HIV-positive patients with primary and secondary syphilis is the same as for HIV-negative patients. Because of concerns about the adequacy of this therapy, a large multicenter trial of therapy of early syphilis in HIV-positive and HIV-negative patients was undertaken to compare standard therapy with enhanced therapy (2.4 million units of benzathine penicillin followed by 2 g of amoxicillin plus 500 mg of probenecid taken orally three times a day for 10 days). In the 1 year of follow-up, no cases of neurosyphilis were observed, suggesting that current recommendations are adequate. Because of ongoing concerns about adequacy of therapy, careful clinical and serologic follow-up should be done at 3, 6, 9, 12, and 24 months.

HIV-infected patients with late latent syphilis, syphilis of unknown duration, and neurosyphilis should be treated like HIV-negative individuals, with follow-up at 6, 12, 18, and 24 months.

Because clinical experience in treating HIV-infected patients with syphilis is based on penicillin regimens, all stages of syphilis should be treated with this drug. If severe allergy exists, the patient should be desensitized to penicillin.

7. Syphilis in Pregnancy

All pregnant women should have a nontreponemal serologic test for syphilis at the time of the first prenatal visit. In women suspected of being at increased risk for syphilis or for populations in which there is a high prevalence of syphilis, another nontreponemal test should be performed during the third trimester at 28 weeks and again at delivery. The serologic status of all women who have delivered should be known before discharge from the hospital. Seropositive women should be considered infected and should be treated unless prior treatment with fall in antibody titer is medically documented.

The preferred treatment is with penicillin in dosage schedules appropriate for the stage of syphilis (see above). Penicillin prevents congenital syphilis in 90% of cases, even when treatment is given late in pregnancy. Tetracycline and doxycycline are contraindicated in pregnancy, and erythromycin is associated with a high risk of failure in the fetus. Women with a history of penicillin allergy should be skin-tested and desensitized if necessary.

The infant should be evaluated immediately, as noted below, and at 6–8 weeks of age.

8. Congenital Syphilis

Congenital syphilis is a transplacentally transmitted infection that occurs in infants of untreated or inadequately treated mothers. The physical findings at birth are quite variable: The infant may have many or only minimal signs or even no signs until 6–8 weeks of life (delayed form). The most common findings are on the mucous membranes and skin—maculopapular rash, condylomas, mucous membrane patches, and serous nasal discharge (snuffles). These lesions are infectious; *T pallidum* can easily be found microscopically, and the infant must be isolated. Other common findings are hepatosplenomegaly, anemia, or osteochondritis. These early active lesions subsequently heal, and if the disease is left untreated it produces the characteristic stigmas of syphilis—interstitial keratitis, Hutchinson's teeth, saddle nose, saber shins, deafness, and central nervous system involvement.

The presence of negative serologic tests at birth in both the mother and the infant usually means that the newborn is free of infection. However, recent infection near the time of delivery may result in negative tests because there has been insufficient time to develop a serologic response. Thus, one must maintain a high index of suspicion in infants who present with delayed onset of symptoms despite negative serologic tests at birth, especially in infants born to high-risk mothers (HIV-positive, illicit drug users).

Augenbraun MH et al: Treatment of syphilis, 1998: nonpregnant adults. Clin Infect Dis 1999;28(Suppl 1):S21. [PMID: 10028107] (Recommended therapies with review of supporting evidence.)

1998 guidelines for treatment of sexually transmitted diseases. MMWR Recomm Rep 1998;47(RR-1):1. [PMID: 9461053] (Comprehensive summary of recommendations.)

■ NON-SEXUALLY TRANSMITTED TREPONEMATOSES

A variety of treponemal diseases other than syphilis occur endemically in many tropical areas of the world. They are distinguished from disease caused by *T pallidum* by their nonsexual transmission, their relatively high incidence in certain geographic areas and among children, and their tendency to produce less severe visceral manifestations. As in syphilis, organisms can be demonstrated in infectious lesions with darkfield microscopy or immunofluorescence but cannot be cultured in artificial media; the serologic tests for syphilis are positive, including the newer tests such as CAPTIA Syph G; the diseases have primary, secondary, and sometimes tertiary stages; and penicillin is the drug of choice. There is evidence that infection with these agents may provide partial resistance to syphilis and vice versa. Treatment with penicillin in doses appropriate to primary syphilis (eg, 2.4 million units of benzathine penicillin G intramuscularly) is generally curative in any stage of the non-sexually transmitted treponematoses. In cases of penicillin hypersensitivity, tetracycline, 500 mg four times a day for 10–14 days, is usually the recommended alternative.

YAWS (Frambesia)

Yaws is a contagious disease largely limited to tropical regions that is caused by *T pallidum* subsp *pertenue*. It is characterized by granulomatous lesions of the skin, mucous membranes, and bone. Yaws is rarely fatal, though if untreated it may lead to chronic disability and disfigurement. Yaws is acquired by direct nonsexual contact, usually in childhood, although it may occur at any age. The "mother yaw," a painless papule that later ulcerates, appears 3–4 weeks after exposure. There is usually associated regional lymphadenopathy. Six to 12 weeks later, similar secondary lesions appear and last for several months or years. Painful ulcerated lesions on the soles are frequent and are called "crab yaws." Late gummatous lesions may occur, with associated tissue destruction involving large areas of skin and subcutaneous tissues. The late effects of yaws, with bone change, shortening of digits, and contractions, may be confused with similar changes occurring in leprosy. Central nervous system, cardiac, or other visceral involvement is rare. See above for therapy.

PINTA

Pinta is a non-sexually transmitted spirochetal infection caused by *Treponema carateum*. It occurs endemically in rural areas of Latin America, especially in Mexico, Colombia, and Cuba, and in some areas of the Pacific. A nonulcerative, erythematous primary papule spreads slowly into a papulosquamous plaque showing a variety of color changes (slate, lilac, black). Secondary lesions resemble the primary one and appear within a year after it. These appear successively, new lesions together with older ones; are commonest on the extremities; and later show atrophy and depigmentation. Some cases show pigmentary changes and atrophic patches on the soles and palms, with or without hyperkeratosis, that are indistinguishable from "crab yaws." Very rarely, central nervous system or cardiovascular disease is observed late in the course of infection. See above for therapy.

ENDEMIC SYPHILIS

Endemic syphilis is an acute or chronic infection caused by an organism indistinguishable from *T pallidum* subsp *endemicum*. It has been reported in a number of countries, particularly in the eastern Mediterranean area, often with local names: bejel in Syria, Saudi Arabia, and Iraq; and dichuchwa, njovera, and siti in Africa. It also occurs in Southeast Asia. The local forms have distinctive features. Moist ulcerated lesions of the skin or oral or nasopharyngeal mucosa are the most common manifestations. Generalized lymphadenopathy and secondary and tertiary bone and skin lesions are also common. Deep leg pain points to periostitis or osteomyelitis. Cardiovascular and central nervous system involvement is rare. See above for therapy.

Engelkens HJ et al: Nonvenereal treponematoses in tropical countries. Clin Dermatol 1999;17:143. [PMID: 10330597]

■ MISCELLANEOUS SPIROCHETAL DISEASES

RELAPSING FEVER

Relapsing fever is endemic in many parts of the world. The main reservoir is rodents, which serve as the source of infection for ticks (eg, ornithodoros). The distribution and seasonal incidence of the disease are determined by the ecology of the ticks in different areas. In the USA, infected ticks are found throughout the West, especially in mountainous areas, but clinical cases are uncommon in humans.

The infectious organism is a spirochete, *Borrelia recurrentis,* though other poorly characterized borrelia-like organisms can cause similar disease. It may be transmitted transovarially from one generation of ticks to the next. The spirochetes occur in all tissues of the tick, and humans can be infected by tick bites or by rubbing crushed tick tissues or feces into the bite wound. Tick-borne relapsing fever is endemic but is not transmitted from person to person. Different species (or strain) names have been given to borrelia in different parts of the world where the organisms are transmitted by different ticks.

When an infected person harbors lice, the lice become infected with borrelia by sucking blood. A few days later, the lice serve as a source of infection for other persons. Large epidemics may occur in louse-infested populations, and transmission is favored by crowding, malnutrition, and cold climate.

Clinical Findings

A. SYMPTOMS AND SIGNS

There is an abrupt onset of fever, chills, tachycardia, nausea and vomiting, arthralgia, and severe headache. Hepatomegaly and splenomegaly may develop, as well as various types of rashes. Delirium occurs with high fever, and there may be various neurologic and psychic abnormalities. The attack terminates, usually abruptly, after 3–10 days. After an interval of 1–2 weeks, relapse occurs, but often it is somewhat milder. Three to ten relapses may occur before recovery.

B. LABORATORY FINDINGS

During episodes of fever, large spirochetes are seen in blood smears stained with Wright's or Giemsa's stain. The organisms can be cultured in special media but rapidly lose pathogenicity. The spirochetes can multiply in injected rats or mice and can be seen in their blood.

A variety of anti-borrelia antibodies develop during the illness; sometimes the Weil-Felix test for rickettsioses and nontreponemal serologic tests for syphilis may also be falsely positive. Infection with *Borrelia recurrentis* can cause false-positive indirect fluorescent antibody and Western blot tests for *Borrelia burgdorferi,* and some cases may be misdiagnosed as Lyme disease. Cerebrospinal fluid abnormalities occur in patients with meningeal involvement. Mild anemia and thrombocytopenia are common, but the white blood cell count tends to be normal.

Differential Diagnosis

The manifestations of relapsing fever may be confused with malaria, leptospirosis, meningococcemia, yellow fever, typhus, or rat-bite fever.

Prevention

Prevention of tick bites (as described for rickettsial diseases) and delousing procedures applicable to large groups can prevent illness. Arthropod vectors should be controlled if possible.

An effective means of chemoprophylaxis has not been developed.

Treatment

A single dose of tetracycline or erythromycin, 0.5 g orally, or a single dose of procaine penicillin G, 400,000–600,000 units intramuscularly, probably constitutes adequate treatment for louse-borne relapsing fevers. Because of higher relapse rates, tick-borne disease is treated with 0.5 g of tetracycline or erythromycin given four times daily for 5–10 days. Jarisch-Herxheimer reactions occur commonly following treatment and may be life-threatening. Treatment with aspirin—but not hydrocortisone—may ameliorate this reaction. The Jarisch-Herxheimer reaction is mediated in part by tumor necrosis factor, and administration of antibody to this cytokine prior to antibiotic therapy is effective in preventing the reaction.

Prognosis

The overall mortality rate is usually about 5%. Fatalities are most common in old, debilitated, or very young patients. With treatment, the initial attack is shortened and relapses are largely prevented.

Dworkin MS et al: Tick-borne relapsing fever in the northwestern United States and southwestern Canada. Clin Infect Dis 1998;26:122. [PMID: 9455520] (Review of 182 cases.)

Johnson WD Jr, Golightly LM: *Borrelia* species: Relapsing fever. In: *Principles and Practice of Infectious Diseases,* 5th ed. Mandell GL, Bennett JE, Dolin R (editors). Churchill Livingstone, 2000.

RAT-BITE FEVER
(Spirillary Rat-Bite Fever, Sodoku)

Rat-bite fever is an uncommon acute infectious disease caused by *Spirillum minus.* It is transmitted to humans by the bite of a rat. Inhabitants of rat-infested slum dwellings and laboratory workers are at greatest risk.

Clinical Findings

A. SYMPTOMS AND SIGNS

The original rat bite, unless secondarily infected, heals promptly, but 1 to several weeks later the site becomes swollen, indurated, and painful; assumes a dusky purplish hue; and may ulcerate. Regional lymphangitis and lymphadenitis, fever, chills, malaise, myalgia, arthralgia, and headache are present. Splenomegaly may occur. A sparse, dusky-red maculopapular rash appears on the trunk and extremities in many cases, and there may be frank arthritis.

After a few days, both the local and systemic symptoms subside, only to reappear again in a few more days. This relapsing pattern of fever for 3–4 days alternating with afebrile periods lasting 3–9 days may persist for weeks. The other features, however, usually recur only during the first few relapses.

B. LABORATORY FINDINGS

Leukocytosis is often present, and the nontreponemal test for syphilis is often falsely positive. The organism may be identified in darkfield examination of the ulcer exudate or aspirated lymph node material; more commonly, it is observed after inoculation of a laboratory animal with the patient's exudate or blood. It has not been cultured in artificial media.

Differential Diagnosis

Rat-bite fever must be distinguished from the rat bite-induced lymphadenitis and rash of streptobacillary fever. Clinically, the severe arthritis and myalgias seen in streptobacillary disease is rarely seen in disease caused by *S minus*. Reliable differentiation requires an increasing titer of agglutinins against *Streptobacillus moniliformis* or identification of the causative organism. Rat-bite fever must also be distinguished from tularemia, rickettsial disease, *Pasteurella multocida* infections, and relapsing fever by identification of the causative organism.

Treatment

Treat with procaine penicillin G, 600,000 units intramuscularly every 12 hours; or tetracycline hydrochloride, 0.5 g every 6 hours for 10–14 days. Give supportive and symptomatic measures as indicated.

Prognosis

The reported mortality rate of about 10% should be markedly reduced by prompt diagnosis and antimicrobial treatment.

Washburn RG: *Spirillum minus* (rat-bite fever). In: *Principles and Practice of Infectious Diseases,* 5th ed. Mandell GL, Bennett JE, Dolin R (editors). Churchill Livingstone, 2000.

LEPTOSPIROSIS

Leptospirosis is an acute and often severe infection that frequently affects the liver or other organs and is caused by *Leptospira interrogans,* which is a diverse organism consisting of 23 serogroups and over 200 serovars. The three most common serovars of infection are *Leptospira icterohaemorrhagiae* of rats, *Leptospira canicola* of dogs, and *Leptospira pomona* of cattle and swine. Several other varieties can also cause the disease, but *L icterohaemorrhagiae* causes the most severe illness. The disease is worldwide in distribution, and the incidence is higher than usually supposed. The leptospires are often transmitted to humans by the ingestion of food and drink contaminated by the urine of the reservoir animal. The organism may also enter through minor skin lesions and probably via the conjunctiva. Recreational cases have followed swimming or rafting in contaminated water, and occupational cases occur among sewer workers, rice planters, abattoir workers, and farmers. Sporadic urban cases have been seen in the homeless exposed to rat urine. The incubation period is 2–20 days.

Clinical Findings

A. SYMPTOMS AND SIGNS

Anicteric leptospirosis is the more common and milder form of the disease and is often biphasic. The initial or "septicemic" phase begins with abrupt fever to 39–40 °C, chills, abdominal pain, severe headache, and myalgias, especially of the calf muscles. There may be marked conjunctival suffusion. Leptospires can be isolated from blood, cerebrospinal fluid, and tissues. Following a 1- to 3-day period of improvement in symptoms and absence of fever, the second or "immune" phase begins. Leptospires are absent from blood and cerebrospinal fluid but are still present in the kidney, and specific antibodies appear. A recurrence of symptoms is seen as in the first phase of disease with the onset of meningitis. Uveitis (which can be unilateral or bilateral and usually involves the entire uveal tract), rash, and adenopathy may occur. A rare but severe manifestation is hemorrhagic pneumonia. The illness is usually self-limited, lasting 4–30 days, and complete recovery is the rule.

Icteric leptospirosis (Weil's syndrome) (usually caused by *L icterohaemorrhagiae*) is the most severe form of the disease, characterized by impaired renal and hepatic function, abnormal mental status, hemorrhagic pneumonia, hypotension, and a 5–10% mortality rate. Symptoms and signs often are continuous and not biphasic.

Pretibial fever, a mild form of leptospirosis caused by *Leptospira autumnalis,* occurred during World War II at Fort Bragg, USA. In pretibial fever, there is patchy erythema on the skin of the lower legs or generalized rash occurring with fever.

Leptospirosis with jaundice must be distinguished from hepatitis, yellow fever, and relapsing fever.

B. LABORATORY FINDINGS

The leukocyte count may be normal or as high as 50,000/μL, with neutrophils predominating. The urine may contain bile, protein, casts, and red cells. Oliguria is not uncommon, and in severe cases uremia may occur. Elevated bilirubin and aminotransferases are seen in 75% and elevated creatinine (> 1.5 mg/dL) in 50%. In cases with meningeal involvement, organisms may be found in the cerebrospinal fluid during the first 10 days of illness. Early in the disease, the organism may be identified by darkfield examination of the patient's blood or by culture on a semisolid medium (eg, Fletcher's EMJH). Cultures take 1–6 weeks to become positive. The organism may also be grown from the urine from the tenth day to the sixth week. Diagnosis is usually made by means of serologic tests, of which several are available. Agglutination tests (microscopic, using live organisms; and macroscopic, using killed antigen) become positive after 7–10 days of illness, peak at 3–4 weeks, and may persist at high levels for many years. Thus, to make a diagnosis, a fourfold or greater rise in titer must be documented. The agglutination tests are cumbersome to perform and require trained personnel. Indirect hemagglutination, enzyme immunosorbent assay (EIA), and ELISA tests are also available. The IgM EIA is particularly useful in making an early diagnosis, as it is positive as early as 2 days into illness, a time when the clinical manifestations may be nonspecific, and it is extremely sensitive and specific (93%). PCR methods (presently investigational) appear to be sensitive, specific, positive early in disease, and able to detect leptospiral DNA in blood, urine, cerebrospinal fluid, and aqueous humor. Serum CK is usually elevated in leptospirosis patients and normal in hepatitis patients.

Complications

Myocarditis, aseptic meningitis, renal failure, and pulmonary infiltrates with hemorrhage are not common but are the usual causes of death. Iridocyclitis may occur.

Treatment

Various antimicrobial drugs, including penicillin and tetracyclines, show antileptospiral activity. Penicillin (eg, 6 million units daily intravenously) is the drug of choice in severe leptospirosis and is especially effective if started within the first 4 days of illness. Jarisch-Herxheimer reactions may occur. Observe for evidence of renal failure, and treat as necessary. Effective prophylaxis consists of doxycycline, 200 mg orally once weekly during the risk of exposure. Doxycycline, 100 mg twice daily for 7 days, is also effective if started early, but this agent is most often used in mild to moderate disease.

Prognosis

Without jaundice, the disease is almost never fatal. With jaundice, the mortality rate is 5% for those under age 30 and 30% for those over age 60.

Katz AR et al: Assessment of the clinical presentation and treatment of 353 cases of laboratory-confirmed leptospirosis in Hawaii, 1974-1998. Clin Infect Dis 2001;33:1834. [PMID: 11692294] (Clinical description of an ongoing outbreak.)

Lomar AV et al: Leptospirosis in Latin America. Infect Dis Clin North Am 2000;14:23. [PMID: 10738671] (Clinical review of diagnosis, manifestations, therapy, and prevention.)

LYME DISEASE
(Lyme Borreliosis)

ESSENTIALS OF DIAGNOSIS

- *Erythema migrans, a flat or slightly raised red lesion that expands with central clearing.*
- *Headache or stiff neck.*
- *Arthralgias, arthritis, and myalgias; arthritis is often chronic and recurrent.*
- *Wide geographic distribution, with most United States cases in the Northeast, mid-Atlantic, Upper Midwest, and Pacific coastal regions.*

General Considerations

This illness, named after the town of Old Lyme, Connecticut, is caused by the spirochete *Borrelia burgdorferi* and is transmitted to humans by ixodid ticks that are part of the *Ixodes ricinus* complex. Four genomic groups of the *B burgdorferi sensu lato* group have been identified: *B burgdorferi sensu stricto,* which causes disease in North America and less commonly in Europe and Asia; *B garinii,* and *B afzelii,* which are the predominant etiologic agents of Lyme disease in Europe and Asia; and the newly named *B bissettii* sp *nov* found in California. Lyme disease is the most common vector-borne disease in the United States and is being reported with increasing frequency, but the true incidence is not known, and overreporting remains a problem. In 2000 there were 17,730 cases reported from 44 states and the District of Columbia, an increase of 8% over 1999. Most cases (over 95%) were reported from the mid-Atlantic, northeastern, and North Central regions of the country. As in years past, cases were reported from states without known enzootic cycles of *B burgdorferi,* raising questions about the accuracy of diagnosis. Overdiagnosis of Lyme disease continues to be a problem. In a Lyme disease clinic at a major teaching hospital in an endemic area, 788 patients were referred over a 4.5-year period. Only 23% were found to have active disease. The remaining patients had adequately treated disease in the past and another concurrent illness (20%) or did not have Lyme disease at all (57%). The consequences of overdiagnosis and overtreatment of Lyme disease are substantial. Individuals with previously treated Lyme disease and another concurrent illness and those without Lyme disease were avid users of the health care system, with multiple office visits to several different physicians resulting in numerous prescriptions for unnecessary antibiotics (approximately 30% of patients received over 100 days of antibiotic therapy) that often caused adverse drug events. In addition, this group of patients seeking a diagnosis of Lyme disease had a significant number of days in which they were unable to perform normal activities and had a high incidence of depression and stress (40–50%). The overreporting and overdiagnosis of Lyme disease is in part explained by the discovery of a nonculturable spirochete in the Lone Star tick (*Amblyomma americanum*). This organism produces a Lyme disease-like illness with a skin lesion very similar to that of erythema migrans. As the Lone Star tick is found in the Midwest and Southern areas where enzootic cycles for *B burgdorferi* have not been reported, cases of Lyme disease reported from these areas are probably due to this newly discovered organism. The vector of Lyme disease varies geographically and is *Ixodes scapularis* (also known as *I dammini*) in the northeastern, North Central, and mid-Atlantic regions of the United States; *Ixodes pacificus* on the West Coast; *Ixodes ricinus* in Europe; and *Ixodes persulcatus* in Asia. The disease also occurs in Australia. Mice and deer make up the major animal reservoir of *B burgdorferi*, but other rodents and birds may also be infected. Domestic animals such as dogs, cattle, and horses can also develop clinical illness, usually manifested as arthritis.

Ticks feed once during each of their three stages of life. Larval ticks feed in late summer, nymphs in the following spring and early summer, and adults during the fall. In the northeastern United States and the mid-Atlantic states, the preferred host for the nymphs and larvae is the white-footed mouse (the black-striped mouse in Europe). This animal is tolerant of infection—a fact that is critical in maintaining infection, since the mouse can remain spirochetemic and transmit the agent to the larvae the following spring after being infected by the nymphal form in early summer. Adult ticks prefer the white-tailed deer as host. Although only 20–25% of nymphs harbor spirochetes compared with 50–65% of adults, most infections occur in the spring and summer (when nymphs are active), and fewer cases occur in the cooler months (October to April), when adults feed. This is probably due to the greater abundance of nymphs; greater human outdoor activity in spring and summer, when nymphs feed; and the fact that adult ticks are larger, easier to detect by the human host, and thus can be removed before disease is transmitted. Less than 1% of larvae are infected with spirochetes, and transmission of the disease through contact with larvae is unlikely. In the Western United States, the *Ixodes pacificus* nymph prefers to feed on lizards, which are not susceptible to infection. It is only the few nymph and larval ticks that feed on wood rats, which can be infected, that are capable of transmitting disease.

The increased incidence of Lyme disease is due in part to the resurgence of the once-decimated deer population, the spread of tick vectors to new areas (infected ixodes ticks have been isolated from migratory birds), and the encroachment of suburbs on once rural areas, bringing humans and ticks into closer proximity. Factors contributing to increased reporting include enhanced provider awareness and better laboratory surveillance.

Under experimental conditions, ticks must feed for 24 hours or longer to transmit infections. Human epidemiologic studies have indicated that the incidence of disease is significantly higher when tick attachment is for longer than 72 hours than if it is less than 72 hours, though rare cases have been documented with attachment of less than 24 hours. In addition, the percentage of ticks infected varies on a regional basis. In the Northeast and Midwest, 15–65% of *I scapularis* ticks are infected with the spirochete; in the Western United States, only 2% of *I pacificus* are infected. These are important epidemiologic features in assessing the likelihood that tick exposure will result in disease. Exposure to *I pacificus* is unlikely to result in disease, since so few ticks are infected, but this is not true of exposure to *I scapularis*. Eliciting a history of brushing a tick off the skin (ie, the tick was not feeding) or removing a tick on the same day as exposure (ie, the tick did not feed long enough) decreases the likelihood that infection will develop, since the vast majority of cases occur when ticks feed for at least 24 hours.

Ixodes ticks are smaller than the more common dog ticks (*Dermacentor variabilis*). Larvae are less than 1 mm in size, and the adult female is 2–3 mm in size, with a red body and black legs. After a blood meal, ticks can reach two to three times their unengorged size. Because the tick is so small, the bite is usually painless and goes unnoticed. After feeding, the tick drops off in 2–4 days. If a tick is found, it should be removed immediately. The best way to accomplish this is to grab the mouth part—not the body—where it enters the skin with a fine-tipped tweezers and pull firmly and repeatedly until the tick releases its hold. Saving the tick in a bottle of alcohol for future identification may be useful, especially if symptoms develop.

Congenital infection has been documented, but the exact frequency and manifestations have not been clearly defined. Similarly, because the organism can be latent, it is not known if women infected prior to becoming pregnant can activate the disease and transmit infection to the fetus. In one retrospective study, 5 of 19 pregnancies complicated by Lyme disease resulted in an adverse outcome, but all of the outcomes were different and could not be conclusively linked to infection. Several serosurveys involving over 2000 pregnant women in endemic areas have not found any association between seropositivity in prospective mothers and the prevalence of congenital malformations, fetal death, and prematurity. Thus, if *B burgdorferi* causes a congenital syndrome like some other spirochetal illnesses, it must be extremely uncommon.

Clinical Findings

The typical clinical description of Lyme disease divides the illness into three stages: stage 1, flu-like symptoms and a typical skin rash (**erythema migrans**); stage 2, weeks to months later, Bell's palsy or meningitis; and stage 3, months to years later, arthritis. The problem with this simplified scheme is that there is a great deal of overlap, and the skin, central nervous system, and musculoskeletal system can be involved early or late. A more accurate classification divides disease into early and late manifestations and specifies whether disease is localized or disseminated.

A. SYMPTOMS AND SIGNS

1. Stage 1, early localized infection—Stage 1 infection is characterized by erythema migrans. About 1 week after the tick bite (range, 3–30 days; median 7–10 days), a flat or slightly raised red lesion appears at the site, which is commonly seen in areas of tight clothing such as the groin, thigh, or axilla. This lesion expands over several days, with central clearing. About 20% of patients either do not have typical skin lesions or the lesions go unnoticed. A flu-like illness with fever, chills, and myalgia occurs in about half of patients. Even without treatment, the symptoms and signs of erythema migrans resolve in 3–4 weeks. Although the classic lesion of erythema migrans is not difficult to recognize, atypical forms can occur that may lead to misdiagnosis. Vesicular, urticarial, and evanescent erythema migrans have been reported, as have lesions that develop central intensification instead of clearing. Similarly, chemical reactions to tick and spider bites, drug eruptions, urticaria, and staphylococcal and streptococcal cellulitis have been mistaken for erythema migrans.

2. Stage 2, early disseminated infection—In stage 2, the spirochete may spread in the patient's blood or lymph to cause a wide variety of symptoms and signs. This usually occurs within days to weeks after inoculation of the organism. The most common manifestations involve the skin, central nervous system, and musculoskeletal system. In about half of patients, secondary lesions develop that are not associated with a tick bite. These lesions are similar in appearance to the primary lesion but are usually smaller. A rare skin lesion (1% of patients) seen primarily in Europe is borrelia lymphocytoma. This presents as a small reddish nodule or plaque on the ear in children and on the nipple in adults. Headache and stiff neck can occur, as well as migratory pains in joints, muscles, and tendons. Fatigue and malaise are common. Generally, the neurologic and musculoskeletal symptoms are intermittent and last only hours to a few days, whereas fatigue is persistent. After hematogenous spread, the organism sequesters itself in certain areas and produces focal symptoms. Some patients experience cardiac (4–10% of patients) or neurologic (10–20% of patients) manifestations. Involvement of the heart includes myopericarditis, with atrial or ventricular arrhythmias and heart block. Neurologic disease is most commonly manifested as aseptic meningitis with mild headache and neck stiffness, Bell's palsy, or encephalitis with irritability, personality change, and forgetfulness that can wax and wane. Even in the absence of symptoms, seeding of the central nervous system can occur. Peripheral neuropathy (sensory or motor), transverse myelitis, and mononeuritis multiplex have also been described. Conjunctivitis, keratitis, and, rarely, panophthalmitis can occur.

3. Stage 3, late persistent infection—Stage 3 infection occurs months to years after the initial infection and again primarily manifests itself as musculoskeletal, neurologic, and skin disease. Up to 60% of patients develop musculoskeletal complaints. Clinical manifestations are quite variable and include (1) joint and periarticular pain without objective findings (perhaps a manifestation of fibromyalgia that may be triggered by Lyme disease); (2) frank arthritis, mainly of large joints, that is chronic or recurrent over years (recurrences become less severe, less frequent, and shorter with time); and (3) chronic synovitis, which may result in permanent disability. The pathogenesis of chronic Lyme arthritis may be an immunologic phenomenon rather than persistence of infection. The observations that individuals with chronic arthritis have an increased frequency of HLA-DR4 gene expression, antibodies to OspA and OspB protein in joint fluid (major outer surface proteins of *B burgdorferi*), lack *B burgdorferi* DNA in synovial fluid as detected by polymerase chain reaction (PCR), and often fail to respond to antibiotics—all support the inference of an immunologic mechanism.

Both the central and the peripheral nervous systems may be involved. Subacute encephalopathy, characterized by memory loss, mood changes, and sleep disturbance, is the most common chronic neurologic manifestation. An axonal polyneuropathy, manifested as distal sensory paresthesias or radicular pain, can occur either alone or, more commonly, in association with encephalopathy. Most of these patients have objective signs of disease when tested by electromyography. A rare form of chronic neurologic dysfunction—leukoencephalitis—presents with cognitive dysfunction, spastic paraparesis, ataxia, and bladder dysfunction. This form of the disease is seen more commonly in Europe than in the United States.

The cutaneous manifestation of late infection, which can occur up to 10 years after infection, is **acrodermatitis chronicum atrophicans.** It has been described mainly in Europe and is due to infection with *Borrelia afzelii,* a species that commonly causes disease in Europe but not the United States. There is usually bluish-red discoloration of a distal extremity with associated swelling. These lesions become atrophic and sclerotic with time and eventually resemble localized scleroderma. At least two cases of diffuse fasciitis with eosinophilia, a rare entity that resembles scleroderma, have been associated with infection with *B burgdorferi.*

B. LABORATORY FINDINGS

The diagnosis of Lyme disease is based on both clinical manifestations and laboratory findings. The National Surveillance Case Definition specifies a person with exposure to a potential tick habitat (within the 30 days just prior to developing erythema migrans) with (1) erythema migrans diagnosed by a physician or (2) at least one late manifestation of the disease and (3) laboratory confirmation as fulfilling the criteria for Lyme disease.

Laboratory confirmation requires detection of specific antibodies to *B burgdorferi* in serum, either by indirect immunofluorescence assay (IFA) or enzyme-linked immunosorbent assay (ELISA); the latter is now preferred, because it is more sensitive and specific. A Western blot assay that can detect both IgM and IgG antibodies is used as a confirmatory test. IgM antibody appears first 2–4 weeks after onset of erythema migrans, peaks at 6–8 weeks, and then declines to low levels after 4–6 months of illness. The presence of IgM antibody in patients with prolonged symptoms persisting for several months is likely to be a false-positive result. IgG occurs later (6–8 weeks after onset of disease), peaks at 4–6 months, and may remain elevated at low levels indefinitely despite appropriate therapy and resolution of symptoms. A two-test approach is now recommended for the diagnosis of active Lyme disease. All specimens positive or equivocal by ELISA or IFA should be tested by Western immunoblot. When Western immunoblot is done during the first 4 weeks of illness, both IgM and IgG should be tested. If a patient with suspected early Lyme disease has negative serologic studies, acute and convalescent titers should be obtained since up to 50% of patients with early disease can be antibody-negative in the first several weeks of illness. A fourfold rise in antibody titer would be diagnostic of recent infection. In patients with later stages of disease, almost all are antibody-positive. False-positive reactions in the ELISA and IFA have been reported in juvenile rheumatoid arthritis, rheumatoid arthritis, systemic lupus erythematosus, infectious mononucleosis, subacute infective endocarditis, syphilis, relapsing fever, leptospirosis, enteroviral and other viral illnesses, and patients with gingival disease (presumably because of cross-reactivity with oral treponemes). False-negative serologic reactions occur early in illness, and antibiotic therapy early in disease can abort subsequent seroconversion. Other investigational tests include an antibody-capture ELISA, which appears to be more specific and sensitive than the routine ELISA or IFA, especially in early disease. It is positive in up to 90% of patients with stage 1 disease. It is difficult to perform and is presently available only in reference and research laboratories. Use of flagellar antigen, which produces an early immune response, to detect antibodies by both ELISA and immunoblotting may improve the ability to detect early disease and is under investigation. Detection of immune complexes (specific antibody directed against *B burgdorferi* anti-gens) may be useful in diagnosing early disease and determining whether positive IgG serology is due to previous infection or active disease.

Caution should be exercised in interpreting serologic tests. Serologic tests are not subject to national standards, and interlaboratory variation of results is a major problem. In addition, some laboratories perform tests that are entirely unreliable and should never be used to support the diagnosis of Lyme disease (eg, the Lyme urinary antigen test). In addition, testing is often done in patients with nonspecific symptoms such as headache, arthralgia, myalgia, fatigue, and palpitations. Even in endemic areas, the pretest probability of having Lyme disease is low in these patients, and the probability of a false-positive test result is greater than that of a true-positive. For these reasons, the American College of Physicians has established guidelines for laboratory evaluation of patients with suspected Lyme disease:

(1) The diagnosis of early Lyme disease is clinical (ie, exposure in an endemic area, with physician-documented erythema migrans), and does *not* require laboratory confirmation. (Tests are often negative at this stage.)

(2) Late disease requires objective evidence of clinical manifestations (recurrent brief attacks of mono- or oligoarticular arthritis of large joints; lymphocytic meningitis, cranial neuritis [Bell's palsy], peripheral neuropathy, or, rarely, encephalomyelitis—but *not* headache, fatigue, paresthesias, or stiff neck alone; atrioventricular conduction defects with or without myocarditis; and laboratory evidence of disease (two-stage testing with ELISA and Western blot, as described above).

(3) Patients with nonspecific symptoms without objective signs of Lyme disease should *not* have serologic testing done. It is in this setting that false-positive tests occur more commonly than true-positives.

(4) The role of serologic testing in neuroborreliosis is unclear, as sensitivity and specificity of cerebrospinal fluid serologic tests have not been determined. However, it is rare for a patient with neuroborreliosis to have positive serologic tests on cerebrospinal fluid without positive tests on serum (see below).

(5) Other tests such as the T cell proliferative assay, PCR testing, and urinary antigen detection have not yet been studied well enough to be routinely used (see discussion below).

Positive cultures for *B burgdorferi* can be obtained early in the course of disease. Aspiration of erythema migrans lesions has yielded positive cultures in up to 30% of cases, whereas culture of a 2-mm punch biopsy is positive in 50–70%. PCR of a skin biopsy is even more sensitive, with positivity rates of 80%. In early disease, blood cultures are positive in up to 50% if large volumes (9 mL) are used, but cerebrospinal fluid is rarely culture-positive. The ability to culture organisms from skin lesions is greatly influenced by antibiotic therapy. Even a brief course of several days will result in negative cultures. Special silver staining of chronically inflamed synovial tissue demonstrates spirochetes in one-third of patients.

PCR is very specific for detecting the presence of borrelia DNA, but sensitivity is variable and depends on which body fluid is tested and the stage of the disease. In general, PCR is more sensitive than culture, especially in chronic disease. Up to 85% of synovial fluid samples are positive in active arthritis. In contrast, 38% of cerebrospinal fluid samples in acute neuroborreliosis are PCR positive, and only 25% are positive in chronic neuroborreliosis. The significance of a positive reaction is unclear. Whether a positive PCR indicates persistence of viable organisms that will respond to further treatment or is a marker for residual DNA (not active infection) has not been clarified. In chronic Lyme arthritis, some have suggested that a positive PCR indicates active infection that requires further therapy, while others have found a positive reaction despite months of therapy, suggesting that the presence of DNA is indicative of an autoimmune arthritis.

The diagnosis of neuroborreliosis is often difficult since clinical manifestations, such as subtle memory impairment, may be difficult to document. Most patients with neuroborreliosis have a history of previous erythema migrans or mono- or polyarticular arthritis, and the vast majority have antibody present in serum. When cerebrospinal fluid is sampled, there may not be evidence of an inflammation (pleocytosis, elevated protein), but localized antibody production, ie, a ratio of cerebrospinal fluid to serum antibody of > 1.0, can often be demonstrated. The role of other tests such as PCR in detection of DNA or ELISA in detecting the presence of OspA antigen is unclear, but in difficult cases these tests can be performed and, if positive, help establish the diagnosis. In addition, many patients with neuroborreliosis will have a peripheral neuropathy that may be detected by electromyography. In the absence of any of the above findings, it is difficult to make the diagnosis of central nervous system borrelia infection.

Nonspecific laboratory abnormalities can be seen, particularly in early disease. The most common are an elevated sedimentation rate of > 20 mm/h seen in 50% of cases and mildly abnormal liver function tests present in 30%. The abnormal liver function tests are transient and return to normal within a few weeks of treatment. A mild anemia, leukocytosis (11,000–18,000/μL), and microscopic hematuria have been reported in 10% or less of patients.

Prevention

Simple preventive measures such as avoiding tick-infested areas, covering exposed skin with long-sleeved shirts and wearing long trousers tucked into socks, wearing light-colored clothing, using repellents, and inspecting for ticks after exposure will greatly reduce the number of tick bites. Environmental controls directed at limiting ticks on residential property would be helpful, but trying to limit the deer, tick, or white-footed mouse populations over large areas is not feasible.

Routine use of prophylactic antibiotics following tick bites is not recommended. Analysis of the cost-effectiveness of prophylactic therapy suggests that antibiotics administered for 2 weeks would be beneficial in preventing illness in endemic areas, where the risk of acquiring disease following a tick bite is 3.6% or greater. However, studies designed to examine the effect of prophylaxis have shown conflicting results. Two studies have shown no benefit of prophylaxis, but one study resulted in a decrease in erythema migrans from 3.2% in patients given placebo to 0.4% in those given a single 200 mg dose of doxycycline following a documented tick bite from *I scapularis*. Since most patients who develop Lyme disease are symptomatic and since treatment of early disease prevents late sequelae, it is reasonable to reserve treatment for patients who develop symptoms rather than to routinely administer prophylactic antibiotics unless the risk is extremely high (endemic area, documented ixodes tick bite, feeding at least 40 hours). Exceptions might include situations where the follow-up is uncertain, the patient is extremely anxious, the patient is a pregnant woman, or the tick was engorged when removed.

A recombinant vaccine using a highly conserved region of *Borrelia burgdorferi* known as outer surface protein A (OspA) has been licensed by the FDA (LYMErix, SmithKline Beecham). In a field study that excluded pregnant women, immunocompromised people, and those with chronic arthritis, almost 11,000 individuals between the ages of 15 and 70 years were immunized with three intramuscular injections at 0, 1, and 12 months. Efficacy in preventing disease was approximately 50% in those receiving two doses and 75% in those receiving all three. (Immunization at 0, 1, and 2 months produces high antibody titers and is likely to afford protection in a shorter time, but it is not currently officially recommended.) Adverse events were minor and included soreness at the site of injection (about 25%) and a flu-like illness with fevers and chills (about 4%). Reactions usually occurred within 48 hours after immunization and only lasted 3–4 days.

Several aspects of the vaccine and its use deserve emphasis. Antibodies decrease rapidly following immunization, and it is likely that boosters will be needed on a regular basis—but the exact frequency has not been determined. The original vaccine study did not include children, but subsequent studies have shown safety and immunogenicity in children between ages 4 and 18. Safety in children younger than 4 or persons older than 70 and in pregnancy is unknown, and the vaccine should not be administered to these individuals. Few or no data are available for vaccine use in immunocompromised individuals, in those with chronic musculoskeletal disease, and in individuals with chronic joint, neurologic, or cardiac disease related to previous Lyme disease. As with any new product, long-term adverse effects are unknown. With this particular product, there are some concerns about causing exacerbations of chronic Lyme arthritis since patients with natural infection who have chronic arthritis have high antibody titers to OspA. Finally, immunization will cause a false-positive ELISA but should not affect the Western blot.

Recommendations for use of the Lyme disease vaccine depend upon two epidemiologic factors—the entomologic risk (the density of ticks in a given area that are infected with *B burgdorferi*) and the human exposure risk (how likely an individual is to come into contact with infected ticks). The Centers for Disease Control and Prevention has stratified the United States into areas of high, moderate, low, and minimal or no risk of infection based on the density of infected ticks in the area. High and moderate risk areas include the northeastern, mid-Atlantic and North Central United States as well as one area on the Western slopes of the Sierra Nevada mountains in Northern California. All other areas are deemed to have low or minimal to no risk. Current recommendations, although somewhat vague and open to interpretation, state that vaccination should be considered for persons who live, work, or spend recreational time in areas of high or moderate risk and whose exposure to tick-infested areas is frequent or prolonged. Vaccination is not recommended for individuals who live or work in high or moderate risk areas if they have minimal or no tick exposure, and it is not recommended for individuals who live in low or minimal risk areas. Immunization should be considered in two additional groups: those who plan to travel to areas of high or moderate risk and who will have frequent or prolonged exposure to tick-infested areas, and individuals with previous uncomplicated Lyme disease who continue to be at risk.

Treatment

Antibiotic sensitivity of *B burgdorferi* has been established in vitro. Tetracycline is effective against the spirochete, but penicillin is only moderately so. Erythromycin is effective in vitro but has been disappointing in clinical trials. Ampicillin, ceftriaxone, azithromycin, cefuroxime, and imipenem are also effective in vitro, but aminoglycosides, ciprofloxacin, and rifampin are not.

Present recommendations for therapy are outlined in Table 34–4. In general, infection confined to skin is treated for 2–3 weeks. For central nervous system disease (with the exception of Bell's palsy), systemic therapy is used. Other organ system involvement usually responds to oral medication. For erythema migrans, oral antibiotic therapy shortens the duration of rash and prevents late sequelae. Doxycycline, 100 mg twice daily, is most commonly used and has the advantage of being active against ehrlichia. Amoxicillin is also effective and is recommended for pregnant or lactating women and for those who cannot tolerate doxycycline. Cefuroxime axetil, 500 mg twice daily, is as effective as doxycycline, 100 mg twice daily, but because

Table 34–4. Treatment of Lyme disease.

Manifestation	Drug and Dosage
Tick bite	No treatment in most circumstances (see text); observe
Erythema migrans	Doxycycline, 100 mg twice daily, or amoxicillin, 500 mg three times daily, or cefuroxime axetil, 500 mg twice daily—all for 3–4 weeks
Neurologic disease Bell's palsy	Doxycycline, or amoxicillin as above for 2–3 weeks
Other central nervous system disease	Ceftriaxone, 2 g IV once daily, or penicillin G, 18–24 million units daily IV in 6 divided doses; or cefotaxime, 2 g IV every 8 hours—all for 2–4 weeks
Cardiac disease First-degree block (PR < 0.3 s)	Doxycycline or amoxicillin as above for 2–3 weeks
High-degree atrioventricular block	Ceftriaxone or penicillin G as above for 2–3 weeks
Arthritis Oral dosage	Doxycycline, or amoxicillin as above for 4 weeks
Parenteral dosage	Ceftriaxone or penicillin G as above for 2–4 weeks
Acrodermatitis chronicum atrophicans	Doxycycline or amoxicillin as above for 4 weeks
"Chronic Lyme disease" or "post-Lyme disease syndrome"	Symptomatic therapy

of its cost it should be considered an alternative choice for those who cannot tolerate doxycycline or amoxicillin or for those in whom the drugs are contraindicated. Erythromycin and azithromycin are less effective, associated with higher rates of relapse, and are not recommended as first-line therapy. Isolated Bell's palsy (without meningitis or peripheral neuropathy) can be treated with doxycycline or amoxicillin for 2–3 weeks. Although therapy does not affect the rate of resolution of the cranial neuropathy, it does prevent development of late manifestations of disease.

The need for a lumbar puncture in patients with seventh nerve palsy is controversial. Some perform lumbar puncture on all patients with Bell's palsy and others only if there are signs or symptoms of meningitis. If meningitis is present, therapy with a parenteral antibiotic is indicated. Ceftriaxone, 2 g intravenously once daily for 14–28 days, is most commonly used, but penicillin, 18–24 million units daily in six divided doses, is equally efficacious. First- and second-degree heart block can be treated with oral agents, but third-degree block should be treated with ceftriaxone or penicillin and the patient should be admitted to the hospital for monitoring.

Therapy of arthritis is difficult because some patients fail to respond to any therapy, and those who do respond may do so slowly. Oral agents (doxycycline or amoxicillin) are as effective as intravenous regimens (ceftriaxone or penicillin). A reasonable approach to the patient with Lyme arthritis is to start with oral therapy and if this fails (persistent or recurrent joint swelling) to re-treat with an oral regimen for an additional 4 weeks or to switch to an intravenous regimen for 2–4 weeks. Re-treatment should be delayed for several months because of the slow resolution of joint symptoms. If arthritis persists after re-treatment, symptomatic therapy with nonsteroidal anti-inflammatory agents is recommended. For severe refractory pain, synovectomy may be required.

Based on the limited published data, therapy of Lyme disease in pregnancy should be the same as therapy in other patients with the exception that doxycycline should not be used.

Clinicians are often confronted with patients with nonspecific symptoms (such as fatigue and myalgias) and positive serologic tests for Lyme disease who request (or demand) therapy for their illness. It is important in managing these patients to remember (1) that the diagnosis of Lyme disease is primarily a clinical one, and nonspecific symptoms alone are not diagnostic; (2) that serologic tests are fraught with difficulty (as noted above), and in areas where disease prevalence is low, false-positive serologic tests are much more common than true-positive tests; and (3) that parenteral therapy with ceftriaxone for 2–4 weeks is costly (approximately $5000) and has been associated with significant adverse effects (cholelithiasis). Parenteral therapy should be reserved for those most likely to benefit, ie, those with cutaneous, neurologic, cardiac, or rheumatic manifestations that are characteristic of Lyme disease. In addition, coinfection may present with an atypical clinical picture, eg, a patient with Lyme disease and ehrlichiosis may present with fever and rash but without the hematologic abnormalities characteristic of ehrlichiosis.

Prognosis

Most patients respond to appropriate therapy with prompt resolution of symptoms within 4 weeks. With adequate therapy, only a small percentage of patients will fail to respond or will develop a late relapse. True treatment failures are thus uncommon, and in most cases re-treatment or prolonged treatment of Lyme disease is instituted because of misdiagnosis or misinterpretation of serologic results rather than inadequate therapy. The terms "chronic Lyme disease" or "post-Lyme disease syndrome" have been used to describe patients with documented Lyme disease who have

been adequately treated but have persistent nonspecific symptoms such as fatigue, arthralgias, and myalgias. These entities are poorly defined, and the patients comprise a heterogeneous group. Although there is a tendency to treat these patients with multiple or prolonged courses of oral or intravenous antibiotics, there are no data suggesting that this is efficacious, and the prolonged use of antibiotics in this setting is emphatically discouraged. It is important to remember also that most areas endemic for Lyme disease are also endemic for babesiosis and ehrlichiosis. Coinfection with the etiologic agents of these diseases may be associated with more severe symptoms than infection with either agent alone and is another possible explanation for failure to respond to therapy directed at Lyme disease.

The long-term outcome of adult patients with Lyme disease is not clear. Joint pain, memory impairment, and poor functional status secondary to pain are common subjective complaints in patients with Lyme disease, but physical examination and neurocognitive testing fail to document the presence of these symptoms as objective sequelae. Similarly, in highly endemic areas, patients with a diagnosis of Lyme disease commonly complain of pain, fatigue, and inability to perform certain physical activities when followed for several years. However, these complaints occur just as commonly in age-matched controls without a history of Lyme disease. Attempts to document chronic cardiac disease in patients treated for Lyme disease also have been unsuccessful. It appears that long-term sequelae of adequately treated disease are uncommon.

Brown SL et al: Role of serology in the diagnosis of Lyme disease. JAMA 1999;282:62. [PMID: 10404913] (Difficulties of making a serologic diagnosis.)

Klempner MS et al: Two controlled trials of antibiotic treatment in patients with persistent symptoms and a history of Lyme disease. N Engl J Med 2001;345:85. [PMID: 11450676]

Nadelman RB et al: Prophylaxis with single-dose doxycycline for the prevention of Lyme disease after an *Ixodes scapularis* tick bite. N Engl J Med 2001;345:79. [PMID: 11450675]

Nichol G et al: Test-treatment strategies for patients suspected of having Lyme disease: A cost-effectiveness analysis. Ann Intern Med 1998;128:37. [PMID: 9424980] (Analyses of common clinical presentations and need to test or treat empirically.)

Poland GA: Prevention of Lyme disease: a review of the evidence. Mayo Clin Proc 2001;76:713. [PMID: 11444404] (Review of environmental, behavioral, antibiotic, and vaccine strategies.)

Rahn DW: Lyme vaccine: issues and controversies. Infect Dis Clin North Am 2001;15:171. [PMID: 11301814] (Review with discussion of unanswered questions.)

Recommendations for the use of Lyme disease vaccine. MMWR Recomm Rep 1999;48(RR-7):1, 21. [PMID: 10371254] (Official recommendations of an Advisory Committee on Immunization Procedures.)

Seltzer EG et al: Long-term outcomes of persons with Lyme disease. JAMA 2000;283:609. [PMID: 10665700] (Cohort study comparing long-term sequelae in patients with and without a diagnosis of Lyme disease.)

Sigal LH et al: A vaccine consisting of recombinant *Borrelia burgdorferi* outer-surface protein A to prevent Lyme disease. N Engl J Med 1998;339:216. [PMID: 9673299] (Safety, efficacy, and adverse events of the Connaught product.)

Steere AC et al: Vaccination against Lyme disease with recombinant *Borrelia burgdorferi* outer-surface lipoprotein A with adjuvant. N Engl J Med 1998;339:209. [PMID: 9673298]

(Full trial describing safety, efficacy, and adverse effects of LYMErix vaccine.)

Steere AC: Lyme disease. N Engl J Med 2001;345:115. [PMID: 11450660] (A review.)

Wormser GP et al: Practice guidelines for the treatment of Lyme disease. Clin Infect Dis 2000;31(Suppl 1):1. [PMID: 10982743]

35

Infectious Diseases: Protozoal & Helminthic

Robert S. Goldsmith, MD, MPH, DTM&H

See www.current-med.com/ch35.html

■ I. PROTOZOAL INFECTIONS

AFRICAN TRYPANOSOMIASIS (Sleeping Sickness)

 ESSENTIALS OF DIAGNOSIS

- History of exposure to tsetse flies, with bite lesion.*

Hemolymphatic stage:*

- Irregular fevers, headaches, joint pains, malaise, pruritus, papular skin rash, edemas.
- Posterior cervical or generalized lymphadenopathy; hepatosplenomegaly.
- Anemia, weight loss.
- Trypanosomes in blood or lymph node aspirates; positive serology.

Meningoencephalitic stage:

- Insomnia, motor and sensory disorders, abnormal reflexes, somnolence to coma.
- Trypanosomes and increased white cells and protein in cerebrospinal fluid.

General Considerations

African trypanosomiasis is caused by *Trypanosoma brucei rhodesiense* and *Trypanosoma brucei gambiense*, both hemoflagellates. The organisms are transmitted by bites of tsetse flies (glossina species), which inhabit shaded areas along streams and rivers. Trypanosomes ingested in a blood meal undergo a developmental period of 18–35 days in the fly; when the fly feeds again on a new mammalian host, the infective stage is injected. Human disease occurs locally throughout trop-

ical Africa from south of the Sahara to about 20° south latitude. *T b gambiense* infections are in the moist sub-Saharan savanna and riverine forests of west and central Africa up to the eastern Rift Valley. *T b rhodesiense* occurs to the east of the Rift Valley in the savannah of east and southeast Africa and along the shores of Lake Victoria.

T b rhodesiense infection is primarily a zoonosis of game animals; humans are infected sporadically. Humans are the principal mammalian host for *T b gambiense;* it is uncertain whether there is an animal reservoir, but domestic animals can be infected. A third trypanosome, *T brucei brucei*, infects only wild and domestic animals.

An estimated 50,000 deaths occur yearly. Of new infections yearly, approximately 100,000 are Gambian but only several hundred Rhodesian. Among visitors to the East African game parks, infections are rare, with about one case a year appearing in the USA.

Clinical Findings

A. SYMPTOMS AND SIGNS

T b rhodesiense infections go through the following three stages, are much more virulent, and untreated patients die within weeks to a year. In *T b rhodesiense* infection, the hemolymphatic stage usually begins within 3–10 days after appearance of the chancre. However, in *T b gambiense* infections, there is generally a long asymptomatic period in which chancres are rare and the hemolymphatic stage may be absent or may go unnoticed; when symptoms do manifest after weeks to years, they are often initially mild and ignored by the patient.

1. The trypanosomal chancre—In *T b rhodesiense* infections, this is a local pruritic, painful inflammatory reaction (3–10 cm) with regional lymphadenopathy that appears about 48 hours after the tsetse fly bite and lasts 2–4 weeks.

2. The hemolymphatic (early) stage—High fever, severe headache, joint pains, and malaise recur at irregular intervals corresponding to waves of parasitemia. Between febrile episodes there are symptom-free periods that last up to 2 weeks. Transient rashes may ap-

---

*Usually absent or unnoticed in *T b gambiense* infections.

pear, often pruritic and papular or circinate. Examination reveals mild enlargement of the liver and spleen, and edema (peripheral, pleural, ascites, etc). Enlarged, rubbery, and painless lymph nodes occur in 75% of patients. In *T b gambiense,* only the posterior cervical group (Winterbottom's sign) may be enlarged. With progression of the disease, there is weight loss and debilitation. Myocardial involvement may appear early in Rhodesian infection, and the patient may succumb to myocarditis before meningoencephalitic signs appear.

3. The meningoencephalitic (late) stage—This stage appears within a few weeks or months of onset of Rhodesian infection but in Gambian sleeping sickness develops more insidiously, starting 6 months to several years after onset. Insomnia, anorexia, personality changes, apathy, and headaches are the early findings. A variety of motor or tonus disorders may develop, including tremors and disturbances of speech, gait, and reflexes; somnolence appears late. The patient becomes severely emaciated and, finally, comatose. Death often results from secondary infection.

B. LABORATORY FINDINGS

Anemia, increased sedimentation rate, thrombocytopenia, and increased serum globulin are common. Eosinophilia is not seen. Definitive diagnosis requires identifying motile organisms in wet films and after Giemsa staining in specimens from blood, the bite lesion aspirates, lymph node aspirates, bone marrow aspirates, or cerebrospinal fluid. Because the number of trypanosomes in blood fluctuates and because they are often are undetectable 3 out of 5 days, specimens should be examined daily for about 15 days, including after concentration by centrifugation of 10–15 mL of heparinized blood, since trypanosomes are concentrated in the buffy coat. Other diagnostic tests with blood are the quantitative buffy coat technique, intraperitoneal inoculation of rodents (sensitive but only effective for *T b rhodesiense*), culture, Millipore filtration, and DEAE-cellulose anion exchange centrifugation. Only soft lymph nodes should be selected for aspiration (25-gauge needle); after the node is gently kneaded, the aspirate is examined immediately for motile organisms. Cerebrospinal fluid shows an increase in lymphocytes and protein; centrifugation to detect the parasite should be done both rapidly and twice, which doubles sensitivity. The fluid should also be inoculated into an experimental animal and cultured. With progression of the disease, organisms are more likely to be found in cerebrospinal fluid than in blood or lymph nodes.

Circulating IgM levels become positive about 12 days after onset of infection and may reach 10–20 times normal, though normal or low levels do not rule out the infection. Titers may fluctuate when brief periods of excess antigens may depress them, often to below detectable levels. In late central nervous system disease, though both circulating antibody and parasitemia may fall below detectable levels, serologic tests of the cerebrospinal fluid may yet prove useful. At any stage, an elevated IgM in the cerebrospinal fluid is pathognomonic for central nervous system infection, though false-negative results occur. Additional immunologic tests include ELISA, immunofluorescent assays, and a field-adapted card agglutination test.

Differential Diagnosis

Trypanosomiasis may be mistaken for a variety of other diseases, including malaria, influenza, pneumonia, infectious mononucleosis, leukemia, lymphoma, the arbovirus encephalitides, and psychosis. Serologic tests for syphilis may be falsely positive in trypanosomiasis.

Treatment

Because all of the drugs used (except eflornithine) are highly toxic (mortality during drug treatment can reach 5–10%), specific detection of the organism is a prerequisite for treatment; immunoassays are insufficient to make the diagnosis.

Suramin and pentamidine do not adequately cross the blood-brain barrier and cannot be used when the central nervous system is involved; melarsoprol and eflornithine, however, do pass the barrier. Melarsoprol causes a reactive encephalopathy in up to 20% of patients; corticosteroids may prevent this. Systemic eflornithine is highly effective and associated with only mild toxicity in early and late *T b gambiense* infections, but it should not be used for *T b rhodesiense* infection, as its efficacy for this parasite is inconsistent. Eflornithine is expensive, and its continued availability (from WHO) is uncertain. In the USA, eflornithine has been approved for topical use to remove facial hair; suramin and melarsoprol are available only from the CDC Drug Service, Centers for Disease Control and Prevention, Atlanta, GA 30333. Telephone: 404-639-3670; 404-639-2888 evenings, weekends, and holidays.

A. EARLY DISEASE, THE HEMOLYMPHATIC STAGE

A drug of choice for both parasites is intravenous suramin (100–200 mg [test dose], then 1 g on days 1, 3, 7, 14, and 21). Alternative drugs of choice only for *T b gambiense* are intravenous eflornithine (see above; 400 mg/kg/d in four divided doses for 14 days, followed by 300 mg/kg/d orally for 3–4 weeks; cure rate 97%) or pentamidine (4 mg/kg/d intramuscularly for 7–10 days; cure rate 93%).

B. LATE DISEASE WITH CENTRAL NERVOUS SYSTEM INVOLVEMENT

Drugs of choice for both parasites are intravenous melarsoprol, 2–3.6 mg/kg/d for 3 days; after 1 week, 3.6 mg/kg for 3 days; repeat after 10–21 days. Relapse rates for Gambian infections, formerly low (5–8%), have markedly increased. Alternative treatments only against *T b gambiense* are eflornithine (as above) or intravenous tryparsamide, 30 mg/kg (maximum: 2 g) every 5 days for 12 injections, plus intravenous suramin, 100–200 mg (test dose), followed by 10 mg/kg every 5 days for 12 injections; the treatment may be repeated in 1 month.

Proper follow-up to ensure detection of the encephalitic stage requires initial cerebrospinal fluid examination, repeat studies at intervals during treatment, 3 months after treatment, and then at 6-month intervals for 2 years.

Prevention

Individual prevention in endemic areas should include wearing long sleeves and trousers, avoiding dark-colored clothing, and using mosquito nets while sleeping. Repellents have no effect. Pentamidine is used in chemoprophylaxis (controversial) only against the Gambian type. In *T b rhodesiense* infection, pentamidine may suppress early symptoms, resulting in late recognition of the disease. Excretion of pentamidine is slow; therefore, one intramuscular injection (4 mg/kg, maximum 300 mg) protects for 3–6 months. The drug is toxic and should only be used for persons at high risk (ie, those with constant, heavy exposure to tsetse flies in areas with known transmission of Gambian disease). Performing serologic tests every 6 months during exposure and for 3 years afterward is the safest method for detecting the disease at an early stage. Gambian control depends on detecting and treating the largely asymptomatic human reservoir.

Prognosis

Most patients—even those with advanced disease—recover following treatment. Relapses are uncommon (about 2%). When therapy is started late, irreversible brain damage or death is common. Most persons with African trypanosomiasis will die if untreated.

Brun R et al: The phenomenon of treatment failures in Human African Trypanosomiasis. Trop Med Int Health 2001 6:906. [PMID: 11703845]

Burri C et al: Efficacy of new, concise schedule for melarsoprol in treatment of sleeping sickness caused by *Trypanosoma brucei gambiense*: a randomized trial. Lancet 2000;355:1419. [PMID: 10791526]

Drugs for parasitic infections: Med Lett Drugs Ther 1998;40:1. [PMID: 9442765] (Important resource for dosages.)

Lejon V et al: Stage determination and follow-up in sleeping sickness. Med Trop (Mars) 2001;61:355. [PMID: 11803826]

AMERICAN TRYPANOSOMIASIS (Chagas' Disease)

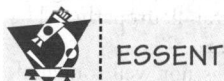

ESSENTIALS OF DIAGNOSIS

Acute stage:

- Inflammatory lesion at site of inoculation; prolonged fever, tachycardia, hepatosplenomegaly, lymphadenopathy, signs of myocarditis.
- Parasites in peripheral blood, positive serologic tests.

Chronic stage:

- Heart failure with cardiac arrhythmias; decreased intensity of heart sounds; episodes of thromboembolism.
- In some regions, dysphagia, severe constipation, and radiologic evidence of megaesophagus or megacolon.
- Positive xenodiagnosis or hemoculture, positive serologic tests, abnormal ECG.

General Considerations

Chagas' disease is caused by *Trypanosoma cruzi*, a protozoan parasite of humans and wild and domestic animals. *T cruzi* occurs only in the Americas; it is found in wild animals and to a lesser extent in humans from southern South America to southern USA. An estimated 16 million people are infected, mostly in rural areas, resulting in about 45,000 deaths yearly. The disease is often acquired in childhood; the proportion of infected persons increases with age. In many countries in South America, Chagas' disease is the most important cause of heart disease. In southern USA, although the organism has been found in triatomine bugs and wild and domestic animals, only five confirmed instances of local transmission have been reported. However, a large number of immigrants from endemic areas of Latin America (particularly Central America) are infected (estimated 50,000–100,000). A handful of infections following blood transfusion have been reported.

T cruzi is transmitted by reduviid (triatomine) bugs infected by ingesting blood from animals or humans who have circulating trypanosomes. Multiplication occurs in the digestive tract of the bug; infective forms are eliminated in feces. Infection in humans occurs through "contamination" with bug feces; the parasite penetrates the skin (generally through the bite wound), mucus membranes, or the conjunctiva. Transmission can also occur by blood transfusion or in utero.

The trypanosomes first multiply close to the point of entry. They then enter the bloodstream as trypanosomes and later invade cells and assume the leishmanial form. The organism has a predilection for myocardium, smooth muscle, and central nervous system glial cells. Multiplication causes cellular destruction, inflammation, and fibrosis.

In South America, a major eradication program based on improved housing, use of residual pyrethroid insecticides, and screening of blood donors has achieved striking reductions in infections in children.

Clinical Findings

A. SYMPTOMS AND SIGNS

Although infection continues for many years—probably for life—as many as 70% of persons remain asymptomatic. The **acute stage,** seen principally in children, lasts 2–4 months and leads to death in up to 10% of cases. The earliest findings are at the site of inoculation either in the eye—Romaña's sign (unilateral bipalpebral edema, conjunctivitis, local lymphadenopathy)—or in the skin—a chagoma (furuncle-like lesion with local lymphadenopathy). Subsequent findings include fever, malaise, headache, hepatomegaly, mild splenomegaly, and generalized lymphadenopathy. Acute myocarditis may lead to biventricular failure, but arrhythmias are rare. Meningoencephalitis is limited to young children and is often fatal.

A **latent period** (indeterminate phase) may last from 10 to 30 years in which the patient is asymptomatic but in which serologic tests and sometimes parasitologic examination confirm the presence of the infection.

The **chronic stage** is usually manifested by cardiac disease in the third and fourth decades of life, characterized by arrhythmias, congestive heart failure (often with prominent right-sided findings), ventricular aneurysms, and systemic or pulmonary embolization originating from mural thrombi. Valvular lesions are absent. Sudden cardiac arrest in young persons may occur and is attributed to ventricular fibrillation. Megacolon and megaesophagus, caused by damage to nerve plexuses in the bowel or esophageal wall, occur in some areas of Chile, Argentina, and Brazil; findings include dysphagia, regurgitation, constipation, sigmoid volvulus, and parotid gland hypertrophy. Megasyndromes can also affect the urinary tract.

In immunosuppressed persons—including infrequent AIDS patients and transplant recipients—latent Chagas' disease may reactivate. Common findings are cardiomyopathy and brain lesions indistinguishable from cerebral toxoplasmosis.

B. LABORATORY FINDINGS

Appropriate selection of tests allows a definitive parasitologic diagnosis in most acute and congenital cases and in up to 40% of chronic ones. In the acute stage, trypanosomes should be looked for (1) by examination of anticoagulated fresh blood or the buffy coat for motile organisms and (2) by examination of the following Giemsa-stained preparations: thick and thin blood films, buffy coat, and the sediment after centrifuging the supernatant of clotted blood. In the chronic stage, the parasite can only be detected by culture or xenodiagnosis. The latter consists of permitting uninfected laboratory-reared bugs of the local major vector to feed on the patients and then examining their intestinal contents for trypanosomes. In both acute and chronic infection, blood should also be cultured using appropriate media and inoculated into laboratory mice or rats 3–10 days old. *Trypanosoma rangeli,* a nonpathogenic blood trypanosome also found in humans in Central America and northern South America, must not be mistaken for *T cruzi.*

Several highly sensitive IgG serologic tests (hemagglutination inhibition, complement fixation, ELISA, immunofluorescence, others) are routinely used and are of presumptive value when positive. However, two or three of these tests should be done because false-positive tests are common, particularly with other infections—including leishmaniasis, malaria, syphilis, and *T rangeli* infection—and with autoimmune diseases. Antibodies of the IgM class are elevated early in the acute stage but are replaced by IgG antibodies as the disease progresses. Maximum titers are reached in 3–4 months; thereafter, titers can remain positive at a low level for life. In chronic infections, when circulating organisms are difficult to find, the polymerase chain reaction and recombinant DNA methods often assess effectiveness of chemotherapy (clearance of parasites), whereas the serologic tests do not. The most important electrocardiographic abnormalities are right bundle branch block and arrhythmias. In certain regions of South America, radiologic examination may show megaesophagus, megacolon, or cardiac enlargement with characteristic apical aneurysms.

Treatment

Treatment, though not ideal, is indicated in acute but not latent infection and is controversial in the chronic stage. Two drugs are used: nifurtimox and benznidazole—both must be used for long periods and are potentially toxic. In acute disease and congenital infections, the drugs are effective in reducing the duration and severity of infection, but cure is achieved in only about 70% of patients. In the chronic phase, although parasitemia may disappear in up to 70% of patients, treatment does not alter the serologic reaction, cardiac function, or progression of the disease. All *T cruzi-*infected persons should be treated with either nifurtimox or benznidazole regardless of clinical status or time since infection. Allopurinol and itraconazole continue under evaluation.

Nifurtimox is given orally in daily doses of 8–10 mg/kg in four divided doses after meals for 90–120 days. It generally produces gastrointestinal complaints, weight loss, tremors, and peripheral neuropathy. Hallucinations, pulmonary infiltrates, and convulsions are rare. In the USA, nifurtimox is available only from the Parasitic Disease Drug Service, Centers for Disease Control, Atlanta 30333 (404-639-3670). Benznidazole—not available in the USA—is given at a dosage of 5 mg/kg/d for 60 days. Its side effects include granulocytopenia, rash, and peripheral neuropathy. The drug is better tolerated by children.

In the chronic stage, digoxin is not well tolerated. The most effective antiarrhythmic drug is amiodarone. Cardiac pacemakers are used for atrioventricular block. Amiodarone and angiotensin-converting enzyme inhibitors may result in better survival in selected patients. In endemic areas, blood should not be used for transfusion unless at least two serologic tests are negative; otherwise, blood can be treated with gentian violet to kill the parasites.

Prognosis

Acute infections in infants and young children are often fatal, particularly when the central nervous system is involved. Adults with chronic heart disease also may ultimately succumb to the disease.

Ben BC: Chagas disease or American trypanosomiasis. Bull WHO 1998;76 Suppl 2:144. [PMID: 10063697]

Leon JS et al: Autoimmunity in Chagas heart disease. Int J Parasitol 2001;31:555. [PMID: 11334942]

Marin Neto JA et al: Chagas' heart disease. Arq Bras Cardiol 1999;72:247. [PMID: 10513039]

Warrell DA: Chagas' disease. Lancet 2001 358:424.[PMID: 11511074]

AMEBIASIS

ESSENTIALS OF DIAGNOSIS

- *Mild to moderate colitis: recurrent diarrhea and abdominal cramps, sometimes alternating with constipation; mucus may be present; blood is usually absent.*
- *Severe colitis: semiformed to liquid stools streaked with blood and mucus, fever, colic, prostration; ileus, perforation with peritonitis, and hemorrhage occur.*
- *Hepatic amebiasis: fever, hepatomegaly, pain, localized tenderness.*
- *Laboratory findings: amebas in stools or in abscess aspirate; serologic tests positive with severe colitis or hepatic abscess, which is readily imaged by ultrasonography or CT scan.*

General Considerations

Though the causative protozoan parasite *Entamoeba histolytica* was once considered a single species with varying virulence, it is now recognized that the entamoeba complex contains two morphologically identical species: (1) *E dispar* (about 90% of the complex), which remains in the colon as a stable commensal that is avirulent and produces an asymptomatic carrier state; and (2) *E histolytica*, which shows varying degrees of virulence ranging from a commensal state in the colon—in which it does not cause disease, yet is potentially invasive—to being invasive of the intestinal wall, resulting in acute diarrhea or dysentery or chronic diarrhea. *E histolytica* may also be carried by the blood to the liver, where it may produce hepatic abscess. Rarely, the lungs, brain, other organs or perianal skin may be infected.

Both *E histolytica* and *E dispar* exist as two forms in the lumen and mucosal crypts of the large bowel: identical-appearing cysts (10–14 μm) and motile trophozoites (12–50 μm). In the absence of diarrhea, trophozoites encyst in the large bowel. Trophozoites passed into the environment die rapidly, but cysts remain viable in soil and water for several weeks to months at appropriate temperature and humidity.

The infections are present worldwide but are most prevalent and severe in subtropical and tropical areas under conditions of crowding, poor sanitation, and poor nutrition. Using the new taxonomy, prevalence estimates have changed. Of 500 million persons worldwide infected with entamoeba, most are infected with *E dispar* and an estimated 10% (50 million) with *E histolytica*. Invasive *E histolytica* may constitute 5 million cases, with mortality in the range of 100,000 per year.

Humans are the only established host and are universally susceptible. Only cysts are infectious, since after ingestion they survive gastric acidity which destroys trophozoites. Transmission occurs through ingestion of cysts from fecally contaminated food or water. Flies and other arthropods also serve as mechanical vectors; to an undetermined degree, transmission results from contamination of food by the hands of food handlers. Where human excrement is used as fertilizer, it is often a source of food and water contamination. Person-to-person contact is also important in transmission; therefore, all household members as well as an infected person's sexual partner should have their stools examined. In communal settings such as mental hospitals (but not child day care centers), prevalence rates as high as 50% have been reported. Amebiasis is rarely epidemic, but urban outbreaks have occurred because of common-source water contamination. Although entamoeba infections occur frequently among homosexuals, in the developed countries these infections are usually due to the *E dispar* and do not require treatment. In AIDS, *E histolytica* infection does not become an opportunistic infection.

Fulminant infections may occur in pregnancy and in young children. Corticosteroids and other immunosuppressive drugs given in error for inflammatory bowel disease may convert a commensal infection into an invasive one.

The characteristic intestinal lesion is the amebic ulcer, which can occur anywhere in the large bowel (including the appendix) and sometimes in the terminal ileum but predominates in the cecum, descending colon, and the rectosigmoid colon—areas of greatest fecal stasis. Trophozoites invade the colonic mucosa by means of their ameboid movement and proteolytic secretions and induce necrosis to form the characteristic flask-shaped ulcers. Ulcers are usually limited to the muscularis, but if penetration to the serous layer occurs, bowel perforation, local abscess, or generalized peritonitis may result. In fulminating cases, ulceration may be extensive, and the bowel becomes thin and friable. Hepatic abscesses range from a few millimeters to 15 cm or larger, usually are single, occur more often in the right lobe (particularly the upper portion), and are more common in men.

Clinical Findings

A. SYMPTOMS AND SIGNS

Amebiasis is classified into intestinal and extraintestinal disease and further subdivided into the clinical syndromes described below. Some patients have an acute onset of severe diarrhea as early as 8 days (commonly 2–4 weeks) after infection. Others may be asymptomatic or have mild intestinal infection for months to several years before either intestinal symptoms or liver abscess appears. Transition may occur from one type of intestinal infection to another, and each may give rise to hepatic abscess, or the intestinal infection may clear spontaneously.

1. Intestinal amebiasis—

a. Asymptomatic infection—In most infected persons, the organism lives as a commensal, and the carrier is without symptoms.

b. Mild to moderate colitis (nondysenteric colitis)—A few stools a day are passed that are semiformed and have no blood. There may be abdominal cramps, flatulence, fatigue, and weight loss; fever is uncommon. Periods of remission and recurrence may last days to weeks or longer; during remissions, the patient may have constipation. Abdominal examination may show distention, hyperperistalsis, and tenderness. In some patients with chronic infection, the colon is thick and palpable, particularly over the cecum and descending colon. Toxic products released as a result of the bowel infection may induce periportal inflammation, mild hepatomegaly, and low-grade liver enzyme abnormalities but without demonstrable trophozoites in the liver.

c. Severe colitis (dysenteric colitis)—As the severity of intestinal infection increases, the number of stools increases, and they change from semiformed to liquid with streaks of blood beginning to appear. With larger numbers of stools, 10–20 or more, little fecal material is present, but blood (fresh or dark) and bits of necrotic tissue become increasingly evident. With increasing severity, the patient may become prostrate and toxic, with fever up to 40.5 °C, and have colic, tenesmus, vomiting, generalized abdominal tenderness, and nonspecific hepatic enlargement and tenderness. Rare complications include appendicitis, bowel perforation, fulminating colitis, massive mucosal sloughing, and hemorrhage. Death may follow.

d. Localized ulcerative lesions of the colon—Bowel ulcerations limited to the rectal area may result in passage of formed stools with bloody exudate. Ulcerations limited to the cecum may induce mild diarrhea and simulate appendicitis. Amebic appendicitis, in which the appendix is extensively involved but not the remainder of the large bowel, is rare.

e. Localized granulomatous lesions of the colon (ameboma)—This occurs as a result of excessive production of granulation tissue in response to amebic infection, either in the course of dysentery or slowly in chronic intestinal infection. These masses may present as an irregular tumor (single or multiple) projecting into the bowel or as an annular constricting mass up to several centimeters in length. Clinical findings (pain, obstructive symptoms, and hemorrhage) and x-ray findings may simulate colonic carcinoma, tuberculosis, or lymphogranuloma venereum. At endoscopy, the mass is deep red and bleeds easily, and biopsy specimens show granulation tissue and *E histolytica;* the number of organisms may be relatively few. Antiamebic drugs are usually adequate treatment; surgical removal of the lesion without prior or immediate postoperative drug therapy is likely to result in death from disseminated disease.

2. Extraintestinal amebiasis—

a. Hepatic amebiasis—Amebic liver abscess, although a relatively infrequent (3–9%) consequence of intestinal amebiasis, is not uncommon given the large number of intestinal infections. A large proportion of patients with liver abscess do not have concurrent intestinal symptoms, nor can they recall having had chronic intestinal symptoms. The onset of symptoms can be sudden or gradual, ranging from a few days to many months. Cardinal manifestations are fever (often high), pain (continuous, stabbing, or pleuritic, and sometimes severe), and an enlarged and tender liver. Patients may also experience malaise or prostration, sweating, chills, anorexia, and weight loss. The liver enlargement may present subcostally, in the epigastrium, as a localized bulging of the rib cage, or, as a result of enlargement against the dome of the diaphragm, it may produce coughing and findings at the right lung base (dullness to percussion, rales, and diminished breath sounds). Intercostal tenderness is common. Localizing signs on the skin may be an area of edema or a point of maximum tenderness. Without prompt treatment, the abscess may rupture into the pleural, peritoneal, or pericardial space or other contiguous organs, and death may follow.

b. Other extraintestinal infections—Skin infections may develop in the perianal area. Metastatic infection may rarely occur throughout the body, particularly the lungs, brain, and genitalia.

B. LABORATORY FINDINGS

1. Intestinal amebiasis—Diagnosis of intestinal amebiasis is made by finding the antigen or the organism in stool. Serologic testing by the indirect hemagglutination test lacks sensitivity in early infections and does not distinguish recent from past infection.

Antigen detection in stools. Where possible, stools should be tested for amebic antigen (the Tech-Lab test is commercially available), which is more sensitive and specific than microscopy. Unlike morphology, which does not distinguish *E histolytica* cysts or trophozoites from nonpathogenic *E dispar,* antigen detection does differentiate the species from each other and from other intestinal protozoa.

Microscopic examination of stools. Standard microscopy of stool specimens is insensitive. Testing three specimens obtained under optimal conditions will generally detect only 80% of entamoeba complex infections; three additional tests will raise the diagnostic rate to 90%. Trophozoites predominate in liquid stools, cysts in formed stools. A standard procedure is to collect three specimens at 2-day intervals or longer, with one of the three obtained after a laxative such as (1) sodium sulfate or phosphate (Fleet's Phospho-Soda), 30–60 g in a glass of water; or (2) bisacodyl 5–15 mL. Oil laxatives should not be used. Because trophozoites rapidly autolyze, stools should be examined within 30 minutes or immediately mixed with a preservative. If the patient has received specific therapy, antibiotics, antimalarials, antidiarrheal preparations (containing bismuth, kaolin, or magnesium hydroxide), barium, or mineral oil, specimen collection should be delayed.

Bowel examination. Colonoscopy is preferred over sigmoidoscopy. The bowel should not be cleansed by laxative or enema as this washes exudate from the ulcers and destroys trophozoites. Typically, there are no findings in mild intestinal disease; in severe disease, ulcers may be found that are 1 mm to 2 cm across, with intact intervening mucosa. If present, exudate should be collected with a glass pipette (not with cotton, to which trophozoites may adhere) or by scraping with a metal curette and examined immediately for motile trophozoites and for *E histolytica* antigen. In some centers, rectal biopsy (from the edge of the ulcer) has enhanced diagnosis; the specimens are best examined by immunofluorescence methods.

Serology. The standard serologic test—the indirect hemagglutination test (a positive titer is 1:128 or a higher dilution)—detects *E histolytica* infections but remains negative in *E dispar* infections. However, because the test remains positive for as long as 10 years after successful treatment, a positive test does not distinguish between past and new infections. In longstanding commensal colon infections with *E histolytica,* the test may become positive. With invasive disease, the test can become positive within a week; with mild colitis, seropositivity may be less than 50%, whereas in dysentery it reaches 85% levels. The agar gel test, though less sensitive, is rapidly conducted and may detect current infection because it becomes negative 3–6 months after eradication of the organism. Other tests for serum antibody include the ELISA and immunofluorescent tests.

Other tests. Detection of trophozoites that contain ingested red blood cells is nearly diagnostic for invasive *E histolytica* but may be confused with the occasional *E dispar* or macrophage that also contains the red blood cells. Many patients with amebic colitis test positive for occult blood, whereas findings for fecal leukocytes are noncontributory. The white blood cell count can reach 20,000/μL or higher in amebic dysentery but is not elevated in mild colitis. A low-grade eosinophilia is occasionally present.

For research purposes, the diagnosis can also be made by isolating the two entamoeba species in culture (this requires specialized techniques) and then differentiating them by isoenzyme analysis, typing with monoclonal antibodies to surface antigens, polymerase chain reaction, or DNA probes.

2. Hepatic abscess—Elevation of the right dome of the diaphragm and the size and location of the abscess can be determined by ultrasonography (usually round or oval nonhomogeneous lesions, abrupt transition from normal liver to the lesion, hypoechoic center with diffuse echoes throughout the abscess), CT (well-defined, round, low-density lesions with an internal, nonhomogeneous structure), MRI, and radioisotope scanning. After intravenous injection of contrast material, CT may show a hyperdense halo around the periphery of the abscess. Gallium scans, only infrequently useful, show a cold spot (sometimes with a bright rim) as opposed to the increased gallium uptake in the center of pyogenic abscesses. Serologic tests are almost always positive (except early in the infection); however, a positive test does not distinguish recent from past infection. Examination of stools for antigen and the organism is frequently negative. The white count ranges from 15,000 to 25,000/μL. Eosinophilia is not present. Liver function test abnormalities, when present, are usually minimal. As CT, MRI, and sonography do not distinguish amebic and pyogenic abscesses, percutaneous aspiration may be indicated; this is best done by an image-guided needle (risks described below). The aspirate is divided into serial 30- to 50-mL aliquots, but only the last sample is examined for amebas, as the organisms are found at the edge of the cyst. Detection of amebic antigen in aspirate appears to be very sensitive.

Differential Diagnosis

Amebiasis should be considered in patients with acute or chronic diarrhea (including cases associated with only mild changes in bowel habits; in patients who have an exposure history, including travel or household or sexual exposure); liver abscess; and annular lesions of the colon. All patients with presumed inflammatory bowel disease should be tested for antibodies, by multiple stool examinations for antigen and the organism, and by colonoscopy with biopsy because of the risk of overwhelming amebic disease if corticosteroid therapy were to be given in the presence of amebiasis. The differential diagnosis of amebic liver abscess includes pyogenic abscess, echinococcal cyst, benign cyst, and hepatocellular carcinoma.

Treatment

The decision to treat is based on a composite of data including (1) finding entamoeba cysts or trophozoites and, when feasible (rarely), differentiating *E histolytica* from *E dispar;* (2) testing for *E histolytica* antigen in stool or hepatic abscess aspirate; and (3) testing for serum antibody, which, if positive, could represent old infection.

The choice of drug depends on the clinical presentation and the site of drug action. Treatment may require the concurrent or sequential use of several drugs. Table 35–1 outlines a preferred and an alternative method of treatment for each clinical type of amebiasis.

The **tissue amebicides** dehydroemetine and emetine act on organisms in the bowel wall and in other tissues but not on amebas in the bowel lumen.

Chloroquine is active principally against amebas in the liver. The **luminal amebicides** diloxanide furoate (not available in the USA), iodoquinol, and paromomycin act on organisms in the bowel lumen but are ineffective against amebas in the bowel wall or other tissues. Oral tetracycline inhibits the bacterial associates of *E histolytica* and thus has an indirect effect on amebas in the bowel lumen and bowel wall but not in other tissues; parenteral antibiotics have little efficacy at any site. Metronidazole (or tinidazole, which is not available in the USA) is unique in that it is effective both in the bowel lumen and in the bowel wall and other

Table 35–1. Treatment of amebiasis.

Clinical Presentation	Drug(s) of Choice	Alternative Drug(s)
Asymptomatic intestinal infection	Diloxanide furoate[1,2]	Iodoquinol (diiodohydroxyquin)[3] or paromomycin[4]
Mild to moderate intestinal disease (nondysenteric colitis)	(1) Metronidazole[5] or tinidazole[1,5] **plus** (2) Diloxanide furoate,[1,2] iodoquinol,[3] or paromomycin[4]	(1) Diloxanide furoate[1,2] or iodoquinol[3] **plus** (2) A tetracycline[6] **followed by** (3) Chloroquine[7] **or** (1) Paromomycin[4] **followed by** (2) Chloroquine[7]
Severe intestinal disease (dysentery)	(1) Metronidazole[5] or tinidazole[1,5] **plus** (2) Diloxanide furoate[1,2] or iodoquinol[3] **or, if parenteral therapy is needed initially:** (1) Intravenous metronidazole[8] until oral therapy can be started; (2) Then give oral metronidazole[5] plus diloxanide furoate[1,2] or iodoquinol[3]	(1) A tetracycline[6] **plus** (2) Diloxanide furoate[1,2] or iodoquinol[3] **followed by** (3) Chloroquine[9] **or, if parenteral therapy is needed initially:** (1) Dehydroemetine[10] or emetine[1,10] **followed by** (2) A tetracycline[6] plus diloxanide furoate[1,2] or iodoquinol[3] **followed by** (3) Chloroquine[9]

(continued)

Table 35–1. Treatment of amebiasis. (continued)

Clinical Presentation	Drug(s) of Choice	Alternative Drug(s)
Hepatic abscess	(1) Metronidazole[5,8] or tinidazole[1,5]	(1) Dehydroemetine[11] or emetine[1,11]
	plus	**followed by**
	(2) Diloxanide furoate[1,2] or iodoquinol[3]	(2) Chloroquine[12]
	followed by	**plus**
	(3) Chloroquine[9]	(3) Diloxanide furoate[1,2] or iodoquinol[3]
Ameboma or extra-intestinal disease	As for hepatic abscess, but not including chloroquine	As for hepatic abscess, but not including chloroquine

[1]Not available in the USA.
[2]Diloxanide furoate, 500 mg three times daily with meals for 10 days.
[3]Iodoquinol (diiodohydroxyquin), 650 mg three times daily for 21 days.
[4]Paromomycin, 25–30 mg/kg (base) (maximum 3 g) in three divided doses after meals daily for 7 days.
[5]Metronidazole, 750 mg three times daily for 10 days. In countries where it is available (not in the USA), tinidazole is preferred over metronidazole as the nitroimidazole component in treatment; although the two drugs are equally effective, tinidazole is given in a shorter course of treatment and is better tolerated. The tinidazole dosage is 800 mg three times daily for 3 days; in severe intestinal disease and hepatic abscess, continue for 5 days.
[6]Tetracycline, 250 mg four times daily for 10 days; in severe dysentery, give 500 mg four times daily for the

first 5 days, then 250 mg four times daily for 5 days. Tetracycline should not be used during pregnancy.
[7]Chloroquine, 500 mg (salt) daily for 7 days.
[8]An intravenous metronidazole formulation is available; change to oral medication as soon as possible. See manufacturer's recommendation for dosage and cautions.
[9]Chloroquine, 500 mg (salt) daily for 14 days.
[10]Dehydroemetine or emetine, 1 mg/kg subcutaneously (preferred) or intramuscularly daily for the least number of days necessary to control severe symptoms (usually 3–5 days) (maximum daily dose for dehydroemetine is 90 mg; for emetine, 65 mg).
[11]Use dosage recommended in footnote 10 for 8–10 days.
[12]Chloroquine, 500 mg (salt) orally twice daily for 2 days and then 500 mg orally daily for 19 days.

tissues, including the central nervous system. However, metronidazole when used alone for bowel infections is not sufficient as a luminal amebicide, for it fails to cure up to 50% of infections.

A. ASYMPTOMATIC INTESTINAL INFECTION

In asymptomatic cyst-passers, if stool antigen and serum antibody tests are negative, it can be presumed that the patient has an *E dispar* infection, which should not be treated. Nevertheless, an unrecognized commensal *E histolytica* infection could be present. Cure rates for *E histolytica* infection with a single course of diloxanide furoate or iodoquinol are 80–85%. Within endemic areas, asymptomatic carriers generally are not treated because of the frequency of reinfection.

B. MILD TO MODERATE INTESTINAL DISEASE

In patients with intestinal symptoms and entamoeba in the stool in whom *E dispar* and *E histolytica* cannot be differentiated, if both stool antigen and serum antibody tests are negative it is possible that the latter tests are false negatives and that an *E histolytica* infection is present. In such cases, it is often best to proceed with anti-*E histolytica* treatment. Metronidazole plus a luminal amebicide is the treatment of choice. Alternatives are set forth in Table 35–1. The minimum dose

of chloroquine needed to destroy trophozoites carried to the liver or to eradicate an undetected early-stage liver abscess is not established.

C. SEVERE INTESTINAL DISEASE

Fluid and electrolyte therapy and opioids to control bowel motility are necessary adjuncts. The latter are used cautiously because of the risk of toxic megacolon.

D. HEPATIC ABSCESS

There is no clinical evidence of metronidazole-resistant *E histolytica*, though it can be induced experimentally. Chloroquine has been included in treatment to avoid rare long-term failures. Regarding rare short-term metronidazole failures, if a satisfactory clinical response does not occur in 3 days, the abscess should be drained for therapeutic purposes and to exclude pyogenic abscess. Continued failure to achieve an adequate clinical response requires changing to the potentially toxic alternative drug dehydroemetine (or emetine) plus chloroquine. Treatment also requires a luminal amebicide (diloxanide furoate or iodoquinol), whether or not the organism is found in the stool. Antibiotics are added for concomitant bacterial liver abscess, although metronidazole itself is highly effective against anaerobic bacteria, a major cause of bacterial liver abscesses. Imaging defects in the liver disappear slowly (range: 3–13 months) after treatment; some calcify.

Most patients treated with metronidazole for an amebic liver cyst do not require therapeutic percutaneous drainage; when needed, the catheter method is preferred. Indications are a large abscess, threatening rupture; the presence of a left lobe abscess (which is associated with a higher rate of severe complications); and the absence of medical response after 3 days of metronidazole therapy. The risks of aspiration or catheter drainage are bacterial superinfection, bleeding, peritoneal spillage, and inadvertent puncture of an infected hydatid cyst.

E. ADVERSE DRUG REACTIONS

Metronidazole often induces transient nausea, vomiting, headache, or a metallic taste in the mouth; if alcohol is taken during or shortly after treatment, a disulfiram-like reaction may occur. Drug interactions with some commonly used drugs (cimetidine, some anticoagulants, phenytoin, phenobarbital, lithium) have been reported. Metronidazole increases the rate of naturally occurring tumors in mice but not in nonrodent species. Prudence dictates that metronidazole be given to pregnant or nursing mothers only if other drugs cannot be used.

Dehydroemetine and emetine cause nausea, vomiting, and pain at the injection site. They are also cardiotoxic, with a narrow range between therapeutic and toxic effects; dehydroemetine may be the safer of the two drugs. The tetracyclines should not be used in pregnancy; erythromycin stearate and paromomycin are alternatives. Paromomycin may cause mild gastrointestinal symptoms, infrequently intense diarrhea, and rarely overgrowth of nonsusceptible organisms. Paromomycin should be used with caution in ulcerated bowel conditions and is not used in the presence of significant renal disease. Iodoquinol produces a mild, transient diarrhea. It should be taken with meals; used with caution in patients with optic neuropathy, renal, or thyroid disease; and discontinued in the event of iodine toxicity (dermatitis, fever). The neurotoxicity seen with extended treatment does not occur at the standard 3-week dosage. Diloxanide usage commonly results in flatulence.

Follow-Up Care

In follow-up, examine at least three stools at 2- to 3-day intervals, starting 2–4 weeks after the end of treatment. For some patients, colonoscopy and reexamination of stools within 3 months may be indicated.

Postdysenteric colitis is an uncommon sequela of severe amebic colitis. Following adequate treatment, diarrhea continues and the mucosa may be reddened and edematous, but no ulcers or organisms are found. Most such cases are self-limited, with permanent remission in weeks to months. Uncommonly, severe and unremitting diarrhea may represent ulcerative colitis triggered by the amebic infection.

Prevention & Control

Prevention requires safe water supplies, sanitary disposal of human feces, adequate cooking of foods, protection of foods from fly contamination, washing hands after defecation and before preparing or eating foods, and, in endemic areas, avoidance of foods that cannot be cooked or peeled. Water supplies can be boiled (briefly) or treated with iodine (0.5 mL tincture of iodine per liter for 20 minutes, or longer if the water is cold); cysts are resistant to standard concentrations of chlorine. Filters are also available to purify drinking water. Disinfection dips for fruits and vegetables are not advised, and no drug is safe or effective in prophylaxis.

Prognosis

The mortality rate from untreated amebic dysentery, hepatic abscess, or ameboma may be high. With chemotherapy instituted early in the course of the disease, the prognosis is good.

Amano K et al: Amebiasis in acquired immunodeficiency syndrome. Intern Med 2001;40:563. [PMID: 11506293]

Clark CG: Amoebic disease. *Entamoeba dispar,* an organism reborn. Trans R Soc Trop Med Hyg 1998;92:361. [PMID: 9850382]

Espinosa-Cantellano M et al: Pathogenesis of intestinal amebiasis: from molecules to disease. Clin Microbiol Rev 2000;13: 318. [PMID: 10756002]

Hanna RM et al: Percutaneous catheter drainage in drug-resistant amoebic liver abscess. Trop Med Int Health 2000;5:578. [PMID: 10995100]

Petri WA et al: Diagnosis and management of amebiasis. Clin Infect Dis 1999;29:1117. [PMID: 10524950]

INFECTIONS WITH PATHOGENIC FREE-LIVING AMEBAS

The pathogenic free-living amebas cause three syndromes: (1) meningoencephalitis, (2) granulomatous encephalitis and other granulomatous lesions, and (3) keratitis.

Primary Amebic Meningoencephalitis

Primary amebic meningoencephalitis is a fulminating, hemorrhagic, necrotizing meningoencephalitis with a limited purulent exudate. It occurs in healthy children and young adults and is rapidly fatal. It is caused by free-living amebas, most commonly by the ameboflagellate *Naegleria fowleri.* Other causes are *Balamuthia mandrillaris* and the acanthamoeba species (see below), both of which may have a predilection for immunocompromised patients.

N fowleri is a thermophilic organism found in fresh and polluted warm lake water, domestic water supplies, swimming pools, thermal water, and sewers. Most patients give a history of exposure to fresh water; dust is also a possible source. Nasal and throat swabs have shown a carrier state, and serologic surveys suggest that inapparent infections occur.

The organism apparently invades the central nervous system through the cribriform plate. The incubation period varies from 2 to 15 days. Early symptoms include headache, fever, and lethargy, often associated with rhinitis and pharyngitis. Vomiting, disorientation, and other signs of meningoencephalitis develop within 1 or 2 days, followed by coma and then death on the fifth or sixth day. No distinctive clinical features distinguish the infection from acute bacterial meningoencephalitis. At autopsy, some victims have a nonspecific myocarditis.

Lumbar or ventricular cerebrospinal fluid contains several hundred to 25,000 leukocytes/μL (50–100% neutrophils) and erythrocytes (up to several thousand/μL). Protein is usually somewhat elevated, and glucose is normal or moderately reduced. If conventional examinations for bacteria and fungi are negative, the fluid is examined for free-living amebas. A wet mount examined by an ordinary optical microscope with the aperture restricted or condenser down will enhance contrast and refractility; a warm stage is not needed. The fluid should not be centrifuged or refrigerated, as this tends to immobilize the amebas (7–14 μm). Their brisk motility distinguishes them from leukocytes of various types, which they closely resemble. Staining, culture, and mouse inoculation should be performed. Serologic testing is only useful epidemiologically; patients die before antibodies are detectable.

Precise species identification is based on morphology, demonstration of flagellate transformation (naegleria only), and various immunologic methods.

Six well-documented survivors of *N fowleri* infection have been reported. One was treated with intravenous and intrathecal amphotericin B and another with a combination of amphotericin B, miconazole, and oral rifampin.

In *B mandrillaris* infections, the usual course is subacute, with death occurring within 1 week to several months. No treatment is available.

Acanthamoeba Infections

A. GRANULOMATOUS LESIONS

Free-living amebas of the genus acanthamoeba are found in soil and in fresh, brackish, and thermal water as trophozoites (15–45 μm) or cysts (10–25 μm). Several species, including *S castellanii* and *A culbertsoni,* cause a number of poorly defined syndromes, especially in debilitated or immunosuppressed patients: (1) subacute and chronic multifocal granulomatous necrotizing encephalitis leading to death in weeks to months, (2) skin lesions (ulcers or hard nodules in which ameba may be detected), and (3) granulomatous dissemination to many tissues. Portals of entry may include the skin, eyes, or respiratory tract. A commensal nasal carrier state is established.

The encephalitis presents with mental status abnormalities, meningismus, and neurologic features of a space-occupying lesion. Focal consolidation on chest films and cerebrospinal fluid lymphocytosis may be present. Antemortem diagnosis has been made by brain biopsy or cerebrospinal fluid wet mounts using specific fluorescent stains. No treatment has been effective, but ketoconazole, miconazole, itraconazole, sulfonamides, clotrimazole, pentamidine, paromomycin, propamidine, neomycin, amphotericin B, or flucytosine can be tried.

B. KERATITIS

Hundreds of cases of acanthamoeba keratitis and some of uveitis have been documented; most were associated with wearing contact lenses, others with penetrating corneal trauma or exposure to contaminated water. Suggestive features include (1) a waxing and waning clinical course over several months with severe ocular pain, photophobia, tearing, blurred vision, and conjunctival injection; (2) partial or 360-degree paracentral stromal ring infiltrate on ophthalmologic examination; (3) recurrent corneal epithelial breakdown; and (4) a corneal lesion refractory to the usual medications. Typically, the keratitis progresses slowly over months and can lead to blindness. The diagnosis can be confirmed by vigorously scraping the cornea with a swab or platinum-tipped spatula. The material is microscopically examined (1) as a wet preparation for cysts and motile trophozoites, (2) after staining, (3) by immunofluorescent techniques, and (4) after being cultured on nonnutrient agar seeded with *E coli.* Isolates can be identified by isoenzyme analysis and DNA profiles and tested for drug sensitivity.

With early treatment, many patients can expect cure and a good visual result. Topical propamidine isethionate (0.1%) with either chlorhexidine digluconate (0.02%), polyhexamethylene biguanide, or neomycin-polymyxin B-gramicidin has been used successfully. Topical miconazole has also been used. Oral itraconazole or ketoconazole can be added for deep keratitis. Use of corticosteroid therapy is controversial. In spite of medical treatment, penetrating keratoplasty is often necessary to excise diseased tissue; corneal grafting can be done after the amebic infection has been eradicated.

Prevention requires immersion of contact lenses in disinfectant solutions or by heat sterilization. The lens should not be cleaned in homemade saline solutions nor be worn while swimming.

Doel I et al: Encephalitis due to a free-living amoeba *(Balamuthia mandrillaris):* case report with literature review. Surg Neurol 2000;53:611. [PMID: 10940434]

Illingworth CD et al: Acanthamoeba keratitis. Surv Ophthalmol 1998;42:493. [PMID: 9635900]

Kidney DD et al: CNS infections with free-living amebas: neuroimaging findings. AJR Am J Roentgenol 1998;171:809. [PMID: 9724321]

McCulley JP et al: The diagnosis and management of Acanthamoeba keratitis. CLAO J 2000;26:47. [PMID: 10656311]

Parija SC et al: *Naegleria fowleri:* a free-living amoeba of emerging medical importance. J Communicable Diseases 1999;31: 153. [PMID: 10916609]

Szénási Z et al: Isolation, identification and increasing importance of "free-living" amoeba causing human disease. J Med Microbiol 1998;47:5. [PMID: 9449945]

BABESIOSIS (Piroplasmosis)

Babesiae are tick-borne protozoal parasites of wild and domestic animals worldwide. Babesiosis in humans (recognized in 1959) is a rare intraerythrocytic infection caused by two babesia species. In Europe, where the infection is caused by *Babesia divergens,* 30 cases have been reported; in the USA, infection is caused by *B microti,* and over 300 cases have been described. Serosurveys and limited confirmations of isolates suggest infection with *B microti* or other species in Taiwan, China, Egypt, South Africa, Mexico, and South America. In the USA, *B microti* infections have been reported from coastal and island areas of northeastern and mid-Atlantic states as well as from Wisconsin, Minnesota, Missouri, Washington, and California. Antibody prevalence of 3–8% in serosurveys indicates a high level of subclinical infection. New babesia species or strains (WA1 and others) have been described in humans in California, Washington, and Georgia. Natural hosts for *B microti* are various wild and domestic animals, particularly the white-footed mouse and white-tailed deer. With extension of the deer's habitat, the range of human infection is increasing as well.

Humans are infected as a result of *Ixodes scapularis* tick bites (mainly nymphal) but also by blood transfusion and perinatally. Coinfections with Lyme disease and probably ehrlichiosis occur. Without passing through an exoerythrocytic stage, *B microti* enters the red blood cell and multiplies, resulting in cell rupture followed by infection of other cells.

The incubation period is 1 week to several months; parasitemia is evident in 2–4 weeks. Patients usually do not recall the tick bite. The illness is characterized by irregular fever, chills, headache, diaphoresis, myalgia, and fatigue but is without malaria-like periodicity of symptoms. Other symptoms may occur including nausea, vomiting, jaundice, arthralgia, and emotional lability. Most patients have a moderate hemolytic anemia, and some have hemoglobinuria, hepatosplenomegaly, or thrombocytopenia. Although parasitemia may continue for months, with or without symptoms, the disease is self-limited, and after several weeks or months most patients recover without sequelae. Splenectomized, older, or immunosuppressed persons are most likely to have severe manifestations; case fatality rates in the USA may reach 5%.

All *B divergens* infections (transmitted by *I ricinus*) have been in splenectomized patients. These infections progress rapidly with high fever, severe hemolytic anemia, jaundice, hemoglobinuria, and renal failure; death rates are over 40%.

Diagnosis is established by identification of the intraerythrocytic parasite (2–3 μm) on Wright- or Giemsa-stained thick and thin blood smears; no gametocytes and no intracellular pigment are seen. A single red cell may contain different stages of the parasite, and parasitemia can exceed 10%. Repeated smears may be necessary. The organism must be differentiated from malarial parasites, particularly *Plasmodium falciparum.* Isolation can be attempted by inoculating patient blood into hamsters or gerbils. Antibody is detectable within 1–4 weeks after onset of symptoms and persists for 6–12 months. Testing with specific antigens in the immunofluorescent test is relatively species-specific, with a titer of 1:256 or greater considered diagnostic; antibody titers against plasmodium are generally low or absent. Detection of specific IgM antibody confirms the diagnosis. The polymerase chain reaction method, where available, is more sensitive for low parasitemias but of equal specificity. The leukocyte count and the serum alkaline phosphatase concentration may be elevated. Imaging studies may detect morphologic changes in the spleen.

No drug treatment is fully satisfactory. Although *B microti* infections in patients with intact spleens are usually self-limiting and can be treated asymptomatically, it is now recommended that all patients—even those mildly ill—should be treated with a 7-day course of quinine (650 mg three times a day) plus clindamycin (1.2 g twice daily intravenously or 650 mg orally three times a day). A secondary mode of treatment is with azithromycin (500 mg twice daily for 3 days followed by 500 mg daily for 7 days) plus either atovaquone (750 mg twice daily for 7–10 days) or quinine (see above). Exchange transfusion with antibiotics has been successful in several severely ill asplenic patients with parasitemia greater than 10%. Management of *B divergens* infection can be attempted with exchange transfusion and clindamycin-quinine therapy.

Hatcher JC et al: Severe babesiosis in Long Island: review of 34 cases and their complications. Clin Infect Dis 2001;32: 1117. [PMID 11283800]

Mylonakis E: When to suspect and how to monitor babesiosis. Am Fam Physician 2001;63:1969. [PMID: 11388711]

Ranque S: The treatment of babesiosis. N Engl J Med 2000;343: 1454. [PMID 11236790]

BALANTIDIASIS

Balantidium coli is a large ciliated intestinal protozoan found worldwide, but particularly in the tropics. Pigs are considered the reservoir host, but the agent has been found in other animals and in insects. The disease is rare in humans, occurring as an acute or chronic infection (sporadic or in outbreaks) resulting from ingestion of cysts passed in stools of humans or swine. In the new host, the cyst wall dissolves and the trophozoite may invade the mucosa and submucosa of the terminal ileum, appendix, and large bowel, causing abscesses and irregularly rounded ulcerations. Many infections are asymptomatic and need not be treated. Chronic recurrent diarrhea, alternating with constipation, is most common, but mild to moderate diarrhea to severe dysentery with bloody mucoid stools, tenesmus, and colic may occur. Rare instances of infection in the lung, liver, and vagina have been reported.

Diagnosis is established by finding trophozoites in liquid stools, cysts in formed stools, or the trophozoite in scrapings or biopsy of ulcers of the large bowel. Specimens must be examined rapidly or placed in preservative.

The treatment of choice is tetracycline hydrochloride, 500 mg four times daily for 10 days. The alternative drug is iodoquinol (diiodohydroxyquin), 650 mg three times daily for 21 days. Occasional success has also been reported with metronidazole (750 mg three times daily for 5 days) or paromomycin (25–30 mg/kg [base] in three divided doses for 5–10 days).

In properly treated mild to moderate symptomatic cases, the prognosis is good, but in spite of treatment, fatalities have occurred in severe infections as a result of intestinal perforation or hemorrhage.

Esteban JH et al: Balantidiasis in Aymara children from the Northern Bolivian Altiplano. Am J Trop Med Hyg 1998; 59:922. [PMID: 9886201]

Garcia LS: Flagellates and ciliates. Clin Lab Med 1999;19:621. [PMID: 10549429] (Review of *Giardia lamblia* and *Balantidium coli*.)

COCCIDIAL & MICROSPORIDIAL INFECTIONS: CRYPTOSPORIDIOSIS, ISOSPORIASIS, CYCLOSPORIASIS, & SARCOCYSTOSIS

Coccidiosis and microsporidiosis are intracellular infections of intestinal epithelial cells by spore-forming protozoa. Various species are the etiologic agents for microsporidiosis (see below). The causes of coccidiosis are *Cryptosporidium parvum, Isospora belli, Cyclospora cayetanensis,* and *Sarcocystis bovihominis* and *S suihominis;* all but the sarcocystis species complete their life cycle in a single host. Many of these infections occur worldwide, particularly in the tropics and in regions where hygiene is poor. They are causes of traveler's diarrhea; endemic childhood gastroenteritis (particularly in malnourished children in developing countries); institutional and community outbreaks of diarrhea; and acute and chronic diarrhea in immunosuppressed patients, including those with AIDS, in whom infection can be life-threatening. Clustering occurs in households, day care centers, and among sexual partners. Diarrhea in non-AIDS patients—sporadic, epidemic, and traveler's—is more likely to be due to cryptosporidia and less often to cyclospora or microsporidia. Diarrhea in AIDS is more commonly due to the microsporidia, *Enterocytozoon bieneusi,* and *En-*

cephalitozoon (formerly *Septata*) *intestinalis,* but cryptosporidium, isospora, and cyclospora are also important causes.

The infectious agents are oocysts (spores) transmitted directly from person to person or by contaminated water or food. Ingested oocysts release sporozoites that invade and multiply in enterocytes, primarily in the small bowel. Liberated merozoites reinvade other cells in the process of asexual intracellular multiplication. Eventually, sexual stages are released; following fertilization, immature oocysts form which are then shed in feces. The oocysts mature on exposure to air and can remain viable in a moist environment for months to years.

The isospora and cyclospora species found in humans appear to be distinct to humans only. Cryptosporidiosis is a zoonosis in which infections in farm animals (cattle, goats, turkeys, and others) can be transmitted to humans; however, most human infections are acquired from humans. Cyclospora and probably isospora require time outside the host to sporulate and become infectious.

Although the small bowel is the usual location of infection, other sites can be involved. Colon infection is common in cryptosporidiosis and has been reported with microsporidiosis. Biliary tract infection in cryptosporidiosis, microsporidiosis, and isosporiasis may result in either a sclerosing, cholangitis-like syndrome or an acalculous cholecystitis. Disseminated disease and corneal infections occur with several microsporidial species.

The pathogenesis of these diarrheas is not well understood. No enterotoxin has been identified. Voluminous secretory or malabsorption diarrhea (including vitamin B_{12}, D-xylose, and fat absorption dysfunction) can result. Although histologic examination of the small bowel can be normal, with intense infection there may be dense inflammatory infiltration accompanied by blunting to atrophy of the villi and crypt hyperplasia. The infections are nonulcerative and noninvasive except for *E intestinalis,* which can be invasive.

Clinical Findings

A. SYMPTOMS AND SIGNS

Generally, the forms of diarrhea caused by the coccidial and microsporidial agents are clinically indistinguishable from each other.

1. In immunocompetent persons, infection varies from no symptoms, to a mild diarrhea with flatulence and bloating, to severe and frequent watery diarrhea in which the onset may be explosive. Mucus may be present in stools, but no microscopic or gross blood. Other findings may include low-grade fever, malaise, anorexia, abdominal cramps, vomiting, and myalgia. These symptoms are generally self-limited, lasting a few days to several weeks (sometimes longer for isosporiasis). Weight loss can be marked. Parasitologic clearance, however, may take several months.

2. In immunologically deficient patients, the diarrhea can be profuse (up to 15 L daily has been reported), with cholera-like watery movements, accompanied by severe malabsorption, electrolyte imbalance, and marked weight loss; fever is uncommon. Mucus is seen in the stools, but blood and leukocytes are seldom present. The diarrhea may recur or persist, and passage of organisms continues for months to indefinitely.

B. LABORATORY FINDINGS

In diagnosis, three stool specimens should be obtained fresh and in preservative over 5–7 days and processed by a variety of flotation or concentration methods to detect the distinctive oocysts (differences are based on size and intracellular location). A modified acid-fast stain is used for cryptosporidia, cyclospora, and isospora; in microsporidiosis, a modified trichrome or Weber stain. The laboratory should be notified that coccidia and microsporidia are being investigated because specific fecal examinations are needed for some of the organisms, especially cyclospora. The organisms can also be detected by duodenal aspiration or biopsy.

Specific Diseases

A. CRYPTOSPORIDIOSIS

The organism is highly infectious (relatively few parasites can induce infection) and readily transmitted in health and day care settings and in households. The incubation period appears to be 5–21 days. Oocysts passed in stools are fully sporulated and infectious; therefore, hospitalized patients should be isolated and stool precautions strictly observed. The prevalence of asymptomatic human carriers in the USA is estimated to be about 1.5%. Outbreaks are of particular concern, as exemplified by the 1993 epidemic in Milwaukee in which 400,000 persons became ill. Since chlorine disinfection of water is not effective, adequate filtration is required. However, because of the oocysts' small size (2–5 μm), filtration is difficult and unreliable (the < 1 μm filters used frequently become obstructed).

In AIDS, infection may involve any part of the gastrointestinal tract, including the biliary tract (sclerosing cholangitis has been described); respiratory tract infection, hepatitis, pancreatitis, lymphadenopathy, and hepatosplenomegaly may occur, as well as multisystem involvement.

In diagnosis, fluorescent microscopy using auramine staining or a monoclonal antibody increases sensitivity and may be as specific as acid-fast staining. Commercially available ELISA tests that detect cryptosporidial antigen in feces appear to have high sensitivity and specificity and provide for ease of use. Other serologic tests are not useful. Stools rarely show white or red blood cells. Blood leukocytosis and eosinophilia are uncommon. Radiologic changes have been reported in the stomach, intestines, and bile ducts in severe disease. In AIDS patients with unexplained diarrhea, the organism should also be looked for in sputum and bronchoalveolar lavage fluid; specimens obtained from lung tissue have sometimes been positive in patients with negative stool specimens.

B. ISOSPORIASIS

I belli oocysts in feces are 20–30 × 10–20 μm. Opinion differs about whether the oocyst can be transmitted directly from person to person by anal-oral sexual contact or if it must pass into the environment and mature to its infectious stage. Outbreaks have occurred in day care centers and mental institutions. The incubation period is 7–11 days. A hemorrhagic ulcerative colitis has been described.

Diagnosis by stool examination is often difficult, for the organisms may be scanty even in the presence of significant symptoms. Because of their buoyancy, oocysts must be looked for just beneath the coverslip of the preparation. Frequently, diagnosis can be made only after duodenal aspiration or duodenal biopsy of multiple specimens. Serologic tests are available.

C. CYCLOSPORIASIS

C cayetanensis oocysts (8–10 μm) must undergo a period of sporulation in the environment before they become infectious. The incubation period appears to be 2–11 days. Transmission is by fecally contaminated food or water; the host range is unknown. The infection has been reported in many parts of the world, in travelers, and as the cause of water and food-borne outbreaks. Oocysts can be identified in stool by examination of wet mounts under phase microscopy, by use of modified acid-fast stains (oocysts are variably acid-fast), microwave-heated safranine staining, or by autofluorescence with ultraviolet light microscopy. Antibodies have been detected, and titers increase during convalescence.

D. SARCOCYSTOSIS

Sarcocystis is a two-host coccidian. Human disease occurs as two syndromes, both rare: (1) an enteric infection in which humans are the definitive host and (2) a muscle infection in which humans are an intermediate host. In the enteric form, sporocysts passed in human feces are not infective for humans but must be ingested by cattle or pigs. Humans become infected by eating poorly cooked beef or pork containing oocysts of *Sarcocystis bovihominis* or *Sarcocystis suihominis,* respectively. Organisms enter intestinal epithelial cells and are transformed into oocysts that release sporocysts into the feces. Clinically, the intestinal infection is often asymptomatic or causes mild but protracted diarrhea; an eosinophilic necrotizing enteritis has been reported. Diagnosis is by stool examination using a flotation method.

The muscle form of sarcocystosis results when humans ingest sporocysts in feces from an infected carnivore that has eaten prey which harbored sarcocysts. The sporocysts liberate sporozoites that invade the intestinal wall and are disseminated to skeletal muscle.

This results in subcutaneous and muscular inflammation lasting several days to 2 weeks and the finding of swellings at these sites, sometimes associated with local erythema, tenderness and myalgia, fever, and eosinophilia. Sarcocysts are often asymptomatic, however, such as those found incidentally at autopsy in cardiac muscle.

E. MICROSPORIDIOSIS

Microsporidia are obligate intracellular protozoans (0.5–2 μm × 1–4 μm) that are pathogens of arthropods, fish, and vertebrates. Many infections are of zoonotic origin from domestic and wild animals, but human-to-human transmission has been documented. Infection is mainly by ingestion of the spores but also by inhalation or finger contamination of the eyes. At least 11 species are known to infect humans; disease is seen mainly in immunoincompetent persons, particular those with AIDS. In chronic AIDS diarrhea, the two most common intestinal parasites are *Enterocytozoon bieneusi* and *Encephalitozoon intestinalis*. These parasites can also cause biliary infection (cholangitis, cholecystitis). In immunocompetent persons, the diarrhea due to these parasites (including traveler's diarrhea) is self-limited. *Encephalitozoon intestinalis, Enterocytozoon cuniculi, Enterocytozoon hellem,* and *Vittaforma corneae* can disseminate to many tissues, including the sinuses, lungs, liver, urinary tract, and brain. In *E cuniculi* infection, MRI has shown contrast-enhancing brain lesions. Most of the above parasites and others have been found as a nonpathogenic carrier state or as a cause of keratoconjunctivitis. Pleistophora species and *Trachipleistophora hominis* cause a myositis associated with high elevations of creatine phosphokinase, lactate dehydrogenase, and myoglobin. Thus, microsporidia should be considered in infections in immunoincompetent persons in whom no other infectious agent can be found.

Microsporidia are detected in feces, body fluids (including duodenal fluid), and tissue biopsies (intestinal epithelium, cornea, conjunctiva, bronchi, and others) by light microscopy using various staining methods, particularly trichrome and Weber's chromotrope-based stains, followed by confirmatory fluorescence staining. Confirmation is sometimes by biopsy followed by electron microscopy or use of molecular methods, such as polymerase chain reaction. Culture is available in specialized laboratories.

Treatment

Most acute infections in immunocompetent persons are self-limited and do not require treatment. Supportive treatment for severe or chronic diarrhea includes fluid and electrolyte replacement and, in chronic cases, parenteral nutrition.

In **isosporiasis,** effective treatment has been described using (1) trimethoprim (160 mg) and sulfamethoxazole (800 mg) (TMP-SMZ) four times daily for 10 days and then twice daily for 3 weeks; or (2)

sulfadiazine, 4 g, and pyrimethamine, 35–75 mg, in four divided doses daily, plus leucovorin calcium, 10–25 mg daily, for 3–7 weeks. In immunocompromised patients, it may be necessary to continue a maintenance dose indefinitely with TMP-SMZ three times weekly or Fansidar once weekly. Efficacy in primary infection has also been reported for furazolidone (400 mg/d for 10 days), roxithromycin, ciprofloxacin, nitrofurantoin, metronidazole, quinacrine, pyrimethamine, albendazole with ornidazole, and diclazuril.

In the treatment of **cyclosporiasis,** TMP (160 mg)-SMZ (800 mg) twice daily for 7 days is effective; in HIV infections, higher doses (four times daily for 10 days) and long-term maintenance (three times weekly) are needed. For patients intolerant of TMP-SMZ, ciprofloxacin can be tried. In **microsporidiosis,** the encephalitozoon species often respond to albendazole (400 mg two or three times daily for several weeks up to 3 months). In *E bieneusi* infection and in the various causes of disseminated disease, albendazole can be tried; although it has not had good success, amelioration may result. For ocular lesions, some infections respond to oral albendazole plus fumagillin eyedrops.

No treatment has been successful for **sarcocystosis** or **cryptosporidiosis.** In cryptosporidiosis, the following have been attempted: roxithromycin (300 mg twice daily for 4 weeks), spiramycin (1 g three times daily for 2 weeks or longer), paromomycin (25–35 mg/kg/d in three or four divided doses; duration uncertain), zidovudine (AZT), azithromycin (600 mg daily), octreotide, eflornithine, letrazuril, and hyperimmune bovine colostrum.

Prevention

Measures to reduce exposure to these organisms are recommended for immunocompromised patients. These include reduced exposure to swimming in fresh water and boiling of drinking water (1 minute) or use of a filter that removes particles over 1 μm in size.

Ambroise-Thomas P: Parasitic diseases and immunodeficiencies. Parasitology 2001;122 (Suppl):S65-71. [PMID: 11442198]

Arness MK et al: An outbreak of acute eosinophilic myositis attributed to human Sarcocystis parasitism. Am J Trop Med Hyg 1999;61:548. [PMID: 10548287]

Bicart-See A et al: Successful treatment with nitazoxanide of *Enterocytozoon bieneusi* microsporidiosis in a patient with AIDS. Antimicrob Agents Chemother 2000;44:167. [PMID: 10602740]

Didier ES: Microsporidiosis. Clin Infect Dis 1998;27:1. [PMID: 9675442]

Franzen C, Muller A: Microsporidiosis: human diseases and diagnosis. Microbes Infect 2001;3:389 [PMID 11369276]

Herwaldt BL: Cyclospora cayetanensis: a review, focusing on the outbreaks of cyclosporiasis in the 1990s. Clin Infect Dis 2000;31:1040. [PMID: 11049789]

Maggi P et al: Effect of antiretroviral therapy on cryptosporidiosis and microsporidiosis in patients infected with human immunodeficiency virus type 1. Eur J Clin Microbiol 2000; 19:213. [PMID: 10795595]

Soave R et al: Cyclospora. Infect Dis Clin North Am 1998;12:1. [PMID: 9494825]

GIARDIASIS

ESSENTIALS OF DIAGNOSIS

- *Most infections are asymptomatic.*
- *In some cases, acute or chronic diarrhea, mild to severe, with bulky, greasy, frothy, malodorous stools, free of blood and pus.*
- *Upper abdominal discomfort, cramps, distention, excessive flatus, and lassitude.*
- *Cysts and occasionally trophozoites in stools.*
- *Trophozoites in duodenal fluid.*

General Considerations

Giardiasis is a protozoal infection of the upper small intestine caused by the flagellate *Giardia lamblia* (also called *G intestinalis* and *G duodenalis*). The parasite occurs worldwide, most abundantly in areas with poor sanitation. In the USA and Europe, the infection is the most common intestinal protozoal pathogen; the USA estimate is of 100,000 to 2.5 million new infections yearly and 5000 hospital admissions. Occurrence is particularly high among children.

The organism occurs in feces as a symmetric, heart-shaped flagellated trophozoite measuring 10–25 × 6–12 μm and as a cyst measuring 11–14 × 7–10 μm. Only the cyst form is infectious by the oral route; trophozoites are destroyed by gastric acidity. Humans are a reservoir for the infection; animals, including dogs, cats, beavers, and other mammals have been implicated but not confirmed as reservoirs or zoonotic sources of infection. Under suitable moist, cool conditions, cysts can survive in the environment for weeks to months. The infectious dose is low, requiring as few as ten cysts.

Cysts are transmitted as a result of fecal contamination of water or food, by person-to-person contact, or by anal-oral sexual contact. Multiple cases are common in households, children's day care centers (often the nidus for spread of organisms to the community), and mental institutions. Outbreaks occur as a result of contamination of water supplies. Giardiasis is a well-recognized problem in special groups including travelers abroad, campers who drink water from USA streams, male homosexuals, and persons with impaired immune states. Giardiasis has not been, however, an opportunistic infection in AIDS.

After the cysts are ingested, trophozoites emerge in the duodenum and jejunum. Infrequently, they cause epithelial damage, atrophy of villi, hypertrophic crypts, and extensive cellular infiltration of the lamina propria; mucosal invasion is rare; hematogenous dissemination does not occur. Hypogammaglobulinemia, low secretory IgA levels in the gut, achlorhydria, and malnutrition favor the development of infection. Gastric giardiasis may represent reflux from the duodenum or localized infection.

Clinical Findings

A. SYMPTOMS AND SIGNS

A large proportion of infected persons (especially children) remain asymptomatic cyst carriers, and their infection clears spontaneously. Giardia should be considered in most cases of diarrhea, especially where it is prolonged and associated with marked weight loss. Syndromes include (1) acute diarrhea, (2) chronic diarrhea, and (3) malabsorption. The incubation period is usually 1–3 weeks but may be longer. The illness may begin gradually or suddenly. The acute phase may last days or weeks, but it is usually self-limited, although cyst excretion may be prolonged. In a few patients, the disorder may become chronic and last for years.

In both the acute and chronic forms, diarrhea ranges from mild to severe; most often it is mild. There may be no complaints other than of one bulky, loose bowel movement a day, often after breakfast. With larger numbers of movements, the stools become increasingly watery but are usually free of blood and pus; they are copious, frothy, malodorous, and greasy. The diarrhea may be daily or recurrent; if recurrent, stools may be normal to mushy during intervening days, or the patient may be constipated. Weight loss is frequent; weakness may occur. Infants and young children may show impaired growth and development. Less common are anorexia, nausea and vomiting, midepigastric discomfort and cramps (often after meals), belching, flatulence, borborygmi, and abdominal distention.

Malabsorption occasionally develops in the acute or chronic stage. Findings may include fat- and protein-losing enteropathy and vitamin A, vitamin B_{12}, and disaccharidase deficiencies and marked weight loss. Certain extraintestinal manifestations (arthritis, anterior uveitis, urticaria) have been attributed to giardiasis infections, but a pathophysiologic relationship has not been established.

B. LABORATORY TESTS

Diagnosis is by identifying antigen in feces, trophozoites in duodenal fluid, or cysts or trophozoites in feces. Using commercial kits, coproantigen detection by ELISA and IFA tests is now the preferred diagnostic test because of its superior sensitivity (80% with one specimen, 93% with two) and high specificity. A second stool specimen should be tested for antigen if the first is negative. Antigen assays and stool examinations are about equal in cost. Antigen detection, however, should be reserved for situations when there is no need to examine feces for other parasitic causes of diarrhea, as among day care children.

Detection of the parasites in feces can be difficult because the number of organisms passed varies considerably from day to day. At the onset of infection, patients may have symptoms for about a week before organisms can be detected; in chronic diarrhea, stool examinations can be persistently negative. Three stool specimens collected at intervals of 2 days or longer should be examined following concentration methods. One specimen will detect 50–75% of cases and three specimens about 90%. Unless the specimens can be submitted within an hour, they should be preserved immediately in a fixative. Purges do not increase the likelihood of finding the organism. Use of barium, antibiotics, antacids, kaolin products, or oily laxatives may temporarily (about 10 days) reduce the number of parasites or interfere with detection. Selected other diagnostic procedures are sometimes warranted: (1) the duodenal string test (Entero-Test), (2) duodenal aspiration (followed by concentration [500 Hz for 5 minutes]), (3) endoscopic brush cytology, or (4) duodenal biopsy (a mucosal imprint for staining should be made before sectioning).

A serum IgM study appears to indicate recently acquired infection, but testing for IgG does not. One-third of infections show a temporary IgA response as well. There is no eosinophilia, and the white blood cell count is normal. Radiologic examination of the small bowel is usually normal.

Treatment

Although controversial, treatment of asymptomatic patients should be considered since they can transmit the infection to others and may occasionally become symptomatic themselves. In selected cases, it may be best to wait a few weeks before starting treatment, as some infections will clear spontaneously. In the presence of a presumptive diagnosis but negative stool specimens, an empirical course of treatment is sometimes indicated.

Treatment is effective with tinidazole, metronidazole, quinacrine, or furazolidone. As none of the agents cure more than 90% of infections (80% for furazolidone), retreatment with an alternative drug may be needed. Single-dose tinidazole (not available in the USA) is the drug of choice because it is as effective as a course of the other drugs. In follow-up, two or more stools are analyzed weekly starting 2 weeks after therapy.

All of these drugs occasionally have unpleasant side effects. The potential for carcinogenicity of furazolidone, metronidazole, and tinidazole appears to be negligible based on over 2 decades of use. Because of its rare potential for severe toxicity, quinacrine should be used only when no other drug is available.

A. TINIDAZOLE

(Not available in the USA.) A dose of 2 g given once has had reported cure rates of 90–100%. Adverse reactions consist of mild gastrointestinal side effects in about 10% of patients; headache and vertigo are less common.

B. METRONIDAZOLE

The dose is 250 mg three times daily for 5–7 days. Metronidazole may cause gastrointestinal symptoms, headache, dizziness, a metallic taste, and candidal overgrowth, in addition to a disulfiram-like reaction in alcohol users. In the USA, metronidazole for giardiasis treatment is only available for off-label use.

C. FURAZOLIDONE

The dose is 100 mg (in suspension) four times daily for 7–10 days. Gastrointestinal symptoms, fever, headache, rash, and a disulfiram-like reaction with alcohol occur. Furazolidone can cause mild hemolysis in glucose-6-phosphate dehydrogenase-deficient persons.

D. QUINACRINE (MEPACRINE)

The dose is 100 mg three times daily after meals for 5–7 days. The drug has a bitter taste. Gastrointestinal symptoms, headache, and dizziness are common; harmless yellowing of the skin is infrequent. Toxic psychosis and exfoliative dermatitis are rare but may be severe. Quinacrine is contraindicated in psoriasis or in persons with a history of psychosis. Although quinacrine is not generally available in the USA, it can be obtained from two pharmacies: 800-247-9767.

E. OTHERS

Albendazole (400 mg daily for 5 days) has shown cure rates that range from 10% to 95%. Reports with **paromomycin** (25–35 mg/kg/d in three divided doses for 7 days) have been mixed; because the drug is not absorbed, it has been proposed for use in pregnancy.

Prevention

There is no effective chemoprophylaxis for giardiasis. Since community chlorination (0.4 mg/L) of water is relatively ineffective for inactivating cysts, filtration is required. For hikers, bringing water to a boil for 1 minute is adequate; halogenation with iodine or filtration with a pore size less than 1 μm can also be used. Relying on iodine halogenation is no longer recommended by the Centers for Disease Control and Prevention. In day care centers, appropriate disposal of diapers and frequent hand washing are essential.

Prognosis

With treatment and successful eradication of the infection, there are no sequelae. Without treatment, severe malabsorption may rarely contribute to death from other causes.

Aziz H et al: A comparison study of different methods used in the detection of *Giardia lamblia*. Clin Lab Sci 2001;14:150. [PMID: 11517624]

Hanson KL et al: Use of an enzyme immunoassay does not eliminate the need to analyze multiple stool specimens for sensitive detection of *Giardia lamblia*. J Clin Microbiol 2001;39:474. [PMID: 11158092]

Gardner TB et al: Treatment of giardiasis. Clin Microbiol Rev 2001;14:114. [PMID: 11148005]

LEISHMANIASIS

Leishmaniasis is infection by species of the genus leishmania. The disease is a zoonosis transmitted by bites of sand flies (2 mm) (phlebotomus [Old World leishmaniasis] and lutzomyia [New World leishmaniasis] species) from the wild animal reservoir (eg, rodents, Canidae, sloths, marsupials) and domestic dogs (they can die from *L infantum* infections) to humans; however, kala azar is transmitted directly from humans to humans. Leishmaniae have two distinct forms in their life cycle: (1) In mammalian hosts, the parasite is found in its amastigote form (Leishman-Donovan bodies, 2×5 μm) within mononuclear phagocytes. When sand flies feed on an infected host, the parasitized cells are ingested with the blood meal. (2) In the sand fly vector, the parasite converts to, multiplies, and is then transmitted during feeding as a flagellated extracellular promastigote (10–15 μm).

Four clinical syndromes occur, with overlap between them, and each syndrome is caused by more than one species. The speciation of leishmaniasis is complex (about 20 species are known to infect humans) and unsettled, and some species, not all of which are noted below, can cause more than one syndrome.

(1) **Visceral leishmaniasis** (kala azar), usually fatal without treatment, is characterized by hepatosplenomegaly and anemia and is caused mainly by the *L donovani* group of agents: *L donovani, L infantum,* and *L chagasi.*

(2) **Old World cutaneous leishmaniasis**—moist or dry cutaneous leishmaniasis—is caused mainly by *L tropica, L major,* and *L aethiopica.* **New World cutaneous leishmaniasis** is caused by the *L mexicana* complex.

(3) **Mucocutaneous leishmaniasis** (espundia), characterized by an initial cutaneous ulcer that is followed in months to years by destructive nasopharyngeal lesions, is caused by the leishmania (viannia) group of agents, principally by *L (V) braziliensis* and rarely by *L (V) panamensis.*

(4) **Diffuse cutaneous leishmaniasis** is a state of deficient cell-mediated immunity, in which the widespread, leprosy-like skin lesions are generally progressive and refractory to treatment. The causative organisms are the *L mexicana* complex in the New World and *L aethiopica* in the Old World.

In tropical and temperate zones, an estimated 12 million persons are infected with leishmaniasis; 1.5–2 million new cases occur yearly, of which more than 1 million are cutaneous and 500,000 visceral disease. The incidence of disease is increasing in many endemic areas. Severity of infection ranges from subclinical or minimally pathologic (self-curing or easily treated cutaneous lesions) to persistent, disfiguring cutaneous and mucocutaneous lesions to potentially fatal visceral disease (about 5000 yearly). Imported infections into the USA each year include about 40 cutaneous infections and several cases of visceral leishmaniasis.

Leishmania results in lifelong latent infection. If immunoparesis supervenes, leishmaniae can become opportunistic pathogens through reactivation or new infection. More than 1000 coinfections with HIV-visceral leishmaniasis have been reported from 25 countries, but the problem is worse in southern Europe (France, Italy, Spain, Portugal), where up to 17% of people with AIDS have coinfections. Coinfections are being increasingly reported with other leishmania species elsewhere in the world. In such cases, diagnostic criteria may be altered (leishmania antibodies become undetectable and, in visceral disease, splenomegaly may not occur); in treatment, drug side effects may exaggerate.

Diagnosis

Definitive diagnosis is by finding (1) the intracellular nonflagellated amastigote in Giemsa-stained biopsies from skin, mucosal lesions, liver, or lymph nodes; or from aspirates from spleen (the most sensitive site, but also a risky procedure), bone marrow, or lymph nodes; or (2) the flagellated promastigote state in culture of these tissue. Occasionally, the organisms are seen in mononuclear cells of Giemsa-stained smears of the buffy coat. Culture requires up to 21 days using specialized media; hamster or Balb/c mouse inoculation of the nose, footpad, or tail base may also be useful and requires 2–12 weeks. Serologic tests (ELISA, direct agglutination, others) and the leishmanin (Montenegro) skin test (not licensed in the USA) may facilitate diagnosis, but none are sufficiently sensitive or specific to be used alone in diagnosis. Polymerase chain reaction and monoclonal antibody tests are under development. Specimens from skin lesions should be obtained through intact skin (cleansed with 70% alcohol) at a raised edge of an ulcer margin. To obtain tissue fluid for staining, press blood out of the site with two fingers, incise a 3-mm slit, and then scrape with the blade. When doing a biopsy, an impression smear is made, a portion is macerated for culture, and the remainder is reserved for pathologic sections. For needle aspiration, sterile preservative-free saline is inserted with a 23- to 27-gauge needle; the aspirate is then cytospun at 800 *g* for 5 minutes.

Treatment

Treatment is less than adequate because of drug toxicity, long courses required, and frequent need for hospitalization. The drug of choice is a pentavalent antimonial, either sodium stibogluconate or meglumine antimoniate; resistance and treatment failures are increasing in frequency. Second line drugs used in cases unresponsive to the antimonials—but potentially more toxic—are amphotericin B and pentamidine. Three new lipid-formulated amphotericins permit a shorter course of treatment with less toxicity and high effectiveness. AmBisome, recently approved for use in the USA, is considered by some workers to be the drug of choice for the treatment of visceral leishmaniasis.

A. SODIUM STIBOGLUCONATE

Sodium stibogluconate is provided as a solution that contains 100 mg of antimony (Sb) per milliliter; only fresh solutions should be used. Treatment is started with a 200-mg Sb test dose followed by 20 mg Sb/kg/d; although dosages greater than 20 mg/kg should not be given, there is no upper limit to the total daily dose. The drug can be administered as a 5% solution intramuscularly (may be locally painful), but intravenous administration is preferred (cough may occur) when the volume is high, as is the case for most adults. Meglumine antimoniate (85 mg Sb/mL) is equal in efficacy and toxicity when used in equivalent Sb doses (20 mg Sb/kg/d). The appropriate volume of drug is mixed with 50 mL of 5% dextrose in water and infused over at least a 10-minute interval. The selected drug is given on consecutive days: 28 days for visceral and mucocutaneous leishmaniasis and 20 days for cutaneous leishmaniasis. In certain regions of the world, because of resistance, longer courses are indicated. Although few side effects occur initially, they are more likely to appear with cumulative doses. Most common are gastrointestinal symptoms, fever, myalgia, arthralgia, phlebitis, and rash; hemolytic anemia, hepatitis, renal and heart damage, and pancreatitis are rare. Patients should be monitored weekly for the first 3 weeks and twice weekly thereafter by serum chemistries, complete blood counts, and electrocardiography. Therapy is discontinued if the following occur: aminotransferases three to four times normal levels or significant arrhythmias, corrected QT intervals greater than 0.50 s, or concave ST segments. Relapses should be treated at the same dosage level for at least twice the previous duration. In the USA, the only drug available is stibogluconate, obtainable from the Parasitic Drug Service, Centers for Disease Control and Prevention, Atlanta, GA 30333 (404-639-3670).

B. AMPHOTERICIN B

For the treatment of visceral leishmaniasis, the parenteral dosage of AmBisome (a liposomal formulation now approved for use in the USA) is 3 mg/kg/d on days 1–5, 14, and 21 and may be repeated; the dosage for immunoincompetent persons is 4 mg/kg/d on days 1–5, 10, 17, 24, 31, and 38. Infusion-related side effects (hypertension, hypotension, dyspnea, thrombophlebitis, fever) and renal toxicity and anemia occur occasionally. The dosage for cutaneous and mucosal leishmaniasis has not been established. Conventional amphotericin B deoxycholate, as given in India, is slow infusion (4–6 hours) of 1 mg/kg daily for 20 days; this dosage achieved 99% cure rates but with side effects as above; an alternative dosage is 0.5–1 mg/kg/d or every second day intravenously for up to 8 weeks.

C. PENTAMIDINE ISETHIONATE

Pentamidine isethionate, 2–4 mg/kg intramuscularly (preferable) or intravenously, is given daily or on alternate days (fifteen doses for visceral and four doses for cutaneous leishmaniasis). For some forms of visceral leishmaniasis, it may be necessary to repeat treatment, but resistance may persist.

D. PAROMOMYCIN (AMINOSIDINE)

Success was limited in cutaneous leishmaniasis when the drug was applied topically (15% paromomycin, 12% methylbenzethonium chloride in soft white paraffin) twice daily for 15 days. The drug is showing promise in parenteral treatment (potentially severely toxic) of refractory visceral leishmaniasis in India and cutaneous disease in Central America.

Prevention & Control

Infection occurs when humans encroach on sand fly habitats—warm, humid microclimates, including rodent burrows, rock piles, or tree holes; these are often in sylvatic areas near forests or semiarid ecosystems. Biting is generally at twilight or at night but may occur in shaded areas during the day. Personal protection may fail but is partially accomplished by clothing (pants, long sleeves) that covers exposed skin, Permethrin applied to clothing, deet repellent (see under Malaria), avoidance of endemic areas (especially at night), use of mosquito coils, and use of fine-mesh sand fly netting for sleeping (may be too warm in tropical areas). Although sand flies can traverse the mesh of standard mosquito nets, insecticide-impregnated nets may prevent this. Often useful in control are destruction of animal reservoir hosts, mass treatment of humans in kala azar-prevalent areas, residual insecticide spraying in domestic and peridomestic areas, and keeping dogs and other domesticated animals out of the house, particularly at night.

Croft SL: Monitoring drug resistance in leishmaniasis. Trop Med Int Health 2001;6:899. [PMID: 11703844]

Davidson RN: Practical guide for the treatment of leishmaniasis. Drugs 1998;56:1009. [PMID: 9878989]

Desjeux P: The increase in risk factors for leishmaniasis worldwide. Trans R Soc Trop Med Hyg 2001;95:239. [PMID: 11490989]

Herwaldt BL: Leishmaniasis. Lancet 1999;354:1191. [PMID: 10513726]

1. Visceral Leishmaniasis (Kala Azar)

Visceral leishmaniasis is infection of the reticuloendothelial system, resulting in fever, hepatosplenomegaly, and pancytopenia. More than 500,000 cases occur yearly. The disease is caused mainly by the *Leishmania donovani* complex: (1) *L donovani* (eastern India, Bangladesh, Southeast Asia, Sudan, Ethiopia, Kenya, scattered foci in sub-Saharan Africa, the central Asian part of Russia, and northern and eastern China); (2) *L infantum* (Mediterranean littoral, Middle East, China, central and southwestern Asia, Ethiopia, Sudan, Afghanistan, Pakistan); and (3) *L chagasi* (South America, Central America, Mexico). The number of cases is increasing, particularly in Sudan, Bangladesh, Brazil, and Nepal. In each locale, the disease has its own peculiar clinical and epidemiologic features. Two other species—*L tropica* in the Middle East, the Mediterranean littoral, Kenya, India, and western Asia and *L amazonensis* in the Amazon Basin—cause visceral leishmaniasis in a few patients, generally in a milder form. Although humans are the major reservoir, animal reservoirs such as the dog, other canids, and rodents are important. The incubation period is usually 4–6 months (range: 10 days to 24 months).

A local nonulcerating nodule at the site of the bite may precede systemic manifestations but usually is inapparent. The onset may be acute (as early as 2 weeks after infection) or insidious. Fever often peaks twice daily, with chills and sweats, weakness, weight loss, cough, and diarrhea. The spleen progressively becomes huge, hard, and nontender. The liver is somewhat enlarged, and generalized lymphadenopathy is common. Hyperpigmentation of skin, especially on the hands, feet, abdomen, and forehead, is marked in light-skinned patients. In blacks, there may be warty eruptions or skin ulcers. Petechiae, bleeding from the nose and gums, jaundice, edema, and ascites may occur. Wasting is progressive; death, often due to intercurrent infection, occurs within months to 1–2 years. In some regions, oral and nasopharyngeal or cutaneous manifestations occur with or without visceral involvement.

In HIV-infected persons—with or without AIDS—visceral leishmaniasis can be an opportunistic infection. Numerous cases have been reported from the Mediterranean area and some from South America. These patients may have a shorter duration of symptoms, no fever or splenomegaly, and a poor response to treatment.

The diagnosis can sometimes be made by demonstrating the organism in buffy coat preparations of blood directly or after culture. More commonly, diagnosis depends on stained smears and culture of aspirates of sternal marrow or iliac crest, liver, enlarged lymph nodes, or spleen. Although splenic aspiration is the most sensitive test, because of its hazard (intra-abdominal bleeding and death) it should be reserved for last and should be performed only by experienced persons; contraindications are a soft spleen in the acute phase, a prolonged prothrombin time, and platelet counts under 40,000/µL. In immunocompetent persons, serologic tests are sensitive (> 90%) but false pos-

itives may occur, especially in malaria and typhoid fever. The direct agglutination IgM test and the ELISAs become positive early; the immunofluorescent IgG test becomes positive in most persons at a titer of 1:256 or higher. After treatment, the tests remain positive for months, though in immunoincompetent persons titers may be low or undetectable. The leishmanin skin test is always negative during active disease and becomes positive months to years after recovery. Other characteristic findings are progressive leukopenia (seldom over 3000/µL after the first 1–2 months), with lymphocytosis and monocytosis, normochromic anemia, and thrombocytopenia. There is a marked increase in total protein up to or greater than 10 g/dL owing to an elevated IgG fraction; serum albumin is 3 g/dL or less. Liver function tests show hepatocellular damage. Proteinuria may be present.

The differential diagnosis includes leukemia, lymphoma, tuberculosis, histoplasmosis, infectious mononucleosis, brucellosis, malaria, typhoid, schistosomiasis, African trypanosomiasis, tropical splenomegaly syndrome, and cirrhosis.

Sodium stibogluconate (20 mg/kg/d for 30 days, sometimes longer) is the drug of choice; however, some prefer lipid formulations of amphotericin B, of which AmBisome (see above for dosages) has become available in the USA. Whereas Mediterranean kala-azar may respond to 10–15 doses of stibogluconate (one per day), the disease in Kenya, Sudan, and India requires at least 30 days of treatment. With incomplete response or relapse, the treatment should be repeated for up to 60 days. Failure of stibogluconate or liposomal amphotericin B should lead to use of pentamidine. Other drugs under evaluation individually or in combination with antimony, pentamidine, or amphotericin B are allopurinol, human gamma interferon, atovaquone, and parenteral paromomycin (aminosidine). In Bihar, India, where the infection is becoming increasingly unresponsive to antimonials (currently 40%), liposomal amphotericin B is usually effective. Miltefosine, a new oral treatment under evaluation, shows high cure rates at a dosage of 100–150 mg daily for 4 weeks. Gastrointestinal side effects are frequent; the drug is contraindicated in pregnancy. It is not available in the USA.

Without treatment, the fatality rate reaches 90%. Early diagnosis and treatment reduces mortality to 2–5%. Relapses (up to 10% in India and 30% in Kenya) are most likely to occur within 6 months after completion of treatment.

Post-kala azar dermal leishmaniasis may appear after apparent cure in the Indian subcontinent and east Africa. It may simulate leprosy, as multiple hypopigmented macules or nodules develop on preexisting lesions. Erythematous patches may appear on the face. Leishmaniae are present in the skin. Antimony treatment should be tried but is often ineffective.

Chiurillo MA et al: Detection of Leishmania causing visceral leishmaniasis in the Old and New Worlds by a polymerase chain reaction assay based on telomeric sequences. Am J Trop Med Hyg 2001;65:573. [PMID: 11716117]

Murray HW: Clinical and experimental advances in treatment of visceral leishmaniasis. Antimicrob Agents Chemother 2001;45:2185. [PMID: 11451673]

Pintado V et al: HIV-associated visceral leishmaniasis. Clin Microbiol Infect 2001;7:291. [PMID: 11442562]

2. Cutaneous Leishmaniasis

Cutaneous swellings appear 2 weeks to several months after sand fly bites and can be single or multiple. Depending on the leishmanial species and host immune response, lesions begin as small papules and develop into nonulcerated dry plaques or large encrusted ulcers with well-demarcated raised and indurated margins. Satellite lesions may be present. The lesions are painless unless secondarily infected. Local lymph nodes may be enlarged. Systemic symptoms are rare, but a low-grade fever of short duration may be present at the onset. For most species, healing usually occurs spontaneously in months to 1–3 years, starting with central granulation tissue that spreads peripherally. Pyogenic complications may be followed by lymphangitis or erysipelas. Contraction of scars can cause deformities and disfigurement, especially if lesions are on the face.

Definitive diagnosis is made by identification of the organisms (see above). Microscopic examination of skin scrapings has limited sensitivity, particularly in chronic infections. Where available, species identification should be done by molecular methods. The skin test becomes positive within 3 months and remains positive for life; false positives occur. Serologic tests are unreliable; they are variably positive in 4–6 weeks, and cross-reactions occur. A PCR technique using boiled dermal scrapings has a sensitivity and specificity of 100% in New World cutaneous leishmaniasis.

The differential diagnosis includes tuberculosis, leprosy, fungal infections, yaws, syphilis, neoplasms, and sarcoidosis.

Diffuse cutaneous leishmaniasis is caused by the *L mexicana* complex and *L aethiopica*. Nonulcerating lesions resembling lepromatous leprosy occur over the entire body. The skin test is negative, but amastigotes are abundant. In spite of repeated doses of antimony, pentamidine, or amphotericin, cures are rare.

Old World Cutaneous Leishmaniasis

Agents of Old World cutaneous leishmaniasis are as follows:

(1) *L tropica* is the agent responsible for an urban infection of dogs and humans. It is found in the Middle East, northwestern India, East Africa, central Asian area of the former Soviet Union, Afghanistan, Pakistan, Turkey, Armenia, Greece, and southern France and Italy. The incubation period is 2 months or longer, and healing is complete in 1–2 years. The lesions of *L tropica* infection tend to be single and dry, to ulcerate slowly or not at all, and to persist for a year or longer. **Leishmaniasis recidivans** is a relapsing form of *L tropica* infection in which the primary lesion nearly heals, lateral spread with central healing follows, and scarring can be extensive; it is associated with hypersensitivity and a strongly positive skin test but scarce amastigotes. Visceral involvement by *L tropica* has been reported rarely (including after troop exposure in Operation Desert Storm) and is relatively resistant to antimony treatment.

(2) *L major* infection causes lesions in dry or desert rural areas and is primarily a disease of desert rodents. Human disease occurs in the Middle East, central Asian area of the former Soviet Union, Arabian peninsula, Afghanistan, and Africa (North, East, and sub-Saharan Africa from Senegal to Sudan and Kenya). The lesions are characterized by multiple, wet, rapidly ulcerating sores with crusting. Spontaneous healing is generally complete in 6–12 months.

(3) *L aethiopica* infection occurs in the Ethiopian and Kenyan highlands. Ulceration is rare; spontaneous healing is slow over several years. An uncommon complication is diffuse cutaneous leishmaniasis, an anergic form with nodular lesions and high parasite count. Treatment has sometimes been successful with sodium stibogluconate plus recombinant interferon gamma.

(4) *L donovani* sometimes causes cutaneous disease with visceral manifestations.

Treatment: Old World leishmaniasis, especially in the Middle East, is generally self-healing in about 6 months and does not metastasize to the mucosa. Thus, it may be justified to withhold treatment if the lesions are small, in an unobtrusive place, and appear to be healing. Parenteral sodium stibogluconate (20–28 days) should be used to treat patients with large or multiple lesions or if the lesions are on cosmetically or functionally important areas (eg, the wrist). Complete healing may not be evident until weeks after the first or second course of treatment. Amphotericin B desoxycholate and pentamidine are used for failures. Pentamidine is often effective against *L aethiopica* lesions and ketoconazole (400–600 mg/d for 4–6 weeks) against *L major* and *L (V) panamensis*. Other treatments for less severe disease are physical measures (local cryotherapy or heat therapy, electrocoagulation, surgical removal) and intralesional injection of sodium stibogluconate. Paromomycin ointment may also be effective against *L tropica*.

New World Cutaneous Leishmaniasis

Agents of New World cutaneous leishmaniasis are as follows:

(1) The *L mexicana* complex: *L mexicana* (Texas—about 20 locally acquired human infections have been reported, Oklahoma, Arizona, Mexico, Central America); *L amazonensis* (Amazonian basin, Venezuela, Panama, Trinidad); *L chagasi* (Central and South America); other species (Venezuela and Dominican Republic).

(2) The leishmania (viannia) group: *L braziliensis* (Central and South America); *L panamensis* (Central

America and northeastern South America); and *L guyanensis* (South America).

L mexicana and *L braziliensis* infections generally result from forest-related activities or from residence in dwellings situated near forests. *P panamensis* is also found in drier habitats. In parts of South America, several leishmania species are now transmitted in domestic environments.

Most New World cutaneous lesions are ulcers, but vegetative, verrucous, or nodular lesions may occur also. *L mexicana* ("chiclero's ulcer") in the Yucatan and Central America produces destructive lesions on the ear cartilage. Up to 80% of *L braziliensis* cutaneous lesions progress to espundia (see below); some *L braziliensis* complex strains also show a chain of palpable local lymph nodes, and some *L mexicana* and South American strains can cause diffuse cutaneous leishmaniasis.

Treatment: In New World *L mexicana* infections from Mexico and Central America, solitary nodules or ulcers in inconspicuous sites generally will heal spontaneously, but metronidazole, 750 mg three times daily for 10 days, can be given. Lesions on the ear, face, or hands should be treated with sodium stibogluconate but usually require only a 12- to 14-day course. Under evaluation are ketoconazole, itraconazole, liposome-encapsulated compounds, combined sodium stibogluconate and allopurinol, and topically applied paromomycin. Cutaneous lesions acquired in regions of mucocutaneous leishmaniasis may be due to *L braziliensis* or *L panamensis* and should be treated with a full course of sodium stibogluconate.

Salman SM et al: Cutaneous leishmaniasis: clinical features and diagnosis. Clin Dermatol 1999;17:291. [PMID: 10384868] (Entire issue devoted to leishmaniasis.)

Soto J et al: Treatment of American cutaneous leishmaniasis with miltefosine, an oral agent. Clin Infect Dis 2001;33:E57. [PMID: 11528586]

Vardy D et al: Efficacious topical treatment for human cutaneous leishmaniasis with ethanolic lipid amphotericin B. Trans R Soc Trop Med Hyg 2001;95:184. [PMID: 11355557]

3. Mucocutaneous Leishmaniasis (Espundia)

Mucocutaneous leishmaniasis occurs in lowland forest areas and is caused by the leishmania (viannia) group of organisms, usually by *L (V) braziliensis* (Central and South America; most cases are in Brazil, Bolivia, and Peru) and rarely by *L (V) panamensis* (Central and northeastern South America) or *L (V) peruviana* (Peru). The initial lesion, single or multiple, is on exposed skin; at first it is papular (can be pruriginous or painful), then nodular, and later may ulcerate or become wart-like or papillomatous. Local healing follows, with scarring within several months to a year. Subsequent naso-oral involvement occurs in a small proportion of patients either by direct extension or, more often, metastatically to the mucosa. It may ap-

pear concurrently with the initial lesion, shortly after healing, or after many years. The mucosa of the anterior part of the nasal septum is generally the first area to be involved. Extensive destruction of the soft tissues and cartilage of the nose, oral cavity, and lips may follow and may extend to the larynx and pharynx. Secondary bacterial infection is common. Regional lymphangitis, lymphadenitis, fever, weight loss, keratitis, and anemia may be present.

Although they are difficult to find, diagnosis is by detecting amastigotes in scrapings, biopsy impressions or histologic sections, or aspirated tissue fluid. Also, the organism grows with difficulty in culture or after inoculation of hamsters; if positive, speciation should be attempted. The leishmanin skin test is useful if it produces a fully developed papule in 2–3 days that disappears after a week. Standard serologic tests are often not useful; a direct agglutination for IgM antibodies may become positive in 4–6 weeks and subsequently an IgG test. The main considerations in the differential diagnosis are paracoccidioidomycosis and other fungal infections, polymorphic reticulosis, Wegener's granulomatosis, lymphoma, and nasopharyngeal carcinoma, yaws, syphilis, and sarcoidosis.

Treatment

Treatment of this condition is difficult; failure rates are high in severe disease even when a full course (28 days) of sodium stibogluconate treatment is used (see above). If repeated and extended antimony treatment fails, amphotericin B desoxycholate or pentamidine is used. Under evaluation are the liposomal formulations of amphotericin B and combined antimony and gamma interferon treatment. Corticosteroids may be needed to control local inflammation due to release of antigens. Antibiotics are usually needed to treat associated bacterial or fungal infections. Successful treatment was recently reported for pentoxifylline plus a pentavalent antimonial drug.

Lessa HA et al: Successful treatment of refractory mucosal leishmaniasis with pentoxifylline plus antimony. Am J Trop Med Hyg 2001;65:87. [PMID: 11508396]

MALARIA

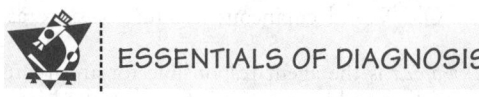

ESSENTIALS OF DIAGNOSIS

- *History of exposure in a malaria-endemic area.*
- *Periodic attacks of sequential chills, fever, and sweating.*
- *Headache, myalgia, splenomegaly; anemia, leukopenia.*
- *Characteristic parasites in erythrocytes, identified in thick or thin blood films.*

• Complications of falciparum malaria: Cerebral findings (mental disturbances, neurologic signs, convulsions), hemolytic anemia, hyperpyrexia, secretory diarrhea or dysentery, dark urine, anuria.

General Considerations

Four species of the genus plasmodium are responsible for human malaria: P vivax, P malariae, P ovale, and P falciparum. Although the disease has been eradicated from most temperate zone countries, it continues to be endemic in many parts of the tropics and subtropics, and imported cases occur in the USA and other countries free of transmission. Malaria is present in parts of Mexico, Haiti, Dominican Republic, Central and South America, Africa, the Middle East, the Indian subcontinent, Southeast Asia, China, and Oceania. P vivax and P falciparum are responsible for most infections and are found throughout the malarious regions; P falciparum is the predominant species in Africa and the only plasmodium in Haiti and the Dominican Republic. P malariae is also widely distributed but is less common. P ovale, although generally rare, seems to replace P vivax in West Africa. P vivax infection is uncommon among blacks because their red blood cells do not have the Duffy factor surface antigen. Annually worldwide, malaria causes clinical illness in about 300 million people and results in 1.5–2.7 million deaths; its greatest impact is on young children, particularly in sub-Saharan Africa. An estimated 30,000 travelers from the developed world are infected yearly with malaria, and several hundred die. The USA experiences each year 1000 or more imported infections with different species; a few cases of locally acquired, mosquito-transmitted infection from an imported case; and an average of four deaths from falciparum malaria. Most of the imported infections are acquired in tropical Africa.

Malaria is transmitted from human to human by the bite of infected female anopheles mosquitoes. Congenital transmission and acquisition by blood transfusion also occurs. Other than the mosquito, there are no animal reservoirs for human malaria.

The mosquito becomes infected by ingesting blood containing the sexual forms of the parasite (micro- and macrogametocytes). After a developmental phase in the mosquito, sporozoites in the salivary glands are inoculated into humans when the mosquito next feeds. The first stage of development in humans, the exoerythrocytic stage, takes place in the liver. In all four infections, the sporozoites invade hepatocytes to mature as tissue schizonts. However, in P vivax and P ovale infections only—but not in induced infections with these parasites—some sporozoites enter hepatocytes to become dormant hypnozoites; activation of the hypnozoites 6–8 months later results in a primary infection or in relapse. When liver schizonts escape from the liver into the bloodstream, they invade red

blood cells, multiply, and 48 hours later (or 72 with P malariae) cause the red cells to rupture, releasing a new crop of parasites (merozoites). Within the bloodstream, this cycle of invasion, multiplication, and red cell rupture may be repeated many times.

In P falciparum and P malariae malaria, the liver infection ceases spontaneously in less than 4 weeks; thereafter, multiplication is confined to the red cells. Thus, 4 weeks after departure from an endemic area, treatment that eliminates these species from the red cells will cure the infection. Cure of P vivax and P ovale malaria, however, requires treatment to eradicate infection from both red cells and liver hypnozoites.

The incubation period after exposure or after stopping chemoprophylaxis is, for P falciparum, approximately 12 days (range: 9–60 days); for P vivax and P ovale, 14 days (range: 8–27 days [initial attacks for some temperate strains may not occur for up to 8 months]); and for P malariae, 30 days (range: 16–60 days). Untreated P falciparum infections can persist for up to 1.5 years but usually end in 6–8 months; P vivax and P ovale infections persist for as long as 5 years; and P malariae infections have lasted for as long as 50 years. Protective immunity results from infection but decays after several years if reinfection does not occur.

Clinical Findings

A. SYMPTOMS AND SIGNS

Typical malarial attacks show sequentially, over 4–6 hours, shaking chills (the cold stage); fever (the hot stage) to 41 °C or higher; and marked diaphoresis (the sweating stage). Associated symptoms may include fatigue, headache, dizziness, gastrointestinal symptoms (anorexia, nausea, slight diarrhea, vomiting, abdominal cramps), myalgia, arthralgia, backache, and dry cough. These symptoms appear to be due in large part to release of tissue necrosis factor and other cytokines during schizogony.

Either from the onset or with progression of the disease, the attacks may show an every-other-day (tertian) periodicity in vivax, ovale, or falciparum malaria or an every-third-day (quartan) periodicity in malariae malaria. Splenomegaly usually appears when acute symptoms have continued for 4 or more days; the liver is frequently mildly enlarged. The patient may be tired between attacks but otherwise feels well. After this primary episode, recurrences are common, each separated by a latent period.

Because of its frequent and severe complications, P falciparum is the more serious infection and causes the most deaths, sometimes within 24 hours. In severe falciparum infections, red blood cell parasitemia is higher than 3–5%. Severe disease results in part from intense sequestration and cytoadherence of parasitized red cells in capillaries and postcapillary venules. Complications include (1) cerebral malaria with edema (headache, mental disturbances, neurologic signs, retinal hemorrhages, convulsions, delirium, coma); (2) hyperpyrexia;

(3) hemolytic anemia; (4) noncardiogenic pulmonary edema; (5) acute tubular necrosis and renal failure—rarely, this is associated with blackwater fever (dark urine), which most commonly is due to severe hemolysis following quinine treatment; (6) acute hepatopathy, with centrilobular necrosis and jaundice; (7) hypoglycemia; (8) cardiac dysrhythmias; (9) gastrointestinal syndromes (including secretory diarrhea and dysentery); (10) lactic acidosis; and (11) water and electrolyte imbalance. The prognosis is poor if more than 20% of infected red cells contain mature parasites or if more than 5% of neutrophils contain pigment. Gram-negative bacteremia may contribute to death.

Immunologic disorders resulting from chronic infection are tropical splenomegaly and nephrotic syndrome (the latter due to *P malariae* only). Malaria infections do not appear to act as an opportunistic infection in AIDS patients, with the possible exception of malaria infection in pregnancy.

B. LABORATORY FINDINGS

The thick and thin blood film, dehemoglobinized and Giemsa-stained or Wright-stained, is the mainstay of diagnosis. Blood should be examined at 8-hour intervals for 3 days, during and between febrile spikes. The newly described quantitative buffy coat method to detect parasitemia is slightly more sensitive than thick smears, but it is expensive and requires fluorescent microscopy.

The number of red cells infected seldom exceeds 2% of the total cells. During paroxysms, there may be transient leukocytosis; leukopenia develops subsequently, with a relative increase in large mononuclear cells. In severe falciparum malaria, parasitemia may reach 30% or higher; mature asexual forms disappear (sequestered in the microcirculation); hepatic function tests often become abnormal; and hemolytic jaundice, thrombocytopenia, and marked anemia with reticulocytosis may develop.

Serologic tests (ELISA and others) are not commonly used in the diagnosis of acute attacks. Antibody becomes detectable only 8–10 days after onset of symptoms—too late to be of use; also, because antibody persists for 10 or more years, it does not distinguish between current and past infection. In rare instances, however, serology may be useful in the differential diagnosis of chronic fevers. Available for field diagnosis for falciparum malaria only is a rapid and simply accomplished dipstick antigen capture assay; sensitivity and specificity range between 75% and 95%. Two fluorescent microscopy methods have high sensitivity, but they do not distinguish between parasitic species. A polymerase chain reaction method is highly specific and sensitive but requires specialized laboratory methods.

Differential Diagnosis

Uncomplicated malaria must be distinguished from a variety of other causes of fever, splenomegaly, anemia,

or hepatomegaly. Often considered are influenza, urinary tract infections, typhoid fever, infectious hepatitis, dengue, kala azar, amebic liver abscess, leptospirosis, and relapsing fever. Malaria complications can mimic many diseases.

Prevention

Prevention is based on evaluating the risk of exposure to infection, preventing mosquito bites, and chemoprophylaxis. Advice should also be given regarding medical care if malaria-like symptoms occur while traveling. All persons who will be exposed should receive chemoprophylaxis. Travelers should be advised that in spite of all precautions, no prophylactic regimen gives complete protection. Fever or other symptoms can develop in malaria as early as 8 days (range: 8–60 days) after exposure or stopping prophylaxis; for *P vivax* infections, the delay may be up to 8–12 months.

A. CONSULTATIVE RESOURCES REGARDING RISKS, CHEMOPROPHYLAXIS, AND TREATMENT

Consultation with a center working on malaria may be necessary to obtain up-to-date information on malaria treatment and risk and prophylaxis by country. A World Health internet source is http://www.who.int/ith/. A source of information and advice in the USA is the Malarial Branch, Centers for Disease Control and Prevention (CDC), Atlanta, Georgia. For recorded information on prophylaxis: fax response, 888-232-3299; Internet, http://www.cdc.gov (choose the Travelers' Health category). For additional information on prophylaxis or for management of acute attacks, phone 770-488-7788; after business hours, 404-639-2888. See also CDC and WHO references, below.

B. RISK OF EXPOSURE

The risk of exposure to mosquitoes may be difficult to estimate since it varies by climate, rainy season, altitude, degree of mosquito control in urban versus rural areas, and according to whether exposure will occur during the time malaria mosquitoes are biting. Travel to urban areas of Central and South America and Southeast Asia entails minimal risk, and chemoprophylaxis is often not recommended for travelers to these areas.

C. PREVENTING MOSQUITO BITES

When out of doors between dusk and dawn (the primary feeding time for anopheles mosquitoes), protective measures should be used: Clothing should cover most of the body, and deet (*N,N*-diethyl-3-methylbenzamide) mosquito repellent should be applied to exposed areas every 3–4 hours. To minimize the slight risk of toxic encephalopathy from deet, it should be applied sparingly and only to exposed skin and outer clothing; avoid high concentrations (over 30%) of the repellent; avoid inhalation and contamination of eyes, mouth, wounds, or irritated skin; and wash skin after coming indoors. The Ultrathon formulation provides a reduced concentration of deet (33%) with extended protection (12 hours). Living quarters should preferably be air-conditioned or be well screened; if screening is not available, mosquito bed nets should be used at night, preferably ones impregnated every 6 months with permethrin (0.2 g/m²) (Permonone). To kill mosquitoes in living quarters, use an antimosquito pyrethrum-containing spray or a powdered insecticide dispenser of pyrethroid tablets or burn pyrethroid mosquito coils. Garments can also be impregnated (sprayed or soaked) with permethrin, which repels for several weeks.

D. Advice Regarding Treatment if Malaria-Like Febrile Symptoms Occur While Traveling

The traveler should insist that blood smears be done and, if negative, repeated at intervals. If malaria is suspected but blood smears cannot be done, malaria treatment should be started empirically.

Emergency ("standby") self-treatment is a recognized resource for individuals who may be exposed to malaria and for whom medical attention cannot be provided expeditiously. Such persons are advised beforehand to carry medication for self-treatment if they develop fever or flu-like symptoms. However, *it is imperative that medical follow-up be sought promptly.* Patients should be given written instructions. The choice among available drugs depends on the anticipated type of exposure to drug-resistant *P falciparum* (see above for areas of resistance and Table 35–3 for dosages): (1) in chloroquine-sensitive areas, for persons who have taken no prophylaxis, use the chloroquine 3-day course of treatment; (2) in chloroquine-resistant areas without Fansidar resistance, use Fansidar (three tablets once only); or (3) in areas with Fansidar resistance, use Malarone (atovaquone plus proguanil) (four tablets daily for 3 days). Mefloquine, halofantrine, and quinine are not recommended because of their toxicity.

Drugs Used in Chemoprophylaxis & Treatment
(Tables 35–2 and 35–3)

A. Drug Classification

By chemical groups, some of the major antimalarial drugs are as follows: **4-aminoquinolines**—chloroquine, hydroxychloroquine, amodiaquine;* **diaminopyrimidines**—pyrimethamine, trimethoprim; **biguanides**—proguanil† (chlorguanide,* chlorproguanil*); **8-aminoquinolines**—primaquine; **cinchona alkaloids**—quinine, quinidine; **sulfonamides**—sulfadoxine, sulfadiazine, sulfamethoxazole; **sulfones**—dapsone; **4-quinoline-carbinolamines**—mefloquine; and **antibiotics**—tetracycline, doxycycline, clindamycin; and others—halofantrine,* artemisinin (qinghaosu)* and its derivatives, and atovaquone.† Pyrimethamine

and proguanil are known as **antifolates,** since they inhibit dihydrofolate reductase of plasmodia. **Drug combinations** used to treat *P falciparum* malaria resistant to chloroquine include Fansidar (pyrimethamine plus sulfadoxine), Maloprim (pyrimethamine plus dapsone), and Malarone (atovaquone plus proguanil). Another drug combination, chloroquine combined with proguanil, has been used in prophylaxis in sub-Saharan Africa but is no longer recommended by the Centers for Disease Control and Prevention.

The effectiveness of antimalarial drugs differs with different species of the parasite and with different stages of the life cycle. Drugs that act in the liver to eliminate developing exoerythrocytic schizonts or latent hypnozoites are called **tissue schizonticides** (primaquine). Those that act on blood schizonts are **blood schizonticides** or **suppressive agents** (eg, chloroquine, amodiaquine, proguanil, pyrimethamine, mefloquine, quinine, quinidine, halofantrine, artemisinin and its derivatives) and atovaquone. **Gametocides** are drugs that prevent infection of mosquitoes by destroying gametocytes in the blood (eg, primaquine for *P falciparum* and chloroquine for *P vivax, P malariae,* and *P ovale*). **Sporonticidal** agents are drugs that render gametocytes noninfective in the mosquito (eg, pyrimethamine, proguanil).

None of the drugs prevent infection (ie, are true **causal prophylactic drugs**). However, proguanil, chlorproguanil, atovaquone and primaquine—and to some extent the antibiotics—prevent maturation of the early *P falciparum*. Blood schizonticides destroy circulating plasmodia and thus prevent malarial attacks (**suppressive prophylaxis**) and, when given weekly for 4 weeks after departure from the endemic area, result in cure of *P falciparum* and *P malariae* infections. Only primaquine destroys the hypnozoites of *P vivax* and *P ovale* and, when given with a blood schizonticide, prevents relapse from infection with these parasites and thus effects **radical cure (terminal prophylaxis).**

B. Parasite Resistance to Drugs

1. *P falciparum* **resistance—**

a. Chloroquine— Strains of *P falciparum* resistant to chloroquine have been confirmed or are probably present in all malarious areas except Haiti, the Dominican Republic, rural areas of Mexico, Central America north and west of the Panama Canal, North Africa, and most of the Middle East (resistance is present, however, in Oman, Yemen, and Iran). Countries with resistance in southern and eastern Africa are Kenya, Malawi, Mozambique, Tanzania, Uganda, and South Africa. In regions of resistance, some strains of *P falciparum* are only partially resistant to the drug, as manifested by temporary subsidence of symptoms and transient decrease or disappearance in asexual parasitemia, followed by return of both after several days to weeks.

b. Pyrimethamine-sulfadoxine (Fansidar)— Fansidar resistance is present at high levels in South-

---

*Not available in the USA but available in some countries.
†Available in the USA but approved for antimalarial use only as the combination drug atovaquone/proguanil (Malarone).

Table 35–2. Prevention of malaria in nonimmune travelers.[1]

TO PREVENT ATTACKS OF ALL FORMS OF MALARIA
AND TO ERADICATE *P FALCIPARUM* AND *P MALARIAE* INFECTIONS[2,3,4]

REGIONS WITH CHLOROQUINE-SENSITIVE *P FALCIPARUM* MALARIA: Central America west of the Panama Canal, the Caribbean, Mexico, and parts of the Middle East and China.

Chloroquine[5]

Dose: Chloroquine phosphate, 500 mg salt (300 mg base) weekly. Give a single dose of chloroquine weekly starting 1 week before entering the endemic area, while there, and for 4 weeks after leaving.

REGIONS WITH CHLOROQUINE-RESISTANT *P FALCIPARUM* MALARIA: All other regions of the world; the frequency and intensity of resistance vary by region.

Mefloquine (preferred method)[6]

Dose: one 250-mg tablet salt (228 mg base) weekly. Give a single dose of mefloquine weekly starting 3 weeks before entering the endemic area, while there, and for 4 weeks after leaving.

Malarone (atovaquone [250 mg] combined with proguanil [100 mg] [alternative method][7]

Dose: One tablet daily. Give one tablet the day before entering the endemic area, daily while there, and daily for 1 week after leaving.

Doxycycline (alternative method)[8]

Dose: 100 mg daily. Give the daily dose for 2 days before entering the endemic area, while there, and for 4 weeks after leaving.

TO ERADICATE *P VIVAX* AND *P OVALE* INFECTIONS[2]

Primaquine[9]

Start primaquine only after returning home, during the last 2 weeks of chemoprophylaxis. Dose: 26.3 mg salt (15 mg base) daily for 14 days. An alternative regimen in regions where chloroquine is effective in prophylaxis is chloroquine phosphate, 500 mg (salt), plus primaquine phosphate 78.9 mg (salt), weekly for 8 weeks.

---

[1]See text for additional information on drug cautions, contraindications, and side effects. For additional information on prophylaxis for specific countries, see the references or call the Centers for Disease Control and Prevention, Atlanta, GA at 770-488-7788 (for fax response: 888-232-3299). The information is also available on the Internet at http://www.cdc.gov (choose the Traveler's Health category).

[2]The blood schizonticides (chloroquine, mefloquine, Malarone, and doxycycline), when taken for 4 weeks (7 days for Malarone) after leaving the endemic area, are curative for sensitive *P falciparum* and *P malariae* infections; primaquine, however, is needed to eradicate the persistent liver stages of *P vivax* and *P ovale*.

[3]A test dose of the selected prophylactic drug should be given before departure to allow for changing to an alternative drug in the event of significant side effects: chloroquine (once weekly for 2 weeks), Malarone (daily for 2 days), doxycycline (daily for 2 days), mefloquine (weekly for 3 weeks). Side effects from mefloquine sometimes do not appear until after the third or later doses.

[4]See text for standby drugs for emergency self-treatment of presumptive malaria; such drugs should be used only when a physician is not immediately available. It is imperative, however, that medical follow-up be sought promptly.

[5]Chloroquine and proguanil can be used by pregnant women.

[6]Because of the high frequency of resistance, mefloquine should not be used in Thailand or adjacent countries; it is now the preferred drug for sub-Saharan Africa. Mefloquine is not recommended in the first trimester of pregnancy or under some other conditions (see text).

[7]Malarone recently became available in the USA. It eradicates falciparum infections after 1 week of postexposure treatment; its efficacy against *P malariae*, however, is undetermined. To eradicate *P vivax* and *P ovale* infections, a course of primaquine is needed, which should be started early in the final week of Malarone treatment. Malarone has not been shown to be safe in pregnancy.

[8]Doxycycline is used in Thailand and adjacent countries and in other regions by persons who cannot tolerate mefloquine or Malarone. It is contraindicated in pregnant women. Take with evening meals. See text for side effects.

[9]Primaquine is indicated only for persons who have had a high probability of exposure to *P vivax* or *P ovale* (see text), and who have not taken the drug for daily prophylaxis. The drug should be taken with food and is contraindicated in pregnancy. Before use, patients must be screened for glucose-6-phosphate dehydrogenase deficiency.

Table 35–3. Treatment of malaria in nonimmune adult populations.

Treatment[1] of Infection With All Species (Except Chloroquine-Resistant *P falciparum*)	Treatment[1] of Infection With Chloroquine-Resistant *P falciparum* Strains
Oral treatment of *P falciparum*[2] or *P malariae* infection Chloroquine phosphate, 1 g (salt)[3,4] as initial dose, then 0.5 g at 6, 24, and 48 hours. **Oral treatment of *P vivax*[5] or *P ovale* infection** Chloroquine[3,4] as above followed by 0.5 g on days 10 and 17 plus primaquine phosphate, 26.3 mg (salt)[3,4] daily for 14 days starting about day 4. **Parenteral treatment of severe attacks** Quinine dihydrochloride[6] or quinidine gluconate.[7] Start oral chloroquine therapy as soon as possible; follow with primaquine if needed.[4]	**Oral treatment** Quinine sulfate, 10 mg/kg 3 times daily for 3–7 days,[8] plus one of the following: (1) doxycycline,[9] 100 mg twice daily for 7 days; (2) clindamycin,[9] 900 mg 3 times daily for 5 days; (3) pyrimethamine, 25 mg twice daily for 3 days, and sulfadiazine, 500 mg 4 times daily for 5 days; (4) tetracycline,[9] 250–500 mg 4 times daily for 7 days; (5) once only, pyrimethamine, 75 mg, and sulfadoxine, 1500 mg (= 3 tablets of Fansidar[10]). or Mefloquine,[11] 750 mg followed after 12 hours by 500 mg.

[1]See text for cautions, contraindications, and side effects of each drug. For advice on management, call the Centers for Disease Control and Prevention (CDC), Atlanta, GA (770-488-7760).

[2]In falciparum malaria, if the patient has not shown a clinical response to chloroquine (48–72 hours for mild infections, 24 hours for severe ones), parasitic resistance to chloroquine should be considered. Chloroquine should be stopped and treatment started with oral quinine plus doxycycline, mefloquine, malarone, or halofantrine.

[3]500 mg chloroquine phosphate = 300 mg base; 26.3 mg of primaquine = 15 mg base.

[4]Chloroquine alone is curative for infection with sensitive strains of *P falciparum* and for *P malariae*, but primaquine is needed to eradicate the persistent liver stages of *P vivax* and *P ovale*. Start primaquine after the patient has recovered from the acute illness; continue chloroquine weekly during primaquine therapy. Patients should be screened for glucose-6-phosphate dehydrogenase deficiency before use of primaquine. An alternative mode for primaquine therapy is combined primaquine, 78.9 mg (salt), and chloroquine, 0.5 g (salt), weekly for 8 weeks.

[5]Strains of *P vivax* resistant to chloroquine have appeared in some regions (see text). For their treatment, give quinine (plus doxycycline or Fansidar), mefloquine, malarone or halofantrine as used to treat *P falciparum* resistant to chloroquine.

[6]Quinine dihydrochloride. As a loading dose, give 20 mg/kg (salt) in 500 mL of 5% glucose solution intravenously slowly over 4 hours; repeat using 10 mg/kg every 8 hours until oral therapy is possible (maximum, 1800 mg/d). If more than 48 hours of parenteral treatment is required, some authorities reduce the quinine dose by one-third to one-half. Blood pressure and ECG should be monitored constantly to detect arrhythmias or hypotension. As severe hypoglycemia may occur, blood glucose levels should be monitored. Extreme caution is required in treating patients with quinine who previously have been taking mefloquine in prophylaxis. In the USA, quinine dihydrochloride is no longer available.

[7]When parenteral quinine is unavailable (as in the USA), quinidine gluconate can be used, administered as a continuous infusion. A loading dose of 10 mg/kg (salt) (maximum, 600 mg) is diluted in 300 mL of normal saline and administered over 1–2 hours, followed by 0.02 mg/kg/min (maximum, 10 mg/kg every 8 hours) by continuous infusion until oral quinine therapy is possible. If more than 48 hours of parenteral treament is required, some authorities reduce the quinidine dose by one-third to one-half. Fluid status, glucose, blood pressure, and ECG should be closely monitored; widening of the QRS interval or lengthening of the QT interval requires discontinuation.

(continued)

east Asia. It is also reported in parts of the Indian subcontinent, the Amazon basin, sub-Saharan Africa, and Oceania. Fansidar shows no cross-resistance with other antimalarial drugs.

c. Pyrimethamine or proguanil—Resistance to either of these drugs when used alone is common in most endemic areas, but the degree and distribution are not accurately known.

d. Mefloquine—Sporadic or low levels of mefloquine resistance have been reported from Southeast and southern Asia and parts of Africa, South America, the Middle East, and Oceania. Along the Thai-Burmese and Thai-Cambodian borders, however, the frequency reaches 30–60%.

e. Quinine and quinidine—Variable degrees of decreased responsiveness have been reported rarely in Southeast Asia (particularly in the border regions of Thailand) and Oceania and apparently in sub-Saharan Africa and Brazil.

f. Halofantrine—A high degree of resistance has been reported in eastern Thailand. Strains resistant to halofantrine are sometimes resistant to mefloquine as well.

g. Malarone—Rare instances of *P falciparum* resistance to Malarone have been reported worldwide.

h. Artemisinin derivatives—There are no known artemisinin-resistant *P falciparum* strains.

2. *P vivax* resistance—

a. Antifolates—Resistance of *P vivax* blood schizonts to pyrimethamine and proguanil, including the pyrimethamine-containing drugs Fansidar and Malo-

Table 35–3. Treatment of malaria in nonimmune adult populations. (continued)

Treatment[1] of Infection With All Species (Except Chloroquine-Resistant *P falciparum*)	Treatment[1] of Infection With Chloroquine-Resistant *P falciparum* Strains
or	or
Parenteral artesunate,[13] artemether,[13] or chloroquine[14] until the patient can take oral chloroquine. Follow with primaquine if the infection is due to–or if there is concurrent infection with–*P vivax* or *P ovale*.	Malarone[9] two tablets twice daily with food for 3 days (each tablet contains atovaquone [250 mg] and proguanil [100 mg])
	or
	Atovaquone/doxycycline, 500 mg/100 mg, twice daily for 3 days
	or
	Artesunate,[13] 4 mg/kg/d for 3 days followed by mefloquine[11] (750 mg followed by 500 mg 12 hours later)
	or
	Halofantrine[12]
	Parenteral treatment of severe attacks Quinine dihydrochloride[6] or quinidine gluconate[7] plus intravenous doxycycline or clindamycin. Start oral therapy with quinine sulfate plus the second drug as soon as possible to complete 7 days of treatment.
	or
	Artemether,[13] or artesunate[13]; followed by mefloquine[11] (750 mg followed by 500 mg 12 hours later)

[8]Although quinine sulfate is usually given for 3 days, it should be continued for 7 days in patients who acquired infections in Southeast Asia and South America, where diminished responsiveness to quinine has been noted.

[9]Contraindicated in pregnant women.

[10]Fansidar should not be used for infections acquired in Southeast Asia, the Amazon Basin, Bangladesh, or Oceania.

[11]Serious side effects are rare. See text for cautions and contraindications. In the USA, a 250 mg tablet of mefloquine contains 228 mg of base; outside the USA, each 275 mg tablet contains 250 mg of base. Mefloquine is hazardous with quinine, quinidine, or halofantrine.

[12]The dosage is 500 mg (salt) every 6 hours for three doses and repeat in 1 week. A possible contraindication is the presence of cardiac conduction abnormalities. Do not use if mefloquine has

been taken in previous 2–3 weeks or with recent use of quinine or quinidine. Not available in the USA.

[13]Not available in the USA. Give artesunate intravenously (2.4 mg/kg on the first day, followed by 1.2 mg/kg daily) or artemether intramuscularly (3.2 mg/kg on the first day, followed by 1.6 mg/kg daily); continue the drug for a minimum of 3 days until the patient can start oral therapy. If parenteral treatment is not available, artemisinin rectal suppositories are being evaluated (40 mg/kg loading dose, then 20 mg/kg at 24, 48, and 72 hours) followed by oral medication.

[14]Give parenteral chloroquine (1) preferably intravenously, 10 mg base/kg in isotonic fluid by constant rate of infusion over 8 hours, followed by 15 mg/kg over the next 24 hours; or (2) intramuscularly or subcutaneously, 3.5 mg base/kg every 6 hours.

prim, has been reported in many areas of the world, particularly Southeast Asia.

b. Primaquine—Partial resistance of some strains of *P vivax* hepatic schizonts to primaquine has been reported in areas of Southeast Asia, (17% failure rate in Thailand), Papua New Guinea (30%), the Amazon Basin, Central America, and Somalia (43% in American military personnel). Treatment is usually successful with a higher dose (30 mg of base daily for 14 days) or a longer course (15 mg of base daily for 28 days).

c. Chloroquine—There are reports from Indonesia and Papua New Guinea of *P vivax* blood schizonts resistant to chloroquine. Decreased susceptibility is also appearing in the Solomon Islands, Myanmar, India, Thailand, Guyana, Brazil, Colombia, and Peru. Mefloquine, halofantrine, or quinine plus doxycycline appear to be effective in treatment.

3. *P ovale* and *P malariae*—These forms have not shown resistance.

C. SELECTED DRUGS: INDICATIONS, LIMITATIONS, AND ADVERSE SIDE EFFECTS

1. Chloroquine phosphate—Chloroquine is the drug of choice in chemoprophylaxis and in treatment for all forms of malaria except for infections due to resistant strains of *P falciparum* and *P vivax* (see above). However, in *P vivax* and *P ovale* infections, primaquine is needed to eradicate the persistent liver phases and thus prevent relapse.

Oral chloroquine is usually well tolerated when used for malaria prophylaxis or treatment and is safe to use in pregnancy. Transient gastrointestinal symptoms, mild headache, pruritus (especially in blacks), dizziness, blurred vision, anorexia, malaise, and urticaria may occur; taking the drug after meals or in divided twice-weekly doses may reduce these side effects.

In parenteral treatment of severely ill patients, quinine, quinidine, or the parenteral artemisinin derivatives are the preferred drugs. If none are available, chloroquine can be given intramuscularly or intravenously. However, parenteral chloroquine can be severely toxic unless it is given in small amounts (3.5 mg [base]/kg) intramuscularly every 6 hours or by slow intravenous infusion.

Rare reactions from oral chloroquine include impaired hearing, psychosis, convulsions, blood dyscrasias, skin reactions, hypotension, and hemolysis in G6PD-deficient persons. When given in large doses for prolonged periods as an anti-inflammatory agent in autoimmune diseases, chloroquine has caused ocular damage. Theoretically, a total cumulative dosage of 100 g (base) may be critical in the development of ocular, ototoxic, and myopathic effects. However, with weekly long-term administration of chloroquine, serious eye damage has not been confirmed; therefore, periodic eye examinations may no longer be indicated. Chloroquine should be used with caution in patients who have histories of liver damage, alcoholism, or neurologic or hematologic disorders. It is contraindicated in patients with psoriasis. Chloroquine suppresses the immune response to the rabies vaccine.

Certain antacids and antidiarrheal agents (kaolin, calcium carbonate, and magnesium trisilicate) should not be taken within about 4 hours before or after chloroquine administration, since they interfere with its absorption.

2. Mefloquine hydrochloride—Mefloquine, a quinoline methanol derivative, is used for oral prophylaxis and treatment of chloroquine-resistant and multidrug-resistant *P falciparum* malaria. In treatment, it is used only for mildly to moderately ill patients; severely ill patients require parenteral treatment with an alternative drug. Mefloquine has strong schizonticidal activity against the four malarial parasites (except for some *P falciparum* strains that are resistant to it)—but it is not active against *P falciparum* gametocytes or the hepatic stages of *P vivax* or *P ovale,* which require a course of primaquine. With weekly doses of mefloquine, the steady state drug level is reached in about 7 weeks, and adverse reactions thus may not appear for 3–7 weeks. The steady state interval can be reduced to 4 days, revealing adverse reactions within a week, by giving an initial course of 250 mg daily for 3 days followed by the standard weekly dose; this, however, is not standard practice.

With the lower doses used in prophylaxis, frequent (25–50%) minor and transient side effects are nausea, vomiting, epigastric pain, diarrhea, headache, dizziness, syncope, and extrasystoles. A small proportion of patients (up to 4%) experience anxiety, mood changes, insomnia, and nightmares. Severe neuropsychiatric symptoms are rare (estimated 1:10,000 to 1:1500). If prophylaxis is continued for more than a year, periodic liver function and ophthalmologic tests should be done. With treatment doses—particularly over 1000 mg—gastrointestinal symptoms and fatigue are more likely to occur, and the frequency of severe neuropsychiatric symptoms (visual disturbances, vertigo, tinnitus, insomnia, restlessness, anxiety, depression, confusion, disorientation, acute psychosis, or seizures) may be of the order of 1:1200. In experimental animals, the drug affects fertility and is teratogenic; it also causes degenerative changes in the epididymis in rats and in the lens and retina of some species. In human males, however, no deleterious effects on spermatozoa were found, and no effects have been noted in the human retina or lens. Because the drug may affect fine motor coordination and spatial orientation, caution in its use is recommended for pilots, drivers, and machinery operators.

Mefloquine is contraindicated in the presence of a cardiac conduction abnormality, liver impairment, or a history of a psychiatric or neurologic disorder, including epilepsy. Also contraindicated is concurrent administration of mefloquine with quinine, quinidine, or halofantrine. If these drugs precede use of mefloquine, 12 hours should elapse before mefloquine is started; however, because of the long elimination half-life of mefloquine (13–26 days), extreme caution is required because of arrhythmias if one of these drugs is used to treat malaria after mefloquine has been taken. Concurrent administration with tetracyclines or ampicillin results in increased mefloquine blood levels.

The development of neuropsychiatric symptoms during prophylaxis is an indication for stopping the drug. Patients taking anticonvulsant drugs (particularly valproic acid and divalproex sodium) may have breakthrough seizures. The drug is no longer contraindicated when beta-blockers and calcium channel blockers are taken. CDC has recently advised that mefloquine can be used throughout pregnancy; nevertheless, its use during the first trimester should be based on risk-benefit assessment. Women of childbearing potential who take mefloquine for antimalarial prophylaxis should preferably avoid conception for the duration of mefloquine usage and for 2 months after the last dose.

Note: The tablet formulation in the USA contains 250 mg of the salt (= 228 mg of base). However, in

Canada and many other countries, the tablets contain 274 mg of the salt (= 250 mg of base). Mefloquine should not be taken on an empty stomach and should be taken with 8 oz of water.

3. Malarone—Malarone—atovaquone 250 mg and proguanil 100 mg—is a fixed-combination oral medication recently approved in the USA for prophylaxis and treatment of multidrug-resistant falciparum malaria, *P vivax,* and *P ovale;* effectiveness against *P malariae* has not been determined. In a limited number of studies in nonimmune adults, Malarone's prophylactic efficacy was 98% against *P falciparum* and 84% against *P vivax.* In treatment, its use is currently limited to uncomplicated malaria; its effectiveness in cerebral and other forms of complicated disease remains to be determined.

Malarone's components, proguanil and atovaquone, used together, are synergistic, but failures are frequent to either component used alone. Because the agents are effective against the liver and blood stages of *P falciparum,* only 7 days of treatment are needed after leaving an endemic area, and primaquine is not required to eradicate a falciparum infection. In *P vivax* and *P ovale* infections, however, in which the components are effective only against the erythrocytic stage, primaquine must be used to eradicate the exoerythrocytic forms. Malarone supersedes Fansidar as the preferred drug for standby treatment (see above).

Malarone appears to be better tolerated than chloroquine or mefloquine. The drug is taken orally with food or milk to increase absorption of atovaquone and to reduce gastrointestinal toxicity (nausea, vomiting, epigastric discomfort). These symptoms may also be reduced by giving the drug in divided doses twice daily. Other side effects include headache, rash, and mild reversible elevations of liver aminotransferases. One case of anaphylaxis has been reported. There are insufficient data to allow Malarone to be used in pregnancy. Concomitant administration of Malarone with rifampin, tetracycline, or metoclopramide is associated with 40–50% reductions in atovaquone plasma levels.

4. Primaquine phosphate—Primaquine is used to prevent relapse by eliminating persistent liver forms of *P vivax* or *P ovale* in patients who have had an acute attack and for individuals returning from an endemic area who have probably been exposed to malaria. However, in persons with a low probability of exposure, it is preferable to avoid primaquine's potential toxicity by not giving the drug. Instead, such patients are advised to seek medical evaluation in the event of malaria-like symptoms, which usually occur within 2 years after infection but can occur up to 4 years after. Because primaquine is effective against the liver stages of all malarial parasites, it has been reevaluated recently for chemoprophylaxis when taken daily. A prophylactic efficacy of 85–95% has been shown against *P falciparum* and *P vivax* with apparent safety in long-term use, though the drug is not licensed for this indi-

cation. Primaquine is sometimes given as a single 45 mg (base) dose to eliminate *P falciparum* gametocytes.

Primaquine is generally well tolerated. Occasional side effects of the drug are gastrointestinal disturbances, headache, dizziness, or neutropenia. Primaquine should not be used in pregnancy (risk of hemolytic disease in the fetus), in autoimmune disorders, or concurrently with quinine.

All patients should be tested for glucose-6-phosphate dehydrogenase (G6PD) deficiency before therapy is begun and followed carefully during treatment; this is because primaquine may cause mild, self-limited hemolysis or marked hemolysis (pallor, weakness, abdominal pain, dark urine) or methemoglobinemia. G6PD deficiency is most common among persons of Mediterranean, African, or certain East Asian extractions. Patients with severe G6PD deficiency (< 10% residual enzyme activity) should not receive primaquine. For individuals with 10–60% residual activity, it is generally safe to give combined primaquine phosphate, 78.9 mg (45 mg base), and chloroquine phosphate, 0.5 g (0.3 g base), weekly for 8 weeks. However, for persons suspected of having the Mediterranean or Canton forms of G6PD deficiency, it may be preferable not to give primaquine but to treat attacks of malaria with chloroquine as they occur.

5. Quinine—Oral quinine sulfate in conjunction with another drug (see Table 35–3) is used to treat malaria due to multidrug-resistant strains of *P falciparum;* however, compliance with the 7-day course is poor because of quinine side effects.

Because quinine is an irritant to the gastric mucosa, it should be taken with food. Mild to moderate quinine toxicity (cinchonism) is manifested by headache, nausea, slight visual disturbances, dizziness, and mild tinnitus. These symptoms may abate as treatment continues and usually do not require discontinuation of treatment. Where available, quinine blood levels can be monitored; desired plasma levels are 5–10 μg/mL. Severe cinchonism requiring temporary or permanent discontinuation of therapy is rare and begins to appear at plasma levels greater than 7 μg/mL; findings include fever, skin eruptions, deafness, marked visual abnormalities (scotomas, diplopia, contracted visual fields, retinal vessel spasticity, optic atrophy, blindness), other central nervous system abnormalities (vertigo, somnolence, confusion, seizures), disturbances in cardiac rhythm or conduction, massive intravascular hemolysis with renal failure (blackwater fever), agranulocytosis, and thrombocytopenia.

Parenteral quinine dihydrochloride is used in the treatment of severe attacks of malaria due to *P falciparum* strains sensitive or resistant to chloroquine. The drug is given intravenously at a slow rate (Table 35–3); rapid infusions may be severely toxic. The drug should be used with extreme caution and only for patients who cannot take the medication orally; appropriate oral therapy should be started as soon as possible. Infusions may cause thrombophlebitis. In the USA, parenteral quinine is no longer available and parenteral quinidine gluconate is used instead.

See references and manufacturers' recommendations for drug interactions (including aluminum-containing antacids, digoxin, anticoagulants, and cimetidine). Quinine is safe to use in pregnancy. Systemic clearance of quinine slows in proportion to the severity of the disease.

6. Quinidine gluconate—Quinidine is the dextrorotatory diastereoisomer of quinine. The two drugs are equally efficacious in parenteral treatment of severe malaria (Table 35–3). The two drugs are also similar with regard to toxicity and drug interactions, but quinidine has a greater cardiosuppressant effect. The principal adverse effect of quinine and quinidine in severe malaria is hypoglycemia, which usually develops after 24 hours of treatment; it is a particular problem in pregnancy.

7. Halofantrine—Halofantrine is a schizonticide for all four malaria species, including multidrug-resistant *P falciparum*. The drug is not active against hepatic stages or gametocytes. It is used only in oral treatment and not for severe malaria. Infrequent to rare, minor side effects are abdominal pain, diarrhea, cough, rash, and pruritus. The drug should not be given from 1 hour before to 3 hours after a meal, because fatty food enhances and results in irregular absorption. Halofantrine is not used for prophylaxis or standby treatment because of this variable bioavailability; because the standard dose prolongs the QT_c interval; and because there have been rare reports of ventricular arrhythmias, sometimes fatal. The drug should not be used in the presence of preexisting cardiac conduction defects, long QT intervals, recent (4 weeks) usage of or concomitant treatment with mefloquine, or treatment with other drugs that prolong the QT interval (ie, quinine, quinidine, chloroquine, tricyclic antidepressants, neuroleptic drugs, terfenadine, astemizole). Because halofantrine is embryotoxic in animals, it should not be given to pregnant women. Halofantrine is widely available abroad; in the USA, however, although approved by the FDA, it has not been marketed.

8. Pyrimethamine-sulfadoxine (Fansidar)—Fansidar is supplied as tablets that contain pyrimethamine (25 mg) and sulfadoxine (500 mg). Fansidar's limitations are that it is effective only against susceptible strains of *P falciparum* (see above); its low efficacy against *P vivax, P ovale,* or *P malariae* and that it is slow-acting. Fansidar is no longer used for weekly prophylaxis because of rare reports of severe cutaneous toxicity and death. However, in single-dose treatment, Fansidar is generally well tolerated. Cutaneous reactions are more common in persons who are HIV-positive.

Current indications for Fansidar are (1) as a single dose (slow-acting) in conjunction with quinine (rapid-acting) in treatment of sensitive strains of acute chloroquine-resistant falciparum malaria and (2) in presumptive self-treatment of malaria (see above).

Fansidar is contraindicated for individuals with known sulfonamide sensitivity and those in the last month of pregnancy (the sulfadoxine component, which has a long half-life, can cause kernicterus in the newborn). The drug should be used with caution in the presence of impaired renal or hepatic function, in patients with G6PD deficiency (hemolysis occurs in some), and in those with severe allergic disorders or bronchial asthma. If folic acid is needed, ingestion should be delayed 1 week to avoid an inhibitory effect on the antimalarial action of Fansidar.

9. Doxycycline—Doxycycline is effective against chloroquine-sensitive and chloroquine-resistant *P falciparum, P vivax,* and (apparently) against *P ovale* and *P malariae*. It is used prophylactically against chloroquine-resistant and mefloquine-resistant falciparum malaria in Thailand and adjacent countries and elsewhere for patients who cannot tolerate mefloquine (Table 35–2). Doxycycline is also used as an adjunct drug with quinine for the treatment of resistant falciparum malaria (Table 35–3). Side effects include infrequent gastrointestinal symptoms (take with meals plus copious amounts of water to avoid esophageal irritation; avoid milk, which reduces absorption); candidal vaginitis (advise carrying a self-treatment antifungal regimen, either vaginal suppositories or cream); and rare photosensitivity (prevention may be achieved by use of sunscreens that absorb ultraviolet radiation and by avoidance of exposure to direct sunlight as much as possible). The drug is contraindicated in pregnancy, in nursing mothers, in children under 8 years of age, and in persons with hepatic dysfunction. No data are available on the long-term use of the drug.

10. Artemisinin (qinghaosu) and its derivatives—Artemisinin and its derivatives are available in some countries but not in the USA. The drugs are effective against all malarial parasites, and artesunate is considered the most rapidly acting. Oil-soluble artemether is administered intramuscularly, whereas water-soluble artesunate is given orally or by intravenous infusion; both drugs are sometimes available as rectal suppositories for use by that route if parenteral administration is not possible. No drug resistance has been reported except for a degree of reduced effectiveness in falciparum malaria resistant to mefloquine. The artemisinin drugs are used only to treat acute malaria, for which they are the most rapidly acting of all schizonticides. They are the only drugs that remain reliably effective against *P falciparum* strains resistant to quinine. They are not effective against the liver stage of vivax and malariae malaria, and because of their short half-lives they cannot be used in prophylaxis. Recrudescences are common, however (up to 50%), when the artemisinin drugs are used alone; therefore, they are usually given with another drug (eg, mefloquine). Mild adverse events—symptoms that also occur in malaria—are headache, gastrointestinal symptoms, pruritus, and fever. Animal studies suggest a potential for embryotoxicity (the drug should be avoided in pregnancy when possible) and central nervous system toxicity (in humans, this has not been documented in prospective studies in more than 10,000 patients).

11. Proguanil—Proguanil (chlorguanide, Paludrine; not available in the USA), 200 mg/d, is a schizonticide against three of the malaria parasites (unknown degree against *P malariae*) and has some causal prophylactic action but it is no longer used alone. Proguanil (100 mg) in combination with atovaquone (250 mg) (Malarone) has recently been approved in the USA for prophylaxis and treatment of multidrug-resistant falciparum malaria. Proguanil (100 mg daily) in combination with chloroquine (0.5 g weekly) for prophylaxis in areas with low-intensity chloroquine-resistant *P falciparum* is no longer recommended in this text. Rarely reported side effects are nausea, vomiting, hair loss, and mouth ulcers. The drug is safe to use in pregnancy; it should not be used in persons with hepatic or renal dysfunction.

Chemoprophylaxis for Nonimmune Populations

See Table 35–2 for methods and dosages and under the individual drugs (above) for details on cautions, contraindications, and toxicities.

Antimalarials should be taken with water at mealtime. The selected drug should be tested for side effects in advance of departure (to allow time for selection of an alternative drug if necessary) and started sufficiently in advance of exposure that a satisfactory prophylactic blood level is achieved. On returning home, primaquine is given to eradicate persistent liver stages of *P vivax* or *P ovale* if there has been significant exposure to these parasites (see above under Primaquine).

A. CHEMOPROPHYLAXIS IN REGIONS WHERE *P FALCIPARUM* IS SENSITIVE TO CHLOROQUINE

1. Drug of choice—Chloroquine prevents attacks for all forms of malaria and is curative for *P falciparum* and *P malariae* when taken for 4 weeks after leaving the endemic area. For persons who cannot tolerate chloroquine, reducing the dose to 250 mg twice weekly or switching to hydroxychloroquine sulfate (400 mg [salt]) can be tried.

2. Alternative drugs—Mefloquine, Malarone, and doxycycline are alternatives to chloroquine. Schizonticides *not used for chemoprophylaxis* are halofantrine (erratic absorption and variable bioavailability), Fansidar (hypersensitivity reactions with rare deaths), amodiaquine (agranulocytosis and toxic hepatitis), pyrimethamine (widespread resistance of both *P falciparum* and *P vivax*), artemisinin and related drugs

(short duration of action), proguanil by itself (resistance), and generally quinine (toxicity).

B. CHEMOPROPHYLAXIS IN REGIONS WHERE *P FALCIPARUM* IS RESISTANT TO CHLOROQUINE

1. Drugs of choice—Mefloquine is preferred, but it has more side effects. Alternative drugs are Malarone and doxycycline.

2. Second alternative drugs—Continuing under evaluation is primaquine (30 mg base) starting 1 day before entering the endemic area, daily while there, and for 7 days afterward. The drug is not licensed for this use in the USA and is contraindicated in pregnancy and in persons with G6PD deficiency. Under evaluation is tafenoquine, an analog of primaquine that is more potent than the parent drug and will require only weekly doses. Under exceptional circumstances, chloroquine and proguanil plus an emergency standby drug (see above) can be considered but are less efficacious—or use of daily quinine.

C. CHEMOPROPHYLAXIS IN SOUTHEAST ASIA

Multidrug *P falciparum* resistance is extensive in Southeast Asia. The drugs of choice are doxycycline and Malarone (limited supporting data). Chloroquine and Fansidar cannot be used throughout the region, and resistance to mefloquine and halofantrine has increased significantly.

D. PROPHYLAXIS FOR PREGNANT WOMEN

Pregnant women should be protected; malaria infection during pregnancy may be particularly severe. Drugs contraindicated in pregnancy are doxycycline, Malarone, and primaquine. Therefore, the best course is weekly chloroquine (or hydroxychloroquine) with or without proguanil. In areas of chloroquine-resistant malaria, mefloquine can be used except in the first trimester. Generally, therefore, travel by pregnant women to resistant areas is not recommended.

E. EMERGENCY SELF-TREATMENT

In selected instances, medication should be provided for emergency self-treatment of breakthrough attacks (see above).

Treatment of Acute Attacks

See under individual drugs and Table 35–3 for dosages.

A. GENERAL CONSIDERATIONS

At times when parasitologic confirmation is not readily available, it may be necessary to start treatment immediately based only on clinical findings. Patients with falciparum infections should be hospitalized. It is important to determine whether a patient has been treated with antimalarials in the previous 1–2 days (3 weeks for mefloquine because of its slow excretion) to avoid the risk of overdose or adverse drug interactions. In the event of mefloquine prophylaxis or treatment failure, it is hazardous—although it may be essential—to use quinine, quinidine, or halofantrine (Table 35–3); under these circumstances, the safest drug to use is artemisinin or one of its derivatives (not available in the USA).

It is essential to determine the density of parasites on the blood smear (as a measure of severity of infection) and to recheck at least twice daily. Within 48–72 hours after start of treatment, patients usually become afebrile and improve clinically; within 48 hours, parasitemia is generally reduced by about 75% (though there may be an initial increase during the first 6–12 hours). If there is no improvement within 48–72 hours for mild infections or 24 hours for severe ones or if there is increasing asexual parasitemia after 1–2 days (in the presence of adequate drug ingestion and retention), parasite resistance to the drug must be assumed and treatment changed.

B. Drug Treatment of All Forms of Malaria Except P falciparum and P vivax Strains Resistant to Chloroquine

(Table 35–3)

1. Elimination of asexual erythrocytic parasites— Infection by all four species of malaria is treated with oral chloroquine. Alternative oral drugs if chloroquine cannot be tolerated are mefloquine, Malarone, quinine sulfate (plus doxycycline, clindamycin, or Fansidar), atovaquone plus doxycycline, or halofantrine.*

If the patient is severely ill, treat with intravenous quinine dihydrochloride* or quinidine gluconate, parenteral preparations of artemisinin derivatives*, or parenteral chloroquine. Start oral therapy with chloroquine as soon as possible.

2. Eradication of P vivax or P ovale infections— This is accomplished with a standard course of primaquine (Table 35–3) except in regions of rare partial resistance, where a higher dosage or longer course of treatment is needed (see above).

3. Elimination of persistent gametocytemia— Gametocytes of P vivax, P ovale, and P malariae can be eliminated by chloroquine. Gametocytes of P falciparum are eliminated by a single dose of 26.3 mg of primaquine salt.

4. Treatment of semi-immunes— Treatment of attacks in semi-immune patients generally requires shorter courses of drug treatment.

C. Drug Treatment of Falciparum Malaria Acquired in Areas Where P falciparum Is Resistant to Chloroquine

Start treatment with oral quinine sulfate and a second drug (Table 35–3) (but not Fansidar if the infection was acquired in an area with Fansidar resistance). Alternative drugs are mefloquine, Malarone, artesunate*

followed by mefloquine, or atovaquone plus doxycycline. In Southeast Asia, mefloquine and halofantrine cannot be used because of multidrug resistance.

If the patient is severely ill, treat with intravenous quinine or quinidine (Table 35–3). A second drug (doxycycline or clindamycin) should also be given parenterally. Oral treatment with quinine plus the antibiotic should be started as soon as possible. An alternative approach is parenteral artesunate* or artemether* followed by mefloquine (not highly effective in Southeast Asia).

D. Special Measures for Management of Severe P falciparum Malaria

(See references for further details.) Severe and complicated falciparum malaria is a medical emergency that requires hospitalization, intensive care with monitoring of electrolytes and acid-base balance, and immediate treatment without waiting for all laboratory results to become available. Indications for parenteral treatment are (1) failure to ingest or retain drugs, (2) cerebral malaria, (3) multiple complications, and (4) peripheral asexual parasitemia of 5% (250,000/μL) or higher. When possible, parenteral treatment should be intravenously, but quinine, artesunate, and chloroquine can be given intramuscularly; chloroquine can also be given subcutaneously. Black urine suggests hemoglobinuria. Renal failure, metabolic acidosis, pulmonary edema, gram-negative sepsis, jaundice, severe anemia, and shock may ensue. Rehydration of the patient should be done with great caution, particularly in the first 24 hours, since overhydration may precipitate noncardiogenic pulmonary edema. In general, 2–3 L of fluid is required the first day, followed by 10–20 mL/kg/d; intake and output should be carefully recorded. After rehydration, the central venous pressure should be maintained at approximately 5 cm of water (pulmonary artery occlusion pressure < 15 mm Hg). Early dialysis may be necessary for renal failure and then sustained for 4–7 days or longer. Blood glucose levels should be monitored every 6 hours during the acute and early convalescent period, since hypoglycemia may be severe, either as a result of the malaria infection or the use of quinine or quinidine; treatment is with 50 mL of 50% dextrose (1–2 mL/kg) followed by maintenance infusion of 5–10% dextrose. Low glucose levels should be rechecked hourly. In cerebral malaria, one should maintain the airway and exclude other treatable causes of coma (hypoglycemia, bacterial meningoencephalitis). The presence of papilledema is a contraindication to lumbar puncture. With convulsions, one should maintain the airway and treat with diazepam (0.15 mg/kg intravenously or 0.5 mg/kg rectally) or with paraldehyde (0.1 mL/kg intramuscularly, preferably dispensed from a glass syringe). The temperature is kept below 38.5 °C using acetaminophen (paracetamol) plus tepid sponging and fanning. Patients with clini-

---

*Not available in the USA but available in some countries.

*Not available in the USA but available in some countries.

cally significant disseminated intravascular coagulation should be treated with fresh whole blood, clotting factors, or platelets as needed. For hematocrits below 20% or hemoglobins below 7 g/dL, transfusion of fresh whole blood or packed cells is required. Bacterial infections are common (eg, pneumonia, cystitis, salmonellosis). Exchange transfusion (5–10 L) should be considered when more than 10% of red blood cells are parasitized (5% if severe dysfunction of other organs is present). Corticosteroids, aspirin, other anti-inflammatory agents, dextran, norepinephrine, and heparin should not be used.

Follow-Up for *P falciparum* Malaria

Blood films should be checked daily until parasitemia clears; check weekly thereafter for 4 weeks to observe for recrudescence of infection.

Prognosis

The uncomplicated and untreated primary attack of *P vivax, P ovale,* or *P falciparum* malaria usually lasts 2–4 weeks; that of *P malariae* about twice as long. Attacks of each type of infection may subsequently recur (once or many times) before the infection terminates spontaneously. With prompt antimalarial therapy, the prognosis is generally good, but in *P falciparum* infections, when severe complications such as cerebral malaria develop, the prognosis is poor even with treatment. It is now recognized that after cerebral malaria, residual neurologic deficits can occur.

Angus BJ: Malaria on the World Wide Web. Clin Infect Dis 2001;33:651. [PMID 11486288]

Atovaquone/Proguanil (Malarone) for malaria. Med Lett Drugs Ther 2000;42:109. [PMID: 11093830]

International Travel and Health: *Vaccination Certificate Requirements and Health Advice.* WHO, 2002.

Kain KC et al: Malaria chemoprophylaxis in the age of drug resistance. I. Currently recommended drug regimens. Clin Infect Dis 2001;33:226. [PMID 11418883]

Lell B et al: Malaria chemoprophylaxis with tafenoquine: a randomized study. Lancet 2000;355:2041. [PMID 10885356]

Losert H et al: Experiences with severe *P falciparum* malaria in the intensive care unit. Intensive Care Med 2000;26:195. [PMID: 10784308]

Newton P et al: Malaria: new developments in treatment and prevention. Annu Rev Med 1999;50:179. [PMID: 10073271]

Management of Severe Malaria: A Practical Handbook, 2nd ed. World Health Organization, 2000.

Prevention of malaria. Med Lett Drugs Ther 2000;42:8. [PMID: 10696232]

Severe falciparum malaria. World Health Organization, Communicable Diseases Cluster. Trans R Soc Trop Med Hyg 2000;94(Suppl 1):S1. [PMID: 11103309] (Diagnosis and management of severe malaria.)

Soto J et al: Primaquine prophylaxis against malaria in non-immune Colombian soldiers: Efficacy and toxicity. A randomized double-blind placebo controlled trial. Ann Intern Med 1998;129:241. [PMID: 9696733]

van Vugt M et al: The treatment of chloroquine-resistant malaria. Trop Doct 1999;29:176. [PMID: 10448249]

Warrell DA: Management of severe malaria. Parasitologia 1999;41:287. [PMID: 10697870]

TOXOPLASMOSIS

 ESSENTIALS OF DIAGNOSIS

Acute primary infection:

- *Fever, malaise, headache, lymphadenopathy (especially cervical), myalgia, arthralgia, stiff neck, sore throat; occasionally, rash, hepatosplenomegaly, retinochoroiditis, confusion; in various combinations.*

- *Positive serologic tests with high and rising IgG and IgM.*

- *Isolation of* Toxoplasma gondii *from blood or body fluids; tachyzoites in histologic sections of tissue or cytologic preparations of body fluids.*

Acute primary or recrudescent infection in immunocompromised patients:

- *Central nervous system mass lesions; retinochoroiditis, pneumonitis, myocarditis less common; sometimes other findings as above.*

- *Positive IgG titers moderately high; IgM antibody usually absent. Tissue diagnosis as above.*

General Considerations

T gondii, an obligate intracellular protozoan, is found worldwide in humans and in many species of animals and birds. The parasite is a coccidian of cats, the definitive host, and exists in three forms: The *trophozoite* (tachyzoite) (3 × 7 μm) is the rapidly proliferating form in tissues and body fluids that causes acute disease. The trophozoites can enter and multiply in most mammalian nucleated cells. The *cyst,* containing viable bradyzoites, is the latent form that can persist indefinitely as a chronic infection and is found particularly in muscle and nerve tissue. The *oocyst* is the form passed only in the feces of the cat family. In the intestinal epithelium of cats, a sexual cycle occurs, with subsequent release of oocysts for 3–14 days; cats may, however, become reinfected and excrete oocysts multiple times. The oocysts, which contain infective sporozoites, are infectious within 12 hours to several days after passage and can remain infective in moist soil for weeks or months.

Human infection results (1) from ingestion of cysts in raw or undercooked meat; (2) from ingestion of oocysts in contaminated food or water, by careless handling of contaminated cat litter, or from soil by soil-eating children; (3) from transplacental transmission of trophozoites; or (4) rarely, from direct inoculation of trophozoites, as in blood transfusion. Reservoirs of human infection are rodents and birds eaten by cats and infected domestic animals used for food. Antibody prevalence rates range from less than 5% in some parts of the world (absence of cats and minimal ingestion of meat) to 15–29% in the USA and over 80% in France.

On ingestion, bradyzoites (from cysts) or sporozoites (from oocysts) invade multiple cells types and propagate as trophozoites; cell death and inflammation follow, but true granulomas do not form.

Clinical Findings

A. Symptoms and Signs

Over 80% of primary infections are asymptomatic. The incubation period for symptomatic persons is 1–2 weeks. Generally, on recovery, both asymptomatic and symptomatic infections persist as chronic latent (cyst) infections. Reactivation occurs almost exclusively in severely immunocompromised patients.

The clinical manifestations of toxoplasmosis may be grouped into four syndromes:

1. Primary infection in the immunocompetent host—Most symptomatic infections are acute, mild, febrile multisystem illnesses that resemble infectious mononucleosis. Lymphadenopathy, usually nontender, particularly of the head and neck, is the most common finding. Other features in various combinations are malaise, myalgia, arthralgia, headache, sore throat, and maculopapular or urticarial rash. Hepatosplenomegaly may occur. Rarely, severe cases are complicated by pneumonitis, meningoencephalitis, hepatitis, myocarditis, and retinochoroiditis. Symptoms may fluctuate, but most patients recover spontaneously within a few months.

2. Congenital infection—Congenital transmission occurs only as a result of infection (generally asymptomatic) in a nonimmune woman during pregnancy. Infection has been detected in up to 1% of women during pregnancy; 15–60% of such infections, the incidence varying by trimester, are transmitted to the fetus, but only a small percentage result in abortions or stillbirths or in active disease in premature or full-term, live-born infants. Though fetal infection may occur in any trimester, it is more severe early in pregnancy. Among all congenital infections, less than 15% show severe brain or eye damage at birth; however, of the apparently normal newborns, more than 85% will develop brain or eye sequelae later in life. Treatment of the mother reduces the congenital infection rate by about 60%. See specialized sources for clinical manifestations and approach to diagnosis.

3. Retinochoroiditis—This develops gradually weeks to years after congenital infection (the preponderant form, which is generally bilateral) or rarely after an acquired infection in a young child (generally unilateral). Acquired infections in older children and adults rarely progress to retinochoroiditis. The inflammatory process persists for weeks to months as focally necrotic retinal lesions (yellow or white patches with blurred margins). Visual defects, which include blurring, central defects, and scotomas, are accompanied by pain and photophobia. Rarely, progression may result in glaucoma and blindness. With healing, white or dark-pigmented scars may result. Panuveitis may accompany retinochoroiditis.

4. Reactivated disease in the immunologically compromised host—Reactivated toxoplasmosis occurs in patients with AIDS, cancer, or those given immunosuppressive drugs. The infection may present in specific organs (brain, lungs, and eye most commonly, but also heart, skin, gastrointestinal tract, and liver) or as disseminated disease. Between 30% and 50% of AIDS patients seropositive for past toxoplasma infection will develop meningeal (uncommon), mass (single or multiple), or diffuse intracerebral toxoplasma lesions, associated with clinical findings of fever, headache, altered mental status, seizures, and focal (or, infrequently, nonfocal) neurologic deficits (see also Chapter 31).

B. Laboratory Findings

Diagnosis depends principally on serologic tests, which are sensitive and reliable. However, diagnosis is occasionally made from tissue (blood, bone marrow aspirates, cerebrospinal fluid sediment, sputum, and other tissues or body fluids or placental tissue) either by (1) demonstration of trophozoites or characteristic histology, (2) isolation of the organism in mice (more sensitive) or in tissue culture (more rapid, 3–6 days), or (3) amplification of *T gondii* DNA by polymerase chain reaction. Interpretation of the results and deciding which patients should be treated or when to advise termination of a pregnancy may require assistance from a reference or research laboratory with large experience in toxoplasmosis.

1. Histology—Cysts or trophozoites may be directly identified in blood (buffy coat from centrifuged heparinized blood), other tissues, or body fluids by staining with standard stains or with specific antibody marked with fluorescein or enzyme. Demonstration of cysts in biopsied tissue does not establish a causal relationship to clinical illness, since cysts may be found in both acute and chronic infections. However, finding tachyzoites confirms active infection. In the placenta, fetus, or newborn, the presence of cysts does indicate congenital infection.

2. Serologic tests—The Sabin-Feldman dye test, indirect hemagglutination, indirect immunofluorescence (IFA), ELISA, and other tests can be done on blood, cerebrospinal fluid, aqueous humor, and other body fluids. The dye test is the standard but is rarely used because of laboratory safety factors; though extremely sensitive and specific, it does not separate IgM from IgG antibody. The ELISA, immunosorbent, and IFA tests do separate IgM and IgG antibody. In the IFA test for IgM, antibody appears 1–2 weeks after start of infection, reaches a peak at 6–8 weeks, and then gradually declines over 6 months. As IgM antibody can persist for up to 5 years, a positive finding does not necessarily represent recent infection; however, a negative finding does rule out acute infection acquired in recent months. Maternal IgM is normally unable to cross the intact placenta; antibody which does pass through a leak has a half-life of only 3–5 days. IgG antibody appears within 1–3 weeks, peaks in 1–2 months, and usually persists at a lower level for life. When positive, it reliably indicates present or past infection; a negative result reliably rules out either time frame.

The following are selected serologic and other findings in specific toxoplasmosis syndromes:

a. Acute infection in immunocompetent persons—The diagnosis is established by seroconversion from negative to positive, by a fourfold rise in serologic titers by any test, or by a single high titer (1:160) of IgM antibody. Acute infection can be diagnosed by detection of tachyzoites in tissue, isolation of organism, or amplification of its DNA in blood or body fluids. The presence of circulating ELISA-IgA also favors the diagnosis of acute infection. A presumptive diagnosis is based on a single IgM titer of over 1:64 and a very high IgG titer (> 1:1000). The diagnosis of acute toxoplasmosis is excluded if the dye test and an IgM test are negative for 3 months after onset of symptoms.

b. Recrudescent infection in immunosuppressed patients—In AIDS patients, toxoplasma can sometimes be isolated from the blood. Alternatively, definitive diagnosis is only by finding toxoplasma organisms in cerebrospinal fluid (Wright-Giemsa stain or by PCR amplification) or by brain biopsy. To avoid the latter, empirical antibiotic treatment is generally started after presumptive evidence is obtained by MRI (the more sensitive test) or CT scan (typically: multiple, isodense or hypodense, ring-enhancing mass lesions). Single-photon emission CT is under evaluation as a highly specific diagnostic method. Antibody titers cannot be depended on, since most patients have IgG titers that reflect past infection, significant rises are infrequent, and IgM antibody is rare. Absence of IgG does not rule out the diagnosis of central nervous system toxoplasmosis. The cerebrospinal fluid may show mild pleocytosis (predominantly lymphocytes and monocytes), elevated protein, and normal glucose. (See also Chapter 31.)

c. Toxoplasmic retinochoroiditis—This is usually associated with stable, usually low IgG titers and no IgM antibody. If IgG antibody in aqueous humor is higher than in the serum, the diagnosis is supported.

d. Congenital infection—The most useful tests for confirmation of fetal infection are ultrasound examination, amniocentesis for detection of toxoplasma DNA in amniotic fluid by PCR, and cordocentesis for detection of IgM-specific antibody. A negative result for IgM antibody does not exclude the diagnosis. Postpartum, a positive IgM after 1 week is diagnostic; IgG antibody, however, is nearly always present if the mother is positive, but that passively transferred antibody disappears in 6–12 months.

3. Other laboratory findings—Leukocyte counts are normal or reduced, often with lymphocytosis or monocytosis with rare atypical cells, but there is no heterophil antibody. Chest radiographs may show interstitial pneumonia. In cerebral imaging studies in HIV-infected persons, toxoplasmosis typically appears as multiple lesions with a predilection for the basal ganglion.

Differential Diagnosis

In acute febrile disease, consider cytomegalovirus infection, infectious mononucleosis, and other causes of pneumonitis, myocarditis, myositis, hepatitis, and splenomegaly. With lymphadenopathy, possibilities include sarcoidosis, tuberculosis, tularemia, lymphoma, cat-scratch disease, and metastatic carcinoma. With brain lesions in the immunosuppressed host, consider lymphoma, tuberculoma, brain abscess, metastatic carcinoma, and fungal lesions.

Treatment

A. APPROACH TO TREATMENT

In immunocompetent hosts, the lymphadenopathic form of the disease is usually not treated unless findings are severe or persistent or there is overt visceral disease. If treatment is started, it should continue for 3–4 weeks and then be reassessed, including testing for acquisition of serologic immunity.

Since most episodes of retinochoroiditis are self-limited, opinions vary on indications for and type of treatment. (See specialized texts.)

Immunocompromised patients with active infection (primary or recrudescent) must be treated. See Chapter 31 for details. Therapy should continue for 4–6 weeks after cessation of symptoms—which may require up to a 6-month course, to be followed by drug prophylaxis as long as immunosuppression persists. In HIV-infected persons, acute toxoplasmosis must be treated followed by continued prophylaxis; in patients who have a positive IgG toxoplasma serology but are asymptomatic, prophylaxis is desirable.

Congenitally infected newborns should be treated; for details on management, see specialized sources.

B. Choice of Drugs

The treatment of choice in nonimmunocompromised patients is pyrimethamine, 25–100 mg once daily, plus either trisulfapyrimidines (4–6 g/d in four divided doses) or sulfadiazine, 1–1.5 g four times daily, continue this treatment for 3–4 weeks. Folinic acid (leucovorin), 10–25 mg with each dose of pyrimethamine, should be given concurrently to avoid bone marrow suppression. Patients should be screened for a history of sulfonamide sensitivity (skin rashes, gastrointestinal symptoms, hepatotoxicity); to prevent crystal-induced nephrotoxicity, good urine output should be maintained (alkalinization with sodium bicarbonate may also be useful). Pyrimethamine side effects include headache and gastrointestinal symptoms. Platelet and white blood cell counts should be performed at least twice weekly. Clindamycin (600 mg four times daily) may be a useful alternative drug; because it concentrates in the choroid, it is also used in the treatment of ocular disease. Atovaquone (750 mg three or four times daily), dapsone, other macrolides, and immunotherapy are under evaluation.

In toxoplasmosis in pregnancy, to decrease the incidence of fetal infection (it is not possible to eliminate all infections), spiramycin is given at a dosage of 3 g daily in four divided doses for 3–4 weeks. Because spiramycin does not reliably cross the placenta, if fetal infection is shown to be already present and fetal treatment is planned, treatment should include sulfadiazine (4 g/d in divided doses) and pyrimethamine (25/mg/d in divided doses plus folinic acid, 5–15 mg/d). The latter two drugs should not be given if the patient is within the first 12–14 weeks of pregnancy, when pyrimethamine can be teratogenic. Spiramycin is not effective in other forms of toxoplasmosis. In the USA, the drug is available from the manufacturer.

For the treatment of central nervous system toxoplasmosis in HIV-infected and immunocompromised persons, see Chapter 31.

Prevention

Freezing of meat to −20 °C for 2 days or heating to 60 °C for 4 minutes kills cysts in tissues. Hands, kitchen surfaces, and cooking utensils must be thoroughly cleaned after contact with raw meat. Under appropriate environmental conditions, oocysts passed in cat feces can remain infective for a year or more. Thus, children's play areas, including sandboxes, should be protected from cat (and dog) feces; hand washing is indicated after contact with soil potentially contaminated by animal feces. Indoor cats should be fed only dry, canned, or cooked meat. Litter boxes should be changed daily, as freshly deposited oocysts are not infective for 48 hours.

Pregnant women should have their serum examined for toxoplasma IgG and IgM antibody. If the IgM test is negative but an IgG titer is present and less than 1:1000, no further evaluation is necessary. Those with negative titers should take measures to prevent infection—preferably by having no further contact with cats and cat litter, by thoroughly cooking meat, and by hand washing after handling raw meat and before eating or touching the face. For seronegative women who continue to have significant environmental exposure, serologic screening should be conducted several times during pregnancy.

Prognosis

The outlook for acute toxoplasmosis in adults is excellent as long as the patient is immunocompetent. In immunosuppressed patients, the disease is usually fatal if untreated; improvement results if treatment is started early, but recrudescence is common. Chronic asymptomatic infection is usually benign.

Derouin F et al: Cotrimoxazole for prenatal treatment of congenital toxoplasmosis. Parasitol Today 2000;16:254. [PMID: 10827434]

Julander I et al: Polymerase chain reaction for diagnosis of cerebral toxoplasmosis in cerebrospinal fluid in HIV-positive patients. Scand J Infect Dis 2001,33:538. [PMID: 11515766]

Kopecky D et al: Knowledge-based interpretation of toxoplasmosis serology test results including fuzzy temporal concepts—the ToxoNet system. Medinfo 2001;10(Part 1):484. [PMID: 11604787]

Luder CG et al: Toxoplasmosis: a persisting challenge. Trends Parasitol 2001;17:460. [PMID 11587941]

■ II. HELMINTHIC INFECTIONS

TREMATODE (FLUKE) INFECTIONS

SCHISTOSOMIASIS (Bilharziasis)

 ESSENTIALS OF DIAGNOSIS

- *Exposure to infection in an endemic area.*
- *Acute phase: Abrupt onset (2–6 weeks postexposure) of abdominal pain, weight loss, headache, malaise, chills, fever, myalgia, diarrhea (sometimes bloody), dry cough, hepatomegaly, and eosinophilia.*
- *Chronic phase: Either (1) diarrhea, abdominal pain, blood in stool, hepatomegaly or hepatosplenomegaly, and bleeding from esophageal varices (Schistosoma mansoni or Schisto-*

soma japonicum *infection*); *or (2) terminal hematuria, urinary frequency, and urethral and bladder pain (Schistosoma haematobium infection).*

- *Depending on species, characteristic eggs in feces, urine, or scrapings or biopsy of rectal or bladder mucosa.*

General Considerations

Schistosomiasis, which infects more than 200 million persons worldwide, induces severe consequences in 20 million persons annually, resulting in up to 200,000 deaths. The disease is caused mainly by three blood flukes (trematodes). *S mansoni,* which causes intestinal schistosomiasis, is widespread in Africa and occurs in the Arabian peninsula, South America (Brazil, Venezuela, Suriname), and the Caribbean (including Puerto Rico but not Cuba). Vesical (urinary) schistosomiasis, caused by *S haematobium,* is found throughout the Middle East and Africa. Asiatic intestinal schistosomiasis, due to *S japonicum,* is important in China and the Philippines, and a small focus is present in Sulawesi, Indonesia, but transmission in Japan has been interrupted. A number of schistosome species of animals sometimes infect humans, including *Schistosoma intercalatum* in central Africa and *Schistosoma mekongi* in the Mekong delta in Thailand, Cambodia, and Laos. In the USA, an estimated 400,000 immigrants are infected, but transmission does not occur because appropriate snail intermediate hosts are absent.

Mammals are important reservoirs for *S japonicum.* Humans are the main reservoir for *S mansoni* and *S haematobium;* the few animal species infected with *S mansoni* are not epidemiologically important.

In the life cycle involving humans, the adult worms live in terminal venules of the bowel *(S mansoni, S japonicum)* or bladder *(S haematobium).* When eggs passed in feces or urine reach fresh water, a larval form is released that subsequently infects snails, the intermediate host. After development, infective larvae (cercariae) leave the snails, enter water, and infect exposed persons through the skin or mucous membranes. After penetration, the cercariae become schistosomula larvae that reach the portal circulation in the liver, where they rapidly mature. After a few weeks, adult worms pair, mate, and migrate mainly to terminal venules of specific veins, where females deposit their eggs. By means of lytic secretions, some eggs reach the lumen of the bowel or bladder and are passed with feces or urine. Others are retained in the bowel or bladder wall, while still others are carried in the circulation to the liver, lung, and (less often) to other tissues.

Except for the allergic response in the acute syndrome (see below), disease is primarily due to delayed hypersensitivity. Antigens released by the eggs stimulate a local T cell-dependent granulomatous response, followed by a strong fibrotic reaction. Live worms produce no lesions and rarely cause symptoms. The type or degree of tissue damage and symptoms varies with the intensity of infection (worm burden), host genetic factors, site of egg deposition, concurrent infection (eg, hepatitis B), and duration of infection.

S mansoni adults migrate to the inferior mesenteric veins of the large bowel and *S japonicum* to the superior and inferior mesenteric veins in the large and small bowel. Ulcers and polyps (common only in Egypt) result from granuloma formation and fibrosis in the bowel wall. Egg accumulation in the liver may result in periportal fibrosis and portal hypertension of the presinusoidal type, but liver function typically remains intact even in advanced disease. Portal-systemic collateralization due to portal hypertension can result in embolization of eggs to the lungs, with subsequent endarteritis, pulmonary hypertension, and cor pulmonale. Because greater numbers of eggs are produced by *S japonicum,* the resulting disease is often more severe.

Adult *S haematobium* mature in the venous plexus of the bladder, ureters, rectum, prostate, and uterus. Ulcers and polyps result from granuloma formation and fibrosis in the bladder wall, and eggshell remnants may calcify. Stricture or distortion of the ureteral orifices or terminal ureters may result in hydroureter, hydronephrosis, and ascending infection. Lesions in the pelvic organs rarely progress to extensive fibrosis and infection. Eggs are carried to the liver or lungs, but severe pathologic changes in these organs are less frequent than in *S mansoni* and *S japonicum* infections.

In size, adult *S mansoni* are 6–13 × 1 mm. The prepatent period—from cercarial penetration until appearance of eggs in feces—is about 50 days. The life span of the worms ranges from 5 to 30 years or more.

Clinical Findings

A. SYMPTOMS AND SIGNS

Although a large proportion of infected persons have light infections (< 100 eggs per gram of feces) and are asymptomatic, an estimated 50–60% have symptoms and 5–10% advanced organ damage. In children, schistosomal infections may contribute to decreased nutritional status and growth retardation. Persons with concomitant AIDS and schistosomiasis can be treated effectively and safely for the latter infection.

1. Cercarial dermatitis—Following cercarial penetration, clinical findings progress from a localized itchy erythematous or petechial rash to macules and papules that last up to 5 days. Most cases occur in fresh or marine water (worldwide) and are due to skin invasion by bird schistosome cercariae, parasites that do not mature in humans and do not cause systemic symptoms. The syndrome is uncommon with human schistosome infections.

2. Acute schistosomiasis (Katayama fever)—This syndrome, primarily an allergic response to the developing schistosomes, may occur with the three schistosomes (rare with *S haematobium*). The syndrome is usually not seen in natives but does occur in travelers, especially to Africa. The incubation period is 2–7 weeks; the severity of illness ranges from mild to (rarely) life-threatening. In addition to fever, malaise, urticaria, diarrhea (sometimes bloody), myalgia, dry cough, leukocytosis, and marked eosinophilia, the liver and spleen may be temporarily enlarged. The patient again becomes asymptomatic in 2–8 weeks. Early in the infection, stool examination may be negative (examinations should be repeated for at least 6 months) but serologic tests positive. Controversy continues about whether praziquantel plus corticosteroids are safe and effective in treatment of acute disease.

3. Chronic schistosomiasis—This stage begins 6 months to several years after infection. In *S mansoni* and *S japonicum* infections, findings include diarrhea, abdominal pain, irregular bowel movements, blood in the stool, a hard enlarged liver, and splenomegaly. With subsequent slow progression over 5–15 years or longer, the following may appear: anorexia, weight loss, weakness, polypoid intestinal tumors, and features of portal and pulmonary hypertension. Immune complex glomerulonephritis may also occur.

In *S haematobium* infection, early symptoms of urinary tract disease are frequency and dysuria, followed by terminal hematuria and proteinuria. Frank hematuria may be recurrent. Sequelae may include bladder polyp formation, cystitis, chronic salmonella infection, pyelitis, pyelonephritis, urolithiasis, hydronephrosis due to ureteral obstruction, renal failure, and death. Severe liver, lung, genital, or neurologic disease is rare. Bladder cancer has been associated with vesical schistosomiasis.

4. Other complications—Portal hypertension may result in a contracted liver, splenomegaly, pancytopenia, esophageal varices, and variceal bleeding. Abnormal liver function, jaundice, ascites, and hepatic coma are end-stage findings. Pulmonary hypertension with cor pulmonale and edema due to right heart failure may supervene. Other large bowel complications include stricture, granulomatous masses, and persistent salmonella infection; colonic polyposis is manifested by bloody diarrhea, anemia, hypoalbuminemia, and clubbing. Transverse myelitis, epilepsy, or optic neuritis may result from collateral circulation of eggs or ectopic worms.

B. LABORATORY FINDINGS

Screening is by testing for eggs (ova) and occult blood in feces and urine (the excretion of which may be irregular and require repeated testing), for protein and leukocytes in urine, and by serology. Ova must be examined for internal detail or by the hatching test to determine that some are alive and that the infection therefore warrants treatment.

1. Eggs—Definitive diagnosis is by finding characteristic live eggs in excreta or mucosal biopsy.

In *S haematobium* infection, eggs may be found in the urine or, less frequently, in the stools. Eggs are sought in urine specimens collected between 9 AM and 2 PM or in 24-hour collections. They are processed either by examination of the sediment or preferably by membrane filtration. Occasionally, eggs are sought by vesical mucosa biopsy.

In *S mansoni* and *S japonicum* infections, eggs may be found in stool specimens by direct examination, but some form of concentration is usually necessary; the Kato-Katz quantitative method is preferred over formal ether concentration. One stool examination can reach 70% sensitivity and four, 92%. If results are negative, rectal mucosal biopsy of inflamed or granulomatous lesions or random biopsy specimens at two or three sites of normal mucosa may yield the diagnosis. Biopsy specimens should be examined as crush preparations between two glass slides and also examined histologically. If eggs are found, a quantitative test should be done after collecting a 24-hour urine or stool; heavy infections are those with counts over 400 eggs per gram.

2. Serologic tests—ELISA, immunoblot, and other tests are used in screening and may detect some egg-negative or ectopic infections. Deficiencies of the tests are that they are commonly negative early in infection and, as they remain positive for long periods of time, do not distinguish active from past infection. The Centers for Disease Control and Prevention uses a "fast ELISA" for screening (sensitivity and specificity = 99%) and a Western blot (specificity = 100%) for confirmation and speciation. Although yet a research tool, evidence is increasing that detection of antigen in blood and urine is a sensitive test, that it can distinguish old from new infection, and that loss of circulating antigen 5–10 days after treatment is indicative of cure. Skin testing is no longer recommended.

3. Other tests—Anemia is common. Eosinophilia, common during the acute stage, usually is absent in the chronic stage. In *S mansoni* and *S japonicum* infections, barium swallow, esophagoscopy, barium enema or colonoscopy, chest x-ray, or an ECG may be indicated. Ultrasound examination of the liver may show the pathognomonic pattern of periportal fibrosis and replaces the need for liver biopsy. The clinical settings in which ultrasonography is most useful are (1) evaluation of portal hypertension, (2) distinguishing schistosomiasis from cirrhosis, and (3) documenting regression of lesions following treatment; in early infections, however, findings are inconsistently present.

In *S haematobium* infection, occult hematuria can often be detected either microscopically or by reagent strip test, particularly if the first portion of the urine specimen is evaluated. In advanced disease, cystoscopy may show "sandy patches," ulcers, and areas of squamous metaplasia; lower abdominal plain films may show calcification of the bladder wall or ureters. Sonography is considered the imaging technique of choice but may fail to show the calcification. CT—which may demonstrate pathognomonic "turtleback" calcifications—intravenous pyelography, and retrograde cystography and pyelography may be useful.

Differential Diagnosis

Early intestinal schistosomiasis may be mistaken for amebiasis, bacillary dysentery, or other causes of diarrhea and dysentery. Later, the various causes of portal hypertension or of bowel polyps must be considered. In endemic areas, vesical schistosomiasis must be differentiated from other causes of urinary symptoms such as genitourinary tract cancer, bacterial infections of the urinary tract, nephrolithiasis, and the like.

Treatment

A. MEDICAL TREATMENT

Treatment should be given only if live ova are identified. The safety and effectiveness of current drugs make it possible to treat all active infections orally, including advanced disease, and without concern for serious side effects. Praziquantel can be used to treat all species; alternative drugs of choice are oxamniquine for S mansoni and metrifonate for S haematobium. Under study are the use of artemisinin and its derivatives for prophylaxis and treatment of acute attacks; the drugs are most useful against juvenile stages of the parasites. Instances of both oxamniquine and praziquantel resistance have been recognized in some localities.

After treatment, periodic laboratory follow-up for continued passage of eggs is essential, starting at 3 months and continuing at intervals for 1 year; if found, viability should be determined, since dead eggs are passed for some months.

1. Praziquantel—Cure rates of 85% and higher are achieved at 6 months for S haematobium, S mansoni, and S japonicum infections, with marked reduction in egg counts (> 90%) in those not cured. Immature schistosomes (2–5 weeks) are largely insensitive to praziquantel.

The praziquantel dosage is 20 mg/kg—give twice in 1 day for S haematobium and S mansoni and three times in 1 day for S japonicum and S mekongi. The dosages should be given at 4- to 6-hour intervals with water after a meal; the tablets should not be chewed.

Mild and transient side effects persisting for hours to 1 day are common and include malaise, headache, dizziness, and anorexia. Less frequent are fatigue, drowsiness, nausea, vomiting, generalized abdominal pain, loose stools, pruritus, urticaria, arthralgia and myalgia, and low-grade fever. Minimal elevations of liver enzymes have occasionally been reported. The drug should not be used in pregnancy, and because of drug-induced dizziness, patients should not drive and should be cautioned if their work requires physical coordination or alertness. In areas where cysticercosis may coexist with a schistosomal infection being treated with praziquantel, treatment is best conducted in a hospital to monitor for death of cysticerci, which may be followed by neurologic complications. Recently reported for praziquantel are comutagenic effects with several mutagens and carcinogens; the authors conclude that the import of these findings needs further study. Reduced susceptibility of S mansoni to praziquantel has been reported from some areas of Africa.

2. Oxamniquine—Oxamniquine is highly effective only in S mansoni infections. For strains in the western hemisphere and western Africa, a dose of 15 mg/kg is given once. Some experts recommend 40–60 mg/kg/d in two or three divided doses for 2–3 days in all of Africa and in the Arabian peninsula. The drug is administered with food; when divided doses are needed, they are separated by 6–8 hours. Cure rates are 70–95%, with marked reduction in egg counts in those not cured. Side effects occur within hours: dizziness is most common; less frequent are drowsiness, nausea and vomiting, diarrhea, abdominal pain, and headache. An orange or red discoloration of the urine may occur. Rarely reported is central nervous system stimulation with behavioral changes, hallucinations, or seizures; patients should be observed for 2 hours after ingestion of the drug for appearance of these findings. Since the drug makes some patients dizzy or drowsy, it should be used with caution in patients whose work or activity requires mental alertness. Instances of parasite resistance to the drug have been reported. Because the drug has shown mutagenic and embryotoxic effects, it is contraindicated in pregnancy.

3. Others—Artemisinin compounds (used in malaria treatment) are being evaluated; because they are particularly active against the migratory stage of the parasite—the schistosomulae—they may be useful in chemoprophylaxis. Metrifonate, effective against S haematobium, has been withdrawn from the market.

B. SURGICAL MEASURES

In selected instances, surgery may be indicated for removal of polyps and for obstructive uropathy. For bleeding esophageal varices, sclerotherapy is the treatment of choice. Whether some patients may benefit from propranolol treatment is under evaluation. As a last resort in patients who have repeated bleeding, shunting procedures (esophagogastric devascularization with splenectomy or distal—but not proximal—splenorenal shunt) are used, though their effectiveness and relative usefulness are not well established. Severe pancytopenia is an indication for splenectomy.

Prognosis

With treatment, the prognosis is excellent in early and light infections. There may be shrinkage or elimination of bladder and bowel ulcerations, granulomas, and polyps and reduction in fibrosis by sonography. In advanced disease with extensive involvement of the intestines, liver, bladder, or other organs, the outlook is poor even with treatment. In endemic areas, mass treatment of children diminishes the risk of developing severely diseased organs, even though reinfection may occur.

Bica I et al: Hepatic schistosomiasis. Infect Dis Clin North Am 2000;14:583. [PMID: 10987111]

Bichler KH et al: Schistosomiasis: a critical review. Curr Opin Urol 2001;11:97. [PMID: 11148754]

Borrmann S et al: Artesunate and praziquantel for the treatment of *Schistosoma mansoni* infections: a double-blind, randomized, placebo-controlled study. J Infect Dis 2001;184:1363. [PMID: 11679932]

Hatz CF. The use of ultrasound in schistosomiasis. Adv Parasitol 2001;48:225. [PMID: 11013757]

Saconato H et al: Interventions for treating schistosomiasis mansoni. Cochrane Database Syst Rev 2000;CD000528. [PMID: 10796552]

Squires N: Interventions for treating schistosomiasis haematobium. Cochrane Database Syst Rev 2000;CD000053. [PMID: 10796476]

FASCIOLOPSIASIS

The large intestinal fluke, *Fasciolopsis buski,* is a common parasite of humans and pigs in central and southern China, Taiwan, Southeast Asia, Indonesia, eastern India, and Bangladesh. When eggs shed in stools reach water, they hatch to produce free-swimming larvae that penetrate and develop in the flesh of snails. Cercariae subsequently escape from the snails and encyst on various water plants. Humans are infected by eating these plants uncooked (usually water chestnuts, bamboo shoots, or caltrops). Adult flukes (length 2–7.5 cm) mature in about 3 months and live in the small intestine attached to the mucosa or buried in mucous secretions. The number of parasites ranges from a few to several thousand.

After an incubation period of 2–3 months, manifestations of gastrointestinal irritation appear in all but light infections. Symptoms in severe infections include nausea, anorexia, upper abdominal pain, and diarrhea, sometimes alternating with constipation. Ascites and edema of the face and lower extremities may occur later; the physiologic mechanism is not understood. Intestinal obstruction, ileus, cachexia, and extreme prostration have been described.

Diagnosis depends on finding characteristic eggs or, occasionally, flukes in the stools. Leukocytosis with moderate eosinophilia is common. No serologic test is available. Because the adult worms live for only 6 months, absence from the endemic area for a longer period makes the diagnosis unlikely.

The drug of first choice is praziquantel, 25 mg/kg three times in 1 day only. The alternative drug is niclosamide (not available in the USA), administered as for taeniasis but given every other day for three doses.

In light infections—even without treatment—the prognosis is good, generally, spontaneous cure occurs within 1 year. In rare cases—particularly in children—heavy infections with severe toxemia have resulted in death from cachexia or intercurrent infection.

Liu LX et al: Liver and intestinal flukes. Gastroenterol Clin North Am 1996;25:627. [PMID: 8863043]

FASCIOLIASIS

Infection by *Fasciola hepatica,* the sheep liver fluke, results from ingestion of encysted metacercariae on watercress or other aquatic vegetables or in water. A wide range of herbivorous mammals are reservoir hosts. The disease in humans probably occurs worldwide but is most prevalent in sheep-raising countries, particularly where raw salads are eaten. The infection has been reported from Europe, mainland USA, Hawaii, the West Indies, the Middle East, China, Siberia, and North, East and South Africa. Eggs of the worm, passed in host feces into fresh water, release a miracidium that infects snails; the snails subsequently release cercariae that in turn encyst as metacercariae on vegetation (some cercariae become metacercariae directly in the water) to complete their life cycle. The leaf-shaped adult flukes measure 3 × 1.5 cm.

In humans, metacercariae excyst, penetrate and migrate through the liver, and mature in the bile ducts, where they cause local parenchymal necrosis and abscess formation. Although the infection is usually mild, three clinical syndromes can develop: acute, chronic latent, and chronic obstructive. The acute illness, associated with migration of immature larvae through the liver, shows an enlarged and tender liver, high fever, leukocytosis, and marked eosinophilia (to 90%). Pain may be present in the epigastrium or right upper quadrant, and the patient may experience headache, anorexia, and vomiting, myalgia, urticaria, and other allergic reactions. Jaundice, cachexia, and prostration may appear in severe illness. Anemia and hypergammaglobulinemia are common; other liver function tests may be abnormal. Early diagnosis is difficult in the acute phase, because eggs are not found in the feces for 3–4 months. The chronic latent phase may be asymptomatic or characterized by hepatomegaly and other acute findings. The chronic obstructive phase takes place if the extrahepatic bile ducts are occluded, producing a clinical picture similar to that of sclerosing cholangitis, biliary cirrhosis, or choledocholithiasis. Occasionally, adult flukes migrate and produce lesions and symptoms in ectopic sites.

Diagnosis is established by detecting characteristic eggs in the feces; repeated examinations may be necessary. Sometimes the diagnosis can only be made by finding eggs in biliary drainage and, in rare instances, only after liver biopsy or at surgical exploration. Exogenous transient fecal carriage can occur as a result of ingestion of egg-containing cow or sheep liver. Ultrasonography and cholangiography may show adult parasites in the gallbladder or ducts. Eosinophilia is characteristic, and hypergammaglobulinemia and abnormal liver function tests may be present. Serologic tests are often useful in presumptive diagnosis, particularly in the acute phase (before eggs have appeared) or in ectopic infection. The ELISA is highly sensitive and specific in detection of both antibody and antigen, particularly in acute infections, but cross-reactions have occurred with schistosomiasis. Successful treatment appears to correlate with a decline in antibody titer. A fecal ELISA is promising.

Evidence is increasing that triclabendazole (Fasinex—available in the USA from Novartis Agribusiness), a veterinary fasciolicide, is the drug of choice. At present, it is used in humans only on an experimental basis; 10 mg/kg given for 2 days with food achieves a cure rate of 80% with an absence of side effects. Instances of *F hepatica* resistance to triclabendazole in domestic animals has been reported. Bithionol (given as for paragonimiasis) is the alternative drug of choice; its deficiencies are its long course, failure rates of up to 50%, and frequent adverse reactions. Albendazole trials continue, but that drug also has shown high failure rates. An initial report suggests high effectiveness with low side-effects for nitazoxanide, a veterinary anthelmintic.

Reports on praziquantel have been variable; generally, it is ineffective even when used for up to 7 days at a dose of 25 mg/kg three times daily with a 4- to 6-hour interval between doses. If triclabendazole, bithionol, or praziquantel is not effective, dehydroemetine or emetine hydrochloride in dosages used for amebic liver abscess may help; both drugs are potentially toxic, but dehydroemetine may be less so. For any of the drugs, the destruction of parasites followed by release of antigen in sensitized patients may evoke symptoms.

Bithionol and dehydroemetine are available in the USA only from the Parasitic Disease Drug Service, Centers for Disease Control, Atlanta, GA 30333.

In endemic areas, aquatic plants should not be eaten raw; washing does not destroy the metacercariae, but cooking will. Drinking water must be boiled (1 minute) or purified.

Dowidar N et al: Endoscopic therapy of fascioliasis resistant to oral therapy. Gastrointest Endosc 1999;50:345. [PMID: 10464682]

Graham CS et al: Imported *Fasciola hepatica* infection in the United States and treatment with triclabendazole. Clin Infect Dis 2001;33:1. [PMID: 11389487]

Mannstadt M et al: Conservative management of biliary obstruction due to *Fasciola hepatica*. Clin Infect Dis 2000;31:1301 [PMID: 11073771]

CLONORCHIASIS & OPISTHORCHIASIS

Infection by *Clonorchis sinensis,* the Chinese liver fluke, is endemic in areas of Japan, Korea, China, Taiwan, Southeast Asia, and the far eastern part of Russia. Over 20 million people are affected. Opisthorchiasis is caused by worms of the genus opisthorchis, generally either *O felineus* (central, eastern, and southern Europe, eastern Asia, Southeast Asia, India) or *O viverrini* (Thailand, Laos, Vietnam). Clinically and epidemiologically, opisthorchiasis and clonorchiasis are identical.

Certain snails are infected when they ingest eggs shed into water in human or animal feces. Larval forms escape from the snails, penetrate the flesh of various freshwater fish, and encyst as metacercariae. Fish-eating wild and domestic mammals—including dogs, cats, and pigs—and humans maintain the life cycle. Human infection results from eating such fish, either raw or undercooked. Pickling, smoking, or drying may not suffice to kill the metacercariae. In humans, the ingested parasites excyst in the duodenum and ascend the bile ducts into the medium and small biliary radicals, but also into the larger ducts and the gallbladder, where they mature and remain throughout their lives (15–25 years), shedding eggs in the bile. In size, the worms are 7–20 × 1.5–3 mm. In the chronic stage of infection, there is progressive bile duct thickening, periductal fibrosis, dilation, biliary stasis, and secondary infection. Little fibrosis occurs in the portal tracts.

Most patients harbor few parasites and are asymptomatic. Among symptomatic patients, an acute and chronic syndrome occurs. Acute symptoms follow entry of immature worms into the biliary ducts and may persist for several weeks. Findings include malaise, low-grade fever, an enlarged, tender liver, pain in the hepatic area or epigastrium, urticaria, arthralgia, leukocytosis, eosinophilia, an elevated serum alanine aminotransferase, and jaundice. The acute syndrome is difficult to diagnose, since ova may not appear in the feces until 3–4 weeks after onset of symptoms.

In chronic infections, findings include weakness, anorexia, epigastric pain, diarrhea, prolonged low-grade fever, intermittent episodes of right upper quadrant pain, localized hepatic area tenderness, and progressive hepatomegaly; liver function tests are normal except in severe cases.

Complications include intrahepatic bile duct calculi that may lead to recurrent pyogenic cholangitis, biliary abscess, or endophlebitis of the portal-venous branches. Although focal initially, this may gradually result in destruction of the liver parenchyma, fibrosis, and, in a few patients, cirrhosis with jaundice and ascites. Chronic cholecystitis, cholelithiasis, and a nonfunctional, enlarged gallbladder may occur. Flukes may also enter the pancreatic duct, causing acute pancreatitis or cholelithiasis. Cholangiocarcinoma has been causally linked with prolonged clonorchis and opisthorchis infection.

Diagnosis is made by finding characteristic eggs in stools (repeated tests may be necessary) or duodenal aspirate (sensitivity approaches 100%). In severe infection, the number of eggs per gram of feces may not reflect the heavy worm burden; and in complete biliary obstruction, eggs can be detected in bile only by needle aspiration or at surgery. In advanced chronic disease, (1) liver function tests will indicate parenchymal damage; (2) CT and sonography may show diffuse dilation of small intrahepatic bile ducts with no or minimal dilation of the large intra- and extrahepatic ducts; and (3) transhepatic cholangiograms may show alternating stricture and dilation of the biliary tree, with worms visualized as filling defects. Where available, of the several evaluated serologic tests, the ELISA is preferred (sensitivity, 77%); however, unless a specific monoclonal antibody is used, cross-reactions are common with other trematode and cestode infections, tuberculosis, and liver cancer. During the chronic stage, leukocytosis varies according to the intensity of infection; eosinophilia may be present.

The drug of choice is praziquantel. With a dosage of 25 mg/kg three times daily for 2 days (with a 4- to 6-hour interval between doses), cure rates over 95% can be anticipated for clonorchis infections. One day of treatment may be sufficient for opisthorchis infections. (For side effects, see Schistosomiasis, above.) Albendazole, at a dosage of 400 mg twice daily for 7 days, appears to be less effective (cures, 40–65%). In relapsing cholangitis, antibiotics are indicated to cover biliary pathogens.

The disease is rarely fatal, but patients with advanced infections and impaired liver function may succumb more readily to other diseases. The prognosis is good for light to moderate infections.

Liu LX et al: Liver and intestinal flukes. Gastroenterol Clin North Am 1996;25:627. [PMID: 8863043]

Pungpak S et al: *Opisthorchis viverrini* infection in Thailand: Studies on the morbidity of the infection and resolution following praziquantel treatment. Am J Trop Med Hyg 1997;56:311. [PMID: 9129534]

PARAGONIMIASIS

Paragonimus westermani, the lung fluke, commonly infects humans (estimated 20 million) throughout the Far East (prevalence in Korea reached 4%); foci are also present in West Africa, South and Southeast Asia, the Pacific Islands, Indonesia, and New Guinea. Many carnivores and omnivores in addition to humans serve as reservoir hosts for the adult fluke (8–16 × 4–8 × 3–5 mm). About a dozen other paragonimus species also infect humans in China, Japan, Mexico, and Central and South America.

Eggs reaching water, either in sputum or feces, hatch in 3–6 weeks. Released miracidia penetrate and develop in snails. Emergent cercariae encyst as metacercariae in the tissues of crabs and crayfish. Human infection results if metacercariae are ingested when the crustaceans are eaten raw or pickled or are crushed and food, vessels, drinking water or fingers become contaminated. The metacercariae excyst in the small intestine and penetrate the peritoneal cavity. Most migrate through the diaphragm and enter the peripheral lung parenchyma; some may lodge in the brain (about 1% of all cases) or at other ectopic sites. In the lungs, the parasite becomes encapsulated by granulomatous fibrous tissue, reaching up to 2 cm in diameter. The lesion, which usually opens into a bronchiole, may subsequently rupture, resulting in expectoration of eggs, blood, and inflammatory cells. Rarely, the eggs may also enter the general circulation and produce ectopic lesions in any tissue. The prepatent period until appearance of expectorated eggs is about 6 weeks. *P szechuanensis* in China has a propensity to migrate and produce subcutaneous nodules.

In pulmonary infections, most persons have light to moderate worm burdens and are asymptomatic. In symptomatic cases, low-grade fever and dry cough are present initially; subsequently, pleuritic pain is common, and a rusty, blood-flecked, viscous sputum or frank hemoptysis may occur. Following slow progression, complications of bronchitis, bronchiectasis, bronchopneumonia, lung abscess, fibrosis, and pleural thickening or effusion may appear.

Only a minority of patients with cerebral infections present with acute disease, usually manifested by meningitis. In chronic central nervous system disease, seizures, cranial neuropathies, or meningoencephalitis may occur; death can follow. Parasites in the peritoneal cavity or the intestinal wall may cause abdominal pain, diarrhea or dysentery, and a palpable tumor mass. Migratory subcutaneous nodules (a few millimeters to 1 cm in diameter) occur with about 10% of *P westermani* infections and up to 60% of *Paragonimus skrjabini* infections.

Pulmonary disease is diagnosed by finding (1) characteristic eggs in sputum (rusty sputum is nearly pathognomonic), feces, bronchoscopic washings, biopsy specimens, or pleural fluid; or (2) adult flukes in subcutaneous nodules or other surgical specimens. If eggs are not found after multiple direct sputum examinations, they may be detectable in a 24-hour sputum collection processed by alkaline sodium hypochlorite concentration. Stool examination for eggs has low sensitivity. Serum and cerebrospinal fluid serologic tests (ELISA, 99% sensitivity, 97% specificity; and immunoblot, 96% sensitivity and 99% specificity) do not differentiate active from prior infection; a newly reported IgM test may do so. Most treated and cured patients become seronegative. An antigen detection assay is promising. Eosinophilia (sometimes to a high level) and low-grade leukocytosis are common. Chest films may show infiltrates, fibrosis, nodules, cavitary lesions, pleural thickening or effusion, or calcifications. By CT, round, low-attenuation cystic lesions (5–15 mm) filled with fluid or gas are seen within the consolidation.

In acute cerebral disease, CT shows multilocular, ring-like enhancement with surrounding low-density areas. In chronic cerebral disease, plain skull films often show round or oval-shaped calcifications, sometimes surrounded by low-density areas. Cerebrospinal fluid may be turgid or bloody, with numerous eosinophils, and eggs may be found. The EEG is almost always abnormal.

Paragonimiasis and tuberculosis must be differentiated, though chest x-ray appearance alone does not make the distinction. Since paragonimus ova are destroyed by Ziehl-Neelsen stain for acid-fast bacilli, the sputum should first be examined for the eggs. The presence of a large number of eosinophils or Charcot-Leyden crystals in sputum suggests paragonimiasis.

In pulmonary paragonimiasis, praziquantel is the drug of choice (25 mg/kg after meals three times daily for 3 days, with a 4- to 6-hour interval between doses). (For side effects, see above under Schistosomiasis.) Bithionol is the alternative drug (30–50 mg/kg, given on alternate days for 10–15 doses [20–30 days]; the daily dose should be divided into a morning and evening dose). Side effects are frequent but generally mild and transient. Gastrointestinal side effects, particularly diarrhea, occur in most patients. Liver function should be tested serially. Bithionol is available in the USA only from the Parasitic Disease Drug Service, Centers for Disease Control, Atlanta, GA 30333. Antibiotics may be necessary for secondary pulmonary infection. Cure rates of over 90% can be anticipated for both praziquantel and bithionol. Triclabendazole, a veterinary fasciolicide, is under investigation at a dosage of 5 mg/kg once daily for 3 days.

In the acute stage of cerebral paragonimiasis, particularly meningitis, praziquantel or bithionol may be effective. With death of parasites, severe local reactions may occur; corticosteroids should therefore be given as in cerebral cysticercosis. In the chronic stage, both surgical removal of the parasites and drug usage are likely to be ineffective in diminishing neurologic symptoms.

Calvopina M et al: Treatment of human pulmonary paragonimiasis with triclabendazole: Clinical tolerance and drug efficacy. Trans R Soc Trop Med Hyg 1998;92:566. [PMID: 9861383]

Nawa Y: Re-emergence of paragonimiasis. Intern Med 2000;39: 353. [PMID: 10830172]

■ CESTODE INFECTIONS

TAPEWORM INFECTIONS
(See also Cysticercosis and Echinococcosis, Below.)

Classification

Six tapeworms infect humans frequently. The large tapeworms are *Taenia saginata* (the beef tapeworm, up to 25 m in length), *Taenia solium* (the pork tapeworm, 7 m), and *Diphyllobothrium latum* (the fish tapeworm, 10 m). The small tapeworms are *Hymenolepis nana* (the dwarf tapeworm, 25–40 mm), *Hymenolepis diminuta* (the rodent tapeworm, 20–60 cm), and *Dipylidium caninum* (the dog tapeworm, 10–70 cm). Four of the six tapeworms occur worldwide; the pork and fish tapeworms have more limited

distribution. Humans are the only definitive host of *T saginata* and *T solium*.

An adult tapeworm consists of a head (scolex), a neck, and a chain of individual segments (proglottids) in which eggs form in mature segments. The scolex is the attachment organ and generally lodges in the upper part of the small intestine.

Multiple infections are the rule for small tapeworms and may occur for *D latum;* however, it is rare for a person to harbor more than one or two of the taeniae.

A. BEEF TAPEWORM

The infection occurs in most countries with beef husbandry but is highly endemic in parts of the Far East, central and eastern Africa, and the central Asian area of the former Soviet Union. Gravid segments of *T saginata* in the human intestine detach themselves from the chain and are passed in feces to soil. When proglottids or eggs are ingested by grazing cattle or other domesticated bovines, the eggs hatch to release embryos that encyst in muscle as cysticerci. Humans are infected by eating raw or undercooked beef containing viable cysticerci, *Cysticercus bovis*. In the human intestines, the cysticercus develops into an adult worm.

B. PORK TAPEWORM

This tapeworm is particularly prevalent in Mexico, Latin America, the Iberian Peninsula, the Slavic countries, Africa, Southeast Asia, India, and China. In the USA and Canada, human infection is rare, usually encountered in persons infected abroad; cysticercosis in hogs is uncommon. The infection is no longer found in northwestern Europe. The life cycle of *T solium* is similar to that of *T saginata* except that pigs ingest human feces containing proglottids and eggs to become the host of the larval stage. Humans become infected when they eat undercooked pork containing viable *C cellulosae*. Humans are also the intermediate host when they become infected with the larval stage (see Cysticercosis, below) by accidentally ingesting eggs in human feces; the eggs are immediately infectious. Transmission of eggs may occur as a result of autoinfection (hand to mouth), direct person-to-person transfer, ingestion of food or drink contaminated by eggs, or (rarely) regurgitation of proglottids into the stomach.

C. FISH TAPEWORM

D latum is found in temperate and subarctic lake regions in many areas of the world, including northern Europe, Canada, Alaska, the Pacific Coast of the USA (the infection may no longer be present in the Great Lakes areas), Japan, Taiwan, Siberia, Manchuria, Australia, and southern South America and southern Africa. Eggs passed in human feces that reach fresh water are taken up first by crustaceans that in turn are eaten by fish, both of which are intermediate hosts.

Human infection results from eating raw or inadequately cooked brackish or freshwater fish, including salmon. Nonhuman reservoir hosts include dogs, bears, and other fish-eating mammals.

D. DWARF TAPEWORM

H nana is the most common cestode. It can reach high prevalence, particularly in children, in regions of the world with poor fecal hygiene and in closed institutions worldwide. Humans are the definitive host of the human strain of the parasite; rodent-adapted strains occur in rodents. The life cycle is unusual in that both larval and adult stages are found in the human intestine, internal autoinfection can occur, and generally there is no intermediate host. Transmission usually results from eggs transferred directly from human to human (the eggs are immediately infective) but sometimes involves fomites, water, or food or the swallowing of fleas or beetles infected with the larval stage. *H nana* infections in children are usually lost spontaneously in adolescence.

E. RODENT TAPEWORM

H diminuta is a common parasite of rodents. Many arthropods (eg, rat fleas, beetles, and cockroaches) serve as intermediate hosts. Humans—most commonly young children—are infected by accidentally swallowing the infected arthropods, usually in cereals or stored products.

F. DOG TAPEWORM

D caninum infection generally occurs in young children in close association with infected dogs or cats. Transmission results from swallowing the infected intermediate hosts, ie, fleas or lice.

Clinical Findings

A. SIGNS AND SYMPTOMS

1. Large tapeworms—Large tapeworm infections are generally asymptomatic. Occasionally, vague gastrointestinal symptoms (eg, nausea, diarrhea, abdominal pain) and systemic symptoms (eg, fatigue, hunger, dizziness) have been attributed to the infections. Vomiting of proglottid segments or obstruction of the bile duct, pancreatic duct, or appendix is rare.

Some persons (mostly Scandinavian residents) who harbor the fish tapeworm develop a macrocytic megaloblastic anemia accompanied by thrombocytopenia and mild leukopenia. Gastric acidity is normal. The anemia is a result of the worm's competing with the host for vitamin B_{12}. Clinical findings are indistinguishable from those of pernicious anemia and include glossitis, dyspnea, tachycardia, and neurologic findings (numbness, paresthesias, disturbances of coordination, impairment of vibration and position sense, and dementia).

2. Small tapeworms—Light infections are generally asymptomatic. Heavy infections, particularly with *H nana*, may cause diarrhea, abdominal pain, anorexia, vomiting, weight loss, and irritability.

B. LABORATORY FINDINGS

Infection by a beef or pork tapeworm is often discovered by the patient finding segments in stool, clothing, or bedding. To determine the species, proglottid segments are either flattened between glass slides and examined microscopically for anatomic detail or differentiated by enzyme electrophoresis of glucose phosphate isomerase. Eggs are only infrequently present in stools, but the perianal cellophane tape test, as used to diagnose pinworm, is sometimes useful in detecting *T saginata* eggs. However, taenia eggs look alike and do not permit species differentiation except by specialized methods. Detection of taenia-specific antigens in stool, currently a research method, may become the most sensitive method for detecting infection.

Fish tapeworm is diagnosed by finding characteristic operculated eggs in stool; repeat examinations and concentration may be necessary. Proglottids are occasionally vomited or passed in feces; their internal morphology is diagnostic. The presence of hydrochloric acid in the stomach differentiates tapeworm anemia from pernicious anemia; in both conditions, the Schilling test is abnormal.

H nana and *H diminuta* infections are diagnosed by finding characteristic eggs in feces; proglottids are usually not seen. *D caninum* infection is diagnosed by detection of proglottids (the size of melon seeds) in feces or after their active migration through the anus.

Serologic tests are not available for tapeworm infections; an ELISA for detection of coproantigens is under evaluation.

Treatment

A. SPECIFIC MEASURES

Although niclosamide (not available in the USA) and praziquantel are both drugs of choice for most tapeworm infections, praziquantel is more effective in hymenolepiasis, and some workers consider it to be somewhat more effective in taeniasis. In areas endemic for neurocysticercosis, a dose of praziquantel of 5 mg/kg or higher carries a small risk of activating the lesions. Niclosamide preferably should not be used in pregnancy.

1. *T saginata* and *D latum*—Praziquantel in a single dose of 10 mg/kg achieves cure rates of about 99%. At this dose, side effects (see under Schistosomiasis, above) are minimal. With a single dose of four tablets (2 g) of niclosamide, cure rates over 90% can be anticipated. The drug is given in the morning before the patient has eaten. The tablets *must be chewed thoroughly* and swallowed with water. Eating may be resumed in 2 hours. Niclosamide usually produces no side effects.

Pre- and posttreatment purges are not used for either drug. The anemia and neurologic manifestations of *D latum* respond to vitamin B_{12} as used in treatment of pernicious anemia.

2. *T solium*—The choice of drugs and methods of treatment are as above. Neither drug kills eggs released from disintegrating segments; therefore, to avoid the theoretical possibility of cysticercosis from hatching eggs, give a moderate purgative 2–3 hours after treatment to rapidly eliminate segments and eggs from the bowel. The patient must be instructed about the need after defecation for careful washing of the hands and perianal area and for safe disposal of feces for 4 days following therapy.

3. *H nana*—Praziquantel, the drug of choice, produces 95% cure rates with a single 25 mg/kg dose. Niclosamide, the alternative drug, produces cure rates of 75% when given at the above dosage for 5–7 days; some workers repeat the course 5 days later.

4. *H diminuta* and *D caninum*—Treatment is with niclosamide or praziquantel in dosages as for *H nana*. Cure rates are not established.

B. Follow-Up Care

In treatment of large tapeworm infections, a disintegrating worm is usually passed within 24–48 hours of treatment. Since efforts are not generally made to recover and identify the scolex, cure can be presumed only if regenerated segments have not reappeared 3–5 months later. If it is preferred that parasitic cure be established immediately, the head (scolex) must be found in posttreatment stools; a laxative is given 2 hours after treatment, and stools must be collected in a preservative for 24 hours. To facilitate examination, toilet paper must be disposed of separately.

Prevention & Prognosis

C cellulosae is killed by cooking at 65 °C or freezing at –20 °C for 12 hours; *C bovis* at 56 °C or –10 °C for 5 days. Pickling is not adequate. Because the prognosis is often poor in cerebral cysticercosis (see below), *T solium* infections must be immediately eradicated.

Ing MB et al: Human coenurosis in North America: Case reports and review. Clin Infect Dis 1998;27:519. [PMID: 9770151]

Shantz P: Tapeworms (cestodiasis). Gastroenterol Clin North Am 1996;25:637. [PMID: 8863044]

CYSTICERCOSIS

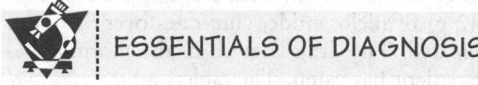

ESSENTIALS OF DIAGNOSIS

- *History of exposure to* Taenia solium *in an endemic region; concomitant or past intestinal tapeworm infection.*
- *Seizures, headache, and other findings of a focal space-occupying central nervous system lesion.*
- *Subcutaneous or muscular nodules (5–10 mm); calcified lesions on x-rays of soft tissues.*
- *Calcified or uncalcified cysts by CT scan or MRI; positive serologic tests.*

General Considerations

Human cysticercosis is infection by the larval (cysticercus) stage of the tapeworm *T solium* (see above). Worldwide, an estimated 20 million persons are infected and 50,000 deaths occur yearly. Antibody prevalence rates to 10% are recognized in some endemic areas.

The natural history of the infection is incompletely known. Cysticerci complete their development within 2–4 months after larval entry and live for months to years. Several factors give rise to symptomatology: Initially, the live larva within a thin-walled cyst (vesicular cyst) is minimally antigenic. When the host immune response or chemotherapy results in gradual death of the cyst, there may be cyst enlargement (colloidal cyst) with mechanical compression, inflammation with pericyst edema, and (sometimes) vasculitis that can result in small cerebral infarcts; increased intracranial pressure and cerebrospinal fluid changes may follow. Subsequently, as the cyst degenerates over 2–7 years, it may disappear or be replaced by a granuloma, calcification, or residual fibrosis. Cysts at different life cycle stages—active (live), transitional, and inactive (dead)—may be present in the same organ. Although some patients develop an intense immune response to the parasite, others show a remarkable tolerance.

Locations of cysts in order of frequency are the central nervous system, subcutaneous tissues and striated muscle, globe of the eye, and, rarely, other tissues. Cysts reach 5–10 mm in soft tissues but may be larger (up to 5 cm) in the central nervous system. Attached to the inner wall of the cyst is an invaginated protoscolex with four suckers and a crown of hooks.

Clinical Findings

A. Signs and Symptoms

1. Neurocysticercosis—In many patients, cysts remain asymptomatic. When symptomatic, the incubation period is highly variable (usually from 1 to 5 years but sometimes shorter). Manifestations are due to mass effect, inflammatory response, or obstruction of the brain foramina and ventricular systems. Neurologic findings are varied and nonspecific, in large part determined by the number and location of the cysts.

a. Acute invasive stage—This rare event, occurring shortly after invasion, results from extensive acute spread of cysticerci to the brain parenchyma. Fever, headache, myalgia, marked eosinophilia, and coma may occur.

b. Parenchymal cysts—Cysticerci can present singly or multiply and may be scattered or in clumps. Findings include epilepsy (focal or generalized), focal neurologic deficits, intracranial hypertension (intense headache, vomiting, papilledema, visual loss), and altered mental status. Seizures usually do not occur until the cyst or cysts have begun to die. Episodic symptoms have been associated with edema around calcified lesions.

c. Subarachnoid space cysts and meningeal cysts—Small to large cysts are generally located in the cortical sulci or basal cisterns. The arachnoid is the principal basal membrane affected. Adhesive arachnoiditis may result in obstructive hydrocephalus, intracranial hypertension, arterial thrombosis leading to transient ischemia or stroke, and cranial nerve dysfunction (most often of the optic nerve).

d. Ventricular cysts—Ventricular cysts may float freely (usually singly) within the ventricles or cerebral aqueduct or may be attached to the ventricular wall. They are usually asymptomatic but can cause increased intracranial pressure as a result of intermittent or total blockage.

e. Racemose cysts—These are rare aberrant forms that are multiple-branched, nonencysted, and lack a scolex; they present as grape-like irregular clusters and may reach over 10 cm in diameter. They generally are found in the ventricular and basal subarachnoid spaces, where they cause marked adhesive arachnoiditis and often obstructive hydrocephalus.

f. Spinal cord cysts—Cysts can be extraspinal or intraspinal and can cause arachnoiditis (meningitis, radiculopathy) or pressure symptoms.

2. Ophthalmocysticercosis—Usually there is a single cyst, free-floating in the vitreous or under the retina. Presenting symptoms include periorbital pain, scotomas, and progressive deterioration of visual acuity. Findings may include disk hemorrhage and edema, retinal detachment, iridocyclitis, and chorioretinitis. MRI but not CT may assist in diagnosis; immunologic tests are negative.

3. Subcutaneous and striated muscle cysticercosis—Subcutaneous cysts are usually asymptomatic; they present as nodules that tend to appear and disappear, or they may die and calcify and be detected on plain radiographs.

B. DIAGNOSTIC CRITERIA AND LABORATORY TESTS

Diagnosis of neurocysticercosis is (1) by CT or MRI detection of brain or spinal cord cystic lesions that show the scolex ("hole-with-dot") image; (2) by visualization of the parasite by ophthalmoscopic examination (subretinal or in the anterior chamber); or (3) by finding the parasite in histologic sections of brain or spinal cord tissue (not usually recommended). A probable diagnosis is based on the presence of various combinations of other major and minor criteria. Highly suggestive of the diagnosis are (1) finding the organism in excisional biopsies of skin or subcutaneous pea-sized nodules or (2) a varied radiologic appearance on brain scans.

1. Imaging—Plain radiographs of muscle may detect oval or linear calcified lesions (4–10 × 2–5 mm). The lesions are usually multiple, sometimes in the hundreds, and the long axes of the cysts are nearly always in the plane of the surrounding muscle fibers. Plain skull films may demonstrate one or more cerebral calcifications (generally 5–10 mm; sometimes 1–2 mm when only the scolex is calcified).

The most useful procedures for examining the skull are imaging initially by nonenhanced CT and then by MRI and enhanced CT. CT patterns include (1) vesicular cysts (viable cysts with no host immune reaction), which are rounded areas of low density with little or no enhancement after contrast medium; (2) colloidal cysts (dead or dying cysts with host immune reaction), which are hypodense or isodense lesions surrounded by edema associated with ring-like or nodular enhancement; and (3) granuloma or calcifications (dead cysts), which are often several millimeters in diameter but variable in size. Signs of increased intracranial pressure and diffuse brain edema may also be seen. A combination of images is often found, owing to different developmental stages. As compared with CT, MRI has superior resolution for vesicular cysts (isodense, similar to cerebrospinal fluid) and for colloidal cysts (hyperdense). However, CT is superior for granulomas and calcifications, the most frequent presentations of cysticercosis, which MRI may miss. The MRI sometimes detects pathognomonic 2- to 4-mm nodules (protoscoleces) within cyst fluid. Intraventricular cysts (isodense) are not seen on routine CT but require intraventricular contrast medium. Spinal cysticercosis is evaluated by CT myelography or MRI.

2. Immunologic tests—With serum, the enzyme-linked immunoelectrotransfer blot (EITB) assay has nearly 100% specificity and 94–98% sensitivity; when used with cerebrospinal fluid, however, both parameters are lower. Additionally, EITB sensitivity drops about 50% if only one or two cysts are present and is also low in patients with only calcified cysts. Where the EITB assay is not available, the older ELISA has a 63% specificity and 65% sensitivity with serum; paradoxically, the ELISA with cerebrospinal fluid has a high specificity (95%) and sensitivity (87%) for both IgM and IgG antibody. In endemic areas, false-positives can occur in patients with previous exposure. Another ELISA test to detect circulating antigen remains under study and may provide a means for distinguishing active from inactive infection and effectiveness of cure.

3. Other laboratory tests—Cerebrospinal fluid typically shows increased protein, decreased glucose, and a cellular reaction of mainly lymphocytes and eosinophils; eosinophilia may be over 20% is diagnostically important. Lumbar puncture is contraindicated in case of increased intracerebral pressure. The EEG may be abnormal. Though the patient usually no longer harbors a tapeworm, all family members should examine their stools over several days for passage of proglottids, and stool specimens should be sent to the laboratory to be examined for proglottids and eggs.

4. Other diagnostic criteria—Other major and minor criteria include (1) an epidemiologic history of tapeworm exposure (travel in an endemic area, tapeworm in a household contact, personal history of tapeworm); (2) spontaneous resolution (disappearance or shrinkage) of a single enhancing lesion or its transformation into a calcified nodule; and (3) resolution of a cyst lesion following therapy.

Differential Diagnosis

The differential diagnosis includes tuberculoma, primary or metastatic tumor, hydatid disease, vasculitis, chronic fungal disorders, pyogenic brain abscess, toxoplasmosis and other parasitic diseases, and neurosyphilis.

Treatment

Medical treatment, which is usually preferable to surgery, is most effective for parenchymal cysts; less effective for intraventricular, subarachnoid, or racemose cysts; and has no effect on and is not needed for granulomatous or calcified cysts. With parenchymal cysts, the evidence is still insufficient to establish that medical treatment is preferable to symptomatic management followed by normal death of the parasites. Some clinicians wait 3 months, with selected patients, to see if cysts will spontaneously disappear without treatment.

Albendazole and praziquantel are both effective in treatment. Albendazole is preferred because its course of treatment is shorter (1 week) than that of praziquantel (2 weeks); because albendazole is less expensive; and because coadministration of albendazole and a steroid (to treat inflammation) results in increased albendazole absorption, whereas combined use of praziquantel and a steroid greatly decreases plasma levels of praziquantel. Both drugs are given with fatty meals which increases absorption fourfold to fivefold. Treatment should be conducted in hospital. In less than a week after starting treatment, inflammatory reactions around dying parasites may be manifested by meningismus, headache (analgesics may be sufficient for mild symptoms), vomiting, hyperthermia, mental changes, and convulsions; decompensation with death is very rare. It remains controversial whether to give steroids concomitantly to avoid or diminish this reaction or to use them only if marked symptoms appear or increase. Even when steroids are given prospectively, the inflammatory reaction may occur. Prednisone, 30 mg/d in two or three divided doses, starting 1–2 days before use of the drug and continuing at diminishing doses for about 14 days afterward, is one regimen. The reaction usually subsides in 48–72

hours, but continuing severity may require steroids in higher dosage and mannitol. Anticonvulsants should be given during drug treatment and probably for an indefinite time afterward.

Cure rates following treatment (disappearance of cysts and clearing of symptoms) ranged up to 88% for albendazole and 50–60% for praziquantel. Of the remaining patients, many have amelioration of symptoms, including intracranial hypertension and seizures.

An ophthalmologic examination should be done; if cysticercocidal drugs are given in the presence of ocular or spinal cysts, irreparable damage can occur.

A. MEDICAL MEASURES

1. Albendazole—The dosage is 400 mg twice daily with a fatty meal. The duration of treatment is unsettled. Eight days may be sufficient for some patients, but a longer course (up to 28 days) is advisable at present; it can be repeated as necessary. Up to 3 months of treatment may be needed for ventricular and subarachnoid cysts. For albendazole side effects, see below under Hydatid Disease.

2. Praziquantel—Give 50–100 mg/kg/d in three divided doses for 15–30 days . Phenytoin, phenobarbital, carbamazepine, cimetidine, and corticosteroids, when administered with praziquantel, reduce serum levels of the latter; high doses of praziquantel have been tried in these circumstances. Ingestion with a high-carbohydrate meal enhances absorption.

B. OTHER MEASURES

Seizures are treated with anticonvulsant drugs. During the acute phase of cysticercotic encephalitis, if intracranial hypertension is present, corticosteroids are used but drug treatment is withheld. Surgery has successfully removed accessible orbital, cisternal, ventricular, cerebral, meningeal, and spinal cord cysts. Obstructive hydrocephalus requires cerebrospinal fluid diversion plus a corticosteroid. Subarachnoiditis and vasculitis are treated with albendazole or praziquantel plus a corticosteroid. Albendazole or praziquantel, when used with ocular or spinal medullary lesions, may cause irreversible damage even when corticosteroids are given.

Prognosis

The fatality rate for untreated neurocysticercosis is about 50%; survival time from onset of symptoms ranges from days to many years. Drug treatment has reduced the mortality rate to about 5–15%. Surgical procedures to relieve intracranial hypertension along with use of steroids to reduce edema improve the prognosis for those not effectively treated with the drugs.

Del Brutto OH et al: Proposed diagnostic criteria for neurocysticercosis. Neurology 2001;57:177. [PMID: 11480424]

Garcia HH et al: Serum antigen detection in the diagnosis, treatment, and follow-up of neurocysticercosis patients. Trans R Soc Trop Med Hyg 2000;94:673. [PMID: 11198654]

Garcia HH et al: Taenia solium cysticercosis. Infect Dis North Am 2000;14:97. [PMID: 10738675]

Salinas R et al: Treating neurocysticercosis medically: a systematic review of randomized, controlled trials. Trop Med Int Health 1999;4:713. [PMID: 10588764]

White AC Jr: Neurocysticercosis: updates on epidemiology, pathogenesis, diagnosis, and management. Annu Rev Med 2000;51:187. [PMID: 10774460]

Zee CS et al: Imaging of neurocysticercosis. Neuroimaging Clin N Am 2000;10:391. [PMID: 10775958]

ECHINOCOCCOSIS
(Hydatid Disease, Hydatidosis)

Human echinococcosis results from parasitism by the larval stage of four echinococcus species of which *E granulosus* (cystic hydatid disease) and *E multilocularis* (alveolar hydatid disease) are the most important. Minor species are the polycystic species, *E vogeli* (polycystic hydatid disease) and *E oligarthrus*, both from Central and South America. Echinococcosis is a zoonosis in which humans are an intermediate host of the larval stage of the parasite. The definitive host is a carnivore (all of which, except for the lion, are Canidae) that harbors the adult tapeworm in the small intestine; the carnivore becomes infected by ingesting the larval form in tissue of the intermediate host. The intermediate hosts, chiefly herbivorous mammals but also humans, become infected by ingesting tapeworm eggs passed in carnivore feces. The larval stage is referred to as a hydatid cyst.

1. Cystic Hydatid Disease (Unilocular Hydatid Disease)

ESSENTIALS OF DIAGNOSIS

- *History of exposure to dogs associated with live-stock in a hydatid-endemic region.*
- *Avascular cystic tumor of liver, lung, or, infrequently, bone, brain, or other organs as detected by imaging procedures.*
- *Symptoms and signs of a space-occupying mass.*
- *Positive serologic tests.*

General Considerations

Human infection with *E granulosus* is common throughout southern South America, the Mediterranean littoral and the Middle East, central Asia, and East Africa. Endemic foci are in eastern Europe, Russia, Australia, New Zealand, India, and the United Kingdom; in North America, foci have been reported from the western USA, the lower Mississippi valley, Alaska, and northwestern Canada.

The pastoral strain—which is more pathogenic to humans—has a transmission cycle in which dogs are the definitive host, and sheep (usually) but also cattle and other domestic livestock are intermediate hosts. However, the strain in horses, pigs, and camels may be of low or no infectivity for humans. The sylvatic, or northern, strain is maintained in wolves and wild ungulates (moose and reindeer) in northern Alaska, Canada, Scandinavia, and Eurasia.

Human infection occurs when eggs passed in dog feces are accidentally swallowed. Liberated embryos penetrate the intestinal mucosa, enter the portal bloodstream, and are carried to the liver where they become hydatid cysts (65% of all cysts). Some larvae reach the lung (25%) and develop into pulmonary hydatids. Infrequently, cysts form in the brain, bones, skeletal muscles, kidneys, spleen, or other tissues. Cysts of the sylvatic strain tend to localize in the lungs.

The cyst wall has three layers: an inner germinal layer that gives rise within the cyst to germinal elements, a supporting intermediate layer, and an outer layer produced by the host. In the liver, cysts may increase in size 1–30 mm in diameter per year and become enormous, but symptoms generally do not develop until they reach about 10 cm. Some cysts die spontaneously; others may persist unchanged for years. Part or all of the inner layer of hepatic and splenic cysts may calcify, which does not necessarily mean cyst death.

Clinical Findings

A. SYMPTOMS AND SIGNS

A liver cyst may remain silent for 10–20 or more years until it becomes large enough to be palpable, to be visible as an abdominal swelling, to produce pressure effects, or (rarely) to produce symptoms due to leakage or rupture. There may be right upper quadrant pain, nausea, and vomiting. The effects of pressure may result in biliary obstruction, with secondary bacterial cholangitis, cirrhosis, and portal hypertension. If a cyst ruptures suddenly, anaphylaxis and death may occur. If fluid and hydatid particles escape slowly, allergic manifestations may result, including a rise in the eosinophil count. Rupture can occur into the pleural, pericardial, or peritoneal space or into the duodenum, colon, or renal pelvis. Dissemination of germinal elements may be followed by the development of multiple secondary cysts. A characteristic clinical syndrome may follow intrabiliary extrusion of cyst contents—jaundice, biliary colic, and urticaria.

Pulmonary cysts cause no symptoms until they leak; become large enough to obstruct a bronchus, causing segmental collapse; or erode into a bronchus and rupture. Brain cysts produce symptoms earlier and may cause seizures or symptoms of increased intracranial pressure. Cysts in the bone marrow or spongiosa do not have a host layer, are irregular in shape, erode osseous tissue, and present as pain or as spontaneous fracture. The bones most often affected are the vertebrae; many of these patients develop epidural extension with compression of the spinal cord and paraplegia. Because 20% of patients have multiple cysts, upon diagnosis each patient should be screened for cysts in the liver, spleen, kidneys, lungs, brain, bones, skin, tongue, vitreous, and other tissues.

B. IMAGING

The method of choice for liver and splenic cysts is sonography (specificity 90%) followed by CT (gives better information about location and depth of cyst). The cysts can also be defined by MRI; scintillation scan and angiography are rarely used. Cysts may present as solitary lesions with interior echoes or as multilocular cysts with daughter cysts. Nearly pathognomonic is the presence within a hydatid cyst of daughter cysts; they must be distinguished, however, from blood clots within the cavity of simple cysts. Spotty calcified densities or a calcified cyst wall may be seen in the liver or spleen. Chest films may show an elevated diaphragm. Pulmonary cysts are best detected by chest films (calcification of the wall is rare); CT and MRI can also be done. An intravenous urogram or bone scan may detect cysts at other sites.

C. LABORATORY FINDINGS

The immunoblot test, where available, is the test of choice (95% specific and 91% sensitive for liver cysts); the arc 5 test is also diagnostic. In both tests, cross-reactions can occur in 5–10% of patients with *T solium* cysticercosis infections. Several other serologic tests (ELISA and indirect hemagglutination and immunofluorescence) are useful for screening, but both false-negative and false-positive results are common. Persons from whom cysts have been completely removed and carriers of dead cysts may become seronegative. In patients with solitary lung cysts, false-negative results occur in up to 50% of infections. Testing for antigen in serum or cyst fluid is under development. The intracutaneous skin tests have been abandoned because of poor specificity.

Eosinophilia is uncommon except after cyst rupture. Liver function tests are usually normal. Confirmation of the diagnosis is possible by examination of cyst contents after surgical removal or cyst aspiration. Although in the past the procedure was contraindicated, ultrasonic-guided percutaneous aspiration of hydatid cysts followed by injection of a scolicidal agent and use of oral albendazole is now being used for diagnosis at some centers (see below).

Differential Diagnosis

Noninfected hydatid cysts of the liver need to be differentiated from simple epithelial cysts and bacterial and amebic abscesses. Hydatid cysts in any site may be mistaken for a variety of malignant and nonmalignant tumors and cysts. In the lung, a cyst may be confused with cavitary tuberculosis. Allergic symptoms arising from cyst leakage may resemble those associated with many other diseases.

Treatment & Prevention

Surgery was formerly the definitive approach to therapy but has now been partially supplanted by anthelmintic treatment. Decision-making between the two modes of treatment must take into account (1) current surgical mortality rates (up to 4%), postoperative complications (10–25%), and recurrence rates after surgery (11–30%); and (2) cure rates after albendazole treatment of about 32%. One approach is to give a course of albendazole to selected asymptomatic patients whose cysts are small and not in danger of rupture. If, after 6–9 months, the cyst has not disappeared or clearly died, it can then be removed surgically.

A. SURGICAL TREATMENT

Operative treatment of liver cysts involves several problems: total removal of all infective components of the cyst, avoiding cyst content spillage, selection of a scolicidal agent to be placed within the cyst, management of communications between the cyst and biliary tract (if present), management of the residual cavity, and minimizing the risk of operation. The main surgical options available for liver cysts are partial hepatic resection, pericystectomy, and cystectomy. Surgery for pulmonary cysts includes extrusion of cysts (Barrett's technique), pericystectomy, and lobectomy. Scolicidal solutions, which include cetrimide (5%), hypertonic saline (20%), silver nitrate (0.5%), ethanol (70–95%), and sodium hypochlorite (3.75%), have come under criticism because of their potential for direct and indirect toxicity (an estimated 20% of cysts are thought to communicate with the biliary tract). Preoperatively, to reduce the risk of recurrence due to spillage, two drugs (taken with meals) are used for 1 month: albendazole, 10 mg/kg/d in two divided doses, and praziquantel, 25 mg/kg/d. Postoperatively, albendazole should be continued for 1 month; the additional use of praziquantel is under evaluation. Pulmonary cysts are treated by surgery plus chemotherapy. The treatment of bone cysts is by combined curettage, lavage, instillation of sterilization substances, and chemotherapy.

B. DRUG TREATMENT

Albendazole is the drug of choice; Mebendazole is no longer recommended in this text for hydatid disease treatment.

1. Albendazole—Albendazole is more readily absorbed than mebendazole; this permits a lower dosage of albendazole to be used, yet its active metabolite, the sulfoxide, reaches effective concentrations in cyst wall and fluid. A current regimen is four tablets (800 mg) daily in divided doses with meals for 3 months; continue for up to 6 months if there is evidence of a response. In multiple studies, apparent cure (shrinkage or disappearance of cysts) was approximately 30%, and improvement was 45%. To be emphasized, however, is that some of these changes result from the natural history of the disease. Relapses occur and should be re-treated, but long-term follow-up results have not been determined. Bone cysts are more refractory and may require a year of treatment. In the 3 month courses, drug side effects include reversible low-grade aminotransferase elevations (15%), leukopenia to 2900/μL (2%), rare gastrointestinal symptoms (including pain at cyst sites), dizziness or headache, alopecia, rash, and pruritus. Anaphylaxis has been reported once and eosinophilia rarely, probably related to cyst fluid leakage. Two deaths attributed to long-term albendazole use have been reported. Liver function tests and complete blood counts should be monitored weekly. The drug is contraindicated in pregnancy.

2. Praziquantel—Praziquantel kills protoscoleces within hydatid cysts but does not affect the germinal membrane. The drug is being evaluated as adjunctive therapy with albendazole both pre- and postsurgery to protect against cyst spillage.

C. PERCUTANEOUS ASPIRATION AND INJECTION OF A SCOLICIDAL AGENT

Under ultrasonic guidance, this approach is indicated in the treatment of accessible cysts in patients who are inoperable or refuse surgery and are not candidates for a chemotherapeutic trial. The procedure is contraindicated for cysts that communicate with the biliary tree, those that are superficially loculated, or those that have thick internal septal divisions. Complications are infection or leakage at the aspiration site followed by an allergic reaction or dissemination of the infection. Several thousand patients have now had the procedure while covered by oral albendazole. One case of anaphylaxis has been reported. Follow-up has not been sufficiently long to permit assessment of therapeutic efficacy or risk of spillage.

D. PREVENTION

In endemic areas, prevention is by prophylactic treatment of pet dogs with 5 mg/kg of praziquantel at monthly intervals to remove adult tapeworms and by health education to prevent feeding of offal to dogs.

Prognosis

About 15% of untreated patients eventually die because of the disease or its complications.

2. Alveolar Hydatid Disease (Multilocular Hydatid Disease)

Alveolar hydatid disease results from infection by the larval form of *Echinococcus multilocularis* and occurs only in the northern hemisphere. The life cycle involves foxes as definitive host and microtine rodents as intermediate host. Domestic dogs and cats can also become infected with the adult tapeworm when they eat infected wild rodents. Human infection is by accidental ingestion of tapeworm eggs passed in fox or dog feces. The disease in humans has been reported in parts of central Europe, much of Siberia, northern Japan, northwestern Canada, and western Alaska. Recent information has extended the Old World range southward to Iran and northern India and China. Increasing numbers of cases have been reported from central North America (eleven USA states and four Canadian provinces). The primary localization of alveolar cysts is in the liver, where they may extend locally or metastasize to other tissues. The larval mass has poorly defined borders and behaves like a neoplasm; it infiltrates and proliferates indefinitely by exogenous budding of the germinative membrane, producing an alveolus-like pattern of microvesicles. Pulmonary involvement is rare, usually occurring by direct extension from the liver. X-rays show hepatomegaly and characteristic scattered areas of radiolucency often outlined by 2- to 4-mm calcific rings. The serologic tests (ELISA and Western blot) are usually positive at high titer and differentiate *E granulosa* from *E multilocularis*. Treatment is by surgical removal of the entire larval mass when possible, accompanied by drug treatment. Ninety percent of patients with nonresectable masses die within 10 years. Long-term drug therapy (5 years to life) is with albendazole (preferred) (800 mg/d in divided doses) or with mebendazole (40 mg/kg/d in divided doses with fatty meals); the drugs inhibit growth of the parasite and have extended patient survival, but larval tissue is not completely destroyed.

Franchi C et al: Long-term evaluation of patients with hydatidosis treated with benzimidazole carbamates. Clin Infect Dis 1999;29:304. [PMID: 10476732]

Pelaez V et al: PAIR as percutaneous treatment of hydatid liver cysts. Acta Trop 2000;75:197. [PMID: 10708659]

Ramos G et al: Hydatid cyst of the lung: Diagnosis and treatment. World J Surg 2001;25:46. [PMID: 11213151]

Saimot AG: Medical treatment of liver hydatidosis. World J Surg 2001;25:15. [PMID: 11213151]

Shantz PM: Advances in clinical management of cystic echinococcosis. Acta Trop 1997;64:1. [PMID: 9095284]

Wagholikar GD et al: Surgical management of liver hydatid. Trop Gastroenterol 2001;22:159. [PMID: 11681113]

■ NEMATODE (ROUNDWORM) INFECTIONS

ANISAKIASIS

Anisakiasis is larval invasion of the stomach or intestinal wall by anisakid nematodes. In the acute form, the infection may mimic surgical abdomen; in the chronic form, mild symptoms may persist for weeks to years.

Definitive hosts are marine mammals, including whales, seals, and dolphins. Eggs discharged with feces are ingested by crustaceans, in which larvae develop that are infective for squids, mackerel, herring, cod, halibut, rockfish, salmon, tuna, and other marine fish. In the fish, in which infection rates can reach 80%, the larvae pass to the musculature and are able to transfer from fish to fish along the food chain, eventually reaching a marine mammal, where they mature into the adult stage.

Humans are infected when they ingest larvae in marine fish or squid eaten raw, undercooked, salted, or lightly pickled. Larvae liberated in the stomach attach to or partially penetrate the gastric or intestinal mucosa (small bowel is more common; colon is rare), resulting in localized ulceration, edema, and eosinophilic granuloma formation; eventually, the parasite dies. Rarely, worms are coughed up and expectorated or penetrate the gut wall, enter the peritoneal cavity, and migrate. Most larvae, however, probably fail to cause infection and are passed in feces. Although the larvae sometimes develop to the adult stages, gravid females are not found in humans.

The infection occurs worldwide, but most cases have been reported in Japan and the Netherlands, with a few in the United States, Scandinavia, Chile, and other fish-eating countries. Regional foods eaten raw such as sashimi in Japan, pickled herring in the Netherlands, and ceviche (seviche) in Latin America are common vehicles of infection.

Clinical Findings

A. SYMPTOMS AND SIGNS

The majority of acute cases present as gastric anisakiasis. Occasionally, acute infection is followed by a chronic course.

1. Acute gastric anisakiasis—Within hours after larval ingestion, the patient experiences nausea, vomiting, and epigastric pain that progressively becomes more severe. Allergic reactions, including rare anaphylaxis, can occur; chest pain and hematemesis are rare.

2. Acute intestinal anisakiasis—Within 1–7 days, colicky pain appears in the lower abdomen, often localized at the ileocecal region, accompanied by diarrhea, nausea, vomiting, diffuse abdominal tenderness, and mild fever.

3. Chronic disease—For weeks to several years, symptoms may continue that mimic gastric ulcer, gastritis, gastric tumor, bowel obstruction, or inflammatory bowel disease.

B. LABORATORY FINDINGS

Stools may show occult blood, but eggs are not produced. Mild leukocytosis and eosinophilia may be present. ELISA and RAST serologic tests may be helpful but are not reliable in chronic disease.

C. IMAGING AND ENDOSCOPY

In acute infection, gastroscopy is preferred because the larvae sometimes can be seen and removed from the stomach. X-rays of the stomach may show a localized edematous, ulcerated area with an irregularly thickened wall, decreased peristalsis, and rigidity. Double contrast technique may show the threadlike larvae. Small bowel x-rays may show thickened mucosa and segments of stenosis with proximal dilation. Ultrasound examination of gastric and intestinal lesions may also be useful.

In the chronic stage, x-rays and endoscopy of the stomach—but not of the bowel—may be helpful. The diagnosis is often made only at laparotomy with surgical removal of the parasite.

Prevention & Treatment

Prevention is by avoidance of ingestion of raw or incompletely cooked squid or marine fish, especially salmon, rockfish, herring, and mackerel; early evisceration of fish is recommended. Larvae within fish may with difficulty be seen as colorless, tightly coiled or spiraled worms in 3-mm whorls or as reddish or pigmented larvae lying open in muscles or viscera. The larvae are killed by temperatures above 60 °C or by freezing at −20 °C for 24 hours (7 days is advised by some workers). Smoking procedures that do not bring the temperature to 60 °C, marinating in vinegar, and salt-curing are not reliable.

There is no drug treatment. Except where larvae can be removed by fiberoptic gastroscopy or colonoscopy, treatment of acute and chronic lesions is limited to symptomatic measures; symptoms generally improve in 1–2 weeks. Surgical excision of the worm may be necessary in severe cases.

Cespedes M et al: Chronic anisakiasis presenting as a mesenteric mass. Abdom Imaging 2000;25:548. [PMID: 10931996]

Daschner A et al: Gastroallergic anisakiasis: borderline between food allergy and parasitic disease—clinical and allergologic evaluation of 20 patients with confirmed acute parasitism by *Anisakis simplex.* J Allergy Clin Immunol 2000;105:176. [PMID: 10629469]

Ido K et al: Sonographic diagnosis of small intestinal anisakiasis. J Clin Ultrasound 1998;26:125. [PMID: 9502034]

Laffon-Leal SM et al: "Cebiche"—a potential source of human anisakiasis in Mexico? J Helminthol 2000;74:151. [PMID: 10881286]

ANGIOSTRONGYLIASIS

1. Angiostrongyliasis Cantonensis (Eosinophilic Meningoencephalitis)

A nematode of rats, *Angiostrongylus cantonensis,* is the causative agent of a form of eosinophilic meningoencephalitis. It has been reported from Hawaii and other

Pacific islands, Southeast Asia, Japan, China, Taiwan, Hong Kong, Australia, Egypt, Madagascar, Nigeria, Bombay, Cuba, Puerto Rico, Bahamas, Brazil, and New Orleans.

Human infection results from the ingestion of infective larvae contained in uncooked food—either the intermediate mollusk hosts (snails, slugs, planarians) or transport hosts that have ingested mollusks (crabs, shrimp, fish). Leafy vegetables contaminated by small mollusks or by mollusk slime may also be the source of infection, as can fingers during collection and preparation of snails for cooking. The mollusks become infected by ingesting larvae excreted in feces of infected rodents, the definitive host.

The incubation period in humans is 1–3 weeks. Ingested larvae (0.5 × 0.025 mm) invade the central nervous system, where, during migration, they may cause extensive tissue damage; at their death, a local inflammatory reaction ensues. The usual clinical findings are those of meningoencephalitis, including severe headache, fever, neck stiffness, nausea and vomiting, and multiple neurologic findings, particularly asymmetric transient cranial neuropathies. Worms in the spinal cord may result in sensory abnormalities in the trunk or extremities; worms have also been seen in the eye.

The spinal fluid characteristically shows elevated protein, eosinophilic pleocytosis, and normal glucose. Occasionally, the parasite can be recovered from spinal fluid. Peripheral eosinophilia with a low-grade leukocytosis is common. A serologic test is available from the Centers for Disease Control and Prevention. CT and MRI may show a central nervous system lesion.

The differential diagnosis includes tuberculosis, coccidioidal or aseptic meningitis, syphilis, lymphoma, gnathostomiasis, cysticercosis, paragonimiasis, echinococcosis, and schistosomiasis japonicum.

No specific treatment is available; however, levamisole, albendazole (400 mg twice daily for 7 days), thiabendazole (25 mg/kg three times daily for 3 days; this dose may be toxic and need to be reduced), mebendazole (100 mg twice daily for 5 days), or ivermectin can be tried. Theoretically, parasite deaths may exacerbate central nervous system inflammatory lesions. Symptomatic treatment with analgesics or corticosteroids may be necessary. The illness usually persists for weeks to months, the parasite dies, and the patient then recovers spontaneously, usually without sequelae. However, fatalities have been recorded.

Prevention is by rat control; by cooking of snails, prawns, fish, and crabs for 3–5 minutes or by freezing them (−15 °C for 24 hours); and by examining vegetables for mollusks before eating. Washing contaminated vegetables to eliminate larvae contained in mollusk mucus is not always successful.

Prociv P et al: Neuro-angiostrongyliasis: unresolved issues. Int J Parasitol 2000;30:1295. [PMID: 11113256]

2. Angiostrongyliasis Costaricensis

Angiostrongylus costaricensis, which causes an eosinophilic ileocolitis, has been identified in humans (predominantly children) in Mexico, Central America, Venezuela, Brazil, and the USA (Texas). The known geographic range of the parasite in rodents (the definitive host) extends from northern South America to Texas. Infection occurs from ingestion of the larvae in the intermediate host (slugs, snails) or from food contaminated by larvae in slug or snail mucus. In humans, the larvae mature in the mesenteric vessels. The inflammatory response to adult worms, larvae, and eggs can be severe, resulting in a marked eosinophilic granulomatous reaction and vasculitis and ischemic necrosis of the intestine. Most cases involve the ileocecal region, appendix, ascending colon, and regional nodes, but other organs can be affected, including the liver and testes. Findings include fever, right lower quadrant abdominal pain and a mass, leukocytosis, and eosinophilia. Some patients have relapsing symptoms that can continue for months. Bowel complications include perforation, bleeding, incomplete or complete obstruction, and infarction. Neither eggs or larvae are passed in stool; a latex agglutination serologic test has been devised. The intra-abdominal mass can mimic tumor. There is no specific treatment; albendazole, thiabendazole, or mebendazole can be tried (as above). Operative treatment is frequently necessary.

Dekumyoy P et al: Angiostrongyliasis: analysis of antigens of *Angiostrongylus costaricensis* adult worms versus IgG from infected patients with *Angiostrongylus cantonensis*. Southeast Asian J Trop Med Public Health 2000;31(Suppl 1):48. [PMID: 11414459]

Kramer MH et al: First reported outbreak of abdominal angiostrongyliasis. Clin Infect Dis 1998;26:365. [PMID: 9580096]

ASCARIASIS

ESSENTIALS OF DIAGNOSIS

- Pulmonary phase: Transient cough, dyspnea, wheezing, urticaria, with eosinophilia and transient pulmonary infiltrates.
- Intestinal phase: Vague upper abdominal discomfort; occasional vomiting, abdominal distention.
- Eggs in stools; worms passed per rectum, nose, or mouth.

General Considerations

Ascaris lumbricoides is the most common of the intestinal helminths; an estimated 1 billion people are infected worldwide. It is cosmopolitan in distribution and is found in high prevalence wherever there are low standards of hygiene and sanitation (including focally in southeastern USA) or where human feces are used as fertilizer. The infection is specific for humans and occurs in all age groups. Heavy worm burdens, however, are usually seen only in children, in whom there may be reduced nitrogen, fat, and D-xylose absorption and reduced mucosal lactate activity resulting in decreased growth rates.

Adult worms live in the upper small intestine. After fertilization, the female produces enormous numbers of eggs that pass in feces. Direct transmission between humans does not occur, as the eggs must remain on the soil for 2–3 weeks before they become infective. Thereafter, they can survive for years. Infection occurs through ingestion of mature eggs in fecally contaminated food and drink. The eggs hatch in the small intestine, releasing motile larvae that penetrate the wall of the small intestine and reach the right heart via the mesenteric venules and lymphatics. From the heart they move to the lung, burrow through the alveolar walls, and migrate up the bronchial tree into the pharynx, down the esophagus, and back to the small intestine. Egg production begins 60–75 days after ingestion of infective eggs. Adult worms (20–40 cm × 3–6 mm) live for 1 year or more.

Clinical Findings

A. Symptoms and Signs

As a result of their migration and induction of hypersensitivity, larvae in the lung cause capillary and alveolar damage, which may result in low-grade fever, nonproductive cough, blood-tinged sputum, wheezing, dyspnea, and substernal pain. There may be urticaria and localized rales. Rarely, larvae lodge ectopically in the brain, kidney, eye, spinal cord, etc, and may cause symptoms referable to those organs.

Small numbers of adult worms in the intestine usually produce no symptoms. With heavy infection, peptic ulcer-like symptoms or vague pre- or postprandial abdominal discomfort may be seen. Adult worms may also migrate with heavy infections; they may be coughed up, vomited, or emerge through the nose or anus. They may also force themselves into the common bile duct, pancreatic duct, appendix, diverticula, and other sites, which may lead to cholangitis, cholecystitis, pyogenic liver abscess, pancreatitis, or obstructive jaundice. With very heavy infestations, masses of worms may cause intestinal obstruction, volvulus, intussusception, or death. During typhoid fever, worms may penetrate the weakened bowel wall. Rare cases of lung abscess or laryngeal obstruction with suffocation have been described. Moderate to high worm loads have been associated with stunting of growth in children. Periodic treatment of children with albendazole for multiple intestinal parasitism has resulted in improved nutrition.

B. Imaging

During the larval migratory phase, chest radiographs may show transitory, patchy, ill-defined asymmetric infiltrations (Löffler's syndrome). Intestinal infection is sometimes established by chance, when radiologic examination of the abdomen (with or without barium) shows the presence of worms. The diagnosis of biliary ascariasis can be made by endoscopic retrograde cholangiopancreatography, which has the therapeutic potential of removing the worms, and by ultrasonography. In intestinal obstruction, plain abdominal films show air-filled levels and multiple linear images of ascarides in dilated bowel loops; ultrasonography can also demonstrate the dilated bowel and worm mass.

C. Laboratory Findings

During the pulmonary phase, eosinophils may reach 30–50% and remain high for about a month; larvae are occasionally found in sputum. During the intestinal phase, diagnosis usually depends upon finding the characteristic eggs in feces. Occasionally, an adult worm spontaneously passed per rectum or orally reveals an unsuspected infection. Serologic tests are not useful; and there is no eosinophilia in the intestinal phase.

Differential Diagnosis

Pulmonary ascariasis with eosinophilia must be differentiated from nonparasitic causes (asthma, Löffler's syndrome, eosinophilic pneumonia, allergic bronchopulmonary aspergillosis), and parasitic causes (tropical pulmonary eosinophilia, toxocariasis, strongyloidiasis, hookworm, paragonimiasis). Ascaris-induced pancreatitis, appendicitis, diverticulitis, etc, must be differentiated from other causes of inflammation of these tissues. Postprandial dyspepsia may simulate duodenal ulcer, hiatal hernia, gallbladder disease, or pancreatic disease.

Treatment

Albendazole and pyrantel pamoate are the treatments of choice. None of the drugs listed below require pre- or posttreatment purges. Stools should be rechecked at 2 weeks and patients re-treated until all ascarids are removed. Ascariasis, hookworm, and trichuriasis infections, which often occur together, may be treated simultaneously by albendazole, mebendazole, or oxantel-pyrantel pamoate.

Treatment with anthelmintics can cause worms to migrate before they die. Because anesthesia stimulates worms to hypermotility, they should be removed in advance in infected patients undergoing elective surgery. In pregnancy, ascariasis should be treated after the first trimester.

Drug treatment should not be used in the migratory phase. In intestinal obstruction or biliary ascariasis, surgery may be avoided by nasogastric suction followed by a standard dose of an anthelmintic given via the tube. In biliary ascariasis, endoscopic removal of the worm under ultrasonographic guidance is often successful; treatment by injection of a solution of albendazole or piperazine into the common duct followed by systemic treatment has also been effective.

A. ALBENDAZOLE

In light infections, a single dose of albendazole (400 mg) results in cure rates over 95%; in heavy infections, however, a 2- to 3-day course is indicated. Side effects, including migration of ascaris through the nose or mouth, are rare. Albendazole is available in the USA though not approved for this indication. The drug is contraindicated in pregnancy.

B. PYRANTEL PAMOATE

Pyrantel pamoate as a single oral dose of 10 mg base/kg (maximum, 1 g) results in 85–100% cure rates. It may be given before or after meals. Infrequent and mild side effects include vomiting, diarrhea, headache, dizziness, and drowsiness.

C. MEBENDAZOLE

Although mebendazole is highly effective when given in a dosage of 100 mg twice daily before or after meals for 3 days, a single 500 mg dose is often sufficient. Gastrointestinal side effects are infrequent. The drug is contraindicated in pregnancy.

D. PIPERAZINE

The dosage for piperazine (as the hexahydrate) is 75 mg/kg body weight (maximum, 3.5 g) for 2 days in succession, giving the drug orally before or after breakfast. For heavy infestations, treatment should be continued for 4 days in succession or the 2-day course should be repeated after 1 week.

Gastrointestinal symptoms and headache occur occasionally; central nervous system symptoms (temporary ataxia and exacerbation of seizures) are rare. Allergic symptoms have been attributed to piperazine. The drug should not be used for patients with hepatic or renal insufficiency or in those with a history of seizures or chronic neurologic disease.

E. LEVAMISOLE

Levamisole, available in the USA but not approved for this indication, is highly effective as a single oral dose of 150 mg. Occasional mild and transient side effects are nausea, vomiting, abdominal pain, headache, and dizziness.

Prognosis

The complications caused by wandering adult worms require that all ascaris infections be treated and eradicated.

Crompton DW: Ascaris and ascariasis. Adv Parasitol 2001;48: 285. [PMID: 11013758]

Dib J et al: Hepato-biliary ascariasis. Gastrointest Endosc 2000; 51:594. [PMID: 10805849]

Gonzalez AH et al: Non-invasive management of *Ascaris lumbricoides* biliary tact migration: a prospective study in 69 patients from Ecuador. Trop Med Int Health 2001;146. [PMID: 11286203]

Misra SP et al: Clinical features and management of biliary ascariasis in non-endemic areas. Postgrad Med J 2000;76:29. [PMID: 10622777]

Ogata H et al: Multilocular pyogenic hepatic abscess complicating *Ascaris lumbricoides* infestation. Intern Med 2000;39:228. [PMID: 10772125]

CUTANEOUS LARVA MIGRANS (Creeping Eruption)

Cutaneous larva migrans, prevalent throughout the tropics and subtropics, including southeastern USA, is caused by larvae of the dog and cat hookworms, *Ancylostoma braziliense* and *Ancylostoma caninum*. A number of other animal hookworms, gnathostomiasis, and strongyloidiasis are rarely also causative agents. Moist sandy soil (eg, beaches, children's sand piles) contaminated by dog or cat feces is a common site of infection. The infection is also reported in travelers to tropical beaches, among whom delayed onset beyond several weeks has been described.

At the site of larval entry, particularly on the hands or feet, up to several hundred minute, intensely pruritic erythematous papules appear. Two to 3 days later, serpiginous eruptions appear as the larvae migrate at a rate of several millimeters a day; the parasite lies slightly ahead of the advancing border. The process may continue for weeks; the lesions may become severely pruritic, vesiculate, encrusted, or secondarily infected. Without treatment, the larvae eventually die and are absorbed.

The diagnosis is based on the characteristic appearance of the lesions and the frequent presence of eosinophilia. Biopsy is usually not indicated.

Mild transient cases may not require treatment. For mild cases, thiabendazole, if available, can be applied topically three times daily for 5 or more days as a 15% cream, which can be formulated in a hygroscopic base using crushed 500 mg tablets. For more severe cases, oral treatment is indicated. Highly effective and nearly free of side effects are ivermectin (200 μg/kg given for 1 or 2 days) and albendazole (400 mg twice daily for 3–5 days or 400 mg daily for 7 days). Thiabendazole, given orally as for strongyloidiasis, is a less satisfactory alternative drug because it has toxic side effects in about one-third of patients. With treatment, progression of the lesions and itching are usually stopped within 48 hours. Antihistamines are helpful in controlling pruritus; antibiotic ointment or oral preparation may be necessary to treat secondary infections.

Albanese G et al: Treatment of larva migrans cutanea (creeping eruption): a comparison between albendazole and traditional therapy. Int J Dermatol 2001;40:67. [PMID: 11277961]

Bouchaud O et al: Cutaneous larva migrans in travelers: a prospective study, with assessment of therapy with ivermectin. Clin Infect Dis 2000;32:523. [PMID: 10987771]

Caumes E: Treatment of cutaneous larva migrans. Clin Infect Dis 2000;30:811. [PMID: 10816151]

DRACUNCULIASIS (Guinea Worm Infection, Dracunculosis, Dracontiasis)

Dracunculiasis is an infection of connective and subcutaneous tissues by the nematode *Dracunculus medinensis*. It occurs only in humans and is a major cause of disability. Since the start of the WHO eradication program, the number of infected persons has declined about 97% from over 3 million to 100,000. Endemic areas have been the Indian subcontinent; West and Central Africa north of the equator (Cameroon to Mauritania, Uganda, and southern Sudan); and Saudi Arabia, Iran, and Yemen. Almost all remaining cases are reported from Africa—75% from Sudan. All ages are affected, and prevalence may reach 60%.

Infection occurs by swallowing water containing the infected intermediate host, the crustacean cyclops (copepods, water fleas). In the stomach, larvae escape from the crustacean and mature in subcutaneous connective tissue. After mating, the male worm dies and the gravid female (60–80 cm × 1.7–2.0 mm) moves to the surface of the body, where its head reaches the dermis and provokes a blister that ruptures on contact with water. Intermittently over 2–3 weeks, whenever the ulcer comes in contact with water, the uterus discharges great numbers of larvae, which are ingested by copepods. Most adult worms are gradually extruded; some worms retract and reemerge; and others die in the tissues, disintegrate, and may provoke a severe inflammatory reaction. Infection does not induce protective immunity.

Clinical Findings

A. SYMPTOMS AND SIGNS

Infection may be at several sites. Patients are asymptomatic during the 9- to 14-month incubation period except in the last 1–2 weeks, when the worm reaches and becomes palpable in the skin and a blister develops around its anterior end. Several hours before the head appears at the skin surface, local erythema, burning, pruritus, and tenderness often develop at the site of emergence. There may also be a 24-hour systemic allergic reaction (pruritus, fever, nausea and vomiting, dyspnea, periorbital edema, and urticaria). After rupture, the tissues surrounding the ulceration frequently become indurated, reddened, and tender. Because most lesions appear on the leg or foot, patients often must give up walking and working for days to several months. Uninfected ulcers heal in 4–6 weeks. The worm rarely reaches ectopic sites.

Secondary infections, including tetanus, are common. Deep "cold" abscesses may result at the sites of dying, nonemergent worms. Ankle and knee joint infections with resultant deformity are common complications.

B. LABORATORY FINDINGS

When an emerging adult worm is not visible in the ulcer or under the skin, the diagnosis may be made by detection of larvae in smears from discharging sinuses. Immersion of an ulcer in cold water stimulates larval expulsion. Eosinophilia is usually present. Skin and serologic tests are not useful. Calcified worms can be recognized on radiographs.

Treatment

All persons in an endemic area should be actively immunized against tetanus.

A. GENERAL MEASURES

The patient should be at bed rest with the affected part elevated. Cleanse the lesion, control secondary infection with topical antibiotics, and change dressings twice daily.

B. MANUAL EXTRACTION

Traditional extraction of emerging worms by gradually rolling them out a few centimeters each day on a small stick is still useful, especially when done along with chemotherapy and use of aseptic dressings. The process appears to be facilitated by placing the affected part in water several times a day. If the worm is broken during removal, however, secondary infection almost always results, leading to cellulitis, abscess formation, or septicemia.

C. ANTHELMINTIC THERAPY

The following drugs have an anti-inflammatory effect but do not kill the adults or the larvae. This effect may alleviate symptoms, reduce duration of infection, facilitate worm removal, or expedite their spontaneous extrusion.

1. Metronidazole, 250 mg three times daily for 10 days, causes only minimal toxicity. (See under Amebiasis.)

2. Mebendazole, 400–800 mg daily for 6 days, can be tried.

3. Thiabendazole, 25 mg/kg twice daily for 2–3 days after meals, frequently causes side effects, sometimes severe (see under Strongyloidiasis, below).

D. SURGICAL REMOVAL

Preemergent female worms can sometimes be surgically removed intact under local anesthesia if not firmly embedded in deep fascia or around tendons.

Prevention & Control

The disease is prevented by use of only noncontaminated drinking water. This can be accomplished either by (1) preventing contamination of community water supplies through use of tube wells, hand pumps, or cisterns or treating water sources with temephos; or (2) filtering water through nets (eg, nylon nets of 100 μm pore size); or (3) boiling water.

Hopkins DR et al: Dracunculiasis eradication: delayed, not denied. Am J Trop Med Hyg 2000;62:163. [PMID: 10813467]

ENTEROBIASIS (Pinworm Infection)

ESSENTIALS OF DIAGNOSIS

- *Nocturnal perianal and vulvar pruritus, insomnia, irritability, restlessness.*
- *Vague gastrointestinal symptoms.*
- *Eggs demonstrable by cellulose tape test; worms visible on perianal skin or in stool.*

General Considerations

Enterobius vermicularis (8–13 × 0.5 mm) is common worldwide. Humans, the only host, can harbor a few to hundreds of worms. Young children are affected more often than adults, and multiple infections occur in households and institutions with young children. High rates have been recorded in homosexual men, but the infection does not become opportunistic in HIV. A second species, *Enterobius gregorii*, has been described in England.

The adult worms inhabit the cecum and adjacent bowel areas, lying loosely attached to the mucosa. Gravid females migrate through the anus to the perianal skin and deposit eggs in large numbers. The eggs become infective in a few hours and may then infect others or be autoinfective if transferred to the mouth by contaminated food, drink, fomites, or hands. After being swallowed, the eggs hatch in the duodenum, and the larvae migrate down to the cecum. Retroinfection occasionally occurs when the eggs hatch on the perianal skin and the larvae migrate through the anus into the large intestine. The development of a mature ovipositing female from an ingested egg requires about 3–4 weeks. Eggs remain viable for 2–3 weeks outside the host. The life span of the worm is 30–45 days.

Clinical Findings

A. SYMPTOMS AND SIGNS

Many patients are asymptomatic. The most common and important symptom is perianal pruritus (particularly at night), due to the presence of the female worms or deposited eggs. Insomnia, restlessness, enuresis, and irritability are common symptoms, particularly in children. Many mild gastrointestinal symptoms have also been attributed to enterobiasis, but the association is difficult to prove. At night, worms may occasionally be seen near the anus. Perianal scratching may result in excoriation and impetigo. Adults sometimes report a "crawling" sensation in the anal area. Rarely, worm migration—including migration through the female genital tract or into the urethra—results in ectopic inflammation (vulvovaginitis, diverticulitis, appendicitis, cystitis) or granulomatous reactions (colon, genital tract, peritoneum, and elsewhere). Colonic ulceration and eosinophilic colitis have been reported.

B. LABORATORY FINDINGS

Diagnosis is made by finding eggs on the perianal skin (eggs are seldom found on stool examination). The most reliable method is by applying a short strip of sealing cellulose pressure-sensitive tape (eg, Scotch Tape) to the perianal skin and then spreading the tape on a slide for low-power microscopic study; toluene is used to clear the preparation. Three such preparations made on consecutive mornings before bathing or defecation will establish the diagnosis in about 90% of cases. Before the diagnosis can be ruled out, five to seven such examinations are necessary. Nocturnal examination of the perianal area or gross examination of stools may reveal adult worms, which should be placed in preservative, alcohol, or saline for laboratory examination. The worms can sometimes be seen on anoscopy. Eosinophilia is rare.

Differential Diagnosis

Pinworm pruritus must be distinguished from similar pruritus due to mycotic infections, allergies, hemorrhoids, proctitis, fissures, strongyloidiasis, and other conditions.

Treatment

A. GENERAL MEASURES

Symptomatic patients should be treated, and in some situations all members of the patient's household should be treated concurrently, since for each overt case there are usually several inapparent cases. Generally, however, treatment of all nonsymptomatic cases is not necessary. Careful washing of hands with soap and water after defecation and again before meals is important. Fingernails should be kept trimmed close and clean and scratching of the perianal area avoided. Ordinary washing of bedding will usually kill pinworm eggs; some workers recommend daily washing.

B. SPECIFIC MEASURES

Treatment with the following drugs should be repeated at 2 and 4 weeks. Albendazole, mebendazole, and pyrantel pamoate are the drugs of choice and can be given with or without food. Albendazole and mebendazole should not be used in pregnancy. Piperazine, although effective, is not recommended because treatment requires 1 week. Thiabendazole is not recommended because it causes frequent side effects which rarely are severe and life-threatening.

1. Albendazole is available in the USA though not approved for this indication. It may reach a 100% cure rate when given as a single 400 mg dose. Abdominal pain and diarrhea are rare.

2. Mebendazole as a single 100 mg dose is also highly effective. It should be chewed for best effect. Gastrointestinal side effects are infrequent.

3. Pyrantel pamoate is highly effective, with cure rates of over 95%. It is administered as a 10 mg (base)/kg (maximum, 1 g) dose. Infrequent side effects include vomiting, diarrhea, headache, dizziness, and drowsiness. In the USA, pyrantel is available as self-medication for pinworm infection.

Prognosis

Although annoying, the infection is benign. Cure is readily attainable with one of several effective drugs. Reinfection is common, especially in children, because of continued exposure outside the home.

Lohiya GS et al: Epidemiology and control of enterobiasis in a developmental center. West J Med 2000;172:305. [PMID: 10832422]

Wu ML et al: *Enterobius vermicularis.* Arch Pathol Lab Med 2000;124:647. [PMID: 10747336]

FILARIASIS

More than 80 million people are infected with lymphatic filariasis in 73 tropical and subtropical countries and an estimated 1 million new persons, mainly children, are infected yearly. The disease is caused by three filarial nematodes: *Wuchereria bancrofti, Brugia malayi,* or *Brugia timori. W bancrofti* is widely distributed in the tropics and subtropics of both hemispheres and on Pacific islands and is transmitted by culex, aedes, and anopheles mosquitoes. *B malayi* is transmitted by mansonia and anopheles mosquitoes of South India, Sri Lanka, Southeast Asia, South China, the northern coastal areas of China, and South Korea.

B timori is found on the southeastern islands of Indonesia.

No animal reservoir hosts are known for *W bancrofti* or *B timori;* cats, monkeys, and other animals may harbor *B malayi.* Mosquitoes become infected by ingesting microfilariae with a blood meal; at subsequent feedings, they can infect new susceptible hosts. Over months, adult worms (females, 8–9 cm × 0.2–0.3 mm) mature and live (up to 2 decades) in or near superficial and deep lymphatics and lymph nodes and produce large numbers of viviparous circulating microfilariae, which may be seen in the blood starting 6–12 months after infection.

Pathologic changes in lymph vessels are due to host immunologic reactions to developing and mature worms. Living microfilariae generally cause no lesions, with the exception of tropical pulmonary eosinophilia. Rapid death of microfilariae, however, does produce findings, and an abscess may form at the site of a dying adult worm.

Dirofilariasis, infection by *Dirofilaria immitis,* the dog heartworm, has been reported in the USA, Japan, and Australia. Nodules have been found in the skin or as solitary 1–4.5 cm (usually 2 cm) "coin" lesions in the periphery of the lungs; they are rarely calcified. The serologic test for filariasis is positive, but there is no microfilaremia. Eosinophilia is seen in 15% of patients.

Other filarial worms. Several other species infect humans—*Mansonella perstans, Mansonella streptocerca,* and *Mansonella ozzardi*—but usually without causing important findings.

Clinical Findings

A. SYMPTOMS AND SIGNS

The incubation period is generally 8–16 months in expatriates but may be longer in indigenous persons. Many infections remain asymptomatic, with or without microfilariae.

1. Acute disease—Episodes of fever (filarial fever), with or without inflammation of lymphatics and nodes, occur at irregular intervals and last for several days. Characteristically, the adenolymphangitis presents as retrograde extension from the affected node (unlike ascending bacterial lymphangitis). With disease progression, epididymitis and orchitis as well as involvement of pelvic, abdominal, or retroperitoneal lymphatics may also occur intermittently. Lymph node enlargement may persist. In travelers, allergic-like findings (hives, rashes, eosinophilia) and lymphangitis and lymphadenitis are more likely to be present.

2. Chronic disease—Obstructive phenomena occur as a result of interference with normal lymphatic flow; this includes hydrocele, scrotal lymphedema, lymphatic varices and elephantiasis, particularly of the extremities, genitals, and breasts. Chyluria may result from rupture of distended lymphatics into the urinary tract. Extrapulmonary manifestations seen in some patients include lymphadenopathy or moderate hepatomegaly or splenomegaly.

3. Occult disease—A small proportion of infected persons develop occult disease, in which the classic clinical manifestations and microfilaremia are not present but microfilariae are present in the tissues.

In **tropical pulmonary eosinophilia,** microfilariae of *W bancrofti* or *B malayi* are sequestered in the lungs but not found in the blood. The condition is characterized by episodic nocturnal coughing or wheezing, dyspnea, low-grade fever, scant expectoration, hypereosinophilia, high filarial antibody titers and IgE levels, diffuse miliary lesions or increased bronchovascular markings on chest films, and a response to diethylcarbamazine treatment (6 mg/kg daily for 21 days). Relapses (in 20%) require re-treatment with up to 12 mg/kg daily for up to 30 days. If untreated, the condition can progress to chronic pulmonary fibrosis.

B. LABORATORY FINDINGS

Diagnosis of active infection is made by finding microfilariae in blood (or hydrocele fluid), a positive antigen test (only available for *W bancrofti*), or by ultrasound. In indigenous persons, microfilariae are rare in the first 2–3 years, abundant as the disease progresses, and again rare in the obstructive stage. In persons from nonendemic areas, inflammatory reactions may be prominent in the absence of microfilariae. Microfilariae of *W bancrofti* are found in the blood chiefly at night (nocturnal periodicity 10 PM to 2 AM), except for a nonperiodic variety in the South Pacific. *B malayi* microfilariae are usually nocturnally periodic but in Southeast Asia may be present at all times, with a slight nocturnal rise. Anticoagulated blood specimens are collected at times related to the periodicity of the local strain. Specimens may be stored at ambient temperatures until examined in the morning by wet film for motile larvae and by Giemsa-stained smears—thick for sensitivity and thin for specific morphology. A formalin-anionic detergent preservative can also be used. If these are negative, the blood specimens should be concentrated by the Knott concentration or membrane filtration technique. Where available, screening for antigenemia for *W bancrofti* should be done. ELISA and immunochromatographic card tests are sensitive (96–100%) and specific (nearly 100%) and thus are particularly useful for amicrofilaremic persons and for daytime examination of blood. A PCR assay has been developed for both *W bancrofti* and *B malayi.*

Live adult worms can be detected by high-frequency ultrasound of the scrotum (up to 80% of infected men) and of the female breast.

Serologic tests may be helpful in screening. A negative test usually rules out present or past infection, but false-positive tests occur with other filarial and helminthic infections, including ascariasis. An indirect hemagglutination titer of 1:128 and a bentonite flocculation titer of 1:5 in combination are considered minimum significant titers. ELISA-IgG and -IgE tests

are also available. Eosinophil counts may be elevated. In differential diagnosis, lymphangiography (potentially damaging to the lymphatics) and radionuclide lymphoscintigraphy may be useful lymphatic imaging methods.

Treatment, Prevention, & Prognosis

Diethylcarbamazine, the drug of choice, rapidly kills blood microfilariae but only slowly kills or injures adult worms. Cure may require multiple 12-day courses (2 mg/kg three times a day after meals, starting with small doses, and gradually increasing over 3–4 days). At this dose, the drug rarely produces direct toxicity. However, adverse immunologic reactions to dying microfilariae and adult worms are common—more so with brugian than with bancroftian filariasis. Reactions are local (lymphadenitis, abscess, ulceration) and systemic (fever, headache, myalgia, dizziness, malaise, and other allergic responses). Antipyretics and analgesics may be helpful. In areas where onchocerciasis or loiasis is also prevalent, special care must be taken not to provoke severe reactions to dying microfilariae of these parasites. Diethylcarbamazine has also been extensively used in mass treatment programs and is being evaluated for prophylaxis. In the USA, the drug is available only from the Parasitic Diseases Drug Service, Centers for Disease Control and Prevention, Atlanta, GA 30333; phone 404-639-3670.

During acute inflammatory episodes, it is controversial whether to treat and whether drug usage will shorten the attack. General measures include rest, antibiotics for secondary infections, use of postural drainage, elastic stockings and pressure bandages for leg edema, and suspensory bandaging for orchitis and epididymitis.

Small hydroceles may benefit from a locally injected sclerosing agent, or surgery may be indicated. To manage elephantiasis, lymphovenous shunt procedures may be useful, combined with removal of excess subcutaneous fatty and fibrous tissue, postural drainage, and physiotherapy.

Ivermectin is effective only as a microfilaricide; it is given as a single 200 µg/kg dose and repeated in 6 months. Diethylcarbamazine, however, must be given to kill the adult worms, which are the cause of the pathologic features. Moxidectin, a new veterinary macrofilaricide, is being tested in humans to evaluate its potential against adult worms.

Albendazole (400 mg once), when combined with ivermectin, may be a better microfilaricide than ivermectin alone, though some studies do not support this. When albendazole (400 mg twice daily) is given for 3 weeks, it has macrofilaricidal action.

Mass treatment programs, in which albendazole is given once yearly with diethylcarbamazine or ivermectin, have been started in ten endemic countries and are being evaluated for their potential to interrupt lymphatic filariasis transmission. Also under evaluation is a remarkable approach to treatment that is based on the recent recognition of wolbachia bacteria as obligate intracellular rickettsial infections of *W bancrofti*. In animal models and in early human studies, antibiotic treatment leads to death of the bacteria and then to loss of worm viability.

The prognosis is good with treatment of early and mild cases (including low-grade lymphedema, chyluria, small hydrocele), but in advanced infection the prognosis is poor.

Chitkara RK et al: Dirofilaria, visceral larva migrans, and tropical pulmonary eosinophilia. Semin Respir Infect 1997;12:138. [PMID: 9195679]

Dreyer G et al: Pathogenesis of lymphatic disease in bancroftian filariasis: a clinical perspective. Parasitol Today 2000;16: 544. [PMID: 11121854]

Haarbrink M et al: Adverse reactions following diethylcarbamazine (DEC) intake in "endemic normals," microfilaremics and elephantiasis patients. Trans R Soc Trop Med Hyg 1999;93:91. [PMID: 10492800]

Ismail MM et al: Long-term efficacy of single-dose combination of albendazole, ivermectin, and diethylcarbamazine for the treatment of bancroftian filariasis. Trans R Soc Trop Med Hyg 2001; 95: 332. [PMID: 11491010]

Plaisier AP et al: Effectiveness of annual ivermectin treatment for *Wuchereria bancrofti* infection. Parasitol Today 2000;16: 298. [PMID: 10858649]

GNATHOSTOMIASIS

Gnathostomiasis, due for the most part to infection by the larval stage of the nematode *Gnathostoma spinigerum*, is rarely caused by other gnathostoma species. Infection is most common in Thailand and Japan but is also reported from Southeast Asia, China, India, Ecuador, Israel, and East Africa. In Mexico, where the gnathostoma species has not been identified, the number of cases is increasing; more than 1000 have been reported in the past 10 years, commonly associated with increased eating of raw freshwater fish, especially a preparation called ceviche. In the USA, though *G spinigerum* has rarely been seen in minks, it has not been reported in humans. Eggs passed in feces of the definitive hosts, wild and domestic dogs and cats, are infective for copepods (water fleas). Ingestion of copepods by secondary hosts results in encysted larvae in their tissues; humans are infected when these larvae are ingested in raw, marinated, or inadequately cooked freshwater fish, chicken or other fowl, frogs, or pork. Infection has also been attributed to ingestion of infected copepods in water.

Within 24–48 hours, larval migration through the intestinal wall can cause acute epigastric pain, vomiting, urticaria, and eosinophilia. The worm then migrates to subcutaneous and other tissues but is unable to mature. Most common is a pruritic subcutaneous swelling up to 25 cm across, occasionally accompanied by stabbing pain. Over weeks to years, the swelling may remain in one area for days or weeks, or move continuously. Occasionally the worm becomes visible under the skin.

Internal organs and the eye may also be invaded. Spontaneous pneumothorax, leukorrhea, hematemesis, hematuria, hemoptysis, paroxysmal coughing, and edema of the pharynx with dyspnea have been reported as complications. Invasion of the brain can result in an eosinophilic meningoencephalitis or subarachnoid hemorrhage. Spinal cord invasion can lead to myelitis or radiculopathy.

Definitive diagnosis is sometimes possible by surgical removal of the worm when it appears close to the skin. Marked eosinophilia is common, except for parasites in the central nervous system. Serodiagnosis by immunoblot assay or ELISA is promising. Skin and other serologic tests are unsatisfactory.

Treatment is with ivermectin (200 µg/kg daily for 1 or 2 days) or with albendazole (400 mg twice daily for 21 days); larval death appears to occur slowly, and cure rates may reach 95%. Courses of prednisolone have provided temporary relief of symptoms.

Nontasut P et al: Comparison of ivermectin and albendazole treatment for gnathostomiasis. Southeast Asian J Trop Med Public Health 2000;31:374. [PMID: 11127342]

Parola P: Gnathostomiasis. Lancet 2001;358:332. [PMID: 11501534]

Ruiz-Maldonado R et al: Human gnathostomiasis. Int J Dermatol 1999;38:56. [PMID: 10065613] (A review of nodular migratory eosinophilic panniculitis.)

HOOKWORM DISEASE

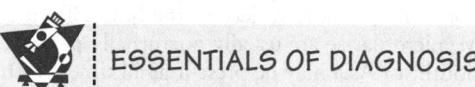

ESSENTIALS OF DIAGNOSIS

Early findings (not commonly recognized):

- *Dermatitis: pruritic, erythematous, papulovesicular eruption at site of larval invasion.*
- *Pulmonary migration of larvae: transient episodes of coughing, asthma, fever, blood-tinged sputum, marked eosinophilia.*

Later findings:

- *Intestinal symptoms: anorexia, diarrhea, abdominal discomfort.*
- *Anemia (iron deficiency): fatigue, pallor, dyspnea on exertion, poikilonychia, heart failure.*
- *Characteristic eggs and occult blood in the stool.*

General Considerations

Hookworm disease, widespread in the moist tropics and subtropics and sporadically in southeastern USA, is caused by *Ancylostoma duodenale* and *Necator americanus*. Probably a quarter of the world's population is infected, and in many areas the infection is a major cause of general debility, retardation of growth and development of children, and increased susceptibility to infection. Prevalence rates can reach 80% in the humid tropics under unsanitary conditions.

In the Western Hemisphere and tropical Africa, necator was the prevailing species, and in the Far East, India, China, and the Mediterranean area, ancylostoma was prevalent, but both species have now become widely distributed. Infection is rare in regions with less than 40 inches of rainfall annually. Humans are the only host for both species.

The adult worms are approximately 1 cm long. Eggs produced by females are passed in the stool and must fall on warm, moist soil if hatching followed by larval development is to take place. Larvae remain infective for hours to about a week, depending on environmental conditions. Following skin penetration, the larvae migrate in the bloodstream to the pulmonary capillaries, break into alveoli, and then are carried by ciliary action upward to the bronchi, trachea, and mouth. After being swallowed, they reach and attach to the mucosa of the upper small bowel; maturation and release of eggs occurs in 6–8 weeks. Ancylostoma infection can also be acquired by ingestion of the larvae in food or water. Adult ancylostoma worms survive about a year; necator, about 3–5 years.

The worms suck blood at their attachment sites. Blood loss is proportionate to the worm burden. A light infection is approximately 1000 eggs per gram of feces (equivalent to about 11 ancylostoma and 32 necator adults); a moderate worm load is 2000–8000 eggs per gram of feces. Iron loss with moderate infection is 1.1 mg/d for *N americanus* and 2.3 mg/d for *A duodenale*, which compares with a basal intake requirement of 0.72 for a typical woman. Over years—and depending upon the host's dietary intake of iron—iron reserves can be depleted and severe anemia can result from moderate infections with 30 or more ancylostoma or 100 or more necator worms.

Clinical Findings

A. SYMPTOMS AND SIGNS

Ground itch, the first manifestation of infection, is a pruritic erythematous dermatitis, either maculopapular or vesicular, that follows skin penetration of the infective larvae. Severity is a function of the number of invading larvae and the sensitivity of the host. Scratching may result in secondary infection. Strongyloidiasis and cutaneous larva migrans must be considered in the differential diagnosis at this stage.

The pulmonary stage, in which there is larval migration through the lungs, may show dry cough, wheezing, blood-tinged sputum, and low-grade fever. The pulmonary migration of ascaris and strongyloides larvae can produce similar findings.

After 2 or more weeks, maturing worms attach to the mucosa of the duodenum and upper jejunum. In heavy infections, worms may reach the ileum. Patients who have light infections and adequate iron intake often remain asymptomatic. In heavy infections, however, there may be anorexia, diarrhea, vague abdominal pain, and ulcer-like epigastric symptoms. Severe anemia may result in pallor, deformed nails, pica, and cardiac decompensation. Marked protein loss may also occur, resulting in hypoalbuminemia, with edema and ascites. There are conflicting reports of malabsorption in some severe infections.

Reduction in worm loads and symptoms after the first decade of life suggests that a moderate degree of immunity develops.

B. LABORATORY FINDINGS

Diagnosis depends upon demonstration of characteristic eggs in feces; a concentration method may be needed. The two species cannot be differentiated by the appearance of their eggs. The stool usually contains occult blood. Hypochromic microcytic anemia can be severe, with hemoglobin levels as low as 2 g/dL, a low serum iron and a high iron-binding capacity, and low serum ferritin. Eosinophilia (as high as 30–60% of a total white blood count reaching 17,000/μL) is usually present in the pulmonary migratory stage of infection but is not marked in the chronic intestinal stage.

Treatment

A. GENERAL MEASURES

The availability of safe anthelmintics makes it possible to treat all patients initially, irrespective of the intensity of infection; nevertheless, it may not be necessary or beneficial to treat light infections. Re-treatment of heavy infections may be necessary at 2-week intervals until the worm burden is reduced to a low level as estimated by semiquantitative egg counts. Eradication of infection is not essential, since light infections do not injure the well-nourished patient and iron loss is replaced if the patient is receiving adequate dietary iron.

If anemia is present, oral ferrous sulfate and a diet high in protein and vitamins are required for at least 3 months after the anemia has been corrected in order to replace iron stores. A dosage schedule for ferrous sulfate tablets (200 mg) is one tablet three times daily for 2 months followed by one tablet daily for 4 months. Parenteral iron is rarely indicated. Blood transfusion may be necessary if anemia is severe.

B. SPECIFIC MEASURES

Mebendazole, pyrantel, and albendazole are highly effective drugs for treatment of both hookworm species; mebendazole or albendazole can be used to treat concurrent trichuriasis, and all three drugs can be used to treat concurrent ascariasis. The drugs are given before or after meals, without purges. For the three drugs, mild gastrointestinal side effects are rare; none should be used in pregnancy. Albendazole and mebendazole should not be given to children under about 1 year of age.

1. Pyrantel pamoate—In *A duodenale* infections, pyrantel given as a single dose, 10 mg (base)/kg (maximum 1 g), produces cures in 76–98% of cases and a marked reduction in the worm burden in the remainder. For *N americanus* infections, a single dose may give a satisfactory cure rate in light infection, but for moderate or heavy infection a 3-day course is necessary. If the species is unknown, treat as for necatoriasis. Mild and transient drowsiness and headache may occur.

2. Mebendazole—When mebendazole is given at a dosage of 100 mg twice daily for 3 days, reported cure rates for both hookworm species range from 35% to 95%. A single 500 mg dose may be sufficient for light infections.

3. Albendazole—Albendazole given orally once only at a dosage of 400 mg results in the cure of 85–95% of patients with ancylostoma infection and markedly reduces the worm burden in those not cured. Because cure rates for single-dose treatments of necator infection were 33–90%, treatment should be continued for 2–3 days, especially in heavy infections. Albendazole is available in the USA, though it is not FDA-approved for this indication.

Prognosis

If the disease is recognized before serious secondary complications appear, complete recovery is the rule following treatment.

Eosinophilic Enteritis

In Australia, *Ancylostoma caninum,* the dog hookworm, has been found to cause abdominal pain, diarrhea, and peripheral eosinophilia.

Crompton DW: The public health importance of hookworm disease. Parasitology 2000;121(Suppl):S39. [PMID: 11386690]

Georgiev VS: Necatoriasis: treatment and developmental therapeutics. Expert Opin Investig Drugs 2000;9:1065. [PMID: 11060728]

LOIASIS

Loiasis is a chronic filarial disease caused by infection with *Loa loa.* The infection occurs in humans and monkeys in rain and swamp forest areas of West Africa from Nigeria to Angola and throughout the Congo river watershed of central Africa eastward to southwestern Sudan and western Uganda. An estimated 3–13 million persons are infected.

The adult worms live in the subcutaneous tissues for up to 12 years. Gravid females release microfilariae into the bloodstream which subsequently are ingested in a blood meal by the vector-intermediate host, female chrysops species, day-biting flies. When the fly feeds again, the larval stage can infect a new host or cause superinfection. The time to worm maturity and detection of new microfilariae is 6 months to several years.

Clinical Findings

A. Symptoms and Signs

Many infected persons are asymptomatic. In symptomatic persons, the worms (females, 4–7 cm × 0.5 mm) are evidenced by their temporary appearance beneath the skin or conjunctiva, by unilateral edema of an extremity, or by Calabar swellings. The latter are subcutaneous edematous reactions, 3–10 cm in diameter, nonpitting and nonerythematous, and at times associated with low-grade fever, local pain, and pruritus. The swellings may migrate a few centimeters for 2–3 days or stay in place before they subside. At irregular intervals, they recur at the same or different sites, but only one appears at a time. When near joints, they may be temporarily disabling. Migration across the eye may be asymptomatic or may produce pain, intense conjunctivitis, and eyelid edema. Dying adult worms may elicit small nodules or local sterile abscesses, and dead worms may result in radiologically detectable calcification.

Microfilariae in the blood do not induce symptoms. Rarely, however, they enter the central nervous system and may cause encephalitis, myelitis, or jacksonian seizures; the larvae can also induce lesions and complications in the retina, heart, lungs, kidneys, and other tissues.

Natives generally have a mild form of the infection or are asymptomatic but are microfilaremic and serologically positive. The disease among visitors, however, is often characterized by more pronounced immunologically mediated symptoms (frequent and debilitating Calabar swellings, elevated leukocyte and eosinophil counts, hypergammaglobulinemia, increased polyclonal IgE) and frequently a positive serologic test but nondetectable microfilaremia.

B. Laboratory Findings

Specific diagnosis is made by finding characteristic microfilariae in daytime (10 AM to 4 PM) blood specimens by concentration methods; in order of increasing sensitivity, they are (1) thick films, (2) Knott's concentration, and (3) Nuclepore filtration. Presumptive diagnosis that permits treatment is based on Calabar swellings or eye migration, a history of residence in an endemic area, and marked eosinophilia (40% or greater). Serologic tests may be positive, but cross-reactions occur with other filarial diseases and sometimes with nematode infections. A polymerase chain reaction test, highly sensitive and specific, can detect the organism in some amicrofilaremic persons.

Treatment & Prognosis

See specialized sources and references for details on proper use of diethylcarbamazine (drug of choice both as a micro- and macrofilaricide), since side effects to dying microfilariae may be severe, and life-threatening encephalitis can occur rarely. The dosage is 50 mg once (day 1), 50 mg three times daily (day 2), 100 mg three times daily (day 3), and 3 mg/kg three times daily (days 4–21). One course of treatment cures about 50% of patients; three courses, 90%. Reactions are more likely with pretreatment microfilaria counts greater than 25/μL. Cytapheresis has been used to reduce parasite loads before starting diethylcarbamazine. Prednisone is sometimes indicated in heavily infected persons to minimize reactions. When ivermectin was used in treatment of 1.1 million persons with onchocerciasis in the presence of endemic loiasis, 28 neurologic reactions occurred (some severe) from death of *Loa loa* microfilariae. The risk of these reactions was high when the *L loa* microfilaria load exceeded 8/μL and very high above 50/μL; albendazole at a dosage of 200 mg twice daily for 3 weeks is being evaluated as a safe way to reduce the level of *L loa* microfilariae. Surgical removal of adult worms from the eye or skin is not recommended.

In the USA, diethylcarbamazine is available only from the Parasitic Diseases Drug Service, Centers for Disease Control and Prevention, Atlanta, GA 30333, telephone 404-639-3670.

Individual protection is facilitated by daytime use of insect repellent and by wearing light-colored clothing with long sleeves and trousers. Diethylcarbamazine prophylaxis, 300 mg weekly, may be useful if the risk of exposure is high. It is not indicated, however, for the casual traveler or for persons who might previously have acquired any of the filarial infections.

Most infections run a benign course, but some are accompanied by severe and temporarily disabling symptoms. The prognosis is excellent with treatment.

Blum J et al: Encephalopathy following *Loa loa* treatment with albendazole. Acta Trop 2001;78:63. [PMID 11164753]

Chippaux JP et al: Impact of repeated large scale ivermectin treatments on the transmission of *Loa loa*. Trans R Soc Trop Med Hyg 1998;92:454. [PMID: 9850408]

Esum M et al: Co-endemicity of loiasis and onchocerciasis in the South West Province of Cameroon: implications for mass treatment with ivermectin. Trans R Soc Trop Med Hyg 2001;95:673. [PMID: 11816443]

ONCHOCERCIASIS

Onchocerciasis is a chronic filarial disease caused by *Onchocerca volvulus*. The advent of the safe drug ivermectin has led to effective treatment and control programs. Mass treatment programs are under way in which the drug is provided free by Merck and Co. Primary findings are subcutaneous nodules that contain adult worms and skin and eye changes that result from dead or dying microfilariae. Heavy infection leads to chronic pruritus, disfiguring skin lesions, visual impairment, and debility. An estimated 18 million persons are infected, of whom 3–4 million have skin disease, 0.3 million are blinded, and 0.5 million severely visually impaired. In hyperendemic areas, more than 40% of inhabitants over 40 years of age are blind. The infection, predominant in West Africa, also occurs in many other parts of tropical Africa and in localized areas of the southwestern Arabian peninsula, southern Mexico, Guatemala, Venezuela, Colombia, and northwestern Brazil. The West African savanna strain is especially associated with severe blinding eye lesions.

Humans are the only important host. The vector and intermediate host are simulium flies, day biters that breed in rivers and fast-flowing streams and become infected by ingesting microfilariae with a human blood meal; at subsequent feedings, they can infect new susceptible hosts.

Clinical Findings

A. SYMPTOMS AND SIGNS

Adult worms, which can live for up to 14 years, typically are in fibrous subcutaneous nodules that are painless, freely movable, and 0.5–1 cm in diameter. Many nodules, however, are deep in the connective and muscular tissues and nonpalpable. The interval from exposure to onset of symptoms can be as long as 1–3 years. Female worms release motile microfilariae into the skin, subcutaneous tissues, lymphatics, and eyes; microfilariae are occasionally seen in the urine but rarely in blood or cerebrospinal fluid. Skin manifestations are localized or cover large areas. Pruritus may be severe, leading to skin excoriation and lichenification; other findings include pigmentary changes, papules, scaling, atrophy, pendulous skin, and acute inflammation. Pruritus may occur in the absence of skin lesions. There may be marked enlargement of femoral and inguinal nodes and generalized lymph node enlargement. Microfilariae in the eye may lead to visual impairment and blindness; findings include itching, photophobia, anterior segment changes (limbitis, punctate and sclerosing keratitis, iritis, secondary glaucoma, cataract), and posterior segment changes (optic neuritis, optic atrophy, chorioretinitis, and other retinal and choroidal findings). Infected visitors, as compared with indigenous persons, may show a more prominent dermatitis despite a low to nondetectable microfiladerma or eosinophilia and an absence of nodules and eye disease.

B. LABORATORY FINDINGS

Diagnosis is by demonstrating microfilariae in skin snips (usually obtained with a punch biopsy instrument), identifying them in the cornea or anterior chamber by slitlamp examination (after the patient has sat with head lowered between knees for 2 minutes) or by nodule aspiration or excision. Skin snips placed in saline are incubated for 2–4 hours before examination, or overnight for low-intensity infections. Adult worms may be recovered in excised nodules, whereas ultrasound has been used to detect nonpalpable onchocercomas and to distinguish them from other lesions (lipomas, fibromas, lymph nodes, foreign body granulomas). Traditional serologic tests are usually positive, but cross-reactions occur with other forms of filariasis, and the tests do not distinguish current from past infection. Immunoblot analysis of IgG4 antibodies and an ELISA appear to be more sensitive than skin snips early in infection, but occasional cross-reactions also occur with other filarial infections. Newly available tests, PCR (on skin snips and urine), and antigen detection (in blood and urine) have the advantage over serology in that they are only positive in people who have active infection; they may also prove useful in monitoring success of treatment. Eosinophilia (15–50%), polyclonal hypergammaglobulinemia, and elevated IgE levels are common. The Mazzotti skin test is no longer recommended because of the potential for dangerous reactions.

Treatment & Prognosis

Drug treatment is with ivermectin (a microfilaricide) as a single oral dose of 150 µg/kg given with water on an empty stomach; the patient should remain fasting for 2 more hours. The number of microfilariae in the skin diminishes markedly within 2–3 days, remains low for about 6 months, and then gradually increases; microfilariae in the anterior chamber of the eye decrease slowly in number over months, eventually disappear, and then gradually return. The optimum frequency of treatment to control symptoms and prevent disease progression remains to be determined. To initiate treatment, three schedules have been proposed: (1) an initial and repeat dose at 6 months, (2) repeated doses at 3-month intervals for a year, or (3) repeated doses at monthly intervals for a total of three doses. Thereafter, treatment is repeated at intervals of 6 months for 2 years and yearly thereafter until the adult worms die, which may take 12–15 years or longer. With the initial treatment only, patients with microfilariae in the cornea or anterior chamber may benefit from several days of prednisone treatment (1 mg/kg/d) to avoid inflammatory eye reactions. Although single-dose ivermectin does not kill the adult worms, with repeated doses, increasing evidence suggests that the drug has a low-level macrofilaricidal action. Adverse reactions, which are more marked with the first dose, are mild in 9% of patients and severe in 0.2%; these include edema (face and limbs), fever, pruritus, lymphadenitis, malaise, and hypotension. Ivermectin does not cause a severe reaction in the eyes or skin as does occur with diethylcarbamazine. Ivermectin should not be used in the presence of concurrent *Loa loa* infections or pregnancy, in children under age 5, or in patients with central nervous system diseases in which increased penetration may occur of ivermectin into the central nervous system (eg, meningitis). In developing countries, ivermectin is available on a compassionate basis from the manufacturer, Merck & Co. In Latin America only, nodulectomy continues to be used for nodules on or near the head.

In comparison studies, ivermectin was as effective as diethylcarbamazine in reducing the number of microfilariae but did so with significantly fewer systemic and ocular adverse reactions. Diethylcarbamazine is no longer recommended by WHO in onchocerciasis therapy. For selected patients in whom repeated ivermectin treatments do not control symptoms, suramin can be given for its macrofilaricidal action; however, because of suramin's toxicity and complex administration, it should only be administered by experts. Amocarzine is under evaluation for its macro- and microfilaricidal actions. Albendazole does not kill microfilariae but interferes with embryogenesis. Doxycycline for 6 weeks has recently been shown to have macrofilaricidal action through its endosymbiont action on bacteria in the parasite.

With treatment, some skin and ocular lesions improve and ocular progression is prevented. The prognosis is unfavorable only for those patients who are seen for the first time with already far-advanced ocular onchocerciasis.

Burnham G: Onchocerciasis. Lancet 1998;351:1341. [PMID: 9643811]

Ejere H et al: Ivermectin for onchocercal eye disease (river blindness). Cochrane Database Syst Rev 2001;(1):CD002219. [PMID: 11279760]

Henry NL et al: Onchocerciasis in a nonendemic population: clinical and immunologic assessment before treatment and at the time of presumed cure. J Infect Dis 2001;183:512. [PMID: 11133386]

Shu EN et al: Community-based ivermectin therapy for onchocerciasis: comparison of three methods of dose assessment. Am J Trop Med Hyg 2001;65:184. [PMID: 11561701]

Vincent JA et al: A comparison of newer tests for the diagnosis of onchocerciasis. Ann Trop Med Parasitol 2000;94:253. [PMID 10884870]

STRONGYLOIDIASIS

 ESSENTIALS OF DIAGNOSIS

- *Pruritic dermatitis at sites of larval penetration.*
- *Diarrhea, epigastric pain, nausea, malaise, weight loss.*
- *Cough, rales, transient pulmonary infiltrates.*
- *Eosinophilia; characteristic larvae in stool specimens, duodenal aspirate, or sputum.*
- *Hyperinfection syndrome: Severe diarrhea, bronchopneumonia, ileus.*

General Considerations

Strongyloidiasis is caused by infection with *Strongyloides stercoralis* (2–2.5 × 30–50 mm). Major symptoms result from adult parasitism, principally in the duodenum and jejunum, or from larval migration through pulmonary and cutaneous tissues. The primary host is humans, but dogs, cats, and primates have been found infected with strains indistinguishable from those of humans. Human infections with *S fulleborni* have been encountered in Papua New Guinea and parts of Africa.

Strongyloidiasis is endemic in tropical and subtropical regions; although the prevalence is generally low, in some areas disease rates exceed 25%. An estimate of total world prevalence is 60 million. In temperate areas, the disease occurs sporadically. In the USA, highest infection rates are found in immigrants from endemic areas, in parts of Appalachia (up to 4%), and in southeastern areas; Puerto Rico is also an endemic area. Multiple infections in households are common, and prevalence may be high in institutions, particularly mental institutions (2–4%). The infection is also prevalent among immunosuppressed persons (see below).

The parasite is uniquely capable of maintaining its life cycle both within the human host and in soil. Infection occurs when filariform larvae in soil penetrate the skin, enter the bloodstream, and are carried to the lungs, where they escape from capillaries into alveoli and ascend the bronchial tree to the glottis. The larvae are then swallowed and carried to the duodenum and upper jejunum, where maturation to the adult stage takes place. The parasitic female, generally held to be parthenogenetic, matures and lives embedded in the mucosa, where its eggs are laid and hatch. Rhabditiform larvae, which are noninfective, emerge, and migrate into the intestinal lumen to leave the host via the feces. The life span of the adult worm may be as long as 5 years.

In the soil, the rhabditiform larvae metamorphose into the infective (filariform) larvae. However, the parasite also has a free-living cycle in soil, in which some rhabditiform larvae develop into adults that produce eggs from which rhabditiform larvae emerge to continue the life cycle.

Autoinfection in humans, which probably occurs at a low rate in most infections, is an important factor in determining worm burden and is responsible for the persistence of infections. Internal autoinfection takes place in the lower bowel when some rhabditiform larvae develop into filariform larvae that penetrate the intestinal mucosa, enter the intestinal lymphatic and portal circulation, are carried to the lungs, and return to the small bowel to complete the cycle. This process is accelerated by achlorhydria, constipation, diverticula, and other conditions that reduce bowel motility. In addition, an external autoinfection cycle can occur as a result of fecal contamination of the perianal area.

Recrudescence of a chronic asymptomatic infection may occur with the immunosuppression accompanying severe infections, corticosteroid treatment, metabolic diseases, severe malnutrition, or malignancy; ex-

acerbation may lead to the hyperinfection syndrome. In the hyperinfection syndrome, autoinfection is greatly increased, resulting in a marked increase in the intestinal worm burden and in massive dissemination of filariform larvae to the lungs and most other tissues, where they can cause local inflammatory reactions and granuloma formation. Occasionally, in the lungs and elsewhere, larvae metamorphose into adults. Penetration of the bowel wall by filariform larvae can result in bacterial or fungal sepsis or meningitis. Hyperinfection is generally initiated under conditions of depressed host cellular immunity, especially in debilitated, malnourished persons and in patients with leukemia or lymphoma or those receiving immunosuppressive therapy, particularly chemotherapy or corticosteroids. Although the hyperinfection syndrome is rare in AIDS, these patients do have a protracted course that is difficult to cure.

Clinical Findings

A. Symptoms and Signs

Up to 30% of infected persons are asymptomatic. The time from larval penetration of the skin by filariform larvae until their appearance in the feces is 3–4 weeks. An acute syndrome can sometimes be recognized in which cutaneous symptoms, usually of the feet, are followed by pulmonary and then intestinal symptoms. Patients usually present, however, with chronic symptoms (continuous or with irregular exacerbations) that can persist for years or for life.

1. Cutaneous manifestations—In acute infection in sensitized patients, there may be focal edema, inflammation, petechiae, serpiginous or urticarial tracts, and intense itching. In chronic infections, both stationary urticaria and larva currens occur, the latter characterized by transient eruptions that migrate in serpiginous tracts.

2. Intestinal manifestations—Symptoms range from mild to severe, the most common being diarrhea, abdominal pain, and flatulence. Anorexia, nausea, vomiting, epigastric tenderness, and pruritus ani may be present; with increasing severity, fever and malaise may appear. Diarrhea may alternate with constipation, and in severe cases the feces contain mucus and blood. The pain is often epigastric in location and may mimic duodenal ulcer. Malabsorption or a protein-losing enteropathy can result from a large intestinal worm burden.

3. Pulmonary manifestations—With migration of larvae through the lungs, bronchi, and trachea, symptoms may be limited to a dry cough and throat irritation or low-grade fever, dyspnea, wheezing, and hemoptysis may occur; asthma is rare. Bronchopneumonia, bronchitis, pleural effusion, progressive dyspnea, and miliary abscesses can develop; the cough may become productive of an odorless, mucopurulent sputum.

4. Hyperinfection syndrome—Intense dissemination of filariform larvae to the lungs and other tissues can result in additional complications, including pleural effusion, pericarditis and myocarditis, hepatic granulomas, cholecystitis, purpura, ulcerating lesions at all levels of the gastrointestinal tract, central nervous system involvement, paralytic ileus, perforation and peritonitis, gram-negative septicemia and meningitis (due to larval carriage of enterobacteria from the colon), cachexia, shock, and death. Nephrotic syndrome is encountered on rare occasions.

B. LABORATORY FINDINGS

1. Detection of eggs and larvae—Eggs are seldom found in feces. Diagnosis, which may be difficult, requires finding the larval stages in feces or duodenal fluid. Rhabditiform larvae may be found in recently passed stool specimens; filariform larvae will be present in specimens held in the laboratory for some hours. Four to six specimens, some unpreserved, should be collected at 2-day intervals or longer (the number of larvae in feces varies from day to day). Since the sensitivity of direct microscopic examination of one specimen is about 30%, it is essential that one-half of the specimens be processed, unpreserved, in the Baermann concentration or agar plate culture methods, the sensitivities of which are high.

The diagnosis can sometimes be made by finding rhabditiform larvae or ova in mucus obtained by means of the duodenal string test or by duodenal intubation and aspiration. Duodenal biopsy is seldom indicated but will confirm the diagnosis in most patients. Rarely, filariform or rhabditiform larvae can be detected in sputum or bronchial washings during the pulmonary phase of the disease or in urine.

2. Serologic and hematologic findings—In chronic low-grade intestinal strongyloidiasis, the white blood cell count is often normal, with a slightly elevated percentage of eosinophils. However, with increasing larval migration, eosinophilia may reach 50% and leukocytosis 20,000/μL. In immunocompromised patients, eosinophilia may not be seen. Mild anemia may be present. Serum IgE immunoglobulins may be elevated. An ELISA is sensitive (85%) and specific (97%), as is Western blot, but cross-reactions can occur with the filaria and other helminthic infections. A positive test indicates current or past infection.

3. Hyperinfection—In the hyperinfection syndrome, there may also be findings of hypoproteinemia, malabsorption, abnormal liver function, and extensive pulmonary opacities. Filariform larvae may appear in the urine. Eosinopenia, when present, is thought to be an unfavorable prognostic sign.

C. IMAGING

Small bowel x-rays may show inflammation, irritability, and prominent mucosal folds; there may also be bowel dilation, delayed emptying, and ulcerative duodenitis. In chronic infections, the findings can resemble those in nontropical and tropical sprue, or there may be narrowing, rigidity, and diminished peristalsis. During pulmonary migration of larvae, chest films are normal or show fine miliary nodules or irregular changing patches of pneumonitis, abscess, or pleural effusion.

Differential Diagnosis

Because of varied signs and symptoms, the diagnosis of strongyloidiasis is often difficult. Eosinophilia plus one or more of the following factors should further enhance consideration of the diagnosis: endemic area exposure, duodenal ulcer-like pain, persistent or recurrent diarrhea, or malabsorption, recurrent coughing or wheezing, and transient pulmonary infiltrates. The duodenitis and jejunitis of strongyloidiasis can also mimic giardiasis, cholecystitis, and pancreatitis. Transient pulmonary infiltrates must be differentiated from tropical pulmonary eosinophilia and Löffler's syndrome. The diagnosis should be considered among the many causes of malabsorption in the tropics and in immunocompromised persons, including HIV-infected patients.

Treatment

Since strongyloides can multiply in humans, treatment should continue until the parasite is eradicated. In follow-up, multiple stool examinations should be done at weekly intervals, preferably by the Baermann concentration method. Patients receiving immunosuppressive therapy should be examined for strongyloidiasis before and at intervals during that treatment. In concurrent infection with strongyloidiasis and ascariasis or hookworm (which is common), eradicate the latter infections first.

The drug of choice in treatment is ivermectin, which appears to be equal in effectiveness to thiabendazole but has far fewer side effects.

A. IVERMECTIN

The dosage is 200 μg/kg; since cure is essential in this disease, a second dose is recommended the next day. Cure rates reported in several studies ranged from 82% to 95%. In the hyperinfection syndrome in immunocompromised patients with or without AIDS, it may be necessary to prolong treatment or change to thiabendazole.

B. THIABENDAZOLE

An oral dose of 25 mg/kg (maximum, 1.5 g per dose) is given after meals twice daily for 2–3 days. Repeat the course in 2 weeks. A 5- to 7-day (or longer) course is needed for disseminated infections. Tablet and liquid formulations are available; tablets should be chewed. Side effects, including headache, weakness, vomiting, vertigo, and decreased mental alertness, occur in as many as 30% of patients and may be severe. These symptoms are lessened if the drug is taken after meals. Other potentially serious side effects occur rarely. Erythema multiforme and the Stevens-Johnson syndrome have been associated with thiabendazole therapy; several fatalities have occurred in children.

C. ALBENDAZOLE

Albendazole is given at a dosage of 400 mg twice daily for 3–7 days and repeated in 1 week; cure rates in several studies ranged from 38% to 95%. In comparative studies, albendazole is less effective than ivermectin.

Prognosis

The prognosis is favorable except in the hyperinfection syndrome and in infections associated with malnutrition, advanced liver disease, immunologic disorders, or the use of immunosuppressive drugs. In selected instances, to control infections that cannot be eradicated, once-monthly treatments can be tried with a 1-day dose of ivermectin or 2-day course of thiabendazole.

Al Samman M et al: Strongyloidiasis colitis: a case report and review of the literature. J Clin Gastroenterol 1999;28:77. [PMID: 9916676]

Hanck C et al: Treatment of strongyloides infections. Gastroenterology 2000;119:1805. [PMID: 11187437]

Link K et al: Bacterial complications of strongyloidiasis: *Streptococcus bovis* meningitis. South Med J 1999;92:728. [PMID: 10414486]

Rodrigues MA et al: Invasive enteritis by *Strongyloides stercoralis* presenting as acute abdominal distress under corticosteroid therapy. Rev Hosp Clin Fac Med Sao Paulo 2001;56:103. [PMID: 11717716]

Siddiqui AA et al: Diagnosis of *Strongyloides stercoralis* infection. Clin Infect Dis 2001;33:1040. [PMID: 11528578]

TRICHINOSIS (Trichinelliosis, Trichinellosis)

ESSENTIALS OF DIAGNOSIS

- *History of ingestion of raw or inadequately cooked pork, boar, or bear.*
- *First week: diarrhea, cramps, malaise.*
- *Second week to 1–2 months: muscle pain and tenderness, fever, periorbital and facial edema, conjunctivitis.*
- *Eosinophilia and elevated serum enzymes; positive serologic tests; larvae in muscle biopsy.*

General Considerations

Trichinosis is caused worldwide by *Trichinella spiralis*. The disease is present wherever pork is eaten but is a greater problem in many temperate areas than in the tropics. In the USA, there has been a marked reduction in prevalence in pigs (rates in commercial pork are nil to 0.01%) and in incidence in humans (fewer than 35 cases are reported yearly). Four other species of trichinella have been recognized in humans: *T nativa* appears to be restricted to Arctic and sub-Arctic regions and *T nelsoni* to tropical Africa. *T pseudospiralis*, reported rarely worldwide, occurs as a persistent muscular infection accompanied by prolonged myalgia, muscular weakness and swelling, elevated muscle enzymes, and asthenia. *T britovi* occurs in temperate areas of Europe.

Human infections occur sporadically or in outbreaks. Infection is usually acquired by eating viable encysted larvae in raw or uncooked pork or pork products. Ground beef has also been a source of infection when adulterated with pork or inadvertently contaminated in a common meat grinder. In some cases, the source of infection is the flesh of dogs (East Asia), horses (France), or wild animals, particularly bears, walruses, bush pigs, foxes, or cougars (USA).

Gastric juices liberate the encysted larvae. They rapidly mature and mate, and the adult female then burrows into the mucosa of the small intestine. Within 4–5 days, the female begins to discharge viviparous larvae (100 × 6 μm) that are disseminated via the lymphatics and bloodstream to most body tissues. Larvae that reach striated muscle encyst and remain viable for months to years; those that reach other tissues are rapidly destroyed. The adult worms (2–3.6 mm × 75–90 μm) survive for up to about 6 weeks.

In the natural cycle, larvae develop into adult worms in the intestines when a carnivore or omnivore ingests parasitized muscle. Pigs generally become infected by feeding on uncooked food scraps or, less often, by eating infected rats. Other reservoir hosts include swine, dogs, cats, rats, and many wild animals, including the wolf, bear, and boar; marine animals in the Arctic; and the hyena, jackal, and lion in the tropics.

Clinical Findings

A. SYMPTOMS AND SIGNS

The incubation period is 2–7 days (range: 12 hours to 28 days). Severity depends upon intensity of infection, tissues invaded, immune status and age of the host (children have less severe infections), and perhaps the strain of the parasite. Findings range from asymptomatic to a mild febrile illness with short-lasting symptoms to a severe progressive illness with multiple system involvement that in rare cases is fatal.

1. Intestinal stage—When present, intestinal symptoms persist for 1–7 days: diarrhea, abdominal cramps, and malaise are the major findings; nausea and vomiting occur less frequently; and constipation is uncommon. Fever, eosinophilia, and leukocytosis are rare during the first week.

2. Muscle invasion stage—This begins at the end of the first week and lasts about 6 weeks. Parasitized muscles show an intense inflammatory reaction. Findings include fever (low-grade to marked); muscle pain and tenderness, edema, and spasm; periorbital and facial edema; sweating; photophobia and conjunctivitis; weakness or prostration; pain on swallowing; dyspnea, coughing, and hoarseness; subconjunctival, retinal, and nail splinter hemorrhages; and rashes and formication. The most frequently parasitized muscles and sites of findings are the masseters, the tongue, the diaphragm, the intercostal muscles, and the extraocular, laryngeal, paravertebral, nuchal, deltoid, pectoral, gluteus, biceps, and gastrocnemius muscles. Inflammatory reactions around larvae that reach tissues other than muscle may result in a broad range of findings, including the development of meningitis, encephalitis, myocarditis, bronchopneumonia, nephritis, and peripheral and cranial nerve disorders.

3. Convalescent stage—This generally begins in the second month but in severe infections may not begin before 3 months or longer. Vague muscle pains and malaise may persist for several more months. Permanent muscular atrophy has been reported.

B. Laboratory Findings

The diagnosis is supported by findings of eosinophilia, elevated serum muscle enzymes (creatine kinase, lactate dehydrogenase, aspartate aminotransferase), and positive serologic tests. There may be a marked hypergammaglobulinemia with reversal of the albumin-globulin ratio. Absence of an elevated sedimentation rate is a useful diagnostic clue. Confirmation of the diagnosis is by detection of larvae in muscle biopsy specimens.

Leukocytosis and eosinophilia appear during the second week. The proportion of eosinophils rises to a maximum of 20–90% in the third or fourth week and then slowly declines to normal over the next few months.

Serologic tests can detect most clinically manifest cases but are not sufficiently sensitive to detect low-level infections (ie, a few larvae per gram of ingested muscle). Circulating antigen can be detected about 2 weeks after infection in heavily infected persons and in 3–4 weeks in light infections. More than one antibody test should be used and then repeated to observe for seroconversion or for a rising titer. The bentonite flocculation (BF) test (positive titer, ≥ 1:5) is highly sensitive and is considered nearly 100% specific. It becomes positive in the third or fourth week, and reaches a maximum titer at about 2 months, and generally reverts to negative in 2–3 years. The immunofluorescence test (positive titer > 16) is also highly sensitive, though less specific than the BF test; it may become positive in the second week. The IgM and IgG ELISAs are also showing high sensitivity and specificity. The intradermal test is no longer recommended, as it may remain positive for years and batches of antigen vary in potency.

Adult worms may be looked for in feces, though they are seldom found. In the second week, there are occasional larvae in blood, duodenal washings, and, rarely, in centrifuged spinal fluid. In the third to fourth weeks, biopsy of skeletal muscle (approximately 1 cm^3) may be definitive (particularly gastrocnemius and pectoralis), preferably at a site of swelling or tenderness or near tendinous insertions. Portions of the specimen should be examined microscopically by compression between glass slides, by digestion, and by preparation of multiple histologic sections. If the biopsy is done too early, larvae may not be detectable. Myositis even in the absence of larvae is a significant finding.

C. Imaging

Chest films during the acute phase may show disseminated or localized infiltrates. Late calcification of muscle cysts cannot be detected radiologically.

Complications

The more important complications are granulomatous pneumonitis, encephalitis, and cardiac failure.

Differential Diagnosis

Because of its protean manifestations, trichinosis may resemble many other diseases. Eosinophilia, muscle pain and tenderness, and fever should lead the physician to consider collagen vascular disorders such as dermatomyositis or polyarteritis nodosa, which is generally accompanied by an elevated sedimentation rate.

Prevention

The frequency and intensity of infection in the USA and other countries have been significantly reduced by public health measures to prevent feeding of uncooked garbage to hogs and by animal inspection (not in the USA). The chief safeguard against trichinosis is adequate cooking of pork to 77 °C or by freezing meat at −17 °C for 20 days (longer if meat is over 15 cm thick). *T nativa* in game is often relatively resistant to freezing. Low doses of gamma irradiation are also effective in killing larvae. *Government inspection of pork is not practiced in the USA as it is in some European countries.*

Treatment

Treatment is principally supportive, since in most cases recovery is spontaneous without sequelae.

A. Intestinal Phase

Though supporting evidence for efficacy is limited, albendazole, because of its relatively high absorption and freedom from adverse reactions, is proposed as the drug of choice in a dosage of 400 mg twice daily for 10 days. Mebendazole is an alternative drug at a dosage of 200–300 mg three times daily for 3 days, followed by 400–500 mg three times daily for 10 days. A third alternative drug is thiabendazole at a dosage of 25 mg/kg (maximum, 1.5 g per dose) twice daily after meals for 3–7 days; side effects, sometimes severe, are common (see Strongyloidiasis, above). Corticosteroids are contraindicated in the intestinal phase.

B. MUSCLE INVASION PHASE

In this stage, severe infections require hospitalization and high doses of corticosteroids (40–60 mg/d for 1–2 days), followed by lower doses for several days or weeks to control symptoms. However, because corticosteroids may suppress the inflammatory response to adult worms, they should be used only when symptoms are severe. Although drug treatment has not been shown to be effective in the muscle invasion stage, albendazole, mebendazole, or thiabendazole can be tried.

Prognosis

Death is rare—sometimes within 2–3 weeks in overwhelming infections, more often in 4–8 weeks from a major complication such as cardiac failure or pneumonia.

Bruschi F et al: New aspects of human trichinellosis: the impact of new Trichinella species. Postgrad Med J 2002;78:15. [PMID: 11796866]

Kociecka W: Trichinellosis: human disease, diagnosis and treatment. Vet Parasitol 2000;93:365. [PMID: 11099848]

Vojnikovic B et al: Severe Trichinellosis cured with pulse doses of glucocorticoids. Coll Antropol 2001;25(Suppl):131. [PMID: 11817004]

Watt G et al: Blinded, placebo-controlled trial of antiparasitic drugs for trichinosis myositis. J Infect Dis 2000;182:371. [PMID: 10882628]

TRICHURIASIS
(Trichocephaliasis, Whipworm)

Trichuris trichiura is a common intestinal parasite of humans throughout the world, particularly in the subtropics and tropics. Persons of all ages are affected, but infection is heaviest and most frequent in children. The slender worms, 30–50 mm in length, attach by means of their anterior whip-like end to the mucosa of the large intestine, particularly to the cecum. Eggs are passed in the feces but require 2–4 weeks for larval development after reaching the soil before becoming infective; thus, person-to-person transmission is not possible. Infections are acquired by ingestion of the infective egg. The larvae hatch in the small intestine and mature in the large bowel but do not migrate through the tissues.

Clinical Findings

A. SYMPTOMS AND SIGNS

Light (fewer than 10,000 eggs per gram of feces) to moderate infections rarely cause symptoms. Heavy infections (30,000 or more eggs per gram of feces) may be accompanied by abdominal cramps, tenesmus, diarrhea, distention, flatulence, and nausea and vomiting. With persistent dysentery and blood loss into the stool, the trichuris dysentery syndrome can appear—particularly in malnourished young children—which is accompanied by anemia, rectal prolapse, clubbing of fingers, growth stunting, and possibly cognitive defects. Adult worms are sometimes seen in stools. Invasion of the appendix, with resulting appendicitis, is rare.

B. LABORATORY FINDINGS

Diagnosis is by identification of characteristic eggs and, sometimes, adult worms in stools. Eosinophilia (5–20%) is common with all but light infections. Charcot-Leyden crystals may be seen in stool. Severe iron deficiency anemia may be present with heavy infections.

Treatment

Patients with asymptomatic light infections do not require treatment. For those with heavier or symptomatic infections, give mebendazole or albendazole. Thiabendazole should *not* be used because it is not effective and because it is potentially toxic. Iron replacement may be needed for anemia.

A. ALBENDAZOLE

Albendazole, given orally at a single dose of 400 mg, has resulted in cure rates of 33–90%, with marked reduction in egg counts in those not cured. Daily treatment for 3 days improves cure rates. Albendazole should not be used in pregnancy.

B. MEBENDAZOLE

A dosage of 100 mg twice daily before or after meals for 3 days results in cure rates of 60–80%, with marked reduction in ovum counts in the remaining patients. It may be therapeutically advantageous for the tablets to be chewed before swallowing. In mild disease, a 500-mg dose may be sufficient, whereas in severe trichuriasis a longer course of treatment (up to 6 days) or a repeat course will often be necessary. Gastrointestinal side effects from the drug are rare. The drug is contraindicated in pregnancy.

Bennett A et al: Reducing intestinal nematode infection: efficacy of albendazole and mebendazole. Parasitol Today 2000;16:71. [PMID: 10652492]

Herman MA et al: Diagnosis and removal of cecal whipworm infection: case report and review. Dig Dis Sci 2000;45:1639. [PMID: 11007117]

Stephenson LS et al: The public health significance of *Trichuris trichiura*. Parasitology 2000;121(Suppl):S73. [PMID: 11386693]

VISCERAL LARVA MIGRANS
(Toxocariasis)

Most visceral larva migrans cases are due to *Toxocara canis,* an ascarid of dogs and other canids; *Toxocara cati* in domestic cats has occasionally been implicated and rarely *Belascaris procyonis* of raccoons. The adult worms live in the intestinal tracts of their respective hosts and release large numbers of eggs in the stool.

The reservoir mechanism for *T canis* is latent infection in female dogs which is reactivated during pregnancy. Transmission from mother to puppies is via the placenta and milk. Most eggs passed to the environment are from puppies (2 weeks to 6 months) and lactating bitches (up to 6 months after parturition). The life cycle of *T cati* is similar, but transplacental transmission does not occur.

Human infections are sporadic and probably occur worldwide. In the USA, antibody seroprevalence is 5–7%. Infection is generally in dirt-eating young children who ingest *T canis* or *T cati* eggs from soil or sand contaminated with animal feces, most often from puppies. Direct contact with infected animals does not produce infection, as the eggs require a 3- to 4-week extrinsic incubation period to become infective; thereafter, eggs in soil remain infective for months to years.

In humans, hatched larvae are unable to mature but continue to migrate through the tissues for up to 6 months. Eventually they lodge in various organs, particularly the lungs and liver and less often the brain, eyes, and other tissues, where they produce eosinophilic granulomas up to 1 cm in diameter.

Clinical & Laboratory Findings

A. Acute Infection

Migrating larvae may induce fever, cough, wheezing, hepatosplenomegaly, and lymphadenopathy. A variety of other findings may occur when other organs are invaded, including myelitis, encephalitis, and carditis. The acute phase may last 2–3 weeks, but resolution of all physical and laboratory findings may take up to 18 months.

Leukocytosis is marked (may exceed 100,000/μL), with 30–80% due to eosinophils. Hyperglobulinemia occurs when the liver is extensively invaded and is a useful clue in diagnosis. An ELISA test is the most specific (92%) and sensitive (78%) serologic test and may permit a presumptive diagnosis, although it does not distinguish acute from prior infection. However, rising or falling titers with twofold differences are consistent with the diagnosis. Nonspecific isohemagglutinin titers (anti-A and anti-B) are usually greater than 1:1024. Chest radiographs may show infiltrates. With central nervous system involvement, the cerebrospinal fluid may show eosinophils. No parasitic forms can be found by stool examination.

Ultrasonography may detect 1-cm hypoechoic lesions in the liver, each with a thread-like hyperechoic line. Specific diagnosis can only be made by percutaneous liver biopsy or by direct biopsy of a granuloma at laparoscopy (mixed inflammatory infiltrate with numerous eosinophils), but these procedures are seldom justified and may not yield larvae.

B. Ocular Toxocariasis

Most cases occur in children, most commonly 5–10 years old, who present with visual impairment in one eye and sometimes leukocoria, squint, and red eye. The principal pathologic entity is eosinophilic granuloma of the retina that resembles retinoblastoma. Until the recent development of the toxocara ELISA test, this resulted in the enucleation of many eyes. Other common clinical findings are peripheral retinochoroiditis, a diffuse, painless endophthalmitis; posterior pole granuloma; and a peripheral inflammatory mass. Uncommonly seen are an iris nodule, optic nerve granuloma, uniocular pars planitis, and a migrating retinal nematode. Ocular toxocariasis, which is generally recognized years after the acute infection, is generally not associated with peripheral eosinophilia, hypergammaglobulinemia, or isohemagglutinin elevation. Serum ELISA tests may be positive, but a negative test does not rule out the diagnosis. If doubt exists about whether a patient with a positive serum ELISA test has toxocariasis or retinoblastoma, examination of the vitreous humor for ELISA antibody and eosinophils can be helpful. High-resolution CT scanning of the orbit should be done.

Prevention, Treatment, & Prognosis

Disease in humans is best prevented by periodic treatment of puppies, kittens, and nursing dog and cat mothers, starting at 2 weeks postpartum, repeating at weekly intervals for 3 weeks and then every 6 months.

A. Acute Infection

Treatment of symptomatic persons is primarily supportive. Although there is no proved specific treatment, the following drugs can be tried: albendazole (400 mg twice daily for 21 days), mebendazole (200 mg twice daily for 21 days), thiabendazole (as used in strongyloidiasis), or ivermectin. Theoretically, release of antigens from dying parasites may exacerbate clinical and laboratory findings. Corticosteroids, antibiotics, antihistamines, and analgesics may be needed to provide symptomatic relief. Symptoms may persist for months but generally clear within 1–2 years. The ultimate outcome is usually good, but permanent neuropsychologic deficits have been seen.

B. Ocular Toxocariasis

Treatment includes oral and subconjunctival corticosteroids, an anthelmintic drug, vitrectomy for vitreous traction and laser photocoagulation. Partial or total permanent visual impairment is rare.

Hartleb M et al: Severe hepatic involvement in visceral larva migrans. Eur J Gastroenterol Hepatol 2001;13:1245. [PMID: 11711784]

Kaplan KJ et al: Eosinophilic granuloma of the liver: a characteristic lesion with relationship to visceral larva migrans. Am J Surg Pathol 2001;25:1316. [PMID: 11688468]

Pawlowski Z: Toxocariasis in humans: clinical expression and treatment dilemma. J Helminthol 2001;75:299. [PMID: 11818044]

Sabrosa NA et al: Nematode infections of the eye: toxocariasis and diffuse unilateral subacute neuroretinitis. Curr Opin Ophthalmol 2001;12:450. [PMID: 11734685]

Infectious Diseases: Mycotic*

36

Richard J. Hamill, MD
See www.current-med.com/ch36.html

Fungal infections have assumed an increasingly important role as use of broad-spectrum antimicrobial agents has increased and the number of immunodeficient patients has risen. Some pathogens (eg, cryptococcus, candida, pneumocystis, fusarium) rarely cause serious disease in normal hosts. Other endemic fungi (eg, histoplasma, coccidioides, paracoccidioides) commonly cause disease in normal hosts but tend to be more aggressive in immunocompromised ones.

CANDIDIASIS

 ### ESSENTIALS OF DIAGNOSIS

- *Common normal flora but opportunistic pathogen.*
- *Gastrointestinal mucosal disease, particularly esophagitis, most common; catheter-associated fungemia occurs in hospitalized patients.*
- *Diagnosis of invasive systemic disease requires tissue biopsy or evidence of retinal disease.*

General Considerations

Candida albicans can be cultured from the mouth, vagina, and feces of most people. Cutaneous and oral lesions are discussed in Chapters 6 and 8, respectively. The risk factors for invasive candidiasis include prolonged neutropenia, recent surgery, broad-spectrum antibiotic therapy, the presence of intravascular catheters (especially when providing total parenteral nutrition), and intravenous drug use. Cellular immun-

odeficiency predisposes to mucocutaneous disease. When no other underlying cause is found, persistent oral or vaginal candidiasis should arouse a suspicion of HIV infection.

Clinical Findings & Treatment

A. MUCOSAL CANDIDIASIS

Esophageal involvement is the most frequent type of invasive mucosal disease. Individuals present with substernal odynophagia, gastroesophageal reflux, or nausea without substernal pain. Oral candidiasis, though often associated, is not invariably present. Diagnosis is best confirmed by endoscopy with biopsy and culture, since radiographically the condition may be difficult to distinguish from esophagitis caused by infection with cytomegalovirus or herpes simplex virus. Therapy depends upon the severity of disease. If patients are able to swallow and take adequate amounts of fluid orally, fluconazole, 100 mg/d (or itraconazole solution, 10 mg/mL, 100 mg/d), for 10–14 days will usually suffice. In the individual who is more ill or has developed esophagitis while taking fluconazole, a 10- to 14-day course of amphotericin B at a dose of 0.3 mg/kg/d intravenously usually results in resolution. Caspofungin acetate at a dosage of 50 mg/d intravenously has equivalent efficacy and is essentially free of significant toxicity. Relapse is common when there is underlying HIV infection.

Vulvovaginal candidiasis occurs in an estimated 75% of women during their lifetime. Risk factors include pregnancy, uncontrolled diabetes mellitus, broad-spectrum antimicrobial treatment, corticosteroid use, and HIV infection. In women with HIV infection, vaginal candidiasis is usually the first and most common opportunistic infection. Symptoms include acute vulvar pruritus, burning vaginal discharge, and dyspareunia. Various topical azole preparations (eg, clotrimazole, 100 mg vaginal tablet for 7 days, or miconazole, 200 mg vaginal suppository for 3 days) are effective. One 150 mg oral dose of fluconazole has been shown to have equivalent efficacy with better patient acceptance.

---

*Superficial mycoses are discussed in Chapter 6.

B. CANDIDAL FUNGURIA

Candidal funguria frequently resolves with discontinuance of antibiotics or removal of bladder catheters. Clinical benefit from treatment of asymptomatic candiduria has not been demonstrated. When symptomatic funguria persists, oral fluconazole, 200 mg/d for 7–14 days, can be used if renal function is normal. Bladder irrigation with amphotericin B (50–200 mg/mL) is rarely indicated, though it may transiently clear candiduria, especially if colonization is confined to the bladder. However, failure to clear the candiduria in this way suggests the presence of upper urinary tract infection. Rare complications of candidal urinary tract infections are ureteral obstruction and dissemination.

C. CANDIDAL FUNGEMIA

Candidal fungemia may represent a benign, self-limited process, but until proved otherwise it should be considered a sign of serious disseminated disease. If fungemia resolves with removal of intravascular catheters, there are often no further complications. The incidence of endophthalmitis may be higher than previously recognized, and a short course of intravenous amphotericin B to a total dose of 200 mg appears to lower this incidence. Such an approach is strongly recommended for patients with candidal fungemia. (See Amphotericin B, Chapter 37.)

If fungemia is documented, if retinal lesions are identified, or if candida is isolated from other sites, the patient is considered to have disseminated disease. Important clinical findings in disseminated candidiasis are fluffy white retinal infiltrates that extend into the vitreous and raised, erythematous skin lesions that may be painful. Though characteristic, these are seen in less than 50% of cases. Other organ system involvement in disseminated disease may include the brain, meninges, and myocardium. Although blood cultures are positive in only about 50% of cases of invasive disease, any positive blood culture for candida should be considered significant. Serologic tests for candida have not proved helpful in differentiating transient fungemia from disseminated disease. Amphotericin B at a dosage of 0.3–0.5 mg/kg/d is one of the agents of choice. Flucytosine, 150 mg/kg/d orally in four divided doses, is added if central nervous system involvement occurs until clinical improvement results. Individuals who do not tolerate amphotericin B may be given fluconazole, 200–800 mg/d intravenously, with equivalent efficacy. Removal or exchange of intravascular catheters substantially decreases the duration of candidemia.

Another form of disseminated disease is hepatosplenic candidiasis. This results from aggressive chemotherapy and prolonged neutropenia in patients with underlying hematologic cancers. Patients typically present with fever and variable abdominal pain weeks after chemotherapy, when neutrophil counts have recovered. Blood cultures are generally negative. Hepatic enzymes reveal an alkaline phosphatase elevation that may be marked. CT scanning of the abdomen shows hepatosplenomegaly, most often with multiple low-density defects in the liver. Diagnosis is established by liver biopsy, histopathology, and culture. Fluconazole, 400 mg daily, or a lipid formulation of amphotericin B is given until clinical and radiographic improvement occurs.

D. CANDIDAL ENDOCARDITIS

Candidal endocarditis rarely is a complication of transient fungemia. It usually results from direct inoculation at the time of valvular heart surgery or repeated inoculation with intravenous drug use. Candidal endocarditis occurs with increased frequency on prosthetic valves in the first few months following surgery. Splenomegaly and petechiae are common, and there is a predilection for large-vessel embolization. Non-albicans species such as *Candida parapsilosis* and *Candida tropicalis* are more often important etiologic agents in endocarditis than in fungemia, which is most often due to *C albicans*. The diagnosis is established definitively by culturing candida from emboli or from vegetations at the time of valve replacement. Valve destruction (usually aortic or mitral) is common, and surgical therapy is necessary in addition to a prolonged course of amphotericin therapy, usually to a total dose of 1–1.5 g intravenously.

It is important to note that non-albicans species of candida now account for over 50% of clinical bloodstream isolates and are often resistant to imidazole antibiotics such as fluconazole. The widespread use of these agents for prophylaxis in immunocompromised patients can lead to the emergence of pathogens such as *Candida krusei*. Dissemination of this organism has been reported in patients undergoing bone marrow transplantation for leukemia. Imidazole-resistant *C albicans* has increased in frequency in immunocompromised patients, particularly in patients with late-stage AIDS receiving chronic suppressive fluconazole.

In all forms of invasive candidiasis, an important element of therapy is reversal of the underlying predisposing factor when possible. In high-risk patients undergoing induction chemotherapy, prophylaxis with fluconazole has been shown to be beneficial.

Kontoyiannis DP et al: Fluconazole vs. amphotericin B for the management of candidaemia in adults: a meta-analysis. Mycoses 2001;44:125. [PMID: 11486448] (Fluconazole is as efficacious as amphotericin B in stable, not severely immunocompromised patients with candidemia.)

Rex JH et al: Practice guidelines for the treatment of candidiasis. Clin Infect Dis 2000;30:662. [PMID: 10770728] (Guidelines assembled by the Infectious Diseases Society of America that discuss therapeutic approaches to invasive and mucosal candidiasis.)

HISTOPLASMOSIS

 ESSENTIALS OF DIAGNOSIS

- *Epidemiologically linked to bird droppings and bat exposure; common along river valleys (espe-*

cially the Ohio River and the Mississippi River valleys).

- Most patients asymptomatic; respiratory illness most common clinical problem.

- Rare patients with normal immune function develop dissemination, with hepatosplenomegaly, lymphadenopathy, and oral ulcers.

- Widespread disease especially common in AIDS or other immunosuppressed states, with poor prognosis.

- Skin test and serology seldom diagnostic; biopsy of affected organs with culture, or urinary polysaccharide antigen most useful in disseminated disease.

General Considerations

Histoplasmosis is caused by *Histoplasma capsulatum,* a dimorphic fungus that has been isolated from soil contaminated with bird or bat droppings in endemic areas (central and eastern USA, eastern Canada, Mexico, Central America, South America, Africa, and southeast Asia). Infection presumably takes place by inhalation of conidia. These convert into small budding cells that are engulfed by phagocytic cells in the lungs. The organism proliferates and is carried hematogenously to other organs.

Clinical Findings

A. SYMPTOMS AND SIGNS

Most cases of histoplasmosis are asymptomatic or mild and thus go unrecognized. Past infection is recognized by the development of a positive histoplasmin skin test and occasionally by pulmonary and splenic calcification noted on incidental x-rays. Symptoms and signs of pulmonary involvement are usually absent even in patients who subsequently show areas of calcification on chest x-ray. Symptomatic infection may present with mild influenza-like illness, often lasting 1–4 days. Moderately severe infections are frequently diagnosed as atypical pneumonia. These patients have fever, cough, and mild central chest pain lasting 5–15 days. Physical examination is usually negative. Radiographic findings during acute illness are variable and nonspecific.

Clinically evident infections occur in several forms: (1) **Acute histoplasmosis** frequently occurs in epidemics, often when soil containing infected bird or bat droppings is disturbed. It is a severe disease manifested by marked prostration, fever, and relatively few pulmonary complaints even when x-rays show pneumonia. The illness may last from 1 week to 6 months but is almost never fatal. (2) **Progressive disseminated histoplasmosis** is usually fatal within 6 weeks or less. Symptoms usually consist of fever, dyspnea, cough, loss of weight, and prostration. Ulcers of the mucous membranes of the oropharynx may be pre-

sent. The liver and spleen are nearly always enlarged, and all the organs of the body are involved, particularly the adrenal glands. (3) **Chronic progressive pulmonary histoplasmosis** is usually seen in older patients with chronic obstructive lung disease. The lungs show chronic progressive changes, often with apical cavities. (4) **Disseminated disease in the profoundly immunocompromised host** often represents reactivation of prior infectious foci or may reflect acute infection. This form is commonly seen in patients with underlying HIV infection—with CD4 cell counts usually < 100 cells/μL—and is characterized by fever and multiple organ system involvement. Chest x-rays may show a miliary pattern. Presentation may be fulminant, simulating septic shock, with death ensuing rapidly unless treatment is provided.

B. LABORATORY FINDINGS

Most patients with progressive pulmonary disease show anemia of chronic disease. Bone marrow involvement may be prominent in disseminated forms with occurrence of pancytopenia. Alkaline phosphatase and marked LDH and ferritin elevations are also common.

In pulmonary disease, sputum culture is rarely positive except in chronic disease; in contrast, blood or bone marrow cultures from immunocompromised patients with acute disseminated disease are positive more than 80% of the time. A urine antigen assay has a sensitivity of greater than 90% for disseminated disease in AIDS patients and can be used to diagnose relapse. The sensitivity of screening immunodiffusion is 50% in acute pulmonary histoplasmosis, and complement fixation titers are positive in about 80% of cases. A combination of these two methods yields a sensitivity of up to 80% in immunodeficient adults.

Treatment

For progressive localized disease and for mild to moderately severe nonmeningeal disseminated disease in immunocompetent or immunocompromised patients, itraconazole, 200–400 mg/d orally is the treatment of choice with an overall response rate of approximately 80%. Duration of therapy ranges from weeks to several months depending upon the severity of illness. Amphotericin B is reserved for individuals who cannot take oral medications; for those who have failed itraconazole therapy; for those with meningitis; and for management of severe disseminated disease in an immunocompromised host. Up to 2.5 g total may need to be given in the latter two situations, though this course of treatment can be abbreviated and oral itraconazole instituted once clinical stabilization has occurred. (See Amphotericin B, Chapter 37.) Patients with AIDS-related histoplasmosis require lifelong suppressive therapy with itraconazole, 200–400 mg/d orally.

Mocherla S et al: Treatment of histoplasmosis. Semin Respir Infect 2001;16:141. [PMID: 11521246] (Amphotericin B or one of the lipid formulations is recommended as initial treatment in seriously ill patients. Itraconazole is used in less severe forms of disease.)

COCCIDIOIDOMYCOSIS

 ESSENTIALS OF DIAGNOSIS

- Influenza-like illness with malaise, fever, backache, headache, and cough.
- Arthralgia and periarticular swelling of knees and ankles.
- Erythema nodosum common.
- Dissemination may result in meningitis, bony lesions, or skin and soft tissue abscesses.
- Chest x-ray findings vary widely from pneumonitis to cavitation.
- Serologic tests useful; spherules containing endospores demonstrable in sputum or tissues.

General Considerations

Coccidioidomycosis should be considered in the diagnosis of any obscure illness in a patient who has lived in or visited an endemic area.

Infection results from the inhalation of arthroconidia of *Coccidioides immitis,* a mold that grows in soil in certain arid regions of the southwestern USA, in Mexico, and in Central and South America.

Fewer than 1% of immunocompetent hosts show dissemination, but among these patients the mortality rate is high.

In HIV-infected people in endemic areas, coccidioidomycosis is a common opportunistic infection. These patients may present with disease manifestations ranging from focal pulmonary infiltrates to widespread miliary disease with multiple organ involvement and meningitis.

Clinical Findings

A. SYMPTOMS AND SIGNS

Symptoms of primary coccidioidomycosis occur in about 40% of infections. Symptom onset (after an incubation period of 10–30 days) is usually that of a respiratory tract illness with fever and occasionally chills. Pleuritic pain is common. Nasopharyngitis may be followed by bronchitis accompanied by a dry or slightly productive cough.

Arthralgia accompanied by periarticular swellings, often of the knees and ankles, is common. Erythema nodosum may appear 2–20 days after onset of symptoms. Persistent pulmonary lesions, varying from cavities and abscesses to parenchymal nodular densities or bronchiectasis, occur in about 5% of diagnosed cases.

Disseminated disease occurs in about 0.1% of white and 1% of nonwhite patients. Filipinos and blacks are especially susceptible, as are pregnant women of all races. Symptoms depend upon the site of dissemination. Any organ may be involved. Pulmonary findings usually become more pronounced, with mediastinal lymph node enlargement, cough, and increased sputum production. Lung abscesses may rupture into the pleural space, producing an empyema. These may also extend to bones and skin, and pericardial and myocardial extension has been occasionally observed. Fungemia may occur and is characterized clinically by a diffuse miliary pattern on chest x-ray and by early death. The course may be particularly rapid in immunosuppressed patients.

Bone lesions most often occur at bony prominences. Meningitis occurs in 30–50% of cases of dissemination. Subcutaneous abscesses and verrucous skin lesions are especially common in fulminating cases. Lymphadenitis may occur and may progress to suppuration. Mediastinal and retroperitoneal abscesses are not uncommon. HIV-infected persons with disseminated disease have a higher incidence of miliary infiltrates, lymphadenopathy, and meningitis, but skin lesions are uncommon.

B. LABORATORY FINDINGS

In primary coccidioidomycosis, there may be moderate leukocytosis and eosinophilia. Serologic testing is useful for both diagnosis and prognosis. The tube precipitin test and an immunodiffusion test detect IgM antibodies and are useful for diagnosis early in the disease process. Historically, a persistent rising complement fixation titer ($\geq 1:16$) has been considered suggestive of disseminated disease; in addition, complement fixation titers can be used to assess the adequacy of therapy. Serum complement fixation titer may be low when there is meningitis but no other disseminated disease. In patients with HIV-related coccidioidomycosis, the false-negative rate may be as high as 30%.

Demonstrable complement-fixing antibodies in spinal fluid are diagnostic of coccidioidal meningitis. These are found in over 90% of cases. Spinal fluid findings include increased cell count with lymphocytosis and reduced glucose. Spinal fluid culture is positive in approximately 30% of meningitis cases. Spherules filled with endospores may be found in biopsy specimens; though they are not infectious, they convert to the highly contagious arthroconidia when grown in culture media. Blood cultures in appropriate media are only rarely positive in disseminated disease.

C. IMAGING

Radiographic findings vary, but patchy, nodular pulmonary infiltrates and thin-walled cavities are most common. Hilar lymphadenopathy may be visible and is seen in localized disease; mediastinal lymphadenopathy suggests dissemination. There may be pleural effusions and lytic lesions in bone.

Treatment

General symptomatic therapy is given as needed for disease limited to the chest with no evidence of progression. For progressive pulmonary or extrapulmonary disease, amphotericin B intravenously has proved effective in some patients (see Chapter 37). Therapy should be continued, with duration of therapy determined by a declining complement fixation titer and a favorable clinical response . For meningitis, treatment consists of the lumbar intrathecal administration of amphotericin B daily in increasing doses up to 1–5 mg/d until the patient is clinically stable. The drug can then be tapered to once every 6 weeks for several years thereafter. Systemic therapy with amphotericin B, 0.6 mg/kg/d intravenously, is generally given concurrently with intrathecal therapy. Once the patient is clinically stable, oral therapy with an azole for an indefinite period is an alternative to intrathecal amphotericin B therapy.

Approximately 75% of patients with mild coccidioidal meningitis who are treated with oral fluconazole at a dosage of 400 mg/d will have a favorable clinical response. Such therapy is suppressive only and must be continued indefinitely, probably lifelong.

Fluconazole, 200–400 mg orally daily, or itraconazole, 400 mg orally daily, may be given for disease in the chest, bones, and soft tissues; however, therapy must be continued for 6 months or longer after the disease is inactive in order to prevent relapse. Response to therapy should be monitored by following the decrease in serum complement fixation titers.

Thoracic surgery is occasionally indicated for giant, infected, or ruptured cavities. Surgical drainage is also useful for soft tissue abscesses and bone disease. Amphotericin B, 1 mg/kg/d intravenously, is advisable following extensive surgical manipulation of infected tissue until the disease is inactive, whereupon therapy may be continued with an azole.

Prognosis

The prognosis for patients with limited disease is good, but persistent pulmonary cavities may cause complications. Nodules, cavities, and fibrotic residuals may rarely progress after long periods of stability or regression. Serial complement fixation titers should be performed after therapy for patients with coccidioidomycosis; rising titers warrant reinstitution of therapy because relapse is likely. Disseminated and meningeal forms still have mortality rates exceeding 50% in the absence of therapy.

Galgiani JN et al: Practice guidelines for the treatment of coccidioidomycosis. Clin Infect Dis 2000;30:658. [PMID: 10770727] (Amphotericin B is the drug of choice for rapidly progressive coccidioidal infections. Itraconazole and fluconazole are effective for more chronic manifestations. Duration of therapy may range from months to years.)

Stevens DA et al: Intrathecal amphotericin in the management of coccidioidal meningitis. Semin Respir Infect 2001;16:263.

[PMID: 11739548] (Description of the methods for intrathecal delivery of amphotericin B for management of coccidioidal meningitis. Lumbar instillation entails fewer patient risks and has not been shown to be inferior to other routes.)

PNEUMOCYSTOSIS
(*Pneumocystis carinii* Pneumonia)

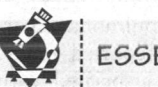 ESSENTIALS OF DIAGNOSIS

- *Fever, dyspnea, nonproductive cough.*
- *Bilateral diffuse interstitial disease without hilar adenopathy by chest x-ray.*
- *Bibasilar crackles on auscultation in many cases; others have no findings.*
- *Reduced partial pressure of oxygen.*
- *P carinii in sputum, bronchoalveolar lavage fluid, or lung tissue.*

General Considerations

Pneumocystis carinii is a fungal organism that has been found in the lungs of a variety of domesticated and wild mammals and is distributed worldwide in humans. Although symptomatic *P carinii* disease is rare in the general population, serologic evidence indicates that asymptomatic infections have occurred in most persons by a young age. The overt infection is an acute interstitial plasma cell pneumonia that occurs with high frequency among two groups: (1) as epidemics of primary infections among premature or debilitated or marasmic infants on hospital wards in underdeveloped parts of the world, and (2) as sporadic cases among older children and adults who have an abnormal or altered cellular immune status. Cases occur generally in patients with cancer or severe malnutrition and debility, in patients treated with immunosuppressive or cytotoxic drugs or irradiation for the management of organ transplants and cancer, and, most commonly, in patients with AIDS (see Chapter 31).

The mode of transmission in primary infection is unknown, but the evidence suggests airborne transmission. Following asymptomatic primary infection, latent and presumably inactive organisms are sparsely distributed in the alveoli. Whether acute infection in older children and adults results from de novo infection or from reactivation of latent infection is unknown.

Pneumocystis pneumonia occurs in up to 80% of AIDS patients not receiving prophylaxis and is a major cause of death. Its incidence increases in direct proportion to the fall in CD4 cells, with most cases occurring at CD4 cell counts below 200/μL. Dissemination of the infection to tissues other than the lung is rare, except in those who have received prophylactic aerosolized pentamidine. In non-AIDS patients receiving immunosuppressive therapy, symptoms frequently begin after corticosteroids have been tapered or discontinued.

Clinical Findings

A. SYMPTOMS AND SIGNS

Findings are usually limited to the pulmonary parenchyma; extrapulmonary disease is reported rarely. In the sporadic form of the disease associated with deficient cell-mediated immunity, the onset is abrupt, with fever, tachypnea, shortness of breath, and usually nonproductive cough. Pulmonary physical findings may be slight and disproportionate to the degree of illness and the radiologic findings; many patients have bibasilar crackles, but others do not. Without treatment, the course is usually one of rapid deterioration and death. Adult patients may present with spontaneous pneumothorax, usually in patients with previous episodes or those receiving aerosolized pentamidine prophylaxis. In the infantile form of the disease, the patient is generally free of fever and may show eosinophilia. Patients with AIDS will usually have other evidence of HIV-associated disease, including fever, fatigue, and weight loss, for weeks or months preceding the illness.

B. LABORATORY FINDINGS

Chest radiographs most often show diffuse "interstitial" infiltration, which may be heterogeneous, miliary, or patchy early in infection. There may also be diffuse or focal consolidation, cystic changes, nodules, or cavitation within nodules. Pleural effusions are not seen. About 5–10% of patients with pneumocystis pneumonia have normal chest films. Patients who have received prophylaxis with aerosolized pentamidine often have atypical chest x-rays, demonstrating upper lobe infiltrates.

Typically, there is reduction in vital and total lung capacity, and the single-breath diffusing capacity for carbon monoxide shows impaired diffusion. Arterial blood gases usually show hypoxemia with hypocapnia. Gallium lung scanning (sensitivity > 95%, specificity 20–40%) shows diffuse uptake; the test should be reserved for those with normal chest films and normal pulmonary function in whom the disease is suspected. Isolated elevation or rising levels of serum LDH are very sensitive but not specific findings for *P carinii*. Lymphopenia with depleted CD4 lymphocytes is common. Serologic tests, including tests to detect antigenemia, are not helpful in diagnosis.

Specific diagnosis depends on morphologic demonstration of the organisms in clinical specimens using specific stains. The organism cannot be cultured. Although patients rarely spontaneously produce sufficient sputum for examination, adequate specimens can be obtained with induced sputum by having pa-

tients inhale an aerosol of hypertonic saline (3%) produced by an ultrasonic nebulizer. Specimens are then stained with Giemsa's stain or methenamine silver, either of which allows detection of cysts. The use of monoclonal antibody with immunofluorescence has increased the sensitivity of diagnosis. If diagnostic results cannot be achieved with induced sputum specimens and the diagnosis of *P carinii* pneumonia is strongly suspected, alternative techniques for obtaining specimens include bronchoalveolar lavage (sensitivity 86–97%) followed if necessary by transbronchial lung biopsy (85–97%). Open lung biopsy and needle lung biopsy are infrequently done. Although conclusions are still preliminary, the polymerase chain reaction (PCR) test for the detection of *P carinii* appears to be sensitive but does not provide more rapid diagnosis.

Treatment
(See Table 31–4.)

It is appropriate to start empiric therapy for *P carinii* pneumonia if the disease is suspected clinically; however, in both AIDS patients and non-AIDS patients with mild to moderately severe disease, continued treatment should be based on a proved diagnosis because of the toxicity of therapy and the possible coexistence of other infections. Both in AIDS patients and in non-AIDS patients with mild to moderately severe disease, oral TMP-SMZ is the preferred agent because of its low cost and excellent bioavailability. Patients suffering from nausea and vomiting or intractable diarrhea should be given intravenous TMP-SMZ. Pentamidine is used if fluid must be restricted or if there is a history of sulfonamide drug sensitivity. Therapy should be continued with the selected drug for at least 5–10 days before one considers changing agents, as fever, tachypnea, and pulmonary infiltrates persist for 4–6 days after starting treatment; some patients have a transient worsening of their disease during the first 3–5 days, which may be related to an inflammatory response secondary to the presence of dead or dying organisms. Early addition of corticosteroids may attenuate this response (Chapter 31). Some clinicians prefer to treat episodes of AIDS-associated pneumocystis pneumonia for 21 days rather than the usual 14 days recommended for non-AIDS cases.

A. TRIMETHOPRIM-SULFAMETHOXAZOLE

The dosage is TMP 20 mg/kg (12–15 mg/kg may decrease side effects without decreasing efficacy) and SMZ 100 mg/kg given orally or intravenously daily in three or four divided doses for 14–21 days. Adverse reactions are generally those of the sulfonamide component. Patients with AIDS have a high frequency of hypersensitivity reactions (approaching 50%), which may include fever, rashes (sometimes severe), malaise, neutropenia, hepatitis, nephritis, thrombocytopenia, and hyperbilirubinemia.

B. Pentamidine Isethionate

This drug is administered intravenously (preferred) or intramuscularly as a single dose of 3 mg (salt) per kilogram per day for 14–21 days. To avoid injection site pain or sterile abscesses, most workers administer the drug only intravenously by diluting it in 250 mL of 5% dextrose in water and giving it slowly over 1 hour. Pentamidine causes side effects in nearly 50% of patients. Occasional reactions include rash, neutropenia, abnormal liver function tests, serum folate depression, hyperkalemia, and hypocalcemia. Hypoglycemia (often clinically inapparent), hyperglycemia, hyponatremia, and delayed nephrotoxicity with azotemia may occur. Rarely, a variety of other severe adverse reactions may occur, including anemia, thrombocytopenia, ventricular arrhythmias, and fatal pancreatitis. Blood glucose levels should be monitored. Inadvertent rapid intravenous infusion may cause precipitous hypotension.

C. Atovaquone

Atovaquone has been FDA-approved for patients with mild to moderate disease who cannot tolerate TMP-SMZ or pentamidine, but failure is reported in 15–30% of cases. Mild side effects are common, but no serious reactions have been reported. The dosage is 750 mg three times daily for 21 days. Because poor gastrointestinal absorption can lead to low serum concentrations and treatment failure, the drug should be taken with food, especially a fatty meal.

D. Other Drugs

Clindamycin, 600 mg three times daily, plus primaquine, 15 mg/d; and dapsone, 100 mg/d, plus trimethoprim 15 mg/kg/d, in three divided doses daily, are alternative oral regimens for mild to moderate disease or for continuation of therapy after intravenous therapy is no longer needed. Trimetrexate, 45 mg/m²/d intravenously, plus high-dose leucovorin has been approved for salvage use in patients not responding to other therapies, but the success rate is less than 25%.

E. Prednisone

In conjunction with antimicrobials, prednisone is given when PaO$_2$ on admission is < 70 mm Hg; its use during the first 72 hours of therapy for severe pneumocystis pneumonia prevents deterioration in oxygenation and improves survival. For dosages and durations of therapy, see the section on corticosteroids in Chapter 31 and the footnote in Table 31–4.

F. Supportive Care

Oxygen therapy is indicated to maintain the oxygen saturation over 90% by pulse oximeter.

Prevention

See Chapter 31 and Table 31–6.

Prognosis

In the absence of early and adequate treatment, the fatality rate for the endemic infantile form of pneumocystis pneumonia is 20–50%; for the sporadic form in immunodeficient persons, the fatality rate is nearly 100%. Early treatment reduces the mortality rate to about 3% in the former and 10–20% in AIDS patients. The mortality rate in other immunodeficient patients is still 30–50%, probably because of failure to make a timely diagnosis. In immunodeficient patients who do not receive prophylaxis, recurrences are common (30% in AIDS).

CRYPTOCOCCOSIS

 ESSENTIALS OF DIAGNOSIS

- Most common cause of fungal meningitis.
- Predisposing factors: Hodgkin's disease, corticosteroid therapy, HIV infection.
- Symptoms of headache, abnormal mental states; meningismus seen occasionally, though rarely in HIV-infected patients.
- Demonstration of capsular polysaccharide antigen in cerebrospinal fluid diagnostic; 95% of HIV-infected patients also have a positive serum antigen.

General Considerations

Cryptococcosis is caused by *Cryptococcus neoformans,* an encapsulated budding yeast that has been found worldwide in soil and on dried pigeon dung.

Infections are acquired by inhalation. In the lung, the infection may remain localized, heal, or disseminate. Immunocompetent hosts rarely develop clinically apparent cryptococcal pneumonia. Progressive lung disease and dissemination most often occur in the setting of cellular immunodeficiency, including underlying hematologic cancer under treatment, Hodgkin's disease, long-term corticosteroid therapy, or HIV infection.

Clinical Findings

A. Symptoms and Signs

Disseminated disease may involve any organ, but central nervous system disease predominates. Headache is usually the first symptom of meningitis. Confusion and other mental status changes as well as cranial nerve abnormalities, nausea, and vomiting may be seen as the disease progresses. Nuchal rigidity and meningeal signs occur about 50% of the time but are uncommon in HIV-infected patients with this complication. Intracerebral mass lesions (cryptococcomas) are rarely seen. Obstructive hydrocephalus may complicate the course.

B. LABORATORY FINDINGS

Spinal fluid findings include increased opening pressure, variable pleocytosis, budding encapsulated fungus cells, increased protein, and decreased glucose, though as many as 50% of AIDS patients have no pleocytosis. Cryptococcal antigen in cerebrospinal fluid and culture establish the diagnosis over 90% of the time. Patients with AIDS often have the antigen in both cerebrospinal fluid and serum, and extrameningeal disease (lungs, blood, urinary tract) is common.

Treatment

In AIDS-related cryptococcal meningitis, oral fluconazole, 400 mg/d for a minimum of 10 weeks, has reasonable efficacy as acute therapy in patients with mild disease. Candidates for initial fluconazole therapy are patients with an intact level of consciousness and a spinal fluid cryptococcal antigen titer of less than 1:128. Higher-risk patients should receive amphotericin B initially. A preliminary study in patients with AIDS suggests that fluconazole plus flucytosine is efficacious for mild cases, but this regimen has not been compared with fluconazole alone.

There has been a trend away from regimens based on prolonged amphotericin B therapy, particularly in HIV-infected patients. However, this agent remains important, especially in severe disease. Amphotericin B, 0.7–1 mg/kg/d intravenously for 14 days, followed by an additional 8 weeks of fluconazole, 400 mg/d orally, have been quite effective, achieving clinical responses and cerebrospinal fluid sterilization in about 70% of patients. Adding flucytosine at this early stage does prevent late relapses but does not substantially contribute to improved cure rates. Flucytosine is administered orally at a dose of 100 mg/kg/d divided into four equal doses and given every 6 hours. Repeated lumbar punctures or ventricular shunting should be performed to relieve high cerebrospinal fluid pressures or if hydrocephalus is a complication. The end points for amphotericin B therapy and for switching to oral fluconazole are a favorable clinical response (decrease in temperature; improvement in headache, nausea, vomiting, and mini-mental status scores) and conversion of cerebrospinal fluid culture to negative.

A similar approach is reasonable for patients with cryptococcal meningitis in the absence of AIDS, though the mortality rate is considerably higher. Because of serious underlying illnesses and generally greater age, this group of patients does not tolerate the higher doses of amphotericin B as well as patients with AIDS. Lipid amphotericin B preparations appear to have equivalent efficacy with reduced nephrotoxicity. Therapy is generally continued until cerebrospinal fluid cultures become negative and cerebrospinal fluid antigen titers are below 1:8.

Maintenance antifungal therapy is important after treatment of an acute episode in HIV-related cases, since otherwise the rate of relapse is greater than 50%. Fluconazole, 200 mg/d, is the maintenance therapy of choice, decreasing the relapse rate approximately tenfold compared with placebo and threefold compared with weekly amphotericin B in patients whose cerebrospinal fluid has been sterilized by the induction therapy. There has been a trend among practitioners in recent years treating patients without AIDS to prescribe a brief course (eg, 3 months) of fluconazole as maintenance therapy following successful therapy for acute illness; recently published guidelines suggest this as an option.

Prognosis

Factors that indicate a poor prognosis include the activity of the predisposing conditions, older age, organ failure, lack of spinal fluid pleocytosis, high initial antigen titer in either serum or cerebrospinal fluid, decreased mental status, and the presence of disease outside the nervous system.

Pappas PG et al: Cryptococcosis in human immunodeficiency virus-negative patients in the era of effective azole therapy. Clin Infect Dis 2001;33:690. [PMID: 11477526] (Fluconazole alone is usually administered to patients with pulmonary disease, while amphotericin B is initially used for central nervous system disease, followed by fluconazole for consolidation. Therapy was successful in 74% of patients.)

Saag MS et al: Practice guidelines for the management of cryptococcal disease. Clin Infect Dis 2000;30:710. [PMID: 10770733] (The choice of treatment for disease due to C neoformans depends on the host's immune status and the anatomic site of infection. Generally, amphotericin B is the drug of choice for CNS infections. Fluconazole is effective for disease at other sites and for maintenance therapy of successfully treated CNS disease.)

ASPERGILLOSIS

Aspergillus fumigatus is the usual cause of aspergillosis, though many species of aspergillus may cause a wide spectrum of disease. Burn eschar and detritus in the external ear canal are often colonized by these fungi. Clinical illness results either from an aberrant immunologic response or tissue invasion.

Allergic bronchopulmonary aspergillosis occurs in patients with preexisting asthma who develop worsening bronchospasm and fleeting pulmonary infiltrates accompanied by eosinophilia, high levels of IgE, and aspergillus precipitins in the blood. It also may complicate cystic fibrosis. The disease characteristically pursues a waxing and waning course with gradual improvement over time, but it may result in saccular bronchiectasis and end-stage fibrotic lung disease. For acute exacerbations, oral prednisone is begun at a dose of 1 mg/kg/d and then tapered slowly over several months. Itraconazole at a dose of 200 mg daily for 16 weeks appears to improve pulmonary function and decrease steroid requirements in these patients.

Invasive manifestations may be seen in immunocompetent adults. These include chronic sinusitis and colonization of preexisting pulmonary cavities (**aspergilloma**). Sinus disease may require long courses of antifungals (itraconazole, 200 mg twice daily, for weeks to months) as well as surgical debridement. Aspergillomas of the lung may be found by incidental radiographic studies but may also present with significant hemoptysis. Intracavitary instillation of amphotericin B and bronchoscopic removal have been tried with little success; several uncontrolled trials have suggested some benefit from itraconazole. The most effective therapy for symptomatic aspergilloma remains surgical resection.

Life-threatening **invasive aspergillosis** most commonly occurs in profoundly immunodeficient patients, particularly those with prolonged severe neutropenia. Patients with very advanced HIV disease may also be at risk for invasive aspergillosis, particularly if they have other risk factors for the disease. Pulmonary disease is most common, with patchy infiltration leading to a severe necrotizing pneumonia. There is often tissue infarction as the organism grows into blood vessels; clues to this are the development of pleuritic chest pain and elevation of serum LDH. AIDS patients are also predisposed to a unique ulcerative tracheobronchitis that may coexist with parenchymal pulmonary disease. At any time, there may be hematogenous dissemination to the central nervous system, skin, and other organs. Early diagnosis and reversal of any correctable immunosuppression are essential. Blood cultures have very low yield. In contrast to allergic aspergillosis, serologic tests have low sensitivities for invasive disease; detection of galactomannan by ELISA has recently been demonstrated to have a sensitivity of 89% and a specificity of 98% for the diagnosis of invasive disease, though multiple determinations may need to be done. Isolation of aspergillus from pulmonary secretions does not necessarily imply invasive disease. Therefore, the mainstay of diagnosis is demonstration of aspergillus in tissue. Biopsy specimens may show branched septate hyphae. Biopsy specimens will not invariably grow the organism.

When severe invasive aspergillosis is considered clinically likely or is demonstrable by laboratory testing, rapid institution of high doses of amphotericin B may be life-saving (see Chapter 37). The total daily dose is rapidly increased to 0.8–1.5 mg/kg/d intravenously as tolerated for the first several weeks of therapy. Thereafter, more traditional doses of 0.6 mg/kg/d are continued until resolution of clinical signs of disease. Itraconazole orally or intravenously at a dosage of 200–400 mg/d has activity against aspergillus, and initial clinical experience is favorable for less severe disease or as a follow-up to amphotericin B therapy. Until more data accumulate, amphotericin B should remain the first-line drug for invasive disease. Some experts believe that lipid preparations of amphotericin B should be used preferentially in this setting because they are better tolerated and can be given at higher doses. Recently, caspofungin acetate, an echinocandin antifungal, has been approved for the treatment of invasive aspergillosis in patients who are refractory to or intolerant of other treatments. The drug is given as a 70 mg intravenous loading dose followed by 50 mg intravenously daily. In critically ill patients who are not responding to conventional antifungal treatment, there may be a role for the addition of caspofungin to amphotericin B therapy. Based on promising results in neutropenic patients with invasive pulmonary aspergillosis, surgical resection warrants further study. The mortality rate of pulmonary or disseminated disease in the immunocompromised patient remains well above 50%, however.

Azoles for allergic bronchopulmonary aspergillosis associated with asthma. Cochrane Database Syst Rev 2001;4:CD001108. [PMID: 11687098] (Itraconazole modifies the immunologic activation associated with allergic bronchopulmonary aspergillosis and improves clinical outcome, at least over a treatment period lasting 16 weeks.)

Maertens J et al. Screening for circulating galactomannan as a noninvasive diagnostic tool for invasive aspergillosis in prolonged neutropenic patients and stem cell transplantation recipients: a prospective validation. Blood 2001;97:1604. [PMID: 11238098])

Stevens DA et al: Practice guidelines for diseases caused by aspergillus. Clin Infect Dis 2000;30:696. [PMID: 10770732] (Amphotericin B or one of the lipid preparations of amphotericin B is the drug of choice for invasive disease; adjunctive therapy—particularly surgery or combination chemotherapy—may be useful in certain situations. Itraconazole has a role in the treatment of other less invasive forms of aspergillosis.)

Walsh TJ et al: Voriconazole compared with liposomal amphotericin B for empirical antifungal therapy in patients with neutropenia and persistent fever. N Engl J Med 2002;346:225. [PMID: 11807146] (There were fewer breakthrough fungal infections, less nephrotoxicity, and fewer infusion-related reactions in patients treated with voriconazole. Transient visual abnormalities occurred in 22% of voriconazole recipients.)

MUCORMYCOSIS

The term mucormycosis (zygomycosis, phycomycosis) is applied to opportunistic infections caused by members of the genera rhizopus, mucor, absidia, and cunninghamella. Predisposing conditions include diabetic ketoacidosis, chronic renal failure, and treatment with steroids or cytotoxic drugs. These organisms appear in tissues as broad, branching nonseptate hyphae. Biopsy with histologic examination is almost always required for diagnosis; cultures are frequently negative. Invasive disease of the sinuses, orbits, and the lungs may occur. Widely disseminated disease has been more commonly seen recently in patients who have received aggressive chemotherapy. The diagnosis should be considered in acidotic diabetic patients with black necrotic lesions of the nose or sinuses or with new cranial nerve abnormalities. Without treatment, cerebral invasion may ensue. A prolonged course of high-dosage amphotericin B (1–1.5 mg/kg/d intravenously) should be started early. Control of diabetes and other underlying conditions, along with extensive repeated surgical removal of necrotic, nonperfused tissue, are essential. Even when these measures are introduced in a timely fashion, the prognosis is poor, with a 30–50% mortality rate for localized disease and higher rates in disseminated cases.

Ribes JA et al: Zygomycetes in human disease. Clin Microbiol Rev 2000;13:236. [PMID: 10756000] (Extensive review of the microbiology, diagnosis, and therapy of infections due to the various zygomycetes.)

BLASTOMYCOSIS

Blastomycosis occurs most often in men infected during occupational or recreational activities out of doors and in a geographically limited area of the south central and midwestern USA and Canada. A few cases have been found in Mexico and Africa.

Pulmonary infection is most common and may be asymptomatic. When dissemination takes place, lesions are most frequently seen on the skin, in bones, and in the urogenital system.

Cough, moderate fever, dyspnea, and chest pain are common. These may resolve or progress, with bloody and purulent sputum production, pleurisy, fever, chills, loss of weight, and prostration. Radiologic studies usually reveal pulmonary infiltrates and enlarged regional lymph nodes, though less commonly than in histoplasmosis or coccidioidomycosis.

Raised, verrucous cutaneous lesions that have an abrupt downward sloping border are usually present in disseminated blastomycosis. The border extends slowly, leaving a central atrophic scar. If left untreated for long periods, they may mimic skin cancer. Bones—often the ribs and vertebrae—are frequently involved. Lesions appear to be both destructive and proliferative on radiography. Epididymitis, prostatitis, and other involvement of the male urogenital system may occur. Central nervous system involvement is uncommon. Cases in HIV-infected persons may progress rapidly, with dissemination common.

Laboratory findings usually include leukocytosis and anemia, though these are not specific. The organism is found in clinical specimens as a thick-walled cell 5–20 μm in diameter that may have a single broad-based bud. It grows readily on culture. Serologic tests are not well standardized.

Itraconazole, 100–200 mg/d orally for at least 2–3 months, is now the therapy of choice for non-meningeal disease, with a response rate of over 80%. Amphotericin B, 0.3–0.6 mg/kg/d intravenously for a total dose of 1.5–2.5 g, is given for treatment failures or cases with central nervous system involvement.

Follow-up for relapse should be regularly made for several years so that therapy may be resumed or another drug instituted.

Chapman SW et al: Practice guidelines for the management of patients with blastomycosis. Clin Infect Dis 2000;30:679. [PMID: 10770729] (Amphotericin B is the drug of choice for life-threatening manifestations of blastomycosis. Itraconazole is the initial treatment of choice for non-life-threatening non-central nervous system blastomycosis.)

Patel RG et al: Clinical presentation, radiographic findings, and diagnostic methods of pulmonary blastomycosis: a review of 100 consecutive cases. South Med J 1999;92:289. [PMID: 10094269] (Patients with pulmonary blastomycosis had symptomatic disease. Air space or interstitial infiltrates or mass-like lesions were demonstrated radiographically. Response to therapy was generally good.)

PARACOCCIDIOIDOMYCOSIS
(South American Blastomycosis)

Paracoccidioides brasiliensis infections have been found only in patients who have resided in South or Central America or Mexico. Long asymptomatic periods enable patients to travel far from the endemic areas before developing clinical problems. Ulceration of the naso- and oropharynx is usually the first symptom. Papules ulcerate and enlarge both peripherally and deeper into the subcutaneous tissue. Differential diagnosis includes mucocutaneous leishmaniasis and syphilis. Extensive coalescent ulcerations may eventually result in destruction of the epiglottis, vocal cords, and uvula. Extension to the lips and face may occur. Eating and drinking are extremely painful. Skin lesions may occur, usually on the face. Variable in appearance, they may have a necrotic central crater with a hard hyperkeratotic border. Lymph node enlargement may follow mucocutaneous lesions, eventually ulcerating and forming draining sinuses; in some patients, it is the presenting symptom. Hepatosplenomegaly may be present as well. Cough, sometimes with sputum, indicates pulmonary involvement, but the symptoms and signs are often mild, even though radiographic findings indicate severe parenchymatous changes in the lungs. The extensive ulceration of the upper gastrointestinal tract may prevent caloric intake and result in cachexia.

Laboratory findings are nonspecific. Serology by immunodiffusion is positive in 98% of cases. Complement fixation titers correlate with progressive disease and fall with effective therapy. The fungus is found in clinical specimens as a spherical cell that may have many buds arising from it. If direct examination does not reveal the organism, biopsy with Gomori staining may be helpful.

Itraconazole, 100–200 mg orally daily, is the treatment of choice and generally results in a clinical response within 1 month and effective control after 2–6 months.

Bethlem EP et al: Paracoccidioidomycosis. Curr Opin Pulm Med 1999;5:319. [PMID: 10461538] (Primary pulmonary infection occurs commonly in the first and second decades of life and usually has a benign, self-limited course. Adult chronic manifestations are usually the result of reactivation of quiescent lesions with diffuse lung infiltrates, with or without systemic disease.)

SPOROTRICHOSIS

Sporotrichosis is a chronic fungal infection caused by *Sporothrix schenckii*. It is worldwide in distribution; most patients have had contact with soil, sphagnum moss, or decaying wood. Infection takes place when the organism is inoculated into the skin—usually on the hand, arm, or foot, especially during gardening.

The most common form of sporotrichosis begins with a hard, nontender subcutaneous nodule. This later becomes adherent to the overlying skin and ulcerates. Within a few days to weeks, similar nodules develop along the lymphatics draining this area, and these may ulcerate as well. The lymphatic vessels become indurated and are easily palpable.

Disseminated sporotrichosis is rare in the immunocompetent host but may present with widespread cutaneous, lung, bone, joint, and central nervous system involvement in immunocompromised patients, especially those with AIDS and alcohol abuse.

Cultures are needed to establish diagnosis. Antibody tests may be useful for diagnosis of disseminated disease, especially meningitis.

Itraconazole, 200–400 mg orally daily for several months, is now the treatment of choice for localized disease and some milder cases of disseminated disease. Because it is inconvenient to take and has unpleasant side effects, saturated solution of potassium iodide (5 drops three times daily, increasing to 40–50 drops three times daily) is considered an alternative to itraconazole for localized lymphocutaneous disease. Amphotericin B intravenously, 1–2 g (see Chapter 37), is used for severe systemic infection. Surgery is usually contraindicated except for simple aspiration of secondary nodules. Joint involvement may require arthrodesis.

The prognosis is good for lymphocutaneous sporotrichosis; pulmonary, joint, and disseminated disease respond less favorably.

Kauffman CA et al: Practice guidelines for the management of patients with sporotrichosis. Clin Infect Dis 2000;30:684. [PMID: 10770730] (Itraconazole is the drug of choice for most forms of sporotrichosis. Meningeal and disseminated forms of sporotrichosis are rare and should be treated with amphotericin B.)

PENICILLIUM MARNEFFEI INFECTIONS

Penicillium marneffei is a dimorphic fungus, endemic in southeast Asia, that causes systemic infection in both healthy and compromised hosts. There have been increasing reports of patients with advanced AIDS presenting with disseminated infections, including travelers returning from southeast Asia. Clinical manifestations include fever, generalized umbilicated papular rash, lymphadenopathy, cough, and diarrhea. Diagnosis is made by identification of the organism on smears or histopathologic specimens or by culture, where the fungus produces a characteristic red pigment. The best sites for isolation of the fungus include the skin, blood, bone marrow, respiratory tract, and lymph nodes. Patients with mild to moderate infection can be treated with itraconazole, 400 mg daily for 8 weeks. Amphotericin B, 0.5–0.7 mg/kg/d, is the drug of choice for severe disease. Because the relapse rate after successful treatment is 30%, maintenance therapy with itraconazole, 200–400 mg daily, is indicated.

Chariyalertsak S et al: A controlled trial of itraconazole as primary prophylaxis for systemic fungal infections in patients with advanced human immunodeficiency virus infection in Thailand. Clin Infect Dis 2002;34:277. [PMID: 11740718] (Primary prophylaxis with itraconazole prevented disease due to *Penicillium marneffei* in patients with AIDS but did not provide a survival benefit.)

Supparatpinyo K et al: A controlled trial of itraconazole to prevent relapse of *Penicillium marneffei* infection in patients infected with the human immunodeficiency virus. N Engl J Med 1998;339:1739. [PMID: 9845708] (Secondary prophylaxis with oral itraconazole is well tolerated and prevents relapses of *P marneffei*.)

CHROMOBLASTOMYCOSIS (Chromomycosis)

Chromoblastomycosis is a chronic, principally tropical cutaneous infection usually affecting young men who are agricultural workers and caused by several species of closely related black molds (fonsecaea species and phialophora species).

Lesions are slowly progressive and occur most frequently on a lower extremity. The lesion begins as a papule or ulcer. Over months to years, papules enlarge to become vegetating, papillomatous, verrucous elevated nodules. Satellite lesions may appear along the lymphatics. There may be secondary bacterial infection. Elephantiasis may result.

The fungus is seen as brown, thick-walled, spherical, sometimes septate cells in potassium hydroxide preparations of pus or skin scrapings, which are quite sensitive for diagnosis. The type of reproduction found in culture determines the species. *Fonsecaea pedrosoi* is the responsible pathogen in the vast majority of cases.

Itraconazole, 200–400 mg/d orally for 6–18 months, achieves a response rate of 65%. Response rates may be improved by the addition of flucytosine to itraconazole. Cryosurgery alone for smaller lesions or combined with itraconazole for larger lesions is beneficial.

Bonifaz A et al: Chromoblastomycosis: clinical and mycological experience of 51 cases. Mycoses 2001;44:1. [PMID:

11398635] (The best results of therapy included cryosurgery for small lesions, with itraconazole for large ones, and sometimes combined therapy.)

MYCETOMA
(Maduromycosis & Actinomycetoma)

Mycetoma is a chronic local, slowly progressive destructive infection that begins in subcutaneous tissues, frequently after localized trauma, and then spreads to contiguous structures. Maduromycosis is the term used to describe mycetoma caused by the true fungi. Actinomycotic mycetoma is caused by nocardia and actinomadura species. The disease begins as a papule, nodule, or abscess that over months to years progresses slowly to form multiple abscesses and sinus tracts ramifying deep into the tissue. Secondary bacterial infection may result in large open ulcers. Radiographs may show destructive changes in the underlying bone. Tissue Gram stain reveals fine branching hyphae with actinomycotic mycetoma. Larger hyphae are seen with fungal mycetoma; the causative species can often be identified by the color of the characteristic grains within the infected tissues.

The prognosis is good for patients with actinomycetoma, since they usually respond well to sulfonamides and sulfones, especially if treated early. Trimethoprim-sulfamethoxazole, 160/800 mg orally twice a day, or dapsone, 100 mg twice daily after meals, has been reported to be effective. Streptomycin, 14 mg/kg/d intramuscularly, may be useful during the first month of therapy. All oral medications must be taken for months and continued for several months after clinical cure to prevent relapse. Debridement assists healing.

The prognosis for maduromycosis is poor, though surgical debridement along with prolonged ketoconazole or itraconazole therapy may result in a response rate of 70%. Amputation is necessary in far-advanced cases.

McGinnis MR: Mycetoma. Dermatol Clin 1996;14:97. [PMID: 8821162] (Review of the biology, clinical aspects, and treatment of mycetoma due to the true fungi.)

OTHER OPPORTUNISTIC MOLD INFECTIONS

Fungi previously considered to be harmless colonizers, including *Pseudallescheria boydii (Scedosporium apiospermum)*, fusarium, paecilomyces, and trichosporon, are emerging as significant pathogens in immunocompromised patients. This occurs most often in patients being treated for hematopoietic malignancies. Infection may be localized in the skin, lungs, or sinuses, or widespread disease may appear with lesions in multiple organs. Colonization of old cavitary disease may cause minimal symptoms or may precede dissemination with meningitis or brain abscesses. Endocarditis occurs more commonly in intravenous drug abusers. Sinus infection may cause bony erosion. Infection in subcutaneous tissues following traumatic implantation may develop as a well-circumscribed cyst or as an ulcer.

Nonpigmented septate hyphae are seen in tissue and are indistinguishable from those of aspergillus when infections are due to *Pseudallescheria boydii* or species of fusarium, paecilomyces, penicillium, or other hyaline molds. Spores or mycetoma-like granules are rarely present in tissue.

Infection by any of a number of black molds is designated as **phaeohyphomycosis.** These black molds (eg, exophiala, bipolaris, cladophialophora, curvularia, alternaria) are common in the environment, especially on decaying vegetation. Human disease due to these agents is rarely encountered but may result in soft tissue abscesses due to traumatic inoculation or may occur as a sequela of chronic sinusitis or profound immunosuppression. In tissues of patients with phaeohyphomycosis, the mold is seen as black or faintly brown hyphae, yeast cells, or both. Culture on appropriate medium is needed to identify the agent. Histologic demonstration of these organisms is definitive evidence of invasive infection; positive cultures must be interpreted cautiously and not assumed to be contaminants in immunocompromised hosts. Some isolates are sensitive to antifungal antibiotics. The differentiation of *Pseudallescheria boydii* and aspergillus is particularly important, since the former is uniformly resistant to amphotericin B but may be sensitive to imidazole antibiotics.

Perfect JR et al: The new fungal opportunists are coming. Clin Infect Dis 1996;22(Suppl 2):S112. [PMID: 8722837] (Review of recently recognized fungal opportunists and suggestions for therapy.)

Revankar SG et al: Disseminated phaeohyphomycosis: review of an emerging mycosis. Clin Infect Dis 2002;34:467. [PMID: 1179717] (The primary risk factor for infection is decreased host immunity. Outcome of antifungal therapy is poor, with an overall mortality rate of 79%.)

ANTIFUNGAL THERAPY

Table 36–1 summarizes the major properties of currently available antifungal agents. A number of lipid-based amphotericin B formulations have recently become available. These agents have shown promise in the treatment of systemic candidiasis, invasive aspergillosis, disseminated histoplasmosis, and cryptococcal meningitis. Their principal advantage appears to be substantially reduced nephrotoxicity, allowing administration of much higher doses. Because of their expense, use of these agents should be reserved for individuals who develop significant nephrotoxicity during amphotericin B therapy. Caspofungin acetate, the first of several agents in the echinocandin class, has recently been approved for use in invasive aspergillosis. These drugs are fungicidal for candida and are active

Table 36–1. Agents for systemic mycoses.

Drug	Dosing	Renal Clearance?	CSF Penetration?	Toxicities	Spectrum of Activity
Amphotericin B	0.3–1.5 mg/kg/d IV	No	Poor	Rigors, fever, azotemia, hypokalemia, hypomagnesemia, renal tubular acidosis, anemia	All major pathogens except pseudallescheria
Amphotericin B lipid complex	5 mg/kg/d IV	No	Poor	Fever, rigors, nausea, hypotension, anemia, azotemia, tachypnea	Same as amphotericin B, above
Amphotericin B colloidal suspension	3–6 mg/kg/d IV	No	Poor	Fever, rigors, nausea, hypotension, azotemia, hypomagnesemia, anemia, tachypnea, thrombophlebitis	Same as amphotericin B, above
Liposomal amphotericin B	3–6 mg/kg/d IV	No	Poor	Fever, rigors, nausea, hypotension, azotemia, anemia, tachypnea, chest tightness	Same as amphotericin B, above
Flucytosine (5-FC)	100–150 mg/kg/d orally in four divided doses	Yes	Yes	Leukopenia,[1] rash, diarrhea, hepatitis, nausea, vomiting	Cryptococcosis,[2] candidiasis,[2] chromomycosis
Ketoconazole	200–800 mg/d orally in one or two doses	No	Poor	Anorexia, nausea, suppression of testosterone and cortisol, rash, headache, hepatic enzyme elevations, hepatic failure[3]	Nonmeningeal histoplasmosis and coccidioidomycosis, blastomycosis, paracoccidioidomycosis, mucosal candidiasis (except urinary)
Fluconazole	100–400 mg/d in one or two doses IV orally	Yes	Yes	Nausea, rash, alopecia, headache, hepatic enzyme elevations[4]	Mucosal candidiasis (including urinary tract), cryptococcosis, histoplasmosis, coccidioidomycosis
Itraconazole	100–400 mg/d orally as single dose or 200–400 mg/d IV in one or two doses	No	Variable	Nausea, hypokalemia, edema, hypertension[3]	Same as ketoconazole plus sporotrichosis, aspergillosis, chromomycosis
Voriconazole	200–400 mg/d orally in two doses or 12 mg/kg IV as loading dose for 2 days followed by 6 mg/kg/d IV in two doses	Yes	Yes	Transient visual disturbances, rash, hepatic enzyme elevations[5]	All major pathogens except zygomycetes and sporotrichosis
Caspofungin acetate	70 mg IV loading dose, followed by 50 mg/d IV in one dose	<50%[6]	Poor	Transient neutropenia; hepatic enzyme elevations when used with cyclosporine	Aspergillosis, candidiasis
Terbinafine	250 mg/d orally in one dose	Yes	Poor	Nausea, abdominal pain, taste disturbance, rash, diarrhea and hepatic enzyme elevations	Dermatophytes, sporotrichosis

[1]Use should be monitored with blood levels to prevent this or the dose adjusted according to creatinine clearance.
[2]In combination with amphotericin B.
[3]Drug interaction with terfenadine, astemizole, or cisapride may produce prolongation of the QT interval, ventricular arrhythmias, and torsade de pointes.
[4]Drug interaction with cisapride may produce prolongation of the QT interval, ventricular arrhythmias, and torsade de pointes.
[5]Administration with drugs that are metabolized by the cytochrome P450 system is contraindicated or requires careful monitoring.
[6]No dosage adjustment required for renal insufficiency; dosage adjustment necessary with moderate to severe hepatic dysfunction.

also against aspergillus. They have relatively few adverse effects. Their exact role in the treatment of invasive fungal diseases needs to be further defined. A new azole, voriconazole, is now available and has excellent activity against aspergillus species. Cytokine therapy (such as with interferon-γ) and use of growth factors such as GM-CSF (sargramostim or molgramostim) have been shown in animal models to increase clearance of fungi and result in better clinical outcomes.

Hoang A: Caspofungin acetate: an antifungal agent. Am J Health Syst Pharm 2001;58:1206. [PMID: 11449878] (Review of the first agent in the echinocandin class to be available for clinical use.)

Robinson RF et al: A comparative review of conventional and lipid formulations of amphotericin. J Clin Pharm Ther 1999;24:249. [PMID: 10475983] (Provides guidelines to aid in the cost-effective use of the lipid preparations of amphotericin B.)

Anti-infective Chemotherapeutic & Antibiotic Agents

37

Richard A. Jacobs, MD, PhD, & B. Joseph Guglielmo, PharmD
See www.current-med.com/ch37.html

Some Principles of Antimicrobial Therapy

The following steps are required in each patient considered for antibiotic therapy. Drugs of first choice and alternative drugs are presented in Table 37–1.

A. ETIOLOGIC DIAGNOSIS

Based on the organ system involved, the organism causing infection can usually be predicted. See Tables 37–2 and 37–3.

B. "BEST GUESS"

One selects an empirical regimen that is likely to be effective against the suspected pathogens.

C. LABORATORY CONTROL

Specimens for laboratory examination are commonly obtained before institution of therapy to determine susceptibility.

D. CLINICAL RESPONSE

Based on clinical response , one evaluates the laboratory reports and consider the desirability of changing the regimen. If the specimen was obtained from a normally sterile site (eg, blood, cerebrospinal fluid, pleural fluid, joint fluid), the recovery of a microorganism in significant amounts is meaningful even if the organism recovered is different from the clinically suspected agent, and this may force a change in treatment. Isolation of unexpected microorganisms from the respiratory tract, gastrointestinal tract, or surface lesions (sites that have a complex flora) may represent colonization or contamination, and cultures must be critically evaluated before drugs are abandoned that were judiciously selected on a "best guess" basis.

E. DRUG SUSCEPTIBILITY TESTS

Some microorganisms are predictably responsive to certain drugs; if such organisms are isolated, they need not be tested for drug susceptibility. For example, most group A hemolytic streptococci and clostridia respond well to penicillin. Other organisms (eg, enteric gram-negative rods) are variably susceptible and require sensitivity testing whenever they are isolated. Organisms that once had predictable susceptibility patterns have now become resistant and require testing. Examples include the pneumococci, which may be resistant to multiple agents, including penicillin, macrolides, and trimethoprim-sulfamethoxazole and the enterococci, which may be resistant to penicillin, aminoglycosides, and vancomycin.

Antimicrobial drug susceptibility tests may be performed on solid media as "disk tests," in broth in tubes, in wells of microdilution plates, or as E-tests. The latter three methods yield results expressed as MIC (minimal inhibitory concentration), and the technique can be modified to give MBC (minimal bactericidal concentration) results. In most infections, the MIC is the appropriate in vitro test to guide selection of an antibacterial agent. When there appear to be marked discrepancies between susceptibility testing and clinical response, the following possibilities must be considered:

1. Selection of an inappropriate drug, drug dosage, or route of administration.

2. Failure to drain a collection of pus or to remove a foreign body.

3. Failure of a poorly diffusing drug to reach the site of infection (eg, central nervous system) or to reach intracellular phagocytosed bacteria.

4. Superinfection in the course of prolonged chemotherapy.

5. Emergence of drug-resistant or tolerant organisms.

6. Participation of two or more microorganisms in the infectious process, of which only one was originally detected and used for drug selection.

7. Inadequate host defenses, including immunodeficiencies and diabetes.

8. Noninfectious causes, including drug fever, malignancy, and autoimmune disease.

F. PROMPTNESS OF RESPONSE

Response depends on a number of factors, including the host (immunocompromised patients respond slower than immunocompetent patients), the site of infection (deep-seated infections such as osteomyelitis and endocarditis respond more slowly than superficial infections such as cystitis or cellulitis), the pathogen

Table 37–1. Drugs of choice for suspected or proved microbial pathogens, 2001.[1]
(± = alone or combined with)

Suspected or Proved Etiologic Agent	Drug(s) of First Choice	Alternative Drug(s)
Gram-negative cocci		
Moraxella catarrhalis	TMP-SMZ,[2] a fluoroquinolone[3]	Cefuroxime, cefotaxime, ceftizoxime, ceftriaxone, cefepime, cefuroxime axetil, an erythromycin,[4] a tetracycline,[5] azithromycin, amoxicillin-clavulanic acid, clarithromycin
Neisseria gonorrhoeae (gonococcus)	Cefixime, ciprofloxacin, or ofloxacin	Ceftriaxone, spectinomycin, cefpodoxime proxetil
Neisseria meningitidis (meningococcus)	Penicillin[6]	Cefotaxime, ceftizoxime, ceftriaxone, ampicillin, chloramphenicol
Gram-positive cocci		
Streptococcus pneumoniae[8] (pneumococcus)	Penicillin[6]	An erythromycin,[4] a cephalosporin,[7] vancomycin, TMP-SMZ,[2] chloramphenicol, clindamycin, azithromycin, clarithromycin, a tetracycline,[5] imipenem, meropenem, quinupristin-dalfopristin, certain fluoroquinolones,[3] linezolid
Streptococcus, hemolytic, groups A, B, C, G	Penicillin[6]	An erythromycin,[4] a cephalosporin,[7] vancomycin, clindamycin, azithromycin, clarithromycin
Viridans streptococci	Penicillin[6] ± gentamicin	Cephalosporin,[7] vancomycin
Staphylococcus, methicillin-resistant	Vancomycin ± gentamicin ± rifampin	TMP-SMZ,[2] minocycline, a fluoroquinolone[3] linezolid, quinupristin-dalfopristin
Staphylococcus, non-penicillinase-producing	Penicillin[6]	A cephalosporin,[8] vancomycin, imipenem, meropenem, a fluoroquinolone,[3] clindamycin
Staphylococcus, penicillinase-producing	Penicillinase-resistant penicillin[9]	Vancomycin, a cephalosporin,[7] clindamycin, amoxicillin-clavulanic acid, ticarcillin-clavulanic acid, ampicillin-sulbactam, piperacillin-tazobactam, imipenem, meropenem, a fluoroquinolone,[3] TMP-SMZ[2]
Enterococcus faecalis	Ampicillin + gentamicin[10]	Vancomycin + gentamicin
Enterococcus faecium	Vancomycin + gentamicin[10]	Quinupristin-dalfopristin, linezolid
Gram-negative rods		
Acinetobacter	Imipenem or meropenem	Minocycline, TMP-SMZ,[2] doxycycline, aminoglycosides,[11] piperacillin, ceftazidime, a fluoroquinolone[3]
Prevotella, oropharyngeal strains	Clindamycin	Penicillin,[6] metronidazole, cefoxitin, cefotetan
Bacteroides, gastrointestinal strains	Metronidazole	Cefoxitin, chloramphenicol, clindamycin, cefotetan, cefmetazole, imipenem, meropenem, ticarcillin-clavulanic acid, ampicillin-sulbactam, piperacillin-tazobactam
Brucella	Tetracycline + rifampin[5]	TMP-SMZ[2] ± gentamicin; chloramphenicol ± gentamicin; doxycycline + gentamicin
Campylobacter jejuni	Erythromycin[4] or azithromycin	Tetracycline,[5] a fluoroquinolone,[3] gentamicin
Enterobacter	TMP-SMZ,[2] imipenem, meropenem	Aminoglycoside, a fluoroquinolone,[3] cefepime
Escherichia coli (sepsis)	Cefotaxime, ceftizoxime, ceftriaxone, ceftazidime, cefepime	Imipenem or meropenem, aminoglycosides,[11] a fluoroquinolone[3]

(continued)

Table 37–1. Drugs of choice for suspected or proved microbial pathogens, 2001.[1] (± = alone or combined with) (continued)

Suspected or Proved Etiologic Agent	Drug(s) of First Choice	Alternative Drug(s)
Gram-negative rods (continued)		
Escherichia coli (uncomplicated urinary infection)	Fluoroquinolones[3], nitrofurantoin	TMP-SMZ,[2] oral cephalosporin, fosfomycin
Haemophilus (meningitis and other serious infections)	Cefotaxime, ceftizoxime, ceftriaxone, ceftazidime	Chloramphenicol, meropenem
Haemophilus (respiratory infections, otitis)	TMP-SMZ[2]	Ampicillin, amoxicillin, doxycycline, azithromycin, clarithromycin, cefotaxime, ceftizoxime, ceftriaxone, cefepime, cefuroxime, cefuroxime axetil, ampicillin-clavulanate
Helicobacter pylori	Amoxicillin + clarithromycin + omeprazole; or tetracycline[5] + metronidazole + bismuth subsalicylate	Clarithromycin + bismuth subsalicylate (Pepto-Bismol) + tetracycline; amoxicillin + metronidazole + bismuth subsalicylate; amoxicillin + clarithromycin
Klebsiella	A cephalosporin	TMP-SMZ,[2] aminoglycoside,[11] imipenem or meropenem, a fluoroquinolone,[3] piperacillin, mezlocillin, aztreonam
Legionella species (pneumonia)	Erythromycin[4] or clarithromycin or azithromycin, or fluoroquinolones[3] ± rifampin	TMP-SMZ,[2] doxycycline ± rifampin
Proteus mirabilis	Ampicillin	An aminoglycoside,[11] TMP-SMZ,[2] a fluoroquinolone,[3] a cephalosporin[7]
Proteus vulgaris and other species (morganella, providencia)	Cefotaxime, ceftizoxime, ceftriaxone, ceftazidime, cefepime	Aminoglycoside,[11] imipenem, TMP-SMZ,[2] a fluoroquinolone[3]
Pseudomonas aeruginosa	Aminoglycoside[11] + antipseudomonal penicillin[12]	Ceftazidime ± aminoglycoside; imipenem or meropenem ± aminoglycoside; aztreonam ± aminoglycoside; ciprofloxacin ± piperacillin; ciprofloxacin ± ceftazidime; ciprofloxacin ± cefepime
Burkholderia pseudomallei (melioidosis)	Ceftazidime	Chloramphenicol, tetracycline,[5] TMP-SMZ,[2] amoxicillin-clavulanic acid, imipenem or meropenem
Burkholderia mallei (glanders)	Streptomycin + tetracycline[5]	Chloramphenicol + streptomycin
Salmonella (bacteremia)	Ceftriaxone, a fluoroquinolone[3]	TMP-SMZ,[2] ampicillin, chloramphenicol
Serratia	Cefotaxime, ceftizoxime, ceftriaxone, ceftazidime, cefepime	TMP-SMZ,[2] aminoglycosides,[11] imipenem or meropenem, a fluoroquinolone[3]
Shigella	A fluoroquinolone[3]	Ampicillin, TMP-SMZ,[2] ceftriaxone
Vibrio (cholera, sepsis)	Tetracycline[5]	TMP-SMZ,[2] a fluoroquinolone[3]
Yersinia pestis (plague, tularemia)	Streptomycin ± a tetracycline[5]	Chloramphenicol, TMP-SMZ[2]
Gram-positive rods		
Actinomyces	Penicillin[6]	Tetracycline,[5] clindamycin
Bacillus (including, anthrax)	Penicillin[6] (ciprofloxacin or doxycycline for anthrax; see Table 33–2)	Erythromycin,[4] tetracycline,[5] a fluoroquinolone[3]
Clostridium (eg, gas gangrene, tetanus)	Penicillin[6]	Metronidazole, chloramphenicol, clindamycin, imipenem or meropenem
Corynebacterium diphtheriae	Erythromycin[4]	Penicillin[6]
Corynebacterium jeikeium	Vancomycin	Ciprofloxacin, penicillin + gentamicin
Listeria	Ampicillin ± aminoglycoside[11]	TMP-SMZ[2]

(continued)

Table 37–1. Drugs of choice for suspected or proved microbial pathogens, 2001.[1]
(± = alone or combined with)

Suspected or Proved Etiologic Agent	Drug(s) of First Choice	Alternative Drug(s)
Acid-fast rods		
Mycobacterium tuberculosis[13]	INH + rifampin + pyrazinamide ± ethambutol or streptomycin	Other antituberculous drugs
Mycobacterium leprae	Dapsone + rifampin ± clofazimine	Minocycline, ofloxacin, clarithromycin
Mycobacterium kansasii	INH + rifampin ± ethambutol	Ethionamide, cycloserine
Mycobacterium avium complex	Clarithromycin or azithromycin + one or more of the following: ethambutol, rifampin or rifabutin, ciprofloxacin	Amikacin
Mycobacterium fortuitum-cheilonei	Amikacin + clarithromycin	Cefoxitin, sulfonamide, doxycycline, linezolid
Nocardia	TMP-SMZ[2]	Minocycline, imipenem or meropenem, sulfisoxazole, linezolid
Spirochetes		
Borrelia burgdorferi (Lyme disease)	Doxycycline, amoxicillin, cefuroxime axetil	Ceftriaxone, cefotaxime, penicillin, azithromycin, clarithromycin
Borrelia recurrentis (relapsing fever)	Doxycycline[5]	Penicillin[6]
Leptospira	Penicillin[6]	Doxycycline[5]
Treponema pallidum (syphilis)	Penicillin[6]	Doxycycline, ceftriaxone
Treponema pertenue (yaws)	Penicillin[6]	Doxycycline
Mycoplasmas	Erythromycin[4] or doxycycline	Clarithromycin, azithromycin, a fluoroquinolone[3]
Chlamydiae		
C psittaci	Doxycycline	Chloramphenicol
C trachomatis (urethritis or pelvic inflammatory disease)	Doxycycline or azithromycin	Ofloxacin
C pneumoniae	Doxycycline[5]	Erythromycin,[4] clarithromycin, azithromycin, a fluoroquinolone[3,14]
Rickettsiae	Doxycycline[5]	Chloramphenicol, a fluoroquinolone[3]

[1]Adapted from Med Lett Drugs Ther 2001;43:69.

[2]TMP-SMZ is a mixture of 1 part trimethoprim and 5 parts sulfamethoxazole.

[3]Fluoroquinolones include ciprofloxacin, ofloxacin, levofloxacin, moxifloxacin, gatifloxacin, and others (see text). Gatifloxacin, levofloxacin and moxifloxacin have the best activity against gram-positive organisms, including penicillin-resistant S pneumoniae and methicillin-sensitive S aureus. Activity against enterococci and S epidermidis is variable. Ciprofloxacin has the best activity against P aeruginosa.

[4]Erythromycin estolate is best absorbed orally but carries the highest risk of hepatitis; erythromycin stearate and erythromycin ethylsuccinate are also available.

[5]All tetracyclines have similar activity against most microorganisms. Minocycline and doxycycline have increased activity against S aureus. Dosage is determined by rates of absorption and excretion of various preparations.

[6]Penicillin G is preferred for parenteral injection; penicillin V for oral administration—to be used only in treating infections due to highly sensitive organisms.

[7]Most intravenous cephalosporins (with the exception of ceftazidime) have good activity against gram-positive cocci.

[8]Intermediate and high-level resistance to penicillin has been described. Infections caused by strains with intermediate resistance may respond to high doses of penicillin, cefotaxime, or ceftriaxone. Infections caused by highly resistant strains should be treated with vancomycin ± rifampin. Many strains of penicillin-resistant pneumococci are resistant to erythromycin, macrolides, TMP-SMZ, and chloramphenicol.

[9]Parenteral nafcillin or oxacillin; oral dicloxacillin, cloxacillin, or oxacillin.

[10]Addition of gentamicin indicated only for severe enterococcal infections (eg, endocarditis, meningitis).

[11]Aminoglycosides—gentamicin, tobramycin, amikacin, netilmicin—should be chosen on the basis of local patterns of susceptibility.

[12]Antipseudomonal penicillins: ticarcillin, piperacillin.

[13]Resistance may be a problem, and susceptibility testing should be done.

[14]Ciprofloxacin has inferior antichlamydial activity compared with newer fluoroquinolones.

Table 37–2. Examples of initial antimicrobial therapy for acutely ill adults pending identification of causative organism.

	Suspected Clinical Diagnosis	Likely Etiologic Diagnosis	Drugs of Choice
(A)	Meningitis, bacterial	Pneumococcus,[1] meningococcus	Cefotaxime,[2] 2–3 g IV every 6 hours, or ceftriaxone, 2 g IV every 12 hours plus vancomycin,10 mg/kg every 8 hours ± rifampin
(B)	Meningitis, bacterial, age > 50	Pneumococcus, meningococcus, *Listeria monocytogenes,*[3] gram-negative bacilli	Ampicillin, 2 g IV every 4 hours, plus cefotaxime or ceftriaxone and vancomycin as in (A)
(C)	Meningitis, postoperative (or posttraumatic)	S aureus, gram-negative bacilli (pneumococcus, in posttraumatic)	Vancomycin, 10 mg/kg every 8 hours, plus ceftazidime, 3 g IV every 8 hours
(D)	Brain abscess	Mixed anaerobes, pneumococci, streptococci	Penicillin G, 4 million units IV every 4 hours, + metronidazole, 500 mg PO every 8 hours, or cefotaxime or ceftriaxone as in (A) + metronidazole 500 mg PO every 8 hours
(E)	Pneumonia, acute, community-acquired, severe	Pneumococci, M pneumoniae, legionella, C pneumoniae	Erythromycin,[4] 0.5 g orally or IV four times daily, or doxycycline, 100 mg IV or orally every 12 hours, plus cefotaxime, 2 g IV every 8 hours (or ceftriaxone, 1 g IV every 24 hours); or a fluoroquinolone[6] alone
(F)	Pneumonia, postoperative or nosocomial	S aureus, mixed anaerobes, gram-negative bacilli	Cefotaxime or ceftriaxone or cefipime, 2 g IV every 8 hours, or piperacillin-tazobactam, 4–5 g IV every 6 hours, with or without tobramycin or ciprofloxacin
(G)	Endocarditis, acute (including IV drug user)	S aureus, E faecalis, gram-negative aerobic bacteria, viridans streptococci	Vancomycin, 15 mg/kg every 12 hours, plus gentamicin, 2 mg/kg every 8 hours
(H)	Septic thrombophlebitis (eg, IV tubing, IV shunts)	S aureus, gram-negative aerobic bacteria	Vancomycin 15 mg/kg every 12 hours plus gentamicin,[5] 2 mg/kg every 8 hours
(I)	Osteomyelitis	S aureus	Nafcillin, 2 g IV every 4 hours, or cefazolin, 2 g IV every 8 hours
(J)	Septic arthritis	S aureus, N gonorrhoeae	Ceftriaxone, 1–2 g IV every 24 hours
(K)	Pyelonephritis with flank pain and fever (recurrent UTI)	E coli, klebsiella, enterobacter, pseudomonas	Ciprofloxacin, 400 mg IV every 12 hours, or levofloxacin, 500 mg IV once daily
(L)	Suspected sepsis in neutropenic patient receiving cancer chemotherapy	S aureus, pseudomonas, klebsiella, E coli	Ceftazidime, 2 g IV every 8 hours, or cefepime, 2 g IV every 8 hours
(M)	Intra-abdominal sepsis (eg, postoperative, peritonitis, cholecystitis)	Gram-negative bacteria, bacteroides, anaerobic bacteria, streptococci, clostridia	Ampicillin, 1–2 g every 6 hours, plus gentamicin, 2 mg/kg every 8 hours, plus metronidazole, 500 mg IV every 8 hours, or piperacillin-tazobactam as in (F) or ticarcillin-clavulanate, 3.1 g IV every 6 hours

[1]Some strains may be resistant to penicillin. Vancomycin should be used with or without rifampin.
[2]Cefotaxime, ceftriaxone, ceftazidime, or ceftizoxime can be used. Most studies on meningitis have been done with cefotaxime or ceftriaxone (see text).
[3]TMP-SMZ can be used to treat *Listeria monocytogenes* in patients allergic to penicillin in a dosage of 15–20 mg/kg of TMP in three or four divided doses.
[4]Other macrolides such as azithromycin or clarithromycin can be used.
[5]Depending on local drug susceptibility pattern, use tobramycin, 5 mg/kg/d, or amikacin, 15 mg/kg/d, in place of gentamicin.
[6]Gatifloxacin, levofloxacin, moxifloxacin.

Table 37–3. Examples of empirical choices of antimicrobials for adult outpatient infections.

Suspected Clinical Diagnosis	Likely Etiologic Agents	Drugs of Choice	Alternative Drugs
Erysipelas, impetigo, cellulitis, ascending lymphangitis	Group A streptococcus	Phenoxymethyl penicillin, 0.5 g orally four times daily.	Erythromycin, 0.5 g orally four times daily, or cephalexin, 0.5 g orally four times daily for 7–10 days; azithromycin, 500 mg on day 1, and 250 mg on days 2–5.
Furuncle with surrounding cellulitis	*Staphylococcus aureus*	Dicloxacillin, 0.5 g orally four times daily for 7–10 days.	Cephalexin, 0.5 g orally four times daily for 7–10 days.
Pharyngitis	Group A streptococcus	Phenoxymethyl penicillin, 0.5 g orally four times daily for 10 days.	Erythromycin, 0.5 g orally four times daily for 10 days; azithromycin, 500 mg on day 1 and 250 mg on days 2–5, or clarithromycin, 500 mg twice daily daily for 10 days.
Otitis media	*Streptococcus pneumoniae, Haemophilus influenzae, Moraxella catarrhalis*	Amoxicillin, 0.5 g orally three times daily for 10 days.	Augmentin,[2] 0.5 g orally three times daily; cefuroxime, 0.5 g orally twice daily; or cefpodoxime, 0.2–0.4 g daily, or doxycycline, 100 mg twice daily or TMP-SMZ,[1] one double-strength tablet twice daily for 10 days.
Acute sinusitis	*S pneumoniae, H influenzae, M catarrhalis*	Amoxicillin, 0.5 g orally three times daily; or TMP-SMZ, one double-strength tablet twice daily for 10 days.	Augmentin,[2] 0.5 g orally three times daily; cefuroxime, 0.5 g orally twice daily; or cefpodoxime, 0.2–0.4 g daily, or doxycycline, 100 mg twice daily for 10 days.
Aspiration pneumonia	Mixed oropharyngeal flora, including anaerobes	Clindamycin, 0.3 g orally four times daily for 10–14 days.	Phenoxymethyl penicillin, 0.5 g orally four times daily for 10–14 days.
Pneumonia	*S pneumoniae, Mycoplasma pneumoniae, Legionella pneumophila, Chlamydia pneumoniae*	Doxycycline, 100 mg twice daily, or erythromycin, 0.5 g four times daily, or clarithromycin, 0.5 g twice daily, for 10–14 days; or azithromycin, 0.5 g on day 1 and 0.25 g on days 2–5.	Amoxicillin, 0.5 g four times daily, or a fluoroquinolone[5] for 10–14 days.
Cystitis	*Escherichia coli, Klebsiella pneumoniae,* proteus species, *Staphylococcus saprophyticus*	Fluoroquinolones,[4] nitrofurantoin.	TMP-SMZ,[1] one double-strength tablet twice daily for 3 days; cephalexin, 0.5 g orally four times daily for 7 days.
Pyelonephritis	*E coli, K pneumoniae,* proteus species, *S saprophyticus*	Fluoroquinolones[4] for 7–14 days	TMP-SMZ,[1] one double-strength tablet twice daily for 7–14 days
Gastroenteritis	Salmonella, shigella, campylobacter, *Entamoeba histolytica*	See Note 3.	
Urethritis, epididymitis	*Neisseria gonorrhoeae, Chlamydia trachomatis*	Cefixime, 400 mg orally once, or ciprofloxacin, 500 mg orally once, for *N gonorrhoeae;* plus doxycycline, 100 mg twice daily for 10 days, or ofloxacin, 300 mg orally twice daily for 10 days.	Ceftriaxone, 250 mg IM once, for *N gonorrhoeae;* plus doxycycline, 100 mg twice daily for 10 days, for *C trachomatis.*

(continued)

Table 37–3. Examples of empirical choices of antimicrobials for adult outpatient infections. (continued)

Suspected Clinical Diagnosis	Likely Etiologic Agents	Drugs of Choice	Alternative Drugs
Pelvic inflammatory disease	*N gonorrhoeae, C trachomatis,* anaerobes, gram-negative rods	Ofloxacin, 400 mg orally twice daily, for 14 days, plus metronidazole, 500 mg orally twice daily, for 14 days.	Cefoxitin, 2 g IM, with probenecid, 1 g orally, followed by doxycycline, 100 mg orally twice daily for 14 days; or ceftriaxone, 250 mg IM once, followed by doxycycline, 100 mg orally twice daily for 14 days.
Syphilis Early syphilis (primary, secondary, or latent of < 1 year's duration)	*Treponema pallidum*	Benzathine penicillin G, 2.4 million units IM once.	Doxycycline, 100 mg orally twice daily for 2 weeks.
Latent syphilis of > 1 year's duration or cardiovascular syphilis	*Treponema pallidum*	Benzathine penicillin G, 2.4 million units IM once a week for 3 weeks (total: 7.2 million units).	Doxycycline, 100 mg orally twice daily, for 4 weeks.
Neurosyphilis	*Treponema pallidum*	Aqueous penicillin G, 12–24 million units/d IV for 10–14 days.	Procaine penicillin G, 2–4 million units/d IM, plus probenecid, 500 mg orally four times daily, both for 10–14 days.

[1]TMP-SMZ is a fixed combination of 1 part trimethoprim and 5 parts sulfamethoxazole. Single-strength tablets: 80 mg TMP, 400 mg SMZ; double-strength tablets: 160 mg TMP, 800 mg SMZ.
[2]Augmentin is a combination of amoxicillin, 250 mg, 500 mg, or 875 mg, plus 125 mg of clavulanic acid.
[3]The diagnosis should be confirmed by culture before therapy. Salmonella gastroenteritis does not require therapy. For sensitive shigella, give TMP-SMZ double-strength tablets twice daily for 5 days; or ampicillin, 0.5 g orally four times daily for 5 days; or ciprofloxacin, 0.5 g orally twice daily for 5 days. For campylobacter, give erythromycin, 0.5 g orally four times daily for 5 days; or ciprofloxacin, 0.5 g orally twice daily for 5 days. For *E histolytica,* give metronidazole, 750 mg orally three times daily for 5–10 days, followed by diiodohydroxyquin, 600 mg three times daily for 3 weeks.
[4]Fluoroquinolones and dosages include ciprofloxacin, 500 mg orally twice daily; ofloxacin, 400 mg orally twice daily; levofloxacin, 500 mg daily; and sparfloxacin, 500 mg as loading dose and then 200 mg once daily. For others see text.
[5]Fluoroquinolones with activity against *S pneumoniae,* including penicillin-resistant isolates, include levofloxacin (500 mg once daily), gatifloxacin (400 mg once daily), sparfloxacin (400 mg on day 1 and then 200 mg once daily), and moxifloxacin (400 mg once daily).

(virulent organisms such as *Staphylococcus aureus* respond more slowly than viridans streptococci; mycobacterial and fungal infections respond slower than bacterial infections), and the duration of illness (in general, the longer the symptoms are present, the longer it takes to respond). Thus, depending on the clinical situation, persistent fever and leukocytosis several days after initiation of therapy may not indicate improper choice of antibiotics but may be due to the natural history of the disease being treated. In most infections, either a bacteriostatic or a bactericidal agent can be used. In some infections (eg, infective endocarditis and meningitis), one must kill the infecting organism to achieve a cure. When potentially toxic drugs (eg, aminoglycosides, flucytosine) are used, serum levels of the drug are measured to avoid toxicity and ensure appropriate dosage. In patients with altered clearance of drugs, the dosage or frequency of administration must be adjusted. Especially in elderly,

morbidly obese patients or those with altered renal function, it is best to measure levels directly and adjust therapy accordingly.

In renal or hepatic failure, the dosage must be adjusted as shown in Table 37–4.

G. DURATION OF ANTIMICROBIAL THERAPY

Generally, effective antimicrobial treatment results in reversal of the clinical and laboratory parameters of active infection and marked clinical improvement. However, varying periods of treatment may be required for cure. Key factors include (1) the type of infecting organism (bacterial infections can be cured more rapidly than fungal or mycobacterial ones), (2) the location of the process (eg, endocarditis and osteomyelitis require prolonged therapy), and (3) the immunocompetence of the patient. Very few studies have examined appropriate length of treatment to effect a cure, and duration of therapy is often arbitrary.

Table 37–4. Use of antimicrobials in patients with renal failure[1] and hepatic failure.

Drug	Principal Mode of Excretion or Detoxification	Approximate Half-Life in Serum Normal	Approximate Half-Life in Serum Renal Failure[2]	Proposed Dosage Regimen in End-Stage Renal Failure Initial Dose[3]	Proposed Dosage Regimen in End-Stage Renal Failure Maintenance Dose	Removal of Drug by Hemodialysis	Dose After Hemodialysis	Dosage in Hepatic Failure
Acyclovir	Renal	2.5–3.5 hours	20 hours	2.5 mg/kg	2.5 mg/kg q24h	Yes	2.5 mg/kg	No change
Ampicillin-sulbactam	Renal	0.5–1 hour	8–12 hours	3 g	1.5 g q8–12h	Yes	1.5 g	No change
Amphotericin B	Unknown	360 hours	360 hours	No change	No change	No	None	No change
Ampicillin	Tubular secretion	0.5–1 hour	8–12 hours	1 g	1 g q8–12h	Yes	1 g	No change
Azithromycin	Renal 20%; hepatic 35%	3–4 hours	Not known	500 mg	250 mg q24h	No	None	Not known[4]
Aztreonam	Renal	1.7 hours	6 hours	1–2 g	0.5–1 g q6–8h	Yes	0.5–1 g	No change
Chloramphenicol	Mainly liver	3 hours	4 hours	0.5 g	0.5 g q6h	Yes	0.5 g	0.25–0.5 g q12h
Clarithromycin	Renal 30%; hepatic > 50%	3–4 hours	15 hours	500 mg	250 mg q12h	No	None	Not known[4]
Clindamycin	Liver	2–4 hours	2–4 hours	0.6 g IV	0.6 g q8h	No	None	0.3–0.6 g q8h
Doxycycline	Renal	15–24 hours	15–24 hours	100 mg	100 mg q12h	No	None	Not known[4]
Ertapenem	Renal	4 hours	20 hours	1 g	0.5 g q24h	Yes	0.15 g	No change
Erythromycin	Mainly liver	1.5 hours	1.5 hours	0.5–1 g	0.5–1 g q6h	No	None	0.25–0.5 g q6h
Famciclovir[5]	Renal	2.5 hours	13–20 hours	500 mg	500 mg q24h	Yes	500 mg	No change
Fluconazole	Renal	30 hours	98 hours	0.2 g	0.1 g q24h	Yes	Give q24h dose	No change
Flucytosine	Renal	3–6 hours	30–250 hours	37.5 mg/kg	25 mg/kg q24h	Yes	25 mg/kg	No change
Foscarnet	Renal	3–8 hours	Not known	90–120 mg	Not known[6]	No	None	No change
Fosfomycin	Renal	6 hours	11–50 hours	NA	NA	NA	NA	No change
Ganciclovir[7]	Renal	3 hours	11–28 hours	1.25 mg/kg	1.25 mg/kg q24h	Yes	Give q24h dose	No change
Imipenem	Glomerular filtration	1 hour	3 hours	0.5 g	0.25–0.5 g q12h	Yes	0.25–0.5 g	No change
Isoniazid	Renal	1–5 hours	2.5 hours	300 mg	300 mg q24h	Yes	None	Not known[4]
Itraconazole	Hepatic	21 hours	25 hours	50–200 mg	50–200 mg q24h	No	None	Not known[4]
Ketoconazole	Hepatic	8 hours	8 hours	200 mg	200–400 mg q24h	No	None	Not known[4]
Meropenem	Renal	1 hour	5–10 hours	1 g	0.5–1 g q24h	Yes	0.5 g	No change

Metronidazole	Liver	6–10 hours	6–10 hours	0.5 g IV	0.5 g q8h	Yes	0.25 g	0.25 g q12h
Mezlocillin	Renal 50–70%; biliary 20–30%	1 hour	3–6 hours	3 g	2 g q6–8h	Yes	1 g	1–2 g q8h
Nafcillin	Liver 80%; kidney 20%	0.75 hours	1.5 hours	1.5 g	1.5 g q4h	No	None	2–3 g q12h
Penicillin G	Tubular secretion	0.5 hours	7–10 hours	1–2 million units	1 million units q8h	Yes	500,000 units	No change
Pentamidine	Not known	6–9 hours	6–9 hours	4 mg/kg	4 mg/kg q24h	No	None needed	No change
Piperacillin and piperacillin + tazobactam	Renal 50–70%; biliary 20–30%	1 hour	3–6 hours	3 g	2 g q6–8h	Yes	1 g	1–2 g q8h
Rifampin	Hepatic	2–5 hours	3–5 hours	600 mg	600 mg q24h	No	None[4]	Not known[4]
Ticarcillin	Tubular secretion	1.1 hour	15–20 hours	3 g	2 g q6–8h	Yes	1 g	No change
Trimethoprim-sulfamethoxazole	Some liver	TMP 10–12 hours; SMZ 8–10 hours	TMP 24–48 hours; SMZ 18–24 hours	320 mg TMP + 1600 mg SMZ	80 mg TMP + 400 mg SMZ q12h	Yes	80 mg TMP + 400 mg SMZ	No change
Trimetrexate	Hepatic	15 hours	Not known	45 mg/m^2	40 mg/m^2 q24h	No	None[2]	Not known
Vancomycin	Glomerular filtration	6 hours	6–10 days	1 g	1 g q6–10d based on serum levels[8]	No	None[2]	No change

[1] For cephalosporins, see text and Table 37–7; for aminoglycosides, see Table 37–8.
[2] Considered here to be marked by creatinine clearance of 10 mL/min or less.
[3] For a 70-kg adult with a serious systemic infection.
[4] Dose adjustment in hepatic failure has not been studied, but because clearance of the drug is principally hepatic, dose reduction may be required.
[5] Pharmacokinetics and dosing are in reference to the active agent, penciclovir.
[6] When creatinine clearance is 30 mL/min, a dose of 60 mg/kg is given once daily. For clearances less than 30 mL/min, the dose has not been established
[7] Oral ganciclovir is same as IV ganciclovir except that the initial dose is 1000 mg, maintenance dose is 500 mg daily, and dose after hemolysis is 500 mg.
[8] When serum levels reach 5–10 µg/mL, another dose should be given.

H. Adverse Reactions and Toxicity

These include (1) hypersensitivity reactions (eg, fever, rashes, anaphylaxis), (2) direct adverse effect or toxicity (eg, diarrhea, vomiting, impairment of renal or hepatic function, neurotoxicity), (3) superinfection by drug-resistant microorganisms, or (4) drug interactions such as the increased INR associated with trimethoprim-sulfamethoxazole added to warfarin.

If the infection is life-threatening and treatment cannot be stopped, the reactions may be managed symptomatically (especially if mild) or another drug may be chosen that does not cross-react with the offending one (Table 37–1). If the infection is less severe, it may be possible to stop all antimicrobials and follow the patient carefully.

I. Route of Administration

Parenteral therapy is preferred for acutely ill patients with serious infections (eg, endocarditis, meningitis, sepsis, severe pneumonia) when dependable levels of antibiotics are required for successful therapy. Certain drugs (eg, fluconazole, rifampin, metronidazole, trimethoprim-sulfamethoxazole, and fluoroquinolones) are so well absorbed that they can be administered orally even in seriously ill patients.

Food does not significantly influence the bioavailability of most oral antimicrobial agents. Exceptions include the tetracyclines and the quinolones, which are chelated by heavy metals. Azithromycin capsules are associated with decreased bioavailability when taken with food and should be given 1 hour before or 2 hours after meals.

A major complication of intravenous antibiotic therapy is catheter infections. Peripheral Teflon catheters are routinely changed every 48–72 hours to prevent phlebitis, and antimicrobial-coated central venous catheters (minocycline and rifampin, chlorhexidine and sulfadiazine) have been associated with a decreased incidence of catheter-related infections. Most of these infections present with local signs of infection (erythema, tenderness) at the insertion site. In the evaluation of a patient with fever who is receiving intravenous therapy, the catheter must always be considered as a potential source. Some small-gauge (20–23F) peripherally inserted silicone or polyurethane catheters (Per Q Cath, A-Cath, Ven-A-Cath, and others) are associated with a very low infection rate and can be maintained for 3–6 months without replacement. Such catheters are ideal for long-term outpatient antibiotic therapy.

J. Cost of Antibiotics

The cost of these agents can be substantial. In addition to the direct cost of purchasing a drug, one must consider the costs of monitoring for toxicity (drug levels, liver function tests, electrolytes, etc), the cost of treating adverse reactions, the cost of treatment failure, and the costs associated with the time required for administering drugs that are given at frequent intervals. Obviously, if several drugs with equal efficacy and toxicity are available, one should choose the least expensive. Table 37–5 lists the costs of commonly used antibiotics.

The Choice of Antibacterial Drugs. Med Lett Drugs Ther 2001;43:69. [PMID: 11518876] (Current recommendations.)

Jorgensen JH: Antimicrobial susceptibility testing: General principles and contemporary practices. Clin Infect Dis 1998;26:973. [PMID: 9564485] (Review of tests available.)

Lampiris HW, Maddix DS: Clinical use of antimicrobial agents. In: *Basic & Clinical Pharmacology,* 8th ed. Katzung BG (editor). McGraw-Hill, 2001.

MacGowan AP: Role of pharmacokinetics and pharmacodynamics: does the dose matter? Clin Infect Dis 2001;33(Suppl 3):S238. [PMID: 11524725]

PENICILLINS

The penicillins are a large group of antimicrobial substances, all of which share a common chemical nucleus (6-aminopenicillanic acid) that contains a β-lactam ring essential to their biologic activity.

Antimicrobial Action & Resistance

The initial step in penicillin action is the binding of the drug to receptors—penicillin-binding proteins—some of which are transpeptidation enzymes. The penicillin-binding proteins of different organisms differ in number and in affinity for a given drug. After penicillins have attached to receptors, peptidoglycan synthesis is inhibited because the activity of transpeptidation enzymes is blocked. The final bactericidal action is the removal of an inhibitor of the autolytic enzymes in the cell wall, which activates the enzymes and results in cell lysis. Organisms that are defective in autolysin function are inhibited but not killed by β-lactam antibiotics ("tolerance"). Organisms that produce β-lactamases (penicillinases) are resistant to some penicillins because the β-lactam ring is broken and the drug is inactivated. Only organisms that are actively synthesizing peptidoglycan (in the process of multiplication) are susceptible to β-lactam antibiotics. Nonmultiplying organisms or those lacking cell walls are not susceptible.

Microbial resistance to penicillins is caused by four factors:

(1) Production of β-lactamases, eg, by staphylococci, gonococci, haemophilus species, and coliform organisms.

(2) Lack of penicillin-binding proteins or decreased affinity of penicillin-binding protein for β-lactam antibiotic receptors (eg, resistant pneumococci, methicillin-resistant staphylococci, enterococci) or impermeability of cell envelope, so that penicillins cannot reach receptors (eg, metabolically inactive bacteria).

(3) Failure of activation of autolytic enzymes in the cell wall; "tolerance," eg, in staphylococci, group B streptococci.

Table 37–5. Approximate costs of antimicrobials.

Drug	Dose per Day[1]	Cost per Unit[2]	Daily Cost of Therapy[3]
	INTRAVENOUS PREPARATIONS		
Acyclovir	15 mg/kg (mucocutaneous herpes)	$32.70/1 g	$32.70
Acyclovir	30 mg/kg (CNS herpes)	$32..70/1 g	$65.40
Amikacin (Amikin, others)	15 mg/kg	$121.25/0.5 g	$242.50
Ampicillin	100 mg/kg	$2.35/2 g	$9.40
Ampicillin plus sulbactam (Unasyn)	3 g q8h	$14.90/3 g (IV)	$44.70
Aztreonam (Azactam)	50 mg/kg	$18.00/1 g	$72.00
Cefazolin (Ancef, others)	50 mg/kg	$1.90/1 g (IV)	$5.70
Cefepime (Maxipime)	500 mg/kg	$16.00/1 g	$48.00
Cefoxitin (Mefoxin)	80 mg/kg	$10.90/1 g	$32.70
Ceftazidime (Fortaz, others)	50 mg/kg	$14.25/1 g	$42.75
Ceftizoxime (Cefizox)	50 mg/kg	$11.40/1 g	$34.20
Ceftriaxone (Rocephin)	30 mg/kg	$50.25/1 g	$50.25
Cefuroxime (Zinacef, others)	60 mg/kg	$13.10/1.5 g	$49.30
Ciprofloxacin (Cipro IV)	0.8 g	$30.00/0.4 g	$60.00
Clindamycin (Cleocin, others)	2400 mg	$25.20/0.6 g	$100.80
Fluconazole (Diflucan IV)	0.2–0.4 g	$95.65/0.2 g $139.80/0.4 g	$95.65–139.80
Foscarnet (Foscavir)	180 mg/kg (induction) 90–120 mg/kg (maintenance)	$76.60 (24 mg/mL × 250 mL = 6000 mg)	$153.20 $76.60–107.00
Ganciclovir (Cytovene IV)	10 mg/kg	$37.10/0.5 g	$74.20
Gatifloxacin (Tequin)	400 mg	$38.00/400 mg	$38.00
Gentamicin	5 mg/kg	$2.50/80 mg	$12.50
Imipenem (Primaxin IV)	50 mg/kg	$30.70/0.5 g	$122.80
Meropenem (Merrem IV)	500 mg/kg	$26.00/0.5 g	$78.00–104.00
Metronidazole (Flagyl, others)	1500 mg	$15.35/0.5 g	$46.05
Mezlocillin (Mezlin)	250 mg/kg	$9.00/2 g	$54.00
Nafcillin	100 mg/kg	$4.40/2 g	$17.60
Penicillin	12 million units	$8.40/1 million units	$100.80

(continued)

Table 37-5. Approximate costs of antimicrobials. (continued)

Drug	Dose per Day[1]	Cost per Unit[2]	Daily Cost of Therapy[3]
INTRAVENOUS PREPARATIONS (continued)			
Piperacillin (Pipracil)	250 mg/kg	$21.20/3 g	$84.80
Piperacillin plus tazobactam (Zosyn)	3.75 g q6–8h	$16.20/3.375 g	$64.80
Ticarcillin (Ticar)	250 mg/kg	$13.50/3 g	$54.00
Ticarcillin-potassium clav-ulanic acid (Timentin)	3.1 g q6h	$15.10/3.1 g	$60.40
Tobramycin	5 mg/kg	$3.70/80 mg	$18.50
Trimethoprim-sulfamethoxazole (Bactrim, Septra)	15 mg/kg TMP	$19.25 (0.48 g TMP in 30 mL)	$38.50
Trimetrexate (Neutrexin)	45 mg/m²	$125.00/25 mg	(Depends on surface area.)
Vancomycin	20–30 mg/kg	$76.40/1 g	$152.80
ORAL PREPARATIONS			
Acyclovir	1000 mg (therapy of herpes)	$1.10/0.2 g	$5.50
Acyclovir	800 mg three times daily (herpes suppression for immunocompromised patient)	$4.20/0.8 g	$12.60
Amoxicillin	20–30 mg/kg	$0.36/0.5 g	$1.00
Ampicillin	20–30 mg/kg	$0.21/0.5 g	$0.63
Augmentin (0.5 g amoxicillin plus 0.125 g clavulanic acid)	30 mg/kg	$4.00/0.5 g	$8.00
Azithromycin (Zithromax)	500 mg as loading dose, then 250 mg/d for 4 days	$7.20/0.25 g	$14.40 load, then $7.20
Azithromycin (Zithromax)	1 g as single dose for C trachomatis infection	$22.30/1 g packet	$22.30/1 g packet
Cefaclor (Ceclor)	20–30 mg/kg	$3.80/0.5 g	$11.40
Cefixime (Suprax)	400 mg	$8.00/0.4 g	$8.00
Cefpodoxime proxetil (Vantin)	400 mg	$4.35/0.2 g	$8.70
Cefprozil (0.5 g) (Cefzil)	15 mg/kg	$7.65/0.5 g	$15.30
Cefuroxime (0.5 g) (Ceftin)	0.5 g twice daily	$8.00/0.5 g	$16.00
Cephalexin (0.5 g) (Keflex, others)	30 mg/kg	$1.25/0.5 g	$5.00
Ciprofloxacin (0.5 g) (Cipro)	0.5–0.75 g twice daily	$5.00/0.5 g	$10.00
Ciprofloxacin (0.75 g) (Cipro)		$5.00/0.75 g	$10.00

(continued)

Table 37–5. Approximate costs of antimicrobials. (continued)

Drug	Dose per Day[1]	Cost per Unit[2]	Daily Cost of Therapy[3]
ORAL PREPARATIONS (continued)			
Clarithromycin (0.25 or 0.5 g) (Biaxin)	250–500 mg twice daily	$4.10/0.5 g	$8.20
Clindamycin (0.3 g) (Cleocin, others)	15 mg/kg	$1.20/150 mg	$9.60
Doxycycline (0.1 g)	3 mg/kg	$0.37/0.1 g	$0.74
Erythromycin (0.5 g)	30 mg/kg	$0.30/0.5 g	$0.90
Famciclovir (0.5 g) (Famvir)	500 mg three times daily	$8.15/0.5 g	$24.45
Fluconazole (0.1 g)	0.1–0.2 g daily	$8.10/0.1 g	$8.10
Fluconazole (0.2 g) (Diflucan)		$13.25/0.2 g	$13.25
Flucytosine (0.5 g) (Ancobon)	150 mg/kg	$8.00/0.5 g	$168.00
Ganciclovir (0.25 g) (Cytovene)	1 g three times daily	$4.60/0.25 g	$55.20
Gatifloxacin (0.4 g) (Tequin)	400 mg	$8.20/0.4 g	$8.20
Itraconazole (0.1 g) (Sporanox)	200–400 mg	$7.75/0.1 g	$15.50–31.00
Ketoconazole (0.2 g) (Nizoral)	0.2–0.4 g	$3.00/0.2 g	$3.00–6.00
Levofloxacin (0.5 g) (Levaquin)	0.5 g daily	$8.90/0.5 g	$8.90
Lomefloxacin (0.4 g) (Maxaquin)	400 mg	$7.00/0.4 g	$7.00
Loracarbef (0.4 mg) (Lorabid)	800 mg	$6.40/0.4 g	$12.80
Metronidazole (0.5 g) (Flagyl)	20 mg/kg	$0.70/0.5 g	$2.10
Moxifloxacin (0.4 g) (Avelox)	400 mg	$9.40/0.4 g	$9.40
Ofloxacin (0.4 g) (Floxin)	400 mg twice daily	$5.45/0.4 g	$10.90
Penicillin VK (0.5 g)	30 mg/kg	$0.10/0.5 g	$0.40
Sparfloxacin (0.2 g) (Zagam)	0.2 g daily	$6.70/0.2 g	$13.40 day 1, then $6.70/daily
Tetracycline (0.5 g)	30 mg/kg	$0.10/0.5 g	$0.40
Trimethoprim-sulfamethoxazole (Bactrim, Septra)	5 mg/kg TMP	$1.10/160 mg TMP and 800 mg SMZ	$2.20
Valacyclovir (0.5 g) (Valtrex)	0.5–1 g three times daily	$3.90/0.5 g	$11.70–23.40
Vancomycin (Vancocin)	125 mg 3 times daily	$5.60/125 mg	$16.80

[1]Doses based on a 70-kg individual with normal renal function.
[2]Approximate (for this table only) cost to pharmacist (average wholesale price, generic when possible) for quantity listed. Source: *Drug Topics Red Book,* March 2002; Vol. 21, No. 3.
[3]Daily cost for intravenous antibiotics includes acquistion cost only and not preparation and administration costs.

(4) The presence of cell wall-deficient (L) forms or mycoplasmas, which do not synthesize peptidoglycans.

1. Natural Penicillins

The natural penicillins include forms of penicillin G for parenteral administration (aqueous crystalline, procaine, and benzathine penicillin G) or for oral administration (penicillin G and phenoxymethyl penicillin [penicillin V]). They are most active against gram-positive organisms and are susceptible to hydrolysis by β-lactamases. They are used for infections caused by susceptible and moderately susceptible pneumococci depending upon the site of infection (however, up to 30–35% of strains now demonstrate intermediate- or high-level resistance to penicillin), streptococci (including anaerobic streptococci), meningococci, non-β-lactamase-producing staphylococci, *Treponema pallidum* and other spirochetes, *Bacillus anthracis* and other gram-positive rods, clostridia, actinomyces, and most anaerobes except β-lactamase-producing strains, eg, *Bacteroides fragilis* (Table 37–1).

Pharmacokinetics & Administration

After parenteral administration, penicillin is widely distributed in tissues. Lower levels are present in the eye, prostate, and central nervous system. However, with acute inflammation of the meninges (eg, in bacterial meningitis) and with appropriate dosing, adequate penetration into the cerebrospinal fluid takes place.

Special dosage forms of penicillin permit delayed absorption to yield low blood and tissue levels for long periods, eg, benzathine penicillin G and procaine penicillin G.

Phenoxymethyl penicillin (penicillin V) is the oral penicillin of choice. It is more acid-stable than oral penicillin G, is better absorbed, and gives higher serum levels.

Most of the absorbed penicillin is rapidly excreted by the kidneys into the urine; small amounts are excreted by other routes. About 10% of renal excretion is by glomerular filtration and 90% by tubular secretion. Tubular secretion can be partially blocked by probenecid to achieve higher systemic levels. Individuals with impaired renal function likewise tend to maintain higher penicillin levels longer, and the dose should be reduced in moderate to severe renal failure. One commonly used formula for calculating the maximum daily dose of penicillin in millions of units in patients with a creatinine clearance of less than 40 mL/min is as follows (see also Table 37–4):

$$\frac{\text{Dosage}}{\text{(millions of units/d)}} = 3.2 + \frac{\text{Creatinine clearance (mL/min)}}{7}$$

Clinical Uses

Most infections caused by organisms sensitive to penicillin will respond to aqueous penicillin G in daily doses of 1–2 million units administered intravenously every 4–6 hours. For life-threatening infections (meningitis, endocarditis), much larger daily doses (18–24 million units) should be given by intermittent intravenous infusion every 4–6 hours in equally divided doses.

Penicillin V is indicated in minor infections such as streptococcal pharyngitis and cellulitis. The usual dose is 1–2 g/d in four equally divided doses.

A single injection of 1.2 million units of benzathine penicillin intramuscularly is satisfactory for treatment of β-hemolytic streptococcal pharyngitis. An injection of 1.2–2.4 million units every 3–4 weeks provides satisfactory prophylaxis for rheumatics against reinfection with group A streptococci. Syphilis is usually treated with benzathine penicillin, 2.4 million units intramuscularly weekly for 1–3 weeks, depending on the stage of the disease (see Table 37–3).

Procaine penicillin is rarely used except as an alternative drug for neurosyphilis (Table 37–3).

2. Extended-Spectrum Penicillins

The extended-spectrum group of penicillins includes the aminopenicillins: ampicillin and amoxicillin; the carboxypenicillins: ticarcillin; and the ureidopenicillins: piperacillin and mezlocillin. These drugs are all susceptible to destruction by staphylococcal (and other) β-lactamases. They tend to be active against many gram-negative rods and have the same activity as natural penicillins against gram-positive bacteria.

Antimicrobial Activity

Ampicillin and amoxicillin are active against most strains of *Proteus mirabilis,* listeria, and non-β-lactamase-producing strains of *Haemophilus influenzae* but inactive against most gram-negative pathogens. Both drugs are active against the pneumococcus, and both are more active than penicillin against *Enterococcus faecalis.*

Ticarcillin extends the activity of ampicillin to include many strains of pseudomonas, serratia, and indole-positive proteus, but it has poor activity against most strains of klebsiella and enterococci and is less active than ampicillin against the pneumococci.

The ureidopenicillins are similar to ticarcillin but exhibit slight differences in activity against gram-negative organisms. Piperacillin and mezlocillin are more active than ticarcillin against *Pseudomonas aeruginosa* and klebsiella, but otherwise their gram-negative spectrum of activity is similar to that of ticarcillin. Similar to ampicillin, mezlocillin and piperacillin are active against *E faecalis.* Piperacillin is more active than ticarcillin against pneumococci. The extended-spectrum penicillins are active against most anaerobes. Ampicillin and amoxicillin are not active against β-lactamase-producing strains of *B fragilis*—in contrast to the other drugs in this class which are active against most (not all) isolates at high concentrations.

Pharmacokinetics & Administration

Ampicillin can be given orally or parenterally. Amoxicillin is absorbed better than ampicillin, resulting in serum levels twice as high as those achieved with ampicillin.

The carboxy- and ureidopenicillins are given intravenously. Increased doses (200–300 mg/kg/d) are required for treatment of infections due to *P aeruginosa*.

Dosage adjustments are required in renal failure and are summarized in Table 37–4.

Clinical Uses

Amoxicillin is given orally for minor infections, such as acute exacerbations of chronic bronchitis, sinusitis, or otitis. Ampicillin is given intravenously for pneumonia, meningitis, bacteremia, or endocarditis.

Amoxicillin is also used as antibacterial prophylaxis to prevent endocarditis. Because of the increased serum and respiratory secretion levels, this agent is valuable in the treatment of moderately penicillin-susceptible pneumococcus. In general, if amoxicillin levels remain above the MIC of the pneumococcus more than 40% of the dosing interval, bacteriologic cure rates approach 85–100%. Although ticarcillin, mezlocillin, and piperacillin have been used as monotherapy, they are more commonly administered in combination with other agents as empirical therapy in the febrile neutropenic patient.

3. Penicillins Combined With β-Lactamase Inhibitors

The addition of β-lactamase inhibitors (clavulanic acid, sulbactam, tazobactam) can prevent inactivation of the parent penicillin by bacterial β-lactamases. Augmentin (amoxicillin, 250 mg, 500 mg, or 875 mg, plus 125 mg of clavulanic acid), Timentin (ticarcillin, 3 g, plus 100 mg of clavulanic acid), Unasyn (ampicillin 1 g plus sulbactam 0.5 g, and ampicillin 3 g plus sulbactam 1.5 g), and Zosyn (piperacillin 3 g plus tazobactam 0.375 g, and piperacillin 4 g plus tazobactam 0.5 g) are available. Augmentin is given orally and the others intravenously. In general, the β-lactamase inhibitors effectively inactivate β-lactamases produced by *S aureus*, *H influenzae*, *Moraxella catarrhalis*, and *Bacteroides fragilis*, thus making Augmentin, Timentin, Unasyn, and Zosyn effective agents for infections with these organisms. In contrast, the β-lactamase inhibitors are variably and unpredictably effective against certain β-lactamases produced by certain aerobic gram-negative bacilli, such as enterobacter, and thus cannot be relied upon to treat these organisms unless specific sensitivity testing is done. Of the available parenteral drugs, Zosyn has the broadest spectrum of activity. Like Unasyn (but not Timentin)

it is active against ampicillin-susceptible enterococci. It has greater in vitro activity against *P aeruginosa* than Timentin and is more active than either Timentin or Unasyn against serratia and klebsiella species.

Augmentin, because of its high cost and gastrointestinal intolerance, is limited to the treatment of refractory cases of sinusitis and otitis that have not responded to less costly agents and is used for therapy and prophylaxis of infections resulting from animal and human bites. The roles of Timentin, Unasyn, and Zosyn include the treatment of polymicrobial infections such as peritonitis from a ruptured viscus, osteomyelitis in a diabetic patient, or traumatic osteomyelitis.

The dosage regimens of these drugs are the same as those of the parent drugs. When Timentin or Zosyn is used to treat pseudomonas infections, dosages of 200–300 mg/kg/d are used. Nonpseudomonal infection can be treated with lower doses (100–200 mg/kg/d).

4. Penicillinase-Resistant Penicillins

Methicillin, oxacillin, cloxacillin, dicloxacillin, nafcillin, and others are relatively resistant to destruction by β-lactamases produced by staphylococci and are limited to the treatment of infections with such organisms. They are less active than natural penicillins against nonstaphylococcal gram-positives; however, they are still adequate in streptococcal infections.

With the exception of methicillin, the primary route of clearance of the above agents is nonrenal—thus, no dosage adjustment is needed in renal insufficiency.

5. Adverse Effects of Penicillins

Allergy

All penicillins are cross-sensitizing and cross-reacting. The responsible antigenic determinants appear to be degradation products of penicillins, particularly penicilloic acid and products of alkaline hydrolysis (minor antigenic determinants) bound to host protein. Skin tests with penicilloyl-polylysine, with minor antigenic determinants, and with undegraded penicillin can identify most individuals with IgE-mediated reactions (hives, bronchospasm). Among positive reactors to skin tests, the incidence of subsequent immediate severe penicillin reactions is high. Although many persons develop IgG antibodies to antigenic determinants of penicillin, the presence of such antibodies is not correlated with allergic reactivity (except for rare instances of hemolytic anemia), and serologic tests have little predictive value. A history of a penicillin reaction in the past is not reliable. Only 15–20% of patients with a history of penicillin allergy have an adverse reaction when challenged with the drug. The decision to administer penicillin or related drugs (other β-lactams) to patients with an allergic history depends upon the severity of the reported reaction, the severity of the infection being treated, and the availability of alternative drugs. For patients with a history of severe reaction (anaphylaxis), alternative drugs should be used. In the rare situations when there is a strong indication for using penicillin (eg, syphilis in pregnancy) despite a history of severe reaction, desensitization can be performed. If the reaction is mild (rash), the patient may be rechallenged with penicillin or may be given another β-lactam antibiotic. (See Chapter 30 for discussion and methods of desensitization.)

Allergic reactions include anaphylaxis, serum sickness (urticaria, fever, joint swelling, angioneurotic edema 7–12 days after exposure), and a variety of skin rashes, oral lesions, fever, interstitial nephritis, eosinophilia, hemolytic anemia, other hematologic disturbances, and vasculitis. The incidence of hypersensitivity to penicillin is estimated to be 1–5% among adults in the USA. Life-threatening anaphylactic reactions are very rare (0.05%). Ampicillin produces maculopapular skin rashes more frequently than other penicillins, but some ampicillin rashes are not allergic in origin. The nonallergic ampicillin rash usually occurs after 3–4 days of therapy, is maculopapular, is more common in patients with coexisting viral illness (especially Epstein-Barr infection), and resolves with continued therapy. Penicillins can induce nephritis with primary tubular lesions association with anti-basement membrane antibodies.

Toxicity

Since the action of penicillin is directed against a unique bacterial structure, the cell wall, it is virtually without effect on animal cells. All penicillins are irritating to the central nervous system, and excessive doses, particularly in renal insufficiency, have been associated with seizures.

Of the oral penicillins, Augmentin is most commonly associated with diarrhea. Nafcillin administered at high doses is associated with a modest leukopenia. High doses of penicillins, particularly ticarcillin, mezlocillin, or piperacillin can inhibit platelet aggregation and produce hypokalemia due to binding of potassium in the kidney.

Craig WA: Pharmacokinetics/pharmacodynamics parameters: Rationale for antibacterial dosing of mice and men. Clin Infect Dis 1998;26:1. [PMID: 9455502] (Review of pharmacologic principles with application of principles to rational dosing.)

Musher DM et al: A fresh look at the definition of susceptibility of *Streptococcus pneumoniae* to beta-lactam antibiotics. Arch Intern Med 2001;161:2538. [PMID: 11718584]

Wright AJ: The penicillins. Mayo Clin Proc 1999;74:290. [PMID: 10090000] (Review of activity, clinical uses, and adverse effects of this class of drugs.)

CEPHALOSPORINS (Tables 37–6 and 37–7)

The cephalosporins are structurally related to the penicillins. They consist of a β-lactam ring attached to a dihydrothiazoline ring. Substitutions of chemical

Table 37–6. Major groups of cephalosporins.

First Generation	Second Generation	Third Generation	Fourth Generation
Cephalothin	Cefamandole	Cefotaxime	Cefepime
Cephapirin	Cefuroxime	Ceftizoxime	
Cefazolin	Cefonicid	Ceftriaxone	
Cephalexin[1]	Ceforanide	Ceftazidime	
Cephradine[1]	Cefaclor[1]	Cefoperazone	
Cefadroxil	Cefoxitin	Cefixime[1]	
	Cefotetan	Cefpodoxime proxetil[1]	
	Cefprozil[1]	Ceftibuten[1]	
	Cefuroxime axetil[1]	Cefdinir[1]	
	Cefmetazole	Cefditoren pivoxil[1]	

[1]Oral agents.

groups at various positions on the basic structure have resulted in a proliferation of drugs with varying pharmacologic properties and antimicrobial activities.

The mechanism of action of cephalosporins is analogous to that of the penicillins: (1) binding to specific penicillin-binding proteins that serve as drug receptors on bacteria, (2) inhibition of cell wall synthesis, and (3) activation of autolytic enzymes in the cell wall that result in bacterial death. Resistance to cephalosporins may be due to poor permeability of the drug into bacteria, lack of penicillin-binding proteins, or degradation by β-lactamases.

Cephalosporins have been divided into four major groups or "generations" (Table 37–6) based mainly on their antibacterial activity: First-generation cephalosporins have good activity against aerobic gram-positive organisms and some community-acquired gram-negative organisms (*P mirabilis, E coli*, klebsiella species); second-generation drugs have a slightly extended spectrum against gram-negative bacteria, and some are active against gram-negative anaerobes; and third-generation cephalosporins are active against most gram-negative bacteria (except enterobacter and citrobacter). Not all cephalosporins fit neatly into this grouping, and there are exceptions to the general characterization of the drugs in the individual classes; however, the generational classification of cephalosporins is useful for discussion purposes. Cefepime is considered a fourth-generation agent because it is more stable against plasmid-mediated β-lactamase and has little or no β-lactamase-inducing capacity. Cefepime compares favorably with ceftazidime with respect to its gram-negative activity; however, its stability versus plasmid-mediated β-lactamase results in improved coverage against enterobacter and citrobacter species. The gram-positive coverage of cefepime approaches that of cefotaxime or ceftriaxone.

Because of their broad spectrum of activity and low toxicity, these drugs are used to treat many infections.

Table 37–7. Pharmacology of the cephalosporins.

Drug	Peak Serum Level (μg/mL) After 1 g IV	Serum Half-Life (min)	Total Daily Dose (mg/kg)	Dosage Interval (hours)	Dosage Adjustments in Renal Failure		
					Moderate (Cl_{cr} 10–50) mL/min	Severe ($Cl_{cr} < 10$ mL/min)	Post-Hemodialysis Dose
Cephalothin, cefapirin	40–60	40	50–200	4–6	1–2 g q6–12h	1 g q12h	1 g
Cefazolin	90–120	90	25–100	8	0.5–1 g q6–12h	0.5 g daily	0.5 g
Cephalexin, cephradine[1]	15–20	50–60	15–30	6	0.25–0.5 g q8–12h	0.25–0.5 g daily	0.5 g
Cefadroxil[1]	15	75	15–30	12–24	1 g daily	0.5 g daily	0.5 g
Cefamandole	60–80	45	75–200	6–8	1 g q12h	1–2 g daily	0.5 g
Cefditoren pivoxil	2–3	90	6	12	0.2 g q12h	0.2 g q12h	None
Cefepime	60–70	120	50–75	8–12	1 g q12h	1 g q24h	1 g
Ceftibuten[1]	20	120	9	12–24	0.4 g daily	0.1–0.2 g daily	0.7 g
Cefuroxime	80–100	80	50	6–12	1 g q12h	1–2 g daily	0.5 g
Cefuroxime axetil[1]	6–8	75	5–15	12	0.5 g q24h	0.25 g daily	0.25 g
Cefonicid	200–250	240	15–30	24	0.5 g daily	1 g q72h	0.25 g
Ceforanide	125	180	15–30	12	1 g daily	1 g q48h	0.25 g
Cefaclor[1]	15–20	50	20–40 children, 10–15 adults	6–8	0.5 g q8–12h	0.25–0.5 g q12–24h	0.25–0.5 g
Cefixime	3–5	180–240	8 (with maximum of 0.4 g/d total)	12–24	0.4 g daily	0.1 g daily	None
Cefpodoxime proxetil[1]	2	150	5	12	0.2 g q24h	0.2 g 3 times/wk after dialysis	0.2 g
Cefprozil[1]	10	90	10–15	12	0.5 g q12–24h	0.25–0.5 g q12–24h	0.5 g
Cefotetan	60–80	150	50–100	8–12	1 g q8–12h	0.5–1 g daily	0.5 g
Cefotaxime	40–60	60	50–75	6–8	1–2 g q6–8h	1–2 g q24h	1–2 g
Cefoxitin	60–80	60	50–100	6–8	1 g q12h	1–2 g daily	0.5 g
Cefmetazole	70–100	60–80	50–100	6–8	1 g q12–24h	1–2 g q24–48h	1 g
Ceftizoxime	80–100	100	50–75	8–12	0.5–1 g q8–12h	0.25–0.5 g q12–24h	0.5 g
Ceftriaxone	150	480	30–50	12–24	1–2 g daily	1–2 g daily	None
Ceftazidime	100–120	120	50–75	8–12	1 g q12h	0.5–1 g daily	0.5 g
Cefoperazone	150	120	30–200	8–12	1–2 g q12h	1–2 g q12h	None
Loracarbef[1]	10	60	10–15	12	0.2 g q24h	0.2 g 3 times/wk after dialysis	0.2 g

[1]Oral agents. Serum levels based on 0.5 g oral dose.

1. First-Generation Cephalosporins

Antimicrobial Activity

These drugs are very active against gram-positive cocci, including penicillin-sensitive pneumococci, viridans streptococci, group A hemolytic streptococci, and *S aureus*. Like all cephalosporins, they are inactive against enterococci and methicillin-resistant staphylococci. Activity against *H influenzae* is poor, and many strains of penicillin-resistant streptococci (both intermediately and highly resistant) are resistant also to first-generation cephalosporins. Among gram-negative bacteria, *E coli, K pneumoniae,* and *P mirabilis* are usually susceptible except for some hospital-acquired strains. There is very little activity against most nosocomial gram-negative rods. Anaerobic cocci are usually susceptible, but *B fragilis* is not.

Pharmacokinetics & Administration

A. ORAL

Cephalexin, cephradine, and cefadroxil are variably absorbed. Cefadroxil, because of its longer half-life, can be given twice daily. Dosage adjustment is required in renal insufficiency.

B. INTRAVENOUS

Cefazolin is preferred over cephalothin and cephapirin because it has a longer half-life, resulting in less frequent dosing. In renal insufficiency, all of these agents require dosage adjustments.

C. INTRAMUSCULAR

Both cephapirin and cefazolin can be given intramuscularly, but pain on injection is less with cefazolin.

Clinical Uses

Oral drugs are sometimes used for treatment of urinary tract infections, and they can be used for minor staphylococcal infections. Oral cephalosporins may also be preferred for minor polymicrobial infections (eg, cellulitis, soft tissue abscess).

Intravenous first-generation cephalosporins are the drugs of choice for surgical prophylaxis in many cases. More expensive second- and third-generation cephalosporins offer no advantage for surgical prophylaxis except where anaerobes play an important role, such as for colorectal surgery or for hysterectomy.

First-generation cephalosporins do not adequately penetrate the cerebrospinal fluid and cannot be used to treat meningitis.

2. Second-Generation Cephalosporins

Second-generation cephalosporins are a heterogeneous group with marked individual differences in activity, pharmacokinetics, and toxicity. In general, all are active against gram-negative organisms also covered by first-generation drugs, but they have an extended gram-negative coverage. Indole-positive proteus and klebsiella (including first-generation cephalosporin-resistant strains) as well as *Moraxella catarrhalis* and neisseria species are usually sensitive. Cefuroxime and cefprozil are active against *H influenzae,* including β-lactamase-producing strains, but have little activity against serratia and *B fragilis*. In contrast, cefoxitin and cefotetan are active against many strains of *B fragilis* and some strains of serratia. end} Against gram-positive organisms, these drugs are generally less active than the first-generation cephalosporins (cefuroxime is an exception). Second-generation agents have no activity against *P aeruginosa* or enterococci.

Pharmacokinetics & Administration

A. ORAL

Only cefaclor, cefuroxime axetil, and cefprozil can be given orally. Cefuroxime axetil is deesterified to cefuroxime after absorption. Its longer half-life permits twice-daily dosing, and absorption is enhanced when it is taken with food (as is not the case with many other oral antibiotics).

B. INTRAVENOUS AND INTRAMUSCULAR

Because of differences in drug half-life and protein binding, peak serum levels achieved and dosing intervals vary greatly for this group of drugs (Table 37–7). Drugs with shorter half-lives (cefoxitin) require higher doses and more frequent dosing than drugs with longer half-lives (cefuroxime, cefotetan). Dosage adjustments are required with renal impairment.

Clinical Uses

Because of their activity against β-lactamase-producing *H influenzae* and *M catarrhalis,* cefprozil and cefuroxime axetil can be used to treat sinusitis and otitis media in patients with mild allergy to ampicillin or amoxicillin or have not responded to treatment with those drugs.

Because of their activity against *B fragilis,* cefoxitin, cefmetazole, and cefotetan can be used to treat mixed anaerobic infections, eg, peritonitis and diverticulitis. However, since 10–15% of *B fragilis* and many enteric gram-negative organisms are resistant to these drugs, for severe life-threatening intra-abdominal infections alternative agents are preferred. Cefoxitin and cefotetan are useful as prophylaxis in colorectal surgery, vaginal or abdominal hysterectomy, and appendectomy because of their activity against *B fragilis*.

3. Third- & Fourth-Generation Cephalosporins

Antimicrobial Activity

Most of these drugs are active against staphylococci (not methicillin-resistant strains) but less so than first-generation cephalosporins. Ceftazidime, however, has notably weak activity against *S aureus* and pneumococci. They have no activity against enterococci but do inhibit most streptococci. Ceftriaxone and cefotaxime offer the most reliable antipneumococcal coverage. A major advantage of these cephalosporins is their expanded gram-negative coverage. In addition to organisms inhibited by other cephalosporins, they are consistently active against *S marcescens,* providencia, haemophilus, and neisseria, including β-lactamase-producing strains. Ceftazidime is effective against *P aeruginosa.* Acinetobacter, citrobacter, enterobacter, and non-aeruginosa strains of pseudomonas are variably sensitive to third-generation cephalosporins, and listeria is uniformly resistant. Activity against *B fragilis* is variable. In contrast to the third-generation agents, cefepime—the only currently available fourth-generation cephalosporin—is active against enterobacter and citrobacter, has activity comparable to that of ceftazidime against *P aeruginosa,* and has gram-positive activity similar to that of ceftriaxone.

Cefixime, cefpodoxime proxetil, cefdinir, cefditoren pivoxil, and ceftibuten, the only oral agents in this group, are more active than cefuroxime axetil but are not as active as parenteral third-generation cephalosporins against gram-negative organisms such as pseudomonas, enterobacter, morganella, and *S marcescens.* The major difference in these drugs is activity against gram-positive bacteria. All are active against *Streptococcus pyogenes* (group A streptococcus). Cefpodoxime proxetil, cefditoren pivoxil, and cefdinir are active against methicillin-sensitive *S aureus,* whereas cefixime and ceftibuten have little activity (none are active against methicillin-resistant strains). Cefdinir, cefixime, cefditoren pivoxil, and cefpodoxime proxetil are active against penicillin-sensitive strains of *Streptococcus pneumoniae* (the pneumococcus), but ceftibuten has marginal activity. None of the oral cephalosporins are reliable against intermediately susceptible or penicillin-resistant *S pneumoniae.* Like other members of this class, these drugs are ineffective against enterococci and *Listeria monocytogenes* infections.

Pharmacokinetics & Administration

The intravenous agents penetrate well into body fluids and tissues and reach levels in the cerebrospinal fluid that exceed those needed to inhibit most pathogens, including gram-negative rods. The half-lives of these drugs are variable, which accounts for the differences in dosing intervals (Table 37–7). Ceftriaxone is eliminated primarily by biliary excretion, and no dosage adjustment is required in renal insufficiency. The other drugs are eliminated primarily by the kidney and thus require dosage adjustments in renal insufficiency.

Clinical Uses

Because of their penetration into the cerebrospinal fluid, intravenous third-generation cephalosporins can be used to treat meningitis. Meningitis due to susceptible pneumococci—strains resistant to penicillin may have high MICs to third-generation cephalosporins and should not be used to treat meningitis caused by highly penicillin-resistant pneumococci—meningococci, *H influenzae,* and susceptible enteric gram-negative rods has been successfully treated. In meningitis in older patients, third-generation cephalosporins should be combined with ampicillin until *L monocytogenes* has been excluded as the etiologic agent. Ceftazidime has been used to treat pseudomonas meningitis. The dosage for meningitis should be at the upper limits of the recommended range, because cerebrospinal fluid levels of these drugs are only 10–20% of serum levels. Ceftazidime or cefepime is frequently administered empirically in the febrile neutropenic patient. Ceftriaxone is indicated for gonorrhea, chancroid, and more serious forms of Lyme disease (see Chapter 34). Because of its long half-life and once-daily dosing requirement, ceftriaxone is an attractive option for the outpatient parenteral therapy of infections due to susceptible organisms.

Cefepime is useful for third-generation cephalosporin–resistant isolates such as enterobacter and citrobacter.

Cefixime, because of its long half-life, can be given once daily. It has limited gram-positive coverage; however, it reliably inhibits *H influenzae* and *M catarrhalis.* Cefdinir and cefpodoxime are the best third-generation oral agents against pneumococci and *S aureus.* Single-dose cefixime and cefpodoxime proxetil are as effective as ceftriaxone for the therapy of genital, rectal, and pharyngeal gonorrhea.

4. Adverse Effects of Cephalosporins

Allergy

Cephalosporins are sensitizing, and a variety of hypersensitivity reactions occur, including anaphylaxis, fever, skin rashes, nephritis, granulocytopenia, and hemolytic anemia. The frequency of IgE cross-allergy between cephalosporins and penicillins approximates 5–10%. Persons with a history of anaphylaxis to penicillins should not receive cephalosporins.

Toxicity

Local pain can occur after intramuscular injection, or thrombophlebitis after intravenous injection. Hypoprothrombinemia is a frequent adverse effect (40–68%) of cephalosporins that have a methylthiotetrazole group (eg, cefamandole, cefmetazole, cefotetan). Prophylactic administration of vitamin K, 10 mg twice weekly, can prevent this complication. Drugs containing the methylthiotetrazole ring can also cause severe disulfiram-like reactions, and use of alcohol or medications containing alcohol (eg, theophylline elixir) must be avoided. Ceftriaxone has been associated with a dose-dependent biliary sludging syndrome and cholelithiasis due to precipitation of drug when its solubility in bile is exceeded. Long term administration of 2 g/d or more is a risk factor for this complication.

Dancer SJ: The problem with cephalosporins. J Antimicrob Chemother 2001;48:463. [PMID: 11581224] (Review of developing resistance patterns associated with cephalosporins.)

Marshall WF et al: The cephalosporins. Mayo Clin Proc 1999;74:187. [PMID: 10069359] (Review of spectrum of activity, clinical use, adverse effects, and mechanisms of resistance.)

OTHER β-LACTAM DRUGS

Monobactams

These are drugs with a monocyclic β-lactam ring that are resistant to β-lactamases and active against gram-negative organisms (including pseudomonas) but have no activity against gram-positive organisms or anaerobes. Aztreonam resembles ceftazidime in its gram-negative activity. Clinical uses of aztreonam are limited because of the availability of third-generation cephalosporins with a broader spectrum of activity and minimal toxicity. Despite the structural similarity of aztreonam to penicillin, cross-reactivity is limited, and it can therefore be used in most patients with penicillin allergy.

Carbapenems

This class of drugs is structurally related to β-lactam antibiotics. Imipenem, the first drug of this type, has a wide spectrum of activity that includes most gram-negative rods (including *P aeruginosa*) and gram-positive organisms and anaerobes, with the exception of *Burkholderia cepacia, Stenotrophomonas maltophilia, E faecium,* and most methicillin-resistant *S aureus* and *S epidermidis.* The half-life of imipenem is 1 hour. Dosage adjustment is required in renal insufficiency.

Meropenem is similar to imipenem in spectrum of activity and pharmacology. It is less likely to cause seizures than imipenem, though the risk of seizures is low with imipenem if dosage is appropriately adjusted for renal insufficiency. Meropenem is associated with less nausea and vomiting than imipenem, a feature of importance when high doses must be used, as in the treatment of pseudomonas infection in patients with cystic fibrosis. The usual dose is 1–2 g every 8 hours. Dosage adjustment in renal insufficiency is required.

Ertapenem is similar to imipenem and meropenem in its activity against aerobic gram-positive and anaerobic organisms but is less active against pseudomonas and acinetobacter. Because of its long half-life (4 hours), it can be administered once daily. The usual dose is 1 g, and adjustments are needed for renal insufficiency.

The carbapenems should not be routinely used as first-line therapy unless the pathogen is multidrug-resistant and is known to be sensitive to these agents. In patients hospitalized for a prolonged period who may have infection with a multidrug-resistant organism, empirical use of carbapenems while awaiting culture results is reasonable. (Ertapenem should not be used if pseudomonas and enterobacter are common nosocomial pathogens.) Pseudomonas may rapidly develop resistance to imipenem and meropenem. In cystic fibrosis, the doubling rate of imipenem resistance is 5–7 days. The use of imipenem or meropenem alone appears to be as effective as combination therapy in the febrile neutropenic patient and all of the carbapenems are as effective as combination therapy in certain polymicrobial infections such as peritonitis and obstetric pelvic infections.

The most common adverse effects of imipenem and meropenem are nausea, vomiting, diarrhea, reactions at the infusion site, and skin rashes. Seizures are more commonly observed with imipenem. Patients allergic to penicillins may be allergic to imipenem and meropenem as well.

Edwards JR et al: Carbapenems: the pinnacle of the beta-lactam antibiotics or room for improvement? J Antimicrob Chemother 2000;45:1. [PMID: 10629005]

Goossens H: MYSTIC (Meropenem Yearly Susceptibility Test Information Collection) results from Europe: comparison of antibiotic susceptibilities between countries and centre types. MYSTIC Study Group (European centres only). J Antimicrob Chemother 2000;46(Suppl T2):39. [PMID: 11065147]

Hellinger WC et al: Carbapenems and monobactams: Imipenem, meropenem, and aztreonam. Mayo Clin Proc 1999;74:420. [PMID: 10221472] (Review of activity, indications and adverse effects.)

ERYTHROMYCIN GROUP (Macrolides)

The erythromycins are a group of closely related compounds characterized by a macrocyclic lactone ring to which various sugars are attached.

Antimicrobial Activity

Erythromycins inhibit protein synthesis by binding to the 50S subunit of bacterial ribosomes. They generally are bacteriostatic and sometimes bactericidal for gram-positive organisms, including most streptococci and corynebacteria in a concentration of 0.02–2 μg/mL. Similar to penicillin, macrolide-resistant *S pneumoniae* is being reported with increased frequency (15–50%), and group A streptococci also can be resistant. Erythromycin-resistant pneumococci are azalide-resistant as well (azithromycin, clarithromycin). Chlamydiae, mycoplasmas, legionella, and campylobacter are susceptible.

Pharmacokinetics & Administration

Preparations for oral use include erythromycin base, erythromycin stearate, estolate, and ethyl succinate. The base is most acid-stable, and the estolate is the best-absorbed; none of the oral preparations have any advantage over others. Erythromycins are excreted primarily nonrenally; only 5% is excreted in the urine, and no adjustment is therefore required in renal failure.

Erythromycin and azithromycin are available for intravenous use, particularly in the treatment of Legionnaires' disease.

Clinical Uses

Macrolides are drugs of choice for infections caused by legionella, mycoplasma, ureaplasma, corynebacterium (including diphtheria and bacteremia), and chlamydia (including ocular and respiratory infections). They are effective in streptococcal and pneumococcal disease in penicillin-allergic patients, though resistance is increasing. They can also be used with neomycin in prophylaxis for bowel surgery. When administered early, erythromycin may shorten the course of campylobacter enteritis. Erythromycins are effective against certain bartonella species (bacillary angiomatosis) and rhodococcus species. In vitro data suggest that macrolides have a direct effect on neutrophil function and the production of cytokines associated with inflammation. Thus, these agents are being evaluated for their anti-inflammatory effects in infectious diseases as well.

Adverse Effects

Nausea, vomiting, and diarrhea may occur after oral or intravenous intake. Erythromycins—particularly the estolate—can produce acute cholestatic hepatitis (fever, jaundice, impaired liver function), probably as a hypersensitivity reaction. Most patients recover, but hepatitis recurs if the drug is readministered. Reversible auditory impairment occurs with large doses (4 g/d or more), particularly in patients with impaired renal or hepatic function. Ototoxicity has been reported with high doses of all agents. Intravenous erythromycin has been associated with prolongation of the QT interval and torsade de pointes—more commonly in women. Erythromycins can increase the effects of oral anticoagulants, digoxin, theophylline, and cyclosporine by inhibiting cytochrome P450.

AZALIDES

Azalides (azithromycin, clarithromycin, dirythromycin, and others) are a group of antibiotics closely related structurally to the macrolides. Like erythromycin, they are active against *Streptococcus pneumoniae*, group A streptococcus, viridans streptococci, *M catarrhalis*, legionella, *Mycoplasma pneumoniae*, and *Chlamydia pneumoniae* and are slightly more active in vitro than erythromycin against *H influenzae* (with azithromycin having better activity than clarithromycin and dirythromycin having activity equivalent to that of erythromycin). They are also active against *Chlamydia trachomatis*, *N gonorrhoeae*, *Ureaplasma urealyticum*,

and *Haemophilus ducreyi*. In addition, these drugs have in vitro activity against a number of unusual pathogens, including atypical mycobacteria (*Mycobacterium avium-intracellulare*, *Mycobacterium chelonei*, *Mycobacterium fortuitum*, *Mycobacterium marinum*), *Toxoplasma gondii*, *Campylobacter jejuni*, *Helicobacter pylori*, and *Borrelia burgdorferi*.

The azalides are more acid-stable than erythromycin, penetrate tissues well, and have a long terminal half-life, with high tissue concentrations that persist for days. The elevated tissue levels associated with azithromycin and clarithromycin could overcome the high incidence of in vitro resistance seen with pneumococci (30%), but clinical observations suggest that the reported resistance translates to clinical failure. Azithromycin, clarithromycin, and dirythromycin are approved for treatment of streptococcal pharyngitis, uncomplicated skin infections, and acute bacterial exacerbations of chronic bronchitis. Because of the long half-life, outpatient treatment with azithromycin is with once-daily dosing for a total of 5 days (500 mg on day 1 and then 250 mg on days 2–5). Clarithromycin is usually administered in a dosage of 250–500 mg twice daily, though an extended-release formulation that is given as a single daily 1000 mg dose has been approved for acute sinusitis and acute exacerbation of chronic bronchitis. Dirythromycin is given as a single daily dose of 500 mg. The azalides are more expensive than erythromycin. However, the less frequent dosing and better tolerability make them superior choices in certain patients.

Azithromycin has also been approved as single-dose therapy (1 g) for chlamydial genital infections. This is much more expensive than 7 days of treatment with doxycycline (Table 37–5), but the assurance of adequate supervised therapy for this infection makes azithromycin preferred therapy in many patients. Azithromycin can also be used as single-dose therapy (1 g) for chancroid, and a single-dose of 1 g is as efficacious as 7 days of doxycycline for nongonococcal urethritis in men and is effective also for incubating syphilis. While a 2 g dose of azithromycin is used for the treatment of gonorrhea, its efficacy is less than that observed with quinolones or ceftriaxone. Furthermore, the incidence of upper gastrointestinal side effects is increased with this dose. The spectrum of activity of the macrolides—particularly their atypical coverage—results in their utility in mild to moderate cases of community-acquired pneumonia; however, penicillin-resistant strains are often resistant to these agents as well. Weekly 1200 mg doses of azithromycin are effective in preventing *Mycobacterium avium* complex infections in HIV-positive patients and in doses of 500 mg daily may be effective in *M avium* complex pulmonary infections in non-HIV-positive patients. Azithromycin may be considered for therapy of dysentery caused by multidrug-resistant shigella. Used as prophylaxis, azithromycin (500 mg weekly) is as effective as benzathine penicillin in preventing upper respiratory tract infections in military recruits, and at a dose of 250 mg daily it is adequate as prophylaxis for malaria (though inferior to doxycycline for multidrug-resistant *P falciparum*). Clarithromycin has been used for the therapy of *M avium* complex infections, usually in combination with other drugs (eg, rifabutin and ethambutol), and can be given daily (500 mg twice daily) or three times weekly (1000 mg) as intermittent therapy. Clarithromycin (500 mg twice daily for 6 months) is effective therapy for disseminated *Mycobacterium chelonei* infections and may be the drug of choice for use against this pathogen. Clarithromycin has also been used in combination regimens for the therapy of *Helicobacter pylori* infections. When clarithromycin is given with omeprazole and amoxicillin or metronidazole, cure rates in excess of 80–90% have been achieved.

Adverse effects of these agents are similar to those of erythromycin, but upper gastrointestinal upset, the major side effect, occurs less often with the azalides. Hepatic enzyme elevations, interstitial nephritis, headache, and dizziness have been reported rarely. Similar to erythromycin, azithromycin and clarithromycin have been associated with dose-dependent ototoxicity. Clarithromycin is similar to erythromycin in its effect on the cytochrome P450 system. Azithromycin appears to affect metabolism of other drugs only minimally.

McConnell SA et al: Review and comparison of advanced-generation macrolides clarithromycin and dirithromycin. Pharmacotherapy 1999;18:404. [PMID: 10212011]

KETOLIDES

Ketolides (such as telithromycin) are similar in structure to macrolides, but they have a broader spectrum of activity and may offer additional benefit in the treatment of community-acquired respiratory infections. They are active against both penicillin-resistant and macrolide-resistant pneumococci and equal to azithromyocin therapeutically against atypical pathogens and *H influenzae*. Upper gastrointestinal adverse events are the complications most commonly associated with these drugs. The dose is 100 mg/d, and no adjustment is needed for renal or hepatic insufficiency.

White RL: Antibiotic resistance: where do ketolides fit? Pharmacotherapy 2002;22(1 Part 2):18S. [PMID: 11791625]

TETRACYCLINE GROUP

The tetracyclines are a large group of drugs with common basic chemical structures, antimicrobial activity, and pharmacologic properties. Microorganisms resistant to this group show extensive cross-resistance to all tetracyclines.

Antimicrobial Activity

Tetracyclines are inhibitors of protein synthesis and are bacteriostatic for many gram-positive and gram-negative bacteria. They are strongly inhibitory for the growth of mycoplasmas, rickettsiae, chlamydiae, spiro-

chetes, and some protozoa (eg, amebas). Their antipneumococcal activity approaches that of the macrolides; almost all *H influenzae* are inhibited. Tetracyclines also have moderate activity against some vancomycin-resistant enterococci. Doxycycline and minocycline are potential options for therapy of staphylococcal infections, including infections with many methicillin-resistant strains. There are marked differences in the susceptibility of different strains of a given species of microorganism. Because of the emergence of resistant strains, tetracyclines have lost much of their former usefulness as broad-spectrum agents, particularly for gram-negative aerobic organisms.

Pharmacokinetics & Administration

Oral bioavailability varies depending upon the drug. Absorption is impaired by dairy products, aluminum hydroxide gels (antacids), and chelation with divalent cations, eg, Ca^{2+} or Fe^{2+}. Consequently, doses of tetracyclines should be staggered at least 2 hours before or after receipt of multivalent cations. Oral bioavailability is moderate with tetracycline and highest with doxycycline and minocycline (95% or more). Lipid solubility of minocycline and doxycycline accounts for their penetration into the cerebrospinal fluid, prostate, tears, and saliva.

Tetracyclines are primarily metabolized in the liver and excreted in bile. All tetracyclines except doxycycline accumulate in renal insufficiency. Thus, doxycycline requires no dosage adjustment in renal failure; in contrast other tetracyclines should be avoided or given in reduced dosage.

For patients unable to take oral medication, some tetracyclines (doxycycline, minocycline) are formulated for parenteral administration in doses similar to the oral ones.

Clinical Uses

Tetracyclines are drugs of choice for infections with chlamydiae, mycoplasmas, rickettsiae, ehrlichia, and vibrio and for some spirochetal infections. Sexually transmitted diseases in which chlamydiae often play a role—endocervicitis, urethritis, proctitis, and epididymitis—should be treated with doxycycline for 7–14 days. Pelvic inflammatory disease is often treated with doxycycline plus cefoxitin or cefotetan. Other chlamydial infections (psittacosis, lymphogranuloma venereum, trachoma) and sexually transmitted diseases (granuloma inguinale) also respond to doxycycline. Other uses include treatment of acne, respiratory infections, Lyme disease and relapsing fever, brucellosis, glanders, tularemia (often in combination with streptomycin), cholera, mycoplasmal pneumonia, actinomycosis, nocardiosis, malaria, infections caused by *M marinum* and *Pasteurella multocida* (typically after an animal bite), and as malaria prophylaxis (including multidrug-resistant *P falciparum*). They also have been used in combination with other drugs for amebiasis, falciparum malaria, and recurrent ulcers due to *H pylori*. Because of generally good activity against pneumococci, *Haemophilus influenzae*, chlamydia, legionella, and mycoplasma, doxycycline should be considered as empirical therapy for outpatient pneumonia.

Minocycline achieves a high concentration in the saliva and can be used for eradication of meningococci in carriers who cannot tolerate rifampin. Minocycline is equally as efficacious as doxycycline for the therapy of nongonococcal urethritis and cervicitis.

Adverse Effects

A. ALLERGY

Hypersensitivity reactions with fever or skin rashes are uncommon.

B. GASTROINTESTINAL SIDE EFFECTS

Diarrhea, nausea, and anorexia are common.

C. BONES AND TEETH

Tetracyclines are bound to calcium deposited in growing bones and teeth, causing fluorescence, discoloration, enamel dysplasia, deformity, or growth inhibition. Therefore, tetracyclines should not be given to pregnant women or children under 6 years of age.

D. LIVER DAMAGE

Tetracyclines can impair hepatic function or even cause liver necrosis, particularly during pregnancy or in the presence of preexisting liver damage.

E. KIDNEY EFFECTS

Demeclocycline can cause nephrogenic diabetes insipidus and has been used therapeutically to treat inappropriate antidiuretic hormone secretion. Tetracyclines may increase blood urea nitrogen when diuretics are administered.

F. OTHER

Tetracyclines—principally demeclocycline—may induce photosensitization, especially in fair-skinned individuals. Minocycline induces vestibular reactions (dizziness, vertigo, nausea, vomiting), with a frequency of 35–70% after doses of 200 mg daily and has also been implicated as a cause of hypersensitivity pneumonitis.

Smilack JD: The tetracyclines. Mayo Clin Proc 1999;74:727. [PMID: 10405705] (Review of clinical indications and adverse effects.)

CHLORAMPHENICOL

Antimicrobial Activity

Chloramphenicol is active against certain rickettsiae. It binds to the 50S subunit of ribosomes and inhibits protein synthesis. It is bacteriostatic for most organisms but is often bactericidal for *S pneumoniae*, *H influenzae*, and *Neisseria meningitidis*. The drug is used minimally because of its toxicity and the availability of alternative agents.

Pharmacokinetics & Administration

Chloramphenicol is widely distributed in tissues, including the eye and central nervous system. Cerebrospinal fluid levels are 70–80% of peak serum levels, and the levels in brain tissue may even exceed those in serum.

Chloramphenicol is metabolized in the liver, and less than 10% is excreted unchanged in the urine. Thus, no dosage adjustment is needed in renal insufficiency. Patients with liver disease may accumulate the drug, and levels should be monitored.

Clinical Uses

Chloramphenicol is a possible choice in the following circumstances: (1) Meningococcal, *H influenzae*, or pneumococcal infections of the central nervous system in patients with a history of anaphylaxis to β-lactam drugs. (2) Anaerobic or mixed infections in the central nervous system, eg, brain abscess. (3) As an alternative to tetracyclines in rickettsial infections, especially in pregnant women, in whom tetracycline is contraindicated.

Adverse Effects

Nausea, vomiting, and diarrhea occur infrequently. The most serious adverse effects pertain to the hematopoietic system. Adults taking chloramphenicol in excess of 50 mg/kg/d regularly exhibit disturbances in red cell maturation within 1–2 weeks. There is anemia, hyperferremia, reticulocytopenia, and the appearance of vacuolated nucleated red cells in the bone marrow. These changes regress when the drug is stopped and are not related to aplastic anemia. The latter is an irreversible consequence of chloramphenicol administration and represents a specific, probably genetically determined individual defect. It occurs in 1:40,000–1:25,000 courses of chloramphenicol treatment.

Kasten MJ: Clindamycin, metronidazole and chloramphenicol. Mayo Clin Proc 1999;74:825. [PMID: 10473362] (Review of clinical uses and adverse effects.)

AMINOGLYCOSIDES

Aminoglycosides are a group of bactericidal drugs sharing chemical, antimicrobial, pharmacologic, and toxic characteristics. At present, the group includes streptomycin, neomycin, kanamycin, amikacin, gentamicin, tobramycin, sisomicin, netilmicin, paromomycin, and spectinomycin. All these agents inhibit protein synthesis in bacteria by attaching to and inhibiting the function of the 30S subunit of the bacterial ribosome. Resistance is based on (1) a deficiency of the ribosomal receptor (chromosomal mutant); (2) the enzymatic destruction of the drug (plasmid-mediated transmissible resistance of clinical importance) by acetylation, phosphorylation, or adenylylation; or (3) a lack of permeability to the drug molecule or failure of active transport across cell membranes. (This can be chromosomal, eg, streptococci are relatively impermeable to aminoglycosides; or plasmid-mediated, eg, in gram-negative enteric bacteria.) Anaerobic bacteria are resistant to aminoglycosides because transport across the cell membrane is an oxygen-dependent energy-requiring process.

All aminoglycosides are more active at alkaline than at acid pH. All are potentially ototoxic and nephrotoxic, though to different degrees. All can accumulate in renal insufficiency; therefore, dosage adjustments must be made in patients with renal dysfunction (see Table 37–8).

Because of their considerable toxicity and the availability of other antibiotics with broad spectrums of activity and fewer adverse effects (eg, cephalosporins, quinolones, carbapenems, β-lactamase inhibitor combinations), aminoglycosides have been used less often in recent years. They are most commonly used to treat resistant gram-negative organisms that are sensitive only to aminoglycosides, or in low doses in combination with β-lactam drugs or vancomycin for their synergistic effect (eg, enterococci, penicillin-resistant viridans streptococci, right-sided *S aureus* endocarditis, *S aureus* and *S epidermidis* prosthetic valve infection). Although aminoglycosides demonstrate in vitro activity against many gram-positive bacteria, they should never be used alone to treat infections caused by these organisms—both because there is no clinical experience with the treatment of such infections and because less toxic alternatives are available.

General Properties of Aminoglycosides

Because of the similarities of the aminoglycosides, a summary of properties is presented briefly.

A. ABSORPTION, DISTRIBUTION, METABOLISM, AND EXCRETION

Aminoglycosides are not absorbed from the gastrointestinal tract. They diffuse poorly into the eye, prostate, bile, central nervous system, and spinal fluid after parenteral injection.

There is no significant metabolic breakdown of aminoglycosides. The serum half-life is 2–3 hours in patients with normal renal function. Excretion is almost entirely by glomerular filtration. Aminoglycosides are removed fairly effectively by hemodialysis but less well by peritoneal dialysis. Continuous hemofiltration is associated with significant aminoglycoside clearance.

B. DOSAGE AND EFFECT OF IMPAIRED RENAL FUNCTION

In persons with normal renal function who have gram-negative infections, the dosage of amikacin is 15 mg/kg/d in a single daily dose; that for gentamicin, tobramycin, or netilmicin is 5 mg/kg injected once daily. A single large daily dose of gentamicin, tobramycin, netilmicin, or amikacin is just as efficacious as—and no more nephrotoxic than—traditional dosing every 8–12 hours. Trough aminoglycoside levels should be undetectable in patients with normal body composition and renal function receiving once-daily dosing. Some clinicians recommend serum level monitoring 12–18 hours after the dose and extending the interval to every 48–72 hours for patients with elevated aminoglycoside levels. Others have suggested maintaining the dosage interval but decreasing the dose. Patients with renal failure, volume overload, or obesity have altered antibiotic clearance or volume of distribution. In patients with abnormal renal function or body composition, once-daily dosing is not recommended and aminoglycoside levels are recommended to guide dosing. In general, peak levels greater than 6 μg/mL are necessary for optimal outcome in the treatment of serious gram-negative infection, including pneumonia. Trough levels of more than

Table 37–8. Dosing of aminoglycosides.[1]

Drug	Creatinine Clearance (mL/min)				
	> 80	**60–80**	**40–60**	**20–40**	**< 20**
Gentamicin, tobramycin, netilmicin	5 mg/kg q24h	1.5–2.5 mg/kg q12h	1.2–1.5 mg/kg q24h	1.2–1.5 mg/kg q12–24h	2 mg/kg as loading dose and then 1–1.5 mg/kg q24–48h
Amikacin	15 mg/kg q24h	4.5–7.5 mg/kg q12h	3.5–4.5 mg/kg q12h	3.5–4.5 mg/kg q12–24h	7.5 mg/kg as loading dose and then 3–4.5 mg/kg q24–48h

[1]Traditional dosing should be guided by serum level measurements (peaks 30 minutes after the end of intravenous infusion and troughs ≤ 30 minutes before the next dose). When a single large daily dose is given, peak levels are not required. Trough levels should be undetectable with high-dose (5 mg/kg) once-daily gentamicin or amikacin. For those patients with creatinine clearances less than 80 mL/min, the dosage ranges in the table are those used to treat gram-negative infections are intended to achieve, for gentamicin, tobramycin, and netilmicin, peak levels of 6–10 mg/L and trough levels of ≤ 2 mg/L; for amikacin, peak levels of 20–30 mg/L and trough levels of ≤ 5 mg/L.

2 μg/mL have been associated with an increased incidence of nephrotoxicity. In patients with normal body composition, once-daily dosing regimens as set forth in Table 37–8 should be followed. Reduced gentamicin doses (1 mg/kg every 8 hours) are recommended when used synergistically with β-lactams or vancomycin in the treatment of serious gram-positive infection (eg, enterococcal endocarditis).

C. ADVERSE EFFECTS

All aminoglycosides can cause ototoxicity and nephrotoxicity. Ototoxicity can be irreversible and is cumulative, presenting as hearing loss (cochlear damage), noted first with high-frequency tones, or as vestibular damage, manifested by vertigo and ataxia. Amikacin appears to be more cochlear toxic than gentamicin, tobramycin, or netilmicin. Nephrotoxicity, which is more common than ototoxicity, is accompanied by rising serum creatinine levels or reduced creatinine clearance. Nephrotoxicity is usually reversible and occurs with similar frequency with gentamicin, tobramycin, amikacin, and netilmicin.

In very high doses, particularly with irrigation of an inflamed peritoneum, aminoglycosides can be neurotoxic, producing a curare-like effect with neuromuscular blockade that results in respiratory paralysis. Calcium gluconate or neostigmine can serve as an antidote to this reaction.

1. Streptomycin

The usual dosage of streptomycin is 15–25 mg/kg/d (about 1 g/d) injected in one or two divided doses intramuscularly. If administered over 30–60 minutes, it can also be given intravenously. Streptomycin exhibits all the adverse effects typically associated with the aminoglycosides; however, it has greater vestibular toxicity and probably less nephrotoxicity when compared with gentamicin.

Resistance emerges so rapidly and has become so widespread that only a few specific indications for this drug remain:

(1) Plague and tularemia.

(2) Endocarditis caused by *Enterococcus faecalis* or viridans streptococci (use in conjunction with penicillin or vancomycin) in strains that are susceptible to high levels of streptomycin (ie, ≤ 2000 μg/mL). Gentamicin may be substituted for streptomycin in this setting.

(3) Active tuberculosis when other less toxic drugs cannot be used.

(4) Acute brucellosis (in combination with tetracycline).

2. Neomycin, Kanamycin, & Paromomycin

These aminoglycosides are closely related, with similar activity and complete cross-resistance. Systemic use has been abandoned because of oto- and nephrotoxicity.

Ointments containing neomycin, often combined with bacitracin and polymyxin, can be applied to infected superficial skin lesions. While the drug mixture covers most staphylococci, streptococci, and gram-negative bacteria likely to be present, the efficacy of topical application is questionable.

In preparation for elective bowel surgery, 1 g of neomycin is given orally every 6–8 hours for 1–2 days (combined with erythromycin, 1 g) to reduce aerobic bowel flora. Action on gram-negative anaerobes is negligible. In hepatic encephalopathy, the coliform bacteria can be suppressed for prolonged periods by oral neomycin, 1 g every 6–8 hours, during reduced protein intake, resulting in diminished ammonia production. Lactulose is more widely used for this indication.

In addition to oto- and nephrotoxicity, which can result from systemic absorption, neomycin or kanamycin can give rise to allergic reactions when applied topically to skin or eye.

Paromomycin, closely related to neomycin and kanamycin, is poorly absorbed after oral administration and has been used mainly to treat asymptomatic intestinal amebiasis and in doses of 25–30 mg/kg/d in three divided doses for 7 days to treat giardiasis in pregnancy. A dosage of 500 mg orally three or four times daily is marginally effective for cryptosporidiosis in AIDS.

3. Amikacin

Amikacin is a semisynthetic derivative of kanamycin. It is relatively resistant to several of the enzymes that inactivate gentamicin and tobramycin. Many gram-negative enteric bacteria—including many gentamicin-resistant strains of proteus, pseudomonas, enterobacter, and serratia—are inhibited. After injection of 500 mg of amikacin every 12 hours (15 mg/kg/d), peak levels in serum are 10–30 μg/mL. In addition to therapy for serious gram-negative infections, amikacin is sometimes included with other drugs for therapy of *M avium* complex and *Mycobacterium fortuitum* complex.

Like all aminoglycosides, amikacin is nephrotoxic and ototoxic (particularly for the auditory portion of the eighth nerve). Its levels should be monitored in patients with renal failure.

4. Gentamicin

With doses of 5 mg/kg/d of this aminoglycoside, serum levels are sufficient for bactericidal effect against many strains of staphylococci, coliforms, and other gram-negative organisms. Enterococci are resistant unless a penicillin or vancomycin is also given. Gentamicin may be synergistic with penicillins active against pseudomonas, proteus, enterobacter, klebsiella, and other gram-negatives. Sisomicin resembles the C1a component of gentamicin.

Indications, Dosages, & Routes of Administration

Gentamicin is used in serious infections caused by gram-negative bacteria. The usual dosage is 5 mg/kg/d intravenously administered once daily. In endocarditis due to viridans streptococci or *E faecalis*, gentamicin in lower synergistic doses (3 mg/kg/d) is combined with penicillin or ampicillin. A single daily dose of 3 mg/kg is just as effective as divided daily doses in the synergistic treatment of endocarditis due to viridans streptococci. In renal insufficiency, the dose should be adjusted as noted above.

5. Tobramycin

Tobramycin closely resembles gentamicin in antibacterial activity, toxicity, and pharmacologic properties and exhibits partial cross-resistance. It may be effective against some gentamicin-resistant pseudomonads but is not used synergistically with penicillin for enterococcal endocarditis. Dosing is the same as for gentamicin. Tobramycin is also given by aerosol (300 mg twice daily) to patients with cystic fibrosis and improves pulmonary function and decreases colonization with pseudomonas without toxicity and without selecting for resistant strains.

Netilmicin shares many characteristics with gentamicin and tobramycin and can be given in a similar dosage. It may be less ototoxic and less nephrotoxic than the other aminoglycosides.

6. Spectinomycin

Spectinomycin is an aminocyclitol antibiotic (related to aminoglycosides) for intramuscular administration. Its sole application is in the treatment of uncomplicated urogenital and anorectal gonorrhea in persons who are hypersensitive to penicillin and who cannot tolerate fluoroquinolones. It is not effective for pharyngeal gonorrhea.

Banerjee D et al: The treatment of respiratory pseudomonas infection in cystic fibrosis—what drug and which way. Drugs 2000; 60: 1053. [PMID: 11129122]

Edson RS et al: The aminoglycosides. Mayo Clin Proc 1999;74:519. [PMID: 10319106]

Mingeot-Leclercq MP et al: Aminoglycosides: activity and resistance. Antimicrob Ag Chemother 1999;43:727. [PMID: 10103173]

POLYMYXINS

The polymyxins are basic polypeptides that are bactericidal for most gram-negative aerobic rods, including pseudomonas. Because of poor distribution into tissues and substantial toxicity (primarily nephrotoxicity and neurotoxicity), systemic use of these agents is limited to infections caused by multidrug-resistant gram-negative organisms that are sensitive only to the polymyxins. Polymyxins B and E (colistin) are the only parenteral agents available. Dosage adjustments are required with renal insufficiency.

ANTITUBERCULOUS DRUGS

Singular problems exist in the treatment of tuberculosis and other mycobacterial infections. The organisms are intracellular, have long periods of metabolic inactivity, and tend to develop resistance to any one drug. Therefore, combined drug therapy is employed to delay the emergence of this resistance. First-line drugs, increasingly used together in all tuberculosis, are isoniazid, ethambutol, rifampin, and pyrazinamide.

See Chapter 9 for a discussion of these medications.

ALTERNATIVE DRUGS IN TUBERCULOSIS TREATMENT

The drugs listed alphabetically below are usually considered only in cases of drug resistance (clinical or laboratory) to first-line drugs.

Aminosalicylic acid (PAS), closely related to *p*-aminobenzoic acid, inhibits most tubercle bacilli but has no effect on other bacteria.

Aminosalicylic acid is readily absorbed from the gastrointestinal tract, and the usual dosage is 8–12 g/d orally. The drug is widely distributed in tissues (except the central nervous system) and rapidly excreted into the urine.

Common side effects include anorexia, nausea, diarrhea, and epigastric pain. Sodium aminosalicylate may be given parenterally. Hypersensitivity reactions include fever, skin rashes, granulocytopenia, lymphadenopathy, and arthralgias.

Clofazimine is a phenazine dye used in the treatment of leprosy and is active in vitro against *M avium* complex and *M tuberculosis*. It is given orally as a single daily dose of 100 mg for treatment of *M avium* complex disease. Its clinical efficacy for the therapy of tuberculosis has not been established. Adverse effects include nausea, vomiting, abdominal pain, and skin discoloration from red-brown to black.

Capreomycin is an injectable agent given intramuscularly in doses of 15–30 mg/kg/d (maximal dose 1 g). Major toxicities include ototoxicity (both vestibular and cochlear) and nephrotoxicity. If the drug must be used in older patients, the dose should not exceed 750 mg.

Cycloserine, a bacteriostatic agent, is given in doses of 15–20 mg/kg (not to exceed 1 g) orally and has been used in re-treatment regimens and for primary therapy of highly resistant *M tuberculosis*. It can induce a variety of central nervous system dysfunctions and psychotic reactions. These may be controlled by phenytoin, 100 mg/d orally, or pyridoxine, 50–100 mg daily.

Ethionamide, like cycloserine, is bacteriostatic and is given orally in a dose of 15–20 mg/kg (maximal dose 1 g). It has been used in combination therapy but produces marked gastric irritation and is the least well tolerated antimycobacterial agent.

The **fluoroquinolones** ofloxacin, ciprofloxacin, and moxifloxacin are active in vitro against *M tuberculosis*, with MICs of 0.25–2 µg/mL. Limited data suggest that these drugs are efficacious in therapy of tuberculosis, particularly in re-treatment regimens. In re-treatment schedules or for infection with resistant organisms, high doses should be used (ciprofloxacin, 750 mg orally twice daily; ofloxacin, 400 mg orally twice daily).

Telenti A et al: Drug-resistant tuberculosis: What do we do now? Drugs 2000;59:171. [PMID: 10730543]

Van Scoy RE et al: Antimycobacterial therapy. Mayo Clin Proc 1999;74:1038. [PMID: 10918872]

SULFONAMIDES & ANTIFOLATE DRUGS

More than 150 different sulfonamides have been marketed at one time or another, the modifications being designed principally to achieve greater antibacterial activity, a wider antibacterial spectrum, greater solubility, or more prolonged action.

Antimicrobial Activity

Sulfonamides are structural analogs of *p*-aminobenzoic acid (PABA) and compete with PABA to block its conversion to dihydrofolic acid. Organisms that utilize PABA in the synthesis of folates and pyrimidines are inhibited. Animal cells and some resistant microorganisms (eg, enterococci) use exogenous folate and thus are not affected by sulfonamides.

Trimethoprim, pyrimethamine, and trimetrexate are compounds that inhibit the conversion of dihydrofolic acid to tetrahydrofolic acid by blocking the enzyme dihydrofolate reductase. These agents have been used alone or (more commonly) in combination with other drugs (usually sulfonamides) to prevent or treat a number of bacterial and parasitic infections. At high doses, all can inhibit mammalian dihydrofolate reductase, but clinically this is a problem only with pyrimethamine and trimetrexate. Folinic acid (leucovorin) is given concurrently with pyrimethamine and trimetrexate to prevent bone marrow suppression.

Sulfonamides alone are rarely used in the treatment of bacterial infection. When used in combination with other drugs, sulfonamides are useful in the treatment of toxoplasmosis and pneumocystosis.

The combination of trimethoprim (TMP) (one part) plus sulfamethoxazole (SMZ) (five parts) is bactericidal for such gram-negative organisms as *E coli*, klebsiella, enterobacter, salmonella, and shigella, though resistance has emerged. It is also active against many strains of serratia, providencia, *Stenotrophomonas maltophilia*, *Burkholderia cepacia* (formerly *Pseudomonas cepacia*), and *Burkholderia pseudomallei*, but not against *P aeruginosa*. It is inactive against anaerobes and enterococci but inhibits most nocardia

and *S aureus* and about 50% *S epidermidis*. *M catarrhalis*, *H influenzae*, *H ducreyi*, *L monocytogenes*, and some atypical mycobacteria are also inhibited by this combination.

Pharmacokinetics & Administration

Trimethoprim-sulfamethoxazole is well absorbed from the gastrointestinal tract and widely distributed in tissues and fluids, including cerebrospinal fluid. For patients who are unable to take oral drugs, intravenous trimethoprim-sulfamethoxazole is available. Dosage adjustment is required for significant renal impairment (creatine clearance ≤ 50 mL/min).

Clinical Uses

Present indications for sulfonamides include the following.

A. URINARY TRACT INFECTIONS

Coliform bacteria, the commonest cause of urinary tract infections, generally remain susceptible to sulfonamides, though resistance of *E coli* has emerged. Short-course therapy (3 days) with double-strength TMP-SMZ (160 mg TMP + 800 mg SMZ) given twice daily is effective therapy for lower urinary tract infections in women who are symptomatic for less than a week. Since TMP is concentrated in the prostate, TMP-SMZ, one double-strength tablet twice daily for 14–21 days, is effective in acute prostatitis. In chronic prostatitis, treatment for 6–12 weeks is indicated. Considering the above resistance trend, the routine use of TMP-SMZ for empirical therapy of urinary tract infections has been questioned. In those areas where resistance of *E coli* is greater than 10–20%, alternative agents should be used as empirical therapy.

B. PARASITIC INFECTIONS

TMP-SMZ is effective for prophylaxis and treatment of pneumocystis pneumonia, cyclospora infection, and *Isospora belli* infection. For therapy of pneumocystis pneumonia, 15–20 mg/kg/d of trimethoprim and 75–100 mg/kg/d of sulfamethoxazole in three or four divided doses is administered intravenously or orally—depending upon the severity of disease—for 3 weeks. The dose for prophylaxis is 160 mg TMP + 800 mg SMZ daily or three times per week. (When given daily, it is also effective prophylaxis against toxoplasmal encephalitis.) *I belli* infection in AIDS has been successfully treated with 160 mg TMP + 800 mg SMZ orally four times daily for 10 days followed by twice-daily administration for 3 weeks. Treatment with 160 mg TMP + 800 mg SMZ three times a week or 500 mg sulfadoxine with 25 mg pyrimethamine once a week has prevented recurrences. Cyclosporiasis is successfully treated with 160 mg TMP and 800 mg SMZ twice daily for 7–10 days. Sulfadiazine with pyrimethamine is also used to treat and prevent recurrence of toxoplasmosis and sulfadoxine plus pyrimeth-amine is used to treat chloroquine-resistant falciparum malaria.

C. BACTERIAL INFECTIONS

Sulfonamides are the drugs of choice for nocardia infections. TMP-SMZ is widely distributed in tissues, penetrates into the cerebrospinal fluid and has been used to treat meningitis caused by gram-negative rods, though third-generation cephalosporins are now preferred. TMP-SMZ is a frequent choice for management of acute sinusitis, otitis media, and infection with susceptible strains of shigella. While it still is used for outpatient respiratory tract infections, the increasing pattern of resistance associated with *S pneumoniae* has decreased its utility. The usual dose for adults is 160 mg TMP + 800 mg SMZ twice daily for 10 days.

TMP-SMZ is effective also for infections with enterobacter, *B pseudomallei* (melioidosis), *Stenotrophomonas maltophilia,* or *Burkholderia cepacia;* in combination with rifampin, for eradication of nasopharyngeal carriage of staphylococci; for prophylaxis against meningococcal disease when susceptible strains predominate; for antibacterial prophylaxis in organ transplant recipients or patients with chronic granulomatous disease; for treatment of *Listeria monocytogenes* meningitis; and perhaps also for management of pulmonary Wegener's granulomatosis.

D. LEPROSY

Certain sulfones are widely used (see below).

Adverse Effects

Adverse reactions to sulfonamides occur in 10–15% of non-AIDS patients (usually a minor rash or gastrointestinal disturbance) and in up to 50% of patients with AIDS (predominantly rash, fever, neutropenia, and thrombocytopenia, often severe enough to require discontinuation of therapy). These drugs have many side effects—due partly to hypersensitivity, partly to direct toxicity—that must be considered whenever unexplained symptoms or signs occur in a patient who may have received these drugs.

A. SYSTEMIC SIDE EFFECTS

Fever, skin rashes, urticaria; nausea, vomiting, or diarrhea; stomatitis, conjunctivitis, arthritis, aseptic meningitis, exfoliative dermatitis; bone marrow depression, thrombocytopenia, hemolytic (in G6PD deficiency) or aplastic anemia, granulocytopenia, leukemoid reactions; hepatitis, polyarteritis nodosa, vasculitis, Stevens-Johnson syndrome; reversible hyperkalemia; and many others have been reported. Because of the risk of Stevens-Johnson syndrome, patients with a previous rash after TMP-SMZ should not receive the drug again.

HIV-positive patients intolerant to TMP-SMZ can often be desensitized. A 70% success rate has been reported after giving 0.004 mg TMP/0.02 mg SMZ as oral suspension and increasing the dose tenfold each hour to achieve a final dose of 160 mg TMP/500 mg SMZ.

B. URINARY TRACT DISTURBANCES

Older sulfonamides were relatively insoluble and would precipitate in urine. The most commonly used sulfonamides presently (sulfisoxazole and sulfamethoxazole) are quite soluble, and the old admonition to force fluids is no longer warranted. Sulfonamides have been implicated in interstitial nephritis. HIV-positive patients receiving high-dose sulfadiazine therapy are predisposed to crystalluria.

SULFONES USED IN THE TREATMENT OF LEPROSY

A number of drugs closely related to the sulfonamides (eg, dapsone) have been used effectively in the long-term treatment of leprosy. The clinical manifestations of both lepromatous and tuberculoid leprosy can often be suppressed by treatment extending over several years. At least 5–30% of *Mycobacterium leprae* organisms are resistant to dapsone, so initial combined treatment with rifampin is advocated. Dapsone, 100 mg daily, is effective therapy for mild to moderate pneumocystis pneumonia in AIDS when combined with trimethoprim, 20 mg/kg/d in four divided doses. At a dose of 50–100 mg daily or 100 mg two or three times a week, it is effective prophylaxis for *P carinii* infection and, when combined with pyrimethamine, 50 mg per week, also prevents toxoplasma encephalitis in HIV-infected patients.

Absorption, Metabolism, & Excretion

All sulfones are well absorbed from the intestinal tract, are distributed widely in all tissues, and tend to be retained in skin, muscle, liver, and kidney. Skin involved by leprosy contains ten times more drug than normal skin. Sulfones are excreted into the bile and reabsorbed by the intestine, prolonging therapeutic blood levels. Excretion into the urine is variable, and the drug occurs in urine mostly as a glucuronic acid conjugate. Some persons acetylate sulfones slowly and others rapidly; this requires dosage adjustment.

Dosages & Routes of Administration

See Leprosy, Chapter 33, for recommendations.

Adverse Effects

The sulfones may cause any of the side effects listed above for sulfonamides. Anorexia, nausea, and vomiting are common. Hemolysis, methemoglobinemia, or agranulocytosis may occur. G6PD levels should be determined prior to initiation of dapsone therapy. If sulfones are not tolerated, clofazimine can be substituted.

SPECIALIZED DRUGS USED AGAINST BACTERIA

1. Bacitracin

This polypeptide is selectively active against gram-positive bacteria. Because of severe nephrotoxicity upon systemic administration, its use has been limited to topical application on surface lesions, usually in combination with polymyxin or neomycin.

2. Mupirocin

Mupirocin (formerly pseudomonic acid) is a naturally occurring antibiotic produced by *Pseudomonas fluorescens* that is active against most gram-positive cocci, including methicillin-sensitive and methicillin-resistant *S aureus* and most streptococci (but not enterococci). It is used topically. It is effective in eliminating staphylococcal nasal carriage in the majority of patients for up to 3 months after application to the anterior nares twice daily for 5 days. However, recurrent colonization occurs (50% at the end of 1 year) and when mupirocin is used chronically over months, resistant organisms can emerge. Monthly application for 5 days each month for up to a year decreases staphylococcal colonization, which in turn lowers the risk of recurrent staphylococcal skin infections. Whether it is more effective than trimethoprim-sulfamethoxazole or dicloxacillin plus rifampin for eradication of staphylococcal nasal carriage is unknown. The other major use of mupirocin is for therapy of impetigo; it is useful in mild disease.

3. Clindamycin

Clindamycin resembles erythromycin (though different in structure) and is active against gram-positive organisms including *S pneumoniae*, viridans streptococci, group A streptococci, and *S aureus*, though resistance has been described in all of these organisms. Enterococci, methicillin-resistant *S aureus*, and most *S epidermidis* isolates are resistant. A dosage of 0.15–0.3 g orally every 6 hours generally is used. It is widely distributed in tissues but not in cerebrospinal fluid. Excretion is primarily nonrenal. Clindamycin is an alternative to erythromycin as a substitute for penicillin. Clindamycin is currently recommended as an alternative drug for prophylaxis against endocarditis following oral procedures in patients allergic to amoxicillin. Clindamycin, 300 mg orally twice daily for 7 days, can be used as an alternative to metronidazole for the therapy of bacterial vaginosis. Topical application of a 2% vaginal cream once or twice daily for 7 days is also effective. Clindamycin is active against most anaerobes, including bacteroides, prevotella, clostridium, peptococcus, peptostreptococcus, and fusobacterium. However, 10–20% of bacteroides isolates are resistant, and alternative agents should be considered for life-threatening anaerobic infections due to these organisms. It is frequently used to treat less severe infections in which anaerobes are significant pathogens (eg, aspiration pneumonia, pelvic and abdominal infections), often in combination with other drugs (aminoglycosides, cephalosporins, fluoroquinolones). In patients with necrotizing pneumonia or lung abscess following aspiration, clindamycin appears to be superior to penicillin. Seriously ill patients are given clindamycin, 600–900 mg (20–30 mg/kg/d) intravenously every 8 hours. It has also been of use in staphylococcal osteomyelitis. Because tissue models document that clindamycin significantly decreases toxin production of a number of organisms, the addition of clindamycin to penicillin for therapy of group A streptococcus toxic shock syndrome has been suggested. In the sulfonamide-allergic patient, high-dose clindamycin therapy (600–1200 mg intravenously every 6 hours or 600 mg orally every 6 hours) in conjunction with pyrimethamine has been used to treat toxoplasmosis of the central nervous system and appears to be as effective as pyrimethamine and sulfadiazine. Clindamycin in combination with primaquine is effective in pneumocystis pneumonia, and clindamycin with quinine is of value for falciparum malaria. While useful in brain abscess, clindamycin is ineffective in meningitis.

Common side effects are diarrhea, nausea, and skin rashes. Bloody diarrhea with pseudomembranous colitis has been associated with the administration of clindamycin and other antibiotics. This antibiotic-associated colitis is due to a necrotizing toxin produced by *C difficile*. The organism is resistant to the antimicrobial, is selected out by its presence, and is favored in its growth and toxin production. *C difficile* is usually susceptible to—and can be treated with—vancomycin or metronidazole given orally, though metronidazole is the drug of choice (see below).

4. Metronidazole

Metronidazole is an antiprotozoal drug (see Chapter 35) that also has striking antibacterial effects against most anaerobic gram-negative bacilli (bacteroides, prevotella, fusobacterium) and clostridium species but has minimal activity against other anaerobic gram-positive and microaerophilic organisms. It is well absorbed after oral administration, is widely distributed in tissues. It penetrates well into the cerebrospinal fluid, yielding levels similar to those in serum. The drug is metabolized in the liver, and dosage reduction is required in severe hepatic insufficiency or biliary dysfunction.

Metronidazole is employed in amebiasis and giardiasis (see Chapter 35) and in the following circumstances:

(1) Trichomonas vaginitis responds to either a single dose (2 g) or to 250 mg orally three times daily for 7–10 days. Bacterial vaginosis responds to a single 2 g dose or to 500 mg twice daily for 7 days. Metronidazole vaginal cream (0.75%) applied twice daily for 5 days is also effective.

(2) In anaerobic infections, metronidazole can be given orally or intravenously, 500 mg three times daily (30 mg/kg/d). It is more predictable against *B fragilis* than clindamycin or second-generation cephalosporins with anaerobic activity.

(3) Metronidazole is less expensive and equally as efficacious as oral vancomycin for the therapy of *C difficile* colitis and is the drug of choice for the disease. A dosage of 500 mg orally three times daily is recommended. If oral medication cannot be tolerated, intravenous metronidazole can be tried at the same dose; however, this route is unproved and usually less effective than the oral one. Because of the emergence of vancomycin-resistant enterococci as a major pathogen and the role of oral vancomycin in selecting for these resistant organisms, metronidazole should be used as first-line therapy for *C difficile* disease.

(4) Preparation of the colon before bowel surgery.

(5) Therapy of brain abscess, often in combination with penicillin or a third-generation cephalosporin.

(6) In combination with clarithromycin and omeprazole for therapy of *H pylori* infections.

Adverse effects include stomatitis, nausea, and diarrhea. Ingestion of alcohol while taking metronidazole can result in a disulfiram reaction. With prolonged use at high doses, reversible peripheral neuropathy can develop. Metronidazole can decrease the metabolism of warfarin and increase the prothrombin time, necessitating monitoring of the prothrombin time and dosage adjustment of warfarin when both drugs are used together. Metronidazole is carcinogenic in certain animal models and mutagenic for certain bacteria, but to date an increased incidence of malignancy has not been confirmed in humans.

Kasten MJ: Clindamycin, metronidazole, and chloramphenicol. Mayo Clin Proc 1999;74:825. [PMID: 10473362] (Clinical review.)

Smilack JD: Trimethoprim-sulfamethoxazole. Mayo Clin Proc 1999;74:730. [PMID: 10405706] (Review of clinical indications and adverse effects.)

5. Vancomycin

This drug is bactericidal for most gram-positive organisms, particularly staphylococci and streptococci, and is bacteriostatic for most enterococci. While active against staphylococci, vancomycin kills more slowly when compared with nafcillin. Although vancomycin has retained activity against staphylococci and streptococci, vancomycin-resistant strains of enterococci (particularly *Enterococcus faecium*) have become a major problem. *Staphylococcus aureus* only intermediately sensitive to the drug has been observed in patients receiving long-term vancomycin therapy. Vancomycin is not absorbed from the gastrointestinal tract. It is given orally only for the treatment of antibiotic-associated enterocolitis. For systemic effect the drug must be administered intravenously (20–30 mg/kg/d in two or three divided doses). An intravenous injection of 10 mg/kg over a period of 20 minutes yields blood levels of 20–30 μg/mL. Vancomycin is excreted mainly via the kidneys. In renal insufficiency, the half-life may be up to 8 days. Thus, only one dose of 0.5–1 g may be given every 4–8 days to a uremic individual undergoing standard chronic hemodialysis. However, vancomycin is cleared via high-flux hemodialysis, necessitating postdialysis dosing. Patients receiving continuous arteriovenous hemofiltration (CAVH) generally required daily dosing. In patients with impaired renal function, the dosing interval is determined by measuring serum levels. When levels decline to 5–15 μg/mL, repeat dosing is required.

Indications for parenteral vancomycin include the following: (1) Severe staphylococcal infections in penicillin-allergic patients; it is the drug of choice for methicillin-resistant *S aureus* and *S epidermidis* infections and for serious infections (pneumonia, meningitis) due to highly resistant *S pneumoniae*. (2) Severe enterococcal infections in the penicillin-allergic patient, usually in combination with an aminoglycoside. (3) Other gram-positive infections in penicillin-allergic patients, eg, viridans streptococcal endocarditis. (4) Surgical prophylaxis in penicillin-allergic patients. (5) For gram-positive infections due to organisms that are multidrug-resistant, ie, *Corynebacterium jeikeium*. (6) Endocarditis prophylaxis in the penicillin-allergic patient undergoing certain genitourinary and gastrointestinal procedures (in combination with an aminoglycoside). (See Table 33–3.)

In antibiotic-associated enterocolitis, vancomycin, 0.125 g, is given orally four times daily.

Vancomycin is irritating to tissues; thrombophlebitis sometimes follows intravenous injection. The drug is infrequently ototoxic when given concomitantly with aminoglycosides or high-dose intravenous erythromycins; it is potentially nephrotoxic when administered with aminoglycosides. Rapid infusion or high doses (1 g or more) may induce diffuse hyperemia ("red man syndrome") and can be avoided by extending infusions over 1–2 hours, by reducing the dose, or by pretreating with a histamine antagonist such as hydroxyzine.

Smith TL et al: Emergence of vancomycin resistance in *Staphylococcus aureus*. Glycopeptide-Intermediate *Staphylococcus aureus* Working Group. N Engl J Med 1999;340:493. [PMID: 10021469]

Wilhelm MP et al: Vancomycin. Mayo Clin Proc 1999;74:928. [PMID: 10488798] (Review.)

STREPTOGRAMINS

Streptogramins are structurally similar to macrolides but do not share cross-resistance with that class. **Pristinamycin** is an oral streptogramin marketed in France for treatment of gram-positive infections. **Synercid** is a combination of two synthetic derivatives of pristinamycin—quinupristin and dalfopristin—in a 30:70 ratio that is administered intravenously. It is bactericidal and inhibits protein synthesis by binding to bacterial ribosomes. In vitro, it has activity against *Moraxella catarrhalis, Haemophilus influenzae,* clostridium, peptostreptococcus, mycoplasma, legionella, and chlamydia. It has no activity against enteric gram-negative bacilli. However, its major clinical use is in the therapy of gram-positive infections, including those due to streptococci (including penicillin-resistant pneumococci) staphylococci (including methicillin-sensitive and methicillin-resistant *S aureus* and *S epidermidis*) and enterococci, including vancomycin-resistant *Enterococcus faecium.* The combination is not reliably active against *E faecalis.* The drug is generally bacteriostatic against the enterococci. The recommended dose is 7.5 mg/kg intravenously every 8 hours. In addition to phlebitis with peripheral administration, the major adverse effect is arthralgias and myalgias that resolve with discontinuation of the drug. It is primarily cleared via the liver; streptogramins inhibit the cytochrome P450 system, resulting in increased levels of cyclosporine and other agents.

Delgado G Jr et al: Quinupristin-dalfopristin: an overview. Pharmacotherapy 2000;20:1469. [PMID: 11130220]

OXAZOLIDINONES

Oxazolidinones represent a new class of antibacterials of which linezolid is the first released. Linezolid is primarily active against aerobic gram-positive pathogens, including penicillin-resistant pneumococci, methicillin-resistant staphylococci and enterococci (both *E faecalis* and vancomycin-sensitive and vancomycin-resistant *E faecium*). Linezolid is bacteriostatic against all of these pathogens. Linezolid-resistant and vancomycin-resistant enterococci and linezolid-resistant *S aureus* may be encountered, however. The oral bioavailability of linezolid is complete, with serum levels approaching those observed with intravenous administration. The drug is eliminated primarily by nonrenal mechanisms. The primary toxicity is bone marrow suppression with long-term therapy, particularly the platelet line. Other adverse effects include tongue discoloration and mild MAO inhibition.

Diekema DJ, Jones RN. Oxazolidinone antibiotics. Lancet 2001;358:1975. [PMID: 11747939] (Review of spectrum, toxicity, and indications.)

Linezolid (Zyvox). Med Lett Drugs Ther 2000;42:45. [PMID: 10859730]

QUINOLONES

The quinolones are synthetic analogs of nalidixic acid that have an exceedingly broad spectrum of activity against many bacteria. The mode of action of all quinolones involves inhibition of bacterial DNA synthesis by blocking the enzyme DNA gyrase.

The earlier quinolones (nalidixic acid, oxolinic acid, cinoxacin) did not achieve systemic antibacterial levels after oral intake and thus were useful only as urinary antiseptics. The newer fluorinated derivatives (norfloxacin, ciprofloxacin, ofloxacin, lomefloxacin, levofloxacin, gatifloxacin, and moxifloxacin) have more potent antibacterial activity, achieve clinically useful levels in blood and tissues, and have low toxicity.

Antimicrobial Activity

A number of fluoroquinolones are in use. Most have quite similar spectrums of activity. In general, these drugs have excellent activity against Enterobacteriaceae but are also active against other gram-negative bacteria such as haemophilus, neisseria, moraxella, brucella, legionella, salmonella, shigella, campylobacter, yersinia, vibrio, and aeromonas. Ciprofloxacin has slightly better activity against *P aeruginosa* than the other fluoroquinolones, but the increasing resistance of *P aeruginosa* to ciprofloxacin limits its utility for infections caused by that organism. None of these agents have reliable activity against *S maltophilia* or *B cepacia*—though the newer drugs are more active against *S maltophilia*—as they are for treating genital tract pathogens such as *Mycoplasma hominis, Ureaplasma urealyticum,* and *C pneumoniae. M tuberculosis* is sensitive to the quinolones, as is *M fortuitum* and *Mycobacterium kansasii.* Although most *M avium* complex organisms are resistant to fluoroquinolones when combined with other antibiotics (ethambutol, rifabutin, and amikacin), ciprofloxacin is effective in treating infections caused by this organism.

In general, the fluoroquinolones are less active against gram-positive than gram-negative organisms, with norfloxacin and lomefloxacin having less activity than ciprofloxacin and ofloxacin and levofloxacin, gatifloxacin, and moxifloxacin the greatest activity. Ciprofloxacin and ofloxacin are active against some strains of *S aureus* and *S epidermidis,* including some methicillin-resistant strains. However, the emergence of ciprofloxacin-resistant strains of staphylococci have limited the use of these drugs as monotherapy of infections caused by these organisms. Enterococci, including *E faecalis, S pneumoniae,* group A, B, and D streptococci, and viridans streptococci, are only moderately sensitive to the older quinolones. Anaerobic bacteria, *T pallidum,* and nocardia are resistant to the earlier fluoroquinolones.

Levofloxacin, gatifloxacin, and moxifloxacin are very similar to the previously described fluoroquinolones with the notable exception of improved activity against streptococci, including penicillin-resistant pneumococci. Gatifloxacin and moxifloxacin also demonstrate activity against many of the significant anaerobic pathogens, including *Bacteroides fragilis* and mouth anaerobes.

Pharmacokinetics & Administration (Table 37–9)

After oral administration, the fluoroquinolones are well absorbed and widely distributed in body fluids

Table 37–9. Pharmacology of the quinolones.

Drug	Peak Serum Levels (µg/mL)	Serum Half-Life (h)	Total Daily Dose	Dosage Adjustments in Renal Failure			
				Dosage Interval (h)	Moderate (Cl$_{cr}$ 10–50 mL/min)	Severe (Cl$_{cr}$ < 10 mL/min)	Posthemo-dialysis Dose
Ciprofloxacin	3–4 (400 mg IV, 500–750 mg PO)	3–6	800–1200 mg (IV), 0.5–1.5 g (PO)	8–12	400 mg q12h	200 mg q12h	None
Gatifloxacin	4–5 (400 mg PO or IV)	7	400 mg	24	200 mg q24h	200 mg q24h	200 mg
Levofloxacin	5–7 (500 mg PO or IV)	6–8	250–500 mg	24	250 mg q24–48h	250 mg q48h	None
Moxifloxacin	3–4 (400 mg PO)	12	400 mg	24	400 mg q24h	400 mg q24h	Not known
Ofloxacin	5–7 (400 mg PO or IV)	6–8	400–800 mg	12	200–400 mg q24h	200 mg q24h	None

and tissues and are concentrated intracellularly. Fluoroquinolones are bound by some heavy metals, and absorption is inhibited when they are given with iron, calcium, and other multivalent cations. Optimal oral bioavailability is achieved if they are given about 1 hour before or 2 hours after meals. The serum half-life ranges from 4 hours (ciprofloxacin) to 12 hours (moxifloxacin). After ingestion of 500 mg, the peak serum level of ciprofloxacin is 2.5 µg/mL and is lower than that of the other quinolones (4–6 µg/mL), but this is offset by ciprofloxacin's slightly greater in vitro activity against most gram-negative organisms. A number of the fluoroquinolones can be administered intravenously, resulting in peak serum levels ranging from 4 to 9 µg/mL. Most are eliminated via mixed renal and nonrenal pathways. As a result, only modest accumulation takes place in the presence of renal insufficiency. Exceptions are ofloxacin, levofloxacin, lomefloxacin, and gatifloxacin, which are primarily dependent upon the kidney for elimination.

Clinical Uses

Because of their broad spectrum of activity and a tendency for some organisms (eg, *P aeruginosa,* staphylococcal species) to develop resistance, these drugs should not be routinely used as first-line therapy when less expensive agents with narrower spectrums are available.

Urinary tract infections caused by trimethoprim-sulfamethoxazole-resistant gram-negative organisms have resulted in quinolones being recognized as one of the drugs of choice in areas with > 10–20% resistance of *E coli* to trimethoprim-sulfamethoxazole.

Because of good penetration into prostatic tissue, quinolones are effective in treating bacterial prostatitis and are alternatives to trimethoprim-sulfamethoxazole (doses for prostatitis are the same as for urinary tract infection, but the duration should be 6–12 weeks).

Quinolones have been approved for use in therapy of certain sexually transmitted diseases. Ofloxacin, 300 mg twice daily for 7 days, is as effective as doxycycline, 100 mg twice daily for 7 days, for the therapy of *C trachomatis* cervicitis, urethritis, and proctitis. It is also effective for nongonococcal urethritis caused by *U urealyticum.* Ciprofloxacin is not effective for the therapy of chlamydial infections or nongonococcal urethritis. In general, the use of quinolones for the therapy of any sexually transmitted disease will be limited by their lack of efficacy in concomitant syphilis. Gonococcal urethritis, cervicitis, pharyngitis, and proctitis can be treated with a single dose of 500 mg of ciprofloxacin, 400 mg of ofloxacin, or 400 mg of enoxacin.

Pelvic inflammatory disease is usually caused by *Chlamydia trachomatis, N gonorrhoeae,* Enterobacteriaceae, or anaerobes. Oral outpatient treatment with ofloxacin, 400 mg twice daily for 14 days, in addition to clindamycin, 450 mg orally four times daily for 14 days, or metronidazole, 500 mg orally twice daily for 14 days, can be used. Epididymitis in young men (< 35 years of age) is caused most commonly by chlamydia and the gonococcus, and outpatient therapy with single-dose ciprofloxacin (500 mg) or ofloxacin (400 mg) followed by doxycycline, 100 mg twice daily for 10 days, is adequate therapy. Alternatively, ofloxacin, 300 mg twice daily for 10 days, can be used. *H ducreyi,* the agent that causes chancroid, is sensitive to quinolones, and ciprofloxacin, 500 mg twice daily, or enoxacin, 400 mg daily for 3 days, can be used as an alternative to erythromycin, azithromycin, or ceftriaxone as therapy for this disease.

N gonorrhoeae resistant to fluoroquinolones has been reported with increasing frequency in the United States. The recommendations cited above for therapy of sexually transmitted diseases in which *N gonorrhoeae* is a potential pathogen may have to be revised since resistance will limit the usefulness of this class of drugs.

Ciprofloxacin and ofloxacin have been successfully used to treat complicated skin and soft tissue infections and osteomyelitis caused by gram-negative organisms. Ciprofloxacin, 500–750 mg twice daily for at least 6 weeks, has been effective therapy for malignant otitis externa.

Because quinolones are the only available oral agents active against campylobacter despite increasing resistance, in addition to the other major bacterial pathogens associated with diarrhea (salmonella, shigella, toxigenic *E coli*), they have been used for the therapy of traveler's diarrhea as well as domestically acquired acute diarrhea. Norfloxacin, ciprofloxacin, and ofloxacin may be effective in eradicating the chronic carrier state of salmonella when therapy is continued for 4–6 weeks.

Ciprofloxacin has been used to eradicate meningococci from the nasopharynx of carriers.

Fluoroquinolones are effective for prophylaxis against gram-negative infections in the neutropenic patient, and intravenous ciprofloxacin in combination with β-lactam antibiotics has been used successfully to treat the febrile neutropenic patient.

Although some clinical studies have suggested that ciprofloxacin is efficacious in the therapy of community-acquired pneumonia, caution should be exercised since the drug has only marginal activity against *S pneumoniae* and *M pneumoniae,* and failures in treating pneumococcal pneumonia have been reported. Newer agents such as levofloxacin, gatifloxacin, and moxifloxacin are more active against the pneumococci, including penicillin-resistant strains, and are useful in the treatment of infections due to these organisms. However, their broad spectrum of activity against resistant aerobic gram-negative pathogens suggests that they should be reserved for the treatment of refractory infections. One setting in which ciprofloxacin is indicated for the therapy of lower respiratory tract infections is in cystic fibrosis, where *P aeruginosa* is the predominant pathogen. However, the increasing rate of resistance to ciprofloxacin has impacted upon use of the drug for this indication.

Ciprofloxacin in combination with other agents has been used to treat *M avium* complex infections, and ciprofloxacin, ofloxacin, and moxifloxacin may be efficacious in the therapy of multidrug-resistant tuberculosis.

Adverse Effects

The most prominent adverse effects of the quinolones are nausea, vomiting, and diarrhea. Occasionally, headache, dizziness, seizures, insomnia, impaired liver function, and skin rashes have been observed as well as more serious reactions such as acute renal failure and anaphylaxis. Severe hepatotoxicity, including liver failure and the need for liver transplantation, has occurred with trovafloxacin use. Although the drug has not been withdrawn, a warning by the FDA has been issued, and trovafloxacin should not be used unless there are no other alternatives. Fluoroquinolones as a class prolong the QT interval; grepafloxacin has been withdrawn from the market as a result of this effect. Quinolones should be used cautiously in patients receiving antiarrhythmics such as amiodarone or in persons with a history of prolonged QT. Ciprofloxacin appears least likely to prolong the QT. Clearance of theophylline may be inhibited by fluoroquinolones (especially enoxacin), and drug levels should be monitored in patients receiving both drugs. Prolongation of the prothrombin time has been observed in some patients receiving stable doses of warfarin after ciprofloxacin has been given, but this interaction is unpredictable and modest. Tendonitis and tendon rupture have been reported with quinolone agents, especially pefloxacin. Risk factors include concomitant glucocorticoid use and hepatic and renal failure. Patients experiencing musculoskeletal symptoms while receiving fluoroquinolones should discontinue therapy.

Gatifloxacin and moxifloxacin: two new fluoroquinolones. Med Lett Drugs Ther 2000;432:15. [PMID: 10705891]

Hooper DC: New uses for new and old quinolones and the challenge of resistance. Clin Infect Dis 2000;30:243. [PMID: 10671323]

Tillotson GS et al: New milestones achieved in fluoroquinolone safety. Pharmacotherapy 2001;21:358. [PMID: 11253861] (Association of toxicities with newer fluoroquinolones.)

Walker RC: The fluoroquinolones. Mayo Clin Proc 1999;74:1030. [PMID: 10918871]

PENTAMIDINE & ATOVAQUONE

Pentamidine and atovaquone are antiprotozoal agents that are primarily used to treat pneumocystis pneumonia. Pentamidine is discussed in Chapters 31 and 35. Atovaquone inhibits mitochondrial electron transport and probably also folate metabolism. It is poorly absorbed and should be given with food to maximize bioavailability. The suspension is significantly better absorbed than the tablet formulation and thus should be used preferentially, especially in high-risk patients (those with diarrhea, malabsorption). It has moderate activity against *P carinii*. In comparative trials with trimethoprim-sulfamethoxazole and pentamidine in the therapy of pneumocystis pneumonia in AIDS, atovaquone, 750 mg orally three times daily for 3 weeks, is less effective than both agents but better tolerated. It has also been used as prophylaxis in AIDS patients at a dosage of 1500 mg daily. Major adverse effects include rash, nausea, vomiting, diarrhea, fever, and abnormal liver function tests. The use of atovaquone is limited to patients with mild to moderate pneumocystis infections who have failed or cannot tolerate other therapies.

URINARY ANTISEPTICS

These drugs exert antimicrobial activity in the urine but have little or no systemic antibacterial effect. Their usefulness is limited to therapy and prevention of urinary tract infections.

1. Nitrofurantoin

Nitrofurantoin is active against the common gram-positive urinary pathogens *Enterococcus faecalis* and *Staphylococcus saprophyticus,* but the drug inhibits only about 50% of *Enterococcus faecium*. It is also used against *E coli* and citrobacter, but activity against proteus, serratia, and pseudomonas is poor. Following oral administration, about 50% of the drug is absorbed, but serum concentrations are very low and tissue levels are undetectable. Levels in the urine reach concentrations of 200–400 μg/mL, which are well above the MICs of susceptible organisms. Because clearance is primarily renal, the amounts of these drugs in the urine are proportionate to the creatinine clearance, and with severe renal insufficiency subtherapeutic levels are present. Given low serum levels, poor tissue penetration, and renal elimination, the use of nitrofurantoin is limited to therapy or prophylaxis of cystitis in patients with normal renal function. Nitrofurantoin should not be used to treat pyelonephritis or prostatitis.

The average daily dose in urinary tract infections is 100 mg orally four times daily, taken with food. The macrocrystal preparation can be given at a dosage of 100 mg twice daily. A single daily dose of 50–100 mg can prevent recurrent urinary tract infections in women.

Oral nitrofurantoin often causes nausea and vomiting. The crystalline formulation is better tolerated than previous preparations. Hemolytic anemia may occur in G6PD deficiency. Other side effects are skin rashes and, uncommonly, peripheral neuropathy. Acute and chronic pulmonary hypersensitivity reactions may occur, and pulmonary fibrosis has occurred with prolonged use.

2. Fosfomycin

Fosfomycin tromethamine is a phosphonic acid derivative useful in the treatment of uncomplicated urinary tract infection. The spectrum of activity includes *E coli, E faecalis,* and other gram-negative aerobic urinary pathogens, but not *P aeruginosa*. Available as a 3 g sachet, fosfomycin may be useful for the single-dose treatment of the above organisms. Like nitrofurantoin, fosfomycin should not be used for systemic infection. However, the increased concentrations in urine allow for its use in uncomplicated bacteriuria. The most frequently reported adverse effects include diarrhea, headache, and nausea.

Gupta K et al: Increasing prevalence of antimicrobial resistance among uropathogens causing acute uncomplicated cystitis in women. JAMA 1999;281:736. [PMID: 10052444]

Nicolle LE et al (editors): Progress in the management of urinary tract infections. J Antimicrob Chemother 2000;46(Suppl 1).

SYSTEMICALLY ACTIVE DRUGS IN URINARY TRACT INFECTIONS

Many antimicrobial drugs are excreted in the urine in high concentrations. For this reason, low and relatively nontoxic dosages of penicillins, cephalosporins, aminoglycosides, quinolones, and trimethoprim-sulfamethoxazole can reach high urinary concentrations and are effective in uncomplicated urinary tract infections.

ANTIFUNGAL DRUGS

Empirical antifungal therapy is rarely instituted except for febrile neutropenic patients. Therapy is reserved for situations in which yeast or mold is seen on KOH preparation or when isolated organisms are thought to be pathogenic. Antifungal sensitivity testing recently has been standardized for yeasts but not for molds and is not routinely recommended. Thus, therapy generally is based on experience and clinical trials and not on susceptibility tests.

1. Amphotericin B

Amphotericin B in vitro inhibits several organisms producing systemic mycotic disease in humans, including aspergillus, histoplasma, cryptococcus, coccidioides, candida, blastomyces, sporothrix, and others. This drug can be used for treatment of these systemic fungal infections. Intraventricular administration may be required in meningitis if systemic therapy fails. *Pseudallescheria boydii* and fusarium are often resistant to amphotericin B.

There is no consensus on how amphotericin B should be administered or on the dosage and the duration of therapy. Most centers no longer use a test dose, since anaphylaxis is extremely rare. The daily dose of amphotericin B for most fungal infections varies from 0.3 mg/kg to 0.7 mg/kg, though infections caused by aspergillus and mucor are often treated with 1–1.5 mg/kg daily.

In meningitis due to fungi other than *Coccidioides immitis,* long-term therapy beyond the initial 8–10 weeks is rarely needed. Combined treatment with flucytosine is beneficial in cryptococcal meningitis and possibly systemic candidiasis. Amphotericin B may have some benefit in naegleria meningoencephalitis.

Amphotericin B in low doses (0.1–0.25 mg/kg/d) has been used prophylactically to prevent invasive fungal infections in bone marrow transplant recipients and may be beneficial in this setting. Whether prophylactic administration is better than early empirical therapy in febrile patients who have not responded to broad-spectrum antibiotics has not been determined.

In patients with Foley catheters in place who have candiduria, amphotericin B bladder irrigations have been used to decrease colony counts. Although the procedure is widely used, the efficacy of amphotericin B bladder irrigation is marginal, and long-term eradication of candiduria following amphotericin B bladder irrigation rarely occurs.

In impaired renal function, the dose of amphotericin B need not be reduced initially. However, if the serum creatinine reaches 2.5–3 mg/dL, either a less nephrotoxic liposomal formulation of amphotericin can be used (see below) or the dose can be temporarily lowered (or even stopped for a few days) until renal function recovers. Amphotericin B is then resumed at about one-half the previous dosage and increased in increments as tolerated. The drug is not removed by hemodialysis, so that no additional drug is needed after dialysis.

The intravenous administration of amphotericin B often produces chills, fever, vomiting, and headache. As a rule, infusions given over 1–2 hours are as well tolerated as those given over 4–6 hours. However, patients who experience infusion-related adverse effects may benefit from slowing the rate of administration. Tolerance may be enhanced by temporary lowering of the dose or premedication with acetaminophen and diphenhydramine. Addition of 25 mg of hydrocortisone to the infusion decreases the incidence of rigors, and meperidine, 25–50 mg, is effective in arresting rigors once they start. Central intravenous administration eliminates the likelihood of thrombophlebitis. Amphotericin B is associated with anemia and is due to impaired iron utilization. Electrolyte disturbances (hypokalemia, hypomagnesemia, distal renal tubular acidosis) also occur. Renal insufficiency can be prevented with salt supplementation. As a result, administration of 0.5–1 L of 0.9% saline prior to infusion of amphotericin B may prevent nephrotoxicity.

The nephrotoxicity of amphotericin has resulted in the development of lipid-based amphotericin B products. Three such products are available: amphotericin B lipid complex (ABLC; Abelcet), amphotericin B colloidal dispersion (ABCD; Amphotec), and liposomal amphotericin B (L-AmB; AmBisome). Complexing amphotericin B with lipid allows larger doses to be administered (1–6 mg/kg, depending on the preparation and the fungal species). All three preparations are associated with less nephrotoxicity than conventional amphotericin B and thus offer benefit for patients who develop renal insufficiency while receiving amphotericin B. Liposomal amphotericin is less nephrotoxic than ABLC. Infusion-related adverse effects are variable, with liposomal amphotericin being associated with the lowest incidence of fevers and chills even when infused over 30–60 minutes. ABCD is associated with the highest rate of infusion toxicity and requires administration over 2.5–3 hours. ABLC is comparable to conventional amphotericin B. All three have significant differences in serum levels, half-life, and tissue penetration. Most of the information on efficacy is gleaned from open-label trials in patients who failed or were intolerant of conventional amphotericin B and who were infected with aspergillus or candida. Most clinical experience has been with L-Am B, as it has been licensed in Europe for several years. L-Am B is approved for therapy in the febrile neutropenic patient, with efficacy equal to that of conventional amphotericin B in success of therapy and prevention of emergent fungal infections. Direct comparative trials between lipid-based preparations are limited.

Drug acquisition costs for all three products are much higher than for conventional amphotericin B.

Whether decreased toxicity and the decreased need to monitor for adverse effects offset these cost differences is not known. A prudent approach is to reserve lipid-based preparations for patients who fail conventional amphotericin B or those who develop renal insufficiency (serum creatinine 2.5–3 mg/dL). The lipid formulations are particularly effective for therapy of visceral leishmaniasis. Short courses (5–10 days) with low doses (2–24 mg/kg depending on which preparation is used) are very effective in eradicating the parasite, probably because of distribution of the drug to the reticuloendothelial system, the major site of parasite invasion.

Ellis D: Amphotericin B: spectrum and resistance. J Antimicrob Chemother 2002;49(Suppl A):7. [PMID: 11801575]

Patel R: Antifungal agents. Part I. Amphotericin B preparations and flucytosine. Mayo Clin Proc 1998;73:1205. [PMID: 9868423]

2. Nystatin

Nystatin has a wide spectrum of antifungal activity but is used almost exclusively to treat superficial candidal infections. It is too toxic for systemic administration, and the drug is not absorbed from mucous membranes or the gastrointestinal tract. Several preparations are available, including oral suspension (100,000 units/mL) and ointments, gels, and creams (100,000 units/g). For oral candidiasis, 500,000 units of suspension is used to rinse the mouth and is retained in the mouth as long as possible before it is swallowed. This is repeated four times a day for at least 2 days after resolution of the infection. Infections of skin are treated with cream or ointment, 100,000 units applied to the affected area twice daily until resolution of the infection. Nystatin is less effective than miconazole and clotrimazole for therapy of vaginal candidiasis.

3. Flucytosine

Flucytosine inhibits some strains of candida, cryptococcus, aspergillus, and other fungi. Dosages of 3–8 g daily (100–150 mg/kg/d) orally produce good levels in serum and cerebrospinal fluid. Clinical remissions of meningitis or sepsis due to yeasts have occurred. However, resistant organisms are selected out rapidly, and flucytosine is therefore not employed as a single drug except in urinary tract infections.

In renal insufficiency, flucytosine may accumulate to toxic levels, and dosage adjustments are needed. Because patients with HIV infection and normal renal function do not tolerate the normal doses of flucytosine (150 mg/kg/d in four divided doses), 75–100 mg/kg/d is recommended. The drug is effectively removed by hemodialysis. Toxic effects include bone marrow depression, abnormal liver function, loss of hair, and others. Bone marrow suppression is caused by conversion of flucytosine to fluorouracil. Combined use of flucytosine and amphotericin B in cryptococcal meningitis and possibly systemic candidiasis has been shown to be of value.

4. Natamycin

Natamycin is a polyene antifungal drug effective against many different fungi in vitro. When it is combined with appropriate surgical measures, topical application of 5% ophthalmic suspension may be beneficial in the treatment of keratitis caused by fusarium, acremonium (cephalosporium), or other fungi. The drug may also be effective in the treatment of oral or vaginal candidiasis. The toxicity after topical application appears to be low.

5. Terbinafine

Terbinafine, an allylamine, inhibits fungal cell membrane function by blocking ergosterol synthesis. Terbinafine is now available topically as well as in 250 mg tablets for oral administration. The recommended dosage is 250 mg daily for 12 weeks for toenail infections and 250 mg daily for 6 weeks for fingernail infections (success rate about 70%). The drug also is active against many strains of candida and aspergillus and has been used in combination with other antifungals for therapy of severe cutaneous infections with these agents. Terbinafine is well tolerated. Most adverse effects are minor (diarrhea, dyspepsia) or transient (taste disturbance). Rare cases of severe hepatic injury have occurred.

6. Antifungal Imidazoles & Triazoles

These antifungal drugs also inhibit synthesis of ergosterol, resulting in inhibition of membrane-associated enzyme activity, cell wall growth, and replication.

Clotrimazole, taken orally in the form of 10 mg troches five times daily, can prevent and treat oral candidiasis. Vaginal tablets inserted daily for 3–7 days are effective for vaginal candidiasis. Topical preparations for treatment of cutaneous dermatophytes are also available. Toxicity precludes systemic use.

Ketoconazole, an imidazole, can be given orally as a single daily dose of 200–600 mg, preferably with food. The dosage remains the same in renal or hepatic failure. Absorption is impaired by antacids and H_2-blockers; coadministration of phenytoin or rifampin can cause enhanced metabolism of ketoconazole and lower plasma levels. The reduction in achievable serum levels in achlorhydria patients has been associated with decreased efficacy in the treatment of HIV-positive patients with esophageal candidiasis.

While ketoconazole previously was used in the treatment of a variety of fungal infections, the improved spectrum of activity, reduced toxicity, and superior pharmacokinetics of newer azoles have reduced ketoconazole to a secondary role.

Adverse effects include nausea, vomiting, skin rashes, and occasional elevations in aminotransferase levels. Although most elevations of liver enzymes are asymptomatic, on rare occasions symptomatic and even fatal hepatitis can occur. Ketoconazole blocks the synthesis of adrenal steroids and testosterone and can cause gynecomastia and impotence. Ketoconazole can also cause increased levels of cyclosporine (and other agents) when administered with this drug, and careful monitoring of serum levels is needed to avoid toxicity.

Fluconazole, a bis-triazole with activity similar to that of ketoconazole, is water-soluble and can be given both orally and intravenously. Absorption of the drug after oral administration is not pH-dependent, in contrast to ketoconazole, and therapeutic serum levels are obtained even when H_2 receptor antagonists are given simultaneously. It penetrates well into the cerebrospinal fluid and eye. The drug has been shown to be effective primarily in therapy of infections with candida, cryptococcus, and blastomyces. *Candida albicans, C tropicalis,* and *C parapsilosus* are usually sensitive to fluconazole, but many other species of candida (*C krusei, C glabrata,* etc) are often resistant. Fluconazole-resistant strains of *C albicans* have been reported and are usually seen in HIV-positive patients on long-term therapy. With the advent of highly active antiretroviral therapy, the rate of fluconazole resistance in *C albicans* has decreased. The drug is inactive against aspergillus, mucor, and pseudallescheria. Fluconazole is effective in oropharyngeal candidiasis and candidal esophagitis in immunosuppressed patients. It is also valuable in vaginal candidiasis, where a single oral dose of 150 mg is 80–90% effective. Response to fluconazole in leukemic patients with hepatosplenic candidiasis has also been observed, as it has in other invasive infections such as peritonitis, wound infection, and pyelonephritis. Fluconazole, 400 mg daily, is as effective as amphotericin B, 0.5–0.6 mg/kg/d, for candidemia in both neutropenic and nonneutropenic patients. Most of these infections are intravenous line-related, and removal of the line is critical to successful therapy. Fluconazole (200 mg/d) is effective as chronic suppressive therapy of cryptococcal meningitis in patients with AIDS and is the drug of choice in this setting. At a dose of 200 mg/d, response rates and overall mortality rates are the same in patients treated with oral fluconazole and with amphotericin B. However, the mortality rate in the first 2 weeks is higher—and it takes longer to sterilize the cerebrospinal fluid— among patients treated with fluconazole than among patients treated with amphotericin. Most clinicians would initiate therapy with amphotericin B for 2 weeks and then switch to oral fluconazole. A dosage of 400 mg of fluconazole daily is effective therapy for coccidioidal meningitis (80% response), but improvement is slow, taking as long as 4–8 months; efficacy has been observed in both non-HIV-infected and HIV-infected individuals. Higher doses (800–1200 mg/d) have been used; however, it is unclear whether they are superior to usual doses. Fluconazole, 400 mg daily, is effective prophylaxis against superficial and invasive fungal infections in bone marrow and liver transplant recipients, but concern has been raised about superinfection with resistant organisms (*Candida krusei, C glabrata,* aspergillus). The same dose of fluconazole has not reduced the incidence of invasive fungal disease in leukemic patients undergoing intensive chemotherapy and has not reduced the need for amphotericin B. Thus, the use of fluconazole as prophylaxis in the neutropenic patient remains controversial. Because the overall incidence of invasive fungal disease in HIV infection is low, universal prophylaxis to prevent disease in a few should be discouraged, especially with the advent of more potent antiretroviral therapy.

Fluconazole is well absorbed after oral administration (80% bioavailability), and serum levels approach those seen after administering the same dose intravenously. In addition, the intravenous preparation is about ten times more expensive than the oral medication. Thus, unless the patient cannot take medication by mouth or has an overwhelming infection, the preferred route of administration is by mouth.

Itraconazole is an oral triazole with antifungal and pharmacologic properties similar to those of ketoconazole. It is moderately well absorbed from the gastrointestinal tract (food increases absorption from 30% to 60%; antacids and H_2 receptor antagonists decrease absorption) and widely distributed in tissues with the notable exception of the central nervous system, where levels in spinal fluid are undetectable. Itraconazole solution is more predictably absorbed than the tablets. While the tablet formulation should be administered with food, the solution is best absorbed on an empty stomach. A parenteral formulation is available, but it is not approved for patients with renal insufficiency (creatinine clearance < 30 mL/min) because of the risk of pancreatic adenocarcinoma. The drug is metabolized by the liver, and no dosage adjustment is needed in renal insufficiency. Itraconazole is very active against most strains of *Histoplasma capsulatum, Blastomyces dermatitidis, Cryptococcus neoformans, Sporotrichum schenkii,* and various dermatophytes. It is also active against some fluconazole-resistant strains of candida, especially *C albicans,* and aspergillus species but inactive against fusarium and zygomycetes. Itraconazole in doses of 200–400 mg/d is effective and approved therapy for localized or disseminated histoplasmosis and is more effective than ketoconazole in AIDS patients with histoplasmosis. It is also effective prophylaxis against recurrent histoplasmosis in these patients and is also effective as secondary prophylaxis against *P marneffei* infection in AIDS patients. Itraconazole is preferred over ketoconazole for therapy of blastomycosis because it is more efficacious and better tolerated. It is also effective in sporotrichosis, dermatophytic infections (including those of the nails), and oral and esophageal candidiasis. Noncomparative clinical trials indicate efficacy in therapy of invasive aspergillosis (55–80%) and coccidioidomycosis (57–94%). In the absence of comparative trials with other agents active against *C immitis* and aspergillus, it is difficult to know if itraconazole should be used as a first-line drug against these organisms, but the oral route of administration makes the drug attractive, particularly in patients who are not critically ill. At doses of 200 mg twice daily, itraconazole increases exercise tolerance and decreases steroid requirements in patients with allergic bronchopulmonary aspergillosis. Itraconazole has been shown to decrease superficial and invasive fungal infections compared with placebo when used as prophylaxis in neutropenic patients. Itraconazole has been approved for onychomycosis. Pulse therapy with 200 mg twice daily for 1 week each month, repeated for 4 consecutive months, is effective in 70% of cases.

Adverse effects are similar to those of ketoconazole and fluconazole, with anorexia, nausea, vomiting, and abdominal pain occurring most commonly. Skin rash has been reported in up to 8% of patients. Hepatitis and hypokalemia occur uncommonly. Drugs that increase hepatic drug-metabolizing enzymes (isoniazid, rifampin, phenytoin, phenobarbital) may increase itraconazole metabolism, and higher doses may be needed when these drugs are administered concurrently with itraconazole. Itraconazole also impairs the metabolism of cyclosporine and can result in toxic levels unless the dosage is adjusted. Like ketoconazole, itraconazole can increase blood levels of digoxin and warfarin.

The usual dosage is 200 mg once or twice daily with meals. Higher dosages (400–600 mg/d) may be required in patients who are immunocompromised and those with severe disease, especially that due to aspergillus. In patients with life-threatening infections, a 600 mg loading dose is given for 3 or 4 days.

Voriconazole is a new triazole antifungal with broad in vitro activity against a number of pathogens, including most species of candida and molds, aspergillus, fusarium, pseudallescheria, and others. It is as efficacious as liposomal amphotericin in the therapy of documented and suspected fungal infections in febrile neutropenic patients, and it is superior to liposomal amphotericin in preventing breakthrough fungemias. Voriconazole is the drug of choice in the treatment of fusarium infections. Unlike itraconazole, oral administration leads to more predictable absorption. The primary toxicity associated with voriconazole is infusion-related but transient alteration in light perception. This usually resolves with subsequent administrations. Visual hallucinations may occur in patients receiving voriconazole.

Martin MV: The use of fluconazole and itraconazole in the treatment of *Candida albicans* infection: a review. J Antimicrob Chemother 1999;44:429. [PMID: 10588302]

Terrell CL: Antifungal agents. Part II: The azoles. Mayo Clin Proc 1999;74:78. [PMID: 9987539]

Walsh TJ et al: Voriconazole compared with liposomal amphotericin B for empirical antifungal therapy in patients with neutropenia and persistent fever. N Engl J Med 2002;346:225. [PMID: 11807146] (Equal efficacy but fewer breakthrough fungemias with voriconazole.)

7. Candins

The echinocandins and pneumocandins represent a new class of antifungals active by inhibition of fungal wall synthesis. They are active against candida, including nonalbicans species, as well as aspergillus species. Candins are not active against cryptococcus or fusarium. Their long pharmacologic half-life confers the advantage of once-daily dosing. Candins are associated with minimal toxicity or adverse effects, and they are not implicated in significant drug interactions. Clinical data in the treatment of aspergillus infections suggest caspofungin, the first candin clinically available, to be associated with success similar to that of other agents active against aspergillus. Caspofungin is indicated for treatment of aspergillus infections in those who fail to respond to or are intolerant of amphotericin and itraconazole.

Caspofungin (Cancidas) for aspergillosis. Med Lett Drugs Ther 2001;43:58. [PMID: 11445777]

De Pauw BE: New antifungal agents and preparations. Int J Antimicrob Agents 2000;16:147. [PMID: 11053798]

ANTIVIRAL CHEMOTHERAPY

Several compounds can influence viral replication and the development of viral disease.

Amantadine is active against influenza A (but not influenza B) and has efficacy both in prophylaxis and therapy of this infection. Yearly immunization against influenza is recommended (see Chapter 30) for disease prevention, but in certain select situations amantadine can be used for this purpose. Amantadine prophylaxis is 70–90% effective and is suggested for the influenza season (6–8 weeks) in patients who cannot be immunized who are at increased risk of developing complications of influenza (those with chronic pulmonary and cardiac diseases, persons over 65 years of age, persons with chronic metabolic diseases such as diabetes mellitus, and chronic renal failure); in medical personnel who cannot receive vaccine but are capable of transmitting influenza to high-risk patients; if vaccine is not available; and if vaccine strains differ from the strain causing an epidemic. Short-term prophylaxis (2 weeks) is indicated if an outbreak occurs before vaccination has been given. In this setting, amantadine will protect against disease while antibody production is induced and will not interfere with antibody production. Because of its modest therapeutic benefit, high-risk patients and others with influenza A may benefit from treatment with amantadine if it is instituted within 48 hours after the onset of symptoms and continued for 1 week. The usual adult dosage is 200 mg orally per day (in persons over 65 years of age, 100 mg). Emergence of influenza A resistant to amantadine and rimantadine has been observed in patients receiving therapy. Considering this resistance, neuraminidase inhibitors such as zanamivir or oseltamivir may be preferable in an outbreak situation. The most marked untoward effects are insomnia, nightmares, and ataxia, especially in the elderly. Amantadine may accumulate and be more toxic in patients with renal insufficiency, and the dosage should be reduced.

Rimantadine, an analog of amantadine, is as effective as amantadine and is associated with fewer central nervous system adverse effects. It is considerably more expensive than amantadine and thus should be considered only in the elderly, in whom central nervous system side effects occur more commonly.

Neuraminidase inhibitors, including zanamivir inhalation and oseltamivir tablets, are available for prevention and treatment of influenza A and B. Like amantadine and rimantadine, they must be administered soon (within 48 hours) after the onset of symptoms to be effective. Zanamivir inhalers are difficult to use for some patients, especially those with asthma and chronic obstructive pulmonary disease, in whom bronchospasm has been reported. Oseltamivir has limited application because of its gastrointestinal side effects. Both drugs are administered twice daily for 5 days when used for therapy. Both agents are significantly more expensive than amantadine and reduce the duration of symptoms by only 1 day and viral shedding by 2 days. The major advantages of neuraminidase inhibitors over amantadine or rimantadine include activity against influenza A and B and a low likelihood of development of resistance, resulting in their preferential use in outbreak settings.

Acyclovir is useful in infections due to herpes simplex and in herpes zoster-varicella infections. In herpes-infected cells, it is selectively active against viral DNA polymerase and thus inhibits virus proliferation. Given intravenously (15 mg/kg/d in three divided doses), it can promote healing of mucocutaneous herpes simplex in immunocompromised patients. It can reduce pain, accelerate healing, and prevent dissemination of herpes zoster and varicella in immunocompromised patients. The usual dosage for varicellazoster infections is 30 mg/kg/d intravenously in three equal doses. The drug has no effect on establishment of latency, frequency of recurrence, or incidence of postherpetic neuralgia. Acyclovir (30 mg/kg/d intravenously in three equal doses) is the drug of choice for herpes encephalitis. Intravenous or oral acyclovir is effective prophylaxis against recurrent mucocutaneous and visceral herpes infections in transplant and other severely immunosuppressed patients. Investigation of the role of intravenous acyclovir in the prevention of cytomegalovirus disease in transplant recipients has yielded conflicting data. Acyclovir appears to be effective in some transplant settings (renal and perhaps bone marrow) but not in others (liver).

Oral acyclovir, 400 mg three times daily, is effective in primary genital herpes simplex infections. Oral acyclovir for recurrent genital herpes reduces viral shedding but has marginal effects on symptoms and is less effective than in primary disease. Suppressive therapy (400 mg twice daily) for 4–6 months reduces the frequency and severity of recurrent genital herpetic lesions. Acyclovir minimally affects symptoms or viral shedding in recurrent herpes labialis and is not generally used for this disease. However, in a dose of 400 mg twice daily, it is effective in preventing recurrent herpes labialis in those with frequent relapses and in preventing sun-induced relapses.

Other uses of oral acyclovir include (1) therapy of acute herpetic keratitis and prevention of recurrences, (2) prevention and treatment of herpetic whitlow, (3) acceleration of healing of herpes zoster in immunocompetent patients if initiated within 48 hours after onset (800 mg five times daily for 7 days), (4) more rapid healing of rash and lessened clinical symptoms of primary varicella in adults and children if instituted within 24 hours after onset of rash and continued for 5–7 days, (5) therapy of herpes proctitis (400 mg five times daily for 10 days), (6) prevention of herpes simplex and cytomegalovirus infections in transplant recipients (in doses of 800 mg four or five times daily), (7) prevention of erythema multiforme that is herpes simplex-related, and (8) prophylaxis against varicella in susceptible household contacts.

Topical 5% acyclovir ointment can shorten the period of pain and viral shedding in herpes simplex mucocutaneous oral lesions in immunosuppressed patients but not in patients with normal immunity. In contrast, acyclovir cream or penciclovir ointment (see famciclovir, below) appears to reduce the duration of pain and viral shedding by approximately 1 day in immunocompetent patients. Oral acyclovir is significantly more efficacious than topical therapy.

The absolute oral bioavailability of acyclovir is 10–30%. Newer agents (famciclovir, valacyclovir; see below) are significantly better absorbed than oral acyclovir and generally can be administered less frequently. Dosage reduction in renal insufficiency is required. For most herpes simplex infections except encephalitis, the intravenous dose is 5 mg/kg per dose. Since hemodialysis reduces serum levels significantly, the daily dose should be given after hemodialysis.

Acyclovir is relatively nontoxic. Precipitation of drug in renal tubules has been described with intravenous acyclovir and can best be avoided by maintaining adequate hydration and urine flow. Central nervous system toxicity manifested by confusion, agitation, tremors, and hallucinations has been reported. Resistance has been described, usually in immunosuppressed patients who have received multiple courses of therapy.

Famciclovir is a prodrug of penciclovir. After oral administration, 75–80% is absorbed and deacetylated in the intestinal wall to the active drug, penciclovir. Penciclovir, like acyclovir, inhibits viral replication by interfering with viral DNA polymerase. Acyclovir-resistant strains of herpes simplex and varicella-zoster virus are also resistant to famciclovir. Famciclovir in a dose of 500 mg three times daily for 7 days accelerates healing of lesions in acute herpes zoster if started within 72 hours after the onset of rash. At a dose of 125 mg twice daily, famciclovir is effective suppressive therapy of recurrent genital herpes.

Valacyclovir is a prodrug of acyclovir that has significantly increased oral bioavailability when compared with acyclovir. After absorption, it is converted to acyclovir and serum levels are three to five times higher than those achieved with acyclovir. Valacyclovir at a dosage of 1 g three times daily is effective therapy for herpes zoster when started within 72 hours after onset of rash and is slightly more effective than acyclovir in relieving zoster-associated pain. It shortens the course of initial episodes of genital herpes (1 g twice daily for 10 days) and is effective prophylaxis for recurrent genital herpes when given as a single 1 g daily dose. At doses of 2 g four times daily, valacyclovir is more effective than placebo in preventing cytomegalovirus infections in seronegative recipients of a kidney from a seropositive donor. The adverse effect profile of valacyclovir is comparable to that of acyclovir. However, HIV-positive patients receiving long-term valacyclovir (8 g/d) for prevention of cytomegalovirus disease have been found to have an increased incidence of thrombocytopenic purpura-hemolytic anemic syndrome.

Foscarnet (trisodium phosphonoformate) is a pyrophosphate analog that inhibits viral DNA polymerase of human herpesviruses (CMV, herpes simplex, varicella-zoster) and the reverse transcriptase of human immunodeficiency virus. The drug is more expensive than ganciclovir, less well tolerated, and more difficult to administer. Therefore, its use is limited to patients who do not respond to ganciclovir or cannot tolerate it. Isolates of CMV resistant to ganciclovir and herpes simplex and varicella-zoster resistant to acyclovir usually are sensitive to foscarnet. Foscarnet appears to be effective for CMV retinitis and has been used successfully in patients who have failed to respond to ganciclovir. Once therapy is stopped, recurrences develop, and lifelong suppressive therapy is required for AIDS patients not receiving highly active antiretroviral therapy. Combination therapy with ganciclovir and foscarnet has been associated with improved efficacy over monotherapy in the treatment of CMV retinitis. While combination therapy reduced progression of disease (eg, retinal changes), no improvement of visual acuity was observed over either drug used alone. Foscarnet has also been used to treat acyclovir-resistant mucocutaneous herpes simplex in AIDS patients as well as varicella cutaneous lesions in AIDS patients who failed to respond to acyclovir. Uncontrolled trials suggest efficacy in CMV gastrointestinal disease, therapy of CMV infection following bone marrow and renal transplantation, and prevention of CMV disease when the drug is given prophylactically to seropositive bone marrow transplant recipients. Oral absorption is poor, and the drug must be given intravenously. The half-life is 3–5 hours, and this is prolonged with renal insufficiency. The usual induction dose is 60 mg/kg every 8 hours, and the dose for maintenance therapy is 120 mg/kg once daily. Adjustments are required for even minimal impairment in renal function (see package insert).

Toxicity is a major drawback to widespread use. The drug can cause severe phlebitis and must be diluted to a concentration of 12 mg/mL to be given peripherally. At higher concentrations, it must be given centrally. Nephrotoxicity, which is dose-dependent and reversible, is its major toxicity. Prehydration with 2.5 L of 0.9% saline may protect against nephrotoxicity. Foscarnet binds divalent cations and hypocalcemia with peripheral neuropathy, seizures and arrhythmias, hypomagnesemia, and hypophosphatemia can occur. Monitoring of electrolytes and renal function is required during therapy. Anemia (20–50%) and nausea and vomiting (20–30%) are other common adverse effects.

Resistance of herpes simplex virus to foscarnet has been described in HIV infection and in association with bone marrow transplantation. Resistance is usually seen in patients who are infected with HIV and either have received foscarnet previously or were receiving suppressive therapy. Isolates may be sensitive to acyclovir.

Cidofovir is a nucleotide analog that is active against all human herpesviruses. The drug has a prolonged pharmacokinetic intracellular half-life, allowing for administration every 1–2 weeks. Phosphorylation of cidofovir to its active form does not depend on viral enzymes. Thus, strains of cytomegalovirus, herpes simplex virus, and herpes zoster virus that are resistant to ganciclovir or acyclovir often are sensitive to cidofovir. Cidofovir delays progression of CMV retinitis in newly diagnosed disease (5 mg/kg weekly for 2 weeks, followed by maintenance of 3–5 mg/kg every other week) and is effective therapy in relapsed disease or in patients who are intolerant of traditional therapy (5 mg/kg every other day). Limited data suggest that direct intravitreal injection (20 μg every 5–6 weeks) of cidofovir is also effective for initial and maintenance therapy. Cidofovir gel (as 3% or 1%) topically applied to mucocutaneous herpetic lesions in AIDS patients unresponsive to oral or intravenous acyclovir provides benefit in healing. The drug is effective in the treatment of AIDS-associated progressive multifocal leukoencephalopathy. Cidofovir is associated with a high incidence of nephrotoxicity, sometimes severe. To avoid this complication, probenecid and intravenous saline are administered with each dose.

Ribavirin aerosol is potentially useful in the treatment of respiratory syncytial virus infections in bone marrow transplant patients. It is not known whether the addition of immune globulin provides additional benefit. Intravenous ribavirin can significantly lower the fatality rate of Lassa fever and has been used as a therapeutic agent for hantavirus pneumonia. However, the benefit in hantavirus infection is unclear. The drug is teratogenic in animals, and pregnant women should not take care of patients receiving the aerosol. Oral ribavirin is used in combination with interferons to treat chronic hepatitis C infections (see Chapter 15).

Ganciclovir is an analog of acyclovir that has broad antiviral activity, including activity against CMV. The drug is efficacious in the therapy of CMV retinitis in AIDS patients, but once therapy is stopped, the relapse rate is high, and long-term maintenance suppressive therapy is required in patients not receiving HAART. CMV pneumonitis therapy with this agent has been disappointing. It has been suggested that the addition of intravenous immunoglobulin or CMV immune globulin to ganciclovir may improve CMV pneumonitis. CMV viremia and hepatitis are often self-limited diseases, and the role of ganciclovir in treating these syndromes awaits clarification. However, because CMV viremia often predicts the presence of invasive disease, it is usually treated when it occurs. Ganciclovir is most efficacious as a prophylactic agent. Administration of ganciclovir for 100–120 days to seropositive bone marrow transplant recipients decreases the incidence of CMV disease. Similar results have been demonstrated in heart and liver transplant recipients treated for 28 days. In renal transplant patients, ganciclovir during periods of maximum immunosuppression (ie, when antilymphocyte antibody therapy is administered for rejection) prevents development of disease in seropositive individuals. Although ganciclovir alone is not effective in the therapy of CMV pneumonia, if the drug is initiated when asymptomatic viral excretion occurs (as determined by a positive culture in bronchoalveolar lavage) in bone marrow transplant patients, there is a marked reduction in the subsequent development of pneumonia. It should be emphasized that regimens employing high-dose intravenous and oral acyclovir have also been shown to be effective in preventing CMV disease following bone marrow, liver, and renal transplants. In practice, most high-risk solid organ transplant recipients receive ganciclovir intravenously for 10–14 days posttransplant followed by 3–4 months of high-dose acyclovir therapy (800 mg four or five times daily adjusted for renal insufficiency), or valacyclovir (8 g/d), or oral ganciclovir (1 g three times daily in donor-positive, recipient-negative transplant patients; see below). Because of the profound immunosuppression associated with bone marrow transplantation, following engraftment (usually at 1 month), intravenous ganciclovir, 5 mg/kg/d three times a week, is given for the first 100–120 days posttransplant, at which time high-dose acyclovir is given for an additional year. An alternative approach in the marrow transplant patient is to follow patients without therapy and to do surveillance for the presence of CMV DNA by antigen detection or PCR. If CMV DNA is detected, therapy with ganciclovir, 5 mg/kg twice daily, is initiated.

The major adverse effect is neutropenia, which is reversible but requires dosage reduction. Thrombocytopenia, disorientation, nausea, rash, and phlebitis occur less commonly.

Oral ganciclovir has poor bioavailability, with maximum absorption of only 6–9% when taken with food. After a dose of 1 g, peak serum levels are about 1 μg/mL (clinical isolates of CMV are inhibited by 0.02–3.5 μg/mL). Controlled clinical studies indicate that the oral drug in a dose of 1 g three times a day is slightly less effective than intravenous ganciclovir, 5 mg/kg daily as maintenance therapy for CMV retinitis (time to progression is 5–12 days shorter in those treated with the oral drug). Thus, in selected populations with peripheral non-sight-threatening lesions, oral ganciclovir maintenance may be convenient and effective therapy compared with long-term intravenous therapy. Because of its poor bioavailability, oral ganciclovir is unlikely to be effective as primary therapy for active CMV infection. The role of oral ganciclovir in prevention of CMV infection following bone marrow or solid organ transplantation has not been well studied, but liver transplant recipients receiving oral ganciclovir, 1 g three times daily for 3 months, appear to have less CMV disease than those receiving placebo.

Oral ganciclovir will probably be replaced by **valganciclovir,** an esterification product of ganciclovir with significantly better oral bioavailability. Administration of 900 mg of valganciclovir results in serum ganciclovir levels equal to that achieved with an intravenous 5 mg/kg dose of ganciclovir. In cytomegalovirus retinitis in AIDS patients, the drug is as efficacious as intravenous therapy. Although widely used for prophylaxis in solid organ transplant recipients, its efficacy in this application has yet to be established.

Lamivudine (3TC), a well-tolerated oral antiviral nucleoside analog used in treatment of HIV infection, is effective against hepatitis B. Once-daily therapy (100 mg) for a year results in clinical, serologic, and histologic improvement in approximately 50% of patients. While lamivudine is useful, development of resistance is common with long-term therapy. Therapy post liver transplantation is associated with a reduced risk of reinfection with hepatitis B.

Human interferons have been prepared from stimulated lymphocytes and by DNA recombinant technology. These agents have antiviral, antitumor, and immunoregulatory properties. The most common uses of these agents include therapy of chronic hepatitis due to hepatitis B, C, and D (see Chapter 15). A long-acting preparation of interferon, peginterferon, has been determined to be superior to conventional interferon. Oral ribavirin in combination with interferon is more effective than interferon monotherapy in the treatment of chronic hepatitis C infection. Interferons are also efficacious in condyloma acuminatum, as prophylaxis against infection in patients with chronic granulomatous disease, and for therapy of a number of malignancies such as hairy cell leukemia, Kaposi's sarcoma in AIDS, chronic myelogenous leukemia, multiple myeloma, renal cell carcinoma, and others, as well as in therapy for relapsing multiple sclerosis. Other potential uses are for therapy of certain intracellular pathogens such as leprosy, atypical mycobacterial infection, toxoplasmosis, and leishmaniasis. Relapse of the underlying disease after cessation of therapy is common but usually responds to reinstitution of drug. Adverse effects are common and include an influenza-like illness with fever, chills, nausea, vomiting, headache, arthralgia, and myalgias. Bone marrow suppression, especially with high-dose therapy, also occurs.

Balfour HH: Antiviral drugs. N Engl J Med 1999;340:1255. [PMID: 10210711] (Review of activity, dosing, clinical indications, and toxicity.)

Cummings KJ et al: Interferon and ribavirin vs interferon alone in the re-treatment of chronic hepatitis C previously nonresponsive to interferon. A meta-analysis of randomized trials. JAMA 2001;285:193. [PMID: 11176813]

Gubareva LV et al: Influenza virus neuraminidase inhibitors. Lancet 2000;355:827. [PMID: 10711940]

Management of herpes virus infections following transplantation. J Antimicrob Chemother 2000;45:729. [PMID: 10837424]

Pegylated interferon (PEG-Intron) for chronic hepatitis C. Med Lett Drugs Ther 2001;43:54. [PMID: 11426190]

Disorders Due to Physical Agents 38

Richard Cohen, MD, MPH, & Brent R.W. Moelleken, MD, FACS
See www.current-med.com/ch38.html

■ DISORDERS DUE TO COLD

Cold tolerance varies considerably among individuals. Factors that increase the likelihood of injury from exposure to cold include poor general physical conditioning, nonacclimatization, advanced age, systemic illness, poor tissue oxygenation, wet or insufficient clothing, previous cold weather injury, and the use of alcohol or other sedative drugs. High wind velocity ("windchill factor") increases the severity of cold injury at low temperatures.

Cold Urticaria

Some persons have a familial or acquired hypersensitivity to cold and may develop urticaria upon even limited exposure to a cold (eg, wind, freezer compartments). The urticaria usually occurs only on exposed areas, but in markedly sensitive individuals the response can be generalized and fatal. Immersion in cold water may result in severe systemic reactions, including shock; histamine release occurs. Familial cold urticaria is an autosomal dominant inflammatory disorder, manifested as a burning sensation of the skin occurring about 30 minutes after exposure to cold. Acquired cold urticaria may be associated with medication (eg, griseofulvin) or with infection. Cold urticaria may occur secondarily to cryoglobulinemia or as a complication of syphilis. Most cases of acquired cold urticaria are idiopathic. For diagnosis, an ice cube is usually applied to the skin of the forearm for 4–5 minutes, then removed, and the area is observed for 10 minutes. As the skin rewarms, an urticarial wheal appears at the site and may be accompanied by itching. Cyproheptadine, 16–32 mg/d in divided doses, is the drug of choice for cold urticaria. As an alternative, a combination of terbutaline, 5 mg three times daily, and aminophylline, 150 mg three times daily, has been recommended.

Raynaud's Phenomenon

See Chapter 12.

ACCIDENTAL SYSTEMIC HYPOTHERMIA

Systemic hypothermia may result from exposure (atmospheric or immersion) to prolonged or extreme cold. The condition may arise in healthy individuals in the course of occupational or recreational exposure or in victims of accidents.

Systemic hypothermia may follow exposure to cool but not cold temperatures when there is altered homeostasis due to debility or disease. In colder climates, elderly and inactive individuals living in inadequately heated housing are particularly susceptible. Patients with cardiovascular or cerebrovascular disease, mental retardation, acute alcoholism, malnutrition, myxedema, hypopituitarism, or use of sedating or tranquilizing drugs are more vulnerable to accidental hypothermia. Prolonged postoperative hypothermia or administration of large amounts of refrigerated stored blood (without rewarming) can cause systemic hypothermia.

Pathogenesis

Systemic hypothermia is a reduction of core (rectal) body temperature below 35 °C. It causes reduced physiologic function—with decreased oxygen consumption and slowed myocardial repolarization, peripheral nerve conduction, gastrointestinal motility, and respirations—as well as hemoconcentration and pancreatitis. Defenses against cold exposure are superficial blood vessel constriction and increased metabolic heat production.

Clinical Findings

Early manifestations of hypothermia include weakness, drowsiness, lethargy, irritability, confusion, shivering, and impaired coordination. A lowered body temperature may be the sole finding; the skin may appear blue or puffy.

The internal (core) body temperature in accidental hypothermia may range from 25 to 35 °C. Oral temperatures are inaccurate; an esophageal or rectal probe that reads as low as 25 °C is required. At core temperatures below 35 °C, the patient may become delirious, drowsy, or comatose and may stop breathing. The pulse and blood pressure may be unobtainable, leading clinicians to believe the patient is dead. Metabolic acidosis, hyperkalemia, pneumonia, pancreatitis, ventricular fibrillation, hypoglycemia or hyperglycemia, coagulopathy, and renal failure may occur. Abnormalities in cardiac rhythm are directly related to the lowering of core temperature; cardiac arrhythmias may occur, especially during the rewarming process. Progression of electrocardiographic abnormalities can also occur, including the pathognomonic J wave of Osborn—prominent in lead II (Figure 38–1). Death in systemic hypothermia usually results from cardiac asystole or ventricular fibrillation.

Treatment
(Figure 38–2)

Patients with mild hypothermia (rectal temperature > 33 °C) who have been otherwise healthy usually respond well to a warm bed or to rapid passive rewarming with a warm bath or warm packs and blankets. A conservative approach is also usually employed in treating elderly or debilitated patients, using an electric blanket kept at 37 °C. Gentle handling and movement of the patient are essential to avoid triggering arrhythmias.

Patients with moderate or severe hypothermia (core temperatures of < 33 °C) do not have the thermoregulatory shivering mechanism and require active rewarming with supportive care. Cardiovascular support, acid-base balance, arterial oxygenation, and adequate intravascular volume should be established prior to rewarming to minimize the risk of organ infarction and "afterdrop" (recurrent hypothermia). The methods and rate of active rewarming are controversial. Successful treatment usually includes a combination of active external and internal methods (see below). Aggressive rewarming should be attempted only by those experienced in the methods. *Once begun, CPR should continue until the patient has been rewarmed to at least 32 °C.* The need for oxygen therapy, endotracheal intubation, controlled ventilation, warmed intravenous fluids, and treatment of metabolic acidosis should be dictated by clinical and laboratory monitoring during the rapid rewarming process. Essential laboratory tests include complete blood count, prothrombin time, partial thromboplastin time, electrolytes, blood urea nitrogen, serum creatinine, liver function tests, amylase, glucose, pH, blood gases, urinalysis, and urine volume. Cardiac rhythm should be monitored, and cardiac, central vascular, or chest trauma or stimulation (catheter, cannulas, etc) should be avoided unless essential because of the risk of inducing ventricular fibrillation. However, patients who are comatose or in respiratory failure should be tracheally intubated. The patient should be evaluated for trauma and peripheral cold injury (eg, frostbite). Antibiotics are not routinely given and should be used only if indicated (neonate, elderly, or immunocompromised patient). Core temperature (esophageal preferred over rectal) should be monitored frequently during and after initial rewarming because of reports of recurrent hypothermia.

A. ACTIVE EXTERNAL REWARMING METHODS

Heated blankets, forced hot air, radiant heat cradles, or warm baths may be used for active external rewarming. Rewarming by a warm bath is best done in a tub of moving water at 40–42 °C, with a rate of rewarming of about 1–2 °C/h. It is easier, however, to monitor the patient and to perform diagnostic and therapeutic procedures when heated blankets are used for active rewarming. Although relatively simple and generally available, active external warming methods may cause marked peripheral dilation that predisposes to ventricular fibrillation and hypovolemic shock and should be accompanied by core rewarming in moderate to severe hypothermia.

Forced air rewarming (38–43 °C) is recommended for clinic or field use when extracorporeal blood rewarming is not available.

B. ACTIVE INTERNAL (CORE) REWARMING METHODS

Internal rewarming is essential for patients with severe hypothermia; extracorporeal blood rewarming (cardiopulmonary, venovenous, or femorofemoral bypass) is the treatment of choice, especially in the presence of cardiac arrest. In the absence of equipment necessary for extracorporeal rewarming, left-sided thoracotomy followed by pericardial cavity irrigation with warmed saline and cardiac massage has been effective in systemic hypothermia < 28 °C. Repeated peritoneal dialysis may be employed with 2 L of warm (43 °C) potassium-free dialysate solution exchanged at intervals of 10–12 minutes until the core temperature is raised to about 35 °C. Parenteral fluids (D_5 normal saline) should be warmed to 43 °C prior to administration. Heated, humidified air warmed to 42 °C through a face mask or endotracheal tube may be administered. Warm colonic and gastrointestinal irrigations are of less value.

Prognosis

With proper early care, more than 75% of otherwise healthy patients may survive moderate or severe systemic hypothermia. Prognosis is directly related to the severity of metabolic acidosis; if the pH is 6.6 or less, the prognosis is poor. The risk of aspiration pneumonia is great in comatose patients. The prognosis is grave if there are underlying predisposing causes or if treatment is delayed.

HYPOTHERMIA OF THE EXTREMITIES

Exposure of the extremities to cold produces immediate localized vasoconstriction followed by generalized vasoconstriction. When the skin temperature falls to

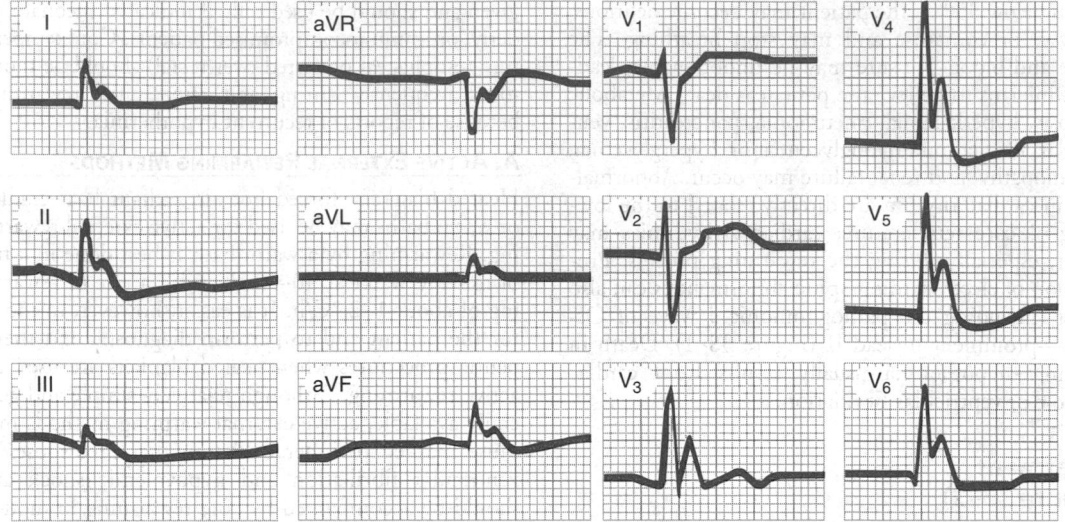

Figure 38–1. Hypothermia. The ventricular rate is 50/min. Atrial activity is not seen. The QRS complexes are narrow and are deformed at their terminal portions by a slurred wave occurring prior to the inscription of the ST–T waves; this is the J wave. The QT interval is prolonged. (Courtesy of R Brindis. Reproduced, with permission from Goldschlager N, Goldman MJ: *Principles of Clinical Electrocardiography*, 13th ed. McGraw-Hill, 1989.)

25 °C, tissue metabolism is slowed, but the demand for oxygen is greater than the slowed circulation can supply, and the area becomes cyanotic. At 15 °C, tissue metabolism is markedly decreased and the dissociation of oxyhemoglobin is reduced; this gives a deceptive pink, well-oxygenated appearance to the skin. Tissue damage occurs at this temperature. Tissue death may be caused by ischemia and thromboses in the smaller vessels or by actual freezing. Freezing (frostbite) does not occur until the skin temperature drops to –4 to –10 °C or even lower, depending on such factors as wind, mobility, venous stasis, malnutrition, and occlusive arterial disease. Neuropathic sequelae such as pain, numbness, tingling, hyperhidrosis, cold sensitivity of the extremities, and nerve conduction abnormalities may persist for many years after the cold injury.

Prevention

"Keep warm, keep moving, and keep dry." Individuals should wear warm, dry clothing, preferably several layers, with a windproof outer garment. Wet clothing, socks, and shoes should be replaced with dry ones. Extra socks, mittens, and insoles should always be carried in a pack in cold or icy areas. Cramped positions, constricting clothing, and prolonged dependency of the feet are to be avoided. Arms, legs, fingers, and toes should be exercised to maintain circulation. Wet and muddy ground and exposure to wind should be avoided. Tobacco and alcohol should be avoided when the danger of frostbite is present.

CHILBLAIN (Erythema Pernio)

Chilblains are red, itching skin lesions, usually on the extremities, caused by exposure to cold without actual freezing of the tissues. They may be associated with edema or blistering and are aggravated by warmth. With continued exposure, ulcerative or hemorrhagic lesions may appear and progress to scarring, fibrosis, and atrophy. Chilblain lupus erythematosus, while clinically similar to ordinary chilblain, can be differentiated by an association with other lupus manifestations or by biopsy.

Treatment consists of elevating the affected part slightly and allowing it to warm gradually at room temperature. Do not rub or massage injured tissues or apply ice or heat. Protect the area from trauma and secondary infection. Prazosin, 1 mg daily, has been recommended for treatment and prevention of recurrence.

FROSTBITE

Frostbite is injury due to freezing and formation of ice crystals within tissues. In mild cases, only the skin and subcutaneous tissues are involved; the symptoms are numbness, prickling, and itching. With increasing severity, deep frostbite involves deeper structures, and there may be paresthesia and stiffness. Thawing causes tenderness and burning pain. The skin is white or yellow, loses its elasticity, and becomes immobile. Edema, blisters, necrosis, and gangrene may appear.

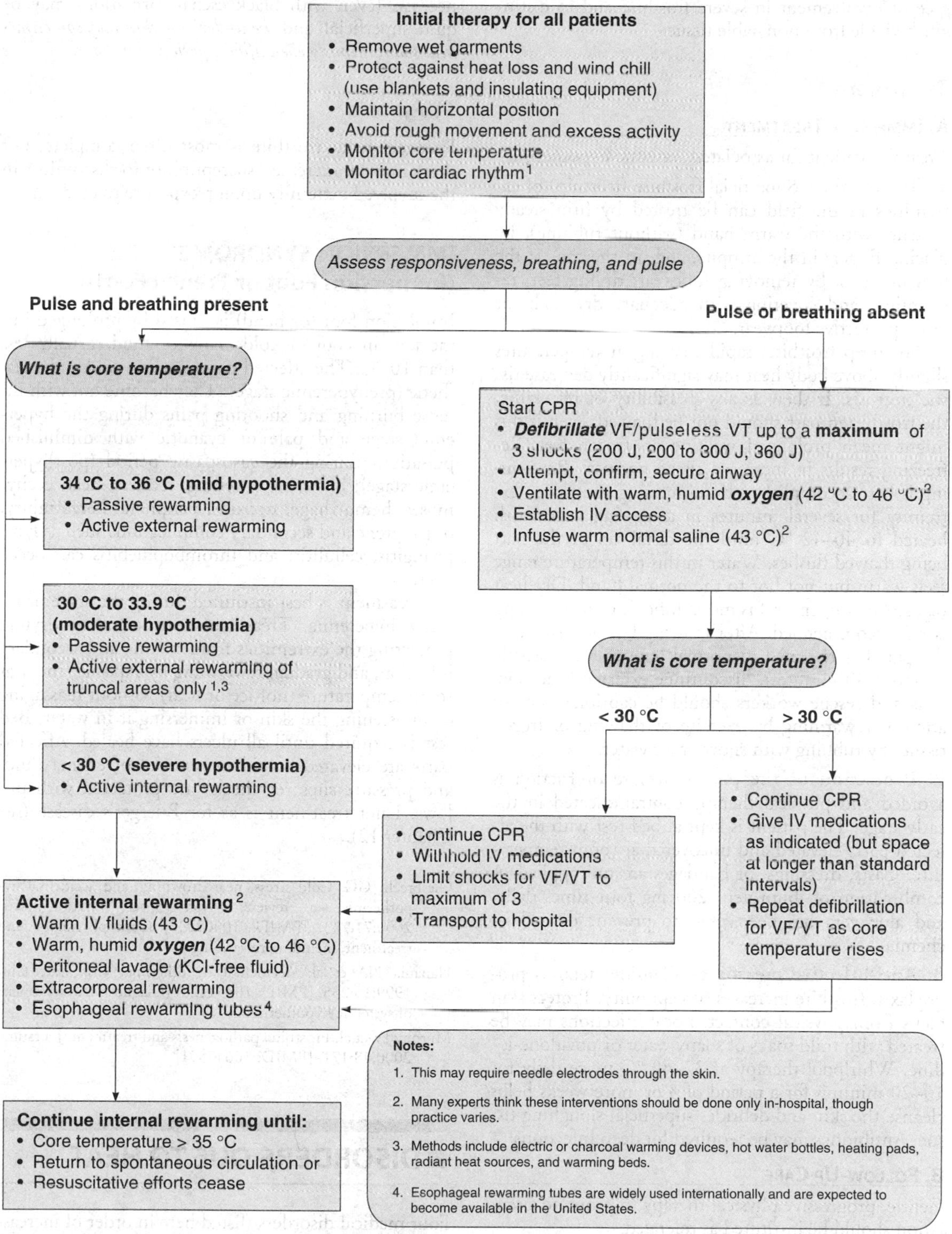

Initial therapy for all patients
- Remove wet garments
- Protect against heat loss and wind chill (use blankets and insulating equipment)
- Maintain horizontal position
- Avoid rough movement and excess activity
- Monitor core temperature
- Monitor cardiac rhythm[1]

↓

Assess responsiveness, breathing, and pulse

Pulse and breathing present ← → **Pulse or breathing absent**

What is core temperature?

34 °C to 36 °C (mild hypothermia)
- Passive rewarming
- Active external rewarming

30 °C to 33.9 °C (moderate hypothermia)
- Passive rewarming
- Active external rewarming of truncal areas only [1,3]

< 30 °C (severe hypothermia)
- Active internal rewarming

Start CPR
- *Defibrillate* VF/pulseless VT up to a **maximum** of 3 shocks (200 J, 200 to 300 J, 360 J)
- Attempt, confirm, secure airway
- Ventilate with warm, humid *oxygen* (42 °C to 46 °C)[2]
- Establish IV access
- Infuse warm normal saline (43 °C)[2]

↓

What is core temperature?

< 30 °C ← → **> 30 °C**

- Continue CPR
- Withhold IV medications
- Limit shocks for VF/VT to maximum of 3
- Transport to hospital

- Continue CPR
- Give IV medications as indicated (but space at longer than standard intervals)
- Repeat defibrillation for VF/VT as core temperature rises

Active internal rewarming [2]
- Warm IV fluids (43 °C)
- Warm, humid *oxygen* (42 °C to 46 °C)
- Peritoneal lavage (KCl-free fluid)
- Extracorporeal rewarming
- Esophageal rewarming tubes [4]

Continue internal rewarming until:
- Core temperature > 35 °C
- Return to spontaneous circulation or
- Resuscitative efforts cease

Notes:
1. This may require needle electrodes through the skin.
2. Many experts think these interventions should be done only in-hospital, though practice varies.
3. Methods include electric or charcoal warming devices, hot water bottles, heating pads, radiant heat sources, and warming beds.
4. Esophageal rewarming tubes are widely used internationally and are expected to become available in the United States.

Figure 38–2. Hypothermia treatment algorithm. (VF, ventricular fibrillation; VT, ventricular tachycardia; J, joules.) (Reproduced, with permission, from American Heart Association. Circulation 2000;102[Suppl I]:I-229.)

MRI with magnetic resonance angiography and triple-phase bone scanning have been used to assess the degree of involvement in severe frostbite and to distinguish viable from nonviable tissue.

Treatment

A. IMMEDIATE TREATMENT

Treat the patient for associated systemic hypothermia.

1. Rewarming—Superficial frostbite (frostnip) of extremities in the field can be treated by firm steady pressure with the warm hand (without rubbing), by placing fingers in the armpits, and, in the case of the toes or heels, by removing footwear, drying feet, rewarming, and covering with adequate dry socks or other protective footwear.

For deep frostbite, rapid thawing at temperatures slightly above body heat may significantly decrease tissue necrosis. If there is any possibility of refreezing, the frostbitten part should not be thawed, even if this might mean prolonged walking on frozen feet. Refreezing results in increased tissue necrosis. Rewarming is best accomplished by immersing the frozen extremity for several minutes in a moving water bath heated to 40–42 °C until the distal tip of the part being thawed flushes. Water in this temperature range feels warm but not hot to the normal hand. Dry heat (eg, stove or open fire) is more difficult to regulate and is not recommended. After thawing has occurred and the part has returned to normal temperature (usually in about 30 minutes), discontinue external heat. Victims and rescue workers should be cautioned not to attempt rewarming by exercise or thawing of frozen tissues by rubbing with snow or ice water.

2. Protection of the part—Pressure or friction is avoided and physical therapy contraindicated in the early stage. The patient is kept at bed rest with the affected parts elevated and uncovered at room temperature. Casts, dressings, or bandages are not applied. A combination of ibuprofen, 200 mg four times daily, and aloe vera has been used to prevent dermal ischemia.

3. Anti-infective measures—Consider tetanus prophylaxis; frostbite increases susceptibility. Protect skin blebs from physical contact. Local infections may be treated with mild soaks of soapy water or povidone-iodine. Whirlpool therapy at 37–40 °C twice daily for 15–20 minutes for a period of 3 or more weeks helps cleanse the skin and debrides superficial sloughing tissue. Antibiotics may be required for deep infections.

B. FOLLOW-UP CARE

Gentle, progressive physical therapy to promote circulation should be instituted as tolerated.

C. SURGERY

Early regional sympathetic blockade can reduce symptoms; sympathectomy (within 36–72 hours) is controversial. In general, other surgical intervention is to be avoided. *Amputation should not be considered until it is definitely established that the tissues are dead.* Tissue necrosis (even with black eschar formation) may be quite superficial, and *the underlying skin may sometimes heal spontaneously even after a period of months.*

Prognosis

Recovery from frostbite is most often complete, but there may be increased susceptibility to discomfort in the involved extremity upon reexposure to cold.

IMMERSION SYNDROME (Immersion Foot or Trench Foot)

Immersion foot (or hand) is caused by prolonged immersion in cool or cold water or mud, usually less than 10 °C. The affected parts are first cold and anesthetic (prehyperemic stage). They become hot with intense burning and shooting pains during the hyperemic stage and pale or cyanotic with diminished pulsations during the vasospastic period (posthyperemic stage); blistering, swelling, redness, heat, ecchymoses, hemorrhage, necrosis, peripheral nerve injury, or gangrene and secondary complications such as lymphangitis, cellulitis, and thrombophlebitis can occur later.

Treatment is best instituted during the stage of reactive hyperemia. Treatment consists of air drying, protecting the extremities from trauma and secondary infection, and gradual rewarming by exposure to air at room temperature (not ice or heat) without massaging or moistening the skin or immersing it in water. Bed rest is required until all ulcers have healed. Affected parts are elevated to aid in removal of edema fluid, and pressure sites (eg, heels) are protected with pillows. Later treatment is as for Buerger's disease (see Chapter 12).

Giesbrecht GG: Cold stress, near drowning, and accidental hypothermia: a review. Aviat Space Environ Med 2000;71:733. [PMID: 10902937] (Pathophysiology and treatment, including rewarming.)

Hanania NA et al: Accidental hypothermia. Crit Care Clin 1999;15:235. [PMID: 10331126] (Diagnosis and treatment of systemic hypothermia.)

Murphy JV et al: Frostbite: pathogenesis and treatment. J Trauma 2000;48:171. [PMID: 10647591]

■ DISORDERS DUE TO HEAT

Four medical disorders (listed here in order of increasing severity) comprise a spectrum of illness that can result from excessive exposure to hot environments: heat syncope, heat cramps, heat exhaustion, and heat stroke. A stable internal temperature requires a balance between heat production and heat loss, which the hypothalamus regulates by initiating changes in muscle tone, vascular tone, and sweat gland function.

Etiology

Conduction (convection)—the direct transfer of heat from the skin to the surrounding air—occurs with diminishing efficiency as ambient temperature rises. The passive transfer of heat from a warmer to a cooler object by radiation accounts for 65% of body heat loss under normal conditions. Radiant heat loss decreases as the temperature of the surrounding environment increases up to 37.2 °C, the point at which heat transfer reverses direction. At normal temperatures, evaporation accounts for approximately 20% of the body's heat loss, but at high temperatures it becomes the major mechanism for dissipation of heat; with vigorous exertion, sweat loss can be as much as 2.5 L/h. This mechanism diminishes as humidity rises.

Health conditions that inhibit sweat production or evaporation and increase susceptibility to heat disorders include obesity, skin disorders (miliaria), reduced cutaneous blood flow, dehydration, malnutrition, hypotension, and reduced cardiac output. Medications that impair sweating include anticholinergics, antihistamines, phenothiazines, tricyclic antidepressants, monoamine oxidase inhibitors, and diuretics; reduced cutaneous blood flow results from use of vasoconstrictors and β-adrenergic blocking agents; and dehydration results from use of alcohol. Illicit drugs—eg, phencyclidine, LSD, amphetamines, and cocaine—can cause increased muscle activity and thus generate increased body heat. Drug withdrawal syndromes or prolonged seizures may have the same effect.

The risk of heat disorder increases with age, impaired cognition, concurrent illness, reduced physical fitness, and insufficient acclimatization.

Prevention

Medical evaluation and monitoring should be used to identify individuals at increased risk of heat disorders. The public should be made aware of the early symptoms and signs of heat disorders. It is not recommended to make salt tablets available for use without medical supervision; close monitoring of fluid and electrolyte intake may be necessary in situations necessitating activity in hot environments. Athletic events should be organized and managed with attention to thermoregulation: the WBGT (wet bulb globe temperature) Index should be monitored, fluid consumption should be encouraged, and medical support should be immediately accessible. Competition is not recommended when the WBGT exceeds 28 °C. Workers should not begin work in hot temperatures without proper acclimatization and should be encouraged to drink water or balanced electrolyte fluids frequently.

Protective cooled suits have been used successfully in industry for prolonged work in environments up to 60 °C.

Acclimatization is achieved by scheduled regulated exposure to hot environments and by gradually increasing the duration of exposure and the work load until the body adjusts by producing sweat of lower salt content in greater amounts at lower ambient temperatures. Acclimatization is accompanied by increased plasma volume, cardiac output, and cardiac stroke volume and a slower heart rate.

SPECIFIC SYNDROMES DUE TO HEAT EXPOSURE

1. Heat Syncope

Sudden unconsciousness can result from cutaneous vasodilation with consequent systemic and cerebral hypotension. Systolic blood pressure is usually less than 100 mm Hg, and there is typically a history of vigorous physical activity for 2 hours or more just preceding the episode. The skin is typically cool and moist, and the pulse is weak.

Treatment consists of rest and recumbency in a cool place, with fluids by mouth (or intravenously if necessary).

2. Heat Cramps

Fluid and electrolyte depletion can result in slow, painful skeletal muscle contractions ("cramps") and severe muscle spasms lasting 1–3 minutes, usually of the muscles most heavily used. Cramping results from salt depletion as sweat losses are replaced with water alone. The skin is moist and cool, and the muscles are tender. There may be muscle twitching. The victim is alert, with stable vital signs, but may be agitated and complaining of pain. The body temperature may be normal or slightly increased. Involved muscle groups are hard and lumpy. There is almost always a history of vigorous activity just preceding the onset of symptoms. Laboratory evaluation may show low serum sodium, hemoconcentration, and elevated urea and creatinine.

The patient should be moved to a cool environment and given oral saline solution (4 tsp of salt per gallon of water) to replace both salt and water. *Because of their slower absorption, salt tablets are not recommended.* The victim may have to rest for 1–3 days with continued dietary salt supplementation before returning to work or resuming strenuous activity in the heat.

3. Heat Exhaustion

Heat exhaustion results from prolonged strenuous activity with inadequate salt intake in a hot environment and is characterized by dehydration, sodium depletion, or isotonic fluid loss with accompanying cardiovascular changes.

The diagnosis is based on prolonged symptoms and a rectal temperature over 37.8 °C, increased pulse(> 150% of the patient's normal)and moist skin.

Symptoms associated with heat syncope and heat cramps may be present. The patient may be quite thirsty and weak, with central nervous system symptoms such as headache, fatigue, and, in cases due chiefly to water depletion, anxiety, paresthesias, impaired judgment, hysteria, and occasionally psychosis. Hyperventilation secondary to heat exhaustion can lead to respiratory alkalosis. Heat exhaustion may progress to heat stroke if sweating ceases.

Treatment consists of patient location in a shaded, cool environment, providing adequate hydration (1–2 L over 2–4 hours), salt replenishment—orally, if possible—and active cooling (fans, ice packs, etc) if necessary. Physiologic saline or isotonic glucose solution should be administered intravenously when oral administration is not appropriate. Intravenous 3% (hypertonic) saline may be necessary if sodium depletion is severe. At least 24 hours of rest is recommended.

4. Heat Stroke

Heat stroke is a life-threatening medical emergency resulting from failure of the thermoregulatory mechanism. Heat stroke is imminent when the core (rectal) temperature approaches 41 °C. It presents in one of two forms: Classic heat stroke occurs in patients with compromised homeostatic mechanisms; exertional heat stroke occurs in healthy persons undergoing strenuous exertion in a thermally stressful environment. Morbidity or even death can result from cerebral, cardiovascular, hepatic, or renal damage.

The hallmarks of heat stroke are cerebral dysfunction with impaired consciousness, high fever, and absence of sweating. Persons at greatest risk are the very young, the elderly (age > 65), chronically infirm, and patients receiving medications (eg, anticholinergics, antihistamines, phenothiazines) that interfere with heat-dissipating mechanisms.

Exertional heat stroke and exertion-related disorders such as rhabdomyolysis are appearing more frequently as complications of participation by unconditioned amateurs in strenuous athletic activities such as marathon and triathlon competition.

Clinical Findings

A. SYMPTOMS AND SIGNS

Heat stroke may present with dizziness, weakness, emotional lability, nausea and vomiting, diarrhea, confusion, delirium, blurred vision, convulsions, collapse, and unconsciousness. The skin is hot and initially covered with perspiration. Later it dries. The pulse is strong initially. Blood pressure may be slightly elevated at first, but hypotension develops later. The core temperature is usually over 41 °C. Hyperventilation can occur, leading to respiratory alkalosis.

Exertional heat stroke may present with sudden collapse and loss of consciousness followed by irrational behavior. Anhidrosis may not be present. Twenty-five percent of heat stroke victims have pro-

dromal symptoms for minutes to hours that may include dizziness, weakness, nausea, confusion, disorientation, drowsiness, and irrational behavior.

B. LABORATORY FINDINGS

Laboratory evaluation may reveal dehydration, leukocytosis, elevated BUN, hyperuricemia, hemoconcentration, acid-base abnormalities (eg, lactic acidosis), and decreased serum potassium, sodium, calcium, and phosphorus; urine is concentrated, with elevated protein, tubular casts, and myoglobinuria. Thrombocytopenia, increased bleeding and clotting times, fibrinolysis, and consumption coagulopathy may also be present. Rhabdomyolysis and myocardial, hepatic, or renal damage may be identified by elevated serum creatine kinase and aminotransferase levels and BUN and by the presence of anuria, proteinuria, and hematuria. Electrocardiographic findings may include ST–T changes consistent with myocardial ischemia.

Treatment

Treatment is aimed at reducing the core temperature rapidly (within 1 hour) and controlling the secondary effects. Evaporative cooling is rapid and effective and is easily performed in most emergency settings. The patient's clothing should be removed and the entire body sprayed with water (15 °C) while cooled or ambient air is passed across the patient's body with large fans or other means at high velocity (100 ft/min). The patient should be in the lateral recumbent position or supported in a hands-and-knees position to expose as much skin surface as possible to the air. Other alternatives include use of cold wet sheets accompanied by fanning or immersion in chilled water. Cardiopulmonary bypass provides rapid cooling but is often not practical.

Immersion in an ice-water bath as initial treatment is no longer preferred because of its patient access limitations and potential for complications of hypotension and shivering. However, it should be considered if core temperature is not decreased rapidly in response to other treatment. Alternatives include hand and forearm immersion in cold water, ice packs (groin, axillas, neck), and iced gastric lavage, though these are much less effective than evaporative cooling.

Treatment should be continued until the rectal temperature drops to 39 °C. The temperature remains stable in most cases, but it should continue to be monitored for 24 hours. Chlorpromazine (25–50 mg intravenously) or diazepam (5–10 mg intravenously) can be given initially and then every 4 hours to control shivering. Antipyretics (aspirin, acetaminophen) have no effect on environmentally induced hyperthermia and are contraindicated.

Hypovolemic and cardiogenic shock must be carefully distinguished, as either or both may occur. Central venous or pulmonary artery wedge pressure should be monitored. Five percent dextrose in half-normal or normal saline should be administered for fluid replacement.

The patient should also be observed for renal failure due to rhabdomyolysis, hypokalemia, cardiac arrhythmias, disseminated intravascular coagulation, and hepatic failure. Hypokalemia frequently accompanies heat stroke but may not appear until rehydration. Maintenance of extracellular hydration and electrolyte balance should reduce the risk of renal failure due to rhabdomyolysis. Fluid administration to ensure a high urine output (> 50 mL/h), mannitol administration (0.25 mg/kg), and alkalinizing the urine (intravenous bicarbonate administration, 250 mL of 4%) are recommended. Fluid output should be monitored through the use of an indwelling urinary catheter.

Because sensitivity to high environmental temperature may persist for prolonged periods following an episode of heat stroke, immediate reexposure should be avoided.

Dehydration, rehydration and exercise in the heat. Int J Sports Med 1998;19(Suppl 2):S89. [PMID: 9766971] (Proceedings of an International Conference. Pathophysiology, diagnosis and treatment of exercise related heat disorders.)

Khosla R et al: Heat related illnesses. Crit Care Clin 1999;15: 251. [PMID: 10331127] (Etiology, pathophysiology, diagnosis, and treatment of heat disorders.)

Montain SJ et al: Fluid replacement recommendations for training in hot weather. Mil Med 1999;164:502. [PMID: 10414066] (Fluid replacement guidelines.)

■ BURNS

The incidence and severity of burn injuries has been declining, with both deaths and acute hospitalizations attributable to burns down about 50%. Over three-fourths of burns involve less than 10% of total body surface area. Aggressive, early (24–72 hours postburn) excision of deeply burned tissues and skin grafting, early enteral feeding—and improved infection control—have contributed to significantly lower mortality rates and shorter hospitalizations. Nonetheless, an estimated 1.25 million burn injuries and 51,000 acute hospitalizations of burn victims occur each year in the United States. Severe burns cause problems in the initial phase from hemodynamic compromise, related injuries such as smoke inhalation or fractures, and associated multiorgan failure and sepsis. Later, secondary scarring and constrictive wounds occur.

Significant quality of life and social functionality can be expected even for severely burned patients.

CLASSIFICATION

Burns are classified by extent, depth, patient age, and associated illness or injury.

Extent

The "rule of nines" (Figure 38–3) is useful for rapidly assessing the extent of a burn. More detailed charts

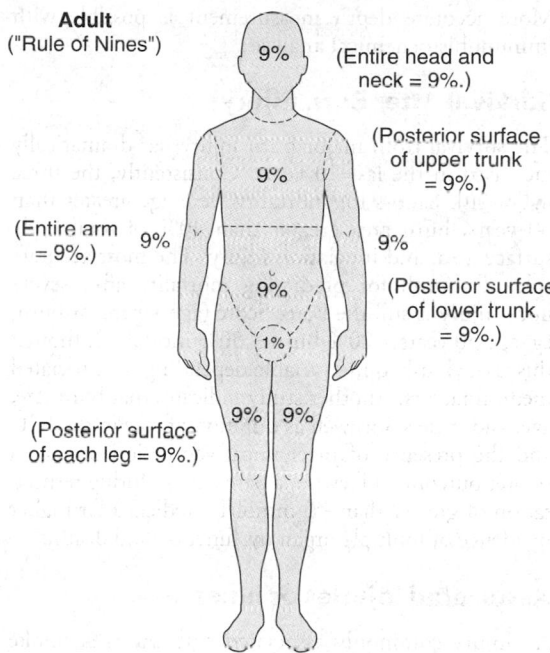

Figure 38–3. Estimation of body surface area in burns.

based on age are available when the patient reaches the burn unit. Therefore, it is important to view the entire patient after cleaning soot to make an accurate assessment, both initially and on subsequent examinations. Only second- and third-degree burns are included in calculating the total burn surface area (TBSA), since first-degree burns usually do not represent significant injury in terms of prognosis or fluid and electrolyte management. However, first- or second-degree burns may convert to deeper burns, especially if treatment is delayed or bacterial colonization or superinfection occurs.

Depth

Judgment of depth of injury is difficult. The **first-degree burn** may be red or gray but will demonstrate excellent capillary refill. First-degree burns are not blistered initially. If the wound is blistered, this represents a partial-thickness injury to the dermis, or a **second-degree burn.** As the degree of burn is progressively deeper, there is a progressive loss of adnexal structures. Hairs can be easily extracted or are absent, sweat glands become less visible, and the skin appears smoother.

The distinction between second- and third-degree burns is unclear and in a sense artificial. Deep second-degree burns are generally treated as full-thickness (third-degree) burns and excised and grafted earlier because of the long time necessary for reepithelialization and the thin, poor quality of the resultant skin.

More accurate depth measurement is possible with immunohistochemical analysis.

Survival After Burn Injury

The survival from major burn injury has dramatically increased in the last 20 years. Consistently, the three major risk factors for mortality were age greater than 60 years, burn area greater than 40% of total body surface area, and inhalation injury. The most accurate rule of thumb for predicting mortality after severe burn injury is still the Baux Score (age + percent burn, eg, age 50 years + 20% burn = 50% mortality), though this is obviously quite variable depending on associated medical factors. Another study indicates that burn size, age, and male sex as well as duration of stay in the ICU and the presence of mechanical ventilation presage a poorer outcome. Likewise, a base deficit during resuscitation of greater than −6 mmol/L predicts a far higher incidence of multiple organ dysfunction and death.

Associated Injuries or Illnesses

An injury commonly associated with burns is smoke inhalation (see Chapter 9). Suspicion of inhalation injury is aroused when the nasal hairs are singed, the mechanism of burn involves closed spaces, the sputum is carbonaceous, or the carboxyhemoglobin level exceeds 5% in nonsmokers. This suspicion should lead the clinician to institute early intubation before airway edema supervenes. The products of combustion, not heat, are responsible for lower airway injury. Electrical injury that causes burns may also produce cardiac arrhythmias that require immediate attention. Pancreatitis occurs in severe burns. Development of hyperamylasemia or hyperlipasemia may signal the development of pancreatic inflammation and subsequent pseudocyst or abscess formation. Prior alcohol exposure may exacerbate the pulmonary components of burn injury.

Toxic epidermal necrolysis (TEN) occasionally occurs following sulfonamide or phenytoin administration (see Chapter 6). If TEN is severe, patients are best transferred to a burn unit and treated as having severe burn injury. Corticosteroid therapy should be avoided.

SYSTEMIC REACTIONS TO BURN INJURY

The actual burn injury is only the incipient event in a cascade of deleterious local tissue and systemic inflammatory reactions leading to multiorgan system failure in the severely burned patient. Locally, substance P, serotonin, prostaglandins E_2 and $F_{2\alpha}$, histamine, platelet-activating factor, nitric oxide, bradykinin, and leukotrienes B_4 and D_4 play a role in the increased local capillary permeability and initiation of the systemic inflammatory cascade. Systemically, levels of interleukin-2, -4, -6, and interferon-gamma (IFN-γ) are elevated in proportion to the severity of the burn injury, perhaps as part of a generalized systemic release of inflammatory mediators. There is often an altered CD4/CD8 (T helper/T suppressor) cell ratio. In addition, in the first 24 hours following a significant burn, there is production of tumor necrosis factor (TNF) and IFN-γ, which in turn stimulate production of the enzyme nitric oxide synthetase in hepatocytes. After 24 hours, lipopolysaccharide (LPS) plays a dominant role in its production. Nitric oxide has been proposed as a mediator of the acute inflammation. Clinical attempts to modify these factors have had mixed success.

INITIAL MANAGEMENT

Airway

The physician or emergency medical technician should proceed as with any other trauma using standard Advanced Trauma Life Support (ATLS) guidelines. The priorities are first to establish an airway, recognizing the frequent necessity to intubate a patient who may appear to be breathing normally but who has sustained an inhalation injury; next, to evaluate the cervical spine and head injuries; and finally, to stabilize fractures. Fluid resuscitation by the Parkland formula (see below) may be instituted simultaneously with initial resuscitation. Endotracheal intubation should be considered for major burn cases regardless of the area of the body involved, because as fluid resuscitation proceeds generalized edema develops, including edema of the soft tissues of the upper airway and perhaps the lungs as well. Chest radiographs are typically normal initially but may develop an acute respiratory distress syndrome picture in 24–48 hours with severe inhalation injury. Supplemental oxygen should be administered. Inhalation injuries should be followed by serial blood gas determination and bronchoscopy. The use of corticosteroids is contraindicated because of the potential for immunosuppression.

Vascular Access

All clothing and jewelry should be removed and an expedient physical examination performed to assess the extent of burn and associated injuries. Simultaneously with the above procedures, venous access must be sought, since the victim of a major burn may develop hypovolemic shock. A percutaneous large-bore (14- or 16-gauge) intravenous line through nonburned skin is preferred. Subclavian lines are avoided in the emergency setting because of the risk of pneumothorax and subclavian vein laceration when such a line is placed in a volume-depleted patient. Femoral lines provide good temporary access during resuscitation. *All lines—without exception—placed in the emergency department should be changed within 24 hours because of the high risk of nonsterile placement.* Distal saphenous cutdown is occasionally necessary. An arterial line is useful for monitoring mean arterial pressure and drawing blood.

FLUID RESUSCITATION

Crystalloids

Generalized capillary leak results from burn injury over more than 25% of total body surface area. This often necessitates replacement of a large volume of fluid.

There are many guidelines for fluid resuscitation. The **Parkland formula** relies upon the use of lactated Ringer's injection. The fluid requirement in the first 24 hours is estimated as 4 mL/kg body weight per percent of body surface area burned. Deep electrical burns and inhalation injury increase the fluid requirement. Adequacy of resuscitation is determined by clinical parameters, including urine output and specific gravity, blood pressure, and central venous catheter or, if necessary, Swan-Ganz catheter readings.

Half the calculated fluid is given in the first 8-hour period. The remaining fluid, divided into two equal parts, is delivered over the next 16 hours. An extremely large volume of fluid may be required. For example, an injury over 40% of the total body surface area in a 70-kg victim may require 13 L *in the first 24 hours.* The first 8-hour period is measured from the hour of injury.

Beta Blockade

Routine beta blockade (propranolol, adjusting dose to decrease resting heart rate by 20%, for up to 4 weeks) may reverse some of the catecholamine-mediated hypermetabolic response after severe burns.

Colloids

Overly aggressive crystalloid administration must be avoided in patients with pulmonary injury, since significant pulmonary edema can develop in patients with normal pulmonary capillary wedge and central venous pressures. In addition, routine colloid administration, commonplace 10 years ago, must now be considered suspect in routine burn resuscitation in view of its deleterious effect on glomerular filtration and its association with pulmonary edema.

Monitoring Fluid Resuscitation

A Foley catheter is essential for monitoring urinary output. *Diuretics have no role in this phase of patient management unless fluid overload has occurred or mannitol diuresis is performed in the case of rhabdomyolysis.*

Escharotomy

As edema fluid accumulates, ischemia may develop under any constricting eschar of an extremity, neck, or trunk if the full-thickness burn is circumferential. Escharotomy incisions through the anesthetic eschar can save life and limb and can be performed in the emergency department or operating room.

Fasciotomy in Electrical Burns & Associated Crush Injuries

When high-voltage electrical injury occurs, extensive deep tissue necrosis is almost invariably present. Deep tissue necrosis leads to profound tissue swelling. Because deep tissue compartments in the arms and legs are contained by unyielding fascia, these compartments must be opened by surgical fasciotomy to prevent further soft tissue, vascular, and nerve death.

Electrical burn injuries remain the most devastating and underrecognized burn injuries, causing amputations (often because of unrecognized compartment syndromes) and acute renal failure, resulting in part from rhabdomyolysis. Prompt recognition of the severity of electrical burns, with early fasciotomy and debridement, may reduce the incidence of such complications.

THE BURN WOUND

Treatment of the burn wound is based on several principles: (1) Protection from desiccation and further injury of those burned areas that will spontaneously reepithelialize in 7–10 days by application of topical antibiotic such as silver sulfadiazine or mafenide acetate. Silver sulfadiazine is currently the most popular topical agent. It is painless, easy to apply, and effective against most strains of pseudomonas. (2) Regular and thorough cleansing of burned areas is a critically important intervention in burn units. Early excision and grafting of burned areas as soon as 24 hours after burn injury or when the patient will hemodynamically tolerate the excision and grafting procedure. The tumescent technique (injection under the burn scar of dilute epinephrine and lidocaine prior to surgery) may reduce blood loss, though lidocaine toxicity must be considered.

Systemic infection remains a leading cause of morbidity among major burn patients, with nearly all burn patients having one or more septicemic episodes during their hospital course. Methicillin-resistant *Staphylococcus aureus,* pseudomonas species, klebsiella species, proteus species, methicillin-resistant *S epidermidis,* and acinetobacter remain commonly cultured microorganisms. Typically, gram-positive organisms predominate early in the clinical course, followed later by gram-negative organisms. Continuous microbiologic surveillance is necessary. There is an increasing trend toward use of prophylactic antibiotics in burn patients. Prophylactic administration of trimethoprim-sulfamethoxazole may help to prevent methicillin-resistant *S aureus* (MRSA) infection in ventilator-dependent burn patients. Systemic infections are manifestations of a globally suppressed immune system. Nitric oxide has been implicated in the depressed lymphoproliferative state in experimental animals. Increasingly, sterile multiple organ failure is regarded as a leading cause of death among severely burned patients.

Wound Closure

The goal of therapy after fluid resuscitation is closure of the wound. Nature's own blister is the best cover to protect wounds that spontaneously epithelialize in 7–10 days (ie, superficial second-degree burns). Where the blister has been disrupted, silver sulfadiazine or skin substitutes can be used. In patients with scald burns—usually no more than superficial partial-thickness (first or superficial second-degree) burns— use of Biobrane dressing is recommended. However, in medium partial-thickness burn wounds or wounds with even minimal contamination, treatment with Biobrane dressing results in a high rate of wound infection. These dressings are temporary and not indicated in deep partial-thickness or full-thickness burns or in burns that are heavily colonized or infected. Cadaver homografts can also serve this purpose if available. Dermal substitutes that have longevity remain elusive, though bovine collagen and elastin-hydrolysate dermal substitute and Integra have shown short-term promise.

Wounds that will not heal spontaneously in 7–10 days (ie, deep second-degree or third-degree burns) are best treated by excision and autograft; otherwise, granulation and infection may develop, and the quality of the skin in regenerated deep partial thickness burns is marginal because of the very thin dermis that emerges.

Cultured keratinocytes remain an option for wound coverage; however, their primary use (lacking a formal dermis) continues to be as a temporary skin substitute establishing the skin barrier.

PATIENT SUPPORT

Burn patients require extensive support. An attempt must be made to maintain normal core body temperature in patients with burns over more than 20% of total body surface area, since the hypermetabolic state of burns is exacerbated by subnormal temperatures. Respiratory injury, sepsis, and multiorgan failure are common. Enteral feedings may be started once the ileus of the resuscitation period has resolved, usually the day after the injury. There is often a markedly increased metabolic rate after burn injury, due in large part to whole body synthesis and increased fatty acid substrate cycles. If the patient does not tolerate low-residue tube feedings, TPN should be started without delay through a central venous catheter. As much as 4000–6000 kcal/d may be required in the postburn period. The metabolic demands are immense. A useful guide is to provide 25 kcal/kg body weight plus 40 kcal per percent of burn surface area. Fat emulsions (Intralipid) given intravenously are useful during the resuscitation period to span the period of ileus. Early experimental data from animal models support the administration of low-fat solutions. Early aggressive enteral nutrition reduces infections, noninfectious complications, length of hospital stay, and mortality. Occasionally, burn patients may develop acute respiratory distress syndrome or respiratory failure unresponsive to maximal ventilatory support. Heroic resuscitative measures are sometimes successfully employed, with use of extracorporeal life support (ECLS), in children who would otherwise die of ARDS, inhalation injury, or pneumonia in the postburn period. Early pulmonary dysfunction after severe burn injury is widely recognized. It is now apparent in children that late and permanent pulmonary dysfunction with later obstructive and restrictive lung disease can result from major burn injury.

Prevention of long-term scars remains a formidable problem in seriously burned patients. The tunable pulse-dye or, more recently, the V-beam laser is emerging as adjunctive treatment to the usual regimen of steroid injections, silicone patches, compression, and scar revision. Permanent sequelae can be avoided by prevention of infection, early aggressive rehabilitation, compressive garments and early psychologic support.

Early burn care and grafting, splinting, and hand therapy are the result of coordinated care by general, hand, and plastic surgeons, therapists, and nurses. Late burn reconstruction is best dealt with by a plastic and reconstructive surgeon. Recent advances in reconstructive burn surgery include the use of microsurgery to perform muscle and fasciocutaneous flaps and tissue expansion. However, complex reconstructive options such as free tissue transfer involve much higher than normal complication rates when performed in the acutely burned patient. In late reconstruction of burns involving the head and neck, tissue expansion is sometimes used instead of conventional skin grafting, since this technique provides skin most similar to that lost because of the burn. After severe hand burns, function may be aided by expedient splinting or axial pin fixation to prevent flexion contractures and facilitate prompt skin grafting and physical therapy. Aggressive microsurgical reconstructions of hand injuries facilitate early motion and improved function of burn injuries to the hand.

Patients who have suffered severe burn injuries can recover to a general health status slightly lower than that of the general population but still have very significant vocational and psychologic problems.

There is research interest in a possible role of antioxidants in early fluid resuscitation in order to prevent free radical-induced tissue damage. Monoclonal antibodies against offending pathogens and growth factors continue to be investigated. Dermal matrix substitutes continue to improve but remain plagued by the lack of a substantial dermis.

Blaha J: Permanent sequelae after burns and tested procedures to influence them. Acta Chir Plast 2001;43:119 [PMID 11789052]

Cumming J et al: Objective estimates of the incidence and consequences of multiple organ dysfunction and sepsis after burn trauma. J Trauma 2001;50:510. [PMID: 11265031]

Dantzer E et al: Reconstructive surgery using an artificial dermis (Integra): results with 39 grafts. Br J Plast Surg 2001;54: 659. [PMID 11728107]

Herndon DN et al: Reversal of catabolism by beta-blockade after severe burns. N Engl J Med 2001;345:1223. [PMID 11680441]

Marik PE et al: Early enteral nutrition in acutely ill patients: a systematic review. Crit Care Med 2001;29:2264. [PMID: 11801821]

Robertson RD et al: The tumescent technique to significantly reduce blood loss during burn surgery. Burns 2001;27:835. [PMID 11718986]

Sheridan RL et al: Long-term outcome of children surviving massive burns. JAMA 2000;283:69. [PMID: 10632282]

van Zuijlen PP et al: Dermal substitution in acute burns and reconstructive surgery: a subjective and objective long-term follow-up. Plast Reconstr Surg 2001;108:1938. [PMID: 11743380]

Wibbenmeyer LA et al: Predicting survival in an elderly burn patient population. Burns 2001;27:583. [PMID 11525852]

Woo SH et al: Optimizing the correction of severe postburn hand deformities with aggressive contracture releases and fasciocutaneous free-tissue transfers. Plast Reconstr Surg 2001; 107:1. [PMID: 11176593]

Yanaga H et al: Cryopreserved cultured epidermal allografts achieved early closure of wounds and reduced scar formation in deep partial-thickness burn wounds (DDB) and split-thickness skin donor sites of pediatric patients. Burns 2001;27:689. [PMID 11600248]

■ ELECTRIC SHOCK

The extent of injury from electroshock is determined by the amount and type of current, the duration and area of exposure, and the pathway of the current through the body. If the current passes through the heart or brain stem, death may occur immediately owing to ventricular fibrillation or apnea. Current passing through skeletal muscle can cause muscle necrosis and contractions severe enough to result in bone fracture. Current traversing peripheral nerves can cause acute or delayed neuropathy. Delayed effects can include damage to the spinal cord, peripheral nerves, bone, kidneys, and gastrointestinal tract and development of cataracts.

With alternating currents (AC) of 25–300 Hz, low voltages (< 220 Hz) tend to produce ventricular fibrillation; high voltages (> 1000 Hz), respiratory failure; intermediate voltages (220–1000 Hz), both. More than 100 mA of domestic house current (AC) of 110 volts at 60 Hz is, accordingly, dangerous to the heart, since it can cause ventricular fibrillation. DC current contact is more likely to cause asystole.

Lightning injuries differ from high-voltage electric shock injuries; lightning usually involves higher voltage, briefer duration of contact, asystole, nervous system injury, and multisystem pathologic involvement.

Electrical burns are of three distinct types: flash (arcing) burns, flame (clothing) burns, and the direct heating effect of tissues by the electric current. The latter lesions are usually sharply demarcated, round or oval, painless yellow-brown areas (Joule burn) with inflammatory reaction. Significant subcutaneous damage can be accompanied by little skin injury, particularly with larger skin surface area electrical contact.

Electric shock may produce loss of consciousness. With recovery there may be muscular pain, fatigue, headache, and nervous irritability. The physical signs vary according to the action of the current. Ventricular fibrillation or respiratory failure—or both—can occur; the patient may be unconscious, pulseless, hypotensive, cold and cyanotic, and without respirations.

Treatment

A. EMERGENCY MEASURES

The victim must be separated from the electric current prior to initiation of CPR or other treatment; the rescuer must be protected. Turn off the power, sever the wire with a dry wooden-handled ax, make a proper ground to divert the current, or separate the victim using nonconductive implements such as dry clothing.

B. HOSPITAL MEASURES

Lightning or unstable electric shock victims should be hospitalized when revived and observed for shock, arrhythmia, thrombosis, infarction, sudden cardiac dilation, hemorrhage, and myoglobinuria. A urinalysis, serum CK and CK-MB, and an electrocardiogram should be obtained immediately. Victims should also be evaluated for blunt trauma, dehydration, skin burns, hypertension, posttraumatic stress, acid-base disturbances, and neurologic damage. Indications for hospitalization include significant arrhythmia or electrocardiographic changes, large burn, loss of consciousness, pulmonary or cardiac symptoms, or evidence of significant deep tissue or organ damage. Extra caution is indicated when the electroshock current has followed a transthoracic route (hand to hand or hand to foot) and in patients with a cardiac history.

To counteract fluid losses and myoglobinuria due to electric shock (not lightning) burns, aggressive hydration with Ringer's lactate should seek to achieve a urine output of 50–100 mL/h.

Prognosis

Complications may occur in almost any part of the body but most commonly include sepsis, gangrene requiring limb amputation, or neurologic, cardiac, cognitive, or psychiatric dysfunction.

Fish RM: Electric injury, Part I: Treatment priorities, subtle diagnostic factors and burns. J Emerg Med 1999;17:977. [PMID: 10595883]

Fish RM: Electric injury, Part II: Specific injuries. J Emerg Med 2000;18:27. [PMID: 10645833] (Diagnosis and treatment of complications and secondary injuries.)

Fish RM: Electric injury, Part III: cardiac monitoring indications, the pregnant patient and lightning. J Emerg Med 2000;18: 181. [PMID: 10699519]

Jain S et al: Electrical and lightning injuries. Crit Care Clin 1999;15:319. [PMID: 10331131] (Epidemiology, pathophysiology, diagnosis, and treatment.)

Occupational Electrical Injury: Proceedings of the 3rd International Conference on Electrical Injury and Safety. Shanghai, China, October 26–28, 1998. Ann N Y Acad Sci 1999;888: 1. [PMID: 10877750] (Diagnosis and treatment of electroshock and electric burn injuries.)

■ IONIZING RADIATION REACTIONS

The extent of damage due to radiation exposure depends on the quantity of radiation delivered to the body, the dose rate, the organs exposed, the type of radiation (x-rays, neutrons, gamma rays, alpha or beta particles), the duration of exposure, and the energy transfer from the radioactive wave or particle to the exposed tissue. The Chernobyl experience suggests that the best biologic indicators of dose are the duration of the asymptomatic latent period (particularly for nausea or emesis), the severity of early symptoms, the rate of decline of the lymphocyte count, and the number and distribution of dicentric chromosomes in peripheral lymphocytes.

The National Committee on Radiation Protection has established the maximum permissible radiation exposure for occupationally exposed workers over age 18 as 0.1 rem* per week for the whole body (but not to exceed 5 rem per year) and 1.5 rem per week for the hands. (For purposes of comparison, routine chest x-rays deliver from 0.1–0.2 rem.) The FDA has recommended 1 Gy as a threshold for skin-absorbed dose from medical fluoroscopy.

Death after acute lethal radiation exposure is usually due to hematopoietic failure, gastrointestinal mucosal damage, central nervous system damage, widespread vascular injury, or secondary infection. The acute radiation syndrome may be dominated by central nervous system, gastrointestinal, or hematologic manifestations depending on dose and survival. Four hundred to 600 cGy of x-ray or gamma radiation applied to the entire body at one time may be fatal within 60 days; death is usually due to hemorrhage, anemia, and infection secondary to hematopoietic injury. Levels of 1000–3000 cGy to the entire body destroy gastrointestinal mucosa; this leads to toxemia and death within 2 weeks. Total body doses above

---

*In radiation terminology, a rad is the unit of absorbed dose and a rem is the unit of any radiation dose to body tissue in terms of its estimated biologic effect. Roentgen (R) refers to the amount of radiation dose delivered to the body. For x-ray or gamma ray radiation, rems, rads, and roentgens are virtually the same. For particulate radiation from radioactive materials, these terms may differ greatly (eg, for neutrons, 1 rad equals 10 rems). In the Système International (SI) nomenclature, the rad has been replaced by the gray (Gy), and 1 rad equals 0.01 Gy = 1 cGy. The SI replacement for the rem is the Sievert (Sv), and 1 rem equals 0.01 Sv.

3000 cGy cause widespread vascular damage, cerebral anoxia, hypotensive shock, and death within 48 hours.

ACUTE (IMMEDIATE) IONIZING RADIATION EFFECTS ON NORMAL TISSUES

Clinical Findings

A. INJURY TO SKIN AND MUCOUS MEMBRANES

Irradiation may cause erythema, epilation, destruction of fingernails, or epidermolysis.

B. INJURY TO DEEP STRUCTURES

1. Hematopoietic tissues—Injury to the bone marrow may cause diminished production of blood elements. Lymphocytes are most sensitive, polymorphonuclear leukocytes next most sensitive, and erythrocytes least sensitive. Damage to the blood-forming organs may vary from transient depression of one or more blood elements to complete destruction.

2. Cardiovascular system—Pericarditis with effusion or constrictive pericarditis may occur after a period of months or even years. Myocarditis is less common. Smaller vessels (the capillaries and arterioles) are more readily damaged than larger blood vessels.

3. Reproductive effects—In males, small single doses of radiation (200–300 cGy) cause temporary aspermatogenesis, and larger doses (600–800 cGy) may cause permanent sterility. In females, single doses of 200 cGy may cause temporary cessation of menses, and 500–800 cGy may cause permanent castration. Moderate to heavy irradiation of the embryo in utero results in injury to the fetus (eg, mental retardation) or in embryonic death and abortion.

4. Respiratory tract—High or repeated moderate doses of radiation may cause pneumonitis, often delayed for weeks or months.

5. Mouth, pharynx, esophagus, and stomach—Mucositis with edema and painful swallowing of food may occur within hours or days after exposure. Gastric secretion may be inhibited by high doses of radiation.

6. Intestines—Inflammation and ulceration may follow moderately large doses of radiation.

7. Endocrine glands and viscera—Hepatitis and nephritis may be delayed effects of therapeutic radiation. The normal thyroid, pituitary, pancreas, adrenals, and bladder are relatively resistant to low or moderate doses of radiation; parathyroid glands are especially resistant.

8. Nervous system—The brain and spinal cord are much more sensitive to acute exposures than the peripheral nerves.

C. SYSTEMIC REACTION (RADIATION SICKNESS)

The basic mechanisms of radiation sickness are not known. Anorexia, nausea, vomiting, weakness, exhaustion, lassitude, and in some cases prostration may occur, singly or in combination. Dehydration, anemia, and infection may follow. Radiation sickness associated with x-ray therapy is most likely to occur when the therapy is given in large dosage to large areas over the abdomen, less often when given over the thorax, and rarely when therapy is given over the extremities.

Prevention

Persons handling radiation sources can minimize exposure to radiation by recognizing the importance of time, distance, and shielding. Areas housing x-ray and nuclear materials must be properly shielded. X-ray equipment should be periodically checked for reliability of output, and proper filters should be employed. When feasible, it is advisable to shield the gonads, especially of young persons. Fluoroscopic examination should be performed as rapidly as possible, using an optimal combination of beam characteristics and filtration, and the beam size should be kept to a minimum required by the examination. Special protective clothing may be necessary to protect against contamination with radioisotopes. In the event of accidental contamination, all clothing should be removed and the body vigorously bathed with soap and water. This should be followed by careful instrument (Geiger counter) check to localize the ionizing radiation.

Emergency Treatment for Radiation Accident Victims

The proliferation of radiation equipment and nuclear energy plants and the increased transportation of radioactive materials necessitate hospital plans for managing patients who are accidentally exposed to ionizing radiation or are contaminated with radioisotopes. The plans should provide for effective emergency care and disposition of victims and materials with the least possible risk of spreading radioactive contamination to health care personnel and facilities.

Treatment

The success of treatment of local radiation effects depends upon the extent, degree, and location of tissue injury. Particulate or radioisotope exposures should be decontaminated in designated confined areas. Serial lymphocyte counts are useful for dose estimation and monitoring of the clinical impact of exposure. For many radioisotopes, chelation, blocking, or dilution therapy is indicated. Treatment of systemic reactions is symptomatic and supportive. Ondansetron, 8 mg orally twice or three times daily, has been recommended for nausea and vomiting. Alternatives include chlorpromazine, 25–50 mg given deeply intramuscularly every 4–6 hours as necessary or 10–25 mg orally every 4–6 hours as necessary; and dimenhydrinate, 50–100 mg, or perphenazine, 4–8 mg, 1 hour before and 1 and 4 hours after radiation therapy has been recommended.

Blood and platelet transfusions, blood stem cell transplantation, bone marrow transplants, antibiotics, fluid and electrolyte maintenance, and other supportive measures may be useful. Recombinant hematopoietic growth factors (filgrastim and sargramostim or molgramostim) have been effective in accelerating hematopoietic recovery.

DELAYED EFFECTS OF EXCESSIVE DOSES OF IONIZING RADIATION

These disorders may occur following excessive ionizing radiation exposure: skin scarring, atrophy, and telangiectasis; cataract, dry eye syndrome, retinopathy; neuropathy, myelopathy, cerebral injury; obliterative endarteritis, coronary artery disease, pericarditis; thyroid disease; pulmonary fibrosis, hepatitis, intestinal stenosis, and nephritis. Neoplastic disease, including leukemia and cancers of the skin, breast, lung, and thyroid, is increased in persons exposed to radiation at relatively low doses (< 0.2 Gy). High-dose radon exposure is associated with an increased risk of lung cancer. Association of ionizing radiation with several other cancers has been reported but not well quantified (salivary glands, skin, stomach, colon, bladder, ovary, and central nervous system). Prenatal irradiation may increase the risk of childhood cancer.

Microcephaly and other congenital abnormalities may occur in children exposed in utero, especially if the fetus was exposed during early pregnancy. Carcinogenesis from low-dose (< 10 rem) exposure to adults has not been demonstrated. However, because of age-related differences in sensitivity to radiation, carcinogenesis following childhood exposures has been observed (eg, Chernobyl and childhood thyroid cancer).

Gusev I et al: *Medical Management of Radiation Accidents.* CRC Press, 2001.

IARC Working group on the evaluation of carcinogenic risks to humans: ionizing radiation, Part I, X- and gamma- radiation and neutrons. Lyon, France, 26 May–2 June 1999. IARC Monogr Eval Carcinog Risks Hum 2000;75(Part 1):1. [PMID: 11203346]

Reeves GI: Radiation injuries. Crit Care Clin 1999;15:457. [PMID: 10331137] (Pathophysiology and treatment.)

■ DROWNING

The asphyxia of drowning is usually due to aspiration of fluid, but it may result from airway obstruction caused by laryngeal spasm while the victim is gasping under water. About 10% of victims develop laryngospasm after the first gulp and never aspirate water ("dry drowning"). The rapid sequence of events after submersion—hypoxemia, laryngospasm, fluid aspiration, ineffective circulation, brain injury, and brain death—may take place within 5–10 minutes. This sequence may be delayed for longer periods if the victim, especially a child, has been submerged in very cold water or if the victim has ingested significant amounts of barbiturates. Immersion in cold water can also cause a rapid fall in the victim's core temperature, so that systemic hypothermia and death may occur before actual drowning.

The primary effect is hypoxia due to perfusion of poorly ventilated alveoli, intrapulmonary shunting, and decreased compliance. *The first requirement of rescue is immediate cardiopulmonary resuscitation.*

A number of circumstances or primary events may precede near drowning and must be taken into consideration in management: (1) use of alcohol or other drugs (a contributing factor in an estimated 25% of adult drownings), (2) extreme fatigue, (3) intentional hyperventilation, (4) sudden acute illness (eg, epilepsy, myocardial infarction), (5) head or spinal cord injury sustained in diving, (6) venomous stings by aquatic animals, and (7) decompression sickness in deep water diving.

Spontaneous return of consciousness often occurs in otherwise healthy individuals when submersion is very brief. Many other patients respond promptly to immediate ventilation. Other patients, with more severe degrees of near drowning, may have frank respiratory failure, pulmonary edema, shock, anoxic encephalopathy, cerebral edema, and cardiac arrest. A few patients may be deceptively asymptomatic during the recovery period—only to deteriorate or die as a result of acute respiratory failure within the following 12–24 hours.

Clinical Findings

A. Symptoms and Signs

The patient may be unconscious, semiconscious, or awake but apprehensive, restless, and complaining of headaches or chest pain. Vomiting is common. Examination may reveal cyanosis, trismus, apnea, tachypnea, and wheezing. A pink froth from the mouth and nose indicates pulmonary edema. Cardiovascular manifestations may include tachycardia, arrhythmias, hypotension, cardiac arrest, and circulatory shock. With prolonged or cold water immersion, hypothermia is likely.

B. Laboratory Findings

Urinalysis shows proteinuria, hemoglobinuria, and acetonuria. Leukocytosis is usually present. The PaO_2 is usually decreased and the $PaCO_2$ increased or decreased. The blood pH is decreased as a result of metabolic acidosis. Chest x-rays may show pneumonitis or pulmonary edema.

Prevention

Prevention consists of avoidance of alcohol during recreational swimming or boating, close supervision of toddlers, swimming lessons early in life, and use of personal flotation devices when boating. All swimming pools should be fenced.

Treatment

A. First Aid

Immediate measures to combat hypoxemia at the scene of the incident—sustained ventilation, oxygenation, and circulatory support—are critical to survival with complete recovery. Hypothermia and cervical spine injury should always be suspected.

1. Standard CPR is initiated if pulse and respirations are absent.

2. *Do not* attempt to drain water from the victim's lungs. The Heimlich maneuver (subdiaphragmatic pressure) should be used only if airway obstruction by a foreign body is suspected. The cervical spine should be immobilized if neck injury is possible.

3. *Do not* discontinue basic life support for seemingly "hopeless" patients until core temperature reaches 32 °C. Complete recovery has been reported after prolonged resuscitation of hypothermic patients.

B. Hospital Care

Careful observation of the patient; continuous monitoring of cardiorespiratory function; serial determination of arterial blood gases, pH, renal function (serum creatinine), and electrolytes; and measurement of urinary output are required. Pulmonary edema may not appear for 24 hours.

1. Ensure optimal ventilation and oxygenation— The danger of hypoxemia exists even in the alert, conscious patient who appears to be breathing normally. Oxygen should be administered immediately at the highest available concentration. Endotracheal intubation and mechanical ventilation are necessary for patients unable to maintain an open airway or normal blood gases and pH. Nasogastric intubation will allow removal of swallowed water and prevention of aspiration. If the victim does not have spontaneous respirations, intubation is required. Oxygen saturation should be maintained at 90% or higher. Continuous positive airway pressure (CPAP) is the most effective means of reversing hypoxia in patients with spontaneous respirations and patent airways. Positive end-expiratory pressure (PEEP) is also effective for treating respiratory insufficiency. Assisted ventilation may be necessary with pulmonary edema, respiratory failure, aspiration, pneumonia, or severe central nervous system injury. Serial physical examinations and chest x-rays should be carried out to detect possible pneumonitis, atelectasis, and pulmonary edema. Bronchospasm due to aspirated material may require use of bronchodilators. Antibiotics should be given only when there is clinical evidence of infection—not prophylactically.

2. Cardiovascular support—Central venous pressure (or, preferably, pulmonary artery wedge pressure) may be monitored as a guide to determining whether vascular fluid replacement and pressors or diuretics are needed. If low cardiac output persists after adequate intravascular volume is achieved, pressors should be given. Otherwise, standard therapy for pulmonary edema is administered.

3. Correction of blood pH and electrolyte abnormalities—Metabolic acidosis is present in 70% of near-drowning victims, but it is usually of minor importance and corrected through adequate ventilation and oxygenation. While controversial, bicarbonate administration (1 meq/kg) has been recommended for comatose patients (see Chapter 21).

4. Cerebral injury—Some near-drowning patients may progress to irreversible central nervous system damage despite apparently adequate treatment of hypoxia and shock. Mild hyperventilation to achieve a $PaCO_2$ of approximately 30 mm Hg is recommended to lower intracranial pressure.

5. Hypothermia—Core temperature should be measured and managed as appropriate (see Systemic Hypothermia, above).

Course & Prognosis

Victims of near drowning who have had prolonged hypoxemia should remain under close hospital observation for 2–3 days after all supportive measures have been withdrawn and clinical and laboratory findings have been stable. Residual complications of near drowning may include intellectual impairment, convulsive disorders, and pulmonary or cardiac disease.

Layon JA, Modell JH: Drowning and Near Drowning. Lung Biology in Health and Disease 1999;132:395. (Pathophysiology and treatment.)

Sachdeva RC: Near drowning. Crit Care Clin 1999;15:281. [PMID: 10331129] (Pathophysiology and treatment.)

■ OTHER DISORDERS DUE TO PHYSICAL AGENTS

DECOMPRESSION SICKNESS & DYSBARIC ILLNESS

Decompression sickness and other disorders related to rapid changes in environmental pressure are hazards for fliers and divers who are involved in recreational diving (eg scuba diving), deep-water exploration, rescue or salvage operations, or construction.

At low depths the greatly increased pressure (eg, at 30 meters [100 feet] the pressure is four times greater than at the surface) compresses the respiratory gases into the blood and other tissues. During ascent from depths greater than 9 meters (30 feet), gases dissolved in the blood and other tissues escape as the external pressure decreases. The appearance of symptoms depends on the depth and duration of submersion; the degree of physical exertion; the age, weight, and physical condition of the diver; and the rate of ascent. The size and number of gas bubbles (notably nitrogen) escaping from the tissues depend on the difference between the atmospheric pressure and the partial pressure of the gas dissolved in the tissues. The release of gas bubbles and (particularly) the location of their release determine the symptoms.

Decompression sickness also occurs among fliers during rapid ascent from sea level to high altitudes when there is no adequate pressurizing protection. Deep-sea and scuba divers may be vulnerable to air embolism if airplane travel is attempted too soon (within a few hours) after diving.

The range of clinical manifestations includes gas bubble formation in the joints ("bends"), cerebral or pulmonary decompression sickness, arterial gas embolism (cerebral, pulmonary), ear and sinus barotrauma, and dysbaric osteonecrosis.

Predisposing factors include exercise, injury, patent foramen ovale, obesity, dehydration, alcoholic excess, hypoxia, some medications (eg, narcotics, antihistamines), and cold. Reported sequelae include hemiparesis, neurologic dysfunction, and bone damage. Asthma, pneumothorax, reduced pulmonary function, lung cysts, or thoracic trauma may be contraindications to diving.

The onset of acute decompression symptoms occurs within 30 minutes in half of cases and almost invariably within 6 hours. Symptoms, which are highly variable, include pain (largely in the joints), headache, fatigue, numbness, confusion, pruritic rash, visual disturbances, nausea, vomiting, loss of hearing, weakness, paralysis, dizziness, vertigo, dyspnea, paresthesias, aphasia, and coma.

Pulmonary decompression sickness ("chokes") presents with burning, pleuritic substernal pain, cough, and dyspnea.

Early recognition and prompt treatment are extremely important. Continuous administration of oxygen is indicated as a first aid measure whether or not cyanosis is present. Aspirin may be given for pain, but narcotics should be used very cautiously, since they may obscure the patient's response to recompression. Rapid transportation to a treatment facility for recompression, hyperbaric oxygen, hydration treatment of plasma deficits, and supportive measures is necessary not only to relieve symptoms but also to prevent permanent impairment. It has been recommended, however, that decompression symptoms be treated whenever they are seen—even up to 2 weeks postinjury—since it is still possible to completely alleviate symptoms. The clinician should be familiar with the nearest compression center. The local public health department or nearest naval facility should be able to provide such information. The National Divers Alert Network at Duke University (DAN; 919-684-8111) provides assistance in the management of underwater diving accidents.

Moon RE: Treatment of diving emergencies. Crit Care Clin 1999;15:429. [PMID: 10331136] (Diagnosis and treatment of barotrauma and decompression disorders.)

Strauss MB et al: Diving medicine: Contemporary topics and their controversies. Am J Emerg Med 2001;19:232. [PMID:11326354] (Treatment of dysbarism related to scuba diving.)

Van Meter K: Medical field management of the injured diver. Respir Care Clin North Am 1999;5:137. [PMID: 10205815] (Emergency assessment, decompression and equipment guidelines.)

MOUNTAIN SICKNESS

Lack of sufficient time for acclimatization, increased physical activity, and varying degrees of health may be responsible for the acute, subacute, and chronic disturbances that result from hypoxia at altitudes greater than 2000 meters (6560 ft). Marked individual differences in tolerance to hypoxia exist. Patients with sickle cell disease are at high risk of painful crises from altitude-induced hypoxemia.

Acute Mountain Sickness

The severity of acute mountain sickness correlates with altitude and rate of ascent. Initial manifestations include headache (most severe and persistent symptom), lassitude, drowsiness, dizziness, chilliness, nausea and vomiting, facial pallor, dyspnea, and cyanosis. Later, there is facial flushing, irritability, difficulty in concentrating, vertigo, tinnitus, visual disturbances, auditory disturbances, anorexia, insomnia, increased dyspnea and weakness on exertion, increased headaches (due to cerebral edema), palpitations, tachycardia, Cheyne-Stokes breathing, and weight loss. More severe manifestations include pulmonary edema and encephalopathy (see below). Voluntary periodic hyperventilation may relieve symptoms. In most individuals, symptoms clear within 24–48 hours, but in some instances, if the symptoms are sufficiently persistent or severe, the patient must be returned to lower altitudes. Definitive treatment is immediate descent, which is essential if reduced consciousness, ataxia, or pulmonary edema occurs. Administration of oxygen, 1–2 L/min, will often relieve acute symptoms. If immediate descent is not possible, portable hyperbaric chambers can provide symptomatic relief depending on altitude and severity. Acetazolamide, 125–250 mg every 12 hours, or dexamethasone, 8 mg initially followed by 4 mg every 6 hours, for as long as symptoms persist, is recommended therapy; they may be used together in severe cases.

Preventive measures include slow ascent—300 meters (984 feet) per day—adequate rest and sleep the day before travel, reduced food intake, and avoidance of alcohol, tobacco, and unnecessary physical activity during travel. Acetazolamide, 125–250 mg every 12 hours, beginning the day before ascent and continuing for 48–72 hours at altitude, may be used as prophylaxis. Dexamethasone, 4 mg every 12 hours beginning on the day of ascent, continuing for 3 days at the higher altitude, and then tapering over 5 days, is an alternative.

Acute High-Altitude Pulmonary Edema

This serious complication usually occurs at levels above 3000 meters (9840 feet). Early symptoms may appear within 6–36 hours after arrival at a high-altitude area: incessant dry cough, shortness of breath disproportionate to exertion, headache, decreased exercise performance, fatigue, dyspnea at rest, and chest tightness. Later, wheezing, orthopnea, and hemoptysis may occur. Recognition of the early symptoms may enable the patient to descend before incapacitating pulmonary edema develops, but strenuous exertion should be avoided. An early descent of even 500 or 1000 meters may result in improvement of symptoms. Physical findings include tachycardia, mild fever, tachypnea, cyanosis, prolonged respiration, and rales and rhonchi. The patient may become confused or comatose, and the clinical picture may resemble severe pneumonia. The white count is often slightly elevated, but the erythrocyte sedimentation rate is usually normal. Chest x-ray findings vary from irregular patchy infiltration in one lung to nodular densities bilaterally or with transient prominence of the central pulmonary arteries. Transient nonspecific electrocardiographic changes, occasionally showing right ventricular strain, may occur. Pulmonary arterial blood pressure is elevated, whereas wedge pressure is normal.

Treatment, which must often be given under field conditions, consists of rest in the semi-Fowler position (head raised) and administration of 100% oxygen by mask at a rate of 4–6 L/min for 15–30 minutes. *Immediate descent (at least 610 meters [2000 feet]) is essential.* Recompression in a portable hyperbaric bag will temporarily reduce symptoms if rapid or immediate descent is not possible. To conserve oxygen, lower flow rates (2–4 L/min) may be used until the victim recovers or can be evacuated to a lower altitude. Treatment for acute respiratory distress syndrome (see Chapter 9) may be required for some patients who have a prolonged course of pulmonary edema. Nifedipine, 10 mg every 4 hours, may provide symptomatic relief. Dexamethasone, 4 mg every 6 hours, has been recommended if central nervous system symptoms are present. Acetazolamide, 125–250 mg every 12 hours, should be administered if acute mountain sickness is suspected. If bacterial pneumonia occurs, appropriate antibiotic therapy should be given.

Preventive measures include education of prospective mountaineers regarding the possibility of serious pulmonary edema, optimal physical conditioning before travel, gradual ascent to permit acclimatization, and a period of rest and inactivity for 1–2 days after arrival at high altitudes. Prompt medical attention with rest and high-flow oxygen if respiratory symptoms develop may prevent progression to frank pulmonary edema. Persons with a history of high-altitude pulmonary edema should be hospitalized for further observation if possible. Pulmonary embolism and high-altitude bronchitis can also occur. Mountaineering parties at levels of 3000 meters (9840 ft) or higher should carry a supply of oxygen and equipment sufficient for several days. Persons with symptomatic cardiac or pulmonary disease should avoid high altitudes.

Acute High-Altitude Encephalopathy

High-altitude encephalopathy appears to be an extension of the central nervous system symptoms of acute mountain sickness (see above). It usually occurs at elevations above 2500 meters (8250 feet) and is more common in unacclimatized individuals. Clinical findings are due largely to hypoxemia and cerebral edema. Severe headaches, confusion, truncal ataxia, staggering gait, focal deficits, nausea and vomiting, and seizures may progress to obtundation and coma. High-altitude retinopathy is a separate but related effect of altitude. It can include dilated vessels, retinal hemorrhage, vitreous hemorrhage, and papilledema.

Treatment is immediate descent for at least 610 meters (2000 feet), continuing until symptoms improve. Oxygen (2–4 L/min) should be administered by mask. Dexamethasone, 4–8 mg every 6 hours, is recommended thereafter. If immediate descent is impossible, a portable hyperbaric chamber should be used until symptomatic improvement occurs.

Subacute Mountain Sickness

This occurs most frequently in unacclimatized individuals and at altitudes above 4500 meters (14,764 feet). Symptoms—dyspnea and cough—are probably due to pulmonary hypertension and secondary congestive heart failure. There are additional problems of dehydration, skin dryness, and pruritus. The hematocrit may be elevated, and there may be electrocardiographic and chest x-ray evidence of right ventricular hypertrophy. Treatment consists of rest, oxygen administration, diuretics, and return to lower altitudes.

Chronic Mountain Sickness (Monge's Disease)

This uncommon condition, consisting of chronic hypoxia and polycythemia in residents of high-altitude communities who have lost their acclimatization to such an environment, is difficult to differentiate from chronic pulmonary disease. The disorder is characterized by somnolence, mental depression, hypoxemia, cyanosis, clubbing of fingers, hemoglobin > 22 g/dL, polycythemia (hematocrit often > 75%), signs of right ventricular failure, electrocardiographic evidence of right axis deviation and right atrial and ventricular hypertrophy, and x-ray evidence of right heart enlargement and central pulmonary vessel prominence. There is no x-ray evidence of structural pulmonary disease. Pulmonary function tests usually disclose alveolar hypoventilation and elevated PCO_2 but fail to reveal defective oxygen transport. There is a diminished respiratory response to CO_2. Almost complete disappearance of all abnormalities eventually occurs when the patient returns to sea level.

Krieger BP et al: Altitude related pulmonary disorders. Crit Care Clin 1999;15:265. [PMID: 10331128] (Pathophysiology, diagnosis, and treatment.)

Ward MP, Milledge JS, West JB: *High Altitude Medicine and Physiology.* Oxford Univ Press, 2000.

MEDICAL EFFECTS OF AIR TRAVEL & SELECTION OF PATIENTS FOR AIR TRAVEL

The decision about whether or not it is advisable for a patient to travel by air depends not only upon the nature and severity of the illness but also upon such factors as the duration of flight, the altitude to be flown, pressurization, the availability of supplementary oxygen and other medical supplies, the presence of health care professionals, and other special considerations. Air carriers in the USA cannot legally allow the use of personal (passenger-supplied) oxygen containers, but most major airlines will supply oxygen upon advance written request from the passenger's physician. Airline policies, charges, and other details must be checked with each carrier. Medical hazards or complications of air travel are uncommon; unless there is some specific contraindication, air transportation may be the best means of moving patients. The medical hazard most likely to be realized is hypoxia. The most common in-flight emergencies are cardiovascular, syncopal, neuropsychiatric, and abdominal. The Air Transport Association of America defines an incapacitated passenger as "one who is suffering from a physical or mental disability and who, because of such disability or the effect of the flight on the disability, is incapable of self-care; would endanger the health or safety of such person or other passengers or airline employees; or would cause discomfort or annoyance of other passengers."

All commercial airlines retain medical consultants to assist their personnel in making decisions regarding the transportation of passengers with noticeable symptoms of sickness or injury. Clinicians may contact these medical consultants by calling or writing the medical departments of major airlines.

Pretravel clinician evaluation is advisable for patients with hospitalization, surgery, emergency care, or medication change within the past 4 weeks. Listed below are the more common contraindications to air travel.

Cardiovascular Disease

A. CARDIAC DECOMPENSATION

Patients in congestive failure should not fly until they are stable or compensated by appropriate treatment; 100% oxygen should be available during the flight.

B. COMPENSATED VALVULAR OR OTHER HEART DISEASE

Patients should not fly above 2400–2800 meters (7874–9186 feet) unless the aircraft is pressurized and oxygen is administered in the cabin at altitudes of 2400 meters (7874 feet) or higher.

C. ACUTE MYOCARDIAL INFARCTION, CONVALESCENT AND ASYMPTOMATIC

At least 3 weeks of convalescence is recommended even for asymptomatic patients; a negative exercise ECG is desirable. Unstable postinfarction patients should not fly. Post PTCA and post CABG patients should not fly until stable and at least 2 weeks after the procedure. Coronary disease patients with severe or poorly controlled hypertension or ventricular ectopy should not fly. Ambulatory, stabilized, and compensated patients tolerate air travel well. Oxygen should be available.

D. ANGINA PECTORIS

Air travel is inadvisable for patients with new-onset severe or unstable angina. In mild to moderate cases of angina, air travel may be permitted in pressurized planes. Oxygen should be available.

E. DEEP VENOUS THROMBOSIS

Patients with deep venous thrombosis should not fly until their anticoagulant therapy is stable and they have no evidence of pulmonary complications. Long flights increase the risk of deep vein thrombosis and resulting embolic disease. Prevention includes avoidance of smoking and alcohol, low-dose aspirin, support hose, and leg exercises and walking during the flight.

Respiratory Disease

A. NASOPHARYNGEAL DISORDERS

Nasal allergies and infections predispose to development of aerotitis. Chewing gum, nasal decongestants (pseudoephedrine timed-release, one 120 mg capsule 30 minutes before departure), appropriate anti-infective treatment, and avoiding sleep on descent may prevent barotitis. (See Barotrauma, Chapter 8.)

B. ASTHMA

Patients with mild asthma can travel without difficulty.

C. CONGENITAL PULMONARY CYSTS

Patients should not travel unless cleared by a physician.

D. TUBERCULOSIS

Patients with active, communicable tuberculosis or pneumothorax should not be permitted to travel by air.

E. OTHER PULMONARY DISORDERS

Breathlessness at rest is a contraindication to air travel. The degree of hypoxemia and hypercapnia should be assessed, and vital capacity should be evaluated. Patients should be able to walk 50 m (164 ft) or climb one flight of stairs without becoming severely dyspneic.

Anemia

Patients with severe anemia (hemoglobin < 8.5 g/dL or red cell count < 3 million/μL) should not travel by air. If hemoglobin is less than 8–9 g/dL, oxygen should be available. Patients with sickle cell disease appear to be particularly vulnerable.

Diabetes Mellitus

Diabetics who do not need insulin or who can administer their own insulin during flight may fly safely. Adjustment of the insulin administration schedule should be discussed prior to travel across time zones.

Patients With Surgical Problems

Patients convalescing from thoracic or abdominal surgery should not fly until 10 days (abdominal) to 21 days (thoracic) after surgery, and then only if the wound is healed and there is no drainage.

Colostomy patients may be permitted to travel by air providing they are nonodorous and colostomy bags are emptied before flight.

Patients with large hernias unsupported by a truss or binder should not be permitted to fly in nonpressurized aircraft because of an increased danger of strangulation of the herniated bowel.

Postsurgical or posttraumatic eye cases require pressurized cabins and oxygen therapy to avoid retinal damage due to hypoxia. Intraocular gas bubbles are a relative contraindication to air travel.

Psychiatric Disorders

Severely psychotic, agitated, or disturbed patients should not be permitted to fly on scheduled airlines even when accompanied by a medical attendant.

Extremely nervous or apprehensive patients may travel by air if they receive adequate sedation before and during flight.

Motion Sickness

Patients subject to motion sickness can be given sedatives or antihistamines (eg, dimenhydrinate, 50 mg every 4–6 hours; promethazine, 25 mg every 6 hours; or meclizine, 25–50 mg every 24 hours) before and during the flight. Small meals of easily digested food before and during the flight may reduce the tendency to nausea and vomiting.

Pregnancy

Pregnant women may be permitted to fly during the first 8 months of pregnancy unless there is a history of complications of pregnancy or premature birth. During the ninth month of pregnancy, air travel is not recommended; if travel is essential, a physician's authorization is required. Infants less than 1 week old should not be flown at high altitudes or for long distances.

Dupont HL, Steffen R: *Textbook of Travel Medicine and Health,* 2nd ed. BC Decker, 2001. (Travel fitness, emergencies, infections, motion sickness, jet lag. and terrorism.)

Stoller JK: Oxygen and air travel. Respir Care 2000;45:214. [PMID: 1077179] (Indications, patient assessment, and practical aspects of oxygen use with air travel.)

Poisoning

Kent R. Olson, MD

See www.current-med.com/ch39.html

39

■ INITIAL EVALUATION OF THE PATIENT WITH POISONING OR DRUG OVERDOSE

Patients with drug overdoses or poisoning may initially present with no symptoms or with varying degrees of overt intoxication. The asymptomatic patient may have been exposed to or may have ingested a lethal dose of a poison but not yet have any manifestations of toxicity. It is always important to (1) quickly assess the potential danger, (2) perform gut decontamination to prevent absorption, and (3) observe the patient for an appropriate interval.

Assess the Danger

If the toxin is known, the danger can be assessed by consulting a text or computerized information resource (eg, Poisindex) or by calling a regional poison control center (Table 39–1). Assessment will usually take into account the dose ingested (in milligrams per kilogram of body weight), the time interval since ingestion, the presence of any clinical signs, preexisting cardiac, respiratory, renal, or liver disease, and, occasionally, specific serum drug or toxin levels. Be aware that the history given by the patient or family may be incomplete or unreliable.

The manufacturer or its local representative may be able to provide information over the phone concerning the toxic ingredients in question and can be contacted directly or via the regional poison control center (Table 39–1).

Gut Decontamination

The choice of gut decontamination procedure depends on the toxin and the circumstances. (See below for more discussion of methods.)

Observation of the Patient

Asymptomatic or mildly symptomatic patients should be observed for at least 4–6 hours. Longer observation is indicated if the ingested substance is a sustained-release preparation or is known to slow gastrointestinal motility or if there may have been exposure to a poison with delayed onset of symptoms (such as acetaminophen, colchicine, or hepatotoxic mushrooms). After that time, the patient may be discharged if no symptoms have developed and adequate gastric decontamination has been provided. Before discharge, psychiatric evaluation should be performed to assess suicidal risk. Intentional ingestions in adolescents should raise the possibility of unwanted pregnancy or sexual abuse.

■ THE SYMPTOMATIC PATIENT

In symptomatic patients, treatment of life-threatening complications takes precedence over in-depth diagnostic evaluation. Patients with mild symptoms may deteriorate rapidly, which is why all potentially significant exposures should be observed in an acute care facility. The following complications may occur, depending on the type of poisoning.

COMA

Assessment & Complications

Coma is commonly associated with ingestion of large doses of antihistamines, barbiturates, benzodiazepines and other sedative-hypnotic drugs, γ-hydroxybutyrate (GHB), ethanol, opioids, phenothiazines, or antidepressants. The most common cause of death in comatose patients is respiratory failure, which may occur abruptly. Aspiration of gastric contents may also occur, especially in victims who are deeply obtunded

Table 39–1. Regional poison control centers.

Regional poison centers operate 24 hours a day, utilizing specially trained and dedicated staff with access to a variety of texts, files, and computerized information resources. They can also provide immediate telephone consultation with a physician specializing in medical toxicology. One contact number, 800–222–1222, can be used for all of these centers.

State or City	Public Number	Other Numbers
ALABAMA		
Birmingham	800-222-1222	205-933-4050
Tuscaloosa	800-222-1222	205-345-0600
ARIZONA		
Phoenix	800-222-1222	602-253-3334
Tucson	800-222-1222	520-626-6016
CALIFORNIA	800-876-4766 (CA only)	800-411-8080 (CA only)
	800-222-1222	(Health Professionals)
COLORADO	800-222-1222	303-739-1123
CONNECTICUT	800-222-1222	860-679-3456
DELAWARE	800-222-1222	215-386-2100
DISTRICT OF COLUMBIA	800-222-1222	202-362-8563 (TTY)
FLORIDA	800-222-1222	800-222-1222
GEORGIA	800-222-1222	404-616-9000
IDAHO	800-222-1222	
ILLINOIS	800-222-1222	
INDIANA	800-222-1222	317-929-2323
KENTUCKY	800-222-1222	800-722-5725
LOUISIANA	800-222-1222	
MARYLAND	800-222-1222	202-625-3333
Baltimore		410-706-7701
MASSACHUSETTS	800-222-1222	617-232-2120
MICHIGAN	800-222-1222	
MINNESOTA	800-222-1222	
MISSOURI	800-222-1222	314-772-5200
		800-366-8888
MONTANA	800-222-1222	
NEBRASKA	800-222-1222	402-955-5555
NEVADA	800-222-1222	775-982-4129
NEW JERSEY	800-222-1222	
NEW MEXICO	800-222-1222	505-272-2222
NEW YORK		
Buffalo	800-222-1222	716-878-7654
Hudson Valley	800-222-1222	914-366-3030
Long Island	800-222-1222	516-663-2650
New York City	800-222-1222	212-340-4494
Rochester	800-222-1222	716-275-3232
Syracuse	800-222-1222	315-476-4766
NORTH CAROLINA	800-222-1222	704-355-4000

(continued)

Table 39–1. Regional poison control centers. (continued)

Regional poison centers operate 24 hours a day, utilizing specially trained and dedicated staff with access to a variety of texts, files, and computerized information resources. They can also provide immediate telephone consultation with a physician specializing in medical toxicology. One contact number, 800–222–1222, can be used for all of these centers.

State or City	Public Number	Other Numbers
OHIO		
Cincinnati	800-222-1222	513-636-5111
Columbus	800-222-1222	614-228-1323
OREGON	800-222-1222	
PENNSYLVANIA		
Hershey	800-222-1222	717-531-6111
Philadelphia	800-222-1222	215-386-2100
Pittsburgh	800-222-1222	
RHODE ISLAND	800-222-1222	617-232-2120
SOUTH DAKOTA	800-222-1222	
TENNESSEE	800-222-1222	615-936-2034
TEXAS	800-222-1222	
UTAH	800-222-1222	
VIRGINIA		
Charlottesville	800-222-1222	
Richmond	800-222-1222	804-828-9123
WASHINGTON STATE	800-222-1222	206-526-2121
WEST VIRGINIA	800-222-1222	
WYOMING	800-222-1222	402-955-5555

or convulsing. Hypoxia and hypoventilation may cause or aggravate hypotension, arrhythmias and seizures. Thus, protection of the airway and assisted ventilation are the most important treatment measures for any poisoned patient.

Treatment

A. Emergency Management

The initial emergency management of coma can be remembered by the mnemonic *ABCD*, for *A*irway, *B*reathing, *C*irculation, and *D*rugs (dextrose, thiamine, and naloxone or flumazenil), respectively (Table 39–2).

1. Airway—Establish a patent airway by positioning, suction, or insertion of an artificial nasal or oropharyngeal airway. If the patient is deeply comatose or if there is no gag or cough reflex, perform endotracheal intubation. These airway interventions may not be necessary if the patient is intoxicated by an opioid or a benzodiazepine and responds rapidly to intravenous naloxone or flumazenil (see below).

2. Breathing—Clinically assess the quality and depth of respiration, and provide assistance if necessary with a bag-valve-mask device or mechanical ventilator. Provide

supplemental oxygen. The arterial blood CO_2 tension is useful in determining the adequacy of ventilation. The arterial blood PO_2 determination may reveal hypoxemia, which may be caused by respiratory arrest, bronchospasm, pulmonary aspiration, or noncardiogenic pulmonary edema. Pulse oximetry provides an assessment of oxygenation but is not reliable in patients with methemoglobinemia or carbon monoxide poisoning.

Table 39–2. Initial management of coma.

A	Airway control
B	Breathing
C	Circulation
D	Drugs (give all three): Dextrose 50%, 50–100 mL IV Thiamine, 100 mg IM or IV Naloxone, 0.45–2 mg IV[1] And consider flumazenil, 0.2–0.5 mg IV[2]

[1]Repeated doses, up to 5–10 mg, may be required.
[2]Do not give if patient has coingested a tricyclic antidepressant or other convulsant drug or has a seizure disorder.

3. Circulation—Measure the pulse and blood pressure, and estimate tissue perfusion (eg, by measurement of urinary output, skin signs, arterial blood pH). Place the patient on continuous electrocardiographic monitoring. Insert an intravenous line, and draw blood for complete blood count, glucose, electrolytes, serum creatinine and liver tests, and possible toxicologic testing.

4. Drugs—

a. Dextrose and thiamine—Unless promptly treated, severe hypoglycemia can cause irreversible brain damage. Therefore, in all comatose or convulsing patients, give 50% dextrose, 50–100 mL by intravenous bolus, unless a rapid bedside blood sugar test is available and rules out hypoglycemia. In alcoholic or very malnourished patients who may have marginal thiamine stores, give thiamine, 100 mg intramuscularly or over 2–3 minutes intravenously.

b. Narcotic antagonists—Naloxone, 0.4–2 mg intravenously, may reverse opioid-induced respiratory depression and coma. If opioid overdose is strongly suspected, give additional doses of naloxone (up to 5–10 mg may be required to reverse potent opioids). *Caution:* Naloxone has a much shorter duration of action (2–3 hours) than most common opioids; repeated doses may be required, and continuous observation for at least 3–4 hours after the last dose is mandatory. Nalmefene, a newer opioid antagonist, has a duration of effect longer than that of naloxone but still shorter than that of the opioid methadone.

c. Flumazenil—Flumazenil, 0.2–0.5 mg intravenously, repeated every 30 seconds as needed up to a maximum of 3 mg, may reverse benzodiazepine-induced coma. *Caution:* Flumazenil has a short duration of effect (2–3 hours), and resedation requiring additional doses is common. Furthermore, flumazenil should not be given if the patient has coingested a tricyclic antidepressant, is a user of high-dose benzodiazepines, or has a seizure disorder—because its use in these circumstances may precipitate seizures.

HYPOTHERMIA

Assessment & Complications

Hypothermia commonly accompanies coma due to opioids, ethanol, hypoglycemic agents, phenothiazines, barbiturates, benzodiazepines, and other sedative-hypnotics and depressants. Hypothermic patients may have a barely perceptible pulse and blood pressure and often appear to be dead. Hypothermia may cause or aggravate hypotension, which will not reverse until the temperature is normalized.

Treatment

Hypothermia treatment is discussed in Chapter 38. Gradual rewarming is preferred unless the patient is in cardiac arrest.

HYPOTENSION

Assessment & Complications

Hypotension may be due to poisoning by many different drugs and poisons. The most common drugs causing hypotension are antihypertensive drugs, beta-blockers, calcium channel blockers, iron, theophylline, phenothiazines, barbiturates, and tricyclic antidepressants. Poisons causing hypotension include cyanide, carbon monoxide, hydrogen sulfide, arsenic, and certain mushrooms.

Hypotension in the poisoned or drug-overdosed patient may be caused by venous or arteriolar vasodilation, hypovolemia, depressed cardiac contractility, or a combination of these effects. The only certain way to determine the cause of hypotension in any individual patient is to insert a pulmonary artery catheter and calculate the cardiac output and peripheral vascular resistance. Alternatively, a central venous pressure (CVP) monitor may indicate a need for further fluid therapy.

Treatment

Most patients respond to empirical treatment (200 mL intravenous boluses of 0.9% saline or other isotonic crystalloid up to a total of 1–2 L. If fluid therapy is not successful, give dopamine, 5–15 µg/kg/min by intravenous infusion in a large peripheral or central line. Consider pulmonary artery catheterization if hypotension persists.

Hypotension caused by certain toxins may respond to specific treatment. For hypotension caused by overdoses of tricyclic antidepressants or related drugs, administer sodium bicarbonate, 150–100 meq by intravenous bolus injection. Norepinephrine is more effective than dopamine in some patients with tricyclic overdose. For beta-blocker overdose, glucagon (5–10 mg intravenously) may be of value. For calcium channel blocker overdose, administer calcium chloride, 1–2 g intravenously (repeated doses may be necessary; doses of 5–10 g and more have been given in some cases).

HYPERTENSION

Assessment & Complications

Hypertension may be due to poisoning with amphetamines, anticholinergics, cocaine, phenylpropanolamine, or monoamine oxidase inhibitors.

Severe hypertension (eg, diastolic blood pressure > 105–110 mm Hg in a person who does not have chronic hypertension) can result in acute intracranial hemorrhage, myocardial infarction, or aortic dissection. Patients often present with headache, chest pain, or encephalopathy.

Treatment

Treat hypertension if the patient is symptomatic or if the diastolic pressure is greater than 105–110 mm

Hg—especially if there is no prior history of hypertension.

Hypertensive patients who are agitated or anxious may benefit from a sedative such as lorazepam, 2–3 mg intravenously. For persistent hypertension, administer phentolamine, 2–5 mg intravenously, or nitroprusside sodium, 0.25–8 µg/kg/min intravenously. If excessive tachycardia is present, add propranolol, 1–5 mg intravenously, or esmolol 25–100 µg/kg/min intravenously. *Caution:* Do not give beta-blockers alone, since doing so may paradoxically worsen hypertension.

ARRHYTHMIAS

Assessment & Complications

Arrhythmias may occur with a variety of drugs or toxins (Table 39–3). They may also occur as a result of hypoxia, metabolic acidosis, or electrolyte imbalance (eg, hyper- or hypokalemia, hypocalcemia), or following exposure to chlorinated solvents or chloral hydrate overdose.

Treatment

Arrhythmias are often caused by hypoxia or electrolyte imbalance, and these conditions should be sought and treated. If ventricular arrhythmias persist, administer lidocaine at usual antiarrhythmic doses. *Caution:* Avoid class Ia agents (quinidine, procainamide, disopyramide), which may aggravate arrhythmias caused by tricyclic antidepressants, calcium channel

Table 39–3. Common toxins or drugs causing arrhythmias.

Arrhythmia	Common Causes
Sinus bradycardia	Beta-blockers, calcium channel blockers, organophosphates, digitalis glycosides, opioids, clonidine, sedative-hypnotics.
Atrioventricular block	Beta-blockers, digitalis glycosides, calcium channel blockers, tricyclic antidepressants, quinidine and other class Ia antiarrhythmics, lithium.
Sinus tachycardia	Theophylline, caffeine, cocaine, amphetamines, phencyclidine, beta-agonists (eg, albuterol), iron, anticholinergics, tricyclic antidepressants, antihistamines.
Wide QRS complex	Tricyclic antidepressants, quinidine and class Ia antiarrhythmics, class Ic antiarrhythmics, phenothiazines (eg, thioridazine), potassium (hyperkalemia).
QT interval prolongation	Lithium, quinidine and other class Ia antiarrhythmics, class III antiarrhythmic drugs, terfenadine, astemizole, thioridazine.

blockers, or beta-blockers. Wide QRS complex tachycardia in the setting of tricyclic antidepressant overdose (or quinidine and other class Ia drugs) should be treated with sodium bicarbonate, 50–100 meq intravenously by bolus injection. (See discussion of tricyclic antidepressant poisoning.)

For tachyarrhythmias induced by chlorinated solvents, chloral hydrate, or sympathomimetic agents, use propranolol or esmolol (see doses given above in hypertension section).

SEIZURES

Assessment & Complications

Seizures may be due to poisoning with many drugs and poisons, including amphetamines, antihistamines, camphor, cocaine, isoniazid, lindane, phencyclidine (PCP), phenothiazines, theophylline, tricyclic antidepressants, and some newer antidepressants (eg, bupropion, venlafaxine).

Seizures may also be caused by hypoxia, hypoglycemia, hypocalcemia, hyponatremia, withdrawal from alcohol or sedative-hypnotics, head trauma, central nervous system infection, or idiopathic epilepsy.

Prolonged or repeated seizures commonly lead to hypoxia, metabolic acidosis, hyperthermia, and rhabdomyolysis.

Treatment

Administer lorazepam, 2–3 mg intravenously over 2 minutes, or—if intravenous access is not immediately available—midazolam, 5–10 mg intramuscularly. If convulsions continue, administer phenobarbital, 15–20 mg/kg slowly intravenously over no less than 30 minutes; or phenytoin, 15 mg/kg intravenously over no less than 30 minutes (maximum infusion rate, 50 mg/min). The drugs may be used together if necessary. Maintenance doses may be required if drug toxicity is expected to last more than 18–24 hours.

Seizures due to a few drugs and toxins may require antidotes or other specific therapies (as listed in Table 39–4).

HYPERTHERMIA

Assessment & Complications

Hyperthermia may be associated with poisoning by amphetamines, atropine and other anticholinergic drugs, cocaine, dinitrophenol and pentachlorophenol, phencyclidine (PCP), salicylates, strychnine, tricyclic antidepressants, and various other medications. Use of serotonin reuptake inhibitors (eg, fluoxetine, paroxetine, sertraline) in a patient taking a monoamine oxidase inhibitor may cause agitation, hyperactivity, and hyperthermia ("serotonin syndrome"). Haloperidol and other antipsychotic agents can cause rigidity and

Table 39–4. Seizures related to toxins or drugs requiring special consideration.[1]

Toxin or Drug	Comments
Isoniazid (INH)	Administer pyridoxine.
Lithium	May indicate need for hemodialysis.
Organophosphates	Administer pralidoxime (2-PAM) and atropine.
Strychnine	"Seizures" are actually spinally mediated muscle spasms and usually require neuromuscular paralysis.
Theophylline	Seizures indicate need for hemodialysis or charcoal hemoperfusion.
Tricyclic antidepressants	Hyperthermia and cardiotoxicity are common complications of repeated seizures; paralyze early with neuromuscular blockers to reduce muscular hyperactivity.

[1]See text for dosages.

hyperthermia (neuroleptic malignant syndrome [NMS]). (See section on schizophrenia and other psychotic disorders in Chapter 25.) Malignant hyperthermia is a rare disorder associated with general anesthetic agents.

Hyperthermia is a rapidly life-threatening complication. Severe hyperthermia (temperature > 40–41 °C) may rapidly cause brain damage and multiorgan failure, including rhabdomyolysis, renal failure, and coagulopathy (see Chapter 38).

Treatment

Treat hyperthermia aggressively by removing all clothing, spraying with tepid water, and fanning the patient. If this is not rapidly effective, as shown by a normal rectal temperature within 30–60 minutes, or if there is significant muscle rigidity or hyperactivity, induce neuromuscular paralysis with a nondepolarizing neuromuscular blocker (eg, pancuronium, vecuronium). Once paralyzed, the patient must be intubated and mechanically ventilated. Absence of visible muscular convulsive movements may give the false impression that brain seizure activity has ceased; however, this must be confirmed by electroencephalography.

Dantrolene (2–5 mg/kg intravenously) may be effective for hyperthermia associated with muscle rigidity that does not respond to neuromuscular blockade (ie, malignant hyperthermia). Bromocriptine, 2.5–7.5 mg orally daily, has been recommended for neuroleptic malignant syndrome. Cyproheptadine, 4 mg orally every hour for three or four doses, has been used to treat serotonin syndrome.

■ ANTIDOTES & OTHER TREATMENT

ANTIDOTES

Give an antidote (if available) when there is reasonable certainty of a specific diagnosis (Table 39–5). Antidotes themselves may have serious side effects. The indications and dosages for specific antidotes are discussed in the respective sections for specific toxins.

DECONTAMINATION OF THE SKIN

Corrosive agents rapidly injure the skin and eyes and must be removed immediately. In addition, many toxins are readily absorbed through the skin, and systemic absorption can be prevented only by rapid action.

Wash the affected areas with copious quantities of lukewarm water or saline. Wash carefully behind the ears, under the nails, and in skin folds. For oily sub-

Table 39–5. Some toxic agents for which there are specific antidotes.[1]

Toxic Agent	Specific Antidote
Acetaminophen	Acetylcysteine
Anticholinergics (eg, atropine)	Physostigmine
Anticholinesterases (eg, organophosphate pesticides)	Atropine and pralidoxime (2-PAM)
Benzodiazepines	Flumazenil (rarely used; see warning in text)
Carbon monoxide	Oxygen
Cyanide	Sodium nitrite, sodium thiosulfate
Digitalis glycosides	Digoxin-specific Fab antibodies
Heavy metals (eg, lead, mercury, iron) and arsenic	Specific chelating agents
Isoniazid	Pyridoxine (vitamin B_6)
Methanol, ethylene glycol	Ethanol (ethyl alcohol) or fomepizole (4-methylpyrazole)
Opioids	Naloxone, nalmefene
Snake venom	Specific antivenin

[1]See text for indications and dosages.

stances (eg, pesticides), wash the skin at least twice with plain soap and shampoo the hair. Specific decontaminating solutions or solvents (eg, alcohol) are rarely indicated and in some cases may paradoxically enhance absorption.

DECONTAMINATION OF THE EYES

Act quickly to prevent serious damage. Flush the eyes with copious amounts of saline (preferred) or water. (If available, instill local anesthetic drops in the eye before beginning irrigation.) Remove contact lenses if present. Direct the irrigating stream so that it will flow across both eyes after running off the nasal bridge. Lift the tarsal conjunctiva to look for undissolved particles and to facilitate irrigation. Continue irrigation for 15 minutes or until each eye has been irrigated with at least 1 L of solution. If the toxin is an acid or a base, check the pH of the tears after irrigation, and continue irrigation until the pH is between 6.5 and 7.5.

After irrigation is complete, perform a careful examination of the eye, using fluorescein and a slitlamp or Wood's lamp to identify areas of corneal injury. Patients with serious conjunctival or corneal injury should be immediately referred to an ophthalmologist.

GASTROINTESTINAL DECONTAMINATION

Removal of ingested poisons is a traditional part of emergency treatment. However, studies indicate that if more than 60 minutes has passed, induced emesis and gastric lavage are relatively ineffective. For small or moderate ingestions of most substances, toxicologists generally recommend activated charcoal alone without prior gastric emptying. Exceptions are large ingestions of anticholinergic compounds and salicylates, which often delay gastric emptying, and ingestion of sustained-release or enteric-coated tablets, which may remain intact for several hours.

Gastric emptying is not generally used for ingestion of corrosive agents or petroleum distillates, because further esophageal injury or pulmonary aspiration may result. However, in certain cases, removal of the toxin may be more important than concern over possible complications. Consult a medical toxicologist or regional poison control center (Table 39–1) for advice.

Emesis

Emesis using syrup of ipecac is a convenient way to partially evacuate gastric contents if given very soon after ingestion (eg, at work or at home). However, it may delay or prevent use of oral activated charcoal and is no longer used in the hospital management of ingestions.

A. INDICATIONS

Induced vomiting may find rare indications in prehospital use but has been virtually replaced by oral activated charcoal.

B. CONTRAINDICATIONS

Induced emesis is contraindicated for drowsy, unconscious, or convulsing patients and for patients who have ingested kerosene or other hydrocarbons (danger of aspiration of stomach contents), corrosive poisons, or rapidly acting convulsants (eg, tricyclic antidepressants, strychnine, camphor).

C. TECHNIQUE

Give syrup of ipecac, 30 mL, followed by an 8-oz glass of water. Repeat in 20 minutes if necessary.

Gastric Lavage

Gastric lavage is more effective for liquid poisons or small pill fragments than for intact tablets or pieces of mushroom. It is most effective when started within 60 minutes after ingestion. However, the lavage procedure may delay administration of activated charcoal and may hasten passage of pills and other toxic material into the small intestine. It is no longer used in the routine management of overdose.

A. INDICATIONS

Gastric lavage is sometimes used after very large ingestions (eg, massive aspirin overdose); for collection and examination of gastric contents for identification of poison; and for convenient administration of charcoal and antidotes.

B. CONTRAINDICATIONS

Do *not* use lavage for stuporous or comatose patients with absent gag reflexes unless they are endotracheally intubated beforehand. Some authorities advise against lavage when caustic material has been ingested; others regard it as essential to remove liquid corrosives from the stomach.

C. TECHNIQUE

In obtunded or comatose patients, the danger of aspiration pneumonia is reduced by placing the patient in a head down, left lateral decubitus position and, if necessary, protecting the airway with endotracheal intubation. Gently insert a lubricated, soft but noncollapsible stomach tube (at least 37–40F) through the mouth or nose into the stomach. Aspirate and save the contents, and then lavage repeatedly with 50–100 mL of fluid until the return fluid is clear. Use lukewarm tap water or saline.

Activated Charcoal

Activated charcoal effectively adsorbs almost all drugs and poisons. Poorly adsorbed substances include iron, lithium, potassium, sodium, cyanide, mineral acids, and alcohols.

A. Indications

Activated charcoal should be used for prompt adsorption of drugs or toxins in the stomach and intestine. Studies show that activated charcoal given alone may be as effective as or more effective than ipecac-induced emesis or gastric lavage.

B. Contraindications

Activated charcoal should not be used for comatose or convulsing patients unless it can be given by gastric tube and the airway is first protected by a cuffed endotracheal tube. This substance is contraindicated also for patients with ileus or intestinal obstruction or those who have ingested corrosives for whom endoscopy is planned.

C. Technique

Administer activated charcoal, 60–100 g orally or via gastric tube, mixed in aqueous slurry. Repeated doses may be given to ensure gastrointestinal adsorption or to enhance elimination of some drugs (see below).

Catharsis

A. Indications

Cathartics are used by some toxicologists for stimulation of peristalsis to hasten the elimination of unabsorbed drugs and poisons and the activated charcoal slurry.

B. Contraindications and Cautions

Do not use mineral oil or other oil-based cathartics. Avoid sodium-based cathartics in patients with hypertension, renal failure, and congestive heart failure and magnesium-based cathartics in those with renal failure.

C. Technique

Magnesium sulfate 10%, 2–3 mL/kg; or sorbitol 70%, 1–2 mL/kg. Sorbitol is commonly used in prepackaged charcoal slurry products.

Whole Bowel Irrigation

Whole bowel irrigation utilizes large volumes of balanced polyethylene glycol-electrolyte solution to mechanically cleanse the entire intestinal tract. Because of the composition of the irrigating solution, there is no significant gain or loss of systemic fluids or electrolytes.

A. Indications

Whole bowel irrigation is particularly effective for massive iron ingestion in which intact tablets are visible on abdominal x-ray. It has also been used for ingestions of sustained-release and enteric-coated tablets as well as drug-filled packets.

B. Contraindications

Same as for cathartics.

C. Technique

Administer the balanced polyethylene glycol-electrolyte solution (CoLyte, GoLYTELY) into the stomach via gastric tube at a rate of 1–2 L/h until the rectal effluent is clear. It is most effective when patients are able to sit on a commode to pass the intestinal contents.

Increased Drug Removal

A. Urinary Manipulation

Forced diuresis is hazardous; the risk of complications (pulmonary edema, electrolyte imbalance) usually outweighs its benefits. Acidic drugs (eg, salicylates, phenobarbital) are more rapidly excreted with an alkaline urine. Acidification (sometimes promoted for amphetamines, phencyclidine) is *not* very effective and is contraindicated in the presence of rhabdomyolysis or myoglobinuria.

B. Dialysis (Hemodialysis or Hemoperfusion)

The indications for dialysis are as follows: (1) Known or suspected potentially lethal amounts of a dialyzable drug (Table 39–6). (2) Poisoning with deep coma, apnea, severe hypotension, fluid and electrolyte or acid-base disturbance, or extreme body temperature changes that cannot be corrected by conventional measures. (3) Poisoning in patients with severe renal, cardiac, pulmonary, or hepatic disease who will not be able to eliminate the toxin by usual mechanisms.

Many of the substances that cannot be removed effectively by aqueous dialysis can be removed by hemoperfusion through specially designed coated charcoal columns. Indications are the same as for dialysis. Peritoneal dialysis may occasionally be employed for acute poisonings when hemodialysis is not available, but it is very inefficient. Dialysis should usually augment rather than replace well-established emergency and supportive measures. Continuous arteriovenous and venovenous hemodiafiltration is of uncertain benefit for elimination of poisons.

C. Repeat-Dose Charcoal

Repeated doses of activated charcoal, 20–30 g every 3–4 hours, may hasten elimination of some drugs (eg, digitoxin, theophylline, phenobarbital) by adsorbing drug excreted into the gut lumen ("gut dialysis"). However, no clinical studies have documented improved outcome using multiple-dose charcoal. Sorbitol or other cathartics should *not* be used with each dose, or resulting large stool volumes may lead to dehydration or hypernatremia.

Table 39–6. Recommended use of hemodialysis (HD) and hemoperfusion (HP) in poisoning.

Poison	Procedure[1]	Indications[2]
Carbamazepine	HP	Seizures, severe cardiotoxicity.
Ethylene glycol	HD	Acidosis, serum level > 50 mg/dL.
Lithium	HD	Severe symptoms; level > 4 meq/L more than 12 hours after last dose.
Methanol	HD	Acidosis, serum level > 50 mg/dL.
Phenobarbital	HP	Intractable hypotension, acidosis despite maximal supportive care.
Salicylate	HD	Severe acidosis, CNS symptoms, level > 100 mg/dL (acute overdose) or > 60 mg/dL (chronic intoxication).
Theophylline	HP or HD	Serum level > 90–100 mg/L (acute) or seizures and serum level > 40–60 mg/L (chronic).
Valproic acid	HD	Serum level > 900–1000 mg/L or deep coma, severe acidosis.

[1]Contact a regional poison control center or a clinical toxicologist before undertaking these procedures.
[2]See text for further discussion of indications.

Krenzelok EP et al: Position statement: ipecac syrup. Am Acad Clin Toxicology; European Association of Poisons Centres and Clinical Toxicologists. J Toxicol Clin Toxicol 1997;35:699. [PMID: 9482425] (There is no evidence from clinical studies supporting the use of ipecac in the management of poisoned patients in the emergency department.)

Position statement and practice guidelines on the use of multi-dose activated charcoal in the treatment of acute poisoning. American Academy of Clinical Toxicology; European Association of Poisons Centres and Clinical Toxicologists. J Toxicol Clin Toxicol 1999;37:731. [PMID: 10584586] (Review. Multidose charcoal is not routinely recommended.)

Tenenbein M: Position statement: whole bowel irrigation. American Academy of Clinical Toxicology; European Association of Poisons Centres and Clinical Toxicologists. J Toxicol Clin Toxicol 1997;35:753. [PMID: 9482429] (Whole bowel irrigation may be considered for toxic ingestions of sustained-release or enteric-coated drugs. If done after the administration of activated charcoal, the binding capacity of charcoal and the osmotic properties of whole bowel irrigations appear to be unchanged.)

Wax PM et al: Prehospital gastrointestinal decontamination of toxic ingestions: a missed opportunity. Am J Emerg Med 1998;16:114. [PMID: 9517681] (Retrospective review of adult ambulance transports for drug overdose found that 30 out of 43 patients who were suitable candidates for oral activated charcoal received it in the ER rather than in the ambulance, which delayed this valuable medical treatment by 82 minutes.)

■ DIAGNOSIS OF POISONING

The identity of the ingested substance or substances is usually known, but occasionally a comatose patient is found with an unlabeled container or refuses or otherwise fails to give a coherent history. By performing a directed physical examination and ordering common clinical laboratory tests, the clinician can often make a tentative diagnosis that may allow empirical interventions or may suggest specific toxicologic tests.

PHYSICAL EXAMINATION

Important diagnostic variables in the physical examination include blood pressure, pulse rate, temperature, pupil size, sweating, and the presence or absence of peristaltic activity. Poisonings with many drugs fit into one of four common syndromes.

Sympathomimetic Syndrome

The blood pressure and pulse rate are elevated, though with severe hypertension reflex bradycardia may occur. The temperature is often elevated, pupils are dilated, and the skin is sweaty, though mucous membranes are dry. Patients are usually agitated, anxious, or frankly psychotic.

Examples: Amphetamines, cocaine, ephedrine and pseudoephedrine, phencyclidine (pupils normal or small), phenylpropanolamine (bradycardia common).

Sympatholytic Syndrome

The blood pressure and pulse rate are decreased and body temperature is low. The pupils are small or even pinpoint. Peristalsis is usually decreased. Patients are usually obtunded or comatose.

Examples: Barbiturates, benzodiazepines and other sedative hypnotics, γ-hydroxybutyrate (GHB), clonidine and related antihypertensives, ethanol, opioids.

Cholinergic Syndrome

Stimulation of muscarinic receptors causes bradycardia, miosis, sweating, and hyperperistalsis as well as bronchorrhea, wheezing, excessive salivation, and urinary incontinence. Nicotinic receptor stimulation may produce initial hypertension and tachycardia as well as fasciculations and muscle weakness. Patients are usually agitated and anxious.

Examples: Carbamates, nicotine, organophosphates, physostigmine.

Anticholinergic Syndrome

Tachycardia with mild hypertension is common, and the body temperature is often elevated. Pupils are widely dilated. The skin is flushed, hot and dry. Peristalsis is decreased, and urinary retention is common. Patients may have myoclonic jerking or choreoathetoid movements. Agitated delirium is frequently seen, and severe hyperthermia may occur.

Examples: Atropine, scopolamine, other naturally occurring and pharmaceutical anticholinergics, amantadine, antihistamines, phenothiazines (hypotension, small pupils), tricyclic antidepressants.

■ CLINICAL LABORATORY TESTS IN MANAGEMENT OF POISONING

The following clinical laboratory tests are recommended for screening of the overdosed patient: measured serum osmolality and osmolar gap, electrolytes, glucose, creatinine, BUN, urinalysis (eg, oxalate crystals with ethylene glycol poisoning, myoglobinuria with rhabdomyolysis), and electrocardiography. Serum acetaminophen and ethanol levels should be determined in all patients with drug overdoses.

OSMOLAR GAP

The osmolar gap is defined and calculation of the gap is described in Table 39–7. It is increased in the presence of large quantities of low-molecular-weight substances, most commonly ethanol. Common poisons associated with increased osmolar gap are acetone, ethanol, ethylene glycol, isopropyl alcohol, methanol, and propylene glycol. **Note:** Severe alcoholic ketoacidosis and diabetic ketoacidoses can also cause an elevated osmolar gap resulting from the production of ketones and other low-molecular-weight substances.

ANION GAP

Metabolic acidosis associated with an elevated anion gap is usually due to an accumulation of lactic acid or other acids (see Chapter 21). Common causes of elevated anion gap in poisoning include carbon monoxide, cyanide, ethylene glycol, medicinal iron, isoniazid, methanol, phenformin, and salicylates.

One should also check the osmolar gap; combined elevated anion and osmolar gap suggests poisoning by methanol or ethylene glycol, though this may also occur in patients with diabetic ketoacidosis and alcoholic ketoacidosis.

Table 39–7. Use of the osmolar gap in toxicology.[1]

The osmolar gap (Δosm) is determined by subtracting the calculated serum osmolality from the measured serum osmolality.

$$\text{Calculated osmolality (osm)} = 2\,[Na^+(meq/L)] + \frac{\text{Glucose (mg/dL)}}{18} + \frac{\text{BUN (mg/dL)}}{2.8}$$

Δosm = Measured osmolality − Calculated osmolality

Serum osmolality may be increased by contributions of circulating alcohols and other low-molecular-weight substances. Since these substances are not included in the calculated osmolality, there will be a gap proportionate to their serum concentration and inversely proportionate to their molecular weight:

$$\frac{\text{Serum concentration}}{\text{(mg/dL)}} = \Delta\text{osm} \times \frac{\text{Molecular weight}}{10}$$

	Molecular Weight	Toxic Concentration	Approximate Corresponding Δosm (mosm/L)
Ethanol	46	300	65
Methanol	32	50	16
Ethylene glycol	60	100	16
Isopropanol	60	150	25

[1]Modified from Saunders CE, Ho MT (editors): *Current Emergency Diagnosis & Treatment,* 4th ed. Originally published by Appleton & Lange. Copyright © 1992 by The McGraw-Hill Companies, Inc. **Note:** Most laboratories use the freezing point method for calculating osmolality. If the vaporization point method is used, alcohols are driven off and their contribution to osmolality is lost.

TOXICOLOGY LABORATORY EXAMINATION

The routine comprehensive toxicology screen (Table 39–8) is of little value in the initial care of the poisoned patient—on the contrary, it is time-consuming, expensive, and frequently erroneous. Specific quantitative levels of certain drugs may be extremely helpful (Table 39–9), however, especially if specific antidotes or interventions (eg, dialysis) would be indicated based upon the results.

If a toxicology screen is required, urine is the best specimen for broad qualitative screening. Blood samples may be saved for possible quantitative testing, but blood is not generally used for screening purposes since it is relatively insensitive for many common drugs, including psychotropic agents, opioids, and stimulants.

Table 39–8. Examples of common drugs screened for in blood and urine in a reference toxicology laboratory.[1,2]

Blood

Acetaminophen	Ethchlorvynol
Alcohols	Glutethimide
Barbiturates	Meprobamate
Benzodiazepines	Phenytoin
Carbamazepine	Salicylates
Carisoprodol	

Urine

Acetaminophen	Meperidine
Alcohols	Meprobamate
Amphetamines	Methadone
Barbiturates	Morphine
Chlorpheniramine	Pentazocine
Cocaine	Phencyclidine
Codeine	Phenothiazines
Dextromethorphan	Propoxyphene
Diphenhydramine	Salicylates
Lidocaine	Tricyclic antidepressants

[1]The urine screen is usually more comprehensive, detecting drugs of abuse (opioids, stimulants), antihistamines, and, in many cases, drugs also found in serum.

[2]Many drugs and poisons are not screened for (eg, limited screens; newer drugs; a variety of drugs and poisons such as cyanide, digitalis, ethylene glycol, isoniazid, theophylline).

ABDOMINAL X-RAYS

A plain film of the abdomen may reveal radiopaque iron tablets, drug-filled condoms, or other toxic material. Studies suggest that few tablets are predictably visible (eg, ferrous sulfate, sodium chloride, calcium carbonate, and potassium chloride). Thus, the x-ray is useful only if positive.

Goldfrank LR (editor): *Goldfrank's Toxicologic Emergencies,* 6th ed. Appleton & Lange, 1998.

Olson KR (editor): *Poisoning and Drug Overdose,* 3rd ed. Appleton & Lange, 1999.

■ TREATMENT OF COMMON SPECIFIC POISONINGS (Alphabetical Order)

ACETAMINOPHEN

Acetaminophen (paracetamol) is a common analgesic found in many nonprescription and prescription products. After absorption, it is metabolized mainly by glucuronidation and sulfation, with a small fraction metabolized via the P450 mixed-function oxidase system to a highly toxic reactive intermediate. This toxic intermediate is normally detoxified by cellular glu-

Table 39–9. Specific quantitative levels and potential therapeutic interventions.[1]

Drug or Toxin	Treatment
Acetaminophen	Specific antidote (acetylcysteine) based on serum level
Carbon monoxide	High carboxyhemoglobin level indicates need for 100% oxygen, consideration of hyperbaric oxygen
Carbamazepine	High level may indicate need for hemoperfusion or hemodialysis
Digoxin	On basis of serum digoxin level and severity of clinical presentation, treatment with Fab antibody fragments (Digibind) may be indicated
Ethanol	Low serum level may suggest nonalcoholic cause of coma (eg, trauma, other drugs, other alcohols). Serum ethanol may also be useful in monitoring ethanol therapy for methanol or ethylene glycol poisoning.
Iron	Level may indicate need for chelation with deferoxamine
Lithium	Serum levels can guide decision to institute hemodialysis
Methanol, ethylene glycol	Acidosis, high levels indicate need for hemodialysis, therapy with ethanol or fomepizole
Methemoglobin	Methemoglobinemia can be treated with methylene blue intravenously
Salicylates	High level may indicate need for hemodialysis, alkaline diuresis
Theophylline	Immediate hemodialysis or hemoperfusion may be indicated based on serum level
Valproic acid	Elevated levels may indicate need to consider hemodialysis

[1]Some drugs or toxins may have profound and irreversible toxicity unless rapid and specific management is provided outside of routine supportive care. For these agents, laboratory testing may provide the serum level or other evidence required for administering a specific antidote or arranging for hemodialysis.

tathione. With acute acetaminophen overdose (> 140 mg/kg, or 7 g in an average adult), hepatocellular glutathione is rapidly depleted and the reactive intermediate attacks other cell proteins, causing necrosis. Patients with enhanced P450 activity, such as chronic alcoholics and patients taking anticonvulsants, are at increased risk of developing hepatotoxicity. Hepatic toxicity may also occur after chronic accidental overuse of acetaminophen—eg, as little as 1 g of acetaminophen every 4–6 hours for 1–2 days in a patient with chronic excessive alcohol use.

Clinical Findings

Shortly after ingestion, patients may have nausea or vomiting, but there are usually no other signs of toxicity until 24–48 hours after ingestion, when hepatic aminotransferase levels begin to increase. With severe poisoning, massive hepatic necrosis may occur, resulting in jaundice, hepatic encephalopathy, renal failure, and death.

The diagnosis of severe poisoning after acute overdose is based on measurement of the serum acetaminophen level. Plot the serum level versus the time since ingestion on the acetaminophen nomogram shown in Figure 39–1. Ingestion of sustained-release products or coingestion of an anticholinergic agent, salicylate, or opioid drug may cause delayed elevation of serum levels and may render the nomogram useless.

Treatment

A. EMERGENCY AND SUPPORTIVE MEASURES

Administer activated charcoal (see p. 1561). Although charcoal may bind the oral antidote acetylcysteine, this is not considered clinically significant.

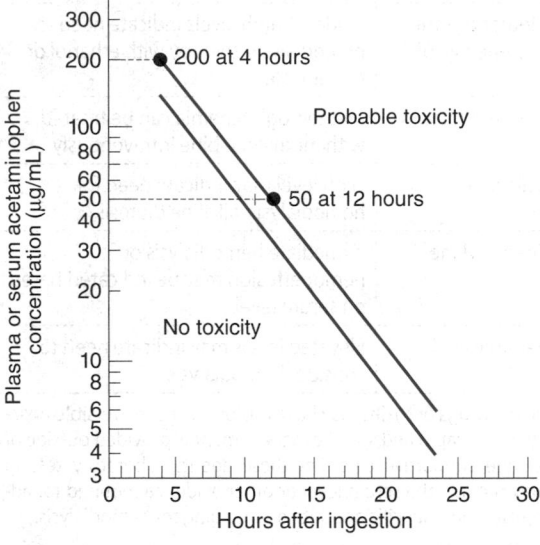

Figure 39–1. Nomogram for prediction of acetaminophen hepatotoxicity following acute overdosage. The upper line defines serum acetaminophen concentrations known to be associated with hepatotoxicity; the lower line defines serum levels 25% below those expected to cause hepatotoxicity. To give a margin for error and for patients at higher risk for hepatotoxicity, the lower line should be used as a guide to treatment. (Modified and reproduced, with permission, from Rumack BH, Matthew H: Acetaminophen poisoning and toxicity. Pediatrics 1975;55:871.)

B. SPECIFIC TREATMENT

If the serum acetaminophen level is higher than the upper toxic line on the nomogram (Figure 39–1), begin treatment with a loading dose of acetylcysteine, 140 mg/kg orally, followed by 70 mg/kg every 4 hours. Dilute the solution to 5% with water, juice, or soda. If vomiting interferes with oral acetylcysteine administration, give the dose by gastric tube and use metoclopramide, 1–2 mg/kg intravenously. The most widely used protocol in the USA continues treatment for 72 hours. However, other regimens have demonstrated equivalent success with 20–48 hours of treatment. Treatment with acetylcysteine is most effective if started within 8–10 hours after ingestion. If the precise time of ingestion is unknown or if the patient is at higher risk of hepatotoxicity (eg, alcoholic, liver disease, chronic use of P450-inducing drugs), then use a lower threshold for initiation of acetylcysteine (ie, the lower nomogram line; in some case reports, a level of 100 mg/L at 4 hours was suggested in very high-risk patients).

Acetylcysteine may also be given intravenously; this is the preferred method in Europe and Canada, but there is no approved parenteral formulation or dosing schedule in the United States. If the patient cannot tolerate acetylcysteine despite antiemetics and administration via a gastric tube, the United States formulation may be given intravenously using a micropore filter and a slow rate of infusion. Call a regional poison control center or medical toxicologist for assistance.

Buckley NA et al: Oral or intravenous N-acetylcysteine: which is the treatment of choice for acetaminophen (paracetamol) poisoning? J Toxicol Clin Toxicol 1999;37:759. [PMID: 10584588] (Intravenous acetylcysteine is preferable but unfortunately is not FDA-approved in the USA.)

Jones AL: Mechanism of action and value of *N*-acetylcysteine in the treatment of early and late acetaminophen poisoning: a critical review. J Toxicol Clin Toxicol 1998;36:277. [PMID: 9711192] (A very good review of the rationale and evidence for the use of *N*-acetylcysteine in patients with acetaminophen poisoning. Highlights the need for lower treatment thresholds in chronic alcoholics and those who take anticonvulsants.)

ACIDS, CORROSIVE (Table 39–10)

The strong mineral acids exert primarily a local corrosive effect on the skin and mucous membranes. Symptoms include severe pain in the throat and upper gastrointestinal tract; bloody vomitus; difficulty in swallowing, breathing, and speaking; discoloration and destruction of skin and mucous membranes in and around the mouth; and shock. Severe systemic metabolic acidosis may occur both as a result of cellular injury and from systemic absorption of the acid.

Severe deep destructive tissue damage may occur after exposure to hydrofluoric acid because of the pen-

Table 39–10. Common corrosive agents.[1]

Category and Examples	Injury Caused
Concentrated alkalies	Penetrating liquefaction necrosis
Clinitest tablets	
Drain cleaners	
Industrial-strength ammonia	
Lye	
Oven cleaners	
Concentrated acids	Coagulation necrosis
Pool disinfectants	
Toilet bowl cleaners	
Weaker cleaning agents	Superficial burns and irritation; deep burns (rare)
Cationic detergents (dishwasher detergents)	
Household ammonia	
Household bleach	
Other	Penetrating, delayed, destructive injury
Hydrofluoric acid	

[1]Reproduced, with permission, from Saunders CE, Ho MT (editors): *Current Emergency Diagnosis & Treatment,* 4th ed. McGraw-Hill, 1992.

etrating and highly toxic fluoride ion. Systemic hypocalcemia and hyperkalemia also may occur after fluoride absorption, even following skin exposure.

Inhalation of volatile acids, fumes, or gases such as chlorine, fluorine, bromine, or iodine causes severe irritation of the throat and larynx and may cause upper airway obstruction and noncardiogenic pulmonary edema.

Treatment

A. INGESTION

Do *not* induce emesis. Dilute immediately by giving a glass (4–8 oz) of milk or water to drink. Do *not* give bicarbonate or other neutralizing agents. Some experts recommend immediate gastric lavage.

Perform flexible endoscopic esophagoscopy promptly to determine the presence and extent of injury. X-rays of the chest and abdomen may reveal the presence of free air in patients with esophageal or gastric perforation. Perforation, peritonitis, and major bleeding are indications for surgery.

B. SKIN CONTACT

Flood with water for 15 minutes. Use no chemical antidotes; the heat of the reaction may cause additional injury.

For hydrofluoric acid burns, soak the affected area in magnesium sulfate solution or apply 2.5% calcium gluconate gel (prepared by adding 3.5 g calcium gluconate to 5 oz of water-soluble surgical lubricant, eg,

K-Y Jelly); then arrange immediate consultation with a plastic surgeon or other specialist. Binding of the fluoride ion may be achieved by injecting 0.5 mL of 5% calcium gluconate per square centimeter under the burned area. (*Caution: Do not use calcium chloride.*)

C. EYE CONTACT

Anesthetize the conjunctiva and corneal surfaces with topical local anesthetic drops (eg, proparacaine). Flood with water for 15 minutes, holding the eyelids open. Check pH with pH 6.0–8.0 test paper, and repeat irrigation, using 0.9% saline, until pH is near 7.0. Check for corneal damage with fluorescein and slitlamp examination; consult an ophthalmologist about further treatment.

D. INHALATION

Remove from further exposure to fumes or gas. Check skin and clothing. Treat pulmonary edema.

ALKALIES
(Table 39–10)

The strong alkalies are common ingredients of some household cleaning compounds and may be suspected by their "soapy" texture. Those with alkalinity above pH 12.0 are particularly corrosive. Clinitest tablets and disk batteries are also a source. Alkalies cause liquefactive necrosis, which is deeply penetrating. Symptoms include burning pain in the upper gastrointestinal tract, nausea, vomiting, and difficulty in swallowing and breathing. Examination reveals destruction and edema of the affected skin and mucous membranes and bloody vomitus and stools. X-ray may reveal the presence of disk batteries in the esophagus or lower gastrointestinal tract.

Treatment

A. INGESTION

Do *not* induce emesis. Dilute immediately with a glass of water. Some gastroenterologists recommend immediate gastric lavage after ingestion of liquid caustic substances to remove residual material.

Immediate endoscopy is recommended to evaluate the extent of damage. If x-ray reveals the location of ingested disk batteries in the esophagus, immediate endoscopic removal is mandatory.

The use of corticosteroids to prevent stricture formation is of no proved benefit and is definitely contraindicated if there is evidence of esophageal perforation.

B. SKIN CONTACT

Wash with running water until the skin no longer feels soapy. Relieve pain and treat shock.

C. EYE CONTACT

Anesthetize the conjunctival and corneal surfaces with topical anesthetic (eg, proparacaine). Irrigate with water or saline continuously for 20–30 minutes, holding the lids open. Check pH with pH test paper, and repeat irrigation, using 0.9% saline, for additional 30-minute periods until the pH is near 7.0. Check for corneal damage with fluorescein and slitlamp examination; consult an ophthalmologist for further treatment.

Hugh TB et al: Corrosive ingestion and the surgeon. J Am Coll Surg 1999;189:508. [PMID: 10549740] (Pathophysiology, presentation, and clinical management of patients with corrosive ingestion injuries.)

Karnak I et al: Combined use of steroid, antibiotics and early bougienage against stricture formation following caustic esophageal burns. J Cardiovasc Surg (Torino) 1999;40:307. [PMID: 10350123] (This protocol was associated with a higher incidence of perforation without preventing stricture formation.)

AMPHETAMINES & COCAINE

Amphetamines and cocaine are widely abused for their euphorigenic and stimulant properties. Both drugs may be smoked, snorted, ingested, or injected. Amphetamines and cocaine produce central nervous system stimulation and a generalized increase in central and peripheral sympathetic activity. The toxic dose of each drug is highly variable and depends on the route of administration and individual tolerance. The onset of effects is most rapid after intravenous injection or smoking. Amphetamine derivatives and related drugs include methamphetamine ("crystal meth," "crank"), methylenedioxymethamphetamine (MDMA, "ecstasy"), ephedrine ("herbal ecstasy"), and methcathinone ("cat"). Nonprescription medications and nutritional supplements may contain stimulant or sympathomimetic drugs such as ephedrine or caffeine (see Theophylline, below): Phenylpropanolamine was recently withdrawn from the market because of an increased incidence of hypertensive intracerebral hemorrhage in young women.

Clinical Findings

Patients may present with anxiety, tremulousness, tachycardia, hypertension, diaphoresis, dilated pupils, agitation, muscular hyperactivity, and psychosis. Metabolic acidosis may occur. In severe intoxication, seizures and hyperthermia may occur. Sustained or severe hypertension may result in intracranial hemorrhage, aortic dissection, or myocardial infarction. Hyponatremia has been reported after MDMA use; the mechanism is not known but may involve excessive water intake, SIADH, or both.

The diagnosis is supported by finding amphetamines, cocaine, or the cocaine metabolite benzoylecgonine in the urine. Blood screening is not sensitive enough to detect these drugs.

Treatment

A. EMERGENCY AND SUPPORTIVE MEASURES

Maintain a patent airway and assist ventilation, if necessary. Treat coma or seizures as described at the beginning of this chapter. Rapidly lower the body temperature (see hyperthermia, above) in patients who are hyperthermic (40 °C). Treat agitation or psychosis with a benzodiazepine such as diazepam, 5–10 mg intravenously (repeated as needed up to 20 mg), or midazolam, 0.1–0.2 mg/kg intramuscularly.

For poisoning by ingestion, perform gastric lavage and administer activated charcoal, or administer activated charcoal alone without prior gut emptying (see p 1561). Do *not* induce emesis, because of the risk of seizures.

B. SPECIFIC TREATMENT

Treat agitation with a sedative such as lorazepam, 2–3 mg intravenously. Treat hypertension with a vasodilator drug such as phentolamine (1–5 mg intravenously) or nifedipine (10–20 mg orally) or a combined α- and β-adrenergic blocker such as labetalol (10–20 mg intravenously). Do *not* administer a pure beta-blocker such as propranolol alone, as this may result in paradoxic worsening of the hypertension as a result of unopposed α-adrenergic effects.

Treat tachycardia or tachyarrhythmias with a short-acting beta-blocker such as esmolol (25–100 μg/kg/min by intravenous infusion). Treat hyponatremia as outlined in Chapter 21.

Albertson TE et al: Methamphetamine and the expanding complications of amphetamines. West J Med 1999;170: 214. [PMID: 10344175] (Review of effects and treatment options for methamphetamine toxicity.)

Haller CA et al: Adverse cardiovascular and central nervous system events associated with dietary supplements containing ephedra alkaloids. N Engl J Med 2000;343:1833. [PMID: 11117974] (Review of 140 adverse event reports submitted to the FDA found hypertension, tachycardia, stroke and seizures resulting in ten deaths.)

Holmes SB et al: Hyponatremia and seizures after ecstasy use. Postgrad Med J 1999;75: 32. [PMID: 10396584] (One of several case reports of profound hyponatremia associated with use of MDMA.)

ANTICOAGULANTS

Warfarin and related compounds (including ingredients of many commercial rodenticides) inhibit the clotting mechanism by blocking hepatic synthesis of vitamin K-dependent clotting factors.

Anticoagulants may cause hemoptysis, gross hematuria, bloody stools, hemorrhages into organs, widespread bruising, and bleeding into joint spaces. The prothrombin time is increased within 12–24 hours (peak 36–48 hours) after a single overdose. After ingestion of brodifacoum and indanedione rodenticides (so-called superwarfarins), inhibition of clotting factor synthesis may persist for several weeks or even months after a single dose.

Treatment

A. EMERGENCY AND SUPPORTIVE MEASURES

Discontinue the drug at the first sign of gross bleeding, and determine the prothrombin time. If the patient has ingested an acute overdose, administer activated charcoal (see p 1561).

B. SPECIFIC TREATMENT

Do not treat prophylactically—wait for the evidence of anticoagulation (elevated prothrombin time). If the prothrombin time is elevated, give phytonadione (vitamin K₁), 5–10 mg subcutaneously or 10–25 mg orally, and additional doses as needed to restore the prothrombin time to normal. Give fresh-frozen plasma as needed to rapidly correct the coagulation factor deficit if there is serious bleeding. If the patient is chronically anticoagulated and has strong medical indications for being maintained in that status (eg, prosthetic heart valve), give much smaller doses of vitamin K (1 mg) and fresh-frozen plasma (or both) to titrate to the desired prothrombin time.

If the patient has ingested brodifacoum or a related superwarfarin, prolonged observation (over weeks) and repeated administration of large doses of vitamin K may be required.

Chua JD et al: Superwarfarin poisoning. Arch Intern Med 1998;158:1929. [PMID: 9759690] (Case series and literature review.)

ANTICONVULSANTS (Carbamazepine, Phenytoin, Valproic Acid)

These drugs are widely used in the management of seizure disorders. In addition, carbamazepine and valproic acid are increasingly used for treatment of mood disorders.

Phenytoin can be given orally or intravenously. Rapid intravenous injection of phenytoin can cause acute myocardial depression and cardiac arrest owing to the solvent propylene glycol; a newer form of phenytoin (fosphenytoin) is available that does not contain this diluent. Phenytoin intoxication can occur with only slightly increased doses because of the small toxic-therapeutic window. Phenytoin intoxication can also occur following acute intentional or accidental overdose. The overdose syndrome is usually mild even with high serum levels. The most common manifestations are ataxia, nystagmus, and drowsiness. Choreoathetoid movements have been described.

Carbamazepine was first used for the treatment of trigeminal neuralgia. It has since become a first-line agent for temporal lobe epilepsy and other seizure disorders. Intoxication causes drowsiness, stupor, and, with high levels, coma and seizures. Dilated pupils and tachycardia are common. Toxicity may be seen with serum levels greater than 20 mg/L, though severe poisoning is usually associated with concentrations greater than 30–40 mg/L. Because of erratic and slow absorption, intoxication may progress over several hours to days.

Valproic acid intoxication produces a unique syndrome consisting of hypernatremia (from the sodium component of the salt), metabolic acidosis, hypocalcemia, elevated serum ammonia, and mild liver aminotransferase elevation. Hypoglycemia may occur as a result of hepatic metabolic dysfunction. Coma with small pupils may be seen and can mimic opioid poisoning. Encephalopathy and cerebral edema can occur.

Treatment

A. EMERGENCY AND SUPPORTIVE MEASURES

For recent ingestions, give activated charcoal orally or by gastric tube. For large ingestions of carbamazepine or valproic acid—especially of sustained-release formulations—consider whole bowel irrigation (see p 1562). Multiple-dose activated charcoal may be beneficial in ensuring gut decontamination for large ingestions and may enhance elimination of absorbed drugs.

B. SPECIFIC TREATMENT

There are no antidotes. Naloxone was reported to have reversed valproic acid overdose in one anecdotal case. Consider hemodialysis (valproic acid) or hemoperfusion (carbamazepine) for massive intoxication (eg, carbamazepine levels > 100 mg/L or valproic acid levels > 1000 mg/L).

Chua HC et al: Elimination of phenytoin in toxic overdose. Clin Neurol Neurosurg 2000;102:6. [PMID: 10717394] (Phenytoin levels declined 4.6–5.9 mg/L per day in patients presenting with levels 34–57.5 mg/L.)

Franssen EJ et al: Valproic acid toxicokinetics: Serial hemodialysis and hemoperfusion. Ther Drug Monit 1999;21:289. [PMID: 10365638] (Case report of coma, hypernatremia, and respiratory failure in a 27-year-old man with a serum valproic acid level of 1414 μg/mL. Hemodialysis clearance was 80 mL/min, compared with 40 mL/min for hemoperfusion.)

Johnson LZ et al: Successful treatment of valproic acid overdose with hemodialysis. Am J Kidney Dis 1999;33:786. [PMID: 10196025] (Case report of effective hemodialysis in the treatment of a patient with a serum valproic acid level of 1380 μg/mL associated with metabolic acidosis, thrombocytopenia, refractory hypotension and coma.)

Schuerer DJ et al: High-efficiency dialysis for carbamazepine overdose. J Toxicol Clin Toxicol 2000;38:321. [PMID: 10866333] (Case report. Carbamazepine level dropped from 27 mg/L to therapeutic range after 4–5 hours of high-efficiency dialysis.)

ARSENIC

Arsenic is found in some pesticides and industrial chemicals. Symptoms of poisoning usually appear within 1 hour after ingestion but may be delayed as long as 12 hours. They include abdominal pain, vomiting, watery diarrhea, and skeletal muscle cramps. Profound dehydration and shock may occur. In chronic poisoning, symptoms can be vague but often include those of peripheral sensory neuropathy. Urinary arsenic levels may be falsely elevated after certain meals (eg, seafood) that contain large quantities of relatively nontoxic organic arsenic.

Treatment

A. Emergency Measures

Perform gastric lavage and administer 60–100 g of activated charcoal (see p 1561).

B. Antidote

For symptomatic patients or those with massive overdose, give dimercaprol injection (BAL), 10% solution in oil, 3–5 mg/kg intramuscularly every 4–6 hours for 2 days. The side effects include nausea, vomiting, headache, and hypertension. Follow dimercaprol with oral penicillamine, 100 mg/kg/d in four divided doses (maximum, 2 g/d), or succimer (DMSA), 10 mg/kg every 8 hours, for 1 week. Consult a medical toxicologist or regional poison control center (Table 39–1) for advice regarding chelation.

Baldwin DR et al: Heavy metal poisoning and its laboratory investigation. Ann Clin Biochem 1999;36(Pt 3):267. [PMID: 10376071]

Graeme KA et al: Heavy metal toxicity, Part I: arsenic and mercury. J Emerg Med 1998;16:45. [PMID: 9472760] (Review of both acute and chronic arsenic and mercury toxicity with recommendations for diagnosis and management.)

Piamphongsant T: Chronic environmental arsenic poisoning. Int J Dermatol 1999;38:401. [PMID: 99323707] (Dermatologic complications of chronic arsenic poisoning.)

ATROPINE & ANTICHOLINERGICS

Atropine, scopolamine, belladonna, diphenoxylate with atropine, *Datura stramonium, Hyoscyamus niger,* some mushrooms, tricyclic antidepressants, and antihistamines are antimuscarinic agents with variable central nervous system effects. The patient complains of dryness of the mouth, thirst, difficulty in swallowing, and blurring of vision. The physical signs include dilated pupils, flushed skin, tachycardia, fever, delirium, myoclonus, ileus, and flushed appearance. Antidepressants and antihistamines may induce convulsions.

Antihistamines are commonly available with or without prescription. Diphenhydramine commonly causes delirium, tachycardia, and seizures. Massive overdose may mimic tricyclic antidepressant poisoning. The nonsedating agents terfenadine and astemizole have caused QT interval prolongation and torsade de pointes (atypical ventricular tachycardia) and were removed from the United States market. Loratadine and fexofenadine have not caused this problem.

Treatment

A. Emergency and Supportive Measures

Administer activated charcoal (see p 1561). Do *not* induce emesis in patients who have ingested antihistamines or antidepressants, because seizures may occur abruptly. Tepid sponge baths and sedation are indicated to control high temperatures (see p 1559).

B. Specific Treatment

For pure atropine or related anticholinergic syndrome, if symptoms are severe (eg, hyperthermia or excessively rapid tachycardia), give physostigmine salicylate, 0.5–1 mg slowly intravenously over 5 minutes, with electrocardiographic monitoring, until symptoms are controlled. Bradyarrhythmias and convulsions are a hazard with physostigmine administration, and it should not be used in patients with tricyclic antidepressant overdose.

Burns MJ et al: A comparison of physostigmine and benzodiazepines for the treatment of anticholinergic poisoning. Ann Emerg Med 2000;35:374. [PMID: 10736125] (Retrospective study of 52 patients found that physostigmine was more effective than benzodiazepines.)

Weiner AL et al: Anticholinergic poisoning with adulterated intranasal cocaine. Am J Emerg Med 1998;16:517. [PMID: 9725971] (Case report.)

BETA-ADRENERGIC BLOCKERS

There are a wide variety of β-adrenergic blocking drugs, with varying pharmacologic and pharmacokinetic properties (see Table 11–6). The most commonly used and most toxic beta-blocker is propranolol. Propranolol competitively blocks β_1 and β_2 adrenoceptors and also has direct membrane-depressant and central nervous system effects.

Clinical Findings

The most common findings with mild or moderate intoxication are hypotension and bradycardia. Cardiac depression from more severe poisoning is often unresponsive to conventional therapy with β-adrenergic stimulants such as dopamine and norepinephrine. In addition, with propranolol and other lipid-soluble drugs, seizures and coma may occur.

The diagnosis is based on typical clinical findings. Routine toxicology screening does not usually include beta-blockers.

Treatment

A. Emergency and Supportive Measures

Initially, treat bradycardia or heart block with atropine (0.5–2 mg intravenously), isoproterenol (2–20 µg/min by intravenous infusion, titrated to the desired heart rate), or an external transcutaneous cardiac pacemaker. Specific antidotal treatment may be necessary (see below).

For ingested drugs, administer activated charcoal (see p 1561).

B. Specific Treatment

If the above measures are not successful in reversing bradycardia and hypotension, give glucagon, 5–10 mg intravenously, followed by an infusion of 1–5 mg/h. Glucagon is an inotropic agent that acts at a different receptor site and is therefore not affected by beta-blockade.

Love JN et al: Acute beta blocker overdose: factors associated with the development of cardiovascular morbidity. J Toxicol Clin Toxicol 2000;38:275. [PMID: 10866327] (Prospective case series found that most patients with serious cardiovascular toxicity had ingested a drug with membrane-stabilizing properties such as propranolol or had coingested a cardiotoxic drug such as a calcium channel blocker.)

Love JN et al: A potential role for glucagon in the treatment of drug-induced symptomatic bradycardia. Chest 1998;114: 323. [PMID: 9674488] (Case series highlighting the effectiveness of glucagon in the treatment of drug-induced symptomatic bradycardia refractory to atropine.)

CALCIUM CHANNEL BLOCKERS

Calcium channel blockers used in the United States include verapamil, diltiazem, nifedipine, nicardipine, amlodipine, felodipine, isradipine, nisoldipine, and nimodipine. These drugs share the ability to cause arteriolar vasodilation and depression of cardiac contractility, especially after acute overdose. Patients may present with bradycardia, AV nodal block, hypotension, or a combination of these effects. With severe poisoning, cardiac arrest may occur.

Treatment

A. EMERGENCY AND SUPPORTIVE MEASURES

Maintain a patent airway and assist ventilation, if necessary. Treat coma, hypotension, and seizures as described at the beginning of this chapter. Treat bradycardia with atropine (0.5–2 mg intravenously), isoproterenol (2–20 µg/min by intravenous infusion), or a transcutaneous or internal cardiac pacemaker.

For ingested drugs, administer activated charcoal (see p 1561). In addition, whole bowel irrigation should be initiated as soon as possible if the patient has ingested a sustained-release product.

B. SPECIFIC TREATMENT

If bradycardia and hypotension are not reversed with these measures, administer calcium chloride intravenously. Start with calcium chloride 10%, 10 mL, or calcium gluconate, 20 mL. Repeat the dose every 3–5 minutes. The optimum (or maximum) dose has not been established, but there are reports of success after as much as 10–12 g of calcium chloride. Calcium is most useful in reversing negative inotropic effects and is less effective for AV nodal blockade and bradycardia. Epinephrine infusion (1–4 µg/min initially) and glucagon, 5–10 mg intravenously, have also been recommended.

Adams BD et al: Amlodipine overdose causes prolonged calcium channel blocker toxicity. Am J Emerg Med 1998;16:527. [PMID: 9725975] (Case report of severe hemodynamic compromise that persisted for 10 days—treated with calcium, glucagon, and other vasopressors.)

Yuan TH et al: Insulin-glucose as adjunctive therapy for severe calcium channel antagonist poisoning. J Toxicol Clin Toxicol 1999;37:463. [PMID: 10465243] (Case series of 5 patients with hypodynamic circulatory shock despite conventional treatment who responded to high-dose insulin plus glucose infusion. This novel treatment is now undergoing a multi-center study.)

CARBON MONOXIDE

Carbon monoxide is a colorless, odorless gas produced by the combustion of carbon-containing materials. Poisoning may occur as a result of suicidal or accidental exposure to automobile exhaust, smoke inhalation in a fire, or accidental exposure to an improperly vented gas heater or other appliance. Carbon monoxide avidly binds to hemoglobin, with an affinity approximately 250 times that of oxygen. This results in reduced oxygen-carrying capacity and altered delivery of oxygen to cells (see also Smoke Inhalation in Chapter 9).

Clinical Findings

At low carbon monoxide levels (carboxyhemoglobin saturation 10–20%), victims may have headache, dizziness, abdominal pain, and nausea. With higher levels, confusion, dyspnea, and syncope may occur. Hypotension, coma, and seizures are common with levels greater than 50–60%. Survivors of acute severe poisoning may develop permanent neurologic deficits. The fetus and newborn may be more susceptible because of high carbon monoxide affinity for fetal hemoglobin.

Carbon monoxide poisoning should be suspected in any person with severe headache or acutely altered mental status, especially in cold weather, when improper heating systems may have been used. Diagnosis depends on specific measurement of the arterial or venous carboxyhemoglobin saturation, although the level may have declined if high-flow oxygen therapy has already been administered. Routine arterial blood gas testing and pulse oximetry are not useful because they may give falsely normal oxyhemoglobin saturation determinations.

Treatment

A. EMERGENCY AND SUPPORTIVE MEASURES

Maintain a patent airway and assist ventilation, if necessary. Remove the victim from exposure. Treat patients with coma, hypotension, or seizures, as described at the beginning of this chapter.

B. SPECIFIC TREATMENT

The half-life of the carboxyhemoglobin complex is about 4–5 hours in room air but is reduced dramatically by high concentrations of oxygen. Administer 100% oxygen by tight-fitting high-flow reservoir face mask or endotracheal tube. Hyperbaric oxygen (HBO) can provide 100% oxygen under higher than atmospheric pressures, further shortening the half-life; it may be useful if immediately available for patients with coma or seizures and in pregnant women, though controlled studies have failed to prove that HBO is superior to high-flow oxygen at normal pressure.

Juurlink DN et al: Hyperbaric oxygen for carbon monoxide poisoning. Cochrane Database Syst Rev 2000:CD002041. [PMID: 10796853] (Review of six randomized controlled trials of HBO therapy failed to show benefit from this treatment. The authors recommend a multicenter, randomized, double-blind controlled trial.)

Scheinkestel CD et al: Hyperbaric or normobaric oxygen for acute carbon monoxide poisoning: a randomised controlled clinical trial. Med J Aust 1999;170:203. [PMID: 10092916] (Randomized trial demonstrating that hyperbaric oxygen treatment compared with normobaric oxygen treatment provided no benefit and may have worsened the outcome of patients with carbon monoxide poisoning.)

Weaver LK: Carbon monoxide poisoning. Crit Care Clin 1999;15:297. [PMID: 10331130]

CHEMICAL WARFARE AGENTS

Nerve agents used in chemical warfare work by cholinesterase inhibition and are most commonly organophosphates. Agents such as **tabun** (dimethylphosphoramidocyanidic acid ethyl ether) and **sarin** (methylphosphonofluoridic acid 1-methylethyl ester) are similar to insecticides such as malathion but are vastly more potent. They may be inhaled or absorbed through the skin. Systemic effects due to unopposed action of acetylcholine include miosis, salivation, abdominal cramps, diarrhea, and muscle paralysis producing respiratory arrest. Inhalation also produces severe bronchoconstriction and copious nasal and tracheobronchial secretions.

Treatment

A. EMERGENCY AND SUPPORTIVE MEASURES

Perform thorough decontamination of exposed areas with repeated soap and shampoo washing. Personnel caring for such patients must wear protective clothing and gloves, since cutaneous absorption may occur through normal skin.

B. SPECIFIC TREATMENT

Give atropine in an initial dose of 2 mg intravenously, and repeat as needed to reverse signs of acetylcholine excess. (Some victims have required several hundred milligrams.) Treat also with the cholinesterase-reactivating agent pralidoxime, 1–2 g intravenously initially followed by 200–400 mg/h. United States military personnel in the Persian Gulf war were equipped with autoinjectable units containing 2 mg of atropine plus 600 mg of the cholinesterase-reactivating agent pralidoxime.

Brennan RJ et al: Chemical warfare agents: emergency medical and emergency public health issues. Ann Emerg Med 1999;34:191. [PMID: 10424921] (Overview of the risk that chemical warfare agents pose to civilians and the necessary preparedness of emergency medical and public health services.)

Okumura T et al: The Tokyo subway sarin attack: Disaster management. Part 2: Hospital response. Acad Emerg Med 1998;5:618. [PMID: 9660290] (Review of hospital planning for chemical disasters based on the author's experience with the Tokyo subway attack.)

Smith KJ: The prevention and treatment of cutaneous injury secondary to chemical warfare agents. Application of these findings to other dermatological conditions and wound healing. Dermatol Clin 1999;17:41. [PMID: 9986995]

CHLORINATED INSECTICIDES (Chlorophenothane [DDT], Lindane, Toxaphene, Chlordane, Aldrin, Endrin)

Lindane (Kwell) and other chlorinated insecticides are central nervous system stimulants that can cause poisoning by ingestion, inhalation, or direct contact. The estimated lethal dose is about 20 g for DDT, 3 g for lindane, 2 g for toxaphene, 1 g for chlordane, and less than 1 g for endrin and aldrin. The manifestations of poisoning are nervous irritability, muscle twitching, seizures, and coma. Arrhythmias may occur. Hepatic and renal damage are reported.

Treatment

Give activated charcoal and consider gastric lavage for large recent ingestions (see p 1561). Repeat-dose activated charcoal may be effective for large ingestions. For seizures, give diazepam, 5–10 mg slowly intravenously, or other anticonvulsants as described on p 1559.

Perform thorough decontamination of exposed areas with repeated soap and shampoo washing. Personnel caring for such patients must be wear protective clothing and gloves, since cutaneous absorption may occur through normal skin.

Nordt SP et al: Acute lindane poisoning in three children. J Emerg Med 2000;18:51. [PMID: 10645838] (Three cases of acute toxicity after inadvertent oral administration of lindane intended for skin application.)

O'Malley M: Clinical evaluation of pesticide exposure and poisonings. Lancet 1997;349:1161. [PMID: 9113024] (Review of pesticide exposure ranging from topical irritant reactions to severe systemic illness.)

CLONIDINE & OTHER SYMPATHOLYTIC ANTIHYPERTENSIVES (Clonidine, Guanabenz, Guanfacine, Methyldopa)

Overdosage with these agents causes bradycardia, hypotension, miosis, respiratory depression, and coma. (Hypertension occasionally occurs after clonidine overdosage, a result of peripheral alpha-adrenergic effects of this drug in high doses.) Symptoms are usually resolved in less than 24 hours, and deaths are rare. Similar symptoms may occur after ingestion of topical nasal decongestants chemically similar to clonidine (oxymetazoline, tetrahydrozoline, naphazoline).

Treatment

A. EMERGENCY AND SUPPORTIVE MEASURES

Give activated charcoal and a cathartic (see p 1561). Maintain the airway and support respiration if necessary. Symptomatic treatment is usually sufficient even in massive overdose. Maintain blood pressure with intravenous fluids. Dopamine can also be used. Atropine is usually effective for bradycardia.

B. SPECIFIC TREATMENT

There is no specific antidote. Although tolazoline has been recommended for clonidine overdose, its effects are unpredictable and it should not be used. Naloxone has been reported to be successful in a few anecdotal and poorly substantiated cases.

Broderick-Cantwell JJ: Case study: accidental clonidine patch overdose in attention-deficit/hyperactivity disorder patients. J Am Acad Child Adolesc Psychiatry 1999;38:95. [PMID: 9893422]

Frye CB et al: Hypertensive crisis and myocardial infarction following massive clonidine overdose. Ann Pharmacother 2000;34:611. [PMID: 10852088] (Case report of acute hypertension after accidental subcutaneous injection of 12.24 mg of clonidine.)

COCAINE

See Amphetamines & Cocaine, above.

CYANIDE

Cyanide is a highly toxic chemical used widely in research and commercial laboratories and many industries. Its gaseous form, hydrogen cyanide, is an important component of smoke in fires. Cyanide-generating glycosides are also found in the pits of apricots and other related plants. Cyanide is generated by the breakdown of nitroprusside, and poisoning can result from rapid high-dose infusions. Cyanide is also formed by metabolism of acetonitrile, found in some over-the-counter fingernail glue removers. Cyanide is rapidly absorbed by inhalation, skin absorption, or ingestion. It disrupts cellular function by inhibiting cytochrome oxidase and preventing cellular oxygen utilization.

Clinical Findings

The onset of toxicity is nearly instantaneous after inhalation of hydrogen cyanide gas but may be delayed for minutes to hours after ingestion of cyanide salts or cyanogenic plants or chemicals. Effects include headache, dizziness, nausea, abdominal pain, and anxiety, followed by confusion, syncope, shock, seizures, coma, and death. The odor of "bitter almonds" may be detected on the victim's breath or in vomitus,

though this is not a reliable finding. The venous oxygen saturation may be elevated (> 90%) in severe poisonings because tissues have failed to take up arterial oxygen.

Treatment

A. EMERGENCY AND SUPPORTIVE MEASURES

Remove the victim from exposure, taking care to avoid exposure to rescuers. For suspected cyanide poisoning due to nitroprusside infusion, stop or slow the rate of infusion. (Metabolic acidosis and other signs of cyanide poisoning usually clear rapidly.)

For cyanide ingestion, administer activated charcoal (see p. 1561). At the scene, induce emesis if charcoal is not immediately available (see p 1561). Although charcoal has a low affinity for cyanide, the usual doses of 60–100 g are adequate to bind typically ingested lethal doses (100–200 mg).

B. SPECIFIC TREATMENT

In the United States, the cyanide antidote package (Taylor Pharmaceuticals) (Table 39–11) contains nitrites (to induce methemoglobinemia, which binds free cyanide) and thiosulfate (to promote conversion of cyanide to the less toxic thiocyanate). Administer amyl nitrite by crushing an ampule under the victim's nose or at the end of the endotracheal tube, and administer 3% sodium nitrite solution, 10 mL intravenously. **Caution:** Nitrites may induce hypotension and dangerous levels of methemoglobin. Also administer 25% sodium thiosulfate solution, 50 mL intravenously (12.5 g).

Beasley DM et al: Cyanide poisoning: pathophysiology and treatment recommendations. Occup Med 1998;48:427. [PMID: 10024740] (Review of the available antidotes for cyanide toxicity.)

Lam KK et al: An incident of hydrogen cyanide poisoning. Am J Emerg Med 2000;18:172. [PMID: 10750924] (Seven cases of HCN gas poisoning.)

Table 39–11. Currently available (prepackaged) cyanide antidotes.[1,2]

Antidote	How Supplied	Dose
Amyl nitrite	0.3 mL (aspirol inhalant)	Break one or two aspirols under patient's nose.
Sodium nitrite	3 g/dL (300 mg in 10 mL vials)	6 mg/kg IV (0.2 mL/kg)
Sodium thio sulfate	25 g/dL (12.5 g in 50 mL vials)	250 mg/kg IV (1 mL/kg)

[1]Reproduced, with permission, from Saunders CE, Ho MT (editors): *Current Emergency Diagnosis & Treatment*, 4th ed. McGraw-Hill, 1992.

[2]In the United States, manufactured by Taylor Pharmaceuticals.

Suchard JR et al: Acute cyanide toxicity caused by apricot kernel ingestion. Ann Emerg Med 1998;32:742. [PMID: 9832674] (Severe cyanide poisoning after ingestion of apricot kernels purchased in a health food store.)

DIGITALIS & OTHER CARDIAC GLYCOSIDES

Cardiac glycosides are derived from a variety of plants and are widely used to treat heart failure and supraventricular arrhythmias. These drugs paralyze the Na^+-K^+ ATPase pump and have potent vagotonic effects. Intracellular effects include enhancement of calcium-dependent contractility and shortening of the action potential duration. Digoxin and ouabain are highly tissue-bound, but digitoxin has a volume of distribution of just 0.6 L/kg, making it the only cardiac glycoside accessible to enhanced removal procedures such as hemoperfusion or repeated doses of activated charcoal.

Clinical Findings

Intoxication may result from acute single exposure or chronic accidental overmedication. After acute overdosage, patients frequently develop nausea and vomiting, bradycardia, hyperkalemia, and atrioventricular block. Patients who develop toxicity gradually during chronic therapy are often hypokalemic and hypomagnesemic owing to concurrent diuretic treatment and more commonly present with ventricular arrhythmias (eg, ectopy, bidirectional ventricular tachycardia, or ventricular fibrillation).

Treatment

A. EMERGENCY AND SUPPORTIVE MEASURES

Maintain a patent airway and assist ventilation, if necessary. Monitor potassium levels and cardiac rhythm closely. Treat ventricular arrhythmias initially with lidocaine (2–3 mg/kg intravenously) or phenytoin (10–15 mg/kg intravenously slowly over 30 minutes) and treat bradycardia initially with atropine (0.5–2 mg intravenously), isoproterenol (1–5 µg/min initially), or a transcutaneous external cardiac pacemaker.

After acute ingestion, administer activated charcoal (see p 1561). Emesis is not recommended because it may enhance vagotonic effects such as bradycardia and AV block.

B. SPECIFIC TREATMENT

For patients with severe intoxication, administer digoxin-specific antibodies (digoxin immune Fab [ovine]; Digibind). Estimation of the Digibind dose is based on the body burden of digoxin calculated from the ingested dose or the steady-state serum digoxin concentration:

1. From the ingested dose—Number of vials = approximately 1.5 × ingested dose (mg).

2. From the serum concentration—Number of vials = serum digoxin (ng/mL) × body weight (kg) × 10^{-2}. *Note:* This is based on the equilibrium digoxin level; after acute overdose, serum levels are falsely high before tissue distribution is complete, and overestimation of the Digibind dose is likely.

3. Empirical dosing of Digibind may be utilized if the patient's condition is relatively stable and an underlying condition (eg, atrial fibrillation) suggests a residual level of digitalis activity. Start with one or two vials and reassess the clinical condition after 20–30 minutes.

Note: After administration of Digibind, serum digoxin levels may be falsely elevated depending on the assay technique.

Miura T et al: Effect of aging on the incidence of digoxin toxicity. Ann Pharmacother 2000;34:427. [PMID: 10772425] (Older age is associated with greater risk of digoxin toxicity.)

Nordt SP et al: Clarithromycin induced digoxin toxicity. J Accid Emerg Med 1998;15:194. [PMID: 9639187] (Case report of digoxin toxicity due to coadministration of clarithromycin.)

Roever C et al: Comparing the toxicity of digoxin and digitoxin in a geriatric population: should an old drug be rediscovered? South Med J 2000;93:199. [PMID: 10701788] (Retrospective review found lower incidence of toxicity in patients using digitoxin compared with digoxin.)

ETHANOL, BARBITURATES, BENZODIAZEPINES, & OTHER SEDATIVE-HYPNOTIC AGENTS

The group of agents known as sedative-hypnotic drugs includes a variety of products used for the treatment of anxiety, depression, insomnia, and epilepsy. Ethanol and other selected agents are also popular recreational drugs. All of these drugs depress the central nervous system reticular activating system, cerebral cortex, and cerebellum.

Clinical Findings

Mild intoxication produces euphoria, slurred speech, and ataxia. Ethanol intoxication may produce hypoglycemia, even at relatively low concentrations. With more severe intoxication, stupor, coma, and respiratory arrest may occur. Death or serious morbidity is usually the result of pulmonary aspiration of gastric contents. Bradycardia, hypotension, and hypothermia are common. Patients with massive intoxication may appear to be dead, with no reflex responses and even absent electroencephalographic activity. Diagnosis and assessment of severity of intoxication are usually based on clinical findings. Ethanol serum levels greater than 300 mg/dL (0.3 g/dL; 65 mmol/L) usually produce coma in persons who are not chronically abusing the drug, but regular users may remain awake at much higher levels. Phenobarbital levels greater than 80–100 mg/L usually cause coma.

Treatment

A. EMERGENCY AND SUPPORTIVE MEASURES

Administer activated charcoal (see p 1561). Repeat-dose charcoal may enhance elimination of phenobarbital, and hemoperfusion may be necessary for patients with severe phenobarbital intoxication, but these procedures are not effective for most other drugs in this group.

B. SPECIFIC TREATMENT

Flumazenil is a benzodiazepine receptor-specific antagonist; it has no effect on ethanol, barbiturates, or other sedative-hypnotic agents. Flumazenil is given slowly intravenously, 0.2 mg over 30–60 seconds, repeated in 0.5 mg increments as needed up to a total dose of 3–5 mg. *Caution:* Flumazenil may induce seizures in patients with preexisting seizure disorder, benzodiazepine addiction, or concomitant tricyclic antidepressant overdose. If seizures occur, diazepam and other benzodiazepine anticonvulsants will not be effective. As with naloxone, the duration of action of flumazenil is short (2–3 hours) and resedation may occur, requiring repeated doses.

Barnett R et al: Flumazenil in drug overdose: randomized, placebo-controlled study to assess cost effectiveness. Crit Care Med 1999;27:78. [PMID: 9934897] (Randomized trial of flumazenil in the empiric treatment of adults with suspected drug overdose and Glasgow Coma Scale score less than 13 failed to demonstrate its cost-effectiveness.)

Mathieu-Nolf M et al: Flumazenil use in an emergency department: a survey. J Toxicol Clin Toxicol 2001;39:15. [PMID: 11327221] (A prospective observational study of 478 patients whose overdose included at least one benzodiazepine failed to show any benefit in the small number of patients [6%] who were treated with flumazenil.)

GAMMA HYDROXYBUTYRATE

Gamma hydroxybutyrate (GHB) has become a popular drug of abuse. It originated as a short-acting general anesthetic and is occasionally used in the treatment of narcolepsy. It gained popularity among bodybuilders for its alleged growth hormone stimulation and found its way into social settings, where it is consumed as a liquid. Symptoms after ingestion include drowsiness and lethargy followed by coma with respiratory depression. Muscle twitching and seizures are sometimes observed. Recovery is usually rapid, with patients awakening within a few hours. Other related chemicals with similar effects include butanediol and gamma-butyrolactone (GBL). A prolonged withdrawal syndrome has been described in some heavy users.

Treatment

For recent ingestions, give activated charcoal orally or by gastric tube. There is no specific treatment. Most patients recover rapidly with supportive care. GHB withdrawal syndrome may require very large doses of benzodiazepines.

Adverse events associated with ingestion of gamma-butyrolactone—Minnesota, New Mexico, and Texas 1998–1999. MMWR Morb Mortal Wkly Rep 1999;48:137. [PMID: 10077458] (GBL is a liquid solvent chemical precursor to GHB; after ingestion, it produces similar effects.)

Chin RL et al: Clinical course of gamma-hydroxybutyrate overdose. Ann Emerg Med 1998;31:716. [PMID: 9624311] (Retrospective review of 88 patients with GHB overdose. Although these patients presented with markedly decreased levels of consciousness, most had spontaneous recovery of consciousness within 5 hours after ingestion. Common findings included coingestion of ethanol and amphetamines, bradycardia, hypothermia, respiratory acidosis, and emesis.)

Zvosec DL et al: Adverse effects, including death, associated with the use of 1,4-butanediol. N Engl J Med 2001;344:87. [PMID: 11150358] (Case series of nine episodes of intoxication by this chemical precursor of GHB. A severe withdrawal syndrome is also described.)

IRON

Iron is widely used therapeutically for the treatment of anemia and as a daily supplement in multiple vitamin preparations. Most children's preparations contain about 12–15 mg of elemental iron (as sulfate, gluconate, or fumarate salt) per dose, compared with 60–90 mg in most adult-strength preparations. Iron is corrosive to the gastrointestinal tract and, once absorbed, has depressant effects on the myocardium and on peripheral vascular resistance. Intracellular toxic effects of iron include disruption of Krebs cycle enzymes.

Clinical Findings

Ingestion of less than 30 mg/kg of elemental iron usually produces only mild gastrointestinal upset. Ingestion of more than 40–60 mg/kg may cause vomiting (sometimes with hematemesis), diarrhea, hypotension, and acidosis. Death may occur as a result of profound hypotension due to massive fluid losses and bleeding, metabolic acidosis, peritonitis from intestinal perforation, or sepsis. Fulminant hepatic failure may occur. Survivors of the acute ingestion may suffer permanent gastrointestinal scarring.

Serum iron levels greater than 350–500 μg/dL are considered toxic, and levels over 1000 μg/dL are usually associated with severe poisoning. A plain abdominal x-ray may reveal radiopaque tablets.

Treatment

A. EMERGENCY AND SUPPORTIVE MEASURES

Maintain a patent airway and assist ventilation if necessary. Treat hypotension aggressively with intravenous crystalloid solutions (0.9% saline or lactated Ringer's solution). Fluid losses may be massive owing to vomiting and diarrhea as well as third-spacing into injured intestine.

Perform whole bowel irrigation to remove unabsorbed pills from the intestinal tract (see p 1562). Activated charcoal is not effective but may be needed if other ingestants are suspected.

B. SPECIFIC TREATMENT

Deferoxamine is a selective iron chelator. It is not useful as an oral binding agent. For patients with established manifestations of toxicity—and particularly those with markedly elevated serum iron levels (eg, greater than 800–1000 μg/dL)—administer 10–15 mg/kg/h by constant intravenous infusion; higher doses (up to 40–50 mg/kg/h) have been used in massive poisonings. Hypotension may occur. The presence of iron-deferoxamine complex in the urine may give it a "vin rosé" appearance. Deferoxamine is safe for use in pregnant women with acute iron overdose. *Caution:* Prolonged infusion of deferoxamine (> 36–48 hours) has been associated with development of acute respiratory distress syndrome (ARDS)—the mechanism is not known.

Siff JE et al: Usefulness of the total iron building capacity in the evaluation and treatment of iron overdose. Ann Emerg Med 1999;33:73. [PMID: 9867890] (Review article, points out the pitfalls of the total iron-binding capacity and recommends it not be used in the estimation of "free iron.")

Tran T et al: Intentional iron overdose in pregnancy—management and outcome. J Emerg Med 2000;18:225. [PMID: 10699527] (Review of 14 publications describing a total of 61 cases found that patients with severe toxicity were more likely to die, spontaneously abort, or deliver preterm.)

ISONIAZID

Isoniazid (INH) is an antibacterial drug used mainly in the treatment and prevention of tuberculosis. It may cause hepatitis in certain patients with chronic use. It produces acute toxic effects by competing with pyridoxal 5-phosphate, resulting in lowered brain γ-aminobutyric acid (GABA) levels. Acute ingestion of as little as 1.5–2 g of isoniazid can cause toxicity, and severe poisoning is likely to occur after ingestion of more than 80–100 mg/kg.

Clinical Findings

Confusion, slurred speech, and seizures may occur abruptly after acute overdose. Severe lactic acidosis—out of proportion to the severity of seizures—is probably due to inhibited metabolism of lactate.

Diagnosis is based on a history of ingestion and the presence of severe acidosis associated with seizures. Isoniazid is not usually included in routine toxicologic screening, and serum levels are not readily available.

Treatment

A. EMERGENCY AND SUPPORTIVE MEASURES

Seizures may require higher than usual doses of benzodiazepines (eg, lorazepam, 3–5 mg intravenously) or administration of pyridoxine as an antidote (see below).

Administer activated charcoal (see p 1561). Do *not* induce emesis, because of the risk of abrupt onset of seizures.

B. SPECIFIC TREATMENT

Pyridoxine (vitamin B$_6$) is a specific antagonist of the acute toxic effects of isoniazid and is usually successful in controlling convulsions that do not respond to benzodiazepines. Give 5 g intravenously over 1–2 minutes or, if the amount ingested is known, give a gram-for-gram equivalent amount of pyridoxine.

Romero JA et al: Isoniazid overdose: recognition and management. Am Fam Physician 1998;57:749. [PMID: 9490997]

Santucci KA et al: Acute isoniazid exposures and antidote availability. Pediatr Emerg Care 1999;15:99. [PMID: 10220077] (A survey of teaching hospitals with emergency medicine or pediatric emergency medicine training programs found that one-third to one-half had insufficient supplies of the antidote pyridoxine.)

Sullivan EA et al: Isoniazid poisonings in New York City. J Emerg Med 1998;16:57. [PMID: 9472761] (Review of 41 patients, 22 of whom presented with seizures. Treatment with pyridoxine is emphasized.)

LEAD

Lead is used in a variety of industrial and commercial products, such as storage batteries, solders, paints, pottery, plumbing, and gasoline and is found in some traditional ethnic medicines. Lead toxicity usually results from chronic repeated exposure and is rare after a single ingestion. Lead produces a variety of adverse effects on cellular function and primarily affects the nervous system, gastrointestinal tract, and hematopoietic system.

Clinical Findings

Lead poisoning often goes undiagnosed initially because presenting symptoms and signs are nonspecific and exposure is not suspected. Common symptoms include colicky abdominal pain, constipation, headache, and irritability. Severe poisoning may cause coma and convulsions. Chronic intoxication can cause learning disorders (in children) and motor neuropathy (eg, wrist drop).

Diagnosis is based on measurement of the blood lead level. Whole blood lead levels less than 10 μg/dL are usually considered nontoxic. Levels between 10 and 25 μg/dL have been associated with impaired neurobehavioral development in children. Levels of 25–50 μg/dL may be associated with headache, irritability, and subclinical neuropathy. Levels of 50–70 μg/dL are associated with moderate toxicity, and levels greater than 70–100 μg/dL are often associated with severe poisoning. Other laboratory findings of lead poisoning include microcytic anemia with basophilic stippling and elevated free erythrocyte protoporphyrin.

Treatment

A. EMERGENCY AND SUPPORTIVE MEASURES

For patients with encephalopathy, maintain a patent airway and treat coma and convulsions as described at the beginning of this chapter.

For recent acute ingestion, give activated charcoal (see p 1561). If a large lead-containing object (eg, fishing weight) is still visible in the stomach on abdominal x-ray, repeated cathartics, whole bowel irrigation, endoscopy, or even surgical removal may be necessary to prevent subacute lead poisoning. (The acidic gastric contents may corrode the metal surface, enhancing lead absorption. Once the object passes into the small intestine, the risk of toxicity declines.)

Conduct an investigation into the source of the lead exposure. Workers with a single lead level greater than 60 μg/dL (or three successive monthly levels greater than 50 μg/dL) or construction workers with any single blood lead level greater than 50 μg/dL must by federal law be removed from the site of exposure. Contact the regional office of the United States Occupational Safety and Health Administration (OSHA) for more information. Several states mandate reporting of cases of confirmed lead poisoning.

B. SPECIFIC TREATMENT

The indications for chelation depend on the blood lead level and the patient's clinical state. A medical toxicologist or regional poison control center (Table 39–1) should be consulted for advice about selection and use of these antidotes.

Note: It is impermissible under the law to treat asymptomatic workers with elevated blood lead levels in order to keep their levels under 50 μg/dL rather than remove them from the exposure.

1. Severe toxicity—Patients with severe intoxication (encephalopathy or levels greater than 70–100 μg/dL) should receive edetate calcium disodium (EDTA), 1500 mg/m^2/kg/d (approximately 50 mg/kg/d) in four to six divided doses or as a continuous intravenous infusion. Some clinicians also add dimercaprol (BAL), 4–5 mg/kg intramuscularly every 4 hours for 5 days.

2. Less severe toxicity—Patients with less severe symptoms and asymptomatic patients with blood lead levels between 55 and 69 μg/dL may be treated with edetate calcium disodium alone in dosages as above. An oral chelator, succimer (dimercaptosuccinic acid, DMSA), is available for use in patients with mild to moderate intoxication. The usual dose is 10 mg/kg orally every 8 hours for 5 days, then every 12 hours for 2 weeks.

Graeme KA et al: Heavy metal toxicity, part II: lead and metal fume fever. J Emerg Med 1998;16:171. [PMID: 9543397] (Review of clinical presentation and management of lead toxicity.)

Jongnarangsin K et al: An unusual cause of recurrent abdominal pain. Am J Gastroenterol 1999;94:3620. [PMID: 10606329] (Case report of lead poisoning from stripping old paint from a Victorian house.)

Lin JL et al: Chelation therapy for patients with elevated body lead burden and progressive renal insufficiency. A randomized, controlled trial. Ann Intern Med 1999;130:7. [PMID: 9890856] (Randomized study demonstrating possible role for lead chelation therapy in patients with chronic renal insufficiency and mildly elevated body lead burden.)

Staudinger KC et al: Occupational lead poisoning. Am Fam Physician 1998;57:719. [PMID: 9490995] (Review of lead poisoning with a special emphasis on the implications of occupational exposures.)

LSD & OTHER HALLUCINOGENS

A variety of substances—ranging from naturally occurring plants and mushrooms to synthetic substances such as phencyclidine (PCP), toluene and other solvents, and LSD—are abused for their hallucinogenic properties. The mechanism of toxicity and the clinical effects vary for each substance.

Many hallucinogenic plants and mushrooms produce anticholinergic delirium (see p 1564), characterized by flushed skin, dry mucous membranes, dilated pupils, tachycardia, and urinary retention. Some plants and mushrooms may contain hallucinogenic indoles such as mescaline and lysergic acid diethylamide (LSD), which typically cause marked visual hallucinations and perceptual distortion, widely dilated pupils, and mild tachycardia. Phencyclidine (PCP), a dissociative anesthetic agent similar to ketamine, can produce fluctuating delirium and coma, often associated with vertical and horizontal nystagmus. Toluene and other hydrocarbon solvents (butane, trichloroethylene, "chemo," etc) cause euphoria and delirium and may sensitize the myocardium to the effects of catecholamines, leading to fatal dysrhythmias.

Treatment

A. EMERGENCY AND SUPPORTIVE MEASURES

Maintain a patent airway and assist respirations if necessary. Treat coma, hyperthermia, and seizures as outlined at the beginning of this chapter. For recent large ingestions, consider giving activated charcoal orally or by gastric tube.

B. SPECIFIC TREATMENT

Patients with anticholinergic delirium may benefit from a dose of physostigmine (see p 1570). However, this drug should not be used if poisoning by tricyclic antidepressants is suspected. Dysphoria, agitation, and psychosis associated with LSD or mescaline intoxication may respond to benzodiazepines (eg, lorazepam, 1–2 mg orally or intravenously) or haloperidol (2–5 mg orally or intravenously). Monitor patients who have sniffed solvents for cardiac dysrhythmias (most commonly premature ventricular contractions, ventricular tachycardia, ventricular fibrillation); treatment with beta-blockers such as propranolol (1–5 mg intravenously) or esmolol (250–500 μg/kg intravenously, then 50 μg/kg/min by infusion) may be more effective than lidocaine.

Dewitt MS et al: The dangers of jimson weed and its abuse by teenagers in the Kanawha Valley of West Virginia. West Virginia Med J 1998;93:182. [PMID: 9274142] (Nine patients treated for ingestion of jimson weed [Datura stramonium].)

Nelson LS et al: Dangerous form of marijuana (letter). Ann Emerg Med 1999;34:115. [PMID: 10409089] (Phencyclidine is sometimes added to marijuana.)

MERCURY

Acute mercury poisoning usually occurs by ingestion of inorganic mercuric salts or inhalation of metallic mercury vapor. Ingestion of the mercuric salts causes a metallic taste, salivation, thirst, a burning sensation in the throat, discoloration and edema of oral mucous membranes, abdominal pain, vomiting, bloody diarrhea, and shock. Direct nephrotoxicity causes acute renal failure. Inhalation of high concentrations of metallic mercury vapor may cause acute fulminant chemical pneumonia. Chronic mercury poisoning causes weakness, ataxia, intention tremors, irritability, and depression. Exposure to alkyl (organic) mercury derivatives from contaminated fish or fungicides used on seeds has caused ataxia, tremors, convulsions, and catastrophic birth defects.

Treatment

A. ACUTE POISONING

There is no effective specific treatment for mercury vapor pneumonitis. Remove ingested mercuric salts by lavage, and administer activated charcoal (see p 1561). For acute ingestion of mercuric salts, give dimercaprol (BAL) at once, as for arsenic poisoning. Unless the patient has severe gastroenteritis, consider succimer (DMSA), 10 mg/kg orally every 8 hours for 5 days and then every 12 hours for 2 weeks. Maintain urine output. Treat oliguria and anuria if they occur.

B. CHRONIC POISONING

Remove from exposure. Neurologic toxicity is not considered reversible with chelation, though some authors recommend a trial of succimer.

Graeme KA et al: Heavy metal toxicity. Part I: Arsenic and mercury. J Emerg Med 1998;16:45. [PMID: 9472760] (Review of mercury toxicity, including exposure, clinical manifestations, diagnosis, and treatment.)

Risher JF et al: Summary report for the expert panel review of the toxicological profile for mercury. Toxicol Ind Health 1999;15:483. [PMID: 10487360]

METHANOL & ETHYLENE GLYCOL

Methanol (wood alcohol) is commonly found in a variety of products, including solvents, duplicating fluids, record cleaning solutions, and paint removers. It is sometimes ingested intentionally by alcoholic patients as a substitute for ethanol and may also be found as a contaminant in bootleg whiskey. Ethylene glycol is the major constituent in most antifreeze compounds. The toxicity of both agents is caused by metabolism to highly toxic organic acids—methanol to formic acid; ethylene glycol to glycolic and oxalic acids.

Clinical Findings

Shortly after ingestion of either of these agents, patients usually appear "drunk." The serum osmolality (measured with the freezing point device) is usually increased, but acidosis is often absent early. After several hours, metabolism to toxic organic acids leads to a severe anion gap metabolic acidosis, tachypnea, confusion, convulsions, and coma. Methanol intoxication frequently causes visual disturbances, while ethylene glycol often produces oxalate crystalluria and renal failure.

Treatment

A. EMERGENCY AND SUPPORTIVE MEASURES

For patients presenting within 30–60 minutes after ingestion, empty the stomach by gastric lavage and administer activated charcoal (see p 1561). (*Note:* Charcoal is not very effective.)

B. SPECIFIC TREATMENT

Patients with significant toxicity (manifested by severe metabolic acidosis, altered mental status, serum methanol or ethylene glycol level > 50 mg/dL, or osmolar gap > 10 mosm/L) should undergo hemodialysis as soon as possible to remove the parent compound and the toxic metabolites.

Ethanol blocks metabolism of the parent compounds by competing for the enzyme alcohol dehydrogenase. The desired serum ethanol concentration is 100 mg/dL. To achieve this, administer a loading dose of approximately 750 mg/kg orally or in a dilute intravenous solution (available from the pharmacy in 5% and 10% solution), and then provide a maintenance infusion of 100–150 mg/kg/h. The infusion will have to be increased to about 175–250 mg/kg/h during hemodialysis to replace dialysis elimination of ethanol. A new antidote, fomepizole (4-methypyrazole), blocks alcohol dehydrogenase and can be used instead of ethanol. A regional poison control center (Table 39–1) should be contacted for indications and dosing.

Barceloux DG et al: American Academy of Clinical Toxicology Practice Guidelines on the Treatment of Ethylene Glycol Poisoning. Ad Hoc Committee. J Toxicol Clin Toxicol 1999;37:537. [PMID: 10497633] (Clinical manifestations, diagnosis, and treatment.)

Brent J et al: Fomepizole for the treatment of ethylene glycol poisoning. N Engl J Med 1999;340:832. [PMID: 10080845] (Fomepizole was effective in preventing renal failure if given early.)

Liu JJ et al: Prognostic factors in patients with methanol poisoning. J Toxicol Clin Toxicol 1998;36:175. [PMID: 9656972]

METHEMOGLOBINEMIA-INDUCING AGENTS

A large number of chemical agents are capable of oxidizing ferrous hemoglobin to its ferric state (methemoglobin), a form that cannot carry oxygen. Drugs and chemicals known to cause methemoglobinemia include benzocaine (a local anesthetic found in some topical anesthetic sprays and a variety of nonprescription products), aniline, nitrites, nitrogen oxide gases, nitrobenzene, dapsone, pyridium, and many others. Dapsone has a long elimination half-life and may produce prolonged or recurrent methemoglobinemia.

Clinical Findings

Methemoglobinemia reduces oxygen-carrying capacity and may cause dizziness, nausea, headache, dyspnea, confusion, seizures, and coma. The severity of symptoms depends on the percentage of hemoglobin oxidized to methemoglobin; severe poisoning is usually present when methemoglobin fractions are greater than 40–50%. Even at low levels (15–20%), victims appear cyanotic because of the "chocolate brown" color of methemoglobin, but they have normal PO_2 results on arterial blood gas determinations. Pulse oximetry gives inaccurate oxygen saturation measurements. Severe metabolic acidosis may be present. Hemolysis may occur, especially in patients susceptible to oxidant stress (ie, those with glucose-6-phosphate dehydrogenase deficiency).

Treatment

A. EMERGENCY AND SUPPORTIVE MEASURES

Administer high-flow oxygen. If the causative agent was recently ingested, administer activated charcoal (see p 1561). Repeat-dose activated charcoal may enhance dapsone elimination (see p 1562).

B. SPECIFIC TREATMENT

Methylene blue enhances the conversion of methemoglobin to hemoglobin by increasing the activity of the enzyme methemoglobin reductase. For symptomatic patients, administer 1–2 mg/kg (0.1–0.2 mL/kg of 1% solution) intravenously. The dose may be repeated once in 15–20 minutes if necessary. Patients with hereditary methemoglobin reductase deficiency or glucose-6-phosphate dehydrogenase deficiency may not respond to methylene blue treatment.

Khan NA et al: Methemoglobinemia induced by topical anesthesia: a case report and review. Am J Med Sci 1999;318:415. [PMID: 10616167] (Case report of severe methemoglobinemia after administration of topical Cetacaine spray for pharyngeal anesthesia.)

Ward KE et al: Dapsone-induced methemoglobinemia. Ann Pharmacother 1998;32:549. [PMID: 9606476]

Wright RO et al: Methemoglobinemia: etiology, pharmacology, and clinical management. Ann Emerg Med 1999;34:646. [PMID: 10533013]

MONOAMINE OXIDASE INHIBITORS (Isocarboxazid, Phenelzine)

Overdoses cause ataxia, excitement, hypertension, and tachycardia, followed several hours later by hypotension, convulsions, and hyperthermia.

Ingestion of tyramine-containing foods may cause a severe hypertensive reaction in patients taking monoamine oxidase inhibitors. Foods containing tyramine include aged cheese and red wines. Hypertensive reactions may also occur with any sympathomimetic drug. Severe or fatal hyperthermia (serotonin syndrome) may occur if patients receiving monoamine oxidase inhibitors are given meperidine, fluoxetine, paroxetine, fluvoxamine, venlafaxine, tryptophan, dextromethorphan, or other serotonin-enhancing drugs. This reaction can also occur with the newer selective MAO inhibitor moclobemide. The serotonin syndrome has also been reported in patients taking selective serotonin reuptake inhibitors in large doses or in combination with other SSRIs, even in the absence of an MAO inhibitor or meperidine.

Treatment

Administer activated charcoal (see p 1561). Treat severe hypertension with nitroprusside, phentolamine, or other rapid-acting vasodilators (see p 1558). Treat hypotension with fluids and positioning, but avoid use of pressor agents if possible. Observe patients for at least 24 hours, since hyperthermic reactions may be delayed. Treat hyperthermia with aggressive cooling; neuromuscular paralysis may be required (see p 1559). Cyproheptadine, 4 mg orally (or by gastric tube) every hour for three or four doses, has been reported to be effective against serotonin syndrome.

Chan BS et al: Serotonin syndrome resulting from drug interactions. Med J Aust 1998;169:523. [PMID: 9861909] (Series of six patients with serotonin syndrome after exposure to combinations of tricyclic antidepressants, selective serotonin uptake inhibitors, selective norepinephrine reuptake inhibitors, or monoamine oxidase inhibitors.)

MUSHROOMS

There are thousands of mushroom species that cause a variety of toxic effects. The most dangerous species of mushrooms are *Amanita phalloides, Amanita verna, Amanita virosa, Gyromitra esculenta,* and the *Galerina* species, all of which contain amatoxin, a potent cytotoxin. Ingestion of even a portion of one mushroom of a dangerous species may be sufficient to cause death.

The characteristic pathologic finding in fatalities from amatoxin-containing mushroom poisoning is acute massive necrosis of the liver.

Clinical Findings
(Table 39–12)

A. SYMPTOMS AND SIGNS

1. Amatoxin-type cyclopeptides—(*Amanita phalloides, Amanita verna, Amanita virosa,* and *Galerina* species.) After a latent interval of 8–12 hours, severe abdominal cramps and vomiting begin and progress to profuse diarrhea, followed in 1–2 days by hepatic necrosis, hepatic encephalopathy, and frequently renal failure. The fatality rate is about 20%. Cooking the mushrooms does not prevent poisoning.

2. Gyromitrin type—(*Gyromitra* and *Helvella* species.) Toxicity is more common following ingestion of uncooked mushrooms. Vomiting, diarrhea, hepatic necrosis, convulsions, coma, and hemolysis may occur after a latent period of 8–12 hours. The fatality rate is probably less than 10%.

3. Muscarinic type—(*Inocybe* and *Clitocybe* species.) Vomiting, diarrhea, bradycardia, hypotension, salivation, miosis, bronchospasm, and lacrimation occur shortly after ingestion. Cardiac arrhythmias may occur. Fatalities are rare.

4. Anticholinergic type—(Eg, *Amanita muscaria, Amanita pantherina.*) This type causes a variety of symptoms that may be atropine-like, including excitement, delirium, flushed skin, dilated pupils, and muscular jerking tremors, beginning 1–2 hours after ingestion. Fatalities are rare.

5. Gastrointestinal irritant type—(Eg, *Boletus, Cantharellus.*) Nausea, vomiting, and diarrhea occur shortly after ingestion. Fatalities are rare.

6. Disulfiram type—(*Coprinus* species.) Disulfiram-like sensitivity to alcohol may persist for several days. Toxicity is characterized by flushing, hypotension, and vomiting after coingestion of alcohol.

7. Hallucinogenic—(*Psilocybe* and *Panaeolus* species.) Mydriasis, nausea and vomiting, and intense visual hallucinations occur 1–2 hours after ingestion. Fatalities are rare.

8. *Cortinarius orellanus*—This mushroom may cause acute renal failure due to tubulointerstitial nephritis.

Treatment

A. EMERGENCY MEASURES

After the onset of symptoms, efforts to remove the toxic agent are probably useless, especially in cases of

Table 39–12. Poisonous mushrooms.

Toxin	Genus	Symptoms and Signs	Onset	Treatment
Amanitin	*Amanita (A phalloides, A verna, A virosa)*	Severe gastroenteritis followed by delayed hepatic and renal failure after 48–72 hours	6–24 hours	Supportive. Correct dehydration. Give repeated doses of activated charcoal orally. Penicillin, thioctic acid, and silibinin are unproved antidotes.
Muscarine	*Inocybe, Clitocybe*	Muscarinic (salivation, miosis, bradycardia, diarrhea)	30–60 minutes	Supportive. Give atropine, 0.5–2 mg intravenously, for severe cholinergic symptoms and signs.
Ibotenic acid, muscimol	*Amanita muscaria* ("fly agaric")	Anticholinergic (mydriasis, tachycardia, hyperpyrexia, delirium)	30–60 minutes	Supportive. Give physostigmine, 0.5–2 mg intravenously, for severe anticholinergic symptoms and signs.
Coprine	*Coprinus*	Disulfiram-like effect occurs with ingestion of ethanol	30–60 minutes	Supportive. Abstain from ethanol for 3–4 days.
Monomethyl-hydrazine	*Gyromitra*	Gastroenteritis; occasionally hemolysis, hepatic and renal failure	6–12 hours	Supportive. Correct dehydration. Pyridoxine, 2.5 mg/kg intravenously, may be helpful.
Orellanine	*Cortinarius*	Nausea, vomiting; renal failure after 1–3 weeks	2–14 days	Supportive.
Psilocybin	*Psilocybe*	Hallucinations	15–30 minutes	Supportive.
Gastrointestinal irritants	Many species	Nausea and vomiting, diarrhea	½–2 hours	Supportive. Correct dehydration.

amatoxin or gyromitrin poisoning, where there is usually a delay of 12 hours or more before symptoms occur and patients seek medical attention. However, induction of vomiting or administration of activated charcoal is recommended for any recent ingestion of an unidentified or potentially toxic mushroom (see p 1561).

B. GENERAL MEASURES

1. Amatoxin-type cyclopeptides—A variety of antidotes (eg, thioctic acid, silibinin, penicillin, corticosteroids) have been suggested for amatoxin-type mushroom poisoning, but controlled studies are lacking and experimental data in animals are equivocal. Aggressive fluid replacement for diarrhea and intensive supportive care for hepatic failure are the mainstays of treatment.

Interruption of enterohepatic circulation of the amatoxin by the administration of activated charcoal and laxatives may be of value. However, by the time this method is employed, most of the amatoxin has already caused cellular damage and has already been excreted. Charcoal hemoperfusion has been recommended but is of unproved value.

Liver transplant may be the only hope for survival in gravely ill patients—contact a liver transplant center early.

2. Gyromitrin type—For gyromitrin poisoning, give pyridoxine, 25 mg/kg intravenously.

3. Muscarinic type—For mushrooms producing predominantly muscarinic-cholinergic symptoms, give atropine, 0.005–0.01 mg/kg intravenously, and repeat as needed.

4. Anticholinergic type—For anticholinergic type, physostigmine, 0.5–1 mg intravenously, may calm extremely agitated patients and reverse peripheral anticholinergic manifestations, but it may also cause bradycardia, asystole, and seizures.

5. Gastrointestinal irritant type—Treat with antiemetics and intravenous or oral fluids.

6. Disulfiram type—For *Coprinus* ingestion, avoid alcohol. Treat alcohol reaction with fluids and supine position.

7. Hallucinogenic type—Provide a quiet, supportive atmosphere. Diazepam or haloperidol may be used for sedation.

8. *Cortinarius*—Provide supportive care and hemodialysis as needed for renal failure.

Broussard CN et al: Mushroom poisoning—from diarrhea to liver transplantation. Am J Gastroenterol 2001;96:3195. [PMID: 11721773]

Yamada EG et al: Mushroom poisoning due to amatoxin. Northern California, winter 1996–1997. West J Med 1998;169: 380. [PMID: 9866444] (Case reports of illness and death after *Amanita phalloides* ingestion.)

OPIOIDS (Morphine, Heroin, Codeine, Propoxyphene, Etc)

Prescription and illicit opioids are popular drugs of abuse and the cause of frequent hospitalizations for overdose. These drugs have widely varying potencies and durations of action; for example, some of the illicit fentanyl derivatives are up to 2000 times more potent than morphine. All of these agents decrease central nervous system activity and sympathetic outflow by acting on opiate receptors in the brain. Tramadol is a newer analgesic that is unrelated chemically to the opioids but acts on opioid receptors.

Clinical Findings

Mild intoxication is characterized by euphoria, drowsiness, and constricted pupils. More severe intoxication may cause hypotension, bradycardia, hypothermia, coma, and respiratory arrest. Pulmonary edema may occur. Death is usually due to apnea or pulmonary aspiration of gastric contents. Propoxyphene may cause seizures and prolongation of the QRS interval. Tramadol, dextromethorphan, and meperidine also occasionally cause seizures. With meperidine, the metabolite normeperidine is probably the cause of seizures and is most likely to accumulate with repeated dosing in patients with renal insufficiency. While the duration of effect for heroin is usually 3–5 hours, methadone intoxication may last for 48–72 hours or longer. Most opioids, with the exception of illicit newer fentanyl derivatives, tramadol, and methadone, are detectable on routine urine toxicology screening. Wound botulism has been associated with skin-popping, especially involving "black tar" heroin.

Treatment

A. EMERGENCY AND SUPPORTIVE MEASURES

Protect the airway and assist ventilation. Administer activated charcoal (see p 1561).

B. SPECIFIC TREATMENT

Naloxone is a specific opioid antagonist that can rapidly reverse signs of narcotic intoxication. Although it is structurally related to the opioids, it has no agonist effects of its own. Administer 0.4–2 mg intravenously, and repeat as needed to awaken the patient and maintain airway protective reflexes and spontaneous breathing. Very large doses (10–20 mg) may be required for patients intoxicated by some opioids (eg, propoxyphene, codeine, fentanyl derivatives). **Caution:** The duration of effect of naloxone is only about 2–3 hours; repeated doses may be necessary for patients intoxicated by long-acting drugs such as methadone. Continuous observation for at least 3 hours after the last naloxone dose is mandatory.

Kaplan JL et al: Double-blind, randomized study of nalmefene and naloxone in emergency department patients with suspected narcotic overdose. Ann Emerg Med 1999;34:42. [PMID: 10381993] (Similar efficacy and safety.)

Passaro DJ et al: Wound botulism associated with black tar heroin among injecting drug users. JAMA 1998;279:859. [PMID: 9516001] (Case series of 26 patients.)

Sporer KA: Acute heroin overdose. Ann Intern Med 1999;130:584. [PMID: 10189329]

PARAQUAT

Paraquat is used as a herbicide. Concentrated solutions of paraquat are highly corrosive to the oropharynx, esophagus, and stomach. The fatal dose after absorption may be as small as 4 mg/kg. If ingestion of paraquat is not rapidly fatal because of its corrosive effects, the herbicide may cause progressive pulmonary fibrosis, with death ensuing after 2–3 weeks. Patients with plasma paraquat levels above 2 mg/L at 6 hours or 0.2 mg/L at 24 hours are likely to die.

Treatment

Remove ingested paraquat by immediate induced emesis, or by gastric lavage if the patient is already in a health care facility. Clay (bentonite or fuller's earth) and activated charcoal are effective adsorbents. Administer repeated doses of 60 g of activated charcoal by gastric tube every 2 hours for at least three or four doses. Charcoal hemoperfusion, 8 hours per day for 2–3 weeks, has been anecdotally reported to be lifesaving, but clinical and animal studies are equivocal. Supplemental oxygen should be withheld unless the P_{O_2} is less than 70 mm Hg because oxygen may contribute to the pulmonary damage, which is mediated through lipid peroxidation.

Yamashita M et al: A long-term follow-up of lung function in survivors of paraquat poisoning. Hum Exp Toxicol 2000;19:99. [PMID: 10773838] (Survivors of paraquat poisoning are often left with significant restrictive pulmonary dysfunction.)

PESTICIDES: CHOLINESTERASE INHIBITORS
(Organophosphates: Parathion, Malathion, etc; Carbamates: Carbaryl, Aldicarb, etc)

Organophosphate and carbamate insecticides are widely used in commercial agriculture and home gardening and have largely replaced older, more environmentally persistent organochlorine compounds such as DDT and chlordane. The organophosphates and carbamates—also called anticholinesterases because they inhibit the enzyme acetylcholinesterase—cause an increase in acetylcholine activity at nicotinic and muscarinic receptors and in the central nervous system. There are a variety of chemical agents in this group, with widely varying potencies. Most of them are poorly water-soluble and are formulated with an aromatic hydrocarbon solvent such as xylene. Most of them are well absorbed through intact skin. Most chemical warfare "nerve agents" (see above) are organophosphates.

Clinical Findings

Inhibition of cholinesterase results in abdominal cramps, diarrhea, vomiting, excessive salivation, sweating, lacrimation, miosis (constricted pupils), wheezing and bronchorrhea, seizures, and skeletal muscle weakness. Initial tachycardia is usually followed by bradycardia. Profound skeletal muscle weakness, aggravated by excessive bronchial secretions and wheezing, may result in respiratory arrest and death. Symptoms and signs of poisoning may persist or recur over several days, especially with highly lipid-soluble agents such as fenthion or dimethoate.

The diagnosis should be suspected in patients who present with miosis, sweating, and hyperperistalsis. Serum and red blood cell cholinesterase activity can be measured in the laboratory and is usually depressed at least 50% below baseline in those victims who have severe intoxication.

Treatment

A. EMERGENCY AND SUPPORTIVE MEASURES

If the agent was recently ingested, empty the stomach by gastric lavage and administer activated charcoal (see p 1561). Do not induce emesis because of the risk of abrupt onset of seizures. If the agent is on the victim's skin or hair, wash repeatedly with soap or shampoo and water. Providers must take care to avoid skin exposure by wearing gloves and waterproof aprons.

B. SPECIFIC TREATMENT

Atropine reverses excessive muscarinic stimulation and is effective for treatment of salivation, wheezing, abdominal cramping, and sweating. However, it does not interact with nicotinic receptors at autonomic ganglia and at the neuromuscular junction and has no effect on muscle weakness. Administer 2 mg intravenously, and give repeated doses as needed to dry bronchial secretions and decrease wheezing; as much as several hundred milligrams of atropine have been given to treat severe poisoning.

Pralidoxime (2-PAM, Protopam) is a specific antidote that reverses organophosphate binding to the cholinesterase enzyme; therefore, it is effective at the neuromuscular junction as well as other nicotinic and muscarinic sites. It should be started as soon as possible, to prevent permanent binding of the organophosphate to cholinesterase. Administer 1–2 g intravenously, and begin a continuous infusion (200–400 mg/h). Constant infusion is more effective because of the short duration of action of single doses. Continue to give pralidoxime as long as there is any evidence of acetylcholine excess. Pralidoxime is of questionable benefit for carbamate poisoning, because carbamates have only a transitory effect on the cholinesterase enzyme.

Lee P et al: Clinical features of patients with acute organophosphate poisoning requiring intensive care. Intensive Care Med 2001;27:694. [PMID: 11398695] (Of 23 patients with acute malathion poisoning who were admitted to the ICU, 74% required mechanical ventilation because of excessive bronchial secretions, altered level of consciousness, pneumonia, or flaccid paralysis. An APACHE II score of 26 or higher was predictive of mortality. Cholinesterase levels were useful in predicting successful weaning of patients from the ventilator.)

Thiermann H et al: Modern strategies in therapy of organophosphate poisoning. Toxicol Lett 1999;107:233. [PMID: 10414801] (Continuous infusion of obidoxime was successful if initiated early.)

PETROLEUM DISTILLATES & SOLVENTS

Petroleum distillate toxicity may occur from inhalation of the vapor or as a result of pulmonary aspiration of the liquid during or after ingestion. Acute manifestations of aspiration pneumonitis are vomiting, coughing, and bronchopneumonia. Some hydrocarbons—ie, those with aromatic or halogenated subunits—can also cause severe systemic poisoning after oral ingestion (Table 39–13). Hydrocarbons can also cause systemic intoxication by inhalation. Vertigo, muscular incoordination, irregular pulse, myoclonus, and seizures occur with serious poisoning and may be due to hypoxemia or the systemic effects of the agents. Chlorinated and fluorinated hydrocarbons (tri-chloroethylene, freons, etc) and many other hydrocarbons can cause ventricular arrhythmias due to increased sensitivity of the myocardium to the effects of endogenous catecholamines.

Treatment
(Table 39–13)

Remove the patient to fresh air. Since aspiration is the primary danger after ingestion of many common products, use of lavage or emesis is not recommended; administration of activated charcoal may be helpful if the preparation contains toxic solutes (eg, an insecticide) or is an aromatic or halogenated product. Observe the victim for 6–8 hours for signs of aspiration pneumonitis (cough, localized rales or rhonchi, tachypnea, and infiltrates on chest radiograph). Corticosteroids are not recommended. If fever occurs, give a specific antibiotic only after identification of bacterial pathogens by laboratory studies. Because of the risk of arrhythmias, use bronchodilators only with caution in patients with chlorinated or fluorinated solvent intoxication.

Chang YL et al: Diverse manifestations of oral methylene chloride poisoning: report of 6 cases. J Toxicol Clin Toxicol 1999;37:497. [PMID: 10465248] (Toxic effects included central nervous system depression, tachypnea, and corrosive gastrointestinal injury. Two patients had mild to moderate elevation of blood carboxyhemoglobin levels.)

Cording CJ et al: A fatality due to accidental PineSol ingestion. J Anal Toxicol 2000;24:664. [PMID: 11043678] (Case report, including postmortem alpha-terpineol levels.)

Table 39–13. Clinical features of hydrocarbon poisoning.[1]

Type	Examples	Risk of Pneumonia	Risk of Systemic Toxicity	Treatment
High-viscosity	Vaseline[2] Motor oil	Low	Low	None.
Low-viscosity, nontoxic	Furniture polish Mineral seal oil Kerosene Lighter fluid	High	Low	Observe for pneumonia. *Do not* induce emesis. *Do not* administer activated charcoal.
Low-viscosity, unknown systemic toxicity	Turpentine Pine oil	High	Variable	Observe for pneumonia. Consider activated charcoal.
Low-viscosity, known systemic toxicity	Camphor Phenol Chlorinated insecticides Aromatic hydrocarbons (benzene, toluene, etc)	High	High	Observe for pneumonia. Give activated charcoal.

[1]Reproduced, with permission, from Saunders CE, Ho MT (editors): *Current Emergency Diagnosis & Treatment*, 4th ed. McGraw-Hill, 1992.
[2]"Vaseline" is one of several proprietary names for petrolatum (petroleum jelly, paraffin jelly).

PHENOTHIAZINES & OTHER ANTIPSYCHOTIC AGENTS (Chlorpromazine, Promazine, Haloperidol, Prochlorperazine, Risperidone, Clozapine, etc)

Chlorpromazine and related drugs are used as antiemetics and antipsychotic agents and as potentiators of analgesic and hypnotic drugs.

Small doses of phenothiazines induce drowsiness and mild orthostatic hypotension in as many as 50% of patients. Larger doses can cause obtundation, miosis, severe hypotension, tachycardia, convulsions, and coma. Abnormal cardiac conduction may occur (particularly with thioridazine), resulting in prolongation of QRS or QT intervals (or both) and ventricular arrhythmias.

With therapeutic or toxic doses, some patients develop an acute extrapyramidal dystonic reaction similar to Parkinson's disease, with spasmodic contractions of the face and neck muscles, extensor rigidity of the back muscles, carpopedal spasm, and motor restlessness. Severe rigidity accompanied by hyperthermia and metabolic acidosis ("neuroleptic malignant syndrome") may occasionally occur and is life-threatening (see Chapters 1 and 25).

Treatment

A. EMERGENCY AND SUPPORTIVE MEASURES

Administer activated charcoal. Consider gastric lavage for massive ingestions. For severe hypotension, treatment with fluids and pressor agents may be necessary. Treat hyperthermia as outlined on p 1559. Maintain cardiac monitoring.

B. SPECIFIC TREATMENT

Hypotension and cardiac arrhythmias associated with widened QRS intervals on the ECG in a patient with thioridazine poisoning may respond to intravenous sodium bicarbonate as used for tricyclic antidepressants.

For extrapyramidal signs, give diphenhydramine, 0.5–1 mg/kg intravenously, or benztropine mesylate, 0.01–0.02 mg/kg intramuscularly. Treatment with oral doses of these agents should be continued for 24–48 hours.

Bromocriptine (2.5–7.5 mg orally daily) may be effective for mild or moderate neuroleptic malignant syndrome. Dantrolene (2–5 mg/kg intravenously) has also been used for muscle contractions but is not a true antidote.

Acri AA et al: Effects of risperidone in overdose. Am J Emerg Med 1998;16:498. [PMID: 9725965] (Case series of 31 patients. Main effects of risperidone overdose included lethargy, dystonia, hypotension, tachycardia, and dysrhythmias.)

Burns MJ: The pharmacology and toxicology of atypical antipsychotic agents. J Toxicol Clin Toxicol 2001;39:1. [PMID: 11327216]

Hustey FM: Acute quetiapine poisoning. J Emerg Med 1999;17:995. [PMID: 10595886] (Case report of acute overdose causing hypotension, tachycardia, coma, and prolonged QTc interval.)

Reith D et al: Features and toxicokinetics of clozapine in overdose. Ther Drug Monit 1998;20:92. [PMID: 9485562] (Presentation of seven cases of clozapine overdose. Anticholinergic effects were minimal, and no reversible ECG changes or biochemical abnormalities were demonstrated.)

QUINIDINE & RELATED ANTIARRHYTHMICS

Quinidine, procainamide, and disopyramide are class Ia antiarrhythmic agents, and flecainide is a class Ic agent. These drugs have membrane-depressant effects on the sodium-dependent channel responsible for cardiac cell depolarization. Manifestations of cardiotoxicity include arrhythmias, syncope, hypotension, and widening of the QRS complex on the ECG (> 100–120 ms). With type Ia drugs, a lengthened QT interval and atypical or polymorphous ventricular tachycardia (torsade de pointes) may occur.

Treatment

A. EMERGENCY AND SUPPORTIVE MEASURES

Administer activated charcoal (see p 1559); consider gastric lavage after large recent overdose. Assist ventilation if needed. Perform continuous cardiac monitoring.

B. SPECIFIC TREATMENT

Treat cardiotoxicity (hypotension, QRS interval widening) with intravenous boluses of sodium bicarbonate, 50–100 meq. Ventricular tachycardia of the torsade de pointes variety may be treated with intravenous magnesium or overdrive pacing.

Corkeron MA et al: Extracorporeal support in near-fatal flecainide overdose. Anaesth Intensive Care 1999;27:405. [PMID: 10470398] (Toxicity of flecainide, a type Ic antiarrhythmic drug, is similar to that of quinidine.)

Reddy VG et al: Chloroquine poisoning: report of two cases. Acta Anaesthesiol Scand 2000;44:1017. [PMID: 10981583]

SALICYLATES

Salicylates (aspirin, methyl salicylate, etc) are found in a variety of over-the-counter and prescription medications. Salicylates uncouple cellular oxidative phosphorylation, resulting in anaerobic metabolism and excessive production of lactic acid and heat, and they also interfere with several Krebs cycle enzymes. A single ingestion of more than 200 mg/kg of salicylate is likely to produce significant acute intoxication. Poisoning may also occur as a result of chronic excessive dosing over several days. Although the half-life of salicylate is 2–3 hours after small doses, it may increase to 20 hours or more in patients with intoxication.

Clinical Findings

Acute ingestion often causes nausea and vomiting, occasionally with gastritis. Moderate intoxication is characterized by hyperpnea (deep and rapid breathing), tachycardia, tinnitus, and elevated anion gap metabolic acidosis. Serious intoxication may result in agitation, confusion, coma, seizures, cardiovascular collapse, pulmonary edema, hyperthermia, and death. The prothrombin time is often elevated owing to salicylate-induced hypoprothrombinemia.

Diagnosis is suspected in any patient with metabolic acidosis and is confirmed by measuring the serum salicylate level. Patients with levels greater than 100 mg/dL (1000 mg/L) after an acute overdose are more likely to have severe poisoning. On the other hand, patients with subacute or chronic intoxication may suffer severe symptoms with levels of only 60–70 mg/dL. The arterial blood gas typically reveals a respiratory alkalosis with an underlying metabolic acidosis.

Treatment

A. Emergency and Supportive Measures

Administer activated charcoal (see p 1559). Gastric lavage followed by administration of extra doses of activated charcoal may be needed in patients who ingest more than 10 g of aspirin. The desired ratio of charcoal to aspirin is about 10:1 by weight; while this cannot always be given as a single dose, it may be administered over the first 24 hours in divided doses every 2–4 hours. Treat metabolic acidosis with intravenous sodium bicarbonate. This is critical because acidosis (especially acidemia, pH < 7.40) promotes greater entry of salicylate into cells, worsening toxicity. Intubation and controlled ventilation may cause sudden and severe deterioration if the pH is allowed to fall.

B. Specific Treatment

Alkalinization of the urine enhances renal salicylate excretion by trapping the salicylate anion in the urine. Add 100 meq (two ampules) of sodium bicarbonate to 1 L of 5% dextrose in 0.2% saline, and infuse this solution intravenously at a rate of about 150–200 mL/h. Unless the patient is oliguric, add 20–30 meq of potassium chloride to each liter of intravenous fluid. Patients who are volume-depleted often fail to produce an alkaline urine (paradoxical aciduria) unless potassium is given.

Hemodialysis may be lifesaving and is indicated for patients with severe metabolic acidosis, markedly altered mental status, or significantly elevated salicylate levels (eg, > 100–120 mg/dL [1000–1200 mg/L] after acute overdose or > 60–70 mg/dL [600–700 mg/L] with subacute or chronic intoxication).

Cohen DL et al: Chronic salicylism resulting in noncardiogenic pulmonary edema requiring hemodialysis. Am J Kidney Dis 2000;36:E20. [PMID: 10977813] (Case report describing pulmonary edema in a 42-year-old woman with chronic salicylate poisoning.)

Higgins RM et al: Alkalinization and hemodialysis in severe salicylate poisoning: Comparison of elimination techniques in the same patient. Clin Nephrol 1998;50:178. [PMID: 9776422] (Alkalinization was very effective, especially in the first 4 hours.)

SEAFOOD POISONINGS

A variety of intoxications may occur after eating certain types of fish or other seafood. These include scombroid, ciguatera, paralytic shellfish, and puffer fish poisoning. The mechanisms of toxicity and clinical presentations are described in Table 39–14. In the majority of cases, the seafood has a normal appearance and taste (scombroid may have a peppery taste).

Treatment

A. Emergency and Supportive Measures
Caution:

Abrupt respiratory arrest may occur in patients with acute paralytic shellfish and puffer fish poisoning. Observe patients for at least 4–6 hours. Replace fluid and electrolyte losses from gastroenteritis with intravenous saline or other crystalloid solution.

For recent ingestions, it may be possible to adsorb residual toxin in the gut with activated charcoal, 50–60 g orally.

B. Specific Treatment

There is no specific antidote for paralytic shellfish or puffer fish poisoning.

1. Ciguatera—There are anecdotal reports of successful treatment of acute neurologic symptoms with mannitol, 1 g/kg intravenously.

2. Scombroid—Antihistamines such as diphenhydramine, 25–50 mg intravenously, and the H_2 blocker cimetidine, 300 mg intravenously, are usually effective. For severe reactions, give also epinephrine, 0.3–0.5 mL of a 1:1000 solution subcutaneously.

Clark RF et al: A review of selected seafood poisonings. Undersea Hyperb Med 1999;26:175. [PMID: 10485519] (Review of the pathophysiology, clinical presentation, and treatment of the most common varieties of seafood poisoning resulting from toxins.)

Crump JA et al: Ciguatera fish poisoning. Postgrad Med J 1999;75:678. [PMID: 10621882]

Field J: Puffer fish poisoning. J Accid Emerg Med 1998;15:334. [PMID: 9785165] (The deadly toxin in this fish can cause rapid onset of muscular paralysis and respiratory arrest.)

SNAKE BITES

The venom of poisonous snakes and lizards may be predominantly neurotoxic (coral snake) or predominantly cytolytic (rattlesnakes, other pit vipers). Neurotoxins cause respiratory paralysis; cytolytic venoms cause tissue destruction by digestion and hemorrhage

Table 39–14. Common seafood poisonings.

Type of Poisoning	Mechanism	Clinical Presentation
Ciguatera	Reef fish ingest toxic dinoflagellates, whose toxins accumulate in fish meat. Commonly implicated fish in the USA are barracuda, jack, snapper, and grouper.	1–6 hours after ingestion, victims develop abdominal pain, vomiting, and diarrhea accompanied by a variety of neurologic symptoms, including paresthesias, reversal of hot and cold sensation, vertigo, headache, and intense itching. Autonomic disturbances, including hypotension and bradycardia, may occur.
Scombroid	Improper preservation of large fish results in bacterial degradation of histidine to histamine. Commonly implicated fish include tuna, mahimahi, bonita, mackerel, and kingfish.	Allergic-like (anaphylactoid) symptoms are due to histamine, usually begin within 15–90 minutes, and include skin flushing, itching, urticaria, angioedema, bronchospasm, and hypotension as well as abdominal pain, vomiting, and diarrhea.
Paralytic shellfish poisoning	Dinoflagellates produce saxitoxin, which is concentrated by filter-feeding mussels and clams. Saxitoxin blocks sodium conductance and neuronal transmission in skeletal muscles.	Onset is usually within 30–60 minutes. Initial symptoms include perioral and intraoral paresthesias. Other symptoms include nausea and vomiting, headache, dizziness, dysphagia, dysarthria, ataxia, and rapidly progressive muscle weakness that may result in respiratory arrest.
Puffer fish poisoning	Tetrodotoxin is concentrated in liver, gonads, intestine, and skin. Toxic effects are similar to those of saxitoxin. Tetrodotoxin is also found in some North American newts and Central American frogs.	Onset is usually within 30–40 minutes but may be as short as 10 minutes. Initial perioral paresthesias are followed by headache, diaphoresis, nausea, vomiting, ataxia, and rapidly progressive muscle weakness that may result in respiratory arrest.

due to hemolysis and destruction of the endothelial lining of the blood vessels. The manifestations of rattlesnake envenomation are mostly local pain, redness, swelling, and extravasation of blood. Perioral tingling, metallic taste, nausea and vomiting, hypotension, and coagulopathy may also occur. Neurotoxic envenomation may cause ptosis, dysphagia, diplopia, and respiratory arrest.

Treatment

A. Emergency Measures

Immobilize the patient and the bitten part in a neutral position. Avoid manipulation of the bitten area. Transport the patient to a medical facility for definitive treatment. Do *not* give alcoholic beverages or stimulants; do *not* apply ice; do *not* apply a tourniquet. The trauma to underlying structures resulting from incision and suction performed by unskilled people is probably not justified in view of the small amount of venom that can be recovered.

B. Specific Antidote and General Measures

1. Pit viper (eg, rattlesnake) envenomation—A new antivenin (CroFab) has replaced the Wyeth horse serum-based product. With local signs such as swelling, pain, and ecchymosis but no systemic symptoms, give 4–6 vials of crotalid antivenin (CroFab) by slow intravenous drip in 250–500 mL saline. Re-peated doses of 2 vials every 6 hours for up to 18 hours has been recommended. For more serious envenomation with marked local effects and systemic toxicity (eg, hypotension, coagulopathy), higher doses and additional vials may be required. Monitor vital signs and the blood coagulation profile. Type and cross-match blood. The adequacy of venom neutralization is indicated by improvement in symptoms and signs, and the rate of swelling slows.

2. Elapid (coral snake) envenomation—Give 1–2 vials of specific antivenom as soon as possible. To locate antisera for exotic snakes, call a regional poison control center (see Table 39–1).

Boyer LV et al: Recurrent and persistent coagulopathy following pit viper envenomation. Arch Intern Med 1999;159:706. [PMID: 10218750] (Thrombocytopenia and hypofibrinogenemia persisted for 2–14 days in this series of 38 patients. None experienced significant spontaneous bleeding.)

Dart RC et al: Efficacy, safety, and use of snake antivenoms in the United States. Ann Emerg Med 2001;37:181. [PMID: 11174237] (CroFab is a new purified, ovine-derived antibody that appears to be as effective as the older horse serum-based product, with fewer side effects such as acute hypersensitivity reactions or serum sickness, although it has a shorter half-life and symptoms may recur.)

Walter F et al: Envenomations. Crit Care Clin 1999;15:353. [PMID: 10331133] (Review of envenomations caused by snakes, spiders and scorpions.

SPIDER BITES & SCORPION STINGS

The toxin of most species of spiders in the USA causes only local pain, redness, and swelling. That of the more venomous black widow spiders (*Latrodectus mactans*) causes generalized muscular pains, muscle spasms, and rigidity. The brown recluse spider (*Loxosceles reclusa*) causes progressive local necrosis as well as hemolytic reactions (rare). Stings by most scorpions in the USA cause only local pain. Stings by the more toxic *Centruroides* species (found in the southwestern USA) may cause muscle cramps, twitching and jerking, and occasionally hypertension, convulsions, and pulmonary edema.

Treatment

A. Black Widow Spider Bites

Pain may be relieved with parenteral narcotics or muscle relaxants (eg, methocarbamol, 15 mg/kg). Calcium gluconate 10%, 0.1–0.2 mL/kg intravenously, may relieve muscle rigidity, though its effectiveness is questionable. Antivenin is available, but because of concerns about acute hypersensitivity reactions it is often reserved for very young or elderly patients or those who do not respond to the above measures. Horse serum sensitivity testing is required. (Instruction and testing materials are included in the antivenin kit.)

B. Brown Recluse Spider Bites

Because bites occasionally progress to extensive local necrosis, some authorities recommend early excision of the bite site, whereas others use oral corticosteroids. Anecdotal reports have claimed success with dapsone and colchicine. An antivenin is being developed. All of these treatments remain of unproved value.

C. Scorpion Stings

No specific treatment is available. For *Centruroides* stings, some toxicologists use a specific antivenom developed in Arizona, but this is neither FDA-approved nor widely available.

Bond GR: Snake, spider, and scorpion envenomation in North America. Pediatr Rev 1999;20:147. [PMID: 10233171]

Heard K et al: Antivenom therapy in the Americas. Drugs 1999;58:5. [PMID: 10439926] (Review of the indications, method of administration, and incidence of adverse reactions for antivenoms in the treatment of envenomations from snakes, spiders, and scorpions.)

THEOPHYLLINE

Theophylline toxicity may be caused by several of its pharmacologic effects, including inhibition of phosphodiesterase and adenosine and release of catecholamines. Theophylline may cause intoxication after an acute single overdose, or intoxication may occur as a result of chronic accidental repeated overmedication or reduced elimination resulting from hepatic dysfunction or interacting drug (eg, cimetidine, erythromycin). The usual serum half-life of theophylline is 4–6 hours, but this may increase to more than 20 hours after overdose. Caffeine and caffeine containing herbal products can produce similar toxicity.

Clinical Findings

Mild intoxication causes nausea, vomiting, tachycardia, and tremulousness. Severe intoxication is characterized by ventricular and supraventricular tachyarrhythmias, hypotension, and seizures. Status epilepticus is common and often intractable to usual anticonvulsants. After acute overdose (but not chronic intoxication), hypokalemia, hyperglycemia, and metabolic acidosis are common. Seizures and other manifestations of toxicity may be delayed for several hours after acute ingestion, especially if a sustained-release preparation such as Theo-Dur was taken.

Diagnosis is based on measurement of the serum theophylline concentration. Acute overdose patients with serum levels greater than 100 mg/L are likely to develop seizures and hypotension. Patients with chronic intoxication may develop serious toxicity at lower levels (ie, 40–60 mg/L).

Treatment

A. Emergency and Supportive Measures

After acute ingestion, administer activated charcoal (see p 1559). Repeated doses of activated charcoal may enhance theophylline elimination by "gut dialysis." Addition of whole bowel irrigation should be considered for large ingestions involving sustained-release preparations.

Hemodialysis (or hemoperfusion) is effective in removing theophylline and is indicated for patients with status epilepticus or markedly elevated serum theophylline levels (eg, > 100 mg/L after acute overdose or > 60 mg/L with chronic intoxication).

B. Specific Treatment

Treat seizures with benzodiazepines (lorazepam, 2–3 mg intravenously, or diazepam, 5–10 mg intravenously) or phenobarbital (10–15 mg/kg intravenously). Phenytoin is not effective. Hypotension and tachycardia—which are mediated through excessive beta-adrenergic stimulation—may respond to beta-blocker therapy even in low doses: Administer esmolol, 25–50 μg/kg/min by intravenous infusion, or propranolol, 0.5–1 mg intravenously.

Polak M et al: Theophylline intoxication mimicking diabetic ketoacidosis in a child. Diabetes Metab 1999; 25:513. [PMID: 10633877] (Case report of a 5-year-old boy with hyperglycemia, glucosuria, ketonuria, low plasma bicarbonate, and tachycardia caused by theophylline poisoning.)

Shannon MW: Comparative efficacy of hemodialysis and hemoperfusion in severe theophylline intoxication. Acad Emerg Med 1997;4:674. [PMID: 9223689] (Hemoperfusion provides a higher theophylline clearance rate than hemodialysis;

however, hemodialysis appears to have comparable efficacy in reducing morbidity.)

Shannon M: Life-threatening events after theophylline overdose: a 10-year prospective analysis. Arch Intern Med 1999;159: 989. [PMID: 10326941] (Review of 356 patients with theophylline intoxication highlighting the substantial morbidity and mortality.)

TRICYCLIC ANTIDEPRESSANTS

Tricyclic and related cyclic antidepressants are among the most dangerous drugs involved in suicidal overdose. These drugs have anticholinergic and cardiac depressant properties ("quinidine-like" sodium channel blockade). Tricyclic antidepressants produce more marked membrane-depressant cardiotoxic effects than the phenothiazines.

Newer antidepressants such as trazodone, fluoxetine, paroxetine, sertraline, bupropion, venlafaxine, and fluvoxamine are not chemically related to the tricyclic antidepressant agents and do not generally produce cardiotoxic effects. However, they may cause seizures in overdoses and they may cause serotonin syndrome (see Monoamine Oxidase Inhibitors, above). Seizures are also reported rarely after therapeutic doses of bupropion.

Clinical Findings

Signs of severe intoxication may occur abruptly and without warning within 30–60 minutes after acute tricyclic overdose. Anticholinergic effects include dilated pupils, tachycardia, dry mouth, flushed skin, muscle twitching, and decreased peristalsis. Quinidine-like cardiotoxic effects include QRS interval widening (> 0.12 s; see Figure 39–2), ventricular arrhythmias, atrioventricular block, and hypotension. Seizures and coma are common with severe intoxication. Life-threatening hyperthermia may result from status epilepticus and anticholinergic-induced impairment of sweating.

The diagnosis should be suspected in any overdose patient with anticholinergic side effects, especially if there is widening of the QRS interval or seizures. For intoxication by most tricyclics, the QRS interval correlates with the severity of intoxication more reliably than the serum drug level.

Treatment

A. EMERGENCY AND SUPPORTIVE MEASURES

Observe patients for at least 6 hours, and admit all patients with evidence of anticholinergic effects (eg, delirium, dilated pupils, tachycardia) or signs of cardiotoxicity (see above).

Administer activated charcoal and consider gastric lavage after recent large ingestions (see p 1559). All of

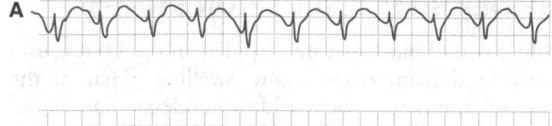
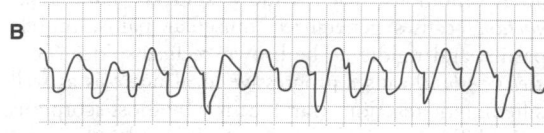
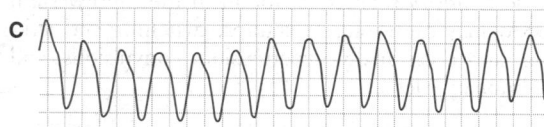

Figure 39–2. Cardiac arrhythmias resulting from tricyclic antidepressant overdose. **A:** Delayed intraventricular conduction results in prolonged QRS interval (0.18 s). **B and C:** Supraventricular tachycardia with progressive widening of QRS complexes mimics ventricular tachycardia. (Reproduced, with permission, from Benowitz NL, Goldschlager N: Cardiac disturbances in the toxicologic patient. In: *Clinical Management of Poisoning and Drug Overdose,* 3rd ed. Haddad LM, Winchester JF [editors]. Saunders, 1998.)

these drugs are highly tissue-bound and are not effectively removed by hemodialysis procedures.

B. SPECIFIC TREATMENT

Cardiotoxic sodium channel-depressant effects may respond to boluses of sodium bicarbonate (50–100 meq intravenously). Sodium bicarbonate provides a large sodium load that alleviates depression of the sodium-dependent channel. Reversal of acidosis may also have beneficial effects at this site. Maintain the pH between 7.45 and 7.50. Alkalinization does not promote excretion of tricyclics.

Harrigan RA et al: ECG abnormalities in tricyclic antidepressant ingestion. Am J Emerg Med 1999;17:387. [PMID: 10452441]

Liebelt EL: Targeted management strategies for cardiovascular toxicity from tricyclic antidepressant overdose: the pivotal role for alkalinization and sodium loading. Pediatr Emerg Care 1998;14:293. [PMID: 9733258] (Pathophysiology, diagnosis, prognosis, and treatment of tricyclic antidepressant overdose.)

Mackway-Jones K: Towards evidence based emergency medicine: best BETs from the Manchester Royal Infirmary. Alkalinisation in the management of tricyclic antidepressant overdose. J Accid Emerg Med 1999;16:139. [PMID: 10191453]

Cancer

40

Hope S. Rugo, MD

See www.current-med.com/ch40.html

This chapter mainly covers the clinical aspects of cancer: prevention, diagnosis, primary treatment, management of complications, and paraneoplastic syndromes. Further information may be obtained by calling the NCI Cancer Information Service at 1-800-4CANCER or accessing NCI's comprehensive cancer information database "Physician Data Query" (PDQ) via the Internet at www.cancernet.nci.nih.gov. PDQ is also available on CD-ROM. The CANCERLIT feature of Medline is a familiar resource for articles about cancer that can be accessed by author or by subject words. A series of oncology practice guidelines compiled by a panel of United States experts and encompassing diagnosis and treatment of a wide variety of cancers as well as pain management is now available on CD-ROM at the National Comprehensive Cancer Network Web site (www.nccn.org). This site also provides a stepwise guide to diagnosis and to treatment options for patients as well as links to a variety of useful sites, including the American Cancer Society.

Many new Web sites are now available for both clinician and patient use. Information includes statistics, treatment, and clinical trial information. Consultations can also be obtained. Web sites can be found by searching for the words "cancer" or "oncology." The American Society of Clinical Oncology has a new information Web site for patients and their families (www.PeopleLivingWithCancer.org) as well as patient guides on subjects such as follow-up care for breast and colorectal cancers, understanding tumor markers, treatment of nausea and vomiting, and advanced lung cancer.

■ INCIDENCE & ETIOLOGY

Cancer is the second most common cause of death in the United States. It is estimated that over 1.3 million new cases of invasive cancer will be diagnosed in the year 2002, with over 550,000 deaths. One out of every two (men) to three (women) individuals in the United States will develop some type of invasive cancer during their lifetime. Table 40–1 summarizes current United States incidence and mortality figures for the ten leading types of cancer. Women have an approximately 1:8 lifetime chance of developing breast cancer, and men have an approximately 1:6 chance of developing prostate cancer. Cancers of the lung, prostate, and breast and of the colon and rectum account for about 55% of all new cancer diagnoses and for over 50% of cancer deaths in the United States. Table 40–2 summarizes the lifetime risk of being diagnosed with or dying from the five leading causes of cancer as well as from all types of cancer. Most rates are now age adjusted to the year 2000 standard million population based on the 2000 census data. The incidence of and the mortality from cancer decreased an average of 1.4% per year from 1994 to 1998 in the United States, with variation by gender and race. This is the first sustained decline in the past 30 years and is attributed to changes in lifestyle as well as improved prevention, early detection, and treatment. However, as the United States population grows and ages and given that the median age at diagnosis of cancer is 68, it is estimated that the number of cancer cases will double by the year 2050. Cancer incidence and mortality vary significantly among racial and ethnic groups, with blacks having the highest rates. Cancers are less likely to be diagnosed when localized; however, stage for stage, 5-year survival rates are lower, suggesting the influence of additional differences such as treatment, pathology, and comorbid conditions. Data from the new census confirms the existence of geographic variability in cancer incidence; for example, breast cancer rates in Marin County in California appear to be among the highest in the United States. The cause of this increase is multifactorial, including socioeconomic status, ethnicity, and perhaps environmental factors.

The cause of most cancers remains unknown. Mutations in DNA sequences leading to abnormal or unregulated expression of proto-oncogenes or deletion of tumor suppressor genes—or both processes—have been linked to abnormal cellular proliferation. Oncogenes encode for cellular growth factor receptors, growth factors, or elements of the proliferative machinery of the cancer cell. Tumor suppressor genes govern regulatory proteins that normally suppress cellular pro-

Table 40–1. Incidence of and mortality from the ten most common cancers in the USA in males and females (all races).

Rank	Men	Incidence[1]	Mortality[1]	Women	Incidence[1]	Mortality[1]
1	Prostate	169	34	Breast	137	29
2	Lung	86	81	Lung	51	41
3	Colorectal	65	26	Colorectal	48	19
4	Bladder	37	8	Uterus[2]	34	7
5	Lymphoma[3]	27	11	Lymphoma[3]	18	8
6	Oropharyngeal[4]	24	7	Ovary	17	9
7	Melanoma	21	4	Melanoma	14	2
8	Leukemia	16	10	Leukemia	9	6
9	Kidney	16	6	Pancreas	10	9
10	Pancreas	13	12	Bladder	10	2

Data obtained from the NCI SEER Program.
[1]Rates are per 100,000, 1995–1999, and are age-adjusted to the 2000 United States population by 5-year age groups.
[2]Uterus includes the cervix and corpus uteri.
[3]Both Hodgkin's disease and non-Hodgkin's lymphoma are included under lymphoma.
[4]Both oropharynx and larynx are included under oropharyngeal.

liferation. Cancer results from these and other mutations, which may be due to environmental exposure, genetic susceptibility, infectious agents, and other factors. Most tumors exhibit chromosomal abnormalities such as deletions, inversions, translocations, or duplications. Although usually nonspecific, certain genetic al-

Table 40–2. Lifetime risks for the five most common cancers.[1]

Cancer	Risk of Diagnosis (%)	Risk of Death (%)
Prostate	16.0	3.1
Breast (women)	13.2	3.1
Lung		
(men)	7.9	7.5
(women)	5.8	4.9
Colorectal		
(men)	6.0	2.4
(women)	5.6	2.4
Bladder (men)	3.4	0.7
Uterus[2]	3.5	0.8
Any cancer		
(men)	43.4	23.9
(women)	38.0	20.4

[1]Data obtained from the National Cancer Institute's SEER program, 1995–1999.
[2]Uterus includes the cervix and corpus uteri.

terations are strongly associated with specific malignancies and in some cases can be used to assess prognosis. In Burkitt's lymphoma, the c-*myc* oncogene is activated by translocation of genetic material from chromosome 8 to chromosome 14. Chronic myelogenous leukemia (CML) is defined by a reciprocal translocation of the long arms of chromosomes 9 and 22, resulting in the generation of a fusion protein (BCR-ABL) with tyrosine kinase activity. In colon cancer, loss of the long arm of chromosome 18 (18q) predicts a poor outcome, whereas mutations in the gene for the type II receptor for transforming growth factor β1 (TGF-β1) with microsatellite instability predict a favorable outcome. In one recent study, 5-year survival following adjuvant chemotherapy for stage III colon cancer was 74% in those who retained the 18q allele and 50% in those with loss of the allele. Five-year survival was 74% for patients whose cancers had both microsatellite instability and a mutated gene for the type II receptor for TGF-β1 and 46% if the tumor did not have the mutation. Genetic mutations in chronic lymphocytic leukemia (CLL) have been shown to occur in up to 82% of cases and strongly predict outcomes. For example, patients with deletions of the short arm of chromosome 17 had a survival of only 2.7 years, whereas those with deletions of the long arm of chromosome 13 had a survival of 11 years. Defining chromosomal aberrations and their association with prognosis will help in designing targeted therapies as well as risk-adapted treatment strategies.

The *P53* gene appears to trigger programmed cell death (apoptosis) as a way of regulating uncontrolled cellular proliferation in the setting of aberrant growth signals. Mutations in the *P53* gene result in loss of the ability of the gene product to bind to DNA, thereby removing its suppressive effect. *P53* can also be inactivated by overexpression of an oncogene whose protein product binds to normal *P53* and prevents its action. This occurs in many soft tissue sarcomas. The Bcl-2 family of proteins act as "arbiters of cell death" with a balance of both "antideath" and "prodeath" activity. Bcl-2 and Bcl-X$_L$ appear to function as "antideath" proteins to prevent programmed cell death of cancer cells; overexpression of these proteins in cancer confers resistance to chemotherapy and radiation therapy. Bcl-2 and Bcl-X$_L$ are overexpressed at a high level (50–100%) on common cancers, including cancers of the breast, colon, prostate, head and neck, and ovary. Agents that target production of these proteins might work to overcome cancer resistance (see section on novel therapies at the end of this chapter). Another control against abnormal cellular proliferation also contributes to cellular aging. As a cell divides and ages, there is progressive shortening of the ends of the chromosomes, or telomeres. A striking correlation between cancer and the overexpression of telomerase (an enzyme capable of preventing the shortening of telomeres) suggests that it might be partially responsible for tumor cell immortality. Telomerase activity is present in about 85% of malignant tumors but absent in most normal somatic tissues. The stage and severity of neuroblastoma, breast cancer, and other cancers have been found to correlate with levels of telomerase activity, indicating a prognostic role of enzyme activity. Normal human cells transfected with the telomerase gene in vitro far exceeded their normal life span and ability to divide, thereby establishing a firmer causal relationship between telomere shortening and cellular senescence. This raises important possibilities for targeting telomerase activity as part of cancer therapy.

The development of cancer is a complicated multistep process that appears to involve the acquisition of an increasing number of genetic mutations, eventually resulting in invasive disease. Clinical examples of this stepwise progression can be found in many common cancers, including breast, colon, and prostate cancers. A history of the benign finding of atypical ductal hyperplasia on breast biopsy is clearly associated with a two- to fourfold increase in the risk of subsequent invasive cancer. Noninvasive breast cancer (ductal carcinoma in situ) is a preinvasive lesion that can progress into invasive cancer if left untreated. Understanding the cascade of genetic changes associated with the progression of benign cells to invasive cancer is a critical step in developing therapies targeted to a specific cancer. These genetic changes can now be mapped by a process called comparative genomic hybridization, this is an intense area of research. DNA microarray studies can detect activation of thousands of genes in a single experiment. The resulting DNA expression profile can be used not only to understand the development of

cancer but also to assess prognosis, predict response to therapy, and direct targeted therapies. Over the last year, studies have associated certain DNA profiles with specific cancer phenotypes, an important first step in this exciting area of research. In non-small cell lung cancer, reduced expression of the adhesion molecule E-cadherin detected by tissue microarray analysis correlated with reduced survival as well as local invasion and regional metastases.

Autoimmune suppression may contribute to the development of cancer. Tumors are allowed to exist by virtue of tolerance—the ability of the tumor to escape the host immune system. The host immune system cannot recognize the tumor as foreign because of an absence of critical immunostimulatory molecules on the tumor itself, resulting in a state of anergy (deletion of tumor-specific lymphocytes) toward the growing cancer. Novel therapies aimed at correcting this immunodeficient state and stimulating the host immune response against tumor cells are now being tested clinically. (See section on Novel Therapies at the end of this chapter.)

Hereditary predisposition to some cancers has been linked to events within a gene and is manifested by a family history of a common cancer occurring frequently—and in a younger than expected age group—or any history of a relatively rare cancer. Examples include familial retinoblastoma, familial adenomatous polyposis, multiple endocrine neoplasia syndromes, and the hereditary breast and ovarian cancer syndromes. Although familial adenomatous polyposis is a rare syndrome, somatic mutations in the affected gene (adenomatous polyposis coli; *APC*) occur in more than 60% of patients with colonic carcinomas and in an equal proportion of patients with adenomas. Genetic mutations associated with an increased risk of developing breast and ovarian cancers appear to be much more common than previously thought and are strongly related to age at diagnosis of cancer. It is estimated that 5–10% of all breast cancers and more than 40% of breast cancers occurring in women under 30 are due to inheritance of an abnormal gene. The risk of ovarian and other cancers is also significantly increased in carriers of these susceptibility genes. A tumor suppressor gene termed *BRCA1* on chromosome 17 has been shown to be mutated in some families with early-onset breast and ovarian cancer. More than 100 mutations have been identified in the *BRCA1* gene, making identification of high-risk individuals difficult. Two population-based studies found that up to 20% of Jewish women with breast cancer at or before the age of 40 and approximately 10% of all women with breast cancer diagnosed before the age of 35 harbor mutations in the *BRCA1* gene. Inheritance of a mutated *BRCA1* gene confers a lifelong risk of approximately 85% for breast cancer and 50% for ovarian cancer. Inheritance of the *BRCA1* gene also appears to increase the risk of developing both colon and prostate cancers. Another susceptibility gene, *BRCA2*, has been associated with an increased risk for male breast cancer as well. There is clearly an association of phenotype and inheritance of susceptibility genes. For a woman diagnosed with breast cancer between the ages of 30 and 34 years, the likelihood of a *BRCA1* mutation is as high as 27% if her tumor is both hormone receptor-negative and of high grade. Carriers of *BRCA* mutations who have children appear to be at higher risk for developing breast cancer by age 40 than carriers who are nulliparous—in contrast to the usual risk factors for sporadic breast cancer. Interestingly— and despite the association of *BRCA1* with an increased risk of hormone receptor-negative breast tumors, recent data confirm that oophorectomy before the age of 40 significantly reduces the risk of breast cancer (up to 75%) and ovarian cancer in women who carry *BRCA1* or *BRCA2* mutations, presumably by decreasing exposure of breast tissue to estrogen. The use of oral contraceptives for more than 5 years appears to significantly reduce the risk of ovarian cancer in mutation carriers, perhaps by regulating ovarian cycling. Compared with sporadic ovarian cancers, those associated with the *BRCA1* mutation appeared to have a better clinical course, with a median survival of 77 months in women carrying the mutation compared with 29 months in controls. Many other less common genes have been identified that increase the risk of breast and other cancers, although clearly there are many yet to be identified. One recent study found that women who have an identical twin sister with breast cancer are at least three times more likely than average to develop cancer. If the twin was diagnosed before age 40, 25% of the remaining siblings developed cancer over the next 20 years. Increased risk in this setting is probably due to a combination of genes that will be more difficult to discern.

With the discovery and cloning of cancer susceptibility genes such as *BRCA1*, commercial testing has been developed for "screening" using linked genetic markers. Tests for genes linked to familial cancer have raised concerns about the impact of positive results on patients. One study has evaluated indications for testing of the *APC* gene. Of the patients tested, 85% were felt to have valid indications for testing. However, only 20% received genetic counseling before the test; only 15% gave informed consent; and in 30% of cases the clinicians misinterpreted the results. It is essential that clinicians recognize the limitations of these tests and that genetic testing be made available in the appropriate setting. Educational programs and publications are available to help educate patients regarding genetic testing. Many cancer centers now have genetic screening and counseling programs. Patients with a strong family history of cancer should be referred to such programs before testing is performed. Early and regular cancer screening is recommended for affected members of the family, and aggressive but relatively effective preventive measures such as prophylactic mastectomy and oophorectomy should also be discussed.

Other familial clusterings of cancer have been described that have not yet been associated with inheritance of a particular gene. Evaluation of participants in a study of colonic polyps revealed an increased risk of colorectal cancer in the siblings and parents of patients with adenomatous polyps, particularly when the adenoma was diagnosed before age 60 or (for a sibling) when a parent had colorectal cancer. This syndrome, referred to as a hereditary nonpolyposis colorectal cancer (HNPCC), has been associated with a germ line mutation of DNA mismatch-repair genes. At least 2% of patients with colorectal cancer had these mutations in one European cohort. Testing for replication errors should be considered in patients under age 50 with colorectal cancer who have a family history of colorectal or endometrial cancer. Family members of patients with this syndrome may benefit from early screening. In addition to the germ-line mutations found in HNPCC, up to 10–15% of sporadic colorectal cancers have somatic mutations in DNA repair genes resulting in microsatellite instability (MSI) or alterations in the size of repetitive nucleotide sequences. These cancers are usually in the right side of the colon and have been associated both with a better prognosis and a striking sensitivity to adjuvant chemotherapy. The HER-2/*neu* oncogene encodes a tyrosine kinase receptor in the epidermal growth factor receptor (EGFR) family and is overexpressed in about 20% of breast cancers; this phenotype is associated with more aggressive cancers, a worse prognosis, and enhanced tumor sensitivity to anthracycline chemotherapy. A recent study found that HER-2/*neu* overexpression in prostate cancer also correlated with a poorer 5-year prognosis, though this result must be validated. Identifying genetic factors that are associated with specific cancer phenotypes may allow effective tailoring of adjuvant chemotherapy.

It is difficult to link exposures to specific carcinogens with the development of cancer, since latency is long and the nature of exposure poorly documented. Environmental carcinogens include chemical carcinogens such as benzene and asbestos, oncogenic viruses such as the human papillomavirus and the Epstein-Barr virus, and physical agents such as ionizing radiation and ultraviolet light.

Certain viral infections may increase the risk of cancer and clearly have a pathogenetic role, such as the association between Epstein-Barr virus infection and endemic Burkitt's lymphoma and non-Hodgkin's lymphoma. Chronic infection with hepatitis B or C viruses increases the risk of hepatocellular carcinoma. Largely owing to the increase in chronic hepatitis, the incidence of hepatocellular carcinoma significantly increased during the 1990s compared with the 1970s. Interestingly, treatment with the antiviral agent interferon alfa following resection of hepatitis C-related hepatocellular carcinoma in a randomized trial appeared to significantly reduce the risk of cancer recurrence. Infection with HIV has been associated with non-Hodgkin's lymphoma, Hodgkin's disease, Kaposi's sarcoma, and cervical and anal cancers. The finding of human herpesvirus-8 (HHV-8) DNA sequences in both AIDS-associated and non-AIDS-associated Kaposi's sarcoma supports a possible causative role of the herpesviruses in the development of some cancers. It appears that HHV-8 is sexually transmitted among men. Antibodies to HHV-8 correlate with the subsequent development of Kaposi's sarcoma, supporting an etiologic role of HHV-8 in this malignancy. The sexually transmitted papillomavirus (HPV) is a major risk factor for the development of cervical carcinoma and anal cancer. The prognosis of cervical cancer is dependent on the oncogenic potential of the associated HPV type, with the worst prognosis associated with HPV18. Typing of the virus strain in each cancer may allow risk-adjusted treatment planning.

An additional cause of cancer is chemotherapy or radiation therapy for a prior malignancy. More aggressive chemotherapeutic and radiation regimens—and especially those combining the two treatment modalities—have been associated with increased rates of both secondary leukemias and solid tumors. The latency period may be short (2–5 years for leukemia) or very long (10–20 years for solid tumors), but the prognosis is uniformly poor. Chemotherapeutic agents known to cause secondary malignancies include alkylating agents (busulfan, cyclophosphamide, mechlorethamine, etc) and topoisomerase II inhibitors (the epipodophyllotoxins [etoposide], anthracyclines [doxorubicin, epirubicin], and anthracenediones [mitoxantrone]). Secondary leukemias are usually associated with chromosomal aberrations involving chromosomes 5 and 7 in alkylator-induced leukemias and myelodysplastic syndromes and the long arm of chromosome 11 (11q23) in epipodophyllotoxin-induced leukemias. Abnormalities of 11q23 involve a specific breakpoint region thought to be involved in DNA transcription. An increase in the rate of secondary acute leukemia has been reported in breast cancer patients treated with dose intensification of cyclophosphamide in combination with doxorubicin (a topoisomerase II active drug) from 1992 to 1994. The incidence is approximately 0.3% in a multicenter study involving over 2500 women with positive axillary nodes. Increased dosages and frequency of administration of anthracyclines, anthracenediones, and the alkylating agent cyclophosphamide have been reported to increase the risk of breast cancer to as high as 3–4%. Prolonged oral exposure to etoposide or alkylator agents can result in a much higher risk of secondary leukemia. Platinum-based chemotherapy for ovarian cancer has been reported to increase the risk of leukemia twofold to eightfold, with larger doses and longer treatment courses associated with higher risks. This risk was significantly higher in women who had also received intravenous melphalan. The risk of certain secondary cancers may be age-dependent. Radiation therapy for Hodgkin's disease increases the risk of breast cancer (including bilateral disease) if the radiation occurred in women under the age of 30. The relative risk of solid tumors and leukemias has been found to increase significantly with younger age at first chemotherapy treatment for Hodgkin's disease. This risk is especially high when chemotherapy and radiation are combined. Nevertheless, the risk of secondary malignancies in children surviving at least 5 years after diagnosis is relatively low at 3.2% 20 years post diagnosis, with the highest risk of mortality remaining primary disease recurrence. The Childhood Cancer Survivor Study (CCSS) is a large prospective study of over 14,000 survivors of childhood cancer designed to characterize the late effects of therapy in this increasing population.

Recent data indicate that the combination of estrogen and progesterone given as long-term hormonal replacement to postmenopausal women may significantly increase the risk of breast cancer over estrogen therapy alone. However, data from the American Cancer Society's Cancer Prevention Study II suggested that long-term estrogen replacement therapy was associated with a higher risk of death from ovarian cancer. Clearly, there is no increased risk associated with short-term (< 5 years) replacement, and cardiovascular and bone density benefits may outweigh these risks in the general population. Further prospective data will be needed to better assess these risks.

Aaltonen LA et al: Incidence of hereditary nonpolyposis colorectal cancer and the feasibility of molecular screening for the disease. N Engl J Med 1998;338:1481. [PMID: 9593786] (By molecular analysis, 2% of 500 patients with colorectal cancer were found to have this syndrome.)

Bremnes RM et al: High-throughput tissue microarray analysis used to evaluate biology and prognostic significance of the E-Cadherin pathway in non-small cell lung cancer. J Clin Oncol 2002;20:2417. [PMID: 12011119] (In this first study of high-throughput tissue microarray analysis for determining prognosis, reduced expression of the tumor adhesion molecules E-cad and catenins is associated with an increase in invasion and regional metastases and reduced survival in non-small cell lung cancer.)

Buys CH: Telomeres, telomerase, and cancer. N Engl J Med 2000;342:1282. [PMID: 10781627] (A brief but readable review of the role of telomerase in cancer and current research.)

Clemons M et al: Estrogen and the risk of breast cancer. N Engl J Med 2001;344:276. [PMID: 11172156] (An excellent review summarizing available data regarding exposure to endogenous and exogenous estrogens and the risk of breast cancer.)

Diller L et al: Breast cancer screening in women previously treated for Hodgkin's disease: a prospective cohort study. J Clin Oncol 2002;20:2085. [PMID: 11956269] (Radiation therapy for Hodgkin's disease clearly increases the risk of subsequent breast cancer; this has important implications for patient education, screening, and prevention.)

Dohner H et al: Genomic aberrations and survival in chronic lymphocytic leukemia. N Engl J Med 2000;343:1910. [PMID: 11136261] (Genetic mutations in chronic lymphocytic leukemia are important independent predictors of disease progression and survival.)

Edwards BK et al: Annual Report to the Nation on the Status of Cancer, 1973–1999, Featuring Implications of Age and Aging on the U.S. Cancer Burden. Cancer 2002;94:2766.

(Death rates for all cancers combined continue to decline in the United States, but the number of cases is expected to increase significantly as the population ages, with double the incidence in 50 years.)

Eng C et al: Genetic testing for cancer predisposition. Annu Rev Med 2001;52:371. [PMID: 11160785] (A review of syndromes identifiable by genetic testing as well as situations in which the results of testing affect medical management.)

Gree DR et al: Evan GI: A matter of life and death. Cancer Cell 2002;1:19. (An understandable review of proliferative and apoptotic pathways that play a role in tumor cell growth and survival.)

Lichtenstein P et al: Environmental and heritable factors in the causation of cancer. N Engl J Med 2000;343:78. [PMID: 10891514] (Inherited genetic factors appear to make a minor contribution to susceptibility to most types of cancers in this registry study of over 44,000 pairs of twins in Sweden, Denmark, and Finland.)

Lombard I et al: Human papillomavirus genotype as a major determinant of the course of cervical cancer. J Clin Oncol 1998;16:2613. [PMID: 8704710] (Invasive cervical cancer with HPV18 or HPV16 sequences has a significantly poorer prognosis than does cancer associated with other HPV sequences.)

Schairer C et al: Menopausal estrogen and estrogen-progestin replacement therapy and breast cancer. JAMA 2000;283:485. [PMID: 10659874] (Data from the Breast Cancer Detection Demonstration Project, a cohort study from 1980 to 1995, suggests that estrogen-progestin increases breast cancer risk over that associated with estrogen alone.)

Soussi T: The p53 tumor suppressor gene: from molecular biology to clinical investigation. Ann N Y Acad Sci 2000;910:121. [PMID: 10911910] (A review of the biology of p53 including pathophysiology, prevalence, and impact on prognosis.)

Statement of the American Society of Clinical Oncology: genetic testing for cancer susceptibility. Adopted on February 20, 1996. J Clin Oncol 1996;14:1730. [PMID: 8622094] (Recommendations for screening.)

Watanabe T et al: Molecular predictors of survival after adjuvant chemotherapy for colon cancer. N Engl J Med 2001;344:1196. [PMID: 11309634] (In patients with locally advanced colon cancer, retention of the long arm of chromosome 18 and microsatellite instability in the presence of a mutated gene for the type II receptor for TGF-β1 predicts a favorable outcome following adjuvant chemotherapy.)

■ PREVENTION OF CANCER

PRIMARY PREVENTION

1. Lifestyle Modifications

Population studies suggest that lifestyle—including tobacco use, diet, and alcohol consumption—accounts for a majority of avoidable cancer deaths in the United States. Other factors, including obesity, parity, and length of lactation, have also been associated with increased cancer risk. Although prostate and breast cancers are the most common malignancies in men and women, respectively, the most common cause of cancer death in both sexes is still lung cancer. Since 1973, there has been only a 10% increase in the incidence of lung cancer in men compared with a 124% increase in women, reflecting a marked increase in the number of women who smoke. Since tobacco-related cancers account for at least 29% of all fatal forms of cancer, smoking cessation is an important area for continued education and prevention efforts. Strategies for helping patients stop smoking are described in Chapter 1. Programs directed both at cessation of smoking and at reversing the social acceptability of cigarette smoking have been more successful than programs encouraging cessation alone. In California and Massachusetts, increasing the excise tax on cigarettes combined with an antismoking campaign resulted in a substantial decrease in the prevalence of adult smoking. In California, this program was responsible for halving of the per capita consumption of cigarettes and translated into a significant decline (almost five times greater than the rest of the United States) in the incidence of lung cancer in both men and women in the state from 1988 to 1997. The decline in women is even more striking when compared with the rest of the United States, where the rate of lung cancer in women is still increasing. The molecular targets for carcinogens such as alcohol and tobacco have not yet been identified. However, an evaluation of tumor samples from over 100 patients with squamous cell carcinoma of the head and neck associated cigarette smoking with genetic mutations in the P53 gene, thought to result in the initiation or progression of this cancer. This supports the epidemiologic evidence that abstinence from smoking is important in preventing head and neck cancer. Cigarette smoking has been linked to cancers of the lung, mouth, pharynx, esophagus, pancreas, kidney, and bladder. In addition, a recent study by the American Cancer Society found a 30–40% increase in the risk of death from colorectal cancer in cigarette smokers, with the increased risk occurring after 20 years of smoking and increasing with the number of cigarettes smoked daily. The risk decreased each year after quitting smoking, indicating that change in this major lifestyle factor can still reduce risk of death from cancer. In addition, a recent study showed that patients who stopped smoking following a diagnosis of small cell lung cancer treated with chemotherapy and radiation had significantly longer 2-year and 5-year survivals than those who continued smoking. A similar prolongation in survival occurs in patients with head and neck cancer who quit smoking following diagnosis. This suggests that ongoing toxicity even in patients already diagnosed with cancer contributes to mortality. However, up to 50% of all lung cancers occur in those who have stopped smoking for at least 1 year, indicating that the carcinogenic effect of cigarette smoking is slow to reverse.

Diet is an important area of intervention for primary cancer prevention. Epidemiologic studies suggest an inverse relationship between fruit and vegetable intake and the risk of common carcinomas, indicating a potential protective role of these dietary components.

A recent case-control study in South Asia found a small reduction in the risk of breast cancer associated with a diet rich in vegetables. High intakes of fat and specific fatty acids have been postulated to increase the risk of breast, colon, prostate, and lung cancer. Linoleic acids in essential fatty acids are the food source for arachidonic acid—and this metabolic pathway has been postulated to play an important role in the development of cancer. However, the Nurses' Health Study, which followed more than 88,000 women for 14 years with food frequency questionnaires every 4 years beginning in 1980, found no evidence that a lower intake of total fat or specific major types of fat decreased the risk of breast cancer. Data from the Nurse's Health Study and other epidemiologic studies suggest that a high consumption of red meat and excess alcohol consumption (probably also in combination with a diet low in possible preventive vitamins such as folate) may increase the risk of colorectal cancer. A meta-analysis published in 1999 evaluated dietary fat intervention studies (published from 1966 through 1998) on serum estradiol levels and fat consumption. These findings did not rule out the possibility that reducing fat consumption below 20% of calories might reduce breast cancer risk by lowering serum estradiol levels. Another study compared the dietary intake of saturated fat of 1665 men with prostate cancer to the diet of an equal number of men without the disease. A high intake of saturated fat increased the risk of prostate cancer in all four major ethnic groups evaluated. There was no increase in prostate cancer among men with the lowest intake of saturated fats. Obesity or a high body mass index has been implicated as a risk factor for breast, colorectal, and lung cancers (in nonsmokers) as well as others. A recent study found that a higher BMI and elevated blood pressure independently increased the risk of renal cell cancer in men. Dietary factors may further increase risk in already high-risk populations. A high intake of saturated fat in 27,111 smokers participating in the Alpha-Tocopherol, Beta-Carotene Cancer Prevention study significantly increased the risk of developing pancreatic cancer, suggesting that diet may be a modifiable factor in the prevention of pancreatic cancer in this population.

A high intake of dietary fiber has long been thought to reduce the risk of colorectal cancer and adenomas. The Nurses' Health Study investigated the intake of dietary fiber in the same population specified above, and no association was found between the intake of dietary fiber and the risk of colorectal cancer or adenomas. A prospective study of over 10,000 men likewise did not find a significant association between fiber intake and the risk of developing adenomas. Two prospective, randomized trials tested the value of a high-fiber, low-fat diet or a high-fiber cereal supplement versus a standard diet in reducing the risk of recurrent colorectal adenomas in men and women with a recent prior diagnosis of adenoma and demonstrated no difference in the risk of recurrent adenoma based on dietary regimens. Other dietary factors such as folate, methionine, and vitamin D may reduce the risk of colorectal malignancy, but this too will require further investigation.

The Women's Health Initiative, begun in 1992, is examining the effects of three distinct interventions: a low-fat eating pattern, hormone replacement therapy, and calcium and vitamin D supplementation on the prevention of cancer, cardiovascular disease, and osteoporosis in 64,500 postmenopausal women of all races. An additional 100,000 women will be enrolled in an observational study. This study will be completed in the year 2007. Other ongoing intervention trials include the Women's Healthy Eating and Living (WHEL) study, which targets women 1–3 years following a diagnosis of breast cancer to assess the affects of a low-fat, high-fiber diet on recurrence and death from cancer.

Given the general lack of specific information linking diet to the risk of cancer, what should we recommend to patients right now? A diet low in saturated fat and rich in whole grains, fruits, and vegetables appears to improve health in a variety of ways—certainly in reducing cardiovascular disease and diabetes and, based on epidemiologic data, reducing the overall risk of cancer. Similarly, weight loss appears to be a prudent recommendation. For more specific diets—in particular, reducing the risk of recurrence of a known cancer or precancer—we will have to wait for more data.

Another lifestyle factor with important implications for primary prevention is exposure to ultraviolet light. Chronic cumulative exposure to solar ultraviolet radiation is the major risk factor for nonmelanomatous skin cancer. Regular use of sunscreen prevents the development of precancerous solar keratoses and results in regression of existing keratoses, although the effect of sunscreens on the incidence of melanoma is not clear. Protection from sunlight and the regular use of sunscreens should be recommended for the primary prevention of skin cancers.

Alberts DS et al: Lack of effect of a high-fiber cereal supplement on the recurrence of colorectal adenomas. N Engl J Med 2000;342:1156. [PMID: 10770980] (A dietary supplement of wheat-bran fiber does not protect against recurrent colorectal adenomas.)

Chow WH et al: Obesity, hypertension, and the risk of kidney cancer in men. N Engl J Med 2000;343:1305. [PMID: 11058675] (A retrospective review of the health records of over 350,000 Swedish men found that a higher body mass index and hypertension were independent risk factors for kidney cancer.)

Holmes MD et al: Association of dietary intake of fat and fatty acids with risk of breast cancer. JAMA 1999;281:914. [PMID: 10078488] (Fat ingestion assessed by periodic dietary questionnaire did not contribute to the risk of breast cancer over a 14 year period.)

Hughes JR: New treatments for smoking cessation. CA Cancer J Clin 2000;50:143. [PMID: 10901738] (A summary of interventions, including physician encouragement and pharmacologic treatment to help patients kick the smoking habit.)

Kup H et al: Tobacco use, cancer causation and public health impact. J Intern Med 2002;251:455. [PMID: 12028500] (Mechanisms of tobacco-induced carcinogenesis and interaction with other factors such as genes, diet, and environmental exposure.)

Schatzkin A et al: Lack of effect of a low-fat, high-fiber diet on the recurrence of colorectal adenomas. N Engl J Med 2000;342:1149. [PMID: 10770979] (A diet low in fat and high in fiber, fruit, and vegetables does not influence the risk of recurrent colorectal adenomas.)

The Women's Health Initiative Study Group: Design of the Women's Health Initiative clinical trial and observational study. Control Clin Trials 1998;19:61. [PMID: 9492970] (A discussion of the design and endpoints of this ongoing important trial scheduled to be completed in 2007.)

2. Chemoprevention

Chemoprevention focuses on the prevention of cancer by administering chemical compounds that interfere with the multistaged carcinogenic process. Better understanding of the biochemical and molecular mechanisms of carcinogenesis has made possible the identification of potential chemopreventive agents. Four risk groups have been identified for intervention: (1) previous cancer patients (to prevent second malignancies), (2) patients with preneoplastic lesions, (3) patients at high risk for malignancy (family history, lifestyle, occupation), and (4) the general population.

Chemicals used in chemoprevention must be nontoxic and well tolerated by otherwise asymptomatic individuals. Because of the long natural history of carcinogenesis, there must also be a method of evaluating the efficacy of chemopreventive agents other than waiting for the development of tumors. Biomarkers, including the premalignant markers such as leukoplakia, colonic polyps, and aberrant crypt formation in the colon, are currently in clinical use. Other less specific surrogate markers for cancer risk such as breast density are also in use as primary end points in prevention studies. Molecular susceptibility markers may become useful; nuclear retinoic acid receptor agonists are under investigation in chemoprevention studies of patients with head and neck cancer.

Retinoids, the natural derivatives and synthetic analogs of vitamin A, are the best-studied chemopreventive agents. NSAIDs—specifically, the selective COX-2 inhibitors—and hormonal agents such as tamoxifen, raloxifene, and finasteride appear to have an important role in prevention of some cancers. Numerous additional investigations include the role of specific dietary components such as vitamins. Ongoing research in this area is assessing the impact and appropriate use of selective NSAIDs, vitamins, and hormonal agents in cancer prevention.

Isotretinoin & Acyclic Retinoids

Retinoids are modulators of epithelial cell differentiation both in vivo and in vitro that are thought to act on nuclear receptors to regulate both cellular growth and differentiation and cell apoptosis.

Isotretinoin has been shown to suppress leukoplakia, a premalignant lesion of the aerodigestive tract. Effectiveness and tolerability of low doses of isotretinoin have been demonstrated. In a randomized maintenance trial, only patients with a demonstrated response to high-dose induction (1.5 mg/kg/d) were placed on low-dose maintenance therapy (0.5 mg/kg/d). The disease progression rate was only 8% compared with a rate of 55% in a separate group taking beta-carotene.

High doses of isotretinoin may prevent the development of second primary tumors in patients with early squamous cell carcinoma of the head and neck. An initial phase III study showed a statistically significant reduction in the incidence of new aerodigestive cancers when isotretinoin versus placebo was given for 1 year following definitive local therapy (4% versus 24%). There were no significant differences in disease recurrence or survival at a median follow-up of 55 months, and 30–40% of patients required reduced dosages or discontinued therapy due to toxicity. A second randomized study using lower doses of a different and probably less active retinoid showed no differences in the incidence of second primary tumors. Based on these preliminary results, three large randomized trials were performed to assess the preventive effects of retinoids on second primary tumors. One trial (Euroscan) studied 2 years of treatment with retinyl palmitate and acetylcysteine in over 2500 patients with either lung cancer or head and neck cancer. No differences were found in the incidence of second primary tumors. A United States intergroup trial studied the use of isotretinoin to prevent second primary tumors following definitive therapy of stage I non-small cell lung cancer. Because of side effects seen with the higher (50- to 100-mg) dose, the drug was given at a dosage of 30 mg/d for 3 years. After a median follow-up of 3.5 years, there was no difference in time to second primary tumor, recurrence, or mortality. Subset analysis suggested that never-smokers might benefit from isotretinoin, whereas there was a higher risk of cancer recurrence and mortality in smokers in the isotretinoin arm. The major toxicity at higher doses includes skin dryness, cheilitis, hypertriglyceridemia, and conjunctivitis. These toxicities require dose reduction or temporary discontinuation of the drug. The third double-blind randomized study investigated the effect of low-dose isotretinoin for 3 years in the prevention of second primary tumors in patients definitively treated for stage I or stage II head and neck cancer. This trial is scheduled to be unblinded and analyzed in late 2002. To date, there has been a significantly higher rate of second primary tumor formation in smokers versus former smokers or never smokers—prospectively proving the impact of active smoking in second primary tumor development. An interesting recent report suggests that nicotine may suppress the antigrowth effects of retinoids in lung cancer cells.

Retinoids have been synthesized that may be more potent chemopreventive agents with less side effects.

The acyclic retinoid polyprenoic acid inhibits chemically induced hepatocarcinogenesis in rats and spontaneous hepatomas in mice. In patients with hepatocellular carcinoma, the rate of recurrent and second primary tumors is high despite curative therapy with surgical resection and ethanol injection therapy. In one study, 89 patients who were free of disease after either method of treatment were randomized to receive either 600 mg/d of polyprenoic acid or placebo for 12 months. After a median follow-up of 38 months, 27% of patients in the polyprenoic acid group versus 49% of the patients in the placebo group had recurrent or new hepatocellular carcinomas, a result which was statistically significant. The difference was even greater in the groups that had secondary hepatomas. Longer follow-up has also shown a survival advantage. At a median of 62 months of follow-up, 75% of the treatment group versus 45% of the placebo group are alive. Toxicity was quite modest (headache, nausea), with none of the side effects usually described with isotretinoin. Three strategies that have been proved to prevent liver carcinogenesis are vaccination against hepatitis B, treatment of chronic active hepatitis C with interferon, and deletion of premalignant and latent malignant cells in the remnant livers of patients undergoing complete resection of hepatocellular carcinomas. The retinamide fenretinide (4-HPR) is a potent apoptosis-inducing synthetic vitamin A analog with significant in vitro activity. Fenretinide appears to reduce the activity of telomerase, which is important in lung carcinogenesis. Expression of telomerase reverse transcriptase (TERT), the catalytic subunit of telomerase, was evaluated on bronchial biopsies in 57 heavy smokers before and after 6 months of treatment with fenretinide or placebo. A 25% reduction in expression of TERT was found in the fenretinide-treated patients. Although clinical follow-up is clearly critical, the hope is that this type of surrogate marker will improve our ability to assess the effectiveness of possible chemopreventive agents and perhaps also identify patients at higher risk for cancer development. A large randomized trial evaluated the effect of fenretinide versus placebo for 5 years to prevent contralateral breast cancer in women aged 30–70 years with a history of resected breast cancer and no other adjuvant therapy. Although no overall effect was observed, subset analysis found a reduction in contralateral and ipsilateral breast cancer rates in premenopausal women. Fenretinide is being studied in randomized trials as a chemopreventive agent in patients with superficial bladder cancer and in women at increased risk for ovarian cancer. Newer and more potent retinoids are being developed and tested in a variety of cancers.

Aspirin & Other NSAIDs

Aspirin and other NSAIDs inhibit tumor growth in experimental systems. Prostaglandin inhibitors reduce the size and number of colon tumors in rats induced by chemicals or radiation by inhibiting cyclooxygenase activity in the arachidonic acid pathway (COX-1 and COX-2). Regular aspirin administration at low doses (16 or more doses of 325 mg per month for at least 1 year) may reduce the risk of fatal colon cancer by as much as 40–50%. Low-dose aspirin may also protect against cancers of the esophagus, stomach, and rectum.

A study evaluating the use of sulindac versus placebo in patients with familial adenomatous polyposis showed reduction of both the number and the size of colorectal adenomas. The effect was incomplete, without complete regression of all polyps in any patient. After the sulindac was discontinued, both polyp size and polyp number increased. A large prospective cohort study was subsequently published evaluating aspirin use and the risk for both colorectal cancer and adenoma in 48,000 male health professionals over a 4-year period. The subsequent risk of developing colorectal cancer and adenomas was lower in men reporting regular use of aspirin (more than twice a week) on the study entry questionnaire even when multiple other variables were taken into account. In the Nurse's Health Study, 90,000 women were evaluated for the risk of colorectal cancer over a 12-year period according to the number of consecutive years of regular aspirin use (two or more 325 mg tablets per week) reported on three consecutive questionnaires. There was a statistically significant decrease in the risk of colorectal cancer after 20 years of consistent aspirin use, with the maximal reduction seen in women who took four to six tablets per week. A slight reduction in risk was seen in women who took aspirin for 10–19 years as well. Known risk factors such as diet did not influence this risk reduction. The Physicians Health Study is the only randomized prospective trial of aspirin (325 mg every other day for 5 years) versus placebo. At the end of the trial, no differences were seen in the frequency of self-reported new colorectal cancers.

The selective COX-2 enzyme inhibitors are the subject of intense research in the area of prevention and treatment of cancer. COX-2 expression is inducible, unlike the constitutive expression of COX-1, and COX-2 up-regulation occurs in most epithelial tumors, including colorectal cancer and cancers of the lung and breast. This up-regulation is thought to be secondary to other initiating events, such as oncogene activation or mutation of a tumor suppressor gene. COX-2 levels increase throughout oncogenesis, and expression appears to promote angiogenesis (new blood vessel growth) and decrease apoptosis (programmed cell death). The COX-2 inhibitors are less toxic and more specific and therefore suitable as chemopreventive agents. One selective COX-2 inhibitor, celecoxib, has been shown to induce regression of polyps in patients with familial adenomatous polyposis at a dosage of 400 mg twice a day for 6 months. Based on these data, celecoxib was approved by the FDA for chemoprevention of polyps in patients with familial adenomatous polyposis. The major side effect of high-dose celecoxib is gastrointestinal bleeding. Celecoxib should not be used for routine chemoprevention of sporadic colorectal cancers. A broad range of cancer prevention studies using COX-2 inhibitors are ongoing through the National Cancer Institute. In addition, because there are in vitro data suggesting antitumor activity of NSAIDs such as antiangiogenic effects, induction of apoptosis, and reduction of proliferation, COX-2 inhibitors are being studied as part of combination therapy of advanced cancers.

Beta-Carotene & Vitamin E

The carotenoids are plant pigments that protect plant cells from damage and were thought to have an antioxidant role in human tissues. Beta-carotene is a carotenoid found in high concentrations in human tissues; its importance as an antioxidant is controversial. A role for beta-carotene and another antioxidant, vitamin E, in the prevention of either premalignant or malignant disease has not been established.

Several randomized studies have evaluated the effect of beta-carotene and vitamin E on the prevention of cancer in high-risk populations. The Alpha-Tocopherol, Beta Carotene (ATBC) Cancer Prevention Study randomized 29,000 Finnish male smokers to receive beta-carotene, vitamin E, both agents, or neither agent for an average of 6 years. A minimal (2%) and statistically insignificant reduction in the incidence of lung cancer was seen in the men who received vitamin E. In contrast, there was a statistically significant 18% higher incidence of lung cancer in the group taking beta-carotene. Vitamin E supplementation reduced prostate cancer incidence by 34% and colorectal cancer by 16%, though only the reduction in prostate cancer incidence was statistically significant. Men in the control group with higher levels of vitamin E or beta-carotene before the study was initiated developed fewer lung cancers, suggesting that other components of foods high in these vitamins may be responsible for the protective effects noted in epidemiologic studies.

The Beta-Carotene and Retinol Efficacy Trial (CARET), a lung cancer chemoprevention study targeting high-risk populations, randomized a total of 18,000 smokers, nonsmokers, and workers with extensive occupational exposure to asbestos to receive either a combination of 30 mg/d of beta-carotene (as an antioxidant) and 25,000 IU/d of retinol (vitamin A—as a tumor suppressor) or placebo. With an average of 4 years and 73,000 person-years of follow-up, the combination of beta-carotene and vitamin A had no benefit on the incidence of lung cancer. In fact, the active treatment group had a 28% higher incidence of lung cancer than the placebo group, and the mortality from all causes and the rate of death from cardiovascular disease were higher by 17% and 26%, respectively. On the basis of these results, this study was stopped early.

The Physician's Health Study randomized 22,000 United States male physicians to receive beta-carotene (50 mg on alternate days) or placebo. The physicians were treated for an average of 12 years; 11% were current smokers and 39% were former smokers at the beginning of the study. In this trial, no evidence either of benefit or of increased risk for cancer was found, with a much longer follow-up than either of the two other studies. There were no differences in the overall incidence of malignant neoplasms, cardiovascular disease, or overall mortality in the group as a whole or in the smokers. One additional randomized study in which a positive effect of beta-carotene supplementation was found evaluated a poorly nourished population group rather than the well-nourished populations described above. Linxian, China, is an area with one of the world's highest rates of esophageal and stomach cancer and a habitually low intake of several nutrients. In nearly 30,000 participants from the general population, the mortality rates from cancer were substantially lower among those who received daily supplementation with a combination of beta-carotene, alpha-tocopherol, and selenium over a 5-year period. A marked reduction in the cancer death rate (13%) was observed in the supplemented group, largely due to a 21% decrease in stomach cancer mortality. Over 85% of cancers arose in the esophagus or stomach, but 31 deaths were caused by lung cancer. The risk of death from lung cancer was reduced by 45% among those receiving supplements, though the numbers were very small (11 versus 20 lung cancer deaths), and only 30% were cigarette smokers. A second study evaluated the effect of supplements, including beta-carotene, on prevention of esophageal and gastric cancers in over 3300 people with esophageal dysplasia. Although esophageal cancer mortality and total cancer mortality were not significantly lower in the supplemented group, the incidence of mortality due to stomach cancer was higher. On repeat endoscopy comparing results 2 and 6 years after randomization, dysplasia had resolved in about two-thirds of patients in both arms at 6 years. These findings underscore the need for placebo-controlled trials in the area of cancer prevention. The NCI is currently collaborating with agencies in China to pursue further chemoprevention studies in this unique population.

In summary, there is no evidence to support the use of beta-carotene in the primary prevention of cancer in well-nourished populations. The major criticism of the large studies conducted to date is that increasing one type of vitamin—even one stereoisomer of a vitamin—does not reflect the vitamin content of a diet high in vegetables. In addition, intake of beta-carotene is a marker of increased fruit and vegetable consumption. The balanced mixture of antioxidants found in a diet rich in fruit and vegetables may be more important and more effective in reducing cancer risk than beta-carotene supplementation. Other micronutrients such as vitamin E may prove more promising.

The Women's Health Study, begun in 1992, is a randomized, double-blind, placebo-controlled trial testing the risks and benefits of vitamin E, beta-carotene, and aspirin in the primary prevention of cancer and cardiovascular disease in 40,000 healthy female health professionals in the USA. Results are expected in 2003.

Calcium & Selenium

Dietary patterns continue to be associated with a risk of colorectal neoplasia. The changes in risk may be contributed to by alterations in bile acids. Calcium appears to bind bile acids in the bowel lumen, inhibiting bile-induced mucosal damage and perhaps carcinogenesis. A modest reduction in the incidence of adenomas in patients taking calcium supplementation has been shown in patients receiving it over a 4-year period. The Selenium and Vitamin E Cancer Prevention Trial (SELECT) is the largest chemoprevention study ever to be undertaken and began in July of 2001. This NCI-sponsored trial will randomize 32,400 men age 50–55 and older to selenium, vitamin E, both, or placebo for 7–12 years. This study is based on the results of the Alpha-Tocopherol Beta-Carotene Cancer Prevention Study, in which vitamin E reduced prostate cancer incidence by 32%, and the selenium and skin cancer trial, in which selenium reduced the incidence of prostate cancer by 63%. Vitamin D induces bile acid breakdown in vitro and may have a role in protection against colon cancer. This effect will need in vivo evaluation.

Tamoxifen

Tamoxifen is a selective estrogen receptor modulator (SERM) with both antiestrogen and proestrogen activity that has an important role in the treatment of both early and advanced breast cancer. Studies of women taking tamoxifen as adjuvant therapy for unilateral breast cancer have shown a 30–40% reduction in the risk of developing a second primary in the opposite breast. The Breast Cancer Prevention Trial (BCPT) is a nationwide trial that randomized 13,400 women at high risk for breast cancer to receive either tamoxifen (20 mg/d) or placebo for 5 years. The trial was stopped at a median follow-up of 4 years due to a striking 50% reduction in the risk of breast cancer in the women taking tamoxifen—89 women taking tamoxifen developed breast cancer, compared with 175 taking placebo. This benefit was restricted solely to the development of estrogen-receptor-positive cancers. In addition to invasive cancer, there was a similar reduction in the risk of noninvasive breast cancer such as ductal or lobular carcinoma in situ. Tamoxifen also decreased the number of bone fractures. Two much smaller European studies that used different parameters to determine risk (and study eligibility) did not show a significant reduction in cancers with the use of tamoxifen. Side effects of tamoxifen include an age-dependent small increase in the risk of endometrial cancer, deep vein thrombosis, and pulmonary embolism. This effect is seen primarily in women over age 50.

The use of tamoxifen for primary prevention of cancer is controversial because of its known secondary effects, primarily the increase in endometrial cancer. This risk is small when compared with the incidence of breast cancer in younger women on placebo in the trial. Even if the incidences of endometrial cancer and breast cancer are considered together, there was still a 30% reduction in the risk of cancer in the women receiving tamoxifen.

Raloxifene

Early results of the MORE (Multiple Outcomes of Raloxifene Evaluation) trial have provided more information regarding prevention of breast cancer. Raloxifene is a novel SERM with estrogenic effects on bone and lipids and estrogen antagonist effects on the breast and uterus. Two different doses of raloxifene or placebo were administered to 7700 postmenopausal women to test the hypothesis that raloxifene would reduce the risk of bone fractures. After 2½ years, a 70% reduction in the risk of breast cancer was found in the women taking raloxifene compared to the women taking placebo. A suggestion of decreased risk of endometrial cancer was also found. The long-term safety and follow-up of raloxifene in these women is ongoing. The effects of raloxifene in women with breast cancer or in women at high risk for developing breast cancer has not been evaluated (see below).

Ongoing Trials in Breast Cancer

The Study of Tamoxifen and Raloxifene (STAR) started in 1999 with a goal of randomizing 22,000 American and Canadian postmenopausal women (age 35 or older) at increased risk of breast cancer to either daily tamoxifen (20 mg/d) or raloxifene (60 mg/d) for 5 years. As of October 2001, 11,307 women had been randomized. This study should answer the question of whether raloxifene is as effective as tamoxifen at reducing the chance of breast cancer—with additional benefits such as fewer side effects. Additional information regarding the STAR trial and eligibility criteria as well as other studies on breast cancer can be found at the NCI clinical trials Web site (http://www.cancertrials.nci.gov) or by calling 800-4-CANCER.

A new class of hormonal agents are now in early clinical trials for primary prevention. The aromatase inhibitors block the peripheral conversion of androstenedione and testosterone to estradiol in menopausal women and are effective in the treatment of metastatic breast cancer. Preliminary data from a large randomized trial (Arimadex and Tamoxifen Alone or in Combination; ATAC) comparing tamoxifen alone with anastrazole alone and with the combination of the two agents as adjuvant therapy for early-stage breast cancer have documented a small but significant reduction from the use of anastrazole alone, particularly in the incidence of second primary cancers of the breast. The combination arm was no better than tamoxifen.

The aromatase inhibitors do not appear to cause either an increased risk of thrombosis or endometrial cancer, making them much more suitable agents for prevention in a healthy population. Further follow-up and results from ongoing prevention trials will be needed to understand the impact of aromatase inhibitors in this area.

Finasteride

Finasteride is a 5α-reductase inhibitor used to treat benign prostatic hyperplasia. This agent inhibits the enzyme responsible for converting testosterone to 5α-dihydrotestosterone, suppressing prostate cell and organ growth. In rats, finasteride prevented macroscopic but not microscopic prostate carcinogenesis—supporting the use of this agent in the prevention of conversion of latent prostate carcinoma to life-threatening disease. The Prostate Cancer Prevention Trial (PCPT) is evaluating the use of finasteride to prevent the development of prostate cancer in men with normal digital rectal examinations and prostate-specific antigen (PSA) concentrations. Eighteen thousand men aged 50 or older have been randomized in this 7-year study to receive either finasteride or placebo. Results are expected in 2004.

Other Current Trials

Additional trials are under way investigating the effect of both diet and pharmacologic agents in the prevention of cancer. These include studies of soy isoflavones, folic acid, dietary fat and fish oils, vitamin supplementation, and others. Dietary agents such as polyprenols in green tea are thought to play a role in chemoprevention and are under investigation. There is great interest in moving the new biologic therapies that target specific pathways important in carcinogenesis into the prevention setting. These include farnesyl transferase inhibitors and agents that block the epidermal growth factor receptor (EGFR).

Further information about ongoing chemoprevention trials can be obtained from the Chemoprevention Branch of the National Cancer Institute (301-496-8563).

Baron JA et al: Calcium supplements for the prevention of colorectal adenomas. N Engl J Med 1999;340:101. [PMID: 9887161] (Calcium supplementation is associated with a moderate reduction in the risk of recurrent colorectal adenomas.)

Brawley OW et al: The future of prostate cancer prevention. Ann N Y Acad Sci 2001;952:145. [PMID: 11795434] (A review of the rationale and design of ongoing chemoprevention trials.)

Chlebowski RT et al: Reducing the risk of breast cancer. N Engl J Med 2000;343:191. [PMID: 10900280] (A review of clinical trials evaluating SERMs as well as surgery for prevention of breast cancer.)

Fisher G et al: Tamoxifen for the prevention of breast cancer: report of the National Surgical Adjuvant Breast and Bowel Project P-1 Study. J Natl Cancer Inst 1998;90:1371. [PMID: 9747868] (Results of the United States primary prevention trial.)

Janne PA et al: Chemoprevention of colorectal cancer. N Engl J Med 2000;342:1960. [PMID: 10874065] (An excellent review of the pathophysiology, clinical data, and directions for future research in this important area.)

Khuri FR et al: The impact of smoking status, disease stage, and index tumor site on second primary tumor incidence and tumor recurrence in the head and neck retinoid chemoprevention trial. Cancer Epidemiol Biomarkers Prev 2001;10:823. [PMID: 11489748] (Patients who continue to smoke and those with a higher stage at presentation have a higher incidence of second primary tumors.)

Kurie JM: The biologic basis of the use of retinoids in cancer prevention and treatment. Curr Opin Oncol 1999;11:497. [PMID: 10550014] (A summary of prevention and treatment trials as well as background on the molecular basis of using retinoids for cancer prevention.)

Prevention of cancer in the next millennium: Report of the chemoprevention working group to the American Association for Cancer Research. Cancer Res 1999;59:4743. [PMID: 10519777] (A review of existing trials and evidence supporting chemoprevention.)

Steinbach G et al: The effect of celecoxib, a cyclooxygenase-2 inhibitor, in familial adenomatous polyposis. N Engl J Med 2000;342:1946. [PMID: 10874062] (Celecoxib 400 mg twice daily for 6 months reduces the number of colorectal polyps in people with familial adenomatous polyposis.)

Sturmer T et al: Aspirin use and colorectal cancer: post-trial follow-up data from the Physicians' Health Study. Ann Intern Med 1998;128:713. [PMID: 9556464]

SECONDARY PREVENTION (Early Detection)

Given the inadequacy of current knowledge concerning the causes of cancer, effective prevention can be achieved for only a minority of malignancies. Other than primary prevention and perhaps chemoprevention, the most effective clinician intervention is early diagnosis. Screening is used for early detection of cancer in otherwise asymptomatic populations. Detection of cancer may be achieved through observation (eg, skin, mouth, external genitalia, cervix), palpation (eg, breast, mouth, thyroid, rectum and anus, prostate, testes, ovaries and uterus, lymph nodes), and laboratory tests and procedures (eg, Papanicolaou smear, sigmoidoscopy or colonoscopy, mammography). Effective screening requires that a test will specifically detect early cancers or premalignancies, be cost-effective, and result in improved therapeutic outcomes. For most cancers, stage at presentation is related to curability, with the highest cure rates reported when the tumor is small and there is no evidence of metastasis. However, for some tumors (eg, lung or ovarian cancer), distant metastases tend to occur early, even from a small primary. More sensitive detection methods such as tumor markers are being developed for many forms of cancer, and some tumor markers, such as PSA, are already a regular (though controversial) part of routine cancer screening (see section on tumor markers). Screening is not useful if no method of early detection exists (eg, cancer of the pancreas) or if there is no apparent localized stage (eg, leukemia).

Cancers for which screening or early detection has led to an improvement in outcome include cancers of the breast, cervix, colon, prostate, oral cavity, and skin. Techniques for early detection for breast cancer include self-examination, clinical examination, and mammography. The benefits of screening mammography have been reviewed in two large recent meta-analyses—these results are highly controversial based on a number of factors. First, several of the large published studies evaluating the value of mammography have serious flaws. Second, mammography increases the detection of the preinvasive lesion ductal carcinoma in situ (DCIS), which has an extremely low 10-year mortality. Lastly, available data suggest that the most significant reduction in mortality obtained from mammographic screening may be in women over the age of 60 (24–33% reduction), with smaller benefits in younger women. The Agency for Healthcare Research and Quality (AHRQ) conducted its own review of the meta-analysis and rated the included studies based on the quality of data and the inclusion of younger age groups as well as other factors. They concluded that there is a demonstrated 20% reduction in the number of breast cancer deaths in women undergoing screening mammography both in the over-50 and under-50 age groups, though the times required in follow-up to see these benefits may be quite different. The AHRQ along with the ACS and the NCI—recently put forth the following recommendations for mammographic screening: Every 1–2 years for women between the ages of 40 and 59, then annually in women 50 years and older. The upper age limit for mammographic screening has not been established.

Both mammography and clinical examination of the breast are associated with a significant number of false-positive results, leading to further testing. Screening mammograms and clinical breast examinations in 2400 women over a 10-year period found that 24% and 13% (respectively) of women had at least one false-positive mammogram or false-positive clinical examination.

In conclusion, the controversy regarding mammographic screening is far from resolved; however, it is the best screening method currently available. Women between the ages of 40 and 49 should be active participants in decisions regarding screening and should have an understanding of known risks and benefits. Despite the sensitivity of mammography, between 15% and 25% of breast cancers are not visible by this radiographic technique; this is particularly true for young women with dense breasts. All clinically suspicious lesions should be biopsied regardless of a negative mammogram. Digital mammography is a newer technique that uses computers and special detectors to produce a digital image displayed on high-resolution monitors. The NCI launched a trial in October 2001 that will include 49,500 women in the United States and Canada in a comparison of digital mammography with standard film mammograms.

Regular screening for cervical cancer (every 3 years in standard risk groups) with Pap tests has been found to decrease the mortality rate in women who are sexually active or are 18 years of age or older. Testing for HPV DNA in high-risk populations may improve early detection and management of cervical cancer, helping to determine which women with low-grade cytologic abnormalities require colposcopic evaluation. Recent data indicate that screening every 2 years with both Pap and HPV testing is more cost-effective than screening with either test alone. Self-collected vaginal swabs for DNA testing may improve screening in areas where cytology is not readily available or in populations where women are hesitant to undergo regular examinations. Routine screening with vaginal Pap smears in women who have previously undergone a hysterectomy for benign gynecologic disease is not useful because of the very low incidence of squamous cell cancers of the vagina.

Annual fecal occult blood testing and screening with sigmoidoscopy every 5 years in people over age 50 decreases the mortality rate from colorectal cancer. An evaluation of over 46,000 people aged 50–80 in the Minnesota Colon Cancer Control study over an 18-year follow-up period showed that either annual or biennial screening of two stool samples significantly reduced the incidence of colorectal cancer when an abnormal fecal blood screen was followed by colonoscopy. Removing polyps detected by colonoscopy reduces the risk of colorectal cancer, and, following polypectomy, colonoscopy is superior to double-contrast barium enema for the detection of recurrent polyps. Even adenomatous polyps 5 mm or less in diameter detected in the rectosigmoid by sigmoidoscopy are markers for more advanced proximal neoplasms. These patients should undergo colonoscopy to evaluate the proximal bowel. However, colonoscopic screening can detect advanced colonic neoplasms in asymptomatic adults even in the absence of distal adenomas. Regular fecal occult blood testing and flexible sigmoidoscopy are still recommended for general screening because of the lower cost and facility of sigmoidoscopy compared with colonoscopy. A novel test to examine stool for DNA alterations that might help to screen for colorectal cancer is in development. Table 1–8 outlines the American Cancer Societies recommendations for cancer screening for standard-risk individuals. Updated guidelines can be obtained at www.cancer.org. It is critical that clinicians involve patients in decisions about whether to order tests for early detection of breast and prostate cancers so that patients will understand the risks and benefits. Unfortunately, screening for ovarian cancer with serum markers (eg, CA 125), transvaginal ultrasound, or pelvic examinations has not been shown to decrease the mortality rate from this disease. A multicenter trial is under way to test whether a multimodality screening program will be more effective than each of these methods alone. Screening for prostate cancer and hepatocellular cancer is discussed in the section on tumor markers.

Recent data from the Women's Health Initiative Observational Study cohort, which represents a large and diverse group of older women, indicates that health insurance type and status are among the most important determinants of cancer screening independent of other factors. Improving coverage of and access to health insurance for older adults in the United States may serve an important role in improving early detection of cancer through screening. Screening is underutilized in minority groups in the United States, especially in inner city and rural areas. This results in the diagnosis of cancers at more advanced stages. Educational and outreach programs should be directed at these underserved areas.

Lieberman DA et al: Use of colonoscopy to screen asymptomatic adults for colorectal cancer. N Engl J Med 2000;343:162. [PMID: 10900274] (Colonoscopy can detect lesions that would not be discovered by sigmoidoscopy.)

Mandel JS et al: The effect of fecal occult-blood screening on the incidence of colorectal cancer. N Engl J Med 2000;343:1603. [PMID: 11096167] (Fecal occult blood screening done annually or biennially with abnormal results followed up with colonoscopy reduces the incidence of colorectal cancer.)

Nystrom L et al: Long-term effects of mammography screening: updated overview of the Swedish randomized trials. Lancet 2002;359:909. [PMID: 11918907] (The analysis of these studies (included in the Cochrane review) indicates that mammographic screening reduces mortality, particularly in women aged 60 and older).

Olsen O et al: Cochrane review on screening for breast cancer with mammography. Lancet 2001;358:1340. [PMID: 11684218] (This controversial meta-analysis of seven large published trials argues that mammographic screening does not result in a significant reduction in breast cancer-specific mortality.)

Sawaya GF et al: Current approaches to cervical cancer screening. N Engl J Med 2001;344:1603. [PMID: 11372013] (A review of current and novel screening approaches for cervical cancer).

Smith RA et al: American Cancer Society Guidelines for the early detection of cancer. CA Cancer J Clin 2000;50:34 (updated 2001;51:38). [PMID: 10735014] (The current ACS guidelines and an explanation of how these guidelines were developed.)

Smith TJ et al: American Society of Clinical Oncology 1998 Update of Recommended Breast Cancer Surveillance Guidelines. J Clin Oncol 1999;17:1080. [PMID: 10071303] (Recommendations for the detection of recurrent cancer based on impact on outcome.)

Wright TC Jr et al: HPV DNA testing of self-collected vaginal samples compared with cytologic screening to detect cervical cancer. JAMA 2000;283:81. [PMID: 10632284] (HPV testing of self collected vaginal swabs is less specific but as sensitive as Pap smears for detecting high-grade cervical disease and may be a way to increase screening in women from areas where cytology is not readily performed.)

SPECIAL TOPICS IN PREVENTION

Patients with a family history of colorectal cancer are at increased risk to develop this disease and should undergo regular screening, which clearly reduces the incidence and mortality from invasive cancer. Guidelines for patients with a risk of hereditary nonpolyposis colon cancer are referenced below. Approximately 10% of breast and ovarian cancers are due to inherited genetic mutations, occurring primarily in women with mutations of *BRCA1* and *BRCA2*. Patients with a family history of breast or ovarian cancer are at higher risk to develop these cancers and require frequent monitoring for early detection, though screening is inadequate to detect early ovarian cancer. Women with a family history of premenopausal or bilateral breast cancer—or any family history of ovarian cancer—should be referred for genetic counseling to better assess their risk of carrying one of the known mutations. Prophylactic oophorectomy after completion of childbearing can decrease but not eliminate the risk of ovarian cancer in high-risk women; there is still a risk of peritoneal cystadenocarcinoma. The actual risk reduction is not known but has been estimated to be about 50%, still leaving women at a substantial risk for ovarian cancer. Bilateral prophylactic oophorectomy also appears to reduce the risk of subsequent breast cancer by up to 75%, presumably because of decreased exposure to ovarian estrogens. Oral contraceptive use for 6 years or more decreased the risk of ovarian cancer by as much as 60% in women with a family history of ovarian cancer. Prophylactic mastectomy has been used for decades to reduce the risk of breast cancer in high-risk women and is associated with a substantial reduction in breast cancer risk. In women at both high and moderate risk of breast cancer based on family history, the incidence of breast cancer (and death from breast cancer) is reduced by at least 90%. Decisions about such prophylactic surgery in high-risk women must be made taking full account of many other factors—clearly, breast or ovarian cancer would not have developed in all women undergoing the procedure. Any patient with a history of dysplasia or premalignant lesions is at high risk for development of invasive cancer and should undergo frequent and thorough screening for subsequent malignancy. Patients at a particularly high individual risk for cancer may require additional screening procedures. Enthusiasm about the ability of spiral CT to image early lung cancers has reawakened interest in screening high-risk individuals with the goal of reducing lung cancer mortality with detection of early, treatable lesions. Randomized trials are required to investigate whether screening for lung cancer with this expensive test can actually reduce mortality rates. At the present time, general guidelines are to consider routine chest x-ray screening on an annual basis for heavy smokers (more than 20 pack years) over the age of 55.

Burke W et al: Recommendations for follow-up care of individuals with an inherited predisposition to cancer. I. Hereditary nonpolyposis colon cancer. Cancer Genetics Studies Consortium. JAMA 1997;277:915. [PMID: 9062331]

Burke W et al: Recommendations for follow-up care of individuals with an inherited predisposition to cancer. II. *BRCA1* and *BRCA2*. Cancer Genetics Studies Consortium. JAMA 1997;277:997. [PMID: 9091675] (Suggestions for screening and prevention in these very high risk groups.)

Henschke CI et al: Early lung cancer action project: overall design and findings from baseline screening. Lancet 1999;354:99. [PMID: 10408484] (Baseline data on risk and survival following diagnosis by incidental x-rays.)

Kauff ND et al: Risk-reducing salpingo-oophorectomy in women with a *BRCA1* or *BRCA2* mutation. N Engl J Med 2002;346:1609. [PMID: 12023992] (Bilateral oophorectomy results in significant reduction—up to 75%—in the subsequent risk of both ovarian and breast cancers in high-risk women.)

Narod SA et al: Oral contraceptives and the risk of hereditary ovarian cancer. N Engl J Med 1999;339:424. [PMID: 9700175] (Oral contraceptives decrease the risk of ovarian cancer in women who carry the *BRCA1* and *BRCA2* mutations.)

Rebbeck TR et al: Prophylactic oophorectomy in carriers of *BRCA1* or *BRCA2* mutations. [PMID: 12023993] N Engl J Med 2002;346:1616.

■ STAGING OF CANCER

Standardized staging for tumor burden at the time of diagnosis is important both for determining prognosis and for making decisions about treatment. The American Joint Committee on Cancer (AJCC) has developed a simple classification scheme that can be incorporated into a form for staging and universally applied. This scheme is designed to encompass the life history of a tumor and is referred to as the TNM system. The untreated primary tumor (T) will gradually increase in size, leading to regional lymph node involvement (N) and, finally, distant metastases (M). The tumor is usually not clinically evident until local invasion or even spread to regional draining lymph nodes has occurred.

TNM staging is used clinically to indicate the extension of cancer before definitive therapy begins. The manner in which staging is accomplished—eg, by clinical examination or pathologic examination of a surgical specimen—must be carefully documented. Certain types of tumors, such as lymphomas and Hodgkin's disease, are usually staged by a different classification scheme that reflects the natural history of this type of tumor spread and helps to direct treatment decisions.

The TNM system allows a numerical assessment of the extent of primary tumor (T), the absence or presence and extent of regional lymph node metastases (N), and the absence or presence of distant metastases (M). The AJCC has just published a new version of the TNM staging criteria with major revisions directed toward providing a standardized method for classifying the extent of cancer at diagnosis and estimating the risk of recurrence and death from cancer. Examples of changes in staging included in the new system are staging melanoma based on the thickness and ulceration of the lesion instead of the level of invasion and the stratification of breast cancer stage based on the number of involved axillary nodes. The new staging system will take effect in January 2003. Details regarding these revisions may be found at the AJCC Web site: www.cancerstaging.net

Traditional staging does not take into account the biology or aggressiveness of a particular tumor and may not allow differentiation of prognostic risk groups. For this reason, specific pathologic characteristics are added into the prognostic evaluation for certain tumors (eg, estrogen and progesterone receptors, grade and proliferative index for breast cancer; histologic grade for sarcoma). Overexpression or underproduction of oncogene products (eg, Her-2/*neu* in breast cancer), infection of cancer cells with specific viral genomes (eg, HPV18 in cervical cancer), and certain chromosomal translocations or deletions (eg, alteration of the retinoic acid receptor gene in acute promyelocytic leukemia) have important prognostic significance and may direct risk-adapted or cancer-specific therapy. As these characteristics become standardized and better understood, they may allow us to identify patients with a poorer prognosis early in the course of disease when the patient might benefit from more aggressive therapy.

AJCC Cancer Staging Manual/ 6th ed. Springer, 2002. (The newly revised bible of TNM staging.)

■ PRIMARY CANCER TREATMENT

The reader is referred to the NCCN Oncology Practice Guidelines: http://www.cancernetwork.com. These guidelines are updated yearly.

SURGERY & RADIATION THERAPY

Most cancers present initially as localized tumor nodules and cause local symptoms. Depending on the type of cancer, initial therapy may be directed locally in the form of surgery or radiation therapy. Surgical excision or local radiation (or both) is the treatment of choice for a variety of potentially curable cancers, including most gastrointestinal and genitourinary cancers, central nervous system tumors, and cancers arising from the breast, thyroid, or skin as well as most sarcomas.

Surgery at presentation has both diagnostic and therapeutic effectiveness, since it permits pathologic staging of the extent of local and regional invasion as well as an opportunity for removal of the primary neoplasm. CT and MRI play an increasing role in noninvasive tumor staging. Based on results of a prospective clinical trial, positron emission tomography (PET) appears to be a more sensitive method than traditional imaging with CT scanning for detecting local and distant metastases in patients with non-small-cell lung cancer. The effect on survival is unknown. PET has also been shown to improve detection of recurrent disease for the purpose of second-look laparotomy and debulking in colon cancer patients with rising levels of carcinoembryonic antigen (CEA). A monoclonal antibody against CEA labeled with technetium Tc 99m (arcitumomab, CEA-Scan) is now approved for imaging of cancers with increased levels of CEA and has been found to be more sensitive and specific than CT scans in the detection of both resectable and nonresectable disease. These newer, more sensitive scans may allow better assessment of resectability before surgery, sparing patients needless surgery but also providing appropriate surgery when cure with local treatment alone is possible.

Although standard surgery for breast cancer has included excision of axillary nodes, this can result in chronic lymphedema, pain, and decreased range of motion of the arm. Sentinel axillary nodes can be detected by injection of radioactive colloid or blue dye into the breast around the tumor or the biopsy cavity. "Hot spots" are then identified with a gamma probe and resected. Biopsy of sentinel nodes can predict the presence or absence of axillary node metastases and direct more aggressive surgery with up to 97% accuracy. However, the procedure is technically challenging and the success rate thus varies with the surgeon. This technique is also used for staging of malignant melanoma. Cryosurgical ablation of localized prostate cancers has been used instead of radiotherapy by some investigators and appears to reduce postablation voiding dysfunction. Radiofrequency ablation (frictional heating) and cryosurgical ablation are being tested as primary treatment of small, localized breast cancers.

Surgery may also play an important role in the treatment of selected patients with limited metastatic cancer. Resection of isolated metastases has been used most commonly for breast cancer with single brain lesions or isolated liver or lung lesions. Removal of isolated liver metastases may result in long-term survival, with 20% of patients living more than 5 years. Additional surgery after subsequent limited recurrence may also result in long-term disease-free survival. Surgical resection of both hepatic and pulmonary metastases may improve survival in appropriately selected colon cancer patients.

For certain tumor sites, complete surgical removal of the tumor can be disfiguring, disabling, or unachievable. Under those circumstances, primary local therapy with ionizing radiation may prove to be the treatment of choice. In other instances, surgery and radiation therapy are used in sequence. For stage I and stage II breast cancer, local incision or "lumpectomy" with axillary node dissection combined with radiation results in equivalent 10-year survivals when compared with the more disfiguring and extensive mastectomy procedure. Despite these well-established data, breast-conserving therapy is still underused in patients with larger tumors, mainly because of surgeon bias. Preoperative or "neoadjuvant" chemotherapy and radiation

therapy allow limb-sparing surgery in osteosarcoma and organ preservation in oropharyngeal cancer, among others.

Radiation therapy is usually delivered as brachytherapy or teletherapy. In brachytherapy, the radiation source is placed close to the tumor. This intracavitary approach is used for many gynecologic or oral neoplasms and occasionally for breast cancer. In teletherapy, supervoltage radiotherapy is usually delivered with a linear accelerator, as this instrument permits more precise beam localization and avoids the complication of skin radiation toxicity. Various beam-modifying wedges, rotational techniques, and other specific approaches are used to increase the radiation dosage to the tumor bed while minimizing toxicity to adjacent normal tissues. Examples of new approaches to minimize radiation to surrounding tissues while maximizing radiation to the cancer include three-dimensional conformal radiation therapy (3D CRT) and intensity modulated radiation therapy (IMRT). Conventional radiation beams are of uniform intensity. In contrast, IMRT's beam intensity is modulated to produce maximum doses where desired and minimal radiation to sensitive surrounding normal tissues. Improved outcomes have been shown for prostate cancer patients receiving IMRT.

Well-oxygenated tumors are more radiosensitive than hypoxic tumors. Hypoxic tumors are often bulky, implying a potential synergistic role of surgical debulking prior to radiotherapy. Radiation therapy is normally delivered in a fractionated fashion over 4–6 weeks, this method appearing to have radiobiologic superiority by permitting time for recovery of normal host tissues (but not the tumor) from sublethal damage during treatment. However, a more accelerated fraction radiation schedule improves local-regional control in patients with head and neck cancer compared with standard fractionated radiation.

For most tumor types, there is a sigmoid curve of increasing rate of control of the local tumor with increasing radiation dose. Radiosensitive tumors usually exhibit radiosensitivity over the dose range of 3500–5000 cGy.

Currently, more than half of all patients with cancer receive radiation therapy during the course of their illness. Radiation therapy is frequently the sole agent used with curative intent for tumors of the larynx (permitting cure without loss of the voice), oral cavity, pharynx, esophagus, uterine cervix, vagina, prostate, skin, Hodgkin's disease, and some tumors of the brain and spinal cord. For more extensive cancers, radiation is combined with surgery (eg, cancer of the breast, ovary, uterus, cervix, urinary bladder, rectum, lung, soft tissue sarcomas, and seminoma of the testis). Following mastectomy for breast cancer, radiation has been shown to reduce the risk of local recurrence from large or high-risk tumors and may increase overall survival by decreasing distant recurrence. Radiation given in combination with chemotherapy may improve long-term disease control. The combination of chemotherapy and radiation therapy for the treatment of invasive carcinoma of the cervix is significantly superior to radiation therapy alone. There is at least a 10% improvement in 3-year survival and a 30–50% reduction in the risk of death from cervical cancer with combination therapy. Twice-daily radiation given concurrently with combination chemotherapy for the treatment of limited small-cell lung cancer results in significantly improved 5-year survival rates compared with any prior treatment results. Twice-daily radiation also appears superior to once-daily treatment for this disease. Radiation combined with chemotherapy for cancer of the rectum or hormone therapy for cancer of the prostate improves survival over treatment with radiation alone, and concurrent radiation and chemotherapy for cancer of the head and neck reduces mortality from that disease compared with either treatment alone. Radiation can also improve disease control when given as an adjuvant to chemotherapy for bulky lymphomas, for non-small cell lung cancer, and for some cancers in children.

Occasionally, chemotherapy is used to sensitize tumor cells to the toxic effects of radiation. Radiation therapy for palliation of pain or dysfunction (eg, bone pain associated with advanced breast or other cancers) may improve the quality of life of patients suffering from incurable malignancies.

Various normal tissues (particularly skin, mucosa, myocardium, spinal cord, bone marrow, and lymphoid system) can exhibit early or late toxicity from radiation therapy. Acute toxicity may include generalized fatigue and malaise, anorexia, nausea and vomiting, local skin changes, diarrhea, and mucosal ulceration of the irradiated area. Radiation of large areas, especially the pelvis and proximal long bones, may result in bone marrow suppression. Radiation of the lungs, heart, and gastrointestinal tract must be approached with appropriate shielding to avoid toxicity such as radiation pneumonitis, congestive heart failure, or radiation gastroenteritis. Long-term toxicity from radiation therapy has significant long-term side effects that must be weighed against its possible benefits. Women under age 60 treated with left-sided adjuvant radiation for breast cancer with 10–15 years of follow-up have a significant increase in risk of death from myocardial infarction. Increased cardiac mortality has also been seen in patients who received radiation at a young age for Hodgkin's disease. Secondary leukemias and solid tumors can be seen after radiation therapy for a wide variety of cancers. This risk is particularly high in patients receiving a combination of both radiation and chemotherapy that includes alkylating agents. Treatment programs now combine less toxic chemotherapy with limited field radiation therapy to limit these fatal long-term side effects in long-term survivors from cancer. Other long-term toxicities include decreased function of the radiation organ (eg, decreased cognitive function after whole brain radiation), myelopathy, osteonecrosis, and hyperpigmentation of the involved skin.

Novel modalities are occasionally used to enhance penetrance into large tumors or to specifically target the site of radiation. Gamma knife radiation allows focused radiation for limited brain metastases and is associated with fewer long-term complications such as cognitive dysfunction compared with whole brain radiation. Regional hyperthermia (40–42 °C) is an adjunct to ionizing irradiation for some tumor sites. The most useful application of hyperthermia to date has been in superficial or easily implantable tumors as well as in relatively bulky hypovascular tumors with some degree of hypoxia. Electron beam therapy has been used effectively to treat superficial tumors in the skin. Radiolabeled antibodies are currently under investigation as a means of delivering high levels of radiation locally to the tumor bed, thereby avoiding systemic toxicity. Ibritumomab tiuxetan is the first radiolabeled antibody to be FDA-approved for the treatment of cancer—specifically, relapsed low-grade non-Hodgkin's lymphoma (see section on Novel Therapies for Cancer Treatment). Increasingly, the primary local therapy of cancer is integrated with systemic therapy, an approach that has proved to be superior for apparently localized tumor types with a high propensity for early metastatic spread and for which anticancer drugs are available.

Chao C et al: Update on the use of the sentinel node biopsy in patients with melanoma: who and how. Curr Opin Oncol 2002;14:217. [PMID: 11880714] (A review of the utility and prognostic importance of the sentinel lymph node biopsy in melanoma.)

Choti MA et al: Trends in long-term survival following liver resection for hepatic colorectal metastases. Ann Surg 2002;235:759. [PMID: 12035031] (Long-term survival following liver resection for colorectal metastases has improved during the last decade, perhaps due to better imaging and selection of patients for surgery.)

Dearnaley DP et al: Comparison of radiation side-effects of conformal and conventional radiotherapy in prostate cancer: a randomised trial. Lancet 1999;353:267. [PMID: 9929018] (Conformational radiotherapy limits radiation to normal tissues and in this study significantly lowered the risk of late radiation-induced proctitis with excellent local tumor control.)

Harris S: Radiotherapy for early and advanced breast cancer. Int J Clin Pract 2001;55:609. [PMID: 11770358] (A broad review of the use of radiation therapy in early and late stage breast cancer as well as a discussion of short and long term side effects.)

Moroz P et al: Status of hyperthermia in the treatment of advanced liver cancer. J Surg Oncol 2001;77:259. [PMID: 11473375] (A review of current results, side effects, and limitations of hyperthermia for this disease.)

Pieterman RM et al: Preoperative staging of non-small-cell lung cancer with positron emission tomography. N Engl J Med 2000;343:254. [PMID: 10911107] (PET scanning improves the rate of detection of local and distant metastases compared with traditional staging in patient with non-small-cell lung cancer.)

Recht A et al: Postmastectomy radiotherapy: Clinical practice guidelines of the American Society of Clinical Oncology. J Clin Oncol 2001;19:1539. [PMID: 11230499] (An expert multidisciplinary panel reviewed published and unpublished information to develop the recommendations, suggestions and expert opinions outlined in this article.)

Thomas GM: Improved treatment for cervical cancer—concurrent chemotherapy and radiotherapy. N Engl J Med 1999;340:1198. [PMID: 10202172] (An editorial summarizing the results of three of the five randomized studies in that issue shows that concurrent radiation and chemotherapy improves survival from invasive cervical cancer.)

SYSTEMIC CANCER THERAPY

Use of cytotoxic drugs, hormones, antihormones, and biologic agents has become a highly specialized and increasingly effective means of treating cancer. Therapy is usually administered by a medical oncologist. Selection of specific drugs or protocols for various types of cancer has traditionally been based on results of prior clinical trials. Many patients are treated on protocols to search for optimal therapy for refractory or poorly responsive malignancies. Treatment may be inadequate or ineffective because of drug resistance of the tumor cells. This has been attributed to spontaneous genetic mutations in subpopulations of cancer cells prior to exposure to chemotherapy. After chemotherapy has eliminated the sensitive cells, the resistant subpopulation grows to become the predominant cell type (Goldie-Coldman hypothesis). This has been the basis of alternating non-cross-resistant chemotherapy regimens.

Molecular mechanisms of drug resistance are now the subject of intense study. In many instances, specific drug resistance results from an amplification in the number of gene copies for an enzyme inhibited by a specific chemotherapeutic agent. A more general form of "multidrug resistance" (MDR) has been described in association with expression of a gene (MDR1) encoding a 170-kDa transmembrane glycoprotein (P-glycoprotein) on tumor cells. This protein is an energy-dependent transport pump that facilitates drug efflux from tumor cells and promotes resistance to a broad spectrum of unrelated cancer drugs. Although a variety of agents have been shown to at least partially and temporarily reverse acquired multidrug resistance in multiple myeloma and lymphoma, the doses of these agents required to overcome drug resistance are associated with serious side effects. MDR modulators will need to be both less toxic and more potent to be clinically useful. PSC 833 is a cyclosporine analog with little of the immunosuppressive effects or renal toxicities of cyclosporine but with five- to tenfold greater MDR-modulating activity. Unfortunately, clinical benefits from adding this agent to chemotherapy have been limited. Both improved response rates and improved survival with a tolerable toxicity profile using novel therapy such as this will have to be demonstrated to prove the effectiveness of this approach.

Variation in drug metabolism due to gene polymorphisms is emerging as a cause of relative resistance or sensitivity to chemotherapeutic agents. In one study, women with breast cancer who had single-nucleotide polymorphisms in the CYP3A4 and CYP3A5 genes were not able to metabolize cyclophosphamide and had a significantly shorter survival than women without this polymorphism. Polymorphisms in CYP have also been shown to increase sensitivity to some environmental carcinogens. With an increased understanding of individual susceptibility or resistance factors, pretreatment evaluation of drug metabolism genes might allow individualization of therapy.

Chemotherapy is used primarily to cure a small percentage of malignancies, as adjuvant therapy to decrease the rate of relapse or improve the disease-free interval, and to palliate symptoms and prolong survival in some patients with incurable malignancies. In addition, chemotherapy is playing an increasing role as preoperative or "neoadjuvant" therapy to reduce the size and extent of the primary tumor, thereby allowing complete excision at the time of surgery. Neoadjuvant (preoperative) chemotherapy results in identical survival when compared with standard postsurgical chemotherapy for breast cancer and allows more limited or complete surgical excision of the primary tumor as well as giving important information about chemosensitivity. Randomized studies now suggest that neoadjuvant chemotherapy may improve survival in patients with esophageal cancer and bladder cancer.

Chemotherapy was first shown to be curative in the treatment of advanced stages of choriocarcinoma in women. It is also curative in Hodgkin's disease, diffuse large-cell and some high-grade lymphomas (including Burkitt's), carcinoma of the testis, some cases of acute leukemia, and embryonal rhabdomyosarcoma. When combined with initial surgery—and in some instances with irradiation—chemotherapy increases the rate of long-term control and cure of breast cancer, cervical cancer, small-cell lung cancer, colon cancer, gastric cancer, esophageal cancer, rectal cancer, and osteogenic sarcomas. Combination chemotherapy provides palliation and prolongation of survival in adults with low-grade non-Hodgkin's lymphoma, mycosis fungoides, multiple myeloma and Waldenström's macroglobulinemia, acute and chronic leukemias, and breast, ovarian, cervical, and small-cell lung carcinoma as well as carcinoid. Patients with incurable tumors who desire aggressive treatment should be referred for experimental therapy in well-designed clinical trials. (See section on Novel Therapies at the end of this chapter.)

High-dose chemotherapy followed by bone marrow transplantation is curative therapy for various types of leukemia, high-risk or relapsed lymphoma, testicular cancer, and occasionally for multiple myeloma. Allogeneic or autologous bone marrow or peripheral blood stem cells with or without ex vivo purging is used depending on the disease. The use of growth factors and blood stem cells has decreased the toxicity and cost of bone marrow transplantation. Autologous transplantation may now be used with low morbidity and mortality on selected patients up to age 70. Dose-intense chemotherapy with autologous bone marrow or peripheral blood stem cell rescue has been intensely studied for the treatment of both high-risk and metastatic breast cancer for the past decade with unfortunately negative or poor-quality data. Details of these studies are presented in the section on adjuvant therapy.

Nonmyeloablative allogeneic peripheral blood stem cell transplantation is now being investigated as immunotherapy for some advanced cancers. This highly toxic and intensive therapy has been shown to result in sustained regression of chemotherapy-resistant metastatic renal cell carcinoma in ten out of nineteen treated patients, with three complete remissions. Tumor response was associated with acquisition of the donor immune system, resulting in a "graft-versus-tumor" effect. Further investigation is required to confirm sustained beneficial effects, reduce toxicity, improve efficacy, and better understand in which diseases this type of therapy can be effective. Chemotherapeutic agents are increasingly being given on different schedules to reduce toxicity and enhance antitumor effects. "Dose-dense" chemotherapy gives smaller doses of chemotherapy agents on a weekly or more frequent schedule. Animal studies have suggested that these dosing regimens may reverse some types of chemotherapy resistance.

While most anticancer drugs are used systemically, there are selected indications for local or regional administration. Regional administration involves direct infusion of active chemotherapeutic agents into the tumor site (eg, intravesical therapy for bladder cancer, intraperitoneal therapy for ovarian cancer, hepatic artery infusion with or without embolization of the main blood supply of the tumor for cancers metastatic to the liver or as primary therapy for hepatocellular carcinoma). These treatments can result in palliation and prolonged survival.

A summary of the types of cancer responsive to chemotherapy and the current treatments of choice is offered in Table 40-3. In some instances (eg, Hodgkin's disease, breast cancer, ovarian and lung cancers), optimal therapy may require a combination of therapeutic resources, eg, radiation plus chemotherapy rather than either modality alone. Patients with stage I or stage II Hodgkin's disease are often treated with radiation alone, avoiding the potential toxicity of systemic chemotherapy. A small percentage of these patients may require chemotherapy later for disease recurrence.

New drugs to treat cancer are under constant development and testing—with the aim of reducing toxicity to normal cells and increasing the toxicity to resistant cancer cells. Several of these newer agents developed over the last decade that are currently available are described in this section. We have entered an exciting new era in the understanding and treatment of malignancies. Molecular techniques have allowed insight into the biologic events resulting in cancer, and these same techniques have developed just the beginning of a cascade of biologic therapies directed toward specific molecular or cellular factors critical to the pathogenesis of cancer growth and survival. Rather than the traditional cytotoxic therapy, newer treatments are more specific, less globally cytotoxic, and are associated with fewer side effects. New biologic therapies are either approved or under investigation for use in the treatment of cancer. The time from development of a novel agent to clinical use and FDA approval has been markedly shortened; in the first half of year 2001, two biologic therapies (imatinib mesylate and alemtuzumab were rapidly approved for use based on marked efficacy with low toxicity for the treatment of two different hematologic malignancies. The next decade will probably see the development of a whole new class of agents and, consequently, a new paradigm for the treatment of cancer.

A purine analog, cladribine (2-chlorodeoxyadenosine; 2-CdA), is used as the primary agent to treat hairy cell leukemia. A 1-week course of therapy results in high and durable remission rates with modest and short-lived toxicity. Repeated courses for disease recurrence are also effective. Pentostatin (2-deoxycoformycin, an adenosine deaminase inhibitor) is also used to treat hairy cell leukemia.

Fludarabine phosphate, another purine analog, has shown improved response rates and progression-free survival compared with oral chlorambucil or combination chemotherapy for chronic lymphocytic leukemia (CLL). Fludarabine is now indicated as first-line therapy for most patients with CLL. Side effects include an increased risk of opportunistic infections as well as very rare problems such as hemolytic anemia and severe bone marrow suppression. Fludarabine is also effective therapy for low-grade lymphomas and Waldenström's macroglobulinemia. Cladribine and pentostatin are also used to treat CLL and the above disorders.

Alemtuzumab is a humanized monoclonal antibody that is approved to treat relapsed or resistant CLL. It targets the CD52 antigen, which is prevalent on the abnormal B lymphocytes found in this common leukemia. In clinical trials of patients with CLL refractory to fludarabine and with prior exposure to alkylating agents, response rates of 33% were seen with a median duration of response of 7 months. Early studies in untreated patients suggest a response rate up to 87% with a high rate of complete responses. Alemtuzumab is given by subcutaneous injection, and side effects include infusion-related events, infections, and bone marrow suppression.

Paclitaxel (Taxol) is a novel agent isolated from the pacific yew tree that has replaced cyclophosphamide as front-line therapy (combined with carboplatin) for the treatment of ovarian cancer. Intraperitoneal instillation may also be helpful for advanced disease. Paclitaxel (and docetaxel; see below) has also been shown to be one of the most effective agents against metastatic breast cancer; it is also effective in AIDS-associated Kaposi's sarcoma and other cancers. The primary toxicities of paclitaxel are hematologic and neurologic.

Table 40–3. Treatment choices for cancers responsive to systemic agents.

Diagnosis	Current Treatment of Choice	Other Valuable Agents and Procedures
Acute lymphocytic leukemia	**Induction:** Combination chemotherapy. *Adults:* Vincristine, prednisone, daunorubicin, and asparaginase. **Consolidation:** Multiagent alternating chemotherapy. Allogeneic bone marrow transplant for young adults or high-risk disease or second remission. CNS prophylaxis with intrathecal methotrexate with or without whole brain radiation. **Remission maintenance:** Methotrexate, thioguanine.	Doxorubicin, cytarabine, cyclophosphamide, etoposide, teniposide, allopurinol,[1] autologous bone marrow transplantation
Acute myelocytic and myelomonocytic leukemia	**Induction:** Combination chemotherapy with cytarabine and an anthracycline (daunorubicin, idarubicin). Tretinoin with idarubicin for acute promyelocytic leukemia. **Consolidation:** High-dose cytarabine. Autologous (with or without purging) or allogeneic bone marrow transplantation for high-risk disease or second remission.	Gemtuzumab ozogamicin (Mylotarg), mitoxantrone, idarubicin, etoposide, mercaptopurine, thioguanine, azacitidine,[2] amsacrine,[2] methotrexate, doxorubicin, tretinoin, allopurinol,[1] leukapheresis, prednisone, arsenic trioxide for acute promyelocytic leukemia
Chronic myelocytic leukemia	Imatinib mesylate (Gleevec), hydroxyurea, alpha interferon. Allogeneic bone marrow transplantation for younger patients.	Busulfan, mercaptopurine, thioguanine, cytarabine, plicamycin, melphalan, autologous bone marrow transplantation,[2] allopurinol[1]
Chronic lymphocytic leukemia	Fludarabine, chlorambucil, and prednisone (if treatment is indicated). Second-line therapy: alemtuzumab (Campath-1H).	Vincristine, cyclophosphamide, doxorubicin, cladribine (2-chlorodeoxyadenosine; CdA), rituximab, allogeneic bone marrow transplant, androgens,[2] allopurinol[1]
Hairy cell leukemia	Cladribine (2-chlorodeoxyadenosine; CdA).	Pentostatin (deoxycoformycin), alpha interferon
Hodgkin's disease (stages III and IV)	**Combination chemotherapy:** doxorubicin (Adriamycin), bleomycin, vinblastine, dacarbazine (ABVD) or alternative combination therapy without mechlorethamine. Autologous bone marrow transplant for high-risk patients or relapsed disease.	Mechlorethamine, vincristine, prednisone, procarbazine (MOPP); carmustine, lomustine, etoposide, thiotepa, autologous bone marrow transplantation
Non-Hodgkin's lymphoma (intermediate to high grade)	**Combination therapy** depending on histologic classification but usually including cyclophosphamide, vincristine, doxorubicin, and prednisone (CHOP) with or without rituximab in older patients. Autologous bone marrow transplantation in high-risk first remission or first relapse.	Bleomycin, methotrexate, etoposide, chlorambucil, fludarabine, lomustine, carmustine, cytarabine, thiotepa, amsacrine, mitoxantrone, allogeneic bone marrow transplantation
Non-Hodgkin's lymphoma (low-grade)	Fludarabine, rituximab, ibritumomab tiuxetan for relapsed or refractory disease	**Combination chemotherapy:** cyclophosphamide, prednisone, doxorubicin, vincristine; chlorambucil, autologous or allogeneic transplantation
Cutaneous T cell lymphoma (mycosis fungoides)	Topical carmustine, electron beam radiotherapy, photochemotherapy, targretin, denileukin diftitox (ONTAK) for refractory disease	Interferon, combination chemotherapy, denileukin diftitox (ONTAK), targretin
Multiple myeloma	**Combination chemotherapy:** vincristine, doxorubicin, dexamethasone; melphalan and prednisone; melphalan, cyclosphosphamide, carmustine, vincristine, doxorubicin, prednisone. Autologous transplantation in first complete or partial remission, mini-allogeneic transplant for poor-prognosis disease. Thalidomide for relapsed or refractory disease	Clarithromycin, etoposide, cytarabine, alpha interferon, dexamethasone, autologous bone marrow transplantation

(continued)

Table 40–3. Treatment choices for cancers responsive to systemic agents. (continued)

Diagnosis	Current Treatment of Choice	Other Valuable Agents and Procedures
Waldenström's macroglobulinemia	Fludarabine **or** chlorambucil **or** cyclophosphamide, vincristine, prednisone. Allogeneic bone marrow transplantation for high-risk young patients.	Cladribine, etoposide, alpha interferon, doxorubicin, dexamethasone, plasmapheresis, autologous bone marrow transplantation
Polycythemia vera, Essential thrombocytosis	Hydroxyurea, phlebotomy for polycythemia	Busulfan, chlorambucil, cyclophosphamide, alpha interferon, radiophosphorus [32]P
Carcinoma of the lung Small cell	**Combination chemotherapy:** cisplatin and etoposide. Palliative radiation therapy.	Cyclophosphamide, doxorubicin, vincristine
Non-small cell[3]	**Localized disease:** cisplatin, vinblastine **Advanced disease:** cisplatin, vinorelbine, docetaxel	Doxorubicin, etoposide, mitomycin, ifosfamide, paclitaxel, radiation therapy
Carcinoma of the head and neck[3]	**Combination chemotherapy:** cisplatin and fluorouracil	Methotrexate, bleomycin, hydroxyurea, doxorubicin, vinblastine
Carcinoma of the esophagus[3]	**Combination chemotherapy:** fluorouracil, cisplatin, mitomycin	Methotrexate, bleomycin, doxorubicin, mitomycin
Carcinoma of the stomach and pancreas[3]	**Stomach:** etoposide, leucovorin,[1] fluorouracil (ELF) **Pancreas:** fluorouracil or ELF, gemcitabine	Carmustine, mitomycin, lomustine, doxorubicin, gemcitabine, doxorubicin, methotrexate, cisplatin, combinations for stomach.
Carcinoma of the colon and rectum[3]	**Colon:** fluorouracil plus levamisole (adjuvant) or with leucovorin and irinotecan or oxaliplatin[2] (advanced) **Rectum:** fluorouracil with radiation therapy (adjuvant)	Capecitabine, methotrexate, mitomycin, carmustine, cisplatin, floxuridine.
Carcinoma of the kidney[3]	Floxuridine, vinblastine, IL-2, alpha interferon; consider mini-allogeneic transplantation[2]	Alpha interferon, progestins, infusional FUDR, fluorouracil
Carcinoma of the bladder[3]	Intravesical BCG or thiotepa. **Combination chemotherapy:** methotrexate, vinblastine, doxorubicin (Adriamycin), cisplatin (M-VAC) or CMV alone	Cyclophosphamide, fluorouracil, intravesical valrubicin, gemcitabine, cisplatin
Carcinoma of the testis[3]	**Combination chemotherapy:** etoposide and cisplatin. Autologous bone marrow transplantation for high-risk or relapsed disease.	Bleomycin, vinblastine, ifosfamide, mesna,[1] carmustine, carboplatin
Carcinoma of the prostate[4]	Estrogens or LHRH analog (leuprolide, goserelin or triptorelin) plus an antiandrogen (flutamide)	Ketoconazole, doxorubicin, aminoglutethimide, progestins, cyclophosphamide, cisplatin, vinblastine, etoposide, suramin[2]; PC-SPES; estramustine phosphate
Carcinoma of the uterus[3]	Progestins or tamoxifen	Doxorubicin, cisplatin, fluorouracil, ifosfamide
Carcinoma of the ovary[3]	**Combination chemotherapy:** paclitaxel and cisplatin or carboplatin	Docetaxel, doxorubicin, topotecan, cyclophosphamide, doxorubicin, etoposide, liposomal doxorubicin
Carcinoma of the cervix[3]	**Combination chemotherapy:** methotrexate, doxorubicin, cisplatin, and vinblastine; or mitomycin, bleomycin, vincristine, and cisplatin with radiation therapy	Carboplatin, ifosfamide, lomustine
Carcinoma of the breast[3]	**Combination chemotherapy:** A variety of regimens are used for adjuvant therapy. For node-positive disease—combinations including doxorubicin or epirubicin and at least one of the following additional drugs: 5-FU, cyclophosphamide, docetaxel, paclitaxel. For node-negative disease—a combination of the drugs listed above or cyclophosphamide, methotrexate, and 5-FU (CMF). For estrogen- or progesterone-positive disease, tamoxifen is given for 5 years regardless of the use of adjuvant chemotherapy.	Trastuzumab (Herceptin) with chemotherapy, paclitaxel, docetaxel, epirubicin, mitoxantrone, topotecan, capecitabine, vinorelbine, thiotepa, vincristine, vinblastine, carboplatin or cisplatin, plicamycin, anastrozole, letrozole, exemestane, fulvestrant, toremifine, progestins

(continued)

Table 40–3. Treatment choices for cancers responsive to systemic agents. (continued)

Diagnosis	Current Treatment of Choice	Other Valuable Agents and Procedures
Choriocarcinoma (trophoblastic neoplasms)[3]	Methotrexate or dactinomycin (or both) plus chlorambucil	Vinblastine, cisplatin, mercaptopurine, doxorubicin, bleomycin, etoposide
Carcinoma of the thyroid gland[3]	Radioiodine (^{131}I)	Doxorubicin, cisplatin, bleomycin, melphalan
Carcinoma of the adrenal gland[3]	Mitotane	Doxorubicin, suramin[2]
Carcinoid[3]	Fluorouracil plus streptozocin with or without alpha interferon	Doxorubicin, cyclophosphamide, octreotide, cyproheptadine,[1] methysergide[1]
Osteogenic sarcoma[3]	High-dose methotrexate, doxorubicin, vincristine	Cyclophosphamide, ifosfamide, bleomycin, dacarbazine, cisplatin, dactinomycin
Soft tissue sarcoma[3]	Doxorubicin, dacarbazine	Ifosfamide, cyclosphosphamide, etoposide, cisplatin, high-dose methotrexate, vincristine
Melanoma[3]	Dacarbazine, alpha interferon, IL-2	Carmustine, lomustine, melphalan, thiotepa, cisplatin, paclitaxel, tamoxifen, vincristine, vaccine therapy (melacine)[2]
Kaposi's sarcoma	Doxorubicin, vincristine alternating with vinblastine or vincristine alone. Palliative radiation therapy.	Alpha interferon, bleomycin, etoposide, doxorubicin
Neuroblastoma[3]	**Combination chemotherapy:** variations of cyclophosphamide, cisplatin, vincristine, doxorubicin, dacarbazine	Melphalan, ifosfamide, autologous or allogeneic bone marrow transplantation

[1]Supportive agent; not oncolytic.
[2]Investigational agent or procedure. Treatment is available through qualified investigators and centers authorized by the National Cancer Institute and Cooperative Oncology Groups.
[3]These tumors are generally managed initially with surgery with or without radiation therapy with or without adjuvant chemotherapy. For metastatic disease, the role of palliative radiation therapy is as important as that of chemotherapy.

Both are dose-dependent—the hematologic toxicity can be ameliorated by the use of myeloid growth factors.

Docetaxel is a synthetic analog of paclitaxel that has also been shown to be highly effective in breast cancer as well as other advanced malignancies, including non-small cell lung cancer and ovarian cancer. Its toxicities include bone marrow suppression and significant peripheral edema. The edema can be treated and generally prevented with steroids.

Vinorelbine, a semisynthetic vinca alkaloid, has been shown to be effective in treating advanced non-small-cell lung cancer. Response rates of 30% have been observed when vinorelbine is used as a single agent against this poorly responsive tumor. Vinorelbine is also used to treat metastatic breast cancer as well as other tumors.

Capecitabine is an oral 5-FU prodrug that is now approved to treat anthracycline- and taxane-resistant breast cancers as well as metastatic colorectal cancer.

Response rates range from 25% to 35%. Treatment can be complicated by a painful, red, and sometimes blistering rash on the palms and soles and severe diarrhea that resolves upon withholding therapy. A variety of other 5-FU prodrugs are in clinical trials but are not yet approved for use. A recent study showed a 3-month improvement in survival using the combination of docetaxel and capecitabine versus docetaxel alone in the treatment of advanced metastatic breast cancer, though there were considerably more side effects in the combination arm. This combination is now FDA-approved, and newer dosing schedules with reduced toxicity are being evaluated.

Gemcitabine, a pyrimidine analog for intravenous use, has been approved to treat pancreatic cancer and non-small-cell lung cancer but is active in other advanced malignancies, including breast cancer.

Topotecan was the first of a class of drugs called camptothecans that inhibit the enzyme topoisomerase I to be FDA-approved for use. It is used to treat advanced ovarian cancer and has shown some efficacy in the treatment of several other tumors.

Irinotecan is highly effective in the treatment of metastatic colorectal cancer. Two randomized studies compared standard therapy (fluorouracil and leucovorin) to standard therapy with irinotecan (the Saltz regimen) in patients with untreated metastatic colorectal cancer. The use of irinotecan resulted in a significantly higher response rate, delayed time to progression, and, in one study, improved survival. Toxicity in the irinotecan arm was also significantly higher, and with longer follow-up mortality was concerningly high at 3.5%. With appropriate management, much of the toxicity appears to be reversible and includes severe diarrhea and neutropenia. Mortality was due either to inflammation of the bowel, leading to sepsis, or to thrombosis. Guidelines have been published to improve management and reduce mortality from this regimen. Results of a phase III randomized trial presented at the annual oncology meetings in 2002 demonstrated prolongation in time to progression using a new regimen to treat metastatic colorectal cancer with the platinum derivative oxaliplatin combined with fluorouracil and leucovorin (FOLFOX4) compared with the Saltz regimen. Oxaliplatin is approved for use in Europe and was expected to be FDA-approved in the United States in 2002 based on the results of this trial. Antitumor responses have been shown using irinotecan to treat non-small cell lung cancer, small cell lung cancer, ovarian cancer, gliomas, and others.

Novel inhibitors of thymidylate synthase are also under study for the treatment of advanced colorectal cancer. Raltitrexed is currently being used in Europe based on early data showing similar efficacy compared with fluorouracil and high-dose leucovorin. Treatment of malignant mesothelioma with the multitargeted antifolate agent pemetrexed—in combination with cisplatin—was recently shown to significantly improve survival from this highly resistant disease when compared with treatment with cisplatin alone. This is the first chemotherapeutic agent that has been shown to alter survival from malignant mesothelioma, a cancer that is rising in incidence due to occupational exposure to asbestos. Pemetrexed must be given with folic acid and vitamin B_{12} supplementation. Liposomal encapsulation of active chemotherapeutic agents may improve drug delivery and decrease systemic toxicity. Two liposomally encapsulated drugs, doxorubicin and daunorubicin, are indicated in the treatment of Kaposi's sarcoma and have shown efficacy in treating many other diseases, including breast cancer and lymphoma.

An increasing number of monoclonal antibodies are used in cancer chemotherapy. Rituximab, a chimeric antibody against the B lymphocyte antigen CD20, is effective therapy for relapsed or resistant low-grade lymphomas and has shown limited usefulness in higher-grade lymphomas as well. Almost 50% of patients with low-grade lymphoma responded with shrinkage of lymph nodes to once-weekly dosing for 4 weeks. Responses lasted a median of over 1 year. Rituximab has been shown to be effective in longer courses lasting 8 weeks and as re-treatment following relapse. A recent study compared standard CHOP chemotherapy with rituximab combined with CHOP as initial therapy for patients aged 60 years or older with diffuse large B cell lymphomas. Response rates, 12-month event-free survival, and overall survival were significantly improved in the combination arm. These results will require further follow-up for confirmation of results in this high-risk older population and in younger patients. Toxicities are generally quite mild, though anaphylaxis (resulting in death) and infusion-related side effects have been reported. The HER-2/neu oncogene (also called c-erbB-2), a gene that encodes a receptor tyrosine kinase, is known to be overexpressed in many human cancers and is associated with tumors with poorer prognoses. In breast cancer, overexpression of HER-2/neu is seen in about 20% of women and is associated with a higher risk of metastatic disease and poorer survival. Trastuzumab (Herceptin) is a recombinant humanized monoclonal antibody directed against the HER-2/neu gene product that is indicated for the treatment of HER-2/neu-expressing metastatic breast cancer. When trastuzumab was used as a single agent to treat anthracycline-resistant breast cancer, the response rate was about 15%, with a median duration of response of over 8 months. However, when trastuzumab was added to first-line chemotherapy for metastatic breast cancer and compared with chemotherapy alone, patients receiving the combination therapy had a response rate of almost 50% with improvement in both remission duration and survival. The most promising combination appears to be trastuzumab and paclitaxel (Taxol) or docetaxel (Taxotere); combinations with other agents, including vinorelbine and gemcitabine, also appear to be effective. The combination of trastuzumab and doxorubicin (Adriamycin) resulted in an increase in subclinical and clinical cardiac toxicity; combinations with anthracyclines should be avoided. Other toxicities of trastuzumab appear to be primarily infusion-related. Ongoing randomized trials are evaluating trastuzumab therapy in combination with neoadjuvant or adjuvant therapy for node-positive breast cancer. In addition, trastuzumab is being tested for use in other HER-2/neu-expressing tumors such as prostate and ovarian cancers.

Another agent approved for the treatment of cutaneous T cell lymphomas (CTCL) such as mycosis fungoides resistant to standard therapy is denileukin diftitox (ONTAK), a recombinant DNA-derived cytotoxic protein composed of amino acid sequences for diphtheria toxin fragments followed by the sequences for interleukin-2 (IL-2). This fusion protein was designed to direct the cytocidal action of diphtheria toxin to cells that express the IL-2 receptor (CD25), such as the tumor cells in CTCL. Thirty percent of patients with advanced CTCL responded to denileukin diftitox in a phase III randomized trial. Toxicity is significant, including acute hypersensitivity reactions—requiring administration of this agent in a close-observation setting—and delayed pulmonary and peripheral edema.

Gemtuzumab ozogamicin is an antibody to CD33 linked to a potent antitumor antibiotic, calicheamicin, that is approved for the treatment of patients over the age of 60 with relapsed or refractory acute myelogenous leukemia (AML). This is the first example of antibody-targeted chemotherapy used clinically. In clinical trials, gemtuzumab ozogamicin resulted in a 31% remission rate in elderly patients with AML in first relapse who could not tolerate standard chemotherapy. Side effects are primarily infusion-related events and bone marrow suppression.

Bisphosphonates inhibit osteoclast activation and may also have antitumor and antiangiogenic effects. In addition to reducing bone pain, pamidronate reduces by approximately 50% the frequency of new skeletal events in breast cancer and prostatic cancer metastatic to bone and in multiple myeloma. Pamidronate must be given intravenously on a monthly basis, with an estimated cost of $775 a month, and may worsen pain for the first few days following the infusion. For this reason, pamidronate therapy may be limited to patients with multiple lytic bone lesions or disease in weight-bearing bones or vertebrae. A new and significantly more potent intravenous bisphosphonate, zoledronic acid, was FDA-approved in early 2002 for the treatment of metastatic bone lesions. Its advantage compared with pamidronate is a shorter infusion time (15 minutes compared with 2 hours or more). Faster-than-indicated infusion rates of this bisphosphonate can result in reversible renal insufficiency. Once-yearly infusions of zoledronic acid have been shown to improve bone mineral density in osteopenic postmenopausal women. Ongoing trials are evaluating the ability of zoledronic acid to prevent bone loss associated with hormonal therapy and chemotherapy in breast and prostate cancers.

Clodronate is an oral bisphosphonate that has been shown to reduce the number of new bone metastases in women with breast cancer. A study of women with a primary diagnosis of breast cancer and microscopic evidence of tumor cells in bone marrow randomized to receive either clodronate, 1600 mg/d for 2 years, or placebo—in addition to standard adjuvant therapy—showed a significant reduction of both osseous metastases as well as mortality. Preliminary results of a larger study of women with operable breast cancer but no other specific high-risk features showed a reduction in the incidence of bone metastases but no difference in visceral metastases or survival. These observations suggest that bisphosphonates may be useful in a very high risk subset of women with primary breast cancer. Clodronate is a less potent bisphosphonate than pamidronate and is currently available only in Europe. A clinical trial testing clodronate in women with node-positive breast cancer is now being conducted in the United States. Zoledronic acid will be tested as adjuvant therapy in the United States as well in women with node-positive breast cancer to see if the results of the clodronate study can be reproduced.

Tretinoin is the first agent designed to target a specific fusion protein caused by a chromosome translocation. This oral agent induces differentiation and decreased proliferation without cytolysis of acute promyelocytic leukemia cells. Use of tretinoin combined with chemotherapy has been shown to improve disease-free and overall survival from this form of leukemia. Arsenic trioxide has been shown to induce remission in 70% of patients with relapsed or refractory acute promyelocytic leukemia (APL). It is indicated both for induction of remission and for consolidation in this high-risk group of patients.

Retinoids modulate the growth and differentiation of a variety of epithelial cells. Bexarotene, a retinoid that selectively activates the retinoid X receptor (RXR), is now FDA-approved to treat cutaneous T cell lymphomas such as mycosis fungoides. Targretin is also in clinical trials for use in a variety of advanced solid tumors including breast cancer.

Several recombinant growth factors have been shown to be effective in the treatment of malignancy. Recombinant alpha interferon has marked antitumor effects in hairy cell leukemia and chronic myelogenous leukemia, moderate effects in lymphomas, in the epidemic (AIDS-associated) form of Kaposi's sarcoma, in multiple myeloma, and as adjuvant therapy for malignant melanoma. Alpha interferon has some utility also in metastatic melanoma, renal cell carcinoma, and carcinoid syndrome. Patients with chronic myelogenous leukemia (CML) may benefit from alpha interferon given with low doses of the chemotherapeutic agent cytarabine and achieve both a hematologic and a cytogenetic remission. Patients with a cytogenic response to interferon and cytarabine (about 30% of treated patients) have a significantly longer survival than patients treated with standard oral chemotherapy. CML is unusual in that almost all cases are associated with a specific reciprocal chromosomal translocation resulting in activation of a tyrosine kinase that is critical to the pathogenesis of the disease. A novel and exciting oral agent, imatinib mesylate, specifically blocks this tyrosine kinase and is approved for clinical use in both early- and late-stage CML. The response in patients with chronic-phase CML was striking, with a 94% hematologic and an 83% cytogenetic response rate. These responses appear to be durable; progression-free survival at 12 months was significantly longer with imatinib mesylate than with the combination of interferon and cytarabine at 97% versus 80% in a recently presented phase III trial. Lower but significant response rates are seen in more advanced disease. The effect of imatinib mesylate on long-term disease control will require further follow-up of treated patients. Imatinib mesylate also inhibits two other tyrosine kinases, receptors encoded by c-kit and platelet derived growth factor (PDGF). Expression of the c-kit receptor is found in high frequency in a relatively uncommon tumor of the gastrointestinal tract, gastrointestinal stromal tumor (GIST). GISTs are highly resistant to chemotherapy, and there is no effective therapy for advanced disease. Imatinib mesylate has demonstrated significant activity in GISTs, with a 60% overall response rate. This drug is also being tested in conditions such as myelofibrosis, chronic myelomonocytic leukemia, prostate cancer, and glioblastoma that express PDGF.

The addition of alpha interferon to systemic chemotherapy for multiple myeloma appears to enhance the degree of cytoreduction achieved as compared with chemotherapy alone; however, toxicity is additive. Use of alpha interferon for myeloma following chemotherapy or autologous bone marrow transplant has prolonged remission duration, though overall survival is not altered. High-dose interferon for about 1 year in patients with malignant melanoma and lymph node metastases has been shown to improve disease-free and overall survival. Combinations of interferon alfa-2b and interleukin-2 given with standard chemotherapy for metastatic melanoma prolongs time to progression and survival (by a median of 2.7 months) but is associated with a significant increase in toxicity. Interleukin-2 treatment is effective in a subset of patients with advanced renal cell carcinoma.

Thalidomide, approved for treatment of lepromatous leprosy, has been found to induce significant responses in advanced and relapsed multiple myeloma. It is now being tested in many clinical trials, and the combination of thalidomide with dexamethasone results in enhanced response.

Newer experimental therapies are discussed briefly at the end of this chapter.

Hormonal therapy also plays an important role in cancer management. Hormonal therapy or ablation is important in treatment and palliation of breast and prostatic carcinoma, while added progestins are useful in suppression of endometrial carcinoma. Women with metastatic breast cancer who show objective improvement with hormonal therapy have tumors that contain cytoplasmic estrogen and progesterone receptors. The selective estrogen response modulator (SERM) tamoxifen has been shown to be effective in prolonging survival in both early-stage and late-stage breast cancer. Tamoxifen has both antiestrogen and proestrogen effects, resulting in side effects that include an increase in the risk of endometrial cancer and thrombosis. Newer SERMs without estrogen-like effects are being developed. Aromatase inhibitors (eg, anastrozole, letrozole) and inactivators (exemestane) block the peripheral conversion of adrenal androgens into estrogens and have been shown to be at least as effective as or more effective than tamoxifen as first-line therapy for metastatic hormone receptor-expressing breast cancer. Aromatase inhibitors are effective only in postmenopausal women and are now being tested in the adjuvant setting. Preliminary data from the ATAC trial comparing the results achieved with tamoxifen alone, with anastrazole alone, and with a combination of the two agents have been presented. At 2.5 years of follow-up, treatment with anastrazole improved disease-free survival and reduced the risk of new breast cancers in the opposite breast. Toxicities were modest. Longer-term follow-up and toxicity data—in particular the impact of aromatase inhibitors on bone mineral density and lipid profiles—must be awaited before this becomes the standard of care for postmenopausal women with early-stage breast cancer. For postmenopausal women who require hormone therapy but are intolerant to tamoxifen, the aromatase inhibitors are a reasonable alternative. A new pure antiestrogen, fulvestrant, has now been FDA-approved as second-line therapy for metastatic hormone receptor-positive breast cancer. This agent is unique in its class and is given by intramuscular injection once a month. Hormonal approaches are also available to treat prostate cancer, though androgen receptors remain difficult to measure. These include the use of estrogen therapy, gonadotropin-releasing hormone agonists (eg, leuprolide), and antiandrogens (eg, bicalutamide, flutamide). The use of leuprolide plus flutamide can be considered as an alternative to orchiectomy but also causes erectile dysfunction. High-dose ketoconazole has been used to rapidly suppress adrenal production of steroids in crises such as cord compression. Use of this agent requires hydrocortisone supplementation.

Table 40–4 sets forth the dosage schedules and toxicities of the most commonly used cancer chemotherapeutic agents. The dosage schedules given are for single-agent therapy. Combination therapy is used for most cancers. Hematologic or other toxicity may limit the therapeutic effectiveness of chemotherapy. It is possible to avoid the need for dose reductions or delay in therapy by using granulocyte colony-stimulating factor (G-CSF; filgrastim) or granulocyte-macrophage colony-stimulating factor (GM-CSF; sargramostim) to stimulate white blood cell recovery. A long-acting pegylated G-CSF (pegfilgrastim) is now FDA approved to reduce the incidence of neutropenic fever associated with chemotherapy. This agent can be given once for every 3-week chemotherapy cycle and in randomized trials was equivalent to 11 doses of filgrastim. Interleukin-11 can be used to reduce the need for delay or dose reductions due to thrombocytopenia; however, the usefulness of this cytokine is quite limited because of its ineffectiveness in severe thrombocytopenia and its toxicity, which includes significant edema.

Coiffier B et al: CHOP chemotherapy plus rituximab compared with CHOP alone in elderly patients with diffuse large-B-cell lymphoma. N Engl J Med 2002;346:280. [PMID: 11807147] (The addition of rituximab to CHOP chemotherapy in elderly patients prolonged survival without significant increase in toxicity.)

Childs R et al: Regression of metastatic renal-cell carcinoma after nonmyeloablative allogeneic peripheral-blood stem-cell

Table 40–4. Single-agent dosage and toxicity of anticancer drugs.

Drug	Dosage	Acute Toxicity	Delayed Toxicity
Alkylating agents			
Mechlorethamine	6–10 mg/m² IV every 3 weeks	Severe vesicant; severe nausea and vomiting	Moderate suppression of blood counts. Melphalan effect may be delayed 4–6 weeks. Excessive doses produce severe bone marrow suppression with leukopenia, thrombocytopenia, and bleeding. Alopecia and hemorrhagic cystitis occur with cyclophosphamide, while busulfan can cause hyperpigmentation, pulmonary fibrosis, and weakness (see text). Ifosfamide is always given with mesna to prevent cystitis. Acute leukemia may develop in 5–10% of patients receiving prolonged therapy with melphalan, mechlorethamine, or chlorambucil; all alkylators probably increase the risk of secondary malignancies with prolonged use. Most cause either temporary or permanent aspermia or amenorrhea.
Chlorambucil	0.1–0.2 mg/kg/d orally (6–12 mg/d) or 0.4 mg/kg pulse every 4 weeks	None	
Cyclophosphamide	100 mg/m²/d orally for 14 days; 400 mg/m² orally for 5 days; 1–1.5 g/m² IV every 3–4 weeks	Nausea and vomiting with higher doses	
Melphalan	0.25 mg/kg/d orally for 4 days every 6 weeks	None	
Busulfan	2–8 mg/d orally; 150–250 mg/course	None	
Estramustine	14 mg/kg orally in 3 or 4 divided doses	Nausea, vomiting, diarrhea	Thrombosis, thrombocytopenia, hypertension, gynecomastia, glucose intolerance, edema.
Carmustine (BCNU)	200 mg/m² IV every 6 weeks	Local irritant	Prolonged leukopenia and thrombocytopenia. Rarely hepatitis. Acute leukemia has been observed to occur in some patients receiving nitrosoureas. Nitrosoureas can cause delayed pulmonary fibrosis with prolonged use.
Lomustine (CCNU)	100–130 mg orally every 6–8 weeks	Nausea and vomiting	
Procarbazine	100 mg/m²/d orally for 14 days every 4 weeks	Nausea and vomiting	Bone marrow suppression, mental suppression, MAO inhibition, disulfiram-like effect.
Dacarbazine	250 mg/m²/d IV for 5 days every 3 weeks; 1500 mg/m² IV as single dose	Severe nausea and vomiting; anorexia	Bone marrow suppression; flu-like syndrome.
Cisplatin	50–100 mg/m² IV every 3 weeks; 20 mg/m² IV for 5 days every 4 weeks	Severe nausea and vomiting	Nephrotoxicity, mild otic and bone marrow toxicity, neurotoxicity.
Carboplatin	360 mg/m² IV every 4 weeks	Severe nausea and vomiting	Bone marrow suppression, prolonged anemia; same as cisplatin but milder.
Structural analogs or antimetabolites			
Methotrexate	2.5–5 mg/d orally; 20–25 mg IM twice weekly; high-dose: 500–1000 mg/m² IV every 2–3 weeks; 12–15 mg intrathecally every week for 4–6 doses	None	Bone marrow suppression, oral and gastrointestinal ulceration, acute renal failure; hepatotoxicity, rash, increased toxicity when effusions are present. **Note:** Citrovorum factor (leucovorin) rescue for doses over 100 mg/m².
Mercaptopurine	2.5 mg/kg/d orally; 100 mg/m²/d orally for 5 days for induction	None	Well tolerated. Larger doses cause bone marrow suppression.
Thioguanine	2 mg/kg/d orally; 100 mg/m²/d IV for 7 days for induction	Mild nausea, diarrhea	Well tolerated. Larger doses cause bone marrow suppression.
Fluorouracil	15 mg/kg/d IV for 3–5 days every 3 weeks; 15 mg/kg weekly as tolerated; 500–1000 mg/m² IV every 4 weeks	None	Nausea, diarrhea, oral and gastrointestinal ulceration, bone marrow suppression, dacryocystitis.

(continued)

Drug	Dosage	Acute Toxicity	Delayed Toxicity
Capecitabine	2500 mg/m² orally twice daily on days 1–14 every 3 weeks	Nausea, diarrhea	Hand and foot syndrome, mucositis.
Cytarabine	100–200 mg/m²/d for 5–10 days by continuous IV infusion; 2–3 g/m² IV every 12 hours for 3–7 days; 20 mg/m² SC daily in divided doses	High-dose: nausea, vomiting, diarrhea, anorexia	Nausea and vomiting; cystitis; severe bone marrow suppression; megaloblastosis; CNS toxicity with high-dose cytarabine.
Temozolamide	150 mg /m² orally for 5 days; repeat every 4 weeks	Headache, nausea, vomiting	Unknown
Androgens and androgen antagonists			
Testosterone propionate	100 mg IM 3 times weekly	None	Fluid retention, masculinization, leg cramps. Cholestatic jaundice in some patients receiving fluoxymesterone.
Fluoxymesterone	20–40 mg/d orally	None	
Flutamide	250 mg 3 times a day orally	None	Gynecomastia, hot flushes, decreased libido, mild gastrointestinal side effects, hepatotoxicity.
Bicalutamide	50 mg/d orally		
Nilutamide	300 mg/d orally for 30 days, then 150 mg/d		
Ethinyl estradiol	3 mg/d orally	None	Fluid retention, feminization, uterine bleeding, exacerbation of cardiovascular disease, painful gynecomastia, thromboembolic disease.
Selective estrogen receptor modulators			
Tamoxifen	20 mg/d orally in 2 divided doses	Transient flare of bone pain, nausea, hot flushes, joint aching	Thromboembolic disease, anovulation, endometrial cancer, cataracts; vaginal bleeding, acne.
Toremifene	60 mg/d orally		
Aromatase inhibitors			
Anastrozole	1 mg orally daily	Hot flushes, joint aching	Thromboembolic disease, vaginal bleeding.
Letrozole	2.5 mg/d orally		
Exemestane	25 mg/d orally		
Pure estrogen receptor antagonist			
Fulvestrant	250 mg IM once a month	Transient injection site reactions	Nausea, vomiting, constipation, diarrhea, abdominal pain, headache, back pain, hot flushes.
Progestins			
Megestrol acetate	40 mg orally 4 times daily	Hot flushes	Fluid retention; rare thrombosis, weight gain.
Medroxyprogesterone	100–200 mg/d orally; 200–600 mg orally twice weekly	None	
GnRH analogs			
Leuprolide	7.5 mg IM (depot) once a month or 22.5 mg every 3 months as depot injection	Local irritation, transient flare of symptoms	Hot flushes, decreased libido, impotence, gynecomastia, mild gastrointestinal side effects, nausea, diarrhea, fatigue.
Goserelin acetate	3.6 mg SC monthly or 10.8 mg every 3 months as depot injection		
Triptorelin pamoate	3.75 mg IM once a month (a 3-month depot formulation also exists)		

(*continued*)

Table 40–4. Single-agent dosage and toxicity of anticancer drugs. (continued)

Drug	Dosage	Acute Toxicity	Delayed Toxicity
Adrenocorticosteroids			
Prednisone	20–100 mg/d orally or 50–100 mg every other day orally with systemic chemotherapy	Alteration in mood	Fluid retention, hypertension, diabetes, increased susceptibility to infection, "moon facies," osteoporosis, electrolyte abnormalities, gastritis.
Dexamethasone	5–10 mg orally daily or twice daily		
Ketoconazole	400 mg orally 3 times daily	Acute nausea	Gynecomastia, hepatotoxicity
Biologic response modifiers			
Interferon alfa-2a Interferon alfa-2b	3–5 million units SC 3 times weekly or daily	Fever, chills, fatigue, anorexia	General malaise, weight loss, confusion, hypothyroidism, retinopathy, autoimmune disease
Aldesleukin (IL-2)	600,000 units/kg IV over 15 minutes every 8 hours for 14 doses, repeated after 9-day rest period. Some doses may be withheld or interrupted because of toxicity. **Caution:** High doses must be administered in an ICU setting by experienced personnel.	Hypotension, fever, chills, rigors, diarrhea, nausea, vomiting, pruritus; liver, kidney, and CNS toxicity; capillary leak (primarily at high doses), pruritic skin rash, infections (can be severe)	Hypoglycemia, anemia.
Peptide hormone inhibitor			
Octreotide acetate	100–600 μg/d SC in 2 divided doses	Local irritant; nausea and vomiting	Diarrhea, abdominal pain, hypoglycemia.
Natural products and miscellaneous agents			
Vinblastine	0.1–0.2 mg/kg or 6 mg/m^2 IV weekly	Mild nausea and vomiting; severe vesicant	Alopecia, peripheral neuropathy, bone marrow suppression, constipation, SIADH, areflexia.
Vincristine	1.5 mg/m^2 (maximum: 2 mg weekly)	Severe vesicant	Areflexia, muscle weakness, peripheral neuropathy, paralytic ileus, alopecia (see text), SIADH.
Vinorelbine	30 mg/m^2 IV weekly	Mild nausea and vomiting, fatigue, severe vesicant	Granulocytopenia, constipation, peripheral neuropathy, alopecia.
Paclitaxel (Taxol)	135 mg/m^2 by continuous infusion over 24 hours every 3 weeks	Hypersensitivity reaction (premedicate with diphenhydramine and dexamethasone), mild nausea and vomiting	Peripheral neuropathy, bone marrow suppression, fluid retention.
Docetaxel (Taxotere)	60–100 mg/m^2 IV every 3 weeks		
Dactinomycin	0.04 mg/kg IV weekly	Nausea and vomiting; severe vesicant	Alopecia, stomatitis, diarrhea, bone marrow suppression.
Daunorubicin	30–60 mg/m^2 daily IV for 3 days, or 30–60 mg/m^2 IV weekly	Nausea, fever, red urine (not hematuria); severe vesicant; acute cardiotoxicity	Alopecia, stomatitis, bone marrow suppression, late cardiotoxicity. Risk of cardiotoxicity increases with radiation, cyclophosphamide.
Idarubicin	12 mg/m^2 daily IV for 3 days		
Doxorubicin	60 mg/m^2 IV every 3 weeks to a maximum total dose of 550 mg/m^2		
Epirubicin	60–100 mg/m^2 IV every 3 weeks		

(continued)

Drug	Dosage	Acute Toxicity	Delayed Toxicity
Liposomal doxorubicin (Doxil)	20 mg/m^2 IV every 3 weeks	Mild nausea	Hand and foot syndrome; alopecia, stomatitis, and bone marrow suppression uncommon.
Liposomal daunorubicin (DaunoXome)	40 mg/m^2 IV every 2 weeks		
Etoposide	100 mg/m^2/d IV for 5 days or 50–150 mg/d orally	Nausea and vomiting; occasionally hypotension	Alopecia, bone marrow suppression, secondary leukemia.
Plicamycin (mithramycin)	25–50 μg/kg IV every other day for up to 8 doses	Nausea and vomiting	Thrombocytopenia, diarrhea, hepatotoxicity, nephrotoxicity, stomatitis.
Mitomycin	10–20 mg/m^2 every 6–8 weeks	Severe vesicant; nausea	Prolonged bone marrow suppression, rare hemolytic-uremic syndrome.
Mitoxantrone	12–15 mg/m^2/d IV for 3 days with cytarabine; 8–12 mg/m^2 IV every 3 weeks	Mild nausea and vomiting	Alopecia, mild mucositis, bone marrow suppression.
Bleomycin	Up to 15 units/m^2 IM, IV, or SC twice weekly to a total dose of 200 units/m^2	Allergic reactions, fever, hypotension	Fever, dermatitis, pulmonary fibrosis.
Hydroxyurea	500–1500 mg/d orally	Mild nausea and vomiting	Hyperpigmentation, bone marrow suppression.
Mitotane	6–12 g/d orally	Nausea and vomiting	Dermatitis, diarrhea, mental suppression, muscle tremors.
Fludarabine	25 mg/m^2/d IV for 5 days every 4 weeks	Nausea and vomiting	Bone marrow suppression, diarrhea, mild hepatotoxicity, immune suppression.
Cladribine (CdA)	0.09 mg/kg/d by continuous IV infusion for 7 days	Mild nausea, rash, fatigue	Bone marrow suppression, fever, immune suppression.
Topotecan	1.5 mg/m^2 IV daily for 5 days every 3 weeks	Nausea, vomiting, diarrhea, headache, dyspnea	Alopecia, bone marrow suppression.
Gemcitabine	1000 mg/m^2 every week up to 7 weeks, then 1 week off, then weekly for 3 out of 4 weeks	Nausea, vomiting, diarrhea, fever, dyspnea	Bone marrow suppression, rash, fluid retention, mouth sores, flu-like symptoms, paresthesias.
Irinotecan	125 mg/m^2 weekly for 4 weeks, then a 2-week rest, then repeat	Flushing, salivation, lacrimation, bradycardia, abdominal cramps, diarrhea	Bone marrow suppression, diarrhea.
Novel therapeutic agents			
Imatinib mesylate (STI571; Gleevec)	400–600 mg/d orally	Mild nausea	Myalgias, edema, bone marrow suppression, abnormal liver function tests.
Alemtuzumab (Campath-1H)	30 mg 3 times a week by SC injection for up to 12 weeks. (Use dose escalation to reduce infusion-related events.)	Severe infusion-related events, injection site irritation	Infections, short-term bone marrow suppression, autoimmune hemolytic anemia.
Gemtuzumab ozogamicin (Mylotarg)	9 mg/m^2 for 2 doses given 14 days apart	Infusion-related events	Profound bone marrow suppression.

(continued)

Table 40–4. Single-agent dosage and toxicity of anticancer drugs. (continued)

Drug	Dosage	Acute Toxicity	Delayed Toxicity
Tretinoin	45 mg/m^2 by mouth daily until remission or for 90 days	Retinoic acid syndrome (fever, dyspnea, pleural or pericardial effusion) must be treated emergently with dexamethasone.	Headache, dry skin, rash, flushing.
Arsenic trioxide	Induction: 0.15 mg/kg IV daily until remission; maximum 60 doses Consolidation: 0.15 mg/kgIV daily for 25 doses	Same as tretinoin	Nausea, vomiting, diarrhea, edema.
Trastuzumab (Herceptin)	Load: 4 mg/kg IV followed by 2 mg/kg weekly	Low-grade fever, chills, fatigue, constitutional symptoms with first infusion	Cardiac toxicity, especially when given with anthracyclines.
Denileukin diftitox (ONTAK)	9–10 µg/kg/d IV for 5 days every 21 days	Hypersensitivity type reactions with first infusion	Vascular leak syndrome, low albumin, increased risk of infections, diarrhea, rash.
Rituximab	375 mg/m^2 IV weekly for 4–8 doses	Hypersensitivity type reactions with first infusion; fever, tumor lysis syndrome (can be life-threatening)	Mild cytopenias, rare red cell aplasia or aplastic anemia, severe mucocutaneous reactions.
Ibritumomab tiuxetan (Zevalin)	0.3–0.4 mCi/kg (not to exceed 32 mCi); dosing must follow rituximab	Rituximab infusion reaction symptom complex	Prolonged and severe myelosuppression, nausea, vomiting, abdominal pain, arthralgias.
Targretin	300 mg/m^2/d/orally	Nausea	Hyperlipidemia, dry mouth, dry skin, constipation, leukopenia, edema.
Supportive agents Allopurinol	300–900 mg/d orally for prevention or relief of hyperuricemia	None	Rash, Stevens-Johnson syndrome; enhances effects and toxicity of mercaptopurine when used in combination.
Mesna	20% of ifosfamide dosage at the time of ifosfamide administration, then 4 and 8 hours after each dose of chemotherapy to prevent hemorrhagic cystitis	Nausea, vomiting, diarrhea	None.
Leucovorin	10 mg/m^2 every 6 hours IV or orally until serum methotrexate levels are below 5×10^{-8} mol/L with hydration and urinary alkalinization (about 72 hours)	None	Enhances toxic effects of fluorouracil.
Amifostine	910 mg/m^2 IV daily, 30 minutes prior to chemotherapy	Hypotension, nausea, vomiting, flushing	Decrease in serum calcium.
Dexrazoxane	10:1 ratio of anthracycline IV, before (within 30 minutes of) chemotherapy infusion	Pain on injection	Increased bone marrow suppression.

(continued)

Table 40–4. Single-agent dosage and toxicity of anticancer drugs. (continued)

Drug	Dosage	Acute Toxicity	Delayed Toxicity
Pilocarpine hydrochloride	5–10 mg orally 3 times daily	Sweating, headache, flushing; nausea, chills, rhinitis, dizziness, and urinary frequency at high dosage.	
Pamidronate	90 mg IV every month	Symptomatic hypoglycemia (rare), flare of bone pain, local irritation	None.
Zoledronic acid	4 mg IV every month		
Epoetin alfa (erythropoietin)	100–300 units/kg IV or SC 3 times a week	Skin irritation or pain at injection site	Hypertension, headache, seizures in patients on dialysis (rare).
Darbopoietin	200 μg SC q week[1]	Injection site pain	Hypertension, thromboses, headache, diarrhea.
Filgrastim (G-CSF)	5 μg/kg/d SC or IV	Mild to moderate bone pain, mild hypotension (rare), Irritation at injection sites (rare)	Bone pain, hypoxia
Pegfilgrastim	6 mg SC each 3-week cycle	Injection site reactions	Bone pain, hypoxia
Sargramostim (GM-CSF)	250 μg/kg/d as a 2-hour IV infusion (can be given SC)	Fluid retention, dyspnea, capillary leak (rare), supraventricular tachycardia (rare), mild to moderate bone pain, irritation at injection sites	
Neumega (IL-11)	50 μg/kg/d SC	Fluid retention, arrhythmias, headache, arthralgias, myalgias	Unknown.
Samarium-153 lexidronam (Sm-153 EDTMP)	1 mCi/kg IV as single dose	None	Hematopoietic suppression.
Strontium-89	4 mCi every 3 months IV	None	Hematopoietic suppression.

[1]Off label

transplantation. N Engl J Med 2000;343:750. [PMID: 10984562] (Nonmyeloablative allogeneic stem cell transplantation resulted in sustained regression of chemotherapy-resistant metastatic renal cell carcinoma.)

Diel IJ et al: Reduction in new metastases in breast cancer with adjuvant clodronate treatment. N Engl J Med 1998;339:357. [PMID: 9691101] (An oral bisphosphonate available in Europe given as adjuvant therapy to women with high-risk breast cancer significantly reduced the risk of developing metastatic breast cancer in bone and viscera at 3 years of follow-up.)

Druker BJ et al: Efficacy and safety of a specific inhibitor of the BCR-ABL tyrosine kinase in chronic myelogenous leukemia. N Engl J Med 2001;344:1031. [PMID: 11287972] (A specific inhibitor of the tyrosine kinase activated in CML is highly effective at inducing hematologic and cytogenetic remissions.)

Eton O et al: Sequential biochemotherapy versus chemotherapy for metastatic melanoma: results from a phase III randomized trial. J Clin Oncol 2002;20:2045. [PMID: 11956264] (Although survival from biochemotherapy was modestly

prolonged, treatment was associated with considerable toxicity.)

Johnston SR: Fulvestrant. Curr Opin Investig Drugs 2002;3:305. [PMID: 12020064]. (A review of this newly FDA approved pure anti-estrogen.)

Kemeny N et al: Hepatic arterial infusion of chemotherapy after resection of hepatic metastases from colorectal cancer. N Engl J Med 1999;341:2039. [PMID: 10615075] (In this randomized study, hepatic arterial infusion of floxuridine with intravenous fluorouracil following liver resection resulted in improved 2-year survival compared with patients receiving intravenous therapy alone.)

Messing EM et al: Immediate hormonal therapy compared with observation after radical prostatectomy and pelvic lymphadenectomy in men with node-positive prostate cancer. N Engl J Med 1999;341:1781. [PMID: 10588962] (Immediate antiandrogen therapy improves survival and reduces the risk of recurrence.)

Rajkumar SV et al: Thalidomide in the treatment of relapsed multiple myeloma. Mayo Clin Proc 2000;75:897. [PMID:

10994824] (A small study confirming the effectiveness of thalidomide in the treatment of multiple myeloma.)

Slamon DJ et al: Use of chemotherapy plus a monoclonal antibody against HER2 for metastatic breast cancer that overexpresses HER2. N Engl J Med 2001;344:783. [PMID: 11248153] (A monoclonal antibody against HER2 combined with chemotherapy prolongs survival in metastatic breast cancer overexpressing HER2.)

ADJUVANT CHEMOTHERAPY FOR MICROMETASTASES

One of the most important roles of cancer chemotherapy is as adjuvant therapy to eradicate or suppress minimal residual disease after local treatment with surgery or irradiation. Failure of local therapy to eradicate tumor is due principally to occult micrometastases of tumor stem cells outside the primary field. These distant micrometastases are more likely to be present in patients with positive lymph nodes at the time of surgery (eg, breast and prostate cancer), in patients with tumors known to have a propensity for early hematogenous spread (eg, osteogenic sarcoma, Wilms' tumor), and in patients with certain pathologic or molecular risk factors (eg, high proliferative index, vascular invasion, oncogene amplification). Given specific risk factors, the risk of recurrent or metastatic disease can be extremely high (> 80%). Only systemic therapy can adequately eradicate micrometastases. Chemotherapeutic regimens that have been shown to be effective in inducing regression of advanced cancers may be curative when combined with surgery for high-risk "early" cancer.

More data are now available to support the use of adjuvant therapy in several neoplasms. Prolongation of survival has been shown for women with breast cancer and negative or positive axillary lymph nodes (stages I, II, and III) from combination chemotherapy following surgical resection; several regimens are used. Node-negative patients are treated with CMF (cyclophosphamide, methotrexate, and fluorouracil), whereas high-risk, node-positive patients are treated with regimens that include anthracyclines (eg, doxorubicin, epirubicin) and in some cases taxanes as well. The SERM tamoxifen and other agents that block the effect of estrogen on the breast cancer cell are used routinely either with or without antecedent chemotherapy if receptors for estrogen or progesterone are present (see preceding section on hormonal therapy). The main challenge in treating women with node-negative (stage I) breast cancer is to identify prognostic factors that distinguish patients at higher risk who are more likely to benefit from adjuvant therapy. Amplification of the HER-2/*neu* oncogene clearly correlates with a poorer prognosis, and these patients appear to have a marked benefit from adjuvant chemotherapy containing anthracyclines. In contrast, patients whose cancers express receptors for estrogen or progesterone have a better prognosis than those whose tumors are hormone receptor-negative. Current research is focusing on the identification of additional and more specific risk factors early in diagnosis that can aid in prognosis and treatment decisions. A study used cytokeratin staining of bone marrow aspirates in women with newly diagnosed breast cancer found a 36% incidence of occult marrow metastases that correlated with a fourfold increased risk of death from breast cancer. This result must be confirmed before it can be used in clinical practice to direct therapy. The goal is to identify patients with high-risk features at the time of diagnosis with localized disease and provide risk-directed (and effective) therapy.

Adjuvant chemotherapy with fluorouracil plus leucovorin is indicated in Dukes B and C (node-positive) colon cancer and has been shown to reduce the risk of cancer recurrence. Many other cancers may be cured with adjuvant chemotherapy, including cancers of the ovary and testes, malignant melanoma, and choriocarcinoma. Still other malignancies are cured when radiation and chemotherapy are used concurrently as described in the section on radiation therapy.

Other tumors that have been shown to respond to adjuvant therapy include gastric, esophageal, and bladder cancers, prostate cancer, osteogenic sarcoma, ovarian cancer, and malignant melanoma. Adjuvant therapy remains investigational for a number of common tumors, including non-small-cell lung cancer and pancreatic cancer. Chemotherapy is given with curative intent often after surgical remission in testicular cancer, non-Hodgkin's lymphoma, and Hodgkin's lymphoma.

Although adjuvant therapy has been shown to reduce the rate of recurrence for some cancers, there is still a high failure rate (up to 60–80% in some high-risk breast cancer despite adjuvant therapy). In most cases, tumor recurrence signifies incurability. The evidence for a dose-response effect of adjuvant chemotherapy for most cancers remains unclear. Although high-dose chemotherapy with either bone marrow or peripheral blood stem cell rescue is curative for some otherwise incurable patients with testicular cancer, efficacy data are lacking for other solid tumors. Research has largely focused on very high doses of chemotherapy for high-risk and metastatic breast cancer; this has translated into thousands of transplants and several randomized clinical trials. Phase II data suggested clinical benefit to this toxic and expensive procedure, but the studies were biased by inappropriate historical controls, rigorous selection criteria, and short follow-up. To date, all randomized studies have failed to show any benefit to high-dose chemotherapy with stem cell rescue compared with intermediate or standard-dose chemotherapy. Two studies performed in South Africa appeared encouraging; however, an onsite review revealed significant scientific misconduct that invalidated all results. At present, high-dose chemotherapy for breast cancer should be performed only in the setting of a properly designed clinical trial; it is still experimental therapy. Bone marrow transplantation for other malignancies is covered in more detail in Chapter 13.

Braun S et al: Cytokeratin positive cells in the bone marrow and survival of patients with stage I, II or III breast cancer. N Engl J Med 2000;342:525. [PMID: 10684910] (Cytokeratin staining of bone marrow aspirates at the time of diagnosis identifies occult metastases in 36% of patients and is unrelated to nodal status. Positive staining correlates with a four-fold increases risk of death from breast cancer.)

Colleoni M et al: Early start of adjuvant chemotherapy may improve treatment outcome for premenopausal breast cancer patients with tumors not expressing estrogen receptors. J Clin Oncol 2000;18:584. [PMID: 10653873] (These data suggest that higher-risk women who start chemotherapy within 20 days of surgery may have improved disease-free survival compared with women who start later.)

Kerr DJ et al: Novel therapeutic strategies for colorectal cancer. Hosp Med 1998;59:617. [PMID: 9829054] (A review of current and experimental treatment for this common cancer.)

Mamounas E et al: Comparative efficacy of adjuvant chemotherapy in patients with Dukes' B versus Dukes' C colon cancer: results from four national surgical adjuvant breast and bowel project adjuvant studies (C-01, C-02, C-03, C-04). J Clin Oncol 1999;27:1349. [PMID: 10334518] (Adjuvant therapy appears to be effective in Dukes B as well as in Dukes C colon cancer; higher risk patients with Dukes B cancer should be identified.)

Stadtmauer EA et al: Conventional-dose chemotherapy compared with high-dose chemotherapy plus autologous hematopoietic stem-cell transplantation for metastatic breast cancer. Philadelphia Bone Marrow Transplant Group. N Engl J Med 2000;342:1069. [PMID: 10760307] (High-dose chemotherapy was no better than conventional chemotherapy in patients with chemotherapy-responsive metastatic breast cancer.)

Weiss R et al: High-dose chemotherapy for high-risk primary breast cancer: an on-site review of the Bezwoda study. Lancet 2000;355:999.[PMID: 10768448] (An on-site review uncovered significant scientific misconduct in this landmark study.)

TOXICITY & DOSE MODIFICATION OF CHEMOTHERAPEUTIC AGENTS

A number of cancer chemotherapeutic agents have cytotoxic effects on rapidly proliferating normal cells in bone marrow, mucosa, and skin. Still other drugs such as the vinca alkaloids and taxanes produce neuropathy, and hormones often have psychologic as well as physical effects. Acute and chronic toxicities of various drugs used to treat cancer are summarized in Table 40–4. Appropriate dose modification may minimize these side effects, so that therapy can be continued with relative safety.

Bone Marrow Toxicity

Depression of bone marrow is usually the most serious limiting toxicity of cancer chemotherapy. Autologous bone marrow or peripheral blood stem cell transplantation or rescue can reduce the myelosuppressive toxicity of high-dose chemotherapy; however, cost and toxicity limit its general use. Growth factors that stimulate myeloid proliferation (eg, granulocyte colony-stimulating factor [G-CSF; filgrastim], the longer acting peg-filgrastim, and granulocyte macrophage stimulating factor [GM-CSF]; sargramostim) or erythroid proliferation (epoetin alfa [erythropoietin]) are now used to ameliorate bone marrow toxicity. G-CSF and GM-CSF have been shown to shorten the period of neutropenia following both standard and high-dose chemotherapy. Mucosal toxicity is reduced as well. The myeloid growth factors are also used to stimulate circulation of stem cells in the peripheral blood either at steady state or during white blood cell recovery following myelosuppressive chemotherapy. These cells are then harvested using an apheresis machine and frozen for later use. When stimulated peripheral blood stem cells are used instead of or in conjunction with bone marrow for autologous transplantation following high-dose chemotherapy and radiotherapy, recovery of both neutrophils and platelets may be hastened by as much as 7–10 days as opposed to the use of bone marrow alone. Recombinant growth factors are expensive and must be used judiciously. Published standard practice guidelines are referenced at the end of this section.

Epoetin alfa (erythropoietin) has been shown to improve anemia associated with malignancy. Patients must have adequate iron stores to respond to this agent, and even patients with marrow infiltration with tumor may benefit. Higher doses are necessary for patients with cancer than for patients with renal failure (100–150 units/kg compared with 50 units/kg). It is useful to check the level of erythropoietin before instituting therapy. Very high levels ($\geq$ 500 ng/mL) predict a poor response. Epoetin alfa may be given as a subcutaneous injection once a week. This dosage schedule is as effective as the traditional three times a week dosing and is much more convenient. For anemia related to cancer chemotherapy or marrow infiltration, a dose of 40,000 units a week is used. Novel erythropoiesis-stimulating protein (NESP; darbepoetin alfa) is now approved to treat anemia associate with renal failure. Its main advantage over epoetin alfa is its longer half-life, which it is hoped will allow for dosing once every 3 weeks to once every 4 weeks. Clinical trials in cancer treatment are ongoing.

Thrombocytopenia remains a problem with high doses of or prolonged exposure to chemotherapeutic agents and may limit therapy. Oprelvekin (recombinant interleukin-11) may be used in treating and preventing chemotherapy-induced thrombocytopenia. It is less effective in treating very severe thrombocytopenia, and its use can be associated with significant fluid retention, arrhythmias, and congestive heart failure.

Commonly used short-acting drugs that affect the bone marrow are the alkylating agents (eg, cyclophosphamide, melphalan, chlorambucil), procarbazine, mercaptopurine, methotrexate, vinblastine, fluorouracil, dactinomycin, anthracyclines, and taxanes. In general, it is preferable to use alkylating agents in intensive "pulse" courses every 3–4 weeks rather than to administer the drugs in continuous daily schedules. This allows for complete hematologic (and immunologic) recovery between courses rather than continuously suppressing the bone marrow with a cytotoxic agent. Pulse therapy reduces side effects to some degree but does not reduce therapeutic efficacy. The standard dosage schedules for tumor response often induce bone marrow suppression. Continuing some drugs in the face of falling blood counts may result in severe bone marrow aplasia with pancytopenia, bleeding, or infection. Simple guidelines for treatment and follow-up can usually prevent this complication.

In patients with normal blood counts as well as normal liver and kidney function, drugs should be started in full dosages. Bone marrow toxicity is cumulative over time, and this must be anticipated during follow-up. Cumulative toxicity from long-term chemotherapy can require cessation of therapy or reduction in dose. Patients with bone marrow involvement may tolerate chemotherapy poorly initially, with improved counts on future cycles as the tumor burden is reduced.

Drug dosage may be modified as a function of the peripheral white blood count or platelet count (or both). These modifications assume that the blood counts are checked shortly before the next course of chemotherapy is to be administered. Dosage modifications are used primarily for repeated courses of oral alkylator or antimetabolite therapy but should be avoided if treatment is given with curative intent. A scheme for dosage modification is presented in Table 40–5. Alternatively, the interval between drug courses can be lengthened, thereby permitting more complete hematologic recovery and repetition of full-dose chemotherapy. Both dosage modification and delay of chemotherapy limit the efficacy of treatment.

Ozer H et al: 2000 update of recommendations for the use of hematopoietic colony-stimulating factors: evidence-based, clinical practice guidelines. J Clin Oncol 2000;18:3558. [PMID: 11032599] (A summary of background data and guidelines.)

Chemotherapy-Induced Nausea & Vomiting

A number of cytotoxic anticancer drugs induce nausea and vomiting. In general, these symptoms are thought to originate in the central nervous system rather than

Table 40–5. A common scheme for dose modification of cancer chemotherapeutic agents.[1]

Granulocyte Count	Platelet Count	Suggested Dosage (% of Full Dose)
> 2000/μL	> 100,000/μL	100%
1000–2000/μL	75,000–100,000/μL	50%
< 1000/μL	< 50,000/μL	0%

[1]In general, dose modification should be avoided to maintain therapeutic efficacy. The use of myeloid growth factors or a delay in the start of the next cycle of chemotherapy is usually effective.

peripherally. Parenteral administration of agents such as doxorubicin, etoposide, or cyclophosphamide is usually associated with mild to moderate nausea and vomiting, whereas nitrosoureas, dacarbazine, and particularly cisplatin cause more severe symptoms. Combination chemotherapy can also cause severe symptoms. Antiemetics clearly reduce and often eliminate nausea and vomiting associated with these drugs and are especially useful in conjunction with cisplatin.

5-Hydroxytryptamine-3 receptor antagonists (ondansetron, granisetron, dolasetron) have now replaced other drugs as the primary agents for the prevention and treatment of emesis from chemotherapy. These drugs are serotonin receptor-blocking agents with few side effects. They are also effective against radiation-induced and postanesthetic emesis and can be useful in the treatment of delayed and refractory nausea and vomiting following chemotherapy. Ondansetron is administered by the parenteral route as a single dose of 32 mg prior to chemotherapy and may be repeated every 24 hours, or it may be given orally at a dose of 8 mg every 8 hours. Lower parenteral doses may be just as effective. Granisetron is given as a single dose of 10 μg/kg intravenously 30 minutes before chemotherapy, or orally at a dose of 1–2 mg per day. The dose of dolasetron is 1.8 mg/kg intravenously or 100–200 mg orally before chemotherapy. The serotonin receptor-blocking agents are more effective when given in conjunction with dexamethasone. Dexamethasone has antiemetic effects when administered at a dosage of 6–10 mg either as a single dose prior to—or both prior to and every 6 hours following—the administration of chemotherapy for two to four total doses.

Substance P appears to have a causative role in chemotherapy-induced nausea. Its biologic actions are mediated through the neurokinin-1 receptor. A novel agent, oral trisubstituted morpholine acetal (L-754,030), is a neurokinin-1 receptor antagonist that is effective in preventing chemotherapy-induced nausea. A randomized trial comparing granisetron and dexamethasone with or without this agent showed a significant reduction in acute emesis following chemotherapy with cisplatin with the three-drug combination. In addition, L-754,030 was effective at preventing delayed emesis from cisplatin.

Other active agents often used in combination as premedication for less emetogenic chemotherapy or as treatment for delayed nausea and vomiting include prochlorperazine, metoclopramide, thiethylperazine, and lorazepam. The phenothiazines (prochlorperazine, thiethylperazine) and metoclopramide can induce extrapyramidal side effects; their incidence is increased with prolonged use. Prochlorperazine is given at a dose of 10 mg orally or intravenously every 6–8 hours. The total dose given over 24 hours should not exceed 40 mg. A 25 mg suppository may be used for patients who are too nauseated to swallow pills without inducing further emesis. Metoclopramide is given at a dose of 10–20 mg orally or intravenously before and then every 6 hours after chemotherapy, usually in combination with dexamethasone. Lorazepam has both antiemetic and sedative effects and is administered at a dose of 0.5–1 mg every 4–6 hours by the sublingual or oral route, making it particularly useful in the outpatient setting. Older patients may experience intolerable psychologic side effects.

Combinations of antiemetics are usually more effective than maximal doses of any one agent to block severe emesis. A typical antiemetic regimen might include ondansetron combined with sublingual lorazepam or prochlorperazine and dexamethasone. For less emetogenic regimens, the serotonin antagonists can be reserved for failure to control nausea with less expensive regimens.

Dronabinol (Δ^9-tetrahydrocannabinol) is effective in some patients at a dose of 5 mg/m^2 prior to and then every 2–4 hours following chemotherapy for a total of four to six doses a day. Dronabinol may cause undesirable side effects such as dysphoria, and it is available only for oral administration. A patient receiving antiemetics (eg, lorazepam, prochlorperazine, metoclopramide) along with chemotherapy on an outpatient basis must be escorted to and from the clinic, since the antiemetics often induce marked sedation and transient impairment of balance and reflexes. Antiemetics are more effective when given prophylactically. Therefore, regular dosing of an agent such as lorazepam or prochlorperazine is recommended after chemotherapy until the emetogenic effects have dissipated. This is dependent on the patient as well as on the type of chemotherapy administered. One problem with all combinations of antiemetic agents is the development of tachyphylaxis over 4–5 days with continuing highly emetogenic chemotherapy. This limits the effectiveness of any regimen. Acute mucosal injury to the upper gastrointestinal tract may complicate nausea associated with chemotherapy or delayed nausea and vomiting. Agents that reduce acid secretion (eg, omeprazole, ranitidine) can be useful adjunctive therapy to the antinausea regimen.

Hesketh PJ et al: Proposal for classifying the acute emetogenicity of cancer chemotherapy. J Clin Oncol 1997;15:103. [PMID: 8996130] (A guide to the emetogenic potential of chemotherapeutic agents.)

Navari RM et al: Reduction of cisplatin-induced emesis by a selective neurokinin-1-receptor antagonist. L-754,030 Antiemetic Trials Group. N Engl J Med 1999;340:190. [PMID: 9917226] (A novel agent significantly reduces delayed emesis and acute emesis from cisplatin chemotherapy in combination with granisetron and dexamethasone.)

Roila F et al: The efficacy and cost-effectiveness of various antiemetic regimens. Curr Opin Oncol 1998;10:310. [PMID: 9702398] (A review of cost and combinations of antiemetic drugs.)

Sartori S et al: Randomized trial of omeprazole or ranitidine versus placebo in the prevention of chemotherapy-induced gastroduodenal injury. J Clin Oncol 2000;18:463. [PMID: 10356831] (Omeprazole is effective in preventing chemotherapy-induced gastroduodenal injury. Both omeprazole and ranitidine reduce the frequency of ulcers and upper gastrointestinal symptoms.)

Gastrointestinal & Skin Toxicity

Chemotherapeutic agents generally act on rapidly proliferating cells, resulting in damage to the normal cells lining the gastrointestinal tract and mouth. This can result in mouth and throat sores, chronic nausea, and diarrhea. Erythema is an early sign of mucosal toxicity. Ulcerations in the mouth due to chemotherapy must be carefully evaluated for the presence of herpes simplex virus. Herpes ulcerations are common in immunosuppressed cancer patients and may be treated with acyclovir or other antiviral agents.. Throat or esophageal pain may be due to either chemotherapy or infection from fungal or viral pathogens. These infections are more common in patients receiving steroids with their chemotherapy regimens. Chemotherapy should be delayed or withheld to allow healing or treatment of infection.

Adequate mouth care with antimicrobial mouthwashes and attention to dental hygiene are essential and may prevent severe toxicity. Common mouthwashes include the microbicidal oral rinse chlorhexidine and a mixture of salt and bicarbonate of soda in warm water, which aids in debridement of dead mucosa. A prophylactic antifungal mouthwash such as nystatin oral suspension may also be used. Certain chemotherapeutic agents can also cause toxicity to the skin, particularly the palms and soles and the skin in the axilla and groin. Common findings are erythema and hyperpigmentation, which may be painful or pruritic. Blistering is uncommon but can occur if chemotherapy is continued after the early signs of skin irritation occur. Toxicities to the gastrointestinal tract and skin may be more serious and harder to treat than bone marrow suppression. Patients receiving drugs that cause these side effects should be monitored closely.

Radiation therapy may cause xerostomia, which can lead to difficulty in swallowing, discomfort, and gum disease. Pilocarpine hydrochloride, 5–10 mg orally three times a day, can relieve symptoms of dry mouth but must be used regularly. Amifostine, a thiol-containing compound that reduces cisplatin-induced nephrotoxicity, has also been shown to reduce acute and chronic xerostomia in patients with head and neck cancers receiving radiation therapy. The dose of amifostine is 200 mg/m^2 intravenously daily 15–30 minutes before irradiation. Side effects include nausea and vomiting.

Radiation therapy to areas that include the gastrointestinal tract can cause diarrhea that resolves gradually with cessation of therapy and healing of normal cells. Topical butyrate appears to improve symptoms of acute radiation proctitis following radiation therapy for malignant pelvic disease. The sodium butyrate is given per rectum. Skin toxicity in the form of erythema and occasionally blistering and exfoliation of the area receiving radiation can also occur. Severe skin toxicity requires holding the radiation doses; the affected area is treated with local application of emollients.

Miscellaneous Drug-Specific Toxicities

The toxicities of individual drugs have been summarized in Table 40–4. Several of these warrant additional mention, since they occur with commonly administered agents, and special preventive measures are often indicated.

A. HEMORRHAGIC CYSTITIS INDUCED BY CYCLOPHOSPHAMIDE OR IFOSFAMIDE

Metabolic products of cyclophosphamide that retain cytotoxic activity are excreted into the urine. Some patients appear to metabolize more of the drug to these active excretory products. If their urine is concentrated, the toxic metabolite may cause severe bladder damage. Patients receiving cyclophosphamide must be advised to maintain a high fluid intake. Early symptoms of bladder toxicity include dysuria and frequency despite the absence of bacteriuria. If microscopic hematuria develops, it is advisable to stop the drug temporarily or switch to a different alkylating agent, increase fluid intake, and administer a urinary analgesic such as phenazopyridine. With severe cystitis, large segments of bladder mucosa may be shed and the patient may have prolonged gross hematuria. Such patients should be observed for signs of urinary obstruction and may require cystoscopy for removal of obstructing blood clots. The risk of developing hemorrhagic cystitis is dose-related and more common in patients who take the drug orally over a prolonged period of time. The cyclophosphamide analog ifosfamide or very high doses of cyclophosphamide can cause severe hemorrhagic cystitis when either is used alone. However, when they are used in conjunction with the neutralizing agent mesna, bladder toxicity can usually be prevented. Mesna is given with the chemotherapeutic agent and in a series of doses over the following 24 hours. Continuous bladder irrigation with 0.9% saline has been used with high-dose cyclophosphamide to prevent hemorrhagic cystitis. This appears to be less effective than mesna and may result in complications from Foley catheter trauma to the urethra, so it is used infrequently in high-risk situations—often in combination with mesna.

B. NEUROPATHY INDUCED BY VINCRISTINE AND OTHER AGENTS

Neuropathy is a toxic side effect that is peculiar to the vinca alkaloid drugs, especially vincristine. A primarily sensory peripheral neuropathy is also commonly caused by two of the newer anticancer therapeutic agents, paclitaxel and vinorelbine. The peripheral neuropathy associated with vincristine can be sensory, motor, autonomic, or a combination of these effects. In its mildest form, it consists of paresthesias of the fingers and toes. Occasional patients develop acute jaw or throat pain after vincristine therapy. This may be a form of trigeminal or glossopharyngeal neuralgia. With continued vincristine therapy, the paresthesias may extend to the proximal interphalangeal joints, hy-

poreflexia can appear in the lower extremities, and weakness may develop in the quadriceps muscle group. At this point, it is wise to discontinue vincristine therapy until the neuropathy has subsided. A useful means of judging whether peripheral motor neuropathy is severe enough to warrant stopping treatment is to have the patient attempt to do deep knee bends or rise from a chair without using the arm muscles. In general, the neuropathy associated with paclitaxel and vinorelbine is mild, well-tolerated, and both dose-sensitive and schedule-sensitive. More frequent dosing of smaller amounts of chemotherapy can reduce this side effect; the neuropathy significantly improves when the chemotherapy is stopped.

Constipation is the most common symptom of autonomic neuropathy associated with vincristine therapy. Patients receiving vincristine should be started on stool softeners and mild cathartics when therapy is begun; otherwise, severe impaction may result as a consequence of an atonic bowel. More serious autonomic involvement can lead to acute intestinal ileus with signs indistinguishable from those of an acute abdomen.

Bladder neuropathies are uncommon but may be severe. Paralytic ileus and bladder atony are absolute contraindications to continued vincristine therapy. The majority of symptoms from vincristine are mild and resolve slowly after therapy has been completed. Docetaxel, cisplatin, carboplatin, and topotecan can also cause peripheral neuropathy, though in general symptoms improve gradually after treatment is stopped.

C. METHOTREXATE TOXICITY AND LEUCOVORIN RESCUE

In addition to standard uses of methotrexate for cancer chemotherapy, this drug is also used in very high doses that could lead to fatal bone marrow toxicity if given without an antidote. High-dose methotrexate therapy with leucovorin rescue is routinely used to treat osteogenic sarcoma, acute lymphocytic leukemia, and some cases of non-Hodgkin's lymphoma, and primary lymphoma of the central nervous system.

The bone marrow and mucosal toxicity of methotrexate can be prevented by early administration of leucovorin (folinic acid). Serum levels of methotrexate are usually monitored and doses of leucovorin adjusted accordingly. Rescue is required for methotrexate doses over 80 mg/m^2 and is usually begun within 4 hours after completing treatment. Up to 100 mg/m^2 of leucovorin is given initially every 6 hours, with further doses adjusted for the serum methotrexate level. Rescue is usually continued orally for 3 days or longer until the serum methotrexate level is below 0.05 μmol/L. Asparaginase can be given as rescue for methotrexate in the treatment of lymphoblastic leukemia. If an overdose of methotrexate is administered accidentally, leucovorin therapy should be initiated as soon as possible, preferably within 1 hour. Intravenous infusion should be employed for larger overdosages to ensure adequate drug delivery. It is generally advisable to give leucovorin repeatedly in this situation.

Vigorous hydration and bicarbonate loading also appear to be important in preventing crystallization of high-dose methotrexate in the renal tubular epithelium. Serum creatinine is determined before beginning therapy and daily thereafter, since methotrexate excretion is slowed by renal insufficiency and toxicity will be enhanced. In high doses, methotrexate can itself cause renal injury. Methotrexate doses are reduced in renal insufficiency. Concomitant use of certain drugs will slow methotrexate excretion, and they are avoided during therapy. These drugs include aspirin, NSAIDs, penicillins, sulfonamides, and probenecid.

D. BUSULFAN TOXICITY

The alkylating agent busulfan, occasionally used for the treatment of myeloproliferative diseases, has curious delayed toxicities, including increased skin pigmentation, a wasting syndrome similar to that seen in adrenal insufficiency, and progressive pulmonary fibrosis. Patients who develop either of the latter two problems should be switched to a different drug (eg, melphalan) when further therapy is needed. The pigmentary changes are innocuous and will usually regress slowly after treatment is discontinued. Long-term treatment with busulfan also results in an increased risk of secondary leukemias.

E. BLEOMYCIN TOXICITY

This antibiotic is used to treat squamous cell carcinoma, Hodgkin's disease, non-Hodgkin's lymphoma, and testicular cancer. Bleomycin can produce edema of the interphalangeal joints and hardening of the palmar and plantar skin. More serious toxicities include an anaphylactic or serum sickness-like reaction and a potentially fatal pulmonary fibrotic reaction (seen especially in elderly patients receiving a total dose of over 300 units). If a nonproductive cough, dyspnea, and pulmonary infiltrates develop, the drug is discontinued, and high-dose corticosteroids are instituted as well as empirical antibiotics pending cultures. Fever alone or with chills is an occasional complication of bleomycin treatment and is not an absolute contraindication to continued treatment. The fever may be avoided by hydrocortisone administration just prior to the injection. Fever alone is not predictive of pulmonary toxicity. About 1% of patients (especially those with lymphoma) may have a severe or even fatal hypotensive reaction after the initial dose of bleomycin. In order to identify and treat such patients, it is wise to administer a test dose of 5 units of bleomycin first and to have adequate monitoring and emergency facilities available. Patients exhibiting a hypotensive reaction should not receive further bleomycin therapy.

F. ANTHRACYCLINE-INDUCED CARDIOMYOPATHY

The anthracycline antibiotics doxorubicin, daunomycin, and idarubicin and the similar drug mitox-antrone both have acute and delayed cardiac toxicity. The problem is greater with doxorubicin because it has a major role and is used in repeated doses in the treatment of sarcomas, breast cancer, lymphomas, acute leukemia, and certain other solid tumors. Studies of left ventricular function and endomyocardial biopsies indicate that changes in cardiac dynamics occur in most patients by the time they have received 300 mg/m^2 of doxorubicin. The *multiple-gated* ("MUGA") radionuclide cardiac scan is the most reproducible noninvasive test for assessing toxicity. Patients should not receive a total dose in excess of 450 mg/m^2, and 1–10% of patients who receive this dose develop cardiomyopathy. Doxorubicin should not be used in patients with intrinsic cardiac disease. Prior chest or mediastinal radiotherapy increases the risk of doxorubicin heart disease at lower total doses. The appearance of a high resting pulse may herald the appearance of cardiac toxicity. Unfortunately, the toxicity may be irreversible at dosage levels above 550 mg/m^2. At lower doses (eg, 350 mg/m^2), the symptoms and signs of cardiac failure generally respond well to medical therapy and cessation of doxorubicin.

Laboratory studies suggest that cardiac toxicity may be due to a mechanism involving the formation of intracellular free radicals in cardiac muscle. Pretreatment with dexrazoxane, an iron chelator that decreases free radical formation, appears to protect the myocardium from anthracycline-induced injury but may also reduce the anticancer efficacy of the anthracycline. Dexrazoxane is useful for the prevention of cardiomyopathy in women with metastatic breast cancer receiving cumulative doxorubicin doses > 300 mg/m^2. Liposomally encapsulated doxorubicin and daunorubicin have been FDA-approved and appear to have minimal cardiac toxicity. Their main use to date has been to treat Kaposi's sarcoma, but they are also effective in the treatment of other anthracycline-sensitive cancers. The anthracycline analog idarubicin has shown efficacy against acute nonlymphocytic leukemia and breast cancer when used in combination with other agents. Idarubicin appears to have a similar potential for causing cardiotoxicity when compared with other anthracyclines, though a maximum lifetime dosage recommendation has not been made. Epirubicin, an anthracycline with lower cardiac toxicity than doxorubicin (but similar gastrointestinal toxicity) is approved for the treatment of breast cancer. A dose of up to 900 mg/m^2 can be tolerated without significant cardiac toxicity. There are no data comparing the effects of doxorubicin with epirubicin, which has been studied primarily in Europe and Canada.

G. CISPLATIN NEPHROTOXICITY AND NEUROTOXICITY

Cisplatin is effective in the treatment of testicular, bladder, and ovarian cancer as well as in several other types of tumor. Nausea and vomiting are common, but nephrotoxicity and neurotoxicity are more serious. Vigorous hydration with or without mannitol diuresis may substantially reduce nephrotoxicity. Renal function must be carefully monitored during cisplatin therapy, as should serum magnesium, which may fall during therapy with this agent. Ototoxicity is a potentially serious neurotoxicity that can result in deafness. Other manifestations include peripheral neuropathy of mixed sensorimotor type that may be associated with painful paresthesias. The neurotoxicity of this drug is delayed and is more common after a total dose of 300 mg/m^2. The second-generation platinum analog carboplatin has been shown to be as effective as cisplatin in ovarian cancer. Carboplatin is less nephrotoxic and causes less severe nausea or vomiting, but it does induce significant myelosuppression along with neurotoxicity. Amifostine, an organic thiophosphate initially developed as a radioprotective agent, is effective in preventing renal toxicity from cisplatin. It is approved to reduce cumulative renal toxicity associated with repeat administration of cisplatin in advanced ovarian cancer. In addition, amifostine may reduce chemotherapy-induced hematologic toxicity and neurotoxicity. Glutathione also appears to be a promising agent in preventing cisplatin neurotoxicity. Glutathione has been given at a dose of 1.5 g/m^2 intravenously before cisplatin administration, then at a dose of 600 mg by intramuscular injection on days 2–5. These supportive measures do not appear to reduce the therapeutic effectiveness of platinum agents.

H. ALPHA INTERFERON TOXICITIES

While alpha interferon is generally tolerated in the standard doses listed in Table 40–4, it has significant toxicity with the higher doses required to treat chronic myelogenous leukemia and malignant melanoma and is more toxic in elderly patients. Even standard doses may be intolerable to some patients. Fever and chills are initial side effects but are infrequent after continued treatment. These symptoms may be ameliorated or prevented by premedication with acetaminophen and bedtime dosing. However, anorexia, fatigue, and weight loss can be cumulative and with time may become severe. These symptoms may be dose- or treatment-limiting. Thirty percent or more of patients are intolerant of interferon therapy even at low doses. In some patients, central nervous system symptoms develop, usually manifested as confusion or somnolence. Interferon causes a reduction in blood counts, but this is usually not clinically important and is part of the desired effect in the treatment of chronic myelogenous leukemia. Interferon-induced side effects are sometimes confused with the symptoms of progressive cancer but usually clear within 1–2 weeks following cessation of interferon therapy.

Borden EC et al: A perspective on the clinical effectiveness and tolerance of interferon-alpha. Semin Oncol 1998;25:3. [PMID: 9482534]

Brizel DM et al: Phase III randomized trial of amifostine as a radioprotector in head and neck cancer. J Clin Oncol 2000;18:3339. [PMID: 11013273] (Amifostine reduced xerostomia but not other side effects of radiation for head and neck cancer.)

Ignoffo R et al (editors): *Cancer Chemotherapy Pocket Guide.* Lippincott-Raven, 1997.

■ EVALUATION OF TUMOR RESPONSE

Inasmuch as cancer chemotherapy can induce clinical improvement, serious toxicity, or both, it is important to critically assess the beneficial effects of treatment in patients with advanced cancer to determine that the net effect is favorable. The most valuable signs to follow during therapy include the following.

TUMOR SIZE

Shrinkage in tumor size can be demonstrated by physical examination, chest film or other x-ray, sonography, or a procedure such as radionuclide bone scanning (breast, lung, prostate cancer). CT scanning is important for the evaluation of tumor size and location and the extent of distant spread for a wide variety of tumors and sites. MRI is now the best noninvasive means of evaluating posterior fossa brain tumors, spinal cord tumors, spinal cord compression, and pelvic disease, but CT scanning remains useful and may provide additional information. Sonography is also helpful in the evaluation of pelvic neoplasms. Gallium scanning can be useful to detect residual disease in lymphomas, but some tumors are not gallium-avid, which limits the usefulness of this test. Positron emission tomography (PET scanning) is an emerging radiographic detection method that depends on metabolic activity for visualization. It appears to be very useful in detection of residual disease in lymphomas and in assessing the extent of disease in several solid tumors. A partial response (PR) is defined as a 50% or greater reduction in the original tumor mass. A complete response (CR) refers to the complete disappearance of detectable tumor. Progression is an increase of more than 25% in the size of the tumor or the appearance of any new lesions. Criteria for measuring responses of solid tumors have been established by the World Health Organization to avoid conflicts and inconsistency in measurements that influence reporting of tumor responses and to lead to more uniform reporting of outcomes of clinical trials. The RECIST criteria are based on measuring the largest single diameter of any tumor mass and include a minimum diameter for measurable lesions. These criteria will be incorporated into all new cancer treatment protocols.

The effectiveness of any agent or combination of agents in the treatment of cancer is determined by the response rates (combination of CR, PR, and, for some aggressive neoplasms, stable disease), response duration, and survival. Treatment efficacy for metastatic or incurable disease is often measured by event free-survival (EFS) or time to progression (TTP). The usefulness of treatment given to prevent recurrence of potentially curable neoplasms is measured by relapse-free survival (RFS) or disease-free survival (DFS) as well as overall survival (OS). The goal of effective palliative therapy for advanced incurable malignancy is to increase survival and improve quality life. Newer agents and new delivery methods have expanded the treatment options and increased their tolerability for some common cancers. Generally, response to therapy is associated with palliation, but it often happens that just stabilization of disease will have the same effect. Tumor response in this setting must be measured against toxicity, and treatment decisions should be made after available options have been discussed with the patient and family. Because patients tend to have unrealistic expectations of the benefits of palliative chemotherapy, clinician-patient communication is critical.

TUMOR MARKERS

A decrease in the quantity of a tumor product or marker substance reflects a reduced amount of tumor in the body. Examples of such markers include paraproteins (abnormal immunoglobulins) in multiple myeloma and macroglobulinemia, human chorionic gonadotropin (hCG) in choriocarcinoma and testicular cancer, prostatic acid phosphatase and PSA in prostatic cancer, urinary steroids in adrenal carcinoma and paraneoplastic Cushing's syndrome, and 5-hydroxyindoleacetic acid (5-HIAA) in carcinoid syndrome.

Tumor-secreted fetal antigens are also used to follow the course and response to treatment of cancers. These include alpha$_1$-fetoprotein (AFP) in hepatocellular carcinoma, testicular cancer, teratoembryonal carcinoma, and in occasional cases of gastric carcinoma; ovarian tumor antigen (CA 125) in ovarian cancer; and carcinoembryonic antigen (CEA) in carcinomas of the colon, lung, breast, and pancreas. CA 15-3 and CA 27.29 may become important in detecting early recurrence of breast cancer but are mainly used to follow response to therapy in metastatic disease. The CA 19-9 radioimmunoassay was just approved to monitor response to therapy of pancreatic cancer. Monoclonal antibodies are now used for measurement of a number of tumor markers and offer the potential of delineating a number of additional markers for diagnostic purposes.

Tumor markers may play an important role in the early detection of some common tumors when combined with good physical examinations. PSA, an immunogenic glycoprotein produced solely by the prostate, is currently the only tumor marker with widespread (and controversial) use in cancer screening. PSA was initially used to indicate tumor bulk and disease progression, but it is now commonly used as a screening tool when paired with the digital rectal examination. The American Cancer Society National Prostate Cancer Detection Project is a multicenter study evaluating the use of PSA, digital rectal examination (DRE), and transrectal ultrasound (TRUS) in a large cohort of healthy men. In this and other studies, the combination of a monoclonal PSA greater than 4 ng/mL and an abnormal digital rectal examination was felt to produce a highly sensitive and specific method for detecting prostate cancer. A large Canadian study showed a significant reduction in death from prostate cancer in men undergoing regular screening. This study randomized more than 46,000 men aged 45–80 years to screening, with PSA (using 3 ng/mL as the upper limit of normal) and digital rectal examination followed by transrectal ultrasound for abnormal test results or for a 10% increase in PSA over 12 months. There was an almost threefold advantage of screening and early treatment to reduce mortality. Annual screening for prostate cancer with digital rectal examination and PSA beginning at age 50 should be offered to men with a life expectancy of at least 10 years. Data obtained from the Prostate, Lung, Colorectal, and Ovarian Cancer (PLCO) Screening Trial and presented at the international oncology meetings in 2002 suggest that the initial PSA level can be used as a guide to the frequency of testing. Thirty thousand men aged 55–74 qualified for inclusion in the trial, and over 90% had normal PSA levels of < 4 ng/mL at baseline. A PSA < 1 ng/mL was associated with only a 1.4% chance of rise over 5 years, and a high percentage of those with a level of 1–2 ng/mL were normal over a period of 2 years. In contrast, 83% of those with an initial screening level of 3–4 ng/mL became abnormal over 5 years. The recommendations are to screen men with an initial level of < 1 ng/mL every 5 years; 1–1.9 ng/mL every 2 years; and ≥ 2 ng/mL yearly. It is estimated that this schedule could reduce PSA testing by 55%, with only a 2.6% risk of missing a positive test. As always, patients need to be involved in the decision to obtain screening PSA testing and should understand the advantages and possible consequences of testing or not testing.

An abnormal PSA or digital rectal examination requires further evaluation by transrectal ultrasound and possible biopsy. The role of PSA screening must be carefully evaluated for each patient and the risks of screening (unnecessary biopsies and surgeries) discussed in detail. The PSA may be elevated in benign prostatic hypertrophy and in prostatitis. Levels in benign disease are usually between 4 and 10 ng/mL; a level greater than 10 ng/mL increases the likelihood of finding cancer. In addition, 25–45% of patients with localized prostate cancer may have a normal PSA value. The increase in screening for prostate cancer over the last few years has markedly increased the reported incidence of this disease, though prostate cancer-specific mortality has been essentially stable. (See Table 40–1.)

Tumor markers may be useful to screen populations at high risk for a specific cancer. A recent study has shown that elevated and altered profiles of AFP can serve as predictive markers for the development of hepatocellular carcinoma in patients with cirrhosis.

Most tumor markers are not specific or sensitive enough to be useful as screening tools owing to their frequent elevation in benign disease and their absence in some cases of malignancy.

In general, tumor markers are used to follow response to therapy of a specific cancer. In diseases where early treatment of recurrence can influence survival (eg, testicular cancer), tumor markers may be used to screen for recurrent disease before it becomes radiographically or clinically evident.

Bast RC et al: 2000 update of recommendations for the use of tumor markers I breast and colorectal cancer: clinical practice guidelines of the American Society of Clinical Oncology. J Clin Oncol 2001;19:1865. [PMID: 11251019] (Updated recommendations based on published literature.)

Doyle C et al: Does palliative care palliate? Evaluation of expectations, outcomes and costs in women receiving chemotherapy for advanced ovarian cancer. J Clin Oncol 2001;19:1266. [PMID: 11230467] (Patient expectations are often unrealistic and objective response rates are low, but palliation with chemotherapy was associated with a substantial improvement in emotional function and quality of life.)

Maggino T: Serum markers as prognostic factors in epithelial ovarian cancer: an overview. Eur J Gynaecol Oncol 2000;21:64. [PMID: 10726623] (A review of the use of tumor markers in ovarian cancer.)

Prostate-specific antigen (PSA) best practice policy. American Urological Association. Oncology (Huntingt) 2000;14:267. [PMID: 10736812] (Recommendations created by a multi-specialty panel in the United States.)

Smith RA et al: American Cancer Society guidelines for the early detection of cancer: update of early detection guidelines for prostate, colorectal, and endometrial cancers. CA Cancer J Clin 2001;51:38. (Updated guidelines for screening.)

GENERAL WELL-BEING, PERFORMANCE STATUS, & SUPPORTIVE CARE

The functional status of the cancer patient at diagnosis (or at the start of treatment) is a major prognostic factor and determinant of outcome with or without tumor-directed therapy. It is therefore important to assess functional status as well as tumor burden and symptoms before deciding on possible anticancer therapy. Functional status or performance status evaluates the patient's ability to perform activities of daily living and is clearly related to tumor burden, tumor site, and the patient's underlying physical condition.

Two scales are commonly used to measure performance status. The Eastern Cooperative Oncology Group (ECOG) scale is a five-point system that is simple and easy to apply to clinical practice. The ECOG scoring system ranges from 0 to 4 as follows: 0, entirely asymptomatic; 1, symptomatic but fully ambulatory; 2, symptomatic and in bed less than 50% of the day; 3, symptomatic and in bed more than 50% of the day but not bedridden; and 4, bedridden. The Karnofsky scale ranges from 100% (asymptomatic and fully functional) through 0% (dead) in steps of 10%. For example, a Karnofsky performance status of 40% implies a patient who is disabled and requires special care and assistance. This patient would be unable to work but would be able to live at home with special assistance. These two systems are often the basis for clinical decisions despite their obvious lack of precision. They are also useful in assessing the impact of therapy and disease progression.

The measures assessing functional status described above do not adequately assess quality of life, a major goal of cancer chemotherapy. Performance status is only one component of quality of life, which is a combination of subjective and objective factors. Factors included in the assessment of general well-being include improved appetite and weight gain and decreased pain as well as improved performance status. In general, cancer patients perceive that they receive inadequate analgesia and have impairment of function because of pain. The adequate use of pain medications is hampered by their sedating side effects. New guidelines for the management of pain and long-acting opioids delivered by a transdermal system may help (eg, fentanyl patch, changed every 3 days). In addition, a short-acting oral transmucosal fentanyl preparation is available that may allow easier titration of analgesia. In addition, sedating effects can sometimes be avoided by adding nonsteroidal anti-inflammatory agents or antidepressants to opioid therapy. Gabapentin can be a useful adjunct to management of pain characterized by nerve compression-like symptoms and can also treat insomnia if given at bedtime. In general, depression is underdiagnosed and undertreated by clinicians; treatment of depression in patients with advanced cancer has been shown to improve functional status. Occasionally, opioids may be given epidurally to relieve severe pain. As with the use of antiemetics, pain medications work better when given prophylactically on a regular schedule rather than as needed for chronic or severe pain. It is only by completely evaluating all of the factors described above that the physician is able to judge whether the net effect of chemotherapy is worthwhile palliation. See Chapters 1 and 5 for further discussions of pain management and care at the end of life.

In addition to opioids, agents that inhibit bone resorption may decrease bone pain and protect against skeletal complications (thereby improving quality of life) in patients with cancer metastatic to bone. Either the bisphosphonate pamidronate or the more potent zoledronic acid is well tolerated; the indications for zoledronic acid are broader and include both lytic and blastic bone lesions in any type of cancer. Pamidronate is given at a dosage of 90 mg intravenously over 2 hours once a month; zoledronic acid, 4 mg intravenously over 15 minutes once a month. In addition to spot radiation, two radioactive agents are available for the palliation of bone pain. Strontium-89 and samarium-153 lexidronam are both given intravenously and have been shown to be effective in reducing bone pain from osteoblastic lesions. The major toxicity is hematopoietic suppression, which may limit the ability to give other palliative therapy. The use of agents such as pamidronate, dronabinol, growth factors such as erythropoietin, and appetite stimulants such as mege-strol acetate (given in dosages ranging from 40 mg orally four times a day up to 800 mg once a day) can improve the quality of life for cancer patients.

As early detection of cancer increases and cancer therapy improves, a growing area of concern is the long-term care of cancer survivors. Careful attention must be paid to psychosocial as well as physical problems resulting from therapy. Chemotherapy often leads to early menopause, depression, sexual difficulties, and osteoporosis, among other problems. Clinician awareness and referral to the appropriate resources is critical for maintaining quality of life in patients who are "survivors."

Berney A et al: Psychopharmacology in supportive care of cancer: a review for the clinician. III. Antidepressants. Support Care Cancer 2000;8.278. [PMID: 10923767] (A review of antidepressants with decision trees for management of patients with advanced cancer.)

Cleary JF: Cancer pain management. Cancer Control 2000;7:120. [PMID: 10783816] (A comprehensive pain management approach integrating pain assessment, opioid therapy, and other modalities.)

Foley KM: Advances in cancer pain. Arch Neurol 1999;56:413. [PMID: 10199328] (An outline of medications and adjunctive therapy to treat cancer pain.)

Mannix K et al: Using bisphosphonates to control the pain of bone metastases: evidence-based guidelines for palliative care. Palliat Med 2000;14:455. [PMID: 11219875] (A review of published data and recommendations for clinical practice.)

Pfeilschifter J et al: Osteoporosis due to cancer treatment: pathogenesis and management. J Clin Oncol 2000;18:1570. [PMID: 10735906] (Pathogenesis, diagnostic tests, prevention, and treatment options are discussed in this review.)

■ CANCER COMPLICATIONS: DIAGNOSIS & MANAGEMENT

ONCOLOGIC EMERGENCIES

Cancer is a chronic disease, but acute emergencies may occur as a consequence of local involvement (spinal cord compression, superior vena cava syndrome, malignant effusions, etc) or generalized systemic effects (hypercalcemia, opportunistic infections, hypercoagulability, hyperuricemia, etc). These complications may be the presenting manifestation of cancer. Two relatively common complications covered elsewhere will not be discussed here: superior vena cava syndrome (Chapter 12) and hypercoagulability (Chapter 13).

Brigden ML: Hematologic and oncologic emergencies. Doing the most good in the least time. Postgrad Med 2001;109:143. [PMID: 11265352] (A review of emergencies focusing on appropriate management.)

Merrill P: Oncologic emergencies. Lippincotts Prim Care Pract 2000;4:400. [PMID: 11261116] (A review of emergencies
oriented to the primary care physician; with differential diagnoses.)

1. Spinal Cord Compression

Spinal cord compression by tumor mass is manifested by back pain, progressive weakness, and sensory loss (usually in the lower extremities). Less commonly, spinal cord disease may present as chest or abdominal pain or as signs of nerve root compression due to the epidural location of the tumor. Bowel and bladder dysfunction are late findings. Spinal cord compression may occur as a complication of metastatic solid tumor, lymphoma, or myeloma. Back pain at the level of the spinal cord lesion occurs in over 80% of cases and may be aggravated by lying down, weight-bearing, sneezing, or coughing. Because back pain may precede the development of neurologic symptoms or signs, it is important to investigate this complaint thoroughly in any patient with cancer.

If neurologic deficits are present at diagnosis, they are usually irreversible, though treatment immediately after symptoms develop may result in partial recovery. Neurologic impairment can progress rapidly. Treatment of early lesions may completely avoid significant compromise. Although patients who present with paralysis may not recover function, they should still be treated for pain relief and to limit the extent of progression. In addition, patients may respond to systemic therapy depending on the specific tumor type.

The diagnosis of spinal cord compression is made by MRI scan with contrast. With this noninvasive and sensitive test, it is possible to obtain detailed views of the area in question as well as sagittal images of the entire spinal cord and vertebral canal. A detailed examination is important for detection and treatment of multiple lesions. Bone radiographs and bone scans are useful for detecting vertebral metastases, but they do not aid in assessing spinal cord compromise.

Leptomeningeal disease, or carcinomatous meningitis, is an uncommon complication occurring in about 3–8% of all cancer patients, though it is being diagnosed more frequently with improved imaging studies and increased longevity in patients with advanced cancer. The most common tumors involving the meninges are cancers of the breast and lung and malignant melanoma. Patients present with varied symptoms, including sequential cranial nerve abnormalities, stroke, and hydrocephalus. The diagnosis is made by finding malignant cells on cerebrospinal fluid cytologic examination or by enhancement of the meninges on gadolinium-enhanced MRI scans. The prognosis is poor, with median survival ranging from 3 months to 6 months despite treatment.

Emergency Treatment

A. SPINAL CORD COMPRESSION

Radiation therapy to the area of spinal cord compression and two adjacent vertebrae above and below the lesion is the treatment of choice. High doses of gluco-corticoids (usually dexamethasone, 10–100 mg intravenously) are administered as soon as the diagnosis is suspected or confirmed. A lower dose (eg, 4–6 mg every 6 hours intravenously or orally) is continued throughout the course of radiation therapy and tapered at or near the end of treatment.

Emergency surgery is indicated (1) for spinal cord compression in the absence of a diagnosis of malignancy, (2) for patients who have already received maximal doses of radiation to the involved area of the spine, and (3) for patients who develop progressive neurologic deficits during radiation whose prognosis warrants aggressive therapy. Chemotherapy is useful in treating lymphomas and multiple myeloma in conjunction with or following completion of radiation therapy.

B. LEPTOMENINGEAL DISEASE

Treatment is by radiation to symptomatic areas (usually whole brain and spinal cord) or with intrathecal chemotherapeutic agents, most commonly methotrexate and cytarabine. For this purpose, an intraventricular reservoir system is recommended. Aggressive therapy (particularly the combination of intrathecal therapy and radiation) can be complicated by necrotizing leukoencephalopathy. Patients with chemotherapy-sensitive cancers and an excellent performance status have the best chance of benefiting from therapy.

Bayley A et al: A prospective study of factors predicting clinically occult spinal cord compression in patients with metastatic prostate carcinoma. Cancer 2001;92:303. [PMID: 11466683]. (Clinical parameters can be used to identify patients at high risk for occult spinal cord compression; treatment can be given before neurologic deficits develop.)

Daw HA et al: Epidural spinal cord compression in cancer patients: diagnosis and management. Cleve Clin J Med 2000;67:497. [PMID: 10902239] (Lower back pain and radiculopathy are the hallmark symptoms of spinal cord compression. Neurologic status at the time of diagnosis is one of the most important prognostic markers.)

Grossman SA et al: Leptomeningeal carcinomatosis. Cancer Treat Rev 1999;25:103. [PMID: 10395835] (A review of the diagnosis, treatment and complications of this disorder.)

Loblaw DA et al: Emergency treatment of malignant extradural spinal cord compression: an evidence-based guideline. J Clin Oncol 1998;16:1613. [PMID: 9552073] (Canadian task force recommendations for emergency management.)

Quinn JA et al: Neurologic emergencies in the cancer patient. Semin Oncol 2000;27:311. [PMID: 10864219] (A review of the presentation and treatment of cord compression, increased intracranial pressure, status epilepticus, and intracerebral hemorrhage related to malignancies.)

2. Hypercalcemia

Hypercalcemia occurs in 10–20% of patients with cancer. Common causes include breast, lung, kidney, and head and neck carcinomas as well as multiple myeloma and lymphoma. Although the majority of cancers associated with hypercalcemia metastasize to the bones, approximately 20% of cases are not associated with bony lesions. The identification of a novel protein called parathyroid hormone-related protein (PTHrP) has revised some previously held views about the pathogenesis of hypercalcemia. Radioimmunoassays have identified this peptide in the serum of approximately two-thirds of cancer patients with hypercalcemia. High levels have been found in patients with hypercalcemia that was previously thought to be due solely to local osteolysis. PTHrP may become a useful tumor marker in normocalcemic patients. In addition, antibodies to PTHrP may be useful as treatment.

The symptoms and signs of hypercalcemia include nausea, vomiting, constipation, polyuria, muscular weakness and hyporeflexia, confusion, psychosis, tremor, and lethargy. Some patients may be asymptomatic. Electrocardiography often shows a shortening of the QT interval. The presence of hypercalcemia does not invariably indicate a dismal prognosis, especially in breast or prostate cancer and multiple myeloma or lymphoma. In the absence of signs or symptoms of hypercalcemia, a laboratory finding of elevated serum calcium should be rechecked to exclude the possibility of laboratory error.

Emergency Treatment

A. HYDRATION

Emergency treatment consists of aggressive intravenous hydration with 3–4 L/d of 0.9% saline followed by diuresis with 10–40 mg of intravenous furosemide. It is essential that the patient be well hydrated before beginning diuretic therapy and that hydration be maintained after diuresis is initiated. Although hydration alone is effective at slowly reducing the calcium level, it is rarely sufficient treatment and can lead to problems with fluid overload.

B. DRUG THERAPY

There are several options for the emergent treatment of hypercalcemia used in conjunction with aggressive hydration.

1. Bisphosphonates—Bisphosphonates are potent inhibitors of osteoclast bone resorption and are currently the most important and least toxic agents for the treatment of cancer-related hypercalcemia. Zoledronic acid is the most potent bisphosphonate available and will replace pamidronate disodium as the treatment of choice for malignant hypercalcemia. A single 15-minute intravenous infusion of 4 mg with adequate hydration produces complete normalization of serum calcium in less than 3 days in 80–100% of patients—with a more rapid onset and duration of effect than pamidronate. Zoledronic acid administration can be repeated as necessary to control hypercalcemia. The most commonly reported side effects have been transient fever, myalgias, and an infusion site reaction. Zoledronic acid has also been found to reduce the incidence of new skeletal lesions and decrease pain from bone disease in cancers with metastatic lesions to bone.

2. Gallium nitrate—For treatment of hypercalcemia, gallium nitrate is given by continuous intravenous infusion at a dose of 100–200 mg/m^2/d for 5 days. Gallium nitrate is superior to calcitonin both in reducing calcium levels acutely and in keeping the levels low after treatment is completed. Renal function must be carefully monitored.

3. Calcitonin—Synthetic salmon calcitonin works immediately to inhibit bone resorption, whereas pamidronate may take 2–3 days to achieve its maximum effect. The usual dose of 4 IU/kg intramuscularly, subcutaneously, or intranasally every 12 hours may be increased to 8 IU/kg every 12 hours after 1–2 days. Calcitonin alone is not effective at lowering serum calcium levels but can be added to pamidronate if necessary to achieve normal calcium levels. Repeated treatment with calcitonin is usually not as effective, and tachyphylaxis usually occurs after 1–3 days of treatment.

4. Other drugs—Prednisone has not been shown to be effective as a single agent to treat hypercalcemia, though it can be used in diseases that are responsive to steroids such as multiple myeloma or lymphoma. Refractory hypercalcemia may be treated with intravenous plicamycin, 25 μg/kg/d for 3 or 4 days. Although often effective, its effect may be short-lived, and its use is often associated with hepatic, renal, and bone marrow toxicity.

C. CHEMOTHERAPY

Patients with breast cancer may develop hypercalcemia as a "flare" associated with bone pain after initiation of estrogen or antiestrogen therapy. These patients often achieve excellent tumor response with continued therapy. Tumors may respond to chemotherapy or radiation therapy, leading to resolution of hypercalcemia. If chronic hypercalcemia persists and is refractory to chemotherapy, pamidronate, and aggressive oral hydration may be tried but are unfortunately rarely effective for long. When the more potent bisphosphonates become available in oral formulations, the management of chronic hypercalcemia may improve.

Berenson JR et al: Bisphosphonates in the treatment of malignant bone disease. Annu Rev Med 1999;50:237. [PMID: 10073275]

Body JJ: Current and future directions in medical therapy: hypercalcemia. Cancer 2000;88:3054. [PMID: 10898351] (A review of the treatment of hypercalcemia of malignancy focusing on bisphosphonate therapy.)

Esbrit P et al: Treatment of malignant hypercalcemia. Expert Opin Pharmacother 2002;3:521 [PMID: 11996631] (A thorough review of etiology and treatment as well as future directions.)

Zolendronate (Zometa). Med Lett Drugs Ther 2001;43:110. [PMID: 11740412] (A review of the newest and most potent bisphosphonate.)

3. Hyperuricemia & Acute Urate Nephropathy

Hyperuricemia can occur both as a complication of rapidly proliferating malignancies or with treatment-associated tumor lysis of hematologic malignancies such as leukemia, lymphoma, and multiple myeloma. Neoplasms with a high nucleic acid turnover such as acute leukemia and lymphoma may present with elevated serum uric acid and associated renal insufficiency. This problem may be compounded by use of thiazide diuretics, which decreases urate excretion. If a patient presents with hyperuricemia, care must be taken to reduce the uric acid before institution of cancer therapy. Patients at risk for tumor lysis syndrome should be followed with twice-daily measurements of uric acid, phosphate, calcium, and creatinine for the first 2–3 days following initiation of chemotherapy. Rapid elevation of serum uric acid can result in acute urate nephropathy caused by uric acid crystallization in the distal tubules, collecting ducts, and renal parenchyma. A serum urate concentration above 15 mg/dL is associated with a high risk of uric acid nephropathy. Gouty arthritis is usually a problem only in patients with a history of gout.

Prophylactic therapy consists of decreasing the production and increasing the renal excretion of uric acid. Allopurinol is a competitive inhibitor of xanthine oxidase and prevents conversion of highly soluble hypoxanthine and xanthine to the relatively insoluble uric acid. Twelve to 24 hours before beginning chemotherapy, a dose of 600 mg is given, followed by 300 mg/d during the period of high risk. Higher doses (up to 900–1200 mg/d) are used when severe hyperuricemia is anticipated following chemotherapy. Patients receiving the purine antagonists mercaptopurine or azathioprine should be given only 25–35% of the calculated dose of chemotherapy if they are also receiving allopurinol, since the latter drug will potentiate both the therapeutic effects and the toxicity of these agents. Renal excretion of uric acid is enhanced by maintaining a high urine flow and by alkalinizing the urine to prevent uric acid crystallization, which occurs at acid pH. The urine can be alkalinized with 6–8 g of oral sodium bicarbonate per day or by adding two or three ampules of sodium bicarbonate to 1 L of D$_5$W by infusion. Alkaline diuresis to maintain a urine pH near 7.0 is required only for prophylaxis in patients expected to have a rapid tumor response with marked hyperuricemia.

Emergency Treatment

Emergency therapy for established severe hyperuricemia consists of (1) hydration with 2–4 L of fluid per day; (2) alkalinization of the urine with 6–8 g of sodium bicarbonate per day; (3) allopurinol, 900–1200 mg/d; and (4) in severe cases, emergency hemodialysis. When severe hyperuricemia is present, adequate therapy may be impossible because of associated renal insufficiency and inadequate urine output. Intravenous allopurinol is available for use in patients unable to tolerate the oral form of this drug. Even if renal failure occurs and dialysis is required, renal function may return to normal after the acute tumor lysis has resolved.

4. Malignant Carcinoid Syndrome

Although tumors of argentaffin cells are uncommon, they are important because they secrete a variety of vasoactive materials. These include serotonin, histamine, catecholamines, prostaglandins, and vasoactive peptides. Carcinoid syndrome is usually associated with carcinoid tumors of the small bowel metastatic to the liver and, less commonly, with primary carcinoid tumors in other sites such as the lung or stomach. These tumors tend to metastasize early but have a relatively indolent course, making control of the syndrome important. Related syndromes occur in patients with pancreatic tumors secreting vasoactive peptides, which can cause severe watery diarrhea (pancreatic cholera).

The manifestations of carcinoid syndrome include facial flushing, edema of the head and neck (especially with bronchial carcinoid), abdominal cramps and diarrhea, bronchospasm, cardiac lesions (tricuspid or pulmonary stenosis or regurgitation), telangiectasias, and increased urinary 5-hydroxyindoleacetic acid (5-HIAA). The most common symptoms are flushing and diarrhea. The diagnosis is made by finding elevated levels of 5-HIAA in a 24-hour urine collection. Patients with symptomatic carcinoid usually excrete more than 25 mg of 5-HIAA per day in the urine. Ideally, all drugs and serotonin-rich foods such as bananas should be withheld for several days before beginning the urine collection.

Emergency Treatment

Emergency therapy for patients with symptomatic bronchial carcinoid includes prednisone, 15–30 mg/d. The associated abdominal cramping and diarrhea of intestinal carcinoids can often be managed by hydration and diphenoxylate with atropine. For severe diarrhea, the H_1 histamine receptor antagonist cyproheptadine (4 mg orally three times daily) or an antiserotonin agent such as methysergide maleate (2 mg orally three times daily until 16 mg has been given) may be effective. Other useful agents include cimetidine and the phenothiazines.

The synthetic peptide somatostatin agonist, octreotide acetate, is the most effective agent for reducing symptoms due to the carcinoid syndrome in association with achieving a reduction in levels of urinary 5-HIAA. The dose of octreotide in carcinoid syndrome is 100–600 μg/d in two to four divided doses by subcutaneous injection. Octreotide is also effective in the treatment of symptoms related to vasoactive intestinal peptide-secreting pancreatic tumors (VIPomas), markedly reducing the watery diarrhea syndrome associated with this neoplasm. The dose of octreotide used to treat patients with VIPomas is 200–300 μg/d in two to four divided doses.

Surgery is important in the treatment of localized carcinoid. Chemotherapy is moderately effective for patients with progressive advanced-stage disease. Active agents include fluorouracil, streptozocin, dacarbazine, cisplatin, doxorubicin, and alpha interferon.

Kulke MH et al: Carcinoid tumors. N Engl J Med 1999;340:858. [PMID: 10080850] (Review of the disease and treatment of complications.)

Fink G et al: Pulmonary carcinoid: Presentation, diagnosis, and outcome in 142 cases in Israel and review of 640 cases from the literature. Chest 2001;119:1647. [PMID: 11399686] (Review of a large series with discussion of diagnosis and treatment.)

OTHER COMPLICATIONS

1. Malignant Effusions

The development of effusions in the pleural, pericardial, and peritoneal spaces may be the presenting sign of some tumors or may cause diagnostic and therapeutic problems in patients with advanced neoplasms. Although the cause of an effusion can be elusive in a newly diagnosed asymptomatic patient, it is rarely difficult in the patient with advanced cancer. Approximately half of undiagnosed effusions in patients not known to have cancer will be malignant. The differential diagnosis includes congestive heart failure, pulmonary embolism, trauma, and infections such as tuberculosis. Direct involvement of the serous surface of the involved space with tumor appears to be the most frequent initiating factor, though many other mechanisms such as obstruction of lymphatic drainage that control the flow of fluid in the pleural space may play a role.

Most patients with pleural or pericardial effusions are symptomatic at presentation with chest pain, shortness of breath, or cough. The diagnosis is made by tapping the involved space. Pericardial effusions are aspirated under fluoroscopic guidance or direct vision through a subxiphoid incision. The fluid should be heparinized and sent for cell count and differential, protein content, lactate dehydrogenase level, and cytologic study. The gross appearance of the fluid is often helpful as well. Bloody effusions are usually due to cancer but occasionally are due to pulmonary embolism, tuberculosis, or trauma. Chylous effusions may be associated with thoracic duct obstruction or may result from enlarged mediastinal lymph nodes in lymphoma. If the cytologic smear is negative on two occasions but the suspicion of tumor is still high, closed pleural biopsy may be helpful.

The management of effusions should be appropriate to the severity of involvement. Treatment of the underlying neoplasm would be ideal but is often not effective in controlling local effusions. Treatment may result in palliation and improve short-term survival when there is substantial pulmonary or cardiac compromise. Diuretics are used as initial treatment for small to moderate-sized peritoneal effusions and as an adjunct to drainage of large effusions to minimize the possibility of reexpansion pulmonary edema that can occur after thoracentesis. Small or loculated effusions may require ultrasonographic localization, but drainage of a large pleural or peritoneal effusion can be accomplished rapidly using an intravenous catheter and phlebotomy tubing connected to a vacuum bottle. Thoracentesis alone controls fewer than 10% of effusions but may be useful in conjunction with systemic chemotherapy for sensitive tumors (eg, lymphoma, small-cell lung cancer, breast cancer). Pleural effusions may occasionally be managed by closed water-seal drainage with a chest tube for 3–4 days, though this procedure is usually performed in conjunction with chemosclerosis (see below). The aim of this procedure is to allow the pleural surfaces to come into close contact and become adherent.

Recurrent symptomatic effusions can often be controlled by drainage followed by chemosclerosis. In this procedure, a chemotherapeutic or nonchemotherapeutic agent is instilled with lidocaine into the involved space. The intended effect is local inflammation and sclerosis to encourage adherence of the serosal surfaces. Several drugs used in the past for this purpose have been abandoned because of severe pain or systemic toxicity, including myelosuppression. Agents currently in use include talc, bleomycin, and the anthracenedione compound mitoxantrone.

Talc poudrage has been used successfully to control malignant pleural effusions and appears to be relatively painless. For these reasons as well as cost considerations, talc is now the sclerosing agent of choice for malignant pleural effusions.

Bleomycin is more effective at controlling pleural effusions than tetracycline; when tetracycline was used, the recurrence rate 90 days after sclerosis was almost double, and the side effects were similar. Tetracycline is no longer manufactured or available for intracavitary instillation. The major side effects of bleomycin are pain, fever, and hypersensitivity reactions.

Mitoxantrone has been reported to be effective in controlling malignant pleural effusions, causing minimal fever and local pain. However, one trial evaluated the effectiveness of mitoxantrone versus chest tube alone and found no differences in response or in duration of response. The instillation of sclerosing agents may best be reserved for patients who fail pleural tube drainage alone.

Sclerosis is generally less useful for the management of malignant ascites, but success has been reported using bleomycin, doxorubicin, thiotepa, and other agents.

Before instilling the sclerosing agent, it is important that the space be drained as thoroughly as possible. For pleural effusions, a small-bore chest tube or pigtail catheter is usually placed and fluid is removed by negative suction until the drainage is under 100 mL per 24 hours and the lung has expanded. Sclerotherapy is ineffective if there is a large residual effusion. Talc is insufflated into the pleural space via a thoracoscope or instilled in a 5 g slurry with iodide via a chest tube. Talc instillation via a thoracoscope under anesthesia can be done quickly, has minimal complications, and appears highly effective. To use chemotherapeutic agents, the patient is premedicated

with an opioid, and 60 units of bleomycin or 30 mg of mitoxantrone in 50–100 mL of 0.9% saline is instilled directly into the chest tube. The chest tube is then clamped, and the patient is placed in different positions every 15 minutes for 4 hours to distribute the agent equally within the pleural space. At the end of this period, the clamp is removed and the chest tube is allowed to drain with suction. After 24 hours, the chest tube is removed from suction, and when the drainage is minimal, the tube is removed. The whole process takes 3–5 days. Occasionally, repeated doses of the sclerosing agent may be required to stop persistent reaccumulation of the effusion.

Surgery is infrequently used for patients with pleural or pericardial effusions who have failed sclerosis and who continue to have a long expected survival. Pleuroperitoneal shunting may have limited value in selected patients with high performance status who can participate actively in pumping the shunt the 100 times on five separate occasions each day required for adequate shunt function and fluid drainage. Pleurectomy has a high complication rate but offers excellent control of effusion in carefully selected patients. For malignant pericardial effusion, a pericardial window or stripping also offers good control with a lower complication rate and may also be performed for constrictive pericarditis following radiation therapy to the chest.

Burrows CM et al: Predicting survival in patients with recurrent symptomatic malignant pleural effusions: an assessment of the prognostic values of physiologic, morphologic, and quality of life measures of extent of disease. Chest 2000;117:73. [PMID: 10631202] (The Karnofsky performance status was predictive of overall survival in patients with recurrent malignant pleural effusions.)

Erasmus JJ et al: Treatment of malignant pleural effusions. Curr Opin Pulm Med 1999;5:250.[PMID: 10407696] (Review of the diagnosis and therapy of malignant pleural effusions.)

Parulekar W et al: Use of small-bore vs large-bore chest tubes for treatment of malignant pleural effusions. Chest 2001;120:19. [PMID: 11451810] (Small-bore catheters appear to be effective in the treatment of malignant effusions and may be associated with less pain and fewer side effects.)

Schulze M et al: Effective treatment of malignant pleural effusion by minimal invasive thoracic surgery: thoracoscopic talc pleurodesis and pleuroperitoneal shunts in 101 patients. Ann Thorac Surg 2001;71:1809. [PMID: 11426752] (The VATS talc pleurodesis can palliate patients with malignant pleural effusions; patients with visceral carcinomatosis may benefit instead from pleuroperitoneal shunting.)

2. Infectious Complications

The reader is referred also to the section on infections in the immunocompromised patient in Chapter 30.

Many patients with cancer have increased susceptibility to both bacterial and opportunistic infections. This may result from impaired host defense mechanisms (eg, Hodgkin's or non-Hodgkin's lymphoma, chronic lymphocytic leukemia, multiple myeloma, acute leukemia or preleukemia) or from the myelosuppressive and immunosuppressive effects of cancer chemotherapy. Impaired host defense mechanisms include defects in neutrophil function, abnormalities in antibody production, depressed cell-mediated immune function, impairment of mechanical barriers by indwelling intravenous catheters, and impairment of mucosal integrity. At least half of the infections seen in neutropenic patients are felt to be endogenous.

The bacterial organisms accounting for the majority of infections in cancer patients include Enterobacteriaceae (klebsiella, enterobacter, serratia, *Escherichia coli*), pseudomonas, staphylococcus, and streptococcus. Other important pathogens include corynebacterium, *Clostridium difficile,* mycobacterium, and legionella. Patients with prolonged neutropenia or those who have undergone bone marrow transplantation are at risk for infections with fungi such as candida, aspergillus, and pneumocystis and with viruses such as herpes zoster, cytomegalovirus, respiratory syncytial virus, and influenza virus. Infections with resistant bacteria, such as vancomycin-resistant enterococcus, are being seen with increasing frequency. The incidence of bacteremia rises dramatically when the white count is less than 1000/μL or when there are fewer than 200 granulocytes per microliter. In patients with neutropenia, hematologic malignancies, or following bone marrow transplantation, infection must be treated emergently and empirically. Although fever may be due to multiple causes, including mucositis, drugs, and the malignancy itself, infection must be the first consideration and may be present even in the absence of fever, especially in patients who are receiving glucocorticoids. Negative cultures in febrile neutropenic patients do not rule out infection, and treatment should be instituted immediately without waiting for culture results to become available. If an indwelling line is present, blood cultures should be drawn from the periphery as well as through the line itself.

Prevention

Details of prevention in immunocompromised hosts are outlined in Chapter 30.

Prophylaxis of infections in high-risk or neutropenic patients can prevent the complications of sepsis. Two randomized clinical trials tested oral versus intravenous antibiotic therapy for hospitalized low-risk febrile patients with neutropenia during cancer chemotherapy. Oral ciprofloxacin plus amoxicillin and potassium clavulanate appeared as effective as intravenous ceftazidime or ceftriaxone and amikacin, indicating that for low-risk patients, outpatient therapy is feasible and safe.

In patients who are severely immunocompromised, some bacterial infections may be prevented with intravenous immune globulin. This is important in patients with chronic lymphocytic leukemia, multiple myeloma, and following bone marrow transplantation if associated immunoglobulin deficiencies are observed.

The availability of recombinant bone marrow growth factors has helped to reduce the morbidity and mortality of infections in immunocompromised hosts. Granulocyte colony-stimulating factor (G-CSF; filgrastim) and granulocyte-macrophage colony-stimulating factor (GM-CSF; sargramostim) have been shown to be effective at reducing the duration of neutropenia and the frequency and severity of infection after myelosuppressive chemotherapy or autologous bone marrow transplantation for nonmyeloid malignancies. These growth factors improve bone marrow tolerance of escalating doses of chemotherapy, allowing higher doses to be given at shorter intervals. G-CSF and GM-CSF have been used to stimulate bone marrow stem cell production in both the circulating blood and in bone marrow cell populations collected for autologous transplantation. Administration of growth factors may improve survival after the failure of autologous or allogeneic bone marrow grafts.

Treatment

Infection management has been aimed at treatment of gram-negative bacterial sepsis, the most rapidly lethal infection. Current concepts have been broadened to include prophylaxis and prevention of the most common infections, including those caused by gram-negative, gram-positive, and fungal pathogens. Until recently, empirical therapy of fever consisted of two- or three-drug combinations, including an aminoglycoside and an antipseudomonal penicillin, with resolution of fever and bacteremia in about 70% of patients. Current results using initial monotherapy with a third-generation cephalosporin such as ceftazidime or cefepime or a combination β-lactam appear to yield similar results. Vancomycin or amphotericin B may be added on the basis of clinical suspicion, culture results, or prolonged fever in the absence of positive cultures. For persistent fevers or clinical deterioration, gram-negative rod coverage should be changed to an agent with a broader spectrum (eg, ciprofloxacin or imipenem). If stenotrophomonas is suspected, trimethoprim-sulfamethoxazole should be added.

Freifeld A et al: A double-blind comparison of empirical oral and intravenous antibiotic therapy for low-risk febrile patients with neutropenia during cancer chemotherapy. N Engl J Med 1999;341:305. [PMID: 10423464] (Empiric oral antibiotics were safe and effective for low-risk patients with febrile neutropenia.)

Garcia-Carbonero R et al: Granulocyte colony-stimulating factor in the treatment of high-risk febrile neutropenia: a multicenter randomized trial. J Natl Cancer Inst 2001;93:31. [PMID:11136839] (Adding G-CSF to antibiotic therapy in patients with high risk febrile neutropenia shortens duration of neutropenia, antibiotic therapy and hospital stay, and decreases hospital costs.)

Walsh TJ et al: Liposomal amphotericin B for empirical therapy in patients with persistent fever and neutropenia. N Engl J Med 1999;340:764. [PMID: 10072411] (Liposomal amphotericin B is as effective as conventional amphotericin B for empirical antifungal therapy and results in less nephrotoxicity and breakthrough fungal infections.)

THE PARANEOPLASTIC SYNDROMES
(Table 40–6)

The clinical manifestations of cancer are usually nonspecific—eg, anorexia, malaise, weight loss, fever—or are due to local effects of tumor growth, either in the primary site or at a distant site. The term "paraneoplasia" has been coined to denote the remote effects of malignancy that cannot be attributed either to direct invasion or metastatic lesions. These syndromes may be the first sign of a malignancy and may affect up to 15% of patients with cancer.

The paraneoplastic syndromes are of considerable clinical importance for the following reasons:

(1) They may accompany relatively limited neoplastic growth and provide an early clue to the presence of certain types of cancer.

(2) The course of the paraneoplastic syndrome usually parallels the course of the tumor. Therefore, effective treatment should be accompanied by resolution of the syndrome, and, conversely, recurrence of the cancer may be heralded by return of systemic symptoms.

(3) The metabolic or toxic effects of the syndrome may constitute a more urgent hazard to life than the underlying cancer (eg, hypercalcemia, hyponatremia).

The paraneoplastic syndromes are usually caused by the secretion of proteins not normally associated with a cancer's normal tissue equivalent. Clinical findings may resemble those of primary endocrine, metabolic, hematologic, or neuromuscular disorders. The mechanisms for such remote effects can be classified into three groups: (1) effects initiated by a tumor product (eg, carcinoid syndrome), (2) effects due to the destruction of normal tissues by tumor products (eg, hypercalcemia due to local secretion of cytokines), and (3) effects due to unknown mechanisms such as unidentified tumor products or circulating immune complexes stimulated by the tumor (eg, osteoarthropathy due to bronchogenic carcinoma and some neurologic syndromes). Even such nonspecific symptoms as fever and weight loss are truly paraneoplastic and are due to the production of specific factors (eg, tumor necrosis factor) by tumor cells or by normal cells in response to the tumor.

Paraneoplastic syndromes associated with ectopic hormone production are the best-characterized entities. Tumor cells secrete a hormone or prohormone that may be of a higher or lower molecular weight than hormones secreted by the more differentiated normal endocrine cell (eg, PTH-related peptide in hypercalcemia, ACTH in Cushing's syndrome, ADH in the syndrome of inappropriate antidiuretic hormone secretion). This ectopic hormone production by cancer cells is believed to result from activation of genes in malignant cells that are normally suppressed in most somatic cells. A single syndrome such as hypercalcemia may be due to more than one of a variety of causes. Effective antitumor treatment usually results in return of the serum calcium to normal, though additional therapy may be required (see Hypercalcemia, above). In some cases, a rapid response to cytotoxic chemotherapy may briefly increase the severity of the paraneoplastic syndrome in association with tumor lysis (eg, hyponatremia with SIADH). Several neurologic paraneoplastic syndromes have been found to be caused by the production of antineuronal antibodies that circulate in the serum and spinal fluid. It is thought that the underlying tumor expresses a similar antigen, resulting in production of a cross-reactive antibody. Treatment of the underlying tumor usually results in only modest improvement of the neurologic deficit. Examples of antineuronal antibodies include the anti-Hu antibody causing sensory neuropathy or encephalitis, associated with small cell cancer of the lung; the anti-Yo antibody causing cerebellar degeneration, associated most often with breast or gynecologic malignancies; the stiff man syndrome, associated with breast cancer; and anti-Purkinje cell antibodies causing cerebellar ataxia, associated with Hodgkin's disease as well as gynecologic, breast, and lung cancers.

Other well-described paraneoplastic syndromes include those involving the skin with or without other organ involvement (eg, dermatomyositis, Sweet's syndrome), hematologic syndromes (eg, polycythemia, thrombocytosis), and those involving the kidneys, the gastrointestinal tract, and the joints.

The most common cancer associated with paraneoplastic syndromes is small-cell cancer of the lung. This is thought to be due to its neuroectodermal origin.

Dropcho EJ: Neurologic paraneoplastic syndromes. J Neurol Sci 1998;153:264. [PMID: 9511883] (A review of the mechanisms and response to therapy; many patients may have irreversible neuronal injury at the time of diagnosis.)

Marmur R et al: Cancer-associate neuromuscular syndromes. Recognizing the rheumatic-neoplastic connection. Postgrad Med 2002;95. [PMID: 11985137]. (An excellent review of neuromuscular syndromes associated with cancer and a discussion of pathogenesis.)

Naschitz JE et al: Rheumatic syndromes: clues to occult neoplasia. Semin Arthritis Rheum 1999;29:43. [PMID: 10488414] (A thorough summary of the literature on cancer-associated rheumatic syndromes.)

Odell WD: Endocrine/metabolic syndromes of cancer. Semin Oncol 1997;24:299. [PMID: 10423692] (A review of the diagnosis and pathologic basis of the endocrine syndromes of cancer.)

Sabir S et al: Cutaneous manifestations of cancer. Curr Opin Oncol 1999;11:139. [PMID: 10188080] (An excellent review of a wide range of cutaneous syndromes associated with cancer.)

Sillevas Smitt P et al: Paraneoplastic cerebellar ataxia due to autoantibodies against a glutamate receptor. N Engl J Med 2000;342:21. [PMID: 10620645] (A new antibody causing ataxia was isolated in two patients with Hodgkin's disease.)

NOVEL THERAPIES
FOR CANCER TREATMENT

The use of cytotoxic drugs against cancer is limited by a number of factors, including toxicity, tumor resistance, and lack of targeted cell death. New strategies are based on increasing and improved knowledge of

Table 40–6. Paraneoplastic syndromes associated with common cancers.

Syndromes; Hormone Excess	Small Cell Lung Cancer	Non-Small Cell Lung Cancer	Breast Cancer	Multiple Myeloma	Gastrointestinal Cancers	Hepatocellular Cancer	Gestational Trophoblastic Disease	Lymphoma	Renal Cell Cancer	Carcinoid	Thymoma	Ovarian Cancer	Prostate Cancer	Myeloproliferative Disease	Adrenocortical Tumors	Cerebellar Hemangioblastomas
Endocrine																
Cushing's syndrome	XX	X														
SIADH	XX	X														
Hypercalcemia	XX	X	X	X				X				X				
Hypoglycemia					X	X										
Gonadotropin excess	XX	X			X		X		X	X						
Hyperthyroidism							X									
Neuromuscular																
Subacute cerebellar degeneration	XX	X			X			X				X				
Sensorimotor peripheral neuropathy	XX	X														
Lambert-Eaton syndrome	XX		X		X							X				
Stiff man syndrome			X									X				
Dermatomyositis/polymyositis	XX	X	X		XX							X		X		

Skin

Dermato-
myositis

Acanthosis
nigricans

Sweet's syn-
drome

Hematologic

Erythrocytosis

Pure red cell
aplasia

Eosinophilia

Thrombocytosis

Coagulopathy

Fever

Amyloidosis

XX = strong association; X = reported association

the molecular events responsible for disordered cellular growth and include antibodies to block receptors, small molecules that inhibit receptor tyrosine kinase-mediated cell signaling, agents directed at suppressing growth of blood vessels that feed cancer growth, vaccines to stimulate immune recognition of cancer cells, cell cycle inhibitors, and gene therapy to turn off signaling pathways or provide a missing tumor suppressor.

One way to block cellular growth is to block growth factor receptors. These receptors cross the cell membrane; the extracellular portion is the ligand-binding site, and the intracellular portion is the receptor tyrosine kinase. Activation of the receptor with ligand phosphorylates the tyrosine kinase and results in cell signaling through a complex series of events. A sketch of the growth factor receptors and various methods to block their activation is presented in Figure 40–1. The epidermal growth factor (EGF) receptor is expressed on most epithelial cells, and activation of the receptor has been shown to promote tumor

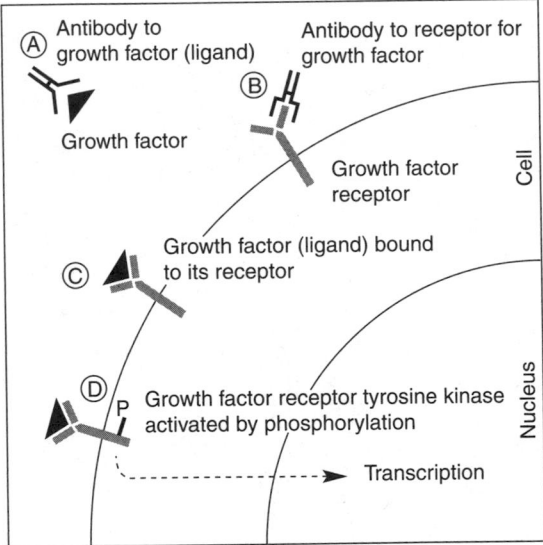

Figure 40–1. Signaling through growth factor receptors can be blocked by antibodies to either the growth factor (ligand) **(A)** (eg, antibody to VEGF; bevacizumab) or to the extracellular portion of the receptor for the growth factor (tyrosine kinase receptor) **(B)** (eg, trastuzumab, cetuximab). The binding of growth factors to their receptors **(C)** can lead to phosphorylation of the intracellular portion of the receptor or the receptor tyrosine kinase **(D).** Phosphorylation activates the receptor and results in many downstream signals in the cell that activate gene transcription, and consequently proliferation. Blockade of receptor phosphorylation—eg, by OSI-774 or ZD1839 (oral tyrosine kinase inhibitors)—interrupts the pathway, with the hoped-for result of blocking tumor growth.

cell growth, proliferation, and survival. Preclinical models have shown that blockade of this receptor results in tumor growth delay or regression and can potentiate radiation and chemotherapy effects. Trastuzumab (Herceptin) is a monoclonal antibody directed against the HER-2/*neu* receptor, one of the EGF family of receptors, and is the only growth factor receptor inhibitor approved for clinical use. Agents that block the EGF receptor are directed against the HER-1 receptor. Three agents targeting the EGF receptor are in clinical trials with encouraging results. Cetuximab (IMC-C225) is a monoclonal antibody that binds to the extracellular domain of the EGF receptor, resulting in inhibition of the receptor tyrosine kinase. Preliminary data indicate that cetuximab potentiates the effect of radiation therapy in head and neck cancer, and this effect is being studied in the setting of an ongoing phase III clinical trial. A phase II trial combined cetuximab with irinotecan in 121 patients with colorectal cancer resistant to both irinotecan and fluorouracil whose tumors expressed the EGF receptor. Twenty-one patients (17%) achieved a partial response, and 37 (31%) had stable disease or a minor response. Two phase III studies comparing cetuximab in combination with irinotecan, fluorouracil, and leucovorin versus irinotecan, fluorouracil, and leucovorin (ie, without cetuximab) to the chemotherapy regimen alone as first-line therapy for metastatic colorectal cancer are accruing patients. OSI-774 and ZD1839 are oral small-molecule tyrosine kinase inhibitors that block EGFR by directly blocking phosphorylation of the intracellular receptor tyrosine kinase. Partial remissions have been seen in a variety of cancers in phase II trials with both agents. A recent trial demonstrated a 9–12% response rate to single-agent ZD1839 therapy in refractory non-small cell lung cancer, with up to 43% of treated individuals experiencing symptom relief. In patients who had failed up to two prior treatments, the response rate rose to about 19%. Toxicity is modest and consists primarily of skin rash and diarrhea. Ongoing trials are evaluating the effect of these agents in combination with standard chemotherapy. ZD1839 has also been shown to inhibit the HER-2/*neu* receptor tyrosine kinase in preclinical models; trials are planned to evaluate the effects of this agent in advanced breast cancers as well.

Angiogenesis (the growth of new blood vessels) is thought to be an essential component of the ability of tumors to invade locally and to metastasize from the primary tumor site. Tumor angiogenesis is regulated by angiogenic stimulators such as vascular endothelial growth factor (VEGF, the ligand for the VEGF receptor) and the newly described inhibitors of angiogenesis, angiostatin and endostatin. There is now intense interest in using inhibitors of angiogenesis to suppress tumor growth and metastases. This type of therapy might avoid the development of chemotherapy resistance and have less toxicity than standard cytotoxic therapy. A recombinant humanized antibody to VEGF (anti-VEGF, rhuMAb VEGF, bevacizumab) has been tested alone and with chemotherapy in colon, breast, and lung cancers. The most promising results have been seen in patients with advanced colon cancer in conjunction with fluorouracil and leucovorin chemotherapy with improved response rates and survival in the anti-VEGF arm. A dose-finding phase II trial in advanced refractory breast cancer found an overall response rate of 11–20% depending on the dose given. Treatment with bevacizumab in patients with renal cell cancer resulted in significant slowing of cancer cell growth, with a 2.5-fold prolongation in time to progression from 2 months to 5 months. Tumor regression was rare, with three partial responses. The antibody was well tolerated in this trial. A large phase III randomized trial using anti-VEGF in combination with chemotherapy versus chemotherapy alone in the treatment of breast cancer has recently been completed; preliminary results are expected at the end of 2002. A second phase III trial in colon cancer should also be concluded in late 2002. Endostatin and angiostatin are potent inhibitors of angiogenesis that appear to be promising. A preclinical study showed that transfer of cells engineered to produce angiostatin into mice inhibited the growth of both the primary tumor and lung metastases from fibrosarcoma. Trials using endostatin to treat patients with advanced malignancy began in late 1999. The results of two phase I dose-escalation trials using recombinant human endostatin (rHE) or angiostatin (rHA) in patients with advanced solid tumors were recently presented. Both agents were associated with minimal side effects at the doses used, but few tumor responses were seen. Tumor blood flow decreased with both agents. Phase II trials are ongoing to assess the antitumor effects of endostatin and angiostatin. Another novel way to suppress angiogenesis is with small molecules that inhibit receptor tyrosine kinases and block VEGF-mediated receptor signaling. Several agents are in clinical trials treating various advanced metastatic cancers, usually in combination with chemotherapy. One agent, SU5416, was found to have unfavorable pharmacokinetics after extensive clinical trials had been conducted; development of this agent has been halted. It is now clear that standard pharmacokinetic studies must be done for novel agents before undertaking large randomized clinical trials. Other oral tyrosine kinase inhibitors that block the VEGF receptors are in early-phase clinical trials with detailed pharmacokinetic assessments. Thalidomide has been shown to have antiangiogenic properties as well as other antitumor effects. Striking responses have been seen in advanced and resistant multiple myeloma. Clinical trials using thalidomide in combination with chemotherapy in multiple myeloma, prostate cancer, and other malignancies are ongoing. An interesting therapy targets matrix metalloproteases that are thought to be important in the ability of cancer cells to metastasize. Unfortunately, phase III results in small-cell lung cancer have been disappointing, indicating at least that the current products are not active enough for clinical use.

Immunotherapy is an exciting area of investigation of the treatment of cancer. The most extensively treated disease with immunotherapeutic modalities is malignant melanoma—for a variety of reasons, including easily identified immunogenic antigens, easy access to tumor cells, and the ability to grow these cells in vitro. Active specific immunotherapy with melanoma vaccines has been evaluated in phase II trials for advanced melanoma as well as in the adjuvant setting with encouraging results. A phase III trial testing the allogeneic melanoma cell lysate vaccine Melacine in 689 patients with intermediate-thickness and clinically node-negative melanoma showed no evidence of improvement in disease-free survival at a median follow-up of 5.6 years among patients receiving the vaccine. Criticisms of the trial include the lack of sentinel node biopsy and lack of ability to detect small differences in recurrence. However, when patients expressing two or more specific HLA class I antigens were evaluated separately, a highly significant benefit was seen in patients receiving adjuvant treatment with Melacine. This suggests that specific HLA types can determine the immune response and disease impact of vaccine strategies. Further studies are ongoing. Identification of a suitable target is critical for the development of any vaccine. Interesting agents in clinical trials include a vaccine directed against human papillomavirus (HPV) to prevent cervical cancer and individualized vaccines directed toward the unique set of B cell tumor antigens that comprise each participating patient's low-grade lymphoma. This type of vaccine has been demonstrated to induce an immune response as well as either stable disease or actual tumor shrinkage in preliminary trials. Other interesting vaccines include monoclonal antibodies directed toward tumor products such as CA-125 for ovarian cancer and CEA for colon cancer.

The field of cancer vaccines is growing rapidly. One type of tumor vaccine in many clinical trials capitalizes on dendritic cells, which are antigen-presenting cells that enhance the response of the immune system to foreign antigens. Dendritic cells may be loaded with a particular abnormal protein to stimulate the immune response to a specific cancer. Early clinical trials in melanoma, multiple myeloma, and other cancers are in progress. One interesting strategy is to target the dendritic cells to a known growth factor present on the tumor cell. A clinical trial using dendritic cells loaded with HER-2/*neu* for the treatment of metastatic breast cancer is evaluating the ability of this type of a vaccine to stimulate a specific immune response in women with advanced breast cancer. In one study, patients with late-stage colorectal cancer were treated with a growth factor, FLT-3 ligand, to expand the number of circulating dendritic cells in vivo. The cells were then harvested, loaded with CEA antigen, and reinfused as a cellular vaccine. Early results in all four patients include tumor response or disease stabilization. A larger trial is planned. This type of therapy might also be useful early in the disease course of an aggressive tumor. Dendritic cell vaccines can be used in conjunction with autologous stem cell transplantation; cells are removed at the time of stem cell harvesting, undergo in vitro stimulation, and are then returned to the patient after completion of chemotherapy and radiation therapy to eradicate bulk tumor.

Several problems with vaccine therapy exist, including the difficulty of generating an immune response in an immunosuppressed cancer patient and the fact that an immune response does not necessarily correlate with tumor response. In order to enhance the immune response to vaccines, growth factors such as GM-CSF are given with the treatment. A GM-CSF gene-modified vaccine is now in clinical trials that produces GM-CSF locally to enhance the immune response. Early results show some evidence of tumor response in non-small-cell lung cancer.

Radiolabeled and toxin-linked antibodies have been used to treat lymphomas with very encouraging results and appear more effective than antibody therapy alone. Ibritumomab tiuxetan is an yttrium 90-labeled antibody to CD20 that has recently been FDA-approved for the treatment of low-grade non-Hodgkin's lymphoma refractory to rituximab or transformed B cell non-Hodgkin's lymphoma. This is the first targeted radioimmunotherapy to be FDA-approved for clinical use. This unique drug consists of an antibody to CD20 bound to tiuxetan; a high affinity chelator for yttrium 90 and indium 111. A recently published randomized controlled trial compared ibritumomab tiuxetan with rituximab in patients with relapsed or refractory low-grade non-Hodgkin's lymphoma or transformed non-Hodgkin's lymphoma. The overall response rate was 80% for the radiolabeled antibody versus 56% for rituximab alone, with a corresponding prolongation in duration of response and time to disease progression. Durable responses were significantly longer in the ibritumomab tiuxetan group. The primary toxicity is reversible but significant myelosuppression. This agent must not be used in patients with impaired marrow function or extensive involvement of marrow with lymphoma. Treatment is given in three steps. On day 1, a dose of rituximab is given followed by indium 111-labeled ibritumomab tiuxetan to determine biodistribution of antibody. One week later, a second dose of rituximab is followed by yttrium 90-labeled antibody. Yttrium 90 is a pure beta emitter with a half-life of 64 hours and a short path length of 5 mm, making it relatively safe to use in clinical practice. A second experimental radiolabeled antibody, tositumomab, is linked to ^{131}I, which requires dosimetry and shielding, making clinical use more cumbersome. Many other antibody combinations are either under development or in preliminary clinical trials.

The arachidonic acid metabolic pathway is thought to be important in the pathogenesis of cancer. COX-2 is overexpressed in many solid tumors, including tumors of the lung, colon, and breast. Higher levels are thought to increase angiogenesis and decrease apoptosis. Multiple clinical trials are under way to evaluate the effects of the COX-2 inhibitor celecoxib in the treatment or prevention of cancer—often in combination with either chemotherapeutic or hormonal agents. One recent small phase II study suggested that celecoxib might improve the response to preoperative chemotherapy in patients with non-small cell lung cancer; this hypothesis needs to be explored in the setting of larger trials.

The goal of gene therapy for cancer is to inhibit the constitutive signals that drive tumor growth. Expanding knowledge about signal transduction has provided multiple possible attack points within this complicated multistep process involving a variety of somatic gene alterations. Although at present it is impossible to deliver therapeutic genes to every cancer cell, bystander effects or the cytotoxic effects produced by engineered cells on nonengineered cells may allow broad effects from a limited number of transduced cells. A variety of approaches are being investigated. These include enhancing the ability of the host immune system to respond to a specific tumor, sensitizing tumor cells to relatively nontoxic drugs or prodrugs, and selective replacement of altered or missing tumor suppressor genes or inactivation of oncogenes. Selective targeting of cells would allow either cell death or return of normal growth patterns without toxicity to nonneoplastic cells. One area of research in active clinical trial is replacement of the missing function of the mutated tumor suppressor gene, *P53*, or to inhibit the function of a dominant oncogene such as *ras*. One approach is to create a vaccine directed against cells with mutant *P53* in order to generate a cytotoxic T cell response to tumor cells expressing the P53 protein. A vaccine made from a disabled adenovirus (the vector or carrier) and the *P53* gene and injected into the arterial circulation is delivered to tumors that have metastasized to the liver with subsequent expression of the *P53* gene. Another unique approach to tumor killing is the use of an adenovirus engineered to selectively kill tumor cells that are lacking *P53* but leave normal cells alone. This agent, ONYX-015, is also in clinical trials both with and without chemotherapy. It appears to be more effective when injected directly into tumors. Results from this and other agents are limited by a variety of problems, including difficulty delivering the agent, identifying tumors that lack *P53*, and production of the novel agent. The Bcl-2 protein, overexpressed in many common solid tumors, is thought to be responsible for blocking apoptosis or natural cell death and appears to confer tumor cell resistance to chemotherapy and radiation therapy. An antisense oligonucleotide that blocks production of the Bcl-2 protein, thereby restoring this principal pathway of cell death, is in clinical trials in combination with chemotherapy in melanoma, multiple myeloma, non-small cell lung cancer, and chronic lymphocytic leukemia. This agent binds to Bcl-2 messenger RNA, causing fragmentation of the protein message. Gene therapy is also being investigated in autologous stem cell transplantation for a variety of malignancies. In this setting, antitumor genes are added to cells that have been removed for transplantation following myeloablative chemotherapy. Trials are ongoing to study this form of therapy in chronic myelogenous leukemia. Multiple other trials, including the introduction of new genes that encode inhibitors of oncogene products or enhance tumor cell immunogenicity, are in progress.

Other areas of investigation include discovery of novel agents that induce apoptosis (programmed cell death), stimulate differentiation, prevent tumor invasion or metastases, and specifically target hormone pathways that stimulate tumor growth. In addition, new antiproliferative agents with improved toxicity profiles and less cross-resistance to known agents are being evaluated or are already in use. Ongoing research is focusing on the identification of new growth factor receptors associated with malignant behavior that can be targeted to suppress cancer growth, such as the HER-2/*neu* receptor targeted by the antibody trastuzumab. The current explosion of clinical trials targeting various pathways of tumor growth as well as ongoing research to identify antigenic targets should lead to a new paradigm for cancer therapy in the coming decades.

Cao Y et al: Expression of angiostatin cDNA in murine fibrosarcoma suppresses primary tumor growth and produces long-term dormancy of metastases J Clin Invest 1998;101:1055. [PMID: 9486976] (Angiostatin appears to result in significant tumor regression in mice.)

Dalgleish AG: Cancer vaccines. Br J Cancer 2000;82:1619. [PMID: 10817493] (Review of clinical trials using vaccines to treat cancers of the prostate, bladder, breast, lung, and kidney.)

Knox SJ et al: Clinical radioimmunotherapy. Semin Radiat Oncol 2000;10:73. [PMID: 10727597] (Reviews the general principles of radioimmunotherapy and its use in the treatment of leukemia, lymphoma, and solid tumors.)

Los M et al: The potential role of antivascular therapy in the adjuvant and neoadjuvant treatment of cancer. Semin Oncol 2001;28:93. [PMID: 11254869] (A review of the conceptual basis of antiangiogenic therapy and their potential roles in the treatment of cancer.)

Sondak VK et al: Adjuvant immunotherapy of resected, intermediate-thickness, node-negative melanoma with an allogeneic tumor vaccine: overall results of a randomized trial of the Southwest Oncology Group. J Clin Oncol 2002; 20:2058. [PMID: 11956266] (This phase III trial in 689 patients with intermediate thickness melanoma with clinically negative nodes found no evidence of improvement in disease free survival in patients treated with adjuvant allogeneic vaccine (Melacine) with a median follow-up of 5.6 years.)

Sosman JA et al: Adjuvant immunotherapy of resected, intermediate-thickness, node-negative melanoma with an allogeneic tumor vaccine: impact of HLA class I antigen expression on outcome. J Clin Oncol 2002;20:2067. [PMID:11956267] (Although vaccine therapy was not beneficial for the trial population as a whole, patients with specific HLA class I antigen expression had a highly significant benefit in terms of disease-free survival when treated with adjuvant vaccine—presumably identifying a subclass with the required

immune phenotype for an immune response to this particular vaccine.)

Witzig TE et al: Randomized controlled trial of yttrium-90-labeled ibritumomab tiuxetan radioimmunotherapy versus rituximab immunotherapy for patients with relapsed or refractory low-grade follicular, or transformed B-cell non-Hodgkin's lymphoma. J Clin Oncol 2002;20:2453. [PMID: 12011122] (Treatment with this radiolabeled antibody improved response rates, response duration, time to progression and the number of durable responses compared to rituximab alone.)

ALTERNATIVE & COMPLEMENTARY THERAPIES FOR CANCER TREATMENT

New areas of cancer therapy are rapidly expanding, and the next decade could bring important changes in the treatment of common malignancies. Many alternatives to traditional cancer therapy exist (one well-known example is shark cartilage, which is widely available and purported to have anti-angiogenic properties), but there is little evidence to support their efficacy or assess their potential toxicity, and at present there is no federal regulation of these products. Agents that are commonly used include green tea, echinacea, essiac tea, flaxseed, mistletoe, and coenzyme Q, as well as others.

It is critical that herbs be tested with the same rigorous standards as chemotherapeutic agents in scientifically based clinical trials. Most herbal preparations are available over the counter, and no information exists regarding the interaction of these herbs with other medications. Many interactions have recently been described between St. John's wort and critical medications such as antiretrovirals, cyclosporine, chemotherapeutic agents, and hormonal agents, among others, that resulted in decreased drug levels due to enhanced metabolism.

A dietary supplement containing a combination of eight Chinese herbs with potent estrogenic activity, PC-SPES, has been tested in prostate cancer. All patients with hormone-sensitive and about 60% of patients with hormone-refractory prostate cancer responded with a decline in PSA; some patients also had improvement in bone scans. Toxicity was modest, including allergic reactions and thromboembolic events in about 4% of patients. Unfortunately, recent laboratory analysis of PC-SPES by the California Department of Health Services found significant contamination of this product with undeclared prescription drugs such as warfarin and alprazolam as well as hormonal agents. Based on these data, the manufacturer of PC-SPES and SPES has voluntarily recalled the products nationwide, and research has been halted. Investigations will need to be repeated if a noncontaminated product is produced, as the finding of hormonal agents in the herbal preparation suggests that the responses seen in published studies could have been due to contaminants instead of the herbs themselves.

Ongoing research is evaluating the effects of herbal combinations on side effects of adjuvant chemotherapy for breast cancer. The NCI is actively supporting research in the field of alternative therapies for cancer through the National Center for Complementary and Alternative Medicine (NCCAM). Additional information on alternative treatment modalities can be found in Chapter 44.

There are now many Web sites devoted to providing information on alternative cancer therapies. NCCAM lists new research and research trials as well as an introduction to alternative medicine. There is also an extensive bibliography. This Web site may be reached at http://nccam.nih.gov. Additional resources can be found at the Cancer Guide Material on Alternative Medicine Web site http://cancerguide.org/alternative.html. The Center for Alternative Medicine Research in Cancer at the University of Texas-Houston Health Science Center (UT-CAM) maintains an excellent Web site with data pertaining to a wide variety of alternative medications and therapies. The site can be reached at http://nccam.nih.gov.

Ernst E: Second thoughts about safety of St John's wort. Lancet 1999;354:2014. [PMID: 10636361] (A discussion of the enzyme-inducing properties of this herbal preparation.)

Jacobson JS et al: Research on complementary/alternative medicine for patients with breast cancer: a review of the biomedical literature. J Clin Oncol 2000;18:668. [PMID: 10653883] (Many studies had encouraging results; none showed a difference in disease progression, though some modalities improved toxicities of therapy.)

Tagliaferri M et al: Complementary and alternative medicine in early-stage breast cancer. Semin Oncol 2001;28:121. [PMID: 11254871] (An excellent review of this widely used treatment modality.)

Vickers AJ et al: Unconventional therapies for cancer and cancer-related symptoms. Lancet 2001;2:226. [PMID: 11905758] (A review of alternative therapies and ongoing research addressing this issue in mainstream medical centers.)

Medical Genetics

41

Reed E. Pyeritz, MD, PhD

See www.current-med.com/ch41.html

The rapid and in some cases spectacular advances in human genetics during the past decade have had important implications for clinical medicine. Familiarity with the fundamental principles of both basic and clinical genetics is now necessary if the clinician is to provide a high standard of care. Virtually all of the 3 billion nucleotides of the human genome have been sequenced. The great hope, of course, is that with this exponential growth in information will come new insights into the causes and pathogenetic mechanisms of human disease, more accurate diagnosis, and effective treatment for many disorders now considered beyond the practitioner's therapeutic reach. Along with this optimistic prospect, however, have come some urgent concerns about (1) the ethical, legal, and sociologic implications of what has been termed "genetic engineering" but is better and more broadly called "molecular medicine"; (2) the problem for medical educators of how best to transmit such an enormous body of information to their students and to primary care practitioners; and (3) the seemingly esoteric nature of much of that information paired with the realization that any one of the obscure facts of medical genetics might achieve clinical relevance at any time.

Gelehrter TD, Collins FS, Ginsburg D: *Principles of Medical Genetics,* 2nd ed. Williams & Wilkins, 1998. (A useful text at the level of a medical student.)

Genetics and disease. Part 3 in: *Harrison's Principles of Internal Medicine,* 15th ed. McGraw-Hill, 2001.

Rimoin DL et al (editors): *Emery and Rimoin's Principles and Practice of Medical Genetics,* 4th ed. Churchill Livingstone, 2002. (Multiauthored compendium covering the basic principles of human genetics, the importance of genetics in medicine, and the diagnosis and management of many genetic disorders.)

■ INTRODUCTION TO MEDICAL GENETICS

Physicians at one time concerned themselves only with what they could discover by bedside evaluation and laboratory investigation. In the parlance of genetics, the patient's symptoms and signs constitute his or her **phenotype.** Now the means are at hand for defining a person's **genotype,** the actual information content inscribed in the 2 meters of coiled DNA present in each cell of the body—or half that amount in every mature ovum or sperm. Virtually all phenotypic characteristics—and this includes diseases as well as human traits such as personality, adult height, and intelligence—are to some extent determined by the genes. The importance of the genetic contribution varies widely among human phenotypes, and methods are only now being developed to identify the genes involved in complex traits and most common diseases. Moreover, the importance of interactions between environment and genotype in producing phenotypes cannot be overstated despite the obscurity of the actual mechanisms.

The billions of nucleotides in the nucleus of a cell are organized linearly along the DNA double helix in functional units called **genes,** and each of the 35,000–50,000 human genes is accompanied by various regulatory elements that control when it is active in producing **messenger RNA (mRNA)** by a process called **transcription.** In most situations, mRNA is transported from the nucleus to the cytoplasm, where its genetic information is **translated** into **proteins,** which perform the functions that ultimately determine phenotype. For example, proteins serve as enzymes that facilitate metabolism and cell synthesis; as DNA binding elements that regulate transcription of other genes; as structural elements of cells and the extracellular matrix; and as receptor molecules for intra- and intercellular communication.

Chromosomes are the vehicles in which the genes are carried from generation to generation. Each chromosome is a complex of protein and nucleic acid in which an unbroken double helix of DNA is coiled and supercoiled into a space many orders of magnitude less than the extended length of the DNA. Within the chromosome there occur highly complicated and integrated processes, including DNA replication, recombination, and transcription. In the nucleus of each somatic cell, humans normally have 46 chromosomes, which are arranged in 23 pairs. One of these pairs, the **sex chromosomes** X and Y, determines the sex of the individual; females have the pair XX and males the pair XY. The remaining 22 pairs are called **autosomes** (Figure 41–1).

In all somatic cells, the 44 autosomes and one of the X chromosomes are transcriptionally active. In males, the active X is the only X; portions of the Y chromosome are also active. In females, the requirement for **dosage compensation** (to be equivalent to the situation in males) is satisfied by inactivation of most of one X chromosome early in embryogenesis.

This process of X chromosomal inactivation, while incompletely understood, is known to be random, so that on average, in 50% of a female's cells, one of the X chromosomes will be active, and in the other 50% the **homologous** member of the pair will be active. The phenotype of the cell is determined by which genes on the chromosomes are active in producing mRNA at any given time.

GENES & CHROMOSOMES

In all genes, information is contained in parcels called **exons,** which are interspersed with stretches of DNA called **introns** that do not encode any information about the protein sequence. However, introns may contain genetic regulatory sequences, and some introns are so large that they encode an entirely distinct gene.

The exact location of a gene on a chromosome is its **locus,** and the array of loci constitutes the **human gene map.** Currently, the chromosomal sites of more than 7730 genes (for which normal or abnormal function has been identified) are known, often to a high degree of resolution. A variation of this map, identifying selected loci known to be involved in human disease, is shown in Figure 41–2. The difference in the higher resolution of the ordering of genes achievable

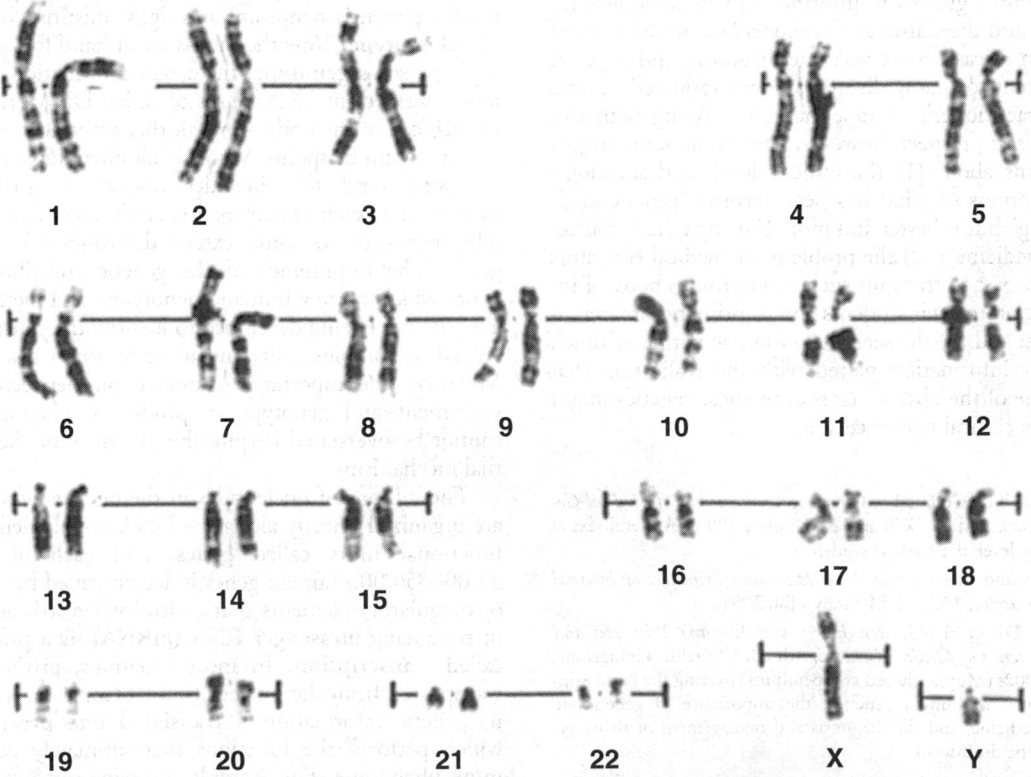

Figure 41–1. Normal karyotype of a human male. Prepared from cultured amniotic cells and stained with Giemsa's stain. About 400 bands are detectable per haploid set of chromosomes.

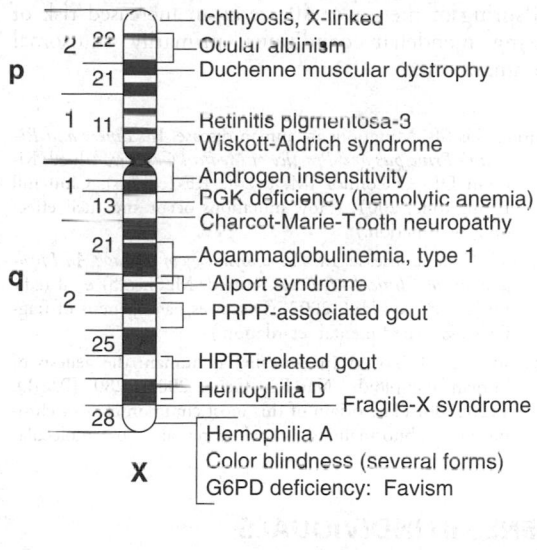

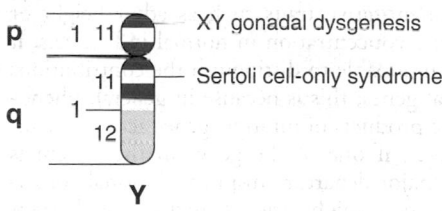

Figure 41–2. A partial "morbid map" of the human genome. Shown next to the ideogram of the human X and Y chromosomes are representative mendelian disorders caused by mutations at that locus. Over 400 genes and phenotypes have been mapped to the X chromosome and 25 to the Y chromosome. (Courtesy of V McKusick and J Strayer.)

by molecular techniques (such as linkage analysis) compared to cytogenetic techniques (such as visualization of small defects) is substantial, though the gap is narrowing. The chromosomes in the "standard" karyotype shown in Figure 41–1 have about 450 visible bands; under the best of cytologic and microscopic conditions, a total of about 1600 bands can be seen. But even in this extended configuration, each band contains dozens—sometimes hundreds—of individual genes. Thus, loss (**deletion**) of a small band will involve loss of many coding sequences and will have diverse effects on the phenotype.

The number and arrangement of genes on homologous chromosomes are identical even though the actual coding sequences of homologous genes may not be. Homologous copies of a gene are termed **alleles.** In comparing alleles, it must be specified at what level of analysis the comparison is being made. When alleles are truly identical—in that their coding sequences are invariant—the individual is **homozygous** at that locus. At a coarser level, the alleles may be functionally identical despite subtle variations in nucleotide se-

quence—with the result either that the proteins produced from the two alleles are identical or that whatever differences there may be in amino acid sequence will have no bearing on the function of the protein. If the individual is being analyzed at the level of the protein phenotype, allelic homozygosity would again be an apt descriptor. However, if the analysis were at the level of the DNA—as occurs in restriction enzyme examination or nucleotide sequencing—then, despite functional identity, the alleles would be viewed as different and the individual would be **heterozygous** for that locus. Heterozygosity based on differences in the protein products of alleles has been detectable for decades and was the first hard evidence concerning the high degree of human biologic variability. In the past decade, analysis of DNA sequences has shown this variability to be much more remarkable—differences in nucleotide sequence between individuals occur about once every 400 nucleotides.

Cantor CR: How will the Human Genome Project improve our quality of life? Nat Biotechnol 1998;16:212. [PMID: 9527989] (Perspective on improved diagnostics, more efficient clinical trials, and gene therapy.)

Collins FS et al: Implications of the Human Genome Project for medical science. JAMA 2001;285:540. [PMID: 11176855] (Prescription for how medical practice will be changed in the next few decades by the sequencing of human DNA.)

Reilly PR et al: We're off to see the genome. Nat Genet 1998;20:15. [PMID: 9731523] (Some of the legal and societal implications of the "human genetics revolution.")

MUTATION

Allelic heterozygosity most often results when different alleles are inherited from the egg and the sperm, but it also occurs as a consequence of spontaneous alteration in nucleotide sequence (**mutation**). Genetic change occurring during formation of an egg or a sperm is called a **germinal mutation.** When the change occurs after conception—from the earliest stages of embryogenesis to dividing cells in the body of the oldest adult—it is termed a **somatic mutation.** As is discussed below, the role of somatic mutation in the etiology of human disease is now increasingly recognized.

The coarsest type of mutation is alteration in the number or physical structure of chromosomes. For example, **nondisjunction** (failure of chromosome pairs to separate) during **meiosis**—the reduction division that leads to production of mature ova and sperms—causes the embryo to have too many or too few chromosomes, a situation called **aneuploidy.** Rearrangement of chromosome arms, such as occurs in **translocation** or **inversion,** is a mutation even if breakage and reunion does not disrupt any coding sequence. Thus, the phenotypic effect of gross chromosomal mutations can range from profound (as in aneuploidy) to nil.

A bit less coarse, but still detectable cytologically, are **deletions** of part of a chromosome. Such mutations almost always alter phenotype, because a number of genes are lost; however, a deletion may involve only a single nucleotide, whereas about 1–2 million nucleotides (1–2 megabases) must be lost before the defect can be visualized by the most sensitive cytogenetic methods short of in situ hybridization. Molecular biologic techniques are needed to detect smaller losses.

Mutations of one or a few nucleotides in exons have several potential consequences. Changes in one nucleotide can alter which amino acid is encoded; if the amino acid is in a critical region of the protein, function might in this way be severely deranged (eg, sickle cell disease). On the other hand, some amino acid substitutions have no detectable effect on function, and the phenotype is therefore unaltered by the mutation. Similarly, because the genetic code is **degenerate** (two or more different three-nucleotide sequences called **codons** encode the same amino acids), nucleotide substitution does not necessarily alter the amino acid sequence of the protein. Three specific codons signal termination of translation; thus, a nucleotide substitution in an exon that generates one of the stop codons usually causes a truncated protein, which is nearly always dysfunctional. Other nucleotide substitutions can disrupt the signals that direct splicing of the mRNA molecule and grossly alter the protein product. Finally, insertions and deletions of one or more nucleotides can have dramatic effects—any change that is not a multiple of three nucleotides disrupts the reading frame of the remainder of the exon—or potentially minimal effects (if the protein can tolerate the insertion or loss of an amino acid).

Mutations in introns may disrupt mRNA splicing signals or may be entirely silent with respect to the phenotype. A great deal of variation in nucleotide sequences among individuals (averaging one difference every few hundred nucleotides) resides within introns. Mutations in the DNA between adjacent genes may also be silent or may have a profound effect on phenotype if regulatory sequences are disrupted. A novel mechanism for mutation, which also helps explain clinical variation among relatives, has been discovered in myotonic dystrophy, Huntington's disease, fragile X mental retardation syndrome, Friedreich's ataxia, and other disorders. A region of repeated trinucleotide sequences close to or within a gene can be unstable in some families; expansion of the number of repeated units within this segment beyond a critical threshold is associated with a more severe phenotype.

Mutations may occur spontaneously or may be induced by such environmental factors as radiation, medication, or viral infections. Both advanced maternal and paternal age favor mutation, but of different types. In women, meiosis is completed only when an egg ovulates, and chromosomal nondisjunction is more common the older the egg. The risk that an aneuploid egg will result increases exponentially and becomes a major clinical worry for women older than their early 30s. In men, mutations of a subtler sort—affecting nucleotide sequences—increase with age.

Offspring of men over 40 are at an increased risk of having mendelian conditions, primarily autosomal dominant ones.

Antonarakis SE: Mutations in human disease. In: *Emery and Rimoin's Principles and Practice of Medical Genetics,* 4th ed. Rimoin DL, O'Connor JM, Pyeritz RE (editors). Churchill Livingstone, 2001. (How mutations occur and their effect on gene function.)

Barsh G: Genetic disease. In: *Pathophysiology of Disease: An Introduction to Clinical Medicine,* 4th ed. McPhee SJ et al (editors): McGraw-Hill, 2002. (Discusses pathogenesis of fragile X-associated mental retardation.)

Hassold T et al: To err (meiotically) is human: the genesis of human aneuploidy. Nat Rev Genet 2001;2:280. [PMID: 11283700] (The origin of this most common class of chromosome abnormalities is being revealed by molecular studies.)

GENES IN INDIVIDUALS

For some quantitative traits such as adult height or serum glucose concentration in normal individuals, it is virtually impossible to distinguish the contributions of individual genes; this is because in general, phenotypes are the products of multiple genes acting in concert. However, if one of the genes in the system is aberrant, a major departure from the "normal" or expected phenotype might arise. Whether the aberrant phenotype is serious (ie, a disease) or even recognized will depend on the nature of the defective gene product and how resilient the system is to disruption. The latter point emphasizes the importance of homeostasis in both physiology and development—many mutations go unrecognized because the system can cope, even though tolerances for further perturbation might be narrowed.

In other words, virtually all human characteristics are **polygenic,** while many of the disordered phenotypes thought of as "genetic" are **monogenic** but still influenced by other loci in a person's genome.

Phenotypes due to alterations at a single gene are also characterized as **mendelian,** after the monk and part-time biologist who studied the reproducibility and recurrence of variation in garden peas. Gregor Mendel showed that some traits were **dominant** to others, which he called **recessive.** The dominant traits required only one copy of a "factor" to be expressed, regardless of what the other copy was, whereas the recessive traits required two copies before expression occurred. In modern terms, the mendelian factors are genes, and the alternative copies of the gene are alleles. Let A be the common (normal) allele and let a be a mutant allele at a locus: If the same phenotype is present no matter whether the genotype is A/a or $a/a,$ the phenotype is dominant, whereas if the phenotype is present only when the genotype is $a/a,$ it is recessive.

In medicine, it is important to keep two considerations in mind: First, dominance and recessiveness are attributes of the phenotype, not the gene; and second, the concepts of dominance and recessiveness depend on how one defines the phenotype. To illustrate both points, consider sickle cell disease. This condition occurs when a person inherits two alleles for β^S-globin, in which the normal glutamate at position 6 of the protein has been replaced by valine; the genotype for the β-globin locus is *HbS/HbS*, compared to the normal *HbA/HbA*. When the genotype is *HbS/HbA,* the individual does not have sickle cell disease, so this condition satisfies the criteria for being a recessive phenotype. But now consider the phenotype of sickled erythrocytes. Red cells with the genotype *HbS/HbS* clearly sickle—but, if the oxygen tension is reduced, so do cells with the genotype *HbS/HbA.* Therefore, sickling is a dominant trait.

A mendelian phenotype is characterized not only in terms of dominance and recessiveness but also according to whether the determining gene is on the X chromosome or on one of the 22 pairs of autosomes. Traits or diseases are therefore called autosomal dominant, autosomal recessive, X-linked recessive, and X-linked dominant.

Beaudet AL: Making genomic medicine a reality. Am J Hum Genet 1999;64:1. [PMID: 9915936] (An enthusiastic perspective on how genetics does and can influence medical care.)

Cook J et al: Mendelian inheritance. In: *Emery and Rimoin's Principles and Practice of Medical Genetics,* 4th ed. Rimoin DL et al (editors). Churchill Livingstone, 2002.

GENES IN FAMILIES

Since the first decade of this century, the patterns of recurrence of specific human phenotypes have been explained in terms of principles first described by Mendel in the garden pea plant. Mendel's second principle—usually referred to as his first*—is called the **law of segregation** and states that a pair of factors (alleles) that determines some trait separates (segregates) during formation of gametes. In simple terms, a heterozygous *(A/a)* person will produce two types of gametes with respect to this locus— one containing only *A* and one containing only *a*, in equal proportions. Offspring of this person will have a 50–50 chance of inheriting the *A* allele and a similar chance of inheriting the *a* allele.

The concepts of genes in individuals and in families can be combined to specify how mendelian traits will be inherited.

---

*Mendel's first law stated that—from the perspective of the phenotype—it mattered not from which parent a particular mutant allele was inherited. For years this principle was thought to be too obvious to be codified as anybody's "law" and was therefore ignored. In fact, however, recent evidence from studies of human disorders suggests that certain genes are "processed" **(imprinted)** as they move through the gonad and that processing in the testis is different from that in the ovary. Thus, not only is this first mendelian principle important, it was incorrect as originally formulated from observations in peas.

Autosomal Dominant Inheritance

The characteristics of autosomal dominant inheritance in humans can be summarized as follows:

(1) There is a vertical pattern in the pedigree, with multiple generations affected (Figure 41–3).

(2) Heterozygotes for the mutant allele show an abnormal phenotype.

(3) Males and females are affected with equal frequency and severity.

(4) Only one parent must be affected for an offspring to be at risk for developing the phenotype.

(5) When an affected person mates with an unaffected one, each offspring has a 50% chance of inheriting the affected phenotype. This is true regardless of the sex of the affected parent—specifically, male-to-male transmission occurs.

(6) The frequency of sporadic cases is positively associated with the severity of the phenotype. More precisely, the greater the **reproductive fitness** of affected persons, the less likely it is that any given case resulted from a new mutation.

(7) The average age of fathers is advanced in the case of isolated (sporadic or new mutation) cases.

Autosomal dominant phenotypes are often age-dependent, less severe than autosomal recessive ones, and associated with malformations or other physical features. They are **pleiotropic** in that multiple, even seemingly unrelated clinical manifestations derive from the same mutation; and **variable** in that expression of the same mutation among people will differ.

Penetrance is a concept associated with mendelian conditions—especially dominant ones—and the term is often misused. It should be defined as an expression of the frequency of appearance of a phenotype (dominant or recessive) when one or more mutant alleles are

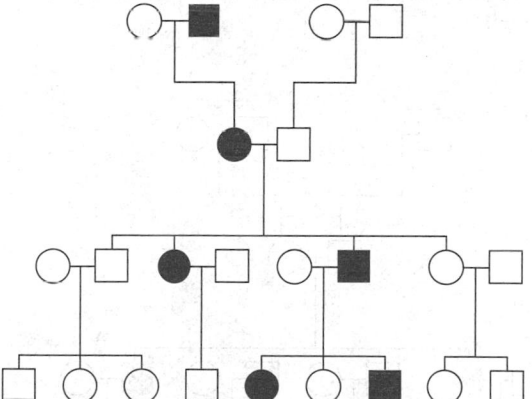

Figure 41–3. A pedigree illustrating autosomal dominant inheritance. Square symbols indicate males and circles females; open symbols indicate that the person is phenotypically unaffected, and filled symbols indicate that the phenotype is present to some extent.

present. For individuals, penetrance is an all-or-none phenomenon—the phenotype is either present (penetrant) or not (nonpenetrant). The term **variability**—not "incomplete penetrance"—should be used to denote differences in expression of an allele.

The most frequent cause of apparent nonpenetrance is insensitivity of the methods for detecting the phenotype. If an apparently normal parent of a child with a dominant condition were in fact heterozygous for the mutation, the parent would have a 50% chance at each subsequent conception of having another affected child. A common cause of nonpenetrance in adult-onset mendelian diseases is death of the affected person before the phenotype becomes evident but after transmission of the mutant allele to offspring. Thus, accurate genetic counseling demands careful attention to the family medical history and high-resolution scrutiny of both parents of a child with a condition known to be a mendelian dominant trait.

When both alleles are expressed in the heterozygote, as in blood group AB, in sickle trait (HbS/HbA), in the major histocompatibility antigens (eg, A2B5/A3B17), or in sickle-C disease (HbS/HbC), the phenotype is called **codominant.**

In human dominant phenotypes, the homozygous state for the mutant allele is almost always more severe than in heterozygotes.

Autosomal Recessive Inheritance

The characteristics of autosomal recessive inheritance in humans can be summarized as follows:

(1) There is a horizontal pattern in the pedigree, with a single generation affected (Figure 41–4).

(2) Males and females are affected with equal frequency and severity.

(3) Inheritance is from both parents, each a heterozygote (carrier) and each usually clinically unaffected.

(4) Each offspring of two carriers has a 25% chance of being affected, a 50% chance of being a carrier, and a 25% chance of inheriting neither mutant allele. Thus, two-thirds of all clinically unaffected offspring are carriers.

(5) In matings between individuals, each with the same recessive phenotype, all offspring will be affected.

(6) Affected individuals who mate with unaffected individuals who are not carriers have only unaffected offspring.

(7) The rarer the recessive phenotype, the more likely it is that the parents are **consanguineous** (related).

Autosomal recessive phenotypes are often associated with deficient activity of enzymes and are thus termed **inborn errors of metabolism.** Such disorders include phenylketonuria, Tay-Sachs disease, and the various glycogen storage diseases and tend to be more severe, less variable, and less age-dependent than dominant conditions.

When an autosomal recessive condition is quite rare, the chance that the parents of affected offspring are consanguineous is increased. As a result, the prevalence of rare recessive conditions is high among inbred groups such as the Old Order Amish. On the other hand, when the autosomal recessive condition is common, the chance of consanguinity between parents of cases is no higher than in the general population (about 0.5%).

Two different *mutant* alleles at the same locus, as in HbS/HbC, form a **genetic compound.** The phenotype usually lies between those produced by either allele present in the homozygous state. Because of the large number of mutations possible in a given gene, many autosomal recessive phenotypes are probably due to genetic compounds. Sickle cell disease is an exception. Consanguinity is strong presumptive evidence for true homozygosity of mutant alleles and against a genetic compound.

X-Linked Inheritance

The general characteristics of X-linked inheritance in humans can be summarized as follows:

(1) There is no male-to-male transmission of the phenotype (Figure 41–5).

(2) Unaffected males do not transmit the phenotype.

(3) All of the daughters of an affected male are heterozygous carriers.

(4) Males are usually more severely affected than females.

(5) Whether a heterozygous female is counted as affected—and whether the phenotype is called "recessive" or "dominant"—depends often on the sensitivity of the assay or of the examination.

(6) Some mothers of affected males will not themselves be heterozygotes (ie, they will be homozygous normal) but will have a germinal mutation. The pro-

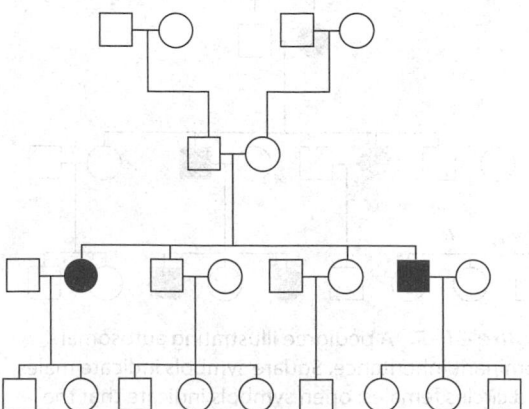

Figure 41–4. A pedigree illustrating autosomal recessive inheritance. (Symbols as in Figure 41–3.)

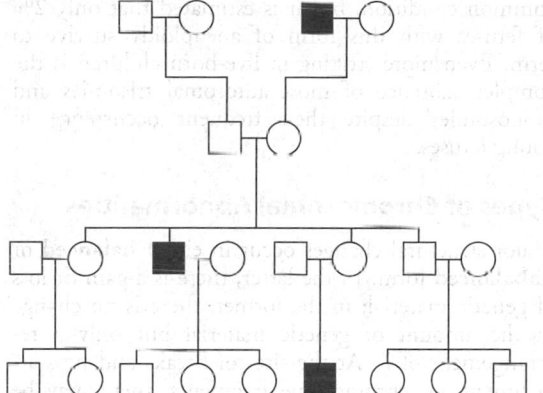

Figure 41–5. A pedigree illustrating X-linked inheritance. (Symbols as in Figure 41–3.)

portion of heterozygous (carrier) mothers is negatively associated with the severity of the condition.

(7) Heterozygous women transmit the mutant gene to one-half of sons, who are affected, and to one-half of daughters, who are heterozygotes.

(8) If an affected male mates with a heterozygous female, half of the male offspring will be affected, giving the false impression of male-to-male transmission. One-half of the female offspring of such matings will be affected as severely as the average hemizygous male; in small pedigrees, this pattern may simulate autosomal dominant inheritance.

The characteristics of X-linked inheritance depend on phenotypic severity. For some disorders, affected males do not survive to reproduce. In such cases, about two-thirds of affected males have a carrier mother; in the remaining third, the disorder arises by new germinal mutation in an X chromosome of the mother. When the disorder is nearly always manifest in heterozygous females (X-linked dominant inheritance), females tend to be affected about twice as often as males; and on average an affected female transmits the phenotype to half of her sons and half of her daughters.

X-linked phenotypes are often clinically variable— particularly in heterozygous females— and suspected of being autosomal dominant with nonpenetrance. For example, Fabry's disease (α-galactosidase A deficiency) may be clinically silent in carrier women or may cause stroke, renal failure, or myocardial infarction by middle age.

Germinal mosaicism occurs in mothers of boys with X-linked conditions. The chance of such a mother having a second affected son or a heterozygous daughter depends on the fraction of her oocytes that carries the mutation. Currently, this fraction is impossible to determine. However, the presence of germinal mosaicism can be detected in some conditions (eg, Duchenne's muscular dystrophy) in a family by analysis of DNA, and this knowledge becomes crucial for genetic counseling.

Nearly 10,500 human genes have been identified through their phenotypes and inheritance patterns in families. This total represents 20–30% of all genes thought to be encoded by the 22 autosomes and 2 sex chromosomes. Victor McKusick coordinates an international effort to catalogue human mendelian variation.

Cook J et al: Mendelian inheritance. In: *Emery and Rimoin's Principles and Practice of Medical Genetics,* 4th ed. Rimoin DL et al (editors). Churchill Livingstone, 2002. (The broad scope of how genes of large effect cause phenotypes and the several known ways in which those phenotypes are expressed variably within families.)

Cummings CJ et al: Fourteen and counting: unraveling trinucleotide repeat diseases. Hum Molec Genet 2000;9:909 [PMID: 10767314] (A succinct review of the 14 degenerative neurologic disorders caused by expansion of a trinucleotide repeat. The complex pathogenetic mechanisms that result from the various mutations are emphasized.)

McKusick VA: *Mendelian Inheritance in Man,* 12th ed. Johns Hopkins Univ Press, 1998. (A catalogue consisting, for each phenotype, of a six-digit identification number—used extensively in the medical literature—a summary statement, and a list of pertinent references. Editions are published periodically, but the catalogue is updated continuously and is computer accessible as Online Mendelian Inheritance in Man [OMIM], accessible through the National Center for Biotechnology Information [http://www.ncbi.nlm.nih.gov/omim]. Six-digit numbers following the names of certain diseases mentioned in this chapter represent their designations in OMIM.)

Wagstaff J: Genetics beyond Mendel. Understanding nontraditional inheritance patterns. Postgrad Med 2000;108:131. [PMID: 11004940] (Reviews other modes of inheritance, including imprinting, trinucleotide repeat expansion, mitochondrial inheritance, and mosaicism.)

DISORDERS OF MULTIFACTORIAL CAUSATION

Many disorders cluster in families but are not associated with evident chromosomal aberrations or mendelian inheritance patterns. Examples include congenital malformations such as cleft lip, pyloric stenosis, and spina bifida; coronary artery disease; type 2 diabetes mellitus; and various forms of neoplasia. They are often characterized by varying frequencies in different racial or ethnic groups, disparity in sexual predilection, and greater frequency (but less than full concordance) in monozygotic than in dizygotic twins. This inheritance pattern is called "multifactorial" to signify that multiple genes interact with various environmental agents to produce the phenotype. The familial clustering is assumed to be due to sharing of both alleles and environment.

For most multifactorial conditions, there is little understanding of which particular genes are involved, how they and their products interact, and in what way different nongenetic factors contribute to the phenotype. For some disorders, biochemical and genetic studies have identified mendelian conditions within the coarse phenotype: Defects of the low-density lipoprotein receptor account for a small fraction of cases of ischemic heart disease (a larger fraction if only patients under age 50 are considered); familial polyposis of the colon predisposes to adenocarcinoma; and some patients with emphysema have inherited deficiency of α_1-proteinase inhibitor. Despite these notable examples, this reductionistic preoccupation with mendelian phenotypes is unlikely to explain the great majority of human disease; but even so, in the last analysis, much of human pathology will prove to be associated with genetic factors in cause, pathogenesis, or both.

Our ignorance about fundamental genetic mechanisms in development and physiology has not completely restricted practical approaches to the genetics of multifactorial disorders. For example, recurrence risks are based on empirical data derived from observation of many families. The risk of recurrence of multifactorial disorders is increased in several instances: (1) in close relatives (sibs, offspring, and parents) of an affected individual; (2) when two or more members of a family have the same condition; (3) when the first case in a family is in the less commonly affected sex (eg, pyloric stenosis is five times more common in boys; an affected woman has a three- to fourfold greater risk of having a child with pyloric stenosis); and (4) in ethnic groups in which there is a high incidence of a particular condition (eg, spina bifida is 40 times more common in Caucasians—and even more frequent among the Irish—than in Asians).

For many apparently multifactorial disorders, enough families have not been examined to have established empirical risk data. A useful approximation of recurrence risk in close relatives is the square root of the incidence. For example, many common congenital malformations have an incidence of 1:2500 to 1:400 live births; the calculated recurrence risks are thus in the 2–5% range—values that correspond closely to experience.

Childs B: *Genetic Medicine.* Johns Hopkins Univ Press, 1999. (An approachable book that lays out a life's perspective on the role of genetics in health and disease.)

CHROMOSOMAL ABERRATIONS

Any deviation from the structure and number of chromosomes as displayed in Figure 41–1 is, technically, a chromosomal aberration. Not all aberrations cause problems in the affected individual, but some that do not may lead to problems in offspring. About 1:200 live-born infants have a chromosomal aberration that is detected because of some effect on phenotype. This frequency increases markedly the earlier in fetal life the chromosomes are examined. By the end of the first trimester of gestation, most fetuses with abnormal numbers of chromosomes have been lost through spontaneous abortion. For example, Turner's syndrome—due to absence of one sex chromosome and the presence of a single X chromosome—is a relatively common condition, but it is estimated that only 2% of fetuses with this form of aneuploidy survive to term. Even more striking in live-born children is the complete absence of most autosomal trisomies and monosomies despite their frequent occurrence in young fetuses.

Types of Chromosomal Abnormalities

Major structural changes occur in either **balanced** or **unbalanced** form. In the latter, there is a gain or loss of genetic material; in the former, there is no change in the amount of genetic material but only a rearrangement of it. At the sites of breaks and new attachments of chromosome fragments, there may be permanent structural or functional damage to one gene or to only a few genes. Despite no visible loss of material, the aberration may nonetheless be recognized as unbalanced through an abnormal phenotype and the chromosomal defect confirmed by molecular analysis of the DNA.

Aneuploidy results from nondisjunction—the failure of a chromatid pair to separate in a dividing cell. Nondisjunction in either the first or second division of meiosis results in gametes with abnormal chromosomal constitutions. In aneuploidy, more or fewer than 46 chromosomes are present (Table 41–1). The following are all forms of aneuploidy: (1) **monosomy,** in which only one member of a pair of chromosomes is present; (2) **trisomy,** in which three chromosomes are present instead of two; and (3) **polysomy,** in which one chromosome is represented four or more times.

If nondisjunction occurs in mitosis, **mosaic** patterns occur in somatic tissue, with some cells having one karyotype and other cells of the same organism another karyotype. Patients with a mosaic genetic constitution often have manifestations of each of the genetic syndromes associated with the various abnormal karyotypes.

Table 41–1. Clinical phenotypes resulting from aneuploidy.

Condition	Karyotype	Incidence at Birth
Trisomy 13	47,XX or XY,+13	1:15,000
Trisomy 18	47,XX or XY,+18	1:11,000
Trisomy 21 (Down's syndrome)	47,XX or XY,+21	1:900
Klinefelter's syndrome	47,XXY	1:600 males
XYY syndrome	47,XYY	1:1000 males
Turner's syndrome	45,X	1:2500 females
XXX syndrome	47,XXX	1:1200 females

Translocation results from an exchange of parts of two chromosomes.

Deletion is loss of chromosomal material.

Duplication is the presence of two or more copies of the same region of a given chromosome. The redundancy may occur in the same chromosome or in a nonhomologous chromosome. In the latter case, a translocation will also have occurred.

An **isochromosome** is one in which the arms on either side of the centromere have the same genetic material in the same order—ie, the chromosome has at some time divided in such a way that it has a double dose of one arm and absence of the other.

In an **inversion**, a chromosomal region becomes reoriented 180 degrees out of ordinary phase. The same genetic material is present, but in a different order.

Ferguson-Smith MA, Andrews T: Cytogenetic analysis. In: *Emery and Rimoin's Principles and Practice of Medical Genetics*, 4th ed. Rimoin DL et al (editors). Churchill Livingstone, 2002. (A review of the indications for and techniques of clinical cytogenetics.)

■ THE TECHNIQUES OF MEDICAL GENETICS

Hereditary disorders affect multiple organ systems and people of all ages. Many disorders are chronic ones, but often there are acute crises. The concerns of patients and families span a wide range of medical, psychologic, social, and economic issues. These characteristics emphasize the need for pediatricians, internists, obstetricians, and family practitioners to provide medical genetics services for their patients. This section reviews the laboratory and consultative services available from clinical geneticists and the indications for their use.

CYTOGENETICS

Cytogenetics is the study of chromosomes by light microscopy. The chromosomal constitution of a single cell or an entire individual is specified by a standardized notation. The total chromosome count is determined first, followed by the sex chromosome complement and then by any abnormalities. The autosomes are all designated by numbers from 1 to 22. A plus (+) or minus (−) sign indicates, respectively, a gain or loss of chromosomal material. For example, a normal male is 46,XY, while a girl with Down's syndrome caused by trisomy 21 is 47,XX,+21, a boy with Down's syndrome caused by translocation of chromosome 21 to chromosome 14 in a sperm or an egg is 46,XY,−14,+t(14;21).

Chromosomal analyses are done by growing human cells in tissue culture, chemically inhibiting mitosis, and then staining, observing, photographing, sorting, and counting the chromosomes. The display of all of the chromosomes is termed the **karyotype** (Figure 41–1) and is the end result of the technical aspect of cytogenetics.

Specimens for cytogenetic analysis can be obtained for routine analysis from the peripheral blood, in which case T lymphocytes are examined; from amniotic fluid for culture of amniocytes; from trophoblastic cells from the chorionic villus; from bone marrow; and from cultured fibroblasts, usually obtained from a skin biopsy. Enough cells must be examined so that the chance of missing a cytogenetically distinct cell line (a situation of mosaicism) is statistically low. For most clinical indications, 20 mitoses are examined and counted under direct microscopic visualization, and two are photographed and karyotypes prepared. Observation of aberrations usually prompts more extended scrutiny and in many cases further analysis of the original culture.

A variety of methods can be used to reveal banding patterns—unique to each pair of chromosomes—in the analysis of aberrations. The number of bands that can be visualized is a function of how "extended" the chromosomes are, which in turn depends chiefly on how early in metaphase (or even in prophase for the most extensive banding) mitosis was arrested. The "standard" karyotype reveals about 400 bands per haploid set of chromosomes, whereas a prophase karyotype might reveal four times that number. As invaluable as extended karyotypes are in certain clinical circumstances, their interpretation is often difficult—in terms of the time and effort required and of ambiguity about what is abnormal, what is a normal variation, and what is a technical artifact. In situ hybridization with DNA probes for specific chromosomes or regions of chromosomes can be labeled and used to identify subtle aberrations. Given proper technique, fluorescent in situ hybridization (FISH) yields sensitivities and specificities of virtually 100%. Some applications are being used routinely and marketed commercially, though the FDA has only recently begun to approve probes for clinical use.

An area of particular relevance is the use of FISH to detect heretofore undetectable deletions in the regions of chromosomes just proximal to their tips (subtelomeric). A remarkable number of patients with unexplained mental retardation or dysmorphology have been found to have such deletions, either because of de novo mutation or because of rearrangements due to balanced parental translocations.

Indications for Cytogenetic Analysis

The current indications are listed in Table 41–2. A wide array of clinical syndromes have been found to be associated with chromosomal aberrations, and analysis of the karyotype is useful any time a patient is discovered to have the manifestations of one of these syndromes. When a chromosomal aberration is re-

Table 41-2. Indications for cytogenetic analysis.

1. Patients with malformations suggestive of one of the recognized syndromes associated with a specific chromosome aberration.
2. Patients of any age who are grossly retarded physically or mentally, especially if there are associated anomalies.
3. Any patient with ambiguous internal or external genitalia or suspected hermaphroditism.
4. Girls with primary amenorrhea and boys with delayed pubertal development. Up to 25% of patients with primary amenorrhea have a chromosomal abnormality.
5. Males with learning or behavioral disorders who are taller than expected (based on parental height).
6. Certain malignant and premalignant diseases (see Tables 41-8 and 41-9).
7. Parents of a patient with chromosome translocation.
8. Parents of a patient with a suspected chromosomal syndrome if there is a family history of similarly affected children.
9. Couples with a history of multiple spontaneous abortions of unknown cause.
10. Couples who are infertile after more common obstetric and urologic causes have been excluded.
11. Prenatal diagnosis (see Table 41-7).

vealed, not only does the patient's physician obtain valuable information about prognosis, but the parents gain insight into the cause of their child's problems and the family can be counseled accurately—and usually reassured—about the risks of recurrence.

Mental retardation is a frequent component of congenital malformation syndromes. Any person with unexplained mental retardation should be studied by chromosomal analysis.

Abnormalities of sexual differentiation can only be understood once the patient's **genetic sex** is clarified. Hormonal therapy and plastic surgery can to some extent determine **phenotypic sex,** but genetic sex is dictated by the complement of sex chromosomes. The best-known example of dichotomy between the genetic sex and phenotypic sex is the **testicular feminization syndrome,** in which the chromosomal constitution is 46,XY but, because of a defect in the testosterone receptor protein (specified by a gene on the Y chromosome), the external phenotype is completely female.

Failure or delay in developing secondary sexual characteristics occurs in **Turner's syndrome** (the most common cause being a form of aneuploidy, ie, monosomy for the X chromosome, 45,X), in **Klinefelter's syndrome** (the most common karyotype is 47,XXY), and in other much rarer chromosomal aberrations.

Tall stature is perhaps the only consistent phenotypic feature associated with having an **extra Y chromosome** (karyotype 47,XYY); most men with this chromosomal aberration lead normal lives, and thus tall stature in a male is itself no indication for chromosomal analysis. However, some evidence suggests that

an increased prevalence of learning difficulties may be associated with this aberration. Furthermore, Klinefelter's syndrome often causes tall stature, albeit with a eunuchoid habitus, and learning and behavioral problems. Thus, the combination of learning or behavioral difficulties and unexpectedly increased height in a male should prompt consideration of cytogenetic analysis.

As discussed below, most tumors are associated with chromosomal aberrations, some of which are highly specific for certain malignancies. Cytogenetic analysis of tumor tissue may assist in diagnosis, prognosis, and management.

Whenever a person is shown to have a chromosome translocation—whether it be balanced and asymptomatic or unbalanced, causing a syndrome—the physician should consider the importance of identifying the source of the translocation. If the proband is a child and the parents are interested in having more children, both parents should be studied cytogenetically. How far the primary physician or consultant should go in tracking a translocation through a family is an unsettled question with legal and ethical as well as medical implications. Certainly the proband (if an adult) or the parents of the proband need to be counseled and the potential risks to relatives discussed. The physician should document, both in the medical record and by correspondence, that the burden of disclosing relevant data to the extended family has been assumed by specific named individuals.

Inability to produce offspring, either through failure to conceive or as a result of repeated miscarriages, is a frustrating and discouraging problem for affected couples and their physicians. Considerable progress in the urologic and gynecologic understanding of infertility has benefited many couples. However, chromosomal aberrations remain an important problem in reproductive medicine, and cytogenetic analysis should be utilized at some stage in extended evaluation. Infertility is common in both Klinefelter's and Turner's syndromes, either of which may be associated with mild external signs—particularly if the chromosomal aberration is mosaic. Any early spontaneous abortion may be due to fetal aneuploidy. Recurrence may be due to parental translocation predisposing to an unbalanced fetal karyotype.

Borgaonkar D: *Chromosomal Variation in Man,* 8th ed. Wiley, 1998. (A comprehensive catalogue; the companion to McKusick's *Mendelian Inheritance in Man.*)

Fan Y-S et al: Detection of submicroscopic aberrations in patients with unexplained mental retardation by fluorescence in situ hybridization using multiple subtelomeric probes. Genet Med 2001;3:416. [PMID: 11715006] (A new approach to diagnosis that is yielding explanations in about 5% of patients who have mental retardation.)

Uhrig S et al: Multiplex-FISH for pre- and postnatal diagnostic applications. Am J Hum Genet 1999;65:448. [PMID: 10417288] (Maximum sensitivity for detecting chromosomal anomalies is obtained by combining standard karyotypic analysis with fluorescent in situ hybridization.)

Wachtel SS et al: FISH and PRINS: competing or complementary technologies? Am J Med Genet 2002;107:97. [PMID: 11807880] (Both of these methods are useful in identifying the cause of syndromes of obscure origin.)

BIOCHEMICAL GENETICS

Biochemical genetics deals not only with enzymatic defects but also with proteins of all functions, including cytoskeletal and extracellular structure, regulation, and receptors. The principal functions of the biochemical genetics laboratory are to determine the presence or absence of proteins, to assess the qualitative characteristics of proteins, and to verify the effectiveness of proteins in vitro. The key elements from the referring clinician's perspective are (1) to indicate what the suspected clinical diagnoses are and (2) to make certain that the proper specimen is obtained and transported to the laboratory in a timely manner.

Indications for Biochemical Investigations

Some inborn errors are relatively common in the general population, eg, hemochromatosis, defects of the low-density lipoprotein receptor, and cystic fibrosis (Table 41–3). Others, while rare across the entire population, are common in certain ethnic groups, such as Tay-Sachs disease in Ashkenazic Jews, sickle cell disease in African-Americans, and thalassemias in populations from around the Mediterranean basin and Asia. Many of these disorders are autosomal recessive, and the frequency of heterozygotes is many times that of the fully expressed disease. Screening for carrier status can be effective if certain requirements are satisfied (Table 41–4). For example, all of the United States and the District of Columbia require screening of newborns for phenylketonuria and often other metabolic diseases. Such programs are cost-effective even

Table 41–4. Requirements for effective screening for inborn errors of metabolism.

1. The disease should be clinically severe or have potentially severe consequences.
2. The natural history of the disease should be understood.
3. Effective treatment should be generally available and depend on early diagnosis for optimal results.
4. The disease incidence should be high enough to warrant screening.
5. The screening test should have favorable specificity (low false-positive rate) and sensitivity (low false-negative rate).
6. The screening test should be available for and used by the entire population at risk.
7. An adequate system for follow-up of positive results should be provided.
8. The economic cost-benefit analysis should favor screening and treatment.

for rare conditions such as phenylketonuria, which occurs in only one of every 11,000 births. Unfortunately, not all disorders that meet the requirements in Table 41–4 are screened for in every state. Furthermore, compliance is highly variable among programs, and follow-up diagnostic tests, management, and counseling are in some cases inadequate. Babies most likely to be missed are those born at home and those discharged before they have digested much milk or formula. In some states, parents can refuse to have their infants studied.

Use of the biochemical genetics laboratory for other than screening purposes must be justified by the need for data on which to base a diagnosis of specific disorders or classes of related disorders. The possibilities are limited only by the extent of knowledge, the enthusiasm of the primary clinician or consultant, the

Table 41–3. Representative inborn errors of metabolism.

General Class of Defect	Example	Biochemical Defect	Inheritance[1]
Aminoacidopathy	Phenylketonuria	Phenylalanine hydroxylase	AR
Connective tissue	Osteogenesis imperfecta type II	α1(I) and α2(I) procollagen	AD
Gangliosidosis	Tay-Sachs disease	Hexosaminidase A	AR
Glycogen storage disease	Type I	Glucose-6-phosphatase	AR
Immune function	Chronic granulomatous disease	Cytochrome b, β chain	XL
Lipid metabolism	Familial hypercholesterolemia	LDL receptor	AD
Mucopolysaccharidosis	MPS II (Hunter's syndrome)	Iduronate sulfatase	XL
Porphyria	Acute intermittent	Porphobilinogen deaminase	AD
Transport	Cystic fibrosis	CF transmembrane conductance regulator	AR
Urea cycle	Citrullinemia	Arginosuccinate synthetase	AR

[1]AR = autosomal recessive; AD = autosomal dominant; XL = X-linked recessive.

willingness of the patient or family to pursue the diagnosis and specimens to be taken, and the availability of a laboratory to examine the specimens.

Though many inborn defects are so subtle they escape detection, there are a number of clinical situations in which an inborn error should be part of the differential diagnosis. The urgency with which the investigation is undertaken will vary depending on the severity of the disorder and the availability of treatment. Table 41–5 lists various clinical presentations.

The possibility of acute metabolic disease of the neonate is the most important indication, because prompt diagnosis and treatment may often make the difference between life and death. The clinical features are nonspecific because the newborn has a limited repertoire of responses to severe metabolic insults. The physician must be both inclusive and systematic in evaluating such ill babies.

Leonard JV et al: Inborn errors of metabolism around the time of birth. Lancet 2000;356:583. [PMID: 10950248] (Proposes a strategy to identify babies at high risk for metabolic defects so that diagnosis and treatment may be started without delay.)

Table 41–5. Manner of presentation of inborn errors of metabolism.

Presentation and Course	Examples
Acute metabolic disease of the neonate	Galactosemia, urea cycle disorders
Chronic disorders with little progression after infancy	Phenylketonuria, hypothyroidism
Chronic disorders with insidious, incessant progression	Tay-Sachs disease
Disorders causing abnormalities of structure	Skeletal dysplasias, Marfan's syndrome
Disorders of transport	Cystinuria, lactase deficiency
Disorders that determine susceptibilities	LDL receptor deficiency, agammaglobulinemia
Episodic disorders	Most porphyrias, glucose-6-phosphate deficiency
Disorders causing anemia	Pyruvate kinase deficiency, hereditary spherocytosis
Disorders interfering with hemostasis	Hemophilia A and B, von Willebrand disease
Congenital disorders with no possibility of reversal	Testicular feminization
Disorders with protean manifestations	Pseudohypoparathyroidism, hereditary amyloidoses
Inborn errors with no clinical effects	Pentosuria, histidinemia

Scriver CR et al (editors): *The Metabolic and Molecular Bases of Inherited Disease*, 8th ed. McGraw-Hill, 2001. (The standard reference work and source of information about most hereditary disorders.)

DNA ANALYSIS

Direct inspection of nucleic acids—often called "molecular genetics" or "DNA diagnosis"—is achieving an increasingly prominent role in a number of clinical areas, including oncology, infectious disease, forensics, and the general study of pathophysiology. A major impact has been in the diagnosis of mendelian disorders. Molecular testing is available for more than 400 separate hereditary conditions. Once a particular gene is shown to be defective in a given condition, the nature of the mutation itself can be determined, often by sequencing the nucleotides and comparing the array with that of a normal allele. One of a variety of techniques can then be used to determine whether that same mutation is present in other patients with the same disorder. Genetic heterogeneity is so extensive that most mendelian conditions are associated with numerous mutations at one locus—or occasionally multiple loci—that produce the same phenotype. Mutations at no less than 26 different genes cause retinitis pigmentosa, and changes in at least seven genes cause familial hypertrophic cardiomyopathy. This fact complicates DNA diagnosis of patients and screening for carriers of defects in specific genes.

A few conditions are associated with relatively few mutations or with only one highly prevalent mutation. For example, all sickle cell disease is caused by exactly the same change of glutamate to valine at position 6 of β-globin, and that substitution in turn is due to a change of one nucleotide at the sixth codon in the β-globin gene. But such uniformity is the exception. In cystic fibrosis, about 70% of heterozygotes have an identical deletion of three nucleotides that causes loss of a phenylalanine residue from a chloride transport protein; however, the remaining 30% of mutations of that protein are diverse (over 800 have been discovered), so that no simple screening test will detect *all* carriers of cystic fibrosis.

Reviews of the current technical status of DNA analysis appear regularly in the medical literature. Polymerase chain reaction (PCR) studies have revolutionized many aspects of molecular biology, and DNA diagnosis has come to involve this technique in many instances. If the sequences of the 10–20 nucleotides at the ends of a region of DNA of interest (such as a portion of a gene) are known, then "primers" complementary to these sequences can be synthesized. When even a minute amount of DNA from a patient (eg, from a few leukocytes, buccal mucosal cells, or hair bulbs) is combined with the primers in a reaction mixture that replicates DNA—and after several dozen cycles are then performed—the region of DNA between the primers will be amplified exponentially. For example, the presence of early HIV infection can be detected after PCR amplification of a portion of the viral genome. A variety of new techniques are being studied in an attempt to permit analysis of many potential genetic variations in one individual in a very short time. For example, "DNA chip arrays," about the size of a microscope cover slip, can contain tens of thousands of specific nucleotide sequences. When an individual's DNA is denatured and allowed to hybridize to the array, pairing of sequences causes a fluorescent signal that can be detected by a laser microscope and recorded and interpreted by a computer.

Indications for DNA Diagnosis

The basic requirement for the use of nucleic acids in the diagnosis of hereditary conditions is that a **probe** be available for the gene in question. The probe may be a piece of the actual gene, a sequence close to the gene, or just a few nucleotides at the actual mutation. The closer the probe is to the actual mutation, the more accurate and the more useful will be the information derived. DNA diagnosis involves one of two general approaches: (1) direct detection of the mutation or (2) linkage analysis, whereby the presence of a mutation is inferred from the nature of a probe DNA sequence remote from the mutation. In the latter approach, as the probe moves farther from the mutation, the chances increase that recombination will have separated the two sequences and confused the interpretation of the data.

Some of the conditions for which direct detection is possible are listed in Table 41-6. Conditions that can be diagnosed only indirectly are also listed; while their number also is increasing, there is a gratifying shift to diagnosis by direct detection as the molecular nature of mutations is defined.

DNA diagnosis is finding frequent application in presymptomatic detection of individuals with age-dependent disorders such as Huntington's disease and adult polycystic kidney disease, screening for carriers of autosomal recessive conditions such as cystic fibrosis and thalassemias, screening for female heterozygotes of X-linked conditions such as Duchenne's muscular dystrophy and hemophilia A and B, and prenatal diagnosis (see below). The full range of indications is undefined at this time. However, primary care providers and specialists alike must be mindful that substantive ethical, psychologic, legal, and social issues remain unresolved. For example, some conditions for which hereditary susceptibility can be readily defined (such as Alzheimer's disease, Huntington's disease, and many cancers) have no effective therapy at this time. For these same conditions, health insurance and life insurance providers may be especially interested in learning who among their current or prospective customers is at higher risk. Some states have enacted legislation to protect people identified as having a heightened genetic risk of disease.

Logistics of DNA Diagnosis

Lymphocytes are a ready source of DNA; 10 mL of whole blood yields up to 0.5 mg of DNA, enough for dozens of analyses based on hybridization, each of which requires only 5 μg. If the analysis is quite narrowly focused on a specific mutation (such as in a family study, in which only one specific nucleotide change is addressed), PCR analysis can often be used and the amount of DNA needed is truly infinitesimal—a few hair bulbs or sperm are adequate. Once isolated, the DNA sample can be divided into aliquots

Table 41–6. Selected DNA probes with current diagnostic applications.

Gene Probe	Disorder	Diagnostic Application
β-Globin	Sickle cell disease Beta thalassemia	Prenatal screening Prenatal screening
α-Globin	Alpha thalassemia Polycystic kidney disease	Prenatal screening Presymptomatic, prenatal screening
Factor VIII	Hemophilia A	Prenatal screening, carrier detection
Dystrophin	Duchenne's muscular dystrophy	Presymptomatic, prenatal screening, carrier detection
α_1-AP	α_1-Antiprotease deficiency	Prenatal screening
Phe hydroxylase	Phenylketonuria	Prenatal screening
CFTR	Cystic fibrosis	Prenatal screening, presymptomatic screening, carrier detection
Trinucleotide repeat (CAG) in huntingtin	Huntington's disease	Presymptomatic screening, prenatal screening
Growth hormone	Growth hormone deficiency	Prenatal screening, carrier detection, early diagnosis
HFE (HLA)	Hemochromatosis	Presymptomatic screening, prenatal screening

and frozen. Alternatively, lymphocytes can be transformed with viruses into lymphoblasts; these cells are immortal, can be frozen, and—whenever DNA is required—can be thawed, propagated, and their DNA isolated. These stored specimens provide access to a person's genome long after the individual dies. This is such an important advantage that many clinical genetics centers and commercial laboratories "bank" DNA from patients and informative relatives even if the samples cannot be put to use immediately. The specimens may later prove invaluable to relatives or to other patients being evaluated. DNA in some instances has become more reliable than the medical records.

Blood for DNA isolation should be drawn in EDTA anticoagulant (lavender-top tubes); blood for lymphoblast culture should be drawn in heparin (green-top tubes). Neither should be frozen. Specimens for DNA isolation can be stored or shipped at room temperature over a period of a few days. Lymphoblast cultures should be established within 48 hours, so prompt shipment is essential. For one or a few specific DNA analyses, some laboratories accept a cotton swab that has been placed between the cheek and gum for a minute (buccal swab); enough cells adhere to the fibers that DNA from the subject can be isolated.

Fetal DNA can be isolated from amniotic cells, from trophoblastic cells taken by chorionic villus sampling, or from either cell type grown in culture. Samples need to be processed promptly but can be shipped by overnight mail and *must not be frozen.*

ASHG statement. Professional disclosure of familial genetic information. The American Society of Human Genetics Social Issues Subcommittee on Familial Disclosure. Am J Hum Genet 1998;62:474. [PMID: 9537923] (Guidelines for dealing with the unavoidable conflicts between confidentiality, opportunities to diagnose relatives, and the law.)

Cunningham GC: The genetics revolution. Ethical, legal, and insurance concerns. Postgrad Med 2000;108:193. [PMID: 10914128] (Discusses the role of primary care physicians in properly educating patients about genetic testing, confidentiality, and access to health insurance.)

Elsas LJ et al: Cancer genetics in primary care. When is genetic screening an option and when is it is the standard of care? Postgrad Med 2000;107:191. [PMID: 10778420] (With the help of qualified genetic professionals, primary care physicians can determine when genetic testing for hereditary cancer is appropriate by taking a complete three-generation family history.)

Grody WW et al: Diagnostic molecular genetics. In: *Emery and Rimoin's Principles and Practice of Medical Genetics,* 4th ed. Rimoin DL et al (editors). Churchill Livingstone, 2002. (Current state of using DNA-based testing for disease.)

Grody WW et al: Report card on molecular testing: Room for improvement? JAMA 1999;281:845. [PMID: 10071008] (An editorial that addresses the quality and proficiency aspects of DNA diagnostics in the United States.)

Maron BJ et al: Impact of laboratory molecular diagnosis on contemporary diagnostic criteria for genetically transmitted cardiovascular diseases: hypertrophic cardiomyopathy, long QT syndrome and Marfan syndrome. Circulation

1998;98:1460. [PMID: 9841131] (A consensus panel concludes that DNA diagnosis has limited applicability for these relatively common hereditary disorders of the cardiovascular system, mainly because the genes are so large and so many mutations cause the disorders.)

Vnencak-Jones CL: Molecular testing for inherited diseases. Am J Clin Pathol 1999;112:S19. [PMID: 10396298] (Review of molecular testing techniques, including mutation analysis of trinucleotide repeats, point mutations, deletions, gene rearrangements, uniparental disomy, and linkage analysis utilized in screening for common inherited diseases.)

PRENATAL DIAGNOSIS

It is possible to diagnose in utero, before the middle of the second trimester, several hundred mendelian disorders, all chromosome aberrations, and a number of congenital malformations that are not mendelian. The first step toward prenatal diagnosis is taken when the expecting couple, the primary care provider, or the obstetrician thinks of the need for it. Recent surveys suggest that even for the most common indication for such service—advanced maternal age—less than half of all women 35 years and older in the United States are offered prenatal testing.

Techniques Used in Prenatal Diagnosis

Prenatal diagnosis depends on the ability to assay the fetus directly (fetal blood sampling, fetoscopy), indirectly (analysis of amniotic fluid, amniocytes or trophoblastic cells, ultrasound), or remotely (analysis of maternal serum). Some of these techniques satisfy the requirements for screening (Table 41–4) and should be offered to all pregnant women; others carry considerable risk and should be reserved for specific circumstances. A few centers are developing preimplantation diagnosis of the embryo; a single cell is plucked from the six- to eight-cell blastocyst, which has been cultured after in vitro fertilization, without harming future development. The chromosomes of the cell can be studied by FISH or the genes by PCR. Another new approach, with considerable potential, is isolation of fetal cells that are circulating in minute numbers in the maternal circulation.

Ultrasound scanning of the fetus is a safe, noninvasive procedure that can diagnose gross skeletal malformations as well as nonbony malformations known to be associated with specific diseases. Some obstetricians routinely perform fetal ultrasound at least once between 12 and 20 weeks of gestation.

Other prenatal diagnostic procedures—fetoscopy, fetography, and amniography—are more invasive and a definite risk to the mother and fetus. They are indicated only if the risk of the suspected abnormality is high and the information cannot be obtained by other means.

All of the cytogenetic, biochemical, and DNA analytic techniques discussed above can be applied to specimens from the fetus. Aside from screening for α-fetoprotein in maternal serum to detect neural tube defects, analysis of fetal chromosomes is the most frequently performed test. Chromosomal analysis can be performed on amniotic cells and on trophoblastic cells grown in culture and directly on any trophoblastic cells that happen to be undergoing mitosis. Amniotic fluid cells are derived chiefly from the fetal urinary system. Amniocentesis can be performed during gestational weeks 16–18 to permit unhurried sample analysis, transmission of results, and reproductive decisions. The time from obtaining the sample to a final reading of the karyotype has now been shortened to an average of 10–14 days, and automated methods may reduce the time a bit further. Abdominal chorionic villus sampling (CVS) for trophoblastic cells (derived embryologically from the same fertilized egg as the fetus) is usually done during gestational weeks 11–13. If the tissue can be analyzed directly, cytogenetic results can be obtained within a few hours; however, the quality of the karyotypes is inferior to that from cultured cells, and most laboratories routinely culture cells and reexamine any suspected abnormalities. The advantage of CVS is that the results are available early in pregnancy, so that termination, if elected, can occur earlier in the pregnancy and the obstetric complications of termination are fewer.

The risk of CVS is somewhat higher than that of amniocentesis, though both are relatively safe. Between 0.5% and 1% of pregnancies are lost as a complication of CVS, whereas less than one in 300 amniocenteses result in fetal loss. Some centers offer "early amniocentesis," performed during gestational weeks 12–14; the magnitude of the risks is similar to that of CVS. These figures are lower than—but are in addition to—the 2–3% spontaneous abortion rate after the first trimester ends.

Indications for Prenatal Diagnosis

The indications for prenatal diagnosis are listed in Table 41–7. A few deserve comment.

Most studies done for advanced maternal age will detect no chromosomal aberration, and the couple will be reassured by this news. However, it is always appropriate to emphasize that the average risk of producing a child with a defect evident at birth, such as a physical malformation or some inborn error of metabolism, is about 3%, and that the risk increases with the age of either parent. Simply examining the chromosomes reduces this risk minimally. On the other hand, unless one of the other indications is present, it is simply not possible to "screen" a pregnancy for most birth defects (neural tube defects being an exception).

Individuals contemplating pregnancy—especially those of Ashkenazic Jewish or other Caucasian ethnicity—should be offered screening for the most common mutations in the *CFTR* gene that cause cystic fibrosis. If both partners are detected as being carriers, prenatal diagnosis of a fetus would be an option for them.

A history for cytogenetic aberrations emphasizes a chromosomal defect in a parent, a family history of a chromosomal defect, or a previous child or conceptus with a defined or undefined chromosomal defect. The factors that render some couples susceptible to repeated episodes of aneuploidy are unclear, and routine prenatal testing is warranted once a defect has occurred.

Cytogenetic analysis of the fetus will of course give information about the sex chromosomes. Some couples do not desire advance knowledge of the sex of their child, and the person transmitting the results to the couple should always address this issue first. On the other hand, some couples *only* want to know the sex of the fetus and plan to terminate the pregnancy if the undesired sex is detected. Virtually no centers in the United States consider sex selection to be an appropriate indication for prenatal diagnosis.

The level of α-fetoprotein in maternal serum changes with gestational age, with the mother's medical status, and with abnormalities of the fetus. If the first two factors can be well controlled, the assay can be used to provide information about the fetus. Levels are expressed as multiples of the median value for a particular gestational age. Higher than normal levels are associated with open neural tube defects (the conditions for which the test was developed), recent or impending fetal demise, gastroschisis, and fetal renal disease. Extremely high levels are highly specific for fetal anomalies—a level three times the median increases 20-fold the risk of meningomyelocele or anencephaly. Low α-fetoprotein levels in maternal serum are associated with fetal trisomy, especially Down's syndrome; the reason for this association remains unclear. The addition of two other analytes in maternal serum—human chorionic gonadotropin (hCG) and unconjugated estriol (uE3)—to the assay for α-fetoprotein (to produce the "triple screen") enhances by several times the ability to detect a fetus with trisomy 21 and trisomy 18. Measuring in the first trimester both serum pregnancy-associated plasma protein A and the translucency of the fetal neck by ultrasound—followed by routine triple screening in the second trimester—improves the rate of detection of Down's syndrome to about 85% while reducing false-positives to about 1%. A positive result on

Table 41–7. Indications for prenatal diagnosis.

Indications	Methods
Advanced maternal age, previous child with chromosome aberration, intrauterine growth delay	Cytogenetics (amniocentesis, chorionic villus sampling)
Biochemical disorder	Protein assay, DNA diagnosis
Congenital anomaly	Ultrasound, fetoscopy
Screening for neural tube defects and trisomy	Maternal serum α-fetoprotein

any of these screening protocols for trisomy should be followed by offering the woman amniocentesis to confirm the diagnosis.

Alfirevic Z: Early amniocentesis versus transabdominal chorion villus sampling for prenatal diagnosis. Cochrane Database Syst Rev 2000;2:CD000077. [PMID: 10796116] (A review of randomised trials reveals that early amniocentesis has an increased risk of complications, including pregnancy loss, while chorion villus sampling is technically more difficult.)

Cunningham GC et al: Cost and effectiveness of the California triple marker prenatal screening program. Genet Med 1999;1:199. (In a state with free maternal serum multiple marker screening, only two-thirds of eligible pregnant women undergo testing.)

Facher JJ et al: Genetic counseling in primary care. What questions are patients likely to ask, and how should they be answered? Postgrad Med 2000;107:59. [PMID: 10728135] (Answers to many commonly asked genetic testing questions.)

Haddow JE et al: Screening of maternal serum for fetal Down's syndrome in the first trimester. N Engl J Med 1998;338:955. [PMID: 9521983] (First-trimester maternal serum screening alone can yield detection rates of about 60% for Down's syndrome with a false-positive rate of 5%.)

Milunsky A (editor): Genetic Disorders and the Fetus, 4th ed. Johns Hopkins Univ Press, 1998. (Multiauthored text that covers methods and specific fetal and maternal disorders.)

Parano E et al: Noninvasive prenatal diagnosis of chromosomal aneuploidies by isolation and analysis of fetal cells from maternal blood. Am J Med Genet 2001;101:262. [PMID: 11424143] (Nucleated fetal cells circulate in the mother's blood and can be used for prenatal diagnosis. These cells are more common when the fetus is aneuploid.)

Saito H et al: Prenatal DNA diagnosis of a single-gene disorder from maternal plasma. Lancet 2000;356:1170. [PMID: 11030304] (Achondroplasia is prenatally diagnosed via PCR of a fetal-derived mutant gene from maternal blood.)

Tongsong T et al: Amniocentesis-related fetal loss: A cohort study. Obstet Gynecol 1998;92:64. [PMID: 9649095] (This study of over 2000 matched pairs found no increase in fetal loss associated with amniocentesis after 15 weeks.)

NEOPLASIA: CHROMOSOMAL & DNA ANALYSIS

Studies of both chromosomes and nucleic acids support Boveri's 1914 hypothesis that cancer is caused by a change in genetic material at the cellular level. Two classes of genes have been discovered that function in neoplastic transformation.

Oncogenes arise from preexisting normal genes (proto-oncogenes) that have been altered by both viral and nonviral factors. As a result, the cells synthesize either normal proteins in inappropriate amounts or proteins that are aberrant in structure and function. Many of these proteins are cellular growth factors or receptors for growth factors. The net result of oncogene activation is unregulated cell division. Mutations that activate oncogenes virtually always arise in somatic cells and are not usually inherited. Although some oncogenes are more likely to be activated in certain tumors, in general the same mutations may be found in neoplasia arising in different cells and tissues.

Tumor suppressor genes can be viewed as the antithesis of oncogenes. Their normal function is to suppress transformation; mutation in both alleles is necessary to obliterate this important function. The first mutant allele at any tumor suppressor gene might arise spontaneously or might be inherited; mutation in the other allele (the "second hit") virtually always arises spontaneously, but by any of a number of molecular mechanisms. These genes show considerably more tumor specificity than do oncogenes; however, while some specific mutations are necessary for certain tumors to arise, no loss of single tumor suppressor function is sufficient. Clearly, a person who inherits one copy of a mutant tumor suppressor gene is at increased risk that in some susceptible cell, at some time during life, the function of that gene will be lost. This susceptibility is inherited as an autosomal dominant trait. For example, mutation in one allele of the P53 locus results in the Li-Fraumeni syndrome (151623), in which susceptibility before age 45 years to sarcomas and other tumors occurs in males and females in successive generations. Inherited mutations in this locus also increase the risk that a second tumor will develop following radiation or chemotherapy for the first tumor, suggesting that the initial treatment may induce a "second hit" in a P53 locus in another tissue. However, inheriting a P53 mutation is not a guarantee that cancer will develop at an early age; much more needs to be learned about the pathogenesis of neoplasia before the genetic counseling of families with a molecular predisposition to cancer is clarified. BRCA1, a gene that predisposes women to breast (114480) and ovarian cancer, is another example of a tumor suppressor gene. Women who inherit one mutant allele of BRCA1 have on average, a 50–80% lifetime risk of developing breast cancer, and the average age of tumor detection is in the fifth decade. Their risk of developing ovarian cancer is variable, but up to 63%.

In selected cases, a patient's DNA can be analyzed for the presence of a mutated gene and thereby assess that individual's risk for developing a tumor. Examples are retinoblastoma (189200), certain forms of Wilms' tumor (194070), breast cancer (114489), and familial colon cancer (114500). To illustrate how noninvasive and sensitive the methodology has become, it is possible to analyze stool for the presence of mutations in tumor suppressor genes that might indicate the presence of a clinically undetected adenocarcinoma of the colon. The analysis—not yet in general use—depends on the ability of the polymerase chain reaction to amplify minute quantities of the mutant DNA present in epithelial cells shed from the tumor.

A third class of genes that predispose to malignancy has been discovered in the past few years. So-called **mutator genes** have joined oncogenes and tumor suppressor genes as risk factors. Mutator genes normally function to repair damage to DNA that occurs from environmental insults such as exposure to carcinogens and ultraviolet irradiation. When a mutator gene is mutated itself, DNA damage accumulates and eventually affects oncogenes and tumor suppressor genes, thereby making cancer more likely. Hereditary nonpolyposis colon cancer (HNPCC) is one familial syndrome due to mutations in one or another of the five mutator genes identified thus far (*MSH2* and *MLH1* being the most commonly responsible for HNPCC).

This exciting work on the molecular nature of oncogenesis was preceded by years of study of the cytogenetics of tumors. Indeed, the retinoblastoma tumor suppressor gene was ultimately isolated because a small number of patients with this tumor have a constitutive deletion of chromosome 13 where this gene maps. Other chromosomal aberrations have been found to be highly characteristic of—or even specific for—certain tumors (Table 41–8). Detection of one of these cytogenetic aberrations can thus aid in diagnosis.

Hematologic malignancies are especially amenable to study because of the relative ease of performing cytogenetic analysis. Such malignancies are associated with over 100 specific chromosomal rearrangements, chiefly translocations. Most of these rearrangements are restricted to a specific type of cancer (Table 41–9), and the remainder occur with many cancers.

In the leukemias, the chromosomal aberration is the basis of one of the subclassifications of the disease. When cytogenetic information is combined with the histologic classification, it is possible to define subsets of patients in which response to therapy, clinical course, and prognosis are predictable. If at the time of diagnosis there are no chromosomal changes in the bone marrow cells, the survival time is longer than if any or all of the bone marrow cells have abnormal cytogenetic characteristics. As secondary chromosomal changes occur, the leukemia becomes more aggressive, often associated with drug resistance and a reduced chance for complete or prolonged remission. The least ominous chromosomal change is numerical alteration without morphologic abnormality.

Table 41–8. Chromosome aberrations associated with representative solid tumors.

Tumor	Chromosome Aberration
Meningioma	del(22)(q11)[1]
Neuroblastoma	del(1)(p36)
Renal cell carcinoma	del(3)(p14.2–p25) or translocation of this region
Retinoblastoma, osteosarcoma	del(13)(q14.1) or translocation of this region
Small cell lung carcinoma	del(3)(p14–p23)
Wilms' tumor	del(11)(p15)

[1]Nomenclature means, "a deletion at band q11 of chromosome 22."

Table 41–9. Chromosomal aberrations associated with representative hematologic malignancies.

Tumor	Chromosomal Aberration
Leukemias	
Acute myeloblastic	t(8;21)(q22;q11)[1]
Acute promyelocytic	t(15;17)(q22;q11–q12)
Acute monocytic	t(10;11)(p15–p11;q23)
Chronic myelogenous	t(9;22)(q34;q11)
Lymphomas	
Burkitt's	t(8;14)(q24.1;q32.3)
B cell	t(1;14)(q42;q43)
T cell	inv, del, and t of 1p13–p12
Premalignancy	
Polycythemia vera	del(20)(q11)

[1]Nomenclature means, "a translocation with the union at band q22 of chromosome 8 and q11 of chromosome 21."

Less cytogenetic information is available for lymphomas and premalignant hematologic disorders than for leukemia. In Hodgkin's disease, studies have been limited by the low yield of dividing cells and the low number of clear-cut aneuploid clones, so that complete chromosomal analyses with banding are available for far fewer patients with Hodgkin's disease than for any other type of lymphoma. In Hodgkin's disease, the modal chromosomal number tends to be triploid or tetraploid. About one-third of the samples have a 14q+ chromosome. In non-Hodgkin's lymphomas, high-resolution techniques of banding detect abnormalities in 95% of cases. Cytogenetic findings are now being correlated with the immunologic and histologic features and with prognosis.

In Burkitt's lymphoma, a solid tumor of B cell origin, 90% of patients have a translocation between the long arm of chromosome 8 and the long arm of chromosome 14, with chromosomal breakage sites being at or near immunoglobulin and oncogene loci.

Instability of chromosomes also predisposes to the development of some malignancies. In certain autosomal recessive diseases such as ataxia-telangiectasia, Bloom's syndrome, and Fanconi's anemia, the cells have a tendency to **genetic instability,** ie, to chromosomal breakage and rearrangement in vitro. These diseases are associated with a fairly high incidence of neoplasia, particularly leukemia and lymphoma.

Some chromosomal aberrations, better known for their effect on phenotype, also predispose to tumors. For example, patients with Down's syndrome (trisomy 21) have a 20-fold increase in the risk of leukemia; 47,XXY males (Klinefelter's syndrome) have a 30-fold increase in the risk of breast cancer; and XY phenotypic females have a heightened risk of developing ovarian cancer, primarily gonadoblastoma.

The indications for cytogenetic analysis of neoplasia continue to evolve. Not all tumors require study. However, in cases of tumors of unclear type (especially leukemias and lymphomas), with a strong family history of early neoplasia, or for certain tumors associated with potential generalized chromosomal defects (present in nonneoplastic cells), cytogenetic analysis should be strongly considered.

Anderlik MR et al: Medicolegal and ethical issues in genetic cancer syndromes. Semin Surg Oncol 2000;18:339. [PMID: 10805956] (Outlines legal and ethical aspects of genetic testing. Examines the physician's duty to the patient's family and discusses informed consent about prophylactic surgery.)

Arver B et al: Hereditary breast cancer: a review. Semin Cancer Biol 2000;10:271. [PMID: 10966850] (*BRCA1* and *BRCA2* genes may lead to up to 10% of breast cancers and predispose to ovarian cancer.)

Boland CR: Molecular genetics of hereditary nonpolyposis colorectal cancer. Ann N Y Acad Sci 2000;910:50. [PMID: 10911905] (Microsatellite instability resulting from mutated mismatch repair genes leads to hereditary nonpolyposis colorectal cancer.)

Fasouliotis SJ et al: *BRCA1* and *BRCA2* gene mutations: decision-making dilemma concerning testing and management. Obstet Gynecol Surg 2000;55:373. [PMID: 10841315] (Reviews the role of genetic testing in identifying women at risk for presymptomatic breast and ovarian cancers, with special attention to the dilemmas presented by interpretation and management options.)

Frank TS: Hereditary cancer syndromes. Arch Pathol Lab Med 2001;125:85. [PMID: 11151059] (A number of syndromes include various forms of neoplasia as prominent features.)

Lindor NM et al: The concise handbook of family cancer syndromes. J Natl Cancer Inst 1998;90:1040. [PMID: 9672254] (Short descriptions of the 35 syndromes involving one or more benign or malignant tumors.)

Peel DJ et al: Characterization of hereditary nonpolyposis colorectal cancer families from a population-based series of cases. J Natl Cancer Inst 2000;92:1517. [PMID: 10995807] (A large population-based study reveals that the prevalence of HNPCC in the general population is likely to be closer to 1% than to 5%.)

Ponder BA: Cancer genetics. Nature 2001;411:336. [PMID: 11357140] (The Human Genome Project suggests a variety of approaches for studying and treating cancer beyond the current focus on single mutant genes.)

Stopfer JE: Genetic counseling and clinical cancer genetics services. Semin Surg Oncol 2000;18:347. [PMID: 10805957] (Trained genetic counselors provide adjuvant services to primary care physicians and oncologists during cancer screening, with emphasis on confirmation of medical and family history, risk assessment, patient education, and supportive counseling.)

Tobias E, Black D: The molecular biology of cancer. In: *Emery and Rimoin's Principles and Practice of Medical Genetics*, 4th ed. Rimoin DL, O'Connor JM, Pyeritz RE (editors). Churchill Livingstone, 2001.

Traverso G et al: Detection of *APC* mutations in fecal DNA from patients with colorectal tumors. N Engl J Med 2002;346:311. [PMID: 11821507] (Mutation of the *APC* gene is frequent and perhaps essential for the development of colon cancer—even nonhereditary forms. Mutations in this gene can be detected in cells sloughed into feces.)

■ SELECTED GENETIC DISORDERS

ACUTE INTERMITTENT PORPHYRIA (176000)

 ESSENTIALS OF DIAGNOSIS

- *Unexplained abdominal crisis, generally in young women.*
- *Acute peripheral or central nervous system dysfunction.*
- *Recurrent psychiatric illnesses.*
- *Hyponatremia.*
- *Porphobilinogen in the urine during an attack.*

General Considerations

Though there are several different types of porphyrias, the one with the most serious consequences and the one that usually presents in adulthood is acute intermittent porphyria, which is inherited as an autosomal dominant, though it remains clinically silent in the majority of patients who carry the trait. Those who develop clinical illness are usually women, with symptoms beginning in the teens or 20s, but in rare cases onset can begin after menopause. The disorder is caused by deficiency of porphobilinogen deaminase activity, leading to increased excretion of aminolevulinic acid and porphobilinogen in the urine. The diagnosis may be elusive if not specifically considered. The characteristic abdominal pain may be due to abnormalities in autonomic innervation in the gut. In contrast to other forms of porphyria, cutaneous photosensitivity is absent in acute intermittent porphyria. Attacks are precipitated by numerous factors, including drugs and intercurrent infections. Harmful and relatively safe drugs for use in treatment are listed in Table 41–10. Hyponatremia may be seen, due in part to inappropriate release of antidiuretic hormone, though gastrointestinal loss of sodium in some patients may contribute.

Clinical Findings

A. SYMPTOMS AND SIGNS

Patients show intermittent abdominal pain of varying severity, and in some instances it may so simulate acute abdomen as to lead to exploratory laparotomy. Since the origin of the abdominal pain is neurologic, there is absence of fever and leukocytosis. Complete

Table 41–10. Some of the "unsafe" and "probably safe" drugs used in the treatment of acute porphyrias.

Unsafe	Probably Safe
Alcohol	Acetaminophen
Alkylating agents	β-Adrenergic blockers
Barbiturates	Amitriptyline
Carbamazepine	Aspirin
Chlorpropamide	Atropine
Chloroquine	Chloral hydrate
Clonidine	Chlordiazepoxide
Dapsone	Diazepam
Ergots	Digoxin
Erythromycin	Diphenhydramine
Estrogens, synthetic	Guanethidine
Food additives	Glucocorticoids
Glutethimide	Hyoscine
Griseofulvin	Ibuprofen
Hydralazine	Imipramine
Ketamine	Insulin
Meprobamate	Lithium
Methyldopa	Naproxen
Metoclopramide	Nitrofurantoin
Nortriptyline	Opioid analgesics
Pentazocine	Penicillamine
Phenytoin	Penicillin and derivatives
Progestins	Phenothiazines
Pyrazinamide	Procaine
Rifampin	Streptomycin
Spironolactone	Succinylcholine
Succinimides	Tetracycline
Sulfonamides	Thiouracil
Theophylline	
Tolazamide	
Tolbutamide	
Valproic acid	

recovery between attacks is usual. Any part of the nervous system may be involved, with evidence for autonomic and peripheral neuropathy. Peripheral neuropathy may be symmetric or asymmetric and mild or profound; in the latter instance, it can even lead to quadriplegia with respiratory paralysis. Other central nervous system manifestations include seizures, psychosis, and abnormalities of the basal ganglia. Hyponatremia may further cause or exacerbate central nervous system manifestations.

B. LABORATORY FINDINGS

Often there is profound hyponatremia. The diagnosis can be confirmed by demonstrating an increased amount of porphobilinogen in the urine during an acute attack. Freshly voided urine is of normal color but may turn dark upon standing in light and air.

Most families have a different mutation in the porphobilinogen deaminase gene causing acute intermittent porphyria. With some effort in research laboratories, mutations can be discovered and used for presymptomatic and prenatal diagnosis.

Prevention

Avoidance of factors known to precipitate attacks of acute intermittent porphyria—especially drugs (sulfonamides and barbiturates, or drugs listed in Table 41–10)—can reduce morbidity. Starvation diets also cause attacks and so must be avoided.

Treatment

Treatment with a high-carbohydrate diet diminishes the number of attacks in some patients and is a reasonable empirical gesture considering its benignity. Acute attacks may be life-threatening and require prompt diagnosis, withdrawal of the inciting agent (if possible), and treatment with analgesics and intravenous glucose and hematin. A minimum of 300 g of carbohydrate per day should be provided orally or intravenously. Electrolyte balance requires close attention. Hematin therapy is still evolving and should be undertaken with full recognition of adverse consequences, especially phlebitis and coagulopathy. The intravenous dosage is up to 4 mg/kg once or twice daily.

Desnick RJ et al: Inherited porphyrias. In: *Emery and Rimoin's Principles and Practice of Medical Genetics*, 4th ed. Rimoin DL et al (editors). Churchill Livingstone, 2002. (Diagnosis and management are stressed.)

Grandchamp B: Acute intermittent porphyria. Semin Liver Dis 1998;18:17. [PMID: 9516674] (A succinct review of the clinical and biochemical features and guidelines for DNA diagnosis.)

Kalman DR et al: Management of acute attacks in the porphyrias. Clin Dermatol 1998;16:299. [PMID: 9554242] (A brief survey of the latest approaches to treating the potentially life-threatening complications of acute intermittent porphyria.)

Sassa S et al: Molecular aspects of the inherited porphyrias. J Intern Med 2000;247:169. [PMID: 10692079] (Discussion of multiple inherited porphyrias and their molecular causes.)

ALKAPTONURIA (203500)

Alkaptonuria is caused by a recessively inherited deficiency of the enzyme homogentisic acid oxidase. This acid derives from metabolism of both phenylalanine and tyrosine and is present in large amounts in the urine throughout the patient's life. An oxidation product accumulates slowly in cartilage throughout the body, leading to degenerative joint disease of the spine and peripheral joints. Indeed, examination of patients in the third and fourth decades shows a slight darkish blue color below the skin in areas overlying cartilage, such as in the ears, a phenomenon called "ochronosis." In some patients, a more severe hyperpigmentation can be seen in the sclera, conjunctiva, and cornea. Accumulation of metabolites in heart valves can lead to aortic or mitral stenosis. A predisposition to coronary artery disease may also be present. While the syndrome causes considerable morbidity, life expectancy is reduced only modestly. Symptoms are more often attributable to spondylitis with back pain, leading to a clinical picture difficult to distinguish from that of ankylosing spondylitis, though on radiographic assessment the sacroiliac joints are not fused in alkaptonuria.

The diagnosis is established by demonstrating homogentisic acid in the urine, which turns black spontaneously on exposure to the air; this reaction is particularly noteworthy if the urine is alkaline or when alkali is added to a specimen. Molecular analysis of the homogentisic acid oxidase gene, recently mapped to chromosome 3, is not necessary for diagnosis.

Treatment of the arthritis is similar to that for other arthropathies. Though in theory rigid dietary restriction might reduce accumulation of the pigment, this has not proved to be of practical benefit.

La Du BN: Alcaptonuria. In: *The Metabolic Basis of Inherited Disease,* 8th ed. Scriver CR et al (editors). McGraw-Hill, 2001. (Clinical and biochemical aspects of one of Garrod's original inborn errors of metabolism.)

Scriver CR: Garrod's foresight; our hindsight. J Inherit Metab Dis 2001;24:93. [PMID: 11405353] (An instructive and sweeping review based on the disorders originally defined as inborn errors by Garrod [including alkaptonuria]. Speaks to how the enhanced knowledge of today can be best used to benefit patients and their families.)

DOWN'S SYNDROME (190685)

Down's syndrome is usually diagnosed at birth on the basis of the typical facial features, hypotonia, and single palmar crease. Several serious problems that may be evident at birth or may develop early in childhood include duodenal atresia, congenital heart disease (especially atrioventricular canal defects), and leukemia. The intestinal and cardiac anomalies usually respond to surgery, and the leukemia generally responds to conservative management. Intelligence varies across a wide spectrum. Many people with Down's syndrome do well in sheltered workshops and group homes, but few achieve full independence in adulthood. An Alzheimer-like dementia usually becomes evident in the fourth or fifth decade and, for those who survive childhood, accounts for a reduced life expectancy. Studies addressing the risk and severity of dementia in relation to the apolipoprotein E genotype have had conflicting results. Cytogenetic analysis should always be performed—even though most patients will have simple trisomy for chromosome 21—to detect unbalanced translocations; such patients may have a parent with a balanced translocation, and there will be a substantial recurrence risk of Down's syndrome in future offspring.

Many pregnancies carrying a fetus with Down's syndrome can be detected in the early second trimester through screening maternal serum for α-fetoprotein and certain hormones ("triple screen") and by detecting increased nuchal thickness on fetal ultrasound.

The risk of bearing a child with Down's syndrome increases exponentially with the age of the mother at conception and begins a marked rise after age 35. By age 45 years, a mother has one chance in 40 of having an affected child. The risk of other conditions associated with trisomy also increases, because of the increased predisposition of older oocytes to nondisjunction during meiosis. There is virtually no risk of trisomy associated with increased paternal age. However, older men do have an increased risk of fathering a child with a new autosomal dominant condition. But because there are so many distinct conditions, the chance of fathering an offspring with any given one is extremely small.

Barsh G: Genetic disease. In: *Pathophysiology of Disease: An Introduction to Clinical Medicine,* 4th ed. McPhee SJ et al (editors). McGraw-Hill, 2002. (Discusses pathogenesis of Down's syndrome.)

Krantz DA et al: First-trimester Down syndrome screening using dried blood biochemistry and nuchal translucency. Obstet Gynecol 2000;96:207. [PMID: 10908764] (Prospective evaluation of first-trimester screening for free beta-hCG, pregnancy-associated plasma protein A, and nuchal translucency detected 87–92% of Down syndrome and 100% of trisomy 18.)

Tolmie JL: Down syndrome and other autosomal trisomies. In: *Emery and Rimoin's Principles and Practice of Medical Genetics,* 4th ed. Rimoin DL et al (editors). Churchill Livingstone, 2002.

Wald NJ et al: Integrated screening for Down's syndrome based on tests performed during the first and second trimesters. N Engl J Med 1999;341:461. [PMID: 10441601] (The authors propose that combining results of maternal serum screening and nuchal translucency obtained in the first trimester with results of standard maternal serum screening in the second trimester improves both sensitivity and specificity of detecting fetuses with Down's syndrome.)

FRAGILE X MENTAL RETARDATION (309550)

This X-linked condition accounts for more cases of mental retardation in males than any condition except Down's syndrome; about one in 2000 males is affected. The first marker for this condition was a small gap, or fragile site, evident near the tip of the long arm of the X chromosome. Subsequently, the condition was found to be due to expansion of a trinucleotide repeat (CGG) near a gene called *FMR1*. All individuals have some CGG repeats in this location, but as the number increases beyond 52, the chances of further expansion during spermatogenesis or oogenesis increase. Being born with one *FMR1* allele with 200 or more repeats results in mental retardation in virtually all men and about 60% of women. The more repeats, the greater the likelihood that further expansion will occur during gametogenesis; this results in **anticipation**, in which the disorder can worsen from one generation to the next.

Affected (heterozygous) women show no physical signs other than early menopause, but they may have learning difficulties or frank retardation. Affected males show macroorchidism (enlarged testes) after puberty, large ears and a prominent jaw, a high-pitched voice, and mental retardation. Some show evidence of a mild connective tissue defect, with joint hypermobility and mitral valve prolapse.

DNA diagnosis for the number of repeats has supplanted cytogenetic analysis for both clinical and prenatal diagnosis. This should be done on any male or female who has unexplained mental retardation.

Jin P et al: Understanding the molecular basis of fragile X syndrome. Hum Mol Genet 2000;9:901. [PMID: 10767313] (A review of the molecular mechanisms leading to the mental retardation seen in fragile X syndrome.)

Kenneson A et al: The female and the fragile X reviewed. Semin Reprod Med 2001;19:159. [PMID: 11480913] (Fragile X is usually thought of as a condition of males. This article reviews the many ways in which female heterozygotes are affected.)

Pesso R et al: Screening for fragile X syndrome in women of reproductive age. Prenat Diagn 2000;20:611. [PMID: 10951469] (A prospective study of antenatal and preconceptional screening reveals that one in 70 women were carriers for fragile X syndrome, suggesting that among women of reproductive age screening should be more widely available.)

Sutherland GR et al: Fragile X syndrome and other causes of X-linked mental handicap. In: *Emery and Rimoin's Principles and Practice of Medical Genetics*, 4th ed. Rimoin DL, O'Connor JM, Pyeritz RE (editors). Churchill Livingstone, 2001.

GAUCHER'S DISEASE
(230800)

Gaucher's disease is inherited as an autosomal recessive. A deficiency of β-glucocerebrosidase causes an accumulation of sphingolipid within phagocytic cells throughout the body. Anemia and thrombocytopenia are common and may be symptomatic; both are due primarily to hypersplenism, but marrow infiltration with Gaucher cells may contribute. Cortical erosions of bones, especially the vertebrae and femur, are due to local infarctions, but the mechanism is unclear. Episodes of bone pain (termed "crises") are reminiscent of those in sickle cell disease. A hip fracture in a patient with a palpable spleen—especially in a Jewish person of Eastern European origin—suggests the possibility of Gaucher's disease. Bone marrow aspirates reveal typical Gaucher cells, which have an eccentric nucleus and PAS-positive inclusions, along with wrinkled cytoplasm and inclusion bodies of a fibrillar type. In addition, the serum acid phosphatase is elevated. Definitive diagnosis requires the demonstration of deficient glucocerebrosidase activity in leukocytes.

Two uncommon forms of Gaucher's disease, called type II and type III, involve neurologic accumulation of sphingolipid and a variety of neurologic problems. Type II is of infantile onset and has a poor prognosis.

Over 200 mutations have been found to cause Gaucher's disease, and some are highly predictive of the neuronopathic forms. Thus, mutation detection, especially in a young person, is of potential value. Only four mutations in glucocerebrosidase account for more than 90% of the disease among Ashkenazic Jews.

Until recently, treatment has been supportive and has included splenectomy for thrombocytopenia secondary to platelet sequestration. The production of a recombinant form of the enzyme glucocerebrosidase (imiglucerase) for intravenous administration on a regular basis now permits a reduction in total body stores of glycolipid and improvement in orthopedic and hematologic manifestations. Unfortunately, the neurologic manifestations of types II and III have not improved with enzyme replacement therapy. The major drawback is the exceptional cost of imiglucerase, which can exceed $350,000 per year for a severely affected patient. Administration of less enzyme (30 units/kg per month) is effective for most adults and reduces the cost to about $100,000–150,000 annually.

Beutler E, Grabowski GA: Gaucher disease. In: *The Metabolic Basis of Inherited Disease*, 8th ed. Scriver CR et al (editors). McGraw-Hill, 2001. (A comprehensive review.)

Charrow J et al: Gaucher disease: Recommendations on diagnosis, evaluation, and monitoring. Arch Intern Med 1998;158:1754. [PMID: 9738604] (Recommendations, developed by consensus, on the major issues involved in managing a person with this highly variable disorder.)

Charrow J et al: The Gaucher registry: demographics and disease characteristics of 1698 patients with Gaucher disease. Arch Intern Med 2000;160:2835. [PMID: 11025794] (The largest database of Gaucher patients with extensive data on the clinical spectrum of disease.)

Koprivica V et al: Analysis and classification of 304 mutant alleles in patients with type 1 and type 3 Gaucher disease. Am J Hum Genet 2000;66:1777-86. [PMID: 10796875] (The largest published survey of mutant alleles in patients with the most common forms of Gaucher's disease found a wide array of mutations and only limited correlation between genotype and phenotype.)

HOMOCYSTINURIA
(236200)

Homocystinuria in its classic form is caused by cystathionine β-synthase deficiency and exhibits an autosomal recessive pattern of inheritance. This results in extreme elevations of plasma and urinary homocystine levels, a basis for diagnosis of this disorder. Homocystinuria is similar in certain superficial aspects to Marfan's syndrome, since patients may show a similar body habitus and ectopia lentis is almost always present. However, mental retardation is often present, and the cardiovascular events are those of repeated venous and arterial thromboses whose precise cause remains obscure. Life expectancy is reduced, especially in untreated and pyridoxine-unresponsive patients; myocardial infarction, stroke, and pulmonary embolism are the most common causes of death. This condition is diagnosed in some states by newborn screening for hypermethioninemia; however, pyridoxine-responsive infants may not be detected. The diagnosis should be suspected in patients in the second and third decades of life who show evidence of arterial or venous thromboses and have no other risk factors. Although many mutations have been identified in the cystathionine β-synthase gene, amino acid analysis of plasma remains the most appropriate diagnostic test. Patients should be studied after they have been off folate or pyridoxine supplementation for at least 1 week. The plasma should be separated promptly from the fresh venous blood specimen.

About one-half of patients have a form of cystathionine β-synthase deficiency that improves biochemically and clinically through pharmacologic doses of pyridoxine and folate. For these patients, treatment from infancy can prevent retardation and the other clinical problems. Patients who are pyridoxine-nonresponders must be treated with dietary reduction in methionine and supplementation of cysteine, also from infancy. The vitamin betaine is also useful in reducing plasma methionine levels by facilitating a metabolic pathway that bypasses the defective enzyme. Patients who have suffered venous thrombosis should be anticoagulated, but there are no studies to support prophylactic use of warfarin or antiplatelet agents.

Mudd H, Levy HL, Skovby F: Disorders of transsulfuration. In: *The Metabolic Basis of Inherited Disease*, 8th ed. Scriver CR et al (editors). McGraw-Hill, 2001. (A comprehensive review of the genetics and clinical features of all of the disorders associated with elevated homocysteine, including the risk of vascular disease in heterozygotes.)

Pyeritz RE: Homocystinuria. In: *McKusick's Heritable Disorders of Connective Tissue*, 5th ed. Mosby, 1993. (Clinical, genetic, and biochemical aspects of an inborn error of metabolism with extensive effects on the extracellular matrix.)

Yap S et al: Vascular outcome in patients with homocystinuria due to cystathionine beta-synthase deficiency treated chronically: a multicenter observational study. Arterioscler Thromb Vasc Biol 2001;21:2080. [PMID: 11742888] (Aggressive measures to reduce plasma homocystine levels have a markedly beneficial impact on reducing occlusive vascular events.)

HOMOCYSTEINE & ARTERIAL OCCLUSIVE DISEASE (603174)

Over the past 5 years, considerable evidence has accumulated to support the 20-year-old observation that patients with clinical and angiographic evidence of coronary artery disease tend to have higher levels of plasma homocysteine than controls without coronary artery disease. The relationship has been extended to cerebrovascular and peripheral vascular diseases. Although this effect was initially thought to be due at least in part to heterozygotes for cystathionine β-synthase deficiency (see above), in fact there is little evidence for this. Rather, the major factor leading to hyperhomocysteinemia is folate deficiency. Pyridoxine (vitamin B_6) and vitamin B_{12} are also important in the metabolism of methionine, and deficiency of any of these vitamins can lead to accumulation of homocysteine. A number of genes influence utilization of these vitamins and can predispose to deficiency. For example, having one—and especially two—copies of an allele that causes thermolability of methylene tetrahydrofolate reductase predisposes to elevated fasting homocysteine levels. However, both nutritional and most genetic deficiencies of these vitamins can be corrected by dietary supplementation of folic acid and, if serum levels are low, vitamins B_6 and B_{12}. In the United States, cereal grains are now fortified with folic acid. Studies are ongoing to determine the long-term utility of routine vitamin supplementation in people at risk for arterial occlusive disease, but many workers in this field recommend, at a minimum, taking 1 mg of folic acid per day. Because patients with end-stage renal disease tend to have marked hyperhomocysteinemia and low serum folate, 5 mg of folic acid per day seems warranted.

Relatively few laboratories currently provide highly reliable assays for homocysteine. Processing of the specimen is crucial to obtain accurate results. The plasma must be separated within 30 minutes; otherwise, blood cells release the amino acid and the measurement will then be artificially elevated.

Aronow WS et al: Increased plasma homocysteine is an independent predictor of new coronary events in older persons. Am J Cardiol 2000;86:346. [PMID: 10922450] (Prospective study of elderly men and women reveals that elevated plasma homocysteine is an independent risk factor for new coronary events [risk ratio 1.073].)

Carmel R, Jacobsen DW (editors): *Homocysteine in Health and Disease*. Cambridge Univ Press, 2001. (Multiauthored text that spans basic and clinical sciences of homocysteine metabolism.)

Knekt P et al: Hyperhomocystinemia: a risk factor or a consequence of coronary heart disease? Arch Intern Med 2001;161:1589. [PMID: 11434790] (Presents an intriguing theory that elevated homocystine levels are not as predictive of occlusive coronary disease as previously thought.)

Makris M: Hyperhomocysteinemia and thrombosis. Clin Lab Haematol 2000;22:133. [PMID: 10931161] (Clinical aspects and treatment of hyperhomocysteinemia.)

Rizvi A et al: The genetics of occlusive arterial disease. In: *Emery and Rimoin's Principles and Practice of Medical Genetics*, 4th ed. Rimoin DL et al (editors). Churchill Livingstone, 2002. (A survey of all known genetic factors that predispose to atherosclerotic disease, with particular attention to homocysteine.)

Stein JH et al: Hyperhomocysteinemia and atherosclerotic vascular disease. Arch Intern Med 1998;158:1301. [PMID: 9645823] (A brief review of the causes of elevated homocysteine.)

KLINEFELTER'S SYNDROME

Boys with an extra X chromosome are normal in appearance before puberty; thereafter, they have disproportionately long legs and arms, a female escutcheon, gynecomastia, and small testes. Infertility is due to azoospermia; the seminiferous tubules are hyalinized. The diagnosis is often not made until a couple is evaluated for inability to conceive. Mental retardation is somewhat more common than in the general population. Many men with Klinefelter's syndrome have learning problems. The risk of breast cancer is much higher in men with Klinefelter's syndrome than in 46,XY men, as is the risk of diabetes mellitus.

Treatment with testosterone after puberty is advisable but will not restore fertility. However, men with Klinefelter's syndrome have had mature sperm aspirated from their testes and injected into oocytes, resulting in fertilization. After the blastocysts were implanted into the uterus of a partner, "natural" children resulted.

Allanson J, Graham G: Sex chromosome abnormalities. In: *Emery and Rimoin's Principles and Practice of Medical Genetics*, 4th ed. Rimoin DL, O'Connor JM, Pyeritz RE. (editors). Churchill Livingstone, 2001.

Palermo GD et al: Births after intracytoplasmic injection of sperm obtained by testicular extraction from men with nonmosaic Klinefelter's syndrome. N Engl J Med 1998;338:588. [PMID: 9475766] (A reproductive option for men previously termed "infertile.")

Smyth CM et al: Klinefelter syndrome. Arch Intern Med 1998;158:1309. [PMID: 9645824] (A concise review of the diagnosis and associated clinical abnormalities of this chromosomal disorder.)

Swerdlow AJ et al: Mortality and cancer incidence in persons with numerical sex chromosome abnormalities. Ann Hum Genet 2001;65.177. [PMID: 11427177] (Men with Klinefelter's syndrome are predisposed to both lung cancer and breast cancer.)

MARFAN'S SYNDROME (154700)

ESSENTIALS OF DIAGNOSIS

- *Disproportionately tall stature, thoracic deformity, and joint laxity or contractures.*
- *Ectopia lentis and myopia.*
- *Aortic dilation and dissection.*
- *Mitral valve prolapse.*

General Considerations

Marfan's syndrome, a systemic connective tissue disease, is inherited as an autosomal dominant. It is characterized by abnormalities of the skeletal system, ocular system, and cardiovascular system. Spontaneous pneumothorax, dural ectasia, and striae atrophicae can also occur. Of most concern is disease of the ascending aorta, which is associated with a dilated aortic root.

Histology of the aorta shows diffuse medial abnormalities. Aortic and mitral valve leaflets are also abnormal and mitral regurgitation may be present as well, often with elongated chordae tendineae, which on occasion may rupture.

Clinical Findings

A. SYMPTOMS AND SIGNS

Affected patients are typically tall, with particularly long arms, legs, and digits (arachnodactyly). However, there can be wide variability in the clinical presentation. Commonly, joint dislocations and pectus excavatum are found. Ectopia lentis may lead to severe myopia and retinal detachment. Mitral valve prolapse is seen in about 85% percent of patients. Aortic root dilation with aortic regurgitation or dissection with rupture can occur. To diagnose Marfan's syndrome, people with an affected relative need features in at least two systems. People with no family history need features in the skeletal system, two other systems, and one of the major criteria of ectopia lentis, dilation of the aortic root, or aortic dissection. Patients with homocystinuria due to cystathionine synthase deficiency also have dislocated lenses; tall, disproportionate stature; and thoracic deformity. They tend to have below normal intelligence, stiff joints, and a predisposition to arterial and venous occlusive disease. Males with Klinefelter's syndrome do not show the typical ocular or cardiovascular features of Marfan's syndrome and are generally sporadic occurrences in the family.

B. LABORATORY FINDINGS

Mutations in the fibrillin gene on chromosome 15 cause Marfan's syndrome. Nonetheless, no simple laboratory test is available to support the diagnosis in questionable cases because related conditions may also be due to defects in fibrillin.

Prevention

There is prenatal and presymptomatic diagnosis for patients in whom the molecular defect in fibrillin has been found and for large enough families in whom linkage analysis using polymorphic markers around the fibrillin gene can be performed.

Treatment

Children with Marfan's syndrome require regular ophthalmologic surveillance to correct visual acuity and thus prevent amblyopia, and annual orthopedic consultation for diagnosis of scoliosis at an early enough stage so that bracing might delay progression. Patients of all ages require echocardiography at least annually to monitor aortic diameter and mitral valve function. All patients should use standard endocarditis prophylaxis. Chronic β-adrenergic blockade, titrated to individual tolerance but enough to produce a negative inotropic effect (atenolol, 1–2 mg/kg), retards the rate of aortic dilation. Restriction from vigorous physical exertion protects from aortic dissection. Prophylactic replacement of the aortic root with a composite graft when the diameter reaches 50–55 mm (normal: < 40 mm) prolongs life. A procedure to spare the patient's aortic valve and replace just the aneurysmal sinuses of Valsalva is showing promise and would also avoid the need for life-long anticoagulation.

Prognosis

People with Marfan's syndrome who are untreated commonly die in the fourth or fifth decade from aortic dissection or congestive heart failure secondary to aortic regurgitation.

Dietz HC, Pyeritz RE: Marfan syndrome and related disorders. In: *The Metabolic Basis of Inherited Disease,* 8th ed. Scriver CR et al (editors). McGraw-Hill, 2001. (Detailed descriptions of the clinical features, management plan, molecular genetics, and pathogenesis of disorders of the microfibril.)

Gott VL et al: Replacement of the aortic root in patients with Marfan's syndrome. N Engl J Med 1999;340:1307. [PMID: 10219065] (The largest published series, demonstrating excellent long-term results from prophylactic surgery.)

Pyeritz RE: The Marfan syndrome. Ann Rev Med 2000;51:481. [PMID: 10774478] (A comprehensive survey of Marfan's syndrome and related conditions.)

Diagnostic Testing & Medical Decision Making

42

C. Diana Nicoll, MD, PhD, MPA, & Michael Pignone, MD, MPH

See www.current-med.com/ch42.html

The clinician's main task is to make reasoned decisions about patient care despite incomplete clinical information and uncertainty about clinical outcomes. While data elicited from the history and physical examination are often sufficient for making a diagnosis or for guiding therapy, more information may be required. In these situations, clinicians often turn to diagnostic tests for help.

■ BENEFITS; COSTS & RISKS

When used appropriately, diagnostic tests can be of great assistance to the clinician. Tests can be helpful for **screening,** ie, to identify risk factors for disease and to detect occult disease in asymptomatic persons. Identification of risk factors may allow early intervention to prevent disease occurrence, and early detection of occult disease may reduce disease morbidity and mortality through early treatment. Optimal screening tests meet the criteria listed in Table 42–1.

Tests can also be helpful for **diagnosis,** ie, to help establish or exclude the presence of disease in symptomatic persons. Some tests assist in early diagnosis after onset of symptoms and signs; others assist in developing a differential diagnosis; others help determine the stage or activity of disease.

Finally, tests can be helpful in **patient management.** Tests can help (1) evaluate the severity of disease, (2) estimate prognosis, (3) monitor the course of disease (progression, stability, or resolution), (4) detect disease recurrence, and (5) select drugs and adjust therapy.

When ordering diagnostic tests, clinicians should weigh the potential benefits against the potential costs and disadvantages:

(1) Some tests carry a risk of morbidity or mortality—eg, cerebral angiogram leads to stroke in 1% of cases.

(2) The potential discomfort associated with tests such as colonoscopy may deter some patients from completing a diagnostic work-up.

(3) The result of a diagnostic test may mandate further testing or frequent follow-up. For example, a patient with a positive fecal occult blood test may incur significant cost, risk, and discomfort during follow-up colonoscopy.

(4) A false-positive test may lead to incorrect diagnosis or further unnecessary testing. Classifying a healthy patient as diseased based on a falsely positive diagnostic test can cause psychologic distress and may lead to risks from unnecessary or inappropriate therapy.

(5) A diagnostic or screening test may identify cases of disease that would not otherwise have been recognized and that would not have affected the patient. For example, early-stage low-grade prostate cancer detected by PSA screening in an 84-year-old man with known severe congestive heart failure will probably not become symptomatic or require treatment during his lifetime.

(6) Total costs may be high, or cost-effectiveness may be unfavorable. An individual test such as MRI of the head can cost more than $1400, and diagnostic tests as a whole account for approximately one-fifth of health care expenditures in the USA. Even relatively inexpensive tests may have poor cost effectiveness if they produce very small health benefits.

■ PERFORMANCE OF DIAGNOSTIC TESTS

TEST PREPARATION

Factors affecting both the patient and the specimen are important. The most crucial element in a properly conducted laboratory test is an appropriate specimen.

Patient Preparation

Preparation of the patient is important for certain tests—eg, a fasting state is needed for optimal glucose and triglyceride measurements; posture and sodium intake must be strictly controlled when measuring

Table 42–1. Criteria for use of screening procedures.

Characteristics of population
1. Sufficiently high prevalence of disease.
2. Likely to be compliant with subsequent tests and treatments.

Characteristics of disease
1. Significant morbidity and mortality.
2. Effective and acceptable treatment available.
3. Presymptomatic period detectable.
4. Improved outcome from early treatment.

Characteristics of test
1. Good sensitivity and specificity.
2. Low cost and risk.
3. Confirmatory test available and practical.

Table 42–2. Properties of useful diagnostic tests.

1. Test methodology has been described in detail so that it can be accurately and reliably reproduced.
2. Test accuracy and precision have been determined.
3. The reference range has been established appropriately.
4. Sensitivity and specificity have been reliably established by comparison with a gold standard. The evaluation has used a range of patients, including those who have different but commonly confused disorders and those with a spectrum of mild and severe, treated and untreated disease. The patient selection process has been adequately described so that results will not be generalized inappropriately.
5. Independent contribution to overall performance of a test panel has been confirmed if a test is advocated as part of a panel of tests.

renin and aldosterone levels; and strenuous exercise should be avoided before taking samples for creatine kinase determinations, since vigorous muscle activity can lead to falsely abnormal results.

Specimen Collection

Careful attention must be paid to patient identification and specimen labeling. Knowing when the specimen was collected may be important. For instance, aminoglycoside levels cannot be interpreted appropriately without knowing whether the specimen was drawn just before ("trough" level) or after ("peak" level) drug administration. Drug levels cannot be interpreted if they are drawn during the drug's distribution phase (eg, digoxin levels drawn during the first 6 hours after an oral dose). Substances that have a circadian variation (eg, cortisol) can be interpreted only in the context of the time of day the sample was drawn.

During specimen collection, other principles should be remembered. Specimens should not be drawn above an intravenous line, as this may contaminate the sample with intravenous fluid. Excessive tourniquet time will lead to hemoconcentration and an increased concentration of protein-bound substances such as calcium. Lysis of cells during collection of a blood specimen will result in spuriously increased serum levels of substances concentrated in cells (eg, lactate dehydrogenase and potassium). Certain test specimens may require special handling or storage (eg, blood gas specimens). Delay in delivery of specimens to the laboratory can result in ongoing cellular metabolism and therefore spurious results for some studies (eg, low serum glucose).

■ TEST CHARACTERISTICS

Table 42–2 lists the general characteristics of useful diagnostic tests. Most of the principles detailed below can be applied not only to laboratory and radiologic

tests but also to elements of the history and physical examination.

Accuracy

The accuracy of a laboratory test is its correspondence with the true value. An inaccurate test is one that differs from the true value even though the results may be reproducible (Figures 42–1A and 1B). In the clinical laboratory, accuracy of tests is maximized by calibrating laboratory equipment with reference material and by participation in external quality control programs.

Precision

Test precision is a measure of a test's reproducibility when repeated on the same sample. An imprecise test is one that yields widely varying results on repeated measurements (Figure 42–1 B). The precision of diagnostic tests, which is monitored in clinical laboratories by using control material, must be good enough to distinguish clinically relevant changes in a patient's status from the analytic variability of the test. For instance, the manual white blood cell differential count is not precise enough to detect important changes in the distribution of cell types, because it is calculated by subjective evaluation of a small sample (100 cells). Repeated measurements by different technicians on the same sample result in widely different results. Automated differential counts are more precise because they are obtained from machines that use objective physical characteristics to classify a much larger sample (10,000 cells).

Reference Range

Reference ranges are method- and laboratory-specific. In practice, they often represent test results found in

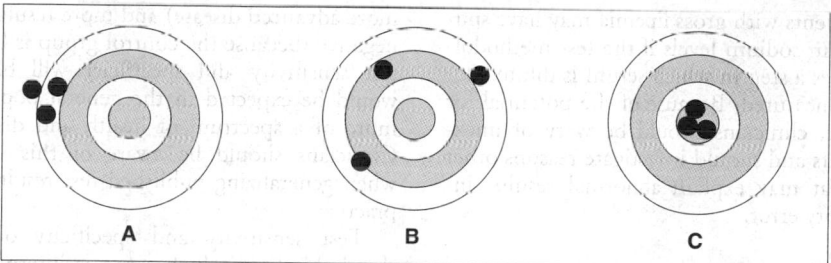

Figure 42–1. Relationship between accuracy and precision in diagnostic tests. The center of the target represents the true value of the substance being tested. Figure "A" represents a diagnostic test which is precise but inaccurate; on repeated measurement, the test yields very similar results, but all results are far from the true value. Figure "B" shows a test which is imprecise and inaccurate; repeated measurement yields widely different results, and the results are far from the true value. Figure "C" shows an ideal test, one that is both precise and accurate.

95% of a small population presumed to be healthy; by definition, then, 5% of healthy patients will have an abnormal test result (Figure 42–2). Slightly abnormal results should be interpreted critically—they may be either truly abnormal or falsely abnormal. The practitioner should also be aware that the more tests ordered, the greater the chance of obtaining a falsely abnormal result. For a healthy person subjected to 20 independent tests, there is a 64% chance that one test result will lie outside the reference range (Table 42–3). Conversely, values within the reference range may not rule out the actual presence of disease since the reference range does not establish the distribution of results in patients with disease.

It is important to consider also whether published reference ranges are appropriate for the patient being evaluated, since some ranges depend on age, sex, weight, diet, time of day, activity status, or posture. For instance, the reference ranges for hemoglobin concentration are age- and sex-dependent. Table 2 of the Appendix contains the reference ranges for commonly used chemistry and hematology tests. Test performance characteristics such as sensitivity and specificity are needed to interpret results and are discussed below.

Interfering Factors

The results of diagnostic tests can be altered by external factors, such as ingestion of drugs; and internal factors, such as abnormal physiologic states.

External interferences can affect test results in vivo or in vitro. In vivo, alcohol increases γ-glutamyl transpeptidase, and diuretics can affect sodium and potassium concentrations. Cigarette smoking can induce hepatic enzymes and thus reduce levels of substances such as theophylline that are metabolized by the liver. In vitro, cephalosporins may produce spurious serum creatinine levels due to interference with a common laboratory method of analysis.

Internal interferences result from abnormal physiologic states interfering with the test measurement. As

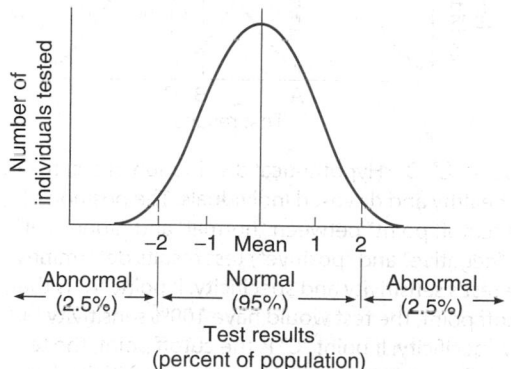

Figure 42–2. The reference range is usually defined as within 2 SD of the mean test result (shown as –2 and 2) in a small population of healthy volunteers. Note that in this example, test results are normally distributed; however, many biologic substances will have distributions that are skewed.

Table 42–3. Relationship between the number of tests and the probability that a healthy person will have one or more abnormal results.

Number of Tests	Probability That One or More Results Will Be Abnormal
1	5%
6	26%
12	46%
20	64%

an example, patients with gross lipemia may have spuriously low serum sodium levels if the test methodology used includes a step in which serum is diluted before sodium is measured. Because of the potential for test interference, clinicians should be wary of unexpected test results and should investigate reasons other than disease that may explain abnormal results, including laboratory error.

Sensitivity & Specificity

Clinicians should use measures of test performance such as sensitivity and specificity to judge the quality of a diagnostic test for a particular disease. Test **sensitivity** is the likelihood that a diseased patient has a positive test. If all patients with a given disease have a positive test (ie, no diseased patients have negative tests), the test sensitivity is 100%. Generally, a test with high sensitivity is useful to exclude a diagnosis because a highly sensitive test will render few results that are falsely negative. To exclude infection with the AIDS virus, for instance, a clinician might choose a highly sensitive test such as the HIV antibody test.

A test's **specificity** is the likelihood that a healthy patient has a negative test. If all patients who do not have a given disease have negative tests (ie, no healthy patients have positive tests), the test specificity is 100%. A test with high specificity is useful to confirm a diagnosis, because a highly specific test will have few results that are falsely positive. For instance, to make the diagnosis of gouty arthritis, a clinician might choose a highly specific test, such as the presence of negatively birefringent needle-shaped crystals within leukocytes on microscopic evaluation of joint fluid.

To determine test sensitivity and specificity for a particular disease, the test must be compared against an independent "gold standard" test that defines the true disease state of the patient. For instance, the sensitivity and specificity of the ventilation-perfusion scan for pulmonary emboli are obtained by comparing the results of scans with the gold standard, pulmonary arteriography. Application of the gold standard examination to patients with positive scans establishes specificity. Failure to apply the gold standard examination following negative scans may result in an overestimation of sensitivity, since false negatives will not be identified. However, for many disease states (eg, pancreatitis), an independent gold standard test either does not exist or is very difficult or expensive to apply—and in such cases reliable estimates of test sensitivity and specificity are sometimes difficult to obtain.

Sensitivity and specificity can also be affected by the population from which these values are derived. For instance, many diagnostic tests are evaluated first using patients who have severe disease and control groups who are young and well. Compared with the general population, this study group will have more results that are truly positive (because patients have more advanced disease) and more results that are truly negative (because the control group is healthy). Thus, test sensitivity and specificity will be higher than would be expected in the general population, where more of a spectrum of health and disease is found. Clinicians should be aware of this **spectrum bias** when generalizing published test results to their own practice.

Test sensitivity and specificity depend on the threshold above which a test is interpreted to be abnormal (Figure 42–3). If the threshold is lowered, sensitivity is increased at the expense of lowered specificity. If the threshold is raised, sensitivity is decreased while specificity is increased.

Figure 42–4 shows how test sensitivity and specificity can be calculated using test results from patients previously classified by the gold standard as diseased or nondiseased.

The performance of two different tests can be compared by plotting the sensitivity and (1 minus the specificity) of each test at various reference range cutoff values. The resulting **receiver operator characteristic (ROC) curve** will often show which test is better; a clearly superior test will have an ROC curve that always lies above and to the left of the inferior test curve, and, in general, the better test will have a larger area under the ROC curve. For instance, Figure 42–5 shows the ROC curves for prostate-specific antigen (PSA) and prostatic acid phosphatase (PAP) in the diagnosis of prostate cancer. PSA is a superior test because it has higher sensitivity and specificity for all cutoff values.

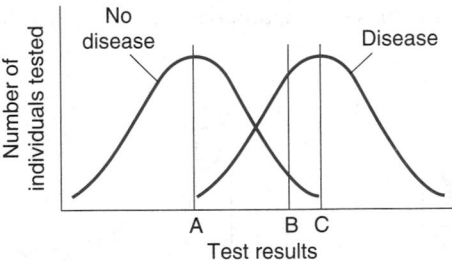

Figure 42–3. Hypothetical distribution of test results for healthy and diseased individuals. The position of the "cutoff point" between "normal" and "abnormal" (or "negative" and "positive") test results determines the test's sensitivity and specificity. If point "A" is the cutoff point, the test would have 100% sensitivity but low specificity. If point "C" is the cutoff point, the test would have 100% specificity but low sensitivity. For many tests, the cutoff point is determined by the reference range, ie, the range of test results that are within 2 SD of the mean of test results for healthy individuals (point "B"). In some situations, the cutoff is altered to enhance either sensitivity or specificity.

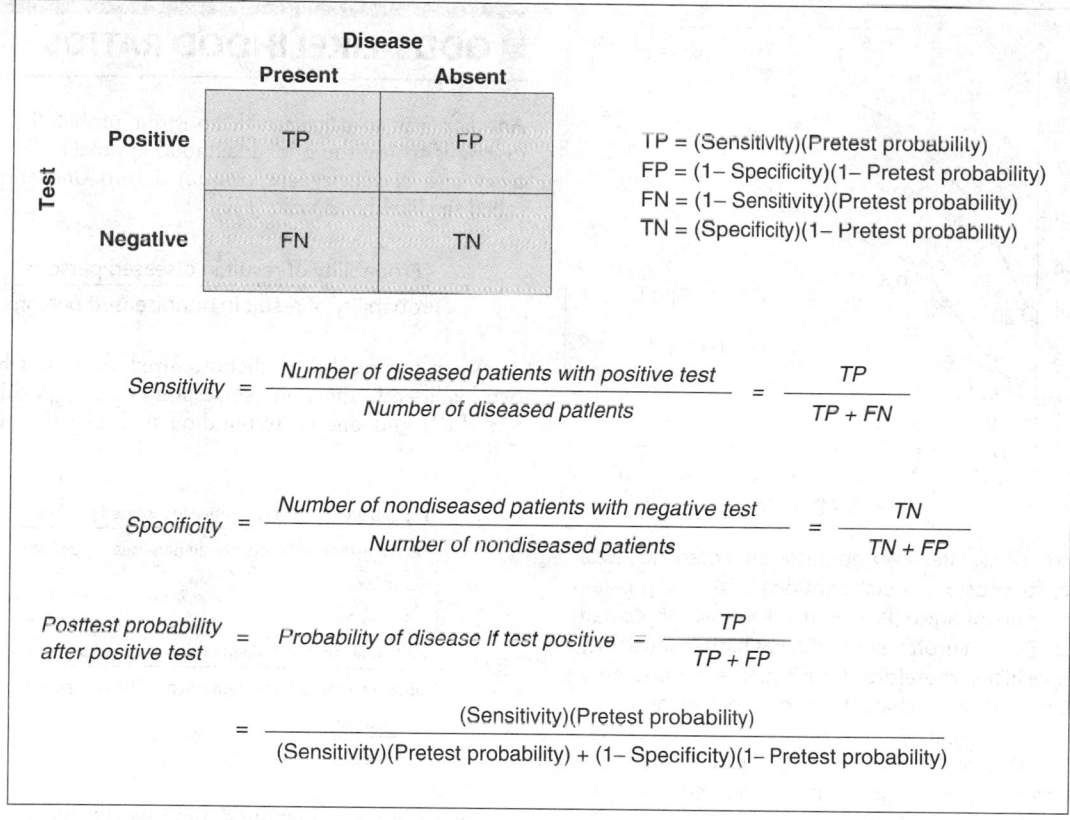

Figure 42–4. Calculation of sensitivity, specificity, and probability of disease after a positive test (posttest probability). (TP, true positive; FP, false positive; FN, false negative; TN, true negative.)

Gilbert R et al: Assessing diagnostic and screening tests: Part 1. Concepts. West J Med 2001;174:405. [PMID: 11381009]

Lijmer JG et al: Empirical evidence of design-related bias in studies of diagnostic tests. JAMA 1999;282:1061. [PMID: 10493205]

Mossman D, Berger JO: Intervals for posttest probabilities: a comparison of 5 methods. Med Decis Making 2001;21:498. [PMID: 11760107]

Omalley AJ et al: Bayesian regression methodology for estimating a receiver operating characteristic curve with two radiologic applications: prostate biopsy and spiral CT of ureteral stones. Acad Radiol 2001;8:713. [PMID: 11508750]

■ USE OF TESTS IN DIAGNOSIS & MANAGEMENT

The value of a test in a particular clinical situation depends not only on the test's sensitivity and specificity but also on the probability that the patient has the disease before the test result is known (**pretest probability**). The results of a useful test will substantially change the probability that the patient has the disease (**posttest probability**). Figure 42–4 shows how posttest probability can be calculated from the known sensitivity and specificity of the test and the estimated pretest probability of disease (or disease prevalence).

The pretest probability of disease has a profound effect on the posttest probability of disease. As demonstrated in Table 42–4, when a test with 90% sensitivity and specificity is used, the posttest probability can vary from 1% to 99% depending on the pretest probability of disease. Furthermore, as the pretest probability of disease decreases, it becomes more likely that a positive test result represents a false positive.

As an example, suppose the clinician wishes to calculate the posttest probability of prostate cancer using the PSA test and a cut-off value of 4 μg/L. Using the data shown in Figure 42–5, sensitivity is 90% and specificity is 60%. The clinician estimates the pretest probability of disease given all the evidence and then calculates the posttest probability using the approach shown in Figure 42–4. The pretest probability that an otherwise healthy 50-year-old man has prostate cancer is equal to the prevalence of prostate cancer in that age group (probability = 10%) and the posttest probability

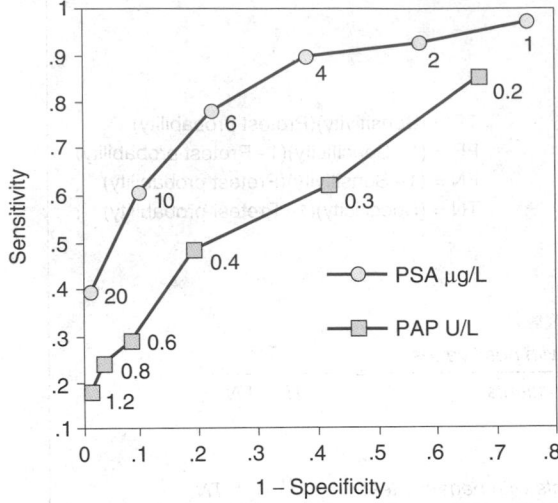

Figure 42–5. Receiver operator characteristic (ROC) curves for prostate-specific antigen (PSA) and prostatic acid phosphatase (PAP) in the diagnosis of prostate cancer. For all cutoff values, PSA has higher sensitivity and specificity; therefore, it is a better test based on these performance characteristics. (Modified and reproduced, with permission, from Nicoll D et al: Routine acid phosphatase testing for screening and monitoring prostate cancer no longer justified. Clin Chem 1993;39:2540.)

after a positive test is only 20%—ie, even though the test is positive, there is still an 80% chance that the patient does not have prostate cancer (Figure 42–6A). If the clinician finds a prostate nodule on rectal examination, the pretest probability of prostate cancer rises to 50% and the posttest probability using the same test is 69% (Figure 42–6B). Finally, if the clinician estimates the pretest probability to be 98% based on a prostate nodule, bone pain, and lytic lesions on spine x-rays, the posttest probability using PSA is 99% (Figure 42–6C). This example illustrates that pretest probability has a profound effect on posttest probability and that tests provide more information when the diagnosis is truly uncertain (pretest probability about 50%) than when the diagnosis is either unlikely or nearly certain.

Table 42–4. Influence of pretest probability on the posttest probability of disease when a test with 90% sensitivity and 90% specificity is used.

Pretest Probability	Posttest Probability
0.01	0.08
0.50	0.90
0.99	0.999

■ ODDS-LIKELIHOOD RATIOS

Another way to calculate the posttest probability of disease is to use the odds-likelihood approach. Sensitivity and specificity are combined into one entity called the likelihood ratio (LR).

$$LR = \frac{\text{Probability of result in diseased persons}}{\text{Probability of result in nondiseased persons}}$$

When test results are dichotomized, every test has two likelihood ratios, one corresponding to a positive test (LR^+) and one corresponding to a negative test (LR^-):

$$LR^+ = \frac{\text{Probability that test is positive in diseased persons}}{\text{Probability that test is positive in nondiseased persons}}$$

$$= \frac{\text{Sensitivity}}{1 - \text{Specificity}}$$

$$LR^- = \frac{\text{Probability that test is negative in diseased persons}}{\text{Probability that test is negative in nondiseased persons}}$$

$$= \frac{1 - \text{Sensitivity}}{\text{Specificity}}$$

For continuous measures, multiple likelihood ratios can be defined to correspond to ranges of results. (See Table 42–5 for an example.)

Lists of likelihood ratios can be found in some textbooks, journal articles, and computer programs (see Table 42–6 for sample values). Likelihood ratios can be used to make quick estimates of the usefulness of a contemplated diagnostic test in a particular situation. The simplest method for calculating posttest probability from pretest probability and likelihood ratios is to use a nomogram (Figure 42–7). The clinician places a straightedge through the points that represent the pretest probability and the likelihood ratio and then reads the posttest probability where the straightedge crosses the posttest probability line.

A more formal way of calculating posttest probabilities uses the likelihood ratio as follows:

Pretest odds × Likelihood ratio = Posttest odds

To use this formulation, probabilities must be converted to odds, where the odds of having a disease are expressed as the chance of having the disease divided by the chance of not having the disease. For instance, a probability of 0.75 is the same as 3:1 odds (Figure 42–8).

To estimate the potential benefit of a diagnostic test, the clinician first estimates the pretest odds of disease given all available clinical information and then multiplies the pretest odds by the positive and negative likelihood ratios. The results are the **posttest**

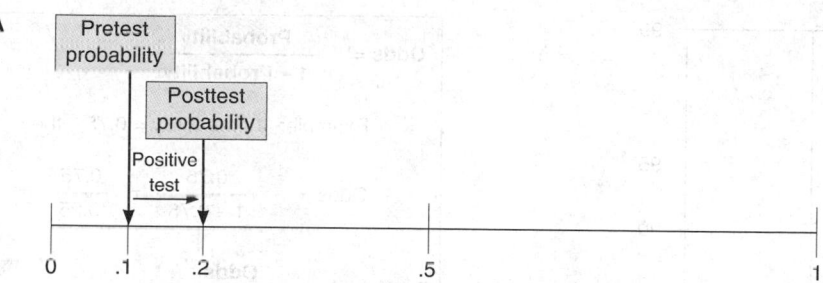

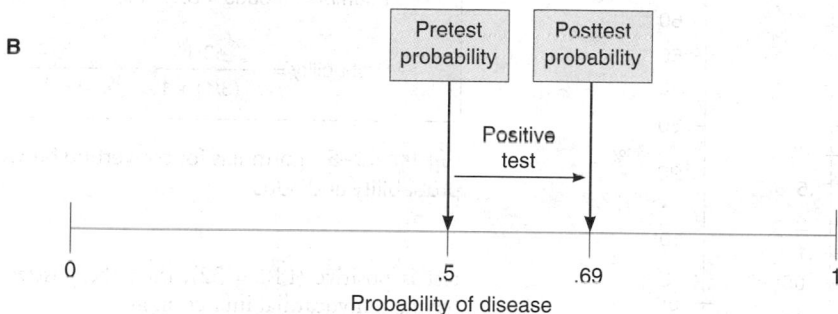

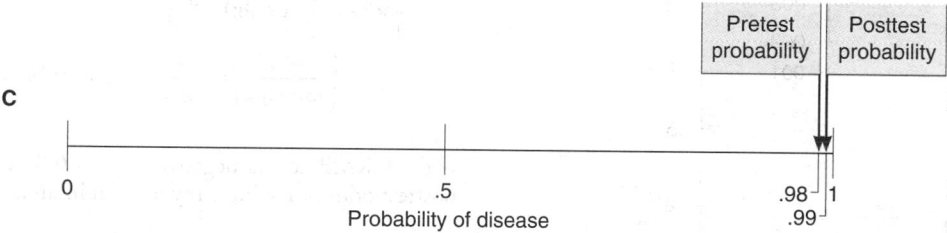

Figure 42–6. Effect of pretest probability and test sensitivity and specificity on the posttest probability of disease. (See text for explanation.)

Table 42–5. Likelihood ratios of serum ferritin in the diagnosis of iron deficiency anemia.[1]

Serum Ferritin (μg/L)	LR for Iron Deficiency Anemia
≥ 100	0.08
45–99	0.54
35–44	1.83
25–34	2.54
15–24	8.83
< 15	51.85

[1]From Guyatt G: Laboratory diagnosis of iron deficiency anemia. J Gen Intern Med 1992;7:145.

Table 42–6. Examples of likelihood ratios.[1]

Target Disease	Test	LR+	LR−
Abscess	Abdominal CT	9.5	0.06
Coronary artery disease	Exercise ECG (1 mm depression)	3.5	0.45
Lung cancer	Chest x-ray	15	0.42
Left ventricular hypertrophy	Echocardiography	18.4	0.08
Myocardial infarction	CK MB	32	0.05
Prostate cancer	Digital rectal examination	21.3	0.37

[1]From: http://www.med.unc.edu/medicine/edursrc/lrmain.htm

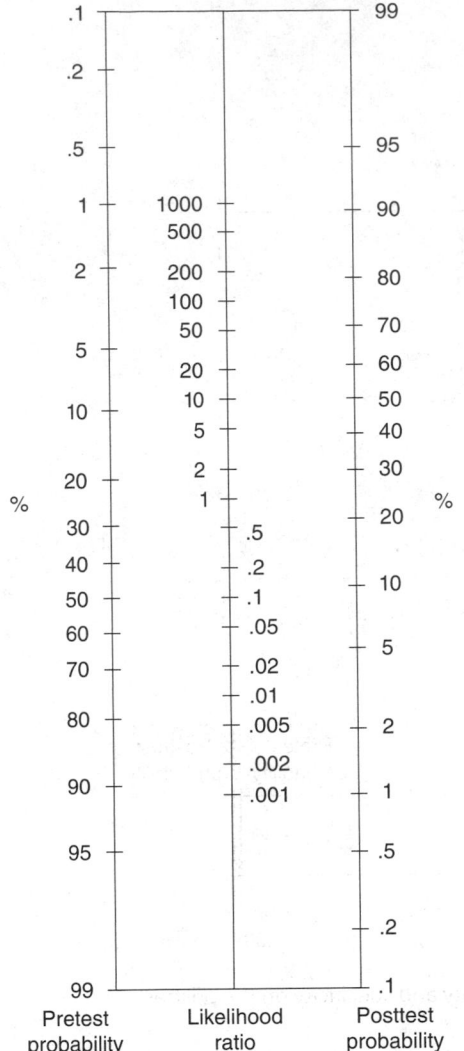

Figure 42–7. Nomogram for determining posttest probability from pretest probability and likelihood ratios. To figure the posttest probability, place a straightedge between the pretest probability and the likelihood ratio for the particular test. The posttest probability will be where the straightedge crosses the posttest probability line.
(Adapted and reproduced, with permission, from Fagan TJ: Nomogram for Bayes theorem. (Letter.) N Engl J Med 1975;293:257.)

$$\text{Odds} = \frac{\text{Probability}}{1 - \text{Probability}}$$

Example: If probability = 0.75, then

$$\text{Odds} = \frac{0.75}{1 - 0.75} = \frac{0.75}{0.25} = \frac{3}{1} = 3:1$$

$$\text{Probability} = \frac{\text{Odds}}{\text{Odds} + 1}$$

Example: If odds = 3:1, then

$$\text{Probability} = \frac{3/1}{(3/1) + 1} = \frac{3}{3 + 1} = 0.75$$

Figure 42–8. Formulas for converting between probability and odds.

test is positive ($LR^+ = 32$), then the posttest odds of having a myocardial infarction are

$$\frac{3}{2} \times 32 = \frac{96}{2} \text{ or 48:1 odds}$$

$$\left(\frac{48/1}{(48/1)+1} = \frac{48}{48+1} = 98\% \text{ Probability} \right)$$

If the CKMB test is negative ($LR^- = 0.05$), then the posttest odds of having a myocardial infarction are

$$\frac{3}{2} \times 0.05 = \frac{0.15}{2} \text{ odds}$$

$$\left(\frac{0.15/2}{(0.15/2)+1} = \frac{0.15}{0.15+2} = 7\% \text{ probability} \right)$$

Sequential Testing

To this point, the impact of only one test on the probability of disease has been discussed, whereas during most diagnostic workups, clinicians obtain clinical information in a sequential fashion. To calculate the posttest odds after three tests, for example, the clinician might estimate the pretest odds and use the appropriate likelihood ratio for each test:

$$\text{Pretest odds} \times LR_1 \times LR_2 \times LR_3 = \text{Posttest odds}$$

When using this approach, however, the clinician should be aware of a major assumption: the chosen tests or findings must be **conditionally independent.** For instance, with liver cell damage, the aspartate aminotransferase (AST) and alanine aminotransferase (ALT) enzymes may be released by the same process and are thus not conditionally independent. If condi-

odds, or the odds that the patient has the disease if the test is positive or negative. To obtain the posttest probability, the odds are converted to a probability (Figure 42–8).

For example, if the clinician believes that the patient has a 60% chance of having a myocardial infarction (pretest odds of 3:2) and the creatine kinase MB

tionally dependent tests are used in this sequential approach, an inaccurate posttest probability will result.

Black ER et al (editors): *Diagnostic Strategies for Common Medical Problems,* 2nd ed. ACP-ASIM, 1999.

Reid MC et al: Academic calculations versus clinical judgments: practicing physicians' use of quantitative measures of test accuracy. Am J Med 1998;104:374. [PMID: 9576412]

Threshold Approach to Decision Making

A key aspect of medical decision making is the selection of a treatment threshold, ie, the probability of disease at which treatment is indicated. Figure 42–9 shows a possible way of identifying a treatment threshold by considering the value (utility) of the four possible outcomes of the treat/don't treat decision.

Use of a diagnostic test is warranted when its result could shift the probability of disease across the treatment threshold. For example, a clinician might decide to treat with antibiotics if the probability of streptococcal pharyngitis in a patient with a sore throat is greater than 25% (Figure 42–10A). If, after reviewing evidence from the history and physical examination, the clinician estimates the pretest probability of strep throat to be 15%, then a diagnostic test such as throat culture ($LR^+ = 7$) would be useful only if a positive test would shift the posttest probability above 25%. Use of the nomogram shown in Figure 42–7 indicates that the posttest probability would be 55% (Figure 42–10B); thus, ordering the test would be justified as it affects patient management. On the other hand, if the history and physical examination had suggested that the pretest probability of strep throat was 60%, the throat culture ($LR^- = 0.33$) would be indicated only if a negative test would lower the posttest probability below 25%. Using the same nomogram, the posttest probability after a negative test would be 33% (Figure 42–10C). Therefore, ordering the throat culture would not be justified as it does not affect patient management.

This approach to decision making is now being applied in the clinical literature.

Kohn MA et al: What white blood cell count should prompt antibiotic treatment in a febrile child? Tutorial on the importance of disease likelihood to the interpretation of diagnostic tests. Med Decis Making 2001;21:479. [PMID: 11760105]

Pauker SG et al: The threshold approach to clinical decision making. N Engl J Med 1980;301:1109. [PMID: 7366635]

Solomon DH et al: The rational clinical examination. Does this patient have a torn meniscus or ligament of the knee? Value of the physical examination. JAMA 2001;286:1610. [PMID: 11585485] (Most recent in an excellent series of articles reviewing the diagnostic test information for different parts of the clinical examination.)

Decision Analysis

Up to this point, the discussion of diagnostic testing has focused on test characteristics and methods for using these characteristics to calculate the probability of disease in different clinical situations. Although useful, these methods are limited because they do not incorporate the many outcomes that may occur in clinical medicine or the values that patients and clinicians place on those outcomes. To incorporate outcomes and values with characteristics of tests, decision analysis can be used.

The basic idea of decision analysis is to model the options in a medical decision, assign probabilities to the alternative actions, assign values (utilities) to the various outcomes, and then calculate which decision gives the greatest value. To complete a decision analysis, the clinician would proceed as follows:

(1) Draw a decision tree showing the elements of the medical decision.

(2) Assign probabilities to the various branches.

(3) Assign values (utilities) to the outcomes.

(4) Determine the expected utility (the product of probability and utility) of each branch.

(5) Select the decision with the highest expected utility.

Figure 42–11 shows a decision tree where the decision to be made is whether to treat without testing, perform a test and then treat based on the test result, or perform no tests and give no treatment. The clinician begins the analysis by building a decision tree showing the important elements of the decision. Once the tree is built, the clinician assigns probabilities to all the branches. In this case, all the branch probabilities can be calculated from (1) the probability of disease before the test (pretest probability), (2) the chance of a positive test if the disease is present (sensitivity), and (3) the chance of a negative test if the disease is absent (specificity). Next, the clinician assigns utility values to each of the outcomes.

After the expected utility is calculated for each branch of the decision tree, by multiplying the utility

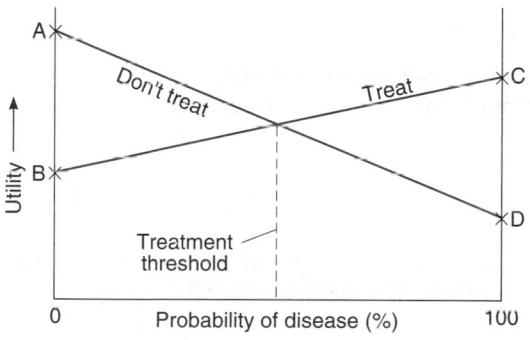

Figure 42–9. The "treat/don't treat" threshold. **A:** Patient does not have disease and is not treated (highest utility). **B:** Patient does not have disease and is treated (lower utility than A). **C:** Patient has disease and is treated (lower utility than A). **D:** Patient has disease and is not treated (lower utility than C).

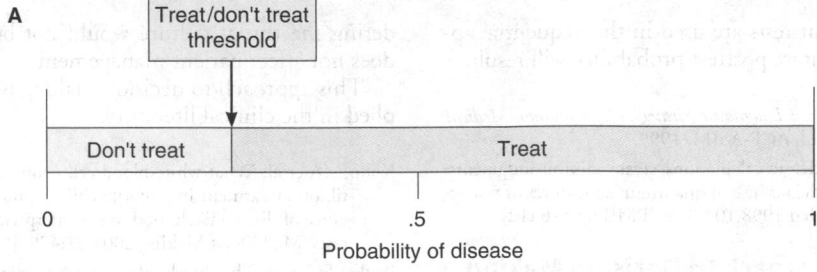

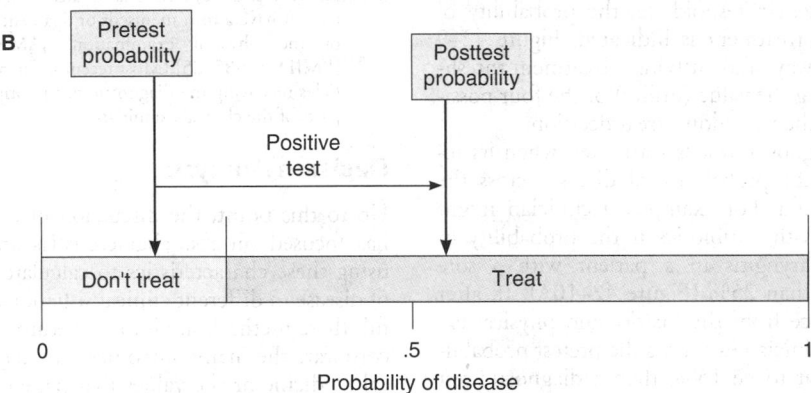

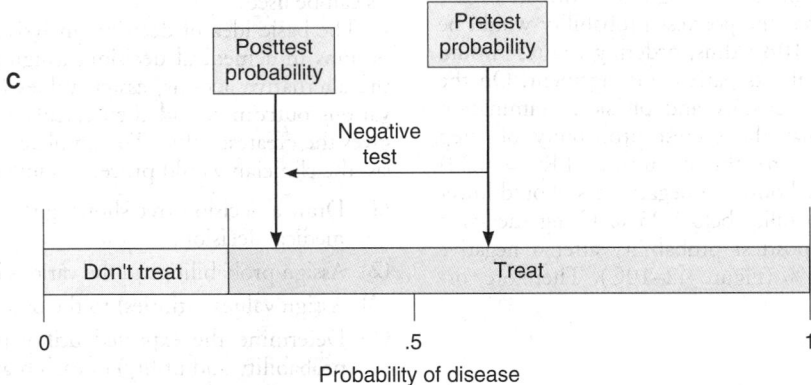

Figure 42–10. Threshold approach applied to test ordering. If the contemplated test will not change patient management, the test should not be ordered. (See text for explanation.)

of the outcome by the probability of the outcome, the clinician can identify the alternative with the highest expected utility.

Although time-consuming, decision analysis can help to structure complex clinical problems and to make difficult clinical decisions.

Detsky AS et al: Primer on decision analysis. Med Decis Making 1997;17:123, 126, 136, 142, 152. [PMID: 9107606, -07, -08, -09, -10] (Five-part series from "getting started" to "working with Markov processes.")

Elwyn G et al: Decision analysis in patient care. Lancet 2001;358:571. [PMID: 11520546]

Evidence-Based Medicine

Evidence-based medicine stresses the use of evidence from clinical research—rather than intuition and pathophysiologic reasoning—as a basis for clinical decision making. Evidence-based medicine relies on the identification of methodologically sound evidence, critical appraisal of research studies, and the dissemi-

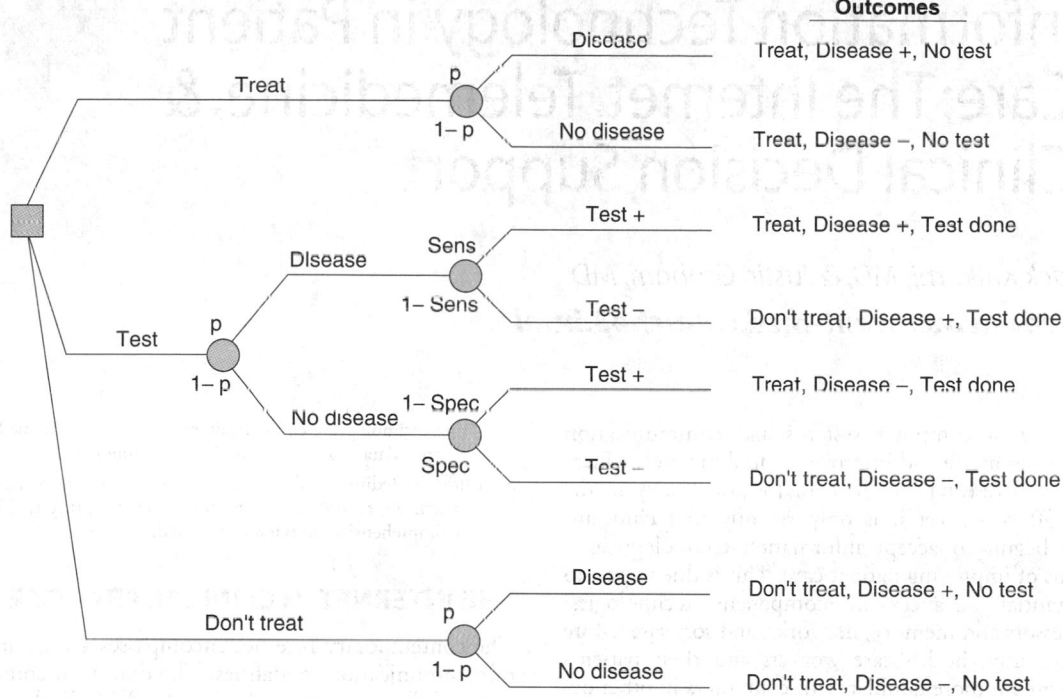

Figure 42–11. Generic tree for a clinical decision where the choices are (1) to treat the patient empirically, (2) to do the test and then treat only if the test is positive, or (3) to withhold therapy. The square node is called a decision node, and the circular nodes are called chance nodes. (p, pretest probability of disease; Sens, sensitivity; Spec, specificity.)

nation of accurate and useful summaries of evidence to inform clinical decision making. Systematic reviews can be used to summarize evidence for dissemination, as can evidence-based synopses of current research Systematic reviews often use meta-analysis—statistical techniques to combine evidence from different studies to produce a more precise estimate of the effect of an intervention or the accuracy of a test.

Clinical practice guidelines are systematically developed statements intended to assist practitioners and patients in making decisions about health care. Clinical algorithms and practice guidelines are now ubiquitous in medicine. Their utility and validity depend on the quality of the evidence that shaped the recommendations, on their being kept current, and on their acceptance and appropriate application by clinicians.

While some clinicians are concerned about the effect of guidelines on professional autonomy and individual decision making, many organizations are trying to use compliance with practice guidelines as a measure of quality of care.

Gillan MG et al: Influence of imaging on clinical decision making in the treatment of lower back pain. Radiology 2001;220:393. [PMID: 11477242]

Guyatt G, Rennie D (editors): *Users' Guides to the Medical Literature: A Manual for Evidence-Based Clinical Practice.* AMA Press, 2002. (A collection of the popular Users Guide to the Medical Literature series from JAMA; provides excellent tools for critical appraisal of the medical literature.)

Jadad AR et al: The Cochrane collaboration: Advances and challenges in improving evidence-based decision making. Med Decis Making 1998;18:2. [PMID: 9456200]

Information Technology in Patient Care: The Internet, Telemedicine, & Clinical Decision Support

43

Rick Kulkarni, MD, & Justin Graham, MD

See www.current-med.com/ch43.html

The use of computer systems and communication tools to enhance and improve medical practice, education, and research has increased exponentially in the past 30 years. Yet it is only recently that clinicians have begun to accept information technology as a means of improving patient care. This is due in part to substantial advances in component technologies: processors and memory, networks, and software. More importantly, health care workers and their patients have grown more familiar with computers in other occupational, commercial, and recreational applications. Therefore, an increasing number of clinicians apply these tools to the practice of medicine.

Modern medicine is very information-intensive. Clinicians regularly synthesize the vast, rapidly growing body of medical literature with detailed, ongoing patient evaluations. They communicate the resulting reams of data to their patients and to other clinicians. Never before has information technology been better suited to assist in these tasks. Modern information systems offer the promise of unprecedented quality, innovation, and efficiency in the delivery of health care. But there are both old pitfalls and new perils to be avoided.

The complex technical and theoretical details underlying medical informatics and computer science are beyond the scope of this chapter. What follows is a brief introduction to topics and resources of general interest in this field, offered to help clinicians care for their patients as information technology becomes an integral part of the patient-clinician relationship.

Committee on Enhancing the Internet for Health Applications: Technical Requirements and Implementation Strategies, Computer Science and Telecommunications Board, National Research Council: *Networking Health: Prescriptions for the Internet.* National Academy Press, 2000. Full text online: http://www.nap.edu/books/0309068436/html/. (Excellent overview by an expert committee of scientists and physicians on the Internet's role in health care.)

Jordan T: *Understanding Medical Information.* McGraw-Hill, 2002. (Introductory text providing clear explanations about basic issues in medical information science.)

Sailors RM et al: Clinical informatics: 2000 and beyond. Proc AMIA Symp 1999:609. [PMID: 10566431] (A brief and basic review of concepts and challenges in medical informa-

tion technology, such as requirements of electronic medical records, data processing, and decision support.)

Shortliffe EH (editor) et al: *Medical Informatics : Computer Applications in Health Care and Biomedicine.* Springer, 2000. (Comprehensive overview of the field.)

THE INTERNET IN CLINICAL PRACTICE

The contemporary Internet encompasses a wide array of communication modalities. The dominant component of the Internet is the World Wide Web. The Web's popularity derives from its ability to rapidly transmit both text and graphics to a user's computer screen through browsers (eg, Microsoft Internet Explorer, Netscape Navigator).

Despite the Web's dominance, other forms of communication on the Internet continue to be vital to the medium's success in facilitating communication. Electronic mail (e-mail) is a text-based form of communication employed by most Internet users in a "store-and-forward" fashion (ie, not processed immediately by the recipient). File transfer protocol (FTP) permits rapid transfer of files from one computer to another through the Internet. User groups make possible congregation and communication between individuals with similar interests.

The individual clinician's interaction with the Internet depends on his or her personal requirements and expectations. Simple store-and-forward modes of communication such as e-mail simplify exchanges with patients and colleagues. Most academic institutions offer to faculty and staff e-mail accounts that can be used without charge. Several online organizations offer free e-mail accounts to the general public.

Activities such as keeping up to date with current events in medicine, learning from electronic journals, and interacting with an institution's Web site for professional activities all require the use of browser software in order to access the Web. Several high-quality medical news Web sites (eg, CNN Health, Doctor's Guide) and an increasing number of online medical journals offering direct access to current and archived issues have made the Internet a valuable resource for physicians. Active participation in online medical communities providing access to searchable reference material and discussion groups (eg, eMedicine.com, MDConsult) add to the overall experience.

Clinicians may consider taking further advantage of the Web by constructing a clinical practice Web site. Although the details of programming and implementing a Web site are complex, the process itself can be straightforward and achievable if the legal implications and the scope of the project are appropriately addressed. Offering clinical information to patients or engaging in the transmission of patient related health information on the Web requires consideration of potential legal pitfalls. Providing medical content can be construed as formal medical advice. General patient education material and online recommendations should be followed by instructions directing patients to first discuss any suggested lifestyle or medication changes with a physician prior to adoption. In addition, the prudent physician should review previously published guidelines on responding to unsolicited e-mail requests for medical guidance. (Refer to the section on Patient-Clinician E-mail Communication, below.) The transfer of health-related information is strictly regulated by federal agencies and federal legislation. (Refer to the section on Legal Aspects of Medical Informatics, below.)

The scope of the clinical practice Web site should also be established prior to embarking on its construction. Programming a small Web site composed of several standard HTML (Hypertext Markup Language) "Web pages" can be accomplished by the individual clinician without a significant expenditure of time spent in learning computer code. Several off-the-shelf HTML editors have greatly simplified HTML programming by providing intuitive, user-friendly work environments. The actual installation of the Web pages onto a computer that "serves" content to the general Internet community can be accomplished by locating an Internet Service Provider (ISP). Professional assistance is recommended for advanced Web activities such as interacting with online databases and implementing interactive Web pages (eg, submission forms, online applications).

[BBC News—Health]

http://news.bbc.co.uk/hi/english/health/default.htm (Current health-related news from a trusted source.)

[CNN—Health]

http://www.cnn.com/HEALTH (A reliable source for clinical content and up-to-date developments.)

[MDConsult]

http://www.mdconsult.com (A comprehensive, fee-based medical information service providing access to fully searchable online medical textbooks, full-text medical journals, patient education material, practice guidelines, drug information, and access to online discussion groups.)

[eMedicine.com]

http://www.emedicine.com (Peer-reviewed, constantly updated compendium of thousands of monographs on clinical topics organized by specialty.)

JAMA patient page: Health and the Internet. JAMA 1998;280: 1380. [PMID: 9794323]

Peters RN et al: Building your own: A physician's guide to creating a Web site. JAMA 1998;280:1365. [PMID: 9794321]

INFORMATION RELIABILITY & QUALITY ASSESSMENT

The contemporary Internet contains a varied and extensive collection of Web sites devoted to the dissemination of health-related information. These Web sites provide a constantly expanding repository of information previously inaccessible to most clinicians and their patients, albeit at a cost. Unfortunately, these sites also frequently offer poor control over the accuracy, timeliness, and reliability of posted information.

Finding useful health-related information on the Internet is time-consuming for the physician unfamiliar with Internet search strategies. Even for those more experienced, location of reliable and useful information depends on one's ability to assemble a short list of potentially useful Web sites and then navigate to those sites and assess their value.

A better alternative is to use Internet health information meta-Web sites that have already rated and reviewed the content. It is the function of meta-Web sites to apply a core set of reviewing criteria to all the primary Web sites they review and rate. The criteria should be based on publisher accountability and applied to all health content Web sites. Table 43–1 sets forth an example of a core set of standards. The weakness of this model is the potential for error if the reviewing meta-Web site uses a flawed rating method.

Several review services provide rating criteria as well as seals of approval that individual Web sites can apply for and display to indicate compliance with established codes of conduct. An excellent example is the Geneva-based Health on the Net Foundation. Other Web sites such as the Current Medical Diagnosis & Treatment Companion Web Page (CMDT-CWP) offer stand-alone reviews and categorical ratings of hundreds of health care-related Web sites without requiring any display of seals of approval. Table 43–2 is an example of a well-constructed rating system currently in use on the CMDT-CWP.

Table 43–1. Core standards for information reliability and quality assessment.

Authorship: The relevant credentials and affiliations of the editors, authors, and contributors should be easily accessible.
Attribution: Detailed reference information for information content should be clearly listed on the entry page of the Web site.
Disclosure: All sponsorships, advertising sources, underwriting, and any other potential conflicts of interest should be prominently and fully disclosed.
Dating: The date of the last critical internal review of the content should be available to the user for review.

Table 43–2. An example of a well-constructed rating system.

Peer-reviewed	Web page claims that other experts in the field have critically evaluated material presented.
MD-oriented	Presentation explicitly designed for health-care professionals.
Patient resources	Substantial material presented here suitable for motivated patients.
Noncommercial	Corporate or for-profit sponsor does not exclusively support Web site. These sites may contain some advertising, however.
Multimedia-enhanced	Easy access to video, audio, animation, high-quality images and other multimedia teaching tools.
Updated regularly	Content was updated within 6 months of researching this guide.

[Current Medical Diagnosis and Treatment—Companion Web Page]

http://www.books.mcgraw-hill.com/medical/lange/cmdt (In addition to concise and informative reviews, a rating based on a six-category instrument (Table 43–2) also follows each Web site; the sites are organized by the textbook's 44 chapters.)

[Health on the Net Foundation Code of Conduct]

http://www.hon.ch/HONcode/Conduct.html (A Geneva-based organization offering health-related Web sites an opportunity to earn a symbol of good conduct if certain criteria are adhered to, including provision of medical information only from medically trained professionals, the precept that all information be provided only as an adjunct to the relationship between a physician and a patient, and the clear identification of all reference sources, funding sources, and "last-modified" details.)

Eysenbach G et al: Towards quality management of medical information on the Internet: Evaluation, labeling, and filtering of information. BMJ 1998;317:1496. [PMID: 91581] (Guide for overcoming the potential inaccuracy of health-related material on the Internet.)

Jadad AR et al: Rating health information on the Internet: navigating to knowledge or to Babel? JAMA 1998;279:611. [PMID: 9486757]

Silberg WM et al: Assessing, controlling, and assuring the quality of medical information on the Internet: Caveant lector et viewor—Let the reader and viewer beware. JAMA 1997;277:1244. [PMID: 9103351]

LEGAL ASPECTS OF MEDICAL INFORMATICS

Today's health care environment includes electronic medical records (EMRs), intranets connecting affiliated health care organizations for sharing patient information, and off-site access protocols for making patient information available to providers. One consequence of these technologies is that the confidentiality of sensitive patient information may be compromised. Although significant strides toward acceptable levels of security have been made in the past several years, questions have been raised regarding the integrity of existing privacy and security measures at both government and third-party institutional levels.

The burden of maintaining a secure electronic health information environment and complying with federally mandated regulations for the secure transmission of patient-related health care information between health care providers and other third-party organizations falls primarily on the health information management specialists at the health care organization. The individual physician must become familiar with the general principles, however, of electronic security to prevent accidental compromise of sensitive information. (See Table 43–3.)

Health care organizations, such as health maintenance organizations and health care clearinghouses, maintain electronic information systems on their patients. Many of these systems will be significantly affected by the implementation of HIPAA (the Health Insurance Portability and Accountability Act). Administered by the Department of Health and Human Services, HIPAA will force health care organizations to standardize their policies on electronic patient information transfer. The expected benefit is an improvement in privacy and security standards as well as transaction and code set standards in electronic data exchange. Further information can be found in the Web sites listed below.

[Current Medical Diagnosis and Treatment—Companion Web Page]

http://www.books.mcgraw-hill.com/medical/lange/cmdt (The CMDT-CWP offers physicians and patients direct access to a large collection of physician-reviewed health-related Web

Table 43–3. Specific methods commonly used to ensure security of electronic patient information.

Authentication: The process of verifying the identity of a user requesting data from the health care information system. Authentication is usually achieved by requesting private information from the user, such as a password or a personal ID number.

Access control: The process of determining the privileges a user has in terms of accessing information and services on the health care information system.

Encryption: Transformation of information into unintelligible data that is only interpretable with a private decryption key.

Audit trails: A record of information access events that is commonly used in health care information systems to deter individual users from system abuses.

Sessions: Persistence of user information designed to ensure user validation and automatic termination at time-outs.

sites. In addition to concise and informative reviews, a rating based on a six-category instrument (Table 43–2) also follows each Web site. The Web sites are organized by the textbook's 44 chapters.)

[Electronic Privacy Information Center—Medical Record Privacy]

http://www.epic.org/privacy/medical/ (An online resource for recent legislative and judicial reports on the topic of medical records privacy. The Web page provides direct links to congressional reports, recent publications in medical and legislative journals, and landmark white papers on the topic.)

[Health Insurance Portability and Accountability Act (HIPAA), Department of Health and Human Services]

http://www.hipaa.com/

http://aspe.hhs.gov/admnsimp/http://www.hhs.gov/

(Act intended to reduce the cost and administrative burdens of health care by standardizing electronic transmission of administrative and financial transactions. Rules on privacy and security ensure that participating providers and organizations adhere to minimum practices.)

[Questions and Answers: Recent Changes in Health Care Law]

http://www.dol.gov/dol/pwba/public/pubs/hippa.pdf (A booklet explaining the new rules, entitled *Questions and Answers: Recent Changes in Health Care Law;* available at the Department of Labor Web site.)

Clayton PD, Boebert WE, DeFriese GH: *For the Record: Protecting Electronic Health Information.* Committee on Maintaining Privacy and Security in Health Care Applications of the National Information Infrastructure, National Research Council, 1997.

O'Brien DG et al: Privacy, confidentiality, and security in information systems of state health agencies. Am J Prev Med 1999;16:351. [PMID: 10493295] (Overview of specific deficiencies in patient information security and privacy standards at the state health agency level.)

Gostin LO: National health information privacy: regulations under the Health Insurance Portability and Accountability Act. JAMA 2001;285:3015. [PMID: 11410101] (A description of the rules issued by the Department of Health and Human Services regarding the interpretation of HIPAA.)

PATIENT-CLINICIAN E-MAIL

Although clinicians have been communicating with their patients by e-mail for several years, this aspect of the patient-provider relationship has come under scrutiny. Electronic communication can extend and complement personal encounters, improve compliance and access to care, and increase the involvement of patients in their own care. However, the nature of e-mail creates legal, ethical, and practical considerations that must be respected by patients and providers alike.

E-mail is more permanent than oral communication and more spontaneous than letters and other written communications. It is by its nature self-documenting. E-mail can be duplicated or forwarded with the press of a button, and copies may linger on intermediate or back-up computer systems long after both the sender and receiver have deleted the originals. It can be easily altered, with or without attribution, by the sender, the recipient, or a third party. E-mail lends itself readily to detailed instructions as well as attachments and links to other information sources.

Electronic communication is well suited for communicating administrative information, medication or dressing instructions, patient education materials, routine laboratory results, appointment reminders, and prescription refills. It can augment home monitoring of a variety of treatment plans, such as diabetic diets or smoking cessation programs. Providers can easily make general announcements to an entire patient practice about issues such as vacation coverage, influenza vaccine availability, or changes in referral procedures (Table 43–4). This new mode of communication should certainly enhance the patient-clinician relationship—although, admittedly, there are few controlled clinical trial reports on outcomes.

E-mail imposes the same legal and ethical obligations that inform other kinds of doctor-patient communication. Providers have a duty to respond promptly to patient inquiries and to maintain strict confidentiality regardless of the technology involved. The very nature of e-mail complicates these issues and presents unfamiliar considerations such as source verification and technical failure. Thus, some experts have advocated obtaining formal informed consent from patients before exchanging e-mails. Providers ought at least come to agreement with their patients about basic policies for exchanges of these messages (Tables 43–5 and 43–6).

Some clinicians have expressed concern that once their e-mail addresses become widely available, they will be deluged by messages from individuals with whom they have no preexisting relationship. Studies have not found e-mail from unfamiliar patients to be burdensome. However, there is currently no consensus on the physician's duty in this situation. Additionally, there may be legal consequences to providing advice to patients who are out of state or abroad and thus possibly beyond the scope of the physician's license. At minimum, physicians should post electronic communica-

Table 43–4. Some suggested uses of patient-provider e-mail.

Patient education
    Medication, diet, or dressing instructions
    Multimedia disease education presentations
    References to appropriate Internet resources
Disease monitoring
    Home glucose, blood pressure, weight, or peak flow
      measurements
    Progress towards smoking cessation
Administrative information
    Referral requests
    Vacation coverage
    Changes in demographic data
Patient requests for prescription refills
Normal laboratory test results and interpretation
Reminders
    Scheduled appointments
    Vaccines or screening tests due
Clarifications, follow-ups, or reinforcement of issues
    discussed in person

Table 43–5. Provider strategies for management of electronic communication.[1]

Use password-protected workstations, digital signatures and encryption for all messages when readily available.

Print all messages, with replies and confirmation of receipt, and place in patient's permanent medical record.

Double-check all "To:" fields prior to sending messages.

Configure automatic reply to acknowledge receipt of messages.

Send a new message to inform patient of completion of request.

Maintain a mailing list of patients, but do not send group mailings where recipients are visible to each other. Use blind copy feature in software.

Create template banner headings and footers giving explicit instructions about how to escalate communication to telephone calls and office visits.

Never forward a patient's message or patient-identifiable information to a third party without the express permission of the patient.

Perform at least weekly backups of mail onto long-term storage.

Commit policy decisions to writing and electronic form.

Avoid anger, sarcasm, harsh criticism, and libelous references to third parties in messages.

[1]Adapted, with permission, from Kane B, Sands DZ: Guidelines for the clinical use of electronic mail with patients. J Am Med Inform Assoc 1998;5:104.

Table 43–6. Suggested elements of a patient-provider agreement for electronic communication.[1]

Establish turnaround time for messages and expressly state that e-mail is not for urgent matters or emergencies.

Provide instructions on how and when to escalate to phone calls, office appointments, and emergency room visits.

Agree on privacy issues and who, besides the addressee, will read messages. Make specific reference to office staff, covering providers, and third-party consultations.

Inform patients about the possibility of electronic eavesdropping by patients' own employers, Internet service providers, and others, such as family, who have access to the same computers or e-mail account.

Establish types of transactions (prescription refill, appointment scheduling, etc) and sensitivity of subject matter (HIV, mental health, etc) permitted over e-mail.

Instruct patients to put category of transaction in subject line of message for filtering: "prescription," "appointment," "medical advice," "billing question."

Request that patients put their name and patient identification number in the body of the message.

Ask that patients use autoreply feature to acknowledge reading provider's message.

Describe how messages will be incorporated into the permanent medical record.

[1]Adapted, with permission, from Kane B, Sands DZ: Guidelines for the clinical use of electronic mail with patients. J Am Med Inform Assoc 1998;5:104.

tion policies addressing unsolicited communication wherever their e-mail addresses can be found.

Kane B et al: Guidelines for the clinical use of electronic mail with patients. J Am Med Inform Assoc 1998;5:104. [PMID: 9452989]

Mandl KD et al: Electronic patient-physician communication: problems and promise. Ann Intern Med 1998;129:495. [PMID: 9735088]

Spielberg AR: On call and online: Sociohistorical, legal, and ethical implications of e-mail for the patient-physician relationship. JAMA 1998;280:1353. [PMID: 9794317]

Spielberg AR: Online without a net: physician-patient communication by electronic mail. Am J Law Med 1999;25:267. [PMID: 10476331](Legal analysis of confidentiality, reimbursement, and malpractice issues.)

INTERACTIVE FORUMS

Informal consultations among clinicians have been common, but limited to the offices and conference rooms of specific health care settings or, periodically, academic meetings. The Internet and its dramatic reduction in barriers to communication has made these continuous and far-reaching.

Many online discussion groups are available for health care providers with similar interests (Table 43–7). Almost all function as electronic bulletin

Table 43–7. Examples of interactive forums.

Newsgroups (accessible at http://groups.google.com)
  sci.med.cardiology
  alt.support.asthma
Web-based forums
  Medical Crossfire
    (http://www.medicalcrossfire.com)
  Physicians Online Discussion Forums
    (http://www.pol.net)
  Medscape Discussions
    (http://www.medscape.com)
Mailing lists
  National Academic Mailing List Service (UK)
    (http://www.jiscmail.ac.uk/category/A.html)
  Program for Monitoring Emerging Diseases (PROMED)
    (http://www.promedmail.org)
  Medical Matrix Internet Medical Resource Mailing List
    (http://listserv.acor.org/archives/mmatrix-l.html)
  Lupus-L Mailing List
    (http://www.hamline.edu/lupus/listproc.html)
Chatrooms
  Talk @ OBGYN.net
    (http://www.obgyn.net/chat_cal/chat_sched.htm)
  Nephrologists' Forum Chatroom
    (http://www.he.net/cgi-bin/cgiwrap/brumley/renal/chat.cgi)

boards, where individuals leave new messages or comments relevant to ongoing discussion "threads" (topics).

Newsgroups (also called Usenet newsgroups) are one of the oldest applications of the Internet, predating the World Wide Web, although today the Web provides a convenient Usenet interface. There are tens of thousands of newsgroups organized in nested series with names like "sci.med.prostate.bph" or "alt.support.crohns-colitis." Newsgroups are open to the general public, are usually unmoderated, and are subject to little or no information quality control. There are many ways to access newsgroups, but perhaps the easiest is to browse through them at "http://groups.google.com."

Web-based forums are usually adjuncts to specific Web sites. They frequently require registration demonstrating appropriate credentials (eg, medical license number), and moderators often monitor postings for veracity and relevance. Thus, Web-based forums generally carry discussions of higher quality among fewer participants.

Mailing lists are discussions delivered directly by e-mail. Any comment posted to the ongoing dialogue is instantly sent to every subscriber throughout the world. Mailing lists can be moderated or unmoderated, private or public, and may have as few as two or as many as tens of thousands of subscribers. High-volume lists, which can average hundreds of postings each day, can be received using digest mode, which gathers the day's postings into a single e-mail message. Subscribing usually involves sending an e-mail message to an address containing "listserv" or "majordomo" with the text containing "Subscribe" followed by the name of the list in question (eg, Stroke-L or Lymenet-L).

The Internet's closest approximation to a face-to-face conversation takes place in chatrooms, where participants take turns typing text visible to the whole group as the discussion unfolds. More advanced chatrooms allow participants to "whisper" private messages to one another. Although as with everywhere on the Internet—it is impossible to verify the identities of those with whom one is communicating, quality chatrooms provide moderators, discussants, or attendants responsible for guiding discussions and omitting noncontributing participants. Most chatrooms of interest to health care providers are hosted by medical Web sites.

TELEMEDICINE

Telemedicine has been defined as "the use of electronic information and communications technologies to provide and support health care when distance separates the participants." The first example was the telephone.

Telemedicine applications of the past 20 years have relied mainly on interactive video to connect patients and referring clinicians in remote locations with spe-

cialists in urban tertiary care centers. Using studio or home video recording equipment, visual and audio information is conveyed either by physical transportation of videotape or other recording media or by more sophisticated, specially designed video conferencing networks.

As broad-bandwidth (high transmission rate) networks have become available, "store-and-forward" telemedicine has become more commonplace, using multimedia e-mail and Web technology to forward medical images, audio, medical records, and laboratory results. By combining these data with real-time synchronous consultations, consultants can now provide comprehensive evaluations from anywhere in the world.

The next generation of telemedicine applications will expand the remote clinician's capabilities beyond diagnosis to therapeutic interventions. Telesurgery, remote psychotherapy, and virtual "home visits" to manage chronic medical problems are all in early development. Multiple Web sites attest to these and even more innovative uses of telemedicine for clinicians to explore (Table 43–8). Telemedicine applications have several limitations. The peer-reviewed literature discussing telemedicine is currently largely limited to pilot projects and short-term outcomes; the few rigorous studies performed to date suggest the efficacy of teleradiology, telepsychiatry, telenursing, transfer of echocardiographic images, and electronic consultations with specialists.

Secondly, given the ease of transmission and duplication of digital information, confidentiality and security must be safeguarded. Although information transfer ignores geographic boundaries, medical licensure does not—especially in the United States, where several states have limited the interstate practice of medicine. Liability and malpractice are thorny and untested issues, as the practice of telemedicine presents a new form of the patient-caregiver relationship and associated hazards, such as technical failures leading to altered or suboptimal data. Finally, health care payer policy is lagging behind the technology. Most insurers

Table 43–8. Examples of current telemedicine applications.

In-flight emergency resuscitation guidance on commercial aircraft
Home fetal monitoring during complicated pregnancies
Monitoring compliance with home drug dispensers
Preoperative screening and postoperative follow-up of patients of surgeons on service missions to developing nations
Remote dermatologic, pathologic, or radiographic consultations
Teleproctoring laparoscopic surgery
Providing specialty care to incarcerated violent criminals
Directly observed therapy (DOT) for tuberculosis

will not yet provide reimbursement to clinicians for telemedicine consultations. Medicare will reimburse teleconsultations that meet a very restrictive set of criteria: the patient must be in an underserved rural area; the referring practitioner, who must be present, earns 25% of the consultation fee; and only teleradiology— and no other form of store-and-forward technology— is used in the consultation.

[National Library of Medicine National Telemedicine Initiative]

http://www.nlm.nih.gov/research/telemedinit.html

[Telemedicine Internet Exchange]

http://tie.telemed.org/

Bratton RL et al: Telemedicine applications in primary care: a geriatric patient pilot project. Mayo Clin Proc 2000;75:365. [PMID: 10761491]

Currell R et al: Telemedicine versus face to face patient care: effects on professional practice and health care outcomes. Cochrane Database Syst Rev 2000;(2):CD002098. [PMID: 10796678]

Kuszler PC: Telemedicine and integrated health care delivery: compounding malpractice liability. Am J Law Med 1999;25:297. [PMID: 10476332] (Legal issues raised by telemedicine.)

Roine R et al: Assessing telemedicine: a systematic review of the literature. CMAJ 2001;165:765. [PMID: 11584564] (A systematic review of the literature from 1966 thru 2000 for telemedicine. Evidence regarding the effectiveness and cost-effectiveness regarding telemedicine is still limited.)

Strode SW et al: Technical and clinical progress in telemedicine. JAMA 1999;281:1066. [PMID: 10188642]

CLINICAL DECISION SUPPORT SYSTEMS

Computers and artificial intelligence systems have played a role in improving the quality of health care delivery to patients for several decades. One specific aspect of their contribution has been in the area of clinical decision support. Advances in enabling technology (eg, the Internet) have led to the dissemination of clinical decision support modalities into the individual practitioner's clinical environment. Two examples are the production of electronic, up-to-date versions of clinical references (ie, medical journals and textbooks) and development of efficient search tools for large bibliographic databases such as Medline.

In contrast to these general clinical modalities, computer-based decision support systems directly assist the clinician in making a decision about a specific patient. These applications incorporate individual patient characteristics into a computerized knowledge base to generate patient-specific assessments or recommendations.

Clinical judgment is dependent on information gathering, accurate assessment of probabilities, and problem-solving skills. Clinicians draw upon their personal knowledge base, accumulated over years of experience, to recognize patterns, anticipate outcomes, and reason heuristically. (Heuristic reasoning uses rules of thumb, eg, "Chest pain in an older man is a myocardial infarction until proved otherwise.")

Health care providers, while adept at these tasks, are subject to limitations and prejudices inherent to humans. Information overload can overwhelm clinicians, forcing them to ignore relevant data. Clinicians are also prone to several human cognitive biases that can hamper decision-making (see Table 43–9).

Immune to human limitations, clinical decision support systems offer an adjunct to the traditional patient care model. They have made possible the sharing of expert knowledge and problem-solving skills from institution to institution in a reliable and reproducible manner. Clinicians can also learn to improve their own decision-making skills by using these systems for feedback, evaluation, and simulations.

Clinical decision support systems perform a variety of functions from providing feedback to actions taken by clinicians to initiating communication between providers upon encountering unusual data. Specific examples of the types of logic used by clinical decision support systems in addition to topical examples are provided in Table 43–10.

Clinical decision support systems save lives and reduce costs. Inpatient order entry systems routinely result in double-digit percentage reductions in costs of patient care without negative effects on outcomes. Drug family checking systems reduce the frequency of adverse drug events by up to 55%. Time-based reminders for preventive care activities increase the percentage of patients who are up-to-date with recommended adult preventive testing schedules, and

Table 43–9. Common biases in human reasoning.

	Definition	Example
Anchoring	Placing unwarranted trust in an initial impression.	Continuing a course of antibiotic therapy for a patient whose "cellulitis" is subsequently found to be local reaction to a deep venous thrombosis
Availability	Assessing probability by the ease with which occurrences come to mind.	No longer prescribing a particular drug after witnessing a rare, idiosyncratic drug reaction in another patient
Representativeness	Believing that patterns, rather than probabilities, are predictive.	Commencing a huge work-up for pheochromocytoma for a patient with paroxysmal hypertension despite the extreme rarity of this tumor

Table 43–10. Functional classes and examples of clinical decision support systems.

Class	Function	Examples
Feedback	Provide feedback by responding to an action taken by the clinician or to new data entered into the system	Drug family checking results in alerts on allergies, drug-drug interactions, and other patient-specific conflicts Parameter checking looks for dosing errors and other parameter discrepancies in patient-specific scenarios (eg, gentamicin dosing in renal failure) Redundant utilization checking alerts physicians to duplicate test orders
Data organization	Organization and presentation of disparate data into logical, intuitive schemas at the point-of-need	Aggregate data trending observes key indicators for large numbers of patients over time (eg, emergence of antibiotic resistance patterns)
Proactive information	Provision of information to the clinician at the point-of-need (eg, clinical pathway on pneumonia when patient with pneumonia being admitted to hospital)	Template and order sets can be provided appropriate to given situations
Intelligent actions	Automation of routine and repeated tasks for the clinician on a regular time schedule (eg, provision of all new laboratory values on current patient list every morning)	Rule-based event detection allows users to create logical rules to be checked when triggering events occur (eg, check glucose level in hyponatremia) Time-based checks to post reminders when expected transactions have not occurred (eg, warfarin order not filled by 8:00 PM)
Communication	Alert clinician and other providers who need to know about unusual data (eg, test results) or communications regarding specific patients	Parameter alerts provide clinicians with key information on panic values Automated e-mails send information to clinicians when provider-patient encounters occur (eg, e-mail to primary doctor when patient evaluated in the emergency department)
Expert advice	Diagnostic and therapeutic advice using a comprehensive knowledge base and a problem-solving method, such as probabilistic reasoning, neural nets, or heuristic rules.	Differential diagnosis and suggestions for further testing generated from patient-specific data. Reducing uncertainty in test interpretation (eg, probability of pulmonary embolism given patient demographics and indeterminate V/Q scan)

automated e-mails increase interprovider communication and satisfaction. Hospital-based providers have accepted use of clinical decision support systems in their daily practice, and such systems are moving also into mainstream clinical practice. Clinicians must investigate how these innovative and rationally developed technologies can be most effective for their specific situations.

Classen DC: Clinical decision support systems to improve clinical practice and quality of care. JAMA 1998;280:1360. [PMID: 9794318]

Grundmeier R, et al: House staff attitudes toward computer based clinical decision support. Proc AMIA Symposium 1999:266. [PMID: 10566362]

Hunt DL et al: Effects of computer-based clinical decision support systems on physician performance and patient outcomes: A systematic review. JAMA 1998;280:1339. [PMID: 9794315]

Teich JM et al: Clinical decision support systems come of age. MD Comput 2000;17:43. [PMID: 10710934] (Structured overview and categorization of clinical decision support systems.)

PERSONAL DIGITAL ASSISTANTS (Handhelds)

Personal digital assistants (PDAs; handhelds) are pocket-sized computing devices used primarily for personal information management. The defining feature of handhelds is their ability to synchronize with a personal computer. The benefits of synchronization include minimization of accidental information loss, ease of information input, and transfer of online information into the device.

The devices are designed for limited data input. Feasible activities on the limited screen size include recording expenses, writing memos, and e-mail composition. Large data entry tasks and image composition are not realistic on the devices themselves but must be accomplished through synchronization of the device with a computer. Additional applications available for the devices included file transfer and backup utilities, investment applications, mapping and navigation tools, digital imagery, and games. Plug-in modules have transformed handhelds in various other devices from cameras to audio players to voice recorders. Higher-end models feature wireless connectivity and integrated cellular functionality, permitting their user to access information on the Web and send and receive e-mail as well as pages.

Clinicians will find handhelds to be particularly useful. To begin, physicians may take full advantage of the personal information management features discussed in the preceding paragraphs. The usefulness of handhelds for physicians is significantly extended beyond this basic functionality through the development of proprietary clinical applications. Specific examples of such functionality are outlined in Table 43–11.

Clinical calculators perform a variety of pertinent clinical functions such as medication calculations (eg, intravenous antibiotic and pressor drip calculations), clinical parameter calculations (eg, fractional excretion of sodium and free water deficit) and physiology calculators (eg, caloric converters, pregnancy estimated date of confinement). Medical databases include collections of useful information on such topics as microbial diseases, immunization schedules, and interpretation of laboratory tests. Drug references provide easy access to comprehensive databases on adult and pedi-

atric drug dosing, regimens, contraindications, adverse reactions, pregnancy and lactation, and mode of metabolism or excretion. Finally, information management applications provide extended functionality through innovative patient charting and clinical management software, procedure and case log, and electronic prescription generators.

[ePocrates]

http://www.epocrates.com. (A commercial Web site offering a free drug database and antimicrobial guide for the Windows CE and Palm OS platforms. The database provides adult and pediatric drug dosing schedules in addition to information on adverse effects, drug interactions, and contraindications.)

[Medscape Mobile]

http://www.medscape.com/Home/Topics/multispecialty/directories/dir-MULT.Mobile.html. (Suite of handheld medical applications including a collection of medical calculators and a drug database with dosing, summary, and interaction information.)

[Software Collections]

http://www.palmgear.com

http://www.handango.com

http://www.pdacortex.com

http://www.pdamd.com

MEDICAL CODING & TERMINOLOGY

Medical classification systems are tools used for bringing semantic and conceptual order to the chaos inherent in the enormously complex practice of medicine. Once thought to be the domain of data analysts and bureaucrats, disease coding and classification have increasingly become important for clinicians to understand. Large epidemiologic studies rely exclusively on disease coding for patient selection and stratification. Political and economic public health decisions are frequently made on the basis of data collected via specialized classification systems. Again, however, disease coding can intrude on the patient-physician relationship if it is allowed to dictate reimbursements, elements of the clinical encounter, documentation, and appropriateness of testing and treatment.

One of the most influential classification systems in use today is the World Health Organization's International Classification of Diseases (Table 43–12). It is currently in its tenth formal revision (ICD-10), though many institutions have not yet upgraded from ICD-9. It divides all of medicine into 21 "chapters," with titles like Diseases of the Digestive System, or External Causes of Morbidity and Mortality. Each chapter is subdivided into blocks, categories, and subcategories, to allow increasing level of detail—nearly 8000 in all. Categorization is inconsistent and incomplete: code outlines can be derived from anatomy, etiology, or epidemiology and frequently end with the category "not elsewhere classified" (NEC) or "not otherwise specified" (NOS). Although ICD was originally designed for epidemiology and health statistics, clinical

Table 43–11. Categorization of medicine-specific personal digital assistant applications.

Category	Example Applications
Clinical calculators	Intravenous antibiotic and pressor drip calculator Fractional excretion of sodium Caloric converter Estimated date of confinement
Medical databases	Microbes, diseases Pediatric immunization schedule Laboratory tests Differential diagnosis generators
Drug references	Adult and pediatric drug dosing guides
Information management	Patient charting and clinical management Procedure and case logs Prescription generators

Table 43–12. Examples of medical coding and terminology classification systems.

ICD-9	786.52 Painful respiration
SNOMED	F-37070 Crushing chest pain & F-37022 & Substernal chest pain & (G-CO40 T-D8 220) & radiating to the left arm
DRG	247, Circulatory disease with MI, w/o invasive investigation or procedure, died
CPT	92980 Transcatheter placement of an intracoronary stent, percutaneous, with or without other therapeutic intervention, any method; single vessel 92981 each additional vessel

MeSH	Cardiovascular diseases [C14]
	  Heart diseases [C14.280]
	    Myocardial ischemia [C14.280.647]
	      Coronary disease [C14.280.647.250]
	        Angina pectoris [C14.280.647.250.125]
	          Angina, unstable [C14.280.647.250.125.150]

modifications (ICD-10-CM) have been created that contain more clinical detail for use with billing, medical review, and reimbursement, raising the number of categories to 50,000. So while ICD-10 may have categories that correspond loosely to the level of information found on a death certificate, ICD-10-CM is able to categorize the fine detail found in that patient's hospital chart.

In an attempt to correlate diagnosis with cost of treatment, the United States Health Care Finance Administration created Diagnosis Related Groups (DRG) (Table 43–12). There are about 500 DRG codes in 23 Major Diagnostic Categories, derived to simplify adult inpatient Medicare billing, each corresponding to a patient's principal diagnosis or procedure and associated with a standardized cost. These correlations can be used to help determine an institution's case-mix or a population's relative severity of illness. Many different ICD codes may fall under a single DRG code—as long as the diseases they represent incur similar inpatient expenses.

There are many other coding systems, each designed for a different purpose (Table 42-12). Current Procedural Terminology (CPT) is a listing of descriptive terms and identifying codes created by the American Medical Association for reporting medical services and procedures—again for billing. The Systematized Nomenclature of Medicine (SNOMED) is a general purpose nomenclature designed to encompass all events in the medical record; unlike CPT, it is intended not for billing but for the standardization of databases, trials, and comparative information. Medical Subject Headings (MeSH) are devised by librarians at the National Library of Medicine to create a loose hierarchy for structuring the medical literature.

Most coding systems are created with very specific purposes in mind, and they usually succeed. However, problems occur when they are applied to tasks for which they were unintended.

[Duke Healthcare Informatics Links to Coding Systems]
http://www.mcis.duke.edu/standards/termcode/codehome.htm
[EICD.com]
http://www.eicd.com. (Online resource for looking up ICD-9 and CPT codes.)
Brett AS: New guidelines for coding physicians' services—a step backward. N Engl J Med 1998;339:1705. [PMID: 9834312] (A strongly worded critique of the inappropriate practice of applying a coding system created for billing to patient encounters.)

Complementary & Alternative Medicine

44

Bradly P. Jacobs, MD, MPH, Ellen F. Hughes, MD, PhD, & Brian M. Berman, MD

See www.current-med.com/ch44.html

The use of complementary and alternative medicine has become common in the United States. To maintain effective clinician-patient communication and ensure responsible clinical practice, it is important that clinicians learn the theory, practice, and scientific evidence associated with these therapies. This chapter provides an overview of four alternative medicine therapies: herbal medicine, nonherbal dietary supplements, acupuncture, and homeopathy.

Background

In 1998 a survey by Eisenberg estimated that over 40% of Americans made more than 600 million visits to alternative medicine practitioners and spent over $27 billion for their services. These visits exceeded the total number of visits to all United States primary care physicians, and the out-of-pocket expenditures were about the same as what the American public pays for all physician services.

Common reasons for seeking this care include acute musculoskeletal strain and conditions such as back pain, anxiety, depression, insomnia, chronic pain, and addiction. A 1998 survey by Astin identified the following predictors for Americans who use this category of care: higher education, poorer health status, having had an experience that caused a change in worldview, a holistic orientation toward life, and identification with a cultural group that has a commitment to women's rights, environmentalism, spirituality, and personal growth psychology.

Of patients using alternative medicine, only 4% use it exclusively. The majority combine it with conventional medicine because they perceive the combination to be superior to either option used alone. In one recent telephone survey, complementary therapies were judged by patients to be more effective for treating headache and back pain, but conventional therapy was considered superior for treatment of hypertension.

Within the conventional medical paradigm, efforts are being made to understand this phenomenon. Most medical schools now offer elective courses, and many are integrating information about these therapies into their required curricula. Special interest groups to discuss the role of alternative medicine have been organized in the Association of American Medical Colleges, the Society of Teachers of Family Medicine, and the American Public Health Association. Private and public hospitals are providing outpatient and inpatient clinical services for people seeking such care. Funding for biomedical research in this field has increased dramatically. The National Institutes of Health established the Office of Alternative Medicine in 1992 with an annual budget of $2 million; in 1998, its role was expanded as the National Center for Complementary and Alternative Medicine (NCCAM). A total of more than $200 million has been budgeted by NIH for research in the field in fiscal year 2002–2003. In 1998, *JAMA* and its ten affiliated *Archives* journals published theme issues including more than 80 articles pertaining to the field.

In 1996, the state of Washington passed legislation requiring insurance companies to reimburse policyholders for all services provided as alternative medicine. Recognizing the large public demand for these services, many United States health insurance companies have expanded benefit packages to include such services for an additional premium. According to data from early 2001, statutory licensure of practitioners exists for chiropractors in all 50 states, for acupuncturists in 42 states, for massage therapists in 32 states, for practitioners of naturopathic medicine in 11 states, and for homeopathic practitioners in 3 states. Insurance coverage is mandated for the costs of chiropractic medicine in 42 states and for costs of acupuncture in 7 states.

The National Institutes of Health classifies the complementary and alternative modalities into five major categories: (1) alternative medical systems (traditional Oriental medicine, acupuncture, Ayurveda, naturopathy, homeopathy, Native American healing, Tibetan medicine, etc); (2) mind-body interventions (meditation, certain uses of hypnosis, dance, art and music therapy, spiritual healing, and prayer); (3) biologic-based therapies (herbal medicines and dietary supplements, special diets, and orthomolecular medicine); (4) manipulative and body-based methods (chiropractic, massage, the Feldenkrais method, other "body work" systems, and aspects of osteopathic medicine such as craniosacral work); and (5) energy therapies (reiki, therapeutic touch, qigong, magnets, and other methods of affecting the "bioelectric field" of the body).

Astin JA: Why patients use alternative medicine: results of a national study. JAMA 1998;279:1548. [PMID: 9605899]

Eisenberg DM et al: Perceptions about complementary therapies relative to conventional therapies among adults who use both: results from a national survey. Ann Intern Med 2001;135:344. [PMID: 11529698]

Eisenberg DM et al: Trends in alternative medicine use in the United States, 1990–1997: results of a follow-up national survey. JAMA 1998;280:1569. [PMID: 9820257]

Levin J, Jonas W: *Essentials of Complementary and Alternative Medicine.* Lippincott Williams & Wilkins, 1999.

■ HERBAL MEDICINES

Epidemiology

The use of herbs for medicinal purposes has increased dramatically over the past decade. One out of three Americans spend a total of $5 billion dollars annually on herbal products, but fewer than half discuss the matter with a conventional health care provider. Consumers hold strong views about the efficacy of the supplements they take. Seventy percent state that they would continue to take their favorite supplement even if a government study claimed it was not effective.

In the 1850s, 80% of medicines in the *United States Pharmacopeia* were derived from plants. Today, approximately 20–30% of the drugs listed in *USP Dictionary* are plant-derived—important examples include atropine, colchicine, digoxin, and many antineoplastic agents.

Herbal medicines have been dispensed for centuries by traditional herbalists who have been involved with their cultivation and preparation as well as assessment of their potency. At present, most herbal products are commercially cultivated, processed in unregulated environments, and sold over-the-counter without the counseling of a qualified health practitioner.

Regulatory Issues

In 1994, the United States Congress passed the Dietary Supplement and Health Education Act (DSHEA). This act limited regulatory control over dietary supplements and herbs. DSHEA classifies vitamins, minerals, herbs, and amino acids as nutritional or dietary supplements. Under DSHEA, supplements can be marketed without proof of safety or efficacy as long as no claim is made for their use in the diagnosis, treatment or cure, or prevention of disease. Manufacturers can, however, make "structure and function" claims that a product enhances a normal body function

or state such as thinking, mood, or immune function. For example, saw palmetto can be marketed to support urinary tract health but not to treat benign prostatic hyperplasia. In contrast to prescription drugs, the FDA must first prove that a herbal preparation is *unsafe* before it can order that a product be taken off the market.

Quality Assurance

Since there are no regulations mandating that herbal manufacturers follow strict quality assurance guidelines, consumers have no guarantee of the safety and efficacy of the products they purchase. They cannot be certain that the plant was accurately identified; that the product is free of microbial, pesticide, and heavy metal contamination; or that all batches will contain the same ingredients in the same strengths. Indeed, a 17-fold difference in the amount of active ingredient was found when six national brands of St. John's wort were tested off the shelf.

The situation is different in Germany, where there is some regulation of herbal medicines. The German Federal Health Agency Commission E was formed in the 1970s to investigate and assess the safety and efficacy of herbal products. More than 400 monographs were produced on 350 herbal preparations, many of which are now available in an expanded English version. Since the United States has no such regulatory system, patients are advised to follow certain guidelines when considering whether to use herbal medicines (Table 44–1).

Product Formulations & Standardization

Herbal formulations include liquids (extracts, tinctures, infusions, and decoctions) and fresh, dried, and powdered preparations. The potency of herbs varies widely depending on which part of the plant is used, where it is cultivated, and what variations there may be in growing conditions and methods of preparation.

To ensure a consistent percentage of the primary active ingredients across batches and brand names, standardized extracts have been developed. Since multiple constituents may have pharmacologic activity, determining the active ingredients for standardization purposes can be a difficult task. The European scientific community has played a significant role in producing high-quality standardized extracts that contain consistent quantities of marker compounds (ideally, the active ingredients) and investigating the most promising ones in clinical trials. This work has laid the foundation for conducting phase 2 and phase 3 clinical trials. The quality of research in the field is improving, but most herbal remedies have not been evaluated in controlled clinical trials.

Safety of Herbal Medicines

Although many medicinal herbs are relatively safe, some have significant toxicity. Herbs themselves can

Table 44–1. Advice to patients using herbal medicines.

Communication
Discuss use of all therapies with your health care provider.

Product Quality
Manufacturers are not required to submit evidence to the FDA or any regulatory body to demonstrate product safety, effectiveness, or product quality.
Ask your primary care provider, a pharmacist, or a trained herbalist regarding the specific herbs you are using.
Use herbs that are standardized to contain a specific quantity of the active ingredients.
Select formulations that have been studied in clinical trials.
Select formulations produced by larger companies. They are more likely to ensure product quality in order to protect their reputation.

Labeling
Look for a seal of approval from an independent testing agency such as NNFA, NSF, or ConsumerLab.
It should state the common and scientific names of herb(s).
It should state the concentration or dose of the herb(s) and provide instructions on dose and frequency.
It should state that the product is "standardized" to contain a certain amount of the active ingredient(s).
It should state the methods used to ensure product quality.
It should state the name and address of the manufacturer.
It should state the batch or lot number and the expiration date.
It should list potential side effects and interactions.

Pregnancy
Few herbs have been studied for safety during pregnancy.
Seek advice from your primary care provider before using herbs during pregnancy.

Interactions
Discuss with your health care provider the safety profile and interactions that may occur when combining herbs and when taking herbs plus drugs.

Reporting
Report any adverse reactions to your state poison control program or the FDA.

---

have unanticipated effects such as hepatotoxicity as seen with chaparral and germander. Ma-huang contains ephedrine and is sold as a component of many weight loss products and in a banned euphoriant called "herbal ecstasy." Over 800 cases of adverse events associated with Ma-huang have been reported to the FDA. (See Ephedra in the specific herbs section for details.) Herbal products may also be intentionally adulterated with prescription drugs or contaminated with harmful substances such as pesticides or heavy metals. Prescription drugs such as prednisone, NSAIDs, antibiotics, and testosterone have been detected in imported Chinese patent medicines. An estimated 15 million adults in 1997 took herbal medi-

cines concurrently with prescription medications, creating a potential risk for adverse drug-herb or drug-supplement interactions. Patients taking St. John's wort along with the drugs indinavir or cyclosporine have lower blood levels of these prescription medicines. St. John's wort has the capacity to induce the cytochrome P450 system, which can lead to increased metabolism (ie, lower blood levels) of prescription medicines that are processed by this system such as warfarin, theophylline, and birth control pills. Proving that a side effect experienced by a patient taking a dietary supplement is caused by that supplement is often difficult. Practitioners should take a detailed history from the patient and, if possible, obtain a sample of the product to facilitate further analysis if needed. All suspected adverse events should be reported to the FDA's Medwatch Program (http://www.fda.gov/medwatch).

Blendon RJ et al: Americans' views on the use and regulation of dietary supplements. Arch Intern Med 2001;161:805. [PMID: 11268222]

Blumenthal M et al: *Herbal Medicine. Expanded Commission E Monographs.* American Botanical Council. Integrative Medicine Communications, 2000.

Fetrow C et al: *Professional's Handbook of Complementary and Alternative Medicine.* Springhouse, 1999.

Fugh-Berman A: Herb-drug interactions. Lancet 2000;355:134. [PMID: 10675182]

Klepser TB et al: Unsafe and potentially safe herbal therapies. Am J Health Syst Pharm 1999;56:125. [PMID: 10030529]

Rotblatt M, Ziment I: *Evidence-Based Herbal Medicine.* Hanley and Belfus, 2001.

Shulz V et al: *Rational Phytotherapy: A Physician's Guide to Herbal Medicine,* 4th ed. Springer, 2001.

REVIEW OF THE EVIDENCE FOR SELECTED HERBAL MEDICINES

Table 44–2 provides an overview of selected herbal medicines.

Garlic

Garlic is one of the most popular herbal remedies and is available in fresh, dried, and powdered forms. The German Federal Health Agency Commission E and the European Scientific Cooperative on Phytotherapy have approved garlic for the treatment of hyperlipidemia and atherosclerosis. Allicin, the ingredient believed responsible for garlic's therapeutic benefit and odor, is highly unstable. Both heat and acid destroy the enzyme allinase, which is necessary to produce allicin, and for that reason garlic is best ingested raw. Garlic is also available over-the-counter in multiple formulations. The best-studied form is an enteric-coated capsule of dehydrated garlic. Freeze-drying helps retain most of the active ingredients found in raw garlic. Enteric coating permits allicin to be re-

Table 44–2. Overview of selected herbal medicines.

	Leading Indications	Active Constituents	Mechanism of Action	Standardized Complex	Dosage	Level of Evidence[1] and Effect Size[2]	Safety[3]	Interaction; Side Effects	Comments	Cost per Day[4]
Echinacea (purple coneflower)	1. Treatment of URIs 2. Prevention of URIs	Isobutyl-amides, chicoric acid, polyenes, alkaloids, and alkylamides	Immunostim-ulant, phagocytosis, cytokines (IL-1, TNF, IFN)	Fresh-pressed juice of *E purpurea* with 2.4% β-1,2-fructo-furanosides, in 20% etha-nol solute	300 mg, or 3 mL q3–4 h	1. B: small 2. C	I	None known: rash, pruritus, nausea	Avoid in immunocompro-mised patients; avoid use > 4 weeks	$0.50–3.60
Ephedra	1. Weight loss 2. Stimulant	Ephedrine alkaloids	Sympathomi-metic		Max: 8 mg/dose; 24 mg/d	1. C: small 2. B: dose-dependent	V (at high doses)	Agitation, arrhythmias, stroke, MI, death	Often combined with caffeine-like herbs	
Garlic (*Allium sativum*)	1. Cholesterol 2. Hypertension 3. Coronary artery disease	Allicin	1. HMG CoA-reductase, 14α-demethylase 2. Unclear 3. Antiplatelet effects	Allicin 0.6–1.3%	600–900 mg qd	1. B: small 2. C: small 3. C	I	None known; bloating, flatulence		$0.12–0.38
Ginkgo biloba (EGB 761, GBE)	1. Dementia 2. Claudication	Flavonoid glycosides, terpenes such as ginkgolide B	PAF inhibition, antioxidant, membrane stabilization	24% flavonoid glycoside	60 mg tid	1. A: moderate 2. A: small	II	May have anticoagulant effect	Use caution if allergic to urusiols (mango rind, sumac-poison ivy, cashew nuts)	$0.35–0.80
Asian ginseng (*Panax ginseng*)	Stamina, aphro-disiac, fertility, "tonic," "energy-booster," "adap-togen"	Ginseno-sides	Unclear	> 2% ginsenosides	200–600 mg qd extract; 1–2 g crude drug	C Multiple studies but few for any given indication.	I	Previous reports of toxicity have been attributed to adulterants		$0.25–0.75

(continued)

Table 44-2. Overview of selected herbal medicines. (continued)

	Leading Indications	Active Constituents	Mechanism of Action	Standardized Complex	Dosage	Level of Evidence[1] and Effect Size[2]	Safety[3]	Interaction; Side Effects	Comments	Cost per Day[4]
Kava (*Piper methysticum*)	Anxiety	Kava lactones	May modulate GABA binding	30–55% kava lactones in USA	70 mg bid–tid kava lactones	B: moderate	II with recent concerns about liver toxicity	With excess use, possible yellow scaling of skin; sedation	Avoid combining with sedatives and alcohol	$0.35–0.60
St. John's wort (*Hypericum perforatum*)	1. Depression: mild to moderate 2. Depression: major	Napthodianthrones (such as hypericum or hyperforin), flavonoids, and xanthones	May modulate neurotransmitters (serotonin, NE, GABA)	Hypericin 0.3% or hyperforin, 3%	300 mg tid	1. A: moderate. 2. B: no better than placebo	I But significant drug-herb interaction	Induces cytochrome P450, leading to lower serum levels of certain drugs	Cyclosporine, protease inhibitors, oral contraceptives, warfarin, digoxin levels reduced	$0.25–0.60
Saw palmetto (*Serenoa repens*)	Benign prostatic hypertrophy	Sterols, free fatty acids	5α-Reductase inhibition; inhibition of DHT binding to androgen receptor	85–95% sterols and fatty acids	160 mg bid	B: moderate	I	Mild GI upset and headaches (rare)	Does not alter PSA levels	$.25–0.60

[1]Level of evidence: A, good evidence; B, some evidence; C, insufficient evidence

[2]Effect size: I, none, small, moderate, large

[3]Safety: I, generally safe; II, relatively safe; III, insufficient evidence; IV, may be harmful; V, clear evidence of harm.

[4]Average range of costs in retail drug stores.

CoA = coenzyme A, DHT = dihydrotestosterone, GABA = gamma-aminobutyric acid, GI = gastrointestinal, HMG = hydroxymethylglutaric acid, IFN = interferon, IL = interleukin, MI = myocardial infarction, NE = norepinephrine, PAF = plateletactivating factor, PSA = prostate-specific antigen, TNF = tumor necrosis factor, leased in the small intestine, thereby enhancing absorption and reducing the breath odor. Over-the-counter preparations are frequently standardized to yield 0.6% allicin.

Garlic appears to have small effects on cholesterol and no effect on blood pressure and glucose levels. The mechanisms of action believed responsible for the lipid-lowering effect include inhibition of HMG-CoA reductase and 14α-demethylase. A recent systematic review by Ackerman funded by the Agency for Health Care Policy and Research identified 36 randomized controlled trials on the use of garlic for the treatment of cardiovascular risk factors. Among the 26 trials evaluating hyperlipidemia, small but statistically significant reductions (16 mg/dL) were found for total cholesterol at 3 months among patients treated with garlic compared with placebo. Among the eight trials with outcomes at 6 months, no significant reductions in lipids were seen with garlic compared with placebo. In a qualitative review of antithrombotic effects, a modest and short-term effect was identified. Because garlic has some activity against platelet activation, there is a theoretical risk of increased bleeding, but there is insufficient evidence to determine a causal association. Effects on glucose and blood pressure were absent to minimal in studies reviewed.

Silagy and Neil reviewed 16 randomized controlled clinical trials representing 952 patients for the treatment of hyperlipidemia with garlic. They found approximately 12% reduction in total cholesterol and triglycerides with doses of 600–900 mg/d of a freeze-dried preparation. This dose was equivalent to one-half to one clove of raw garlic per day. They also performed a meta-analysis of garlic for the treatment of hypertension and found a pooled mean blood pressure reduction of 8 mm Hg systolic and 5 mm Hg diastolic between groups. A more recent meta-analysis of 13 randomized controlled trials by Stevenson showed less of a lipid-lowering effect of garlic. Total cholesterol decreased approximately 6%; analyses of trials limited to high quality found no difference in cholesterol levels between garlic and diet control.

Garlic is well tolerated and apparently safe for chronic use. In addition to the well-known breath and body odor, common side effects include gastrointestinal upset, nausea, and flatulence.

A more than 50% reduction in blood levels of saquinavir after garlic supplementation was reported recently. The mechanism of action of this significant herb-drug interaction may be induction of the cytochrome P450 system by the herb, as has been noted also with St. John's wort. Garlic supplementation causes a decrease in platelet aggregation, but the clinical significance of this observation is not clear.

Ackermann RT et al: Garlic shows promise for improving some cardiovascular risk factors. Arch Intern Med 2001;161:813. [PMID: 11268223]

Neil H et al: Garlic powder in the treatment of moderate hyperlipidaemia: a controlled trial and meta-analysis, J R Coll Physicians Lond 1996;30:329 [PMID: 8875379]

Piscitelli SC et al: The effect of garlic supplements on the pharmacokinetics of saquinavir. Clin Infect Dis 2002;34:234. [PMID: 11740713]

Silagy C et al: Garlic as a lipid lowering agent: a meta-analysis. J R Coll Physicians Lond 1994;28:39. [PMID: 8169881]

Stevinson C et al: Garlic for treating hypercholesterolemia. A meta-analysis of randomized clinical trials. Ann Intern Med 2000;133:420. [PMID: 10975959]

St. John's Wort (*Hypericum perforatum*)

St. John's wort is used in the treatment of mild to moderate depression. Multiple constituents identified as potential active ingredients include naphthodianthrones, flavonoids, and xanthones. Most preparations are standardized to hypericin content (a naphthodianthrone), but recent data indicate that there are other active ingredients as well, including hyperforin. The highest concentration of active ingredients is found in the flowering tops. The precise mechanisms of action are not known. Irreversible MAO-inhibitory activity noted in vitro has not been observed in vivo. Other postulated mechanisms include selective inhibition of serotonin, γ-aminobutyrate, norepinephrine, and dopamine reuptake in the central nervous system.

Over the past decade, randomized controlled clinical trials, systematic reviews, and meta-analyses have shown that St. John's wort is more effective than placebo and as effective as tricyclic agents for the treatment of mild to moderate depression. In Linde's review of 23 randomized controlled trials with 1757 subjects, hypericin-treated patients did significantly better than those receiving placebo (OR – 2.7; 95% CI, 1.8–4.0) and as well as those receiving antidepressants such as imipramine 50–75 mg/d, maprotiline 75 mg/d, desipramine 100–150 mg/d, and amitriptyline 30 mg/d (OR = 1.1; 95% CI, 0.9–1.3). Side effects occurred in over 50% of patients taking conventional antidepressants compared with 20% of patients taking St. John's wort. A recent Cochrane Collaboration systematic analysis of 27 randomized controlled trials with almost 2300 patients confirmed Linde's earlier findings. A recent review of commonly used herbs by Ernst also concludes that St. John's wort is effective in treating mild to moderate depression. In contrast, two recent studies conclude that St. John's wort is no more effective than placebo in the treatment of major depressive symptoms. In one trial, 340 patients with major depression were randomized to receive St. John's wort, sertraline, or placebo. After 8 weeks of treatment, no differences were observed—using the Hamilton and Beck depression scales—in patients taking St. John's wort, the SSRI, or placebo. St. John's wort is generally well tolerated. Side effects are not common and include mild headache, photosensitivity, gastrointestinal upset, and restlessness. Patients are advised to avoid taking St. John's wort in addition to prescription antidepressants, as there have been case reports of serotonin syndrome. St. John's wort also induces the cytochrome P450 system (isozyme CYP

34A), which may lower the blood levels of other drugs that are metabolized by this system (eg, ethinyl estradiol, warfarin, cyclosporine, and indinavir). Several cases of cardiac and renal organ rejection have been reported in patients whose previously stable level of cyclosporine was lowered after initiation of St. John's wort. Of further concern is that this herb-drug interaction may persist even after St. John's wort is discontinued. A 40% decrease in serum levels of the chemotherapeutic agent irinotecan noted in five patients taking concurrent St. John's wort persisted for 3 weeks after St. John's wort was discontinued.

Ernst E: The risk-benefit profile of commonly used herbal therapies: Ginkgo, St. John's Wort, Ginseng, Echinacea, Saw Palmetto, and Kava. Ann Intern Med 2002;136:42. [PMID: 11777363]

Gaster B et al: St. John's wort for depression: a systematic review. Am J Med 2000;160:152. [PMID: 10647752]

Hypericum Depression Trial Study Group: Effect of *Hypericum perforatum* (St John's wort) in major depressive disorder: a randomized controlled trial. JAMA 2002;287:1807. [PMID: 11939866]

Linde K et al: St. John's wort for depression: an overview and meta-analysis of randomised clinical trials. BMJ 1996;313:253. [PMID: 8704532]

Shelton RC et al: Effectiveness of St John's wort in major depression. A randomized controlled trial. JAMA 2001;285:1878. [PMID: 11308434]

Whiskey E et al: A systematic review and meta-analysis of *Hypericum perforatum* in depression: a comprehensive clinical review. Int Clin Psychopharmacol 2001;16:239. [PMID: 11552767]

Ginkgo

The dried leaf of the ginkgo tree has been used medicinally for thousands of years. More than 400 studies over the past 30 years have investigated ginkgo's ability to improve blood flow in a variety of conditions, including memory impairment, dementia, peripheral vascular disease, and tinnitus. The German Commission E has approved a standardized form of ginkgo leaf extract (Egb761) for the treatment of cognitive impairment and intermittent claudication. Multiple pharmacologically active compounds have been isolated from ginkgo, including flavonoid glycosides and terpene lactones (ginkgolides). The flavonoids have antioxidant and free radical scavenging ability. The terpene lactones (especially ginkgolide B) have platelet-activating factor antagonist activity. In addition, ginkgo extracts activate certain central neurotransmitters, including the cholinergic system, which may contribute to their beneficial effects on memory and cognition. Egb761—the formulation that has been studied most extensively—is standardized to contain 24% flavonoid glycosides and 6% terpene lactones.

A 1998 review identified 50 trials that assessed ginkgo's efficacy on cognitive function in the elderly. Because the vast majority of trials did not require a definitive diagnosis of dementia or Alzheimer's disease,

only four trials involving 424 patients met study entry criteria for meta-analysis. Results showed a modest improvement in cognitive function when compared with the placebo group—comparable to the effect of donazepil on dementia. The longest of these studies (1 year) showed stabilization of cognitive and functional abilities in 309 demented patients treated with Egb761 compared with placebo, with no differences in adverse outcomes. The NIH has recently funded investigators at the University of Pittsburgh to determine whether ginkgo taken over 5 years can prevent or delay the development of dementia in 3000 patients 75 years of age or older.

In general, ginkgo is well tolerated. Allergic skin reactions, gastrointestinal disturbances, and headache occur in fewer than 2% of patients. There are theoretical concerns about a risk of increased bleeding because antiplatelet activating factor activity has been demonstrated in vitro. Seven cases of increased bleeding have been reported (two patients were also taking aspirin or warfarin). Although no bleeding complications have been reported in any clinical trials and causality has not been clearly established, caution should be exercised when combining ginkgo with anticoagulants.

Gingko has also been evaluated for its effect on intermittent claudication. In a recent meta-analysis of eight randomized, placebo-controlled, double-blinded trials involving 418 patients, there was a modest treatment effect in the increase of pain-free walking distance in favor of ginkgo over placebo.

Ernst E: The risk-benefit profile of commonly used herbal therapies: Ginkgo, St. John's Wort, Ginseng, Echinacea, Saw Palmetto, and Kava. Ann Intern Med 2002;136:42. [PMID: 11777363]

Jacobs BP et al: Ginkgo biloba: A living fossil. Am J Med 2000;108:341. [PMID: 11014729]

Kleijnen J et al: Ginkgo biloba for cerebral insufficiency. Br J Clin Pharmacol 1992;34:352. [PMID: 1457269]

LeBars PL et al: A placebo-controlled trial of an extract of Ginkgo biloba for dementia. North American EGb Study Group. JAMA 1997;278:1327. [PMID: 9343463]

Pittler MH et al: Ginkgo biloba extract for the treatment of intermittent claudication: a meta-analysis of randomized trials Am J Med 2000;108:276. [PMID: 11014719]

Oken B et al: The efficacy of Ginkgo biloba on cognitive function in Alzheimer disease. Arch Neurol 1998;55:1409. [PMID: 9823823]

Echinacea

Echinacea ranks among the top-selling herbs in the United States, accounting for more than $300 million in sales annually. In the 1920s, echinacea tincture was a popular anti-infective agent until the discovery of antibiotics. Three of nine echinacea species are currently used for the treatment and prevention of upper respiratory infections. Above-ground parts and roots of *Echinacea purpurea* and the roots of *E pallida* and *E angustifolia* are used for medicinal purposes. Several active ingredients have been identified, including polysaccharides, glycoproteins, alkaloids, and flavonoids. In vitro and animal studies suggest that these ingredients cause stimulation of the immune system (natural killer cells, macrophages, and cytokine activity) and that they possess anti-inflammatory, free radical-scavenging, and antiviral activity.

Two high-quality systematic reviews have evaluated 13 double-blind, randomized, controlled trials of echinacea for prevention or treatment of the common cold. The quality of most clinical trials has been limited by use of multiple products and doses (including formulations containing multiple herbs) and the lack of rigorous methodology. In both reviews, there was modest benefit of echinacea compared with placebo for the acute treatment of upper respiratory infections. Subjects reported reduced symptoms or shortened duration of a viral upper respiratory tract when the herb was started within several days after onset of cold symptoms and continued for 8–10 days. There is not sufficient evidence to support the use of echinacea to prevent upper respiratory infections. Four large European trials of echinacea for that purpose showed positive trends but no statistically significant efficacy of the herb compared with placebo. Similar findings were reported in a recent double-blind trial of 117 adults who were challenged with rhinovirus after taking a United States echinacea product or placebo for 2 weeks.

In general, echinacea is well tolerated, with few reported adverse events. Rare allergic reactions have been reported (especially in patients with ragweed allergies), and there was a single case of recurrent erythema nodosum. The German Commission E recommends that patients who are pregnant, have autoimmune disease, or who are immunocompromised not take echinacea because of its immune-stimulating effects. The Commission also recommends that its use be limited in others to less than 4 weeks. The data supporting these recommendations are not clear.

Barrett B et al: Echinacea for upper respiratory infection. J Fam Pract 1999;48:628. [PMID: 10496642]

Grimm W et al: A randomized controlled trial of the effect of fluid extract of *Echinacea purpurea* on the incidence and severity of colds and respiratory infections. Am J Med 1999; 106:138. [PMID: 10230741]

Melchart D et al: Echinacea for preventing and treating the common cold. Cochrane Database Syst Rev 2000(2): CD000530. [PMID: 10796553]

Turner RB et al: Ineffectiveness of echinacea for prevention of experimental rhinovirus colds. Antimicrob Agents Chemother 2000;44:1708. [PMID: 10817735]

Kava

Kava is prepared from the dried rhizome of the *Piper methysticum* plant. Traditionally, it was used to prepare a ceremonial drink in the South Pacific islands. Its present-day uses include the treatment of anxiety, stress, and insomnia. The active ingredients (kavapyrones) have central muscle-relaxing properties and anticonvulsant activity. The precise anxiolytic mechanism of action is not fully understood but may involve enhanced binding of γ-aminobutyric acid in the central nervous system.

A recent systematic review and meta-analysis of seven German randomized, double-blind, placebo-controlled trials concluded that kava was more effective than placebo in relieving anxiety. The longest study involved 101 German outpatients randomized to kava or placebo for 6 months. Compared with placebo, kava-treated patients had progressively lower Hamilton anxiety scale scores at 3 and 6 months. In two shorter trials, kava also relieved acute anxiety more effectively than placebo. In one study, 59 patients were given two doses of kava prior to surgery. In the second study, 20 women were given kava for 1 week while awaiting the results of a breast biopsy. In one head-to-head 6-week European study—there was no placebo group—kava was as effective in relieving anxiety in 172 patients as oxazepam, 5 mg three times daily, or bromazepam, 3 mg three times daily.

Kava has been well tolerated in clinical trials. Fewer than 2.3% of patients report gastrointestinal complaints, drowsiness, tremor, headache, or allergic skin reactions. There are several case reports of patients feeling sedated, disoriented, or ataxic after consuming high doses of kava (or kava in combination with alcohol or prescription drugs that act on the central nervous system). These include two "driving under the influence" arrests of patients who had consumed 8–16 cups of a kava beverage. Kava may have dopamine antagonist properties. Three patients using European kava preparations developed extrapyramidal dystonic reactions or worsening Parkinson's disease. A reversible kava dermopathy (dry, flaky, yellow skin, ataxia, partial hearing loss, and weight loss) has been reported in South Pacific Islanders who consume kava at doses 100 times higher than recommended.

In November 2001, the German government reported 29 cases of hepatitis, cirrhosis, and liver failure possibly associated with the use of kava. Although 18 of these reports were in patients who were also taking medications with known or potential liver toxicity, one case involved a previously healthy 50-year-old man who was not taking prescription medications or alcohol who required a liver transplant. As a result, kava products have been taken off the market in Switzerland and Germany. Warnings about possible hepatic toxicity have been issued to patients with acute or chronic liver disease.

Escher M et al: Hepatitis associated with Kava, a herbal remedy for anxiety. BMJ 2001;322:139. [PMID: 11159570]

Pittler MH et al: Efficacy of kava extract for treating anxiety: systematic review and meta-analysis. J Clin Psychopharmacol 2000;20:84. [PMID: 10653213]

Volz HP et al: Kava-kava extract WS 1490 versus placebo in anxiety disorders—A randomized placebo-controlled 25 week outpatient trial. Pharmacopsychiatry 1997;30:1. [PMID: 9065962]

Ginseng

Ginseng root has been used for medicinal purposes in Asia for over 2000 years. There are three major forms of ginseng in use today. *Panax ginseng,* known as Asian ginseng, is commonly used in the United States. *Panax quinquefolius,* known as American ginseng, is cultivated in the United States and exported to China. *Eleutherococcus senticosus,* known as Siberian ginseng, is not a member of the panax genus. The German Commission E monograph on ginseng root approves its use as "a tonic to counteract weakness and fatigue, as a restorative for declining stamina and impaired concentration, and as an aid to convalescence." Extracts are made from dried roots and contain ginsenosides. Over 25 ginsenosides have been isolated, each with unique and sometimes oppositional effects on the cardiovascular, central nervous, and immune systems. The mechanisms of action have not been clearly delineated.

There is an extensive body of scientific literature on this subject, with over 4000 books and papers published. Multiple indications have been studied using different ginseng species, often with poor methodologic rigor. One European study identified 57 randomized controlled trials of ginseng in the world's literature, but only 16 studies were of good enough quality to be included in their systematic review. Insufficient evidence was available to support or refute the use of ginseng for any of the purported indications, including improvement of physical performance, cognitive functioning, and quality of life. One recent study suggests that American ginseng may attenuate postprandial glycemia in both normal and diabetic subjects.

Ginseng is well tolerated, with few adverse effects. Earlier reports of "ginseng abuse syndrome" and other toxicities are now attributed to adulterants found in earlier unregulated over-the-counter ginseng products. Indeed, 13 out of 21 ginseng products recently evaluated for quality and purity failed because they contained unacceptable levels of pesticides or heavy metals or inadequate concentrations of ginsenosides.

Ong YC et al: Panax (ginseng)—panacea or placebo? Molecular and cellular basis of its pharmacological activity. Ann Acad Med Singapore 2000;29:42. [PMID: 10748963]

Vogler BK et al: The efficacy of ginseng. A systematic review of randomised clinical trials. Eur J Clin Pharmacol 1999;55: 567. [PMID: 10541774]

Vuksan V et al: American ginseng (*Panax quinquefolius* L) reduces postprandial glycemia in nondiabetic and subjects with type 2 diabetes. Arch Intern Med 2000;160:1009. [PMID: 10761967]

Saw Palmetto

Traditionally, the fruit of the dwarf palm tree *(Serenoa repens)* was used by Native Americans for urinary complaints. Saw palmetto is now widely used to treat benign prostatic hyperplasia. In some European countries, herbal medicine is first-line therapy for that problem. Saw palmetto lipophilic extract is prepared from the berries of this palm indigenous to the southeastern United States. The principal active ingredients are sterols and free fatty acids. The mechanism of action is unclear; but there is evidence for inhibition of 5α-reductase activity and dihydrotestosterone binding at the androgen receptor.

A recent systematic review of saw palmetto extracts for the treatment of benign prostatic hyperplasia identified 18 randomized controlled trials involving 2939 patients. Although most studies were of short duration (mean of 9 weeks) and included small numbers of patients, symptoms and flow rates improved in men taking saw palmetto relative to those taking placebo. In two large, well-designed trials, saw palmetto extract appears to be as effective as finasteride. Two small European studies suggest that the herb is slightly less effective than prazosin and alfuzosin, an alpha-adrenergic antagonist not available in the United States. A recent 6-month double-blind, placebo-controlled trial of 44 men showed slightly (not statistically significant) greater reduction in prostatic hyperplasia symptoms in those taking a herbal blend containing saw palmetto, nettle root, pumpkin seed, and lemon bioflavonoid extracts and beta-carotene. Prostate biopsies taken before and after treatment demonstrated a decrease in the percentage of epithelium in the transition zone of the prostate from 17.8% to 10.7% ($P < .01$) in saw palmetto-treated men versus no change in the placebo group.

This herb is very well tolerated, with only mild and rare gastrointestinal symptoms being reported. Erectile dysfunction is more prevalent among persons using finasteride compared with saw palmetto (4.9% versus 1.1%; $P < .01$). Saw palmetto has not been shown to reduce prostate size or lower the serum level of prostate-specific antigen. No herb-drug interactions have been reported.

The University of California at San Francisco is conducting a randomized controlled trial funded by the NIH to evaluate the long-term efficacy of this herb for benign prostatic hyperplasia.

Marks LS et al: Effects of a saw palmetto herbal blend in men with symptomatic benign prostatic hyperplasia. J Urol 2000;163:1451. [PMID: 10751856]

Wilt TW et al: Saw palmetto extracts for treatment of benign prostatic hyperplasia. JAMA 1998;280:1604. [PMID: 9820264]

Ephedra (Ma-huang)

The dried young stems of *Ephedra sinica* have been used for thousands of years in traditional Oriental medicine to treat respiratory disorders, especially bronchospasm and congestion. Ephedra is widely marketed for its stimulant and appetite suppressant effects (alone or in combination with caffeine-like herbs). Ephedra's alkaloids are structurally similar to amphetamines. Sympathomimetic side effects include tremors, severe hypertension, seizures, and arrhythmias. These may lead to myocardial infarction, stroke, and death. Over 800 cases of adverse events, including more than 20 deaths, have been reported to the FDA. Samenuk et al reviewed 926 cases of possible Ma-huang toxicity reported between 1995 and 1997. In 37 patients, use of this herb was temporally related to stroke, myocardial infarction, or sudden death. Underlying heart disease was not a prerequisite for adverse events, and the toxic effects were not limited to massive doses. The FDA has advised patients with hypertension, glaucoma, seizure disorders, and coronary artery disease to avoid using this product. It is contraindicated also in patients with anxiety, mania, or thyroid disease and in those taking other stimulants or who are pregnant. Because it may increase steroid clearance, it may reduce the effectiveness of prednisone. The recommended maximum daily dose of ephedra is 24 mg.

Haller CA, Benowitz NL: Adverse cardiovascular and central nervous system events associated with dietary supplements containing ephedra alkaloids. N Engl J Med 2000;343:1833. [PMID: 11117974]

Samenuk D et al: Adverse cardiovascular events temporally associated with ma huang, an herbal source of ephedrine. Mayo Clin Proc 2002;77:12. [PMID: 11795249]

■ DIETARY SUPPLEMENTS

Sales of dietary supplements have increased dramatically over the past decade. The Dietary Supplement Health Education Act of 1994 has made it possible for manufacturers to sell dietary supplements directly to the public without FDA approval or oversight. Consequently, in the United States, there are no quality assurance regulations that pertain to these products. Reports of adulteration and contamination are available, but the magnitude of this problem remains unknown. Furthermore, there have been several reports of the dose printed on the label being different from the actual dose provided. (See section on herbal medicines, above, for further details on regulatory and quality assurance issues and advice for patients to follow when purchasing these products.) Table 44–3 provides an overview of selected dietary supplements commonly used in the United States today.

S-Adenosylmethionine (SAMe)

S-Adenosylmethionine is an endogenous compound that serves as a methyl group donor for hundreds of compounds, including neurotransmitters, fatty acids, nucleic acids, proteins, and membrane phospholipids. Endogenous production is dependent on vitamin B_{12} and folic acid metabolism. Primary uses of the drug are the treatment of depression, osteoarthritis, fibrositis, alcoholic liver disease, and migraine headaches. Originally discovered in the 1950s, SAMe was not synthesized as a stable compound that could be made commercially available until the 1970s. It is available by prescription throughout Europe. The mechanism of action is unclear for most conditions. Based on clinical trial data from over 22,000 patients, SAMe is well-tolerated and safe. Side effects include nausea, flatulence, headache, and anxiety. A phase 4 open-label clinical trial involving over 20,000 patients followed for 8 weeks found that 87% of the cohort reported good to very good tolerance with SAMe. There are no significant drug-herb interactions, although a case of serotonin syndrome in a patient taking SAMe with clomipramine has been reported.

Early studies suggesting that SAMe may be helpful in treating depression were limited by short duration and poor methodology. SAMe may affect multiple neurotransmitters; increased levels of serotonin, 5-hydroxyindoleacetic acid, and dopamine as well as inhibition of norepinephrine reuptake have been noted after SAMe administration. A meta-analysis published in 1994 identified 11 trials comparing SAMe with tricyclic antidepressants and 13 trials comparing either oral or parenteral formulations of SAMe with placebo. SAMe was found to be as effective as tricyclic antidepressants and superior to placebo in the treatment of depression. A 50% improvement in the Hamilton Rating Scale for Depression was reported by 38% of patients taking SAMe compared with 22% of those taking placebos. Furthermore, SAMe was better-tolerated and had a more rapid onset of clinical effect than tricyclic antidepressants. Overall, there is moderate evidence to support the use of SAMe for the treatment of depression.

SAMe appears to have analgesic and anti-inflammatory properties and was studied extensively in the 1980s for the treatment of osteoarthritis. The mechanism of action for these effects is unknown. SAMe appears to enhance native proteoglycan production in vitro, and in animal studies it is associated with higher proteoglycan content in cartilage and a reduction in surgically induced osteoarthritis following partial meniscectomy. A multicenter randomized, double-blind, placebo-controlled trial involving over 734 patients compared treatment with naproxen (750 mg daily), SAMe (1200 mg daily), and placebo over 30 days. Investigators found that SAMe was as effective as naproxen and superior to placebo. Patient lack of tolerability, number of patients reporting side effects, and frequency of occult blood identified in stool were higher in the naproxen-treated group compared with the SAMe or placebo groups. Other studies have shown similar efficacy when SAMe is compared with piroxicam 20 mg/d, ibuprofen 1200 mg/d, and indomethacin 150 mg/d, although many of these studies are of poor methodologic quality. SAMe appears to be better tolerated than and as effective as NSAIDs, but it

Table 44-3. Overview of selected dietary supplements.

	Leading Indications	Mechanism of Action	Dosage	Level of Evidence[1] and Effect Size[2]	Safety[3]	Interactions; Side Effects	Comments	Cost per Day[4]
S-Adenosyl-methionine (SAMe, SAM)	1. Depression, 2. Osteoarthritis, 3. Alcohol-related liver disease	Universal methyl donor	200–800 mg bid	1. C: moderate 2. C: moderate 3. C	I	None; may precipitate mania in persons with bipolar affective disorder		$2.00–$8.00
Dehydroepi-androsterone (DHEA, DHEAS)	1. Depression, dysthymia 2. Lupus 3. Adrenal insufficiency 4. Aging	1. Unknown 2. Unknown 3. Replacement 4. Replacement	50 mg qd	1. B: small 2. B: moderate 3. B: small 4. C	IV (with long-term use)	None reported; androgenic effects	Theoretical concerns that long-term use may result in hormone-dependent malignancies	$0.25–0.50
Glucosamine sulfate and chondroitin	Osteoarthritis	Proteoglycan production	Glucosamine 500 mg tid; chondroitin 400 mg tid	A: moderate	I	None reported; rare reports of constipation, diarrhea, drowsiness	Insulin resistance not seen in clinical trials	$0.35–0.95
Coenzyme Q_{10} (ubiquinone, ubidecarenone, Co-Q_{10})	Congestive heart failure, angina pectoris, acute myocardial infarction, periodontal disease	ATP production, membrane stabilization	50–100 mg bid; goal is to achieve serum level of 2.1 μg/mL	C	I	Patients taking statins noted to have lower serum levels of Co-Q_{10}	Fat-soluble, so absorption improved when taken with meals	$1.50–2.50

[1] Level of evidence: A, good evidence; B, some evidence; C, insufficient evidence

[2] Effect size: none, small, moderate, large

[3] Safety: I, generally safe; II, relatively safe; III, insufficient evidence; IV, may be harmful; V, clear evidence of harm.

[4] Average range of costs in retail drug stores.

requires a longer course of treatment to obtain the desired effects. Although many early studies used a parenteral form of SAMe, only an oral formulation is available in the United States, and it is expensive ($50–$150 per month) and has poor bioavailability.

Studies of alcohol-fed baboons suggest that SAMe increases glutathione levels and attenuates liver injury. There is some evidence that SAMe increases glutathione levels in humans as well. Investigators performed a multicenter clinical randomized, double-blind, placebo-controlled trial involving 123 patients with alcoholic liver cirrhosis treated with SAMe or placebo for 2 years. Combined mortality and liver transplantation rate was 30% in the placebo group compared with 16% in the SAMe group (P = .08). When Child class C subjects (n – 8) were excluded, respective rates were 29% and 12% (P = .03). This study provides support for SAMe supplementation in alcoholic liver disease.

Berger R et al: A new medical approach to the treatment of osteoarthritis. Report of an open phase IV study with ademetionine (Gumbaral). Am J Med 1987;83:84. [PMID: 3318446]

Bressa GM: *S*-adenosyl-l-methionine (SAMe) as antidepressant: meta-analysis of clinical studies. Acta Neurol Scand Suppl 1994;154:7. [PMID: 7941964]

Caruso I et al: Italian double-blind multicenter study comparing *S*-adenosylmethionine, naproxen and placebo in the treatment of degenerative joint disease. Am J Med 1987;83:66. [PMID: 3318442]

Mato JM et al: *S*-Adenosylmethionine in alcoholic liver cirrhosis: a randomized, placebo-controlled, double-blind, multicenter clinical trial. J Hepatol 1999;30:1081. [PMID: 10406187]

Dehydroepiandrosterone (DHEA)

DHEA and its sulfate ester, DHEAS, are secreted by the adrenal cortex. In healthy individuals there is a 25% decrease in serum DHEA levels per decade until age 70, when levels are at 20–30% of lifetime peak levels. Low DHEA levels have been reported in people who are critically ill, suffering from major burns, or depressed and in premenopausal women with breast cancer. Low levels with advanced age and in conditions of stress have been cited in the popular press as evidence that DHEA supplementation would be beneficial.

The mechanism of action of DHEA remains unknown. Preliminary evidence suggests that DHEA supplementation might be useful in depression, dysthymia, systemic lupus erythematosus, and adrenal insufficiency.

Animal studies suggest that DHEA and DHEAS have excitatory effects on the central nervous system, which may account for their influence on mood and sense of well-being. A 6-week clinical trial randomized 22 subjects with major depression to DHEA or placebo and found DHEA to be superior as measured by a 50% reduction from baseline using the Hamilton Depression Scale. Another study by Bloch found similar improvements using multiple well-validated instruments for the treatment of midlife dysthymia in a randomized double-blind crossover pilot study involving 15 patients.

Low DHEA levels in men and women with systemic lupus erythematosus suggest that DHEA may play a causative role. Twenty-eight patients with mild to moderate disease were randomized to DHEA or placebo for 3 months. DHEA-treated subjects had fewer flares and assessed their disease to be less severe.

Women with adrenal insufficiency have unmeasurable DHEA serum levels. Treatment with DHEA in a 4-month randomized, double-blinded, placebo-controlled crossover study was associated with improvements in mood, well-being, and libido.

Side effects of DHEA include acne, deepening of the voice, and facial hair growth, but no serious adverse events have been reported. The long-term effects of DHEA supplementation remain unknown. The safety issue of most concern is that DHEA—as a potent precursor of sex steroids—may increase the risk of estrogen- or androgen-dependent malignancies. Therefore, if supplementation is used, patients should be monitored closely. Furthermore, patients at high-risk for prostate, ovarian, breast, or uterine cancer should be counseled against DHEA supplementation.

Arlt W et al: Dehydroepiandrosterone replacement in women with adrenal insufficiency. N Engl J Med 1999;341:1013. [PMID: 10502590]

Bloch M et al: Dehydroepiandrosterone treatment of midlife dysthymia. Biol Psychiatry 1999;45:1533. [PMID: 10376113]

Huppert FA et al: Dehydroepiandrostenedione (DHEA) supplementation for cognition and well-being. Cochrane Database Syst Rev 2000;CD000304. [PMID: 10796526]

Kroboth PD et al: DHEA and DHEA-S: A review. J Clin Pharmacol 1999;39:327. [PMID: 10197292]

Van Vollenhoven R et al: Dehydroepiandrosterone in systemic lupus erythematosus. Results of a double-blind, placebo-controlled, randomized clinical trial. Arthritis Rheum 1995;38:1826. [PMID: 8849355]

Wolkowitz O et al: Double-blind treatment of major depression with dehydroepiandrosterone. Am J Psychiatry 1999;156:646. [PMID: 10200751]

Glucosamine & Chondroitin

Glucosamine and chondroitin have been used in Europe alone and in combination to treat osteoarthritis since the 1980s. These compounds are substrates for the production of articular cartilage. Glucosamine stimulates the production of glycosaminoglycans, leading to increased synthesis of cartilage. Chondroitin may help maintain articular fluid viscosity, inhibit enzymes that break down cartilage, and stimulate cartilage repair. Glucosamine is prepared commercially from crustacean shells. Chondroitin is extracted from bovine tissues such as cow trachea.

A meta-analysis by McAlindon and coworkers identified 15 randomized, double-blind, placebo-controlled trials involving 1710 patients with knee or hip osteoarthritis. Summary estimates found glucosamine and chondroitin to have moderate to large effects for treating osteoarthritis symptoms. Most trials were of poor to fair quality, and publication bias probably exaggerated the benefits. However, at least a modest degree of efficacy can perhaps be assumed. A Cochrane Review of 16 double-blind, randomized controlled trials of glucosamine for osteoarthritis showed that glucosamine was superior to placebo.

Glucosamine not only reduces the symptoms of osteoarthritis but may also slow the progression of the disease. Reginster and coworkers randomized 212 patients with osteoarthritis of the knee to receive either 1500 mg/d of glucosamine or placebo. After 3 years, patients taking glucosamine reported a 24% reduction in symptoms versus a 10% increase in the placebo group. X-rays revealed that the treatment patients experienced a loss of only 0.06 mm joint space versus 0.31 mm in the placebo group after 3 years. Glucosamine was very well-tolerated and did not elevate serum glucose levels. No drug-herb interactions have been reported. An NIH-funded multicenter trial is under way to evaluate glucosamine and chondroitin sulfate (alone and in combination) in more than 1000 patients compared with celecoxib and placebo. In summary, clinical trial literature suggests that glucosamine with or without chondroitin is well tolerated, safe, and effective in the treatment of osteoarthritis, with fewer side effects than NSAIDs.

McAlindon RE et al: Glucosamine and chondroitin for the treatment of osteoarthritis: A systematic quality assessment and meta-analysis. JAMA 2000;283:1469. [PMID: 10732937]

Reginster JY et al: Long-term effects of glucosamine sulphate on osteoarthritis progression: a randomized, placebo-controlled clinical trial. Lancet 2001;357:251. [PMID: 11214126]

Towheed TE et al: Glucosamine therapy for treating osteoarthritis. Cochrane Database Syst Rev 2001;(1):CD0022946. [PMID: 11279782]

Coenzyme Q_{10} (Ubidecarenone)

Coenzyme Q_{10} (also known as ubiquinone-10), is a lipid-soluble endogenous provitamin. The compound resides in the lipid layer of the mitochondria and plays a crucial role in oxidative phosphorylation for ATP production. It has also been observed to have effects on membrane stabilization, free radical scavenging, and calcium-dependent slow channels. Deficiencies in coenzyme Q_{10} have been observed among patients with congestive heart failure, renal failure, male infertility, and periodontal disease and in those taking HMG-CoA reductase inhibitors.

Studies of coenzyme Q_{10} for the prevention and treatment of cardiovascular disease have had mixed results. Earlier trials studying patients with congestive heart failure demonstrated fewer disease exacerbations, reduced hospitalizations, improved ejection fraction and quality of life measurements. Morisco and colleagues in 1993 reported a reduction in congestive heart failure exacerbations and number of hospitalizations in a yearlong multicenter randomized, double-blind, placebo-controlled study of 651 patients with class III and class IV congestive heart failure. A

methodologically more rigorous study performed by Watson and coworkers in 1999 showed that coenzyme Q_{10} had no effect on ejection fraction, hemodynamic parameters, or quality of life. A more recent study of 55 patients with class III and class IV congestive heart failure receiving standard medical therapy also showed no benefit of coenzyme Q_{10} on ejection fraction, peak oxygen consumption, or exercise duration. Other studies have evaluated coenzyme Q_{10} for acute myocardial infarction, angina, diabetes, and periodontal disease. Although several medical conditions are associated with coenzyme Q_{10} deficiency, there is insufficient evidence to support or refute the use of coenzyme Q_{10} to improve outcomes for any particular condition.

Because coenzyme Q_{10} is lipophilic, it is often formulated with vegetable oil or vitamin E to enhance its absorption. Its bioavailability is also enhanced when it is taken with meals, especially fat-rich foods. No serious adverse events have been reported with coenzyme Q_{10} use, and it is generally well tolerated. No significant drug-herb interactions have been reported, but coenzyme Q_{10} is chemically similar to vitamin K and so may reduce the effectiveness of warfarin. Although coenzyme Q_{10} supplementation appears to be safe, it is relatively expensive.

Khatta M et al: The effect of coenzyme Q_{10} in patients with congestive heart failure. Ann Intern Med 2000;132:636. [PMID: 11074912]

Morisco C et al: Effect of coenzyme Q_{10} therapy on patients with congestive heart failure: a long-term multicenter randomized study. Clin Investig 1993;71(8 Suppl):S134. [PMID: 8241697]

Watson P et al: Lack of effect of coenzyme Q on left ventricular function in patients with congestive heart failure. J Am Coll Cardiol 1999;33:1549. [PMID: 10334422]

■ ACUPUNCTURE

In acupuncture, certain locations on the surface of the body are stimulated, often with needles, to treat illness and promote health. Practitioners trained in Oriental medicine believe that a vital energy called chi (pronounced "chee") circulates in the body through 12 main pathways called meridians. Each meridian is named after a particular organ or "official," but the term actually relates to the energetic function more than the structure or anatomy of the organ. There are both surface and internal projections for each meridian. The surface projections contain sites called acupuncture points. Oriental medicine practitioners insert needles into these points to influence the body's chi to restore health.

History

The earliest reference to acupuncture can be traced to a text on Chinese medicine called *The Yellow Em-*

peror's *Classic of Internal Medicine* (the *Huang Ti Nei Ching*), which dates from the second century BC. This text is often referenced to support the authenticity of a particular practice or theory and is used as part of the curriculum in training colleges. Acupuncture spread through much of Asia and by the sixteenth century Jesuit missionaries had brought the practice to Europe. As early as 1912, William Osler described its use in the first edition of *The Principles and Practice of Medicine.* "For lumbago," he wrote, "acupuncture is, in acute cases, the most efficient treatment." Research and enthusiasm in the United States grew dramatically in 1971 when James Reston wrote an article describing his experience with acupuncture for postoperative analgesia after undergoing an appendectomy while in China.

Mechanism of Action

Acupuncture for analgesia stimulates the muscle's small-diameter nerve fibers that enter the dorsal horn of the spinal cord. An impulse is then sent to other levels within the spinal cord, the midbrain, and the hypothalamic-pituitary system, which then release neurotransmitters that cause analgesia. Therefore, when practitioners place a needle in the region of pain, all three centers are activated to provide an analgesic effect. When practitioners place needles in locations distant from the pain site, only the midbrain and hypothalamic-pituitary systems are activated. Although this theory implies that sham acupuncture may be as effective as real acupuncture, experimentally induced acute pain studies in animals and humans have consistently shown that real point stimulation is far superior to sham. These conflicting findings have prevented sham acupuncture from being widely accepted as an appropriate control. The 1998 NIH Consensus Statement on Acupuncture strongly recommends that future acupuncture research focus on finding such a control. A study of functional brain MRI imaging of healthy volunteers identified preferential activation of the hypothalamus and nucleus accumbens and deactivation of the rostral part of the anterior cingulate cortex, amygdala, and hippocampal complex among patients receiving active needling compared with minimally stimulated controls. Chronic pain studies, however, have shown less consistent results.

Despite extensive histologic studies, investigators have been unable to identify unique anatomic structures or physiologic effects at acupuncture points. Despite these shortcomings, our understanding of the mechanism of action of acupuncture for the treatment of pain is superior to our understanding of the mechanism of action for many drugs in widespread use today.

Stux G, Hammerschlag R (editors): *Clinical Acupuncture: Scientific Basis.* Springer, 2000.

Stux G, Pomeranz B: *Basics of Acupuncture,* 4th ed. Springer, 1998.

Wu MT et al.: Central nervous pathways for acupuncture stimulation: localization of processing with functional MR imaging of the brain—preliminary experience. Radiology 1999;212:133. [PMID: 10405732]

Training, Licensure, & Regulation

Acupuncture educational programs are accredited by the Accreditation Commission for Acupuncture and Oriental Medicine (ACAOM). Typical acupuncture training for nonphysicians in the United States requires completion of an accredited 4-year (2500 hours) master's degree training program. In order to become a licensed acupuncturist (LAc), one must pass a national and, frequently, state board examination. Although many states do not require physicians to obtain additional training, most states require a minimum of 200 hours of training in an accredited program. There are currently over 10,000 licensed acupuncture practitioners and 3000 physician acupuncturists in the United States. In 22 of the 40 states that license, register, or certify acupuncturists, these practitioners are permitted to work independently.

Clinical Practice

In the United States and Europe, Oriental medicine-trained practitioners conduct a comprehensive multisystem history, observation, and physical examination during the initial consultation. Examination consists of palpation of the abdomen and selected acupuncture points; examination of the tongue to assess color, shape, and coating; and palpation of the pulse along the wrist at three locations on both arms to assess its quality, rhythm, and strength. Treatment by the **classic acupuncture method** is based on the belief that each patient presents with a unique constellation of symptoms and signs. What this means is that ten patients presenting with migraine headaches may receive ten different treatments. Western-style practitioners will conduct a conventional examination and include variable components of the Oriental medicine approach depending on the individual's depth of training. Treatment is based on the **formula acupuncture method,** which utilizes a fixed combination of acupuncture points for a given medical diagnosis such that a cohort of migraine sufferers will be treated in the same way.

Treatment involves inserting four to fifteen needles at selected acupuncture points for 10–30 minutes—though certain schools leave the needles in place for only a few seconds to minutes. Needles are approximately 37-gauge, stainless steel, and disposable. Needles are stimulated with electricity, heat, or manually. Follow-up consultations last from 20 minutes to 45 minutes.

Patients can expect to see the practitioner weekly or bimonthly for 4–10 weeks, followed by less frequent visits as the condition improves.

Adverse Events

In current practice in the United States and Europe, acupuncture is generally considered safe, associated with a very low incidence of adverse events. Precautions useful for avoiding serious adverse events are listed in Table 44–4. The most frequent problems are vasovagal or sedating reactions such as presyncope, syncope, and drowsiness. These are easily prevented by having the patient lie flat on the table, monitoring patients during the initial visit, and permitting the patient to remain in the office until a normal state of awareness is achieved. Serious complications in the literature over the past 30 years have been due to the reuse of needles between patients, leading to transmission of infection such as hepatitis B and C or HIV, and needling the thorax in patients with emphysema, leading to pneumothorax. There have also been case reports of unusual serious adverse events, including endocarditis in patients with prosthetic heart valves who had small indwelling needles in place for several days, cardiac tamponade after needling directly over the heart, spinal cord trauma from deep insertion or migration of cut or broken retained needles, and pacemaker malfunction during acupuncture with electrical stimulation.

Most surveys estimate that the frequency of adverse events is 1:100,000 to 1:10,000. A 14-year review of the world literature identified 193 complications and concluded that acupuncture is generally safe except for patients with emphysema, in whom the risk of pneumothorax is significant. Another review identified 300 complications reported in the literature over a 30-year period. With more than 10 million acupuncture visits in the United States annually, the frequency approximates one per million visits.

CLINICAL USES OF ACUPUNCTURE

In the United States, acupuncture is frequently used to treat acute non-life-threatening conditions or chronic conditions that conventional medicine is unable to treat effectively (Table 44–5). What follows is a survey of some conditions for which patients frequently seek acupuncture care.

Stroke Rehabilitation

A 2001 systematic review of randomized controlled trials of acupuncture for stroke rehabilitation identified nine trials, including 538 subjects meeting study entry criteria. Six of out nine trials found acupuncture superior to control interventions, but study quality was poor. These findings suggest that acupuncture appears promising for the treatment of stroke, but studies of high quality are needed to confirm these preliminary findings.

Park J et al: Effectiveness of acupuncture for stroke: a systematic review. J Neurol 2001;248:558. [PMID: 11517996]

Chronic Pain

A 1989 meta-analysis of randomized controlled trials of acupuncture for chronic pain identified 14 trials meeting study entry criteria with five studies on low back pain, five studies on head and neck pain, and three studies on other types of chronic pain. Only two studies used inert medical placebo, with the remainder using sham acupuncture, transcutaneous electrical nerve stimulation (TENS), or continued standard medical care. Heterogeneity was present across trials as well as in all subgroups. With this limitation, the overall risk difference was statistically significant in favor of acupuncture ($P < .01$). In sensitivity analyses, individualized treatments (classic acupuncture) were superior to placebo; however, standardized treatments (formula acupuncture) were not more effective than placebo. Overall, although this review concluded that acupuncture was superior to control group intervention, serious methodologic issues were present. A criterion-based review of 51 controlled trials of acupuncture for the treatment of chronic pain found 24 trials reporting results favoring acupuncture. Using a 100-point quality scale, only 11 trials scored at least 50 points. The investigators concluded that poor study quality made it impossible to arrive at definitive conclusions.

Overall, there is some evidence suggesting benefit of acupuncture for persons with chronic pain when compared with placebo and insufficient evidence to suggest acupuncture is superior to standard medical care or sham acupuncture. The ability to make definitive recommendations regarding efficacy for chronic pain is hampered by poor methodologic study quality, which includes possible insufficient frequency and duration of acupuncture treatments.

Ezzo J: Is acupuncture effective for the treatment of chronic pain? A systematic review. Pain 2000;86:217. [PMID: 10812251]

Patel M et al: A meta-analysis of acupuncture for chronic pain. Int J Epidemiol 1989;18:900. [PMID: 2695475]

Table 44–4. How to avoid preventable adverse events associated with acupuncture.[1]

Make certain that only sterile disposable needles are used.

When press-in needles are used, make certain that sterile technique is employed.

Make certain that the patient is lying flat during the treatment.

Make certain that the practitioner counts the number of needles used before and after treatment.

Exert caution when patients are taking anticoagulants.

Avoid electrical stimulation in patients with pacemakers.

Exert caution when needling the thorax in patients with emphysema.

---

[1]Modified, with permission, from Rampes H: Adverse reactions to acupuncture. In: *Medical Acupuncture: A Western Scientific Approach.* Filshie J, White A (editors). Churchill Livingstone, 1998.

Table 44–5. Overview of acupuncture literature for selected medical conditions.

	Condition	Study	Inclusion Criteria	No. of Studies	No. of Patients	Measures	Results
Park, 2001	Stroke rehabilitation	Systematic review	RCTs, All types of stroke.	9	538	Scandinavian and Chinese stroke scales, Barthel Index, Nottingham Health Profile, motor function, balance and days in hospital	Overall, acupuncture appears promising for stroke rehabilitation. 6/9 trials favoring acupuncture compared with control. Future studies require higher study quality to confirm these findings.
Patel, 1989	Chronic pain	Meta-analysis	RCTs published in English from 1970 to 1989 listed in Index Medicus	14	558 plus 182 in crossover studies	Positive report of pain relief; otherwise, not specified	Positive result overall and for head-neck pain. Heterogeneity across trials was present. However, inconclusive due to potential for bias resulting from poor study quality.
ter Riet, 1990	Chronic pain	Systematic review	Controlled trials. Needles used. "Chronic" mentioned in title or abstract or pain > 6 months.	51	N/A	Positive report of pain relief; otherwise, not specified	No pooled analysis due to heterogeneity. 24/51 trials favoring acupuncture compared with control. However, inconclusive because of poor study quality.
Ezzo, 2000	Chronic pain	Systematic review	RCTs published in English. Pain > 3 months.	47	N/A	Positive report of pain relief; otherwise, not specified	Inconclusive
van Tulder, 1999	Low back pain	Systematic review	RCTs, Acute or chronic low back pain.	11	542	Pain relief	Inconclusive
Ernst, 1998	Low back pain	Meta-analysis	RCTs, Any type of low back pain.	9	377	Pain relief	Overall, acupuncture is superior to control. However, subgroup analysis found no difference between real and sham acupuncture.
Smith, 2000	Back and neck pain	Systematic review	RCTs, Chronic neck and back pain.	13	N/A	Pain relief	No convincing evidence for efficacy of acupuncture in relieving back and neck pain.
Ernst, 1997	Osteoarthritis	Systematic review	Controlled trials, Symptomatic disease.	13	437	Pain relief	Inconclusive. Overall, the literature is conflicting. There is limited evidence to suggest real acupuncture is not more effective than sham acupuncture.

(continued)

Table 44–5. Overview of acupuncture literature for selected medical conditions. (continued)

	Condition	Study	Inclusion Criteria	No. of Studies	No. of Patients	Measures	Results
Ernst, 1998	Acute dental pain	Systematic review	Controlled trials.	16	941	Pain relief	Definitive conclusion that acupuncture is superior to sham and placebo-controlled acupuncture. Evidence for use as adjunctive therapy.
Melchart, 1999	Recurrent headache	Systematic review	RCTs, quasi-RCTs.	26	1151	Any one clinical outcome related to headache, eg, pain intensity, global assessment.	Overall, the data support acupuncture for the treatment of recurrent headaches. 8/16 found real acupuncture superior to sham acupuncture, 4/16 found a trend favoring real acupuncture.
Linde, 2000	Asthma	Systematic review	Randomized and quasi-randomized trials	7	174	All subjective and objective outcomes	There is insufficient evidence to make recommendations about the value of acupuncture for chronic asthma.
Lee, 1999	Postoperative nausea and vomiting	Meta-analysis	RCTs Trials stimulating P6 acupuncture point by needling, manual pressure, or electricity.	19	N/A	Number of nausea, vomiting or both 0–6 h or 0–48 h after surgery.	Equal benefit compared with first-line antiemetics. Clear benefit compared with placebo.
Vickers, 1996	Nausea and vomiting from surgery, cancer chemotherapy, and pregnancy	Systematic review	Controlled trials. Trials stimulating P6 acupuncture point by needling, manual pressure, or electricity.	33	2456	Number and duration of vomiting episodes. Symptom-free days. Nausea score	Clear evidence of benefit for all conditions excluding while subjects are under anesthesia.
White, 2000	Tobacco addiction	Meta-analysis	RCTs	18	Complete Abstinence	Abstinence at first treatment, 6 months, 12 months	Negative at all time intervals.
ter Riet, 1990	Addiction to tobacco, heroin, and alcohol	Systematic review	Controlled trials.	22	N/A	Statement of efficacy	Inconclusive due to poor study quality.

RCT = randomized controlled trial.

ter Riet G et al: Acupuncture and chronic pain: a criteria based meta-analysis. J Clin Epidemiol 1990;43:1191. [PMID: 2147032]

Low Back Pain

Ernst et al performed a meta-analysis on acupuncture in the treatment of low back pain and identified 30 trials, of which nine met inclusion criteria involving 377 patients. The summary odds ratio was 2.3 (95% CI, 1.3–4.1) favoring acupuncture compared with various control groups. Subgroup analysis limited to four trials using sham acupuncture as the control group found real and sham acupuncture to have similar effectiveness. Investigators concluded that acupuncture is an effective treatment for low back pain; however, larger studies using sham acupuncture are needed to distinguish between the specific effects of treatment at correct acupuncture points and the nonspecific effects of needling.

Van Tulder et al performed a systematic review using 11 randomized controlled trials on acupuncture for low back pain—none of which studied acute back pain. The quality of the studies was poor, and pooled analyses were not performed because of heterogeneity across trials. Overall, the reviewers found acupuncture equally effective as trigger point injection, TENS, and sham acupuncture. More recently, Smith performed a systematic review on acupuncture as a treatment for chronic neck and back pain that included 13 randomized controlled trials, five of which reported positive results. Studies with better methodologic quality were more likely to show negative results.

In summary, the literature is contradictory, with results from a meta-analysis favoring acupuncture and results from a systematic review finding no clear evidence for effectiveness. There is insufficient evidence on which to base a claim that acupuncture is superior to inert placebo or standard medical care for the treatment of low back pain.

Ernst E et al: Acupuncture for back pain: a meta-analysis of randomized controlled trials. Arch Intern Med 1998;158:2235. [PMID: 9818803]

Smith LA et al: Teasing apart quality and validity in systematic reviews: an example from acupuncture trials in chronic neck and back pain. Pain 2000;86:119. [PMID: 10779669]

van Tulder MW et al: The effectiveness of acupuncture in the treatment of acute and chronic low back pain. A systematic review within the framework of the Cochrane Collaboration Back Review Group. Spine 1999;24:1113. [PMID: 10361661]

Osteoarthritis

A systematic review performed by Ernst in 1997 found 13 trials that met study entry criteria. The majority of trials used formula acupuncture. Seven of the 13 trials reported positive results; however, overall the methodologic quality was poor. Among randomized trials, five out of ten were positive. When sham acupuncture was used as the control group, only one out of five trials were positive. The reviewers concluded that acupunc-

ture was not clearly superior to control interventions and that the literature was of poor quality.

A more recent methodologically rigorous randomized controlled trial involved 73 patients treated for 12 weeks with acupuncture or conventional care. Subjective scores were recorded using the Western Ontario and McMaster Universities Osteoarthritis Index (WOMAC) and the Lequesne Index. Acupuncture was superior to control intervention based on the WOMAC and Lequesne scores. No adverse events were reported. Investigators concluded that acupuncture for osteoarthritis appeared safe and effective when compared with standard care.

In conclusion, there is limited evidence suggesting that acupuncture is more effective than conventional care alone. An NIH-funded multicenter randomized controlled trial currently under way at the University of Maryland will more definitively assess efficacy and long-term outcomes.

Berman BM et al: A randomized trial of acupuncture as adjunctive therapy in osteoarthritis of the knee. Rheumatology (Oxford) 1999;38:346. [PMID: 10388713]

Ernst E: Acupuncture as a symptomatic treatment of osteoarthritis. A systematic review. Scand J Rheumatol 1997;26:444. [PMID: 9433405]

Acute Dental Pain

The NIH consensus development statement on acupuncture states, "There is evidence of efficacy for postoperative dental pain." A review in 1999 identified 16 controlled trials of acupuncture for the treatment of acute dental pain. Among the eight randomized and at least partially blinded trials, seven showed benefit. Among the seven trials using sham control, six showed benefit. Subsequent to this review, a randomized, double-blind, placebo acupuncture-controlled trial involving 39 patients evaluated acupuncture for the treatment of postsurgical dental pain. Controls experienced a similar tap sensation next to the acupuncture sites to produce a noticeable sensation; however, needle insertion was not performed. Patients receiving acupuncture scored more favorably than controls on multiple outcomes. There is thus sufficient evidence to recommend the use of acupuncture as effective adjunctive treatment for the treatment of acute dental pain. Multiple studies have demonstrated its efficacy when compared with sham acupuncture.

Ernst E et al: The effectiveness of acupuncture in treating acute dental pain: a systematic review. Br Dent J 1998;184:443. [PMID: 9617000]

Lao L et al: Evaluation of acupuncture for pain control after oral surgery: a placebo-controlled trial. Arch Otolaryngol Head Neck Surg 1999;125:567. [PMID: 10326816]

Headache

Melchart et al performed a systematic review in 2002 to evaluate the treatment of acupuncture for recurrent headaches. That group identified 26 randomized and quasi-randomized trials involving 1151 subjects in which 16 trials studied migraine headaches, six studied tension headaches, and 4 studied mixed headaches. Of the 16 trials that used sham acupuncture, 8 found real acupuncture superior to sham acupuncture and four found a trend in favor of real acupuncture. Two trials found no difference between groups, and two trials were uninterpretable. In the remaining 10 trials, control groups varied, and conflicting results were reported. Overall, investigators felt there was evidence that acupuncture is effective in the treatment of recurrent headaches; however, more research is needed to ascertain which headaches would be most responsive to acupuncture treatment.

Melchart D et al: Acupuncture for idiopathic headache. Cochrane Database Syst Rev 2001;(1):CD001218. [PMID: 11279710]

Melchart D et al: Acupuncture for recurrent headaches: a systematic review of randomized controlled trials. Cephalalgia 1999;19:779. [PMID: 10595286]

Asthma

Linde performed a systematic review of randomized and possibly randomized clinical trials that evaluated the effects of acupuncture for the treatment of asthma. Seven trials met study entry criteria, including 174 participants. All trials compared real acupuncture with sham acupuncture. Among the three trials that measured postexpiratory flow rates, there was no difference between the real and sham acupuncture groups. The authors conclude that there is insufficient evidence that acupuncture has a significant treatment effect for people with asthma. No research has evaluated the efficacy of acupuncture as part of a comprehensive treatment program. Among trials reporting positive results, benefit was primarily identified in subjective rather than objective measures. Since asthma can be a life-threatening condition and effective standard medical therapy exists, acupuncture should be used, if at all, only as an adjunct to conventional therapy.

Jobst KA: Acupuncture in asthma and pulmonary disease: an analysis of efficacy and safety. J Altern Complement Med 1996;2:179. [PMID: 9395653]

Linde K et al: Acupuncture for chronic asthma. Cochrane Database Syst Rev 2000;(2):CD000008. [PMID: 10796465]

Nausea & Vomiting

Based on multiple randomized controlled trials, there is strong evidence demonstrating effectiveness of acupuncture in the treatment of pregnancy-induced, chemotherapy-induced, and postoperative nausea and vomiting. One review identified 33 trials using a particular acupuncture point (P6) for treatment of nausea and vomiting. None of the four trials in which acupuncture was given while the patient was under general anesthesia demonstrated a positive effect.

Among the remaining 29 trials, 27 identified real acupuncture as being more effective than sham acupuncture or placebo control. In subgroup analyses, all five studies evaluating acupuncture for cancer chemotherapy-induced nausea and vomiting were positive. Six out of seven studies for pregnancy-induced symptoms were positive. Among trials in which acupuncture was performed while the subjects were not under general anesthesia, 16 out of 17 studies of treatment for postoperative nausea and vomiting were positive. In sensitivity analyses, 11 out of the 12 high-quality trials involving over 2000 patients identified acupuncture as superior to control. A subsequent review on studies of treatment for postoperative nausea and vomiting reported acupuncture to be equivalent to first-line antiemetics in preventing early and late vomiting. The NIH consensus development panel on acupuncture stated, "There is clear evidence that needle acupuncture is efficacious for adult postoperative and chemotherapy induced nausea and vomiting and probably for the nausea of pregnancy."

Lee A et al.: The use of nonpharmacologic techniques to prevent postoperative nausea and vomiting: a meta-analysis. Anesth Analg 1999;88:1362. [PMID: 10357346]

Shen et al: Electroacupuncture for control of myeloablative chemotherapy-induced emesis. JAMA 2000;284:2755. [PMID: 11105182]

Vickers AJ: Can acupuncture have specific effects on health? A systematic review of acupuncture antiemesis trials. J R Soc Med 1996;89:303. [PMID: 8758186]

Nicotine, Heroin, Cocaine, & Alcohol Addiction

There is good evidence suggesting that acupuncture is not effective in maintaining abstinence from nicotine addiction. Systematic reviews have identified multiple trials of sufficient quality to determine that there is no evidence to support its use. In a randomized trial comparing electroacupuncture and sham control for nicotine withdrawal symptoms, there was no difference in nicotine withdrawal symptoms or abstinence rates at day 14. The NIH consensus development statement acupuncture states, "There is evidence that acupuncture does not demonstrate efficacy for cessation of smoking."

Despite insufficient evidence to support its use, auricular acupuncture is in widespread use throughout American drug treatment facilities. Although heroin, alcohol, and cocaine addiction studies have frequently reported positive outcomes, serious methodologic flaws are present. For example, an 8-week clinical trial randomized 82 methadone-maintained cocaine-dependent subjects to auricular acupuncture, placebo needle insertion, or no-needle relaxation control. Intention-to-treat analyses showed patients assigned to acupuncture were significantly more likely to remain abstinent from cocaine use. However, analyses did not adjust for the 50% versus 20% dropout rate in the acupuncture and relaxation groups, respectively. Until scientifically rigorous studies can demonstrate efficacy, acupuncture should not be used as monotherapy in the treatment of these addictions.

Avants SK et al: A randomized controlled trial of auricular acupuncture for cocaine dependence. Arch Intern Med 2000;160:2305. [PMID: 10927727]

ter Riet G et al: A meta-analysis of studies into the effect of acupuncture on addiction. Br J Gen Pract 1990;40:379. [PMID: 2148263]

White A et al: Acupuncture for smoking cessation. Cochrane Database Syst Rev 2000;(2):CD000009. [PMID: 10796466]

■ HOMEOPATHY

Christian F.S. Hahnemann is credited with devising the system of homeopathy in 1790. Three main principles of homeopathy include the "law of similars," the use of dilute concentrations of medicines, and "potentization." The second and third principles remain the most controversial for many scientists and conventionally trained physicians. The law of similars is also known as the principle of "like cures like"; it is derived from the observation that a homeopathic medicine when given to a healthy volunteer will produce a constellation of symptoms similar to those it will cure in an ill patient. Since the 1800s, the process of testing medicines on healthy volunteers to record the symptoms provoked (known as "provings") has been recorded and compiled to create several materia med icas.

The second principle, the use of dilute concentrations of medicine, entails serially diluting and "succussing" (shaking) a substance to concentrations in which there is little probability of any molecules remaining in solution. Yet homeopathic physicians affirm that these remedies remain pharmacologically active and allude to allergy desensitization and immunization as sharing similar approaches to homeopathy, ie, in that both use low doses of potentially toxic substances to achieve beneficial clinical effects. Potentization is based on the claim that once a medicine is at low concentration, the more dilute the solute the more potent the effect.

The World Health Organization states that homeopathy is the second most used medical system internationally, with over $1 billion in expenditures for such therapy. Twenty to 30 percent of French and German physicians use homeopathy in clinical practice. In Great Britain, five homeopathic hospitals are part of the National Health System, and over 30% of generalists use homeopathy. In the United States, there are more than 500 physicians and 5000 nonphysicians using homeopathy in clinical practice, and 2.5 million Americans currently use homeopathic medicines—of which two-thirds are self-prescribed—spending more than $250 million annually.

Mechanisms of Action

Although there are several mechanisms under investigation, none are well validated.

Adverse Events

Given the low concentration of homeopathic medicines, the probability of adverse events is remote. However, adverse events have been reported from ingestion of large quantities of remedies containing heavy metals. Indirect adverse events may occur—eg, if children do not receive immunizations because certain homeopathic physicians advise parents against this practice.

Training, Licensure, & Regulation

Homeopathic educational programs are accredited by the Council for Homeopathic Education. There are two levels of training for homeopaths. The Primary Care Certificate in Homeotherapeutics requires 60–100 hours of course work and passage of a written examination. The more advanced level, the Diplomate in Homeotherapeutics (DHt), requires an additional 3 years of clinical practice. There is comprehensive homeopathic training which involves 3 or more years of part-time to full-time study. Nonphysicians may practice homeopathy within the scope of practice of their specific profession. The American Board of Homeotherapeutics governs certification for physicians; the Homeopathic Association of Naturopathic Physicians governs naturopaths; and the Council for Homeopathic Certification governs all other practitioners.

The *Homeopathic Pharmacopoeia of the United States* was included in the original Food and Drug Act of 1938, which classified these medicines as drugs. Currently, the Food and Drug Administration considers these medicines as nonprescription products. Unlike the practice in Great Britain and Europe, there is little oversight of the manufacturing of these products.

Clinical Encounter

The initial consultation takes about 1–1½ hours, with significant time spent on obtaining a detailed history. Attention is given to the physical, mental, and emotional symptoms, overall personality type, and any internal or external factors that influence the presenting symptoms, such as emotions, wind, season of the year, and reactions to different foods. The symptom inventory is then matched to an appropriate remedy taken from the materia medica. Follow-up visits may last for a few minutes to 40 minutes. During the follow-up visit, the practitioner determines if there has been improvement in symptoms, no change, or aggravation of symptoms. The latter scenario, if transient, is viewed as the first sign of recovery.

Clinical Uses

Homeopathic physicians are trained to treat a broad range of conditions in the primary care and specialty setting. In clinical practice, however, practitioners frequently treat patients with chronic conditions that conventional medicine cannot adequately address, including arthritis, allergies, autoimmune diseases, or non-life-threatening acute conditions such as viral infections or minor trauma. Parents may take their children to homeopathic physicians for recurrent conditions such as otitis media and allergies with the goal of avoiding repetitive antibiotic, steroid, or chronic conventional medications.

Research

Over 180 controlled trials and over ten reviews have been published on the effects of homeopathy compared with placebo. The majority of trials are published in non-English language journals and are frequently not listed in Medline. A few methodologically rigorous reviews have been published in English (Table 44–6). The majority of systematic reviews have pooled trials on homeopathy regardless of the medical condition being treated. These reviews have found that patient outcomes in homeopathic treatment groups were superior to placebo group outcomes. Since many of the trials do not provide in-depth reports on the treatment encounter, it remains unclear whether these positive effects are specific to the homeopathic remedy itself or to nonspecific effects that occur as part of the treatment encounter. Since few trials have been independently replicated, there is insufficient evidence to determine if treatment effects found for a single medical condition are reproducible by independent investigators.

A 1991 systematic review identified 107 controlled clinical trials and found 77% reported a positive result. Since 84 out of 107 trials scored < 55 points on a 100-point quality scale, high-quality studies were ana-

Table 44–6. Overview of English language homeopathy systematic reviews.

	Condition	Inclusion Criteria	No. of Studies	Measures	Results	Conclusions
Kleijnen, 1991	No limitation	Controlled trials	107	Vote-count	All trials: 81/107 positive High quality: 15/22 positive Majority of trials received low-quality scores, but effect remained after adjustment.	Positive findings; however, no definitive conclusions due to poor study quality of majority of trials
Linde, 1997	No limitation	Double-blind or RCTs	89	Pooled summary estimates	Overall: OR[3] = 2.45 (95% CI 2.0–2.9) High-quality: OR = 1.7 (95% CI 1.3–2.1) Publication-bias correction: OR = 1.8 (95% CI 1.0–3.1) Seasonal allergies[1]: OR = 2.0 (95% CI 1.5–2.7) Postoperative ileus[2]: effect-size difference = –0.22 SD (95% CI –0.33 to –0.03)	Positive findings. Unable to determine if homeopathy is effective for any single clinical condition under a priori defined criteria.
Cucherat, 2000	No limitation	RCTs with clearly defined primary outcome.	16	Pooled summary estimate	Overall: p-value = 0.000036 High quality trials: $P = .08$	Positive findings overall. Study quality is inversely associated with probability of obtaining a statistically significant result.
Barnes, 1997	Postoperative ileus	RCTs	6	Pooled summary estimates	Time to first flatus: 7.4 hours earlier favoring homeopathy ($P < .05$). Effect remained after adjustment for study quality.	Clinically meaningful effect with reservation due to variable study quality of trials.

[1]Not independent investigators.
[2]Different remedies used.
[3]OR = odds ratio; CI = confidence interval.
RCT = randomized controlled trial.

lyzed separately. Sixty-eight percent of high-quality trials favored patients in the homeopathy-treated group compared with placebo. A 1997 systematic review identified 89 double-blind or randomized placebo-controlled trials and found the overall combined odds ratio was 2.45 (95% CI, 2.0–2.9) favoring patients in the homeopathy-treated group. Analyses restricted to high-quality studies found similar statistically significant results with an odds ratio of 1.66 (95% CI, 1.3–2.1); this effect persisted after adjustment for publication bias. Pooled analysis of four multicenter trials by the same investigator evaluating the effects of *Galphimia glauca* for seasonal allergies found an odds ratio of 2.0 (95% CI, 1.5–2.7) for improvement in ocular and nasal symptoms at 4 weeks.

A meta-analysis conducted in 2000 identified 118 randomized controlled clinical trials of which 16 satisfied inclusion criteria. Investigators reported that patients receiving homeopathic remedies compared with placebo were significantly more likely to have improved treatment outcomes (*P* = .00003); however, analyses limited to the five high-quality studies revealed only a trend for improvement (*P* = .08). Overall, there is some evidence that homeopathy is more effective than placebo; however, multiple high-quality studies of individual conditions are needed to validate these findings.

Chapman E: Homeopathy. In: *Essentials of Complementary and Alternative Medicine.* Jonas W, Levin J (editors). Lippincott Williams & Wilkins, 1999.

Cucherat M et al: Evidence of clinical efficacy of homeopathy: a meta-analysis of clinical trials. Eur J Clin Pharmacol 2000; 56:27. [PMID: 10853874]

Jonas W: Neuroprotection from glutamate toxicity with ultra-low dose glutamate. Neuroreport 2001;12:335. [PMID: 11209946]

Kleijnen J et al: Trials of homoeopathy. BMJ 1991;302:316. [PMID: 1825800]

Linde K et al: Are the clinical effects of homeopathy placebo effects? A meta-analysis of placebo-controlled trials. Lancet 1997;350:834. [PMID: 9310601]

Reilly D et al: Is evidence for homoeopathy reproducible? Lancet 1994;344:1601. [PMID: 7983994]

Vickers AJ: Homoeopathic Oscillococcinum for preventing and treating influenza and influenza-like syndromes. Cochrane Database Syst Rev 2000;(2):CD001957. [PMID: 10796675]

Appendix: Therapeutic Drug Monitoring & Laboratory Reference Ranges

C. Diana Nicoll, MD, PhD, MPA

Table 1. Therapeutic drug monitoring.[1,2]

Drug	Effective Concentrations	Half-Life (hours)	Dosage Adjustment	Comments
Amikacin	Peak: 20–30 mg/L; trough: < 10 µg/mL	2–3 ↑ in uremia	↓ in renal dysfunction	Concomitant kanamycin or tobramycin therapy may give falsely elevated amikacin results by immunoassay.
Amitriptyline	95–250 ng/mL	9–46		Drug is highly protein-bound. Patient-specific decrease in protein binding may invalidate quoted range of effective concentration.
Carbamazepine	4–12 mg/L	10–15		Induces its own metabolism. Metabolite 10,11-epoxide exhibits 13% cross-reactivity by immunoassay.
Cyclosporine	50–400 µg/L (ng/L) whole blood	6–12	Need to know specimen and methodology used	Cyclosporine is lipid-soluble (20% bound to leukocytes; 40% to erythrocytes; 40% in plasma, highly bound to lipoproteins). Binding is temperature-dependent, so whole blood is preferred to plasma or serum as specimen. High-performance liquid chromatography (HPLC) or monoclonal fluorescence polarization immunoassay measures cyclosporine reliably; polyclonal fluorescence polarization immunoassays cross-react with metabolites, so the therapeutic range used with those assays is higher. Anticonvulsants and rifampin increase metabolism. Erythromycin, ketoconazole, and calcium channel blockers decrease metabolism.
Desipramine	100–250 ng/mL	13–23		Drug is highly protein-bound. Patient-specific decrease in protein binding may invalidate quoted range of effective concentration.
Digoxin	0.8–2 ng/mL	42 ↑ in uremia, CHF	↓ in renal dysfunction, CHF, hypothyroidism ↑ in hyperthyroidism	Bioavailability of digoxin tablets is 50–90%. Specimen must not be drawn within 6 hours of dose. Dialysis does not remove a significant amount. Hypokalemia potentiates toxicity. Digitalis toxicity is a clinical and *not* a laboratory diagnosis. Digibind (digoxin-specific antibody) therapy of digoxin overdose can interfere with measurement of digoxin levels depending on the digoxin assay. Elimination reduced by quinidine, verapamil, and amiodarone.
Ethosuximide	40–100 mg/L	Child: 30 Adult: 50		Levels used primarily to assess compliance. Toxicity is rare and does not correlate well with plasma concentrations.

(continued)

Table 1. Therapeutic drug monitoring.[1,2] (continued)

Drug	Effective Concentrations	Half-Life (hours)	Dosage Adjustment	Comments
Gentamicin	Peak: 4–8 mg/L; trough: < 2 mg/L	2–5 ↑ in uremia (7.3 on dialysis)	↓ in renal dysfunction	Draw peak specimen 30 minutes after end of infusion. Draw trough just before next dose. In uremic patients, carbenicillin may decrease gentamicin half-life from 46 hours to 22 hours.
Imipramine	180–350 mg/L	10–16		Drug is highly protein-bound. Patient-specific decrease in protein binding may invalidate quoted range of effective concentration.
Lidocaine	1–5 mg/L	1.8 ↔ in uremia, CHF; ↑ in cirrhosis	↓ in CHF, liver disease	Levels increased with cimetidine therapy. CNS toxicity common in the elderly.
Lithium	0.7–1.5 mmol/L	22 ↑ in uremia	↓ in renal dysfunction	Thiazides and loop diuretics may increase serum lithium levels.
Methotrexate		8.4 ↑ in uremia	↓ in renal dysfunction	7-Hydroxymethotrexate cross-reacts 1.5% in immunoassay. To minimize toxicity, leucovorin should be continued if methotrexate level is > 0.1 μmol/L at 48 hours after start of therapy. Methotrexate > 1 μmol/L at > 48 hours requires an increase in leucovorin rescue therapy.
Nortriptyline	50–140 ng/mL	18–44		Drug is highly protein-bound. Patient-specific decrease in protein binding may invalidate quoted range of effective concentration.
Phenobarbital	10–40 mg/L	86 ↑ in cirrhosis	↓ in liver disease	Metabolized primarily by the hepatic microsomal enzyme system. Many drug-drug interactions.
Phenytoin	10–20 mg/L; 5–10 mg/L in uremia, hypoal-buminemia	Dose-dependent		Metabolite cross-reacts 10% in immunoassay. Metabolism is capacity-limited. Increase dose cautiously when level approaches therapeutic range, since new steady-state level may be disproportionately higher. Drug is very highly protein-bound; protein binding is decreased in uremia and hypoalbuminemia.
Primidone	5–10 mg/L	8		Phenobarbital cross-reacts 0.5%. Metabolized to phenobarbital. Primidone/phenobarbital ratio > 1:2 suggests poor compliance.
Procainamide	4–8 mg/L	3 ↑ in uremia	↓ in renal dysfunction	30% of patients with plasma levels of 12–16 μg/mL have electrocardiographic changes; 40% of patients with plasma levels of > 16 μg/mL have severe toxicity.
Quinidine	1–4 mg/L	7 ↔ in CHF; ↑ in liver disease	↓ in liver disease, CHF	Effective concentration is lower in chronic liver disease and nephrosis, where binding is decreased.
Salicylate	150–300 mg/L	Dose-dependent		
Theophylline	5–20 mg/L	9	↓ in CHF, cirrhosis, and with cimetidine	Caffeine cross-reacts 10%. Elimination is increased 1½–2 times in smokers. 1,3 Dimethyl uric acid metabolite increased in uremia and, because of cross-reactivity, may cause an apparent slight increase in serum theophylline.

(continued)

Table 1. Therapeutic drug monitoring.[1,2] (continued)

Drug	Effective Concentrations	Half-Life (hours)	Dosage Adjustment	Comments
Tobramycin	Peak: 5–10 mg/L; trough: < 2 mg/L	2–3; ↑ in uremia	↓ in renal dysfunction	Tobramycin, kanamycin, and amikacin may cross-react in immunoassay.
Valproic acid	55–100 mg/L	13–19		95% protein-bound. Decreased binding in uremia and cirrhosis.
Vancomycin	Trough: 5–15 mg/L	6 ↑ in uremia	↓ in renal dysfunction	Toxicity in uremic patients leads to irreversible deafness. Keep peak level < 30–40 mg/L to avoid toxicity.

↔ = unchanged; ↑ = increase(d); ↓ = decrease(d); CHF = congestive heart failure.
[1]Modified and reproduced, with permission, from Nicoll D et al: *Pocket Guide to Diagnostic Tests,* 3rd ed. McGraw-Hill, 2000.
[2]Use red-topped tube (not marbled) for therapeutic drug monitoring. In general, the specimen should be drawn just before the next dose (trough).

Table 2. Reference ranges for commonly used tests.[1,2]

		Current metric units × Conversion factor = SI units SI units ÷ Conversion factor = Current metric units			
Test	Specimen	Conventional Units	Conversion Factor	SI Units[2]	Collection[3]
Acetaminophen	Serum	10–20 mg/L **Panic:** > 50 mg/L	66.16	66–132 µmol/L	Marbled Gold SST
Acetoacetate	Serum or urine	Negative		Negative	Marbled or urine container Gold SST
Adrenocorticotropic hormone (ACTH)	Plasma	9–52 pg/mL (laboratory-specific)	0.22	2–11 pmol/L	Siliconized glass or plastic lavender
Alanine aminotransferase (ALT, SGPT, GPT)	Serum	7–56 units/L (laboratory-specific)	0.02	0.14–1.12 µkat/L (laboratory-specific)	Marbled Gold SST
Albumin	Serum	3.4–4.7 g/dL	10.00	34–47 g/L	Marbled Gold SST

Aldosterone	Serum	Salt-loaded (120 meq Na+/d):
		   Supine: 3–10 ng/dL
		   Upright: 5–30 ng/dL
		Salt-depleted (20 meq Na+/d):
		   Supine: 12–36 ng/dL
		   Upright: 17–137 ng/dL
			27.74	83–277 pmol/L
				139–831 pmol/L
				
				332–997 pmol/L
				471–3795 pmol/L
					Gold SST

	Urine	Salt-loaded (120 meq Na+/d for 3–4 days):
		   1.5–12.5 µg/24 h
		Salt-depleted (20 meq Na+/d for 3–4 days):
		   18–85 µg/24 h
			2.77	4.2–34.6 nmol/d
				
				49.9–235.5 nmol/d
					Boric acid

Alkaline phosphatase	Serum	41–133 units/L (method- and age-dependent)	0.02	0.7–2.2 µkat/L (method- and age-dependent)	Marbled Gold SST
Ammonia (NH₃)	Plasma	18–60 µg/dL	0.59	11–35 µmol/L	Green (iced)
Amylase	Serum	20–110 units/L (laboratory-specific)	0.02	0.33–1.83 µkat/L (laboratory-specific)	Marbled Gold SST

(continued)

Table 2. Reference ranges for commonly used tests.[1,2] (continued)

| | | Current metric units × Conversion factor = SI units | | | |
| | | SI units ÷ Conversion factor = Current metric units | | | |

Test	Specimen	Conventional Units	Conversion Factor	SI Units[2]	Collection
Angiotensin-converting enzyme (ACE)	Serum	12–35 units/L (method-dependent)	16.67	< 590 nkat/L (method-dependent)	Marbled Gold SST
Antithrombin III (AT III)	Plasma	84–123% (qualitative) 22–39 mg/dL (quantitative)			Blue
α_1-Antitrypsin	Serum	110–270 mg/dL	0.01	1.1–2.7 g/L	Marbled Gold SST
Aspartate aminotransferase (AST, SGOT, GOT)	Serum	0–35 units/L (laboratory-specific)	0.02	0–0.58 μkat/L (laboratory-specific)	Marbled Gold SST
Basophil count	Whole blood	$0.01–0.12 \times 10^3/\mu L$	1.00	$0.01–0.12 \times 10^9/L$	Lavender
Bilirubin	Serum	Total: 0.1–1.2 mg/dL Direct (conjugated to glucuronide): 0.1–0.5 mg/dL Indirect (unconjugated): 0.1–0.7 mg/dL	17.10	2–21 μmol/L < 8 μmol/L < 12 μmol/L	Marbled Gold SST
Blood urea nitrogen (BUN)	Serum	8–20 mg/dL	0.36	2.9–7.1 mmol/L	Marbled Gold SST
C-peptide	Serum	0.8–4.0 ng/mL	1.00	0.8–4.0 μg/L	Iced (fasting) Gold SST
Calcitonin	Plasma	Male: 0-11.5 pg/mL Female: 0.46 pg/ml	1.00	Male: 0-11.5 ng/L Female: 0-4.6 nq/L	Green Gold SST
Calcium (Ca^{2+})	Serum	8.5–10.5 mg/dL **Panic:** < 6.5 or > 13.5 mg/dL	0.25	2.1–2.6 mmol/L	Marbled Gold SST
Calcium (ionized)	Serum	4.6–5.3 mg/dL	0.25	1.15–1.32 mmol/L	Green (Anaerobic)
Calcium (U_{Ca})	Urine	100–300 mg/d	0.025	2.5–7.5 mmol/d	Urine bottle containing hydrochloric acid
Carbon dioxide, partial pressure (P_{CO_2})	Whole blood	32–48 mm Hg	0.13	4.26–6.38 kPa	Heparinized syringe (iced)
Carbon dioxide (CO_2), total (bicarbonate)	Serum	22–32 meq/L **Panic:** < 15 or > 40 meq/L	1.00	22–32 mmol/L **Panic:** < 15 or > 40 mmol/L	Marbled Gold SST
Carboxyhemoglobin (HbCO)	Whole blood	< 9% of total hemoglobin (Hb)	0.01	< 0.09 fraction of total hemoglobin	Green
Carcinoembryonic antigen (CEA)	Serum	0–5 ng/mL	1.00	0–5 μg/L	Marbled Gold SST
CD4 T cell count	Whole blood	359–1725 cells/μL			Lavender (CBC and differential and % CD4 required)
Ceruloplasmin	Serum	20–60 mg/dL (laboratory-specific)	10.00	200–600 mg/L	Marbled Gold SST
Chloride (Cl⁻)	Serum	101–112 meq/L	1.00	101–112 mmol/L	Marbled Gold SST

(continued)

Table 2. Reference ranges for commonly used tests.[1,2] (continued)

		Current metric units × Conversion factor = SI units SI units ÷ Conversion factor = Current metric units			
Test	**Specimen**	**Conventional Units**	**Conversion Factor**	**SI Units**[2]	**Collection**
Cholesterol	Serum	Desirable: < 200 mg/dL Borderline: 200–239 mg/dL High risk: > 240 mg/dL	0.03	Desirable: < 5.2 mmol/L Borderline: 5.2–6.1 mmol/L High risk: > 6.2 mmol/L	Marbled Gold SST
Chorionic gonadotropin, β-subunit (β-hCG), quantitative	Serum	Males and nonpregnant females: undetectable or < 5 mU/mL	1.00	Males and nonpregnant females: undetectable or < 5 units/L	Marbled Gold SST
Complement C3	Serum	64–166 mg/dL	10.00	640–1660 mg/L	Marbled Gold SST
Complement C4	Serum	15–45 mg/dL	10.00	150–450 mg/L	Marbled Gold SST
Complement CH50	Serum	(laboratory-specific)			Red
Cortisol	Serum	8:00 AM: 5–20 µg/dL	27.59	140–550 nmol/L	Marbled Gold SST
Cortisol (urinary free)	Urine	10–110 µg/24 h	2.76	30–300 nmol/d	Urine bottle containing boric acid
Creatine kinase (CK)	Serum	32–267 units/L (method-dependent)	0.02	0.53–4.45 µkat/L (method-dependent)	Gold SST
Creatine kinase MB (CKMB)	Serum	< 16 units/L or < 4% of total CK (laboratory-specific) Mass units: 0–7 µg/L	0.04	< 0.27 µkat/L	Marbled Gold SST
Creatinine (Cr)	Serum	0.6–1.2 mg/dL	83.3	50–100 µmol/L	Marbled Gold SST
Creatinine clearance (Cl_{Cr})	See Collection column.	Adults: 90–140 mL/min/1.73 m^2 BSA	0.017	1.5–2.3 mL/s/1.73 m^2 BSA	Carefully timed 24-hour urine and simultaneous serum or plasma creatinine sample
Cryoglobulins	Serum	< 0.12 mg/dL			Red (at 37 °C)
Eosinophil count	Whole blood	$0.04–0.5 \times 10^3$/µL	1.00	$0.04–0.5 \times 10^9$/L	Lavender
Erythrocyte count (RBC count)	Whole blood	$4.7–6.1 \times 10^6$/µL	1.00	$4.7–6.1 \times 10^{12}$/L	Lavender
Erythrocyte sedimentation rate	Whole blood	Male: < 10 mm/h Female: < 15 mm/h (laboratory-specific)		Same	Lavender
Erythropoietin (EPO)	Serum	5–20 mU/mL	1.00	5–20 units/L	Marbled Gold SST
Ethanol	Serum	mg/dL Legal "driving under the influence" in many states is defined as > 80 mg/dL (> 17 mmol/L)	0.217	mmol/L	Marbled Gold SST

(continued)

Table 2. Reference ranges for commonly used tests.[1,2] (continued)

| | | Current metric units × Conversion factor = SI units | | | |
| | | SI units ÷ Conversion factor = Current metric units | | | |
Test	Specimen	Conventional Units	Conversion Factor	SI Units[2]	Collection
Factor VIII assay	Plasma	40–150% of normal (varies with age)			Blue
Fecal fat	Stool	Random: < 60 droplets of fat per high-power field 72-hour: < 7 g/d			Qualitative: Random stool sample Quantitative: 72-hour collection following 2-day dietary fat regimen
Ferritin	Serum	Male: 16–300 ng/mL Female: 4–161 ng/mL	1.00	Male: 16–300 µg/L Female: 4–161 µg/L	Marbled Gold SST
α-Fetoprotein (AFP)	Serum	0–15 ng/mL	1.00	0–15 µg/L	Marbled Gold SST
Fibrin D-dimers	Plasma	Negative			Blue
Fibrinogen (functional)	Plasma	175–433 mg/dL **Panic:** < 75 mg/dL	0.01	1.75–4.3 g/L	Blue
Folic acid (red cells)	Whole blood	165–760 ng/mL	2.27	370–1720 nmol/L	Lavender
Follicle-stimulating hormone (FSH)	Serum	Female: Follicular phase 4–13 mU/mL Luteal phase 2–13 mU/mL Midcycle 5–22 mU/mL Postmenopausal 30–138 mU/mL Male: 1–10 mU/mL (laboratory-specific)	1.00	Female: 4–13 units/L 2–13 units/L 5–22 units/L 30–138 units/L Male: 1–10 units/L (laboratory-specific)	Marbled Gold SST
Free erythrocyte proto-porphyrin (FEP)	Whole blood	< 35 µg/dL (method-dependent)			Lavender
Fructosamine	Serum			1.6–2.6 mmol/L	Marbled Gold SST
Gamma-glutamyltrans-peptidase (GGT)	Serum	9–85 units/L (laboratory-specific)	0.02	0.15–1.42 µkat/L (laboratory-specific)	Marbled Gold SST
Gastrin	Serum	< 100 pg/mL (laboratory-specific)	1.00	< 100 ng/L	Marbled Gold SST
Glucose	Serum	60–110 mg/dL **Panic:** < 40 or > 500 mg/dL	0.055	3.3–6.1 mmol/L	Marbled (fasting) Gold SST
Glucose-6-phosphate dehydrogenase (G6PD) screen	Whole blood	5–14 units/g Hb	0.02	0.1–0.28 µkat/L	Lavender
Glutamine	CSF	6–15 mg/dL **Panic:** > 40 mg/dL	68.5	411–1028 µmol/L	Collect CSF in a plastic tube

(continued)

Table 2. Reference ranges for commonly used tests.[1,2] (continued)

Test	Specimen	Conventional Units	Conversion Factor	SI Units[2]	Collection
		Current metric units × Conversion factor = SI units **SI units ÷ Conversion factor = Current metric units**			
Glycated (glycosylated) hemoglobin (HbA$_{1c}$)	Serum	3.9–6.9% (method-dependent)			Lavender
Growth hormone (GH)	Serum	0–5 ng/mL	1.00	0–5 µg/L	Marbled Gold SST
Haptoglobin	Serum	46–316 mg/dL	0.01	0.5–3.2 g/L	Marbled Gold SST
HDL cholesterol	Serum	Male: 27–67 mg/dL Female: 34–88 mg/dL	0.026	0.7–1.73 mmol/L 0.88–2.28 mmol/L	Marbled Gold SST
Helicobacter pylori antibody	Serum	Negative			Marbled Gold SST
Hematocrit (Hct)	Whole blood	Male: 39–49% Female: 35–45% (age-dependent)	0.01	Male: 0.39–0.49 Female: 0.35–0.45	Lavender
Hemoglobin A$_1$c (See Glycated Hemoglobin)	Serum				
Hemoglobin A$_2$ (HbA$_2$)	Whole blood	1.5–3.5% of total hemoglobin	0.01	0.015–0.035	Lavender
Hemoglobin electrophoresis	Whole blood	HbA: > 95% HbA$_2$: 1.5–3.5%			Lavender
Hemoglobin, fetal (HbF)	Whole blood	Adult: < 2% (varies with age)			Lavender
Hemoglobin, total (Hb)	Whole blood	Male: 13.6–17.5 g/dL Female: 12.0–15.5 g/dL **Panic:** ≤ 7 g/dL (age-dependent)	10.00	Male: 136–175 g/L Female: 120–155 g/L	Lavender
Hemosiderin	Urine	Negative			Urine container
HIV viral load	Plasma	Negative			Lavender
β-Hydroxybutyrate	Serum	0.5–3 mg/dL	0.096	0.05–0.3 mmol/L	Marbled Gold SST
5-Hydroxyindoleacetic acid (5-HIAA)	Urine	2–8 mg/24 h	5.23	10–40 µmol/d	Urine bottle containing hydrochloric acid
IgG index	Serum and CSF	0.29–0.59 ratio			Marbled Gold SST and plastic tube for CSF
Immunoglobulins (Ig)	Serum	IgA: 78–367 mg/dL IgG: 583–1761 mg/dL IgM: 52–335 mg/dL	0.01	IgA: 0.78–3.67 g/L IgG: 5.83–17.6 g/L IgM: 0.52–3.35 g/L	Marbled Gold SST
Insulin, immunoreactive	Serum	6–35 µU/mL	7.18	42–243 pmol/L	Marbled Gold SST
Insulin-like growth factor-1	Plasma	123–463 ng/mL (age- and sex-dependent)	1.0	123–463 µg/L	Marbled Gold SST
Iron (Fe^{2+})	Serum	50–175 µg/dL	0.18	9–31 µmol/L	Marbled Gold SST

(continued)

Table 2. Reference ranges for commonly used tests.[1,2] (continued)

		Current metric units × Conversion factor = SI units SI units ÷ Conversion factor = Current metric units			
Test	**Specimen**	**Conventional Units**	**Conversion Factor**	**SI Units[2]**	**Collection**
Iron-binding capacity, total (TIBC)	Serum	250–460 µg/dL	0.18	45–82 µmol/L	Marbled Gold SST
Lactate dehydrogenase (LDH)	Serum	88–230 units/L (laboratory-specific)	0.02	1.46–3.82 µkat/L (laboratory-specific)	Marbled Gold SST
Lactic acid (lactate)	Venous blood	0.5–2.0 meq/L	1.00	0.5–2.0 mmol/L	Gray
LDL cholesterol	Serum	< 130 mg/dL	0.026	< 3.37 mmol/L	Marbled Gold SST
Lead (Pb)	Whole blood	Child: < 25 µg/dL Adult: < 40 µg/dL	0.05	Child: < 1.21 µmol/L Adult: < 1.93 µmol/L	Navy
Lecithin/sphingomyelin (L/S) ratio	Amniotic fluid	> 2.0 (method-dependent)			Collect in a plastic tube
Leukocyte alkaline phosphatase (LAP)	Whole blood	40–130 Based on 0 to 4+ rating of 100 PMNs stained for alkaline phosphatase			Green
Leukocyte (white blood cell) count, total (WBC count)	Whole blood	4.8–10.8 × 10³/µL **Panic:** < 1.5 × 10³/µL	1.00	4.8–10.8 × 10⁹/L	Lavender
Lipase	Serum	0–160 units/L (laboratory-specific)	0.02	0–2.66 µkat/L (laboratory-specific)	Marbled Gold SST

Luteinizing hormone (LH)	Serum	Female:
		  Follicular phase 1–18 mU/mL
		  Luteal phase 0.4–20 mU/mL
		  Midcycle 24–105 mU/mL
		  Postmenopausal 15–62 mU/mL
		Male: 1–10 mU/mL
		(laboratory-specific)
			1.00	1–18 units/L
				
				0.4–20 units/L
				
				24–105 units/L
				
				15–62 units/L
				Male: 1–10 units/L
				(laboratory-specific)
					Marbled Gold SST

Lymphocyte count	Whole blood	0.8–3.5 × 10³/µL	1.00	0.8–3.5 × 10⁹/L	Lavender
Magnesium (Mg²⁺)	Serum	1.8–3.0 mg/dL **Panic:** < 0.5 or > 4.5 mg/dL	0.41	0.75–1.25 mmol/L	Marbled Gold SST
Mean corpuscular hemoglobin (MCH)	Whole blood	26–34 pg			Lavender
Mean corpuscular hemoglobin concentration (MCHC)	Whole blood	31–36 g/dL	10.00	310–360 g/L	Lavender
Mean corpuscular volume (MCV)	Whole blood	80–100 fL			Lavender
Metanephrines	Urine	0.3–0.9 mg/24 h	5.46	1.6–4.9 µmol/d	Urine bottle containing hydrochloric acid

(continued)

Table 2. Reference ranges for commonly used tests.[1,2] (continued)

		Current metric units × Conversion factor = SI units SI units ÷ Conversion factor = Current metric units			
Test	**Specimen**	**Conventional Units**	**Conversion Factor**	**SI Units[2]**	**Collection**
Methemoglobin (MetHb)	Whole blood	< 1% of total hemoglobin	0.01	< 0.01 fraction of total hemoglobin	Green
Methylmalonic acid	Serum	0–0.05 mg/L	8.475	0–0.4 μmol/L	Marbled Gold SST
Monocyte count	Whole blood	$0.2–0.8 \times 10^3/\mu L$	1.00	$0.2–0.8 \times 10^9/L$	Lavender
Neutrophil count	Whole blood	$2.2–8.6 \times 10^3/\mu L$	1.00	$2.2–8.6 \times 10^9/L$	Lavender
Osmolality	Serum	275–293 mosm/kg H_2O **Panic:** < 240 or > 320 mosm/kg H_2O	1.00	275–293 mmol/kg H_2O	Marbled Gold SST
	Urine	Random: 100–900 mosm/kg H_2O	1.00	Random: 100–900 mmol/kg H_2O	Urine container
Oxygen, partial pressure (Po_2)	Whole blood	83–108 mm Hg	0.13	11.04–14.36 kPa	Heparinized syringe (iced)
Parathyroid hormone (PTH)	Serum	Intact PTH: 11–54 pg/mL (laboratory-specific)	0.11	Intact PTH: 1.2–5.7 pmol/L (laboratory-specific)	Red
Partial thromboplastin time, activated (PTT)	Plasma	25–35 seconds (range varies) **Panic:** ≥ 60 seconds			Blue
pH	Whole blood	Arterial: 7.35–7.45 Venous: 7.31–7.41			Heparinized syringe (iced)
Phosphorus	Serum	2.5–4.5 mg/dL **Panic:** < 1.0 mg/dL	0.32	0.8–1.45 mmol/L	Marbled Gold SST
Platelet count (Plt)	Whole blood	$150–450 \times 10^3/\mu L$ **Panic:** $< 25 \times 10^3/\mu L$	1.0	$150–450 \times 10^9/L$ **Panic:** $< 25 \times 10^9/L$	Lavender
Platelet-associated IgG	Whole blood	Negative			Lavender
Porphobilinogen (PBG)	Urine	Negative			Protect from light
Potassium (K^+)	Serum	3.5–5.0 meq/L **Panic:** < 3.0 or > 6.0 meq/L	1.00	3.5–5.0 mmol/L	Marbled Gold SST
Prolactin (PRL)	Serum	< 20 ng/mL	1.00	< 20 μg/L	Marbled Gold SST
Prostate-specific antigen (PSA)	Serum	0–4 ng/mL	1.00	0–4 μg/L	Marbled Gold SST
Protein C	Plasma	71–176%			Blue
Protein electrophoresis	Serum	Adults: Albumin: 3.3–4.7 g/dL α_1: 0.1–0.4 g/dL α_2: 0.3–0.9 g/dL β_2: 0.7–1.5 g/dL γ: 0.5–1.4 g/dL	10.00	 33–47 g/L 1–4 g/L 3–9 g/L 7–15 g/L 5–14 g/L	Marbled Gold SST
Protein S (antigen)	Plasma	76–178%			Blue

(continued)

Table 2. Reference ranges for commonly used tests.[1,2] (continued)

		Current metric units × Conversion factor = SI units SI units ÷ Conversion factor = Current metric units			
Test	**Specimen**	**Conventional Units**	**Conversion Factor**	**SI Units**[2]	**Collection**
Protein, total	Serum	6.0–8.0 g/dL	10.00	60–80 g/L	Marbled Gold SST
Prothrombin time (PT)	Whole blood	11–15 seconds **Panic:** ≥ 30 seconds (laboratory-specific)			Blue
Red blood cell count	Whole blood	$4.7–6.1 \times 10^6/\mu L$	1.00	$4.7–6.1 \times 10^{12}/L$	Lavender
Red cell volume	Whole blood	25–35 mL/kg			Green
Renin activity (PRA)	Plasma	High-sodium diet (75–150 meq Na^+/d): Supine: 0.2–2.3 ng/mL/h Standing: 1.3–4.0 ng/mL/h) Low-sodium diet (30–75 meq Na^+/d): Standing: 4.0–7.7 ng/mL/h)			Lavender
Reptilase clotting time	Plasma	13–19 seconds			Blue
Reticulocyte count	Whole blood	$33–137 \times 10^3/\mu L$	1.00	$33–137 \times 10^9/L$	Lavender
Russell's viper venom clotting time (dilute) (RVVT)	Plasma	24–37 seconds			Blue
Salicylate (aspirin, others)	Serum	20–30 mg/dL **Panic:** > 35 mg/dL	10.00	200–300 mg/L	Marbled/ Gold SST
Sodium (Na^+)	Serum	135–145 meq/L **Panic:** < 125 or > 155 meq/L	1.00	135–145 mmol/L	Marbled Gold SST
Testosterone	Serum	Male: 175–781 ng/dL Female: 10–75 ng/dL	0.0347	Male: 6–27 nmol/L Female: 0.3–2.6 nmol/L	Marbled Gold SST
Thrombin time	Plasma	8–12 seconds (laboratory-specific)			Blue
Thyroglobulin	Serum	3–42 ng/mL	1.00	3–42 µg/L	Marbled Gold SST
Thyroid-stimulating hormone (TSH)	Serum	0.4–6 µU/mL	1.00	0.4–6 mU/L	Marbled Gold SST
Thyroid-stimulating hormone receptor antibody (TSH-R Ab [stim])	Serum	< 130% of basal activity. Based on cAMP generation in thyroid cell tissue culture.			
Thyroxine, free (FT_4)	Serum	9–24 pmol/L (varies with method)			Marbled Gold SST
Thyroxine (T_4), total	Serum	5–11 µg/dL	12.80	64–142 nmol/L	Marbled Gold SST

(continued)

Table 2. Reference ranges for commonly used tests.[1,2] (continued)

Test	Specimen	Conventional Units	Conversion Factor	SI Units[2]	Collection
Current metric units × Conversion factor = SI units **SI units ÷ Conversion factor = Current metric units**					
Thyroxine index, free (FT$_4$I)	Serum	6.5–12.5			Marbled Gold SST
Transferrin	Serum	190–375 mg/dL	0.01	1.9–3.75 g/L	Marbled Gold SST
Triglycerides	Serum	< 165 mg/dL	0.01	< 1.65 g/L	Marbled Gold SST (fasting)
Triiodothyronine (T$_3$), total	Serum	95–190 ng/dL	0.015	1.5–2.9 nmol/L	Marbled Gold SST
Troponin-I (cTnI)	Serum	< 0.05 ng/mL			Marbled Gold SST
Uric acid	Serum	Male: 2.4–7.4 mg/dL Female: 1.4–5.8 mg/dL	59.48	Male: 140–440 μmol/L Female: 80–350 μmol/L	Marbled Gold SST
Vanillylmandelic acid (VMA)	Urine	2–7 mg/24 h	5.05	10–35 μmol/d	Urine bottle containing hydrochloric acid
Vitamin B$_{12}$	Serum	140–820 pg/mL	0.74	100–600 pmol/L	Marbled Gold SST
Vitamin B$_{12}$ absorption test (Schilling test)	24-hour urine	Excretion of > 8% of administered dose			Urine bottle
Vitamin D, 25-hydroxy (25[OH]D)	Serum	10–50 ng/mL	2.5	25–125 nmol/L	Marbled Gold SST
Vitamin D, 1,25-dihydroxy (1,25[OH]$_2$D)	Serum	20–76 pg/mL	2.4	48–182 pmol/L	Marbled Gold SST
White blood cell count	Whole blood	4.8–10.8 × 10^3/μL	1.00	4.8–10.8 × 10^9/L	Lavender

[1]The reference ranges given here in conventional units and in SI units are from several large medical centers. Always use the reference ranges provided by your clinical laboratory, since ranges may be method-dependent.
[2]Reference: Young DS: Implementation of SI units for clinical laboratory data. Ann Intern Med 1987;106:114; JAMA Instructions for Authors, JAMA 1997;278:74.
[3]Gold SST = gold serum separator tube.

Commonly Used Specimen Collection Tubes

Tube Color	Tube Contents	Typical Use
Lavender	EDTA	Complete blood count
Gold or marbled	Serum separator	Serum chemistry tests
Red	None	Blood banking (serum); therapeutic drug monitoring
Blue	Citrate	Coagulation studies
Gray	Inhibitor of glycolysis (sodium fluoride)	Lactic acid
Green	Heparin	Plasma studies
Yellow	Acid citrate	HLA typing
Navy	Trace metal free	Trace metals (eg, lead)

Index

NOTE: Page numbers in **boldface** type indicate a major discussion. A *t* following a page number indicates tabular material and *f* following a page number indicates a figure. Drugs are listed under their generic names. When a drug trade name is listed, the reader is referred to the generic name.

for bronchiectasis, 243
for COPD, 240
for cystic fibrosis, 245
prevention of postoperative pulmonary complications and, 34
spirometry after administration of, 221
Bronchogenic carcinoma, 267–272. *See also* Lung cancer
Bronchoprovocation testing. *See* Bronchial provocation testing
Bronchopulmonary mycosis/aspergillosis, allergic, 243, 1488–1489
Bronchoscopy, 223. *See also* Bronchoalveolar lavage
in bronchial obstruction, 224
in hemoptysis, 218
in lung cancer, 268
for respiratory secretion analysis
in pneumonia, 254, 255
in pulmonary infiltrates in immunocompromised host, 256
in tuberculosis, 257
in solitary pulmonary nodule, 266
Bronchospasm/bronchoconstriction
in anaphylactic transfusion reaction, 520
in anaphylaxis, 765
cough and, 217
in desensitization therapy, 233, 1271
exercise-induced, 225
mediator inhibitors for, 230
short-acting beta-adrenergic agents for, 233
in near drowning victim, 1550
in pulmonary edema, 391
Brown-Séquard syndrome, 989
Brown spider bites, 132, 1587
Brown tumors of bone, in hyperparathyroidism, 1111
Bruce protocol, for exercise electrocardiography, 338
Brucella abortus/melitensis/suis, (brucellosis), 1376–1377, 1496t
Bruch's membrane, in age-related macular degeneration, 161
Brudzinski sign, in meningococcal meningitis, 1367
Brugia
malayi, 280, 1468, 1469
timori, 1468
Bruits
carotid, 445
in cerebrovascular occlusive disease, 445
cranial, in arteriovenous malformation, 967
in heart disease, 314
in subclavian steal syndrome/transient ischemic attacks, 959, 960
Brush border enzyme deficiency, 585. *See also* Lactase deficiency
Bruxism, earache and, 185
BSE. *See* Bovine spongiform encephalopathy
Buboes
in lymphogranuloma venereum, 625, 1388
in plague, 1378
Buccal swab, for DNA analysis, 1656
Buckle, scleral, for retinal detachment, 160
Budd-Chiari syndrome (hepatic vein obstruction), 545, 546, 653–654
Budesonide
for asthma, 231t
for inflammatory bowel disease, 603
Crohn's disease, 603, 607
Buerger's disease (thromboangiitis obliterans), 451–452
Raynaud's disease/phenomenon and, 451
Buffalo hump obesity, in Cushing's syndrome, 1067, 1126
Bulbar palsy, progressive, 990
Bulbar poliomyelitis, 1319, 1320

Bulbocavernous reflex, 906, 920
Bulbospinal neuronopathy, X-linked, 991
Bulimia nervosa, 1229–1230
with anorexia nervosa (bulimarexia), 1229, 1230
Bullectomy, for COPD, 242
Bulletin boards, electronic, 1682–1683, 1682t
Bullous impetigo, in HIV infection/AIDS, 1283
Bullous pemphigoid, 123
Bullous (blistering) skin disorders, 87t, 121–123. *See also specific type*
chemotherapy causing, 1623
drugs causing, 145t
radiation therapy causing, 1623
Bumetanide
for cardiac failure, 384
infarct-associated, 356
for hypertension, 417t
lithium interactions and, 1045
for pulmonary edema, 391
Bumex. *See* Bumetanide
BUN. *See* Blood urea nitrogen
Bundle branch block, 377
ventricular tachycardia and, 374
Buprenorphine, 67
Bupropion, 1037, 1041t
for antidepressant-induced sexual dysfunction, 1039
for depression, 1037, 1041t
for neuropathic pain, 73, 73t
overdose/toxicity of, seizures/serotonin syndrome caused by, 1588
for rapid cyclers, 1037
for smoking cessation, 5, 10t
Burkholderia (Pseudomonas) mallei, 1497t
Burkholderia (Pseudomonas) pseudomallei (melioidosis), 1497t
infection in drug users caused by, 1257
Burkitt's lymphoma, 499, 500
chromosomal abnormalities in, 499, 1590, 1659, 1659t
Epstein-Barr virus in, 1312, 1592
Burn blister, 1543, 1546
Burn surface area, estimating, 1543, 1543f
Burning/scratching, of eye, 146
Burns, 1543–1547
chemical. *See* Chemical injury
depth of, 1543–1544
electrical, 1544, 1547
fasciotomy in, 1545
extent of, 1543, 1543f
flash, 1547
Joule, 1547
management of
fluid resuscitation in, 1545
initial, 1544
patient support and, 1546
wound care, 1545–1546
psychiatric/psychologic problems associated with hospitalization and, 1065
smoke inhalation and, 293–294, 1544
survival after, 1544
Burow's solution, for weepy dermatoses, 85
Bursitis, 798–799
Buruli ulcer, 1385
Bush tea, hepatic veno-occlusive disease caused by, 653
Buspar. *See* Buspirone
Buspirone, 1013t
for aggressive/violent behavior, 1050
for anxiety, 1013t, 1014–1015
for depression/dementia in elderly, 50
for obsessive-compulsive disorders, 1015
Busulfan, 1614t
toxicity of, 1614t, 1625
Butane, 1577
Butenafine, 83t
Butoconazole, for vaginal candidiasis, 703

Butorphanol, 67
for cluster headache, 948
Butterfly rash, in systemic lupus erythematosus, 810
Butyrate, for radiation-induced toxicity, 1623
Butyrophenones
abnormal movements caused by, 982
for nausea and vomiting, 525–526
relative potency/side effects of, 1029t
for schizophrenia/psychotic disorders, 1027, 1028, 1028t, 1029t
Bypass grafting
for abdominal aortic aneurysm, 437
antibiotic prophylaxis for, 39
for aortic dissection, 441
coronary artery. *See* Coronary artery bypass grafting
for erectile dysfunction, 443, 925
for lower extremity occlusive disease, 443–444
for popliteal aneurysms, 439
for Raynaud's disease/phenomenon, 454
for renal artery aneurysm, 440
for renal artery stenosis, 449, 885
for thoracic aortic aneurysm, 438
Bypass surgery, for obesity, 1226–1227
Bystander effects, gene therapy in cancer and, 1640

C3
in bullous pemphigoid, 123
in focal segmental glomerular sclerosis, 894
in herpes (pemphigoid) gestationis, 123
laboratory reference range for, 1714t
in membranous nephropathy, 893
in pemphigus, 122
in postinfectious glomerulonephritis, 888
C3b
in autoimmune hemolytic anemia, 483
in cold agglutinin disease, 484
in paroxysmal nocturnal hemoglobinuria, 479
C4, laboratory reference range for, 1714t
C282Y gene, in hemochromatosis, 651, 652
nonalcoholic fatty liver disease and, 644
C$_{cr}$. *See* Creatinine clearance
c-erbB-2. *See* HER2/neu oncogene
c-kit receptor
in gastrointestinal stromal tumors, 583, 1613
imatinib mesylate inhibition of, 1612–1613
c-myc gene, in Burkitt's lymphoma, 499, 1590
C-peptide, laboratory reference range for, 1713t
C-reactive protein, in atherosclerosis, 333
C (constant) region, immunoglobulin, 770
C urea breath testing. *See* Urea breath testing
$^{13}C/^{14}C$-xylose test, in bacterial overgrowth, 589
Ca. *See* Calcium
CA 15-3, in breast cancer, 682
CA 19-9
in cholangiocarcinoma, 664, 665
in pancreatic and periampullary carcinoma, 672
CA 27-29, in breast cancer, 682
CA 125, in ovarian tumors, 714, 716t
response to chemotherapy evaluated by, 1627
as screening tool, 1601
Cabergoline, for hyperprolactinemia, 1081
CABG. *See* Coronary artery bypass grafting
Cachectin. *See* Tumor necrosis factor
Cachexia
in heart disease, 313
malignant, in diabetes mellitus, 1182
Cadexomer iodine, for stasis dermatitis, 463
Cadmium, tubulointerstitial disease caused by, 897

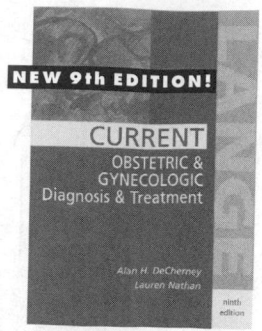
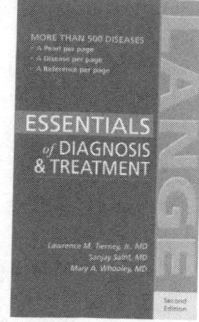
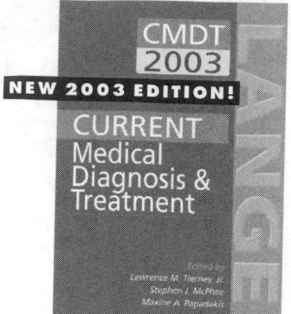
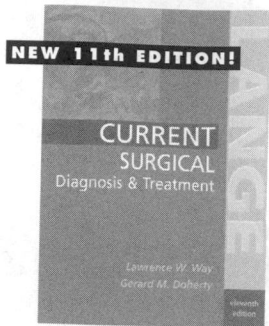
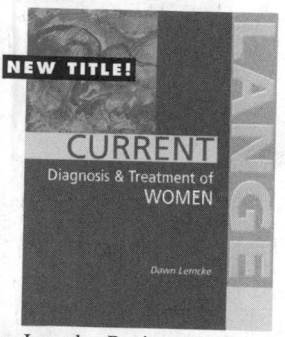
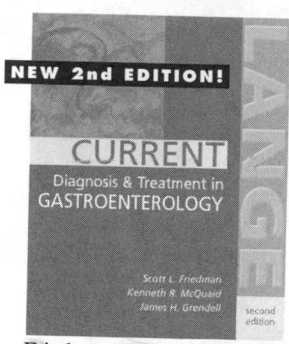
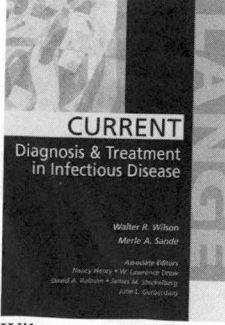
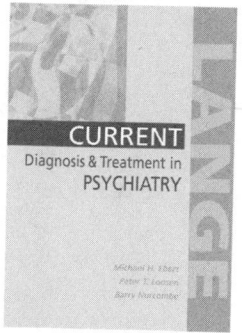
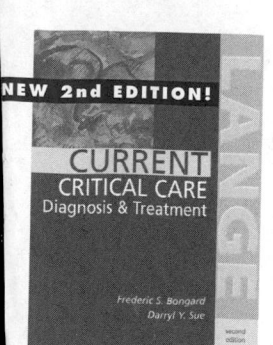
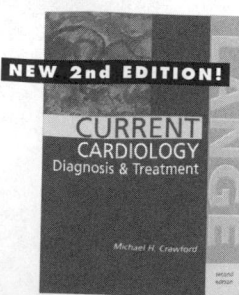
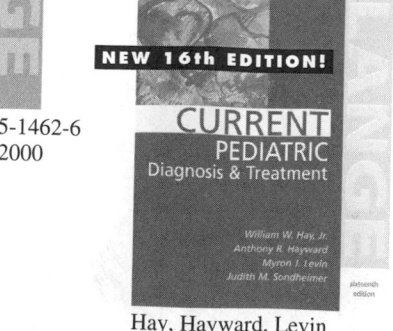